18000

D1643938

Wylie and Churchill-Davidson's

A Practice of Anesthesia

SEVENTH EDITION

Wylie and Churchill-Davidson's

A Practice of Anesthesia

SEVENTH EDITION

Edited by

Thomas E J Healy BSc (Hons) MD LLM MSc FRCA
Emeritus Professor of Anaesthesia and Head of the University Department of Anaesthesia
University of Manchester
and
Honorary Consultant Anaesthetist
Manchester Royal Infirmary, Withington Hospital, and Hope Hospital
Manchester, UK

Paul R Knight MD PhD
Professor of Anesthesiology and Microbiology
Vice Chairman for Research (Department of Anesthesiology)
Witebsky Center for Microbial Pathogenesis and Immunology
and
The Veterans' Administration Medical Center of Buffalo
Buffalo, NY, USA

Section Editors

Mark Lema MD PhD
Professor of Anesthesiology and Chair
Department of Anesthesiology
University at Buffalo, School of Medicine
Buffalo, NY, USA

Peter J Cohen MD JD
Adjunct Professor of Law
Georgetown University Law Center
Washington, DC, USA

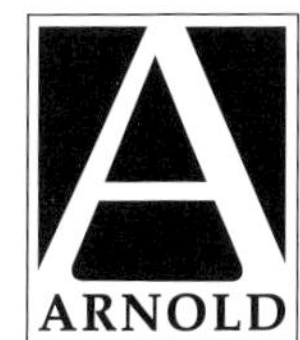

A member of the Hodder Headline Group
LONDON

First published in Great Britain in 1960 by Lloyd-Luke (Medical Books) Ltd
Second Edition 1966
Third Edition 1972
Fourth Edition 1978
Fifth Edition 1984
Sixth Edition 1995
Seventh Edition published in 2003
by Arnold, a member of the Hodder Headline Group,
338 Euston Road, London NW1 3BH

http://www.arnoldpublishers.com

Distributed in the United States of America by
Oxford University Press Inc.,
198 Madison Avenue, New York, NY10016
Oxford is a registered trademark of Oxford University Press

British Library Cataloguing in Publication Data
A catalogue record for this book is available from the British Library

Library of Congress Cataloging-in-Publication Data
A catalog record for this book is available from the Library of Congress

ISBN 0 340 73130 3

1 2 3 4 5 6 7 8 9 10

Commissioning Editor: Serena Bureau
Development Editor: Layla Vandenbergh
Project Manager: Lindsey Williams
Production Controller: Deborah Smith

Typeset in 9 on 11 pt Minion by Prepress Projects Ltd, Perth, Scotland
Printed and bound in India by Ajanta Offset & Packaging Ltd

As I now cross the threshold into retirement I dedicate this book, in gratitude, to all the members of my loving family for their unfailing support, to my colleagues, my teachers and my patients for all that they have taught me during almost 40 years in anaesthesia and for all the memories that I now treasure.

T E J H

I would like to dedicate this book to my best friend and wife, Dana, and our parents, Paul and Elizabeth, and Guido and Anna, for giving the time and patience to raise us to be what we are, and also to our sons, Patrick and Sean, and their wives, Kathy and Elizabeth Jr, for presenting us with terrific grandchildren, Kelsey, Patrick Jr, and Calvin. I am truly blessed to have the support of a family like this.

P K

Contents

Contributors

Anthony R Absalom MB ChB FRCA ILTM
Consultant, Anaesthesia and Intensive Care, Norfolk and Norwich University Hospital, Norwich, UK

Anthony P Adams MB BS PhD FANZCA FRCA LRCP MRCS DA
Emeritus Professor of Anaesthetics, University of London, and Consultant Emeritus to the Army, Guy's Hospital, London, UK

Michael G Adragna MD
Assistant Professor of Clinical Anesthesiology, State University of New York at Buffalo, Buffalo, NY, USA

Simon P Allison MD FRCP
Director of Clinical Nutrition Unit and Professor of Clinical Nutrition, Queen's Medical Centre, Nottingham, UK

John M Anderton MB ChB DObst RCOG FRCA (retired)
Emeritus Consultant Anaesthetist, Manchester Royal Infirmary, Manchester, UK

Douglas R Bacon MD MA
Associate Professor of Anesthesiology, Mayo Clinic, Rochester, MN, USA

Anis S Baraka MD FRCA
Professor and Chair, Department of Anesthesiology, American University of Beirut, Lebanon

Janet Barrie MB ChB FRCA
Consultant Anaesthetist, Royal Oldham Hospital, Oldham, UK

Anna M Batchelor MB ChB FRCA
Consultant, Anaesthesia and Intensive Care Medicine, Royal Victoria Infirmary, Newcastle upon Tyne, UK

David G Bjoraker MD
Associate Professor of Anesthesiology, University of Florida College of Medicine, Gainesville, FL, USA

Timothy Black MD
Anesthesiologist, Valley Anesthesiology Consultants Ltd, and Attending Staff at Good Samaritan Medical Center and Phoenix Children's Hospital, Phoenix, AZ, USA

James G Bovill MD PhD FCARCSI
Department of Anaesthesiology, Leiden University Medical Centre, Leiden, The Netherlands

T Andrew Bowdle MD PhD
Professor of Anesthesiology and Pharmaceutics and Chief, Cardiothoracic Anesthesiology, University of Washington, Seattle, WA, USA

The Lord Brennan of Bibury QC LLB
Matrix Chambers, Gray's Inn, London, UK

M Keith Bresland MB ChB
Consultant Anaesthetist, Darlington Memorial Hospital, Darlington, UK

Jay B Brodsky MD
Professor, Department of Anesthesia, Stanford University Medical Center, Stanford, CA, USA

Angella Bryan BSc MSc PhD SRCS
Department of Anaesthesia, Manchester Royal Infirmary, Manchester, UK

Ross Bullock MD PhD
Reynolds Professor of Neurosurgery and Director, Neuroscience Intensive Care Unit, Medical School of Virginia, Richmond, VA, USA

Iain T Campbell MD FRCA
Honorary Professor of Human Physiology, Liverpool John Moores University, Liverpool, formerly Reader in Anaesthesia, University of Manchester and Consultant Anaesthetist, South Manchester University Hospitals NHS Trust, Manchester, UK

Enrico M Camporesi MD
Professor and Chair, Department of Anesthesiology, and Professor of Physiology, State University of New York Upstate Medical University Syracuse, NY, USA

Jonathan D Cardy MBBS BSc FRCA
Consultant, Anaesthesia and Intensive Care Medicine, West Suffolk Hospital NHS Trust, Bury St Edmunds, UK

Irshad H Chaudry PhD
Professor, Departments of Surgery, Microbiology, Physiology, and Biophysics, Vice Chairman, Department of Surgery, and Director, Center for Surgical Research, University of Birmingham at Alabama, Birmingham, AL, USA

Peter T-L Choi MD MSc FRCPC
Assistant Professor, Departments of Anesthesia and Clinical Epidemiology and Biostatistics, McMaster University, Ontario, Canada

Tobias Clausen MD
Anesthesiologist, Department of Anesthesiology and Intensive Care Medicine, Martin-Luther-University Halle-Wittenberg, Halle (Saale), Germany

Thomas H Clutton-Brock MB ChB MRCP FRCA
Senior Lecturer in Anaesthesia and Intensive Care Medicine, Queen Elizabeth Hospital, Birmingham, UK

Peter J Cohen MD JD
Adjunct Professor of Law, Georgetown University Law Center, Washington, DC, USA

Bruce A Crider MD
Assistant Professor of Anesthesiology, University of Michigan Medical Center, Ann Arbor, MI, USA

Anthony J Cunningham MD FFARCSI FANZCA FRCPC
Clinical Vice-Dean, Medical Faculty, Professor of Anaesthesia, Royal College of Surgeons in Ireland, Education and Research Centre, Beaumont Hospital, Dublin, Ireland

Albert Dahan MD PhD
Associate Professor, Department of Anaesthesiology, Leiden University Medical Center, Leiden, The Netherlands

Oscar A de Leon-Casasola MD
Professor of Anesthesiology, University at Buffalo, School of Medicine, and Vice-Chair for Clinical Affairs, Department of Anesthesiology, University at Buffalo, Chief of Pain Medicine, Roswell Park Cancer Institute, Buffalo, NY, USA

David M Dewan MD
Professor of Anesthesia, Head of Section, Obstetric and Gynecologic Anesthesia, Wake Forest University School of Medicine, Winston-Salem, NC, USA

François Donati PhD MD FRCPC
Professor, Department of Anesthesiology, University of Montréal, Montréal, Québec, Canada

Noreen Dowd MD FFARCSI Dip Intens. Care
Consultant Anaesthetist, St James's Hospital, Dublin, Ireland

D John Doyle MD PhD
Department of Anesthesiology, The Cleveland Clinic Foundation, Cleveland, OH, USA

Michel Y Dubois MD
Director, New York University Pain Program, and Professor of Anesthesiology, New York University School of Medicine, New York, NY, USA

Roderic G Eckenhoff MD
Austin Lamont Professor of Anesthesia, Director for Research, Department of Anesthesia, University of Pennsylvania Health System, Philadelphia, PA, USA

David F Evans BA PhD FAGIP
Visiting Professor of Gastrointestinal Physiology and Consultant Clinical Physiologist, St Bartholomew's and the Royal London School of Medicine and Dentistry, London, UK

Muzaffar H Faroqui MBBS FRCA
Consultant Anaesthetist, Queen Elizabeth Hospital, Birmingham, UK

Rachel A Farragher MB FCARCSI
Clinical Fellow in Obstetric Anesthesia, Brigham and Women's Hospital, Harvard Medical School, Boston, MA, USA

Brendan T Finucane MB BCh FRCPC FRCA
Professor and Program Director, Department of Anesthesiology and Pain Medicine, University of Alberta, Edmonton, Alberta, Canada

Leonard L Firestone MD
Director, Innovative Durg Delivery Systems, Inc., New York, NY, USA

Susan Firestone MD
Director, Cardiac Anaesthesia, Children's Hospital of Pittsburgh and the University of Pittsburgh, Pittsburgh, PA, USA

Malcolm Fisher MB ChB MD FJFICM FANZCA FRCA
Head, Intensive Care Unit, Royal North Shore Hospital of Sydney, and Clinical Professor, Departments of Anaesthesia and Medicine, University of Sydney, Sydney, Australia

Pierre Foëx MD (Geneva) MA DPhil FRCA FANZCA FMedSci
Emeritus Nuffield Professor of Anaesthetics, University of Oxford, and Honorary Consultant Anaesthetist, Oxford Radcliffe Hospitals, Oxford, UK

Christopher Gharibo MD
Assistant Professor of Anesthesiology, Medical Director, Bellevue Pain Treatment Center, and Assistant Professor of Anesthesiology, New York University School of Medicine, New York, NY, USA

Brenda Golianu MD
Assistant Professor of Anesthesia, Stanford University School of Medicine, Stanford, CA, USA

Heidi V Gordon MD
Attending Anesthesiologist, Cooper Hospital, Camden, NJ, USA

Charles E Granger MB BS BSc FRCA
Consultant in Anaesthesia and Intensive Care, Royal Lancaster Infirmary, Lancaster, UK

Thaddeus H Grasela PharmD PhD
President, Cognigen Medical Research, Buffalo, NY, USA

Betty L Grundy MD
Courtesy Professor of Anesthesiology, University of Florida College of Medicine, Gainesville, FL, USA

Carl L Gwinnutt MB BS FRCA
Consultant Anaesthetist, Hope Hospital, Salford, UK

P Jane Halsall MB ChB FRCA
Associate Specialist in Anaesthesia and Honorary Research Fellow, Malignant Hyperthermia Investigation Unit, Academic Unit of Anaesthesia, St James's University Hospital, Leeds, UK

Charles Hantler MD
Professor of Anesthesiology at Washington University School of Medicine, St Louis, MO, USA

Nigel J N Harper MB ChB FRCA
Consultant in Anaesthesia and Intensive Care, Department of Anaesthesia, Manchester Royal Infirmary, Manchester, UK

Thomas E J Healy BSc (Hons) MD LLM MSc FRCA
Emeritus Professor of Anaesthesia, University of Manchester, and Honorary Consultant Anaesthetist, Manchester Royal Infirmary, Withington Hospital, and Hope Hospital, Manchester, UK

John A Henry MB BS FRCP FFAEM
Professor of Accident and Emergency Medicine, St Mary's Hospital, London, UK

Penelope B Hewitt MB BS (Lond) LRCP MRCS (Eng) DA (Eng) FRCA
Emeritus Consultant Anaesthetist, Guy's and St. Thomas' Hospital Trust, London, UK

Philip M Hopkins MD MB BS FRCA
Professor of Anaesthesia, Malignant Hyperthermia Unit, Academic Unit of Anaesthesia, St James's University Hospital, Leeds, UK

Michael B Howie MD
Professor and Chair, Department of Anesthesiology, and Professor and Pharmacy Director, Cardiovascular Anesthesia, Ohio State University, Columbus, OH, USA

Christopher J Hull MB BS DA FRCA
Professor of Anaesthesia, University of Newcastle, and Honorary Consultant Anaesthetist, Royal Victoria Infirmary, Newcastle upon Tyne, UK

Jennifer M Hunter MB ChB PhD FRCA
Professor of Anaesthesia, University of Liverpool, Liverpool, UK

Peter Hutton BSc PhD MB ChB FRCA FRCP
Past President, Royal College of Anaesthetists, and Henry Hill Hickman Professor of Anaesthesia, University of Birmingham, Birmingham, UK

David James MB BS FRCA
Consultant in Anaesthesia, Guy's and St Thomas' Hospital Trust, London, UK

Michael F M James MB ChB PhD FRCA FCA(SA)
Professor and Head, Department of Anaesthesia, University of Cape Town, Western Cape, South Africa

J Gareth Jones MD FRCP FRCA FANZCA
University of Cambridge, Department of Anaesthesia, Addenbrooke's Hospital, Cambridge, UK

Keith C Judkins MB ChB FRCA
Consultant Anaesthetist, Pinderfields Hospital, Wakefield, Medical Director, Mid Yorkshire Hospitals NHS Trust, and Senior Lecturer, University of Leeds School of Medicine, Leeds, UK

Douglas Justins MB BS FRCA
Consultant in Anaesthesia and Pain Management, Guy's and St Thomas' Hospital Trust, London, UK

Gavin N C Kenny BSc (Hons) MD FRCA FANZCA
Professor and Head, University Department of Anaesthesia, University of Glasgow, Glasgow, UK

Judy R Kersten MD
Professor of Anesthesiology, Pharmacology and Toxicology, The Medical College of Wisconsin, Milwaukee, WI, USA

E F Klein Jr MD FCCM
Professor of Anesthesiology, University of Arkansas for Medical Sciences, Little Rock, AR, USA

Michal T Kluger MB ChB DA DipDHM FRCA FANZCA
Specialist Anaesthetist, Waitemata Health, North Shore Hospital, Auckland, New Zealand

Paul R Knight MD PhD
Professor of Anesthesiology and Microbiology, Vice Chairman for Research (Department of Anesthesiology), Witebsky Center for Microbial Pathogenesis and Immunology, and The Veterans' Administration Medical Center of Buffalo, Buffalo, NY, USA

Bhavani Shankar Kodali MD
Associate Professor, Harvard Medical School, Boston, MA, USA

Elliot J Krane MD
Professor of Anesthesia and Pediatrics, Stanford University School of Medicine, Stanford, CA, USA

Donald A Kroll MD PhD
Staff Anesthesiologist, Memphis Veterans' Affairs Medical Center, and Professor of Anesthesiology, University of Tennessee, Memphis, TN, USA

Carlos Kurek MD
Assistant Professor, Department of Anesthesiology, State University of New York at Buffalo, and Director, Critical Care Unit, The Veterans' Administration Medical Center of Buffalo, Buffalo, NY, USA

Allen H Lebovits PhD
Co-Director, New York University Pain Management Center, and Associate Professor, Departments of Anesthesiology and Psychiatry, New York University School of Medicine, New York, NY, USA

Michael Lee MBBS
Specialist Registrar in Anaesthesia, Addenbrooke's Hospital, Cambridge, UK

Mark J Lema MD PhD
Professor of Anesthesiology and Chair, Department of Anesthesiology, University at Buffalo, School of Medicine, Buffalo, NY, USA

Jerrold Lerman MD FRCPC FANZCA
Clinical Professor of Anesthesiology, Department of Anesthesiology, Children's Hospital of Buffalo, Buffalo, NY, USA

J Lance Lichtor MD
Professor, Department of Anesthesia, University of Iowa, Iowa City, IA, USA

Roderick A Little PhD FRCPath
Professor of Surgical Science, University of Manchester, Manchester, UK

W David Lord BSc (Hons) MB ChB FRCA
Consultant Paediatric Anaesthetist, Regional Paediatric Burns Unit, Central Manchester and Manchester Children's University Hospitals, Manchester, UK

Mirjana Lovrincevic MD
Assistant Professor, Department of Anesthesiology and Pain Medicine, The University at Buffalo and Roswell Park Cancer Institute, Buffalo, NY, USA

Philip D Lumb MB BS FCCM
Professor and Chairman, Department of Anesthesiology, Keck School of Medicine of University of Southern California, Los Angeles, CA, USA

Ian McConachie MB ChB FRCA
Consultant Anaesthetist, Blackpool Victoria Hospital, Blackpool, UK

John McGeachie MB ChB FRCA
Consultant Anaesthetist, The Royal Oldham Hospital, Oldham, UK

Gretl A McHugh MSc BNurs (Hons) RGN RHV
Research Fellow, School of Nursing, Midwifery and Health Visiting, University of Manchester, Manchester, UK

James D Martin MD
Attending Physician, Emergency Medicine, Affiliated Health Services, Mount Vernon, WA, USA

George H Meakin MB ChB MD FRCA
Senior Lecturer in Paediatric Anaesthesia, University of Manchester, and Honorary Consultant Anaesthetist, Royal Manchester Children's Hospital, Manchester, UK

James B Mayfield MD
Medical Director, Perioperative Services, and Vice Chairman, Anesthesiology and Perioperative Medicine, Medical College of Georgia, Augusta, GA, USA

Rajinder K Mirakhur MD PhD FRCA FFARCSI
Professor of Anaesthetics and Intensive Care Medicine, The Queen's University of Belfast, Belfast, UK

David H Morison MB ChB FRCPC
Professor Emeritus, McMaster University, Ontario, Canada

Andrew J Mortimer BSc MD FRCA
Consultant in Anaesthesia and Intensive Care, Wythenshawe Hospital, Manchester, UK

Stanley Muravchick MD PhD
Professor of Anesthesia and Interim Chair, Hospital of the University of Pennsylvania, Philadelphia, PA, USA

Frank L Murphy MD (dec.)
Associate Professor of Anesthesia, The Hospital of the University of Pennsylvania, Philadelphia, PA, USA

Nader D Nader MD PhD FCCP
Associate Professor of Anesthesiology, Surgery, Pathology, and Anatomical Sciences, University at Buffalo, Buffalo, NY, USA

Norah N Naughton MD
Clinical Associate Professor and Director, Obstetric Anesthesiology, University of Michigan Medical Center, Ann Arbor, MI, USA

Kenneth E Nelson MD
Assistant Professor, Department of Anesthesia, Forsyth Memorial Hospital – Women's Center, Winston-Salem, NC, USA

Peter Nightingale FRCA MRCP
Consultant Anaesthetist, University Hospital of South Manchester, Manchester, UK

Jerry P Nolan FRCA
Consultant in Anaesthesia and Critical Care, Royal United Hospital, Bath, UK

Martin L Norton MSPH MD DAn JD
Active Emeritus Professor, Medical Education, Emeritus Professor, Anesthesiology, Emeritus Associate Professor, Otorhinolaryngology, The University of Michigan Medical Center, Ann Arbor, MI USA

Niall O'Keeffe MB BCH BAO FRCA
Consultant Anaesthetist, Manchester Royal Infirmary, Manchester, UK

Fredrick K Orkin MD MBA MSc
Anesthesiologist, Pennsylvania State Milton S. Hershey Medical Center, and Professor of Anesthesiology and of Health Evaluation Sciences, The Pennsylvania State University, Hershey, PA, USA

Charles W Otto MD FCCM
Professor of Anesthesiology, Associate Professor of Medicine, University of Arizona College of Medicine, Tucson, AZ, USA

Paul S Pagel MD PhD
Professor of Anesthesiology, Director of Cardiac Anesthesia, Department of Anesthesiology, The Medical College of Wisconsin, Milwaukee, WI, USA

Mark Patrick BSc MB BS FRCA
Consultant Anaesthetist, University Hospital of South Manchester, Manchester, UK

Barbara J Pleuvry BPharm MSc PhD MRPharmS
Senior Lecturer in Anaesthesia and Pharmacology, University of Manchester, Manchester, UK

Brian J Pollard BPharm MB ChB MD FRCA
Professor of Anaesthesia, University of Manchester, Honorary Consultant Anaesthetist to Central Manchester and Manchester Children's University Hospitals NHS Trust, and Honorary Consultant Anaesthetist to the University Hospitals of South Manchester, Manchester, UK

Saifudin Rashiq MB FRCPC
Assistant Professor, Department of Anesthesiology and Pain Medicine, University of Alberta, Edmonton, Alberta, Canada

Michael F Roizen MD FACP FFARCS
Professor of Anesthesiology and Medicine, State University of New York Upstate, Syracuse, NY, USA, and Professor of Anesthesia and Critical Care Medicine, University of Chicago, Chicago, IL, USA

Carl E Rosow MD PhD
Associate Professor of Anaesthesia, Harvard Medical School, and Anesthetist, Department of Anesthesia and Critical Care, Massachusetts General Hospital, Boston, MA, USA

W Lawrence Roy MD FRCP
Associate Professor, Department of Anaesthesia, University of Toronto, and Anaesthetist-in-Chief, The Hospital for Sick Children, Toronto, Ontario, Canada

Anthony Rubin MB BChir MRCS LRCP
Consultant Anaesthetist, Wellington Eye Unit, London, UK

William B Runciman MB ChB FANZCA FRCA FHKCA PhD
Professor and Head, Department of Anaesthesia and Intensive Care, Royal Adelaide Hospital and University of Adelaide, Adelaide, Australia

Andrew R A Rushton FRCA
Consultant Anaesthetist, Derriford Hospital, Plymouth, UK

Timothy W Rutter Mb ChB FRCA
Associate Chair for Clinical Affairs, UH, Clinical Director of University Hospital Operating Rooms, Department of Anesthesiology, University of Michigan Medical Center, Ann Arbor, MI, USA

David Sage MB ChB Obstet FANZCA
Chief Medical Officer, Auckland District Health Board, and Honorary Assistant Professor in Anaesthesiology, University of Auckland, Auckland, New Zealand

M Ramez Salem MD
Chair, Department of Anesthesiology, Advocate Illinois Masonic Medical Center and Clinical Professor of Anesthesiology, University of Illinois College of Medicine, Chicago, IL, USA

Martin G Schwacha PhD
Assistant Professor of Surgery and Microbiology, University of Alabama, Birmingham, AL, USA

Steven L Shafer MD
Staff Anesthesiologist, Palo Alto VA Healthcare System, Professor of Anesthesia, Stanford University School of Medicine, and Adjunct Professor of Biopharmaceutical Science, University of California at San Francisco, San Francisco, CA, USA

Maire P Shelly MB ChB FRCA
Wythenshawe Hospital, Department of Postgraduate Medicine and Dental Education, University of Manchester, Manchester, UK

J Robert Sneyd MD FRCA
Professor of Anaesthesia and Associate Dean, Peninsula Medical School, Plymouth, UK

Dirk G Snijdelaar MD
Department of Anesthesiology, University Medical Centre, Nijmegen, The Netherlands

Caren M Stalburg MD FACOG
Clinical Assistant Professor, Division of Women's Health, Department of Obstetrics and Gynecology, University of Michigan Health System, Ann Arbor, MI, USA

Roger Stedman MB ChB FRCA
Consultant, Anaesthesia and Intensive Care, Birmingham Heartlands and Solihull NHS Trust, Birmingham, UK

Alan R Tait PhD
Associate Professor, Director of Clinical Research, Department of Anesthesiology, University of Michigan Health System, Ann Arbor, MI, USA

Stephen R Thom MD PhD
Chief of Hyperbaric Medicine and Professor of Emergency Medicine, Institute for Environmental Medicine, University of Pennsylvania Health System, Philadelphia, PA, USA

Mark L Thomas MB ChB BSc MB BChir FRCA
Consultant Anaesthetist, Great Ormond Street Hospital, London, UK

Gavin M M Thoms MBChB FRCA FFPHM MSc
Consultant Anaesthetist, Manchester Royal Infirmary, and Senior Research Fellow (Hon), University of Manchester, Manchester, UK

Wolfgang G Toller MD DEAA
Associate Professor of Anesthesiology, The Medical College of Wisconsin, Milwaukee, WI, USA, and Department of Anesthesiology, University of Graz, Austria

Kevin K Tremper PhD MD FRCA
Robert B Sweet Professor and Chair, University of Michigan Medical Center, Ann Arbor, MI, USA

James R Trudell PhD
Professor of Chemistry in Anesthesia, Department of Anesthesia and Program for Molecular and Genetic Medicine, Stanford School of Medicine, Stanford, CA, USA

Robert B Truog MD
Professor of Anesthesia (Pediatrics), Children's Hospital, ICU Boston, MA, USA

John M Turner MA MB ChB FRCA
Consultant in Neuroanaesthesia and Neurocritical Care, Addenbrooke's Hospital, and Associate Lecturer in the Faculty of Clinical Medicine, University of Cambridge, Cambridge, UK

Shermeen B Vakharia MD
Assistant Professor, Department of Anesthesiology, State University of New York Upstate Medical University, Syracuse, NY, USA

Christopher J Vallis BSc MB BS FRCA FRCPCH DCH
Consultant Paediatric Anaesthetist, Royal Victoria Infirmary, Newcastle upon Tyne, UK

David B Waisel MD
Associate Professor of Anesthesia, Children's Hospital, and Assistant Professor of Anesthesia, Harvard Medical School, Boston, MA, USA

Cynthia A Walawander MA
Executive Vice President, Cognigen Medical Research, Buffalo, NY, USA

Denham S Ward MD PhD
Professor and Chair Emeritus, Department of Anesthesiology, Strong Health System, University of Rochester, Rochester, NY, USA

David C Warltier MD PhD
Professor and Vice Chairman of Anesthesiology, Pharmacology and Toxicology, and Medicine, Division of Cardiovascular Diseases, The Medical College of Wisconsin, Milwaukee, WI, USA

Leila G Welborn MD
Professor of Anesthesiology and Pediatrics, George Washington University, and Operating Room Clinical Director, Children's National Medical Center, Washington, DC, USA

David J Wilkinson MBBS DRCOG FRCA Hon FCARCSI
Boyle Department of Anaesthesia, St Bartholomew's Hospital, London, UK

Anthony Wilton BSc MSc PhD FRCP
Consultant Physician, Department of Diabetes/Endocrinology/General Medicine, Ymddiriedolaeth GIG, Gogledd Orllewin Cymru (North West Wales NHS Trust), Bangor, Wales, UK

Leon D Wright MD
Carroll County General Hospital, Westminster, MD, USA

Homer Yang MD CCFP FRCPC
Chairman, Department of Anesthesia, McMaster University, Ontario, Canada

René Zellweger MD
Associate Professor, Division of Trauma Surgery, University of Zurich, Zurich, Switzerland

Preface

In this, the seventh edition of this text and the first in the twenty-first century, it is important that we should take stock and that we should recognize, with pride, the immeasurable contribution that the discovery of anesthesia has made to mankind.

Dr T B Boulton and Dr D J Wilkinson, in the sixth edition, described how the practice of modern anesthesia evolved from the demonstration by the dentist William Thomas Morton at Massachusetts General Hospital in Boston, USA, on "Ether Day," Friday, 16 October 1846, that the inhalation of ether vapor could abolish the pain of surgery.[1] News of this great discovery spread quickly from America to Scotland and to England. On 19 December 1846, ether was used for the first time by Mr James Robinson in London for a dental extraction and by Dr William Scott in Dumfries for an amputation. Two days later, Robert Lister, a famous London surgeon, carried out an above-the-knee amputation; again ether was used.

> To place a value on this, mankind's greatest discovery, we need occasionally to remember the horror and desolation of conscious patients strapped to operating tables undergoing amputation of limbs or, perhaps, the ripping open of their abdomens as, in the case of women patients, for removal of ovaries. We can, I sense, hear even yet the screams of those who suffered, if we listen hard enough.[2]

In response to the above letter, Captain P R D Kimm OBE Royal Navy reached back across the bridge which spans the river of time and wrote the following:

> … my maternal grandmother, Kate Mayes née Munns (1870–1957), remembered as a child having seen dental booths on the market square in Northampton where the populace gathered round to laugh and cheer as "dentists" pulled the teeth of their unfortunate victims. She never forgot the sight – or the sound – and I never have forgotten her stories …

His wife also tells her anesthetic story:

> I was 4 years old in 1932 when I walked into a room where a whole lot of people were washing their hands, and I was told to get up onto a table in the middle of the room. I was wearing a pair of pink jersey pyjamas with green cuffs and collar. I couldn't reach the table, so they gave me a stool. Then suddenly a whole lot of hands were holding me down, and a great big white thing with a horrid smell was pressed down onto my face. I was absolutely terrified.

A similar experience also occurred to PRK during his first anesthetic:

> I was 6 years old when I was wheeled on a gurney through the halls of the hospital to a corridor and left alone for over an hour. I was then taken into a room and asked to crawl onto another narrow bed. Suddenly, my arms were pinned to my side by someone hugging me and another held down my legs. A mask was placed on my face with a great deal of pressure. I remember a terrible smell and trying to hold my breath in order to prevent breathing that pungent air. I felt as though I was being suffocated. The experience was so terrible that if today I met the anesthesiologists who were responsible for my first anesthetic I would go out my way to be very impolite to them.

These glimpses into the past, more distant and more recent, remind us how we were, but through them we also gain the experience not only to know but also to understand more clearly the important place that anesthesia plays in clinical care and our responsibility to do better, to take no short cuts, and to do our best for all our patients all the time. All our patients are sombody's somebody and, like ourselves, have feelings and experience fear.

It is now 43 years since Dr W D Wylie and Dr H C Churchill-Davidson, with the need to always do the best, edited the first edition of this now classic textbook of anesthesia. The first paragraph of the preface on that occasion drew attention to important concepts, which still remain with us:

> Physiological and pharmacological principles now govern the choice of anaesthetic drugs and techniques and although many patents can safely be dealt with by routines born of experience, a sound understanding of the background of a particular patient enables the proper and best choice to be made.

In the sixth edition attention was drawn to the advances in monitoring techniques that opened new windows on the patient and, combined with ever-present vigilance, made it possible for us to improve still more our patients' security during anesthesia and surgery. The introduction of many new opportunities for surgical intervention, ranging from transplantation of major organs to the implantation of automatic cardiac defibrillators, and to surgery performed on the fetus *in utero*, have been made possible only with the ever-advancing skill and knowledge of the anesthesiologist. Surgery will always stand on the shoulders of anesthesia, and for this reason the science of anesthesiology has the essential responsibility to strive continuously to push forward its own frontiers of knowledge and practice.

This seventh edition has been replanned by the new editorial team, which includes Professor Peter Cohen, co-editor of the sixth edition, who is now editor of the section Anesthesia and Society. It is very appropriate that Peter, who first suggested the title as a section heading for the sixth edition and is now a professor of law at Georgetown University, should take the responsibility for this section, which includes chapters on stress and bereavement care. We think that this section is a first for a textbook for anesthesiologists.

Anesthesiologists have now established an important niche in the management of pain both chronic and acute. There is an increasing need for the skills and knowledge that have been gained since many readers qualified to be shared with them. We are grateful to Professor

Mark Lema, an expert in pain management, for accepting the task of expanding the presentation of this subject. He is editor of the section Pain Management.

The subjects covered in the other sections offer the flavor of the practice of anesthesia, both general and specialized, thereby remaining close to the founding editors' intentions. The authorship, as in the sixth edition, is truly international, although the majority of the authors work in the USA or the UK. A number of the chapters were co-written by authors from The Netherlands, Australasia, South Africa, Canada, Germany, Ireland, Austria, Switzerland, and Lebanon.

We believe that this edition meets the needs of all trainees in anesthesia who are preparing to approach the entrance to the examination hall, but it is also designed to meet the needs of consultants or attending physicians, who may sometimes find themselves involved in clinical situations with which they have less familiarity. We have not in this edition limited the reference lists and hope that these, some of which are extensive, will prove useful.

We have been saddened by the deaths of those authors who worked so hard for the successful sixth edition and who were personal friends, and of Derek Wylie and Harry Churchill-Davidson, who were among the most highly respected British anesthesiologists of their generation. We are grateful for the permission of the editor of *The Times* of London to print their obituaries here.

We are also grateful to all the authors who, in spite of busy professional lives, have given so much time in writing and keeping their chapters up to date during a prolonged gestation period. We could not have produced this book without their specialized skills, their generosity, and their time. We are also thankful to the anesthesiologists who, at our request, reviewed the sixth edition and have given us many useful suggestions for the preparation of the current textbook. Their advice has been extremely valuable in the preparation of the seventh edition.

We must place on record our appreciation and gratitude for the advice and help given to us by Sarah Desouza, Serena Bureau, and Layla Vandenbergh of Arnold and Lindsey Williams of Prepress Projects Ltd, who smoothed even the most turbulent moments, bringing the many manuscripts together to form a cohesive whole. The completion of this textbook owes much to their never faltering advice and hard work.

The editors of the sixth edition, T E J Healy and P K Cohen, would like to congratulate all the authors who contributed to the sixth edition, which was awarded First Prize at The British Medical Association Medical Book Competition, for books in a surgical subject 1996.

T E J H and P R K

REFERENCES

1. Boulton TB, Wilkinson DJ The origins of modern anaesthesia. In: Healy TEJ, Cohen P (eds). *Wylie and Churchill-Davidson's A Practice of Anaesthesia*, 6th edn. London: Arnold, 1995.
2. Healy TEJ. Painless Surgery Pioneers Praised. *The Times*, 19 December 1996.

Preface to the sixth edition

It is over three decades since the First Edition of Wylie and Churchill-Davidson's *A Practice of Anaesthesia* was published. During these years, there have been fundamental changes in medicine, anaesthesia and society. Evolution, with its attendant progress and problems, is clearly evident in this, the Sixth Edition. Manifesting this vast increase in our knowledge, the number of chapters has increased by 50 per cent. No one nation, practice or academic institution has a monopoly of truth; the editors and contributors reflect the significant international and multidisciplinary nature of our specialty.

The book is directed both to the consultant or attending physician and to the registrar or resident in training; it should be of major assistance in giving the senior trainee and examination candidate the opportunity to gain a broad view of anaesthesia as a discipline. As surgery and those allied medical disciplines that require the assistance of anaesthesia have advanced, so has the complexity of the anaesthetic techniques that are required.

Since the appearance of the First Edition, new areas for surgical intervention have been born, ranging from transplantation of major organs to implantation of automatic cardiac defibrillators to surgery performed on the fetus *in utero*. Advances in monitoring techniques have opened new windows on the patient and, combined with ever-present vigilance, have granted us the opportunity to increase our patients' security during anaesthesia.

Our understanding and appreciation of anaesthesia at a molecular level has burgeoned. Knowledge of drug–receptor interactions is increasing rapidly. Use of the fundamental tools of genetic research to examine mechanisms of drug action is flourishing.

The first section introduces the reader to the history and theories of anaesthesia. Since the practice of anaesthesia cannot be separated from certain fundamental scientific principles, these are dealt with in depth. In addition to areas of obvious parochial focus, we have invited contributions dealing with topics of general importance such as operating room transmission of infection, hyperbaric medicine and the role of computers.

In the second section, we move into the theatre and examine the impact of disease and patient status on our practice. The broad areas of the anaesthetist's involvement throughout the perioperative period is apparent.

There is a necessary overlap between the second and third sections; the latter present a comprehensive and up-to-date discussion of the subspecialties of anaesthesia and the application of our practice to specific pathological conditions.

Finally, the last section illustrates the important and exciting ways our specialty interacts with society as a whole. Medicolegal principles (both in the UK and in the USA), quality and medical ethics are thoroughly discussed.

Thomas E J Healy
Manchester, UK

Peter J Cohen
Bethesda, Maryland, USA

Obituaries

DEREK WYLIE

Dr Derek Wylie, anaesthetist and former Dean of St Thomas' Hospital Medical School, died on September 29 [1998] aged 79. He was born on October 24, 1918.

As practitioner, researcher, lecturer and author, Derek Wylie made a notable contribution to the development of the specialism of anaesthesia within the National Health Service. He sat on many specialist bodies, and was also Dean of St Thomas' Medical School. In the later part of his life, as part of his work for the Medical Defence Union, he helped to tackle medical negligence.

William Derek Wylie was born in Huddersfield and educated at Uppingham School, Gonville and Caius College, Cambridge and St Thomas' Hospital Medical School qualifying in 1943. Initially he intended to become a physician and held junior appointments as casualty officer, house physician and resident anaesthetist, during which time he became a member of the Royal College of Physicians. In 1945, he joined the RAF Volunteer Reserve, and served as physician in England, Palestine and Aden before demobilisation in 1947.

Two vacancies for honorary anaesthetists in St Thomas' were advertised in 1946 and although he was still in Palestine, Wylie was encouraged by the senior anaesthetist at the hospital to apply for one of these posts. His application was successful but he faced a difficult decision because acceptance meant abandoning his physician's training. There was no guarantee of financial security for a trainee physician at that time, so Wylie, who was recently married and with a child on the way, decided to accept the post even though his experience of the speciality was minimal.

He started work at St Thomas' in 1948, and quickly brought himself up to date with what was then a very limited speciality, although major changes were taking place as new drugs became available and new ideas emerged. Wylie realised the importance of these developments and saw that it was vital to train young doctors to become the anaesthestists for the new NHS. The old-fashioned administering of anaesthetics by GPs was being phased out as developing surgical techniques depended upon more advanced anaesthesia.

Wylie wrote many papers, and in 1953 he published *The Practical Management of Pain in Labour*. He also carried out some clinical research, and lectured in Britain and overseas. The textbook *A Practice of Anaesthesia*, which he wrote with Harry Churchill-Davidson, was widely translated and is still current under a different editorship.

In 1963 Wylie was appointed president of the anaesthetic section of the Royal Society of Medicine, and he served as honorary treasurer, 1964–70. He was elected to the board of the Faculty of Anaesthetists (now the Royal College of Anaesthetists) in 1960, and was Dean from 1967 to 1969. He was president of the Association of Anaesthetists of Great Britain and Ireland from 1980 to 1982, and also president of the sixth European Congress of Anaesthesiologists.

He sat on many committees at St Thomas', and in 1974 he was elected Dean of the Medical School, a post which he filled with distinction. When he had completed his term of office in 1979, he retired from the Health Service to devote his time to the study of medical negligence and its prevention.

This was a longstanding interest. He had been a member in the early 1950s of a committee set up by the Association of Anaesthetists of Great Britain and Ireland to investigate the causes of deaths associated with anaesthesia; this was probably the first national investigation of its kind. He went on to join the council of the Medical Defence Union in 1962, and served as its president, 1982–88, during which time he developed his view that the union should play a significant part in preventing medical practice that might lead to claims of negligence; with this in mind he set up the union's journal. He was the recipient of many honours.

He is survived by his wife Margaret, a Nightingale nurse, whom he married in 1945, and by two daughters and a son. Another son died in 1984.

Times Newspapers Limited
London, 29 October 1998

HARRY CHURCHILL-DAVIDSON

Harry Churchill-Davidson, anaesthetist, died on October 15 [1995], aged 73. He was born on April 25, 1922.

A whole generation of anaesthetists will instantly recognise the name of Harry Churchill-Davidson. It was he and his lifelong friend Derek Wylie who were the authors of an internationally acclaimed textbook for anaesthetists entitled *A Practice of Anaesthesia*. It ran to five editions and included contributions from other authors far and wide. His contribution to British anaesthesia was unique in that he recognised the great potential of the newly developing media and capitalised on their ability to disseminate wider understanding.

Harry Cunningham Churchill-Davidson was educated at Charterhouse and Trinity College, Cambridge, qualifying in medicine as the war ended. He represented the university at soccer and squash but, these being the war years, he was not accorded a Blue.

He served in the RAMC in Malaya during his National Service and returned to embark upon his medical career at St Thomas' Hospital, London, where he remained as a consultant anaesthetist until his retirement in 1986. He also held consultant posts at the Chelsea Hospital for Women and at the Brompton Hospital.

The art of anaesthesia was rapidly developing into a science and "C-D", as he was generally known, was eager to be part of this new era. He wrote extensively on the use of muscle-relaxant drugs, and did much to establish the reputation of British anaesthesia in many parts of the world. In the United States his lecturing skills were in demand and he delivered lectures at several celebrated medical centres.

Positions in his department were eagerly sought and his ceaseless drive and enthusiasm were to fire the imagination and ambition of scores of young anaesthetists. He was a very approachable man, with an enthusiasm for life.

He was president of the anaesthetist section of the Royal Society of Medicine and served 25 years on the board of the Faculty of Anaesthetists. It was a matter of great personal satisfaction to him when the faculty was granted independent Royal College status.

He is survived by his wife Yvonne and their two daughters and a son.

Times Newspapers Limited
London, 10 November 1995

Great moments in the history of anesthesiology

DOUGLAS R BACON AND DAVID J WILKINSON

The history of anesthesiology is a rich mosaic of interwoven events around the world that have created and defined the specialty. From the days of the ancient Greeks and Romans to the computerized operating rooms of the twenty-first century, the care of patients undergoing surgery has been and remains challenging. Only during the last century and a half has there been consistent and reliable pain relief for those seeking a cure through the surgeon's knife. It was the introduction of general anesthesia in 1846, combined with the description of aseptic technique in the second half of the nineteenth century, that permitted increasingly extensive and complex operations to be performed. The story of anesthesia is rich and varied – driven in part by surgical needs, but at the same time often ignored or undervalued by surgeons.

Many individuals and organizations helped to create the infrastructure that the specialty currently enjoys. The organizations were key to the development of anesthesiology for, through their scientific meetings, they brought together concerned individuals to discuss problems of mutual interest. The pioneering spirit of many of these physicians was crucial to solving patient care issues and making anesthesia safe. Some of these individuals are the bright stones which stand out in the mosaic; others are the contrast that makes the image understandable. One without the other fails to give a complete picture. It is hoped that the historical highlights in this chapter will form an impression of the roots of anesthesiology, even as the tree is cultivated.

No short chapter of this nature can provide a full history of our specialty. Those who seek more should search out one of the many sources of further information available, some examples of which are provided in the Appendix.

PREHISTORY – BEFORE 16 OCTOBER 1846

Most conventional histories of anesthesiology begin with the events surrounding the first public demonstration of ether anesthesia, yet the quest for surgical anesthesia goes back much further and is not necessarily rooted in Western medicine. Over time, many different agents have been used to achieve anesthesia.

The physician Dioscorides, in the first century AD, noted that mandragora, a drug prepared from the bark and leaves of the mandrake plant by boiling in wine and straining, could be used "... in the case of persons ... about to be cut or cauterized, when they wish to produce anesthesia."[1] Mandragora was still being used to anesthetize patients as late as the seventeenth century.

During the Middle Ages, the soporific sponge was developed to provide pain relief during surgery. According to published reports of the time, mandrake leaves, along with black nightshade, poppies, and other herbs, were boiled and cooked onto a sponge. The sponge was then reconstituted in hot water, and placed under the patient's nose prior to surgery. Such sponges would have contained morphine and scopolamine in varying amounts, drugs still clinically used in anesthesia.[2] In addition to use of the "sleeping sponge," Europeans attempted to relieve pain by hypnosis, by the ingestion of alcohol, herbs, and extracts of botanical preparations, and by the topical application of pressure or ice. While it is difficult to see how the inhalation of what are essentially nonvolatile agents within the "soporific sponge" could have had any effect, the recipes for "dwale" are much more believable. This combination of black henbane (*Hyoscyamus niger*), opium poppy (*Papaver somniferum*), and hemlock (*Conium maculatum*) would have been potent, and a variety of mixtures are described in medieval manuscripts.[3] Recent pharmacological archeology has demonstrated the presence of seeds of these plants in the drains of Soutra Hospital in the border region between Scotland and England, together with bone fragments that suggest surgical activity.[4] Dwale has much to commend it as the original anesthetic agent.

During the Renaissance, local anesthesia, in the form of the application of cold water and ice, was introduced. In the mid-seventeenth century, Marco Aurelio Severino described "refrigeration anesthesia," which involved placing snow in parallel lines across the incisional plane; the site became insensate within minutes. The technique failed to gain popularity, probably because of the challenge of maintaining stores of snow year-round.[5] However, during the Winter War between Finland and the Soviet Union in 1939–40, refrigeration anesthesia was extensively utilized.[6]

Diethyl ether had been known for centuries prior to its first public use for the induction of surgical anesthesia. Although it may first have been compounded by an eighth-century Arabian philosopher, Jabir ibn Hayyam, or by Raymond Lully, an alchemist in the thirteenth century, it was certainly known in the sixteenth century to both Valerius Cordus and Paracelsus, who prepared it by distilling sulfuric acid (oil of vitriol) with fortified wine to produce an oleum vitrioli dulce (sweet oil of vitriol). Paracelsus observed that it caused chickens to fall asleep and awaken unharmed. He must have been aware of its analgesic qualities, because he recommended that it could be used to treat painful illnesses, although there is no evidence that his suggestion was followed. In 1540, Valerius Cordus recommended it as a medication to be taken in wine for the relief of whooping cough and other respiratory diseases. Interestingly, neither of these physicians was able to "make the connection" between relief of painful conditions and possible use in surgery.

For three centuries thereafter, this simple compound remained a therapeutic agent with only occasional medicinal use. Some of its properties were examined by distinguished British scientists, including Robert Boyle, Isaac Newton, and Michael Faraday, but without sustained interest. Its only routine application came as an inexpensive recreational drug among the poor of Britain and Ireland, who sometimes drank an ounce or two of ether when taxes made gin prohibitively expensive.[7] An American variation of this practice was conducted by groups of students, who held ether-soaked towels to their faces at nocturnal "ether frolics."

Another agent used in a similar manner to ether is nitrous oxide. Known for its ability to induce lightheadedness and often inhaled by those seeking a thrill, it was not used as frequently as was ether because it was more difficult to prepare and store. Nitrous oxide was produced by heating ammonium nitrate in the presence of iron filings. The evolved gas was passed through water to eliminate toxic oxides of nitrogen before being stored.

Nitrous oxide was first prepared in 1773 by Joseph Priestley, an English clergyman and scientist. Humphry Davy (Fig. 1) performed a brilliant series of investigations of several gases at the Pneumatic Institute, founded by Thomas Beddoes in the city of Bristol. Davy focused much of his attention on nitrous oxide, which he and his associates inhaled. Davy used these experiments to measure the rate of uptake of nitrous oxide and its effect on respiration and other central nervous system actions. These results were combined with research on the physical properties of the gas in a 580-page book published in 1800, *Nitrous Oxide*. This impressive treatise is now best remembered for a few incidental observations: Davy's comments that nitrous oxide transiently relieved a severe headache, obliterated a minor headache, and briefly quenched an aggravating toothache. The most frequently quoted passage was a casual entry, "As nitrous oxide in its extensive operation appears capable of destroying physical pain, it may probably be used with advantage during surgical operations in which no great effusion of blood takes place."[8] Although Davy did not pursue this prophecy, perhaps because he was set on a career in basic chemical research, he did coin the persisting sobriquet for nitrous oxide, "laughing gas." The affection with which Davy is held in many anesthetic circles is perhaps misplaced. He made a dramatic discovery and was uniquely placed to develop and promulgate it and yet he abandoned the concept except perhaps for recreational use.

Another English physician, Henry Hill Hickman (Fig. 2), in 1823 and 1824 sought an inhaled anesthetic to relieve the pain of surgery. He might have succeeded if he had used nitrous oxide or ether, but the mice and dogs he studied inhaled high concentrations of carbon dioxide. Carbon dioxide has some anesthetic properties, as shown by the absence of response to an incision in the animals of Hickman's study. Hickman's concept was correct, his choice of agent unfortunate. Hickman lacked either the conviction or perhaps the resources to pursue his investigations on patients; he was unable to persuade his colleagues in England or France to attempt to duplicate his work in man and committed suicide at a young age. His seminal work was ignored by the medical profession for decades.

DISCOVERY: CLARKE, LONG, AND WELLS

William E Clarke may have given the first true ether anesthetic in Rochester, New York, in January 1842. From techniques learned as a chemistry student in 1839, Clarke entertained his companions and fellow medical students with nitrous oxide and ether. "... Clarke diligently propagated this convivial method among his fellow students. Emboldened by these experiences, in January, 1842, having returned to Rochester, he administered ether, from a towel, to a young woman named Hobbie, and one of her teeth was then extracted without pain by a dentist named Elijah Pope."[9] Clarke's medical school professors believed that the anesthetic state was due to hysteria, and he was advised to conduct no further anesthetic experiments.[10]

There is no doubt that 2 months later, on 30 March 1842, Crawford Williamson Long (Fig. 3) administered ether on a towel for surgical

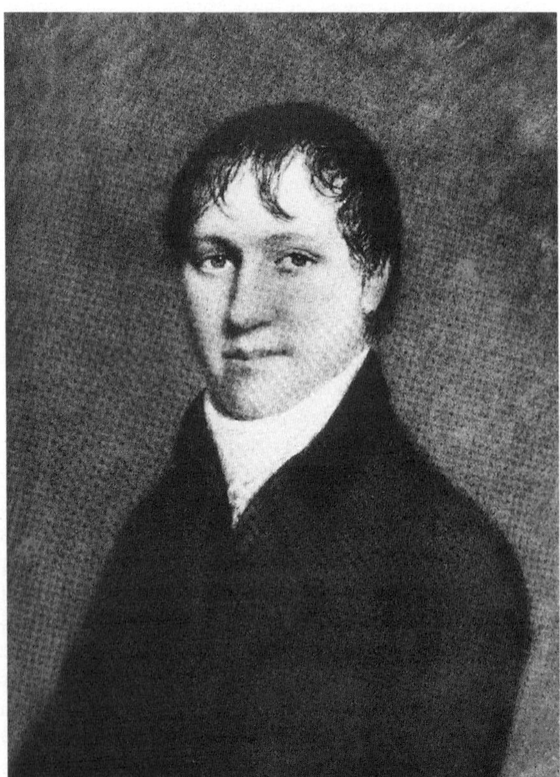

Figure 1 *Humphry Davy (image courtesy of the Wood Library-Museum).*

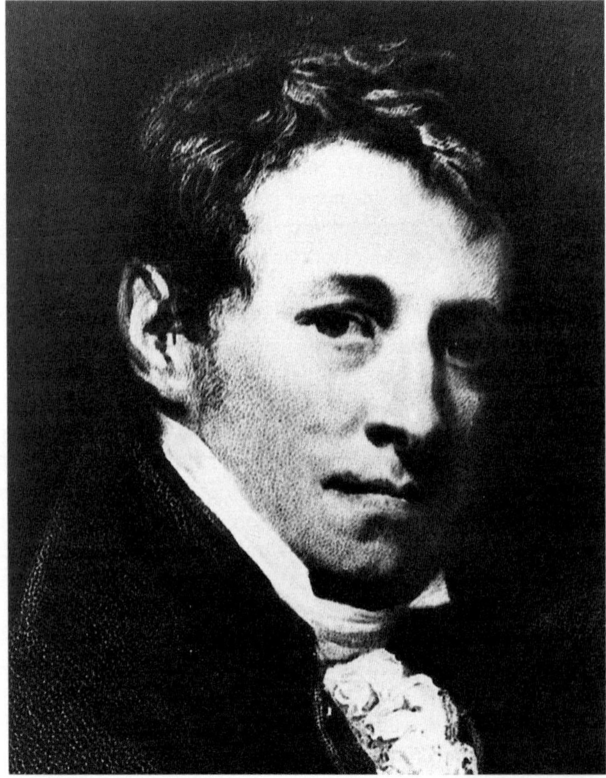

Figure 2 *Henry Hill Hickman (image courtesy of the Wood Library-Museum).*

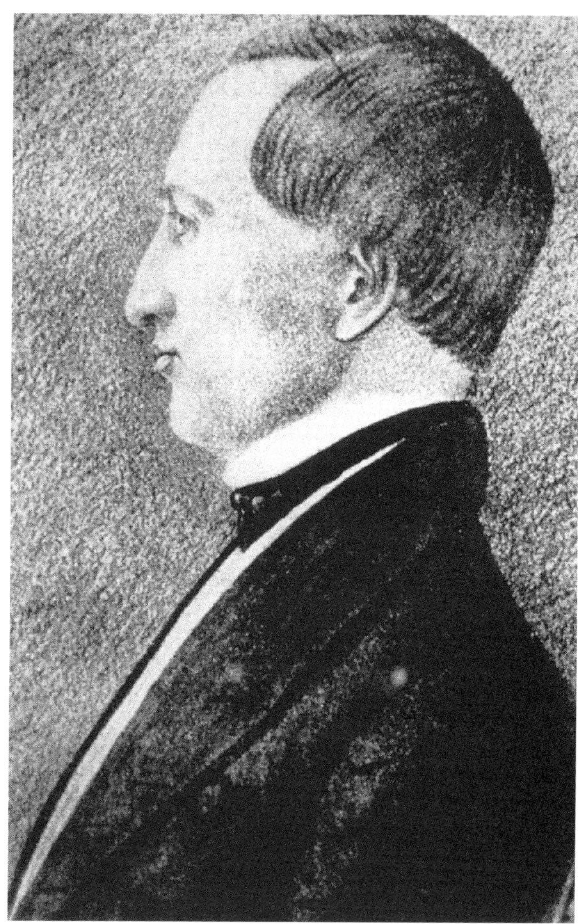

Figure 3 *Crawford Williamson Long (image courtesy of the Wood Library-Museum).*

anesthesia in Jefferson, Georgia. His patient, James M Venable, was a young man who had enjoyed ether's exhilarating effects, for he reported in a certificate that he had previously inhaled it frequently and was fond of its use. Venable had two small tumors on his neck but refused to have them excised because he dreaded the pain associated with surgery. Knowing that Venable was familiar with ether's action, Dr Long proposed that ether might alleviate pain and gained his patient's consent to proceed. After inhaling ether from the towel, Venable reported that he was unaware of the removal of the tumor.[11] As a rural physician with a very limited surgical practice, Crawford Long had few opportunities to administer ether anesthesia, but he did study its effects. He wished to prove that insensibility to pain was caused by ether and was not simply a reflection of the individual's pain threshold or the result of self-hypnosis. When ether was withheld during amputation of the second of two toes, his patient reported great pain and strenuously proclaimed a preference for ether. When asked in 1849, long after the public demonstration of ether at Harvard University, why he failed to publish the results of his work, Long explained that he practiced in an isolated environment and had few opportunities for surgical or dental procedures. Thus, with a limited number of cases, he did not wish to mislead his professional colleagues.

In contrast to the limited opportunities for surgery presented to rural practitioners in the mid-nineteenth century, urban dentists regularly met patients who refused restorative treatment because of fear of the pain inflicted by the procedure. From a dentist's perspective, pain was not so much life-threatening as it was livelihood-threatening. A few dentists searched for new techniques of effective pain relief. Horace Wells (Fig. 4), of Hartford, Connecticut, recognized what others had ignored, the analgesic potential of nitrous oxide. On 10 December

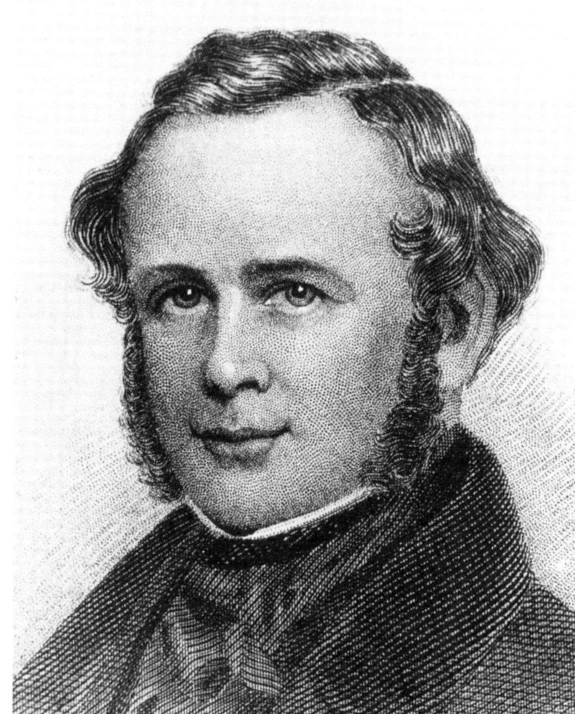

Figure 4 *Horace Wells (image courtesy of the Wood Library-Museum).*

1844, when he attended a lecture–exhibition by an itinerant "scientist," Gardner Quincy Colton, who prepared nitrous oxide and encouraged members of the audience to inhale the gas. Wells observed that a young man, Samuel Cooley, was unaware that he had injured his leg while under the influence of nitrous oxide. Sensing that nitrous oxide might also relieve the pain of dental procedures, Wells contacted Colton and boldly proposed an experiment. The following day, Colton gave Wells nitrous oxide before a fellow dentist, William Riggs, extracted a tooth.[12] When Wells awoke, he declared that he had not felt any pain and termed the experiment a success. Colton taught Wells how to prepare nitrous oxide, which the dentist administered with success. His apparatus probably resembled that used by Colton. The patient placed a wooden tube in his mouth through which he rebreathed nitrous oxide from a small bag filled with the gas.[13]

A few weeks later, in January 1845, Wells attempted a public demonstration in Boston at the Harvard Medical School. He had planned to anesthetize a patient for an amputation, but, when the patient refused surgery, a dental anesthetic for a medical student was substituted. Wells, perhaps influenced by a large and openly critical audience, began the extraction without an adequate level of anesthesia, and the trial was judged a failure. The exact circumstances of Wells' failure are not known. His less than enthusiastic patient may have refused to inhale the anesthetic. Alternatively, Wells may have lost part of his small supply of nitrous oxide, which could have occurred if the patient involuntarily removed his lips from the mouthpiece or if his nostrils were not held shut. It might have been that Wells did not know that nitrous oxide lacks sufficient potency to serve predictably as an anesthetic without supplementation. In any event, the student cried out, and Wells was jeered by his audience. No-one offered Wells even conditional encouragement or recognized that, even though his presentation had been flawed, nitrous oxide might represent a valuable therapeutic advance.[13]

The disappointment disturbed Wells deeply, and, although he continued to use nitrous oxide in his dental practice for some time, his life became unsettled. While profoundly distressed, and under arrest in the Toombs prison in New York City, Wells committed suicide in 1848.

Wells was an important pioneer of anesthesia as he was the first person to recognize the anesthetic qualities of nitrous oxide.[13]

A DISCOVERY – SURGICAL ANESTHESIA!

A second New Englander, William Thomas Green Morton (Fig. 5), briefly shared a dental practice with Horace Wells in Hartford. Wells' daybook shows that he gave Morton a course of instruction in anesthesia, but Morton apparently moved to Boston without paying for his lessons. In Boston, Morton continued his interest in anesthesia and, after learning from Charles Jackson that ether dropped on the skin provided analgesia, began experiments with inhaled ether. The volatility of the ether permitted effective inhalation. The concentrations required for surgical anesthesia were low and patients did not become hypoxic when breathing air. Ether also possessed a unique property among all inhaled anesthetics: the quality of providing surgical anesthesia without causing respiratory or cardiovascular depression. These properties, combined with a slow rate of induction, allowed a high margin of safety when physicians were attempting to master the new art of administering an inhaled anesthetic.[14]

After anesthetizing a pet dog, Morton's confidence in this wonder drug increased and he began to anesthetize patients in his dental office. As a result of his success, he received an invitation to give a public demonstration in the Bullfinch amphitheater of the Massachusetts General Hospital. On Friday 16 October 1846, Morton secured permission to administer an anesthetic to Edward Gilbert Abbott before the surgeon, John Collins Warren, excised a vascular lesion from the left side of Abbott's neck. Morton was late in arriving, and Warren was at the point of proceeding when Morton fortunately turned up. The dentist had been obliged to wait for an instrument-maker to complete his inhaler, which consisted of a large glass bulb containing a sponge soaked with colored ether and a spout, which was to be placed in the patient's mouth. An opening on the opposite side of the bulb allowed air to enter and to be drawn over the ether-soaked sponge with each breath.

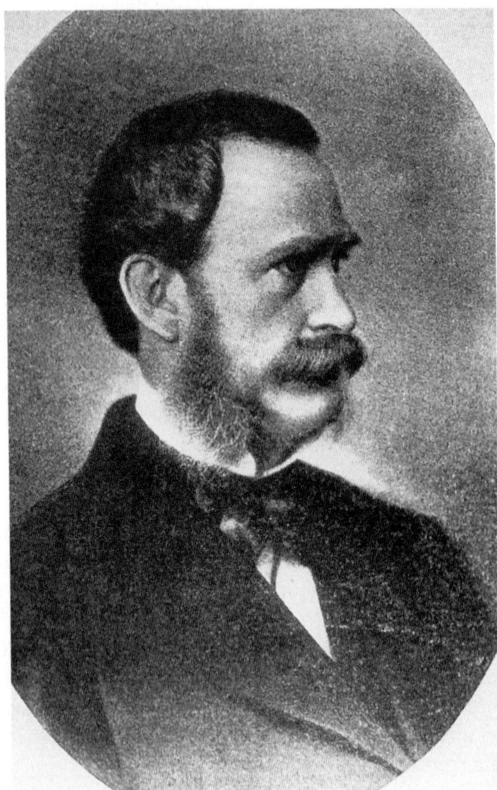

Figure 5 *William Thomas Green Morton (image courtesy of the Wood Library-Museum).*

Abbott took the inhaler in his mouth. Surgery proceeded. Gilbert Abbott later reported that he was aware of the operation but had experienced no pain. At the moment that the procedure ended, Warren turned to his audience and allegedly announced, "Gentlemen, this is no humbug."[15] Oliver Wendell Holmes soon suggested the term "anesthesia" to describe this state of temporary insensibility. William Morton's demonstration of ether was a seminal event, in part because it took place in a public arena and in part because of the very revolutionary nature of what had happened. The centuries-long chain of surgical pain had been cut by a few breaths of ether but the "good news" took weeks, months, and even years to become fully accepted.[16]

America's greatest contribution to nineteenth-century medicine had been realized, but almost immediately the event was shrouded in subterfuge and conflict. Some weeks passed before Morton admitted that the active component of the colored fluid, which he had called "Letheon," was the familiar drug diethyl ether. Morton, Wells, and Jackson, and their supporters soon became caught up in a contentious, protracted, and fruitless debate who should be credited with the discovery, popularly termed "the ether controversy." In short, Morton had applied for a patent for Letheon,[17] and when this was granted tried to extract royalties for the use of ether as an anesthetic. Eventually, the matter came before the United States Congress; the House of Representatives voted to grant Morton a large sum of money for the discovery, but the Senate quashed the deal.

When the details of Morton's anesthetic technique became public knowledge, the information was transmitted to the rest of the world. By December, the first procedures under anesthesia had been performed in Britain, and by January continental Europe was experimenting with this new American invention. Within 6 months of the first public demonstration, anesthetics were being administered in Australia.[18] There can be little doubt that the enthusiasm shown in Western Europe for painless surgery through ether anesthesia ensured that what was initially considered to be a doubtful procedure had a platform on which its subsequent development could build. But even though surgery could now be performed painlessly, the frequency of operations did not rise rapidly. Several years would pass before anesthesia was universally recommended as many senior surgeons believed that pain was part of the healing process. And the other surgical demon, infection, would await the great discoveries of the second half of the nineteenth century; only then, with pain and infection conquered, did complex surgical intervention assume a prominent role in medical care.

A "BLESSING" TO OBSTETRICS

James Young Simpson (Fig. 6), a successful obstetrician in Edinburgh, Scotland, had been among the first to use ether for the relief of the pain of labor, having spent the Christmas of 1846 with the London surgeon Robert Liston, who told him of its efficacy in achieving painless surgery. However, the effect of ether was slow in onset, and in the domiciliary practice of obstetrics at that time there was the added risk of explosion when ether was administered in a room containing an open fire. Simpson therefore sought a more pleasant, rapid-acting anesthetic. Simpson and his junior associates experimented by inhaling samples of several volatile chemicals collected by local apothecaries. David Waldie suggested chloroform, which had first been prepared in 1831. At a dinner party in Simpson's home on the evening of 4 November 1847, the assembled group sampled the chloroform. They promptly fell unconscious, and when they awoke they were delighted at their success. Simpson quickly set about encouraging the use of chloroform. Within

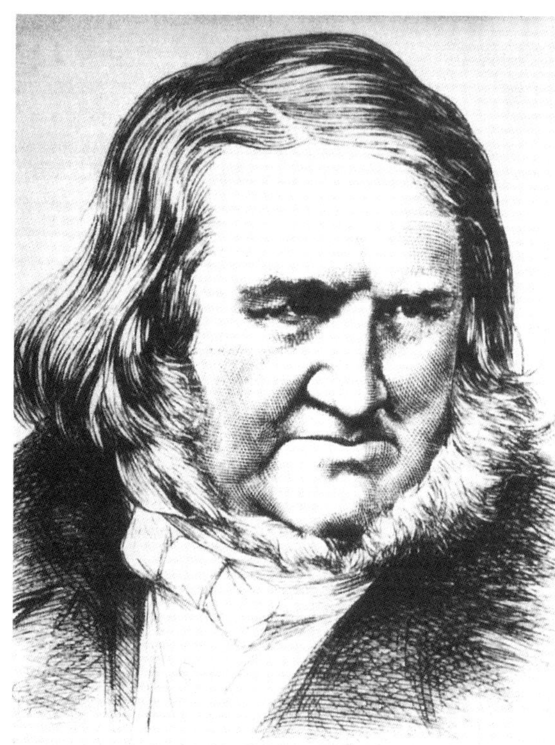

Figure 6 *James Young Simpson (image courtesy of the Wood Library-Museum).*

2 weeks, he had dispatched his first account of its use to *The Lancet*. Although Simpson introduced chloroform with alacrity, boldness, and enthusiasm, and was later to become a vocal defender of the use of anesthesia for women in labor, he administered few anesthetics himself. His goal was simply to improve a patient's comfort during his operative or obstetric activities.[19]

The relief of obstetric pain had significant social ramifications, particularly in the nineteenth century, and made anesthesia during delivery a controversial subject. Simpson himself argued against the prevailing view that relief of the pain of childbirth was contrary to God's will. The pain of the parturient was perceived as both a component of punishment and a means of atonement for Original Sin. Less than a year after administering the first anesthesia during childbirth, Simpson addressed these concerns in a pamphlet entitled "Answers to the Religious Objections Advanced Against the Employment of Anaesthetic Agents in Midwifery and Surgery and Obstetrics." In this work, Simpson recognized the Book of Genesis as being the root of this sentiment, and noted that God promised to relieve the descendants of Adam and Eve of the curse. Additionally, Simpson asserted that labor pain is an outcome of scientific and anatomical causes, and not the result of religious condemnation. He stated that the upright position humans assumed during labor required strong pelvic muscles to support the abdominal contents. As a result, he argued, the uterus necessarily developed strong musculature – with such great contractile power that it caused pain – to overcome the resistance of the pelvic floor.[19]

The response to Simpson's assertions was variable. While he was criticized for these ideas by fellow physician Samuel Ashwell in an editorial published in *The Lancet*, many other physicians commented favorably, including some who had opposed obstetric anesthesia for medical reasons. All in all, Simpson's pamphlet probably did not have much impact in terms of changing the prevailing viewpoints about pain control during labor, but he did verbalize many concepts that his contemporaries were debating at the time.[19] It was John Snow (Fig. 7), an English contemporary of the Simpson, who achieved fame as an obstetric anesthetist by treating Queen Victoria.

Queen Victoria's consort, Prince Albert, interviewed John Snow before he was called to Buckingham Palace at the request of the Queen's obstetrician to administer chloroform during delivery of what was to be her penultimate child. During the delivery, Snow administered analgesic doses of chloroform on a folded handkerchief, a technique that was soon termed *chloroform à la reine*. Victoria abhorred the pain of labor and enjoyed the relief that chloroform provided; she wrote in her journal, "Dr. Snow gave that blessed chloroform and the effect was soothing, quieting, and delightful beyond measure."[20] After the Queen, who was head of the Church of England, endorsed obstetric anesthesia, the religious debate over the appropriateness of the use of anesthesia in labor terminated abruptly. Four years later, during delivery of her last child, Queen Victoria was determined to have chloroform and Snow again administered the anesthetic. Snow's daybook states that, by the time he arrived, Prince Albert had begun the anesthetic and had given his wife "a little chloroform." This may be the only time in history that a queen has had a prince as her anesthetist.

THE EARLY PIONEERS

John Snow was already a respected physician when the news of ether anesthesia reached Britain in December 1846. He took an interest in anesthetic practice and was soon invited to work with many of the leading surgeons of the day. He was not only adept at administering

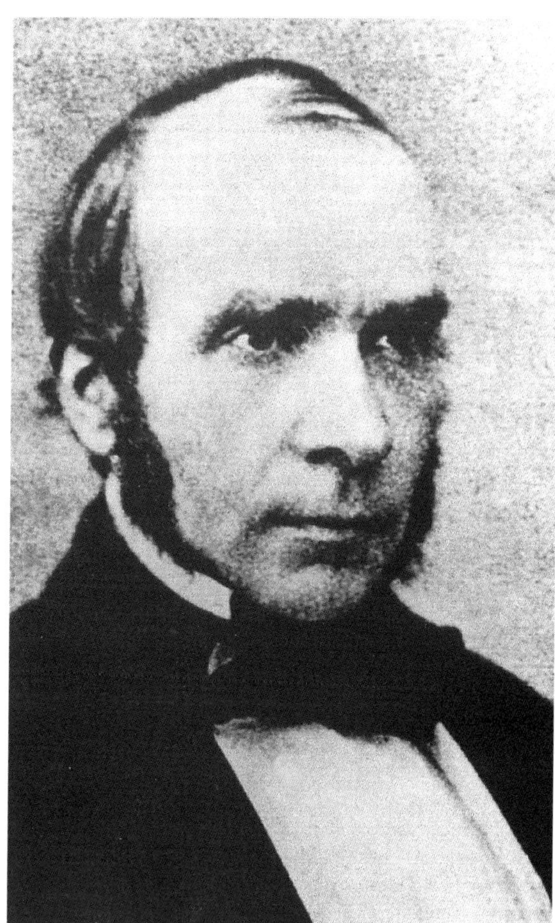

Figure 7 *John Snow (image courtesy of the Wood Library-Museum).*

anesthesia but was also a remarkably keen observer. Snow's innovative description of the stages or degrees of ether anesthesia based on the patient's responsiveness was not improved on for another 70 years.

Snow developed anesthetic apparatus. He soon realized the inadequacies of ether inhalers into which the patient rebreathed through a mouthpiece. After practicing anesthesia for only 2 weeks, Snow designed the first of his series of ingenious ether inhalers.[21] His best-known apparatus featured unidirectional valves within a malleable, well-fitting mask of his own design, which closely resembles the form of a modern face mask. The face piece was connected to the vaporizer by a breathing tube, which Snow deliberately designed to be wider than the human trachea so that even rapid respirations would not be impeded. A metal coil within the vaporizer ensured that the patient's inspired breath was drawn over a large surface area to promote the uptake of ether. The device also incorporated a warm water bath to maintain the volatility of the agent. Snow, in contrast to Morton, Wells, and Jackson, did not attempt to capitalize on his invention; rather he encouraged others to duplicate his work. He closed his account of the preparation of the inhaler with the generous observation, "There is no restriction respecting the making of it."[22]

The following year, John Snow introduced an agent-specific chloroform inhaler. At the same time, he initiated what was to become an extraordinary series of experiments that were remarkable both in their scope and in the manner in which they anticipated sophisticated research performed a century later. Snow realized that successful anesthetics must not only abolish pain but also prevent movement. He anesthetized several species of animals with varying concentrations of ether and chloroform to determine the concentration required to prevent movement in response to a sharp stimulus. Despite the limitations of technology in 1848, this element of his work anticipated the modern concept of minimum alveolar concentration (MAC).[23] Snow assessed the anesthetic action of a large number of potential anesthetics, and, although he did not find any to rival chloroform or ether, he determined a relation between solubility, vapor pressure, and anesthetic potency that was not fully appreciated until after World War II, when Charles Suckling employed Snow's principles in developing halothane. He also fabricated an experimental closed-circuit device in which the subject (Snow himself) breathed oxygen while the exhaled carbon dioxide was absorbed by potassium hydroxide. Snow published two remarkable books *On the Inhalation of the Vapour of Ether* (1847) and *On Chloroform and Other Anaesthetics* (1858), which was almost completed when he died of a stroke at the age of 45.

Snow's investigations were not confined to anesthesia. His memory is also respected by specialists in infectious and tropical diseases for his proof through an epidemiological study in 1854 that cholera was transmitted by water. At that time, before the development of microbiology by Louis Pasteur and Robert Koch, most physicians in North America and Europe attributed the mysterious recurring epidemics of cholera to the contagion of "fecalized air." For many years, however, Snow had believed that, because the disease affected the gastrointestinal tract, the causative agent must be ingested rather than inhaled. In 1854, he found an opportunity to prove his thesis when cholera visited his section of London and caused the deaths of more than 500 people near his residence. Snow determined that the water supply for these persons had been the Broad Street pump. He prepared what would come to be appreciated as the first epidemiological survey to prove his contention. With that information, he was able to encourage the parish authorities to remove the pump handle so that residents were obliged to find other sources of water. The prompt end of this already resolving epidemic was attributed to his action. The existence of the John Snow Public House in Broadwick Street in London's Soho area commemorates these events and acts as the meeting house for the John Snow Society, whose members are anesthetists and public health physicians.

NINETEENTH-CENTURY BRITISH ANESTHESIA – AFTER JOHN SNOW

The pattern of fortuitous discovery of anesthetic agents that brought nitrous oxide, diethyl ether, and chloroform forward between 1844 and 1847 continued for decades. The next inhaled anesthetics to be used routinely, ethyl chloride and ethylene, were also discovered as a result of unexpected observations. Ethyl chloride and ethylene were first formulated in the eighteenth century, and had been examined as anesthetics in Germany soon after the discovery of ether's action, but were ignored for decades. Ethyl chloride retained some use as a topical anesthetic and counterirritant. It was so volatile that the skin transiently "froze" after ethyl chloride was sprayed upon it. Its rediscovery as an anesthetic came in 1894, when a Swedish dentist, Hjalmar Carlson, sprayed ethyl chloride into a patient's mouth to "freeze" a dental abscess. Carlson was surprised to discover that his patient suddenly lost consciousness. Ethyl chloride became a commonly employed inhaled anesthetic in several countries. Throughout the remainder of the nineteenth century, the "American invention" excited interest everywhere.

Joseph Clover became the leading anesthetist in London following the death of John Snow in 1858. Clover was a talented clinician and skillful inventor, but he never performed research or wrote to the extent that Snow did. If he had written a text, he might be better remembered, but most physicians have little knowledge of Clover beyond identifying the familiar photograph in which he is seen anesthetizing a seated man while palpating his patient's pulse. Clinicians now accept Clover's monitoring of the pulse as a simple routine of prudent practice, but in Clover's time this was a contentious issue. Prominent Scottish surgeons scorned Clover's emphasis on the action of chloroform on the heart. Baron Lister and others preferred that senior medical students give anesthetics and urged them to "strictly carry out certain simple instructions, among which is to never touch the pulse, in order that their attention may not be distracted from the respiration."[24] Lister also counseled, "it appears that preliminary examination of the chest, often considered indispensable, is quite unnecessary, and more likely to induce the dreaded syncope, by alarming the patients, than to avert it."[24] Little progress in anesthesia could come from such reactionary statements.

In contrast, Clover had observed the effect of chloroform on animals and urged other anesthetists to monitor the pulse at all times and to discontinue the anesthetic temporarily if any irregularity or weakness in the strength of the pulse was observed. He earned a loyal following among London surgeons, who accepted him as a dedicated specialist. Clover was the first anesthetist to administer chloroform in known concentrations through the Clover bag. He obtained a 4.5% concentration of chloroform in air by pumping a measured volume of air with a bellows through a warmed evaporating vessel containing a known volume of liquid chloroform. The apparatus featured inspiratory and expiratory valves of ivory supported by springs. A flap valve in the face mask permitted the dilution of the anesthetic with air. In 1868, Clover reported no deaths among 1802 anesthetics using his device, but he later reviewed a fatality in searching detail. He attributed the death to an unrecognized error in calculating the volume of air diluting the chloroform.[25] After 1870, Clover favored administration of nitrous oxide and ether in sequence and designed a very complex apparatus for this purpose. The Clover portable regulating ether inhaler was the first of a series of elegant metal and glass inhalers that remained in regular use right up to the 1960s and maybe even later. An Ombredanne inhaler of this type was found as standard issue for combat anesthesia in one South American country in the 1980s.

In addition to his work with anesthetic agents, Clover was very adept in managing the airway. He was the first Englishman to urge the now universal practice of thrusting the patient's jaw forward to overcome obstruction of the upper airway by the tongue. Despite the limitation of working before the first tracheal tube was used in anesthesia, Clover published a landmark case report in 1877. His patient had a tumor of the mouth that obstructed the airway completely in spite of performing the jaw thrust maneuver once the anesthetic was begun. Clover averted disaster by inserting a small curved cannula of his own design through the cricothyroid membrane. He continued anesthesia via the cannula until the tumor was excised. Clover, the model of the prepared anesthesiologist, remarked, "I have never used the cannula before although it has been my companion at some thousands of anaesthetic cases."[26]

Every element of Clover's records and his published accounts reflect a consistent dedication to patient safety coupled with a prudent ability to anticipate potential difficulties and to prepare an effective response beforehand. In this respect, his manner was very much like that of his successor, the first English anesthetist to be knighted, Sir Frederick Hewitt. Hewitt gained the first of his London hospital anesthesia appointments in 1884. He earned a reputation as a superb and inventive clinician and came to be considered the leading British practitioner of anesthesia in the next 30 years. Hewitt engineered modifications of portable ether and nitrous oxide inhalers and, recognizing that nitrous oxide and air formed a hypoxic mixture, designed the first anesthetic apparatus to deliver oxygen and nitrous oxide in variable proportions. He was also influential in ensuring that anesthesia was taught in all British medical schools. His book, *Anaesthetics and Their Administration*, which first appeared in 1893 and continued through five editions, is considered the first true modern textbook of anesthesia. In 1908, Hewitt developed an important appliance that would assist all anesthesiologists in managing an obstructed upper airway. He called his oral device an "air-way restorer," thus introducing the practice of inserting an airway to help ventilation during an anesthetic.

LATE NINETEENTH-CENTURY ANESTHESIA IN AMERICA

American clinicians of the second half of the nineteenth century failed to achieve the lasting recognition gained by their British colleagues. Several factors contributed to this disparity. Snow, Clover, and Hewitt were unique men of genius who did not have contemporaries in America. Ether remained the dominant anesthetic in America, where the provision of anesthesia was a task often delegated to medical students, junior house officers, nurses, and nonprofessionals. The subordinate status of anesthesia was reflected in American art. Thomas Eakins' great studies *The Gross Clinic* of 1876 and *The Agnew Clinic* of 1889 present the surgeon as the focus of attention, whereas the person administering the anesthetic is barely discernible among the supporting figures.

During this period, however, Americans led the revival of nitrous oxide. Gardner Q Colton, the "professor" who had first demonstrated the use of nitrous oxide to Horace Wells, developed the Colton Dental Association after he returned from the California gold rush. He opened offices in several eastern cities equipped with nitrous oxide generators and, perhaps profiting from Wells' unhappy experience, larger breathing bags of 30 L capacity. By 1869, his advertisements carried the intriguing slogan "31½ Miles Long." Colton had asked each patient to sign a scroll, which then contained the names of 55 000 patients who had experienced painless extractions of teeth without hazard. He proposed that if this great number of patients were to march past in single file, the line would extend for 31½ miles.[27]

Colton gave brief exposures of nitrous oxide undiluted with air or oxygen, which raised concern that the gas was acting as an asphyxiant. The following year a Chicago surgeon, Edmund Andrews, experimented with an oxygen–nitrous oxide mixture and proved that nitrous oxide does not cause anesthesia by depriving the brain of oxygen. Although the oxygen–nitrous oxide mixture was safer, he identified a disadvantage to its use that was unique to that time, when patients were attended in their homes. The large bag was conspicuous and awkward to carry whenever Andrews walked along busy streets. He observed that "In city practice, among the higher classes, however, this is no obstacle as the bag can always be taken in a carriage, without attracting attention."[28] Four years later, Andrews was delighted to report the availability of liquefied nitrous oxide compressed under 750 lb of pressure, which allowed a supply sufficient for three patients to be carried in a single cylinder. Despite Andrews' early enthusiasm, few American surgeons relied on nitrous oxide until it was used in combination with regional anesthesia, the last great contribution to anesthetic practice achieved in the late nineteenth century.

THE DISCOVERY OF REGIONAL ANESTHESIA IN THE NINETEENTH CENTURY

Cocaine, an extract of the coca leaf, was the first effective local anesthetic. Its property of numbing mucous membranes and exposed tissues had been known for centuries in Peru, where folk surgeons performing trephinations of the skull chewed coca leaves and allowed their saliva to fall onto the surfaces of the wound. This was a unique situation in anesthesia; there are no other examples of both operator and patient routinely sharing the effects of the same drug. After Albert Niemann refined the active alkaloid and named it cocaine, it was used in experiments by a few investigators. It was noted that cocaine provided topical anesthesia and even produced local insensibility when injected, but these observations were not applied in clinical practice until 1884, when the significance of the action of cocaine was realized by Carl Koller (Fig. 8), a Viennese surgical intern.[29]

Carl Koller appreciated what others had failed to recognize because of his past experience and his ambition to practice ophthalmology at a time when many operations on the eye were still being performed without anesthesia. Almost four decades after the discovery of ether, general anesthesia by mask had several limitations for ophthalmologic surgery. The anesthetized patient could not cooperate with the surgeon and the anesthesiologist's apparatus interfered with surgical access. Also, at that time, many surgical incisions on the eye were not closed, as fine sutures were not yet available while the high incidence of vomiting following the administration of ether or chloroform threatened the extrusion of the internal contents of the globe, with the risk of permanent blindness.

Koller, while a medical student, had worked in a laboratory in Vienna, looking for a topical ophthalmic anesthetic to overcome the limitations of general anesthesia. Unfortunately, the suspensions of morphine, chloral hydrate, and other drugs that he tried were not effective. In 1884, his friend, Sigmund Freud, became interested in the cerebrum-stimulating effects of cocaine and gave Koller a small sample in an envelope, which he placed in his pocket. When the envelope leaked, a few grains of cocaine stuck to Koller's finger, which he casually licked with his tongue. It became numb. At that moment, Koller realized that he had found the object of his search. He dashed to the laboratory and made a suspension of cocaine crystals. He and Gustav Gartner, a laboratory associate, observed its anesthetic effect on the eyes of a frog, a rabbit, and a dog before they dropped the solution onto their own corneas. To their amazement, their eyes were insensitive to the touch of a pin.[29]

As an intern Carl Koller could not afford to attend the Congress of German Ophthalmologists in Heidelberg on 15 September 1884, but, after a friend read his article, a revolution in ophthalmic surgery and other surgical disciplines began. Within the next year, more than 100 articles supporting the use of cocaine appeared in European and American medical journals. Despite this gratifying success, Koller was not able to pursue his goal of gaining a residency position in Vienna. After a duel provoked by an anti-Semitic slur, Koller left Austria and, after studying briefly in The Netherlands and Britain, emigrated in 1888

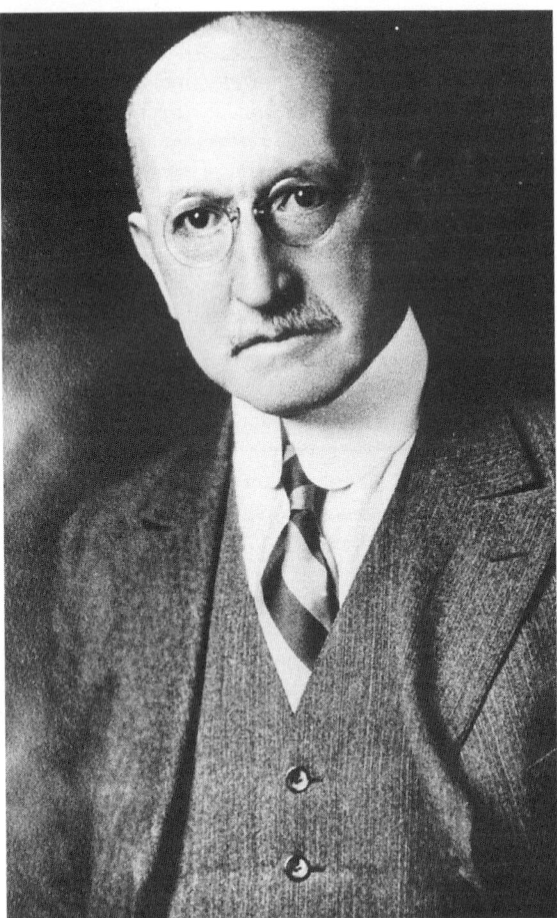

Figure 8 *Carl Koller (photograph courtesy of the Wood Library-Museum).*

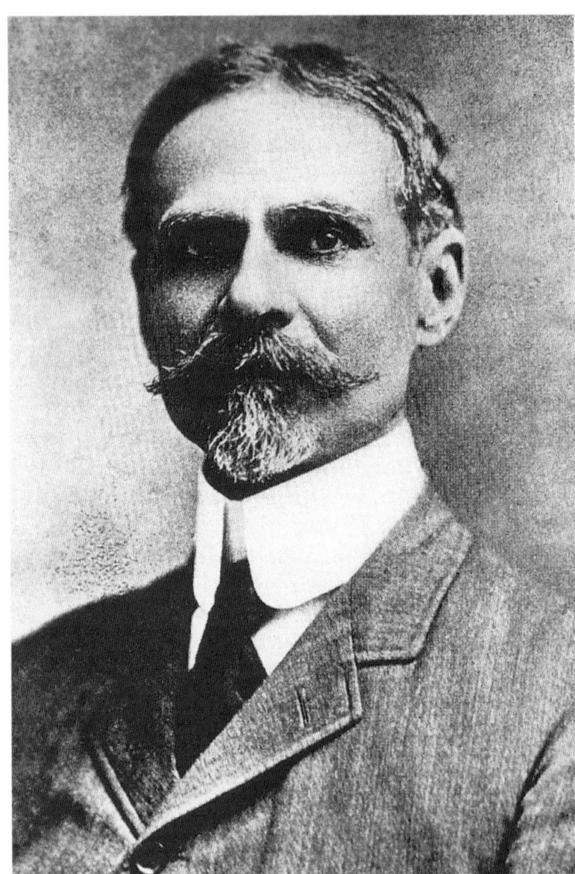

Figure 9 *Leonard Corning (photograph courtesy of the Wood Library-Museum).*

to New York, where he practiced ophthalmology for the remainder of his career.

American surgeons quickly developed new applications for cocaine. Its efficacy in anesthetizing the nose, mouth, larynx, trachea, rectum, and urethra was described in October 1884. The next month, the first reports were published of its subcutaneous injection. In December 1884, two young surgeons, William Halsted and Richard Hall, described blocks of the sensory nerves of the face and arm. Halsted even performed a brachial plexus block, but did so under direct vision while the patient received an inhaled anesthetic. Unfortunately, self-experimentation with cocaine was hazardous as both surgeons became addicted. Addiction was an ill-understood but frequent problem in the late nineteenth century, especially when cocaine and morphine were present in many patent medicines.[30]

Other local anesthetic techniques were attempted before the end of the nineteenth century. The term "spinal anesthesia" was coined in 1885 by Leonard Corning (Fig. 9), a neurologist who had observed Hall and Halsted. Corning wanted to assess the action of cocaine as a specific therapy for neurological problems. After first assessing its action in a dog, producing a blockade of rapid onset that was confined to the animal's rear legs, he administered cocaine to a man "addicted to masturbation." Corning administered one dose without effect, then, after a second dose, the patient's legs "felt sleepy." The man had impaired sensibility in his lower extremity after about 20 minutes. He left Corning's office "none the worse for the experience."[31] Although Corning does not refer to the escape of cerebrospinal fluid (CSF) in either case, it is likely that the dog had a spinal anesthetic and that the man had an epidural anesthetic. No therapeutic benefit was described, but Corning closed his account and his attention to the subject by suggesting that cocainization might in time be "a substitute for etherization in genito-urinary or other branches of surgery."[32]

Two other authors, August Bier (Fig. 10) and Theodor Tuffier, described authentic spinal anesthesia, with mention of cerebrospinal fluid, injection of cocaine, and an appropriately short onset of action. When the original articles by Bier, Tuffier, and Corning were compared, one author came to the conclusion that Corning's injection was extradural, and Bier merited the credit for introducing spinal anesthesia.[31]

Fourteen years passed before spinal anesthesia was performed in surgery. In the interval, Heinrich Quincke of Kiel, Germany, described his technique of lumbar puncture. He proposed that it was most safely performed at the level of the third or fourth lumbar interspace, because an entry at that level would be below the termination of the spinal cord. Quincke's technique was used in Kiel by a surgical colleague, August Bier, for the first deliberate cocainization of the spinal cord in 1899. Six patients received small doses of cocaine intrathecally, but, because some cried out during surgery while others vomited and experienced headaches, Bier considered it necessary to conduct a clinical experiment.[33]

Professor Bier allowed his assistant, Dr Hildebrandt, to give him a lumbar puncture, but, after the needle penetrated the dura, Hildebrandt could not fit the syringe to the needle and a large volume of spinal fluid escaped. The pair were at the point of abandoning the study when Hildebrandt volunteered to be the subject of a second attempt. This time they experienced remarkable success. Twenty-three minutes later, Bier noted: "A strong blow with an iron hammer against the tibia was not felt as pain. After twenty-five minutes: Strong pressure and pulling on a testicle were not painful."[33] They celebrated their success with wine and cigars. That night, both developed violent headaches, which they attributed at first to their celebration. Bier's headache was relieved

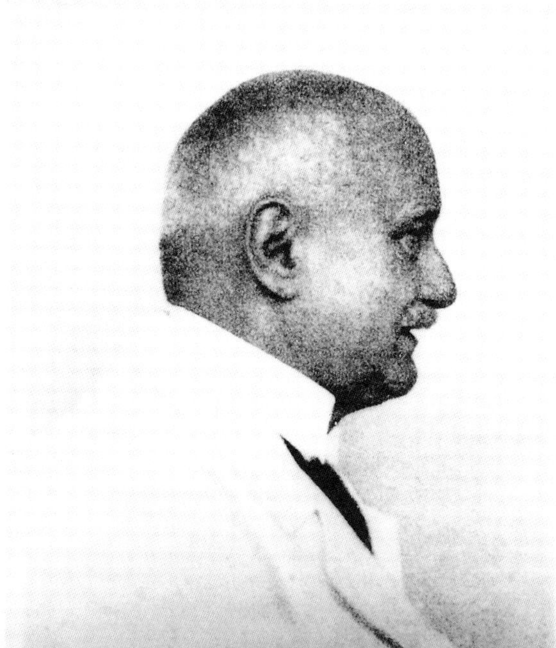

AUGUST BIER
Bonn, Germany
Who had the temerity to have cocaine injected into his own spine in order to prove a theory.

Figure 10 *August Bier (photograph courtesy of the Wood Library-Museum).*

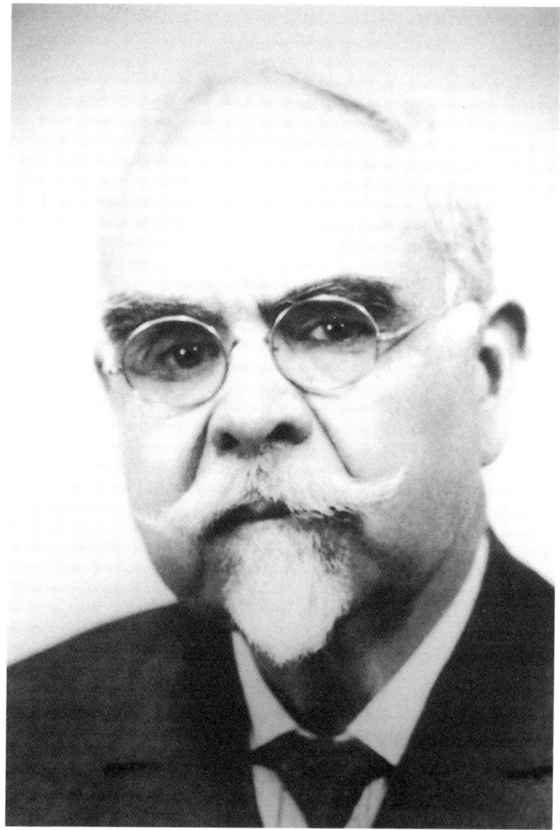

Figure 11 *Rudolph Matas (photograph courtesy of the Wood Library-Museum).*

after 9 days of bedrest. The house officer did not have the luxury of continued rest; Bier noted that Hildebrandt "felt very poor the next morning but with great physical effort he was able to do his work, which consisted mainly in operating and dressing of wounds." Bier postulated that their headaches were due to the loss of large volumes of CSF and urged that this be avoided if possible. The high incidence of complications following lumbar puncture with wide-bore needles and the toxic reactions attributed to cocaine explain his later loss of interest in spinal anesthesia.[33]

Surgeons in several other countries soon adopted the practice of spinal anesthesia. Many of their observations are still relevant. The first series from France of 125 cases was published by Theodor Tuffier, who later advised that the anesthetic solution should not be injected until CSF was seen. The first American report was by Rudolph Matas (Fig. 11) of New Orleans, whose first patient developed postanesthetic meningismus, a then frequent complication, that was overcome in part by the use of hermetically sealed sterile solutions recommended by E W Lee of Philadelphia and sterile gloves as advocated by Halsted. During 1899, Dudley Tait and Guidlo Caglieri of San Francisco performed experimental studies in animals and therapeutic spinal anesthesia in orthopedic patients.[34] They encouraged the use of fine needles to minimize the escape of CSF and urged that the skin and deeper tissues be infiltrated beforehand with local anesthesia, as had been urged earlier by William Halsted and the foremost advocate of infiltration anesthesia, Carl Ludwig Schleich of Berlin.[35] An early American specialist in anesthesia, Ormond Goldan, published an anesthesia record appropriate for recording the course of "intraspinal cocainization" in 1900. In the same year, Heinrich Braun learned of a newly described extract of the adrenal gland, epinephrine, which he used to prolong the action of local anesthetics with great success. Braun developed several new nerve blocks, coined the term "conduction anesthesia," and is remembered by European writers as the "father of conduction anesthesia." Braun was the first person to use procaine, which, along with stovaine, was one of the first synthetic local anesthetics produced to reduce the toxicity of cocaine. Further advances in spinal anesthesia followed the introduction of these and other synthetic local anesthetics.

Before 1907, several anesthesiologists were disappointed to observe that spinal anesthesia was frequently incomplete. Most believed that the drug spread solely by local diffusion until this phenomenon was investigated by Arthur Barker, a London surgeon.[35] Barker constructed a glass tube shaped to follow the curves of the human spine and used it to demonstrate the limited spread of colored solutions that he had injected through a T-piece in the lumbar region. Barker applied this observation to use solutions of stovaine made hyperbaric by the addition of 5% glucose, which worked in a more predictable fashion. After the injection was complete, Barker placed his patient's head on pillows to contain the anesthetic below the nipple line. Lincoln Sise acknowledged Barker's work in 1935 when he introduced the use of hyperbaric solutions of pontocaine. John Adriani advanced the concept further in 1946 when he used a hyperbaric solution to produce "saddle block" or perineal anesthesia. Adriani's patients remained seated after injection as the drug descended to the sacral nerves.

Tait, Jonnesco, and other early masters of spinal anesthesia used a cervical approach for thyroidectomy and thoracic procedures, but this radical approach was supplanted in 1928 by the lumbar injection of hypobaric solutions of "light" nupercaine by G P Pitkin. Although hypobaric solutions are now usually limited to patients in the jack-knife position, their former use for thoracic procedures demanded skill and precise timing. Enthusiasts of hypobaric anesthesia devised formulas in an attempt to predict the time in seconds needed for a warmed solution of hypobaric nupercaine to spread in patients of varying size from its site of injection in the lumbar area to the level of the fourth thoracic dermatome. At this point, the patient was suddenly tipped head down so that the drug would not affect the innervation of the diaphragm and larynx. Among the accepted risks of the hypobaric technique was a prompt and total sympathetic blockade, which occurred so predictably that "wise" clinicians advised their residents, "Don't bother taking the blood pressure! I know that it will be down."

The recurring problem of inadequate duration of single-injection spinal anesthesia led a Philadelphia surgeon, William Lemmon, to devise an apparatus for continuous spinal anesthesia in 1940.[36] Lemmon began with the patient in the lateral position. The spinal tap was performed with a malleable silver needle, which was left in position. As the patient was moved into the supine position, the needle was inserted through a hole in the mattress and table. Additional injections of local anesthetic could be performed as required. Malleable silver needles also found a less cumbersome and more common application in 1942, when Waldo Edwards and Robert Hingson encouraged the use of Lemmon's needles for continuous caudal anesthesia in obstetrics. In 1944, Edward Tuohy of the Mayo Clinic introduced two important modifications to the continuous spinal techniques. He developed the now familiar Tuohy needle as a means of improving the ease of passage of lacquered silk ureteral catheters through which he injected incremental doses of local anesthetic.[37]

OTHER TWENTIETH-CENTURY CONTRIBUTIONS TO REGIONAL ANESTHESIA

Surgery on the extremities lent itself to other regional anesthesia techniques. At first, these were combined with general anesthesia. In 1902, Harvey Cushing coined the phrase "regional anesthesia" for his technique of blocking either the brachial or sciatic plexus under direct vision during general anesthesia to reduce anesthesia requirements and provide postoperative pain relief.[38] Fifteen years before his publication, a similar approach had been energetically advanced to reduce the stress and shock of surgery by George Crile, another dedicated advocate of regional and infiltration techniques during general anesthesia.

An intravenous regional technique with procaine was reported in 1908 by August Bier, the surgeon who had pioneered spinal anesthesia. Bier injected procaine into a vein of the upper limb between two tourniquets. Even though the technique is termed Bier's block, it was not used for many decades, until it was reintroduced 55 years after its first use by Mackinnon Holmes, who modified the technique by exsanguination before applying a single proximal cuff. Holmes used lidocaine, the very successful amide local anesthetic synthesized in 1943 by Lofgren and Lundquist of Sweden.[39]

Several investigators achieved upper extremity anesthesia by percutaneous injections of the brachial plexus. In 1911, based on his intimate knowledge of the anatomy of the axillary area, Hirschel promoted a "blind" axillary injection. In the same year, Kulenkampff described a supraclavicular approach in which the operator sought out paresthesias of the plexus while keeping the needle at a point superficial to the first rib and the pleura. The risk of pneumothorax with Kulenkampff's approach led Mulley to attempt blocks more proximally using a lateral paravertebral approach, the precursor of which is now popularly known as the Winnie block.

Heinrich Braun wrote the earliest textbook of local anesthesia, which appeared in its first English translation in 1914. After 1922, Gaston Labat's (Fig. 12) *Regional Anesthesia* dominated the American market. Labat migrated from France to the Mayo Clinic, where he served briefly before taking a permanent position at the Bellevue Hospital in New York, where he worked with Hippolite Wertheim. They formed the first American Society for Regional Anesthesia in 1926. After Labat's death, Emery A Rovenstine was recruited to Bellevue to continue Labat's work. Rovenstine created the first American clinic for the treatment of chronic pain, where he and his associates refined techniques of lytic and therapeutic injections, and used the American Society of Regional Anesthesia to further knowledge of pain management across the United States.[40]

The development of the multidisciplinary pain clinic was one of many contributions to anesthesiology made by John J Bonica, a renowned teacher of regional techniques. During his periods of military, civilian, and university service at the University of Washington, John Bonica formulated a series of improvements in the management of patients with chronic pain. His text, *The Management of Pain*, now in its second edition, is regarded as a classic of the literature of anesthesia.[41]

EPIDURAL ANESTHESIA

In 1949, Martinez Curbelo of Havana, Cuba, used Tuohy's needle and a ureteral catheter to administer the first continuous epidural anesthetic. Silk and gum elastic catheters were difficult to sterilize and sometimes caused dural infections until they were superseded by disposable plastic catheters. However, deliberate single-injection peridural anesthesia had been practiced occasionally for decades before continuous techniques brought it greater popularity. At the beginning of the twentieth century, two French clinicians experimented independently with caudal anesthesia. A neurologist, Jean Athanase Sicard, applied the technique for a nonsurgical purpose, the relief of back pain while Fernand Cathelin used caudal anesthesia as a less dangerous alternative to spinal anesthesia for repair of a hernia. He also demonstrated that the epidural space terminated in the neck by injecting a solution of India ink into the caudal canal of a dog. The lumbar approach was first used solely

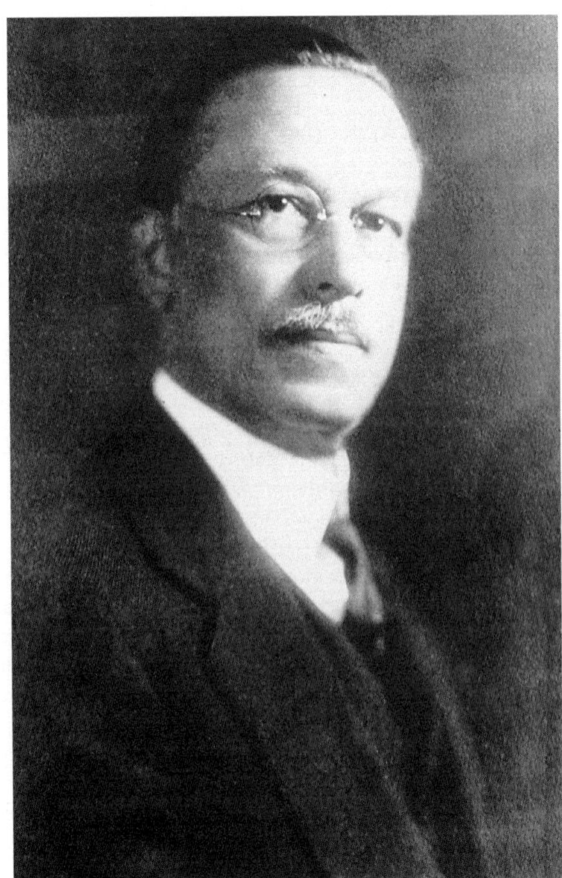

Figure 12 *Gaston Labat (photograph courtesy of the Wood Library-Museum).*

for multiple paravertebral nerve blocks before the Pagés–Dogliotti single-injection technique became accepted. As they worked separately, the technique carries the names of both men. Captain Fidel Pagés conducted an elegant demonstration of segmental single-injection peridural anesthesia in 1921, but died soon after his paper appeared in a Spanish military journal.[42] Ten years later, Achille M Dogliotti of Turin, Italy, wrote a classical paper that resulted in the epidural technique becoming well known.[43] Whereas Pagés used a tactile approach to identify the epidural space, Dogliotti identified it by the loss of resistance technique that is still being taught.

INTUBATION OF THE LARYNX

Medical history abounds with occasions on which the trachea was intubated either via a tracheostomy or through the larynx in an attempt to provide an airway for an asphyxiated or dead animal or human. Few of these have any bearing on anesthetic practice and are merely interesting interludes in the development of various techniques. At the time that anesthesia was introduced, the only regular intubation of the trachea that was taking place was in the resuscitation of asphyxiated neonates. The work of the Humane Societies in promoting intubation for drowned people[44] had been abandoned over fears of creating pneumothoraces through overzealous use of bellows.[45] Joseph O'Dwyer's pioneering work with intubation of the larynx in children with diphtheria[46] paved the way for the acceptance of intubation in medical practice, and the brief adoption of tracheal tubes by McEwen in Glasgow,[47] and the more lasting work of Kuhn[48] in Germany, ensured that Sir Ivan Magill and Rowbotham's work in the 1920s gained rapid acceptance.[49] The addition of an inflatable cuff to this rubber tube by Ralph Waters (Fig. 13) and Arthur Guedel paved the way for closed-circuit anesthesia and true isolation of the airway.[50]

Control of the airway was to be one of the defining moments for anesthesia. It permitted surgery in fields hitherto denied to surgeons and allowed the development of long-term ventilation for the critically ill. Following the work of Magill and others of that era, and in spite of many subsequent refinements, it was not until the introduction of the laryngeal mask airway by Brain in the late 1980s that any major advance in airway care occurred.

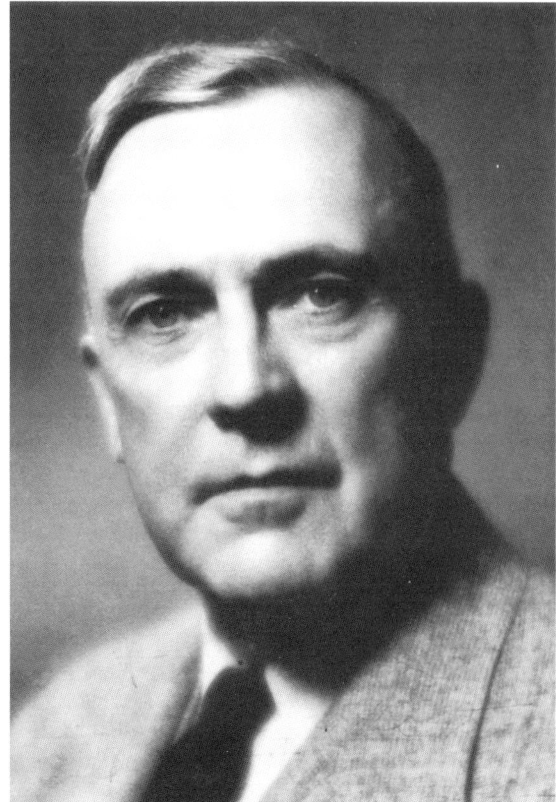

Figure 13 *Ralph Waters (photograph courtesy of the Wood Library-Museum).*

INTRAVENOUS INDUCTION AGENTS

Although Cyprian Ore used intravenous chloral hydrate[51] and Burkhardt induced anesthesia with intravenous ether and chloroform,[52] it was not until the use of intravenous barbiturates by Bardet[53] and Bumm[54] in the 1920s that intravenous induction became a practical possibility. Amytal was popular for a while, especially in the USA,[55] but popular acceptance of such a technique was limited until the introduction of evipan by Weese in the early 1930s.[56] However, the "great moment" was the introduction of thiopentone, and this drug soon became the "gold standard" against which all subsequent anesthetic induction agents are compared. Waters[57] and John Lundy[58] (Fig. 14) used thiopentone independently in the same year (1935), and the new revolution in anesthesia had started.

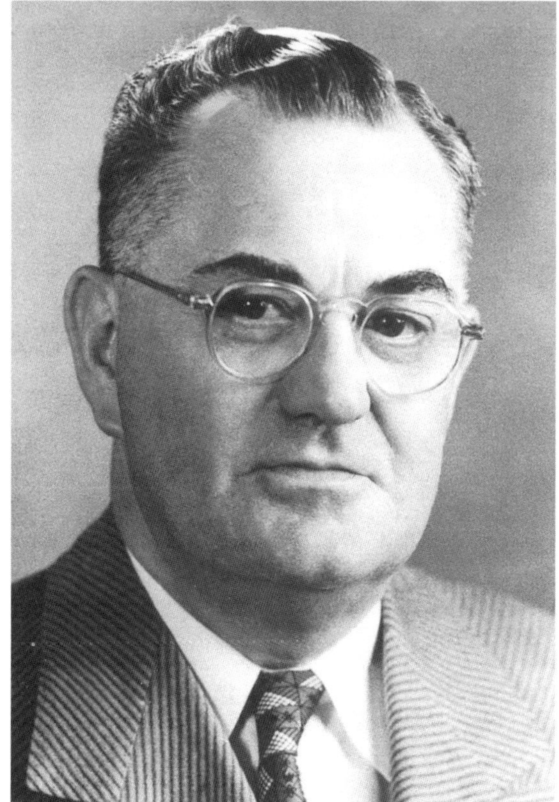

Figure 14 *John Lundy (photograph courtesy of the Wood Library-Museum).*

THE INTRODUCTION OF MUSCLE RELAXANTS

Prior to the introduction of the muscle relaxant curare into modern anesthetic practice by Harold Griffith (Fig. 15) and Enid Johnson in 1942,[59] the only method of producing muscle relaxation for surgery was with deep inhalational anesthesia or the use of local anesthesia in central blockade. Although Boem in Germany and de Caux[60] in London had administered muscle relaxants during anesthesia prior to this, their work was not taken further because of the problems of obtaining standard preparations of curare. In the UK, Cecil Gray and Halton in Liverpool took up the use of curare and popularized it across Europe.[61] Their paper aptly predicted the way forward when they wrote that "we venture to say we have passed yet another milestone," and the subsequent introduction of a myriad of relaxants up to the present day could fill another book.

THE INTRODUCTION OF HALOTHANE

The initial use of ether and nitrous oxide and the subsequent use of chloroform gave the emerging specialty a strong basis on which to build. Inhalational anesthesia has remained the bedrock on which all developments have been based. Many anesthetic agents have been introduced for inhalational use and all have had their advantages and disadvantages. Those used for the longest time have included ethyl chloride, trichloroethylene, and methoxyflurane, but it was the introduction of halothane in the mid-1950s that simplified the induction and maintenance of anesthesia. Halothane was first described by the research chemist Raventos[62] after preliminary work by Fergusson and Suckling at the ICI Laboratories, in Alderley Edge, England, and was introduced into anesthetic practice by Michael Johnstone at Manchester Royal Infirmary.[63] The introduction of this new agent was also to change vaporizer technology, as a more accurate method of administration was required for this and subsequent agents. Halothane's smooth induction, combined with its relatively pleasant smell and potent action, made it the ideal agent for the next two decades. Halothane is only now being fully supplanted by new agents such as sevoflurane.

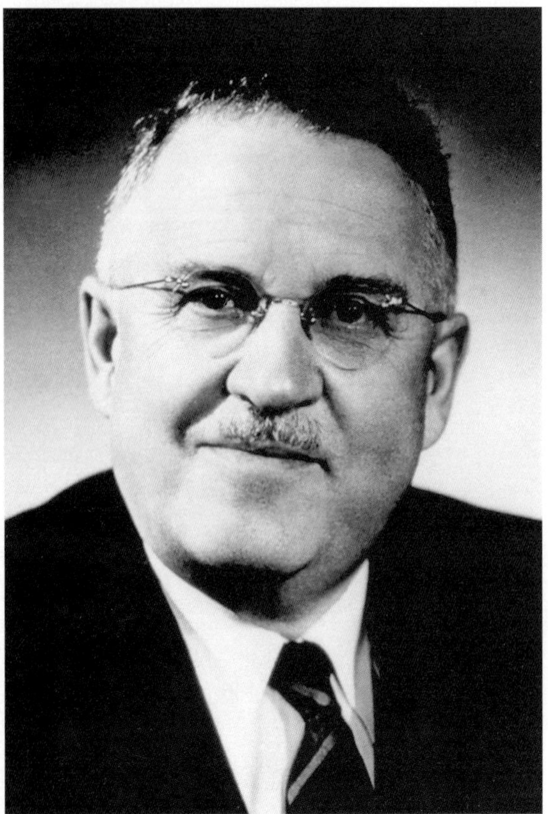

Figure 15 *Harold Griffith (photograph courtesy of the Wood Library-Museum).*

THE RISE OF PROFESSIONALISM

As the twentieth century began, professional organizations in anesthesiology began to emerge. In 1893, the London Society of Anaesthetists was founded by F W Silk of King's College Hospital.[64] This organization, whose stated purpose was "for the study of anesthetics and to promote and encourage friendly relations amongst members," also worked hard to encourage the idea that instruction on how to give an anesthetic should be a compulsory part of undergraduate medical training. These political activities were successful, but further work of this nature ceased when the Society joined with over 20 similar specialist organizations to form the Royal Society of Medicine in 1909. The Section of Anaesthetics of this organization held clinical sessions at the annual meeting of the British Medical Association from 1912 onwards. In 1923, a new outlet for clinical research anesthesia in emerged with the publication of a new independent journal of anesthesia, the *British Journal of Anaesthesia*. Its first editor was Hyman Cohen, who was a New Yorker and had both UK and USA qualifications. It is likely that he knew of Francis Hoeffer McMechan's work in the USA, and his first editorial in the new journal includes a plea for the formation of a British Society of Anaesthesia.

In the USA, formation of a professional organization for physician anesthetists did not take place until after the turn of the century. Adolph Erdmann brought together 11 of his colleagues on 6 October 1905 at the Long Island College Hospital in Brooklyn, New York. For the next 6 years, the original members and other physicians interested in the specialty gathered to exchange techniques and read papers describing their experiences with anesthesia. In 1911, James Gwathmey moved the society meetings to Manhattan and the name of the organization changed to the New York Society of Anesthetists. Larger numbers of physicians became interested in the problems of anesthesia and, by 1912, the group petitioned the American Medical Association (AMA) to form a section on anesthesia within the AMA to study the problems within the field.

The petition was defeated by the House of Delegates but, out of the frustration at the failure, the first national anesthesia organization in American was formed, the Associated Anesthetists of America (AAA). James Gwathmey of New York was elected President and Francis Hoeffer McMechan of Cincinnati was elected Secretary-Treasurer. The following year, McMechan organized a 1-day session for the group in Minneapolis during the AMA national meeting. Ten papers were presented. Most dealt with clinicians' experience with different forms of anesthesia.[65] The most important outcome of this meeting was the sense of community it fostered in the physician anesthetists, and the formation, at last, of a national organization to give voice to their concerns.

Within 2 years, fate had delivered a crushing blow to McMechan. His joints were so severely affected by rheumatoid arthritis that he could no longer practice. However, this catastrophe turned out to be a blessing for the specialty, as McMechan turned his considerable talents toward editing and organizing anesthesiology. By 1926, McMechan had created a North American organization that truly covered the continent. The AAA had been transformed into the Associate Anesthetists of the United States and Canada (AAUSC). The regional groups that McMechan had helped organize, the Canadian Society, the Pacific Coast Association, the Eastern Society, and the Southern Association, joined the Mid-Western Association as members of the AAUSC. In addition, McMechan in 1922 formed a truly international society dedicated to the pursuit of research in anesthesiology, the International Anesthesia Research Society (IARS) (Fig. 16). This group published the first journal in the world devoted exclusively to anesthesiology, *Current Researches in Anesthesia and Analgesia*, predating the British counterpart by 1 year.[66]

In the 13 years between the first AAA meeting and the joint meeting of the AAUSC, several other remarkable accomplishments had been achieved by McMechan. The first truly international meeting, between the AAUSC and the Section on Anaesthetics of the British Medical Association, was held in England in 1925. John Henry Evans, President of the Board of Governors of the IARS, was present, and so impressed the British that an issue of the *British Journal of Anaesthesia* was dedicated to him. In 1926, McMechan held the Congress of Anesthetists in a joint conference with the Section on Anaesthetics of the British Medical Association. Subsequently, he traveled throughout Europe, giving lectures and networking with physicians in the field. Upon his final return to America, he became gravely ill and was confined to bed for 2 years. However, hard work and constant travel paid dividends. By 1929, McMechan's IARS included members not only from North America, but from several European countries as well as Japan, India, Argentina, and Brazil.[67]

In the 1930s, McMechan expanded his mission from organizing anesthesiologists to promoting the academic aspects of the specialty. In 1931, work began on what would become the International College of Anesthetists (Fig. 17). This body began to award fellowships in 1935. For the first time, physicians were recognized as specialists in anesthesiology. The certification qualifications were universal, and fellows were recognized as specialists in several countries.[68] Although the criteria for certification were not strict, the College was a success in raising the standards of anesthesia practice in many nations. On 29 June 1939, McMechan finally succumbed to illness, and the anesthesia world lost its tireless leader and advocate.

Other Americans participated in the promotion of organized anesthesiology. Ralph Waters participated in the evolving anesthesia society; his greatest contribution to the specialty was raising its academic standards. After completing his internship in 1913, he entered medical practice in Sioux City, Iowa, where he gradually limited his practice to anesthesia. His personal experience and extensive reading were supplemented by the only postgraduate training available, a 1-month course conducted in Ohio by E I McKesson. At that time, the custom of becoming a self-proclaimed specialist in medicine and surgery was not uncommon. Waters, who was frustrated by low standards, and who would eventually have a great influence by establishing both anesthesia residency training and the formal examination process, recalled that

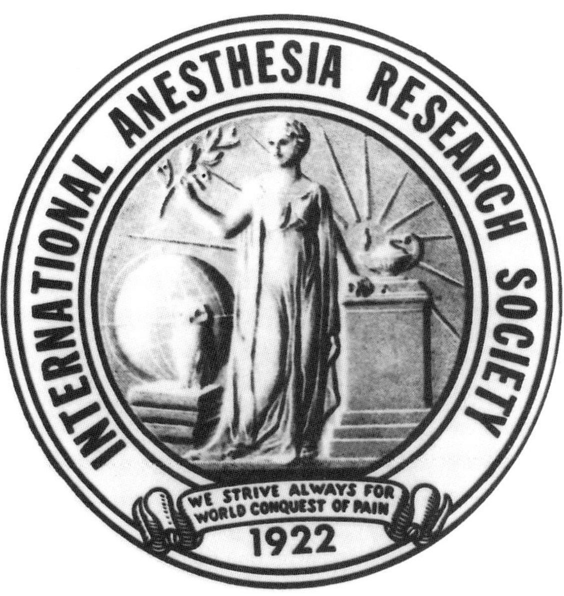

Figure 16 *Seal of the IARS (image courtesy of the Wood Library-Museum).*

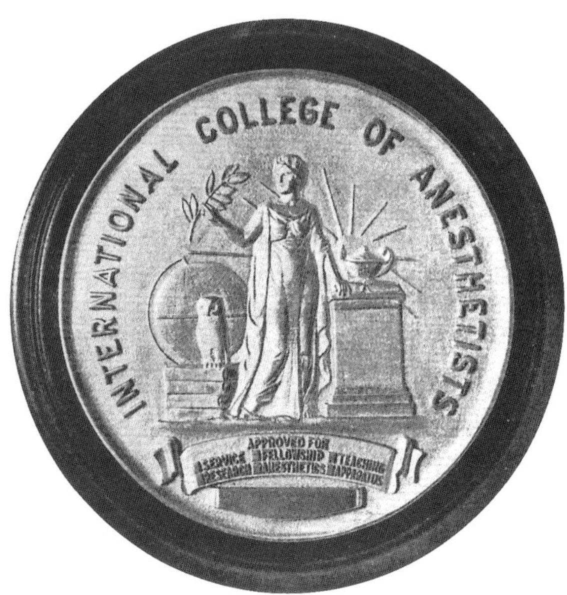

Figure 17 *Seal of the International College of Anesthetists (image courtesy of the Wood Library-Museum).*

before 1920, "The requirements for specialization in many Midwestern hospitals consisted of the possession of sufficient audacity to attempt a procedure and persuasive power adequate to gain the consent of the patient or his family."[69]

In 1925, Waters relocated to Kansas City. The larger city allowed him to initiate his freestanding outpatient surgical facility, The Downtown Surgical Clinic, which featured one of the first postanesthetic recovery rooms. In 1927, Erwin Schmidt, professor of surgery at the University of Wisconsin's medical school, encouraged Dean Charles Bardeen to recruit Waters.

In accepting the first American academic position in anesthesia, Waters described four objectives that have since been adopted by many other academic departments. His goals were as follows: "(1) to provide the best possible service to patients of the institution; (2) to teach what is known of the principles of Anesthesiology to all candidates for their medical degree; (3) to help long-term graduate students not only to gain a fundamental knowledge of the subject and to master the art of administration, but also to learn as much as possible of the effective methods of teaching; (4) to accompany these efforts with the encouragement of as much cooperative investigation as is consistent with achieving the first objectives."[69]

Ralph Waters' personal and professional qualities impressed talented young men and women, who sought residency posts in his department. He encouraged residents to initiate research interests, in which they collaborated with two pharmacologists, Arthur Loevenhart and Chauncey Leake. Anesthesia records were coded onto punch cards to form a database. Morbidity and mortality meetings also originated in Madison. In more casual times, a practitioner could complain, "The patient died because he did not take a good anesthetic." Alternatively, the death might be attributed to a mysterious force such as "status lymphaticus," of which Arthur Guedel, a master of sardonic humor, observed, "Certainly status lymphaticus is at times a great help to the anesthetist. When he has a fatality under anesthesia with no other cleansing explanation he is glad to recognize the condition as an entity."[70] Through the instruction received from Ralph Waters and his colleagues, anesthesiologists in training learned to accept responsibility for their actions.

The University of Wisconsin became a regular destination for other specialists. In 1929, Ralph Waters helped John Lundy organize the anesthesia "Travel Club," whose members were leading American or Canadian teachers of anesthesia. Even during the lean years of the Depression, international guests also visited. For Geoffrey Kaye of Australia, Torsten Gordt of Sweden, Robert Macintosh, and Michael Nosworthy of England, and scores of others, Waters' department was their final stop.

Ralph Waters trained 60 residents during the 22 years he was the "chief," who declared themselves the "Aqualumni" in his honor. Thirty-four "Aqualumni" took academic positions, and, of these, 14 became chairmen of departments of anesthesia. Sixty-five years after Waters arrived in Madison, more than 80 chairmen or former chairmen of academic departments could trace their professional lineage back to Ralph Waters.[71] His enduring legacy was once recognized by the dean who had recruited him in 1927, Charles Bardeen, who observed, "Ralph Waters was the first person the University hired to put people to sleep, but, instead, he awakened a worldwide interest in anesthesia."

Waters also energetically supported the growth of physician anesthesia organizations. He supported Paul Wood's drive to change the name of the New York Society of Anesthetists to reflect its national role. In 1936, the American Society of Anesthetists was formed from the New York Society in an effort to show the AMA that a national anesthesia society favored certification of specialists in the field. Combined with the American Society of Regional Anesthesia, whose president was Emery Rovenstein, the American Board of Anesthesiology (ABA) (Fig. 18) was organized as a board subordinate to the American Board of Surgery. With McMechan's death in 1939, the AMA favored independence for the ABA, largely through the efforts of John Lundy, and in 1940 this was granted.[68]

A few years later, the officers of the American Society of Anesthetists were challenged by M J Seifert, who wrote, "An Anesthetist is a technician and an Anesthesiologist is the specific authority on anesthesia and anesthetics. I cannot understand why you do not term yourselves the American Society of Anesthesiologists?"[72] Ralph Waters was declared the first president of the newly named ASA in 1945. In that year, when World War II ended, 739 (37%) of 1977 ASA members were in the armed forces.

Meanwhile, in the UK, similar forces were at work to develop and strengthen the emerging profession of anesthesia. In 1932, Henry Featherstone of Birmingham founded the Association of Anaesthetists of Great Britain and Ireland (AAGBI). This new organization was to be the focus of the majority of all new developments within the specialty for the next 50 years. It was an independent body and its council was elected by UK and Irish anesthetists from among their own ranks. Those attending the first meeting of the Association reads like a "who's who" of anesthesia at that time: Featherstone, Shipway, Boyle, Magill, Howard Jones, Mennell, Hughes, Daly, Chaldecott, Hill, Hadfield, Clausen, and Hewer. These men would shape the future of the specialty within the British Isles and throughout the world.[73]

One of the first functions of the AAGBI was to initiate the creation of a Diploma in Anaesthetics that was awarded by the Conjoint Examining Board in England under the aegis of the Royal College of Physicians of London and the Royal College of Surgeons of England. The first examination was held in 1935. There was soon dissatisfaction over the single examination to represent specialist status in anesthesia, and a two-part examination was introduced in 1947. At the same time, the Association set up the Faculty of Anaesthetists within the Royal College of Surgeons of England, and this new body took over the running of the Diploma from the Conjoint Board. The new Faculty continued to work in close cooperation with the Association, and many notable anesthetists served on both Councils. The Faculty later evolved into a full College within the Royal College of Surgeons in 1988 and received a Royal Charter and full independent College status as a Royal College in 1992.[73]

In 1948, at the inception of the National Health Service, the efforts of the AAGBI ensured that anesthesia obtained full specialist recognition and consultant status, with full parity with surgeons and physicians. This single advance was to ensure that the specialty had both the status and respect it needed to continue its development into the twenty-first century.[73]

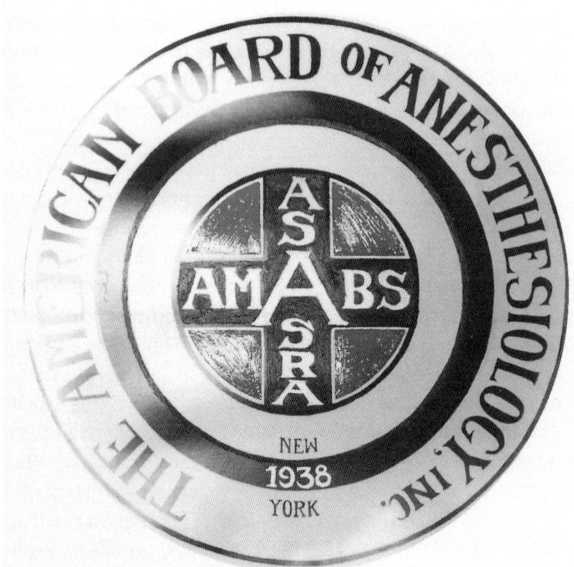

Figure 18 *Seal of the American Board of Anesthesiology (image courtesy of the Wood Library-Museum).*

THE WORLD FEDERATION

As Europe and the rest of the world recovered from the effects of World War II, a long-held dream of many anesthesiologists came to fruition. Beginning in the late 1930s, Robert Monod had been discussing with Francis Hoeffer McMechan and many others the possibility of a worldwide society for anesthesiologists. McMechan had suggested that a European Congress be held in Paris in 1940. There was support for such a meeting from British, American, Italian, and Mexican anesthesiologists. However, the German offensive and subsequent capture of Paris destroyed these plans.[67]

After the war, Monod continued his campaign for a world society. Another Frenchman, Marcel Thalheimer, joined Monod in discussions about the organization, first in London and later in Paris. Jean Dalafresnaye, Secretary of the Council for International Organizations of Medical Societies of the United Nations Educational, Scientific and Cultural Organization, soon joined the discussions. He suggested that a committee be formed with the charge of soliciting support from various anesthesia organizations.[74]

In 1952, the committee met in Brussels. Interestingly, the meeting was jointly sponsored by the IARS and the Council for International Organization of Medical Societies. Several important conclusions emerged from that meeting. First, there was sufficient interest to move forward with an international organization. Secondly, with over 20 different countries responding, there was enough concentration to move the organization forward. A constitution was drafted and sent to the various countries for study. Finally, an invitation to a World Congress of Anesthesiologists was proposed by the Dutch for The Hague in 1955. Another committee meeting was set for 1954 to finalize the preliminary plans.[67]

Plans were finalized for the Congress the following year. The

Federation's constitution was completed and sent to the House of Delegates at the Congress for approval. The First World Congress the following year was a great success with attendees from across the world. A 320-page volume of the papers presented was produced, supported by the IARS. Subsequently, the World Federation of Societies of Anesthesiologists (WFSA) has continued to grow in membership and to help "developing" nations with both technology and education, making the world of anesthesiology a smaller place indeed.[67]

CONCLUSIONS

Great moments in anesthesia are often appreciated only with hindsight. It is rare for those involved with great decisions or discoveries to understand fully the contribution that they have made. Each great moment is held in the eye of the beholder to have great significance, but that may not be so for others, who will have different perceptions and contexts on which they base their "great moments." This chapter is very much related to the development of anesthesia in the operating theatre in the USA and UK. To develop the concept to include the whole world, as well as the development of resuscitation, intensive care medicine, pain management, obstetric care, trauma care, patient transfer, etc., all of which have fundamental anesthesia input, would require several textbooks in their own right. The authors recognize the limitations of the "great moments" that they have recounted here and encourage their readers to look further within their spheres of interest to trace the further "great moments" that can be drawn into our specialty in due course.

REFERENCES

1. Dioscorides. On mandragora, Dioscorides opera libra. In: Bergman N (ed.). *The Genesis of Surgical Anesthesia*. Park Ridge, IL: Wood Library-Museum, 1998: 11.
2. Infusino M, Viole O'Neill Y, Calmes S. Hog beans, poppies, and mandrake leaves – a test of the efficacy of the soporific sponge. In: Atkinson RS, Boulton TB (eds). *The History of Anaesthesia*. London: Parthenon Publishing Group, 1989: 39.
3. Voigts LE, Hudson RP. A drynke pat men callen dwale to make a man to slepe whyle men kerven him – a surgical anesthetic from Late Medieval England. In: Campbell S, Hall B, Klausner D (eds). *Health, Disease and Healing in Medieval Culture*. New York: St Martin's Press, 1992; 34–56.
4. Moffat B. The seeds of narcosis in medieval medicine. *Hist Anaesth Soc Proc* 1998; **22:** 7–12.
5. Bacon DR. Regional anesthesia and chronic pain therapy: a history. In: Brown DL (ed.). *Regional Anesthesia and Analgesia*. Philadelphia, PA: WB Saunders,1996: 10–22.
6. Robinson V. *Victory Over Pain*. New York, NY: Henry Schumann, 1946: 40.
7. Strickland R. Ether drinking in Ireland. *Mayo Clin Proc* 1996; **71:** 1015.
8. Davy H. *Researches Chemical and Philosophical Chiefly Concerning Nitrous Oxide or Dephlogisticated Nitrous Air, and Its Respiration*. London: J Johnson, 1800: 533.
9. Lyman HM. *Artificial Anaesthesia and Anaesthetics*. New York: William Wood, 1881: 6.
10. Stetson JB. William E. Clarke and the discovery of anesthesia. In: Fink BR, Morris L, Stephen CR (eds). *The History of Anesthesia: Third International Symposium Proceedings*. Park Ridge, IL: The Wood Library-Museum of Anesthesiology Press, 1992.
11. Long CW. An account of the first use of sulphuric ether by inhalation as an anaesthetic in surgical operations. *South Med Surg J* 1849; **5:** 705.
12. Smith GB, Hirsch NP. Gardner Quincy Colton: pioneer of nitrous oxide anesthesia. *Anesth Analg* 1991; **72:** 382.
13. Wolfe R. *I Awaken to Glory*. Boston, MA: The Francis A. Countway Library of Medicine, 1994: 1–72.
14. Greene NM. A consideration of factors in the discovery of anesthesia and their effects on its development. *Anesthesiology* 1971; **35:** 515.
15. Duncum BM. *The Development of Inhalation Anaesthesia*. London, Oxford University Press, 1947: 110.
16. Boulton TB, Wilkinson DJ. The origins of modern anaesthesia. In: Healy TEJ, Cohen PJ (eds). *Wylie and Churchill-Davidson's A Practice of Anaesthesia*, 6th edn. London: Edward Arnold, 1995: 3–35.
17. Morton WTG. Patent application for Letheon. Park Ridge, IL: Wood Library-Museum of Anesthesiology Collection.
18. Wilson G. *One Grand Chain*. Melbourne: The Australian and New Zealand College of Anaesthetists, 1995: 1–40.
19. Caton D. *What a Blessing She Had Chloroform*. New Haven, CT: Yale University Press, 1999: 103–6.
20. Journal of Queen Victoria. In: Strauss MB (ed.). *Familiar Medical Quotations*. Boston, MA: Little, Brown, 1968: 17.
21. Calverley RK. An early ether vaporizer designed by John Snow, a treasure of the Wood Library-Museum of Anesthesiology. In: Fink BR, Morris LE, Stephen CR (eds). *The History of Anesthesia*. Park Ridge, IL: Wood Library-Museum, 1992: 91.
22. Snow J. *On the Inhalation of the Vapour of Ether* (reprinted by the Wood Library-Museum). London: J Churchill, 1847: 23.
23. Snow J. *On Chloroform and Other Anesthetics* (reprinted by the Wood Library-Museum). London: J Churchill, 1858: 58.
24. Duncum BM. *The Development of Inhalation Anaesthesia*. London: Oxford University Press, 1947: 538–40.
25. Calverley RK. J. T. Clover. A giant of Victorian anaesthesia. In: Rupreht J, van Lieburg MJ, Lee JA, Erdmann W (eds). *Anaesthesia: Essays on Its History*. Berlin: Springer-Verlag, 1985: 21.
26. Clover JT. Laryngotomy in chloroform anesthesia. *Br Med J* 1877; **1:** 132.
27. Colton Dental Association (advertisement from the Public Ledger and Transcript, Philadelphia, December 4, 1869, Reynolds Historical Library, University of Alabama in Birmingham).
28. Andrews E. The oxygen mixture, a new anaesthetic combination. *Chicago Med Examin* 1868; **9:** 656.
29. Becker HK. Carl Koller and cocaine. *Psychoanal Q* 1963; **32:** 332.
30. Olch PD, William S. Halstead and local anesthesia: contributions and complications. *Anesthesiology* 1975; **42:** 479–86.
31. Marx G. The first spinal anesthesia: who deserves the laurels? *Reg Anesth* 1994; **19:** 429.
32. Corning JL. Spinal anaesthesia and local medication of the cord. *New York Med J* 1885; **42:** 485.
33. Bier AKG. Experiments in cocainization of the spinal cord, 1899. In: Faulconer A, Keys TE (trans.). *Foundations of Anesthesiology*. Springfield, IL: Charles C Thomas, 1965: 854.
34. Larson MD. Tait and Caglieri. The first spinal anesthetic in America. *Anesthesiology* 1996; **85:** 913–19.
35. Lee JA. Arthur Edward James Barker, 1850–1916: British pioneer of regional anaesthesia. *Anaesthesia* 1979; **34:** 885.
36. Lemmon WT. A method for continuous spinal anesthesia: a preliminary report. *Ann Surg* 1940; **111:** 141.
37. Tuohy EB. Continuous spinal anesthesia: its usefulness and technic involved. *Anesthesiology* 1944; **5:** 142.
38. Cushing H. On the avoidance of shock in major amputations by cocainization of large nerve trunks preliminary to their division: with observations on blood-pressure changes in surgical cases. *Ann Surg* 1902; **36:** 321.
39. Bier A. A new method of producing local anesthesia of the extremities. *Arch Klin Chir* 1908; **86:** 1007–16.
40. Bacon DR, Darwish H. Emery Rovenstine and regional anesthesia. *Reg Anesth* 1997; **22:** 273–9.
41. Bonica JJ (ed.). *The Management of Pain*, 2nd edn. Philadelphia, PA: Lea & Febiger, 1990.
42. Pagés F. Metameric anesthesia, 1921. In: Faulconer A, Keys TE (trans.). *Foundations of Anesthesiology*. Springfield, IL: Charles C Thomas, 1965: 927.
43. Fink BR. History of local anesthesia. In: Cousins MJ, Bridenbaugh PO (eds). *Neural Blockade*. Philadelphia, PA: JB Lippincott, 1980: 12.
44. Cogan T. Memoirs of the Society instituted at Amsterdam in favour of drowned persons. For the years 1767, 1768, 1769, 1770 and 1771. London, 1773.
45. Leroy J. Recherches sur l'asphyxie. *J Physiol Exp Pathol* 1872; **7:** 45–65.
46. O'Dwyer J. Intubation of the larynx. *New York Med J* 1885; **42:** 145–7.
47. Macewen W. Clinical observations on the introduction of tracheal tubes by the mouth instead of performing tracheotomy or laryngotomy. *Br Med J* 1880; **2:** 122–4.
48. Kuhn F. *Die Perorale Intubation*. Berlin: Karger, 1911.
49. Magill IW. Endotracheal anaesthesia. *Proc Roy Soc Med* 1929; **22:** 83–7.
50. Guedel AE, Waters RM. A new intratracheal catheter. *Curr Res Anesth Analges* 1928; **7:** 238–9.
51. Ore PC. Des injections intraveneuses de chloral. *Bull Soc Chir Paris* 1872; **1:** 400–2.

52. Burkhardt L. Die intravenose narkose mit Aether und Chloroform. *Munsch Med Wosschr* 1909; **2:** 2365–9.
53. Bardet D. Sur l'utilisation, comme anesthisique general, d'un product nouveau le diethyl diallyl barbiturate de diethylamine. *Bull Gen Ther (Paris)* 1921; **1:** 27–30.
54. Bumm R. Intravenose narkosen mit Barbitur-Saurederivaten. *Klin Wschr* 1927; **6:** 725–6.
55. Zerfas LG, McCallum JTC. The analgesic and anesthetic properties of sodium isoamyl-ethyl barbiturate. *J Indiana Med Assoc* 1929; **22:** 47–50.
56. Weese H, Scharpff W. Evipan ein neuartiges einschlafmittel. *Dtsch Med Wschr* 1932; **58:** 1205–7.
57. Pratt TM, Tatum AL, Hathaway HR, Waters RM. Sodium ethyl (I-methyl butyl) thiobarbiturate. *Am J Surg* 1936 [ns]; **31:** 464–6.
58. Lundy JS. Intravenous anesthesia; preliminary report on the use of two new thiobarbiturates. *Proc Mayo Clin* 1935; **10:** 536.
59. Griffith HR, Johnson GE. The use of curare in general anaesthesia. *Anesthesiology* 1942; **3:** 418–20.
60. Wilkinson DJ. Dr F P de Caux – the first user of curare for anaesthesia in England. *Anaesthesia* 1991; **46:** 49–51.
61. Gray TC, Halton J. A milestone in anaesthesia (d-tubocurarine chloride)? *Proc Roy Soc Med* 1946; **39:** 400–10.
62. Raventos J. The action of fluothane: a new volatile anaesthetic. *Br J Pharmacol* 1955; **2:** 394–7.
63. Johnstone M. The human cardiovascular responses to fluothane. *Br J Anaesth* 1956; **28:** 392–410.
64. Rushman GB, Davies NJH, Atkinson RS. *A Short History of Anaesthesia*. Oxford: Butterworth-Heinemann, 1996: 188.
65. Program from the First meeting of the Associated Anesthetists of America. Park Ridge, IL: Albert Miller Collection, Wood Library-Museum.
66. Seldon TH. Francis Hoeffer McMechan. In: Volpitto PP, Vandam LD (eds). *Genesis of American Anesthesiology*. Springfield, IL: Charles C Thomas, 1982: 5.
67. Bacon DR. The World Federation of Societies of Anesthesiologists: McMechan's final legacy? *Anesth Analg* 1997; **84:** 1131.
68. Bacon DR, Lema MJ. To define a specialty: a brief history of the American Board of Anesthesiology's first written examination. *J Clin Anesthesiol* 1992; **4:** 489–97.
69. Waters RM. Pioneering in anesthesiology. *Postgrad Med* 1948; **4:** 265.
70. Guedel AE. *Inhalation Anesthesia: A Fundamental Guide*. New York: Macmillan, 1937: 129.
71. Bacon DR , Ament R. Ralph Waters and the beginnings of academic anesthesiology in the United States: the Wisconsin template. *J Clin Anesth* 1995; **7:** 534–43.
72. Little Jr DM, Betcher AM. *The Diamond Jubilee 1905–1980*. Park Ridge, IL: American Society of Anesthesiologists, 1980: 8.
73. Boulton TB. *The Association of Anaesthetists of Great Britain and Ireland 1932–1992 and the Development of the Speciality of Anaesthesia*. London: Association of Anaesthetists of Great Britain and Ireland, 1999.
74. Griffith HR. History of the World Federation of Societies of Anesthesiologists. *Anesth Analg* 1963; **42:** 389–97.

APPENDIX

Anesthesia History Association
2121 Northview Lane NE
Rochester
MN 55096-6905
USA

History of Anaesthesia Society
Department of Anaesthesia
West Suffolk Hospital
Hardwick Lane
Bury St Edmunds
Suffolk IP33 2QZ
UK

Wood Library-Museum of Anesthesiology
520 N Northwest Highway
Park Ridge
IL 60068-2573
USA

Museum and Archive
Association of Anaesthetists of Great Britain and Ireland
21 Portland Place
London W1B 1PY
UK

PART I

Anatomy, Physiology, Pathophysiology, and Basic Pharmacology

1

Drug–receptor interactions

BRIAN J POLLARD

Applied pharmacology is central to the practice of anesthesia. Following intravenous administration of a drug, the onset of effect is rapid and usually immediate. Unwanted effects also appear with similar rapidity. It is essential therefore for the anesthesiologist to be aware of all of the desired effects and also the possible side-effects of every agent administered.

Consider the two sequential events that have occurred, namely administration of the drug and its effect. The observed effect is not the drug itself but the response of the body (or certain parts of the body) to the presence of the drug. The drug must therefore have exerted an effect on the cells or organs as an intermediate stage to bring about the observed response. But what component of the cell is affected and what is the nature of the interaction?

THE HISTORIC DEVELOPMENT OF THE CONCEPT OF RECEPTORS

At the end of the nineteenth century, the nature of this interaction was receiving a great deal of interest. Two schools of thought existed – one supported the concept of a physical nature and the other supported the concept of a chemical nature. Supporters of the first hypothesis held the view that drugs exerted their effects by altering certain physical properties of cells, such as surface tension or osmotic pressure. Supporters of the chemical hypothesis regarded the action of a drug as being mediated by the formation of a chemical union with some structure either on or within a cell. The answer to the question came from pioneering work at the beginning of the twentieth century from Langley[1–3] and Ehrlich.[4]

Langley's studies centered on the nervous system, particularly with respect to the effects of cholinomimetic compounds on the stimulation of secretion and their antagonism by atropine. These studies led him to suggest that "there is some substance or substances in the nerve endings or gland cells with which both atropine and pilocarpine are capable of forming compounds."[1] He called these "specific receptive substances." He hypothesized that these substances were present around the nerve ending and also that they were capable of receiving or transmitting stimuli.[2] This was later shown to be true. It is interesting to note that, during the course of his studies, he examined the alkaloid nicotine and concluded that it was able to form a complex with specific receptive substances on skeletal muscle.[3]

At around the time that Langley was studying the nervous system, Ehrlich was working with stains and dyes on biological tissues. Several early investigations into immunologic mechanisms are also attributed to Ehrlich.[4] Ehrlich's work led him to formulate the theory that surface groups on cells could exhibit specific binding properties with toxin molecules. He called these groups "receptors;" therefore, it is Ehrlich who should be given the credit for coining the term "receptor." However, credit for establishing the drug receptor theory must be accorded to A J Clarke.

The early work of A J Clarke centered on the actions of the glycoside strophanthin. He concluded that strophanthin acted on the outside of the heart cells without entering them. His initial thoughts were that this action was likely to be of a physical nature.[5] However, his subsequent work on the quantitative relation between the concentration and action of acetylcholine led him to reconsider this hypothesis. In these later studies, he examined the responses of tissue to a range of concentrations of acetylcholine. The concentration of acetylcholine and the effect produced by that concentration can be plotted graphically and expressed mathematically as:

$$x = ky/(100 - y)$$

where x is the concentration of acetylcholine, y is the effect expressed as a percentage of the maximum possible effect, and k is a constant.

The simplest explanation for this relation would be a reversible monomolecular reaction between two entities, in this case the drug and a single binding site on the cell. Another crucial piece of information was also provided by Clarke. He discovered that there was no relation between the amount of drug entering a cell and the effect produced. This made it likely that the interaction was taking place on the surface of the cell. Calculations of the number of molecules that became attached to each cell led him to conclude that they could only be occupying a very small area of the cell surface – an area insufficient to exert any significant physical effect.[6,7] Previous views had therefore to be revised, leading to the conclusion that drugs were acting on a small number of sites on the surface of cells.

Although the concept of receptors on the surface of cells was soon established, receptors remained a theoretical entity until the 1970s, when advanced techniques of electron microscopy allowed them to be visualized. Simultaneous advances in biochemistry allowed receptors to be isolated and purified. In certain instances, it became possible for receptors to be removed and reinserted into artificial lipid membranes for further electrophysiologic examination.[8] Of similar, if not greater, importance was the development of immunologic binding techniques by which it is possible to raise antibodies to receptors in small animals, usually rabbits.[9,10]

The discovery of toxins that would attach to receptors also assisted research, e.g. in neuromuscular transmission. The toxins α-bungarotoxin and β-bungarotoxin from the Taiwanese banded krait, *Bungarus multicinctus*, have been described previously. α-Bungarotoxin blocks neuromuscular transmission by binding specifically and irreversibly to acetylcholine receptors.[11] The application of radiolabeled α-bungarotoxin to the neuromuscular junction results in its localization almost exclusively to the crests of the folds on the postjunctional membrane.[12] The implication of this observation was that the receptors were located on the shoulders of the folds – a fact that has since been confirmed.

It must be noted that, despite the widespread acceptance of the receptor theory of drug action and the conclusion that drugs did not act by physical mechanisms, there are a small number of substances which probably do act (at least in part) by physical means. One example of this is the effect of the gaseous and volatile general anesthetic agents that is thought, at least in part, to be a nonspecific action on cell membranes. Certain agents that induce anesthesia may also act through receptor systems (e.g. barbiturates and benzodiazepines).

DEFINITION AND CLASSIFICATION OF RECEPTORS

A receptor is an entity which binds to a drug or a transmitter substance and puts into action a chain of events that leads to an effect (or part of an effect if it is necessary to exceed a threshold). It must be remembered that there are also nonreceptor sites which will bind drugs, e.g. plasma proteins. When a drug binds to a nonreceptor site, there is no effect. Although these sites possess an affinity for the drug and will bind the drug, they are not receptors in the classic sense. The term "acceptor" is often used in this context. It must be noted that the presence and concentration of inactive acceptor sites may considerably influence the action of a drug either by removing it from the active biophase, thus decreasing the expected effect or by acting as a storage site and potentially prolonging the effect. For greater detail concerning these pharmacokinetic factors, see Chapter 2.

The characteristic properties of receptors are those of sensitivity, selectivity, and specificity. Drugs acting on receptors produce marked effects in very low concentrations (sensitivity). Responses are produced only by a narrow range of chemical substances which possess very similar chemical groupings (selectivity). The response of a cell of a particular type to an agonist which is acting on the same set of receptors is always the same because it is determined by the cells themselves (specificity).

Receptors are commonly classified according to the target systems to which they relate, e.g. cholinergic, adrenergic. It must be remembered that the transmitter or mediator may be a hormone, a neurotransmitter, or another cellular messenger. Although this classification is logical and is commonly used, there are a number of inadequacies. Detailed studies with more selective agonists and antagonists have revealed many subdivisions in most classifications, e.g. cholinergic muscarinic M_1, M_2, M_3; adrenergic α_1, α_2, β_1, β_2.

A second method of classification which might be appropriate relates to the anatomic location of the receptors. Most receptors are extracellular (e.g. acetylcholine receptors), although receptors may be intracellular (e.g. local anesthetics on sodium channels of nerves). The tissue supporting the receptors could also be used to categorize receptors in an anatomic sense, e.g. most cholinergic muscarinic receptors lie on smooth muscle or glandular tissues whereas a particular subtype of cholinergic nicotinic receptors lies on striated muscle.

Following advances in molecular biology, a third method of classifying receptors has become available relatively recently. These advances have enabled the isolation and study of single receptors to be performed. Subsequent studies have delineated the actual amino acid sequence for some receptor systems. Receptors could therefore be classified in a very detailed manner, according to their individual characteristics and even the gene sequence encoding the receptor. Such detail is at present principally a research tool.

CHEMICAL BONDS INVOLVED IN THE ACTIONS OF DRUGS

In view of the existence of receptors to which drugs attach, it is appropriate to consider the forms by which these bond together. Receptors and drugs form chemical bonds, which can be divided into two principal types – covalent and electrostatic – both of which may exhibit further subdivisions.

Covalent bonds

These are strong bonds, formed by the mutual sharing of electrons from the outer electron shells (orbits) surrounding two different atoms. A good example is the bond between carbon and hydrogen (C–H), in which the single electron from the hydrogen atom is shared with an electron from the carbon. This effectively gives the hydrogen two electrons in that shell, which increases its stability. If three more hydrogen atoms (or other suitable groups) each share one electron, the result will be that the carbon has eight, which is the stable number in that shell. Carbon has a valency of four, and readily takes part in covalent bonding. Double bonds are formed by the sharing of two pairs of electrons, and triple bonds by the sharing of three pairs of electrons. If the two atoms involved in the bonding are identical, the whole entity is electrically neutral. However, when two dissimilar atoms are involved, the electron sharing will not be exactly equal; this will result in one atom having a very small positive charge and the other having an identical negative charge. This dipole can be amplified by adjacent atoms or groups such that a significant charge may appear at certain points. This has the effect of creating dipoles of sufficient magnitude to enable molecules to create bonds by electrostatic forces. Examples of drugs acting through covalent bonds are the organophosphate anticholinesterases ecothiopate and dyflos.

Electrostatic bonds

These bonds are formed by the attraction of opposing electrical charges. The extent to which molecules may attach to one another (e.g. a drug to a receptor) depends upon the actual charges involved. When the charges are weak, for example when created by unequal distribution of electrons in a covalent bond, then the bonds will be weak. It will be possible for molecules to attach to one another only when they can align themselves closely. It might therefore be expected that such bonds are involved in drug–receptor binding because the shape of most drugs is very specific and complementary to their receptors.

By gaining an extra proton (hydrogen atom) or losing a proton, certain molecules may become positively or negatively charged respectively. Such ionization creates more powerful charges, and the formation of these charges depends upon the pH of the medium and the pK_a of the molecule. Strong charges appear to be concerned with nonspecific drug binding at nonreceptor sites as well as with binding.

Weaker ionic bonds can exist, such as hydrogen bonding. A hydrogen bond results from the existence of an identical dipole or a covalent bond involving a hydrogen atom. Hydrogen bonds are very weak and principally serve as reinforcements for other types of ionic bonds. The importance of hydrogen bonds in biological systems is considerable. The macromolecular structure of DNA and similar proteins depends upon the presence of large numbers of hydrogen bonds.

van der Waals bonds are even weaker and arise from distortion of the outer electron orbits of atoms held in close proximity. They provide very weak electrostatic links which serve to reinforce other bonding and help to stabilize certain structural conformations or interactions.

RELATION BETWEEN STRUCTURE AND ACTIVITY

It has been demonstrated that drugs act at receptors and that these receptors are specific entities on the surface of cells. There is a large number of different receptors, each with its own individual family of related drugs. In general, there is little or no cross-reactivity between drugs in these separate families, e.g. tubocurarine has an action at the nicotinic acetylcholine receptor and diazepam at the benzodiazepine receptor. Neither of these agents has any effect on the other receptor. Tubocurarine and diazepam differ considerably in their chemical structure, and it might therefore be expected that the characteristics and shape of the molecule are relevant to activity at a receptor. A molecule of a certain shape and/or size is required in order for an effect to appear on a particular receptor system. However, the whole molecule is not necessarily involved. For example, pancuronium, vecuronium, and atracurium have the same effect as tubocurarine on the nicotinic acetylcholine receptor, whereas midazolam, temazepam, and lorazepam all affect the benzodiazepine receptor. The actual chemical structure of each individual component of each series differs, but there are similarities within the molecules. It would thus appear logical to infer that there must be some component part of each molecule which is common to a series and which possesses the ability to combine with the receptor. That moiety on benzodiazepines must be different from that on the cholinergic agonists. Therefore, a particular structure has an activity at certain receptors, and this is the basis of the study of the relation between structure and activity.

A good analogy for the action of a drug on a receptor is that of a lock (receptor) and key (drug) system. The analogy, although crude, does demonstrate some important concepts, as follows:

- The drug is capable of "unlocking" the response.
- The lock (receptor) has specificity toward a particular key (drug).
- The lock may be turned by other keys that, although not identical to the correct key, have certain similarities (master keys or "skeleton" keys).
- The key may operate other locks either by accident or by design.
- The lock may be "jammed" by attempting to insert the wrong key. The resulting physical obstruction would prevent the correct key from being used (a pharmacologic response may be blocked by an appropriate drug).

The study of the relation between structure and activity has enabled us to infer a number of factors with respect to the receptor molecules themselves. For example, information concerning the number of binding sites and their spatial configuration, the probable nature of the binding forces, and the requirements for activation may be deduced. Although the relation between structure and activity continues to be important in the elucidation of receptor structure, newer methods have been developed. Recently introduced computational techniques that involve advanced graphics are of particular importance. These enable predictions to be made about the energies between bonds and the conformations of the bound versus unbound states of drug–receptor complexes. Advances in recombinant DNA technology enable the primary structures of certain receptors to be elucidated and copied. X-ray crystallography and nuclear magnetic resonance imaging have also played a vital role. To better understand the relation between structure and activity, it is appropriate to examine some well-understood examples.

The various subtypes of acetylcholine receptors are well understood and provide a suitable example. Although a number of acetylcholine receptors exist, they were originally subdivided into two broad categories – nicotinic and muscarinic. This subdivision was determined following the observation of the agonist activities of the two alkaloids nicotine and muscarine at acetylcholine receptors. Further subdivisions on the basis of antagonist activity have since been made.

If the structure of acetylcholine is examined, it can be seen that there is a cationic center (positively charged nitrogen) near one end. Toward the other end of the molecule are two oxygen atoms, one of which exists as a carbonyl group (C=O) and the other as an ester link (–O–C–) (Fig. 1.1). Both of these oxygen atoms have the potential to take part in hydrogen bonding to other groups (which may be on a receptor). If the structure of acetylcholine is compared with that of nicotine (Fig. 1.2), both of which are potent agonists at the nicotinic acetylcholine receptor, structural similarities can be seen. The distance between the positive nitrogen and a group capable of hydrogen bonding is 0.59 nm. This second group need not be the same in both molecules, but it must behave in a similar fashion. In acetylcholine it is the carbonyl group, and in nicotine it is the nitrogen in the pyridine ring.

Acetylcholine is a potent agonist at the muscarinic acetylcholine receptor (it is the transmitter). Muscarine is also a potent agonist at that receptor. A comparison of the structures of acetylcholine and muscarine also reveals a similarity (Fig. 1.3). In this case, the distance separating the positive nitrogen and a group capable of hydrogen bonding (an oxygen atom in each case) is 0.44 nm. Acetylcholine is therefore capable of activating two different receptor systems. A closer inspection would reveal that the acetylcholine molecule is not aligned in exactly the same way in both of these situations. It must be remembered that the acetylcholine molecule is a very flexible molecule and can be conformed in a number of different shapes. This factor is very important in the relation between structure and activity. Two molecules whose apparent structures differ

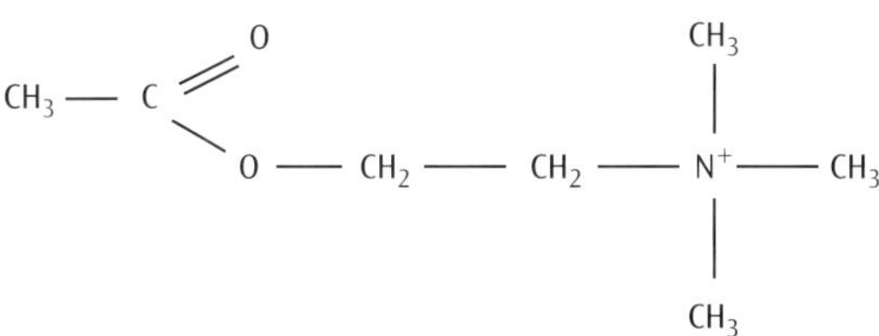

Figure 1.1 *The structural formula of acetylcholine.*

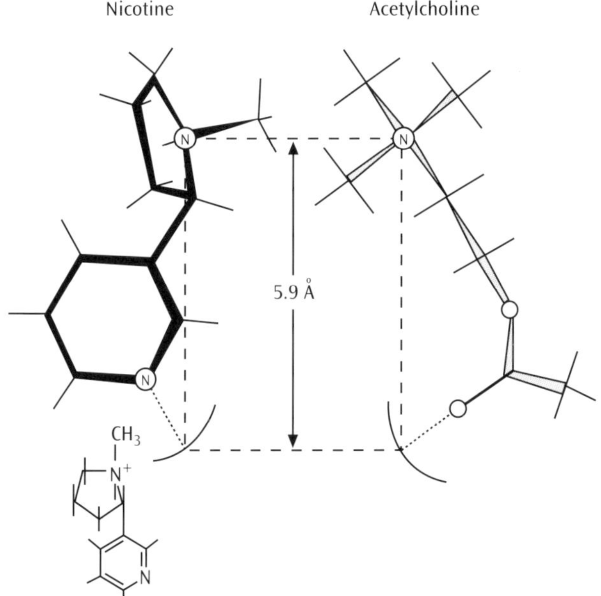

Figure 1.2 *The structural formula of nicotine, demonstrating its structural similarity to acetylcholine. (Reproduced with permission from Paton.[13])*

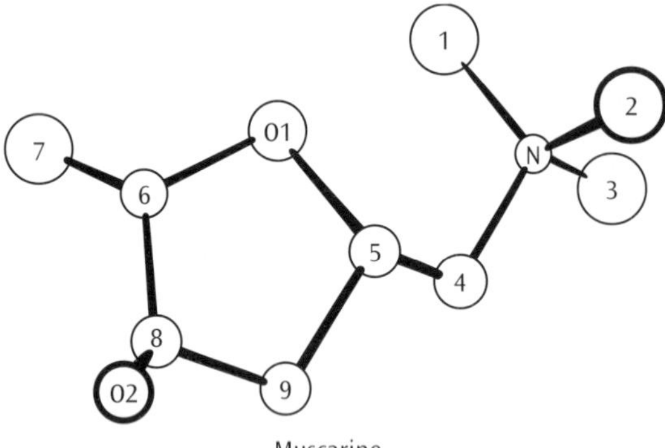

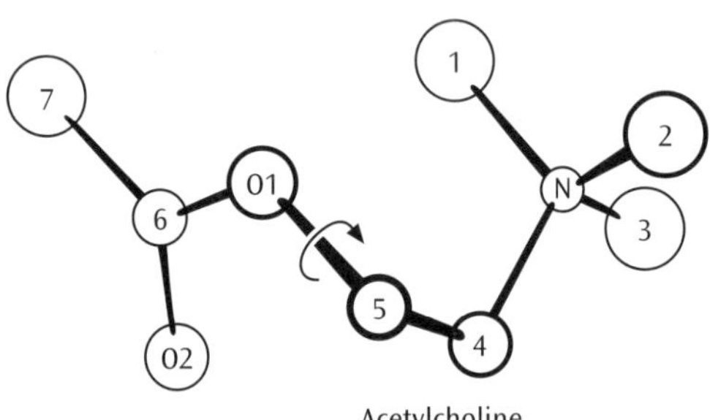

Figure 1.3 *The structural formula of muscarine, demonstrating its structural similarity to acetylcholine. (Reproduced with permission from Ramsey and Forster.[14])*

greatly may each have potent action at the same receptor because a part of each molecule can be manipulated into a certain similar shape.

Consider the antagonists at the nicotinic acetylcholine receptor. The original antagonist at the skeletal muscle nicotinic receptor was tubocurarine (the active constituent of curare, the South American Indian arrow poison). When it was found to contain two positively charged nitrogen groups, the hypothesis was advanced that perhaps other compounds which possessed two positively charged nitrogen groups might also exhibit neuromuscular-blocking activity. A variety of such compounds was then examined for this activity. Of considerable interest was the polymethylene-bismethonium family, described by Paton and Zaimis[15,16] (Fig. 1.4). A series of different compounds was tested, the only difference being variations in the length of the $-CH_2-$ chain. Two distinct phenomena were observed. Both autonomic ganglion block and neuromuscular block could be produced, but the optimum for ganglion block was at a chain length of 6 (hexamethonium) and that for neuromuscular block at a chain length of 10 (decamethonium). The polymethylene-bismethonium compounds are long flexible molecules. It might therefore be imagined that they could conform themselves into almost any configuration, and thus fit almost any receptor system that required the presence of two positively charged nitrogen atoms at a fixed distance. This will, of course, be limited by the electrostatic repulsion between the two positive forces, thereby limiting the number of possible conformations.

Care must be taken when inferring action at a receptor system from the simple existence of a certain group, or groups, in a chemical structure. Not every molecule with two positively charged nitrogen atoms is a neuromuscular blocker, nor does every neuromuscular blocker have two positively charged nitrogen atoms. There may also be more than one mechanism at work. Decamethonium weakly stimulates the receptor before blocking, and at higher concentrations blocks the receptor channel. This latter action does not occur at the acetylcholine recognition site and is noncompetitive in nature.[17] A similar noncompetitive action has also been demonstrated for hexamethonium.[18]

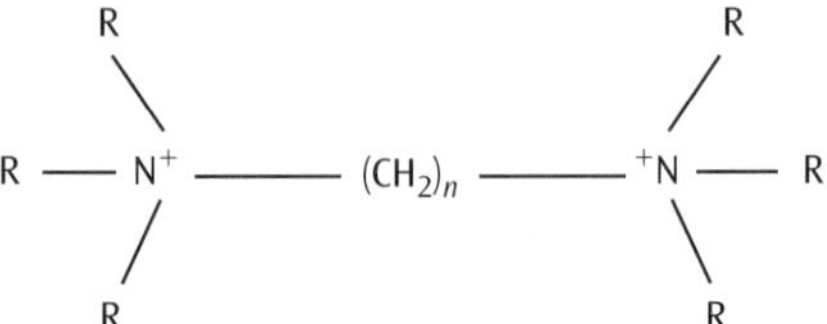

Figure 1.4 *The general structural formula of the methonium series, as examined by Paton and Zaimis.[16] In hexamethonium,* n = 6; *in decamethonium,* n = 10.

ISOMERISM

The preceding discussions have centered around simple molecular structures. Few drugs in clinical use have a simple structure, with the possible exception of the volatile and gaseous anesthetic agents. Although certain simple molecules can demonstrate isomerism, it is more common with complex molecules.

It is important first to consider terminology. Several important descriptive terms exist to define molecules; these terms may also be used to describe the relation between molecules and receptors. The word isomer differentiates between two unique molecular entities that are composed of the same chemical constituents. Isoflurane and enflurane are examples of isomers (Fig. 1.5). A particular form of isomerism is stereoisomerism. Stereoisomers are substances in which the constituent atoms or groups differ with respect to their spatial arrangement. These fall into two principal groups: geometric isomers and optical isomers. Many molecules which exhibit geometric isomerism contain a double bond or a heterocyclic (nonaromatic) ring system, although this is not a prerequisite for geometric isomerism. Because a double bond is rigid and does not permit rotation, a molecule containing a double bond has the potential to exist in two different forms – cis and trans (Fig. 1.6A and B). A simple heterocyclic ring is also a relatively rigid structure, although it can exist in two basic configurations – "chair" and "boat" (Fig. 1.7). In addition, because the ring structure is relatively rigid, if certain groups protrude onto the upper surface while others do so onto the lower surface, further asymmetry is introduced (Fig. 1.7). Therefore, it should be appreciated that two molecules of apparently identical chemical structure can exist in more than one actual configuration and that these configurations are not interchangeable. Furthermore, they may behave as quite different substances with different physicochemical properties.

Returning to the concept of receptors, it is clear that many receptors are very specific and will combine only with agents that possess a certain pattern of constituent atoms in exact locations. It is not difficult

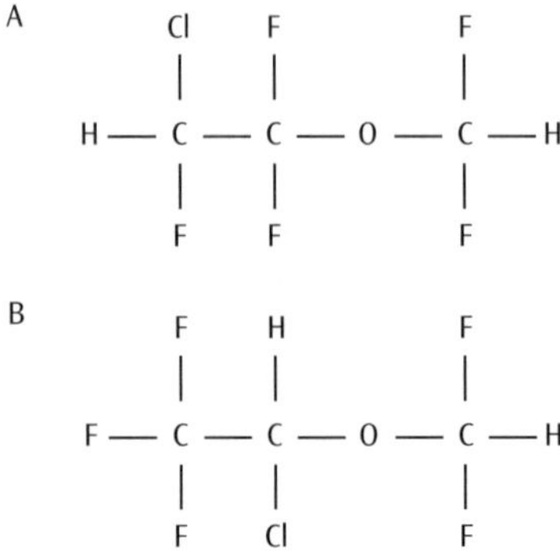

Figure 1.5 *The structural formulae of enflurane (A) and isoflurane (B) to show isomerism.*

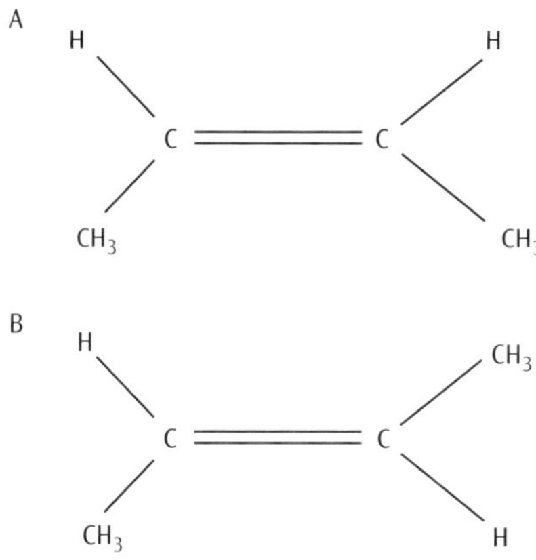

Figure 1.6 *A simple molecule (butene) containing a double bond between two carbon atoms that demonstrates geometric isomerism. The rigidity of the double bond results in two possible structural configurations. (A) Both methyl groups are on the same side – the cis form. (B) The methyl groups are on opposite sides – the trans form.*

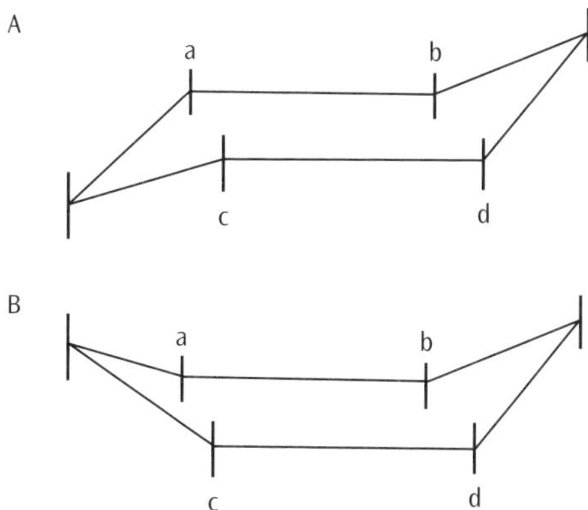

Figure 1.7 *A simple heterocyclic six-carbon ring showing (A) chair and (B) boat configurations. Each of the unlabeled bonds would contain a hydrogen atom. The molecules also demonstrate further asymmetry because the additional groups a and b protrude from the upper surface of the molecule and the groups c and d from the lower surface.*

to recognize that only one of the geometric isomers of a drug might be able to combine with a particular receptor whereas the other isomer is inactive. The nature of the synthetic manufacturing process for a drug usually results in the production of roughly equal numbers of each possible structure, although certain molecules are capable of conversion from one form to another under certain circumstances. Therefore, an injected drug is usually a mixture of all possible isomers, only one of which is active.

Further evidence with respect to the relation between structure and activity for certain drugs may be obtained by observation of the activity of individual stereoisomers of a drug. If there is a specific biological receptor involved, then the activity of the various isomers should differ. If there is no difference, then it is likely either that the action of the drug is not taking place through the medium of a specific receptor system or that the receptor has only one or two loci and thus attachment of a drug is less specific.

A particular form of isomerism – optical isomerism – has received a great deal of attention. Optical isomers are a particular subset of stereoisomers in which at least two of the isomers are optically active. The term chirality (right- or left-handedness) is often used in this context. Molecules which possess a chiral center exist in two forms (enantiomers) that cannot be distinguished with respect to the majority of their physical or chemical properties, e.g. melting point, boiling point, and lipid solubility. A chiral molecule has at least one isomeric center, which is usually a carbon atom (Fig. 1.8), but phosphorus, sulfur, and nitrogen can also form chiral centers. A mixture of equal portions of each enantiomer is a racemic mixture. If more than one chiral center is present in the molecule, four or more different configurations can exist, and these are termed diastereoisomers. Diastereoisomers may have different chemical and physical properties.

The usual difference between a pair of chiral isomers concerns their ability to rotate a plane of polarized light. The "L" or "−" isomer rotates the plane to the left (anticlockwise), and the "D" or "+" rotates it to the right (clockwise). The capacity to rotate the plane of polarized light is a function of the electronic properties of the molecule, and this has confused organic chemists. A second convention was therefore developed – the R–S convention. The groups around the chiral center are sized according to atomic number and, depending upon the order, the molecule is assigned the R (rectus) or S (sinister) designation.[19] Usually, but not always, the particular R and S configurations correlate with a particular direction of light rotation. In general terms, when one enantiomer in a series shows a certain pharmacologic activity, the equivalent enantiomer of other compounds in that series will also be an active enantiomer, i.e. if the D(+) form of one substance is the active one, it will be the D(+) form of all others in that series that will also be active.

Biologic systems are principally constructed from chiral molecules – most amino acids are in the L-form and most sugars are in the D-form. It is not surprising therefore that many drugs which possess one or more asymmetric centers exhibit a high degree of stereoselectivity in their interaction with receptors. Stereoselectivity in the action of drugs, not only on receptors but also with respect to ion channels and enzymes, is well established.[20]

Traditionally, physicians and pharmacologists alike have tended to regard every drug as a single agent that would produce a single effect. This is not necessarily the case when administering a racemic mixture. A racemic mixture in reality contains a number of "drugs," each with the potential to behave in a different fashion. Several different pharmacologic outcomes are therefore possible depending upon the pharmacologic action of each individual enantiomer.

1. All activity could reside in one isomer, with the other(s) being completely inactive. It might not be unexpected for all activity to reside in one enantiomer because of the necessity for a particular molecular configuration of drug for attachment to the receptor. However, it is unusual for the other isomer to be completely inactive. The antihypertensive agent α-methyldopa is one of the few examples of a drug in which the desired effect is confined to one optical isomer, the L-isomer.[21]
2. All activity could reside in one isomer while the other(s) have alternative pharmacologic action(s). Possible alternative actions

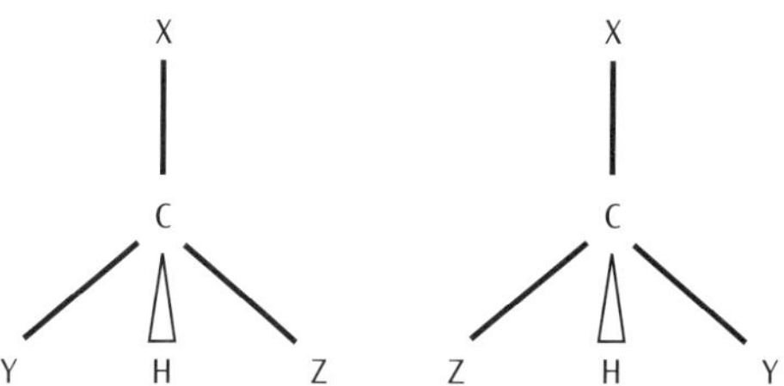

Figure 1.8 *A simple chiral molecule. The two forms can be seen to be mirror images of one another.*

might include antagonism to the action of the first isomer, totally unrelated actions, or potentially toxic effects. Labetalol is both an α- and β-adrenoceptor antagonist and is a good example of a drug in this category. Labetalol is a mixture of four diastereoisomers by virtue of its two chiral centers. The RR isomer has β-blocking activity, whereas the SR isomer is an α-blocker. The RS and SS forms are thought to be inactive.[22] L-Dopa is another example. During the development of L-dopa, it was noted that there were a number of serious side-effects, which included granulocytopenia. Detailed studies revealed that these were confined to the D-isomer and not the L-isomer. Therefore, it was the L-isomer which was marketed and not the racemic mixture. With respect to anesthetic drugs, ketamine, which is a chiral molecule, is marketed as a racemic mixture. The S(+) enantiomer is approximately three to four times more potent than the R(–) enantiomer, and the unwanted side-effects appear to be principally associated with the R(–) enantiomer. Therefore, development of the S(+) enantiomer alone might have led to a more acceptable anesthetic agent.

3 Both (all) isomers could have the same qualitative action, but with different potencies. This is a common situation. Propranolol, verapamil, and warfarin are all examples of drugs that fall into this category. It might be thought that the use of racemic mixtures of these agents would present very few problems, but this may not always be the case. Drugs tend to be stereoselective not only in their interactions with receptors but also in their binding to plasma proteins, their metabolism, and their interactions with other drugs. If the pharmacokinetic disposition of the isomers is different, the pharmacodynamic action can vary quite markedly between patients, and even within the same patient on different occasions.

4 Both (all) isomers could be equal in activity. This situation is uncommon but should be expected because of the selectivity of receptors for drugs. The two isomers of promethazine have equal antihistamine activity. The isomers of propranolol show an interesting phenomenon in which their effect on insulin secretion is not selective (all of these have an effect) yet their β-blocking action is highly selective, being confined to one isomer.

There is insufficient space in this chapter to discuss the many other considerations of the isomers of drugs. The different isomers of a drug may differ in respect of absorption, plasma protein binding, distribution, metabolism, renal clearance, drug interactions, and pharmacogenetics. The existence of any of these factors is likely to affect the actions of a drug given in a racemic mixture. It is also possible for certain drugs to undergo conversion *in vivo* between isomers (e.g. ibuprofen). Pharmacologists and the drug companies are recognizing more and more the advantages of using single isomers rather than a racemic mixture. However, the separation of one isomer may be complex and, in many instances, not commercially viable. It is becoming apparent that decisions about safety and efficacy of a compound should extend to understanding the actions and pharmacokinetics of each component enantiomer. It is likely that we will see more drugs presented as single isomers for clinical use in the future.

QUANTITATIVE ASPECTS OF DRUG–RECEPTOR INTERACTIONS

This section considers the interpretation of the relation between drug concentration and observed response. The simplest model is derived from the law of mass action and assumes that two entities (molecules) are combining in a reversible manner to form a third. With respect to drug–receptor interactions, one entity is the drug and the other the receptor.

In its simplest form, the combination of a drug with a receptor may be expressed by the following equation:

$$[\text{Drug}] + [\text{Receptor}] \rightarrow [\text{Drug–receptor complex}]$$

Unless the drug forms a completely irreversible union with the receptor – an uncommon result – the drug–receptor complex can dissociate again into its two component parts. The equation should really therefore be bidirectional:

$$[\text{D}] + [\text{R}] \underset{K_{21}}{\overset{K_{12}}{\Longleftrightarrow}} [\text{DR}] \rightarrow \text{Effect}$$

The rate of reaction is the same as the rate of formation of the drug–receptor complex (K_{12}) and depends upon both the concentration of drug, [D], and the concentration of receptors, [R]. The rate of dissociation of the drug–receptor complex (K_{21}) depends upon its concentration, [DR]. The rates of these two reactions can therefore be summarized as follows:

$$\text{Rate of formation (forward reaction)} = K_{12}\,[\text{D}]\,[\text{R}]$$

$$\text{Rate of dissociation (reverse reaction)} = K_{21}\,[\text{DR}]$$

When steady state is reached,

$$K_{12}\,[\text{D}]\,[\text{R}] = K_{21}\,[\text{DR}]$$

therefore

$$[\text{D}]\,[\text{R}]/[\text{DR}] = K_{21}/K_{12} = K_{\text{d}}$$

The ratio K_{21}/K_{12} is usually replaced by the single term K_{d}, the dissociation constant.

Although K_{d} is known as the dissociation constant, theoretically it may be more correct to describe it as the association constant because it has been defined in terms of the association of the two components – drug and receptor – and not their dissociation. Because of this, some authors use the symbol K for the association constant and it is important to be aware of this potential confusion. The dissociation constant is the reciprocal of the association constant:

$$K = 1/K_{\text{d}}$$

It must be noted that, in this scheme, several assumptions have been made. It has been assumed that the reaction is totally reversible, that all receptor sites have an equal affinity for the drug, that binding to some receptor sites does not affect the binding to others, and that there are no other nonspecific binding sites present. Clearly, this is an "ideal" situation and not one which pertains in many clinical circumstances.

A pharmacologist would next determine the degree of binding of drugs to receptors using a variety of techniques. These may include the use of radioactively labeled drugs or nuclear magnetic resonance spectroscopy. Complex kinetic analyses can then be used in order to further elucidate the extent of drug–receptor binding or to calculate the dissociation constant. Such theoretical considerations are not relevant to the clinical anesthesiologist. There are, however, many similarities between some of those more sophisticated analyses and the quantitative evaluation of drug effect. Receptor binding is very important in respect of the characterization of receptors at the molecular level. It is the ability of a receptor to produce an effect that distinguishes the true receptor from any other binding site. The principal means by which many drug receptors are defined is by the measurement of the response. The quantification of the responses is central to understanding how receptors initiate their response.

Agonists

An agonist is a substance that combines with a receptor to produce a response, e.g. acetylcholine.

Mathematical rearrangement of the equation of the law of mass action (above) allows interpretation. At equilibrium, the sum of the total number of free receptors [R] and the total number of bound receptors [DR] must equal the overall total of available receptors, which is denoted by the term $[R_{tot}]$.

Thus,

$$[R_{tot}] = [R] + [DR]$$

Rearranging,

$$[R] = [R_{tot}] - [DR]$$

Substituting for $[R]$ in the law of mass action equation results in the following:

$$K_d = [D]\,[R_{tot} - DR]/[DR]$$

This can be further rearranged to provide the following ratio of bound to total receptors:

$$[DR]/[R_{tot}] = [D]/(K_d + [D])$$

It should be clear that when all of the receptors, $[R_{tot}]$, are occupied by agonist, the maximum effect (E_{max}) will be produced. When no receptors are occupied, there will be no effect. Between these two extremes, the effect (E) will be in proportion to the concentration of receptor occupied [DR].

Thus,

E_{max} is proportional to $[R_{tot}]$

and

E is proportional to [DR]

therefore

$$E/E_{max} = [DR]/[R_{tot}]$$

Substituting this equation in the earlier equation,

$$E/E_{max} = [DR]/[R_{tot}] = [D]/K_d + [D]$$

Rearranging this equation produces the following result:

$$E = E_{max}\,[D]/K_d + [D]$$

Although it may not be immediately obvious, this is the equation describing the rectangular hyperbola (Fig. 1.9). This equation may be examined with respect to the different parts of the curve. When there is no agonist present at the beginning of the curve, there will be no effect, i.e. when $[D] = 0, E = 0$.

When the effect is at 50% of maximum,

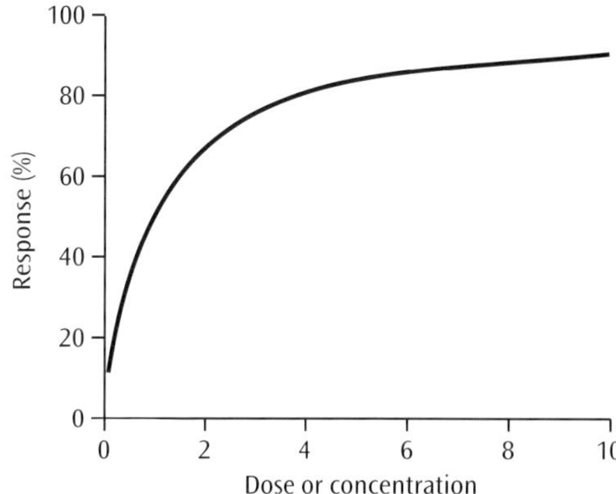

Figure 1.9 *A relation between dose and response.*

$$E/E_{max} = 0.5$$

Substituting in the above equation, at 50% maximum effect:

$$[D]/K_d + [D] = 0.5$$

therefore

$$[D] = K_d$$

The dissociation constant, K_d, is equal to the concentration of drug required to produce an effect that is 50% of maximum.

When [D] is very large, [D] will be very much greater than K_d, and E will almost equal E_{max}, i.e. high concentrations of drug produce effects that are close to the maximum effect.

When [D] is very low, [D] is very much less than K_d, and then E is approximately equal to:

$$[D] \times E_{max}/K_d$$

or, to put it more simply, at low concentrations of agonist, the effect E becomes almost directly proportional to the agonist concentration. It should now be clear why the relation between agonist combination and effect has the shape of a rectangular hyperbola.

Let us return to the basic equation:

$$[DR]/[R_{tot}] = [D]/K_d + [D]$$

The proportion of receptors occupied by drug is given by the function

$$[DR]/[R_{tot}]$$

Responses measured will depend upon the actual proportion of receptors occupied and the term $[DR]/[R_{tot}]$ was replaced earlier by the expression E/E_{max}, which is the measured effect and can therefore be denoted by r, the response.

Then,

$$r = [D]/K_d + [D]$$

Rearranging,

$$[D] = K_d\,(r/1 - r)$$

This equation is immediately seen to be directly analogous to that derived by A J Clarke when he showed that:

$$x = (\text{constant} \times y)/(100 - y)$$

where x is the concentration of drug and y is response as a percentage of maximum possible response.

It is common to express the relation between drug concentration and measured effect graphically. When the measured effect is plotted against the concentration of drug, the resulting rectangular hyperbola (Fig. 1.9) is particularly difficult to construct and to use. It is therefore common to display the data as the logarithm of the dose (or logarithm of the concentration of drug) against the response, the response being expressed as a percentage of the maximum response. This yields a sigmoid-shaped graph (Fig. 1.10). This transformation is particularly useful because the section from approximately 20% to 80% of maximal response is converted to a straight line, allowing a more precise estimate of the ED_{50} (or EC_{50}). Additional advantages of this semilogarithmic plot are that it is possible to visualize effects over a wide range of drug doses (concentrations) and also to more easily compare the effects of different agonists and antagonists. Theoretically, if two agonists are acting in exactly the same way on a receptor system, their log dose–response curves must be parallel; if they are not parallel, their mechanism of action is unlikely to be the same. However, the converse does not apply, in that parallel curves do not imply an identical mechanism of action.

The log dose–response graph is difficult to use outside the range 20–80% of maximum response because it is not linear outside this range. If data can be confined to that central linear part, then statistical analysis becomes much simpler. Logarithms can be taken of both sides of the equation above and yield the following result:

$$\log [D] = \log K_d + \log (r/1 - r)$$

Thus, a graph of log [D] against log $(r/1 - r)$ will produce a straight line, the intercept of which gives the value for log K_d. This relation is known as the Hill plot (named after A V Hill). Strictly speaking, the relation should be:

$$N \times \log [D] = \log K_d + \log (r/1 - r)$$

If the agonist and receptor combine on a 1:1 basis, then N (the slope of the line) should be unity. This is often the case, but not always so.

The term log $(r/1 - r)$ is also referred to as the logit (or logistic) transformation and is commonly used in biological data handling. The logit transformation has the effect of extending the ends of the scale of r and allows points to be plotted out to approximately 1% and 99% of maximum response. The corresponding logits for values of r of 0, 0.5, and 1 are $-\infty$, 0, and $+\infty$ respectively.

When considering biological responses, as the concentration of agonist rises, a point will be reached when an effect begins; this effect

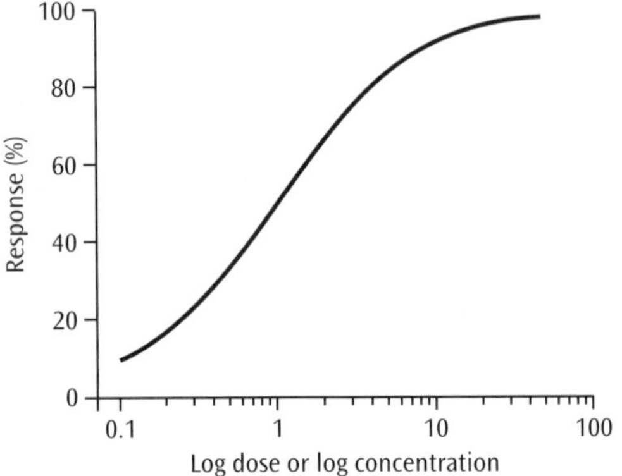

Figure 1.10 *A relation between log dose and response.*

increases until a maximum effect is obtained. The two extreme points of 0% and 100% must be excluded for two reasons:

1 Infinity cannot be plotted on a graph.
2 Theoretically, the concentration to just give 100% can be determined but that same value of 100% would also be produced by concentrations of agonist of greater than that to just produce 100%.

There is an alternative approach, namely that of probit analysis. This considers the response as being the result of a statistical summation of the probabilities that any individual drug and receptor will combine to initiate an effect. The response axis is replaced by an axis which represents the proportion (or percentage) of positive receptor interactions for that given dose and response. As the concentration of agonist rises, the proportion (or rate) of receptor interactions increases until the 50% response point is reached. The proportional increase for each unit increase in dose then declines with further increases in dose, although the total number of receptors occupied must be increasing. The frequency distribution of quantal responses to many drugs has been shown to be described by such a normal (Gaussian) distribution. Conversion of a response to its probit value requires complex mathematical methods, and it is easier to use either a table of probit values or graph paper that is marked with a probit scale. Corresponding probits for values of r of 0, 0.5, and 1 are $-\infty$, 5, and $+\infty$ respectively. The effect of probit analysis is almost identical with that of logit analysis in that it expands the ends of the scale of response and converts the sigmoid relation between log concentration and response to a straight line. The same limitations also apply to the points of 0% and 100% as to logit analysis.

One further technique is occasionally applied to biological data, namely arcsine transformation (alternatively known as the angular transformation or inverse sine transformation). The equation $y = \sin^{-1}x$ is applied to the data, where x is the square root of the original variable. As the original variable increases from 0 to 1, y increases from 0° to 90°, and equal changes in x correspond to greater changes in y toward the ends of the scale. Therefore, the result is to convert a sigmoid curve (which might be regarded as having the appearance of a section of a sine wave) into a straight line.

Theories underlying the drug–receptor interaction

There are two principal theories underlying the interaction between drugs and receptors, namely the occupation theory and the rate theory. The occupation theory of drug action holds that the observed response is a direct function of the number of receptors occupied by the drug. The rate theory recognizes that receptors have to be occupied by drug for the effect to be produced, but holds that the drug is constantly binding with and dissociating from the receptors in a dynamic fashion. The response should then be a function of the rate of occupation of receptors by the agonist.

The occupation theory has its origins in the work of A J Clarke, who showed that there were many situations in which the effect of a drug was linearly proportional to receptor occupancy. In addition, the maximum response is reached when all of the receptors are occupied by agonist molecules. The occupation theory can readily explain the shape of the relation between dose and response from the equations already described above. However, there are some discrepancies. When the behavior of a partial agonist is considered, why does it not result in a maximum response with the same magnitude as that which follows the use of a full agonist? The number of receptors is the same, and when the drug is in great excess surely all (or almost all) of the receptors are occupied by drug. It is necessary to postulate that the drug possesses both agonist and antagonist actions, and the original descriptive term of "dualist" is an apt description. This discrepancy has to be explained by introducing the term "intrinsic activity." Full agonists have an intrinsic activity of 1; antagonists have an intrinsic activity of 0; and partial agents lie between these two. This explanation is regarded with skepticism by some pharmacologists. An additional problem for the occupation theory follows work from Stephenson,[23] who showed that there were some experimental situations in which the response was not exactly proportional to the fraction of receptors occupied.

The rate theory of drug action was advanced by Paton in 1961.[13] This theory can also be shown mathematically to predict the same shapes of graph as the occupation theory for the relations between dose and response and log dose and response. The dissociation constant K_d also remains equal to the concentration of agonist at half-maximum response. However, the time curve of a response under the rate theory differs from that predicted by the occupation theory. At time 0, as the drug is administered, [DR] is 0. According to the rate theory, the response should immediately rise to a transient peak and then decrease exponentially and very rapidly to a plateau (equilibrium response). It is the equilibrium response that is the measured response. Theoretically, the plateau responses are the same as those predicted by the occupation theory. The peak response, according to the rate theory, may considerably exceed the maximum possible response calculated using the occupation theory. It is hard to reconcile these theoretical considerations, and the existence of these instantaneous maximum values is almost impossible to test experimentally.

The points of difference between the two theories of drug action have therefore to be regarded with a certain degree of caution. The only firm conclusion that can be drawn is that one theory holds for certain drug–receptor interactions and the other for different interactions.

Antagonists

An antagonist is a substance that inhibits or blocks the action of an agonist, e.g. tubocurarine is an antagonist to acetylcholine at the neuromuscular junction. Antagonism of a drug's effect can take place in a number of ways. It may be competitive or noncompetitive, reversible or irreversible. It may or may not take place at the same receptor and may involve more than one process simultaneously. Each has its own characteristic features.

Competitive antagonism

Competitive antagonists simply compete with agonists for a common receptor binding site. There are two reactions taking place simultaneously and these are illustrated as follows:

$$[\mathrm{D}] + [\mathrm{R}] \overset{K_D}{\Longleftrightarrow} [\mathrm{DR}] \rightarrow \text{Response}$$

$$\uparrow\downarrow$$

$$[\mathrm{I}] + [\mathrm{R}] \underset{K_I}{\Longleftrightarrow} [\mathrm{IR}]$$

The receptor concentration is common to both equations, i.e. both reactions involve the same receptor pool. The extent of the competitive antagonism depends on both the concentration of agonist and its dissociation constant, and also upon the concentration of antagonist [I] and its dissociation constant K_I. In the presence of the competitive inhibitor, the fractional occupation of receptors by drug, [DR], will decrease as a proportion of the maximum number of receptors available, $[\mathrm{DR}_{max}]$. Here, $[\mathrm{DR}_{max}]$ is equal to the maximum available concentration of drug–receptor complexes and is the same as $[\mathrm{R}_{tot}]$.

Because the nature of the interactions is competitive, increasing the concentration of agonist, [D], still produces the same maximum response, but at a lower concentration in the absence of the antagonist. A large excess of agonist drives the equations in the direction that favors a normal response, and the combination of antagonist with receptor is reduced to a level at which there is no discernible effect from the agonist. Plots of the log dose of agonist against response produce a family of parallel sigmoid curves, one for each dose (concentration) of antagonist. These are displaced further to the right as the concentration of competitive antagonist increases (Fig. 1.11).

Noncompetitive antagonism

Noncompetitive antagonists attach to the receptor, or to a nearby group, and prevent the receptor from initiating the response whether or not it is activated. The mathematical equations which describe noncompetitive reactions might be similar to those described below:

$$[\mathrm{D}] + [\mathrm{R}] \overset{K_D}{\Longleftrightarrow} [\mathrm{DR}] \rightarrow \text{Response}$$

$$\uparrow\downarrow$$

$$[\mathrm{I}] + [\mathrm{R}] \overset{K_I}{\Longleftrightarrow} [\mathrm{RI}] \quad \text{(inactivated receptor)}$$

$$\uparrow\downarrow$$

$$[\mathrm{D}] + [\mathrm{RI}] \overset{K_D}{\Longleftrightarrow} [\mathrm{RI}] \quad \text{(no response)}$$

The two equations at the top are very similar in appearance to the equations for the competitive inhibitor above. However, a third reaction can take place in which drug [D] can combine with inactivated receptor [RI] with the same K_d as it combines with normal receptors, but no response is produced. Note that all these equations are reversible and are all interlinked.

The antagonist does not necessarily alter the ability of the drug (agonist) to combine with the receptor and the drug can, therefore, combine with either the normal receptor or the inactivated receptor. The presence of the antagonist has effectively reduced the number of available receptors, and because the response depends upon the number of receptors activated, the maximum possible response is reduced. The greater the concentration of noncompetitive antagonist present, the greater will be the reduction in possible maximum response. The drug should still combine with the receptor (whether normal or inactivated) with the same affinity (K_d remains the same). Other characteristics of the graph, for example the ED_{50}, will be the same, i.e. the dose to cause 50%

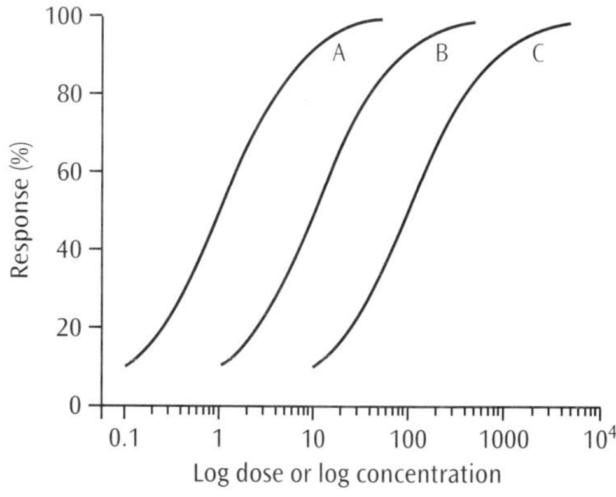

Figure 1.11 *A family of log dose–response lines. Curve A represents the effect of agonist alone. In the presence of a competitive antagonist, there is a parallel shift to the right (B). As the concentration of competitive antagonist is further increased, the line moves further to the right (C).*

of the maximum response is the same although it is 50% of a maximum that is different from that in the absence of antagonist. Increasing the concentration of agonist will have no effect on the maximum response obtainable. Plots of the log dose of agonist against response produce a family of curves similar to those in Fig. 1.12. It can be seen that graphic analysis can be used to discriminate easily between competitive and noncompetitive antagonism.

Irreversible antagonism

It was assumed that the competitive and noncompetitive mechanisms described above involved reversible reactions. When an antagonist reacts in an irreversible manner with a receptor, the receptors so bound are likely to be permanently removed from the receptor pool. Under these circumstances, it may be necessary to await the formation of new receptors. In the mean time, a normal relation between log dose and response will be apparent, but the maximum possible response will be reduced. A family of curves similar to those in Fig. 1.12 for a noncompetitive antagonist will result.

Nonreceptor antagonism

Antagonism may result from a mechanism that is unrelated to blockade of drug receptors. Examples include inhibition of a second-messenger system that is activated by the receptor, or an alteration in cellular excitability by another means. This type of antagonism is sometimes referred to as physiologic antagonism. It must be remembered that it is possible for some antagonists not to act by one mechanism alone, but by several different mechanisms simultaneously.

CONCLUSION

The theories and studies of drug–receptor interactions are central to the study of pharmacology. They are central to the action of any drug or any system in the body, and it is essential that every anesthesiologist has a clear understanding of these receptor–drug interactions. It is partly for these reasons that questions about drug–receptor interactions are very common during postgraduate examinations in anesthesia.

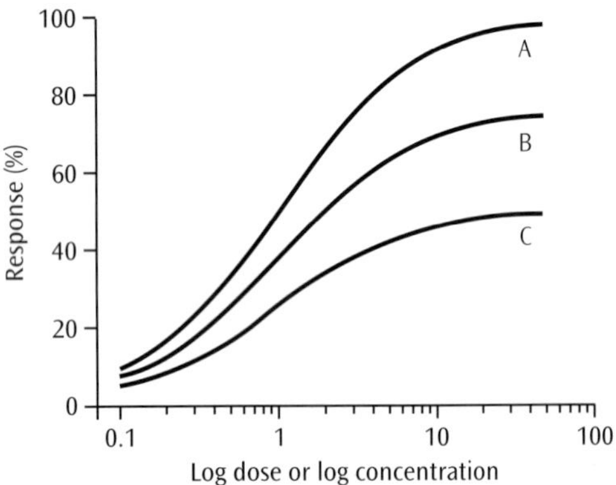

Figure 1.12 *A family of dose–response lines. Curve A represents the effect of agonist alone. In the presence of increasing concentrations of a noncompetitive antagonist, the overall shape of the line is retained, but the maximum possible response is progressively reduced (B and C).*

A broad view of the subject has been taken in this chapter, limiting the discussion to some of the most important aspects. The reader is encouraged to consult any of the common pharmacology texts for further details with respect to this complex, but fascinating, subject.

REFERENCES

1. Langley JN. On the physiology of salivary secretion. Part II. On the mutual antagonism of atropin and pilocarpin, having especial reference to their relations in the sub-maxillary gland of the cat. *J Physiol* 1878; **1:** 339–69.
2. Langley JN. Croonian Lecture 1906 – On nerve endings and on special excitable substances in cells. *Proc R Soc Lond B* 1906; **78:** 170–94.
3. Langley JN. On the contraction of muscle chiefly in relation to the presence of "receptive" substances. Part 4. The effect of curare and of some other substances on the nicotine response of the sartorius and gastrocnemius muscles of the frog. *J Physiol* 1909; **39:** 235–95.
4. Ehrlich P. On immunity with special reference to cell life. *Proc R Soc Lond B* 1900; **66:** 424–48.
5. Clarke AJ. The factors determining tolerance of glucosides of the digitalis series. *J Pharmacol Exp Ther* 1913; **4:** 399–424.
6. Clarke AJ. The reaction between acetyl choline and muscle cells. *J Physiol* 1926; **61:** 530–46.
7. Clarke AJ. The reaction between acetyl choline and muscle cells. Part II. *J Physiol* 1927; **64:** 123–43.
8. Boheim G, Hanke W, Barrantes FJ, *et al.* Agonist activated ionic channels in acetylcholine receptor reconstituted into planar lipid bilayers. *Proc Natl Acad Sci USA* 1981; **78:** 3586–90.
9. Conti-Tronconi B, Tzartos S, Lindstrom J. Monoclonal antibodies as probes of acetylcholine receptor structure. 2. Binding to native receptor. *Biochemistry* 1981; **20:** 2181–91.
10. James RW, Kato AC, Rey M-J, Fulpius BW. Monoclonal antibodies directed against the neurotransmitter binding site of nicotinic acetylcholine receptor. *FEBS Lett* 1980; **120:** 145–8.
11. Lee CY. Chemistry and pharmacology of polypeptide toxins in snake venoms. *Annu Rev Pharmacol* 1972; **12:** 265–86.
12. Fertuk HC, Salpeter MM. Localization of acetylcholine receptor by ^{125}I-labeled alpha-bungarotoxin binding at mouse motor end plate. *Proc Natl Acad Sci USA* 1974; **71:** 1376–80.
13. Paton WDM. A theory of drug action based on the rate of combination. *Proc R Soc Lond B* 1961; **154:** 21–69.
14. Ramsey W, Forster R. Conformations of acetyl choline. *Nature* 1968; **219:** 1156–7.
15. Paton WDM, Zaimis EJ. Curare-like action of polymethylene bis-quaternary ammonium salts. *Nature* 1948; **161:** 718–19.
16. Paton WDM, Zaimis EJ. The pharmacological actions of polymethylene bis trimethylammonium salts. *J Pharmacol* 1949; **4:** 381.
17. Adams PR, Sakmann B. Decamethonium both blocks and opens end-plate channels. *Proc Natl Acad Sci USA* 1978; **75:** 2994–7.
18. Gurney AM, Rang HP. The channel blocking action of methonium compounds on rat submandibular ganglion cells. *Br J Pharmacol* 1984; **82:** 623–31.
19. IUPAC. Tentative rules for the nomenclature of organic chemistry, Section E. Fundamental stereochemistry. *J Org Chem* 1970; **35:** 2849–67.
20. Timmermans PBMWM. Stereoselectivity in various drug fields. In: Ariens EJ, Sondijn W, Timmermans PBMWM (eds). *Stereochemistry and Biological Activity of Drugs.* Oxford: Blackwell Scientific Publications, 1983: 161–80.
21. Gillespie L, Oates JA, Grant JR, Sjoerdsma H. Clinical and chemical studies with α-methyldopa in patients with hypertension. *Circulation* 1962; **25:** 281–91.
22. Brittain RT, Drew GM, Levy GP. The alpha and beta adrenoceptor blocking properties of labetalol and its individual stereoisomers. *Br J Pharmacol* 1982; **77:** 105–14.
23. Stephenson RP. A modification of receptor theory. *Br J Pharmacol* 1956; **11:** 379–93.

2

Principles of pharmacokinetics

STEVEN L SHAFER

Pharmacokinetics is the study of the what the body does to a drug. It examines the processes by which drugs distribute into body tissues, reach the site of action, and are eliminated from the body. Pharmacokinetics will be introduced with a discussion of the underlying physiologic properties of the body: volumes of distribution and clearance. From these we will develop the mathematic formulae used to relate drug concentrations to the route and dose of administration. The equations are intended as a reference for clinicians and scientists. For the most part, it is not necessary to memorize equations to understand the basic principles of pharmacokinetics. The essential point is to understand the shapes of the functions. Envisioning the general shape of the mathematic relations, rather than worrying about the equations, will lead to intuitive understanding about the role of pharmacokinetics in clinical anesthetic practice.

THE PHYSIOLOGICAL BASIS OF PHARMACOKINETICS

The basic pharmacokinetic concepts are volume and clearance. These are illustrated in Fig. 2.1. The volume of distribution, seen at the top of Fig. 2.1, represents the apparent dilution of a drug from the concentrated form in the syringe to the far more dilute concentration in the blood. Clearance, the process that removes drug from the volume, is illustrated at the bottom of this figure. Clearance has units of flow: volume per unit time. If the clearing organ shown at the bottom of Fig. 2.1 removes all the drug that flows into it, clearance is simply the flow in the pipe.

The time required to remove the drug from the body is determined by the ratio of volume to clearance. This is often reported as the half-life, which is the time required to remove half of the drug from wherever it is being measured (usually the plasma). If the volume increases, as shown at the top of Fig. 2.2, then it takes longer to remove drug from the body. In other words, the half-life increases. If the clearance increases, as shown at the bottom of Fig. 2.2, then drug is removed from the body more quickly. In this case, the half-life decreases. We will now explore the concepts of volume and clearance more carefully, understanding how physiology and experimental considerations influence these concepts.

Pharmacokinetics are dependent on the reference point: what, *exactly*, is being measured? Are we measuring drug concentrations in plasma, blood, urine, or tissues? If they are blood samples, are they venous, mixed venous, arterial, or effluent from a particular organ? Are we measuring total drug or free (unbound) drug? If the drug is a racemic mixture, are we distinguishing enantiomers, or just measuring total drug concentration? While the fundamental concepts are the same regardless of site, the actual numbers and the physiological implications are site dependent. Pharmacokinetic relativity! Unless stated otherwise, we will assume that the site of observation is the arterial plasma, and we are measuring total drug concentration.

Volume of distribution

The concept of volume comes directly from the definition of concentration: amount divided by volume:

$$\text{Concentration} = \text{Amount/Volume} \tag{2.1}$$

A

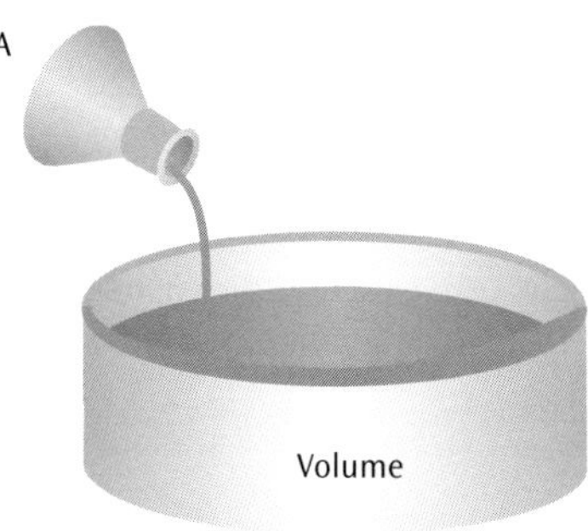

B

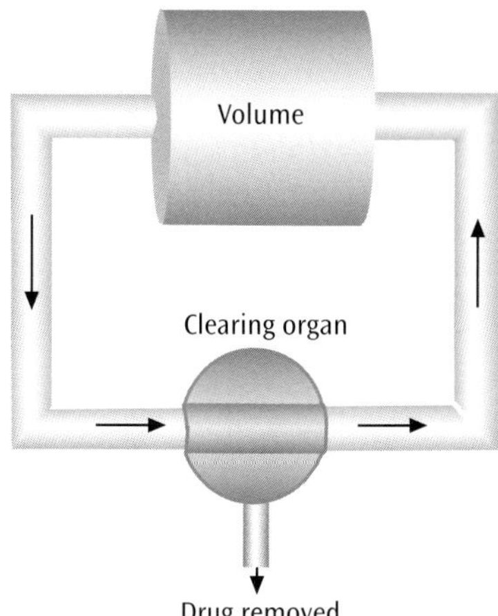

Figure 2.1 *(A) The volume of distribution, represented as the volume of a tank into which the drug is poured. The volume of distribution is the apparent volume into which the drug has been diluted, based on the measured concentration. (B) Clearance, represented as the plasma flow to a tissue that completely eliminates the drug.*

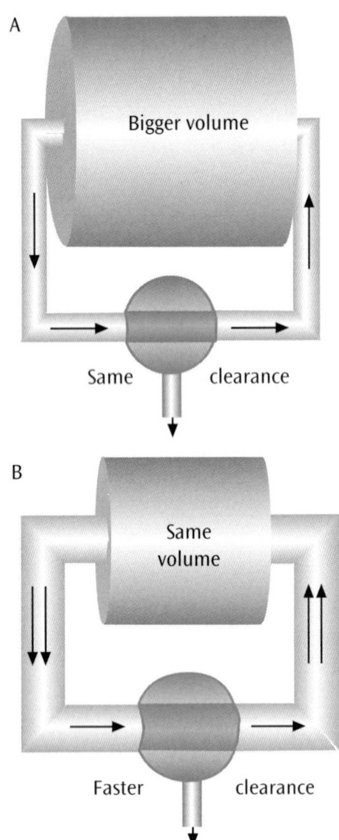

Figure 2.2 *Relation between volume, clearance, and half-life. (A) Compared with Fig. 2.1, the volume is increased, which increases half-life because it takes longer to clear the drug from the volume. (B) The clearance is increased, which reduces half-life because the drug can be cleared more readily from the volume.*

If we assume that the drug added in Fig. 2.1 is thoroughly mixed in the tank of fluid, we can determine the volume of the tank from the known amount of drug added and the observed concentration:

$$\text{Volume} = \text{Amount (or dose)/Concentration} \quad (2.2)$$

The utility of measuring this volume term is that it can be used to calculate the expected drug concentration from any arbitrary bolus dose, using equation 2.1. Additionally, it suggests an important concept: if you double the dose, you double the concentration. This is the principle of "linearity."

Unfortunately, the body is much more complex than the simple tank shown in Fig. 2.1. The apparent dilution of drug depends on exactly where the drug is sampled (arterial vs. mixed venous vs. peripheral venous), what is measured (blood vs. plasma), and the time that the measurement is taken. For this reason, "volume" is actually several related concepts.

Central volume of distribution

The central volume of distribution, V_1, is the initial dilution volume that explains the arterial concentration immediately after an intravenous bolus. This volume reflects the plasma volume of the heart, the great vessels, and the venous volume of the upper arm (assuming that is where the drug was given). It also reflects any uptake into the pulmonary parenchyma prior to the blood reaching the arterial circulation. The central volume in the case of drugs directly metabolized in the plasma (e.g. succinylcholine, remifentanil) reflects the metabolism of the drug en route from the venous site of injection to the arterial sampling catheter, which appears pharmacokinetically as dilution of the drug into a larger space. If we are measuring plasma, then the central volume also reflects the drug taken up by the red cells.

The concept of central volume is the most problematic of the pharmacokinetic concepts that will be introduced in this chapter. To be blunt, it does not exist. However, as George Box[1] observed, "All models are wrong. Some models are useful." Central volume is often a useful model. The concept of the central volume is based on a notion that the arterial concentration instantaneously peaks at time 0 following a bolus injection, and then continuously declines. Of course, this does not happen. The concentration of drug in the arterial blood immediately after intravenous injection is 0. Time is required for the blood to flow from the venous to the arterial circulation. This creates a lag time of 20–40 s from injection to appearance of drug on the arterial side. Over the next 30–60 s, there are also several oscillations reflecting very rapid recirculation of the drug through the heart and lung. Thus, there is a lag time, and about 1 min of oscillations, before the concentrations settle down into the time-course predicted by conventional pharmacokinetic models. To create a model that shows this time-course requires modeling the components between the venous site of injection and the arterial site of sampling. Models for this have been described by Henthorn, Avram, and Krejcie,[2,3] with recent contributions from Ludbrook and colleagues.[4] Thus, the central volume is not a real volume at all, but rather is the backward extrapolation of the concentration vs. time curve from its peak at about 30–60 s to the *y*-axis. It can be thought of as the initial concentration, had circulation been infinitely fast. It is also the *y* intercept for a curve that adequately describes the concentrations from roughly 30–60 s onwards, but fails seriously prior to that.

Why is the central volume of distribution a useful, if incorrect, concept? The central volume is the core of a model that accurately explains the entire time-course of drug concentration in the body, except during the first 30–60 s. The concept of an initial mixing volume greatly simplifies dosing calculations, even those performed by a computer. Indeed, at the time of writing this chapter, all pharmacokinetically based dosing guidelines for anesthetic drugs are based on models that assume a central volume of distribution.

Study design markedly influences the magnitude of the central volume. For example, a pharmacokinetic study with arterial samples (as all such studies should be performed) will have higher initial concentrations than a study with venous samples because drug is removed by the hand and forearm tissues prior to reaching the arm veins. The higher concentrations imply a smaller central volume. The central volume of distribution is also influenced by the timing of blood samples. When one begins to gather samples at 30 s, a high peak is observed initially, which if extrapolated backward to the *y*-axis predicts a small central volume. When blood sampling starts at 5 min, much of the initial rapid decrease in concentration is missed. Therefore, the backward extrapolation assumes much smaller initial concentrations, and hence a much larger volume for the central compartment. The central volume is also influenced by pulmonary uptake of the drug. For example, alfentanil is far less lipophilic than sufentanil, and, as a result, less is taken up on first pass through the lungs,[5] therefore the initial concentrations following bolus injection are higher. This results in a lower apparent dilution of the drug, and thus a lower V_1. Fentanyl is avidly taken up by the lungs,[6] also resulting in a large V_1 compared with alfentanil.

The decreased total body water and redistribution of cardiac output in elderly patients results in a smaller V_1 and higher initial plasma concentrations. This has been documented for thiopental,[7,8] propofol,[9] and remifentanil.[10]

Volume of distribution at steady state

The volume of distribution at steady state ($V_{d(ss)}$) is the volume that relates the plasma drug concentration to the total amount of drug in the body at steady state. By definition, steady state occurs only during an intravenous infusion, once the rate of elimination matches the rate of drug administration and the net rate of transfer between body tissues is 0. If the total amount of drug in the body, $X_{total\ drug}$, and the concentration of drug in the plasma, C_{plasma}, are known, rearrangement of the definition of concentration (amount/volume; equation 2.1) enables a volume term relating these to be derived:

$$V_{d(ss)} = X_{total\ drug}/C_{plasma} \tag{2.3}$$

$V_{d(ss)}$ is larger than the central volume because it includes peripheral volumes of distribution that accumulate drug during and after drug administration. These peripheral volumes represent body tissues other than the plasma. The sizes of the peripheral volumes of distribution reflect the tissue solubility of a drug, relative to its solubility in plasma. The more soluble a drug is in peripheral tissues, relative to plasma, the larger the apparent peripheral volumes of distribution. The true solubility of drugs in peripheral tissues is usually not known. Therefore, the solubility of the drug is assumed to be the same everywhere. Although not technically correct, this assumption simplifies the mathematics of $V_{d(ss)}$, which now simply equals the sum of the sizes of the central volume and the distribution volumes. This assumption does not influence our ability to characterize what happens in the plasma over time. However, it does lead to very large volumes of distribution for drugs that are highly soluble in tissues (e.g. 5000 L for propofol).

Since the magnitudes of the peripheral volumes are determined at steady state, the flow to the tissues will not affect the size of the peripheral volumes. Tissue blood flow influences only how long it takes for the peripheral volumes of distribution to equilibrate with the central volume of distribution.

If the tissue solubility of a drug depends on simple physiochemical constants, then it would seem likely that volumes of distribution would be consistent between individuals. However, changes in body habitus and composition do occur, and these affect peripheral volumes of distribution. For example, casual observation of elderly individuals reveals several obvious physiologic changes associated with age: (1) lean body mass decreases with age, (2) body fat increases with age, and (3) total body water decreases with age.[11] These changes in body habitus and muscle and fat distribution might be expected to produce changes in the volumes into which drugs distribute. In a study of several benzodiazepines, lipid solubility was found to predict the $V_{d(ss)}$.[12] Since the lipid content of elderly patients is higher than that of young patients, one might reasonably expect that elderly patients would have larger peripheral volumes of distribution. An increased volume of distribution, with increased duration of drug effect, has been documented in elderly individuals for trazodone[13] and nitrazepam.[14] However, as indicated above, the partitioning of drugs between body tissues is dictated by the physicochemical properties of the drug itself, and thus the partitioning, per unit of tissue, is not influenced by age.[15]

Some readers may have heard about a V_z or V_β, the apparent volume of distribution during the terminal half-life. This is the apparent volume that relates the drug concentration to the total amount of drug in the body during the terminal log-linear phase of drug elimination. V_z is a worthless concept as far as anesthetic drugs are concerned.

Clearance

Clearance is the body's ability to remove drug from the observation site. Generally, clearance applies to blood or plasma, reflecting the design of most pharmacokinetic studies in which blood or plasma is the sampled tissue. Clearance has units of flow: volume per unit time. There are many ways of thinking about clearance, all equally valid. The simplest concept is that clearance is the flow of plasma from which drug has been completely removed. At the bottom of Fig. 2.1, the eliminating organ removes all of the drug from the fluid that flows into the organ. In this case, clearance is simply the plasma flow to and from the organ, indicated by the arrows placed on the pipes.

Clearance describes an intrinsic capability of the body, i.e. the volume of fluid or tissue that can be cleared of drug per unit time. Assuming linear clearance (true for nearly all anesthetic drugs), the clearance is the same whether the amount of drug in the body is 0, 1 mg, 10 mg, or 10 000 mg. The actual rate of removal of drug is the drug concentration multiplied by the clearance. For example, if the body has a clearance of $1\ L\ min^{-1}$ for a particular drug, the actual rate of drug removal will be 0 if no drug is present in the body, $1\ mg\ min^{-1}$ if the drug concentration is $1\ mg\ L^{-1}$, $100\ mg\ min^{-1}$ if the plasma drug concentration is $100\ mg\ L^{-1}$, and so on.

Hepatic clearance

Nearly all drugs used in anesthesia are cleared by hepatic biotransformation. The liver metabolizes drugs through oxidation, reduction, hydrolysis, or conjugation. Oxidation and reduction occur in the cytochrome P450 system. Routes of oxidative metabolism include hydroxylation, dealkylation, deamination, desulfuration, epoxidation, and dehalogenation. These enzymes can be induced by exposure to certain drugs, increasing the liver's intrinsic metabolic capacity. They can also be inhibited by drugs or hepatic disease. The P450 system of greatest interest to anesthesiologists is P450 3A4. This enzyme is responsible for metabolizing fentanyl, alfentanil, sufentanil, midazolam, and lidocaine (lignocaine). Cytochrome P450 2D6 is responsible for the conversion of codeine, a prodrug, to morphine, the analgesic. About 5–10% of individuals have a genetic variant of cytochrome P450 2D6 that renders them unable to convert codeine to morphine. The P450 system is also involved in glucuronidation. Conjugation and hydrolysis often occur outside of the P450 system. The effect of conjugation is to transform hydrophobic molecules into water-soluble molecules by the addition of polar groups, and thus render the molecules easier to excrete via the kidneys. The metabolites generated by the liver are generally inactive, although some drugs (e.g. morphine, midazolam) have metabolites that are highly potent. Genetic polymorphism can occur in all of these pathways, and this accounts for part of the variability in clearance in the population.[16]

When the metabolic rate is proportional to concentration, clearance is constant over the range of concentrations used clinically. The rate of drug metabolism by the liver, R, can be calculated as the difference between the drug concentration flowing into the liver and the drug concentration flowing from the liver, multiplied by the rate of blood flow:

$$\text{Rate of drug metabolism} = R = \dot{Q}(C_{inflow} - C_{outflow}) \tag{2.4}$$

where $\dot{Q}$ is hepatic blood flow (about $1.4\ L\ min^{-1}$ in an adult), C_{inflow} is the drug concentration in the arterial blood perfusing the liver (ignoring the portal circulation for simplicity), and $C_{outflow}$ is the concentration in the venous blood draining the liver. This is simply a way of stating the mass balance of drug across the liver: the rate of metabolism must be the rate of drug going into the liver, $\dot{Q} \times C_{inflow}$, minus the rate of drug leaving the liver, $\dot{Q} \times C_{outflow}$. As described above, the rate of drug metabolism is also the clearance of the drug multiplied by the arterial concentration. We can add this to equation 2.4:

$$\text{Rate of drug metabolism} = R = \dot{Q}(C_{inflow} - C_{outflow}) = C_{inflow} \times \text{Clearance} \tag{2.5}$$

We can determine the clearance by dividing all of the terms in equation 2.5 by the concentration of drug flowing into the liver:

$$\text{Clearance} = \text{Rate of drug metabolism}/C_{\text{inflow}}$$
$$= \dot{Q}[(C_{\text{inflow}} - C_{\text{outflow}})/C_{\text{inflow}}] \quad (2.6)$$

Equation 2.6 offers two definitions of clearance, each of which merits additional comments:

$$\text{Clearance} = \text{Rate of drug metabolism}/C_{\text{inflow}} \quad (2.7)$$

Equation 2.7 tells us that clearance is the proportionality constant that relates drug metabolism to the drug concentration. A high ratio (high clearance) means that there is a high level of metabolism, whereas a low ratio (low clearance) means that metabolism is at a low level, even at high inflowing drug concentrations. If the liver is completely efficient, then the rate of drug metabolism will equal the rate at which drug is flowing into the liver ($\dot{Q} \times C_{\text{inflow}}$), the rate of outflow ($\dot{Q} \times C_{\text{outflow}}$) will be 0, and clearance will then equal hepatic blood flow, $\dot{Q}$

$$\text{Clearance} = \dot{Q}[(C_{\text{inflow}} - C_{\text{outflow}})/C_{\text{inflow}}] \quad (2.8)$$

Equation 2.8 introduces the concept of extraction ratio. The extraction ratio is the ratio between the amount of drug that flows into the liver and the amount of drug extracted (i.e. cleared) by the liver. The extraction ratio can be calculated as:

$$\text{Extraction ratio (ER)} = (C_{\text{inflow}} - C_{\text{outflow}})/C_{\text{inflow}} \quad (2.9)$$

Referring back to equation 2.8, we see that clearance equals the liver blood flow multiplied by the extraction ratio, $\dot{Q} \times \text{ER}$. In this sense, Fig. 2.1 is misleading because it suggests that clearance is the same as the flow of blood to the organ. This is only true if the extraction ratio is 1, i.e. the blood is completely cleared of drug. Otherwise, clearance is the flow multiplied by the extraction ratio.

Propofol is an example of a drug that is nearly all removed as it passes through the liver, thereby resulting in an extraction ratio of 1 (i.e. 100%). For drugs such as propofol, the clearance is simply liver blood flow. Clearly, any reduction in liver blood flow will reduce clearance for drugs with high extraction ratios. Such drugs are therefore said to be "flow dependent." Another way to think about flow-dependent drugs is that the capacity of the liver to metabolize "flow-dependent" drugs vastly exceeds the usual flow of drug to the liver at typical clinical concentrations.

Changes in hepatic function per se will have little impact on the clearance of flow-dependent drugs. For example, it is occasionally suggested that "tolerance" to propofol (if it occurs at all) may be caused by enzymatic induction. The suggestion is absurd because the liver already metabolizes all the propofol that flows to it. More enzymatic capacity would not increase propofol clearance. If there is "tolerance" to propofol, either hepatic blood flow has increased or, more likely, this is the result of a pharmacodynamic effect (e.g. the potency has *decreased*).

For many drugs (e.g. alfentanil), the extraction ratio is considerably less than 1. Clearance of drugs with low extraction ratios is limited by the capacity of the liver to take up and metabolize the drug. These drugs are said to be "capacity dependent." Any change in the capacity of the liver to metabolize such drugs, as might result from liver disease or enzymatic induction, will affect clearance. However, changes in liver blood flow, as might be caused by the anesthetic state itself, usually have little influence on the clearance because the liver only metabolizes a fraction of the drug it is exposed to.

Figure 2.3 relates changes in clearance to changes in liver blood flow for drugs with extraction ratios ranging from 0.1 to 1.[17] The extraction ratios are calculated at a liver blood flow of 1.4 L min^{-1}. For drugs with an extraction ratio of nearly 1 (e.g. propofol), the clearance changes

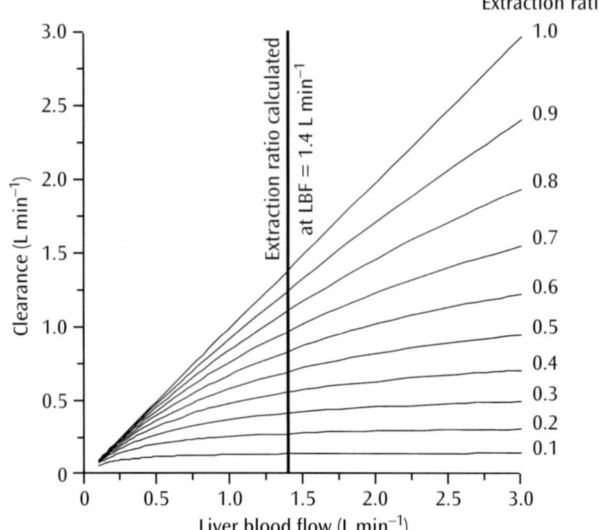

Figure 2.3 *Changes in clearance as a function of changes in liver blood flow for drugs with extraction ratios ranging from 0.1 to 1, calculated at an hepatic blood flow ($\dot{Q}$) of 1.4 L min^{-1}. The clearance of drugs with high extraction ratios changes with liver blood flow, whereas the clearance of drugs with low extraction ratios is limited by the intrinsic metabolic capacity, and thus remains nearly constant with changing liver blood flow. (Adapted from Wilkinson and Shand.[17])*

linearly with liver blood flow. However, drugs with a low extraction ratio (e.g. alfentanil) show almost no change in clearance with changes in liver blood flow.

Liver volume, blood flow, and metabolic capacity decrease with advancing age.[18,19] Intrinsic hepatic metabolic capacity also decreases with age. Additionally, hepatic enzymes can be induced by other drugs or substances in the environment. Such induction can increase the clearance of capacity limited drugs (i.e. drugs with low hepatic extraction ratios). Smoking can induce liver enzymes, particularly in young patients.[20] As patients age, the liver becomes more refractory to enzyme induction, and clearance decreases. This has been found to partly explain the reduced clearance of lorazepam in elderly individuals.[21] Lastly, drugs themselves can alter hepatic blood flow. For example, halothane decreases liver blood flow in dogs by 60%.[22,23]

Renal clearance

The kidneys use two mechanisms to clear drug from the body: filtration at the glomerulus and excretion into the tubules. For drugs less than 5000 Da, the filtration clearance is the glomerular filtration rate multiplied by the free fraction of drug. Tubular excretion is the net balance between active secretion of drug into the tubules and reabsorption of drug from the tubules. The glomerular filtration rate is typically approximated using creatinine clearance, which can be predicted from age and weight:[24]

Men:

$$\text{Creatinine clearance}\left(\text{mL min}^{-1}\right) = \frac{\left(140 - \text{age}\left(\text{years}\right)\right) \times \text{weight}\left(\text{kg}\right)}{72 \times \text{serum creatinine}\left(\text{mg\%}\right)}$$

Women: 85% of the above (2.10)

Equation 2.10 confirms that age is an independent factor in the prediction of creatinine clearance.[25] Creatinine clearance is thus decreased in elderly subjects, even in the presence of a normal serum creatinine. Clinically, this applies to only a single drug in the anesthetic pharmacopeia – pancuronium. About 85% of the pancuronium dose is excreted by the kidney.[26] Thus, equation 2.10 indicates the need to reduce the dose of pancuronium in elderly patients, even if the serum creatinine is normal.

Distribution clearance

Drug is permanently cleared from the body by metabolic or renal clearance. Drug can be removed temporarily from the plasma by the distribution clearance. Distribution clearance is the transfer of drug between the plasma and the peripheral tissues. It is a function of tissue blood flow and the permeability of the capillary walls to the drug. Tissue blood flow varies nonlinearly with cardiac output. The flow to some tissues such as the brain and heart is well preserved across a wide range of cardiac outputs. This selective preservation of flow comes at the expense of other tissues, which may have a profound decrease in blood flow even with modest decreases in cardiac output. The relation between distributional clearance and cardiac output is complex, and depends on the tissues involved in the clearance process. Drugs can also raise or lower cardiac output, or alter the distribution of cardiac output. In particular, virtually all hypnotics reduce cardiac output.[27–34] Several studies have suggested that opioids can alter the pharmacokinetics of propofol.[35,36] This may result from alterations in cardiac output when opioids are combined with propofol, thereby exacerbating the sympatholytic effects of propofol. Age, per se, is associated with very modest changes in cardiac output in the absence of hypertension, coronary artery disease, valvular heart disease, or other cardiovascular pathology.[37,38] If cardiac output, and hence intercompartmental clearance, is reduced, the plasma concentrations will be higher during drug administration. When administration is stopped, the effects of changes in distributional clearance are complex.[39] In general, plasma concentrations will decrease more rapidly following prolonged infusions when intercompartmental clearance is decreased.

The permeability of the vascular wall and tissue membranes to the drug is the other component of tissue clearance. In general, permeability is a function of lipophilicity. A highly lipophilic drug such as propofol can be expected to have a very high distribution clearance, for it crosses cell membranes readily. A highly hydrophilic drug such as glycopyrrolate is expected to have a slower distribution clearance because of the difficulty in crossing cell membranes.

Protein binding

Virtually all anesthetic drugs are bound to plasma proteins. The relation between drugs and their binding proteins can be described by the law of mass action:

$$[\text{Free drug}] + [\text{Unbound protein binding sites}] \underset{k_{off}}{\overset{k_{on}}{\rightleftharpoons}} [\text{Bound drug}]$$

where [free drug] is the free drug concentration, [unbound protein binding sites] is the concentration of the *available unbound protein binding sites*, [bound drug] is the concentration of drug bound to plasma proteins, k_{on} is the rate constant for binding, and k_{off} is the rate constant for dissociation of bound drug from the plasma proteins. At equilibrium (which happens very quickly), we can solve for k, the ratio of k_{on}/k_{off}, as:

$$k = \frac{k_{on}}{k_{off}} = \frac{[\text{Bound drug}]}{[\text{Free drug}][\text{Unbound protein binding site}]} \quad (2.11)$$

Anesthetic drugs are sufficiently potent that there are many times more protein binding sites than anesthetic molecules looking for a site to bind. For practical purposes, [unbound protein binding sites] can be reasonably approximated by n[protein], where [protein] is the plasma concentration of the binding protein and n is the number of binding sites per protein molecule. Since n, the number of binding sites per molecule, is constant, we can just include it in our rate constant k, by defining the association rate constant, k_a as:

$$k_a = [\text{Bound drug}]/([\text{Free drug}]\,[\text{Protein}]) \quad (2.12)$$

Let us define f_u as the free fraction of drug:

$$f_u = [\text{Free drug}]/([\text{Bound drug}] + [\text{Free drug}]) \quad (2.13)$$

Combining equations 2.12 and 2.13, we can calculate f_u in terms of the unbound drug concentration:

$$f_u = 1/(k_a\,[\text{Protein}] + 1) \quad (2.14)$$

Equation 2.14 reveals that the fraction bound to plasma protein depends on the protein concentration alone and not on the drug concentration, within the approximation that [bound drug] $<<n$[protein] as described above. The association constant, k_a, reflects the affinity of the drug for the plasma. This should not change in the presence of disease. However, [protein] can change with disease, age, other drugs, etc. What would be the influence of a 50% decrease or a 100% increase in protein concentration? The mathematics of this are described elsewhere.[40] For drugs that are not bound (free fraction = 1.0), there is no relation between free fraction and protein concentration. For drugs with a free fraction of 90% in normal plasma, there will be a small change in free drug concentration with changes in protein concentration. For drugs which are highly protein bound (e.g. free fraction = 10%), there is an almost linear change in free drug concentration with changes in protein concentration. As the binding approaches 100% (free drug $\rightarrow$ 0.0), the relation between change in protein concentration and change in free fraction becomes inversely proportional. Note that there is never a greater than proportional change in free drug concentration with change in plasma concentration. For example, the *most* that a 10% change in protein concentration would produce is a 10% change in free drug concentration, and that would only be the case if the drug were nearly 100% bound to plasma proteins.

The above paragraph describes what happens in a test tube of plasma, but the *in vivo* situation is more complex. It is the free (e.g. unbound) drug that equilibrates between the plasma and the tissues. If protein binding is decreased, then the driving concentration gradient increases between the plasma and the peripheral tissues. Equilibrium is achieved between the plasma and the tissue free drug concentrations at a lower total plasma drug concentration. This lower concentration gives the *appearance* that the drug has distributed into a larger total space. Thus, decreased protein binding causes an increase in the *apparent* volume of distribution.

However, at steady state the free concentration is the same everywhere in the body, and is determined by the solubility of the drug in all body tissues. For lipophilic drugs, only a trivial fraction is bound in the plasma, the vast majority of drug being bound in body tissues. Thus, a change in plasma protein binding causes only a trivial change in the free concentration at steady state. A change in protein binding may thus change the free drug concentration immediately after bolus injection, but following equilibration with peripheral tissues the free plasma drug concentration is not greatly affected by changes in protein binding.

Changes in protein binding may also affect the clearance of drugs. If a drug has a high extraction ratio, the liver is going to remove nearly all of the drug flowing to it, regardless of the extent of protein binding. However, if the drug has a low hepatic extraction ratio, an increase in the free fraction of drug will result in an increase in the driving gradient, with an associated increase in clearance.

Protein binding also affects the apparent potency of a drug, when compared with the total plasma drug concentration. An increase in free fraction increases the driving pressure to the site of drug effect (see below), and thus increases the concentration at the effect site. Thus, decreased protein binding may decrease the dose required to produce a given drug effect even in the absence of pharmacokinetic changes.

Albumin and α_1-acid glycoprotein are the primary sites of protein binding. Albumin concentration decreases with advancing age, hepatic disease, and malnutrition. In contrast, α_1-acid glycoprotein concentration increases with advancing age, and also with acute disease. The effects of age and disease on protein binding depend on which protein binds the drug. For example, since diazepam primarily binds to albumin, the free fraction increases in elderly patients, and this has been shown to correlate with reduced dose requirements,[41,42] probably resulting from the apparent increase in steady-state potency due to the increased free fraction. In contrast, lidocaine binds primarily to α_1-acid glycoprotein, and in elderly patients increased α_1-acid glycoprotein reduces the free fraction, which may contribute to the reduced clearance.[42]

Stereochemistry

The last physiological concept to introduce is stereochemistry. Many anesthetic drugs are fictitious, such as thiopental, fentanyl, and midazolam. These are chiral drugs, and are supplied as racemic mixtures. The pharmacokinetics and pharmacodynamics of the enantiomers need not be identical.[43] The body is a chiral environment. Drugs interact stereospecifically with enzymes, proteins, and receptors. When a racemic mixture is given, it is as if two different drugs have been infused. However, drug assays are usually insensitive to chirality. Thus, the concentration measured is actually a mixture of two separate drugs, each of which may have unique pharmacokinetic (PK) and pharmacodynamic (PD) characteristics.

Mather and coworkers have studied the PK and PD of the enantiomers of bupivacaine,[44] mepivacaine,[45] and prilocaine.[46] The enantiomers of ketamine have been extensively studied,[47,48] in the hope that the S(+) isomer will provide the hypnosis and analgesia associated with ketamine without the undesirable psychotomimetic effects. Recent data by Persson and coworkers suggest little difference in therapeutic windows between (*S*)- and (*R*)-ketamine.[49]

Physiologically based pharmacokinetic models

So far, we have considered the physiological underpinnings of pharmacokinetics: what happens in tissues and plasma that influences the time-course of concentrations in the body. We can apply this approach tissue by tissue, slowly building up a model of all the organs and their "plumbing." This produces a physiologically based model of pharmacokinetics, and these models can be used to predict the time-course of concentration changes in the plasma and in all body tissues. Ebling *et al.*[50] have produced physiologically based pharmacokinetic models for each tissue that describe the pharmacokinetics of thiopental in rats. Björkman *et al.*[51] have produced similar models for fentanyl and alfentanil in rats. In this latter work, it was demonstrated that, if the individual tissue volumes and blood flows were scaled from rats to humans, the resulting model could accurately describe the observed time-course of fentanyl and alfentanil in humans. This illustrates the potential utility of physiologically based pharmacokinetic models.

An enormous effort is required to characterize experimentally models that may be applied to individual tissues. These models are also mathematically cumbersome and do not offer a better prediction of *plasma* drug concentration than models that group the tissues into a few compartments, based on plasma concentration data alone. Einstein observed that "Everything should be made as simple as possible, but not simpler."[52] If the goal is to understand the *mechanism* of pharmacokinetic behavior, then compartmental models are too simple. However, our goal in this chapter is clinical: we want to understand the relation between dose and concentration. For this purpose, detailed physiological models are needlessly complex, and simple compartmental models will perform adequately.

The most simple of the classic pharmacokinetic models is the "one-compartment" pharmacokinetic model with a single volume and clearance, shown at the top of Fig. 2.4. The clearance is $k \times V$, as will be explained when we develop the mathematics of pharmacokinetic models in the next section. Most equations used to calculate dosage regimens (initial bolus dose and maintenance infusion rates) are based on a one-compartment model. As we will see below, dosage regimens calculated using one-compartment concepts lead to absurd recommendations for anesthetic drugs. This is because the "one-compartment" model is too simple for anesthetic drugs. For most drugs, pharmacokinetic behavior suggests that the human body is made up of several tanks connected together by pipes, as shown in Fig. 2.4 (top right, two-compartment model; bottom, three-compartment model). These are the multicompartment models that were alluded to earlier. In both the two-compartment model and the three-compartment model, V_1 is the central volume. The other volumes are the peripheral volumes.

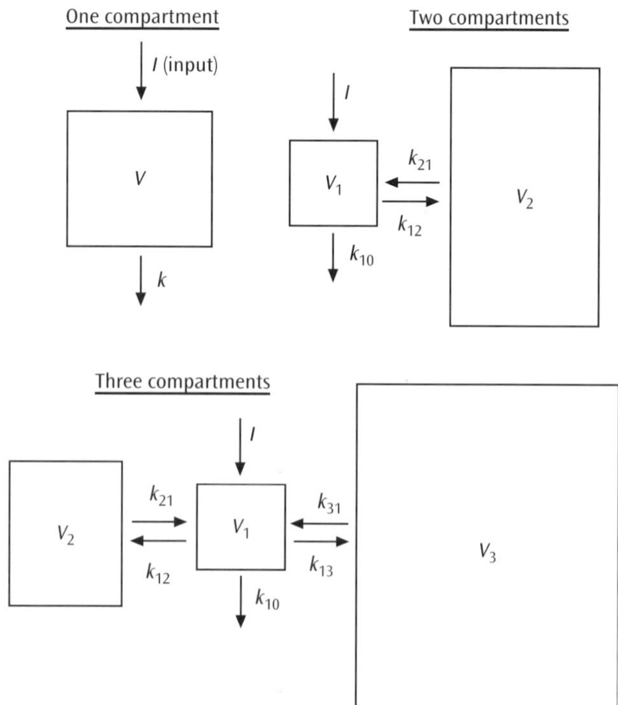

Figure 2.4 *One-, two-, and three-compartment pharmacokinetic models. Drug is administered into a central compartment, from which it is cleared by metabolism or renal elimination. Drug also distributes into peripheral volumes of distribution in the two- and three-compartment pharmacokinetic models.*

The sum of the all volumes is the volume of distribution at steady state, $V_{d(ss)}$. The clearance leaving the central compartment for the outside is the "central" or "metabolic" clearance. If there were renal clearance, that would also be a component of central clearance. The clearances between the central compartment and the peripheral compartments are called "intercompartmental clearances."

What do the volumes and clearances estimated by pharmacokinetic modeling mean? It is likely that the central (or "metabolic") clearance estimated by pharmacokinetic modeling has a true physiological basis. It is also conceivable that the $V_{d(ss)}$ has a physiological basis: the partitioning of drug into all body tissues at steady state.

For three-compartment models, it is tempting to speculate that the rapidly equilibrating volume (V_2) corresponds to the vessel-rich group and the slowly equilibrating volume (V_3) corresponds to the fat and vessel-poor group. In fact, many authors discuss drugs in exactly this way. This may provide some insight, particularly for highly lipophilic drugs for which a large V_3 may be explained by extensive distribution of the drug into fat. However, the volumes and clearances developed in pharmacokinetic models are mathematical constants derived from equations that describe the plasma drug concentrations over time. With the possible exception of clearance and $V_{d(ss)}$, the volumes and intercompartmental clearances estimated using pharmacokinetic modeling *are not direct measures of anatomic structures or human physiology*. In fact, the physiologically based models of volumes and clearances do not yield tissues that can be readily grouped into anything resembling a compartmental pharmacokinetic model. This is not to imply that there is no physiological basis for the compartmental models, but rather that the relation between mathematically derived volumes and clearances and underlying physiological responses is complex. The reader is encouraged to maintain a healthy skepticism about the literal "truth" of the compartmental models used in pharmacokinetics.

MATHEMATICAL PRINCIPLES OF COMPARTMENTAL PHARMACOKINETICS

First-order processes

Many processes in life happen at a constant rate, such as the power consumption of a clock, the water flowing from the end of a garden hose, or the speed of a car on a freeway. These are examples of zero-order processes. The rate for a zero-order process is simply:

$$dx/dt = k \quad (2.15)$$

Equation 2.15 states simply that the rate, dx/dt, is a constant, k. If x represents an amount of drug and t represents time, the units of k are amount/time. If we want to know the value of x at time t, $x(t)$, we can find it as the integral of equation 2.15 from time 0 to time t:

$$x(t) = x_0 + kt \quad (2.16)$$

where x_0 is the value of x at time 0. This is, of course, the equation of a straight line with a slope of k and an intercept of x_0.

Other processes occur at a rate proportional to the amount. The rate at which we pay interest on a loan is proportional to the amount of the loan. A 10% interest rate means that the interest payment is the outstanding balance multiplied by 0.10. Similarly, the rate at which water flows out of a bathtub is proportional to the amount of water in the tub, and the rate at which the planet's population grows is proportional to the size of the population. These are examples of first-order processes. Compared with a zero-order process, the rate of a first-order process is just modestly more complex:

$$dx/dt = kx \quad (2.17)$$

Here, the units of k are simply 1/time, since x already includes the units for the amount. If we want to know the value of x at time t, $x(t)$, we can find it as the integral of the equation from time 0 to time t:

$$x(t) = x_0 e^{kt} \quad (2.18)$$

where x_0 is the value of x at time 0. If $k > 0$, $x(t)$ increases exponentially. If $k < 0$, $x(t)$ decreases exponentially. In pharmacokinetics, the exponent is generally negative, i.e. concentrations decrease over time. However, to simplify tabulating pharmacokinetic parameters, it is customary to remove the minus sign from k, and express it explicitly in the equation. Thus, the equation we will explore is:

$$x(t) = x_0 e^{-kt} \quad (2.19)$$

The graph in Fig. 2.5A shows the relation between x and time, as described by equation 2.19. Such a graph might describe the amount of drug in the plasma after an intravenous bolus. If we take the natural

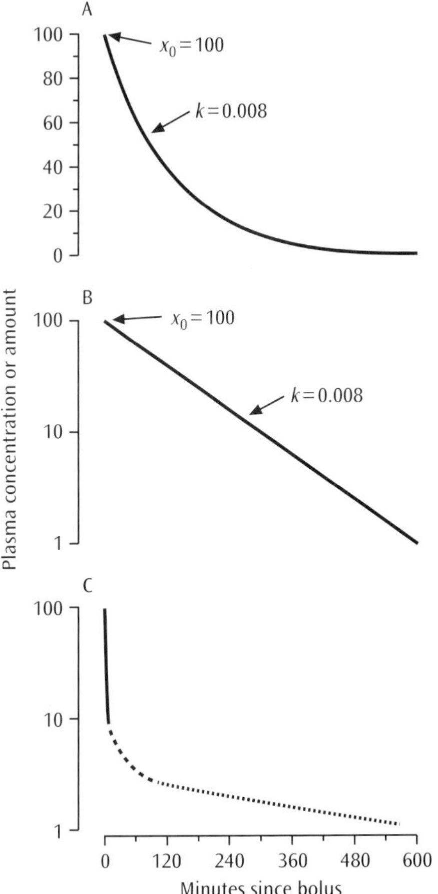

Figure 2.5 *(A) The relation between time and amount is a first-order process. The amount decreases continuously at a rate proportional to the residual amount. (B) The relation between time and amount, with amount represented logarithmically on the y-axis. The relation becomes linear, with an intercept of ln(x_0) and a slope of −k. (C) The relation between time and amount usually observed for intravenous anesthetic drugs. Although the y-axis is logarithmic, there is still an initial rapid decay, followed by a slower log-linear decay. This suggests multicompartment pharmacokinetics.*

logarithm (expressed as "ln" in equations) of both sides of equation 2.19, we get:

$$\ln(x(t)) = \ln(x_0 e^{-kt}) \quad (2.20)$$
$$= \ln(x_0) + \ln(e^{-kt})$$
$$= \ln(x_0) - kt$$

This is the equation for a straight line, in which the y-axis is the natural log of x, the y intercept is the log of x at time 0, and the slope of the line is $-k$. This is why first-order processes are usually plotted using the logarithm of the amount vs. time: the graphs become straight lines, as shown by the graph in Fig. 2.5B. However, this is only a straight line when there is a single exponential term, as in equation 2.20. When there are multiple exponentials, even a logarithmic representation will show curvature, as seen in the graph in Fig. 2.5C.

In the case of a single exponential, as in equation 2.20, we may ask how long will it take for x (e.g. amount or concentration) to decrease by 50%? We can relate the slope of the line ($-k$) to the change in x and t as follows:

$$k = \frac{\Delta \ln(x)}{\Delta t} = \frac{\ln(x) - \ln\left(\frac{x}{2}\right)}{t_{1/2}} \quad (2.21)$$

where $t_{1/2}$ is the "half-life," the time required for a 50% decrease in x. We can simplify the numerator to:

$$\ln(x_1) - \ln\left(\frac{x}{2}\right) = \ln\left(\frac{x}{\left(\frac{x}{2}\right)}\right) = \ln(2) \approx 0.693 \quad (2.22)$$

Thus, the relation between the slope, k, and the half-life, $t_{1/2}$, reduces to:

$$k = 0.693/t_{1/2} \quad (2.23)$$

If $t_{1/2}$, the time it takes for the concentration to fall by 50%, is measured, the exponent, k, may be calculated. The time it will take for x to fall by 50% may be calculated if we know k, the exponent in equation 2.19:

$$t_{1/2} = 0.693/k \quad (2.24)$$

The one-compartment model

What connection do first-order processes and exponential equations have with pharmacokinetics? To answer this, we return to the simple one-compartment model and analyze it mathematically. We start with a tank, as in Fig. 2.1. Into this tank we pour an amount of drug, x. The concentration of drug in the tank, C, is the amount of drug present, x, divided by the volume of the tank, V.

The fluid in the tank flows out at a constant rate, Cl (for clearance), as in Fig. 2.1B. For our purposes, the clearing organ will be 100% efficient (extraction ratio = 1) so that the flow from the clearing organ to the tank maintains a constant fluid volume. The rate at which drug (x) flows out at time t is simply the rate of fluid flow, Cl, multiplied by the concentration of drug in the fluid at time t, C. To express this more formally, the rate at which drug flows out of the tank is:

$$\text{Rate of drug elimination} = dx/dt = \text{Cl}\,C \quad (2.25)$$

Is this a first-order process? Substituting x/V for C in equation gives:

$$\text{Elimination rate} = dx/dt = \text{Cl}\,C \quad (2.26)$$
$$= \text{Cl}(x/V)$$
$$= (\text{Cl}/V)x$$

Since Cl/V is a constant, and this constant is multiplied by x, the amount, this is a first-order process. As such, the constant Cl/V must equal k, the rate constant, in equations 2.17–2.24. The relation Cl/V = k suggests a very simple interpretation of the rate constant. Consider the inverse: V/Cl = 1/k. The left side, V/Cl, is simply the amount of time it would take for the flow, Cl, to fill up the volume, V. Thus, k is nothing more than the inverse of the time required to fill the volume with a given flow.

Combining the above definition of k with the relation between k and half-life in equation 2.24 yields a more quantitative view of the relationships among volume, clearance, and half-life than originally presented when describing Fig. 2.2:

$$t_{1/2} = 0.693(V/\text{Cl}) \quad (2.27)$$

An increase in volume yields a proportional increase in half-life, whereas an increase in clearance yields an inversely proportional decrease in half-life. Also, if the volume and clearance are known, we can calculate both k, the rate constant, and the half-life as 0.693/k.

If the amount of drug at time t, $x(t)$, equals $x_0 e^{-kt}$ (equation 2.19), dividing through by V, the volume, yields:

$$C(t) = C_0 e^{-kt} \quad (2.28)$$

where C_0 is the concentration at time 0. Equation 2.28 is the commonly used expression relating concentration to time, initial plasma concentration, and the rate constant. It defines the "concentration vs. time" curve for a one-compartment model, and has the log linear shape seen in Fig. 2.5A.

We can calculate the flow, Cl, in several ways. First, if we know V and k, then Cl = kV. However, a more general solution is to consider the integral of the concentration vs. time curve, known in pharmacokinetics as the area under the curve (AUC). Remembering that the instantaneous rate of elimination of a drug is C multiplied by clearance (equation 2.25), the total amount of drug eliminated must be the integral of the instantaneous rate of elimination from time 0 to infinity:

$$\text{Amount of drug eliminated} = \int_0^\infty \text{Cl} \times C(t)\,dt$$
$$= \text{Cl} \times \int_0^\infty C(t)\,dt \quad (2.29)$$
$$= \text{Cl} \times \text{AUC}$$

If the drug has complete bioavailability, as happens with intravenous doses, then all the drug is eventually eliminated. Thus, "amount of drug eliminated" is equivalent to "total dose." Substituting "total dose" for "amount of drug eliminated" and rearranging equation 2.29 gives:

$$\text{Cl} = \text{Total dose/AUC} \quad (2.30)$$

If a drug is infused at a rate of I (for Input) into a person who has no drug in their body, the plasma concentration will continue to rise as long as the rate of drug entering the body, I, exceeds the rate at which drug leaves the body, $C \times$Cl. When $I = C \times$Cl, i.e. drug is entering and leaving the body at the same rate, the body is at steady state. This raises two questions: (1) what is the eventual concentration? and (2) how long will it take until $I = C \times \text{Cl}$?

To answer the first question, consider that when the body is in equilibrium the rate of drug entering must equal the rate of drug leaving. From equation 2.7, we know that rate of metabolism at steady state is:

$$\text{Rate of metabolism} = C_\infty \text{Cl} \quad (2.31)$$

where C_∞ is the concentration at steady state (time = infinity). At steady state, the drug infusion rate must equal the rate of metabolism (or it would not be steady state). Thus, the infusion rate at steady state is:

$$I = C_\infty \text{Cl} \quad (2.32)$$

where I is the rate of the drug infusion. Equation 2.32 can be rearranged to solve for the concentration at steady state, C_∞:

$$C_\infty = I/\text{Cl} \quad (2.33)$$

Thus, the steady-state concentration during an infusion is the rate of drug input divided by the clearance. This relation, $C = I/\text{Cl}$, is satisfyingly similar to the equation describing the concentration following a bolus injection, $C = x_0/V$. This suggests another way to consider volume and clearance: volume relates initial concentration to the size of the initial bolus and clearance relates steady-state concentration to the infusion rate. One consequence is that the initial concentration following a bolus is independent of the clearance, and the steady-state concentration during a continuous infusion is independent of the volume.

It takes infinitely long to reach steady state because the steady-state concentration is asymptotically approached, but never reached. However, it is possible to determine how long it will take to reach any given fraction of the steady-state concentration. We start with the rate of change in x, the amount of drug in the compartment:

$$\text{d}x/\text{d}t = I - kx(t) \quad (2.34)$$

where I is the rate of drug entering the body, $x(t)$ is the amount of drug present at time t, and $kx(t)$ is the rate of drug leaving the body (by definition because elimination is a first-order process). To find $x(t)$, it is necessary to integrate this from time 0 to time t, knowing that $x_0 = 0$ (i.e. starting with nothing in the body). The result is:

$$x(t) = (I/k)(1 - e^{-kt}) \quad (2.35)$$

If we divide both sides of equation 2.35 by volume, we get:

$$x(t)/V = [I/(kV)(1 - e^{-kt})] \quad (2.36)$$

$$C(t) = (I/\text{Cl})(1 - e^{-kt})$$

How long will it take to reach 50% of the steady-state amount, $C_\infty/2$? From equation 2.33, we know that $C_\infty/2 = I/(2\,\text{Cl})$. Substituting $I/(2\,\text{Cl})$ for $C(t)$ in equation 2.36, we get:

$$I/(2\,\text{Cl}) = (I/\text{Cl})(1 - e^{-kt}) \quad (2.37)$$

Solving equation 2.37 for t, we get: $\ln(2)/k$. We previously showed that the half-life, $t_{1/2}$, following a bolus injection was $\ln(2)/k$. Again, there is a satisfying parallel between boluses and infusions: with an infusion, the time to reach 50% of the steady-state concentration is one half-life. We can similarly show that we will reach 75% of the steady-state concentration following two half-lives, 88% following three half-lives, 94% following four half-lives, and 97% following five half-lives. By four to five half-lives, we consider that the patient is at steady state.

Multicompartment models

The above covers most of the standard pharmacokinetic equations for a single compartment. Unfortunately, none of the drugs used in anesthesia can be accurately characterized by one-compartment models. Distribution of anesthetic drugs into and out of peripheral tissues plays a crucial role in the time-course of the anesthetic drug effect. To describe intravenous anesthetics, we must extend the one-compartment model to account for this distribution.

Following a bolus of an intravenous drug, the plasma concentrations over time actually resemble the graph in Fig. 2.5C. Although it is plotted on a log vertical scale, the relation is not a straight line. This curve has the characteristics common to most drugs when given by intravenous bolus. First, the concentrations decline continuously over time. Second, the rate of decline is initially steep, but continuously becomes less steep (i.e. the slope increases continuously), until we get to a portion which is "log linear."

The behavior seen in the graph in Fig. 2.5C can be explained in terms of a hydraulic model, as seen in Fig. 2.6.[53] In this model, there are three tanks, corresponding (from left to right) to the slowly equilibrating peripheral compartment, to the central compartment (the plasma, into which drug is injected), and to the rapidly equilibrating peripheral compartment. The horizontal pipes represent intercompartmental clearance or (for the pipe draining onto the page) metabolic clearance. The volumes of each tank correspond to the volumes of the compartments for fentanyl. The cross-sectional areas of the pipes correlate with the systemic and intercompartmental clearances of fentanyl. The height of water in each tank corresponds to drug concentration.

Using this hydraulic model, we can follow the processes that decrease drug concentration over time following a bolus injection. Initially, drug flows from the central compartment to both peripheral compartments through intercompartmental clearance, and then out of the model onto the page through metabolic clearance. Because there are three places for the drug to go, the central compartment concentration decreases very rapidly. At the transition between the solid line and the dashed line in

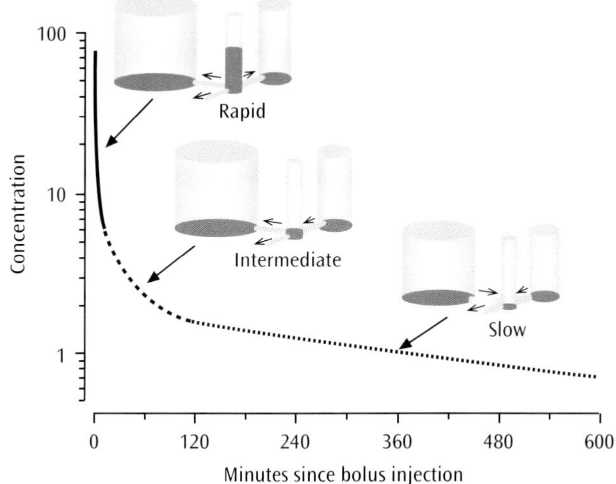

Figure 2.6 *The concentrations over time from Fig. 2.5 with a hydraulic representation of a three-compartment model superimposed. The central tank represents the central compartment (plasma), and the height of the water in each tank represents the apparent concentration. (Adapted from Youngs and Shafer.[53])*

Fig. 2.6, there is a change in the role of the most rapidly equilibrating compartment. At this transition, the central compartment concentration falls below the concentration in the rapidly equilibrating compartment, and the direction of flow between them is reversed. After this transition (dashed line), there is a slower rate of decrease because drug levels only fall by flow into the slowly equilibrating compartment and by metabolic clearance. The return of drug from the rapidly equilibrating compartment also slows the rate of decrease in plasma concentration. Once the concentration in the central compartment falls below *both* the rapidly and slowly equilibrating compartments (Fig. 2.6, dotted line), the only method of decreasing the plasma concentration is systemic clearance (e.g. metabolic and renal clearance). The return of drug from both peripheral compartments to the central compartment greatly slows the rate of decrease in plasma drug concentration.

Curves that continuously decrease over time with a continuously *increasing* slope, i.e. Fig. 2.5C and Fig. 2.6, can be described by a sum of exponentials. In pharmacokinetics, one way of denoting this sum of exponentials is to say that the plasma concentration over time is:

$$C(t) = Ae^{-\alpha t} + Be^{-\beta t} + Ce^{-\gamma t} \tag{2.38}$$

where t is the time since the bolus, $C(t)$ is the drug concentration following a bolus dose, and A, α, B, β, C, and γ are parameters of a pharmacokinetic model. A, B, and C are termed coefficients, whereas α, β, and γ are termed exponents or, occasionally, hybrid rate constants. Following a bolus injection, all six of the parameters in equation will be greater than 0. If the drug is given orally, or is absorbed from a depot, then the sum of the coefficients is necessarily 0, reflecting that there is no drug in the body at the start of absorption.

So, why use equation 2.38 and deal with exponents? The most important reason is that equation 2.38 describes the data. Compartmental models are empirical: the models describe the mathematical link between the dose and the observed concentrations, not the underlying physiology. The second reason is that polyexponential models permit us to use most of the one-compartment ideas with some generalization. The third reason is that equation 2.38 can be mathematically transformed into a model of volumes and clearances that has an appealing, if not necessarily accurate, physiological flavor, as seen in Fig. 2.6. Lastly, equation 2.38 has convenient mathematical properties. For example, the integral of equation 2.38, the AUC, is readily calculated as $A/\alpha + B/\beta + C/\gamma$.

When the pharmacokinetics have multiple exponents, each exponent is associated with a half-life. Thus, a drug described by three exponents has three half-lives: two rapid half lives, calculated as $0.693/\alpha$ and $0.693/\beta$, and a terminal half-life (sometimes called the "elimination half-life"), calculated as $0.693/\gamma$. The half-life of a drug is often mentioned in the literature. Unless it is stated otherwise, the half-life will be the terminal half-life, i.e. 0.693/smallest exponent. It is now well established that the terminal exponent is of zero clinical interest for anesthetic drugs and has been replaced by the alternative concepts of recovery time,[54] context-sensitive half-times,[55] or, more generally, decrement times.[39]

Constructing pharmacokinetic models represents a trade-off between accurately describing the data, having confidence in the results, and mathematical tractability. Adding exponentials to the model usually provides a better description of the observed concentrations, but at a cost of decreased confidence in the individual parameter estimates and increased mathematic complexity. This is why most models are limited to two or three exponential terms.

Multicompartment models can have several representations. One is the polyexponential form, with coefficients and exponents. An alternative form has volumes for each compartment, plus systemic and distributional clearances. The third form is the volume of the central compartment and "micro-rate constants." These parameters, expressed as k_{ij}, define the rate of drug transfer from compartment i to compartment j as a fraction of the amount of drug in each compartment, just as k did for the one-compartment model. Compartment 0 is a compartment outside the model, so k_{10} is the micro-rate constant for those processes acting through biotransformation or elimination that irreversibly remove drug from the central compartment (compartment 1). The intercompartmental micro-rate constants (k_{12}, k_{21}, etc.) describe the exchange of drug between the central and peripheral compartments. Each compartment has at least two micro-rate constants, one for drug entry and one for drug exit. The micro-rate constants for one-, two-, and three-compartment models can be seen in Fig. 2.4. The differential equations describing the rate of change for the amount of drugs in compartments 1, 2, and 3 follow directly from the definition for micro-rate constants. For the two-compartment model, the differential equations for the two compartments, including an infusion of rate I, are:

$$\begin{aligned} dx_1/dt &= I + x_2k_{21} - x_1k_{10} - x_1k_{12} \\ &= I + x_2k_{21} - x_1(k_{10} + k_{12}) \\ dx_2/dt &= x_1k_{12} - x_2k_{21} \end{aligned} \tag{2.39}$$

For the three-compartment model, the differential equations for the three compartments are:

$$\begin{aligned} dx_1/dt &= I + x_2k_{21} + x_3k_{31} - x_1k_{10} - x_1k_{12} - x_1k_{13} \\ &= I + x_2k_{21} + x_3k_{31} - x_1(k_{10} + k_{12} + k_{13}) \\ dx_2/dt &= x_1k_{12} - x_2k_{21} \\ dx_3/dt &= x_1k_{13} - x_3k_{31} \end{aligned} \tag{2.40}$$

For the one-compartment model, k was both the rate constant and the exponent. For multicompartment models, the relationships are far more complex. The interconversion between the micro-rate constants and the exponents becomes exceedingly complex as more exponents are added because every exponent is a function of every micro-rate constant and vice versa. Readers interested in such interconversions can find them in the Excel spreadsheet "convert.xls," which can be downloaded from http://anesthesia.stanford.edu/pkpd.

Plasma–effect site equilibration

If we are to understand the relation between dose and concentration, we must understand the processes that account for the time delay between the drug concentrations in the plasma and at the site of drug effect. If one observes the drug concentration and the drug effect, as in Fig. 2.7, there is a clear delay between the rise and fall of drug concentration in the plasma and the onset and offset of drug effect. This delay or "hysteresis" represents the time required for drugs to transit into the "biophase," also called the "effect site," and exert their effects upon the site of biological action. The concentration of drug in the biophase cannot be measured. First, it is usually inaccessible, at least in human subjects. Second, even if we could take tissue samples, the drug concentration in the microscopic environment of the receptive molecules will not be the same as the concentration grossly measured in, for example, ground brain or cerebrospinal fluid. Although it is not possible to measure drug concentration in the biophase, using rapid measures of drug effect we can characterize the time-course of drug effect. Knowing the time-course of drug effect, we can characterize the apparent rate of drug flow into and out of the biophase. Knowing these rates, we can characterize the drug concentra-

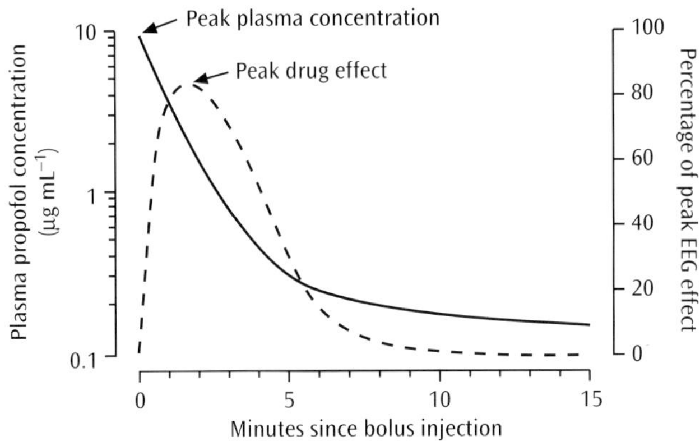

Figure 2.7 *The plasma concentrations and percentage drug effect following an intravenous bolus, based on a PK/PD model of propofol,*[9,59] *showing the delay between peak plasma concentrations and peak drug effect.*

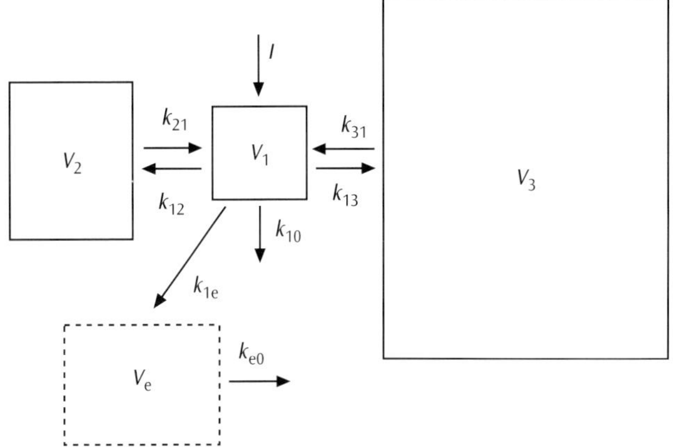

Figure 2.8 *A three-compartment pharmacokinetic model with an effect site.* k_{e0} *is the equilibration rate constant for the effect site. Although this usually indicates metabolism at the effect site, the model does not change if it is directed back into the* V_1*, as shown by the dotted line.* V_e*, the volume of the effect site, is negligible with respect to* V_1*.*

tion in the biophase in terms of the steady-state plasma concentration that would produce the same effect.

We can model hysteresis by adding an "effect" site to our basic compartmental pharmacokinetic model, as shown in Fig. 2.8.[56,57] The effect compartment is defined as being such a tiny compartment that it receives almost no drug from the central compartment, and thus has no influence on the plasma pharmacokinetics. The rate constant k_{e0} defines the elimination from the effect site, which determines the time-course of blood–brain equilibration. k_{1e} is the rate constant for drug flow from the plasma to the effect site. It is not immediately obvious that k_{1e} has no influence on the rate of plasma–effect site equilibration, but that is the case.[40,57]

If a constant plasma concentration is maintained, the time required for the biophase concentration to reach 50% of the plasma concentration ($t_{1/2}\,k_{e0}$) can be calculated as $0.693/k_{e0}$. Following a bolus dose, the onset of drug effect is a function of *both* the plasma pharmacokinetics and k_{e0}. For drugs with a very rapid decline in plasma concentration following a bolus (e.g. adenosine, with a half-life of several seconds), the effect site concentration will peak within several seconds of the bolus regardless of k_{e0}. This happens because the plasma concentrations very quickly drop to such low levels that there is no longer a driving gradient into the brain. For drugs with a rapid k_{e0} and a slow decrease in concentration following bolus injection (e.g. pancuronium), the time to peak effect site concentration will be determined more by the k_{e0} than by the plasma pharmacokinetics. k_{e0} has been characterized for many drugs used in anesthesia. Equilibration between the plasma and the effect site is rapid for thiopental,[7] propofol,[58,59] and alfentanil;[60] intermediate for fentanyl[60] and sufentanil[61] and the nondepolarizing muscle relaxants;[56,62–64] and slow for morphine and ketorolac.

Figure 2.9 shows the plasma and effect site concentrations following boluses of fentanyl, alfentanil, or sufentanil as a percentage of initial plasma concentration.[54] The rapid plasma–effect site equilibration (large k_{e0}) of alfentanil causes the effect site concentration to peak about 90 s after bolus injection. At the time of this peak, about 63% of the alfentanil will have distributed into peripheral tissues or been eliminated from the body. For sufentanil, the effect site peaks 5–6 min after the bolus. At the time of the peak, over 80% of the initial bolus of sufentanil will have been distributed into the tissues or eliminated. As a result of the slower equilibration with the effect site, relatively more sufentanil than alfentanil must be injected into the plasma, which slows the rate of drug offset from a sufentanil bolus compared with an alfentanil bolus.

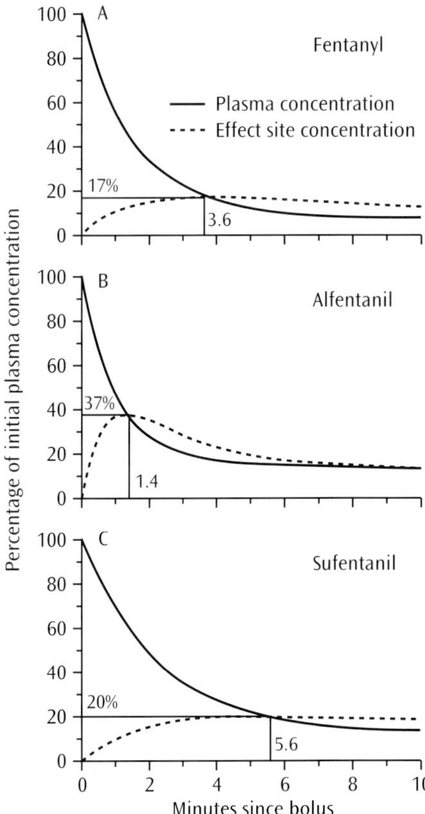

Figure 2.9 *The plasma and effect site concentrations, as a percentage of initial plasma concentration, following a bolus of fentanyl, alfentanil, and sufentanil. Alfentanil has a more rapid* $t_{1/2}\,k_{e0}$*, which produces a more rapid rise in effect site concentration and also reduces the bolus dose required to reach the desired drug effect (more "bang" for the bolus). (Adapted from Shafer and Varvel.*[54]*)*

CLINICAL APPLICATION OF PHARMACOKINETICS

Onset of drug effect

Most anesthetics start with a bolus dose of intravenous drug. Returning to equation 2.1, the definition of concentration is amount divided by volume. We can rearrange the definition of concentration to find the amount of drug required to produce any desired target concentration, C_T, for a known volume:

$$\text{Bolus} = C_T \times V \qquad (2.41)$$

Many introductory pharmacokinetic texts suggest using this formula to calculate the "loading bolus" required to achieve a given concentration. The problem is that there are several volumes: V_1 (central compartment); V_2 and V_3 (the peripheral compartments); and $V_{d(ss)}$, the sum of the individual volumes. V_1 is usually much smaller than $V_{d(ss)}$, and thus it is commonly stated that the loading dose should be something between:

$$\text{Bolus} = C_T \times V_1 \qquad (2.42)$$

and

$$\text{Bolus} = C_T \times V_{d(ss)} \qquad (2.43)$$

Consider the dose of fentanyl required to attenuate the hemodynamic response to intubation when combined with thiopental. The target concentration is approximately 3 ng mL^{-1}. The V_1 and $V_{d(ss)}$ for fentanyl are 13 L and 360 L respectively. According to equations 2.42 and 2.43, an appropriate dose of fentanyl to attenuate the hemodynamic response is between 39 µg (3 ng mL^{-1} × 13 L) and 1080 µg (3 ng mL^{-1} × 360 L). This is not much of a recommendation!

The usual dosing guidelines for bolus injection, as presented above, are oriented toward producing a specific plasma concentration. Since the plasma is not the site of drug effect, it is illogical to base the calculation of the initial bolus on a plasma concentration. Once we know the k_{e0} of an intravenous anesthetic, we can design a dosing regimen that yields the desired concentration at the site of drug effect. In Fig. 2.9, we can see the relative plasma and effect site concentrations following an intravenous (i.v.) bolus of fentanyl (Fig. 2.9A). The plasma concentration decreases continuously, while the effect site concentration rises until it reaches the plasma concentration; at this point, both decrease continuously. To avoid overdosing the patient, we should select the bolus that produces the desired peak concentration in the effect site.

The decline in plasma concentration between the initial concentration following the bolus (amount/V_1) and the concentration at the time of peak effect can be thought of as a dilution of the bolus into a yet larger volume, the volume of distribution at peak effect, $V_{d(\text{peak effect})}$, which can be calculated as:

$$V_{d(\text{peak effect})} = \text{Bolus dose}/C_{\text{peak effect(plasma)}} \qquad (2.44)$$

where $C_{\text{peak effect(plasma)}}$ is the plasma concentration at the time of peak effect. Equation 2.44 may be rearranged to calculate the loading dose necessary to produce any desired target concentration, C_T, at the time of peak effect:

$$\text{Bolus dose} = C_T \times V_{d(\text{peak effect})} \qquad (2.45)$$

The $V_{d(\text{peak effect})}$ for fentanyl is 75 L. To produce a peak fentanyl effect site concentration of 3.0 ng mL^{-1} requires 225 µg, which will produce a peak effect in 3.6 min. This is a clinically reasonable suggestion, particularly when compared with the useless suggestion based upon V_1 and $V_{d(ss)}$.

Maintenance of drug effect

The rate at which a drug exits from the body is the systemic clearance, Cl, multiplied by the plasma concentration (equation 2.5). To maintain a steady target concentration, C_T, the drug must be delivered at the same rate that drug is exiting the body. Thus, the infusion rate to maintain a target concentration, C_T, is often presented as:

$$\text{Maintenance infusion rate} = C_T \times \text{Cl} \qquad (2.46)$$

Drugs with multicompartment pharmacokinetics, which includes all of the drugs used in anesthetic practice, are distributed into the peripheral tissues for many hours until steady state is reached. Equation 2.46 is only correct after the peripheral tissues have equilibrated with the plasma, which requires many hours. At all other times, this maintenance infusion rate will be too slow.

However, in some situations, this simple maintenance rate calculation may be acceptable when combined with a bolus based on $V_{d(\text{peak effect})}$. For drugs with a prolonged delay between the bolus dose and peak effect, much of the distribution of drug into the tissues may have occurred by the time the effect site concentration reaches a peak. In this case, the maintenance infusion rate, calculated as $C_T \times \text{Cl}$, may be fairly accurate because $V_{d(\text{peak effect})}$ was sufficiently higher then V_1 to account for much of the distribution of drug into peripheral tissues. This is probably the reason why the principle of using a loading dose followed by a simple maintenance infusion works modestly well for theophylline. However, for most anesthetic drugs, equilibration between the plasma and effect site is sufficiently rapid that we must take into account the accumulation of drug in peripheral tissues when designing infusion regimens.

This leads us to consider a more sophisticated approach to the design of infusion rates to maintain target concentrations for drugs with multicompartment pharmacokinetics. Since the net flow of drug into peripheral tissues decreases over time, the infusion rate required to maintain any desired concentration also decreases over time. If the initial bolus has been based on $V_{d(\text{peak effect})}$, no infusion need be administered until the effect site concentration peaks. Following the peak in effect site concentration, the equation to maintain the desired concentration is (unfortunately):

$$\text{Maintenance infusion rate} = C_T \times V_1 (k_{10} + k_{12} e^{-k_{21} t} + k_{13} e^{-k_{31} t}) \qquad (2.47)$$

The infusion rate calculated by the above equation is initially rapid, and the rate decreases over time. At equilibrium ($t \to \infty$), the infusion rate decreases to $C_T \times V_1 \times k_{10}$, which is the same as $C_T \times \text{Cl}$ (equation 2.46). Few anesthesiologists would choose to mentally solve this equation during administration of an anesthetic. Fortunately, there are simple techniques that can be used in place of solving such a complex expression. Most involve nomograms or simple guidelines, as can be found in several widely available references.[40,65] The essential point is that the rate of drug administration must be continuously titrated downward during anesthesia to avoid overdosing the patient as drug accumulates.

Offset of drug effect

In anesthesia, the offset of drug effect governs awakening from the anesthetic state. As mentioned previously, the terminal half-life sets an upper limit on how long it will take the plasma concentrations to fall by

50%. For drugs described by multicompartment pharmacokinetics, the actual time for the plasma concentrations to fall by 50% is always faster than that – and is often *much* faster.

The rate at which drug concentration decreases is dependent on both elimination and distribution of the drug from the central compartment. A drug that has been distributed into peripheral tissues is partly sequestered from the plasma. A gradient must be established between the concentration in the central compartment and that in the peripheral tissues before a net flow will be established between the peripheral tissues and the plasma. The contribution of distribution, elimination, and sequestration toward the rate of decrease of drug concentration varies according to the duration of drug delivery. As a result, the time for the drug concentration to decrease by a set percentage varies according to the duration of drug administration.

Because half-lives tell us almost nothing about the time required for the concentrations to fall by 50%,[54] Hughes *et al.*[55] introduced the term "context-sensitive half-time" to describe the time required for a 50% decrease in plasma concentration following infusions of varying duration. The "context" is the duration of an infusion that maintains a steady drug concentration. The "context-sensitive half-time" has been generalized to the concept of the "decrement time"[39]. Figure 2.10 shows the context-sensitive effect site decrement times of 20%, 50%, and 80% when an infusion is terminated for four opioids (fentanyl, alfentanil, sufentanil, and remifentanil[10,54]) and for three hypnotics (thiopental,[8] midazolam,[66] and propofol[9,59]) in anesthesia practice. It is instructive to compare the times required for a 50% decrease in effect site concentration for alfentanil and sufentanil (Fig. 2.10C). The terminal half-lives for these drugs are 2 h and 9 h respectively. Although sufentanil has a terminal half-life that is nearly five times longer than that of alfentanil, the sufentanil concentrations will fall much faster than the alfentanil concentrations for infusions of less than 8 h duration. Thus, the terminal half-life is grossly misleading. The same is true for remifentanil, for which effect site concentrations fall by 50% in less than 4 min, regardless of infusion duration and despite a measured half-life that exceeds 50 min.[10,67]

The clinical setting determines the percentage decrease necessary to produce a given change in drug effect. For example, in the case of a very light anesthetic, so light that just a 20% decrease in opioid concentration would result in emergence from anesthesia, Fig. 2.10A demonstrates that any of these opioids would result in rapid emergence, even though sufentanil and fentanyl have fairly long terminal half-lives. Conversely, in the case of a very deep anesthetic (e.g. an opioid anesthetic for cardiac surgery), an 80% decrease in concentration may be required for the patient to awaken. Figure 2.10E suggests that if an 80% decrease in opioid concentration is necessary at the end of anesthesia, then alfentanil and remifentanil will assure a much more rapid awakening than sufentanil (if the anesthesia is prolonged for more than 3 h) or fentanyl.

One cannot predict the shapes of these decrement curves a priori. Only with computer simulations can the time-course of recovery following administration of drugs described by multicompartment

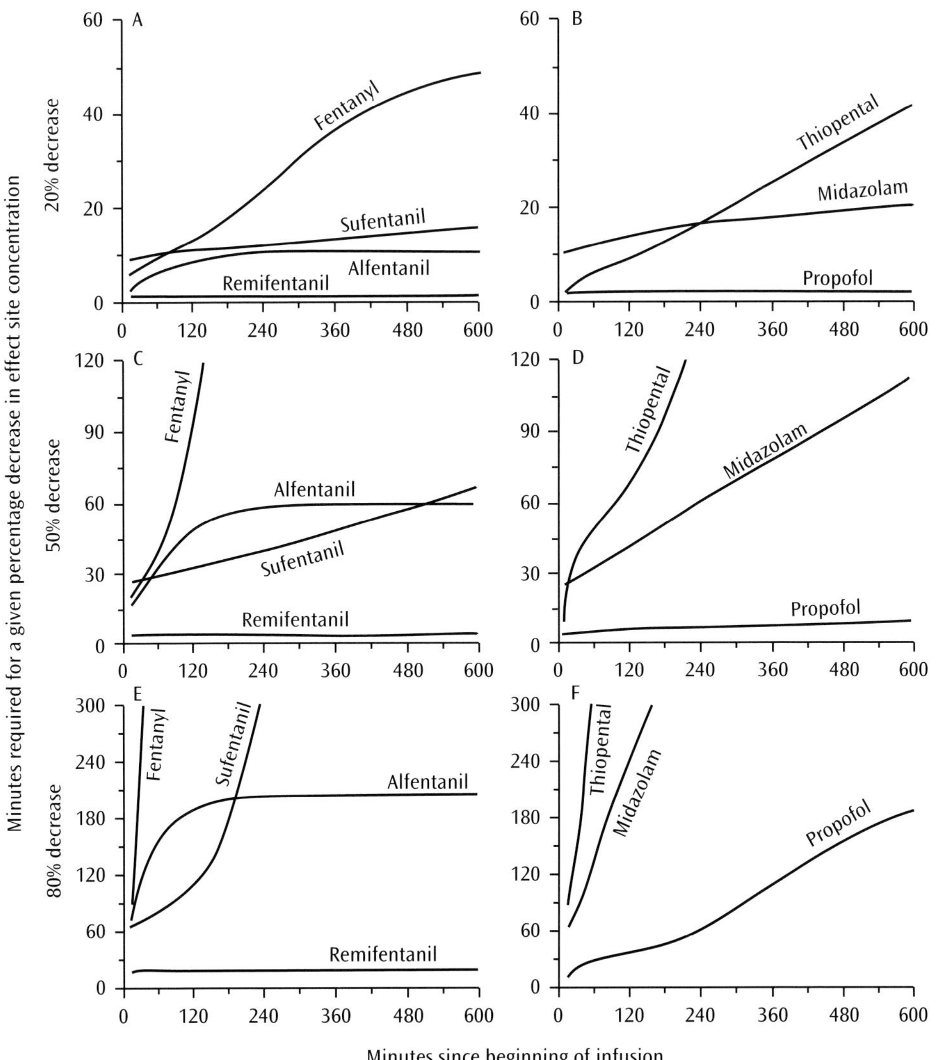

Figure 2.10 *(A, C, E) The relation between infusion duration and the time required for decreases in effect site concentration of 20%, 50%, and 80% when an infusion is terminated for fentanyl, alfentanil, sufentanil, and remifentanil. The time for the 50% decrease is similar to the "context-sensitive half-time" except that it describes the time-course in the effect site rather than the plasma. Adapted from Shafer and Varvel[54] and Minto* et al.*[10] (B, D, F) The relation between infusion duration and the time required for decreases in effect site concentration of 20%, 50%, and 80% when an infusion is terminated for thiopental,[8] midazolam,[66] and propofol.[9,59]*

pharmacokinetics, which includes almost all anesthetic drugs, be predicted. These concepts have been further expanded by Bailey[68] with the introduction of the mean effect time to integrate pharmacokinetics and pharmacodynamics for quantal measures of drug effect.

CONCLUSIONS

There has been a revolution in pharmacokinetics over the last decade. Most of us were taught pharmacokinetics in medical school that were based on the one-compartment model. These concepts are now grossly outdated and have been replaced by newer concepts that are more accurate and that provide useful dosing guidelines. Additionally, implementation of pharmacokinetic concepts no longer requires extensive training in mathematics and clinical pharmacology because simulation programs have become widely available. Clinicians can easily download programs from the World Wide Web and use them to design drug dosing regimens and simulate the time-course of anesthetic drugs. At present, four programs – STANPUMP, STELPUMP, RUGLOOP, and IVA-SIM – are freely available at http://anesthesia.stanford.edu/pkpd. These programs can be used to experiment with the ideas contained in this chapter, as well as to design drug doses tailored to individual situations based on our present knowledge of the pharmacokinetics of anesthetic drugs.

REFERENCES

1. Box G. Robustness in the strategy of scientific model building. In: Launer RL, Wilkerson, GN (eds). *Robustness in Statistics*. New York: Academic Press, 1979: 201–36.
2. Henthorn TK, Avram MJ, Krejcie TC, *et al*. Minimal compartmental model of circulatory mixing of indocyanine green. *Am J Physiol* 1992; **262** (3 Pt 2): H903–10.
3. Krejcie TC, Henthorn TK, Shanks CA, Avram MJ. A recirculatory pharmacokinetic model describing the circulatory mixing, tissue distribution and elimination of antipyrine in dogs. *J Pharmacol Exp Ther* 1994; **269:** 609–16.
4. Ludbrook GL, Upton RN, Grant C, Martinez A. The effect of rate of administration on brain concentrations of propofol in sheep. *Anesth Analg* 1998; **86:** 1301–6.
5. Boer F, Bovill JG, Burm AG, Mooren RA. Uptake of sufentanil, alfentanil and morphine in the lungs of patients about to undergo coronary artery surgery. *Br J Anaesth* 1992; **68:** 370–5.
6. Roerig DL, Kotrly KJ, Vucins EJ, *et al*. First pass uptake of fentanyl, meperidine, and morphine in the human lung. *Anesthesiology* 1987; **67:** 466–72.
7. Homer TD, Stanski DR. The effect of increasing age on thiopental disposition and anesthetic requirement. *Anesthesiology* 1985; **62:** 714–24.
8. Stanski DR, Maitre PO. Population pharmacokinetics and pharmacodynamics of thiopental: the effect of age revisited. *Anesthesiology* 1990; **72:** 412–22.
9. Schnider TW, Minto CF, Gambus PL, *et al*. The influence of method of administration and covariates on the pharmacokinetics of propofol in adult volunteers. *Anesthesiology* 1998; **88:** 1170–82.
10. Minto CF, Schnider TW, Egan TD, *et al*. Influence of age and gender on the pharmacokinetics and pharmacodynamics of remifentanil. I. Model development. *Anesthesiology* 1997; **86:** 10–23.
11. Forbes GB, Reina JC. Adult lean body mass declines with age: some longitudinal observations. *Metabolism* 1970; **19:** 653–63.
12. Greenblatt DJ, Arendt RM, Abernethy DR, *et al*. In vitro quantitation of benzodiazepine lipophilicity: relation to in vivo distribution. *Br J Anaesth* 1983; **55:** 985–9.
13. Greenblatt DJ, Friedman H, Burstein ES, *et al*. Trazodone kinetics: effect of age, gender, and obesity. *Clin Pharmacol Ther* 1987; **42:** 193–200.
14. Greenblatt DJ, Abernethy DR, Locniskar A, *et al*. Age, sex, and nitrazepam kinetics: relation to antipyrine disposition. *Clin Pharmacol Ther* 1985; **38:** 697–703.
15. Scavone JM, Friedman H, Greenblatt DJ, Shader RI. Effect of age, body composition, and lipid solubility on benzodiazepine tissue distribution in rats. *Arzneimittelforschung* 1987; **37:** 2–6.
16. Meyer UA. Drugs in special patient groups: clinical importance of genetics in drug effects. In: Melmon KL, Morelli HF, Hoffman BB, Nierenberg DW (eds). *Clinical Pharmacology*. New York: McGraw-Hill, 1991.
17. Wilkinson GR, Shand DG. Commentary: a physiological approach to hepatic drug clearance. *Clin Pharmacol Ther* 1975; **18:** 377–90.
18. Wynne HA, Cope LH, Mutch E, *et al*. The effect of age upon liver volume and apparent liver blood flow in healthy man. *Hepatology* 1989; **9:** 297–301.
19. Wood AJ, Vestal RE, Wilkinson GR, *et al*. Effect of aging and cigarette smoking on antipyrine and indocyanine green elimination. *Clin Pharmacol Ther* 1979; **26:** 16–20.
20. Vestal RE, Wood AJ. Influence of age and smoking on drug kinetics in man: studies using model compounds. *Clin Pharmacokinet* 1980; **5:** 309–19.
21. Greenblatt DJ, Allen MD, Locniskar A, *et al*. Lorazepam kinetics in the elderly. *Clin Pharmacol Ther* 1979; **26:** 103–13.
22. Kien ND, Reitan JA, White DA, *et al*. Hemodynamic responses to alfentanil in halothane-anesthetized dogs. *Anesth Analg* 1986; **65:** 765–70.
23. Thulin L, Andreen M, Irestedt L. Effect of controlled halothane anaesthesia on splanchnic blood flow and cardiac output in the dog. *Acta Anaesthesiol Scand* 1975; **19:** 146–53.
24. Cockcroft DW, Gault MH. Prediction of creatinine clearance from serum creatinine. *Nephron* 1976; **16:** 31–41.
25. Danziger RS, Tobin JD, Becker LC, *et al*. The age-associated decline in glomerular filtration in healthy normotensive volunteers. Lack of relation to cardiovascular performance. *J Am Geriatr Soc* 1990; **38:** 1127–32.
26. Upton RA, Nguyen TL, Miller RD, Castagnoli Jr N. Renal and biliary elimination of vecuronium (ORG NC 45) and pancuronium in rats. *Anesth Analg* 1982; **61:** 313–16.
27. Waxman K, Shoemaker WC, Lippmann M. Cardiovascular effects of anesthetic induction with ketamine. *Anesth Analg* 1980; **59:** 355–8.
28. Bennett GM, Stanley TH. Cardiovascular effects of fentanyl during enflurane anesthesia in man. *Anesth Analg* 1979; **58:** 179–82.
29. Westenskow DR, Jordan WS, Hodges MR, Stanley TH. Correlation of oxygen uptake and cardiovascular dynamics during N_2O-fentanyl and N_2O-thiopental anesthesia in the dog. *Anesth Analg* 1978; **57:** 37–41.
30. Liu W, Bidwai AV, Stanley TH, Isern-Amaral J. Cardiovascular dynamics after large doses of fentanyl and fentanyl plus N_2O in the dog. *Anesth Analg* 1976; **55:** 168–72.
31. Mallow JE, White RD, Cucchiara RF, Tarhan S. Hemodynamic effects of isoflurane and halothane in patients with coronary artery disease. *Anesth Analg* 1976; **55:** 135–8.
32. Lappas DG, Buckley MJ, Laver MB, *et al*. Left ventricular performance and pulmonary circulation following addition of nitrous oxide to morphine during coronary-artery surgery. *Anesthesiology* 1975; **43:** 61–9.
33. Fairfield JE, Dritsas A, Beale RJ. Haemodynamic effects of propofol: induction with 2.5 mg kg^{-1}. *Br J Anaesth* 1991; **67:** 618–20.
34. Brismar B, Hedenstierna G, Lundh R, Tokics L. Oxygen uptake, plasma catecholamines and cardiac output during neurolept-nitrous oxide and halothane anaesthesias. *Acta Anaesthesiol Scand* 1982; **26:** 541–9.
35. Pavlin DJ, Coda B, Shen DD, *et al*. Effects of combining propofol and alfentanil on ventilation, analgesia, sedation, and emesis in human volunteers. *Anesthesiology* 1996; **84:** 23–37.
36. Cockshott ID, Briggs LP, Douglas EJ, White M. Pharmacokinetics of propofol in female patients. Studies using single bolus injections. *Br J Anaesth* 1987; **59:** 1103–10.
37. Rodeheffer RJ, Gerstenblith G, Becker LC, *et al*. Exercise cardiac output is maintained with advancing age in healthy human subjects: cardiac dilatation and increased stroke volume compensate for a diminished heart rate. *Circulation* 1984; **69:** 203–13.
38. Katori R. Normal cardiac output in relation to age and body size. *Tohoku J Exp Med* 1979; **128:** 377–87.
39. Youngs EJ, Shafer SL. Pharmacokinetic parameters relevant to recovery from opioids. *Anesthesiology* 1994; **81:** 833–42.
40. Shafer S. Principles of pharmacokinetics and pharmacodynamics. In: Longnecker DE, Tinker JH, Morgan GE (eds). *Principles and Practice of Anesthesiology*, 2nd edn. St. Louis: Mosby, 1997: 1159–1210.
41. Macklon AF, Barton M, James O, Rawlins MD. The effect of age on the pharmacokinetics of diazepam. *Clin Sci* 1980; **59:** 479–83.
42. Davis D, Grossman SH, Kitchell BB, *et al*. The effects of age and smoking on the plasma protein binding of lignocaine and diazepam. *Br J Clin Pharmacol* 1985; **19:** 261–5.
43. Ariens EJ. Stereochemistry, a basis for sophisticated nonsense in pharmacokinetics and clinical pharmacology. *Eur J Clin Pharmacol* 1984; **26:** 663–8.
44. Rutten AJ, Mather LE, McLean CF. Cardiovascular effects and regional clearances of i.v. bupivacaine in sheep: enantiomeric analysis. *Br J Anaesth* 1991; **67:** 247–56.

45. Mather LE. Disposition of mepivacaine and bupivacaine enantiomers in sheep. *Br J Anaesth* 1991; **67:** 239–46.
46. Tucker GT, Mather LE, Lennard MS, Gregory A. Plasma concentrations of the stereoisomers of prilocaine after administration of the racemate: implications for toxicity? *Br J Anaesth* 1990; **65:** 333–6.
47. White PF, Ham J, Way WL, Trevor AJ. Pharmacology of ketamine isomers in surgical patients. *Anesthesiology* 1980; **52:** 231–9.
48. White PF, Schuttler J, Shafer A, *et al.* Comparative pharmacology of the ketamine isomers. Studies in volunteers. *Br J Anaesth* 1985; **57:** 197–203.
49. Persson J, Hasselstrom J, Maurset A, *et al.* Pharmacokinetics and non-anagesic effects of S- and R-ketamines in healthy volunteers with normal and reduced metabolic capacity. *Eur J Clin Pharmacol* 2002; **57:** 869–75.
50. Ebling WF, Wada DR, Stanski DR. From piecewise to full physiologic pharmacokinetic modeling: applied to thiopental disposition in the rat. *J Pharmacokinet Biopharm* 1994; **22:** 259–92.
51. Bjorkman S, Wada DR, Stanski DR, Ebling WF. Comparative physiological pharmacokinetics of fentanyl and alfentanil in rats and humans based on parametric single-tissue models. *J Pharmacokinet Biopharm* 1994; **22:** 381–410.
52. Olson RW. *The Art of Creative Thinking*. New York: HarperCollins, 1986.
53. Youngs EJ, Shafer SL. Basic pharmacokinetic and pharmacodynamic principles. In: White PF (ed.). *Textbook of Intravenous Anesthesia*. Baltimore, MD: Williams & Wilkins, 1997: 10–26.
54. Shafer SL, Varvel JR. Pharmacokinetics, pharmacodynamics, and rational opioid selection. *Anesthesiology* 1991; **74:** 53–63.
55. Hughes MA, Glass PS, Jacobs JR. Context-sensitive half-time in multicompartment pharmacokinetic models for intravenous anesthetic drugs. *Anesthesiology* 1992; **76:** 334–41.
56. Hull CJ, Van Beem HB, McLeod K, *et al.* A pharmacodynamic model for pancuronium. *Br J Anaesth* 1978; **50:** 1113–23.
57. Sheiner LB, Stanski DR, Vozeh S, *et al.* Simultaneous modeling of pharmacokinetics and pharmacodynamics: application to d-tubocurarine. *Clin Pharmacol Ther* 1979; **25:** 358–71.
58. Billard V, Gambus PL, Chamoun N, *et al.* A comparison of spectral edge, delta power, and bispectral index as EEG measures of alfentanil, propofol, and midazolam drug effect. *Clin Pharmacol Ther* 1997; **61:** 45–58.
59. Schnider TW, Minto CF, Shafer SL, *et al.* The influence of age on propofol pharmacodynamics. *Anesthesiology* 1999; **90:** 1502–16.
60. Scott JC, Stanski DR. Decreased fentanyl and alfentanil dose requirements with age. A simultaneous pharmacokinetic and pharmacodynamic evaluation. *J Pharmacol Exp Ther* 1987; **240:** 159–66.
61. Scott JC, Cooke JE, Stanski DR. Electroencephalographic quantitation of opioid effect: comparative pharmacodynamics of fentanyl and sufentanil. *Anesthesiology* 1991; **74:** 34–42.
62. Glavinovic MI, Law Min JC, Kapural L, *et al.* Speed of action of various muscle relaxants at the neuromuscular junction binding vs. buffering hypothesis. *J Pharmacol Exp Ther* 1993; **265:** 1181–6.
63. Rupp SM, Castagnoli KP, Fisher DM, Miller RD. Pancuronium and vecuronium pharmacokinetics and pharmacodynamics in younger and elderly adults. *Anesthesiology* 1987; **67:** 45–9.
64. Stanski DR, Ham J, Miller RD, Sheiner LB. Pharmacokinetics and pharmacodynamics of D-tubocurarine during nitrous oxide-narcotic and halothane anesthesia in man. *Anesthesiology* 1979; **51:** 235–41.
65. Glass PS, Shafer SL, Reves JG. Intravenous anesthesia delivery systems. In: Miller RD (ed.). *Anesthesia*, 5th edn. New York: Churchill Livingston, 1999.
66. Zomorodi K, Donner A, Somma J, *et al.* Population pharmacokinetics of midazolam administered by target controlled infusion for sedation following coronary artery bypass grafting. *Anesthesiology* 1998; **89:** 1418–29.
67. Egan TD, Lemmens HJ, Fiset P, *et al.* The pharmacokinetics of the new short-acting opioid remifentanil (GI87084B) in healthy adult male volunteers. *Anesthesiology* 1993; **79:** 881–92.
68. Bailey JM. Technique for quantifying the duration of intravenous anesthetic effect. *Anesthesiology* 1995; **83:** 1095–103.

3

Physics and measurement in anesthesia

NIGEL J N HARPER AND ANGELLA BRYAN

UNITS OF MEASUREMENT

The System of International Units

The System of International Units (SI units) is a metric system that was developed to facilitate standardization between disciplines and between countries. SI units are divided into fundamental or base units and derived units. There are seven fundamental units: time, length, mass, temperature, number of atoms or molecules, light intensity, and electric current. Examples of fundamental and derived units are given in Tables 3.1 and 3.2.

Indicial symbols (e.g. $kg\,m^{-3}$) are preferred to the solidus notation (kg/m^3). Because the quantities described by the fundamental or base units may not be of the same order of magnitude as the quantities that are of direct relevance to our physical surroundings, it is often necessary to use a multiplication factor as a prefix. For example, the unit of pressure, the pascal, is too small to be used in physiologic measurements and so the kilopascal (kPa) is commonly used. One bar is the same in value as 10^5 Pa. Standard atmospheric pressure (one atmosphere) is equal to 101.325 kPa or 760 mmHg. One kilopascal is approximately equal to 10.2 cmH_2O. The only acceptable prefixes in SI are in multiples of 10^3 or 10^{-3} (Table 3.3).

Universal constants

All units of measurement can be related to physical constants that describe properties of the physical world and therefore cannot vary. Examples are the wavelength of light, the speed of sound in a vacuum, the universal gas constant, and pi.

Table 3.1 *SI units of measurement: base and supplementary units*

Quantity	Unit	Symbol
Length	Meter	m
Mass	Kilogram	kg
Time	Second	s
Electric current	Ampere	A
Temperature	Kelvin	K
Amount of substance	Mole	mol
Luminous intensity	Candela	cd
Plane angle	Radian	rad
Solid angle	Steradian	sr

MATHEMATICAL CONCEPTS

Scalars and vectors

A physical property that has a magnitude but not a direction, for example temperature, is a scalar quantity. Properties that have a magnitude and a direction, for example force, distance, and electrical current, are vectors.

An obvious example of the use of vectors in medicine is the representation of the electrical activity of the heart by resolution into several vectors or "leads." The electrical axis of the heart can be calculated from the relative amplitude of any two frontal leads. It is convenient to take leads s1 and aVF because they are at right angles to each other. The amplitude

Table 3.2 *SI units of measurement: derived units*

Quantity	Unit	Symbol
Velocity	Meter per second	$m\,s^{-1}$
Acceleration	Meter per second squared	$m\,s^{-2}$
Force	Newton	N ($m\,kg\,s^{-2}$)
Pressure	Pascal	Pa ($N\,m^{-2}$)
Energy, work, quantity of heat	Joule	J (N m)
Power	Watt	W ($J\,s^{-1}$)
Quantity of electricity	Coulomb	C (A s)
Potential difference (e.m.f.)	Volt	V ($W\,A^{-1}$)
Electrical resistance	Ohm	Ω
Electric conductance	Siemens	S (Ω^{-1})
Capacitance	Farad	F ($C\,V^{-1}$)
Magnetic flux	Weber	Wb (V s)
Magnetic flux density	Tesla	T ($Wb\,m^{-2}$)
Inductance	Henry	H (Ω s)
Magnetic field strength	Ampere per meter	($A\,m^{-1}$)
Activity of radionuclide	Becquerel	Bq (s^{-1})
Luminous flux	Lumen	lm (cd sr)
Luminance	Candela per square meter	$cd\,m^{-2}$
Illuminance	Lux	lx ($lm\,m^{-2}$)
Heat capacity (entropy)	Joule per kelvin	$J\,K^{-1}$
Specific heat capacity	Joule per kilogram kelvin	$J\,kg^{-1}\,K^{-1}$
Thermal conductivity	Watt per meter kelvin	$W\,m^{-1}K^{-1}$
Surface tension	Newton per meter	$N\,m^{-1}$

Table 3.3 *SI units of measurement: multiples*

Prefix	Symbol	Multiplier
Kilo	k	10^3
Mega	M	10^6
Giga	G	10^9
Tera	T	10^{12}
Milli	m	10^{-3}
Micro	μ	10^{-6}
Nano	n	10^{-9}
Pico	p	10^{-12}
Femto	f	10^{-15}
Atto	a	10^{-18}

of the S-wave is subtracted from the amplitude of the R-wave to give the net amplitude of the QRS complex in leads s1 and aVF. A rectangle is constructed, the sides of which represent the relative amplitudes of s1 and aVF. The diagonal of the rectangle represents the cardiac vector. The ratio of the two sides of the rectangle (avF/s1) equals the tangent of the angle, θ, of the cardiac axis clockwise from the horizontal.

Functions

If a change in one variable is necessarily associated with a change in another, their relation can be described mathematically by a function. If y is a function of x, then x is the independent variable and y is the dependent variable. Graphical plots of some common functions are described in Fig. 3.1.

Linear functions

If a plot of the dependent variable against the independent variable is a straight line, the relation of the variables is proportional. An example would be current (dependent variable) passing through a resistance, which is proportional to the voltage (independent variable). A proportional relation can be described by a linear function, where x is the independent variable and y is the dependent variable (Fig. 3.1A). The proportionality may be direct or inverse:

$$f(x) \propto x \text{ (in graphical form } y \propto x)$$

or, if a constant of proportionality (a) is added:

$$f(x) = ax \text{ (in graphical form } y = ax)$$

If the value of the dependent variable is not zero when the value of the independent value is zero, i.e. there is an intercept on the y-axis, this situation can be described by the function:

$$f(x) = ax + b \text{ (in graphical form } y = ax + b)$$

where b is the value of the intercept.

Quadratic functions

Quadratic functions contain the term x^2:

$$f(x) = ax^2 + bx + c$$

They commonly describe the storage or dissipation of energy, for example kinetic energy ($\frac{1}{2}mv^2$). The inverse square law governs the relation between radiated electromagnetic energy and the distance from its source. The curve described by a quadratic function is a parabola (Fig. 3.1B).

Exponential functions

An exponential change is one in which the rate of change of a variable at any time depends on the value of that variable at that particular time. The value of an exponential change approaches zero (for a negative exponential) or a maximum value (for a positive exponential) but reaches it only at infinity. An exponential relation can be converted to a straight-line relation by plotting the values of y on a logarithmic axis.

Exponentials can be described in three categories: tear-away; washout (die-away), and washin.

In a *tear-away* exponential function, the value of the variable *rises* at an increasing rate in direct proportion to its actual value (Fig. 3.1C). The rate of change of y depends on the value of y and a constant:

$$dy/dt = ky$$

Multiplying both sides of the equation by dt/y, integrating both sides with respect to t, and taking antilogs of each side:

$$y = y_0 e^{kt}$$

where y_0 is the initial value of the variable y at time zero, e is the base of natural logarithms (2.71828), and k is a rate constant that is specific for each individual exponential change (the reciprocal of k is the time constant; see below). The size of a bacterial colony, for example, may double in each 20-min period. In theory, there is no limit to the eventual size of the variable.

In a *washout* (die-away) exponential function, the value of the variable *falls* at a decreasing rate in proportion to the distance it still has to fall (Fig. 3.1D). Examples are passive expiration, the fall in arterial P_{CO_2} after a stepwise increase in ventilation, the fall in concentration of (the majority of) drugs with time (second-order kinetics), the discharge of a capacitor through a resistor, the decay of radioactivity, and the fall in plasma concentration during the measurement of organ flow by obtaining a dye dilution curve:

$$dy/dt = -ky$$

$$y = y_0 e^{-kt}$$

The *washin* exponential function is the reverse of the washout function. The value of the variable rises toward a limit at a rate that progressively decreases in proportion to the distance it still has to rise. As time progresses, the rate of change falls toward zero, at which time the variable has a value of y_∞. Thus,

$$dy/dt = k(y_\infty - y)$$

and, at any one time:

$$y = y_\infty(1 - e^{-kt})$$

Typical examples of a washin exponential change are the uptake of inhalational agents and the increase in arterial P_{CO_2} after a stepwise decrease in ventilation.

Half-time and time constant

If the original rate of change were to be continued, the time that would then be required to complete the change is $1/k$ or the time constant of that particular exponential (Fig. 3.1E). After one time constant, the

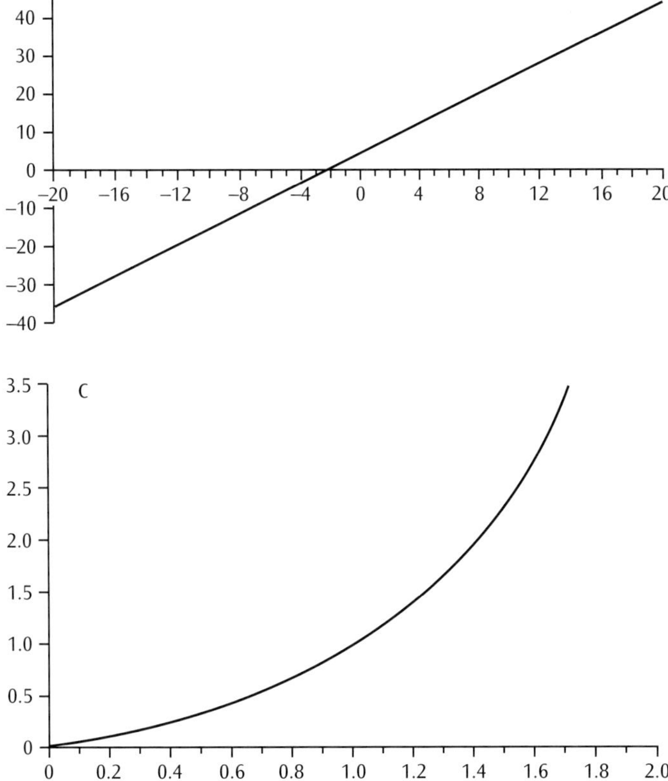

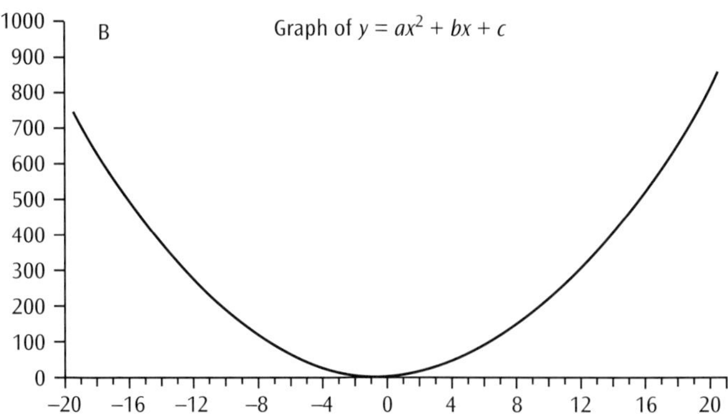

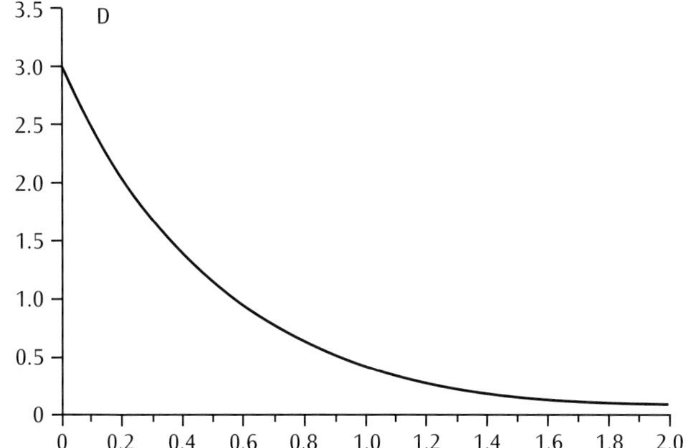

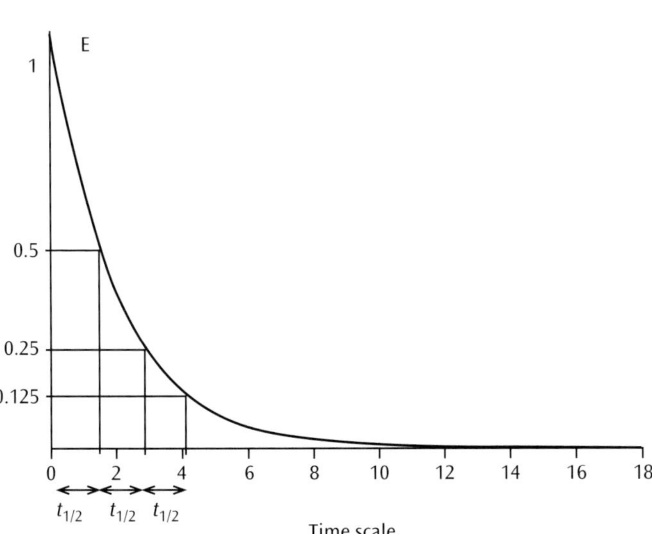

Figure 3.1 *Functions. (A) A proportional relation can be described by a linear function, where* x *is the independent variable and* y *is the dependent variable. (B) The curve described by a quadratic function is a parabola. (C) A* tear-away *exponential function. The value of the variable* rises *at an increasing rate in direct proportion to its actual value. (D) A* washout *(die-away) exponential function. The value of the variable* falls *at a decreasing rate in proportion to the distance it still has to fall. (E) The time constant of an exponential function. If the original rate of change were to continue, the time that would then be required to complete the change is 1/k or the time constant of that particular exponential. After one time constant, the value of the variable will have fallen to approximately 37% (1/e) of its original value; after two time constants to approximately 13.5% ($1/e^2$) of its original value; after three time constants to approximately 5% ($1/e^3$); and after four time constants approximately 1% ($1/e^4$) of its original value.*

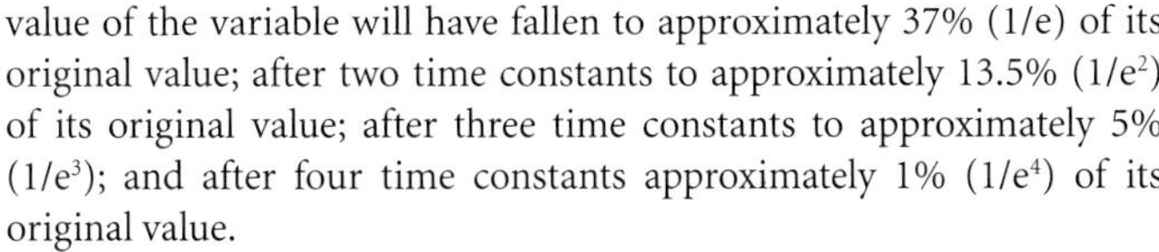

value of the variable will have fallen to approximately 37% (1/e) of its original value; after two time constants to approximately 13.5% ($1/e^2$) of its original value; after three time constants to approximately 5% ($1/e^3$); and after four time constants approximately 1% ($1/e^4$) of its original value.

The time constant of an exponential change equals the product of compliance and resistance. This concept has direct applications in pulmonary physiology. For example, during inflation of the lung, a time constant of 0.3 s results from a compliance of 0.05 L cmH$_2$O^{-1} and a resistance of 6 cmH$_2$O L^{-1} s.

The half-time of an exponential is the time that would be taken for the value of the variable to fall to 50% of its original value (or to increase by a factor of 2), i.e. the time taken for *y* to decrease to *y*/2 (or to increase to 2*y*). The half-time is easy to measure from a graphical plot provided that the value of *y* at time zero is known. When measuring the plasma half-time of a drug, it is necessary to back-extrapolate on a log concentration versus time curve to obtain the value at time zero. For a particular exponential, the relation between the time constant and the half-life is constant:

$$\text{Half-time} = 0.693 \times \text{time constant } (\tau)$$
$$t_{1/2} = 0.69\tau$$

Integration

Integration is an operation that is used to calculate the area under a curve between any two values of *x*, for example the measurement of FEV$_1$, the forced expired volume in 1 s. A continuous measurement of expired flow is obtained from a pneumotachograph (Fig. 3.2). Volume can be obtained from flow using the general equation volume equals flow multiplied by time:

$$V = Qt$$

However, the flow of expired air changes with time, and this simple approach will not suffice. The volume of air expired between two points in time may be calculated by integrating the flow curve between these two points (time zero and 1 s). If the flow curve is divided into a large number of thin vertical strips of equal width, then each can be considered as a tall, thin rectangle. Because the strips are narrow, the flow can be considered to be constant during each brief interval of time. For each strip the volume of air expired during that short time is equal to the flow multiplied by the time:

$$\delta V = Q(t) \times \delta t$$

The total expired volume is simply the sum of the individual rectangular strips:

$$\delta V = \Sigma Q(t) \times \delta t$$

The process of integration assumes that the strips are infinitely narrow:

$$\text{Volume expired} = \int_{t=t_1}^{t=t_2} Q(t) \times dt$$

The values of t_1 and t_2 relate to the defined starting time and the finishing time of the integration process: in the case of FEV_1, $t_1 = 0$ and $t_2 = 1$ s. If, for a different purpose, it is desired to produce a continuous tracing of tidal volume from the continuous output of a pneumotachograph, this can easily be accomplished electronically. In a similar way,

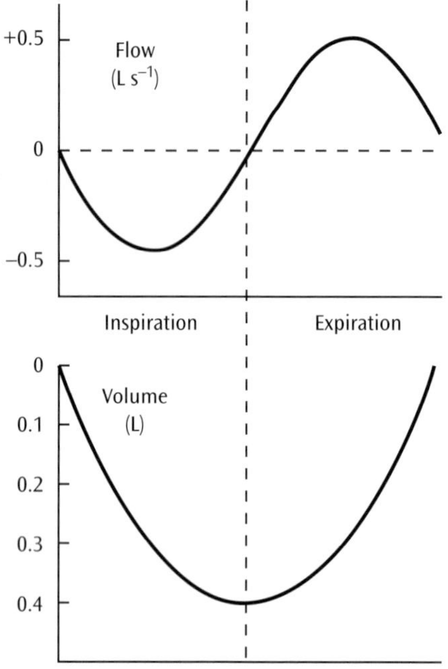

Figure 3.2 *The volume of inspired and expired gas (lower plot) can be derived by integrating the flow signal from a pneumotachograph (upper plot). (After West JB.* Respiratory Physiology – The Essentials. *Baltimore: Williams & Wilkins, 1974.)*

the mean blood pressure can be derived from a continuous arterial blood pressure recording and displayed on a vital signs monitor.

Differentiation

Differentiation results in a function that defines the gradient of a curve at any point. Differentiation is the reverse of integration. The integral of acceleration is velocity: if velocity is differentiated, the result is acceleration. If flow is integrated, the result is volume: if volume is differentiated, the result is flow. If it is desired to obtain a flow tracing from a spirometer, a device that measures expired volume, a similar approach is used whereby time is divided into very small, equal intervals, each of which has the duration δt. The average flow during this small time interval is equal to the gradient of the flow versus time graph:

$$\text{Average flow} = \delta V/\delta t$$

The time interval is now permitted to become infinitely short so that the average flow becomes an instantaneous flow:

$$\text{Instantaneous flow} = dV/dt$$

Electronic differentiation is used to calculate the velocity of blood flow from continuous measurements of pressure.

PROPERTIES OF MATTER

Mechanics

Mass and weight

The mass of an object is an intrinsic property related to the number of molecules it contains. The weight of an object is the result of gravitational force. Thus, the weight of a mass m is mg.

Momentum

Momentum is defined as mass × velocity (units kg m s^{-1}). Because velocity is a vector (see above), momentum is a vector. The principle of conservation of momentum states that when no resultant force acts on a system of bodies the total momentum of the system remains unchanged.

Force

The unit of force is the newton (N). One newton is equivalent to 10^5 dynes. One newton will give a mass of 1 kg an acceleration of 1 m s^{-2}. Force is proportional to mass × acceleration. Force is commonly measured by a strain gauge transducer. In physiology, the contraction of a muscle can be described as isometric or isotonic. In an isotonic contraction, the muscle shortens against a constant load. An isometric contraction is not associated with a reduction in the length of the muscle. During an isometric contraction, a force is being applied, but this force is resisted by an equal opposing force so that there is no net change in muscle length. As work is the product of force and distance (see below), work is performed by isotonic contraction but not by isometric contraction. The relation between force and acceleration is utilized when accelerometry is used to monitor the action of muscle relaxant drugs during anesthesia. The acceleration transducer is taped to the thumb of the patient. Because the mass of the thumb is constant, the force of contraction of the adductor pollicis muscle is reflected in a proportional change in the acceleration of the thumb that is conveniently measured by the accelerometric transducer.

Newton's laws of motion are:

1 An object stays at rest or at a uniform velocity unless acted upon by a resultant force.
2 The change in momentum per unit time is proportional to the resultant force, and in the same direction.
3 Action and reaction are equal and opposite.

Work, energy, and power

The work done by a force is defined as the product of the force (N) and the distance moved by the force in the direction of the force (m). One joule (J) of work is done when a force of 1 N moves its point of application by 1 m in the direction of the force.

Energy is the capacity of a body to do work. Energy can be thought of as stored work or, alternatively, as work that has been used up to produce a change in a system. The unit of energy is also the joule. One joule is equivalent to 0.239 calories. The basal metabolic rate is approximately 2000 kcal per day or 8.4 MJ.

The principle of conservation of energy states that energy cannot be created or destroyed: it can only be changed from one form of energy to another.

Kinetic energy is the energy contained within a body by virtue of its motion:

$$\mathrm{KE} = \tfrac{1}{2}mv^2$$

Potential energy is the energy possessed by a body because if its height (h) in relation to gravitational attraction (g):

$$\mathrm{PE} = mgh$$

Heat energy and chemical energy are special examples of energy. The energy consumption of the body can be calculated approximately by measuring the oxygen consumption and using the value of 20.17 kJ (4.82 kcal) per liter of oxygen consumed.

Power is the rate of doing work. If work is done at 1 J s^{-1}, the power consumption is 1 watt (W). Power is proportional to the product of force and velocity.

Heat

A knowledge of the physics of heat is useful in anesthesia in many unrelated but important areas, for example the maintenance of body temperature, the theory of anesthetic vaporizers, and the effects of compressing or decompressing medical gases.

Temperature scales

Centigrade scale

Any temperature scale depends on calibration to two fixed points. The fixed points of the centigrade scale are the temperature of melting pure ice (the ice point), defined as 0 °C, and the temperature of steam at one standard atmosphere of pressure (the steam point), defined as 100 °C.

Celsius scale

This scale uses the same fixed points but it is based on the properties of an ideal gas. A constant-volume gas thermometer is used, which serves as a standard against which other types of thermometer can be calibrated.

Absolute (or thermodynamic) scale

The fixed points are absolute zero [zero kelvin (K) or −273.15°C] and the triple point of water.

Types of thermometer

Four types of thermometer are commonly used: mercury in glass, platinum resistance, thermocouple, and thermistor (Table 3.8, p. 00).

Heat capacity

The specific heat capacity (c) of a substance is defined as the heat (Q) necessary to raise the temperature of *unit mass* by 1 degree without change of state:

$$\Delta Q = mc\Delta\theta$$

where θ is temperature change (K or °C).

The heat capacity (C) of an object is the heat necessary to raise its temperature by 1 degree without change of state:

$$C = mc$$

where m is the mass of the object.

Anesthetic vaporizers are made from materials of a high specific heat capacity so that, by continuously transferring heat to the liquid anesthetic agent, the fall in temperature consequent on vaporization is minimized for as long as possible.

Latent heat

The specific latent heat of vaporization of a substance is the heat necessary to change its state from liquid to vapor of unit mass of material *without change of temperature*. Specific latent heat of fusion applies to the change of state from solid to liquid. Specific heat of sublimation applies to the change of state from solid directly to vapor.

Heat transfer

There are three methods of heat transfer. *Convection* occurs when there is bulk motion of liquid or gas that carries heat with it. Hotter liquid or gas rises by convection. *Radiation* involves emission or absorption of electromagnetic radiation. It is governed by Stefan's law: radiated power (W) is proportional to the product of surface emissivity (e), the surface area (A), and the fourth power of the *absolute* temperature (T):

$$W \propto eAT^4$$

Conduction takes place in solids and fluids regardless of any bulk motion and requires only a temperature gradient.

LIGHT AND THE ELECTROMAGNETIC SPECTRUM

Light is electromagnetic radiation within the visible waveband part of the electromagnetic spectrum (Fig. 3.3). It is radiation with wavelength in the range 400–780 nm and has the properties of all electromagnetic waves. These properties are:

1 Electromagnetic waves consist of varying electric and magnetic fields. The two fields are perpendicular to each other and to the direction of travel of the wave. Each wave vibrates at the same frequency.
2 All electromagnetic waves travel at the same speed in a vacuum and that is 2.998×10^8 m s^{-1}.

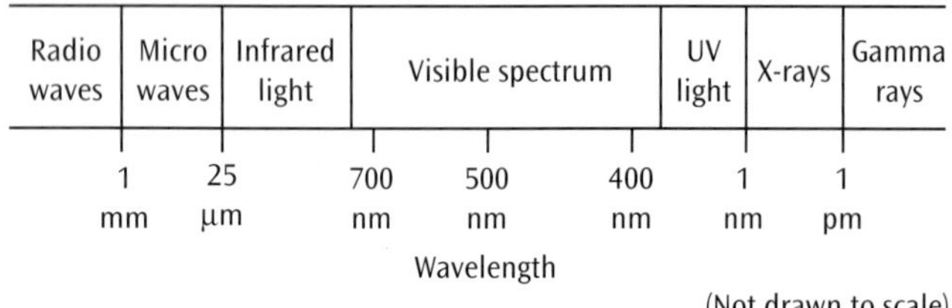

Figure 3.3 *The electromagnetic spectrum. In the human eye, three types of cones are maximally sensitive at 419 nm (blue), 531 nm (green), and 559 nm (red).*

3 Electromagnetic waves are unaffected by electric and magnetic fields.
4 They travel in straight lines within the limits set by diffraction.
5 They are capable of being polarized.
6 They can be used to produce interference effects.

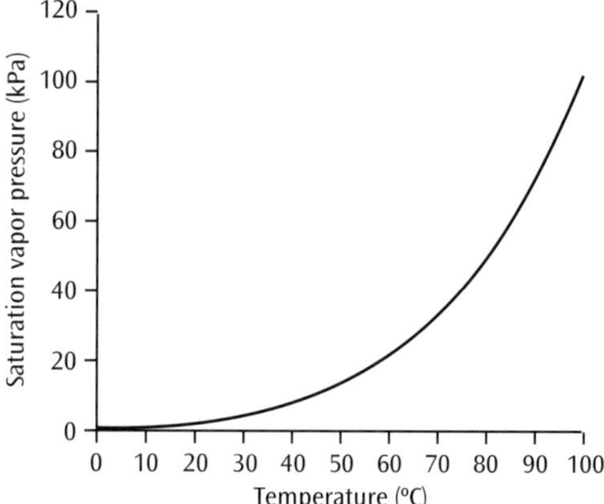

Figure 3.4 *If, in a closed container, there is a vapor and some of the parent liquid is at the bottom of the container, then the vapor is said to be saturated and its pressure is known as the saturated vapor pressure. The saturated vapor pressure is dependent only on the temperature.*

GASES

Gases are characterized by having no inherent boundaries: they expand to fill whatever container they are put into, however large or irregular. The molecules in a gas continually undergo collisions with other gas molecules and with the walls of the container. The term "vapor" is often used synonymously with the term "gas." However, there is a difference: if the container is progressively pressurized a vapor will begin to return to the liquid phase whereas a gas will not, provided that the temperature remains above the critical temperature of that particular substance. A gas can be thought of as a vapor that is above its critical temperature. A substance cannot exist as a liquid above its critical temperature, however much pressure is applied to it: it has to exist as a gas.

Vapor pressure

If a closed container contains a vapor with some of the parent liquid at the bottom of the container, then the vapor is said to be saturated and its pressure is known as the saturated vapor pressure. The molecules in the vapor phase are in a dynamic equilibrium with the molecules in the liquid phase. The vapor is saturated when the number of molecules leaving the surface of the liquid by evaporation is equal to the number leaving the vapor phase and condensing as liquid. If an attempt were to be made to increase the pressure in the container artificially, using a pump, more molecules would leave the vapor phase and condense as liquid until equilibrium is re-established at exactly the same pressure as before. The saturated vapor pressure is dependent only on the temperature (Fig. 3.4).

The higher the saturated vapor pressure of a substance, the more volatile it is. The saturated vapor pressure of isoflurane at 20 °C is 32 kPa (0.32 bar) so that the maximum concentration of vapor that can be obtained is approximately 32%. Desflurane is very much more volatile, and its saturated vapor pressure at 20 °C is 88.5 kPa: in other words, it is very nearly at boiling point (22.8 °C) at room temperature. In contrast, the vapor pressure of the obsolete agent trichlorethylene is only 1.1 kPa at 20 °C and the maximum concentration available for anesthesia was only approximately 1%.

Partial pressure

Because there is so much space between gas molecules, when more than one gas occupies a container each gas behaves as though it were the only gas present. Each gas therefore exerts its own pressure on the walls of the container and the total pressure exerted on the walls of the container is equal to the sum of the individual pressures. The partial pressure of a gas is its contribution to the total pressure of the mixture of gases. Dalton's law states that the contribution that each gas makes to the total pressure is proportional to the number of molecules of that gas. Oxygen constitutes 21% of the atmosphere, therefore its partial pressure is 0.21 bar or $21/100 \times 760 = 159.6$ mmHg (or torr).

Humidity

The gases supplied by pipeline or cylinder are almost completely dry. An exception is pipeline medical air, which may carry residual water from the hospital compressor plant. Alveolar air is saturated with water at 37 °C and contains approximately 6% water by volume: this approximates to a vapor pressure of 6.3 kPa (47 mmHg). Circle breathing systems preserve humidity, and a variety of active and passive humidifiers are used during anesthesia and in the intensive care unit.

Absolute humidity is defined as the amount of water vapor contained in a given volume of gas at a given temperature and pressure. The units are grams of water per cubic meter of gas ($g\,m^{-3}$).

Relative humidity is the amount of water vapor present in a volume of gas *expressed as a percentage of the maximum amount possible at that temperature*. Relative humidity is expressed as a percentage at a specified temperature. Operating room air normally has a relative humidity of 50% at 20 °C; in other words, only half of the amount that would be present if the air were fully saturated with water vapor at 20 °C. Alveolar air has a relative humidity of 100% at 37 °C.

Dew point

As gas cools, the saturated vapor pressure of water vapor falls to the point at which condensation begins. The dew point of a water-containing gas is the temperature to which the gas must be lowered for water to condense from it. At the point when condensation just begins, the partial pressure of water vapor is equal to the saturated vapor pressure. This principle is used in Regnault's hygrometer, which measures absolute humidity. Relative humidity can then be inferred from knowledge of the water content of fully saturated air at various temperatures. Humidity is normally measured using an electronic (resistance or capacitance) transducer.

Pressure

Pressure is proportional to force divided by area. For a given force, a greater pressure can be generated if the force is applied over a small area. It is a common observation that a greater pressure can be applied via a 2-cm^3 syringe than a 10-cm^3 syringe. This principle is also utilized in the pressure-regulating valve (Fig. 3.5).

The SI unit is the kilopascal (kPa), corresponding to newtons per square meter. Conversion factors are given in Table 3.4.

Pressure is commonly measured using a manometer, a Bourdon gauge, an aneroid gauge, or an electronic transducer incorporating several strain gauges (see Fig. 3.8).

The gas laws

Avogadro's law states that equal volumes of any gases at the same pressure and temperature contain equal numbers of molecules. The volume of a gas is therefore proportional to the number of molecules present. One kilomole of any ideal gas will occupy 22.71 m^3 at 1 bar and 0 °C. Because the molecular weights of all the inhalational anesthetic agents are similar, 1 mL of the liquid agent will produce approximately the same volume of saturated vapor, actually about 200 mL of vapor.

The pressure of a gas in a leakproof rigid container results from collisions between the molecules of the gas and the container. The pressure depends on the volume of the container, the number of molecules of gas. and the temperature. This relation is described by the universal gas law:

$$PV = nRT$$

where P is pressure, V is the volume of the container, n is the number of moles of the gas, and T is the absolute temperature. R is the universal gas constant, the value of which is 8314.3 J $kmol^{-1}$ K^{-1}. This law applies only to ideal gases in which the forces between molecules are negligible and the size of the molecules is negligible.

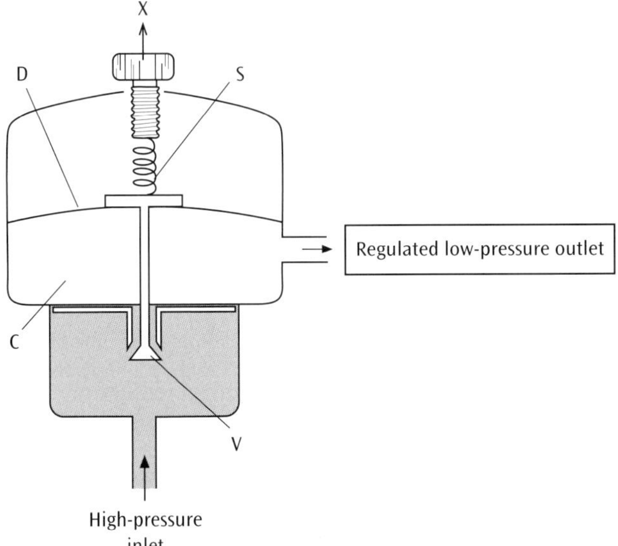

Figure 3.5 *A simplified pressure regulator. Gas at high (unregulated) pressure enters the lower chamber (C), from which its passage into the upper (regulated) chamber is controlled by a valve (V). The characteristics of the pressure regulator are governed by the ratio of the surface areas of the valve seat and the diaphragm (D) as well as the tension in the spring (S), which is adjusted by the screw X. [After Ward C (ed.).* Ward's Anaesthetic Equipment, *4th edn. Philadelphia: WB Saunders, 1998.]*

Table 3.4 *Conversion factors between units of pressure*

Unit of pressure	Conversion factor
1 kilopascal (kPa)	7.5 mmHg 10.2 cmH_2O
1 standard atmosphere	760 mmHg 1033 cmH_2O 10 m sea water (sg 1.033)
1 mmHg (≅ torr)	1.36 cmH_2O

Boyle's law states that, for a given mass of gas, provided that the temperature is kept constant, the volume varies inversely with the pressure:

$$P \propto 1/V$$

Charles's law states that, for a given mass of gas at constant pressure, the volume varies directly with the absolute temperature:

$$V \propto T$$

Solubility of gases in liquids

The amount of gas that will dissolve in a liquid depends on the temperature and pressure as well as the nature of the particular gas and liquid. More gas will dissolve in a cold liquid at a high pressure. The solubility of a gas can be quantified using the Bunsen coefficient or the Ostwald coefficient. The Ostwald coefficient is the volume of gas (at the temperature and pressure of the solution) that is dissolved by unit volume of liquid. Because the coefficient represents one volume divided by another, it is dimensionless:

$$\beta = V/v$$

The solubility of anesthetic gases and vapors is usually described using their Ostwald coefficients. Solubility of gases may also be expressed as the mass of the gas that will dissolve in unit volume of liquid. Henry's law states that the mass of a gas dissolved in a liquid at a constant temperature is proportional to the pressure of the gas at equilibrium:

$$m = hpv$$

where m is the mass of the gas, h is a constant for a combination of a specified gas and a specified liquid at a particular temperature, p is the partial pressure of the gas, and v is the volume of gas dissolved.

Henry's law may also be interpreted as stating that the partial pressure exerted by a gas in solution is proportional to the concentration of gas molecules in the solution.

Gas flow

Gases and liquids both behave as fluids. Flow can be characterized by taking a very small element of a fluid and describing its movement in terms of speed and direction. A line along which a fluid element moves is called a flowline. A stable flowline, in which all the elements follow the same path, one after the other, is called a streamline. Stable flow is described as laminar (or streamlined) and unstable flow is described as turbulent. Streamlines cannot exist in areas of turbulence. Both stable and unstable flow can exist within a fluid.

Viscosity

For a given pressure difference between the ends of a tube, the rate of flow of a fluid through the tube will depend on the viscosity of the fluid: a more viscous fluid will flow more slowly. This is because fluid friction exists between layers of the fluid which move at different speeds. In the center of the tube the fluid moves rapidly, whereas the layer adjacent to the walls of the tube is almost stationary. The layers of fluid need to slide against each other in order for flow to take place. The sliding effect causes a drag or shearing action between the layers. This can be quantified as shear stress, which represents the drag effect per unit area of the surface over which the fluid is flowing. In general, liquids become less viscous as their temperature is raised, and gases become more viscous. The unit of viscosity is the poise. The coefficient of viscosity η is the tangential stress T in a fluid required to produce unit velocity gradient across the fluid.

$$T=\eta dv/dx$$

The coefficient of viscosity is often simply stated as viscosity. A fluid is said to be Newtonian if its viscosity is constant irrespective of the magnitude of the velocity gradient (shear rate) between its layers. Blood is non-Newtonian because its viscosity becomes less as the shear rate increases, thus facilitating flow through small vessels.

Laminar flow

Laminar flow (see above) through a tube is governed by the Hagen–Poiseuille equation:

$$Q=P\pi r^4/8\eta l$$

where Q is flow, P is the pressure difference across the tube, r is the radius of the tube, η is the viscosity of the fluid, and l is the length of the tube. This equation explains why the flow through an intravenous cannula can be increased 16 times by doubling its diameter. It also explains why the flow through an i.v. line is halved if its length is doubled.

The pneumotachograph is a device that uses the Hagen–Poiseuille equation to calculate flow by measuring the pressure difference across a tube in which the flow is deliberately made laminar. The majority of mechanical ventilators in common use employ this technique for measuring the flow of inspired and expired gases.

Turbulent flow

If the pressure difference across a tube is progressively increased, the velocity of a fluid flowing through the tube also increases until a critical point is reached when the flow changes from laminar to turbulent. This is the critical velocity. Turbulent flow is associated with eddies that increase the viscous drag. At the point at which the flow becomes turbulent there is a dramatic increase in the pressure difference across the tube that is required to maintain the flow at the same value – in other words, turbulent flow is less efficient than laminar flow. Turbulent flow is more dependent on the density of the fluid and less dependent in its viscosity. The likelihood that flow will be laminar or turbulent in any particular circumstances can be established by calculating the Reynolds number (Re). If the Reynolds number is less than 2000, then flow through a tube is likely to be laminar; if greater than 2000, flow is likely to be increasingly turbulent.

$$Re=vl/\mu$$

where v is the mean flow velocity, l is the length of the tube, and μ is the kinematic viscosity, which is the ratio of the viscosity to the density of the fluid.

In physiology, flow in the tracheobronchial tree and the circulation is predominantly laminar. Turbulent flow occurs in the larger airways and at the aortic root and cardiac valves.

Flow through an orifice

When gas is forced through an orifice, flow is proportional to the density of the gas and the square of the velocity. The rotameter that is used to measure gas flows in anesthesia machines presents an interesting demonstration of both orifice flow and laminar flow. Crucially, the bobbin of the rotameter rotates in a glass tube that is wider at the top than at the bottom. At the bottom of the tube, the length of the bobbin is much greater than the annular space between the bobbin and the wall of the tube; as a result, flow is predominantly laminar and the viscosity of the gas is important when determining the pressure drop across the bobbin and hence the height to which it rises. At greater flows, the bobbin rises and the annular space becomes relatively less small in relation to the length of the bobbin. The annular space now increasingly resembles an orifice and the pressure drop across the bobbin, becomes increasingly dependent on the density of the gas. If back-pressure is exerted on a rotameter, the density of the gas increases and the bobbin is observed to fall. The actual flow is actually only slightly less than that indicated by the bobbin. The back-pressure effect can be minimized by positioning the control valve on the outlet side of the flowmeter. In circumstances of high environmental pressure, for example in a hyperbaric chamber, the density of the gas is increased and a rotameter will read high, especially at greater flows.

The Venturi effect

If the diameter of a tube is made smaller at some point in its length and the flow through the tube is held constant, the velocity of the gas in the narrowed segment must increase. The increase in kinetic energy that enables the gas to flow faster can only be achieved by converting some of its potential energy, and this potential energy can only be derived from the pressure within the tube. Thus, in the narrowed segment, the gas flows faster and the pressure is reduced (Fig. 3.6).

Bernouille's equation relates the pressure gradient across a tube and the velocity of the gas flowing through it:

$$P+\rho gH+\tfrac{1}{2}\rho v^2=\text{constant}$$

where ρ is the density of the gas, P is the pressure, and h is the height measured from a fixed point, i.e. the pressure is approximately proportional to the square of the flow rate.

The most common application of this principle in medicine is found in the fixed-performance Venturi oxygen mask. High-pressure oxygen from a cylinder or pipeline is accelerated through a small-diameter tube in the base of the mask. At the point at which the tube emerges inside the mask, the pressure is reduced to below atmospheric and air is

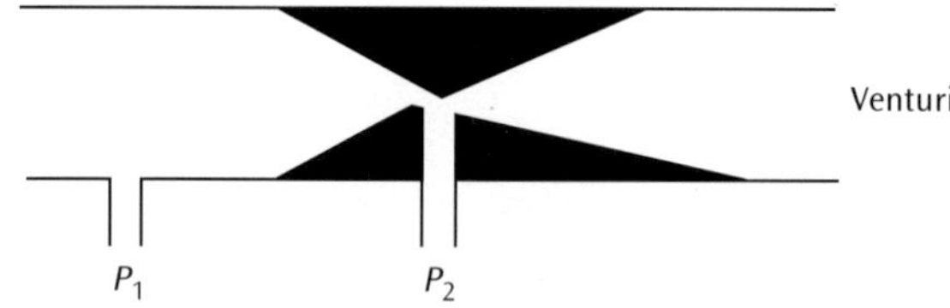

Figure 3.6 *The velocity of the gas increases at the narrowed segment of a Venturi. The increase in the kinetic energy of the gas at this point can be achieved only at the expense of some of its potential energy. As a result, the pressure P_2 is less than pressure P_1. [After Ward C (ed.).* Ward's Anaesthetic Equipment, *4th edn. Philadelphia: WB Saunders, 1998.]*

entrained which is mixed with the oxygen feed in the body of the mask. The concentration of oxygen received by the patient depends on the flow of oxygen and the diameter of the Venturi. The Venturi principle can also be used as a generally applicable device to calculate the flow of gas by measuring the pressure drop in a narrowed segment in a specially constructed and calibrated tube.

Other devices that are used to measure the flow of gases include the thermistor flowmeter (cooled by the flow of gas) and the moveable-pointer peak flowmeter (a variable-orifice flowmeter).

Ultrasonic flowmeter

The ultrasonic flowmeter measures the velocity of flow in liquids by detecting the phase shift (Doppler) or the interval between pulses of ultrasound transmitted through the fluid. This device is widely used to measure flow in blood vessels and in the heart. If the cross-sectional area of the vessel is known or can be measured either directly or by ultrasound, the flow through the vessel can be calculated from the velocity.

The Fick principle

This principle is widely used in medicine to measure widely differing physiological flow parameters. A substance is added or subtracted from the flow that it is desired to measure. The Fick principle states that the flow of liquid in a given period of time is equal to the amount of substance entering or leaving the stream in the same period of time, divided by the concentration difference before and after the point of entry or exit. Two forms of indicator dilution technique can be used to measure blood flow. In the first, an indicator is injected at a constant rate upstream and its concentration is measured from a downstream sample after mixing has taken place.

Flow = rate of infusion of indicator/concentration of indicator in blood

Nontoxic dyes such as indocyanine green have historically been used for physiological measurements of blood flow. Radioactive tracers may also be used.

The direct Fick principle is the basis of the calculation of cardiac output from measurements of the steady-state oxygen consumption of the body as follows:

Cardiac output = oxygen consumption/arteriovenous oxygen content difference

Oxygen consumption is measured over a fixed period of time using a volumetric method or indirectly by measuring the inspired and expired volumes and oxygen concentrations. The arteriovenous oxygen content difference is calculated by subtracting the mixed venous (pulmonary artery) oxygen content from the arterial oxygen content. This technique is beset by many sources of measurement error.

In the second technique, a slug of indicator is injected and the concentration of the indicator is sampled *continuously* downstream. In the commonly used thermodilution measurement of cardiac output, a bolus of cold saline is injected into the right atrium and a thermistor continuously measures the temperature of the blood downstream in the pulmonary artery. The cardiac output is inversely proportional to the area under the plot of temperature with time and is calculated using a modified Stewart–Hamilton equation, the denominator of which is the integral of the change in blood temperature. A modification of this technique uses a special catheter that pulse-heats blood in the right side of the heart and detects the rise in temperature in the pulmonary artery. In this way, an almost continuous estimation of cardiac output can be estimated.

ELECTRICITY

Units of charge and current

An electric current consists of a flow of charged particles. In metal conductors, this flow of charge is mainly carried by electrons. The quantity of charge carried by 6.3×10^{18} electrons is called 1 coulomb (C). In other types of conductors, flow is carried by ions.

The current which flows when 1 C passes each point in a circuit every second is given by:

1 ampere = 1 coulomb per second (1 A = 1 C/s)

The definition of an *ampere* is that steady current which, when flowing in each of two infinitely long, parallel straight conductors, which have negligible areas of cross-section and are 1 m apart in a vacuum, causes each conductor to exert a force of 2×10^{-7} N on each meter of the other.

Kirchoff suggested the following laws to apply to any electrical circuit:

1 The sum of the currents entering a junction equals the sum of the currents leaving it.
2 The sum of all the potential differences around a circuit equals the e.m.f. of the battery.

The electromotive force (e.m.f.), E, of a battery is defined as 1 volt if it gives 1 joule of electrical energy to each coulomb of charge passing through it. That is:

1 volt = 1 joule per coulomb (1 V = 1 J/C)

The potential difference (p.d.) across a device in a circuit is 1 V if it changes 1 J of electrical energy into other forms of energy (e.g. heat and light) when 1 C passes through it. If W J are changed when Q C pass, the p.d., V, across the device is:

$$V = W/Q$$

Cells and batteries

When a battery drives current round a circuit, some of the electrical energy carried by the charge is needed to get the current through the battery itself. The energy is changed to heat in the battery and there is therefore less energy available to drive each coulomb around the rest of the circuit. Therefore, for each coulomb, assuming that energy is conserved:

Energy supplied by the battery = Energy changed in devices + Energy "lost" inside battery

A battery consists of two or more cells joined in series to give a greater e.m.f. than one cell alone.

Potential

It is usual to consider the p.d. between two points in a circuit, although at times you have to deal with the potential at a point. To do this we choose one point in the circuit as having zero potential, i.e. 0 V, ground, common, or earth.

Resistance

Conductors oppose the flow of current. The resistance, R, in ohms (Ω) is defined by:

$$R = V/I$$

where V is the p.d. across the conductor in volts and I is the resulting current in amperes.

Ohm's law

For metals, carbon, and some alloys, V/I is a constant, i.e. the current through a conductor is directly proportional to the p.d. across it if the temperature is constant. Ohmic or linear conductors obey this law. The resistance of a nonohmic or nonlinear conductor varies with the p.d., and their I–V graph is curved, e.g. for a semiconductor diode. The total resistance of a series of resistors, R_{total} (e.g. R_1, R_2, R_3), in a circuit (i.e. one current path) is given by:

$$R_{total} = R_1 + R_2 + R_3$$

The total resistance of resistors in parallel, Rtotal (a choice of current paths), is given by:

$$R_{total} = 1/R = 1/R_1 + 1/R_2$$

Energy and power

The rate at which energy is supplied is measured in watts and

$$\text{Power} = \text{current} \times \text{voltage}$$

$$P = IV = I^2R = V^2/R$$

Resistance and temperature

If the temperature of a conductor rises, the resistance increases if it is a metal but decreases if it is a pure semiconductor or carbon. The change is given by the temperature coefficient, α, defined by:

$$\alpha = \frac{R_\theta - R_0}{R_0 \times \theta}$$

where R_θ and R_0 are the resistances at θ and 0 °C; for metals α is positive, for semiconductors and carbon it is negative.

Resistivity

The resistance, R, of a conductor is directly proportional to its length, l, and inversely proportional to its cross-sectional area, A, i.e.

$$R = \rho l/A$$

where ρ is called the resistivity of the material.

Resistors

The resistor component has to dissipate the heat it produces so for each component there is a maximum power it can dissipate measured in watts, its power rating. Various types exist, such as molded carbon resistors, which are common and cheap and made of carbon and clay. They typically dissipate about 0.5 W. Wire wound resistors have a length of nichrome wire wound on a former of ceramic and covered with a thin protective coating of cement. They can handle high power and can be made more accurately than the molded type. Some resistors are of the high-stability type, which essentially means they keep the same value (as much as possible) whatever the conditions, i.e. despite changes in temperature, dampness, storage, application of heat during soldering, high operating voltages, etc. Color bands indicate resistance value and tolerance. Most resistors are linear devices, obeying Ohm's law. Exceptions are semiconductor devices, Zener diodes, voltage-dependent resistors, and human tissue.

Direct current

A steady flow of electrons along a wire or through a component under the influence of a potential difference is considered to be direct current (d.c.).

Alternating current

Alternating current (a.c.) describes a flow of electrons first in one direction and then in the opposite direction along a wire. A graph of a.c. against time may appear at its simplest as a sine wave. The practical value of an alternating current is not its peak value but the root-mean-square (r.m.s.) value. This is defined as that steady current which produces the same heating effect per second in a given resistance. As the heat produced depends on the square of the current, the r.m.s. value can be calculated by taking the square root of the average of all the values of I^2 during a cycle. Thus,

$$I_{rms} = \sqrt{(\text{average value of } I^2)} = \sqrt{(\tfrac{1}{2}I_0^2)} = 0.707I_0$$

where I_0 is the peak value of the current.

Capacitance

Capacitance is a measure of the ability of an object (two conductors separated by an insulator or dielectric) to hold an electric charge [SI unit: coulomb (C) = A (amps) × s (seconds)].

The capacitance depends on the permittivity, area, and thickness. One coulomb (1 A flowing for 1 s) will charge a 1-farad capacitor to a potential of 1 volt. Hence,

$$V = Q/C$$

There are many types of capacitor with different values, ranging from 10 pF to 10 000 μF; the simplest is an air-filled capacitor of 5–500 pF. If larger capacities are required, then the air is replaced by a dielectric which will store electrical energy by distortion of its molecular structure and so increase the capacity of the capacitor. The choice of capacitor depends on the voltage ratings and quality as well as value of capacitance required. The quality of the capacitor also determines its performance at high frequencies. A perfect capacitor will have an opposition to a current flow (termed reactance), which drops inversely in proportion to the frequency of the alternating voltage applied, i.e.:

$$\text{Reactance of capacitor in a.c. circuit} = 1/(2\pi fC)$$

where f is frequency of the alternating voltage and C is capacitance.

Inductance

An inductor consists of a number of turns of wire wound as a coil around a core of magnetic material (or air). The measure of the ability of the coil to give rise to a back-e.m.f. is the *self-inductance* of the coil, i.e.:

$$E = -L\mathrm{d}I/\mathrm{d}t$$

where E is the back-e.m.f. induced in the coil, L is the self-inductance measured in henrys (H), and $\mathrm{d}I/\mathrm{d}t$ is the rate of change of current in the coil. This is Lenz's law.

Inductors are in many ways the opposite of capacitors: they can be used to block changing voltages and yet pass steady or d.c. voltages. In medical equipment inductors are used in transformers, as chokes in power supplies, and in high-frequency circuits, where they can be used to form tuned circuits with capacitors, e.g. surgical diathermy, ultrasound, and telemetry equipment:

$$\text{Reactance of an inductor in an a.c. circuit} = 2\pi fL$$

where f is frequency of alternating supply and L is inductance.

Mutual inductance

When two coils are in close proximity, the current in one coil will have an associated changing magnetic field that induces an e.m.f. in the second. The flux linkage in the second due to the current in the first is called *mutual inductance* and is measured in henrys.

The ratio of the voltage across each coil is equal to the ratio of the number of turns of the coil. Examples include power supplies and an isolation transformer which has a 1:1 ratio of output voltage to input voltage.

Impedance

The opposition which an alternating current circuit offers to current flow is called the impedance of the circuit. Impedance has resistive and reactive components. The unit of impedance is the ohm.

If there is a linear relation between current (I) and p.d. (V), then impedance is resistive only as in a d.c. circuit. The reactive component is indicated by a phase difference between I and V from a combination of capacitors and inductors in an alternating current circuit and where there is a dependence on frequency.

A capacitor can transmit a.c. but not d.c. An inductor passes low-frequency I more easily than high-frequency I.

Resistance–capacitance combination as a high-pass filter

By applying a sinusoidal input voltage, at low frequencies the impedance is large and the circuit will produce a high attenuation of the input signal. However, at high frequencies the impedance of the capacitor is small and so the attenuation will be small. This simple passive circuit is called a high-pass circuit because it allows high-frequency signals to be passed but attenuates low-frequency signals.

MEASUREMENT SYSTEMS

The basic components of a physiological recording or measurement system which constitutes a patient monitoring system can be considered as units of black boxes. Some of the quantities to be measured, for instance the electrical activity of the heart (ECG), exist as an electrical signal. Other quantities, such as blood pressure, cardiac output, and oxygen saturation, require a transducer so that a corresponding electrical voltage can be processed.

The quantity to be measured is interfaced from the patient to the recording device by a transducer or sensor, which is the first essential component of a monitoring system. The complete system will consist of an isolated connection to the patient, signal conditioning in terms of amplifiers and filters, and an analog-to-digital converter before collection and storage on a processor and a display or recording component.

Transducers

A sensor is a device that detects changes in physical stimuli and produces a resultant measurable signal. A transducer is a device which can change energy from one form to another and will normally consist of a sensing element and the necessary circuitry.

A wide range of transducers and sensors are available. They are classified according to the physical property that is utilized (transduction method) or the quantity that is measured. The following types of signal are important for measurement purposes: mechanical (displacement, force, velocity, acceleration, pressure), thermal, light, sound, electrical, magnetic, and chemical. Many of the methods used to convert physiological events to electrical signals depend on the measurement of dimensional changes such as variations in resistance, inductance, capacitance, or the magnetic linkage between two or more coils. Thermocouples, both piezoelectric and photovoltaic, are self-generating, requiring no external generating energy source.

A displacement transducer emits an electrical output that is proportional to a change in position. They can be used for both direct (e.g. change in volume and shape of cardiac vessels and heart chambers) and indirect measurements (e.g. movement of microphone diaphragm to monitor heart murmurs). Figure 3.7 shows translational, single, and multiturn displacement sensors utilizing potentiometers.

Resistive transducers

The variation in resistance can be used to monitor change in temperature, as in thermistors and thermoresistors which will be discussed later in this chapter, and also change in mechanical displacement using either a potentiometer device or a strain gauge for example the measurement of pressure.

Strain gauges

In a strain gauge, the resistance of the wire is proportional to its length and resistivity and inversely proportional to its cross-sectional area when it is strained within its elastic limit.

The gauge factor is useful for the comparison of different strain gauge materials and is found by dividing change in resistance by change in length. The gauge factor for semiconductor materials is approximately 60 times that of metals. A single crystal of silicon with a small amount of impurity has a resistance that changes with strain. The most common type of pressure transducer consists of a diaphragm, with the pressure to be measured causing movement of the diaphragm that is detected by a strain gauge (Fig. 3.8A). The resistance of such systems, particularly semiconductor devices, is temperature dependent, so a compensatory arrangement in the form of a Wheatstone bridge (Fig. 3.8B) is often included. Two strain gauges are attached close to the center of the diaphragm and two are attached to the periphery. In the former, resistance increases with applied pressure whereas, in the latter, resistance decreases as applied pressure increases and the bridge will be unbalanced by the change, However, as all four branches will change with temperature to the same degree, the output is unaffected.

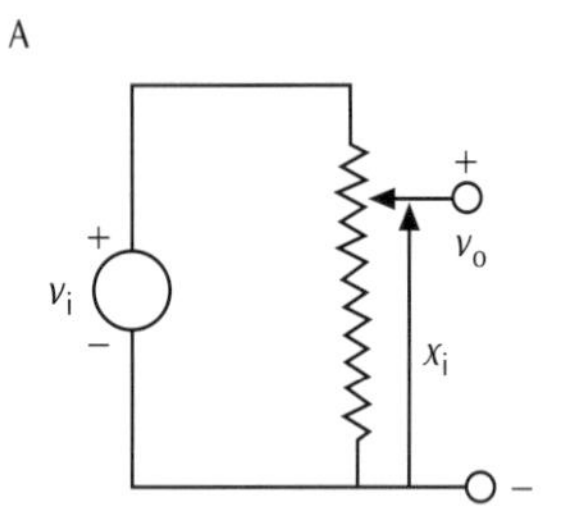

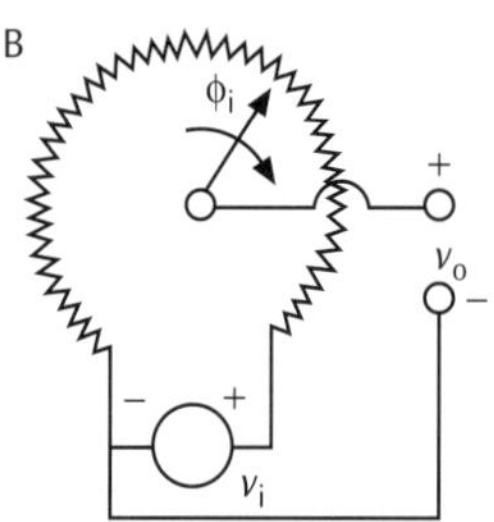

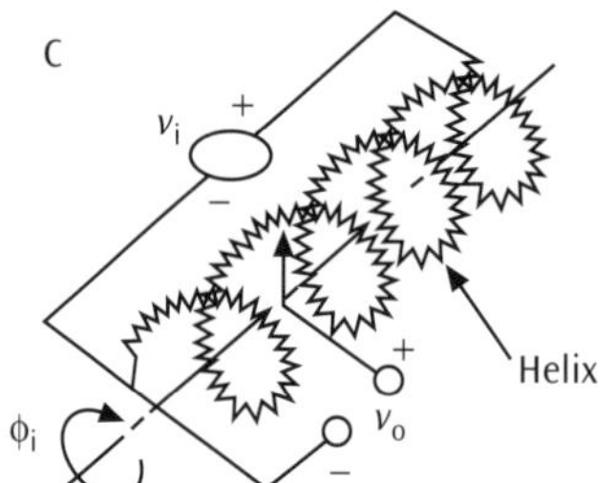

Figure 3.7 *Translational (A) and rotational (B, single turn; C, multiturn) displacement sensors. These devices measure a voltage drop across a divided resistance as in a potentiometer. (After Doebelin EO.* Measurement Systems: Application and Design. *New York: McGraw-Hill, 1990.)*

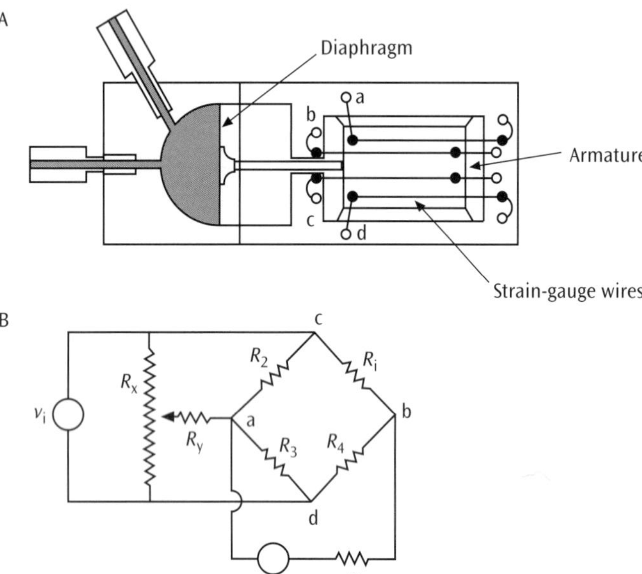

Figure 3.8 *Strain gauge transducer to measure pressure. (A) A Wheatstone bridge arrangement is attached to the diaphragm of the transducer to measure its displacement from the applied pressure. Two arms of the bridge are attached to the center of the diaphragm, where the resistance will increase with pressure, and the other two are at the periphery, where the resistance will decrease. The bridge arrangement allows for temperature changes, which will be compensated for by each arm of the bridge and not at the output. (B) The equivalent circuit where resistance R_1=strain gauge wire b, R_2=a, R_3=d, R_4=c. The bridge is balanced using resistor R_x and potentiometer R_y. The applied voltage is v_i and Δv_o is the output voltage on the voltmeter (internal resistance, R_i). [After Webster JG (ed.).* Medical Instrumentation. Application and Design. *New York: Wiley, 1998.]*

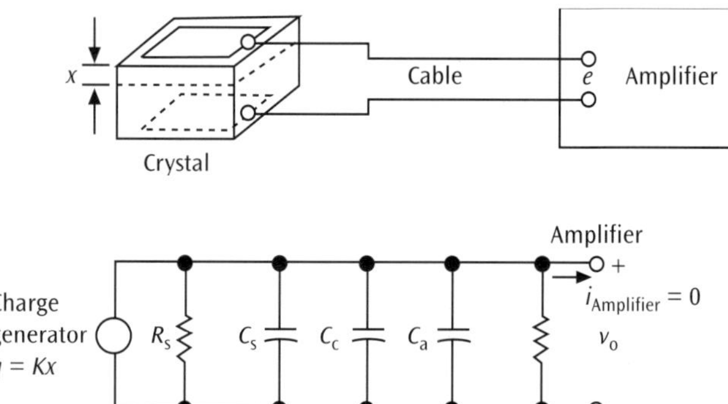

Figure 3.9 *Circuit diagram of piezoelectric transducer measurement system with crystal and amplifier. R_s is the sensor resistance and C_s, C_c, and C_a are the capacitances of the sensor, cable, and amplifier respectively. (After Doebelin EO.* Measurement Systems: Application and Design. *New York: McGraw-Hill, 1990.)*

Piezoelectric transducers

Piezoelectric materials generate an electric charge, and hence potential, when mechanically strained or squeezed in specific directions. This is because when particular crystals are distorted there is relative displacement of negative and positive charges and charge is redistributed, causing opposite polarity on opposite sides of the crystal (Fig. 3.9). The charge in a piezoelectric transducer is proportional to the piezoelectric constant of the material and the stress that is applied.

Some devices utilize quartz crystals, but manufactured ceramics produce a higher piezoelectric constant.

Direct measurement of arterial pressure

The direct measurement of blood pressure is most commonly made clinically by coupling the arterial pressure to an external transducer via a liquid-filled catheter arrangement. A silicon chip in a disposable tubing system incorporates a Wheatstone bridge arrangement of strain gauges etched into the diaphragm. Alternatively, the pressure may be detected by a sensor at the catheter tip, which eliminates the effect of the liquid-connected external system and thus allows a high-frequency measurement response.

The arterial blood pressure may be changing fairly rapidly, so the catheter–transducer system should be capable of faithfully reproducing the pressure change. The diaphragm of the pressure transducer fixed to the external end of the catheter will have a resonant frequency of several kilohertz (i.e. if it is struck it will "ring" at the resonant frequency). However, the addition of a fluid-filled dome drastically reduces the resonant frequency, and the addition of a fluid-filled catheter, which has slightly elastic walls, reduces the resonant frequency even further. The combination of transducer and catheter has an increased gain at the resonant frequency, and the result is that the output of the transducer oscillates following any abrupt change in pressure. This both distorts the waveform and results in inaccurate measurements of systolic and diastolic blood pressure. The basic sine-wave components of any complex waveform can be dissected into an infinite sum of sine and cosine functions of the correct frequency and phase which when added together give the original complex time-varying waveform, which can be identified by the mathematical technique called Fourier analysis. The blood pressure pulse can be divided into its fundamental component (which is at the pulse frequency and the greatest amplitude), and also its significant harmonics. When comparing the original waveform, a reasonably good reproduction is found from the fundamental frequency and the first 10 harmonics. When the representative harmonic components are known, then the bandwidth requirements of the instrumentation system can be specified. For example, the bandwidth requirements for a heart rate of 120 beats min^{-1} (or 2 Hz) would be 20 Hz ($120 \times 10/60$ for the 10th harmonic), so the system must produce a linear response up to 20 Hz.

To detect a more rapid change in pressure requires a greater number of harmonics and a higher frequency response. Errors in amplitude of the recorded waveform are minimal if the resonant frequency of the system is much greater than the significant harmonics, as with a catheter-tip transducer. A disposable fluid-filled catheter system has a much lower resonant frequency, of the order of 100 Hz. When the resonant frequency is less than the important harmonics, attenuation due to damping may occur. If a single step change in pressure is introduced to a catheter–transducer system, then the response depends on the degree of damping (Fig. 3.10A). If D is the damping coefficient or factor then, if there is no damping ($D = 0$), the system oscillates at its natural frequency for a prolonged period of time. If the damping is increased slightly (e.g. $D = 0.2$), then the amplitude falls quickly, overshoots the baseline, and then oscillates with decreasing amplitude. The relation between the damped resonant frequency, f_d, and the natural resonant frequency, f_0, is given by:

$$f_d = f_0\sqrt{(1 - D^2)}$$

where D is the damping coefficient.

Distortion of a blood pressure waveform is apparent in either the underdamped or overdamped case (Fig. 3.10B). In the underdamped case, the systolic elements are emphasized and the amplitude of the response is elevated. In the overdamped case, the true frequency is underestimated and the high frequencies are damped out with a slow response time. In the optimal case, the amplitude is within the bounds of accuracy with a reasonable response time.

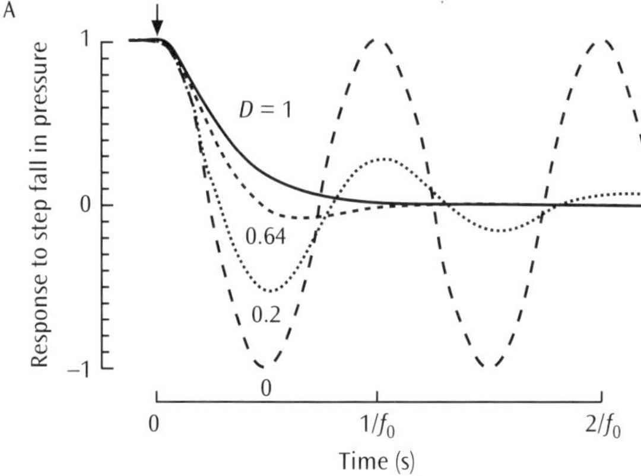

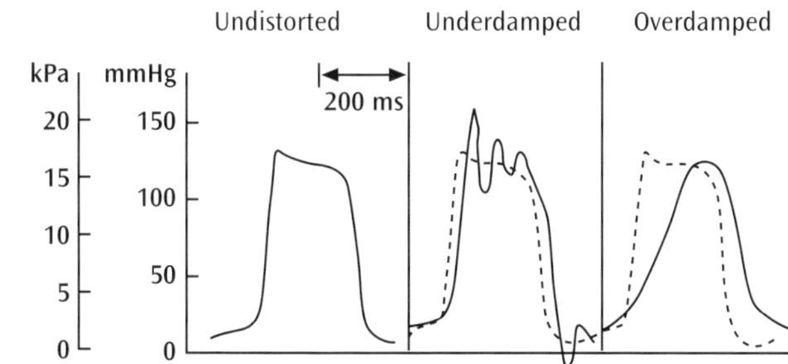

Figure 3.10 *The effect of damping in a transducer measurement system. (A) The effect of damping coefficients on a step change in pressure introduced into the system. (B) Underdamping emphasizes the high-frequency elements in the measurement of blood pressure and overdamping underestimates the true frequency. [After Webster JG (ed.).* Medical Instrumentation. Application and Design. *New York: Wiley, 1998.]*

Electrodes

Electrodes are sensors that detect electrochemical reactions at the interface with the patient's skin. Disposable, self-adhesive, ECG surface electrodes are of the Ag/AgCl type, consisting of a silver metal base coated electrolytically with a layer of ionic compound, silver chloride, and pregelled with electrolyte gel. This type of electrode is electrochemically stable and reduces polarization potentials, which cause signal distortion. Surface electrodes are subject to movement artefacts, which in turn disturb the electrochemical equilibrium between the electrode and skin and so cause a change in electrode potential. Electrode gel minimizes this by moving the metal and electrolyte away from the skin so that movement of the electrode does not disturb the metal–electrolyte junction and the potential is not changed. Electrode gel contains Cl^- as the principal anion in order to maintain good contact. Impedance at the electrode–skin barrier is important in order that stray induced currents from external sources, appearing at the electrode–skin interface are kept to a minimum. Impedance has components of resistance, capacitance, and inductance, making it frequency dependent. Many techniques have been used to reduce electrode–skin impedance and motion artefacts, such as "light" abrasive skin preparation. Degreasing the skin with acetone or alcohol is the minimum skin preparation technique employed prior to application of electrodes.

Gas electrodes

Blood gas analysis systems allow the measurement of the partial pressures of oxygen and carbon dioxide in addition to the pH in a sample of blood. The heparinized sample is passed across four electrodes at the same time in a stabilized temperature environment; the fourth electrode is a reference electrode.

Oxygen electrode

The principle of the Clark-type, polarographic electrode for the measurement of the partial pressure of oxygen (Po_2) in a blood sample involves the electrolytic reduction of oxygen at a cathode constructed of glass-coated platinum (Fig. 3.11).

The platinum electrode is charged negatively with respect to a suitable reference electrode, ($Ag/AgCl_2$) in a solution containing oxygen. At the cathode, the oxygen combines with water and the additional electrons to give hydroxyl ions in a reduction process:

$$O_2 + 2H_2O + 4e^- \rightarrow 2H_2O + 4e^- \rightarrow 4OH^-$$

The hydroxyl ions are buffered by the electrolyte (e.g. potassium chloride):

$$4OH^- + 4KCl \rightarrow 4KOH = 4Cl^-$$

At the anode of the Po_2, oxidation or loss of electrons occurs. The electrons in the process are provided by the silver anode and chloride ions, which form silver chloride:

$$4Ag + 4Cl^- \rightarrow 4AgCl + 4e^-$$

The Clark electrode has an oxygen-permeable, plastic membrane covering the tip of the cathode. As the polarizing voltage increases, the current flow reaches a plateau at about 0.6 to 0.8 V. This minimizes interference resulting from electrochemical reactions with other gases and provides sufficient voltage to drive the reaction. There is a linear relation between the current generated and the concentration of oxygen in the solution. The dependence on temperature is overcome by using

Figure 3.11 *Clark* Po_2 *polarographic electrode. (After Shapiro BA, Peruzzi WT, Templin R. Clinical Application of Blood Gases. St. Louis: Mosby, 1993.)*

a precise operating temperature such as with an electronic heat source. The system is calibrated with two gases, one containing no oxygen and the other containing a known amount of oxygen.

pH electrode

In this electrode two solutions of differing pH (one of known pH) are placed on either side of a glass membrane to generate a potential difference or voltage change (Fig. 3.12).

There are two reference electrodes, made of Ag/AgCl and Hg/Hg_2Cl_2 (calomel). The circuit is completed with a salt bridge of potassium chloride solution and a pH-meter detects the voltage difference between that of the specimen and the reference, $(V_S - V_R)$, which is related to the pH value according to the Nernst equation:

$$pH_S = pH_R + (V_S - V_R)/2.3026T(F/R)$$

where pH_s and pH_R are the pH values of the specimen and reference solutions, F is the Faraday constant, T is the absolute temperature, and R is the molar gas constant. A constant operating temperature or a correction factor is necessary because, according to this relation, the pH is also dependent on temperature. Calibration of known pH solutions is also necessary.

Pco_2 electrode

Within this electrode, first developed by Stowe and later by Severinghaus in the late 1950s, the carbon dioxide gas undergoes a reaction that produces hydrogen ions, as in:

$$CO_2 + H_2O \rightarrow H_2CO_3 \rightarrow H^+ + HCO_3^-$$

The difference in potential so produced is measured in a way similar to that produced by the pH electrode. The relation between Pco_2 and pH is linear over the range of 10–90 mmHg (1.3–12 kPa). The electrode has two chambers, one for the specimen and the other containing the Ag/AgCl reference and measuring electrode assembly (Fig. 3.13).

In this case, the pH electrode is contained in a bicarbonate solution and saline, which replenishes the solution at the electrode tip. The pH-sensitive glass is separated from the sample by a rubber or Teflon semipermeable membrane. This allows the diffusion of carbon dioxide until the concentration of gas is the same in both chambers. Any net movement of carbon dioxide, and hence hydrogen ion movement, is detected by a pH-meter, which has been previously calibrated with known concentrations of gas in solution.

Electrical isolation

An isolation barrier is necessary for the safe connection of a patient to a mains-powered monitor involving the attachment of electrodes. If the patient connection exists as an *applied part*, then the electrode assembly connects directly to the *patient circuit*. These terms are defined under the safety requirements for medical electrical equipment, which will be discussed further. However, the safety implication for the amplifier circuitry is that the *patient circuit* is electrically isolated from the amplifying equipment and the connection provides no path to ground. This isolation barrier is often provided by an isolation transformer and a frequency modulator. After passing through a transformer with a low primary to secondary ratio, the modulated carrier is demodulated and the original signal is recovered. This isolated input means that the potential of the patient is *floating* and the patient is isolated from earth

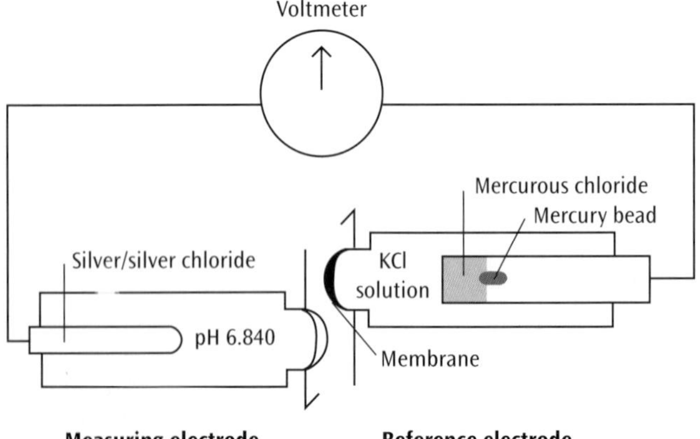

Figure 3.12 *pH electrode principles. (After Shapiro BA, Peruzzi WT, Templin R.* Clinical Application of Blood Gases. *St. Louis: Mosby, 1993.)*

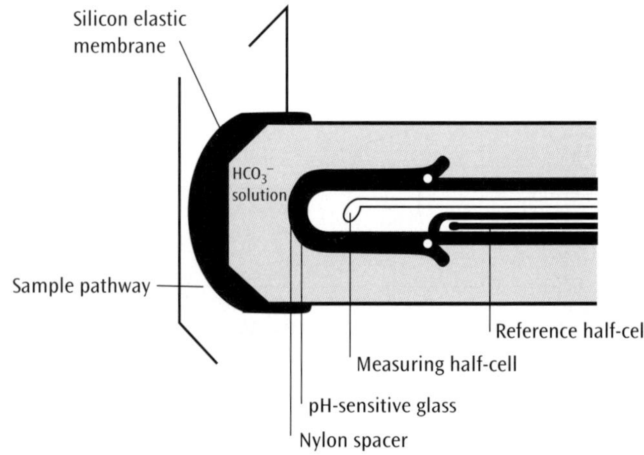

Figure 3.13 Pco_2 *electrode. (After Shapiro BA, Peruzzi WT, Templin R.* Clinical Application of Blood Gases. *St. Louis: Mosby, 1993.)*

and the mains equipment under a single fault condition and protected by an allowable patient leakage current according to safety standards. For electrical safety requirements, isolation preamplifiers are used for direct patient connection providing a high impedance between the patient connector and the mains supply. This can be provided either by transformer isolation or by optical isolation. In transformer isolation, the voltage ratio is 1:1 and there is no earth-seeking path in the event of current flow under a fault condition. In optical isolation, there is a light-emitting diode (LED) on the source side and a photodetector (often a diode) on the output side; voltage is converted to a stream of pulses by the LED, which is detected and converted back to a voltage by the photodiode (frequency to voltage conversion).

Amplifier design

Several important aspects of amplifier design are critical to the collection of physiological data. The amplifier should be situated close to the patient during recordings in order to minimize noise, which can come from many sources and appears as mains interference across the input terminals (Fig. 3.14A and B). Sources of interference include the patient, the environment, and the instrumentation being used in the patient environment. Particularly common is interference due to electrostatic or electromagnetic induction from mains or radiofrequency sources. As a result of induced currents from an electrostatic source, the patient can act as a plate of a capacitor, which may have as the other plate the a.c. source potential or objects such as other equipment, the operating table, or people nearby. These capacitative-linked electrostatic potentials will vary as the potential path to ground varies with the object, and they may appear as 50 Hz interference at the input of the amplifier. In addition, interference occurs close to cables carrying alternating current because of the constantly changing flux linkage across a conductor within its field and an electromagnetically induced current flowing at the same frequency as the source would be produced. Further 50 Hz interference can be introduced by earth-loop interference, whereby two earth points have slightly different potentials and a leakage current can flow because of the potential difference between the two.

Finally, radiofrequency, i.e. >100 kHz, can enter the recording system by a number of routes: through the mains, mixed with 50 Hz current; directly, as when the patient is touched by the active electrode of surgical diathermy, when it is detected by the recording electrodes; or propagated through the air, e.g. if a diathermy probe is activated when held in the air its lead acts as a radiotransmitting aerial and the interference is received by the patient lead. All of these interference effects can all be accentuated by high electrode impedance. If the electrode impedance is low, then the induced current due to the interference will not cause a significant potential drop at the amplifier input, which will be exhibited as 50 Hz interference on the input signal. Good amplifier design aims to reduce interference; all biological amplifiers are of a differential type with a high common mode rejection ratio (CMRR). The CMRR is a measure of how well the amplifier rejects any interference or *common mode* signal that will appear at both input terminals of a differential amplifier. The amplifier amplifies the difference between the voltage appearing at the two input terminals so that the common mode signal is rejected. CMRR is defined as:

$$\text{CMRR} = \frac{\text{amplifier gain for a signal voltage}}{\text{amplifier gain for a common mode voltage}}$$

Expressed in decibels:

$$\text{CMRR (dB)} = 20\log_{10}(\text{CMRR})$$

Another feature of a biological amplifier that ensures faithful reproduction of the signal of interest is the high input impedance of the amplifier. The high input impedance of at least 10 MΩ ensures that most of the signal voltage is presented at the input of the amplifier. If the input impedance was not much higher than the skin and tissue impedance, then a high proportion of the signal voltage would be lost as a result of the potential drop across the electrodes and the signal voltage at the input to the amplifier would be much less.

A

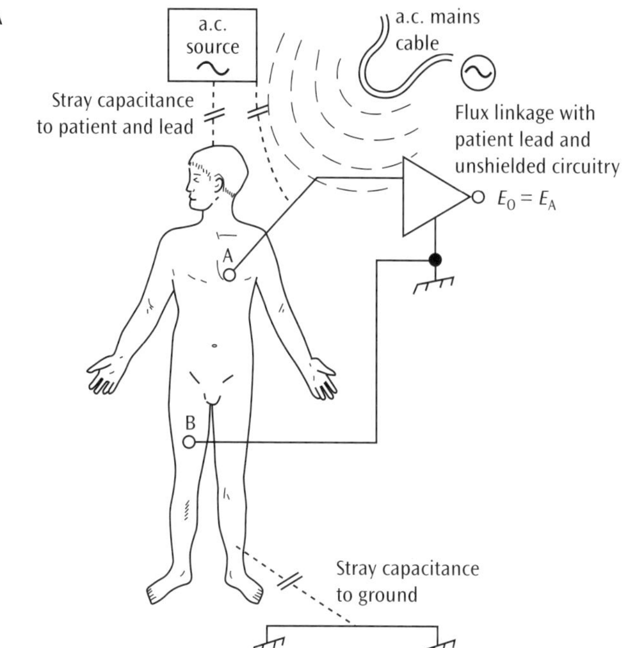

B

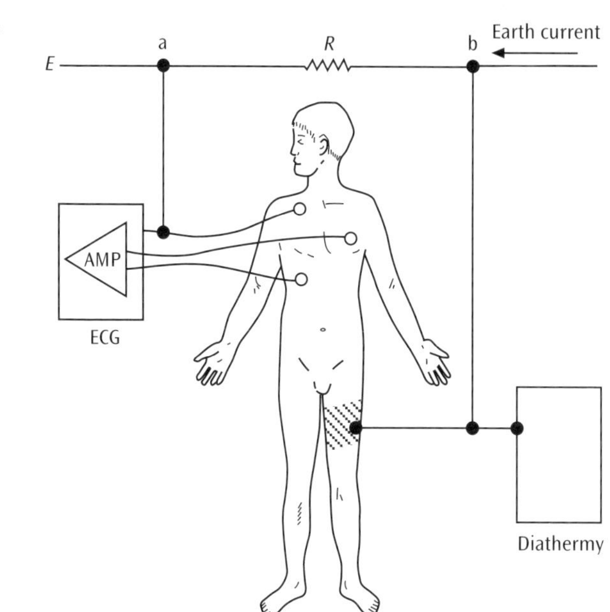

Figure 3.14 *Electromagnetic and electrostatic origins of noise. (A) Noise arising from an electrostatic or electromagnetic source will appear at the input to a biological amplifier. (B) Interference caused by an earth loop when a patient is connected to the earth connections (a and b) of two monitoring devices. The potential difference appears across the patient and hence the input to the amplifier. (After Sykes MK, Vickers MD, Hull CJ.* Principles of Measurement and Monitoring in Anaesthesia and Intensive Care. *Oxford: Blackwell Scientific Publications, 1991.)*

The basic building block of an amplifier is an operational amplifier (op-amp). An ideal op-amp has infinite gain, infinite input impedance, zero output impedance, an infinite frequency response, and zero noise contribution. The properties of a circuit containing a practical op-amp are determined by the properties of a negative feedback loop. There are two inputs: the inverting input (–) and the noninverting input (+). In a biologic or medical amplifier, the differential configuration is used, in which the output voltage, V_{out}, is proportional to $(V_1 - V_2) \times$gain, where V_1 and V_2 are two inputs. The common mode voltage, V_c, is that voltage common to both inputs that is normally an interference signal which is counteracted when used in this mode.

In practice, an instrumentation amplifier consists of many op-amp stages in order to obtain high gain with low resistance values and high input impedance with superior rejection of common mode signals.

In summary, a bioelectrical amplifier has the following characteristics:

1 single-ended output but differential input;
2 high common mode rejection ratio;.
3 an extremely high input impedance;
4 variable gain adequate for the job intended;
5 frequency response suitable for the application;
6 zero suppression [a feature that allows shift about the zero baseline by nulling offsets inherent in the signal and which permits small varying signals superimposed on a larger d.c. signal (or d.c. offset) to be processed in the amplifier using the full gain of the amplifier for the small varying signal only].

Filters

Filters are used in medical devices such as ECG, EMG or EEG monitoring equipment in order to separate one signal from another or from any associated noise. Fourier showed that any signal waveform can be split into its component waveforms and can be considered as a summation of sine waves. For instance, the ECG is a periodic signal of which the lowest frequency component is the heart rate, e.g. 1 Hz (60 min^{-1}). Fourier analysis shows that biggest component is ≈ 17 Hz and that the components above 100 Hz have negligible amplitude. An ECG amplifier must be able to handle frequency components between 1 and 100 Hz; in addition, it must amplify the components equally and preserve the relative phase of the components. In addition, in order to prevent aliasing of the signal being measured, that is erroneously measuring the sampled signal, the rate of digitization must be at least twice the highest frequency expected in the sample. This is termed the Nyquist frequency. As any frequency above the Nyquist frequency will be recorded as an artifact, it is necessary to filter the signal with an anti-aliasing hardware high-pass filter to ensure that only frequencies below this optimum frequency pass into the recording system.

There are four basic types of filter: low-pass filters pass only frequencies within their pass band and attenuate higher frequencies; high-pass filters disregard d.c. signals and signals of low frequency; and bandpass and bandstop filters have upper and lower frequency limits that define the pass or reject band respectively, e.g. notch filters which reject mains frequency (50 Hz/60 Hz). The simplest form of low-pass filter comprises a resistor and capacitor. In practice, it is impossible to construct a sharp-edged frequency cut-off point on a filter – there is always a degree of "roll-off." The more R–C combinations, the steeper the roll-off-specification. For instance, a filter may be specified as a flat response between 0.14 and 50 Hz, allowing 3 dB attenuation at 0.05 and 100 Hz. The unit bel represents the drop in amplitude, e.g. 1 bel represents 10-fold, 2 bels 100-fold, etc. based on logarithmic scale. The most commonly quoted roll-off is –3 dB, which represents a drop in amplitude of 30%. Filters that use resistors, capacitors, and op-amps are called active filters (power gain).

Filters are chosen to allow faithful reproduction of the signal, for instance passing high-frequency components will give more information but may cause drifting of the baseline of the signal. In this case, it is necessary to compromise fidelity with stability in some bioelectric monitors.

Analog-to-digital converter

An analog-to-digital converter (ADC) converts the analog physiological waveform into a binary number by sampling at regular intervals and storing an integer value whose magnitude is proportional to that of the waveform at a particular time interval. The resolution of the converted number depends on the number of bits in the binary number that is produced. Hence, eight-bit resolution produces numbers in the range 0–255, 12-bit 0–4095 and 16-bit, 0–65 535; the greater the number of bits, the more sensitive the measurement.

The ADC comprises a digital-to-analog converter (DAC), a binary counter, a clock, some control logic, and a single comparator. The counter is clocked into the DAC, the output of which is a ramp voltage. If the ramp is stopped when it is equal in amplitude to the voltage to be digitized then the output of the counter is the corresponding binary number.

Sampling frequency is also important when considering the accuracy of the ADC. Although a relatively low sampling frequency may faithfully reproduce a slowly varying waveform, it may be inadequate for one containing higher frequency components. The accuracy of the integer amplitude of the digitized output depends on how quickly or slowly the analog signal changes between recording intervals: more data points (and hence a higher sampling rate) are required to identify rapidly changing parts of the sampled signal than with a slowly varying waveform, in which case inherent detail will not be lost if there is a greater interval between samples.

Electrical safety

There are internationally agreed standards of construction for patient-connected electrical equipment to protect the patient and operator from lethal currents and voltages. In the UK, the British Standards Institution has detailed the principal requirements for the safety of medical electrical equipment to be used in conjunction with patients in British Standard European Norm (BS EN) 60601-1:1993 (this incorporates the older BS5724 Section 1.1:1992 in order to cover new European guidelines). Its international equivalent is IEC (International Electrotechnical Commission) 601-1: 1988 *Medical Electrical Equipment, Part 1: General Requirements for Safety (Amendments 1991 and 1995).* There is essentially no difference between the documents. CE marking on equipment means that it has been constructed to all three guidelines and has been enforceable to all commercially available medical equipment since June 1998. The standard demands that, generally, the failure of a single component in a protective system should not cause a hazard, e.g. a short circuit, isolation breakdown, or missing connection on the mains plug.

IEC 601–1 recognizes two classes of equipment that may be powered from the mains supply. The relevant symbols can be seen in the Appendix. Basic protection against electric shock is provided by different methods of construction, depending on the class of the equipment (Fig. 3.15). These are:

Class I: Equipment which has earthed metal parts. The connection to mains earth prevents accessible parts becoming live in the event of failure of basic insulation inside the equipment. An example of this would be mains-powered equipment enclosed in a metal case connected to mains earth via the earth conductor of the mains lead (Fig. 3.15A).

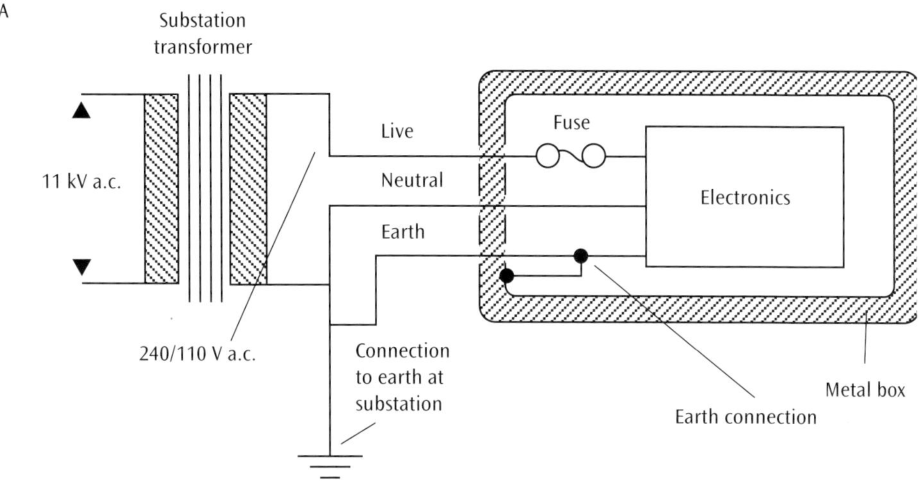

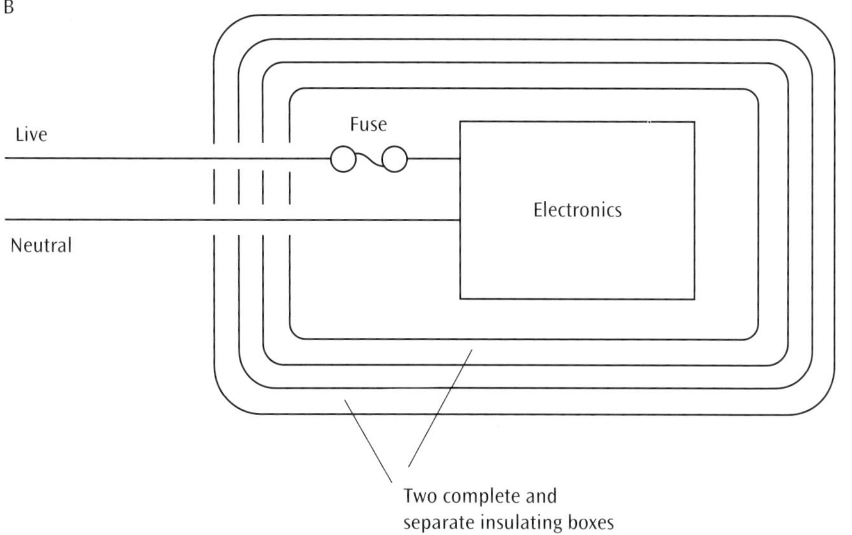

Figure 3.15 *Electrical safety circuit design. (A) Class I equipment as defined by IEC 601-1. Exposed metal parts are earthed. There is an earth connection to the mains and also a fuse in the live connection. (B) Class II equipment as defined by IEC 601-1. All electrical parts are double insulated and there is no earth lead. (After Brown BH, Smallwood RH, Barber DC,* et al. Medical Physics and Biomedical Engineering. *Bristol and Philadelphia: Institute of Physics Press, 1999.)*

Class II: Equipment which has no provision for protective earthing. Protection against electric shock is achieved using insulation in addition to the basic insulation. Examples of this would be mains-powered equipment enclosed in a metal case with a layer of supplementary insulation between its case and its live parts, i.e. double-insulated equipment or, alternatively, mains-powered equipment enclosed in a plastic case with reinforced insulation between metal controls and live parts, i.e. all-insulated equipment (Fig. 3.15B).

IEC 601–1 also recognizes three types of equipment depending on the degree of patient protection against electric shock that it provides. They are:

Type B: Equipment that has no "applied parts," i.e. does not intentionally come into contact with patients, or which has applied parts (e.g. patient connections) that are earth or earth referenced. This type of equipment may be used in electrically "safe" environments or where it is unlikely to come into contact with patients.

Type BF: Equipment which has electrically isolated ("floating") patient applied part(s). This type of equipment is preferred over type B if it is likely to come into contact with patients.

Type CF: Equipment that also has electrically isolated applied part(s). This class of equipment provides a very high degree of patient protection from electric shock. It is primarily intended for applications that involve conductive pathways to a patient's heart.

All mains-powered medical equipment, whether type B, BF, or CF, may be of class I or class II construction, but the standard is specific in respect of the allowable *earth leakage* and *patient leakage* currents for each type under normal working conditions and under single-fault conditions.

Earth leakage current is defined as that current flowing from the mains-powered part of the equipment through the insulation to the protective earth conductor. Patient leakage current is that current flowing from the applied part via the patient to earth. There is a risk of causing electrocution by the initiation of a persistent, grossly abnormal cardiac rhythm, usually ventricular fibrillation, if a mains frequency current is allowed to pass through the patient in such a way that a sufficiently high current passes through the heart muscle itself. These currents, if in the range of 100 μA and allowed to pass through the ventricular endocardium under certain specialized circumstances, such as with cardiac catheters, may induce fibrillation, termed *microshock*. All equipment used in a high-risk microshock situation should be of type CF, but battery-operated equipment is preferred. Surfaces are coated with resistive material to increase the safety from accidental contact. True earth-free systems are recommended (Fig. 3.16). It is important then that allowable leakage currents under such conditions are much more stringent than with the other types of equipment. The allowable earth leakage and patient leakage currents for the different types of equipment are:

B or BF	100 μA normal conditions	500 μA on a single fault
CF	10 μA normal conditions	50 μA on a single fault

In the USA, the Underwriters Laboratories (UL) proposes to adopt the international standard, IEC 601-1, including its specification for leakage current limits. This has been supported by the Health Industry Manufacturers Association (HEMA), the National Electrical Manufacturers Association (NEMA), and the US Food and Drug Administration (FDA).

Faithful reproduction of a biological potential

Faithful reproduction of a biological potential requires the system to have amplitude and phase linearity and sufficient bandwidth to encompass the inherent frequencies in the signal being recorded. These criteria are met by the design of the black box components as previously described; the complete system must amplify the signal components equally and preserve the relative phase of the components. The recording system should be capable of linearly reproducing an input signal without causing an overloading and hence distortion. In addition, the component harmonics of the signal must be processed in the system without introducing any phase advance or lag so that the phase relation to the fundamental of the input signal is preserved. As discussed above, an adequate frequency response encompasses not only the fast-changing components of the waveform but also those below the fundamental frequency. In addition, the signal to noise ratio and the effect of hysteresis should be kept to a minimum.

Factors to be considered in electrophysiological recordings

An ECG records the largest of the biological potentials, normally of the order of 1 mA, and requires a system with a bandwidth of 0.5–100 Hz. An EMG amplifier must be able to handle all of the component waveforms, which would be expected to lie between 2 and 10 kHz. Most of the signal content is between 1 and 50 Hz, and filters are included in the circuitry between amplification and signal processing in order to reproduce the signal faithfully. One problem is that the normal frequency of the mains is 50 Hz in the UK and 60 Hz in the USA. This can be overcome by use of a "notch" filter. However, these are to be avoided in EMG studies because of their effect on the EMG content at this frequency. The choice of electrode also affects the frequency response of the signal; needle electrodes will record much higher frequencies, of the order of 10 kHz, compared with an upper frequency response of 1 kHz for surface electrodes, of duration between 2 and 15 ms and an amplitude from 100 μV to 2 mV. EEG recordings are inherently difficult because of the size and amplitude of a normal EEG, which is 10–300 μV and a frequency content 0.5–40 Hz (δ, < 4 Hz; θ, 4–8 Hz; α 8–13 Hz; β, > 13 Hz).

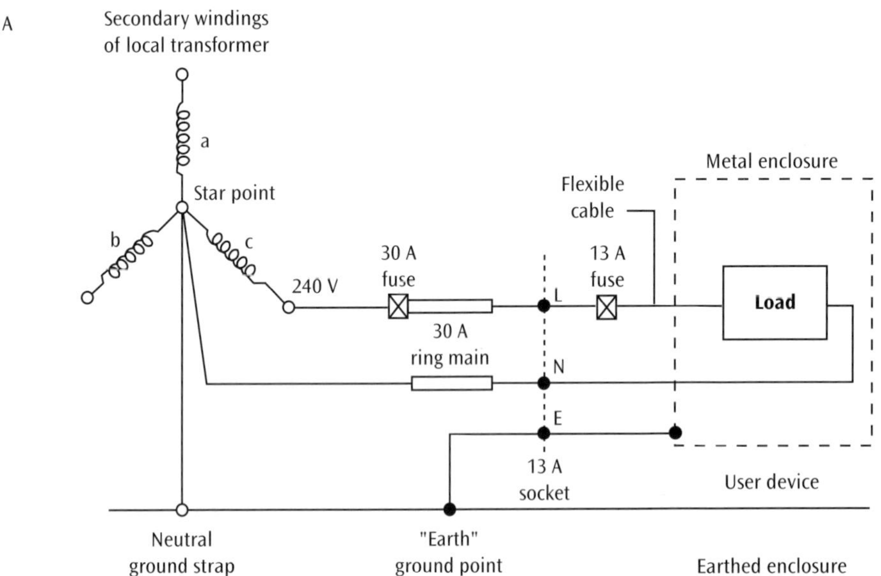

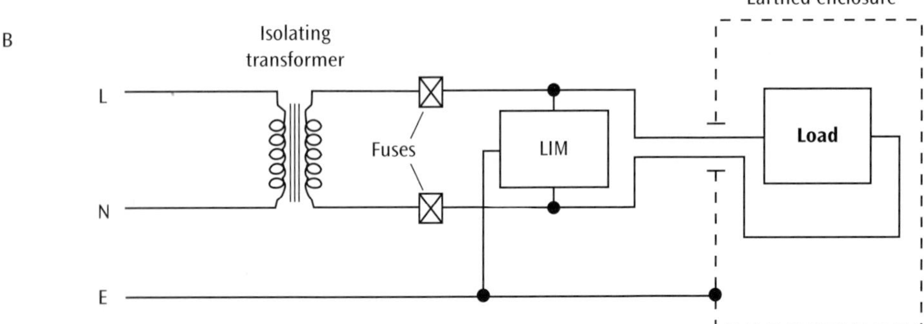

Figure 3.16 *Comparison of normal mains supply and earth-free systems. (A) Normal mains supply showing the connection of the three-phase 11-kV supply to the star point and neutral mains connection. (B) Isolated transformer "earth-free" system with a LIM (line isolation monitor). In this system there is no pathway to ground through the mains supplied at the wall unless there is a fault in the secondary circuit, for which the LIM acts as a warning. (After Sykes MK, Vickers MD, Hull CJ.* Principles of Measurement and Monitoring in Anaesthesia and Intensive Care. *Oxford: Blackwell Scientific Publications, 1991.)*

MEDICAL LASERS

Laser is an acronym for *l*ight *a*mplification by *s*timulated *e*mission of *r*adiation.

Visible light is nonionizing radiation (wavelength ~ 10^{-6} m) and is part of the electromagnetic spectrum (Fig. 3.3). Photons, the fundamental units of light, are produced by *spontaneous emission*, the energy of which is the difference between energy levels of an atom when an electron falls from higher to lower level (Fig. 3.17A). The production of a laser beam requires an active substance in which lasing action can occur, and this substance must in a condition such that there are more atoms contain electrons at higher energy levels than at lower levels; this condition is termed *population inversion*.

Lasers are named after the medium that produces the light, e.g. CO_2, argon. Different media emit characteristic colors. A gas, liquid, or crystal medium is energized (pumped) by a suitable source (light, electric discharge, radiofrequency). The input of the pumping energy raises electrons to higher energy levels in more atoms and more quickly than spontaneous decay can return them to their original level. This produces a surplus of excited atoms, and further photons from spontaneous decay stimulate the excited atom to emit an identical photon. The photons produced fuse in time and space to produce a coherent output and give rise to the term "*stimulated emission*" (Fig. 3.17B).

When atoms are raised from a low energy (ground state) to a higher energy (excited state), they must absorb radiation of wavelength, λ_e, given by:

$$\lambda_e = ch/\Delta E$$

where c is the speed of light in a vacuum, h is Planck's constant, and ΔE is the energy difference between the ground and excited states.

Lasers have been used extensively in medicine in the following areas: ophthalmology, gynecology, otorhinolaryngology, surgery, neurosurgery, urology, plastic surgery, dermatology, and dentistry.

The basic components of a laser delivery tube or chamber are the active laser medium source, an outside energy source, optics, and a delivery system (Fig. 3.18). The lasing medium is contained in a cavity between a partially reflecting mirror and a totally reflecting mirror.

The number of photons is amplified on each traverse as they are reflected back and forth in the laser tube before being allowed to escape as a laser beam through the partially reflecting mirror. The outside energy source required to pump the medium comes from either an electrical or radiofrequency source. There is a focusing lens to direct the laser beam to the delivery system, which could be, for example, a handpiece, microscope or colposcope adapter or endoscope coupler.

The resulting laser beam is monochromatic (consisting of one wavelength and hence color), collimated (nondivergent and parallel), and coherent (synchronized as a result of the characteristic single wavelength). For three reasons, laser light can be effectively focused to precise spots of energy and applied to tissue.

The interaction of laser light with biological material can be described in terms of reflection, scattering, transmission, and absorption. In addition, Table 3.5 shows the characteristic types, which have a particular tissue reaction and depth of thermal damage.

Absorption causes the conversion of light energy to heat energy. The carbon dioxide laser is the most easily absorbed by water, and hence tissue, which makes it the most useful for cutting and vaporization of small vessels, such as its use as a laser scalpel or for ablating cells. The Nd: YAG laser [yttrium aluminum garnet doped with neodymium (Nd^{3+})] scatters its light over a broader volume of tissue, causing coagulation at depths of about 5 mm in tissue. It will vaporize at a higher power but leaves a crater of coagulation at the base. Argon and KTP (potassium titanyl phosphate, 532 nm) lasers produce superficial coagulation, causing necrosis at 0.5–2 mm depth. Argon is selectively absorbed by red pigments and so has been used for removing port wine stains and for coagulating blood. Vaporization of tissue occurs when the fluid is heated to above 100 °C; steam and cellular debris are produced as a laser plume.

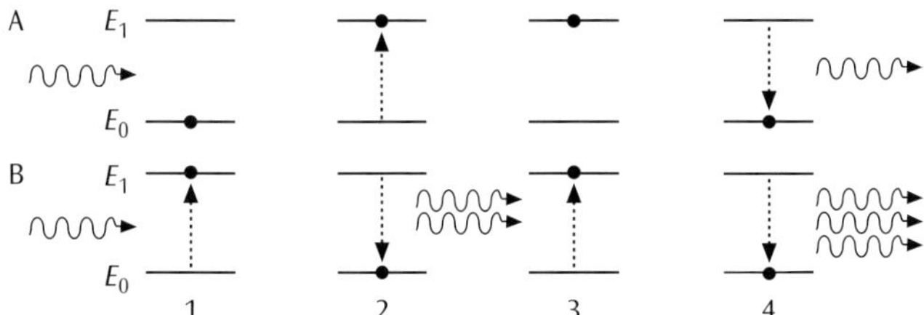

Figure 3.17 *Comparison of spontaneous and stimulated emission of photons. (A) Spontaneous emission. Energized electrons decay back to their original orbit with the spontaneous production of a photon. (B) Stimulated emission. Energized electrons in a substance which has undergone population inversion in which most of the atoms are in an excited state. Each interaction with an atom stimulates the emission of another photon with the same wavelength and phase and direction.*

Laser safety considerations

Laser products are grouped in to four classes according to degree of hazard (Table 3.6); the higher the class number, the more stringent the safety measures required. The eye is the organ most likely to sustain laser damage, so the operator should wear protective goggles and the patient's eyes should also be protected.

Each hospital using lasers should appoint a laser protection officer and maintain a register of authorized users. The safety requirements for a particular working area and safe working practice are typically defined locally and include safety procedures and operator/staff responsibilities for each laser. In addition, general safety measures such as displaying warning signs in laser-controlled areas and the institution of key-operated laser controls should be implemented.

There are special considerations when lasers are used in the operating room. The use of lasers in or around patient airways necessitates special measures, including the use of laser-proof endotracheal tubes, the use of wet fire-retardant drapes around the operation site, and the use of nonreflective surgical instruments.

Mandatory European requirements are stated in The Health & Safety at Work Act 1974 and the Safety Standards in IEC 60825:2001 – *Radiation Safety of Laser Products, Equipment Classification Requirements and Users' Guide*. A further document is DoH (MDA) 1996 – *Guidance on the Safe Use of Lasers in Medical and Dental Practice*. In the USA, the regulation on lasers is known as 21 CFR 1040.10. This is out of step with

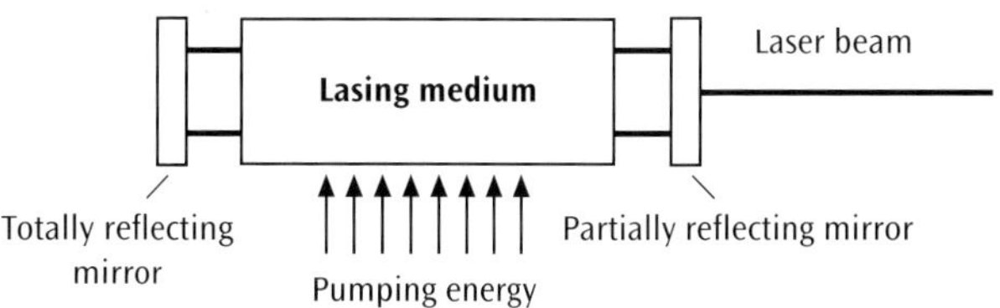

Figure 3.18 *Basic components of a laser delivery tube. Light produced by stimulated emission of photons is reflected between the mirrors until the beam leaves the chamber through the partially reflective mirror.*

Type	Color	Wavelength (nm)	Power (W)	Depth of absorption (mm)
CO_2	Infrared	10 600	25	0.1–0.2
Argon	Blue/green	488/515	5	1–2
Nd:YAG	Infrared	1064	100	3–5

Table 3.5 *Characteristics of commonly used lasers*

Class	Safety measure
1	Inherently safe in all conditions. Few medical lasers fall within this category
2	Low-power devices emitting light in the visible range, 400–700 nm. Output power limited to 1 mW
3A	Lasers operating in the visible range up to 5 mW
3B	Emit in range 180 nm to 1 mm. Power up to 0.5 W according to wavelength
4	High-power devices operating in any part of the spectrum. Potential fire hazard

Table 3.6 *Classes of lasers according to degree of hazard*

the IEC/ EN standard but a notice in May 2001 was issued by the US FDA, which now accepts IEC classification and labeling.

SURGICAL DIATHERMY

Surgical diathermy units consist of high-voltage (approximately 1500 V), high-frequency (500 kHz to 1.5 MHz) current generators. They operate by cutting tissue cleanly or by coagulating blood vessels or may incorporate a blend feature that cuts and coagulates in one go (Fig. 3.19).

There are two types: monopolar or bipolar. The monopolar type contains two electrodes. The main cutting electrode is a small needle-shaped electrode in which the current density is high because of the small contact area; this causes localized heating and cutting of the tissue. The other electrode is the patient return plate, a large electrode attached to the thigh. The current density in this electrode is much lower and is dissipated over the large contact area; no heating occurs at this point and thus there is no tissue damage. A power of up to 400 W is used for cutting and up to 200 W for coagulation or a blend.

Bipolar diathermy units are used to seal and coagulate small vessels, with power levels limited to 50 W. The active and return electrodes are the same size, usually the two blades of a forceps electrode. The vessels are held between the points of the electrodes and are sealed when the coagulator is activated.

Some precautions are necessary for the safe use of these devices. In monopolar diathermy, if the large return plate (low-impedance path to earth) is not firmly attached to the patient, localized heating can occur at the points where the plate is in contact with the patient and burns may result. Burns may also occur at the site of ECG electrodes in these circumstances.

All diathermy units are manufactured to IEC601-1 and have inbuilt safety features to minimize the risks of problems occurring. These include plate voltage and plate earth monitoring. In the former, an alarm will sound if the return plate is poorly connected to the patient and also if the plate is disconnected. In the latter, the impedance between the patient and earth is monitored so that an alarm sounds if the patient accidentally comes into contact with something earthed. In the case of the bipolar configuration, an alarm will sound if the impedance between the parts of the forceps is too high.

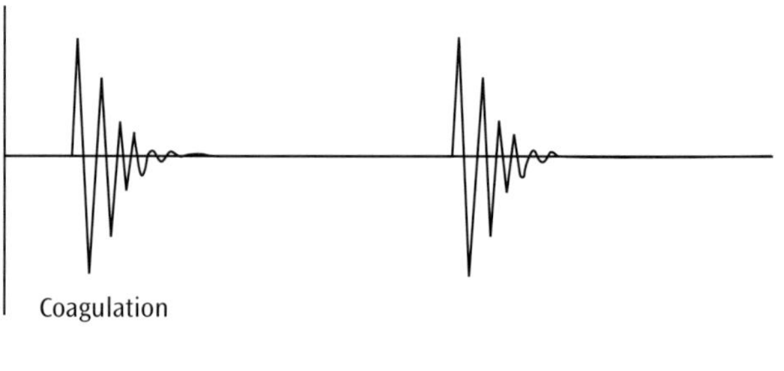

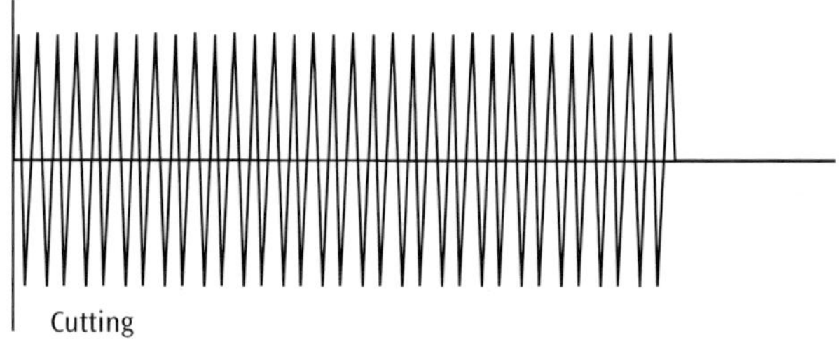

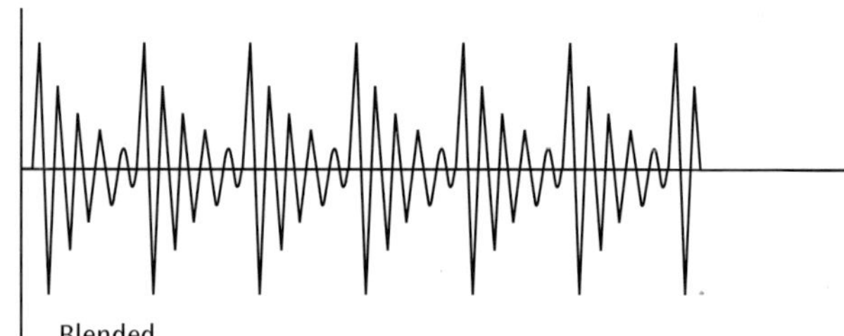

Figure 3.19 *Surgical diathermy waveforms. The different waveforms are shown for coagulation, cutting, and a blend of both.*

STIMULATORS

The nerve stimulators used in the operating room or intensive care unit are usually small and battery operated (9 V) for safety and ease of use. Mains-powered stimulators are usually part of an EMG recording system. They deliver monophasic, square pulses of width 0.1–0.3 ms as a constant-current output, adjusting the current as an ohmic relation according to the perceived electrode–skin impedance at the time of stimulation. Biphasic pulses and increased width of stimulus beyond the refractory period of the nerve may cause repetitive action potentials. The output is generally expected to be variable to a maximum of between 50 and 70 mA, delivering 200–400 V through a 2.5–3 kV load. There are two factors to be considered in the specification: the current required for supramaximal stimulation and the skin-electrode impedance, which influences the stimulator output. Supramaximal stimulation occurs when all the nerve fibers are activated; it ensures a consistent stimulus effect in an individual subject and enables a graded decrement in response to be attributed to neuromuscular block. Supramaximal stimulation is achieved by increasing the stimulating current until a level is reached at which there is no further increase in amplitude of the muscle response. This threshold of current output has been quoted as being in the range 15–40 mA in 75% of patients using surface electrodes and stimulating the ulnar nerve.

CARDIAC DEFIBRILLATORS

A defibrillator is a stimulator that delivers an electric shock to the myocardium of the heart in order to re-establish a normal cardiac rhythm by terminating ventricular fibrillation and arrhythmias. Defibrillation is achieved by passing current either through electrodes placed directly on the heart or through large-area, thoracic electrodes. A short current pulse is produced by discharging a capacitor through the electrodes. The delivered energy is given by:

$$\text{Delivered energy (J)} = \tfrac{1}{2} I^2 R t$$

where I is the peak current, R is the chest impedance, and t is the duration of the waveform. The delivered energy may be as high as 400 J when using chest electrodes. As the resistance of a human thorax is about 50 V, defibrillators are rated on the ability to deliver energy through this value of resistance. The energy stored in the capacitor is given by:

$$\text{Energy} = CV^2/2$$

where C is the capacitance and V is the voltage to which it is charged. The value of capacitors in defibrillators ranges from 10 to 50 µF, so that the voltage must range from 2 to 9 kV in order to deliver energies in this region. In practice, the capacitor is discharged through an inductor, which gives a characteristic discharge pulse shape that significantly reduces the peak voltage to the patient and lengthens the pulse duration so as to prevent defibrillation.

Defibrillators are of three types: manual, semiautomatic, and automatic. Manual defibrillators incorporate an ECG monitor and usually have a synchronicity selector, which synchronizes delivery of the waveform at the peak of the R-wave in atrial fibrillation or cardioversion of ventricular tachycardia. The operator decides if a defibrillatory shock is indicated, and the strength of the shock is set manually. Semiautomatic defibrillators analyze the ECG and indicate whether defibrillation is appropriate, alerting the operator by sound or screen message before they then make the decision to give a predetermined shock. Automatic defibrillators analyze cardiac rhythms and deliver a shock to a patient in ventricular fibrillation without the need for any further operator action. They are designed to be used by first aid personnel and lay people in order to promote early defibrillation, but the safety aspects of such devices are crucial as these give relatively untrained users the ability to deliver lethal shocks. These devices are small, light, durable, and are capable of being stored ready charged for prolonged periods of time.

The delivered energy from a capacitor used to depolarize the myocardium is normally 200 or 360 J. Optimal depolarization of the myocardium depends on the current delivered, which in turn depends on body size, electrode position, energy of the shock, and the impedance of the tissues of the thorax. Delivered energy is less than the stored energy in the capacitor, normally rated as that energy delivered to a 50-Ω resistor. Improved defibrillator design incorporates battery enhancement and the use of impedance-compensating and voltage-adjusting waveforms, as in automatic external defibrillators. The impedance compensation method of waveform adjustment allows an appropriate effective shock dose that reduces the risk of refibrillation within the patient. Biphasic defibrillation waveforms have been found to have distinct advantages over monophasic waveforms. Monophasic waveforms are either damped sinusoidal (Lown) or truncated exponential. Biphasic waveforms, in which the current flows in both positive and negative directions through the heart, are attracting interest following research findings using implantable cardioverter defibrillators. This type of waveform allows defibrillation to be achieved at lower energy levels than with monophasic waveforms. This implies that devices can be developed which are more compact and portable because of the lower battery requirements and cause less damage to the myocardium at the time of application. Some commercially available biphasic defibrillators are now licensed for use in the UK and USA (American Heart Association class IIb recommended) and deliver a 150-J biphasic shock with equivalent efficacy to 200-J or 360-J monophasic shocks.

CARDIAC PACEMAKERS

A cardiac pacemaker is a type of stimulator that delivers electrical pulses to electrodes at the surface of the heart in order to reproduce the action potentials that provide the pumping action. There are two types: asynchronous pacemakers, which produce a constant train of pulses of a fixed frequency regardless of the heart activity, and synchronous pacemakers, which produce pulses in the absence of any intrinsic depolarization of the heart.

Pacemakers are also either unipolar or bipolar, which refers to the relative position of the electrodes. In a unipolar configuration, an electrode is placed on the heart with the other indifferent electrode situated elsewhere on the body; it requires negative directional pulses from the source. In the bipolar configuration, both electrodes are within the heart. Unipolar systems allow external checking on the outer electrode but tend also to be more susceptible to external electromagnetic interference.

The generic pacemaker code describes pacemaker function in five letters (Table 3.7). The first three letters describe the mode of pacing. The first letter indicates the chamber being paced; this is either atrium

Table 3.7 *Generic pacemaker code*

	I	II	III	IV	V
Category	**Chamber(s) paced**	**Chamber(s) sensed**	**Response to sensing**	**Programmability, rate modulation**	**Antitachycardia functions**
	O = None	O = None	O = None	O = None	O = None
	A = Atrium	A = Atrium	T = Triggered	P = Simple programmable	P = Pacing
	V = Ventricle	V = Ventricle	I = Inhibited	M = Multiprogrammable	S = Shock
	D = Dual (A + V)	D = Dual (A + V)	D = Dual (T + I)	C = Communicating	D = Dual (P + S)
				R = Rate modulation	

(A), ventricle (V), dual (D) (i.e. A + V), or neither (O). The second letter indicates the chamber in which the activity is sensed (A, V, D, or O), and the third describes the response of the pacemaker [none (O), triggered (T), inhibited (I), or dual (D) (i.e. T + I)]. The fourth letter describes special programmability, rate modulation, and the fifth antitachycardia functions.

The asynchronous modes are VOO, AOO, and DOO; in these cases, cardiac stimulation is independent of the intrinsic activity of the heart and paces at a fixed rate. Stimulation may compete with the normal heart rhythm and induce atrial flutter or fibrillation, so these modes are used only to test the pacing function or to check pacemaker-mediated tachycardias.

Synchronous or demand modes are atrial (AAI and AAT) or ventricular (VVI and VVT) or dual chamber (VAT, VDD, DVI, DDD). The atrial demand mode is utilized in patients with sinus node dysfunction caused by atrioventricular conduction defect or sick sinus syndrome: the electrode is situated in the right atrium and the ventricle is depolarized through the atrioventricular conduction system. In ventricular demand mode, the right ventricle is the site of the sensing and pacing; this is the mode used mostly to treat bradycardia. Dual-chamber pacing modes provide a synchronized atrioventricular depolarization. The DVI mode paces both the atrium and ventricle with a preset atrioventricular interval after sensing the atrium. The DDD modes senses both chambers.

Other pacemakers sense external stimuli, such as increased heart rate due to the demand of exercise, and increase the pacer rate appropriately. These sensors, which are usually piezoelectric or accelerometers, detect changes with, for example, respiration, QT interval, muscle activity, central temperature, movement, or transthoracic electrical impedance. Rate-adaptive pacemakers are indicated by the letter in the fourth position, e.g. VVIR, DVIR, DDDR. Antitachycardia pacemakers are relatively uncommon as treatment with radiofrequency ablation methods is available.

The asynchronous pacemaker is the simplest design and involves a free-running constant stream of pulses from a logic circuit or microprocessor triggered from a timing circuit. They can be either constant voltage, usually 5–6 V with a pulse width of 500–600 μs, or constant current, 8–10 mA with a pulse width of 1–1.2 ms.

Synchronous pacemakers, which provide intermittent stimulation, fall into two categories, the demand type and the atrial-synchronous type. Demand pacemakers are similar to synchronous pacemakers but have a feedback loop in the circuit which detects the natural ECG signal and uses it to reset the timing circuit so that it remains in standby mode for the appropriate interval or provides a stimulus if the heart has not produced one itself.

Atrial-synchronous circuits detect atrial contraction corresponding to the natural pacemaker of the heart at the sinoatrial node. They are designed to stimulate the atrium to contract and then provide a stimulus to the atrioventricular node, which in turn will stimulate the ventricles after an appropriate delay. Thus, these pacemakers mimic the natural process involved in initiating the heart's pumping action. These functions are carried out by microprocessors in the pacemaker. The newer types of pacemakers, which incorporate control systems to cope with the demands of a changing heart rate brought about by physiological changes, utilize electrocardiogram analysis algorithms; sensors differentiate between physiological and pathological changes in hemodynamic behavior and adapt the voltage to the controller accordingly.

The leads used with pacemakers usually consist of a helical coil of multistranded wire molded into silicone rubber or a polyurethane cylinder. This coil design is mechanically strong, as it needs to be to withstand the heart's pumping action. The multistrands allow conduction to be maintained should some of the integrity of the wire be lost. The silicone construction allows flexibility and maintains electrical insulation. The electrode construction requirements are similar; they are usually constructed from platinum or its alloys, stainless steel, carbon, or titanium. They must withstand the same rigorous treatment from the heart's mechanical action and also be inherently stable so that they do not deteriorate over time. In addition, they should be of material that does not cause any tissue interaction or scarring when *in situ*.

ELECTRONIC MEASUREMENT OF TEMPERATURE

Most clinical temperature monitoring devices use platinum resistance, mercury in glass, thermocouples or thermistors to measure temperature (Table 3.8).

Thermocouples

Thomas J Seebeck (1821) discovered that an electromotive force (e.m.f.) exists across a junction of two dissimilar metals as a result of the diffusion of electrons across the junction in unequal numbers. Jean P Peltier (1834) is accredited with the discovery that as the diffusion increases with temperature so does the potential between the metals. The net Peltier e.m.f. is proportional to the temperatures difference between the two junctions. The net e.m.f. is proportional to the difference between the squares of the absolute junction temperatures (Thomson effect). The net e.m.f. at the junction is a function of the difference in temperature of the two junctions and the properties of the two metals. One junction is held at a constant known temperature for reference in order to determine the unknown temperature. Increased sensitivity is achieved by connecting a number of thermocouples in series. A direct readout of the thermocouple voltage can be achieved using a digital voltmeter. The advantages of thermocouples are their fast response time (~ 1 ms), small size (they can be inserted into catheters), and long-term stability.

Table 3.8 *Thermometer properties*

Type	Thermometric property	Advantages	Disadvantages
Mercury in glass (−39 °C to 450 °C)	Length of column of mercury	Portable Direct reading	Fragile
Platinum resistance (−180 °C to 1150 °C)	Electrical resistance of platinum coil (measured by Wheatstone bridge)	Very accurate Wide thermal range	Slow response time
Thermocouple (−250 °C to 1150 °C)	EMF produced between dissimilar metals (copper and constantan or iron and constantan) (constantan is 60% copper and 40% nickel)	Small Very sensitive Rapid response time	Less accurate than platinum resistance
Thermistor	Semiconductor. Resistance falls as temperature rises		Nonlinear. May require recalibration after a period of time

They can be made to have an accuracy better than 0.01 °C with careful design and are superior to thermistors for accurate measurement. Their disadvantages are the small output voltage, low sensitivity, and the need for a reference temperature (which is often supplied with a semiconductor reference element).

Thermistors

Thermistors are semiconductor devices made from ceramic materials which have a high negative temperature coefficient. The resistance of thermistors decreases as temperature increases and increases as temperature decreases, and the change may be as great as 5% for each degree centigrade increase in temperature. Thermistors are small, so that they may be placed in hyperdermic needles or in catheter tips. They are usually glass-encapsulated beads when used clinically so as to protect the element without significantly affecting the thermal response time. They are also very stable devices. A bridge circuit and a differential amplifier used to complete the temperature measuring device give high sensitivity and good accuracy and can be used to measure minute differences in temperature. The circuit gives a linear output change with temperature by applying a constant voltage to the thermistor and monitoring its current output. For use in neonates the thermal contact with skin can be monitored by applying a 14-s pulse every 4.5 min and measuring the resultant temperature rise.

FURTHER READING

Blum LJ, Coulet PR. *Biosensor Principles and Applications*. New York, NY: Marcel Dekker, 1991.

Carr JJ, Brown JM. *Introduction to Biomedical Equipment Technology*, 2nd edn. Englewood Cliffs, NJ: Prentice Hall,1993.

Geddes LA, Baker LE. *Principles of Applied Biomedical Instrumentation*. New York, NY: Wiley, 1989.

Sykes MK, Vickers MD, Hull CJ. *Principles of Measurement and Monitoring in Anaesthesia and Intensive Care*. Oxford: Blackwell Scientific Publications, 1991.

Webster JG (ed.). *Medical Instrumentation. Application and Design*. New York: Wiley, 1998.

APPENDIX

Markings on medical electrical equipment according to IEC601-1: 1988 Medical Electrical Equipment, Part I: *General Requirements for Safety (Amendments 1991 and 1995).*

Note There is no symbol for class I equipment

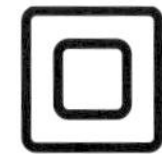

Class II equipment

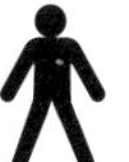

Type B equipment

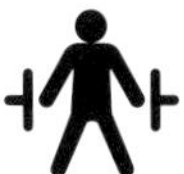

Type B with defibrillator protection

Type BF equipment

Type BF with defibrillator protection

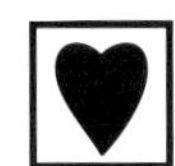

Type CF equipment

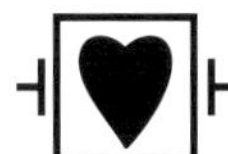

Type CF with defibrillator protection

4

Statistics for the anesthesiologist

NADER D NADER, CYNTHIA A WALAWANDER, AND THADDEUS H GRASELA

Information is abundant in today's world. Statistics can and should be used as a vehicle to turn quantitative information into knowledge, thereby assisting clinicians in the important medical decision-making process. No individual patient is a statistic, but understanding what has happened in a population of patients can guide clinicians in diagnosing and treating individual patients and, importantly, provides a basis on which to talk to patients about choices and decisions involved in their medical care. If all treatments or diagnosis decisions were clear cut, probability and statistics would not be necessary. However, every individual is unique, and variation and uncertainty exist in every situation, "except for death and taxes" (according to Benjamin Franklin). The science of probability and statistics simply quantifies the degree of uncertainty and helps to identify sources of variation that may affect the outcome for a patient in order to minimize the random causes of variation that are uncontrollable. The basic science of statistics and probability is a valuable tool in the armamentarium of every clinician.

DATA TYPES

Quantitative information is the basis of probability and statistics. Numbers and factual information can take on several data formats (e.g. discrete, continuous) and, depending on the format of the data, the analysis and interpretation will vary. Data are described as discrete if they form a scale comprising distinct numbers with gaps in between; examples include the number of surgical procedures performed, race, and gender. Continuous data can take any value within an interval and there are no gaps between numbers; examples include patient height and the length of a surgical procedure. A patient can undergo surgery for 1.567 h (continuous data) but cannot undergo 1.567 surgical procedures (only one or two); thus, numbers of procedures must be discrete data. Further, discrete data can be subclassified into nominal or ordinal data, and continuous data can be subclassified into interval or ratio data.

Nominal data are defined as categories without order, and one category does not have more weight than another. Eye color and comorbidities (e.g. a patient either has hypertension or does not) are examples of nominal data. Both types of data can be represented by numbers, and this conversion is necessary when using a statistical software package for analysis (i.e. 0 = no hypertension, 1 = hypertension exists; or 1 = blue eyes, 2 = brown eyes, etc.).

Ordinal data have an order, but the difference between consecutive data points is not necessarily constant. Physical status as defined by the American Society of Anesthesiologists (ASA) is ordinal. The difference between ASA class 1 and 2 is not necessarily equal to the difference between ASA class 3 and 4. Similarly, case classification such as emergent, urgent, or elective assumes that an emergent case is higher risk than an urgent case, but the difference in risk is not quantifiable.

Both interval and ratio data are ordered and there is equal distance between consecutive data points. Interval data that lie on a scale that includes an absolute zero are called ratio data. Temperature values in kelvin are considered to be ratio data because a zero temperature has physical significance and because a temperature of 20 kelvin is twice as warm as a temperature of 10 kelvin. Height, weight, and surgery duration are also considered to be ratio data. Interval data do not have to be relative to the zero point. Temperature values measured in degrees Celsius are not relative to the zero point, i.e. 20 °C is not twice as warm as 10 °C but the difference between 10 °C and 11 °C is the same as the difference between 20 °C and 21 °C.

PROBABILITY

Probability is the chance of a particular event happening. If the probability of postoperative nausea and vomiting (PONV) were found to be 0 (PONV never happens) or 1 (PONV always happens) there would no interest in further study of PONV from a statistical viewpoint. If the probability of occurrence of PONV is found to lie somewhere between 0 and 1, then statistical uncertainty exists and further study to identify who will or will not experience PONV or what medication might reduce the probability of developing PONV will be of value. Thus, when reporting probability values it is important to report the characteristics of the patient sample in which the probability was determined. For instance, did the PONV event occur within a certain time period after surgery or were the patients all undergoing a specific surgical procedure?

POPULATION, SAMPLES, AND SAMPLING

As over 12 million surgical procedures are performed annually in the USA alone,[1] to determine the number of patients in the USA who experience PONV each year would be a daunting task. The first question to ask is whether the 12 million patients undergoing surgical procedures in the USA is truly the target group or population of interest. It might be the case that target group is in fact women in the USA or patients who have been administered a particular opiate regardless of where in the world they are. Correctly identifying the population of interest is the first step in a sound statistical analysis. Once the population is identified, a sample or a subgroup of the population is selected to calculate the portion of patients who experience a particular event. Ways of selecting a sample of patients and how to determine the number of patients who should be sampled are discussed later in this chapter. Once the sample is selected, it is easy to calculate the frequency of occurrence of PONV by dividing the number of patients in the sample who experienced PONV by the total number of patients in the sample. Almost certainly, the rate of PONV in the sample of patients selected will not be exactly the same as the percentage in the true population, but it will be close. Defining "likely" or "close to" with more precision in the face of uncertainty is an important objective of statistics.

To illustrate this, one can test several samples from a population and calculate the percentage of interest for each sample. A simple experiment is to pull random samples of M&M's from a 1-lb bag. Randomly select 10 M&M's (sample), count how many are brown (event), and work out the percentage of the sample which are brown. Return the M&M's to the bag once the percentage of brown sweets has been calculated. Repeat this process 100 times. Determine the number of samples with 0–10 brown M&M's and plot the results on a graph (Fig. 4.1). As shown in the figure, even when the population is well defined, the samples drawn will present a variety of results. Defining the center and spread of the distribution is the basis for understanding the precision of the sample drawn and in determining statistical significance. The mean of the distribution of samples was 2.8 brown M&M's per sample. In the entire bag of M&M's from which the samples were drawn, there were 140 brown sweets out of a total of 530 (26.4%); in other words, the true number of brown M&M's in every 10 is 2.6 compared with a value of 2.8 obtained by sampling.

DISTRIBUTION SHAPE

The most common measures used to describe the central tendency of a frequency distribution are mean, median, and mode. The arithmetic mean is obtained by summing the measured value for each observation across observations then dividing by the total number of observations and is algebraically represented in equation 4.1.

$$\bar{x} = \frac{\sum_{i=1}^{N} x_i}{N} \quad (4.1)$$

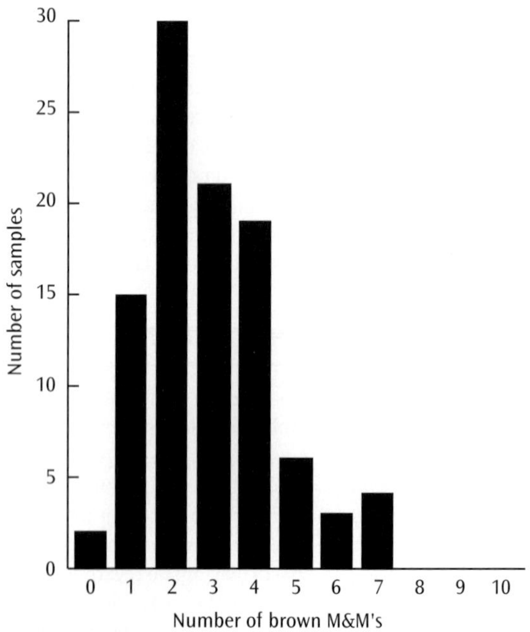

Figure 4.1 *Frequency distribution of M&M's across 100 samples.*

where $\bar{x}$ is the arithmetic mean, N is total number of observations, x_i is the random variable representing the values measured in the sample, and Σ is the symbol for summing across the N observations in the sample. The arithmetic mean is also commonly known as the balancing point of the distribution. Imagine balancing a pencil on your finger. The point at which the pencil meets your finger and the pencil is balanced is considered the mean point.

The median is a nonparametric method of measuring the center of a distribution. Nonparametric data are data for which the shape of the relative frequency distribution is unknown. Several parametric distributions are discussed later in the chapter. The calculation of the median is based on the ranking of the data and not the actual values of the data. The data are sorted in ascending order and the median is defined as the value above which half of the data points fall and below which half fall. The median is less affected by extreme variation in data and is generally used when outliers are present. The mode is defined as the most frequently occurring value of the data. If the mean, median, and mode are the same value, the greatest density of the distribution is located in the center of the range of values and it is a called symmetric distribution. If the median is smaller than the mean, the distribution is right skewed as a result of large observations (possible outliers) on the data scale. If the median is larger than the mean, then the distribution is left skewed.

To complete our understanding of the shape of a distribution, it is necessary to examine the spread of the distribution. The amount of variation around the distribution center is important in order to understand the precision of the mean or median. Understanding the sources of variation allows one to reduce variation and increase precision of the point estimate. It is possible for two different distributions to have the exact same center but for the amount of variation around the center to be extremely different. Common measures of the distribution spread are the range, variance, and standard deviation. Range is usually used for nonparametric data and refers to the difference between the minimum and the maximum data value. The interquartile range is the difference between the first quartile (the value below which 25% of data fall and above which 75% of the data fall) and the third quartile (the value below which 75% of the data fall and above which 25% of the data fall) and comprises the middle 50% of the data. The sample variance is the sum of the deviations from the center of the distribution squared and divided by the total number of observations minus 1 and is algebraically represented in equation 4.2. The sample standard deviation is simply the square root of the sample variance. The standard error of the mean is the sample standard deviation divided by the square root of the total number of observations.

$$s^2 = \frac{\sum_{i=1}^{N} \left(x_i - \bar{x}\right)^2}{N} \quad (4.2)$$

A point estimate such as the mean or median alone does not provide a full description of the data. When describing a distribution, reporting of the point estimate should always be accompanied by a measure of spread. For example, data can be described nonparametrically using the median and range. Alternatively, parametric data can be displayed using the mean ± standard deviation or the standard error of the mean. The standard deviation is used to describe variability of a distribution, whereas the standard error is used to describe the precision of the point estimate. Another summary measure useful in describing the precision of the estimate is the coefficient of variation, which is the ratio of the sample standard deviation to the sample mean.

Visual representation of a frequency distribution will help in understanding the data being examined. There are several ways of graphing data. A histogram, as shown in Fig. 4.1, can be used to represent discrete or continuous data. With discrete data, the classifications or categories of the data are presented on the x-axis or horizontal axis. The relative frequency of the category is presented on the y-axis. With continuous data, the range of data must be determined, and from this equal intervals are identified and plotted along the x-axis. The relative frequency is the number of occurrences of data within the defined intervals divided by the total number of data points. Boxplots are used to display non-parametric data in graph form. Such plots display the minimum, first quartile, median, third quartile, and maximum value of a distribution, as shown in Fig. 4.2. Plotting boxplots of comparison groups is a good visual aid to identify differences between groups.

The box represents the first quartile, median, and third quartile. The lines extend to the minimum and maximum duration.

PROBABILITY DISTRIBUTIONS

A percentage is calculated based on one sample and hence differs slightly from a probability, in that a percentage achieves the limit of a probability when a very large number of samples are used to calculate the result. This concept applies similarly to the relation between a frequency distribution and a probability distribution. Probability distributions are usually denoted in terms of a random variable. The random variable, usually represented by a capital italic letter such as X, is an observed value that occurs as a result of an experiment. Therefore, the values of a random variable cannot be determined with certainty before the performance of the experiment. When calculating the mean age of a random sample of patients ($\bar{x}$) the random variable X represents the age of each patient in the sample of patients observed. The probability associated with all the possible values of a random variable in a population is called the probability distribution. The mean of a probability distribution is the correlate of the mean of a frequency distribution and is represented by the Greek letter μ. Similarly, the variance of the probability distribution is represented by the Greek letter σ. Probability distributions have been extensively studied, and there are several standard models which apply to many models in nature. These distributions are used in a variety of statistical tests and are described below.

Binomial distribution

The binomial distribution is a discrete probability distribution. The binomial distribution determines the probability of an outcome after repeated, independent, identical experiments. Each experiment has two possible outcomes and the probability of the outcome remains the same for all experiments. For example, the probability that 9 out of 10 patients will have a right-dominant blood supply given that the probability of blood supply to the sinus node from the right coronary artery is 0.55 and from the left coronary artery is 0.45 can be determined using the binomial distribution. The algebraic notation of the binomial distribution is described in equation 4.3.

$$\frac{n!}{r!(n-r)!} \times p^{r} \times q^{(n-r)} \tag{4.3}$$

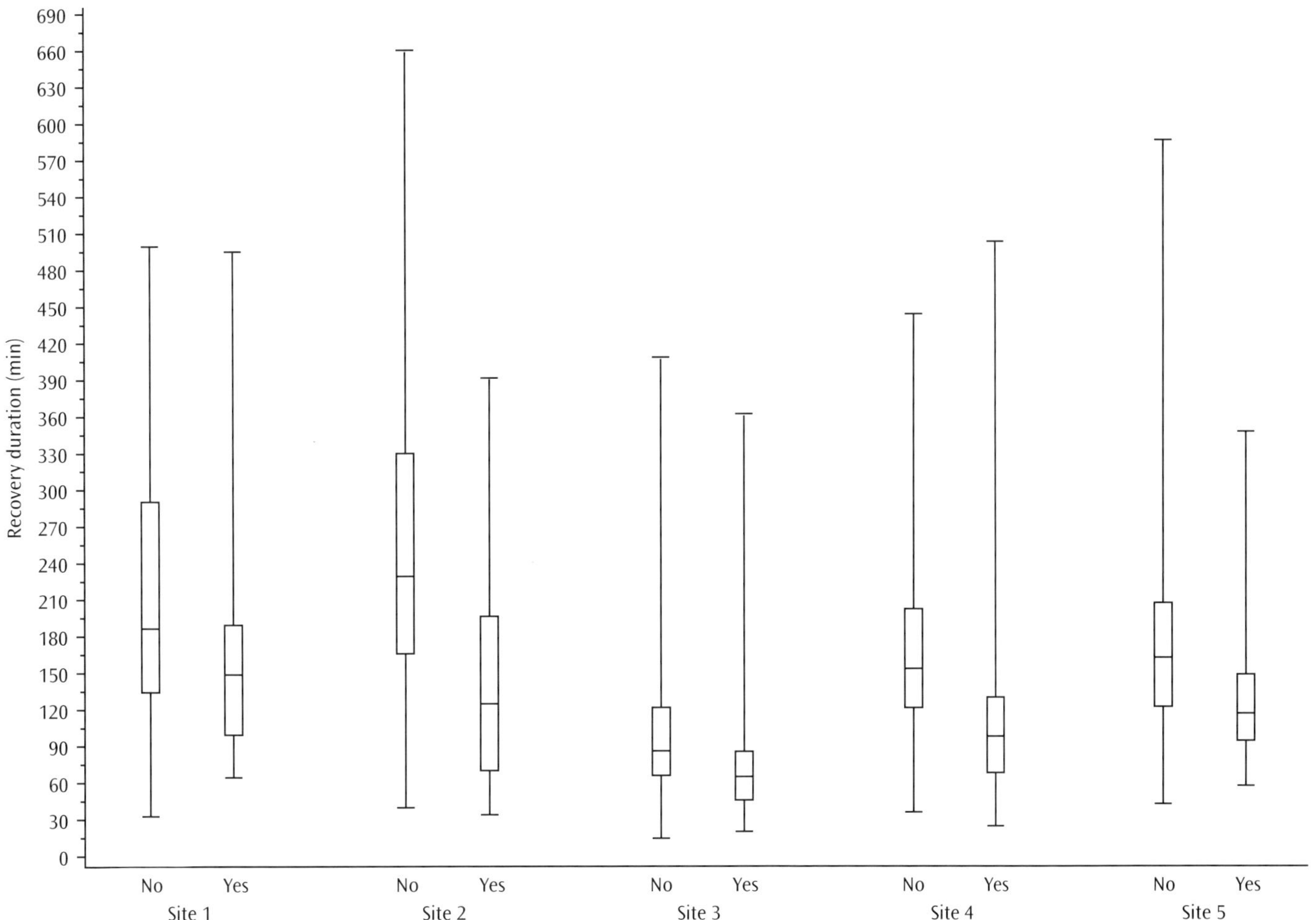

Figure 4.2 *Boxplots of total recovery duration in patients receiving a general anesthetic and stratified by facility and whether the patient bypassed the postanesthesia care unit. No, Yes – patients bypassed the PACU.*

where $n!$ is n factorial, which is the product of integers from 1 to n, i.e. 4 factorial $= 1 \times 2 \times 3 \times 4$; n is the number of trials; r is the number of favorable outcomes; p is the probability of the favorable outcome occurring; and q is $(1-p)$. The above example results in a probability of 0.026 that nine patients will have a right-dominant blood supply, and the calculation is shown in equation 4.4.

$$\frac{10!}{9! \times (10-9)!} \times 0.55^9 \times 0.45^1 = 0.026 \text{ probability} \qquad (4.4)$$

The mean of the binomial distribution is calculated by multiplying the number of experiments by the probability of a favorable outcome ($n \times p$) and the variance is calculated by multiplying the number of experiments by the probability of a favorable outcome by the probability of a negative outcome ($n \times p \times q$). When a large number of experiments are performed and the probability of outcome is approximately 0.5, the binomial distribution approximates a normal distribution. There are also several derivatives of the binomial distribution, such as the geometric distribution (used when addressing the question that probability of the first success will occur on the xth trial), the hypergeometric distribution (used when the independent experiment assumption is not true), and the Poisson distribution (used when the probability of the outcome is very small). The Poisson distribution will approximate the binomial distribution when the number of trials becomes infinitely large and the probability of outcomes approaches zero.

Normal distribution

The normal distribution generally describes continuous data and is referred to as a probability density function. The normal distribution is the foundation for much of statistical theory and has several distinguishing characteristics, as described in Table 4.1.

From the normal distribution for small sample sizes, several sampling distributions can be derived and are heavily utilized in statistical inference. The chi-squared distribution, the t-distribution, and the F-distribution are the most common distributions used in statistical inference. The t-distribution is used when the population mean and standard deviation are unknown, but a sample mean and standard deviation are known. The F-distribution is used when the variances of two population samples are being compared. The F-distribution is the square of the t-distribution when the number of degrees of freedom is 1. The chi-squared distribution is commonly used when making inferences on categorical outcomes. When samples sizes are less than 30, the F-distribution and the chi-squared distribution no longer have the symmetry of the normal distribution. When samples sizes are greater than 30, these sampling distributions are approximated by the normal distribution.

Table 4.1 *Characteristics of a normal distribution*

The shape of the normal distribution is a bell curve
The curve is symmetric and has no skew (deviation of the distribution curve to the extreme right or left) or kurtosis (vertical flatness of distribution curve)
The tails of the curve never reaches the x-axis, although the tails approach zero
The values of mean, median, and mode are equal
When the mean = 0 and the standard deviation = 1, the distribution is referred to as the standard normal distribution
When the distribution has a normal distribution the following assumption applies: Mean ± 1 standard deviation represents approximately 68% of the data Mean ± 2 standard deviations represents approximately 95% of the data Mean ± 3 standard deviations represents approximately 99% of the data

STATISTICS

Statistics is a branch of mathematics dealing with the collection, analysis, interpretation, and presentation of masses of numerical data and can be defined into three categories: descriptive, estimation, and inferential.

Descriptive statistics

Descriptive statistics are exploratory in nature, and are used when the goal is to determine the type of data collected and to provide a visual inspection of the data. Summary statistics are calculated to make comparisons with relevant data in the literature. Data are graphically displayed to determine the underlying assumptions of the data and to determine if any outliers exist.

An outlier may be an error. In the case of a discrete variable, if the only possible values are yes or no, represented by 1 or 0, and a value of 2 exists in the dataset, it is clear that the correct value needs to be identified or it should be set to missing if the true value cannot be retrieved. With continuous data, outlier detection is often more controversial. Assume that a dataset contains a value of 550 lb (250 kg) for the weight of a man and that the next largest weight is 310 lb (140 kg). Although 550 lb is a large weight and an outlier, it may be an actual weight. To determine whether this value is an outlier, assess the other data in relation to this patient to determine whether this is a possible true value (history of hypertension or diabetes, not a pediatric patient, etc.) or refer back to the original source of the data. An outlier should be removed from the analysis only if there is assurance that something is wrong with the data, and this should be well documented. Another common practice in epidemiologic analyses, when the number of patients in a study is often large, is to replace values above either the 95th or 99th percentile with a missing value, without exploring reasons for the nature of observation. However, it is essential when doing this to analyze the data including the outliers and then to perform another analysis without the outliers and report differences between the analyses. The extent of missing data in a dataset must be reported and evaluated for potential bias. In an exploratory analysis, multidimensional data analyses should be performed either graphically or in tabular format to determine serendipitous results. In descriptive analyses, the main concern is not to determine statistical significance, but to understand what type of data were collected, to assess distributional assumptions, and to determine if any problems with the data exist.

Statistical estimation

Statistical estimation often involves calculating confidence intervals around a point estimate using the sampling distributions described above. An example of a point estimate can be the mean of the population, the difference between the means of two populations, the ratio of the means of two populations, or some other variant. The calculation of the confidence interval is generally as described in equation 4.5:

$$\text{mean} \pm (\text{standard error of the mean} \times \text{critical value of the distribution}) \qquad (4.5)$$

A 95% confidence interval for a point estimate consists of lower and upper limits, and the limits are defined such that in repeated sets of samples of the same size 95% of all such intervals would be expected to contain the point estimate. If the sample size is greater than 30, the critical values used in calculating confidence intervals assuming a normal distribution are as provided in Table 4.2.

Statistical inference

Statistical inference, the logical basis by which conclusions regarding populations are drawn from results obtained in a sample, is what is commonly seen in the medical literature. Statistical inference tests hypotheses. In statistical inference there are two types of variables. The response or dependent variable is the outcome predicted from other factors. The other factors are generally referred to as predictor or independent variables. A dependent variable is the alteration of mean arterial blood pressure in response to increasing doses of propofol (independent variable). Statistical inference requires the design of a research study.

RESEARCH STUDY DESIGN

Research designs can be broadly classified into experimental and observational. Both methods are discussed in this chapter. In designing a research study, there are key issues to be addressed, and these are given in Table 4.3. It is important in any research study to abide by the good clinical practice guidelines.[2]

Randomization and blinding

The most common experimental design in medicine is the randomized controlled clinical trial, in which a group of patients is assigned to receive an experimental drug while another group of patients, who have similar characteristics, receive a placebo or alternative treatment. The decision to use the experimental drug or alternative treatment is based on a randomization scheme. By randomly assigning subjects to a group, researchers can reduce the potential for differences between groups which may bias the study in some systematic way. If both groups have similar characteristics, the outcome of the factor being tested is the only uncontrolled factor, hence the term controlled clinical trial. A trial can be blinded (the patients do not know which treatment they have received) or double blinded (neither the patients nor the members of the research team know the treatment received). Blinding attempts to eliminate conscious or unconscious bias in conducting or interpreting the results of a study. The knowledge that a subject is to receive a particular treatment may create a bias in assignment of treatment or the consequent treatment course. A study is typically blinded until after the statistical analyses have been performed. As a general principle, the person assigning the treatment based on a randomization scheme should not have anything else to do with the study. The double-blind, randomized controlled clinical trial is the gold standard experimental design for clinical trials.

Trial designs

Different trial designs will necessitate different procedures for generating randomization schemes. Several experimental trial designs exist, including parallel groups, crossover designs, factorial designs, and sequential designs. The parallel group design is the simplest. In this design, a sequential list of subjects and treatment is generated and the treatment assignment is made. In the parallel design, subjects are allocated to one of multiple treatment arms and a between-group analysis is performed using a t-test, or an analysis of variance test when the outcome measure is continuous.

Table 4.2 *Critical values of the normal distribution*

α	Critical value
0.05	1.645
0.025	1.96
0.01	2.326
0.005	2.576

In a crossover design, a single patient receives multiple treatments that are separated by a washout period. In essence, each subject is serving as his or her own control. If the study design includes only two treatment arms, then all patients will receive both treatments. However, there are several variations of this design. If there are more than two treatments, a subject may still receive all treatments or may receive only a subset of the treatments based on the randomization scheme. A randomization scheme similar to the parallel group design is used, except that a patient is randomized to receive treatment A followed by treatment B or vice versa. A paired analysis or repeated measures analysis is typically performed for these trial designs. A major advantage of this design is that fewer subjects are needed. This pairing or matching process also reduces variability and increases the statistical power. A disadvantage of the trial design is the potential carry-over effect between treatments. Extra care is necessary to understand this carry-over effect and to assure that it does not affect the study results.

A factorial design can take many forms. Factorial designs are often selected when an interaction between experimental factors is of interest or when there is interest in controlling for confounding factors. As anesthetic regimens consist of multiple agents, a factorial design would be a beneficial approach. For example, hemodynamic changes in 83 ASA class I or II patients were monitored after induction using either thiopental or etomidate. Patients were grouped into 12 groups, by induction agent, pretreatment drug, and maintenance anesthetic technique.[3] This design allows the evaluation of two experimental variables and their interaction. The randomization scheme for these designs is constructed using randomized blocks. Subjects are stratified into groups or blocks based on certain characteristics and then the treatment is randomly assigned to the subject. There are several randomization schemes that can be used, such as the nested design or Latin square design. A variant of the two-factor analysis of variance test is used for analysis.

Sequential trial designs allow the potential for performing interim analyses. This type of design is typically used for large, long-term studies. However, if safety is a concern, a sequential trial design should be considered to allow the opportunity of curtailing a trial early if too many adverse events occur or, conversely, if a treatment is so beneficial that not giving the treatment to all patients would be unethical.

Multicenter studies must take special care with their randomization schemes. Often, each center is given its own randomization scheme as it is recruiting subjects from its own geographic region.

HYPOTHESIS TESTING

Although closely related to estimating confidence intervals, hypothesis testing has a slightly different orientation. When developing a confidence interval, sample data are used to estimate what is a likely set of values for the point estimate of interest. When performing a statistical test, sample data are used to test whether the estimated value for the point estimate is different enough from the hypothesized value to conclude that the null hypothesis is unlikely to be true. The null hypothesis is the statement of no difference between treatment groups. Table 4.4 shows the steps involved in hypothesis testing.

Based on the test statistic, a corresponding P-value is obtained, most commonly from one of the sampling distributions described above or the normal distribution. The P-value quantifies how unlikely the

Table 4.3 *Questions to answer before designing a research study*

What is the hypothesis of interest and has it been studied before?
What is the outcome being measured?
How many groups will be compared?
Will the comparator group be treated with a placebo or an already accepted standard treatment?
What is the expected difference in magnitude of effect between the groups?
What data need to be collected and how difficult are they to collect?
What patients will be included or excluded from the study?
How many subjects are required to measure the expected magnitude of effect?
How difficult will it be to recruit subjects for the study?
How long will a subject be on the treatment?
What statistical tests will be used to analyze the results?
Are there financial constraints?
Where will the study be performed?
Which audience will be reading and interpreting the study results?

Table 4.4 *Hypothesis testing*

Check the assumptions concerning the properties of the underlying variable(s) being measured that are needed to justify the use of the statistical test being considered
State the null hypothesis and the alternative hypothesis
Specify the significance level
Specify the test statistic to be used and its distribution under the null hypothesis
Form the decision rule of rejection and not rejecting the null hypothesis
Compute the value of the test statistic from the observed data
Draw your conclusions concerning rejection or nonrejection of the null hypothesis

observed results would be if the null hypothesis were true. The uncertainty present in statistics results in two types of errors in regards to hypothesis testing. as shown in Table 4.5. A type I error (alpha: α) occurs if the true state supports the null hypothesis but based on the observed data the alternative hypothesis is chosen. A type II error (beta: β) occurs if the true state supports the alternative hypothesis but the observed data support the null hypothesis. For a fixed sample size, the alpha and beta errors are inversely related. If a type I error is being guarded against by selecting a small rejection region, then the nonrejection area (β) will be large. Conversely, if a small nonrejection area (β) is selected, the rejection area will become larger (α). Increasing the sample size and fixing the type I error will generally decrease the type II error.

The correct sample size to be used in a study can be calculated using four parameters: the expected outcome of the experiment, the variability of the outcome, the type I error rate (α), and the power of the test. Power refers to the probability of avoiding a type II error ($1-\beta$), or the probability that the true state and the observed data both support the alternative hypothesis. Based on these parameters, a sample size is calculated. The exact formula for calculating the sample size is dependent on the statistical test being utilized. Many computer programs are available today for calculating the sample size and will not be discussed here. In medical studies, the significance level (α) is almost always defined as 0.05. When evaluating a study, it is important to calculate the power of the study, which can be calculated using the sample size formula and solving for the power of the test. The goal of a good experimental study is to be able to repeat the test and obtain similar results. To achieve this goal, controlling not only the α level, but also the power, is essential. If, based on the significance level, it is decided that the results are statistically significant but the power is low, then the sample statistic is unreliable and the reproducibility of the experiment is questionable.

By controlling for type I and type II errors, assigning treatments randomly to subjects, and blinding the study, the research design has a higher likelihood of producing valid and reliable results. There are other sources of bias that must be taken into consideration because they may affect the external validity of the statistical results. Selection or randomization bias, in which there is a systematic pattern to selecting patients for a treatment, is an example. For instance, patients with a higher risk profile might be more likely to get the gold standard treatment instead of the experimental drug or vice versa. Publication or commercially motivated bias is slanting the results, whether consciously or not, to please the affected audience. There are several other problems to avoid. An inappropriate trial design may not give the information needed to evaluate the outcome being studied. Incorrect statistical tests lead to misinterpretation of the study results. Deviation from the study protocol will render a study invalid unless these deviations have been approved by the principal investigator and written into the protocol as an addendum. A written, well-planned, sound research design is the foundation for any research study. It is wise to have the research design reviewed by a multidisciplinary group of colleagues, including a statistician or a clinician with extensive experience of statistics in the area of the research study.

STATISTICAL TESTS

Chi-squared test

The chi-squared test is the most commonly used statistical test to analyze ordinal or nominal data. The foundation of the chi-squared test is a 2×2 contingency table, i.e. a table with two columns and two rows. The word "contingency" indicates that the values in each cell of the table are contingent on what is happening at the marginals. Marginals are defined as the row totals or the column totals. As an example, the use of succinylcholine (suxamethonium) and its association with malignant hyperthermia was evaluated. A multicenter study revealed that a total of 10 000 patients undergoing general anesthesia received succinylcholine as a part of their anesthetic induction. Another 20 000 patients who were included in the study did not receive succinylcholine as a part of their anesthetic plan. The 2×2 table shown in Table 4.6 reports the incidence of malignant hyperthermia among patients exposed and not exposed to succinylcholine. The count of patients fitting into each of the defined cells is the observed value. The expected value is derived by multiplying the row marginal by the column marginal and dividing it by the total number of subjects. The chi-squared statistic is the sum of individual chi-squared values. The chi-squared statistic is calculated by squaring the ratio of the observed value minus the expected value and dividing by

Table 4.5 *Errors in hypothesis testing*

	True state	
Observed data	**No difference**	**Difference**
No difference	Correct decision $1-\alpha$	False negative Type II error $=\beta$
Difference	False positive Type I error $=\alpha$	Correct decision $1-\beta=$ power

Table 4.6 *Contingency table of the effect of succinylcholine on malignant hyperthermia*

		Malignant hyperthermia	Normal response	Total
Received succinylcholine	Observed	20	9980	10 000
	Expected	8	9992	
Did not receive succinylcholine	Observed	4	19 996	20 000
	Expected	16	19 984	
Total		24	29 976	30 000

the expected value, as shown in equation 4.6. The value obtained for the chi-squared statistic is cross-referenced to the tables of the chi-squared distribution to determine a *P*-value.

$$\sum \left(\frac{\left(O_{ij} - E_{ij}\right)^2}{E_{ij}} \right) \tag{4.6}$$

where O is the observed value, E is the expected value, i is the number of rows or categories of the factor being compared, and j is the number of columns. The chi-squared statistic for the above example is calculated in equation 4.7.

$$\chi^2 = \frac{(20-8)^2}{8} + \frac{(4-16)^2}{16} + \frac{(9980-9992)^2}{9992} + \frac{(19\,996-19\,984)^2}{19\,984} = 27.02\ (P<0.001) \tag{4.7}$$

$$\chi^2 = 18 + 9 + 0.0144 + 0.0072 = 27.02\ (P<0.001) \tag{4.8}$$

The larger the difference between the observed and expected value for any particular cell, the larger the contribution to the chi-squared statistic and the higher likelihood of achieving a *P*-value <0.05. The cell with the highest chi-squared value is contributing most to the association between the two variables. In this case, the association between patients administered succinylcholine who experienced malignant hyperthermia, for whom the individual chi-squared statistic is 18, is strongest.

As a general rule of thumb, if the chi-squared test statistic is larger than the number of cells in the table (four in this case), the difference is statistically significant. If there are more than two rows or two columns, the number of degrees of freedom will change and hence the critical value to define statistical significance will change. The degrees of freedom are calculated by multiplying the number of rows minus 1 ($r-1$) by the number of columns minus 1 ($c-1$).

When reporting the percentages from a contingency table, it is important to consider what the denominator of the percentage should be. If the question of interest is whether there is a difference in the incidence of malignant hyperthermia, the percentages calculated should be 20/10 000 = 0.2% compared with 4/20 000 = 0.02%. If the researcher is interested in determining differences in the characteristics between the population of patients with or without malignant hyperthermia then the marginal percentages to calculate would be 20/24 = 83.3% and 9980/29 976 = 33.3%.

The first set of percentages suggests that the incidence of malignant hyperthermia is low, but is higher among patients administered succinylcholine. The second set of figures suggests that a high proportion of patients who suffered malignant hyperthermia received succinylcholine but that, even among patients without malignant hyperthermia, one-third received succinylcholine. Understanding the percentages in a contingency table will help in interpreting the relationship between the two factors.

Continuity adjustment – Yates' correction

Because the chi-squared distribution or normal distribution (depending on sample size) is being used to represent discrete data, Yates proposed using a continuity correction. The continuity correction will appear to reduce the significance level. It is recommended that the Yates correction be used when calculating the chi-squared statistic for any 2×2 table. No similar correction factor exists for tables larger than 2×2.

Fisher's exact test

One of the assumptions for the chi-squared test is that the expected value of each cell is greater than 5. If this is invalid, the chi-squared test statistic will be biased. To eliminate the source of bias, the Fisher's exact test, which gives the exact probability of a 2×2 table, can be used to determine statistical significance. The Fisher's exact test uses the hypergeometric distribution. As the total count in each cell increases, the probabilities from the Fisher exact test and the chi-squared test become nearly identical.

Student's *t*-test

The *t*-test is one of the most commonly employed statistical tests and is used in all industries. There are several formulations of the *t*-test, including a one-sample *t*-test, a two-sample *t*-test, a paired *t*-test, and corresponding nonparametric tests.

In a one-sample test, an investigator may be evaluating the null hypothesis of whether the duration of stay in the postanesthesia care unit is 60 min for inpatients administered general anesthesia. To calculate the *t*-statistic, equation 4.9 is used:

$$t\text{-statistic} = \frac{(\bar{x}-60)}{s/\sqrt{n}} \tag{4.9}$$

Assuming that the sample size (n) is 177, the mean duration ($\bar{x}$) is 73.98 min, and the standard deviation (s) is 34.5 min, the test statistic would have a value of 5.33 and the critical value defined for statistical significance is 1.96. In this case, the test statistic is larger than the critical value and therefore the null hypothesis of no difference is rejected. Most computer programs will provide the test statistic along with the exact *P*-value.

A special case for the one-sample *t*-test is the crossover trial design in which each subject serves as his or her own control. The t-test performed for this trial design is referred to as a paired t-test. Although there are two target groups (before and after an intervention), the statistical analysis requires that only one population be tested. The difference between the "before" and "after" values of the sample is calculated. The test statistic compares the mean of the sample with zero. The numerator of the test statistic would be the mean of the differences minus zero and the standard error would be the sample standard deviation of the differences divided by the square root of the total number of observations. If the test statistic is larger than the critical value, the null hypothesis is rejected.

In the parallel trial design, the calculation of the test statistic differs from that of the one-sample test depending on whether or not it can be assumed that the two population variances are equal. If the two populations are assumed to have equal variances, the standard error is based on pooled variances. If the two populations are assumed to have unequal variances, the standard error is calculated using separate variances. Computer programs provide P-values using both of these standard errors. The numerator of the test statistic is calculated by taking the difference of the two sample means. If the sample variance is large relative to the sample mean, the ability to detect a difference between samples will be small. The smaller the sample variances, the smaller will be the detectable difference.

In the t-tests described above, it was assumed that the population distribution of the samples was normally distributed. If this is not a valid assumption, the test statistic will be biased. There are several events that are measured for which the assumption of a normal distribution would be invalid. For instance, duration of surgical procedure or duration of stay in the postanesthesia care unit is more likely to have a log normal distribution than a normal distribution because of the small number of patients who will always have a longer stay in each of these units. It is possible to take the log of the values to make the assumption of a normal distribution valid. More often, it is the case that the distribution is unknown and therefore it is not possible to transform the data. If this is the case, using a nonparametric test is a viable alternative. Nonparametric statistical tests base their test statistic on rank-ordered data instead of the original data. A test statistic is calculated that is a function of the rank sum and of the count of subjects for each group. The corresponding nonparametric test to the one-sample t-test is the Wilcoxon one-sample test, and the corresponding test for two samples is the Wilcoxon rank sum test. The critical values are obtained from the normal probability density distribution. In the event that a nonparametric test or a parametric test is applicable, the parametric test will be more powerful.

Parallel trial designs can also evaluate more than two groups. One analysis strategy for multiple groups could be to perform multiple t-tests. This strategy is not the best strategy because multiple t-tests are likely to magnify the type I error rate. If multiple t-tests are performed, it is advisable to use the Bonferroni correction on the α level by dividing the α level by the number of comparisons to be made. An alternative strategy is to use the analysis of variance (ANOVA), which is the preferred analytical methodology for comparing more than two groups.

Analysis of variance

Analysis of variance (ANOVA) examines the effect of one or several nominal variables on a continuous or dependent variable. In medicine, researchers are rarely interested in only two groups of patients. Frequently, more than two treatments are compared, multiple measurements need to be collected over a period time, or multiple factors of a population may be of interest. For these situations, ANOVA can be used.

Although in the ANOVA or the t-test it appears that the means among groups are being compared, the comparisons are made using estimates of the sample variances. Again, a key component of statistics is identifying and controlling for sources of variation. The test statistics for ANOVA are based on a ratio of variances. In general, the numerator is the variability between the means of the samples and the denominator is the variability among all the members within the samples. This is true even in the calculation of the test statistic for t-tests.

A one-way fixed-effects analysis of variance model is an extension of the two-sample t-test. Similar assumptions are applied: random samples are selected, a value for the dependent variable is recorded for each subject selected, the dependent variable is normally distributed for each population, and the variance of the dependent variable is the same in each population. The null hypothesis is $H_0: \mu_1 = \mu_2 = \mu_3 = \ldots = \mu_k$ and is tested using the F-sampling distribution using the appropriate degrees of freedom. The test statistic compares the variability between groups with the variability within groups and is calculated as shown in equation 4.10. If the variability between the means is much greater than the variability within samples, the test statistic will become large and lead to the rejection of the null hypothesis.

$$F = \frac{\text{mean sum of squares between groups}}{\text{mean sum of squares within groups}} = \frac{\dfrac{\sum_{i=1}^{k} n_i\left(\bar{y}_i - \bar{y}\right)^2}{k-1}}{\dfrac{\sum_{i=1}^{k}\left[\sum_{j=1}^{n}\left(y_{ij} - \bar{y}_i\right)^2\right]}{N-k}} \qquad (4.10)$$

The F-statistic gives an overall significance level between groups. It does not specify what groups differ. Several multiple comparison procedures can be used to determine which groups differ. The names of a few of these procedures are the least significant difference method, the Tukey method, and the Scheffé method. The choice of which of these procedures to use depends on how many groups are being compared, whether the comparisons were preplanned or unplanned, and the number of subjects in each group.

The two-way ANOVA is the next level of complexity. The repeated-measure design is a special case of the two-way ANOVA. Using the paired t-test is one way to analyze the results of a repeated-measures design. The other way is to use the two-way ANOVA, which differs from the paired t-test in that it uses the principles of randomized blocking. In randomized blocking, homogeneous groups of subjects or objects are grouped together to form a block and then the various treatments are assigned at random to the subjects within each block. Based on this approach, the F-test statistic is calculated differently. Instead of comparing two components of variability (between treatments and within samples), as in the one-way ANOVA, the two-way ANOVA breaks the variability into three components (between treatments, between blocks, and within samples). Blocking is generally carried out because there is a belief that there will be differences between the blocks. One additional assumption for the two-way randomized block design is that an interaction between the block and treatment does not exist, i.e. the true extent to which treatments differ is the same regardless of block considered. Two F-statistics calculated are presented in equations 4.11 and 4.12. The first F-statistic is comparing the means of the treatment groups relative to the unaccounted for variability or random error.

$$F_1 = \frac{\text{mean sum of squares between treatments}}{\text{mean sum of squares within groups}} \qquad (4.11)$$

$$F_2 = \frac{\text{mean sum of squares between blocks}}{\text{mean sum of squares within groups}} \quad (4.12)$$

There are several variants of ANOVA, and the differences in the test statistics are related to the definition and testing of the components of variability. If the assumption of normality is invalid, there are corresponding nonparametric ANOVA models. For any one study design, there may be several appropriate ways of analyzing the data. It is important to keep in mind the effect being measured and the distributional assumption of the test. Dexter[4] carried out a literature review of several studies that used different statistical tests to compare the effect of various doses of analgesics among patient groups. Based on these data, data from his own institution, and simulated data, the chi-squared test, *t*-test, and parametric and nonparametric ANOVA were compared. Overall, differences among the tests were small for this series of simulated data. The assumptions of statistical tests are very important when choosing and interpreting the results of a test; however, as shown in this simulation study, several statistical tests are sufficiently robust, confirming that if the assumptions are not flagrantly invalid the results of the statistical test will be valid.

Correlation

The previously discussed statistical tests evaluate the relation of interval data with nominal data or ordinal/nominal data with ordinal/nominal data. In the event that an investigator wants to look at the relation between two mutually dependent variables, such as systolic and diastolic blood pressure, a correlation coefficient is used. If the relation between the factors is nonlinear, the correlation coefficient will be biased.

The correlation coefficient differs from a linear regression relation (discussed below) in that in a linear regression one variable is considered the dependent variable and one variable is considered the independent variable. For the correlation coefficient both variables are essentially considered dependent variables. A correlation analysis looks for the relation between two variables, not necessarily whether one variable is predictive of the other variable.

PHARMACOEPIDEMIOLOGY

Pharmacoepidemiology is a relatively new area of research that combines epidemiology research methods, such as the case-control study or a prospective cohort study research designs, with biostatistics and principles of clinical pharmacology to determine the risk of adverse events, therapeutic failure, or other outcomes in patient populations and to identify patient characteristics associated with a higher likelihood of these events.

In a cohort study, the incidence of an adverse event in a group of patients exposed to a drug is compared with the incidence in a group of patients who are not exposed to the drug. A cohort study is similar to the design of a clinical trial with the important exception that the enrollment of patients into the various treatment or exposure groups is not randomized. Both groups are initially free from the outcome interest and are monitored to determine the number of adverse events that occur over a specified period. The incidence of the adverse event in the exposed group is computed as the number of new cases of the adverse event detected in the exposed group divided by the total number of patients in the exposed groups.

In a case–control study, patients with the disease of interest (cases) and patients without the disease (control subjects) are identified and differences in exposures between the two groups are compared. Because incidence cannot be computed in a case–control study, the odds ratio is used to assess the probability of the outcome given the exposure.

Both the cohort and case-control study methodologies can serve as a scientific framework for studying patient outcome to drug therapy and are well used as the basis for performing outcome management evaluations. The wealth of experience with these approaches in other settings can serve to help in the design, analysis, and interpretation of studies of adverse events or other patient outcome measures in the anesthesia setting.[5]

In a pharmacoepidemiologic study, it is necessary to select random subjects who will be monitored to minimize selection bias. The experimental trial designs differ in that the patient is randomly allocated to a treatment regimen. In epidemiologic studies, investigators do not allocate treatment to a patient; rather they select patients who are already on a treatment plan. Therefore, a sampling plan is constructed to select subjects. Several methods are applicable in the clinical setting, including simple random sampling, systematic sampling, and stratified random sampling. Briefly, in simple random sampling, every subject in the sampling frame has an equal chance of being selected. Systematic sampling is one of the most widely used sampling methods. As an example, assume that a quality assurance audit is being performed on anesthetic records. As it is not known in advance what the total number of records is, in an ongoing initiative, simple random sampling cannot be used. However, as it is known how many will be available over a certain time period, systematic sampling allows one to choose every *k*th record over a period of time. For example, every 30th record for the month. Simple and systematic random sampling require sampling from the whole. Stratified sampling allows the sampling frame to be broken down into strata, and within each stratum subjects are selected using either simple random sampling or systematic sampling. Sampling is as important in epidemiologic studies as randomization is in experimental trial designs.

Clinical significance vs. statistical significance

In pharmacoepidemiology, the process of analyzing data is the same as in experimental trial designs. First, an exploratory analysis should be performed, followed by univariate statistical tests; more commonly performed in epidemiologic studies are multivariable analyses. The odds ratio and the relative risk are two summary statistics that help in assessing the strength of the univariate relation being evaluated between categorical variables, regardless of the research design. When calculating a test statistic or *P*-value, a large sample size may produce a *P*-value that represents a highly statistically significant relation. However, if you look closer and determine the value of the relative risk or odds ratio, the relation may not be clinically significant. Use of both the *P*-value and one of these two summary measures will give a better perspective for understanding the study results.

Relative risk

In a cohort study, the incidence of an event in a group of patients exposed to a drug is compared with the incidence in a group of patients who are not exposed to the drug and the ratio of the two incidences is the relative risk. The magnitude of the relative risk is an indicator of the likelihood of experiencing the event based on exposure. A relative risk > 1.0 indicates an increased risk and a relative risk < 1.0 indicates a decreased risk of the event. In a population of patients undergoing general anesthesia lasting longer than 90 min, the risk of postoperative nausea and/or vomiting was nearly twice as high in women as in men, as shown in Table 4.7.

Table 4.7 *Relative risk*

	Postoperative nausea/vomiting			
	No	Yes	Relative risk	*P*-value
Women	*a* 2420 (81.6)	*b* 545 (18.4)	1.96	<0.001
Men	*c* 1532 (90.6)	*d* 159 (9.4)		

Relative risk $= [b/(a+b)]/[c/(c+d)]$.
Odds ratio $= (a \times d)/(b \times c)$.

Odds ratio

The odds ratio is a summary measure of the probability of an outcome occurring given the exposure and is commonly used in case–control studies. Using Table 4.7, the odds ratio is calculated as $[(a\times d)/(b\times c)]$. If the odds ratio is 1, there is no association between the risk factor and the outcome. If the odds ratio is not 1, there is an association between the risk factor and the outcome. It has been shown that the odds ratio provides an approximation of the relative risk when the incidence of disease is small. It is possible to compute 95% confidence intervals and perform hypothesis testing on the relative risk and odds ratio.

Multivariate analysis

Multivariate analysis examines the influence of multiple risk factors acting simultaneously. The dependent variable (the outcome) is a function of the independent (predictor) variables. Two important concepts that can be explored in multivariate analyses are confounding and interaction or effect modification, which may take place when exploring multiple risk factors. A confounding variable is a variable that is associated with both the exposure and the outcome and which independently affects the risk of developing the outcome. Thus, the observed association between the exposure and outcome may be due to differences between the exposed and nonexposed groups that have little to do with the exposure. Uncontrolled confounding is one of the major issues when assessing the validity of study results. It can result in over- or underestimation of the regression model coefficients for an exposure and can even change the direction of the effect. Interaction occurs when the relation between the outcome and exposure is different at different levels of exposure. A regression model can be built using several different methods. Predictor variables can be added or removed from the model using forward, backward, or stepwise strategies. In backward selection, all variables are included in the model and the variable with the least significant *P*-value is removed from the model. This is repeated until all nonsignificant variables are removed from the model. In forward selection, one variable is entered at a time, based on the correlation with the dependent variable, and evaluated for significance. Stepwise selection is a variation of forward selection method in that at each step the variable is evaluated for entry and removal from the model.

A number of multivariate data analysis techniques are available to investigate the association between multiple patient factors and outcome while simultaneously controlling for confounding factors. The specific type of multivariate analysis to be used is dependent on the nature of the outcome under study. If the outcome is a continuous variable and the error terms are normally distributed, multiple linear regression may be used. The patient outcome of interest in many medical studies is often dichotomous and not continuous; that is, an event occurs or it does not, the patient has successful therapeutic outcome or does not. In this setting, logistic regression analysis represents an appropriate method for estimating the magnitude of the association between drug exposure and the outcome while adjusting for the effects of other patient characteristics that may be confounding factors or effect modifiers. Although less common in the field of surgery and anesthesia, an outcome of interest can be dependent on time, such as survival rate of a person with cancer or the amount of time it takes to alleviate chronic pain given two different treatment regimens. This type of analysis is performed with survival analysis models.

It is important to be cautious about results obtained from a regression analysis or, more generally, from any form of analysis seeking to quantify an association among two or more variables in a nonexperimental research design. Although the statistical computations used to produce an estimated measure of association may be correct, the estimate itself may be biased. Several examples of bias have been discussed earlier in this chapter and apply to regression analysis as well. Also, in regression analysis, the finding of a statistically significant association in a particular study (no matter how well the study was done) does not establish a causal relation. In epidemiology, the criteria used to assess a causal relation are strength of association, dose–response effect, lack of temporal ambiguity, consistency of findings across studies, biological and theoretical plausibility of the hypothesis, coherence of the evidence, and specificity of the association. The best way to determine a causal relation is through an experimental study design. However, if an experimental design is not practical, epidemiologic studies using regression analyses may be a logical and practical way to address the issue of association and then further contemplate the results to assess causality.

In addition to the advantages of being able to evaluate the effect of multiple factors simultaneously on an outcome measure, several practical advantages may result from the use of regression models. The results of any one of the regression models described can be converted to a scoring system that can be used in clinical practice to determine the probability of outcome for an individual patient based on individual factors. Second, the results of the regression models can be used to risk adjust the incidence of a patient outcome when comparing the incidence of patient outcomes across providers or across institutions.

Linear regression

In linear regression, the dependent variable is continuous and it is assumed that the dependent observations are statistically independent of one another, that the variance of the dependent variable is the same for any category of the predictor values, and that, for any fixed value of the predictor value, the dependent variable is normally distributed. The independent variables are a linear function of the dependent variable. Linear regression is an extension of ANOVA in that regression allows nominal, ordinal, and interval data as independent variables.

$$y=\beta_0+\beta_1x_1+\beta_2x_2+\ldots+\beta_mx_m \tag{4.13}$$

In the simple case of one dependent variable and one independent variable, the equation is that of a straight line, $y=\beta_0+\beta_1x_1$, where β_0 is the intercept or where the regression line crosses the vertical axis and β_1 is the slope of the line or the amount of change in the dependent variable for a unit change in the independent variable.

The linear regression model is most commonly estimated using the least-squares method to choose the best-fitting model that minimizes the sum of squares of the distances between the observed responses and those predicted by the fitted model. The interpretation of the coefficient in multiple linear regression is the same as in the simple case when all other factors are held constant.

Logistic regression

In logistic regression analysis, the dependent variable is defined to be the natural logarithm (ln) of the odds of the outcome. The independent variables can be represented by a linear function. Using notation, $P(y)$ is the probability of the outcome and $P(y)/[1 - P(y)]$ represents the "odds" of the outcome. In logistic regression, the log odds is the dependent variable and is expressed as a linear function of the independent predictor variables as shown in equation 4.14:

$$\ln\left[\frac{P(y)}{1-P(y)}\right] = \beta_0 + \beta_1 x_1 + \beta_2 x_2 + \ldots + \beta_m x_m \quad (4.14)$$

This equation can be rewritten to give the probability of developing the outcome, as shown in equation 4.15:

$$P(y) = \frac{1}{1+e^{-(\beta_0+\beta_1 x_1+\beta_2 x_2+\ldots+\beta_m x_m)}} \quad (4.15)$$

In equation 4.15, $P(y)$ is the probability of developing the outcome and the βs are coefficients of the model relating predictor variables to the probability of the event. The predictor variables can be either continuous, such as age or weight, or categorical, such as gender or the presence of another concurrent illness. The coefficients can be converted to odds ratios that provide an estimate of the relative risk when the incidence of the outcome is low. When the independent variable is categorical, the exponential of the coefficient gives the odds ratio. When the independent variable is continuous, such as is the case with drug concentrations, the exponential of the corresponding β gives the magnitude of the increase or decrease in the log odds produced by a unit change in the independent variable, for example drug concentrations, when all other factors are held constant.

Survival analysis

Survival analysis is another type of regression model and is used when the outcome being evaluated is the time to when an event occurs. Time to when a patient can return to work after an elective surgical procedure or time to when a patient is wheelchair bound as a result of chronic pain are examples of when survival analysis would be utilized. As with many medical measures, the response times can be very skewed. Within a given study period, it may be possible to track the number of days that is takes for a patient to resume working after elective surgery, but it could be the case that the study is over and one or more patients have not yet returned to work. Survival analysis methodology accounts for this situation by "censoring" the event. Censoring occurs when some information about the time to an event is available, but the time is not exact. Censoring may be required when a study ends before the defined event occurs, a person is lost to follow-up during the study, or a person withdraws from the study because of death or other morbidity.

The two functions that are used in survival analysis are the survivor function and the hazard function. The survivor function gives the probability that a person survives longer than some specified time. The hazard function is a rate ranging from zero to infinity and gives the instantaneous potential per unit of time for the event to occur, given that the individual has survived up to time t. The survivor function focuses on the event not happening, whereas the hazard function focuses on the event occurring.

As in linear and logistic regression modeling, there is a measure of the effect for survival analysis models. The exponential of the regression coefficient is equivalent to the hazard ratio. The hazard ratio, although different from the odds ratio described under logistic regression, does have a similar interpretation. A hazard ratio of 1 has no effect. A hazard ratio of 10 indicates that the exposed group has 10 times the hazard of the unexposed group.

If the baseline hazard rate for an event is known, a parametric model can be used in the survival analysis model. An example would be the time to death after cardiac surgery. A decreasing Weibull distribution (i.e. a parametric probability distribution) would be used because the potential for dying after surgery usually decreases as the time after surgery increases. Common parametric distributions used in survival analysis are the exponential, Weibull, and log normal distributions. However, more commonly used is a nonparametric approach called Cox's proportional hazard model. In Cox's proportional hazard model the baseline hazard is unknown, but reasonable estimates of the regression coefficients are obtainable. This model is a robust model when time to an event information is available and censoring of patients occurs.

Risk adjustment

Measuring patient outcomes in today's healthcare system is being mandated by governing agencies such as the Joint Commission of Healthcare Organizations and Healthcare and Finance Administration. Comparing outcome measures between clinicians or between institutions is often desired. Risk adjustment attempts to take into consideration the amount of risk that a patient's health brings to the medical event being measured that is not related to the event or was a pre-existing condition of the patient but may have a positive or negative impact on patient outcome.

Defining risk is the most controversial aspect of risk adjustment. Different outcomes will involve different types of risk. Opinions may vary on what risk is involved and how to account for this risk. There are several measures in surgery and anesthesia that define different levels of severity of a case: ASA classification, Apache score (Acute Physiology Age Chronic Health Evaluation), and New York State coronary artery bypass graft (CABG) surgery risk assessment score. For each of these scores, the patient characteristics or procedures that defined the risk that contributed to the severity score were either agreed upon by a consensus from experts in the field and literature reviews or derived through empirical regression models described in previous paragraphs. Ideally, a combination of the two methods are used. These scores are used in adjusting the incidence of patient outcome across clinicians or institutions.

In New York, a "home-grown" risk adjustment strategy was developed for mortality as a result of cardiac revascularization procedures. The factors incorporated in the model were developed by a multidisciplinary group of professionals consisting of cardiac surgeons, cardiologists, and epidemiologists. This committee formulated a cardiac surgical report form requiring information on risk that was easily collected and quantifiable, including ventricular ejection fraction, >90% narrowing of the left main coronary artery, diabetes mellitus requiring medication, and whether the CABG was a reoperation. Twenty-eight hospitals forwarded this information to a central processing office, and a logistic regression model was used to develop the mortality prediction models. The blinded reporting of the results in *JAMA* were meant for scientific discussion. However, in New York State there was public clamor for not only institution names, but also physician-specific morality rates and the physicians' names to be revealed. After review by the New York State Supreme Court, 140 physicians' names and their CABG mortality rates were released for public consumption 1 year later. Despite the uproar regarding the release of these data, there has been an increase in acceptance of this type of data even among the surgeons. One year later, CABG mortality dropped by 36% despite apparent increases in the severity of cases. This fall in mortality rates has been attributed by some to quality improvement measures put into place as a result of the release of information, although there is no objective evidence to confirm this theory.

When deciding how risk should be defined it is necessary first to ask what is the purpose behind the risk adjustment. No risk adjustment model will serve all purposes and, depending on whether one is predicting resource consumption or comparing clinical outcomes, very different risk adjustment models may be developed and used. Other considerations to take into account are the source of the data and the reliability of the data. If the source of the data for risk adjustment of a clinical outcome measure is a claims database, it is necessary to list the limitations of such a database. Data should be reliable in the sense that if multiple clinicians reviewed the risk factors the same conclusions would be drawn. Although there are limitations in the methodology of risk adjustment and defining risk, and controversy will always surround risk adjustment, when applied across groups of patients risk adjustment does facilitate interpretation of outcome information and prompts quality improvement measures.

Continuous quality improvement

Variation in medicine is natural and expected as every individual and disease state is unique. However, when there is a systematic deviation from what is considered natural variation, it is important to understand why there is deviation and to improve the quality of the process. The objective of continuous quality improvement (see also Chapter 84) is not to find and assign blame for errors or inefficiencies, but rather to change care processes that allow error or inefficiencies to happen. Joseph Juran, an international pioneer in total quality management, developed the total quality management (TQM) system, which strives to plan, control, and improve processes that continually deliver optimal outcomes, known as the "Juran trilogy." By measuring and analyzing outcomes, unintended or inappropriate variability in practice patterns can be identified. Heavy investment by healthcare organizations in information systems makes this type of measurement a real possibility, offering real-time accounting of what actually happens in healthcare and what it costs. After an outcome with unintended variation is identified, a multidisciplinary team develops a plan, usually in terms of a clinical practice guideline or standard operating procedure, to re-engineer the process involved. Implementation of the plan should actually change and improve day-to-day practice and clinical outcomes. Routine feedback on change in clinical outcomes and benchmarking of the clinical outcomes across clinicians or facilities will provide the basis for ongoing modifications to refine and enhance the process and to demonstrate improvements objectively.

Ultimately, every organization has its own set of areas that have excessive variability or problems, and hence the TQM approach will need to be tailored to individual healthcare organizations, but from these initiatives best practices are established that become standards for all healthcare organizations. An example of a continuous quality improvement initiative that led to a paradigm shift in ambulatory surgery was the realization that patients undergoing ambulatory surgery and receiving anesthetic agents with short-acting, faster emergence pharmacokinetic and pharmacodynamic properties were able to bypass the postanesthesia care unit and be transferred from the operating room to the second-stage recovery unit without any adverse effect on patient outcome.[6]

TQM looks at a population view of patient care, but it is relevant to everyday clinical practice. In today's era of accountability, clinicians are expected to justify the type of care they provide and the cost-effectiveness of that care. To make this possible, organizations need to describe, evaluate, and improve their care processes and their outcomes. Although TQM is often referenced to the assembly line in the auto industry, in healthcare one may perceive TQM as a second cousin to the principles and methodology of epidemiology. Epidemiology assesses risk, care, outcomes, and comparison of patient groups, these being similar concepts to TQM.

EVALUATING STATISTICAL SOFTWARE

Computers and the availability of several statistical software packages have made it possible for both the novice data analyst and the full-time statistician/mathematician to carry out simple to complex statistical analyses. With the proliferation of statistical software packages, selecting the most appropriate software may be one of the more difficult tasks. Available statistical software packages include general packages, such as S-Plus, SPSS, Minitab, SAS, Statistica, Systat, and Microsoft Excel, and specialized packages such as EpiInfo and Treeage. When selecting a statistical software package there are several criteria to take into consideration.

The most important criterion to look for in a statistical software package is the validity and quality of the statistical methods utilized. The Food and Drug Administration has written a guidance on statistical principles for clinical trials which incorporates a section on integrity of data and computer software validity.[7] Selecting a popular, commercialized software package that has documentation on the statistical methodology will usually satisfy this criterion but does not guarantee complete accuracy.

Other factors to take into consideration are the ability to and ease of entering raw data into the software package, the ability to export the data or results, the ability to manage and manipulate data, the types of statistical procedures needed, the ability to save and rerun analyses, graphing ability, presentation of results, friendliness of the graphical–user interface, computer hardware availability, ability to upgrade the software package, technical support, and price. Developing a matrix of needs required from a statistical software package and comparing that list of needs across statistical software packages can guide the decision-making process of software selection.

MANUSCRIPT WRITING/READING

Research is complete only when the results are shared with the professional community. Although such sharing is achieved in a variety of formal and informal ways, the traditional medium for communicating research results is the peer-reviewed journal. The scholarly journal is the repository of the accumulated knowledge of a field. The literature distills success and failures, information, and perspectives contributed by numerous investigators over many years. Familiarity with the literature allows an investigator to avoid needlessly repeating work that has been done previously, to build on existing work, and in turn to contribute something new. A literature built of meticulously prepared, carefully reviewed contributions fosters the growth of the medical field. Thus, performing a thorough literature search is an essential prerequisite for experimental design and manuscript writing.

When evaluating a study presented in a peer-reviewed journal, several questions should prompt a critical review of the relevance of the

Table 4.8 *Questions to pose when evaluating a study*

Who is the target population and does the sample selected represent the target population?
Will the results extrapolate to the population?
How was the research designed: a controlled clinical trial, double-blind, prospective cohort, retrospective?
Does the research design properly answer the study questions?
Where was the study conducted: preclinical environment, one surgical center, multiple surgical centers?
What type of therapy was administered and to what groups?
What patients were included or excluded from the study?
Were the patients appropriately assigned to the treatment groups using a randomization scheme or a sampling plan?
What is the outcome measure?; is it clearly defined?
How were the statistics calculated and were they the appropriate statistics?
How many patients were studied and are the statistics convincing based on the number of patients studied?
Was the interpretation drawn from the results and was it valid?
And, finally, so what does it mean to my patients, is it clinically relevant, and does it add to the literature?

study methods and results. The basic questions should be who?, what?, where?, when?, why?, how?, how many?, and so on. Table 4.8 lists specific questions.

Clinical science is not exact and is often fraught with controversy. There is no right answer to any of the questions listed above. The point of the questions is to expand the knowledge of the clinician when an article is being critically reviewed. Taking the knowledge gained, integrating it with other research, or designing new studies to target an area that may have been lacking in an existing study, and ultimately continually building on the wealth of knowledge that is available, are the reasons for critically evaluating a study.

CONCLUSION

The accessibility of computers and the progression to miniaturized, high-powered computers is only in its infancy and, because of this, the field of statistics is continually expanding as new methodologies take advantage of new technologies. Statistics will play a much different role in the future as this progression continues. Imagine entering information on your patient's history, the level of risk you and the patient are willing to accept, the quality of life the patient is willing to tolerate, and current medical status into a wireless hand-held device and having alternative treatment modalities for the patient appear before your eyes based on the experience and data from tens of thousands of patients with similar conditions; the device might then rank the options best suited for your patient, and all within the matter of a couple of minutes. Statistics promises to become even more important as mass customization of pharmaceuticals and other treatment modalities are made available. As years pass, statistics will become more user friendly, but understanding the basics of statistics and probability will always be essential.

REFERENCES

1. Johnstone RE. Costs of anesthesia. *Anesth Analg* 1993; **76:** 840–8.
2. Spriet A, Dupin-Spriet T. *Good Practice of Clinical Drug Trials*, 2nd edn. Basle: Karger, 1994.
3. Giese JL, Stockham RJ, Stanley TH, *et al*. Etomidate versus thiopental for induction of anesthesia. *Anesth Analg* 1985; **64:** 871–6.
4. Dexter F. Analysis of statistical test to compare doses of analgesics among groups. *Anesthesiology* 1994; **81:** 610–15.
5. Grasela TH, Watkins D, Hug Jr CC, *et al*. The role of pharmacoepidemiology research in postmarketing surveillance and anesthesia practice/critical care medicine. *Anesth Analg* 1993; **77:** S44–50.
6. Apfelbaum JL, Walawander CA, Grasela TH, *et al*. Eliminating intensive postoperative care in same-day surgery patients using short-acting anesthetics. *Anesthesiology* 2002; **97:** 66–74.
7. Department of Health and Human Services and the Food and Drug Administration. *International Conference on Harmonization: Guidance on Statistical Principles for Clinical Trials.* Federal Register, Vol. 63, No. 179, Wednesday, September 16, 1998. 49583–98.

FURTHER READING

Introductory statistics

Colton T. *Statistics in Medicine*. Boston: Little, Brown, 1974.

Last JM. *A Dictionary of Epidemiology*, 2nd edn. New York: Oxford University Press, 1988.

Marriott FHC. *A Dictionary of Statistical Terms*, 5th edn. New York: Longman Scientific & Technical, 1990.

Phillips DS. *Basic Statistics for Health Science Students*. San Francisco: W. H. Freeman and Company, 1978.

Wonnacott TH, Wonnacott RJ. *Introductory Statistics*, 3rd edn. New York: John Wiley & Sons, 1977.

Zar JH. *Biostatistical Analysis*. Englewood Cliffs, NJ: Prentice-Hall, 1974.

Introductory probability

Evans M, Hastings N, Peacock B. *Statistical Distributions*, 2nd edn. New York: John Wiley & Sons, 1993.

Freund JF, Walpole RE. *Mathematical Statistics*, 3rd edn. Englewood Cliffs, NJ: Prentice-Hall, 1980.

Exploratory statistics

Chamber JM, Cleveland WS, Kleiner B, Tukey PA. *Graphical Methods for Data Analysis*. Pacific Grove, CA: Wadsworth & Brooks/Cole Publishing Company, 1983.

Tufte ER. *The Visual Display of Quantitative Information*. Cheshire, CT: Graphic Press, 1983.

Tukey JW. *Exploratory Data Analysis*. Reading, MA: Addison-Wesley Publishing Company, 1977.

Research design

Iber FL, Riley WA, Murray PJ. *Conducting Clinical Trials*. New York: Plenum Medical Book Company, 1987.

Levy PS, Lemeshow S. *Sampling of Populations: Methods and Applications*. New York: John Wiley & Sons, 1991.

Marks RG. *Analyzing Research Data: The Basics of Biomedical Research Methodology*. Belmont, CA: Lifetime Learning Publications, 1982.

Riegelman RK, Hirsch RP. *Studying a Study and Testing a Test: How to Read the Medical Literature*, 2nd edn. Boston: Little, Brown, 1989.

Spriet A, Dupin-Spriet T. *Good Practice of Clinical Drug Trials*, 2nd edn. Basle: Karger, 1994.

Statistical inference and experimental design

Armitage P. *Sequential Medical Trials*, 2nd edn. Oxford: Blackwell Scientific Publications, 1975.

Cochran WG, Cox GM. *Experimental Designs*, 2nd edn. New York: John Wiley & Sons, 1957.

Fleiss JL. *Statistical Methods for Rates and Proportions*, 2nd edn. New York: John Wiley & Sons, 1981.

Oakes M. *Statistical Inference*. Chestnut Hill, MA: Epidemiology Resources, 1986.

Winer BJ. *Statistical Principles in Experimental Design*, 2nd edn. New York: McGraw-Hill, 1971.

Nonparametric statistics

Lehmann EL. *Nonparametrics: Statistical Methods Based on Ranks*. Oakland, CA: Holden-Day, 1975.

Multivariable analyses

Draper N, Smith H. *Applied Regression Analysis*, 2nd edn. New York, NY: John Wiley & Sons, 1981.
Hosmer DW, Lemeshow S. *Applied Logistic Regression*. New York, NY: John Wiley & Sons, 1989.
Kleinbaum DG. *Survival Analysis: A Self-learning Text*. New York, NY: Springer-Verlag, 1996.
Kleinbaum DG, Kupper LL, Muller KE. *Applied Regression Analysis and Other Multivariable Methods*, 2nd edn. Boston, MA: PWS-KENT Publishing Company, 1988.
Schumacher GE. *Therapeutic Drug Monitoring*. Norwalk, CT: Appleton & Lange, 1995.
Strom BL. *Pharmacoepidemiology*, 2nd edn. Chichester, UK: John Wiley & Sons, 1994.

Cost, quality, and risk adjustment

Gold MR, Siegel JE, Russell LB, Weinstein MC. *Cost-effectiveness in Health and Medicine*. New York, NY: Oxford University Press, 1996.
Goonan KJ. *The Juran Prescription: Clinical Quality Management*. San Francisco, CA: Jossey-Bass Publishers, 1995.
Iezzoni LI. *Risk Adjustment for Measuring Health Care Outcomes*. Ann Arbor, MI: Health Administration Press, 1994.
Spilker B. *Quality of Life and Pharmacoeconomics in Clinical Trials*, 2nd edn. Philadelphia, PA: Lippincott-Raven, 1996.
Weinsten MC, Fineberg HV. *Clinical Decision Analysis*. Philadelphia, PA: W. B. Saunders Company, 1980.

5

Pulmonary physiology and pathophysiology

JONATHAN D CARDY AND J GARETH JONES

This chapter describes (1) the flow of gas through the conducting airways from the atmosphere to the alveoli, (2) how the regional distribution of gas depends on lung volume, (3) the exchange of gas between the alveoli and pulmonary blood, and (4) the control of breathing. We combine a discussion of these normal processes with an outline of how general anesthesia, or other pathophysiologic derangements relevant to anesthesiologists, may disturb these processes.

FLOW IN TUBES

Human airways are short and branch repeatedly. They are collapsible, they may be lined with a viscoelastic liquid, and gas flow in the lumen is constantly changing direction. Intrapulmonary airways are distensible. Their caliber depends on the way that the surrounding alveoli, acting like springs, couple their walls to the pleural surface (Fig. 5.1). Because of gravity, these "springs" give a vertical gradient of lung elastic recoil pressure, which is greater at the top than at the bottom of the lung.

Flow in long straight tubes

Gas flow through such a branched system is complex, so we must first consider flow slowly increasing through a long straight tube. Initially, this is *laminar*, but it then becomes *turbulent*, with the pressure drop down the tube (ΔP) depending on the type of flow:

Laminar flow: $\Delta P \propto \dot{V}\mu / r^4$

Turbulent flow: $\Delta P \propto \dot{V}^2 \rho / r^5$

where V is gas flow and r is tube radius. For air, viscosity (μ) = 0.000181 poise at 20 °C, and density (ρ) = 0.00113 g cm^{-3}.

Under laminar conditions, airway resistance ($\Delta P/\dot{V}$) is proportional to gas viscosity, but with turbulent flow the resistance depends on gas density. Thus, helium (ρ = 0.00017 g cm^{-3} at 0 °C) reduces resistance only under turbulent flow conditions.

The type of flow depends on the Reynolds number (*Re*), which is the ratio of inertial (density dependent) forces to viscous forces. This is calculated from $Re = \rho D v/\mu$, where v is gas velocity (cm s^{-1}) and D is tube diameter (cm). An instructive experiment is to measure the pressure drop across a straight tube whose diameter is similar to that of the trachea (1.7 cm). To ensure laminar flow, a long (> 50 × diameter) tube of the same bore leading smoothly into the "tracheal segment" must be used. The air flow rate and pressure drop should be displayed simultaneously as an *x–y* plot. *The pressure drop at tidal flow rates is very small.* If flow is gradually increased, a pattern similar to that in Fig. 5.2 will be seen. Laminar flow is associated with a *linear* increase in pressure. Transitional flow is the wobbly stage before turbulent flow is established.

Branched, curved, and short tubes

Contrast this with flow through a tube of the same total length but which branches at 75° at one end into two daughter tubes with the same total cross-sectional area as the parent (Fig. 5.2). At no stage is flow laminar. At the same Reynolds numbers (i.e. the same flow rate), there is a nonlinear pressure–flow relation at all flows, with a considerably greater

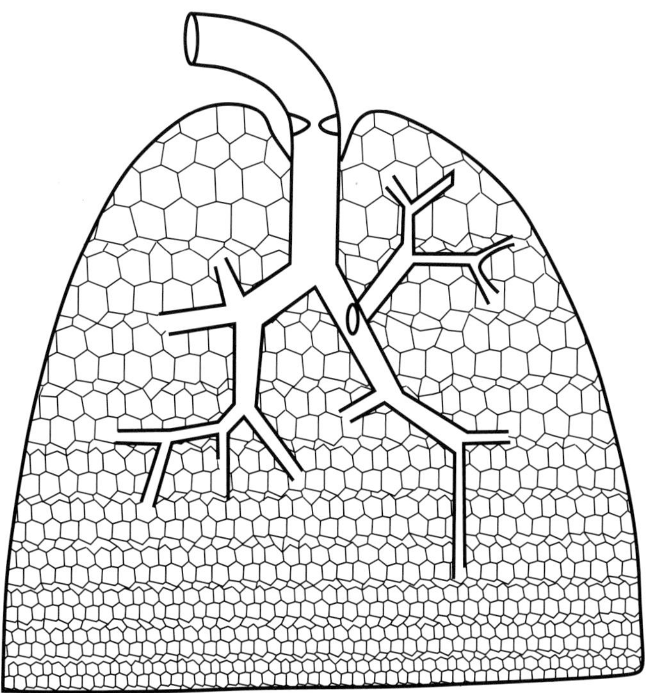

Figure 5.1 *Diagram of the conducting airways coupled by the alveoli to the chest wall. Gravity produces a continuous vertical gradient of alveolar size, shown as three horizontal slices.*

Figure 5.2 *Comparison of the pressure–flow curves in a straight tube that is the size of the trachea and a similar tube branching at 75° into two bronchi. The transitional change from laminar to turbulent flow is shown by a sudden instability in pressure.*

pressure drop than in the straight tube even at low Reynolds numbers. A similar result is seen if a straight tube is progressively bent, e.g. a tracheal tube; the greater the bend the larger the pressure drop per unit flow.

In fully developed *laminar* flow, the velocity profile is parabolic (Fig. 5.3). This means that the velocity is high at the center of the tube but zero at the wall. In long straight tubes, flow is laminar if *Re* is between 0 and 2000. If *Re* is between 2000 and 4000, flow may be *transitional* – any perturbation can change it from laminar to turbulent. If *Re* is greater than 4000, flow is always turbulent.

At *Re* of about 1500, flow in a straight tube should be laminar, but it takes a finite distance – the entrance length ($EL = 0.03 \times D \times Re$) – for a gas to establish the fully parabolic velocity profile associated with laminar flow (Fig. 5.3). The entrance length for the trachea ($D = 1.7$ cm) at this flow is 77 cm; however, the tracheal is only 12 cm long, so fully developed laminar flow is never achieved. Similarly in branching airways, the distances between junctions are shorter than the entrance length and even with *Re* as low as 50 the pressure drop is greater than would be expected in fully developed laminar flow.

The Bernoulli effect

Reducing cross-sectional area in part of a tube causes a considerable drop in pressure as the gas velocity increases ($\Delta P \propto \rho \Delta v^2$, where Δv = velocity change). This Bernoulli effect may produce a subatmospheric pressure, causing the walls of the tube to flutter if they are sufficiently compliant. This mechanism underlies snoring and expiratory flow limitation.

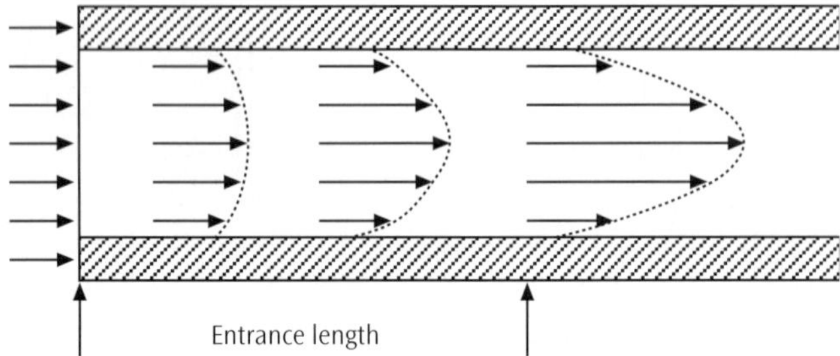

Figure 5.3 *Flow entering a tube, showing the entrance length needed to produce a fully developed parabolic velocity profile.*

UPPER RESPIRATORY TRACT

Flow patterns

The upper airway extends from the lips and nares to below the larynx. It has a right-angled bend and its cross-sectional area varies considerably along its length. The geometry and flow have been examined using a hollow transparent cast[1] with dye in a water-filled model or with smoke in an air flow model at the same Reynolds number. In a simple glass model with water flow at a *Re* of only 1000, flow patterns are very complex (Fig. 5.4). Flow streams *across* the axis of the tube and there are vortices at the cords. In quiet inspiratory flow, turbulence produced at the larynx produces large-scale disturbances that, because of short entrance lengths, persist as eddies even into sublobar bronchi.

Reducing the density of inspired gas using helium is of benefit in large airway obstruction (e.g. tracheal stenosis, tracheomalacia) where there may be a strong Bernoulli effect. The concentration of helium must be nearly 80%. It is not useful where the flow limitation lies in the small airways where Reynolds numbers are low and flow is viscosity dependent (e.g. asthma). The viscosity of helium is greater than air and in these circumstances resistance will increase.

The laryngopharyngeal wall

The patency of this muscular tube is maintained by an increase in the tone in the intrinsic muscles of the pharynx and larynx. This is normally initiated just prior to diaphragmatic contraction and resists the tendency of the airway to collapse when pressure in the lumen falls below atmospheric. Similar neural control mechanisms are involved in

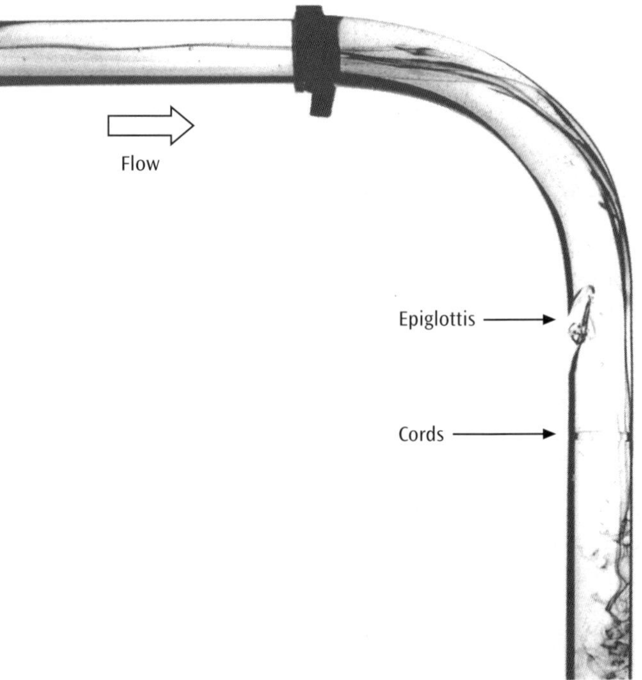

Figure 5.4 *The flow pattern in a glass model of the upper airway seen on "inspiration" at a Reynolds number of 1000. Note the dye stream in the center of the tube before the bend. At the bend, this flows around and across the axis of the tube to the outer part of the bend with eddy formation below the "cords."*

phonation as well as in preventing aspiration of liquid or particulate material into the lower airway.

Although it is important that the respiratory tract be kept patent, the human airway can be quickly narrowed through most of its length. This has advantages in swallowing, phonation, and coughing. Unfortunately, the mechanisms that maintain patency are deranged or abolished by intracranial pathology, sedative drugs (including alcohol), and during sleep, general anesthesia, or coma. The anatomy and pathophysiology of the upper airway have been reviewed.[2,3] Recent advances in the neural control of the airways have been well described.[4,5]

Upper airway patency

Magnetic resonance imaging (MRI) is the best method for visualizing upper airway dimensions in life.[6] The pharynx is divided into three parts: the nasopharynx, the oropharynx, and the laryngopharynx. The nasopharynx produces nitric oxide in high concentrations.[7] If this is bypassed by a tracheal tube, pulmonary vasoconstriction may result. The main pharyngeal muscles are the superior, middle, and inferior constrictors. The *motor nerve* supply to the pharynx and soft palate is from the cranial part of the accessory nerve via the pharyngeal branch of the vagus nerve. The *sensory innervation* is by the glossopharyngeal and vagus nerves.

The oropharynx and nasopharynx are the parts of the upper airway most liable to flutter on inspiration. The resulting subatmospheric pressure collapses the hypotonic pharyngeal wall, which relies on muscular tone to maintain patency. There is centrally mediated phasic electromyographic (EMG) activity on inspiration in the genioglossus in humans[8] with a magnitude that is directly related to negative intrapharyngeal pressure.[9] The afferent side of this reflex originates in mechanoreceptors in the pharynx and larynx that respond to subatmospheric pressure. Airway obstruction (snoring) may occur when airflow due to diaphragmatic contraction begins in the absence of, or just before, activation of the upper airway musculature.

Loss of consciousness and upper airway obstruction

Sedation, sleep, anesthesia, and coma all reduce or abolish the tone in the upper airway and impair ventilatory drive. Brouillette and Thach[10] showed that the closing pressure of the pharynx is about 80 cmH_2O when awake but only a few cmH_2O when sedated. Inspiration and expiration in awake patients do not alter the sagittal airway configuration, but in anesthetized patients inspiratory efforts tend to cause pharyngeal collapse.

Most adults have a significant but variable increase in upper airway resistance during sleep. This increases from a normal awake value of about 1 $cmH_2O\,L^{-1}\,s$ to about 5 $cmH_2O\,L^{-1}\,s$ in young, lean, nonsnorers, but may exceed 60 $cmH_2O\,L^{-1}\,s$ in a heavy snorer. Upper airway resistance varies markedly during sleep and changes from breath to breath. This is due to change in posture, neck flexion, depth of sleep, and respiratory drive.

Does the tongue obstruct the upper airway?

For many years it was assumed that the tongue was the major cause of upper airway obstruction in unconscious patients. Different regions of collapse have been identified. When the patient is supine, the tongue moves posteriorly and has been implicated in obstruction especially in edentulous patients. However, the tongue does not usually occlude the oropharynx, and ultrasound imaging suggests that during sodium thiopental (thiopentone) induction, even if anesthesia is maintained at a very light level, airway obstruction may occur despite minimal movements of the main mass of the tongue.[11]

What about the soft palate?

At induction of general anesthesia, airway occlusion has been shown at the level of the soft palate, but not the tongue.[6,12] Boidin,[13] using a flexible fiberoptic endoscope, has implicated the epiglottis to a greater extent than the tongue or soft palate as the major site of obstruction of the airway during anesthesia. However, the epiglottis, when moving posteriorly as muscle tone reduces, does not always touch the posterior pharyngeal wall.[12] MRI of the upper airway in awake and sedated patients showed a reduction in the anteroposterior (AP) diameter of the pharynx in sedated patients, particularly at the level of the epiglottis and soft palate.[14] General anesthesia with propofol also showed a reduced AP diameter at the level of the soft palate, but with increased diameters at the level of the tongue and epiglottis. Therefore, there may be more than one site of upper airway closure;[6,12] the most recent studies implicate structures other than the tongue.

Head extension

Extension of the head[15] and the application of continuous positive airway pressure (CPAP) will restore airway patency. Mathru *et al.*[6] showed that CPAP increased pharyngeal volume during propofol anesthesia. In contrast, negative pressure applied to the upper airway may cause central apnea.

Laryngeal reflexes – effect of propofol and opioids

Since the classic description of human laryngospasm by Fink,[16] the anesthesia literature has been largely without clinical investigation into this topic until the paper by Tagaito *et al.*[17] They studied patients anesthetized with propofol who had a laryngeal mask *in situ*. The larynx was examined using a fiberoptic laryngoscope and the flow through the mask was measured. The vocal cords were stimulated by spraying with water.

With propofol alone, laryngeal stimulation caused vigorous reflex responses such as expiration, reflex spasmodic panting, coughing, apnea, and laryngospasm. An important finding was that increasing doses of fentanyl reduced, in a dose-dependent manner, the incidence of all these responses except for apnea with laryngospasm. The fact that vigorous airway reflexes were elicited under baseline propofol anesthesia shows that the manual infusion scheme of propofol anesthesia[18] is not effective in suppressing these reflexes arising from the larynx despite the fact that the patients could tolerate the laryngeal mask airway in the hypopharynx. This suggests the possibility that vagal receptors rapidly adapt to a constant stimulation of the mask but not to the intermittent (every 6 min) stimulation of the larynx. The original paper by Tagaito *et al.*[17] should be consulted because of the beautiful serial color photography of the larynx before and after stimulation. A further study[19] showed that opioids reduce laryngeal spasm and cough during induction of anesthesia with desflurane.

Midazolam and upper airway obstruction

In normal subjects, midazolam can cause obstruction between the nasal cavity and just below the tip of the soft palate, i.e. the velopharynx, which is the oropharynx posterior to the soft palate. Midazolam sedation causes an increase in resistance of the nasal passage, snoring, or complete obstruction. This was abolished by using flumazenil.[20]

The larynx as regulator of lung volume

Expiratory flow is controlled by the larynx (and by the diaphragm) so as to exert a braking effect and maintain functional residual capacity (FRC). This is particularly important in the newborn, in whom alveoli are prone to collapse at low lung volume. Tracheal intubation bypasses this function and would partly explain why the FRC is reduced during anesthesia.

Two models of snoring

Huang *et al.*[21] described two sites – the *palate* and the *pharynx* – where snoring is generated. The first site involves airflow over and under the hard and soft palates, similar to an airplane wing but with the trailing edge of the soft palate freely mobile. Above a critical gas velocity, the soft palate starts to flutter, striking the pharyngeal walls. The length and flexibility of the soft palate affects the critical flow speed for flutter to occur. Increasing the palatal tone or reducing its length will increase the critical speed. This may be achieved by uvulopalatopharyngoplasty.

The second site involves the Bernoulli effect in the hypotonic pharynx, where airflow causes narrowing and a subsequent increase in flow velocity then further narrowing at an accelerating rate until wall collapse occurs. This is followed by reopening at an even faster rate. Reduced palatal or pharyngeal tone from whatever cause predisposes to unstable airway conditions and airflow obstruction. Postoperative hypoxemia has been attributed to upper airway obstruction with or without snoring. However, snoring can occur in normal people without causing hypoxemia.

LOWER RESPIRATORY TRACT

Dichotomous branching

Weibel[22] used a plastic cast of an excised human lung to describe the branching geometry of the airways below the larynx. Weibel's model simplified the conducting airways into a series of *symmetrical* branching tubes with each parent tube dividing into two daughter branches of smaller but identical caliber and length.[22,23] The 23 divisions or generations begin at the trachea (generation 0) and finish at the alveolar sacs (generation 23). The trumpet model shows the initial branches are for bulk flow and the terminal branches to the alveoli are for gaseous diffusion (Fig. 5.5). In reality, the flow transition from turbulent to diffusive mixing is gradual and branching is *asymmetrical*.[24]

The caliber of the lower respiratory tract is controlled by (1) autonomic nerve action on smooth muscle,[25,26] (2) change in lung volume, (3) gravity, (4) expiratory effort, and (5) a host of chemical mediators of bronchial muscle contractility.[27] All of these are susceptible to the effects of general anesthesia.

Nerve supply of the airways

The parasympathetic innervation is via the vagus nerve. *Afferents* arise from three types of receptors: (1) slowly adapting stretch receptors are found in the airway wall and may influence the rate and depth of respiration; (2) rapidly adapting irritant receptors are found throughout the mucosa and respond to chemical and mechanical stimuli to initiate the cough reflex; (3) J-receptors are adjacent to pulmonary capillaries and respond to pulmonary edema. *Efferent* fibers cause bronchoconstriction and glandular secretion. Five subtypes of muscarinic receptors have been isolated (M_{1-5}), of which three have been demonstrated in the human airway.[28] M_3 receptors mediate bronchoconstriction and mucus secretion. M_2 receptors are at the prejunctional nerve terminals of postganglionic fibers and cause feedback inhibition of acetylcholine (ACh) release. M_3 receptors are found at parasympathetic ganglia, but their role is uncertain. Sympathetic innervation of the airway is very sparse and may modulate parasympathetic action. Circulating catecholamines mediate most of the effects of the sympathetic nervous system on the airways via β_2-receptors. Sympathetic activity causes bronchodilation via smooth muscle relaxation, inhibits release of inflammatory mediators, and increases mucus clearance.

A third neural system has been described which involves nonadrenergic–noncholinergic (NANC) fibers with both constricting and dilating mechanisms.[29,30] Nitric oxide is the major transmitter for these fibers, causing smooth muscle relaxation and dilation in the pulmonary vasculature. Substance P and other tachykinins are responsible for smooth muscle contraction.

Structure and function

The patency of the trachea is maintained by a series of C-shaped cartilages in the posterior membrane containing smooth muscle under vagal

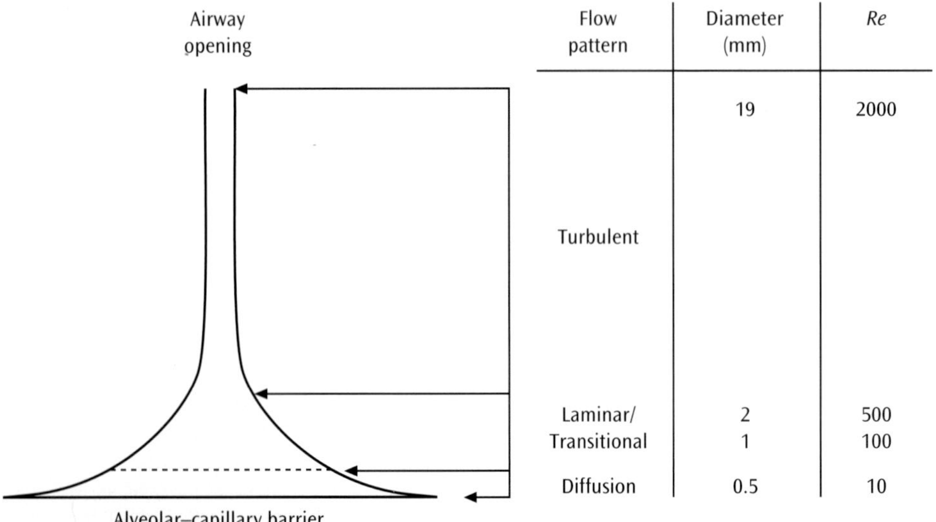

Figure 5.5 *The "trumpet model" of branching airways. The cross-sectional area increases from a few cm² in the trachea to >80 m² at the alveolar–capillary barrier. The diameter and the flow pattern of the airways at each generation is shown.* Re, *Reynolds number.*

control. With normal tone, the trachea has a closing pressure greater than 100 cmH_2O, but after vagal blockade the posterior membrane is lax and the trachea collapses at much lower transmural pressures.[31] Severe airway obstruction is seen when the cartilages are weakened in tracheomalacia and sometimes following retrosternal thyroidectomy.

The intrapulmonary bronchi (diameter 1–3 mm) have discrete plates rather than rings of cartilage. Their caliber is determined by intrinsic smooth muscle activity as well as by the forces applied by the surrounding lung acting radially around the bronchus (lung elastic recoil pressure). Smooth muscle contraction, interstitial edema, and mucous plugging can easily obstruct these airways.

The bronchioles (diameter 0.5–1 mm) lack any cartilaginous support and their caliber is determined by intrinsic smooth muscle and lung elastic recoil. At this point, the total cross-sectional area increases abruptly and gas velocity decreases proportionately, giving Reynolds numbers of less than 10 during tidal breathing (Fig. 5.5). Despite their small size, these air passages constitute only about 10% of the total airway resistance owing to their large cumulative cross-sectional area. This section of the airway culminates in the terminal bronchioles (generation 16), which are the smallest airways without alveoli. From here on, gaseous diffusion dominates gas transport from the respiratory bronchioles to the alveolar wall.

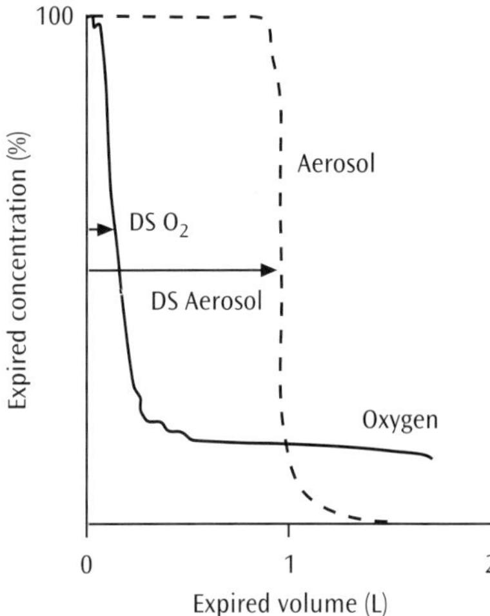

Figure 5.6 *Fowler's single-breath method to compare the size of the dead space (DS) measured with a 1-L breath of oxygen containing an insoluble aerosol. The oxygen dead space (DS O_2) is much smaller than that measured with aerosol (DS Aerosol), which does not mix with alveolar gas.*

Gaseous diffusion between the respiratory bronchioles and the alveoli

During tidal breathing, gas velocity in the trachea is about 200 cm s^{-1}, but this falls abruptly as the cross-sectional area increases. The fresh gas interface moving along the airways becomes almost stationary in the respiratory bronchioles when mass flow gives way to gaseous diffusion as the dominant process of gas movement.[32]

The importance of diffusive mixing in determining the size of the dead space is illustrated in an experiment similar to Fowler's single-breath test. A subject takes a 1-L breath of oxygen that contains a 0.5-μm-diameter insoluble aerosol (di-2-ethylhexylsebacate), which has a concentration that can be measured optically. These "giant molecules" are too large to diffuse into alveolar gas. The expired breath is analyzed for both oxygen and aerosol concentration. About 100 mL of pure oxygen is expired (part of the dead space volume); the remainder of the expired oxygen is mixed with alveolar gas. In contrast, almost all of the 1 L of aerosol is expired unmixed with alveolar gas into which it has diffused. Thus, the dead space for a 1-L breath of aerosol is 1 L[33] (Fig. 5.6).

The alveoli

The alveoli in the alveolar ducts and air sacs (generations 20–23) are the basic units of gas exchange, of which there are about 300 million in the normal adult human lung. About 50% of alveoli arise from alveolar sacs; the remainder arise from the respiratory bronchioles and alveolar ducts. Each alveolus is approximately 300 μm in diameter, but alveolar size varies with the degree of lung inflation and position in the lung – those in the upper lung being the largest and those in the base the smallest (see Fig. 5.1). Note that, by dividing the terminal airways into a vast number of alveoli, the total area available for gas exchange is 5–10 000 times greater than a single sphere with the same volume as the thoracic cavity. In emphysema, the alveolar spaces are larger but the total alveolar surface area is greatly decreased.

The alveolar wall

The alveolar epithelium and capillary endothelium make up the blood–gas interface or barrier, which is exceedingly thin with a large surface area (50–100 m^2). It is therefore very well suited for gas exchange. The alveolar wall includes the alveolar epithelium, the capillary endothelium with the basement membrane of each, and a very thin interstitial space in between (Fig. 5.7A).

The alveolar wall forms a blood–gas diffusion distance of less than 0.4 μm in most places and a barrier of 1–2 μm where the nuclei and supporting structures lie. It is an extraordinary bioengineering structure, but almost no attention has been given to its mechanical properties. These have been recently reviewed by West.[34] The alveolar epithelium is composed mainly of type 1 squamous epithelial cells arranged in very thin sheets. The tight junctions between these cells are shown in Fig. 5.7A. These cells are originally derived from type 2 alveolar cells, which are found in the angles of the junctions in the alveolar septae. They are not only the precursors of type 1 cells but also produce surfactant, which they extrude onto the alveolar surface[27,35] (Fig. 5.7B).

GASEOUS DIFFUSION ACROSS THE ALVEOLAR–CAPILLARY BARRIER

Fick's law

Oxygen and carbon dioxide cross the blood–gas barrier by passive diffusion along a concentration gradient. Fick's law states that the rate of transfer of a gas through a tissue is proportional to its area and to the partial pressure gradient of the gas and is inversely proportional to the tissue thickness. The diffusion constant depends on the solubility of the gas and is inversely proportional to the square root of its molecular weight. Because of its high solubility, CO_2 diffuses about 20 times faster than O_2 through biological tissues.

Capillary transit times

The transit time for a red cell through the pulmonary capillaries at rest is about 0.75 s.[31] The lung is so efficient that the hemoglobin is fully saturated with oxygen in 0.25 s. The equilibration time is increased if the concentration gradient is decreased, e.g. by altitude or a hypoxic gas mixture reducing alveolar oxygen tension.

A

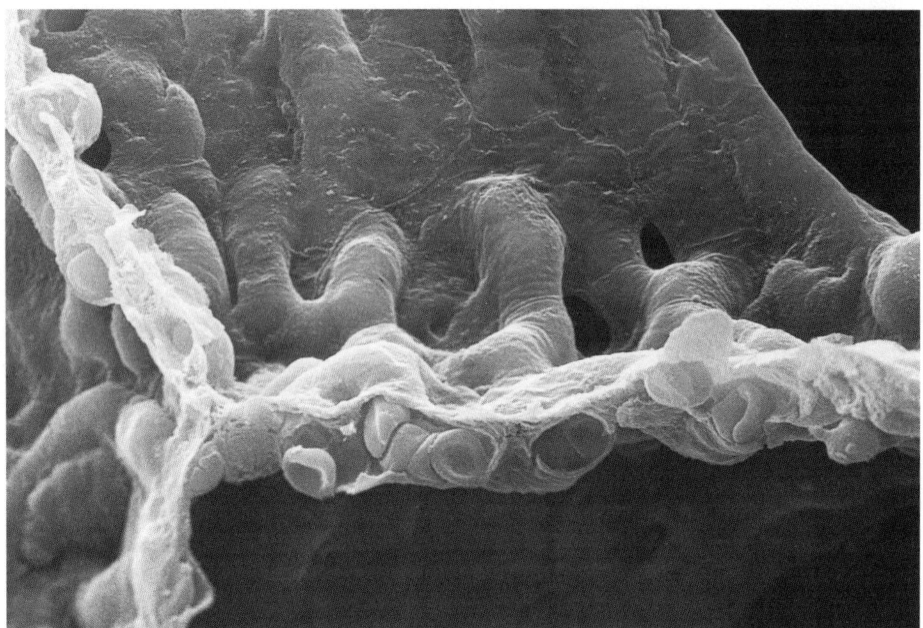

B

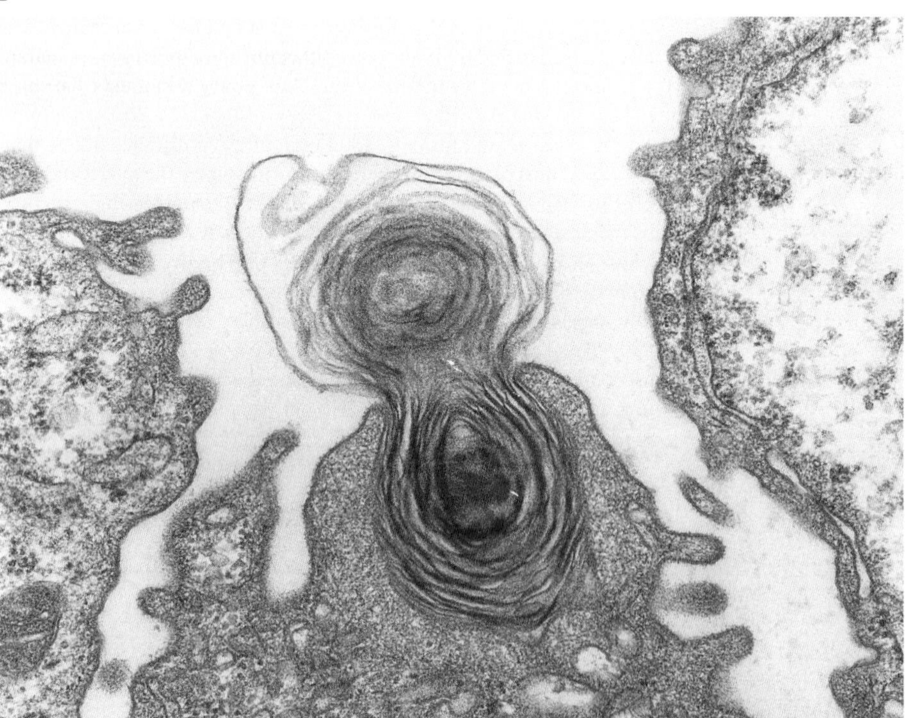

Figure 5.7 *(A) Scanning electron microscope image of the alveolar capillary barrier (courtesy of Professor E. Weibel). Note the lines on the alveolar surface marking the junction between the type I cells. (B) Surfactant being extruded from an alveolar type II cell (courtesy of Professor Mary Williams).*

Differences in uptake of nitrous oxide, carbon monoxide, and oxygen

When nitrous oxide crosses the blood–gas barrier, no combination with hemoglobin takes place. Its partial pressure in blood rises rapidly and equilibration occurs when the red cell is only about one-tenth of its way along the capillary. The amount of nitrous oxide taken up by the blood depends only on the pulmonary blood flow and not at all on the diffusion properties of the blood–gas barrier. Thus, for nitrous oxide, transfer is perfusion dependent.

Carbon monoxide, in contrast, is avidly bound to hemoglobin, which can take up a large amount of this gas with little increase in partial pressure. During red cell transit through the capillary, no back-pressure develops, and carbon monoxide continues to move rapidly into the blood. The limiting factor here is not blood flow but the diffusion properties of the blood–gas barrier, i.e. the alveolar surface area.

The situation for oxygen lies somewhere between nitrous oxide and carbon monoxide. Oxygen binds with hemoglobin, but much less avidly than with carbon monoxide. Also, the oxygen partial pressure of mixed venous blood entering pulmonary capillaries is about 5.3 kPa (40 mmHg) compared with the alveolar tension of about 13.3 kPa (100 mmHg). Under normal conditions, the transfer of oxygen is perfusion limited, as for nitrous oxide. However, if diffusion properties of the blood–gas barrier are impaired, for example by acute respiratory distress syndrome (ARDS), then diffusion equilibration may not occur by the end of the capillary.

Carbon monoxide transfer

In emphysema, the alveolar surface area for gas exchange is considerably reduced. This can be quantified by measuring the diffusion capacity of the lung using a low concentration of carbon monoxide. Fick's equation may be rewritten as the diffusing capacity of the lung (D_L), which incorporates area, thickness, and diffusion properties of the tissue and gas concerned. Because of the high affinity of hemoglobin for this gas, the partial pressure of carbon monoxide in the capillary blood is minute. The term transfer factor may be used, which is a measurement that reflects the magnitude of the alveolar surface area.

FLOW IN THE TRACHEOBRONCHIAL TREE

Narrowing the lumen with a layer of liquid

The conducting airway is normally lined with a very thin layer of liquid. If the layer of fluid on the airway wall is thicker than 1 mm, there is a much greater increase in resistance when airflow becomes turbulent than in a dry-walled tube of the same diameter lumen.[36] This is called two-phase gas–liquid flow. The degree of gas–liquid interaction depends on the gas velocity and on the thickness and viscosity of the liquid layer. *Two-phase flow is the fundamental mechanism whereby a cough clears the airway of mucus.* However, fluid of a high viscosity may not separate if the critical flow rate for detachment is not achieved; this liquid may remain on the wall, causing a persistent increase in resistance which may lead to respiratory muscle fatigue.[37,38]

Effort-independent flow in collapsible airways

The resistance to flow through a tube is pressure drop divided by flow. How, then, can the resistance of the lungs be inferred when flow *alone* is measured (e.g. as in flow–volume loops or $FEV_{1.0}$)? This is the result of "effort-independent flow" (Fig. 5.8). In Fig. 5.8 (left), a normal subject has made a set of flow–volume curves, each with increasing expiratory effort, from total lung capacity (TLC) to residual volume (RV). Up to a point, increasing effort results in an increase in flow. These data have been replotted at one particular lung volume (Fig. 5.8, middle), showing that above a certain effort, indicated by pleural pressure, flow remains constant – *effort-independent flow.* Effort-independent flow is determined only by *three variables*: (1) lung elastic recoil pressure, (2) resistance of small upstream airways, and (3) compliance of the compressed downstream segment.

Some patients with severe airway obstruction have an alarming airflow pattern in which maximum expiratory effort gives a small peak followed by an even *lower* flow than during tidal breathing (Fig. 5.8, right, shaded loop). This is *negative effort dependence* (see also Fig. 5.8, middle panel).

What happens during maximum expiratory flow? There is a sudden large rise in pleural and alveolar pressure. The latter exceeds pleural pressure by an amount equal to lung elastic recoil pressure. There is a very large pressure drop from the alveoli to the mouth (Fig. 5.9, dashed line). At the equal pressure point (EPP), the pressure inside the airway equals the pleural pressure outside. The upstream airways, i.e. those between the alveoli and the EPP, are fully patent. Downstream of EPP, the pressure in the airways is less than that outside (pleural pressure), and these airways may collapse depending on their compliance. Effort independence is due to a choke point or *flow-limiting segment* (FLS) downstream of EPP and acts like a Starling resistor. The caliber of this segment maintains a constant flow independent of the driving pressure. This is the basis of *the wave speed theory*. During a cough, the compressed segment of the airway moves upstream towards the alveoli.[31,39] If the collapse extends too far upstream (in patients with emphysema with low elastic recoil or in patients with bronchitis or asthma with small airway obstruction), the maximum expiratory flow may be even lower than tidal flow (Fig. 5.8) and the shear rate will be too low to clear mucus. Note that the flow volume curve is especially useful in the preoperative assessment of thyroid patients who may have tracheal compression. In this case, the flow curve loses its peak and is flat throughout expiration.

Cough, regional lung emptying, and physiotherapy

Foreign material and chemical irritants stimulate rapidly adapting receptors in the larynx and tracheobronchial tree. After a moderately

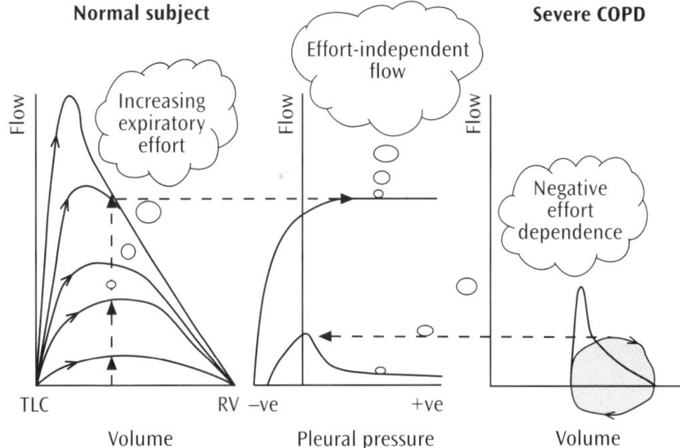

Figure 5.8 *Effort-dependent and -independent flow. (Reproduced by courtesy of The Royal College of Anaesthetists from reference 39.)*

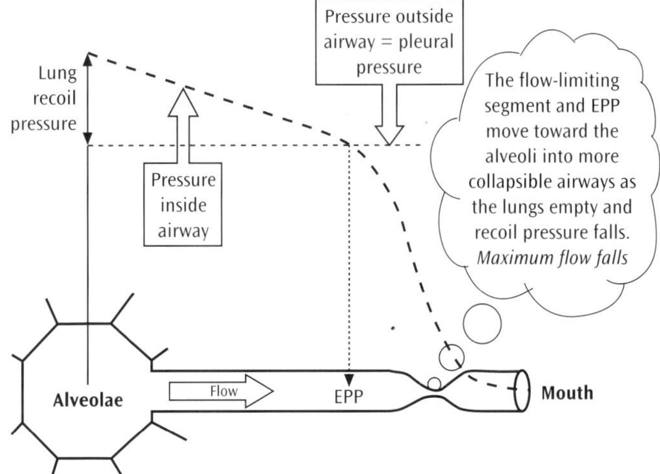

Figure 5.9 *The equal pressure point (EPP) and flow-limiting segment move upstream during maximum expiratory flow. (Reproduced by courtesy of The Royal College of Anaesthetists from reference 39.)*

deep breath, adduction of the vocal cords closes the larynx. Contraction of the respiratory and abdominal muscles generates a high intrathoracic pressure (up to 100 cmH_2O) and then the vocal cords and epiglottis open suddenly, allowing air to escape at high velocity. Shear forces generated by rapid airflow detach mucus, which is expelled by two-phase flow. During a cough, there is a progressive collapse of the airway, beginning at the upper end of the trachea then moving upstream past the carina toward the smaller airways, particularly those in the dependent lung.[37] This closure of dependent airways during a cough causes preferential emptying of the *upper* lung. The narrow moving segment is the site of maximum gas velocity, high *Re*, and very high resistance with maximum gas–liquid interaction and airway clearance.

LUNG VOLUMES AND DISTRIBUTION OF VENTILATION

Lung volumes

Functional residual capacity (FRC) is determined by (1) the balance between the outward pull of the structures of the thoracic cage (chest wall muscle tone, abdominal viscera), (2) the inward elastic recoil of the lung parenchyma, and (3) intrathoracic blood volume. FRC is affected by changes in *posture*. The lung volumes can be measured using the methods shown in Table 5.1.

Anatomic dead space

Originally measured by pouring wax into the lungs of corpses, the anatomic dead space ($V_{D.ANAT}$) corresponds to the volume of airways from the mouth to the terminal bronchioles in which bulk flow rather than diffusion predominates, i.e. nonalveolated airways. The anatomic dead space is about 150 mL (1 mL per cm height). The physiologic dead space ($V_{D.PHYS}$), consists of the $V_{D.ANAT}$ *plus* the alveolated parts of the lung which are ventilated but not perfused. The size of the anatomic dead space is determined by (1) lung volume, (2) tidal volume, (3) airway geometry, and (4) time. Lung volume is a determining factor because the airways increase in diameter as the lungs distend. The dependence on time and tidal volume follows from the fact that alveolar gas will diffuse into dead space gas with time.[40] If an infinite amount of time elapses, alveolar gas will diffuse throughout the airways and the dead space will fall to 0.

Physiologic dead space

Bohr's method uses the principle that all expired CO_2 comes from perfused alveoli and none comes from nonperfused alveoli and conducting airways. The Bohr equation, $V_D/V_T = (P_aCO_2 - P_{\bar{E}}CO_2)/P_aCO_2$, derives physiologic dead space. Many examination candidates forget how to derive the mixed expired CO_2 ($P_{\bar{E}}CO_2$). *Remember that expired air is sampled in a Douglas bag and subsequently analyzed with a CO_2 detector.*

The causes of an increase in physiological dead space include:

1 hypovolemia, hemorrhage;
2 pulmonary embolism;
3 impaired gas exchange (COPD, ARDS);
4 mechanical ventilation.

Table 5.1 *Measuring subdivisions of lung volume*

Volume	Method
V_T, ERV, IC, VC	Spirometer
FRC, RV, TLC	Helium dilution, body plethysmograph, multibreath nitrogen washout
Anatomic dead space	Fowler's single-breath method
Physiologic dead space	Bohr's method
Closing capacity	Modification of Fowler's method

V_T, tidal volume; ERV, expiratory reserve volume; IC and VC, inspiratory and vital capacity; FRC, functional residual capacity; RV, residual volume; TLC, total lung capacity.

The single-breath test

The single-breath test gives information about (1) anatomical dead space (Fig. 5.10; phase I and II), (2) uniformity of regional ventilation (Fig. 5.10; slope of phase III), and (3) closing volume (Fig. 5.10; phase IV). Either Fowler's method (measuring nitrogen, the residual gas) or a tracer gas (e.g. argon, helium, or xenon-133) can be used.

Fowler's method

A single vital capacity breath of oxygen is taken followed by a slow expiration to residual volume. Expired *nitrogen* concentration is plotted against expired *volume* (Fig. 5.10). Phase I, the first part of the expirate, is dead space and contains no nitrogen as pure oxygen is washed out of the conducting airways. In phase II, the nitrogen content rises steeply as the concentration gradient across the terminal bronchioles is sampled. *The anatomic dead space is the expired volume needed to reach the mid-point of phase II* (see also Fig. 5.6). The slope of phase III is a function of uniformity of regional ventilation. Phase IV shows the volume at which dependent airways close. With severe obstructive airway disease, the very uneven regional distribution of ventilation makes it impossible to distinguish among phases II, III, and IV owing to the steepness of the alveolar plateau. Because of poor alveolar gas mixing, such patients also require two or three times longer to oxygenate the lungs prior to induction of anesthesia.

Argon method

A small volume (100 mL) of argon is inspired from the residual volume and is washed into the lung with a vital capacity breath of air. Because of the effect of gravity, different horizontal lung segments (Fig. 5.11, a–g) fill and empty at different rates, depending on lung volume. The onion skin model (Fig. 5.11) shows that *when a subject breathes within the closing volume* the change in regional ventilation is greatest in the

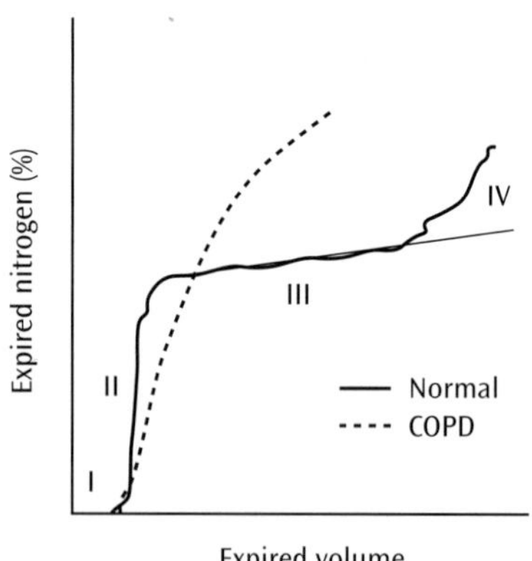

Figure 5.10 *Fowler's method to show the four phases of the alveolar plateau in a normal subject. A line is drawn through phase III to show the start of phase IV. Compare this with the pattern seen in a patient with chronic obstructive airway disease (COPD).*

upper lung (Fig. 5.11, a) and least in the lower region (Fig. 5.11, g), where airways have closed. When a subject is breathing above closing volume, this pattern reverses. The argon–air maneuver washes a very high tracer gas concentration into the top of the lung with very little at the base. The subsequent slow maximum expiration is analyzed for argon to produce a trace such as that shown in Fig. 5.11. The ripples are due to the heart pressing on the lower zone airways during systole. Note that these ripples are like the CO_2 ripples on an anesthetic monitor screen, but these are not usually synchronous with the electrocardiogram trace because the two signals have a different time base. At some point near RV is the onset of closing volume (CV), as the dependent airways close and the vertical gradient of emptying reverses.

Gravity and regional ventilation

The alveolar plateau (phase III) of expired nitrogen, argon, or CO_2 always slopes upwards. The opposite is the case for the alveolar oxygen plateau. Arguments have raged for many years about the mechanism of the slope in phase III and whether airways actually close in phase IV. The onion skin model was elucidated by Milic-Emili *et al.*[41] using ^{133}Xe.

An esophageal balloon is used to infer pleural pressure during a slow inspiration from RV to TLC. The pleural pressure in the upper part of the lung is more negative (−10 cmH_2O) than in the lower part of the lung (−2 cmH_2O). This is because the elastic recoil pressure is greater at the top of the lung; consequently, the top of the lung lies on the flatter upper part of the compliance curve and the bottom of the lung lies on the steep lower part of the curve (Fig. 5.12). The alveoli and conducting airways are more distended at the top of the lung than at the bottom, but because the lower lung is more compliant more ventilation passes to the bottom than to the top. Jere Mead used a Slinky spring to model alveolar distension and regional ventilation. The upper part of the spring is more distended than the lower part, but the lower part moves more than the upper when the spring is slowly oscillated in a vertical plane.

If FRC falls (e.g. after induction of anesthesia), basal airways close; this pattern reverses when more ventilation passes to the top of the lung as the dependent lung becomes more atelectatic.

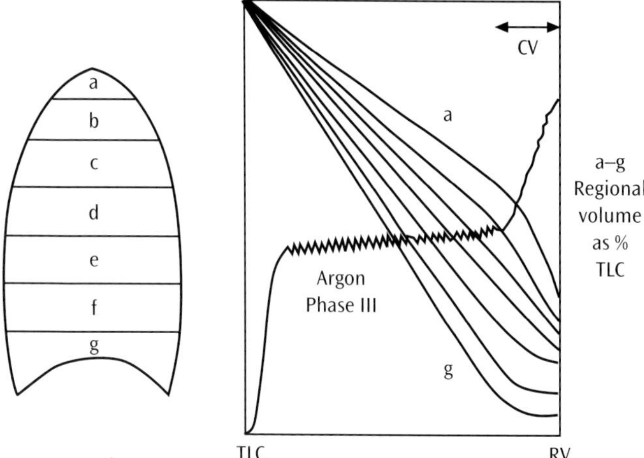

Figure 5.11 *The onion skin model of regional ventilation. Different horizontal lung slices (a–g) fill and empty at different rates owing to the effect of gravity on regional lung compliance. TLC, total lung capacity; RV, residual volume; CV, closing volume.*

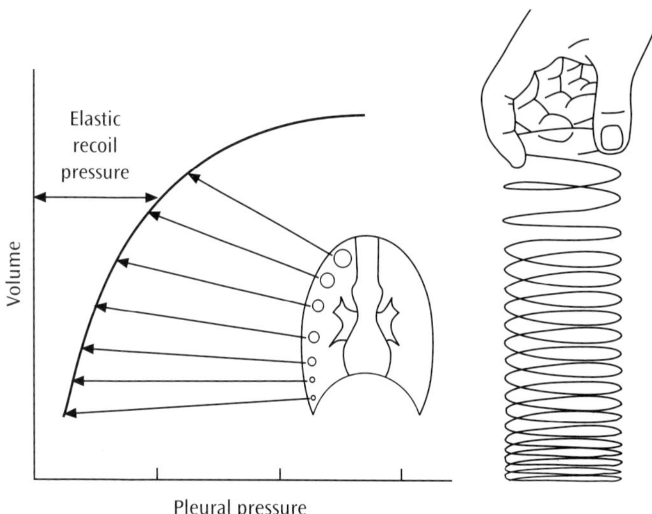

Figure 5.12 *Effect of gravity on regional lung compliance can be compared to a Slinky spring (after Jere Mead). The bottom of the spring (and the lung) is much more compliant than the top. Note that, like the spring, the airways are more distended at the top (see Fig. 5.1).*

Effect of change in gravitational force and posture on regional ventilation

So far the effect of normal gravitational force on regional ventilation has been discussed. If gravitational force increases during acceleration[32] in a human centrifuge or if the lung becomes heavier because of pulmonary edema, closing volume will increase[42,43] progressively until only the uppermost parts of the lung are ventilated. If the patient lies down or is inverted, a similar vertical gradient of ventilation is seen.

On the basis of our studies in the human centrifuge, we suggested, more than 30 years ago, that if gravitational force falls to 0 then in theory all the alveoli will be similar in size and ventilation will be distributed evenly over the whole lung.[44] This has recently been confirmed experimentally.[45]

Lung volume and airway resistance

Lung volume is an important determinant of airway resistance. On taking a deep inspiration, the airway caliber increases as the lung expands. Conversely, when breathing out to residual volume, the airways progressively narrow. Airway resistance is usually measured in a body plethysmograph and is derived from the pressure drop across the airway divided by the flow rate:

$$R = \Delta P / \dot{V}$$

The plethysmograph is impractical in anesthetized patients, and we have studied the effect of changing lung volume using *forced oscillation*. This uses a piston pump with a stroke volume of 50 mL to produce an oscillating air flow at 3 Hz. Pressure and flow are measured at the mouth as lung volume is slowly reduced to RV, producing the curves shown in Fig. 5.13. This produces a hyperbolic relation between airway resistance and lung volume which can be measured relatively easily in either awake or anesthetized paralyzed subjects.[46] The reciprocal of resistance is conductance, which has a linear relation with volume as shown.

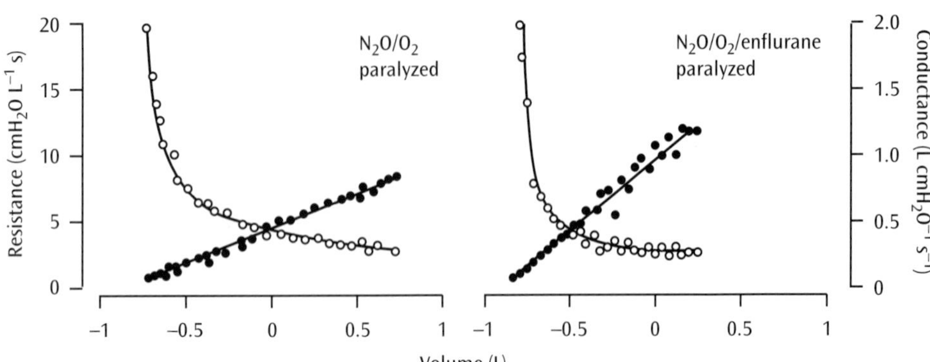

Figure 5.13 *The forced oscillation method can be used to measure airway resistance (open circles) in anesthetized patients. The reciprocal of resistance is conductance (filled circles). The shape of the resistance–volume curve and the slope of the conductance curve are measures of bronchomotor tone. Enflurane is a bronchodilator.*

The shape of the resistance curve and slope of conductance are changed by bronchoactive drugs (histamine or β-agonists) or volatile anesthetics. The gradient of the conductance plot gives a convenient descriptor of airway caliber. Bronchodilators increase the gradient, whereas bronchoconstrictors decrease it. The effect of administering a volatile anesthetic to a previously paralyzed patient is interesting because, in addition to a change in the shape of the curve, the FRC also changes. The latter can only be explained by a change in intrathoracic blood volume and has been discussed at length elsewhere.[47]

The effect of anesthetic drugs on bronchomotor tone

An excellent review on the basic mechanisms of general anesthetic action on airway smooth muscle has recently been published.[48] In this review, the techniques most often referred to for measuring airway caliber are high-resolution computed tomography, superfine bronchoscopic techniques, and isolated smooth muscle. Halothane, enflurane, isoflurane, sevoflurane, desflurane, sodium thiopental, ketamine, and propofol all relax airway smooth muscle *in vitro*. High concentrations of benzodiazepines have similar effects. The effects of these agents on *in vivo* airway caliber may not all reflect *in vitro* activity. Desflurane and isoflurane may induce constriction. Propofol has occasionally been reported to induce bronchospasm.

Volatile inhalational anesthetic agents

There is no doubt that volatile agents reduce airway resistance in man. The forced airflow oscillation method of measuring airways conductance in anesthetized humans, described above, shows that halothane, enflurane, and, to a lesser extent, isoflurane all caused a decrease in bronchomotor tone.[46,49]

Intravenous anesthetic agents

Therapeutic doses of sodium thiopental leave airway reflexes largely intact so that vagally mediated reflex bronchoconstriction to airway instrumentation can be expected. Propofol suppresses airway reflexes to a greater degree than sodium thiopental. Conti *et al.*[50] noted a consistent decrease in airway resistance after propofol administration to patients with chronic obstructive airways disease. Hence, propofol may be indicated as an alternative to sodium thiopental for patients with pre-existing bronchial hyper-reactivity. The bronchodilator effects of ketamine have been noted since its introduction into clinical practice and are attributed to a direct relaxant effect on bronchial smooth muscle, inhibition of vagal pathways, and sympathomimetic effects due to increases in endogenous catecholamines. Recently, it was shown in sheep that ketamine and propofol reduce bronchoconstriction produced by vagal stimulation or methacholine through neurally mediated effects.[51]

Muscle relaxants

Both tubocurarine and atracurium are potent inducers of histamine release. However, in normal subjects, significant increases in airway tone after tubocurare administration have not been demonstrated, although some patients with pre-existing lung disease did show an increase in airway tone. Simpson *et al.*[52] studied changes in specific airway conductance after tubocurare, pancuronium, and atracurium administered to normal patients. Overall, there was a significant decrease in conductance only after atracurium, whereas a decrease in conductance after tubocurare was shown in only one out of eight patients. Note that patients who had cutaneous flushing did not show a decrease in conductance and vice versa.

Anticholinesterase drugs can provoke airway constriction by inhibiting the destruction of endogenous acetylcholine at parasympathetic nerve terminals. This effect is largely dismissed by most authors as being prevented by concurrent administration of anticholinergic agents, although the use of neostigmine in asthmatics has been cautioned against. However, even in normal subjects, reversal of neuromuscular block using neostigmine and either atropine or glycopyrolate is associated with a significant increase in airway resistance.

Opioids

Morphine causes histamine release from mast cells. However, only in patients with pre-existing bronchial hyperactivity does histamine release appear to cause a clinical problem. Any potentially adverse effects of histamine can be avoided by using fentanyl or other similar synthetic opioids. Nevertheless, even in paralyzed patients, fentanyl administration ($5\,\mu g\,kg^{-1}$) can cause an increase in respiratory resistance which can be partly reversed by atropine.[53] Meperidine (pethidine) may be the opioid of choice for patients with hyper-reactive airways.

Nonsteroidal anti-inflammatory drugs (aspirin-induced asthma)

The use of nonsteroidal anti-inflammatory drugs (NSAIDs) in anesthetic practice has greatly increased in recent years, with obvious benefits in analgesia. In the majority of patients, NSAIDs have no apparent effect on the airways, but in asthmatic patients they can cause severe airway problems, even after only one dose.[54] Aspirin-induced asthma (AIA) affects 8–20% of adult asthmatics, but is rare in asthmatic children. Individuals with AIA are intolerant of other NSAIDs, with the ability to cause symptoms being directly related to their potency as inhibitors of cyclo-oxygenase. NSAIDs that do not inhibit cyclo-oxygenase, such as sodium salicylate and choline magnesium trisilicate, are well tolerated by patients with AIA.

Antileukotrienes

Leukotriene receptor antagonists are the first novel class of drugs to treat asthma to become available over the last three decades. They have a unique profile in that they are a hybrid of both a bronchodilator and an anti-inflammatory drug. Antileukotrienes such as montelukast and zafirlukast[55,56] may be taken as a tablet either once or twice daily. They show a good antiasthmatic activity over a wide spectrum of asthma severity, resulting in improvement in lung function, asthma symptoms, and β_2-agonist use. In addition, they protect against antigen- and exercise-induced bronchoconstriction and can decrease asthma exacerbations. They are particularly effective in the subgroup of patients with aspirin-intolerant asthma. The use of antileukotriene agents in severe and steroid-dependent asthma has not been studied.

CHANGES IN THE LUNG DURING GENERAL ANESTHESIA

Reading the ventilator pressure gauge in the paralyzed patient

The changes seen on the ventilator pressure gauge reflect the mechanical properties of the lung and chest wall.[57] If the rib cage were opened and the lungs inflated, a lung compliance curve such as that shown in Fig. 5.14A would be seen. However, if we were to remove the lungs and just inflate the closed chest, we would see a pattern such as that shown in Fig. 5.14B, in which a subatmospheric pressure (P_{neg}) must be applied to collapse the chest wall to zero volume. If lungs (L) and chest wall (CW) were restored and inflated with a ventilator, the chest wall and lung pressure curves must be added to give the ventilator gauge pressure, P_{aw} (Fig. 5.14C). From these curves, it can be seen that during mechanical ventilation:

$$P_{pl} = P_{aw} - P_L = P_{CW}$$

i.e. the chest wall curve gives the pleural pressure (P_{pl}) at any lung volume during mechanical ventilation. This pressure, which is above atmospheric for most of the curve, interferes with venous return and thus cardiac output. For this reason, it is obvious from Fig. 5.14C that the change in P_{aw} read off the ventilator pressure gauge *overestimates* the pleural pressure at a given lung volume.

Effect of general anesthesia on lung function

General anesthesia produces:

1 a fall in FRC;
2 a fall in lung compliance;
3 more uneven distribution of ventilation;
4 increased physiologic dead space;
5 increased $P_{(A-a)}O_2$.

General anesthesia, with or without neuromuscular blockade, causes a reduction in FRC, probably as a result of a fall in muscle tone in the chest wall and a shift in intrathoracic blood volume.[47] The reduction in lung volume is associated with an increase in airway resistance because of the hyperbolic relation between lung volume and airway resistance (Fig. 5.13). Dependent atelectasis may occur, and the tidal volume may encroach into the closing volume. If the lung is already at minimum volume, the application of mechanical ventilation, particularly with the addition of PEEP (positive end-expiratory pressure), may reverse some of these effects.

For volatile agents, the increase in airway resistance is offset to some extent by a reduction in bronchomotor tone. The consequence of a reduced FRC and dependent airway narrowing is the development of impaired gas exchange due to extensive atelectasis in the dependent part of the lung. This was first shown using computed tomography (CT) by Hedenstierna *et al.*[58] and provided a convincing explanation for the ubiquitous abnormality in gas exchange which occurred during anesthesia. In particular, the extent of atelectasis, measured from the area on the CT scan, correlated very closely with the degree of $\dot{V}_A/\dot{Q}$ abnormality, as measured by the multiple inert gas elimination test (MIGET).

The impairment of gas exchange induced by general anesthesia is, in the vast majority of cases, trivial. Dependent lung atelectasis

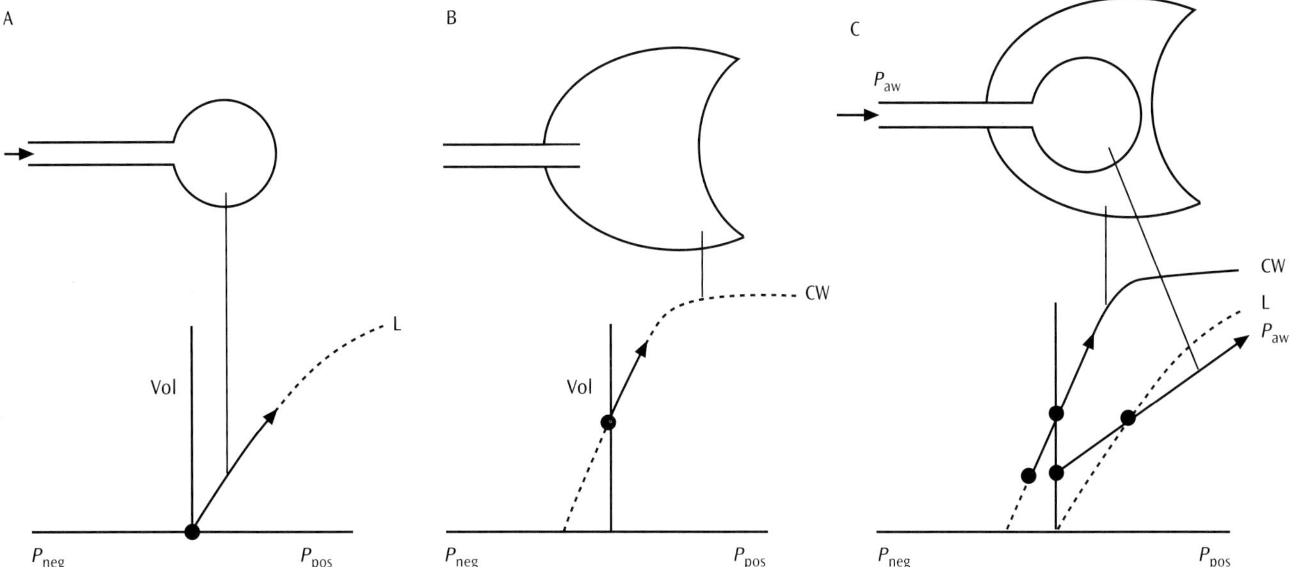

Figure 5.14 *The mechanical properties of the lung (L) and chest wall (CW) in paralyzed patients can be inferred from the ventilator pressure gauge (see text).*

induced during anesthesia can be re-expanded by a series of large lung inflations. In general, the degree of atelectasis was reduced significantly only at airway pressures of 30–40 cmH_2O maintained for 5 s and was accompanied by a decrease of pulmonary shunt with normalization of oxygen saturation.[59] Thus, if a patient shows a persistently reduced S_pO_2 during anesthesia, it is worth carrying out a series of hyperinflations; it is a common observation that the S_pO_2 will rise into the normal range. In patients undergoing thoracotomy, it has been shown that including nitrogen in the inspired gas and either avoiding the use of nitrous oxide or using a lower concentration of N_2O than is present standard practice prevents the formation of atelectasis.[60] Hedenstiena and Rothen[61] suggested three mechanisms that might cause atelectasis during anesthesia: compression of alveoli, absorption of alveolar gas, and loss of surfactant. Joyce and Williams[62] showed that preoxygenation increased the rate of gas uptake from unventilated regions and was a more important determinant of the time to collapse than whether there was N_2 or N_2O in the anesthetic mixture. Increasing the F_IO_2 during anesthesia reduced the time to collapse.

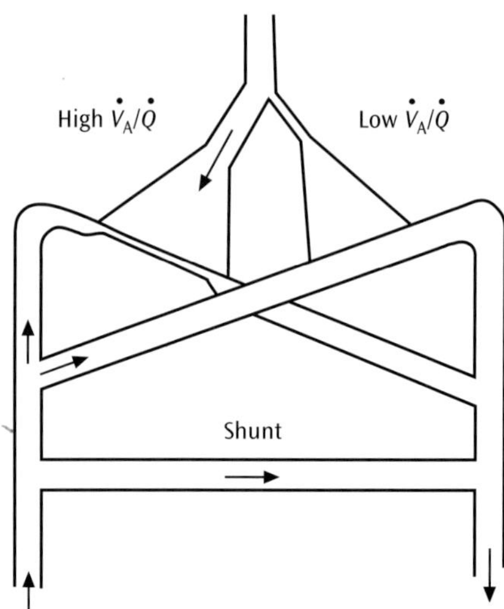

Figure 5.15 *A three-compartment gas exchange model showing shunt and high- and low-$\dot{V}_A/\dot{Q}$ regions.*

GAS EXCHANGE

Methodology

When FRC falls after induction of anesthesia, the airways in the dependent lung become even narrower and ventilation is redirected to the upper lung as basal alveoli collapse. The dependent lung is the site of severely impaired gas exchange, which causes an increase in the alveolar–arterial oxygen gradient, $P_{(A-a)}O_2$. Complete closure of airways to alveoli that are still perfused causes a $\dot{V}_A/\dot{Q}$ of 0, also referred to as a *physiologic shunt*. In contrast, the complete occlusion of a vessel to normally ventilated alveoli gives a $\dot{V}_A/\dot{Q}$ of infinity, which is a *physiologic dead space*. Between these extremes there may be any number of compartments with variable $\dot{V}_A/\dot{Q}$ values that cause a progressive impairment of oxygen exchange. The $\dot{V}_A/\dot{Q}$ ratios of these compartments are likely to be log-normal in distribution. The MIGET uses six to eight gases of different solubility, ranging from sulfur hexafluoride ($\lambda = 0.008$) to acetone ($\lambda = 374$), to calculate the $\dot{V}_A/\dot{Q}$ distribution.[63–66] This technique, which is invasive and requires complex gas analysis using gas chromatography, is available in only a handful of laboratories throughout the world.

A more easily used method, shown in Fig. 5.15, is the three-compartment model, which describes high and low $\dot{V}_A/\dot{Q}$ as well as shunt. The three compartments are (1) a physiologic shunt, (2) a low $\dot{V}_A/\dot{Q}$ region, which will increase the $P_{(A-a)}O_2$ gradient, and (3) a high $\dot{V}_A/\dot{Q}$ region, which will increase physiologic dead space but have little effect on $P_{(A-a)}O_2$.

How to measure oxygen exchange noninvasively

Zetterström[67] reviewed an alphabet soup of indices of pulmonary oxygen exchange. These included $P_{(A-a)}O_2$, $P_{(A-a)}O_2/P_aO_2$, P_aO_2/P_AO_2, and P_aO_2/F_IO_2. Although these are widely used in clinical practice, he concluded that none of them gave a satisfactory description of pulmonary oxygen exchange except the invasive measurement of *shunt fraction*, which is calculated from the equation

$$\dot{Q}_s/\dot{Q}_t = (C_{c'}O_2 - C_aO_2)/(C_{c'}O_2 - C_{\bar{v}}O_2)$$

Here, $\dot{Q}_s$ is the physiologic shunt, $\dot{Q}_t$ is the total cardiac output, $C_{c'}O_2$ is the pulmonary capillary oxygen content, C_aO_2 is the arterial content, and $C_{\bar{v}}O_2$ is the mixed venous oxygen content. $C_{c'}O_2$ has to be derived from the alveolar PO_2 (P_aO_2) using the *alveolar air equation*. At its simplest, this is $P_AO_2 = P_IO_2 - P_aCO_2/R$. The other measurements are made using the co-oximeter.

Noninvasive measure of oxygen exchange

A simple method has been described for deriving shunt and low $\dot{V}_A/\dot{Q}$ using only a pulse oximeter and varying inspired oxygen concentration to produce a P_IO_2 vs. S_pO_2 diagram.[66,68–70] The curve relating inspired oxygen partial pressure (P_IO_2) to oxyhemoglobin saturation (S_pO_2) reflects the shape of the oxygen dissociation curve and can be used to derive *shunt* and *low* (<0.5) $\dot{V}_A/\dot{Q}$ (Fig. 5.16). The shape and position of the P_IO_2 vs. S_pO_2 curve varies considerably among patients, with different degrees of shunt and $\dot{V}_A/\dot{Q}$ abnormality. *An increase in shunt produces a downward displacement of the curve whereas a decrease in $\dot{V}_A/\dot{Q}$ shifts the curve to the right.* Both downward and leftward shifts usually occur together when gas exchange is impaired.

The P_IO_2 vs. S_pO_2 curve gives:

1 shunt;
2 low $\dot{V}_A/\dot{Q}$;
3 a predictor of postoperative hypoxemia.

The shape and position of the curve is sensitive to hemoglobin concentration and cardiac output. These values, if known, can be entered into the computer algorithm.[68]

Effect of thoracotomy on shunt and low $\dot{V}_A/\dot{Q}$

An example of an acute change in curve position during anesthesia is shown in Fig. 5.17A. This figure shows a patient studied before, during, and after thoracotomy for esophageal surgery.[71] After induction of anesthesia, the inspired oxygen is varied to give a range of S_pO_2 values from 92% to 99%. Note how much the F_IO_2 has to be reduced in a normal person to reduce S_pO_2. During thoracotomy the curve moves downward, representing an increase in *shunt* from 4.2% to 17.8%, and to the right, representing a considerable increase in the P_IO_2/P_AO_2 gradient from 5.2 kPa (40 mmHg) to 24 kPa (180 mmHg). This is a measure of *low* $\dot{V}_A/\dot{Q}$ and shows that the $\dot{V}_A/\dot{Q}$ falls from 0.8 to 0.2. Note that at the end of surgery the gas exchange returns almost to baseline conditions.

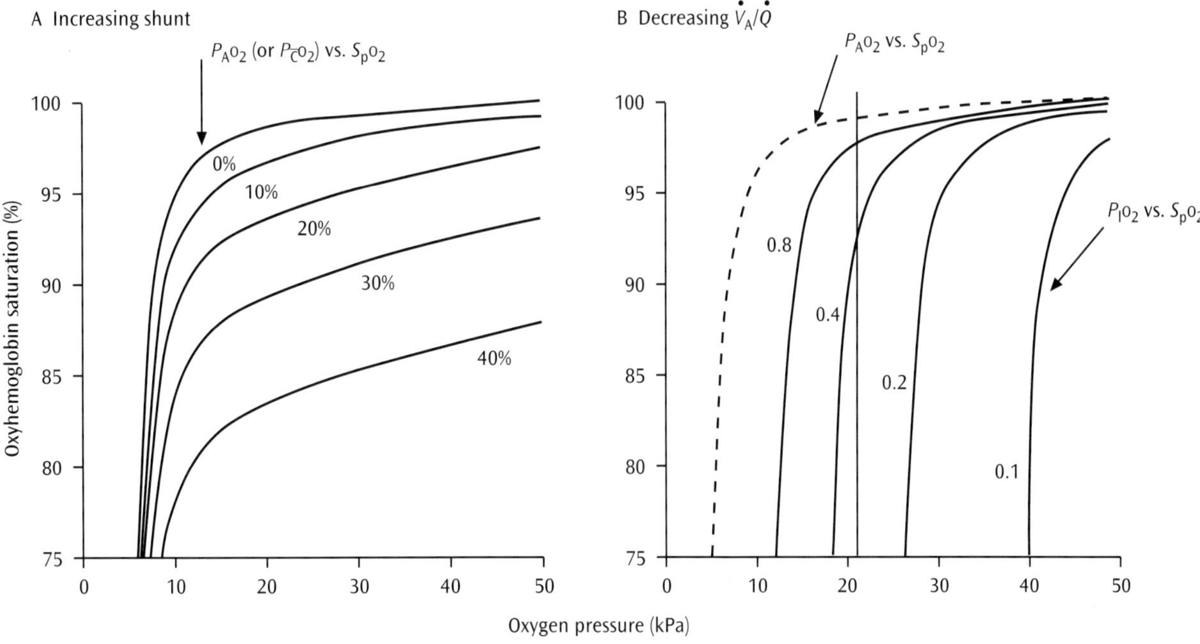

Figure 5.16 *(A) Increasing right to left shunt (0–40%) moves the P_{IO_2} vs. S_{pO_2} curve downwards. (B) Decreasing $\dot{V}_A/\dot{Q}$ (0.8–0.1) produces a rightward displacement of the curve.*

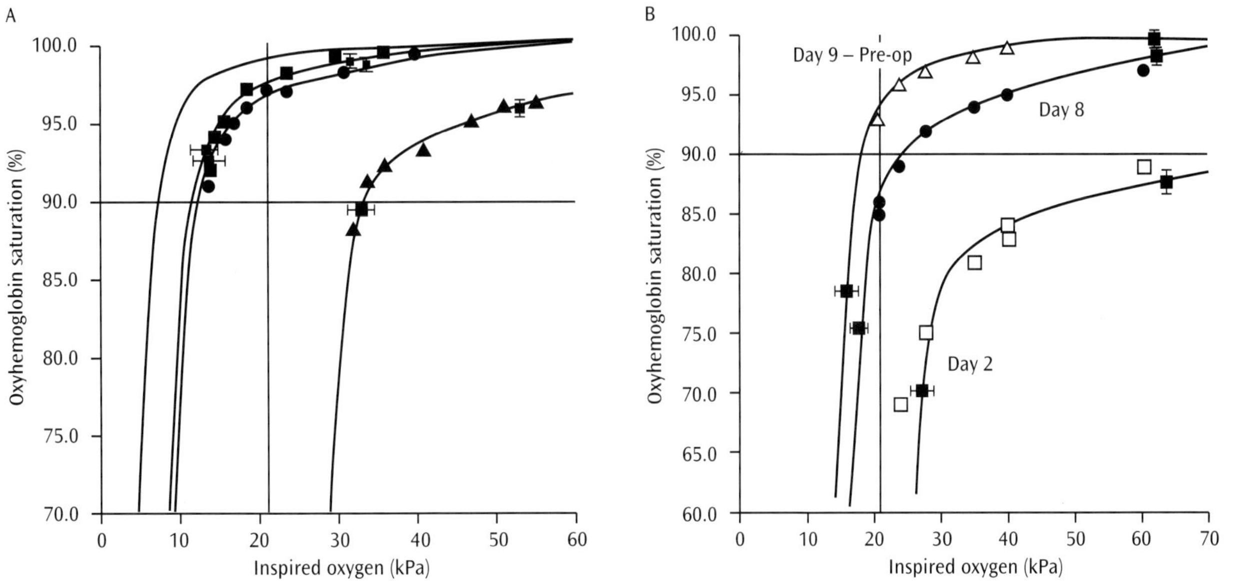

Figure 5.17 *(A) Effect of thoracotomy on the P_{IO_2} vs. S_{pO_2} curve. Filled squares, post induction; filled triangles, chest opened; filled circles, end of operation. (B) Effect of fat embolism on the P_{IO_2} vs. S_{pO_2} curve (see text).*

Effect of fat embolism

This approach can also be used to demonstrate the effects of fat embolism on gas exchange.[72] Following a road traffic accident, a 27-year-old patient sustained a fractured femur and was found to be very hypoxemic.[72] Operation was postponed to the day after admission, when he was found to have a considerable shunt (40%) and very low $\dot{V}_A/\dot{Q}$ (0.2) (Fig. 5.17B). Operation was further postponed, and 8 days after admission shunt had fallen to 16% and $\dot{V}_A/\dot{Q}$ had risen to 0.4. Both of these values were very abnormal. He was operated on 9 days after admission, when he still had a significantly reduced $\dot{V}_A/\dot{Q}$, although his shunt had returned to normal. Postoperatively, his shunt and $\dot{V}_A/\dot{Q}$ became significantly worse then gradually returned to normal.

Prediction of postoperative hypoxemia

The most important cause of postoperative hypoxemia is the combination of (1) a reduced $\dot{V}_A/\dot{Q}$ introduced intraoperatively and (2) impaired postoperative ventilatory control induced by opioids. As we have seen above, a reduced $\dot{V}_A/\dot{Q}$ shifts the P_{IO_2} vs. S_{pO_2} curve to the right so that the steep part of this curve becomes a tangent to the inspired oxygen pressure. In this circumstance, opioid administration causes a further shift to the right and this causes a profound fall in oxygen saturation.

To demonstrate this, postoperative oxygen saturation was measured continuously overnight *with patients breathing air*. All the oxygen saturation values were plotted as a series of distribution curves every 30 min on the first postoperative night[69,73] (Fig. 5.18). Patient A – with

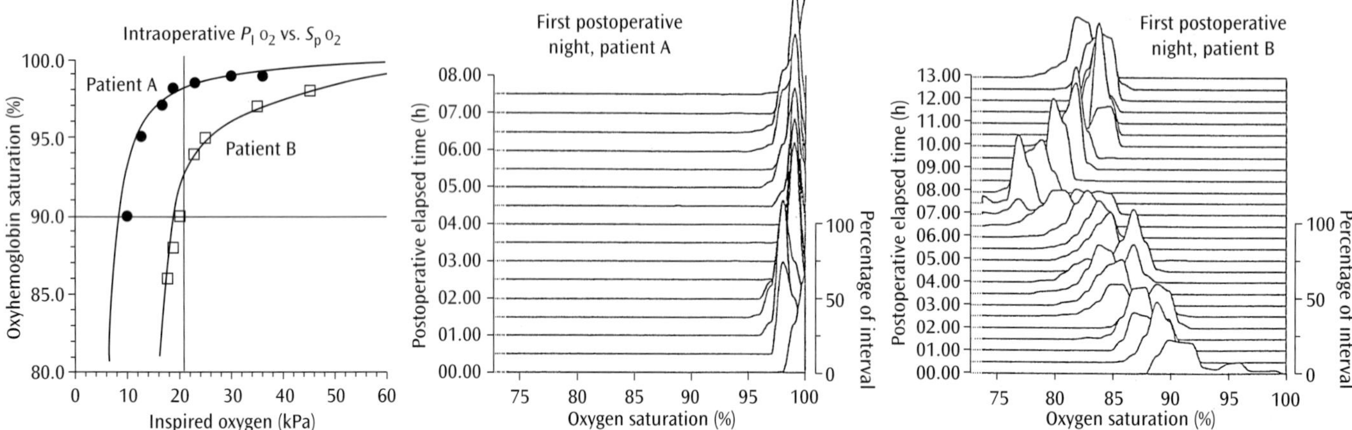

Figure 5.18 *Intraoperative P_Io_2 vs. S_po_2 curves predict postoperative hypoxemia when patients breathe air. Left: The P_Io_2 vs. S_po_2 curve measured by varying P_Io_2 in a normal patient (A) and a patient with reduced $\dot{V}_A/\dot{Q}$ (B). The latter curve is shifted to the right. Middle: The S_po_2 distribution pattern measured throughout the first postoperative night in patient A. Each curve shows cumulative S_po_2 values for each 30-min period. Right: Severe postoperative hypoxemia in patient B caused by the right shift of the P_Io_2 vs. S_po_2 curve (see text).*

normal intraoperative gas exchange, as shown by the normal position of the P_IO_2 vs. S_pO_2 curve – had a postoperative S_pO_2 distribution pattern which remained in a narrow, overlapping range around 97% throughout the measuring period. In contrast, patient B, whose P_IO_2 vs. S_pO_2 curve is shifted to the right because of a reduction in $\dot{V}_A/\dot{Q}$, had widely scattered distribution curves with long periods of hypoxemia with S_pO_2 falling to less than 75%.

A fall in $\dot{V}_A/\dot{Q}$, causing a shift in the P_IO_2 vs. S_pO_2 curve to the right, is a very important factor in predisposing patients to sleep-related hypoxemia. For example, in patient B, a small rise (1 kPa, 7.5 mmHg) of $P\text{CO}_2$ following morphine administration or during sleep apnea produced a large fall in oxygen saturation (> 10%), whereas in patient A, with a normal P_IO_2 vs. S_aO_2 curve, a similar rise in $P\text{CO}_2$ had a trivial effect on S_aO_2.[69,73]

Recommendations for postoperative oxygen therapy[69]

1 Give a known concentration of oxygen and record this value.
2 Monitor all patients in the recovery room using pulse oximetry.
3 Reduced $\dot{V}_A/\dot{Q}$, and therefore increased likelihood of hypoxemia, is likely (1) in obese patients when the body mass index (BMI) > 27 kg m^{-2}, (2) following upper abdominal or thoracic surgery, and (3) in patients with obstructive airway disease.
4 Patients taking opioids, especially if they have a reduced $\dot{V}_A/\dot{Q}$, are at increased risk of hypoxemia, particularly during sleep.
5 Other risk factors indicating oxygen therapy are (1) hypovolemia, (2) hypotension, (3) myocardial and cerebral ischemia, and (4) sickle cell disease.
6 Continue oxygen administration until S_pO_2 is > 93% or has returned to stable preoperative values.
7 Of those patients with severe obstructive airway disease, 10% rely on a hypoxic ventilatory drive and caution is required in the administration of oxygen. Nevertheless, tissue oxygenation is paramount.

PULMONARY CIRCULATION AND MICROCIRCULATION

The pulmonary arteries follow the airways down to the terminal bronchioles where they ramify to form a dense pulmonary capillary bed in close proximity to the alveolar walls. The bronchial circulation, which comes from the systemic circulation, supplies the airway walls down to the level of the terminal bronchioles. This blood does not enter the alveolar capillary network but drains into the pulmonary veins and mixes with the oxygenated blood. The pulmonary arterial pressure [mean pulmonary artery pressure (MPAP) = 2 kPa (15 mmHg)] is much lower than its systemic counterpart [mean artery pressure (MAP) = 12 kPa (90 mmHg)]. Under normal conditions, the PAP is just sufficient to raise blood to the lung apex; however, if PAP were reduced by acute blood loss, or if alveolar pressure were increased by application of PEEP or CPAP, then the physiological dead space at the apex would increase. The gradient of increased perfusion down the lung does not compensate for the gradient of ventilation in the same direction. Thus, $\dot{V}_A/\dot{Q}$ is much higher at the top of the lung than at the bottom.

Control of the pulmonary circulation

Under hypoxic conditions there is pulmonary vasoconstriction (HPV); this contrasts with the systemic circulation, in which hypoxemia causes vasodilation. The alveolar $P\text{O}_2$ is the prime stimulus, with the pulmonary arterial $P\text{O}_2$ having a lesser effect. Eisenkraft[74] has shown that HPV has no clinical significance in compensating for a reduced $\dot{V}_A/\dot{Q}$ and influencing the arterial $P\text{O}_2$ in patients. This was recently endorsed by Conacher.[75]

Nitric oxide is a potent vasodilator that can be delivered to the pulmonary vasculature without causing systemic vasodilation. It has been extensively used in patients with pulmonary vascular disease, pulmonary hypertension, and various gas exchange abnormalities. Its use in the routine treatment of acute lung injury and the acute respiratory distress syndrome cannot be recommended. Treatment of the latter with sodium nitroprusside, hydralazine, prostaglandin E_1, or prostaglandin I_2 (prostacyclin) has not been shown to be beneficial.[76]

Fluid balance in the lung

It is essential that the alveoli remain free of fluid to maintain efficient gas exchange. This is a considerable feat considering that almost the entire cardiac output passes within about 0.3 μm of the alveolar lumen. To some extent, fluid exchange across the capillary wall obeys Starling's law, but note that *surface tension* and *active ion transport* are of crucial importance (Fig. 5.19). The Starling equation is:

$$\text{Net fluid out} = K_f[\Delta P - (\Sigma\sigma \times \Delta\pi)]$$

Here, the force expelling fluid from the capillary into the alveolar or interstitial space is the capillary hydrostatic pressure minus the alveolar or interstitial space pressure (ΔP). The force pulling fluid back into the capillary is the difference between the colloid osmotic pressure of the proteins in the blood and those in the interstitial or alveolar fluid ($\Delta\pi$). This is modified by the reflection coefficient (σ) and the filtration coefficient (K_f). In the normal lung, $\Delta\pi$ exceeds ΔP by about 3.2 kPa (24 mmHg). This is the critical wedge pressure above which pulmonary edema will develop in left-sided heart failure.

The reflection coefficient is a measure of the leakiness of the wall to various solutes. Independent consideration should be given to the alveolar epithelium and the capillary endothelium, which have different reflection coefficients.[77] The reflection coefficient of the epithelium for protein is 1, and that for the endothelium is 0.6. This means that protein cannot permeate the epithelium but it can leak through the endothelium into the interstitial space, causing a lymph flow of about 20 mL h^{-1}. The different types of junction between epithelial cells and between endothelial cells explain why the solute permeation of epithelial junctions is about 10 times less than that of the endothelium. This low permeability and its ability to actively transport sodium also explains the very large osmotic pressure (several atmospheres) that can be developed across the epithelial part of the barrier. However, the high resistance of the epithelium may rapidly break down under the mechanical distension of fluid or overdistension of the lung or epithelial injury. In these circumstances, the Starling equation modifies to:

$$\text{Net fluid out} = K_f \times \Delta P$$

When this occurs there is no force opposing the net flow of fluid out of the capillaries into the alveolar space. Thus, in acute lung injury there is no point in trying to manipulate plasma colloid osmotic pressure because there is no effective semipermeable membrane in the lung for it to operate across.

Fluid that permeates the capillary wall tends to track through the alveolar interstitium into the perivascular and peribronchial spaces where most of the lymph vessels are found. In early pulmonary edema, these spaces become engorged with fluid. This interstitial edema does not hinder gas exchange as the alveoli remain "dry." With worsening edema, fluid begins to cross the alveolar epithelium and enter the alveolar spaces, gradually filling them and preventing ventilation so that no gas exchange can occur.

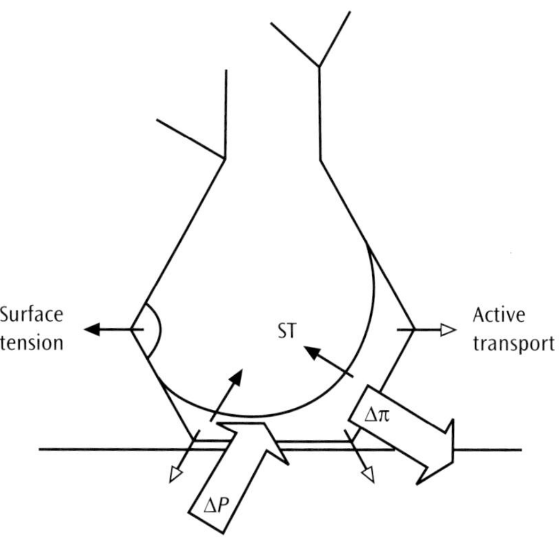

Figure 5.19 *Diagrammatic representation of an alveolus and capillary to show how the balance of pressures is maintained to preserve an air-filled alveolar space. If the alveolus floods, a high surface tension (ST) can exert a considerable force and draw more water into the lumen.*

Surface tension and ion transport

Two important factors which influence fluid flux from capillary to alveolar lumen are not included in the Starling equation. These are surface tension and ion transport (Fig. 5.19). Some of the controversial roles of surfactant have been previously summarized.[78] The surface tension of the liquid lining the alveoli can develop large forces, making the whole system unstable with a tendency to collapse. Surfactant secreted by the type II pneumocytes markedly reduces the surface tension of this liquid layer, causing the stability of the alveoli to be enormously increased. A much greater pressure is required to open a collapsed alveolus than is needed to expand it once opened. Thus, surfactant greatly reduces the work of breathing. Hills[79–81] has been one of the most provocative workers in this field. He proposed that, under normal conditions, there is either an aqueous layer (hypophase) between the surfactant layer and the epithelial wall or large parts of the alveolar surface may be dry with surfactant bound directly to the alveolar surface. One of the implications of the latter is that surfactant may act as a water repellent. Any droplets of water which accumulate on the airway wall have convex surfaces and the surface tension of this surface creates a hydrostatic pressure which "pumps" water out of the lumen into the interstitium. In a thoughtful editorial, Dorrington and Young[82] criticized some of these proposals. More than a decade ago, Hill's proposal that (cationic) surfactant binds to the anionic alveolar surface, providing an essentially dry layer without an aqueous subphase, was also criticized.[83] Although type II cells have extensive anionic sites, the type I cells, which make up most of the alveolar surface, have none. However, Hills may be right in that after extensive lung damage, as in ARDS, the type I cells are replaced by anionically charged type II cells, and this may be of crucial importance in the way that surfactant helps to restore the normal mechanical properties of the alveoli. Nevertheless, it has also been shown that endotoxin can alter the charge distribution of the alveolar surface and permit the permeation of charged tracer molecules, which are retained by the normal lung.[84,85]

Active transport of both protein and electrolyte are important in maintaining the large concentration gradient of solute across the barrier which, if the reflection coefficient is near unity, results in a highly protective gradient of osmotic pressure that keeps the alveoli free of fluid. Active transport of electrolyte is so effective that, even if liquid with a protein concentration twice that of plasma is instilled into the alveoli, it will be pumped out against the colloid osmotic pressure gradient.[86]

Acute respiratory distress syndrome

The pathophysiology of ARDS is fundamentally a breakdown in the integrity of the alveolar capillary barrier, particularly of the epithelium, and a reduction in the reflection coefficient of both epithelium and endothelial components. This causes an increased flux of protein into the alveolar space, which itself denatures surfactant and promotes further flooding and alveolar collapse. Although an increased solute permeability of the alveolar barrier is a cardinal feature of ARDS, it must be pointed out that PEEP itself and even 50% oxygen can increase solute permeability.[87]

The characteristic features of ARDS are protein-rich pulmonary edema with pulmonary artery wedge pressure <2.4 kPa (18 mmHg), dyspnea, and impaired gas exchange. There are large numbers of precipitating clinical conditions which initiate barrier injury. These can be subdivided into chemical, physical, microbiologic, and host defense. These can initiate a huge variety of mediators of lung injury.

From the outset, the treatment of ARDS made the condition a strong candidate for an iatrogenic disease. The first cases were described during the Vietnam war (Da Nang lung), when massive fluid overload was in vogue. Because this made gas exchange worse, very high oxygen concentrations were then needed. This caused oxygen toxicity and increased the pulmonary edema that was caused by fluid overload. This initiated the era of super PEEP, which caused fatal barotrauma by exceeding Hooke's law and made the injury to the alveolar epithelium worse. Then followed a search for one or more mediators of lung injury, each of which could be blocked by the thoughtful use of laboratory science. All of these approaches failed. The final solution was the use of extracorporeal circulation to maintain life while nature cured the disease. We are now entering a more conservative era of treatment that is reducing mortality.[88] This is summarized as:

1 Thirty percent of the alveoli in ARDS are normally aerated, although these structures may also show changes if investigated by electron microscope (EM).
2 The pressure–volume curve (Fig. 5.20) shows a high opening pressure (P_1) and a second pressure (P_2) above which ventilator pressures injure the lung. If ventilator pressures fall below P_T, lung injury also occurs.
3 To avoid exceeding Hooke's law and injuring the lung, use a tidal volume of 6 mL kg^{-1} and do not exceed a plateau pressure of 32 cmH_2O. Plateau pressures less than this do not seem beneficial.
4 Recommendations in (3) may result in hypoventilation, so correct respiratory acidosis with bicarbonate.
5 Research into mediators has not resulted in any identifiable improvement in outcome.
6 With regard to fluid restriction, a review article[76] has recommended "maintain[ing] the intravascular volume at the lowest level that is consistent with adequate systemic perfusion." This is now being formally evaluated by a National Institutes of Health (NIH) study.

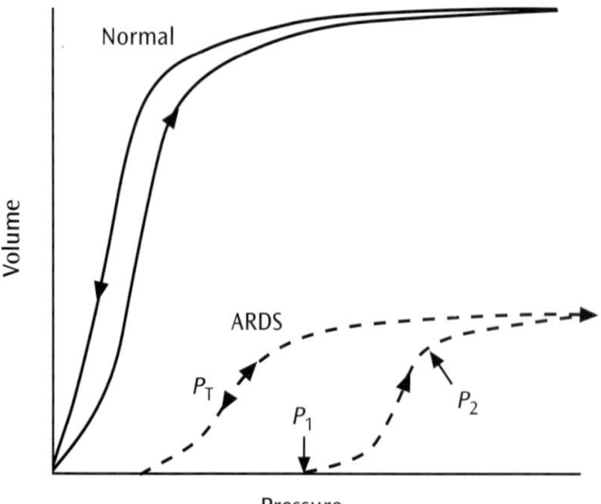

Figure 5.20 *Lung pressure–volume curves in a normal person compared with a patient with ARDS. The latter needs a very high opening pressure* P_1 *and only a small further increase in lung volume* P_2 *leads to barotrauma. Pressure* $\geq P_T$ *is ideal for tidal ventilation. Arrows indicate inflation and deflation.*

GAS TRANSPORT

Oxygen

When breathing air, the oxygen reserve in a 3-L FRC is about 500 mL. The blood stores about 850 mL of oxygen. Increasing the inspired oxygen fraction ($F_{I}O_2$) increases oxygen stores in the FRC to nearly 3 L and increases dissolved oxygen, but this has little effect on the volume bound to hemoglobin as it is nearly fully saturated when breathing air. Oxygen is carried to the tissues by means of being dissolved in the plasma and bound to hemoglobin (Hb). The amount dissolved depends on the partial pressure and solubility, giving 0.003 mL per 100 mL blood for each mmHg of PO_2. Blood substitutes such as perfluoronated hydrocarbons have a high oxygen solubility and can carry as much oxygen as blood at high oxygen tensions. Unlike Hb, these compounds have a linear PO_2 vs. content relation. In theory, 1 g of Hb can combine with 1.39 mL of oxygen (Hoffman coefficient). In reality, this amount is less (1.34–1.36 mL) because *in vivo* the heme group of a small fraction of hemoglobin is oxidized to methemoglobin, which is unable to release its oxygen to the tissues. Nitrites and sulfonamides oxidize hemoglobin, as can a congenital deficiency in the enzyme methemoglobin reductase. If the oxygen capacity of hemoglobin is 1.36 mL g^{-1}, 15 g of hemoglobin can combine with 20.4 mL of oxygen – the oxygen content. The oxygen saturation of Hb ($S_{a}O_2$) is expressed as a percentage of the oxygen capacity:

$$O_2 \text{ content} = (1.36 \times \text{Hb} \times SO_2/100) + (0.003 \times PO_2)$$

$$O_2 \text{ content} = O_2 \text{ bound to Hb} + O_2 \text{ dissolved in plasma}$$

where the O_2 content is given as mL O_2 per 100 mL blood, Hb is given as g per 100 mL, and PO_2 is given as mmHg.

Oxyhemoglobin dissociation curve

The shape of the curve (Fig. 5.16) confers important physiologic advantages. The flat upper portion implies that small changes in alveolar oxygen (breath holding, moderate altitude) have little deleterious effect on full oxygen saturation of blood. At alveolar oxygen tensions of less than 70 mmHg (9.3 kPa), small reductions in capillary oxygen tension result in large reductions in hemoglobin oxygen content, which facilitates the unloading of oxygen from hemoglobin to supply the tissues. The position of the oxyhemoglobin dissociation curve (ODC) is conventionally described by the term P_{50}, which is the oxygen tension required for 50% saturation of hemoglobin and is normally 27 mmHg (3.6 kPa). The P_{50} may shift to the right or left under certain physiologic conditions (Table 5.2).

A right shift means that more oxygen is unloaded at a given PO_2. Most of the effect of altering PCO_2 can be attributed to the associated change in the hydrogen ion concentration (Bohr effect). Conditions associated with a right shift in the ODC are found in active tissues, so that hemoglobin gives up its oxygen more easily where it is needed most. The compound 2,3-DPG is an endproduct of red cell metabolism and is increased in anemia, thyrotoxicosis, and chronic hypoxia (lung disease and high altitude). Stored blood has depleted 2,3-DPG and is less effective at oxygen delivery.

Carboxyhemoglobin

The affinity of hemoglobin for carbon monoxide is 240 times greater than its affinity for oxygen. Carboxyhemoglobin will tie up a large amount of hemoglobin, making it unavailable for oxygen carriage.

Table 5.2 *Factors causing a shift of the oxyhemoglobin dissociation curve*

Left shift	Right shift
↓ $[H]^+$	↑ $[H]^+$
↓ $P\text{CO}_2$	↑ $P\text{CO}_2$
↓ Temperature	↑ Temperature
↓ 2,3-DPG	↑ 2,3-DPG

DPG, diphosphoglycerate.

Carbon monoxide causes a left shift in the ODC, thus further interfering with oxygen unloading. Smokers may have up to 25% of their hemoglobin bound to carbon monoxide, thus reducing the oxygen content of the blood. Carbon monoxide poisoning is easy to miss if not looked for specifically (using a CO oximeter) and requires prompt treatment with 100% oxygen or hyperbaric oxygen to encourage formation of oxyhemoglobin by competition for binding sites.

Carbon dioxide transport

The capacity of the body to store carbon dioxide, unlike oxygen, is very large – an adult being able to store well over 100 L. The major store is bicarbonate in the bones. Hyperventilation will cause the arterial $P\text{CO}_2$ to fall faster than hypoventilation will cause it to climb. In respiratory arrest, the arterial $P\text{CO}_2$ increases by 0.4–0.8 kPa (3–6 mmHg) min^{-1}. The plasma carries CO_2 in three forms: in plasma proteins to form carbamino compounds; in water to form carbonic acid; and as bicarbonate ions when carbonic acid dissociates. Most of the CO_2 in plasma passes into the red blood cells, where some stays in solution, some binds to hemoglobin, forming carbamino-hemoglobin, but most forms carbonic acid and then dissociates into bicarbonate and hydrogen ions. This reaction is very fast within the red blood cell owing to the presence of carbonic anhydrase. The chloride (or Hamburger) shift is when bicarbonate diffuses out of the cell into the plasma and is accompanied by chloride ions to retain electrical neutrality. The result is that most of the carbon dioxide produced in the tissues is carried in the blood as the bicarbonate ion.

CONTROL OF BREATHING

Objectives of the controller

Breathing is regulated as if it were a negative feedback control system.[89] If the system is disrupted from its controlled state, receptors detect changes in $P_a\text{CO}_2$, $P_a\text{O}_2$, or stretch in the lung/chest wall. These receptors transmit signals via their afferents to the central controller, which institutes corrective action by changing ventilation. Two control objectives are to minimize the work of the respiratory muscles and to maintain the acid–base environment of the brain. The outputs can be combined to give: *minute ventilation* and the *timing and volume* of each breath.

Minute ventilation

In awake subjects, a small increase in $P_a\text{CO}_2$ from normal leads to a marked increase in ventilation. In contrast, a reduction in $P_a\text{O}_2$ needs to be very much larger for the control mechanism to alter ventilation. These variables are influenced by the state of consciousness of the individual. During sleep, there is a decrease in ventilation which is accompanied by an increase in $P_a\text{CO}_2$.

Resting ventilation is set at the intersection of two curves (Fig. 5.21). In Fig. 5.21, curve A is the metabolic hyperbola whose position is determined by CO_2 production, and curve B is the linear plot of minute ventilation to $P_a\text{CO}_2$ (set by the respiratory control system). The point of intersection of the two determines the *set point of the system*, i.e. the levels of normal ventilation per minute and $P_a\text{CO}_2$. Either of the two relations that determine the set point can be altered. Thus, narcotics shift the control system response line to *the right* and *reduce its slope* (curve D). This results in a new system set point that has a reduced minute ventilation and an elevated $P_a\text{CO}_2$.

In the case of a spontaneously breathing anesthetized patient, passive hyperventilation of the patient by the anesthesiologist will reduce $P_a\text{CO}_2$ to point E, where the subject stops breathing. This is called the apneic threshold. This does not occur in fully awake subjects, who after a period of hyperventilation continue to breathe with $P_a\text{CO}_2$ values well below the apneic threshold at point C. However, subjects sedated with nitrous oxide who are able to obey commands become apneic if their $P_a\text{CO}_2$ falls below the apneic threshold at point C.[90] This has important implications for postoperative patients and those sedated with other drugs.

Timing, volume, and the Hering–Breuer reflex

It is well known that minute ventilation (V_m) is obtained by multiplying tidal volume (V_T) by respiratory rate (f), so do not be alarmed by the following:

$$V_m = V_T \times f = (V_T/T_I) \times (T_I/T_{tot})$$

When T_{tot} is the duration of one breath in seconds, then frequency (f) is $60/T_{tot}$, and the inspiratory time is T_I. With a little bit of effort, you can see that ventilation is now described by two terms, one reflecting the average inspiratory *flow rate*, V_T/T_I, and the other relating to *timing*, T_I/T_{tot}. The latter is simply the fraction of the respiratory cycle that is taken up by inspiration.

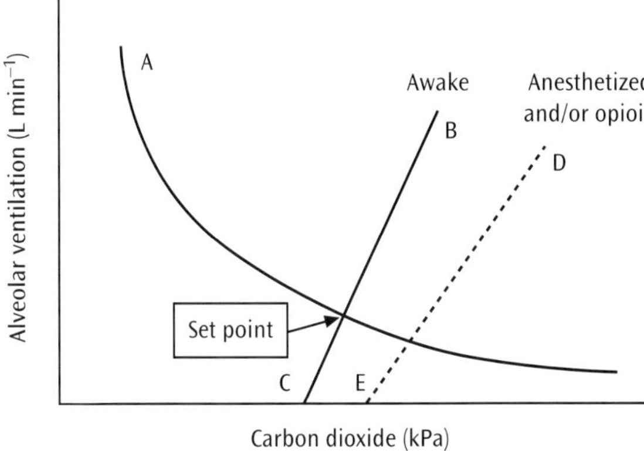

Figure 5.21 *There are two curves relating* $P\text{CO}_2$ *to ventilation. Curve A is the result of changing ventilation primarily (the metabolic hyperbola) and curve B results from changing* $P\text{CO}_2$ *primarily. Curve D is seen after opioid administration. The point of intersection determines the set point of the systems (see text). The apnea threshold (points C or E) is reached if a sedated or anesthetized subject is passively hyperventilated.*

Time thresholds and volume thresholds control ventilation

When ventilation is increased by gradually raising inspired CO_2, the relation between tidal volume (V_T) and T_I exhibits two regions (Fig. 5.22). In region I, inspiratory time is determined by a time threshold and the T_I values are constant. Because CO_2 increases inspiratory flow rate, tidal volume also increases by up to about 1.5–2 times the normal value with the same inspiratory time (T_I). The increase in respiratory frequency is brought about by a reduction in T_E. In region I, tidal volume can increase at constant T_I until it reaches the Hering–Breuer volume threshold.[91] This brings ventilation into region II. In region II, any further increase in tidal volume is limited by the Hering–Breuer threshold. Tidal volume is now inversely related to T_I, and in this region minute ventilation increases because of an increase in tidal volume and an increase in frequency, which is also due to a decrease in T_I.

Hering–Breuer reflex in man and animals

In both awake and anesthetized humans, region I-type behavior extends the normal V_T range by up to twice. The Hering–Breuer threshold is higher in awake subjects than in awake animals. When animals are anesthetized, the Hering–Breuer reflex has a much lower volume threshold and is much more important in controlling tidal volume. Consequently, region I behavior is not seen in anesthetized animals; instead, as V_T increases, T_I decreases.

With T_I remaining constant during tidal breathing, it is the operation of a *central timing mechanism* that sets a tidal volume in humans that is characteristic of region I behavior. Sensory inputs traveling up the vagus nerves from pulmonary stretch receptors are responsible for the hyperbolic relation between V_T and T_I that is characteristic of region II behavior.

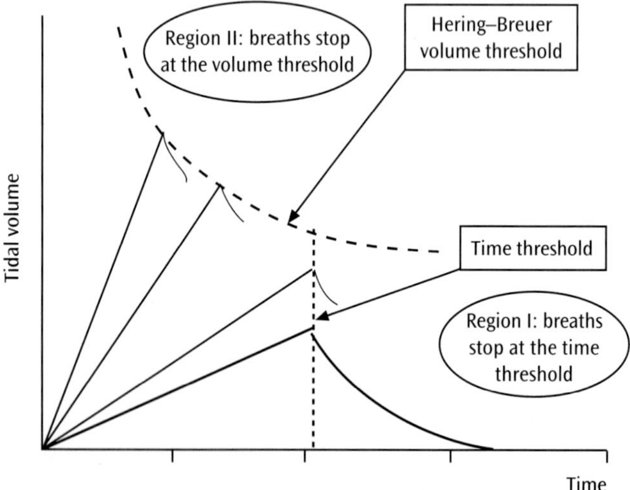

Figure 5.22 *The relation between inspiratory time, tidal volume, and the Hering–Breuer volume threshold. With normal breathing, tidal volume does not reach the Hering–Breuer threshold, giving a constant* T_I. *With increased ventilatory drive, the Hering–Breuer threshold is reached, giving an inverse relation between* V_T *and* T_I.

CENTRAL ORGANIZATION OF RESPIRATORY CONTROL

Voluntary ventilation is governed by the cortex, and automatic ventilation is governed by the brainstem. The spinal cord exerts a further regulation. The brainstem center for automatic ventilation lies bilaterally in the ventral medulla, surrounding the motor nuclei of the vagus and glossopharyngeal nerves. This is called the ventral respiratory group (VRG), whose function is to drive intercostal, abdominal, and laryngeal muscles, with only a small part of its output going to the diaphragm. The VRG is responsible for both inspiratory and expiratory activity.

On each side of the dorsal part of the medulla is the dorsal respiratory group (DRG), where the respiratory rhythm is generated. The DRG is the first processing station for afferent information from pulmonary stretch receptors, laryngeal receptors, and peripheral chemoreceptors. It also provides the principal respiratory drive to the diaphragm and is the only driver to the VRG. Part of the information in its sensory input is fed to the apneustic center (APC) just rostral to DRG, and it is this center which normally switches off inspiration. The classic model represents this rhythm generator in terms of reciprocal inhibition of two groups of respiratory neurons – one inspiratory and the other expiratory.

The rate and depth of ventilation can be modulated either by changes in the cortical input or by a change in input from central and peripheral receptors, which include the following:

- Peripheral chemoreceptors at the bifurcation of the common carotid arteries and in the ascending arch of the aorta and branches. These show a progressive increase in activity as P_aO_2 falls below 13.5 kPa (101 mmHg). This response can be linearized by plotting chemoreceptor drive against O_2 saturation. The fact that the peripheral chemoreceptors are also stimulated by a decrease in blood pressure and increased sympathetic activity suggests that changes in local blood flow are important. These chemoreceptors are also stimulated by the pH effects of changing $P\text{CO}_2$.
- Central chemoreceptors lie near the ventral lateral surface of the medulla and sense changes in $P\text{CO}_2$ from the changes in brain extracellular fluid pH. The ventilatory responses to acute nonrespiratory acidosis or alkalosis are not mediated by central chemoreceptors but by peripheral chemoreceptors. The respiratory response to change in $P\text{CO}_2$ is linear between $P\text{CO}_2$ values of 2.7 and 8.0 kPa (20 and 56 mmHg).

The lung and chest wall receptors

There are three types of *lung receptor* mediating responses in the vagus nerve: stretch receptors, irritant receptors, and J receptors. The *chest wall receptors* include the Golgi tendon organs, joint receptors, and the muscle spindles. Impulses from these pass centrally in the phrenic or intercostal nerves. The feedback between intercostal afferents and the laryngeal musculature and synchronization is important to avoid obstructive apnea.

Fine control of ventilatory muscles – response to loading

The tonic and phasic output of the spinal neural network is distributed via motor neurons to the intercostals, diaphragm, and the musculature of the abdomen, neck, larynx, and tongue. The tonic component to the chest wall maintains a constant resting lung volume, whereas the phasic output changes lung volume when activity switches from inspiratory to expiratory firing. In general, expiration is passive, but there may be a carry-over of some phasic inspiratory muscle activity into expiration, thus exerting a braking effect on the expired breath. This system must permit the respiratory musculature to adapt to sudden unanticipated breathing loads or to control the postural activity of the ventilatory and other muscles against predictable loads such as gravitational force.

A large part of this load compensatory mechanism lies in the muscle spindle system. This is highly susceptible to depression by sleep and general anesthesia and is responsible for the relaxation in most muscle groups seen in anesthetized patients. However, the diaphragm has few muscle spindles compared with the muscles of the neck, abdominal wall, or intercostal spaces. Sensory information from the diaphragm is mediated mainly by the Golgi tendon organ system via type Ib afferent fibers. This difference in proprioceptive control of diaphragm and other muscles of respiration may explain the differences in response of the two muscle groups during general anesthesia, i.e. phasic and tonic activity in the intercostals is lost but diaphragmatic contraction is spared even with high concentrations of anesthetic agents.

Chest wall

The chest wall is divided into rib cage, diaphragm, and abdominal wall. The chest wall has two functions: *supportive* and *ventilatory.* The *supportive function* maintains the shape and volume of the lungs so that the inward elastic recoil of the lungs and the outward recoil of the rib cage and gravitational force are in balance. This supportive function also prevents paradoxical movement from rib cage to abdomen. The *ventilatory function* is used to assess the output of the respiratory control system. General anesthesia normally results in a reduction in tidal volume and an increase in breathing frequency. The reduction in tidal volume may be largely due to a loss of rib cage contribution, but diaphragm function is retained. This leads to paradoxical movement of the chest wall and is one of the oldest signs of depth of anesthesia, being included in the Guedel stages of ether anesthesia. The slightest obstruction to breathing during anesthesia results in greatly exaggerated paradoxical ventilation as the diaphragm pulls the rib cage inwards.[92] The best evidence of airway obstruction can be obtained from simultaneous monitoring of either intrathoracic and abdominal pressures or rib cage and abdominal (and thus diaphragmatic) movement. The latter method, using lightweight inductance belts, is a simple technique that can be applied in anesthetic practice, with a plot of rib cage vs. abdominal movement.

The evaluation of central respiratory drive

Measuring respiratory drive and timing can be carried out during resting breathing or with challenge tests. The latter examine the ventilatory response to either chemical or mechanical loading.

Chemical loading

The inter-relation between $P\text{CO}_2$ and ventilation is shown in Fig. 5.21. Increase in the inspired $P\text{CO}_2$ by rebreathing 7% CO_2 in oxygen from a 5-L spirometer produces the curve shown at B or D. Curve D illustrates the well-known central depressant effect of 10 mg morphine in a subject with normal lungs.[93] Inhalation and intravenous anesthetics are potent respiratory depressants. Equivalent anesthetic doses [1 MAC (minimal alveolar concentration)] of the following agents all reduce alveolar ventilation and increase $P\text{CO}_2$ in the order: cyclopropane < methoxyflurane < halothane < isoflurane < enflurane.[94,95] Ether is a notable exception, producing no noticeable respiratory depression at an equivalent anesthetic concentration. Sodium thiopental, methohexitone, and propofol are all respiratory depressants.

Halothane has been the most extensively studied anesthetic agent. It has been assumed until recently that the ventilatory depressant effect of halothane was due to a central effect on the respiratory center. Tusiewicz *et al.*[96] showed that the normal increase in ventilation in response to rising $P\text{CO}_2$ in awake subjects is mainly the result of a large increase in rib cage contribution to ventilation with a much smaller increase in diaphragm contribution. The contraction of rib cage musculature is quickly depressed by general anesthetics, but the diaphragmatic response to increased carbon dioxide is little affected. The net effect, including paradoxical chest movement, leads to a reduction in total ventilatory response to CO_2.

Hypoxia

More than 20 years ago, Knill and coworkers[94,95] showed that chemoreceptors are very sensitive to the effects of halothane, enflurane, and isoflurane. The hypoxic response is abolished by subanesthetic concentrations (0.1 MAC) long before the CO_2 response is attenuated. More recently, Temp *et al.*[97] failed to repeat the findings of Knill and coworkers, but later Nagyova *et al.*[98] confirmed Knill's results and also showed that propofol depressed the hypoxic ventilatory response. The question of whether the depressant effect of anesthetic agents in low doses on the acute hypoxic ventilatory response is clinically important remains controversial. Robotham[99] argues that a patient may be at risk with a depressed ventilatory response to hypoxia with even 0.1 MAC halothane, enflurane, or isoflurane. Goodman[100] suggests that, for most patients, complete loss of the hypoxic response does not matter.

REFERENCES

1. Olson DE, Sudlow MF, Horsfield K, Filley GF. Convective patterns of flow during inspiration. *Arch Intern Med* 1973; **131:** 51–7.
2. Stevens JJWM, Jones JG. Functional anatomy and pathophysiology of the upper airway. In: Jones JG, Hanning CD (eds). *International Practice and Research*, vol. 9. London: Baillière Tindall, 1995: 213–34.
3. Jones JG, Hanning CD. The upper airway. In: Jones JG, Hanning CD (eds). *Clinical Anaesthesiology. International Practice and Research*, vol. 9. London: Baillière Tindall, 1995: 213–401.
4. Nishino T. Physiological and pathophysiological implications of upper airway reflexes in humans. *Jpn J Physiol* 2000; **50:** 3–14.
5. Jordan D. Central nervous pathways and control of the airways. *Respir Physiol* 2001; **125:** 67–81.
6. Mathru M, Esch O, Lang J, *et al.* Magnetic resonance imaging of the upper airway. *Anesthesiology* 1996; **84:** 273–9.
7. Gerlach H, Rossaint R, Pappart D, *et al.* Autoinhalation of nitric oxide after endogenous synthesis in nasopharynx. *Lancet* 1994; **343:** 518–19.
8. Sauerland EK, Sauerland BAT, Orr WC, Hairston LE. Non-invasive electromyography of human geniolglossal (tongue) activity. *Electromyogr Clin Neurophysiol* 1981; **21:** 279–86.
9. Horner RL, Guz A. Some factors affecting the maintenance of upper airway patency in man. *Respir Med* 1991; **85** (Suppl. A): 27–30.
10. Brouillette RT, Thach BT. A neuromuscular mechanism maintaining extrathoracic airway patency. *J Appl Physiol* 1979; **46:** 772–9.
11. Abernethy LJ, Allan PL, Drummond GB. Ultrasound assessment of position of the tongue during induction of anaesthesia. *Br J Anaesth* 1990; **65:** 744–8.
12. Nandi PR, Charlesworth CH, Taylor SJ, *et al.* Effect of anaesthesia on the pharynx. *Br J Anaesth* 1991; **66:** 157–62.
13. Boidin MP. Airway patency in the unconscious patient. *Br J Anaesth* 1985; **57:** 306–10.
14. Shorten GD, Opie NJ, Graziott P, *et al.* Assessment of upper airway anatomy in awake, sedated and anaesthetised patients using magnetic resonance imaging. *Anaesth Intensive Care* 1994; **22:** 165–9.
15. Sivarajan M, Joy JV. Effects of general anaesthesia and paralysis on upper airway changes due to head position in humans. *Anesthesiology* 1996; **85:** 787–93.
16. Fink BR. The etiology and treatment of laryngeal spasm. *Anesthesiology* 1956; **17:** 569–77.
17. Tagaito Y, Isono S, Nishino T. Upper airway reflexes during a combination of propofol and fentanyl anaesthesia. *Anesthesiology* 1998; **88:** 1459–66.

18. Roberts FL, Dixon J, Lewis GTR, *et al.* Induction and maintenance of propofol anaesthesia. A manual infusion scheme. *Anaesthesia* 1988; **43** (Suppl.): 14–17.
19. Kong CF, Chew STH, Ip-Yam PC. Intravenous opioids reduce airway irritation during induction of anaesthesia with desflurane in adults. *Br J Anaesth* 2000; **85:** 364–7.
20. Oshima T, Masaki Y, Toyooka H. Flumazenil antagonises midazolam-induced airway narrowing during nasal breathing in humans. *Br J Anaesth* 1999; **82:** 698–702.
21. Huang I, Quinn SJ, Ellis PSM, Ffowcs Williams JE. Biomechanics of snoring. *Endeavour* 1995; **19:** 96–100.
22. Weibel ER. *Morphometry of the Human Lung*. Berlin: Springer Verlag, 1963.
23. Weibel ER. *The Pathway for Oxygen*. Cambridge: Harvard University Press, 1984.
24. Horsfield K, Cumming G. Functional consequences of airway morphology. *J Appl Physiol* 1968; **24:** 384–90.
25. Widdicombe J. Airway receptors. *Respir Physiol* 2001; **125:** 3–15.
26. Canning BJ, Fisher A. Neural regulation of airway smooth muscle tone. *Respir Physiol* 2001; **125:** 113–27.
27. Rogers DF. Motor control of airway goblet cells and glands. *Respir Physiol* 2001; **125:** 129–44.
28. Barnes PJ. Muscarinic receptor subtypes in airways. *Eur Respir J* 1993; **6:** 328–31.
29. Thomson NC, Dagg KD, Ramsey SG. Humoral control of airway tone. *Thorax* 1996; **51:** 461–4.
30. Barnes PJ. Neural control of airway smooth muscle. In: Crystal RG, West JB, Weibel ER, Barnes PJ (eds). *The Lung. Scientific Foundations*, 2nd edn. Philadelphia: Lippincott-Raven Publishers, 1997: 1269–85.
31. Jones JG, Fraser RB, Nadel JA. Prediction of maximum expiratory flow rate from area-transmural pressure curve of compressed airway. *J Appl Physiol* 1975; **38:** 1002–11.
32. Paiva M, Engel LA. Theoretical studies of gas mixing and ventilation distribution in the lung. *Physiol Rev* 1987; **67:** 750–96.
33. Cumming G, Horsfield K, Jones JG, Muir DCF. The influence of gaseous diffusion on the alveolar plateau at different lung volumes. *Respir Physiol* 1967; **2:** 386–98.
34. West JB. Pulmonary capillary stress failure. *J Appl Physiol* 2000; **89:** 2483–9.
35. Rooney SA. The surfactant system and lung phospholipid biochemistry. *Am Rev Respir Dis* 1985; **131:** 439–60.
36. Clarke SW, Jones JG, Oliver DR. Resistance to two-phase gas-liquid flow in airways. *J Appl Physiol* 1970; **29:** 464–71.
37. Selsby D, Jones JG. Some physiological and clinical aspects of chest physiotherapy. *Br J Anaesth* 1990; **64:** 621–31.
38. King M. Role of mucus viscoelasticity in clearance by cough. *Eur J Respir Dis* 1987; **71** (Suppl. 153): 165–72.
39. Jones JG. Flow–volume loops, flow limiting segments and wave speed. *Bull R Coll Anaesth* 2003; **17:** 850–2.
40. Cumming G, Jones JG, Horsfield K. Inhaled argon boluses in man. *J Appl Physiol* 1969; **27:** 447–51.
41. Milic-Emili J, Henderson JAM, Dolovich MB, *et al.* Regional distribution of inspired gas in the lung. *J Appl Physiol* 1966; **21:** 749–59.
42. Lemen R, Jones JG, Graf P, Cowan G. Closing volume change in Alloxan-induced pulmonary edema in anesthetized dogs. *J Appl Physiol* 1975; **39:** 235–9.
43. Jones JG, Lemen R, Graf P. Changes in airway calibre following pulmonary venous congestion. *Br J Anaesth* 1978; **50:** 743–52.
44. Jones JG, Clarke SW, Glaister DH. Effect of acceleration on regional lung emptying. *J Appl Physiol* 1969; **26:** 827–32.
45. Frerichs I, Dudykevych T, Hinz J, *et al.* Gravity effects on regional lung ventilation determined by functional EIT during parabolic flights. *J Appl Physiol* 2001; **91:** 39–50.
46. Jordan C, Lehane JR, Jones JG, *et al.* Specific conductance using forced airflow oscillation in mechanically ventilated human subjects. *J Appl Physiol* 1981; **51:** 715–24.
47. Jones JG. Anaesthesia and atelectasis; the role of VTAB and the chest wall. *Br J Anaesth* 1987; **59:** 949–53.
48. Yamakage M. Effects of anaesthetic agents on airway smooth muscles. *Br J Anaesth* 2002; **88:** 624–7.
49. Heneghan CPH, Bergman NA, Jordan C, *et al.* Effect of isoflurane on bronchomotor tone in man. *Br J Anaesth* 1986; **58:** 24–8.
50. Conti G, Dell'utri D, Vilardi V, *et al.* Propofol induces bronchodilatation in mechanically ventilated chronic obstructive pulmonary disease patients. *Acta Anaesthesiol Scand* 1993; **37:** 105–9.
51. Brown RH, Wagner EM. Mechanisms of bronchoprotection by anesthetic induction agents. *Anesthesiology* 1999; **90:** 822–8.
52. Simpson DA, Wright DJ, Hammond JE. Influence of tubocurarine, pancuronium and atracurium on bronchomotor tone. *Br J Anaesth* 1985; **57:** 753–7.
53. Cohendy R, Lefrant JY, Laracine M, *et al.* Effect of fentanyl on ventilatory resistance during barbiturate anaesthesia. *Br J Anaesth* 1992; **69:** 595–8.
54. Szczeklik A. The cyclo-oxygenase theory of aspirin-induced asthma. *Eur Respir J* 1990; **3:** 588–93.
55. Lipworth BJ. Leukotriene-receptor antagonists. *Lancet* 1999; **356:** 57–62.
56. Wenzel SE. Antileukotriene drugs in the management of asthma. *JAMA* 1998; **280:** 2068–9.
57. Grummitt RM, Jones JG. The physiology of artificial ventilation. *Curr Anaesth Crit Care* 1989; **1:** 3–10.
58. Hedenstierna G, Standberg A, Brismar B, *et al.* Functional residual capacity, thoracoabdominal dimensions and central blood volume during general anaesthesia with muscle paralysis and mechanical ventilation. *Anesthesiology* 1985; **62:** 247–54.
59. Rothen HU, Sporre B, Engberg G, *et al.* Influence of gas composition on recurrence of atelectasis after a re-expansion maneuver during general anaesthesia. *Anesthesiology* 1995; **82:** 832–5.
60. Browne DRG, Rochford J, O'Connell U, Jones JG. The incidence of post-operative atelectasis in the dependent lung following thoracotomy: the value of added nitrogen. *Br J Anaesth* 1970; **47:** 340–6.
61. Hedenstiena G, Rothen HU. Atelectasis formation during anesthesia: causes and measures to prevent it. *J Clin Monitor Comput* 2001; **16:** 329–35.
62. Joyce CJ, Williams AB. Kinetics of absorption atelectasis during anesthesia: a mathematical model. *J Appl Physiol* 1999; **86:** 114–15.
63. Wagner PD, Saltzman HA, West JB. Measurement of continuous distributions of ventilation perfusion ratios: theory. *J Appl Physiol* 1974; **36:** 588–99.
64. Wagner PD, Naumann PF, Laravuso RB. Simultaneous measurement of eight foreign gases in blood by gas chromatography. *J Appl Physiol* 1974; **36:** 600–5.
65. Dueck R. Gas exchange. In: Jones JG (ed.). *Effects of Anesthesia and Surgery on Pulmonary Mechanisms and Gas Exchange. International Anesthesiology Clinics*, Vol. 22. Boston: Little, Brown, 1984: 13–28.
66. Roe PG, Jones JG. Analysis of factors which affect the relationship between inspired oxygen partial pressure and arterial oxygen saturation. *Br J Anaesth* 1993; **71:** 488–94.
67. Zetterström H. Assessment of the efficiency of pulmonary oxygenation. The choice of oxygenation index. *Acta Anaesthesiol Scand* 1988; **32:** 579–84.
68. Sapsford DJ, Jones JG. The P_IO_2 vs SpO_2 diagram: a non invasive measure of pulmonary oxygen exchange. *Eur J Anaesthesiol* 1995; **12:** 375–86.
69. Jones JG, Jones SE. Discriminating between the effect of shunt and reduced V_A/Q on arterial oxygen saturation is particularly useful in clinical practice. *J Clin Monitor Comput* 2001; **16:** 337–50.
70. Smith HL, Jones JG. Non-invasive assessment of shunt and ventilation/perfusion ratio in neonates with pulmonary failure. *Arch Dis Child (Fetal Neonatal Edn)* 2001; **85:** F127–F132.
71. de Gray L, Rush EM, Jones JG. A non-invasive method for evaluating the effect of thoracotomy on shunt and ventilation perfusion inequality. *Anaesthesia* 1997; **52:** 630–5.
72. Burnstein RM, Newell JP, Jones JG. Sequential changes in gas exchange following traumatic fat embolism. *Anaesthesia* 1998; **53:** 369–81.
73. Roe PG, Gadelrab R, Sapsford D, Jones JG. Intra-operative gas exchange and postoperative hypoxaemia. *Eur J Anaesthesiol* 1997; **14:** 203–10.
74. Eisenkraft JB. Effects of anaesthetics on the pulmonary circulation. *Br J Anaesth* 1990; **65:** 63–78.
75. Conacher ID. 2000 – Time to apply Occam's razor to failure of hypoxic pulmonary vasoconstriction during one lung ventilation. *Br J Anaesth* 2000; **84:** 434–6.
76. Ware L, Matthay MA. The acute respiratory distress syndrome. *N Engl J Med* 2000; **342:** 1334–49.
77. Barrowcliffe M, Jones JG. The pathophysiology and treatment of adult respiratory distress syndrome. In: Kaufman L (ed.). *Anaesthesia Review 5.* Edinburgh: Churchill Livingstone, 1988: 182–95.
78. Jones JG, Somerville ID. Lung surfactant: composition, physiology and replacement therapy. In: Kaufman L (ed.). *Anaesthesia Review 6.* Edinburgh: Churchill Livingstone, 1989: 185–202.
79. Hills BE. The role of lung surfactant. *Br J Anaesth* 1990; **65:** 13–29.
80. Hills BE An alternative view of the role(s) of surfactant and the alveolar model. *J Appl Physiol* 1999; **87:** 1567–83.
81. Scarpelli EM, Hills BE. Opposing views on the alveolar surface, alveolar models, and the role of surfactant. *J Appl Physiol* 2000; **89:** 408–12.

82. Dorrington KL, Young JD. Development of the concept of a liquid pulmonary alveolar lining layer. *Br J Anaesth* 2001; **86:** 614–17.
83. Barrowcliffe MP, Jones JG. Solute permeability of the alveolar capillary barrier. *Thorax* 1987; **42:** 1–10.
84. Barrowcliffe MP, Zanelli GD, Ellison D, Jones JG. Clearance of charged and uncharged dextrans from normal and injured lungs. *J Appl Physiol* 1990; **68:** 341–7.
85. Barrowcliffe MP, Zanelli GD, Jones JG. Pulmonary clearance of radiotracers after positive end-expiratory pressure or acute lung injury. *J Appl Physiol* 1989; **66:** 288–94.
86. Carter EP, Wang Y, Campbell AR, *et al.* Resolution of alveolar edema. In: Matthay MA, Ingbar DH (eds). *Pulmonary Edema*. New York: Marcel Dekker, 1998: 431–55.
87. Barrowcliffe MP, Jones JG. Pulmonary clearance of ^{99m}Tc-DTPA in the diagnosis and evolution of increased permeability pulmonary oedema. *Anaesth Intensive Care* 1989; **17:** 422–32.
88. Tobin MJ. Culmination of an era in research on the acute respiratory distress syndrome. *N Engl J Med* 2000; **342:** 1360–1.
89. Berger AJ. Control of breathing. In: Murray JF, Nadel JA (eds). *Textbook of Respiratory Medicine*. Philadelphia: WB Saunders/Harcourt Brace Jovanovich, 1988: 149–66.
90. Northwood D, Sapsford DJ, Jones JG, *et al.* Nitrous oxide sedation causes post-hyperventilation apnoea. *Br J Anaesth* 1991; **67:** 7–12.
91. Clark FJ, von Euler C. On the regulation of depth and rate of breathing. *J Physiol (Lond)* 1972; **222:** 267–95.
92. Jones JG, Faithfull D, Jordan C, Minty B. Rib cage movement during halothane anaesthesia in man. *Br J Anaesth* 1979; **51:** 399–407.
93. Jordan C, Lehane JR, Robson PJ, Jones JG. A comparison of the respiratory effects of meptazinol pentazocine and morphine. *Br J Anaesth* 1979; **51:** 497–502.
94. Knill RL, Clement JL. Variable effects of anaesthetics on the ventilatory response to hypoxaemia in man. *Can Anaesth Soc* 1982; **29:** 93–9.
95. Knill RL, Gelb AW. Ventilatory response to hypoxia and hypercapnia during halothane sedation and anesthesia in man. *Anesthesiology* 1978; **49:** 244–51.
96. Tusiewicz K, Bryan AC, Froese AB. Contributions of changing rib cage–diaphragm interactions to the ventilatory depression of halothane anaesthesia. *Anesthesiology* 1977; **47:** 327–37.
97. Temp JA, Henson LC, Ward DS. Subanaesthetic isoflurane and the ventilatory response to hypoxaemia. *Anesthesiology* 1993; **78:** 1190–2.
98. Nagyova B, Dorrington KL, Robbins PA. Effect of low-dose enflurane on the ventilatory response to hypoxia in humans. *Br J Anaesth* 1994; **72:** 509–14.
99. Robotham JL. Do low-dose inhalational anesthetic agents alter ventilatory control. *Anesthesiology* 1994; **80:** 723–6.
100. Goodman NW. Volatile agents and the ventilatory response to hypoxia. *Br J Anaesth* 1994; **72:** 503–5.

6

Respiratory pharmacology

DENHAM S WARD AND ALBERT DAHAN

Adequate gas exchange may be matched with the systemic circulation; however, it is necessary to coordinate the functioning of the lung (including the conducting airways, the pulmonary circulation, and the gas exchanging regions), the ventilatory pump (diaphragm and chest wall), and the central ventilatory controller with its afferent inputs and neural connections to the respiratory muscles. The control of breathing is influenced by drugs with side-effects that can cause or relieve pulmonary dysfunction and drugs that can be used to treat pulmonary dysfunction caused by disease or surgical and anesthetic procedures. This chapter is organized on the basis of respiratory system structure and function, and in it the significant effects of pharmacologic agents used in anesthesia for the control of ventilation both in normal individuals and in patients with respiratory compromise are discussed. The chapter is designed to enable the reader to understand the respiratory pharmacology of common drugs and conditions as they relate to anesthesiology. Further information concerning the general physiology and pharmacology of the regulation of breathing can be found in authoritative monographs.[1,2]

METABOLIC CONTROL OF VENTILATION

The central respiratory centers

Experiments with animals, generally cats, have provided most of the information about the anatomy and physiology of central respiratory centers. Although early studies required destruction or sectioning of brain areas, more recent studies have provided greater detail and information concerning these anatomical structures. Some noninvasive techniques, such as functional magnetic resonance imaging (MRI), have also provided data from human studies. Extracellular recordings of neural spike trains have allowed primary classification of neurons as inspiratory, if they fire in synchrony with the phrenic nerve discharge, and expiratory, if they fire during phrenic nerve silence. There are many variations in these basic patterns that permit numerous subclassifications.[3]

The medulla is the site of the primary rhythm-generating groups of neurons. The dorsal respiratory group (DRG) is a morphologically homogeneous group of neurons with primarily inspiratory-related discharge. The larger, more heterogeneous group of neurons with a variety of respiratory-related discharge patterns has been referred to as the ventral respiratory group (VRG). These two respiratory groups of neurons are sufficient to generate a basic respiratory rhythm.[4] The neurons in these centers synapse with motor and premotor neurons of the phrenic nerve as well as with motor neurons of the intercostal and pharyngeal/laryngeal muscles. The afferent projections from the central and peripheral chemoreceptors also connect with these medullary centers. Other central neurons seem to have important respiratory-related roles. In the pons, a group of neurons seems to influence inspiratory duration. This group of neurons, previously referred to as the "pneumotaxic center," is now called the pontine respiratory group (PRG).[5]

The respiratory centers in the pons and medulla create normal ventilatory patterns and can provide appropriate ventilatory adjustments in response to chemoreflexes. However, except in states such as sleep and general anesthesia, the respiratory muscles are frequently under the control of other regions of the brain. This permits the ventilatory system to be used for functions other than breathing. Some functions are voluntary acts, such as speech, singing, breath-holding, and hyperventilation, and others are autonomic acts, e.g. coughing, sneezing, hiccupping, and vomiting. There are also connections from the cortex and the limbic systems to the respiratory muscles.[6] Cortical connections can bypass the brainstem respiratory centers, which explains the mechanism by which anesthesiologists can stimulate patients to breath voluntarily even when narcosis causes respiratory depression or apnea. There are also connections from the cortex to the respiratory centers (in the brainstem), either directly or via the limbic system, which bring about the changes in respiration seen with emotional stress.[7]

All of these various autonomic functions, conscious commands, emotions, stress, and pain influence the level of ventilation. In addition, during anesthesia, many drugs are used to provide anxiolysis, analgesia, muscle relaxation, and loss of consciousness. Understanding the control of breathing in the clinical environment requires an understanding of these interactions.

Central chemoreceptors

Although the precise chemoreceptor cells in the brainstem have not been identified and located with certainty,[8-10] they appear to be close to the surface of the brainstem. However, they are on the brain side of the blood–brain barrier, so they are not accessible to drugs and ionized substances that only cross the blood–brain barrier in a limited manner. These factors make it impossible to identify those drugs that act only on the central chemoreceptors. It is generally assumed that most centrally acting respiratory drugs have a site of action on the central respiratory centers and not on the central chemoreceptors alone.

Peripheral chemoreceptors

The carotid bodies provide the only peripheral chemoreceptor efferent input to the central ventilatory controller in humans.[11] Rather than a simple sensory transducer, their function includes significant neural processing. Although this processing may contribute to the stability of the ventilatory control system, it also provides an opportunity for many drugs to affect the process. The carotid bodies provide the major ventilatory stimulating effect of hypoxia,[12] and also provide a response to changes in arterial pH and $P\text{CO}_2$. Drugs that alter the hypoxic ventilatory response are often thought of as acting on the peripheral chemoreceptors; however, because the afferent input from the carotid bodies is modified by the central neural controller, human studies have not always been able to detail the sole site of action at the peripheral chemoreceptor. The results from studies must often be interpreted in light of animal studies that provide direct measurement of the carotid sinus nerve (see below) discharge rate.

The peripheral chemoreflex loop refers to the reflex loop between the peripheral chemoreceptors in the carotid bodies and pulmonary ventilation.[13] This loop consists of: the peripheral chemoreceptors that sense the chemical composition of arterial blood; the connection, i.e. the carotid sinus nerve, between these receptors and the brainstem; centers involved in the processing of afferent input from peripheral chemoreceptors; brainstem centers that integrate respiratory input from peripheral and central chemoreceptors, hypothalamus, cortex, and subcortical brain areas, proprioreceptors in joints and muscles, etc.; and the neuromechanical link between brainstem and ventilation (this includes the phrenic nucleus, the phrenic nerve, and diaphragm; spinal motoneurons, intercostal nerves, and intercostal muscles; lungs and airways) that eventually determines the chemical composition of arterial blood. The integrity of all parts of the peripheral and central chemoreflex loops (see below) is needed for an appropriate normal response to pulmonary and systemic pathology and to maintain the chemical equilibrium of the body in wakefulness and sleep.

The carotid bodies are two small organs (4–6 mm^3) located bilaterally near the bifurcation of the common carotid artery.[11] The blood flow to the carotid bodies is the highest of any organ in the body ($2\,\text{L}\,\text{min}^{-1}\,100\,\text{g}^{-1}$ tissue), and the resulting small arterial to venous $P\text{O}_2$ permits the carotid bodies to sense changes in arterial blood. The carotid bodies contain two cell types: chemoreceptor, or type I, cells and nonchemoreceptor, or type II, cells. The full function of the type II cells is unknown. Stimulation of the chemoreceptor cells (stimulation is caused by a decrease in arterial $P\text{O}_2$, a decrease in pH, or an increase in arterial $P\text{CO}_2$) results in an immediate increase in breathing activity (see below). Type I cells make contact with the carotid sinus nerve, a branch of the glossopharyngeal nerve which connects the carotid bodies to the respiratory centers in the brainstem. Transduction of chemical stimuli into the type I cells and neurotransmission at the chemoreceptor cell–carotid sinus nerve synapse is complex. Type I cells have oxygen-sensitive K^+ channels that are believed to be involved in oxygen (O_2) sensing. Hypoxia inhibits outward potassium currents in these cells and causes a reduction in the membrane potential, whereas carbon dioxide (CO_2) activates type I cells by an intracellular reduction in pH. Thus, $P\text{O}_2$ and pH (H^+) are the stimuli sensed by these chemoreceptor cells. Type I cells contain various neurotransmitters, second messengers, and modulators that are involved in the process of carotid sinus nerve activation. The most important (inhibitory) neurotransmitter is dopamine, which is released by the type I cells into the synapse and acts at the postsynaptic D_2-receptor. Other transmitters include 5-hydroxytryptamine (5-HT), acetylcholine (ACh), norepinephrine (noradrenaline), and opioid peptides. Nitric oxide (NO) and carbon monoxide (CO) are thought to be involved in the signal transduction–neurotransmission process. Exogenously administered agents that act at D_2, ACh, 5-HT, or opioid receptors, or agents that interact with NO or CO, interfere with normal chemoreceptor sensitivity.

Central processing of afferent input from peripheral chemoreceptors is not yet fully understood, but it involves, in addition to various neurotransmitters: various sites in the brainstem, particularly the nucleus tractus solitarius in the DRG; areas in the VRG; and the locus ceruleus, which is related to arousal.[14] Recent studies suggest an important, but not exclusive, role for the excitatory neurotransmitter glutamate and the *N*-methyl-D-aspartate (NMDA) receptor in the process of central transmission of carotid body input to the central nervous system and the respiratory motor neurons.

MEASURING THE METABOLIC CONTROL OF VENTILATION

Hypercapnic ventilatory response

Carbon dioxide is a powerful stimulus to ventilation. The stimulus (end-tidal CO_2)–response (minute ventilation, $\dot{V}_m$ is the symbol for minute ventilation and can be either inspired or expired minute ventilation depending on which is measured) relation is used to test regulation of breathing and assess the effects of disease and/or pharmacologic agents on the ventilatory control system.[15,16] The ventilatory response to inspired CO_2 is a popular test because of its clinical importance and because the relation $\dot{V}_m/P_{ET}\text{CO}_2$ is linear and easily obtained. However, the measured $P_{ET}\text{CO}_2$ stimulus may not always quantitatively reflect the actual stimulus at the chemoreceptor sites, and it may sometimes be necessary to obtain arterial $P\text{CO}_2$ values when large end-tidal to arterial $P\text{CO}_2$ gradients are anticipated (e.g. in patients with chronic obstructive pulmonary disease). Furthermore, various nonchemical respiratory stimuli, such as discomfort, fear, and pain, may influence the measured ventilatory response. Pure chemical or metabolic control of breathing can be measured only when all disturbing influences are removed. Experimentally, this is very difficult or impossible to achieve. Furthermore, these other influences are often clinically very important and, therefore, these additional drives to breathe must be taken into account.

In awake humans, the conscious drive to breathe and other stabilizing influences on respiration maintain breathing when CO_2 tensions are below resting values (Fig. 6.1), even at levels of extreme hypocapnia. This results in a flattening of the CO_2 response curve at lower CO_2 levels, sometimes referred to as a dogleg or hockey stick. Only when consciousness is lost, as with sleep or anesthesia, does apnea consistently occur with hypocapnia, i.e. the dogleg disappears and a true apneic threshold is found. When assessing CO_2 drive, it is important to ensure that all the data points used in the analysis are on the linear part of the CO_2 response curve and not on the flat CO_2-independent portion.

At $P_{ET}\text{CO}_2$ levels above resting, the relationship between minute ventilation ($\dot{V}_m$) and $P_{ET}\text{CO}_2$ is expressed as:

$$\dot{V}_m = S(P_{ET}\text{CO}_2 - B) \tag{6.1}$$

where S ($\text{L}\,\text{min}^{-1}\,\text{mmHg}^{-1}$, or $\text{L}\,\text{min}^{-1}\,\text{kPa}$) is the ventilatory CO_2 sensitivity (also referred to as the slope or gain of the ventilatory response to CO_2) and B (mmHg or kPa) is the apnea or "set" point (also called apneic threshold) or the value of $P_{ET}\text{CO}_2$ when the response curve is extrapolated to the *x*-axis, i.e. ventilation is 0 (dashed line in Fig. 6.1). The value of S shows large intra- and intersubject variability. Apart from genetic variability, S depends on sex, female and male sex hormones, age, physical training, circadian rhythm, behavioral state, underlying disease, ambient O_2 tension, and acid–base status. In healthy young humans, the value of S ranges from at least 1 up to $3\,\text{L}\,\text{min}^{-1}\,\text{mmHg}^{-1}$ and

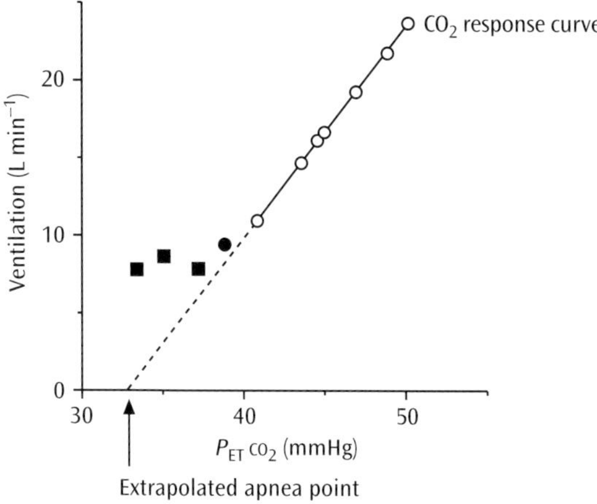

Figure 6.1 *The ventilatory response of a healthy human to CO_2. The filled circle is resting ventilation. Open circles are steady-state data points obtained at various inspired CO_2 levels. The ventilatory CO_2 sensitivity is obtained by linear regression analysis of the data points on the linear part of the response curve. The slope of the curve represents the CO_2 sensitivity (S in equation 6.1). Extrapolation of the CO_2 response curve to the x-axis yields the so-called apnea point or apneic threshold. Note that hyperventilation will decrease $P_{ET}CO_2$, but subsequent ventilation remains sustained (filled squares) in awake, unsedated subjects.*

it is most likely that many people have values outside these without any apparent abnormality. Once accustomed to the measurement apparatus, the repeatability of *S* may be greatly improved in single individuals when tests are performed in a single session.

The experimental data points used in determining the relation between ventilation and CO_2 shown in Fig. 6.1 and equation 6.1 can be determined by several methods. The fundamental technique is one of making steady-state measurements, with steady-state in this case meaning that the input ($P_{ET}CO_2$) and the output ($\dot{V}_m$) do not change over time as data points are recorded. The technique involves the sequential inhalation of gas mixtures with different constant CO_2 concentrations (e.g. 3%, 5%, and 8%), and then waiting until constant values of $P_{ET}CO_2$ and $\dot{V}_m$ are obtained. This may mean that more than 20 min is required to obtain a single point. When steady state has been reached, data points are obtained, usually by averaging the breath-to-breath data over 1–2 min to reduce the effects of normal fluctuations in breathing, and the linear relationship between end-tidal CO_2 and ventilation is determined (see Fig. 6.1). The steady-state method is time-consuming and therefore unpleasant for the subject. A reliable but faster technique is the so-called dynamic end-tidal forcing technique.[17–19] Using sophisticated apparatus, the $P_{ET}CO_2$ is increased rapidly by computer-controlled manipulation of the inspired gas concentrations. This technique has the advantage that, in addition to providing a value for steady-state CO_2 sensitivity within 5–7 min, it also provides CO_2 sensitivities and the dynamics of central and peripheral chemoreceptors separately (see below). Although this technique requires sophisticated apparatus and data analysis, it is the method of choice if one wants to assess the effects of anesthetics and opioids on the control of breathing.

Various nonsteady-state techniques have been developed to assess CO_2 response quickly without complex apparatus. The most popular method is Read's rebreathing technique, which he first described in 1967.[18] This technique uses a 4- to 6-L bag primed with 7% CO_2 in O_2. The subject breathes a hyperoxic gas mixture and, at the end of a maximum expiration, the breathing circuit is connected to the primed bag; rebreathing is then continued for 8–10 min. Under these conditions, rebreathing is initiated close to the mixed venous CO_2 tension, and a rapid CO_2 equilibrium is established among the lung, the rebreathing bag, the mixed venous blood, and the arterial blood, but not with the brain tissue P_{CO_2}.[19] Experimentally, the increases in ventilation and end-tidal P_{CO_2} are linear over time. Only central chemoreceptor CO_2 sensitivity, i.e. *S* in equation 6.1, is obtained by linear regression of $\dot{V}_m$ on $P_{ET}CO_2$ because the peripheral chemoreceptors are silenced by hyperoxia. Resting $P_{ET}CO_2$ values and metabolism differ among subjects and conditions, therefore the initial increase, "the step," in $P_{ET}CO_2$, at the start of rebreathing, and the subsequent slow rise, "the ramp," in $P_{ET}CO_2$ vary between subjects as well as between different conditions, such as rest versus exercise, acid–base disturbances, and administration of opioids. Variations in step size and ramp speed will affect by themselves the values of *S* and *B* independently of the effect of the treatment on *S* and *B*. Note that the steady-state technique is not step size and ramp speed dependent. This indicates that, although determination of CO_2 response using rebreathing techniques is relatively simple, interpretation of the results is often complex, especially when the effects of respiratory depressants are examined.[20]

Drugs may alter the ventilatory response to CO_2 by altering the slope, i.e. increasing or decreasing *S*, or by altering the position of the curve relative to the *x*-axis by increasing or decreasing *B*, the apneic point. A decrease in the slope or a rightward shift of the response curve indicates respiratory depression, whereas respiratory stimulation results in the opposite. For example, inhalational anesthetics decrease the slope of the response curve, indicating that a higher level of CO_2 is needed to reach a certain ventilation level. The carboanhydrase inhibitor acetazolamide, used to treat mountain sickness, reduces the threshold of *B*, the apneic point, without affecting *S*. This indicates that lower levels of CO_2 are needed to reach a certain ventilation level, i.e. ventilatory stimulation.

An increase in arterial CO_2 tension increases ventilation by stimulating both peripheral and central chemoreceptors. Various methods have been employed to quantify the separate contributions of the central and peripheral chemoreceptors to total minute ventilation. In humans, the dynamic end-tidal forcing technique was developed to achieve this noninvasively.[17,21,22] After applying a stepwise increase in $P_{ET}CO_2$, the ventilatory response shows an initial rapid increase followed by a slower one. Steady-state ventilation is reached after about 7 min (Fig. 6.2). Peripheral chemoreceptors respond quickly to changes in CO_2 stimulation (time constant 1–3 s), and respond more quickly than central chemoreceptors (delay time between start of inhalation of CO_2 to ventilatory response is about 6 s). The response of central chemoreceptors to CO_2 stimulation is slower (time constant about 2 min) and has a delay time of about 12 s.[17,23] Using a mathematical model of the respiratory controller, these differences in dynamics are used to separate the total ventilatory response to CO_2 into peripheral and central contributions. In awake humans, the contribution of the peripheral and central chemoreceptors to CO_2-stimulated ventilation is 30% and 70% in normoxia respectively. The time constant of the central response is partly the result of the cerebral blood flow-dependent wash-in of CO_2 and partly the result of the central neuronal dynamics, which have a stabilizing influence on breathing by damping ventilatory responses when chemical and nonchemical respiratory stimuli are suddenly withdrawn. For example, removal of acute pain, which causes hyperventilation and relative hypocapnia, is not followed by apnea, but ventilation is maintained at a level much higher than expected for the arterial or end-tidal P_{CO_2} value.[24]

Because of the positive interactive effects of O_2 and CO_2 at peripheral chemoreceptors, the ventilatory CO_2 sensitivity of the peripheral component (S_p) increases with hypoxia and decreases with hyperoxia. The value of S_p increases from 0.6 in normoxia to 1 L min^{-1} mmHg^{-1} in mild hypoxia (inspired O_2 concentration 14%) in healthy young volunteers.[17] During hyperoxia, apart from the decrease in S_p (to 0.08 L min^{-1} mmHg^{-1}), the CO_2 response curve is shifted to the left, i.e. the value of the apneic point decreases, because of the stimulatory

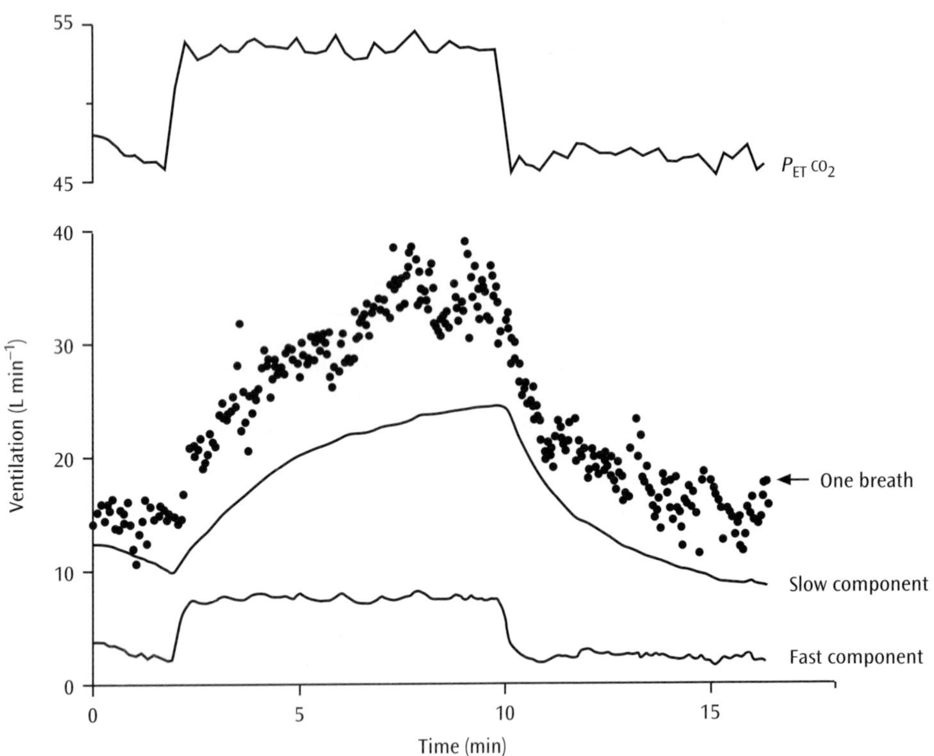

Figure 6.2 *The dynamic ventilatory response to a stepwise increase and decrease in $P_{ET}CO_2$. Each data point (filled circles) represents one breath. Note that, after the step into and out of hypercapnia, ventilation initially changes rapidly, followed by a slower change. A mathematical model of the respiratory controller is used to separate the total response into a fast component from peripheral chemoreceptors and a slow component from central chemoreceptors.*

effects of hyperoxia on ventilation.[17] Chronic metabolic acidosis and alkalosis also affect the position of the CO_2 response curve, with metabolic acidosis reducing the threshold of the apnea point and metabolic alkalosis increasing the value of the apnea point. The values of the CO_2 sensitivities of central and peripheral chemoreceptors are not affected. Acute moderate metabolic acidosis affects ventilation mainly through stimulation of the peripheral chemoreceptors.[24] Note, however, that, because of conversion of acid into CO_2, stimulation of the central chemoreceptors occurs as cerebrospinal fluid (CSF) acidifies during prolonged metabolic acidosis.

Hypoxic ventilatory response

The acute hypoxic response is caused by the hypoxic drive of the peripheral chemoreceptors in the carotid bodies.[12] The measured increase in ventilation due to hypoxia is not linear when the increase is expressed as a function of the arterial Po_2.[25] Instead, a curvilinear response is seen in which the ventilation increases greatly after the P_ao_2 is reduced below 60 mmHg (8 kPa) (Fig. 6.3). Another problem is that $P_{ET}o_2$ is not a good measurement of P_ao_2 even in normal subjects because of the variable effects of shunts. However, ventilation does bear a linear relation to decreases in saturation, and pulse oximeter-measured saturation (S_po_2) is often used as the measured independent variable (Fig. 6.4).

$$\dot{V}_m = G(100 - S_po_2) + \dot{V}_o \qquad (6.2)$$

The acute hypoxic response may be expressed as the difference in ventilation between peak and baseline $\dot{V}_m$ (L min^{-1}) or as $\Delta\dot{V}_m/\Delta S_po_2$ (L min^{-1} %$^{-1}$) represented by G in equation 6.2. The slope or gain is independent of the saturation level, to levels that cause no neuronal damage. However, the gain depends on the level of CO_2 because of the strong interaction of hypercapnia with hypoxia. Thus, it is very important that $P_{ET}CO_2$ is carefully controlled during an hypoxic test, or the hypocapnia resulting from increased hypoxic ventilation will reduce ventilatory drive and result in an underestimation of the hypoxic ventilatory gain.

In the typical clinical situation, a subject's hypoxic increase in ventilation will be blunted by the resulting hypocapnia as long as adequate gas exchange is possible. With hypoxia and hypercapnia, owing to failure of gas exchange, there is maximal stimulation to breathe (asphyxial response). The most important tests to study ventilatory response in the laboratory are step and ramp hypoxic tests; both of these tests achieve arterial hypoxemia from a reduction in inspired O_2 concentration.

In healthy adult volunteers, when mild hypoxia (arterial Hbo_2 saturation of approximately 80%) is suddenly imposed and the hypoxic stimulus and $P_{ET}CO_2$ are kept constant over 15–30 min (step hypoxic test), the temporal profile of the ventilatory response is biphasic.[26,27] When isocapnia is maintained, a desaturation to 80% causes $\dot{V}_m$ to increase rapidly, peaking within 5 min to 75–100% above the normoxic baseline and followed subsequently by a slow decrease (hypoxic ventilatory decline), reaching a steady state after 15–25 min (Fig. 6.3).[26,27] Steady-state ventilation is 50–75% of the peak hypoxic ventilatory response. The acute hypoxic response is underestimated when isocapnia is not maintained (poikilocapnia) because of CO_2 washout from body stores and a subsequent decrease in stimulation of the central chemoreceptors.[28] During mild hypoxia (inspired O_2 concentration 12–14%), the increase in ventilation is transient, and eventually ventilation may be essentially the same as when breathing air owing to the combined effects of accommodation and hypocapnia. Newborns, unlike adults, show little or no initial hyperventilatory response to hypoxia[29] but do show a hypoxic decline, which may result in a decrease in ventilation below the normoxic baseline. During prolonged mild poikilocapnic hypoxia, newborns show an increased time spent in apnea with severe desaturation occurring.[30]

At present, the mechanism and location of the generation of slow ventilatory decline remain controversial. Possible mechanisms include: (1) a decrease in peripheral chemoreceptor discharge with sustained hypoxia; (2) an hypoxia-induced increase in cerebral blood-flow wash-out of acid metabolites (CO_2 and or H^+), with a resulting decrease in central chemoreceptor drive and $\dot{V}_m$; and (3) central accumulation of inhibitory neuromodulators/transmitters such as γ-aminobutyric acid (GABA), adenosine, lactic acid, dopamine, or neuronal nitric

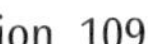

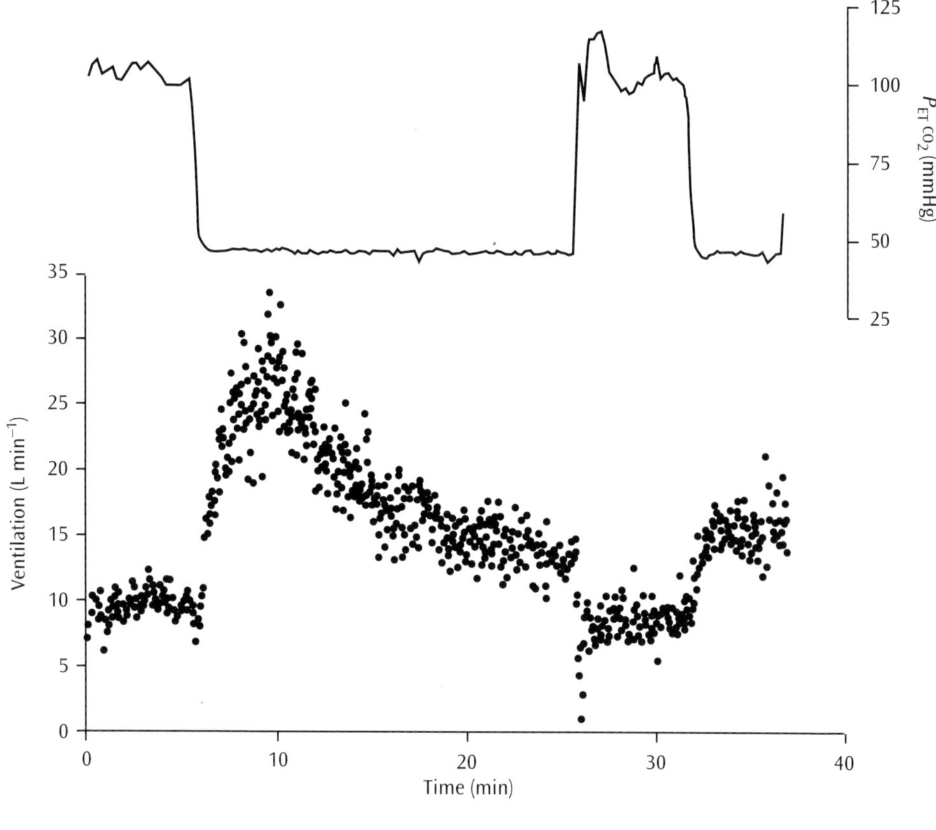

Figure 6.3 *The ventilatory response in a young healthy volunteer to 20 min of isocapnic hypoxia ($P_{ET}O_2$ = 50 mmHg), 5 min of normoxia ($P_{ET}O_2$ = 110 mmHg), and another 5 min of hypoxia ($P_{ET}O_2$ = 50 mmHg). Each filled circle represents one breath. The solid line is the $P_{ET}O_2$ waveform. Note the biphasic response to 20 min of isocapnic hypoxia: the peak response occurs in the fifth minute of hypoxia; the subsequent slow ventilatory decline results in steady-state ventilation after 15 min. The hypoxic exposure after 20 min of hypoxia and 5 min of normoxia results in a ventilatory response less than half the response after air breathing. (Adapted from Dahan* et al.[27]*)*

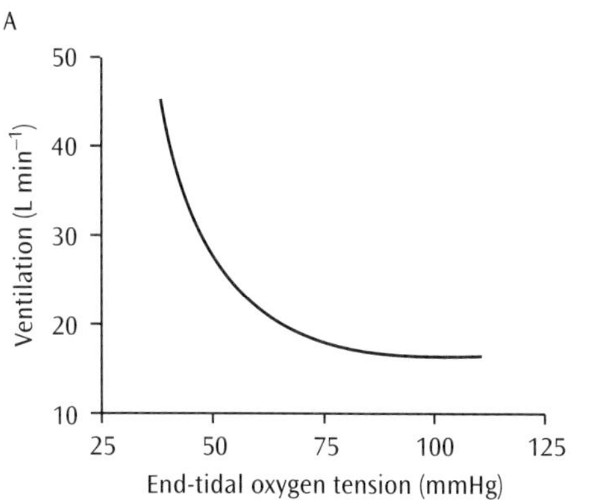

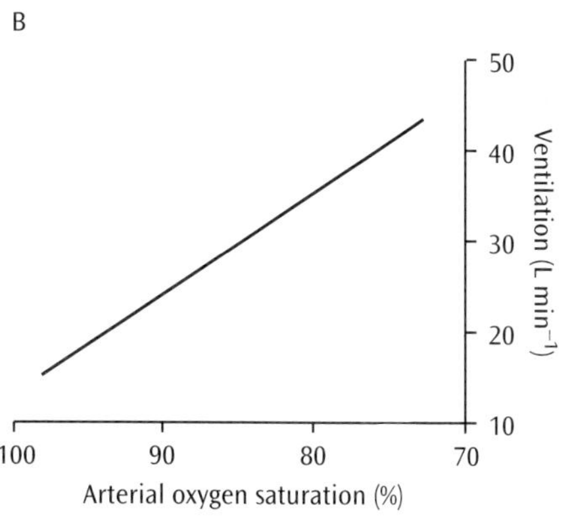

Figure 6.4 *The $P_{ET}O_2$–$\dot{V}_m$ relationship (A) and the arterial HbO_2 saturation–$\dot{V}_m$ relationship (B). Saturation data are commonly derived from pulse oximetry.*

oxide synthase, causing a net depressant effect on the respiratory centers in the central nervous system (CNS).[31] Studies with anesthetized animals indicate the importance of factor 2 in the development of hypoxic ventilatory decline,[32] whereas awake human studies point toward factor 3 as its most important cause.[26,27] An interesting and clinically relevant finding is that the depressive effects of prolonged (> 15 min) hypoxia persist beyond the time of hypoxic exposure.[26,27] When hypoxia is reintroduced after 15 min of hypoxia and 5 min of air breathing, the acute hypoxic response is smaller than when hypoxia is introduced after only air breathing (see Fig. 6.4). This observation favors a prominent role for factor 3. At the termination of sustained hypoxia, neurotransmitter turnover is not immediate and, therefore, the depressant effects of hypoxia wane slowly. When the carotid bodies are removed or the peripheral response is silenced by low-dose dopamine, no hypoxic ventilatory decline is observed.[27,33] This indicates that central hypoxia (i.e. within the CNS) by itself is insufficient to cause the decline. The increased peripheral input to the CNS during hypoxia may activate the build-up of inhibitory neurotransmitters in the CNS. This hypothesis is further strengthened by the observation that the magnitude of the hypoxic ventilatory decline is proportionally related to the size of the initial response.[26,27] Subjects with large acute hypoxic responses have large declines. Increasing the size of the acute response by pharmacologic intervention will also increase the magnitude of the resultant decline. The identity of the neurotransmitters that are involved remains unresolved. Pharmacologic studies point toward a major role for $GABA_A$ and adenosine receptors.[34,35] Evidently, at deeper levels of hypoxia (S_pO_2 < 80%), inhibition of hypoxic ventilation is also related to the direct inhibition of respiratory neuronal networks.[31]

The performance of the step hypoxic test, described above, requires sophisticated apparatus. A simpler and more popular method is to induce hypoxia by rebreathing a specific gas mixture from a balloon, resulting in the gradual exposure to hypoxia over 8–10 min with variable absorption of CO_2 by soda lime in the circuit.[36] The resultant ventilatory response is a mixture of the two opposing effects of hypoxia and, as a consequence, when compared at identical S_pO_2 levels, a smaller value for the hypoxic sensitivity results (differences in ventilation) than with a step hypoxic test.[37] When studying the influence of pharmacologic agents on the ventilatory response to a ramp hypoxic test, problems of interpretation may occur when the agents affect both the acute hypoxic response and decline. For example, when the acute response remains unaffected but the decline is increased (as occurs with benzodiazepines such as midazolam),[35] the result of a ramp hypoxic test suggests a reduced hypoxic drive, whereas the step hypoxic test would indicate potentiation or facilitation of the central depressant effects with an intact peripheral hypoxic drive.

When the acute hypoxic response is affected by drugs, the site of action may be at any location within the peripheral chemoreflex loop. This loop consists of the peripheral chemoreceptors at the carotid bodies, sinus nerve, respiratory integrating centers in the brainstem, and neuromechanical link between brainstem and respiratory and upper airway muscles. Thus, it is difficult to draw conclusions regarding the sites of action of drugs (central or peripheral) acting on this response in humans. Studies must be interpreted in the light of animal studies that provide information such as the direct measurement of the sinus nerve discharge rate. Although extrapolation of animal studies is appealing, species differences, surgical trauma induced in animal experiments, and the anesthesia needed to perform animal experiments make comparison between human and animal studies often difficult, if not impossible.

Breathing oxygen-enriched air transiently decreases $\dot{V}_m$ owing to a decrease in peripheral chemoreceptor activity.[38] Although the decrease in $\dot{V}_m$ is small, short-lived, and variable among subjects (5–30% reduction in $\dot{V}_m$ lasting 30–120 s in only 60% of the population), the simplicity of this test has made it a popular tool for the study of peripheral chemoreceptor drive. When hyperoxia is continued, $\dot{V}_m$ increases, especially when isocapnia is maintained. The magnitude of the ventilatory increase depends on the inspired O_2 concentration, with greater responses at higher inspired concentrations.[39] The mechanisms of the response incorporate the increase in brain tissue $P\text{CO}_2$ resulting from the reduction in the Haldane effect, the reduced cerebral blood flow, and the central release of excitatory agents such as glutamate or nitric oxide.[40]

NONMETABOLIC VENTILATORY CONTROL: PAIN, CONSCIOUSNESS, AND SLEEP

Apart from the chemical or the metabolic control of breathing, i.e. control of breathing dependent on the chemical composition of the arterial blood and CSF, various other systems influence breathing, particularly during wakefulness.[41,42] These nonchemoreceptor-related systems, including pain related and behavioral, have nonchemoreceptor-related inputs that modulate or may even temporarily override the metabolic system. Although pain may interact with respiratory centers in the pons and medulla, the behavioral effects may either directly control motoneurons from higher centers (i.e. cortical or limbic) via corticospinal pathways or interact with centers in the medulla via the reticular system.[6,7,42] Behavioral control of breathing allows for adjustment of breathing in specific situations such as speaking, singing, reading aloud, eating, and diving. When pain and behavioral control are absent, for example during nonrapid eye movement (NREM) sleep and anesthesia, the ventilatory control system becomes critically dependent on $P_a\text{O}_2$ and $P_a\text{CO}_2$.

Noxious stimulation clearly modulates the ventilatory control system. Pain and surgical stimulation act as respiratory stimulants in awake, sedated, and anesthetized states.[43–45] Pain also reverses the depression of minute ventilation associated with anesthetics and opioids.[45,46] The respiratory effects of the pharmacological treatment of patients with acute or chronic pain should therefore always be viewed as a balance between the stimulatory effects of any inadequately treated pain and the depressant effects of the agents used. It is generally possible to achieve adequate pain relief, both acute and chronic, safely without dangerous respiratory depression by the proper titration of analgesic drugs. In the postoperative period, adequate treatment of pain may improve gas exchange.

When pain occurs in awake patients, there is an increase in breathing frequency and mean inspiratory flow, with little effect on tidal volume.[24] The resultant increase in minute ventilation leads to a reduction in $P_a\text{CO}_2$ (Fig. 6.5). The mechanisms by which noxious stimulation modulates ventilatory control may be dependent on the intensity of such stimulation and the location of nociception. For example, when pain from injuries to the upper extremities is blocked by axillary brachial plexus block anesthesia, the ventilatory response to hyperoxic hypercapnia is reduced by more than 20%.[47] This suggests that pain from the upper body, at least, interacts with ventilatory control via the central chemoreflex loop. On the other hand, experimental pain induced by activation of cutaneous nociceptors with electrical stimulation of the lower extremities causes a chemoreflex-independent increase in tonic ventilatory drive, i.e. CO_2 and hypoxic ventilatory responses are shifted to higher $\dot{V}_m$ levels.[45] The mechanism for these apparent differences has not been resolved.

During anesthesia and conscious sedation, the influence of pain and surgical stimulation on breathing is qualitatively not very different from that during wakefulness. In spontaneously breathing anesthetized patients, surgical stimulation causes an increase in mean inspiratory flow and a (transient) increase in respiratory frequency,[24,43–45] whereas the chemoreflex-related responses to hypoxia and hypercapnia remain unaltered (Fig. 6.5).[43–45] These findings indicate that pain is unable to reverse anesthetic-induced impairment of chemoreflex-related responses. From a clinical point of view, what matters most is whether a patient maintains an adequate minute ventilation. Since pain increases ventilatory drive, it may be able to partly offset the anesthetic-induced loss of chemoreceptor drive.

The above indicates that removal of residual pain by local or regional anesthesia may be dangerous for patients with acute pain who have been treated with opioids. Indeed, several reports show profound and life-threatening respiratory depression when regional anesthesia causes pain relief in patients treated with opioids.[44] Clearly, the goal of complete pain relief should not be forgotten, but interaction of the various modes of pain treatment with the control of breathing always needs to be remembered.

The pathways by which pain increases ventilatory drive remain speculative, but a direct effect of nociceptive afferents on the respiratory centers in the brainstem seems the most plausible mechanism. The central neuronal network involved in the control of pain transmission is close to and overlaps neurons involved in respiratory control, especially in the rostral ventral medulla, lateral medulla, and pons. Stimulation of neurons involved in both respiratory function and pain regulation or the overspill of activity from one set of neurons to another may cause an increase in $\dot{V}_m$. Brain sites involved include the reticular activating network in the medulla and the locus ceruleus.[48,49]

Ventilation in both NREM sleep and anesthesia, in the absence of pain and the typical stimuli associated with wakefulness, becomes critically dependent on peripheral and central chemoreceptor stimulation. Stimulation through the $P_a\text{CO}_2$ level becomes especially important in sustaining adequate ventilation; this is in sharp contrast to the awake state, in which active hyperventilation to even severe hypocapnia is not associated with apnea. This CO_2-independent ventilatory drive is called the wakefulness drive to breathe and gives the CO_2 response curve its dogleg form (see Fig. 6.6). During NREM sleep, breathing is regular and ventilatory responses to CO_2 are intact or mildly depressed, causing a modest reduction of $\dot{V}_m$ and an increase in arterial $P_a\text{CO}_2$. Hypocapnia to a level 3–6 mmHg (0.4–0.8 kPa) below resting levels causes apnea.[50] Interestingly, recent studies indicate that normocapnic mechanical ven-

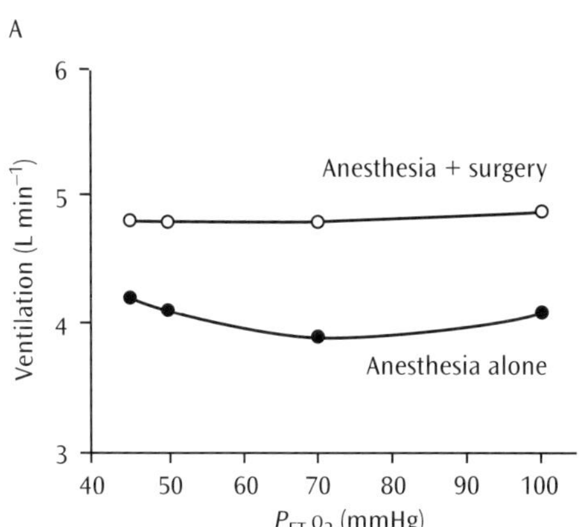

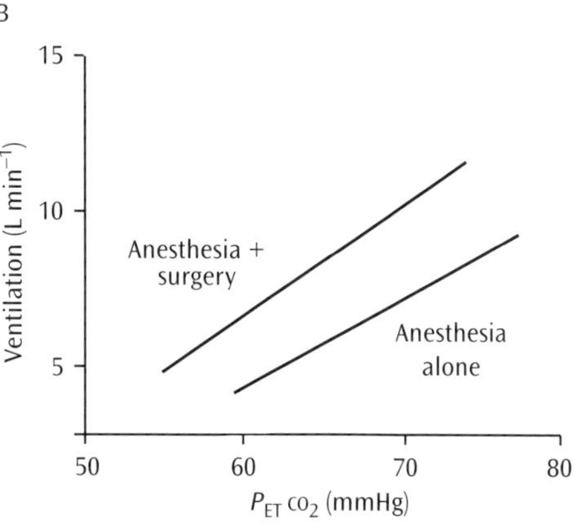

Figure 6.5 *The influence of enflurane anesthesia (1.1 MAC) on the ventilatory response to hypoxia (A) and hypercapnia (B) before and during surgery. Note the abolishment of the hypoxic ventilatory response by anesthesia. Noxious stimulation, as occurs during surgery, did shift the O_2 and CO_2 ventilatory response curves to higher ventilation levels without affecting the relative increase in ventilation from hypercapnia. The parallel shift in response curves results from a chemoreflex-independent ventilatory drive as a result of noxious stimulation. (Adapted from Lam* et al.*[139]).*

tilation at high tidal volumes may be associated with apnea in sleeping and also in awake subjects[51,52] – a phenomenon which may be important when patients are being weaned from mechanical ventilation and which is possibly related to nonvagally mediated inhibitory neuromechanical feedback mechanisms involving pulmonary stretch receptors. P_aCO_2 levels higher than those at which apnea occurs are necessary to terminate the apnea.

As in NREM sleep, hypocapnia during general anesthesia is associated with apnea at the apneic threshold (point 2, Fig. 6.6). Much higher PCO_2 levels are required to terminate apnea and stimulate respiratory activity (point 4, Fig. 6.6).[53] Delay in the initiation of respiration during the emergence from anesthesia is often related to the *relative* hypocapnia induced by mechanical ventilation during the anesthestic. The hypocapnia is relative to the rightward-shifted CO_2 response curve (see legend to Fig. 6.6). Breathing is initiated at a PCO_2 level (point 4 in Fig. 6.6) higher than the level at which it was terminated (point 2, Fig. 6.6). In contrast to NREM sleep, general anesthesia is associated with severely depressed responses to hypercapnia and hypoxia, resulting in high P_aCO_2 levels with depressed ventilation despite the reduction in brain and body metabolism. How much the loss of consciousness per se contributes to respiratory depression and how much is due to the specific effects of anesthetics remains unknown. As discussed above, apart from causing unconsciousness, anesthetics affect the ventilatory control system at various parts of the body. Afferents, chemoreceptors and afferent neural pathways, suprapontine centers and their pathways, central command, respiratory centers in the brainstem and pons, and efferents are all affected. However, there is some evidence that sedation itself affects ventilatory control. At identical blood propofol concentrations but variable levels of sedation/hypnosis, as measured by the electroencephalogram (EEG) bispectral index, human subjects show a sigmoidal relation between the level of sedation/hypnosis and depression of peripheral chemoreflex-related drives (Fig. 6.7).[54]

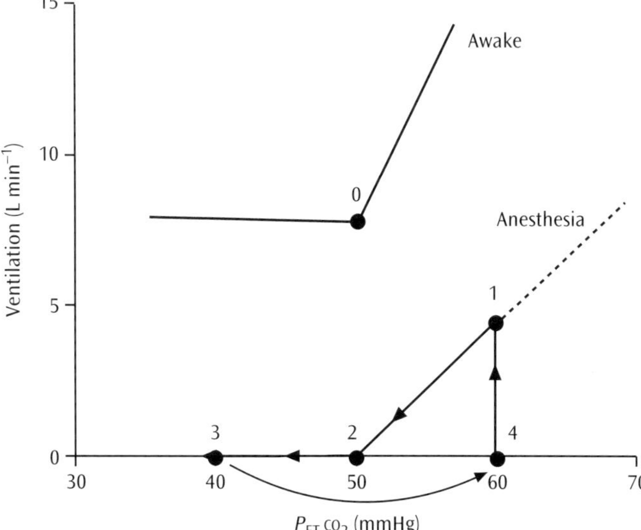

Figure 6.6 *The influence of hypocapnia on ventilation in the awake state and after consciousness has been lost. In the awake state, the CO_2 response curve has a "dogleg" shape (see text). Even at deep hypocapnia, owing to voluntary hyperventilation, ventilation is sustained. When consciousness is lost, hypocapnia (e.g. as a result of mechanical ventilation) causes apnea at the apneic threshold (point 2). Further hyperventilation causes a further reduction in PCO_2 (point 3). Breathing is initiated at a PCO_2 level (point 4) higher than the level at which it was terminated (point 2). Point 0, awake resting ventilation; point 1, anesthetized resting ventilation.*

The administration of opioids perioperatively results in alterations in the structure of sleep. During the first postoperative night, rapid eye movement (REM) sleep is virtually absent, followed during nights 2–4 by a rebound increase in REM sleep.[55] Activation of the opioid μ-receptors is thought to be the cause of the altered sleep architecture.[56] REM sleep is associated with a raised tendency to upper airway muscle hypotonia and to periods of hypopnea and apnea. The frequency of hypoxic events during the second and third postoperative nights is consequently increased threefold.[57] Since REM sleep is associated with changed cardiovascular responses, such as hypertension and tachycardia, it is not surprising that cardiovascular complications are traditionally felt to be related to the second and third postoperative nights. The respiratory depression induced by opioids is augmented during natural sleep and anesthesia-induced sedation. Forrest and Bellville[58] measured the displacement of the CO_2 response curve and observed a rightward shift of 4 mmHg (0.5 kPa) during morphine alone, 7 mmHg (0.9 kPa) during sleep alone, but about 20 mmHg (2.7 kPa) during sleep and morphine.

DRUGS ACTING ON CENTRAL NERVOUS SYSTEM NEUROTRANSMITTER SYSTEMS

There are many neurotransmitter systems involved in creating the required pulmonary ventilation, including generation of the neural respiratory rhythm, modulation of that rhythm by various factors determining the instantaneous ventilatory drive, and the transmission of that drive to the muscles of ventilation.[59] An increased understanding of these neurotransmitter systems has helped to define the mechanisms of drug action during anesthesia; however, many drugs used in anesthesia act on multiple neurotransmitter systems, or else their dominant effect

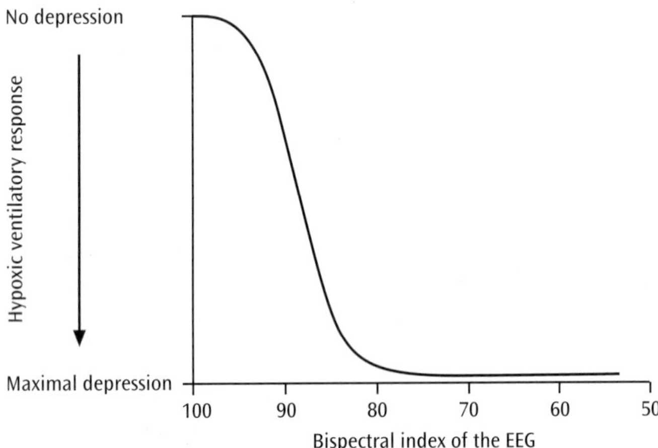

Figure 6.7 *Influence of the level of sedation/hypnosis, as measured by the bispectral index (BIS) of the EEG (x-axis), on the ventilatory response to hypoxia at similar blood propofol concentrations (target = 1000 ng mL^{-1}) in healthy volunteers. The maximal depressed responses, occurring at BIS values < 80, were about 50% of control. (Adapted from Nieuwenhuijs* et al.[54]*)*

is not completely understood. Because the effects of most anesthetic drugs on synaptic transmission will extend throughout the nervous system, respiratory effects of these drugs can be complex. Often, an effect on part of the ventilatory control system, i.e. the peripheral chemoreceptors, may not be apparent unless special tests are performed or clinical situations encountered, e.g. hypoxia. Thus, an understanding of the ventilatory control system in its entirety is needed in order to put the specific ventilatory effects of anesthetic agents in their proper context. In particular, the balance between metabolic, chemoreceptor-driven drives and nonchemoreceptor-related drives, e.g. pain or arousal, may be difficult to assess clinically or in the laboratory. This section will discuss, within a framework of the most relevant neurotransmitter system, drugs commonly used in anesthesia. In some cases, the localization and effects of a particular drug are quite well known, for example the effect of a benzodiazepine acting on the GABA receptor, whereas in other cases knowledge of the drug's effect at a receptor level is fragmentary and speculative, e.g. effects of inhalational anesthetics on the intramembrane portion of proteins making up the GABA receptor. The classification of drugs in this section by possible neurotransmitter system effects must take into account the many effects of these drugs – both known and unknown. The sections in this book dealing with the specific pharmacology of these agents provide more detailed information about their general pharmacology.

Drugs acting at opioid receptors

Animal studies demonstrate that endogenous opioids and receptors are found in the carotid bodies[60] and in the respiratory centers.[61] Local exogenous placement of opioid agonists in the carotid bodies,[60] respiratory centers (DRG and VRG),[3] and close to the central chemoreceptors produces severe respiratory depression.[61] However, roles for endogenous opioid neurotransmitters, for example enkephalins and endorphins, have not been clearly determined during normal breathing. The best evidence indicates that they play little or no role under most conditions. Even during ventilatory depression caused by sustained hypoxia (see above), naloxone, a pure μ-receptor antagonist, does not increase ventilation.[62]

Opioids are perhaps the most common drugs given in the perioperative period; only a few patients undergoing a painful procedure do not receive a dose of one opioid or another. Severe pain can be adequately treated with opioids, but their dose-related ventilatory depression limits the dose that can be administered acutely. However, in general, acute pain does not need to be left inadequately treated for fear of ventilatory compromise.[63] Although many opioids are commonly used in clinical practice – morphine, meperidine (pethidine), and the fentanyl family, i.e. fentanyl, alfentanil, sufentanil, and remifentanil, being the most common – their primary effects, for both pain relief and respiratory depression, are through their effects on the CNS mediated at the μ opioid receptor.[61,64] However, opioids possess different pharmacokinetic characteristics extending from their different physiochemical properties, for example lipid solubilities, which result in pronounced differences in the severity and time-course of any respiratory depression.

The clinically obvious effect of opioids is a dose-related reduction in ventilatory effort; this results in hypercapnia – as shown by an increased arterial and end-tidal $P\text{CO}_2$ – which is due to a reduction in both tidal volume and respiratory frequency.[65,66] Although clinically the respiratory rate is often used as a measure of the degree of narcotization, tidal volume is affected to at least the same degree, and in some circumstances to a greater extent. This increase in resting CO_2 indicates that the hypercapnic ventilatory response line is shifted to a higher CO_2 level. This is owing to the line being shifted to the right, but in addition a decrease in the response slope may also be present (increases in *B* and decreases in *S* in equation 6.1). The degree to which a reduction in the slope is found may depend on the opioid dose, the level of sedation induced, and the testing method (see above discussion on measuring the hypercapnic ventilatory response). Sleep and morphine have been found to synergistically produce a marked reduction in the slope of the hypercapnic ventilatory response;[58] presumably, this is also true for other opioids.

Opioids also reduce the hypoxic ventilatory response. Weil *et al.*[67] were the first to study the effects of morphine on the ventilatory response that is induced by a gradual decrease in arterial oxygenation. When compared with the reduction in hypercapnic response (see Santiago *et al.*,[66] who compared the effects of morphine on hypercapnic, hypoxic, and exercise-induced increases in ventilation in the same subjects), the decrease in hypoxic response seems to be of approximately the same magnitude. This implies that the opioid effect occurs primarily after integration of the peripheral and central drives, e.g. in the respiratory centers. Like morphine, alfentanil also reduces the acute hypoxic ventilatory response[68,69] as well as increases the relative depression in ventilation caused by sustained hypoxia.[69]

Interestingly, there may be a difference between the respiratory effects of opioids in men and women. Women seem to have a relatively larger reduction in responsiveness to CO_2 (in equation 6.1, the slope is reduced whereas the apneic threshold is unaffected) and to hypoxia (ventilation difference in equation 6.2), whereas men have a smaller reduction in hypercapnic and hypoxic sensitivities but a significant increase in apneic threshold, i.e. the CO_2 response line is shifted to higher $P_{ET}\text{CO}_2$ levels.[16,23] These sex-related differences reside in the peripheral chemoreflex loop and are equivalent to sex-related differences in opioid-mediated analgesia.[16,23]

After it was discovered that the anterior horn of the spinal cord contains opioid receptors that modulate pain pathways, epidural or intrathecal opioids have been utilized to provide pain relief with a potential for less respiratory depression. Opioids given into the spinal canal may potentially cause respiratory depression by their systemic absorption or by their cephalad migration through the CSF. Clinically significant respiratory depression has been found with the use of both spinal and epidural opioids.[70,71] Bailey *et al.*[72] extensively studied the effects of different doses of intrathecal morphine in healthy volunteers. Using intrathecal doses of 0.2–0.6 mg morphine, they found that respiratory depression peaked at 6–10 h following injection; for the 0.6-mg doses, $P_{ET}CO_2$ reached a maximum of 50 mmHg (6.7 kPa). They recommended that doses larger than 0.4 mg should be used with caution. This delayed respiratory depression indicates slow cephalad spread. Because morphine is hydrophilic, it will be retained in the CSF more than lipophilic compounds such as sufentanil. Retained morphine eventually circulates throughout the cerebrospinal fluid.

Drugs that provide a mixed agonist and antagonist effect at the μ-receptor are commonly used clinically. Although these drugs appear to have limited respiratory depression owing to antagonist effects, their maximum analgesic effect is also limited (ceiling effect).

The pure μ-receptor opioid antagonist naloxone approximately equally reverses both the ventilatory depression and the analgesia produced by opioids.[46] Naloxone has a relatively short duration of action compared with many opioids, thus the possibility of renarcotization with respiratory depression must be borne in mind whenever this drug is used.

Drugs affecting amino acid neurotransmitter systems – GABA and glutamate

Inhalational anesthetics

As a group, inhalational anesthetics affect ventilatory control at many sites, most likely through different mechanisms of action. They cause ventilatory depression by abolishing the peripheral chemoreceptor drive, by depressing respiratory integration centers in the brainstem, by general depression of the central nervous system, and by suppressing the function of the intercostal muscles and diaphragm. Although patients often still breathe adequately with minimal CO_2 retention at concentrations that provide surgical anesthesia,[73,74] animal studies indicate that at high concentrations [a minimal alveolar concentration (MAC) greater than 2] complete cessation of respiratory activity occurs, irrespective of the CO_2 tension.

At anesthetic concentrations, halothane, enflurane, isoflurane, desflurane, and sevoflurane all cause a dose-dependent increase in respiratory rate (see Fig. 6.8), which is related to a direct stimulatory effect on the respiratory rhythm generator in the brainstem, and a reduction in tidal volume. These effects – together with the increase in dead space ventilation, increased $\dot{V}/\dot{Q}$ mismatch, and increased shunt – result in an increase in arterial and end-tidal $P\text{CO}_2$ (Fig. 6.8). Painful stimuli or the addition of nitrous oxide (with a reduction in the inhalational anesthetic to keep a constant MAC) reduces the arterial $P\text{CO}_2$ somewhat. At greater than 1 MAC, the overall effect of the inhalational anesthetic is a 30–50% depression of resting minute ventilation.[73,74] At 1 MAC, the ventilatory response to hypercapnia is severely depressed and the response to hypoxia is abolished.[75]

The general decrease in ventilatory drive caused by inhalational anesthetics does not produce an equal reduction to all muscles of respiration, but rather produces significantly different effects on the diaphragm and chest wall muscles.[76,77] Although the diaphragm is the principal muscle of ventilation, coordination with other ventilation muscles (e.g. intercostal muscles) is needed to produce a normal breathing pattern. Caudad movement of the diaphragm produces an increase in intrathoracic volume through the displacement of abdominal contents, whereas intercostal muscle activation permits ribcage expansion. Warner *et al.*[77] found that 1 MAC halothane significantly reduced hypercapnic ventilatory sensitivity; this reduction was primarily through a reduction in the ribcage contribution (see Fig. 6.9).

Knill and Gelb[75] showed that during halothane anesthesia (1.1 MAC) the gradual development of mild to moderate hypoxia ($P_{ET}O_2$ = 7 kPa or 53 mmHg) in hypercapnic patients did not cause an increase in ventilation but reduced $\dot{V}_m$ by more than 30%. This lack of ventilatory stimulation may be due to the development of hypoxic ventilatory decline when the peripheral chemoreceptor drive is reduced by the inhalational agent. This contrasts sharply with the normal synergistic interaction between the two stimuli (hypoxia and hypercapnia), which causes brisk ventilatory responses in awake individuals. This experimental finding is important clinically since it shows that, during anesthesia, the development of even mild hypoxia will *reduce* ventilation despite

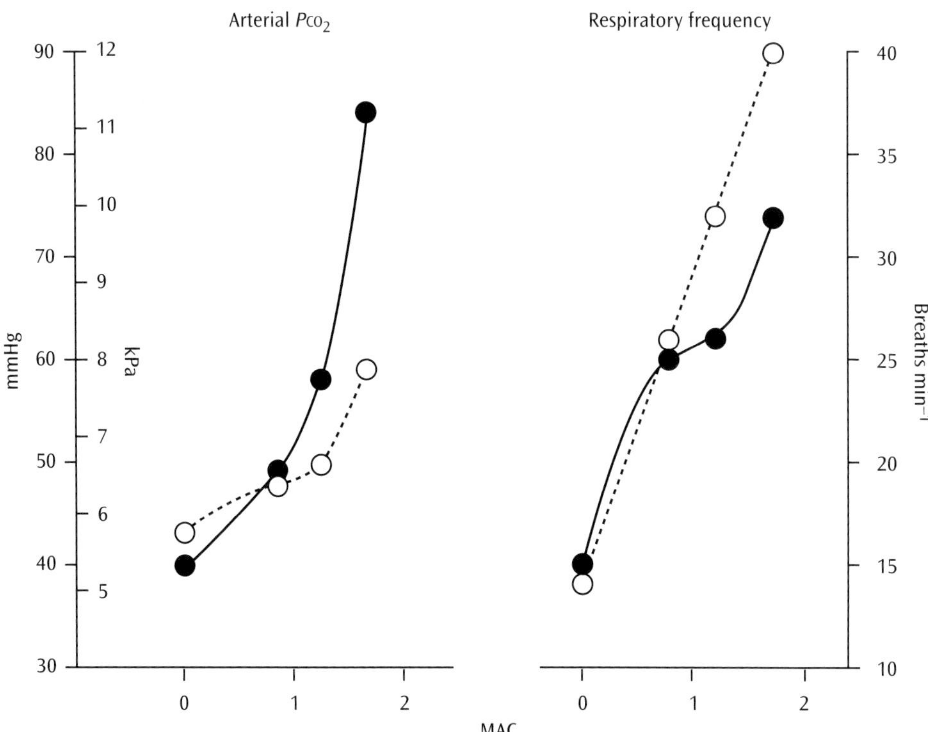

Figure 6.8 *Effect on arterial* $P\text{CO}_2$ *(left) and respiratory frequency (right) of adding* N_2O *to desflurane at equi-MAC values. Note the nearly 30 mmHg difference in arterial* $P\text{CO}_2$ *between 1.7 MAC desflurane and 1.7 MAC desflurane plus* N_2O*. Filled circles are desflurane in oxygen; open circles are desflurane plus 60%* N_2O *in oxygen. (Adapted from Lockhart* et al.[102]*)*

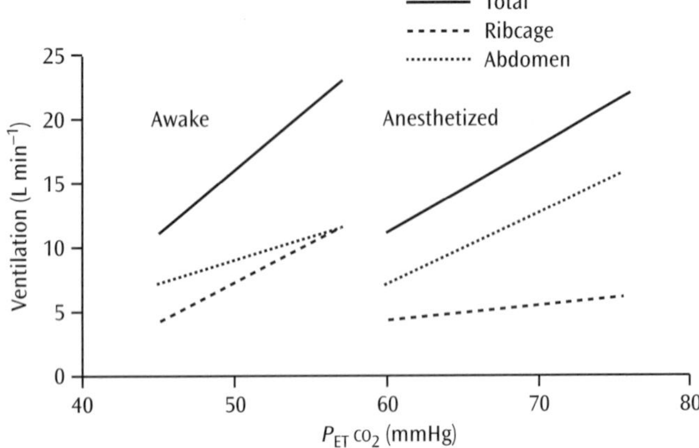

Figure 6.9 *Hypercapnic ventilatory response divided into ribcage and abdominal/diaphragm responses using respiratory impedance plethysmography in one subject awake and with 1.0 MAC halothane anesthesia. (From Warner* et al.[77] *with permission)*

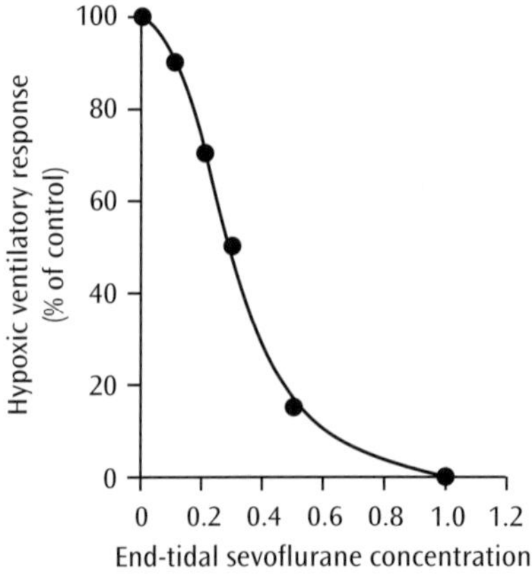

Figure 6.11 *The steep dose–response curve of sevoflurane measured in one subject. On the x-axis, the end-tidal sevoflurane concentration; on the y-axis, the hypoxic ventilatory response as a percentage of control (control response is 100%). An inhibitory sigmoid E_{max} function is plotted to the data. The IC_{50} (end-tidal sevoflurane concentration causing 50% inhibition of the hypoxic response) is 0.3%.*

overt hypercapnia. Recent studies indicate that this also applies to the postanesthesia recovery period.[78]

At subanesthetic concentrations, inhalational anesthetics have little or no effect on resting respiratory variables such as respiratory rate and tidal volume. Their effect on the peripheral chemoreceptor-related response to hypoxia varies between agents (see Fig. 6.10). At 0.1 MAC, while the subject remains alert,[79–81] halothane reduces the ventilatory response to isocapnic hypoxia by about 70%; 35% depression is seen with isoflurane and sevoflurane; and virtually no depression is observed with desflurane.[25,45,78,82,83] Halothane, isoflurane, and sevoflurane exhibit steep dose–response curves (Fig. 6.11), and at concentrations greater than 0.15 MAC the response to hypoxia is depressed by more than 50%. This is clinically important because the tissue concentration of halothane, isoflurane, and enflurane may remain above 0.1 MAC for some time in the postoperative period. Owing to their rapid removal from the body, sevoflurane and desflurane are less likely to contribute to the postoperative depression of the hypoxic response. The absence of depression of the hypoxic response with 0.1-MAC desflurane is due to an increase in the respiratory rate with hypoxia, which offsets the reduced tidal volume response. Possibly, desflurane (in combination with hypoxia) activates receptors which, at high inspired desflurane concentrations, induce airway irritation and sympathetic activation.[84] Note that all anesthetics (including desflurane) at 0.1 MAC block the synergistic interaction of hypoxia and hypercapnia, which indicates an action at the carotid bodies.[25]

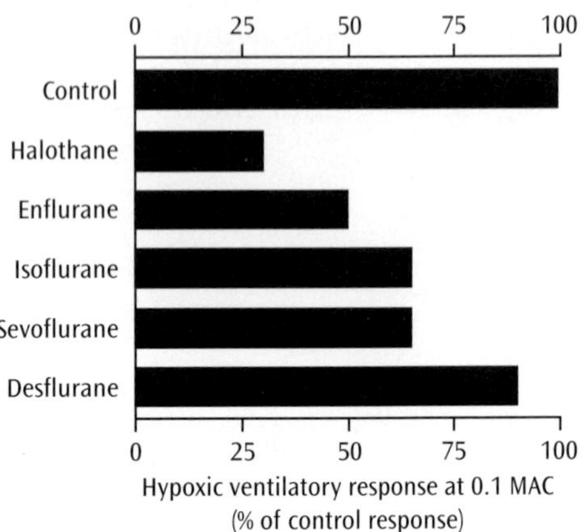

Figure 6.10 *The influence of inhalational anesthetics at 0.1 MAC on the ventilatory response to isocapnic hypoxia in healthy volunteers. Values are percentage of control; the control response is 100%. Note that halothane causes the most depression, desflurane the least. (Data are from references 25, 45, 78, and 82.)*

Benzodiazepines

Clinically, benzodiazepines are frequently administered preoperatively to reduce anxiety and as intraoperative sedation in surgical procedures where analgesia is provided by local or regional anesthesia. Diazepam and midazolam are the most commonly used agents. Except for occasions when midazolam is used as an induction agent, patients are commonly breathing spontaneously. Benzodiazepines act through a specific receptor on the GABA receptor complex; activation of this receptor increases activity of GABA at this inhibitory site.

Given alone, either diazepam or midazolam has minimal but variable effects on resting ventilation as well as on hypercapnic and hypoxic ventilatory responses.[85,86] Bailey *et al.*[85] found that 0.1 mg kg^{-1} of diazepam increased resting $P_{ET}CO_2$ consistently but had a variable effect on the slope of the CO_2 response, with some subjects consistently showing an increase in the slope. The respiratory effects of midazolam are similar to those seen with diazepam. Gross *et al.*[86] gave 0.2 mg kg^{-1} of midazolam, a higher dose than is commonly used for preoperative anxiolysis, and found that when most subjects become unresponsive to verbal stimulation (average of 3.5 min after injection) the slope of their CO_2 response is depressed by 35% and is still depressed by 25% after 15 min. Because of the experimental design, the change in resting CO_2 could not be estimated.

Similar variable effects of benzodiazepines were found on the hypoxic ventilatory response.[87–89] Alexander and Gross[87] studied the influence of 0.1 mg kg^{-1} of midazolam on the response to isohypercapnic ($P_{ET}CO_2$ = 50 mmHg, 6.7 kPa) hypoxia (approximated S_pO_2 = 75%) and found the slopes of the ventilatory response decreased from 1.5 to 0.7 L min^{-1} %$^{-1}$. Interestingly, none of their subjects had overt airway obstruction with this dose, but two of the nine subjects required prompting to breathe deeply to stabilize their saturation above 90% when they were breathing room air.

Flumazenil is a specific benzodiazepine antagonist that acts at the benzodiazepine receptor on the GABA receptor complex. Although it clearly quickly reverses sedation and even unconsciousness caused by benzodiazepines, the completeness of its reversal of benzodiazepine-induced ventilatory depression has been questioned. This may in part be due to the variable effects on ventilatory control caused by benzodiazepines themselves and also to the effects of the presence or absence of wakefulness (see above). Flögel *et al.*[90] gave flumazenil during a computer-controlled infusion of midazolam (constant predicted plasma level). This midazolam infusion reduced the slope of the CO_2 response and the ventilation at constant $P_{ET}CO_2$ levels of both 46 mmHg (6 kPa)and 58 mmHg (7.7 kPa). Large doses of flumazenil (1, 3, and 10 mg) reversed sedation and ventilatory depression at 46 and 58 mmHg. However, ventilatory measurements returned to preflumazenil levels of depression more quickly than the subjects became resedated. In a clinical study in which diazepam was given by multiple bolus injection over 1–3 h in patients undergoing procedures using local anesthesia (total dose 1.6±0.8 mg kg^{-1}), Mora *et al.*[88] found that, although each patient became awake and alert, only five of 10 subjects had significant depression of the hypoxic response and only one of these patients had complete reversal after 1 mg flumazenil. In a more controlled study of volunteers, Blouin *et al.*[89] found that, with midazolam titrated to a level of sedation resulting in the subjects being just arousable to a loud verbal command (0.6–0.2 mg kg^{-1}), the hypoxic response was depressed by 50–55%. Flumazenil, 1-mg bolus, caused a significant increase in hypoxic response (Fig. 6.12). These studies all seem to indicate that, although flumazenil is probably effective in reversing the ventilatory depression caused by midazolam, the effect does not last as long as the reversal of the sedation.

Propofol

Because of its rapid recovery profile, propofol has become the most commonly used induction agent. When patients are immediately manually ventilated after induction, given muscles relaxants, intubated, and mechanically ventilated for the duration of the anesthetic and surgery, the ventilatory effects of the intravenous induction agent are of little clinical importance. However, with the frequent use of spontaneous ventilation using a laryngeal mask airway (LMA), the ventilatory effects of the induction agent have become more important.

The measurement of ventilatory effects during induction of anesthesia often results in comparison of the different ventilatory drives. Before induction, wakefulness drives may be the dominant factors, with few effects seen from the metabolic control mediated via the chemoreflex loops. Induction of anesthesia removes the wakefulness factors, and immediately chemoreflex loops must support total ventilatory drive. Apnea after induction may result from several factors, including a loss of ventilatory drive that is associated with wakefulness at a time when there is little metabolic chemoreflex stimulation (i.e. hyperoxia and hypocapnia) as well as depression of chemoreflexes by the induction agent.

In patients preoxygenated with 35% F_IO_2, 2.5 mg kg^{-1} of propofol caused apnea in all subjects (duration 1–2 min, median 88 s); in some patients, this was long enough to cause a significant desaturation.[91] Blouin *et al.*[92] used a forced hypercapnic technique and found that ventilation was significantly reduced for 15 min following 2.5 mg kg^{-1} propofol (Fig. 6.13). The slope of the CO_2 response is depressed for a longer period with propofol than with thiopental. When propofol is infused and titrated to a constant subanesthetic level, a significant depression of hypoxic ventilatory response occurs.[93] In this study, the $P_{ET}CO_2$ was maintained at approximately 6 mmHg (0.8 kPa)above the subject's baseline; thus, some of the ventilatory depression probably resulted from a reduction in the hypercapnic ventilatory response.

Barbiturates

Thiopental is used as an induction drug primarily for longer lasting cases; thus, the ventilatory depression caused by an induction dose of thiopental may be of less clinical interest. However, induction doses of thiopental will frequently cause a significant apneic period,[91,94,95] particularly in a premedicated patient who has been hyperventilated with 100% O_2 to a degree of mild hypocapnia prior to induction. Yet, even during hypercapnia induced by breathing an increased level of inspired CO_2, 3.5 mg kg^{-1} of thiopental reduces ventilation by 37% when $P_{ET}CO_2$ is 60 mmHg (8 kPa) and by 49% when $P_{ET}CO_2$ is 49 mmHg(6.5 kPa).[96] This ventilatory depression lasted approximately 15 min.

Etomidate

Etomidate appears to cause less respiratory depression than barbiturates when used as an induction agent.[97] Interestingly, there is a similar reduction in the slope of the hypercapnic response but there is an upward shift (toward higher ventilation), indicating that perhaps etomidate causes some nonchemoreflex-mediated ventilatory stimulation.

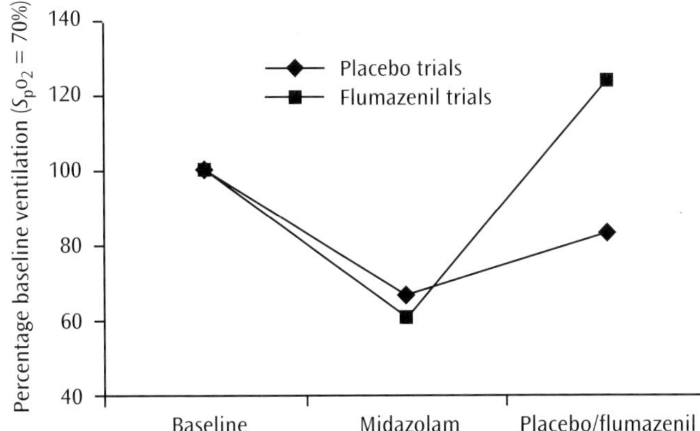

Figure 6.12 *Changes in the acute hypoxic response following midazolam titrated to responsiveness to loud verbal command. Midazolam reduced hypoxic sensitivity, which was reversed by 1 mg flumazenil. The slight increase in hypoxic sensitivity following placebo was due to the waning effect of midazolam. (From Blouin* et al.[89] *with permission.)*

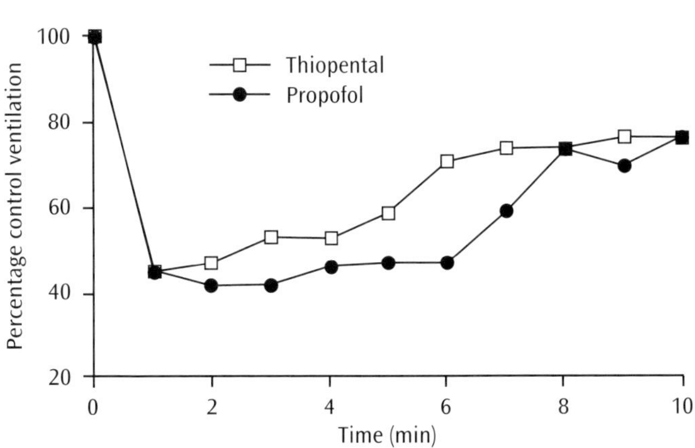

Figure 6.13 *Comparison of the effects of thiopental (4 mg kg^{-1}) with propofol (2.5 mg kg^{-1}) on minute ventilation at $P_{ET}CO_2$ of 46 mmHg. Values are means ± SEM. (From Blouin* et al.[92] *with permission.)*

Drugs affecting the *N*-methyl-D-aspartate receptor system for excitatory amino acids

Nitrous oxide (N_2O) and ketamine possess some similar clinical characteristics. Both agents increase the catecholamine levels in blood, resulting in an increase in peripheral resistance, cardiac output, and cerebral blood flow. Both also cause analgesia and amnesia, increase the incidence of postoperative nausea and vomiting, and have secondary psychomimetic effects. With respect to ventilatory control, N_2O and ketamine behave in a similar fashion, causing, at least at the levels used clinically, little or no effect on the ventilatory responses to CO_2 and hypoxia. The mechanism used by these agents may be inhibition of the glutamate-requiring NMDA receptors.[98] Both agents may also interact with μ-opioid receptors.[20,99] Opioid-induced ventilation changes may involve a reduction in glutamatergic transmission,[3] making interpretation more difficult.

Nitrous oxide

Nitrous oxide is a weak inhalational anesthetic (MAC = 105%) that is used as a sedative/analgesic for dental procedures, for pain relief during labor, or as an adjuvant during general anesthesia. When given at 1 MAC (in a hyperbaric chamber), N_2O causes an increase in respiratory rate, reduces tidal volume, and depresses the hypercapnic ventilatory response.[100] At subanesthetic concentrations, N_2O does not change ventilatory responses to hypercapnia or acute hypoxia.[101] Interestingly, the ventilatory response to hypoxia is better sustained with N_2O than without, indicating that N_2O counteracts the development of hypoxic ventilatory decline (Fig. 6.14).[101] As an adjuvant to inhalational anesthesia with halogenated agents such as sevoflurane, desflurane, and isoflurane, N_2O posses both MAC and ventilatory-sparing effects. The decrease in ventilation and the increase in $P_{ET}CO_2$ seen with the inhalational anesthetics is reduced when nitrous oxide is added[102] (see Fig. 6.8). The mechanism of action of the respiratory effects of nitrous oxide is probably related in part to its stimulation of the sympathetic system.

At subanesthetic concentrations, N_2O renders overall control of ventilation somewhat unstable, especially as consciousness is lost. At 30% inspired concentration, N_2O induces frequent central and obstructive sleep apneas.[103] During N_2O sedation, a short episode of hypocapnia due to hyperventilation is followed by apnea and desaturation.[104] These findings are important to all patients sedated with N_2O, including those sedated with a mix of 50% N_2O in 50% O_2 (Entonox) during labor.

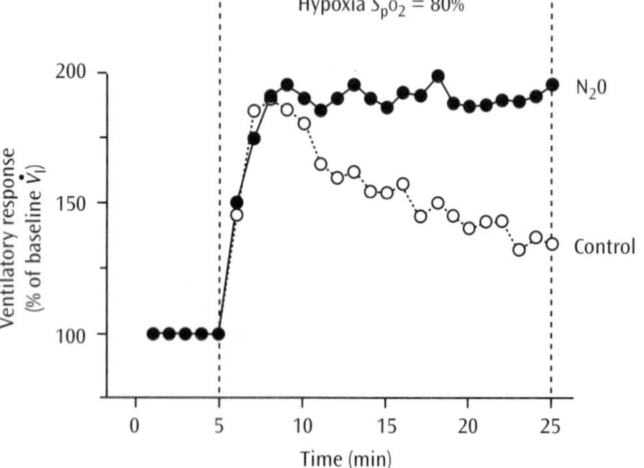

Figure 6.14 *Influence of subanesthetic N_2O on the ventilatory response to sustained isocapnic hypoxia. Nitrous oxide does not affect the acute hypoxic response. The ventilatory response to sustained hypoxia is better sustained with N_2O than without. (Adapted from Dahan and Ward.[101])*

Ketamine

Ketamine is a phencyclidine that produces dissociation between the cortex and the limbic system. This action causes analgesia and loss of awareness of the environment; however, visceral reflexes and muscle tone are maintained. Despite a general preservation of ventilation, airway reflexes are suppressed, thus aspiration may occur. Ketamine is associated with several undesirable side-effects, such as increased saliva production, delirium, cardiovascular stimulation, and increased cranial pressure, all of which may alter ventilation.

In children, an initial intravenous (i.v.) dose of 2 mg kg^{-1} followed by a 40 μg kg^{-1} min^{-1} infusion causes no effect on $P_{ET}CO_2$, respiratory frequency, tidal volume, resting minute ventilation, or the slope of the ventilatory response to CO_2.[105] At higher doses, ketamine does produce significant respiratory depression and apnea. In adults, the results of respiratory studies are mixed. Bourke and colleagues[106] have compared the respiratory effects of ketamine with those of morphine and morphine plus ketamine. Ketamine alone (cumulative i.v. dose 3 mg kg^{-1}) causes a small dose-dependent decrease in resting ventilation (maximum decrease 10%) which lasts for 90 min after the last dose. The slope of the CO_2 response curve is not changed. Morphine interacts with ketamine in an additive fashion with respect to depression of resting ventilation and the slope of the CO_2 response curve.

Adrenergic receptor system

α_2-Adrenergic agonists

Agonists at the α_2-adrenergic receptor, initially developed because of their central antihypertensive effects, have also been found to have analgesic, anesthetic, and sedative properties. The site of action in the CNS may include the locus ceruleus, which is also related to the respiratory centers. The respiratory effects of clonidine, and the more selective and potent α_2-agonist dexmedetomidine, have been studied in humans. Neither drug seems to depress resting ventilation or elevate arterial CO_2 more than would be expected from the decrease in arousal or the sleep that is induced.[107,108] Similarly, the effect on the CO_2 response was minimal for both clonidine[109] and dexmedetomidine.[108] When oral clonidine was combined with an opioid, no synergistic effect on the hypercapnic ventilatory response was found.[109]

Dopamine agonists and antagonists

Dopamine is frequently used for surgical patients and seriously ill patients in the intensive care unit (ICU) to increase cardiac output, support blood pressure, and improve renal blood flow. Intravenous dopamine at intermediate (3–5 μg kg^{-1} min^{-1}) and high (> 5 μg kg^{-1} min^{-1}) doses activates β- and α-adrenergic receptors, causing an increase in cardiac contractility and systemic vascular resistance. At low doses (0.5–3 μg kg^{-1} min^{-1}), dopaminergic receptors (D_2-receptors) are preferentially activated and primarily cause renal vasodilatation. Apart from the kidneys, dopaminergic receptors are present in various other organs, including the carotid bodies. Endogenous and exogenous dopamine inhibits the carotid bodies. Dopamine at 3 μg kg^{-1} min^{-1} blunts the ventilatory response to hypoxia and reduces the response to hypercapnia, which is entirely due to an effect within the peripheral chemoreflex loop at the carotid bodies.[27,110]

Dopamine receptor antagonists such as droperidol, domperidone, and haloperidol reverse the effects of exogenous dopamine on carotid bodies. Droperidol and haloperidol have a strong sedative effect by acting on central dopaminergic receptors and cause what has been termed a neuroleptic state. The blockade of D_2-receptors at the carotid bodies will result in loss of the inhibitory influence of endogenous dopamine; as a consequence, dopamine antagonists will cause increases in responses mediated via peripheral chemoreflexes (e.g. the hypoxic ventilatory response).[110,111]

DRUG INTERACTIONS

Although very few patients who require anesthesia, or even merely sedation and analgesia, receive only a single drug, few studies detail the respiratory effects of drug combinations. Combinations of drugs are used to achieve all elements of anesthesia: sedation, anxiolysis, analgesia, and amnesia. Frequently, an analgesic, most commonly an opioid, will be combined with a sedative/anxiolytic drug such as midazolam or propofol for a patient undergoing a procedure with conscious sedation. The ventilatory effects in this situation are particularly important because the training of personnel providing conscious sedation may be less than that of personnel who ordinarily provide general anesthesia. (As of 27 June 1989, the US Department of Health and Human Services had reports of 86 deaths associated with midazolam. All but three occurred outside the operating room.[112]) During general anesthesia with an inhalational anesthetic, an opioid is usually included as part of the anesthetic regimen. This may be in the form of a preinduction dose of fentanyl or the titration of a longer-acting drug such as morphine toward the conclusion of the anesthetic, in order to provide analgesia during the immediate recovery period. The goal of these drug combinations is to provide the desired effects with no increase – and, hopefully, a decrease – in respiratory side-effects. However, very few studies guide the selection of drug combination by taking into account their effects on the control of ventilation.

Drug interactions, especially if synergistic, may be particularly important when patients are expected to return to spontaneous ventilation in the immediate postoperative period. Ventilation during this time will be driven by metabolic (i.e. chemoreceptor) inputs, pain, and the level of arousal to different degrees, while also being affected by the residual effects of intraoperative anesthetics and muscle relaxants as well as any analgesic drugs given for control of postoperative pain. Obviously, these many drug interactions, although clinically very important, are difficult to sort out scientifically. The anesthesiologist must be alert to potential unexpected ventilatory depression or airway obstruction in the immediate postoperative period.

Opioids are frequently combined with centrally acting dopamine antagonists, i.e. in low doses for improved analgesia and in higher doses as part of a neuroleptic anesthetic. These agents are thought to potentiate the analgesic effects of the opioid and to provide sedation, and they may counter the emetogenic effects of the opioid. As discussed above, neuroleptic drugs increase the hypoxic ventilatory response through an effect on dopamine receptors in the carotid bodies. Olson *et al.*[113] found that adding prochlorperazine to morphine did not change resting hypercapnia or depression of the hypercapnic response, but the asphyxial response (hypercapnic hypoxia) was increased.

During regional anesthesia or procedures not painful enough to require general anesthesia, an opioid is frequently combined with a benzodiazepine. Fentanyl and midazolam is a particularly common clinical combination. As mentioned above, this combination may have resulted in a significant number of clinical complications.

Bailey *et al.*[112] studied this combination in 12 healthy male volunteers by comparing the ventilatory effects of $2\,\mu g\,kg^{-1}$ fentanyl with $0.05\,mg\,kg^{-1}$ midazolam, with the combined drug doses being the same. The CO_2 response was unaffected by midazolam, and midazolam did not potentiate the depression caused by fentanyl (Fig. 6.15). However, although no subject receiving only midazolam became hypoxic ($S_{p}O_2$ < 90% for over 10 s), 6 of the 12 receiving only fentanyl and 11 of 12 subjects receiving the drug combination had an hypoxic episode. Half of the subjects had an episode of apnea (cessation of respiratory effort for > 15 s) after receiving the drug combination whereas no apnea followed either drug given alone. This study clearly illustrated the potentially severe respiratory consequences that could occur after a drug combination.

Opioids are also frequently combined with infused propofol to provide sedation and analgesia during painful procedures or during regional anesthesia. The combination of a propofol infusion and an alfentanil infusion on pharmacokinetics and various pharmacodynamic effects, including ventilation, has been examined.[114] Interestingly, adding alfentanil to propofol increases the average propofol and alfentanil plasma concentrations over those expected with either one given alone. This observation shows that synergism can be pharmacokinetic as well as pharmacodynamic. Although there appears to be an enhancement of propofol sedation by alfentanil as well as alfentanil-induced analgesia by propofol, there is little increase in ventilatory depression. With propofol alone, ventilation decreases mildly with no increase in $P_{ET}CO_2$. With the combination of alfentanil and propofol, $P_{ET}CO_2$ rises to the same level (approximately 48 mmHg, 6.4 kPa) seen with only alfentanil. Propofol alone does not cause desaturation and the hypercapnic response curve is depressed by only 22%; however, the effective highest infusion rate in this study is only approximately $43\,\mu g\,kg^{-1}\,min^{-1}$. Alfentanil alone causes a 41% decrease in the hypercapnic response and the combination leads to 56% decrease.

EFFERENT CONTROL OF THE RESPIRATORY MUSCLES

Whether the dominant neural drive to breathe originates from hypoxia, hypercapnia, pain, anxiety, or conscious volitional control, it must be translated into effective movement of air into and out of gas-exchanging regions of the lung. This requires coordinated effort of the diaphragm, other chest wall muscles, and laryngeal and pharyngeal muscles. The motor neurons of some respiratory muscles must also respond to other inputs that utilize these muscles for nongas-exchanging functions such as talking, singing, sneezing, coughing, hiccupping, vomiting, and helping to maintain erect posture. Patency of the upper airway is maintained by the activation of muscles positioning the soft palate, pharynx, tongue, and larynx when inspiration results in negative airway pressure. The

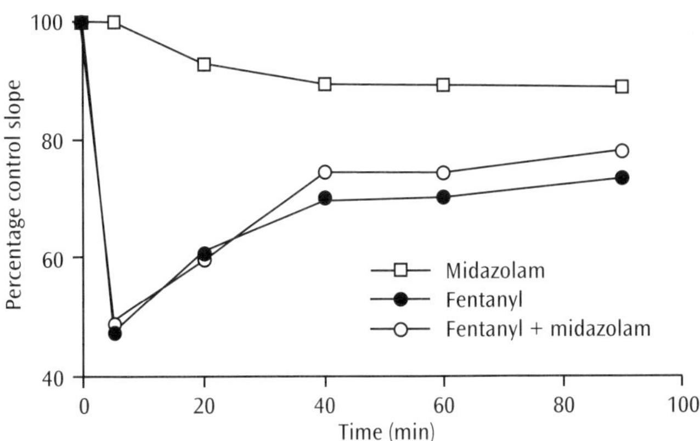

Figure 6.15 *The time-course of the change in the slope of the CO_2 response curve ($L\,min^{-1}\,mmHg^{-1}$) after $2\,\mu g\,kg^{-1}$ fentanyl, $0.05\,mg\,kg^{-1}$ midazolam, or the combination. The addition of midazolam did not significantly decrease the response over fentanyl alone. (From Bailey* et al.[112] *with permission.)*

physiology of the control of these muscle groups is very complex and not completely understood (for a comprehensive review of upper airway physiology, see Mathew and Sant'Ambrogio[115]) and depression of their activation by anesthesia drugs can result in partial or complete airway obstruction. Airway obstruction by these mechanisms may result in hypoxia more quickly than the hypoventilation caused by depression of metabolic chemoreflexes.

Upper airway patency during anesthesia

It is clinically obvious that sedation, analgesia, and anesthesia cause an increased propensity for upper airway obstruction even when there is sufficient ventilatory drive. Levels of anesthesia permitting adequate ventilation with an airway device in place (e.g. endotracheal tube or LMA) can result in complete apnea owing to upper airway obstruction if the device is removed. Although this is an obvious clinical observation, the pharmacology of upper airway obstruction is much less well studied than that of the chemoreflex loops. Maintaining an open airway is a fundamental skill learned by an anesthesiologist. Various maneuvers (e.g. jaw thrust) and devices (e.g. oral airway, LMA, and endotracheal tube) are used to keep the airway open. Although classically it is believed that the primary obstruction site is at the base of the tongue, recent data indicate that the soft palate and the epiglottis are at least as important.

The primary site of upper airway obstruction may be the soft palate.[116,117] Following induction of anesthesia with thiopental, Nandi *et al.*[117] have found that, during the initial postinduction apnea, there is significant posterior movement of the soft palate, tongue, and epiglottis, but obstruction occurs most commonly at the level of the soft palate. During subsequent spontaneous ventilation under enflurane and N_2O, placement of the head in a neutral position results in the collapse of the pharynx. Mathru *et al.*[116] have evaluated the upper airway with MRI during anesthesia with propofol as the sole agent, and have found that the soft palate seems to be the principal site of airway obstruction. The many sites of obstruction are similar to those found in sleep apnea patients, and are indicative of the complex interactions required to maintain a patent airway.[118]

There are also frequent periods of airway obstruction in the postoperative recovery period. In a study of 18 473 patients in the recovery room, 6.9% have required prolonged support of their upper airways in order to prevent obstruction.[119] Catley *et al.*[120] have found that patients who receive postoperative morphine rather than regional anesthesia for their pain relief have hypoxemic episodes during sleep that are related to obstructive apneas or obstructive breathing. Hypoxemic episodes that are related to slow respiratory rate or central apnea are rare.

Obstructive sleep apnea is very common, particularly in the male population.[121] These patients have frequent episodes of obstructive apnea during sleep. When severe, the frequent arousals cause sufficient disruption of the nocturnal sleep pattern that daytime hypersomnolence occurs. Risk factors include obesity, a history of snoring, and male gender or postmenopausal age for females. These patients are at risk for cardiovascular complications, including hypertension and myocardial infarction.[122] The anesthetic management of these patients can be quite difficult;[123] they are a risk for severe hypoxemia during sleep, particularly when postoperative opioids are required.[124] The use of epidural opioids may also be problematic in patients with sleep apnea.[125]

Ventilatory effects of spinally administered drugs

The administration of drugs into the CSF, directly via intrathecal injection or through epidural administration, can potentially cause significant respiratory effects. The medication can diffuse cephalad in the CSF and can affect central chemoreceptors and medullary ventilatory controllers. Also, in the case of epidural administration, significant systemic absorption can occur with subsequent delivery to other parts of the ventilatory control system. The effects of opioids given epidurally or intrathecally have been discussed earlier in this chapter. However, when local anesthetics are used, the effects of selective blocking of both efferent and afferent signals related to ventilation must be considered.

Intrathecal injection limits systemic absorption because of the small amount used, but lipophilic compounds (e.g. sufentanil[126]) may still have significant plasma levels. Blockade to high thoracic dermatomes with local anesthetics effectively removes ventilatory drive to the intercostal muscles and afferent input from the sympathetic nervous system entering the spinal cord in the thoracic dermatomes. There may be some "deafferation" effects with a decrease of sensory stimulus in the reticular activating system, resulting in altered drives to the ventilatory controllers. However, resting ventilation and hypercapnic sensitivity seem to be unaltered.[127,128]

The ventilatory effects of epidural anesthesia with lidocaine (lignocaine) must also include the effects of systemic lidocaine as there is significant systemic absorption from the relatively large epidural doses used. Because lidocaine has both depressant and stimulant actions on the central nervous system, it is not surprising that different ventilatory effects from systemic administration of lidocaine have been observed. Gross *et al.*[129] have found that, although a bolus of lidocaine (1.5 $mg\,kg^{-1}$) causes transient ventilatory depression lasting approximately 2 min, an infusion of 60 $\mu g\,kg^{-1}\,min^{-1}$ leads to an increase in hypercapnic sensitivity. However, the acute hypoxic ventilatory response is variably depressed.[130] Labaille *et al.*[131] have found that epidural lidocaine results in a similar increase in hypercapnic sensitivity to intravenous lidocaine.

Ventilatory effects of neuromuscular blocking drugs

Neuromuscular blocking drugs affect ventilation by preventing the neural drive of the respiratory centers from being translated effectively into coordinated muscular action and, in addition, have effects on the metabolic chemoreflex loops themselves. Nondepolarizing muscle relaxants (such as vecuronium and pancuronium) act at cholinergic receptors by reversible competition with acetylcholine. Nicotinergic and muscarinergic receptors are also found in the carotid bodies.

Blockade of cholinergic receptors at the carotid bodies, occurring with clinical and subclinical doses of nondepolarizing relaxants, disturbs the normal carotid body hypoxic response. Relaxation of the adductor pollicis muscle to a train-of-four ratio of 0.7 is associated with normal tidal volume, $P_{ET}CO_2$, maximal inspiratory muscle force,[132] and an intact ventilatory response to (hyperoxic) hypercapnia; yet, the ventilatory response to hypoxia is severely blunted.[133] This is most likely related to an effect of muscle relaxants at the carotid bodies. However, as the hypoxic drive is associated with relatively more diaphragmatic activity,[134] a selective effect of muscle relaxants at the diaphragm cannot be excluded.

Mild neuromuscular blockade, as measured by a train-of-four between 0.7 and 0.9, is associated with pharyngeal dysfunction and reduced resting tonus in the upper esophageal sphincter muscle of awake volunteers.[135] This may result in impaired airway protection and an increased risk of stomach contents aspiration as well as upper airway obstruction. Such a degree of muscle relaxation correlates with the ability to sustain a "head lift" for 5 s; Pavlin *et al.*[132] have found that greater levels of blockade resulted in airway obstruction in normal subjects partially paralyzed with curare. However, D'Honneur *et al.*[136] have used vecuronium in volunteers to a train-of-four of 0.5 and found no effect on the upper airway, even using a negative airway pressure of $-40\,cmH_2O$ as stimulation. However, this may not be true in patients recovering from the effects of other anesthetic drugs, in addition to the partial paralysis. Thus, it would appear to be prudent to ensure a reversal to at least 0.8–0.9 in order to be confident of adequate upper airway function.

SUMMARY

The administration of drugs required by anesthesiologists to produce adequate anesthesia renders the ventilatory control system less able to respond to physiologic stresses involved in the perioperative period. This is related not only to the direct effects of anesthetics, sedatives, hypnotics, and analgesics at peripheral or central sites but also to changes in the behavioral state of the patient and possible mechanical effects of the surgery itself. As a result, all perioperative patients are at risk for respiratory depression. Although dramatic ventilatory depression or airway obstruction resulting in significant hypoxemia remain important clinical problems, appropriate drug selection and monitoring have done much to reduce the mortality associated with anesthetic drugs. However, significant morbidity may result from, for example, transient hypoxemia during sleep in the postoperative period.[137,138] Just as the brain integrates input from the chemoreceptors and other nonmetabolic stimuli in order to determine the appropriate ventilation, the anesthesiologist must integrate all the information about drug effects on the various components of the ventilatory control system in order to provide safe anesthesia.

REFERENCES

1. Dempsey JA, Pack AI. Regulation of breathing. In: Lenfant C (ed.). *Lung Biology in Health and Disease.* Vol. 79, 2nd edn. New York: Marcel Dekker, 1995.
2. Cherniack NS, Widdicombe JG. The respiratory system. In: Fishman A (ed.). *Handbook of Physiology*, vol. II. Bethesda, MD: American Physiology Society, 1986.
3. Bianchi AL, Denavit-Saubié M, Champagnat J. Central control of breathing in mammals: neuronal circuitry, membrane properties, and neurotransmitters. *Physiol Rev* 1995; **75:** 1–45.
4. von Euler C. Neural organization and rhythm generation. In: Crystal RG, West JB, Barnes PJ, *et al.* (eds). *The Lung: Scientific Foundations.* New York: Raven Press, 1991: 1307–18.
5. Duffin J, Ezure K, Lipski J. Breathing rhythm generation: focus on the rostral ventrolateral medulla. *News Physiol Sci* 1995; **10:** 133–40.
6. Orem J, Trotte RH. Behavioral control of breathing. *News Physiol Sci* 1994; **9:** 228–32.
7. Munschauer FE, Mador MJ, Ahuja A, Jacobs L. Selective paralysis of voluntary but not limbically influenced automatic respiration. *Arch Neurol* 1991; **48:** 1190–2.
8. Nattie EE, Wood J, Mega A, Goritski W. Rostral ventrolateral medulla muscarinic receptor involvement in central ventilatory chemosensitivity. *J Appl Physiol* 1989; **66:** 1462–70.
9. Coates EL, Li A, Nattie EE. Widespread sites of brain stem ventilatory chemoreceptors. *J Appl Physiol* 1993; **75:** 5–14.
10. Sato M, Severinghaus JW, Basbaum AI. Medullary CO_2 chemoreceptor neuron identification by c-fos immunocytochemistry. *J Appl Physiol* 1992; **73:** 96–100.
11. Gonzalez C, Almaraz L, Obeso A, Rigual R. Carotid body chemoreceptors: from natural stimuli to sensory discharges. *Physiol Rev* 1994; **74:** 829–98.
12. Vizek M, Pickett CK, Weil J. Biphasic ventilatory response of adult cats to sustained hypoxia has central origin. *J Appl Physiol* 1987; **63:** 1658–64.
13. Dejours P. Chemoreflexes in breathing. *Physiol Rev* 1962; **42:** 335–58.
14. Erickson JT, Millhorn DE. Hypoxia and electrical stimulation of the carotid sinus nerve induce fos-like immunoreactivity within catecholaminergic and serotoninergic neurons of the rat brainstem. *J Comp Neurol* 1994; **348:** 161–82.
15. Kikuchi Y, Okabe S, Tamura G, *et al.* Chemosensitivity and perception of dyspnea in patients with a history of near-fatal asthma. *N Engl J Med* 1994; **330:** 1329–34.
16. Dahan A, Sarton E, Teppema L, Olievier C. Sex-related differences in the influence of morphine on ventilatory control in humans. *Anesthesiology* 1998; **88:** 903–13.
17. Dahan A, DeGoede J, Berkenbosch A, Olievier ICW. The influence of oxygen on the ventilatory response to carbon dioxide in man. *J Physiol (Lond)* 1990; **428:** 485–99.
18. Read DJC. A clinical method for assessing the ventilatory response to carbon dioxide. *Aust Ann Med* 1967; **16:** 20–32.
19. Dahan A, Berkenbosch A, DeGoede J, *et al.* On a pseudo-rebreathing technique to assess the ventilatory sensitivity to carbon dioxide in man. *J Physiol (Lond)* 1990; **423:** 615–29.
20. Bourke DL, Warley A. The steady-state and rebreathing methods compared during morphine administration in humans. *J Physiol (Lond)* 1989; **419:** 509–17.
21. Swanson GD, Bellville JW. Step changes in end-tidal CO_2: methods and implications. *J Appl Physiol* 1975; **39:** 377–85.
22. Bellville JW, Whipp BJ, Kaufman RD, *et al.* Central and peripheral chemoreflex loop gain in normal and carotid body-resected subjects. *J Appl Physiol* 1979; **46:** 843–53.
23. Sarton E, Teppema L, Dahan A. Sex differences in morphine-induced ventilatory depression reside within the peripheral chemoreflex loop. *Anesthesiology* 1999; **90:** 1329–38.
24. Sarton E, Dahan A, Teppema L, *et al.* Influence of acute pain induced by activation of cutaneous nociceptors on ventilatory control. *Anesthesiology* 1997; **87:** 289–96.
25. Dahan A, Sarton E, van den Elsen M, *et al.* Ventilatory response to hypoxia in humans. *Anesthesiology* 1996; **85:** 60–8.
26. Easton PA, Slykerman LJ, Anthonisen NR. Recovery of the ventilatory response to hypoxia in normal adults. *J Appl Physiol* 1988; **64:** 521–8.
27. Dahan A, Ward DS, van den Elsen M, *et al.* Influence of reduced carotid body drive during sustained hypoxia on hypoxic depression of ventilation in humans. *J Appl Physiol* 1996; **81:** 565–72.
28. Berkenbosch A, DeGoede J. Effects of brain hypoxia on ventilation. *Eur Respir J* 1988; **1:** 184–90.
29. Haddad JS, Priestly JG. Hypoxia and respiratory control in early life. *Annu Rev Physiol* 1984; **46:** 629–43.
30. Parkins KJ, Poets CF, O'Brien LM, *et al.* Effect of exposure to 15% oxygen on breathing patterns and oxygen saturation in infants: interventional study. *Br Med J* 1998; **316:** 887–91.
31. Neubauer JA, Melton JE, Edelman NH. Modulation of respiration during brain hypoxia. *J Appl Physiol* 1990; **68:** 441–51.
32. Ward DS, Berkenbosch A, DeGoede J, Olievier CN. Dynamics of the ventilatory responses to central hypoxia in cats. *J Appl Physiol* 1990; **68:** 1107–13.
33. Kimura H, Tanaka M, Nagano K, *et al.* Possible role of the carotid body responsible for hypoxic ventilatory decline in awake humans. In: Dahan A, Teppema L, Van Beek JHGM (eds). *Physiology and Pharmacology of Cardio-Respiratory Control.* Dordrecht: Kluwer Academic, 1998: 11–18.
34. Easton PA, Anthonisen NR. Ventilatory response to sustained hypoxia after pretreatment with aminophylline. *J Appl Physiol* 1988; **64:** 1445–50.
35. Dahan A, Ward DS. Effect of i.v. midazolam on the ventilatory response to sustained hypoxia in man. *Br J Anaesth* 1991; **66:** 454–7.
36. Weil JV, Bryne-Quinn E, Sodal IE, *et al.* Hypoxic ventilatory drive in normal man. *J Clin Invest* 1970; **49:** 1061–72.
37. Temp JA, Henson LC, Ward DS. Effect of a subanesthetic minimum alveolar concentration of isoflurane on two tests of the hypoxic ventilatory response. *Anesthesiology* 1994; **80:** 739–50.
38. Dejours P, Labrousse Y, Raynaud J, Teillac A. A stimulus oxygène chemoréflexe de la ventilation à basse altitude (50 m) chez l'homme. *J Physiol* 1957; **49:** 115–20.
39. Becker HF, Polo O, McNamara SG, *et al.* Effect of different levels of hyperoxia on breathing in healthy subjects. *J Appl Physiol* 1996; **81:** 1683–90.
40. Gozal D. Potentiation of hypoxic ventilatory response by hyperoxia in the conscious rat: putative role of nitric oxide. *J Appl Physiol* 1998; **85:** 129–32.
41. Fink BR. Influence of cerebral activity in wakefulness on regulation of breathing. *J Appl Physiol* 1961; **16:** 15–20.
42. Shea SA. Behavioral and arousal-related influences on breathing in humans. *Exp Physiol* 1996; **81:** 1–26.
43. Lam AM, Clement JL, Knill RL. Surgical stimulation does not enhance ventilatory chemoreflexes during enflurane anaesthesia in man. *Can J Anaesth* 1980; **27:** 22–8.
44. Rosenberg M, Tobias R, Bourke D, Kamat V. Respiratory responses to surgical stimulation during enflurane anesthesia. *Anesthesiology* 1980; **52:** 163–5.
45. Sarton E, Dahan A, Teppema L, *et al.* Acute pain and central nervous system arousal do not restore impaired hypoxic ventilatory response during sevoflurane sedation. *Anesthesiology* 1996; **85:** 295–303.

46. Borgbjerg FM, Nielsen K, Franks J. Experimental pain stimulates respiration and attenuates morphine-induced respiratory depression: a controlled study in human volunteers. *Pain* 1996; **64:** 123–8.
47. Bourke DL. Respiratory effects of regional anesthesia during acute pain. *Reg Anesth* 1993; **18:** 361–5.
48. Casey KL. Somatosensory responses of bulboreticular units in awake cat: relation to escape-producing stimuli. *Science* 1971; **173:** 77–80.
49. Dobbins EG, Feldman JL. Brainstem network controlling descending drive to phrenic motoneurons in rat. *J Comp Neurol* 1994; **347:** 64–86.
50. Skatrud JB, Dempsey JA. Interaction of sleep state and chemical stimuli in sustaining rhythmic ventilation. *J Appl Physiol* 1983; **55:** 813–22.
51. Leevers AM, Simon PM, Dempsey JA. Apnea after normocapnic mechanical ventilation during NREM sleep. *J Appl Physiol* 1994; **77:** 2079–85.
52. Leevers AM, Simon PM, Xi L, Dempsey JA. Apnoea following normocapnic mechanical ventilation in awake mammals: a demonstration of control system inertia. *J Physiol* 1993; **472:** 749–68.
53. Nishino T, Kochi T. Effects of surgical stimulation on the apnoeic thresholds for carbon dioxide during anaesthesia with sevoflurane. *Br J Anaesth* 1994; **73:** 583–6.
54. Nieuwenhuijs D, Sarton E, Teppema L, *et al.* Propofol for monitored anesthesia care: implications on hypoxic control of cardiorespiratory responses. *Anesthesiology* 2000; **92:** 46–54.
55. Knill RL, Moote CA, Skinner MI, *et al.* Anesthesia with abdominal surgery leads to intense REM sleep during the first postoperative week. *Anesthesiology* 1990; **73:** 52–61.
56. Cronin A, Keifer JC, Baghdoyan HA, Lydic R. Opioid inhibition of rapid eye movement sleep by a specific mu receptor agonist. *Br J Anaesth* 1995; **74:** 188–92.
57. Rosenberg J, Wildschiodtz G, Pedersen MH, *et al.* Late postoperative nocturnal episodic hypoxaemia and associated sleep pattern. *Br J Anaesth* 1994; **72:** 145–50.
58. Forrest Jr WH, Bellville JW. The effect of sleep plus morphine on the respiratory response to carbon dioxide. *Anesthesiology* 1964; **25:** 137–41.
59. Ward DS, Temp JA. Neuropharmacology of the control of ventilation. In: Biebuyck J, Lynch C, Maze M, *et al.* (eds). *Anesthesia: Biologic Foundations*. Philadelphia: Lippincott-Raven, 1997: 1367–94.
60. Kirby GC, McQueen DS. Characterization of opioid receptors in the cat carotid body involved in chemosensory depression in vivo. *Br J Pharmacol* 1986; **88:** 889–98.
61. Lipp J. Possible mechanisms of morphine analgesia. *J Clin Neuropharmacol* 1991; **14:** 131–47.
62. Kagawa S, Stafford MJ, Waggener TB, Severinghaus JW. No effect of naloxone on hypoxia-induced ventilatory depression in adults. *J Appl Physiol* 1982; **52:** 1030–4.
63. US Government. *Acute Pain Management. Operative or Medical Procedures and Trauma*. Washington, DC: Public Health Service, 1992.
64. Pasternak GW. Pharmacological mechanisms of opioid analgesics. *Clin Neuropharmacol* 1993; **16:** 1–18.
65. Dripps RD, Comroe JH. Clinical studies on morphine. I. The immediate effect of morphine administered intravenously and intramuscularly upon the respiration of normal man. *Anesthesiology* 1945; **6:** 462–8.
66. Santiago TV, Johnson J, Riley DJ, Edelman NH. Effects of morphine on ventilatory response to exercise. *J Appl Physiol* 1979; **47:** 112–18.
67. Weil JV, McCullough RE, Kline JS, Sodal IE. Diminished ventilatory response to hypoxia and hypercapnia after morphine in normal man. *N Engl J Med* 1975; **292:** 1103–6.
68. Gross JB, Blouin RT, Zandsberg S, *et al.* Effect of flumazenil on ventilatory drive during sedation with midazolam and alfentanil. *Anesthesiology* 1996; **85:** 713–20.
69. Cartwright CR, Henson LC, Ward DS. Effects of alfentanil on the ventilatory response to sustained hypoxia. *Anesthesiology* 1998; **89:** 612–19.
70. Chaney MA. Side effects of intrathecal and epidural opioids. *Can J Anaesth* 1995; **42:** 891–903.
71. Camporesi EM, Nielsen CH, Bromage PR, Durant PAC. Ventilatory CO_2 sensitivity after intravenous and epidural morphine in volunteers. *Anesth Analg* 1983; **62:** 633–40.
72. Bailey PL, Rhondeau S, Schafer PG, *et al.* Dose–response pharmacology of intrathecal morphine in human volunteers. *Anesthesiology* 1993; **79:** 49–59.
73. France CJ, Plumer MH, Eger EI, Wahrenbrock EA. Ventilatory effects of isoflurane (Forane) or halothane when combined with morphine, nitrous oxide and surgery. *Br J Anaesth* 1974; **46:** 117–20.
74. Eger EI, Dolan WM, Stevens WC, *et al.* Surgical stimulation antagonizes the respiratory depression produced by Forane. *Anesthesiology* 1972; **36:** 544–9.
75. Knill RL, Gelb AW. Ventilatory responses to hypoxia and hypercapnia during halothane sedation and anesthesia in man. *Anesthesiology* 1978; **49:** 244–51.
76. Warner DO, Warner MA, Ritman EL. Human chest wall function while awake and during halothane anesthesia. I. Quiet breathing. *Anesthesiology* 1995; **82:** 6–19.
77. Warner DO, Warner MA, Ritman EL. Human chest wall function while awake and during halothane anesthesia. II. Carbon dioxide rebreathing. *Anesthesiology* 1995; **82:** 20–31.
78. Dahan A, van den Elsen M, Berkenbosch A, *et al.* Influence of a subanesthetic concentration of halothane on the ventilatory response to step changes into and out of sustained isocapnic hypoxia in healthy volunteers. *Anesthesiology* 1994; **81:** 850–9.
79. Temp JA, Henson LC, Ward DS. Does a subanesthetic concentration of isoflurane blunt the ventilatory response to hypoxia? *Anesthesiology* 1992; **77:** 1116–24.
80. Robotham JL. Do low-dose inhalational anesthetic agents alter ventilatory control? *Anesthesiology* 1994; **80:** 723–6.
81. van den Elsen MJLJ, Dahan A, Berkenbosch A, *et al.* Does subanesthetic isoflurane affect the ventilatory response to acute isocapnic hypoxia in healthy volunteers? *Anesthesiology* 1994; **81:** 860–7.
82. van den Elsen M, Dahan A, DeGoede J, *et al.* Influences of subanesthetic isoflurane on ventilatory control in humans. *Anesthesiology* 1995; **83:** 478–90.
83. Sarton E, van der Wal M, Nieuwenhuijs D, *et al.* Sevoflurane-induced reduction of hypoxic drive is sex-independent. *Anesthesiology* 1999; **90:** 1288–93.
84. Weiskopf RB, Eger EI, Daniel M, Noorani M. Cardiovascular stimulation induced by rapid increases in desflurane concentration in humans results from activation of tracheopulmonary and systemic receptors. *Anesthesiology* 1995; **83:** 1173–8.
85. Bailey PL, Andriano KPP, Goldman M, *et al.* Variability of the respiratory response to diazepam. *Anesthesiology* 1986; **64:** 460–5.
86. Gross JB, Smith L, Smith TC. Time course of ventilatory response to carbon dioxide after intravenous diazepam. *Anesthesiology* 1982; **57:** 18–21.
87. Alexander CM, Gross JB. Sedative doses of midazolam depress hypoxic ventilatory responses in humans. *Anesth Analg* 1988; **67:** 377–82.
88. Mora CT, Torjman M, White PF. Effects of diazepam and flumazenil on sedation and hypoxic ventilatory response. *Anesth Analg* 1989; **68:** 473–8.
89. Blouin RT, Conrad PF, Perreault S, Gross JB. The effect of flumazenil on midazolam-induced depression of the ventilatory response to hypoxia during isohypercarbia. *Anesthesiology* 1993; **78:** 635–41.
90. Flögel CM, Ward DS, Wada DR, Ritter JW. The effects of large-dose flumazenil on midazolam-induced ventilatory depression. *Anesth Analg* 1993; **77:** 1207–14.
91. Spens HJ, Drummond GB. Ventilatory effects of eltanolone during induction of anaesthesia: comparison with propofol and thiopentone. *Br J Anaesth* 1996; **77:** 194–9.
92. Blouin RT, Conrad PF, Gross JB. Time course of ventilatory depression following induction doses of propofol and thiopentathal. *Anesthesiology* 1991; **75:** 940–4.
93. Blouin RT, Seifert HA, Babenco D, *et al.* Propofol depresses the hypoxic ventilatory response during conscious sedation and isohypercapnia. *Anesthesiology* 1993; **79:** 1177–82.
94. Taylor MB, Grounds RM, Mulroony PD, Morgan M. Ventilatory effects of propofol during induction of anaesthesia. *Anaesthesia* 1986; **41:** 816–20.
95. Grounds RM, Maxwell DL, Taylor MB, *et al.* Acute ventilatory changes during I.V. induction of anaesthesia with thiopentone or propofol in man. *Br J Anaesth* 1987; **59:** 1098–102.
96. Gross JB, Zebrowski ME, Carel WD, *et al.* Time course of ventilatory depression after thiopental and midazolam in normal subjects and in patients with chronic obstructive pulmonary disease. *Anesthesiology* 1983; **58:** 540–4.
97. Choi SD, Spaulding BC, Gross JB, Apfelbaum JL. Comparison of the ventilatory effects of etomidate and methohexital. *Anesthesiology* 1985; **62:** 442–7.
98. Jevtovic-Todorovic V, Todorovic SM, Mennerick S, *et al.* Nitrous oxide (laughing gas) is an NMDA antagonist, neuroprotectant and neurotoxin. *Nature Med* 1998; **4:** 460–3.
99. Gillman MA. Analgesic (subanesthetic) nitrous oxide interacts with the endogenous opioid system: a review of the evidence. *Life Sci* 1986; **39:** 1209–21.
100. Winter PM, Hornbein TF, Smith G, *et al.* Hyperbaric nitrous oxide anesthesia in man: determination of anesthetic potency (MAC) and cardiorespiratory effects. Paper presented at the ASA Meeting, 1972.

101. Dahan A, Ward DS. Effects of 20% nitrous oxide on the ventilatory response to hypercapnia and sustained isocapnic hypoxia in man. *Br J Anaesth* 1994; **72:** 17–20.
102. Lockhart SH, Rampil IJ, Yasuda N, *et al.* Depression of ventilation by desflurane in humans. *Anesthesiology* 1991; **74:** 484–8.
103. Beydon L, Goldenberg L, Heyer MP, *et al.* Sleep apnea-like syndrome induced by nitrous oxide inhalation in normal men. *Respir Physiol* 1997; **108:** 215–74.
104. Northwood D, Sapsford DJ, Jones JG, *et al.* Nitrous oxide sedation causes post-hyperventilation apnoea. *Br J Anaesth* 1991; **67:** 7–12.
105. Hamza J, Ecoffey C, Gross JB. Ventilatory response to CO_2 following intravenous ketamine in children. *Anesthesiology* 1989; **70:** 422–5.
106. Bourke DL, Malit LA, Smith TC. Respiratory interactions of ketamine and morphine. *Anesthesiology* 1987; **66:** 153–6.
107. Benhamou D, Veillette Y, Narchi P, Ecoffey C. Ventilatory effects of premedication with clonidine. *Anesth Analg* 1991; **73:** 799–803.
108. Belleville JP, Ward DS, Bloor BC, Maze M. Effects of intravenous dexmedetomidine in humans. I. Sedation, ventilation and metabolic rate. *Anesthesiology* 1992; **77:** 1125–33.
109. Bailey PL, Sperry RJ, Johnson GK, *et al.* Respiratory effects of clonidine alone and combined with morphine, in humans. *Anesthesiology* 1991; **74:** 43–8.
110. Ward DS, Bellville JW. Effect of intravenous dopamine on hypercapnic ventilatory response in human. *J Appl Physiol* 1983; **55:** 1418–25.
111. Bascom DA, Clement ID, Dorrington KL, Robbins PA. Effects of dopamine and domperidome on ventilation during isocapnic hypoxia in humans. *Respir Physiol* 1991; **85:** 319–28.
112. Bailey PL, Pace NL, Ashburn MA, *et al.* Frequent hypoxemia and apnea after sedation with midazolam and fentanyl. *Anesthesiology* 1990; **73:** 826–30.
113. Olson LG, Hensley MJ, Saunders NA. The effects of combined morphine and prochlorperazine on ventilatory control in humans. *Am Rev Respir Dis* 1986; **133:** 558–61.
114. Pavlin DJ, Coda B, Shen DD, *et al.* Effects of combining propofol and alfentanil on ventilation, analgesia, sedation and emesis in human volunteers. *Anesthesiology* 1996; **84:** 23–37.
115. Mathew OP, Sant'Ambrogio G. Respiratory function of the upper airway. In: Lenfant C (ed.). *Lung Biology in Health and Disease*. Vol. 35. New York: Marcel Dekker, 1988.
116. Mathru M, Esch O, Lang J, *et al.* Magnetic resonance imaging of the upper airway. *Anesthesiology* 1996; **84:** 273–9.
117. Nandi PR, Charlesworth CH, Taylor SJ, *et al.* Effects of general anaesthesia on the pharynx. *Br J Anaesth* 1991; **66:** 157–62.
118. Hudgel DW. Mechanisms of obstructive sleep apnea. *Chest* 1992; **101:** 541–9.
119. Hines R, Barash PG, Watrous G, O'Connor T. Complications occurring in the postanesthesia care unit: a survey. *Anesth Analg* 1992; **74:** 503–9.
120. Catley DM, Thorton M, Jordan C, *et al.* Pronounced, episodic oxygen desaturation in the postoperative period: its association with ventilatory pattern and analgesic regimen. *Anesthesiology* 1985; **63:** 20–8.
121. Young T, Paeta M, Dempsey J, *et al.* The occurrence of sleep-disordered breathing among middle-aged adults. *N Engl J Med* 1993; **328:** 1230–73.
122. Parish JM, Shepard JW. Cardiovascular effects of sleep disorders. *Chest* 1990; **97:** 1220–6.
123. Boushra NN. Anaesthetic management of patients with sleep apnoea syndrome. *Can J Anaesth* 1996; **43:** 599–616.
124. Rosenberg J, Kehlet H. Postoperative episodic oxygen desaturation in the sleep apnoea syndrome. *Acta Anaesthesiol Scand* 1991; **35:** 368–9.
125. Ostermeier AM, Roizen MF, Hautkappe M, *et al.* Three sudden postoperative respiratory arrests associated with epidural opioids in patients with sleep apnea. *Anesth Analg* 1997; **85:** 452–60.
126. Lu JK, Schafer PG, Gardner TL, *et al.* The dose–response pharmacology of intrathecal sufentanil in female volunteers. *Anesth Analg* 1997; **85:** 372–9.
127. Eisele J, Trenchard D, Burki N, Guz A. The effect of chest wall block on respiratory sensation and control in man. *Clin Sci* 1968; **35:** 23–33.
128. Steinbrook RA, Concepcion M, Topulos GP. Ventilatory responses to hypercapnia during bupivacaine spinal anesthesia. *Anesth Analg* 1988; **67:** 247–52.
129. Gross JB, Caldwell CB, Shaw LM, Laucks SO. The effect of lidocaine on the ventilatory response to carbon dioxide. *Anesthesiology* 1983; **59:** 521–5.
130. Gross JB, Caldwell CB, Shaw LM, Apfelbaum JL. The effect of lidocaine infusion on the ventilatory response to hypoxia. *Anesthesiology* 1984; **61:** 662–5.
131. Labaille T, Clergue F, Samii K, *et al.* Ventilatory response to CO_2 following intravenous and epidural lidocaine. *Anesthesiology* 1985; **63:** 179–83.
132. Pavlin EG, Holle RH, Schoene RB. Recovery of airway protection compared with ventilation in humans after paralysis with curare. *Anesthesiology* 1989; **70:** 381–5.
133. Eriksson LI, Sato M, Severinghaus JW. Effect of a vecuronium-induced partial neuromuscular block on hypoxic ventilatory response. *Anesthesiology* 1993; **78:** 693–9.
134. Takasaki Y, Orr D, Popkin J, *et al.* Effect of hypercapnia and hypoxia on respiratory muscle activation in humans. *J Appl Physiol* 1989; **67:** 1776–84.
135. Erikson LI, Sundman E, Olsson R, *et al.* Functional assessment of the pharynx at rest and during swallowing in partially paralyzed humans. *Anesthesiology* 1997; **87:** 1035–43.
136. D'Honneur G, Lofaso F, Drummond GB, *et al.* Susceptibility to upper airway obstruction during partial neuromuscular block. *Anesthesiology* 1998; **88:** 371–8.
137. Rowlingson JC. Just when we thought we understood patient-controlled analgesia. *Anesth Analg* 1999; **89:** 3–6.
138. Stone JG, Cozine KA, Wald A. Nocturnal oxygenation during patient-controlled analgesia. *Reg Anesth* 1999; **89:** 104–10.
139. Lam AM, Knill C, Knill RL. Surgical stimulation does not enhance ventilatory chemoreflexes during enflurane anaesthesia in man. *Can J Anaesth* 1980; **27:** 22–8.

7

Cardiac physiology and pathophysiology

WOLFGANG G TOLLER, PAUL S PAGEL, JUDY R KERSTEN, AND DAVID C WARLTIER

A thorough knowledge of cardiac physiology and pathophysiology is essential for the clinical anesthesiologist. This chapter will summarize the structure and function of the heart and describe several of the major pathologic conditions that affect it.

STRUCTURE OF THE CARDIAC CELL

Left ventricular (LV) myocardium is composed of individual cardiac myocytes arranged in a functional syncytium. The myocytes are connected longitudinally in both end-to-end and end-to-side configurations. The typical cardiac muscle cell is electrically and mechanically connected to approximately seven other myocytes.[1] The direction of this interconnecting network of muscle cells is dependent on the depth within the LV wall, and there is a general orientation of myocytes at any given depth. Collagen fibers surround these cells and form an interstitial architectural framework. A rich coronary vascular network supplies approximately one capillary per muscle cell to facilitate rapid exchange of oxygen (O_2), carbon dioxide (CO_2), and metabolic substrates.

Sarcolemma

Each myocyte is separated from the extracellular space by a plasma membrane known as the sarcolemma. The sarcolemma not only forms the cardiac cell membrane but also invaginates into the myoplasm to form a system of transverse (T) tubules (Fig. 7.1). The T-tubules greatly increase the surface area between the intra- and extracellular environments. Adjacent myocardial cells are connected end to end by a thickened portion of the sarcolemma, termed an intercalated disk, that allows electrical, chemical, and physical communication between individual cells. The hydrophobic phospholipid bilayer composing the sarcolemma is essentially impermeable to charged molecules. Formation and maintenance of a membrane potential and generation of action potentials are primarily achieved through embedded membrane proteins. These proteins function as ion channels, ion pumps (e.g. Na^+,K^+-ATPase), ion exchangers (e.g. Na^+/Ca^{2+} and Na^+/H^+), and regulatory structures or signaling receptors.

Contractile apparatus

The sarcomere represents the basic functional unit of the contractile apparatus. The sarcomere contains thick filaments composed of myosin, thin filaments containing actin, and the regulatory proteins troponin (composed of C, I, and T subunits) and tropomyosin (Fig. 7.2). Individual sarcomeres are joined end to end to form myofibrils. Multiple myocytes are arranged longitudinally to form a myofiber with interconnections to other cardiac muscle cells to form a functional syncytium. Interaction between actin and myosin filaments produces muscle contraction after electrical activation. Contraction of cardiac muscle cells depends on changes in the structure of the myofilaments. Individual actin and myosin molecules do not actually shorten in length, but are arranged so that actin filaments slide along adjacent myosin filaments. This process requires adenosine triphosphate (ATP).

Sarcoplasmic reticulum

The sarcoplasmic reticulum (SR) is a dense intracellular membranous network that consists of a phospholipid bilayer with intrinsic membrane proteins. The SR contains two major regions (Fig. 7.1): (1) the sarcotubular network that surrounds the contractile protein bundles and (2) the subsarcolemmal cisternae that come in close contact with the sarcolemma and the T-tubules. The SR plays a key role in excitation–contraction coupling because this structure is involved in the regulation of intracellular Ca^{2+} during systole and diastole. The SR contains a high concentration of calsequestrin, a protein that reversibly binds Ca^{2+}. The Ca^{2+} stored within the SR lumen during cardiac muscle relaxation is released into the myoplasm through a specialized Ca^{2+} release channel ("ryanodine sensitive") that is activated by Ca^{2+} influx through voltage-dependent Ca^{2+} channels in the sarcolemma immediately after membrane depolarization. Diastolic SR uptake of Ca^{2+} from the myoplasm is energy dependent and requires an ATP-dependent Ca^{2+} pump (Ca^{2+}-ATPase) that is closely regulated by the protein phospholamban. Phosphorylation of phospholamban enhances SR Ca^{2+} uptake and increases the rate of myocardial relaxation.[2]

Mitochondria

Myocardial mitochondria occupy 30–40% of the total myocyte volume and are organized in rows between the myofilaments near the T-tubules. This location optimizes access to O_2 and metabolic substrates from the extracellular space while simultaneously providing an immediate supply of ATP to the myofilaments. Myocytes contain a large number of mitochondria because of the continuous high rate of energy consumption. Mitochondria also regulate intracellular Ca^{2+} concentration by a Ca^{2+}/H^+ exchanger that exploits a proton gradient across the inner and

Figure 7.1 *Ultrastructure of the cardiac cell demonstrating invaginations of the sarcolemma (T-tubules), numerous mitochondria, and network of sarcoplasmic reticulum with a sarcotubular network that surrounds the contractile protein bundles. Contractile proteins are arranged in a regular array of thick and thin filaments. The Z-line connects adjacent sarcomeres. The I-band extends from the Z-line toward the center of the sarcomere and delineates the region of the sarcomere occupied primarily by thin filaments. The A-band represents the region of the sarcomere occupied by the thick filaments into which thin filaments extend from either side. Reproduced with permission.*

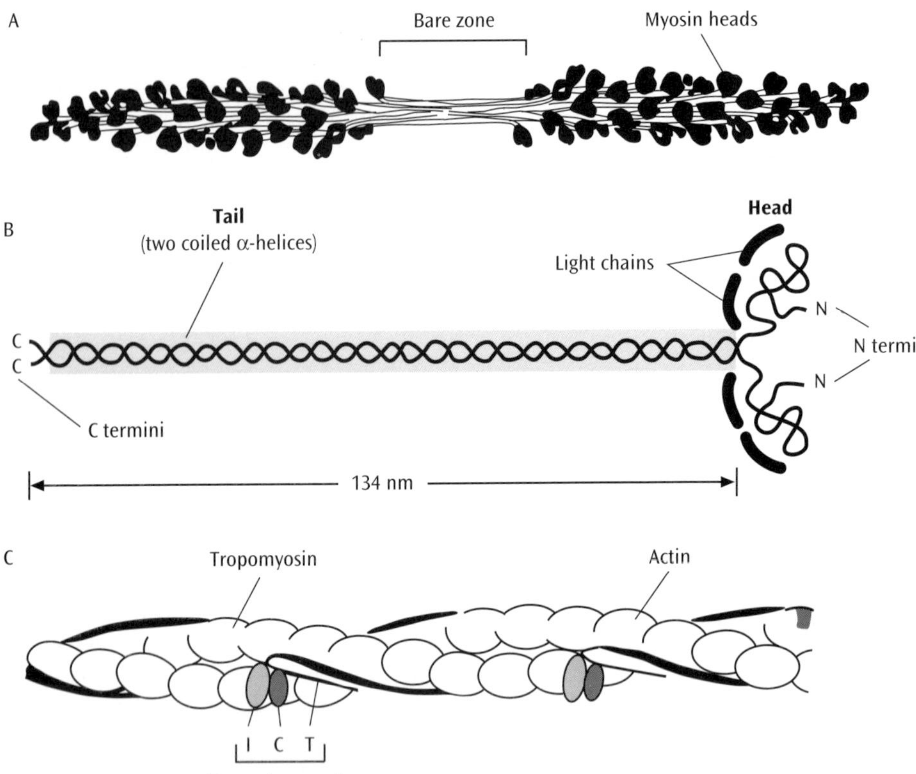

Figure 7.2 *Schematic diagram of a myosin filament (A) from skeletal muscle, a myosin molecule showing two heavy chains and four light chains (B), and an actin filament showing the position of tropomyosin and the troponin complex along the actin filament (C). Reproduced with permission.*

outer membranes. This Ca^{2+}/H^+ exchanger helps to maintain normal intracellular Ca^{2+} concentrations in pathologic conditions associated with intracellular Ca^{2+} overload (e.g. acute myocardial ischemia).

Nucleus

Cardiac myocytes usually contain a single nucleus, although binucleate and multinucleate cells are also occasionally found. Nuclei are located near the center of the cell. Almost all of the genetic information required for each myocyte to maintain and repair its structure is contained within the nucleus.

ELECTRICAL ACTIVITY OF THE CARDIAC CELL

Resting membrane potential

Myocytes from different regions of the heart have unique electrical characteristics that establish resting membrane potential, automaticity, and signal conduction. The resting membrane potential is primarily determined by the electrochemical gradient for K^+ across the sarcolemma and is maintained by a sarcolemmal Na^+,K^+-ATPase that concentrates K^+ within the myocyte. Two opposing forces are involved in the movement of K^+ across the sarcolemma (Fig. 7.3). A chemical force

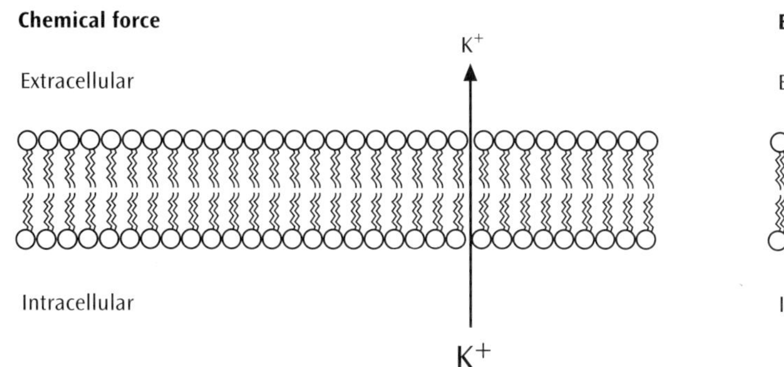

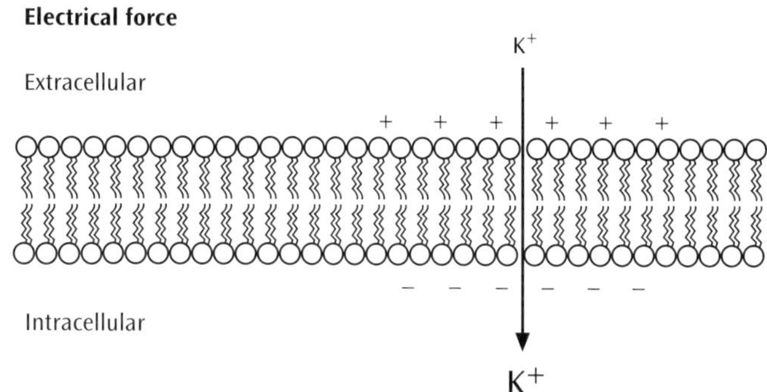

Figure 7.3 *The resting membrane potential is based primarily on the K^+ equilibrium potential. A concentration gradient drives K^+ out of the cell (chemical force). Because the sarcolemma is impermeable to large protein anions, an electrical force is created that resists further outward diffusion of K^+. The balance of these chemical and electrical forces determines the K^+ equilibrium potential.*

based on the K^+ concentration gradient results in outward diffusion of K^+. Outward movement of K^+ down its concentration gradient cannot be balanced by simultaneous outward diffusion of large negatively charged protein anions or organic phosphates because the sarcolemma is impermeable to these species. Consequently, the myoplasm becomes more negatively charged, an action that tends to reverse movement of K^+ down its concentration gradient. Thus, when K^+ diffuses out of a cell, this creates an electrical potential across the membrane that tends to retard subsequent extracellular diffusion of this ion. The membrane potential at which the electrical forces maintaining intracellular K^+ concentration balance the chemical forces resulting in outward diffusion of K^+ is termed the equilibrium (Donnan) potential and may be calculated using the modified Nernst equation: $E_m = -61.5 \log K_i/K_o$, where E_m is the electrical potential, and K_i and K_o are the internal and external K^+ concentrations respectively. The calculated equilibrium potential for K^+ is −95 mV when K_i and K_o equal 140 and 4 mM respectively. In contrast to ventricular myocytes, atrial cells have a more positive resting potential, whereas nodal cells have no defined resting potential.

Action potential

The phases of the cardiac action potential (Fig. 7.4) are associated with changes in Na^+, K^+, and Ca^{2+} ion permeabilities of the sarcolemma. Sodium and Ca^{2+} channels are closed and K^+ channels are open during diastole. Sarcolemmal depolarization occurs at a threshold potential of −65 mV and triggers a sequence of events that follow an all-or-none response. Each depolarization causes a very small amount of the extracellular Na^+ to be exchanged for intracellular K^+. Initiation of a propagated depolarization wave requires a threshold stimulus, whereas an insufficient depolarization stimulus renders the sarcolemma refractory to a subsequent depolarization until the resting potential has been restored by ion pumps and exchangers within the membrane.

Phase 0 (rapid upstroke)

Membrane depolarization causes a rapid inward Na^+ current. An increase in permeability of the sarcolemmal Na^+ channels and a rapid influx of extracellular Na^+ at a threshold potential (−65 mV) displaces the membrane potential toward the Na^+ equilibrium potential (+50 mV), whereas K^+ permeability simultaneously declines. In contrast to atrial and ventricular myocytes, nodal cells lack functional Na^+ channels and depolarization depends on a slower increase of Ca^{2+} channel permeability. Na^+ channels remain refractory to subsequent stimulation until their resting conformation has been re-established. Inactivation of Na^+ channel permeability represents the end of phase 0.

Phase 1 (early repolarization)

Rapid decreases in Na^+ channel permeability and simultaneous transient increases in outward K^+ and Cl^- currents produce early repolarization. Depression of these outward K^+ and Cl^- fluxes during early repolarization has been linked to arrhythmogenic prolongation of the action potential in areas of myocardium immediately adjacent to infarction.[3]

Phase 2 (plateau)

After the rapid membrane voltage changes associated with phase 0 and phase 1, membrane potential remains approximately 0 mV for a relatively prolonged duration. A balance between slow inward Ca^{2+} and outward K^+ currents mediates the plateau phase of the action potential. Membrane conductance to all ions is also relatively low during this phase.

Phase 3 (repolarization)

Inactivation of Ca^{2+} channels and a simultaneous increase in outward K^+ current through K^+ channels produces a net outward movement of positive charge and repolarization of the sarcolemmal membrane.

Phase 4 (resting membrane potential or diastolic depolarization)

During this final phase of action potential, the membrane potential of ventricular myocytes remains at the resting membrane potential (Fig. 7.4A) until the cell is stimulated again. In contrast, sinus and atrioventricular node cells slowly gain positive charge during phase 4 (Fig. 7.4B). This time-dependent diastolic depolarization gradually raises the membrane potential from the maximum diastolic potential to the threshold and accounts for spontaneous depolarization observed in atrial and nodal cardiocytes.

Conduction of action potentials

Precise, synchronous coordination of cardiac muscle contraction is required for efficient mechanical action of the heart. Contraction of each myocyte is triggered when an action potential sweeps over the sarcolemmal membrane. Active depolarization in one region of the sarcolemma produces local ion currents and passively depolarizes adjacent areas to the voltage threshold, subsequently propagating the depolarization stimulus. Propagation of action potentials between myocytes is achieved through gap junctions that are less resistant to transmission of electrical current. Thus, the number of gap junctions between adjacent myocytes is a major determinant of conduction veloc-

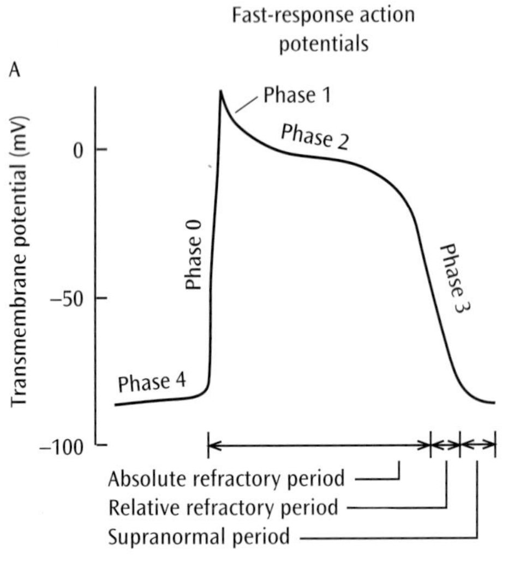

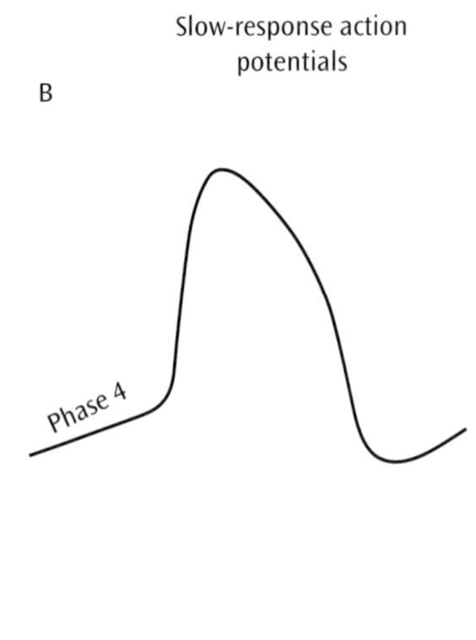

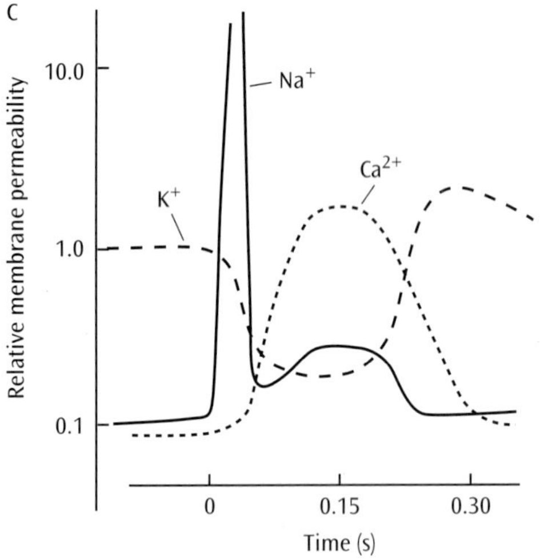

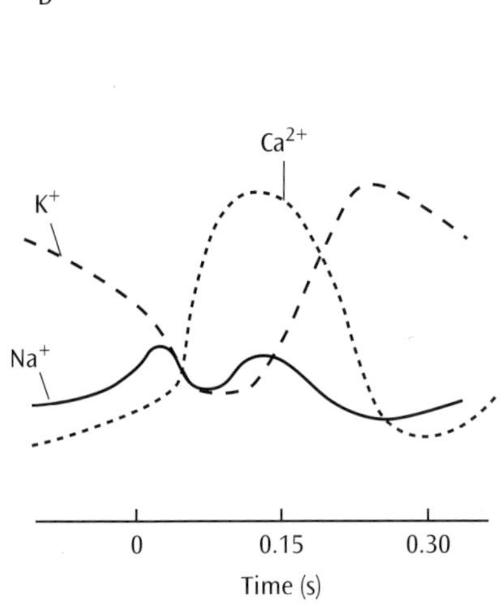

Figure 7.4 *Time-course of the action potential in working myocytes (A) and in cells with pacemaker activity (B). Note the spontaneous diastolic depolarization (phase 4) and the lack of the plateau (phase 2) in cardiac pacemaker cells. The corresponding ionic flows are shown in C and D. Reproduced with permission.*

ity in cardiac muscle. Permeability of myocardial gap junctions has been shown to be dependent on ATP[4] and cyclic adenosine monophosphate (cAMP)-dependent protein kinases.[5] Alterations in gap junction permeability may be partially responsible for demarcation of viable from necrotic tissue after myocardial infarction and contribute to conduction abnormalities leading to malignant ventricular arrhythmias under these conditions.[6]

MECHANICAL ACTIVITY OF THE CARDIAC CELL

Excitation–contraction coupling

The sequence of intracellular events that begins when an action potential depolarizes the sarcolemmal membrane and ends with myofilament contraction is classically defined as excitation–contraction coupling. Recent evidence also suggests that myocardial relaxation may play an important role in excitation–contraction coupling. The most important ionic event during cardiac muscle contraction is the rise in myoplasmic Ca^{2+} mediated by the SR after sarcolemmal depolarization. This event, known as Ca^{2+}-induced Ca^{2+} release, is triggered by highly localized entry of Ca^{2+} through voltage-dependent sarcolemmal Ca^{2+} channels (L-type). The amount of Ca^{2+} that enters the myocyte through voltage-dependent Ca^{2+} channels during sarcolemmal depolarization is very small when compared with that released by the SR, but this Ca^{2+} also contributes to contractile activation. During systole, Ca^{2+} binds to the troponin C subunit and causes a conformational change in the troponin–tropomyosin regulatory complex that allows the actin and myosin filaments to interact. Calcium also interacts with the myofibrils and causes the formation of cross-bridges between actin and myosin. In the presence of ATP, these contractile proteins are propelled against each other by a ratchet-like mechanism to shorten each sarcomere. The degree of myocardial contraction is determined by the rate and extent of Ca^{2+} release into the myoplasm from voltage-dependent Ca^{2+} channels and the SR.

Relaxation of cardiac muscle is primarily mediated by the rate and extent of dissociation of Ca^{2+} from the contractile apparatus and the activity of a specific Ca^{2+}-ATPase in the SR membrane that resequesters Ca^{2+} from the myoplasm into the SR lumen. This Ca^{2+}-ATPase is regulated by the membrane protein phospholamban. Activation of phospholamban by protein kinase A or Ca^{2+}/calmodulin-dependent kinase enhances the activity of the Ca^{2+}-ATPase. Abnormal activity of the Ca^{2+}-ATPase or phospholamban contributes to delays in myocardial relaxation and may produce LV diastolic dysfunction.

Alterations in plasma K^+ and Ca^{2+} concentrations may have profound effects on excitation–contraction coupling. Although a reduction in plasma K^+ has little effect on myocardial contractility, large increases in K^+ (>7 mequiv L^{-1}) can produce sustained sarcolemmal depolarization resulting in cardiac arrest. Decreased plasma Ca^{2+} concentrations cause diminished contractile force. Conversely, increases in extracellular Ca^{2+}

produce small increases in contractility but may also result in cardiac arrest at very high concentrations because the SR Ca^{2+}-ATPase is overwhelmed and myocardial relaxation cannot occur (e.g. Ca^{2+} paradox).

Mechanics of cardiac muscle *in vitro*

Studies of isolated papillary muscles (Fig. 7.5) have provided important insight about the functional characteristics of the intact heart.[7] In this experimental setting, loading conditions and stimulation frequency of cardiac muscle can be rigidly controlled and precisely altered, allowing not only for specific assessment of functional consequences of changes in these parameters but also for strict definition of intrinsic myocardial contractility. Several variables are used to characterize myocardial contractile function *in vitro*, including the magnitude and rate of development (+d*F*/d*t*) of exerted force (tension), the velocity and extent of muscle shortening, and the time-course of occurrence of these events after electrical activation.[8] Analysis of the responsiveness of isolated myocardium to four major physiologic determinants establishes the basis for an understanding of the intact heart as a muscular pump. These inherent characteristics of cardiac muscle include the effects of variable stretch prior to the onset of contraction (preload), the responsiveness of cardiac muscle to increased load imposed after contraction has begun (afterload), the effects of acute changes in stimulation rate on myocardial function, and, finally, the intrinsic strength of the contractile apparatus independent of preload, afterload, and heart rate, a property termed myocardial contractility.

Preload is defined as the initial stretch of the myocardium before contraction. The tension developed by isolated contracting myocardium is greater if the muscle has been previously stretched.[8] Preload-dependent increases in developed tension can also be demonstrated at the ultrastructural level.[9,10] Increases in the length of a single sarcomere elicit increases in tension until the sarcomere becomes overstretched. This phenomenon was initially attributed to geometrically improved actin–myosin overlap.[9] However, length-dependent enhanced tension development in isolated cardiac muscle probably results from an increased affinity of troponin C for activator Ca^{2+} at greater sarcomere lengths, resulting in enhanced contractility.[11,12]

The influence of afterload on cardiac muscle mechanics *in vitro* can be studied using a small modification[8] of the isolated papillary muscle preparation. A desired starting muscle length is obtained by the addition of preload. A stop, positioned on the lever–fulcrum system connecting the papillary muscle to the preload, prevents further stretching of the muscle prior to contraction. Additional weight is then added to the preload, but the stop prevents further stretch of the muscle. This additional weight will not influence the muscle until after contraction has begun. At constant preload, an increase in afterload results in declines in the degree of shortening, the velocity of shortening, and the total time of contraction. Velocity of shortening varies inversely with applied afterload, creating a "force–velocity" curve (Fig. 7.6). The velocity of shortening at zero afterload [maximum velocity of shortening (V_{max})] and the intercept of the force–velocity curve at maximal force during isometric contraction (P_0) can be extrapolated from the force–velocity relation.[7] V_{max} is related to the turnover rate of actin–myosin cross-bridges,[13] a function of actin–myosin ATPase activity.[14] The value of P_0 is proportional to the total number of cross-bridges[13] and is also directly related to the affinity of the contractile complex for Ca^{2+}.[11,12]

Myocardial contractility (inotropic state) is defined as the inherent strength of the contractile apparatus independent of stimulation (heart) rate and loading conditions. In the isolated papillary muscle, contractility can be precisely characterized because preload and afterload can be rigidly controlled. Under these conditions, increases in peak developed tension and velocity of muscle shortening indicate enhanced inotropic state.[7] For example, administration of norepinephrine (noradrenaline) to the isolated papillary muscle shifts the velocity of the shortening–afterload curve upwards and to the right, resulting in increased velocity of shortening at any given afterload. In contrast, myocardial depressants such as volatile anesthetics shift the force–velocity curve to the left.

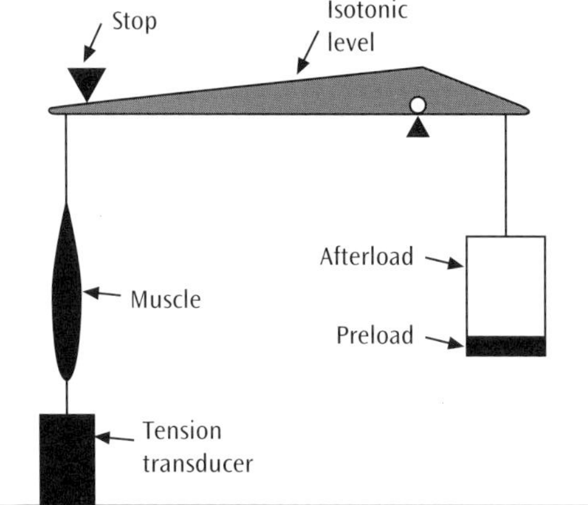

Figure 7.5 *Schematic illustration of the isolated papillary muscle preparation. The muscle is attached at the lower end via a tension transducer whereas the upper end is attached to a lever system that is allowed to move. A small weight, termed "preload," is placed at the distal end of the lever. Preload stretches the muscle to a length consistent with its resting length–tension relation. A stop is then positioned above the tip of the lever. Additional weight is then added to the preload but the stop prevents further stretch on the muscle. This additional weight will not influence the muscle until contraction has begun ("after" load). The papillary muscle is suspended in a tissue bath and stimulated by electrodes placed longitudinally against the muscle (removed for clarity). Reproduced with permission.*

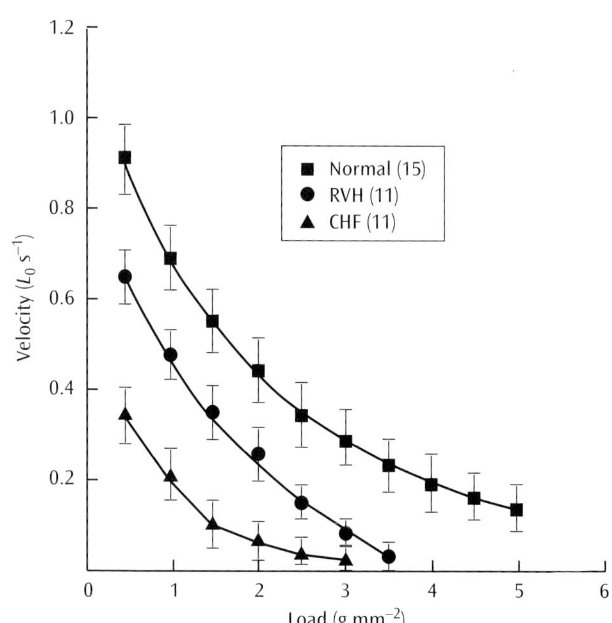

Figure 7.6 *Force–velocity relations in normal cat papillary muscle (squares), right ventricular hypertrophy (RVH) (circles), and congestive heart failure (CHF) (triangles). Reproduced with permission.*

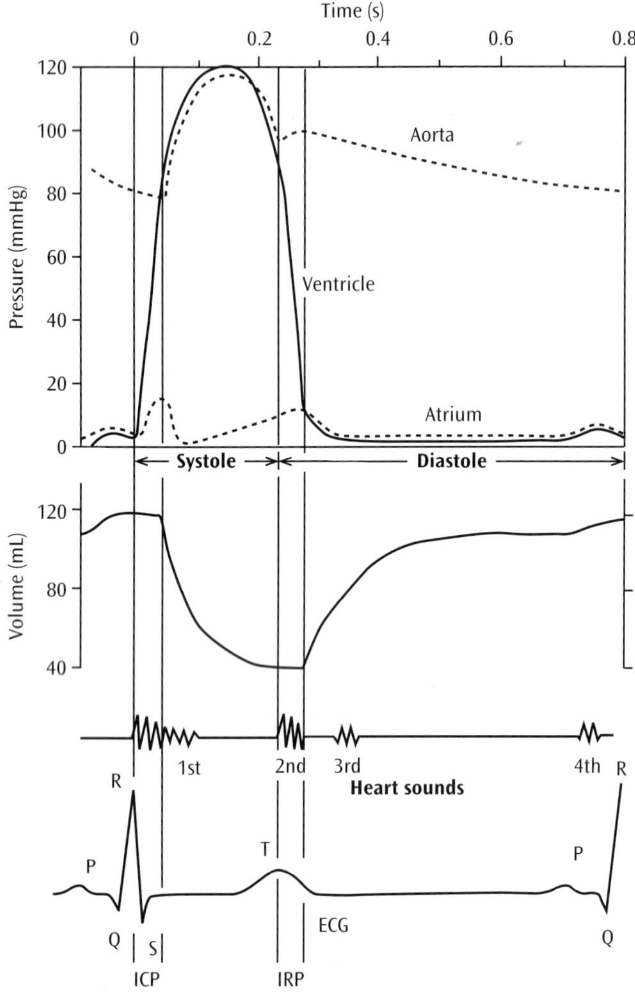

Figure 7.7 *The cardiac cycle. Left ventricular pressure, aortic pressure, and left atrial pressure are correlated with ventricular volume, heart sounds, venous pulse, and the electrocardiogram. Reproduced with permission.*

THE CARDIAC CYCLE

The LV cardiac cycle is a complex combination of electrical, mechanical, and valvular events (Fig. 7.7). LV systole begins with the initial rise of LV pressure and closure of the mitral valve (isovolumic contraction) after LV depolarization. When LV pressure exceeds aortic pressure, the aortic valve opens and ejection occurs. Equilibration of LV and aortic pressures at end-systole produce closure of the aortic valve and, subsequently, LV pressure falls (isovolumic relaxation). When LV pressure falls below left atrial (LA) pressure, the mitral valve opens and LV filling occurs. Systole and diastole compose approximately one- and two-thirds of the cardiac cycle, respectively, during sinus rhythm. Substantial reductions in the duration of diastole occur at higher heart rates that affect LV filling and coronary perfusion.

Left atrial pressure waveform

The LA pressure waveform consists of three major deflections. After the electrocardiographic P-wave of atrial depolarization, the left atrium contracts, causing the "a" wave in late diastole. LV isovolumic contraction causes a retrograde pressure wave to be transmitted to the left atrium, resulting in the "c" wave. LA filling occurs during systole and continues into early diastole before LA pressure exceeds LV pressure. There is a slow increase in LA pressure that accounts for the "v" wave of the LA pressure waveform because the mitral valve remains closed. LA systole is responsible for approximately 15–20% of total LV filling under normal conditions. However, the contribution of the LA to LV filling may be greater in disease states characterized by reduced LV compliance (e.g. myocardial ischemia, pressure overload hypertrophy).

Left ventricular pressure waveform

Isovolumic contraction occurs between closure of the mitral valve and opening of the aortic valve, during which time LV volume remains constant. The upstroke of the LV pressure waveform reaches a maximum during isovolumic contraction and is often used to estimate myocardial contractility (LV $+dP/dt_{max}$). After LV pressure exceeds aortic pressure, the aortic valve opens and rapid ejection of blood from the left ventricle into the aorta occurs. Approximately two-thirds of the total LV stroke volume empties into the aorta during the period of rapid ejection. Ejection slows in late systole and ceases when the aortic valve closes (end-systole). Thus, reductions in LV volume are greatest during the first third of ejection and decrease in an exponential fashion until end-systole. Normal LV end-diastolic and end-systolic volumes (EDV and ESV respectively) are 120 and 40 mL respectively. Thus, stroke volume (EDV – ESV) is 80 mL and ejection fraction $[(EDV - ESV) \times 100 \times EDV^{-1}]$ is 67%.[15] Diastole is composed of four major components. After aortic valve closure, a rapid fall in LV pressure occurs at constant LV volume (isovolumic relaxation). When LV pressure falls below LA pressure, the mitral valve opens and rapid LV filling begins. Rapid LV filling contributes approximately 75% of LV stroke volume under normal conditions. Rapid LV filling is followed by a slower filling phase (diastasis) that is primarily determined by pulmonary venous return. The final phase of diastole is atrial systole.[16]

LEFT VENTRICULAR PRESSURE–VOLUME RELATIONS

The pressure–volume diagram

Simultaneous measurement of time-dependent LV pressure and volume waveforms in Cartesian coordinates results in the creation of an LV pressure–volume diagram. This diagram may be used to illustrate various phases of the cardiac cycle and determine several indices of LV systolic and diastolic function. Initially described by Frank,[17] the changes in LV pressure with respect to volume occur in a counterclockwise fashion over time. The cardiac cycle begins at end-diastole (Fig. 7.8, point A). The time period between mitral valve closure and aortic valve opening is the first phase of the LV pressure–volume diagram. This abrupt increase in LV pressure with little change in LV volume describes isovolumic contraction. The aortic valve opens and systolic ejection begins when pressure within the left ventricle exceeds that in the aorta (Fig. 7.8, point B). LV volume rapidly declines as blood is ejected into the aorta. The aortic valve closes at end ejection when LV pressure declines below aortic pressure (Fig. 7.8, point C). A rapid decrease in LV pressure with little change in volume (isovolumic relaxation) then occurs. Isovolumic relaxation ends with the opening of the mitral valve as LV pressure falls below LA pressure (Fig. 7.8, point D). The LV pressure–volume diagram is completed as large increases in LV volume occur with minimal increases in LV pressure during rapid LV filling, diastasis, and atrial systole.

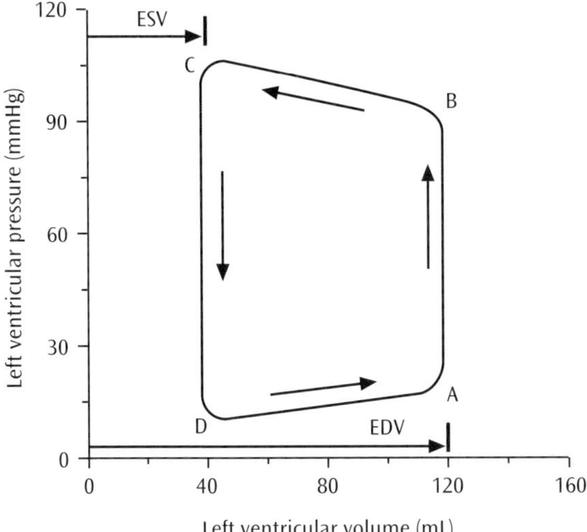

Figure 7.8 *Schematic left ventricular pressure–volume diagram. The cardiac cycle proceeds in a counterclockwise direction (arrows). A, end-diastole; B, aortic valve opening; C, aortic valve closure; D, mitral valve opening. Segments AB, BC, CD, and DA represent isovolumic contraction, ejection, isovolumic relaxation, and diastolic filling respectively. End-diastolic volume (EDV) and end-systolic volume (ESV) can be identified as the lower right (A) and upper left (C) corners of the diagram, allowing rapid calculation of stroke volume and ejection fraction. The area of the loop defines stroke work. Reproduced with permission.*

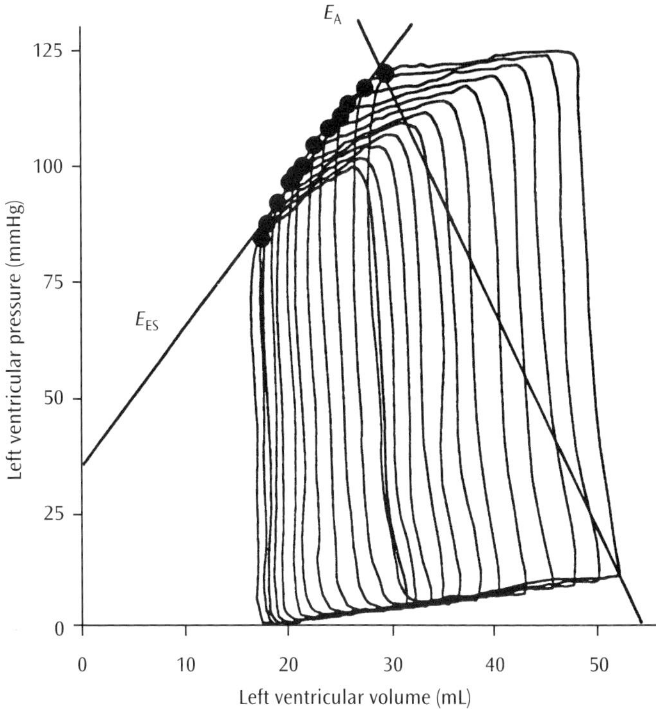

Figure 7.9 *Left ventricular (LV) pressure–volume diagrams during inferior vena caval occlusion in a dog. The LV maximal elastances of each pressure–volume diagram are used to calculate the slope (E_{es}) of the end-systolic pressure–volume relation, a relatively load-independent index of myocardial contractility* in vivo. *Effective arterial elastance (E_a) is determined as the ratio of end-systolic arterial pressure and stroke volume during steady-state hemodynamic conditions. In the pressure–volume plane, E_a represents the magnitude of the slope connecting end-systole to end-diastole. The ratio of E_{es} to E_a defines LV–arterial coupling. Reproduced with permission.*

Interpretation of LV pressure–volume diagrams

Analysis of LV pressure–volume diagrams offers several advantages over simple time plots of pressure and volume waveforms.[18] Determination of EDV and ESV can be identified as the lower right (Fig. 7.8, point A) and upper left (Fig. 7.8, point C) corners of the diagram and allow simple calculation of stroke volume and ejection fraction. The area within the diagram defines LV stroke work (kinetic energy) for each cardiac cycle. A series of LV pressure–volume diagrams of consecutive cardiac cycles can be obtained during transient mechanical or pharmacological alterations in preload or afterload (Fig. 7.9). This nested set of diagrams can be used to estimate the contractile state of the left ventricle. Sagawa *et al.*[19] described the end-systolic pressure–volume relation (ESPVR) as a linear relation whose slope was shown to be directly related to inotropic state. A set of LV pressure–volume diagrams also yields a linear Frank–Starling analog termed "preload recruitable stroke work" (PRSW)[20] that relates stroke work of each cardiac cycle to the corresponding end-diastolic volume (Fig. 7.10). PRSW also provides useful information about the contractile state of the heart *in vivo*.[21] The end-diastolic pressure–volume relation (EDPVR) may also be determined from a series of diagrams, providing an estimate of diastolic LV compliance. Incomplete isovolumic relaxation resulting from acute myocardial ischemia shifts the EDPVR upward consistent with reduced LV compliance.

LV pressure–volume diagrams have been constructed in humans in the cardiac catheterization laboratory and during cardiac surgery using an impedance catheter positioned within the left ventricle to measure continuous LV volume. For example, Kass and coworkers[22] have obtained sets of LV pressure–volume diagrams and examined the influence of percutaneous transluminal coronary artery angioplasty (PTCA) on LV function in patients with coronary artery disease. Coronary occlusion during PTCA decreased the slope of the ESPVR, effects that were rapidly reversible upon reperfusion. The authors[22] suggested that monitoring LV pressure–volume diagrams may be used clinically to assess adequacy of PTCA in this patient population.

LEFT VENTRICULAR SYSTOLIC FUNCTION

The primary functions of the left ventricle are to propel blood into the high-pressure arterial vasculature during systole and to collect blood from the low-pressure venous circulation during diastole. Systolic function describes LV mechanical performance between the onset of isovolumic contraction and end ejection. The amount of blood ejected by the left ventricle into the aorta during each cardiac cycle is the stroke volume and is determined by four major factors: preload, afterload, myocardial contractility, and heart rate.

Preload

In the intact left ventricle, preload is defined as the volume of blood contained in the LV cavity at end-diastole (EDV). This volume establishes the passive stretch on each LV myofibril immediately before isovolumic contraction. This definition in the intact heart accurately reflects the concept of preload in isolated cardiac muscle, but measurement of continuous LV volume and EDV during the cardiac cycle is difficult. LV

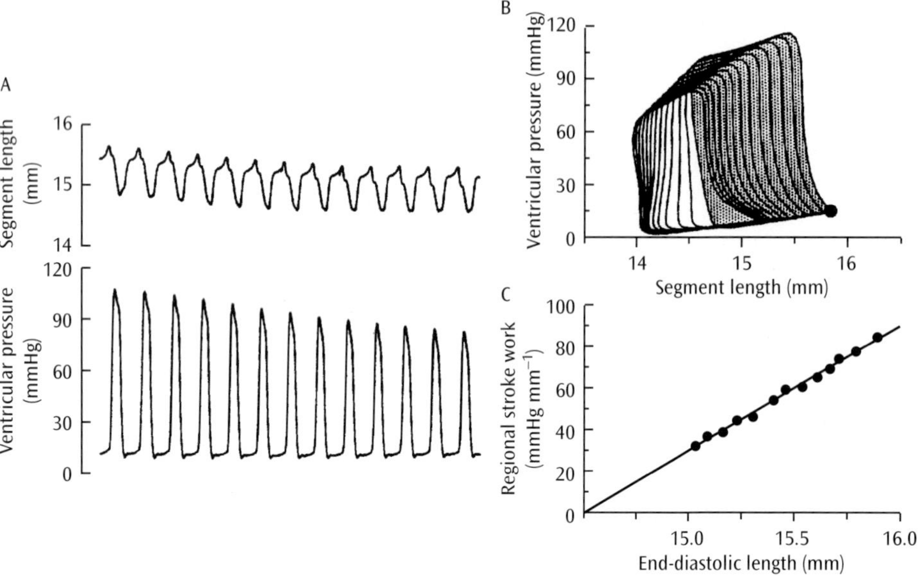

Figure 7.10 *Continuous left ventricular (LV) pressure and segment length waveforms (A) and resultant pressure–length diagrams (B) in a chronically instrumented dog. Pressure–length diagrams were generated by abrupt occlusion of the inferior vena cava, resulting in decreases in LV pressure for 13 consecutive cardiac cycles. The area of each diagram (shaded area), corresponding to regional stroke work, was plotted against the corresponding end-diastolic segment length (solid circle) for each loop (B). A linear regression analysis was then used to define the relation between regional stroke work and end-diastolic length (C, preload recruitable stroke work). Reproduced with permission.*

volume may be assessed using three-dimensional arrays of implanted sonomicrometry crystals or a conductance catheter placed within the LV chamber in experimental animals; however, these techniques have limited applicability in humans. Continuous LV dimension and end-diastolic dimension may be evaluated using transthoracic or transesophageal echocardiography, providing a useful noninvasive technique for clinically quantifying LV preload. Despite the widespread application of echocardiographic methods for assessing preload, LV EDV is frequently not quantified and often other estimates of preload are used in the clinical setting. LV end-diastolic pressure (LVEDP) can be invasively measured in the cardiac catheterization laboratory or during cardiac surgery. LVEDP is related to EDV via the nonlinear end-diastolic pressure–volume relation (EDPVR). However, LVEDP may be a poor reflection of EDV during pathologic conditions characterized by decreases in LV compliance. Other estimates of LV volume and pressure are based on measurements further "upstream" from the left ventricle. LA pressure, pulmonary capillary occlusion and pulmonary artery arterial diastolic pressures, and right atrial pressure are all indirect indicators of LV volume that are influenced by the functional integrity of the structures that separate their measurement site from the left ventricle itself (Fig. 7.11). Thus, the correlation between these "upstream" measures of preload and LVEDV may be poor in patients with compromised LV function, pulmonary disease, or right ventricular (RV) failure.

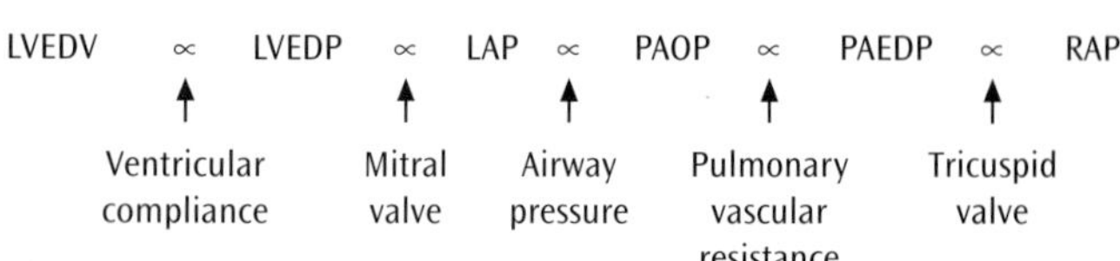

Figure 7.11 *Summary of factors that alter estimates of left ventricular end-diastolic volume (LVEDV) "upstream" from the left ventricle. LVEDP, left ventricular end-diastolic pressure; LAP, left atrial pressure; PAOP, pulmonary artery occlusion pressure; PAEDP, pulmonary artery end-diastolic pressure; RAP, right atrial pressure. Reproduced with permission.*

Afterload

Resistance to LV ejection by the arterial vasculature provides a qualitative definition of afterload *in vivo*. Several models of afterload have been proposed based on the multiple factors that are involved in this description. In one approach, afterload is described as LV wall stress at end-systole, when the forces driving LV ejection are equal to the arterial inertial forces that resist it. Wall stress (σ) is quantified using the law of Laplace: $\sigma = (P \times r)/2h$, where P is LV pressure, r is LV radius, and h is LV wall thickness. LV wall stress reaches its maximum during the first phase of ejection, and subsequently decreases because increases in wall thickness and decreases in chamber size occur despite continued increases in LV pressure during the remainder of ejection.[23] Peak LV wall stress is a major determinant in the development of LV hypertrophy during chronic pressure overload conditions, such as essential hypertension and aortic stenosis. The integral of systolic LV wall stress over time is also a major determinant of myocardial O_2 demand.[24] LV end-systolic wall stress defines the force that ultimately limits LV fiber shortening and determines the degree of LV emptying for any given contractile state.

Afterload may also be defined by the elastic interaction between arterial vasculature and the left ventricle (Fig. 7.9).[25] Using the slope of the ESPVR derived from LV pressure–volume diagrams, LV chamber elastance (E_{es}) is defined as the ratio of changes in pressure to volume at end-systole. The arterial vasculature is considered as a second elastic chamber quantified by effective arterial elastance (E_a; the ratio of end-systolic pressure to stroke volume). The relation between E_{es} and E_a defines the stroke volume that can be transferred from the left ventricle to the arterial system and describes the mechanical balance between these elastic elements in a model of left ventricle–arterial coupling.

Another approach to afterload defines this variable as the forces external to the left ventricle (impedance) present in a viscoelastic arterial circulation that oppose ejection of a viscous fluid (blood). Aortic input impedance is a dynamic characteristic of the arterial vasculature and is defined as the ratio of aortic pressure to aortic blood flow. Aortic input impedance incorporates the pulsatile nature of aortic blood flow and the presence of arterial wave reflection independent of LV performance. Calculation of aortic input impedance is very difficult even under controlled experimental conditions and requires simultaneous high-fidelity measurement of aortic pressure and blood flow. The magnitude of aortic input impedance depends primarily on peripheral arterial resistance, an index of afterload that assumes steady state rather than pulsatile aortic pressure and blood flow. Arterial resistance is determined as a single quotient of aortic pressure and flow, in contrast to aortic input impedance, which generates a frequency-dependent spectrum of variable resistance to LV ejection that incorporates aortic compliance. The assumption of steady-state arterial resistance forms the basis for use of systemic vascular resistance (SVR) as the most common clinical measure of afterload: SVR = (MAP – RAP) × 80/CO, where MAP is mean arterial pressure, RAP is right atrial pressure, and CO is cardiac output. SVR calculations parallel LV end-systolic wall stress measurements in a variety of clinical conditions but may underestimate the magnitude of changes in resistance to LV outflow.

Myocardial contractility

Myocardial contractility is relatively easy to measure in isolated cardiac muscle because loading conditions can be precisely controlled, but contractile state is considerably more difficult to quantify in the intact heart. All indices of inotropic state *in vivo* developed to date, including those based on LV pressure–volume diagrams, have some degree of dependence on heart rate and LV loading conditions. Thus, evaluation of myocardial contractility must consider not only the properties of the myocardium but also the impact of changes in heart rate and systemic and pulmonary hemodynamics that affect LV preload and afterload.

The mechanical behavior of the left ventricle can be described using a model of time-varying elastance. This concept characterizes the left ventricle as an elastic chamber whose elasticity (ratio of pressure to volume) becomes maximal at end-systole. The maximum elastance of a series of LV pressure–volume diagrams obtained at various loads is linear and determines the ESPVR. The slope (E_{es}) of the ESPVR has been used to quantify contractile state of the left ventricle relatively independent of alterations in heart rate and loading conditions. This LV pressure–volume analysis is also useful for the description of diastolic function, left ventricle–arterial coupling, and myocardial energetics. Applications of ESPVR to the invasive examination of systolic function have been made in experimental animals, in the cardiac catheterization laboratory, and during cardiac surgery in humans.

Another index of contractility derived from LV pressure–volume diagrams is based on the Frank–Starling relation. Increases in LV preload produce direct increases in cardiac output and LV stroke work by optimizing sarcomere length,[10] actin–myosin overlap,[9] and Ca^{2+} sensitivity of the contractile apparatus.[11] Preload recruitable stroke work (PRSW) relates the preload (EDV) of each LV pressure–volume diagram to the LV stroke work (area of each diagram) performed during each cardiac cycle (Fig. 7.10). The slope of the linear PRSW is a quantitative index of contractile state. PRSW may be calculated from the same series of LV pressure–volume diagrams used to determine ESPVR and has been successfully applied as a contractile index under a variety of pathologic conditions in both experimental and clinical settings.

Because ESPVR and PRSW require invasive measurement of continuous LV pressure and volume, these techniques have limited clinical applicability. The most commonly measured clinical index of global myocardial contractility is ejection fraction (the ratio of stroke volume to EDV). Ejection fraction can be calculated using a variety of noninvasive methods, including echocardiography and radionuclide ventriculography. Ejection fraction is 67% in normal patients and is reduced in patients with LV dysfunction. Ejection fraction is only moderately affected by changes in preload in the presence of normal mitral and aortic valve function, but decreases linearly with increases in LV afterload and also varies inversely with heart rate. Thus, ejection fraction is a relatively insensitive index of contractility. Ejection fraction may also be misleading in the presence of regional myocardial ischemia, mitral or aortic valve pathology, and LV hypertrophy or dilation.

Another frequently reported index of contractility is the maximum rate of increase of LV pressure ($+dP/dt_{max}$). LV $+dP/dt_{max}$ requires invasive measurement of LV pressure, is often recorded in the cardiac catheterization laboratory, and is a very sensitive index of contractile state. LV $+dP/dt_{max}$ is considered to be independent of LV afterload because the peak rate of increase of LV pressure occurs before opening of the aortic valve. However, $+dP/dt_{max}$ is influenced by LV preload, and alterations in $+dP/dt_{max}$ during increases in contractility may be indistinguishable from those induced by concomitant increases in preload. LV $+dP/dt_{max}$ may also be influenced by LV mass, chamber geometry, valvular dysfunction, and regional myocardial ischemia.

Heart rate

Myocardial contractility increases in direct response to increases in heart rate – an effect known as the Bowditch staircase or "treppe." This "force–frequency" relation was initially described in isolated cardiac muscle and has also been demonstrated in the intact heart. The "force–frequency" effect plays a role in matching of cardiac output to venous return during exercise, but tachycardia itself has little effect on overall cardiac performance under resting conditions. In contrast, rate-dependent increases in contractile state are especially important in failing myocardium. Enhanced venous return and pulmonary congestion resulting from intravascular volume expansion, increased venous tone, and depression of contractility may also be compensated by increases in heart rate despite concomitant reductions in diastolic filling time. Tachycardia also increases cardiac output in conditions that limit LV filling (e.g. constrictive pericarditis, cardiac tamponade). Contractility eventually becomes reduced at extremely high heart rates (greater than 175 beats min^{-1}) associated with tachyarrhythmias. Tachycardia of this magnitude also limits the extent to which cardiac output can increase because substantial reductions in diastolic duration and LV filling occur.

LEFT VENTRICULAR DIASTOLIC FUNCTION

Cardiac function during diastole has become the focus of intense experimental and clinical research in recent years because diastolic function significantly influences the overall mechanical performance of the heart. Abnormalities in LV diastolic function can usually be directly linked to systolic dysfunction, but heart failure may result from primary diastolic dysfunction in the absence of, or before the appearance of, systolic dysfunction in a variety of diseases, including ischemic heart disease, hypertrophic obstructive cardiomyopathy, and pressure or volume overload hypertrophy.[26] In fact, many patients with congestive heart failure directly related to diastolic dysfunction have normal systolic performance.[27,28] LV diastolic function is determined by myocardial relaxation, LV compliance, and the physical properties of the pulmonary veins, left atrium, mitral valve, and pericardium (Fig. 7.12).

As discussed above, diastole is usually divided into four phases: isovolumic relaxation, rapid LV filling, diastasis, and atrial systole. LV isovolumic relaxation (Fig. 7.13, point 1) occurs when the LV pressure falls below aortic pressure (closure of the aortic valve) and ends when LV pressure falls below LA pressure (opening of mitral valve). Isovolumic relaxation is an energy-dependent process, requiring ATP for the clearance of Ca^{2+} from the myoplasm by sarcolemmal and SR Ca^{2+} pumps. Isovolumic relaxation can be invasively measured by the maximal rate of decay of LV pressure ($-dP/dt$) or by a time constant (τ) of relaxation. Relaxation can also be quantified noninvasively by

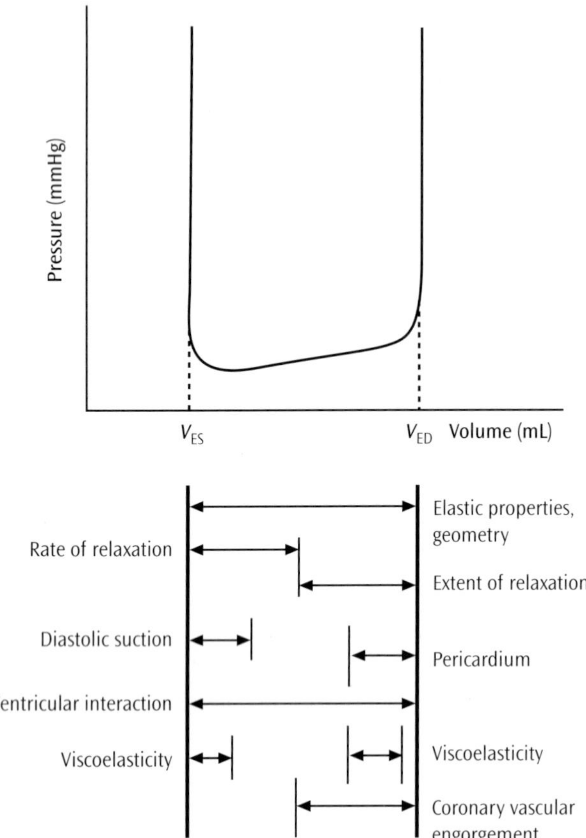

Figure 7.12 *Properties of the left ventricle that contribute to the rate, timing, and extent of left ventricular (LV) filling. Myocardial elasticity and geometry (size and wall thickness) are important throughout diastole. During early diastole, active relaxation and recoil of elastic energy (diastolic suction) stored in the myocardium during systole determine the left atrial–LV pressure gradient and early LV filling rate. Late in diastole, LV/right ventricular interaction and pericardial forces become important determinants of LV filling. Viscoelastic properties of the myocardium are important during rapid LV filling and during atrial systole. Coronary vascular engorgement also plays a role in determining the extent of filling in late diastole.* V_{es}*, end-systolic volume;* V_{ed}*, end-diastolic volume. Reproduced with permission.*

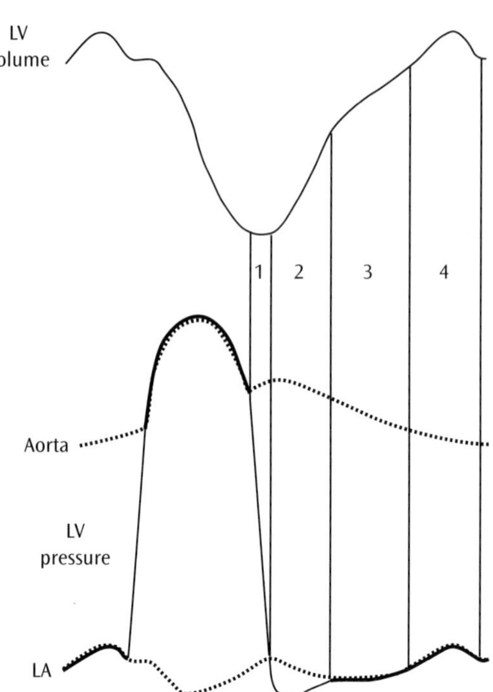

Figure 7.13 *Left ventricular (LV) volume and pressure and aortic and left atrial (LA) pressure during the various phases of diastole. 1, Isovolumic relaxation; 2, rapid LV filling; 3, diastasis (slow ventricular filling); 4, atrial systole. Reproduced with permission.*

determining isovolumic relaxation time (IVRT) derived from Doppler transthoracic or transesophageal echocardiography.

Rapid LV filling (Fig. 7.13, point 2) occurs after the mitral valve opens and blood flows from the left atrium to the left ventricle. Despite the fact that rapid LV filling composes only one-third of diastole, the vast majority (60–80%) of total LV stroke volume enters the left ventricle during this phase. LV pressure and volume curves may diverge in the initial portion of rapid LV filling because LV pressure continues to decrease as relaxation is completed during simultaneous expansion of LV volume. This process has been described as "diastolic suction" and aids rapid LV filling, especially during exercise and hypovolemia.[29] After completion of rapid LV filling, LV and LA pressures equalize and a relatively small amount of additional LV filling continues that originates from pulmonary venous return. Diastasis or slow LV filling (Fig. 7.13, point 3) usually contributes less than 5% of the total LV stroke volume, and may be substantially limited or abolished during increases in heart rate. Atrial systole is the final phase of diastole (Fig. 7.13, point 4).

Diastolic LV filling is typically measured noninvasively using Doppler echocardiography to evaluate transmitral blood flow velocity patterns (Fig. 7.14). Under normal conditions, the transmitral flow

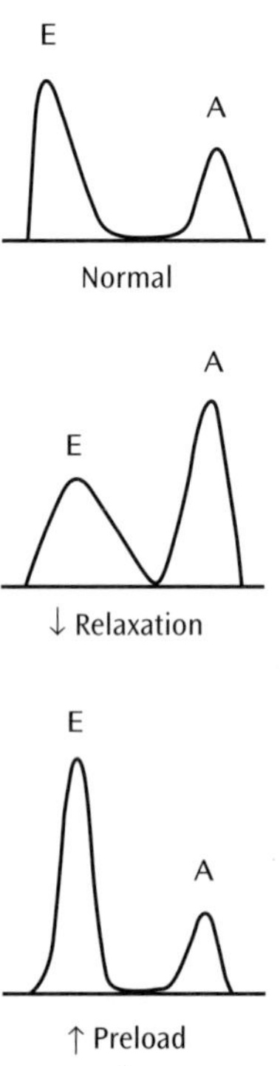

Figure 7.14 *Schematic diagram of transmitral blood flow velocity under normal conditions (top), during impaired myocardial relaxation secondary to severe left ventricular (LV) hypertrophy (middle), and during end-stage heart failure (increased LV end-diastolic and left atrial pressures; bottom). An early and late peak of blood flow velocity occur during rapid LV filling (E-wave) and atrial systole (A-wave) respectively. A reversal of the E/A ratio occurs during conditions characterized by impaired relaxation, indicating enhanced atrial contribution to LV filling. Large increases in E-wave velocity are observed during evolving heart failure because LV compliance progressively decreases.*

velocity profile reveals two peaks corresponding to a larger early (E) filling wave and a smaller atrial systole (A) wave. During pathological processes that delay relaxation, the relative significance of early LV filling may be diminished (decreased E wave) and atrial systole may be augmented (increased A wave), yielding a reversal of the E/A ratio.[30] This filling pattern may be artificially restored ("pseudonormalization")[31] in end-stage heart failure as LV compliance continues to decrease and LV end-diastolic pressure increases.

RIGHT VENTRICULAR FUNCTION

The right ventricle is a crescent-shaped chamber that receives blood from the right atrium and propels it into the low-pressure pulmonary circulation. The right ventricle is composed of specific inflow and outflow tracts that have embryologically distinct origin, resulting in unique structure[32] and response to autonomic nervous system activity. Myocardial contraction of the right ventricle is different from the left ventricle. Because the interventricular septum predominantly contributes to LV function, the contracting septum bulges into the right ventricle cavity during systole. Contraction of the right ventricular (RV) inflow and outflow tracts follows a sequential pattern, establishing regional pressure differences within the right ventricle during systole and accounting for the peristaltic action of this pump.[33] True isovolumic relaxation does not occur in the right ventricle.[34] Instead, ejection of blood from the outflow tract into the pulmonary artery continues after the inflow tract has begun to relax.[35]

THE CORONARY CIRCULATION

Anatomy of coronary arteries and veins

The coronary ostia arise from their respective sinuses of Valsalva above the expanse of the aortic valvular cusps so that they are not completely shielded during systole. While the left main coronary artery tends to arise from the left sinus of Valsalva at an acute angle and to travel parallel to the aortic wall, the right coronary artery (RCA) arises nearly perpendicular from the right sinus of Valsalva. The RCA remains surrounded by abundant adipose tissue throughout its course within the right atrioventricular (AV) groove, mainly supplying the RV wall, right atrium, and the LV posterior surface. The origin of the posterior descending artery (PDA) determines the blood supply to the inferior portion of the left ventricle and the inferior third of the interventricular septum, and thereby defines "coronary dominance." In 70% of hearts, this PDA branch arises from the RCA. Elements of the cardiac conduction system, including sinus node,[36] AV node, and bundle of His, are usually supplied by the RCA.

The left main coronary artery extends for several centimeters past the left coronary ostia before dividing into the left anterior descending coronary artery (LAD) and left circumflex coronary artery (LCCA). The LAD courses down within the anterior interventricular sulcus and, after wrapping around the apex, ascends a variable distance along the posterior interventricular sulcus. The majority of the interventricular septum is supplied by branches of the LAD (septal perforating arteries), as are the right and left anterior bundle branches of the LV conduction system. Diagonal branches of the LAD supply the LV anterior wall and small RV branches may provide blood to the RV anterior wall. The LCCA travels within the left atrioventricular sulcus and provides blood to the lateral LV free wall (obtuse marginal branches). By continuing around the left ventricle to reach the posterior interventricular sulcus, the LCCA usually terminates at or before the "crux of the heart," where the plane of the interventricular septum crosses the plane of the atrioventricular sulcus. In a minority of patients (10%), the LCCA gives rise to the PDA and supplies the inferior third of the interventricular septum, and thereby establishes "left coronary dominance." In the remaining 20% of patients, both the RCA and the LCCA supply this region, resulting in a shared coronary dominance.[37]

The major epicardial coronary arteries communicate with one another by small collateral arteries, which usually do not provide substantial blood flow between them. These coronary collateral vessels may dilate and provide an important pathway for blood flow beyond a coronary artery stenosis, however. These functional collaterals may develop between two different coronary arteries, between branches of the same coronary artery, or within the same branch via the vasa vasorum. The epicardial coronary arteries give rise to intramural penetrating arteries that extend perpendicularly from subepicardium to subendocardium, providing extensive collateral capillary networks throughout the transmural thickness of the myocardium.

Venous drainage for the coronary circulation occurs by an extensive intercommunicating network of veins. The majority of LV venous return drains into the coronary sinus located in the posterior atrioventricular sulcus, where it empties into the right atrium. Minor portions of the venous drainage directly enter the right atrium, or the right and left ventricle via the thebesian veins.[38] These direct venous conduits to the left ventricle contribute to the normal physiologic arteriovenous shunt. Anastomoses occur frequently between all coronary venous channels.

Determinants of myocardial oxygen consumption

Ventricular myocardium consumes approximately 10 mL O_2 per 100 g of muscle per minute under resting conditions. Myocardial O_2 consumption may increase over 300% during exercise. Heart rate, wall tension, and contractile state determine myocardial O_2 consumption. Tachycardia causes a direct increase in myocardial O_2 consumption by increasing the number of LV contractions per minute and enhancing inotropic state. Tachycardia may also be detrimental to myocardial O_2 supply because diastolic filling of the coronary circulation may become limited. Thus, tachycardia is especially dangerous in patients with coronary artery disease because increases in myocardial O_2 demand cannot be appropriately matched by increases in supply.

The law of Laplace indicates that LV wall tension is directly related to LV pressure and radius and inversely proportional to wall thickness. As LV pressure, radius, and wall thickness vary throughout the cardiac cycle, wall tension varies from diastole to systole. Increases in wall tension during systole (afterload) and diastole (preload) cause direct increases in myocardial O_2 consumption. Thus, myocardial O_2 consumption increases during pathologic conditions that increase systolic (e.g. hypertension, aortic stenosis) and diastolic (e.g. aortic or mitral regurgitation) wall stress. Increases in wall thickness (concentric or eccentric LV hypertrophy) occur as a compensatory response to chronically elevated wall stress. However, although LV hypertrophy directly reduces wall stress, hypertrophied myocardium is also more susceptible to ischemia because the increased muscle mass requires higher myocardial O_2 consumption under resting conditions and during exercise.

Factors that increase myocardial contractility, including endogenous stimulation of the sympathetic nervous system or exogenous administration of positive inotropic drugs, result in substantial increases in myocardial O_2 consumption. However, changes in cardiac output alone do not necessarily reflect alterations in contractility or increased myocardial O_2 consumption. For example, cardiac output increases during a pure reduction in LV afterload, and myocardial O_2 consumption remains unchanged despite increases in LV stroke volume and stroke work. In contrast, increases in cardiac output resulting from tachycardia, enhanced inotropic state, or increased preload will cause simultaneous increases in myocardial O_2 consumption. Thus, β-adrenoceptor antagonists and nitrates have been a mainstay in the treatment of patients with coronary artery disease because these drugs reduce myocardial O_2 consumption by decreasing heart rate and preload respectively.

Regulation of coronary blood flow

The resting coronary blood flow in an adult man is approximately 225 mL min^{-1}, representing about 5% of total cardiac output. Peak coronary flow occurs during early diastole after LV isovolumic relaxation because extravascular compression of the coronary microcirculation is minimal. Coronary blood flow to the left ventricle continues throughout diastole and is determined by coronary perfusion pressure, calculated as the difference of diastolic arterial pressure and LV end-diastolic pressure. Thus, the amount of blood flow in the coronary vasculature is directly related to the pressure gradient across the coronary circulation. Alterations in transmural myocardial blood flow distribution occur primarily as a consequence of changes in vascular resistance. Several factors affect blood flow (Q) through a vessel, as determined by Poiseuille's equation: $Q = \Delta P \pi r^4 / 8L\eta$, where ΔP is pressure difference; r is inside radius of the vessel; L is vessel length; and η is fluid viscosity. The vessel radius is raised to the fourth power in Poiseuille's equation and is clearly the most important determinant of blood flow. Accordingly, decreases in coronary vascular resistance occur as a result of increases in vessel diameter and opening of new vascular channels. Because small coronary arteries and arterioles determine the majority of vascular resistance, it is likely that overall regulation of coronary flow occurs by changes in caliber of these vessels. Alterations in blood viscosity caused by changes in plasma protein concentration or hematocrit also play a small role in determining overall coronary vascular resistance.

The coronary circulation is autoregulated and coronary blood flow remains nearly constant when coronary perfusion pressure ranges between 50 and 120 mmHg (6.7 and 16 kPa).[39] Blood flow becomes pressure-dependent above or below this autoregulation range because maximal vasoconstriction or vasodilation of the coronary circulation occurs. Rapid, accurate control of transmural myocardial blood flow is primarily established by local metabolism and is relatively unaffected if external humoral and autonomic nervous system regulation is removed.[40] Several mediators,[41,42] including adenosine, O_2, CO_2, nitric oxide, endothelin, and prostaglandins, have been implicated in the local regulation of coronary blood flow.

The coronary circulation is innervated by sympathetic and parasympathetic nerves, whose stimulation produces both direct and indirect effects on the coronary vasculature. Activation of the sympathetic nervous system causes vasoconstriction by direct α_1-adrenoceptor stimulation and indirect metabolic vasodilation resulting from increases in heart rate and myocardial contractility mediated by β_1-adrenoceptors. The indirect increase in coronary blood flow is mediated by enhanced myocardial O_2 consumption and is of greater importance in determining the response to increases in sympathetic tone than the direct α_1-adrenoceptor effect on the coronary vasculature itself. Antagonism of β-adrenoceptors prevents the increase in coronary flow secondary to tachycardia and enhanced contractility[43] and allows α_1-adrenoceptor stimulation of the coronary circulation to occur unopposed. There is also a varied distribution of α-adrenoceptor subtypes in the coronary circulation. Although α_1-adrenoceptors are uniformly present in the coronary circulation, α_2-adrenoceptors are primarily located in coronary arterioles of less than 100 μm in diameter.[44]

Myocardial O_2 consumption is the most important factor that affects coronary blood flow. The myocardium extracts 70–75% of coronary arterial O_2 content under resting conditions. As a result, coronary venous O_2 content is very low and myocardial O_2 extraction (Do_2) cannot significantly increase from its resting value during exercise. Consequently, increases in myocardial O_2 consumption (Vo_2) must be accompanied by appropriate increases in coronary blood flow because $Vo_2 = Q \times Do_2 \times 10$, where Q is coronary blood flow. Thus, coronary blood flow and metabolism are very closely matched and coronary venous O_2 content remains constant over a wide range of myocardial O_2 consumption.[45]

THE CARDIAC CONDUCTION SYSTEM

The electrical activity of the heart is responsible for coordinating the sequence of myocardial contraction and relaxation. Efficient pumping action is based on a precise coordination of contraction of individual myocytes. Spontaneous generation and distribution of coordinated impulses is achieved through a specifically adapted system of excitation and conduction.

Sinus node

The sinus node is located in an epicardial position at the confluence of the superior vena cava, right atrial appendage, and lateral wall of the right atrium. The sinus node contains specialized myocytes (P cells) that act as the intrinsic cardiac pacemaker. Automaticity is based on the unstable resting membrane potential ("phase 4" depolarization) that these cells exhibit after repolarization. The membrane potential reaches a maximum negative value, but then spontaneously begins to slowly depolarize towards the threshold value, creating the next action potential. Sinus node action potentials have a slow upstroke of depolarization, reflecting the lack of functional Na^+ channels. The absence of an inward Na^+ current is due in part to the high resting potential of the sinus node, which inactivates the Na^+ channels. As a result, the upstroke of the sinus node action potential is due primarily to an inward Ca^{2+} current. The sinus node pacemaker is modulated by autonomic nervous system activity. Blood supply to the sinus node is provided by the sinus nodal artery, which usually originates from the RCA but may also arise from the LCCA.[36]

Atrial internodal pathways

The action potential spreads through the atrial wall in a wave centered about the sinus node. Conduction of the electrical impulse between the sinus and AV nodes may be facilitated by three conducting pathways, designated the anterior (Bachman), middle (Wenckebach), and posterior (Thorel) internodal tracts, but these pathways lack definitive histologic evidence. Bachman tract fibers also branch off to the left atrium to produce LA contraction. Atrial conduction velocity is approximately 1 m s^{-1}, and the sinus node impulse reaches the AV node 0.08 s after generation under normal conditions.

Atrioventricular node

The AV node is located in the medial right atrial subendocardium at the base of the atrial septum immediately above the coronary sinus. Propagation of the impulse through the AV node is slow (0.05 m s^{-1}) in comparison with other parts of the conduction system and is responsible for the 0.15-s delay between atrial and ventricular depolarization. This delay allows completion of atrial contraction and emptying before the initiation of ventricular contraction. Blood supply to the AV node is derived from the AV nodal artery, which most often arises from RCA.

Bundle of His and Purkinje fibers

The bundle of His arises from the distal portion of the AV node and bifurcates at the top of the interventricular septum. By virtue of its position in the interventricular septum, the bundle of His lies adjacent to the annuli of the aortic, mitral, and tricuspid valves. The right bundle branch originates from the distal end of the bundle of His. The right bundle branch courses around the RV cavity to reach the free RV wall from the right side of the ventricular septum. The left bundle fans out widely within the subendocardium of the left side of the interventricular septum shortly after it separates from the common bundle. The left bundle separates into two major divisions (the anterior–superior and posterior–inferior fascicles) approximately midway to the LV apex. These fascicles continue to the origin of the papillary muscles and adjacent myocardium. The right and left bundle branches give rise to a highly redundant subendocardial network of Purkinje fibers that distribute the action potential to each ventricular myocyte. Impulse conduction velocity in the bundle of His and its branches is approximately 3 m s^{-1}.

PATHOPHYSIOLOGY

Cardiovascular disease is one of the leading causes of death following anesthesia and surgery.[46] The clinical risk factors for perioperative cardiac morbidity and mortality are diverse and include advanced age, documented or occult coronary artery disease, previous myocardial infarction, and congestive heart failure. Hypertension, diabetes mellitus, peripheral vascular disease, valvular heart disease, hypercholesterolemia, cigarette smoking, previous coronary artery bypass graft (CABG) surgery or PTCA, and cardiovascular drug therapy are also considered important risk factors that affect cardiovascular outcome.

CORONARY ARTERY DISEASE

Clinical presentation

Patients with acute myocardial ischemia resulting from coronary artery disease may be asymptomatic or exhibit symptoms of chest pain or pressure, progressive dyspnea on exertion, and fatigue. Syncope and sudden cardiac death may also be the initial presenting signs of coronary artery disease. Myocardial ischemia can be present without chest pain in up to 30% of patients, especially in those with diabetes mellitus, chronic renal insufficiency, and advanced age. Enhanced O_2 demand associated with increased myocardial workload in the presence of coronary stenoses is responsible for symptoms in patients with angina pectoris. In contrast, patients with unstable angina have symptoms that occur with increasing frequency and severity or at rest. The transition from stable to unstable angina is frequently associated with thrombosis complicating an atheroma.[47,48] Disruption of the atherosclerotic plaque usually provides the thrombogenic stimulus under these circumstances.[49]

Coronary atherosclerosis and thrombosis

A number of important risk factors have been specifically identified that predict an increased susceptibility to coronary atherosclerosis. These include hypertension, diabetes mellitus, hypercholesterolemia, obesity, cigarette smoking, and a positive family history of coronary artery disease.[50] Several mechanisms may convert a stable atherosclerotic plaque to an unstable highly thrombogenic lesion, producing angina, infarction, or sudden death. Platelet attachment to an atherosclerotic plaque or plaque rupture with exposure of thrombogenic collagen may produce thrombus formation, converting a partially occluded coronary artery into one that is severely stenosed or totally occluded.[48,51] The coronary perfusion pressure–blood flow relation is disturbed in myocardium supplied by an atherosclerotic coronary artery because pressure distal to the stenosis may be substantially less than diastolic arterial pressure. The resistance to blood flow increases and the pressure gradient across the narrowed vessel becomes greater with stenosis severity. The hemodynamic consequences of multiple serial stenoses in the same coronary artery are profound, and distal stenoses of lesser severity "downstream" from a proximal lesion may disproportionally diminish coronary blood flow in the ischemic zone.[52] Resting coronary blood flow is maintained at normal levels until stenosis severity reaches greater than a 90% reduction in vessel cross-sectional area, but the ability of flow to increase in response to increases in myocardial O_2 demand or vasodilators is substantially reduced at an area of only 60%.[53] Atherosclerosis dramatically alters metabolic, humoral, and autonomic nervous system control of the coronary circulation. Endothelium-dependent relaxation in epicardial arteries and coronary microvessels is also impaired by atherosclerotic disease.[54]

Coronary collateral circulation

Coronary collateral blood vessels develop as a consequence of chronic myocardial ischemia resulting from coronary artery disease. Enlarged collateral vessels supply enhanced blood flow to the myocardium perfused by a stenosed or occluded coronary artery.[55,56] These coronary collateral vessels are primarily located in the subendocardium in human hearts.[57] The protective role of coronary collaterals has been demonstrated in several clinical studies,[58–60] and the extent of injury after myocardial infarction has been shown to be inversely related to the degree of collateral blood flow arising from interarterial anastomoses distal to the occluded segment.[61] Recent experimental and clinical evidence indicates that coronary collateral development may be regulated by the coordinated action of growth factors, including basic fibroblastic growth factor (bFGF) and vascular endothelial growth factor (VEGF). These data suggest that gene therapy may play an important future role in the treatment of coronary artery disease.[62,63]

Coronary steal

The redistribution of coronary collateral blood flow away from ischemic to normal myocardium is known as coronary "steal" (Fig. 7.15). This phenomenon may occur in response to vasodilators (e.g. dipyridamole, adenosine) independent of changes in systemic hemodynamics.[64] Perfusion of collateral-dependent myocardium depends on the driving pressure at the origin of the collateral vessels. Arterioles in the collateral-dependent zone are relatively dilated in comparison with vessels in surrounding normal regions, and collateral blood flow will decrease in direct proportion to reductions in perfusion pressure because normal autoregulatory responses have been exhausted. Coronary steal has important pathophysiologic consequences and may cause an increase in myocardial infarct size[65] in susceptible patients with "steal prone" coronary artery anatomy.[66]

Mechanical consequences of myocardial ischemia

Acute myocardial ischemia results from increased demand for or inadequate supply of O_2 and is accompanied by impairment of LV systolic and diastolic function. Depending on the underlying cause of the myocardial O_2 supply–demand mismatch, the extent of ischemia may be restricted to a small region or involve the majority of the left

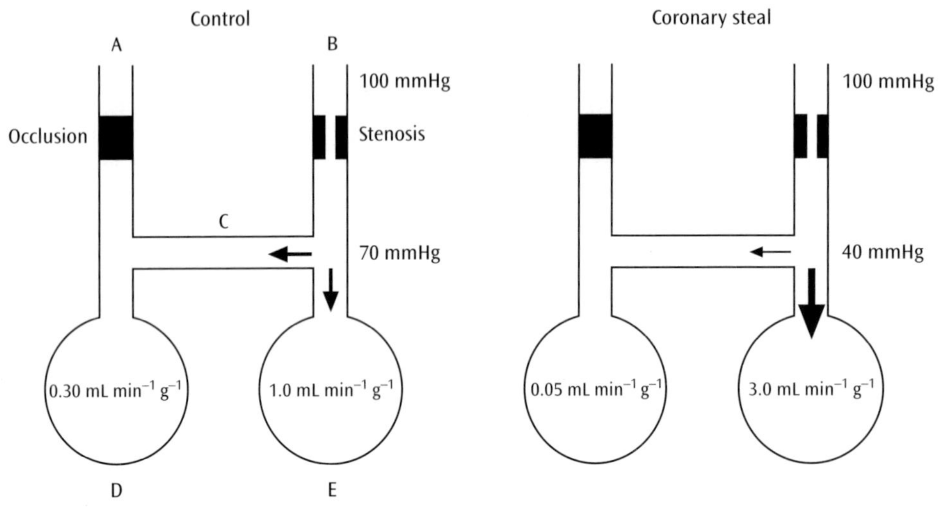

Figure 7.15 *Schematic diagram of coronary circulation illustrating the mechanism of vasodilator-induced coronary steal. Tissue (D) previously supplied by coronary artery (A) is perfused via collaterals (C) whose artery of origin (B) contains a proximal stenosis. Collateral vessels are maximally dilated in the control state and during coronary steal. During vasodilation, perfusion pressure at the origin of the collateral vessels is reduced from 70 to 40 mmHg (9.3 to 5.3 kPa), resulting in decreased perfusion of ischemic tissue (D). In contrast, vasodilation of the artery of origin (B) distal to the stenosis causes an increase in blood flow to tissue (E) supplied by the stenotic artery and coronary steal has occurred. Reproduced with permission.*

ventricle. Ischemia frequently affects the cardiac conduction system and produces malignant ventricular arrhythmias. Ischemia is associated with profound metabolic consequences, including insufficient O_2 to support oxidative phosphorylation, intracellular acidosis,[67] accumulation of toxic metabolites, and intracellular Ca^{2+} overload. The primary metabolic disturbance in ischemic myocardium is the blockade of aerobic synthesis of high-energy phosphates and a shift to anaerobic metabolism,[68] resulting in a rapid decline of intracellular concentrations of ATP and creatine phosphate.[69]

The abrupt decrease in coronary blood flow during acute coronary artery occlusion causes a nearly simultaneous contractile dysfunction.[70] The noncontracting ischemic region bulges outward during systole (dyskinesis) because this zone passively expands in response to developed LV systolic pressure generated by surrounding normal myocardium. These changes in regional systolic function are accompanied by LV dilation, consistent with thinning and expansion of the acutely ischemic segment and enhanced preload and contractility in the remaining functional zones.[71] Abnormalities in LV diastolic function also occur because ATP-dependent elimination of Ca^{2+} from the myoplasm is profoundly reduced. Intracellular Ca^{2+} accumulation during diastole causes impaired relaxation, reduced LV compliance, and shifts the end-diastolic pressure–volume relation upward. Thus, acute pulmonary edema resulting from myocardial ischemia may occur as a direct consequence of diastolic dysfunction.[26]

Reperfusion injury

Reperfusion of ischemic myocardium within 20–30 min of coronary artery occlusion alleviates the physiologic abnormalities of ischemia but may be associated with prolonged contractile dysfunction without tissue necrosis,[72] a phenomenon known as "stunned" myocardium (Fig. 7.16).[73] Postischemic contractile dysfunction persists from hours to days and is directly affected by the extent of coronary collateral perfusion during the coronary artery occlusion.[72] Recovery of diastolic function may follow a more prolonged time-course,[74] despite restoration of systolic function. Several factors have been implicated in the development of stunned myocardium, including intracellular Ca^{2+} overload,[75] depletion of high-energy phosphates,[76] production of O_2-derived free radicals by ischemic myocytes or infiltrating neutrophils,[72,77,78] reduction in myofilament Ca^{2+} sensitivity,[79] and myocyte excitation–contraction uncoupling.[80] Recent findings indicate that neutrophil migration and activation play a central role in contractile dysfunction in stunned myocardium.[81] Reperfusion may also be associated with malignant ventricular arrhythmias,[82] resulting from α-adrenoceptor stimulation[83] and disturbances of Ca^{2+} and K^+ homeostasis.[84]

Postischemic, reperfusion injury plays an important role in the natural history of ischemic heart disease because spontaneous reperfusion of ischemic myocardium after thrombosis or coronary vasospasm is known to occur frequently in patients with coronary artery disease. In addition, patients with acute myocardial ischemia may undergo coronary artery reperfusion through interventions such as thrombolytic therapy, angioplasty, and emergency coronary artery bypass graft surgery to salvage myocardium at risk for infarction. Delayed recovery of myocardial function also occurs in O_2 demand-induced ischemia in the presence of a fixed coronary artery stenosis.[85]

Prolonged coronary artery occlusion (30 min to 3 h) followed by reperfusion results in severe, persistent contractile dysfunction. Myocardium within the central ischemic zone may become infarcted, but some viable myocardium still remains and partial recovery of function eventually occurs over a time-course of several weeks. Rapid restoration of coronary blood flow decreases infarct size and accelerates the process of partial functional repair, but reperfusion itself may also cause further tissue injury.[86] Chronic myocardial ischemia resulting from continuous, partial reductions in myocardial perfusion produces sustained depression of contractile function without infarction, a phenomenon termed "myocardial hibernation."[87] Dysfunction during hibernation may result from the precarious matching of the limited energy supply to contractile function. Marked enhancement of systolic performance from reversal of hibernation often occurs after coronary artery bypass graft surgery.

Myocardial infarction and ventricular remodeling

Infarction causes a series of changes in regional and global LV function produced by scar formation in the infarcted region and compensatory hypertrophy of remaining viable myocardium in surrounding normal regions.[88,89] Extensive remodeling of the left ventricle results from this segmental hypertrophy. Heart failure may also develop late after a large myocardial infarction because of decompensation of the remodeled myocardium in the absence of further ischemic injury.[90]

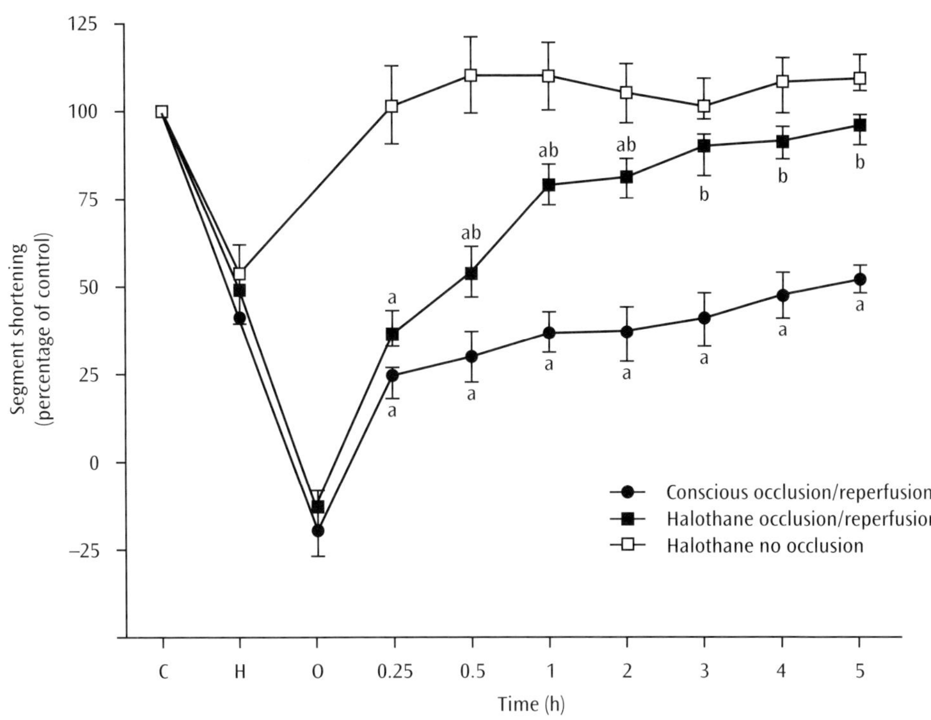

Figure 7.16 *Segment-shortening data during coronary artery occlusion (O) and at various times after reperfusion in conscious and halothane (H)-anesthetized dogs. Anesthetized dogs were allowed to emerge from anesthesia after the onset of reperfusion. At various time intervals, comparisons are made with anesthetized dogs allowed to emerge from halothane anesthesia that did not undergo coronary artery occlusion and reperfusion. Recovery of function of stunned myocardium is improved in dogs anesthetized with halothane. Note that the control state (C) indicates awake, unsedated state in each group. a, Significant difference from emergence without prior occlusion; b, significant difference from conscious occlusion. Reproduced with permission.*

Ischemic preconditioning

Ischemic preconditioning is a process by which a brief ischemic stimulus confers myocardial protection against subsequent sustained periods of coronary artery occlusion.[91] This increased tolerance to further ischemia occurs concomitant with reduced cellular metabolism during the ischemic episode and delayed onset of irreversible cell injury, and limits the extent of myocardial infarction. The mechanisms of ischemic preconditioning remain incompletely understood, but K_{ATP} channel opening[92] and adenosine subtype 1 (A_1) receptors[93] have been shown to play important roles. Ischemic preconditioning affords an immediate protection against infarction, which lasts approximately 2 h.[91] The existence of a second, more prolonged window of myocardial protection after a period of ischemia has also been suggested.[94]

LEFT VENTRICULAR HYPERTROPHY

Prolonged exposure of the left ventricle to pressure or volume overload causes hypertrophy that develops in a pattern specific to the inciting stress.[95,96] Increases in LV systolic wall stress and concentric LV thickening result from long-standing pressure overload (e.g. hypertension, aortic stenosis, aortic coarctation). Elevated diastolic wall stress and progressive LV dilation are observed in eccentric LV hypertrophy associated with chronic volume overload (e.g. aortic or mitral regurgitation). The mechanisms responsible for hypertrophy are controversial,[97] but enhanced systolic or diastolic wall stress appear to stimulate sarcomere synthesis in parallel or in series with pre-existing contractile units in pressure and volume overload respectively (Fig. 7.17).[96] Hypertrophy is an important compensatory response to chronic overload states that partially restores wall stress toward normal and improves overall cardiac performance. However, depression of myocardial contractility eventually contributes to the onset of heart failure. The degree of myocardial depression observed in hypertrophic states depends on the time-course, severity, and etiology of the increased load. Rapidly developing pressure or volume overload results in early myocardial damage, LV dilation, and acute heart failure. In contrast, gradually increased load allows contractile function to be relatively maintained. However, it is important to recognize that persistent elevation of wall stress places the hypertrophied myocytes at greater risk of ischemia, dysfunction, and cellular death.[98] Hypertrophy-induced depression of contractility can be reversed in both pressure and volume overload conditions by sustained pharmacologic treatment[99] or appropriately timed surgical intervention.[100] Profound abnormalities in LV diastolic function are also observed in patients with LV hypertrophy. Delayed isovolumic relaxation and decreased LV compliance are typical findings, and diastolic dysfunction plays an important role in the development of congestive heart failure late in the natural history of pressure or volume overload hypertrophy.

CARDIOMYOPATHIES

Hypertrophic obstructive cardiomyopathy

Hypertrophic obstructive cardiomyopathy (HOCM) is characterized by selective hypertrophy of the interventricular septum. During systole, thickening of the hypertrophied septum partially obstructs the LV outflow tract and creates a pressure gradient between the LV cavity and the aorta. The anterior leaflet of the mitral valve is often drawn into the LV outflow tract by Venturi forces, contributing to the outflow tract obstruction[101] and producing severe mitral regurgitation in mid- to late systole. Thus, the findings of "eject, obstruct, leak" are typical echocardiographic or angiographic observations in patients with HOCM. The outflow tract obstruction also causes hypertrophy of the remaining left ventricle, contributing to the profound diastolic dysfunction[102] that occurs early in this disorder. Abnormalities in relaxation occur concomitant with decreased LV compliance and impaired LV filling. The histology in HOCM reveals disordered myocyte and interstitial architecture within the interventricular septum. Patients with HOCM are also more susceptible to the development of malignant ventricular arrhythmias and sudden cardiac death.[103]

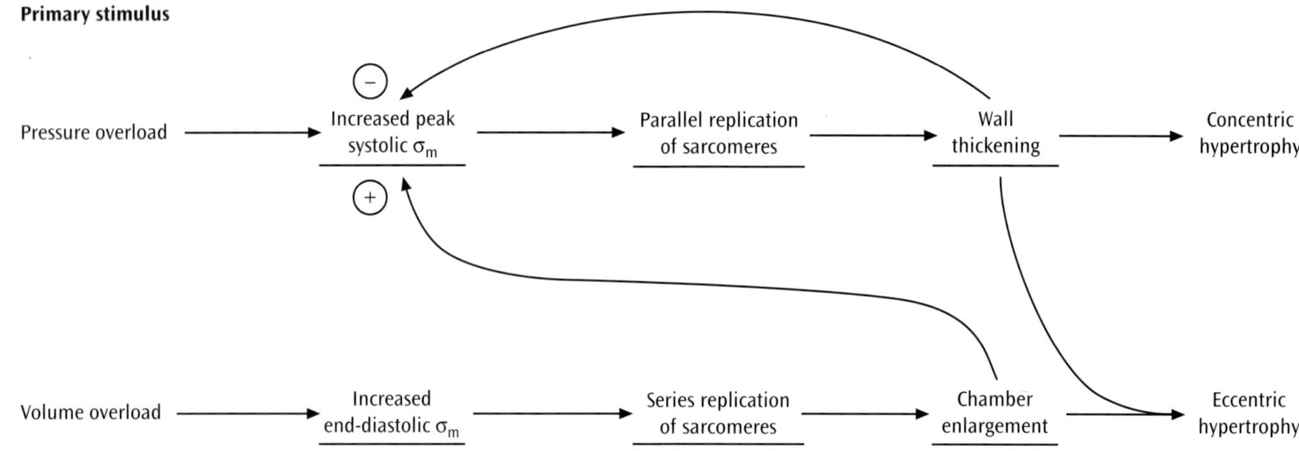

Figure 7.17 *Hypothesis relating wall stress and patterns of ventricular hypertrophy. Reproduced with permission.*

Dilated cardiomyopathy

Heart failure in patients with dilated cardiomyopathy occurs as a result of pump failure. As the LV ejection fraction falls, volume overload occurs concomitant with marked elevations in LV wall stress. Compensatory hypertrophy is usually inadequate to normalize wall stress. Dilated cardiomyopathy may develop without identifiable cause (e.g. idiopathic), after myocardial infarction, following an infectious process (e.g. myocarditis), or as a consequence of chronic alcohol abuse.[104,105] Dilation of the mitral valve annulus and reduced LV compliance result in centrally directed mitral regurgitation and pulmonary congestion. Ventricular failure often involves both cardiac chambers.[106]

Restrictive cardiomyopathy

Restrictive cardiomyopathy may occur as a consequence of eosinophilia, amyloid infiltration, hemochromatosis, or Fabry's disease. Restrictive cardiomyopathy is characterized by endocardial interstitial fibrosis and myocyte hypertrophy of the LV inflow tract and apex. The LV outflow tract is rarely affected. Marked endomyocardial hypertrophy may eventually lead to apical obliteration. While cardiac contractile function often remains relatively normal until late in the disease, severe LV diastolic dysfunction characterized by incomplete relaxation, restricted LV filling, and elevated filling pressures occurs.[107] In addition, mitral regurgitation, atrial dilation,[108] and conduction defects (e.g. bundle branch blocks) are common findings in patients with restrictive cardiomyopathy. The elevated filling pressures that occur in early diastole result in pulmonary hypertension and RV failure.

VALVULAR HEART DISEASE

Disruption of the anatomic integrity of the cardiac valves may result in either stenosis or regurgitation. Morphologic changes in size or shape of the left ventricle, right ventricle, or aorta may also precipitate functional or structural alterations in these valves.

Aortic stenosis

Stenosis of the aortic valve may develop as a result of age, or as a consequence of congenital (e.g. bicuspid valve), rheumatic, or infectious disease (e.g. endocarditis). A pressure gradient across the aortic valve is the pathognomonic finding in aortic stenosis as the left ventricle attempts to overcome the partial obstruction to LV ejection. Increased LV systolic and diastolic pressure and prolongation of LV ejection time also occur.[109] The stenotic aortic valve affects the morphology of the LV pressure waveform, progressively delaying peak ejection into late systole in severe disease (valve area $\leq 0.7\,cm^2$). Thus, peak systolic LV wall stress is delayed and mean systolic wall stress is greater than that predicted from the augmented LV pressure alone.[110] Compensatory concentric LV hypertrophy lowers wall stress by increasing wall thickness, but also produces diastolic dysfunction characterized by delayed relaxation and reduced compliance.[111] These changes in diastolic mechanics also produce an increase in LVEDP.[112]

A syncopal episode during exercise is often the presenting symptom in aortic stenosis because cardiac output cannot increase to maintain arterial pressure during exercise-induced declines in SVR. Angina may occur in conjunction with aortic stenosis in the presence or absence of coronary artery disease.[113] LV hypertrophy with concomitant increases in myocardial O_2 demand[114] may exceed the ability of the coronary vasculature to supply O_2, even in the absence of coronary stenoses. Coronary perfusion pressure is reduced as a result of increased LVEDP and reduced flow into coronary ostia owing to excessively rapid flow through the constricted aortic valve orifice (Venturi effect). Mechanical compression of intramural coronary vessels and the increased duration of left ventricular ejection are also contributing factors in the development of angina in patients with aortic stenosis. Clearly, coexisting coronary artery disease may precipitate myocardial ischemia more rapidly in the presence of aortic stenosis and LV hypertrophy.[115] Cardiac arrhythmias are also frequently observed in patients with severe aortic stenosis.[116] Progressive LV systolic and diastolic dysfunction contributes to the onset of congestive heart failure in end-stage aortic stenosis.

Aortic regurgitation

Loss of valvular support produced by trauma or aortic root dissection or new structural damage produced by endocarditis rapidly results in congestive heart failure in acute aortic regurgitation. The sudden increase of LV end-diastolic volume produced by regurgitation shifts the operating region of the left ventricle to the right along the end-diastolic pressure–volume relation and LVEDP rises precipitously.[117] This pressure is transmitted to the left atrium and pulmonary circulation, resulting in acute pulmonary edema and RV dysfunction. The increase in LVEDP may also decrease coronary perfusion pressure and compromise coronary blood flow. Early closure of the mitral valve resulting from reflux of blood from the aorta to the left ventricle may also compromise "forward" flow in acute aortic regurgitation.[118]

Chronic aortic regurgitation subjects the left ventricle to volume overload, resulting in increased LV volume and compensatory eccentric LV hypertrophy. The compensatory LV dilation increases stroke volume and systolic arterial pressure until late in the natural history of the disease. Regurgitant blood flow back into the LV through the incompetent valve reduces the aortic diastolic pressure and contributes to the increase in pulse pressure observed in patients with this disease.[119] LV compliance initially remains normal; however, as contractile function begins to decline, diastolic dysfunction also occurs and compliance decreases.[120–122] Regurgitation-induced declines in aortic diastolic pressure directly reduce coronary perfusion pressure and may further compromise O_2 delivery to the hypertrophied myocardium. Vasodilators will reduce the regurgitant volume and improve forward flow by decreasing SVR,[123] but may also further compromise coronary perfusion. LV dilation may also widen the mitral valve annulus and lead to secondary mitral regurgitation.[124] Patients may remain asymptomatic for many years during the initial phases of the clinical course of chronic aortic regurgitation.

Mitral stenosis

Rheumatic fever is the most common cause of mitral stenosis.[125] Most patients typically remain asymptomatic for two to three decades before they present with heart failure or new-onset atrial fibrillation. Mitral stenosis is a disease defined by diastolic dysfunction. Narrowing of the mitral valve area below 2 cm^2 causes partial obstruction to LV filling and results in a pressure gradient across the valve. Increases in LA pressure occur as the disease progresses, eventually leading to pulmonary hypertension and RV dysfunction. The mitral valve pressure gradient is initially observed during early diastole and atrial systole, but eventually becomes present throughout diastole as the stenosis severity increases. This diastolic pressure gradient maintains blood flow from the left atrium to the left ventricle. LV ejection fraction and cardiac output may be markedly reduced as a result of relative LV underloading[126] and the residual effects of rheumatic myocarditis. LV isovolumic contraction may also be attenuated to some degree because the persistent left atrium to left ventricle pressure gradient prevents closure of the mitral valve during early systole. Tachycardia may have especially deleterious effects on cardiac output because the mechanical obstruction to LV filling prevents compensatory increases in stroke volume.[127] LA enlargement occurs as a consequence of elevated pressure and supraventricular arrhythmias, including premature atrial contractions, paroxysmal atrial tachycardia, atrial flutter, and atrial fibrillation, may be observed. Loss of atrial systole with the onset of atrial fibrillation may precipitate acute pulmonary edema in severe mitral stenosis.[128]

Mitral regurgitation

Acute mitral regurgitation may occur during myocardial ischemia in the base of the heart,[129–131] papillary muscle dysfunction, chordae tendinae rupture,[132] or infectious endocarditis. In severe, acute mitral regurgitation, a large regurgitant volume is ejected into the left atrium during LV systole.[133] Volume overload of both the left atrium and left ventricle produce striking elevations of LA and LV end-diastolic pressures because compensatory dilation of these chambers cannot occur. As a result, acute pulmonary edema and severe dyspnea ensue. Forward LV stroke volume is markedly diminished because of the sudden onset of regurgitation into the low-pressure left atrium, resulting in hypotension and cardiogenic shock.[134]

Clinical progression in patients with chronic mitral regurgitation is usually gradual, permitting adaptive compensatory mechanisms associated with volume overload hypertrophy. Chronic mitral regurgitation most frequently results from myxomatous degeneration of one or both mitral leaflets but may also occur as a consequence of myocardial ischemia, congenital or rheumatic heart disease, or endocarditis. The major pathophysiologic finding is partial ejection of the LV stroke volume into the low-pressure left atrium through the incompetent mitral valve.[135] The left atrium gradually dilates and accommodates this extra volume load. As a result, there may be a minimal or moderate increase in LA pressure. Eccentric hypertrophy occurs in response to chronic volume overload. As a result of this dilation, the left ventricle may eject two or more times its normal stroke volume.[136] Chronic LA and LV dilation produce increased compliance of these chambers. Thus, LA and LV pressures may remain relatively normal despite large volumes until late in the natural history of the disease. Because the left ventricle ejects blood into both the left atrium and the aorta, LV ejection is rapid and an "enhanced" ejection fraction may be erroneously measured. However, depression of myocardial contractility and reductions in cardiac output occur later in the clinical course. Chronic LA overload frequently causes atrial arrhythmias. The predominant clinical symptoms are fatigue and exercise intolerance.

Tricuspid regurgitation

Tricuspid annular dilation resulting from RV chamber enlargement associated with chronically elevated pulmonary arterial pressures is the most frequent cause of tricuspid regurgitation. Thus, patients with mitral stenosis or chronic, severe mitral regurgitation may present with secondary tricuspid insufficiency due to pulmonary hypertension.[137–139] Carcinoid syndrome,[140] infectious endocarditis associated with intravenous drug abuse,[141] rheumatic or congenital (e.g. tricuspid valve prolapse,[142] Ebstein's anomaly[143]) heart disease, transvenous pacemakers and catheters,[144] and cardiac trauma[145,146] may also produce tricuspid regurgitation independent of other cardiac pathology. Isolated tricuspid regurgitation is usually well tolerated and does not produce significant hemodynamic compromise because the right atrium and vena cavae are very compliant structures capable of tolerating the regurgitant volume with minor increases in pressure. However, patients with secondary tricuspid regurgitation resulting from pulmonary hypertension frequently present with signs and symptoms of RV failure including exercise intolerance, hepatic congestion, ascites, and peripheral edema. Under these conditions, forward blood flow from the vena cavae into the right atrium during RV systole may be attenuated or even reversed, and cardiac output declines because adequate RV filling cannot occur and LV preload subsequently becomes reduced. Increased RV pressure observed during pulmonary hypertension also further restricts LV filling by displacing the interventricular septum toward the LV cavity.

PERICARDIAL DISEASE

Functional anatomy of the pericardium

The pericardium is a closed, relatively noncompliant mediastinal space composed of visceral and parietal layers that contains the heart and proximal great vessels. The pericardium normally contains between 15 and 20 mL of serous fluid and serves several important functions. The pericardium provides ligamentous structure to the heart and great vessels, thereby preventing their abnormal displacement within the thoracic cavity. The pericardium maintains LV and RV compliance by resisting abrupt dilation of these cardiac chambers.[147] The pericardium also reduces cardiac friction during contraction and relaxation and provides an important barrier to inflammatory processes occurring in adjacent, external structures. The pressure within the pericardium is determined by the compliance of this structure and the volume of fluid it contains. Under normal conditions, intrapericardial pressure is negative and equal to pleural pressure. Abrupt increases in intrapericardial volume are associated with pronounced elevations in intrapericardial pressure because the pericardium is relatively inelastic (Fig. 7.18). However, intrapericardial volume may expand slowly and intrapericardial pressure rise gradually if fluid accumulation within the pericardial space occurs over time (e.g. weeks to months).[148]

Pericardial tamponade

The atria and right ventricle are low-pressure, high-compliance chambers whose filling may be compromised by increases in pressure within the relatively noncompliant pericardium. Pericardial tamponade may occur as a result of blunt or penetrating chest trauma, aortic dissection, rapidly enlarging pericardial effusions (e.g. infectious disease, neoplasm, or connective tissue disorders), or after cardiac surgery. Tamponade occurs when intrapericardial pressures rises to a sufficient degree to impede venous return to the right side of the heart. This functional hypovolemia leads to reductions in LV preload, hypotension, and shock. LV filling during diastole is also compromised because LV compliance is reduced by elevated intrapericardial pressure. Equalization of left and right ventricular end-diastolic pressures, diastolic pulmonary arterial and capillary occlusion pressures, and right atrial pressure and exaggeration of the respiratory effects on LV filling (pulsus paradoxus) are frequently observed in pericardial tamponade.[149] Compensatory tachycardia and enhanced myocardial contractility result from sympathetic nervous system activation and serve to partially preserve cardiac output. Acute myocardial ischemia may also be observed in tamponade because pronounced reductions in coronary perfusion pressure occur[150] concomitant with increases in myocardial O_2 consumption.

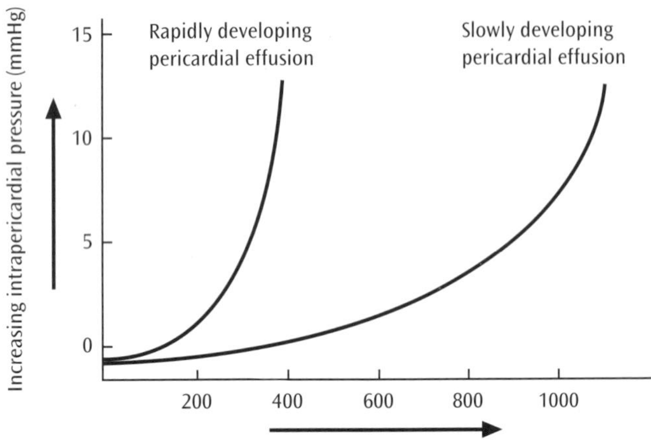

Figure 7.18 *The rate of fluid accumulation is an important determinant of changes in intrapericardial pressure. The compliance markedly decreases during a rapidly developing pericardial effusion. In contrast, a slowly developing effusion may be hemodynamically tolerated because of gradual expansion of the pericardium. Reproduced with permission.*

Constrictive pericarditis

Constrictive pericarditis may result from an infectious (e.g. tuberculosis) or neoplastic (e.g. lung or breast carcinoma) disease, connective tissue disorder, or chronic renal failure, or may appear as sequelae of myocardial infarction (Dressler's syndrome), cardiac surgery, or thoracic radiation therapy. Constrictive pericarditis is characterized by a fibrous, thickened, and inelastic pericardium that may be adherent to the external surface of the heart. Hemodynamic abnormalities associated with constrictive pericarditis are based on restricted LV and RV filling that occurs primarily during diastasis and atrial systole. In contrast to the findings in pericardial tamponade, early filling is relatively preserved in constrictive pericarditis and cardiac output may be maintained until the latter stages of the disease.[151] The RV pressure waveform often demonstrates a "square root" morphology because RV pressure rises precipitously during completion of early filling and subsequently remains relatively constant until RV systole occurs. Patients with constrictive pericarditis most often complain of progressive dyspnea and exercise intolerance and may present with signs of RV decompensation including peripheral edema, hepatic congestion, ascites, and jugular venous distension.

ARRHYTHMIAS AND CONDUCTION ABNORMALITIES

Arrhythmias are among the most frequently reported perioperative cardiovascular abnormalities (60–80%).[152,153] These arrhythmias are usually of limited duration, produce minimal hemodynamic effects, and do not require pharmacologic treatment. However, if malignant supraventricular or ventricular arrhythmias occur, cardiac performance may be seriously compromised. A recent multicenter study demonstrated that hemodynamically significant arrhythmias were responsible for up to 40% of all severe perioperative adverse outcomes.[154] Factors determining these adverse events include the ventricular rate, the duration of the tachyarrhythmias, and the functional cardiac impairment.[155] Bradyarrhythmias, especially those with loss of atrial activity, may have a profound impact on patients with LV dysfunction.[156] Arrhythmias are usually categorized by abnormalities in impulse formation or propagation. Impulse formation defects include altered automaticity of primary and latent pacemakers or triggered activity from early or delayed afterdepolarizations.[157] Abnormalities of impulse propagation include conduction blockade and re-entry of the cardiac impulse. Complex arrhythmias may be produced by combinations of abnormalities of impulse formation and propagation.

Abnormalities of impulse formation

Altered normal automaticity

The sinus node pacemaker may fail in disease states or fire very rapidly or slowly during enhanced activity of the sympathetic or parasympathetic nervous system respectively. Pacemakers in the His–Purkinje system may control cardiac rhythm as escape pacemakers. Under these conditions, sinus bradycardia or AV block reduces propagation of supraventricular impulses to a rate lower than the intrinsic rate His–Purkinje pacemakers. Myocardial ischemia or drugs that affect chronotropic state may also increase the rate of firing of His–Purkinje pacemakers.

Afterdepolarizations and triggered activity

Afterdepolarizations are defined as secondary depolarizations that occur after repolarization has begun. Triggered activity is single or repetitive firing of a cell or group of cells initiated by an afterdepolarization.

Triggered activity itself is not excitatory, but depends on the preceding action potential and afterdepolarization to initiate the process. Early afterdepolarizations often arise from the plateau of the action potential, but may also occur during the rapid phase of repolarization. Conditions that cause striking delays in repolarization, including hypokalemia, slow pacing rates, and drug toxicity, predispose for the occurrence of early afterdepolarizations. Early afterdepolarizations may also stimulate sustained rapid firing of Purkinje fibers. Ventricular myocardium will often respond to early afterdepolarizations in the adjacent Purkinje fibers because the Purkinje fiber action potential is longer than that in ventricular muscle. The torsades de pointes form of ventricular tachycardia is common in patients who display clinical conditions known to produce early afterdepolarizations.[158] Delayed afterdepolarizations are small depolarizations that occur after the cell has repolarized. This behavior is present under normal circumstances (e.g. coronary sinus myocytes[159]), and may also be observed in other cardiac cell types under abnormal conditions.[160] Delayed afterdepolarizations are typically too small to reach the threshold voltage, but their amplitude varies dynamically with changes in heart rate or firing pattern. As heart rate increases or stimulation becomes more premature, the delayed afterdepolarization may become larger and may provoke rapid firing or triggered activity after the threshold voltage is reached. Factors known to increase the amplitude of delayed afterdepolarizations include rapid pacing, premature activation, increased plasma catecholamine concentrations, and digitalis toxicity.[161]

Abnormalities of impulse propagation

Atrioventricular block

Impaired AV conduction includes four forms of AV block. First-degree AV block is present when the PR interval is greater than 0.21 s. Second-degree AV block is divided into Mobitz type I (Wenckebach) and Mobitz type II block. Progressive prolongation of the PR interval with the appearance of dropped beats is the characteristic finding of Wenckebach block. In contrast, Mobitz II block displays dropped beats without PR interval prolongation. Interruption of the AV bundle before its bifurcation produces third-degree or complete heart block. Under these conditions, the ventricles are no longer activated by impulses propagated from the atria.

Bundle branch blocks

Impulses that depolarize the left ventricle or right ventricle in patients with bundle branch block do not reach the ventricular myocardium via the rapidly conducting His–Purkinje system. Instead, the impulse that activates myocardium affected by bundle branch block is delayed because it must cross the interventricular septum through more slowly conducting ventricular myocardium. This delay in the spread of the wave of depolarization over the ventricle prolongs and deforms the QRS complex.

Re-entrant arrhythmias

The conditions that permit re-entry arrhythmias are slowed conduction and unidirectional block in some portion of the circuit (Fig. 7.19). A unidirectional block may be permanent or dynamic. The exceedingly long refractory period of cardiac muscle tends to prevent re-entry. Unless an impulse is propagated for a prolonged period, cells in the circuit will remain refractory. Conduction delay or block is usually asymmetrical in a segment of Purkinje fiber and impulses entering a depolarized zone may propagate back to re-excite the portion of fiber from which they originate.

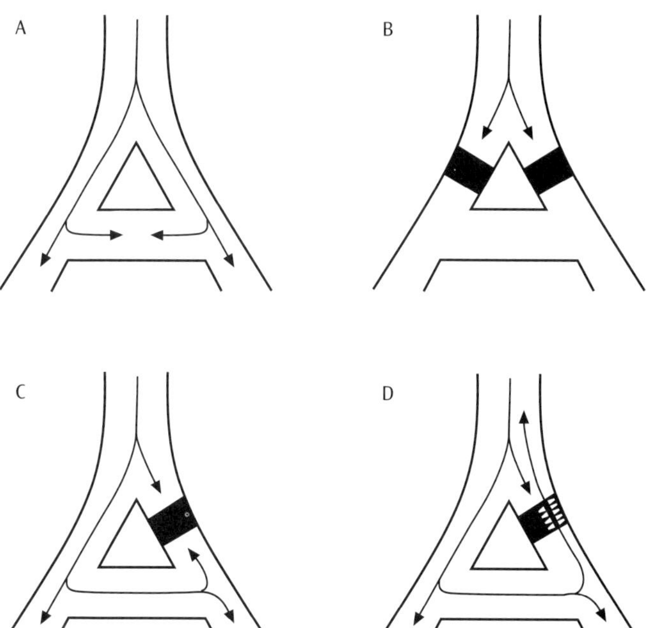

Figure 7.19 *Mechanism of re-entry arrhythmias. Under normal conditions (A), the depolarization wave is extinguished at the zone of collision between the two major bundle branches. Blockade of both branches (B) or the presence of a bidirectional block (C) does not produce re-entry. A unidirectional block with slowed conduction in some portion of the circuit (D) must be present for re-entry to occur. Impulse propagation in the antegrade direction is blocked but retrograde impulse waves re-enter and re-excite the portion of fiber from which they originate if this portion of the conduction system is allowed to recover from a refractory state.*

Anomalous connections between atria and ventricles may cause re-entrant arrhythmias and are observed in the pre-excitation syndromes. In patients with Wolff–Parkinson–White (WPW) syndrome, a functional accessory pathway causes a short PR interval and a wide QRS complex, and premature activation of the ventricles occurs because this accessory pathway conducts more rapidly than the AV node. Thus, conduction of sinus impulses uses both the AV node and the accessory pathway in this disorder. Reciprocating tachycardias in WPW syndrome may be triggered when an impulse entering the ventricles by way of the AV node (antegrade) is propagated back into the atria via the accessory pathway (retrograde). Most supraventricular tachycardias in patients with WPW are initiated by premature atrial contraction. Conduction through an accessory pathway involves Na^+ channel activation, allowing rapid impulse transmission from the atria to the ventricles. Thus, patients with pre-excitation who develop atrial fibrillation are at risk of sudden cardiac death because rapid conduction of the disorganized atrial impulses into the ventricles through an accessory pathway may produce ventricular tachycardia or fibrillation.

REFERENCES

1. Sommer JR, Jennings RB. Ultrastructure of cardiac muscle. In: Fozzard H, Haber E, Jennings, R, *et al.* (eds). *The Heart and Cardiovascular System: Scientific Foundations.* New York: Raven Press, 1992: 3–50.
2. Wegener AD, Simmerman HK, Lindemann JP, Jones LR. Phospholamban phosphorylation in intact ventricles. Phosphorylation of serine 16 and

threonine 17 in response to beta-adrenergic stimulation. *J Biol Chem* 1989; **264:** 11468–74.

3. Lue WM, Boyden PA. Abnormal electrical properties of myocytes from chronically infarcted canine heart. Alterations in V_{max} and the transient outward current. *Circulation* 1992; **85:** 1175–88.
4. Sugiura H, Toyama J, Tsuboi N, *et al.* ATP directly affects junctional conductance between paired ventricular myocytes isolated from guinea pig heart. *Circ Res* 1990; **66:** 1095–102.
5. De Mello WC. Effect of isoproterenol and 3-isobutyl-1-methylxanthine on junctional conductance in heart cell pairs. *Biochim Biophys Acta* 1989; **1012:** 291–8.
6. Zipes DP. Genesis of cardiac arrhythmias: electrophysiological considerations. In: Braunwald E (ed.). *Heart Disease: A Textbook of Cardiovascular Medicine*, 5th edn. Philadelphia: WB Saunders, 1997: 548–92.
7. Sonnenblick EH. Force–velocity relations in mamillian heart muscle. *Am J Physiol* 1962; **202:** 931–9.
8. Sonnenblick EH. Implications of muscle mechanics in the heart. *Fed Proc* 1962; **21:** 975–90.
9. Gordon AM, Huxley AF, Julian FJ. The variation in isometric tension with sarcomere length in vertebrate muscle fibres. *J Physiol* 1966; **184:** 170–92.
10. Lakatta EG. Starling's law of the heart is explained by an intimate interaction of muscle length and myofilament calcium activation. *J Am Coll Cardiol* 1987; **10:** 1157–64.
11. Kentish JC, ter Keurs HE, Ricciardi L, *et al.* Comparison between the sarcomere length–force relations of intact and skinned trabeculae from rat right ventricle. Influence of calcium concentrations on these relations. *Circ Res* 1986; **58:** 755–68.
12. Allen DG, Kentish JC. Calcium concentration in the myoplasm of skinned ferret ventricular muscle following changes in muscle length. *J Physiol* 1988; **407:** 489–503.
13. Murphy R. Contraction of muscle cells. In: Berne RM, Levy MN (eds). *Physiology*. St. Louis: CV Mosby, 1983: 359–86.
14. Brenner B. Effects of Ca^{2+} cross-bridge turnover kinetics in skinned single rabbit psoas fibers. *Proc Natl Acad Sci USA* 1988; **85:** 3265–9.
15. Fifer MA, Grossman W. Measurement of ventricular volumes, ejection fraction, mass, wall stress, and regional wall motion. In: Grossman W, Baim DS (eds). *Cardiac Catheterization, Angiography, and Intervention*, 4th edn. Philadelphia: Lea & Febiger, 1991: 300–18.
16. Smith JJ, Kampine JP. *Circulatory Physiology – the Essentials*, 3rd edn. Baltimore: Williams & Wilkins, 1990.
17. Frank O. Die Grundform des arteriellen Pulses. *Z Biol* 1898; **37:** 483–526.
18. Sagawa K, Maughan L, Suga H, Sunagawa K. *Cardiac Contraction and the Pressure–Volume Relationship*. New York: Oxford University Press, 1988.
19. Sagawa K, Suga H, Shoukas AA, Bakalar KM. End-systolic pressure/volume ratio: a new index of ventricular contractility. *Am J Cardiol* 1977; **40:** 748–53.
20. Glower DD, Spratt JA, Snow ND, *et al.* Linearity of the Frank–Starling relationship in the intact heart: the concept of preload recruitable stroke work. *Circulation* 1985; **71:** 994–1009.
21. Pagel PS, Kampine JP, Schmeling WT, Warltier DC. Comparison of end-systolic pressure–length relations and preload recruitable stroke work as indices of myocardial contractility in the conscious and anesthetized, chronically instrumented dog. *Anesthesiology* 1990; **73:** 278–90.
22. Kass DA, Midei M, Brinker J, Maughan WL. Influence of coronary occlusion during PTCA on end-systolic and end-diastolic pressure–volume relations in humans. *Circulation* 1990; **81:** 447–60.
23. Gould KL, Lipscomb K, Hamilton GW, Kennedy JW. Relation of left ventricular shape, function and wall stress in man. *Am J Cardiol* 1974; **34:** 627–34.
24. Weber KT, Janicki JS. Myocardial oxygen consumption: the role of wall force and shortening. *Am J Physiol* 1977; **233:** H421–30.
25. Sunagawa K, Maughan WL, Burkhoff D, Sagawa K. Left ventricular interaction with arterial load studied in isolated canine ventricle. *Am J Physiol* 1983; **245:** H773–80.
26. Grossman W. Diastolic dysfunction and congestive heart failure. *Circulation* 1990; **81:** III1–7.
27. Zile MR, Brutsaert DL. New concepts in diastolic dysfunction and diastolic heart failure. Part I. Diagnosis, prognosis, and measurements of diastolic function. *Circulation* 2002; **105:** 1387–93.
28. Zile MR, Brutsaert DL. New concepts in diastolic dysfunction and diastolic heart failure. Part II. Causal mechanisms and treatment. *Circulation* 2002; **105:** 1503–8.
29. Sabbah HN, Stein PD. Pressure–diameter relations during early diastole in dogs. Incompatibility with the concept of passive left ventricular filling. *Circ Res* 1981; **48:** 357–65.
30. Pearson AC, Labovitz AJ, Mrosek D, *et al.* Assessment of diastolic function in normal and hypertrophied hearts: comparison of Doppler echocardiography and M-mode echocardiography. *Am Heart J* 1987; **113:** 1417–25.
31. Appleton CP, Hatle LK, Popp RL. Relation of transmitral flow velocity patterns to left ventricular diastolic function: new insights from a combined hemodynamic and Doppler echocardiographic study. *J Am Coll Cardiol* 1988; **12:** 426–40.
32. Armour JA, Pace JB, Randall WC. Interrelationship of architecture and function of the right ventricle. *Am J Physiol* 1970; **218:** 174–9.
33. Meier GD, Bove AA, Santamore WP, Lynch PR. Contractile function in canine right ventricle. *Am J Physiol* 1980; **239:** H794–804.
34. Myhre ES, Slinker BK, LeWinter MM. Absence of right ventricular isovolumic relaxation in open-chest anesthetized dogs. *Am J Physiol* 1992; **263:** H1587–90.
35. Pouleur H, Lefevre J, Van Mechelen H, Charlier AA. Free-wall shortening and relaxation during ejection in the canine right ventricle. *Am J Physiol* 1980; **239:** H601–13.
36. Kyriakidis MK, Kourouklis CB, Papaioannou JT, *et al.* Sinus node coronary arteries studied with angiography. *Am J Cardiol* 1983; **51:** 749–50.
37. Bittl JA, Levin DC. Coronary arteriography. In: Braunwald E (ed.). *Heart Disease: A Textbook of Cardiovascular Medicine*, 5th edn. Philadelphia: WB Saunders, 1997: 240–72.
38. Katz AM. Structure of the heart and cardiac muscle. In: Katz AM (ed.). *Physiology of the Heart*, 2nd edn. New York: Raven Press, 1992: 15.
39. Mosher P, Ross JJ, McFate PA, Shaw RF. Control of coronary blood flow by an autoregulatory mechanism. *Circ Res* 1964; **14:** 250–9.
40. Bassenge E, Heusch G. Endothelial and neuro-humoral control of coronary blood flow in health and disease. *Rev Physiol Biochem Pharmacol* 1990; **116:** 77–165.
41. Broten TP, Romson JL, Fullerton DA, *et al.* Synergistic action of myocardial oxygen and carbon dioxide in controlling coronary blood flow. *Circ Res* 1991;**68:**531–42.
42. Rubio R, Berne RM. Release of adenosine by the normal myocardium in dogs and its relationship to the regulation of coronary resistance. *Circ Res* 1969; **25:** 407–15.
43. Hamilton FN, Feigl EO. Coronary vascular sympathetic beta-receptor innervation. *Am J Physiol* 1976; **230:** 1569–76.
44. Chilian WM, Layne SM, Eastham CL, Marcus ML. Heterogeneous microvascular coronary alpha-adrenergic vasoconstriction. *Circ Res* 1989; **64:** 376–88.
45. Feigl EO. Coronary physiology. *Physiol Rev* 1983; **63:** 1–205.
46. Mangano DT. Perioperative cardiac morbidity. *Anesthesiology* 1990; **72:** 153–84.
47. Gutstein DE, Fuster V. Pathophysiology and clinical significance of atherosclerotic plaque rupture. *Cardiovasc Res* 1999; **41:** 323–33.
48. Falk E, Shah PK, Fuster V. Coronary plaque disruption. *Circulation* 1995; **92:** 657–71.
49. Davies MJ. Stability and instability: two faces of coronary atherosclerosis. The Paul Dudley White Lecture 1995. *Circulation* 1996; **94:** 2013–20.
50. Stamler J, Berkson DM, Lindberg HA. Risk factors: their role in the etiology and pathogenesis of the atherosclerotic diseases. In: Wissler RW, Geer JC, Kaufman N (eds). *The Pathogenesis of Atherosclerosis*. Baltimore: Williams & Wilkins, **1972:** 41–119.
51. Yeghiazarians Y, Braunstein JB, Askari A, Stone PH. Unstable angina pectoris. *N Engl J Med* 2000; **342:** 101–14.
52. Warltier DC, Buck JD, Brooks HL, Gross GJ. Coronary hemodynamics and subendocardial perfusion distal to stenoses. *Int J Cardiol* 1983; **4:** 173–83.
53. Warltier DC, Hardman HF, Gross GJ. Transmural perfusion gradients distal to various degrees of coronary artery stenosis during resting flow or at maximal vasodilation. *Basic Res Cardiol* 1979; **74:** 494–508.
54. Kuo L, Davis MJ, Cannon MS, Chilian WM. Pathophysiological consequences of atherosclerosis extend into the coronary microcirculation. Restoration of endothelium-dependent responses by L-arginine. *Circ Res* 1992; **70:** 465–76.
55. Topol EJ, Ellis SG. Coronary collaterals revisited. Accessory pathway to myocardial preservation during infarction. *Circulation* 1991; **83:** 1084–6.
56. Hirai T, Fujita M, Nakajima H, *et al.* Importance of collateral circulation for prevention of left ventricular aneurysm formation in acute myocardial infarction. *Circulation* 1989; **79:** 791–6.
57. Schaper W, Gorge G, Winkler B, Schaper J. The collateral circulation of the heart. *Prog Cardiovasc Dis* 1988; **31:** 57–77.
58. Forman MB, Collins HW, Kopelman HA, *et al.* Determinants of left ventricular aneurysm formation after anterior myocardial infarction: a clinical and angiographic study. *J Am Coll Cardiol* 1986; **8:** 1256–62.

59. Juilliere Y, Danchin N, Grentzinger A, *et al.* Role of previous angina pectoris and collateral flow to preserve left ventricular function in the presence or absence of myocardial infarction in isolated total occlusion of the left anterior descending coronary artery. *Am J Cardiol* 1990; **65:** 277–81.
60. Sedlis SP, Cohen KH, Sequeira JM, el-Sherif N. Preservation of left ventricular function in patients with total occlusion of the left anterior descending coronary artery and wide-caliber distal vessel filling by collateral vasculature. *Cathet Cardiovasc Diagn* 1988; **15:** 139–42.
61. Warltier DC, Zyvoloski MG, Gross GJ, Brooks HL. Importance of retrograde coronary flow in the prediction of experimental myocardial infarct size. *Cardiology* 1986; **73:** 333–46.
62. Kersten JR, Pagel PS, Chilian WM, Warltier DC. Multifactorial basis for coronary collateralization: a complex adaptive response to ischemia. *Cardiovasc Res* 1999; **43:** 44–57.
63. Epstein SE, Fuchs S, Zhou YF, *et al.* Therapeutic interventions for enhancing collateral development by administration of growth factors: basic principles, early results and potential hazards. *Cardiovasc Res* 2001; **49:** 532–42.
64. Becker LC. Conditions for vasodilator-induced coronary steal in experimental myocardial ischemia. *Circulation* 1978; **57:** 1103–10.
65. Warltier DC, Gross GJ, Brooks HL. Coronary steal-induced increase in myocardial infarct size after pharmacologic coronary vasodilation. *Am J Cardiol* 1980; **46:** 83–90.
66. Buffington CW, Davis KB, Gillispie S, Pettinger M. The prevalence of steal-prone coronary anatomy in patients with coronary artery disease: an analysis of the Coronary Artery Surgery Study Registry. *Anesthesiology* 1988; **69:** 721–7.
67. Allen DG, Orchard CH. Myocardial contractile function during ischemia and hypoxia. *Circ Res* 1987; **60:** 153–68.
68. Schwaiger M, Neese RA, Araujo L, *et al.* Sustained nonoxidative glucose utilization and depletion of glycogen in reperfused canine myocardium. *J Am Coll Cardiol* 1989; **13:** 745–54.
69. Koretsune Y, Corretti MC, Kusuoka H, Marban E. Mechanism of early ischemic contractile failure. Inexcitability, metabolite accumulation, or vascular collapse? *Circ Res* 1991; **68:** 255–62.
70. Serruys PW, Wijns W, van den Brand M, *et al.* Left ventricular performance, regional blood flow, wall motion, and lactate metabolism during transluminal angioplasty. *Circulation* 1984; **70:** 25–36.
71. Goto Y, Igarashi Y, Yamada O, *et al.* Hyperkinesis without the Frank–Starling mechanism in a nonischemic region of acutely ischemic excised canine heart. *Circulation* 1988; **77:** 468–77.
72. Bolli R, Marban E. Molecular and cellular mechanisms of myocardial stunning. *Physiol Rev* 1999; **79:** 609–34.
73. Braunwald E, Kloner RA. The stunned myocardium: prolonged, postischemic ventricular dysfunction. *Circulation* 1982; **66:** 1146–9.
74. Charlat ML, O'Neill PG, Hartley CJ, *et al.* Prolonged abnormalities of left ventricular diastolic wall thinning in the "stunned" myocardium in conscious dogs: time course and relation to systolic function. *J Am Coll Cardiol* 1989; **13:** 185–94.
75. Marban E, Koretsune Y, Corretti M, *et al.* Calcium and its role in myocardial cell injury during ischemia and reperfusion. *Circulation* 1989; **80:** IV17–22.
76. Reimer KA, Hill ML, Jennings RB. Prolonged depletion of ATP and of the adenine nucleotide pool due to delayed resynthesis of adenine nucleotides following reversible myocardial ischemic injury in dogs. *J Mol Cell Cardiol* 1981; **13:** 229–39.
77. Engler R, Covell JW. Granulocytes cause reperfusion ventricular dysfunction after 15-minute ischemia in the dog. *Circ Res* 1987; **61:** 20–8.
78. Hammond B, Hess ML. The oxygen free radical system: potential mediator of myocardial injury. *J Am Coll Cardiol* 1985; **6:** 215–20.
79. Marban E. Myocardial stunning and hibernation. The physiology behind the colloquialisms. *Circulation* 1991; **83:** 681–8.
80. Krause SM, Jacobus WE, Becker LC. Alterations in cardiac sarcoplasmic reticulum calcium transport in the postischemic "stunned" myocardium. *Circ Res* 1989; **65:** 526–30.
81. Simpson PJ, Todd RFD, Mickelson JK, *et al.* Sustained limitation of myocardial reperfusion injury by a monoclonal antibody that alters leukocyte function. *Circulation* 1990; **81:** 226–37.
82. Manning AS, Hearse DJ. Reperfusion-induced arrhythmias: mechanisms and prevention. *J Mol Cell Cardiol* 1984; **16:** 497–518.
83. Sheridan DJ, Penkoske PA, Sobel BE, Corr PB. Alpha adrenergic contributions to dysrhythmia during myocardial ischemia and reperfusion in cats. *J Clin Invest* 1980; **65:** 161–71.
84. Opie LH. Role of calcium and other ions in reperfusion injury. *Cardiovasc Drugs Ther* 1991; **5:** 237–47.
85. Homans DC, Sublett E, Dai XZ, Bache RJ. Persistence of regional left ventricular dysfunction after exercise-induced myocardial ischemia. *J Clin Invest* 1986; **77:** 66–73.
86. Kloner RA, Przyklenk K, Whittaker P. Deleterious effects of oxygen radicals in ischemia/reperfusion. Resolved and unresolved issues. *Circulation* 1989; **80:** 1115–27.
87. Braunwald E, Rutherford JD. Reversible ischemic left ventricular dysfunction: evidence for the "hibernating myocardium." *J Am Coll Cardiol* 1986; **8:** 1467–70.
88. Frangogiannis NG, Smith CW, Entman ML. The inflammatory response in myocardial infarction. *Cardiovasc Res* 2002; **53:** 31–47.
89. Maytin M, Colucci WS. Molecular and cellular mechanisms of myocardial remodeling. *J Nucl Cardiol* 2002; **9:** 319–27.
90. Pfeffer MA, Braunwald E. Ventricular remodeling after myocardial infarction. Experimental observations and clinical implications. *Circulation* 1990; **81:** 1161–72.
91. Murry CE, Jennings RB, Reimer KA. Preconditioning with ischemia: a delay of lethal cell injury in ischemic myocardium. *Circulation* 1986; **74:** 1124–36.
92. Auchampach JA, Grover GJ, Gross GJ. Blockade of ischaemic preconditioning in dogs by the novel ATP dependent potassium channel antagonist sodium 5-hydroxydecanoate. *Cardiovasc Res* 1992; **26:** 1054–62.
93. Yao Z, Gross GJ. A comparison of adenosine-induced cardioprotection and ischemic preconditioning in dogs. Efficacy, time course, and role of K_{ATP} channels. *Circulation* 1994; **89:** 1229–36.
94. Baxter GF, Ferdinandy P. Delayed preconditioning of myocardium: current perspectives. *Basic Res Cardiol* 2001; **96:** 329–44.
95. Lorell BH, Carabello BA. Left ventricular hypertrophy: pathogenesis, detection, and prognosis. *Circulation* 2000; **102:** 470–9.
96. Grossman W, Jones D, McLaurin LP. Wall stress and patterns of hypertrophy in the human left ventricle. *J Clin Invest* 1975; **56:** 56–64.
97. Moalic JM, Charlemagne D, Mansier P, *et al.* Cardiac hypertrophy and failure – a disease of adaptation. Modifications in membrane proteins provide a molecular basis for arrhythmogenicity. *Circulation* 1993; **87:** IV21–6.
98. Hunter JJ, Chien KR. Signaling pathways for cardiac hypertrophy and failure. *N Engl J Med* 1999; **341:** 1276–83.
99. Pfeffer JM, Pfeffer MA, Mirsky I, Braunwald E. Regression of left ventricular hypertrophy and prevention of left ventricular dysfunction by captopril in the spontaneously hypertensive rat. *Proc Natl Acad Sci USA* 1982; **79:** 3310–14.
100. Bonow RO, Dodd JT, Maron BJ, *et al.* Long-term serial changes in left ventricular function and reversal of ventricular dilatation after valve replacement for chronic aortic regurgitation. *Circulation* 1988; **78:** 1108–20.
101. Shah PM, Taylor RD, Wong M. Abnormal mitral valve coaptation in hypertrophic obstructive cardiomyopathy: proposed role in systolic anterior motion of mitral valve. *Am J Cardiol* 1981; **48:** 258–62.
102. Maron BJ, Spirito P, Green KJ, *et al.* Noninvasive assessment of left ventricular diastolic function by pulsed Doppler echocardiography in patients with hypertrophic cardiomyopathy. *J Am Coll Cardiol* 1987; **10:** 733–42.
103. McKenna WJ. The natural history of hypertrophic cardiomyopathy. *Cardiovasc Clin* 1988; **19:** 135–48.
104. Gavazzi A, De Maria R, Parolini M, Porcu M. Alcohol abuse and dilated cardiomyopathy in men. *Am J Cardiol* 2000; **85:** 1114–18.
105. Piano MR. Alcoholic cardiomyopathy: incidence, clinical characteristics, and pathophysiology. *Chest* 2002; **121:** 1638–50.
106. Rahko PS, Orie JE. The clinical presentation and laboratory evaluation of congestive and ischemic cardiomyopathies. *Cardiovasc Clin* 1988; **19:** 75–119.
107. Katritsis D, Wilmshurst PT, Wendon JA, *et al.* Primary restrictive cardiomyopathy: clinical and pathologic characteristics. *J Am Coll Cardiol* 1991; **18:** 1230–5.
108. Wilmshurst PT, Katritsis D. Restrictive cardiomyopathy. *Br Heart J* 1990; **63:** 323–4.
109. Harpole DH, Jones RH. Serial assessment of ventricular performance after valve replacement for aortic stenosis. *J Thorac Cardiovasc Surg* 1990; **99:** 645–50.
110. Danielsen R, Nordrehaug JE, Vik-Mo H. Clinical and haemodynamic features in relation to severity of aortic stenosis in adults. *Eur Heart J* 1991; **12:** 791–5.
111. Diver DJ, Royal HD, Aroesty JM, *et al.* Diastolic function in patients with aortic stenosis: influence of left ventricular load reduction. *J Am Coll Cardiol* 1988; **12:** 642–8.
112. Murakami T, Hess OM, Gage JE, *et al.* Diastolic filling dynamics in patients with aortic stenosis. *Circulation* 1986; **73:** 1162–74.
113. Hakki AH, Kimbiris D, Iskandrian AS, *et al.* Angina pectoris and coronary

artery disease in patients with severe aortic valvular disease. *Am Heart J* 1980; **100:** 441–9.

114. Smucker ML, Tedesco CL, Manning SB, *et al.* Demonstration of an imbalance between coronary perfusion and excessive load as a mechanism of ischemia during stress in patients with aortic stenosis. *Circulation* 1988; **78:** 573–82.
115. Marcus ML, Doty DB, Hiratzka LF, *et al.* Decreased coronary reserve: a mechanism for angina pectoris in patients with aortic stenosis and normal coronary arteries. *N Engl J Med* 1982; **307:** 1362–6.
116. Klein RC. Ventricular arrhythmias in aortic valve disease: analysis of 102 patients. *Am J Cardiol* 1984; **53:** 1079–83.
117. Belenkie I, Rademaker A. Acute and chronic changes after aortic valve damage in the intact dog. *Am J Physiol* 1981; **241:** H95–103.
118. Downes TR, Nomeir AM, Hackshaw BT, *et al.* Diastolic mitral regurgitation in acute but not chronic aortic regurgitation: implications regarding the mechanism of mitral closure. *Am Heart J* 1989; **117:** 1106–12.
119. Iskandrian AS, Hakki AH, Manno B, *et al.* Left ventricular function in chronic aortic regurgitation. *J Am Coll Cardiol* 1983; **1:** 1374–80.
120. Bonow RO. Left ventricular structure and function in aortic valve disease. *Circulation* 1989; **79:** 966–9.
121. Siemienczuk D, Greenberg B, Morris C, *et al.* Chronic aortic insufficiency: factors associated with progression to aortic valve replacement. *Ann Intern Med* 1989; **110:** 587–92.
122. Starling MR, Kirsh MM, Montgomery DG, Gross MD. Mechanisms for left ventricular systolic dysfunction in aortic regurgitation: importance for predicting the functional response to aortic valve replacement [see comments]. *J Am Coll Cardiol* 1991; **17:** 887–97.
123. Greenberg BH, DeMots H, Murphy E, Rahimtoola SH. Mechanism for improved cardiac performance with arteriolar dilators in aortic insufficiency. *Circulation* 1981; **63:** 263–8.
124. Borow KM, Marcus RH. Aortic regurgitation: the need for an integrated physiologic approach. *J Am Coll Cardiol* 1991; **17:** 898–900.
125. Kinare SG, Kulkarni HL. Quantitative study of the mitral valve in chronic rheumatic heart disease. *Int J Cardiol* 1987; **16:** 271–84.
126. Gash AK, Carabello BA, Cepin D, Spann JF. Left ventricular ejection performance and systolic muscle function in patients with mitral stenosis. *Circulation* 1983; **67:** 148–54.
127. Leavitt JI, Coats MH, Falk RH. Effects of exercise on transmitral gradient and pulmonary artery pressure in patients with mitral stenosis or a prosthetic mitral valve: a Doppler echocardiographic study. *J Am Coll Cardiol* 1991; **17:** 1520–6.
128. Stott DK, Marpole DG, Bristow JD, *et al.* The role of left atrial transport in aortic and mitral stenosis. *Circulation* 1970; **41:** 1031–41.
129. Izumi S, Miyatake K, Beppu S, *et al.* Mechanism of mitral regurgitation in patients with myocardial infarction: a study using real-time two-dimensional Doppler flow imaging and echocardiography. *Circulation* 1987; **76:** 777–85.
130. Balu V, Hershowitz S, Zaki Masud AR, *et al.* Mitral regurgitation in coronary artery disease. *Chest* 1982; **81:** 550–5.
131. Rankin JS, Feneley MP, Hickey MS, *et al.* A clinical comparison of mitral valve repair versus valve replacement in ischemic mitral regurgitation. *J Thorac Cardiovasc Surg* 1988; **95:** 165–77.
132. Roberts WC, Braunwald E, Morrow AG. Acute severe mitral regurgitation secondary to ruptured chordae tendineae: clinical, hemodynamic, and pathologic considerations. *Circulation* 1966; **33:** 58–70.
133. Carabello BA. The pathophysiology of mitral regurgitation. *J Heart Valve Dis* 2000; **9:** 600–8.
134. Yoran C, Yellin EL, Becker RM, *et al.* Dynamic aspects of acute mitral regurgitation: effects of ventricular volume, pressure and contractility on the effective regurgitant orifice area. *Circulation* 1979; **60:** 170–6.
135. Eckberg DL, Gault JH, Bouchard RL, *et al.* Mechanics of left ventricular contraction in chronic severe mitral regurgitation. *Circulation* 1973; **47:** 1252–9.
136. Urabe Y, Mann DL, Kent RL, *et al.* Cellular and ventricular contractile dysfunction in experimental canine mitral regurgitation. *Circ Res* 1992; **70:** 131–47.
137. Glancy DL, Marcus FI, Cuadra M, *et al.* Isolated organic tricuspid valvular regurgitation. Causes and consequences. *Am J Med* 1969; **46:** 989–96.
138. Waller BF. Etiology of pure tricuspid regurgitation. *Cardiovasc Clin* 1987; **17:** 53–95.
139. Cohen SR, Sell JE, McIntosh CL, Clark RE. Tricuspid regurgitation in patients with acquired, chronic, pure mitral regurgitation. I. Prevalence, diagnosis, and comparison of preoperative clinical and hemodynamic features in patients with and without tricuspid regurgitation. *J Thorac Cardiovasc Surg* 1987; **94:** 481–7.
140. Lundin L, Norheim I, Landelius J, *et al.* Carcinoid heart disease: relationship of circulating vasoactive substances to ultrasound-detectable cardiac abnormalities. *Circulation* 1988; **77:** 264–9.
141. Cannon NS, Cabbs CS. Infective endocarditis in drug addicts. In: Kaye D (ed.). *Infective Endocarditis*. Baltimore: University Park Press, 1**976:** 111–27.
142. Froom P, Krivisky M, Ribak J, *et al.* Systolic tricuspid leaflet prolapse in asymptomatic young men [see comments]. *Clin Cardiol* 1989; **12:** 697–700.
143. Giuliani ER, Fuster V, Brandenburg RO, Mair DD. Ebstein's anomaly: the clinical features and natural history of Ebstein's anomaly of the tricuspid valve. *Mayo Clin Proc* 1979; **54:** 163–73.
144. Stewart D, Leman RB, Kaiser J, Mann DL. Catheter-induced tricuspid regurgitation. Incidence and clinical significance. *Chest* 1991; **99:** 651–5.
145. Bertrand S, Laquay N, El Rassi I, Vouhe P. Tricuspid insufficiency after blunt chest trauma in a nine-year-old child. *Eur J Cardiothorac Surg* 1999; **16:** 587–9.
146. Gayet C, Pierre B, Delahaye JP, *et al.* Traumatic tricuspid insufficiency. An underdiagnosed disease. *Chest* 1987; **92:** 429–32.
147. Lee JM, Boughner DR. Mechanical properties of human pericardium. Differences in viscoelastic response when compared with canine pericardium. *Circ Res* 1985; **57:** 475–81.
148. Freeman GL, LeWinter MM. Pericardial adaptations during chronic cardiac dilation in dogs. *Circ Res* 1984; **54:** 294–300.
149. Reddy PS, Curtiss EI, O'Toole JD, Shaver JA. Cardiac tamponade: hemodynamic observations in man. *Circulation* 1978; **58:** 265–72.
150. Wechsler AS, Auerbach BJ, Graham TC, Sabiston Jr DC. Distribution of intramyocardial blood flow during pericardial tamponade. Correlation with microscopic anatomy and intrinsic myocardial contractility. *J Thorac Cardiovasc Surg* 1974; **68:** 847–56.
151. Gaasch WH, Peterson KL, Shabetai R. Left ventricular function in chronic constrictive pericarditis. *Am J Cardiol* 1974; **34:** 107–10.
152. Katz RL, Bigger Jr JT. Cardiac arrhythmias during anesthesia and operation. *Anesthesiology* 1970; **33:** 193–213.
153. Bertrand CA, Steiner NV, Jameson AG, Lopez M. Disturbances of cardiac rhythm during anesthesia and surgery. *JAMA* 1971; **216:** 1615–17.
154. Forrest JB, Rehder K, Cahalan MK, Goldsmith CH. Multicenter study of general anesthesia. III. Predictors of severe perioperative adverse outcomes. *Anesthesiology* 1992; **76:** 3–15.
155. Atlee JL. Perioperative cardiac dysrhythmias: diagnosis and management. *Anesthesiology* 1997; **86:** 1397–424.
156. Brutsaert DL, Sys SU, Gillebert TC. Diastolic failure: pathophysiology and therapeutic implications. *J Am Coll Cardiol* 1993; **22:** 318–25.
157. Atlee JL, Bosnjak ZJ. Mechanisms for cardiac dysrhythmias during anesthesia. *Anesthesiology* 1990; **72:** 347–74.
158. el-Sherif N, Bekheit SS, Henkin R. Quinidine-induced long QTU interval and torsade de pointes: role of bradycardia-dependent early afterdepolarizations. *J Am Coll Cardiol* 1989; **14:** 252–7.
159. Wit AL, Cranefield PF. Triggered and automatic activity in the canine coronary sinus. *Circ Res* 1977; **41:** 434–45.
160. Gilmour Jr RF, Heger JJ, Prystowsky EN, Zipes DP. Cellular electrophysiologic abnormalities of diseased human ventricular myocardium. *Am J Cardiol* 1983; **51:** 137–44.
161. Kass RS, Tsien RW, Weingart R. Ionic basis of transient inward current induced by strophanthidin in cardiac Purkinje fibres. *J Physiol* 1978; **281:** 209–26.

8

Drugs acting on the cardiovascular system

PIERRE FOËX

ADRENERGIC AGONISTS AND ANTAGONISTS

Adrenergic receptors

Catecholamines produce a wide range of effects mediated by the activation of adrenoceptors. These receptors have been subclassified into α- and β-receptors, themselves subdivided into α_1- and α_2-receptors and β_1- and β_2-receptors respectively.[1–4] Dopaminergic receptors have also been subdivided into two subtypes: the presynaptic D_2- and the postsynaptic D_1-receptors.

α- and β-adrenoceptors are membrane receptors with seven membrane-spanning domains linked to guanine nucleotide binding regulatory proteins (G-proteins).[5] The G-proteins are involved in the activation of one or more second-messenger effector systems such as adenylate cyclase, phospholipases, potassium and calcium ion channels, and the sodium/proton (Na^+/H^+) antiport. α-Adrenoceptors should be subdivided into at least four subtypes (α_{1A}, α_{1B}, α_{2A}, α_{2B}). This subdivision is becoming clinically relevant as α_2-adrenoceptor agonists (clonidine, azepexole, dexmedetomidine) play a role in anesthesia, pain relief, and ischemia prevention.

Receptors have two main characteristics: (1) affinity for a specific molecule (the transmitter) and (2) triggering of a chain of reactions leading to a physiologic response. Chemicals other than the natural transmitters may bind to the receptor and cause either activation (agonists) or inactivation (antagonists). Receptors may be located on the cell membrane, in the cytoplasm, or at the surface of intracellular organelles. The wide variety of locations of adrenergic receptors (Table 8.1) explains the multiplicity of the effects of adrenergic stimulation.

Table 8.1 *Location of adrenergic receptors*

Location	Subtype of receptor
Heart	β_1, β_2, α_1
Blood vessels	α_1, α_2, β_1, β_2
Lungs (bronchi)	β_2, β_1, α_1
Gut	α_1, β_1
Uterus	α_1, β_2
Eye	α_1, β_2
Skin	α_1
Liver	α_1
Kidney	β_1, α_2
Pancreas	β_2, α_2
Adipose tissue	β_1
Platelets	α_2

Desensitization of adrenergic receptors causes a reduction in the efficacy of an agonist for the receptor. It may occur because of uncoupling of the receptor G-protein, sequestration of the receptors into intracellular vesicles, or destruction of the receptors. The last is termed downregulation. With low catecholamine background activity, the number of receptors increases (upregulation). Conversely, exposure to high catecholamine concentrations (chronic cardiac failure, pheochromocytoma) decreases the number of receptors (downregulation). This also occurs after administration of exogenous catecholamines and their derivatives.[6] Chronic β-adrenoceptor blockade causes an increase in β-adrenoceptor density. This may contribute to the rebound hypertension and worsening of myocardial ischemia that are observed after abrupt withdrawal of β-adrenoceptor blockade.[7]

Postsynaptic α_1- and β_1-receptors are sensitive to norepinephrine (noradrenaline), whereas presynaptic receptors are sensitive to epinephrine (adrenaline). Because of these differences in sensitivity, α_1- and β_1-receptors behave as transmitter receptors, whereas presynaptic α_2- and β_2-receptors behave as hormonal receptors.

In usual situations, cardiovascular regulation is influenced mostly by activation of sympathetic nerve endings (α_1- and β_1-receptors). However, in stress situations, epinephrine is liberated and there is intense stimulation at α_2- and β_2-receptors.

Three types of drugs interact with the receptors: agonists, partial agonists, and antagonists. Most of the interactions are competitive. In the presence of an antagonist, the dose–response curve to the agonist is displaced to the right (Fig. 8.1). Partial agonists exert a stimulating effect on the receptors and prevent the association of agonists with the receptors.

Adrenergic agonists

Norepinephrine, epinephrine, and dopamine are naturally occurring catecholamines that, with their structurally related synthetic derivatives, appear to act on at least five types of receptors (Table 8.2). Stimulation of the postsynaptic α_1-receptors causes peripheral arteriolar constriction and venoconstriction. Stimulation of the presynaptic α_2-receptors decreases the release of the neurotransmitter. β_1-Receptor stimulation is responsible for most of the cardiac effects and β_2-receptor stimulation for most of the peripheral effects of β-adrenergic stimulation. However, β_2-receptors are also found in the myocardium. They constitute 15% of the population of β-adrenoceptors in ventricular muscle and 25% in atrial muscle. Finally, specific dopaminergic receptors in the renal, mesenteric, coronary, and cerebral vascular beds are the mediators of

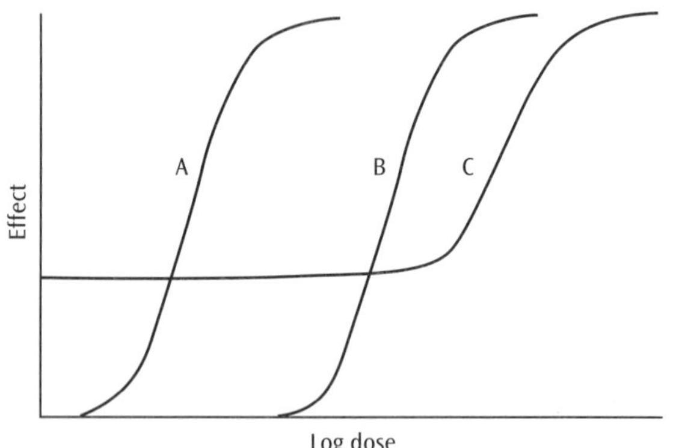

Figure 8.1 *Dose–response curves: effects of pure antagonists and partial agonists. A, Dose–response to a pure agonist; B, dose–response in the presence of an antagonist; C, dose–response in the presence of a partial agonist.*

Table 8.2 *Major sites of action of adrenergic agonists*

	Receptors				
Drug	α_1	α_2	β_1	β_2	**Dopaminergic**
Norepinephrine	+++	+++	+	+	
Epinephrine	+	+	+	+	
Isoprenaline			+	+	
Dopamine					
LD					+
MD			+		
HD	+		+		
Dobutamine			+	(+)	
Salbutamol				+	

Norepinephrine (noradrenaline); epinephrine (adrenaline).
LD, low dose (< 5 μg kg^{-1} min^{-1}); MD, doses between 5 and 15 μg kg^{-1} min^{-1}; HD, doses in excess of 15 μg kg^{-1} min^{-1}.
(+), Weak effect; +, moderate effect; +++, very strong effect.

dopamine-induced vasodilation. This response is most pronounced in the mesenteric and renal arteriolar territories. The hemodynamic effects of adrenergic receptor stimulation are summarized in Table 8.3.

With the exception of salbutamol and low-dose dopamine, which are used to obtain either bronchodilation or peripheral or splanchnic and renal vasodilation, catecholamines are predominantly used to increase the inotropic state of the myocardium and to increase arterial pressure. Unless the drug causes vasodilation (e.g. isoprenaline, dobutamine, and dopexamine), arterial pressure increases because of the improved performance of the cardiac pump and/or peripheral vasoconstriction.

Catecholamines and their derivatives are used in the treatment of cardiogenic shock following myocardial infarction, in the treatment of cardiac failure following cardiac surgery, in the treatment of circulatory failure complicating septicemia, to improve cardiac performance during artificial ventilation with positive end-expiratory pressure, and, at times, to increase cardiac output above the normal range to improve oxygen delivery and oxygen consumption. As increases in inotropy are usually associated with increases in heart rate, myocardial oxygen consumption may increase markedly. In patients with coronary heart disease, this may cause myocardial ischemia.

Hemodynamic profile of the catecholamines

The hemodynamic profile of some of the catecholamines used in clinical practice is summarized in Fig. 8.2; usual doses are listed in Table 8.4. For most of the catecholamines, administration by continuous infusion is necessary because of their very short duration of action.

Table 8.3 *Cardiovascular effects of adrenergic receptor stimulation*

Receptor	Effects
α_1	Peripheral vasoconstriction Venoconstriction Increased inotropy
α_2	Presynaptic sympathetic inhibition Vasoconstriction
β_1	Positive chronotropy Positive inotropy Increased atrioventricular conduction Increased myocardial excitability
β_2	Peripheral vasodilation Presynaptic sympathetic stimulation Positive chronotropy Increased atrioventricular conduction
DA_1	Renal vasodilation Mesenteric vasodilation
DA_2	Presynaptic dopaminergic inhibition

Norepinephrine

The main hemodynamic effects of norepinephrine are α-adrenoceptor-mediated arteriolar vasoconstriction, venoconstriction and β_1-adrenoceptor-mediated positive inotropy, which result in increases in arterial pressure while cardiac output may increase or decrease. In response to the increase in arterial pressure, there is a baroreceptor-mediated bradycardia. Renal, hepatic, and muscle blood flows are generally reduced. However, in septic shock, normalization of hemodynamic activity by norepinephrine improves renal function.[8] The effects of norepinephrine on the myocardium are a combination of increased afterload (vasoconstriction), increased preload (venoconstriction), and increased contractility. The last is caused by increased myoplasmic calcium and by an increase in the sensitivity of the contractile proteins to calcium. When the coronary arteries are narrowed, coronary blood flow may increase because of the increase in aortic diastolic pressure, thus improving myocardial metabolism and myocardial performance. However, oxygen demand may still exceed supply. Norepinephrine is used increasingly frequently in septic shock, when peripheral vascular resistance is greatly reduced. Norepinephrine is also used to prevent hypotension during venodilator therapy with glyceryl trinitrate. In congestive heart failure, the inotropic response may be reduced because of β-receptor "downregulation," and cardiac output may decrease.

Epinephrine

Epinephrine acts on the peripheral α- and β-adrenoceptors and on the cardiac β-receptors. The increase in myocardial contractility is accompanied by an increase in heart rate, cardiac automaticity, and atrioventricular node conduction. Because epinephrine causes less vasoconstriction and hypertension than norepinephrine, the direct chronotropic effect (β_1-adrenoceptor stimulation) is less inhibited by baroceptor reflexes. At low doses, cardiac stimulation is predominant and systemic vascular resistance may decrease because of vasodilation in skeletal muscle, whereas at high doses α_1-mediated vasoconstriction becomes important. Renal blood flow and glomerular filtration rate are reduced by epinephrine. The development of epinephrine-induced tachycardia and arrhythmias may compromise coronary perfusion.

Isoprenaline

Isoprenaline acts on the β_1- and β_2-adrenoceptors. Its effects include increases in inotropy, chronotropy, atrioventricular conduction, automaticity, and peripheral and pulmonary vasodilation. Large increases in cardiac output are obtained, facilitated by the unbridled chronotropic

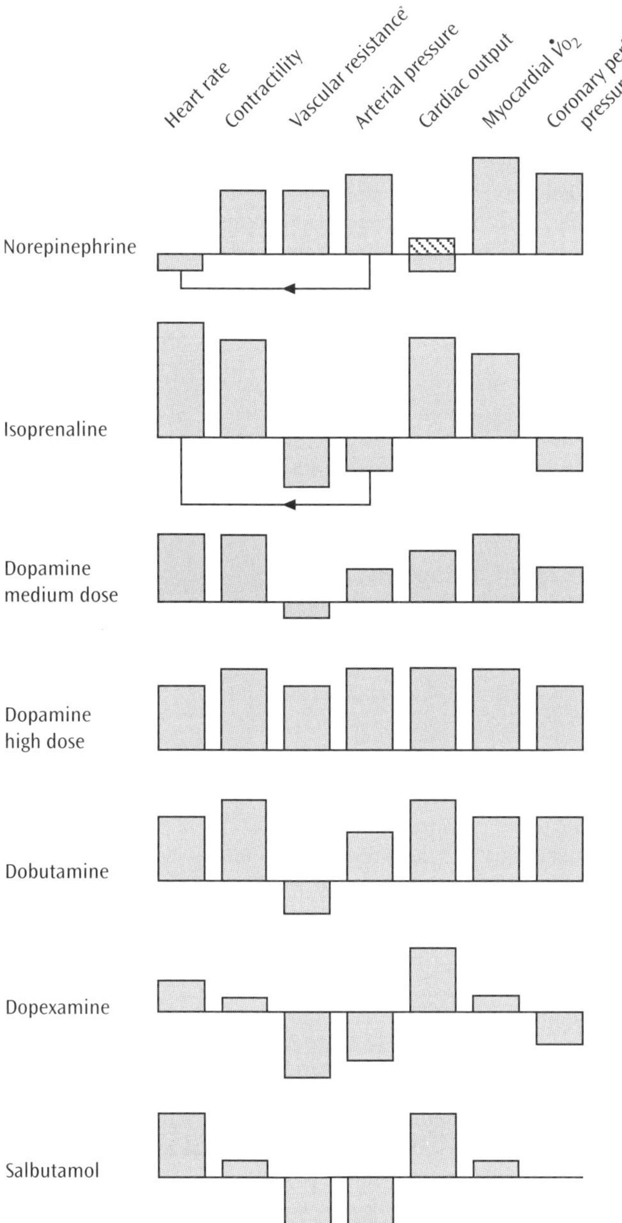

Figure 8.2 *Hemodynamic profile of some catecholamines and their derivatives.*

response, contributed to by a reflex increase secondary to arterial hypotension. Because of the tachycardia and reduced aortic diastolic pressure, coronary perfusion may be adversely affected and, in the presence of coronary artery disease, myocardial ischemia can develop. Indeed, experimentally, isoprenaline has been shown to increase the size of myocardial infarction and the extent of S–T segment elevation. Thus, isoprenaline is contraindicated in the treatment of circulatory failure caused by myocardial ischemia or infarction. However, when circulatory failure is associated with bradycardia, isoprenaline is useful, particularly in the emergency treatment of heart blocks. In addition, isoprenaline may be advantageous when patients exhibit exaggerated responses to the α-adrenoceptor-mediated effects of epinephrine, norepinephrine, and dopamine.[9]

Dopamine

The effects of dopamine on the circulation are dose dependent (see Table 8.2). In low doses, dopamine acts predominantly on dopaminergic receptors in the renal and mesenteric vasculature, increasing blood flow, glomerular filtration, and natriuresis. With higher doses of dopamine, β_1-adrenoceptor stimulation becomes predominant, myocardial contractility is enhanced, and both cardiac output and arterial pressure increase. The elevation of arterial pressure tends to lessen the chronotropic response to β_1-receptor stimulation. As dopamine maintains or improves the coronary perfusion pressure, the risk of myocardial ischemia is less than with isoprenaline. At the highest doses, α_1-adrenoceptor-mediated peripheral vasoconstriction occurs.

Table 8.4 *Usual doses of catecholamines*

Drug	Infusion rate ($\mu g\,kg^{-1}\,min^{-1}$)
Norepinephrine	0.01–0.07
Epinephrine	0.06–0.18
Isoprenaline	0.02–0.18
Dopamine	
Dopaminergic effect	1–5
β_1 effect	5–15
α and β effects	>15
Dobutamine	2–40
Salbutamol	0.2–0.5
Dopexamine	2.5–10.0

Dobutamine

This β_1-adrenoceptor agonist causes less β_2-receptor stimulation than isoprenaline, and much less α-adrenoceptor stimulation than norepinephrine. Dobutamine does not exert any effect on the dopaminergic receptors. For an equivalent enhancement of contractility, dobutamine causes less tachycardia than isoprenaline. Enhancement of left ventricular performance is reflected in reductions of left ventricular end-diastolic pressure and volume, which enhance coronary perfusion. However, oxygen demand may still outstrip oxygen supply and dobutamine may increase myocardial ischemia. Dobutamine is an effective inotropic agent in the treatment of circulatory failure after cardiac surgery and is also very useful for patients with low cardiac output syndromes. As dobutamine causes an inotropic response associated with vasodilation, it represents the model of an "inodilator." Thus, other drugs offering the same therapeutic profile, i.e. the phosphodiesterase inhibitors, are often evaluated with reference to dobutamine.[10] Dobutamine is used extensively in conjunction with echocardiography or radionuclide angiography and scintigraphy to elicit reversible ischemia in patients suspected of coronary artery disease.

Arbutamine

Adenosine, dipyridamole, and dobutamine are widely used to mimic certain aspects of the circulatory response to exercise such as tachycardia, coronary vasodilation, and positive inotropy, which provoke reversible ischemia and elicit cardiac functional changes in patients with coronary artery disease. Recently, dobutamine has become the agent of choice, yet it does not always cause enough tachycardia to induce ischemia and its positive inotropic properties can make the diagnosis of wall motion abnormalities equivocal in some patients. Arbutamine has been developed as a stress agent and exhibits similar affinities for β_1-, β_2-, and α_1-adrenoceptors. Its affinity characteristics place arbutamine between isoprenaline and dobutamine. The effects of arbutamine last only marginally longer than those of isoprenaline and dobutamine.[11]

Dopexamine

Dopexamine hydrochloride is a potent β_2-adrenoceptor agonist with activity at dopaminergic DA_1- and DA_2-receptors. As it is a potent inhibitor of the uptake-1 process, it potentiates the actions of endogenous catecholamines. Dopexamine possesses one-third of the potency of dopamine on DA_1-receptors. Dopexamine causes renal and splanchnic vasodilation and increases natriuresis. Experimental studies suggest that dopexamine increases the likelihood of recovery of renal function in hemorrhagic shock.[12] The reduced vascular resistance contributes to moderate increases in cardiac output and heart rate.[13]

The inotropic activity of dopexamine is probably the result of β_2-adrenoceptor stimulation as its activity on the β_1-adrenoceptor is very weak. In chronic heart failure, β_1-adrenoceptors, but not β_2-adrenoceptors, are downregulated. This reduces the efficacy of β_1-adrenoceptror agonists but does not prevent the inotropic effect of dopexamine.

The place of dopexamine in intensive care appears to be in patients with low-output circulatory failure associated with an elevated vascular resistance. Improvement in oxygen delivery to the splanchnic region contributes to a reduction in the risk of multiple organ failure. A comparison of dopexamine, dopamine, and dobutamine is shown in Table 8.5.

Salbutamol

Salbutamol is a β_2-adrenoceptor agonist with selectivity for bronchial and vascular smooth muscle. The major effect of salbutamol on the cardiovascular system is to cause peripheral vasodilation. This facilitates left ventricular ejection and reduces ventricular wall stress. Salbutamol causes increases in heart rate. This may result from stimulation of the cardiac β_2-adrenoceptors and reflexes elicited by systolic hypotension. As salbutamol causes a greater increase in heart rate than other peripheral vasodilators, its usefulness in the treatment of circulatory failure associated with ischemic heart disease is limited. However, salbutamol is useful in the face of protracted vasoconstriction.

Phenylephrine

Phenylephrine is a relatively selective α_1-adrenoceptor agonist. It has weak α_2-agonist activity and some activity at β-adrenoceptors. As phenylephrine causes dose-dependent vasoconstriction, arterial pressure rises and there is reflex bradycardia. Cardiac output is slightly decreased, renal and splanchnic blood flows are markedly reduced. Phenylephrine may be used to counteract the hypotension of spinal or epidural anesthesia.

Ephedrine

Ephedrine increases the release of norepinephrine and has weak α- and β-adrenoceptor agonist properties. Ephedrine increases blood pressure by peripheral vasoconstriction and cardiac stimulation. The effects of ephedrine are variable. Ephedrine continues to be used routinely in the prevention or treatment of hypotension resulting from regional anesthesia.

Clonidine

Clonidine is an α_2-agonist that causes presynaptic α_2-mediated inhibition of norepinephrine release from nerve terminals, reduces renin secretion, and acts on medullary pathways involved in vasomotor control. This may be the most important mechanism of clonidine in the control of hypertension. Clonidine has been used successfully in the prevention of the large variations in arterial pressure observed during anesthesia and surgery,[14] and has been shown to minimize the release of epinephrine and norepinephrine.[15] Clonidine causes sedation, decreases the minimum alveolar concentration of inhalational anesthetics, and reduces opioid requirements.[16] These effects suggest that α_2-adrenoceptors may play a role in the mechanisms of anesthesia and pain relief, possibly as a result of altered ion fluxes.

Dexmetedomidine

Dexmetedomidine is a more selective α_2-agonist than clonidine; it is a full agonist known to reduce the requirements for opioids, thiopentone, and inhalation anesthetics. In doses of 1 or 2 mg kg^{-1}, dexmetedomidine causes a decrease in plasma catecholamines in healthy volunteers, associated with reductions in mean arterial pressure and cardiac output.[17] Such doses cause sedation and result in loss of responsiveness in most subjects. This is associated with minimal ventilatory depression.[18]

Mivazerol

Mivazerol is a relatively new selective α_2-adrenoceptor agonist. It possesses both sympatholytic and anti-ischemic properties. The latter result from the prevention of tachycardia and hypertension and cause a decrease in the incidence of perioperative myocardial ischemia[19] and an improvement of the total exercise duration in patients with angina.

Table 8.5 *Comparison of dopexamine, dopamine, and dobutamine*

Receptors	α	β_1	β_2	DA_1	DA_2	Uptake-1 inhibition
Dopexamine	0	(+)	+++	++	+	+++
Dopamine	+++	++	(+)	+++	++	++
Dobutamine	++	+++	++	0	0	+

0, No effect; (+), weak effect; +, moderate effect; ++, strong effect; +++, very strong effect.

Adrenoceptor antagonists

β-Adrenoceptor antagonists

As a group, β-adrenoceptor antagonists exhibit five main characteristics:

1 They are competitive antagonists at the β-receptors.
2 They may exhibit receptor subtype selectivity.
3 They may exhibit partial agonist activity.
4 They possess, at very high doses, "quinidine-like activity."
5 They may cause an increase in the number of β-receptors, when administered over a prolonged period of time.

Competitive antagonism

Beta-blockers displace the dose–response curve to isoprenaline or dobutamine to the right. Because they are competitive, their effects can be reversed by the administration of large doses of β-adrenoceptor agonists.

Receptor subtype selectivity

The structure of the β-adrenoceptor antagonists is relatively similar to that of the sympathomimetic amines. Some β-adrenoceptor antagonists have greater affinity for the cardiac (β_1) than for the peripheral (β_2) adrenoceptors. Propranolol is considered nonselective, since it is almost equally as effective in blocking β_1- and β_2-adrenoceptors. Similarly, nadolol, oxprenolol, pindolol, and timolol are nonselective β-adrenoceptor antagonists. Cardioselective antagonists (acebutolol, atenolol, metoprolol) act predominantly on the β_1-adrenoceptors, reducing the positive inotropic and chronotropic responses to isoprenaline without inhibiting peripheral vasodilation and bronchodilation. Nevertheless, when large doses of β_1-adrenoceptor blockers are administered, they eventually block both β_1- and β_2-receptors.

Partial agonist activity

Partial agonists stimulate β_1- or β_1- and β_2-adrenoceptors, an effect previously called intrinsic sympathomimetic activity. However, their presence at receptor sites prevents the effect of other agonists.[20] Partial agonists increase heart rate and contractility. Typical examples include acebutolol, oxprenolol, pindolol, and xamoterol. They cause less resting bradycardia and, in the case of borderline heart failure, may be better tolerated than pure antagonists (Table 8.6).

Membrane stabilization

Membrane stabilization is caused by inhibition of sodium transport. With the exception of atenolol and nadolol, the β-adrenoceptor antagonists cause some membrane stabilization in the heart and, therefore, resemble quinidine but only at concentrations that are considerably greater than those required to obtain adequate clinical β-adrenoceptor blockade.

Upregulation of β-adrenoceptors

Prolonged administration of β-adrenoceptor blockers causes an increase in the number of β-adrenoceptors. This upregulation may be partly responsible for the adverse effects of the abrupt withdrawal of β-adrenoceptor blockers.

Antiarrhythmic action

The major antiarrhythmic effect of β-adrenoceptor blockade is the prevention of the arrhythmogenic effect of the endogenous and exogenous catecholamines. Membrane stabilization is probably of little importance. However, increased duration of the action potential contributes to the antidysrrhythmic efficacy of sotalol.[21] As β-adrenoceptor blockers decrease heart rate and contractility, thereby reducing myocardial oxygen consumption, they are also effective in the treatment of ischemia-related arrhythmias.

Absorption and elimination

Lipophilic beta-blockers (metoprolol, pindolol, propranolol, timolol) are almost completely absorbed from the gastrointestinal tract. The more hydrophilic beta-blockers (atenolol, nadolol) are absorbed to a much lesser extent (25–50%). Because of degradation in the gut wall and liver (first-pass effect), bioavailability may be as low as 25% (nadolol) or between 50% and 100% (pindolol). The most lipophilic drugs have the highest bioavailability.[22,23]

Although data on bioavailability are very important when oral administration is to be replaced by intravenous administration, in practice it is necessary to titrate the intravenous administration to obtain the desired effect.

Hemodynamic effects of β-adrenoceptor blockade

All β-adrenoceptor blockers reduce heart rate and cardiac output because they reduce the effect of β_1-receptor stimulation on the heart. Their effects are more pronounced when sympathetic activity is exaggerated and less pronounced when it is depressed. β_2-Adrenoceptor blockade increases peripheral vascular resistance as it leaves α-adrenoceptor stimulation unopposed. With the administration of partial agonists, changes in heart rate and cardiac output are of smaller magnitude than with pure antagonists. However, during exercise, the heart rate and cardiac output increase less than in the absence of beta-blockade; this offers protection against ischemia.

Effect on respiratory function

β-Adrenoceptor blockade may increase airway obstruction, especially when nonselective antagonists are used, and may also decrease the ventilatory response to CO_2.

Table 8.6 *Classification of the β-adrenoceptor blockers*

	Cardioselective (β_1)	Nonselective (β_1 and β_2)
Pure antagonists	Atenolol Metoprolol	Nadolol Propranolol Sotalol Timolol Esmolol Labetalol[a]
Partial agonists	Acebutolol Practolol	Alprenolol Oxprenolol Pindolol

a. Labetalol is also an α-adrenoceptor blocker.

Reversal of β-adrenoceptor blockade

Reversing the effect of β-adrenoceptor blockade is seldom warranted. However, bradycardia may cause concern and this may be treated with atropine. If it becomes necessary to increase the inotropic state of the myocardium, β-adrenoceptor agonists are effective, but the doses required may be 5–20 times the usual doses. When nonselective β-adrenoceptor antagonists have been administered, large doses of the nonselective agonist isoprenaline are effective. However, when cardioselective β_1-adrenoceptor antagonists have been administered, a β_1-agonist, such as dobutamine, should be used.

Withdrawal syndrome

Sudden withdrawal of β-adrenergic blockade may be dangerous. The syndrome of withdrawal consists of development of ventricular arrhythmias, worsening of angina, myocardial infarction, and even sudden death. This may reflect β-adrenoceptor upregulation.

Cardiac protection by β-adrenoceptor blockers

β-Receptor blockers improve the stability of the cardiovascular system and protect the myocardium in patients with coronary heart disease,[24,25] hypertensive heart disease, dysrhythmias, or obstructive cardiomyopathies.

Beta-blockers and cardiac failure

Despite advances in the treatment of heart failure, the rates of morbidity and mortality remain high, even though patients are treated with angiotension-converting enzyme inhibitors. Beta-blockers seem to work by blocking the overstimulated sympathetic nervous system. Adrenergic and renin–angiotensin systems are activated in heart failure. Beta-blockers prevent some of their effects and protect the heart against the consequences of high levels of circulatory catecholamines, thereby reducing the overall energy expenditure of the heart. They reduce mortality in patients with heart failure after myocardial infarction or chronic left ventricular failure. The greatest effect may be on sudden death.[26] However, beta-blockers are not easy to use in the setting of heart failure, and must be very carefully titrated as some patients may "decompensate" during titration.

β-Adrenoceptor antagonists in anesthesia

It has been demonstrated that β-adrenoceptor blockade causes only modest reductions in cardiac output under anesthesia for hypertensive patients, while decreasing the incidence of arrhythmias and myocardial ischemia after laryngoscopy and intubation. It is been recommended that their administration be continued until the day of surgery,[27,28] and postoperatively (if necessary by the intravenous route).

β-Adrenoceptor antagonists may be used deliberately in order to prevent anesthesia-related dysrhythmias (laryngoscopy, endotracheal intubation, bronchoscopy, dental surgery, cardiac and vascular surgery, neurosurgery, surgery of the thyroid gland, pheochromocytoma, administration of catecholamines). They are also used to prevent or limit the tachycardia that is associated with induced hypotension, and to prevent or treat anesthesia- and surgery-related hypertensive crises caused by sympathetic overactivity. Even a single dose of a beta-blocker given as premedication decreases the incidence of episodes of myocardial ischemia.[29]

It is beyond the scope of this chapter to discuss the small differences that exist between different β-adrenoceptor blockers, with the exception of esmolol because of its very short duration of action.

Esmolol is a relatively selective β_1-receptor antagonist. It undergoes rapid hydrolysis by esterases.[30,31] Hydrolysis by erythrocyte esterases reduces the terminal half-life of esmolol to 9.2 min. Onset of blockade occurs in about 5 s, with a maximum reached after about 1 min. Esmolol is 50-fold less potent than propranolol and sixfold less potent than metopolol.[32,33] Infusion of esmolol 50–200 $\mu g\,kg^{-1}\,min^{-1}$ causes a degree of blockade similar to that of 3–6 mg propranolol.

Perioperative tachycardia and hypertension are the main indications for esmolol.[34] In patients undergoing coronary artery surgery, esmolol given throughout the early phases of surgery decreases the cardiocirculatory effects of induction of anesthesia, intubation, sternotomy, and aortic dissection.[35] Esmolol is also effective in the control of postoperative hypertension following coronary artery bypass surgery. A possible adverse effect of esmolol is hypotension. It is dose related and resolves within 30 min with the reduction of the dosage.

Ultrashort-acting β-adrenoceptor blockade is a useful therapeutic modality when sympathetic overactivity is limited in time. Moreover, the rapid reversibility of beta-blockade may make esmolol safer than longer acting beta-blockers in the perioperative period.

α-Adrenoceptor antagonists

α-Adrenoceptor antagonists are used in the treatment of hypertensive emergencies, and in the long-term treatment of arterial hypertension and chronic cardiac failure.

With the exception of phenoxybenzamine, the α-adrenoceptor antagonists are competitive blockers. They can exhibit selectivity for the postsynaptic α_1-receptors (prazosin) or the presynaptic α_2-receptors (yohimbine). Phenoxybenzamine and phentolamine are nonselective α-receptor antagonists, whereas labetalol blocks α_1-, β_1-, and probably β_2-receptors. The administration of α-adrenoceptor antagonists causes peripheral vasodilation in addition to some venodilation. The resulting arterial hypotension causes baroreceptor-mediated increases in sympathetic activity.

Phenoxybenzamine

Phenoxybenzamine is a nonselective, noncompetitive, α-adrenoceptor antagonist with a slow onset of action. The marked vasodilation produced by phenoxybenzamine is useful in the short-term preservation of human kidneys for transplantation. The major place for phenoxybenzamine was, and still is, in the treatment and preoperative preparation of patients suffering from pheochromocytoma, usually in association with β-adrenoceptor blockers.[36] However, doxazocin is also used in the preparation of patients for surgery for such tumors.

Phentolamine

Phentolamine is a weak, nonselective, competitive, α-adrenoceptor antagonist. Less potent than phenoxybenzamine, phentolamine causes vasodilation mostly by a direct effect on vascular smooth muscle. It has a rapid onset of action and its effects last for approximately 15–30 min. In patients suffering from myocardial infarction and chronic heart failure, phentolamine increases stroke volume and decreases the pulmonary capillary wedge pressure. The occurrence of tachycardia may be a significant disadvantage. Phentolamine can abolish α-adrenoceptor-mediated coronary artery spasm. In patients with pheochromocytoma, phentolamine is effective in the treatment of paroxysmal hypertension during operative manipulations of the tumor. Phentolamine, administered as a bolus dose or by continuous infusion, may be used to control intra- and postoperative hypertension and also to control the perfusion pressure during extracorporeal circulation for cardiac surgery.

Prazosin

Prazosin is a selective, competitive, α_1-adrenoceptor blocker that reduces arterial and venous tone. Because α_2-receptors are not blocked, the negative feedback effect of norepinephrine on its own release is not inhibited. This explains why tachycardia and renin stimulation do not occur. The major side-effects of prazosin are postural hypotension and occasionally a precipitous decrease in arterial pressure after the first dose. Prazosin is used in the treatment of congestive cardiac failure and has been shown to increase cardiac output and decrease the pulmonary capillary wedge pressure.

Doxazocin

This quinazoline derivative possesses selective postjunctional α_1-adrenoceptor antagonist activity. It has no effect on presynaptic α_2-adrenoceptors. Doxazocin causes a parallel rightward shift of the dose–response curve to phenylephrine. The long half-life of doxazocin allows for once-daily administration to control arterial hypertension.

Labetalol

Labetalol differs from other adrenergic receptor antagonists in that it blocks both α- and β-adrenoceptors. As an α-blocker, it is less potent than phentolamine; as a beta-blocker, it is much less potent than propranolol. Labetalol does not block the presynaptic α_2-receptors, but blocks both β_1- and β_2-receptors. Labetalol produces a decrease in arterial pressure because of the simultaneous reductions in systemic vascular resistance and cardiac output. Labetalol is effective and provides smooth control of arterial pressure in hypertensive emergencies.

Thymoxamine

Thymoxamine is an α_1-selective antagonist. Although it may be effective in the treatment of circulatory failure after cardiac surgery, most of the literature relates to the treatment of peripheral vascular disease. Thymoxamine improves regional peripheral blood flow after oral, intravenous, or intra-arterial administration.

CHOLINERGIC AGONISTS AND ANTAGONISTS

Cholinergic agonists

These drugs may either bind to the cholinergic receptors (direct action) or inhibit the action of the enzyme cholinesterase, thus increasing the concentration of endogenous acetylcholine.

Muscarinic agonists appear to stimulate the enzyme guanylate cyclase, increase potassium fluxes across the cell membrane, and increase the turnover of inositol phospholipids in cell membranes.

Nicotinic agonists modify the conformation of the nicotinic receptors so that sodium and potassium ions are allowed to diffuse down their concentration gradients: depolarization of the nerve cell or neuromuscular endplate occurs.

By increasing the membrane permeability to potassium in atrial muscle and in sinoatrial and atrioventricular nodes, and by decreasing the slow calcium current, cholinergic agonists reduce the pacemaker rate and decrease the conduction velocity. The mechanisms of peripheral arteriolar and venous dilation by acetylcholine involve the release of nitric oxide by vascular endothelium.

Edrophonium is the only cholinergic stimulant used for its cardiovascular effects, as it may convert supraventricular tachyarrhythmias into sinus rhythm. The vagolytic effect of edrophonium has been used to convert atrial tachycardia to sinus rhythm. It is used as an intravenous bolus dose of 10–20 mg.

Cholinergic antagonists

These can be subdivided into antimuscarinic and antinicotinic agents. The latter comprise ganglion-blocking and neuromuscular-blocking drugs.

Muscarinic receptor-blocking agents cause tachycardia at moderate and high doses, whereas at low doses they may cause bradycardia because of central vagal stimulation. Atrioventricular conduction increases, and any parasympathetically mediated depression of cardiac performance is abolished. Sympathetic cholinergic vasodilation is blocked by muscarinic antagonists.

Atropine

Atropine is effective in preventing or abolishing the bradycardia associated with vagal discharge, irrespective of its cause. It is also effective in preventing the bradycardia associated with the administration of anticholinesterases to reverse neuromuscular blockade, and in preventing or abolishing the bradycardia associated with direct carotid sinus stimulation.

Glycopyrronium

Glycopyrronium has a longer duration of action than atropine and provides prolonged cardiac protection against the muscarinic effects of neostigmine. The onset of action of both glycopyrronium and neostigmine are similar, and the heart rate remains stable when they are administered together. Glycopyrronium does not penetrate the blood–brain barrier, and this minimizes the risk of central anticholinergic syndrome.

GANGLIONIC BLOCKING AGENTS

Drugs that block this subtype of nicotinic receptors exert powerful cardiovascular effects because they block both sympathetic and parasympathetic transmissions. Ganglion blockade may be caused by depolarizing drugs that stimulate before blocking transmission (nicotine) or by nondepolarizing drugs that block transmission without causing any stimulation. Hexamethonium, trimetaphan, and pentolinium are competitive nondepolarizing ganglion blockers. Their effects on the circulation depend on the level of sympathetic activity. Usually, the capacitance vessels are more sensitive to ganglion blockers than the resistance vessels, and blood pooling on assuming the erect position is a major determinant of orthostatic hypotension. Myocardial contractility reduces because of reduced sympathetic activity, whereas heart rate increases because of reduced vagal tone. Cerebral blood flow is maintained but renal blood flow decreases.

Hexamethonium

Hexamethonium is a selective nicotinic receptor antagonist. Tachyphylaxis develops rapidly because of the dominance of the muscarinic pathway when the nicotinic pathway is blocked.

Pentolinium

Pentolinium is more potent and longer acting than hexamethonium. As well as reducing sympathetic activity it appears to reduce plasma renin activity.

Trimetaphan

Trimetaphan is a competitive ganglion-blocking drug that exhibits some direct vasodilation. Interruption of sympathetic outflow produces vasodilation. The latter is relatively slow in both onset and recovery. The association of parasympathetic blockade results in mydriasis and tachycardia. Mydriasis makes neurologic assessment difficult; this is an important drawback during neurosurgery. Tachyphylaxis makes it difficult to achieve a stable blood pressure reduction.

ANTIARRHYTHMIC DRUGS

Electrophysiology

The electrophysiological classification of the antiarrhythmic drugs introduced by Vaughan-Williams[37] subdivides antiarrhythmics into four or five classes (see Table 8.7).

Class I

Drugs in this class interfere with the fast sodium inward current. They are subclassified into three groups. Class 1a drugs depress conduction of both sinus beats and premature beats and prolong the duration of the action potential. Class 1b drugs depress conduction of premature beats and conduction through ischemic tissue; they shorten the duration of the action potential. Class 1c drugs cause marked depression in conduction of both normal and premature beats, without altering the duration of the action potential.

Class II

Cardiac arrhythmias can be initiated or exacerbated by stress or emotions: thus, drugs with antisympathetic effects, such as β-adrenoceptor blockers, have antiarrhythmic properties. In addition, some β-blockers have class I action on cardiac muscle and some prolong the duration of the action potential.

Class III

Class III drugs prolong the duration of the action potential by selectively decreasing potassium ion conductance.[38] They are very effective in prolonging atrial refractoriness and abolishing an experimentally induced circus movement.[39] It is still unclear whether the antiarrhythmic effect is solely due to the increased duration of the action potential since most agents possess other actions such as antiadrenergic activity.

Class IV

Class IV is now divided into IVa and IVb. The antiarrhythmic effects of class IVa drugs result from the blockade of the second inward current carried by calcium ions.[40] Blockade of the calcium channels produces a slowing of conduction and prolongs the refractoriness within sinus and atrioventricular nodes. The sinus rate decreases, the *P–R* interval is lengthened, and there is a reduced ventricular response to atrial arrhythmias. Calcium antagonists (especially verapamil and diltiazem but not nifedipine and its analogs) are effective in terminating episodes of paroxysmal supraventricular tachycardia. They slow the ventricular response in atrial flutter and fibrillation and, less reliably, control multifocal atrial tachycardia.

In the ischemic myocardium, the second inward current could take over the depolarizing function, so that slow action potentials may conduct impulses at low velocity, encouraging the development of re-entry. This is prevented by calcium channel blockers.

The main side-effect of calcium antagonists is hypotension. The association of calcium channel blockers with beta-blockers or disopyramide may cause severe cardiac depression in patients with poor left ventricular function.

The antiarrhythmic effects of class IVb drugs result from the opening of ATP-dependent potassium channels. This causes hyperpolarization of the cells.

Table 8.7 *The Vaughan-Williams classification of antiarrhythmic drugs*

	Class I (Na^+ channel blockers)	Class II (beta-blockers)	Class III (K^+ channel blockers)	Class IV (Ca^{2+} channel blockers)	
1a	Quinidine Procainamide Disopyramide	Beta-blockers	Amiodarone Bretylium tosylate Sotalol Clofilium	IVa	Verapamil Diltiazem Bepridil
1b	Lidocaine Phenytoin Mexiletine			IVb	Adenosine Nicorandil
1c	Flecainide Tocainide Encainide Propaphenone				

Lidocaine (lignocaine).

Class V

This class of drugs includes specific bradycardic agents.[41] Alinidine has a selective bradycardic action on the sinoatrial node because it reduces the slope of slow diastolic depolarization. It does not block the sodium channels, does not have a negative inotropic action, and does not block the positive inotropic effect of the β-adrenoceptors.[42] The effect of alinidine may be mediated by reducing the chloride current.

Antiarrhythmic drugs within the Vaughan-Williams classification

Class Ia

Quinidine

Quinidine slows down conduction in the bundle of His, decreases the rate of diastolic depolarization, and prolongs the effective refractory period. It is effective in the prophylaxis of supraventricular dysrhythmias, particularly those involving re-entry, and in the treatment of ventricular tachycardia. It facilitates cardioversion and maintenance of sinus rhythm following cardioversion.[43]

Procainamide

Procainamide is particularly effective in the treatment of ventricular arrhythmias. The negative inotropic action of procainamide may cause cardiac failure. Procainamide is also used to maintain sinus rhythm after cardioversion.

Disopyramide

Disopyramide is effective in patients with atrial and ventricular arrhythmias. Negative inotropy is more pronounced in patients with pre-existing heart failure. Disopyramide is successful in maintaining patients in sinus rhythm after conversion of atrial fibrillation,[44] and in the treatment of supraventricular tachycardia associated with Wolff–Parkinson–White syndrome.

All three drugs increase sinus rate because of their anticholinergic properties and a reflex-mediated increase in sympathetic tone. However, caution should be exercised as the heart rate may slow in patients with pre-existing sinus node disease and in patients with transplanted hearts.

Class Ib

Lidocaine (lignocaine)

Lidocaine (lignocaine) is the first-line drug for the treatment of ventricular arrhythmias associated with acute myocardial infarction, for the treatment of digitalis toxicity, and, together with cardioversion, for the treatment of ventricular fibrillation. Neurologic side-effects have been well documented, ranging from paresthesiae, drowsiness, nausea, and confusion to convulsion and respiratory arrest,[45] especially in the elderly. In patients with poor left ventricular function, circulatory failure may occur, and in those with conduction disorders there is the risk of heart block.

Mexiletine

Mexiletine is available for oral and intravenous administration, and is effective in the treatment of ventricular arrhythmias especially after myocardial infarction. However, overall mortality may be increased.[46] Arrhythmias (sinus bradycardia, atrial fibrillation, and heart blocks) may occur.

Tocainide

Tocainide is available in oral and intravenous forms. Its therapeutic indications are the same as those for mexiletine.[47] However, the relatively high incidence of neutropenia and of interstitial pneumonitis precludes its use as a first-choice drug.

Class Ic

Flecainide

Flecainide is an oral antiarrhythmic with a mean elimination half-life of 14 h. Flecainide is effective in the control of supraventricular tachycardias. However, the drug is arrhythmogenic and raises the threshold for both defibrillation and ventricular pacing.

Encainide

The overall drug action is that of its metabolites *O*-demethyl encainide and 3-methoxy-*O*-demethyl encainide.[48] Encainide is effective in the control of ventricular dysrhythmias but may not be effective in the prevention of sustained ventricular tachycardia.

Propafenone

Propafenone is effective in the treatment of ventricular and supraventricular arrhythmias. It has some β-blocking activity in addition to class Ic effects.

Class II agents

β-Adrenoceptor blockers are effective in the treatment of arrhythmias caused by increased sympathetic activity. They are also effective in the management of arrhythmias associated with myocardial infarction. These arrhythmias are due to a number of factors, including increases in plasma catecholamines, leakage of potassium owing to hypoxia, a rise in free fatty acids, and alterations in action potential duration (shortened by hypoxia; lengthened by acidosis), all of which enhance the heterogeneity of repolarization.

Beta-blockers cause significant reductions in sinus rate and decrease the number of both supraventricular and ventricular arrhythmias.[49]

This is associated with a reduction in the incidence of ventricular fibrillation, and a reduction in mortality.[50] Beta-blockers may also reduce the risk of cardiac rupture.[51]

Class III agents

Amiodarone

Amiodarone is a potent antiarrhythmic agent used in the control and prophylaxis of most supraventricular and ventricular arrhythmias.[52] Amiodarone has noncompetitive antiadrenergic actions, resulting from the inhibition of the coupling of β-receptors with the regulatory unit of the adenylate cyclase complex.[53] In addition, amiodarone reduces the density of β-adrenoceptors. Amiodarone is unique in its slow hepatic metabolism, resulting in an elimination half-life of 26–107 days.[54]

The hemodynamic effects of amiodarone include reductions in heart rate, blood pressure, and systemic and coronary vascular resistances. In patients with normal ventricular function or only mild left ventricular dysfunction, intravenous amiodarone exerts a mild negative inotropic effect associated with peripheral vasodilation.[55] The negative inotropy is more prominent in patients with moderate or severe left ventricular dysfunction.[56] However, continuous infusions of doses up to 1000 mg per day are well tolerated even by patients with severe left ventricular dysfunction.

Oral amiodarone is highly effective in paroxysmal and persistent atrial fibrillation. It is also effective in the management of drug-resistant paroxysmal supraventricular tachycardias and in the prevention of the recurrence of tachycardia in Wolff–Parkinson–White syndrome.[57]

Oral amiodarone is highly effective in the treatment of ventricular arrhythmias even when other antiarrhythmic drugs have failed.[54] These advantages must be balanced against potentially serious side-effects. The most serious complication is pulmonary toxicity, resulting in diffuse bilateral interstitial changes accompanied by patchy alveolar infiltrates, and mild hypoxemia.[58]

As amiodarone contains iodine (75 mg for each 250-mg tablet) and is deiodinated *in vivo*, excess iodine may cause hypothyroidism. Microdeposits of the drug or its metabolites in the cornea occur during long-term therapy with amiodarone.

Amiodarone reduces both the renal and nonrenal elimination of digoxin.[59] As amiodarone prevents the development of ventricular ectopic activity, digoxin toxicity is characterized by sinus arrest and gastrointestinal symptoms.

Serious arrhythmias may occur when class I antiarrhythmics are used together with amiodarone, therefore their dosage should be reduced. Additive suppressive effects on sinus and atrioventricular nodes may occur with β-adrenoceptor blockers and calcium antagonists.

Sotalol

This nonselective β-adrenoceptor antagonist reduces the time-dependent outward K^+ current activated during the plateau of the action potential resulting in a dose-dependent increase in the action potential duration of atrial, ventricular, and Purkinje fibers.[60]

Sotalol reduces heart rate and cardiac output. The class III effects of sotalol are not unique. Other β-adrenoceptor blockers have a "chronic class III effect" that may reduce the incidence of sudden death after myocardial infarction.[61]

Clofilium

This quaternary ammonium is a highly selective and potent class III agent. It prolongs the cardiac action potential duration and increases ventricular and atrial refractoriness without altering the conduction velocity in normal or ischemic myocardium. Clofilium does not act on α- and β-adrenoceptors. Its electrophysiologic effects are enhanced by halothane, which facilitates the development of ventricular arrhythmias, particularly when bradycardia is present.[62]

Bretylium

Bretylium causes an immediate release of norepinephrine from adrenergic terminals, and subsequently prevents the further release of norepinephrine. In addition, bretylium prolongs the duration of the cardiac action potential and, in very high doses, blocks both sodium and potassium channels. The antiarrhythmic and antifibrillatory activity of bretylium is such that it has been termed a "pharmacologic defibrillator." The main indication is the treatment of ventricular arrhythmias resistant to conventional treatment.[63]

Class IVa agents

Verapamil

Verapamil reduces vascular smooth muscle tone, decreases myocardial contractility, and is effective in the control of supraventricular arrhythmias. Intravenous boluses (2.5 mg repeated if necessary after 30 s) of verapamil [under electrocardiograph (ECG) monitoring] are effective in the control of the ventricular rate in atrial fibrillation but may cause hypotension. Conduction defects are a contraindication.

Diltiazem

Diltiazem acts as an arteriolar dilator with less negative inotropy than verapamil. It is used more in the treatment of myocardial ischemia than in the treatment of supraventricular arrhythmias.

Bepridil

Bepridil is a calcium antagonist that slows intramyocardial conduction velocity and increases the QTc interval and refractoriness.[64] These effects suggest class III activity, although studies have shown bepridil to block sodium and calcium but not potassium channels.[65]

Class IVb agents

Adenosine

Adenosine is an endogenous nucleoside with an extremely short half-life. The main antiarrhythmic effects of adenosine are mediated by A_1-receptors linked to an inhibitory guanine binding protein and are characterized by a negative chronotropic effect on the sinus node and negative dromotropic effect on atrioventricular conduction.[66] Adenosine is effective in terminating paroxysmal supraventricular tachycardias involving the atrioventricular node as it blocks the anterograde limb of re-entrant circuits. As the duration of action is short, adverse reactions are also short lived. This is an advantage over other drugs as the success rate in terminating paroxysmal supraventricular tachycardias is high.[67]

Nicorandil

Nicorandil is a nicotinamide nitrate. It acts both as a nitrate and as an activator of ATP-dependent potassium channels.[68] Both its coronary vasodilating and its antiarrhythmic properties result from hyperpolarization of vascular smooth muscle and cardiac cells. It causes coronary vasodilation and is effective in the management of ischemia-induced dysrhythmias.[69,70]

Antiarrhythmics outside the Vaughan-Williams classification

Cardiac glycosides

Cardiac glycosides cause an increase in K^+ conductance associated with a slowly developing decrease in the action potential duration, whereas resting membrane potential and action potential amplitude are essentially unchanged.[71] Shortening of the action potential duration by toxic doses of cardiac glycosides contributes to their arrhythmogenicity because the refractory period is reduced.

By contrast, the antiarrhythmic effects of cardiac glycosides are essentially mediated by the autonomic nervous system.[72] The vagomimetic effects of cardiac glycosides may be due to the sensitivity of the baroreceptors being increased, to activation of the vagal centers, to inhibition of the peripheral sympathetic effects on the heart, or to increased sensitivity to acetylcholine.

Atrial fibrillation is one of the most common dysrhythmias. It occurs in 2–5% of patients over 60 years of age; it increases the risk of both stroke and mortality.

Atrial fibrillation and atrial flutter are the most frequent indications for cardiac glycosides. Atrial flutter is frequently converted into atrial fibrillation, and recent atrial fibrillation may revert to sinus rhythm over a few hours. This effect may be facilitated by the addition of disopyramide.[73] The main advantage of digoxin is its weak positive inotropic action. This may play an important role when the myocardium is compromised, and any negative inotropic drug would further impair cardiac function to an unacceptable extent.

There is no evidence that prophylactic preoperative digitalization of patients with marginal cardiac failure is of any benefit, but appropriate digoxin therapy to maintain normal heart rates (55–70 beats min^{-1}) in patients with atrial fibrillation is very important. Patients in atrial fibrillation who present for urgent surgery with heart rates over 100 beats min^{-1} should not be treated with intravenous digoxin, but should have their heart rates *cautiously* slowed under ECG control by intravenous cardioselective β-adrenoceptor antagonists.[74]

Perioperative management of arrhythmias

The first step in the treatment of arrhythmias occurring during anesthesia and surgery is *not* the administration of antiarrhythmic drugs but the correction of factors which may have contributed to their development, such as hypoxia, hypercarbia, hypocarbia, metabolic acidosis, or inadequate depth of anesthesia. Once these factors have been corrected, most arrhythmias disappear. If they persist, treatment is indicated when the circulation is impaired, or when the arrhythmia is likely to develop into a life-threatening type.

Hypokalemia poses difficult problems. Chronic hypokalemia is usually accompanied by intracellular potassium deficiency so that the ratio of intracellular to extracellular potassium concentration may remain normal or near normal. Rapid potassium replacement may worsen the electrophysiology of the myocardium.[75] If chronic hypokalemia is accompanied by arrhythmias, surgery should be postponed and correction of potassium depletion should be achieved over several days and not attempted over a few hours. Acute hypokalemia, however, should be corrected before anesthesia and surgery.

With hyperkalemia, the risks of further increases in potassium concentration causing life-threatening arrhythmias are such that correction should be attempted. In the case of chronic renal failure, hemodialysis may be necessary before surgery. During anesthesia, arrhythmias may occur when large volumes of stored blood are given rapidly, causing sudden and severe hyperkalemia. The intravenous administration of calcium may be necessary to suppress these arrhythmias. Other measures, such as the administration of sodium bicarbonate, may be necessary to cause a shift of potassium into the cells. In addition, glucose and insulin may be needed.

Supraventricular arrhythmias

Sinus bradycardia caused by vagal stimulation is frequently accompanied by hypotension and responds well to intravenous atropine or glycopyrrolate. If atropine is ineffective, it may be necessary to administer a β_1-receptor agonist (dobutamine or isoprenaline).

Supraventricular tachyarrhythmias can be controlled by β-adrenoceptor blockers, calcium channel blockers, and digitalis. Verapamil and diltiazem are effective in the treatment of supraventricular tachycardias. However, they reduce the inotropic state of the myocardium; their administration during anesthesia with halogenated anesthetics may cause exaggerated myocardial depression. However, they can be used successfully because the beneficial effects of bringing the heart rate to within the normal range may outweigh the detrimental effect on the circulation caused by myocardial depression. If calcium channel blockers are used, they should be given in small doses to achieve the desired effect by titration. In the absence of hypokalemia, digitalis may be preferred to calcium blockers or β-adrenoceptor blockers when the quality of the myocardium is poor.

Ventricular arrhythmias

Lidocaine is the drug of choice for the intraoperative treatment of acute ventricular arrhythmias (ventricular premature beats and ventricular tachycardia). The usual dose is 1 mg kg^{-1} body weight followed by an infusion to maintain blood levels between 2 and 5 mg L^{-1}. High concentrations may cause myocardial and central nervous system depression. Isolated ventricular premature beats may not require treatment. However, treatment is necessary if they are frequent, assume the R on T configuration, or appear in salvos.

When ventricular arrhythmias are obviously caused by sympathetic overactivity, β-adrenoceptor blockade is the treatment of choice. A small initial dose should be followed by further small incremental doses to achieve control of the arrhythmia.

Ventricular tachycardia is probably best treated with cardioversion when it impairs the circulation. In some patients, ventricular fibrillation may occur and prove resistant to electroconversion. In this situation, bretylium tosylate may either restore a normal rhythm (acting as a "pharmacologic defibrillator") or facilitate the conversion of ventricular fibrillation into a normal rhythm.

INOTROPES

The first step in the management of low output states is to optimize the ventricular filling. If this fails to restore cardiac output, inotropic drugs and vasodilators may be necessary. As catecholamines and their derivatives have already been discussed (see Adrenergic agonists), this section will deal with cardiac glycosides, phosphodiesterase inhibitors, calcium entry promoters, and calcium sensitizers.

Cardiac glycosides

Cardiac glycosides are used in the management of congestive heart failure, particularly when associated with atrial fibrillation. Cardiac glycosides decrease the activity of the membrane-bound enzyme Na^+K^+ (Mg^{2+}-dependent) adenosine triphosphatase (ATPase). This increases the cytosolic sodium ion concentration.[76] The uninhibited fraction of the sodium pump is stimulated, thus increasing the rate of exchange of calcium. Increases in both cytosolic free Ca^{2+} and the cellular calcium transients suggest increased exchange and releasability of calcium from cellular stores.[77] The combined inotropic–bradycardic action of digitalis is unique and the weak inotropy of digoxin is useful in the treatment of congestive cardiac failure, improving survival when added to vasodilators and diuretics. In acute left ventricular failure, however, diuretics and more powerful inotropes such as dobutamine, dopamine, amrinone, or enoximone have superseded digitalis, unless failure is associated with valvular disease and atrial fibrillation.

Cardiac glycosides may accumulate in patients with poor renal function. This may be accentuated following anesthesia and surgery because of the alterations in renal function associated with the stress response to surgery. Digitalis toxicity may be precipitated during anesthesia if the patient is hyperventilated and made hypocapnic because acute hypocapnia causes hypokalemia. There is a particular risk in patients taking diuretics, in whom the plasma K^+ concentration will already be at the lower limit of normal (3.5 mmol L^{-1}).

Phosphodiesterase inhibitors

Phosphodiesterase (PDE) is the enzyme responsible for the breakdown of cyclic AMP into 5-AMP. Inhibition of this enzyme results in an increase in the concentration of cyclic AMP and, in turn, in the activation of protein kinases. This increases calcium entry through calcium L-channels, resulting in an increase in myoplasmic Ca^{2+}. Phosphodiesterase inhibitors increase cardiac contractility and reduce peripheral vascular resistance,[78,79] hence they can be regarded as inodilators.

Until 1978, the only oral inotropic agents for use in patients with chronic heart failure were the digitalis glycosides. In 1978, the first clinical report on the inotropic effect of amrinone, a drug selective for the myocardial phosphodiesterase (PDE-III or -IV), was published and amrinone was hailed as a "new digitalis."

Bipyridine derivatives

Amrinone exerts hemodynamic effects similar to dobutamine. Given intravenously, it increases cardiac output by 30–70% in patients with heart failure without changing the heart rate and blood pressure. The lack of effect on heart rate and blood pressure is an advantage over the sympathomimetic amines. Amrinone has no significant effect on cardiac conduction but decreases the atrial and atrioventricular functional refractory periods. Amrinone is effective in patients with poor left ventricular function after cardiopulmonary bypass, in patients with borderline ventricular function undergoing noncardiac surgery, and in patients after myocardial infarction. In addition, amrinone reverses the depressant effect of halothane in isolated heart papillary muscle.[80] Long-term administration of amrinone is complicated by a high incidence of side-effects, particularly thrombocytopenia and ventricular arrhythmias; in addition, the therapeutic results appear to be variable.

Milrinone causes more vasodilation than amrinone, resulting in marked reduction in left ventricular end-diastolic pressure and arterial hypotension. Beneficial in patients with systemic or pulmonary congestion, the inotropic potential of milrinone is limited to patients with high filling pressures. Milrinone may be particularly useful in patients who are relatively insensitive to catecholamines because of β-adrenoceptor downregulation.[81]

In small clinical studies, milrinone was found to be much less toxic than amrinone. However, the Prospective Randomized Milrinone Survival Evaluation has shown milrinone to increase mortality by approximately 30%.[82] Although it was widely accepted that depression of cyclic AMP was responsible for the reduced performance of the chronically failing heart, the disappointing effects of the phosphodiesterase inhibitors and of the partial β-adrenoceptor agonist xamoterol suggest that reduced cAMP may be an adaptive response to protect myocardial cells from further injury. Thus, the short time gains of enhanced inotropy do not necessarily predict better outcome.[83]

Imidazoline derivatives

Enoximone and piroximone are imidazolines with known PDE inhibitory properties. Their effects are similar to those of dobutamine, but they cause greater reductions in pulmonary wedge pressure.

Enoximone is active both intravenously and orally. It has a very favorable inotropic–chronotropic dose ratio (less than 0.1) and a wide margin of safety. The positive inotropic effect is accompanied by vaso- and venodilation. Enoximone is effective in the treatment of low output states following cardiac surgery,[84] and reverses the negative inotropy of verapamil.[85]

Long-term treatment with enoximore increases exercise tolerance, left ventricular function and exercise time.[86] This long-term effect, however, is not always observed and the place of enoximone is mainly in the short-term treatment of exacerbations of cardiac failure, or during the waiting period for cardiac transplantation.[87]

Piroximone increases cardiac output, reduces pulmonary and systemic vascular resistance, and improves contractility. Although increases in contractility may increase the risk of myocardial ischemia, piroximone has been shown to increase the anginal threshold in patients with coronary heart disease.

Calcium sensitizers

Sensitivity of troponin C to calcium is decreased by ischemia, hypoxia, and acidosis, resulting in depression of contractility. By contrast, sensitivity is increased by α-adrenoceptor stimulation[88] and by some phosphodiesterase inhibitors. The advantage of drugs increasing the sensitivity of troponin C to calcium is that they do not increase myoplasmic calcium. Therefore, they neither facilitate arrhythmias nor increase the energy requirements associated with outward calcium transport.

Pimobendan

Pimobendan, a benzimidazole derivative, is a weak phosphodiesterase inhibitor (20–30% of the inhibition obtained by milrinone) that sensitizes troponin C to calcium. The addition of pimobendan to standard therapy for heart failure increases exercise tolerance and peak oxygen uptake. In the long term, the effects of pimobendan compare favorably with those of enalapril.[89] Pimobendan has been confirmed to improve both acute and chronic heart failure. At variance with adrenergic agonists and PDE-III inhibitors, which mediate their effects by a cAMP-dependent mechanism causing an increase in myoplasmic calcium, pimobendan and other calcium sensitizers mediate their effects (at least in part) by increasing the sensitivity of the contractile elements to calcium. This may be related to changes in calcium binding to troponin C or to direct effects on the actin–myosin complex. However, the long-term safety of calcium sensitizers has not been determined.

Levosimendan

Levosimendan is a very promising calcium sensitizer. Administered as an intravenous infusion it improves function in patients with decompensated heart failure. Its effects outlast the duration of the infusion because of an active metabolite with prolonged half-life.[90] A multicenter study has confirmed the efficacy of levosimendan in patients with heart failure. It suggests that levosimendan is more effective than dobutamine.[91]

Calcium entry promoters

While many calcium antagonists (nifedipine, nimodipine, nicardipine) are antagonists at the nitrendipine receptors, thereby reducing calcium entry into the cells, calcium entry promoters are agonists at these receptors. New drugs with a selective effect on cardiac cells are being developed.

CALCIUM ANTAGONISTS

Calcium ions play a decisive role in the electrical activity of the heart, in the excitation–contraction coupling of skeletal, cardiac, and vascular smooth muscle, and in the release of neurotransmitters at the presynaptic junctions.

Calcium current

The slow (calcium) inward current (I_{si}) is distinct from the sodium current, underlies impulse conduction in nodal tissue, and is responsible for the plateau phase of the action potential. It is increased by adrenergic agonists, ischemia, and hypoxia. The slow inward current plays an important role in the development of arrhythmias. Ischemia inactivates sodium channels so that electrical activation is initiated by the calcium current. This causes delays in impulse propagation that facilitate re-entry.

The calcium channels have two separate mechanisms. One, on the extracellular side of the sarcolemmal membrane, is voltage dependent. The other, on the cytoplasmic side of the channel, is less voltage dependent and appears to be regulated by cyclic nucleotides such as cyclic AMP and cyclic GMP. Voltage dependence means that when the cell is depolarized the gate is open, and when the cell is repolarized the gate is closed. Nucleotide dependence means that a critical phosphorylation reaction at the inner gate of the Ca^{2+} channel determines the state of the gate.[92]

Voltage-operated channels can be divided into three subtypes: L, N, and T.[93] Transient calcium currents are carried by channels with a short mean lifetime and a low conductance (T-channels). Other channels have a long mean lifetime and a large conductance (L-channels), whereas some channels (N-channels) have intermediate characteristics. In cardiac muscle, the major pathway for calcium entry is through L-channels.[94]

In smooth muscle, particularly arterial muscle cells, L- and T-channels,[95] as well as receptor-operated and stretch-operated channels, have been described.[96] Calcium binds with calmodulin. The calcium–calmodulin complex activates myosin light chain kinase, which catalyses the phosphorylation of the myosin light chain. This initiates shortening of vascular smooth muscle.

Specific blockade of the slow channels

The chemical heterogeneity of the calcium antagonists suggests that they act at different receptor sites that are functionally linked with the calcium L-channels (Table 8.8). Recently, a new class of calcium antagonists was described. They selectively block T-type calcium channels, unlike other calcium antagonists which block L-type channels. Mibefradil belongs to this class of drugs and relaxes coronary arteries without depressing contractility and decreases heart rate. It is effective in the control of arterial hypertension and has antianginal and anti-ischemic effects.[97]

Cardiovascular effects of the calcium antagonists

The selective inhibition of the transmembrane influx of Ca^{2+} is responsible for the depression of sinus automaticity, atrioventricular conduction, and vascular tone.

Calcium antagonists protect the ischemic myocardium by reducing heart rate and contractility while inducing vasodilation, all of which decrease oxygen consumption. At the same time, they decrease coronary vascular resistance and thus facilitate oxygen supply. Moreover, calcium blockers prevent coronary spasm. As calcium overload plays an important role and contributes to permanent damage in totally ischemic muscle, calcium channel blockers minimize the cellular damage caused by ischemia.[98]

Table 8.8 *Classification of calcium antagonists*

Selective for slow Ca^{2+} channels	
I	Verapamil and derivatives (verapamil, gallopamil, anipamil)
II	Dihydropyridines (nifedipine, nicardipine, nimodipine, nisoldipine, nitrendipine)
III	Diltiazem
Nonselective for slow Ca^{2+} channels	
IV	Diphenylpiperazines (cinnarazine, flunarizine)
V	Prenylamine derivatives (prenylamine, fendiline)
VI	Others (bepridil, caroverine, perhexiline)

Therapeutic indications

Myocardial ischemia

The potency of the calcium antagonists as coronary dilators is of greatest benefit in the treatment of vasospastic and unstable angina. Calcium antagonists are also effective in the treatment of effort-induced angina. However, in patients with severe left ventricular dysfunction or congestive cardiac failure, negative inotropy may be exaggerated.

Arterial hypertension

Calcium antagonists reduce arterial pressure in direct proportion to the degree of hypertension. Nifedipine is effective in the treatment of malignant hypertension complicated by encephalopathy and left ventricular failure.

Congestive heart failure

Afterload reduction by nifedipine and nicardipine is associated with improved subendocardial perfusion and left ventricular relaxation.[99]

Hypertrophic cardiomyopathy

The major effect of calcium antagonists is to improve relaxation, so that the relation between pressure and volume during diastole becomes more normal.

Cerebral artery vasospasm

Vasospasm is commonly associated with subarachnoid hemorrhage and trauma. Nifedipine and nimodipine are effective in blocking experimental vasospasm. Nimodipine improves the functional prognosis after rupture of an intracranial aneurysm.[100] However, increases in intracranial pressure may occur in patients following head injury.

Interactions between calcium antagonists and anesthesia

Interactions with verapamil and diltiazem

Halothane, enflurane, isoflurane, and propofol cause dose-dependent depression of contractile performance, may modify atrioventricular conduction, and may cause peripheral vasodilation. These effects reflect a reduction in Ca^{2+} fluxes across the cell membrane and within the cells.[101,102] Thus, potentiation of cardiac depression, vasodilation, and slowing of conduction may be expected in the presence of calcium antagonists.[103,104]

The observation of left ventricular apical dysfunction when administration of verapamil is combined with isoflurane or halothane is intriguing but as yet unexplained;[105,106] this is probably caused by exaggerated disruption of calcium fluxes.

Interactions with nifedipine

Nifedipine causes peripheral vasodilation and may increase cardiac output.[107] However, during high-dose fentanyl anesthesia, the increase in cardiac output may be associated with hypotension.[108] By contrast, during anesthesia with halothane or enflurane, left ventricular performance decreases with the administration of nifedipine and cardiac output may be reduced.

Protection against perioperative ischemia

Diltiazem has been used successfully as an intravenous infusion to reduce the frequency of ischemic S–T segment depression in patients with ischemic heart disease undergoing noncardiac surgery and anesthetized with fentanyl and nitrous oxide.[109] In contrast, oral medication with calcium antagonists alone did not seem to prevent the development of ischemia in patients undergoing cardiac surgery, whereas β-adrenoceptor blockade was effective.[110]

Need for inotropic support

When exaggerated cardiovascular depression results from the association of calcium antagonists and inhalational anesthetics, an intravenous (i.v.) bolus dose of calcium increases the inotropic state of the myocardium and restores cardiac output and arterial pressure for approximately 5 min. However, intravenous calcium is ineffective in reversing atrioventricular conduction disorders.[111]

Catecholamines are not always effective in the treatment of severe calcium antagonist overdose, probably because calcium fluxes are too heavily blocked and therefore myoplasmic calcium cannot be elevated. Glucagon, a polypeptide hormone which exerts positive inotropic and chronotropic actions independent of β-adrenoceptors or norepinephrine depletion, may offer a useful alternative to calcium and catecholamines.[112] Amrinone has also been shown to reverse the effects of verapamil in several experimental models.[113]

ANGIOTENSIN-CONVERTING ENZYME INHIBITORS

Renin, angiotensin, and aldosterone play a role in the development of hypertension as well as in the regulation of fluids and electrolytes. Conversion of angiotensin I into angiotensin II involves the angiotensin-converting enzyme (ACE), which can be inhibited by ACE inhibitors. The same enzyme is responsible for the breakdown of bradykinin into inactive metabolites. Thus, ACE inhibitors prevent the formation of a potent vasoconstrictor (angiotensin II) and facilitate the accumulation of a potent vasodilator (bradykinin). ACE inhibitors may exert some of their effects by preventing the interaction between angiotensin and sympathetic activity, thus reducing sympathetic tone and norepinephrine release. Interactions with other vasoactive substances may also contribute to the vaso- and venodilation of the ACE inhibitors and explain their efficacy in patients with normal renin levels. Currently, 10 ACE inhibitors are available in the UK. Their antihypertensive efficacy is similar for all compounds. However, many modern agents are suitable for once-daily dosage. This maximizes compliance.

- *Captopril* is a stable inhibitor of ACE.[114] Its sulfhydryl moiety has been implicated in various side-effects (skin rash, loss of sense of taste).
- *Enalapril*, an *N*-carboxyalkyl dipeptide, is devoid of the sulfhydryl group and is metabolized into a highly potent ACE inhibitor – enalaprilat.[115] The latter is more potent than captopril.
- *Lisinopril* is the lysine derivative of enalaprilat and is also a nonsulfur-containing compound. Lisinopril is a potent ACE inhibitor that is effective both in reducing mean arterial pressure in hypertensive patients and in the treatment of congestive heart failure. In patients with heart failure, lisinopril appears to cause a greater improvement in exercise performance than captopril.[116]
- *Ramipril*, another ACE inhibitor, has been shown in the Heart Outcomes Prevention Evaluation (HOPE) to exert protective effects in patients at risk for cardiac events, even though they did not present with left ventricular dysfunction. The mechanism of this protection may be a reduction in the rate of progression of atherosclerosis.[117]

Cardiovascular effects

ACE inhibitors cause a decrease in blood pressure principally by decreasing systemic vascular resistance while cardiac output remains unchanged or increases. The absence of reflex tachycardia has been attributed to resetting of the baroreflex. Prolonged treatment of hypertension with ACE inhibitors can lead, after a few months, to a regression of left ventricular hypertrophy.[118]

Angiotensin-converting enzyme inhibitors in congestive heart failure

More than 2 000 000 people in the USA are thought to suffer from congestive heart failure (CHF), and new cases develop at a rate of 2 per 1000 population per year.[119] The overall mortality exceeds 50% in 5 years from the initial diagnosis and, for patients with refractory symptoms, it is about 20% per year.

The clinical syndrome of CHF is caused by the inability of cardiac output to meet the demands of peripheral tissues. This activates neural and humoral factors, leading to increases in sympathetic tone, circulating catecholamines, and plasma renin activity, which results in vasoconstriction that further reduces stroke volume.

Conventional treatment of heart failure with cardiac glycosides and diuretics may aggravate vasoconstriction, whereas vasodilators improve cardiac performance by reducing afterload. ACE inhibitors cause significant reductions in systemic and pulmonary pressures with a marked decrease in pulmonary wedge pressure. Heart rate tends to fall while stroke volume and cardiac output increase markedly.[120] Vasodilation is more marked in the renal circulation, with the rise in renal blood flow accounting for 50% of the increase in cardiac output.[121] Arteriolar dilation is accompanied by relaxation of venous tone. Exercise capacity is improved by about 20% and the mortality of patients with CHF is reduced. In postmyocardial infarction patients, ACE inhibitors reduce the progression of heart failure and increase survival. Such benefits have been demonstrated in numerous studies.[122] Similar benefits have been demonstrated in patients with asymptomatic left ventricular dysfunction and in those with established heart failure.[123] Widespread use of ACE inhibitors in these groups of patients prolongs lives and reduces hospitalization for congestive heart failure. Data are available from randomized trials of ACE inhibitor therapy in over 98 000 patients. ACE inhibitors reduce 30-day mortality by 7% and the incidence of nonfatal cardiac failure by 4%, but at the price of an excess of persistent hypotension and renal dysfunction.[122] One of the advantages of ACE inhibitors after myocardial infarction is their beneficial effect on remodeling of the heart.[124]

Angiotensin-converting enzyme inhibitors in hypertension

ACE inhibitors were originally developed for the treatment of hypertension. Their efficacy is well established and they are now used as alternative first-line therapies where beta-blockers or diuretics are either contraindicated or ineffective. ACE inhibitors are particularly beneficial in patients with left ventricular hypertrophy, diabetes, or renal functional impairment. ACE inhibitors have been shown in double-blind randomized studies to be more effective than beta-blockers in reducing the left ventricular mass index,[125] a surrogate endpoint for morbid events in hypertension treatment trials.

Although the greatest antihypertensive efficacy may be expected in high-renin hypertension, many low-renin patients respond to ACE inhibitors. At variance with other vasodilators, ACE inhibitors do not cause sodium and fluid retention. A first-dose hypotensive effect has been noted, especially in patients with high plasma renin activity. Low-dose captopril and enalapril are effective in a large proportion of patients with uncomplicated hypertension and have few side-effects.

Renovascular hypertension

Because of the increased renin production from the kidneys in patients with a significant renal artery stenosis, renovascular hypertension is very responsive to ACE inhibitors. Abrupt, profound hypotension is likely to occur in response to the first dose of an ACE inhibitor. This extreme responsiveness can be used as a test of the surgical curability of renovascular hypertension. However, there is a serious risk of deterioration of renal function when lesions are bilateral, when renal function is marginal, or when atherosclerotic lesions are extensive. The concurrent use of a loop diuretic increases the risk of renal failure.

Chronic renal failure

In hypertensive patients with chronic renal failure, ACE inhibitors may be effective and may increase renal function. However, acute or insidious renal failure may also develop, especially when they are administered with a loop diuretic.

The ultimate aim in reducing blood pressure is the prevention of vascular disease, especially in the coronary and cerebral arteries. Also important is the prevention of reduced arterial compliance, which increases the workload of the heart and increases the rate at which left ventricular hypertrophy develops.[126] Pressure reduction with ACE inhibitors (and calcium antagonists) is associated with an increase in vascular compliance and a reduction in cardiac hypertrophy. Moreover, the reduction in both angiotensin II and sympathetic activity improves coronary blood flow.[127]

Side-effects of angiotensin-converting enzyme inhibitors

Severe hypotension may occur in patients with high plasma renin activity, especially after the first dose of captopril or enalapril. Drug-induced renal insufficiency occurs mostly in patients with renal artery stenosis and is usually reversible after discontinuation of ACE inhibitors. Hyperkalemia may occur because of the inhibition of aldosterone; in patients with renal insufficiency, hyperkalemia may reach life-threatening levels. Moreover, potassium-sparing diuretics and prostaglandin synthetase inhibitors can induce uremia and excessive potassium retention when associated with ACE inhibitors.

Relatively little is known about the modification of the effects of anesthesia by ACE inhibitors. Some studies suggest that chronic treatment of arterial hypertension with enalapril accentuates the hypotensive effect of anesthesia.[128] Hypotension is attributed to a reduction in preload (corrected by moderate volume loading) and peripheral vascular resistance (corrected by phenylephrine). In patients undergoing cardiac surgery, vascular responsiveness has been found to be profoundly reduced by preoperative ACE inhibitor treatment.

ANGIOTENSIN II RECEPTOR ANTAGONISTS

The indications for angiotensin II receptor antagonists are the same as for ACE inhibitors. A number of drugs have been developed such as losartan, valsartan, and candesartan. An advantage of angiotensin II receptor antagonists is that they do not cause coughing (a frquent side-effect of ACE inhibitors). They are effective in the treatment of arterial hypertension[129] and congestive cardiac failure.[130] It is recommended to stop their administration the day before surgery because of reports of refractory hypertension.[131]

VASODILATORS

Several groups of vasodilators have already been discussed in the sections on adrenergic agonists and antagonists (α-adrenoceptor blockers, α_2-adrenoceptor agonists, β_2-adrenoceptor agonists, ganglion-blocking agents), calcium channel blockers, and ACE inhibitors.

The role of the endothelium is important to the understanding of modern concepts of the control of vascular tone. The endothelial cells of the vascular system modulate vascular tone by releasing vasodilator and vasoconstrictor substances such as endothelium-derived relaxing factor (EDRF), endothelins (potent vasoconstrictors), prostaglandin I_2 (prostacyclin; a vasodilator), and thromboxane (a vasoconstrictor).

Nitric oxide

Endogenous nitric oxide

The discovery that nitric oxide is a vasodilator stems from observations that the vasodilator effect of acetylcholine requires the integrity of the vascular endothelium. This suggested to Furchgott and Zawadzki[132] that the effect of acetylcholine was mediated by an endothelium-derived relaxing factor, now known to be nitric oxide (NO) or an NO-containing species such as nitrosothiol.

Glyceryl trinitrate, sodium nitroprusside, nitrosothiols, and molsidomine release NO and can be considered as prodrugs. They do not need an intact endothelium to cause vasodilation, hence their efficacy in diseases in which endothelial function is impaired (hypertension, atherosclerosis, vasospastic disorders).

Exogenous nitric oxide

Because NO binds rapidly with hemoglobin, inhaled NO exerts its effects on the pulmonary but not the systemic vasculature.[133] This makes it unique because all other pulmonary vasodilators cause some systemic vasodilation. In addition, within the lungs NO dilates vessels only in the ventilated areas whereas other vasodilators dilate vessels throughout the lungs, including the poorly ventilated areas, thus increasing venous admixture.[134] Beneficial effects of NO have been reported in acute respiratory distress syndrome, after mitral valve surgery in patients known to have long-standing pulmonary hypertension, and after cardiac transplantation. Because of possible toxicity, concentrations should be kept as low as possible, in the range of 40–180 parts per million (p.p.m.).

Nitrates

Nitroglycerin (glyceryl trinitrate) was first used in angina pectoris by William Murrel in 1879. More recently, nitrates have gained popularity in the management of congestive heart failure. Nitrates improve left ventricular dynamics, decreasing preload and increasing cardiac output.[135,136] Nitrate tolerance has been documented in animal models and, to a lesser extent, in humans.[137] This is particularly important as far as transdermal nitroglycerin patches are concerned.

Nitroglycerin and organic nitrates are relaxants of vascular smooth muscle in virtually all vascular beds. Their effect involves NO and other nitrosothiols. The latter activate guanylcyclase (cGMP), the common pathway for smooth muscle relaxation, via a decrease in intracellular free calcium, possibly caused by enhanced calcium extrusion from the cytolsol.[138]

Vascular effects of nitrates

At low concentrations, nitrates are potent venodilators. Blood flow to the extremities is increased and there is venous pooling in the splanchnic circulation, whereas blood volume is reduced in the lungs, heart, and liver. Reductions in right and left ventricular filling pressures improve right and left ventricular failure. However, in the presence of a relatively low preload, nitrates may decrease cardiac output.

At relatively low concentrations, nitrates increase arterial conductance and compliance. The diameter of vessels increases, and the impedance of the vascular tree is reduced. The increase in pulse pressure may cause pounding headaches. High concentrations of nitrates cause arteriolar dilation and hypotension. This, in turn, may elicit reflex sympathetic activation.

Nitrates cause dilation of the epicardial conductance coronary arteries. They enhance collateral flow[139] and have the ability to dilate eccentric stenoses, particularly the eccentric stenoses that possess sufficient smooth muscle.[140] Moreover, they reduce the myocardial compressive forces in patients with high left ventricular end-diastolic pressure. Nitrates are effective in reversing and preventing vasospasm.

Ischemic heart disease

Nitrates remain the "gold standard" for antianginal activity. Few patients with exercise angina fail to obtain relief from nitroglycerin because of the combined systemic and coronary actions of the drug. Long-acting, as opposed to short-acting, nitrates are of proved value for patients with relatively frequent anginal attacks, the most convincing evidence being for isosorbide dinitrate.[141] However, long-acting nitrates are not recommended for patients who experience fewer than two or three episodes of angina per week because tolerance develops.

Nitrate therapy is particularly effective for stable angina associated with impaired systolic function, left ventricular enlargement, or a history of left ventricular failure. In contrast, nitrate therapy should not be used as monotherapy for patients with stable angina associated with arterial hypertension.

Patients with a variable angina threshold benefit from nitrates because excessive coronary vascular tone is a determinant of anginal syndrome. Intravenous nitroglycerin is very effective,[142] later replaced by oral long-acting nitrates (isosorbide dinitrate) or nitroglycerin ointment. Nitrates are effective probably because adrenergically increased vascular tone plays a major role in unstable angina. For the same reason, nitrates are particularly effective for vasospastic angina.[143]

Congestive heart failure

Nitrates are unique in the treatment of congestive cardiac failure because of their efficacy in reducing ventricular preload. Although venodilation occurs with low doses in the normal heart, higher doses may be necessary to achieve adequate preload reduction in the face of cardiac failure. Nitrate therapy results in long-term improvement of exercise capacity.[144] In patients with cardiac failure, nitrates do not appear to cause hypotension. The greatest efficacy is in patients with large hearts and ejection fractions less than 40%, and in those with mitral regurgitation. The combination of nitrates and vasodilators (isosorbide dinitrate plus hydralazine) has been shown to decrease mortality compared with placebo or a vasodilator alone.[145]

Short-acting drugs

Sublingual nitroglycerin and isosorbide dinitrate, as aerosol sprays, are the major formulations for acute episodes of angina. Isosorbide dinitrate has a slower onset of action and lasts longer than nitroglycerin. Buccal or transmucosal nitroglycerin provide immediate and sustained release for several hours.

Intravenous nitroglycerin is adsorbed onto plastic tubing. However, little difference in efficacy has been found between polyvinylchloride (conventional) and special delivery sets made of polyethylene.

Long-acting drugs

Buccal or transmucosal nitroglycerin may ensure delivery of the drug for up to 6 h. Oral isosorbide dinitrate has a half-life of 1–2 h and is metabolized into two active compounds: 2- and 5-isosorbide mononitrate; 5-isosorbide mononitrate is almost completely bioavailable, is not metabolized by the liver, and has a half-life of 3–4 h.

Topical or dermal nitrates have been shown to be effective in angina and congestive cardiac failure. Nitroglycerin ointment may exert beneficial effects for up to 3–6 h as they deliver therapeutic plasma nitroglycerin concentrations.[146] In order to avoid tolerance, nitrate-free intervals of 6–8 h are necessary.

Transdermal disks or patches of nitroglycerin, which consist of nitroglycerin bound to a silicone matrix, allow for the very slow release of the drug across the skin. There is considerable controversy about this formulation, in terms of both doses to be given and risk of tolerance. The latter may be avoided by nitroglycerin-free intervals of 10–12 h.

Prostanoids: prostaglandin I_2 (prostacyclin) and prostaglandin E_1

These prostanoids are powerful vasodilators. While prostaglandin I_2 (prostacyclin) exerts its effects on both the systemic and pulmonary vasculatures, prostaglandin E_1 exerts its effects predominantly on the pulmonary vessels. Prostaglandin I_2 can be used in patients with acute peripheral ischemia and in patients with pulmonary hypertension in order to decrease the right ventricular afterload. Because of the systemic effects of prostaglandin I_2, norepinephrine is usually needed to prevent a substantial reduction in systemic arterial pressure. This has also been found to be necessary during administration of prostaglandin E_1.[147]

Endothelin antagonists

The endothelial cells generate vasoconstrictor substances known as endothelins.148 Three isoforms have been identified, each with 21 amino acids. Their vasoconstricting power is 10 times that of angiotensin II, and their duration of action is much longer. As the systemic, renal, coronary, and pulmonary vasoconstrictor effects of endothelin are enhanced by the NO inhibitor *N*(G)-monomethyl-L-arginine (L-NMMA), it is suggested that endothelin and NO are in balance. Imbalance may be responsible for the development of atherosclerosis, congestive heart failure, essential hypertension, and pulmonary hypertension. The inhibition of the effects of endothelin by calcium channel blockers such as nifedipine suggests that endothelin may be an agonist at nitrendipine receptors.[149]

ANTIHYPERTENSIVE THERAPY

For the purpose of making treatment decisions, hypertension can be defined as blood pressure equal to or greater than 160–190 mmHg (21.3–25.3 kPa), as recorded in the sitting position on several occasions. Isolated systolic hypertension is defined as a systolic blood pressure greater than 160 mmHg with diastolic pressure up to 90 mmHg (12 kPa). Between the ages of 65 and 74 years, the prevalence of hypertension is 50% and increases further above this age.[150] Isolated systolic hypertension increases from 5% at age 60 years to 24% at 80 years.[151] The absolute risk of complications is higher among elderly patients than in their younger counterparts. Even in the elderly, treatment of hypertension confers substantial advantages: mortality, cardiovascular events, and strokes being reduced by 12%, 20%, and 36% respectively. A Medical Research Council Trial[152] has shown that, in mild hypertension, stroke rate and incidence of all cardiovascular events are decreased by treatment. Diuretics reduce stroke rate more than beta-blockers, but they are ineffective in reducing coronary events.[153] The question of the level of diastolic blood pressure at which treatment is justified has been answered by the Hypertension Detection and Follow-up Program Cooperative Group.[154] After 5 years of intensive stepped care, all-cause mortality was 16.9% lower in well-controlled patients than in less rigorously treated patients; the highest difference (20.3% reduction in mortality) was in the group with diastolic pressure between 90 and 104 mmHg (12 and 13.9 kPa). Such data support the view that antihypertensive therapy should be initiated when diastolic pressure exceeds 90 mmHg.

From the question of whether hypertension should be treated, the focus of research has moved toward the question of how patients should be treated. The main issues are how low to aim for the blood pressure and which drug to choose. Taking into consideration the results of large recent trials involving a variety of drugs, including ACE inhibitors (captopril), the conclusion is that drugs other than diuretics and/or beta-blockers should be selected infrequently.[155] However, in clinical practice, patient outcome is far worse than might be predicted from clinical trials. Ineffective monotherapies, failure to titrate doses, changing treatments, or selecting additional therapy when target blood pressure is not achieved, together with poor patient compliance, explain this discrepancy. In addition, there is evidence that hypertension results from a complex interaction between lifestyle-related factors (high-salt diet, obesity, stress) and genetic susceptibility. In the face of such heterogeneity, the response to treatment is also heterogeneous. Combining antihypertensive drugs that act on different pathophysiologic mechanisms is likely to improve the overall efficacy of blood pressure control. As treatment may elicit counter-regulatory responses to single drugs, combinations with agents that block such reflex responses is also likely to be beneficial. Finally, combined therapy may be better tolerated than escalation of the dose with monotherapy.[156]

Diuretics

Diuretics are inexpensive, easy to administer, and effective in a high proportion of patients and over prolonged periods of time.

Thiazide-type diuretics

The antihypertensive effect of thiazide-type diuretics reaches a plateau at relatively low doses with which hypokalemia is usually limited to a reduction of 0.4–0.6 mmol L^{-1}. Magnesium depletion may also occur and may contribute to arrhythmias. Impaired glucose tolerance and hyperuricemia are observed; diabetes and gout may develop.

Potassium-sparing diuretics

These are usually given in association with thiazide-type diuretics to patients with thiazide-induced hypokalemia. There is a risk of hyperkalemia, particularly in patients with renal failure, diabetes, or hypoaldosteronism. This risk is enhanced by the concomitant administration of nonsteroidal anti-inflammatory drugs, ACE inhibitors, and potassium supplements. The most commonly used diuretics in this group are amiloride, spironolactone, and triamterene.

Loop diuretics

These are not used for the treatment of hypertension except in the presence of chronic renal insufficiency or of an edematous state (chronic heart failure, nephrotic syndrome, cirrhosis). The antihypertensive effect is dose dependent and does not have the ceiling effect of the thiazides.

A meta-analysis of 10 randomized trials of beta-blockers compared with diuretics in the management of hypertension in the elderly revealed that diuretics were superior to beta-blockers with regard to all endpoints. The odds ratios for all cerebrovascular events were 0.61 [confidence interval (CI) 0.51–0.72], fatal stroke 0.67 (CI 0.49–0.90), coronary heart disease 0.74 (CI 0.64–0.85), cardiovascular mortality 0.75 (CI 0.04–0.87), and all-cause mortality 0.86 (CI 0.77–0.96). Beta-blockers only reduced the odds ratio for cerebrovascular events to 0.75 (CI 0.57–0.98). Therefore, in the elderly, diuretics remain the first-line therapy.[157]

Adrenergic receptor antagonists

β-Adrenoceptor antagonists

β-Adrenoceptor antagonists are effective in the long-term treatment of hypertension as monotherapy and in the management of cardiac conditions associated with arterial hypertension (supraventricular tachyarrhythmias, hypertrophic cardiomyopathy, angina). Beta-blockers reduce blood pressure by decreasing cardiac output. This may explain the reduced exercise tolerance and cold extremities. Fatigue, depression, insomnia, vivid dreams, bronchospasm, Raynaud's phenomena, and cold extremities are side-effects of beta-blockade. Hydrophilic beta-blockers (acebutolol, atenolol, nadolol) are less likely to cause central nervous system (CNS) side-effects than lipophilic ones. Selective beta-blockers do not prolong insulin-induced hypoglycemia as much as nonselective blockers.[158]

Beta-blockers appear to be less effective in the elderly than in younger patients. Young patients with a hyperkinetic circulation respond particularly well to beta-blocker monotherapy. Patients with angina, hypertrophic cardiomyopathy, or supraventricular arrhythmias also benefit most.

α-Adrenoceptor antagonists

Nonselective α-adrenoceptor antagonists such as phenoxybenzamine and phentolamine have been superseded by selective α_1-adrenoceptor blockers, such as prazosin, terazosin, and doxazosin. They reduce peripheral vascular resistance and increase vascular capacitance; they do not interfere with the feedback control on norepinephrine release. Diastolic pressure is well controlled by α_1-blockers.[159] Syncopal episodes are rare (less than 1%). The risk of first-dose effect (orthostatic hypotension leading to syncope), particularly in the elderly, can be reduced by giving a small initial dose at bedtime. In patients with diabetes, asthma, and peripheral vascular disease, α_1-blockers may offer advantages over thiazides and beta-blockers.

Prazosin

A selective α_1-receptor antagonist that is effective singly or in association with other drugs. There is little increase in sympathetic activity or plasma renin activity. Sodium and water retention do occur and the efficacy of prazosin is enhanced by the addition of a diuretic.[160] Prazosin may be given in association with beta-blockers, α-methyldopa, and direct vasodilators. As prazosin causes little change in the glomerular filtration rate, it can be used safely in renal hypertension.[161]

Terazosin

A long-acting, selective α_1-blocker with a half-life of 12 h that is less potent than prazosin and has a slower onset of action.[162] Terazosin is effective in the control of hypertension as monotherapy. It is also used as a complement to beta-blockers and diuretics.[163] The first-dose phenomenon (severe orthostatic hypotension) is less pronounced than with prazosin.

α- and β-adrenoceptor antagonists

Labetalol is useful in the treatment of all grades of hypertension. It reduces vascular resistance. Heart rate and cardiac output do not increase because of beta-blockade.[164] Orthostatic hypotension may occur. Although afterload is reduced by labetalol, great care should be exercised with patients in cardiac failure.

Calcium antagonists

Diltiazem, nifedipine, nicardipine, and verapamil decrease blood pressure in hypertensive patients by vasodilation. Nifedipine is the most potent vasodilator. Its administration causes an increase in heart rate unless a beta-blocker is added. This association is well tolerated, whereas that of verapamil or diltiazem with a beta-blocker may result in disorders of conduction and marked cardiac depression.

Nifedipine is effective in the treatment of hypertensive crises (encephalopathy, intracranial hemorrhage, acute left ventricular failure, and aortic dissection) associated with blood pressures exceeding 200/120 mmHg (26.7/16 kPa). Small doses or oral or sublingual nifedipine may be effective in 5–60 min as they reduce systemic and pulmonary pressures and improve cardiac output.[165] The advantages of nifedipine are: (1) rapid oral absorption (sublingual administration is not faster than bite–swallow capsules); (2) relatively long duration of action (3–5 h); (3) blood pressure reduction as a function of the initial level of hypertension, maintenance of cardiac output, and coronary vasodilation.

Verapamil

Verapamil reduces vascular resistance. Activation of the sympathetic nervous system occurs, but its effects on the myocardium are minimized by the negative inotropy and chronotropy of verapamil.

Angiotensin-converting enzyme inhibitors

Captopril and enalapril are particularly useful in patients with hypertension and left ventricular dysfunction. Low-dose diuretics associated with an ACE inhibitor achieve control in 75% of patients with mild hypertension.[166]

The acute antihypertensive response to an ACE inhibitor is a function of the pretreatment plasma renin activity, but this relation is no longer obvious during long-term therapy.[167] As the frequency of renal artery disease increases with age, the possibility of renovascular hypertension should be borne in mind when ACE inhibitors are given to elderly patients because their administration may precipitate acute renal failure.

Hypotension may occur in patients with renovascular hypertension, high renin essential hypertension, diuretic pretreatment, and congestive cardiac failure. Low doses of captopril (6.25–12.5 mg) or enalapril (2.5 mg) should be given in the early phase of treatment.

Centrally acting sympatholytic agents

Clonidine and methydopa are α_2-receptor agonists that decrease blood pressure by reducing sympathetic efferent discharge. This is often accompanied by lethargy and fatigue. As there is an association between sympathetic activity and the development of left ventricular hypertrophy, centrally acting sympatholytic agents may be expected to prevent or cause regression of hypertrophy.[168] Such a regression is desirable since left ventricular hypertrophy increases cardiovascular mortality.[169]

Other antihypertensive drugs

Direct vasodilators

The most commonly used direct vasodilators are hydralazine and minoxidil. The mechanism of hydralazine-induced vasodilation includes the opening of high-conductance Ca^{2+}-activated potassium channels.[170] Long-term administration of hydralazine may cause systemic lupus erythematoid (SLE) syndrome. Minoxidil is the most powerful, and a loop diuretic is needed to prevent vasodilator-induced edema. A major side-effect of minoxidil is hirsutism.

Serotonin antagonists

The effects of serotonin on the circulation are mediated by two subtypes of the receptor – S_1 and S_2. The diversity of vascular responses is influenced by the distribution of receptor subtypes. Vasoconstriction is largely mediated by S_2-receptors on platelets and endothelial cells. Moreover, activation of S_2-receptors amplifies the effects of histamine, angiotensin, prostaglandin $F_{2\alpha}$, and norepinephrine.[171] Direct effects of serotonin on the heart and the circulation include increases in cardiac contractility, cardiac output, and pulmonary vascular resistance. However, S_1-receptor activation in the endothelium causes the release of endothelial-derived relaxing factor, prostaglandin I_2, and vasoactive intestinal peptide (VIP). Inhibition of the release of norepinephrine results in systemic vasodilation.[172,173]

In the elderly and in hypertensive patients, serotonin activity is increased. This could cause an increase in the tone of the capacitance vessels. More importantly, damaged vessels (a common feature of atherosclerosis) lose their protective endothelial barrier and their S_1-receptor-mediated vasodilation. In addition, serotonin could contribute to hypertension by an increase in aldosterone secretion.[174]

Ketanserin

Ketanserin is a highly selective S_2-antagonist. Its administration decreases peripheral vascular resistance by antagonizing the effects of S_2-receptor activation on vessels and platelets. It also unmasks the effect of S_1-receptor activation on blood vessels and on the release of norepinephrine (unopposed inhibition). Some of the effects of ketanserin may be due to α-adrenergic blockade.

Ketanserin lowers systolic and diastolic pressures. The main mechanism is systemic vasodilation, resulting in increases in renal, splanchnic, cerebral, and cutaneous blood flow but not cardiac output.

It is especially effective in the elderly, in whom serotonergic stimulation plays an important role.[175] The effects of ketanserin are augmented by association with β-adrenergic blockers. Side-effects include orthostatic hypotension, sleep disturbances and anxiety, fatigue, and sedation.[176] Ketanserin can be administered orally and intravenously.

Imidazoline receptor agonists

Stimulation of imidazoline receptors and the development of selective imidazoline agonists, especially moxonidine, allows control of the blood pressure with fewer side-effects (drowsiness and sedation) than with α_2-adrenoceptor stimulation. Blood pressure reduction is similar to that observed with the other major classes of alternative first-line antihypertensive drugs.[177] Moxonidine is at least as well tolerated as the other first-line antihypertensive agents, exhibiting a relative lack of interference with quality of life. At variance with clonidine, moxonidine does not present the risk of rebound hypertension on discontinuation of therapy. As a result of the reduction in sympathetic outflow, moxonidine administration causes regression of left ventricular hypertrophy.

HYPERTENSIVE EMERGENCIES

Perioperative hypertension

β-Adrenoceptor blockers blunt the hypertensive responses to some of the stimuli encountered during anesthesia and surgery. Calcium channel blockers (nifedipine, nimodipine, nicardipine) also minimize the risk of hypertensive responses to anesthetic and surgical maneuvers largely by reducing vascular resistance. In addition, they may reduce the release of catecholamines.

The adrenergic responses may be decreased by the administration of an α_2-adrenoceptor agonist used as a premedicant. Premedication with clonidine has been shown to minimize the increase in plasma norepinephrine during surgery of the abdominal aorta and to decrease the blood pressure and heart rate variability in treated hypertensive patients undergoing anesthesia and surgery.[14,178,179]

Postcardiac surgical hypertension

Hypertension occurs in 30–60% of patients after cardiac surgery.[180] The risks of postoperative hypertension include cerebrovascular accidents, disruption of suture lines, dissection of the aorta, and myocardial ischemia.

Neurohormonal changes include elevated catecholamines, renin, angiotensin, and vasopressin. They persist for several days after surgery, especially if tracheal intubation is maintained or if sedation and pain relief are inadequate. Postoperative hypertension is more common in hypertensive patients and in those with a high ejection fraction, which is indicative of good left ventricular function.[181]

The main hemodynamic disturbance is an increase in systemic vascular resistance, hence the efficacy of a rapidly acting vasodilator such as sodium nitroprusside with which arterial pressure is easily titrated to the desired level. Excessive reductions in diastolic arterial pressure and coronary steal may cause myocardial ischemia. Because of these risks, nitroglycerin is often used rather than nitroprusside, and is particularly effective when filling pressures are abnormally high.

In some patients, hypertension is associated with a hyperdynamic circulation and responds well to β-adrenoceptor blockers. In this respect, the ultrashort-acting beta-blocker esmolol given as a continuous infusion is particularly useful. Blood pressure may be titrated, cardiac output is usually only minimally reduced, diastolic pressure is well maintained, heart rate is reduced, and pulmonary shunting is not increased.[182]

Combined α- and beta-blockade with labetalol or nicardipine is effective. Once blood pressure control has been achieved, buccal or sublingual nifedipine medication may be practical. Associations of drugs may prove more effective than single drugs. Ketanserin has been shown to reduce the sodium nitroprusside requirements and to improve the quality of blood pressure control.[183]

Hypertensive emergencies in patients with intracranial disease

Marked hemodynamic fluctuations occur during neurosurgical procedures, including excessive responses to laryngoscopy, intubation, skin incision, handling of brain structures, and extubation. As autoregulation of cerebral blood flow is disturbed both before and after surgery in neurosurgical patients, hypertensive episodes may be accompanied by marked increases in cerebral blood flow and in intracranial pressure. Prevention of hypertensive episodes is a prerequisite for a safe perioperative outcome.[184]

As hypertensive episodes during surgery and during emergence from anesthesia may occur in a very high percentage of patients, antihypertensive drugs are often required. The choice of the drug must take into consideration its effect on the cerebral circulation.

Most conventional hypertensive agents, such as sodium nitroprusside, nitroglycerin, hydralazine, and trimetaphan, impair cerebral autoregulation and may increase cerebral blood flow and cerebral blood volume. Of the β-adrenoceptor blockers, esmolol may be more effective and more easily controlled than the others.[34] Labetalol does not alter intracranial pressure and compliance. Urapidil, an α_1-adrenoceptor blocker with some β_1-blocking efficacy and a central hypotensive activity,[185] is effective in the control of hypertensive episodes and does not increase the intracranial pressure even in patients with brain tumors.[186]

REFERENCES

1. Ahlquist RP. A study of the adrenotropic receptors. *Am J Physiol* 1948; **153:** 586–600.
2. Arnold A, McAuliff JP, Ludena FP, *et al.* Lipolysis and sympathomimetic amines. *Fed Proc* 1966; **25:** 500.
3. Lands AM, Arnold A, McAuliff JP, *et al.* Differentiation of receptor systems activated by sympathomimetic amines. *Nature* 1967; **215:** 597–8.
4. Langer SZ. Presynaptic regulation of catecholamine release. *Biochem Pharmacol* 1974; **23:** 1793–800.
5. Schwinn DA. Adrenoceptors as models for G protein-coupled receptors: structure, function and regulation. *Br J Anaesth* 1993; **71:** 77–85.
6. Van Tits LJH, Michel MC, Grosse-Wilde H, *et al.* Catecholamines increase lymphocyte β_2-adrenergic receptors via a β_2-adrenergic, spleen-dependent process. *Am J Physiol* 1990; **258:** E191–E202.
7. Aarons RD, Nies AS, Gal J, *et al.* Elevation of beta-adrenergic receptor density in human lymphocytes after propranolol treatment. *J Clin Invest* 1980; **65:** 949–57.
8. Martin C, Eon B, Saux P, *et al.* Renal effects of norepinephrine used to treat septic shock patients. *Crit Care Med* 1990; **18:** 282–5.
9. Lesch M. Inotropic agents and infarct size. Theoretical and practical considerations. *Am J Cardiol* 1976; **37:** 508–13.
10. Mager G, Klocke RK, Hopp H-W, Hilger HH. Phosphodiesterase III inhibition or adrenoreceptor stimulation: milrinone as an alternative to dobutamine in the treatment of severe heart failure. *Am Heart J* 1991; **121:** 1974–82.
11. Young M, Pan W, Wiesner J, *et al.* Characterisation of arbutamine: a novel catecholamine stress agent for diagnosis of coronary artery disease. *Drug Dev Res* 1994; **32:** 19–28.
12. Chintala MS, Lockandwala MF, Jandhyala BS. Protective effect of dopexamine hydrochloride in renal failure after acute haemorrhage in anaesthetized dogs. *J Auton Pharmacol* 1990; **10** (Suppl. 1): 95–102.
13. Smith GW, O'Connor SE. An introduction to the pharmacologic proper-

ties of Dopacard (dopexamine hydrochloride). *Am J Cardiol* 1988; **62:** 9C–17C.

14. Quintin L, Viale JP, Hoen JP, *et al.* Oxygen uptake after major abdominal surgery: effect of clonidine. *Anesthesiology* 1991; **74:** 236–41.
15. Hayashi Y, Maze M. Alpha$_2$-adrenoceptor agonists and anaesthesia. *Br J Anaesth* 1993; **71:** 108–18.
16. Ghignone M, Calvillo O, Quintin L. Anesthesia and hypertension: the effect of clonidine on perioperative hemodynamics and isoflurane requirements. *Anesthesiology* 1987; **67:** 3–10.
17. Bloor BC, Ward BS, Belleville JP, Maze M. Effects of intravenous dexmetedomidine in humans. *Anesthesiology* 1992; **77:** 1134–42.
18. Belleville JP, Ward DS, Bloor BC, Maze M. Effects of intravenous dexmetedomidine in humans. *Anesthesiology* 1992; **77:** 1125–33.
19. McSPI–Europe Research Group. Perioperative sympatholysis. Beneficial effects of the alpha$_2$-adrenoceptor agonist mivazerol on haemodynamic stability and myocardial ischemia. *Anesthesiology* 1997; **86:** 346–63.
20. Ablad B, Brogard M, Ek L. Pharmacologic properties of H56/28 a beta-adrenergic receptor antagonist. *Acta Pharmacol Toxicol (Copenhagen)* 1967; **25** (Suppl. 2): 9–40.
21. Bennett DH. Acute prolongation of myocardial refractoriness by sotalol. *Br Heart J* 1982; **47:** 521–6.
22. Regardh C-G. Pharmacokinetics of β-adrenoceptor antagonists. In: Poppers PJ, van Dijk B, van Elzakker AHM (eds). *β-Blockade and Anaesthesia*. Rijswijk, The Netherlands: Astra Pharmaceutica, 1982: 29–45.
23. Feely J, de Vane PJ, Maclean D. Beta-blockers and sympathomimetics. *Br Med J* 1983; **286:** 1043–7.
24. Yusuf S, Ramsdale D, Peto R, *et al.* Early intravenous atenolol treatment in suspected acute myocardial infarction. *Lancet* 1980; **2:** 273–6.
25. Hjalmarson A. International beta-blocker review in acute and postmyocardial infarction. *Am J Cardiol* 1988; **61:** 26B–29B.
26. CIBIS II Investigators and Committees. The cardiac insufficiency Bisoprolol Study II (CIBIS-II): a randomised trial. *Lancet* 1999; **353:** 9–13.
27. Prys-Roberts C, Foëx P, Biro GP, Roberts JG. Studies of anaesthesia in relation to hypertension. V. Adrenergic beta-receptor blockade. *Br J Anaesth* 1973; **45:** 671–81.
28. Foëx P. Alpha- and beta-adrenoceptor antagonists. *Br J Anaesth* 1984; **56:** 751–65.
29. Stone JG, Foëx P, Sear J, *et al.* Myocardial ischemia in untreated hypertensive patients: effect of a single small oral dose of a beta-blocker. *Anesthesiology* 1988; **68:** 495–500.
30. Gorcyski RJ. Basic pharmacology of esmolol. *Am J Cardiol* 1985; **56:** 3F–13F.
31. Quon CY, Stampfli HF. Biochemical properties of blood esmolol esterase. *Drug Metab Drug Dispos* 1989; **13:** 420–4.
32. Reynolds RD, Gorczynski RJ, Quon CY. Pharmacology and pharmacokinetics of esmolol. *J Clin Pharmacol* 1986; **26** (Suppl. A): A3–A14.
33. Zaroslinski J, Borgman RJ, O'Donnell JP, *et al.* Ultra-short acting beta-blockers: a proposal for the treatment of the critically ill patient. *Life Sci* 1982; **31:** 899–907.
34. Cucchiara RF, Benefiel DJ, Matteo RS, *et al.* Evaluation of esmolol in controlling increases in heart rate and blood pressure during endotracheal intubation in patients undergoing carotid endarterectomy. *Anesthesiology* 1986; **65:** 528–31.
35. Newsome LR, Roth JV, Hug CC, Nagle D. Esmolol attenuates hemodynamic responses during fentanyl–pancuronium anesthesia for aortocoronary bypass surgery. *Anesth Analg* 1986; **65:** 451–6.
36. Hull CJ. Phaeochromocytoma. Diagnosis, preoperative preparation and anaesthetic management. *Br J Anaesth* 1986; **58:** 1453–68.
37. Vaughan-Williams EM. Relevance of cellular to clinical electrophysiology in interpreting antiarrhythmic drug action. *Am J Cardiol* 1989; **64:** 5J–9J.
38. Snyders DJ, Katzung BG. Clofilium reduces the plateau potassium current in isolated cardiac myocytes. *Circulation* 1985; **72-III:** 233.
39. Feld GK, Vankatesh N, Singh BN. Pharmacologic conversion and suppression of experimental canine atrial flutter: differing effects of D-sotalol, quinidine and lidocaine and significance of changes in refractoriness. *Circulation* 1986; **74:** 197–204.
40. Singh BN, Vaughan Williams EM. A fourth class of antiarrhythmic agents? Effects of verapamil on ouabain toxicity, on atrial and ventricular intracellular potentials, and on other features of cardiac function. *Cardiovasc Res* 1972; **6:** 109–19.
41. Kobinger W. Specific bradycardic agents. In: Vaughan Williams EM (ed.). *Antiarrhythmic Drugs*. Berlin: Springer-Verlag, 1989: 423–52.
42. Millar JS, Vaughan Williams EM. Pacemaker selectivity. Effects on rabbit atria of ionic environments and of alinidine, a possible anion channel antagonist. *Cardiovasc Res* 1981; **15:** 335–50.
43. Grande P, Sonne B, Pedersen A. A controlled study of digoxin and quinidine in patients DC reverted from atrial fibrillation to sinus rhythm. *Circulation* 1986; **74** (Suppl. II): 101.
44. Karlson BW, Thorstensson I, Abjorn C. Disopyramide in the maintenance of sinus rhythm after electroconversion of atrial fibrillation: a placebo-controlled one year follow-up study. *Circulation* 1986; **74** (Suppl. II): 101.
45. Turner WM. Lidocaine and psychotic reactions. *Ann Intern Med* 1982; **97:** 149–50.
46. Impact Research Group. International mexiletine and placebo antiarrhythmic coronary trial. 1. Report on arrhythmia and other findings. *J Am Coll Cardiol* 1984; **4:** 1184–1193.
47. Pottage A. Clinical profiles of newer class I antiarrhythmic agents – tocainide, mexiletine, encainide, flecainide and lorcainide. *Am J Cardiol* 1983; **52:** 24c–31c.
48. Elharrar V, Zipes D. Effects of encainide and metabolites (MJ14030 and MJ9444) on canine cardiac Purkinje and ventricular fibers. *J Pharmacol Exp Ther* 1982; **220:** 440–7.
49. Rossi PRF, Yusuf S, Ramsdale D, *et al.* Reduction of ventricular arrhythmias by early intravenous atenolol in suspected acute myocardial infarction. *Br Med J* 1983; **286:** 506–10.
50. Yusuf S, Peto R, Lewis J, *et al.* Beta blockade during and after myocardial infarction: an overview of the randomized trials. *Prog Cardiovasc Dis* 1985; **27:** 335–71.
51. Julian D, Chamberlain D, Sandoe E, *et al.* Mechanisms for the early mortality reduction produced by beta blockade started early in acute myocardial infarction. *Lancet* 1988; **1:** 921–3.
52. Singh BN, Collett JT, Chew CYC. New perspectives in the pharmacologic therapy of cardiac arrhythmias. *Prog Cardiovasc Dis* 1980; **22:** 243–301.
53. Gagnol JP, Devos C, Clinet M, Nokin P. Amiodarone: biochemical aspects and hemodynamic effects. *Drugs* 1985; **29** (Suppl. 5): 1–10.
54. Rotmensch HH, Belhassen B. Amiodarone in the management of cardiac arrhythmias: current concepts. *Med Clin North Am* 1988; **72(2):** 321–58.
55. Kosinski EJ, Albin JB, Young E, *et al.* Hemodynamic effects of intravenous amiodarone. *J Am Coll Cardiol* 1984; **4:** 565–70.
56. Bellotti G, Silva LA, Esteves Filho A, *et al.* Hemodynamic effects of intravenous administration of amiodarone in congestive heart failure from chronic Chagas' disease. *Am J Cardiol* 1983; **52:** 1046–9.
57. Feld GK, Nademanee K, Weiss J, *et al.* Electrophysiologic basis for the suppression by amiodarone of orthodromic supraventricular tachycardias complicating pre-excitation syndromes. *J Am Coll Cardiol* 1984; **3:** 1298–307.
58. Rakita L, Sobol SM, Mostow N, Wrobel T. Amiodarone pulmonary toxicity. *Am Heart J* 1983; **106:** 906–15.
59. Fenster PE, White Jr NW, Hanson CD. Pharmacokinetics evaluation of the digoxin-amiodarone interaction. *J Am Coll Cardiol* 1985; **5:** 108–12.
60. Carmeliet E. An electrophysiologic and voltage-clamp analysis of the effects of sotalol on isolated cardiac muscle and Purkinje fibers. *J Pharmacol Exp Ther* 1985; **232:** 817–25.
61. Norwegian Multicentre Study Group. Timolol-induced reduction in mortality and reinfarction in patients surviving acute myocardial infarction. *N Engl J Med* 1981; **304:** 801–7.
62. Steinberg MI, Smallwood JK. Clofilium and other class III agents. In: Vaughan Williams EM (ed.). *Antiarrhythmic Drugs*. Berlin: Springer-Verlag, 1989: 399–412.
63. Frame VB, Wang HH. Importance of interaction with adrenergic neurons for antifibrillatory action of bretylium in the dog. *J Cardiovasc Pharmacol* 1986; **8:** 336–45.
64. Lynch JJ, Rahwan RG, Lucchesi BR. Antifibrillatory actions of bepridil and butyl-MDI, two intracellular calcium antagonists. *Eur J Pharmacol* 1985; **111:** 9–15.
65. Yatani A, Brown AM, Schwartz A. Bepridil block of cardiac calcium and sodium channels. *J Pharmacol Exp Ther* 1986; **237:** 9–17.
66. Rankin AC, Brooks R, Ruskin JN, McGovern BA. Adenosine and the treatment of supraventricular tachycardia. *Am J Med* 1992; **92:** 655–64.
67. Hood MA, Smith WM. Adenosine versus verapamil in the treatment of supraventricular tachycardia: a randomized double-crossover trial. *Am Heart J* 1992; **123:** 1543–9.
68. Richer C, Pratz J, Mulder P, *et al.* Cardiovascular and biological effects of K^+ channel openers, a class of drugs with vasorelaxant and cardioprotective properties. *Life Sci* 1990; **47:** 1693–705.
69. Schlepper M, Thormann J, Berwing K, *et al.* Effects of nicorandil on regional perfusion and left ventricular function. *Cardiovasc Drugs Ther* 1995; **9** (Suppl. 2): 203–11.
70. Vegh A, Gyorgyi K, Papp JG, *et al.* Nicorandil suppressed ventricular arrhythmias in a canine model of myocardial ischaemia. *Eur J Pharmacol* 1996; **305:** 163–8.

71. Herzig S, Lüllmann H. Effects of cardiac glycosides at the cellular level. In: Vaughan Williams EM (ed.). *Antiarrhythmic Drugs*. Berlin: Springer-Verlag, 1989: 545–63.
72. Gillis RA, Quest JA. The role of the nervous system in the cardiovascular effects of digitalis. *Pharmacol Rev* 1980; **31:** 19–97.
73. Gavaghan TP, Feneley MP, Campbell TJ, Morgan JJ. Atrial tachyarrhythmias after cardiac surgery: results of disopyramide therapy. *Aust NZ J Med* 1985; **15:** 27–32.
74. Gorven AM, Cooper GM, Prys-Roberts C. Haemodynamic disturbances during anaesthesia in a patient receiving calcium channel blockers. *Br J Anaesth* 1986; **58:** 357–60.
75. Wong KC, Kawamura R, Hodges MR, Sullivan SP. Acute intravenous administration of potassium chloride to furosemide pretreated dogs. *Can Anaesth Soc J* 1977; **55:** 203–11.
76. Lee CO, Abete P, Pecker M, *et al.* Strophantidin inotropy: role of intracellular sodium ion activity and sodium–calcium exchange. *J Mol Cell Cardiol* 1985; **17:** 315–30.
77. Morgan JP. The effects of digitalis on intracellular calcium transients in mammalian working myocardium as detected with aequorin. *J Mol Cell Cardiol* 1985; **17:** 1065–75.
78. Evans DB. Overview of cardiovascular physiologic and pharmacologic aspects of selective phosphodiesterase peak III inhibitors. *Am J Cardiol* 1989; **63:** 9A–11A.
79. Naccarelli GV, Goldstein RA. Electrophysiology of phosphodiesterase inhibitors. *Am J Cardiol* 1989; **63:** 34A–40A.
80. Komai M, Rusy BF. Inotropic effect of amrinone in rabbit papillary muscle: reversal of myocardial depressant effect of halothane. *Can J Physiol Pharmacol* 1984; **62:** 1382–6.
81. Colucci WS, Wright RF, Jaski BE, *et al.* Milrinone and dobutamine in severe heart failure: differing hemodynamic effects and individual patient's responsiveness. *Circulation* 1986; **73** (Suppl. 3): 175–83.
82. Packer M, Carver JR, Rodeheffer RJ, *et al.* Effect of oral milrinone on mortality in severe chronic heart failure. *N Engl J Med* 1991; **325:** 1468–75.
83. Curfman GD. Inotropic therapy for heart failure – and unfulfilled promise. *N Engl J Med* 1991; **325:** 1509–10.
84. Gonzalez M, Desager J-P, Jacquemart J-L, *et al.* Efficacy of enoximone in the management of refractory low-output states following cardiac surgery. *J Cardiothorac Anesth* 1988; **2:** 409–18.
85. Dage RC, Kariya T, Hsieh CH, *et al.* Pharmacology of enoximone. *Am J Cardiol* 1987; **60:** 10C–14C.
86. Treese N, Erbel R, Pilcher J, *et al.* Long-term treatment with oral enoximone for chronic congestive heart failure: the European experience. *Am J Cardiol* 1987; **60:** 85C–90C.
87. Loisance D, Sailly JC. Cost-effectiveness in patients awaiting transplantation receiving intravenous inotropic support. *Eur J Anaesth* 1993; **10** (Suppl. 8): 9–13.
88. Endoh M, Hiramoto T, Ischihata A, *et al.* Myocardial α_1-adrenoceptors mediate positive inotropic effect and changes in phosphatidylinositol metabolism. *Circ Res* 1991; **68:** 1179–90.
89. Katz SD, Kubo SH, Jessup M, *et al.* A multicentre randomized, double-blind placebo-controlled trial of pimobendan, a new cardiotonic and vasodilator agent in patients with severe congestive heart failure. *Am Heart J* 1992, **123:** 95–102.
90. Kivikko M, lehtonen L, Colucci WS. Sustained hemodynamic effects of intravenous levosimendan. *Circulation* 2003; **107:** 81–6.
91. Follath F, Cleland JG, Just H, *et al.* Efficacy and safety of intravenous levosimendan compared with dobutamine in severe low-output heart failure (the LIDO study): a randomised double-blind trial. *Lancet* 2002; **60:** 196–202.
92. Tsien RW. Calcium channels in excitable membranes. *Annu Rev Physiol* 1984; **45:** 341–58.
93. Spedding M. Three types of Ca^{2+} channel explain discrepancies. *Trends Pharmacol Sci* 1987; **8:** 115–16.
94. Morad M, Cleeman L. Role of Ca^{2+} channel in development of tension in heart muscle. *J Mol Cell Cardiol* 1987; **19:** 527–53.
95. Benham CD, Hess P, Tsien RW. Two types of calcium channels in single smooth muscle cells from rabbit ear artery studied with whole-cell and single-channel recordings. *Circ Res* 1987; **61** (Suppl. I): 10–16.
96. Lansman JB, Hallam TJ, Rink TJ. Single stretch-activated ion channels in vascular endothelial cells as mechanotransducers? *Nature* 1987; **325:** 811–13.
97. Brogden RV, Markham A. Mibefradil. A review of its pharmacodynamic and pharmacokinetic properties and therapeutic efficacy in the management of hypertension and angina pectoris. *Drugs* 1997; **54:** 774–93.
98. Nayler WG, Panagiotopoulos S, Elz JS, Sturrock WJ. Fundamental mechanism of action of calcium antagonists in myocardial ischemia. *Am J Cardiol* 1987; **59:** 75B–83B.
99. Burlew BS, Gheorghiade M, Jafri SM, *et al.* Acute and chronic hemodynamic effects of nicardipine hydrochloride in patients with heart failure. *Am Heart J* 1987; **114:** 793–804.
100. Petruk KC, West M, Mohr G, *et al.* Nimodipine treatment in poor-grade aneurysm patients. Results of a multicenter double-blind placebo-controlled trial. *J Neurosurg* 1988; **66:** 505–17.
101. Terrar DA, Victory JGG. Effects of halothane on membrane currents associated with contraction in single myocytes isolated from guinea-pig ventricle. *Br J Pharmacol* 1988; **94:** 500–8.
102. Puttick RM, Terrar DA. Effects of propofol and enflurane on action potentials, membrane currents and contraction of guinea-pig isolated ventricular myocytes. *Br J Pharmacol* 1992; **107:** 559–65.
103. Reves JG, Kissin I, Lell WA, Tosone S. Calcium entry blockers: uses and implications for anesthesiologists. *Anesthesiology* 1982; **57:** 504–18.
104. Atlee JL, Hamann SR, Brownlee SW, Kreigh C. Conscious state comparisons of the effects of the inhalation anesthetics and diltiazem, nifedipine, or verapamil on specialized atrioventricular conduction times in spontaneously beating dog hearts. *Anesthesiology* 1988, **68:** 519–28.
105. Videcoq M, Arvieux CC, Ramsay JG, *et al.* The association isoflurane–verapamil causes regional myocardial dysfunction. *Anesthesiology* 1987; **67:** 635–41.
106. Ramsay JG, Cutfield GR, Francis CM, *et al.* Halothane–verapamil causes regional myocardial dysfunction in the dog. *Br J Anaesth* 1986; **58:** 321–6.
107. Coriat P, Pamela F, Godet G, *et al.* Prevention des poussées hypertensives après chirurgie carotidienne. Interêt de la nifedipine et du diltiazem. *Ann Fr Anesth Reanim* 1986; **5:** 278–86.
108. Griffin RM, Dimich I, Jurado R, Kaplan JA. Haemodynamic effects of diltiazem during fentanyl-nitrous oxide anaesthesia. *Br J Anaesth* l988; **60:** 655–9.
109. Godet G, Coriat P, Baron JF, *et al.* Prevention of intraoperative myocardial ischemia during noncardiac surgery with intravenous diltiazem: a randomized trial versus placebo. *Anesthesiology* 1987; **66:** 241–5.
110. Slogoff S, Keats AS. Does chronic treatment with calcium entry blocking drugs reduce perioperative myocardial ischemia? *Anesthesiology* l988; **68:** 676–80.
111. Lehot JJ, Leone B, Foëx P. Calcium reverses global and regional myocardial dysfunction caused by the combination of verapamil and isoflurane. *Acta Anaesth Scand* 1987; **31:** 441–7.
112. Zaritsky AL, Horowitz M, Chernow B. Glucagon antagonism of calcium channel blocker-induced myocardial dysfunction. *Crit Care Med* 1988; **16:** 246–51.
113. Makela VHM, Kapur PA. Amrinone and verapamil–propranolol induced cardiac depression during isoflurane anesthesia in dogs. *Anesthesiology* 1987; **66:** 792–7.
114. Cushman DW, Ondetti MA. Inhibitors of angiotensin converting enzyme for treatment of hypertension. *Biochem Pharmacol* 1980; **29:** 1871–7.
115. Vlasses PH, Larijani GE, Conner DP, Ferguson RH. Enalapril, a nonsulfhydryl angiotensin-converting enzyme inhibitor. *Clin Pharmacol* 1985; **4:** 27–40.
116. Power ER, Chiaramida A, DeMaria AN, *et al.* A double-blind comparison of lisinopril with captopril in patients with symptomatic congestive heart failure. *J Cardiovasc Pharmacol* 1987; **9** (Suppl. 3): S82–S88.
117. Sleight P. Angiotensin II and trials of cardiovascular outcomes. *Am J Cardiol* 2002; **89** (2A): 11A–16A.
118. Dunn FG, Oigman W, Ventura HO, *et al.* Enalapril improves systemic and renal hemodynamics and allows regression of left ventricular mass in essential hypertension. *Am J Cardiol* 1984: **53:** 105–8.
119. Franciosa JA. Epidemiologic patterns, clinical evaluation, and long-term prognosis in chronic congestive heart failure. *Am J Med* 1986; **80** (Suppl. 2B): 14–21.
120. Romankiewicz JA, Brogden RN, Heel RC, *et al.* Captopril: an update review of its pharmacological properties and therapeutic efficacy in congestive heart failure. *Drugs* 1983; **25:** 6–40.
121. Packer M, Medina N, Yushak M, Meller J. Hemodynamic patterns of response during long-term captopril therapy for severe chronic heart failure. *Circulation* 1983; **68:** 803–12.
122. ACE Inhibitor Myocardial Infarction Collaborative Group. Indication for ACE inhibitors in the early treatment of acute myocardial infarction: systematic overview of individual data from 100,000 patients in randomised trials. *Circulation* 1998; **97:** 2202–12.
123. Garg R, Yusuf S. Overview of randomised trials of angiotension-converting enzyme inhibitors on mortality and morbidity in patients with heart failure. Collaborative Group on ACE inhibitor trials. *JAMA* 1995; **273:** 1450–6.
124. Ball SG, Hall AS. Who should be treated with angiotension-converting

enzyme inhibitors after myocardial infarction. *Am Heart J* 1996; **132:** 244–50.
125. Schmieder RE, Schlaich MP, Klingbeil AU, Martus P. Update on reversal of left ventricular hypertrophy in essential hypertension (a meta-analysis of all randomised double-blind studies until December 1996). *Nephrol Dial Transplantation* 1998; **13:** 564–9.
126. Safar ME. Focus on the large arteries in hypertension. *J Cardiovasc Pharmacol* 1985; **7** (Suppl. 2): S1–S4.
127. Magrini F, Shimizu M, Roberts N, *et al.* Converting enzyme inhibition and coronary blood flow. *Circulation* 1987; **75** (Suppl. I): 168–74.
128. Colson P, Saussine M, Seguin JR, *et al.* Hemodynamic effects of anesthesia in patients chronically treated with angiotensin converting enzyme inhibitors. *Anesth Analg* 1992; **74:** 805–8.
129. Dickstein K. The role of losartan in the management of patients with heart failure. *Clin Ther* 2001; **23:** 1456–77.
130. Doba N, Tomiyama T. Drugs, heart failure and quality of life: what are we achieving? What should we be trying to achieve? *Drugs Aging* 1999; **14:** 153–63.
131. Brabant SM, Bertrand M, Eyraud, *et al.* The hemodynamic effects of anesthetic induction in vascular surgical patients chronically treated with angiotensin II receptor agonists. *Anesth Analg* 1999; **89:** 1388–92.
132. Furchgott RF, Zawadzki JV. The obligatory role of endothelial cells in the relaxation of arterial smooth muscle. *Nature* 1980; **288:** 373–6.
133. Moncada S, Palmer PMJ, Higgs EA. Nitric oxide: physiology, pathophysiology and pharmacology. *Pharmacol Rev* 1991; **43:** 108–42.
134. Frostell C, Fratacci MD, Wain JC, *et al.* Inhaled nitric oxide. A selective pulmonary vasodilator reversing hypoxic pulmonary vasoconstriction. *Circulation* 1991; **83:** 2038–47.
135. Cohn JN, Franciosa JA. Vasodilator therapy of cardiac failure (first of two parts). *N Engl J Med* 1977; **297:** 27–31.
136. Cohn JN, Franciosa JA. Vasodilator therapy of cardiac failure (second of two parts). *N Engl J Med* 1977; **297:** 254–8.
137. Cowan JC. Nitrate tolerance. *Int J Cardiol* 1986; **12:** 1–19.
138. Popescu LM, Foril CP, Hinescu M, *et al.* Nitroglycerin stimulates the sarcolemma Ca^{2+} extrusion of coronary smooth muscle cells. *Biochem Pharmacol* 1985; **34:** 1857–60.
139. Cohen MV, Downey JM, Sonnenblick EH, Kirk ES. The effects of nitroglycerin on coronary collaterals and myocardial contractility. *J Clin Invest* 1973; **52:** 2836–47.
140. Brown G, Bolson E, Petersen RB, *et al.* The mechanisms of nitroglycerin action. Stenosis vasodilatation as a major component of drug response. *Circulation* 1981; **64:** 1089–97.
141. Dalal JJ, Yao L, Parker JO. Nitrate tolerance: influence of isosorbide dinitrate on the haemodynamic and antianginal effects of nitroglycerin. *J Am Coll Cardiol* 1983; **2:** 115–20.
142. Conti CR, Hill JA, Feldman RL, *et al.* Nitrates for treatment of unstable angina pectoris and coronary vasospasm. *Am J Med* 1983; **74** (Suppl. 6B): 28–32.
143. Ginsburg R, Lamb I, Schroeder JS, *et al.* Randomized double-blind comparison of nifedipine and isosorbide dinitrate therapy in variant angina pectoris due to coronary arterial spasm. *Am Heart J* 1982; **103:** 44–9.
144. Leier CV, Huss P, Magorien RD, Unverferth DV. Improved exercise capacity and differing arterial and venous tolerance during chronic isosorbide dinitrate therapy for congestive heart failure. *Circulation* 1983; **67:** 817–22.
145. Cohn JN, Archibald DG, Ziesche S, *et al.* Effect of vasodilator therapy on mortality in chronic congestive heart failure. Results of a Veterans Administration Cooperative Study. *N Engl J Med* 1986; **374:** 1547–52.
146. Armstrong PW, Armstrong JA, Marks LS. Pharmacokinetic–hemodynamic studies of nitroglycerin ointment in congestive heart failure. *Am J Cardiol* 1980; **46:** 670–6.
147. Vincent JL, Leon M, Berre J, *et al.* Addition of enoximone to adrenergic agents in the management of severe heart failure. *Crit Care Med* 1992; **20:** 1102–6.
148. Yanagisawa M, Kurihara H, Kimura S, *et al.* A novel potent vasoconstrictor peptide produced by vascular endothelial cells. *Nature* 1988; **332:** 411–15.
149. Kramer BK, Nishida M, Kelly RA, Smith TW. Endothelins. *Circulation* 1991; **85:** 350–6.
150. Prescott-Clarke P, Primatesta P. *Health Survey for England 1996: a Survey Carried out on Behalf of the Department of Health.* London: Stationery Office, 1998 (series HS, no.6).
151. Staessen J, Armery A, Fagard R. Isolated systolic hypertension in the elderly. *J Hypertens* 1990; **8:** 393–405.
152. Medical Research Council Working Party. MRC trial of treatment of mild hypertension: principal results. *Br Med J* 1985; **291:** 97–102.
153. Greenberg G, Thompson SG, Brennan PJ. The relationship between smoking and the response to antihypertensive treatment in mild hypertensives in the Medical Research Council's trial treatment. *Int J Epidemiol* 1987; **16:** 25–30.
154. Hypertension Detection and Follow-up Program Cooperative Group. Persistence of reduction in blood pressure and mortality in the Hypertension Detection and Follow-up Program. *JAMA* 1988; **259:** 2113–22.
155. Cutler J. Which drug for treatment of hypertension. *Lancet* 1999; **353:** 604–5.
156. Sever P. Additional therapy versus monotherapy in the treatment of hypertension. *Br J Cardiol* 1999; **6:** 24–34.
157. Messerli FA, Grossman E, Goldbourt U. Are beta-blockers efficacious as first-line therapy for hypertension in the elderly? A systematic review. *JAMA* 1998; **279:** 1903–7.
158. Wright AD, Barber SC, Kendall MJ, Poole PH. Beta-adrenoceptor blocking drugs and blood sugar control in diabetes mellitus. *Br Med J* 1979; **1:** 159–61.
159. Grimm RH. Alpha$_1$-antagonists in the treatment of hypertension. *Hypertension* 1989; **13** (Suppl. I): I131–I136.
160. Colucci WS. New developments in alpha-adrenergic receptor pharmacology: implications for the initial treatment of hypertension. *Am J Cardiol* 1983; **51:** 639–43.
161. Gunnells Jr JC. Treating the patient with mild hypertension and renal insufficiency. *Am J Cardiol* 1983; **51:** 651–6.
162. Kynch J. Pharmacology of terazocin. *Am J Med* 1986; **80** (Suppl. 5B): 12–19.
163. Chrysant SG. Experience with terazocin administered in combination with other antihypertensive agents. *Am J Med* 1986; **80** (Suppl. 5B): 55–61.
164. MacCarthy EP, Bloomfield SS. Labetalol: a review of its pharmacology, pharmacokinetics, clinical uses, and adverse effects. *Pharmacotherapy* 1983; **3:** 193–217.
165. Takekoshi N, Murakami E, Murakami H, *et al.* Treatment of severe hypertension and hypertensive emergency with nifedipine, a calcium antagonistic agent. *Jpn Circ J* 1981; **45:** 852–60.
166. Weinberger MH. Comparison of captopril and hydrochlorothiazide alone and in combination in mild to moderate essential hypertension. *Br J Clin Pharmacol* 1982; **14:** 127S–131S.
167. Hodson GP, Isles CG, Murray GD, *et al.* Factors related to first dose hypotensive effect of captopril; prediction and treatment. *Br Med J* 1983; **286:** 832–4.
168. Fouad FM, Nakashima Y, Tarazi RC, Salcedo EE. Reversal of left ventricular hypertrophy in hypertensive patients treated with methyldopa. *Am J Cardiol* 1982; **49:** 795–801.
169. Pooling Project Research Group. Relationship of blood pressure, serum cholesterol, smoking habit, relative weight, and ECG abnormalities to incidence of major coronary events; final report of the Pooling Project. *J Chronic Dis* 1978; **31:** 201–306.
170. Bang L, Nielsen-Kudsk JE, Gruhn N, *et al.* Hydralazine-induced vasodilatation involves opening of high conductance Ca^{2+}-activated K^+ channels. *Eur J Pharmacol* 1998; **361:** 43–9.
171. Houston D, Vanhoutte P. Serotonin and the vascular system: role in health and disease and implications for therapy. *Drugs* 1986; **31:** 149–63.
172. Vanhoutte PM, Luscher TF. Serotonin and the blood vessel wall. *J Hypertens* 1986; **4** (Suppl. 1): S29–S35.
173. Breuer J, Meschig R, Breuer H, Arnold G. Effects of serotonin on the cardiopulmonary circulatory system with and without 5-HT$_2$-receptor blockade by ketanserin. *J Cardiovasc Pharmacol* 1985; **7** (Suppl. 7): s23–s25.
174. Mantero F, Rocco S, Opocher G, *et al.* Effect of ketanserin in primary aldosteronism. *J Cardiovasc Pharmacol* 1985; **7** (Suppl. 7): s172–s175.
175. De Cree J, Hoing M, De Ryck M, Symoens J. The acute antihypertensive effect of ketanserin increases with age. *J Cardiovasc Pharmacol* 1985; **7** (Suppl. 7): s126–s127.
176. Breckenridge A. Ketanserin – a new antihypertensive agent. *J Hypertens* 1986; **4** (Suppl. 1): s13–s16.
177. Van Zwieten PA. Central imidazoline (I$_1$) receptors as targets of centrally-acting antihypertensives: monoxidine and rilmenidine. *J Hypertens* 1997; **15:** 117–25.
178. Engleman RM, Haag B, Lemeshow S, *et al.* Mechanism of plasma catecholamine increases during coronary artery bypass and valve procedures. *J Thorac Cardiovasc Surg* 1983; **86:** 608–15.
179. Ghignone M, Noe C, Calvillo O, Quintin L. Anesthesia for ophthalmic surgery in the elderly: the effects of clonidine on intraocular pressure, perioperative hemodynamics, and anesthetic requirements. *Anesthesiology* 1988; **68:** 707–16.

180. Gray RJ. Postcardiac surgical hypertension. *J Cardiothorac Anesth* 1988; **2:** 678–82.
181. Roberts AJ, Niarchos AP, Subramanian VA, *et al.* Systemic hypertension associated with coronary artery bypass surgery. Predisposing factors, hemodynamic characteristics, humoral profile, and treatment. *J Thorac Cardiovasc Surg* 1977; **74:** 846–59.
182. Gray RJ, Bateman TB, Czer LSC, *et al.* Comparison of esmolol and nitroprusside for acute post-cardiac surgical hypertension. *Am J Cardiol* 1987; **59:** 887–92.
183. Hodsman NBA, Colvin JR, Kenny GNC. Effect of ketanserin on sodium nitroprusside requirements, arterial pressure control and heart rate following coronary artery bypass surgery. *Br J Anaesth* 1989; **52:** 527–31.
184. Van Aken H, Cottrell JE, Anger C, Puchstein C. Treatment of intraoperative hypertensive emergencies in patients with intracranial disease. *Am J Cardiol* 1989; **63:** 43C–47C.
185. Van Zwieten PA, De Jonge A, Wilffert B, *et al.* Cardiovascular effects and interaction with adrenoceptor of urapidil. *Arch Int Pharmacodyn Ther* 1985; **276:** 180–1.
186. Van Aken H, Puchstein C, Sicking K, Koning H. Antihypertensive treatment with urapidil does not increase ICP in patients. *Intensive Care Med* 1986; **12:** 106–107.

9

The physiology of oxygen transport and red cell transfusion

TIMOTHY W RUTTER AND KEVIN K TREMPER

It has long been recognized that the maintenance of optimal oxygen delivery is the core concern in anesthesia and critical care medicine.[1] Although the delivery of oxygen to the cell mitochondria is a continuous process, it may be regarded as occurring in four phases.[2] During the first phase, the mechanical act of breathing causes gas to pass into the alveoli by the mechanism of breathing. Gas exchange then takes place between the oxygen in the alveoli and the bloodstream; the oxygenated blood is then transported to the tissues; and, finally, diffusion between the bloodstream tissue capillaries and the cell mitochondria occurs. The complicated process is necessary in order to maintain the adequate end-capillary oxygen tension necessary for aerobic metabolism and has evolved to deal with the limitations of oxygen delivery to cells living in a normal aqueous environment and with an enormous oxygen consumption. These limitations arise from the slow process of molecular diffusion of gases in liquids and the low solubility of oxygen in water. For multicellular organisms, the diffusion gradient deteriorates as the diffusion distance increases. Henry's law states that the amount of oxygen dissolved in solution is proportional to its partial pressure ($P\text{O}_2$). Therefore, arterial blood at a $P\text{O}_2$ of 100 mmHg (13.3 kPa) contains only 0.3 mL O_2 per dL. It is apparent that a human would be unable to maintain aerobic metabolism in the mitochondria by employing pure molecular diffusion over long distances in a water-based environment. The solution has been the development of a far more efficient oxygen transport system, the cardiovascular system, and the blood, using hemoglobin to increase the oxygen-carrying capacity of this aqueous solution (Fig. 9.1).

The need for this efficient oxygen transport system is reinforced by the small stores of oxygen in the body,[3,4] approximately 20 mL kg^{-1}. The functional residual capacity of adult lungs contains approximately 400 mL of oxygen, which can be increased by approximately 2.35 L by inspiring 100% oxygen. In addition, arterial blood contains an oxygen reserve of approximately 1000 mL. The tissues, interstitial fluid, and myoglobin probably account for further storage of 200 mL of oxygen. Oxygen stores in the blood, from the perspective of oxygen utilization, are of limited value because they have to maintain the pressure gradients between the alveoli and the mitochondria, and in an emergency they are rapidly consumed in the absence of an oxygen supply.[5,6] Failure of oxygen transport results in hypoxia, inadequate tissue oxygenation caused by either an inadequate blood flow (ischemia) or a low arterial oxygen content (Table 9.1).

If hypoxemic hypoxia is due to a low arterial oxygen content, this may be the result of a decrease in hemoglobin, $P\text{O}_2$, or saturation of the hemoglobin molecule ($S_a\text{O}_2$). The amount of oxygen, therefore, that is delivered to the tissues depends on the blood flow (cardiac output) and on the quantity of oxygen that is carried by the blood (O_2 content). These two variables determine systemic oxygen transport. Within this context, the way in which variations in blood volume and blood component replacement therapy alter this vital function of oxygen delivery will be discussed.

This makes the physiology of O_2 transport significant from another point of view. Anesthesiologists transfuse more than half of the 20 million units of blood and blood components administered each year in the USA. Although this life-saving treatment is accomplished with very little acute mortality, the risk of transmitting infectious agents with significant morbidity and mortality is present with every unit. [The risk of transmitting acquired immune deficiency syndrome (AIDS) has been estimated to be between 1:100 000 and 1:1 000 000 per unit.] The more commonly transmitted virus is non-A/non-B hepatitis, now known as hepatitis C. This virus has been associated with disease transmission at a rate of approximately 1% per unit, with nearly half of these patients developing clinical hepatitis and up to one-third going on to chronic disease.[7] Even with the recent introduction of an assay for the antibody to hepatitis C, there will still be a significant rate of disease transmission owing to the latency of seroconversion.[8] Six months after clinical hepatitis, as many as 40% of patients have not seroconverted.[8] These factors must be part of the decision-making process in choosing how and when to replace blood. The importance of maintaining oxygen transport while minimizing risk to the patient requires careful consideration by the practicing anesthesiologist.

THE PHYSIOLOGIC DETERMINANTS OF OXYGEN TRANSPORT

The importance placed on the physiology of oxygen transport is reflected by the number of variables used to measure the efficiency of the oxygen delivery system and the number of monitoring systems that have been developed to assess oxygen transport.[9,10]

OXYGEN TENSION: INSPIRED, ALVEOLAR, AND ARTERIAL

One of the simplest ways of quantifying pulmonary function with respect to oxygenation is to examine the alveolar–arterial oxygen tension difference (A–a gradient). To do this, the alveolar oxygen tension

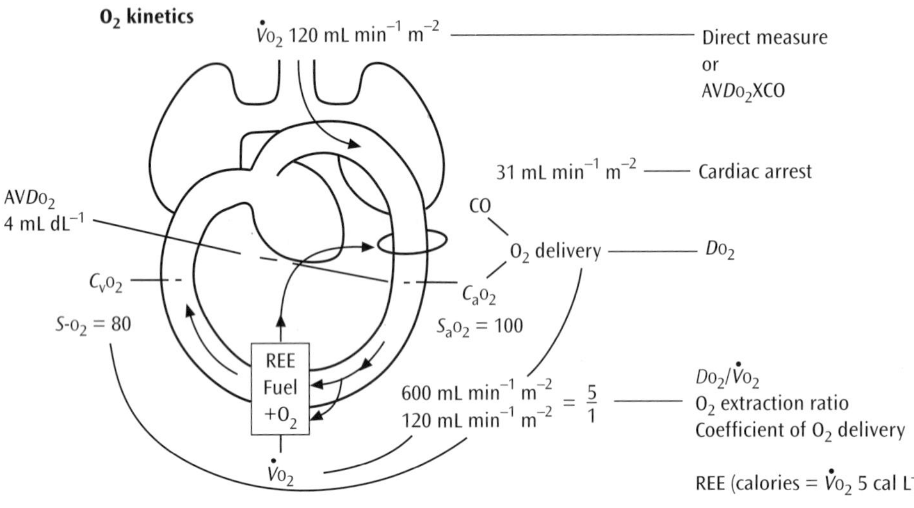

Figure 9.1 *Schematic representation of oxygen transport physiology depicting oxygen uptake in the lungs and oxygen delivery to the cardiovascular system.* $\dot{V}O_2$*, oxygen consumption; AVD*O_2*, arterial–venous oxygen content difference; CO, cardiac output;* DO_2*, oxygen delivery; REE, resting energy expenditure.*

must first be estimated using the "alveolar gas equation:"

$$P_AO_2 = F_IO_2\,(P_b - 6.3) - P_aCO_2 \times F$$

$$[P_AO_2 = F_IO_2\,(P_b - 47) - P_aCO_2 \times F]$$

in which P_AO_2 is alveolar oxygen tension measured in kPa(mmHg); F_IO_2 is the fraction inspired oxygen; P_b is the barometric pressure measured in kPa (mmHg); 6.3 kPa (47 mmHg) is the vapor pressure of water at body temperature (37 °C); P_aCO_2 is arterial PCO_2, used to estimate alveolar PCO_2, kPa (mmHg); and F is the respiratory exchange ratio.

The normal value for P_AO_2 is 13.26 kPa (102 mmHg) at sea level. Note that the normal P_AO_2 will decrease with increasing altitude (decreasing P_b), increasing P_aCO_2 and with decreasing F_IO_2. Consequently, a hypercapnic patient at high altitude would have a substantially lowered P_AO_2. A patient in Denver, Colorado, with a P_aCO_2 of 7.8 kPa (60 mmHg) would be expected to have a P_aO_2 of only 6.76 kPa (52 mmHg). Once the P_AO_2 is estimated, pulmonary function can be roughly assessed by obtaining P_aO_2 from an arterial blood sample and calculating an A–a gradient (normal value 0.65–1.3 kPa; 5–10 mmHg). Unfortunately, the A–a gradient itself is a function of F_IO_2, increasing to approximately 13 kPa (100 mmHg) at an F_IO_2 of 1.0. For this reason, the arterial–alveolar ratio (P_aO_2/P_AO_2 or a/A ratio ≈ 0.7) is also used to assess pulmonary function. This a/A ratio is less dependent on F_IO_2 than the A–a gradient. As with many other physiological variables, the expected "normal" value of P_aO_2 changes with the patient's age. The following expression has been used to predict an expected P_aO_2 as a function of age:

$$\text{"Normal" } P_aO_2 \approx 13 - 0.04 \times \text{age (years) kPa}$$

$$= [100 - 0.3 \times \text{age (years) mmHg}]$$

Table 9.1 *Classification of hypoxia*

Ischemic hypoxia	↓Blood flow, normal C_aO_2
Hypoxemic hypoxia	C_aO_2
Hypoxic hypoxemia	↓P_aO_2, S_aO_2, normal Hb
Anemic hypoxemia	↓Hb, normal P_aO_2, S_aO_2
Toxic hypoxemia	↓S_aO_2, normal P_aO_2 (i.e. MetHb or COHb)

This expression assumes that the patient is breathing room air at sea level and is normocapnic.

Arterial hypoxemia (hypoxic hypoxemia) can be produced by three mechanisms: decreased P_AO_2, right-to-left pulmonary shunt, or pulmonary diffusion barrier. If P_AO_2 is adequate, the most common cause of hypoxemia in perioperative patients is an increased pulmonary shunt ($\dot{Q}_{sp}/\dot{Q}_t$). Since the calculation of pulmonary shunt is based on oxygen content and oxygen transport, variables have been defined.

OXYGEN CONTENT

The oxygen content of the blood is that quantity of oxygen contained in the red cell added to the quantity dissolved in the plasma, and is defined as the volume of oxygen in milliliters carried in 1 dL of blood. It is normally calculated from the equation:

$$C_aO_2 = \text{Hb} \times 1.37 \times S_aO_2 + 0.023 \times P_aO_2 \text{ kPa}$$

$$(C_aO_2 = \text{Hb} \times 1.37 \times S_aO_2 + 0.0034 \times P_aO_2 \text{ mmHg})$$

where a signifies an arterial blood sample; C_aO_2 is the arterial oxygen content in mL dL^{-1} of blood; Hb is the hemoglobin concentration in g dL^{-1} of blood; 1.37 is the volume of oxygen in milliliters carried by 1 g of fully saturated hemoglobin; S_aO_2 is the fractional hemoglobin saturation; 0.023 and 0.0034 are the solubility coefficients of oxygen in plasma (mL of oxygen per dL plasma, in kPa or mmHg respectively); and P_aO_2 is equal to the arterial oxygen tension measured in kPa or mmHg. The red cells' contribution to oxygen content is, therefore, governed by the concentration of active hemoglobin and by the ability of hemoglobin to combine with oxygen, i.e. the saturation. The saturation depends on the partial pressure of oxygen and the position of the oxygen dissociation curve (Fig. 9.2).

Fractional hemoglobin saturation (S_aO_2) is defined as the ratio of oxyhemoglobin to total hemoglobin:

$$S_aO_2 = \text{HbO}_2/(\text{HbO}_2 + \text{Hb} + \text{metHb} + \text{COHb})$$

where HbO_2 is oxyhemoglobin, Hb is reduced hemoglobin, metHB is methemoglobin, and COHb is carboxyhemoglobin. Multiwavelength co-oximeters are required to measure the saturation. Another term that is frequently used to describe hemoglobin saturation is functional

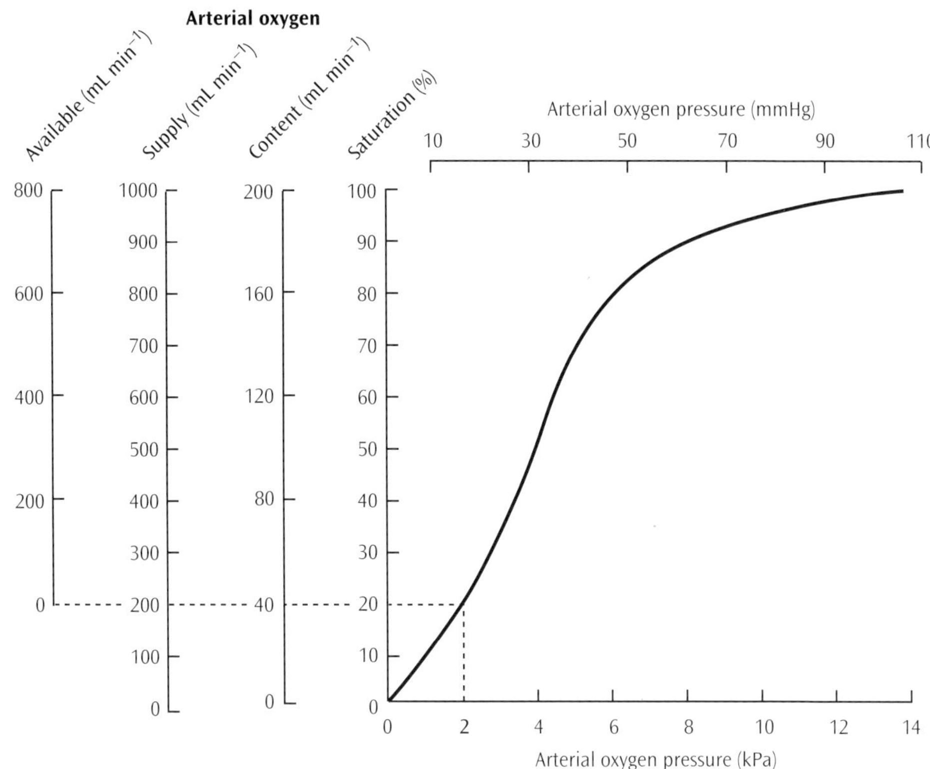

Figure 9.2 *O_2 dissociation curve and O_2 supply. The "content" scale shows the O_2 content ($mL\,L^{-1}$ blood) assuming a normal Hb concentration of 14.5 $g\,dL^{-1}$. The "supply" scale gives the systemic O_2 flow per minute assuming a cardiac output of 5 $L\,min^{-1}$. The available scale allows for the fact that many vital tissues cannot extract the last 20% of oxygen from hemoglobin because they cannot tolerate a capillary Po_2 value below about 2–2.6 kPa (15–20 mmHg). Note that when the arterial Po_2 lies on the steep portion of the curve, a small increase in tension, for example from a Po_2 value of 3.3 to 5.3 kPa (25–40 mmHg), causes a large increase in saturation (from 40% to 70%) and a large increase in available O_2 (from 200 to 500 $mL\,min^{-1}$).*

saturation, which ignores the presence of methemoglobin and carboxyhemoglobin:

$$\text{fn}S_aO_2 = HbO_2/(HbO_2 + Hb)$$

This functional hemoglobin saturation is that provided by blood gas analysis and estimates of saturation from P_aO_2 and the oxyhemoglobin dissociation curve (Fig. 9.2). Because methemoglobin and carboxyhemoglobin do not carry oxygen, only fractional saturation should be used when accurately calculating oxygen content.

With a hemoglobin level of 15 g and normal values of P_aO_2 and S_aO_2, the arterial oxygen content is 20 $mL\,dL^{-1}$ blood, 20 vol%, or 9 $mmol\,L^{-1}$. Normal oxygen content of blood is very similar to that of room air at sea level.

OXYGEN DELIVERY

The total quantity of oxygen delivered to the tissues per minute is a function of the oxygen content and the cardiac output (Fig. 9.2). This overall flow rate of oxygen to the tissues is called the O_2 delivery.[11–13] With a normal cardiac output of 5 $L\,min^{-1}$ for a 70-kg adult, this will result in a normal O_2 delivery of 44.5 $mmol\,min^{-1}$ O_2 or 1000 $mL\,min^{-1}$ O_2. Since the normal cardiac output (CO) depends on the size of the patient, cardiac output is commonly indexed to body surface area (BSA) (CI = CO/BSA $L\,min^{-1}\,m^{-2}$) using a normal cardiac index (CI) of 3 $L\,min^{-1}\,m^{-2}$ of O_2 delivery, as shown in the following equation:

$$O_2\ \text{delivery} = C_aO_2 \times CI \times 10\ mL\,min^{-1}\,m^{-2}\ O_2$$

In an adult patient with a normal CI of 3 $L\,min^{-1}\,m^{-2}$, the oxygen delivery index would be 600 $mL\,min^{-1}\,m^{-2}$ O_2 or approximately 27 $mmol\,min^{-1}\,m^{-2}$ O_2.

This measure of the oxygen delivery index is a value of total oxygen transport, but may be misleading as it does not take into consideration the regional variations in oxygen transport to specific organ systems.

AVAILABLE OXYGEN (see Fig. 9.2)

The concept of available oxygen implies that a proportion of the oxygen supply cannot be extracted. This is determined by the need to maintain the diffusion gradients and requires a working pressure at the capillary level of approximately 2 kPa (15 mmHg). Thus, 150–200 mL of the total O_2 delivery represents the core tissue requirement below which aerobic metabolism cannot occur. The level of oxygen supply above this lower limit necessary to prevent anaerobic metabolism is of considerable importance in the management of the critically ill.[14–16]

OXYGEN CONSUMPTION (Vo_2)

Approximately one-fifth to one-fourth of all the oxygen delivered to the periphery is consumed in maintaining the metabolic functions of the body. This represents an oxygen consumption of 150 $mL\,min^{-1}\,m^{-2}$ or 6.7 $mmol\,min^{-1}\,m^{-2}$ O_2. Human tissue consumes approximately 5 mL of oxygen for every deciliter of blood flow, and since the normal arterial oxygen content is 20 $mL\,dL^{-1}$ of blood, 75% of the oxygen remains in the venous blood returning to the heart. The mixed venous oxygen saturation, is therefore 75%. The oxygen consumption (Vo_2) can be calculated by multiplying the arterial venous oxygen content difference of approximately 5 vol% (2.2 $mmol\,L^{-1}$) by the cardiac output:

$$\text{Oxygen consumption} = (C_aO_2 - C_vO_2) \times CO$$

As with the oxygen delivery, the consumption may be indexed to adult body size so that the equation becomes:

$$\text{Oxygen consumption index} = (C_aO_2 - C_vO_2) \times CI$$

$$Vo_2 = (20\ mL\,dL^{-1} - 15\ mL\,dL^{-1}) \times L\,min^{-1}\,m^{-2} \times 10\ dL\,L^{-1}$$

$$Vo_2 = 150\ mL\,min^{-1}\,m^{-2}$$

This relation between oxygen consumption, the arterial venous oxygen content difference, and the cardiac output was first described by Fick and predicts that any increase in oxygen demand requires an increase in cardiac output if the arterial–venous difference is to remain constant.[17]

MIXED VENOUS OXYGEN TENSION, SATURATION, AND CONTENT

As we are unable to measure the mitochondrial or working tissue $P\text{O}_2$ in clinical practice, the mixed venous $P\text{O}_2$ is the basis on which to judge the adequacy of tissue oxygenation.[18,19] This has been measured by sampling expired air during rebreathing[20] or, as is the practice today, by sampling mixed venous blood via a pulmonary artery catheter.[21,22] The normal value in humans is 5–6 kPa (39 mmHg). The normal mixed venous oxygen content of $C_{\bar{v}}\text{O}_2$ of 12–15 vol% corresponds to a mixed venous hemoglobin saturation, $S_{\bar{v}}\text{O}_2$, of 72–78%. The oxygen extraction ratio is the relation between the consumption of oxygen and its delivery, as shown in the following equation:

$$\text{O}_2 \text{ extraction} = [(C_a\text{O}_2 - C_{\bar{v}}\text{O}_2) \times \text{CI}]/C_a\text{O}_2 \times \text{CI}$$

The normal extraction ratio of 25% indicates a wide margin of safety built into the oxygen delivery system. If the O_2 delivery decreases, the extraction ratio from arterial blood will increase, thus lowering the $C_{\bar{v}}\text{O}_2$. An increase in $\dot{V}\text{O}_2$ will produce the same result if there is not a compensatory increase in O_2 delivery. From Fick's equation, it can be seen that, if $C_a\text{O}_2$ and $V\text{O}_2$ are constants, $C_{\bar{v}}\text{O}_2$ (also $P_{\bar{v}}\text{O}_2$ and $S_{\bar{v}}\text{O}_2$) will follow changes in cardiac index. However, in acute care settings with hemorrhage and rapid fluid resuscitation, there are dynamic changes in oxygen content and $V\text{O}_2$ that negate the usefulness of $S_{\bar{v}}\text{O}_2$ monitoring as an early indicator of low cardiac output states.[23,24] In addition, as it is a mean value for all blood returning to the heart, it does not represent regional variations in flow, which may distort its true significance.[25–27] When tissue perfusion limits oxygen supply, there is a redistribution of blood flow from tissues with low oxygen extraction to tissues with high oxygen extraction, ensuring oxygen supply to the heart and brain (Table 9.2).

Small contributions from these sources to venous return may lead to normal or falsely elevated readings for $S_{\bar{v}}\text{O}_2$. Normal or elevated $S_{\bar{v}}\text{O}_2$ values may also occur in high-output states, large left-to-right shunts, and in cases of cyanide poisoning. The $S_{\bar{v}}\text{O}_2$ does not measure oxygen consumption, cardiac output, or systemic oxygen delivery, but is a valuable guide to the ratio of oxygen delivery to consumption[28,29] and, with the above caveats, $S_{\bar{v}}\text{O}_2$ is considered by many to be a reliable monitor in acute care settings.[30,31]

MIXED VENOUS OXYGEN PULMONARY SHUNT AND HYPOXEMIA

The concept of "absolute" intrapulmonary shunt assumes that blood flowing through the lung is divided into two streams: one with "ideal" oxygenation producing a $P\text{O}_2$ equal to $P_A\text{O}_2$, and another which picks up no oxygen and has a $P\text{O}_2$ equal to $P_{\bar{v}}\text{O}_2$. Given this assumption, an oxygen flow balance can be calculated for the left heart as follows:

Oxygen flow in = oxygen flow out

Ideal O_2 + shunt O_2 = O_2 delivery

$$C_A\text{O}_2 \times \dot{Q}_{\text{ideal}} + C_{\bar{v}}\text{O}_2 \times \dot{Q}_{\text{sp}} = C_a\text{O}_2 \times \dot{Q}_t$$

In the above equation, $C_A\text{O}_2$ is calculated from the oxygen content equation, assuming the $P\text{O}_2$ equals the $P_A\text{O}_2$. "Ideal" represents the pulmonary blood flow of that ideally oxygenated blood. $\dot{Q}_{\text{sp}}$ is the shunt blood flow and $\dot{Q}_t$ equals the total cardiac output. Because $\dot{Q}_t$ equals the sum of $\dot{Q}_{\text{ideal}}$ and $\dot{Q}_{\text{sp}}$, $\dot{Q}_t - \dot{Q}_{\text{sp}}$ can be substituted into the above equation for $\dot{Q}_{\text{ideal}}$. After algebraic rearrangement, the ratio of shunt blood flow to total blood flow ($\dot{Q}_{\text{sp}}/\dot{Q}_t$) can be calculated:

$$\dot{Q}_{\text{sp}}/\dot{Q}_t = [(C_A\text{O}_2 - C_a\text{O}_2)/(C_A\text{O}_2 - C_{\bar{v}}\text{O}_2)] \times 100$$

In actuality, pulmonary shunt is not usually produced by two distinct blood flows. Pulmonary blood perfuses lung units with various ventilation to perfusion ratios, resulting in less than ideal oxygen uptake. Pulmonary shunt is a useful concept and a useful method of quantifying decreased pulmonary function with respect to oxygenation. It is often referred to as venous admixture because the shunt blood is venous blood being admixed to the alveolar oxygenated blood. This terminology emphasizes the importance of venous oxygenation on the ultimate arterial oxygenation in the presence of a pulmonary shunt (Fig. 9.3).

During anesthesia, some causes of hypoxemia are obvious (ventilator disconnect, airway obstruction, etc.) while others are not (low $P_{\bar{v}}\text{O}_2$ in the presence of a pulmonary shunt). The larger the $\dot{Q}_{\text{sp}}/\dot{Q}_t$, the greater the effect $P_{\bar{v}}\text{O}_2$ has on $P_a\text{O}_2$, for example at 100% shunt $P_{\bar{v}}\text{O}_2$ is $P_a\text{O}_2$, and the less effect increasing $F_I\text{O}_2$ will have on increasing $P_a\text{O}_2$. Furthermore, any lowering of $P_{\bar{v}}\text{O}_2$ will lower $P_a\text{O}_2$ in the presence of a shunt. As discussed earlier, $P_{\bar{v}}\text{O}_2$ ($C_{\bar{v}}\text{O}_2$, $S_{\bar{v}}\text{O}_2$) decreases if there is a decrease in O_2 delivery (i.e. a decrease in $C_a\text{O}_2$ or CO) or increase in $V\text{O}_2$. As $\dot{Q}_{\text{sp}}/\dot{Q}_t$ invariably increases under anesthesia, blood loss is common [decreasing hematocrit (Hct), i.e. $C_a\text{O}_2$], and most anesthetic agents depress myocardial function

Table 9.2 *Distribution of blood flow*

Basal tissue exchange			**Blood flow**		
Tissue	**Arteriovenous oxygen (vol%)**	**$P_{\bar{v}}\text{O}_2$ [kPa (mmHg)]**	**Basal (mL min^{-1})**	**Exercise (mL min^{-1})**	**Cardiac failure (mL min^{-1})**
Heart	11.4 (11)[a]	3.0 (23)	250 (4)[b]	1000	300
Muscle	8.4 (30)	4.4 (34)	1200 (21)	22 000	1200
Brain	6.3 (20)	4.3 (33)	750 (13)	750	50
Splanchnic (liver)	4.1 (25)	5.6 (43)	1400 (24)	300	800
Kidney	1.3 (7)	7.3 (56)	1100 (19)	250	350
Skin	1.0 (2)	7.8 (60)	500 (9)	600	50
Other			600	100	200
Total flow			5800	25 000	34 000
Oxygen uptake			240	2000	300

a. Percentage of oxygen delivery.
b. Percentage of total cardiac output.

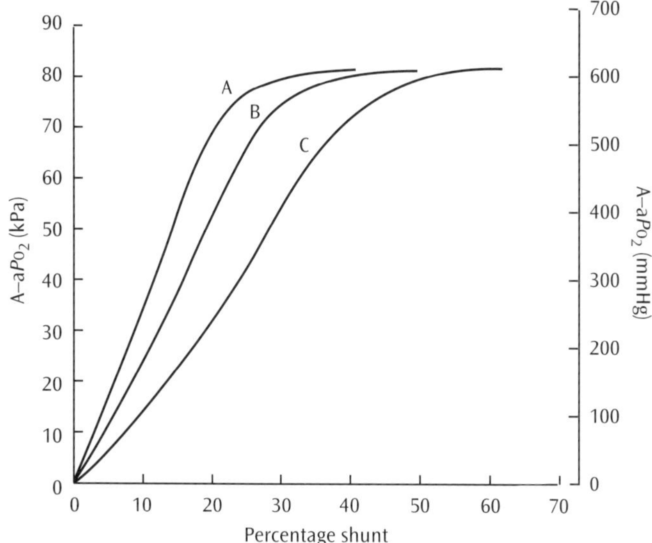

Figure 9.3 *Relation between A–a Po_2 and percentage left–right shunt when breathing oxygen. Hb = 15 g dL^{-1}; Pco_2 = 5.3 kPa (40 mmHg). Curves are drawn for three arteriovenous content differences. A, 3.13 mmol L^{-1} (7 vol%); B, 2.23 mmol L^{-1} (5 vol%); C, 1.34 mmol L^{-1} (3 vol%).*

(decreasing CO), the stage is set for hypoxemia even in the presence of adequate ventilation with high concentrations of oxygen. Because of the potentially severe consequences of unrecognized hypoxemia, continuous oxygen monitoring has become a standard of care.[10]

HEMOGLOBIN AND OXYGEN TRANSPORT

The tetrameric protein hemoglobin, a respiratory pigment, is of crucial importance in the transport of oxygen and carbon dioxide by the blood. Heme is a tetrapyrrole ring with a central iron atom and globin is an unbranched chain of amino acid units. The hemoglobin molecule is formed in the cytoplasm and the principal species in the normal adult is HbA. This denotes that the structural formula of the four globin chains is $\alpha_2\beta_2$. Other hemoglobin species may be present, but usually in smaller amounts. Hemoglobin F ($\alpha_2\gamma_2$), which is found in the neonate, has the property of binding oxygen more tightly than adult hemoglobin, thus its suitability for transport of oxygen in the fetus, i.e. higher saturation or lower Po_2. Hemoglobin F is gradually replaced by adult hemoglobin over the first few months of life.

The ability of hemoglobin to function as an oxygen transporter depends on the tetrapyrrole ring with a central iron atom that is able to reversibly bind oxygen. This function is used in a variety of subcellular mechanisms, including the myoglobin and cytochrome systems. The hemoglobin molecule combines with four molecules of oxygen which, in theory, equals 1.39 mL g^{-1} of hemoglobin or 0.062 mmol g^{-1} Hb. There are small amounts of methemoglobin and carboxyhemoglobin normally present, and a more usual figure for the oxygen combining power would be 0.059 mmol L^{-1} g^{-1} or 1.34 mL g^{-1} Hb.[32,33]

Blood, therefore, contains approximately 200 mL O_2 per liter or 9 mmol L^{-1}. The oxygen equilibrium curve for hemoglobin under normal physiological conditions is sigmoidal (Fig. 9.2). This results from the specific characteristics of the hemoglobin molecule, which are due to a heme–heme interaction.[34] This interaction allows the oxygenation of one subunit of the hemoglobin molecule to alter the oxygen affinity of the other subunits. This interaction also depends on the configuration of the globin chains. The further recruitment of subunits within the hemoglobin molecule for oxygen combination will occur at a lower partial pressure of oxygen than would otherwise be required, e.g. the rapidity with which the fourth subunit of hemoglobin combines with oxygen occurs at approximately 300 times the rate for the first subunit.[35] Perhaps more importantly, oxygen release from the hemoglobin will occur in the same way, i.e. the release of oxygen from the first hemoglobin subunit facilitates release of further oxygen.[36] This enhancement of oxygen uptake and release is the cause of the sigmoidal shape of the oxygen dissociation curve and defines the percentage saturation of hemoglobin at any partial pressure of oxygen.

The importance of the shape of the curve is several-fold. The rapid descent allows a large fraction of oxygen to be released to the tissues, as blood flows through them, with a modest drop in the partial pressure of oxygen. As the partial pressure of oxygen falls from an arterial level of 13.0 kPa (100 mmHg) to a venous level of 5.2 kPa (40 mmHg), 25% of the oxygen is released. However, as the pressure further decreases to 2.6 kPa (20 mmHg), an additional 25% is released, approximately doubling the original amount (Fig. 9.4). The relatively high "head of oxygen pressure" at the tissue level in microvascular beds provides sufficient oxygen partial gradient pressure to ensure diffusion of oxygen to cells at the periphery.

The position of the curve is defined by the P_{50} (Fig. 9.5), which is the partial pressure of oxygen at which the hemoglobin is 50% saturated. The P_{50} at pH 7.4 is approximately 3.5 kPa or 26.6 mmHg. When the curve shifts to the right, the P_{50} will increase, and it decreases when the curve shifts to the left. These alterations in the position of the curve greatly affect the rate at which oxygen can be delivered to the cells from capillaries. These factors are particularly important in the region of the venous Po_2, on the rapidly descending portion of the sigmoidal curve, where a right shift leads to a much lower venous saturation; therefore, for any given arterovenous oxygen partial pressure difference, there is much greater oxygen content difference.

The important factors determining the position of the curve are shown in Table 9.3.

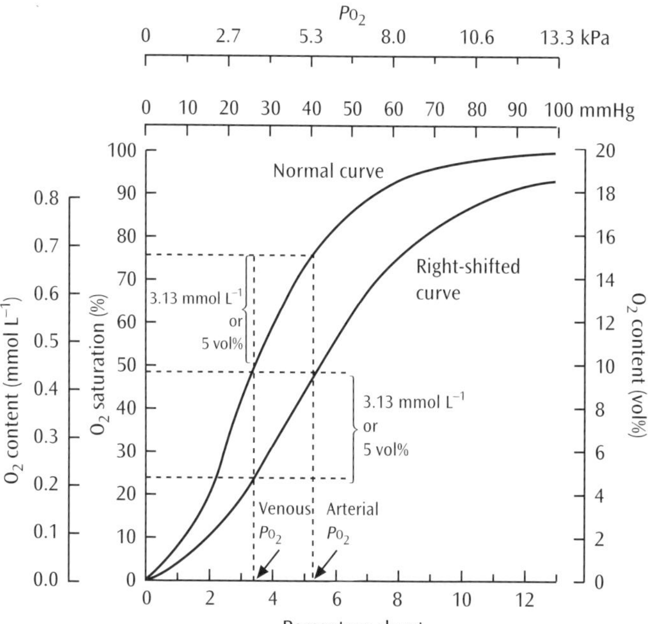

Figure 9.4 *The effect of a rightward shift of the dissociation curve when the arterial Po_2 is on the steep part of the curve. There is no increase in oxygen delivery when P_{50} is increased.*

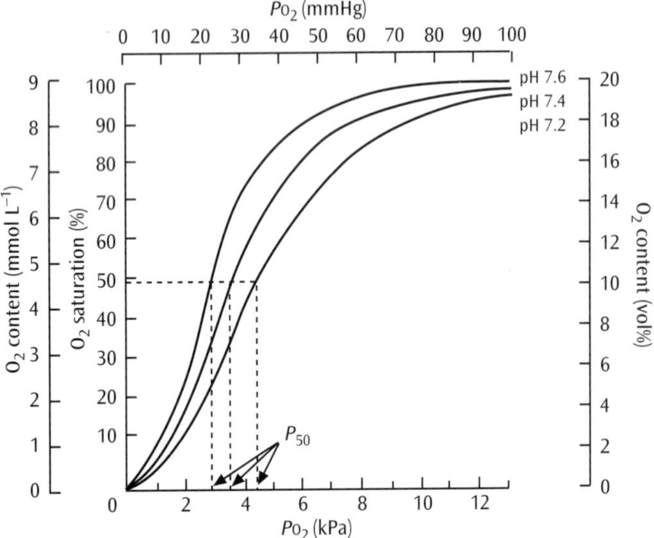

Figure 9.5 *Normal dissociation curves. The position of the curve is determined by the P_{50}.*

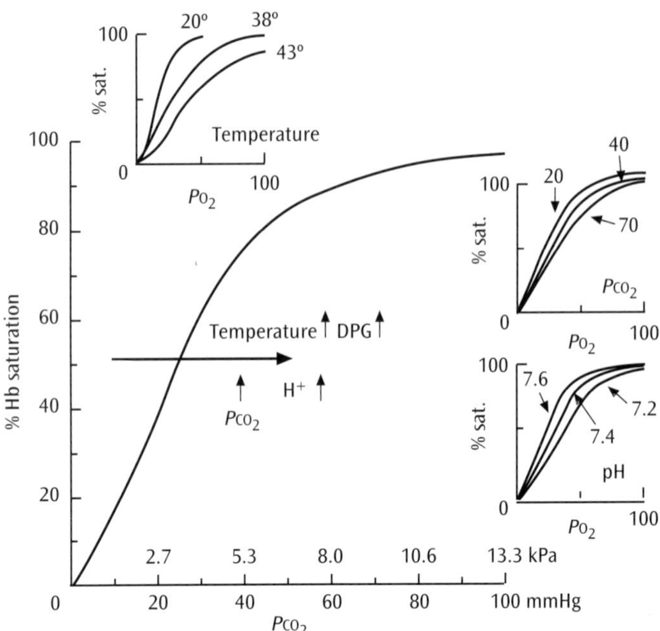

Figure 9.6 *Rightward shift of the O_2 dissociation curve by increase of H^+, Pco_2, temperature, and 2,3-diphosphoglycerate (DPG).*

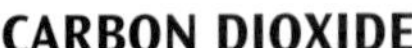

CARBON DIOXIDE

The change in oxygen affinity resulting from an alteration in carbon dioxide concentration was first described by Bohr, and has come to be known as the Bohr effect (Fig. 9.6). This effect, which is independent of the effect due to the change in the pH brought about by the presence of carbon dioxide, is the result of an interaction between carbon dioxide and the end-terminal amino acid groups of the β-chain of the hemoglobin molecule.[37] When carbon dioxide binds, affinity for oxygen by the molecule is reduced. The converse is also true. Hemoglobin is, therefore, intimately involved not only in the transport of oxygen to the periphery but also in the transfer of carbon dioxide to the lungs, where it is excreted. However, although the alteration in the P_{50} brought about by an increase in the partial pressure of carbon dioxide in the bloodstream is not of significant proportions under normal physiological conditions, it may be important in situations in which oxygen is low or in conditions that lead to a low level of 2,3-diphosphoglycerate (2,3-DPG).[38]

Table 9.3 *Some causes of shifts of the O_2–hemoglobin dissociation curve*

P_{50} decreased	P_{50} increased
By direct action	By direct action
Decreased [H⁺]	Increased [H⁺]
Decreased Pco_2	Increased Pco_2
Decreased temperature	Increased temperature
Abnormal Hb	Abnormal Hb
Fetal Hb	
Carboxyhemoglobin	
Methemoglobin	
By decreasing DPG	By increasing DPG
Increased [H⁺]	Decreased [H⁺]
Decreased thyroid hormone	Thyroid hormone
Hyperoxia	Hypoxemia
Panhypopituitarism	Congestive heart failure
Blood storage	Hepatic cirrhosis

HYDROGEN ION

The change in the position of the oxygen saturation curve or, more specifically, the alteration of oxygen affinity as a result of an increasing hydrogen ion concentration is also known as the Bohr effect, but should probably be more specifically called the hydrogen ion Bohr effect (Fig. 9.6). A reduction in the pH from 7.4 to 7.3, i.e. an increase in the hydrogen ion concentration of approximately 10 nmol L^{-1}, will increase P_{50} by approximately 0.3 kPa (3 mmHg). The molecular mechanism for the Bohr effect is the interaction between the hydrogen ions and specific amino acid residues on the globin moiety, causing an alteration in their tertiary structure, such that the affinity for oxygen is changed.[37] There is, therefore, a reciprocal relation between the hydrogen ion and oxygen binding of hemoglobin.

TEMPERATURE

In addition to the effect of carbon dioxide and hydrogen ion concentration on the affinity of hemoglobin for oxygen, alterations in body temperature will also cause an alteration in the position of the oxygen dissociation curve according to the equation:

$$(\Delta \log P_{50})/\Delta T = 0.023$$

Under these circumstances, an increase in temperature of approximately 5 °C will increase the P_{50} by approximately 0.9 kPa (7 mmHg).[37]

These effects of carbon dioxide, hydrogen ion concentration, and temperature have almost instantaneous effects on the position of the dissociation curve shown in Fig. 9.6. From the point of view of maintaining homoeostasis, these effects are beneficial to the organism. They enable hemoglobin to transport carbon dioxide to the lungs for excretion, and increase the buffering power of hemoglobin for the hydrogen ion. Under certain circumstances, the amount of acid produced may be extremely large. In actively exercising muscle, for example, this buffering capacity is able to "soak up" the hydrogen ion concentration with very little change in the erythrocyte or plasma pH and allow it to be transported to the kidneys for excretion. In addition, the relation between carbon dioxide, hydrogen ion concentration, and temperature allows oxygen to be delivered more effectively at the periphery to tissues with raised metabolic activity, thus facilitating aerobic metabolism.

2,3-DIPHOSPHOGLYCERATE

Further changes in the position of the oxygen dissociation curve result from the products of metabolism within the red cell, namely adenosine triphosphate (ATP) and 2,3-diphosphoglycerate (2,3-DPG) (Fig. 9.6). Changes in 2,3-DPG concentration are the most important and are often seen in chronic hypoxemia, heart disease, and anemia. Patients who have sickle cell anemia have a chronic right shift of the oxygen dissociation curve, associated with changes in 2,3-DPG concentration, which probably allows them to withstand the deleterious effects of anemia relatively well. 2,3-DPG is a metabolic product of anaerobic metabolism, with a normal intraerythrocyte concentration of 15 μmol g^{-1} Hb. It is able to bind with the β-chains when hemoglobin is in its deoxygenated form and increases oxygen availability.[39]

Increasing the 2,3-DPG concentration to twice the basal erythrocyte concentration leads to an increase in the P_{50} from 3.3 to 4.9 kPa (25 to 37 mmHg), thereby favoring oxygen release.[36] The mechanism of action by which the levels of 2,3-DPG increase P_{50} depends on the level of intracellular hydrogen ion. This may result from increased intracellular levels of reduced hemoglobin or from an overall increase in the hydrogen ion concentration of whole blood. However, in acute situations, the pH and 2,3-DPG interact to determine oxygen affinity.[40]

Any change in the hydrogen ion concentration produces an alteration in oxygen affinity and a delayed and opposite effect via 2,3-DPG. Any increase in the hydrogen ion concentration will move the curve to the right, which results in an intracellular diminution of the 2,3-DPG concentration, restoring the oxygen dissociation curve to its original position. The converse effect is true in alkalosis. As the effects on hydrogen ion concentration are more immediate and those of 2,3-DPG more long acting, the presence of an acidosis or alkalosis, and its attendant alteration in the oxygen dissociation curve, may alter oxygen affinity for some time until 2,3-DPG compensation occurs. In patients who have an otherwise normal physiological environment, such a change may not be of great consequence. However, in patients with altered blood flow, the consequences may be more severe. An example of this would be the vasoconstrictor effect of alkalosis on specific organ systems, such as the brain and heart, diminishing the oxygen available to those tissues.[38]

Changes in the levels of 2,3-DPG in the erythrocyte can be of importance in transfusion physiology. During the storage of red cells, there is a reduction in the levels of 2,3-DPG to extremely low levels at approximately 1–2 weeks. This reduction will occur at a slower rate in citric phosphate dextrose solution than in acid citrate dextrose blood. Frozen cells retain 2,3-DPG to a greater extent than normally stored cells. Blood that has been stored in liquid form and subsequently transfused into the patient has an alteration in its oxygen affinity as shown by a decrease in the P_{50}, which returns to normal over a period of 24–48 h. The transfusion of small amounts of stored blood may be of minimal consequence, physiologically, to a patient; however, massive transfusions of blood to patients who have altered tissue blood flow may produce marked changes in oxygen transport and oxygen affinity such that oxygen delivery may be impaired.

OXYGEN TRANSPORT FROM THE BLOOD TO THE MITOCHONDRIA

The regulation of oxygen transport between the systemic capillary blood and the tissue cell is brought about by simple diffusion in the same manner that gas exchange occurs in the lungs. Fick's law of diffusion describes the process of the molecular transport down a concentration gradient:

$$J = (\mathrm{d}c)/{-D}\,\mathrm{d}x$$

where J equals mass flux or rate of transport of the diffusing gas (oxygen) through a plane. D, diffusivity, is the diffusion constant in units of $cm^2\,s^{-1}$; dc and dx represent the concentration gradient, where c is the concentration of oxygen as a function of distance x. To determine the volume of oxygen being transported, we can multiply this equation by the surface area through which transport takes place. Additionally, to use oxygen partial pressure, the solubility constant (α) of oxygen in water must be included. The above equation changes to:

$$\mathrm{mL\ O_2/min} = AD\alpha\ [(P_1 - P_2)/\Delta x]$$

where Δx is the diffusion distance; P_1 and P_2 the partial pressure of oxygen at the capillary wall and the mitochondria respectively; and A is the surface area through which transport takes place, i.e. the surface areas of the capillary walls. Because the diffusion distances and the area of transport are often difficult to measure, the term permeability has been substituted for the combination of area (A), diffusivity (D), solubility (α), and diffusion distance (x):

$$(AD\alpha)/)P = \Delta x$$

The diffusion constant, D, for all gases diffusing in liquids is in the range of $10^{-5}\,cm^2\,s^{-1}$ and is inversely proportional to the square of the molecular weight of the gas. The diffusion constant therefore depends on the type of tissue through which it is diffusing, and also the gas being transferred. In the lung, the size of the tissue bed and thickness of the blood–gas barrier are favorable to diffusion. In the tissues, the size of the tissue bed varies significantly in terms of density of capillaries per unit tissue size and, therefore, the distance for gas diffusion will vary proportionately. Thus, oxygen delivery is flow dependent and will increase as recruitment of capillaries occurs, as in actively exercising muscle.

The composition of the interstitial fluid spaces is important. The presence of edema will increase the diffusion distance, diminish the rate of oxygen delivery, and produce an unfavorable balance between supply and demand for oxygen. As the oxygen diffuses away from the capillary, it is consumed, and the partial pressure of oxygen within the tissue will fall. At a critical point, the $P\mathrm{O}_2$ reaches a level at which all the delivered oxygen is utilized by the tissues and oxygen delivery is unable to meet demands. This appears to occur when $P\mathrm{O}_2$ is approximately 0.4 kPa (3 mmHg), which would appear to be the working pressure for the diffusion of oxygen intracellularly to the mitochondria. The presence of a significantly higher partial pressure of oxygen at the arterial end of the capillary ensures that these diffusion gradients remain intact, that aerobic metabolism can continue, and that tissue anoxia will not occur.

BLOOD VOLUME

The central role of the circulating blood volume for the maintenance of oxygen delivery has been stressed. Therefore, perioperative fluid management is of critical importance in the case of the surgical patient requiring detailed evaluation by the anesthesiologist. The blood makes up a unique proportion of the extracellular fluid volume, being composed of extracellular water contained in the plasma and intracellular water within the erythrocytes. In the normal adult, the blood volume approximates 5000 mL, of which 60% is made up of the plasma and 40% contained within the formed elements and constitutes the hematocrit. Compartmental analysis to measure these two fractions by "tagged red cells" or dye dilution allows calculation of total blood volume, although this is of limited practical clinical value:

$$\text{Blood volume} = \text{plasma volume} \times [100/(100 - 0.87 \times \text{hematocrit})]$$

The blood volume (more specifically the plasma volume) represents a small fraction (5%) of the total body water, but it is the precise regulation of this key portion that determines well-being (Fig. 9.7).

The homeostatic mechanism is volume driven such that the loss of red cells will be compensated for by an increase in the plasma volume until such time as the red cell mass can be reconstituted; likewise, any alteration in plasma proteins. The reconstitution of the blood volume from interstitial and intracellular fluid reserves depends on the transcapillary forces that make up the Starling equilibrium (Fig. 9.8).

The Starling equilibrium (Fig. 9.8) is in fact a disequilibrium, whereby approximately 2 mL min^{-1} of fluid is lost from the intravascular space to the interstitium owing to a positive filtration coefficient of 0.87 mL min^{-1} kPa^{-1} (6.67 mL min^{-1} $mmHg^{-1}$) for the whole body. This sensitive homoeostatic mechanism allows major changes in transcapillary fluid exchange for relatively minor alterations in applied pressure in order to react rapidly to any challenges to loss of blood volume. However, in the case of acute hemorrhage, this may take many hours to complete, requiring that the circulating blood volume be maintained, as opposed to absolute blood volume. The concentration of hemoglobin at which the cardiac index begins to rise varies according to the age and physiological state of the patient (Fig. 9.9).

THE REGULATION OF OXYGEN TRANSPORT

Therefore, a number of variables determine oxygen delivery in the adult patient. These are the concentration of hemoglobin, the oxygen saturation, the cardiac output, and the ability to onload oxygen in the lung and offload oxygen at the periphery. The $P_{a}O_2$, which is one of the factors that governs hemoglobin saturation, may be followed as a measure of adequate oxygen delivery to the tissues and used to guide therapy. However, a patient can have serious physiological derangements in O_2 delivery and yet retain a normal $P_{a}O_2$; hemorrhagic anemia, which may be acute or chronic, is a prime example. In either case, the oxygen content of the blood will be reduced but the oxygen delivery may be markedly different depending on the ability of the organism to mount a satisfactory response. This may be determined by several factors, including age. Hemoglobin production is under the control of the kidneys, where an unfavorable balance in the supply and demand for oxygen by renal tissue leads to the production of erythropoietin. These changes occur slowly and can approximately double the rate of red cell production from 1% to 2% per day. Further, in chronic anemia, the oxyhemoglobin curve is shifted to the right, the degree depending on the cause and being proportional to the severity of the anemia.[42] This is due to an increase in the concentration of intraerythrocyte 2,3-DPG.[43,44] The normal physiological response to anemia is to increase cardiac output, thereby tending to normalize O_2 delivery.[45,46] The concentra-

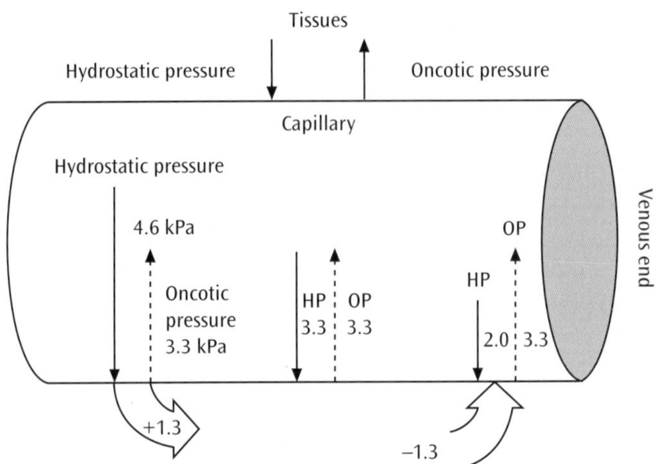

Figure 9.8 *Schematic representation of a normal capillary depicting the forces involved in the Starling equilibrium. At the arterial end, hydrostatic pressure (HP) exceeds oncotic pressure (OP) and there is a net efflux of capillary fluid. At the venous end, hydrostatic pressure is reduced and the oncotic pressure causes a reabsorption of interstitial fluid. Pressure values are in kPa. (Adapted from Guyton.[41])*

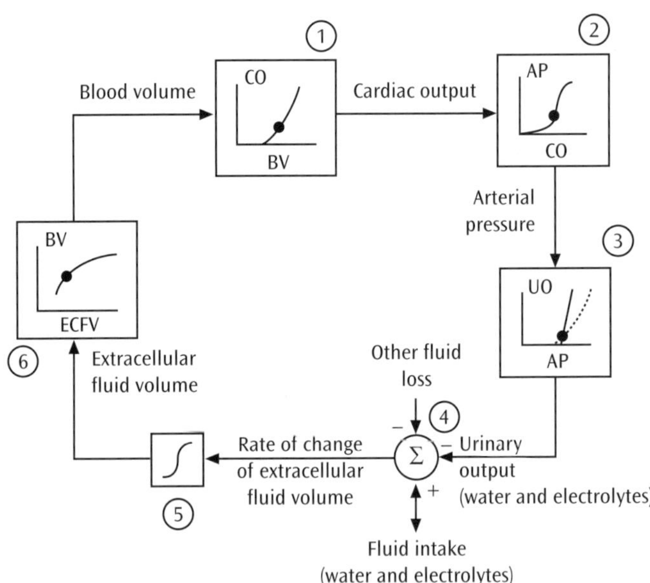

Figure 9.9 *Basic feedback mechanism for control of blood volume and extracellular fluid volume (the points on each of the curves represent normal values). CO, cardiac output; BV, blood volume; AP, arterial pressure; UO, urinary output; and ECFV, extracellular fluid volume.*

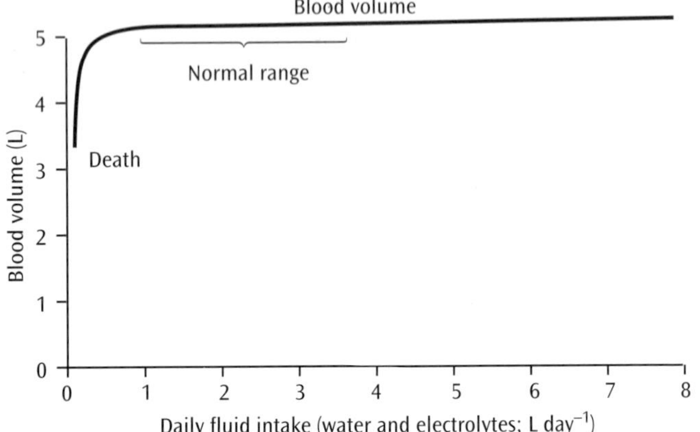

Figure 9.7 *Effect on blood volume of marked changes in daily fluid intake. Note the precision of blood volume control in the normal range.*

tion of hemoglobin at which the cardiac index begins to rise varies according to the physiological state and age, but is usually in the range of 8–9 g Hb dL^{-1} blood.[35] At these levels, the fall in oxygen content can be compensated for by a moderate increase in the P_{50}, as shown in Fig. 9.10. In this figure, arteriovenous content difference is an indirect measure of cardiac output, i.e. cardiac output increases as arteriovenous content difference decreases.

Below these levels, oxygen demand must be met either by increasing cardiac output or by increasing oxygen extraction and allowing the mixed venous oxygen content to fall (Fig. 9.10). Conversely, if the cardiac output is low, as measured by the $C_{(a-v)}O_2$ difference, the ability to tolerate even moderate anemia is compromised, and further reductions in Hb will lead to a further increase in the $C_{(a-v)}O_2$.

After acute surgical hemorrhage, a patient who is anemic may receive a large amount of stored blood with an increased affinity for oxygen, and simultaneously have a diminished circulating blood volume with a low cardiac output. This patient may have a significant reduction in oxygen delivery (DO_2), an increase in oxygen extraction, and an extremely tenuous balance between supply of oxygen and its demand by the tissues for oxidative phosphorylation (Fig. 9.11).

The importance of this $\dot{V}O_2/DO_2$ ratio can be further appreciated in hypermetabolic states, as found in thermal injuries when oxygen demand may outstrip oxygen delivery and oxygen delivery reserves (Fig. 9.12). The kinetics of oxygen transport require that there be complex and as yet poorly understood compensatory mechanisms to autoregulate DO_2 and VO_2. Figure 9.13 indicates that in acute-onset anemia DO_2 can only be met by an increase in cardiac index; likewise, any fall in oxygen content due to acute hypoxia (Fig. 9.14). The increase in cardiac index maintains the normal $DO_2/\dot{V}O_2$ ratio of 4:1 and ensures that aerobic metabolism can continue. However, an acute reduction in cardiac index cannot induce any beneficial response to facilitate oxygen delivery. Instead, oxygen demand must be met by an increase in oxygen extraction, with a consequent decrease in the $DO_2/\dot{V}O_2$ ratio (Fig. 9.15).

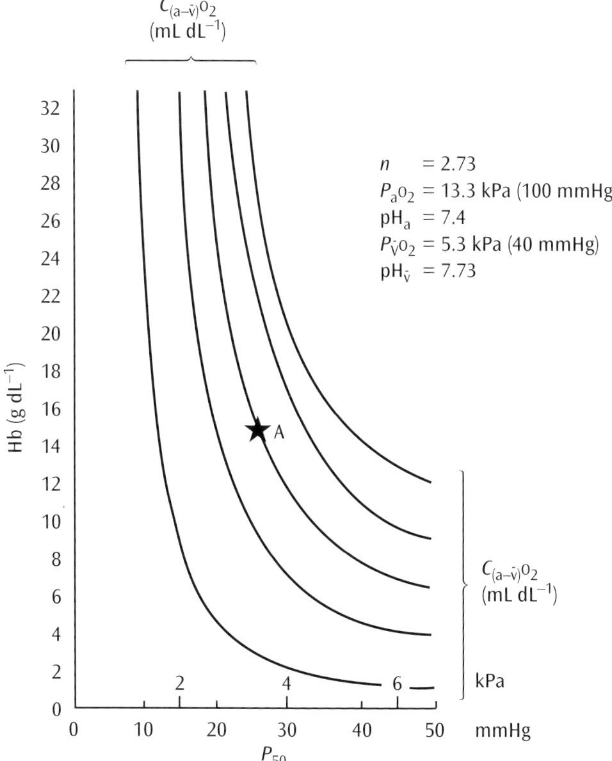

Figure 9.10 *The relation between hemoglobin concentration (Hb) and P_{50} at different levels of cardiac output, expressed as arteriovenous content differences, $C_{(a-\bar{v})}O_2$. Point A represents normal values for these three variables. Normal arterial and mixed venous PO_2 and pH and an oxygen–hemoglobin equivalent of 1.34 mL g^{-1} have been assumed.*

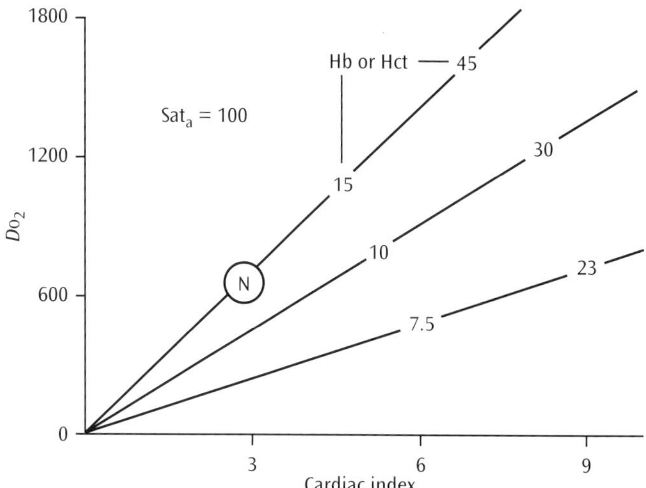

Figure 9.11 *The relation between oxygen delivery (DO_2) and changes in hemoglobin concentrations (Hb) or hematocrit (Hct) at normal saturation and changes in the cardiac index (CI). N, normal range.*

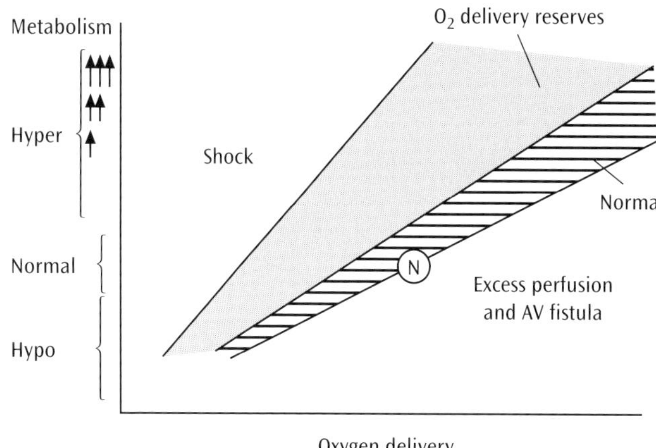

Figure 9.12 *The relation between oxygen delivery (DO_2) and oxygen consumption ($\dot{V}O_2$) with increasing oxygen demand. N represents the balance between the delivery of oxygen and consumption with maintenance of a normal $DO_2/\dot{V}O_2$ ratio. Hyperbolic states deplete oxygen delivery reserves and the normal $DO_2/\dot{V}O_2$ ratio to a point beyond which compensatory mechanisms can no longer provide adequate oxygenation and a state of shock is said to exist.*

The actual $DO_2/\dot{V}O_2$ ratio at which oxygen consumption becomes supply dependent is a matter of conjecture, but a 2:1 ratio is often regarded as a critical point.[14,15,47] Several studies indicate that below this level anaerobic metabolism, with its attendant production of lactic acid, occurs.[48–50]

However, the significance of oxygen delivery values may differ depending on how they are produced, i.e. variations in content versus variations in flow and distribution of flow. Several studies have demonstrated lactate acidosis without mixed venous desaturation.[51,52] Lactate

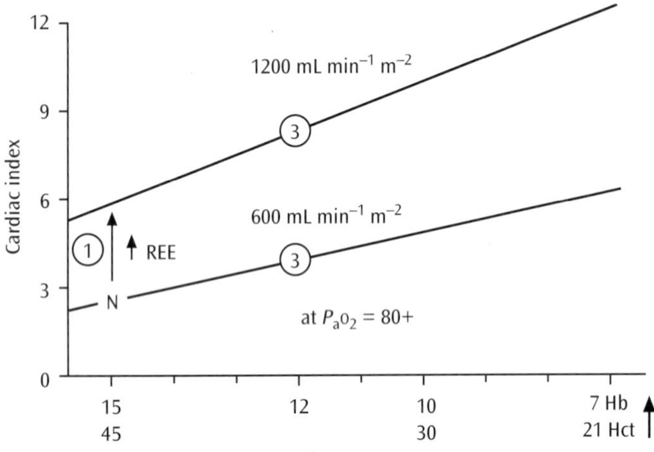

Figure 9.13 *Relation between the cardiac index (CI) and the hemoglobin (Hb) or hematocrit (Hct) curve at normal saturation. N represents the "normal" change in CI with increasing anemia. 3, increasing metabolic expenditure (REE) shifts the curve to a higher level of cardiac index (1) in order to match oxygen delivery to increasing demand. This effect is accentuated by increasing anemia.* P_aO_2 *is measured in mmHg.*

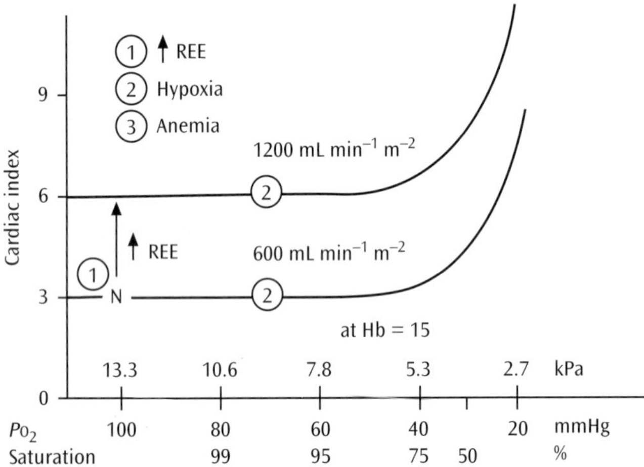

Figure 9.14 *Relation between the cardiac index (CI) and the partial pressure of oxygen (*PO_2*) and the saturation of hemoglobin at a normal hemoglobin concentration (Hb = 15), at two different levels of metabolic expenditure (REE).*

acidosis and lactate ratio have also been demonstrated to be relatively insensitive to changes in hemoglobin until there is less than 6.9 g dL^{-1}, and P_aO_2 until it is less than 5.3 kPa (40 mmHg).[53,54]

In clinical practice, when there is increased oxygen consumption it remains independent of oxygen delivery as long as there is a proportionate increase in oxygen delivery and the ratio $DO_2/\dot{V}O_2$ is greater than 2 (Fig. 9.15). This is seen in shock, trauma, infection, and sepsis, where oxygen consumption may be increased to as much as 20%. In the severely traumatized septic or burned patient, this may clearly exceed 100%.[15,55] If the $DO_2/\dot{V}O_2$ ratio falls below the threshold level, a state of supply dependency is considered to exist. In Fig. 9.15, this threshold, i.e. the "knee" on the curve, occurs at approximately 330 mL mm^{-2} per minute of DO_2 if the VO_2 is 160 mL mm^{-2} min^{-1}.[56]

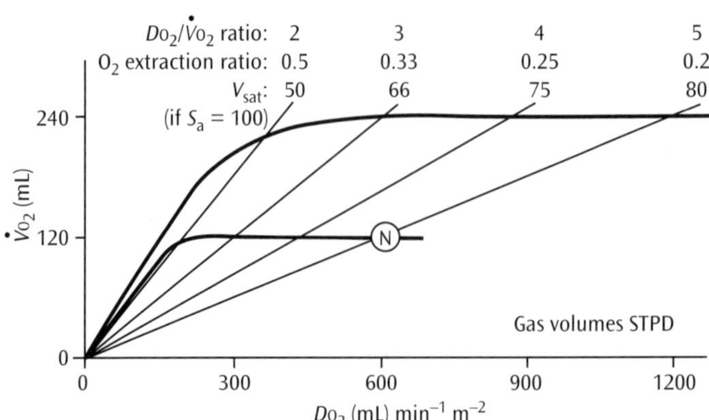

Figure 9.15 *Relation between oxygen consumption (*$\dot{V}O_2$*) and oxygen delivery (*DO_2*) with changes in oxygen delivery to oxygen consumption ratios (*$DO_2/\dot{V}O_2$*), oxygen extraction ratios, and changes in mixed venous saturation. N represents the point on a normal curve with a* $DO_2/\dot{V}O_2$ *ratio of 5. In both normal and increased metabolic states, as the* $DO_2/\dot{V}O_2$ *ratio approaches 2, the oxygen consumption (*$\dot{V}O_2$*) becomes supply dependent.*

Below these levels of DO_2, increasing oxygen extraction cannot compensate for the decrease in oxygen supply and oxygen debt is incurred. Over time, organ system failure occurs and a state of circulatory shock is considered to exist. The biphasic response to the challenge of anemia, hypoxia, or falling cardiac output has been questioned.[16] It has been the view of some authors that in the severely ill, such as in patients with adult respiratory distress syndrome (ARDS), a condition of supply dependency exists at all levels of oxygen delivery.[57,58] The methodology of these experiments has been challenged on the basis of a lack of independence of the measurements made. Specifically, the need to measure oxygen consumption and oxygen delivery separately and not from the same variables, i.e. C_AO_2, C_vO_2, and cardiac output. In the studies in which the measurements have been independently confirmed, the biphasic response for varying $DO_2/\dot{V}O_2$ ratios has been demonstrated.[29,48]

OXYGEN TRANSPORT TRANSFUSION THERAPY

Taking these matters into account, how should the anesthesiologist approach blood component replacement therapy in clinical practice? As the hematocrit decreases, the tissues may: extract more oxygen if blood flow remains constant; increase blood flow if the volume of oxygen extracted is to remain constant; increase capillary recruitment; or decrease oxygen consumption. Blood flow usually increases owing to an increase in stroke volume in normovolemic anemia; however, in hypovolemic anemia, there is an increase in heart rate and possibly stroke volume. The increase in stroke volume reflects the decrease in end-systolic volume as the myocardium operates against a diminished impedance. Since blood viscosity decreases with hematocrit and decreases with increasing flow rate (blood is a non-Newtonian fluid), normovolemic anemia decreases cardiac afterload (systemic vascular resistance). This assumes that intravascular volume is maintained and there is ample cardiac reserve. The effect of viscosity on flow is predicted by Poiseuille's law:

$$F = [(P_1 - P_2)\pi r^4]/8\mu L$$

where F is the flow, $P_1 - P_2$ is the pressure drop, μ is the viscosity, and L is the length of the tube. From this equation, it can be seen that flow is very sensitive to vessel radius (r) as well as to changes in length, pressure drop, and viscosity. What is not obvious in this equation is that viscosity is not a constant but decreases with increasing flow during progressive anemia. The change in flow with viscosity will also reflect the total cross-sectional area of the vascular bed, such that the profound effect of viscosity on flow is greatest in the postcapillary venules.

However, the $P_{\bar{V}}O_2$ at which DO_2 becomes critical in normovolemic anemia is considerably higher than in hypoxic hypoxemia or ischemic hypoxia, which would indicate that the $P_{\bar{V}}O_2$ does not accurately reflect tissue oxygenation in this circumstance. This is interpreted as a limitation on oxygen extraction at lower levels of hematocrit owing to significant reductions in the erythrocyte capillary transit time offsetting beneficial rheological effects of hemodilution.

BLOOD COMPONENT REPLACEMENT

Indications for red blood cell transfusion

With this in mind, what are the indications for red blood cell transfusion? Although there is great concern over the risk and expense of blood transfusions, it is interesting to note that there are relatively few studies that have evaluated the benefits of a red cell transfusion. Much of the early literature is composed of noncontrolled studies and case reports documenting the degree of anemia that patients have tolerated. The following section will review the literature relating to the indications for red blood cell transfusion. This will be followed by the published standards regarding transfusion of blood and blood components.

The general indication for a red cell transfusion is whenever there is physiologic evidence of inadequate oxygen-carrying capacity resulting in tissue hypoxia. Since we do not have a readily available monitor of all the tissues for the presence of hypoxia, we rely on monitors which provide information regarding inadequacy of oxygen supply to target organs, most commonly the heart. Because progressive anemia requires increased cardiac output to maintain oxygen delivery, the heart is the organ which may be considered at most risk during severe anemia.

Recently, there have been studies which evaluate the consequences of progressive normovolemic anemia in healthy humans. Lieberman *et al.*[59] followed changes in oxygen delivery and oxygen consumption in a group of healthy subjects during progressive anemia to hemoglobin levels of 4.7 g dL^{-1}. At this degree of anemia, the oxygen delivery was decreased by approximately 30% while the oxygen consumption was maintained. To simulate anemia in patients with impaired cardiac function, the subjects were then treated with infusions of esmolol, which further decreased oxygen delivery but still did not produce a drop in oxygen consumption but merely an increase in oxygen extraction.[59]

The second study by the same group looked at the incidence of myocardial ischemia associated with similar degrees of anemia.[60] They found that there was a 5% incidence of reversal ischemia which did not result in hemodynamic compromise in these healthy subjects.[60] Nearly all the clinical literature regarding severe anemia has resulted from caring for patients who refuse blood transfusions on religious grounds.

Some of the first reports were associated with the early testing of the perfluorochemical blood substitute Fluosol-DA 20%.[61,62] It was noted from these clinical trials that patients with good cardiopulmonary function tolerated severe normovolemic anemia down to hematocrits as low as 10%.[61] In general, patients with hematocrits much below 10% did not survive. Therefore, it is clear from the volunteer studies and the limited clinical evidence that healthy patients can tolerate normovolemic anemia to hemoglobin values around 5 g dL^{-1} given there are no other confounding variables such as heart disease or dilutional coagulopathy. For patients at risk of cardiac disease, studies became available in the 1990s.

In 1993, Nelson *et al.*[63] followed S–T segment changes and symptoms perioperatively in patients undergoing vascular surgery. Figure 9.13 illustrates this group's findings. It was noted that the incidences of *S–T* segment changes did not increase significantly until the hematocrit fell below 28%. A few years letter, Hogue *et al.*[64] published similar data on patients undergoing radical prostatectomies. They found a similar increase in the incidence of S–T segment changes with hematocrits less than 28% which was accentuated in patients with heart rates greater than 100 (Fig. 9.15).[64] In 1997, Herbert *et al.*[65] reviewed the intensive care unit (ICU) mortality in patients as a function of hematocrit. Their data also confirmed that, in this ICU population, mortality increased when the hematocrit dropped below approximately 28% in patients with cardiac disease.[65] None of these studies was controlled or randomized as they were more observational in nature.

The first and only prospective randomized study of sufficient power was published in 1999, again by Herbert and colleagues.[66] In this study,[66] patients admitted to intensive care units who met entrance criteria were randomized to either receive blood transfusions when their hemoglobin levels reached 10 g dL^{-1} and maintain the hemoglobin between 10 and 12 g dL^{-1} or to wait until the hemoglobin reached 7 g dL^{-1} and maintain the hemoglobin between 7 and 9 g dL^{-1}. This study enrolled 835 patients and concluded that there was no difference in inhospital and 30-day mortality level between the two groups. In fact, if the patients were stratified by Apache (Acute Physiology Age Chronic Health Evaluation score), the patients with the lower Apache scores ($\leq$20) did better if they did not receive a blood transfusion.[66] For patients with clinically significant heart disease, the 30-day mortality level was similar in both high- and low-hematocrit groups. When all of these studies are considered, it is difficult to come to a definitive conclusion regarding which hematocrit requires a transfusion in the perioperative period, but much of the data would suggest that patients with heart disease would do better with hemoglobin levels greater than 9 g dL^{-1}.

In March 1996, a task force of the American Society of Anesthesiologists published practice guidelines for blood component therapy (Table 9.4).[67] These guidelines were the result of a review of the world literature as of 1996. Therefore, the conclusions do not include some of the studies referenced above but still are very reasonable guidelines on which to base one's practice. Although they allow for a wide range of clinical decision-making, they do mandate that decisions be based on the measurement of hematocrit and that, when one chooses to transfuse outside the recommended range, it is important to document the reasons for that transfusion in the medical record. The same is true for treating patients with platelets, fresh-frozen plasma, and cryoprecipitate. The indications for blood transfusions has recently been reviewed by Goodnough *et al.*[68]

Current risks

The current risks of a transfusion of blood or blood components can be categorized as infections, reactions, and immune suppression (Table 9.5). Although there are a variety of infectious agents, those that elicit most concern are associated with acquired immune deficiency syndrome (AIDS) and hepatitis. Other viral agents, as well as bacterial infections, continue to produce significant complications but are either more treatable or relatively infrequent.[68] It has also been demonstrated that the acute febrile reaction associated with many transfusions is mediated through cytokine release from white cells, which also carry the cytomegalovirus virus (CMV).[68] Another problem with residual white cells left in platelets and packed red cells is alloimmunization to platelets.[69] Although this is not a frequent problem, when it occurs it causes a bleeding diathesis owing to the ineffectiveness of the platelet transfusion. Although somewhat controversial, it has been recommended that all cellular components be leukocyte depleted.[70] This costs an additional $30–35 per unit but is becoming the standard in many institutions.

Table 9.4 *ASA transfusion guidelines*

	Usually indicated	Not usually indicated
RBCs	$<6\,g\,dL^{-1}$	$>10\,g\,dL^{-1}$
FFP	PT/PTT > 1.5 times normal	PT/PTT < 1.5 times normal
Platelets	< 50 000	> 100 000
Cryoprecipitate	Fibrinogen <80–$100\,mg\,dL^{-1}$	Fibrinogen >80–$100\,mg\,dL^{-1}$

RBCs, red blood cells; FFP, fresh-frozen plasma; PT, prothrombin time; PTT, partial thromboplastin time.

Table 9.5 *Risks of blood transfusions*

	Incidence per unit
Infection – viral	
Hepatitis A	1:1 000 000
Hepatitis B	1:30 000 to 1:250 000
Hepatitis C	1:30 000 to 1:150 000
HIV	1:200 000 to 1:2 000 000
HTLV types I and II	1:250 000 to 1:2 000 000
Parvovirus B19	1:10 000
Infection – bacterial	
Red cells	1:500 000
Platelets	1:12 000
Acute hemolytic reaction (mortality)	1:250 000 to 1:1 000 000

Table 9.5 lists the current estimated incidences of viral contamination associated with human immunodeficiency virus (HIV), human T-cell leukemia virus (HTLV), hepatitis C, hepatitis B, and parvovirus B19.[69,71] With the advent of more comprehensive testing and donor screening, it is impressive that the incidence of HIV has been reduced to nearly 1:1 000 000.[72] It is estimated that there are 12–15 units of HIV-contaminated blood in the 12 million units collected annually in the USA. Completely eliminating this virus from the blood supply may be impossible.

Hemolytic transfusion reactions resulting in death occur, at a rate of approximately 1:500 000.[73] Most of these are attributed to clerical errors, i.e. not checking the patient's name with the unit of blood.[73]

As noted in Table 9.5, the incidence of hepatitis B and C have also been dramatically reduced recently.[71] Many of the patients who contract hepatitis C will develop chronic active hepatitis, and ultimately cirrhosis or hepatocellular carcinoma. The mean duration between blood transfusion and symptomatic liver disease is 20 years.[74] Tong *et al.*[74] followed a group of patients with hepatitis C who presented with fatigue or hepatomegaly. In that group, 50% were noted to have cirrhosis and 10% had or subsequently developed hepatocellular carcinoma.

Several technologies have become available to treat fresh-frozen plasma to inactivate lipid-encapsulated viruses (hepatitis A and B as well as HIV).[75,76] The product currently available is referred to as plasma SD (solvent detergent treated) and is free of the abovementioned viral pathogens, but unfortunately it may have an increased incidence of nonlipid-encapsulated viruses, such as parvovirus B19. Since plasma SD is produced in a pooled fashion from 2500 donors, the estimated incidence of parvovirus infection is high. Parvovirus causes fifth disease, which is one of the viral exanthems of childhood. Although most patients survive this viral syndrome without severe adverse sequelae, parvovirus does attack the erythroid precursor cells, thereby causing anemia 10 days to 2 weeks post infection. This would appear to be a very unfortunate consequence in the immediate postoperative period for a patient who has just suffered surgical blood loss. For that reason, it may not be beneficial to use plasma SD in surgical patients until this product can be made parvovirus free.

One of the more recent concerns about allogeneic blood is its potential as an immunosuppressive agent. It has been noted that this effect is related to the exposure of leukocytes within the red cell unit. The concern is that this immunosuppressive process would lead to an increased incidence of postoperative infections and in cancer patients an increased incidence of tumor recurrence. It is difficult to analyze this question retrospectively since patients who require more allogeneic blood clearly have larger procedures and therefore would be expected to have more postoperative complications. Several prospective studies have tried to clarify this immunosuppressive effect of blood transfusions on outcome. Most studies have either found no difference in either group or a slight suggestion of an increased incidence of both complications.[68] Leukocyte-depleted red cells have also been used but were unable to demonstrate a difference in outcome. Other studies have found improved results with leukocyte-depleted red cells. Although the topic of universal white cell depleted red cells remains controversial and would be a very expensive option, data would suggest that we should consider moving in that direction.[68]

Methods of reducing the need for allogeneic blood transfusions

Owing to the risks and expenses associated with blood transfusions, a variety of techniques have been employed to try to reduce the need for allogeneic blood and blood components. These include autologous predonation, intraoperative hemodilution, induced hypotension, perioperative cell salvage, and pharmacologic interventions in the coagulation cascade. Recently, the effectiveness of preoperative autologous donation and intraoperative hemodilution has been called into question. Each of these techniques as well as the controversies surrounding them will be described below. This topic has also been recently reviewed by Goodnough *et al.*[77]

Preoperative autologous donation

Since the mid-1980s, the popularity of preoperative autologous blood donation has progressively increased. It has become routine at many medical centers for elective procedures which may require a blood transfusion. Its advantages appear obvious: avoiding transfusion reactions (excluding clerical error) and disease transmission (excluding bacterial contamination) and possibly stimulating red cell production. It also "adds" to the blood supply. Overall, it was seen as a safer alternative, especially in the eyes of the public.

In recent years, the practice of autologous blood donation has been scrutinized with respect to both cost and safety. Because of the timing and additional clerical effort, autologous blood is more costly than bank blood. Since unused autologous blood is discarded, approximately 50% of this cost produces no benefit. As the safety of the blood supply improves, the potential benefits of autologous blood diminish. Taking all of this into account, studies have estimated the cost-effectiveness of autologous blood in terms of dollars per potential year of life saved for various surgical procedures.[78,79] For a total hip replacement, the cost per potential year of life saved is $235 000, whereas for a total abdominal hysterectomy it may be as much as $1 358 000, and for a prostatectomy as much as $23 643 000 per year of life saved![77] For coronary artery bypass surgery, the cost per year of life saved is approximately $500 000 with the assumption that there is no morbidity associated with the autologous donation process and the time delay required for that process.[80] To put these costs per year of life saved in perspective, it is estimated that coronary bypass surgery for a patient with left main coronary disease costs $6000 per year of life saved, Pap smears cost $11 000 per year of life saved, and treating hypertension with captopril costs $79 000 per year of life saved.[80]

It would appear that the autologous blood donation process has passed the point of providing cost-effective value to health. Even if one is not concerned with cost, more recent studies have brought into question the benefits of autologous blood transfusion, i.e. it may not improve safety but actually may increase risk. When a patient donates preoperative blood, it is expected that they will generate additional red cells between the time of donation and the time of surgery. Unfortunately, this may not be the case. Recent studies have found that patients who donate blood preoperatively arrive on the day of surgery relatively anemic and therefore have an increased chance of requiring at least their autologous blood if not bank blood. Since even their own blood has the same clerical risks and bacterial contamination risks as bank blood, this adds additional risks.

Kanter *et al.*[81] studied 263 patients undergoing elective total abdominal hysterectomy between 1993 and 1994. The 140 patients who donated an average of 2 units of blood arrived on the day of surgery with a hematocrit of 35%, whereas the 123 patients who did not donate preoperatively had a preoperative hematocrit of 40%.[81] Eighteen percent of the patients in the autologous group required a blood transfusion, two of whom required bank blood. In the group that did not predonate, only one patient received a transfusion. Crosby *et al.*[82] found similar results in patients undergoing reduction mammoplasties. For these two procedures, it appears predonating autologous blood increases the patient's overall risk of having an adverse outcome as a result of a blood transfusion.[81,82]

Since the erythropoietic response appears to be sluggish in most patients providing autologous blood, several studies have looked at combining preoperative donation with treatment with synthetic erythropoietin (Epogen).[83] It has been demonstrated that, if patients received treatments of Epogen during the preoperative donation process, they would increase their red cell production but may or may not reduce their need for allogeneic blood transfusions.[84] This therapy costs approximately $1500 per patient, thereby making a procedure that is already very ineffective on a cost–benefit analysis dramatically worse.

It has always been assumed that the process of donating blood itself was innocuous and was not considered as part of the risk. Popovsky *et al.*[85] recently reviewed the incidence of clinical problems associated with voluntary donation and autologous donation. They defined a very severe outcome as an incident associated with the blood donation which required hospitalization. For volunteer donors, there was one very severe outcome per approximately 200 000 donations, whereas in the autologous group there was one for every 16 783 donations.[85] The most common very severe outcome was vasovagal symptoms, but 12% of patients had angina severe enough to require hospitalization. It is therefore clear that donating autologous blood is not without some risk, especially in those patients who are older and have heart disease. Given the fact that there may be little or no benefit and potentially an increased risk with autologous donation, it would appear that the practice should be comprehensively reviewed.[77]

Intraoperative hemodilution

Preoperative phlebotomy and isovolemic hemodilution have also been recommended as a method to save intraoperative red cell loss.[86] The assumption is that blood is retrieved from the patient prior to surgical blood loss with an isovolemic exchange using either crystalloid or colloid. Blood is kept in the operating room and maintained at room temperature, thereby maintaining platelet activity. For patients with good cardiac function, the normal compensation is increased stroke volume with a relative maintenance of blood pressure and heart rate as the patient becomes hemodiluted. When the surgical blood loss begins the patient bleeds "anemic" blood, thereby saving the patient's fresh whole blood in the room to be transfused at the end of the procedure. This practice has been advocated as an effective way to reduce the need for banked blood.[86–88]

Recently, this practice has been called into question by two studies which calculated the potential savings using a mathematical model.[89,90] To determine the theoretical maximal blood savings, the model requires the patient's initial hematocrit, the hematocrit at the end of hemodilution, the patient's estimated blood volume (estimated from body weight), and the surgical blood loss during the procedure. Given these data and the assumption that the patient does not benefit unless at least 1 unit is saved (i.e. the risk of transfusion is the same for a partial unit as for the total unit), it would appear unlikely to reduce the number of banked units using hemodilution. For example, if a patient starts with a hematocrit of 40% and has a minimum safe hematocrit of 25%, 5 units of blood would have to be withdrawn from the patient and the procedure would be required to have 2500 mL of blood lost to save 1 unit of bank blood. If crystalloid were used to hemodilute, this would require 7.5 L of crystalloid to be given during the hemodilution process in addition to the 1 L or so required for the overnight fast prior to the skin incision. It could be argued that the risk associated with collecting 5 units of hemodilution blood would outweigh the potential benefit of 1 unit of bank blood. If the surgical blood loss was less than 2500 mL, then no benefit could be achieved, but the anesthesiologist would be required to retransfuse those 5 units of blood without fluid overloading the patient. Of course, if the patient's initial hematocrit is less than 40%, the potential of saving blood is more remote. On the other hand, if one is willing to hemodilute to a hematocrit of 15% the potential savings may be realized. Overall, from a clinical perspective, these mathematical models predict that the probability of saving bank blood by using the technique of hemodilution highly unlikely.

How is it that the literature reports repeated successes using this technique? The answer lies in the design of the studies used to evaluate its hemodilution. In fact, there are very few controlled studies using transfusion criteria evaluating hemodilution. Many of the studies reporting success have no control group at all.[91] Others use different hematocrit triggers for transfusion in the hemodilution group compared with the nonhemodilution group.[91] The one retrospective study which used consistent criteria in both groups found an average of only 95 mL savings in the hemodilution group and only a 204-mL saving in the best patient.[88] This volume of blood saving is consistent with the mathematical models and would not save a single unit of banked blood.

Although hemodilution has been reported to be a less costly alternative than other techniques of blood conservation, it would also appear to have little or no value. It is clear that the practice of withdrawing 1 or 2 units in an attempt to save red cell loss is highly unlikely to provide any clinical benefit.

Perioperative cell salvage

In 1860, Brainard[92] reported using operative shed blood for retransfusion in a patient undergoing a leg amputation. Since then, cell salvage has become a routine part of perioperative care for a variety of surgical procedures. The technique can be divided into two types: retransfusion of washed blood and retransfusion of unwashed blood. Intraoperative cell salvage devices usually wash blood, thereby providing a product which is the patient's own red cells suspended in normal saline.

Retransfusion of unwashed blood is frequently used in the postoperative setting, when blood is collected from drains and the defibrinated blood is retransfused along with fibrin degradation products and other debris.

Intraoperative cell salvage has been demonstrated to be a cost-effective technique of reducing allogeneic blood exposure. A recent meta-analysis by Huët *et al.*[93] reviewed the literature for orthopedic and cardiac procedures. They concluded that administration of both washed and unwashed blood was effective for orthopedic surgical procedures, but the retransfusion of unwashed shed blood in cardiac surgery was marginally effective at best.[93]

Salvaged blood has the obvious advantages of avoiding the risks associated with allogeneic blood as well as being readily available. Owing to the cost of the disposables at the authors' institution, the device is used whenever 2 or more units may be collected during the surgical procedure. The cost–utility ratio has been reported to be approximately $120 000 per quality adjusted year of life saved.[94,95] This is high compared with the cost–utility ratio of other medical therapies, e.g. cardiac surgery for left main disease is $6000 per year of life saved.[94,95]

There are several relative contraindications for the use of cell salvage blood. These include bacterial contamination, malignant cell contamination, and sickle hemoglobin.[93] The first two relative contraindications have been recently reviewed by Thomas.[96] With respect to bacterial contamination, there is evidence that even when blood is collected in a clean surgical field the sucker tip may be culture positive. From an outcomes perspective, there is no evidence that salvaged blood is associated with an increased postoperative infection rate, even if there is clear soiling in the surgical field. There appears to be clear agreement that salvaged blood should be used in cases of trauma where significant blood loss is occurring.

Although there are concerns that salvaged blood may increase the spread of malignant cells and ultimately increase the incidences of disseminated malignancies, this has not been reported. All the studies to date have demonstrated that the use of salvage blood does not change the overall tumor recurrence rate.[96] In fact, it has been found that malignant cells are found circulating in the blood prior to the incision and increase during manipulation of the tumor. Of course, the long-term follow-up for malignancies may involve decades, therefore a definitive statement is difficult to make. Experimentally, it has been confirmed that irradiating shed blood will effectively eliminate cancer cells.[97] In spite of the clinical evidence, cancer surgery is still considered a relative contraindication to cell salvage.

Pharmacologic methods of reducing blood loss

The fibrinolytic enzyme system functions as a defense mechanism against the excess deposition of fibrin. The fibrinolytic system acts in balance with the coagulation system through a series of activators and inhibitors. The key substance in the fibrinolytic system is plasminogen, which when activated releases the proteinase plasmin, which cleaves peptide bonds in fibrin, producing fibrinolysis.

Over the past decade, research has been directed toward purifying substances which activate fibrinolysis [streptokinase, urokinase, tissue plasminogen activator (TPA), etc.] and other substances which inhibit the fibrinolytic system. Synthetic inhibitors of fibrinolysis include ε-aminocaproic acid and tranexamic acid. Aprotinin is a naturally occurring serine proteinase inhibitor of human plasmin, trypsin, and tissue kallikrein. In recent years, these drugs have been investigated for use in the treatment of postoperative bleeding disorders, e.g. bleeding associated with a cardiac bypass and prostatic surgery.

ε-Aminocaproic acid and tranexamic acid, the two synthetic agents, act at the same binding site on plasminogen and exert their inhibitory effect. Tranexamic acid is approximately seven times as potent as ε-aminocaproic acid, and therefore can be used in lower doses with fewer side-effects. The usual dose of tranexamic acid is 0.5–1 g (10–15 mg kg^{-1}) intravenously two or three times daily immediately following urological surgery, for 2–3 days. An ε-aminocaproic acid dose of 2.5 g before and after bypass has been demonstrated to reduce blood loss following cardiopulmonary bypass by 10–20%.[98,99] Although one might be concerned about an increased risk of thrombotic complications, none was noted in these studies. These drugs are contraindicated in patients with suspected disseminated intravascular coagulation (DIC) or in patients in whom fibrinolysis is necessary to prevent potentially fatal thrombosis.

Aprotinin has been found to significantly reduce blood loss following cardiopulmonary bypass.[100,101] Its mechanism involves antifibrinolytic activity and a platelet activity protective effect during cardiac bypass. Royston *et al.*[100] first reported that high-dose aprotinin decreased blood loss in patients undergoing repeat open heart surgery from 1500 mL in the control group to 280 mL in the aprotinin group. The dose of aprotinin was 280 mg prior to sternotomy followed by an infusion of 70 mg h^{-1} with an additional 280 mg added to the pump prime solution. This reduction in blood loss has been confirmed by many other controlled blinded studies.[101]

Aprotinin also substantially increased the activated clotting time (ACT), when the usual celite activator is used.[102] It has been recommended that, when the celite activator is used in the ACT device to assess the adequacy of heparinization, the ACT be greater than 750 s (instead of greater than 400 s) before extracorporeal circulation is initiated.[102] The prolonged ACT is an interaction between celite, heparin, and aprotinin and falsely increases the ACT value. It has recently been demonstrated that, if kaolin is used as the activator in determining the ACT, normal ACT values should be used.

Desmopressin acetate (DDAVP) is a synthetic analog of L-arginine vasopressin (antidiuretic hormone). This also increases von Willebrand's factor, increases factor VIII activity, and has some nonspecific enhancement of platelet function. It has also been reported[103] to decrease postcardiac bypass blood loss at a dose of 0.3 μg kg^{-1}. In spite of initial enthusiasm for its use, follow-up studies have not found a significant reduction in blood loss with DDAVP treatment. DDAVP is indicated in the prophylactic treatment of patients with hemophilia A and type I von Willebrand's disease. It is not effective in types II, III, or V (von Willebrand's disease).[104]

Blood substitutes

Two types of products have been developed that can supplement oxygen transport and therefore act as "blood substitutes." Neither of these products performs all the functions of blood, but both can supplement oxygen transport temporarily until blood is available or until blood is not needed. The two approaches to producing oxygen-transporting liquids have been emulsions of perfluorocarbons (PFC emulsions) and solutions of hemoglobin (Hb).

Hb solutions are produced from either outdated human blood or bovine blood by lysing the red cells and purifying the Hb. When Hb is removed from the red cell, the tetrameric structure quickly breaks down to dimers, which are small enough to be diuresed by the kidney. To prevent this diuresis, Hb dimers must be either attached to a larger molecule, cross-linked with another dimer producing a tetramer, or polymerized to produce a tetramer or larger molecule. Hemoglobin can also be produced using recombinant techniques. The current products in clinical testing use polymerization and cross-linking.[105,106]

When Hb leaves the red cells, it also loses its 2,3-DPG and the P_{50} of the oxyhemoglobin dissociation curve, which is normally in the range of 27 mmHg, drops to the range of 12 mmHg. This lowering of the P_{50} diminishes the release of oxygen to the tissues. Therefore, these products modify Hb to increase the P_{50} into the range of 28–32 mmHg. Bovine

Hb has a P_{50} in the range of 30 mmHg without 2,3-DPG, and therefore requires no modification to increase its P_{50}.[107]

It was observed in early studies that transfusions with Hb solutions caused pulmonary and systemic hypertension. More recently, it was recognized that this effect is due to nitric oxide scavenging by the Hb as it passes through the microcirculation, thereby increasing vasomotor tone and consequently resistance. It appears that Hb in solution is more efficient in scavenging nitric oxide than Hb encapsulated in red blood cells. Most of the clinical studies have noted an increase in systemic blood pressure and pulmonary artery pressure when the current investigational products are transfused.[105]

Two randomized studies have compared treating patients with Hb solutions with red blood cells. Gould *et al.*[106] randomized 44 trauma patients to receive up to 6 units of the Hb solution, PolyHeme, or red blood cells (RBCs). At the end of the first day, the patients who received PolyHeme required significantly less bank blood than those who had been resuscitated with bank blood alone – 6.8 units versus 10.4 units. There was no difference in overall outcome. A second study by Lamy *et al.*[107] randomized cardiac surgical patients to receive either 3 units of Hb solution or 3 units of RBCs immediately after bypass surgery. On postoperative day 7, 19% of the Hb group had received no bank blood, whereas all the patients in the other group received bank blood.

Perfluorocarbons are inert, immiscible liquids which have an oxygen solubility of approximately 20 times that of normal plasma. These inert liquids are emulsified in aqueous electrolyte solutions, forming a suspension of small (0.1 μm) particles. PFC emulsions have also been used to try to reduce the amount of bank blood during elective surgery. Spahn *et al.*[108] conducted a study in which perfluorochemical emulsions were used in conjunction with acute normovolemic hemodilution. After hemodilution, patients were randomized into four groups: two received different concentrations of PFCs while the third received autologous blood and the fourth received colloid. The study followed the need for oxygen carriage by surpassing the specific transfusion trigger of having the mixed venous $P\text{O}_2$ below 38 mmHg. The doses of PFC emulsion reversed the trigger in more patients and for a longer duration than blood or colloid, although this reversal lasted for only 2–3 h. This study did not demonstrate any reduction in overall blood utilization.[108]

Both of these blood substitutes have the limitations of short duration of potential benefit (12–24 h). PFC emulsion has the additional limitation that to be effective it requires high $P_a\text{O}_2$. Each of these products has some adverse consequences: hypertension with the Hb solution and a drop in platelet count with the PFC emulsion. At this point it is difficult to determine whether either of these products will be suitable as a replacement for blood if it is available, but either may be useful as a product which provides a temporary supplement to oxygen transport. For a more comprehensive review of the topic, please refer to recent reviews of this topic by Wahr.[109]

REFERENCES

1. Barcroft J. Presidential address on anoxaemia. *Lancet* 1920; **2:** 485–9.
2. Nunn JF. *Applied Respiratory Physiology.* London: Butterworth, 1987.
3. Cross CE, Packer BS, Altman M, *et al.* The determination of total body exchangeable oxygen stores. *J Clin Invest* 1968; **47:** 2402–10.
4. Finch CA, Lenfant MD. Oxygen transport in man. *N Engl J Med* 1972; **286** (8): 407–15.
5. DeHaan EJ. Cell respiration. *Folia Med Neerl* 1970; **13:** 90–100.
6. Baue AE, Soyeed MM. Alterations in the functional capacity of mitochondria in hemorrhagic shock. *Surgery* 1970; **68:** 40–7.
7. Alter MJ, Pascell RM, Shih JW, *et al.* Detection of antibody C virus in prospectively followed transfusion recipients with acute and chronic non-A, non-B hepatitis. *N Engl J Med* 1989; **321:** 1494.
8. Alter MJ, Hadler SL, Judson FN, *et al.* Risk factors for acute non-A, non-B hepatitis in the United States and association with hepatitis C virus infection. *JAMA* 1990; **264:** 2231.
9. Tremper KK, Barker SJ. Monitoring of oxygen. In: Lake C (ed.). *Clinical Monitoring.* London: WB Saunders, 1990.
10. Eichorn JM, Cooper JB, Cullen DJ, *et al.* Standards for patient monitoring during anesthesia at Harvard Medical School. *JAMA* 1986; **1256:** 1017–20.
11. Richards DW. *The Circulation in Traumatic Shock in Man. Harvey Lectures* 1943–44; **39:** 217.
12. Nunn JF, Freeman J. Problems of oxygenation and oxygen transport during hemorrhage. *Anaesthesia* 1964**; 19:** 206.
13. Sullivan SF. Oxygen transport. *Anesthesiology* 1972; **37:** 140.
14. Bartlett RH. Critical care. In: Greenfield LJ, Mulholland MW, Oldham KT, Zelenock GB (eds). *Surgery, Scientific Principles and Practice.* Philadelphia: JB Lippincott, 1993: 195–222.
15. Bartlett RH. Critical care and metabolism. *Bull Am Coll Surg* 1989; **74:** 10–15.
16. Cain SM. Acute lung injury. Assessment of tissue oxygenation. *Crit Care Clin* 1986; **2:** 537–50.
17. Wade OC, Bishop JM. *Cardiac Output and Regional Blood Flow.* Oxford: Blackwell Scientific Publications, 1962.
18. Cain SM. Oxygen transport and consumption. In: Tinker J, Zapel WM (eds). *Care of the Critically Ill Patient*, 2nd edn. Berlin: Springer Verlag, 1992: Chapter 5.
19. Barcroft J. *Features in the Architecture of Physiological Function.* Cambridge: Cambridge University Press, 1938: 71.
20. Cerretelli P, Cruiz JC, Fashi LE, *et al.* Determination of mixed venous O_2 and CO_2 tensions and cardiac output by rebreathing method. *Respir Physiol* 1966; **1:** 258–64.
21. Scheinmann MM, Brown MA, Rapaport E. Critical assessment of use of central venous oxygen saturation as a mirror of mixed venous oxygen in severely ill cardiac patients. *Circulation* 1969; **40:** 165–72.
22. Muir AL, Kirby BJ, King AJ, *et al.* Mixed venous oxygen saturation in relation to cardiac output in myocardial infarctions. *Br Med J* 1970; **4:** 276–8.
23. Norfleet EA, Watson CB. Continuous mixed venous oxygen saturation measurement: a significant advance in hemodynamic monitoring? *J Clin Monitoring* 1965; **1:** 245–58.
24. Birman H, Hag A, Hew E, *et al.* Continuous monitoring of mixed venous oxygen saturation in hemodynamically unstable patients. *Anesthesiology* 1984; **86:** 753–6.
25. Carron CC, Snyder JV. Hyperdynamic severe intravascular sepsis depends on fluid resuscitation in cynomolgus monkey. *Am J Physiol* 1982; **243:** R131–41.
26. Miller MJ. Tissue oxygenation in clinical medicine: an historical review. *Anesth Analg* 1982; **61:** 527–35.
27. Lee MD, Wright F, Barber R, Stanley L. Central venous oxygen saturation in shock. *Anesthesiology* 1972; **36:** 472–8.
28. Zwischenberger JB, Colley RD, Kirsh MM, *et al.* Does continuous monitoring of mixed venous oxygen saturation accurately reflect oxygen delivery and oxygen consumption following coronary artery bypass grafting? *Surgical Forum* 1986; **37:** 66–8.
29. Cilley RE, Polley TZ, Swischenberger JB, *et al.* Independent measurement of oxygen consumption and oxygen delivery. *J Surg Res* 1988; **47:** 242–7.
30. Nelson LD. Continuous venous oscimetry in surgical patients. *Ann Surg* 1986; **203:** 329–33.
31. Shenaq SA, Casar G, Ott H, Crawford ES. Continuous monitoring of mixed venous oxygen saturation during aortic surgery. *Chest* 1987; **97:** 796–9.
32. Cregory IC. The oxygen and carbon monoxide capacities of foetal and adult blood. *J Physiol (Lond)* 1974; **236:** 625.
33. Von Hufner CG. Neue Versuche zur Bestimmung der Sauerstoff Capacitah des Blut Forbstoffs. *Arch Anat Physiol Abt* 1984; 130.
34. Adair GS. The hemoglobin system vs. The oxygen dissociation curve of hemoglobin. *J Biol Chem* 1925; **63:** 529.
35. Gillies IDS. Anaemia and anaesthesia. *Br J Anaesth* 1974; **46:** 589.
36. Perutz MF. Stereochemistry of cooperative efforts in hemoglobin. *Nature (London)* 1970; **228:** 726.
37. Woodson RD. Hemoglobin structure and oxygen transport. *Principles of Transfusion Medicine.* Baltimore: Williams and Wilkins, 1991.
38. Bellingham AJ, Deto JC, Lenfant C. Regulatory mechanisms of oxygen affinity in acidosis and alkalosis. *J Clin Invest* 1971; **50:** 700.
39. Hamasaki N, Asakura T, Minakami S. Effect of oxygen tension of glycolysis in human erythrocytes. *J Biochem (Tokyo)* 1970; **68:** 157–61.
40. Rapaport S. The regulation of glycolysis in mammalian erythrocytes. *Essays Biochem* 1965; **1:** 69–103.
41. Guyton AC. Capillary dynamics and exchange of fluid between the blood and interstitial fluid. *Textbook of Medical Physiology*, 6th edn. Philadelphia: WB Saunders, 1981: 363.

42. Torrance J, Jacobs P, Restrepo A, *et al.* Intraerythrocytic adaptation to anemia. *N Engl J Med* 1970; **283:** 165.
43. Greenwald I. A new type of phosphoric acid compound isolated from blood, with some remarks on the effect of substitution of the rotation of L-glycergic acid. *J Biol Chem* 1925; **63:** 339.
44. Bluesch R, Bluesch RE. The effect of organic phosphates from the human erythrocyte on the allosteric properties of hemoglobin. *Biochem Biophys Res Commun* 1967; **26:** 162.
45. Sharpey Schafer EP. Cardiac output in severe anemia. *Clin Sci* 1944; **5:** 125.
46. Murray JF. Anemia and cardiac function. *UCLA Forum Med Sci* 1970; **10:** 309.
47. Bartlett RH, Dechert RE. Oxygen kinetics: pitfalls in clinical research. *J Crit Care* 1990; **5** (2): 77–80.
48. Cilley RE, Scharenberg AM, Bongiorno PF, *et al.* Low oxygen delivery produced by anemia, hypoxia and low cardiac output. *J Surg Res* 1991; **51:** 425–33.
49. Simmons DH, Alpas AP, Tashkin DP, Coulson A. Hyperlactemia due to arterial hypoxemia or reduced cardiac output or both. *J Appl Physiol* 1978; **45:** 195–202.
50. Kasnitz P, Druger GL, Yorra F, Simmons DH. Mixed venous oxygen tension and hyperlactemia. *JAMA* 1976; **236:** 570–4.
51. DaLuz PL, Cavanilles JM, Michaels S, *et al.* Oxygen delivery, anoxic metabolism and hemoglobin oxygen affinity (P_{50}) in patients with acute myocardial infarction and shock. *Am J Cardiol* 1975; **36:** 148–54.
52. Cohen RD, Simpson R. Lactate metabolism. *Anesthesiology* 1975; **43:** 661–73.
53. Seibert DJ, Ebaugh Jr FG. Assessment of tissue anoxemia in chronic anemia by the arterial lactate pyruvate ratio and excess lactate formation. *J Lab Clin Med* 1967; **69:** 177–82.
54. Green NM, Talner NS. Blood lactate pyruvate and lactate pyruvate ratios in congenital heart disease. *N Engl J Med* 1964; **270:** 1331–6.
55. Wolf GT, Coter S, Perel A, Manny J. Dependence of oxygen consumption of cardiac output in sepsis. *Crit Care Med* 1987; **15:** 198–203.
56. Shibutani K, Kamatsu T, Kubal K, *et al.* Critical level of oxygen delivery in anesthetized man. *Crit Care Med* 1983; **11:** 640–3.
57. Danek SJ, Lynch JP, Weg JG, Dantzker DR. The dependence of oxygen uptake on oxygen delivery in the adult respiratory distress syndrome. *Am Rev Respir Dis* 1980; **122:** 387–95.
58. Gutierez G, Pohil RJ. Oxygen consumption is linearly related to oxygen supply in critically ill patients. *J Crit Care* 1986; **1** (1): 45–53.
59. Lieberman JA, Weiskopf RB, Kelley SD, *et al.* Critical oxygen delivery in conscious humans is less than 7.3 ml $O_2 \times kg^{-1} \times min^{-1}$. *Anesthesiology* 2000; **92:** 407–13.
60. Leung JM, Weiskopf RB, Feiner J, *et al.* Electrocardiographic ST Segment changes during acute, severe isovolemic hemodilution in humans. *Anesthesiology*, 2000; **93:** 1004–1010.
61. Tremper KK, Friedman AE, Levine EM, *et al.* The preoperative treatment of severely anemic patients with a perfluorochemical oxygen-transport fluid, Fluosol-DA. *N Engl J Med*, 1982; **307:** 277–83.
62. Gould SA, Rosen AL, Sehgal LR, *et al.* Fluosol-DA as a red-cell substitute in acute anemia. *N Engl J Med*, 1986; **314:** 1653–6.
63. Nelson AH, Fleisher LA, Rosenbaum SH. Relationship between postoperative anemia and cardiac morbidity in high-risk vascular patients in the intensive care unit. *Crit Care Med* 1993; **21:** 860–6.
64. Hogue CW, Goodnough LT, Monk TG. Perioperative myocardial ischemic episodes are related to hematocrit level in patients undergoing radical prostatectomy. *Transfusion Pract* 1998; **38:** 924–31.
65. Herbert PC, Wells G, Tweeddale M, *et al.* Does transfusion practice effect mortality in critically ill patients? *Am J Respir Crit Care Med* 1997; **155:** 1618–23.
66. Herbert PC, Wells G, Blajchman MA, *et al.* A multicentered randomized controlled clinical trial of transfusion requirements in critical care. *N Engl J Med* 1999; **340:** 409–17.
67. Practice guidelines for blood component therapy. A report by the American Society of Anesthesiologists Task Force on Blood Component Therapy. *Anesthesiology* 1996; **84:** 732–47.
68. Goodnough LT, Brecher ME, Kanter MH, AuBuchon JP: Transfusion medicine. First of two parts – blood transfusion. *N Engl J Med*, 1999; **340** (6): 438–47.
69. The Trial to Reduce Alloimmunization to Platelets Study Group. Leukocyte reduction and ultraviolet B irradiation of platelets to prevent alloimmunization and refractoriness to platelet transfusions. *N Engl J Med* 1997; **337:** 1861–915.
70. Balajachman MA. Transfusion-associated immunomodulation and universal white cell reduction: are we putting the cart before the horse. *Transfusion* 1999; **39:** 665–70.
71. Schreiber GB, Busch MP, Kleinman SH, Korelitz JJ. The risk of transfusion transmitted viral infections. *N Engl J Med* 1996; **34:** 1685–90.
72. Remis RS, Delage G, Palmer RWH. Risk of HIV infection from blood transfusion in Montreal. *Can Med Assoc J* 1997; **157:** 375–82.
73. Linden JV, Kaplan HS. Transfusion errors: cause and effects. *Transfusion Med* 1994; **8:** 169–83.
74. Tong MJ, el-Farra NS, Reikes AR, Co RL. Clinical outcomes after transfusion associated hepatitis C. *N Engl J Med* 1995; **332:** 1463–6.
75. Williamson LM, Allain JP. Virally inactivated fresh frozen plasma. *Vox Sang* 1995; **69:** 159–65.
76. Klein HG, Dodd RY, Dzik WH, *et al.* Current status of solvents/detergent-treated plasma. *Transfusion* 1998; **38:** 102–7.
77. Goodnough LT, Brecher ME, Kanter MH, AuBuchon JP. Transfusion medicine. Second of two parts – blood conservation. *N Engl J Med*, 1999; **340** (7): 525–33.
78. Etchason J, Petz L, Keeler E, *et al.* Cost-effectiveness of preoperative autologous donations. *N Engl J Med* 1995; **332:** 719–24.
79. Birkmeyer JD, Goodnough LT, AuBuchon JP, *et al.* The cost-effectiveness of preoperative autologous donation for total hip and knee replacement. *Transfusion* 1993; **33:** 544–51.
80. Birkmeyer JD. Cost-effectiveness of preoperative autologous donation in coronary bypass grafting. *Ann Thor Surg* 1994; **57:** 161–9.
81. Kanter NH, vanMaanen D, Anders KH, *et al.* Preoperative autologous blood donations before elective hysterectomy. *JAMA* 1996; **276:** 798–801.
82. Crosby ET, Murphy P, Benoit PR. Routine pre-deposited autologous blood is not warranted before breast reduction surgery. *Can J Surg* 1995; **38:** 309–13.
83. Goodnough LT. Clinical application of recombinant erythropoietin in the perioperative period. *Hematol Oncol Clin North Am* 1994; **8:** 1011–20.
84. Goodnough LT, Price TH, Friedman MJ, *et al.* A phase II trial of recombinant human erythropoietin therapy in non anemic orthopaedic patients, subjected to removal of blood for autologous use: dose response, toxicity and efficacy. *Transfusion* 1994; **34:** 66–71.
85. Popovsky MA, Whitaker B, Arnold NL. Severe outcomes of allogenic and autologous blood donation: frequency and characterization. *Transfusion* 1995; **35:** 734–7.
86. Stehling L. Autotransfusion and hemodilution. In: Miller RD (ed.). *Anesthesia*, 3rd edn. New York: Churchill Livingstone, 1990: 1501–3.
87. The National Blood Resource Education Program Expert Panel. The use of autologous blood. *JAMA* 1990; **263:** 414–17.
88. Goodnough LT, Grishaber JE, Monk TG, Catalona WJ. Acute preoperative hemodilution in patients undergoing radical prostatectomy: a case study analysis of efficacy. *Anesth Analg* 1994; **78:** 932–7.
89. Feldman JM, Roth JV, Bjoraker DG. Maximum blood savings by acute normovolemic hemodilution. *Anesth Analg* 1995; **80:** 108–13.
90. Brecher ME, Rosenfeld M. Mathematical and computer modeling of acute normovolemic hemodilution. *Transfusion* 1994; **34:** 176–9.
91. Bryson GL, Laupacis A, Wells GA, *et al.* Does acute normovolemic hemodilution reduce perioperative allogeneic transfusion? A meta-analysis. *Anesth Analg* 1998; **86:** 9–15.
92. Brainard DMD. Amputation of the thigh for disease of the knee joint: transfusion of blood. *Chicago Med J* 1860; **18:** 116–17.
93. Huët C, Salmi LR, Fergusen D, *et al.* A meta-analysis of the effectiveness of cell salvage to minimize perioperative allogenic blood transfusion in cardiac and orthopaedic surgery. *Anesth Analg* 1999; **89:** 861–9.
94. Huber TS, McGorray SP, Carlton LC, *et al.* Intraoperative autologous transfusion during elective infrarenal aortic reconstruction: a decision analysis model. *J Vasc Surg* 1997; **25:** 984–94.
95. Laupacis A, Feeny D, Detsky AS, Tugwell PX. How attractive does new technology have to be to warrant adoption and utilization: tentative guidelines for using clinical and economic evaluations. *Can Med Assoc J* 1992; **146:** 473–81.
96. Thomas MJG. Infected and malignant fields are an absolute contraindication to intraoperative cell salvage: fact or fiction? *Transfusion Med* 1999; **9:** 269–78.
97. Hansen E, Knuechel R, Altmeppen J, Taeger K. Blood irradiation for intraoperative autotransfusion in cancer surgery: demonstration of efficient elimination of contaminating tumor cells. *Transfusion* 1999; **39:** 608–15.
98. Del Rossi AI, Cernaiann AC, Botros S, *et al.* Prophylactic treatment of post perfusion bleeding using EACA. *Chest* 1989; **96:** 27.
99. Harrow JC, Hlavacek J, Strong MD, *et al.* Prophylactic tranexamic acid decreases bleeding after cardiac operations. *J Thor Cardiovasc Surg* 1990; **99:** 70.
100. Royston D, Bidstrup BP, Taylor KM, Sapsford RN. Effects of aprotinin on

need for blood transfusion after repeat open heart surgery. *Lancet* 1987; **2:** 1289.

101. Royston D. High-dose aprotinin therapy: a review of the first five years' experience. *J Cardiothor Vasc Anesth* 1992; **6:** 76.
102. Wang JS, Lynn CY, Hung WT, Carp RB. Monitoring of heparin induced anticoagulation with kaolin-activated clotting time in cardiac surgical patients treated with aprotinin. *Anesthesiology* 1992; **77:** 1080–4.
103. Salzman EW, Weinstein MJ, Weintraub RM, *et al.* Treatment with desmopressin acetate to reduce blood loss after cardiac surgery. *N Engl J Med* 1986; **314:** 1402.
104. Mannucci PM. Desmopressin: a nontransfusional form of treatment for congenital and acquired bleeding disorders. *Blood* 1988; **72:** 1449.
105. Kasper SM, Grune F, Walter M, *et al.* The effects of increased doses of bovine hemoglobin on hemodynamics and oxygen transport in patients undergoing preoperative hemodilution for elective abdominal aortic surgery. *Anesth Analg* 1998; **87:** 284–91.
106. Gould SA, Moore EE, Hoyt DB, *et al.* The first randomized trial of human polymerized hemoglobin as a blood substitute in acute trauma and emergent surgery. *J Am Coll Surg* 1998; **187:** 113–20.
107. Lamy ML, Daily EK, Brichant JF, *et al.* Randomized trial of diaspirin cross linked hemoglobin solutions as an alternative to blood transfusion after cardiac surgery. *Anesthesiology* 2000; **92:** 646–56.
108. Spahn DR, van Brempt R, Theilmeier G, *et al.* Perflubron emulsion delays blood transfusions in orthopaedic surgery. *Anesthesiology* 1999; **91:** 1195–208.
109. Wahr JA, Tremper KK. Blood substitutes. In: Fleisher LA, Prough DS (eds). *Problems in Anesthesia*. Philadelphia: Lippincott, Williams and Wilkins, 2000; 82–93.

10

Hemostasis

DAVID G BJORAKER

THE PHYSIOLOGY OF HEMOSTASIS

Hemostasis includes all the mechanisms by which excessive bleeding is stopped and by which undesired thrombosis is prevented, thus allowing the blood to remain liquid and flowing in an intact vasculature. In the perioperative period, excessive bleeding is prevented by maintaining or restoring vascular integrity, by providing sufficient coagulation factor activity so that the coagulation cascade produces ample fibrin, and by maintaining adequate platelet function. Excessive thrombosis in the postoperative period is controlled by antithrombotic systems that limit fibrin accumulation in the vasculature: antithrombin, protein C/protein S, tissue factor pathway inhibitor, and fibrinolysis.

Prohemostatic mechanisms

Vascular integrity

When the vasculature is damaged, immediate physiologic responses are set into play to close off a leak and initiate repair. Local vasoconstriction mediated by thromboxane, serotonin, and diminished nitric oxide occurs in normal vascular beds, but often not in malignant tissue and atherosclerotic vessels. Vasoconstriction not only directly reduces the supply of blood to the vascular leak but also shunts flow into adjacent nonconstricted vessels. Similarly, adjacent tissue swelling also reduces flow to vessels that are damaged. The exposure of collagen and microfibrils in the subendothelial layer of the injured vessel wall permits platelet adhesion and initiates the formation of a platelet plug.

Unfortunately, subtle damage to the vascular endothelium, such as that caused by handling or retracting vessels, may initiate a hemostatic response that can lead to thrombus formation and generate activated circulating platelets that are prone to respond too hastily at other sites. More obvious interruptions of the endothelium, such as suture lines in newly anastomosed vessels or prosthetic vascular grafts, cause a vigorous hemostatic response which if unopposed will result in thrombosis.

In the perioperative period, uncorrected breaches of vascular integrity requiring surgical exploration and ligation are often diagnosed by excluding platelet and coagulation cascade deficiencies and fibrinolytic excess. Fibrin glue, derived from products rich in fibrinogen such as cryoprecipitate mixed with thrombin, have been used extensively as vascular sealants and adhesives.[1] Fibrin glue is now commercially available, as are other materials which promote the hemostatic response of small vessels such as thrombin spray, absorbable gelatin sponges (Gelfoam), and oxidized, cross-linked, and microfibrillar collagen (Surgicel, Angiostat, and Avitene respectively).

The platelet plug

Platelets are circulating biconvex disks, approximately 2–4 µm in diameter, that are fragments of megakaryocyte cytoplasm. The normal maturation cycle of a platelet is about 4 days before they are shed and released from the bone marrow. They have a circulation half-life of 9–10 days, which is significantly reduced in circumstances of high consumption such as extensive atherosclerosis, cardiac valve dysfunction, or surgery.

The platelet cell surface contains important glycoprotein (GP) receptors that mediate their hemostatic response.[2,3] Initially, platelets may adhere to the injured vessel by the GPIb receptor to von Willebrand factor (vWF), the GPIa/IIa or GPIV receptors to collagen, the GPIc/IIa receptor to laminin or fibronectin, or the GPIV receptor to thrombospondin. Low concentrations of vWF or abnormal vWF is responsible for the platelet dysfunction known as von Willebrand's disease. GPIIb/IIIa is the receptor for fibrinogen, which is always required to be occupied for platelets to aggregate. It is exposed to the circulation only after platelet activation and is the main site of platelet-to-platelet adherence.

Platelets have four main hemostatic functions: (1) formation of a temporary vascular plug later reinforced by fibrin, (2) exposure of a phospholipid surface (platelet factor 3, PF3) to serve as a reaction site for the coagulation cascade, (3) release of active biochemicals (Table 10.1), and (4) mechanical clot retraction. Fortunately, platelets passively agglutinate and actively aggregate because their small size requires large numbers to actually plug a significant vascular leak. A chemical reaction involving actin and myosin within the platelet causes it first to become spherical, then spicular, then to spread into contorted forms during which release occurs through an open canalicular system, and finally to contract the fibrin mesh. During this platelet response, organelles such as the alpha and dense granules release their contents and their phospholipid surfaces that were previously hidden become exposed to the circulation. Although phospholipid membranes are ubiquitous, these negatively charged membranes rich in phosphatidylserine and phosphatidylinositol are optimal for PF3 activity.

As cytoplasmic fragments, platelets do not contain a nucleus, but do contain organelles filled with locally and systemically active biochemicals (Table 10.1) that are released during clotting. Many of these substances can trigger or enhance the response of other platelets, thereby creating a positive feedback phenomenon. Adenosine diphos-

Table 10.1 *Biochemical platelet-release products*

α-granule
β-Thromboglobulin (βTG)
Platelet-derived growth factor (PDGF)
Platelet factor 4 (PF4)
von Willebrand factor (vWF)
Dense granules (δ-granules)
Adenosine diphosphate (ADP)
Adenosine triphosphate (ATP)
Calcium ion (Ca^{2+})
Epinephrine (adrenaline)
Serotonin
Platelet cytoplasm
Fibrinogen
Prostaglandin intermediates
Thrombospondin
Thromboxane A_2 (TXA_2)
Tissue factor pathway inhibitor (TFPI)

phate (ADP) is an important release product that serves as an activator of other platelets; however, its rapid removal by red blood cells prevents uncontrolled propagation of its effect. Thromboxane A_2, a product of the cyclo-oxygenase pathway, is also released and causes potent vasoconstriction and activation of other platelets.

Several substances generated by the vascular endothelium downregulate platelet response. Prostaglandin I_2 (prostacyclin; PGI_2), synthesized in the endothelial cell, is a cyclo-oxygenase product of arachidonic acid. It is a potent vascular dilator and blocks platelet aggregation by increasing platelet cyclic adenosine monophoshate (cAMP) levels. Nitric oxide (NO) is also a potent vascular dilator that inhibits both platelet adhesion and aggregation by increasing intraplatelet cyclic guanosine monophosphate (cGMP).

Fibrin polymerization

Classically, the coagulation cascade (Fig. 10.1) is divided into the intrinsic and extrinsic pathways, which both lead to a common pathway that produces an insoluble cross-linked fibrin polymer. The resulting mesh of fibrin strands reinforces the platelet plug and is commonly referred to as a clot. The intrinsic pathway contains all of the factors within the blood that are necessary for clot formation beginning with factor XII (Table 10.2), which is usually activated by surface contact or contact with negatively charged activated platelet membrane. The extrinsic pathway, which requires an extravascular tissue factor (TF), plays the greater role in initiating clot formation *in vivo*. Both pathways converge to activate factor X (Fig. 10.1).

A more recent unified concept of the coagulation cascade involves three steps: initiation, amplification, and propagation.[4] During the initiation phase, TF – a phospholipid – from an injury site combines with circulating activated factor VII (VIIa). Unlike other activated factors, factor VIIa is commonly present in the circulation. The factor VIIa/TF complex activates a small amount of factor IX, which then converts a small amount of factor X to Xa, eventually forming a small amount of thrombin (factor IIa). If this thrombin is not neutralized by antithrombin III or thrombomodulin, the amplification phase begins. Thrombin activates factor XI in the intrinsic system, enhances conversion of the cofactors factor VIII and factor V to their active forms, and promotes platelet activation and aggregation. Once the factor Va, factor VIIIa, and factor IXa complexes are assembled on the platelet surface, the formation of factor Xa, thrombin, and fibrin proceeds explosively.

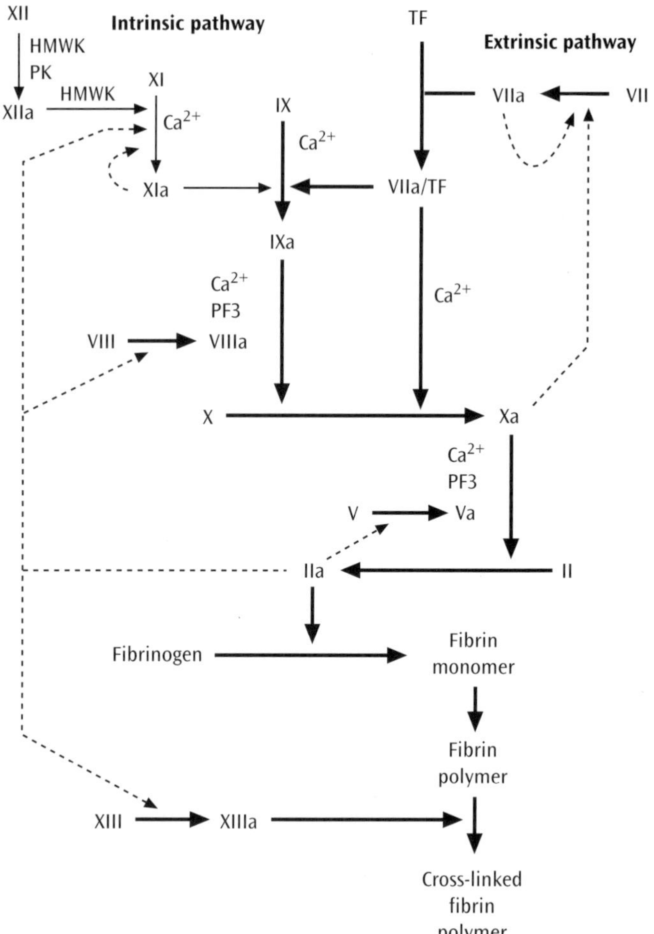

Figure 10.1 *The coagulation cascade. Major pathways are designated by bold arrows, minor pathways by narrow arrows, and feedback pathways by dotted arrows. See Table 10.2 for factor names. HMWK, high-molecular-weight kininogen; PK, prekallikrein; TF, tissue factor; PF3, platelet factor 3; Ca^{2+}, calcium ion.*

Table 10.2 *Synonyms of the Roman numeral-designated coagulation factors*

Factor	Synonym
I	Fibrinogen
II	Prothrombin
III	Platelet factor III; thromboplastin; tissue extract
IV	Calcium ion (Ca^{2+})
V	Labile factor; proaccelerin; accelerator globulin
VI	(Not now used)
VII	Stable factor; proconvertin; autoprothrombin I
VIII	Antihemophilic factor A; antihemophilic globulin
IX	Antihemophilic factor B; Christmas factor
X	Stuart–Prower factor
XI	Antihemophilic factor C; plasma thromboplastin antecedent (PTA)
XII	Hageman factor
XIII	Fibrin-stabilizing factor

Activated factors are designated by the suffix "a," e.g. factor VIIa.

The circulating coagulation factors XII, XI, X, IX, VII, and II are serine proteases or cleavage enzymes which are activated by the activated factors preceding them in the coagulation cascade. Factors V and VIII are not proteolytic enzymes themselves, but coenzymes. Both are labile and depleted in stored bank blood but are present in fresh-frozen plasma (FFP). Fibrinogen is a nonenzymatic, soluble protein. Phospholipids such as PF3 and TF bind the calcium cation (Ca^{2+}), which in turn binds serine proteases to the phospholipids by its double positive charge. The amino acids of the serine protease side chains do not intrinsically contain the necessary double negative charge until carboxylated by vitamin K. Vitamin K acts on each of the four serine proteases that must bind to platelet phospholipid (factors IX, X, and II) or tissue phospholipid (factor VII). These four factors are known as the vitamin K-dependent factors or hepatic factors.

Antithrombotic mechanisms

Antithrombin III

Antithrombin III (ATIII) is the major inhibitor of activated serine protease coagulation factors.[5] In addition to thrombin (factor IIa), it will inhibit factors IXa, Xa, XIa, XIIa, and XIIIa and plasmin by forming a complex with the serine protease near its active site, thus attenuating their proteolytic capability. When heparin binds to ATIII, the active protease site is further compromised. Endogenous heparin and heparan sulfate on the vascular wall bind ATIII, thereby scavenging thrombin and other circulating activated serine proteases.

ATIII is a single-chain α_2-glycoprotein that is synthesized in the liver. If congenitally absent, severe or fatal thrombosis occurs. More commonly, congenitally low levels of 50–60% of normal are associated with renal vein thrombosis, unexpected peripheral vascular thrombosis, and pulmonary emboli after age 20 years. Acquired ATIII deficiency can occur in a number of medical conditions, including disseminated intravascular coagulopathy (DIC), sepsis, oral contraceptive use, and with chronic heparin administration.

Protein C and protein S

Protein C is a glycoprotein synthesized in the liver, where it undergoes vitamin K-dependent carboxylation.[6] Under normal conditions, thrombin slowly reacts with protein C, generating activated protein C (APC). APC is a physiologic anticoagulant that works by inactivating membrane-bound factors Va and VIIIa. Thrombomodulin is a glycosaminoglycan on the surface of the endothelial cell that forms a high-affinity bond with thrombin. If thrombin is complexed with thrombomodulin, it rapidly activates protein C. So, thrombin is inactivated by virtue of it complexing with thrombomodulin and APC is formed, which down-regulates thrombin formation by inactivating Va and VIIIa.

Protein S is also a vitamin K-dependent glycoprotein that is synthesized in the liver, in megakaryocytes, and in vascular endothelial cells. It serves as a cofactor for APC by increasing the affinity of APC for negatively charged phospholipids such as PF3. Membrane-bound APC–protein S complexes on the surface of platelets facilitate Va and VIIIa degradation.

Tissue factor pathway inhibitor

Tissue factor pathway inhibitor (TFPI) is an endogenous regulator of the extrinsic pathway.[7,8] It is a multivalent plasma protease blocker that inhibits the factor VIIa/TF complex. It circulates in plasma, where it is either bound to lipoproteins or contained by platelets. The 10% of TFPI in platelets is subject to release when activation occurs. TFPI that is bound to glycosaminoglycans on endothelial cells may be released by heparin. TFPI also has inhibitory activity against factor Xa.

Fibrinolysis

Fibrin formation that occurs despite the antithrombin III, protein C/protein S, and TFPI systems is rapidly degraded by the fibrinolytic system. Activation of the fibrinolytic system is achieved by the conversion of an inactive circulating and fibrin-bound zymogen, plasminogen, to plasmin, a serine protease (Fig. 10.2).[9,10] Plasmin cleaves fibrinogen and noncross-linked fibrin to indistinguishable fibrin and fibrinogen degradation products. Degradation of factor XIII cross-linked fibrin yields the additional D-dimer fragment.

There are two dominant physiologic plasminogen activators produced by the vascular endothelium. Tissue plasminogen activator (tPA) is continuously released into the circulation and metabolized by the liver. Prourokinase is converted to urokinase by a reaction accelerated by plasmin. Both tPA and urokinase are serine proteases that cleave plasminogen to yield plasmin. Thrombin and the intrinsic pathway active factors can also convert plasminogen to plasmin.

Plasminogen activator inhibitors (PAI) control the conversion of plasminogen to plasmin by forming irreversible complexes with the active sites of tPA and urokinase. PAI-1 is the physiologic modulator of tPA activity, whereas PAI-2 inhibits urokinase. Additionally, PAI-3 and the protease nexin also function as plasminogen activator inhibitors. Added control of fibrinolytic activity is provided by α_2-antiplasmin, which is a circulating, rapid, and efficient inactivator of plasmin.

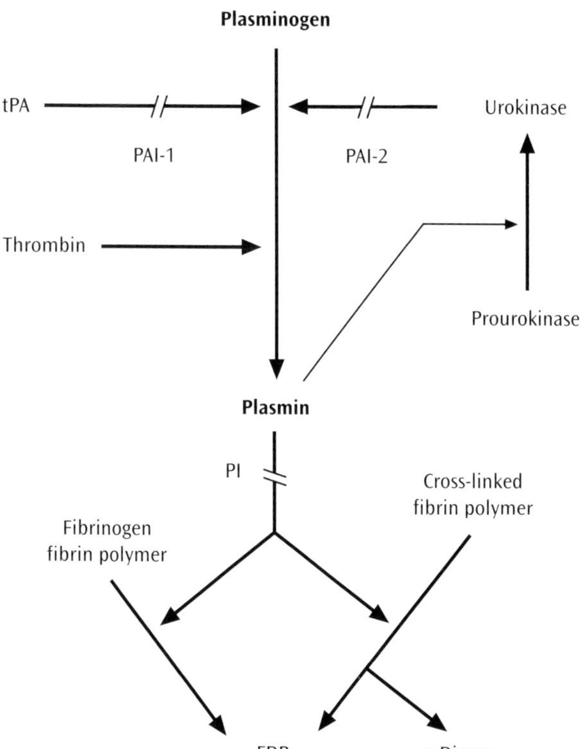

Figure 10.2 *The fibrinolytic system. Major pathways are designated by bold arrows and minor pathways by narrow arrows. Breaks in an arrow represent a major inhibitory site. tPA, tissue plasminogen activator; PAI, plasminogen activator inhibitor; PI, plasmin inhibitors, e.g. α_2-antiplasmin; FDP, fibrin and fibrinogen degradation products; D-dimer, D-dimer fragment containing fibrin degradation products.*

MONITORING HEMOSTASIS

Although most of the hemostasis-monitoring techniques in daily use during the perioperative period are well established and time tested, substantial progress has occurred in point-of-care testing and platelet function analysis. A traditional panel of hemostasis tests will be reviewed and techniques of particular interest to anesthesiologists will be presented: the activated clotting time, the thrombelastograph, whole blood prothrombin time and partial thromboplastin time, and platelet function analysis.

Blood must be properly anticoagulated and analyzed within minutes because it will clot shortly after removal from the vascular system and labile constituents deteriorate. Assay systems that require blood to clot or platelets to function are generally anticoagulated with anionic citrate, which chelates enough calcium ion (Ca^{2+}) to radically delay clotting. In the laboratory, Ca^{2+} is added to exactly replace what was chelated by the citrate in the sample tube. If either the concentration of citrate is excessive because the sampling tube was underfilled or the concentration is low because of overfilling, a timed assay system will be artifactually prolonged. Extremes of overfilling or recent systemic administration of calcium chloride to the patient may result in the specimen clotting. The volume of blood added to vacuum sample tubes must be carefully observed because a tube may have partially lost its original vacuum and underfilling will result. Ethylene diamine tetra-acetic acid (EDTA) chelates Ca^{2+} more completely and is used for complete blood counts, including platelet counts.

Ideally, a sample obtained from a patient should come from a free-flowing uncontaminated stream of blood directly into the anticoagulant. Blood obtained during a difficult venipuncture contains enough tissue thromboplastin to alter results and activate platelets. If an indwelling catheter is not used, a two-syringe collection technique should be employed, i.e. after the vein is punctured using a scalp vein needle, an initial aliquot is withdrawn without needle movement and discarded and then a second aliquot is withdrawn for testing. When specimens are obtained from an indwelling catheter, three times the volume between the catheter tip and the sampling port should first be removed before the sample is collected. Heparin flush solutions used to prevent catheter thrombosis are generally 2–5 U mL^{-1} heparin, and blood gas syringes are often prepared with 1000 U mL^{-1} heparin. Either heparin flush or a small heparin droplet left in a sampling port can significantly distort hemostasis test results.

The hemostasis panel

The prothrombin time (PT) assesses the extrinsic coagulation pathway. A tissue thromboplastin reagent, Ca^{2+}, and plasma are mixed in a clot-timing instrument and the clot formation in seconds is reported. In recent years, the international normalized ratio[11] (INR) is also reported – 1.0 being normal. The INR is calculated as: $INR = (PT\ ratio)^{ISI}$, where PT ratio is the patient's PT in seconds divided by the PT of normal donor pooled plasma; ISI is the International Sensitivity Index of the thromboplastin reagent used in a specific coagulometer. The manufacturer of the reagent assigns the ISI to each reagent batch after assaying it against a reference thromboplastin. The INR should not vary by reagent or equipment, but only by changes in the patient's hemostatic capacity.

INR increases will occur with factor V, VII, or X deficiency of either congenital or acquired etiology. Only approximately 30% of the normal concentration of these factors will maintain a normal INR. Hypofibrinogenemia will influence the INR when levels are below 80 mg dL^{-1}, as will a severe deficiency of factor II, prothrombin. Coumarin therapy, vitamin K deficiency, liver disease, circulating anticoagulants, and DIC are associated with an increase in INR. Small levels of heparin do not increase INR, but large doses such as those administered intraoperatively do.

The activated partial thromboplastin time (aPTT) assesses the intrinsic coagulation pathway. A phospholipid PF3 substitute, an activator of factor XII, Ca^{2+}, and plasma are mixed in a clot-timing instrument and the clot formation in seconds is reported. Approximately 30% of the normal concentration of factors V, VIII, IX, X, XI, and XII will produce a normal aPTT value. Congenital and acquired intrinsic factor deficiencies, warfarin therapy, liver disease, circulating anticoagulants, specific factor inhibitors, and DIC are associated with aPTT prolongation. Although very sensitive to heparin, the degree of aPTT prolongation in response to heparin varies considerably with the phospholipid and activator reagent used.

There are several commercial systems available for point-of-care whole blood PT and aPTT analysis. Because the available PT reagent and aPTT reagent products vary widely, existing laboratory normal ranges for the plasma assays used in a hospital's main laboratory cannot be applied to the point-of-care whole blood systems. Normal ranges should be established separately for the whole blood techniques. The cause of reported poor correlations between whole blood and plasma assays of PT and aPTT have not been adequately explained.

The thrombin time (TT) assesses only the late portion of the common pathway – the clotting of fibrinogen. Thrombin reagent, Ca^{2+}, and plasma are mixed in a clot-timing instrument and the clot formation in seconds is reported. Thrombin time is usually not used as a screening assay, but can be used with a calibration curve to accurately measure circulating heparin levels. However, as a screening assay, TT prolongation may indicate hypofibrinogenemia or fibrin(ogen) degradation products (FDP) interfering with the polymerization of sufficient insoluble fibrin to trigger the assay endpoint. A similar interference by high levels of FDPs may occur during PT and aPTT determination.

Clottable fibrinogen concentration can be measured by a modification of the TT in which the plasma is diluted 10-fold before the thrombin and Ca^{2+} are added. The time to detectable clot formation is converted to mg dL^{-1} fibrinogen concentrations using a calibration curve. Decreased levels of fibrinogen are seen in hereditary hypofibrinogenemia as well as in acquired disorders such as DIC, primary and secondary fibrinolysis, and liver disease. Increased concentrations occur with inflammatory disorders, pregnancy, and in women taking oral contraceptives. Fibrinogen can also be measured immunologically. There can be a substantial difference between clottable fibrinogen and antigen-reactive fibrinogen in dysfibrinogenemias and liver disease.

The platelet count is usually measured by the Coulter principle, in which a known volume of a highly diluted solution of platelets passes one platelet at a time through an orifice, thus altering an electric field across the orifice in proportion to the cell size. Each field disturbance is counted within a designated size range and then corrected for dilution. The usual normal count is approximately 150 000–350 000 platelets per μL. Platelet volumes are often reported: large platelets are recently released from the megakaryocyte, while mature platelets lose volume. Red blood cells are lysed for most electronic counters because the sizes of microcytic red cells and large platelets overlap unpredictably. EDTA anticoagulant has been known to cause a pseudothrombocytopenia by agglutinating platelets, thus making their size too large for the defined platelet range. Confirmation of low or suspicious counts can be obtained by examination of the patient's whole blood smear. With a new two-dimensional analysis, both the volume and refractive index of apparent platelets are measured on a cell-by-cell basis, permitting true platelets to be distinguished from red cell fragments and debris, microcytic red cells, and red cell ghosts.[12]

Bleeding time is the classic,[13] apparently simple method of *in vivo* platelet function testing that has now been largely discredited.[14] With a commercial spring-loaded disposable lancet, reproducible incisions are made on the volar aspect of the forearm while the venous pressure is adjusted using a minimally inflated blood pressure cuff. The time from incision until no additional blood is shed is the bleeding time, normally less than 6 min. Platelet counts less than 100 000 μL^{-1} can be expected to prolong bleeding time. Unfortunately, accuracy of bleeding time is greatly dependent on the technician's precise control of detail and is labor intensive. Hypothermia prolongs bleeding time. Straining and movement prolong bleeding time, such as occurs during labor or with a Valsalva maneuver. Interpatient variability is also influenced by skin type, vessel wall collagen composition, vWF concentration, vWF multimer size, and the ratio of endothelial prostacyclin production to platelet thromboxane production. Skin bleeding time does not correlate with bleeding time in other types of tissue. Even when accurately performed, an individual value is not specifically or accurately related to the patient's platelet function as measured by other means. Epidemiologic studies do show that anemia, female gender, and older age are associated with longer bleeding times. Other methods of platelet function assessment should now be used.[14]

Activated clotting time

Because of the apparent simplicity of the activated clotting time (ACT), its nearly linear response to heparin concentration, and its low sensitivity to large amounts of heparin, the ACT is widely used to manage large-dose heparin administration during intraoperative vascular occlusion, cardiopulmonary bypass, hemodialysis, and cardiac catheterization.[15] However, the ACT is not sufficiently sensitive to assess mild coagulation factor deficiencies or small anticoagulant effects, such as residual heparin.

A minimum ACT is usually chosen to define adequate anticoagulation for cardiopulmonary bypass; however, the selection of that endpoint is imprecise. In 1975 Bull *et al.*[16] determined an endpoint of 480 s; in 1978 Young *et al.*[17] recommended 400 s; other target values of similar magnitude are often used today without regard for the differences in ACT methods. Different activating substances are in clinical use, such as kaolin, ellagic acid, Celite, siliceous earth, diatomaceous earth, and glass beads. Factors important in contact activation all vary, such as activator chemistry, preparation, batch-to-batch consistency, and effective surface area. In addition, the degree of mixing of blood with the activator provided manually by the operator or by the incubating device is not standardized. The ACT is temperature dependent and requires proper thermostatic control during incubation. The sensitivity of the mechanism used to detect the onset of fibrin formation is also variable.

Although the utility of ACT monitoring of heparinization during cardiopulmonary bypass has been questioned, ACT prolongation does demonstrate that heparin was successfully administered and that errors have not occurred, such as a mislabeled syringe, an incorrect heparin dose, and an injection into a nonfunctioning intravenous catheter. In addition, congenital and acquired deficiencies of antithrombin III will be uncovered as apparent heparin resistance. Both hemodilution and hypothermia prolong the ACT during cardiopulmonary bypass and cause the heparin concentration–ACT correlation to diverge. Inhibition of platelet activation also results in prolongation of the ACT.

Although the ACT can be used to estimate the current amount of heparin circulating prior to administering protamine,[16] the blood temperature at that time must be considered. The ACT can be restored to preheparinization levels in the 37 °C assay, but the still hypothermic patient may continue to bleed. The restoration of ACT to preheparinization levels is most reliably achieved if the initial control ACT is obtained after sternotomy.

Thrombelastography

The thrombelastograph (TEG) is a pre-World War II instrument that has gained acceptance in the management of hemostatic problems during liver transplantation, cardiopulmonary bypass, and other major surgery. Although the TEG does provide an assessment of the global interaction of the cellular and the soluble coagulation factor components of hemostasis, it is an *in vitro* analysis that does not include all the relevant components of *in vivo* hemostasis such as interactions with the endothelium.[18]

Nonanticoagulated whole blood is usually analyzed, but the TEG may also analyze recalcified citrated blood or plasma. Blood is placed in a disposable oscillating plastic cuvette and the movement of a cylindrical plastic piston which is suspended in the cuvette is displayed (Fig. 10.3). As fibrin strands form and adhere to both the cuvette and piston surfaces, the magnitude of the movement of the piston increases, yielding a pattern that is usually characterized by five parameters (Fig. 10.3).[19] Any defects in platelet function, the intrinsic system, or other interference in polymerization of fibrin alter the shape of the normal trace (Fig. 10.4).

Platelet function analyzers

In addition to the maximum amplitude (ma) value of the thrombelastograph, other point-of-care objective measurements of platelet function in the perioperative period have become available and several more are under development. Considerable experience has been accumulated with the Dade Platelet Function Analyzer (PFA-100), the Medtronic Hemostatus, and the Array Medical Ichor-Plateworks system.

The PFA-100 uses a disposable cartridge system that contains a membrane coated with collagen–epinephrine (adrenaline) or collagen–ADP.[20] Recalcified citrated whole blood is aspirated from the cartridge's sample reservoir through a capillary tube and microscopic aperture in the coated membrane. The biochemical coatings on the membrane and high shear forces cause platelets to adhere, activate, and aggregate at the aperture. The time required for a stable platelet plug to progressively form and occlude the aperture is called the "closure time." This assay is designed to be analogous to the bleeding time, but much more reliable, reproducible, and less labor intensive.[21] The PFA-100 is similar to the Thrombostat 4000 device developed in Europe.

The Hemostatus is a platelet-sensitive ACT that uses a disposable cartridge system which requires the Medtronic Hepcon/HMS instrument.[22,23] The assay measures simultaneous kaolin ACTs with progressively increasing concentrations of platelet-activating factor (PAF). Two of six assay wells contain no PAF and the others contain 1.25, 6.25, 12.5, and 150 nmol L^{-1} PAF. A clot ratio (CR) is reported for the PAF channels that is defined as the difference between the control ACT and the ACT in that channel divided by the control ACT. When functioning platelets are present, PAF accelerates the ACT in a dose-related fashion. Thus, if platelet function is poor, then the CR in channel 6 should approach 0; if excellent, then CR increases (0.51 in a population of normal patients).

The Ichor-Plateletworks system consists of the automated eight parameter Ichor cell counter and the Plateletworks sampling kit, which contains both a baseline collection tube and one of two types of platelet-aggregating agonist tubes. The user collects an EDTA anticoagulated whole blood specimen on which the Ichor counter performs a complete blood count including a platelet count. A second platelet count is then performed on a citrate anticoagulated whole blood specimen that is treated with a platelet-aggregating agent, either ADP or calf collagen. The aggregating agonist causes responsive, functioning platelets to clump and not be counted within the platelet size range. Platelet aggregation is calculated by the formula:

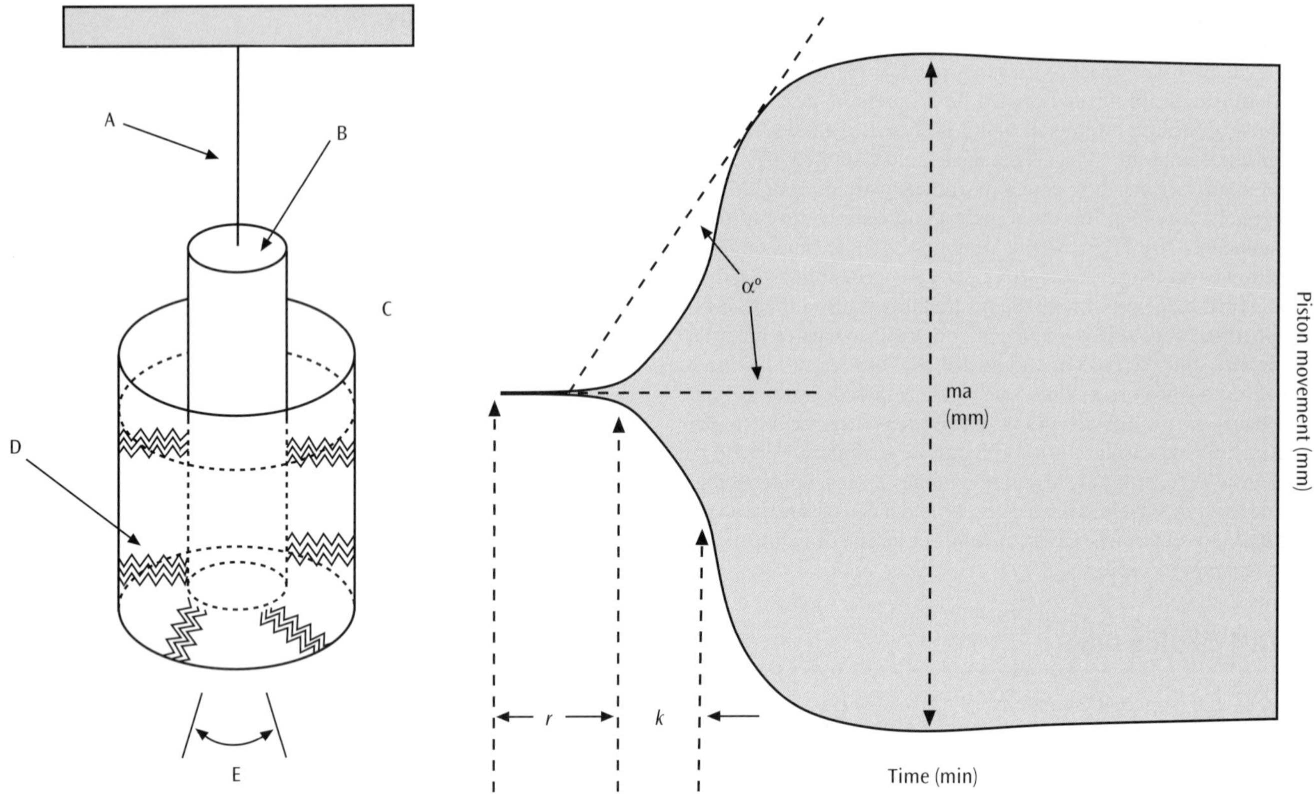

Figure 10.3 *Thrombelastograph schematic. A cylindrical plastic piston (B) is suspended from a torsion wire (A) into a plastic specimen cuvette (C) allowing 1 mm of blood between the piston and cuvette surfaces. The cuvette repeatedly twists through an arc of 1/12 radian (9.5°) (E), one cycle taking 10 s including a 1-s pause at each extreme of rotation. Initially, when the blood is a liquid suspension of cells, none of the cuvette movement is transferred to the piston. As fibrin strands (D) form and adhere to both the cuvette and piston surfaces, the piston begins to twist with the cuvette, thus generating a signal. When the movement amplitude is 2 mm,* r *is determined. The* r*-value or reaction time is the time to onset of fibrin formation and correlates with other assays of the intrinsic pathway. The* k*-value is the time between 2 and 20 mm amplitude and α is the angle in degrees from the onset of piston movement to the shoulder of the trace; both reflect the rate of fibrin formation. The ma value indicates clot firmness and is dependent on functioning platelets and fibrinogen concentration. The* a_{60} *value (not illustrated) is the amplitude 60 min after ma and indicates fibrinolysis if* a_{60} *is less than 85% of the ma value.*

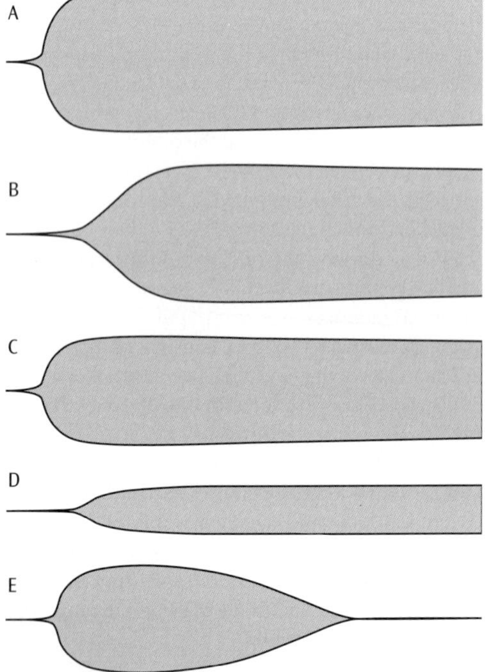

Figure 10.4 *Characteristic thrombelastograph patterns. (A) Normal thrombelastographic pattern. (B) Factor deficiency or moderate anticoagulation is characterized by prolongations of* r *and* k*, reduction of α, but maintenance of ma and* a_{60}*. (C) Moderate platelet deficiency is characterized by preservation of* r *and* k*, but a reduction in ma. (D) Severe platelet deficiency results in marked increases in* r *and* k *and reductions in α and ma. (E) If fibrinolysis is present,* a_{60} *is less than 85% of ma 1 h after ma or full clot dissolution occurs.*

Percent aggregation = 100 × (Baseline count – agonist count)/ baseline count

In healthy volunteers, the normal percent aggregation range (mean ± standard deviation) for the collagen agonist was 63–87% and for the ADP agonist was 80–97%. Carville *et al.* confirmed the correlation of classic platelet aggregometry to the Ichor-Plateletworks assay for collagen and ADP ($r = 0.90$ and $r = 0.96$, respectively).[24] This correlation is maintained when the whole blood specimen is obtained from a heparinized patient. Comparison of traditional ADP aggregometry and the Plateletworks ADP assay for three *in vitro* dosage levels of three GP IIb/IIIa inhibitors produced strong correlations, $r = 0.91$ for tirofiban, $r = 0.88$ for eptifibatide, and $r = 0.79$ for abciximab.[25] A major benefit of the Ichor-Plateletworks methodology in the operating room is that a platelet count and an index of platelet function are both rapidly available.

AVAILABLE TREATMENT MODALITIES

The flourishing inventory of products available to treat hemostatic disorders can be divided into three groups: replacement therapeutics derived from blood, antithrombotic pharmaceuticals, and prohemostatic pharmaceuticals. Indications for treatment of the surgical patient must take into account the site of potential bleeding; intracranial, paraspinal, and ocular locations are particularly high risk.

Replacement therapeutics

Fresh-frozen plasma

Fresh-frozen plasma (FFP) is the noncellular fraction of whole blood remaining after red cell and platelet concentrates have been separated. Its administration, therefore, carries the infectious risks of whole blood. The 200- to 250-mL unit of citrate anticoagulated plasma is frozen immediately after separation in order to stop the rapid decline in the labile coagulation factors V and VIII. Once a unit is thawed, it should be refrigerated and infused within 4 h to avoid a substantial decrease in factors V and VIII.

The main indication for FFP is to increase clotting factors in patients with a deficiency demonstrated by laboratory testing or with a significant increase in INR or aPTT.[26] FFP is not indicated for volume expansion, for nutritional support, or for maintenance of colloid oncotic pressure. When vitamin K-dependent coagulation factors (II, VII, IX, and X) are depressed after coumarin derivatives, emergent correction may be accomplished by FFP infusion; however, discontinuation of oral anticoagulants and administration of vitamin K_1 is preferred when time permits. Patients with antithrombin III (ATIII) deficiency who have heparin resistance can be treated by replacement of ATIII through FFP administration.

Cryoprecipitate

When FFP is thawed at 4 °C, some plasma proteins will remain precipitated. When solubilized by further warming, this cryoprecipitate becomes 20–25 mL of plasma containing 30–60% of the factor VIII and 25% of the fibrinogen in a unit of blood. Factor XIII, vWF, and fibronectin are also present in high concentration. Cryoprecipitate treatment may provide sufficient replacement of factor VIII in patients with mild hemophilia A and in patients deficient in factor VIII who require only minor surgery provided that factor VIII antibody titers are low. Active bleeding or major surgery in patients with von Willebrand's disease may be treated with cryoprecipitate or desmopressin. Cryoprecipitate can also provide replacement therapy for fibrinogen and factor XIII deficiency. Because anti-A, anti-B, and Rh antibodies may be contained in the cryoprecipitate, blood type compatibility is observed. Large quantities of cryoprecipitate can result in an impractical volume and may increase fibrinogen concentrations to several times normal.

Platelet transfusion

The need for platelet transfusions should not be based on the platelet count alone, but also on the clinical circumstance and direct observation of the surgical field. Many of the drugs taken chronically or administered in the perioperative period are inhibitors of platelet function, e.g. nonsteroidal anti-inflammatory drugs (NSAIDs), calcium channel blockers, local anesthetics, and antibiotics. Intraoperative techniques, such as cardiopulmonary bypass, veno-venous bypass, and autotransfusion, activate and damage platelets, returning to the circulation a cell which may contribute to an electronic platelet count but which is not capable of normal function. If the hemostatic system is otherwise normal and platelet function is intact, the minimum counts of 50 000 μL^{-1} for minor surgery and 100 000 μL^{-1} for major surgery are probably appropriate if the surgical site is high risk (intracranial, paraspinal, or ocular). When a regional anesthetic technique is considered, the same preoperative limits as for major surgery at a high-risk site should be observed. Often, diffuse oozing in the surgical field and a marginal platelet count may require platelet transfusion. Ideally, intraoperative evaluation of platelet count and function should confirm the need for platelet transfusion; however, objective assessment of platelet function in the operating room is in its infancy.

Prophylactic transfusion of platelets for massive blood transfusion or cardiopulmonary bypass is not acceptable.[27] The risks of platelet transfusion are the same as for blood transfusion, magnified by the multiple donor exposures that are necessary to increase the platelet count to effective levels when single-donor units are used. If bacterial contamination has occurred during blood collection, bacteremia is likely because of bacterial multiplication during platelet storage at room temperature. Platelet alloimmunization may make the patient refractory to platelet transfusion or may result in late thrombocytopenia. Leukocyte reactions, such as febrile responses, also occur.

Platelets separated from citrate-anticoagulated blood into the commonly used polyvinylchloride transfer packs can only be stored at 22 °C for 5 days with constant gentle agitation. The *in vivo* recovery of platelets stored for 72 h is 50%, with a typical survival of 7.3 days.[28] For each 450 mL of collected blood, at least 5.5×10^{10} platelets should be recovered and resuspended in 50–70 mL of plasma, representing a 40–85% yield. Transfused platelets sustain a biochemical storage lesion which impairs function and is not instantly corrected by infusion.

An initial dose of platelets to achieve a 50 000–100 000 μL^{-1} platelet count, depending on the clinical circumstance, may be estimated by anticipating a 5000–10 000 increase in count when administering one unit of platelet concentrate to an adult. One unit per 10 kg body weight is another often used dosage guideline. The age and quality of the platelet preparation and the rapidity of platelet consumption may greatly alter the efficacy of the treatment. Rapid administration of platelets after, rather than during, brisk blood loss will improve the efficacy of the transfusion. Once single-donor platelets are pooled, the combined product should be infused within 4 h.

The transfusion of the equivalent of several units of platelets collected from a single donor is possible with plateletpheresis. Continuous centrifugation equipment can process 3–4 L of blood in less than 2 h and harvest $4–6 \times 10^{11}$ platelets. Although the cost is high, when prolonged platelet transfusion support is planned, the number of exposures to blood donors is decreased and alloimmunization is reduced. The preoperative collection of autologous platelets by plateletpheresis may be efficacious in select circumstances, such as redo coronary artery bypass graft (CABG), extensive cancer surgery, or difficult hepatic resections. Although donor exposure is reduced with the pheresis product, one must be confident that the donor's platelets are fully functional.

Antihemophilic factor concentrates

Antihemophilic factor concentrates are indicated for the treatment of active bleeding and prior to major surgery in patients with severe factor VIII deficiency (hemophilia A).[29] Although only 10% of normal factor VIII levels prevent spontaneous hemorrhage, prior to major surgery factor VIII should be increased to 100% of normal and confirmed by laboratory analysis.[30] A minimum maintenance level of factor VIII of 30% of normal should be continued for 7–14 days postoperatively. Since antibodies to factor VIII occur in approximately 10% of patients who have had prior factor VIII administration, factor VIII antibody levels should also be measured before and throughout the course of replacement. If antibody levels are high, treatment with activated prothrombin complex concentrates or recombinant factor VIIa may be required. In the absence of antibodies, the level increases immediately and decays with a half-life of 9–15 h. The risk of transmission of human immunodeficiency virus (HIV), hepatitis C, and other viral diseases when factor VIII concentrates are produced from human pooled plasma is now greatly limited by donor testing, solvent–detergent treatment, and pasteurization. Purity has also been greatly improved by monoclonal antibody-affinity chromatography. Recombinant factor VIII products are now available, pure, and virus free; however, treatment of a single hemorrhage is extremely expensive and may not solve the problem of antibody formation to the treatment material over the long term.

Prothrombin complex concentrates

Factor IX or prothrombin complex concentrates (PCCs) are indicated for treatment of factor IX deficiency (hemophilia B, Christmas disease) when the deficiency is severe and the bleeding risk is too great to use fresh-frozen plasma alone.[29] Five percent of normal factor IX levels are required to prevent spontaneous hemorrhage, and only 20–30% of normal for hemostasis in severe trauma and major surgery if factor IX deficiency is the single deficit. These patients are generally treated with high purity products that are processed by immunoaffinity or chromatography techniques to greatly reduce the other hepatic factors (II, VII, and X) that may also be present in PCC. Virus transmission with currently available PCC preparations is now very unlikely. The half-life of infused factor IX is approximately 24 h.

Activated PCCs are occasionally indicated for the treatment of severe factor VIII deficiency when factor VIII antibodies prevent effective levels from being achieved.[29] The potency of the preparation is determined by its ability to normalize clotting time in factor VIII deficient plasma containing factor VIII antibodies. Autoplex (Baxter/Hyland) is a complex of factor II and factor Xa and FEIBA (Immuno) contains significant activated factors VII and IX. Both should be administered only for factor VIII deficiency with high factor VIII antibodies and with the consultation and advice of a hematologist experienced in treating hemophilia. Hemodynamic instability may occur during infusion, and simultaneous blockade of the fibrinolytic system may result in severe thrombotic complications.

Recombinant activated factor VII

In the early 1980s, plasma-derived factor VIIa was demonstrated to be effective in treating hemophilic patients with inhibitors to factor VIII and factor IX. By the late 1990s, recombinant factor VIIa (NovoSeven) was approved for such a treatment role. Off-label use of recombinant factor VIIa in trauma[31] and surgery-related coagulopathy has suggested a promising role as a rescue therapy in patients with penetrating trauma, poorly controlled intra-abdominal hemorrhage, and prior massive transfusion with an ungoing uncontrolled coagulopathy. Apparently, recombinant factor VIIa enhances hemostasis at the injury site and does not appear to promote systemic activation of the entire hemostatic system. Intravascular thrombosis and organ microthrombosis have not been major postoperative complications that have disqualified factor VIIa use, but patients deserve close monitoring for thrombotic findings. Significant practical issues include decision criteria for when conventional therapy should be supplemented, contraindications to factor VIIa as a rescue therapy, proper dosing for rescue therapy, and the extremely high cost of a course of treatment. Forthcoming controlled clinical studies that enhance the current case report literature should be enlightening.

Antithrombin III concentrate

Human antithrombin III concentrate is now available for the treatment of patients with congenital antithrombin III deficiency when they have a thrombotic event or when they are at increased risk of having a thrombotic episode such as with surgery or pregnancy. Its use in some acquired antithrombin III deficiencies, DIC, and sepsis is under investigation and results appear to be promising.[32,33] ATIII levels should be measured before treatment and shortly after to confirm ATIII deficiency, to calculate the required dose, and to determine the recovery of administered ATIII in an individual patient's plasma. Trough levels of ATIII should be measured before each 24-h dose and kept in the range of 80–120% of normal. The half-life of ATIII is approximately 22 h, but may be decreased with bleeding, surgery, acute thrombosis, or heparin administration. Concurrent dosing of heparin should be decreased.

Antithrombotic pharmaceuticals

Antithrombin agents

Standard heparin (SH) is a heterogeneous group of anionic glycosaminoglycans that have a molecular weight between 5000 and 30 000 Da, with an average of approximately 15 000 Da. Commercial preparations are derived from porcine intestinal mucosa or beef lung and are prepared as sodium or calcium salts. Small amounts of heparin combined with ATIII inhibit thrombosis by inactivating factor Xa. When larger amounts are available, the heparin–ATIII complex inactivates thrombin (factor IIa) and factors IXa, Xa, XIa, XIIa, and XIIIa and plasmin.

Administration is by intermittent intravenous (i.v.) injection, i.v. infusion, deep subcutaneous (s.c.) injection, or intranasal spray. Oral administration is ineffective, and intramuscular (i.m.) injection is associated with hematoma formation. After s.c. administration, peak plasma levels are reached 2–4 h after injection, but may vary considerably. Owing to its strong anionic nature, it is rapidly protein bound and has an anticoagulant half-life of approximately 90 min, but this varies widely. A typical bolus dosage prior to temporary vascular occlusion is 100 U kg^{-1}, and before extracorporeal circulation is 300 U kg^{-1}.

The primary complication of heparin is hemorrhage, with particular concern for the intracranial, paraspinal, and ocular sites where minute quantities of blood can produce devastating injury. While the concurrent use of SH and neuraxial regional anesthesia is not absolutely contraindicated, following guidelines (Table 10.3) and careful attention to procedural details is warranted.[34] Heparin resistance is frequently encountered early in acute thrombotic processes and is usually mediated by a consumption-related decrease in ATIII level. The apparently contradictory practice of administering FFP, which contains ATIII, and heparin may be required to achieve adequate anticoagulation. Although SH does not cross the placenta, its chronic use during pregnancy is related to a dose- and duration-dependent maternal osteoporosis.[35]

Another potential major complication is heparin-associated thrombocytopenia (HAT; heparin-induced thrombocytopenia, HIT).[36–38] While historically thrombocytopenia was common and related to the questionable purity of heparin preparations, a reported incidence of 0–30% remains. The usual platelet response to bolus heparin administration is modest hypotension and transient reversible platelet aggregate formation.[39] HAT does rarely occur catastrophically with bolus administration, causing copious large platelet aggregates that clog the pulmonary and peripheral circulation with massive release of the compounds listed in Table 10.1. With aggressive resuscitation, these largely reversible aggregates do dissipate and the patient may survive. Another pattern of platelet response is the "white clot syndrome," in which irreversible platelet aggregation produces a platelet-rich thrombus and thrombocytopenia. In addition, heparin antibodies may also interact with heparin-like molecules on the endothelial surface, thus injuring the endothelium and further increasing the risk of thrombosis. Clinical manifestations can include skin necrosis, gangrene of the extremities, myocardial infarction, pulmonary embolism, and stroke. The least severe platelet response is thrombocytopenia (less than 100 000 μL^{-1}) without thrombosis. All forms of HAT require immediate discontinuation of heparin and its future avoidance.

In contrast with SH, low-molecular-weight heparin (LMWH) molecular size is reduced, e.g. for enoxaparin to 2000–8000 Da with an average of 4500 Da. LMWHs are prepared from SH by fractionation, enzymatic degradation, or chemical modification, but are still heterogeneous and differ somewhat in biologic properties from product to product.[40,41] Internationally, there are approximately a dozen LMWH commercial products, with four approved in the USA: enoxaparin, ardeparin, dalteparin, and tinzaparin. Subcutaneous absorption of LMWH is nearly complete; consequently, only one injection per day is usually required rather than two for SH.

The aPTT, thrombin clotting time, and ACT cannot be used to monitor LMWH antithrombotic effect because of their low anti-factor IIa activity; however, prolongation would signify a high likelihood of bleeding. Unfortunately, the converse – an aPTT, thrombin clotting time,

Table 10.3 *Recommendations for neuraxial anesthesia and anticoagulation (modified from the 1998 and 2002 American Society of Regional Anesthesia Consensus Statements)*

Standard heparin[34]

1 Subcutaneous SH (mini-dose) prophylaxis is not a contraindication to NAB. Delay SH until after NAB. After 4 days of SH, confirm that HIT has not occurred
2 Intraoperative SH for vascular surgery with NAB considerations:
 a Avoid if other coagulopathies present
 b Delay SH for 1 h after NAB performed
 c Remove catheter 1 h before dose and 2–4 h after dose
 d Use minimal local anesthetics postoperatively in order to monitor motor function
 e Blood in the needle or difficult needle placement does not mandate cancellation
3 When full anticoagulation for cardiac surgery is done after NAB, there should be early postoperative confirmation and monitoring of sensory and motor function
4 Avoid NAB with a protracted therapeutic SH infusion or if other anticoagulants or fibrinolytics are combined with SH. If systemic SH is begun with an epidural in place, delay catheter removal for 2–4 h following discontinuation and measure an aPTT
5 Neuraxial bleeding risk is increased by concurrent SH and antiplatelet agents, LMWH, or oral anticoagulants

Low-molecular-weight heparin[43]

1 Monitoring anti-factor Xa level is not predictive of bleeding and unnecessary
2 Concurrent SH, oral anticoagulants, or platelet inhibitors increase the risk of neuraxial bleeding
3 Blood in the needle or catheter does not necessitate postponement; however, LMWH initial dosage should not be given for 24 h
4 If LMWH given preoperatively, single-dose spinal safest NAB. Perform NAB 10–24 h after LMWH dose depending on agent and dosage. Avoid NAB, if LMWH given 2 h preoperatively
5 For postoperative LMWH thromboprophylaxis when NAB used: initiate LMWH 24 h postoperatively, 2 h after catheter removal

Oral anticoagulants[56]

1 Discontinue chronic oral anticoagulants and measure INR prior to NAB
2 Concurrent SH, LMWH, or platelet inhibitors increase the risk of neuraxial bleeding
3 Preoperative initiation of warfarin: if the initial dose was more than 24 h earlier or the second dose was given, check the INR before NAB
4 Patients receiving low dose warfarin (approximately 5 mg day^{-1}) for more than 36 h and epidural analgesia should have their INR monitored daily and before catheter removal
5 Remove neuraxial catheters when the INR < 1.5
6 Repeat testing of sensory and motor function in patients receiving warfarin during epidural analgesia. The analgesic solution should minimize sensory and motor block. Continue neurologic testing after catheter removal for 24 h or longer if the INR > 1.5 when the catheter was removed
7 If a neuraxial catheter is present, withhold or reduce warfarin if INR > 3

Platelet inhibitors[57]

1 No specific platelet function test is suggested. Medical history recommended
2 NSAIDs alone and NAB are compatible
3 The effects of more potent platelet inhibitors, e.g. ticlopidine, clopidogrel, and GP IIb/IIIa inhibitors, should be allowed to dissipate before NAB
4 Concurrent use with SH, LMWH, or oral anticoagulants may increase the risk of neuraxial bleeding

Fibrinolytics[67]

1 Patient evaluation before NAB must determine if the patient did receive or will receive fibrinolytics
2 NAB should not be performed after fibrinolytics except in highly unusual circumstances
3 When SH or platelet inhibitors are used with fibrinolytics the risk of neuraxial bleeding from NAB is potentiated
4 If NAB does occur near fibrinolytic administration, perform neurologic monitoring at least each 2 h. If a catheter is placed, analgesic infusions should minimize sensory and motor blockade
5 Confirm adequate fibrinogen and low FDP levels for neuraxial catheter removal after fibrinolytics

SH, standard heparin; NAB, neuraxial block; HIT, heparin-induced thrombocytopenia; aPTT, activated partial thromboplastin time; LMWH, low-molecular-weight heparin; NSAIDs, nonsteroidal anti-inflammatory drugs; INR, international normalized ratio; FDP, fibrin and fibrinogen degradation products.

and ACT measurement within the normal range – does not guarantee that there will be no bleeding. Anti-factor Xa assays can verify effect. Because of the less complicated, dose-independent clearance and more predictable anticoagulant response than SH, laboratory monitoring is generally not required to a establish a therapeutic antithrombotic effect.

LMWH has a higher anti-factor Xa activity and lower anti-factor IIa activity than SH, which is generally believed to mean greater antithrombotic activity and lower anticoagulant activity. For example, if the ratio of anti-factor Xa to anti-factor IIa activity for SH is defined as 1:1, then for enoxaparin the ratio is 3.35:1. This ratio and, therefore, dosage regimens are unique to each LMWH product. At one time, the lower anti-factor IIa activity of LMWH was thought to directly correlate with less clinical bleeding, but such a concept was too simplistic. LMWH does have a lesser effect on platelet function and a reduced incidence of HAT compared with SH. Fondaparinux is a synthetic and specific inhibitor of factor Xa used for thromboprophylaxis by sc. administration in hip and knee replacement surgery that does not have anti-factor IIa or platelet effects. Its sustained antithrombotic effect, early postoperative dosing requirement, and lack of antagonists suggest extreme caution with respect to use with neuraxial anesthesia.

The compatibility of LMWH heparin with regional anesthesia has been of great concern to anesthesiologists. In a retrospective review, Bergqvist *et al.*[42] found that 9013 patients in reported controlled studies of LMWH efficacy had epidural or spinal anesthesia without difficulty. They estimated that by 1992 over 1 million patients had experienced the combination of LMWH and regional anesthesia without apparent neurologic sequelae. Unfortunately, the US experience was not as good, and by 1997 the manufacturer of enoxaparin warned that concurrent use of indwelling epidural catheters and enoxaparin was not safe (Table 10.3).[43]

Although several approaches to the management of cardiopulmonary bypass (CPB) without heparin have been developed, all are associated with an increased risk of thrombosis during CPB, a greater use of blood products, and a less rapid return to normal hemostasis after CPB.[37,38] If an allergy to heparin without thrombocytopenia or to chlorocresal – a preservative often used in heparin formulation – is present, heparin of a different biologic source, heparin free of chlorocresal, and pharmacologic immune prophylaxis with methylprednisolone and histamine blockers may be all that is required. However, if HAT is strongly suspected or has been confirmed in the laboratory, management of CPB with a heparin substitute or with its platelet-aggregating effect inhibited are logical approaches. Heparin with iloprost, an analog of the more potent platelet inhibitor prostaglandin I_2, has been used successfully.[44] Another prostaglandin, PGE_1, has also been used successfully with heparin and aspirin; however, hypotension and profound vasodilation were present.[45] Attempted use of LMWH compounds for CPB have often been associated with thrombosis, excessive bleeding, difficult dosing, and slow reversal.

If heparin is to be completely avoided, heparin-coated catheters and CPB circuit components, pressure line flush solutions, and heparinized flush solutions on the surgical field should all be eliminated. In addition, a large surface area oxygenator with differential pressure monitoring can warn of early fibrin deposition without sudden oxygenator failure. The development of synthetic direct-acting thrombin inhibitors, such as argatroban, may simplify CPB without heparin; until these are available, ancrod, danaparoid, or recombinant hirudin may be used.

Ancrod is a protease that removes fibrinopeptide A from fibrinogen, thus resulting in end-to-end linkage rather than cross-linkage during fibrin polymerization. The resulting friable material is rapidly removed from the circulation, thus permitting CPB to proceed successfully. Reduction in circulating fibrinogen to less than 50 mg dL^{-1} prior to CPB is achieved by an infusion of 1.6 U kg^{-1} over 12–24 h preoperatively.[46,47] The ACT will remain normal initially because even the friable "fibrin" can trigger the ACT endpoint. However, during CPB, fibrinolytic activity increases markedly, thus promoting the rapid clearance of any insoluble fibrin and also prolonging the ACT. Continuous monitoring of fibrinogen provides assurance that clotting will be prevented. Ancrod is generally not required intraoperatively because the low concentration of fibrinogen is not rapidly normalized in the absence of transfusion and is further diluted during CPB. At the end of CPB, cryoprecipitate administration will elevate fibrinogen to normal levels and fibrin formation will return.

Danaparoid[48] is a low molecular weight heparinoid derived from pork mucosa that consists of a combination of heparan sulfate, dermatan sulfate, and chondroitin sulfate. The ratio of anti-factor Xa to anti-factor IIa activity for danaparoid is greater than 22:1, and it has minimal platelet effects. ACT and aPTT are not effective monitoring assays. For CPB, the measurement of anti-factor Xa levels will indicate adequate dosing if a 1.5–2 U mL^{-1} range is achieved. Currently, a regimen of 3 U mL^{-1} in the CPB prime and an initial dose of 125 U kg^{-1} prior to initiating CPB is recommended. If the CPB period will exceed 1 h, 7 U kg^{-1} h^{-1} is infused and discontinued 45 min before terminating CPB. Because the elimination half-life is greater than 24 h and it is mainly eliminated by the kidneys, normalization of hemostasis is often slow. Protamine has minimal effect; however, residual danaparoid elimination by plasmapheresis can be effective.[49]

Recombinant hirudin (e.g. lepirudin) is a genetically engineered polypeptide derived from leech anticoagulant that is a highly specific direct inhibitor of thrombin. For CPB, a 0.25 mg kg^{-1} i.v. bolus prior to CPB followed by a 0.15 mg kg^{-1} h^{-1} infusion has been used with a 0.2 mg kg^{-1} dose in the CPB prime.[50,51] An aPTT of greater than 100 s has been associated with marginal anticoagulation, but an aPTT greater than 200 s appears to be adequate. Potzsch *et al.*[52] recommend a whole blood ecarin clotting time owing to its greater linearity with respect to r-hirudin blood levels. There is no antagonist to r-hirudin; however, the 30- to 60-min elimination half-life permits early normalization in patients with normal renal function.

Coumarin derivatives

Unlike heparin, coumarins (dicumarol and warfarin) and indandiones (anisindione) are not direct-acting anticoagulants because, when added to native whole blood, the blood will still clot. Their action is indirect because their oral administration interferes with the hepatic synthesis of vitamin K-dependent clotting factors, resulting in an *in vivo* depletion of clotting factors VII, IX, X, and II. The coumarin derivatives are indicated for prophylaxis and treatment of thrombosis in thrombophlebitis, atrial fibrillation, pulmonary embolization, acute myocardial infarction, mechanical prosthetic valves, and valvular heart disease.

Although oral absorption is rapid and complete, activity is more related to the kinetics of the vitamin K-dependent clotting factors. Altered nutritional intake, diarrhea, gastrointestinal motility, malabsorption, or hepatic dysfunction may substantially change vitamin K clotting factor synthesis. Also, since oral anticoagulants are highly plasma bound, other drugs may displace them from binding sites, thus altering activity. This high degree of pharmacodynamic variability requires individualized dosing and adjustment using prothrombin time.[53] When the INR is within the therapeutic range, hemorrhage may still occur.

The anesthesiologist's major concern for patients receiving coumarin derivatives preoperatively is how to readjust therapy sufficiently that hemorrhage is prevented. The site(s) of potential bleeding, the absence of concurrent hemostatic deficiencies, and the current INR must be considered. For minor surgery, an INR at the low end of the therapeutic range would be acceptable if combined with local measures for hemostasis. For example, dental extraction may require no readjustment because local hemostatic measures are particularly effective. For moderately extensive surgery, a reduced therapeutic level may be considered.[54] For example, the therapeutic range for tissue heart valve embolic prophylaxis is for the INR to be between 2 and 3; this may be reduced to 1.5 or 1.6 for the procedure. Appreciate that changes in perioperative nutritional intake, malabsorption, hepatic function, or drug administrations may substantially alter the INR. For major surgery, coumarin derivatives are usually discontinued, allowing the INR to normalize and s.c. or i.v. heparin is started.[55] During the operative procedure, the heparin is stopped or antagonized and restarted postoperatively as soon as the surgeon believes that bleeding is unlikely. Rapid correction of the INR with vitamin K or FFP administration is rarely required and may complicate the smooth resumption of anticoagulation with oral agents after surgery. For regional anesthesia with neuraxial block in patients receiving coumarin derivatives chronically, the INR should be normalized (Table 10.3).[56] A greater problem is the use of coumarin derivatives for prophylaxis against postoperative venous thrombosis and the use of neuraxial catheters for postoperative pain control (Table 10.3).[56]

Platelet inhibitors

Thrombi in the veins consist mainly of fibrin and red cells, whereas arterial thrombi are mainly composed of aggregated platelets. Theoretically, platelet inhibitors should be more effective at reducing the risk of arterial thrombi in patients. Dextran and low-potency oral platelet inhibitors such as aspirin, dipyridamole, and, historically, sulfinpyrazone made up the limited clinical armamentarium prior to 1990. The oral agents ticlopidine, clopidogrel, and cilostazol were incorporated into clinical use as potent specific antiplatelet agents in the 1990s. Parenteral infusions of extremely potent platelet GPIIb/IIIa blockers abciximab, eptifibatide, and tirofiban became available in the late 1990s.

Even with adequate numbers of platelets, the platelet inhibitors may leave patients vulnerable not only to excessive blood loss at the time of surgery but also to major surgical complications and morbidity. Preoperative signs of platelet inhibition include petechiae in the extremities; ecchymoses from minimal injury; episodes of epistaxis, hematuria, conjuctival hemorrhages, and gastrointestinal bleeding; and excessive bleeding after minor trauma or surgery. Many drugs used in the perioperative period – such as calcium channel blockers, local anesthetics, some antibiotics, and drugs that modulate nitric oxide – have inhibitory effects. Platelet-inhibiting drugs may have an additive or even synergistic effect on bleeding in the surgical patient. Neuraxial regional anesthesia in the presence of aspirin and NSAIDs does not appear to be a major problem (Table 10.3).[57] Data on the new oral agents and the GPIIb/IIIa inhibitors are insufficient to permit the cavalier use of neuraxial blockade in the presence of these drugs.

Dextrans are highly linear glucose polymers that are fractionated by molecular weight to obtain a narrow distribution of molecular weights. The two commonly used solutions are 10 g dL^{-1} dextran 40 and 6 g dL^{-1} dextran 70, which are 40 000 Da, i.e. low molecular weight, and 70 000 Da, i.e. high molecular weight, respectively. Dextran 40 infusion is used both for volume expansion and for prophylaxis of deep vein thrombosis, pulmonary emboli, and premature closure of recent arterial anastomoses. Dextran 70 is used as a volume expansion solution. Dextran dosages greater than 15 mg kg^{-1} may prolong bleeding time in patients with normal hemostasis. The decreased aggregation and adhesion of platelets results in attenuated platelet effectiveness. A blood clot formed in the presence of dextran has greater porosity and fewer, but thicker, fibrin strands, making it more susceptible to lysis. Dextran may also interfere with procedures for blood typing and cross-matching.

Severe anaphylactoid reactions, which are more frequent with dextran 70 than with dextran 40, have been a major concern with dextran use, even in the absence of prior exposure to dextrans. Prophylaxis is now possible by administration of 0.3 mL kg^{-1} of 15 g dL^{-1} dextran 1 within 15 min of beginning dextran infusion. Dextran 1 functions as a monovalent hapten binding to only one of the two available sites on dextran-reacting immunoglobulins, thus preventing the bridge formation required for the large immune complexes which trigger anaphylactoid reactions.

Aspirin is the most commonly used medicinal agent because of its effective analgesic, antipyretic, anti-inflammatory, and, more recently appreciated, antiplatelet properties. The antihemostatic action of aspirin is largely due to acetylation of cyclo-oxygenase (COX),[58] a trait not shared by salicylates. It is approximately 150- to 200-fold more potent an inhibitor of the COX-1 antithrombotic isoform than the COX-2 anti-inflammatory isoform. Even at very low aspirin dosages, the COX inhibition in platelets is irreversible because platelets cannot resynthesize cyclo-oxygenase. Platelet thromboxane A_2, a potent platelet aggregatory compound, can no longer be produced by COX metabolism of arachidonic acid. In the vascular endothelial cell, the synthesis of prostaglandin I_2, a potent antiaggregatory platelet inhibitor and also a product of COX acting on arachidonic acid, is blocked. However, it is resynthesized in the endothelial cell within a few hours. This shift in the thromboxane–prostaglandin I_2 balance results in prolongation of the bleeding time by 1.5–3 times, even at low aspirin dosages. At very high aspirin dosages, the continuing acetylation of COX in the endothelial cells may mitigate the increase in bleeding time by aspirin.

Occasional aspirin users rarely have bleeding problems, because noncyclo-oxygenase-dependent pathways in the platelet are unaffected by aspirin. For example, any substantial production of thrombin during clotting will immediately precipitate a full platelet response. However, the modulation of platelet function by aspirin in the presence of other hemostatic deficiencies may be clinically synergistic and potentiate the other defects. To be completely free of the effects of aspirin before surgery, the entire population of platelets would need to be replaced, which is normally a 10-day cycle. If normal platelet production is assumed and the aspirin exposure of megakaryocytes is appreciated, then a minimum of 3–5 days would be required to produce adequate numbers of platelets with COX capability.

Dipyridamole, originally introduced as a vasodilator, is administered orally often in combination with aspirin as an antiplatelet aggregatory agent. It inhibits platelet phosphodiesterase, thus building up platelet cytoplasmic cAMP and decreasing cytoplasmic Ca^{2+}. It also inhibits the red blood cell uptake of adenosine, an inhibitor of platelet reactivity, and inhibits the formation of thromboxane A_2 by blocking thromboxane synthetase. Also, prostaglandin I_2 released by the endothelium may be increased by dipyridamole. Alone, it minimally alters bleeding time, but does act synergistically with aspirin and other anticoagulants to significantly prolong bleeding time. Recovery of normal platelet function is rapid once dipyridamole is discontinued.

NSAIDs (Table 10.4), except aspirin and COX-2-specific drugs, reversibly attenuate platelet function by inhibition of COX-1 while the active drug is present. Although NSAIDs generally have mixed and variable COX-1 and COX-2 inhibitory capability, the maintenance of normal hemostasis is predominantly a COX-1 function. The NSAID COX-1 hemostatic defect is usually subclinical except in the presence of other hemostatic defects, such as oral anticoagulants, or during clinical hemostatic challenges, such as surgery. NSAIDs with half-lives greater than 6 h – etodolac, sulindac, naproxen, nabumetone, piroxicam, and oxaprozin – are associated with increased blood loss after total hip arthrodesis and should be discontinued five half-lives before the procedure.[59] Parenteral ketorolac for analgesia after tonsillectomy has been associated with a 70% increase in blood loss intraoperatively,[60] and an increase in the incidence of postoperative bleeding from 3–4% without ketorolac to 14–17% when it is administered.[60,61] Ketorolac has also been associated with a case of spinal hematoma after spinal anesthesia.[62] In

Table 10.4 *Nonsteroidal anti-inflammatory drugs (NSAIDs)*

	Generic name	Half-life (h)	Trade name
Salicylates	Aspirin	2–20	Acuprin, Anacin, Aspergum, Aspirtab, Empirin, Ecotrin, and many others
	Buffered aspirin	2–10	Ascriptin, Bufferin, Buffex, Buffinol
	Choline salicylate	4–16	Arthropan
	Choline magnesium salicylate	9–17	Tricosal, Trisilate
	Diflunisal	8–12	Dolobid
	Magnesium salicylate	4–16	Doan's tablets, Magan, Mobidin
	Salsalate	3–16	Salflex, Disalcid
Nonsalicylates	Diclofenac	2	Arthrotec, Cataflam, Voltaren
	Etodolac	7–8	Lodine
	Fenoprofen	3	Nalfon
	Flurbiprofen	6	Ansaid
	Ibuprofen	2	Advil, Motrin, Nuprin, Rufen
	Indomethacin	5	Indocin
	Ketoprofen	3	Actron, Orudis, Oruvail
	Ketorolac	2	Toradol
	Meclofenamate	2	Meclomen
	Mefenamic acid	2–4	Ponstel
	Nabumetone	24	Relafen
	Naproxen	13–15	Aleve, Anaprox, Naprelan, Naprosyn
	Oxaprozin	45	Daypro
	Piroxicam	50	Feldene
	Sulindac	8	Clinoril
	Tolmetin	3	Tolectin
Cyclo-oxygenase 2 (COX-2)-specific nonsalicylates	Celecoxib	11	Celebrex
	Meloxicam	15–20	Mobic
	Rofecoxib	10	Vioxx
	Valdecoxib	8–11	Bextra

the usual therapeutic dose regimens, COX-2-specific inhibitors have no significant effect on bleeding time or platelet aggregation.

Ticlopidine and clopidogrel are potent oral antiplatelet agents that both cause irreversible blockade of ADP-induced platelet–fibrinogen binding and resulting platelet aggregation. Ticlopidine should be discontinued 12–14 days prior to surgery and clopidogrel 7 days prior to surgery because both drugs significantly prolong bleeding time. Clopidogrel has now largely replaced ticlopidine because ticlopidine has been associated with thrombotic thrombocytopenic purpura, neutropenia, and agranulocytosis. Clopidogrel is commonly used after coronary artery stent insertion.

Cilostazol is a phosphodiesterase III inhibitor approved for the treatment of claudication. It increases platelet cytoplasmic cAMP, thus inhibiting platelet aggregation, and causes peripheral vasodilation and increased heart rate. A reduced survival rate of patients with class III–IV congestive heart failure has been noted with cilostazol. Discontinuation is not associated with rebound ischemia and platelet function can be normalized within a day.

Parenteral platelet GPIIb/IIIa receptor inhibitors are the most potent platelet inhibitors currently available. They are infused in the acute coronary syndromes of unstable angina and non-Q-wave myocardial infarction and in patients undergoing percutaneous coronary angioplasty. Patients with these conditions may suddenly require surgery for an emergency CABG. GPIIb/IIIa inhibitors prevent the binding of fibrinogen and vWF to the platelet, thereby blocking aggregation. The blockade is reversible following discontinuation of the GPIIb/IIIa inhibitor infusion. Tirofiban has a 2-h elimination half-life and eptifibatide a 2.5-h half-life; however, both clearances are reduced in renal insufficiency. The oldest GPIIb/IIIa inhibitor, abciximab, will block platelet aggregation for 24–48 h after discontinuation, but to some degree may be present on platelets for up to 10 days. Tirofiban and eptifibatide will be substantially eliminated by the end of CPB, if infusion is discontinued as soon as surgery is decided upon. The persistence of abciximab is a much greater problem that required platelet transfusions in 52% of patients (placebo 32%) and surgical re-exploration for bleeding in 12% of patients (placebo 3%) in one series.[63] Scrupulous heparin management, multiple platelet transfusions, and a low threshold for surgical re-exploration are usually required for these patients. Neuraxial blockade should not be performed until the GPIIb/IIIa block has dissipated.

Fibrinolytics

Patients will occasionally require urgent or emergent surgery after treatment with the plasminogen activators because of the acceptance of thrombolytic therapy for treating acute coronary thrombosis and its expanding indications for other conditions. The major hemostatic problems that follow thrombolytic therapy are not related to residual activators because they are eliminated within minutes or hours. Circulating antiplasmins rapidly block fibrinolysis once the activator is no longer administered. Anistreplase, streptokinase, urokinase, reteplase, and alteplase have elimination half-lives of 100, 83, 20, 15, and 2–3 min respectively. Local infusions of these plasminogen activators also have major systemic effects and should not be underestimated.

The major source of hemostatic difficulty is defective fibrin polymerization because of the presence of FDPs. FDPs can continue to be a problem for 24 h after termination of activator administration because of their very high levels after induced thrombolysis, even though their elimination half-life is approximately 3 h. Their interaction can terminate the developing fibrin polymer, yielding a mechanically defective fibrin mesh composed of a few large-diameter broken strands rather than a tight mesh of abundant fine strands.[64] Platelet aggregation suppression by FDPs and some reduction in concentrations of fibrinogen, factor V, and factor VIII also contribute to impaired hemostasis. The plasminogen that is most effective in clot dissolution is that which is present within the fibrin matrix during clot formation. Clots formed during periods of low circulating plasminogen are very resistant to subsequent thrombolysis, such as during thrombolytic therapy when plasminogen is rapidly consumed. Therefore, post-thrombolysis heparin is a component of most thrombolytic regimens.

The prevention of intraoperative hemorrhage after thrombolysis will be aided by even a modest delay in the start of the surgical procedure. If residual anistreplase or streptokinase effect is still likely, aminocaproic acid or aprotinin can be used to antagonize active fibrinolysis. Although Hill *et al.*[65] reported more bleeding in their emergency myocardial revascularization group than in their elective surgery group, they observed no difference in the bleeding tendency of the five patients who received aminocaproic acid after treatment with streptokinase and the 10 who did not. After the activator is eliminated, procoagulant replacement using FFP and cryoprecipitate may be started. Mantia *et al.*[66] did note a greater need for FFP and cryoprecipitate in their streptokinase-treated CABG patients, although blood loss and red cell concentrate transfusion were not different. Neuraxial blockade is best avoided immediately after thrombolytic therapy (Table 10.3).[67]

Several patient care considerations after thrombolysis can reduce morbidity. The electrocardiogram should be monitored diligently for reperfusion arrhythmias. Coughing and Valsalva maneuvers and arterial hypertension should be avoided. Intramuscular injections should not be used and the patient should be padded thoroughly. Arterial and venous blood sampling should be carried out through indwelling catheters. Diagnostic arterial puncture sites may also be used for monitoring and sampling. Lower extremity blood pressure cuffs may embolize dissolving clots.

Prohemostatic pharmaceuticals

Vitamin K

Phytonadione, vitamin K_1, is indicated for the restoration of vitamin K-dependent hepatic factors II, VII, IX, and X.[68,69] Clinical conditions include the treatment of coumarin anticoagulant-induced prothrombin deficiency, hypoprothrombinemia due to antibiotics or salicylates, hypoprothrombinemia due to insufficient absorption or synthesis of vitamin K, and prophylaxis or therapy of hemorrhagic disease of the newborn. When extensive hepatocellular destruction is responsible for hypoprothrombinemia, vitamin K therapy will not be effective but is often attempted. Adults with anticoagulant-induced prothrombin deficiency should receive 2.5–10 mg orally or parenterally; however, up to 50 mg i.v. may be required for a severe deficiency. The INR will show detectable improvement within 1–2 h of parenteral administration and significant reduction within 12–14 h. The prophylactic dosage in newborns is 0.5–1.0 mg i.m. within 1 h of birth or 25 µg orally daily; however, excessive dosages have been associated with hemolysis, hyperbilirubinemia, and kernicterus in premature infants. For the treatment of bleeding or preoperative preparation in the neonate, 1.0 mg i.m. or s.c. is required. Failure of a newborn to respond may suggest the presence of another congenital hemostatic deficit.

Phytonadione can be used in tablet form or as a parenteral solution. Hypersensitivity reactions, including anaphylaxis, may occur without prior exposure, therefore oral administration is preferred if time permits and biliary obstruction is not present. If parenteral administration is necessary, s.c. or i.m. injection is preferred. When administration is i.v., the infusion rate should be less than 1 mg min^{-1}, but severe reactions may still occur. Since potential thrombotic complications may occur during the temporary period of resistance to the reinstitution of coumarin drugs, prophylactic low-dose heparinization may be required until a therapeutic INR is re-established.

Heparin antagonists

Protamine sulfate is a polycationic protein that is infused to antagonize excess circulating heparin at the completion of cardiovascular diagnostic and surgical procedures.[70] Protamine can remove polyanionic heparin from the heparin–antithrombin III complex, thus returning the antithrombin III to its basal activity and permitting fibrin formation. The action of protamine is immediate, and unbound protamine is rapidly cleared from the circulation by nonspecific binding and by rapid renal excretion. Occasionally, evidence of the heparin effect recurs 30 min to 18 h after initial protamine administration. This "heparin rebound" can be treated with additional protamine doses. The efficacy of protamine for reversal of heparin is dependent on the type of heparin used: 1 mg reverses 90 units of lung tissue heparin and 115 units of intestinal mucosa heparin.

Severe hypersensitivity reactions to protamine, including anaphylaxis, do occur. Most reports of allergic reactions to protamine do not implicate prior protamine exposure as a causative factor.[71] However, exposure to protamine also occurs through the use of NPH insulin (isophane or protamine zinc insulin), and diabetic patients receiving daily s.c. injections of insulin-containing protamine do have a 40- to 50-fold greater risk of severe reactions to i.v. protamine.[72,73]

Although with the rapid administration of protamine sulfate (over less than 3 min) a transient decrease in mean arterial pressure occurs, the usual hemodynamic response to protamine sulfate is not remarkable.[15] However, severe hypotension in patients can occasionally occur and lead to considerable clinical difficulty. This unusual hemodynamic response may be due to predisposing unfavorable hemodynamic conditions or to factors evident in only a few patients. In a study of vascular surgery patients receiving 0.5 mg kg^{-1} min^{-1} protamine sulfate, five cases of severe hypotension, 24 torr or greater reduction in mean arterial pressure, occurred in 24 patients, three of whom required vasopressor treatment. This high incidence in patients who received much lower doses of protamine than given after CPB may suggest a greater sensitivity in patients undergoing noncardiac vascular surgery procedures or a reduced sensitivity in patients after CPB.

Transient thrombocytopenia and leukopenia are common consequences of protamine administration. Protamine sulfate has been shown to aggregate human platelets *in vitro*. *In vivo*, severe protamine-induced pulmonary platelet sequestration occurs in animals; however, in humans, hepatic not pulmonary sequestration of platelets labeled with indium-111 occurred.[74] The degree of reversibility and clinical significance of the protamine-induced platelet aggregates is not known. When a severe protamine reaction occurs, the pulmonary responses are compatible with transient pulmonary vascular vasoconstriction and obstruction of the pulmonary circulation. Pulmonary artery pressures may increase. The airway pressure increases, compliance decreases, the dead space to tidal volume ratio increases, and arterial Po_2 decreases.[75]

Protamine itself does have anticoagulant activity, but excess protamine does not have a clinically important effect on the procoagulant cascade. However, protamine does unfavorably alter platelet function by binding to heparin, which in turn binds to the platelet surface.[76] Clinically, administration of the lowest adequate level to antagonize circulating heparin is beneficial.[77] When protamine is to be administered, using the ACT allows the circulating level to be estimated and an appropriate protamine dose to be calculated.[16]

Alternatives to the administration of protamine that are not clinically available include polybrene, heparinase, platelet factor IV, and membrane-bound heparin chelators or inactivators. Of course, not antagonizing the heparin at all is possible, but requires meticulous surgical technique, blood product conservation methods, and patience.

Fibrinolytic inhibitors

Aminocaproic acid

Aminocaproic acid (ε-aminocaproic acid, EACA) inhibits fibrinolysis by inhibition of plasminogen activators and, to a lesser extent, by direct antiplasmin activity. For primary fibrinolysis, an initial adult loading dose of 5 g i.v. is followed by 1–1.25 g h^{-1}, but not to exceed 30 g in 24 h. Dosage reduction is required if urine output cannot be maintained because most of the drug is recovered unmetabolized in the urine. Surgery of the lower genitourinary tract, particularly of the prostate, has been associated with primary fibrinolysis successfully treated with aminocaproic acid. Aminocaproic acid administration to patients with secondary fibrinolysis, such as with DIC, can result in indiscriminate thrombus formation in capillary beds, causing microinfarcts, and in major vessels, causing organ ischemia and potentially a fatal outcome. However, its administration in DIC with concurrent heparin treatment may be appropriate.

During oral surgery in hemophilia A patients, aminocaproic acid has been used in addition to factor VIII replacement therapy to prevent the ongoing local fibrinolysis and fibrin replacement that occurs during clot development, thereby enhancing the efficacy of the replacement therapy. Survival of transfused factor VIII in hemophilic patients is increased[78] and factor VIII inhibitor activity is reduced.[79]

During cardiothoracic surgery, sternal splitting and cardiopulmonary bypass have been associated with enhanced fibrinolytic activity. Although a reduction in postcardiopulmonary bypass blood loss by aminocaproic acid was demonstrated more than 25 years ago,[80] a recent resurgence of interest and use has occurred owing to the efficacy, but at great expense, of aprotinin. A meta-analysis comparing aminocaproic acid and aprotinin[81] in cardiac surgery suggests that total blood loss, postoperative transfusions, and the number of patients requiring transfusion are reduced substantially and similarly. Neither drug increased the risk of postoperative myocardial infarction or overall mortality. Based on pharmacokinetic analysis, Butterworth *et al.*[82] recommended a loading infusion of 50 mg kg^{-1} over 20 min followed by a maintenance infusion of 25 mg kg^{-1} h^{-1} to maintain a stable blood level; however, renal insufficiency requires a significant reduction. Administration for excessive postoperative chest tube drainage, during extracorporeal membrane oxygenation, and to offset increased bleeding associated with aspirin ingestion before cardiac surgery have also been advocated.

In liver transplantation, during the final stages of excision of the failing liver and during the anhepatic period, fibrinolysis due to the accumulation of endogenous tPA may cause problematic bleeding.[83] As little as 1–2 g of aminocaproic acid may attenuate bleeding and correct fibrinolysis evident on the thrombelastograph. Large doses and the continuing inhibition of fibrinolysis after the new hepatic graft is perfused may leave the patient vulnerable to portal vein or hepatic artery thrombosis.

Tranexamic acid

Tranexamic acid is a synthetic amino acid that is a competitive inhibitor of plasminogen activation and, at high concentrations, an inhibitor of plasmin. It is much more potent than aminocaproic acid and has a terminal half-life of approximately 2 h. To prevent hypotension, i.v. infusion should not exceed 100 mg min^{-1}. Because tranexamic acid is filtered by the glomerulus and excreted in the urine 95% unchanged, a dosage reduction is required for patients with renal insufficiency.

Tranexamic acid has an efficacy comparable with aprotinin in reducing postoperative bleeding and perioperative transfusion for cardiac surgery, but at a fraction of the cost.[84–86] Dosage recommendations vary; however, in a dose–response study,[87] a loading dose of 10 mg kg^{-1} and a maintenance infusion of 1 mg kg^{-1} h^{-1} was recommended. Higher dosage regimens (10-fold greater loading dose) and regimens including tranexamic acid in the CPB pump prime have been used. Tranexamic acid has not been implicated in increasing the risk of postoperative myocardial infarction or overall thrombotic problems. Administration for excessive postoperative chest tube drainage, to offset increased bleeding associated with preoperative aspirin ingestion, and topically into the pericardial cavity have also been proposed.

Other off-label applications of tranexamic acid have been shown to reduce operative blood loss. In liver transplantation, an advantage over aminocaproic acid for reducing blood transfusion was observed.[88] In orthopedic surgery, blood loss may be reduced for both total knee and total hip arthrodesis; however, the severe thrombotic risks associated with these procedures and the relatively limited amount of blood loss involved suggest that it should be reserved for orthopedic cases with special hemostatic problems.

Aprotinin

Aprotinin is a polypeptide proteinase inhibitor isolated from bovine lung that can inhibit human trypsin, plasmin, kallikrein, and other proteinases. Kallikrein inhibition – the interaction of aprotinin with the intrinsic coagulation pathway – requires about four times the dose that is required for plasmin inhibition. Aprotinin is indicated for prophylactic use to reduce perioperative blood loss and blood transfusion in patients undergoing CPB for repeat CABG surgery. Use in primary CABG surgery should be reserved for high bleeding risk cases such as severe haemostatic defects and when transfusion is unacceptable or suitable blood products are unavailable. The incidence of acute hypersensitivity is less than 0.5%, if no prior exposure has occurred. However, repeated use in multiple cardiopulmonary bypass procedures may result in a much higher incidence of hypersensitivity reactions.

A high-dose and a low-dose regimen have been used, each consisting of a loading dose, a maintenance infusion, and a pump prime dose. With both adult regimens, a 1.4-mg (10 000 kallikrein inhibitor units, KIU) test dose is infused i.v. into a central line 10 min before the loading dose. The loading dose of 280 mg or 140 mg is infused over 20–30 min prior to sternotomy. The same amount is added to the pump prime fluid. The maintenance infusion of 70 mg h^{-1} or 35 mg h^{-1} is continued until surgery is complete. No significant benefit of one regimen over the other has consistently been shown with respect to postoperative blood loss or transfusion requirements.[89]

Plasmin has also been implicated as one of the causes of platelet dysfunction after cardiopulmonary bypass. The vWF and fibrinogen receptors are both damaged by plasmin proteolysis, resulting in impaired platelet adhesion and aggregation respectively. Aprotinin protects platelets during CPB, preserves their number, and shortens postoperative bleeding times. Preservation of platelet function may also be indirectly aided by prevention of the dysfunction caused by fibrinolysis and the kallikrein system activation of complement and neutrophils. Both the intrinsic cascade system and platelets are protected from contact activation in the aprotinin-treated patient.

The effectiveness of aprotinin in reducing blood loss and transfusion requirements in surgery requiring CPB is well established.[90] The high-dose regimen is more effective in reducing postoperative blood loss than either aminocaproic acid or desmopressin, but in some studies it is similar to tranexamic acid. The low-dose regimen reduces postoperative blood loss in a similar manner to aminocaproic acid and tranexamic acid. The effectiveness of aprotinin in pediatric patients is less impressive.[91] Also, the use of aprotinin in congenital heart disease may be limited because of renal toxicity in patients with prior renal damage and thrombosis resulting from the combination of polycythemia and the prothrombotic tendency of aprotinin. Intraoperative use of aprotinin in adult patients undergoing liver transplantation significantly reduced blood-transfusion requirements without increasing thromboembolic events.[92]

Blocking the fibrinolytic system with aprotinin could put new coronary grafts and poorly perfused nonrevascularized coronary microvasculature at risk. In a controlled study, Cosgrove *et al.*[93] found a 17.5% and 14.3% incidence of perioperative myocardial infarction with his high- and low-dose aprotinin regimens, respectively, compared with an 8.9% increase in the placebo-treated group. Acute vein graft thrombosis was found in 6 out of 12 grafts at postmortem examination in the aprotinin group and in 0 out of 5 in the control group.[93] However, heparinization was probably inadequate because their target ACT endpoint was too low. Subsequently, the occurrence of myocardial infarction, mortality, and internal mammary artery bypass graft occlusion has been shown not to be adversely affected by aprotinin;[94] however, the patency rate of saphenous vein grafts may be reduced.[89] Perioperative thrombophlebitis and thromboembolism are also potential risks.

Aprotinin is eliminated almost entirely in the urine as inactive metabolites. It is rapidly filtered by the glomerulus, then taken up by the proximal renal tubular epithelial cells, and slowly inactivated and excreted. Because of rapid accumulation in the kidney, possible renal toxicity has been extensively studied. Transient reductions in sodium reabsorption and potassium excretion for up to 3 h after infusion have been reported, but in normal kidneys typically no permanent damage occurs. However, prior renal damage, perhaps extreme hypothermia, and extraordinary dosages may be risk factors for permanent damage.

Aprotinin prolongs the ACT and the aPTT. All activating substances appear to be attenuated by aprotinin; however, kaolin activation may be less affected. Because aprotinin is overall prothrombotic, reducing heparin dosages as a result of aprotinin prolongation of the ACT may increase the incidence of postoperative graft thrombosis and thromboembolic phenomena. Aprotinin should not be considered as a heparin-sparing agent, i.e. standard heparin dosages should not be reduced. The ACT for cardiopulmonary bypass should be maintained at longer than 750 s using a Celite method or longer than 480 s using a kaolin method. Alternatively, the heparin concentration should be maintained at $> 2.7\ \mathrm{U\,mL^{-1}}$ using heparin/protamine titration.[89]

Desmopressin

Desmopressin (DDAVP, 1-desamino-8-D-arginine vasopressin) is a synthetic analog of endogenous arginine vasopressin or antidiuretic hormone (ADH). It was synthesized not only to attenuate the pressor effect of vasopressin but also to maintain its antidiuretic effect. DDAVP also mobilizes factor VIII, vWF, and tPA from peripheral endothelial cell sites. Clinically, therapeutic increases in factor VIII and vWF have been shown to be useful in mild hemophilia A and in von Willebrand's disease, respectively, although tachyphylaxis is great owing to depletion of peripheral stores of factor VIII and vWF.

DDAVP administration at dosages suitable for the treatment of hemostasis deficits will also cause a potent antidiuretic effect that will persist for 8–20 h. Urine output is reduced, urine osmolality is increased, and plasma osmolality is decreased. Repeated dosages and failure to adjust fluid regimens can result in water intoxication, severe hyponatremia, and *grand mal* seizures, particularly in children under the age of 2 years.

Since severe hypotension during infusion can occur because of vasodilation, DDAVP should be administered over at least 15 min with monitoring of the blood pressure. Although the substances released from the endothelial cells are known to increase within 30 min and peak by 90–120 min, the relative quantity and distribution of factor VIII, vWF, and tPA released with repeated administrations is unclear, but markedly declines when DDAVP is administered every 12–24 h. Clinically, tPA-induced fibrinolysis is apparently not a problem, but most clinical studies of DDAVP efficacy have ignored the fibrinolytic response.

Some patients treated with $0.3\ \mu\mathrm{g\,kg^{-1}}$ DDAVP may experience improvement of postcardiopulmonary bypass platelet dysfunction and other primary platelet disorders, presumably through an increase in vWF. Also, the size distribution of vWF multimers is shifted toward the more effective larger sizes after DDAVP administration. The initial report of DDAVP efficacy by Salzman *et al.*[95] was of a group of patients undergoing valve replacement or repeat CABG. They reported a 40% reduction in blood loss and a 34% reduction in transfusions. Many subsequent studies, typically with patients undergoing their first CABG, failed to show DDAVP to be effective in reducing blood loss. On subsequent reflection, Salzman *et al.*[96] concluded "that there is no benefit from the use of desmopressin in patients who have adequate hemostasis without it and in whom bleeding is not greater than the norm."

When substantial blood loss and platelet dysfunction are expected, such as with complicated cardiac surgical cases, prophylactic DDAVP may be efficacious,[97] but not of the same magnitude as the fibrinolytic inhibitors. A meta-analysis study indicated a reduction in postoperative blood loss by only 9% and no reduction in transfusion requirements.[98] However, if only trials resulting in the largest one-third of blood loss were considered, then DDAVP reduced postoperative blood loss by 34%.[98] Use as a successful rescue therapy in CABG patients with excessive postoperative bleeding can also be effective. It may be possible to identify those patients for whom DDAVP could be beneficial by platelet testing preoperatively.[22]

Owing to the relatively low risk of a single administration, use in patients with evidence of platelet dysfunction during vascular and noncardiac surgery should be considered.[97,99] DDAVP may be effective in treating the platelet dysfunction associated with renal failure and hepatic cirrhosis. It may also improve platelet function if there is a qualitative defect due to aspirin, other platelet-inhibiting drugs, or from a congenital platelet deficiency. However, for patients with normal hemostasis, DDAVP is unlikely to reduce surgical bleeding.

REFERENCES

1. Martinowitz U, Saltz R. Fibrin sealant. *Curr Opin Hematol* 1996; **3:** 395–402.
2. Coller BS. Platelets and thrombolytic therapy. *N Engl J Med* 1990; **322:** 33–42.
3. Ferguson JJ, Waly HM, Wilson JM. Fundamentals of coagulation and glycoprotein IIb/IIIa receptor inhibition. *Am Heart J* 1998; **135:** S35–42.
4. Roberts HR, Lozier JN. New perspectives on the coagulation cascade. *Hosp Pract* 1992; **27:** 97–105, 109–12.
5. Rosenberg RD, Bauer KA, Marcum JA. Protease inhibitors of human plasma. Antithrombin-III "the heparin–antithrombin system." *J Med* 1985; **16:** 351–416.
6. Rick ME. Protein C and protein S. Vitamin K-dependent inhibitors of blood coagulation. *JAMA* 1990; **263:** 701–3.
7. Sandset PM. Tissue factor pathway inhibitor (TFPI) – an update. *Haemostasis* 1996; **26** (Suppl. 4): 154–65.
8. Petersen LC, Valentin S, Hedner U. Regulation of the extrinsic pathway system in health and disease: the role of factor VIIa and tissue factor pathway inhibitor. *Thromb Res* 1995; **79:** 1–47.
9. Collen D. The plasminogen (fibrinolytic) system. *Thromb Haemostasis* 1999; **82:** 259–70.
10. Gaffney PJ, Edgell TA, Whitton CM. The haemostatic balance – Astrup revisited. *Haemostasis* 1999; **29:** 58–71.
11. Robert A, Chazouilleres O. Prothrombin time in liver failure: time, ratio, activity, percentage, or International Normalized Ratio? *Hepatology* 1996; **24:** 1392–4.

12. Stanworth SJ, Denton K, Monteath J, Patton WN. Automated counting of platelets on the Bayer ADVIA 120 analyzer. *Clin Lab Haematol* 1999; **21:** 113–17.
13. Harker LA, Slichter SJ. The bleeding time as a screening test for evaluation of platelet function. *N Engl J Med* 1972; **287:** 155–9.
14. Bjoraker DG. Monitoring platelet function. In: Lake CL, Johnson JO (eds): *Advances in Anesthesia*. St. Louis, MO: Mosby, 2001: 73–106.
15. Jobes DR. Safety issues in heparin and protamine administration for extracorporeal circulation. *J Cardiothor Vasc Anesth* 1998; **12** (2 Suppl. 1): 17–20.
16. Bull BS, Huse WM, Brauer FS, Korpman RA. Heparin therapy during extracorporeal circulation. II. The use of a dose–response curve to individualize heparin and protamine dosage. *J Thorac Cardiovasc Surg* 1975; **69:** 685–9.
17. Young JA, Kisker CT, Doty DB. Adequate anticoagulation during cardiopulmonary bypass determined by activated clotting time and the appearance of fibrin monomer. *Ann Thorac Surg* 1978; **26:** 231–40.
18. Bjoraker DG. The thrombelastograph D coagulation analyzer. *Anesthesiol Rev* 1991; **18** (4): 34–40.
19. Hartert H, Schaeder JA. The physical and biological constants of thrombelastography. *Biorheology* 1962; **1:** 31–9.
20. Mammen EF, Comp PC, Gosselin R, *et al.* PFA-100™ system: a new method for assessment of platelet dysfunction. *Semin Thromb Hemostasis* 1998; **24:** 195–202.
21. Marshall PW, Williams AJ, Dixon RM, *et al.* A comparison of the effects of aspirin on bleeding time measured using the Simplate™ method and closure time measured using the PFA-100™, in healthy volunteers. *Br J Clin Pharmacol* 1997; **44:** 151–5.
22. Despotis GJ, Levine V, Filos KS, *et al.* Evaluation of a new point-of-care test that measures PAF-mediated acceleration of coagulation in cardiac surgical patients. *Anesthesiology* 1996; **85:** 1311–23.
23. Ereth MH, Nuttall GA, Klindworth JT, *et al.* Does the platelet-activated clotting test (HemoSTATUS®) predict blood loss and platelet dysfunction associated with cardiopulmonary bypass? *Anesth Analg* 1997; **85:** 259–64.
24. Carville DG, Schleckser PA, Guyer KE, *et al.* Whole blood platelet function assay on the ICHOR point-of-care hematology analyzer. *J Extra Corpor Technol* 1998; **30:** 171–7.
25. Sackett E, Nuttall GA, Ereth MH, Oliver Jr WC. Validation of the Plateletworks™ point of care platelet function analyzer. *Anesth Analg* 2000; **90** (2S): S86.
26. Office of Medical Applications of Research, National Institutes of Health. Consensus Conference. Fresh frozen plasma: indications and risks. *JAMA* 1985; **253:** 551–3.
27. Office of Medical Applications of Research, National Institutes of Health. Consensus Conference. Platelet transfusion therapy. *JAMA* 1987; **257:** 1777–80.
28. Scott EP, Slichter SJ. Viability and function of platelet concentrates stored in CPD-Adenine (CPDA-1). *Transfusion* 1980; **20:** 489–97.
29. DiMichele D. Hemophilia 1996: new approach to an old disease. *Pediatr Clin North Am* 1996; **43:** 709–36.
30. Ellison N. Diagnosis and management of bleeding disorders. *Anesthesiology* 1977; **47:** 171–80.
31. Martinowitz U, Kenet G, Segal E, *et al.* Recombinant activated factor VII for adjunctive hemorrhage control in trauma. *J Trauma* 2001; **51:** 431–9.
32. Schwartz RS, Bauer KA, Rosenberg RD, *et al.* Clinical experience with antithrombin III concentrate in treatment of congenital and acquired deficiency of antithrombin. *Am J Med* 1989; **87** (Suppl. 3B): 53S–60S.
33. Bucur SZ, Levy JH, Despotis GJ, *et al.* Uses of antithrombin III concentrate in congenital and acquired deficiency states. *Transfusion* 1998; **38:** 481–98.
34. Liu SS, Mulroy MF. Neuraxial anesthesia and analgesia in the presence of standard heparin. *Reg Anesth Pain Med* 1998; **23** (6 Suppl. 2): 157–63.
35. Bjoraker DG. Hemostasis and blood transfusion in the obstetrical patient. *Curr Opin Anesthesiol* 1990; **3:** 412–17.
36. Slaughter TF, Greenberg CS. Heparin-associated thrombocytopenia and thrombosis. Implications for perioperative management. *Anaesthesiology* 1997; **87:** 667–75.
37. Cummins D, Hill E. Heparin-induced thrombocytopenia. *Semin Cardiothorac Vasc Anesth* 1997; **1:** 349–65.
38. Shorten GD, Comunale ME. Heparin-induced thrombocytopenia. *J Cardiothorac Vasc Anesth* 1996; **10:** 521–30.
39. Bjoraker DG, Ketcham TR. Hemodynamic and platelet response to the bolus intravenous administration of porcine heparin. *Thromb Haemostasis* 1983; **49:** 1–4.
40. Hirsh J, Levine MN. Low molecular weight heparin. *Blood* 1992; **79:** 1–17.
41. Hoppensteadt D, Walenga JM, Fareed J. Low molecular weight heparins. An objective overview. *Drugs Aging* 1992; **2:** 406–22.
42. Bergqvist D, Lindblad B, Matzsch T. Low molecular weight heparin thromboprophylaxis and epidural/spinal anaesthesia – is there a risk? *Acta Anaesth Scand* 1992; **36:** 605–9.
43. Horlocker TT, Wedel DJ. Neuraxial block and low-molecular-weight-heparin: balancing perioperative analgesia and thromboprophylaxis. *Reg Anesth Pain Med* 1998; **23** (6 Suppl. 2): 164–77.
44. Addonizio Jr VP, Fisher CA, Kappa JR, Ellison N. Prevention of heparin-induced thrombocytopenia during open heart surgery with iloprost (ZK36374). *Surgery* 1987; **102:** 796–807.
45. Shorten G, Comunale ME, Johnson RG. Management of cardiopulmonary bypass in a patient with heparin-induced thrombocytopenia using prostaglandin E_1 and aspirin. *J Cardiothorac Vasc Anesth* 1994; **8:** 556–8.
46. Teasdale SJ, Zulys VJ, Mycyk T, *et al.* Ancrod anticoagulation for cardiopulmonary bypass in heparin-induced thrombocytopenia and thrombosis. *Ann Thorac Surg* 1989; **48:** 712–13.
47. O-Yurvati AH, Laub GW, Southgate TJ, McGrath LB. Heparinless cardiopulmonary bypass with ancrod. *Ann Thorac Surg* 1994; **57:** 1656–8.
48. Magnani HN. Heparin-induced thrombocytopenia (HIT): an overview of 230 patients treated with orgaran (Org 10172). *Thromb Haemostasis* 1993; **70:** 554–61.
49. Schmahl KS, Ganjoo AK, Harloff MG. Orgaran (Org 10172) for cardiopulmonary bypass in heparin-induced thrombocytopenia: role of adjunctive plasmapheresis. *J Cardiothorac Vasc Anesth* 1997; **11:** 262–3.
50. Latham P, Revelis AF, Joshi GP, *et al.* Use of recombinant hirudin in patients with heparin-induced thrombocytopenia with thrombosis requiring cardiopulmonary bypass. *Anesthesiology* 2000; **92:** 263–6.
51. Koster A, Kuppe H, Hetzer R, *et al.* Emergent cardiopulmonary bypass in five patients with heparin-induced thrombocytopenia type II employing recombinant hirudin. *Anesthesiology* 1998; **89:** 777–80.
52. Potzsch B, Madlener K, Seelig C, *et al.* Monitoring of r-hirudin anticoagulation during cardiopulmonary bypass – assessment of the whole blood ecarin clotting time. *Thromb Haemostasis* 1997; **77:** 920–5.
53. Triplett DA. Current recommendations for warfarin therapy. Use and monitoring. *Med Clin North Am* 1998; **82:** 601–11.
54. Kitchens CS. A stuck pig – even on warfarin – doesn't always bleed. *Chest* 1999; **115:** 1492–3.
55. Kearon C, Hirsh J. Management of anticoagulation before and after elective surgery. *N Engl J Med* 1997; **336:** 1506–11.
56. Enneking FK, Benzon H. Oral anticoagulants and regional anesthesia: a perspective. *Reg Anesth Pain Med* 1998; **23** (6 Suppl. 2): 140–5.
57. Urmey WF, Rowlingson J. Do antiplatelet agents contribute to the development of perioperative spinal hematoma? *Reg Anesth Pain Med* 1998; **23** (6 Suppl. 2): 146–51.
58. Schror K. Aspirin and platelets: the antiplatelet action of aspirin and its role in thrombosis treatment and prophylaxis. *Semin Thromb Hemostasis* 1997; **23:** 349–56.
59. Connelly CS, Panush RS. Should nonsteroidal anti-inflammatory drugs be stopped before elective surgery? *Arch Intern Med* 1991; **151:** 1963–6.
60. Splinter WM, Rhine EJ, Roberts DW, *et al.* Perioperative ketorolac increases bleeding after tonsillectomy in children. *Can J Anaesth* 1996; **43:** 560–3.
61. Judkins JH, Dray TG, Hubbell RN. Intraoperative ketorolac and post-tonsillectomy bleeding. *Arch Otolaryngol Head Neck Surg* 1996; **122:** 937–40.
62. Gerancher JC, Waterer R, Middleton J. Transient paraparesis after postdural puncture spinal hematoma in a patient receiving ketorolac. *Anesthesiology* 1997; **86:** 490–4.
63. Lincoff AM, LeNarz LA, Despotis GJ, *et al.* Abciximab and bleeding during coronary surgery: results from the EPILOG and EPISTENT trials. Improved long-term outcome with abciximab GP IIb/IIIa blockade. Evaluation of platelet IIb/IIIa inhibition in stenting. *Ann Thorac Surg* 2000; **70:** 516–26.
64. Bang NU, Fletcher AP, Alkjaersig N, Sherry S. Pathogenesis of the coagulation defect developing during pathological plasma proteolytic ("fibrinolytic") states. III. Demonstration of abnormal clot structure by electron microscopy. *J Clin Invest* 1962; **41:** 935–48.
65. Hill RF, Kates RA, Davis D, Reves JG. Anesthetic implications for the management of patients with acute myocardial infarction: a matched cohort study of patients undergoing emergency myocardial revascularization. *J Cardiothorac Anesth* 1988; **2:** 23–9.
66. Mantia AM, Lolley DM, Stullken Jr EH, *et al.* Coronary artery bypass grafting within 24 hours after intracoronary streptokinase thrombolysis. *J Cardiothorac Anesth* 1987; **1:** 392–400.
67. Rosenquist RW, Brown DL. Neuraxial bleeding: fibrinolytics/thrombolytics. *Reg Anesth Pain Med* 1998; **23** (6 Suppl. 2): 152–6.
68. Shearer MJ. Vitamin K. *Lancet* 1995; **345:** 229–34.

69. Taylor CT, Chester EA, Byrd DC, Stephens MA. Vitamin K to reverse excessive anticoagulation: a review of the literature. *Pharmacotherapy* 1999; **19:** 1415–25.
70. Wakefield TW, Stanley JC. Intraoperative heparin anticoagulation and its reversal. *Semin Vasc Surg* 1996; **9:** 296–302.
71. Horrow JC. Protamine: a review of its toxicity. *Anesth Analg* 1985; **64:** 348–61.
72. Stewart WJ, McSweeney SM, Kellett MA, *et al.* Increased risk of severe protamine reactions in NPH insulin-dependent diabetics undergoing cardiac catheterization. *Circulation* 1984; **70:** 788–92.
73. Gottschlich GM, Gravlee GP, Georgitis JW. Adverse reactions to protamine sulfate during cardiac surgery in diabetic and non-diabetic patients. *Ann Allergy* 1988; **61:** 277–81.
74. Heyns AD, Lotter MG, Badenhorst PN, *et al.* Kinetics and in vivo redistribution of ^{111}Indium-labelled human platelets after intravenous protamine sulphate. *Thromb Haemostasis* 1980; **44:** 65–8.
75. Morel DR, Zapol WM, Thomas SJ, *et al.* C5a and thromboxane generation associated with pulmonary vaso- and broncho-constriction during protamine reversal of heparin. *Anesthesiology* 1987; **66:** 597–604.
76. Ellison N, Edmunds Jr LH, Colman RW. Platelet aggregation following heparin and protamine administration. *Anesthesiology* 1978; **48:** 65–8.
77. Guffin AV, Dunbar RW, Kaplan JA, Bland Jr JW. Successful use of a reduced dose of protamine after cardiopulmonary bypass. *Anesth Analg* 1976; **55:** 110–13.
78. Weiss AE, Webster WP, Strike LE, Brinkhous KM. Survival of transfused factor VIII in hemophilic patients treated with epsilon aminocaproic acid. *Transfusion* 1976; **16:** 209–14.
79. Ghosh K, Shetty S, Pathare A, Mohanty D. Epsilon-aminocaproic acid inhibits the activity of factory VIII inhibitors in patients with severe haemophilia A in vivo and in vitro. *Acta Haematol* 2000; **103:** 67–72.
80. McClure PD, Izsak J. The use of epsilon-aminocaproic acid to reduce bleeding during cardiac bypass in children with congenital heart disease. *Anesthesiology* 1974; **40:** 604–8.
81. Munoz JJ, Birkmeyer NJ, Birkmeyer JD, *et al.* Is epsilon-aminocaproic acid as effective as aprotinin in reducing bleeding with cardiac surgery?: a meta-analysis. *Circulation* 1999; **99:** 81–9.
82. Butterworth J, James RL, Lin Y, *et al.* Pharmacokinetics of epsilon-aminocaproic acid in patients undergoing aortocoronary bypass surgery. *Anesthesiology* 1999; **90:** 1624–35.
83. Kang Y, Lewis JH, Navalgund A, *et al.* Epsilon-aminocaproic acid for treatment of fibrinolysis during liver transplantation. *Anesthesiology* 1987; **66:** 766–73.
84. Casati V, Guzzon D, Oppizzi M, *et al.* Tranexamic acid compared with high-dose aprotinin in primary elective heart operations: effects on perioperative bleeding and allogeneic transfusions. *J Thorac Cardiovasc Surg* 2000; **120:** 520–7.
85. Wong BI, McLean RF, Fremes SE, *et al.* Aprotinin and tranexamic acid for high transfusion risk cardiac surgery. *Ann Thorac Surg* 2000; **69:** 808–16.
86. Nuttall GA, Oliver WC, Ereth MH, *et al.* Comparison of blood-conservation strategies in cardiac surgery patients at high risk for bleeding. *Anesthesiology* 2000; **92:** 674–82.
87. Horrow JC, Van Riper DF, Strong MD, *et al.* The dose–response relationship of tranexamic acid. *Anesthesiology* 1995; **82:** 383–92.
88. Dalmau A, Sabate A, Acosta F, *et al.* Tranexamic acid reduces red cell transfusions better than epsilon-aminocaproic acid or placebo in liver transplantation. *Anesth Analg* 2000; **91:** 29–34.
89. Peters DC, Noble S. Aprotinin: an update of its pharmacology and therapeutic use in open heart surgery and coronary artery bypass surgery. *Drugs* 1999; **57:** 233–60.
90. Royston D. Aprotinin versus lysine analogues: the debate continues. *Ann Thorac Surg* 1998; **65** (Suppl. 4): S9–19.
91. Westaby S. Aprotinin in perspective. *Ann Thorac Surg* 1993; **55:** 1033–41.
92. Porte RJ, Molenaar IQ, Begliomini B, *et al.* Aprotinin and transfusion requirements in orthotopic liver transplantation: a multicentre randomized double-blind study. EMSALT Study Group. *Lancet* 2000; **355:** 1303–9.
93. Cosgrove III DM, Heric B, Lytle BW, *et al.* Aprotinin therapy for reoperative myocardial revascularization: a placebo-controlled study. *Ann Thorac Surg* 1992; **54:** 1031–8.
94. Rich JB. The efficacy and safety of aprotinin use in cardiac surgery. *Ann Thorac Surg* 1998; **66** (Suppl. 5): S6–11.
95. Salzman EW, Weinstein MJ, Weintraub RM, *et al.* Treatment with desmopressin acetate to reduce blood loss after cardiac surgery. A double-blind randomized trial. *N Engl J Med* 1986; **314:** 1402–6.
96. Salzman EW, Weinstein MJ, Reilly D, Ware JA. Adventures in hemostasis. Desmopressin in cardiac surgery. *Arch Surg* 1993; **128:** 212–17.
97. Mannucci PM. Desmopressin (DDAVP) in the treatment of bleeding disorders: the first 20 years. *Blood* 1997; **90:** 2515–21.
98. Cattaneo M, Harris AS, Stromberg U, Mannucci PM. The effect of desmopressin on reducing blood loss in cardiac surgery – a meta-analysis of double-blind, placebo-controlled trials. *Thromb Haemostasis* 1995; **74:** 1064–70.
99. Clagett GP. Desmopressin, hemostasis, and vascular surgery. *Semin Vasc Surg* 1996; **9:** 340–6.

11

Control of circulation

M RAMEZ SALEM AND ANIS S BARAKA

The use of circulatory adjustments to achieve a desirable hemodynamic state is a cornerstone of perioperative anesthetic management. These maneuvers are mostly accomplished by physiologic and pharmacologic manipulations and, thus, are within the purview of the anesthesiologist. The broad spectrum of circulatory adjustments in the anesthetized patient will be highlighted by focusing on some of the circulatory measures intended to reduce blood loss and the management of perioperative hypertension.

CIRCULATORY MEASURES TO REDUCE BLOOD LOSS

The control of hemorrhage during surgical operations and the maintenance of adequate circulating blood volume constitute fundamental tenets of sound practice. Such control, however, is not always feasible. Persistent oozing may turn a simple operation into a difficult one. The volume of blood lost from a wound depends on the number and sizes of vessels cut (which depends on the size of the incision and the vascularity of the tissues), the rate of blood flow from the transected vessels, and the effectiveness of hemostasis.[1]

Surgical and anesthetic technique

Although blood loss can be controlled by meticulous surgical technique and prompt surgical intervention, certain factors can increase bleeding in anesthetized patients. These include light anesthesia, hypertension, systemic or regional increases in venous pressure, hyperdynamic circulation, and hypercapnia. Bleeding may increase during light anesthesia because of selective increases in skin and muscle blood flows and peripheral vasodilation, concomitant with increased cardiac output (CO). Coughing, bucking, increased airway resistance, airway obstruction, venous obstruction, inadequate muscular relaxation, positive end-expiratory pressure (PEEP), improper positioning, fluid overload, and congestive heart failure can all cause a generalized rise in central venous pressure and increased venous oozing.

Partial or complete obstruction to the inferior vena cava (IVC) owing to improper prone positioning will increase venous pressure distal to the obstruction.[2] This causes blood to be diverted into the vertebral venous plexuses, leading to increased oozing during spinal surgery. A rise in intra-abdominal pressure (due to increased muscle tone, external pressure on the abdomen, massive gastric inflation, coughing, bucking, airway obstruction, and increased airway pressure) increases IVC pressure and oozing. Conversely, complete relaxation of the diaphragm and the abdominal musculature decreases intra-abdominal pressure and IVC pressure, reducing bleeding during spinal surgery. Monitoring hemodynamic responses, neuromuscular function, and ventilation should provide the information to alert the anesthesiologist to these problems.

General compared with regional anesthesia

It is a common perception that regional anesthesia reduces bleeding in lower abdominal and lower limb surgery. Decreased arterial and/or venous pressure, often associated with regional anesthesia, seem to be the logical explanation. However, some investigators believe that this advantage of regional anesthesia can be achieved even if blood pressure is maintained at normal levels, and despite increased arterial flow.[1] Commonly studied procedures comparing general with regional anesthesia are transurethral resection of the prostate (TURP), cesarean section, and hip surgery.

Blood loss during TURP ranges[3,4] between 2.6 and 4.6 $mL\,min^{-1}$. Some studies of TURP found no significant difference in perioperative blood losses between general and regional anesthesia,[5–7] whereas others showed that blood losses are substantially greater in patients receiving general anesthesia.[8] Other factors influencing blood loss include weight of resected tissue, resection time, and the presence of infection.[3–5] Postoperative bleeding may also occur secondary to release of urokinase from prostatic tissue, which activates plasminogen to plasmin, causing fibrinolysis.[3,4,7]

In elective cesarean sections, Gilstrap *et al.*[9] found increased blood loss during general anesthesia with halogenated drugs compared with general anesthesia with nitrous oxide alone or regional anesthesia. Another study found no differences in blood loss between epidural anesthesia, general anesthesia with "low-dose" halothane–nitrous oxide, or nitrous oxide–opioid anesthesia.[10] Others found that the proportion of patients undergoing elective cesarean section with a decrease in hematocrit of 5% or more was greater in patients undergoing general anesthesia supplemented with halogenated drugs than in those undergoing regional anesthesia.[11]

Most investigators found no differences in intraoperative blood losses between spinal and general anesthesia during hip fracture procedures.[8,12] In total hip arthroplasty, epidural anesthesia is accompanied by reduced blood loss compared with general anesthesia.[13] However, no differences were found in hemoglobin levels up to 2 weeks postoperatively.[14,15]

Although there is no uniform agreement on the role of anesthetic choice in influencing blood loss, some conclusions may be drawn: (1)

factors other than the anesthetic influence blood loss; (2) by causing uterine relaxation, inhalation anesthetics increase blood loss following loss of a fetus; (3) the decreased blood loss sometimes observed during spinal or epidural anesthesia may be attributed to decreased arterial and/or venous pressure.

Posture

The physiology of posture can be learned from the giraffe.[16] Because its head is far above the heart, the task of supplying the giraffe with oxygenated blood demands a remarkably high blood pressure. At heart level, blood pressure is approximately 34.6/21.3 kPa (260/160 mmHg). However, the pressure that perfuses the brain is the same in giraffes, humans, and most other animals (Fig. 11.1).[16,17]

In individuals in the supine position, the arterial and venous pressures are the same in various parts of the body. Moving from the supine to the standing position results in considerable changes in arterial pressures. Parts above the heart are perfused at lower pressures, whereas parts below the heart are perfused at higher pressures. Similar changes are seen in the veins. In the standing position, the venous pressure is near zero above the heart and is subatmospheric in the cerebral sinuses.[18] Below the heart level, the venous pressure increases progressively, reaching its highest level in the feet.

Tilting produces a gradient of about 0.27 kPa (2 mmHg) for each 2.5 cm (1 inch) of vertical height, above which the arterial pressure is recorded. It produces increases of the same magnitude below the heart. In an individual of average height (172 cm), the difference between arterial pressure at the head and that at the feet could be 16 kPa (120 mmHg) in the standing position.[18] Because of their small stature, gravitational effects on arterial and venous pressures are less in children than in adults.[19] With vertical tilting, twice as much blood can accumulate in the legs, and even larger volumes can be accommodated in the abdomen. Tilting also increases the capillary pressure in dependent parts, and, if prolonged, increased filtration results in tissue edema, ultimately reducing blood volume.

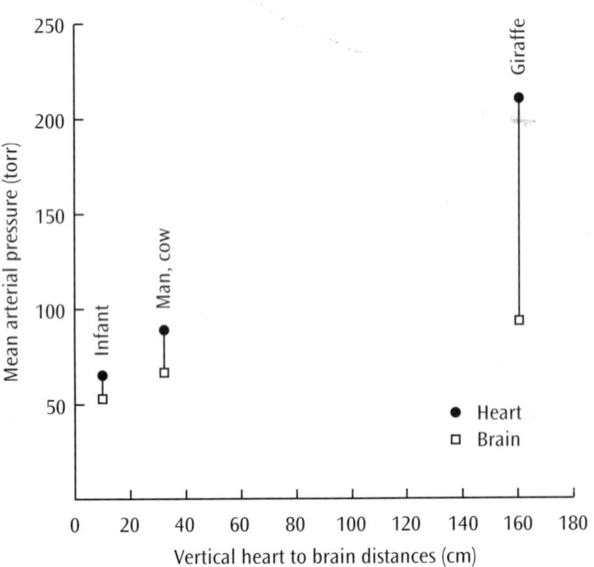

Figure 11.1 *Mean arterial pressure at the heart and brain levels in various animals and man. Although there is an appreciable difference between mean arterial pressure in the giraffe and in man at the heart level, the pressure perfusing the brain is the same in both species. (Modified with permission from Warren.[16])*

In awake individuals, tilting initiates baroreceptor reflex activity, which leads to increased production of catecholamines and plasma renin activity, inducing the formation of the vasoconstrictor angiotensin II with aldosterone and sodium and water retention. Increased sympathetic activity constricts the capacitance vessels, maintaining venous return, whereas constriction of the resistance vessels minimizes the decrease in arterial pressure. These mechanisms are evident 15–30 min after tilting. In the normal subject, little change occurs in arterial pressure at the heart level during tilting or standing, although heart rate may increase. Anesthetic drugs and ganglionic and β-adrenergic blocking drugs interfere with these compensatory mechanisms. Consequently, head-up (or foot-down) tilt in the anesthetized patient will favor arterial hypotension in the upper parts and venous pooling in the lower parts of the body.

Positioning the patient so that the operative site is placed uppermost is a widely practiced maneuver to decrease blood loss. The tilt varies from 10° to 25° in head and neck procedures to 90° in sitting position craniotomy. When head-up tilt is used, pressure gradients should be taken into account to assure adequate cerebral perfusion. Either an estimate of the pressure gradient is calculated by measuring the vertical distance between the heart and the brain [gradient (mmHg) = distance (inches) × 2] or the pressure transducer (in case of arterial cannulation) is positioned at the brain level.

Induced hypotension

Historical background

The concept of intentional induction of hypotension to decrease blood loss and improve operative conditions for intracranial surgery was first proposed by Cushing in 1917.[20] Gardner[21] reported on the deliberate decrease in blood pressure in patients undergoing difficult neurosurgical procedures by arteriotomy.[22] The blood removed was kept in heparinized bottles and reinfused at the end of the procedure. The many complications ("irreversible shock," tissue hypoxemia, acidosis, and overheparinization) indicated that the boundaries of physiologic trespass were broken down, and the technique was quickly abandoned. Griffiths and Gillies[23] advocated the use of high spinal analgesia to induce hypotension and to produce relatively bloodless conditions.[22] The major advancement with normovolemic hypotension was achieved when ganglionic blockade was combined with foot-down tilt. Enderby[23] described the new method as "controlled circulation with hypotensive drugs and posture to reduce bleeding in surgery." The enthusiastic initial reception was followed by reports of unexplained morbidity and mortality.[24]

After investigations using hexamethonium (C_6), attention was drawn to pentolinium, which proved superior to other drugs.[22] The knowledge that triethylsulfonium salts, such as the quaternary and bisquarternary ammonium ions, possess ganglionic blocking activity culminated in the synthesis of trimethaphan, which offered a new dimension in the control of blood pressure by continuous infusion. Its short action was surpassed only by sodium nitroprusside (SNP), introduced into clinical practice in 1962.[25] The introduction of halothane allowed an easier and gentler induction of hypotension with and without ganglionic blockade.[22] This milestone in vascular control was responsible for a marked improvement in safety. β-Adrenergic blocking drugs were introduced to treat tachycardia.[26,27] The 1970s witnessed the introduction of nitroglycerin[28] and labetalol[29] as hypotensive drugs and the wider use of induced hypotension in pediatric surgery.[19,30] Advances in knowledge of the physiology and pharmacology of induced hypotension, as well as in the application of the newer monitoring methods, have contributed to the evolution and safety of this technique. Induced hypotension has also been referred to as deliberate or controlled hypotension.

Uses of hypotensive drugs

Hypotensive drugs are used to achieve one or more of the following goals:[17] (1) reduction of blood loss, (2) facilitation of vessel surgery, and (3) improvement of myocardial performance by reducing the preload and afterload. When hypotensive drugs are used to reduce blood loss, the blood pressure is deliberately lowered to hypotensive levels to achieve the desired response. In contrast, when these drugs are used to facilitate vessel surgery or to enhance myocardial performance, the goal is to "control" the blood pressure so as to prevent an unwanted rise or to maintain a slightly hypotensive state.

Reduction of blood loss

By producing a relatively dry operative field, induced hypotension improves visualization and allows the accurate delineation of lesions.[31] There is less trauma inflicted on nerves, vessels, and delicate tissues. Hypotension may increase the viability of pedicles and grafts and may diminish the incidence of postoperative hematoma, sepsis, and fibrosis. There is less need for (or avoidance of) allogeneic blood transfusion. In certain operations, the need for infiltration with epinephrine (adrenaline)-containing solution may be eliminated, thereby allowing delicate surgery to be performed without distorting the anatomy. Induced hypotension may also decrease operative time.[30] Reports on blood loss with induced hypotension vary and may depend on the site of operation, posture, drugs and techniques used, level of blood pressure, heart rate, and the experience of the surgeon and the anesthesiologist. In this regard, hypotensive anesthesia is not the answer to poor surgical technique and, as Enderby put it, "good surgical technique skillful enough to match the high standards of hypotensive anesthesia is essential if any real advantages are to accrue to the patient."[23]

Facilitation of vessel surgery

By keeping large vessels soft and preventing progressive stretching of their walls, blood pressure control makes suturing or clipping easier.[31] It also minimizes trauma to diseased vessels and helps prevent aortic dissection. Common applications include coarctectomy,[32] aortic surgery,[33–35] clipping of an intracranial aneurysm,[36,37] or arteriovenous malformation, excision of vascular tumors, and operations for portal hypertension.[38] Hypertension after cardiopulmonary bypass can increase the potential for bleeding from suture lines and, thus, should be prevented and treated.

Improvement of myocardial performance

The reader is referred to Chapter 45.

Techniques of induced hypotension

Many hypotensive techniques have been described previously,[39–41] most of which rely on a combination of physiologic and pharmacologic components. A reliable intravenous line and basic monitoring, including accurate blood pressure measurements, should be established. Hypotension is initiated only after tracheal intubation and after a steady anesthetic state is obtained. This may be achieved with either an opioid–nitrous oxide–oxygen mixture supplemented with a muscle relaxant and/or a low concentration of a volatile anesthetic. Most practitioners prefer to control ventilation, although some prefer spontaneous ventilation. Hypotension is induced gradually using a hypotensive drug given at least 10 min before surgery commences (if hypotension is required before the incision is made) while the patient is in the horizontal position. A β-adrenergic blocking drug may be given before the hypotensive drug is administered. A comparison of five hypotensive drugs is shown in Table 11.1.

After the effect of the drug(s) is assessed, the patient is then tilted (head up or foot down). A hypotensive response may not be evident in the horizontal position, but subsequent tilting decreases the arterial pressure as a result of peripheral venous pooling. The patient should not be tilted too quickly as cerebral autoregulation requires several minutes.[42,43] A further decrease in arterial pressure can be obtained by a gradual increase in the anesthetic concentration. This is particularly useful when head-up tilt is not possible (hip and back surgery).

Some anesthesiologists prefer to initiate hypotension by deepening the anesthetic level or relying on posture without the use of hypotensive drugs.[37,44,45] Others prefer the use of small doses of β-adrenergic blocking drugs or combinations of drugs with the inhalational anesthetic. All these variations and modifications are acceptable. Although the dose-related depression of the cardiovascular function by inhalation anesthetics is well documented, some qualitative and quantitative differences exist.[46,47] In healthy individuals, both halothane and enflurane have minimal effects on the systemic vascular resistance (SVR), and the hypotension is secondary to a dose-dependent decrease in left ventricular function. Isoflurane causes hypotension by decreasing the SVR, whereas the CO is preserved because of the associated decrease in afterload.[37,48] The intravascular volume status contributes to the decrease in CO during isoflurane anesthesia. Halothane has little effect on heart rate, whereas enflurane and isoflurane produce an increase in heart rate. The newer anesthetics sevoflurane and desflurane have effects which are similar to those of isoflurane.[49] Because of the impairment of the myocardial contractile function by inhalation anesthesia, the use of these drugs as the sole means of inducing hypotension is not recommended for all patients.[50]

With increasing inhalation anesthetic concentration, cerebral autoregulation is impaired and cerebral blood flow (CBF) increases. The intracranial pressure (ICP) may also increase owing to the increased intracranial volume. Even low concentrations of inhalation anesthetics may provoke increases in ICP in patients with a reduced intracranial compliance, and cerebral edema may occur, especially if the blood pressure is allowed to increase.[51] Because of these potential undesirable effects, inhalation anesthetics should not be used as the sole means of inducing hypotension in patients with intracranial lesions.

Isoflurane [up to 1 MAC (minimal alveolar concentration)] produces a concentration-related depression of cerebral metabolism, whereas the physiological relations between flow and pressure and between flow and metabolism are preserved. With higher concentrations, the vasodilator effect predominates: autoregulation is impaired and CBF increases.[48,52,53] However, the use of isoflurane seems to offer certain advantages over other techniques for induced hypotension.[54,55] It influences the global cerebral oxygen supply–demand ratio favorably. At low cerebral perfusion pressure (CPP), the cerebral metabolic rate for oxygen is better preserved, and this suggests that isoflurane may afford cerebral protection during profound hypotension. It has been found that isoflurane-induced hypotension increased both brain edema and neurologic deficits in dogs with cryogenic brain lesions, in contrast with dogs given labetalol.[56] Using sensitive biochemical markers of brain cell injury, similar effects were found in patients undergoing normotensive as well as hypotensive isoflurane anesthesia.[57,58] Thus, induced hypotension did not seem to contribute to these adverse effects. Combining isoflurane with other drugs which have β- or combined α- and β-adrenergic receptor blocking activity attenuates the undesirable effects of isoflurane used as the sole hypotensive drug.[59] For more than 10 years, the authors have used the combination of isoflurane and labetalol as the main hypotensive technique with very satisfactory results.

Historically, PEEP was used to fine-tune hypotension to the desired level.[22] However, with the availability of potent inhalation anesthetics and hypotensive drugs, there seems to be no need to resort to its use.

Mode of action of hypotensive drugs

Induced hypotension (in normovolemic patients) can be produced by either a reduction in CO or a decrease in SVR. The precapillary arterioles contain relatively large amounts of smooth muscle and, thus,

Table 11.1 *Comparison of five hypotensive drugs*

Characteristic	Pentolinium tartrate (unavailable in USA)	Trimethaphan camphorsulfonate	Sodium nitroprusside	Nitroglycerin	Labetalol
Onset of action	Gradual onset, slow recovery	Rapid onset, usually rapid recovery	Rapid onset, very rapid recovery	Rapid onset, moderately slower recovery	Gradual onset, slower recovery
Duration	Long acting	Short acting; may be prolonged with halothane and propranolol	Evanescent action; prolonged with cyanide toxicity	Short acting	Long acting
Method of administration	Single injection	i.v. drip (0.2% in 5% D/W solution)	i.v. drip (0.01% solution)	i.v. drip (0.01% in 5% D/W or 0.9% NaCl)	i.v. injection, repeated in increments
Mode of action	Ganglionic blockade	Ganglionic blockade, direct effect, a-adrenergic blockade, histamine release?	Direct effect (resistance and capacitance vessels)	Direct effect, capacitance vessels predominantly	α- and β-adrenoceptor antagonist
Tachycardia	Occurs in children, less likely in adults	Occur in children, less likely in adults	Very common	May occur in children, unlikely in adults	None, usually slight bradycardia
Cardiac output	May remain unchanged, increase, or decrease, depending on posture (venous pooling), changes in heart rate, preload and afterload, anesthetics, other myocardial depressant drugs, ventilation, intravascular volume status				Slight decrease
Blood–brain barrier	Minimal or no derangement	Minimal or no derangement	Pronounced dysfunction	Probably same as sodium nitroprusside	Probably none
Metabolism	Excreted unchanged	Unclear, inhibits plasma cholinesterase but not metabolized by it	Metabolized to cyanide and thiocyanate	Degraded rapidly in the liver	Degraded in the liver
Stability	Stable	Unstable; kept refrigerated	Available as powder, unstable when reconstituted, protect from light, use within 12 h	Stable; colorless, absorbed by plastics, use high-density polyethylene drip set	Stable
Dose	0.2 $mg\,kg^{-1}$	Total i.v. dose should not exceed 10 $mg\,kg^{-1}$	Initial dose 0.5–1.5 $mg\,kg^{-1}\,min^{-1}$; dose usually <8 $mg\,kg^{-1}\,min^{-1}$; total dose not to exceed 1.5 $mg\,kg^{-1}$ in 4 h	10–20 $mg\,kg^{-1}\,min^{-1}$	0.2–0.4 $mg\,kg^{-1}$ followed by increments
Histamine release	None	Histamine release related to administration rate	Unknown	Unknown	Unknown
Rebound hypertension	Does not occur	Does not occur	Occurs in absence of β-blockade	Does not occur	Does not occur
Intracranial pressure	Unknown	Variable, but may decrease	Increases in early stages, less than with trimethaphan	Increases, greater than with trimethaphan	Does not increase

D/W, dextrose in water. From Salem.[194]

are the major determinants of resistance. As SVR is inversely related to arteriolar caliber by approximately the fourth power of the radius, relatively small changes in intraluminal diameter have profound effects on SVR.[60]

Hypotensive drugs may be classified into ganglionic blocking drugs (e.g. pentolinium, trimethaphan), direct-acting vasodilators (e.g. SNP, nitroglycerin, hydralazine, adenosine, prostaglandin E_1), α-adrenergic blocking drugs (e.g. phentolamine, urapidil, nicergoline), β-adrenergic blocking drugs (e.g. propranolol, esmolol), drugs with combined α- and β-adrenergic blocking actions (e.g. labetalol), and calcium channel-blocking drugs (e.g. verapamil, nicardipine).

Ganglionic blocking drugs

Ganglionic blocking drugs compete with acetylcholine for the nicotinic receptors on the autonomic postjunctional ganglionic membrane. Since most organs are reciprocally innervated by sympathetic and parasympathetic nerves, the overall effect of autonomic blockade depends on the predominance of one or the other system at the end-organ. The arterioles and venules of the skin and splanchnic viscera have predominantly sympathetic vasoconstrictor innervation, so ganglionic blockade produces vasodilation, increased venous capacitance, and hypotension. In contrast, the iris, ciliary muscle, gastrointestinal tract, urinary bladder, and sweat glands are all under predominantly parasympathetic control, and, therefore, ganglionic blockade produces mydriasis, cycloplegia, constipation, urinary retention, and abolition of sweating. These side-effects are of no consequence after intravenous use during anesthesia, except mydriasis and cycloplegia, which may be misinterpreted in the postoperative neurologic assessment. The hypotensive action of trimethaphan has been attributed to ganglionic blockade, a direct effect on vascular smooth muscle, α-adrenergic blockade, and histamine release.[61]

Direct-acting vasodilator drugs

Direct-acting vasodilator drugs fall into two categories: (1) nitric oxide dependent and (2) nitric oxide independent. Nitric oxide (NO) is produced in cardiac and vascular endothelial cells from the amino acid L-arginine in a reaction requiring the constitutive enzyme nitric oxide synthase.[62–65] Nitric oxide production is stimulated by increases in intracellular calcium in response to the interaction of a chemical agent in the blood, for example bradykinin or acetylcholine, with its specific membrane receptor, or by increases in shear stress. It diffuses into the underlying vascular smooth muscle, where it stimulates production of cyclic guanosine monophosphate, thus causing vascular relaxation. The vasodilating effects of SNP and nitroglycerin have been explained by their ability to provide exogenous NO.[66] Inhaled NO has been used as a treatment for pulmonary hypertension.[67]

Sodium nitroprusside exerts its hypotensive action primarily by decreasing SVR whereas the venous effect is minimal, so that CO is maintained. In contrast, nitroglycerin has little effect on arteriolar resistance vessels at lower concentrations, but exhibits relatively pronounced effects on the venous capacitance vessels, which results in decreased venous return, decreased ventricular filling pressures, and, ultimately, reduced CO.[60]

Adenosine

Adenosine, a metabolic endproduct of adenosine triphosphate (ATP), is an endogenous vasodilator that has been implicated in local regulation of several vascular beds, including the heart and brain. Although ATP has been used as a hypotensive drug, its effect has been attributed to the arterial adenosine concentration.[68] Intravenous infusion of adenosine produces hypotension that is rapidly obtained, easily controlled, short-lasting, and not accompanied by rebound hypertension when the infusion is discontinued.[68–70] The hypotensive effect results entirely from a sharp decrease in SVR, with minimal effect on the venous vascular bed because of the rapid degradation of adenosine or the decreased sensitivity of the venous vascular bed for adenosine. Because it increases the coronary blood flow and decreases the afterload, adenosine influences the myocardial oxygen supply–demand balance favorably. However, patients with coronary artery disease may develop signs of myocardial ischemia during hypotension. Increased CO has been noted. [Although decreased heart rate occurs (probably because of direct depressive effect on the sinoatrial node) in dogs, this finding has not been consistent in humans.] Adenosine inhibits renin release and therefore prevents the activation of the renin–angiotensin system. β-Adrenergic blocking drugs are usually not needed to control the heart rate. Adenosine-induced hypotension is not associated with any cardiovascular, hematologic, central nervous system, renal, or hepatic toxicity. However, adenosine dilates cerebral vessels, increases ICP, and impairs cerebral autoregulation.[69,71] Other potential adverse features include its paradoxical ability to cause renal vasoconstriction and heart block.[69,71]

Prostaglandin E_1

Prostaglandin E_1 (PGE_1) has a potent vasodilator effect on the pulmonary and systemic vascular beds. Despite its vasodilator properties, PGE_1 infusion causes only slight hypotension in conscious patients because of the concomitant increase in CO secondary to its positive inotropic effect and the reflex increase in heart rate. PGE_1 infusion (100–150 ng kg^{-1} min^{-1}) has been successfully used to induce hypotension.[72] Resistance was encountered in some patients.[73] Blood pressure returns to within 15% of normal 15 min after the infusion is stopped. Increase in plasma renin activity occurs during PGE_1 infusion, presumably because of the fall in pressure rather than a direct effect on the kidney. PGE_1 also causes increases in renal blood flow, urine flow, and sodium excretion.[73] Although an inhibitory effect on both platelet aggregation and thrombus formation has been described, PGE_1 in clinical doses has no discernable effect on platelet aggregation.

β-Adrenergic blocking drugs

Treatment with a β-adrenergic blocking drug prevents the increase in heart rate, CO, plasma renin activity, and catecholamine levels and blocks rebound hypertension after cessation of SNP infusion. Furthermore, the dose requirements of SNP are decreased by approximately 40%. Propranolol given in small increments up to 60 μg kg^{-1}, before or after the hypotensive drug, prevents tachycardia and facilitates the control of blood pressure.[19] It is preferable to give it before rather than after the onset of tachycardia, when a much larger dose may be needed. Being a nonselective β-adrenergic blocking drug, propranolol blocks both β_1 (predominantly the heart) and β_2 (predominantly blood vessels and bronchial smooth muscles) receptors. With propanolol, increased airway resistance in normal subjects and the occurrence of bronchospasm in asthmatics led to the development of more selective β_1-adrenergic blocking drugs. Table 11.2 lists the currently available β-adrenergic blocking drugs that can be used as adjutants to induced hypotension.

Some clinicians have found esmolol-induced hypotension to be more effective than SNP in producing better operative conditions.[74,75] Because of the ability to produce severe myocardial depression,[76] these drugs should probably be used mostly as adjuvants rather than as the sole hypotensive agent.[77] The advantages of esmolol are its rapid onset, titration of action, short duration, and cardioselectivity. The drug may be given in a loading dose of 500 μg kg^{-1} min^{-1} for 2–4 min and continued by constant infusion[78] at a rate of 300 μg kg^{-1} min^{-1}.

Labetalol

Labetalol acts as a competitive antagonist at both α_1- and β-adrenergic receptors. Its pharmacologic properties include selective blockade of α_1-adrenergic receptors, blockade of β_1- and β_2-adrenergic receptors, partial agonist activity at β_2 receptors, and inhibition of neural uptake of norepinephrine (noradrenaline; cocaine-like effect).[79] The potency of labetalol for β-adrenergic blockade is one-fifth to one-tenth of that

Table 11.2 *Dose, cardioselectivity, and elimination half-life data of currently available β-adrenergic blocking drugs*

Drug	Dose	Cardioselectivity (β_1)	Elimination half-life
Propranolol	0.06 mg kg^{-1}	0	4 h
Practolol	0.15 mg kg^{-1}	+	10 h
Metoprolol	0.15 mg kg^{-1}	+	3–4 h
Esmolol	Loading dose 0.5 mg kg^{-1} min^{-1} followed by 300 mg kg^{-1} min^{-1} (constant infusion)	+	10 min
Labetalol	0.2–0.4 mg kg^{-1} depending upon background anesthetic, additional increments until desired effect is achieved	0 (has α-, β_1-, and β_2-adrenergic blocking properties)	3.5–4.5 h

From Salem.[194]

for α-adrenergic blockade: 10 mg labetalol is equivalent to 2 mg of propranolol at β_1-receptors, 0.75 mg of propranolol at β_2-receptors, and 2 mg of phentolamine (a pure α_1-antagonist) at α-receptors. In patients anesthetized with inhalation anesthetics, labetalol reduces blood pressure gradually (over 5–10 min) by decreasing SVR with either no change in heart rate or with bradycardia and a slight or no decrease in CO.[29,80,81] Its hypotensive effect is less pronounced when given with intravenous rather than with inhalation anesthetics. Because of its long elimination half-life (3–6 h), it may be the preferred drug when prolonged hypotension is required. In contrast, its prolonged action may mask the adrenergic response to acute blood loss in the early postoperative period. Labetalol is given in an initial dose of 0.2–0.4 mg kg^{-1}. Incremental doses (half the initial dose) may be repeated after 5–10 min until the desired hypotension is obtained. Advantages over SNP include absence of tachycardia, no increase in CO, no rebound hypertension, no increase in intrapulmonary shunt, and no increase in ICP.

Calcium channel blocking drugs

Nicardipine and verapamil exert their hypotensive effects primarily by decreasing SVR. Because verapamil produces myocardial depression and delays atrioventricular conduction, it is not recommended for inducing hypotension. Nicardipine has been successfully utilized as a hypotensive drug.[82–84] It vasodilates the peripheral, coronary, and cerebral vessels while maintaining the CO without tachycardia. Careful titration (10–250 μg kg^{-1} h^{-1}) is mandatory because it has an "increasing effect" over time and because the hypotension may be resistant to conventional treatment.

Hydralazine

Hydralazine is a direct arteriolar vasodilator. It decreases blood pressure within 10 min by reducing SVR, without changing CO. Reflex tachycardia tends to accompany the decrease in blood pressure. The hypotensive effect is more pronounced when hydralazine is given with an inhalation anesthetic.[85] ICP increases following the administration of hydralazine, but rebound hypertension does not occur.[85] Hydralazine is more commonly used as an antihypertensive drug in the perioperative period, although the long duration (more than 3 h) may be unwanted.

Fenoldopam

Fenoldopam is a pure dopamine $(D)_1$-receptor antagonist with selective coronary, renal, mesenteric, and peripheral arteriolar vasodilator action. Mild reflex tachycardia usually occurs with its use. The maximal response is usually achieved in 10–20 min. Fenoldopam is given by a continuous infusion (0.1–0.6 μg kg^{-1} min^{-1}). Unlike other hypotensive drugs, fenoldopam has renal vasodilation and natriuretic actions which maintain or increase urine flow during hypotension. There is a growing consensus that these properties may constitute a renal protective effect.[86]

Hemodynamic effects of hypotensive drugs

Tachyphylaxis and tachycardia

Since the introduction of hypotensive agents into anesthetic practice, failure to maintain the desired hemodynamic changes has been observed. This phenomenon (tachyphylaxis) is best described as diminished response despite repeated administration of the drug. Resistance to hypotensive drugs is usually associated with tachycardia and is seen frequently in children and young adults but is very rare in the elderly.

Several mechanisms have been postulated to explain tachycardia and/or tachyphylaxis. Sodium nitroprusside-induced hypotension is associated with increases in heart rate, CO, activation of the renin–angiotensin system, and release of catecholamines.[87–89] In contrast, ganglionic blockade results in less of an increase in circulating catecholamines and no activation of the renin–angiotensin axis.[88,90] The increased heart rate with ganglionic blocking drugs probably results from parasympathetic blockade, which may be prominent in children because of increased vagal tone.[17,91] In response to the initial hypotension, reflex tachycardia, mediated through the baroreceptors, occurs with most hypotensive agents, and results in an increased CO and a rise in blood pressure. As a result of sympathetic activation, renin is released from the juxtaglomerular apparatus in the kidney. This acts on α_2-globulin from the liver to produce the decapeptide angiotensin I, which is converted in the lungs to the octapeptide angiotensin II, a potent vasoconstrictor.

Stimulation of the sympathetic and the renin–angiotensin systems may adversely affect the operative course during hypotension. The increased CO can cause bleeding. Rebound hypertension may occur following abrupt termination of the SNP infusion. This is most likely to be due to an increase in SVR secondary to unopposed activation of the sympathetic and renin–angiotensin responses. The consequences of rebound hypertension include wound bleeding, hematoma formation, cerebral edema, cerebrovascular accidents, disrupted cerebral autoregulation, increased myocardial oxygen demand, and pulmonary edema. The varying sensitivities of vessels to catecholamines in different vascular beds may cause major changes in the distribution of blood flow, as well as a redistribution of blood flow within organs. Very high levels of circulating catecholamine and angiotensin II may have deleterious effects on myocardial and renal tubular cells and may adversely affect arterial and capillary function.[92]

Techniques advocated to prevent and treat tachycardia/tachyphylaxis are shown in Table 11.3. The simplest effective means is the judicious use of a β-adrenergic blocking drug. Other alternatives include pretreatment with saralasin, an angiotensin II competitive antagonist, and with captopril, an oral angiotensin-converting enzyme inhibitor.[93,94] Pretreatment with captopril results in lower dosage requirements and prevents rebound hypertension. A 10:1 mixture of trimethaphan (250 mg) and SNP (25 mg) in a solution of 5% dextrose in water has been advocated.[95,96] The mixture produces hypotension with smaller doses of SNP

Table 11.3 *Techniques to prevent tachyphylaxis to hypotensive drugs*

Halothane – other inhalation anesthetics (inactivates the baroreceptor response)
Avoiding fluid overload
Omitting belladonna drugs (or decreasing dosage)
Preoperative sedation and i.v. opioids
Use of a β-adrenergic blocking drug
Pretreatment with angiotensin II competitive antagonist
Pretreatment with angiotensin-converting enzyme inhibitor
Combining hypotensive drugs
Premedication with clonidine

Modified from Salem.[194]

and trimethaphan than when either drug is used separately (synergistic effect). When the mixture is used, the dose of SNP is approximately one-third to one-fifth of the amount required when SNP is used alone, and blood pressure returns gradually without rebound hypertension.

Clonidine, an α_2-adrenoceptor agonist, reduces the requirement for isoflurane (by 60%)[97,98] and SNP (by 45%) and substantially reduces the need for labetalol during induced hypotension. By its central effect within the medulla and hypothalamus, clonidine blocks the increased central adrenergic activity concomitant with the use of hypotensive drugs. Other actions include the inhibition of renin release in the kidney and a reduction in vasopressin release. The recommended dose is 4–8 μg kg^{-1} given orally 2 h prior to surgery.

Effects on cardiac output and regional blood flows

The cardiovascular effects of hypotensive drugs may be modified by many factors: the anesthetic and adjuvant drugs, posture, degree of hypotension, intrathoracic pressure, acid–base status, circulating blood volume, age, and change in preload and afterload.

Cardiac output Vasodilators alter the CO through changes in stroke volume and heart rate. They decrease afterload by lowering arterial impedance and reduce preload by increasing venous compliance. Depending on the ventricular function, as defined by the Frank–Starling mechanism and the relative effect on the preload and afterload, stroke volume may rise, remain constant, or even decline (Fig. 11.2).[99] Decreased afterload shifts the curve to the left. If preload remains constant, stroke volume will increase. If the decrease in afterload is associated with a decrease in preload, then stroke volume may remain constant. A decrease in preload without a decrease in afterload will result in decreased stroke volume.

In anesthetized humans, SNP-induced hypotension is associated with either increased or unchanged CO. In contrast, nitroglycerin, because of its effect on venous capacitance and venous pressure, decreases ventricular filling pressure and, ultimately, reduces CO.[28,60] Hypotension secondary to ganglionic blockade has variable effects on CO.

Hypotension associated with "shock states" may be followed by irreversible organ damage. In contrast, induced hypotension rarely, if ever, is followed by organ damage. In theory, as long as mean arterial blood pressure exceeds the sum of colloid osmotic pressure plus venous pressure, the circulation should be adequate for tissue needs. This calculation suggests that a pressure of 4.3 kPa (32 mmHg) is satisfactory. However, this value is probably below the safe level for two reasons. First, it ignores specific blood flow requirements. The critical closing pressure varies from organ to organ and from individual to individual. Second, it ignores the limitations set by disease. In view of these factors, the mean arterial blood pressure should *not* be allowed to fall below 6.7 kPa (50 mmHg) in healthy patients unless there is a definite indication or unless additional measures are used to ensure adequate organ protection.

Coronary circulation The main factor affecting coronary perfusion is the aortic diastolic pressure. During induced hypotension, reduced

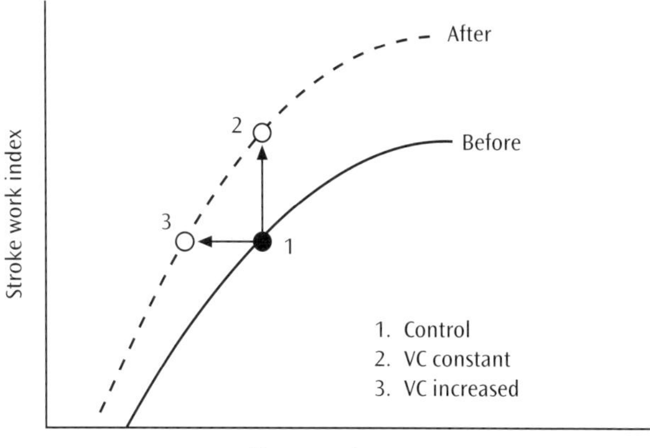

Figure 11.2 *Effect of a vasodilator on the Frank–Starling relation. Decreased afterload shifts the curve (solid line) to the left (dashed line). If transmural pressure (preload) remains constant, cardiac output increases; if the decrease in afterload is also associated with decreased preload (transmural pressure), cardiac output remains constant. VC, venous compliance. (Reproduced with permission from Fahmy and Laver.[99])*

myocardial work secondary to decreased afterload requires less coronary blood flow. A decrease in the heart rate-systolic pressure product as an index of myocardial oxygen demand has been observed during induced hypotension.[17,99] Unless severe hypotension occurs, the decreased coronary perfusion during induced hypotension is adequate. This may explain the lack of electrocardiographic evidence of myocardial ischemia during induced hypotension.[19]

Some investigators have combined induced hypotension with acute normovolemic hemodilution, so as to minimize or eliminate the use of allogeneic blood requirement. Animal studies showed that myocardial oxygen supply versus demand are well maintained with the combined technique.[70,100] However, diminished coronary vasodilator reserve suggested increased vulnerability to ischemia if the additional stresses of augmented cardiac work demand or impaired arterial oxygenation were superimposed. These animal studies lead us to emphasize the importance of preoperative evaluation of patients, experience, and vigilant monitoring when hypotension and hemodilution are combined.

Cerebral circulation With progressive decreases in blood pressure, a corresponding decrease occurs in cerebrovascular resistance, maintaining normal CBF. In the healthy unanesthetized human, CBF is virtually constant as long as mean blood pressure remains between 6.7 and 20 kPa (50 and 150 mmHg). Below or above these levels, flow becomes pressure dependent. This autoregulatory mechanism is compromised in disease states, by anesthetics, and after head trauma.[101] Chronic hypertension raises the lower limit of blood pressure, below which CBF is no longer autoregulated; CBF may fall at pressures higher than those in normotensive patients.[102] With a significant reduction in CBF, other compensatory mechanisms come into play, including widening of the arteriovenous oxygen difference.

Knowledge of the patient's preoperative blood pressure may be helpful when deciding on the lower limit of hypotension. In normotensive patients, cerebral ischemia is not expected to occur until mean CPP is decreased by 65% (a 40% reduction during which flow is unchanged because of autoregulation, plus a 25% reduction during which CBF falls linearly). Employing a conservative margin of safety by dividing the calculated allowable reduction in half, the minimum acceptable mean CBF would be 67% of the mean normal preoperative CPP. Common practice, however, dictates a greater reduction in CPP by assuming a lower safe blood pressure.

In normotensive individuals, CBF changes linearly with changes in P_aCO_2. At P_aCO_2 levels between 2.7 and 9.3 kPa (20 and 70 mmHg), a 0.13-kPa (1-mmHg) change in P_aCO_2 produces a corresponding 2.6% change in CBF. With progressive hypotension, this relation becomes progressively flatter, so that at a mean arterial blood pressure below 6.7 kPa (50 mmHg) CBF does not respond to changes in P_aCO_2.[103] However, clinical evidence in man indicates that cerebral vascular response to CO_2 continues at moderate levels of induced hypotension.[42,104] Therefore, unless indicated, hypocapnia should be avoided.

Based on animal studies using profound hypotension, it is often argued that one hypotensive drug may be better than another in preserving CBF and function. For example, it was found in dogs subjected to hypotension [CPP decreased from 10.7 to 4 kPa (80 to 30 mmHg)] that CBF was maintained with SNP, whereas with trimethaphan, it progressively decreased.[105] In another study, dysfunction of the blood–brain barrier was found to be more pronounced with SNP than with trimethaphan.[106]

Sodium nitroprusside can abolish cerebral autoregulation and increase CBF.[107] Increases in ICP are mostly seen during the early stages of SNP infusion,[108] especially during rapid infusion rates.[109] Hypocapnia tends to attenuate SNP-induced increases in ICP. Similar increases occur during nitroglycerin-induced hypotension.[110] In contrast, trimethaphan does not usually result in increased ICP except when intracranial compression is severe.[108]

Spinal cord blood flow and function With the popularity of induced hypotension for the operative correction of scoliosis, there has been concern that hypotension may decrease spinal cord blood flow and predispose to spinal cord injury, particularly during instrumentation.[111,112] The spinal cord exhibits autoregulation between mean pressures of 50 and 150 mmHg (6.7 and 20 kPa).[112] This allows normal spinal cord metabolism during hypotension. It has been suggested that the hypotension and direct pressure on the spinal cord may have an additive effect leading to impairment of spinal cord function.[113,114] Hypotension increases the effects of compression, whereas intentional hypertension reverses somatosensory-evoked potential (SSEPs) changes caused by compression. Changes in SSEPs at normotension have also been observed in patients undergoing spinal distraction, but have been resolved with slight increases in blood pressure. Based on findings in a canine study, trimethaphan, despite its favorable effect on hemodynamic responses, may not be the drug of choice for induced hypotension during scoliosis surgery.[115] However, these findings have not been documented in man.

The above studies do not document the deleterious effects of well-conducted normovolemic hypotension on spinal cord function. However, they emphasize that: (1) hemorrhagic hypotension could result in a severe reduction in spinal cord blood flow and an alteration in spinal cord function, (2) spinal distraction (even without hypotension) may result in an alteration in spinal cord function, (3) changes in SSEPs noted during hypotension may return to normal after blood pressure is increased, and (4) monitoring of spinal cord function is recommended whenever the spinal cord is potentially at risk of injury or interruption to its blood supply.

Clinically, anesthetic requirements are reduced during induced hypotension. In a canine study, the MAC of an inhalation anesthetic was found to be decreased by one-third.[116] If deep anesthesia is used during scoliosis surgery, a more prolonged time may be needed to successfully perform the wake-up test. Furthermore, these higher concentrations of the inhalation anesthetic can interfere with SSEP monitoring.

Renal circulation Renal blood flow, normally autoregulated over a range of arterial pressures between 80 and 180 mmHg (7.5 and 24 kPa), is abolished during anesthesia.[101] Decreases in renal blood flow occur with moderate decreases in arterial pressures. Below 60 mmHg (8 kPa), renal blood flow may decrease to the point where urine flow ceases. If induced hypotension does not decrease the renal blood flow below the critical value for the kidney, it is unlikely that renal damage will ensue. Renal medullar tissue oxygenation, an index of tissue viability, remains adequate despite a significant reduction in endogenous creatinine clearance during induced hypotension.[117] Since glomerular filtration rate is also not autoregulated during anesthesia, monitoring the urine output may be useful, especially during prolonged hypotension.

Hepatic and other regional blood flows A 40% decrease in arterial pressure by SNP results in a decrease in portal pressure (44%) and portal blood flow (25%) and an increase in hepatic arterial blood flow (13%).[118] Sodium nitroprusside decreases portal sinusoidal resistance, does not interfere with the ability of the liver to increase hepatic arterial blood flow (in conditions of insufficient portal circulation), and does not lead to hepatic hypoxia.

Induced hypotension and the dry operative field

Controversy surrounds the relative importance of blood pressure and CO (or blood flow at the operative site) in producing a dry operative field. Some authors maintain that a reduction in CO is essential to reduce bleeding and that, even when blood pressure is low, bleeding is not necessarily reduced unless there is a concomitant fall in CO.[17,90,119] Others found that blood pressure was the important factor in determining blood loss even if the blood flow was increased.[120,121]

A relatively dry operative field and improved operative conditions are not automatically achieved at a predetermined hypotensive level. The skillful anesthesiologist should ascertain that induced hypotension has achieved its objective and that improved operative conditions have in fact resulted. Decreased blood pressure or other hemodynamic adjustments may be needed to improve the operative field. In orthopedic operations where most bleeding is of venous origin, blood loss is less with nitroglycerin than with SNP at similar levels of hypotension.[28] Lower venous pressure associated with nitroglycerin may be partly responsible for the decreased blood loss. These findings have not been confirmed in children.[91]

The requirement of a relatively bloodless field in some procedures (scoliosis surgery) may depend on decreased CO, decreased blood flow at the operative site, or both. In contrast, when hypotension is used to facilitate surgery on large vessels, the reduced vessel tension, not necessarily the decreased blood flow, is required. Therefore, a technique that does not decrease CO may be preferred in these situations.

Both SNP and nitroglycerin infusions lead to prolongation of bleeding times in a dose-dependent manner. When the dose of SNP exceeds 3 $\mu g\,kg^{-1}\,min^{-1}$, a dose-related inhibition of platelet aggregation occurs.[122] The prolonged bleeding time with nitroglycerin seems to result from vasodilation and increased venous capacitance rather than inhibition of platelet aggregation.[123] In contrast, trimethaphan has no effect on platelet function.[124]

Safety factors of induced hypotension

Onset and degree of hypotension

Hypotension should be induced slowly over a period of 10–15 min. Time is needed for the cerebral, coronary, and renal vasculature to dilate maximally in the face of a lowered head of pressure, so as to maintain adequate perfusion. If the blood pressure is allowed to decrease too acutely, a sharp decrease in mixed venous oxygen saturation ($S_{\bar{v}}O_2$) and mixed venous oxygen content ($C_{\bar{v}}O_2$) may occur, reflecting inadequate tissue oxygenation.[125] Cardiac arrest and other complications during the induction of hypotension have been related to a too rapid decrease in pressure.

Because of individual variations, the blood pressure should not be lowered to a "predetermined" level. The desired level of hypotension depends on the age, condition, and posture and on the surgical requirement. The anesthesiologist should look for warning signs, including a very dry operative field and dark venous blood. These signs are indications to raise the blood pressure. Central venous or jugular venous oxygen tension below 4 kPa (30 mmHg) indicates tissue hypoxia, and the blood pressure should be increased. Unusually high $S_{\bar{v}}O_2$ may be an early sign of cyanide toxicity (if SNP is used). If the blood pressure falls too low, attempts should be made to raise the blood pressure by decreasing the head-up tilt, slowing the infusion of the hypotensive drug, lightening the anesthetic, and speeding up the intravenous fluids. Vasopressors are best avoided unless an uncontrollable decrease in pressure occurs.

Maintenance of near normal P_aCO_2 and acid–base balance

Unless hypocapnia is required to reduce the ICP, a near normal arterial carbon dioxide tension (P_aCO_2) should be maintained. Hypocapnia decreases the CO, decreases the coronary, cerebral, and spinal cord blood flows, may alter drug action (by altering blood pH), decreases both ionized calcium and serum potassium concentrations, causes leftward shift of the oxyhemoglobin dissociation curve, may increase the oxygen consumption, and may inhibit hypoxic pulmonary vasoconstriction (HPV). If adequate oxygenation is maintained, metabolic acidosis is not a feature of well-managed hypotensive technique.

The redistribution of pulmonary blood during induced hypotension may lead to an alteration in alveolar ventilation and perfusion ratios. Eckenhoff *et al.*[104] demonstrated that the alveolar dead space may increase to as much as 80% of the tidal volume in hypotensive adults in the head-up position with a raised airway pressure. Further studies in adults showed that the increase in alveolar dead space is less than previously thought.[126] Data from pediatric patients suggest that it does not increase during hypotension, even with the head-up tilt.[19] Others have found that hypotension with SNP caused no change in pulmonary dead space in adequately hydrated patients who were operated on in the prone position.[127]

The effect of induced hypotension on the magnitude of change in the alveolar dead space has been re-evaluated by assessing the arterial to end-tidal CO_2 partial pressure difference [$P_{(a-ET)}CO_2$].[128] The increase in $P_{(a-ET)}CO_2$ was noted only in older patients and was attributed to changes in pulmonary function that were due to age and pulmonary disease. The increase in alveolar dead space during induced hypotension may have been overemphasized and may be of significance only in elderly patients or when both PEEP and head-up tilt are used.

Oxygenation

An increase in the difference between alveolar and arterial oxygen tensions [$P_{(A-a)}O_2$] may occur during hypotension.[129,130] This may be explained by: (1) increased intrapulmonary shunt ($\dot{Q}_s/\dot{Q}_t$) and/or (2) decreased CO.

Increased intrapulmonary shunt Changes in functional residual capacity and closing volume during anesthesia and surgery contribute to airway closure, trapping of gas distal to the closure, and alveolar collapse. This local alveolar hypoxia is normally offset (to a degree) by reflex HPV that directs blood from hypoxic areas of the lung to adequately ventilated alveoli. Blunting or inhibition of this reflex has been noted with pulmonary hypertension, inhalation anesthetics, and vasodilators.[131] Although inhibition of HPV occurs with all vasodilators, it is greater with SNP than with nitroglycerin. Inhibition of HPV is associated with a decrease in pulmonary vascular resistance and pulmonary artery pressure and results in increased $\dot{Q}_s/\dot{Q}_t$.

Decreased cardiac output Decreased CO is accompanied by an increased extraction of oxygen by the tissues, resulting in decreased mixed venous oxygen tension ($P_{\bar{v}}O_2$) and $C_{\bar{v}}O_2$. Any portion of blood with decreased $C_{\bar{v}}O_2$ that passes through hypoventilated or nonventilated areas ($\dot{Q}_s/\dot{Q}_t$) will contribute to a greater decrease in arterial oxygen tension (P_aO_2). A decrease in CO during induced hypotension can result in a relevant decrease in P_aO_2, significant only in the presence of regional atelectasis.[132]

A high inspired oxygen fraction (F_IO_2) during induced hypotension is recommended. It tends to compensate for the portion of venous admixture contributed by ventilation–perfusion imbalance. It has been shown that during induced hypotension the lactate-pyruvate ratio does not increase when the P_aO_2 is kept above 40 kPa (300 mmHg),[133] and that the jugular bulb oxygen tension ($P_{JB}O_2$) rises significantly when F_IO_2 is altered from 0.4 to 1.0.[42] These findings stress the importance of using high F_IO_2, monitoring oxygenation, and avoiding profound decreases in CO.

Monitoring

In addition to routine monitoring (electrocardiograph, pulse oximetry, capnography), accurate recording of the blood pressure is essential during induced hypotension. Although various methods have been used, direct measurement via arterial cannulation allows continuous blood pressure measurements and arterial blood sampling. A variety of automated noninvasive devices may be used as a backup system for direct arterial pressure measurement. Central venous access permits measurement of central venous blood gases, which is a fairly accurate estimation of mixed venous blood gases.

Contraindications

Relative contraindications to induced hypotension include: (1) inexperience, (2) infants (see below), (3) pregnancy, (4) significant reduction in oxygen delivery, (5) systemic diseases compromising major organ function, (6) renal, cerebral, or coronary artery disease, (7) children with cardiac shunts, (8) patients with sickle cell disease, (9) uncorrected polycythemia, and (10) ganglionic blocking drugs in patients with narrow-angle glaucoma.

At one time, almost all systemic diseases were considered absolute contraindications to induced hypotension. With this stringent rule, many patients were denied the benefits of the technique. Many of these absolute contraindications are now regarded as relative. Inexperience and unfamiliarity with the technique constitute the most important contraindication. Age is not a contraindication to induced hypotension. Except for infants, in whom blood pressure may be difficult to measure accurately, the technique need not be withheld. Significant reduction in oxygen delivery to the tissues (including anemia, low fixed CO, and severe lung disease) may contraindicate induced hypotension. The presence of severe or acute cardiac, cerebral, or renal disease is likely to constitute a contraindication. In the presence of renal artery stenosis, hypotension may cause further decrease in the perfusion pressure to the kidney. In children with cardiac shunts, reduction of SVR may increase right-to-left shunting and cause hypoxemia. In patients with sickle cell disease, a decrease in $P_{\bar{v}}O_2$ [<4 kPa (30 mmHg)] due to decreased CO may trigger a crisis. Uncorrected polycythemia may increase sludging and thrombosis. Diabetes is not a contraindication to induced hypotension if blood sugar levels are controlled perioperatively. β-Adrenergic blockade may lower the blood sugar level through its actions on carbohydrate metabolism, although not seriously with the small doses given. The pupillary dilation caused by trimethaphan is short lived, but may be misinterpreted in the immediate postoperative period as cerebral ischemia.

Cyanide toxicity

Sodium nitroprusside has the molecular formula $Na_2[Fe(CN)_5NO] \times 2H_2O$. Although cyanide ($CN^-$) released from the SNP molecule is transformed mostly into relatively nontoxic products, it can be toxic and an excessive amount of CN^- can cause death.[134–136] There are four pathways for the disposal of this free CN^- (Fig. 11.3):

1 *Conversion to cyanomethemoglobin.* One of every five CN^- ions is normally converted to cyanomethemoglobin.
2 *Binding to cytochrome oxidase.* Cyanide binds to mitochondrial cytochrome oxidase, inhibiting oxidative phosphorylation. The subsequent anaerobic metabolism leads to acidosis.
3 *Conversion to cyanocobalamin.* In the presence of adequate hydroxocobalamin, CN^- becomes cyanocobalamin. This is probably not an important pathway in normal humans.
4 *Conversion to thiocyanate.* Transformation of CN^- to thiocyanate is the major metabolic pathway for CN^- in humans. It occurs in the liver and kidney, is catalyzed by the enzyme rhodenase, and requires B_{12a} as a cofactor. Added thiosulfate speeds the reaction, which is slowly reversible.

The mechanism of CN^- intoxication with SNP overdose is interference with aerobic metabolism, the major pathway of high-energy phosphate production.[134,137] Free CN^- inhibits the reoxidation of reduced cytochrome oxidase by oxygen, and, by crossing cell and mitochondrial membranes, rapidly inhibits the electron transport system. The consequences of CN^- intoxication are decreased oxygen utilization, decreased CO_2 production via inhibition of the Krebs cycle and increased production of anaerobic metabolites. Metabolic acidosis and deterioration in the central nervous and cardiovascular systems ensue. The combination of tissue hypoxia with normal or elevated $P_{\bar{v}}O_2$ levels is the hallmark of cytotoxic hypoxia produced by CN^-.[135]

Detection of cyanide toxicity

The clinical manifestations of CN^- intoxication during anesthesia[138] are shown in Table 11.4. In children, three abnormal responses have been recognized suggesting impending CN^- intoxication:[139] (1) a requirement for high doses of SNP (> 10 μg kg^{-1} min^{-1}), (2) tachyphylaxis which is apparent 30–60 min after the start of the infusion, and (3) resistance apparent within 5–10 min after the start of the infusion. The incidence of these abnormal responses may be as high as 30%. Tachyphylaxis may or may not be associated with concurrent metabolic acidosis. The severity of acidosis is usually proportional to the CN^- level. Cardiovascular collapse may ensue and may not respond to cardiopulmonary resuscitation, but a dramatic response may be seen after the administration of sodium thiosulfate.

Early laboratory recognition of CN^- intoxication poses difficulties because of the absence of specific tests. The lethal blood CN^- level in humans is approximately 500 μg dL^{-1}, whereas lethal blood thiocyanate levels can be as low as 340 μg dL^{-1}; however, this varies with the rate of CN^- release as well as with the total dose. Measurement of blood levels of CN^- or thiocyanate does not reflect the magnitude of CN^- released. Thus, nonspecific laboratory tests are relied upon as indicators of CN^- intoxication. The most sensitive metabolic indicators in a dog model of CN^- are blood pH, blood lactate (or lactate/pyruvate) levels, $P_{\bar{v}}O_2$ or $S_{\bar{v}}O_2$, sagittal sinus oxygen tension (reflecting decreased cerebral oxygen uptake), cerebral metabolic rate for oxygen, and brain lactate (or lactate/pyruvate).[135] Of these, arterial pH and gas tensions as well as $P_{\bar{v}}O_2$ or $P_{JB}O_2$ are easily obtained and should be measured when CN^- intoxication is suspected. "Bright" venous blood should alert the anesthesiologist to the possibility of early CN^- intoxication.

Prevention of cyanide toxicity

Cyanide intoxication associated with the use of SNP is a preventable complication. The total projected dose should not exceed 1.5 mg kg^{-1} for short exposures or 0.5 mg kg^{-1} h^{-1} for prolonged exposures. Infusion rates exceeding 10 μg kg^{-1} min^{-1} are contraindicated. When SNP infusion is first given, the initial rate should be adjusted to deliver 0.5–1 μg kg^{-1} min^{-1} by a microdrop or infusion pump. The patient's response to the infusion should be monitored constantly, especially during the first 30 min. Frequent (half-hourly) arterial acid–base determinations are recommended during SNP infusion. In addition, CN^- antidote therapy should be available. If either a constant requirement for administration of high doses of SNP or tachycardia is noted, a β-adrenergic blocking drug should be administered and the inhaled anesthetic concentration increased. A rapid response is usually noted after these measures are instituted, and the SNP dose can be decreased. If resistance is still detected (within 5–10 min), the infusion should be abandoned and a different hypotensive drug given.

Use of sodium nitroprusside during hypothermic cardiopulmonary bypass

Sodium nitroprusside infusions are occasionally given during cardiopulmonary bypass (CPB) to achieve uniform perfusion with cooling, to control blood pressure, and to speed rewarming. Concern over accumulation of CN^- with the administration of SNP during hypothermic CPB has been raised. Hypothesized causes include hypothermic inhibition

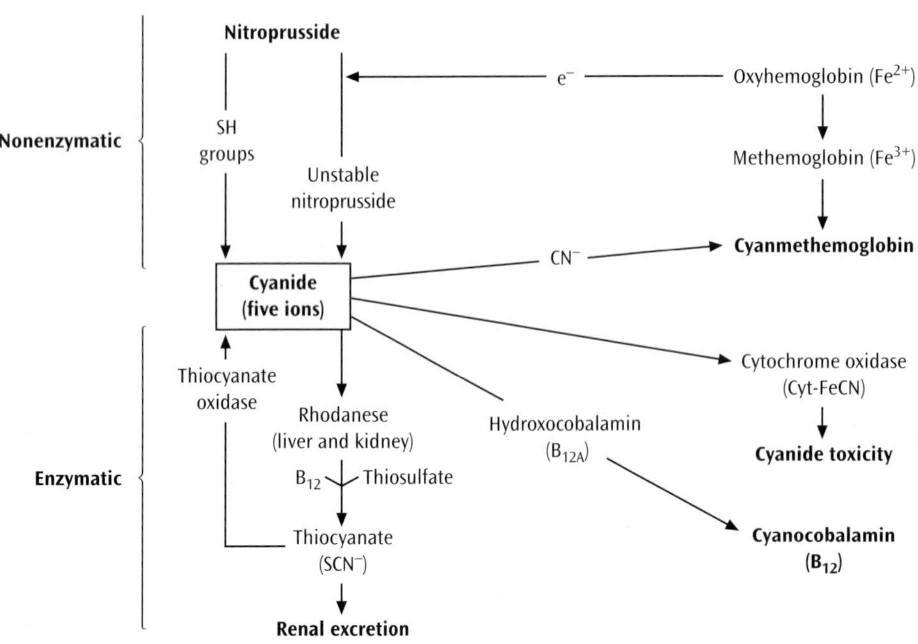

Figure 11.3 *Metabolism of sodium nitroprusside. (Modified with permission from Tinker and Michenfelder.[134])*

Table 11.4 *Clinical manifestation of cyanide toxicity*

Increased requirements for sodium nitroprusside
Metabolic acidemia
Progressive hypotension with narrow pulse pressure
Refractory hypotension unresponsive to fluids and vasopressors but responsive to thiosulfate
Cardiovascular collapse
Bright venous blood
Increased $S_{\bar{v}}O_2$ and $P_{\bar{v}}O_2$

From Salem.[194]

of the rhodanese enzyme system, insufficient thiosulfate levels, and decreased hepatic blood flow.[140,141] Alteration of hepatic blood flow is an unlikely cause because the decrease is only 20% during normal flow CPB.[142] Several studies have demonstrated the increase in CN^- levels with SNP infusion during hypothermic CPB in a dose-dependent manner, although with considerable patient-to-patient variability.[140–142] However, CN^- levels quickly returned to baseline after discontinuation of the infusion without an increase in SCN^- levels and without evidence of CN^- toxicity.

Treatment of cyanide toxicity

The rational approach in the treatment of CN^- toxicity is to prevent the CN^- from binding to cytochrome oxidase. Sodium thiosulfate can afford complete protection against CN^- and complete detoxification if three times more thiosulfate than CN^- is present. Sodium thiosulfate ensures the plentiful supply of sulfhydryl radicals needed to form thiocyanate from CN^-. Since the kidneys rapidly eliminate thiosulfate, a high level of plasma thiosulfate is best maintained by constant infusion. A bolus injection of 30 mg kg^{-1} followed by a continuous infusion of 60 mg kg^{-1} h^{-1} appears to be the most effective antidote against CN^- toxicity.[143]

Hydroxocobalamin (vitamin B_{12a}) has been advocated as a treatment for cyanide intoxication.[144,145] It prevents an increase in the CN^- concentration in erythrocytes when given prophylactically with large doses of SNP. The recommended dose is a 50-mg kg^{-1} bolus, plus 100 mg kg^{-1} h^{-1}.[143] In addition to these specific antidotes, correction of acidosis and fluid replacement are important in the management of CN^- intoxication. If the patient is bleeding, blood transfusion may help to "exchange the blood volume" and thus eliminate CN^-.

Complications

Data collected from single institutions where induced hypotension is commonly practiced offer more realistic assessments of morbidity and mortality. In a single series of over 25 000 procedures using induced hypotension, the technique posed no greater risks than those associated with normotensive techniques.[146] The complications observed in another study fit into one of the following categories:[125] (1) cardiac arrest and hypotension, (2) temporary or permanent neurologic deficits, (3) reactionary hemorrhage, and (4) failure of the technique. Critical analysis of the cases revealed that most complications could be attributed to faulty technique, including rapid induction of hypotension, maintenance of low pressure for long periods, excessive head-up tilt, underestimation of blood loss, failure to detect important warning signs, hypocapnia, hypoxemia, improper use of drugs, and improper selection of patients.[125]

Although there is no evidence that hemorrhage occurs more often after induced hypotension, the following procedures should be adopted: (1) allow a gradual return of pressure without vasopressors, (2) obtain reasonable hemostasis before closure, (3) apply pressure dressings whenever the procedure involves a wide superficial surface area, and (4) prevent coughing and straining in the early postoperative period.

Before the patient is transferred to the recovery room, airway patency and oxygenation should be assessed. Respiratory and cardiovascular monitoring should be continued. Attention should be paid to hemodynamic stability, adequacy of blood volume, temperature, and positioning. Head-up tilt is commonly used in the postoperative period, as long as it does not cause hypotension. Sudden movements and shivering should be avoided. Skilled nursing care is essential. If narcotics are needed, the dose requirement may be decreased and should be tailored to the individual patient.

PERIOPERATIVE HYPERTENSION

Perioperative hypertension is defined as a systolic pressure 5.3 kPa (40 mmHg) greater than baseline, 20% greater than the patient's normal value, or greater than 26.7 kPa (200 mmHg). Mechanisms of perioperative hypertension are likely to be multifactorial.[147–149] Causes of preoperative, intraoperative, and postoperative hypertension are listed in Table 11.5.

Preoperative hypertension

Essential hypertension

Essential hypertension is the commonest cause of perioperative hypertension. Hypertensive patients are at increased risk of perioperative hypertension. According to the World Health Organization, the accepted upper limit of normal blood pressure in the adult is 18.8/12 kPa (140/

Table 11.5 *Perioperative hypertension*

Preoperative
Primary (essential) hypertension
Secondary
Renal hypertension
Vascular
Pyelonephritis, glomerulonephritis
Diabetic nephropathy
Endocrinal hypertension
Pheochromocytoma
Hyperadrenocorticism (Cushing's disease)
Primary aldosteronism
Vascular
Coarctation of the aorta
Pregnancy-induced hypertension
Intracranial hypertension
Intraoperative
Light anesthesia
Tracheal intubation and extubation
Surgical stimulation
Catecholamines
Endogenous release secondary to light anesthesia, hypercapnia, and hypoxemia
Exogenous administration
Hypercarbia
Retention secondary to hypoventilation
Insufflation during laparoscopic procedures
Excessive CO_2 production
Postoperative
Postoperative pain
Emergence excitement
Shivering and hypothermia
Bladder distension
Hypoxemia and/or hypercapnia
Excessive fluid resuscitation
Preoperative withdrawal of antihypertensive medications

90 mmHg), rather than 21.3/12.6 kPa (160/95 mmHg). Systolic blood pressure levels above 18.7 kPa (140 mmHg) and diastolic levels above 12 kPa (90 mmHg) are associated with increased risk of cardiovascular disease. The degree of end-organ damage and increased mortality is related to both the severity of the hypertension and the length of disease without treatment.[150]

Classification of patients

Patients may be classified into three categories. (1) Normotensive patients can develop intraoperative hypertension secondary to activation of the sympathetic nervous system by separate stimuli such as anxiety, pain, light level of anesthesia, hypercapnia and hypoxemia. "Physiological" hypertension represents a warning sign and should encourage the anesthesiologist to treat the underlying cause. (2) Normotensive patients with left ventricular hypertrophy have an abnormal blood pressure increase during exercise and an exaggerated hypertensive response to "physiological" stimuli. (3) Essential hypertension, untreated or improperly treated, often shows marked hyperactivity to perioperative stress. Baseline blood pressure higher than 24/14.7 kPa (180/110 mmHg) is considered a contraindication to elective surgery.[147,151]

Morbidity

The most widely cited study of the risk for hypertensive patients who undergo anesthesia and surgery was published by Goldman and Caldera.[152] They found that 8% of patients who were normotensive before operation and not receiving any therapy had perioperative hypertensive episodes. In contrast, hypertensive patients who were normotensive when taking antihypertensive therapy, patients who remained hypertensive despite therapy, and patients with untreated hypertension had incidences of 27%, 25%, and 20% perioperative hypertension respectively.

Mild to moderate hypertension does not increase the risks of major morbid events. Hypertension may affect perioperative morbidity through the extent of end-organ damage. Left ventricular hypertrophy, which signifies a long-standing poorly controlled hypertension, can increase the risk of myocardial ischemia from imbalances in myocardial oxygen supply and demand.[147,151] The hemodynamic derangements of essential hypertension include increased SVR. Any stimulation that results in increased catecholamine release, such as tracheal intubation, results in a greater increase in SVR and blood pressure in the hypertensive patient. Furthermore, the increased thickness of the arterial wall contributes to a greater increase in blood pressure with vascular contraction, and a greater decrease in blood pressure with vascular relaxation, than in the normotensive patient.[148] In hypertensive patients, systemic vasoconstriction is associated with decreased blood volume. In addition, autoregulation curves are shifted to the right.[153] This applies to the cerebral, coronary, and renal circulation. Thus, acute lowering of the blood pressure in response to intravenous drugs and inhalation anesthetics must be safeguarded. A useful guide is that a 25% decrease in the mean arterial pressure reaches the lower limit of autoregulation, and that the systolic blood pressure should not be decreased to a level lower than the patient's diastolic pressure.

Patients with pre-existing hypertension appear to be at an increased risk of perioperative circulatory instability.[154–157] This may be related to decreased sensitivity of the baroreceptor reflex.[158] The arterial baroreflex operates as a rapid control system to adjust CO and SVR in order to maintain arterial pressure around a homeostatic "set point." Reduced baroreceptor sensitivity impairs the compensatory response and results in greater hemodynamic fluctuations. Improved baroreflex function and less perioperative hemodynamic variability are most likely closely related.

Preoperative administration of β-adrenergic antagonists can reduce intraoperative hemodynamic instability and myocardial ischemia in hypertensive patients. Preoperative administration of a single dose of a β-adrenergic blocking drug, such as atenolol, effectively attenuates increases in heart rate associated with tracheal intubation and emergence.[159] Mangano *et al.*[160] reported decreased mortality at 6 months after discharge when atenolol was administered intravenously (i.v.) (5 or 10 mg before and every 12 h after surgery) or orally (50 or 100 mg once per day up to 1 week after surgery) to patients with, or at risk for, coronary artery disease, including hypertension.,

Two of the most recent developments in antihypertensive drugs involve angiotensin II receptor antagonists and centrally acting drugs.[147,161] The prototype of the former drug class is losartan, which acts by displacing angiotensin II from the AT_1 receptor. The centrally acting antihypertensive drugs such as clonidine act on α_2-adrenoceptors and I_1-imiadazoline receptors located in the pontomedullary region, in or around the vasomotor center, and reduce sympathetic activity. Clonidine, an α_2-adrenergic agonist,[162] and β-adrenergic blocking drugs improve the sympathovagal balance by decreasing the basal sympathetic outflow and maintaining the vagally mediated baroreflex control of heart rate, resulting in better perioperative hemodynamic control. Patients receiving β-adrenergic blocking drugs or α_2-adrenergic agonists such as clonidine are at risk of perioperative hypertensive crisis or myocardial ischemia if the drug used is discontinued preoperatively.[163]

Guidelines for management of the hypertensive patient

1 Preoperative management of hypertensive patients should be optimized and maintained. A diastolic blood pressure above 14.7 kPa (110 mmHg) is considered a contraindication for elective surgery.
2 Pre-existing left ventricular hypertrophy and/or left ventricular failure are major risk factors.
3 Well-controlled hypertensive patients are at less risk of adverse cardiovascular events, during and after surgery, than are poorly controlled or untreated patients.
4 Intraoperative hypertension is usually a response to laryngoscopy and intubation or to surgical stimulation.
5 Sympathetic overactivity is the main cause of such adverse events; therefore, a β-adrenergic blocking drug or α_2-adrenergic agonist can be beneficial.
6 Epidural block during surgery is well tolerated hemodynamically, and can contribute to the suppression of excess sympathoadrenal activity.

Intraoperative hypertension

The most frequent causes of intraoperative hypertension are direct rigid laryngoscopy, tracheal intubation and extubation, and surgical stimuli under a light level of anesthesia.[147–149] These maneuvers provoke marked sympathetic and hormonal responses that may result in hypertension, tachycardia, and even cardiac arrhythmias. These undesirable hemodynamic responses are more exaggerated during a rapid sequence induction/intubation technique. The rise in blood pressure and heart rate occurs about 15 s after the start of laryngoscopy and becomes maximal after 30–45 s. Thus, limiting laryngoscopy to 15 s or less can minimize blood pressure elevation. Although transient, such responses may be potentially dangerous in patients with cardiac or cerebrovascular disease. Tracheal intubation-induced hypertension and tachycardia may be associated with decreases in left ventricular ejection fraction and myocardial ischemia,[164] particularly in patients with coronary artery disease.

Various pharmacologic drugs administered 1–2 min prior to laryngoscopy can blunt the stress response to laryngoscopy and intubation. These include low-dose fentanyl,[165,166] sufentanil (5–7 $\mu g\,kg^{-1}$),[167,168] or alfentanil (30–100 $\mu g\,kg^{-1}$)[164] 1 min before laryngoscopy; lidocaine (lignocaine) either intravenously (1.5 mg kg^{-1}) or topically,[169–172] α- or β-adrenergic blocking drugs such as esmolol (up to 1–2 mg kg^{-1}), or labetalol (0.15–0.3 mg kg^{-1}) or nitroglycerin (50–100 μg). SNP (0.5–1.0 μg kg^{-1} min^{-1}) may also be used for prophylaxis or for management of hypertensive crisis.

Drugs administered during a rapid sequence induction of anesthesia may influence the circulatory response to laryngoscopy and tracheal intubation. In patients undergoing emergency cesarean section and in asthmatic or hypovolemic patients, ketamine (1.5 mg kg^{-1}) may be used.[173] However, ketamine (sympathetic effect) can result in hypertension and tachycardia. Because propofol (15–2.5 mg kg^{-1}) causes slightly less variation in blood pressure than thiopental, greater depression of laryngeal reflexes, and less adduction of the vocal cords than thiopental, its use during rapid sequence induction has gained popularity.[174,175] Although etomidate (0.4 mg kg^{-1}) has minimal cardiac effects, its use has been associated with hypertension and tachycardia during laryngoscopy and with intubation when used for rapid sequence induction in patients with cardiac disease.[167]

Surgical stimulation under light levels of anesthesia can trigger perioperative hypertension. A balanced technique of anesthesia involving the use of nitrous oxide–oxygen, neuromuscular block, and an opioid may not effectively block the sensory input from the surgical field, and a higher concentration of an inhalation anesthetic may be necessary to prevent the rise of blood pressure. Combined epidural and light general anesthesia may effectively block the sensory input from the surgical site. Lumbar or thoracic segmented epidural blocks during abdominal or thoracic surgery are well tolerated hemodynamically, and contribute to the suppression of excess sympathoadrenal activity. Studies have suggested that intraoperative epidural anesthesia and postoperative analgesia have the potential to reduce significantly perioperative myocardial morbidity following major surgery in a high-risk patient population.[176]

Hydration of the hypertensive patient is indicated prior to induction of anesthesia because these patients may be vasoconstricted and volume depleted. Adequate hydration can attenuate the fluctuations in blood pressure often seen during anesthesia ("roller-coaster" anesthesia record). For best results, hydration overnight is preferred.

Acute postoperative hypertension

A history of hypertension is the most common factor associated with acute postoperative hypertension. Other causes include pain, emergence excitement, hypoxemia, hypercapnia, reaction to the tracheal tube, full bladder, hypothermia, shivering, preoperative withdrawal of antihypertensive medication, and administration of drugs that cause an increase in blood pressure. Relative hypervolemia, secondary to overhydration, can contribute to postoperative hypertension when the effects of general anesthesia, or the effects of sympathetic blockade following spinal or epidural anesthesia, have worn off.

Anticipation and prevention of postoperative hypertension, which usually occurs during emergence, extubation, and the first hour after general anesthesia, are important. The use of opioids and antihypertensive drugs such as low-dose labetalol or esmolol, before extubation, are usually effective in attenuating the hyperdynamic state. Nicardipine (bolus or continuous infusion) may be useful when β-adrenergic blocking drugs are contraindicated, such as in the presence of acute reactive airway disease.

The treatment of postoperative hypertension depends on the etiology, severity, and the clinical scenario.[148] The cause of hypertension should be sought and treated accordingly. The drug choice and methods of administration (bolus or intravenous infusion) depend on the urgency to control the blood pressure, the patient's heart rate, the cardiac status, the presence of other diseases, available means of blood pressure monitoring (direct vs. indirect), the site where the patient is being treated (i.e. operating room, recovery room or, intensive care unit), whether the patient is an inpatient or outpatient, and familiarity with the drug.[148,177] Aggressive management is warranted to protect vascular anastamoses or to prevent intracranial bleeding.

Scenarios associated with perioperative hypertension

Pregnancy-induced hypertension (PIH)

Pregnancy-induced hypertension occurs in 5–15% of all pregnancies and encompasses a range of disorders, including gestational hypertension, pre-eclampsia, and eclampsia.[178] The three principal mechanisms proposed for the etiology of PIH are vasospasm caused by an abnormal sensitivity of vascular smooth muscle to catecholamines, an antigen–antibody reaction between fetal and maternal tissues, and an imbalance in the production of thromboxane A and prostacylin leading to vasoconstriction.

Definitive treatment of PIH is delivery of the baby and placenta. Until delivery is possible, therapy should be directed at treating major organ dysfunction. Therapy includes magnesium, sulfate, and antihypertensive drugs such as hydralazine. A continuous lumbar epidural technique can be used for vaginal delivery after performing coagulation studies, and prehydration of the patient with 1–2 L of lactated Ringer's solution. If general anesthesia is administered, blood pressure increases following direct laryngoscopy and tracheal intubation. Hydralazine (10 mg i.v.) administered 10–15 min before induction of anesthesia, or nitroglycerin (1–2 mg kg^{-1}) just before laryngoscopy, can attenuate the hypertensive response.[179,180]

Carotid endarterectomy

Hemodynamic instability frequently follows carotid endarterectomy (CEA).[181] The carotid sinus reflex plays an important role in perioperative hemodynamic instability following CEA. Arterial mechanoreceptors are located in the media and adventitia of the common carotid artery near its bifurcation; they have a threshold of pressure below which they are inactive. In a normotensive patient, the threshold pressure is approximately 8.7–9.3 kPa (65–70 mmHg). The threshold is reset by hypertension. The activity of these receptors increases as blood pressure rises to about 24 kPa (180 mmHg). Impulses from these receptors are conducted via the carotid sinus nerve to the glossopharyngeal nerve on to the solitary tract nucleus, resulting in a lower sympathetic tone and an increase in vagal tone, with subsequent vasodilation and bradycardia. Hypotension associated with CEA may result from increased activity of the carotid sinus reflex; after CEA, the undamped pressure wave produces increased mechanoreceptor stimulation and reflex hypotension.

The mechanism of postoperative CEA hypertension is rather complex.[181] Probably, preoperative hypertension is the most important determinant. The carotid sinus is also believed to be involved to some extent. Patients who sustain damage to the carotid sinus nerve during dissection are at risk of perioperative hypertension. In addition, significant increases in jugular vein renin and norepinephrine are observed in patients developing hypertension, suggesting that intraoperative cerebral ischemia in patients with inadequate collateral cerebral circulation may also occur. Impaired cerebral autoregulation in chemically ischemic brain regions may predispose patients to an intracerebral hemorrhage after restoration of normal CBF. Defective autoregulation in the ipsilateral hemisphere has been demonstrated after CEA.[182,183] Therefore, blood pressure should be controlled to normal, or even below normal, levels after CEA.[148]

Aortic cross-clamping

Cross-clamping the descending aorta, particularly the thoracic segment, consistently increases the mean arterial pressure above the cross-clamp by approximately 40%. This rise can be complicated by a decrease in the cardiac index and an increase in pulmonary capillary wedge pressure. The arterial pressure below the cross-clamp decreases to approximately 15% of the value before clamping.[184] See Chapter 45.

Paradoxical hypertension after aortic coarctation repair

Surgical repair of coarctation of the aorta results in a syndrome of paradoxical hypertension in 10–60% of patients.[185] Two phases of hypertension have been observed: the immediate phase, which occurs during the first 24 h, and the delayed phase, occurring 2–3 days postoperatively.[186] The obstruction to flow in coarctation is distal to the ascending aortic and carotid baroreceptors and proximal to the blood supply to the kidneys and gastrointestinal tract. This situation can lead to unusual responses by the autonomic nervous system. The etiology of the immediate phase is believed to be a reflex in nature. Before the repair, the baroreceptors are adapted to a greater stretch because of the concomitant hypertension, but after the repair there is no longer the same degree of stretch. This is interpreted by the baroreceptors, as hypotension and reflex mechanisms act to increase the blood pressure.[186]

The etiology of the delayed phase is probably related both to a reflex and to humoral and mechanical factors. Stimulation of the sympathetic nerve fibers in the adventitia of the aorta results in the release of norepinephrine, causing vasoconstriction,[187] as well as stimulation of the juxtaglomerular cells activating the renin–angiotensin system.[188] Increased postoperative plasma norepinephrine may persist for as long as 6 months after coarctectomy.[187] Shunting of blood from the mesenteric arteries leads to mesenteric arteritis and is proportional to the degree of rise in blood pressure.

Liver transplantation

Hypertension during stage III, after revascularization, of liver transplantation is a frequent occurrence. It is associated with a decrease in vasopressin levels and an increase in atrial natriuretic peptide and plasma renin.[189,190] See Chapter 53.

Portal triad clamping

Portal triad clamping (PTC) causes significant hemodynamic changes in humans. SVR increases by 40%; mean arterial pressure increases by 15%; and cardiac index decreases by 15%. Combined occlusion of the portal vein and hepatic artery reduces venous return to the heart and decreases CO. A neurogenic-induced vasoconstriction elicited in the splanchnic venous system secondary to surgical stimulation may be a major factor in the increase in SVR and mean arterial pressure.[191]

Pheochromocytoma

Pheochromocytoma is a catecholamine-secreting tumor, which originates in the adrenal medulla or in chromoffin tissue along the paravertebral sympathetic chain. More than 95% of all pheochromocytomas are found in the abdominal cavity, and about 90% originate from the adrenal medulla. Hypertensive crisis during surgery is frequent if the patient is inadequately prepared by α-adrenergic blocking drugs. Hypertension can occur during laryngoscopy and intubation of the trachea. However, the most dramatic increase in blood pressure occurs during manipulation of the tumor.[192] See Chapter 54.

Autonomic hyper-reflexia

Autonomic hyper-reflexia appears in patients with chronic spinal cord transection. The reflex response can be initiated by cutaneous or visceral stimulation below the level of spinal cord transection. Distension of a hollow viscous such as the bladder is a common stimulus. The incidence of autonomic hyper-reflexia depends on the level of transection; 85% of patients with cord transection above T6 will exhibit the reflex. Surgery is a potent stimulus to the development of autonomic hyper-reflexia. Impulses will elicit reflex sympathetic activity over the splanchnic outflow tract, resulting in excessive vasoconstriction below the level of cord transection associated with hypertension and reflex bradycardia.[193]

REFERENCES

1. Mclintic AJ, Todd JG. Induced hypotension. In: Healy TEJ, Cohen PJ (eds). *Wylie and Churchill-Davidson's A Practice of Anesthesia*, 6th edn. London: E. Arnold, 1995.
2. Relton JE, Hall JE. An operation frame for spinal fusion. A new apparatus designed to reduce haemorrhage during operation. *J Bone Joint Surg (Br)* 1967; **49:** 327.
3. Hatch PD. Surgical and anaesthetic considerations in transurethral resection of the prostate. *Anaesth Intensive Care* 1987; **15:** 203.
4. Agin C. Anesthesia for transurethral prostate surgery. *Int Anesthesiol Clin* 1993; **31:** 25.
5. McGowan SW, Smith GFN. Anaesthesia for transurethral prostatectomy. *Anaesthesia* 1980; **35:** 847.
6. Nielsen KK, Andersen K Asbjorn J, *et al.* Blood loss in transurethral prostatectomy: epidural versus general anaesthesia. *Int Urol Nephrol* 1987; **19:** 287.
7. Smyth R, Cheng D, Asokumar B, Chung F. Coagulopathies in patients after transurethral resection of the prostate: spinal versus general anesthesia. *Anesth Analg* 1995; **81:** 680.
8. McKenzie PJ, Wishhart HY Dewar KMS, *et al.* Comparison of the effects of spinal anaesthesia and general anaesthesia on postoperative oxygenation and perioperative mortality. *Br J Anaesth* 1980; **52:** 49.
9. Gilstrap LC III, Hauth JC, Hankins GDV, Patterson AR. Effect of type of anesthesia on blood loss at cesarean section. *Obstet Gynecol* 1987; **69:** 328.
10. Hood DD, Holubec DM. Elective repeat cesarian section. *J Reprod Med* 1990; **35:** 368.
11. Andrews WW, Ramin SM, Maberry MC, *et al.* Effect of type of anesthesia on blood loss at elective repeat cesarean section. *Am J Perinatol* 1992; **9:** 197.
12. Sorenson RM, Pace NL. Anesthetic techniques during surgical repair of femoral neck fractures: a meta-analysis. *Anesthesiology* 1992; **77:** 1095.
13. Modig J, Borg T, Karlström G, *et al.* Thromboembolism after total hip replacement: role of epidural and general anesthesia. *Anesth Analg* 1983; **62:** 174.
14. Hole A, Terjesen T, Breivik H. Epidural versus general anesthesia for total hip arthroplasty in elderly patients. *Acta Anaesthesiol Scand* 1980; **24:** 279.
15. Chin SP, Abou-Madi MN, Eurin B, *et al.* Blood loss in total hip replacement: extradural v. phenoperidine analgesia. *Br J Anaesth* 1982; **54:** 491.
16. Warren JV. The physiology of the giraffe. *Sci Am* 1974; **231:** 96.
17. Salem MR, Toyama T, Wong AY, *et al.* Haemodynamic responses to induced arterial hypotension in children. *Br J Anaesth* 1978; **50:** 489.
18. Hainsworth R. Arterial blood pressure. In: Enderby GEH (ed.). *Hypotensive Anaesthesia*. London: Churchill Livingstone, 1985.
19. Salem MR, Wong AY, Bennett EJ, Mani M. Deliberate hypotension in infants and children. *Anesth Analg* 1974; **53:** 975.
20. Cushing H. *Tumors of the Nervus Acusticus*. Philadelphia: WB Saunders, 1917.
21. Gardner WS. The control of bleeding during operation by induced hypotension. *JAMA* 1946; **132:** 572.
22. Enderby GEH. Historical review of the practice of deliberate hypotension. In: Enderby GEH (ed.). *Hypotensive Anaesthesia*. London: Churchill Livingstone, 1985.
23. Enderby GEH. Controlled hypotension with hypotensive drugs and posture to reduce bleeding in surgery. Preliminary results with pentamethonium iodide. *Lancet* 1950; **1:** 1145.
24. Hampton LJ, Little DM. Complications associated with the use of "controlled hypotension" in anesthesia. *Arch Surg* 1953; **67:** 549.
25. Moraca PP, Bitte EM, Hale DE, *et al.* Clinical evaluation of sodium nitroprusside as a hypotensive agent. *Anesthesiology* 1962; **23:** 193.
26. Hellewell J, Potts MW. Propranolol during controlled hypotension. *Br J Anaesth* 1966; **38:** 794.
27. Salem MR, Ivankovich AD. The place of beta adrenergic blocking drugs in the deliberate induction of hypotension. *Anesth Analg* 1970; **49:** 427.

28. Fahmy NR. Nitroglycerine as a hypotensive drug during general anesthesia. *Anesthesiology* 1978; **49:** 17.
29. Scott DB, Buckley FP, Littlewood DG, *et al.* Circulatory effects of labetalol during halothane anaesthesia. *Anaesthesia* 1978; **33:** 145.
30. McNeil TW, DeWald RL, Kuo KN, *et al.* Controlled hypotensive anesthesia in scoliosis surgery. *J Bone Joint Surg (Am)* 1974; **56:** 1167.
31. Larson AG. Deliberate hypotension. *Anesthesiology* 1964; **24:** 682.
32. Dalal FY, Bennett EJ, Salem MR, El-Etr AA. Anaesthesia for coarctation. A new classification for rational anaesthetic management. *Anaesthesia* 1974; **29:** 704.
33. Zaidan JR, Guffin AV, Perdue G, *et al.* Hemodynamics of intravenous nitroglycerin during aortic clamping. *Arch Surg* 1982; **117:** 1285.
34. Gelman S, McDowell H, Varner PD, *et al.* The reason for cardiac output reduction following aortic-crossclamping. *Am J Surg* 1988; **155:** 578.
35. Gelman S. The pathophysiology of aortic cross-clamping and unclamping. *Anesthesiology* 1995; **82:** 1026.
36. Lagerkranser M, Gordon E, Rudehill A. Cardiovascular effects of sodium nitroprusside in cerebral aneurysm surgery. *Acta Anaesthesiol Scand* 1980; **24:** 426.
37. Lam AM, Gelb AW. Cardiovascular effects of isoflurane-induced hypotension for cerebral aneurysm surgery. *Anesth Analg* 1983; **62:** 742.
38. Sood S, Jayalaxmi TS, Vijayaraghavan S, Nundy S. Use of sodium nitroprusside induced hypotension for reducing blood loss in patients undergoing lienorenal shunts for portal hypertension. *Br J Anaesth* 1987; **74:** 1036.
39. Adams AP. Techniques of vascular control for deliberate hypotension during surgery. *Br J Anaesth* 1975; **47:** 777.
40. Salem MR. Therapeutic uses of ganglionic blocking drugs. *Int Anesthesiol Clin* 1978; **16:** 171.
41. Green DW. Techniques for deliberate hypotension. In: Enderby GEH (ed.). *Hypotensive Anaesthesia*. London: Churchill Livingstone, 1985.
42. Salem MR, Kim Y, Shaker M. The effect of alteration of inspired oxygen concentration on jugular-bulb oxygen tension during deliberate hypotension. *Anesthesiology* 1970; **33:** 358.
43. Patel H. Experience with the cerebral function monitor during deliberate hypotension. *Br J Anaesth* 1981; **53:** 639.
44. Thompson GE, Miller RD, Stevens WC, Murray WR. Hypotensive anesthesia for total hip arthroplasty: a study of blood loss and organ function (brain, heart, liver, kidney). *Anesthesiology* 1978; **48:** 91.
45. Diaz JH, Lockhart CH. Hypotensive anaesthesia for craniectomy in infancy. *Br J Anaesth* 1979; **51:** 233.
46. Calverley RK, Smith NT, Jones CW, *et al.* Ventilatory and cardiovascular effects of enflurane anesthesia during spontaneous ventilation in man. *Anesthesiology* 1978; **57:** 610.
47. Merin RG. Are the myocardial functional, metabolic effects of isoflurane really different from those of halothane and enflurane? *Anesthesiology* 1981; **55:** 398.
48. Van Aken H, Cottrell JE. Hypotensive anesthesia and its effect on the cardiovascular system. In: Altura BM, Halevey S (eds). *Cardiovascular Actions of Anesthetics and Drugs Used in Anesthesia*, 5th edn. Basel: Karger, 1986.
49. Harkin CP, Pagel PS, Kersten JR, *et al.* Direct negative inotropic and lusitropic effects of sevoflurane. *Anesth Analg* 1994; **81:** 156.
50. Prys-Roberts C, Lloyd JW, Fisher A, *et al.* Deliberate profound hypotension induced with halothane. Studies of haemodynamics and pulmonary gas exchange. *Br J Anaesth* 1974; **46:** 105.
51. Grosslight K, Forster R, Colohan AR, Bedford RF. Isoflurane for neuroanesthesia. Risk factors for increases in intracranial pressure. *Anesthesiology* 1985; **65:** 533.
52. Madsen JB, Cold GE, Hansen ES, *et al.* Cerebral blood flow and metabolism during isoflurane-induced hypotension in patients subjected to surgery for cerebral aneurysms. *Br J Anaesth* 1987; **59:** 1204.
53. Van Aken H, Fitch W, Graham DI, *et al.* Cardiovascular and cerebrovascular effects of isoflurane-induced hypotension in the baboon. *Anesth Analg* 1986; **65:** 565.
54. Newberg LA, Milde JH, Milchenfelder JD. Systemic and cerebral effects of isoflurane-induced hypotension in dogs. *Anesthesiology* 1984; **60:** 541.
55. Newman B, Gelb AW, Lam AM. The effect of isoflurane-induced hypotension on cerebral blood flow and cerebral metabolic rate for oxygen in humans. *Anesthesiology* 1986; **64:** 307.
56. Bendo AA, Kozlowski PB, Capuano C, *et al.* Cerebral edema formation in dogs following hypotension induced with isoflurane and labetalol. *Acta Anaesthesiol Belg* 1993; **44:** 103.
57. Enlund M, Ahlstedt B, Revenas B, *et al.* Adverse effects on the brain in connection with isoflurane-induced hypotensive anesthesia. *Acta Anaesthesiol Scand* 1989; **33:** 413.
58. Enlund M, Mentell O, Engström C, *et al.* Occurrence of adenylate kinase in cerebrospinal fluid after isoflurane anesthesia and orthognathic surgery. *Upsala J Med Sci* 1996; **101:** 97.
59. Toivonen J, Virtanen H, Kaukinen S. Labetalol attenuates the negative effects of deliberate hypotension induced by isoflurane. *Acta Anaesthesiol Scand* 1992; **36:** 84.
60. Longnecker DE. The microvascular response to hypotensive drugs. In: Enderby GEH (ed.). *Hypotensive Anaesthesia*. London: Churchill Livingstone, 1985.
61. Fahmy NR, Soter NA. Effects of trimethaphan on arterial blood histamine and systemic hemodynamics in humans. *Anesthesiology* 1985; **62:** 562.
62. Palmer RM, Ferrige AG, Moncada S. Nitric oxide release accounts for the biological activity of endothelium-derived relaxing factor. *Nature* 1987; **327:** 524.
63. Rees DD, Palmer RM, Hodson HF. A specific inhibitor of nitric oxide formation from L-arginine attenuates endothelium-dependent relaxation. *Br J Pharmacol* 1989; **96:** 418.
64. Rees DD, Palmer RMJ, Moncada S. Role of endothelium-derived nitric oxide in regulation of blood pressure. *Proc Natl Acad Sci USA* 1989; **86:** 3375.
65. Moncada S, Palmer RMJ, Higgs EA. Nitric oxide: physiology, pathophysiology, and pharmacology. *Pharmacol Rev* 1991; **43:** 110.
66. Kruszyna H, Kruszyna R, Smith RP, Wilcox DE. Red blood cells generate nitric oxide from directly acting, nitrogenous vasodilators. *Toxicol Appl Pharmacol* 1987; **91:** 429.
67. Rich GF, Lowson SM, Johns RA, *et al.* Inhaled nitric oxide selectively decreases pulmonary vascular resistance without impairing oxygenation during one-lung ventilation in patients undergoing cardiac surgery. *Anesthesiology* 1994; **80:** 57.
68. Sollevi A, Lagerkranser M, Irestedt L, *et al.* Controlled hypotension with adenosine in cerebral aneurysm surgery. *Anesthesiology* 1984; **61:** 400.
69. Lagerkranser M, Irestedt L, Sollevi A, Andreen M. Central and splanchnic hemodynamics in the dog during controlled hypotension with adenosine. *Anesthesiology* 1984; **60:** 547.
70. Crystal GJ, Rooney MW, Salem MR. Myocardial blood flow and oxygen consumption during isovolemic hemodilution alone and in combination with adenosine-induced controlled hypotension. *Anesth Analg* 1988; **67:** 539.
71. Van Aken H, Puchstein C, Anger C, *et al.* Changes in intracranial pressure and compliance during adenosine triphosphate-induced hypotension in dogs. *Anesth Analg* 1984; **63:** 381.
72. Carlson LA, Ekelund LG, Orö L. Circulatory and respiratory effects of different doses of prostaglandin E_1 in man. *Acta Physiol Scand* 1969; **75:** 161.
73. Goto F, Otani E, Kato S, Fujita T. Prostaglandin E_1 as a hypotensive drug during general anesthesia. *Anaesthesia* 1982; **37:** 530.
74. Blau WS, Kafer ER, Anderson JA. Esmolol is more effective than sodium nitroprusside in reducing blood loss during orthognathic surgery. *Anesth Analg* 1992; **75:** 172.
75. Boezaart AP, van der Merwe,J Coetzee A. Comparison of sodium nitroprusside- and esmolol-induced controlled hypotension for functional endoscopic sinus surgery. *Can J Anaesth* 1995; **42:** 373.
76. Ornstein E, Young WL, Ostapkovich N, *et al.* Deliberate hypotension in patients with intracranial or arteriovenous malformations: esmolol compared with isoflurane and sodium nitroprusside. *Anesth Analg* 1991; **72:** 639.
77. Edmondson R, Del Valle O, Shah N, *et al.* Esmolol for potentiation of nitroprusside-induced hypotension: impact on the cardiovascular, adrenergic, and renin–angiotensin systems in man. *Anesth Analg* 1989; **69:** 202.
78. Menkhaus PG, Reves JG, Kissin I, *et al.* Cardiovascular effects of esmolol in anesthetized humans. *Anesth Analg* 1985; **64:** 327.
79. Hoffman BB, Lefkowitz RJ. Adrenergic receptor antagonists. In: Goodman Gilman A, Rall TW, Nies AS, Taylor P (eds). *Goodman and Gilman's The Pharmacological Basis of Therapeutics*, 8th edn. New York: McGraw-Hill, 1990.
80. Fahmy NR, Bottros MR, Charchafieh J, *et al.* A randomized comparison of labetalol and nitroprusside for induced hypotension. *J Clin Anesth* 1989; **1:** 409.
81. Goldberg ME, McNulty SE, Azad SS, *et al.* A comparison of labetalol and nitroprusside for inducing hypotension during major surgery. *Anesth Analg* 1990; **70:** 537.
82. Flamm ES, Adams Jr HP, Beck DW, *et al.* Dose-escalation study of intravenous nicardipine in patients with aneurysmal subarachnoid hemorrhage. *J Neurosurg* 1988; **68:** 393.

83. Bernard J-M, Passuti N, Pinaud M. Long-term hypotensive technique with nicardipine and nitroprusside during isoflurane anesthesia for spinal surgery. *Anesth Analg* 1992; **75:** 179.
84. Hersey SL, O'Dell NE, Lowe S. Nicardipine versus nitroprusside for controlled hypotension during spinal surgery in adolescents. *Anesth Analg* 1997; **84:** 1239.
85. James DJ, Bedford RF. Hydralazine for controlled hypotension during neurosurgical operations. *Anesth Analg* 1982; **61:** 1016.
86. Aronson S, Goldberg LI, Roth S, *et al.* Preservation of renal blood flow during hypotension induced by fenoldopam in dogs. *Can J Anaesth* 1990; **37:** 380.
87. Khambatta HJ, Stone JG, Kahn E. Propranolol alters renin release during nitroprusside induced hypotension and prevents hypertension on discontinuation of nitroprusside. *Anesth Analg* 1981; **60:** 569.
88. Knight PR, Lane GA, Hensinger RN, *et al.* Catecholamine and renin–angiotensin response during hypotensive anesthesia induced by sodium nitroprusside or trimethaphan camsylate. *Anesthesiology* 1983; **59:** 248.
89. Fahmy NR, Mihelakos PT, Battit GE, Lappas DG. Propranolol prevents hemodynamic and humoral events after abrupt withdrawal of nitroprusside. *Clin Pharmacol Ther* 1984; **36:** 470.
90. Knight PR, Lane GA, Nicholls MG, *et al.* Hormonal and hemodynamic changes induced by pentolinium and propranolol during surgical correction of scoliosis. *Anesthesiology* 1980; **53:** 127.
91. Yaster M, Simmons RS, Tolo VT, *et al.* A comparison of nitroglycerin and nitroprusside for inducing hypotension in children: a double-blind study. *Anesthesiology* 1986; **65:** 175.
92. Gavras H, Kremer D, Brown JJ, *et al.* Angiotensin and norepinephrine induced myocardial lesions: experimental and clinical studies in rabbits and man. *Am Heart J* 1975; **89:** 321.
93. Delaney TJ, Miller Jr ED. Rebound hypertension after sodium nitroprusside prevented by saralasin in rats. *Anesthesiology* 1980; **52:** 154.
94. Fahmy NR, Gavras HP. Impact of captopril on hemodynamic and hormonal effects of nitroprusside. *J Cardiovasc Pharmacol* 1985; **7:** 869.
95. Wildsmith JA, Sinclair CJ, Thorn J, *et al.* Haemodynamic effects of induced hypotension with a nitroprusside-trimethaphan mixture. *Br J Anaesth* 1983; **55:** 381.
96. Fahmy NR. Nitroprusside vs. a nitroprusside-trimethaphan mixture for induced hypotension: hemodynamic effects and cyanide release. *Clin Pharmacol Ther* 1985; **37:** 264.
97. Woodcock TE, Millard RK, Dixon J, Prys-Roberts C. Clonidine premedication for isoflurane-induced hypotension. *Br J Anaesth* 1988; **60:** 388.
98. Maroof M, Khan RM, Bhatti TH. Clonidine premedication for induced hypotension with total intravenous anaesthesia for middle ear microsurgery. *Can J Anaesth* 1994; **41:** 164.
99. Fahmy NR, Laver MB. Hemodynamic response to ganglionic blockade with pentolinium during N_2O-halothane anesthesia in man. *Anesthesiology* 1976; **44:** 6.
100. Crystal GJ, Salem MR. Myocardial and systemic hemodynamics during isovolemic hemodilution alone and combined with nitroprusside-induced controlled hypotension. *Anesth Analg* 1991; **72:** 227.
101. Strunin L. Organ perfusion during controlled hypotension. *Br J Anaesth* 1975; **47:** 793.
102. Lassen NA. Physiology of cerebral blood flow. *Br J Anaesth* 1976; **48:** 719.
103. Harper AM, Glass HI. Effects of alterations in the arterial carbon dioxide tension on the blood flow through the cerebral cortex at normal and low arterial blood pressures. *J Neurol Neurosurg Psychiatry* 1965; **28:** 449.
104. Eckenhoff JE, Enderby GEH, Larson A, *et al.* Human cerebral circulation during deliberate hypotension and head-up tilt. *J Appl Physiol* 1963; **18:** 1130.
105. Stoyka WW, Schutz H. The cerebral response to sodium nitroprusside and trimetaphan controlled hypotension. *Can Anaesth Soc J* 1975; **22:** 275.
106. Ishikawa T, Funatsu N, Okamoto K, *et al.* Blood–brain barrier function following drug-increased hypotension in the dog. *Anesthesiology* 1983; **59:** 526.
107. Ivankovich AD, Miletich DJ, Albrecht RF, Zahed B. Sodium nitroprusside and cerebral blood flow in the anesthetized and unanesthetized goat. *Anesthesiology* 1976; **44:** 21.
108. Turner JM, Powell D, Gibson RM, McDowall DG. Intracranial pressure changes in neurosurgical patients during hypotension induced with sodium nitroprusside or trimetaphan. *Br J Anaesth* 1977; **49:** 419.
109. Marsh ML, Aidinis SJ, Naughton KVH, *et al.* The technique of nitroprusside administration modifies the intracranial pressure response. *Anesthesiology* 1979; **51:** 538.
110. Rogers MC, Hamburger C, Owen K, Epstein MH. Intracranial pressure in the cat during nitroglycerin-induced hypotension. *Anesthesiology* 1979; **51:** 227.
111. Grundy BL, Nash Jr CL, Brown RH. Arterial pressure manipulation alters spinal cord function during correction of scoliosis. *Anesthesiology* 1981; **54:** 249.
112. Jacobs HK, Lieponis JV, Bunch WH, *et al.* The influence of halothane and nitroprusside on canine spinal cord hemodynamics. *Spine* 1982; **7:** 35.
113. Brodkey JS, Richards DE, Blasingame JP, Nulsen FE. Reversible spinal cord trauma in cats: additive effects of direct pressure and ischemia. *J Neurosurg* 1972; **37:** 591.
114. Ponte A. Postoperative paraplegia due to hypercorrection of scoliosis and drop of blood pressure. *J Bone Joint Surg (Am)* 1974; **56:** 444.
115. Kling TF, Wilton N, Hensinger RN, Knight PR. The influence of trimethaphan (Arfonad)-induced hypotension with and without spine distraction on canine spinal cord blood flow. *Spine* 1986; **11:** 219.
116. Rao TLK, Jacobs K, Salem MR, Santos P. Deliberate hypotension and anesthetic requirements of halothane. *Anesth Analg* 1981; **60:** 513.
117. Behnia R, Martin A, Koushanpour E, Brunner EA. Trimethaphan-induced hypotension: effect on renal function. *Can Anaesth Soc J* 1982; **29:** 581.
118. Gelman S, Ernst EA. Hepatic circulation during sodium nitroprusside infusion in the dog. *Anesthesiology* 1978; **49:** 182.
119. Enderby GEH. Blood pressure and bleeding. In: Enderby GEH (ed.). *Hypotensive Anaesthesia*. London: Churchill Livingstone, 1985.
120. Amaranath L, Cascorbi HF, Singh-Amaranath AV, Frankmann DB. Relation of anesthesia to total hip replacement and control of operative blood loss. *Anesth Analg* 1975; **54:** 641.
121. Sivarajan M, Amory DW, Everett GB, Buffington C. Blood pressure, not cardiac output, determines blood loss during induced hypotension. *Anesth Analg* 1980; **59:** 203.
122. Hines R, Barash PG. Infusion of sodium nitroprusside induces platelet dysfunction. *Anesthesiology* 1989; **70:** 611.
123. Lichtenthal PR, Rossi EC, Louis G, *et al.* Dose-related prolongation of the bleeding time by intravenous nitroglycerin. *Anesth Analg* 1985; **64:** 30.
124. Hines R. Preservation of platelet function during trimethaphan infusion. *Anesthesiology* 1990; **72:** 834.
125. Salem MR. Deliberate hypotension is a safe and accepted anesthetic technique. In: Eckenhoff JE (ed.). *Controversy in Anesthesiology*. Philadelphia: WB Saunders, 1979.
126. Askrog VF, Pender JW, Eckenhoff JE. Changes in physiological dead space during deliberate hypotension. *Anesthesiology* 1964; **25:** 774.
127. Khambatta HJ, Stone JG, Matteo RS. Effect of sodium nitroprusside-induced hypotension on pulmonary deadspace. *Br J Anaesth* 1982; **54:** 1197.
128. Salem MR, Paulissian R, Joseph NJ, *et al.* Effect of deliberate hypotension on arterial to peak expired carbon dioxide tension difference. *Anesth Analg* 1988; **67:** S194.
129. Stone JG, Khambatta HJ, Matteo RS. Pulmonary shunting during anesthesia with deliberate hypotension. *Anesthesiology* 1976; **45:** 508.
130. Casthely PA, Lear S, Cottrell JE, Lear E. Intrapulmonary shunting during induced hypotension. *Anesth Analg* 1982; **61:** 231.
131. Benumof JL, Wahrenbrock EA. Blunted hypoxic pulmonary constriction by increased lung vascular pressure. *J Appl Physiol* 1975; **38:** 846.
132. Cheney FW, Colley PS. The effect of cardiac output on arterial blood oxygenation. *Anesthesiology* 1980; **52:** 496.
133. Robinson JS. Hypotension without hypoxia. *Int Anesthesiol Clin* 1967; **5:** 467.
134. Tinker JH, Michenfelder JD. Sodium nitroprusside: pharmacology toxicology and therapeutics. *Anesthesiology* 1976; **45:** 340.
135. Michenfelder JD. Cyanide release from sodium nitroprusside in the dog. *Anesthesiology* 1977; **46:** 196.
136. Verner IR. Techniques for deliberate hypotension: direct acting vasodilators. In: Enderby GEH (ed.). *Hypotensive Anaesthesia*. London: Churchill Livingstone, 1985.
137. Michenfelder JD, Tinker JH. Cyanide toxicity and thiosulfate protection during chronic administration of sodium nitroprusside in the dog. *Anesthesiology* 1977; **47:** 441.
138. Davies DW, Greiss L, Kadar D, Steward DJ. Sodium nitroprusside in children: observations on metabolism during normal and abnormal responses. *Can Anaesth Soc J* 1975; **22:** 553.
139. Greiss L, Tremblay NAG, Davies DW. The toxicity of sodium nitroprusside. *Can Anaesth Soc J* 1976; **54:** 249.
140. Moore RA, Geller EA, Gallagher JD, Clark DL. Effect of hypothermic cardiopulmonary bypass on nitroprusside metabolism. *Clin Pharmacol Ther* 1985; **37:** 680.
141. Lundquist P, Rosling H, Tyden H. Cyanide release from sodium nitroprusside during coronary bypass in hypothermia. *Acta Anaesthesiol Scand* 1989; **33:** 686.
142. Przybylo, HJ Stevenson GW, Schanbacher P, *et al.* Sodium nitroprusside

metabolism in children during hypothermic cardiopulmonary bypass. *Anesth Analg* 1995; **81:** 952

143. Ivankovich AD, Braverman B, Kanuru RP, *et al.* Cyanide antidotes and methods of their administration in dogs. *Anesthesiology* 1980; **52:** 210.
144. Posner MA, Tobey RE, McElroy H. Hydroxocobalamin therapy of cyanide intoxication in guinea pigs. *Anesthesiology* 1976; **44:** 157.
145. Cottrell JE, Casthely P, Brodie JD, *et al.* Prevention of nitroprusside-induced cyanide toxicity with hydroxocobalamin. *N Engl J Med* 1978; **298:** 809.
146. Lindop MJ. Complications and morbidity of controlled hypotension. *Br J Anaesth* 1975; **47:** 799.
147. Skarvan K. Perioperative hypertension: new strategies for management. *Curr Opin Anesthesiol* 1998; **11:** 29.
148. Domino KB. Perioperative hypertension. *Am J Anesthesiol* 1999; **26:** 259
149. Rose DK, Cohen MM, DeBoer DP. Cardiovascular events in the postanesthesia care unit. *Anesthesiology* 1996; **94:** 771.
150. The Sixth Report of the Joint National Committee on Prevention, Detection, Evaluation and Treatment Of High Blood Pressure. *Arch Intern Med* 1988; **148:** 1023.
151. Devereux RB, Roman MJ. Hypertensive cardiac hypertrophy; pathophysiologic and clinical characteristics. In: Laragh JH, Brenner BM (eds). *Hypertension: Pathophysiology, Diagnosis and Management*, 2nd edn. New York: Raven Press, 1995: 409.
152. Goldman L, Caldera DL. Risks of general anesthesia and elective operation in the hypertensive patient. *Anesthesiology* 1979; **50:** 285.
153. Strandgaard S. Autoregulation of cerebral blood flow in hypertensive patients. The modifying influence of prolonged antihypertensive treatment on the tolerance to acute, drug-induced hypotension. *Circulation* 1976; **53:** 720.
154. Prys-Roberts C, Meloche R, Foex P. Studies of anaesthesia in relation to hypertension. I. Cardiovascular responses to treated and untreated patients. *Br J Anaesth* 1971; **43:** 122.
155. Prys-Roberts C. Anesthesia and hypertension. *Br J Anaesth* 1984; **56:** 711.
156. Goldman L. Risk in noncardiac surgery: an update. *Anesth Analg* 1995; **80:** 810.
157. Howell SJ, Sear YM, Yeates D, *et al.* Hypertension, admission blood pressure and perioperative cardiovascular risk. *Anaesthesia* 1996; **51:** 1000.
158. Parlow JL, Begou G, Sagnard P, *et al.* Cardiac baroreflex during the postoperative period in patients with hypertension: effect of clonidine. *Anesthesiology* 1999; **90:** 681.
159. Stone JG, Foex P, Sear JW, *et al.* Myocardial ischemia in untreated hypertensive patients: effect of a single small dose of a beta-adrenergic blocking agent. *Anesthesiology* 1988; **68:** 495.
160. Mangano DT, Layung EL, Wallace A, Tateo I. Effect of atenolol on mortality and cardiovascular morbidity after noncardiac surgery. Multicenter study of Perioperative Ischemia Research Group. *N Engl J Med* 1996; **335:** 1713.
161. Van Zwieten PA. Centrally acting antihypertensive: a renaissance of interest. Mechanisms and haemodynamics. *J Hypertens* 1997; **15** (Suppl. 1): S53.
162. Engelman E, Lipszyc M, Gilbart E, *et al.* Effects of clonidine on anesthetic drug requirements and hemodynamic response during aortic surgery. *Anesthesiology* 1989; **71:** 178.
163. Prichard BN, Walden RJ. The syndrome associated with the withdrawal of beta-adrenergic receptor blocking drugs. *Br J Clin Pharmacol* 1982; **13** (Suppl. 2): 337S.
164. Chraenmer-Jorgensen B, Hoilund-Carlsen PF, Bjerre-Jepsen K, *et al.* Does alfentanil preserve left ventricular pump function during rapid sequence induction of anaesthesia? *Acta Anaesthesiol Scand* 1992; **36:** 362.
165. Dahlgren N, Messeter K. Treatment of stress response to laryngoscopy and intubation with fentanyl. *Anaesthesia* 1981; **36:** 1022.
166. Martin DE, Rosenberg H, Aukburg SJ, *et al.* Low-dose fentanyl blunts circulatory responses to tracheal intubation. *Anaesthesia* 1982; **61:** 680.
167. Butterworth IV JF, Bean VE, Royster RL. Sufentanil is preferable to etomidate during rapid-sequence anesthesia induction for aortocoronary bypass surgery. *J Cardiothorac Anesth* 1989; **3:** 396.
168. Licina MG, Newsome LR, Reeder DA, *et al.* Sufentanil and succinylcholine for rapid-sequence anesthetic induction and tracheal intubation: hemodynamic and hormonal responses. *J Cardiothorac Anesth* 1990; **4:** 318.
169. Denlinger JK, Ellison N, Ominsky AJ. Effects of intratracheal lidocaine on circulatory responses to tracheal intubation. *Anesthesiology* 1974; **41:** 409.
170. Stoelting RK. Circulatory changes during direct laryngoscopy and tracheal intubation: influence of duration of laryngoscopy with or without prior lidocaine. *Anesthesiology* 1977; **47:** 381.
171. Stoelting RK. Blood pressure and heart rate changes during short-duration laryngoscopy for tracheal intubation: influence of viscous or intravenous lidocaine. *Anesth Analg* 1978; **57:** 197.
172. Hamill JF, Bedford RF, Weaver DC, Colohan AR. Lidocaine before endotracheal intubation: intravenous or laryngotracheal? *Anesthesiology* 1981; **55:** 578.
173. Baraka AS, Sayyid SS, Assaf BA. Thiopental-rocuronium versus ketamine-rocuronium for rapid-sequence intubation in parturients undergoing cesarean section. *Anesth Analg* 1997; **84:** 1104.
174. MacKenzie H, Grant IS. Comparison of the new emulsion formulation of propofol with methohexitone and thiopentone for induction of anaesthesia in day cases. *Br J Anaesth* 1985; **57:** 725.
175. Beck GN, Masterson GR, Richard J, Bunting P. Comparison of intubation following propofol and alfentanil with intubation following thiopentone and suxamethonium. *Anaesthesia* 1993; **48:** 876.
176. Yeager MP, Glass DD, Neff RK, Brinck-Johnsen T. Epidural anesthesia and analgesia in high-risk surgical patients. *Anesthesiology* 1987; **66:** 729.
177. Calhoun DA, Oparil S. Treatment of hypertensive crisis. *N Engl J Med* 1990; **323:** 1177.
178. Cunningham FG, Lindheimer MD. Hypertension in pregnancy. *N Engl J Med* 1992; **326:** 927.
179. Snyder SW, Wheeler AS, James III FM. The use of nitroglycerin to control severe hypertension of pregnancy during cesarean section. *Anesthesiology* 1979; **51:** 563.
180. Wright JP. Anesthetic considerations in preeclampsia-eclampsia. *Anesth Analg* 1983; **62:** 590.
181. Bove EL, Fry WJ, Gross WS, Stanley JC. Hypotension and hypertension as consequences of baroreceptor dysfunction following carotid endarterectomy. *Surgery* 1979; **85:** 633.
182. Solomon RA, Loftus CM, Quest DO, Correll JW. Incidence and etiology of intracerebral hemorrhage following carotid endarterectomy. *J Neurosurg* 1986; **64:** 29.
183. Jorgensen LG, Schroeder TV. Defective cerebrovascular autoregulation after carotid endarterectomy. *Eur J Vasc Surg* 1993; **7:** 370.
184. Symbas PN, Mender LM, Drucker MH, *et al.* Cross clamping of the descending aorta: hemodynamic and neurohumoral effects. *J Thorac Cardiovasc Surg* 1983; **85:** 300.
185. Fox S, Pierce WS, Waldhausen JA. Pathogenesis of paradoxical hypertension after coarctation repair. *Ann Thorac Surg* 1980; **29:** 134.
186. Sealy WC. Coarctation of the aorta and hypertension. *Ann Thorac Surg* 1967; **3:** 15.
187. Benedict CR, Grahame-Smith DG, Fisher A. Changes in plasma catecholamines and dopamine beta-hydroxylase after corrective surgery for coarctation of the aorta. *Circulation* 1978; **57:** 598.
188. Rocchini AP, Rosenthal A, Barger AC, *et al.* Pathogenesis of paradoxical hypertension after coarctation resection. *Circulation* 1976; **54:** 382.
189. Aggarwal S, Kang Y, Freeman JA, *et al.* Postreperfusion syndrome: cardiovascular collapse following hepatic reperfusion during liver transplantation. *Transplant Proc* 1987; **19** (Suppl. 3): 54.
190. Lawless S, Ellis D, Thompson A, *et al.* Mechanisms of hypertension during and after orthotopic liver transplantation in children. *J Pediatr* 1989; **115:** 372.
191. Lentschener C, Franco D, Bouaziz H, *et al.* Hemodynamic changes associated with portal triad clamping are suppressed by prior hepatic pedicle infiltration with lidocaine in humans. *Br J Anaesth* 1999; **82:** 691.
192. Hull CJ. Phaeochromocytoma. Diagnosis, preoperative preparation and anaesthetic management. *Br J Anaesth* 1986; **58:** 1453.
193. Lambert DH, Deane RS, Mazuzan Jr JE. Anesthesia and the control of blood pressure in patients with spinal cord injury. *Anesth Analg* 1982; **61:** 344.
194. Salem MR. Blood conservation. In: Motoyama EK, Davis PJ (eds). *Anesthesia for Infants and Children*. St Louis: CV Mosby, 1996.

12

Monitoring the central nervous system

ANTHONY R ABSALOM, BETTY L GRUNDY, AND MICHAEL LEE

Monitoring the central nervous system is an essential part of general anesthesia, but is commonly effected by direct clinical assessment with no special equipment or techniques or by monitoring of surrogate markers such as heart rate or blood pressure. The effects of anesthetic agents on the brain and spinal cord are usually evaluated to determine whether anesthesia is adequate for proposed diagnostic or therapeutic interventions. Additional monitoring may be needed in several situations, particularly when general anesthesia or coma limits full clinical evaluation of neurological function. This chapter addresses monitoring methods and techniques that are useful in the operating room or critical care unit when the functional integrity of structures and pathways in the central nervous system may be at risk. Monitors of function, pressure, flow, and metabolism are discussed.

CLINICAL NEUROLOGICAL ASSESSMENT

When feasible and appropriate, clinical assessment of neurological function in the awake patient is highly cost-effective. This is commonly used with high-risk patients when procedures can be satisfactorily completed under local or regional anesthesia.

Local or regional anesthesia

Clinical evaluation of the alert patient is particularly important during certain procedures. In some of these, management of systemic medication may be critical. For example, narcotic administration during radiofrequency lesioning for trigeminal neuralgia may prevent appropriate localization if the patient's typical pain cannot be reproduced by stimulation. Benzodiazepines can hamper or preclude evaluation of parkinsonian tremor and its improvement during stereotactic thalamotomy. Similarly, benzodiazepines may interfere with cortical mapping of language areas during resection of nearby tumors.[1]

Techniques for minimizing discomfort are therefore tailored to facilitate each procedure. Radiofrequency lesioning of the fifth cranial nerve is usually accompanied by intermittent small doses of propofol, which allow rapid recovery. This permits testing for the blink reflex, typical symptoms of neuralgia, or possible sensory loss. Vasoactive drugs may be needed during this procedure to control cardiovascular responses to painful stimulation. Stereotactic procedures for movement disorders are usually performed with either no medication or minimal doses of a short-acting narcotic. Benzodiazepines are specifically avoided during functional neurosurgery for movement disorders.

Intraoperative mapping of cortical language areas, craniotomy, and even tumor resection can often be accomplished with local anesthesia alone[2] or with monitored sedation provided by low-dose propofol infusion[3,4] – with or without narcotics, such as remifentanil,[5] fentanyl,[6] and sufentanil – and midazolam.[7] Awake craniotomy for surgery for epilepsy has been performed with various combinations of sedatives and narcotics – propofol and fentanyl have been used for children[8] and for adolescents (in combination with midazolam).[9] Remifentanil has also been used for sedation.[10]

Clinical evaluation of the alert patient under regional anesthesia is a highly cost-effective method of monitoring brain function during carotid endarterectomy (CEA). It remains the most reliable technique for identification of ischemia,[11] and there is some evidence that it is associated with improved outcomes when compared with general anesthesia.[11,12] Sedation must be minimal so that the patient is indeed alert. This approach allows observation of the precise time of onset of neurological deficits and, secondarily, may be useful in determining the probable cause of each deficit.[13,14] In alert patients needing a shunt, the usual manifestation of severe ischemia is complete loss of consciousness within seconds of test occlusion of the carotid artery. When ischemia is less severe and the onset of symptoms less abrupt, symptoms can often be completely alleviated by raising the arterial blood pressure. This maneuver may avoid the need to use a shunt, which is associated with an increased risk of intraoperative embolism.

In a series of 359 patients having CEA with selective shunting under cervical plexus block, only 14 (4%) had neurological deterioration during test occlusion of the carotid artery and had shunts inserted.[14] Only one patient in this series had a postoperative deficit that could be attributed to cerebral hypoperfusion during carotid occlusion. The other 20 postoperative deficits were related to arterial hypotension, thromboembolism, or reperfusion.

Wake-up test

The "wake-up test" is another clinical monitoring technique that requires no special equipment.[15,16] In a cooperative patient, it can provide definite evidence of intact motor function, whereas the most frequently used electrophysiological monitoring techniques reflect primarily dorsal column function. A major disadvantage of the test is that it can be used only intermittently and infrequently. It also presents some risks of its own. Spontaneous inspiration may produce air embolism, and movement during wake-up may result in injury, accidental extubation, or dislocation of orthopedic instrumentation. Controlled ventilation and adequate analgesia help to prevent complications during the wake-up test. Although some centers still consider it to be the "gold standard" test, most clinicians will only apply this test if electrophysiological monitoring is unavailable or if it is showing deterioration in cord function. When used, appropriate emotional support should be given to the patient preoperatively, intraoperatively, and postoperatively to minimize the possibility of subsequent psychological problems.

The Glasgow coma scale[17] and classifications of patients with aneurysms and subarachnoid hemorrhage[18,19] are used virtually universally in critical care units. These clinical assessments are discussed elsewhere in this volume.

ELECTROPHYSIOLOGICAL MONITORING: GENERAL CONSIDERATIONS

The electroencephalogram (EEG) and evoked potentials (EPs) are valuable tools for assessing the functional integrity of the nervous system when clinical neurological examination is limited by altered states of consciousness. These can be used to monitor neural structures and pathways at risk; to identify specific parts of the brain during stereotactic procedures or open craniotomy; to identify cranial and peripheral nerves and evaluate their functional integrity; and to monitor responses to interventions and treatments that affect neurological function.[20–22] Prompt recognition of changes in the functional integrity of the nervous system may allow therapeutic interventions by the anesthesiologist or surgeon, or both, to decrease the risk of neurological injury.

Electrophysiological monitoring of the nervous system may be useful in the operating room or critical care unit when four conditions are met:[21]

1. A part of the nervous system amenable to monitoring must be at risk or otherwise require identification or assessment that cannot be carried out clinically.
2. Equipment and personnel must be available to record and interpret waveforms.
3. Appropriate sites must be available for recording (and for stimulation for EPs).
4. If the monitoring is to serve any practical purpose for the individual patient, there must be some possibility of intervening to improve function if deterioration is detected.

When EEG or EP monitoring is undertaken in the operating room, the active cooperation of the anesthesiologist is necessary. Close communication between the anesthesiologist and the monitoring team is essential, so that normal and reversible changes due to anesthetic drugs and manipulations can be distinguished from changes that should prompt corrective action to preserve neurological function. Some important therapeutic interventions, such as manipulation of arterial blood pressure, are the direct responsibility of the anesthesiologist. Monitoring of EPs that are particularly sensitive to anesthetics, such as motor EPs or those sensory EPs emanating from the cerebral cortex, may be impossible without the active cooperation of the anesthesiologist.

In many settings, the anesthesiologist is primarily responsible for EEG or EP monitoring in the operating room. An expert technologist is needed for reliable and continuous monitoring, but a physician must take responsibility for interpreting changes in the context of all that is happening to a patient physiologically and pathophysiologically. Only in this way can appropriate interventions be carried out in a timely fashion. Serious errors in interpretation of EP changes, with resulting inappropriate management of patients and potentially devastating outcomes, can occur even in experienced hands if the interpretation of EEG or EPs is carried out by a physician who is outside the operating room and who is not fully aware of all concurrent events.

Although no large-scale prospective randomized clinical trials have shown that electrophysiological monitoring (or any other monitoring) changes patient outcome, numerous controlled experiments in animals have demonstrated an association between EEG or EP changes and permanent neurological injury. Documented risks of injury to the nervous system during certain neurosurgical, orthopedic, and vascular operations, combined with knowledge of pathophysiological aspects of these injuries, support the concept of intraoperative monitoring. The collective body of knowledge linking the association between intraoperative EEG or EP changes and neurological outcome continues to strengthen the case for intraoperative electrophysiological monitoring during procedures associated with known risks to the nervous system.

Reports of so-called "false-positive" and "false-negative" results with intraoperative electrophysiological monitoring are naturally of concern to physicians considering the use of these techniques. However, these terms are not always appropriate. The goal of EP monitoring is continual optimization of function during periods of recognized risk so that the possibility of lasting damage is minimized. Untoward intraoperative events that can be detected with EEG or EP monitoring, although uncommon, may be of devastating proportions. Analysis of published reports suggests that most reports of so-called "false-negative" results in intraoperative EP monitoring may be due to inappropriate application of techniques, technical difficulties, and erroneous interpretation of EP changes in the operating room.[23]

ELECTROENCEPHALOGRAPHY

The EEG represents the ongoing spontaneous electrical activity of the brain. Signals recorded from the scalp consist of shifting dipole fields, which are generated by the graded summation of excitatory and inhibitory postsynaptic potentials in cortical neurons.[24,25] The only cells in a position to generate these dipole fields at the cortical surface or scalp are the pyramidal cells found in layers 2, 3, and 5 of the cerebral cortex. These cells and their long dendritic trees are oriented perpendicularly to the cortical surface. A depth electrode inserted into this region shows a phase reversal midway through the granular layer.

EEG activity is often described in terms of nominal frequencies: δ (< 4 Hz); θ (4 to less than 8 Hz); α (8–13 Hz); and β (> 13 Hz). Widely differing conditions can produce similar frequencies: δ activity is typical of metabolic encephalopathy or cerebral ischemia, but is also seen during deep stages of sleep and with deep anesthesia; θ activity is common in children and adolescents and during anesthesia; α rhythm is the characteristic EEG pattern in the alert but relaxed adult with eyes closed and is most prominent in occipital leads. Normal α rhythm breaks up when eyes are opened or during mental activity, such as mental arithmetic. Not all α frequencies constitute normal α rhythms. Frequencies in this range that spread over the entire head and do not react to stimulation such as eye opening are seen during halothane anesthesia and in α coma. α coma, typically seen after an injury of the brainstem, may be irreversible. Frequencies in the β range are typical of intense mental activity, but are also produced by low doses of hypnotics or benzodiazepines. Activity in this range may also be seen after an initial small dose of thiopentone (thiopental) or propofol, but may also persist, particularly in frontal areas, up to 2 weeks after discontinuation of ambulatory doses of diazepam.

EEG activity is altered by anesthetic agents and by changes in cerebral blood flow, P_{aO_2}, P_{aCO_2}, hematocrit, and temperature.[26] Thus, the frequency ranges of EEG activity are never diagnostic of a particular state of the brain and require interpretation within the clinical context.

Methods

Recording

Electrodes are required to convert ionic currents into electronic currents. An electrode placed on the scalp primarily records activity arising within a 2- to 2.5-cm radius. Correct localization and careful application of electrodes are important, even though standard locations are often modified to meet the needs of a specific situation. Scalp electrodes are positioned according to designations of the International Ten Twenty System[27] (Fig. 12.1).

Electrodes must be securely attached to minimize artifact from movement. Various types of electrodes are available. Options for EEG recordings include metal cup, hypodermal, corkscrew electrodes, and self-adhesive disposable silver/silver chloride electrodes. The lowest impedance and highest signal quality is achieved with the use of metallic cups attached to the scalp by means of collodion and filled with conductive gel. In our institution, metal cups embedded in a Teflon cap are used. For prolonged recording, cup electrodes may be sealed with plastic tape or collodion to prevent drying of the electrode gel. Skin is prepared by rubbing with alcohol, then with dry gauze. An abrasive salt gel on a cotton-tipped applicator is used to lightly abrade the skin, reducing impedance to transmission of the electrophysiological signals. With cup electrodes, a blunt-tipped needle is used to place gel inside the cup and may also be used for additional light abrasion of the skin if necessary to obtain sufficiently low impedances. The time required for attachment of metal cups is a distinct disadvantage.

Electrodes designed for electrocardiographic (ECG) recording are often suitable for locations without hair, but careful attention to skin preparation and electrode impedances is required. Those with large conductive areas and that are resistant to drying are best. "Self-prepping" disposable EEG electrodes, which have become available in recent years, need little or no skin preparation.[29]

Subdermal needle electrodes, usually platinum, are easily inserted and can be used within the sterile surgical field. Because the surface of needle electrodes is small, impedances tend to be higher than with cup or disk electrodes. Corkscrew subdermal electrodes, similar to fetal scalp electrodes, are more secure than the usual needle electrodes but are also more uncomfortable. They may be inserted with local refrigeration anesthesia obtained with a volatile spray such as ethyl chloride.

Regardless of the type of electrode, impedances must always be measured and should be low and matched. We prefer impedances of 1–3 kΩ, although 5–10 kΩ may be acceptable for EEG if the impedances between recording electrodes are matched. These higher impedances often prove unsatisfactory for EP monitoring in the operating room or critical care unit. More attention is required for EEG or EP electrodes than for ECG electrodes because the signals are much smaller. Whereas the ECG signal amplitude is of the order of *millivolts*, that of the EEG is *microvolts* and that of the far-field EP a few hundred *nanovolts*.

Signal processing, display, and measurement

Once acquired, the analog EEG signals are amplified, digitized, and filtered to minimize frequencies outside the range of interest (usually 0.5–70 Hz in the diagnostic laboratory; 1–30 Hz in the operating room or critical care unit). The traditional diagnostic EEG recording consists of a paper strip chart showing 16–32 channels as a plot of voltage against time (Fig. 12.2). This representation is in the time domain. Multiple channels are required to show regional activity of the brain.

Numerous techniques for signal processing have been developed to facilitate data compression and interpretation. When these are used, the unprocessed analog signal must still be monitored to exclude artifacts. A method of signal processing commonly used in commercially available monitors is power spectral analysis.[25,31] This mathematically converts the EEG signal from the time domain to the frequency domain (Fig. 12.3). This technique forms the basis for display of the compressed spectral array (CSA) and the density-modulated spectral array (DSA) (Fig. 12.4). Quantitative measurements derived from the power spectrum, such as the peak power frequency (PPF), the median power frequency (MPF), and the spectral edge frequency (SEF), give a simple quantitative estimate of EEG activity, but much of the information contained in the original signal is lost.[32,33] Aperiodic analysis, which depends on measurements of amplitude and frequency in the time domain,[34] is relatively simple and is better than spectral analysis at preserving information on varying EEG patterns such as burst suppression or epileptic activity.

Power spectral analysis assumes that component frequencies in the EEG are independent and do not interact. This is not strictly true. Like the weather, the EEG is actually a deterministic chaotic process sensitively dependent on initial conditions, even though a given sample may appear to be random or stochastic.[36–38]

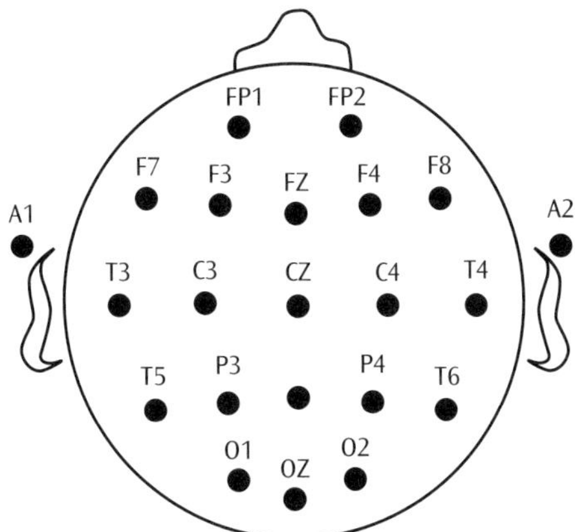

Figure 12.1 *Electrode positions designated by the International Ten Twenty system. The letters indicate anatomical regions of the brain (F, frontal; C, central; P, parietal; O, occipital; A, auricular). Even numbers are to the right of the midline, odd numbers to the left, and Z represents the midline. (From Grundy,[28] with permission.)*

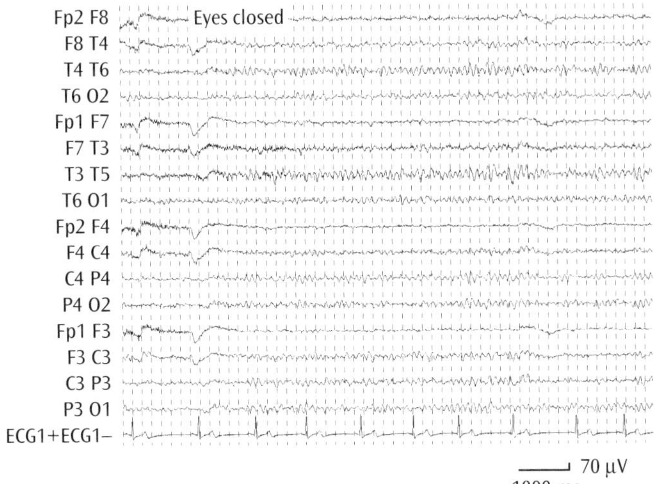

Figure 12.2 *Traditional 16-lead EEG recording from an awake 30-year-old woman. The recording shows predominantly α activity. The large number of leads and complexity of the patterns make traditional EEG recordings difficult to interpret for most anesthesiologists (who do not have special training in neurophysiology).*

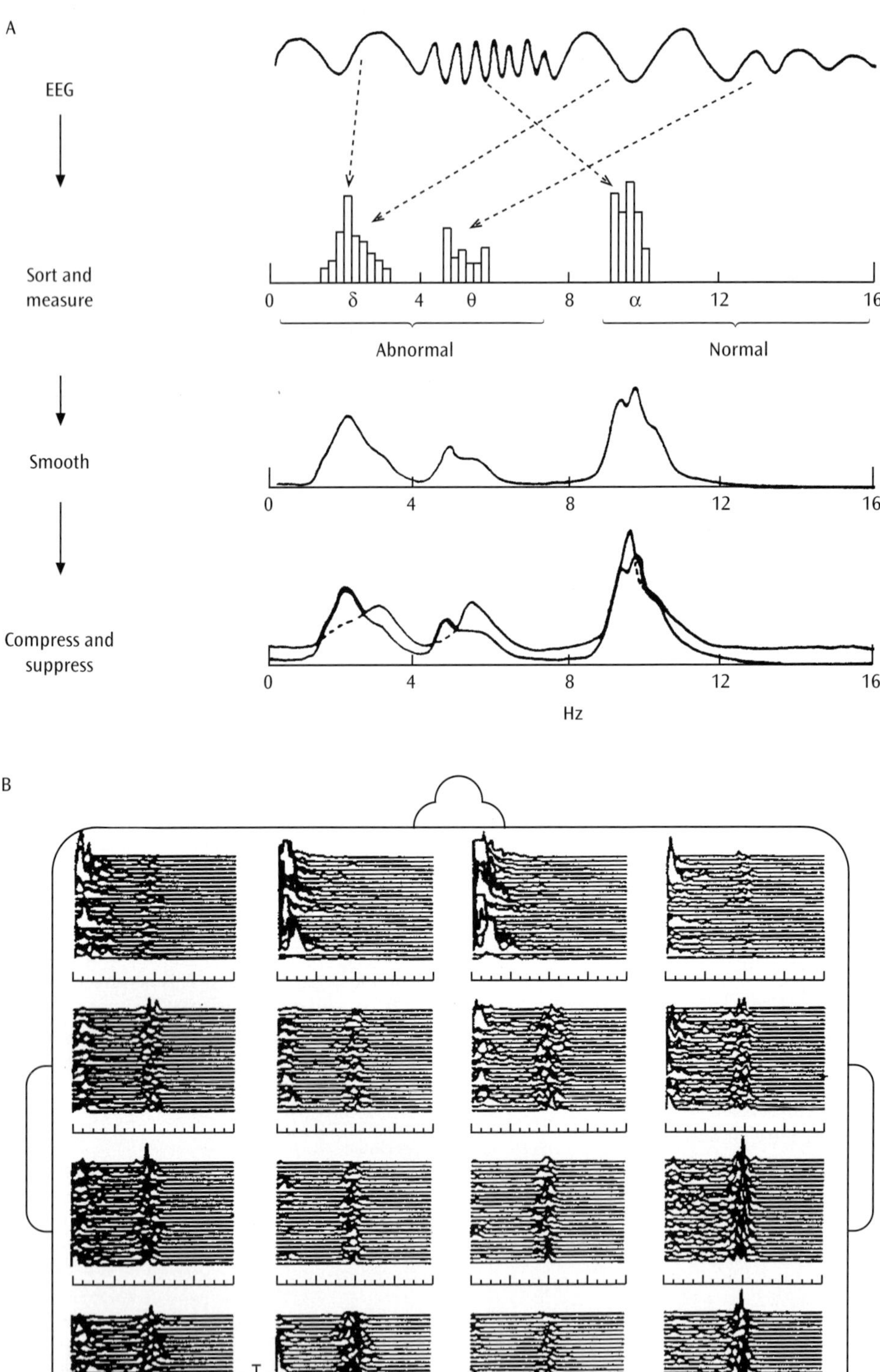

Figure 12.3 *The compressed spectral array (CSA) as popularized by Bickford. (A) Signal processing. (B) A 16-channel CSA recorded from a patient with a right occipital tumor. Note the attenuation of activity in the right occipital leads. The slow activity in frontal leads actually represents eye blinks rather than δ frequency EEG. (From Bickford,[35] with permission.)*

Bispectral analysis[25] analyzes coherence between any two components of the spectral array and thus reflects some nonlinear characteristics of the EEG. Commercially available monitors (Aspect Medical Systems, Newton, USA) are approved by the Food and Drug Administration (FDA) and European Union (EU) for use in the operating room and intensive care as monitors of hypnosis. These calculate and display the bispectral index (BIS), which is the weighted sum of three subparameters – based on time domain, frequency domain, and bispectral EEG analysis.[25] Although there is a large body of literature on the use of the BIS as a measure of hypnosis, relatively little is know about the utility of this measure in the compromised brain.

Clinical applications

Both traditional multichannel EEG recording and automated EEG signal analysis are used in the operating room and the critical care unit. Monitoring during carotid endarterectomy and EEG recording as an

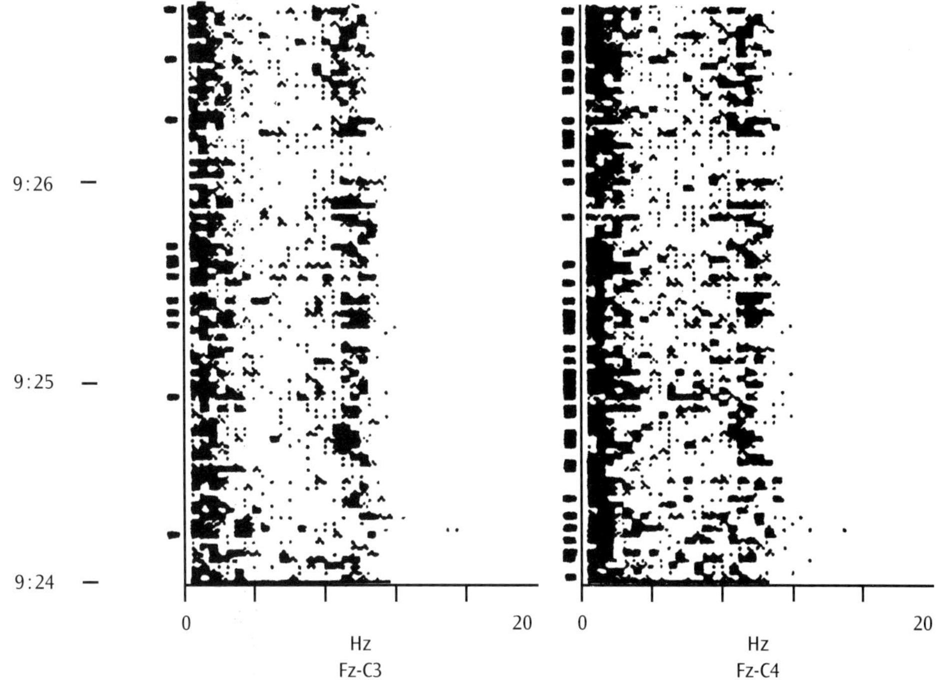

Figure 12.4 *The density-modulated spectral array (DSA). This display shows information also derived by power spectral analysis. It uses varying shades of gray rather than "mountains and valleys" to indicate the intensity of EEG activity at various frequencies. This two-channel tracing depicts bimodal activity, with predominant amplitudes in the δ and α frequency ranges, somewhat more intense on the right. (From Grundy,[28] with permission.)*

adjunct to other tests in the diagnosis of brain death are historically most well established.

EEG monitoring during carotid endarterectomy

Carotid cross-clamping during carotid endarterectomy carries a significant risk of cerebral ischemia, and it has been known for a long time that cerebral ischemia is associated with changes in the EEG.[39–42] As yet, no single EEG-based parameter has been shown to reliably predict ischemia. However, power spectral displays generally show abrupt and obvious changes if ischemia develops and electrodes have been placed within the ischemic area.[39,43,44] These changes may indicate the need for efforts to improve cerebral perfusion and oxygenation, such as insertion of a shunt, raising the arterial pressure, or adjusting retractors within the surgical field. Selective vascular shunting based on major EEG changes has been shown to be associated with a large reduction in stroke incidence when compared with unshunted, unmonitored cases.[45]

Despite this, monitoring of brain activity during carotid endarterectomy (CEA) is not universal and is surrounded by controversy.[46–48] Some surgeons always use a shunt; some never use a shunt; and some use selective shunting based on monitoring of neurological function in the awake patient, distal carotid stump pressures, EEG, somatosensory-evoked potentials (SEPs), cerebral blood flow, or cerebral blood flow velocity. In most large reported series, serious morbidity and mortality are in the range of 2% or less. Although a few teams with reasonably low rates of serious neurological morbidity after CEA do not use brain monitoring of any kind, it is clear that some patients who have marked, but potentially treatable, changes in brain function intraoperatively go on to suffer severe and permanent neurological deficits.[40,49]

Shunt insertion is not without risk – risks include embolization, malfunction, and limitation of the exposure of the artery.[50] EEG monitoring can identify those patients (the majority) who are able to tolerate cross-clamping and do not need a shunt.[51] However, changes in the electrical activity of the brain during CEA do not invariably indicate permanent injury.[49] Once electrical activity is affected, the EEG cannot be used to determine whether cells are dying or are merely in the "ischemic penumbra," with sufficient flow to maintain cellular integrity of neurons but insufficient flow to support electrical activity.[52,53] When EEG monitoring is used to select those patients who will have a shunt inserted, some will have ischemic cerebral segments that are merely in the "ischemic penumbra" and these patients may have shunts inserted unnecessarily. However, it should be remembered that the risk of shunting is clearly less than the risk of omitting a shunt when marked EEG changes are caused by severe and permanent brain injury.[49]

A report of 176 CEA procedures carried out with EEG monitoring without shunting describes EEG changes in 55 patients (with major changes in 22 of the 55).[49] Five (9%) of the 55 with EEG changes had related neurological deficits upon awakening from anesthesia. Two patients had severe and permanent brain damage – both showed major EEG changes within 20 s of carotid occlusion. During episodes of major EEG change, activity in the range 8–15 Hz was markedly attenuated or absent, and δ activity at 1 Hz or less was at least doubled (Fig. 12.5). Thus, 9% of the patients with marked EEG changes had related neurological injuries. By contrast, among the 121 patients with no intraoperative EEG changes, there were no new deficits on awakening from anesthesia.

Optimal EEG monitoring during CEA requires multiple channels, usually 16, to detect regional changes in brain activity. Further, it requires constant and knowledgeable observation of the EEG. An unassisted anesthesiologist is quite unable to accomplish this. Such an individual can, however, monitor two or four symmetrical EEG channels with electrodes placed over the watershed areas of the middle cerebral arteries. Although focal changes will be missed, major catastrophic ischemia can be detected. Two-channel EEG monitoring during 103 operations prompted shunt insertion in 14 patients.[54] None of these 14 suffered new ischemic injuries, but six of the unshunted patients awoke postoperatively with new neurological deficits. Seventy other patients having CEA under cervical plexus block anesthesia also had two-channel EEG monitoring. Aperiodic analysis of the two channels was less reliable than clinical neurological assessment in detecting intraoperative ischemic events.[55] In two other series, neither the four-channel density-modulated spectral array[56] nor a set of 18 quantitative descriptors of the EEG power spectrum[57] adequately substituted for the 16-channel EEG interpreted by a neurologist. Elsewhere, EEG power changes were found to be more sensitive than variations in spectral edge frequency as indicators of intraoperative cerebral ischemia.[58]

The largest series of CEA procedures monitored with 16-channel

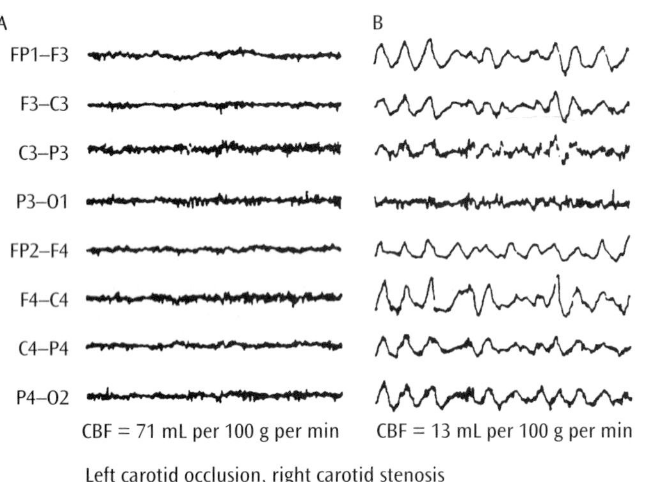

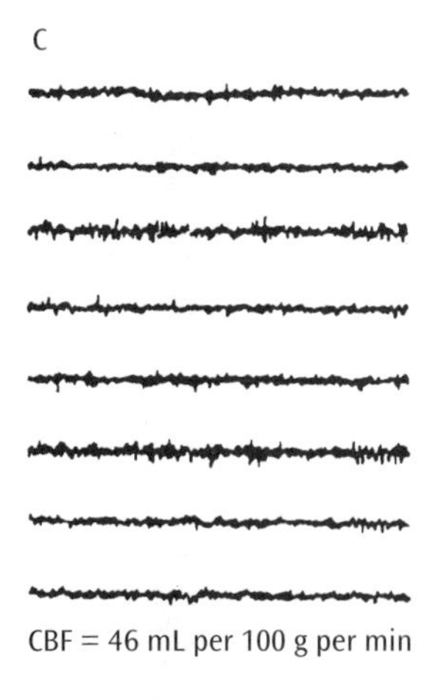

Figure 12.5 *EEG changes during carotid endarterectomy. Paper speed is 15 mm s^{-1}. The typical changes of ischemia are seen with carotid occlusion and correlated with the dramatic fall in cerebral blood flow. Placement of a temporary shunt restores a satisfactory level of cerebral blood flow and returns the EEG to near its preocclusion pattern. CBF, cerebral blood flow. (From Blume and Sharbrough,[30] with permission.)*

EEG is that at the Mayo Clinic,[40] where several thousand patients have been operated upon under general anesthesia with selective shunting based on continuous EEG monitoring and intermittent measurements of regional cerebral blood flow. In this series, no patient awakened with a major new neurological deficit that was not anticipated by intraoperative EEG changes. These patients were monitored continuously from before induction of anesthesia until awakening from anesthesia permitted clinical neurological assessment.

Such continuous monitoring is important for reliable results. Monitoring limited to the period of carotid occlusion and reperfusion will miss a large proportion of insults. Studies reporting patients operated on under regional anesthesia show that only a small percentage of perioperative neurological injuries occur during carotid occlusion when selective shunting is used.[13,14]

EEG monitoring during cardiac surgery

Few of the reported studies in this controversial area describe interventions made on the basis of EEG data; most were attempts to predict outcome and were therefore of very limited use in patient management.

In an early series of 75 patients having EEG monitoring during cardiac surgery, all 15 patients who had clinically important episodes of hypotension during cardiopulmonary bypass developed EEG changes (slowing and/or loss of amplitude).[59] When the changes were transient (seven patients), no postoperative neurological deficits were seen, whereas persistent changes (eight patients) were associated with postoperative neurological deficits.

Despite the recognized limitations of spectral analysis, particularly of a limited number of channels, these techniques can provide valuable information about global cerebral function. Timely warning may lead to prompt restoration of adequate cerebral perfusion or institution of other protective measures. EEG has also been used to determine safe levels of hypothermia for circulatory arrest[60] and to detect burst suppression produced by thiopentone when this drug is given before aortic unclamping in an attempt to protect the brain.[61]

While some studies have shown dramatic improvements in rates of postoperative neuropsychological dysfunction when physicians intervened on the basis of EEG changes,[62,63] others have failed to show an improvement.[64] Unfortunately, the above-mentioned reports, attributing a positive effect on outcome to interventions based on EEG changes, used sequential groups of patients rather than randomization. With no strong evidence of benefit to patients, it is hardly surprising that EEG monitoring during cardiopulmonary procedures is not in widespread use.

EEG monitoring during intracranial surgery

Recordings directly from the surface of the brain or from depth electrodes are essential for determining the extent of resection when epileptogenic foci are removed.

During intracranial vascular neurosurgery, simultaneous monitoring of EEG and EPs may be particularly helpful. Thiopentone may be given as a protective measure before temporary occlusion of key intracranial arteries, and EEG recording is used to detect burst suppression at a time when EPs can still be recorded.[65] High-dose barbiturate anesthesia, with or without mild hypothermia, may also be used to prevent or treat cerebral edema after surgery for arteriovenous malformation. Titration of effective doses in these settings is greatly facilitated by EEG monitoring. Both EEG and EPs can be recorded from the same electrodes.

Electroencephalography in the critical care unit

An important application of EEG monitoring in critical care is for detection of epileptic activity. When muscle relaxants are administered to assist ventilation, or when alterations in consciousness may be caused by continual epileptic activity without motor manifestations, EEG monitoring may be useful to confirm or exclude the presence of seizure activity.[66] Seizure activity is easily detected on the EEG, even by inexperienced users,[67] and the presence of status epilepticus should prompt rapid and aggressive treatment to prevent further neurological activity. A predictable sequence of EEG changes is seen during untreated status epilepticus.[68] Patterns include discrete electrographic seizures, followed by waxing and waning seizure activity, continuous seizure, continuous seizure with flat periods, and, finally, periodic epileptiform discharges on a relatively flat background.

EEG monitoring can provide useful prognostic information in various circumstances. In coma due to head injury, EEG patterns reflect the degree of rostrocaudal neurological deterioration. Loss of such EEG characteristics as sleep-like activity, alternating patterns, and reactivity to stimulation indicates an unfavorable prognosis.[69] In eclamptic women, the EEG may be more sensitive than computed tomography (CT) in detecting the extent of brain pathology,[70] and in neonates treated with extracorporeal membrane oxygenation for severe respiratory failure, EEG seizure activity indicates a significantly increased rate of adverse outcomes.[71] Bursts of slow waves seen in patients with subarachnoid hemorrhage from ruptured aneurysms are highly predictive of angiographic vasospasm.[72]

BIS monitoring is showing promise as a useful method for assessing the adequacy of sedation in intensive care patients.[73,74] In a recent study, the BIS was shown to correlate significantly with clinical scores of neurological status in awake, unsedated critically ill patients, in whom neurological dysfunction was caused either by a primary neurological problem (15 patients) or by critical illness caused by non-neurological problems.[75] Overall, little is known about the usefulness of BIS monitoring for patients with neurological injuries.

In some countries, such as France and the USA, EEG recording and measurement of cerebral blood flow are commonly used to help confirm the diagnosis of brain death. Technical guidelines for EEG recording in suspected brain death were published by the American Electroencephalographic Society in 1994.[76] BIS recording, using a single self-adhesive strip containing three or four electrodes, is easier to perform than traditional multichannel EEG monitoring and is showing some promise as a method for predicting the onset of brain death.[77]

Whatever method is used, rigorous technical standards must be met during both recording and interpretation, and repeated recordings may be indicated. Electrocerebral inactivity can be produced by drug overdose and/or hypothermia even in a normal brain, whereas absent cerebral perfusion is always associated with brain death.[78] Tests for the absence of cerebral blood flow have thus largely replaced EEG recordings for the purpose of confirming brain death in many centers.

EVOKED POTENTIALS (EPs)

Evoked potentials (EPs) are the electrophysiological responses of the nervous system to sensory, electrical, magnetic, or cognitive stimulation. They reflect the functional integrity of structures from which potentials arise and of pathways traversed between the site of stimulation and the neural generators of the evoked electrophysiological activity.

Classifications of evoked potentials

EPs are classified primarily according to the *type of stimulation* used to elicit electrophysiological signals. Although EPs are most often elicited by sensory or electrical stimulation, event-related potentials can also be evoked by movement, thought processes, or other identifiable events. Different types of stimulation activate different parts of the nervous system. Additional useful classifications of EPs are according to the *poststimulus latency* of an evoked peak or complex, the *distance separating the neural generator from the recording electrode*, and the *neural structures from which EP waveforms are thought to arise.* A framework for the classification of EPs useful to the anesthesiologist is outlined in Table 12.1.

Type of stimulation

The modes of stimulation to be considered here include *somatosensory, auditory, visual, trigeminal, cognitive*, and *motor.* All these except cognitive EPs have been used in the operating room, but only somatosensory, motor, and auditory stimulation are in routine clinical use for intraoperative monitoring.

Poststimulus latency

The time between application of a stimulus and the occurrence of a peak or complex in the EP waveform, the *poststimulus latency*, is measured in milliseconds (ms). This latency is characterized as *short* (< 10–15 ms for brainstem auditory EPs or < 40 ms for somatosensory EPs), *intermediate or middle* (usually 20–120 ms), or *long* (usually 120–500 ms).

Short-latency sensory EPs are subcortical in origin or represent only initial cortical activity, are less variable than later potentials, and are less affected by anesthetic agents. When recorded from scalp electrodes, short-latency subcortical EPs are far-field potentials and of smaller amplitude than the ongoing EEG. Short-latency EPs may be near-field potentials, with greater amplitudes and better signal-to-noise ratios, when recorded directly over a peripheral source. For example, an electrode placed on the skin at Erb's point records a near-field short-latency potential from the brachial plexus. In recording short-latency potentials, rapid stimulus rates can be used with relatively little loss of signal. This is because recovery from each individual stimulus is faster than for potentials of intermediate or long latency, presumably because fewer synapses are involved.

Sensory EPs of intermediate latency are near-field potentials when recorded from the scalp and are therefore of greater amplitude than short-latency potentials. They arise from the primary sensory areas of the cerebral cortex and associated areas. Recording can be carried out with fewer repetitions of the stimulus than needed for far-field short-latency potentials, but slower stimulus rates must be used. These EPs are affected by anesthetics to a greater extent than short-latency EPs, but to a lesser extent than long-latency potentials. Reliable monitoring can be achieved during general anesthesia.

Long-latency EPs such as the P300 are thought to reflect cognitive function or physiological responses to pain. Their current usefulness is in research rather than in clinical monitoring.

The *central conduction time (CCT)* and *conduction velocity (CV)* are measurements derived from poststimulus latencies of EP components. These facilitate quantitative comparisons of EPs over time, between sites, and among populations of normal and abnormal patients. CCT is calculated by measuring the poststimulus time intervals between EP peaks generated in peripheral or cranial nerves, cervical spinal cord, or brainstem, and later peaks generated in midbrain, thalamus, or primary sensory cortex. Right-to-left asymmetries in CCT are particularly helpful diagnostically, as well as in the operating room and critical care unit. Conduction velocity for a peripheral or cranial nerve can be estimated from the poststimulus latency of evoked electrical activity and the measured distance between the stimulus site and the record-

Table 12.1 *Classifications of EPs*

Mode of stimulation (for intraoperative EP monitoring)
Sensory
- Somatosensory: electrical current
- Auditory: clicks or tones, delivered by ear-insert transducers
- Visual: flash, delivered by light-emitting diodes mounted on opaque goggles over closed eyes
- Trigeminal: electrical current

Motor: electrical current or magnetic transients
- Neurogenic (recorded at a nerve)
- Myogenic (recorded at a muscle)

Poststimulus latency
Short (< 10 ms for BAEPs, < 40 ms for SEPs)
Intermediate (approximately 20–120 ms)
Long (approximately 120–500 ms)

Stimulation frequency
Transient
Steady state

Distance from neural generator to recording electrode
Near-field-evoked potentials
Far-field-evoked potentials

Purported neural generators
Cerebral cortex
Subcortical structures of the brain
Spinal cord
Cranial nerve, peripheral nerve of nerve plexus
Sensory receptor

EP, evoked potential; BAEPs, brainstem auditory-evoked potentials; SEPs, somatosensory-evoked potentials.

ing electrode. Spinal cord CV can be estimated from the time interval between EPs detected by different pairs of electrodes placed at intervals along the spine or, intraoperatively, from electrodes on the cord or in the epidural space.

Distances separating neural generators from recording electrodes

Near-field potentials are those recorded from electrodes within a few centimeters (perhaps 2–3 cm) of their sites of origin. Near-field EPs recorded from the scalp are of cortical origin and have voltages similar to those of the ongoing EEG. Only 32–128 individual responses need be averaged to make the near-field intermediate-latency cortical EPs apparent. Near-field potentials can also be recorded from electrodes placed over peripheral nerves or from invasive electrodes placed intraoperatively directly on or near structures such as the spinal cord or auditory nerve. In near-field recording, the EP waveform is markedly affected by electrode location. Polarity inversion between bipolar channels localizes the signal of interest to the electrode that is common to both channels. This kind of localization is essential for cortical mapping to identify the sensorimotor strip during craniotomy. Another practical application of this phenomenon lies in the fact that inappropriate placement of electrodes can make EP recording difficult or impossible.

By contrast, *far-field EPs* are relatively little affected by small changes in electrode position. Signals travel by volume conduction to electrodes far removed from their anatomic sites of origin. Because signal strength decreases with distance, far-field potentials are much smaller than near-field potentials. They are far smaller than the background EEG, so that hundreds or thousands of individual responses must be averaged to extract the EP signal from the "noise" of the ongoing EEG.

Neural structures from which EPs arise

Cortical EPs, like the spontaneous EEG, arise in the pyramidal cells of the cerebral cortex. Several types of cortical EPs are known. Those recorded over the primary sensory receiving areas are *primary specific responses*.

These potentials are complex but consistent, can be produced by either meaningful or nonmeaningful stimuli, and show little habituation. Waveforms arising in regions adjoining the primary sensory areas may have secondary waves not seen in the primary specific complex, habituate quickly, and are called *secondary specific responses*. *Nonspecific responses*, also called *late* or simply *event-related responses*, can be recorded widely from the frontal and temporal regions regardless of the mode of sensory stimulation. They habituate rapidly with monotonous stimulation, but are enhanced when the stimulus is meaningful or the subject focuses attention on the stimulus. Shifts in the surface negative potential of the cerebral cortex that depend on some relation between a signal and a subsequent action or decision by the subject are *contingent responses*. The best known of these is the *contingent negative variation* (CNV) – a gradual increase in the surface negativity seen over the frontal areas of the brain for 15–30 s between a conditional warning stimulus and an unconditional signal that requires decision or action by the subject. *Antecedent and imaginary responses* can be recorded over the frontal cortex for about a second before voluntary movement and can be produced by intent alone even when no movement occurs. Of these cortical responses, only the primary specific response is of interest for intraoperative monitoring.

Subcortical potentials reflect some combination of ascending volleys in sensory axons and firing or potential shifts of neurons in subcortical nuclei. Both auditory and somatosensory EPs reflect activity arising in the medulla, pons, and thalamus, as well as thalamocortical radiations.

Potentials generated by the spinal cord and spinal nerve roots can be recorded invasively or noninvasively, but noninvasive recordings are small in amplitude and thousands of repetitions must usually be averaged. EPs can be recorded from the *brachial plexus* by using a surface electrode at Erb's point, and similar potentials can be recorded from electrodes overlying the *lumbar plexus*.

Nerve action potentials (NAPs) and the evoked *electromyogram* (EMG) are used in nerve conduction studies to evaluate the function of peripheral nerves. An electrode placed on or near a peripheral nerve detects a triphasic potential when the nerve is depolarized. An initial positive deflection is recorded as the potential approaches the electrode. With the net flow of positive ions into the nerve, depolarization and a dominant negative potential occur, followed by a small positive deflection as the area of depolarization moves away from the electrode. An electrode placed on the proximal cut end of a peripheral nerve detects only a large positivity.

The *M-wave* is the directly evoked muscle action potential produced by stimulation of a peripheral motor or mixed nerve. The latency of its onset is the time required for action potentials in the fastest conducting fibers that are stimulated to reach nerve terminals and activate the muscle. When the recording electrode is directly over the muscle endplate, the M-wave is biphasic (negative/positive) and latency measurement is most accurate. If recording is not directly over the endplate, the M-wave is triphasic (positive/negative/positive) and onset latency is less precise. With supramaximal stimulation, the area of the negative phase of the M-wave is directly proportional to the number of muscle fibers depolarized, but this area is also influenced by the distance separating the muscle from the recording electrode.

Late muscle responses to stimulation of peripheral nerves include the H-reflex, the F-wave, and the axon "reflex" (Fig. 12.6). These responses are particularly useful for the diagnosis of abnormalities in the proximal segments of peripheral nerves, such as Guillain–Barré syndrome, thoracic outlet syndrome, and lumbar disk disease with radiculopathy. The *H-reflex* is the electrophysiological equivalent of the clinical deep tendon reflex. To record the H-reflex, the posterior tibial nerve is stimulated in the popliteal fossa with the cathode positioned proximally to avoid anodal block. The active recording electrode is placed over the soleus muscle and the indifferent electrode over the Achilles tendon. The H-reflex is a monosynaptic response served by the same pathways traversed by deep tendon reflexes. Because the stimulus is electrical rather than a muscle stretch, the response is not affected by alterations in muscle spindle sensitivity. Afferent Ia fibers carry the impulse through the dorsal horn of the lumbar spinal cord and synapse with motor neurons that innervate the soleus–gastrocnemius muscle complex. An efferent NAP in the motor nerve generates a compound muscle action potential (CMAP) that is recorded as the H-reflex. The H-reflex can be consistently recorded only from the soleus muscle in adults, and the amplitude and latency fluctuate widely with the level of excitability of the central nervous system. During the first 24 h after spinal cord injury, both the H-reflex and deep tendon reflexes are depressed. The tendon reflexes remain depressed for weeks. By contrast, the H-reflex rapidly recovers[79] and, after recovery from spinal shock, shows a marked increase in amplitude.[80] This reflects the recognized increase in excitability of central reflexes in chronic spinal cord injury.

The *F-wave* (Fig. 12.6) can be easily recorded from most distal skeletal muscles. When a motor nerve is stimulated, impulses are transmitted not only distally (to activate muscle, producing the M-wave) but also antidromically. If the cathode of the stimulating pair is placed proximally to the anode along the nerve, to avoid proximal anodal block, a few anterior horn cells will be activated and produce orthodromic potentials along the same nerve. These late potentials produce a small muscle response 20–50 ms after stimulation, actual latencies depending on the distance between the site of stimulation and the spinal cord. Because the F-wave provides a rough measure of conduction in central segments of motor fibers, it is particularly useful

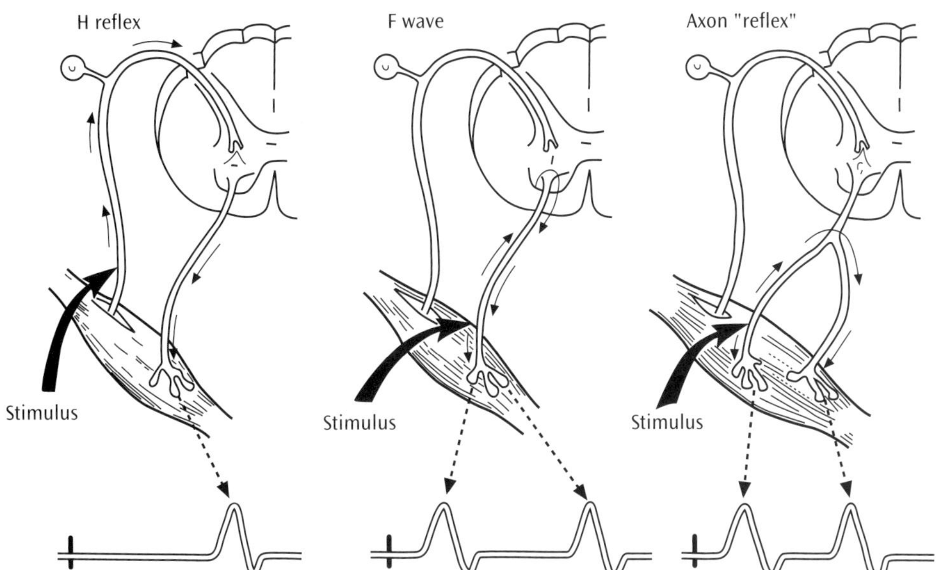

Figure 12.6 *Late muscle responses following peripheral nerve stimulation. See text for explanation. (From Daube,[81] with permission.)*

in the diagnosis of Guillain–Barré syndrome. Central nerve segments may be predominantly involved in the early stages of this disease.[82,83]

The *axon "reflex"* is an abnormal response seen in pathological states when an axon branches in the peripheral nerve. Electrical stimulation distal to the site of branching produces a late muscle response through the abnormal axon branch (Fig. 12.6). Other delayed responses can be seen when some axons are conducting more slowly than others or with irritability of peripheral nerves and repetitive firing after each stimulation.

Potentials generated by sensory receptors include the electrocochleogram and electroretinogram, which are of greater interest to otologists and ophthalmologists, respectively, than to anesthesiologists. In clinical monitoring of auditory and visual EPs, these potentials from sensory receptors can be used to document satisfactory stimulation when later waveforms are abnormal or cannot be recorded.

Methods for monitoring evoked potentials

Equipment

An EP monitoring system has three main components: a system for generating the EP; a system for acquiring, filtering, and amplifying the resulting electrophysiological signals; and a computer to control stimulation and recording, process the acquired electrophysiological signals, and store and display them for measurement and evaluation. Guidelines for EP recording[84] and for intraoperative monitoring of EPs[85] have been suggested by the American Electroencephalographic Society.

For adequate quality control, it is necessary to be able to observe the unprocessed signal (after initial filtering and amplification) and to suspend recording when the signal contains excessive noise. The available options for automatic artifact rejection, although these are very helpful, depend on amplitude criteria and may allow artifacts not exceeding certain limits to be included in the signal. A common offender is the bipolar cautery. Similarly, the automatic artifact rejection may exclude physiological EEG or EP signals under certain conditions and must be reset or turned off to permit recording.

Most workers consider at least two channels to be necessary for effective EP monitoring, and at least four channels highly desirable. Other desirable features for EP systems used for monitoring in the operating room or critical care unit include the capacity to display and store several waveforms, automatic counting and display of the number of repetitions accepted and rejected in an average, and automatic storage of stimulus and recording parameters with each waveform. Accurate documentation is greatly facilitated and human errors in data collection are minimized by placing as much of the monitoring as possible under program control.

Stimulation

When sensory stimuli are used, they are applied at regular intervals, usually at a noninteger rate to avoid synchronization with electrical mains supply. For several reasons, methods used for stimulation in the operating room differ in some respects from those used in the diagnostic electrophysiology laboratory. The unconscious patient is neither able to warn of impending injury nor able to cooperate with testing procedures. Special precautions are necessary for electrical safety and to avoid interfering with or contaminating the sterile surgical field. Some operations provide opportunities for invasive stimulation and recording that are not available in the diagnostic laboratory. Specific techniques for stimulation to elicit EP are detailed below.

Signal processing

A broad range of signal processing techniques have been applied to EP data,[86] but only *averaging* is in widespread clinical use. After each stimulus, the EEG is recorded for a set period of time (a "sweep"). After acquisition, the analog EEG signal is digitized. The recording interval after a stimulus must be sufficiently long to include the required components of the EP, which are "buried" in the "noise" of the background EEG and other electrical activity. As the EP signal is time-locked to a regular stimulus whereas EEG activity is to some extent random, averaging of multiple sweeps of EEG activity increases the signal-to-noise ratio by the square root of the number of sweeps averaged. The averaged digital signal is then converted to an analog waveform for display and measurement.

Other methods of signal analysis have been applied to EP signals. However, if the EP waveform cannot be seen in the usual average, more complex signal processing may yield spurious results. Even traditional filtering and smoothing, when carried to excess with noisy waveforms, can lead to erroneous interpretation of EPs and possible mismanagement of patients. Highly processed noise may resemble EP waveforms while bearing no relation to electrophysiological activity.

Up to 2000 or more sweeps may be required to extract an EP signal using averaging. This is time-consuming, and for situations in which the neurological status is varying, such as on the intensive care unit or in the operating room, changes occurring during a small number of sweeps will be missed. The system will also take a relatively long time to detect more permanent changes. Autoregressive modeling with exogenous input is a newer technique of signal analysis that has the potential to produce a sweep-by-sweep estimate of the EP, and has been applied to visual-evoked potentials (VEPs) in the laboratory setting[87] and auditory-evoked potentials (AEPs) during general anesthesia.[88,89] This method of analysis is employed in a commercially available anesthetic depth monitor ("Aline," Alaris Medical Systems, Basingstoke, UK).

Evoked potentials are customarily recorded in the time domain as plots of voltage against time. They are then described in terms of the poststimulus latencies and peak-to-peak amplitudes. Identification of peaks is by visual pattern recognition by a trained observer. Peaks should not be automatically identified by the maximum deflection within a given time window. Prolonged latencies may be caused by neurological abnormalities, but are also affected by other factors such as anesthetic drugs and the length of the nerve being stimulated. Barring such explanations, however, prolonged absolute or interpeak latencies indicate delayed conduction. Particular patterns of latency change can help localize abnormalities.

EP amplitudes are usually measured from peak to peak, rather than from baseline to peak, in order to minimize the effects of underlying low-frequency activity or baseline drift. Amplitudes are more variable than latencies and have therefore been less often examined in diagnostic testing or monitoring. Amplitude changes, however, may be more sensitive than latency changes as indicators of abnormal function.[90,91] Differences in the amplitudes of EPs elicited by stimulation at different sites may be diagnostically important.[92]

Numerous methods have been suggested for quantitative characterization of EPs, including, among others, measurement of component wave areas,[93] power spectral analysis,[94] noise estimation,[95] correlation analysis,[96] stepwise discriminate analysis,[97] significance probability mapping,[98] and parametric predictive modeling.[99] Other statistical techniques have also been employed. Color or gray-scale mapping of EPs ("brain mapping") has also been popularized.

Steady-state EPs are produced by stimulation at sufficiently high rates to cause overlapping of the responses to successive stimuli.[100] As the stimulation frequency increases, the amplitude of the evoked responses increases. In the case of auditory EPs, in normal conscious subjects, the frequency at which the peak amplitude of this waveform is found is approximately 40 Hz. A sinusoidal response develops owing to superimposition of the two main waves of the transient EP – P_a and P_b.[101]

The sinusoidal waveform produced is characterized by measuring the amplitude and phase angle of the response relative to the train of stimuli. Steady-state EPs can also be analyzed by using Fourier analysis to compute the power spectra for trains of responses evoked at each of several stimulus frequencies. Ratios between the power spectra recorded over symmetrical areas of the right and left hemispheres of the brain should be less than 2.0 in normal subjects. The coherent frequency, the frequency in the steady-state EP at which the greatest proportion of power resides in the fundamental frequency, has been shown to correlate with depth of sedation and cognitive function in normal volunteers.[102] Although steady-state EPs seem inherently attractive for monitoring because they can be rapidly recorded and quantitatively measured, little experience has been gained with this technique in the operating room or intensive care unit.

Interpreting evoked potentials

Once EP peaks are identified by pattern recognition, precise interpretation depends on reproducible quantitative representation of data and statistical characterization of appropriate databases. EPs vary with gender and age, so that normal data should be established separately for males and females in each age group. Once a normal data set is established, and the 95% and 99% tolerance limits for quantitative measurements are determined, each EP recording can be classified as normal, abnormal, or technically inadequate. Normal data sets have been published, but if these published normal values are used it is important to show that the techniques and values in the literature can be reproduced in the individual laboratory.[84]

In the operating room, each patient serves as his own control. Successful monitoring can be performed even when baseline EPs are abnormal, so long as reproducible signals can be obtained. The degree and duration of EP change consistent with preservation of function in the monitored pathway are not precisely known. EP values consistent with recovery vary according to the pathway being monitored, the nature of the underlying pathophysiology, and other factors that are not fully defined. We do not know whether complete obliteration of the brainstem auditory-evoked potential (BAEP) signals may be compatible with preservation of neurological function when the insult is retraction of the auditory nerve and the EP changes are reversible in the operating room.[103,104] By contrast, obliteration of somatosensory-evoked potentials (SEPs) during operations on the aorta for more than 15–30 min may be associated with recovery of dorsal column function but permanent loss of motor function.[105]

Confounding variables such as changes in body temperature, anesthetic agents, and arterial tensions of respiratory gases must be considered when interpreting intraoperative EP changes. Monitoring is greatly facilitated when the anesthesiologist can maintain a steady state both pharmacologically and physiologically during critical monitoring periods.

SOMATOSENSORY-EVOKED POTENTIALS (SEPs)

The most widely used EPs in the operating room, as in the diagnostic laboratory, are the SEPs. These potentials are used to monitor brain, spinal cord, and peripheral nerves.

Neurophysiology

Electrical stimulation of a somatosensory nerve preferentially activates the largest sensory fibers in the peripheral nerve (group I). These fibers subserve vibratory and proprioceptive sensation, and NAPs can easily be recorded over proximal segments of the nerve. According to a somewhat simplified classic description, the cell bodies of the first-order neurons lie in the dorsal root ganglion, with distal axons in the peripheral nerve and proximal axons coursing through the dorsal nerve root, entering the dorsal root entry zone of the cord at its medial division, and continuing cephalad in the posterior funiculus, or dorsal columns, of the cord. The fasciculus cuneatus conducts impulses from the upper extremity and thorax; it is lateral to the fasciculus gracilis, which lies next to the dorsal median septum and carries fibers from the lower extremity. The first-order neurons of the somatosensory system synapse uncrossed in the nucleus gracilis and nucleus cuneatus of the lower medulla. Second-order neurons pass through the decussation of the medial lemniscus in the lower medulla and ascend as the medial lemniscus to the thalamus, where they synapse with third-order neurons in the ventral posterolateral nucleus of the thalamus. Axons of the third-order neurons lie in the thalamocortical radiations and project through the posterior limb of the internal capsule to the postcentral gyrus of the parietal lobe. Classically, this pathway is considered to be traversed by the SEPs. In actual fact, however, only a small number of the lumbosacral dorsal root fibers in the fasciculus gracilis reach the upper cervical cord, and even fewer fibers in the fasciculus cuneatus reach the medulla. The pathway as classically described, with direct conduction of the first-order neuron to the dorsal column nuclei, is greatly oversimplified. Interneuronal relays along this pathway are common.[106,107]

Even with intervening synapses, EPs produced by stimulation of the upper extremity seem to be conducted predominantly ipsilaterally in the dorsal columns. By contrast, EPs elicited by stimulation of the lower extremity may be carried to a substantial extent in the lateral funiculus.[108] Stimulation of the posterior tibial nerve with intensity set at a subject's motor threshold activates group I fibers that synapse and ascend in the dorsal spinocerebellar tract. The fibers synapse in nucleus Z at the spinomedullary junction. The impulse is then transmitted to the ventral posterolateral thalamic nucleus and through the thalamocortical radiations to the primary sensory cortex.[109] Studies of spinal cord lesions in the monkey, cat, and dog are consistent with SEP conduction in all quadrants of the spinal cord but predominantly in the ipsilateral dorsal lateral funiculus.[110]

A number of reproducible waveforms are generated as the SEP impulse is transmitted from the peripheral nerve to the brain. The NAP shows a triphasic form, as described above. Additional potentials, probably composed of NAP and excitatory postsynaptic potentials, are generated where the nerve roots enter the cord. Recordings from the skin over the spine or directly from the spinal cord sometimes show an initial triphasic spike, probably produced by primary afferent activity. Subsequent slow activity, the N-wave, has been attributed to cellular activity in Rexed's laminae III and V of the dorsal horn, with an early deflection which is also presynaptic and is thought to reflect activity in afferent terminals. A subsequent slow positive wave is related to primary afferent depolarization, a process by which axoaxonic synapses are thought to produce presynaptic inhibition.[107]

Figure 12.7 shows an intermediate-latency SEP after median nerve stimulation, as recorded in a four-channel array for intraoperative monitoring. Purported neural generators of the short-latency SEPs are outlined in Table 12.2. Peaks in EPs are usually labeled N for negative or P for positive, with a following number designating the nominal poststimulus latency. A negative peak recorded over the contralateral sensory cortex approximately 20 ms after stimulation of the median nerve at the wrist is thus called N20. It seems to be the initial cortical component of the SEPs, although some observers believe that it arises in the thalamus or thalamocortical radiations. All observers agree that the following positivity, with a latency of about 23 25 ms, arises in the somatosensory cortex.

In far-field recordings, new deflections are generated whenever the impulse enters a new and different volume conductor (base of finger or thumb; wrist; shoulder; spinal cord; foramen magnum). The moment the impulse reaches a boundary, current density changes suddenly in the two adjacent conducting media, giving rise to an apparent standing potential.[111] This mechanism probably plays an important role in the generation of early positive waves recorded from the scalp with a noncephalic reference. These early positive waves are obscured in frontally referenced recordings and are not of concern during intraoperative monitoring of SEPs.

A popular technique for measuring central conduction time (CCT)[112] uses the negativity recorded from the skin overlying the spine of the second cervical vertebra referenced to FZ or FPZ, as a benchmark for subcortical activity. The N20 is used as the indicator of cortical activity, and the CCT is the time required for impulse transmission between these two points. If the cervical potential is indistinct or unavailable, and the initial cortical positivity is clearer than the N20, it is often practical to substitute a measurement of elapsed time between the Erb's point potential and the initial cortical positivity.

In clinical neurology, abnormal SEPs are seen when demyelinating diseases, tumors, infarcts, or other structural abnormalities disrupt the conducting pathway.[113,114] Cortical SEPs are altered in patients with focal lesions of the somatosensory system at any point along the neuraxis, whether lesions are in the peripheral nerve, nerve plexus, spinal cord, brainstem, midbrain, or cortex. SEPs are particularly helpful in the diagnosis of multifocal or diffuse lesions, such as multiple sclerosis.

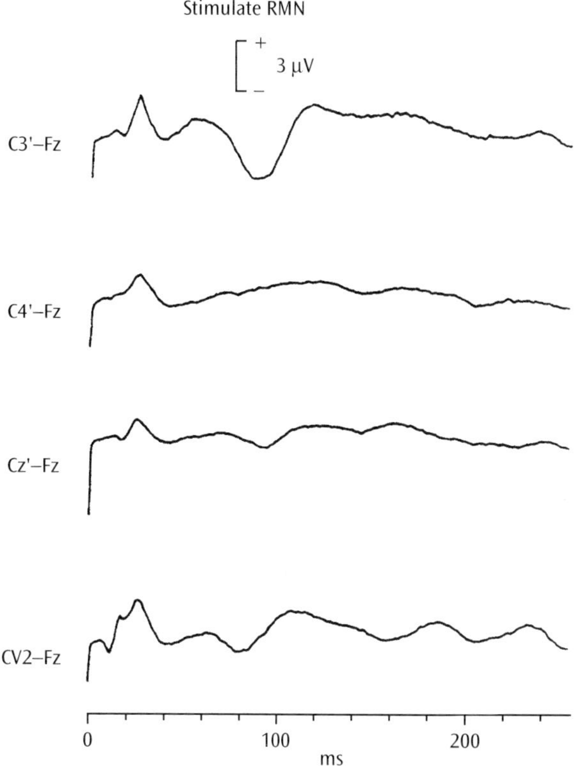

Figure 12.7 *Normal intermediate-latency SEPs recorded during anesthesia. The same electrode montage can be used to record activity elicited by stimulation of either median nerve or the posterior tibial nerve. The last tracing, recorded from the skin overlying the spine of the second cervical vertebra, is often easier to record during anesthesia than in the awake patient because muscle activity is suppressed. If the site is not available, does not give satisfactory responses, or is rostral to the likely points of injury intraoperatively, NAPs should be recorded at each site to document signal input. RMN, right median nerve. (From Grundy,[21] with permission.)*

Methods

Somatosensory stimulation

Somatosensory EPs can be elicited by stimuli that are electrical, mechanical, thermal, or magnetic. *Electrical stimulation* is most commonly used in both the diagnostic laboratory and the operating room. Electrical current is easy to apply, measure, and control. It is delivered to a sensory or mixed nerve via surface or subdermal electrodes. The median and ulnar nerves at the wrist, the posterior tibial nerve at the ankle, and the common peroneal nerve at the knee are mixed nerves commonly stimulated for diagnostic or monitoring purposes. Sometimes, the sural nerve is also tested. When peripheral nerves are stimulated, it is best to stimulate each extremity singly in turn. Stimulation of pathways not at risk from the surgical procedure helps to distinguish operative effects on EPs from effects of systemic factors such as changes in temperature, anesthetic agents, or arterial tensions of respiratory gases. Simultaneous stimulation of nerves in both lower extremities (bilateral stimulation) gives larger responses than stimulation of a single nerve, but unilateral lesions of the cord can be missed.[115]

Table 12.2 *Purported generators of short-latency somatosensory-evoked potentials*

Peak	Generator
N9	Brachial plexus
N11	Spinal roots or dorsal columns
N13,14	Spinal cord gray matter or dorsal columns
N14,15	Brainstem and/or thalamus
N20	Primary somatosensory cortex

Stimulation: median nerve; recording: clavicle, mastoid process, second cervical vertebra, primary somatosensory cortical area; reference electrode: Fz or non-cephalic. (Early cortical waves are obscured in frontally referenced recordings.) (From Grundy,[21] with permission.)

For most clinical SEP monitoring, electrode pairs are placed on the skin over peripheral nerves. Electrical current flowing between the two electrodes depolarizes the nerve at the cathode (−). For sensory stimulation, the cathode is placed proximal to the anode. This is because some axons may be hyperpolarized at the anode (+) and, at least theoretically, this hyperpolarization might block proximal transmission of the impulse ("anodal block"). Stimulators delivering constant currents are preferable to those giving constant voltages. It is the current that actually stimulates the nerve, and constant-current stimulators automatically adjust voltage to compensate for changes in electrode impedance so that the stimulus is kept constant. Stimulation of a mixed nerve – sufficient to produce a motor twitch – is called supramaximal, and it is often stated that further increases in current produce no change in the SEPs. In actual practice, however, it is clear that additional current usually produces augmentation of SEP amplitude. For clinical testing, some practitioners use the lowest current that produces a visible motor twitch; others use the highest current easily tolerated by the patient. A reasonable compromise that provides a level of reproducibility is use of a current equal to the sum of sensory and motor thresholds to electrical stimulation. In any case, the actual stimulus intensity used should be recorded, and it should be kept constant during critical monitoring periods. During anesthesia, the current is often increased to some arbitrary level such as 20 mA.

When a mixed nerve is stimulated, the signal ultimately reaching the central nervous system is complex and somewhat dispersed over time.[116] The signal includes not only orthodromic sensory impulses but also antidromic motor impulses and subsequent sensory impulses due to the muscle contraction produced by orthodromic motor impulses. Pure sensory stimulation can be performed with ring electrodes on the fingers, and cutaneous receptors can be stimulated with surface electrodes to test sensory function in specific dermatomes. Dermatomal SEPs can be used to localize radiculopathies diagnostically or in the operating room. Pure somatosensory stimulation produces SEPs that are smaller and less reproducible than those produced by electrical stimulation of mixed nerve trunks, and this technique is used only for special indications in the operating room or critical care unit.

The spinal cord can be directly stimulated by epidural or subarachnoid electrodes.[117] When recording is also from within the spinal canal, very rapid rates of stimulation can be used (30–50 Hz). This is because few if any synapses are involved and recovery from each individual stimulus is rapid. Very large amplitudes are achieved (100–150 μV), so only 50–100 repetitions need to be averaged. Direct spinal stimulation is nonspecific and involves multiple pathways, but is in common use in Europe and Japan and is considered to be remarkably safe.[118] Nonspecific stimulation of the cauda equina has also been described. Because of the nonspecific stimulation of multiple pathways, unilateral cord injury could be missed with either of these methods.[115]

Mechanical stimulation can be used to evoke SEPs,[119] but this technique is less reproducible than electrical stimulation and is essentially experimental. Late cortical EPs produced by *laser heat stimulation* are thought to represent a psychophysiological pain response.[120] Each painful stimulus, however, produces a second-degree burn. The potentials are large enough for single responses to be seen with special filtering techniques, so repeated stimulation and averaging of the response are not necessary. Thermal stimulation is valuable for pain research but not practical for clinical application.

Magnetic stimulation does not require electrode contact. Nerve trunks can be stimulated by time-varying magnetic fields.[121,122] Magnetic stimulation is more comfortable than electrical, but techniques for adequately reproducible localization are not yet fully developed.

Recording

Selection and arrangement of electrode locations for recording depend on the pathways to be monitored and the number of channels available. Signals are recorded over peripheral nerves, plexi, spine, and scalp. Various invasive techniques have been described, with electrodes placed intraoperatively in bone,[123] interspinous ligament,[124,125] epidural space,[126,127] and subarachnoid space.[128] SEPs recorded from electrodes placed stereotactically in the depths of the brain can be used to localize subcortical structures for diagnostic or therapeutic purposes,[129,130] but these applications have been largely displaced by modern stereotactic localization based on CT radiological techniques or magnetic resonance imaging.

Clinical experience with SEP monitoring

Operations for scoliosis

SEPs were the first EPs made practical for routine intraoperative monitoring when they were used for spinal cord monitoring during scoliosis surgery.[131] It is thus not surprising that the largest collective experience with intraoperative EP recording is with scoliosis surgery. Scoliosis correction is generally a cosmetic, elective procedure, but newer instrumentation methods can cause huge distraction forces on the vertebral column and spinal cord, potentially resulting in permanent neurological injury. A report by the Scoliosis Research Society in 1975 indicated an incidence of spinal cord injury of the order of 1% for operations involving Harrington rod instrumentation, and even higher when sublaminar wiring was used.[132,133] Therefore, orthopedic surgeons were the most enthusiastic early users of SEP monitoring in the operating room.

Since then, numerous investigators have described their experiences with SEP monitoring during orthopedic procedures on the spine.[123,128,134–139] All observers report that the majority of patients monitored during spine surgery show either no clinically important changes or changes that are only transient. Cortical SEPs are very sensitive to intraoperative changes in spinal cord function. Postoperative neurological deficits are almost always associated with persistent intraoperative SEP changes.

In a multicenter survey of over 50 000 operations monitored with SEPs, the overall incidence of neurological deficits was 0.55%, and the negative predictive value of SEPs was 99.93%.[136] False-negative results are thus very rare, but when they do occur they are usually caused by anterior lesions, lesions that developed after spinal cord monitoring stopped, or lesions in regions not amenable to monitoring (such as nerve roots). In the same survey, the positive prediction value of SEPs was only 42%. Therefore, there were a large number of "false positives;" however, some of these were probably not false positives, but true positives where the deterioration in the SEP prompted appropriate and successful action to improve spinal cord perfusion, thereby preventing a postoperative neurological deficit. Possible reasons for "true false positives" include a recent bolus of anesthetic drug and spinal cord concussion.[140]

In most centers, the threshold for intervention is a > 10% reduction in the latency of P1 or a > 50% decrease in cortical P1/N1 peak-to-peak amplitude.[141,142] It should be borne in mind that spontaneous variability in the SEP amplitude can be as high as 50%.[143] Despite this, and the fact that these criteria for intervention have not been subjected to prospective studies, they were shown to predict lower limb deficits in early SEP studies when no interventions were made.[144]

Reported interventions made on the basis of SEP changes during spinal surgery have included readjustment of spinal instrumentation, reversal of induced hypotension, decreases in the amount of surgical correction of the deformity, and removal of bone grafts. When sudden changes are seen in SEPs during spinal surgery, an immediate wake-up test should be performed if at all possible. When SEPs are monitored continuously and are stable, many teams omit wake-up tests.

Simultaneous stimulation of both lower extremities can lead to false-negative results.[145] SEPs elicited by stimulation of either lower extremity can be easily recorded from the same midline electrodes on the scalp. If injury occurs to one side of the cord while the other side continues to function, bilateral stimulation can produce unaltered SEPs, whereas stimulation of each lower extremity separately would clearly show the loss of signal during stimulation of the extremity ipsilateral to the injury.[115]

Operations for spinal injury

The wake-up test may be dangerous for the patient with an acutely injured and severely unstable spine because uncontrolled movement might produce additional serious injury to the spinal cord. SEP monitoring therefore seems attractive as an aid to intraoperative management of these patients. In a series of 295 patients undergoing surgery for stabilization of traumatic unstable spinal injuries, SEP monitoring was associated with a reduction in neurological injury rate from 6.9% to 0.7%.[146]

Other operations within the spinal canal

SEP monitoring has been used during resection of spinal cord tumors and other lesions impinging on the spinal canal.[126,127,147–149] SEPs are often abnormal or absent preoperatively in symptomatic patients; if reproducible waveforms cannot be obtained during anesthesia, monitoring cannot be performed. Interactions among pathophysiological factors, anesthetic effects, and stimulus and recording techniques are incompletely understood, but some clinical guidelines may prove useful. Slowing the rate of stimulation to the range of 0.9–3.1 Hz may be helpful, as may increasing the stimulus current and/or duration. Omission of inhaled anesthetics may also be useful. Opioid analgesics and intravenous anesthetic agents have only minor effects on SEP amplitude and latency. A propofol/opioid combination is commonly used for induction and maintenance of anesthesia. Etomidate amplifies cortical SEPs[150] and may be an appropriate anesthetic agent in this setting, although the problem of adrenocortical suppression should be borne in mind[151,152] and steroid supplements may be required.

If reproducible waveforms can be recorded, even though these may be abnormal, useful monitoring can be achieved. Several reports even describe improvement in SEPs with decompression of the spinal cord. SEP monitoring has been used by several investigators during resection of spinal arteriovenous malformation.[144,153] This seems particularly useful when large feeding vessels are available for test occlusion or when resection can be stopped if marked SEP changes occur.

Some neurosurgeons consider SEP recording indispensable during surgery for the relief of intractable pain by placing deliberate lesions in the dorsal route entry zone of the cord.[23,107] The appropriate segment for lesioning is located by using stimulation of peripheral nerves at multiple levels with monopolar recording from the cord. Unwanted numbness in the lower extremities, formerly the most frequent complication of this procedure, can usually be avoided by monitoring cortical SEPs elicited by stimulation of the posterior tibial nerve at the ankle or the peroneal nerve at the knee.

Good results have been reported when monitoring evoked spinal potentials during surgery for scoliosis.[128] This technique proved less satisfactory during surgery for spinal cord tumors. During resection of six extramedullary and 14 intramedullary spinal cord tumors, an epidural electrode caudal to the level of the tumor was used to stimulate the cord and potentials were recorded from an epidural electrode rostral to the tumor.[154] Although a decreased amplitude of the evoked spinal potential after removal of the tumor was fairly specific for cord injury (five out of six patients with decreased amplitude had a postoperative deficit), the sensitivity was poor. Four patients (20%) developed postoperative deficits despite having stable spinal cord EPs throughout the operation. Of these four, two had intramedullary tumors and experienced postoperative symptoms consistent with unilateral spinal cord damage. Thus, despite the high amplitude of the evoked spinal cord potential, the reproducible waveforms, and the robust character of this potential during anesthesia, the investigators concluded that this technique was insufficiently sensitive to monitor patients with spinal cord tumors.

Operations on the aorta

The spinal cord may suffer ischemic injury during operations to the thoracic or abdominal aorta, or even during angiography. The blood supply to the anterior two-thirds of the cord consists of a single artery that traverses the entire anterior aspect of the cord. The anterior spinal artery is supplied by branches of the vertebral arteries and numerous tributaries, including the thyrocervical trunk and several radicular branches in the thoracic and lumbar regions. Usually, one radicular branch is larger than the others and more critical for cord perfusion. This vessel arises as a left intercostal branch, between T9 and L2 in most patients, and is known as the greater medullary artery or the artery of Adamkiewicz. Two posterior spinal arteries, also arising from the vertebral arteries, supply the posterior one-third of the cord.

Occlusion of the anterior spinal artery causes infarction of the anterior part of the cord, with loss of sensation to pain, temperature, and crude touch below the lesion. If the lesion extends far enough posteriorly, bilateral spastic paralysis results. When the posterior spinal arteries continue to function, a patient with anterior spinal artery occlusion may be paraplegic while position and vibration sense, as well as SEPs, are preserved.

The incidence of neurological deficits after abdominal aortic aneurysm surgery is in the order of 0.16–0.25%.[155,156] The risk of cord injury is even greater during operations for large, complex thoracoabdominal abnormalities of the aorta – in one large series the incidence of neurological deficits was 16%.[157] In patients with aortic coarctation, the risk of paraplegia is lower, probably because the collateral blood supply to the cord is better.

Axonal conduction of action potentials requires little energy expenditure and is therefore relatively resistant to cord ischemia, resulting in a delay between onset and detection of ischemia of between 8 and 18 min.[158] Simple cross-clamping will cause obliteration of the SEP in 17 ± 8 min.[159] This delay – and the fact that SEPs largely reflect the status of the dorsal columns, supplied by the posterior spinal arteries – naturally poses questions about the possible usefulness of SEP monitoring during surgery on the aorta, when the anterior spinal artery perfusion is most at risk.

Several experimental studies of compromised aortic flow have included SEP monitoring.[160–165] Microsphere studies of cord perfusion in dogs[162–164] showed that maintenance of distal aortic pressure at or above 70 mmHg (9.3 kPa) kept spinal cord blood flow and SEPs within an acceptable range, whereas distal aortic pressures below 40 mmHg (5.3 kPa) abolished SEPs.[166] Occlusion of a critical intercostal artery in other animals markedly decreased cord perfusion and abolished

SEPs.[166] When cord perfusion was restored 5 min after SEP loss, no paraplegia resulted. By contrast, when aortic occlusion was maintained for 10 min after SEP loss, two-thirds of the animals were paraplegic postoperatively.[167]

If the duration of aortic clamping in humans is < 30 min, the incidence of neurological damage is low. The probability of paraplegia after 30 min of occlusion increases linearly, to almost 90% after 60 min.[168] The cases described in the literature to date suggest that marked change or loss of SEPs for longer than a critical period, probably somewhere between 15 and 45 min, may be associated with paraplegia. If SEPs recover intraoperatively during this type of surgery but alteration or obliteration has lasted beyond the critical period (which probably differs somewhat from patient to patient), the patient can be expected to have paraplegia with preservation of both dorsal column function and SEPs.

Intraoperative SEP changes and postoperative neurological deficits are rare for patients with distal pressures greater than 60 mmHg (8 kPa) during aortic occlusion.[159,163,169] Distal aortic pressures less than 40 mmHg (5.3 kPa), or interruption of intercostal artery flow, are associated with SEP loss, and SEP loss for more than 30 min is associated with a high incidence of paraplegia.[105,159,163,170,171]

Methodological issues cloud the conclusions reached in one report of an attempt to assess the impact of distal aortic perfusion and SEP monitoring on outcomes of 198 operations for thoracoabdominal aneurysm.[172] First, patients were not randomized to have surgery with or without these adjuncts. The patients who did not have distal aortic perfusion and SEP monitoring were those in whom these measures could not be used for either technical or administrative reasons. Second, SEPs were not monitored until completion of the operation. It is not unlikely that SEPs may have deteriorated after monitoring was stopped in the three patients who had immediate postoperative neurological deficits despite lack of intraoperative SEP change. Another factor complicating the analysis of these results is the fact that 11 of the 20 neurological deficits began between 12 h and 21 days after the initial postoperative examination. Despite the methodological limitations in this report, there was an association between level of intraoperative SEP change and final neurological outcome. However, the high rate of false negatives (13%) and false positives (67%) limited the influence of combined SEP and distal aortic perfusion monitoring on neurological outcome.

Of 1509 patients having thoracoabdominal aortic operations performed by a single surgeon between 1960 and 1991,[157] 234 had paraplegia or paraparesis postoperatively (16%). Factors associated with spinal cord injury were total aortic clamp time, extent of aortic repair, aortic rupture, patient age, proximal aortic aneurysm, and history of renal dysfunction. During the more recent years, survival rates improved but rates of paraplegia changed little. Late onset of paraplegia was related to postoperative complications, particularly respiratory failure and hypotension. A separate report describing variables predictive of outcome in 832 of these same patients[173] showed that the use of atriofemoral bypass eliminated the increased risk associated with prolonged aortic occlusion times. The authors of this analysis concluded that the two most important factors for patients who were paraplegic or paraparetic postoperatively were the degree and duration of spinal cord ischemia and failure to successfully reimplant critical intercostal arteries.

Reports describing aggressive approaches to preservation of spinal cord function during surgery on the thoracoabdominal aorta suggest that progress is being made. A multimodality protocol used for 42 patients included complete intercostal reimplantation whenever possible, cerebrospinal fluid drainage to improve spinal cord perfusion pressure, maintenance of proximal hypertension during aortic occlusion, moderate hypothermia, high-dose barbiturates, and avoidance of hyperglycemia.[174] Mannitol, steroids, and calcium channel blockers were also used to minimize reperfusion injury. None of the 42 patients managed with this protocol had postoperative spinal cord injuries, compared with 6% of 108 historical control patients. More recently, the same group used atriofemoral bypass with local cooling of intercostal and visceral arteries during segmental resection of high-risk thoracoabdominal aneurysms.[175] Each segment of the aorta was perfused with cold crystalloid prior to occlusion and attempts were made to reimplant all pairs of intercostal arteries from T8 to L2. Warm ischemia of each segment was therefore limited to 30 min. Seven of the 23 patients described in this report had dissections or ruptures that necessitated emergency surgery and only one of these seven was paraplegic postoperatively – a remarkably low incidence in these very high-risk patients. Another approach to regional hypothermia of the spinal cord during aortic surgery was tested in rabbits.[176] With normothermia, 40% of the animals were paraplegic after 20 min of ischemia, 75% after 40 min, and 100% after 60 min. Perfusion of the lumbar epidural space with isotonic saline at 5 °C prevented any spinal cord injury even after 60 min of ischemia.

In a series of 22 patients monitored during surgery for coarctation,[105] one patient had abrupt and reproducible loss of SEPs upon test occlusion of the aorta. Because of this, the patient had subclavian aortic bypass

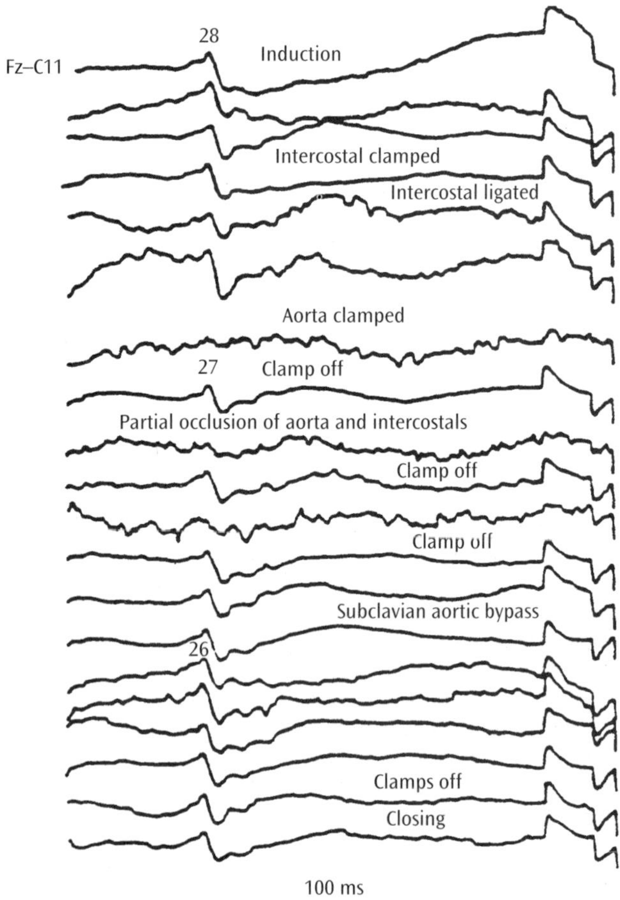

Figure 12.8 *SEP during aortic surgery. Potentials were elicited by stimulation of the posterior tibial nerve during thoracotomy for repair of an aortic coarctation. The cervical spinal-evoked potential disappeared during test occlusion of the aorta but returned promptly when the clamp was removed. The same phenomenon was seen during two subsequent attempts at aortic clamping. The surgeon elected to perform a subclavian aortic bypass rather than the usual patch-graft repair, which requires complete aortic occlusion. SEPs were normal during the rest of the procedure. There was no neurological deficit postoperatively. (A 1-µV, 9-ms calibration pulse is shown at the end of each waveform.) (From Friedman[23] with permission.)*

rather than resection of the coarctation (Fig. 12.8). SEPs recovered after full restoration of flow, and the patient suffered no neurological injury.

Simultaneous recordings from scalp electrodes and electrodes placed over the third lumbar vertebra showed that, during ischemia of a peripheral nerve produced by occlusion of the abdominal aorta or femoral artery, the lumbar spinogram could disappear rapidly while cortical potentials were preserved.[177] Presumably, a desynchronized afferent volley from the partially ischemic peripheral nerve was not adequate to produce a lumbar potential but was sufficient for amplification at the cortical level.

Motor EPs (MEPs) are less sensitive than SEPs for reliably predicting motor function after aortic occlusion in animals.[178] Spinal EPs may also be less sensitive than cortical SEPs for detecting clinically important spinal cord ischemia. Postoperative paraparesis has been described postoperatively in a patient who had well-maintained spinal EPs throughout aortic cross-clamping.[179]

SEP monitoring may be helpful during spinal angiography and embolization. In a series of 41 patients, injection of contrast material rapidly reduced SEP amplitudes.[180] Improved SEPs after embolization correlated with improved clinical function. One patient in this group suffered irreversible SEP loss and a new neurological deficit.

SEP monitoring during carotid endarterectomy

The middle cerebral artery is the artery most often embolized in patients having carotid endarterectomy (CEA), and its watershed areas are the most at risk from cerebral hypoperfusion during carotid occlusion. The primary cortical response to stimulation of the median nerve at the wrist arises in the area at risk, so that SEP monitoring is potentially useful for detecting ischemia, for indicating the need for shunting, and for predicting postoperative outcome. However, there is considerable debate about this issue, largely centered around the criteria for assessment of ischemia and the reliability of SEP monitoring compared with standard EEG monitoring.

In a series of 675 CEA procedures, SEPs had a diagnostic sensitivity of 60% in the prediction of neurological outcome, and a specificity of 100%.[181] SEPs,[182] as in the case of EEGs,[183] have detected otherwise unsuspected shunt occlusions. A report published in 1991 showed that shunting in those patients demonstrating complete loss of SEPs during occlusion was associated with an improved outcome.[184] In the latter study involving 400 operations, 17 patients had complete loss of SEPs during carotid occlusion. Of these, seven did not have a shunt inserted and five (71%) of them had postoperative neurological deficits; however, of the 10 patients who did have shunts inserted, only three (30%) had neurological deficits after surgery.

Some of the apparent discrepancies among reports of EEG and SEP monitoring during CEA may be related to the fact that there is no consensus on criteria for abnormality of either. This problem is clearly illustrated by a report of 193 CEA procedures under general anesthesia that compared SEPs according to different criteria.[185] An increase in central conduction time of > 20% from the anesthetic baseline control recording was 100% sensitive and 89% specific for early postoperative neurological morbidity. When a criterion of amplitude reduction of > 50% was used, sensitivity was 86% and specificity 96%. For complete loss of the cortical response, sensitivity was 71% and specificity 99%. A high level of sensitivity in detecting possible ischemic injury is far more important than specificity when attempting to prevent neurological injury. Most clinicians would prefer a criterion with sensitivity as close to 100% as possible (no undetected brain injuries) even at the cost of a lower level of specificity.

A few studies have directly compared SEP and EEG monitoring during CEA under general anesthesia. Results were not uniform. One study concluded that conventional EEG and SEP monitoring had similar sensitivity and specificity.[186] However, evaluation of this result is difficult in light of the fact that SEPs were monitored only before, during, and for 15 min after carotid occlusion rather than continuously from before induction of anesthesia until awakening. Also, no shunt was used in any patient regardless of EEG or SEP changes.

Other authors have argued that SEP monitoring is a sufficiently reliable predictor of the need for shunting, and can be used as the primary monitoring modality.[187–189] However, in another study, SEP monitoring was found to be less sensitive than 16-channel EEG recording for detecting intraoperative cerebral ischemia.[190] In this study, selective shunting was used in a series of 53 CEA procedures, during which EEG evidence of ischemia was seen in 23 patients during carotid occlusion; only 10 of these had an increase of ≥ 0.1 ms in SEP latency and only one of the 23 had a ≥ 50% decrement in SEP amplitude.

Another comparison of EEGs and SEPs during CEA included 151 operations and found that SEP monitoring was a useful supplement to conventional EEG monitoring.[191] No change was seen in either EEG or SEPs upon carotid occlusion in 120 cases. In 16 cases, cortical SEPs were severely depressed; these were the only cases in which a bypass shunt was used. Fifteen patients with more moderate SEP changes had no shunts, and none of these 15 had new neurological deficits postoperatively. Two deficits were seen in patients who had marked SEP abnormalities as well as EEG changes, and one occurred in a patient with no reported change in EEG or SEPs.

Most intraoperative SEP monitoring examines only subcortical and initial cortical activity, usually through the initial cortical positivity. This peak is normally seen 20–25 ms after stimulation of the median nerve at the wrist. SEPs of intermediate latency, thought to arise in immediately adjacent areas of the cortex, may be more sensitive to cerebral ischemia than the short-latency SEPs most often used for monitoring during CEA.[192]

Taken together, the most reliable methods of brain monitoring during CEA seem to be clinical assessment of the alert patient operated upon under regional anesthesia and 16-channel analog EEG, continuously monitored by a knowledgeable observer from before induction of anesthesia until the patient is sufficiently awake for postoperative neurological assessment. When neither of these techniques is available, SEP or more limited EEG monitoring can provide valuable information to guide intraoperative management.

SEP monitoring during cardiac surgery

Fewer investigations have been carried out with EP monitoring during cardiac surgery than during CEA. Hypothermia increases the latencies of all major components of the SEPs.[193] Late components are more markedly affected than early components. Brachial plexus injury related to self-retaining sternal retractors can be detected with SEPs elicited by stimulation of the median or ulnar nerve.[194]

All cortical SEP activity was lost at 18 °C in nine profoundly hypothermic infants. SEPs recovered in an average time of 30 min after rewarming.[195] One infant had a prolonged time to recovery of SEPs after rewarming and went on postoperatively to develop seizures. Two babies with normal recovery of SEPs had cortical blindness. This suggests that EEGs or multimodal EPs may be preferable for monitoring patients during cardiopulmonary bypass. SEPs would not be expected to reflect function of the occipital cortex.

SEP and nerve conduction studies in peripheral nerve surgery

Management of injuries to peripheral nerves or the brachial plexus is greatly facilitated by intraoperative recording of EPs and NAPs.[23,196–198]

The most important contribution of electrophysiological monitoring in this setting is determination of the type of injury to the peripheral nerve: neurapraxia, axonotmesis, or neurotmesis. Neurapraxia is a reversible injury; the variable loss of distal function usually improves within days or weeks without surgical intervention. Intraoperatively, the most important distinction is between axonotmesis, in which axons and myelin are interrupted but the surrounding connective tissue is preserved, and neurotmesis, when not only the axons and myelin but also the surrounding connective tissue elements are disrupted. During surgery 2–3 months after injury, the appearance of either lesion is usually that of a "neuroma-in-continuity." The distinction between the two types of injury in this case cannot normally be made by either visual inspection or observation of the muscle response to proximal nerve stimulation. No muscle contraction will be produced in either case. It is the distinction between neurotmesis and axonotmesis, however, that determines the appropriate operative treatment. With neurotmesis, no natural pathway exists for regeneration of the nerve, and so the intervening neuroma should be resected and the cut ends of the nerve reanastomosed. By contrast, in axonotmesis, the natural pathway already provided for regeneration of the nerve is far superior to the pathway provided by reanastomosis. In this situation, only neurolysis should be carried out.

This dilemma can be resolved electrophysiologically. In the axonotmetic injury, sufficient nerve regrowth (about 1 mm day^{-1}) will have occurred for conduction of NAPs across the neuroma incontinuity. Thus, transmission of the NAPs indicates an axonotmetic lesion, whereas failure of transmission determines that the lesion is neurotmetic. Sensory fibers can be tested by stimulation just distal to the neuroma and recording cortical SEPs.

SEP monitoring during intracranial surgery

Recordings of SEPs from multiple electrodes placed directly on the surface of the cerebral cortex can be used to locate precisely the rolandic fissure during resection of lesions in adjacent areas.[199,200] The fissure is identified by a phase reversal of the N20 component.[139] Recordings from depth probes can also be used to identify the locations of deep cortical structures during surgery for Parkinson's disease and other movement disorders.[130] More frequently, SEPs recorded from scalp electrodes are used to monitor the adequacy of brain perfusion during surgery for intracranial aneurysms or arteriovenous malformations (AVMs). Studies in baboons have shown that SEPs elicited by stimulation of the median nerve begin to deteriorate at cerebral blood flow levels of approximately 15 mL per 100 g per min.[201] Neuronal injury, however, does not occur until flows fall to 10 mL per 100 g per min or lower.[202] Thus, SEP monitoring can warn of cerebral ischemia before irreversible damage occurs. When induced hypotension is planned, SEPs can be monitored during a trial of hypotension prior to placement of brain retractors so that pressures below those that alter the SEPs can subsequently be avoided to minimize cortical injury from retractors.[203]

Reduction in SEP amplitude, increasing central conduction time, or loss of the cortical response can be used as guides for manipulating arterial blood pressure, timing temporary vascular occlusion, or repositioning imperfectly placed aneurysm clips.[204,205] If EPs are lost during temporary occlusion of an intracranial artery, postoperative neurological deficit will be less likely if flow can be established within 10–12 min.[206,207]

Ischemia in areas not monitored by the EP recordings may not be detected.[204] In areas of the cerebral cortex adjacent to but not within the monitored pathway, ischemia will not be detected unless it is so severe that it extends to areas within the monitored pathway. SEP monitoring is most valuable during surgery for aneurysms of the middle cerebral artery[205] or internal carotid artery.[207]

By contrast, undetected injury is relatively frequent during surgery for aneurysms at the tip of the basilar artery. Here, ischemia of motor pathways can occur whereas somatosensory pathways are unaffected. The ischemia is sometimes sufficiently severe to extend into the somatosensory pathway and alter SEPs, but unpredictable motor deficits are particularly likely in patients with aneurysms at the basilar bifurcation. Unfortunately, this is the most common location of aneurysms in the posterior circulation, leading to a recommendation that both BAEP and SEP monitoring are performed during surgery on the posterior circulation. In a study published in 1994, it was found that by using both modalities the false-negative rate was 20%, compared with 60% if only the BAEP data was considered and 47% if only SEP monitoring had been performed.[208]

Most SEP monitoring for intracranial vascular surgery has been carried out with median nerve stimulation. For anterior communicating and anterior cerebral artery aneurysms, however, posterior tibial nerve stimulation is more appropriate. The leg and foot areas of the cortex are at greatest risk during these procedures. SEPs elicited by stimulation of the posterior tibial nerve have been used to determine the safety of sacrificing an enlarged anterior cerebral artery that was the main feeding vessel of a large AVM.[209]

SEP changes with positioning

SEP changes related to positioning have been detected incidentally, indicating brachial plexus compression. In two patients, peripheral and cortical SEP components were lost when patients were placed in the park-bench position for neurosurgical procedures.[210] As both peripheral components and cortical waveforms were affected, it was evident that the problem was peripheral in nature. SEPs were restored by positioning an axillary roll under one patient and repositioning the arm of the other. This maneuver restored the SEPs so that the surgical procedure could be monitored, and it almost certainly prevented compression injuries of the brachial plexus.

Transient loss of cortical SEPs, with preserved cervical potentials, has been seen when positioning a patient with a large posterior fossa tumor that displaced the brainstem.[211] The reversible SEP changes were attributed to transient brainstem ischemia, and so the patient's position was modified to one that did not obliterate the cortical SEPs. Unfortunately, SEP loss occurred after about 2 h of surgery and the patient was left with a profound hemiparesis.

SEP monitoring in the critical care unit

SEPs can provide information of diagnostic and prognostic value in patients with head trauma.[212–216] Central conduction time (CCT) measurement is particularly useful in comatose patients.[214] The extent of CCT prolongation is usually correlated with the extent of injury, and decreases with clinical recovery. Only in patients with supratentorial injuries, however, are nearly normal SEPs correlated with good outcomes.[217] When the primary injury is in the brainstem, prolonged CCT may be found in patients who make good recoveries. Patients who die or have severe disability may initially have normal CCT on one side but absent cortical SEPs on the other. In one series of patients with severe head injuries (Glasgow coma scale ≤ 7), EP measurements predicted outcome more accurately than did motor findings, intracranial pressure measurements, or pupillary light reaction.[218]

In children with mild to moderately severe closed head injuries, long-latency SEP findings were correlated with long-term deficits in school performance.[219] A comparison of SEPs and MEPs in 140 patients with head injury and 73 with nontraumatic coma showed that SEPs were better predictors of outcome than were MEPs.[220] All the patients in this series with bilaterally absent cortical SEPs died, whereas all with bilaterally preserved SEPs and CCT ≤ 6.5 ms survived. Approximately one-third of the patients in this series had bilaterally preserved electromyographic responses to transcranial stimulation but died. Asymmetries in CCT between the two hemispheres are usual in head-injured patients and are the most important criterion for recognizing the onset of cerebral ischemia.

CCT is also prolonged in patients comatose from nontraumatic causes,[221] although experience is less in these patients than in patients with head injuries. Central hypothermia prolongs CCT,[214] but hypothermia of the limbs with central normothermia may not.[222] During barbiturate coma with EEG silence or marked burst suppression, CCT can be recorded but is prolonged.[65,214]

In patients who have suffered cardiac arrest, SEP measurements correlate well with outcomes.[223-225] Absence of cortical or thalamocortical activity after a cardiac arrest, while Erb's point or cervical recordings are intact, portends a poor outcome. If these findings persist for several days after cardiopulmonary arrest, it is very likely that the patient will die or remain in a persistent vegetative state. Intermediate-latency SEPs elicited by stimulation of the median nerve (erroneously called long-latency potentials in the report) were 100% accurate in predicting good versus poor outcomes among 66 patients who were successfully resuscitated from cardiac arrest but were still unconscious and mechanically ventilated.[225] In a recent study of outcome after cardiac arrest, long-latency SEPs were found to be better at predicting outcome than emergency physician review of clinical data.[226] The N70 peak was found between 74 and 116 ms in all 17 patients with good outcomes. In the 49 patients with poor outcomes, the N70 was either absent ($n = 35$) or delayed to a latency between 121 and 171 ms ($n = 14$). Among 57 asphyxiated infants, normal SEPs recorded within 3 days of birth were associated with normal outcomes at 18–24 months.[227]

SEP latencies and regional cerebral blood flow measurements in patients with grade IV aneurysms differed statistically from those of patients in all other grades.[228,229] CCT measurements can be used in the critical care unit to detect the onset of vascular spasm and monitor its course.[112,230] In baboons subjected to ligation of the middle cerebral artery, CCT and regional cerebral blood flow showed a highly significant correlation.[201]

SEP monitoring may be particularly helpful in infants or comatose patients with known or suspected injuries of the spinal cord because clinical assessment of cord function is severely hampered by inability of the patient to cooperate. The most important prognostic sign for spinal cord recovery is whether any function exists shortly after injury as this can be associated with considerable recovery over many months. Electrophysiological tests are also important for detecting peripheral nerve injuries in patients who have injuries of the spinal cord or who are comatose. Electrophysiological evaluation of the patient with spinal cord injury has been reviewed.[231]

SEPs are normal in psychogenic unresponsiveness. In the locked-in syndrome, the SEPs are variable – for lesions restricted to motor pathways they can be normal, whereas lesions involving the somatosensory pathways will cause marked changes.[232]

BRAINSTEM AUDITORY-EVOKED POTENTIALS (BAEPS)

Basic neurophysiology

The first 10–15 ms of the auditory-evoked potential is subcortical in origin (Table 12.3), and is referred to as the brainstem auditory-evoked potential (BAEP). BAEPs consist of a series of positive and negative waves that can be recorded in the far field from the vertex and ear, or from the vertex and a noncephalic reference (Fig. 12.9). They provide no information about the functional integrity of the cerebral cortex.

When sound waves strike the tympanic membrane, vibrations are transmitted through the middle ear by way of the ossicular chain to reach the inner ear. Pressure is applied to the cochlear fluid by means of stapes footplate displacement at the oval window. The fluid-filled chambers of the snail-shaped cochlea are separated by the basilar membrane, which supports the inner and outer hair cells in rows. When it is stimulated by sound waves, the basilar membrane moves like a traveling wave that starts at the base of the cochlea and moves toward the apex. The distance traversed from the base of the cochlea toward the apex is a function of the frequency of the stimulating sound, with low-frequency sounds traveling a greater distance than high-frequency sounds and therefore reaching farther toward the apex. The basilar membrane at the base of the cochlea responds mainly to very high frequencies, whereas that at the apex responds to low frequencies. The mechanical stimulus of membrane motion is transduced by the receptor cells (inner and outer hair cells) into a form that can excite the auditory neurons that innervate them. Each inner hair cell connects to several nerve fibers, while one nerve fiber supplies several outer hair cells. The electrocochleogram (ECochG) consists of the responses of the cochlea and auditory nerve to sound. It includes the cochlear microphonic and summating potential, which originate in the cochlear receptor cells, as well as the compound action potential of the extracranial portion of the auditory nerve.

Table 12.3 *Purported generators of brainstem auditory-evoked potentials*

Peak	Generator
I	Acoustic nerve
II	Intracranial acoustic nerve and/or cochlear nucleus (medulla)
III	Superior olive (pons)
IV	Lateral lemniscus (pons)
V	Inferior colliculus (midbrain)
VI	Medial geniculate (thalamus)
VII	Thalamocortical radiations

Listed peaks are positive at the vertex. See text for references. From Grundy,[21] with permission.

The first-order afferents of the auditory system are the spiral ganglion cells in the cochlea. Their central processes form the auditory portion of the eighth cranial nerve. These units discharge spontaneously but increase their discharges above the baseline rate in response to sounds. They synapse in the cochlear nuclear complex, where most of the afferents are ipsilateral but some units are also affected by inputs from the contralateral ear. Wave I of the BAEP arises from the extracranial portion of the auditory nerve. Wave II arises from the intracranial portion of the auditory nerve and/or the cochlear nucleus (medulla).

The central portion of the auditory pathway is complex. The neurons

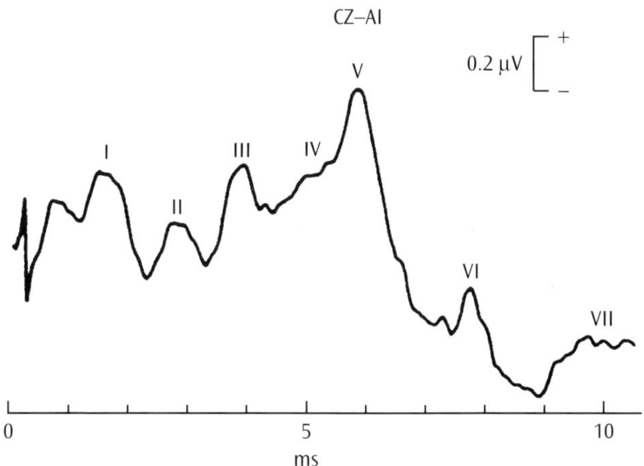

Figure 12.9 *A normal BAEP recorded during anesthesia, with the vertex positive, i.e. the grid 1 electrode is placed on the vertex and the grid 2 electrode on the earlobe. Activity which is positive (+) at the vertex is shown as an upward deflection.*

of the cochlear nuclear complex receive considerable nonprimary input from other neurons in the cochlear nucleus as well as from the superior olivary complex and the lateral lemniscus. The neurons of the cochlear nucleus connect to several nuclei on both sides, including the nuclei of the superior olivary complex through the nucleus of the trapezoidal body and the inferior colliculus through the lateral lemniscus. The inferior colliculus transmits impulses to the medial geniculate body and thence to the auditory cortex. Wave III of the BAEP is thought to arise primarily in the superior olivary complex (pons); wave IV from the lateral lemniscus (pons); wave V from the inferior colliculus (midbrain); wave VI from the medial geniculate (thalamus); and wave VII from the thalamocortical radiations. Waves VI and VII are inconsistent and are not routinely studied. These designations are clinically useful, although they represent considerable simplification of the actual situation. For example, it seems clear that each component of the BAEP, as recorded from the vertex and ear, represents some combination of afferent volleys in nerve fibers with nerve action potentials that may arise in more than one site.

Methods

Auditory stimulation

Ideally, baseline EPs will be recorded preoperatively with the same techniques and stimulators that are to be used intraoperatively. Pure-tone audiometry and testing of speech discrimination before anesthesia and operation are thought to be essential by a few authors. At the very least, the ear canals and tympanic membranes should be examined with an otoscope.

Because many patients have some hearing loss preoperatively, broadband filtered clicks are preferable to tones unless pure-tone audiograms have been carried out preoperatively to test hearing at the frequencies to be used for monitoring. Clicks with predominant frequencies near 2000 Hz minimize the effects of high-frequency hearing loss on EPs. This is particularly important in elderly patients.

Most clinicians prefer to set the intensity of auditory stimulation in relation to the individual patient's hearing threshold. Transducers should be regularly calibrated, so that actual stimulus intensity is known in "decibels peak equivalent sound pressure level" (dB pe SPL or dBSPL). The patient's auditory threshold ("sensation level;" SL) for the stimulus to be used should be tested, and stimuli 60–70 dB greater are used for intraoperative EP monitoring (60–70 dBSL). "Hearing level" (HL) refers to the mean sensation level established in a group of normal subjects with the equipment to be used for monitoring. A stimulus intensity set according to HL or dBSPL might be inadequate for a patient with partial hearing loss. Conductive hearing loss, if compensated for by increased stimulus intensity, produces little change in BAEP. By contrast, abnormalities of the eighth nerve or of central auditory pathways typically produce marked changes in the BAEP.

In the operating room, stereo headphones are usually impractical because they interfere with access to the surgical field during operations that pose risks of injury to auditory pathways. Transducers attached to molded ear inserts are ideal because the acoustic signal is delivered directly to the ear canal and cannot be obstructed by compression of soft tubing or earpieces. However, this transducer produces artifact in the nearby ear electrode, which can obscure as much as 2 ms of the initial portion of the BAEP when single-polarity stimuli are used. The stimulus artifact can be satisfactorily reduced by using clicks or tones of alternating polarity, i.e. the initial sound pressure alternates between positive (compression) and negative (rarefaction) so that the stimulus artifact in the averaged EPs cancels out.

To avoid the stimulus artifact when single polarity clicks are used, foam ear inserts can be connected with plastic tubing to speakers a few centimeters from the ear. Rarefaction clicks have been most widely used, but compression clicks are also satisfactory. In a proportion of normal subjects, rarefaction clicks are converted to compression clicks while traversing the ear canal. Click polarity is less important than keeping the stimulus constant throughout monitoring.

When speakers are removed from the ear by even a few centimeters of tubing, allowance must be made in measuring EP peaks for the time elapsed during transmission of the click or tone through the tube connecting the speaker to the earpiece. Manufacturers should specify the duration of this time delay; it can also be directly measured in an audiology laboratory. Because changes from the individual patient's baseline values are the parameters of interest for monitoring, it is best to record baseline BAEP with the same transducers to be used intraoperatively.

Recording

Recording in at least two channels, with at least periodic stimulation of the ear contralateral to the site of surgery, is helpful not only for quality control but also for help in identifying peaks when waveforms are abnormal or unusual. If central auditory conduction time is prolonged, and wave V (Fig. 12.9) is not well seen, sweep times should be lengthened to 15 or even 20 ms so that a delayed but recordable peak will not be missed. BAEP waveforms shown in this chapter show vertex positivities (or ear negativities) as upward deflections.

Intraoperatively, it is possible to record the compound nerve action potential directly from the auditory nerve in the surgical field. With the recording electrode directly on the nerve, the action potential is in the near field and is of greater amplitude than when recorded from surface electrodes. Although this technique is popular with some electrophysiologists, others find that it adds little to information gained noninvasively. Physical movement of the electrode causes noise that interferes with recording, but many fewer sweeps must be averaged to demonstrate the action potential recorded directly from the nerve.

Clinical experience with BAEP monitoring

BAEPs are used to monitor the functional integrity of the auditory nerve and brainstem in patients having neurosurgical procedures in the posterior cranial fossa, and in comatose patients in critical care units.

Intraoperative BAEP monitoring

BAEPs are used extensively during surgery in the posterior fossa. They are useful because the cochlear nerve is extremely sensitive,[233] is often involved in posterior fossa tumors, and is at risk during microvascular decompression of other cranial nerves.

In a series of 54 neurosurgical operations in the cerebellopontine angle,[104] intraoperative alterations in BAEPs were reported in 37 cases. An increase in wave V latency of 1.5 ms was considered abnormal, and more than half the patients in this series had changes of this magnitude or greater. In 22 of the 54 operations, BAEP changes were related to retraction of the cerebellum or brainstem. These changes progressed to virtual obliteration in six cases. Changes were also seen with the combination of relative hypotension and hypocapnia and with positioning for retromastoid craniectomy. In six cases, the BAEP was virtually obliterated with positioning.[104,234] Except for two patients in whom the auditory nerve was deliberately sacrificed, the BAEP returned toward normal when the head was returned to a neutral position at the end of the procedure and hearing was preserved.

In 32 of the 37 cases in this series during which BAEP changes were reported intraoperatively, waveforms recovered well toward baseline in the operating room.[104] In the remaining five patients, hearing was diminished preoperatively and BAEPs recorded before the induction of anesthesia were abnormal but reproducible. Two of these patients lost the BAEP prior to surgical incision, perhaps because of local ischemia related to anesthesia and positioning in already compressed nerves. One patient underwent sectioning of the eighth nerve as treatment for tinnitus, and in the four others the eighth nerve had to be cut during resection of large acoustic neuromas. All five patients with irreversible loss of the BAEP were deaf in the affected ear after operation. In all 54 cases, the presence or absence of BAEP at the end of anesthesia correctly predicted the presence or absence of auditory function postoperatively.

In another report, intraoperative BAEP recordings correctly predicted postoperative function of the auditory nerve after surgery in the cerebellopontine angle.[235] Out of 66 patients, 10 developed delays greater than 1.5 ms in "BAEP latencies" (peak or peaks not specified). These patients had diminished hearing postoperatively that recovered within 30 days. All six patients who had irreversible loss of the BAEP afterwave I had profound hearing loss postoperatively. Of these six, five had an apparently intact eighth nerve. Another patient had extensive cortical damage despite normal BAEP intraoperatively. In light of the fact that BAEPs are entirely subcortical in origin, this is not surprising.

Deafness is a recognized risk of surgery for microvascular decompression of cranial nerves.[103,104] Before the introduction of BAEP monitoring, ipsilateral hearing loss during this surgery was reported in 1–4% of patients having decompression of the fifth cranial nerve for trigeminal neuralgia, and partial hearing loss occurred in as many as 20% of these patients.[236] The risk of damaging the auditory nerve is greatest during surgery to decompress the seventh cranial nerve for treatment of hemifacial spasm, because of the proximity of the seventh and eighth nerves, but this risk can be reduced with the use of BAEP monitoring.[237,238]

In 21 patients monitored during microvascular decompression of cranial nerves,[239] prolongations of the absolute latencies of waves I, III, and V as well as I–III and I–V interpeak latencies were predictable with retraction of the cerebellum. Transient obliteration of BAEP occurred in four cases, and the surgeons were warned only for disappearance of the BAEP.

The BAEP is an exquisitely sensitive monitor of auditory function. When cranial nerve function is primarily at risk, warning can perhaps be withheld until the BAEP is lost. In contrast, because the brainstem is far more sensitive to ischemia and hypoxia than the cranial nerve, earlier warning might be chosen when the brainstem or its perfusion is primarily at risk. Clearly, BAEPs do not necessarily reflect function in all areas of the brainstem. This was illustrated in a report of a brainstem stroke during microvascular decompression while BAEPs were normal intraoperatively.[240] Postoperatively, however, auditory function was intact.

A number of reports have shown an improvement in hearing outcome when BAEP monitoring is used in attempts to preserve hearing during removal of acoustic neuromas.[241–243] A comparison of 90 patients who had BAEP monitored with 90 unmonitored historical controls, matched for tumor size and preoperative hearing, showed that in patients with tumors < 2 cm in size monitoring was associated with a greater likelihood that hearing would be preserved and a greater likelihood that preserved hearing would be usefu l.[242]

BAEPs are very small-amplitude signals. The large number of sweeps or recordings that need to be averaged before a useful signal can be obtained, and this delay while the signal is acquired, can reduce the sensitivity of the technique to neural injury. Cochlear microphonics, and recordings directly from the intracranial portion of the eighth cranial nerve, can provide valuable additional information during monitoring of the auditory system. Both produce large amplitude signals and thus have a faster response time. Cochlear microphonics are recorded directly from the inner ear, and provide information about cochlear viability,[244] whereas cochlear nerve action potentials are recorded from the intracranial portion of the eighth nerve.[245] These recordings may be superior to BAEP monitoring for monitoring and predicting postoperative hearing.[246,247]

BAEP in critical care

Brain-injured and comatose patients have been monitored in the intensive care unit with BAEP recordings. In 30 patients with severe head injuries, all those patients who recovered had normal BAEP throughout the clinical course, whereas patients who were severely disabled or vegetative had at least transient BAEP abnormalities.[248] In another 85 patients who were comatose after head trauma, BAEP findings also correlated with outcome status.[217] Both primary and secondary brainstem lesions affected BAEP. Most of the patients who died or survived with severe disabilities had abnormal BAEPs and abnormal SEPs.

BAEPs may not be helpful in predicting outcome from anoxic coma, as brainstem auditory pathways are more resistant to hypoxia than the cortex. They may thus remain normal, or in the case of postanoxic cochlear dysfunction they may disappear only to reappear a day later.[249]

In 53 comatose patients who had simultaneous BAEP and intracranial pressure recordings, acute increases in intracranial pressure to levels greater than 40 mmHg (5.3 kPa) were not always followed by changes in BAEP.[250] In these patients, prolongation of BAEP brainstem transmission time in response to elevations in intracranial pressure was almost always followed by brain death, while lack of BAEP change in association with increases in intracranial pressure was associated with a high probability of survival.

When no BAEP can be recorded from a comatose patient, it is necessary to demonstrate that the peripheral hearing mechanism is functional, as peripheral injuries to the auditory system are common in head injury. This can be done by showing presence of wave I of the BAEP or by recording the electrocochleogram or cochlear microphonic. If none of these can be recorded, the patient might simply be deaf.

Midlatency auditory-evoked potentials (AEPs) have been used extensively for assessment of anesthetic depth in the operating room.[89,251,252] More recently, midlatency AEPs have been used to assess sedation in the intensive care unit.[253] Event-related long-latency AEPs have been used to assess potential attention,[254] and predict outcome from traumatic coma.[255]

VISUAL-EVOKED POTENTIALS (VEPs)

Relatively little experience has been gained with monitoring VEPs in the operating room and intensive care unit. This may be partly explained by the remarkable complexity of the visual system and by logistic considerations.

Neurophysiology

Parallel processing in multiple channels is a key characteristic of the visual system.[256] At least seven parallel channels of ganglion cells are thought to process visual formation in the primate retina. Different classes of neurons specialize in recognizing particular features of visual stimuli such as luminance, contrast, and color-specific groups of neurons in the retina project to separate specialized brain regions, beginning with different laminae of the lateral geniculate body (LGB). Impulses are transmitted from the LGB to area 17 in the occipital cortex, and thence along multiple pathways to areas 18, 19, and the midtemporal areas. The inferior temporal cortex is another important area for visual processing, and multiple links exist between different areas. It has been estimated that more than half the cerebral cortex is devoted primarily to visual function in primates, and presumably in man, with at least nine visiotopically organized areas. Thus, visual responses involve large areas of the temporal and parietal lobes as well as the occipital lobe.

Different kinds of stimuli can be used to activate preferentially particular structures in the retina and associated visual pathways. For example, in a patient with impaired night vision, full-field flash stimulation would be used to evaluate the rod retinal receptor system, whereas a pattern-reversal VEP, the most sensitive electrophysiological test for function of the optic nerve, would be appropriate for a patient with suspected multiple sclerosis. In retrochiasmatic disorders, VEPs elicited by full-field pattern stimulation may be normal even in the presence of dense homonymous hemianopia. Attempts to detect unilateral retrochiasmatic lesions with hemifield VEPs have met with varying success.

Methods

VEPs are widely distributed over the occipital and parietal areas. They can be recorded from multiple locations between the vertex and inion, with a reference anterior to the vertex or off the head.

In the diagnostic laboratory, the visual system is most often stimulated with a reversing chessboard pattern on a television screen. The reversing pattern activates edge receptors in the retina, and the potentials produced are more sharply defined, with better reproducibility within and among subjects, than the VEPs produced by flash stimulation (Figs 12.10 and 12.11). Designation of the type of stimulus is important for interpretation,[84] as the different methods of stimulation produce different VEP responses. For pattern-reversal VEPs (P-VEPs or PREPs), various check sizes are used and are described as the number

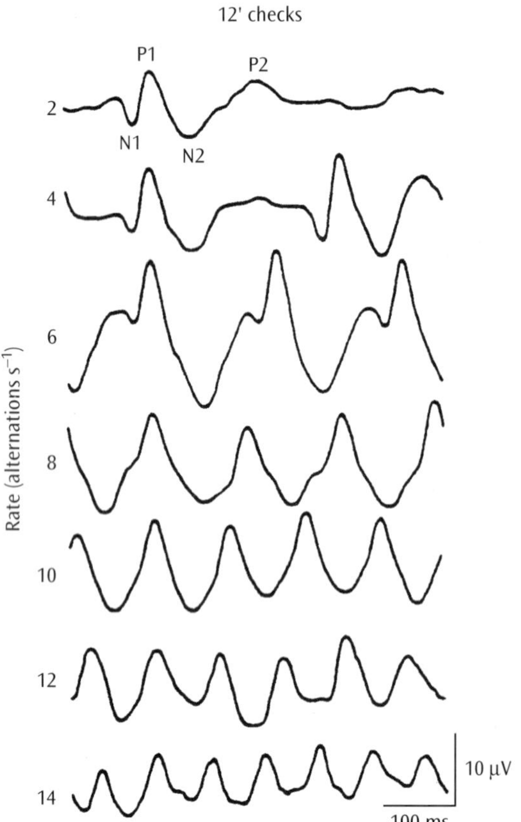

Figure 12.10 *Pattern reversal visual-evoked potentials elicited by stimulation at different alternation rates. The alternation rate per second is shown to the left of the records. Note the change from transient to steady-state VEPs at eight alternations per second. (From Sokol,[257] with permission.)*

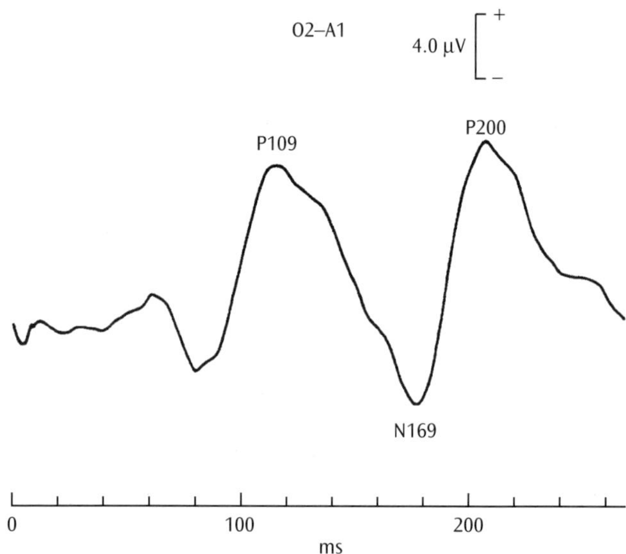

Figure 12.11 *Flash-evoked potential elicited by stimulation through closed eyelids, as for intraoperative VEP monitoring. (From Grundy,[28] with permission.)*

of degrees of visual arc subtended by a single square. Because the test requires the subject's cooperation, P-VEPs cannot be recorded in anesthetized or comatose patients.

Flashes of light can be used to evoke VEPs (Fig. 12.11). Stroboscopic flash is sometimes used in the laboratory or intensive care unit, but because of limited access to the patient's eyes stroboscopic flash is rarely used in the operating room. Arrays of light-emitting diodes (LEDs) can also be used to elicit VEPs (LED-VEPs). The color of the diodes should be noted, although it seems that any color flash through closed eyelids will be perceived as red.

In the operating room, LED arrays mounted in swimmer's goggles are most often used for visual stimulation. A bland ophthalmic ointment and clear tape should be used to protect the eyes under the goggles, and great care must be taken to assure that the goggle housing does not slip off the bony ridge of the orbit to compress the globe of the eye. Prolonged pressure on the eye can produce central retinal artery thrombosis and permanent untreatable blindness in that eye. VEPs are of greatest interest during surgery at the optic chiasm, in the anterior cranial fossa, and in the retrobulbar area, but these operations place the surgical field and the visual stimulators in immediate proximity. In such cases, any change in the VEPs that does not resolve immediately should prompt a careful check of the position of the visual stimulator.

Some investigators have obtained promising results with small LEDs mounted on scleral caps or contact lenses of the sort that are commonly used to protect the eye during major craniofacial operations.[258] A disadvantage of this stimulator is that it might pose some risk of injury to the eye, particularly when the eye (and contact lens) is not accessible for inspection intraoperatively. Better visual stimulators are needed.

For best results with VEP monitoring in the operating room or critical care unit, the pupils should be maximally dilated. The visual response is directly related to "retinal illuminance," the amount of light reaching the retina. This cannot be completely standardized when eyes are closed, but the pupillary constriction seen with narcotics can severely limit the quality of VEP recording. When mydriatic agents are used to dilate the pupil artificially, the ocular signs of neurological deterioration are temporarily lost. If the patient is awakened immediately after surgery for clinical neurological evaluation and is doing well, the dilated pupils may not be a serious problem. Otherwise, confusion about the patient's status could result. Individualized decisions must be made in consultation with the surgeon and anesthesiologist.

Clinical applications of VEP monitoring

Applications are essentially limited to procedures that might affect the anterior visual pathways or optic chiasm, such as operations in the anterior cranial fossa or on the pituitary gland. Because of the exquisite sensitivity of VEPs to anesthetic agents, meaningful monitoring is possible only with careful maintenance of a pharmacological steady state and avoidance of high concentrations of volatile inhaled anesthetics. Several interesting observations have been reported, including intraoperative improvement in abnormal VEPs followed by improved visual fields postoperatively.[22]

Somewhat more work has been carried out with VEPs in the critical care unit. In a series of 57 asphyxiated term infants who had SEPs and VEPs recorded during the first 3 days of life, abnormal VEPs were always followed by abnormal neurological outcomes.[227] In the same series, normal SEPs virtually guaranteed a normal outcome. Outcome prediction was better with both VEPs and SEPs than with either alone. Abnormal VEPs were also reliable predictors of unfavorable outcomes after head injury.[218] Steady-state VEPs recorded during neurosurgical procedures or in the intensive care unit showed changes within seconds of surgical and/or medical decompression of intracranial hypertension.[259]

MOTOR-EVOKED POTENTIALS (MEPS)

Motor pathways can be stimulated with electrical current or magnetic transients applied to peripheral or cranial nerves or nerve roots, to the spinal cord, or to the motor strip of the cerebral cortex. Motor nerve conduction studies are important in both the diagnostic laboratory and the operating room. Intraoperatively, direct stimulation is used to identify branches of the facial nerve or other motor nerves.

Monitoring of motor pathways in the spinal cord is of particular interest during operations that pose risks of injury to anterior segments of the cord with little effect on the posterior cord. SEPs are conducted predominantly in the dorsal columns, and in chronic injury or with isolated microsurgical or vascular insults to the anterior cord, SEPs and posterior cord function may remain intact while motor function is lost. Intraoperative insults to the anterior cord, however, are almost always accompanied by at least temporary alterations in posterior column function and SEPs. The "wake-up test"[15,16] is a reliable and simple method for testing motor function, but during some operations this test is not feasible.

Neurophysiology

The full length of a central motor pathway can be monitored electrophysiologically by stimulating the motor cortex transcranially either electrically or magnetically and recording nerve action potentials (NAPs) in peripheral nerves or evoked compound muscle action potentials (CMAPs) from muscles. For stimulation of the spinal cord, electrodes can be placed into the epidural or subarachnoid space blindly, with fluoroscopic control, or under direct vision.

When the motor pathways are stimulated at the level of the cervical spinal cord or lower, recording of peripheral NAPs may be misleading. Recordings from peripheral nerves following rostral stimulation of the spinal cord (the so-called "neurogenic motor-evoked potential") were initially thought by some observers to reflect the function of motor pathways.[260] Subsequent studies in animals, however, showed that the sciatic nerve response to spinal cord stimulation was abolished by dorsal column transection.[261] Antidromic sensory impulses recorded from peripheral nerves might be mistaken for motor NAPs because some sensory nerve fibers traverse these pathways from the periphery to the cervical cord with no intervening synapses. If antidromic sensory potentials were mistaken for motor potentials, serious misinterpretations might be made and injury to the patient could result. This is not a problem with cortical motor stimulation because no sensory nerves pass between points of stimulation and recording without intervening synapses.

Methods

Guidelines for the clinical application of electrical and magnetic stimulation of the brain, spinal cord, and nerve roots were produced by the International Federation of Clinical Neurophysiology and published in 1994.[262] Traditional stimulation of motor nerves in the surgical field is by placing the cathode in nearby subcutaneous tissue while the exploring anode is held in the surgeon's hand. Noninvasive stimulation of peripheral nerves is similar to that used for eliciting SEPs, except that the cathode is distal to prevent anodal block. The spinal cord can be stimulated by subarachnoid or epidural electrodes or by electrodes placed directly on the spinal cord. Evoked muscle activity can be monitored by direct observation or by recording the CMAPs. Inadvertent mechanical stimulation of the facial nerve by instruments in the surgical field produces electromyographic activity that can be used to provide audible feedback to the surgeon. This is similar to detection of unintended mechanical stimulation of spinal nerve roots during laminectomy by observation of the resulting muscle contractions.

Monitoring of the muscle activity evoked by any of these methods requires avoidance of complete neuromuscular blockade. Whether partial blockade lessens the reliability of MEP monitoring is not known. Complete resolution of this question would require extensive studies that considered, among other factors, the differing susceptibilities of different muscles to neuromuscular-blocking agents. Recording of peripheral NAPs avoids the requirement for preservation of neuromuscular transmission. Only with cortical stimulation, however, can one be sure that the recorded NAP is motor rather than sensory.

Initial reports of transcranial electrical stimulation described an anodal plate 3 cm by 5.5 cm attached to the scalp over the motor cortex, with a curved 4-cm disk electrode on the hard palate as the cathode.[263] Biphasic pulses of about 20 mA were applied for 0.75–1 ms at 17–28 Hz. Averaged EPs were recorded directly from the spinal cord after 250–500 stimuli. Movement was seen only at the higher levels of stimulation. Intraoperative monitoring was carried out using currents of 20–40 mA and 5–25 Hz, applied for several milliseconds. Multiple cathodal plates or a headband around the base of the skull permit stimulation with lower current levels. Although no seizure activity was described after this type of stimulation, hypertension and tachycardia were produced in some patients, but could usually be minimized by reducing the rate and duration of stimulation.

High voltages are required to transmit the necessary current across the skin and skull to the motor cortex. Single shocks of 500–700 V and 1000 mA have been used to demonstrate slowed conduction in patients with multiple sclerosis, and no apparent adverse effects have been reported.[264] The risk of cortical injury is reduced by minimizing current density using lower currents and larger electrodes.

A major disadvantage of MEPs is their sensitivity to anesthetic agents. Small changes can lead to large alterations in amplitude, and even low doses of inhalational anesthetic agents may obliterate MEPs.[265] Attempts to provide adequate anesthesia without abolishing these potentials suggest that intravenous anesthesia with nitrous oxide in concentrations no greater than 50–60% may be the most suitable.[266–268]

This problem can be overcome by direct electrical stimulation of the motor cortex, but this is only suitable for monitoring during surgery involving open craniotomy.[269] Modern methods of direct stimulation involve initial localization of the motor cortex using median or tibial nerve SEPs,[270,271] after which 1-cm^2 silver plate electrodes are placed on and around the area of the cortex that showed the largest P20/N30 response. Short trains of 1–5 high-frequency (200–800 Hz) monopolar pulses are administered. Each pulse lasts between 0.2 and 0.5ms.

Repeated electrical stimulation of the cerebral cortex with current densities sufficient to elicit after-discharges can produce an epileptic focus that continues to fire in the absence of further stimulation. In experimental animals, electrical stimulation, continued beyond the production of after-discharges, is used to produce a new epileptic focus in previously normal cortex. This phenomenon is called "kindling." During clinical electrocorticography, the EEG is monitored for after-discharges following direct cortical stimulation. If after-discharges are seen, subsequent stimulation can be reduced or eliminated so that kindling is prevented. Although seizures can be produced in epileptics, there are no reports of kindling due to direct electrical cortical stimulation in the clinical setting. Calculations of current densities at the surface of the cerebral cortex during transcranial electrical stimulation suggest that these are near those current densities achieved during direct cortical stimulation.

Large variations in MEP amplitude between and within patients have been noticed, and even 80% decreases of amplitude have been unreliable in predicting adverse outcome.[272] The problems of variability and of the deleterious effects of general anesthesia can be dealt with by using high-frequency multipulse transcranial stimulation. When short trains of brief stimuli (50 µs each, with an interstimulus interval of 2–3 ms) are applied, the descending motor impulses overcome the synaptic inhibition caused by anesthetic agents, and temporal summation of the excitatory postsynaptic potential amplifies the myogenic responses. This technique has been successfully used in several investigations.[273–275] In these investigations, the endpoints were latency and amplitude of myogenic MEPs. "Threshold-level" repetitive transcranial electrical stimulation is now in common use and differs in that the primary outcome is the minimum stimulus energy required to produce a barely perceptible muscle contraction.[276] Trains of three or four stimuli, each with a duration of 50 µs, separated by 2- or 3-ms intervals are applied at gradually increasing intensity, starting at 100 V, and with a maximum of 500 V. A reduction in threshold of > 100 V in any muscle group is considered significant.

Transcranial magnetic stimulation is less well localized than electrical stimulation. In addition to exciting neurons that generate descending motor potentials, it activates excitatory intracortical axon collaterals to neighboring pyramidal cells.[277] Inhibitory neurons projecting to the same pyramidal cells are also activated.[278] At low rates of stimulation (0.3–1 Hz), these connections balance each other and no horizontal spread of excitation is seen. With stimulation at higher frequencies, of which recently available stimulators are capable, the faster conduction in myelinated monosynaptic excitatory collaterals outstrips the slower conduction of inhibitory potentials. Temporal summation of excitatory postsynaptic potentials thus proceeds more rapidly than temporal summation of inhibitory postsynaptic potentials. The imbalance between excitatory and inhibitory corticocortical connections can produce widespread horizontal activation of the cortex sufficient that re-entering self-generating activity causes a seizure, even in subjects with no predisposing factors.

Studies in normal volunteers revealed that the number of transcranial magnetic stimuli required to produce excitatory spread fell as stimulus frequency and intensity increased.[279] These investigators derived parameters estimating a maximum number of stimuli that could be given at various rates and intensities. According to their estimates, magnetic stimulation at 25 Hz and 200% threshold can be safely applied for only four impulses.

It should also be noted that many commercially available magnetic stimulators produce noise sufficient to impair hearing in both patient and physician.[280,281] Susceptibility to noise-induced hearing loss may be increased by the effects of muscle relaxants on the protective middle ear acoustic reflex.[282] Three out of nine volunteers in one study had decreased hearing after only 240 s of rapid transcranial magnetic stimulation.[279] This had resolved 4 h later. Violent propulsion of ferromagnetic objects within the field of the magnetic stimulator is an ever-present possibility, even though the field is relatively small.

Precautions for transcranial magnetic stimulation at rates of 1 Hz or faster have been suggested, based on studies in normal conscious volunteers.[279] Both patient and physician should wear earplugs. Precautions must be taken to prevent burns from metal electrodes that can be overheated by magnetic pulses. Subjects should be informed of the possibility of seizures, particularly when there is a family history of seizure activity. As EEG after-discharges are not sufficiently reliable to predict a risk of seizures occurring, spreading muscle activity that increases with continued stimulation should be considered the first sign of epileptogenic activity. With adequate precautions and adherence to guidelines safety is within acceptable limits.[283]

Transcranial magnetic stimulation is also very sensitive to the anesthetic agents. In a study of the effects of intravenous agents of magnetically stimulated MEPs, after induction of anesthesia MEPs were only obtained in 14% of patients in whom anesthesia was induced with propofol, compared with 20% in the thiopentone group, 53% in the methohexitone group, and 57% in the etomidate group.[284] Another study confirmed that propofol impairs the signal, and that volatile anesthetic agents can obliterate the signal. The authors thus recommended that an etomidate–fentanyl–nitrous oxide technique is used.[285] Although neuromuscular blockade can be used, it must be carefully titrated to levels of around 70–80% blockade.[272,285]

Complications with transcranial electrical stimulation are rare, but include tongue laceration caused by contraction of the masseter and temporalis muscles[274] and mandibular fracture caused by biting movements on the endotracheal tube.[276]

Clinical applications of MEP monitoring

Monitoring of motor activity elicited by stimulation of cranial or motor nerves is well accepted and straightforward. Such monitoring is considered indispensable during operations on peripheral nerves and during mastoidectomy or procedures in the posterior cranial fossa. Auditory monitoring of electromyographic activity inadvertently produced by surgical instruments can rapidly alert the surgeon to possible impending injury of the facial nerve.[286,287] Six out of 10 patients so monitored during partial neuromuscular blockade had marked decreases in CMAPs intraoperatively and postoperatively had severe impairment of facial nerve function.[288] The cranial nerves that supply the extraocular muscles can be monitored during cranial base surgery by stimulating within the surgical field and recording from subdermal electrodes placed near the extraocular muscles.[289]

Much of the current work is on refinements in technique, rather than on the benefits of MEP monitoring on outcome. Evaluation of studies of MEPs is made complicated by the large number of permutations between methods available. For example, for electrically stimulated MEPs, stimuli can be applied via the scalp or directly to the cortex or spine, while recordings may be taken from the spine, epidural space, or a peripheral nerve (neurogenic MEPs), from a muscle (myogenic MEPs), or simply from observation of motor response. Another complicating factor is the lack of consensus on warning or action criteria.

Early studies of MEPs and spinal cord potentials produced by transcranial stimulation of the motor cortex provided some disappointing information. These potentials are exquisitely sensitive to anesthetic agents (Fig. 12.12), particularly when slower stimulation frequencies are used.[290] An initial report of MEP monitoring in 98 cases indicated that

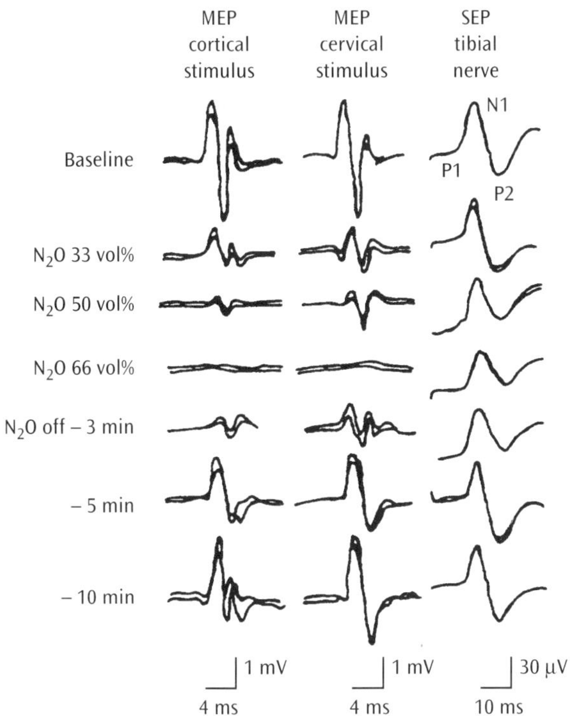

Figure 12.12 *Changes in rodent motor and somatosensory EPs produced by nitrous oxide. MEPs represent the electromyographic activity elicited by cortical and cervical stimulation. SEPs were recorded from cortical electrodes after stimulation of the tibial nerve. (From Zentner and Ebner,[290] with permission.)*

responses to stimulation of the motor cortex that were recorded from the spinal cord were relatively resistant to anesthetics but changed so little in amplitude and latency with injury conditions that their use was compromised.[291] In a study in 27 dogs, MEPs elicited by direct electrical stimulation of the motor cortex and recorded over the lumbar spinal cord were compared with SEPs elicited by stimulation of the sciatic nerve and recorded over the thoracic spinal cord.[178] The dogs were subjected to 60 min of occlusion of the proximal descending aorta. Twenty dogs developed cord injuries. SEPs were found to be more sensitive to ischemic spinal cord injury than MEPs: SEPs changed in 19, whereas MEPs were lost in only nine of the 20 dogs with cord injury. However, MEPs were more specific. SEPs were lost in three of the seven dogs that remained neurologically normal, whereas MEPs were unchanged in all seven.

More recent reports using newer electrical transcranial stimulation techniques show more encouraging results and much greater sensitivity to cord injury, and some groups now report sensitivity that is similar to or better than that obtained with SEPs.[292] Good sensitivity has also been reported with magnetic stimulation.[268,293]

In a recently published series of 194 patients monitoring with both SEPs and threshold-level transcranial electrical stimulation, there were no false-negative and no false-positive MEP studies with regard to postoperative motor outcome, whereas with SEPs there were four false positives and three false negatives with regard to sensory function.[276] Many groups now recommend that both modalities are used when spinal cord function is at risk.[276,294–296]

MEP monitoring deserves investigation during surgery for aneurysms at the bifurcation of the basilar artery. Unpredictable motor deficits are particularly likely in these patients, as motor areas are much closer than sensory pathways to the artery in question and may become ischemic while sensory pathways are spared and SEPs unchanged.

There is a paucity of published literature on the ability of MEPs to predict outcome from coma. In one study, MEPs and SEPs were recorded in 60 patients with traumatic coma and 35 patients with nontraumatic coma.[297] All patients in both groups with bilaterally absent cortical SEPs died. When SEPs were preserved bilaterally and central conduction times were 6.5 ms or less, all patients survived. By contrast, 31% of patients with traumatic coma and 39% with nontraumatic coma had bilaterally preserved MEPs to transcranial stimulation but died. Only the bilateral absence of MEPs was associated with certain death.

In 22 other patients who had coma of diverse etiology, MEPs were closely related to outcomes and appeared to be better predictors than the Glasgow coma scale.[298] However, of the six patients in this group who had bilaterally absent MEPs, one made a good recovery. Outcome prediction in this series was improved by using both SEPs and MEPs.

Six patients with severe chronic tetraparesis caused by head injury (three cases), basilar thrombosis (two cases), or global hypoxia (one case) had normal MEP thresholds and latencies following transcranial magnetic stimulation.[299] MEP amplitudes were greater than normal. These findings did not correlate with the clinical severity of paresis, particularly the severe paresis of the muscles from which MEPs were recorded – the thenar and abductor hallucis muscles. Despite the different underlying causes of the tetraparesis in these patients, all were shown using CT scans to have diffuse atrophy of cerebral white matter. Thus, intact conduction of the fastest corticospinal efferents is not sufficient for normal voluntary muscle strength.

INTRACRANIAL PRESSURE (ICP) MONITORING

Neurons and glia require perfusion with oxygenated blood in order to function and survive. The cranial vault is a relatively closed space and therefore subject to increases in pressure if the volume of any its contents rises beyond the limit of compensatory mechanisms. Monitoring of intracranial pressure in patients with mass lesions or intracranial catastrophes may facilitate appropriate clinical management when intracranial pressure levels are so high that they threaten cerebral perfusion.

Physiology

Cerebrospinal fluid (CSF) makes up only about 150 mL of the 1650-mL volume of the central nervous system contained within the cranial vault and the spinal column. Normally, about 500 mL of CSF is produced daily by the choroid plexus within the ventricles of the brain. This fluid circulates to the cisterna magna and the subarachnoid space before being absorbed by arachnoid villi in the sagittal venous sinus. Normal intracranial pressure (ICP) is usually less than 15 mmHg (2 kPa). Small changes in volume can be compensated for by movement of CSF out of the cranial vault into the spinal canal, but larger changes cannot. With an expanding supratentorial lesion, rostrocaudal deterioration in neurological function may be seen. If this process continues unabated, cerebral perfusion pressure falls, the brainstem and cerebellar tonsils herniate through the foramen magnum, and death results. Pressure differences between compartments of the intracranial vault can lead to other herniation syndromes, such as upward transtentorial herniation due to a rapidly expanding hematoma in the posterior fossa or uncal herniation beneath the falx with rapid formation of an intracerebral hematoma. Thus, pressure is not necessarily uniform throughout the cranial vault.

In the normal situation, small increases in intracranial volume produce only small and transient changes in intracranial pressure. As the limits of compensation are approached, however, intracranial compliance is decreased and a small change in volume can cause a marked change in ICP (Fig. 12.13). Moment-to-moment changes in intracranial

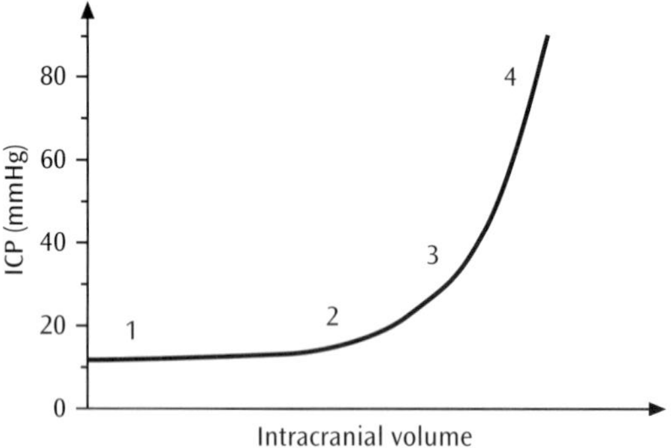

Figure 12.13 *Idealized pressure–volume curve for the intracranial vault. (From Shapiro,[300] with permission.)*

volume are often explained by changes in cerebral blood flow and blood volume. Autoregulation maintains cerebral blood flow constant between mean arterial pressures of approximately 50 and 150 mmHg (6.7 and 20 kPa), whereas cerebral blood flow is quite sensitive to either hypoxia or changes in the arterial partial pressure of carbon dioxide. ICP normally shows fluctuations with moment-to-moment changes in arterial blood pressure and respiration. Changes in ICP with hypercapnia or hypoxia can be dangerous in patients with decreased intracranial compliance. Patients with intracranial hypertension may show intermittent plateau waves, during which ICP is sustained for several minutes at levels of 50–100 mmHg (6.7–13.3 kPa). This is a dire prognostic sign.

Methods

Devices for monitoring ICP have been developed over the last 30 years. The ideal monitoring technique is accurate, reliable, cost-effective, and causes minimal patient morbidity.[301] The devices themselves can be classified according to whether the transducer is located within the cranial vault or externally.[302] Two devices using external fluid-coupled transducers will be discussed: the ventricular catheter and subarachnoid screw or bolt.

Measurement of ventricular fluid pressure by means of a catheter inserted into the lateral ventricle through a burr hole, fluid coupled to an external transducer, is the standard with which other methods are compared. First used by Guillaume and Janny[303] and later by Lundberg,[304] more than three decades of experience have now shown this technique to be relatively safe, even if it is the most invasive of the methods currently in use for continuous monitoring of ICP. It has the potential therapeutic advantage of lowering ICP by drainage of CSF. After subgaleal or subcutaneous tunneling, the catheter is attached to a strain gauge transducer and collecting system. Alternatively, the ventricular catheter may be attached to a subcutaneous reservoir, which is then tapped with a small needle for pressure measurement. When intracranial hypertension has produced small slit-like ventricles or when mass lesions have distorted the normal anatomy of the lateral ventricles, placement of a ventricular catheter may be difficult. The average rate of bacterial colonization of the catheter is 5%.[301] This increases significantly after 5 days of implantation.[305] However, the incidence of clinically significant intracranial infection is low.[306,307]

The subarachnoid screw or bolt (Fig. 12.14) is another fluid-coupled ICP monitor with an external transducer system.[308] A threaded hollow screw is inserted through a burr hole just far enough for its unthreaded tip to protrude about a millimeter beyond the inner surface of the dura. The screw is then linked to the external transducer through a saline-filled tube. Small leaks and frequent obstruction are the most common problems with this device.

ICP devices with transducers placed in the epidural space were widely used but are seldom indicated now. They are of questionable accuracy and technically difficult to place.[310–312]

The Ladd intracranial pressure monitor (Fig. 12.15) detects changes in ICP by deflection of a mirror which in turn alters return of fiberoptically transmitted light.[313,314] An external monitor detects the change in returned light and activates a servosystem which increases the air pressure in the intracranial transducer just enough to return the mirror to its original position. The ICP is equal to the counterbalance in air pressure generated by the monitor. This transducer can be placed in either the epidural or the subdural space. It has the relative disadvantage that it cannot be calibrated or zeroed *in vivo*. Also, it provides no waveforms for visual monitoring. Erroneous readings may be due either to air leaks or to fractures in the fiberoptic cable. With epidural placement, falsely high readings can be produced if the sensor is not exactly parallel with the dura or if prolonged use causes a change in the compliance of the dura.

The Gaeltec ICP monitor (Fig. 12.16) contains a strain gauge transducer at its tip with one side connected to the atmosphere by a rigid tube and the other reflecting ICP through a thin membrane.[315,316] The transducer generates an electrical signal that can be easily visualized on an external monitor. This transducer can be zeroed, *in vivo*, by injecting 0.3 mL of air to open the potential space between the transducer and the overlying membrane, equalizing pressure on the two sides of the strain gauge. The Gaeltec transducer is most often used in the epidural position, but its design permits subdural placement as well. Although this transducer can fail by either breakage of electrical connections or ruptures in the intracranial membrane, these problems are easily identified by failure to zero properly. Pneumocephalus has been detected following repeated attempts to zero this device after the membrane was ruptured.[317]

Intraparenchymal monitoring has recently been introduced for assessment of ICP. The Camino intracranial pressure monitor probe (Fig. 12.17) consists of a fiberoptic cable with a miniature transducer at the tip.[318] ICP is calculated following recording of a phase shift of an externally generated laser beam reflected off a pressure-sensitive diaphragm at the tip of the catheter. The probe is much smaller than those previously described for use in epidural or subdural ICP measurements. It can be inserted through a ventricular catheter or into brain parenchyma. The transducer can be calibrated but not zeroed *in vivo*. The Camino system is safe, accurate, and reliable. Comparisons of readings from this monitor with values from an intraventricular catheter have for the most part shown very close correspondence.[318,319] There is, however, potential for significant ICP measurement drift.[320,321]

Clinical applications of ICP monitoring

Monitoring of ICP is recommended for all patients who are comatose as a result of head injuries, even when initial CT shows no signs of intracranial hypertension.[323,324] Multimodality monitoring, including such measurements as blood flow velocity in the middle cerebral artery, jugular bulb venous oxygenation saturation, cerebral oximetry, and brain tissue oxygen monitoring, discussed below, add valuable information. Cerebral perfusion pressure, derived from ICP and intra-arterial pressure, is widely used and considered to be the most important monitoring parameter in patients with severe head injuries.[324–326]

Monitoring of ICP is also valuable in nontraumatic coma. It has been considered essential for managing patients having liver transplantation for fulminant hepatic failure.[327] In Reye's syndrome, which is characterized by brain swelling, there is evidence that ICP monitoring and a management protocol similar to that used for severe head injury can reduce mortality and morbidity.[328]

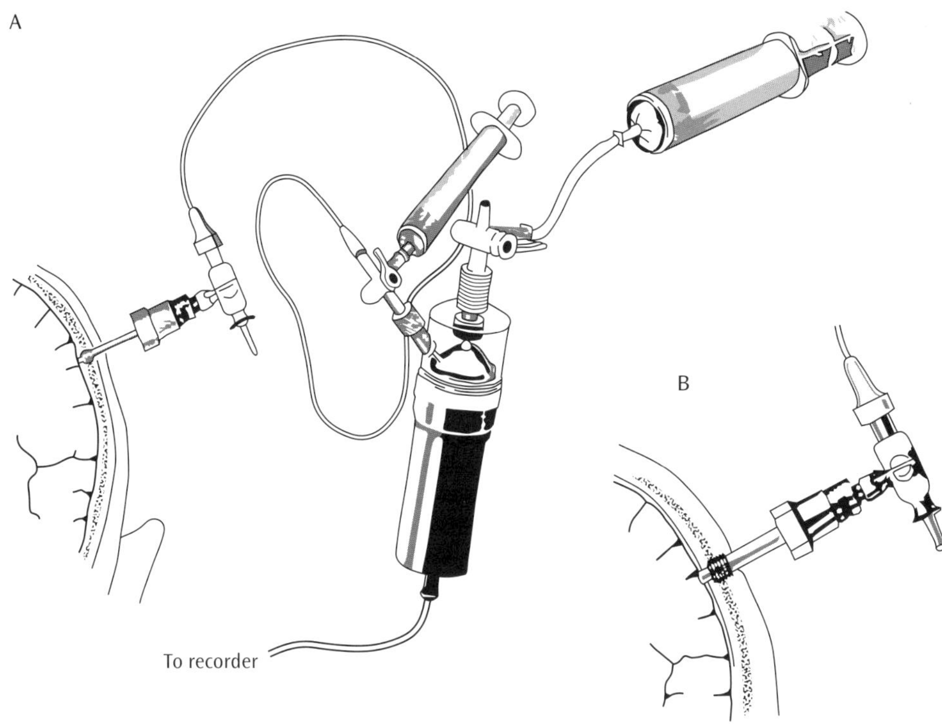

Figure 12.14 *(A) Subarachnoid intracranial pressure bolt. The device is screwed into a twist drill hole in the skull. The dura is incised and curetted up into the hole. (B) The tip of the bolt lies in the subarachnoid space. (From Warner and Sokoll,[309] with permission.)*

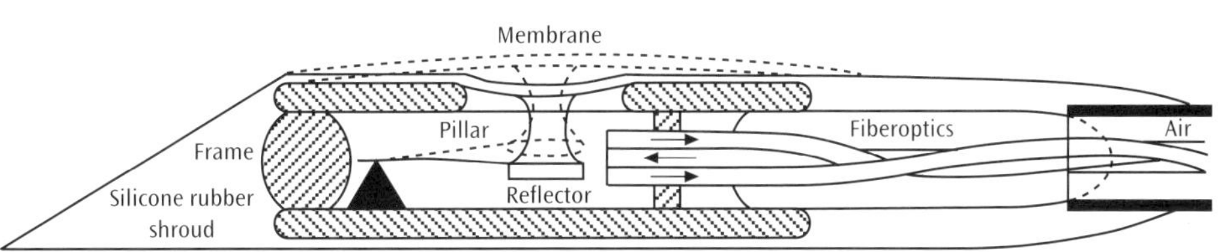

Figure 12.15 *Cross-section of the original Ladd intracranial pressure transducer. Deflection of mirror by ICP diminishes the amount of light transmitted along the fiberoptic columns. Counterbalancing air pressure maximizes light transmission when equal to ICP. (From Levin,[313] with permission.)*

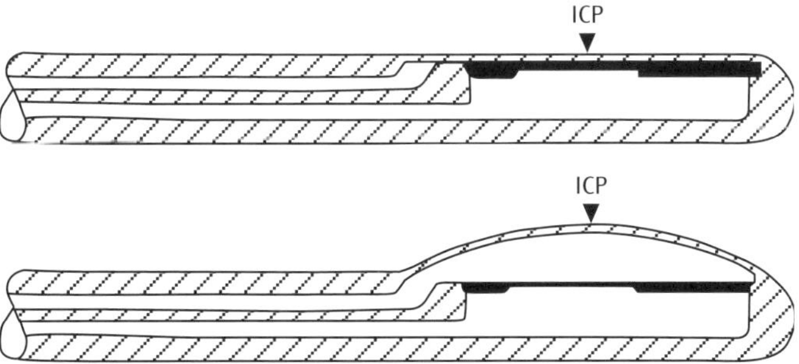

Figure 12.16 *Cross-section of Gaeltec intracranial pressure device. The top view shows how the transducer at the tip measures the difference between pressure transmitted across the membrane and atmospheric pressure. In the bottom view, the zero determination is made* in vivo *by injecting 0.3 mL air to equalize pressure across the transducer. (From Barnett and Chapman,[302] with permission.)*

CEREBRAL BLOOD FLOW (CBF)

The brain uses aerobic metabolism exclusively for energy production. Accordingly, the brain is critically dependent on the continuous delivery of oxygen and glucose to sustain cellular energy production. Resting CBF in the awake patient is approximately 50 mL per 100 g brain tissue per min.[329] As CBF decreases, neuronal dysfunction and injury occur. At levels of 16–18 mL per 100 g per min, cortical electrical function fails, as evidenced by attenuation in EEG and SEP recordings.[330] At levels of approximately 10 mL per 100 g per min or less, rapid changes in intracellular and extracellular ion concentrations occur, as well as the development of intracellular acidosis. Persistence of CBF at levels below this threshold for maintaining ionic balance will result in membrane disruption, irreversible neuronal injury, and cell death.[331]

Only a few of the numerous methods available for measuring or estimating CBF or oxygenation are practical in the operating room and the critical care unit. Positron emission tomography (PET), single-photon emission CT (SPECT), stable xenon CT, and magnetic resonance techniques, with few exceptions, require that the patient be transported to another part of the hospital. Although they can be used repeatedly, they cannot be used continuously at the bedside.

TRANSCRANIAL DOPPLER SONOGRAPHY (TCD)

Doppler ultrasound has been used extensively for noninvasive measurement of blood flow velocity in the heart and extracranial vascular tree. However, the skull is relative impermeable to ultrasound in conventional frequency ranges, and this initially hampered measurement of intracranial blood flow. In 1982, Aaslid and colleagues first described the use of Doppler ultrasound to record blood flow velocity in the basal cerebral arteries.[332]

The governing principle of the technique is application of the Doppler effect to blood flow. Doppler shift is defined as the difference between the ultrasound frequency emitted and the frequency that returns. In the case of blood cells flowing through an artery, the

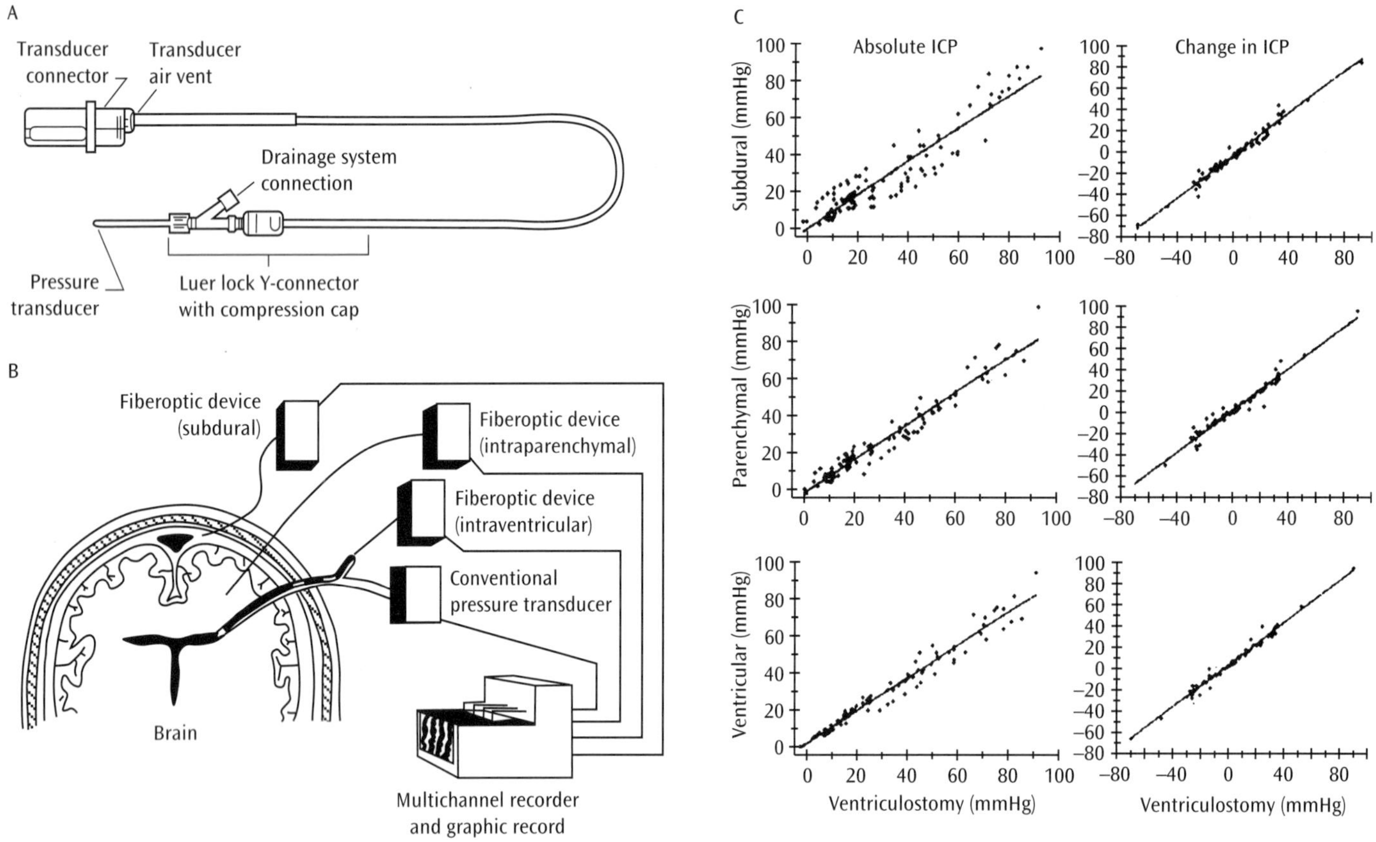

Figure 12.17 *The nonpneumatic fiberoptic Camino intracranial pressure monitor. (A) The intracranial transducer. (B) Set-up of Camino system for monitoring at different intracranial locations in dogs. (From Crutchfield* et al.,[322] *with permission.)*

ultrasonic beam is reflected in a spectrum of frequencies, as the blood cells in a cross-section of blood vessels are moving at different velocities. Spectral analysis of the frequency spectrum of the reflected beam permits calculation of systolic and diastolic blood flow velocities. (Figs 12.18 and 12.19)

TCD is most commonly performed through the temporal window (Fig. 12.20), where the skull is relatively thin, but can be performed using transorbital, suboccipital, or submandibular approaches. Using the transtemporal approach, flow velocity can be measured in the middle cerebral artery, the carotid siphon, and the anterior communicating artery. Posterior angulation will also permit insonation of elements in the posterior circulation. Commercial devices use a 2-MHz pulse range-gated transducer, which allows adjustment of the depth of interrogation.

TCD monitoring offers the following advantages. It monitors CBF continuously, is noninvasive, inexpensive, does not involve the use of ionizing radiation, and is easily usable in the operating room or critical care unit at the bedside.

It is, however, a far from ideal method of assessing cerebral blood flow.[334] The signal cannot be acquired in all subjects. The image must be obtained through areas in the skull which have no trabeculae "windows." Up to 15–40% of studied individuals do not have adequate windows.[335] The incidence of inability to record the signal is also greater with advancing age and in women. In addition, the angle of insonation must be less than 30° in order to improve the accuracy of the result. The orientation of the vessel path may preclude such a small angle. Maintaining a constant angle on follow-up studies is not possible. Most importantly, TCD measures velocity not flow.[336] The use of velocity to estimate flow depends on the critical assumption that the cross-sectional area of the insonated vessel and the viscosity of blood flowing through the vessel remains constant. Attempts to address these issues, such as calculating the pulsatiliy index as a reflection of cerebrovascular resistance, remain controversial.[337,338]

TCD monitoring is used during carotid endarterectomy (CEA) for detecting cerebral ischemia. Clinical experience with the technique has generally been favorable.[339] Controversy continues to surround issues such as the relation between absolute CBF and flow velocity under various clinical conditions, and whether predictions regarding CBF derived from monitoring flow velocity in large cerebral vessels correlate with perfusion at a regional, microvascular level.

In contrast with the use of TCD as a monitor of CBF flow during CEA, TCD is a sensitive method for detecting cerebral emboli that may accompany carotid manipulation, cross-clamping, and shunt inser-

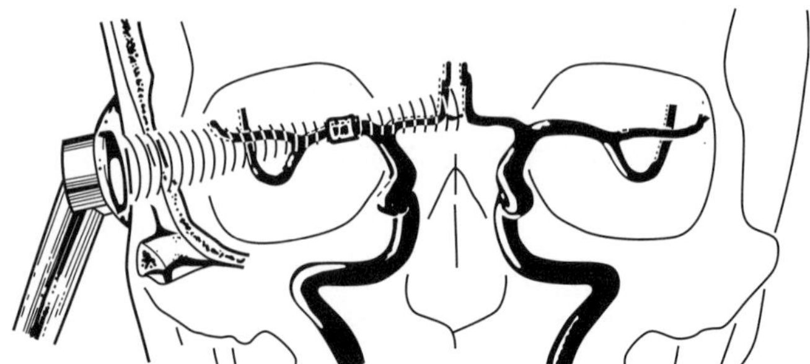

Figure 12.18 *Frontal view of the TCD probe directed toward the middle cerebral artery (MCA). The cylinder around the MCA indicates the observation region (sampling volume) for the Doppler recording. The distance from the middle of the cylinder to the probe corresponds to the depth setting. (From Aaslid* et al.,[332] *with permission.)*

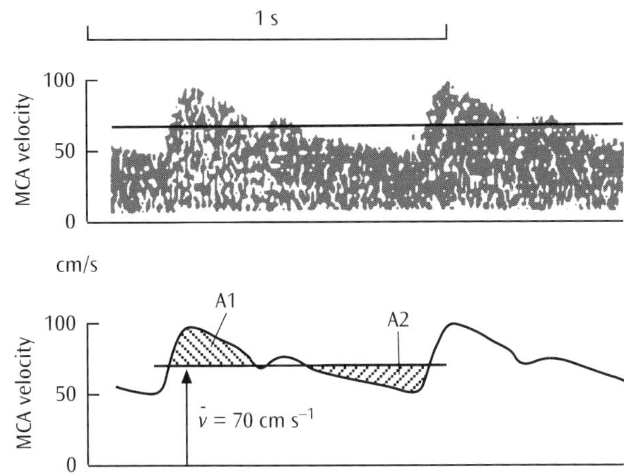

Figure 12.19 *Spectral display of the Doppler signal from the middle cerebral artery (MCA). The horizontal line through the spectra represents a cursor that can be moved up or down the display by the operator. The spectra are shown above and an outline of them below. The cursor was placed so that the areas A1 and A2 were judged equal, and the corresponding velocity was calculated by using the Doppler equation. (From Aaslid* et al.,[332] *with permission.)*

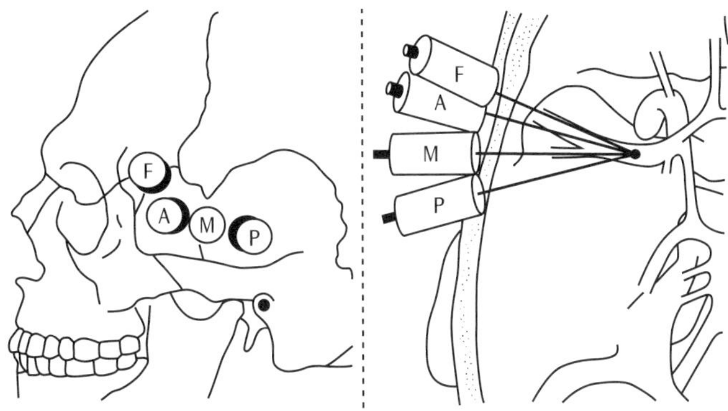

Figure 12.20 *Temporal sites for transcranial Doppler probe insonation of the middle cerebral artery: the frontal (F), anterior (A), middle (M), and posterior (P) windows are depicted. (From Newell and Aaslid,[333] with permission.)*

tion.[340] Several prospective studies have demonstrated that the number of emboli detected during carotid dissection correlate with the risk of adverse neurological outcome and radiologic evidence of cerebral injury.[341,342] TCD has also been used to detect shunt malfunction during CEA.

TCD monitoring of CBF can be performed during nonpulsatile normothermic or hypothermic cardiopulmonary bypass. A decline in neuropsychological function following cardiopulmonary bypass has been related to the number of emboli detected.[343] Cerebral microembolization therefore represents an important mechanism of perioperative brain injury during certain operations. There are, however, few validation studies that correlate TCD signals with known emboli.[344] A consensus committee report has been published, providing identifying criteria for Doppler-detected emboli, for TCD users.[345]

In critical care units, there is considerable experience with the use of TCD for the detection of cerebral vasospasm following subarachnoid hemorrhage.[346,347] In this setting, one assumes that blood flow either remains constant or decreases so that an increase in velocity indicates a narrowing of blood vessels rather than increased flow.

Other applications of TCD include confirmation of cerebral death,[348] detection of intracranial hemorrhage in head injuries, and assessing CBF and its autoregulation in pathological states such as acute stroke[349,350] and infective meningitis.[351,352]

LASER DOPPLER FLOWMETRY (LDF)

LDF is similar to TCD in that it uses the principle of Doppler shift to calculate flow velocity. In contradistinction, LDF fibers measure velocity in the microvessels of a very small volume of tissue, rather than a large artery. Coherent light from a laser source (usually helium neon) is carried to the probe via a fiberoptic cable. The probe is placed on the brain area of interest, and the laser waves penetrate the tissue. When light strikes moving red blood cells in brain parenchyma, a Doppler shift is produced and light is reflected back to the probe. A photodetector quantifies the reflected light and this is analyzed by a microprocessor. The final output is a graphical representation of pulsatile blood flow.[353] The device is inexpensive, lightweight, small enough to be inserted through the same site as an intracranial pressure monitor, and provides continuous flow measurement to a discrete area of the brain. There are several drawbacks to this device, however. Owing to difficulties in calibration and data handling, measured flow is expressed in arbitrary LDF units. An unsolved problem is the definition of LDF signal threshold below which cerebral ischemia occurs.[354] Other disadvantages are that it is invasive, analyzes a very small volume of tissue, (often less than 3 mm^3), and is susceptible to blood clots obscuring laser light transmission. Further, this technique is subject to significant movement artifacts, by either probe or patient movement.[355]

LDF has found applications in neuroanesthesia[356] and intensive care[357] in the management of intracranial aneurysm and head injury. However, it is still largely a research tool, useful for studying rapid changes in regional cerebral blood flow.[358]

XENON-133 CLEARANCE TECHNIQUE

In the 1950s and 1960s, radioactive inert gases such as ^{133}Xe came into use for the determination of cerebral blood flow. Xenon was chosen for the following reasons: superior uptake into brain tissue, improved accuracy of cerebral blood flow measurements, low radiation exposure, and elimination of inhaled gas.

Xenon may be administered via the carotid artery, by intravenous injection,[359] or by inhalation.[360] It equilibrates between the blood and the brain tissue after a sufficient period of administration. Once the administration of xenon is completed, arterial blood containing no xenon will wash out the xenon from the brain tissue into the venous blood. The xenon is cleared from the brain tissue at a rate that is dependent upon the quantity of blood that is perfusing the brain providing that the partition coefficient remains constant.[361] Arterial xenon concentration is estimated by arterial blood sampling or by measuring end-tidal xenon concentrations.[362] Multiple radiation detectors are used to measure uptake and clearance of radioactivity over the brain allowing for continuous measurement of regional blood flow. The data from these techniques are used to construct a xenon clearance curve from which global and regional cerebral blood flow can be calculated. The values of CBF using the xenon techniques have been shown to correlate well with cerebral blood flow values using the Kety–Schmidt method[363] and microsphere technique.[364] Furthermore, blood flow can be separated into gray and white matter flows. The invasive method of cerebral blood flow measurement also allows for calculation of global cerebral metabolic rate of oxygen ($CMRO_2$) as well as global cerebral vascular resistance.

The accuracy of the xenon clearance technique can be influenced by numerous factors. Recirculation of xenon from extracerebral tissues or decreased clearance from the lungs results in falsely low calculations of CBF.[362,365–367] The orientation and external placement of scintillation counters results in poor spatial resolution of gray and white matter,[368] "interhemispheric cross-talk,"[369] and "look through."[367] The partition coefficient and relative weights of gray and white matter vary regionally[370] and cannot be determined. Under conditions of low blood flow, there is an overlap of gray and white matter blood flows and xenon clearance rates (compartmental slippage), resulting in a falsely high CBF.[369] Xenon itself may modify the accuracy of CBF measurements via direct effects on CBF.[371–373]

The xenon clearance technique has been used as a method for intraoperative measurement of CBF in CEA.[374] These measurements are however expensive and require technical support. Hence, use of the technique has been limited to only a few centers. Reductions in measured CBF have been correlated with evidence of ischemic EEG changes.[40,375] However prospective studies using neurological outcome as the yardstick for evaluating the efficacy of CBF measurements during CEA have failed to demonstrate a consistent correlation.

CEREBRAL OXYGENATION

Jugular venous oxygen saturation (S_jO_2)

The measurement of oxygen tension or saturation in blood drawn intermittently from the jugular bulb to monitor cerebral oxygenation is not a new technique.[376] This method fell into disuse after it became clear that regional ischemia, even when severe, was often missed.[377] Continuous monitoring of S_jO_2 is now possible through the availability of flexible oximetric fiberoptic catheters. This has revived interest in the technique.

Based on the Fick principle, the $CMRO_2$ is the product of CBF and cerebral arteriovenous oxygen content difference ($AVDO_2$). Just as mixed venous oximetry reflects the balance between systemic oxygen consumption and cardiac output, so S_jO_2 reflects the balance between cerebral oxygen consumption and CBF. When oxygen delivery is greater than oxygen demand, as in hyperemia, $AVDO_2$ will decrease and S_jO_2 will increase. During periods of global cerebral hypoperfusion, more oxygen will be extracted from the blood, $AVDO_2$ will widen, and S_jO_2 will decrease.

The use of the catheter is safe and associated with few complications.[378] It provides an easily repeatable bedside measure of global cerebral blood flow, $CMRO_2$, and $AVDO_2$. However, there are technical limitations to this technique relating to the catheter.[379] Proper placement in the jugular bulb may be difficult both to obtain and to maintain. Falsely low saturations have been reported secondary to catheter coiling and to changes in head position.[380] Abutment of the catheter against the vessel wall produces low light intensity from the tip. Catheters have been reported to require high maintenance and frequent recalibration.

Noncatheter-related limitations of this method have also been described. The jugular venous bulb must drain only intracerebral structures for the calculation to yield reliable results. Extracerebral blood contaminant within the bulb and a rapid rate of withdrawal of blood cause underestimation of CBF.[381]

Blood from each hemisphere cross-drains into the contralateral jugular vein. Clinically significant variation in the jugular bulb oxygen saturations between the two sides has been demonstrated in a number of head-injured patients. However, it was not possible to predict which jugular vein would show the greater desaturation.[382] The right jugular vein is usually chosen for the purpose of continuous jugular venous oximetry because cannulation is both simpler and safer, although ipsilateral placement is preferred when there are lateralizing lesions. Trial compression of the internal jugular veins has been suggested to assess the relative effect on intracranial pressure produced in an attempt to judge which internal jugular vein has the greater flow.[382]

Clinical applications

Traumatic brain injury is an area where S_jO_2 monitoring has been found to be useful.[383] Episodes of S_jO_2 desaturation in patients with severe head injury have been correlated with poor neurological outcome.[384] Oximetry may be useful for optimizing hyperventilation, head-tilt, and blood pressure in the management of raised intracranial pressure in these patients.

Jugular bulb oximetry may similarly guide intraoperative management of blood pressure and ventilation in patients undergoing craniotomy.[385] Its use during cardiopulmonary bypass has shown that S_jO_2 desaturation occurs during rewarming.[386] This has been correlated with a worse postoperative outcome. However, the interpretation of S_jO_2 during hypothermic cardiopulmonary bypass is complex, and the underlying physiologic principles are not fully understood.

Near-infrared spectroscopy (NIRS)

NIRS is a noninvasive technique for continuous measurement of intracerebral oxygen saturation using reflected near-infrared light.[387,388] There are several commercially available NIRS instruments used to derive cerebral oxygen saturation (Fig. 12.21).

Multiple narrow-band wavelengths of light, generated either by refraction and filtering light from an incandescent source or by multiple lasers, are delivered by fiberoptic strands to the skin surface and directed through the segment of the brain. In neonates and infants, the scalp and skull are thin enough and the head small enough that the delivering fiberoptic bundle (optode) can be placed over the temporal area on one side of the head and the collecting fibers over the opposite temple. The intervening tissues scatter the light considerably, but most of the absorption of light in this pathway is by oxyhemoglobin, deoxyhemoglobin, and oxidized cytochrome aa_3. Their absorption spectra were determined in animal experiments. After signal processing and mathematical analyses, data are displayed on channels that represent oxyhemoglobin, deoxygenated hemoglobin, total volume of hemoglobin, and cytochrome aa_3.

Older instruments display relative rather than absolute units. An approximate quantification, however, can be obtained by calculating the length of the differential light path. The mean distance traveled by the photons is determined by measuring the time of flight of a light pulse traversing the head from one fiberoptic bundle to the other. The differential path length (mean distance traveled by the photons divided by the interoptode distance) is used to estimate quantitative values for oxyhemoglobin, deoxygenated hemoglobin, total volume of hemoglobin, and cytochrome aa_3. These values can only be valid for that part of tissue traversed by the light beam. Newer instruments used in adults use specially resolved spectrometry. Multidistance measurements of optical attenuation negate the need for estimating the path length.

Preterm neonates are ideal candidates for NIRS monitoring.[389,390] Term infants, older children, and adults have thicker skulls and larger heads that limit transmission of the photons. When the distance between the temples is greater than 7–9 cm, the light transmitter and receiver must be placed closer together. In this case, light is reflected rather than transilluminated.

Special problems hamper interpretation of reflectance NIRS. Because the thickness of scalp and skull vary considerably, appropriate focusing to facilitate separation of the superficial tissue signals from signals reflected from brain tissue is quite uncertain. Also, only a small wedge of cortex can be monitored, compared with a much greater segment of the frontal lobes in preterm neonates. When values are derived

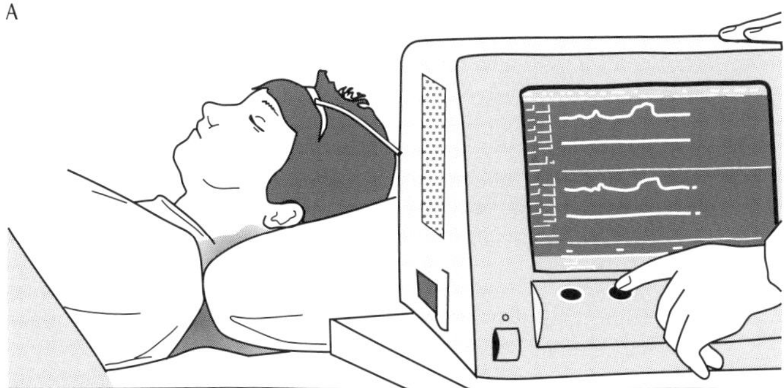

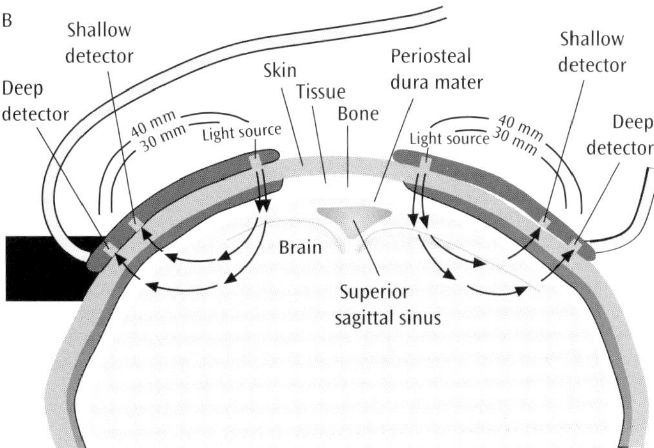

Figure 12.21 *(A) The INVOS 4100 uses two wavelengths of length in the near-infrared range from a light-emitting diode (LED) and measures the ratio of oxyhemoglobin (Hbo_2) to total hemoglobin (HbT), which is the percentage value of regional cerebral oxygenation saturation. (B) Two detectors located 30 and 40 mm from the LED allow the removal of the extracranial contribution of scattered light by application of a subtraction algorithm. The proximal detector receives less of a signal from the deeper brain tissue, whereas the distal detector measures the saturation of all of the tissue, including the skin, muscle tissue, skull, and brain. If the signal detected by the proximal detector is subtracted from that of the distal detector, the ratio of the two can give a mean value for cerebral saturation. (Redrawn with permission from Hamamatsu, Billerica, MA, USA, and Somanetics, Troy, MI, USA.)*

from reflected rather than transilluminated light, it is not possible to determine with certainty how much light reached the brain. This complicates estimates based on absorption, which are derived from measurements of light returned to the collecting optode. Furthermore, there is a suggestion that cerebral oximetry is affected significantly by changes in extracranial blood flow.[391]

Although NIRS has been reported to accurately reflect changes in jugular mixed venous oxyhemoglobin saturations in normal patients,[392] the technique suffers from a lack of agreement as to how criteria of cerebral oxygenation for various commercial monitors are established. Because the measurement technique and algorithms differ between instruments, there appears to be little agreement between their indices of cerebral oxygenation.[393] It has been studied as a monitor of cerebral ischemia in patients undergoing carotid endartectomy.[394,395] But there are still, to date, limited clinical data that evaluate cerebral oximetry as a predictor of adverse neurological outcome during carotid endartectomy.[396] Its use in the management of head injuries has been described,[397,398] but some studies have demonstrated limited clinical value for patients with severe head injury.[399] The information provided at present by near-infrared spectroscopy[400,401] can only be interpreted within a specific clinical context (Table 12.4).

Brain tissue oxygen tension monitoring

During the late 1990s the Neurotrend Cerebral Tissue Monitoring System (Fig. 12.22), an invasive monitor of brain tissue oxygen partial pressure, underwent several clinical trials during the late 1990s that resulted in FDA approval in 1999. The sensor (Fig. 12.23), a 0.5-mm-diameter catheter, is placed alone or in combination with an intracranial

Table 12.4 *Factors causing near-infrared spectroscopy changes*

Parameter	Factor causing a decrease
Oxyhemoglobin	A decrease in oxygen saturation
	Decreased cerebral blood flow
	Decreased oxyhemoglobin concentration
Deoxyhemoglobin	An increase in oxygen saturation
	Removal of obstruction to cerebral venous return
	Decreased inflow of desaturated blood
	Decreased deoxyhemoglobin concentration
Blood volume	A decrease in cerebral blood flow
	Removal of obstruction to cerebral venous return
	Decrease amount of hemoglobin
Cytochrome aa_3 oxidation	Decreased oxygen availability
	Decreased metabolic activity
	Increased electrons on respiratory chain

Increases in oxyhemoglobin, deoxyhemoglobin, blood volume, and cytochrome aa_3 oxidation occur with the opposite conditions. (From Brazy,[390] with permission.)

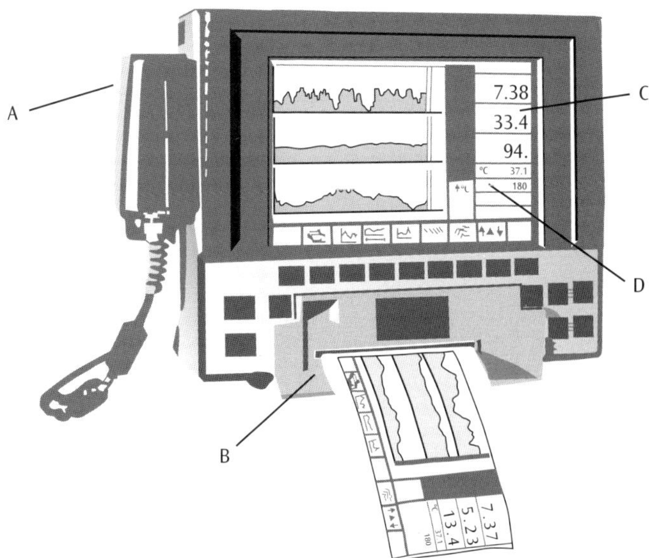

Figure 12.22 *The Codman Neurotrend Cerebral Tissue Monitoring System. Local brain tissue temperature, pH, Po_2, Pco_2 are monitored continuously. (A) Patient data module; portable and removable patient data module allows for patient transfers without loss of calibration or data. (B) Thermal printer module; thermal printer provides hard copy of information. (C) Large electroluminescent display; the monitor can be customized by the user to display real-time trending graphs or numbers according to needs. (D) Twenty-four-hour trend analysis; trended information provides immediate feedback to guide and confirm therapy, allowing the clinician to intervene before a crisis occurs. (Redrawn from Andrews,[402] with permission.)*

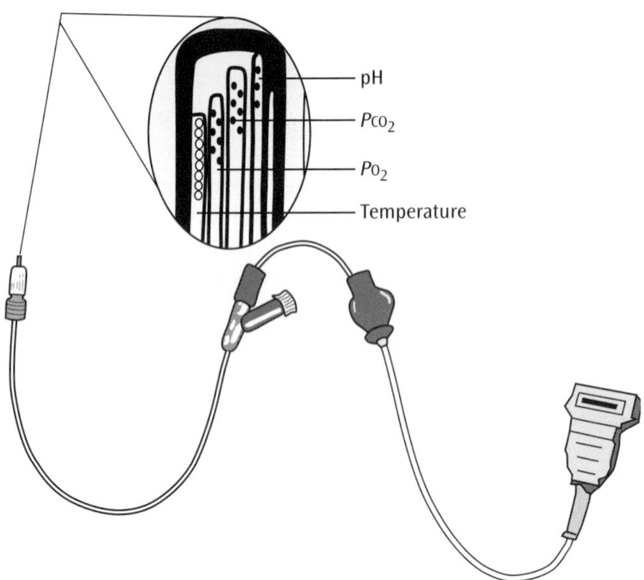

Figure 12.23 *The multiparameter sensor probe of the Neurotrend System, approximately 0.5 mm in diameter. (Redrawn from Andrews,[402] with permission.)*

pressure monitor probe in viable brain tissue (usually the frontal cortex, to a depth of 2–3 cm). Fluorescent dyes chosen to respond to oxygen, carbon dioxide, and hydrogen ion, or, alternatively, in the case of oxygen, a Clark electrode, and a temperature sensor are included within the catheter.

Monitoring of oxygen partial pressure in brain tissue ($P_{ti}O_2$) reflects the balance between oxygen delivery and consumption by the brain tissue investigated. It has been used in the early detection of brain tissue hypoxia and to direct therapy in severely head-injured patients.[403–405] There remains debate as to where best to place the probe in these patients and the value of $P_{ti}O_2$ below which the brain is critically ischemic. Because the technique is new, the role of $P_{ti}O_2$ measurements in the effort to minimize the risk of secondary ischemic brain damage requires further definition.[406]

CONCLUSIONS

New developments in monitoring technology, in concert with our rapidly growing understanding of the function and malfunction of the central nervous system, offer exciting new ways of monitoring the brain and spinal cord. Many of these methods are still experimental, but some provide important information that may well have a dramatic effect on the outcome of patient care in the operating room and critical care unit. Nevertheless, clinical assessment of the awake patient, when this is possible and reasonable, is still the most important technique available for monitoring the central nervous system. The additional methods described in this chapter become important primarily, although not solely, when clinical assessment is severely constrained by anesthesia or coma.

REFERENCES

1. Haglund MM, Berger MS, Shamseldin M, *et al.* Cortical localization of temporal lobe language sites in patients with gliomas. *Neurosurgery* 1994; **34:** 567–76.
2. Signorelli F, Guyotat J, Isnard J, *et al.* The value of cortical stimulation applied to the surgery of malignant gliomas in language areas. *Neurol Sci* 2001; **22:** 3–10.
3. Ebel H, Ebel M, Schillinger G, *et al.* Surgery of intrinsic cerebral neoplasms in eloquent areas under local anesthesia. *Minim Invasive Neurosurg* 2000; **43:** 192–6.
4. Silbergeld DL. Intraoperative transdural functional mapping. Technical note. *J Neurosurg* 1994; **80:** 756–8.
5. Hans P, Bonhomme V, Born JD, *et al.* Target-controlled infusion of propofol and remifentanil combined with bispectral index monitoring for awake craniotomy. *Anaesthesia* 2000; **55:** 255–9.
6. Meyer FB, Bates LM, Goerss SJ, *et al.* Awake craniotomy for aggressive resection of primary gliomas located in eloquent brain. *Mayo Clin Proc* 2001; **76:** 677–87.
7. Danks RA, Aglio LS, Gugino LD, Black PM. Craniotomy under local anesthesia and monitored conscious sedation for the resection of tumors involving eloquent cortex. *J Neurooncol* 2000; **49:** 131–9.
8. Soriano SG, Eldredge EA, Wang FK, *et al.* The effect of propofol on intraoperative electrocorticography and cortical stimulation during awake craniotomies in children. *Paediatr Anaesth* 2000; **10:** 29–34.
9. McDougall RJ, Rosenfeld JV, Wrennall JA, Harvey AS. Awake craniotomy in an adolescent. *Anaesth Intensive Care* 2001; **29:** 423–5.
10. Herrick IA, Craen RA, Blume WT, *et al.* Sedative doses of remifentanil have minimal effect on ECoG spike activity during awake epilepsy surgery. *J Neurosurg Anesthesiol* 2002; **14:** 55–8.
11. McCleary AJ, Maritati G, Gough MJ. Carotid endarterectomy; local or general anaesthesia? *Eur J Vasc Endovasc Surg* 2001; **22:** 1–12.
12. Love A, Hollyoak MA. Carotid endarterectomy and local anaesthesia: reducing the disasters. *Cardiovasc Surg* 2000; **8:** 429–35.
13. Peitzman AB, Webster MW, Loubeau JM, *et al.* Carotid endarterectomy under regional (conductive) anesthesia. *Ann Surg* 1982; **196:** 59–64.
14. Steed DL, Peitzman AB, Grundy BL, Webster MW. Causes of stroke in carotid endarterectomy. *Surgery* 1982; **92:** 634–41.
15. Vauzelle C, Stagnara P, Jouvinroux P. Functional monitoring of spinal cord activity during spinal surgery. *Clin Orthop* 1973; **93:** 173–8.
16. Sudhir KG, Smith RM, Hall JE, Hansen DD. Intraoperative awakening for early recognition of possible neurologic sequelae during Harrington-rod spinal fusion. *Anesth Analg* 1976; **55:** 526–8.
17. Teasdale G, Jennett B. Assessment of coma and impaired consciousness. A practical scale. *Lancet* 1974; **2:** 81–4.
18. Botterell EH, Lougheed WM, Scott JW, Vandewater SL. Hypothermia, and interruption of carotid, or carotid and vertebral circulation, in the surgical management of intracranial aneurysms. *J Neurosurg* 1956; **13:** 1–42.
19. Hunt WE, Hess RM. Surgical risk as related to time of intervention in the repair of intracranial aneurysms. *J Neurosurg* 1968; **28:** 14–20.
20. Kapoor RK, Kumar R, Misra PK, *et al.* Brainstem auditory evoked response (BAER) in childhood bacterial meningitis. *Indian J Pediatr* 1996; **63:** 217–25.
21. Grundy BL. Monitoring of sensory evoked potentials during neurosurgical operations: methods and applications. *Neurosurgery* 1982; **11:** 556–75.
22. Grundy BL. Intraoperative monitoring of sensory-evoked potentials. *Anesthesiology* 1983; **58:** 72–87.
23. Friedman WA, Theisen GJ, Grundy BL. Electrophysiologic monitoring of the nervous system. In: Stoelting RK, Barash PG, Gallagher TJ (eds). *Advances in Anesthesia.* Chicago, IL: Year Book Medical Publishers, 1988: 213–89.
24. Speckmann E-J, Elger CE. Introduction to the neurophysiological basis of the EEG and DC potentials. In: Niedermeyer E, Lopes Da Silva F (eds). *Electroencephalography: Basic Principles, Clinical Applications, and Related Fields.* Baltimore, MD: Williams & Wilkins, 1993: 15–26.
25. Rampil IJ. A primer for EEG signal processing in anesthesia. *Anesthesiology* 1998; **89:** 980–1002.
26. Kochs E. Monitoring of the central nervous system. *Acta Anaesthesiol Scand Suppl* 1996; **109:** 60–1.
27. Jasper HH. The ten-twenty electrode system of the International Federation. *Electroencephalogr Clin Neurophysiol* 1958; **10:** 371–3.
28. Grundy BL. Electrophysiologic monitoring: electroencephalography and evoked potentials. In: Newfield P, Cottrell JE (eds). *Neuroanesthesia: Handbook of Clinical and Physiologic Essentials.* Boston, MA: Little, Brown and Company, 1991: 30–58.
29. Thogersen B, Ording H. Bispectral index monitoring: comparison of two types of electrode. *Anaesthesia* 2000; **55:** 242–6.
30. Blume WT, Sharbrough FW. EEG monitoring during carotid endarterectomy and open heart surgery. In: Niedermeyer E, Lopes Da Silva F (eds). *Electroencephalography: Basic Principles, Clinical Applications, and Related Fields.* Baltimore, MD: Williams & Wilkins, 1993: 747–56.
31. Lopes Da Silva F. EEG analysis: theory and practice. In: Niedermeyer E, Lopes Da Silva F (eds). *Electroencephalography: Basic Principles, Clinical Applications, and Related Fields.* Baltimore, MD: Williams & Wilkins, 1993: 1097–123.

32. Nuwer MR. Quantitative EEG. II. Frequency analysis and topographic mapping in clinical settings. *J Clin Neurophysiol* 1988; **5:** 45–85.
33. Nuwer MR. Quantitative EEG. I. Techniques and problems of frequency analysis and topographic mapping. *J Clin Neurophysiol* 1988; **5:** 1–43.
34. Demetrescu M. The aperiodic character of the EEG: a new approach to data analysis and condensa. *Physiologist* 1975; **18:** 189.
35. Bickford RG. Computer analysis of background activity. In: Redmond A (ed.). *EEG Informatics: a Didactic Review of Methods and Applications of EEG Data Processing*. Amsterdam: Elsevier, 1977: 215–32.
36. Fell J, Roschke J, Beckmann P. Deterministic chaos and the first positive Lyapunov exponent: a nonlinear analysis of the human electroencephalogram during sleep. *Biol Cybern* 1993; **69:** 139–46.
37. Law SK, Nunez PL, Wijesinghe RS. High-resolution EEG using spline generated surface Laplacians on spherical and ellipsoidal surfaces. *IEEE Trans Biomed Eng* 1993; **40:** 145–53.
38. Pradhan N, Dutt DN. A nonlinear perspective in understanding the neurodynamics of EEG. *Comput Biol Med* 1993; **23:** 425–42.
39. Chiappa KH, Burke SR, Young RR. Results of electroencephalographic monitoring during 367 carotid endarterectomies. Use of a dedicated minicomputer. *Stroke* 1979; **10:** 381–8.
40. Sundt Jr TM, Sharbrough FW, Piepgras DG, *et al.* Correlation of cerebral blood flow and electroencephalographic changes during carotid endarterectomy: with results of surgery and hemodynamics of cerebral ischemia. *Mayo Clin Proc* 1981; **56:** 533–43.
41. Tolonen U, Sulg IA. Comparison of quantitative EEG parameters from four different analysis techniques in evaluation of relationships between EEG and CBF in brain infarction. *Electroencephalogr Clin Neurophysiol* 1981; **51:** 177–85.
42. Tolonen U. Quantitative 99mTechnetium cerebral circulation time in brain infarction. Its relation to clinical findings, electroencephalograms and conventional radionuclide studies. *Acta Neurol Scand* 1981; **64:** 337–52.
43. Rampil IJ, Holzer JA, Quest DO, *et al.* Prognostic value of computerized EEG analysis during carotid endarterectomy. *Anesth Analg* 1983; **62:** 186–92.
44. Krul JM, Ackerstaff RG, Eikelboom BC, Vermeulen FE. Stroke-related EEG changes during carotid surgery. *Eur J Vasc Surg* 1989; **3:** 423–8.
45. Nuwer MR. Intraoperative electroencephalography. *J Clin Neurophysiol* 1993; **10:** 437–44.
46. Rosenthal D, Stanton Jr PE, Lamis PA. Carotid endarterectomy. The unreliability of intraoperative monitoring in patients having had stroke or reversible ischemic neurologic deficit. *Arch Surg* 1981; **116:** 1569–75.
47. Green RM, Messick WJ, Ricotta JJ, *et al.* Benefits, shortcomings, and costs of EEG monitoring. *Ann Surg* 1985; **201:** 785–92.
48. Kresowik TF, Worsey MJ, Khoury MD, *et al.* Limitations of electroencephalographic monitoring in the detection of cerebral ischemia accompanying carotid endarterectomy. *J Vasc Surg* 1991; **13:** 439–43.
49. Blume WT, Ferguson GG, McNeill DK. Significance of EEG changes at carotid endarterectomy. *Stroke* 1986; **17:** 891–7.
50. Jansen C, Moll FL, Vermeulen FE, *et al.* Continuous transcranial Doppler ultrasonography and electroencephalography during carotid endarterectomy: a multimodal monitoring system to detect intraoperative ischemia. *Ann Vasc Surg* 1993; **7:** 95–101.
51. Redekop G, Ferguson G. Correlation of contralateral stenosis and intraoperative electroencephalogram change with risk of stroke during carotid endarterectomy. *Neurosurgery* 1992; **30:** 191–4.
52. Astrup J, Symon L, Branston NM, Lassen NA. Cortical evoked potential and extracellular K+ and H+ at critical levels of brain ischemia. *Stroke* 1977; **8:** 51–7.
53. Symon L, Lassen NA, Astrup J, Branston NM. Thresholds of ischaemia in brain cortex. *Adv Exp Med Biol* 1977; **94:** 775–82.
54. Tempelhoff R, Modica PA, Grubb Jr RL, *et al.* Selective shunting during carotid endarterectomy based on two-channel computerized electroencephalographic/compressed spectral array analysis. *Neurosurgery* 1989; **24:** 339–44.
55. Silbert BS, Koumoundouros E, Davies MJ, Cronin KD. Comparison of the processed electroencephalogram and awake neurological assessment during carotid endarterectomy. *Anaesth Intensive Care* 1989; **17:** 298–304.
56. Kearse Jr LA, Martin D, McPeck K, Lopez-Bresnahan M. Computer-derived density spectral array in detection of mild analog electroencephalographic ischemic pattern changes during carotid endarterectomy. *J Neurosurg* 1993; **78:** 884–90.
57. Young WL, Moberg RS, Ornstein E, *et al.* Electroencephalographic monitoring for ischemia during carotid endarterectomy: visual versus computer analysis. *J Clin Monit* 1988; **4:** 78–85.
58. Hanowell LH, Soriano S, Bennett HL. EEG power changes are more sensitive than spectral edge frequency variation for detection of cerebral ischemia during carotid artery surgery: a prospective assessment of processed EEG monitoring. *J Cardiothorac Vasc Anesth* 1992; **6:** 292–4.
59. Stockard JJ, Bickford RG, Myers RR, *et al.* Hypotension-induced changes in cerebral function during cardiac surgery. *Stroke* 1974; **5:** 730–46.
60. Coselli JS, Crawford ES, Beall Jr AC, *et al.* Determination of brain temperatures for safe circulatory arrest during cardiovascular operation. *Ann Thorac Surg* 1988; **45:** 638–42.
61. Metz S, Slogoff S. Thiopental sodium by single bolus dose compared to infusion for cerebral protection during cardiopulmonary bypass. *J Clin Anesth* 1990; **2:** 226–31.
62. Arom KV, Cohen DE, Strobl FT. Effect of intraoperative intervention on neurological outcome based on electroencephalographic monitoring during cardiopulmonary bypass. *Ann Thorac Surg* 1989; **48:** 476–83.
63. Edmonds Jr HL, Griffiths LK, van der LJ, *et al.* Quantitative electroencephalographic monitoring during myocardial revascularization predicts postoperative disorientation and improves outcome. *J Thorac Cardiovasc Surg* 1992; **103:** 555–63.
64. Grote CL, Shanahan PT, Salmon P, *et al.* Cognitive outcome after cardiac operations. Relationship to intraoperative computerized electroencephalographic data. *J Thorac Cardiovasc Surg* 1992; **104:** 1405–9.
65. Drummond JC, Todd MM, Schubert A, Sang H. Effect of the acute administration of high dose pentobarbital on human brain stem auditory and median nerve somatosensory evoked responses. *Neurosurgery* 1987; **20:** 830–5.
66. Brenner RP. The electroencephalogram in altered states of consciousness. *Neurol Clin* 1985; **3:** 615–31.
67. Nuwer MR. Quantitative EEG analysis in clinical settings. *Brain Topogr* 1996; **8:** 201–8.
68. Treiman DM. Generalized convulsive status epilepticus in the adult. *Epilepsia* 1993; **34** (Suppl. 1): S2–11.
69. Rumpl E. [Electro-neurological correlations in early stages of posttraumatic comatose states. I. The EEG at different stages of acute traumatic secondary midbrain and bulbar brain syndrome (author's transl)]. *EEG EMG Z Elektroenzephalogr Elektromyogr Verwandte Geb* 1979; **10:** 148–57.
70. Moodley J, Bobat SM, Hoffman M, Bill PL. Electroencephalogram and computerised cerebral tomography findings in eclampsia. *Br J Obstet Gynaecol* 1993; **100:** 984–8.
71. Streletz LJ, Bej MD, Graziani LJ, *et al.* Utility of serial EEGs in neonates during extracorporeal membrane oxygenation. *Pediatr Neurol* 1992; **8:** 190–6.
72. Rivierez M, Landau-Ferey J, Grob R, *et al.* Value of electroencephalogram in prediction and diagnosis of vasospasm after intracranial aneurysm rupture. *Acta Neurochir (Wien)* 1991; **110:** 17–23.
73. Kaplan LJ, Bailey H. Bispectral Index (BIS) monitoring of ICU patients on continuous infusion of sedatives and paralytics reduces sedative utilization and cost. *Critical Care* 2000; **4:** S110.
74. Riker RR, Fraser GL. Monitoring sedation, agitation, analgesia, neuromuscular blockade, and delirium in adult ICU patients. *Semin Respir Crit Care Med* 2001; **22:** 189–98.
75. Gilbert TT, Wagner MR, Halukurike V, *et al.* Use of bispectral electroencephalogram monitoring to assess neurologic status in unsedated, critically ill patients. *Crit Care Med* 2001; **29:** 1996–2000.
76. Guideline Three. Minimum technical standards for EEG recording in suspected cerebral death. American Electroencephalographic Society. *J Clin Neurophysiol* 1994; **11:** 10–3.
77. Vivien B, Paqueron X, Le Cosquer P, *et al.* Prediction of brain-death onset using Bispectral Index (BIS) in severe comatose patients. *Eur J Anaesthesiol* 2001; **18:** A75.
78. Goodman JM, Heck LL. Confirmation of brain death at bedside by isotope angiography. *JAMA* 1977; **238:** 966–8.
79. Diamantopoulos E, Zander OP. Excitability of motor neurones in spinal shock in man. *J Neurol Neurosurg Psychiatry* 1967; **30:** 427–31.
80. Little JW, Halar EM. H-reflex changes following spinal cord injury. *Arch Phys Med Rehabil* 1985; **66:** 19–22.
81. Daube J. Nerve conduction studies. In: Aminoff MJ (ed.). *Electrodiagnosis in Clinical Neurology*. New York, NY: Churchill Livingstone, 1992: 283–326.
82. Kimura J, Butzer JF. F-wave conduction velocity in Guillain–Barré syndrome. Assessment of nerve segment between axilla and spinal cord. *Arch Neurol* 1975; **32:** 524–9.
83. King D, Ashby P. Conduction velocity in the proximal segments of a motor nerve in the Guillain–Barré syndrome. *J Neurol Neurosurg Psychiatry* 1976; **39:** 538–44.
84. Guideline Nine. Guidelines on evoked potentials. American Electroencephalographic Society. *J Clin Neurophysiol* 1994; **11:** 40–73.
85. Guideline Eleven. Guidelines for intraoperative monitoring of sensory

evoked potentials. American Electroencephalographic Society. *J Clin Neurophysiol* 1994; **11:** 77–87.

86. Grundy BL. Sensory-evoked potentials. In: Boulton AA, Baker GB, Boisvert DPJ (eds). *Neuromethods-8*. Clifton, NJ: Humana Press, 1988: 375–433.
87. Liberati D, Cerutti S, Di Ponzio E, *et al*. The implementation of an autoregressive model with exogenous input in a single sweep visual evoked potential analysis. *J Biomed Eng* 1989; **11:** 285–92.
88. Jensen EW, Lindholm P, Henneberg SW. Autoregressive modeling with exogenous input of middle-latency auditory-evoked potentials to measure rapid changes in depth of anesthesia. *Methods Inf Med* 1996; **35:** 256–60.
89. Struys MM, Jensen EW, Smith W, *et al*. Performance of the ARX-derived auditory evoked potential index as an indicator of anesthetic depth: a comparison with bispectral index and hemodynamic measures during propofol administration. *Anesthesiology* 2002; **96:** 803–16.
90. Achor LJ, Starr A. Auditory brain stem responses in the cat. I. Intracranial and extracranial recordings. *Electroencephalogr Clin Neurophysiol* 1980; **48:** 154–73.
91. Achor LJ, Starr A. Auditory brain stem responses in the cat. II. Effects of lesions. *Electroencephalogr Clin Neurophysiol* 1980; **48:** 174–90.
92. Desmedt JE, Noel P. Average cerebral evoked potentials in the evaluation of lesions of the sensory nerves and of the central somatosensory pathways. In: Desmedt JE (ed.). *New Developments in Electromyography and Clinical Neurophysiology*. Basle: S. Karger, 1973: 352–71.
93. Anthony PF, Durrett R, Pulec JL, Hartstone JL. A new parameter in brain stem evoked response: component wave areas. *Laryngoscope* 1979; **89:** 1569–78.
94. Boston JR. Spectra of auditory brainstem responses and spontaneous EEG. *IEEE Trans Biomed Eng* 1981; **28:** 334–41.
95. Wong PK, Bickford RG. Brain stem auditory evoked potentials: the use of noise estimate. *Electroencephalogr Clin Neurophysiol* 1980; **50:** 25–34.
96. Keller I, Madler C, Schwender D, Poppel E. Analysis of oscillatory components in perioperative AEP-recordings: a nonparametric procedure for frequency measurement. *Clin Electroencephalogr* 1990; **21:** 88–92.
97. Donchin E, Herning RI. A simulation study of the efficacy of stepwise discriminant analysis in the detection and comparison of event related potentials. *Electroencephalogr Clin Neurophysiol* 1975; **38:** 51–68.
98. Duffy FH, Bartels PH, Burchfiel JL. Significance probability mapping: an aid in the topographic analysis of brain electrical activity. *Electroencephalogr Clin Neurophysiol* 1981; **51:** 455–62.
99. Cerutti S, Chiarenza G, Liberati D, *et al*. A parametric method of identification of single-trial event-related potentials in the brain. *IEEE Trans Biomed Eng* 1988; **35:** 701–11.
100. Galambos R, Makeig S, Talmachoff PJ. A 40-Hz auditory potential recorded from the human scalp. *Proc Natl Acad Sci USA* 1981; **78:** 2643–7.
101. Plourde G, Stapells DR, Picton TW. The human auditory steady-state evoked potentials. *Acta Otolaryngol Suppl* 1991; **491:** 153–9.
102. Andrade J, Sapsford DJ, Jeevaratnum D, *et al*. The coherent frequency in the electroencephalogram as an objective measure of cognitive function during propofol sedation. *Anesth Analg* 1996; **83:** 1279–84.
103. Grundy BL, Lina A, Procopio PT, Jannetta PJ. Reversible evoked potential changes with retraction of the eighth cranial nerve. *Anesth Analg* 1981; **60:** 835–8.
104. Grundy BL, Jannetta PJ, Procopio PT, *et al*. Intraoperative monitoring of brain-stem auditory evoked potentials. *J Neurosurg* 1982; **57:** 674–81.
105. Kaplan BJ, Friedman WA, Alexander JA, Hampson SR. Somatosensory evoked potential monitoring of spinal cord ischemia during aortic operations. *Neurosurgery* 1986; **19:** 82–90.
106. Higgins AC, Pearlstein RD, Mullen JB, Nashold Jr BS. Effects of hyperbaric oxygen therapy on long-tract neuronal conduction in the acute phase of spinal cord injury. *J Neurosurg* 1981; **55:** 501–10.
107. Nashold Jr BS, Ovelmen-Levitt J, Sharpe R, Higgins AC. Intraoperative evoked potentials recorded in man directly from dorsal roots and spinal cord. *J Neurosurg* 1985; **62:** 680–93.
108. Gugino V, Chabot RJ. Somatosensory evoked potentials. *Int Anesthesiol Clin* 1990; **28:** 154–64.
109. Pereon Y, Bernard JM, Delecrin J, Passuti N. Could neurogenic motor evoked potentials be used to monitor motor and somatosensory pathways during scoliosis surgery? *Muscle Nerve* 1995; **18:** 1214–5.
110. Snyder BG, Holliday TA. Pathways of ascending evoked spinal cord potentials of dogs. *Electroencephalogr Clin Neurophysiol* 1984; **58:** 140–54.
111. Kimura J, Mitsudome A, Yamada T, Dickins QS. Stationary peaks from a moving source in far-field recording. *Electroencephalogr Clin Neurophysiol* 1984; **58:** 351–61.
112. Symon L, Hargadine J, Zawirski M, Branston N. Central conduction time as an index of ischaemia in subarachnoid haemorrhage. *J Neurol Sci* 1979; **44:** 95–103.
113. Chiappa KH, Ropper AH. Evoked potentials in clinical medicine (first of two parts). *N Engl J Med* 1982; **306:** 1140–50.
114. Chiappa KH, Ropper AH. Evoked potentials in clinical medicine (second of two parts). *N Engl J Med* 1982; **306:** 1205–11.
115. Friedman WA, Richards R. Somatosensory evoked potential monitoring accurately predicts hemi-spinal cord damage: a case report. *Neurosurgery* 1988; **22:** 140–2.
116. Burke D, Skuse NF, Lethlean AK. Cutaneous and muscle afferent components of the cerebral potential evoked by electrical stimulation of human peripheral nerves. *Electroencephalogr Clin Neurophysiol* 1981; **51:** 579–88.
117. Erwin CW, Erwin AC. Up and down the spinal cord: intraoperative monitoring of sensory and motor spinal cord pathways. *J Clin Neurophysiol* 1993; **10:** 425–36.
118. Loughnan BA, Fennelly ME. Spinal cord monitoring. *Anaesthesia* 1995; **50:** 101–2.
119. Pratt H, Starr A. Mechanically and electrically evoked somatosensory potentials in human: scalp and neck distributions of short latency components. *Electroencephalogr Clin Neurophysiol* 1981; **51:** 138–47.
120. Bromm B, Treede RD. Pain related cerebral potentials: late and ultralate components. *Int J Neurosci* 1987; **33:** 15–23.
121. Zarola F, Rossini PM. Nerve, spinal cord and brain somatosensory evoked responses: a comparative study during electrical and magnetic peripheral nerve stimulation. *Electroencephalogr Clin Neurophysiol* 1991; **80:** 372–7.
122. Kunesch E, Knecht S, Classen J, *et al*. Somatosensory evoked potentials (SEPs) elicited by magnetic nerve stimulation. *Electroencephalogr Clin Neurophysiol* 1993; **88:** 459–67.
123. Brown RH, Nash Jr CL. Current status of spinal cord monitoring. *Spine* 1979; **4:** 466–70.
124. Lueders H, Gurd A, Hahn J, *et al*. A new technique for intraoperative monitoring of spinal cord function: multichannel recording of spinal cord and subcortical evoked potentials. *Spine* 1982; **7:** 110–15.
125. Hahn JF, Lesser R, Klem G, Lueders H. Simple technique for monitoring intraoperative spinal cord function. *Neurosurgery* 1981; **9:** 692–5.
126. Macon JB, Poletti CE. Conducted somatosensory evoked potentials during spinal surgery. Part 1. Control conduction velocity measurements. *J Neurosurg* 1982; **57:** 349–53.
127. Macon JB, Poletti CE, Sweet WH, *et al*. Conducted somatosensory evoked potentials during spinal surgery. Part 2. Clinical applications. *J Neurosurg* 1982; **57:** 354–9.
128. Tamaki T, Tsuji H, Inoue S, Kobayashi H. The prevention of iatrogenic spinal cord injury utilizing the evoked spinal cord potential. *Int Orthop* 1981; **4:** 313–17.
129. Birk P, Riescher H, Struppler A, Keidel M. Somatosensory evoked potentials in the ventrolateral thalamus. *Appl Neurophysiol* 1986; **49:** 327–35.
130. Daube JR. Recent applications of electrophysiologic monitoring during surgery. *Electroencephalogr Clin Neurophysiol Suppl* 1987; **39:** 231–49.
131. Nash Jr CL, Lorig RA, Schatzinger LA, Brown RH. Spinal cord monitoring during operative treatment of the spine. *Clin Orthop* 1977; **126:** 100–5.
132. MacEwen GD, Bunnell WP, Sriram K. Acute neurological complications in the treatment of scoliosis. A report of the Scoliosis Research Society. *J Bone Joint Surg Am* 1975; **57:** 404–8.
133. Mostegl A, Bauer R. The application of somatosensory-evoked potentials in orthopedic spine surgery. *Arch Orthop Trauma Surg* 1984; **103:** 179–84.
134. Bradshaw K, Webb JK, Fraser AM. Clinical evaluation of spinal cord monitoring in scoliosis surgery. *Spine* 1984; **9:** 636–43.
135. Veilleux M, Daube JR, Cucchiara RF. Monitoring of cortical evoked potentials during surgical procedures on the cervical spine. *Mayo Clin Proc* 1987; **62:** 256–64.
136. Nuwer MR, Dawson EG, Carlson LG, *et al*. Somatosensory evoked potential spinal cord monitoring reduces neurologic deficits after scoliosis surgery: results of a large multicenter survey. *Electroencephalogr Clin Neurophysiol* 1995; **96:** 6–11.
137. Forbes HJ, Allen PW, Waller CS, *et al*. Spinal cord monitoring in scoliosis surgery. Experience with 1168 cases. *J Bone Joint Surg Br* 1991; **73:** 487–91.
138. Ashkenaze D, Mudiyam R, Boachie-Adjei O, Gilbert C. Efficacy of spinal cord monitoring in neuromuscular scoliosis. *Spine* 1993; **18:** 1627–33.
139. Friedman WA, Grundy BL. Monitoring of sensory evoked potentials is highly reliable and helpful in the operating room. *J Clin Monit* 1987; **3:** 38–44.
140. Albanese SA, Spadaro JA, Lubicky JP, Henderson NA. Somatosensory cor-

tical evoked potential changes after deformity correction. *Spine* 1991; **16:** S371–S374.

141. Brown RH, Nash Jr CL, Berilla JA, Amaddio MD. Cortical evoked potential monitoring. A system for intraoperative monitoring of spinal cord function. *Spine* 1984; **9:** 256–61.
142. York DH, Chabot RJ, Gaines RW. Response variability of somatosensory evoked potentials during scoliosis surgery. *Spine* 1987; **12:** 864–76.
143. Lubicky JP, Spadaro JA, Yuan HA, *et al.* Variability of somatosensory cortical evoked potential monitoring during spinal surgery. *Spine* 1989; **14:** 790–8.
144. Grundy BL, Nelson PB, Doyle E, Procopio PT. Intraoperative loss of somatosensory-evoked potentials predicts loss of spinal cord function. *Anesthesiology* 1982; **57:** 321–2.
145. Molaie M. False negative intraoperative somatosensory evoked potentials with simultaneous bilateral stimulation. *Clin Electroencephalogr* 1986; **17:** 6–9.
146. Mavroudakis N, Vandesteene A, Brunko E, *et al.* Spinal and brain-stem SEPs and H reflex during enflurane anesthesia. *Electroencephalogr Clin Neurophysiol* 1994; **92:** 82–5.
147. McPherson RW, North RB, Udvarhelyi GB, Rosenbaum AE. Migrating disc complicating spinal decompression in an achondroplastic dwarf: intraoperative demonstration of spinal cord compression by somatosensory evoked potentials. *Anesthesiology* 1984; **61:** 764–7.
148. Schramm J, Kurthen M. Recent developments in neurosurgical spinal cord monitoring. *Paraplegia* 1992; **30:** 609–16.
149. Cioni B, Meglio M, Moles A, *et al.* Spinal somatosensory evoked potential monitoring during microsurgery for syringomyelia: case reports. *Stereotact Funct Neurosurg* 1991; **57:** 123–9.
150. McPherson RW, Sell B, Traystman RJ. Effects of thiopental, fentanyl, and etomidate on upper extremity somatosensory evoked potentials in humans. *Anesthesiology* 1986; **65:** 584–9.
151. Wagner RL, White PF. Etomidate inhibits adrenocortical function in surgical patients. *Anesthesiology* 1984; **61:** 647–51.
152. Watt I, McLedingham I. Mortality among multiple trauma patients admitted to an intensive therapy unit. *Anaesthesia* 1994; **39:** 973–81.
153. Owen MP, Brown RH, Spetzler RF, *et al.* Excision of intramedullary arteriovenous malformation using intraoperative spinal cord monitoring. *Surg Neurol* 1979; **12:** 271–6.
154. Koyanagi I, Iwasaki Y, Isu T, *et al.* Spinal cord evoked potential monitoring after spinal cord stimulation during surgery of spinal cord tumors. *Neurosurgery* 1993; **33:** 451–9.
155. Joseph MG, Langsfeld MA, Lusby RJ. Infrarenal aortic aneurysm: unusual cause of paraparesis. *Aust NZ J Surg* 1989; **59:** 743–4.
156. Noirhomme P, Buche M, Louagie Y, *et al.* Ischemic complications of abdominal aortic surgery. *J Cardiovasc Surg (Torino)* 1991; **32:** 451–5.
157. Svensson LG, Crawford ES, Hess KR, *et al.* Experience with 1509 patients undergoing thoracoabdominal aortic operations. *J Vasc Surg* 1993; **17:** 357–68.
158. Kobrine AI, Evans DE, Rizzoli HV. The effects of ischemia on long-tract neural conduction in the spinal cord. *J Neurosurg* 1979; **50:** 639–44.
159. Cunningham Jr JN, Laschinger JC, Spencer FC. Monitoring of somatosensory evoked potentials during surgical procedures on the thoracoabdominal aorta. IV. Clinical observations and results. *J Thorac Cardiovasc Surg* 1987; **94:** 275–85.
160. Hitchon PW, Lobosky JM, Wilkinson TT, *et al.* Direct spinal cord stimulation and recording in hemorrhagic stock. *Neurosurgery* 1985; **16:** 796–800.
161. Coles JG, Wilson GJ, Sima AF, *et al.* Intraoperative detection of spinal cord ischemia using somatosensory cortical evoked potentials during thoracic aortic occlusion. *Ann Thorac Surg* 1982; **34:** 299–306.
162. Laschinger JC, Cunningham Jr JN, Isom OW, *et al.* Definition of the safe lower limits of aortic resection during surgical procedures on the thoracoabdominal aorta: use of somatosensory evoked potentials. *J Am Coll Cardiol* 1983; **2:** 959–65.
163. Laschinger JC, Cunningham Jr JN, Nathan IM, *et al.* Experimental and clinical assessment of the adequacy of partial bypass in maintenance of spinal cord blood flow during operations on the thoracic aorta. *Ann Thorac Surg* 1983; **36:** 417–26.
164. Laschinger JC, Cunningham Jr JN, Nathan IM, *et al.* Intraoperative identification of vessels critical to spinal cord blood supply – use of somatosensory evoked potentials. *Curr Surg* 1984; **41:** 107–9.
165. Laschinger JC, Cunningham Jr JN, Cooper MM, *et al.* Prevention of ischemic spinal cord injury following aortic cross-clamping: use of corticosteroids. *Ann Thorac Surg* 1984; **38:** 500–7.
166. Laschinger JC, Cunningham Jr JN, Baumann FG, *et al.* Monitoring of somatosensory evoked potentials during surgical procedures on the thoracoabdominal aorta. III. Intraoperative identification of vessels critical to spinal cord blood supply. *J Thorac Cardiovasc Surg* 1987; **94:** 271–4.
167. Laschinger JC, Cunningham Jr JN, Cooper MM, *et al.* Monitoring of somatosensory evoked potentials during surgical procedures on the thoracoabdominal aorta. I. Relationship of aortic cross-clamp duration, changes in somatosensory evoked potentials, and incidence of neurologic dysfunction. *J Thorac Cardiovasc Surg* 1987; **94:** 260–5.
168. Katz NM, Blackstone EH, Kirklin JW, Karp RB. Incremental risk factors for spinal cord injury following operation for acute traumatic aortic transection. *J Thorac Cardiovasc Surg* 1981; **81:** 669–74.
169. Cunningham Jr JN, Laschinger JC, Merkin HA, *et al.* Measurement of spinal cord ischemia during operations upon the thoracic aorta: initial clinical experience. *Ann Surg* 1982; **196:** 285–96.
170. Krieger KH, Spencer FC. Is paraplegia after repair of coarctation of the aorta due principally to distal hypotension during aortic cross-clamping? *Surgery* 1985; **97:** 2–7.
171. Mizrahi EM, Crawford ES. Somatosensory evoked potentials during reversible spinal cord ischemia in man. *Electroencephalogr Clin Neurophysiol* 1984; **58:** 120–6.
172. Crawford ES, Mizrahi EM, Hess KR, *et al.* The impact of distal aortic perfusion and somatosensory evoked potential monitoring on prevention of paraplegia after aortic aneurysm operation. *J Thorac Cardiovasc Surg* 1988; **95:** 357–67.
173. Svensson LG, Crawford ES, Hess KR, *et al.* Variables predictive of outcome in 832 patients undergoing repairs of the descending thoracic aorta. *Chest* 1993; **104:** 1248–53.
174. Hollier LH, Money SR, Naslund TC, *et al.* Risk of spinal cord dysfunction in patients undergoing thoracoabdominal aortic replacement. *Am J Surg* 1992; **164:** 210–13.
175. Fehrenbacher JW, McCready RA, Hormuth DA, *et al.* One-stage segmental resection of extensive thoracoabdominal aneurysms with left-sided heart bypass. *J Vasc Surg* 1993; **18:** 366–70.
176. Vanicky I, Marsala M, Galik J, Marsala J. Epidural perfusion cooling protection against protracted spinal cord ischemia in rabbits. *J Neurosurg* 1993; **79:** 736–41.
177. Fava E, Bortolani EM, Ducati A, Ruberti U. Evaluation of spinal cord function by means of lower limb somatosensory evoked potentials in reparative aortic surgery. *J Cardiovasc Surg (Torino)* 1988; **29:** 421–7.
178. Elmore JR, Gloviczki P, Harper CM, *et al.* Failure of motor evoked potentials to predict neurologic outcome in experimental thoracic aortic occlusion. *J Vasc Surg* 1991; **14:** 131–9.
179. Ihaya A, Morioka K, Noguchi H, *et al.* [A case report of descending thoracic aortic aneurysm associated with anterior spinal artery syndrome despite no marked ESP changes]. *Kyobu Geka* 1990; **43:** 843–6.
180. Berenstein A, Young W, Ransohoff J, *et al.* Somatosensory evoked potentials during spinal angiography and therapeutic transvascular embolization. *J Neurosurg* 1984; **60:** 777–85.
181. Horsch S, De Vleeschauwer P, Klenidis K. Intraoperative assessment of cerebral ischemia during carotid surgery. *J Cardiovasc Surg (Torino)* 1990; **31:** 599–602.
182. Sasaki T, Takeda R, Ogasawara T, *et al.* [Monitoring of somatosensory evoked potentials during extracranial revascularization]. *Neurol Med Chir (Tokyo)* 1989; **29:** 280–4.
183. Artru AA, Strandness Jr DE. Delayed carotid shunt occlusion detected by electroencephalographic monitoring. *J Clin Monit* 1989; **5:** 119–22.
184. Schweiger H, Kamp HD, Dinkel M. Somatosensory-evoked potentials during carotid artery surgery: experience in 400 operations. *Surgery* 1991; **109:** 602–9.
185. Russ W, Thiel A, Moosdorf R, Hempelmann G. [Somatosensory evoked potentials in obliterating interventions of the carotid bifurcation]. *Klin Wochenschr* 1988; **66** (Suppl. 14): 35–40.
186. Lam AM, Manninen PH, Ferguson GG, Nantau W. Monitoring electrophysiologic function during carotid endarterectomy: a comparison of somatosensory evoked potentials and conventional electroencephalogram. *Anesthesiology* 1991; **75:** 15–21.
187. Tiberio G, Floriani M, Giulini SM, *et al.* Monitoring of somatosensory evoked potentials during carotid endarterectomy: relationship with different haemodynamic parameters and clinical outcome. *Eur J Vasc Surg* 1991; **5:** 647–53.
188. Amantini A, Bartelli M, de Scisciolo G, *et al.* Monitoring of somatosensory evoked potentials during carotid endarterectomy. *J Neurol* 1992; **239:** 241–7.
189. Haupt WF, Horsch S. Evoked potential monitoring in carotid surgery: a review of 994 cases. *Neurology* 1992; **42:** 835–8.
190. Kearse Jr LA, Brown EN, McPeck K. Somatosensory evoked potentials sensitivity relative to electroencephalography for cerebral ischemia during carotid endarterectomy. *Stroke* 1992; **23:** 498–505.

191. Fava E, Bortolani E, Ducati A, Schieppati M. Role of SEP in identifying patients requiring temporary shunt during carotid endarterectomy. *Electroencephalogr Clin Neurophysiol* 1992; **84:** 426–32.
192. Markand ON, Dilley RS, Moorthy SS, Warren Jr C. Monitoring of somatosensory evoked responses during carotid endarterectomy. *Arch Neurol* 1984; **41:** 375–8.
193. Markand ON, Warren CH, Moorthy SS, *et al.* Monitoring of multimodality evoked potentials during open heart surgery under hypothermia. *Electroencephalogr Clin Neurophysiol* 1984; **59:** 432–40.
194. Hickey C, Gugino LD, Aglio LS, *et al.* Intraoperative somatosensory evoked potential monitoring predicts peripheral nerve injury during cardiac surgery. *Anesthesiology* 1993; **78:** 29–35.
195. Coles JG, Taylor MJ, Pearce JM, *et al.* Cerebral monitoring of somatosensory evoked potentials during profoundly hypothermic circulatory arrest. *Circulation* 1984; **70:** 96–102.
196. Kline DG, Judice DJ. Operative management of selected brachial plexus lesions. *J Neurosurg* 1983; **58:** 631–49.
197. Kaplan BJ, Gravenstein D, Friedman WA. Intraoperative electrophysiology in treatment of peripheral nerve injuries. *J Fla Med Assoc* 1984; **71:** 400–3.
198. Murase T, Kawai H, Masatomi T, *et al.* Evoked spinal cord potentials for diagnosis during brachial plexus surgery. *J Bone Joint Surg Br* 1993; **75:** 775–81.
199. Allison T. Localization of sensorimotor cortex in neurosurgery by recording of somatosensory evoked potentials. *Yale J Biol Med* 1987; **60:** 143–50.
200. Suzuki A, Yasui N. Intraoperative localization of the central sulcus by cortical somatosensory evoked potentials in brain tumor. *J Neurosurg* 1992; **76:** 867–70.
201. Hargadine JR, Branston NM, Symon L. Central conduction time in primate brain ischemia – a study in baboons. *Stroke* 1980; **11:** 637–42.
202. Branston NM, Strong AJ, Symon L. Extracellular potassium activity, evoked potential and tissue blood flow. Relationships during progressive ischaemia in baboon cerebral cortex. *J Neurol Sci* 1977; **32:** 305–21.
203. Hargadine JR. Intraoperative monitoring of sensory evoked potentials. In: Rand DW (ed.). *Microneurosurgery*. St Louis: CV Mosby, 1985: 92–110.
204. Friedman WA, Kaplan BL, Day AL, *et al.* Evoked potential monitoring during aneurysm operation: observations after fifty cases. *Neurosurgery* 1987; **20:** 678–87.
205. Friedman WA, Chadwick GM, Verhoeven FJ, *et al.* Monitoring of somatosensory evoked potentials during surgery for middle cerebral artery aneurysms. *Neurosurgery* 1991; **29:** 83–8.
206. Symon L, Momma F, Murota T. Assessment of reversible cerebral ischaemia in man: intraoperative monitoring of the somatosensory evoked response. *Acta Neurochir Suppl (Wien)* 1988; **42:** 3–7.
207. Mizoi K, Yoshimoto T. Permissible temporary occlusion time in aneurysm surgery as evaluated by evoked potential monitoring. *Neurosurgery* 1993; **33:** 434–40.
208. Manninen PH, Patterson S, Lam AM, *et al.* Evoked potential monitoring during posterior fossa aneurysm surgery: a comparison of two modalities. *Can J Anaesth* 1994; **41:** 92–7.
209. Grundy BL, Nelson PB, Lina A, Heros RC. Monitoring of cortical somatosensory evoked potentials to determine the safety of sacrificing the anterior cerebral artery. *Neurosurgery* 1982; **11:** 64–7.
210. Mahla ME, Long DM, McKennett J, *et al.* Detection of brachial plexus dysfunction by somatosensory evoked potential monitoring – a report of two cases. *Anesthesiology* 1984; **60:** 248–52.
211. McPherson RW, Szymanski J, Rogers MC. Somatosensory evoked potential changes in position-related brain stem ischemia. *Anesthesiology* 1984; **61:** 88–90.
212. Greenberg RP, Mayer DJ, Becker DP, Miller JD. Evaluation of brain function in severe human head trauma with multimodality evoked potentials. Part 1. Evoked brain-injury potentials, methods, and analysis. *J Neurosurg* 1977; **47:** 150–62.
213. Greenberg RP, Becker DP, Miller JD, Mayer DJ. Evaluation of brain function in severe human head trauma with multimodality evoked potentials. Part 2. Localization of brain dysfunction and correlation with posttraumatic neurological conditions. *J Neurosurg* 1977; **47:** 163–77.
214. Hume AL, Cant BR. Central somatosensory conduction after head injury. *Ann Neurol* 1981; **10:** 411–19.
215. Kawahara N, Sasaki M, Mii K, Takakura K. Reversibility of cerebral function assessed by somatosensory evoked potentials and its relation to intracranial pressure – report of six cases with severe head injury. *Neurol Med Chir (Tokyo)* 1991; **31:** 264–71.
216. Firsching R, Frowein RA. Multimodality evoked potentials and early prognosis in comatose patients. *Neurosurg Rev* 1990; **13:** 141–6.
217. Rumpl E, Prugger M, Gerstenbrand F, *et al.* Central somatosensory conduction time and acoustic brainstem transmission time in post-traumatic coma. *J Clin Neurophysiol* 1988; **5:** 237–60.
218. Anderson DC, Bundlie S, Rockswold GL. Multimodality evoked potentials in closed head trauma. *Arch Neurol* 1984; **41:** 369–74.
219. Ruijs MB, Keyser A, Gabreels FJ, Notermans SL. Somatosensory evoked potentials and cognitive sequelae in children with closed head-injury. *Neuropediatrics* 1993; **24:** 307–12.
220. Zentner J, Rohde V. The prognostic value of somatosensory and motor evoked potentials in comatose patients. *Neurosurgery* 1992; **31:** 429–34.
221. Hume AL, Cant BR, Shaw NA. Central somatosensory conduction time in comatose patients. *Ann Neurol* 1979; **5:** 379–84.
222. Cant BR, Shaw NA. Central somatosensory conduction time: method and clinical applications. In: Cracco RQ, Bodis-Wollner I (eds). *Evoked Potentials*. New York, NY: Alan R Liss, 1986: 58–67.
223. Brunko E, Zegers dB. Prognostic value of early cortical somatosensory evoked potentials after resuscitation from cardiac arrest. *Electroencephalogr Clin Neurophysiol* 1987; **66:** 15–24.
224. Rothstein TL, Thomas EM, Sumi SM. Predicting outcome in hypoxic-ischemic coma. A prospective clinical and electrophysiologic study. *Electroencephalogr Clin Neurophysiol* 1991; **79:** 101–7.
225. Madl C, Grimm G, Kramer L, *et al.* Early prediction of individual outcome after cardiopulmonary resuscitation. *Lancet* 1993; **341:** 855–8.
226. Madl C, Kramer L, Domanovits H, *et al.* Improved outcome prediction in unconscious cardiac arrest survivors with sensory evoked potentials compared with clinical assessment. *Crit Care Med* 2000; **28:** 721–6.
227. Taylor MJ, Murphy WJ, Whyte HE. Prognostic reliability of somatosensory and visual evoked potentials of asphyxiated term infants. *Dev Med Child Neurol* 1992; **34:** 507–15.
228. Symon L, Wang AD, Silva IE, Gentili F. Perioperative use of somatosensory evoked responses in aneurysm surgery. *J Neurosurg* 1984; **60:** 269–75.
229. Rosenstein J, Wang AD, Symon L, Suzuki M. Relationship between hemispheric cerebral blood flow, central conduction time, and clinical grade in aneurysmal subarachnoid hemorrhage. *J Neurosurg* 1985; **62:** 25–30.
230. Wang AD, Cone J, Symon L, Silva IE. Somatosensory evoked potential monitoring during the management of aneurysmal SAH. *J Neurosurg* 1984; **60:** 264–8.
231. Grundy BL, Friedman W. Electrophysiological evaluation of the patient with acute spinal cord injury. *Crit Care Clin* 1987; **3:** 519–48.
232. Towle VL, Maselli R, Bernstein LP, Spire JP. Electrophysiologic studies on locked-in patients: heterogeneity of findings. *Electroencephalogr Clin Neurophysiol* 1989; **73:** 419–26.
233. Yingling CD. Intraoperative monitoring of cranial nerves in skull base surgery. In: Jackler RJ and Brackman DE (eds) *Neurotology*. St Louis: Mosby, 1994: 967.
234. Grundy BL, Procopio PT, Jannetta PJ, *et al.* Evoked potential changes produced by positioning for retromastoid craniectomy. *Neurosurgery* 1982; **10:** 766–70.
235. Raudzens PA, Shetter AG. Intraoperative monitoring of brain-stem auditory evoked potentials. *J Neurosurg* 1982; **57:** 341–8.
236. van Loveren H, Tew Jr JM, Keller JT, Nurre MA. A 10-year experience in the treatment of trigeminal neuralgia. Comparison of percutaneous stereotaxic rhizotomy and posterior fossa exploration. *J Neurosurg* 1982; **57:** 757–64.
237. Auger RG, Piepgras DG, Laws Jr ER. Hemifacial spasm: results of microvascular decompression of the facial nerve in 54 patients. *Mayo Clin Proc* 1986; **61:** 640–4.
238. Moller AR, Jannetta PJ. Monitoring auditory functions during cranial nerve microvascular decompression operations by direct recording from the eighth nerve. *J Neurosurg* 1983; **59:** 493–9.
239. Friedman WA, Kaplan BJ, Gravenstein D, Rhoton Jr AL. Intraoperative brain-stem auditory evoked potentials during posterior fossa microvascular decompression. *J Neurosurg* 1985; **62:** 552–7.
240. Piatt Jr JH, Radtke RA, Erwin CW. Limitations of brain stem auditory evoked potentials for intraoperative monitoring during a posterior fossa operation: case report and technical note. *Neurosurgery* 1985; **16:** 818–21.
241. Glasscock III ME, Hays JW, Minor LB, *et al.* Preservation of hearing in surgery for acoustic neuromas. *J Neurosurg* 1993; **78:** 864–70.
242. Harper CM, Harner SG, Slavit DH, *et al.* Effect of BAEP monitoring on hearing preservation during acoustic neuroma resection. *Neurology* 1992; **42:** 1551–3.
243. Fischer G, Fischer C, Remond J. Hearing preservation in acoustic neurinoma surgery. *J Neurosurg* 1992; **76:** 910–17.
244. Levine A. Monitoring auditory evoked potentials during cerebellopontine angle surgery: relative value of electrocochleography, brainstem auditory evoked potentials, and cerebellopontine angle recordings.

In: Schramm J, Moller AR (eds). *Intraoperative Neurophysiological Monitoring*. Berlin: Springer-Verlag, 1991: 193.

245. Nedzelski JM, Chiong CM, Cashman MZ, *et al.* Hearing preservation in acoustic neuroma surgery: value of monitoring cochlear nerve action potentials. *Otolaryngol Head Neck Surg* 1994; **111:** 703–9.
246. Lenarz T, Ernst A. Intraoperative monitoring by transtympanic electrocochleography and brainstem electrical response audiometry in acoustic neuroma surgery. *Eur Arch Otorhinolaryngol* 1992; **249:** 257–62.
247. Silverstein H, McDaniel A, Norrell H, Haberkamp T. Hearing preservation after acoustic neuroma surgery with intraoperative direct eighth cranial nerve monitoring. Part II. A classification of results. *Otolaryngol Head Neck Surg* 1986; **95:** 285–91.
248. Facco E, Munari M, Casartelli LM, *et al.* Serial recordings of auditory brainstem responses in severe head injury: relationship between test timing and prognostic power. *Intensive Care Med* 1988; **14:** 422–8.
249. Sohmer H, Freeman S, Gafni M, Goitein K. The depression of the auditory nerve-brain-stem evoked response in hypoxaemia – mechanism and site of effect. *Electroencephalogr Clin Neurophysiol* 1986; **64:** 334–8.
250. Garcia-Larrea L, Artru F, Bertrand O, *et al.* The combined monitoring of brain stem auditory evoked potentials and intracranial pressure in coma. A study of 57 patients. *J Neurol Neurosurg Psychiatry* 1992; **55:** 792–8.
251. Gajraj RJ, Doi M, Mantzaridis H, Kenny GN. Analysis of the EEG bispectrum, auditory evoked potentials and the EEG power spectrum during repeated transitions from consciousness to unconsciousness. *Br J Anaesth* 1998; **80:** 46–52.
252. Doi M, Gajraj RJ, Mantzaridis H, Kenny GN. Relationship between calculated blood concentration of propofol and electrophysiological variables during emergence from anaesthesia: comparison of bispectral index, spectral edge frequency, median frequency and auditory evoked potential index. *Br J Anaesth* 1997; **78:** 180–4.
253. Schulte-Tamburen AM, Scheier J, Briegel J, *et al.* Comparison of five sedation scoring systems by means of auditory evoked potentials. *Intensive Care Med* 1999; **25:** 377–82.
254. Engelhardt W, Dierks T, Pause M, *et al.* P300-mapping – a neurophysiological tool to quantify cerebral dysfunction after coronary artery bypass grafting. *Eur J Cardiothorac Surg* 1995; **9:** 12–17.
255. Kane NM, Curry SH, Rowlands CA, *et al.* Event-related potentials – neurophysiological tools for predicting emergence and early outcome from traumatic coma. *Intensive Care Med* 1996; **22:** 39–46.
256. Celesia GG. Visual evoked potentials in clinical neurology. In: Aminoff MJ (ed.). *Electrodiagnosis in Clinical Neurology*. New York, NY: Churchill Livingstone, 1992: 467–90.
257. Sokol S. Visual evoked potentials. In: Aminoff M (ed.). *Electrodiagnosis in Clinical Neurology*. New York: Churchill Livingstone, 1992: 441–66.
258. Stechison MT. Neurophysiologic monitoring during cranial base surgery. *J Neurooncol* 1994; **20:** 313–25.
259. Zaaroor M, Pratt H, Feinsod M, Schacham SE. Real-time monitoring of visual evoked potentials. *Isr J Med Sci* 1993; **29:** 17–22.
260. Owen JH, Bridwell KH, Grubb R, *et al.* The clinical application of neurogenic motor evoked potentials to monitor spinal cord function during surgery. *Spine* 1991; **16:** S385–S390.
261. Su CF, Haghighi SS, Oro JJ, Gaines RW. “Backfiring” in spinal cord monitoring. High thoracic spinal cord stimulation evokes sciatic response by antidromic sensory pathway conduction, not motor tract conduction. *Spine* 1992; **17:** 504–8.
262. Rossini PM, Barker AT, Berardelli A, *et al.* Non-invasive electrical and magnetic stimulation of the brain, spinal cord and roots: basic principles and procedures for routine clinical application. Report of an IFCN committee. *Electroencephalogr Clin Neurophysiol* 1994; **91:** 79–92.
263. Levy WJ, York DH, McCaffrey M, Tanzer F. Motor evoked potentials from transcranial stimulation of the motor cortex in humans. *Neurosurgery* 1984; **15:** 287–302.
264. Cowan JM, Rothwell JC, Dick JP, *et al.* Abnormalities in central motor pathway conduction in multiple sclerosis. *Lancet* 1984; **2:** 304–7.
265. Kalkman CJ, Drummond JC, Ribberink AA. Low concentrations of isoflurane abolish motor evoked responses to transcranial electrical stimulation during nitrous oxide/opioid anesthesia in humans. *Anesth Analg* 1991; **73:** 410–15.
266. Zentner J. Noninvasive motor evoked potential monitoring during neurosurgical operations on the spinal cord. *Neurosurgery* 1989; **24:** 709–12.
267. Jellinek D, Platt M, Jewkes D, Symon L. Effects of nitrous oxide on motor evoked potentials recorded from skeletal muscle in patients under total anesthesia with intravenously administered propofol. *Neurosurgery* 1991; **29:** 558–62.
268. Jellinek D, Jewkes D, Symon L. Noninvasive intraoperative monitoring of motor evoked potentials under propofol anesthesia: effects of spinal surgery on the amplitude and latency of motor evoked potentials. *Neurosurgery* 1991; **29:** 551–7.
269. Kawaguchi M, Sakamoto T, Ohnishi H, *et al.* Intraoperative myogenic motor evoked potentials induced by direct electrical stimulation of the exposed motor cortex under isoflurane and sevoflurane. *Anesth Analg* 1996; **82:** 593–9.
270. Taniguchi M, Cedzich C, Schramm J. Modification of cortical stimulation for motor evoked potentials under general anesthesia: technical description. *Neurosurgery* 1993; **32:** 219–26.
271. Cedzich C, Taniguchi M, Schafer S, Schramm J. Somatosensory evoked potential phase reversal and direct motor cortex stimulation during surgery in and around the central region. *Neurosurgery* 1996; **38:** 962–70.
272. Lang EW, Beutler AS, Chesnut RM, *et al.* Myogenic motor-evoked potential monitoring using partial neuromuscular blockade in surgery of the spine. *Spine* 1996; **21:** 1676–86.
273. Kalkman CJ, Ubags LH, Been HD, *et al.* Improved amplitude of myogenic motor evoked responses after paired transcranial electrical stimulation during sufentanil/nitrous oxide anesthesia. *Anesthesiology* 1995; **83:** 270–6.
274. Jones SJ, Harrison R, Koh KF, *et al.* Motor evoked potential monitoring during spinal surgery: responses of distal limb muscles to transcranial cortical stimulation with pulse trains. *Electroencephalogr Clin Neurophysiol* 1996; **100:** 375–83.
275. Pechstein U, Cedzich C, Nadstawek J, Schramm J. Transcranial high-frequency repetitive electrical stimulation for recording myogenic motor evoked potentials with the patient under general anesthesia. *Neurosurgery* 1996; **39:** 335–43.
276. Calancie B, Harris W, Brindle GF, *et al.* Threshold-level repetitive transcranial electrical stimulation for intraoperative monitoring of central motor conduction. *J Neurosurg* 2001; **95:** 161–8.
277. DeFelipe J, Conley M, Jones EG. Long-range focal collateralization of axons arising from corticocortical cells in monkey sensory-motor cortex. *J Neurosci* 1986; **6:** 3749–66.
278. Stefanis C, Jasper H. Recurrent collateral inhibition in pyramidal tract neurons. *J Neurophysiol* 1964; **27:** 855–77.
279. Pascual-Leone A, Houser CM, Reese K, *et al.* Safety of rapid-rate transcranial magnetic stimulation in normal volunteers. *Electroencephalogr Clin Neurophysiol* 1993; **89:** 120–30.
280. Counter SA, Borg E, Lofqvist L. Acoustic trauma in extracranial magnetic brain stimulation. *Electroencephalogr Clin Neurophysiol* 1991; **78:** 173–84.
281. Counter SA, Borg E, Lofqvist L, Brismar T. Hearing loss from the acoustic artifact of the coil used in extracranial magnetic stimulation. *Neurology* 1990; **40:** 1159–62.
282. Counter SA, Borg E. Acoustic middle ear muscle reflex protection against magnetic coil impulse noise. *Acta Otolaryngol* 1993; **113:** 483–8.
283. Padberg AM, Bridwell KH. Spinal cord monitoring: current state of the art. *Orthop Clin North Am* 1999; **30:** 407–33.
284. Taniguchi M, Nadstawek J, Langenbach U, *et al.* Effects of four intravenous anesthetic agents on motor evoked potentials elicited by magnetic transcranial stimulation. *Neurosurgery* 1993; **33:** 407–15.
285. Gugino LD, Aglio LS, Segal ME. Use of transcranial magnetic stimulation for monitoring spinal cord motor pathways. *Semin Spinal Surg* 1997; **9:** 315–36.
286. Harner SG, Daube JR, Ebersold MJ. Electrophysiologic monitoring of facial nerve during temporal bone surgery. *Laryngoscope* 1986; **96:** 65–9.
287. Harner SG, Daube JR, Ebersold MJ, Beatty CW. Improved preservation of facial nerve function with use of electrical monitoring during removal of acoustic neuromas. *Mayo Clin Proc* 1987; **62:** 92–102.
288. Lennon RL, Hosking MP, Daube JR, Welna JO. Effect of partial neuromuscular blockade on intraoperative electromyography in patients undergoing resection of acoustic neuromas. *Anesth Analg* 1992; **75:** 729–33.
289. Jannetta PJ, Moller MB, Moller AR, Sekhar LN. Neurosurgical treatment of vertigo by microvascular decompression of the eighth cranial nerve. *Clin Neurosurg* 1986; **33:** 645–65.
290. Zentner J, Ebner A. Nitrous oxide suppresses the electromyographic response evoked by electrical stimulation of the motor cortex. *Neurosurgery* 1989; **24:** 60–2.
291. Levy Jr WJ. Clinical experience with motor and cerebellar evoked potential monitoring. *Neurosurgery* 1987; **20:** 169–82.
292. Padberg AM, Wilson-Holden TJ, Lenke LG, Bridwell KH. Somatosensory- and motor-evoked potential monitoring without a wake-up test during idiopathic scoliosis surgery. *Spine* 1998; **23:** 1392–400.
293. Herdmann J, Lumenta CB, Huse KO. Magnetic stimulation for monitoring of motor pathways in spinal procedures. *Spine* 1993; **18:** 551–9.

294. Burke D, Hicks RG. Surgical monitoring of motor pathways. *J Clin Neurophysiol* 1998; **15:** 194–205.
295. Nagle KJ, Emerson RG, Adams DC, *et al.* Intraoperative monitoring of motor evoked potentials: a review of 116 cases. *Neurology* 1996; **47:** 999–1004.
296. Owen JH, Sponseller PD, Szymanski J, Hurdle M. Efficacy of multimodality spinal cord monitoring during surgery for neuromuscular scoliosis. *Spine* 1995; **20:** 1480–8.
297. Zentner J, Ebner A. [Somatosensory and motor evoked potentials in the prognostic assessment of traumatic and non-traumatic comatose patients]. *EEG EMG Z Elektroenzephalogr Elektromyogr Verwandte Geb* 1988; **19:** 267–71.
298. Facco E, Baratto F, Munari M, *et al.* Sensorimotor central conduction time in comatose patients. *Electroencephalogr Clin Neurophysiol* 1991; **80:** 469–76.
299. Netz J, Homberg V. Intact conduction of fastest corticospinal efferents is not sufficient for normal voluntary muscle strength: transcranial motor cortex stimulation in patients with tetraplegia. *Neurosci Lett* 1992; **146:** 29–32.
300. Shapiro HM. Intracranial hypertension: therapeutic and anesthetic considerations. *Anesthesiology* 1975; **43:** 445–71.
301. The Brain Trauma Foundation. The American Association of Neurological Surgeons. The Joint Section on Neurotrauma and Critical Care. Recommendations for intracranial pressure monitoring technology. *J Neurotrauma* 2000; **17:** 497–506.
302. Barnett GH, Chapman PH. Insertion and care of intracranial pressure monitoring devices. In: Ropper AH, Kennedy SF (eds). *Neurological and Neurosurgical Intensive Care.* Rockville, MD: Aspen Publishers, 1988: 43–55.
303. Guillaume I, Janny P. Manometrie intracranie et continue. Interact de la methode et premiers resultats. Rev Neurol (Paris) 1951; **85:** 953–5.
304. Lundberg N. Continuous recording and control of ventricular fluid pressure in neurosurgical practice. *Acta Physchiatr Scand* 1960; **36** (Suppl.): 149.
305. Paramore CG, Turner DA. Relative risks of ventriculostomy infection and morbidity. *Acta Neurochir (Wien)* 1994; **127:** 79–84.
306. Mayhall CG, Archer NH, Lamb VA, *et al.* Ventriculostomy-related infections. A prospective epidemiologic study. *N Engl J Med* 1984; **310:** 553–9.
307. Narayan RK, Kishore PR, Becker DP, *et al.* Intracranial pressure: to monitor or not to monitor? A review of our experience with severe head injury. *J Neurosurg* 1982; **56:** 650–9.
308. Vries JK, Becker DP, Young HF. A subarachnoid screw for monitoring intracranial pressure. Technical note. *J Neurosurg* 1973; **39:** 416–19.
309. Warner DS, Sokoll MD. Monitoring intracranial pressure. In: Blitt CD (ed.). *Monitoring in Anesthesia and Critical Care Medicine*, 2nd edn. New York: Churchill Livingstone, 1990: 532.
310. Powell MP, Crockard HA. Behavior of an extradural pressure monitor in clinical use. Comparison of extradural with intraventricular pressure in patients with acute and chronically raised intracranial pressure. *J Neurosurg* 1985; **63:** 745–9.
311. Czech T, Korn A, Reinprecht A, *et al.* Clinical evaluation of a new epidural pressure monitor. *Acta Neurochir (Wien)* 1993; **125:** 169–72.
312. Schwartz N, Matuschka H, Meznik A. The Spiegelberg device for epidural registration of the ICP. *Unfallchirurg* 1992; **95:** 113–17.
313. Levin AB. The use of a fiberoptic intracranial pressure monitor in clinical practice. *Neurosurgery* 1977; **1:** 266–71.
314. Marcotty SF, Levin AB. A new approach in epidural intracranial pressure monitoring. *J Neurosurg Nurs* 1984; **16:** 54–9.
315. Barlow P, Mendelow AD, Lawrence AE, *et al.* Clinical evaluation of two methods of subdural pressure monitoring. *J Neurosurg* 1985; **63:** 578–82.
316. Roberts PA, Fullenwider C, Stevens FA, Pollay M. *Intracranial Pressure*, V. Berlin: Springer-Verlag, 1983: 104–5.
317. Gentleman D, Mendelow AD. Intracranial rupture of a pressure monitoring transducer: technical note. *Neurosurgery* 1986; **19:** 91–2.
318. Ostrup RC, Luerssen TG, Marshall LF, Zornow MH. Continuous monitoring of intracranial pressure with a miniaturized fiberoptic device. *J Neurosurg* 1987; **67:** 206–9.
319. Yablon JS, Lantner HJ, McCormack TM, *et al.* Clinical experience with a fiberoptic intracranial pressure monitor. *J Clin Monit* 1993; **9:** 171–5.
320. Bavetta S, Norris JS, Wyatt M, *et al.* Prospective study of zero drift in fiberoptic pressure monitors used in clinical practice. *J Neurosurg* 1997; **86:** 927–30.
321. Artru F, Terrier A, Gibert I, *et al.* Monitoring of intracranial pressure with intraparenchymal fiberoptic transducer. Technical aspects and clinical reliability. *Ann Fr Anesth Reamin* 1992; **11:** 424–9.
322. Crutchfield JS, Narayan RK, Robertson CS, Michael LH. Evaluation of a fiberoptic intracranial pressure monitor. *J Neurosurg* 1990; **72:** 482–7.
323. The Brain Trauma Foundation. The American Association of Neurological Surgeons. The Joint Section on Neurotrauma and Critical Care. Indications for intracranial pressure monitoring. *J Neurotrauma* 2000; **17:** 479–91.
324. Marion DW, Spiegel TP. Changes in the management of severe traumatic brain injury: 1991–1997. *Crit Care Med* 2000; **28:** 16–18.
325. Matta B, Menon D. Severe head injury in the United Kingdom and Ireland: a survey of practice and implications for management. *Crit Care Med* 1996; **24:** 1743–8.
326. The Brain Trauma Foundation. The American Association of Neurological Surgeons. The Joint Section on Neurotrauma and Critical Care. Intracranial pressure treatment threshold. *J Neurotrauma* 2000; **17:** 493–5.
327. Ascher NL, Lake JR, Emond JC, Roberts JP. Liver transplantation for fulminant hepatic failure. *Arch Surg* 1993; **128:** 677–82.
328. Jenkins JG, Glasgow JF, Black GW, *et al.* Reye's syndrome: assessment of intracranial monitoring. *Br Med J (Clin Res Ed)* 1987; **294:** 337–8.
329. Langfitt TW, Obrist WD (eds). *Cerebral Blood Flow.* New York: McGraw-Hill, 1985: 1167–73.
330. Meyer KL, Dempsey RJ, Roy MW, Donaldson DL. Somatosensory evoked potentials as a measure of experimental cerebral ischemia. *J Neurosurg* 1985; **62:** 269–75.
331. Ogawa A, Sato H, Sakurai Y, Yoshimoto T. Limitation of temporary vascular occlusion during aneurysm surgery. Study by intraoperative monitoring of cortical blood flow. *Surg Neurol* 1991; **36:** 453–7.
332. Aaslid R, Markwalder TM, Nornes H. Noninvasive transcranial Doppler ultrasound recording of flow velocity in basal cerebral arteries. *J Neurosurg* 1982; **57:** 769–74.
333. Newell DW, Aaslid R (eds). *Transcranial Doppler.* New York: Raven Press, 1992.
334. Bass A, Krupski WC, Schneider PA, *et al.* Intraoperative transcranial Doppler: limitations of the method. *J Vasc Surg* 1989; **10:** 549–53.
335. White DN, Curry GR, Stevenson RJ. The acoustic characteristics of the skull. *Ultrasound Med Biol* 1978; **4:** 225–52.
336. Murkin JM, Lee DH. Noninvasive measurement of cerebral blood flow: techniques and limitations. *Can J Anaesth* 1991; **38:** 805–8.
337. Steinmeier R, Laumer R, Bondar I, *et al.* Cerebral hemodynamics in subarachnoid hemorrhage evaluated by transcranial Doppler sonography. Part 2. Pulsatility indices: normal reference values and characteristics in subarachnoid hemorrhage. *Neurosurgery* 1993; **33:** 10–18.
338. Pourcelot L. Present and future of diagnostic ultrasound. In: Donald J, Levis S (eds). Rotterdam: Kooyker Scientific Publication, 1976: 141–7.
339. Dunne VG, Besser M, Ma WJ. Transcranial Doppler in carotid endarterectomy. *J Clin Neurosci* 2001; **8:** 140–5.
340. Spencer MP, Thomas GI, Nicholls SC, Sauvage LR. Detection of middle cerebral artery emboli during carotid endarterectomy using transcranial Doppler ultrasonography. *Stroke* 1990; **21:** 415–23.
341. Ackerstaff RG, Jansen C, Moll FL, *et al.* The significance of microemboli detection by means of transcranial Doppler ultrasonography monitoring in carotid endarterectomy. *J Vasc Surg* 1995; **21:** 963–9.
342. Jansen C, Ramos LM, van Heesewijk JP, *et al.* Impact of microembolism and hemodynamic changes in the brain during carotid endarterectomy. *Stroke* 1994; **25:** 992–7.
343. Stump DA, Rogers AT, Hammon JW, Newman SP. Cerebral emboli and cognitive outcome after cardiac surgery. *J Cardiothorac Vasc Anesth* 1996; **10:** 113–18.
344. Spencer MP. Detection of embolism with Doppler ultrasound: a review. *Echocardiography* 1996; **13:** 519–28.
345. Consensus Committee of the 9th International Cerebral Hemodynamic Symposium. Basic identification criteria of Doppler microembolic signals. Stroke 1995; **26:** 1123.
346. Lysakowski C, Walder B, Costanza MC, Tramer MR. Transcranial Doppler versus angiography in patients with vasospasm due to a ruptured cerebral aneurysm: a systematic review. *Stroke* 2001; **32:** 2292–8.
347. Mariak Z, Krejza J, Swiercz M, *et al.* Accuracy of transcranial color Doppler ultrasonography in the diagnosis of middle cerebral artery spasm determined by receiver operating characteristic analysis. *J Neurosurg* 2002; **96:** 323–30.
348. Hassler W, Steinmetz H, Gawlowski J. Transcranial Doppler ultrasonography in raised intracranial pressure and in intracranial circulatory arrest. *J Neurosurg* 1988; **68:** 745–51.
349. Camerlingo M, Casto L, Censori B, *et al.* Transcranial Doppler in acute ischemic stroke of the middle cerebral artery territories. *Acta Neurol Scand* 1993; **88:** 108–11.

350. Gahn G, von Kummer R. Ultrasound in acute stroke: a review. *Neuroradiology* 2001; **43:** 702–11.
351. Goh D, Minns RA. Cerebral blood flow velocity monitoring in pyogenic meningitis. *Arch Dis Child* 1993; **68:** 111–19.
352. Haring HP, Rotzer HK, Reindl H, *et al.* Time course of cerebral blood flow velocity in central nervous system infections. A transcranial Doppler sonography study. *Arch Neurol* 1993; **50:** 98–101.
353. Bonner RF, Nossal R. Principles of laser flowmetry. In: Shepherd AP, Oberg PA (eds). *Laser Doppler Blood Flowmetry*. Boston, MA: Kluwer Academic, 1990: 17.
354. Obeid AN, Barnett NJ, Dougherty G, Ward G. A critical review of laser Doppler flowmetry. *J Med Eng Technol* 1990; **14:** 178–81.
355. Bolognese P, Miller JI, Heger IM, Milhorat TH. Laser-Doppler flowmetry in neurosurgery. *J Neurosurg Anesthesiol* 1993; **5:** 151–8.
356. Arbit E, DiResta GR. Application of laser Doppler flowmetry in neurosurgery. *Neurosurg Clin North Am* 1996; **7:** 741–8.
357. Vinas FC. Current applications of laser Doppler in the neurosurgical intensive care unit. *Crit Rev Neurosurg* 1999; **26 (1):** 28–33.
358. Steinmeier R, Bondar I, Bauhuf C, Fahlbusch R. Laser Doppler flowmetry mapping of cerebrocortical microflow: characteristics and limitations. *Neuroimage* 2002; **15:** 107–19.
359. Ingvar DH, Lassen NA. Quantitation of regional cerebral blood flow in man. *Lancet* **2:** 806–7.
360. Mallet BL, Veall M. Investigation of cerebral blood flow in hypertension using radioactive xenon inhalation. *Lancet* 1963; **27:** 1081.
361. Kety SS. The theory and applications of exchange of inert gas at the lungs and tissues. *Pharmocol Rev* 1951; **3:** 1–41.
362. Obrist WD, Thompson HK, King CH, Wang HS. Determination of cerebral blood flow by inhalation of 133-xenon. *Circ Res* 1967; **20:** 124–33.
363. Lassen NA, Munck O. The cerebral blood flow in man determined by the use of radioactive krypton. *Acta Physiol Scand* 1954; **33:** 30–49.
364. Marcus ML, Bischof CJ, Heistad DD. Comparison of microsphere and Xenon-133 clearance method in measuring skeletal muscle and cerebral blood flow. *Circ Res* 1981; **48:** 748–61.
365. Veall N, Mallett BL. Regional cerebral blood flow determination by 133-Xe inhalation and external recording: the effect of arterial recirculation. *Clin Sci* 1966; **30:** 353–69.
366. Hansen M, Jakobsen M, Enevoldsen E, Egede F. Problems in cerebral blood flow calculation using xenon-133 in patients with pulmonary diseases. *Stroke* 1990; **21:** 745–50.
367. Obrist WD, Thompson Jr HK, Wang HS, Wilkinson WE. Regional cerebral blood flow estimated by 133-xenon inhalation. *Stroke* 1975; **6:** 245–56.
368. Cannon PJ, Sciacca RR, Brust JC, *et al.* Measurement of regional cerebral blood flow with ^{133}xenon and a multiple-crystal scintillation camera. *Stroke* 1974; **5:** 371–83.
369. Blauenstein UW, Halsey Jr JH, Wilson EM, *et al.* ^{133}Xenon inhalation method. Analysis of reproducibility: some of its physiological implications. *Stroke* 1977; **8:** 92–102.
370. Olesen J, Paulson OB, Lassen NA. Regional cerebral blood flow in man determined by the initial slope of the clearance of intra-arterially injected ^{133}Xe. *Stroke* 1971; **2:** 519–40.
371. Giller CA, Purdy P, Lindstrom WW. Effects of inhaled stable xenon on cerebral blood flow velocity. *AJNR Am J Neuroradiol* 1990; **11:** 177–82.
372. Hartmann A, Dettmers C, Schuier FJ, *et al.* Effect of stable xenon on regional cerebral blood flow and the electroencephalogram in normal volunteers. *Stroke* 1991; **22:** 182–9.
373. Plougmann J, Astrup J, Pedersen J, Gyldensted C. Effect of stable xenon inhalation on intracranial pressure during measurement of cerebral blood flow in head injury. *J Neurosurg* 1994; **81:** 822–8.
374. Zampella E, Morawetz RB, McDowell HA, *et al.* The importance of cerebral ischemia during carotid endarterectomy. *Neurosurgery* 1991; **29:** 727–30.
375. Sundt Jr TM, Sharbrough FW, Anderson RE, Michenfelder JD. Cerebral blood flow measurements and electroencephalograms during carotid endarterectomy. *J Neurosurg* 1974; **41:** 310–20.
376. Meyerson A, Halloran D, Hirsch HL. Technique for obtaining blood from the internal jugular vein and carotid artery. *Arch Neuro Psychiatr* 1927; **17:** 807–9.
377. Larson CP, Ehrenfield WK, Wade JG, Wylie EJ. Jugular venous oxygen saturation as an index of adequacy of cerebral oxygenation. *Surgery* 1967; **62:** 31–9.
378. Coplin WM, O'Keefe GE, Grady MS, *et al.* Thrombotic, infectious, and procedural complications of the jugular bulb catheter in the intensive care unit. *Neurosurgery* 1997; **41:** 101–7.
379. Dearden NM, Midgley S. Technical considerations in continuous jugular venous oxygen saturation measurement. *Acta Neurochir Suppl (Wien)* 1993; **59:** 91–7.
380. Schneider GH, von Helden GH, Franke R, *et al.* Influence of body position on jugular venous oxygen saturation, intracranial pressure and cerebral perfusion pressure. *Acta Neurochir Suppl (Wien)* 1993; **59:** 107–12.
381. Matta BF, Lam AM. The rate of blood withdrawal affects the accuracy of jugular venous bulb. Oxygen saturation measurements. *Anesthesiology* 1997; **86:** 806–8.
382. Stocchetti N, Paparella A, Bridelli F, *et al.* Cerebral venous oxygen saturation studied with bilateral samples in the internal jugular veins. *Neurosurgery* 1994; **34:** 38–43.
383. Feldman Z, Robertson CS. Monitoring of cerebral hemodynamics with jugular bulb catheters. *Crit Care Clin* 1997; **13:** 51–77.
384. Gopinath SP, Robertson CS, Contant CF, *et al.* Jugular venous desaturation and outcome after head injury. *J Neurol Neurosurg Psychiatry* 1994; **57:** 717–23.
385. Matta BF, Lam AM, Mayberg TS, *et al.* A critique of the intraoperative use of jugular venous bulb catheters during neurosurgical procedures. *Anesth Analg* 1994; **79:** 745–50.
386. Croughwell ND, Frasco P, Blumenthal JA, *et al.* Warming during cardiopulmonary bypass is associated with jugular bulb desaturation. *Ann Thorac Surg* 1992; **53:** 827–32.
387. Villringer A, Chance B. Non-invasive optical spectroscopy and imaging of human brain function. *Trends Neurosci* 1997; **20:** 435–42.
388. Wahr JA, Tremper KK, Samra S, Delpy DT. Near-infrared spectroscopy: theory and applications. *J Cardiothorac Vasc Anesth* 1996; **10:** 406–18.
389. Adcock LM, Wafelman LS, Hegemier S, *et al.* Neonatal intensive care applications of near-infrared spectroscopy. *Clin Perinatol* 1999; **26:** 893–903.
390. Brazy JE. Cerebral oxygen monitoring with near infrared spectroscopy: clinical application to neonates. *J Clin Monit* 1991; **7:** 325–34.
391. Germon TJ, Kane NM, Manara AR, Nelson RJ. Near-infrared spectroscopy in adults: effects of extracranial ischaemia and intracranial hypoxia on estimation of cerebral oxygenation. *Br J Anaesth* 1994; **73:** 503–6.
392. McCormick PW, Stewart M, Goetting MG, *et al.* Noninvasive cerebral optical spectroscopy for monitoring cerebral oxygen delivery and hemodynamics. *Crit Care Med* 1991; **19:** 89–97.
393. Yoshitani K, Kawaguchi M, Tatsumi K, *et al.* A comparison of the INVOS 4100 and the NIRO 300 near-infrared spectrophotometers. *Anesth Analg* 2002; **94:** 586–90.
394. Samra SK, Dy EA, Welch K, *et al.* Evaluation of a cerebral oximeter as a monitor of cerebral ischemia during carotid endarterectomy. *Anesthesiology* 2000; **93:** 964–70.
395. Cho H, Nemoto EM, Yonas H, *et al.* Cerebral monitoring by means of oximetry and somatosensory evoked potentials during carotid endarterectomy. *J Neurosurg* 1998; **89:** 533–8.
396. de Letter JA, Sie HT, Thomas BM, *et al.* Near-infrared reflected spectroscopy and electroencephalography during carotid endarterectomy – in search of a new shunt criterion. *Neurol Res* 1998; **20** (Suppl. 1): S23–S27.
397. Gopinath SP, Robertson CS, Contant CF, *et al.* Early detection of delayed traumatic intracranial hematomas using near- infrared spectroscopy. *J Neurosurg* 1995; **83:** 438–44.
398. Kirkpatrick PJ, Smielewski P, Czosnyka M, *et al.* Near-infrared spectroscopy use in patients with head injury. *J Neurosurg* 1995; **83:** 963–70.
399. Muellner T, Schramm W, Kwasny O, Vecsei V. Patients with increased intracranial pressure cannot be monitored using near infrared spectroscopy. *Br J Neurosurg* 1998; **12:** 136–9.
400. Lewis SB, Myburgh JA, Thornton EL, Reilly PL. Cerebral oxygenation monitoring by near-infrared spectroscopy is not clinically useful in patients with severe closed-head injury: a comparison with jugular venous bulb oximetry. *Crit Care Med* 1996; **24:** 1334–8.
401. Ter Minassian A, Poirier N, Pierrot M, *et al.* Correlation between cerebral oxygen saturation measured by near- infrared spectroscopy and jugular oxygen saturation in patients with severe closed head injury. *Anesthesiology* 1999; **91:** 985–90.
402. Andrews RJ. Monitoring for neuroprotection. New technologies for the new millennium. *Ann NY Acad Sci* 2001; **939:** 101–13.
403. van Santbrink H, Maas AI, Avezaat CJ. Continuous monitoring of partial pressure of brain tissue oxygen in patients with severe head injury. *Neurosurgery* 1996; **38:** 21–31.
404. Zauner A, Doppenberg EM, Woodward JJ, *et al.* Continuous monitoring of cerebral substrate delivery and clearance: initial experience in 24 patients with severe acute brain injuries. *Neurosurgery* 1997; **41:** 1082–91.
405. Menzel M, Doppenberg EM, Zauner A, *et al.* Increased inspired oxygen concentration as a factor in improved brain tissue oxygenation and tissue lactate levels after severe human head injury. *J Neurosurg* 1999; **91:** 1–10.
406. van den Brink WA, van Santbrink H, Steyerberg EW, *et al.* Brain oxygen tension in severe head injury. *Neurosurgery* 2000; **46:** 868–76.

13

Molecular mechanisms of general anesthetic action

JAMES R TRUDELL

Recent developments in neurophysiology, molecular genetics, and computational chemistry have the potential to advance our knowledge of molecular theories of anesthesia. Recent research results have not supported theories that postulate a general anesthetic-induced change in properties of nerve membranes. Instead, they have pointed to anesthetic action at specific sites in transmembrane ion channels.[1] We will review the recent data that have caused rejection of mechanisms based on the Meyer–Overton hypothesis.[2,3] We will discuss theories of anesthesia based on changes in bulk properties in membrane lipids and then consider theories based on interaction of anesthetics with specific sites on transmembrane proteins, in particular ligand-gated ion channels. Finally, we will consider the potential of future developments, including X-ray structures of ion channels and preparation of transgenic animals that may be resistant to anesthetic drugs.

EVIDENCE FOR MEYER–OVERTON HYPOTHESIS

Some of the most pervasive hypotheses concerning anesthetic action were based on the Meyer–Overton correlation. At the turn of the twentieth century, the chemists Meyer and Overton independently measured the ease with which anesthetics dissolve in olive oil, octanol, and other "membrane-like" substances.[2,3] The excellent correlation of anesthetic potency with solubility in olive oil led to the hypothesis that anesthesia commenced when anesthetic molecules reached a concentration of approximately 50mmol per mol of lipid membrane. Subsequent studies proposed that, by becoming incorporated into and expanding the volume of the neuronal membrane to a critical level, general anesthetics alter the physical properties of the membrane lipid bilayer.[4–8] The changes resulted in increased fluidity (decreased order parameter) in the membrane, leading to alteration of the function of the neuron in some unspecified way.[9,10] However, clinical concentrations of inhaled anesthetics increased membrane fluidity by amounts too small to affect intrinsic membrane proteins without some other form of amplification of the effect.[11] Considerable amplification of the effect of anesthetics could be provided by the capacity of anesthetics to strongly alter the phase transition temperatures of pure phospholipids (the temperature at which compounds shift from "fluid" to "gel" phase).[12,13] Moreover, biological membranes have areas of solid-phase phospholipids surrounded by regions of fluid-phase lipids – a condition termed "lateral phase separation." The demonstration that anesthetics decreased lateral phase separations in mixtures of phospholipids[14] provided a potential mechanism of anesthetic action because such changes remove lateral compressibility (the force exerted by the lipid matrix) from intrinsic membrane proteins.[8]

The following sections will discuss why the concept of anesthetic action in a lipid phase is no longer fashionable. This occurred because too many exceptions to the Meyer–Overton correlation have been established, and experiments involving subtle alterations of protein structure have shown that specific amino acids in ion channels determine sensitivity to anesthetics. Nevertheless, interaction of ligand-gated ion channels with the membrane phospholipid bilayer remains of interest for molecular theories of anesthesia for two reasons: (1) results with substitutions of select portions of several ion channels have consistently shown that the transmembrane domains (portions of proteins that span the nerve membrane), which are bounded by phospholipids, contain the sites relevant to anesthetic action; (2) models of the cavities within the subunits that make up ion channel proteins often require phospholipids to form one "wall" or boundary of the cavities. In these cases, there will be an interaction between the anesthetic molecules and the lipids, even though the anesthetics are formally "bound" to a site on a protein. In addition, several reports describe interactions between transmembrane proteins and the surrounding phospholipid bilayer.[15–19] However, these lipid-based hypotheses cannot explain how changes in bulk properties of the membrane result in alterations in function of neural proteins.[11,20,21] In addition, these simple hypotheses have made few useful predictions that can be tested.

EVIDENCE AGAINST THE MEYER–OVERTON CORRELATION

Hypotheses based on this correlation have failed to accurately predict several key experimental observations. For example, several compounds are known to be nonanesthetics, even though their lipid solubilities are such that the Meyer–Overton correlation predicts that they should be anesthetics.[22,23] Eger and coworkers[22,24] have described several families of compounds that deviate from the Meyer–Overton correlation. The most striking deviations from the Meyer–Overton hypothesis are provided by the nonanesthetics (now often referred to as "nonimmobilizers" because they do affect recall and learning[24,25]). A clear difference between anesthetics and nonimmobilizers also occurs at the level of the nicotinic acetylcholine receptor,[26] and even at the interface between tryptophan amino acids of the gramicidin channel and the surrounding phospholipid membrane.[27] Second sets of molecules that deviate from the Meyer–Overton correlation are called "transitional compounds."

These compounds do produce anesthesia, but at concentrations that are much higher than predicted by the Meyer–Overton correlation. In a given series of halogenated compounds, the extent of halogenation and the percentage of halogens that are fluorines increase in this order: anesthetics, transitional compounds, and nonanesthetics.[28] The potencies of transitional compounds and nonanesthetics correlate poorly with their oil–gas partition coefficients.

Nonanesthetics

The nonanesthetics provide ideal candidates for molecular modeling because a change in a single atom (e.g. changing hydrogen to fluorine) can cause an anesthetic to become a transitional compound or a transitional molecule to become a nonanesthetic. A powerful test of any hypothesis that involves interactions at anesthetic-binding sites can be made by requiring that the hypothesis explain this step-function in activity that is caused by substitution of a single atom.

Anesthetic stereoisomers

The differential potency of anesthetic stereoisomers has been explored for clues about putative anesthetic binding sites.[29–33] The recent availability of stereoisomers with over 90% enantiomeric purity has allowed demonstration of small effects, approximately a factor of 1.5 difference in potency in specific receptors and in animals.[34] Although there has been some interest in exploring this effect to produce more efficacious anesthetic drugs,[35] the main value has been reinforcement of the concept that the site of anesthetic action is on a protein.[32,36] In this regard, although it is true that the C-2 carbon of the glycerol backbone of phospholipids is optically active,[37] there are few structure–activity data on interaction of lipids with optically active drugs.

SITES OF ANESTHETIC ACTION

The study of general anesthetics is complicated by the fact that anesthesia is a complex behavioral phenomenon. A recent review of anesthesia included several behavioral "endpoints," including hypnosis, amnesia, analgesia, depression of sympathetic/autonomic reflexes, and immobility in response to a noxious stimulus.[38] The most common behavioral endpoint in animal or human studies of inhaled anesthetic potency is the measurement of minimal alveolar concentration (MAC), a vapor-phase concentration that prevents response of 50% of subjects to a noxious stimulus.[39] Thus, MAC measures an ability to produce immobility, but not necessarily hypnosis or amnesia. This simple endpoint is useful because it can be applied to experiments on nonhuman subjects, such as mice and rats.

Anesthetic effects (MAC, learning, and memory) may occur at different sites

Eger and coworkers[39] have introduced the concept of "MAC awake," which more specifically relates to hypnosis. MAC awake is defined as the concentration of inhaled anesthetic at which 50% of patients fail to respond to verbal command. This cognitive function is more sensitive to lower anesthetic concentrations than to movement in response to mechanical stimulation, and so MAC awake is lower than MAC.[39] Recent studies have shown that the effect of anesthetics on learning and memory occur at lower anesthetic concentrations and involve different receptors from those characterized by MAC.[24,25]

There are different anatomic sites for anesthetic action

An additional complication for definitions of sites of anesthetic action is that details of anesthetic effects on synaptic transmission vary owing to the anatomic and neurochemical complexity of the central nervous system (CNS). For example, studies of synaptic transmission in the hippocampus by MacIver and Roth[40] and in the spinal cord by Collins *et al.*[41] find evidence for both presynaptic and postsynaptic effects of general anesthetics. Glutamate is the main excitatory transmitter in the CNS, γ-aminobutyric acid (GABA) is the main inhibitory transmitter in the brain, and glycine the main inhibitory transmitter in the spinal cord.[42] Acetylcholine (ACh), serotonin, dopamine, and norepinephrine (noradrenaline) play important modulatory roles in the brain. As a result, anesthesia could be a combination of blockade of excitatory synaptic transmission (either pre-or postsynaptic) and enhancement of inhibitory synaptic transmission.

A surprising finding is that MAC – the absence of response to a noxious stimulus – is primarily mediated by anesthetic action in the spinal cord. This point has been demonstrated by ingenious experiments using decerebrate rats[43] as well as in goats in which the blood circulation to the brain was isolated from the spinal column.[44] Of course, memory and learning are still thought to reside in the brain.

USE OF MAC AS AN ENDPOINT IN RESEARCH ON ANESTHETIC MECHANISMS

Advantages of vapor phase concentration (1 atm) compared with concentration in solution (1 M)

The choice of units for measuring anesthetic potency is very controversial.[45] It should be emphasized that the problem is not simply a matter of converting between units of concentration. The choice of units has large effects on the rank order of potency.[46] For example, when expressed in aqueous concentration units (molar), ethanol is much less potent than halothane. However, when expressed in vapor-phase concentration units (% by volume or fraction of 1 atm), ethanol is more potent than halothane. The difference stems from the high solvation energy of some anesthetics in water.[47] When these anesthetics are considered to move from the aqueous phase to some, as yet unknown, site of anesthesia, much energy is consumed to desolvate the molecules before they can occupy the putative anesthetic site. As a result, they are less potent when measured in the aqueous phase.

Advantages of MAC (% in vapor phase) compared with chemical potential (% saturation)

Even when anesthetic concentration is expressed in the vapor phase, there is controversy about the best units.[6,23,47,48] The issue is whether to use concentrations units (e.g. % by volume) or to express concentration as the chemical potential of a gas. The chemical potential of a gas is approximately equal to the ratio of its vapor pressure in the test system to the saturated vapor pressure of the pure liquid at the same temperature. Ferguson[6] proposed that the latter units were more correct because, at equilibrium, the chemical potential of a gas is the same in all phases in a system: gas, liquid, cell membranes, or proteins. The advantage of expressing potency as the chemical potential is that many anesthetics achieve 1 MAC at the same chemical potential.[6,23] This distinction has important implications in that, much like the Meyer–Overton correlation, it suggests that anesthetic potency is a property of the anesthetic and not the binding site in the CNS.

ESSENTIAL PROPERTIES OF A SITE OF ANESTHETIC ACTION

The discussion above suggests that we should discuss some well-known properties of conventional anesthetics and some properties that seem essential for anesthetic binding sites. Almost all compounds that are anesthetics show an extraordinarily close correlation between potency and lipid solubility. This correlation extends over a 100000-fold range of potency; over this range, the product of MAC and lipid solubility varies by only threefold.[20,22,49] Almost all inhaled anesthetics interact additively,[50–52] and those that deviate probably do so unremarkably.[53,54] This additivity had been studied extensively by the Eger group[22,55] and underlies their determination of the potencies of transitional and non-anesthetic compounds. Additivity of the anesthetic effect of molecules having very different shapes and volumes (e.g. the halocyclobutanes and the halogenated methylethyl ethers) requires that either the sites be flexible[52,56] or that there be many sites and that occupancy of any of them is additive. All anesthetic compounds act within a few seconds of reaching the brain, and reversal of the anesthetic state occurs rapidly with elimination of the anesthetic from the brain. A corollary of rapid reversal (and of the high 0.1 to 1 mM aqueous concentrations needed to produce anesthesia with many conventional anesthetics) is that the affinity or binding energy of anesthetics for their "receptor" sites is low.

Nonanesthetics (nonimmobilizers) do not compete with anesthetics at the sites of anesthetic action. Some nonanesthetics, for example perfluorotoluene,[57] are remarkably potent convulsants, yet none of the nonanesthetics increases the MAC requirement for conventional anesthetics such as desflurane.[24,57,58] Nevertheless, nonanesthetics are not lacking in ability to affect neuronal receptors because, to act as convulsants, they presumably must bind to some sites other than those that produce an anesthetic state.[24]

CONSENSUS FOR A SITE OF ANESTHETIC ACTION

The debate over lipid versus protein sites of anesthetic action was strongly influenced by the demonstration of inhibitory effects of many general anesthetics on the enzyme firefly luciferase.[21,59] Not only is this water-soluble protein inhibited by anesthetics but also the potency for inhibition corresponds to anesthetic potency for a wide variety of compounds. As a result, despite the attractiveness of phospholipid membranes for fulfilling requirements of the Meyer–Overton correlation, there is now a consensus that anesthetics act in or on sites in neural proteins.

NEURONAL ION CHANNELS AS SITES OF ANESTHETIC ACTION

Molecular biology has provided compelling evidence that the sites at which anesthetics affect ion channels are agent specific, with distinct volume requirements. Recently, several groups have defined some receptor subunits that are sensitive to volatile anesthetics (e.g. $GABA_{A\alpha2}$) as well as other receptor subunits that are not sensitive to anesthetics (e.g. $GABA_{\rho1}$). Chimeric receptors were made by replacing short amino acid sequences of the $GABA_{A\alpha2}$ receptor with corresponding sequences from the $GABA_{\rho1}$ receptor.[60] In this manner, the parts of the $GABA_A$ receptor that are targets of anesthetic were identified. Progress has been rapid in this area, and now there are several examples of single amino acid mutations that confer such sensitivity.[60–63] A recent review summarizes these results.[1]

LIGAND-GATED ION CHANNELS AS SITES OF ANESTHETIC ACTION

As a result of the evidence described above, there is a growing consensus that ligand-gated ion channels are a primary target for inhalational anesthetics.[64] However, despite intense effort, there is no basis for selecting one of these receptors as the critical site. In fact, the available evidence suggests that anesthesia may be a combination of effects at a wide spectrum of ligand-gated ion channels. The following are examples of some of the ligand-gated ion channels known to be affected by anesthetics.[1]

GABA receptors

General anesthetic agents (including barbiturates, propofol, and isoflurane) also enhance the inhibitory effects of GABA on neuronal activity. These actions occur within the clinically relevant concentration range. Since GABA is a ubiquitous inhibitory transmitter in the brain, $GABA_A$ receptors may fulfill many of the criteria for the candidate target sites for amnesia, hypnosis, and unconsciousness.[65]

Glycine receptors

Glycine receptors are located mainly in the spinal cord[66] and so are candidates for involvement in the immobilizing actions of some inhaled anesthetics.[41,44]

Acetylcholine receptors

Several general anesthetics have activity on acetylcholine receptors of the muscarinic type (mAChRs).[67,68] Recent work has also demonstrated the existence of neuronal-type nicotinic acetylcholine receptors (nAChRs). Although the neuronal nAChRs have considerable sequence homology with mAChRs, they have distinct subunit composition, pharmacology, and physiology. The neuronal nAChRs are found throughout the brain, where they modulate synaptic transmission.[69] Activation of presynaptic neuronal nAChRs by nicotine or acetylcholine increases neurotransmitter release, and such an effect in the hippocampus may underlie the well-known positive effects of nicotine on memory. Flood and coworkers[70] have recently shown that some of these neuronal nAChRs are sensitive to inhibition by inhaled anesthetics, such as isoflurane. Harris and coworkers[71] have shown that human neuronal nAChRs expressed in oocytes are inhibited by approximately 70% by 1 MAC concentrations of inhalational anesthetics, but are not inhibited by either of two nonimmobilizers.

Is there a single most sensitive channel?

Clinical anesthesia is possible partly because anesthetic drugs affect a subset of neuronal functions associated with hypnosis, inhibition of motion in response to a noxious stimulus, and ablation of autonomic responses, whereas respiration and circulation are less affected. As a result, it has been postulated that there must be differential sensitivity to anesthetic drugs. Therefore, a single most sensitive receptor that would explain all anesthetic action has been sought. Much effort has been expended in this search and, indeed, some examples have been found.[72] However, the evidence that many families of receptors are strongly affected at clinically useful concentrations of anesthetics, as well as different pharmacophysiologic profiles of anesthetics, make it seem unlikely that a single site or receptor will be found.

SPECIFIC SITES OF ANESTHETIC ACTION

Specific amino acids in transmembrane segments define anesthetic potency

As reviewed above, many general anesthetics act potently and specifically at several receptors of the ligand-gated ion channel gene superfamily in the CNS, including the inhibitory $GABA_A$ and glycine receptors and the neuronal nicotinic acetylcholine receptors (for reviews, see references 1 and 21). This subfamily of receptors is composed of variations on a common structural theme. Five polypeptide subunits combine to form a functional receptor; each subunit has a characteristic transmembrane domain in which four segments traverse the cell membrane, looping back and forth between the extracellular surface of the cell membrane and the cytoplasmic surface. Using the techniques of site-directed mutagenesis, Mihic and coworkers,[60] Harrison and coworkers,[73] and Harris and coworkers[1] have described two amino acid residues in complementary positions on the $GABA_A$ (serine-270 and alanine-291) and glycine (serine-267 and alanine-288) receptors that are essential for volatile anesthetic potentiation of the inhibitory GABA and glycine signals.

The proposal that the closed to open transition of an ion channel is the critical event, and that the site of action of anesthetics is in the transmembrane region, has turned out to be a good starting point to define the molecular mechanisms of anesthesia. The single amino acid mutations described above have shown that transmembrane regions 2 and 3 (TM2 and TM3) of the $GABA_A$ receptors subunits[60] and TM4 of the glutamate receptor subunits[74] govern sensitivity and specificity toward anesthetic agents. Mutations at these sites often have two effects: (1) they alter activation and gating by their normal agonists; and (2) they mediate the extent that anesthetic agents potentiate the effect of the concentration of agonist associated with activation of 10% of the receptors in a given group (ED_{10}).

Using mutations in ligand-gated ion channels to test and refute the Meyer–Overton hypothesis

We have reviewed substantial evidence for specific anesthetic binding sites in proteins. However, in each of the experimental test systems used, the vapor or aqueous concentrations of anesthetics that delivered a molecule of anesthetic to the "specific" binding site also delivered the 50mmol per mol of lipid concentration to the surrounding membrane, as predicted by the Meyer–Overton hypothesis.[2,3] In order to make a rigorous test of the "specific" binding site theories, it would be necessary to saturate the "specific" sites without a corresponding concentration of anesthetic molecules in the "nonspecific" sites. To accomplish this, the amino acid residue that confers the largest change in glycine agonist potency in the α_1-glycine receptor[60] (serine-267) was replaced with a cysteine residue. It was then demonstrated that propanethiol was a reversible anesthetic both in rats and at the α_1-glycine receptor expressed in oocytes. There was a particular advantage in expressing a glycine receptor with the serine-267 to cysteine mutation in oocytes and using propanethiol as an anesthetic: it was possible to chemically oxidize the propanethiol molecule to form a covalent bond to the sulfur group of cysteine-267. In a typical experiment, the anesthetic effect of propanethiol was established; next, the oxidant (iodine) was added; finally, all the "nonspecific" concentration of propanethiol was washed away, leaving a single molecule of propanethiol at the putative "specific" binding site. The anesthetic effect of the propanethiol remained, demonstrating that the "nonspecific" membrane concentration of anesthetic was unnecessary.[75]

FUTURE DIRECTIONS

Structural analysis of ion channels

There has been rapid progress in the structural analysis of transmembrane proteins by X-ray diffraction. In addition to low-resolution images of the acetylcholine receptor,[76] there are now high-resolution images of the potassium channel, the bacterial stretch receptor,[77] and the aspartate receptor.[78] However, the structures of the more complicated ligand-gated ion channels are more difficult to assess. As discussed above, the predicted pentameric structure of the receptor–ion channel complex, with each of the five subunits having four transmembrane segments, makes it difficult to express and crystallize these proteins. However, when these channels are known to atomic resolution, it will be possible to visualize the exact sites where anesthetic drugs bind.[79,80]

Molecular modeling to define properties of binding sites

Molecular modeling is an excellent way to visualize putative binding sites in ligand-gated ion channels.[1,63,81] Molecular modeling relies on a set of potential functions that describe all properties of a molecule: van der Waals radii of all atoms, bond lengths between atoms, bond angles, and stretching forces of these bonds and angles.[82] Considerable progress had been made in defining how specific mutations (e.g. replacement of amino acids at serine-267 and alanine-288 in the glycine receptor or serine-270 and alanine-291 in the $GABA_A$ receptor) could alter the binding affinity for anesthetic molecules.[24,63,73,74,83] One of the goals of molecular modeling is to resolve the question about whether the specific amino acids described above define a true binding site for anesthetic drugs or whether they cause allosteric changes in ion channel structure that allow remotely bound anesthetic molecules to have an effect.

The volume occupied by anesthetics has become an increasingly important aspect of their specificity and potency.[73] Raines *et al.*[84] compared straight chain alkanols with corresponding cycloalkanemethanols with the same number of carbons. They investigated the anesthetic "cut-off" length – the number of carbon atoms at which a molecule either ceases to increase in potency with chain length or loses anesthetic potency altogether. They concluded that "Cutoff was not related to molecular length, but does correlate with molecular volume." A similar conclusion was reached by Wick *et al.*[63] using double mutations on adjacent transmembrane α-helices. They suggested that the "cut-off" length of long-chain alcohols was increased when the molecular volume of either of those amino acid residues forming a putative binding site was decreased.[63] Molecular modeling has been used to calculate the molecular volume of internal cavities in proteins.[85,86] The ability to calculate cavity volumes will be of value as more site-directed mutations are made in ligand-gated ion channels in an effort to understand the possible role of these cavities as binding sites for anesthetic molecules.[73]

The families of multisubunit transmembrane ion channels offer particularly suitable structural motifs for testing a mechanism of action based on binding of anesthetic molecules to sites in the transmembrane region of α-helices. Noncovalent bonds – the same weak bonds that hold anesthetics in their binding sites – hold together the subunits of transmembrane ion channels that form a central pore that can open to conduct ions across the nerve membrane.[65] The subunits exist in a low dielectric transmembrane environment and are sensitive to the composition of the membrane[87,88] as well as to the presence of anesthetic compounds.[89,90] An example of molecular modeling applied to understanding putative binding sites for anesthetic drugs is shown in Fig. 13.1. A model of one of the five subunits of the glycine receptor–ion channel complex is shown. The four segments that are predicted to traverse the membrane (transmembrane segments, TM1–4) are shown.[1,83,91] There is a strong consensus that the second of the four sequences of amino acids identified as transmembrane segments (TM2) is an α-helix. Five of these TM2 α-helices, one from each subunit, form the lining of the ion channel. The structural homology between the transmembrane domains of the glycine, $GABA_A$, and nicotinic acetylcholine receptors is so high that it is possible to use this common model to combine experimental results of site-directed mutations in all three of these families of receptors.

Expression and reconstitution of mutant ion channels

At present, the effects of specific site directed mutations are tested by injecting the modified DNA into oocytes and performing electrophysiology on the expressed ion channels.[92] A future goal is to express milligram amounts of the proteins and reconstitute the proteins into a stable membrane-like environment. It will be possible to perform nuclear magnetic resonance (NMR) or electron spin resonance (ESR) spectroscopy on such preparations. These techniques will detect differences in the structure of the ion channels during transitions between the resting, open, closed, and desensitized cycle. Such experiments could determine the specific changes in structure and function caused by anesthetic molecules. The appropriate spectroscopic tools are already available to analyze the resulting conformational changes.[93–95]

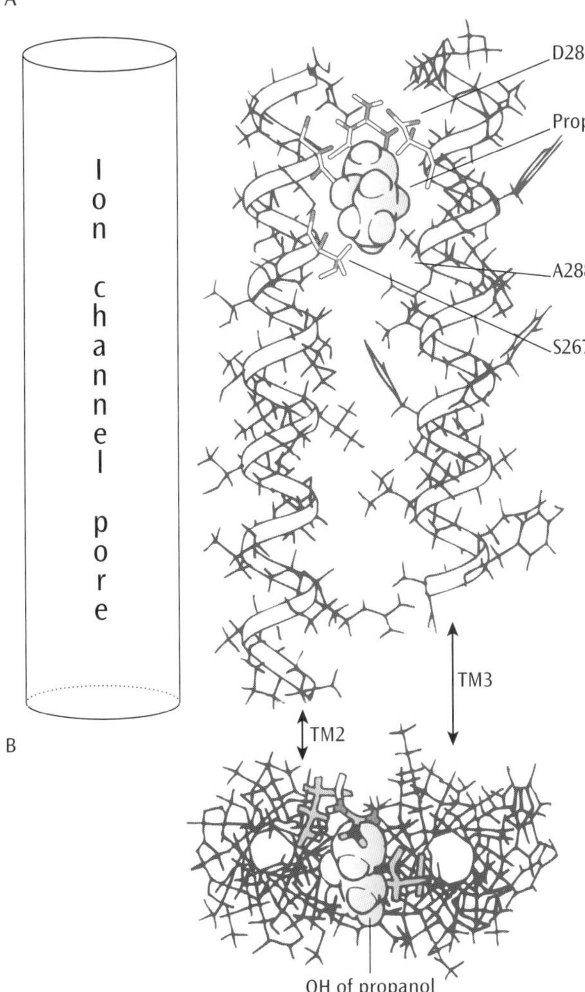

Figure 13.1 *Two antiparallel α-helices that form one subunit of the α_1-glycine receptor. In this superfamily of ligand-gated receptors, five subunits are arranged around a central pore to form an ion channel. Transmembrane α-helix 2 (TM2) lines the pore of the ion channel and TM3 is known to be proximate to TM2, but is not exposed to the pore. The amino acid residues indicated by arrows are: aspartic acid-284 (D284), alanine-288 (A288), and serine-267 (S267). The last two residues have been shown to regulate sensitivity to many anesthetic drugs. In this case, one molecule of propanol is shown in the putative binding site. (A) Two α-helices from the side; the extracellular space is to the top and the cytoplasm of the cell is to the bottom. (B) The same α-helices but rotated 90° about the y-axis. The reader is looking down from the extracellular side of the nerve membrane and the ion channel pore is to the left.*

Defining important receptors with transgenic mice

The ability of site-directed mutations to affect sensitivity to anesthetics in ligand-gated receptors expressed in oocytes suggests that these receptors may be important to anesthesia. However, more conclusive proof of relevance would be to produce the same mutations in a whole animal and demonstrate the same control of sensitivity to anesthetics. Initial experiments of this type have already taken place. For example, Homanics and coworkers[96] recently created and tested several different mouse strains in which specific $GABA_A$ receptor subunit genes have been selectively "knocked out" by genetic recombination. In that the $GABA_{\rho l}$ subunit is insensitive to anesthetic drugs,[60] it follows that animals with their normal $GABA_A$ subunits replaced with $GABA_{\rho l}$ should be insensitive to anesthetics. Providing that the mutations are not lethal to the animal, gene knockout studies of this sort may help to define sites of anesthetic action at the molecular level.

SUMMARY

In the last decade, there has been a paradigm shift from nonspecific "membrane binding" sites to specific binding sites for anesthetic molecules within transmembrane ion channels. Rapid progress in molecular biology has allowed the demonstration that alterations in specific regions of proteins, and even single amino acids, can modulate sensitivity to anesthetic drugs. Structural homology between domains in ligand-gated receptors that mediate anesthetic sensitivity suggests that a common structural motif may confer the response. It may soon be possible to test the relevance of mutations in putative anesthetic binding sites by expressing the mutations in transgenic animals.

REFERENCES

1. Yamakura T, Bertaccini E, Trudell JR, Harris RA. Anesthetics and ion channels: molecular models and sites of anesthetic action. *Annu Rev Pharmacol Toxicol* 2001; **41:** 23–51.
2. Meyer HH. Zur theorie der alkoholnarkose. I. Mit welch Eigenshaft der Anasthetika bedingt ihre narkotische Wirkung? *Arch Exp Path Pharmakol (Naunyn Schmiedebergs)* 1899; **42:** 109–137.
3. Overton E. *Studien uber die narkose zugleich ein beitrag zur allgemeinen pharmacologie.* Jena: Verlag von Gustav Fischer, 1901.
4. Mullins LJ. Some physical mechanisms in narcosis. *Chem Rev* 1954; **54:** 289–323.
5. Miller KW, Paton WDM, Smith EB. Site of action of general anaesthetics. *Nature* 1965; **206:** 574–7.
6. Ferguson J. The use of chemical potentials as indices of toxicity. *Proc R Soc Lond (Biol)* 1939; **127:** 387–404.
7. Miller KW, Paton WDM, Smith RA, Smith EB. The pressure reversal of general anesthesia and the critical volume hypothesis. *Mol Pharmacol* 1973; **9:** 131–43.
8. Trudell JR. A unitary theory of anesthesia based on lateral phase separations in nerve membranes. *Anesthesiology* 1977; **46:** 5–10.
9. Trudell JR, Hubbell WL, Cohen EN. The effect of two inhalation anesthetics on the order of spin-labeled phospholipid vesicles. *Biochim Biophys Acta* 1973; **291:** 321–7.

10. Pang K-YY, Braswell LM, Chang L, *et al.* The perturbation of lipid bilayers by general anesthetics: a quantitative test of the disordered lipid hypothesis. *Mol Pharmacol* 1980; **18:** 84–90.
11. Trudell JR. Biophysical concepts in molecular mechanisms of anesthesia. In: Fink BR (ed.). *Progress in Anesthesiology*, vol. 2. New York: Raven Press, 1980: 261–70.
12. Trudell JR, Payan DG, Chin JH, Cohen EN. Pressure-induced elevation of phase transition temperature in dipalmitoylphosphatidylcholine bilayers: an electron spin resonance measurement of the enthalpy of phase transition. *Biochim Biophys Acta* 1974; **373:** 436–43.
13. Galla HJ, Trudell JR. Asymmetric antagonistic effects of an inhalation anesthetic and high pressure on the phase transition temperature of dipalmitoyl phosphatidic acid bilayers. *Biochim Biophys Acta* 1980; **599:** 336–40.
14. Trudell JR, Payan DG, Chin JH, Cohen EN. The antagonistic effect of an inhalation anesthetic and high pressure on the phase diagram of mixed dipalmitoyl-dimyristoylphosphatidylcholine bilayers. *Proc Natl Acad Sci USA* 1975; **72:** 210–13.
15. Woolf TB, Roux B. Molecular dynamics simulation of the gramicidin channel in a phospholipid bilayer. *Proc Natl Acad Sci USA* 1994; **91:** 11631–5.
16. Hu W, Lee KC, Cross TA. Tryptophans in membrane proteins: indole ring orientations and functional implications in the gramicidin channel. *Biochemistry* 1993; **32:** 7035–47.
17. Urry DW, Sandorfy C. *Chemical Modulation of Transmembrane Protein Structure and Function: Drug and Anesthetic Effects on Membrane Structure and Function*. New York: Wiley-Liss, 1991: 91–131.
18. Takeuchi H, Nemoto Y, Harada I. Environments and conformations of tryptophan side chains of gramicidin A in phospholipid bilayers studied by Raman spectroscopy. *Biochemistry* 1990; **29:** 1572–9.
19. Koeppe II RE, Killian JA, Greathouse DV. Orientations of the tryptophan 9 and 11 side chains of the gramicidin channel based on deuterium nuclear magnetic resonance spectroscopy. *Biophys J* 1994; **66:** 14–24.
20. Miller KW. The nature of the site of general anesthesia. *Int Rev Neurobiol* 1985; **27:** 1–61.
21. Curry S, Lieb WR, Franks NP. Effects of general anesthetics on the bacterial luciferase enzyme from *Vibrio harveyi*: an anesthetic target site with differential sensitivity. *Biochemistry* 1990; **29:** 4641–52.
22. Koblin DD, Chortkoff BS, Laster MJ, *et al.* Polyhalogenated and perfluorinated compounds that disobey the Meyer–Overton hypothesis. *Anesth Analg* 1994; **79:** 1043–8.
23. Suckling CW. Some chemical and physical factors in the development of fluothane. *Br J Anaesth* 1957; **29:** 466–72.
24. Eger II EI, Koblin DD, Harris RA, *et al.* Hypothesis: inhaled anesthetics produce immobility and amnesia by different mechanisms at different sites. *Anesth Analg* 1997; **84:** 915–18.
25. Kandel L, Chortkoff BS, Sonner J, *et al.* Nonanesthetics can suppress learning. *Anesth Analg* 1996; **82:** 321–6.
26. Raines DE. Anesthetic and nonanesthetic halogenated volatile compounds have dissimilar activities on nicotinic acetylcholine receptor desensitization kinetics. *Anesthesiology* 1996; **84:** 663–71.
27. Tang P, Hu J, Liachenko S, Xu Y. Distinctly different interactions of anesthetic and nonimmobilizer with transmembrane channel peptides. *Biophys J* 1999; **77:** 739–46.
28. Targ AG, Yasuda N, Eger II EI, *et al.* Halogenation and anesthetic potency. *Anesth Analg* 1989; **68:** 599–602.
29. Xu Y, Tang P, Firestone L, Zhang TT. ^{19}F nuclear magnetic resonance investigation of stereoselective binding of isoflurane to bovine serum albumin. *Biophys J* 1996; **70:** 532–8.
30. Kendig JJ, Trudell JR, Cohen EN. Halothane stereoisomers: lack of stereospecificity in two model systems. *Anesthesiology* 1973; **39:** 518–24.
31. Tomlin SL, Jenkins A, Lieb WR, Franks NP. Stereoselective effects of etomidate optical isomers on gamma-aminobutyric acid type A receptors and animals. *Anesthesiology* 1998; **88:** 708–17.
32. Dickinson R, Franks NP, Lieb WR. Can the stereoselective effects of the anesthetic isoflurane be accounted for by lipid solubility? *Biophys J* 1994; **66:** 2019–23.
33. Dickinson R, White I, Lieb WR, Franks NP. Stereoselective loss of righting reflex in rats by isoflurane. *Anesthesiology* 2000; **93:** 837–43.
34. Eger II EI, Koblin DD, Laster MJ, *et al.* Minimum alveolar anesthetic concentration values for the enantiomers of isoflurane differ minimally. *Anesth Analg* 1997; **85:** 188–92.
35. Moody EJ, Harris BD, Skolnick P. The potential for safer anaesthesia using stereoselective anaesthetics. *Trends Pharmacol Sci* 1994; **15:** 387–91.
36. Moody EJ, Knauer C, Granja R, *et al.* Distinct loci mediate the direct and indirect actions of the anesthetic etomidate at GABA(A) receptors. *J Neurochem* 1997; **69:** 1310–13.
37. Marsh D. *CRC Handbook of Lipid Bilayers*. Boca Raton: CRC Press, 1990.
38. Urban BW, Friederich P. Anesthetic mechanisms in-vitro and in general anesthesia. *Toxicol Lett* 1998; **100:** 9–16.
39. Eger II EI, Saidman L, Brandstater B. Minimum alveolar anesthetic concentration: a standard of anesthetic potency. *Anesthesiology* 1965; **26:** 756–63.
40. MacIver MB, Roth SH. Anesthetics produce differential actions on membrane responses of the crayfish stretch receptor neuron. *Eur J Pharmacol* 1987; **141:** 67–77.
41. Collins JG, Kendig JJ, Mason P. Anesthetic actions within the spinal cord: contributions to the state of general anesthesia. *Trends Neurosci* 1995; **18:** 549–53.
42. Krasowski MD, Harrison NL. General anaesthetic actions on ligand-gated channels. *Cell Mol Life Sci* 1999; **55:** 1278–303.
43. Rampil I, Mason P, Yasuda N, *et al.* Anesthetic potency (MAC) is independent of forebrain structures in the rat. *Anesthesiology* 1993; **78:** 707–12.
44. Borges M, Antognini JF. Does the brain influence somatic responses to noxious stimuli during isoflurane anesthesia? *Anesthesiology* 1994; **81:** 1511–15.
45. Franks NP, Lieb WR. Molecular and cellular mechanisms of general anaesthesia. *Nature* 1994; **367:** 607–14.
46. Dickinson R, Franks NP, Lieb WR. Thermodynamics of anesthetic/protein interactions. *Biophys J* 1993; **64:** 1264–71.
47. Abraham MH. Thermodynamics of solution of homologous series of solutes in water. *J Chem Soc Faraday Trans 1* 1984; **80:** 153–81.
48. Ionescu P, Eger II EI, Trudell JR. Direct determination of oil/saline partition coefficients. *Anesth Analg* 1994; **79:** 1056–8.
49. Taheri S, Halsey MJ, Liu J, *et al.* What solvent best represents the site of action of inhaled anesthetics in humans, rats, and dogs? *Anesth Analg* 1991; **72:** 627–34.
50. Miller SL, Eger II EI, Lundgren C. Anaesthetic potency of CF4 and SF6 in dogs. *Nature* 1969; **221:** 468–9.
51. Cullen S, Eger II EI, Cullen B, Gregory P. Observations on the anesthetic effect of the combination of xenon and halothane. *Anesthesiology* 1969; **31:** 305–9.
52. Goto T, Nakata Y, Ishiguro Y, *et al.* Minimum alveolar concentration-awake of Xenon alone and in combination with isoflurane or sevoflurane. *Anesthesiology* 2000; **93** (5): 1188–93.
53. Cole DJ, Kalichman MW, Shapiro HM, Eger II EI. Does 1+1=2? – A continuing debate. *Anesth Analg* 1990; **70:** 126–7.
54. Gonsowski CT, Eger II EI. Nitrous oxide minimum alveolar concentration in rats is greater that previously reported. *Anesth Analg* 1994; **79:** 710–12.
55. Koblin DD, Eger II EI, Johnson BH, *et al.* Are convulsant gases also anesthetics? *Anesth Analg* 1981; **60:** 464–70.
56. Morton A, Matthews BW. Specificity of ligand binding in a buried nonpolar cavity of T4 lysozyme: linkage of dynamics and structural plasticity. *Biochemistry* 1995; **34:** 8576–88.
57. Fang Z, Sonner J, Laster MJ, *et al.* Anesthetic and convulsant properties of aromatic compounds and cycloalkanes: implications for mechanisms of narcosis. *Anesth Analg* 1996; **83:** 1097–104.
58. Fang Z, Laster MJ, Ionescu P, *et al.* Effects of inhaled nonimmobilizer, proconvulsant compounds on desflurane minimum alveolar concentration in rats. *Anesth Analg* 1997; **85:** 1149–153.
59. Kamaya H, Ueda I, Eyring H. Combined effects of dissociable and undissociable local anesthetics upon ATP-induced firefly bioluminescence. *Proc Natl Acad Sci USA* 1976; **73:** 1868–71.
60. Mihic SJ, Ye Q, Wick MJ, *et al.* Sites of alcohol and volatile anaesthetic action on GABA(A) and glycine receptors. *Nature* 1997; **389:** 385–9.
61. Dildy-Mayfield JE, Eger II EI, Harris RA. Anesthetics produce subunit-selective actions on glutamate receptors. *J Pharmacol Exp Ther* 1996; **276:** 1058–65.
62. Mihic SJ, Whiting PJ, Harris RA. Anaesthetic concentrations of alcohols potentiate GABAA receptor-mediated currents: lack of subunit specificity. *Eur J Pharmacol* 1994; **268:** 209–14.
63. Wick MJ, Mihic SJ, Ueno S, *et al.* Mutations of GABA and glycine receptors change alcohol cutoff: Evidence for an alcohol receptor? *Proc Natl Acad Sci USA* 1998; **95:** 6504–9.
64. Belelli D, Pistis M, Peters JA, Lambert JJ. General anesthetic action at transmitter-gated inhibitory amino acid receptors. *Trends Pharmacol Sci* 1999; **20:** 496–502.
65. Tanelian DL, Kosek P, Mody I, MacIver MB. The role of the $GABA_A$ receptor/chloride channel complex in anesthesia. *Anesthesiology* 1993; **78:** 757–76.
66. Rajendra S, Lynch JW, Schofield P. The glycine receptor. *Pharmacol Ther* 1997; **73:** 121–46.
67. Firestone LL, Sauter J-F, Braswell LM, Miller KW. Actions of general

anesthetics on acetylcholine receptor-rich membranes from torpedo californica. *Anesthesiology* 1986; **64:** 694–702.

68. Forman SA, Miller KW, Yellen G. A discrete site for general anesthetics on a postsynaptic receptor. *Mol Pharmacol* 1995; **48:** 574–81.
69. Devay P, Qu X, Role L. Regulation of nAChR subunit gene expression relative to the development of pre- and postsynaptic projections of embryonic chick sympathetic neurons. *Dev Biol* 1994; **162:** 56–70.
70. Flood P, Ramirez-Latorre J, Role L. Alpha 4 beta 2 neuronal nicotinic acetylcholine receptors in the central nervous system are inhibited by isoflurane and propofol, but alpha 7-type nicotinic acetylcholine receptors are unaffected. *Anesthesiology* 1997; **86:** 859–65.
71. Cardoso RA, Yamakura T, Brozowski SJ, *et al.* Human neuronal nicotinic acetylcholine receptors expressed in xenopus oocytes predict efficacy of halogenated compounds that disobey the Meyer–Overton rule. *Anesthesiology* 1999; **91:** 1370–7.
72. Violet JM, Downie DL, Nakisa RC, *et al.* Differential sensitivities of mammalian neuronal and muscle nicotinic acetylcholine receptors to general anesthetics. *Anesthesiology* 1997; **86:** 866–74.
73. Jenkins A, Greenblatt EP, Bertaccini E, *et al.* Measuring a general anesthetic binding cavity in the GABAa receptor. *J Neurosci* 2001; **21** (RC136): 1–4.
74. Minami K, Wick MJ, Stern-Bach Y, *et al.* Sites of volatile anesthetic action on kainate (GluR6) receptors. *J Biol Chem* 1998; **273:** 8248–55.
75. Mascia MP, Trudell JR, Harris RA. Specific binding sites for alcohols and anesthetics on ligand-gated ion channels. *Proc Natl Acad Sci USA* 2000; **97:** 9305–10.
76. Unwin N. Projection structure of the nicotinic acetylcholine receptor: distinct conformations of the alpha subunits. *J Mol Biol* 1997; **257:** 586–96.
77. Chang G, Spencer RH, Lee AT, *et al.* Structure of the MscL homolog from mycobacterium tuberculosis: a gated mechanosensitive ion channel. *Science* 1998; **282:** 2220–6.
78. Ottemann KM, Xiao W, Shin YK, Koshland Jr DE. A piston model for transmembrane signaling of the aspartate receptor. *Science* 1999; **285:** 1751–4.
79. Conti E, Franks NP, Brick P. Crystal structure of firefly luciferase throws light on a superfamily of adenylate-forming enzymes. *Structure* 1996; **4:** 287–98.
80. Bhattacharya AA, Curry S, Franks NP. Binding of the general anesthetics propofol and halothane to human serum albumin. High resolution crystal structures. *J Biol Chem* 2000; **275:** 38731–8.
81. Davies LA, Klein ML, Scharf D. Molecular dynamics simulation of a synthetic four-alpha-helix bundle that binds the anesthetic halothane. *FEBS Lett* 1999; **455:** 332–8.
82. Trudell JR, Bertaccini E. Evaluation of forcefields for molecular mechanics/dynamics calculations involving halogenated anesthetics. *Toxicol Lett* 1998; **100:** 413–19.
83. Bertaccini E, Trudell JR. Molecular modeling of the transmembrane regions of ligand-gated receptors. Int Rev Neurobiol 2001; **48:** 141–6.
84. Raines DE, Korten SE, Hill WAG, Miller KW. Anesthetic cutoff in cycloalkanemethanols. A test of current theories. *Anesthesiology* 1993; **78:** 918–27.
85. Blaber M, Baase WA, Gassner N, Matthews BW. Alanine scanning mutagenesis of the alpha-helix 115–123 of phage T4 lysozyme: effects on structure, stability and the binding of solvent. *J Mol Biol* 1995; **246:** 317–30.
86. Liang J, Edelsbrunner H, Woodward C. Anatomy of protein pockets and cavities: measurement of binding site geometry and implications for ligand design. *Protein Sci* 1998; **7:** 1884–97.
87. Bhushan A, McNamee MG. Correlation of phospholipid structure with functional effects on the nicotinic acetylcholine receptor. A modulatory role for phosphatidic acid. *Biophys J* 1993; **64:** 716–23.
88. Ben-Tal N, Honig B. Helix–helix interactions in lipid bilayers. *Biophys J* 1996; **71:** 3046–50.
89. Wu J, Voss J, Hubbell WL, Kaback HR. Site-directed spin labeling and chemical crosslinking demonstrate that helix V is close to helices VII and VIII in the lactose permease of *Escherichia coli*. *Proc Natl Acad Sci USA* 1996; **93:** 10123–7.
90. Covarrubias M, Vyas TB, Escobar L, Wei A. Alcohols inhibit a cloned potassium channel at a discrete saturable site. *J Biol Chem* 1995; **270:** 19408–16.
91. Bertaccini E, Trudell JR. Prediction of the secondary structure of an anesthetic site of action in the glycine alpha 1 receptor subunit. *Anesthesiology* 1999; **91:** A363.
92. Bello EA, Schwinn DA. Molecular biology and medicine. *Anesthesiology* 1996; **85:** 1462–78.
93. Xu Y, Hu J, Zubrzycki I, Tang P. NMR structures of M2 segment of human glycine receptor and its anesthetic-insensitive mutant. *Anesthesiology* 1999; **91:** A356.
94. Todd AP, Cong J, Levinthal F, *et al.* Site-directed mutagenesis of colicin E1 provides specific attachment sites for spin labels whose spectra are sensitive to local conformation. *Proteins* 1989; **6:** 294–305.
95. Xu Y, Firestone L. Use of nuclear magnetic resonance and electron paramagnetic resonance in anesthesia research. In: Yaksh TL (ed.). *Anesthesia: Biologic Foundations*. Philadelphia: Lippincott-Raven, 1997: 375–97.
96. Homanics GE, Quinlan JJ, Mihalek RM, Firestone LL. Alcohol and anesthetic mechanisms in genetically engineered mice. *Front Biosci* 1998; **3:** 548–58.

14

Nerve conduction and local anesthetic action

SAIFUDIN RASHIQ AND BRENDAN T FINUCANE

HISTORY OF LOCAL ANESTHESIA[1]

Surgical treatment is as old as mankind itself, and for much of that time no attempt was made to ablate the pain of treatment. The French surgeon Ambrose Paré obtained limited local anesthesia by mechanical compression of nerve trunks, and during the sixteenth and seventeenth centuries other European surgeons followed suit. The isolation of cocaine from coca leaves by Niemann in 1860 set the stage for the first real advances in local anesthesia as we understand it today. Carl Koller, the young Viennese ophthalmologist, performed an impressive series of experiments on himself and his colleagues using a suspension of cocaine powder in distilled water. News of Koller's work spread rapidly, and cocaine solution was injected and applied topically by a wide variety of practitioners in different areas of the body. The systemic toxic effect of cocaine proved to be the rate-limiting step in this development. Nonetheless, the unpalatable side-effects of general anesthesia, as practiced at the turn of the nineteenth century, made the search for better local anesthetics a subject of interest for many.

Einhorn synthesized procaine in 1904.[1] The safety profile of this drug was much better than cocaine, and this made it the drug of choice, despite its short duration of action, for the now established technique of infiltration anesthesia. The 1930s saw the arrival of dibucaine and tetracaine, which despite being much longer acting still proved to be toxic in large volumes. Furthermore, these compounds, like their predecessors, were unstable at high temperature and thus could not be autoclaved.

The synthesis of lidocaine (lignocaine) in 1943 by Löfgren and Lundqvist[1] was the next great step forward in the subject. This drug was stable at high temperatures and, moreover, did not have metabolites that could be implicated in allergic reactions. Considerable commercial interest was aroused by news of this discovery, and competition for the patent was intense. Lidocaine became the prototype of a new class of local anesthetic agents – the amides. It is still the most widely used local anesthetic for general clinical purposes today. The late 1950s saw the synthesis of mepivacaine, prilocaine, and bupivacaine. These agents all offered the clinician something in terms of differential potencies, durations, and side-effect profiles. The introduction into clinical practice of bupivacaine in 1963 was the start of a prolonged period of clinical value for this long-acting local anesthetic agent. Concerns about its potential cardiotoxicity in certain circumstances provided the impetus for the development of ropivacaine, the newest local anesthetic, which became available generally to clinicians in most countries in 1997.

Clinicians continue to demand better local anesthetics, and it is likely that this will be an area of fruitful research for some time to come. An agent which provides complete sensory blockade while sparing motor fibers would be particularly useful in obstetrics and for postoperative pain control. Ultralong-acting local anesthetic agents would find application in the management of chronic pain states. Along with these and other clinical disease states are the ongoing requirements for drugs that are stable, safe, and procurable at reasonable cost.

NERVE CONDUCTION

Structure and function of the axon

The vast amount of sensory and motor information that flows between and within the peripheral and central nervous systems is carried by nerve axons. Axons are elongated parts of nerve cells, the bodies of which may be in the brain, in the spinal cord, or outside them. Out of every 1000 axons, 999 lie entirely within the central nervous system. With a few exceptions, the general structure and function of the axon is the same whether it is large or small, peripheral or central.[2]

Axons are grouped together by Schwann cells. These protect the axon and supply nutrients to it. In addition, each axon may or may not be wrapped in a helical sheet of myelin(Figs 14.1 and 14.2). The presence of myelin is a major factor in determining the maximum velocity at which a given axon can transmit an electrical signal. Most unmyelinated axons are less than 1 µm in diameter. They lie submerged in longitudinal troughs in the Schwann cell's surface. A Schwann cell may be associated with as many as 100 individual unmyelinated axons, or in some cases it may be confined to the support of just one.

Myelinated axons are conspicuously different. Their course is punctuated by short segments, approximately 1 µm in length, that are free of the myelin sheath that otherwise surrounds them. These are the nodes of Ranvier. The distance between the nodes ranges from 200 to 2000 µm – the greater distances being associated with thicker axons. The nodes of Ranvier show several forms of morphological specialization – including the presence of voltage-sensitive sodium channels, such as are necessary for action potential conduction, and a high concentration of mitochondria in order to provide energy for the nerve conduction process.

One Schwann cell and the axons to which it is directly related are wrapped in a layer of permeable connective tissue called the endoneurium. Several of these units are further bundled together within a sheet of squamous cells known as the perineurium. This layer is more

Figure 14.1 *Transversely sectioned dorsal root of adult cat (× 13 000), showing myelinated axons (M) and multiple unmyelinated axons within a Schwann cell unit which are distributed singly (×) or in groups (*). Circled axons are outside the Schwann cell cytoplasm. E, endoneural space.*

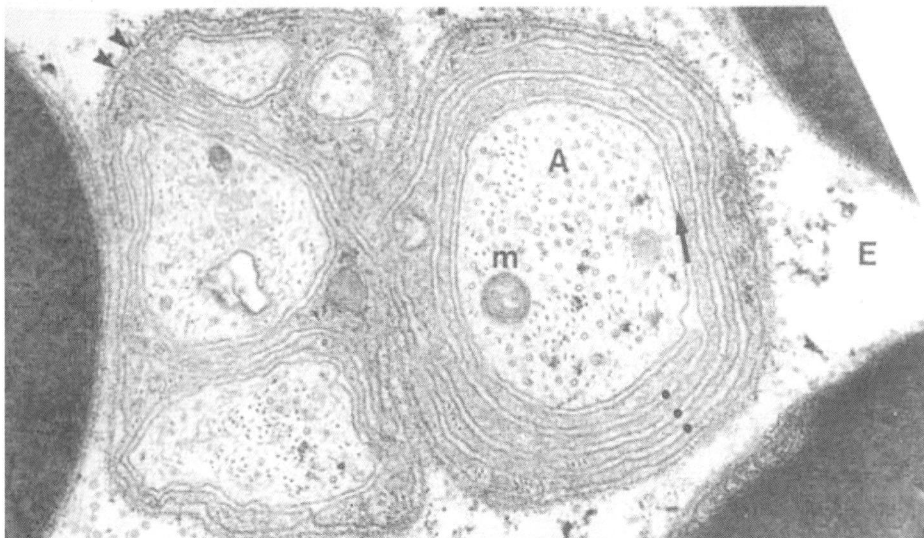

Figure 14.2 *Five unmyelinated axons (× 55 000), showing axoplasm (A) and mitochondrion (m). The axons are surrounded by helically wrapped Schwann cell cytoplasm. Arrow, periaxonal space; E, endoneural space.*

resistant than the endoneurium to the passage of chemical molecules. The perineural bundles are themselves organized into the nerves that can be seen with the naked eye. The outermost covering of such a nerve is a connective tissue layer called the epineurium. This layer protects the nerve from external damage, yet it is more permeable than the perineurium. It also contains the nerve's blood vessels.

A nerve may contain motor, sensory, or autonomic fibers in variable proportion. In 1930, Erlanger and Gasser classified nerve fibers according to their diameter and function (Table 14.1).

The axon has two functions.

1 The axoplasm, the solid internal portion of the axon, is responsible for the transport of chemical signals and cytoplasmic materials. This transport takes place in both directions and occurs at low speeds – typically 1–400 mm day^{-1}.
2 Of more interest to the clinician using local anesthetics is the function of the membranous layer surrounding the axoplasm, known as the axolemma. This layer is analogous to the cell membrane of other cells in that it regulates the flow of nutrients and other substances in and out of the cell; in addition, it has a complex apparatus to enable it to transmit nerve signals.

The nerve cell at electrical rest

At any given moment in time, any given point on an axon is in one of three states: it may be resting, it may be actively involved in electrical signal propagation, or it may be refractory.[4]

At rest, the inside of the axon has an electrical potential difference of −70 mV compared with the outside. This is known as the resting membrane potential. This state is necessary for the cell membrane to receive and transmit the action potential. However, in order to maintain this polarized state, the nerve cell must resist the natural tendencies of opposing electrical charges to neutralize each other (Fig. 14.3).

The axoplasm is rich in proteins and organic acids. These molecules have a net negative electrical charge but are too large to pass through the cell membrane. Concentration gradients exist across the cell membrane for both sodium and the potassium ions. These gradients favor the influx of sodium into the cell and the movement of potassium out of the cell. However, a specialized protein structure which straddles the cell membrane, known as the sodium–potassium ion pump, moves sodium out into the extracellular fluid and potassium into the cell against their respective concentration gradients. This is an energy-dependent process requiring adenosine triphosphate (ATP).

Table 14.1 *Classification and physiologic characteristics of nerve fibers*[3]

	$A\alpha$	$A\beta$	$A\gamma$	$A\delta$	B	C
Function	Motor	Touch/pressure	Proprioception/ motor tone	Pain/temperature	Preganglionic autonomic (sympathetic	Pain/temperature
Myelin	+++	+++	++	++	+	–
Diameter (mm)	12–20	5–12	5–12	1–4	1–3	0.5–1
Conduction speed ($m\,s^{-1}$)	70–120	30–70	30–70	12–30	14.8	1.2

+++, Heavily myelinated; ++, moderately myelinated; +, lightly myelinated; –, nonmyelinated.

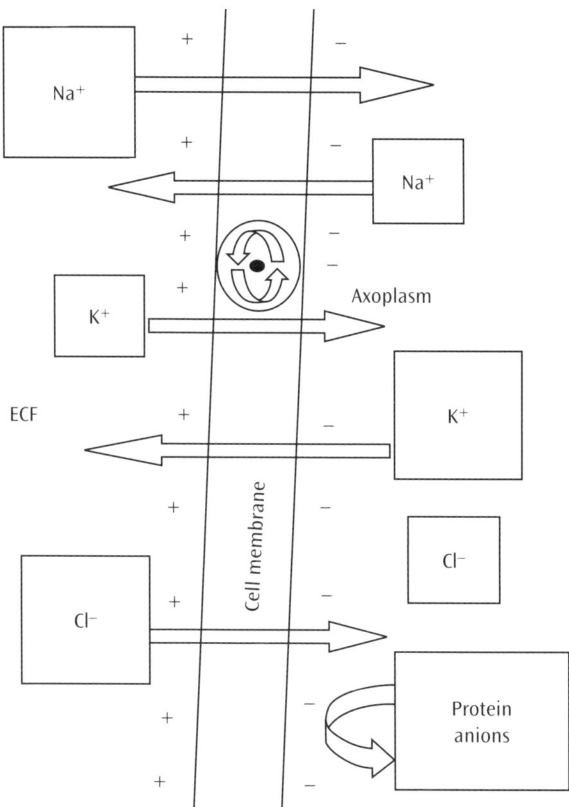

Figure 14.3 *Maintenance of the resting membrane potential. The cell membrane separates the cell contents or axoplasm from the extracellular fluid (ECF). Sodium, potassium, and chloride concentrations are proportional to box size. These ions diffuse across the membrane down concentration gradients, subject to the specific permeability of the membrane to each ion. The sodium–potassium ion pump in the membrane exchanges intracellular sodium for extracellular potassium. Negatively charged protein anions inside the cell are too large to pass through the membrane.*

Not all ions are equally important for the maintenance of the resting membrane potential. Each ion contributes to the aggregate potential difference across the cell membrane based on the ratio of its concentration inside the cell to that outside and also based on the permeability of the cell membrane to that particular ion.

Action potential

The mechanism by which a nerve cell transmits electrical signals is known as the action potential. The cell maintains its resting membrane potential largely irrespective of minor fluctuations in potential differences that occur outside it. However, if the potential difference across the cell membrane rises to a critical level (approximately –40 mV for most cells),[5] there is a sudden increase in the permeability of the cell membrane to the passage of the sodium ion. The permeability of the membrane to the passage of any ion is directly proportional to the importance of that ion in determining transmembrane potential at any moment in time, the net effect of this change in permeability is for the cell to approach the transmembrane potential of the sodium ion. This is approximately +50 mV. The transmembrane potential therefore rises toward this goal. In addition, the rise in transmembrane potential is accompanied by further increases in sodium ion permeability. Thus, a feedback loop is created by which the influx of sodium facilitates further sodium influx.

Clearly, this unstable condition cannot be allowed to continue indefinitely; indeed, within a few hundred milliseconds, the sodium channel becomes inactivated (Fig. 14.4). Net sodium transport decreases dramatically. At this point, a less rapid but more sustained change occurs in the permeability of the cell to the passage of the potassium ion. Potassium flows along its concentration gradient from the inside to the outside of the cell, taking positive charge with it. The loss of positive ions from inside the cell causes a fall in the electrical potential of the axoplasm below neutral. Indeed, the change in potassium conductance is sustained for sufficient time for the net potential difference across the membrane to reach –75 mV, somewhat below the resting membrane potential. This hyperpolarization, combined with the inactive sodium ion channel, is responsible for the brief refractory period that each

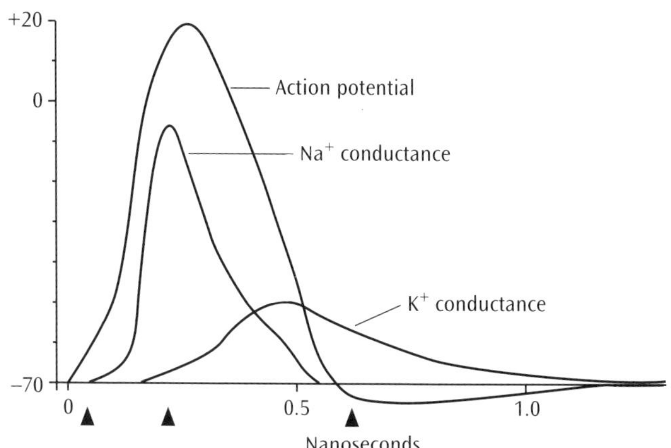

Figure 14.4 *Action potential. Depolarization of adjacent membrane segments results in brief but large changes in ion permeability, resulting in an influx of sodium followed by an efflux of potassium then return to equilibrium.*

segment of neuron is required to undergo following generation of an action potential.

Owing to the myelin sheath, myelinated axons are able to transmit an action potential more rapidly than unmyelinated axons. Depolarization at a node of Ranvier results in the transmission of the change in potential difference directly to the next node of Ranvier along the nerve without having to depolarize all of the axolemma in between. This has two advantages, namely that impulse conduction occurs more rapidly and that less energy is required.

Molecular actions of local anesthetics

Local anesthetics work by interfering with the normal functioning of the sodium ion channel.[6] The exact mechanism by which this takes place is the subject of ongoing research.[7]

Local anesthetics in clinical use are weak bases with pK_a values between 7.5 and 9.5. Thus, at physiological pH, most of the drug exists in a protonated form and a much smaller fraction exists as a neutral species. Conceptually, the sodium channel is a protein embedded in a lipid-rich bilayer. Unprotonated local anesthetic species are hydrophobic; therefore, they are preferentially absorbed into the membrane itself. These molecules move easily and rapidly through the membrane to arrive at the sodium channel. Conversely, protonated species must traverse the water- and electrolyte-rich matrix of the intracellular and extracellular spaces.

Once at the sodium channel, it appears that the local anesthetic molecule can act at one of a variety of sites.[3] The fact that local anesthetics inhibit active sodium channels more than those that are inactive[8] has enabled the modulated receptor hypothesis to be postulated.[9] This hypothesis holds that the sodium channel passes through a cycle of different shapes corresponding to different functional states. The ability of a local anesthetic molecule to bind to any given sodium channel is said to be a function of the position of that sodium channel in its cycle and also to be a dynamic process such that channels are rapidly occupied and unoccupied during a single action potential (Fig. 14.5).[7]

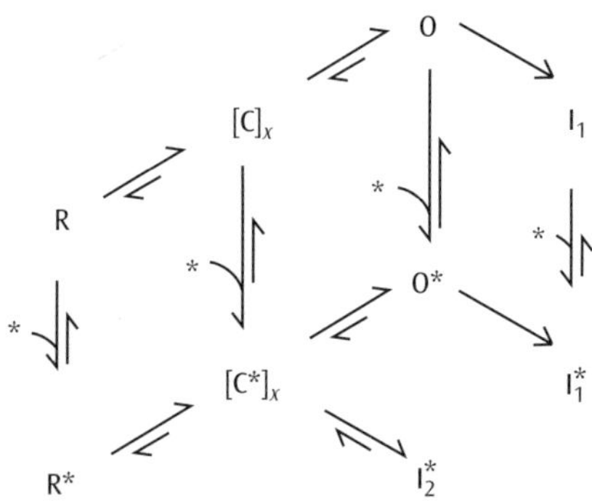

Figure 14.5 *The revised modulated receptor model. Each letter represents a state of the sodium channel. R, resting; C_x, any one of several intermediate, closed states between R and O, which is the open, ion-conducting state; I_1, an inactivated (nonopenable) state that is formed from O; I_2, a different inactivated state that is formed from the anesthetic-bound C* states, without going through O. The vertical arrows indicate binding reactions of a local anesthetic molecule (asterisk). States C, O, and I have higher affinities for anesthetics than does R. The $[C^*]_x \rightarrow I_2^*$ reaction may account for much of the resting, tonic-blocking activity of local anesthetics, and thus favor the neutral, more hydrophobic drugs. Anesthetic-binding reactions of O and I conformations are activated by rapid depolarization (e.g. action potentials), with the former being faster than the latter. Charged drugs bound to O* and I_1 and I_2* dissociate slowly, accounting for much of the phasic blocking behavior.*

CHEMISTRY AND PHARMACOLOGY OF LOCAL ANESTHETIC AGENTS

Structure of local anesthetic agents

All local anesthetics share three important structural elements (Table 14.2). These are: aromatic or benzene rings that confer lipophilicity; an amino group, which by accepting a charged hydrogen ion can form water-soluble bonds; and some form of hydrocarbon chain linking the two. The central hydrocarbon chain can contain a variety of different moieties, but the agents are generally classified into one of two groups depending on whether this central chain contains an ester linkage or an amide linkage. Cocaine, the alkaloid that served as the prototypical local anesthetic for the second half of the nineteenth century, is an ester. Other esters include amethocaine, benzocaine, butamben, chloroprocaine, procaine, and tetracaine. Amide local anesthetics are usually more common in contemporary clinical practice. They include lidocaine, bupivacaine, etidocaine, mepivacaine, prilocaine, and ropivacaine. The classification of local anesthetics as either esters or amides is important because, unlike amides, ester local anesthetics are metabolized to a varying extent by plasma enzymes. In rare cases of true local anesthetic allergy, if a local anesthetic agent is needed, an agent from the structural class other than that which contains the offending drug may be contemplated.

All local anesthetic drugs except ropivicaine are racemic mixtures. Ropivicaine is unique in that it is produced in a pure chiral form. This is important because the components of any given racemic mixture will have different potencies and toxicities. One of the advantages of ropivicaine in clinical use is that it has less systemic toxicity than other local anesthetic agents with similar durations of action.

Factors affecting movement of local anesthetic molecules

Clinicians inject or apply local anesthetics as close to the intended site of action as possible. What happens to the drug molecules, and indeed to the patient, after the drug has been applied is a function both of the proficiency with which the block was performed and of the chemistry and pharmacology of the local anesthetic in question.

The drug must first move from the site of application to the area immediately outside the target nerve. This may be a very short distance, such as when local anesthetic is applied to mucus membranes, or may involve some bulk flow through subcutaneous or other tissues, as in the case of a radial nerve block at the wrist. The factors governing the first stage of a local anesthetic's journey are the concentration gradient, mass, degree of ionization, and solubility.[10]

The concentration gradient down is primarily a function of the quantity of local anesthetic injected: greater concentrations or larger volumes of a given drug will cause therapeutic concentrations to be achieved at the nerve more rapidly. According to the theory of drug diffusion, the larger the drug molecule, the more difficulty it will have in moving rapidly through the extracellular space. In fact, the speed of drug movement is more closely related to the square root of the size of the molecule. Local anesthetics have approximately the same molecular

Table 14.2 *Chemical structure and physicochemical and pharmacological properties of the commonly used local anesthetics*

Agent	Chemical configuration: Aromatic lipophilic	Intermediate chain	Amine hydrophilic	Physicochemical properties: Molecular weight (base)	pK_a (25°C)	Partition coefficient	Protein binding (%)
Esters							
Procaine	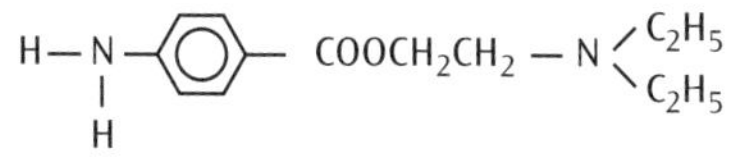 $H-N(H)-$⌬–	$COOCH_2CH_2-$	$-N(C_2H_5)(C_2H_5)$	236	8.9	0.02	6
Amethocaine	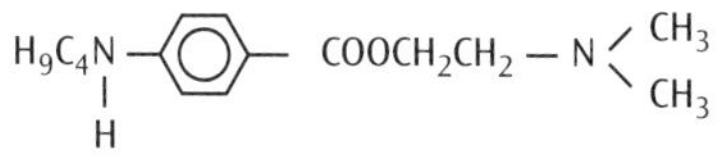 $H_9C_4N(H)-$⌬–	$COOCH_2CH_2-$	$-N(CH_3)(CH_3)$	264	8.5	4.1	76
Chloroprocaine	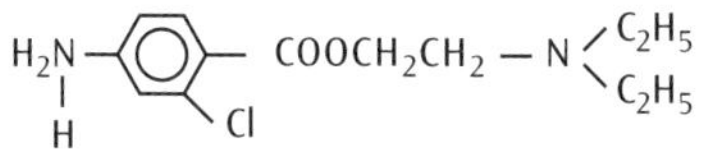 $H_2N(H)-$⌬(Cl)–	$COOCH_2CH_2-$	$-N(C_2H_5)(C_2H_5)$	271	8.7	0.14	–
Amides							
Prilocaine	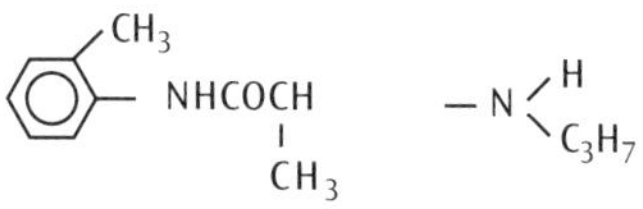 ⌬(CH_3)–	$NHCOCH(CH_3)$	$-N(H)(C_3H_7)$	220	7.9	0.9	55
Lidocaine	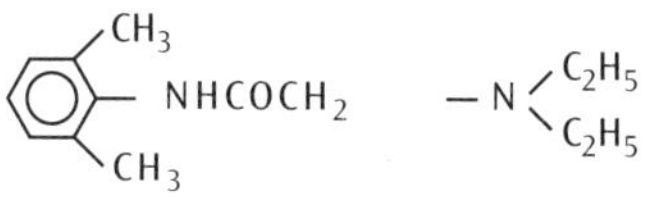 ⌬(CH_3)(CH_3)–	$NHCOCH_2$	$-N(C_2H_5)(C_2H_5)$	234	7.9	2.9	64
Mepivacaine	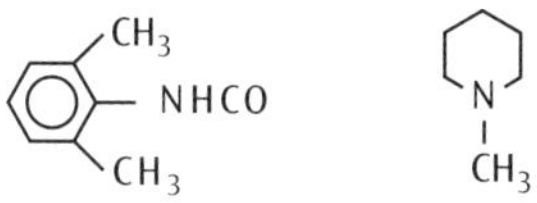 ⌬(CH_3)(CH_3)–	NHCO	⬡N–CH_3	246	7.6	0.8	78
Bupivacaine	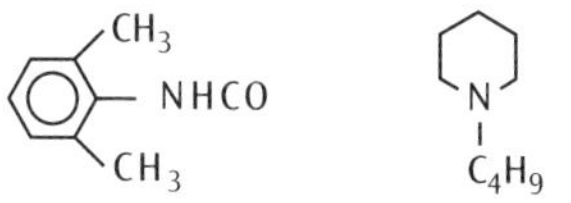 ⌬(CH_3)(CH_3)–	NHCO	⬡N–C_4H_9	288	8.1	27.5	96
Etidocaine	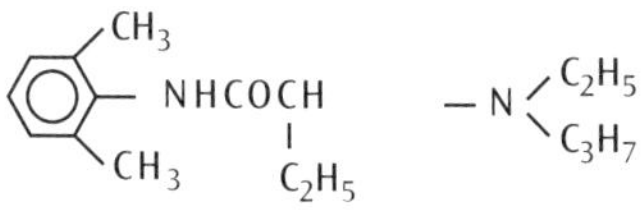 ⌬(CH_3)(CH_3)–	$NHCOCH(C_2H_5)$	$-N(C_2H_5)(C_3H_7)$	276	7.7	141	94
Ropivacaine	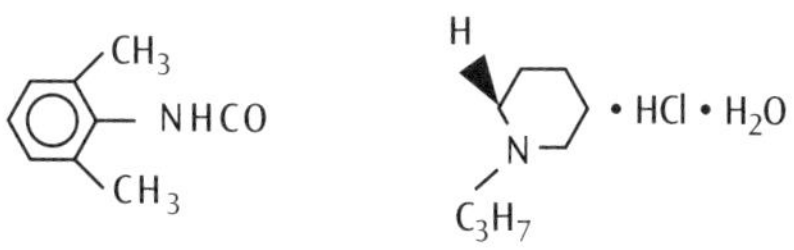 ⌬(CH_3)(CH_3)–	NHCO	(H)⬡N–C_3H_7 • HCl • H_2O	275	8.1	6.1	94

Lidocaine (lignocaine).
Adapted with permission from Covino.[23]

weights (of the order of 250 Da); therefore, this factor does not play an important role in the differences in the speed of onset of the block.[10]

Ionization is much more important. Local anesthetics are buffers and will respond to changes in nascent hydrogen ion concentration by changing the ratio of unionized to ionized moieties. This equilibrium can be predicted by the pK_a of the drug, as described by the Henderson–Hasselbach equation. The pK_a of a local anesthetic is the pH at which 50% of its molecules are in the ionized and 50% are in the unionized forms. The higher the pH, the more strongly the drug acts as a base; therefore, less of it will be unionized at normal body pH. It is the unionized, lipid-soluble moiety that can penetrate most rapidly the lipid-rich barriers protecting the axon. This is also observed clinically. Tetracaine, for example, has a pK_a of 8.46. As it is a strong base and therefore exists mostly in the ionized form at physiological pH, one would predict that tetracaine would penetrate the body tissues slowly; indeed, the clinical utility of tetracaine is confined primarily to circumstances in which large lipid barriers are not encountered, such as direct topical anesthesia of the cornea and conjunctiva or spinal anesthesia. Lidocaine, on the other hand, has a pK_a of 7.91, which is much closer to that of the body's tissues; therefore, lidocaine is much less ionized once injected. This agent is more extensively and effectively used for infiltration nerve block for this reason.

Although pure local anesthetics are bases, commercial preparations of these drugs are produced as (hydrochloride) salts, with pH values in the range 3–7. One would predict that these acidic solutions would take longer to penetrate the nerve than those with pH values closer to that of the local anesthetic in question. Furthermore, it can be predicted that alkalinization of the local anesthetic solution with sodium bicarbonate prior to its injection will result in a greater proportion of the local anesthetic molecules being in the unionized state, thereby increasing the number of molecules that can penetrate the nerve sheath.[11] Clinical studies have confirmed this prediction. Alkalinized solutions of local anesthetic accelerate the onset of local anesthesia.[12–14]

Elimination

As soon as the local anesthetic reaches its target site, elimination begins by natural processes. Initially, a small amount of local metabolism by plasma and tissue enzymes takes place. This is greater for the esters than for amides, but has minimal clinical significance.[15] The predominant mechanism by which a local anesthetic block is terminated is by absorption of the drug into the systemic circulation and its subsequent metabolism and excretion. The kinetics of this process vary to some extent from drug to drug, but more importantly the kinetics vary greatly with the anatomic site of injection. For example, local anesthetics are more rapidly absorbed the intercostal space than from the caudal or epidural space or from the brachial plexus sheath. These agents are very slowly absorbed following sciatic, femoral, and peripheral nerve block (Fig. 14.6).

These relative speeds of absorption are determined by the vascularity of the site in question and by the amount of local fat that can bind the injectate and slow its absorption into the blood stream. Nevertheless, different drugs given at the same site will result in different plasma concentrations. Ionization and solubility play some role in this process. However, of greater importance are factors such as the dose of drug, the speed of injection,[17] the presence or absence of additives such as bicarbonate and epinephrine (adrenaline), the effects of concomitant end-organ disease, and the effect of the surgical lesion on homeostasis. Interestingly, plasma local anesthetic levels do not correlate well with age, body habitus, or gender.[10]

Local anesthetics are bound to plasma proteins. Binding to α_1-acid glycoprotein is rapid, but a quantitatively more important contribution is made by plasma albumin.[18] This binding reduces the amount of free

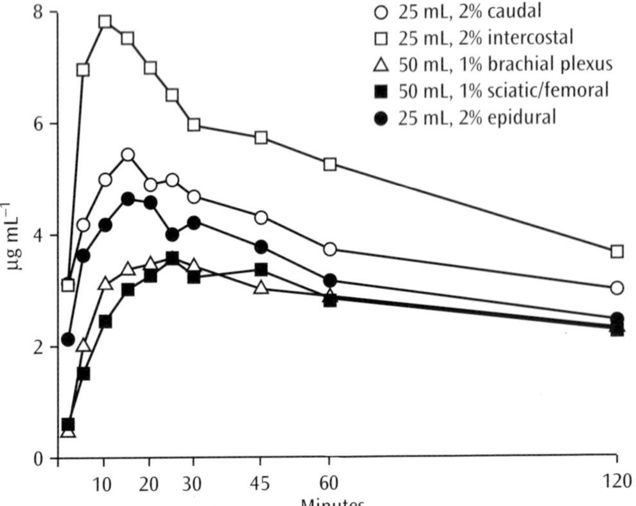

Figure 14.6 *Plasma concentrations of mepivacaine after a single injection of 500 mg. (Adapted with kind permission from Tucker* et al.[16]*)*

local anesthetic and, thus, the incidence of systemic adverse effects. The first organ to which absorbed local anesthetic flows is the lung. The lung plays an important role in reducing plasma local anesthetic levels, primarily by virtue of its enormous blood supply and surface area.[19] Lung tissue has a lower pH than plasma, and thus favors the transformation of local anesthetic into its ionized form. The potent protective effect of the lung is graphically illustrated by observing the consequences of direct injection of even small amounts of local anesthetic into a vessel that bypasses the lung, such as might occur when anesthetic is accidentally injected into the vertebral artery as a complication of stellate ganglion block.

Local anesthetic metabolism takes place primarily in the liver.[20] A variety of metabolic processes are involved, including hydroxylation, dealkylation, and hydrolysis. The liver handles local anesthetic drugs in the same way as it handles other exogenous substances, and the rate of metabolism is dependent on the hepatic extraction ratio and hepatic blood flow (see Chapter 2). There is no strong relation between a local anesthetic drug's class, potency, or solubility and rate of hepatic metabolism.

Ester local anesthetics are also subject to the effects of plasma pseudocholinesterase and red cell esterases.[21] For most local anesthetics, the products of both plasma and hepatic metabolism have few important pharmacological effects. In addition, a small fraction of the injected dose is subject to direct renal excretion. Some of the systemic local anesthetic may be secreted in gastric juice or transferred across the placenta. As might be expected, the time required to eliminate a dose of local anesthetic from the body entirely depends on a number of patient factors. As a general rule, major end-organ disease increases the total body residence time of a given dose of local anesthetic. The concomitant administration of other drugs changes the metabolism and excretion of local anesthetics, based largely on predictable effects on competitive plasma protein binding, hepatic blood flow, and competition for intrahepatic enzyme pathways.

LOCAL ANESTHETIC TOXICITY

When used carefully and in appropriate doses, local anesthetics are extremely safe. Complications are almost exclusively associated with the injection of excessive quantities, overly rapid injection, or the inadvertent intravascular injection of a dose.

Central nervous system toxicity

Central nervous system (CNS) axons, which subserve all central control pathways, have sodium channels analogous to those described above. If sufficient drug is absorbed centrally, higher functions will be impaired. The pathways most susceptible to local anesthetic effects are cortical inhibitory pathways. When these are blocked, excitatory pathways are permitted to work unopposed, and this results in the excitatory motor phenomena that are usually witnessed in the initial stage of local anesthetic toxicity.[22] Involuntary motor activity progressing to generalized tonic clonic seizures are the usual clinical signs. Smaller toxic doses give rise to subjective feelings of light-headedness, disorientation, and tinnitus. All of these effects will be modified if the patient has received other drugs with an effect on the CNS. As a general rule, the more potent the local anesthetic, the smaller the systemic dose required to produce CNS complications. Any concomitant factor that may be expected to decrease the seizure threshold will increase the likelihood of such a toxic reaction. Of particular relevance is the effect of mild hypercarbia, as may be observed when sedation is given before ordering a regional block. There is a strong correlation between arterial CO_2 tension and the propensity for a given dose of local anesthetic to result in convulsions

(Table 14.3). Among the postulated explanations for this phenomenon are that increasing arterial CO_2 tension increases cerebral blood flow, delivering a greater dose of local anesthetic more rapidly to the brain. Additionally, the decrease in intracellular pH favors the formation of protonated local anesthetic species, which are subsequently trapped within the neuron. Finally, the decreased ability of plasma proteins to bind local anesthetics in an acidic environment may increase available drug for diffusion into the brain.[24]

Although excitatory CNS phenomena are significant events which require treatment, much of their importance arises from the fact that they may presage the development of cardiovascular sequelae.

Cardiovascular toxicity

For all local anesthetics, a greater dose is required to produce cardiovascular complications than to cause CNS effects. However, the ratio between the respective levels required varies from drug to drug. For obvious reasons, research in this area has been mostly confined to animal models. For lidocaine, more than seven times as much drug as is necessary to cause convulsions must be given in the case of sheep before irreversible cardiovascular collapse occurs. The ratio for bupivacaine is less than four times.[25]

Local anesthetics adversely affect the heart in two ways. They cause arrhythmias and act as negative inotropes.[26] The arrhythmogenic effects of local anesthetics are a direct result of their effects on cardiac sodium channels. Both lidocaine and bupivacaine decrease the speed with which the cell membrane begins to depolarize. Bupivacaine binds more strongly to cardiac sodium channels than lidocaine, leading to a prolonged inhibition of normal conduction. Spontaneous recovery from the direct cardiac effects of bupivacaine is slower in the presence of tachycardia. Recovery from lidocaine occurs much more readily. High doses of lidocaine usually cause bradyarrhythmia.

The negative inotropic effects of local anesthetics occur in direct proportion to their potency. A rise in pulmonary artery pressure is also seen. Ropivacaine has a greater safety window than bupivacaine from the cardiovascular point of view, and doses of some 25% more may be used. However, if cardiovascular collapse results from the use of a local anesthetic in common current clinical use, resuscitation is still likely to be easiest if lidocaine was the drug used.[27] A fall in tissue pH, such as one would expect to accompany cardiovascular collapse, makes the prognosis worse after bupivacaine but not after lidocaine.

Allergy

True allergy to local anesthetic drugs is extremely rare. When meeting a patient with a past history of such experience, more often than not careful history-taking will reveal that the patient suffered the systemic effects of an inadvertent intravascular injection. Subjective CNS phenomena or the cardiovascular effect of an additive such as epinephrine are often the cause. In addition, most commercially prepared local anesthetics contain one or more preservatives. Methylparaben is commonly used for this purpose. It shares a similar chemical structure with *p*-aminobenzoic acid. This latter compound is the metabolite of ester local anesthetics that caused a greater occurrence of allergic phenomena prior to the widespread use of amides. Other potentially culpable preservatives in local anesthetic solutions include hydroxybenzene and metabisulfite. Metabisulfite is used to stabilize local anesthetic solutions that contain epinephrine.

Methemogolobinemia and prilocaine

The use of large doses of prilocaine is associated with the potential development of a unique side-effect. The patient appears to be cyanotic, yet has normal oxygen saturation. This phenomenon is known as methemogolobinemia. The mechanism is a result of the metabolism of prilocaine to orthotoludine by the liver.[28] Orthotoludine oxidizes hemoglobin to methemoglobin. The effect on oxygen-carrying capacity is not large in a healthy adult patient. It can be of significance in infants, for which reason the use of prilocaine is generally avoided. The condition is readily treatable with intravenous methylene blue.

Management of toxic local anesthetic effects

Most toxic episodes arising from the use of local anesthetics can be prevented by careful selection of drug, its concentration, and its dose, by slow fractionated injections with adequate time in between each aliquot, and by careful aspiration to rule out the possibility of direct intravascular injection. Noninvasive monitoring, intravenous access, supplemental oxygen, and constant verbal communication with the patient all help to detect such a complication at its earliest stages, enabling prompt treatment to be provided.[23] Nonetheless, even the most meticulous approach does not guarantee that major complications will not occur.

The treatment of an acute toxic reaction to local anesthetic follows the general principles of resuscitation. Airway maintenance and ventilation of the lungs with oxygen is paramount. Adequate circulation must be maintained and may require the use of parenteral fluids and/or inotropes. The ability to treat malignant arrhythmias should be immediately available.

If a patient suffers a persistent convulsion, they may require pharmacological intervention with a rapidly acting barbiturate (e.g. thiopental 1–2 mg kg^{-1}) or a benzodiazepine (midazolam 0.05–0.1 mg kg^{-1}). The concomitant administration of a muscle relaxant and endotracheal intubation may also be required.

CLINICAL CHARACTERISTICS OF LOCAL ANESTHETICS IN CURRENT USE (Table 14.4)

Lidocaine

Lidocaine is the amide local anesthetic with the longest pedigree and may be the most widely used in general clinical medicine. It works

Table 14.3 *Effect of* P_{CO_2} *on the convulsive threshold* (CD_{100}) *of various local anesthetics in cats*[23]

	CD (mg kg^{-1})		
Agent	P_{CO_2} **(25–40 mmHg)**	P_{CO_2} **(65–81 mmHg)**	**Change in** CD_{100} **(%)**
Procaine	35	17	51
Mepivacaine	18	10	44
Prilocaine	22	12	45
Lidocaine	15	7	53
Bupivacaine	5	2.5	50

25–40 mmHg = 3.3–5.3 kPa; 65–81 mmHg = 8.7–10.8 kPa.

Table 14.4 *Clinical profile of local anesthetic agents*

Agent	Concentration (%)	Speed of onset	Usual duration when infiltrated (h)	Customary maximum single dose (mg kg^{-1})	pH of plain solutions	Comments
Amides						
Lidocaine	0.5–1.0	Fast	1.0–2.0	5[a]	6.5	Can be given by almost any route. Lidocaine is the standard agent for general purpose use
Prilocaine	0.5–3.0	Fast	1.0–2.0	7	4.5	A good alternative to lidocaine when large doses are anticipated because of its lower toxicity. Not available for intrathecal use. Risk of methemoglobinemia in small children or when very high doses are used
Mepivacaine	0.5–4.0	Fast	1.5–3.0	6[a]	4.5	Works for longer than lidocaine. Useful when vasopressor additives are contraindicated
Bupivacaine	0.25–0.75	Route dependent	2.0–4.0	3[a]	4.5–6	Widely used when longer durations of block are required. Epidurals and particularly peripheral nerve blocks are established much more slowly than lidocaine. Some motor sparing at lower concentrations. More toxic than the other amides
Ropivacaine	0.2–1.0	Fast	2.0–4.0	4		Lower toxicity enables higher dosing than bupivacaine. Better preservation of motor function at lower doses. Not available for spinal use
Etidocaine	0.5–1.5	Fast	2.0–4.0	5[a]	4.5	Profound motor blockade. Best used for surgical anesthesia. Not available for interfetal use
Esters						
Procaine	1.0–10.0	Slow	0.5–1.0	12	5–6.5	High incidence of allergic phenomena. Low cost is its only advantage over newer agents
Chloroprocaine	1.0–3.0	Fast	0.5–1.0	10[a]	2.7–4	Very potent but poorly soluble drug. Modern use confined to spinals and topical application to the eye
Cocaine	4.0–10.0	Slow	0.5–1.0	2		Potent vasoconstrictor. Useful topical agent in nasal surgery and topical anesthesia of the airway. Potent sympathomimetic, potentially addictive and unavailable in some jurisdictions
Benzocaine	Up to 20	Slow	0.5–1.0	3		Useful only for topical anesthesia
Butamben	5% suspension	Slow	Several weeks		6	Highly insoluble drug. Special vehicle allows slow conversion from suspension to solution. Some suggestion of preferential activity against pain rather than motor and sensory fibers. Not available for general clinical use

a. 33–50% more drug may safely be given if epinephrine (adrenaline) is added.

rapidly and reliably to give motor and sensory blockade. It can be used by virtually any route and is a standard antiarrhythmic agent when given intravenously. In many circumstances, the effective duration, which ranges between 45 min and 3 h, can be too short. Nonetheless, it is likely to remain the local anesthetic of choice for general purpose use for some time.

Bupivacaine

Bupivacaine has been the long-acting local anesthetic of choice in both North America and Europe. Dilute solutions of 0.125% or less have been widely used to provide sensory analgesia without motor blockade, as in obstetric epidurals. Higher concentrations of bupivacaine can produce profound motor and sensory blockade that is ideal for surgical anesthesia. Depending on the site of injection and dose, bupivacaine is effective for 6–18 h. The anesthetic onset time is somewhat longer than lidocaine, yet it is still rapid enough for general clinical purposes. Unfortunately, a number of fatal cardiovascular collapses have accompanied bolus injection of the 0.75% concentration of bupivacaine in obstetrics. The use of more dilute solutions of this agent has led to a considerable decrease in the frequency of these cardiovascular toxic events.

Ropivacaine

Ropivacaine is a new amide local anesthetic that was developed specifically to address the issue of toxicity. This drug has a greater margin of safety than bupivacaine, partly because it is marketed as a pure form of the S enantiomer. Ropivacaine behaves much like bupivacaine in clinical use, with a suggestion that low concentrations of ropivacaine preferentially block sensory fibers to a greater degree than the older local anesthetic drugs. This agent is also the only local anesthetic that is specifically approved for use by infusion. Advantage may be taken of its lesser toxic risk by the use of more concentrated solutions. Currently, the maximum available concentration of ropivacaine is 1%.

Chloroprocaine

Chloroprocaine is a derivative of procaine that is noteworthy for its low toxicity and rapid onset of effect. Concentrations as high as 3% may be used to block sensory and motor fibers rapidly. The drug has a short duration of action, making it an obvious choice for short procedures. The popularity of chloroprocaine as an agent for use in the epidural space has been marred by problems allegedly resulting from preservatives in the solution. Inadvertent intrathecal injection of chloroprocaine has been associated with several reports of permanent neurological impairment. Studies reveal that this is most likely due to the preservative bisulfate. The product has been repackaged using ethylene diamine tetra-acetic acid (EDTA); however, although this has solved the problem of neurotoxicity, an increased incidence of severe low back pain has resulted. Minimization of the dose of EDTA chloroprocaine to less than 25 mL in the epidural space appears to reduce this complication.

Tetracaine

Tetracaine is an extremely potent ester local anesthetic. Its physicochemical characteristics result in a prohibitively slow onset following infiltration and peripheral nerve blockade. However, the drug has enjoyed continued popularity as an agent for intrathecal injection and for topical anesthesia of the eye. Topical application must be carried out judiciously because of the potential for systemic effects.

Cocaine

The use of cocaine as a local anesthetic for clinical purposes is limited by its toxicity and by legislative proscriptions on its use according to whether it is an illicit recreational substance in some jurisdictions. In some countries, however, cocaine is still used because of its unique ability to provide topical anesthesia and profound vasoconstriction. It is therefore useful for local anesthesia for intranasal surgery and for preparation of the airway prior to awake endotracheal intubation.

Emla

Emla consists of 2.5% lidocaine and 2.5% prilocaine, which, when combined, form an oily paste that can be directly applied to the skin. This compound has become widely used as a preparatory step for painful procedures, such venipuncture, especially in children. The unique physical properties of this mixture create a steep concentration gradient across the epidermis that forces local anesthetic into the deeper layers. The compound must be applied to the site of the procedure at least 45 min, and preferably 2 h, beforehand. The mixture causes slight vasoconstriction, which can make venipuncture more difficult. Nevertheless, the evidence that this compound reduces venipuncture pain is strong. Although the quantity of prilocaine in the Emla cream is quite small, Emla is generally avoided in very small children (under 6 months of age) because of the potential risk for methemoglobinemia.

Mepivacaine

Mepivacaine is an amide local anesthetic with a potency roughly equal to that of lidocaine. This agent is somewhat less toxic than lidocaine and has less vasodilator effect. It cannot be applied topically and tends to accumulate in the fetus, thus limiting its usefulness in obstetrics. Mepivacaine has been used extensively for dental anesthesia and has been found to be reliable for this purpose.

Etidocaine

The hallmark of etidocaine is its profound capacity to block motor fibers. This makes it a useful drug in the operating room, but this property becomes a liability when the goal is to give sensory blockade without motor weakness. This local anesthetic acts more rapidly than bupivacaine but lasts approximately as long.

SUMMARY

Understanding the mechanisms of local anesthetic action and the physical and pharmacological characteristics of currently available local anesthetics enables the clinician to select the best drug for each clinical situation. Local and regional anesthesia have continued to be popular with clinicians and patients despite the enormous improvements in general anesthesia during the last century of practice.

A survey of the medical landscape today shows that judicious application of local anesthetic-based techniques has revolutionized certain aspects of surgery. In many countries, virtually all ophthalmic surgery is carried out using local or regional blockade. The absence of debilitating side-effects has facilitated increased surgical efficiency. This desire to make maximal use of shrinking clinical facilities has made anesthesiologists re-examine the use of general anesthesia in many cases. Orthopedic surgery of all types for both in- and outpatients can be performed under local and regional anesthesia with shorter discharge times and lower anesthetic-associated morbidity. In many cases, judiciously administered local or regional anesthesia can have a beneficial effect far beyond the operating room. Common surgical complications such as thromboembolism can be diminished by the intraoperative use of spinal anesthesia for joint replacement surgery. Evidence is emerging that the wider use of such techniques would reduce surgical mortality in certain patient groups. Furthermore, an emerging body of evidence suggests that the choice of regional anesthesia as either the primary technique or a supplemental modality can enhance the body's ability to defend itself against metastasis and infection following surgery for cancer.

The local anesthetic drugs that we use now, and the means that we use to administer them, bear little resemblance to the tools used in pioneering regional anesthesia a century ago. As the science of local anesthesia evolves, better agents will eclipse those currently available. Nonetheless, patients, surgeons, and anesthesiologists will always be attracted to a means of making surgery acceptable to the patient without suffering, while exerting minimal effects on the rest of the body and protecting it against the systemic effects of surgical incursion. For that reason, the future of local and regional anesthesia seems assured.

REFERENCES

1. Brown DL, Fink BR. History of neural blockade and pain management. In: Cousins MJ, Bridenbaugh PO (eds). *Neural Blockade in Clinical Anesthesia and Management of Pain*, 3rd edn. Philadelphia: Lippincott-Raven, 1998.
2. Berthold C-H, Rydmark M. Morphology of normal peripheral axons. In: Waxman SG, Kocsis JD, Stys PK (eds). *The Axon: Structure, Function and Pathophysiology*. New York: Oxford University Press, 1995: 13–48.
3. Strichartz GR. Neural physiology and local anesthetic action. In: Cousins MJ, Bridenbaugh PO (eds). *Neural Blockade in Clinical Anesthesia and Management of Pain*, 3rd edn. Philadelphia: Lippincott-Raven, 1998.
4. Ritchie JM. Physiology of axons. In: Waxman SG, Kocsis JD, Stys PK (eds). *The Axon: Structure, Function and Pathophysiology*. New York: Oxford University Press, 1995: 68–96.
5. Netter FM. Physiology and functional neuroanatomy. In: Brass A, Dingle RV (eds). *Nervous System: Anatomy and Physiology*. Summit, NJ: Ciba-Geigy, 1983: 151–219.
6. Hille B. The common mode of action of three agents that decrease the transient change in sodium permeability in nerves. *Nature* 1966; **210:** 1220.
7. Ragsdale DD, McPhee JC, Scheuer T, Catterall WA. Molecular determinants of state-dependent block of Na^+ channels by local anesthetics. *Science* 1994; **265:** 1724.
8. Courtney KR. Structure–activity relations for frequency-dependent sodium channel block in nerve by local anesthetics. *Pharmacology* 1980; **213:** 114.
9. Hille B. Local anesthetics: hydrophilic and hydrophobic pathways for the reaction. *J Gen Physiol* 1977; **69:** 497.
10. Tucker GT, Mather LE. Properties, absorption, and disposition of local anesthetic agents. In: Cousins MJ, Bridenbaugh PO (eds). *Neural Blockade in Clinical Anesthesia and Management of Pain*, 3rd edn. Philadelphia: Lippincott-Raven, 1998.
11. Turner D, Williams S, Heavner J. Pleural permeability to local anesthetics – the influence of concentration, pH, and local anesthetic combinations. *Reg Anesth* 1989; **14:** 128.
12. McClure JH, Scott DB. Comparison of bupivacaine hydrochloride and carbonated bupivacaine in brachial plexus block interscalene technique. *Br J Anaesth* 1981; **53:** 523.
13. Cousins MJ, Bromage PR. A comparison of the hydrochloride and carbonated salts of lignocaine for caudal analgesia in outpatients. *Br J Anaesth* 1971; **43:** 1149.
14. Bromage PR, Burfoot ME, Crowell DE, Truant AP. Quality of epidural blockade. III. Carbonated local anaesthetic solutions. *Br J Anaesth* 1967; **39:** 197.
15. Skou JC. Local anaesthetics. III. Distribution of local anaesthetics between the solid phase/aqueous phase of peripheral nerves. *Acta Pharmacol Toxicol (Kbh)* 1954; **10:** 297.
16. Tucker GT, Moore DC, Bridenbaugh PO, *et al.* Systemic absorption of mepivacaine in commonly used regional block procedures. *Anesthesiology* 1972; **37:** 277.
17. Scott DB, Jebson PJR, Braid DP, *et al.* Factors affecting plasma levels of lignocaine and prilocaine. *Br J Anaesth* 1972; **44:** 1040.
18. Denson DD, Coyle DE, Thompson G, Myers JA. Alpha$_1$-acid glycoprotein and albumin in human serum bupivacaine binding. *Clin Pharmacol Ther* 1984; **35:** 409.
19. Tucker GT, Boas RA. Pharmacokinetic aspects of intravenous regional anesthesia. *Anesthesiology* 1971; **34:** 538.
20. Tucker GT. Pharmacokinetics of local anaesthetics. *Br J Anaesth* 1986; **58:** 717.
21. Kuhnert BR, Kuhnert PM, Philipson EH, *et al.* The half-life of 2-chloroprocaine. *Anesth Analg (Cleve)* 1986; **65:** 273.
22. Tanaka K, Yamasaki M. Blocking of cortical inhibitory synapses by intravenous lidocaine. *Nature* 1966; **209:** 207.
23. Covino BG, Wildsmith JAW. Clinical pharmacology of local anesthetic agents. In: Cousins MJ, Bridenbaugh PO (eds). *Neural Blockade in Clinical Anesthesia and Management of Pain*, 3rd edn. Philadelphia: Lippincott-Raven, 1998.
24. Englesson S, Grevsten S. The influence of acid–base changes on central nervous system toxicity of local anaesthetic agents: II. *Acta Anaesthesiol Scand* 1974; **18:** 88.
25. Morishima HO, Peterson H, Finster M, *et al.* Is bupivacaine more cardiotoxic than lidocaine? *Anesthesiology* 1983; **59:** A409.
26. Lieberman NA, Harris RS, Katz RI, *et al.* The effects of lidocaine on the electrical and mechanical activity of the heart. *Am J Cardiol* 1968; **22:** 375.
27. Thigpen JW, Kotelko DM, Shnider SM, *et al.* Bupivacaine cardiotoxicity in hypoxic-acidotic sheep. *Anesthesiology* 1983; **59:** A204.
28. Hjelm M, Holmdahl MH. Biochemical effects of aromatic amines. II. Cyanosis, methaemoglobinaemia and Heinz-bocy formation induced by a local anaesthetic agent (prilocaine). *Acta Anaesthesiol Scand* 1965; **9:** 99.

15

Physiology of neuromuscular transmission and monitoring neuromuscular block

FRANÇOIS DONATI AND RAJINDER K MIRAKHUR

The introduction of neuromuscular blocking agents into clinical anesthesia in 1942 was one of the milestones in the history of the specialty.[1] These drugs are used to provide a relaxed, immobile surgical field without the need for large doses of hypnotics and opioid drugs. Thus, the cardiovascular side-effects of these anesthetic agents can be minimized, allowing very sick patients the benefit of surgery.

The use of neuromuscular blocking agents has always been controversial. In 1954, Beecher and Todd[2] reported an increased mortality associated with the use of neuromuscular blocking drugs. In the 1980s, many reports of postoperative residual paralysis were published, and in one study inadequate reversal of neuromuscular blockade was found to be the leading cause of unanticipated intensive care unit (ICU) admissions.[3] More recently, inadequate reversal was found to be associated with an increased incidence of atelectasis postoperatively.[4] In addition, the vast majority of cases of intraoperative awareness have been reported when neuromuscular blocking agents were used.

These problems have arisen because neuromuscular blocking agents have a unique mechanism of action. They have little or no effect on the central nervous system, but they block neurotransmission at the interface between peripheral nerve and skeletal muscle. In particular, respiratory muscles, including those of the upper airway, are affected. Thus, administration of neuromuscular blocking drugs implies the need to sustain ventilation until neuromuscular recovery is complete. The type of receptor present at the neuromuscular junction is of the nicotinic cholinergic type. Most modern drugs are specific for this receptor, with limited effects on other cholinergic receptors, found in the peripheral nervous system at the autonomic ganglia and the parasympathetic effector organs. All neuromuscular blocking agents have a quaternary ammonium structure, are ionized at physiological pH, and therefore penetrate the blood–brain barrier poorly.

PHYSIOLOGY OF EXCITABLE CELLS

Resting potential

Nerve and muscle are excitable tissue, that is they respond to an electrical current. Active, ATP-driven ionic transport systems pump potassium (K^+) into the cell and sodium (Na^+) out. Because the lipid bilayer is more permeable to K^+ than to Na^+, K^+ leaks out of the cell more than Na^+ gets in, thus creating a slight excess of positive charges on the outside and a slight deficit on the inside. Thus, at rest, the inside of an excitable cell has a negative electrical potential (typically −90 mV) with respect to the outside. This is the resting potential.

Sodium channels

The membrane of excitable cells contains sodium channels, which are voltage gated, i.e. they open and close in response to a change in electrical potential. The channels are made up of three protein subunits, called α, β_1, and β_2. The α-subunit has the shape of a doughnut which is thicker than the membrane itself. The intracellular portion of the channel is larger than the extracellular portion. The β-subunits each lie on the outside of the α-subunit. They are smaller than the α-subunit and they occupy only the external half of the membrane. The overall size of the sodium channel is approximately 13.5 nm in thickness and 10 nm in its largest diameter. Its molecular weight is 300 000 Da.[5]

At rest, the sodium channel is closed, i.e. the hole in the center of the doughnut is not patent. When a depolarization occurs, i.e. when the inside of the cell is made less negative, a conformational change occurs which results in opening of the channel. Only sodium ions are allowed to go through. Thus, an inward movement of Na^+ ions occurs, driven by favorable concentration and electrical gradients, and this makes the inside of the cell more positive. The process stops after 1–2 ms, when sodium channels become inactivated. Inactivation is stopped in turn when membrane potential is brought back to its resting value. Many isoforms of the sodium channel exist. Their differences are of little significance here.

Potassium channels

Although inactivation of sodium channels plays a role, complete restoration of the resting potential is accomplished because of the activation of potassium channels, which open when the inside of the cell becomes electrically positive. These channels are selective for K^+ ions, which exit the cell down a concentration and electrical gradient. Also, the excitability of the resting cell can be modified by potassium channels. Opening them produces a hyperpolarization, and the cell becomes less excitable. A large number of isoforms have been described for potassium channels, and they play complex roles within the central and the peripheral nervous system.

Calcium channels

The concentration of Ca^{2+} is many times greater outside than inside the cell. This concentration gradient is maintained thanks to efficient systems to transport the ion outside the cell, to sequester it inside intracellular organelles, and to make proteins which bind Ca^{2+}. The trigger that produces opening of the calcium channels is normally depolarization of the cell, which normally occurs with sodium channel opening. The effect of calcium channel activation is a transient and localized rise in Ca^{2+} concentration. The usual effect is binding to specific proteins involved in neurotransmitter secretion, contraction, etc. There are many types and subtypes of calcium channels.

Action potential

In muscle, depolarization occurs through the action of acetylcholine at the endplate. Peripheral nerve is normally activated at the spinal cord, where the cell body integrates inputs from various sources within the central nervous system. Depolarization can also occur through electrical stimulation, as is commonly administered during neuromuscular monitoring. Stimulators provide a brief impulse of current, which flows through tissue between two electrodes applied to the skin. In this case, it is best to apply the negative electrode nearest the nerve, in order to make the outside of the nerve fiber more negative (and the inside more positive) than normal. When depolarization is established over a patch of excitable membrane, sodium channels are activated, which makes the inside of the cell more positive. This depolarization spreads to a neighboring segment of membrane, triggering the activation of more sodium channels, and so on, until the end of the cell is reached. After a short time, the process is terminated by inactivation of sodium channels and activation of potassium channels. The event which follows depolarization is like a wave, called the action potential, which spreads throughout the excitable cell.

NEUROMUSCULAR JUNCTION

Motor unit

A single nerve fiber branches and joins 5–2000 muscle fibers,[6] all included into the same muscle. The nerve fiber plus the muscle fibers it innervates form the motor unit. There is no electrical connection between nerve and muscle. Although the inside of nerve and muscle cells are good electrical conductors, their membranes act as insulators, making electrical transmission from cell to cell impossible.

Synapse and endplate

Neuromuscular transmission is thus accomplished by the release of a chemical, acetylcholine, at the nerve terminal or synapse. This specialized structure is in close approximation with an area of the muscle membrane, the endplate, which contains receptors that are sensitive to acetylcholine. In so-called tonic muscles, there are many endplates per fiber, located at a short distance from each other, and the intensity of contraction can be graded, depending on how many endplates are depolarized. The extraocular muscles and possibly some laryngeal muscle fibers function this way in humans. Virtually all other human muscles, however, contract in an all-or-none fashion. Short fibers have only one endplate, but long muscle fibers many have 2–6 endplates, separated by long distances, typically 100 mm.[7] However, these long muscles also have an all-or-none mode of action and depend on the spread of an action potential to trigger a contraction.

Structure

In mammals, the neuromuscular junction is typically oval shaped, approximately 20–30 μm across, and forms a depression in the muscle fiber. The nerve terminal is in close approximation with, but physically separated from, the endplate by a space called the synaptic cleft. Acetylcholine-containing vesicles, approximately 45 nm across, are arranged in rows on the nerve terminal side. These high-density vesicular areas are called active zones. The synaptic cleft is very narrow, approximately 100 nm across, which amounts to only 0.3–0.5% of the diameter of the neuromuscular junction itself. It contains a basal membrane, fibrous strands linking nerve and muscle, and the enzyme acetylcholinesterase.

On the muscle side, the endplate features a large number of folds. The crests of the folds lie opposite the active zones of the nerve terminal and contain a high density of acetylcholine receptors. The number of acetylcholine receptors per endplate varies across species and from one muscle to the next, but a typical number is 10 million, for a density of 10 000 to 20 000 per μm^2 of endplate.[8] Deep in the folds, the endplate membrane contains a high density of sodium channels. Acetylcholinesterase can also be found in the folds, but this enzyme is not membrane-bound.

ACETYLCHOLINE SYNTHESIS, STORAGE, AND RELEASE (Fig. 15.1)

Synthesis

The neurotransmitter acetylcholine is made up in the nerve terminal from acetyl coenzyme A (acetyl CoA) and choline. Both constituents are abundant in the body. The enzyme which catalyzes the reaction is cathecol-*O*-methyltransferase (COMT).

Storage

When formed, acetylcholine is incorporated into vesicles against a concentration gradient. These 45-nm vesicles are bound by a lipid bilayer membrane analogous to cell membrane, into which regulatory proteins and channels are embedded. Each vesicle contains approximately 10 000 acetylcholine molecules. Most vesicles are clustered near the synaptic membrane opposite to the endplate, but only a small proportion of them are in a position to be released immediately.[9] The rest of the vesicles form a large reserve, which can replenish the immediately releasable pool when needed, i.e. during high rates of stimulation.

Presynaptic receptors

It is likely that presynaptic acetylcholine receptors play a role in mobilizing vesicles from the reserve to the immediately releasable position. These positive-feedback receptors are most likely of the nicotinic type, and are blocked by small doses of nondepolarizing agents.[10] With high-frequency stimulation, the number of vesicles released decreases progressively, accounting for the rundown, or fade, seen with these drugs. This phenomenon is observed with frequencies greater than 0.1 Hz, with a plateau between 2 and 50 Hz.[11] Presynaptic receptors also bind agonists such as succinylcholine. This presynaptic action accounts for fasciculations and the effectiveness of pretreatment with small doses of nondepolarizing agents.

Release

The release process involves many steps, all of which are regulated by

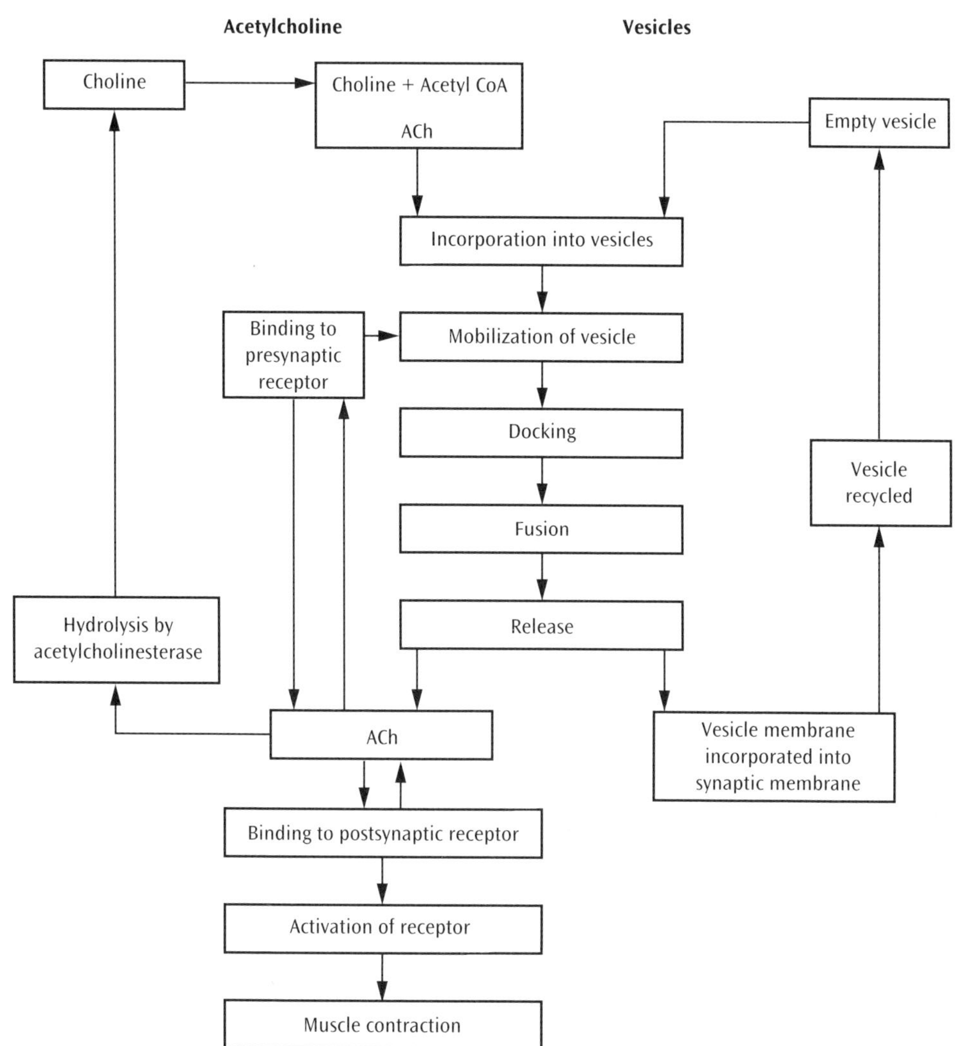

Figure 15.1 *Schematic representation of acetylcholine synthesis, storage, and release, with turnover of vesicles.*

vesicular or synaptic membrane proteins. The vesicle has to unbind from the storage position, and binds to a docking protein on the inside of the synaptic membrane. There then occurs fusion of the vesicular and synaptic membranes, allowing the contents of the vesicle (acetylcholine) to empty into the synaptic cleft. The extra part of membrane is then recycled to make a new vesicle. This process is normally triggered by the invasion of the nerve terminal by an action potential, which opens the calcium channels that are strategically located near the active zones, i.e. in very close proximity to the immediately releasable vesicles. This local increase in the intracellular calcium concentration changes the binding affinities of most of the proteins [synaptotagmin, synaptobrevin, synaptosome associated protein (SNAP), etc.] involved in the release process.[12] An action potential normally triggers the release of 200–500 vesicles, i.e. 1–2.5 million acetylcholine molecules are extruded into the synaptic cleft. Magnesium competes with calcium for entry into the nerve terminal but has less effect on the regulatory proteins. As a result, magnesium diminishes greatly transmitter release.

CHOLINERGIC RECEPTORS (FIG. 15.2)

Structure

The nicotinic receptor at the endplate is made up of five protein subunits, two of which, called α, are the same. One of the likely configurations, looking clockwise from the outside of the endplate membrane, is α, ε, α, δ, and β. The α-subunit is the smallest of the five, and is made up of 437 amino acids adding up to a weight of 40 000 Da. The other subunits range in molecular weight between 50 and 70 000 Da. All five subunits have four membrane domains, that is their string of amino acids traverse the membrane four times, both ends being on the extracellular side. The five units are arranged to form a rosette, or more accurately a funnel, the thickness of which exceeds that of the endplate membrane. The larger end of the funnel is on the outside. The hole in the funnel is lined by the second membrane domain of each subunit. The acetylcholine binding site is on both α subunits, on the extracellular side, between the amino end and the first membrane domain.[8,12]

Function

At rest, the receptor is closed, i.e. the membrane domains lining the hole in the center touch each other at one point to prevent passage of ions. When two acetylcholine molecules bind to each α-subunit simultaneously, a conformational change in the proteins occurs and a passageway is created between the inside and the outside of the cell. Passage through the receptor is nonselective, and movement of ions is determined by their electrical and concentration gradients. Sodium ions are thus more likely to enter the cells than potassium ions are likely to exit, because Na^+ ions are driven by a favorable electrical gradient (negative inside)

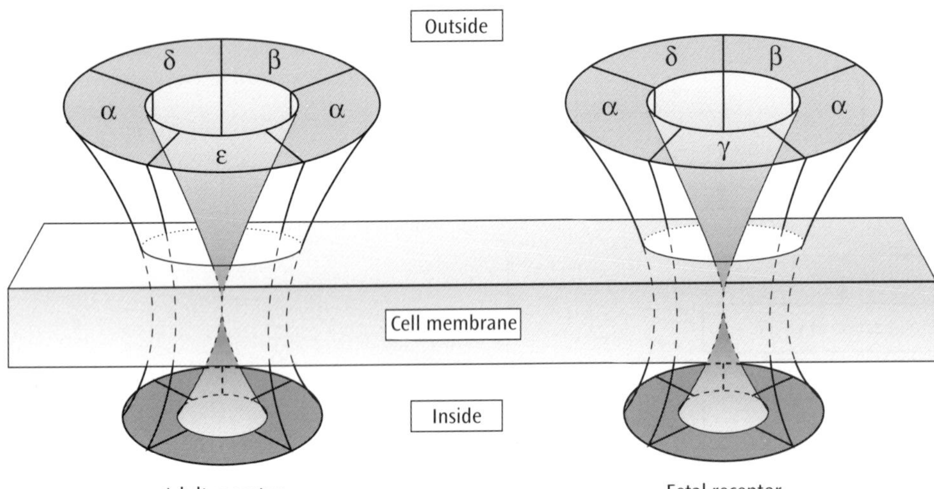

Figure 15.2 *The acetylcholine receptor at the neuromuscular junction is made up of five subunits arranged in the form of a rosette. Each subunit crosses the membrane entirely. Two of these units are identical (α). Normal adult junctional receptors differ from fetal or extrajunctional receptors by the presence of the ε-subunit instead of the γ-subunit. There is general agreement in the literature that the position of the ε- or the γ-subunit is between the two α-subunits. The relative position of the β- and δ-subunits was taken from the Corringer* et al.,[54] *although some workers consider that the order is inverted compared with that shown.*

and concentration gradient (less inside) (Fig. 15.3). Thus, a depolarization occurs. Each receptor has an open time of approximately 1 ms, irrespective of how long acetylcholine remains bound. During that time, approximately 10 000 Na^+ ions can go through, giving rise to a depolarization of approximately 0.3 μV.

It has been calculated that a single vesicle can open approximately 1500 receptors, requiring 3000 acetylcholine molecules in the process. This implies that, of the 10 000 molecules released, only 30% actually participate in receptor activation, the rest being either destroyed by acetylcholinesterase or binding solo instead of in pairs to a receptor. Thus, a single vesicle can depolarize the endplate by about 0.5 mV. When a nerve is stimulated, 200 of these vesicles can be released simultaneously, but only 20–30 mV (corresponding to 40–60 vesicles) is required to reach the threshold, i.e. for an action potential to be generated in the muscle cell. Thus, the amount of acetylcholine released is far in excess of that required for transmission.

Types of receptors

Cholinergic receptors are broadly classified as muscarinic and nicotinic, determined by their specific affinity for muscarine and nicotine receptors respectively. In the peripheral nervous system, nicotinic receptors are found postsynaptically at the neuromuscular junction and autonomic ganglia. Muscarinic receptors are found at postganglionic parasympathetic nerve endings. However, both nicotinic- and muscarinic-type receptors are found presynaptically at the neuromuscular junction.[13] There are many types of nicotinic receptors, but muscle contains only two of these varieties. During development, so-called fetal-type receptors can be found more or less evenly spread throughout the muscle fiber membrane. These receptors have a γ-subunit instead of an ε subunit between both α-subunits (Fig. 15.2). Innervation produces clustering of the receptors in one area of the membrane (the endplate), just beneath the contact with nerve, a change in receptor type at the endplate from the fetal (with a γ-subunit) to the adult (with an ε subunit) form, and an increase in complexity of the endplate, with the appearance of many folds.[14,15] In extrajunctional areas, there is persistence of fetal-type receptors, but their density is reduced. In humans, the conversion from fetal to adult receptors is almost complete by birth, but the final architecture is not present until the end of the first year of life. Maintenance of a large density gradient between junctional and extrajunctional areas depends on the presence of innervation. Denervation causes loss of adult-type receptors at the junction and an increase in fetal-type receptors elsewhere on the muscle membrane.[16]

POSTSYNAPTIC EVENTS

Electrical activity

When receptors simultaneously open in response to nerve stimulation, an ingoing Na^+ current produces depolarization at the endplate. Sodium channels present at and near the endplate become activated; the depolarization spreads to adjacent areas of the muscle fiber, activating sodium channels and allowing the depolarization to propagate away from the endplate in two directions to both ends of the muscle fiber.[17] The process ends when sodium channels become inactivated, potassium channels become activated and potassium flows out, and the potential inside the muscle cell returns to normal. This action potential typically propagates at a speed of 3–5 m s^{-1} (3–5 mm ms^{-1}),[18] so it takes 5–7 ms to spread through a small (5 cm) muscle such as the adductor pollicis, which has a neuromuscular junction in the center.

The electromyogram (EMG) is the sum of the electrical activity produced by adjacent fibers in a muscle. When a nerve is stimulated in an unparalyzed patient, all muscle fibers generate an action potential simultaneously. The surface EMG is best recorded by placing one electrode over the mid-portion of the muscle, where the endplate is located, and the second electrode at one end of the muscle. A potential difference, the action potential between both electrodes, is recorded as it travels down the muscle. The size, shape, and duration of the EMG depend on the geometry of the muscle and the position of the electrodes and their location with respect to the muscle. In hand muscles, an amplitude of 10 mV and duration of 5 ms are typical.[19] The activity of the adductor pollicis, the first dorsal interosseous, and the muscles of the hypothenar eminence, all innervated by the ulnar nerve, have been used. During partial paralysis, there is failure of neurotransmission at some of the endplates, and the size of the EMG is reduced proportionally.

Mechanical activity

A muscle action potential triggers a chain of events leading to contraction. Briefly, calcium channels are activated on the membrane of intracellular organelles called the sarcoplasmic reticulum and of the

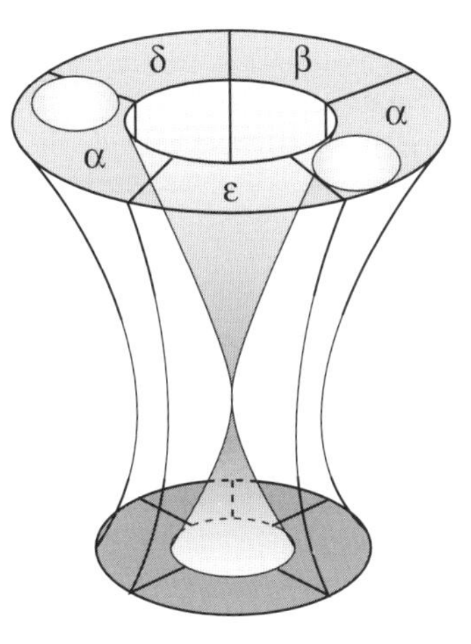

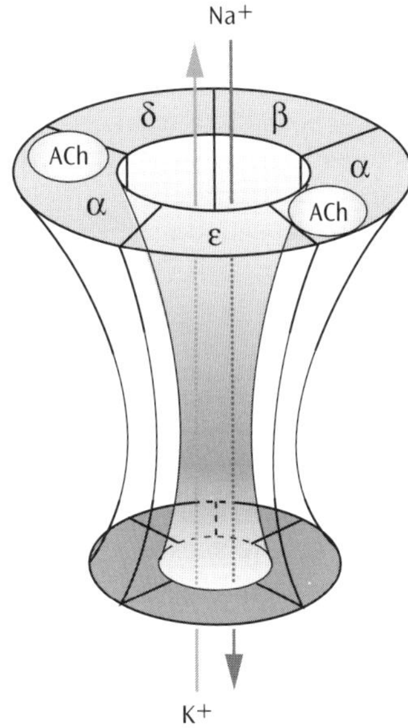

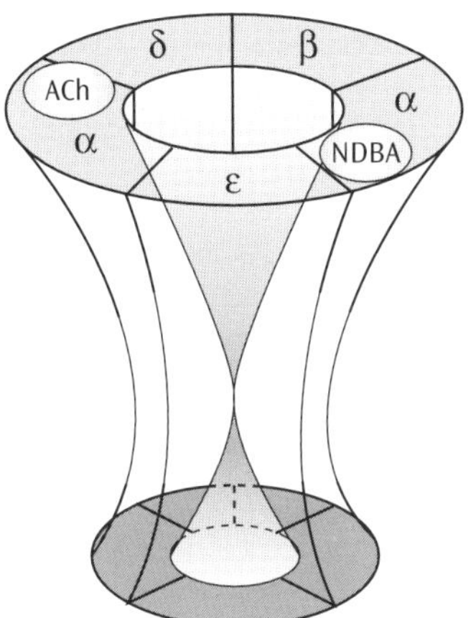

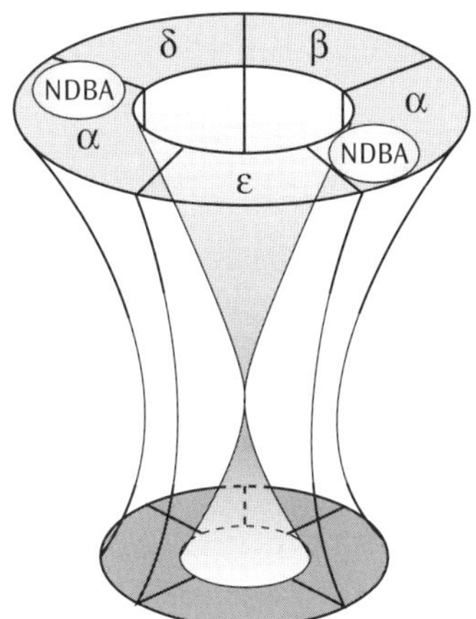

Figure 15.3 *Function of the acetylcholine receptor. At rest, the receptor is closed (top left). When two acetylcholine (ACh) molecules bind to specific recognition sites on the α-subunit, a conformational change occurs, the inside of the receptor opens sufficiently to let ions through (top right). This process is prevented if both (bottom right) or even only one (bottom left) of the binding sites is occupied by a nondepolarizing blocking agent (NDBA).*

muscle fiber itself. The net effect is an immediate increase in intracellular calcium ions. These bind to troponin, a protein which in the resting state prevents actin and myosin filaments from bridging. The effect of calcium is to remove this troponin-induced inhibition and allow interaction between actin and myosin. A muscle contraction results. If all fibers of a muscle are activated at the same time, as occurs when a nerve is stimulated in an unparalyzed patient, a twitch can be observed or measured. Muscle contraction is said to be isometric if shortening of the muscle is prevented, that is if an obstacle is present. In this case, force is generated, and this force can be measured by a force transducer or appreciated semiquantitatively by the clinician's hand.

A twitch is an event that typically lasts 150 ms and is characterized by a relatively fast rising phase and a more slowing declining relaxation phase. It is thus more prolonged than the EMG and occurs slightly later. If a second contraction occurs before the end of the relaxation phase, a second twitch will add to the first one. This fusion or addition process can be seen with stimulation frequencies greater than approximately 10 Hz. At frequencies > 30 Hz, it is impossible to distinguish individual responses and the phenomenon is called tetanus. Stimulation frequencies of up to 100 Hz have been used. When higher rates of stimulation (> 200 Hz) are used, failure of transmission at the neuromuscular junction may occur.

Acceleration

If no restriction is placed on muscular movement, or if the muscle contracts against a fixed load, the contraction is isotonic. It is then possible to measure movement or acceleration. Accelerometers are small sensors of negligible weight which are sensitive to acceleration, which in turn is proportional to force, according to Newton's law.[20]

Sound

It has been known for a long time that contracting muscle emits low-frequency sounds. However, the origin of these sounds is controversial. A low-frequency component (< 20 Hz, which is below the threshold of human hearing) is probably generated by bulk movement induced by bulging of the muscle. In addition, a higher frequency component probably originates from the vibrations of a muscle under tension, just as the string of a violin produces vibrations. These sounds can be heard by placing a stethoscope over the adductor pollicis and stimulating the ulnar nerve. Practical applications are now being considered.[21]

Fate of acetylcholine

Once bound to two acetylcholine molecules, the receptor stays open for 1–2 ms, irrespective of the time that acetylcholine stays bound. The neurotransmitter comes off the receptor very quickly and is broken down very efficiently by acetylcholinesterase. Usually, acetylcholine does not have the opportunity to bind twice. Inhibition of acetylcholinesterase allows acetylcholine a more prolonged presence within the synaptic cleft and the opportunity to bind repeatedly with receptors.

DENERVATION

The normal distribution of receptors is maintained on the muscle fiber by nerve activity. If incoming nerve impulses cease completely, as occurs with denervation, or, to a lesser extent, if this traffic diminishes significantly, more fetal-type (γ) receptors will appear extrajunctionally as the normal inhibition to their proliferation, the presence of activity at the nerve ending, is removed. This phenomenon starts within 24 h following denervation. If some activity is maintained or returns at the neuromuscular junction, an upregulation of receptors normally occurs and leads to a higher density of receptors at the endplate. When a nerve is completely cut, nerve atrophy occurs, which leads to the destruction of the endplate architecture, with loss of receptor density.

Complete denervation does not affect the mechanism of action of nondepolarizing drugs, because there is no longer neurotransmission at the junction. However, there is usually resistance to the effect of these drugs at normal synapses because of three factors. Upregulation usually occurs because of the effect of the disease or the immobility it produces. After a few days of administration of neuromuscular blocking agents, upregulation is also observed. Secondly, the numerous extrajunctional receptors act as binding sites for the neuromuscular blocking drugs, preventing some drug molecules from reaching their intended target, the neuromuscular junction. Finally, there might be an increase in plasma protein binding of neuromuscular blocking agents. One or more of these mechanisms explain the resistance observed in spinal cord transection, burns, stroke, etc.

The effect of the depolarizing drug succinylcholine is different, because this drug is an agonist that binds and activates extrajunctional receptors. Thus, a large inward movement of Na^+ ions and, more significantly, a large outward flow of K^+ ions occurs, producing hyperkalemia. The normal serum K^+ increase is 0.5–1.0 mequiv L^{-1}. In cases of burns and cord transection, the increase might be several times greater and cause cardiac arrest.[22]

EFFECT OF DRUGS

Nondepolarizing agents

Nondepolarizing neuromuscular blocking drugs are competitive antagonists of acetylcholine. They bind to the same site on the receptor, and their affinity for each of the acetylcholine recognition sites on the α-subunit is probably different. Nevertheless, binding to only one of the α-subunits is sufficient to prevent opening of the receptor (Fig. 15.3). However, the neuromuscular junction is particularly resistant to the effect of nondepolarizing agents because of the wide margin of safety of neuromuscular transmission, as implied above. Animal receptor occlusion experiments have suggested that as many as 70% of all receptors need to be occupied before blockade is detectable, i.e. before neurotransmission fails in the most sensitive fibers, and as many as 92% have to be occupied before total paralysis occurs.[23] It must be emphasized here that these numbers, obtained in the tibialis muscle of the cat, are muscle specific and species specific. For example, the margin of safety is greater in the diaphragm than in peripheral muscle in cats, and greater in cats than in dogs.[24] There is a suggestion that the margin of safety might be smaller in humans,[25] and is certainly greatly reduced in myasthenia gravis. The practical consequence of the margin of safety effect, irrespective of its actual magnitude, is that neuromuscular blockade occurs over a narrow margin, and the difference in dosage between inadequate and too much paralysis is small.

Nondepolarizing neuromuscular blocking drugs also have presynaptic effects, probably mediated through nicotinic receptors located at the nerve terminal, the function of which is normally to provide positive feedback during high-frequency stimulation. These receptors, which are different from the postsynaptic variety, are blocked by relatively small doses of nondepolarizing drugs. This effect accounts for the fade observed with train-of-four or tetanic stimulation.

Depolarizing agents

The mechanism of action of depolarizing agents such as succinylcholine is still poorly understood, and the net effect of these drugs is probably a summation of many interactions, which are muscle, species, dose, and time dependent. These drugs are agonists at the nicotinic receptor; as in the case of acetylcholine, they produce depolarization at the endplate. However, metabolism is not as rapid as for acetylcholine, so binding to the receptor is prolonged, and this produces desensitization, i.e. unresponsiveness of the receptor. Another reason for the flaccid paralysis induced by depolarizing drugs might be that sodium channels become inactivated by sustained depolarization, which prevents the action potential from propagating in muscle.[26]

Succinylcholine also has presynaptic action. Binding to presynaptic receptors depolarizes nerve terminals, and action potentials may be generated and travel backwards to invade neighboring branches, thus producing contraction in a whole motor unit.[27] Fasciculations are probably due to this mechanism rather than a transient excitation of the endplate receptors, because small doses of nondepolarizing agents are effective in preventing this phenomenon. Another possibility is the special sensitivity of intrafusal fibers (muscle spindles) to succinylcholine, which may produce muscular contractions via the gamma afferents.

Finally, the reasons for the change in nature of the succinylcholine block (from phase I to phase II) with time and dose, from a depolarizing to a nondepolarizing type, is not well understood. Although the features of phase II block and of competitive block are similar, the mechanisms of action might be quite different.

Reversal agents

Neostigmine, pyridostigmine, and edrophonium all have acetylcholinesterase-inhibiting activity.[28] These drugs are not competitive antagonists of nondepolarizing drugs, but tip the balance in favor of neurotransmission by making more acetylcholine available for longer periods of time. Thus, the agonist acetylcholine can compete with the nondepolarizing blocking agents. This indirect mechanism explains why reversal drugs have a ceiling effect, which is reached when 100% inhibition acetylcholinesterase is achieved.[29]

Reversal agents certainly have other effects, but it is unclear how much they contribute to their ability to reverse blockade. These drugs certainly have direct agonist, acetylcholine-like, effects, on pre- and postsynaptic receptors. They can produce desensitization, and this might be the mechanism for the neuromuscular block and weakness observed in healthy, unparalyzed subjects. They have been reported to cause channel block, and this is especially a feature of edrophonium. The relative importance of these mechanisms is unknown, but prior inhibition of acetylcholinesterase activity does not abolish all action of neostigmine.[30]

Different muscles

Muscles of the body do not respond in a uniform manner to neuromuscular blocking drugs. Differences are found with respect to rate of onset, maximum blockade and duration of action, which do not always parallel each other. Onset is governed chiefly by the rate of access of drug molecules to the neuromuscular junction, which in turn is largely determined by blood flow. In contrast, maximum blockade is a function of the sensitivity of the muscle to the drug. At least in the case of intermediate and long-acting drugs, recovery occurs because plasma concentrations fall below a critical threshold. Thus, duration of action depends chiefly on the sensitivity of the muscle. However, blood flow is important in determining recovery for short-acting drugs.

Respiratory muscles

Among the muscles that have clinical significance, resistance to the action of neuromuscular blocking agents is greatest in the diaphragm, the most important muscle of respiration, and the laryngeal adductors, which close the glottis, i.e. maximum blockade for any dose tends to be less than for peripheral muscle, and duration of action is relatively brief.[31,32] However, because blood flow is greater in centrally located muscles than at the periphery, onset of blockade occurs earlier at the diaphragm and at the larynx. The most sensitive muscles of the respiratory system are those that keep the upper airway patent. For example, the geniohyoid can be partially blocked by small doses of atracurium or vecuronium, and recovery occurs relatively slowly.[33] Onset is rapid, because the muscle is centrally located and has a large blood flow. The same conditions can be found at the masseter[34] and pharyngeal muscles involved in swallowing.[35] Other respiratory muscles have been poorly studied, but fragmental evidence suggests that their response is intermediate between that of the diaphragm and that of the upper airway.

Adductor pollicis

The behavior of other muscles is of little interest clinically, unless those muscles are used for monitoring. Of these, the adductor pollicis is of special importance because it constitutes the gold standard on which all pharmacologic data on neuromuscular blocking drugs are based. In addition, this hand muscle is frequently accessible for clinical monitoring. Compared with all the respiratory muscles mentioned above, onset is slower at the more peripherally located adductor pollicis. The adductor pollicis muscle appears to be a good reflection of paralysis of the upper airway muscles, especially when considering recovery.[33] The diaphragm recovers earlier.

Other peripheral muscles

There are slight differences between the muscles of the hand with respect to their response to neuromuscular blocking drugs. Muscles of the hypothenar eminence, which are innervated by the ulnar nerve, are usually slightly more resistant, and recover earlier, than the adductor pollicis.[36] The response of the first dorsal interosseous, which moves the index finger toward the thumb, is very similar to that of the adductor pollicis.[37] Of the muscles of the foot, the flexor hallucis longus, innervated by the posterior tibial nerve, has received the most attention. As expected, onset is slow. Maximum blockade and recovery are close to those of the adductor pollicis.

Muscles around the eye

The facial nerve is often stimulated to monitor neuromuscular blockade and, until recently, it has been considered that all muscle movements observed around the eye were due to the action of the orbicularis oculi. It appears that the response of the upper eyelid, which is due to the action of the palpebral part of the orbicularis oculi, is similar to that of the adductor pollicis, whereas the muscle controlling movement of the eyebrow is quite resistant to the effect of neuromuscular blocking agents.[38] This movement is likely to be the effect of the corrugator supercilii rather than the orbicularis oculi. Irrespective of the actual muscle in question, maximum blockade and recovery parallel those of the diaphragm and the laryngeal adductor muscles.[38] A summary of the effect of nondepolarizing drugs on different muscles is presented in Table 15.1.

MONITORING

Neuromuscular blocking drugs have a very narrow therapeutic index, and there is wide interindividual variability. Thus, there are excellent theoretical reasons to monitor their effect in all patients. Moreover, the equipment required for monitoring is inexpensive, simple to use, and noninvasive. The usefulness of monitoring has been questioned because residual paralysis is difficult to detect when using visual and tactile methods,[39] and because in some studies residual paralysis could not be prevented by monitoring.[40] The correct and systematic use of monitoring has been associated with fewer instances of residual paralysis in some studies,[41] but, also, monitoring neuromuscular function can help manage relaxation during onset, maintenance, and recovery.

Stimulators

To test the state of the neuromuscular junction, a nerve must be stimulated. The most convenient way is to apply two electrodes on the skin near the nerve in question and apply an electrical current. It is unnecessary to use needle electrodes to obtain a better response, as most present-day stimulators can provide sufficient output to deliver enough current density in the vicinity of the nerve. In addition, virtually all commercially available stimulators are of the constant-current variety, which means that the current delivered through a relatively high-resistance skin is the same as that which goes through needles implanted beneath the epidermis. To avoid injury and infection, the use of needles should be replaced by EKG-type electrodes. The position of the electrodes is important. The negative electrode should be placed where the nerve is most superficial and the positive electrode 5–10 cm away from it along the path of the nerve. For the ulnar nerve, a negative electrode at the wrist and a positive electrode 10 cm proximal offers an optimal arrangement.

To depolarize an axon sufficiently for an action potential (or nerve impulse) to be generated, a certain threshold has to be reached. The applied current must be of a certain magnitude and held there for a long enough time. There is no advantage in applying a current for more than 0.2–0.3 ms, because a plateau is reached. This is the current impulse duration of most stimulators. Some stimulators have briefer current durations (0.1 ms). A current of greater magnitude is then required. A nerve trunk is made up of many axons of different sizes and different distances from the stimulating electrodes, which implies that not all the axons may respond to a given current. The relation between response and current applied is typically sigmoidal.[42] Low currents do not stimulate any axons and the response is zero. As the current increases, the number of axons responding increases continuously until all axons

Table 15.1 *Relative effect of nondepolarizing neuromuscular blocking agents on different muscles in humans*

Muscle	Onset	Maximum blockade	Duration
Muscles that are resistant			
Diaphragm	Fast	Shallow	Short
Laryngeal adductors	Fast	Shallow	Short
Corrugator supercilii (eyebrow muscle)	Fast	Shallow	Short
Muscles that are intermediate			
Abdominal	Fast	Intermediate	Intermediate
Intercostals	Fast	Intermediate	Intermediate
Muscles of the hypothenar eminence	Slow	Intermediate	Long
Muscles that are sensitive			
Adductor pollicis	Slow	Deep	Long
First dorsal interosseous	Slow	Deep	Long
Flexor hallucis (foot)	Slow	Deep	Long
Geniohyoid	Fast	Very deep	Long
Other upper airway	Fast	Very deep	Long
Orbicularis oculi	Fast	Deep	Long

are stimulated and a plateau is reached. The stimulation is then said to be supramaximal. A partial response is the result of submaximal stimulation. For most applications in anesthesia, better results are obtained with supramaximal stimulation, which is 30–60 mA at the wrist and 20–30 mA when the facial nerve is stimulated. For awake patients, supramaximal stimulation may be painful.

Characteristics of nondepolarizing blockade

Stimulators feature different monitoring modalities to take advantage of the special characteristics of nondepolarizing blockade. When high-frequency stimulation is applied, fade of the response is observed. At least 10 s must elapse between two successive pulses to allow the junction to recover. Fade increases with frequency until 2 Hz, when a plateau is reached until 50 Hz. More fade is seen at 100 Hz than at 50 Hz. At 2 Hz, twitches are distinct and easily separated from each other. Fade reaches its maximum value by the fourth impulse, thus the interest in the train-of-four modality, which consists of four impulses separated by 0.5 s. With nondepolarizing blockade, a decrement, or fade, is seen after the first response (Table 15.1).

Tetanic stimulation (30–100 Hz) is also characterized by fade. In addition, intense stimulation is followed by a period during which the response to single twitch or train-of-four stimulation is exaggerated. This phenomenon is called post-tetanic facilitation, and has been attributed to the temporary displacement of nondepolarizing blocking molecules from the endplate by the acetylcholine released during the tetanic stimulation. The mechanism is unclear, as it seems unlikely that such an effect might be manifest for as long as 2 min. The technique of post-tetanic count (PTC), designed to monitor profound blockade, is based on the post-tetanic facilitation. When there is no response to single twitch or train-of-four nerve stimulation, a 5-s, 50-Hz tetanus can be applied, followed by stimulation at 1 Hz. The number of visible twitches observed, or post-tetanic count, is inversely related to the depth of blockade.[43] Post-tetanic facilitation must not be confused with post-tetanic potentiation, which is an augmented height of the twitch after tetanic stimulation in the absence of neuromuscular blocking agents, and is not usually seen in humans.

Finally, nondepolarizing blockade is reversed by anticholinesterase agents. When conditions are correct, depolarizing agents can also antagonize nondepolarizing blockade. The dose of the depolarizing agent must be small enough not to produce a block in its own right, and blockade should be relatively intense (Table 15.2).

Characteristics of depolarizing blockade

During phase I block, train-of-four and tetanic fade are not observed. There is no post-tetanic facilitation. Anticholinesterase agents do not antagonize, but potentiate, depolarizing blockade. This effect is separate from the inhibitory action of neostigmine and pyridostigmine on plasma cholinesterase, which accentuates succinylcholine effect by inhibiting its metabolism. Edrophonium has little effect on plasma cholinesterase activity, yet it potentiates succinylcholine blockade. With increasing time (30–60 min) and dose (5–7 $mg\,kg^{-1}$), the characteristics of succinylcholine block change.[44] Train-of-four fade and tetanic fade become apparent and anticholinesterase agents accelerate recovery. Thus, phase II block has all the characteristics of nondepolarizing blockade (Table 15.2).

Recording the effect

Once stimulating electrodes are in place, the most convenient and easiest way to assess the response is to observe it by visual and tactile means. For the adductor pollicis, it is recommended to hold the thumb in one's hand and disregard the response of other muscles of the hand. There is less train-of-four fade during onset than during recovery, so it is best to wait for disappearance of the response before tracheal intubation is attempted. The preferred site for monitoring onset is the eyebrow, because of its laryngeal-like neuromuscular blocking profile. During surgery, the train-of-four response at the adductor pollicis is the most convenient modality. Adequate relaxation is usually obtained when there are one or two visible twitches, which corresponds to 80–99% first-twitch depression, and train-of-four count made by visual or tactile means is quite accurate.[45] However, keeping relaxation at that level does not guarantee absence of movement of the diaphragm or abdominal muscles, because of the greater resistance of these muscles compared with the adductor pollicis. Profound relaxation may be monitored by observing the response of the eyebrow to facial nerve stimulation, or by using PTC.

During recovery it might be difficult to detect residual blockade. Many studies have demonstrated that tactile identification of fade is virtually impossible for train-of-four ratios or T4/T1 (height of the fourth twitch compared with that of the first) as low as 0.3–0.4. The ability to detect tetanic fade at 50 Hz is no better.[46] The situation can be improved by a different modality, called double burst stimulation (DBS), which consists of two sets of three 50-Hz impulses generated

Characteristic	Depolarizing block	Nondepolarizing block
Effect on single twitch height	Depression	Depression
Train-of-four fade	Absent	Present
Tetanic fade	Absent	Present
Post-tetanic facilitation	Absent	Present
Effect of anticholinesterase agents	Potentiation of block	Reversal of block
Effect of nondepolarizing drugs	Less blockade	More blockade

Table 15.2 *Characteristics of depolarizing and nondepolarizing blockade*

750 ms apart, each giving a mini-tetanic response.[47] During recovery from nondepolarizing block, the ability to detect DBS fade is better than for train-of-four fade and extends to T4/T1 ratios of 0.5–0.6. Several other methods can be used alone or together to improve the range of detection of residual paralysis. Tetanic stimulation at 100 Hz has been reported to extend it to T4/T1 ratios of 0.8–0.9[48] (Fig. 15.4). Assessing the response of the index finger (first dorsal interosseous) improves detection rates for both train-of-four and DBS modes.[49] Paradoxically, using submaximal stimulation also makes detection of fade easier.[50]

All these methods are obsolete unless a reliable objective method is used. Unfortunately, monitoring devices that measure force or EMG are cumbersome, expensive, or both. Accelerometry is less expensive and more convenient, provided the thumb is free to move. Unfortunately, the resting T4/T1 is usually greater than 100% with this method, so the interpretation of recovery may be difficult.

Relation with respiratory function

Traditionally, a T4/T1 ratio of 70% has been considered to correspond to full return of respiratory function. This contention was largely based on a study performed in six healthy awake volunteers who were asked to perform expiratory force, inspiratory force, and vital capacity maneuvers while their T4/T1 ratio was measured at the thumb and *d*-tubocurarine was being infused.[51] More recent evidence based on several lines of evidence suggests that, although some individuals might have recovered when T4/TI = 70%, complete return of respiratory function in all patients does not occur until T4/TI = 80–90%. Some patients with a T4/T1 ratio > 70% in the recovery room have been found to have clinical signs of weakness (failure to lift the head, grip the investigator's finger firmly, or protrude the tongue).[52] In addition, depression of the respiratory response to hypoxia (but not to hypercapnia) has been demonstrated, at least for vecuronium, at T4/T1 < 90%.[53] Function of the upper airway is also abnormal for T4/T1 < 90%, as the ability to swallow is impaired and laryngeal aspiration is a common occurrence.

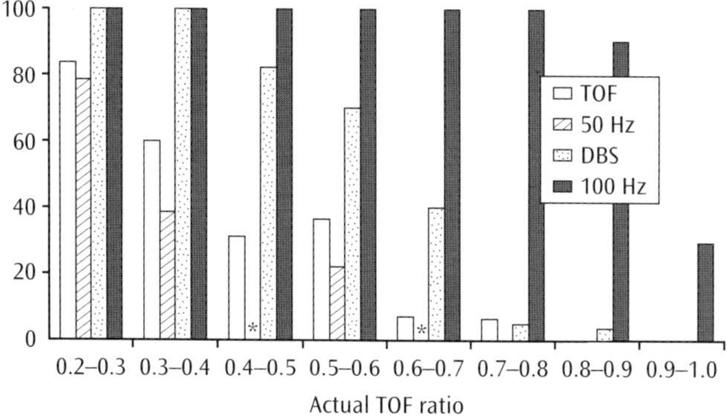

Figure 15.4 *Detection rate using visual and tactile means, with train-of-four (TOF), tetanic stimulation at 50 Hz (50 Hz), double burst (DBS) or tetanic stimulation at 100 Hz (100 Hz), versus actual (measured) train-of-four ratio. Detection rate is the percentage of observers who correctly identified fade. Data from references 46–48. *No data available.*

Clinical signs

A variety of clinical signs have been proposed to complement neuromuscular monitoring in evaluating neuromuscular recovery. The ability to lift the head for 5 s has been considered to a indicate complete recovery. However, pain makes this test difficult to perform in patients with an abdominal incision. In this case, hand grip or tongue protrusion might be tried. However, recent evidence suggests that none of these tests is particularly sensitive. For example, head lift could be performed with a T4/T1 ratio of 67%, well below the desired cut-off point of 90%. The most sensitive test was the ability to hold a tongue depressor between one's teeth against force exerted by the anesthesiologist to pull it out. A mean T4/T1 ratio of 86% was required for this test (Fig. 15.5). Unfortunately, this maneuver cannot be performed in patients without teeth.

Special situations

The method of monitoring described above applies to patients devoid of neuromuscular disease, with an intact and relatively warm extremity. Local cooling potentiates neuromuscular blockade, especially if skin temperature falls below 32 °C, thus overestimating the intensity of the blockade. The response of an extremity affected by trauma, collagen or vascular disease such as rheumatoid arthritis, scleroderma, polyneuropathy, or diabetes is unpredictable, so a normal site should be chosen as much as possible. Disuse tends to produce resistance to nondepolarizing drugs, so the risk of overdosage is present if the involved extremity is used for monitoring. For example, the unaffected side is preferred for patients with stroke as the other side is resistant to nondepolarizing agents.

CONCLUSION AND SUMMARY

Information flows from peripheral nerve to muscle as a result of the neurotransmitter acetylcholine, which is synthesized, packaged into vesicles, and released at the nerve terminal. The postsynaptic receptor is activated if two molecules of acetylcholine bind simultaneously. Control of the release process occurs via presynaptic receptors. Acetylcholine is rapidly destroyed by acetylcholinesterase. Neuromuscular blocking agents interfere with the action of acetylcholine at the interface between peripheral nerve and muscle. Their central effects are negligible. Two types of drugs can be distinguished. Nondepolarizing agents compete with acetylcholine for the same receptor sites but do not activate the receptor. Their effect can be antagonized by inhibitors of acetylcholinesterase, which increase the amount of acetylcholine available. Depolarizing agents are agonists, i.e. they mimic the effect of acetylcholine, but prolonged exposure to the receptor produces paralysis via desensitization. Onset of action of neuromuscular blocking agents is faster in centrally located muscles than in peripheral muscle.

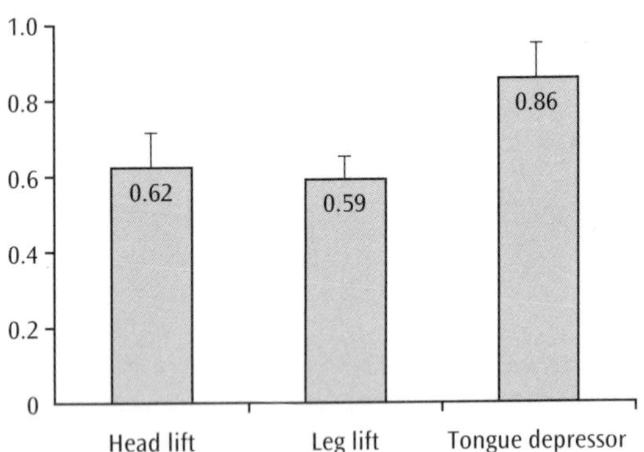

Figure 15.5 *Correlation between actual train-of-four-ratio and clinical tests. The measured train-of-four ratio was correlated with head lift, leg lift, and holding a tongue depressor between one's teeth in volunteers receiving mivacurium. Data from Kopman* et al.[52]

The diaphragm and vocal cord muscles are resistant to the effect of neuromuscular blocking agents, while muscles of the upper airway are particularly sensitive. Because of the variability in response between one patient and the next, monitoring is essential.

REFERENCES

1. Griffith HR, Johnson GE. The use of curare in general anesthesia. *Anesthesiology* 1942; **3:** 418–20.
2. Beecher HK, Todd DP. Study of deaths associated with anesthesia and surgery based on a study of 599, 548 anesthesias in 10 institutions 1948–1952 inclusive. *Ann Surg* 1954; **140:** 2–35.
3. Lunn JN, Hunter AR, Scott DB. Anaesthesia-related surgical mortality. *Anaesthesia* 1983; **38:** 1090–6.
4. Berg H, Roed J, Viby-Mogensen J, *et al.* Residual neuromuscular block is a risk factor for postoperative pulmonary complications. A prospective, randomised, and blinded study of postoperative pulmonary complications after atracurium, vecuronium and pancuronium. *Acta Anaesthesiol Scand* 1997; **41:** 1095–103.
5. Sato C, Ueno Y, Asai K, *et al.* The voltage-sensitive sodium channel is a bell-shaped molecule with several cavities. *Nature* 2001; **409:** 1047–51.
6. Enoka RM, Fuglevand AJ. Motor unit physiology: some unresolved issues. *Muscle Nerve* 2001; **24:** 4–17.
7. Paul AC. Muscle length affects the architecture and pattern of innervation differently in leg muscles of mouse, guinea pig, and rabbit compared to those of human and monkey muscles. *Anat Rec* 2001; **262:** 301–9.
8. Boonyapisit K, Kaminski HJ, Ruff RL. Disorders of neuromuscular junction ion channels. *Am J Med* 1999; **106:** 97–113.
9. Van der Kloot W, Molgo J. Quantal acetylcholine release at the vertebrate neuromuscular junction. *Physiol Rev* 1994; **74:** 899–991.
10. Langer SZ. 25 years since the discovery of presynaptic receptors: present knowledge and future perspectives. *Trends Pharmacol Sci* 1997; **18:** 95–9.
11. Lee C, Katz RL. Fade of neurally evoked compound electromyogram during neuromuscular block by d-tubocurarine. *Anesth Analg* 1977; **56:** 271–275.
12. Naguib M, Flood P, McArdle JJ, Brenner HR. Advances in neurobiology of the neuromuscular junction: implications for the anesthesiologist. *Anesthesiology* 2002; **96:** 202–31.
13. Meir A, Ginsburg S, Butkevich A, *et al.* Ion channels in presynaptic nerve terminals and control of transmitter release. *Physiol Rev* 1999; **79:** 1020–64.
14. Sanes JR, Lichtman JW. Development of the vertebrate neuromuscular junction. *Annu Rev Neurosci* 1999; **22:** 389–442.
15. Marques MJ, Conchello JA, Lichtman JW. From plaque to pretzel: fold formation and acetylcholine receptor loss at the developing neuromuscular junction. *J Neurosci* 2000; **20:** 3663–75.
16. Martyn JA, White DA, Gronert GA, *et al.* Up- and down-regulation of skeletal muscle acetylcholine receptors. Effects on neuromuscular blockers. *Anesthesiology* 1992; **76:** 822–43.
17. Wood SJ, Slater CR. The contribution of postsynaptic folds to the safety factor for neuromuscular transmission in rat fast- and slow-twitch muscles. *J Physiol (Lond)* 1997; **500 (Pt 1):** 165–76.
18. Malmstrom JE, Lindstrom L. Propagation velocity of muscle action potentials in the growing normal child. *Muscle Nerve* 1997; **20:** 403–10.
19. Kalli I. Effect of surface electrode position on the compound action potential evoked by ulnar nerve stimulation during isoflurane anaesthesia. *Br J Anaesth* 1990; **65:** 494–9.
20. Viby-Mogensen J, Jensen E, Werner M, Nielsen HK. Measurement of acceleration: a new method of monitoring neuromuscular function. *Acta Anaesthesiol Scand* 1988; **32:** 45–8.
21. Hemmerling TM, Donati F, Beaulieu P, Babin D. Phonomyography of the corrugator supercilii muscle: signal characteristics, best recording site and comparison with acceleromyography. *Br J Anaesth* 2002; **88:** 389–93.
22. Gronert GA. Cardiac arrest after succinylcholine: mortality greater with rhabdomyolysis than receptor upregulation. *Anesthesiology* 2001; **94:** 523–9.
23. Paton WD, Waud DR. The margin of safety of neuromuscular transmission. *J Physiol* 1967; **191:** 59–90.
24. Waud BE, Waud DR. The margin of safety of neuromuscular transmission in the muscle of the diaphragm. *Anesthesiology* 1972; **37:** 417–22.
25. Wood SJ, Slater CR. Safety factor at the neuromuscular junction. *Prog Neurobiol* 2001; **64:** 393–429.
26. Bowman WC. Block by depolarization. *Acta Anaesthesiol Scand* 1994; **38:** 529–32.
27. Hartman GS, Fiamengo SA, Riker WFJ. Succinylcholine: mechanism of fasciculations and their prevention by d-tubocurarine or diphenylhydantoin. *Anesthesiology* 1986; **65:** 405–13.
28. Bevan DR, Donati F, Kopman AF. Reversal of neuromuscular blockade. *Anesthesiology* 1992; **77:** 785–805.
29. Bartkowski RR. Incomplete reversal of pancuronium neuromuscular blockade by neostigmine, pyridostigmine, and edrophonium. *Anesth Analg* 1987; **66:** 594–8.
30. Sherby SM, Eldefrawi AT, Albuquerque EX, Eldefrawi ME. Comparison of the actions of carbamate anticholinesterases on the nicotinic acetylcholine receptor. *Mol Pharmacol* 1985; **27:** 343–8.
31. Kirov K, Motamed C, Dhonneur G. Differential sensitivity of abdominal muscles and the diaphragm to mivacurium. *Anesthesiology* 2001; **95:** 1323–8.
32. Donati F, Meistelman C, Plaud B. Vecuronium neuromuscular blockade at the adductor muscles of the larynx and adductor pollicis. *Anesthesiology* 1991; **74:** 833–7.
33. D'Honneur G, Guignard B, Slavov V, *et al.* Comparison of the neuromuscular blocking effect of atracurium and vecuronium on the adductor pollicis and the geniohyoid muscle in humans. *Anesthesiology* 1995; **82:** 649–54.
34. Smith CE, Donati F, Bevan DR. Differential effects of pancuronium on masseter and adductor pollicis muscles in humans. *Anesthesiology* 1989; **71:** 57–61.
35. Sundman E, Witt H, Olsson R, *et al.* The incidence and mechanisms of pharyngeal and upper esophageal dysfunction in partially paralyzed humans: pharyngeal videoradiography and simultaneous manometry after atracurium. *Anesthesiology* 2000; **92:** 977–84.
36. Kopman AF. The relationship of evoked electromyographic and mechanical responses following atracurium in humans. *Anesthesiology* 1985; **63:** 208–11.
37. Harper NJ. Comparison of the adductor pollicis and the first dorsal interosseous muscles during atracurium and vecuronium blockade: an electromyographic study. *Br J Anaesth* 1988; **61:** 477–8.
38. Plaud B, Debaene B, Donati F. The corrugator supercilii, not the orbicularis oculi, reflects rocuronium neuromuscular blockade at the laryngeal adductor muscles. *Anesthesiology* 2001; **95:** 96–101.
39. Viby-Mogensen J, Jensen NH, Engbaek J, *et al.* Tactile and visual evaluation of the response to train-of-four nerve stimulation. *Anesthesiology* 1985; **63:** 440–3.
40. Pedersen T, Viby-Mogensen J, Bang U, *et al.* Does perioperative tactile evaluation of the train-of-four response influence the frequency of postoperative residual neuromuscular blockade? *Anesthesiology* 1990; **73:** 835–9.
41. Fruergaard K, Viby-Mogensen J, Berg H, el-Mahdy AM. Tactile evaluation of the response to double burst stimulation decreases, but does not eliminate, the problem of postoperative residual paralysis. *Acta Anaesthesiol Scand* 1998; **42:** 1168–74.
42. Kopman AF, Lawson D. Milliamperage requirements for supramaximal stimulation of the ulnar nerve with surface electrodes. *Anesthesiology* 1984; **61:** 83–5.
43. Viby-Mogensen J, Howardy-Hansen P, Chraemmer-Jorgensen B, *et al.*

Posttetanic count (PTC): a new method of evaluating an intense nondepolarizing neuromuscular blockade. *Anesthesiology* 1981; **55:** 458–61.

44. Donati F, Bevan DR. Potentiation of succinylcholine phase II block with isoflurane. *Anesthesiology* 1983; **58:** 552–5.
45. O'Hara DA, Fragen RJ, Shanks CA. Comparison of visual and measured train-of-four recovery after vecuronium-induced neuromuscular blockade using two anaesthetic techniques. *Br J Anaesth* 1986; **58:** 1300–2.
46. Dupuis JY, Martin R, Tessonnier JM, Tetrault JP. Clinical assessment of the muscular response to tetanic nerve stimulation. *Can J Anaesth* 1990; **37:** 397–400.
47. Drenck NE, Ueda N, Olsen NV, *et al.* Manual evaluation of residual curarization using double burst stimulation: a comparison with train-of-four. *Anesthesiology* 1989; **70:** 578–81.
48. Baurain MJ, Hoton F, Dernovoi BS, D'Hollander AA. Influence and relative sensitivities of 50-Hz and 100-Hz tetanic stimuli on subsequent tetanic fade ratios in patients receiving vecuronium. *Anesth Analg* 1996; **82:** 139–42.
49. Saitoh Y, Nakazawa K, Makita K, *et al.* Evaluation of residual neuromuscular block using train-of-four and double burst stimulation at the index finger. *Anesth Analg* 1997; **84:** 1354–8.
50. Brull SJ, Silverman DG. Visual assessment of train-of-four and double burst-induced fade at submaximal stimulating currents. *Anesth Analg* 1991; **73:** 627–32.
51. Ali HH, Wilson RS, Savarese JJ, Kitz RJ. The effect of tubocurarine on indirectly elicited train-of-four muscle response and respiratory measurements in humans. *Br J Anaesth* 1975; **47:** 570–4.
52. Kopman AF, Yee PS, Neuman GG. Relationship of the train-of-four fade ratio to clinical signs and symptoms of residual paralysis in awake volunteers. *Anesthesiology* 1997; **86:** 765–71.
53. Eriksson LI. The effects of residual neuromuscular blockade and volatile anesthetics on the control of ventilation. *Anesth Analg* 1999; **89:** 243–51.
54. Corringer JP, Le Norève N, Changeux JP. Nicotinic receptors at the amino acid level. *Annu Rev Pharmacol Toxicol* 2000; **40:** 431–58.

16

Motor physiology of the gastrointestinal tract

DAVID F EVANS

INTRODUCTION

The gastrointestinal (GI) tract is the largest and most diverse organ in the human body. The whole organ system is compartmentalized, with major differences in structure and function, and it is appropriate to discuss each compartment as a separate system but understanding that any individual section depends on the others for the normal functioning of the organ as a whole.

For the anesthesiologist, the GI tract is seen as an important organ for nutritional purposes, particularly in the intensive care situation, as an aid for drug delivery, when oral delivery is not possible, and as a clinical hazard, when aspiration of gastric contents endangers the respiratory tract or when postoperative paralytic ileus threatens recovery after surgery.

This chapter will deal with the tubular alimentary tract, which forms a continuum from the mouth to the anus. Some mention will be made of the hepatobiliary–pancreatic system but only in the context of anesthetic practice.

MOUTH AND PHARYNX

The mouth and pharynx are not normally regarded as part of the GI tract but for the purposes of this section will be seen as the first stage of the journey of ingested nutrient as it passes through the gut. The primary purpose of the mouth and pharynx is to introduce nutrient into the esophagus. This process also involves the reduction of the particle size of food by mastication and the lubrication and mixing of the food bolus with saliva, itself containing amylase. The result of this process is to present a reasonably homogeneous mixture of nutrients in an appropriate form, which is further processed by the stomach.

Physiologically, in terms of the digestive function of the mouth, after appropriate mastication by the teeth, the food bolus, mixed with enzymatic salivary secretions, is maneuvered into the hypopharynx and the long journey through the GI tract begins.

For the anesthesiologist, the mouth and larynx are of primary importance as the entrance point for the introduction of endotracheal tubes for the purpose of controlling the breathing during general anesthesia. In this case, the esophagus is regarded as alien territory, unless a nasogastric tube is also being introduced. Otherwise, the pharyngoesophageal system is a potential hazard for aspiration of toxic gastric contents into an unprotected airway.

ESOPHAGUS

The primary function of the esophagus is to transport ingested nutrient from the mouth to the stomach. Its physiologic activity is simple in some respects but complex in others. Its pathology relates to abnormalities of organic and nonorganic (functional) diseases, which result in impairment of its primary function (i.e. transport). This includes the most common motility disorder in gastroenterology, reflux of gastric content back into the esophagus caused by failure of the antireflux mechanism (ARM). For the anesthesiologist, the esophagus is a structure to be avoided during insertion of endotracheal tubes, and regurgitation threatens aspiration of gastric contents, thereby endangering the airways and pulmonary system. It is also a route by which nutrient can be delivered in the critically ill patient, when normal conscious eating is impossible and parenteral nutrition is undesirable.

Structure

The esophagus is a muscular tube, approximately 25 cm in length, which connects the pharynx to the stomach. The esophagus lies in loose connective tissue in the posterior mediastinum. The distal 3–5 cm is normally intra-abdominal, having passed through the diaphragmatic hiatus in the left hemidiaphragm formed by the crura, just anterior to the aorta and posterior to the left lobe of the liver. The esophagus terminates at the gastroesophageal junction (GEJ) or cardia. Internally, the squamous epithelium also terminates close to the GEJ where it joins the columnar-lined epithelium of the stomach (Z line) (Fig. 16.1).

Histologically, the esophagus can be separated into the following regions:

1 The innermost layer, the mucosa, consists of nonkeratinized stratified epithelium, lamina propria, and muscularis mucosae. Mucus-secreting glands are also present close to the GEJ. There are no other secreted substances within the esophageal mucosa as its entire function relates to maintaining a state of emptiness.
2 The submucosa contains connective tissue, blood vessels, and mucous glands.
3 The muscularis layer contains two layers of muscle – an inner circular layer and an outer longitudinal layer. This is similar to, and in keeping with, the remainder of the GI tract. The most proximal 5% of the esophageal body, distal to the upper sphincter, is composed entirely of striated muscle fibers. The next 35–40% is mixed striated

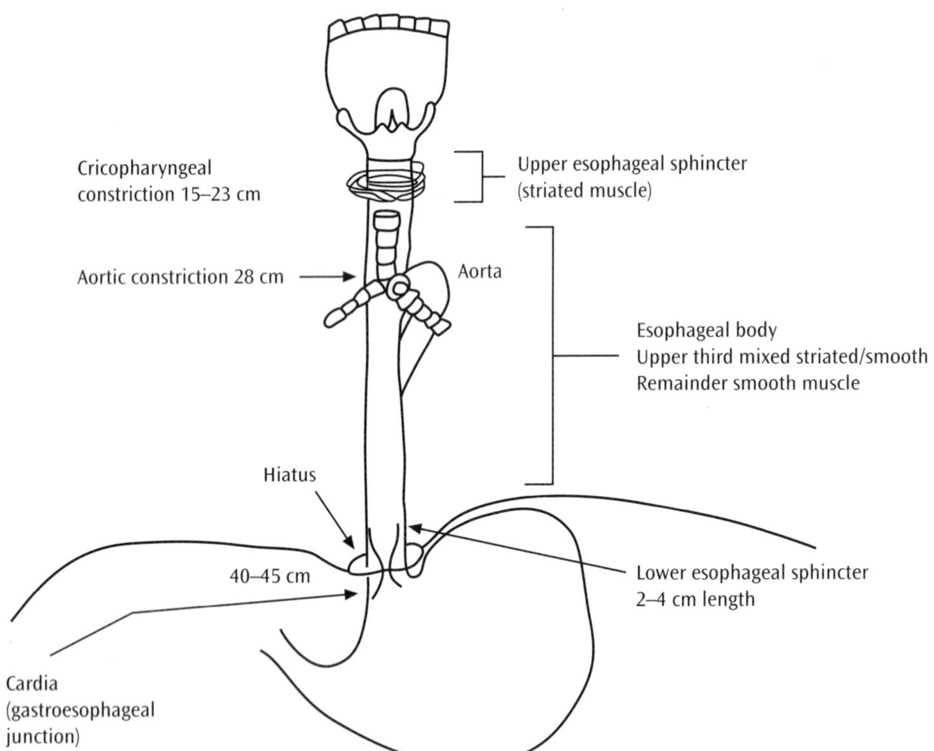

Figure 16.1 *Normal structure of the esophagus.*

and smooth muscle, with an increasing proportion of smooth to striated muscle moving distally. The most distal 35–40% is composed entirely of smooth muscle fibers.[1,2] The outer adventitial layer is composed of connective tissue that merges with adjacent structures within the thorax.

4 Extrinsic innervation is via the vagus nerve,[3,4] which forms a plexus of mixed sympathetic and parasympathetic nerve fibers on the outer surface of the esophagus, which coalesce in the distal third to form the anterior and posterior vagal trunks. Intrinsic innervation is controlled by the two ganglionated neural plexi.[5,6] The submucosal, or Meissner's, plexus lies between the submucosa and circular muscle layer and the myenteric, or Auerbach's, plexus lies between the circular and longitudinal muscle layers. The function of the submucosal plexus is mainly control of secretion and blood flow in the epithelium and submucosa. The myenteric plexus controls motor function, including sphincter activity during deglutition. Until recently, the importance of the myenteric plexus has been underestimated. It is now recognized that this system contains the motor programming that effectively controls motor function within the gut. It is the major neural network in the GI tract and the terms "enteric nervous system" and "the little brain in the gut" are commonly used to describe it. Extrinsic neural modulation is also via these nerve plexi, and this is important in the regulation of deglutitive reflex activity.[7,8]

The esophageal sphincters

The esophagus contains two sphincters. The upper esophageal sphincter (UES) is situated at the junction of the pharynx and esophageal body and lies behind the hyoid bone. It is a slit-like structure, having a high resting pressure [6.7–13.3 kPa (50–100 mmHg)] manometrically, predominantly in the anterior and posterior orientation with lower pressures laterally. Functionally, the UES protects the esophagus from the oral cavity and prevents aerophagia and esophagopharyngeal reflux. The cricopharyngeus muscle forms the major part of the upper esophageal sphincter and sustains a tonic contraction of around 13.3 kPa (100 mmHg) except during deglutition, when it relaxes to accommodate a swallowed bolus. For the anesthesiologist, the UES is the barrier to the passage of a nasogastric tube, which is often passed after induction of anesthesia for aspiration of gastric contents. As normal deglutition is suppressed during anesthesia, it is important to pass the nasogastric tube carefully through the UES because it is possible to perforate the cricopharyngeal region with a nasogastric sump tube, particularly if a stiffener is required to aid the procedure. Cricopharyngeal perforation would obviously lead to major preoperative and postoperative complications.

The lower esophageal sphincter (LES) is found at the GEJ and within the hiatus. Anatomically and histologically, no major distinction is evident at the LES and the remainder of the muscle layers, although there is slight thickening of the wall in this region. Functionally, a high-pressure zone exists in the most distal 2–5 cm of the circular smooth muscle. The LES exhibits both radial and axial asymmetry from extrinsic and intrinsic influences and also shows diurnal, postural, and prandial variations in pressure. Many external factors have been demonstrated to affect the overall pressure in the LES and esophageal body motility and these are illustrated in Table 16.1.

The LES acts as nonreturn valve and is a weak sphincter with an intrinsic pressure of only 1.3–3.3 kPa (10–25 mmHg). The LES is a major component of the ARM and is under both neural and hormonal control. The intrinsic basal tone has to resist reflux of gastric contents under the challenge of a wide range of intrathoracic [up to −8 kPa (−60 mmHg)] and intra-abdominal [up to 13.3 kPa (100 mmHg)] pressures. Not surprisingly, LES dysfunction is very common.

Normal deglutition

Swallowing can be initiated voluntarily or as part of a reflex following stimulation of the mouth and pharynx. However, once initiated the act of swallowing becomes an involuntary act. The sensory nerves for this reflex are the glossopharyngeal and superior laryngeal branches of the

Table 16.1 *Factors affecting lower esophageal sphincter (LES) efficiency*

Anatomical factors
Angle of His
Diaphragmatic crus
Mucosal rosette
LES vagal reflex
Hiatus hernia
Esophageal factors
Salivary flow (as an aid to acid clearance)
LES pressure
LES length
Intra-abdominal length
Esophageal motility
Peristaltic efficiency
Contractile amplitude and force
Gastric and intestinal factors
Acid and pepsin secretion
Gastric motility
Gastric emptying
Pyloric function
Small intestinal motility and transit

vagus. Stimuli reach the swallowing center in the medulla and pons, where swallowing is coordinated. Efferent impulses travel via the fifth, seventh, tenth, eleventh, and twelfth cranial nerves as well as the motor neurons from C1 to C3.

There are three phases to normal swallowing.

Oral phase

In the first phase, food is broken up and lubricated with saliva by mastication. The bolus is moved into the posterior oropharynx by the tongue and forced into the hypopharynx.

Pharyngeal phase

In the second phase, simultaneously with the posterior movement of the tongue, the soft palate is raised to close off the nasopharynx to prevent nasal regurgitation. The hyoid is pulled upwards, elevating the larynx, to bring the epiglottis under the tongue. This backward tilt of the epiglottis covers the opening of the larynx and, with the adduction of the vocal cords and the inhibition of respiration, prevents the passage of food into the airway. The pressure in the hypopharynx rises abruptly during swallowing to reach at least 8 kPa (60 mmHg). A differential develops between the pressure in the pharynx and the subatmospheric pressure in the intrathoracic esophagus, which results in movement of the bolus into the esophagus when the cricopharyngeus muscle relaxes. Once the bolus enters the esophagus proper, the cricopharyngeus closes with the immediate closing pressure of twice the resting pressure [20–26.6 kPa (150–200 mmHg)]. The peristaltic wave in the proximal esophageal body is initiated at the time of the highest cricopharyngeal pressure to prevent reflux into the pharynx. As the peristaltic wave progresses distally, the UES returns to its resting pressure.

Esophageal phase

The pharyngeal activity in swallowing initiates the third, i.e. the esophageal, phase. The transmission of the food bolus from the distal esophagus into the stomach is accomplished over a pressure gradient of 0.7–6.7 kPa (5–50 mmHg) below atmospheric pressure in the thorax to 0.7–4 kPa (5–30 mmHg) above atmospheric pressure in the abdomen. A primary peristaltic wave is initiated by a pharyngeal swallow and consists of an occlusive pressure rise varying from 4 to 8 kPa (30 to 60 mmHg). The peak wave of contraction moves down the esophagus at a velocity ranging from 2 to 5 cm s^{-1} and reaches the distal esophagus between 4 and 10 s after the initial pharyngeal stimulus. Once the bolus reaches the lower esophagus, a further peristaltic wave may be initiated by a reflex secondary to lower esophageal distension, and this is termed secondary peristalsis. At the time the bolus is approaching the stomach, and after the initial pharyngeal stimulus, the LES relaxes completely to the level of the gastric baseline pressure to allow the passage of luminal content. The relaxation phase is present for up to 4 s. The LES undergoes an after-contraction with a pressure rise of up to 6.7–13.3 kPa (50–100 mmHg) in some cases before returning to its basal tone of 2–2.7 kPa (15–20 mmHg). It has been suggested that the after-contraction functions as a clearing contraction to ensure that any remaining content is moved into the stomach. Table 16.2 lists the normal physiologic pressure values derived from manometry for the normal swallowing sequence.

A third type of contraction can sometimes be present in the esophageal body and this is termed a tertiary contraction. These contractions may be seen as isolated contractions at any site in the esophageal body and are not preceded by a voluntary swallow or secondary peristalsis. The function of tertiary contractions is unknown but may be related to localized stimulation of stretch or chemoreceptors in the wall. Figure 16.2 illustrates the different patterns of esophageal body motility detectable by manometry.

Gastroesophageal reflux

The majority of episodes of gastroesophageal reflux (GER) occur during transient periods of LES relaxation. Transient relaxations of the LES (TLESRs) were first described by Dent *et al.*[9] and are termed "inappropriate" as they are not preceded by a corresponding primary peristaltic wave in the esophageal body, initiated by a voluntary swallow. TLSERs have been shown to account for a significant proportion of GER. During anesthesia, in the early postoperative period, and in the unconscious critically ill patient under sedation and on a ventilator, GER can cause major problems. It is therefore important to have a basic knowledge of the mechanisms that prevent GER and how to manage reflux if it occurs.

Table 16.2 *Pressures developed in the esophagus*

Lower esophageal sphincter (LES)	
LES position	37–50 cm from nares (depends on age, gender, and height)
LES pressure	8–25 mmHg
LES length	2–4 cm
Intra-abdominal length	1–3 cm
LES relaxation	< 5 mmHg above gastric baseline
Upper esophageal sphincter (UES)	
UES position	15–23 cm from nares
UES pressure	25–120 mmHg (highest in anterior/posterior orientation)
UES length	2–4 cm
Esophageal body	
Contractile amplitudes	30–160 mmHg
Duration	2–6 s
Propagation velocity	1.8–7.0 cm s^{-1}
Wave type	Monophasic or biphasic
Wave properties	At least 80% peristaltic (primary or secondary)

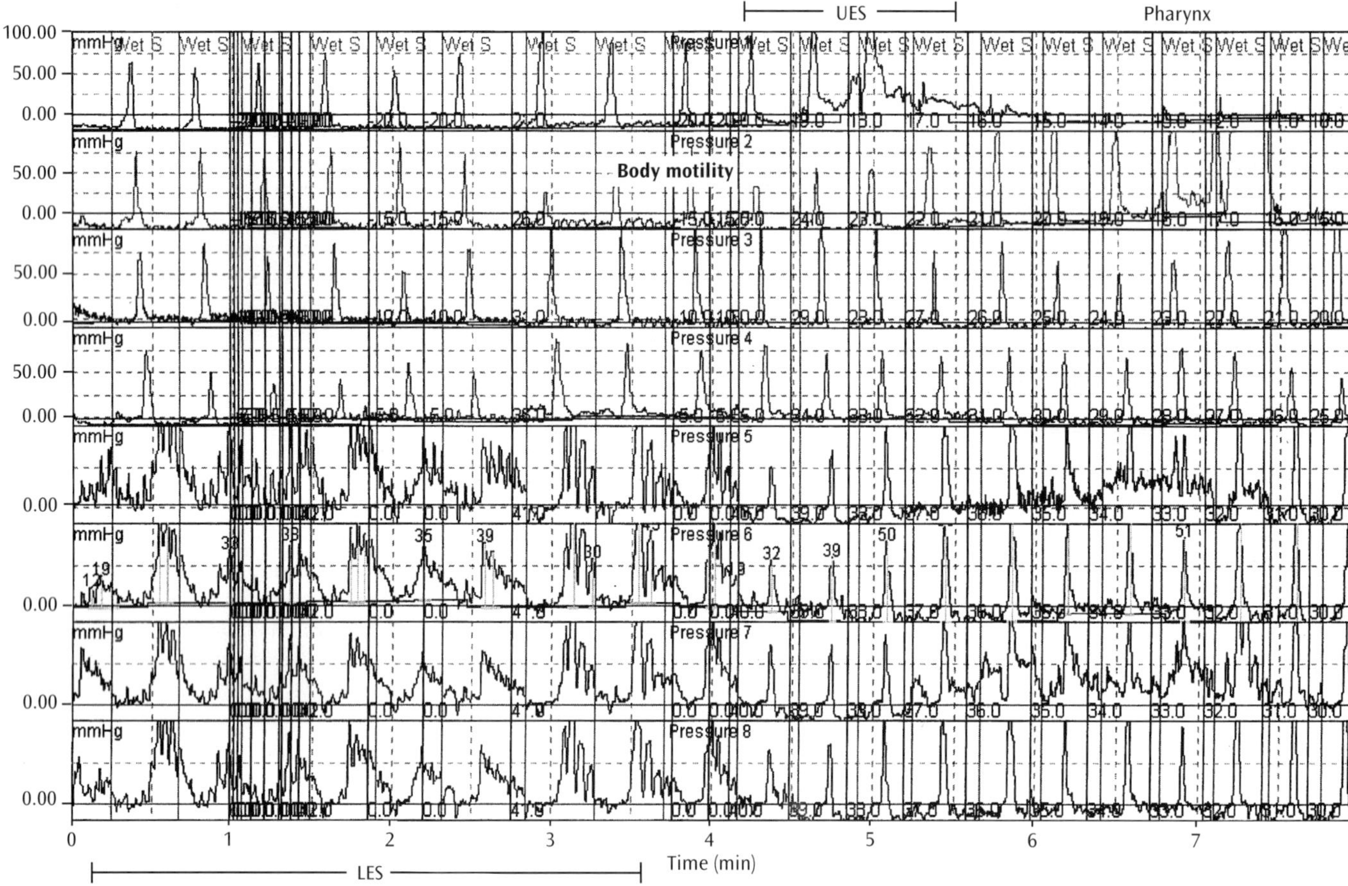

Figure 16.2 *Normal motor activity in the human esophagus. LES, lower esophageal sphincter; UES, upper esophageal sphincter.*

Although the LES in itself is an important barrier to GER, it is one of only a number of other factors that are likely to be important in the overall ARM. Failure of one or more of these factors may result in reflux, which may give rise to symptoms precipitating the disease entity of gastroesophageal reflux disease (GERD).

The following factors have been considered to be important for maintaining an effective reflux barrier. Although some have been unequivocally proved to be important in the reflux control, others, despite being based on sound physiologic principles, have not been adequately defined or the order of their importance classified. Table 16.3 summarizes these factors.

Managing gastroesophageal reflux for the anesthesiologist

Physical management

Posture and gravity In the absence of normal deglutition and a loss of LES tone, which can be a feature in the unconscious patient, GER of gastric and small intestinal secretions may be a significant risk, particularly during minor surgery when the airway may not be protected with an endotracheal tube. This may apply in many day-case procedures or when the laryngeal mask is used and a short-acting intravenous anesthetic agent or light anesthesia with inhalational agents is employed.

Gastric factors The content of the stomach has a major influence on the volume of gastric acid secretion and is therefore important in the control of GER, which can be controlled to a degree by minimizing acid secretion. It is therefore important to maintain a low volume of chyme in the gastric compartment within the constraints of any enteral feeding regime.

Table 16.3 *Putative factors that prevent gastroesophageal reflux (GER)*

Lower esophageal sphincter (LES)
Total length
Intra-abdominal length (hiatus hernia)
Intrinsic pressure
Inappropriate transient lower esophageal sphincter relaxation
Esophageal body
Contractile amplitude
Peristaltic efficiency (clearance time/velocity)
Gastric and intestinal
Acid secretion
Gastric motility/emptying (stasis leads to secondary GER)
Gastric pressure
Pyloric stenosis
Small intestinal dysmotility
Gravity and pressure differentials
Intra-abdominal pressure (IAP; increased in obesity)
Intrathoracic pressure (ITP; increased in airways disease and exercise)
Ratio IAP/ITP

The factors under consideration are therefore related to this:

1 maintenance of normal gastric motility (see below), particularly gastric emptying;
2 optimizing gastric load during enteral feeding;
3 adjustment to rate and timing of feeds (intermittent vs. continuous and optimum flow rate);
4 manipulation of nutritional content (liquid better than solid; reduc-

tion of lipid content; choice of high-energy, low-volume feeds; and smaller molecular size of nutritional content);
5 repositioning of gastric feeding tubes in the jejunum when gastric stasis is suspected.

These simple measures will help the throughput of gastric content and avoid the problems of gastric stasis and GER. When intestinal stasis is evident due to a postoperative ileus, parenteral feeding must be considered in the nutritional care of the critically ill patient.

Pharmacologic

Gastric acid secretion The effect of GER may also be reduced by pharmacologic reduction of gastric secretions. This is most easily achieved by inhibition of gastric acid secretion by either H_2-receptor antagonists (ranitidine, famotidine) or proton pump inhibitors (omeprazole, lansoprazole, rabeprazole, pantoprazole). These substances can be administered intravenously when oral dosing is compromised. An additional benefit of acid inhibition is prevention of peptic ulceration of the stomach and duodenum, a complication which is not uncommon in the intensive care setting.

STOMACH AND SMALL INTESTINE

Although the stomach and small intestine are anatomically and physiologically very different, they act effectively as a single functional unit in terms of digestion and motility, with many shared and linked mechanisms.

Stomach

Anatomy

The stomach shows wide diversity between species, both anatomically and functionally, depending on diet and feeding patterns. In man, the stomach undertakes a reservoir function for ingested food, a grinding and milling function, reducing the particle size of swallowed materials, and also acts as a regulator, controlling the volume and caloric value of chyme entering the small intestine. Apart from low-molecular-weight substances, water, and alcohol, the stomach plays no major role in absorption of nutrients.[10]

Anatomically, the stomach is a dynamic reservoir with a resting capacity of about 500 mL in man. In keeping with the rest of the GI tract, the stomach is composed of the same tissue layers in its walls as the esophagus but with some modifications determined by specific functions. The mucosa is modified and contains columnar-type mucosa with specialized glands in the submucosa to aid digestion. The muscle layers are also modified in three distinct regions to reflect their function.

The three functional regions are as follows. The fundus acts as a reservoir and receptively relaxes to up to three times its resting capacity to accommodate ingested food. The gastric body, or corpus, contains most of the glands related to secretory function but its motor function also acts to mill and grind particles to a smaller size. The most distal part of the stomach is the antrum. This is a powerful muscular pump, which drives small aliquots of chyme into the duodenum across the pyloric sphincter. The antrum is also able to "sample" chyme within its lumen and retropel larger particles (> 3–5 mm) back into the gastric body for further processing.

Secretions

The primary secretions of the stomach are hydrochloric acid (HCl) from the parietal cells of oxyntic glands. The stomach therefore acts as a powerful bactericide, effectively sterilizing ingested nutrients that are contaminated with bacteria. The HCl also activates the proteolytic enzyme pepsin. Pepsinogens produced by the chief cells in the gastric wall are activated and act optimally at pH 2. Gastrin, an important GI hormone, which in the stomach is responsible for control of acid secretion and in the small intestine helps to modulate gastroduodenal motility, is produced by the G cells found in the gastric antrum. Details of other minor but important secretory functions can be found elsewhere (see Further reading).

Small intestine

Anatomy

The small intestine contains the same basic structures as the rest of the gut. It has, however, undergone extensive development in terms of secretory and absorptive capacity (by comparison with the esophagus, for example).[11]

Secretory function is primarily related to enzyme production to aid digestion of ingested nutrient (this also involves the pancreas and hepatobiliary system). Other secretory substances include a whole host of gastrointestinal peptides, which act as regulatory substances as part of normal digestive and motor functions. Details of these mechanisms are beyond the scope of this chapter and may be found elsewhere (see Further reading).

The second major small intestine activity is absorption of nutrient molecules extracted from the intestinal chyme during the process of digestion. This is effected by different mechanisms, depending on the composition of the molecular structures and size of molecules, but in essence the three major components of food (carbohydrate, fat, and protein) are all handled differently. Again, the scope of this chapter cannot cover these mechanisms in detail; suffice to say that the anesthesiologist in the critical care situation will be wise to understand the potential problems arising from impaired digestion and malabsorption. This is particularly important when artificial enteral feeding regimes are a requirement.

Motor physiology

Stomach

The two muscle layers have a number of functions and can act in different ways. Unlike the esophagus, the stomach has three motor functions. The first is to reduce the particle size of chyme to one small enough to be acceptable to the duodenum. The second is to retropel particles that are too large (> 3–5 mm) back into the gastric body and fundus. The third is to propel chyme into the duodenum at a controlled rate such as to allow optimum digestive efficiency without overloading the absorptive process.

Gastric smooth muscle is myogenic and a pacemaker exists in the muscle syncytium, in an as yet ill-defined region of the gastric body.[12] The pacemaker in man oscillates at just three cycles per minute and this determines the maximum rate of gastric smooth muscle contraction. This rate is only achieved during maximal muscular contractions in the fed state or phase III of the migrating motor complex.

Motility state of the stomach and small intestine

Fasting and fed state

There are predominantly two functional states that commonly exist in the stomach and small intestine in most mammal species, including man.

The migrating motor complex In the interdigestive, or fasting, state a cyclical motor pattern with a periodicity of around 2 h is present. This is called the migrating motor complex (MMC) and was first observed at the turn of the twentieth century[13] but only accurately classified in 1969 by Szurzsewski.[14] The MMC consists of three distinct motor patterns. Phase I is a period of total motor silence lasting around 60 min. Phase II is a period of intermittent contractility of the muscle wall of the gut and this lasts for around 40–50 min. This is followed by a short burst of intense motor activity with a frequency maximum within that part of the gut (e.g. 12 cycles per minute in man in the duodenum). This is known as the phase III period and lasts for only around 5–10 min. Figure 16.3 shows an example of a normal MMC cycle in the stomach and proximal small intestine in man.

The MMC has been labeled by Code[15] as the gut "housekeeper." Its function is to sweep intraluminal debris and basal secretions from the stomach and small intestine into the colon, a sort of GI tract "spring clean," every 2 h when fasted.

The MMC acts as the controller of the basic enteric programs that maintain normal states of transit of intraluminal content. The origin of the MMC lies within the myenteric plexus of the gut; this neural network can be found between the circular and longitudinal muscle layers. Perturbation of the MMC can be affected normally by feeding or pathologically by neuronal damage, such as in enteric neuropathy,[16] or with some pharmacologically active substances including some anesthetic agents and analgesics.[17,18]

The MMC is interrupted by food.[19] In carnivores and omnivores, the presence of significant quantities of nutrient in the gastrointestinal lumen switches the interdigestive motor patterns into a prandial phase. The motor activity is modified (see below), gastrointestinal secretions, blood flow, hormones, and other substances required for the digestive phase are recruited, and the whole of the GI tract adopts a different state. The period of disruption of the MMC has been shown to be related to the volume, caloric content, and chemical composition of the meal and in man is variable between about 2 and 6 h.[20] Herbivores, such as cattle and sheep, do not abolish their MMC patterns during feeding because of the way in which they feed. The grazing animal eats continuously in order to take in sufficient nutrient to sustain life. This is because the energy value of grass and other vegetative foodstuffs is low per unit volume in comparison with meat. Consequently, the caloric load to the gut is not sufficient to switch off the MMC pattern and it therefore continues even during the prandial state.[21]

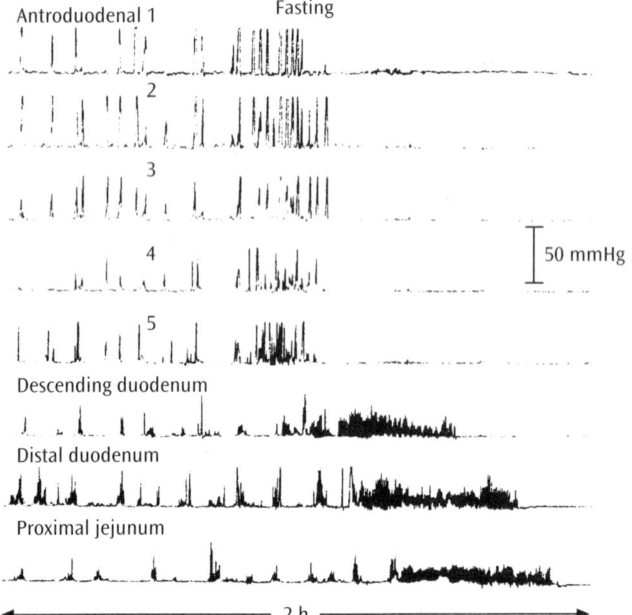

Figure 16.3 *The migrating motor complex of the stomach and small intestine in man.*

Motility during fed state Food entering the stomach undergoes partial and mechanical breakdown prior to its further digestion in the small intestine. The stomach relies on coordinated contraction of its smooth muscle walls to propel chyme into the small intestine, although liquids can be passively emptied by a pressure gradient across the pylorus. Gastric motility comprises two major types: mixing and peristaltic waves. In order to facilitate mechanical and chemical breakdown of ingested food, the stomach has the ability to mix its contents with secretions produced by the gastric wall, including acid and pepsin, which initiate the process of digestion. When the mixture has attained the appropriate consistency suitable for passage into the duodenum, a series of antral peristaltic waves propel small quantities of chyme across the pylorus, which opens to accommodate the passage. Any impairment of contractility or coordination may lead to gastric stasis. As volume and pressure rise in the stomach (caused by secretion and chemical breakdown) GER can be a consequence and reflux symptoms may be induced. Prandial antral gastric motility is seen as bursts of variable contractions with a maximum frequency of three contractions per minute. These contractions continue with decreasing amplitude until the digestive phase is completed, when there is a reversion to phase I (quiescence) of the MMC.

Motility of the small intestine in the prandial state switches from the phasic cycle of the MMC to a variable state, in which contractions are intermittent, with bursts of propulsive activity mixed with segmental, localized mixing contractions. The rate and amplitude of contractions are variable and relate to the nature of the luminal content. The appearance of the contractions is not dissimilar to phase II of the MMC (Fig. 16.4). During the later period of the prandial phase, the motor pattern reduces in intensity and reverts to the interdigestive state (as is seen in the stomach) and hence the whole cycle is repeated through successive states of eating and resting. During sleep, the MMC continues to cycle but the phasic states are modified, with changes to the proportions and length of the phases and cycle length.[22]

For the anesthesiologist, motor function of the stomach and small intestine should be considered in three main groups: preoperatively, in which normal function might be impaired as a result of organic or functional abnormalities;[23] immediately postoperatively, in which ileus might be problematic in initiating normal food regimes; [24,25] and, in the long term, in groups in which the GI tract is of paramount importance in relation to maintaining nutritional levels to sustain and support normal recovery.

Ileus

Interruption of the normal function of the enteric nervous system may be temporary and is often evident after laparotomy (postoperative ileus) or chronically after gastrointestinal or other infections. This leads to loss of normal function, with reduced transit, pain, and, in its most serious presentation, as pseudo-obstruction or long-term paralytic ileus.

During anesthesia, particularly in combination with laparotomy, motor function of the GI tract is reduced or even ceases completely and this state can continue for a significant period after recovery. In the most severe cases the loss of gut motor activity can continue for many days and even weeks and this is then called paralytic ileus. The delay in restoration of normal nutrition leads to a slow postoperative course and requires parenteral nutrition in extreme cases.

The cause of ileus is unknown but the condition well recognized.[26] Research into the phenomenon is scanty, but the few studies that have been performed show complete abolition of gastric and colonic motility and gross depression of small intestinal activity.[27,28] In the small intestine, a similar pattern is seen with the infusion of opiates,[18] and clearly

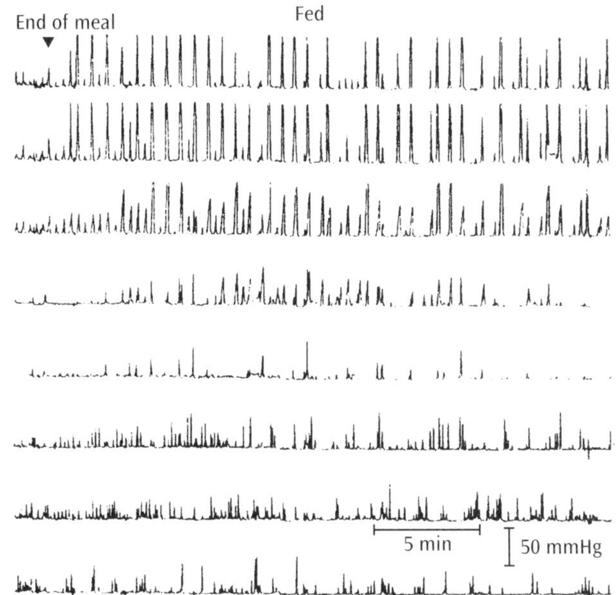

Figure 16.4 *Prandial motility of the stomach and small intestine in man.*

the administration of analgesia during anesthesia may well be a factor in the extent and severity of the ileus.

Return of gut motor activity after surgery appears to be ordered in that the small intestine seems to recover first in around 4–10 h. This is followed by gastric function, and it seems that the colon is the last part to regain motor activity.[28] Clinically, detection of the return of normal motility is an important marker to signal the resumption of normal feeding. The simplest and most widely used technique is the return of bowel sounds, which are easily detected by auscultation of the abdomen.[29] However, bowel sounds may emanate from any part of the gut so this is really a rather crude tool and may not be sufficient in cases of severe paralytic ileus. Other techniques using microphones and surface vibration analysis have been advocated but none has been widely adopted.[30]

COLON

The colon forms the most distal part of the GI tract, excluding the rectum and anus, and provides a number of important functions.

Anatomy

The colon is a sacculated tube about 1.5 m in length in man, with a variable diameter of about 6–8 cm in the cecum and 3–4 cm in the rectosigmoid region. Unlike the other parts of the GI tract, colonic circular muscle is arranged in pockets or haustra and the longitudinal muscle is arranged in three distinct bands called taeniae coli, thus giving it its characteristic shape.

Physiology

Physiologically, the colon is responsible for the final stages of digestion and absorption of a number of important substances. The colon is colonized by up to 150 species of harmless bacteria, which reduce long-chain complex carbohydrates, derived from plant and vegetable sources, to short-chain fatty acids, which can then be absorbed and utilized for energy. This process is brought about by bacterial fermentation, mainly in the cecum and proximal colon.[31] The colon also reabsorbs a number of recyclable substances including water, bile acids, vitamins, and electrolytes. As the luminal content progresses distally, it becomes dehydrated and laden with dead bacteria and other waste products of digestion and finally enters the rectum as semisolid feces. The journey through the GI tract is almost complete.

Motor function

Passage of colonic effluent is a slow, intermittent activity with a wide range of transit times. Ceco-anal transit times can be as little as a few minutes or as long as 100 h or more. Typically, normal colonic transit times are in the order of a few tens of hours. Motor activity in the colon is mainly responsible for this variation. Although our knowledge about colonic motility is scanty, motor function has been shown to possess prandial and interdigestive phases [colonic motor complexes (CMCs)[32] and circadian and prandial variations in motility states[33]].

Motor contractions in the colon can be divided into three functional types; these are all segmental contractions, in which isolated wall motor activity has little effect on either antegrade or retrograde movement. The first type of contractions are often regarded as mixing waves. They are infrequent or even absent during sleep, but increase during wakefulness, being at a maximum shortly after a meal.[33] The second type are peristaltic contractions, which move colonic contents in short bursts toward the rectum. The third type are giant contractions, which arise in the cecum and sweep colonic contents into the rectum more rapidly than peristalsis. These occur infrequently (only once or twice per day) and are associated with the urge to defecate.

RECTUM AND ANUS

The rectum and anus act as the final reservoir in the GI tract and, as such, play a minimal role, in terms of function, in the digestive process. One should not however ignore the importance of this part of the gut in clinical medicine. Neoplasia of the rectum and functional and organic disorders of defecation are an important part of the medical and surgical gastroenterologist's workload.

For the anesthesiologist, the rectum offers a useful route for the assimilation of drugs when other routes are unavailable. Many drugs in the form of suppositories may be administered rectally; this is particularly useful when patients are unconscious and the normal routes of injection are undesirable.

SUMMARY

An understanding of the physiology of the gastrointestinal tract is useful for clinicians as baseline information in order to be able to assess pathological changes brought about by diseases, drugs, and surgery. Our understanding of gut physiology is far from complete but, over the past 20–30 years, research, particularly into gut motor function, has helped the clinician to understand more about gut pathophysiology and has led the way to a more structured approach to treatments. This chapter has highlighted the areas of particular interest to anesthesiologists but there are a number of specialized textbooks dedicated to gastrointestinal motility and neurogastroenterology that would be of interest to those who seek further knowledge (see Further reading).

REFERENCES

1. Meyer GW, Austin RM, Brady CE, Castell DO. Muscle anatomy of the human oesophagus. *J Clin Gastroenterol* 1986; **8:** 13.
2. Arey LB, Tremaine MJ. The muscle content of the lower oesophagus of man. *Anat Rec* 1933; **56:** 315–20.
3. Cannon WB. Oesophageal peristalsis after bilateral vagotomy. *Am J Physiol* 1907; **19:** 436–44.
4. Roman C, Gonelli J. Extrinsic control of digestive tract motility. In: Johnson LR (ed.). *Physiology of the Gastrointestinal Tract*, 2nd edn. New York: Raven Press, 1987: 507–53.
5. Mukhopadyhyay AK, Weisbrodt NW. Neural organisation of esophageal peristalsis: role of the vagus nerve. *Gastroenterology* 1975; **68:** 444–7.
6. Christensen J. The innervation and motility of the esophagus. *Front Gastrointest Res* 1978; **3:** 18–32.
7. Diamant NE, Sharkawy TY. Neural control of oesophageal peristalsis: a conceptual analysis. *Gastroenterology* 1977; **72:** 546–56.
8. Furness JB, Costa M. Arrangement of the enteric plexuses. In: Furness JB and Costa M (eds). *The Enteric Nervous System*. London: Churchill Livingstone, 1987: 6–25.
9. Dent J, Hollaway RH, Toouli J, Dodds WJ. Mechanism of lower oesophageal sphincter incompetence in patients with symptomatic gastro-oesophageal reflux. *Gut* 1988; **29:** 1020–8.
10. Smout A. The stomach – clinical physiology. In: Wingate DL, Phillips S (eds). *Functional Disorders of the Gut*. London: Harcourt Brace, 1998: 196–215.
11. Husebye E. Clinical physiology of the small bowel. In: Wingate DL, Phillips S (eds). *Functional Disorders of the Gut*. London: Harcourt Brace, 1998: 240–69.
12. Stern RM. A brief history of the electrogastrogram. In: Stern RM, Koch KL (eds). *Electrogastrography: Methodology, Techniques and Validation*. New York: Praeger, 1985: 3.
13. Boldyreff WN. Le travail periodique de l'appareil digestif en dehors de la digestion. *Arch Des Biol* 1905; **11:** 1–157.
14. Szurzsewski JH. A migrating electric complex of the canine small intestine. *Am J Physiol* 1969; **217:** 1757–63.
15. Code CF, Marlett JA. The interdigestive and myoelectric complex of the stomach and small bowel of dogs. *J Physiol* 1975; **246:** 289–309.
16. Summers RW, Anuras S, Green J. Jejunal manometry patterns in health, partial intestinal obstruction and pseudo-obstruction. *Gastroenterology* 1983; **85:** 1290–300.
17. Healy TEJ, Foster GE, Evans DF, Syed A. Effect of some IV anaesthetic agents on canine gastrointestinal motility. *Br J Anaesth* 1981; **53:** 229–33.
18. Benson MJ, Roberts JP, Rogers J, *et al.* Small bowel motility following major intra-abdominal surgery. The effect of opiates and cisapride. *Gastroenterology* 1994; **106:** 924–36.
19. Wingate DL. Backwards and forwards with the migrating motor complex. *Am J Dig Dis* 1981; **26:** 641–66.
20. Evans DF. The disruption of the migrating motor complex by meals of varying calorific value. PhD thesis. Nottingham University, 1983.
21. Ruckebusch Y, Bueno L. The effect of feeding on the motility and the stomach and small intestine of pigs. *Br J Nutr* 1976; **35:** 397–405.
22. Finch PM, Ingram DM, Hestridge JD, Catchpole BN. Relationship of fasting gastro-duodenal motility to the sleep cycle. *Gastroenterology* 1982; **83:** 605–12.
23. Hirsch S, de Obaladia N, Petermann M, *et al.* Nutritional status of surgical patients and the relationship of nutrition to post-operative outcome. *J Am Coll Nutr* 1992; **11:** 21–24
24. Reimers KJ, Carlson SJ, Lombard KA. Selection of optimal lipid sources in enteral and parenteral nutrition. *Nutr Clin Pract* 1992; **7:** 152–65.
25. Anderson JD, Moore FA, Moore EE. Enteral feeding in the critically ill patient. *Nutr Clin Pract* 1992; **7:** 117–22.
26. Renik J, Greenwald DA, Brandt LJ. Delayed gastric emptying and post-operative ileus after non-gastric abdominal surgery. *Am J Gastroenterol* 1997; **92:** 751–62.
27. Catchpole BN, Duthie HL. Post-operative gastrointestinal complexes. In: Duthie HL (ed.). *Gastrointestinal Motility in Health and Disease*. Lancaster: MTP Press, 1978: 33–42.
28. Morris DL, Clark AG, Evans DF, Hardcastle JD. Triple radiotelemetric pill study of post-operative ileus. *Dig Surg* 1987; **4:** 160–3.
29. Anon. Interpreting abnormal abdominal sounds. *Nursing* 2000; **30:** 28
30. Gimondo P, Mirk P. A new method of evaluating small intestinal motility using duplex Doppler ultrasonography. *J Roentgenol* 1997; **168:** 187–92.
31. Clausen R. Production and oxidation of short-chain fatty acids in the human colon. *Dan Med Bull* 1998; **45:** 51–75.
32. Rao SC, Leistikow J, Ackerson K, *et al.* Colonic motility patterns in healthy humans: a 24 h ambulatory study. *Gastroenterology* 1998; **114:** G3384.
33. Narducci F, Bassotti G, Gaburri M, Morelli A. Twenty four hour manometric recording of colonic motor activity in healthy man. *Gut* 1987; **28:** 17–25.

FURTHER READING

Evans DF, Buckton GK. *Handbooks in Gastroenterology.* Vol I. *The Oesophagus*. Oxford: Blackwell Science, 1997.

Kamm M, Lennard-Jones J. *Gastrointestinal Transit*. Stroud, Glos.: Wrightson Biomedical, 1991.

Kumar D, Christensen J. *Clinical Gastroenterology*. London: Churchill Livingstone, 1996.

Kumar D, Wingate DL. *An Illustrated Guide to Gastrointestinal Motility*. London: Churchill Livingstone, 1993.

Sanford PA. *Digestive System Physiology*. London: Edward Arnold, 1982.

Smout A, Akkermans L. *Motility of the Gastrointestinal Tract*. Stroud, Glos.: Wrightson Biomedical, 1994.

Wingate DL, Phillips S. *Functional Disorders of the Gut*. London: Churchill Livingstone, 1998.

17

The physiology of the liver

MUZAFFAR H FAROQUI

ANATOMY AND PHYSIOLOGY

Macroscopic anatomy

The liver is the largest single organ in the body, with an average weight of 1.5 kg in adults. Its large vascular capacity makes it an important reservoir of blood, storing 10–15% of total blood volume.[1] Seventy percent of this is distributed to the venous system, 20% to the arterial system, and 10% to the capillaries.[2] The liver occupies the right hypochondrium and is divided into a large right and a smaller left lobe. Its domed upper surface separates it from the pleura, lungs, pericardium, and heart. The inferior (visceral) relations include the abdominal esophagus, stomach, duodenum, hepatic flexure of colon, right kidney, and the suprarenal gland. Anteriorly, the lower ribs and the anterior abdominal wall cover the liver. These relations are shown in Fig. 17.1.[3]

The biliary system is formed by the condensation of fine bile capillaries, which originate in the liver lobules. The right and left hepatic ducts join in the porta hepatis to give rise to the common hepatic duct, which in turn joins the cystic duct to form the common bile duct (CBD) about 2.5 cm above the duodenum (Fig. 17.2). The CBD then passes behind the duodenum to open at a papilla on its medial aspect. The arrangement shown in Fig. 17.2 is the most common, although there are variations. The gall bladder acts as a bile concentrator and reservoir normally holding about 50 mL of bile.

Histology

The architectural unit of the liver is the hepatic lobule. Each lobule, measuring approximately 1 mm across, consists of a hexagonal arrangement of hepatocytes. At its center each hexagon has a small central vein (a tributary of the hepatic vein), and along its edge are portal triads. Each portal triad is surrounded by a connective tissue sheath called the perivascular fibrous capsule and contains a branch of portal vein, a branch of hepatic artery (perilobular arteriole), and an interlobular bile ductule. A portal lobule, on the other hand, consists of the adjoining parts of three hepatic lobules, which center on and surround a portal triad. Under normal anatomical conditions, the hepatic lobular structure predominates, but this can be changed to a portal lobular structure by alteration in the relative pressure in the portal and hepatic venous systems.[4]

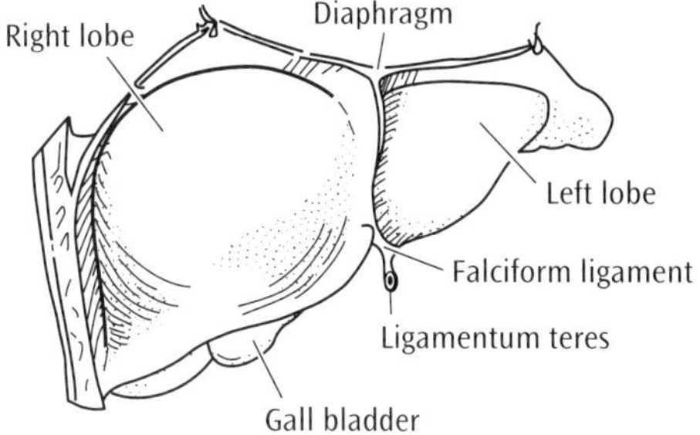

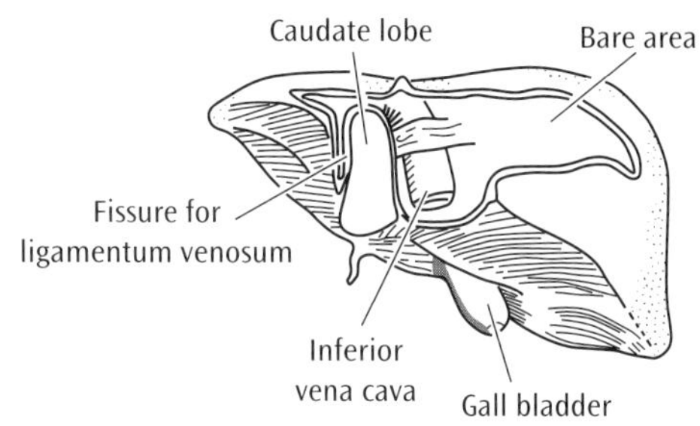

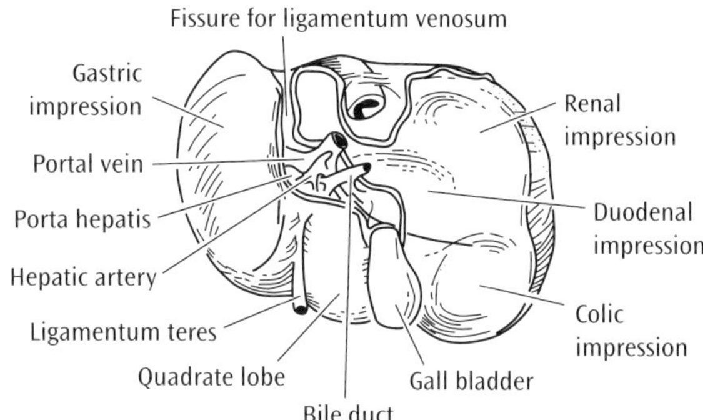

Figure 17.1 *The topographical anatomy of the liver. (Reproduced, with permission, from Ellis.[3])*

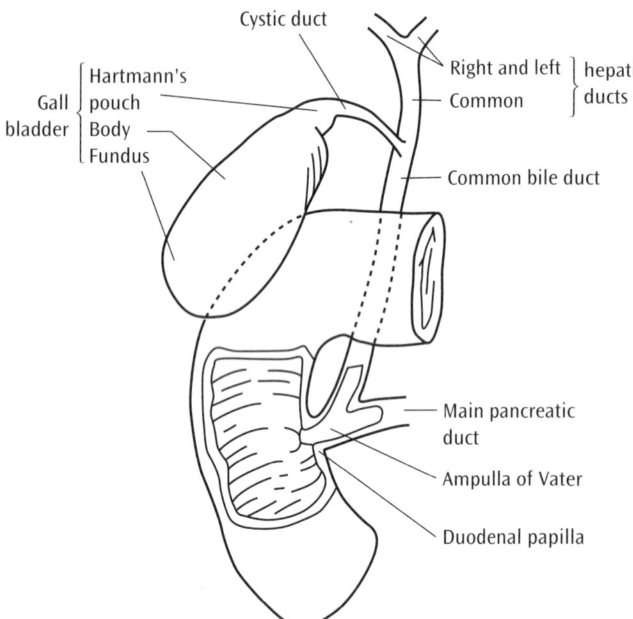

Figure 17.2 *The gall bladder and its duct system. (Reproduced, with permission, from Ellis.[3])*

Hepatocytes have a spheroid nucleus and the cytoplasm has numerous ribosomal clusters, many of which are attached to endoplasmic reticulum. There are high concentrations of mitochondria, lysozymes, and a well-developed Golgi complex, suggesting high metabolic activity. Periportal hepatocytes receive blood rich in oxygen and nutrients and are thought to be responsible for oxidative metabolism and synthesis of glycogen. Centrilobular hepatocytes receive blood that has already bathed periportal areas and thus has lower oxygen saturation. These cells have a high content of cytochrome P450 and are responsible for biotransformation of drugs, chemicals, and toxins. Cells between these two sites are intermediate in oxygen supply and function. Between the hepatocytes that are arranged radially around a central vein are vascular sinusoids. These sinusoids transfer blood from the perilobular arterioles and the portal vessels to the center of the lobule, where it drains via the central vein to the hepatic vein.

Some of the cells lining the venous sinusoids are hepatic macrophages (Kupffer cells) of the reticuloendothelial system. These phagocytose bacteria passing to the liver from the gastrointestinal (GI) tract via the portal vessels; they also phagocytose endotoxins, denature foreign proteins, and remove ferritin and hemosiderin.[5] During fetal life, the liver acts as one of the main hemopoietic organs, producing both red and white blood cells in the mesenchyme covering the endothelium of the sinusoids.[4] These hemopoietic cells, except in congenital hemolytic anemia, disappear once bone marrow takes over the function.

Blood supply

Hepatic blood flow at rest is approximately 25% of the cardiac output (1100–1800 mL min^{-1}). This is roughly around 100 mL per min per 100 g of hepatic tissue. The two major sources of blood supply are the hepatic artery and the portal vein. The hepatic artery delivers about 30% of the total liver blood flow and 40–50% of the total liver oxygen supply. Flow rate within the hepatic artery is controlled by a sphincter mechanism (see below).[4]

The portal vein is formed from a number of venous tributaries (splenic vein, superior mesenteric vein, left and right gastric veins, cystic vein, and paraumbilical vein), and enters the liver via the porta hepatis.[4] The portal vein provides 70% of the total liver blood flow but only 50–60% of the oxygen supply. Depending on the metabolic activity of the GI tract, the portal venous blood has an oxygen saturation of 60–75%. Being a valveless system the resistance to flow is only 6–10% of that in the hepatic artery. Portal pressure is dependent upon the pressure within the liver and the tone of the sphincter-like sections of the hepatic vein. Sinusoids effectively act as hepatic capillaries, allowing blood from the hepatic arterial and the portal venous systems to merge. From the sinusoids the blood flows to the central vein and drains into the inferior vena cava on the posterior surface of the liver via the upper and lower hepatic veins.

Flow within the liver is dependent upon the pressure gradient across the sinusoids. Normally, the pressure is 35 mmHg (4.7 kPa) in the hepatic arterioles, 5–13 mmHg (0.7–1.7 kPa) in the portal vein, and 6 mmHg (0.8 kPa) in the hepatic vein.[5]

The nerve supply to the liver comes from the hepatic plexus, which is derived from branches of the celiac plexus, the right and the left vagus nerves, and the right phrenic nerve. It has afferent and efferent sympathetic and parasympathetic functions. The termination of many fibers is not known with certainty but some control the gall bladder and sphincter of Oddi.[4]

Measurement techniques

There are three main techniques for measurement of hepatic blood flow: clearance of substances with a high hepatic extraction, clearance of radiolabeled particles, and the indicator dilution method. Several agents with a high hepatic extraction ratio [e.g. lidocaine (lignocaine), colloidal particles, and indocyanine green] have been used for the measurement of total liver blood flow, although the indocyanine infusion technique is regarded as the most reliable.[6] Assuming a normal reticuloendothelial system, radiolabeled particles such as gold-198 can be used to measure blood flow.[7] With indicator dilution techniques the measurement is independent of hepatic function. Iodinated serum albumin is injected into the spleen and its flow through the liver is then estimated either using continuous sampling from one of the hepatic veins or using external γ-scintillation counting.[8] Other invasive methods include square-wave electromagnetic flow probe implantation for measuring hepatic artery and portal venous blood flow.[9]

Control of hepatic blood flow

Many factors influence hepatic blood flow. These are summarized in Table 17.1.[10] The regulatory mechanisms can be classed as intrinsic and extrinsic.

Intrinsic regulation

Intrinsic regulation influences the liver blood flow and is independent of the nerves and vasoactive substances carried in circulation and can be broadly grouped as autoregulation and arteriovenous reciprocity.

Autoregulation ensures that the local blood flow remains constant in spite of changes in the systemic arterial pressure. However, autoregulation of the arterial flow occurs down to a pressure of about 80 mmHg; (10.7 kPa) below this, the flow becomes pressure dependent.[11,12] In the portal venous system the relation between pressure and flow is linear, thereby suggesting the absence of autoregulation.[13] In congestive heart failure there is a reduction in both hepatic arterial and portal venous flow.[11,12]

Arteriovenous reciprocity is a phenomenon by which decreases in portal venous flow reduce hepatic arterial resistance and hence increase arterial flow and vice versa.[14] Changes in arterial flow do not, however, result in similar reciprocal responses in the portal venous system. Although the exact mechanism is unknown, it is thought to depend upon locally produced adenosine.[15] Other factors, for example neural,

Table 17.1 *Factors influencing hepatic blood flow*

Increase liver blood flow	Decrease liver blood flow
Hypercapnia	IPPV + PEEP
Acute hepatitis – viral; alcoholic	Surgery
	Hypocapnia; hypoxia
Supine posture	Upright posture
Food	Cirrhosis
Drugs	α-Adrenostimulation
β-Adrenostimulation	β-Adrenoceptor blockade
Phenobarbital	Ganglion blockade
Other enzyme-inducing drugs	Cimetidine, ranitidine
	Vasopressin
	Anesthetics – volatile and intravenous

Reproduced, with permission, from Sear.[10] IPPV, intermittent positive-pressure ventilation; PEEP, positive end-expiratory pressure.

myogenic, and metabolic, as well as the oxygen content or pH of the portal blood may also influence this response.[16] Total occlusion of one inflow circuit reduces the resistance to flow in the other by approximately 20%;[17] therefore, these changes do not fully compensate with respect to oxygen delivery. With portal hypertension the liver becomes dependent upon hepatic arterial flow.[5]

Extrinsic regulation

Surgery Depending upon its exact nature, surgery can have a variety of effects. Clamps and packs within the abdomen can directly affect the blood flow but, in addition, mesenteric traction[18] and the standard "surgical stress" of laparotomy reduce splanchnic blood flow in a variable manner.[19] Surgical intervention rather than anesthesia is the main determinant of splanchnic blood flow; the type of anesthesia then modulates these surgical effects.[20–23]

Ventilation During spontaneous ventilation there is a steady venous return from the inferior vena cava,[24] but with intermittent positive-pressure ventilation (IPPV) the rise in intrathoracic pressure during inspiration produces a rise in resistance. IPPV, particularly with large tidal volumes or high expiratory pressures, decreases splanchnic blood flow.[25,26] The reductions in mesenteric arterial and portal venous blood flow have been found to parallel reductions in cardiac output.[27,28] Although high-frequency positive-pressure ventilation does not alter liver blood flow under normal conditions, as soon as airway pressure is raised, hepatic blood flow is reduced.[29]

Hypoxia The response to hypoxia is determined by a balance between a direct depression of cardiac output and an indirect effect due to release of catecholamines. In addition, the overall effect is further modified by depth and type of anesthesia.

Hypercapnia and hypocapnia Hypercapnia causes vasodilation of vascular beds as a direct effect of carbon dioxide together with systemic sympathoadrenal stimulation. In the liver, hypercapnia increases portal blood flow, with little change in the hepatic artery flow.[30,31] Hypocapnia can reduce total hepatic flow by over 30%.[32]

Hemorrhage Hemorrhage produces a greater fall in portal venous than in hepatic arterial flow. Sympathetic stimulation following acute hemorrhage reduces liver blood flow, resulting in the mobilization of 50–80% of the reservoir blood into the systemic circulation.[2,10,33]

Hormones Both α- and β-receptors are present in the hepatic arterial bed but the portal venous system has only α-receptors.[34] At physiologic concentrations dopamine has no effect on liver hemodynamic activity, whereas epinephrine (adrenaline) induces vasoconstriction initially followed by β-receptor stimulation leading to vasodilatation. In contrast, the portal bed can only vasoconstrict in response to epinephrine stimulation of α-receptors. Glucagon causes a graded and long-lasting vasodilatory effect, which can be used to reverse the hepatic arterial vasoconstriction of a wide range of physiological stimuli.[35] Angiotensin II results in a profound vasoconstriction of both hepatic arterial and portal vessels and a reduction in the mesenteric flow, which leads to a substantial reduction in the overall liver blood flow.[35] Vasopressin is used to alleviate portal hypertension as it induces significant splanchnic vasoconstriction, leading to a reduction in venous outflow into the portal system and hence a reduction in inflow resistance.[36]

Anesthesia and liver blood flow

Anesthetics can alter splanchnic blood flow by a direct effect on the splanchnic vasculature, by neural and humeral mechanisms, and by alterations in the systemic hemodynamic activity. The reader is referred to a detailed review by Gelman and Frenette.[37] Overall, a majority of anesthetics decrease the total splanchnic blood flow and in so doing can alter the ratio of hepatic artery to portal venous flow.[38]

The direct effect of halothane on intestinal vasculature is vasodilatation,[39] but its more general effect of lowering the arterial pressure and cardiac output are the over-riding influences on hepatic blood flow. If, however, the fall in cardiac output or blood pressure is less than 30%, hepatic artery flow is well maintained.[40–42]

Halothane anesthesia also has an effect on other drugs administered simultaneously, causing a reduced clearance of lidocaine, verapamil, propranolol, and fentanyl.[40–42] The effects of enflurane on liver blood flow, like those of halothane, are dominated by changes in cardiac output and arterial blood pressure.[43,44]

Isoflurane, halothane, and enflurane dilate the intestinal vasculature and decrease its oxygen uptake.[39,40] Hepatic artery flow is substantially preserved during isoflurane anesthesia, possibly because of preserved autoregulation or from the profound vasodilatory effect of isoflurane on the hepatic vessels.[41–46] Isoflurane has been shown to increase hepatic artery blood flow at both one and two minimum alveolar concentrations (MACs), in contrast with halothane.[42] Experiments in miniature pigs demonstrated that isoflurane is the optimal inhalational agent for providing a balance between hepatic oxygen supply and demand.[47] Compared with other anesthetics, isoflurane is the only anesthetic that preserves hepatic arterial blood flow in cirrhotic rats.[48] In man, an increase in hepatic blood flow with isoflurane anesthesia has been demonstrated using a pulsed Doppler technique.[49]

In comparative trials of halothane, isoflurane, and sevoflurane, the hepatic oxygen supply–uptake ratio was poorest with sevoflurane, which suggests that it is not the drug of choice if the liver is likely to be subject to physiologic insult.[37,50] Nitrous oxide alone causes little change in cardiac output or blood pressure, which possibly explains why the hepatic circulation is not disturbed significantly when nitrous oxide is used in trained animals without any baseline anesthesia or surgical intervention.[37,46]

Both animal and human studies with barbiturates have shown conflicting results.[37,51,52] In chronically cannulated sheep, Runciman and colleagues[52] found that hepatic blood flow was reduced by 17% during propofol anesthesia; Diedericks and colleagues[53] attributed similar results to the fall in cardiac output.

Morphine in small doses causes dilatation of the intestinal vasculature, but higher doses lead to vasoconstriction.[54] In the pig model, fentanyl alone increased both hepatic oxygen supply and extraction with little subsequent change in hepatic venous blood oxygen content.[23,37] Alfentanil, on the other hand, decreased hepatic artery blood flow to a greater extent than it reduced mean arterial pressure or cardiac output.[55]

It is difficult to draw any conclusions about the total liver blood flow because no simultaneous portal blood flow measurements were made.

Neuromuscular-blocking drugs such as pancuronium and vecuronium have little effect on splanchnic circulation, but agents with autonomic ganglion-blocking properties, histamine release, myocardial depression, etc. all exert an indirect influence via their effect on cardiac output and arterial blood pressure.[37]

Both spinal and epidural anesthesia produce a fall in hepatic blood flow that parallels the reduction in systemic blood pressure.[56–60]

HEPATIC DRUG METABOLISM

Drug metabolism occurs mainly in the liver, although some drugs are metabolized in the kidney and to some extent in the lung, skin, and intestine. The liver transforms pharmacologically active lipophilic substances into hydrophilic excretion products by a combination of non-synthetic and conjugative reactions. However, some of the intermediate products can be pharmacologically active also and account for some of the toxic side-effects. The relevance of biotransformation to anesthesia has been the subject of review articles,[61,62] as has the influence of liver disease and drug disposition.[63–65]

Factors affecting drug disposition in liver disease include altered blood flow (usually reduced), portasystemic shunting, impaired metabolic capacity, and abnormal binding.[65]

The metabolic processes involved in drug biotransformation can be divided into two phases: phase I and phase II reactions.

Phase I reactions

Phase I reactions alter the existing functional groups of a drug molecule to make it water soluble. Oxidation (hydroxylation) accounts for most of the phase I reactions and is carried out by the cytochrome P450 system, located mainly in the smooth endoplasmic reticulum of the centrilobular cells. Genetic and environmental factors are considered important in individualizing a person's P450, leading to considerable variation in drug handling.[66,67] Table 17.2 shows some examples of phase I reactions.

Phase II reactions

Phase II metabolism consists of conjugation reactions occurring primarily in the cytosolic fraction of hepatocytes. The conjugation of polar compounds occurs by the attachment of endogenous hydrophilic groups to pre-existing or newly formed –OH, –COOH, $–NH_2$, or –SH groups. Although phase II reactions usually follow phase I reactions, phase II reactions can, if the substrates are already polar, act directly on drugs. The most common phase II reaction is glucuronidation.[68] This is particularly important in the metabolism of morphine. The primary metabolite of morphine (morphine 6-glucuronide) may be responsible for the majority of its actions.[68,69] With a few exceptions, phase II reactions produce inactive water-soluble compounds. Table 17.2 gives a few examples.

Clearance

The clearance of a drug (Cl) is defined as the volume of blood from which the drug is removed in unit time. Hepatic clearance is often simply represented as:[61]

$$\mathrm{Cl} = QE$$

where Q is the liver blood flow and E is the extraction ratio (i.e. the proportion of drug extracted in one pass through the liver). Drug metabolism is therefore controlled by blood flow (as described above) or the metabolic capacity of the liver. Drugs may be classified into three groups depending upon their hepatic metabolism: "high-risk," "limited risk," and "low-risk" drugs.[65] The degree of risk depends largely on the dependence of drug metabolism on liver blood flow.

Factors affecting hepatic drug extraction are: the activity of enzyme systems, the fraction of free drug in the plasma, and the rate at which drug is presented to the liver. When the extraction ratio is very high, clearance approaches liver blood flow. With a lower extraction ratio, the clearance depends on the rate of metabolism and is independent of liver blood flow.[62] Drugs can therefore be classed as flow-limited drugs ($E > 0.7$), for which clearance depends on liver blood flow, and capacity-limited drugs ($E < 0.3$), for which clearance depends on the rate of hepatic metabolism. Examples of these effects are given in Table 17.3.

Protein binding

The fraction of a drug that is unbound diffuses freely to reach receptor sites and takes part in pharmacologic reactions. A reduction in protein binding, from 95% to 90% for a normally highly bound drug, results in a doubling of the free fraction, whereas for a poorly bound drug a reduction from 10% to 5% has much less effect. Consequently, those drugs with extensive binding to proteins will have a clearance that is affected by changes in binding, but those with less extensive binding will not be significantly affected. Examples of the protein binding of drugs relevant to anesthesia are shown in Table 17.4.[61,70] The effects of protein binding are included in Table 17.3.

Table 17.2 *Some examples of phase I and II reactions*

Reaction	Example	Product
Phase I		
Hydroxylation	Phenobarbital to *p*-hydroxyphenobarbital	Inactive
N-demethylation	Imipramine to desipramine	Active
Hydrolysis	Aspirin (acetylsalicylic acid) to salicylic acid	Active
Desulfuration	Thiopental sodium to pentobarbital	Active
Phase II		
Glucuronidation	Acetaminophen (paracetamol)	Inactive
	Morphine	Active
Sulfation	Minoxidil	Active
Acetylation	Procainamide	Active
	Sulfanilamide	Inactive

Reproduced, with permission, from Jorm and Stamford.[61]

Table 17.3 *Effect of extraction ratio and protein binding on elimination of drugs by the liver*

	Approximate extraction ratio (*E*)	Protein binding (%)	Comments on effects of liver disease
Flow-limited drugs			
Labetalol	0.85	40	Changes in liver blood flow and intrinsic clearance associated with liver disease affect these drugs. The shunting of blood around the liver has important effects on the bioavailability of the drugs
Lidocaine (lignocaine)	0.60	65	
Morphine	0.75	35	
Propranolol	0.65	95	
Verapamil	0.80	92	
Flow/enzyme-sensitive drugs			
Acetaminophen (paracetamol)	0.30	20	Changes in liver blood flow, free intrinsic clearance, and free fraction of drug in blood may be important for this class of drugs
Chlorpromazine	0.30	95	
Meperidine	0.50	70	
Methohexital	0.53	–	
Metoprolol	0.56	10	
Quinidine	0.27	85	
Ranitidine	0.28	15	
Capacity-limited, binding-insensitive drugs			
Antipyrine (phenazone)	0.05	10	This class of drugs is most sensitive to changes occurring in the free intrinsic drug clearance with liver disease
Caffeine	0.04	31	
Hexobarbital	0.15	47	
Theophylline	0.05	62	
Capacity-limited, binding-sensitive drugs			
Chlordiazepoxide	0.02	96	This class of drugs will be influenced by changes in the free fraction of drug in blood and free intrinsic drug clearance. The overall change in drug clearance will be governed by which one of these factors changes the most as a result of the disease process
Diazepam	0.02	97	
Phenytoin	0.03	92	
Warfarin	0.005	99	

Reproduced, with permission, from Eagle and Strunin.[62]

Table 17.4 *Plasma protein binding of some drugs used in anesthesia*

0% ← **Binding** → **100%**

Induction agents

Ketamine

Etomidate

Methohexital

Midazolam

Propofol

Thiopental

Local anesthetics

Bupivacaine

Etidocaine

Mepivacaine

Lidocaine

Narcotic analgesics

Alfentanil

Fentanyl

Lofentanil

Meperidine

Codeine

Morphine

Sufentanyl

Muscle relaxants

Alcuronium

Pancuronium

Vecuronium

Tubocurarine

Low ← Danger of displacement reaction → High

Data from Kien *et al.*[55] and Howden *et al.*[64]

Table 17.5 *The characteristics of drug disposition in normal subjects and recommendations for dose adjustment in patients with liver disease for a variety of drugs available to anesthesiologists*

Drug	Protein binding (%)	Volume of distribution (V_d) (L kg^{-1})	Half-life ($t_{1/2}$) (h)	Hepatic/renal elimination	Effect of liver disease on drug disposition	Adjustment of dose
Drugs commonly used in anesthetic practice						
Thiopental	85	2.3	9.0	> 99% hepatic; < 1% renal	$t_{1/2}$ (u); V_d (u); Cl (u); f_p (i)	Uncertain; may need to decrease dose
Methohexitone	–	61	2.0	> 90% hepatic; < 10% renal	No data; assume Cl (d); $t_{1/2}$ (i)	Probably decrease dose
Succinylcholine	–	–	0.1	Plasma pseudocholinesterase	$t_{1/2}$ (u); Cl (u)	Single dose unchanged
Atracurium	–	0.16	0.33	Hofmann elimination; autometabolism	$t_{1/2}$ (u); V_d (i); Cl (u); long $t_{1/2}$ of metabolite	Decrease dose if long-term use
Pancuronium	0.416	3.5	1.5		$t_{1/2}$ (i), V_2 (i), Cl (d)	Increase loading dose
Cimetidine	20	1.1	2.3	40% hepatic; 60% renal	$t_{1/2}$ (u); V_d (i) or (d) or (u); Cl (u) or (d); f_p changes assumed unimportant. Drug associated with increased incidence of mental confusion in cirrhotic patients	Decrease dose in severe liver disease
Ranitidine	–	1.2	2.7	50% renal; 30% hepatic	$t_{1/2}$ (i); Cl (d)	Changes seen only with advanced disease
Narcotics						
Meperidine	65	4.5	4.5	>95% hepatic; <5% renal	$t_{1/2}$ (i); V_d (u); Cl (d) 50%; f_p (u)	Decrease oral dose by 50% in cirrhosis or acute viral hepatitis
Morphine	35	3.7	2.0	90% GI tract and liver; 10% renal glucuronidation	$t_{1/2}$(u); V_d (u); Cl (u); f_p (u), by some reports; f_p (i)	None, but avoid in severe liver disease
Alfentanil	90	0.28	1.5	99% hepatic; 1% renal	$t_{1/2}$ (i); V_d (u); Cl (d); f_p (i) (dose dependent)	Decrease dose
Fentanyl	80	3.5	4.0	92% hepatic; 8% renal	$t_{1/2}$ (u); V_d (u); Cl (u)	None
Sufentanyl	90	4.0	4.1		$t_{1/2}$ (u); V_d (u); Cl (u)	None
Cardiovascular						
Atenolol	< 5	0.55	6.5	10% hepatic; 90% renal	$t_{1/2}$ (u); V_d (u); Cl (u)	None
Digitoxin	95	0.60	180	70% hepatic; 30% renal	$t_{1/2}$ (u) or (d); Cl (i) or (u); f_p (i)	None
Digoxin	30	6.0	35	30% hepatic; 70% renal	Appears negligible	None
Disopyramide	80 nonlinear	1.0	8	45% hepatic; 55% renal	No data; would not expect a tremendous change in liver disease	Probably slight decrease
Labetalol	50	11.5	3.0	> 95% hepatic; < 5% renal	$t_{1/2}$ (u); V_d (d); Cl (u) or (d); f_p (?)	Decrease oral dose; decrease i.v. dose to much smaller extent
Lidocaine	65 nonlinear	1.1	2.0	97% hepatic; 3% renal	$t_{1/2}$ (i); V_d (i) or (u); Cl (d) ~ 50%; f_p (?) Low therapeutic ratio Decrease in Cl depends on severity of disease	Decrease dose by 50% in severe liver disease
Lorcainide	70	12.9	8.0	98% hepatic; 2% renal	$t_{1/2}$ (i); V_d (u); Cl (d) 29%; f_p (i) slightly. Cl_{int} exhibits a very large decrease	Decrease dose
Metoprolol	10	3.2	4.0	95% hepatic; 5% renal	$t_{1/2}$ (i); V_d (i) slightly; Cl (d) 23%; f_p (?)	Decrease dose slightly
N-Acetyl-procainamide	10	1.4	8.0	20% hepatic; 80% renal	No data; except little change unless renal function altered	None

Nifedipine	98	1.0	3.0	100% hepatic	$t_{1/2}$ (i); V_d (u); Cl (d)	Decrease dose
Pindolol	57	6.2	3.5	70% hepatic; 30% renal	Not affected by AVH Cirrhosis Cl (d) slightly and renal excretion of drug increased	Some decrease in severe liver disease
Prazosin	97	1.3	3.0	95% hepatic; 5% renal	No data – would expect $t_{1/2}$ (i); Cl (d); f_p (i)	Decrease dose
Procainamide	15	2.2	3.0	45% hepatic; 55% renal	$t_{1/2}$ (i); V_d (?); Cl (?) probably decreased slightly	Some minor decrease in dose
Propranolol	95	4.0	4.0	>95% hepatic; <5% renal	$t_{1/2}$ (i); V_d (i); Cl (d) ~ 60%; f_p (i) Tremendous decrease in Cl_{int} Flow/enzyme limited in cirrhosis	Decrease dose depending on extent of damage
Quinidine	85	3.0	6.0	80% hepatic; 20% renal	$t_{1/2}$ (i); V_d (i); Cl (u); f_p (i); Cl_{int} decreased significantly	Decrease dose
Furosemide	95	0.15	1.0	35% hepatic; 65% renal	$t_{1/2}$ (i) or (u); V_d (i) or (u); Cl (u); f_p (i); the change in f_p decrease in Cl_{int} of liver	None or slight decrease in severe cases
Sedative/hypnotic						
Diazepam	99	1.2	45	> 97% hepatic; < 3% renal	$t_{1/2}$ (i); V_d (i); Cl (d) 50%; f_p (i); AVH and cirrhosis increase $t_{1/2}$ Large therapeutic index – safe	Single dose, no change; chronic, decrease dose
Lorazepam	90	1.3	12.0	> 98% hepatic; < 2% renal Extensive glucuronidation	$t_{1/2}$ (i); V_d (i); Cl (u); f_p (i); neither AVH nor cirrhosis affects drug dosing	None
Midazolam	–	1.3	1.6	> 95% hepatic; < 5% renal	$t_{1/2}$ (i); V_d (i) slightly; Cl (d)	Decrease dose
Oxazepam	90	1.6	6.0	>95% hepatic; <1% renal Extensive glucuronidation	$t_{1/2}$ (i); V_d (u); Cl (u); f_p (u); neither AVH nor cirrhosis alters disposition significantly	None

Reproduced, with permission, from Eagle and Strunin.62 AVH, acute viral hepatitis; Cl, clearance; Cl_{int} internal clearance; (d), decreased; fp, plasma fraction; GI, gastrointestinal; (i), increased; i.v., intravenous; (u), unchanged.

Drug metabolism and liver disease

In patients with end-stage liver disease or gross hepatocellular damage the effect of drugs is unpredictable and often dramatic. The majority of patients seen in anesthetic practice are, however, well compensated with preservation of hepatocellular function. Despite this, dosage modification has been suggested for cirrhotic patients in whom the response to drugs differs considerably from other noncirrhotic patients. Table 17.5 summarizes the information on drugs used in routine anesthetic practice.[61,62] Patients with alcohol-induced cirrhosis may require a higher dose of thiopentone, probably because of redistribution of the drug.[62] In cirrhotic patients, "resistance" to curare, possibly owing to sequestration of the drug in the liver and spleen with an increased volume of distribution, has been described. More recently, pancuronium and vecuronium have shown an increased half-life in cirrhosis.[71,72] Atracurium, on the other hand, is not affected by cirrhosis.[73]

Opioid pharmacokinetics has been studied extensively in patients with cirrhosis. Following a single-dose administration, the elimination half-lives of fentanyl and sufentanil are unaffected,[74,75] but both the elimination half-life and the plasma-free fraction of alfentanil are increased.[76] Morphine appears to be safe in well-compensated cirrhosis with normal renal function. This may be because the glucuronide pathway is spared until late in liver disease.[77] Meperidine (pethidine), in contrast, has a markedly prolonged half-life.[78] Unpredictable and enhanced effects may result in patients with cirrhosis when opioids or other central nervous system (CNS) depressants are administered. This is related to receptor density changes and an altered permeability of the blood–brain barrier, especially in patients with end-stage disease. Benzodiazepine sensitivity, as a result of altered pharmacologic responsiveness rather than derangement of pharmacokinetics, has been reported.[79]

Volatile anesthetics undergo metabolism to both volatile and nonvolatile metabolites by both oxidative and reductive pathways.[62] Although there are good animal models demonstrating the metabolic pathways, their relevance to damage in humans is not clear.[80] All available data suggest that when volatile anesthetics are administered to patients with liver disease the outcome after operation is related to the extent of pre-existing damage and surgical trauma and that no one anesthetic agent or technique has been shown to be safer than another.[62]

LIVER FUNCTION TESTS

The assessment of liver and biliary function should include a complete history, thorough physical examination, and appropriate laboratory tests. Biochemically, the liver has a large functional reserve and it needs to be significantly compromised before there will be any clinical manifestations. The one exception to this is obstructive jaundice, which is caused by extrahepatic pathology. Both anesthesia and surgery may affect liver function adversely and occult disease may only become manifest postoperatively. A thorough assessment of alcohol or drug intake, exposure to toxins, history of blood transfusion or inoculation injury, family history of liver disease, etc. should be sought. Likewise, physical examination should focus on detecting the presence of jaundice, spider naevi, ascites, collateral portal circulation, and signs of hepatic encephalopathy. Liver disease often affects other organs such as the kidney, heart, lungs, and brain and their assessment is as important as that of liver itself.

The liver takes part in a variety of metabolic and synthetic processes. Liver function tests reflect these in the myriad of results returned from the laboratory. Table 17.6 shows typical laboratory results along with the normal ranges.[81] Minor asymptomatic changes in liver function test values are not uncommon[82,83] and can be related to alcohol intake, obesity, or diabetes. However, serial abnormal tests suggest hepatocellular damage. The combination of elevated bilirubin, aspartate aminotransferase (AST), alkaline phosphatase (AP), and alanine aminotransferase (ALT) has a predictive accuracy of over 90% for the presence of liver disease.[81] AST and ALT are raised not only with hepatocellular damage and necrosis but also after trauma and myocardial infarction. A carefully taken history and a thorough physical examination should help in the true diagnosis. The quest for a single marker to determine the degree of liver damage in specific pathologies has led to the use of glutathione-*S*-transferase to assess damage due to anesthetic agents.[84,85] γ-Glutamyltranspeptidase rises after alcohol- and drug-induced liver damage[86] and ALP increases early in biliary obstruction. Enzyme assays may signify loss of cellular integrity but do not indicate the residual metabolic or the synthetic capacity of the liver. In acute liver failure, following an initial rise in enzymes, a fall may indicate total cellular failure rather than recovery.

When the serum concentration of bilirubin rises above 20 μmol L^{-1} there is usually sufficient bilirubin sequestered in the tissues to cause jaundice. The serum bilirubin can be divided into conjugated and unconjugated fractions but the laboratory does not normally assay them separately. An increase in the unconjugated fraction (which cannot enter the urine and produces acholuric jaundice) results from an abnormal bilirubin load (hemolysis) or from a biochemical defect at, or proximal to, the site of conjugation on the smooth endoplasmic reticulum of the hepatocytes. The latter is typified in Gilbert's disease, a benign condition of intermittent jaundice affecting 5% of the population.

An elevated serum-conjugated bilirubin is always evidence of liver pathology and indicates defective excretion via the normal route into the biliary tree. Once conjugated, bilirubin is water soluble and can enter the urine. Traditional teaching suggests that disordered liver function test results, interpreted with the conjugated–unconjugated bilirubin ratio, can identify the problem to be pre-, intra-, or posthepatic. Although neat in theory, this can rarely be achieved in practice because parenchymal disease ultimately possesses an obstructive component and obstructive disease produces cellular dysfunction.

Defective excretion may occur either within the bile canaliculi and small ducts in the liver (intrahepatic cholestasis) or within the main bile ducts between the liver and the duodenum (extrahepatic cholestasis). Extrahepatic obstruction results from gallstones, strictures, and neoplasia of the bile duct and head of the pancreas. Intrahepatic cholestasis may, for instance, occur as a result of widespread hepatocellular damage (viral, alcohol, or cirrhosis), cellular reactions around the ductules from drug reactions (e.g. phenothiazines), and inflammatory reactions around the intralobular and septal bile ducts (primary biliary cirrhosis, ascending cholangitis). Pathologies that have a significant inflammatory or autoimmune component may have the bilirubin level dramatically reduced by steroid therapy.

In the presence of biliary obstruction, intravenous cholangiography will not afford adequate images. In recent years, ultrasound has become the most valuable imaging technique for characterizing the cause of cholestasis and for determining the pathway for further specialized tests. These tests include computed tomography (CT) scanning, magnetic resonance imaging (MRI) scanning, and invasive procedures such as angiography, endoscopic retrograde cholangiopancreatography (ERCP) (with or without papillotomy), and percutaneous transabdominal cholangiography.

The levels of albumin and the prothrombin ratio can index the synthetic ability of the liver. A serum albumin level of less than 25 g L^{-1} indicates substantial liver damage provided nephrotic syndrome and excessive protein loss from gastrointestinal disease have been excluded. Most of the clotting factors are synthesized in the liver, and the syntheses of factors II, VII, IX, and X depends on vitamin K. Deficiency of these prolongs the prothrombin time. This is expressed as the international normalized ratio (INR), which is unity when there is no abnormality.

Table 17.6 *Liver function tests*

Test	Normal range	If abnormal, may indicate
Aspartate aminotransferase	10–40 U L^{-1}	Hepatocellular damage/necrosis
Alanine aminotransferase	10–37 U L^{-1}	Hepatocellular damage/necrosis
Alkaline phosphatase	35–100 U L^{-1}	Cholestasis
γ-Glutamyl transpeptidase	11–64 U L^{-1}	Alcohol- or drug-related damage
Serum albumin	30–44 g L^{-1}	Decreased synthetic function
Prothrombin time	1.0–1.3 INR	Decreased synthetic function
Serum bilirubin		
Total	4–17 μmol L^{-1}	Assessment of jaundice/primary biliary cirrhosis
Unconjugated	< 0.3 μmol L^{-1}	Gilbert's disease
5′-Nucleotidase	1–18 U L^{-1}	Cholestasis
Total serum bile acids	0–6 μmol L^{-1}	Cholestasis/portasystemic shunt
Serum iron	8–31 μmol L^{-1}	Increased ferritin and transferritin suggests hemochromatosis
Transferritin saturation	< 50%	–
Ferritin	10–250 μg L^{-1}	–
Ceruloplasmin	1.1–2.9 μmol L^{-1}	Low with low copper suggests Wilson's disease
Serum copper	11–24 μmol L^{-1}	–
α_1-Antitrypsin	25–64 μmol L^{-1}	Low in deficiency disease
α-Fetoprotein	<0.29 nmol L^{-1}	Increased in hepatoma

Reproduced, with permission, from Strunin.[96] INR, international normalized ratio.

In obstructive jaundice, vitamin K is not absorbed from the intestine in the absence of bile salts. Parenteral vitamin K begins to act within a few hours and usually will return the prothrombin time to normal within 24 h. If it remains elevated (vitamin K resistant), this indicates cellular damage, the hepatocytes being unable to synthesize the clotting factors in the presence of active substrate. In these circumstances, fresh-frozen plasma will correct the clotting defect temporarily and allow diagnostic procedures (e.g. liver biopsy) to be undertaken.

Liver biopsy will demonstrate definitive evidence of cirrhosis. Cirrhosis is the final result of many conditions and represents the endpoint in the sequence of cellular necrosis, fibrosis, and nodular regeneration with distortion of the architecture. Histologically, there are further subdivisions based on the nodule size and the location of the fibrosis but the functional result is the same.

All patients with hepatic disease should be screened for hepatitis. α-Fetoprotein is raised in 70–90% of patients with primary hepatocellular carcinoma (which is also a valuable postoperative marker of recurrence). Over 90% of patients with primary biliary cirrhosis will have antinuclear antibodies in the serum. Patients with Wilson's disease have low levels of copper and ceruloplasmin, and those with hemochromatosis have increased concentrations of ferritin and transferritin.

THE LIVER IN PREGNANCY

During normal pregnancy the liver does not alter significantly in size, weight, or its blood flow. However, the finding of an enlarged liver should lead to a presumptive diagnosis of liver disease. The proportion of cardiac output delivered to the liver falls from 35% in the nonpregnant state to about 29% in late pregnancy. Serum alkaline phosphatase levels rise slowly during early gestation with a sharp rise in the last trimester; a concentration of twice the normal is not uncommon at term. In contrast, serum transaminases (AST, ALT) are unaffected during pregnancy and are reliable indicators of hepatocellular damage. Serum cholinesterase levels are reduced by up to 30% but prolonged neuromuscular block with suxamethonium is rare.[87] When this does occur in those with a normal genotype, it rarely lasts more than 20 min.[88]

In severe cases of hyperemesis gravidarum, the serum transaminase level may rise by up to twice normal but jaundice is rare. Hepatic dysfunction is not severe and death due to hepatic failure has not been reported. Transaminase levels return to normal once vomiting subsides.

Intrahepatic cholestasis of pregnancy

Although less than 1% of pregnant women develop signs and symptoms of this disorder, it is second only to viral hepatitis as a cause of jaundice in pregnancy. The distinct possibility exists, however, that this disorder of liver function has been poorly recognized and therefore under-reported.[89] Intrahepatic cholestasis of pregnancy is of unknown etiology and should be considered in any pregnant patient with pruritus and jaundice.[90] The diagnosis is confirmed with the elevation of serum bile acids by 10–100 times.[89] AST and ALT levels may vary from being normal to rising to four times normal. Prolonged prothrombin time can be treated with vitamin K. Although the maternal prognosis is excellent, several studies report an increased incidence of premature labor, fetal distress, and neonatal death.[90]

Acute fatty liver of pregnancy

This is a rare and serious disorder of unknown etiology with symptoms appearing in late pregnancy. The estimated incidence is one case per million pregnancies.[91] An association between acute fatty liver of pregnancy, the HELLP syndrome (described below), and a recessively inherited fatty acid oxidation disorder – long-chain 3-hydroxyacyl-CoA dehydrogenase deficiency – has been demonstrated.[92] Symptoms appear suddenly in the third trimester and include abdominal pain, anorexia, nausea, vomiting, fatigue, headaches, and fever. This rapidly progresses to bleeding, right upper quadrant tenderness, jaundice, renal failure, and encephalopathy. Investigations reveal an elevated bilirubin level as well as raised transaminase levels. Coagulation disorders range from a prolonged prothrombin time to disseminated intravascular coagulation. Serum creatinine rises with renal failure and life-threatening hypoglycemia may be present. Hepatic failure develops within a few days with marked coagulopathy and a high risk of postpartum hemorrhage.[90] Treatment of coagulation disorders as described elsewhere is essential. Since the disease runs a relentless course until after delivery, prompt delivery is advisable as soon as the diagnosis is made.

Toxemia and HELLP syndrome

Mild abnormalities in liver function have been reported in only 10% of patients with pre-eclampsia. However, a combination of hemolysis, elevated liver enzymes and a low platelet count, termed HELLP syndrome, was first described in 1982.[93] It has been argued that this is "merely a cluster of signs seen in some patients with hypertensive disorders of pregnancy."[94] The incidence of the disease is reported to be between 0.17% and 0.85% of all live births; in 20% of the patients there is no hypertension and in about 30% of the cases the syndrome appears post partum.[95] Symptoms include epigastric and right upper quadrant pain, nausea, and vomiting. Fibrin deposits in the hepatic sinusoids lead to their occlusion, necrosis, and periportal hemorrhage. In severe cases, focal and even diffuse necrosis together with subcapsular and/or intrahepatic hemorrhage may be encountered. Abdominal paracentesis, ultrasound, or CT scanning aids diagnosis. Treatment goals include correction of hypovolemia, coagulopathy, and management of other aspects of pre-eclampsia. Intrahepatic hemorrhage may be treated conservatively but capsular rupture requires surgical intervention. Despite improved diagnosis and management, maternal mortality remains high at 50–60% and fetal mortality around 60%.[90]

REFERENCES

1. Campra JL, Reynolds TB. The hepatic circulation. In: Arias IM, Jakoby WB, Popper H, *et al.* (eds): *The Liver: Biology and Pathobiology*. New York: Raven Press, 1988: 911.
2. Greenway CV, Lautt WW. Hepatic circulation. In: Schultz SG (ed.). *Handbook of Physiology*. 6. *The Gastrointestinal System*. Bethesda, MD: American Physiological Society, 1989: 1519.
3. Ellis H. *Clinical Anatomy*, 5th edn. Oxford: Blackwell Scientific Publications, 1974: 92–4.
4. Warwick R, Williams PL. *Gray's Anatomy*, 35th edn. London: Longman, 1973: 1302–14.
5. Sear JW. Anatomy and physiology of the liver. *Baillière's Clin Anaesthesiol* 1992; **6**: 697–727.
6. Caesar J, Sheldon S, Chiandussi L, *et al.* The use of indocyanine green in the measurement of hepatic blood flow and as test of hepatic function. *Clin Sci* 1961; **21:** 43.
7. Szabo G, Benyo I, Sandor J, *et al.* Estimation of hepatic blood flow in the dog with the Xe and hydrogen washout, Au-colloid uptake techniques and with the electromagnetic flowmeter. *Res Exp Med (Berl)* 1976; **169:** 69.
8. Reichman S, Davis WE, Storaasli JP, *et al.* Measurement of hepatic blood flow by indicator dilution techniques. *J Clin Invest* 1958; 37: 1848.
9. Hopkinson BR, Schenk WG. The electromagnetic measurement of liver blood flow and cardiac output in conscious dogs during feeding and exercise. *Surgery* 1968; **63:** 970–5.
10. Sear JW. Hepatic physiology. *Curr Anaesth Crit Care* 1990; 1: 196–203.
11. Lutz J, Pieper U, Bauereisen E. Appearance and size of veno-vasomotor reactions in the liver circulation. *Pflugers Arch* 1968; **299:** 311–25.
12. Hanson KM, Johnson PC. Local control of hepatic arterial and portal venous flow in the dog. *Am J Physiol* 1966; **211:** 712–20.
13. Richardson PDI, Withrington PG. Pressure–flow relationships and effects of noradrenaline and isoprenaline on the hepatic arterial and portal venous vascular beds of the dog. *J Physiol* 1978; **282:** 451–70.
14. Lautt WW. Mechanism and role of intrinsic regulation of hepatic arterial blood flow: the hepatic arterial buffer response. *Am J Physiol* 1985; **249:** G549–56.
15. Lautt WW, Legare DJ, d'Almeide MS. Adenosine as putative regulator of hepatic arterial flow (the buffer response). *Am J Physiol* 1985; **248:** H331–8.
16. Gelman S, Ernst E. Role of pH, Pco_2 and O_2 content of portal blood in hepatic circulatory autoregulation. *Am J Physiol*, 1977; **233**: E255–62.
17. Richardson PDI, Withrington PG. Pressure flow relationships and the effects of noradrenaline and isoprenaline on the simultaneously perfused hepatic arterial and portal venous vascular beds of dogs. *J Physiol* 1978; **282:** 451–70.
18. Seltzer JL, Ritter DE, Starsnic MA, Marr AT. The hemodynamics response to traction on the abdominal mesentery. *Anesthesiology* 1985; **63:** 96–9.
19. Gelman S. Disturbances in hepatic blood flow during anesthesia and surgery. *Arch Surg* 1976; **111:** 881–3.
20. Clarke RSJ, Doggart JR, Lavery T. Changes in liver function after different types of surgery. *Br J Anaesth* 1976; **48:** 119–28.
21. Bohrer SL, Rogers EL, Koehler RC, Traystman RJ. Effect of hypovolemic hypotension and laparotomy on splanchnic and hepatic arterial blood flow in dogs. *Curr Surg* 1981; **38:** 325–8.
22. Harper MH, Collins P, Johnson BH, *et al.* Postanesthetic hepatic injury in rats: influence of alterations in hepatic blood flow, surgery, and anesthesia time. *Anesth Analg* 1982; **61:** 79–82.
23. Gelman S, Dillard E, Bradley EL. Hepatic circulation during stress and anesthesia with halothane, isoflurane or fentanyl. *Anesth Analg* 1987; **66:** 936–43.
24. Moreno AH, Burchell AR. Respiratory regulation of splanchnic and systemic venous return in normal subjects and in patients with hepatic cirrhosis. *Surg Gynecol Obstet* 1982; **154:** 257–67.
25. Manney J, Justice R, Hetchman HB. Abnormalities in organ blood flow and its distribution during end-expiratory pressure. *Surgery* 1979; **85:** 425–32.
26. Halden E, Jakobson S, Janeras L, Norlen K. Effects of positive and end-expiratory pressure on cardiac output distribution in the pig. *Acta Anaesthesiol Scand* 1982; **26:** 403–8.
27. Bonnet F, Richard C, Glaser P, *et al.* Changes in hepatic flow induced by continuous positive pressure ventilation in critically ill patients. *Crit Care Med* 1982; **10:** 703–5.
28. Brendenberg CE, Paskanik AM. Relation of portal haemodynamics to cardiac output during mechanical ventilation with PEEP. *Ann Surg* 1983; **198:** 218–22.
29. Gioia FR, Harris AP, Traystman RJ, Rogers MC. Organ blood flow during high frequency ventilation at low and high airway pressure in dogs. *Anesthesiology*,1986; **65:** 50–5.
30. Thompson IA, Fitch W, Hughes RL, Campbell D. Effect of increased concentrations of carbon dioxide during halothane anaesthesia on liver blood flow and hepatic oxygen consumption. *Br J Anaesth* 1983; **55:** 1231–7.
31. Fujita Y, Takayuki S, Akiyuki O. Effects of hypocapnia and hypocarbia on splanchnic circulation and hepatic function in the beagle. *Anesth Analg* 1989; **69:** 152–7.
32. Cooperman LH, Warden JC, Price JC. Splanchnic circulation during nitrous oxide anaesthesia and hypocarbia in normal man. *Anesthesiology* 1968; **29:** 254–8.
33. Carneiro JJ, Donald DE. Changes in liver blood flow and blood content in dogs during direct nerve activity. *Circ Res* 1977; **40:** 150–8.
34. Richardson PDI, Withrington PG. Liver blood flow. 2. Effects of drugs and hormones on liver blood flow. *Gastroenterology* 1981; **81:** 356–75.
35. Richardson PDI, Withrington PG. Glucagon inhibition of hepatic arterial responses to hepatic nerve stimulation. *Am J Physiol* 1977; **233:** H647.
36. Richardson PDI, Withrington PG. Effects of intra-arterial and intra-portal injections of vasopressin on the hepatic arterial and portal venous vascular beds of the dog. *Circ Res* 1978; **43:** 496.
37. Gelman S, Frenette L. Effects of anaesthetics on liver blood flow. *Baillière's Clin Anaesthesiol* 1992; **6:** 729–50.
38. Strunin L. The splanchnic, hepatic and portal circulation. In: Prys-Roberts C (ed.). *The Circulation in Anaesthesia*. Oxford: Blackwell Scientific Publications, 1980: 241–51.
39. Tverskoy M, Gelman S, Fowler KC, Bradley EL. Intestinal circulation during inhalation anesthesia. *Anesthesiology* 1985; **62:** 462–9.
40. Tranquilli WJ, Manohar M, Parks CM, *et al.* Systemic and regional blood flow distribution in unanesthetized swine and swine with halothane + nitrous oxide, halothane, or enflurane. *Anesthesiology* 1982; **56:** 369–79.
41. Gelman S, Fowler KC, Smith LR. Regional blood flow during isoflurane and halothane anesthesia. *Anesth Analg* 1984; **63:** 557–65.
42. Gelman S, Fowler KC, Smith LR. Liver circulation and function during isoflurane and halothane anesthesia. *Anesthesiology* 1984; **61:** 726–30.
43. Frink E, Morgan S, Coetzee A, *et al.* The effects of sevoflurane, halothane, enflurane and isoflurane on hepatic blood flow and oxygenation in chronically instrumented greyhound dogs. *Anesthesiology* 1992; **76:** 86–90.
44. Hughes RL, Campbell D, Fitch W. Effects of enflurane and halothane on liver blood flow and oxygen consumption in the greyhound. *Br J Anaesth* 1980; **52:** 1079–86.
45. Miller C, Fitch W, Thompson A. Effect of isoflurane on the canine hepatic circulation and hepatic oxygen balance. *Br J Anaesth* 1990; **65:** 698–703.
46. Lundeen G, Manohar M, Parks C. Systemic distribution of blood flow in

swine while awake and during 1.0 and 1.5 MAC isoflurane anesthesia with and without 50% nitrous oxide. *Anesth Analg* 1983; **62:** 499–512.
47. Nagano K, Gelman S, Parks D, Bradley L. Hepatic oxygen supply uptake relationships and metabolism during anesthesia in miniature pigs. *Anesthesiology* 1990; **72:** 902–10.
48. Debaene B, Goldfard G, Braillon A, *et al.* Effects of ketamine, halothane, enflurane and isoflurane on systemic and splanchnic haemodynamics in normovolemic and hypovolemic cirrhotic rats. *Anesthesiology* 1990; **76:** 86–90.
49. Payen D, Gatecel C, Dupuy P, *et al.* Effects of isoflurane vs. halothane on human arterial hepatic blood flow (AHBF) and portal vein blood flow (PVBF) after surgical stress. *Anesthesiology* 1988; **69** (3A): A77.
50. Fujita Y, Kumura K, Hamada H, Takaori M. Comparative effects of halothane, isoflurane and sevoflurane on the liver with hepatic artery ligation in the beagle. *Anesthesiology* 1991; **76:** 86–90.
51. Thompson IA, Fitch W, Hughes RL, *et al.* Effects of certain i.v. anaesthetics on liver blood flow and hepatic oxygen consumption in the greyhound. *Br J Anaesth* 1986; **58:** 69–80.
52. Runciman WB, Mather LE, Selby DG. Cardiovascular effects of propofol and of thiopentone anaesthesia in the sheep. *Br J Anaesth* 1990; **65:** 353–9.
53. Diedericks J, Sear JW, Foex P. The effect of propofol on hepatic blood flow. *Anesthesiology* 1990; **73:** A624.
54. Tverskoy M, Gelman S, Fowler KC, Bradley EL. Influence of fentanyl and morphine on intestinal circulation. *Anesth Analg* 1985; **64:** 577–84.
55. Kien ND, Reitan JA, White DA, *et al.* Hemodynamic responses to alfentanil in halothane-anesthetized dogs. *Anesth Analg* 1986; **65:** 765–70.
56. Kennedy W, Everett G, Cogg L, Allen G. Simultaneous systemic and hepatic hemodynamic measurements during high epidural anesthesia in normal patients. *Anesth Analg* 1971; **50:** 1069–77.
57. Hendolin H, Penttilla M. Liver enzymes after retropubic prostatectomy in patients receiving continuous lumbar epidural or general anesthesia. *Ann Clin Res* 1982; **14:** 1–6.
58. Grieg T, Andreen M, Irestedt L. Hemodynamics and oxygen consumption in the dog during high spinal epidural block with special reference to the splanchnic region. *Acta Anaesthesiol Scand* 1983; **27:** 211–17.
59. Loft S, Boel J, Kyst A, *et al.* Increased hepatic microsomal enzyme activity after surgery under halothane or spinal anesthesia. *Anesthesiology* 1985; **62:** 11–16.
60. Kennedy WF, Everett GB, Cobb LA, *et al.* Simultaneous systemic and hepatic hemodynamic measurements during high spinal anesthesia in normal man. *Anesth Analg* 1970; **49:** 1016–24.
61. Jorm CM, Stamford JA. Hepatic metabolism of xenobiotics with reference to anaesthesia. *Baillière's Clin Anesthesiol* 1992; **6**: 751–79.
62. Eagle CJ, Strunin L. Drug metabolism in liver disease. *Curr Anaesth Crit Care* 1990; **1:** 204–12.
63. Arns PA, Wedlund PJ, Branch RA. Adjustment of medications in liver failure. In: Chernow B (ed.). *The Pharmacologic Approach to the Critically Ill Patient*. Baltimore, MD: Williams & Wilkins, 1988: 85–111.
64. Howden CW, Birnie GG, Brodie MJ. Drug metabolism in liver disease. *Pharmacol Ther* 1989; 40: 439–74.
65. Hayes PC. Liver disease and drug disposition. *Br J Anaesth* 1992; **68:** 459–61.
66. Watkins PB. Role of cytochromes P450 in drug metabolism and hepatotoxicity. *Semin Liver Dis* 1990; **10:** 235–50.
67. Andersson T. Omeprazole drug interaction studies. *Clin Pharmacokinet* 1991; 21: 195–212.
68. Mulder GJ. Glucuronidation and its role in regulation of biological activity of drugs. *Annu Rev Pharmacol Toxicity* 1992; **32:** 25–49.
69. Portenoy RK, Thaler HT, Inturrisi CE, *et al.* The metabolite morphine 6-glucuronide contributes to the analgesia produced by morphine infusion in patients with pain and normal renal function. *Clin Pharmacol Ther* 1992; **51:** 422–31.
70. Wood M. Plasma drug binding: implications for anesthesiologist. *Anesth Analg* 1986; **65:** 786–804.
71. Lebrault C, Berger JL, D'Hollander AA, *et al.* Pharmacokinetics and pharmacodynamics of vecuronium (ORG NC45) in patients with cirrhosis. *Anesthesiology* 1985; **62:** 601–5.
72. Duvaldestin P, Saada J, Berger JL, *et al.* Pharmacokinetics, pharmacodynamics, and dose–response relationship of pancuronium in control and elderly subjects. *Anesthesiology* 1982; **56:** 36–40.
73. Ward S, Neill EA. Pharmacokinetics of atracurium in acute hepatic failure (with acute renal failure). *Br J Anaesth* 1983; **55:** 1169–72.
74. Hammerer JP, Schaeffler P, Couture E, Duvaldestin P. Fentanyl pharmacokinetics in anaesthetized patients with cirrhosis. *Br J Anaesth* 1982; **54:** 1267–70.
75. Chauvin M, Ferrier C, Haberer JP, *et al.* Sufentanil pharmacokinetics in cirrhosis. *Anesth Analg* 1989; **68:** 1–4.
76. Ferrier C, Marty J, Buffered Y, *et al.* Alfentanil pharmacokinetics in patients with cirrhosis. *Anesthesiology* 1985; **62:** 480–4.
77. Patwardhan RV, Johnson RF, Hoympa A, *et al.* Morphine metabolism in cirrhosis. *Gastroenterology* 1981; **81:** 1006–11.
78. McHorse TS, Wilkinson GR, Johnson RF, Shenker S. Effect of acute viral hepatitis in man on the disposition and elimination of meperidine. *Gastroenterology* 1975; **68:** 775–80.
79. Branch RA, Morgan MH, James J, Reid AE. Intravenous administration of diazepam in patients with chronic liver disease. *Gut* 1976; **17:** 975–83.
80. Stock JGL, Strunin L. Unexplained hepatitis following halothane. *Anesthesiology* 1985; **63:** 424–39.
81. Henry DA, Kitchingman G, Langman MJS. 14C-aminopyrine breath analysis and conventional biochemical tests as predictors of survival in cirrhosis. *Dig Dis Sci* 1985; **30:** 813–18.
82. Schemel WH. Unexpected hepatic dysfunction found by multiple laboratory screening. *Anesth Analg* 1976; **55:** 810–14.
83. Hulcrantz R, Glauman H, Lindberg G, Nilsson LH. Liver investigation in 149 asymptomatic patients with moderately elevated activities of serum aminotransferases. *Scand J Gastroenterol* 1986; **21:** 109–13.
84. Hussey AJ, Aldridge LM, Paul D, *et al.* Plasma glutathione-S-transferase concentrations: a measure of hepatocellular integrity following a single anaesthetic with halothane, enflurane or isoflurane. *Br J Anaesth* 1988; **60:** 130–5.
85. Murray JM, Trinick TR. Hepatic function and indocyanine green clearance during and after prolonged anaesthesia with propofol. *Br J Anaesth* 1992; **69:** 643–4.
86. Gluud C, Anderson I, Dietrichson O, *et al.* Gamma-glutamyl-transferase, aspartate aminotransferase and alkaline phosphatase as markers of alcoholic consumption in outpatient alcoholics. *Eur J Clin Invest* 1981; **11:** 181–6.
87. Schnider SM. Serum cholinesterase activity during pregnancy, labor and puerperium. *Anesthesiology* 1965; **26:** 335–9.
88. Blitt CD, Petty WC, Albertenst EE, Wright BJ. Correlation of plasma cholinesterase activity and duration of action of succinylcholine during pregnancy. *Anesth Analg* 1977; **56:** 78–83.
89. Lunzer M, Barnes P, Blyth J, O'Halloran M. Serum bile acid concentrations during pregnancy and their relationships to obstetric cholestasis. *Gastroenterology* 1986; **91:** 825–9.
90. Lunzer MR. Jaundice in pregnancy. *Baillière's Clin Gastroenterol* 1989; **3:** 467–83.
91. Kaplan MM. Acute fatty liver of pregnancy. *N Engl J Med* 1985; **313:** 367–70.
92. Ibdah JA, Yang Z, Bennett MJ. Liver disease in pregnancy and fetal fatty acid oxidation defects. *Mol Genet Metab* 2000; **71:** 182–9.
93. Weinstein L. Syndrome of hemolysis, elevated liver enzymes and low platelet count: a severe consequence of hypertension in pregnancy. *Am J Obstet Gynecol* 1982; **142:** 159–67.
94. MacKenna J, Dover NL, Brame RG. Pre-eclampsia associated with haemolysis, elevated liver enzymes and low platelets – an obstetric emergency? *Gynaecology* 1983; **62:** 751–4.
95. Rath W, Faridi A, Dudenhausen JW. HELLP syndrome. *J Perinat Med* 2000; **28:** 249–60.
96. Strunin L. Preoperative assessment of hepatic function. *Baillière's Clin Anaesthesiol* 1992; **6**: 781–93.

18

Renal physiology, fluids, and electrolytes

SHERMEEN B VAKHARIA AND ENRICO M CAMPORESI

The kidneys play an important role in the regulation of extracellular fluid composition and volume as well as the excretion of metabolic waste products. Unlike the cardiac and pulmonary systems, which are closely monitored in the operative period, the monitoring of the kidneys is often limited to urine volume measurements. This contrasts with the fact that renal failure occurring in the perioperative period carries significant morbidity and mortality. Patients with pre-existing renal impairment are more vulnerable to the development of acute renal failure in the perioperative period. Accurate preoperative assessment of renal function and optimal perioperative fluid, hemodynamic, and drug management may consequently reduce the occurrence of perioperative renal failure.

ANATOMY AND PHYSIOLOGY OF THE RENAL SYSTEM

The kidneys are paired structures located in the retroperitoneal space at the level of the twelfth thoracic to the third lumbar vertebrae. The functional unit of the kidneys is the *nephron.* The nephron is made up of: (1) the glomerulus; and (2) the renal tubule, which consists of the Bowman's capsule, proximal convoluted tubule, loop of Henle, distal convoluted tubule, and cortical connecting tubule, which leads to the collecting duct (Fig. 18.1). The *cortical nephrons* have short loops of Henle, which are surrounded by a network of capillaries. Twenty-five percent of the nephrons are *juxtamedullary nephrons,* which have long loops of Henle, which are surrounded by the vasa recta, and play an essential role in the formation of concentrated urine (Fig. 18.2).[1]

RENAL BLOOD FLOW AND GFR

In a normal 70-kg man, the kidneys receive about 1200 mL min^{-1} of blood or 21% of cardiac output. The proportion of renal blood flow going to the renal cortex is 85–90%; The glomerular capillaries filter 10–20% of the plasma flowing through the kidney, with the average glomerular filtration rate (GFR) being 125 mL min^{-1} in a healthy adult. GFR is influenced by the glomerular filtration pressure (glomerular hydrostatic pressure minus the sum of glomerular oncotic pressure and Bowman's capsule pressure).

Autoregulation

Renal blood flow is autoregulated to remain constant between mean arterial blood pressures of 60 and 160 mmHg (8 and 21.3 kPa). Two mechanisms appear to regulate glomerular blood flow: (1) the myogenic reflex, which causes the afferent arteriole to constrict or dilate with changes in blood pressure; and (2) feedback control of glomerular blood flow involving the juxtaglomerular apparatus (JGA). In hypotensive states, the JGA responds to renal tubular fluid composition by signaling to the arteriole to dilate as well as triggering the renin–angiotensin system, leading to efferent arteriolar constriction. As a result, glomerular pressure increases and thus glomerular filtration increases. In the absence of autoregulation, small increases in arterial blood pressure can result in large fluid and sodium losses. Therefore, normal kidneys regulate blood flow and hence GFR over a wide range of arterial blood pressures. In disease states in which autoregulation is impaired, small periods of hypotension can significantly affect renal blood flow. Although the GFR is autoregulated, the final urine output is affected by several other factors and is not autoregulated with changes in blood pressure (Fig. 18.3).

TUBULAR PROCESSING OF WATER AND ELECTROLYTES

Tubular resorption, unlike glomerular filtration, is a highly selective process.

Approximately 65% of the filtered sodium is reabsorbed in the proximal convoluted tubule, mostly by an adenosine triphosphatase (ATPase)-driven pump. Chloride follows passively, as does water along its osmotic gradient. Thus, the osmolarity of the filtrate does not change in the proximal convoluted tubule. Bicarbonate, potassium, and calcium are also reabsorbed into the peritubular capillaries. Glucose and amino acids are completely reabsorbed in the proximal convoluted tubule by secondary active transport coupled with sodium. When blood glucose levels exceed the resorption threshold (180 mg mL^{-1}), glucose appears in the urine.

The descending loop of Henle is highly permeable to water and only moderately permeable to solutes. About 20% of filtered water is reabsorbed in this part of the tubule. The ascending loop of Henle is impermeable to water and only electrolytes are reabsorbed into the medullary interstitium, thus decreasing the osmolarity of the fluid within the tubule. Especially important is the active reabsorption of sodium, chloride, and potassium. Calcium, bicarbonate, and magnesium are also reabsorbed. The solute reabsorption and the diffusion of urea from the medullary collecting ducts maintain a highly osmolar medullary interstitium. As additional filtrate enters from the descending loop of Henle into the ascending loop of Henle, additional solutes are pumped into the medullary interstitium, causing ion trapping and further increasing medullary interstitial osmolarity.

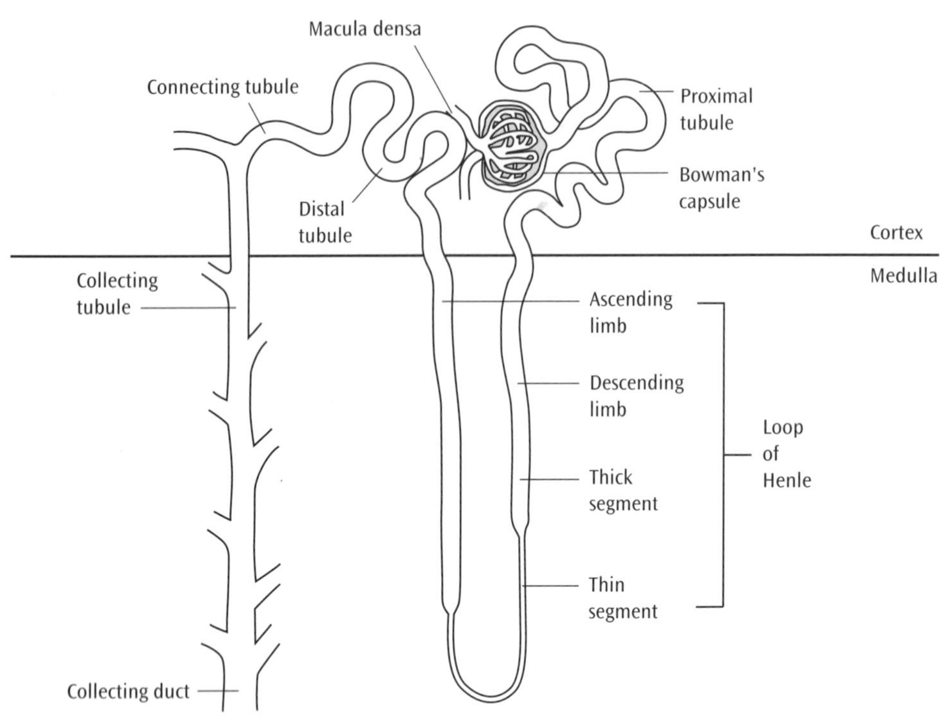

Figure 18.1 *Anatomy of the nephron (with permission from Guyton and Hall,[1] p. 318).*

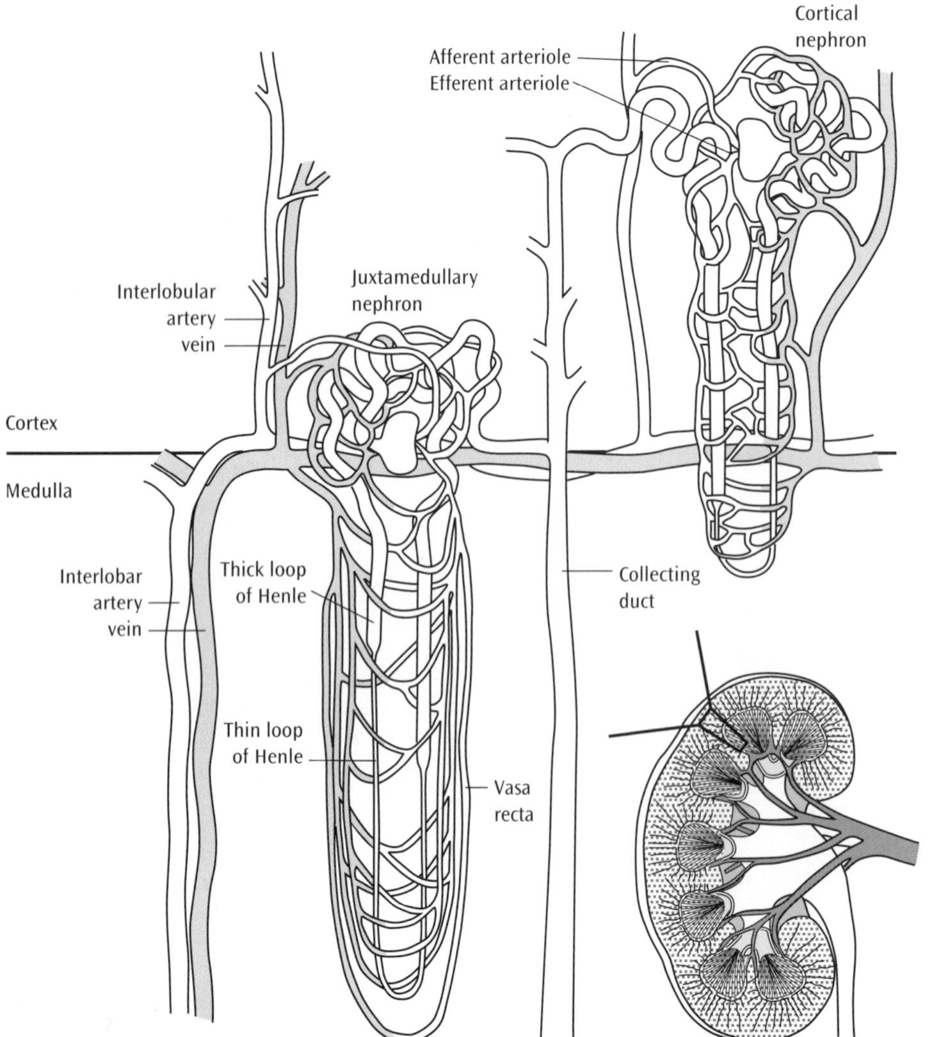

Figure 18.2 *Schematic representation of cortical and juxtamedullary nephrons and their blood supply.*

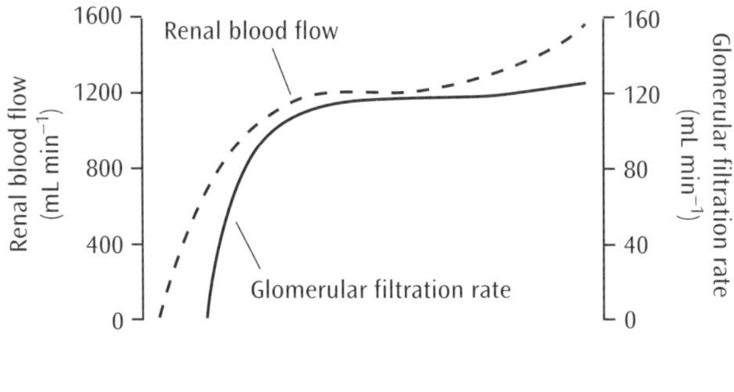

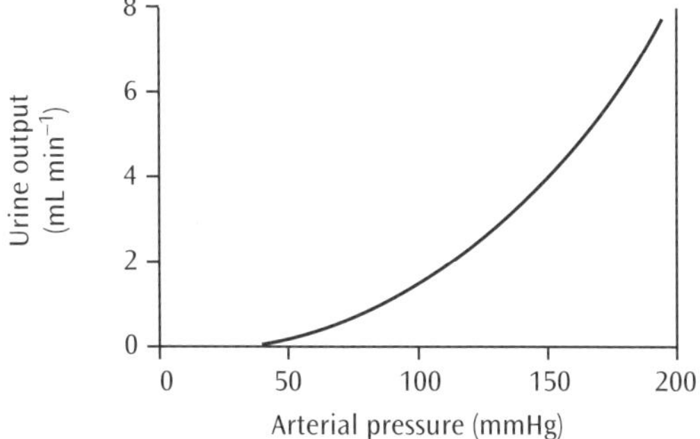

Figure 18.3 *Renal blood flow and glomerular filtration rate are autoregulated with changes in arterial blood pressure but the final urine output is not autoregulated (with permission from Guyton and Hall,[1] p. 327).*

The U-shaped vasa recta surrounding these loops of Henle are permeable to solutes and have sluggish blood flow. As they descend in the hyperosmolar medulla, solutes move in and water moves out, thus concentrating the blood in the vasa recta. As they ascend, solutes move out and water moves in to the vasa recta. Thus, there is little net dilution of the concentration of medullary interstitial fluid. The vasa recta, therefore, act as countercurrent exchangers and prevent medullary hyperosmolarity from being dissipated. This medullary hyperosmolarity is important for the formulation of concentrated urine at the level of the medullary collecting duct. During a period of volume depletion or increased sympathetic tone, the cortical blood flow is preferably redistributed to the "salt and water" conserving juxtamedullary nephrons.[2] This region of the kidney is particularly susceptible to ischemic injury, because of its sluggish medullary blood flow, in situations in which renal perfusion is decreased.[3]

The tubular fluid then enters the early distal convoluted tubule with an osmolarity of approximately 100 mosmol L^{-1}. The very first part of the distal convoluted tubule forms the juxtaglomerular apparatus, which is involved in feedback control of GFR in the same nephron. Following this, the early distal tubule, which has properties similar to those of the ascending loop of Henle, further dilutes this fluid.

The late distal convoluted tubule and the cortical collecting duct continue to absorb solutes and also become highly permeable to water only in the presence of high concentrations of antidiuretic hormone (ADH). Large amounts of water are reabsorbed in the presence of ADH and swept away by cortical peritubular capillaries, thus preserving the medullary interstitial hyperosmolarity. At this level of the nephron sodium reabsorption and potassium secretion is controlled by aldosterone. The late distal convoluted tubule and the cortical collecting ducts also play an important role in acid–base regulation of body fluids by secreting hydrogen ions and reabsorbing bicarbonate ions. The medullary collecting duct determines the final concentration of the urine. Under the influence of ADH, the medullary collecting duct becomes permeable to water as it traverses the hyperosmolar medullary interstitium. Water is reabsorbed and solutes are concentrated in the urine. H^+ ions are also secreted by medullary collecting ducts. Thus, two important factors in the formation of concentrated urine are: (1) the presence of ADH; and (2) the high osmolarity of medullary interstitium.

HORMONAL CONTROL OF RENAL TUBULAR FUNCTION

Antidiuretic hormone

Antidiuretic hormone (ADH), also known as vasopressin, plays an important role in the conservation of fluid and excretion of concentrated urine. In hypovolemic states, arterial baroreceptor and atrial receptor reflexes stimulate ADH release from the posterior pituitary gland. Tubular actions of ADH, as discussed earlier, increase water reabsorption. In the absence of ADH, the water permeability of the distal convoluted tubule, the collecting tubule, and the collecting ducts is greatly reduced leading to excretion of large amounts of diluted urine. Under stressful situations, high circulating levels of ADH cause cortical vasoconstriction, thereby diverting the blood to the renal medulla.

Renin–angiotensin–aldosterone system

Renin is secreted by the juxtaglomerular cells in response to hypotension. Renin cleaves renin substrate to form angiotensin I, which on passage through the lungs is converted to angiotensin II. Angiotensin II, by a direct action and by an efferent arteriolar constricting effect, leads to sodium and water reabsorption. Angiotensin II, like sympathetic stimulation, causes the zona glomerulosa cells to secrete aldosterone. Aldosterone acts on the distal convoluted tubule and collecting ducts to cause sodium and water retention and potassium secretion.[4]

Atrial natriuretic peptide

Distension of cardiac atria as in response to hypervolemia leads to the release of atrial natriuretic peptide (ANP), which blocks sodium and water reabsorption especially in the collecting ducts. It also increases GFR, and causes vasodilation in an attempt to return the blood volume to normal. ANP opposes the effects of the renin–angiotensin–aldosterone system and ADH.[5,6]

Prostaglandins

Prostaglandins produced by the kidney cause renal arteriolar dilation and sodium and water excretion. Under stressful situations, or during hypotension and hypovolemia, renal prostaglandins play an important role in maintaining renal blood flow.[7,8] Administration of cyclo-oxygenase inhibitors under such conditions can have adverse effects on renal perfusion and damage the kidney. Cyclo-oxygenase inhibitors do not have this deleterious effect under conditions of normovolemia and adequate renal blood flow.

Parathyroid hormone

Parathyroid hormone (PTH) acts on the thick ascending loop of Henle and the proximal and distal convoluted tubules to increase calcium and magnesium reabsorption and inhibit phosphate reabsorption.

SIGNIFICANCE OF PERIOPERATIVE RENAL DYSFUNCTION

Acute renal failure

Prerenal and *renal* factors play an important role in the development of perioperative renal failure. Urine output is frequently reduced in the surgical patient as a result of the stress responses leading to sympathetic activation and elevation of angiotensin II, aldosterone, and ADH levels. Neurohumoral activation causes redistribution of the renal blood flow from the renal cortex to the medulla, sodium and water reabsorption, and a resulting decrease in urine output. Intrinsic renal mechanisms tend to preserve renal perfusion and renal failure rarely occurs. Acute deterioration in renal function under anesthesia is usually multifactorial, *renal ischemia* being the most common cause. Decreased renal perfusion due to coexisting diseases (atherosclerotic diseases, aortic dissection, diabetes, congestive heart failure, pre-existing renal disease) intravascular volume contraction, cardiopulmonary bypass, and aortic cross-clamping increase the risk of acute renal insufficiency.[9–11]

Exposure to neophrotoxins may contribute to perioperative renal dysfunction. Nonoliguric renal failure associated with the nephrotoxic effects of the fluoride ions has been associated with the use of fluorinated volatile anesthetic agents (further details are described later in this chapter in the section on volatile anesthetic agents). The two other commonly used nephrotoxic agents in the perioperative period are aminoglycoside antibiotics and radiocontrast agents.[12,13] Aminoglycoside nephrotoxicity is enhanced in the presence of hypotension, volume depletion, and advanced age.[12,14,15] Administration of radiocontrast agents to patients with chronic renal insufficiency appears to cause further deterioration in renal function, especially in the presence of diabetes and fluid restriction.[14,16] Nonsteroidal anti-inflammatory drugs (NSAIDs) can also induce reversible renal insufficiency in the presence of hemodynamic abnormalities, primary renal disease, and advanced age.[17] Finally, *postrenal* obstructive uropathy is a rare cause of perioperative renal impairment.

Acute decline in renal function occurring preoperatively needs to be thoroughly investigated and reversed, if possible, prior to performing elective surgery in order to avoid exposure to several other perioperative factors that may lead to sustained or worsening renal failure. The incidence of perioperative renal failure is raised in patients with pre-existing renal dysfunction. Perioperative morbidity and mortality in patients correlate directly with the increase in the degree of renal impairment.[10] The prognosis is worse for patients requiring postoperative dialysis. One explanation for this poor prognosis is the multiple organ insult that is present in these critically ill surgical patients, of which acute renal failure is only one of the manifestations.[18] Dialysis appears to have little effect in altering the cause of acute renal failure in critically ill surgical patients.[11]

Renal insufficiency and end-stage renal disease

Patients with chronic renal failure presenting for anesthesia may have two distinct stages of renal impairment: (1) *renal insufficiency* or *decreased renal reserve*; and (2) *end-stage renal disease (ESRD)*, which requires dialysis as renal function is no longer sufficient to sustain life.

Since preoperative renal insufficiency has been repeatedly shown to be an important predictor of postoperative renal dysfunction,[10,19] management of patients with pre-existing renal disease should be designed to preserve the existing renal function and to prevent further deterioration. These strategies include maintenance of adequate intravascular volume and myocardial function. The use of invasive monitors, prevention of hypotension, avoidance of nephrotoxic agents, and the use of adjuncts to maintain GFR and avoid renal damage should be aggressively considered.

Patients with ESRD suffer multiple organ and system abnormalities that make the perioperative management of these patients a challenge. Diabetes and hypertension, which are often the cause of the renal impairment, may be present. Fluid balance becomes critical in the perioperative period.

The *metabolic acidosis* commonly observed is hyperchloremic. In advanced stages, acidosis may be associated with an increased anion gap. Acidosis depresses neuromuscular responsiveness and myocardial contractility and is also accompanied by a rise in extracellular, and hence serum, potassium levels. Dialysis helps to restore the pH to near normal values.

Electrolyte abnormalities are commonly encountered in patients with chronic renal disease. The hyperkalemia observed in ESRD is due to the rise in total body potassium. K^+ levels above 5.5 mequiv L^{-1} generally occur when GFR falls below 10 mL min^{-1}. Tubular insensitivity to aldosterone may be present. Hyperkalemia may be so severe that the patient responds only transiently to drug therapy and dialysis is generally required to lower the serum potassium levels. Hyponatremia, though not common, may be seen in patients with fluid retention or inadequate dietary intake. Serum magnesium is often elevated in patients with GFR less than 10 mL min^{-1}. Hypermagnesemia can cause hypotension, central nervous system depression, and potentiation of the action of neuromuscular blocking agents. However, the magnesium level in these patients is rarely high enough to produce significant clinical effect unless magnesium-containing antacids have been administered. Hyperphosphatemia, hypocalcemia, and subsequently elevated PTH lead to renal osteodystrophy. Calcium deposition occurs in soft tissues and also in arteries causing further impairment of autoregulation, as well as increasing the risk of coronary artery disease.

Hemopoietic disorders

Normochromic normocytic anemia is found almost universally and appears to be multifactorial. Decreased red cell production, as a result of the lack of erythropoietin synthesis by the failing kidney, appears to be the most prominent cause of anemia.[20,21] Other contributing factors include iron and folate deficiency, heavy metal toxicities, and the shortened lifespan of red cells due to a high concentration of uremic toxins. Moreover, red cell loss may be accelerated by bleeding caused by uremic gastroenteritis and platelet function disorders. The decreased oxygen-carrying capacity in these patients is overcome by an increase in cardiac output and an increase in 2,3-diphosphoglycerate. The higher levels of 2,3-diphosphoglycerate shifts the oxyhemoglobin dissociation curve to the right, facilitating oxygen delivery to the tissues. Human recombinant erythropoietin is sometimes used to treat the anemia of end-stage renal disease.[22] Hypertension may occur as a side-effect of erythropoietin therapy.

Prolongation of bleeding time (BT) is the most common hemostatic defect in patients with chronic renal failure. This appears to be due to abnormal platelet function rather than decreased number of platelets or von Willenbrand factor defects. Platelet dysfunction is only partially corrected by dialysis.[21] Desmopressin (DDAVP), cryoprecitate, and conjugated estrogens have also been used to correct the bleeding disorder.

Functional abnormalities of white blood cells in uremic patients include decreased leukocyte chemotaxis, phagocytosis, and diminished bactericidal activity. Cell-mediated immune defects and hypogammaglobinemia predispose patients with chronic renal failure and dialysis to life-threatening infections and sepsis.[21]

Cardiovascular abnormalities

Ischemic heart disease is a leading cause of death in nonsurgical patients with chronic renal failure.[23] The high incidence of coronary artery disease is partly attributed to the presence of hypertension, hyperlipidemia, glucose intolerance, and accelerated atherosclerotic problems in uremic patients.[24,25] Volume expansion, hypertension, anemia, arteriovenous (AV) fistula, acidemia, and myocardial dysfunction all contribute to the development of congestive heart failure in these patients. Pericardial disease, with or without an effusion, can occur in two distinct clinical situations: (1) in inadequately dialyzed patients in whom dialysis may result in resolution of the pericarditis; and (2) in well-dialyzed patients, 20% of whom can develop tamponade.[26] Acute pericardial tamponade may be life-threatening, requiring immediate drainage. Arrhythmias can occur in the presence of abnormal potassium and calcium levels. Conduction abnormalities from calcium deposition have also been described.

Neurologic manifestations may be central (uremic encephalopathy, cerebrovascular disease) or peripheral (sensorimotor neuropathy). Autonomic nervous system dysfunction may also occur in ESRD. Clinical manifestations may include labile blood pressure, inability to tolerate dialysis, and gastroparesis. Overt manifestations of autonomic neuropathy do not reverse on dialysis.

The most commonly reported *gastrointestinal disorders* in uremic patients include gastroenteritis and motility disorders. Other manifestations of ESRD are listed in Table 18.1.

In general, patients with ESRD undergo more surgical procedures than other patients: 80–90% of operations performed in these patients are to establish vascular access for dialysis and generally carry a low mortality rate.[27] However, invasive procedures, especially cardiac and emergency surgeries, are fraught with a high incidence of perioperative death.[28]

Table 18.1 *Uremic syndrome – grouping of symptoms*

Neurologic
Drowsiness, decreased cognitive function
Encephalopathy
Seizures
Sensorimotor peripheral neuropathy
Autonomic dysfunction
Cardiovascular
Hypertension
Atherosclerosis
Dysrhythymias
Congestive heart failure
Pericarditis
Cardiomyopathy
Pulmonary
Pulmonary edema
Pneumonitis
Pleuritis
Hematologic
Anemia
Platelet dysfunction
Cellular and humoral immune defects
Fluids and electrolytes
Metabolic acidosis
Hypervolemia
Hyperkalemia
Hyponatremia
Hypocalcemia
Hypermagnesemia
Hyperphosphatemia
Endocrinologic
↑ Parathyroid hormone
Carbohydrate intolerance
Hyperlipidemia
Testicular/ovarian dysfunction
Gastrointestinal
Anorexia, nausea, vomiting
Gastroenteritis
Upper gastrointestinal bleeding
Motility disorders
Pancreatitis
Ascitis

Evaluation of renal function

Standard tests for renal function evaluate GFR and renal tubular function. These functions are often affected simultaneously. It is important to realize that most of these tests are insensitive in detecting early renal dysfunction in the perioperative period. Comparing the results with those of previous tests is helpful in the detection of any deterioration in renal function.

TESTS OF GLOMERULAR FUNCTION

Blood urea nitrogen (BUN) and *creatinine* are among the most commonly performed tests. Abnormalities usually indicate late renal dysfunction. Urea is filtered and partially absorbed by the kidneys. BUN is not a sensitive index of GFR as several factors affect its production and excretion. Low-flow states, such as congestive heart failure and dehydration, cause increased resorption of filtered urea, leading to elevated levels of BUN. A high-protein diet, gastrointestinal bleeding, catabolic states as in sepsis, and trauma can all lead to marked elevations in BUN levels, even in patients with normal renal function. On the other hand, in overhydration and liver disease (decreased urea synthesis) BUN levels may remain within the normal range despite a significant reduction in GFR. However, BUN greater than 50 mg dL^{-1} indicates renal disease unless proved otherwise.

A constant daily amount of creatinine is produced in normal individuals from the creatine found in muscle. Creatinine is excreted mostly by filtration and mainly by the kidneys. Muscular individuals may have high normal creatinine values whereas individuals with reduced muscle mass may have creatinine values in the normal range despite a significant reduction in GFR, as occurs in the elderly. Since creatinine excretion almost conclusively depends on the GFR, a 50% reduction in GFR would double the serum creatinine[29] (Fig. 18.4). Hence following the trend is more useful than are isolated measurements. The urine–plasma urea ratio and urine–plasma creatinine index were initially introduced as methods of evaluating patients with suspected acute tubular necrosis (ATN). These ratios have been subsequently shown to lack reliability.[30]

Creatinine clearance, as determined by 24-h urine collection, gives a more accurate estimate of GFR. Abbreviated 2-h creatinine clearance appears to correlate well with the traditional method.[31] Creatinine clearance may be used to distinguish ATN from prerenal azotemia. A creatinine clearance of < 25 mL min^{-1} over 1 h appears to be a reliable early predictor of renal impairment in the postoperative period.[32] Creatinine clearance may be estimated preoperatively from the serum creatinine levels with reasonable accuracy using the following formula:

$$\text{Creatinine clearance} = [(140 - \text{age}) \times \text{body weight in kg}] / [72 \times \text{serum creatinine}]$$

Tests of tubular function

Urine specific gravity and osmolality are used to assess the concentrating capacity of renal tubules. For each 0.01 increase in urine specific gravity, the urine osmolality increases by approximately 400 mosmol kg^{-1} of H_2O above plasma osmolality ($\pm$ 200 mosmol kg^{-1} of H_2O).[33] If tubular

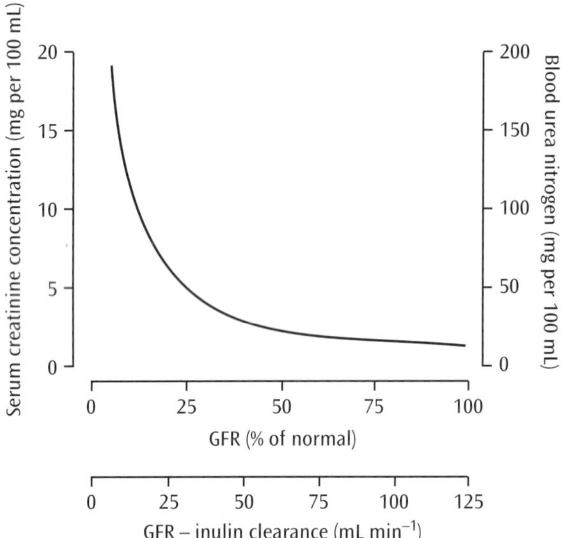

Figure 18.4 *Relation between glomerular filtration rate (GFR) and serum creatinine and blood urea nitrogen concentrations. This curve represents average values from the clinical assessment of renal function (with permission from Valtin,[29] p. 206).*

damage occurs, as in ATN, urine osmolality and specific gravity will be low (< 350 mosmol kg^{-1} of H_2O and 1.010 respectively) as compared with prerenal azotemia, in which urine osmolality and specific gravity are elevated (> 500 mosmol kg^{-1} of H_2O and 1.030 respectively). The concentrating ability of renal tubules may also be affected by lack of ADH (diabetes insipidus) or nephrogenic diabetes insipidus, which can occur with fluoride nephrotoxicity, osmotic diuretics, hypokalemia, and hypercalcemia.

Urinary sodium of > 40 mequiv L^{-1} or fractional excretion of sodium (FE_{Na}) > 1.0 occurs as a result of a fall in the concentrating capacity of the renal tubules and is indicative of ATN. On the other hand, in prerenal azotemia ADH-induced sodium reabsorption leads to a decrease in urinary sodium to < 20 mequiv L^{-1} or FE_{Na} to < 1.0. Although these tests of tubular function have some diagnostic value, they are of little value in the early prediction of renal failure.[30]

Urine output

Measurement of urine output is important in certain situations in which anuria can develop due to impaired renal blood flow or urinary tract obstruction. However, urine output is not always a reliable indicator of the adequacy of renal perfusion. This is especially true intraoperatively, when several other factors such as fluctuating levels of renin, aldosterone, ADH, catacholamines, and other hemodynamic variations are involved. Intraoperative oliguria, as opposed to anuria, is not a reliable sign of pending renal dysfunction and does not correlate with changes in BUN, serum creatinine, creatinine clearance, or with histologic evidence of ATN.[27,34]

Other tests of renal function include evaluation for hematuria, proteinuria and analysis of urinary sediment. Proteinuria and red cell casts are indicative of glomular disease. Tubular cells, tubular cell casts, and granular casts are seen in the urinary sediment in ATN. Intravenous tests, urography, renal ultrasound, and renal biopsy may also be performed to diagnose renal pathology.

ANESTHESIA, SURGERY, AND THE KIDNEY

General anesthesia and renal function

Anesthesia in general results in a decrease in renal blood flow and a small reduction in GFR. This in turn may decrease the elimination of polar substances. In patients with already compromised renal function, anesthesia may lead to the prolongation of certain drug effects.

Volatile anesthetic agents

Hemodynamic changes associated with volatile anesthetic agents produce dose-dependent reductions in renal blood flow, GFR, and hence urine output. This reduction in GFR and renal blood flow can be attenuated by preoperative hydration, which presumably helps to maintain better renal perfusion.[35] Volatile anesthetics do not interfere with the autoregulation of renal blood flow.

The second untoward effect is due to fluoride ion nephrotoxicity resulting from the metabolism of fluorinated volatile anesthetic agents. Fluoride-induced nephrotoxicity depends on the volatile agent used and the duration of exposure. It is manifested by an inability to concentrate urine in response to ADH, leading to polyuria, hypernatremia, and increased serum osmolality. Postoperative renal failure from the nephrotoxic effects of fluoride ions are associated with the use of methoxyflurane.[36,37] Metabolism of enflurane is associated with the production of substantially lower levels of fluoride ions,[38] although prolonged administration of enflurane [9.6 h at minimum alveolar concentration (MAC)] has been shown to decrease concentrating ability.[39] Excretion of fluoride is dependent on GFR; however, a study including a large series of patients with chronic renal disease failed to show any adverse renal effects after enflurane administration.[40] Nevertheless, there are reports of renal failure following enflurane anesthesia.[41–43] Obesity is associated with higher fluoride ion production following enfurane anesthesia,[44] but a higher incidence of renal failure has not been reported in these patients. Similarly, despite elevated plasma inorganic fluoride levels after sevoflurane anesthesia, there are no reports of clinically significant nephrotoxicity, even after repeated administration.[45] This may be due to the lack of renal biotransformation of sevoflurane as compared with methoxyflurane.[46] Halothane, isoflurane, and desflurane do not undergo significant defluorination.[39,47,48]

Intravenous anesthetic agents

Central nervous system depressant effects of intravenous anesthetic agents are exaggerated in patients with renal failure for various reasons:

1 increased unbound drug levels, due to low serum albumin, or displacement by nitrogenous waste products;[49,50]
2 higher drug concentration in the central nervous system as a result of an altered blood–brain barrier in uremia;[51]
3 acidosis, which may also increase the nonionized form of the drugs whose pK is close to the physiologic value.[52]

Thiopental is extensively protein bound and the induction dose of thiopental may be reduced in uremic patients. The central nervous system effects of thiopental also appear to be prolonged in proportion to the degree of uremia.[53]

The hemodynamics and pharmacokinetics of a single bolus or infusion of propofol do not appear to be altered in uremic patients.[54] Although the free fraction of etomidate is increased in patients with renal failure, this does not appear to have any significant clinical effect.[55] Ketamine may be associated with a deterioration in coexisting hypertension[56] and cause tachycardia in patients in whom renal disease is associated with hypertension or coronary artery disease. Therefore, ketamine should be avoided. Benzodiazepines are used by anesthesiologists as sedatives and occasionally induction agents. An increased free fraction of these drugs, due to decreased protein binding, increased central nervous system sensitivity, and an accumulation of renal active metabolites can occur in patients with ESRD, thereby prolonging the clinical effect of benzodiazepines.[57,58]

The decreased protein binding of morphine in patients with renal failure may result in a higher plasma free drug level. Also, a potent active metabolite, morphine 6-glucuronide can accumulate in these patients predisposing them to respiratory depression.[57,59] Repeated doses of meperidine are not recommended because of the risk of nervous system toxicity due to the accumulation of its renal excreted metabolite normeperidine. Fentanyl has a short half-life and its metabolites are inactive. Therefore, it appears to be a good choice in patients with renal disease.[57] Except for a slightly decreased protein binding, the free drug volume of distribution and clearance of alfentanil appear to be unaffected by the presence of chronic renal failure.[60] Postoperative respiratory depression has been reported in a patient with chronic renal failure receiving sufentanyl.[61]

Muscle relaxants

Depolarizing neuromuscular blocking agents

Succinylcholine is the agent of choice for rapid-sequence induction. A dose of 1 mg succinylcholine per kg body weight results in the serum potassium inreasing by 0.5–0.7 mequiv L^{-1} in normal patients.[62,63] This rise in serum potassium is not exaggerated in patients with renal failure, with the exception of some cases associated with uremic neuropathy.[64] Therefore, in the majority of patients with renal failure, a single dose of succinylcholine is considered safe provided that serum potassium level is below 5.5 mequiv L^{-1}. The duration of action of succinylcholine does not appear to be significantly prolonged in renal failure.

Nondepolarizing neuromuscular blocking agents

The short-acting nondepolarizing muscle relaxant mivacurium is metabolized by plasma cholinesterase at a slower rate than succinylcholine. As plasma cholinesterase levels are reduced in ESRD, the duration of neuromuscular blockade is prolonged.[65] In comparison with healthy patients, anephric patients require much lower mivacurium infusion rates to produce the same degree of muscle relaxation.[66]

The intermediate-acting nondepolarizing muscle relaxants, atracurium and its derivative cisatracurium, appear to be the neuromuscular blocking agents of choice for ESRD patients. These agents undergo Hofmann's degradation with only minimal excretion by the kidney in healthy individuals. ESRD does not prolong the clinical effect of these neuromuscular blocking agents,[67,68] even when given by a constant infusion over several days. The risk of seizures from laudanosine accumulation has not been reported, even after continuous infusion of atracurium in patients with multiorgan failure.[69]

Approximately 20–30% of vecuronium is excreted by the kidney. Potentiation of neuromuscular blockade with vecuronium has been reported in patients with renal failure,[70] therefore in patients with ESRD the normal intubation and maintenance doses need to be reduced and the dosing interval increased. Furthermore, a continuous infusion is not recommended in anephric patients because of the accumulation of the active metabolite 3-desacetyl vecuronium.[71] Rocuronium, which has a rapid onset of action, exhibits great variability in the duration of neuromuscular blockade in patients with ESRD.[72]

The longer-acting nondepolarizing muscle relaxants, such as *d*-tubocurarine, metocurine, pancuronium, doxacurium, and pipercuronium, have all been shown to have an increased elimination half-life, reduced clearance, and a prolonged duration of blockade in patients with ESRD,[73–76] and are generally avoided in such patients.

Both anticholinergic drugs (atropine, glycopyrrolate) and the anticholinesterase drugs (neostigmine and edrophonium) undergo significant renal excretion. Therefore, the duration of action of these drugs will also be prolonged in patients with renal failure.

Regional anesthesia and renal function

Epidural and spinal anesthesia both result in decreases in GFR and renal plasma flow, which appear to parallel the decreases in mean arterial pressure and peripheral vascular resistance as a consequence of sympathetic blockade.[77] These changes, however, are of little clinical significance in adequately hydrated normotensive patients. Impaired coagulation in uremic patients may be a concern while performing regional anesthesia.

Brachial plexus blockade is often performed to allow construction of AV fistulas. An earlier suggestion that the duration of brachial plexus anesthesia was reduced in patients with ESRD has not been supported by more recent studies.[78,79] No difference in the speed of onset and duration of anesthesia was found compared with normal controls. Even though the plasma clearance of local anesthetics appears to be unaffected by the presence of renal failure,[80] metabolic acidosis and hyperkalemia may increase susceptibility to local anesthetic toxicity.[81]

SURGERY AND RENAL FUNCTION

Surgical stress response occurs even in well-anesthetized patients, leading to elevated plasma levels of catacholamines, angiotensin, aldosterone, and ADH. Urine output is frequently reduced as a result. Blood loss, fluid shifts, and occult fluid loss may lead to a prerenal oliguric state. Intrarenal redistribution of blood away from the outer cortex occurs under such situations. Injury or vasospasm of the renal artery during the surgery may further decrease renal blood flow.

Certain surgical procedures may, in particular, impose ischemic risk to the kidney. Such procedures involve either complete or partial interruption of renal blood flow, as occurs during aortic surgery and cardiopulmonary bypass. Infrarenal aortic cross-clamping causes a reduction in renal blood flow which may lead to renal dysfunction.[82] Emboli, both particulate and gaseous, cross-clamp time, and intraoperative hemodynamic instability[11] may contribute to ischemic renal injury. Renal hypoperfusion during cardiopulmonary bypass for cardiac surgery causes renal dysfunction in up to 5% of patients.[10,83] Duration of cardiopulmonary bypass, pre-existing renal disease, and left ventricular dysfunction appear to correlate with renal injury. Patients having emergency surgery, especially trauma victims, appear to be at a high risk of renal failure.

There are no conclusive outcome data regarding the prophylactic role of mannitol or "renal dose" dopamine in preventing renal dysfunction after aortic surgery. Mannitol has been shown to reduce subclinical renal injury following infrarenal aortic aneurysm repair.[84] Renal dose dopamine appears to improve renal blood flow, GFR, and creatinine clearance.[85] Other agents that increase renal blood flow, such as ANP, prostaglandin E, and calcium channel blockers, are currently being investigated for their prophylaxis against acute renal failure (ARF).

ANESTHETIC IMPLICATIONS IN RENAL DISEASE

Preoperative evaluation

Preoperative evaluation of patients with renal insufficiency includes assessment of the stability of renal function and detection of any acute deterioration from baseline. In anephric patients, the aim is detection and preoperative management of the systemic abnormalities that commonly occur in these patients. Problems with previous general anesthetic procedures (residual postoperative weakness, excessive bleeding, etc.) should be noted. The patient's weight and vital signs should be correlated with the dialysis records. This, as well as the time that has elapsed from the previous hemodialysis treatment, gives an indication of the extracellular fluid volume status. Previous records also suggest the range of blood pressures and heart rate that the patient can tolerate. The site of a functional AV fistula should be noted. Particular attention should be paid to the following laboratory tests.

Hemoglobin/hematocrit

Hematocrit values on the low side, between 25% and 30%, are routinely encountered in patients with ESRD and appear to be tolerated well.[86] Red cell transfusions are associated with several disadvantages (viral infections, hyperkalemia, volume overload, etc.) and are not routinely indicated for these patients. The preoperative hematocrit value should be compared with values in the dialysis records and any significant acute decrease should be investigated. If anemia is poorly tolerated (as in the case of an acute decrease in hematocrit or in the presence of associated systemic disease, e.g. cardiac disease), blood transfusion should not be withheld for the fear of sensitization to histocompatibility antigens. Anemic patients with ESRD may not be able to tolerate blood loss in excess of 500 mL.

Electrolyte and acid–base status

Potassium, sodium, bicarbonate, and BUN should be checked on the day of the surgery. Hyperkalemia (>5.5 mequiv L^{-1}), hyponatremia (<125 mequiv L^{-1}), hypoalbuminemia, and acidosis (low bicarbonate levels) all indicate inadequate dialysis in anephric patients. Hyperkalemia is the most serious electrolyte abnormality in patients with renal failure. Even if dialysis has been performed within 24 h of surgery, serum potassium should be measured before induction of anesthesia as hyperkalemia can occur rapidly. When surgery cannot be delayed until hemodialysis is accomplished, administration of intravenous glucose with insulin, or calcium, may be useful in decreasing transiently the extracellular potassium levels and maintaining normal cardiac function. Hyperventilation after intubation can also lower serum potassium levels by about 0.5 mequiv L^{-1} for every 10 mmHg (1.3 kPa) decrease in P_aCO_2. In emergency situations, if severe acidosis exists, intravenous bicarbonate should be given very slowly to partially correct the acidosis, keeping in mind that rapid correction may precipitate overt symptoms of hypocalcemia. If serum bicarbonate levels are very low (12–15 mequiv L^{-1}), other causes of anion gap acidosis should be sought (e.g. ketoacidosis). Decreased excretion of glucose by the kidneys can make blood glucose control a challenge, particularly in diabetic patients. Furthermore, an increase in blood glucose level leads to a concomitant elevation of serum potassium levels.[87]

Patients with BUN levels >100 mg dL^{-1} also have a higher incidence of serious bleeding complications in the perioperative period.[88] Dialysis performed 12–24 h preoperatively helps to remove waste products and excess fluid and to correct hyperkalemia, hyponatremia, and acidosis.

Coagulation profile

Hemodialysis partially corrects platelet dysfunction and should be performed within 24 h of the planned surgical procedure. In a patient with a history of bleeding, administration of desmopressin (0.3 μg kg^{-1} intravenously over 30 min or intranasal spray at 3μg kg^{-1}) may also be considered. It may shorten the BT for up to 4 h. If a prolonged effect is desired, especially before elective surgery, conjugated estrogens may be given. Repeated daily administration of conjugated estrogens for 2–4 days decreases BT within 6 h and for up to 3–14 days.[21] Cryoprecipitate is rarely used because of the risk of infection. Prothrombin time (PT) and partial thromboplastin time (PTT) are normal in patients with chronic renal failure and any abnormalities in PT or PTT should be investigated.

Electrocardiography

Evidence of myocardial ischemia should be sought. Electrocardiogram (ECG) in patients with renal failure often reveals cardiac enlargement, arrhythmias, conduction abnormalities, and arrhythmias due to electrolyte disorders and drug toxicities (e.g. digitalis).

Chest radiograph

A chest radiograph must always be obtained in a patient with chronic renal failure. Evidence of pulmonary congestion or edema, infection, or pleural or pericardial effusion should be sought.

PREMEDICATION

Sedatives and *anxiolytics* may be considered, but caution must be exercised when these are used in patients with ESRD. Benzodiazepines are among the most common sedative premedicants used by anesthesiologists. If benzodiazepines are used in patients with renal dysfunction, the dose should be reduced and repeated doses should be avoided to prevent excessive and prolonged sedation.

Metoclopramide may be used preoperatively to counteract the delayed gastric emptying in uremic patients. The use of cytoprotective agents is also recommended to prevent the development of perioperative stress ulcers. Among the H_2-receptor blocking agents, ranitidine is the preferred agent, although the dose needs to be appropriately reduced. Particulate antacids should be avoided just prior to induction.

Steroid cover may be indicated in the perioperative period for patients already on chronic steroid therapy. As the long-term use of steroids can impair the stress response, a higher dose of steroids may be required in the perioperative period.

Antimuscarinic agents such as *atropine* and *glycopyrrolate* are both excreted to a certain extent by the kidneys, and their effect can be prolonged in renal failure. Therefore, their use for premedication should be restricted to specific indications (bronchoscopy, fiberoptic intubation, oral surgery). Only a minimal amount of scopolamine is excreted by the kidney and its use may be considered in patients with impaired renal function.[52]

VENOUS ACCESS

In patients on immunosuppression therapy and in those with ESRD, strict aseptic techniques should be used during intravenous cannulation to avoid the complications of infection. Patients undergoing dialysis also have a higher incidence of blood-borne infections (i.e. hepatitis).[89] Therefore, anesthesiologists must take appropriate protective measures to avoid becoming infected. Intravenous cannulas should not be inserted at the extremity of the AV fistula. Patients with previous central venous hemodialysis cannulas may develop stenosis of those vessels, making future central venous access at those sites difficult.

MONITORS

The ECG is helpful for detecting ischemia and conduction abnormalities or arrhythmias, especially those associated with hyperkalemia. Care should be taken not to place the blood pressure cuff on the same extremity as the AV fistula. AV fistulas should be protected to minimize the risk of thrombosis. Monitoring AV fistula patency during the intraoperative period has also been recommended. Arterial cannulation for blood pressure monitoring may be required in unstable patients. If arteries need to be preserved for AV fistula creation, dorsalis pedis or temporal artery cannulation may be performed. Optimal fluid management may require central venous or pulmonary artery pressure monitoring. A peripheral nerve stimulator is useful when the dose of muscle relaxants is altered in order to avoid prolonged neuromuscular blockade.

INDUCTION

Uremic patients often have an exaggerated hypotensive response on induction, regardless of their volume status. Ascertaining adequate intravascular volume status prior to induction decreases this hypotensive response. Rapid-sequence induction is the preferred method because of delayed gastric emptying and the risk of aspiration. If succinylcholine is contraindicated, a nondepolarizing muscle relaxant that does not depend on the kidney for clearance may be used. Largnyoscopy should be brief. Prolonged periods of apnea may lead to respiratory acidosis, which may then exacerbate the hyperkalemia. After intubation, compensatory hyperventilation in acidotic patients may protect against dangerous levels of hyperkalemia.[90] Inhalational induction has been described[91] but is generally not preferred.

MAINTENANCE OF ANESTHESIA

Anesthesia is generally maintained with the combination of nitrous oxide and a volatile inhalational anesthetic agent. Enflurane and sevoflurane are best avoided in patients with impaired renal function. This avoids the possibility of further a deterioration in renal function from the nephrotoxic effects of inorganic fluoride. However, in anephric patients this is not an issue. An opioid, such as fentanyl, and an intermediate-acting muscle relaxant, preferably atracuricum or cisatracuricum, may be used in conjunction with inhalational agents.

Maintenance of anesthesia by mask should be avoided because of the gastrointestinal effects of uremia mentioned earlier. Mechanical ventilation should be adjusted to avoid hypoventilation as respiratory acidosis can accentuate hyperkalemia. On the other hand, hyperventilation may also be undesirable in anemic patients. Respiratory alkalosis resulting from hyperventilation shifts the oxyhemoglobin dissociation curve to the left, thus effecting the unloading of oxygen to the tissues. An increase in the intrathoracic pressure during mechanical ventilation can decrease cardiac output. This can cause further deterioration in renal function by decreasing perfusion to the kidneys, which already have limited reserve. This untoward effect of mechanical ventilation can be avoided by making appropriate adjustment in respiratory rate, tidal volume, and IE ratio. Intraoperative hypertension can generally be controlled by adjusting the depth of anesthesia with a volatile agent. If this is not effective, then vasodilators, such as nitroprusside or hydralazine, may be used. Cyanide toxicity following nitroprusside infusion is unlikely in patients with renal failure.[92] This is probably because of the decreased renal excretion of thiosulfate, which facilitates conversion of cyanide to thiocyanate. Occasionally, hypotension refractory to volume repletion may occur in dialysis patients. This is generally due to autonomic dysfunction and is treated with norepinephrine.[93]

In patients with pre-existing renal impairment, the goal should be the preservation of renal function. Oliguria should be recognized and treated promptly to avoid the development of ARF. If anuria occurs intraoperatively, mechanical obstruction of the urinary catheter should be ruled out. A rapid intravenous bolus of 500 mL of 0.9% saline should be administered. If intravenous volume is judged to be adequate, a small dose of furosemide (0.1 $mg\,kg^{-1}$) may sometimes be effective if oliguria is due to ADH release. If urine output does not increase in response to intravascular fluid administration, invasive monitors may need to be used (central venous line or pulmonary artery catheter) to adequately assess the intravascular volume status and cardiac output. Once the filling pressures are optimized, dopamine at 1–2 $mg\,kg^{-1}\,min^{-1}$ may increase renal blood flow and urine output.[85,94] Higher doses of dopamine (5 $mg\,kg^{-1}\,min^{-1}$) may be used to improve cardiac performance and indirectly improve urine output. Furosemide, dopamine, and mannitol are generally used, either alone or in combination, during procedures involving reduction or interruption of blood flow to the kidneys.

POSTOPERATIVE CARE

The recovery room nurse should be informed of the site of an AV fistula to prevent inadvertent placement of a blood pressure cuff on the same arm. If hypertension is due to hypervolemia, hemodialysis is indicated. However, vasodilators may be used until hemodialysis can be performed.

Hyperkalemia usually occurs in the first 24 h postoperatively and is one of the most common complications in patients under dialysis. Serum potassium levels should be obtained in the recovery room. Continuous ECG monitoring is helpful for the detection of ischemia and conduction abnormalities related to electrolyte disturbances.

Recurarization, though rare, should be considered if the patient shows signs of skeletal muscle weakness. It usually improves with a small additional dose of anticholinesterase agent combined with an anticholinergic agent.

Parenteral opioids should be used with caution because of the increased central nervous system sensitivity to its depressant effects. Patient-controlled analgesia (PCA) with fentanyl, is the preferred method of pain control for patients with compromised renal function. Regional techniques for postoperative analgesia may also be used in the absence of coagulation abnormalities.

REFERENCES

1. Guyton AC, Hall JE. Urine formation by the kidneys. In: Guyton AC, Hall JE (eds). *Textbook of Medical Physiology,* 9th edn. Philadelphia, PA: WB Saunders, 1996: 315–48.
2. Barger AC, Herd JA. The renal circulation. *N Engl J Med* 1971; **284:** 482–90.
3. Brezis M, Rosen S. Hypoxia of the renal medulla: its implications for disease. *N Engl J Med* 1995; **332:** 647–55.
4. Mirenda JV, Grissom TE. Anesthetic implications of the renin–angiotensin system and angiotensin-converting enzyme inhibitors. *Anesth Analg* 1991; **72:** 667–83.
5. Espiner EA. Physiology of naturetic peptides. *J Intern Med* 1994; **235:** 527–41.
6. Awazu M, Ichikawa I. Biological significance of atrial natriuretic peptide in the kidney. *Nephron* 1993; **63:**1–14.
7. Mene P, Dunn MJ. Vascular, glomerular and tubular effects of angiotensin II, kinins, and protaglandins. In: Seldin DW, Giesbisch G (eds). *The Kidney: Physiology and Pathophysiology*, 2nd edn. New York: Raven Press, 1992: 1205–48.
8. Satosh S, Zimmerman, BG. Influence of renin–angiotensin system on the effect of prostaglandin synthesis inhibitors in the renal vasculature. *Circ Res* 1975; **36** (Suppl. 1): 89–96.
9. Badr KF, Ichikawa I. Prerenal failure: a deleterious shift from renal compensation to decompensation. *N Engl J Med* 1988; **319:** 623–9.
10. Abel RM, Buckley MJ, Austen WG, *et al.* Etiology, incidence and prognosis of renal failure following cardiac operations. *J Thorac Cardiovasc Surg* 1976; **71:** 323–33.
11. Olsen PS, Schroeder T, Perko MJ, *et al.* Renal failure after operation for abdominal aortic aneurysm. *Ann Vasc Surg* 1990; **4:** 580–3.
12. Moore RD, Smith CR, Lipsky JJ, *et al.* Risk factors for nephrotoxicity in patients with aminoglycosides. *Ann Intern Med* 1984; **100:** 352–7.
13. Byrd L, Sherman RL. Radiocontrast-induced acute renal failure. A clinical and pathophysiological review. *Medicine* 1979; **58:** 270–9.

14. Shusterman N, Strom BL, Murray TG, *et al.* Risk factors and outcome of hospital-acquired acute renal failure. *Am J Med* 1987; **83:** 65–71.
15. Meyer RD. Risk factors and comparison of clinical nephrotoxicity of amioglycosides. *Am J Med* 1986; **80** (Suppl. 6B):119–25.
16. Berkseth RO, Kjellstrand CM. Radiologic contact-induced nephropathy. *Med Clin North Am* 1984; **68:** 351–70.
17. Stillman MT, Napier J, Blackshear JL. Adverse effects of nonsteroidal anti-inflammatory drugs on the kidney. *Med Clin North Am* 1984; **68:** 371–85.
18. Wardle EN. Acute renal failure and multiorgan failure. *Nephron* 1994; **66:** 380–5.
19. Novis BK, Roizen MF, Aronson S, Thisted RA. Association of preoperative risk factors with postoperative acute renal failure. *Anesth Analg* 1994; **78:** 143–9.
20. Fisher JW. Mechanisms of the anemia of chronic renal failure. *Nephron* 1980; **25:** 106–11.
21. Zachee P, Vermylen J, Boogaerts MA. Hematologic aspects of end-stage renal failure. *Ann Hematol* 1994; **69:** 33–40.
22. Hambley H, Mufti GH. Erythropoetin: an old friend revisited. *Br Med J* 1990; **300:** 621–2.
23. Broyer M. Demography of dialysis and transplantation in Europe, 1984. Report from the European Dialysis and Transplant Association Registry. *Nephrol Dial Transplantation* 1986; **1:** 1–8.
24. Lindner A, Charra B, Sherrard DJ, Scribner BH. Accelerated atherosclerosis in prolonged maintenance hemodialysis. *N Engl J Med* 1974; **290:** 697–701.
25. Rostand SG, Gretes JC, Kirk KA, *et al.* Ischemic heart disease in patients with uremia undergoing maintenance hemodialysis. *Kidney Int* 1979; **16:** 600–11.
26. Kuruvila KC, Schrier RW. Chronic renal failure. *Int Anesth Clin* 1984; **22:** 101–20.
27. Palder SB, Kirkman RL, Whittemore AD, *et al.* Vascular access for hemodialysis: patency rates and results of revision. *Ann Surg* 1985; **202:** 235–9.
28. Pinson CW, Schuman ES, Gross GF, *et al.* Surgery in long term dialysis patients: experience with more than 300 cases. *Am J Surg* 1986; **151:** 567–71.
29. Valtin H. Clinical assessment of renal function. In: Valtin H (ed.). *Renal Dysfunction: Mechanisms Involved in Fluid and Solute Imbalance.* Boston: Little, Brown & Co, 1979: 199–226.
30. Kellen M, Aronson S, Roizen MF, *et al.* Predictive anddiagnostic tests of renal failure: a review. *Anesth Analg* 1994; **78:** 134–42.
31. Sladen RN, Endo E, Harrison T. Two hour versus 22-hour creatinine clearance in critically ill patients. *Anesthesiology* 1987; **67:** 1013–6.
32. Shin B, Mackenzie CF, Helrich M. Creatinine clearance for early detection of post traumatic renal dysfunction. *Anesthesiology* 1986; **64:** 605–9.
33. Preibe H. Evaluation of renal function. *Int Anesthesiol Clin* 1984; **22:** 121–35.
34. Knos CB, Berry AJ, Isaacson IJ, Weitz FI. Intraoperative urinary output and postoperative blood urea nitrogen and creatinine levels in patients undergoing aortic reconstructive surgery. *J Clin Anesth* 1989; **1:** 181–5.
35. Barry KG, Mazze RI, Schwartz FD. Prevention of surgical oliguria and renal hemodynamic suppression by sustained hydration. *N Engl J Med* 1964; **270:** 1371–7.
36. Cousins MJ, Mazze RI. Methoxyflurane nephrotoxicity – a study of dose response in man. *J Am Med Assoc* 1973; **225:** 1611–6.
37. Crandell WB, Pappas SG, MacDonald A. Nephrotoxicity associated withmethoxyflurane anesthesia. *Anesthesiology* 1966; **27:** 591–607.
38. Cousins MJ, Greenstein LR, Hitt BA, Mazze RI. Metabolism and renal effects of enflurane in man. *Anesthesiology* 1976; **44:** 44–53.
39. Mazze RI, Calverley RK, Smith T. Inorganic fluoride nephrotoxicity: prolonged enflurane and halothane anesthesia in volunteers. *Anesthesiology* 1977; **46:** 265–71.
40. Creasser C, Stoelting RK. Serum inorganic fluoride concentration during and after halothane, fluroxene and methoxyflurane anesthesia in man. *Anesthesiology* 1973; **39:** 537–40.
41. Eichhorn JH, Hedley-Whyte J, Steinman TI, *et al.* Renal failure following enflurane anesthesia. *Anesthesiology* 1976; **45:** 557–60.
42. Loehning RW, Mazze RI. Possible nephrotoxicity from enflurane in a patient with severe renal disease. *Anesthesiology* 1974; **40:** 203–5.
43. Hartnett MN, Lane W, Bennett WM. Non-oliguric renal failure and enflurane. *Ann Intern Med* 1974; **81:** 560.
44. Miller MS, Gandolfi AJ, Vaughan RW, Bentley JB. Disposition of enflurane in obese patients. *J Pharmacol Exp Ther* 1980; **215:** 292–6.
45. Nishiyama T, Hanaoka K. Inorganic fluoride kinetics and renal and hepatic function after repeated sevoflurane anesthesia. *Anesth Analg* 1998; **87:** 468–76.
46. Kharasch ED, Hankins DC, Thummel KE. Human kidney methoxyflurane and sevoflurane metabolism. Intrarenal fluoride production as a possible mechanism of methoxyflurane nephrotoxicity. *Anesthesiology* 1995; **82:** 689–99.
47. Mazze RI, Cousins, MJ, Barr GA. Renal effects and metabolism of isoflurane in man. *Anesthesiology* 1974; **40:** 536–42.
48. Koblin DD. Characteristics and implications of desflurane metabolism and toxicity. *Anesth Analg* 1992; **75:** S10–S16.
49. Ghoneim MM, Pandya H. Plasma protein binding of thiopental in patients with impaired renal or hepatic function. *Anesthesiology* 1975; **42:** 545–9.
50. Burch PG, Stanski DR. Decreased protein binding and thiopental kinetics. *Clin Pharmacol Ther* 1982; **32:** 212–17.
51. Freeman RB, Sheff MF, Maher JF, Schreiner GE. The blood–cerebrospinal fluid barrier in uremia. *Ann Intern Med* 1962; **56:** 233–40.
52. Müller MC. Anesthesia for the patient with renal dysfunction. *Int Anesthesiol Clin* 1984; **22:** 169–87.
53. Dundee JW, Richards RK. Effect of azotemia upon the action of intravenous barbiturate anesthesia. *Anesthesiology* 1954; **15:** 333–46.
54. Kirvela M, Olkkola KT, Rosenberg PH, *et al.* Pharmacokinetics of propofol and hemodynamic changes during induction of anesthesia in uraemic patients. *Br J Anesth* 1992; **68:** 178–82.
55. Carlos R, Calvo R, Erill S: Plasm protein binding of etomidate in patients with renal failure or hepatic cirrhosis. *Clin Pharmacokinet* 1979; **4:** 144–8.
56. White PF, Way WL, Trevor AJ. Ketamine – its pharmacologic and therapeutic uses. *Anesthesiology* 1982; **56:** 119–36.
57. Sears JW. Kidney transplants: induction and analgesic agents. *Int Anesthesiol Clin* 1995; **33:** 45–68.
58. Schmith VD, Piraino B, Smith RB, Kroboth PD. Aprazolam in end-stage renal disease. II. Pharmacodynamics. *Clin Pharmacol Ther* 1992; **51:** 533–40.
59. Sear JW, Hand CW, Moore RA, McQuay HJ. Studies on morphine disposition: influence of renal failure on the kinetics of morphine and its metabolites. *Br J Anaesth* 1989; **62:** 28–32.
60. Chauvin M, Lebrault C, Levron JC, Duvaldestin P. Pharmacokinetics of alfentanyl in chronic renal failure. *Anesth Analg* 1987; **66:** 53–6.
61. Wiggum DC, Cork RC, Weldon ST, *et al.* Post operative respiratory depression and elevated sufentanil levels in a patient with chronic renal failure. *Anesthesiology* 1985; **63:** 708–10.
62. Koide M, Waud BE. Serum potassium concentrations after succinylcholine in patients with renal failure. *Anesthesiology* 1972; **36:** 142–5.
63. Miller RD, Way WL, Hamilton WK, Layzer RB. Succinylcholine induced hyperkalemia in patients with renal failure. *Anesthesiology* 1972; **36:** 138–41.
64. Walton JD, Farman JV. Suxamethonium hyperkalemia in uraemic neuropathy. *Anaesthesia* 1973; **28:** 666–8.
65. Mangar D, Kirchhoff GT, Rose PL, Castellano FC. Prolonged neuromuscular block with mivacurium in a patient with end-stage renal disease. *Anesth Analg* 1993; **76:** 866–7.
66. Phillips BJ, Hunter JM. The use of mivacurium chloride by constant infusion in the anephric patient. *Br J Anaesth* 1992; **68:** 492–8.
67. Fahey MR, Rupp SM, Fisher DM, *et al.* The pharmacokinetics and pharmacodynamics of atracurium in patients with and without renal failure. *Anesthesiology* 1984; **61:** 699–702.
68. Boyd AH, Eastwood NB, Parker CJ, Hunter JM. Pharmacodynamics of the 1'R *cis* 1R *cis* isomer of atracurium (S1W89) in health and chronic renal failure. *Br J Anaesth* 1995; **74:** 400–4.
69. Shearer ES, O'Sullivan EP, Hunter JM. Clearance of atracurium and laudanosine in the urine and by continuous venovenous filtration. *Br J Anaesth* 1991; **67:** 569–73.
70. Lynam DP, Cronnelly R, Castagnoli KP, *et al.* The pharmacodynamics and pharmacokinetics of vecuronium in patients anesthetized with isoflurane with normal renal function or with renal failure. *Anesthesiology* 1988; **69:** 227–31.
71. Segredo V, Matthay MA, Sharma ML, *et al.* Prolonged neuromuscular blockade after long term administration of vecuronium in two critically ill patients. *Anesthesiology* 1990; **72:** 566–70.
72. Cooper RA, Maddineni VR, Mirakhur RK, *et al.* Time course of neuromuscular effects and pharmacokinetics of rocuronium bromide (ORA 9426) in patients with chronic renal failure. *Br J Anaesth* 1993; **71:** 222–6.
73. Riordan DD, Gilbertson AA. Prolonged curarization in a patient with renal failure. *Br J Anaesth* 1971; **43:** 506–8.
74. Smith CE, Hunter JM. Anesth for renal transplantation: relaxants and volatiles. *Int Anesthesiol Clin* 1995; **33** (2):69–92.
75. Cook DR, Freeman JA, Lai AA, *et al.* Pharmacokinetics and pharmacody-

namics of doxacurium in normal patients and in those with hepatic or renal failure. *Anesth Analg* 1991; **72:** 145–50.
76. Caldwell JE, Canfell PC, Castagnoli KP, *et al*. The influence of renal failure on the pharmacokinetics and the duration of action of pipercuronium bromide in patients anesthetized with halothane and nitrous oxide. *Anesthesiology* 1989; **70:** 7–12.
77. Kennedy Jr WF. Effects of spinal and peridural blocks on renal and hepatic functions. *Clin Anesth* 1969; **2:** 109–21.
78. Martin R, Beauregard L, Tétrault JP. Brachial plexus blockade and chronic renal failure. *Anesthesiology* 1988; **69:** 405–6.
79. McEllistrem RF, Schell J, O'Malley K, *et al*. Interscalene brachial plexus blockade with lidocaine in chronic renal failure – a pharmacokinetic study. *Can J Anaesth* 1989; **36:** 59–63.
80. Thomson PD, Rowland M, Melmon KL. The influence of heart failure, liver disease and renal failure on the disposition of lidocaine in man. *Am Heart J* 1971; **82:** 417–21.
81. Gould DB, Aldrete JA. Bupivicaine cardiotoxicity in a patient with renal failure. *Anesthesiol Scand* 1983; **27:** 18–21.
82. Welch M, Knight DG, Carr HM, *et al*. Influence of renal artery blood flow on renal function during aortic surgery. *Surgery* 1994; **115:** 46–51.
83. Hilberman M, Myers BD, Carrie BJ, *et al*. Acute renal failure following cardiac surgery. *J Thorac Cardiovasc Surg* 1979; **77:** 880–8.
84. Nicholson ML, Baker DM, Hopkinson BR, Wenham PW. Randomized controlled trial of the effect of mannitol on renal reperfusion injury during aortic aneurysm surgery. *Br J Surg* 1996; **83:** 1230–3.
85. Carcoana OV, Hines RL. Is renal dose dopamine protective or therapeutic? Yes. *Crit Care Clin* 1996; **12:** 677–85.
86. Lundin AP, Stein RA, Brown CD, *et al*. Fatigue, acid–base and electrolyte changes with exhaustive treadmill exercise in hemodialysis patients. *Nephron* 1987; **45:** 57–62.
87. Goldfarb S, Cox M, Singer I, Goldberg M. Acute hyperkalemia induced by hyperglycemia; hormonal mechanisms. *Ann Intern Med* 1976; **84:** 426–32.
88. Schreiner GE, Maher JF. The patient with chronic renal failure and surgery. *Am J Cardiol* 1963; **12:** 317–23.
89. Zeldis JB, Depner TA, Kuramoto IK, *et al*. The prevalence ofhepatitis C virus antibodies among hemodialysis patients. *Ann Int Med* 1990; **112:** 958–60.
90. Goggin MJ, Joekes AM. Gas exchange in renal failure. *Br Med J* 1971; **2:** 244–8.
91. Logan DA, Howie HB, Crawford J. Anesthesia and renal transplantation: 56 cases. *Br J Anesthesiol* 1974; **46:** 69–72.
92. Tinker JH, Michenfelder JD. Increased resistance to nitroprusside-induced cyanide toxicity in anuric dogs. *Anesthesiology* 1980; **50:** 40–7.
93. Kersh ES, Kronfield SJ, Unger A, *et al*. Autonomic insufficiency in uremia as a cause of hemodialysis-induced hypotension. *N Engl J Med* 1974; **290:** 650–3.
94. Henderson IS, Beattie TJ, Kennedy AC. Dopamine hydrochloride in oliguric states. *Lancet* 1980; **2:** 827–8.

19

Acid–base balance

MICHAEL G ADRAGNA AND E F KLEIN Jr

ACIDS AND BASES

A thorough understanding of acid–base balance in the human body is of vital importance to a clinician, for it is both an indicator of current processes occurring in a patient as well as an almost real-time predictor of the utility of critical therapies provided for that patient. Acid–base balance has a modifying effect on almost every drug we use and thus is fundamental to the scientific practice of medicine. Unfortunately, most clinicians find acid–base instruction and clinical use only marginally comprehensible and have often shied away from it whenever possible. This is partly because pH is defined and measured as the negative logarithm of the hydrogen ion concentration and in great part because of the widespread use of multiple, complex, overlapping, and often clinically irrelevant terms to describe acid–base status, such as "negative base excess," "bicarbonate," "standard bicarbonate," and "alkali reserve," as well as simply "pH." Similarly, "proton," "hydrogen ion," and "H^+" all mean the same thing.

The Bronsted–Lowry definition of acids and bases provides a simple and workable understanding of acid–base balance. In the simplest terms, acids are proton (H^+) donors and bases are proton (H^+) acceptors, i.e. an acid is a substance from which a proton can be removed and a base is a substance that can remove a proton from an acid. In solution, an acid (HA) will dissociate and form a hydrogen ion (H^+) and a base (A^-), as a result of the principle of mass action. This principle states that the products of a reaction on one side of the equation are proportional to the products of the reaction on the other side:

$$\mathrm{HA} \rightleftharpoons \mathrm{H^+} + \mathrm{A^-} \qquad (19.1)$$

The degree to which a certain acid will dissociate in solution is constant for that specific acid and is known as the dissociation constant. This can be expressed in the following formula:

$$\mathrm{HA} \underset{k_2}{\overset{k_1}{\rightleftharpoons}} \mathrm{H^+} + \mathrm{A^-} \qquad (19.2)$$

wherein the dissociation constant (k) determines the point at which equilibrium is reached in a specific equation.

Therefore, if k_1 is larger than k_2, the reaction will proceed preferentially toward the right and will result in more H^+ and A^- than HA. If, conversely, k_2 is larger, then there will be more HA than the amount of H^+ and A^- formed.

Henderson described it thus:

$$[\mathrm{H^+}] = K\,([\mathrm{HA}]/[\mathrm{A^-}]) \qquad (19.3)$$

where $K = k_1/k_2$, demonstrating that the hydrogen concentration [H^+] depends upon the dissociation constant K and the *ratio* of HA to A^-. Some years later, Hasselbalch modified Henderson's equation into a negative logarithm, solving for pH:

$$\mathrm{pH} = \mathrm{p}K_a + \log([\mathrm{A^-}]/[\mathrm{HA}]) \qquad (19.4)$$

where p = –log. pK_a is the negative logarithm of the dissociation constant of the acid and is the pH at which the acid is 50% dissociated, i.e. it is the pH at which there are equal concentrations of HA and A^- in the solution. The term pK_a serves to describe the strength of the acid, as stronger acids would dissociate more completely, weaker ones less so. However, since pH and pK_a are expressed numerically as the negative logarithms of the hydrogen ion concentrations, stronger acids have a lower numeric value and weaker ones a higher value. For example, lactic acid (pK_a = 3.9) is a stronger acid than carbonic acid (pK_a = 6.1) because, at any given pH, lactic acid will be more dissociated and therefore will release more H^+ than carbonic acid.

Acids and bases are defined not on the basis of their charges but upon their abilities to donate or accept protons (H^+), and, in fact, they may be positively or negatively charged, or may be neutral. Whether a substance acts as an acid (donating a proton) or a base (accepting a proton) depends on the concentration of that substance in solution (the pH) and the degree of dissociation of the substance (the pK).

THE pH SYSTEM

The pH system is a source of confusion for a great many clinicians. Unlike concentrations of most ions, which are usually expressed in a linear, positive numeric scale, pH is neither of these. The pH scale is logarithmic, not linear, and the number used to express pH becomes smaller as the H^+ concentration becomes greater. This seemingly counterintuitive system makes sense from an electrochemical point of view, but as clinicians we are trained to think in another manner and often find this very awkward. However, once understood, the concept is quite workable in the clinical setting. Some points to remember when considering the logarithmic vs. linear scales are:

1 The negative logarithmic scale means that there is a tenfold change

in hydrogen ion concentration for every one unit change in pH. As the pH decreases, the hydrogen ion concentration increases. Example: a solution with a pH of 4 has 10 times the hydrogen ion concentration of a solution with a pH of 5 and 100 times the hydrogen ion concentration of a solution with a pH of 6.

2 The same numeric changes along different portions of the pH scale create vastly different *nanomolar* concentrations of hydrogen ions, depending upon where on the scale those changes occur. Example: a change in pH from 5 to 6 requires a 100-fold greater ionic concentration change than a change in pH from 7 to 8.

3 While a nanomolar scale would be easier to visualize, the use of the pH system is deeply ingrained in the medical and scientific community and is the standard with which we function.

CLINICAL MEASUREMENT OF ACID–BASE STATUS

Clinical acid–base balance depends heavily upon the chemistry of buffers. A buffer is a solution containing both a weak acid (HA) and its base (A^-), having the ability to resist a change in pH upon addition of a strong acid or base. The buffer pair of greatest import in the extracellular fluid is carbonic acid (H_2CO_3) and bicarbonate (HCO_3^-). By convention, the interaction of this buffer pair serves as the basis for measurement of acid–base balance.

When CO_2 is added to water, the following reaction occurs:

$$H_2O + CO_2 \rightleftharpoons H_2CO_3 \rightleftharpoons H^+ + HCO_3^- \quad (19.5)$$

The initial reaction of CO_2 and H_2O producing carbonic acid is slow, requiring several minutes to reach equilibrium, and would be inadequate to enable gas exchange in the pulmonary capillaries if it were not for the accelerating effect of the catalytic enzyme carbonic anhydrase. This enzyme is found in tissue and erythrocytes but not in the plasma.

The second part of the above reaction shows the carbonic acid dissociating freely into bicarbonate and H^+. About 96% of the carbonic acid dissociates at physiologic pH.

Inserting the carbonic acid–bicarbonate reaction into the Henderson–Hasselbalch equation, we obtain:

$$pH = pK_a + \log([HCO_3^-]/[H_2CO_3]) \quad (19.6)$$

Since carbonic acid continuously and almost completely dissociates into H^+ and HCO_3^-, it is very difficult to measure accurately. Fortunately, it is fairly easy to accurately measure the amount of dissolved CO_2 in solution instead, described as α-P_{CO_2} [α is the solubility coefficient for CO_2, or 0.23 mmol L^{-1} kPa^{-1} (0.03 mmol L^{-1} mmHg^{-1}) at 37 °C]. Under physiologic conditions, the pK_a for this reaction is 6.1, although it is variable with temperature and pH. The equation for this reaction in plasma at 37 °C is:

$$pH = 6.1 + \log([HCO_3^-]/0.23\,P_{CO_2}) \quad (19.7)$$

There are several reasons for which this formula is clinically useful for the measurement of acid–base disturbances:

1 The formula includes acid–base disturbances caused by both metabolic (HCO_3^-) and respiratory (P_aCO_2) disorders. While the two disturbances *in vivo* are intimately intertwined and disturbances of one usually affect the other, a distinction between them is useful in characterizing most primary acid–base imbalances.

2 The value of any one of the single components of the Henderson–Hasselbalch equation (pH, P_{CO_2}, or HCO_3^- may be calculated if the values of the other two components are known. Commonly, serum bicarbonate is often a calculation derived from measurements of pH and P_aCO_2.

3 Most important is the fact that pH is determined not by the absolute values of HCO_3^- or P_{CO_2} but by the *ratio* of one to the other. Under normal conditions, the HCO_3^- is 24 mmol L^{-1}, the P_aCO_2 is 5.3 kPa (40 mmHg), and the ratio can be described. Multiplying the P_aCO_2 of 5.3 kPa by its coefficient of solubility in plasma (0.23 mmol L^{-1} kPa^{-1} or 0.03 mmol L^{-1} mmHg^{-1}), one obtains the ratio of 24/1.2 or 20:1. Since pH equals p*K* (6.1) plus log 20 (1.3), normal pH therefore equals 7.4. Increasing the ratio, either by increasing HCO_3^- or by decreasing P_aCO_2, results in a higher pH (alkalosis). Conversely, decreasing the ratio by a loss of HCO_3^- or an increase in P_aCO_2 results in a lower pH and therefore acidosis. Keep in mind that if both the HCO_3^- and the P_aCO_2 are increased (or decreased) *proportionally* to each other, the pH remains normal. This is the basis by which homeostasis is maintained in the face of changing levels of either HCO_3^- or P_aCO_2, i.e. as one of these factors either increases or decreases, homeostatic mechanisms modify the other one of these factors to maintain the normal ratio of one to the other.

PRODUCTION OF ACIDS

Volatile

Almost all acids in the body are created by metabolic processes, both normal and abnormal. Most acid is created by the formation of carbon dioxide in the mitochondria as an endproduct of carbohydrate metabolism. This gas is produced at an average rate of 200 mL min^{-1} or 288 L day^{-1}. The net daily production of acid in the form of carbon dioxide is 12 960 mequiv (the term mmol L^{-1} is not usually used for a gas). This gas is eliminated via the lungs, and therefore is referred to as "volatile" or "respiratory" acid.

Nonvolatile

Most metabolic or "nonvolatile" acids are created by protein degradation. Sulfuric acid (H_2SO_4) is a product of cysteine and methionine metabolism, hydrochloric acid (HCl) is a product of lysine, arginine, and histidine, and phosphoric acid ($H_2PO_4^-$) is derived from the normal metabolism of dietary phosphate. Some of this acid load is offset by the bicarbonate (HCO_3^-) production resulting from the metabolism of aspartate, glutamate, and some organic ions, such as citrate. The sum of these metabolic acids and bases results in a net balance of about 70 mmol day^{-1} of acid, or approximately 1 mmol kg^{-1} day^{-1}.

Although lactic acid is often used as a clinical marker of anaerobic metabolism from hypoxia, poor perfusion, or other disturbance of tissue oxygenation, it is important to realize that about 1400 mmol of lactic acid is produced each day normally, principally by skeletal muscle, red blood cells, and the skin. This lactic acid is then converted in the liver to form CO_2 and H_2O. A smaller amount of lactate is cleared by the kidney through renal excretion, oxidation, or conversion by gluconeogenesis.

Normal metabolism creates lactic acid, pyruvic acid, acetoacetic acid, and β-hydroxybutyric acid, and these acids are normally further degraded to CO_2 and H_2O. Derangements in their production or elimination can be seen in various disease states, such as diabetic ketoacidosis, anaerobic metabolism, etc. Inorganic acids (and others that are not degraded to CO_2) are excreted by the kidney and account for a normal loss of 1 mequiv kg^{-1} day^{-1} of H^+.

ACID–BASE HOMEOSTASIS

Acid–base homeostasis requires both elimination of acid and production or recovery of base to balance that small portion of acid that is normally not eliminated.

Despite these regulating mechanisms, the H^+ concentrations compatible with life can vary 10-fold from 16 to 160 nmol L^{-1} (pH 6.8–7.8). No other ion in the body has such a wide range of variability. The normal range of H^+ ion concentration is 35–40 nmol L^{-1} (pH 7.35–7.44).

There are three mechanisms that maintain this homeostasis:

1 buffering;
2 compensation;
3 correction.

Buffering is the use of a chemical buffer in the body to immediately minimize the change in pH due to an acid or base.

Compensation is the attempt to restore the HCO_3^-/P_aCO_2 ratio to normal by alteration of a nonderanged variable. For example, the retention of HCO_3^- would result in a downward adjustment of ventilation so as to retain CO_2 and maintain a normal acid–base ratio.

Correction refers to homeostasis regained simply by correction of the primary metabolic derangement responsible for the abnormality in pH.

Buffering systems

The normally narrow range of H^+ in the body is largely a result of the buffering systems of the body. These buffers are typically weak acids (H buffers) and their salts (Na buffers) with an ability to resist or minimize the change in H^+ with the addition of a stronger acid or base. Strong acids (HCl, for example) are buffered by the salts of a weak acid, as shown below:

$$\begin{aligned} &HCl + Na\ buffer \rightleftharpoons H^+ + Cl^- + Na^+ + \\ &Buffer^- \rightleftharpoons H\ buffer + NaCl \end{aligned} \quad (19.8)$$

In this example, the HCl is largely dissociated and the H^+, which it releases by its dissociation, combines with the dissociated buffer ion to produce the weak acid H buffer. Because H buffer is a weaker acid than HCl, it is less dissociated and therefore less H^+ is released by its dissociation than if the HCl was present alone in the solution without a buffer.

In the same way, a strong base such as sodium hydroxide (NaOH) is buffered by a weak acid:

$$\begin{aligned} &NaOH + H\ buffer \rightleftharpoons Na^+ + OH^- + H^+ + \\ &Buffer^- \rightleftharpoons Na\ Buffer + H_2O \end{aligned} \quad (19.9)$$

If it were not for the buffer, the dissociated OH^- from the strong base NaOH would combine with H^+, decreasing the concentration of H^+ and thereby raising the pH. Because the Na buffer is a weaker base than NaOH, it is less dissociated and thereby causes less of a change in the H^+ concentration.

To be maximally effective, a buffering system must be large enough to be able to buffer a large amount of H^+ and have a pK_a close to the initial pH of the solution to be buffered. Weaker acids and their salts are more effective buffers against strong acids and strong bases. Whereas there are many buffering systems in the body, the most important buffers are:

1 carbonic acid–bicarbonate;
2 hemoglobin;
3 protein;
4 phosphate.

The carbonic acid–bicarbonate buffer is predominant in the extracellular fluid, whereas the hemoglobin, protein, and phosphate buffer systems are more important intracellularly.

Carbonic acid–bicarbonate system

Carbonic acid and its salt (usually $NaHCO_3$ in the extracellular fluid and $KHCO_3$ or $Mg(HCO_3)_2$ intracellularly) is a major buffer of metabolic acid or alkali. This system buffers metabolic acid and base only, and does not function to buffer respiratory acid. This buffering process is indicated below:

$$HCl + NaHCO_3 \rightleftharpoons NaCl + H_2CO_3 \rightleftharpoons NaCl + H_2O + CO_2 \quad (19.10)$$

Adding strong acid to the bicarbonate buffer system ultimately converts the acid to CO_2, which is then eliminated by ventilation. Since CO_2 is in equilibrium with the HCO_3^-, excretion of the CO_2 via the lungs also consumes a corresponding amount of HCO_3^- from the body. It is clinically important to note that the change in HCO_3^- in the body reasonably reflects the amount of H^+ added to or removed from the system in a short time, at least until other (slower) systems have had time to compensate.

A strong base such as NaOH may also be buffered by carbonic acid:

$$NaOH + H_2CO_3 \rightleftharpoons NaHCO_3 + H_2O \quad (19.11)$$

In this case, the continuous supply of CO_2 needed to maintain adequate amounts of H_2CO_3 would come from normal metabolic processes.

The carbonic acid–bicarbonate system functions to buffer metabolic acid and base only. It does not buffer respiratory acid. If CO_2 is added to a bicarbonate buffer *in vitro*, H^+ and HCO_3^- are produced in equal amounts:

$$CO_2 + H_2O + NaHCO_3 \rightleftharpoons H^+ + HCO_3^- + NaHCO_3 \quad (19.12)$$

Despite the fact that the bicarbonate buffer has a lower pK_a relative to physiologic pH and is a small part of the body's buffering components, this system plays a major role in maintaining the acid–base balance in the body. The efficacy of the bicarbonate buffer is equivalent to that of all the others combined as a result of the respiratory and metabolic regulation of CO_2 and HCO_3^-.

Hemoglobin system

Hemoglobin (Hb) is the predominant noncarbonic buffer in the extracellular fluid and buffers both respiratory and metabolic acids. Hemoglobin buffers and transports CO_2 by two methods.

First, it allows CO_2 to combine directly with the terminal amino acids of the hemoglobin molecule to form carbamino compounds. This method of CO_2 transport accounts for 15–25% of the total CO_2 carried in the blood. A very small amount is also carried by the plasma proteins.

Second, CO_2 is catalyzed within the erythrocyte by carbonic anhydrase to produce H^+ and HCO_3^-. The H^+ produced by carbamino formation and by carbonic acid degradation (as well as from dissociation of a metabolic acid) is buffered by hemoglobin, which exists within the erythrocyte as a weak acid (HHb) and its potassium salt (KHb). Because hemoglobin is a weaker acid (pK_a 6.8) than carbonic acid (pK_a 6.1), H^+ is buffered by hemoglobin and HCO_3^- is increased proportionally. This is described by the formula:

$$H^+ + HCO_3^- + KHb \rightleftharpoons HHb + K^+HCO_3^- \quad (19.13)$$

When H^+ is buffered in the erythrocyte, the corresponding increase in HCO_3^- causes a diffusion of HCO_3^- into the plasma along the concentration gradient. As HCO_3^- diffuses out of the cell, chloride (Cl^-) moves intracellularly to maintain electrical neutrality. This entrance of chloride (Cl^-) into the erythrocyte in response to the outward migration of HCO_3^- is referred to as the "chloride shift." Therefore, while most of the H^+ is buffered within the cell, most of the change in HCO_3^- is seen in the plasma.

The Haldane effect, for our purposes, explains that reduction (deoxygenation) of hemoglobin makes it a weaker acid. Therefore, the buffering capacity of hemoglobin is increased in the reduced (deoxygenated) state. This explains the ability of hemoglobin to carry more CO_2 as carbamino compounds and increases the availability of buffer sites for H^+. Upon reaching the lung and becoming oxygenated, the hemoglobin becomes a stronger acid and the opposite is now true: CO_2 is released from the carbamino groups and H^+ is released from the hemoglobin to react with $KHCO_3$, as described below:

$$HHb + O_2 + K^+ + HCO_3^- \rightleftharpoons KHbO_2 + H_2O + CO_2 \quad (19.14)$$

As the CO_2 diffuses out of the erythrocyte and is eliminated by the lung, a diffusion gradient is created for HCO_3^- causing it to diffuse back into the cell in exchange for Cl^-, and the cycle just described begins once again.

Protein buffers

In addition to hemoglobin, other plasma proteins are effective buffers, both because of the large total concentration of proteins in the body and because the pK_a of some proteins approximates 7.4. Although most amino acids are bound by peptide linkages, some have free acid radicals in the form of ·COOH, which can liberate H^+ to buffer excess base:

$$\cdot COOH + OH^- \rightleftharpoons -COO^- + H_2O \quad (19.15)$$

Other amino acids have free basic radicals, commonly in the form of $\cdot NH_3OH$, to buffer acid:

$$\cdot NH_3OH + H^+ \rightleftharpoons -NH_3^+ + H_2O \quad (19.16)$$

The protein buffer system is predominantly intracellular, where concentrations of protein are generally greater than in the extracellular fluid. Approximately three-quarters of the body's buffering capacity is intracellular. However, this system also participates in the buffering of extracellular fluid, thanks in great part to the ability of CO_2 (and to a lesser extent H^+ and HCO_3^-) to diffuse across the cell membrane.

Phosphate buffer

The largest inorganic buffer is the phosphate buffer system. Its importance is predominantly intracellular, it has a pK_a of 6.8, and it functions in a manner similar to that of the bicarbonate buffer.

The phosphate system buffers a strong acid as seen below:

$$HCl + Na_2HPO_4 \rightleftharpoons NaH_2PO_4 + NaCl \quad (19.17)$$

while the buffering of a strong base is described as follows:

$$NaOH + NaH_2PO_4 \rightleftharpoons Na_2HPO_4 + H_2O \quad (19.18)$$

These conversions of strong acids or bases to weaker ones result in the liberation of less H^+ and therefore smaller changes in pH.

This system has little effect in the extracellular environment, because the concentrations of the buffer are less than 10% of the bicarbonate system. Furthermore, phosphate buffer concentrations are highest within the cell, and its pK_a is about the same as the intracellular pH, estimated at 6.9, thereby increasing its buffering potential. For similar reasons, this buffer is particularly important in the renal tubular fluid. In the renal tubules, phosphate is greatly concentrated and the renal tubular fluid is much more acidic than plasma, having a pH closer to the pK_a of the phosphate buffer system.

Inter-relation of buffers

The buffering capacity of the body is greater than the sum of the various intracellular and extracellular buffers because of the common link of the hydrogen ion and the inter-relation of the various buffer systems. When any metabolic factor causes a change in H^+, it initiates a cascade of changes in all the buffer systems, as they effectively buffer one another. This inter-relation between the carbonic and noncarbonic buffers also distorts the relation between HCO_3^- and P_aCO_2 as respective markers of metabolic and respiratory imbalances. For example, in a pure bicarbonate system, the change in HCO_3^- is equivalent to the amount of metabolic acid or base added. However, because of the concurrent effect of noncarbonic buffers, the change in HCO_3^- is not as great as would otherwise be expected. Similarly, alterations in $P\text{CO}_2$ do not change the HCO_3^- in an isolated bicarbonate buffer. The noncarbonic buffers will buffer CO_2 and result in a change in HCO_3^-. Greater concentrations of noncarbonic buffers will result in more buffering of H^+, for a given change in CO_2, and a greater change in HCO_3^-. Therefore, the mixed buffer solutions of the body interact in a manner such that:

1 HCO_3^- is a useful marker of metabolic acid changes but not in a linear fashion.
2 Changes in HCO_3^- are dependent upon respiratory acid–base variations.

Compensation

In addition to buffering of acid–base disturbances, homeostasis is also maintained by pulmonary and renal excretion of acids and bases. Alterations in pH stimulate homeostatic mechanisms that restore the ratio of HCO_3^-/P_aCO_2 to maintain a normal pH.

Ventilation

Respiratory compensation of acid–base disturbance is limited to CO_2 excretion by the lungs. The respiratory drive is controlled by chemosensitive areas primarily in the medulla and to a lesser extent in the carotid bodies. While both areas do respond to changes in H^+ and CO_2 ions, H^+ is the predominant mediator affecting the medullary center.

Changes in blood P_aCO_2 rapidly cause changes in cerebrospinal fluid (CSF) $P\text{CO}_2$, which is quickly converted to carbonic acid and dissociated into H^+. However, because of the limited buffering capacity of the CSF, the concentration of H^+ in the CSF is greater than it would be in the interstitial fluid.

Ventilation also serves to compensate for metabolic acid–base disturbances. Decreasing HCO_3^- with its concomitant decrease in pH will stimulate an increase in ventilation (despite normal or low P_aCO_2 levels), such as to maintain a normal ratio of HCO_3^-/P_aCO_2. Conversely, an increase in HCO_3^- decreases pulmonary ventilation and causes an elevation in P_aCO_2. If the decrease in ventilatory drive is so powerful as to also cause hypoxia, the ventilatory center will be stimulated by the effects of low O_2 on the carotid bodies.

Renal elimination

The major function of the kidney in acid–base homeostasis is the recovery of HCO_3^- produced by the titration of acid against the buffer systems of the body. The amount of HCO_3^- filtered by the kidney (and virtually all reabsorbed) is approximately 4320 mmol day^{-1} (24 mmol L^{-1} × 180 L day^{-1}). H^+ is titrated into the tubular fluid, and carbonic anhydrase catalyzes the production of H_2O and CO_2 (which is rapidly reabsorbed). Carbonic anhydrase within the cell converts the CO_2 back into HCO_3^-, which exits into the peritubular blood. Additionally, the kidneys generate new HCO_3^-, by the metabolism of glutamine in the proximal tubules, producing CO_2 and NH_3. The NH_3 is secreted into the tubular fluid as a buffer, and combines with H^+ to form NH_4^+, and the CO_2 combines with H_2O to form HCO_3^-, which is then absorbed. If the kidney is unable to excrete NH_4^+, the retention of the NH_4 negates the benefit of the new HCO_3^- generation.

In addition to recovering HCO_3^-, the kidneys excrete an amount of acid equal to its daily production, or approximately 70 mmol L^{-1} day^{-1}. Before being excreted, these free acids are first buffered by the weaker acids ammonia (NH_3/NH_4^+) and phosphate ($HPO_4^{2-}/H_2PO_4^-$), and, to a lesser degree, other buffer species in the renal tubular fluid. Both the excretion of acid and the resorption of HCO_3^- depend on the active secretion of H^+ into the tubular fluid. The amount of H^+ secreted is regulated by changes in the plasma HCO_3^-, plasma pH, and P_{CO_2}. During times of systemic acidosis, (from loss of HCO_3^- or an increased $P_{a}CO_2$), the reduction of intracellular pH stimulates the release of H^+ into the tubular fluid, thereby increasing the recovery of HCO_3^-. The metabolism of glutamine is also stimulated by intracellular acidosis. However, the increased production of new HCO_3^- and NH_4 requires synthesis of enzymes and may take up to several days for complete adaptation. Conversely, metabolic and respiratory alkalosis inhibits resorption of HCO_3^- in the kidney by reduction of H^+ secretion. Since renal H^+ secretion occurs simultaneously with Na^+ reabsorption for electrical balance, the process is also affected by aldosterone. Increasing aldosterone stimulates reasorption of Na^+ and excretion of H^+ into the tubular fluid, causing an increased resorption of HCO_3^-. The opposite effect occurs with decreased levels of aldosterone.

METHODS OF ASSESSMENT OF ACID–BASE BALANCE

Acid–base imbalances do occur in the body, despite the efficacy of the buffer and compensatory mechanisms. Measurement of pH and $P_{a}CO_2$ and the calculation of HCO_3^- are necessary to determine the primary disorder causing the imbalance, the degree of compensation occurring, and the most useful therapy. There are several methods used to measure these parameters, but because of the complex inter-relations between the acid–base buffer systems and the compensatory mechanisms, these methods of measurement all suffer in varying degrees from the same flaw: the loss of precision inherent in the simplification of a complex process. There are both *in vivo* and *in vitro* methods.

In vitro

The Henderson–Hasselbalch equation for carbonic acid–bicarbonate is a most convenient method for measuring acid–base disorders. Several different methods are utilized to correct for the presence of other buffers, thus allowing one to evaluate the entire system as though it was a bicarbonate buffer. They include the alkali reserve, standard bicarbonate, the Astrup method, and the buffer base and base excess systems.

The alkali reserve, standard bicarbonate, and Astrup method are of historical interest, but are no longer in use in clinical practice. The buffer base and base excess systems take different approaches to the description and *in vitro* analysis of acid–base disorders, and they do attempt to compensate for the buffering capacity of noncarbonic buffer systems. To do so, the dual buffer system is converted to the equivalent of a carbonic acid–bicarbonate buffer, in which the change in HCO_3 directly reflects a change in H^+ of the system. However, they suffer from inaccuracies in the estimation of the magnitude of an acid–base disorder, and cannot account for either the acute interaction between buffer systems or the changes related to compensatory mechanisms. Therefore, there is a greater utility in the *in vivo* titration curves.

In vivo

In vivo titration curves are derived from the collation of normal human values of pH, $P_{a}CO_2$ and HCO_3^- in acute and chronic disorders. Clinical sample values are then compared with these values and the deviation from them may be characterized and quantified for both acute and chronic disorders. This method is superior to the *in vitro* methods because it recognizes that changes occur in both HCO_3^- and $P_{a}CO_2$ in both acute and chronic acid–base disturbances.[1] This is because changes in pH due to a specific cause are not only buffered but initiate compensation by other homeostatic mechanisms and thus present a very dynamic scenario.

In vivo evaluation of respiratory acidosis

With an acute increase in $P_{a}CO_2$, the increase in carbonic acid results in an increase in both H^+ and HCO_3^-. Acutely, each 1.3 kPa (10 mmHg) rise in $P_{a}CO_2$ results in an increase in HCO_3^- of 0.08 mmol L^{-1} and an increase in H^+ of 8 nmol L^{-1}. Although the relation between $P_{a}CO_2$ and H^+ is linear, conversion to the logarithmic pH scale distorts this association. As an approximate conversion, each 1.3 kPa (10 mmHg) rise in $P_{a}CO_2$ produces a pH decrease of about 0.07 units, within the $P_{a}CO_2$ range of 4–8 kPa (30–60 mmHg). This generalization is less accurate as the $P_{a}CO_2$ deviates further from normal.

Renal compensation for the respiratory acidosis results in excretion of H^+ and reabsorption of HCO_3^-, raising the pH but not completely normalizing it. As the ratio of HCO_3^- to $P_{a}CO_2$ approaches normal, the change in HCO_3^- is greater and the change in pH is less than for an acute disturbance. Therefore, under conditions of chronic hypercapnia with renal compensation, each 1.3 kPa (10 mmHg) increase in $P_{a}CO_2$ results in a HCO_3^- rise of 4 mmol L^{-1}, and an increase in H^+ of 3.2 nmol L^{-1}, or an approximate 0.03 unit decrease in pH.

In vivo evaluation of respiratory alkalosis

Under conditions of acute hyperventilation and hypocapnia, the levels of carbonic acid are reduced and H^+ and HCO_3^- are decreased. An acute decrease of 1.3 kPa (10 mmHg) in the $P_{a}CO_2$ results in a decrease in HCO_3^- of 2 mmol L^{-1}. For each 1.3 kPa (10 mmHg) decrease in $P_{a}CO_2$, H^+ decreases by 8 mmol L^{-1} (an equivalent magnitude of change as in respiratory acidosis, but the opposite in direction), and the pH increases by approximately 0.08 units.

Renal compensation for chronic hypocapnia causes a decrease in tubular H^+ secretion and diminished HCO_3^- reabsorption. As plasma HCO_3^- decreases, the ratio of HCO_3^- to $P_{a}CO_2$ approaches normal, and the change in pH is less than with an acute respiratory alkalosis. In the chronic compensated respiratory alkalosis, each 1.3 kPa (10 mmHg) decrease in $P_{a}CO_2$ is associated with a 6 mmol L^{-1} decrease in HCO_3^- and a decrease in H^+ of 1.7 nmol L^{-1}, corresponding to a pH increase of approximately 0.03 units.

In vivo evaluation of metabolic acidosis

Excess metabolic acid in the system produces an almost immediate increase in alveolar ventilation. Peripheral chemoreceptors in the carotid bodies stimulate ventilatory drive, resulting in a decrease in P_aCO_2 and attenuation of the fall in pH. Although reduction in P_aCO_2 is rapid, the respiratory response is only capable of a 50–75% compensation for the metabolic acidosis (i.e. an uncorrected metabolic acidosis which would reduce the pH to 7.0 is normally compensated to a pH of 7.2–7.3). *In vivo* measurements of the normal response to metabolic acidosis show that the P_aCO_2 is decreased by 0.15 kPa (1.1 mmHg) for each 1 mmol L^{-1} reduction in HCO_3^-. An alternative method of predicting P_aCO_2 associated with a pure metabolic acidosis uses the formula:

$$\text{Predicted } P_aCO_2\ (\text{kPa}) = (0.2 \times [HCO_3^-]) + 1.06\ (\pm 0.27)$$

or

$$\text{Predicted } P_aCO_2\ (\text{mmHg}) = (1.5 \times [HCO_3^-]) + 8\ (\pm 2) \qquad (19.19)$$

Because the respiratory compensation ameliorates the change in pH, *in vivo* measurements show that, for each 4 mmol L^{-1} decrease in HCO_3^-, the pH decreases by 0.08 units. Owing to the logarithmic nature of the pH system, this generalization becomes less accurate as the HCO_3^- is further from normal.

In vivo evaluation of metabolic alkalosis

The normal compensatory response to a pure metabolic alkalosis is a rapid depression of respiratory drive, resulting in an increase in P_aCO_2 as an attempt to restore the ratio of HCO_3^-/P_aCO_2 to normal. This compensation may be limited if hypoxemia results from hypoventilation, particularly in the patient breathing room air. It appears that the respiratory stimulus from hypoxemia is stronger than the compensatory depression due to alkalosis, and oxygenation is often maintained despite a metabolic alkalosis.

Although less well compensated than other acid-base disturbances, hypercapnia can occur in the presence of metabolic alkalosis, and the following formula is used to predict the resultant P_aCO_2:

$$\text{Predicted } P_aCO_2\ (\text{kPa}) = (0.9 \times [HCO_3^-]) + 2.67\ (\pm 0.27)$$

or

$$\text{Predicted } P_aCO_2\ (\text{mmHg}) = (0.7 \times [HCO_3^-]) + 20\ (\pm 2) \qquad (19.20)$$

Utilizing *in vivo* titration curves

There are three basic steps in the evaluation of acid-base disorders using the *in vivo* titration curve data.

1 *Evaluate the arterial pH.* Normal arterial pH values range from 7.35 to 7.45; acidemia is defined as an arterial pH of less than 7.35, and alkalemia is defined as an arterial pH of greater than 7.45. The primary disturbance of acid-base balance will shift the pH in the direction of that disorder (i.e. a metabolic acidosis will produce an acidemia). While compensatory mechanisms will minimize the alteration in pH, these are unable to restore it to completely normal values. Note that a normal pH does not preclude the presence of an acid-base disturbance: two concurrent disorders of equal magnitude but opposite direction (as in metabolic acidosis and respiratory alkalosis) may result in a normal pH.
2 *Evaluate the markers for the etiology of the primary disturbance.* In general, P_aCO_2 is used as a descriptor of respiratory disorders, and HCO_3^- serves as an indicator of metabolic disturbances. As an example, consider the blood gas sample: pH 7.30, $P_aCO_2 = 4.53$ kPa, (34 mmHg), $HCO_3^- = 19$ mmol L^{-1}. The low P_aCO_2 describes a respiratory alkalosis, and the reduction in HCO_3^- concentration suggests a metabolic acidosis. Because the pH is acidemic, the primary etiology will usually be the metabolic acidosis. The reduction in P_aCO_2 may be a compensatory measure and should be evaluated as follows.
3 *Compare the observed values with those predicted.* In the previous example of a metabolic acidosis, the HCO_3^- value is reduced by 5 mmol L^{-1}. The predicted respiratory response is a 0.15 kPa (1.1 mmHg) reduction in P_aCO_2 for each 1 mmol L^{-1} decrease in HCO_3^-. This should reduce the P_aCO_2 by 0.75 kPa (5.5 mmHg), to a level of 4.55 kPa (34.1 mmHg). This example describes an appropriate respiratory compensation for a metabolic acidosis.

CLINICAL EFFECTS OF ACID–BASE DERANGEMENTS

Any acid–base disturbance in the body, whether metabolic (H^+ and HCO_3^-) or respiratory (P_aCO_2), is met with the previously described buffer and compensation mechanisms and is directed toward normal. Acute or severe disturbances can outpace or overwhelm those homeostatic mechanisms and result in a variety of clinical responses.

The following discussion will generally focus on acidosis, the most frequently found acid–base disturbance, but this is not to diminish the importance of alkalosis, which can be even more harmful than acidosis in some instances.

While acid–base abnormalities have been quite extensively studied, the organ-specific effects of these changes are, at best, difficult to predict because of the myriad of inter-relations present in any specific patient during these changes. Despite this disclaimer, however, it can be broadly stated that organ function is optimal in the normal pH range and decreases outside this range. Some of these changes and effects are summarized in Tables 19.1 and 19.2.

Cardiovascular effects

Heart rate

As pH decreases from 7.4 toward 7.1, the heart rate increases as a result of the indirect effect of epinephrine released from the adrenal medulla in response to acidemia.[2] Without catecholamine release (as in the isolated heart preparation or a sympathetically blocked patient), the effect of acidemia is bradycardia, and the effect is more pronounced below a pH of 7.1. The decrease in heart rate is thought to be due to increased vagal tone and accumulation of acetylcholine (ACh) as a result of the decreased metabolism of ACh in the acidic environment.[3,4] Clinically, in the normal patient, both respiratory and metabolic acidosis will cause an increase in heart rate, followed later by a decrease in heart rate as the depressant effect described above overcomes the initial cardioacceleration due to sympathetic activation.

Cardiac rhythm

Both atrial and ventricular dysrhythmias are more common under conditions of acid–base derangements. It cannot be stated with certainty whether it is the change in pH alone or the change in extracellular potassium levels (which are closely related to pH) that serves as the mechanism for the dysrhythmias. A change of 0.1 pH units can cause the serum potassium level to change as much as 0.5–1.5 mmol L^{-1} in the opposite direction. In the acidotic state, the high H^+ concentration causes a reduction in intracellular potassium, which in turn alters the resting membrane potential of the cardiac conduction system. Arrhythmogenicity will also be affected by pH-related changes in calcium, magnesium, and catecholamine levels. Most studies support

Table 19.1 *Predicted changes in acid–base abnormalities* in vivo

Clinical status	Primary alteration	Associated alterations	
	P_aCO_2 kPa (mmHg)	HCO_3^- mmol L^{-1}	pH units
Respiratory acidosis			
Acute	+ 1.33 (10)	+0.8	–0.07
Chronic	+ 1.33 (10)	+4.0	–0.03
Respiratory alkalosis			
Acute	–1.33 (10)	–2.0	+0.08
Chronic	–1.33 (10)	–6.0	+0.03
	HCO_3^- mmol L^{-1}	P_aCO_2 kPa (mmHg)	pH units
Metabolic acidosis	–4	–0.6 (4.4)	–0.08
Alternatively	Predicted P_aCO_2 (kPa) = $(0.2 \times [HCO_3^-]) + 1.06 (\pm 0.27)$ Predicted P_aCO_2 (mmHg) = $(1.5 \times [HCO_3^-]) + 8 (\pm 2)$		
Metabolic alkalosis	Predicted P_aCO_2 (kPa) = $(0.9 \times [HCO_3^-]) + 2.67 (\pm 0.27)$ Predicted P_aCO_2 (mmHg) = $(0.7 \times [HCO_3^-]) + 20 (\pm 2)$		

Table 19.2 *Summary of clinical effects of acid–base imbalance*

	Decreased pH			Increased pH		
	Direct	Indirect	Clinical	Direct	Indirect	Clinical
Cerebral blood flow	+	+	+	–	0	–
Heart rate	–	+	+	0	0	0
Cardiac inotropy	–	+	0	0	0	0
Systemic arterial tone	–	+	–	+	0	+
Systemic venous tone	+	+	+	0	0	0
Pulmonary artery tone	+	+	+	0	–	–
Airway tone	–	+	+	+	–	+
Uterine blood flow	+	–	0	–	0	–
Renal blood flow	+	–	–	0	0	0
Ionized Ca^{2+}	+	0	+	–	0	–
Serum potassium	+	0	+	–	0	–

–, Decreases; +, increases; 0, variable or no effect.

the belief that the threshold for ventricular fibrillation is lowered by decreasing pH and increased by increasing pH.[5–7]

Under anesthesia with volatile agents, spontaneous ventilation will result in a respiratory acidosis. The resting P_aCO_2 with halothane at 1.25 minimum alveolar concentration (MAC) will be 6.13 kPa (46 mmHg); with isoflurane at 1.25 MAC it will be 6.93 kPa (52 mmHg); and with enflurane at 1.25 MAC it will be 8.26 kPa (62 mmHg).

The increasing level of circulating catecholamines and decrease in pH may cause an increase in ventricular ectopy. Of the volatile anesthetics, halothane lowers the arrhythmogenic threshold the most because of sensitization of the myocardium to catecholamine effects. In healthy patients, this is of little clinical significance. However, when the ventilatory depression inherent in the volatile anesthetics is compounded by effects of other disease states such as obstructive lung disease, poor neuromuscular function, or other drugs which depress ventilation, the P_aCO_2 may rise dramatically and cause significant dysrhythmias.

Myocardial contractility

Acidosis causes a depression of contractility in the isolated heart.[3,8] This direct depression is thought to be due to either impairment of calcium entry into the cells and/or the decreased release of calcium from the intracellular storage sites.[9,10] However, acidosis also causes an increase in circulating catecholamines, which will stimulate the heart in the intact patient. This catecholamine-driven stimulus overcomes the direct depressant effect of acidosis and results in a net increase in inotropy, at least until the pH falls below 7.0,[2,3] below which point the depressant effects of acidosis predominate and there is a net decrease in inotropy. Patients with sympathetic blockade or those taking calcium channel blockers will demonstrate a decrease in contractility at a relatively milder change in pH.

Alkalosis can also produce a mild elevation in contractility by increasing the responsiveness of the myocardium to circulating catecholamines. This occurs at the expense of greater coronary oxygen extraction. Alkalosis causes an increase in coronary vascular resistance and also shifts the oxyhemoglobin dissociation to the left, thereby providing less oxygen to the myocardium. At equal cardiac workloads, coronary sinus lactate levels are higher in the alkalotic patient, suggesting greater oxygen extraction and smaller myocardial oxygen reserve. Unbound plasma calcium is also decreased during alkalosis, possibly reducing contractility further.

Cardiac output

Mild acidemia-induced increases in catecholamine levels will elevate cardiac output as a result of both increased heart rate and contractility, as well as decreased arterial vascular tone (afterload) and increased venous tone (preload). This combination of increased preload, contractility, and heart rate along with decreased afterload serves to increase cardiac output only up to a point. As the pH decreases to near 7.0, the cardiac depressant effects of acidemia are greater than the cardiac stimulus provided by the increased catecholamine levels, and the cardiac output will fall because of a reduction in both heart rate and contractility. Decreased cardiac output in the presence of increased venous return may result in congestive heart failure.

Systemic vascular effects

The direct effect of increasing acidemia on systemic (nonpulmonary) arterial vasculature is vasodilation.[11] However, this effect varies substantially, depending upon whether the decrease in pH is due to respiratory or metabolic acidosis, and is much more pronounced during respiratory acidosis. This is because CO_2 crosses the cell membranes more readily than bicarbonate and thus it can enter the cell easily. Intracellularly, CO_2 is converted to carbonic acid, which then dissociates to H^+ and HCO_3^-. The resultant decrease in intracellular pH is the mechanism responsible for the decrease in vascular smooth muscle tone. In metabolic acidosis, on the other hand, the limited diffusibility of the acid (compared with CO_2) into the cell decreases the intracellular pH to a lesser degree. Mild degrees of metabolic acidosis may even result in vasoconstriction due to the release of catecholamines caused by the acidemia. This vasoconstriction will continue until the pH falls to below 7.2, at which point vasodilation would again be expected.[12] Alkalosis tends to produce vasoconstriction (except for the pulmonary vasculature). Therefore, because of the multiple factors that determine cardiac output, and because of the varying effects different degrees of acid–base imbalance have on each of them, systemic blood pressure may or may not change until extremes of imbalance are reached.

Individual vascular beds respond differently to acid–base variations because of the varying contributions of direct and indirect effects of the acidemia or alkalemia. Metabolic acidosis will *directly* dilate arterial vessels of the skin and skeletal musculature, the renal and splanchnic beds, and the uterine and coronary arteries. Respiratory acidosis has the same effect, but to a greater degree on the vasculature of the kidney, gastrointestinal tract, and uterus. However, because of the indirect effects mediated by the sympathoadrenal axis, both types of acidosis result in clinical vasoconstriction of the renal and splanchnic beds, with variable changes in the other aforementioned vascular beds. In contrast to this, the direct response of the pulmonary vasculature to metabolic or respiratory acidosis is vasoconstriction.

While coronary vascular resistance is closely tied to myocardial oxygen demand, it is very difficult to define the coronary response to acid–base changes in the intact patient. This is because of the effects of heart rate, contractility, preload, and afterload on the oxygen demand, and these factors themselves are affected by acid–base imbalance. However, in the isolated heart, the coronary vasculature responds to acidosis by dilation and to alkalosis by constriction.[13,14] Therefore, hyperventilation can reduce coronary blood flow significantly, thus increasing myocardial ischemia and coronary sinus lactate levels.

The venous system is one of the few vascular beds in which acidosis produces constriction both directly and indirectly, i.e. directly by an increase in H^+ concentration and indirectly by such H^+ concentration having stimulated an increase in catecholamine levels.[15] Acidosis, therefore, creates an increase in venous return to the heart, which may increase cardiac work (especially in an acid environment), thereby impairing myocardial contractility.

Respiratory effects

Minute ventilation

The respiratory response to acidosis is to increase minute ventilation (V_E). This is accomplished by a substantial increase in tidal volume and a slight increase in respiratory rate (Kussmaul respirations). The rise in V_E is about twice as great if the fall in pH is caused by a rise in CO_2 than if the same fall in pH is caused by an increase in metabolic acidosis. Most (80%) of this change in V_E is due to the effect on the medullary chemoreceptors, while a lesser percentage of the change in V_E is due to the stimulus originating from peripheral chemoreceptors in the carotid bodies.[16,17] While the carotid receptors are stimulated by changes in both pH and P_aCO_2, the medullary receptors are stimulated by the passage of CO_2 across the blood–brain barriers and the subsequent increase in H^+ in the CSF. This reduction in pH at the medullary level, either from respiratory or from metabolic causes, stimulates the efferent respiratory drive to increase V_E.

The increase in V_E is greater with respiratory acidosis than with metabolic acidosis because the CO_2 diffuses more rapidly across the blood–brain barrier than does metabolic acid, and thus stimulates the medullary centers more quickly. The normal CO_2 response curve shows that respiratory acidosis will increase the V_E by 15–23 L min^{-1} for each 1 kPa increase in P_aCO_2 (or 2–3 L min^{-1} for each 1 mmHg increase in P_aCO_2). This increase in ventilation peaks at a P_aCO_2 of about 13.3 kPa (or 100 mmHg), and further increases in P_aCO_2 will cause respiratory depression. Volatile anesthetic agents decrease the slope of the response to CO_2 in a dose-dependent fashion.

Airway resistance

Acid–base disturbances modify changes in airway tone by both the local effect of CO_2 and the indirect effects of sympathoadrenal stimulation. Increased P_aCO_2, by means of intracellular diffusion, increases H^+ and causes smooth muscle relaxation, while the indirect effects of hypercapnia cause bronchoconstriction by means of vagal stimulation. It is this bronchoconstrictive effect that predominates in the intact patient and results predictably in increased airway resistance, decreased tracheal volume, and increased resistive work of breathing.[18] Bronchoconstriction is minimized or abolished by atropine or vagotomy.[19] Conversely, hypocapnia produces a direct bronchoconstrictive effect, which may be partially offset by a centrally mediated bronchodilatory action. However, the bronchoconstrictive effect is clinically predominant and is useful in the matching of ventilation to blood flow in normal lungs and in pathologic conditions such as pulmonary embolism.

Oxygen transport depends on both cardiac output and oxygen-carrying capacity; and acid–base imbalance has an impact on each of these variables. The Bohr effect describes the decreased affinity of hemoglobin for oxygen as the H^+ increases. This shifts the oxygen–hemoglobin dissociation curve to the right and results in increased availability of oxygen to the tissues. Conversely, alkalosis increases the affinity of hemoglobin for oxygen and increases its absorption in the lung. In the normal patient, this has the overall effect of increasing the efficiency of hemoglobin-mediated oxygen delivery to the tissues, since its oxygen affinity is greater in the normally somewhat alkalotic lung and lesser in the more acidotic tissue. The rightward shift of the oxyhemoglobin dissociation curve in acidosis occurs immediately, but within 12–36 h the concentration of 2,3-diphosphoglycerate (2,3-DPG) falls and restores the oxygen affinity, shifting the oxygen dissociation curve back to the left.[20] The 2,3-DPG concentration decreases because glycolysis is impaired in an acid environment and the glycolytic intermediates in the 2,3-DPG production become depleted.

The response of the pulmonary vasculature to pH changes is the opposite of that in the other vascular beds, in that resistance is increased in acidosis and decreased in alkalosis.[21–23] While there is some evidence that an increase in P_aCO_2 may cause a small increase in vasodilation as in other tissues, this effect is over-ridden in acidosis by vasoconstriction of the pre- and postcapillary sphincters of the pulmonary vascular bed.[24] When compared with hypoxic pulmonary vasoconstriction, the vasoconstriction caused by acidosis is small, although an acidotic environment will greatly enhance the normal hypoxic vasoconstrictor response.[25] Acidosis will increase both the pulmonary artery pressure and resistance, as a result not only of capillary sphincter constriction, but also of an increase in venous return secondary to acidosis-induced venoconstriction. Furthermore, the catecholamine-mediated increase in cardiac output, caused by mild acidemia, produces an increase in pulmonary blood flow and further increases pulmonary artery pressures.

Gastrointestinal effects

Studies of splanchnic vasculature have yielded conflicting data. Some animal studies have shown that respiratory acidosis increases splanchnic blood flow and the increase persists after sympathetic blockade. This increase does not occur with metabolic acidosis. This suggests that CO_2 directly reduces the intracellular pH of the vessel endothelium to produce vasodilation.[26] However, Epstein *et al.* found that respiratory acidosis caused an increase in splanchnic vascular resistance.[27] The differences between these two studies may reflect vasoconstriction overwhelming local vasodilation.

Isolated gastric and esophageal tissue have decreased spontaneous rate and amplitude of intrinsic neural discharge when bathed in an acid medium.[28] These effects may be magnified by concurrent derangements of potassium, magnesium, and calcium. Clinically, this may correlate with the vague abdominal pain, nausea, and vomiting often seen with acidosis.

Renal effects

While renal vascular response to acidosis depends on the balance of direct and systemic factors, the clinical outcome of this balance is vasoconstriction. Mild respiratory acidosis may leave renal vascular resistance unchanged or slightly diminished, but as acidosis worsens, the renal vascular resistance increases and renal blood flow decreases. Metabolic acidosis increases renal vascular resistance much more than an equal change in pH resulting from an increase in P_aCO_2.[29,30] This is probably due to the ability of CO_2 to cross the cell membrane and reduce the intracellular pH. Direct vasodilation is not found in pure metabolic acidosis, and therefore the catecholamine-mediated vasoconstriction acts unopposed.

Uteroplacental effects

Acid–base imbalance affects the fetus directly through the placenta and indirectly by means of changes in placental blood flow. CO_2 diffuses readily across the placenta, and maternal changes in P_aCO_2 cause fetal changes in the same direction. Passage of H^+ and HCO_3^- is much slower and therefore a metabolic acidosis or alkalosis will cause little change in fetal pH for several hours. Changes in fetal pH produce similar effects in fetal organ function as seen in adults. The direct effect of acidosis on uterine circulation is vasodilation, with respiratory acidosis having slightly greater vasodilator effect than metabolic acidosis. Severe hypercapnia, however, has little overall effect on uterine blood flow because of the vasodilatory effect of high P_aCO_2 being effectively opposed by the vasoconstrictor effects of sympathoadrenal stimulation.[31] The direct effect of alkalosis is vasoconstriction of the uterine vessels. Respiratory alkalosis produces a significantly greater reduction in uteroplacental blood flow than metabolic alkalosis for a given change in pH. Alkalosis also causes a leftward change in the maternal oxygen–hemoglobin dissociation curve, increasing the affinity of maternal hemoglobin for oxygen, and therefore decreasing the quantity of oxygen available to the fetus. The combination of vasoconstriction and decreased oxygen delivery seen in severe alkalosis (pH > 7.65) will cause fetal hypoxemia and metabolic acidosis.[32,33] In milder respiratory alkalosis (as in active labor), placental blood flow is maintained and the low maternal P_aCO_2 equilibrates across the placenta. This increases fetal pH and changes the fetal oxygen–hemoglobin dissociation curve to the left, increasing oxygen uptake by fetal hemoglobin, thereby resulting in a higher fetal oxygen saturation than in a maternal metabolic alkalosis of the same degree.

Neuroendocrine effects

The cerebrovascular response to P_aCO_2 is similar to other vascular beds. A rise in P_aCO_2 results in vasodilation and increased cerebral blood flow. An increase in P_aCO_2 to 10.6 kPa (80 mmHg) will approximately double the cerebral blood flow, whereas reducing the P_aCO_2 to 2.7 kPa (20 mmHg) will halve the blood flow. There is no further reduction in blood flow at a P_aCO_2 of less than 2.7 kPa, probably due to accumulation of lactic acid in the periarteriolar tissue, which causes local vasodilation, thereby limiting cerebral vasoconstriction.[34]

Neurologic changes from acid–base imbalance are due predictably to the ability of CO_2 to cross the blood–brain barrier. This causes changes in the pH of the CSF, which impairs neuronal function and may lead to mental status changes and coma.[35] As with other vascular beds, the clinical effects are more pronounced in respiratory derangements because of the increased blood–brain barrier permeability to CO_2 rather than to metabolic acids.

Respiratory acidosis can also decrease body temperature, partly by impairment of central thermoregulation,[36] but also by causing cutaneous vasodilation (thus increasing cutaneous heat loss) and decreased rate of cellular metabolism.

The primary neuroendocrine response to acidosis is an increase in the level of circulating catecholamines. Epinephrine release from the adrenal glands and norepinephrine from nerve terminals causes direct stimulation of the sympathetic nervous system.[37,38] Norepinephrine synthesis is also increased to match the increased rate of catecholamine release. In mild acidosis, the elevated catecholamine levels tend to counteract the depressant effects of acidemia on organ systems. However, as the pH falls, the cellular response to catecholamine stimulation decreases, and the depressant effect of acidosis on cellular function becomes more apparent despite increased catecholamine levels.[39]

Electrolyte effects

Calcium

Calcium exists in three forms in plasma. Approximately 50% is nonionized and bound to plasma proteins (and thus unavailable for diffusion into the tissues). Five percent of the calcium is diffusible but bound to other plasma components (such as citrate), and 45% of the plasma calcium is in the ionized, chemically active form. During periods of acidosis, hydrogen ions compete for the negatively charged binding sites on albumin, displacing calcium and increasing the proportion of serum ionized calcium. Conversely, alkalosis causes an increase in available protein binding sites, a reduction in ionized calcium concentrations, and clinical hypocalcemia.[40] This causes tetany or mild disturbances in cardiac contractility. Although nomograms are available to estimate ionized calcium concentrations based upon measurements of total calcium, albumin, and pH, the only accurate method of assessing free calcium is direct measurement of ionized calcium.

Potassium

Serum potassium and pH levels are usually reciprocal, i.e. when pH falls, serum K^+ rises. In acidemia, hydrogen ions enter the cell along the concentration gradient, and potassium ions move into the extracellular fluid to maintain intracellular electrical neutrality. Whereas previous assessments implied that each 0.1 unit change in pH caused a 0.6 mmol L^{-1} change in potassium ion concentration, we now know that this relation is nonlinear.[41] Furthermore, it can be influenced by other factors known to affect potassium homeostasis, including catecholamines, aldosterone, insulin, and the nonlinearity of the pH system itself.

THERAPY OF ACID–BASE DISORDERS

While clinical imbalances of acid–base homeostasis can be measured readily, the decision of how (or even if) to treat an imbalance remains one of continuing controversy. Logically, one could expect that therapy to correct such imbalances would benefit a patient, but such is not always the case. In general, it is usually wise to treat the cause of the imbalance, but if time or the severity or nature of the disease process does not allow, then specific treatment may be warranted.

Alkalosis

While troublesome, clinically significant alkalosis is less frequent and ominous than acidosis. Increased blood pH decreases serum potassium and ionized calcium levels, and it can potentiate the arrhythmias seen with digitalis toxicity. Metabolic alkalosis can be classified as either chloride responsive or chloride resistant in nature, depending upon the measurement of urinary chloride levels. Urinary chloride values of less than 10 mmol L^{-1} are usually caused by intravascular volume depletion, for example by diuretic use, hyperemesis, nasogastric suctioning, or diarrhea. Alkalosis and hypovolemia will respond to or correct with the administration of a salt-containing solution. For example, sodium chloride will usually restore intravascular volume and promote bicarbonate excretion, correcting the alkalosis. Administration of potassium chloride is also needed to correct the alkalosis and restore concomitant hypokalemia, which may be exacerbated or unmasked as the pH falls. The hypokalemia must be corrected because, in the hypokalemic state, the kidneys will switch from the usual sodium–potassium ion exchange to a sodium–hydrogen ion exchange to promote potassium retention. This alteration will result in acidification of the urine, thereby maintaining alkalosis.

Chloride-resistant alkalosis, demonstrated by urinary chloride levels greater than 20 mmol L^{-1}, is less common, and is usually due to mineralocorticoid excess, thiazide or loop diuretics, or potassium supplementation. These patients usually are normovolemic or hypervolemic, have normal urine sodium and chloride levels, and do not respond to the administration of chloride salts. Therapy, therefore, is centered around resolving the underlying disorder. Carbonic anhydrase inhibitors such as acetazolamide can effectively treat metabolic alkalosis by decreasing the renal reabsorption of filtered sodium and bicarbonate, producing a net loss of bicarbonate.

Respiratory alkalosis results from alveolar ventilation exceeding the requirements of current CO_2 production. Among the more common etiologies of respiratory alkalosis are pregnancy (mild, chronic alkalosis), hepatic failure, hypoxemia with $P_{a}O_2$ of less than 8 kPa (60 mmHg), pulmonary embolism, head injury, neurologic disorders, acute anxiety, and certain forms of toxicity, both pharmacologic and infectious. In general, therapy is directed at correcting the underlying etiology. Under general anesthesia using controlled ventilation, minute ventilation high enough to cause decreased $P_{a}CO_2$ will result in respiratory alkalosis leading to minor hypokalemia, decreased Ca^{2+} due to increased protein binding, decreased cerebral blood flow, and a leftward shift in the oxygen–hemoglobin dissociation curve.

Acidosis

Respiratory acidosis

Respiratory acidosis is caused by the retention of carbon dioxide as a result of an imbalance between its rate of production and its rate of excretion through the lungs. This is most commonly the result of a decrease in minute ventilation due to trauma, neurologic impairment, respiratory depressant drugs, lung disease, muscle relaxants, or muscle diseases. However, it can also be seen in cases of unusually high carbon dioxide production as in cases of malignant hyperthermia or thyroid storm. Therapy for respiratory acidosis is generally directed toward removing the cause of the imbalance, and occasionally requires the use of mechanical ventilation.

Metabolic acidosis

Metabolic acidosis is generally more serious than respiratory acidosis, not because the acidosis is worse, but because the etiology of the acidosis is frequently more life-threatening. Treating this etiology of low blood pH is often much more complex than treating respiratory acidosis. Decreased oxygen delivery to the tissues will cause the development of metabolic acidosis, which if severe enough can result in cardiac arrest. Alkali therapy in cardiac arrest has been debated for decades. In the 1970s, sodium bicarbonate ($NaHCO_3$) was given early and regularly during a resuscitative effort. In the 1980s, bicarbonate administration was guided by the results of arterial blood gas analysis, and in the 1990s there were warnings against the routine administration of bicarbonate during cardiac arrest.[42]

There are several reasons for the hesitation to use sodium bicarbonate freely to correct metabolic acidosis,[43] (see Chapter 73 on management of cardiac and respiratory arrest) and among them are:

1 During cardiac arrest, both respiratory and metabolic acidosis develops rapidly in the tissue. Hypercapnia results from inadequate pulmonary excretion of carbon dioxide, and lactic acidosis results from anaerobic metabolism. While the administration of sodium bicarbonate may raise the measured pH in the blood, the reaction:

$$NaHCO_3 + H^+ \rightleftharpoons H_2CO_3 \rightleftharpoons CO_2 + H_2O \qquad (19.21)$$

indicates that the sodium bicarbonate will be changed to carbon dioxide and water. In fact, one 50-mL ampule of $NaHCO_3$ will be converted to the equivalent of 200 mL of CO_2, the same amount as produced by the basal metabolism of a normal adult in 1 min. This sudden increase in the CO_2 in the blood reverses the diffusion gradient and, since the CO_2 is more readily diffusible across the cell membrane than is the H_2CO_3, it will easily enter the cell and cause intracellular (cytoplasmic) acidosis. This internal hypercapnia will compound the existing lactic acidosis,[44] further reducing intracellular pH[45] and decreasing myocardial contractility, thereby exacerbating an already compromised low-flow cardiac output state.

2 The CO_2 thus produced in the blood also easily crosses the blood–brain barrier and causes a disproportionate acidosis of the CSF.[46]

3 The administration of a 50-mL ampule of sodium bicarbonate will increase the serum osmolarity by 3 mmol L^{-1} in the normal adult.[47]

4 $NaHCO_3$ administration can cause an extracellular alkalosis, with a resulting shift in the oxygen–hemoglobin dissociation curve to the left and thus a reduced oxygen transfer to the tissue. The alkalosis will also reduce serum ionized calcium by 25% and can decrease myocardial contractility.[48,49]

5 The hemodynamic effects of the administration of sodium bicarbonate are unpredictable, and increases in cardiac output may be due to increases in intravascular volume rather than changes in pH. One study demonstrated that correction of pH by bicarbonate did not increase the efficacy of catecholamine infusions.[50]

6 In animals, $NaHCO_2$ will reduce hepatic clearance of lactic acid, possibly as a result of hepatocellular dysfunction due to increased intracellular CO_2 and acidosis.[51]

Until increased knowledge permits a definitive basis upon which to make clinical decisions regarding acid–base disturbances, the following guidelines are offered:

a Treat the underlying disorder, whenever possible.

b Adjust controlled ventilation to assist in pH balance.

c Remain wary of potential side-effects, especially in low-flow states.

d Recall that at extremes of pH, buffering is very limited and small changes in H^+ concentration may have profound effects on pH. At serum bicarbonate levels of 10–12 mmol L^{-1}, the benefit of avoiding the physiologic impairment of extreme acidosis may be worth the risk of the judicious and slow administration of a buffer.

SUMMARY

Multiple factors contribute to the clinical effects of acid-base imbalances in patients. This vastly complicates the therapy of such disturbances and makes it difficult to develop a clear, simple therapeutic plan. Despite this, there are several cardinal points that the clinician can use to guide therapy:

1 The direct effects of mild alkalemia or acidemia are overshadowed by the stimulation of the sympathoadrenal axis.

2 As alkalemia or acidemia increases, their direct depressant effects upon the organs begin to predominate over the stimulating effects of the sympathoadrenal axis.

3 Since CO_2 diffuses into cells so readily, respiratory alkalosis or acidosis will have a greater and more acute clinical effect than the same acute change in pH caused by metabolic disturbances. Hypoxic myocardial contractility is more closely related to cellular P_aCO_2 than to serum pH.

4 The price of bicarbonate administration in metabolic acidosis is the initial acute increase in blood P_aCO_2 and the subsequent decrease in intracellular pH due to diffusion of CO_2 into the cell before that cellular pH later rises.

5 If time and pH permit, the best therapy is usually the correction of the cause of the underlying metabolic derangement.

REFERENCES

1. Brackett NC, Cohen JJ, Schwartz WB. Carbon dioxide titration curve of normal man. The effect of increasing degrees of acute hypercapnia on acid–base equilibrium. *N Engl J Med* 1965; **272:** 6–12.
2. Wildenthal K, Mierzwiak DS, Myers RW, Mitchell JH. Effects of acute lactic acidosis on left ventricular performance. *Am J Physiol* 1968; **214:** 1352–9.
3. Mitchell JH, Wildenthal K, Johnson Jr RL. The effects of acid–base disturbances on cardiovascular and pulmonary function. *Kidney Int* 1972; **1:** 375–89.
4. Clowes GA, Hopkins A, Simeone F. Comparison of physiological effects of hypercapnia and hypoxia in production of cardiac arrest. *Ann Surg* 1955; **142:** 446–51.
5. Gerst PH, Fleming WH, Malm JR. A quantitative evaluation of the effects of acidosis and alkalosis upon the ventricular fibrillation threshold. *Surgery* 1966; **59:** 1050–60.
6. Rogers RM, Spear JF, Moore EN, *et al.* Vulnerability of canine ventricle to fibrillation during hypoxia and respiratory acidosis. *Chest* 1973; **63:** 986–94.
7. Kerber RE, Pandian NG, Hoyt R, *et al.* Effect of ischemia, hypertrophy, hypoxia, acidosis, and alkalosis on canine defibrillation. *Am J Physiol* 1983; **244:** H825–H831.
8. Pannier JL, Brutsaert DL. Contractility of isolated cat papillary muscle and acid–base changes. *Arch Int Pharmacodynam Ther* 1968; **172:** 244–6.
9. Katz AM. Contractile proteins of the heart. *Physiol Rev* 1970; **50:** 63–158.
10. Williamson JR, Safer B, Rich T, et al. Effects of acidosis on myocardial contractility and metabolism. Acta Med Scand 1976; **587** (Suppl.): 95–112.
11. Kontos HA, Richardson DW, Patterson Jr JL. Vasodilator effect of hypercapnic acidosis on human forearm blood vessels. *Am J Physiol* 1968; **215:** 1403–5.
12. Downing SE, Talner NS, Gardner TH. Cardiovascular responses to metabolic acidosis. *Am J Physiol* 1965; **208:** 237–42.
13. McElroy WT, Gerdes AJ, Brown EB Jr. Effects of CO_2, bicarbonate, and pH on the performance of isolated perfused guinea pig hearts. *Am J Physiol* 1958; **195:** 412–16.
14. Daugherty Jr RK, Scott JB, Dabney JM, Haddy FJ. Local effects of O_2 and CO_2 on limb, renal, and coronary vascular resistances. *Am J Physiol* 1967; **213:** 1102–10.
15. Sharpey-Schafer EP, Semple SJG, Halls RW, Howarm S. Venous constriction after exercise and its relation to acid–base changes in venous blood. *Clin Sci* 1965; **29:** 397–406.
16. Biscoe TJ. Carotid body: structure and function. *Physiol Rev* 1971; **51:** 437–95.
17. Wollman H, Smith TC, Stephen GW, *et al.* Effects of extremes of respiratory and metabolic alkalosis on cerebral blood flow in man. *J Appl Physiol* 1968; **4:** 60–5.
18. Daly MdeB, Lambertsen CJ, Schweitzer A. The effects upon bronchial musculature of altering the oxygen and carbon dioxide tensions of blood perfusing the brain. *J Physiol* 1953; **119:** 292–341.
19. Nadel JA, Widdicombe JG. Effect of changes in blood gas tensions and carotid sinus pressure on tracheal volume and total lung resistance to airflow. *J Physiol* 1962; **163:** 13–33.
20. Chanutin A, Curnish RR. Effect of organic and inorganic phosphates on the oxygen equilibrium of human erythrocytes. *Arch Biochem Biophysiol* 1967; **121:** 96–102.
21. Duke HN, Killick EM, Marchant JV. Changes in pH of the perfusate during hypoxia in isolated perfused cat lungs. *J Physiol* 1960; **153:** 413–22.
22. Bergofsky EH, Lehr DE, Fishman AP. The effect of changes in hydrogen ion concentration on the pulmonary circulation. *J Clin Invest* 1962; **41:** 1492–502.
23. Tenny SM. Sympatho-adrenal stimulation by carbon dioxide and the inhibitory effect of carbonic acid on epinephrine response. *Am J Physiol* 1956; **187:** 341–6.
24. Barer GR, Shaw JW. Pulmonary vasodilator and vasoconstrictor actions of carbon dioxide. *J Physiol (London)* 1971; **213:** 633–45.
25. Shubrooks Jr SJ, Schneider B, Dubin H, Turino, GM. Acidosis and pulmonary hemodynamics in hemorrhagic shock. *Am J Physiol* 1973; **225:** 225–9.
26. McGinn FP, Mendel D, Perry PM. The effects of alterations of CO_2 and pH on intestinal blood flow in the cat. *J Physiol (London)* 1967; **192:** 669–80.
27. Epstein RM, Wheeler HO, Frumin MH, *et al.* The effect of hypercapnia

on estimated hepatic blood flow, circulating splanchnic blood volume, and hepatic sulfobromophthalein clearance during general anesthesia in man. *J Clin Invest* 1961; **40:** 592–8.
28. Schulze-Delrieu K, Lepsien G. Depression of mechanical and electrical activity in muscle strips of opossum stomach and esophagus by acidosis. *Gastroenterology* 1982; **82:** 720–4.
29. Stone JE, Wells J, Draper WB, Whitehead RW. Changes in renal blood flow in dogs during the inhalation of 30 percent CO_2. *Am J Physiol* 1958; **194:** 115–19.
30. Norman JN, MacIntyre J, Shearer JR, *et al.* Effect of carbon dioxide on renal blood flow. *Am J Physiol* 1970; **219:** 672–6.
31. Blechner JN, Stenger VG, Eitzman DV, Prystowski H. Effects of maternal metabolic acidosis on the human fetus and newborn infant. *Am J Obstet Gynecol* 1967; **99:** 46–54.
32. Moya F, Morishima HO, Shnider JM, James LS. Influence of maternal hyperventilation on the newborn infant. *Am J Obstet Gynecol* 1965; **91:** 76–84.
33. Motoyama EK, Rivard G, Acheson F, Cook CD. The effects of changes of maternal pH and PCO_2 on the PO_2 of fetal lambs. *Anesthesiology* 1967; **28:** 891–903.
34. Berne RM, Winn HR, Rubio R. The local regulation of cerebral blood flow. *Prog Cardiovasc Dis* 1981; **24:** 243–60.
35. Posner JB, Plum F. Spinal fluid pH and neurologic symptoms in systemic acidosis. *N Engl J Med* 1967; **277:** 605–13.
36. Schaefer KE, Messier AA, Morgan C, Baker 3rd GT. Effect of chronic hypercapnia on body temperature regulation. *J Appl Physiol* 1975; **38:** 900–6.
37. Nahas GG, Steinsland OS. Increased rate of catecholamine synthesis during respiratory acidosis. *Respir Physiol* 1968; **5:** 108–17.
38. Nahas GG, Ligou JC, Mehlman B. Effects of pH changes on O_2 uptake and plasma catecholamine levels in the dog. *Am J Physiol* 1960; **198:** 60–6.
39. Hornbein TF, Griffo ZJ, Roos A. Quantitation of chemoreceptor activity: interrelation of hypoxia and hypercapnia. *J Neurophysiol* 1961; **24:** 561–8.
40. Moore EW. Ionized calcium in normal serum ultrafiltrates, and whole blood determined by ion-exchange electrodes. *J Clin Invest* 1970; **49:** 318–34.
41. Goodkin DA, Narins RG. Quantitation of serum potassium changes during acute acid–base disturbances. In: Whelton PK, Whelton A (eds). *Potassium in Cardiovascular and Renal Medicine.* New York: Marcel Dekker, 1986: 67–78.
42. Albarran-Sotelo R, Atkins JM, Bloom RS, *et al.* Cardiovascular pharmacology I. In: Cummins RO (ed.). *Advanced Cardiovascular Life Support.* Dallas, TX: American Heart Association, 1997: 7.14–7.15.
43. Young GP. Reservations and recommendations regarding sodium bicarbonate administration in cardiac arrest. *J Emerg Med* 1988; **6:** 321–3.
44. Weil MH, Rackow EC, Trevino R, *et al.* Difference in acid–base state between venous and arterial blood during cardiopulmonary resuscitation. *N Engl J Med* 1986; **315:** 153–6.
45. Bishop RL, Weisfeldt ML. Sodium bicarbonate administration during cardiac arrest. Effect on arterial pH, Pco_2, and osmolality. *J Am Med Assoc* 1976; **235:** 506–9.
46. Berenyi K, Wolk M, Killip T. Cerebrospinal fluid acidosis complicating therapy of experimental cardiopulmonary arrest. *Circulation* 1975; **52:** 319–24.
47. Mattar JA, Weil MH, Shubin H, Stein L. Cardiac arrest in the critically ill. II. Hyperosmolal states following cardiac arrest. *Am J Med* 1974; **56:** 162–8.
48. Pedersen KO. Binding of calcium to serum albumin. II. Effect of pH via competitive hydrogen and calcium ion binding to the imidazole groups of albumin. *Scand J Clin Lab Invest* 1972; **29:** 75–83.
49. Lang RM, Fellner SK, Neumann A, *et al.* Left ventricular contractility varies directly with blood ionized calcium. *Ann Intern Med* 1988; **108:** 524–9.
50. Cooper DJ, Walley KR, Wiggs BR, Russell JA. Bicarbonate does not improve hemodynamics in critically ill patients who have lactic acidosis. A prospective, controlled study. *Ann Intern Med* 1990; **112:** 492–8.
51. Arieff AI, Leach W, Park R, Lazarowitz VC. The systemic effects of $NaHCO_3$ in experimental lactic acidosis in dogs. *Am J Physiol* 1982; **242:** F586–F591.

20

Calcium and magnesium

MICHAEL F M JAMES

Calcium and magnesium are the major divalent cations in the body. The two elements are chemically related, both being classified as alkaline earths in group 2 (IIa) in the periodic table and occupying adjacent periods. Both ions are of importance for skeletal and muscular integrity, with calcium being the most important structural mineral in the body. Although these structural roles are critical, it is the metabolic and regulatory functions of these two substances that have attracted most recent attention. Both ions also have the potential to be used as pharmacologic agents for various therapeutic purposes.

CALCIUM

Calcium (atomic weight 40.3) is present in the human body in greater amounts than any other mineral, with the average human body containing about 1100 g of calcium. Calcium is found in all tissues of the body, but by far the majority is in the skeleton (about 1 kg in the average adult man). The greater proportion of bone calcium is bound in the hydroxyapatite and is necessary for structural integrity; a smaller pool of approximately 100 mmol of readily exchangeable calcium exists, which can be rapidly released into the circulation as required. The total plasma concentration of calcium is approximately 2.5 mmol L^{-1}, divided almost equally into a protein-bound component and a freely diffusible, ionized fraction (Table 20.1); a small additional quantity is complexed with HCO_3^-, phosphate, and citrate. The ionized calcium fraction (Ca^{2+}) is responsible for a wide range of physiological functions including blood coagulation, activation of calcium-dependent enzymes, and the release of neurotransmitters and hormones. Intracellular calcium is a critical controller of muscle contraction, metabolic processes, and an array of other intracellular functions. Although the quantity of intracellular calcium is quite large (approximately 275 mmol in the average adult), most of this is bound to intracellular proteins or sequestered in intracellular organelles, such as the endoplasmic reticulum and the mitochondria. Consequently, the free, cytosolic calcium concentration is extremely low.

Regulation of plasma calcium concentration

Despite large movements of calcium across the three major organ systems involved in calcium exchange – the gut, the kidney, and the bone – the plasma concentration of calcium is remarkably constant. The plasma calcium concentration is regulated by the interaction of four factors – Ca^{2+} itself, parathyroid hormone (PTH), calcitonin, and vitamin D in its active form of 1,25-dihydroxy-vitamin D_3, also known as calcitriol (Fig. 20.1).

The calcium receptor

The discovery of an extracellular, G-protein-coupled, calcium-sensing receptor (CaR) has helped to clarify some of the mechanisms by which calcium and its regulating factors interact.[1] The CaR represents the first example of a G-protein-coupled, cell-surface receptor to be described in mammals that responds to inorganic ions rather than molecules. The response range of this receptor is in the millimolar concentration for both Ca^{2+} and Mg^{2+}, as opposed to the nanomolar to micromolar response range of the intracellular calcium receptors.[2] However, this response range is in the physiologically relevant concentration of these ions in extracellular fluid. The CaR has been demonstrated in several organ systems including the parathyroid gland and the kidney – where it coordinates regulation of the extracellular ionized calcium concentration ($[Ca^{2+}]_o$) – as well as in the thyroidal C-cells, brain, and gastrointestinal tract, where its regulatory function has yet to be fully elucidated.[3,4] Activation of the CaR by Ca^{2+} results in CaR-mediated activation of second-messenger systems such as phospholipases and cyclic adenosine monophosphate (cAMP) and leads to altered function in the target cells.

The CaR system regulates parathyroid secretion, with an increase in $[Ca^{2+}]_o$ inhibiting the release of PTH. The production of PTH is also controlled by the PTH gene, and expression of this gene is regulated by calcium, phosphate, and vitamin D.[5] Mutations of this gene produce abnormalities of Ca^{2+} homeostasis, leading to congenital disorders of calcium metabolism.[6] It is also possible that estrogen may exert its effects on calcium metabolism through a regulatory action on the PTH gene. The relation between $[Ca^{2+}]_o$ and parathyroid hormone release is a very tight one with a steep dose–response curve. Remarkably small changes in the circulating concentration of either Ca^{2+} or Mg^{2+} are sensed by the CaR and produce corresponding changes in the secretion of PTH.[7] The steepest part of the response curve occurs over a range of changes in the free Ca^{2+} concentration of 0.25 mmol. Magnesium has approximately one-third of the effect of that of calcium on the release of PTH.

Parathyroid hormone

PTH is an 84-amino-acid peptide with a molecular weight of 9500 Da and a half-life in the circulation of 2–3 min.[8] PTH regulates $[Ca^{2+}]_o$ (and $[Mg^{2+}]_o$) by direct effects on the bone and the kidney and indirect actions (via calcitriol production) on the gut. When the Ca^{2+} concentration in the plasma falls, a number of events occur. In response to sudden

Table 20.1 *Concentrations and units of measurement of the divalent cations*

	Total plasma concentration	Ionized fraction	Other units
Calcium	2.2–2.7 mmol L^{-1}	0.9–1.1 mmol L^{-1}	1 mmol L^{-1} = 2 mequiv L^{-1} = 4 mg 100 mL^{-1}
Magnesium	0.75–1.2 mmol L^{-1}	0.47–0.70 mmol L^{-1}	1 mmol L^{-1} = 2 mequiv L^{-1} = 2.4 mg 100 mL^{-1}

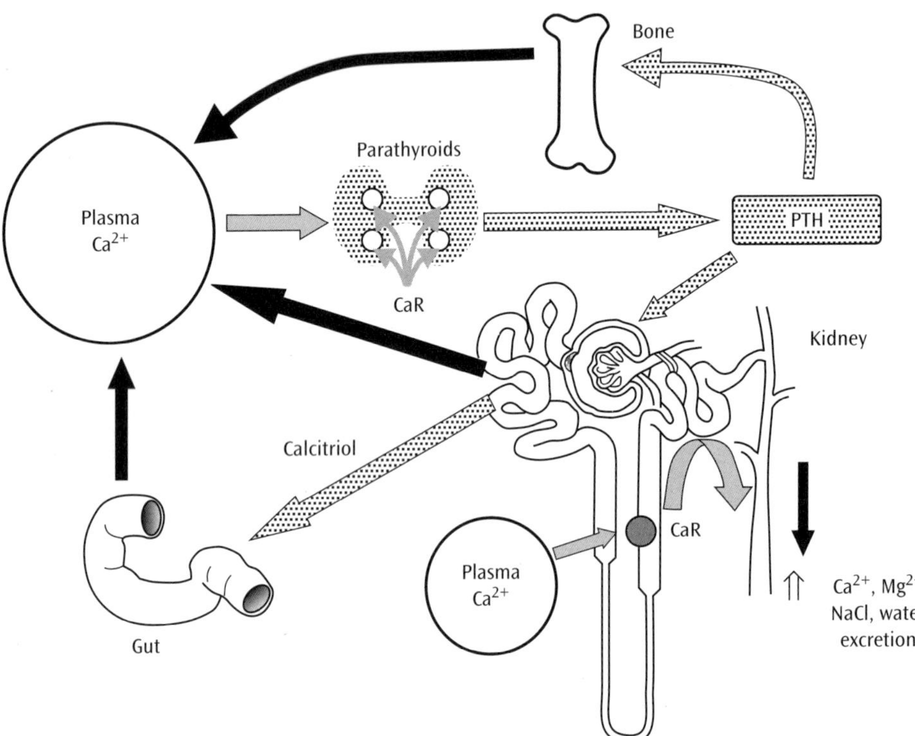

Figure 20.1 *Control of plasma calcium. Ionized calcium (Ca^{2+}) acts on the extracellular calcium receptor (CaR) in the parathyroid glands to inhibit the release of parathyroid hormone (PTH), while low plasma Ca^{2+} stimulates the release of PTH. PTH acts on bone to release calcium and on the kidney to reabsorb calcium. PTH also stimulates the conversion of vitamin D to calcitriol, which, in turn, stimulates the uptake of calcium from the gut. Elevated Ca^{2+} acts on the CaR in the thick ascending limb of the loop of Henle to inhibit sodium and water reabsorption, resulting in diuresis, together with calcium and magnesium loss. Black arrows indicate movement of calcium; gray arrows indicate actions of calcium; hatched arrows indicate hormone effects.*

reductions in the plasma Ca^{2+} concentration (such as can be produced by the infusion of citrate-containing blood), calcium in the rapidly exchangeable pool of bone is swiftly mobilized. This minimizes short-term fluctuations in plasma calcium concentration. At the same time, there is a rapid increase in the concentration of PTH,[9] which stimulates osteoblastic activity directly, with indirect stimulation of osteoclastic activity[8] resulting in an increase in bone turnover with a slower, but more sustained, release of calcium into the circulation.

PTH also influences the excretion of calcium in the kidneys and absorption of calcium from the gut. In the kidney, PTH acts on the thick ascending limb of the loop of Henle and in the distal convoluted tubule to increase reabsorption of Ca^{2+}. In the proximal tubule, PTH inhibits the reabsorption of inorganic phosphate, thus increasing phosphate excretion. PTH also stimulates the conversion of vitamin D from 25-hydroxy-cholecalciferol to the vastly more active 1,25-dihydroxy-cholecalciferol (calcitriol) in the kidney. Calcitriol acts on intestinal epithelial cells, causing the opening of calcium channels, allowing the influx of calcium into these cells. Calcitriol is also thought to activate calcium-binding proteins known as calbindins, which are structurally similar to troponin C and facilitate the absorption of calcium from the intestinal lumen and then the active transport of calcium out of the luminal cells and into the circulation. Calcitriol may also have an effect on osteoclast activity.

Parathyroid hormone-related protein is a 141-amino-acid peptide, functionally similar to PTH, which is produced by certain malignant tumors, particularly squamous cell tumors of the head and neck and also tumors arising from kidney, breast, and lymphoid tissue. It is responsible for the majority of the hypercalcemia associated with malignancy.

Renal control of calcium

Renal control of calcium (and magnesium) excretion is also influenced directly by the plasma Ca^{2+} (and Mg^{2+}) concentration through the CaR, which is located on the thick ascending limb of the loop of Henle. Stimulation of the CaR reduces tubular NaCl reuptake, as well as Ca^{2+} and Mg^{2+} reabsorption, with consequent increases in water excretion. Increased peritubular Ca^{2+} may also act on the CaR to reduce the magnitude of antidiuretic hormone (ADH)-stimulated water reabsorption in the collecting duct, further encouraging diuresis. Thus, elevated plasma concentrations of Ca^{2+} or Mg^{2+} enhance the excretion of both cations, as well as increasing sodium and water clearance through the kidney.[2] This mechanism explains the well-known diuretic effect of both Ca^{2+} and Mg^{2+}, and may have relevance in reducing the likelihood of renal stone formation by decreasing the urinary concentration of calcium.

Calcitonin

The third hormone involved in calcium regulation is calcitonin, which is a linear polypeptide produced by the parafollicular cells of the thyroid gland. Calcitonin secretion is regulated by the plasma Ca^{2+} concentration and the hormone acts on bone to suppress osteoclastic activity. It also enhances renal excretion of calcium, sodium, phosphate,

> *Plasma calcium control*
>
> - Parathyroid hormone controls plasma calcium concentration by regulating calcium release from bone and reabsorption from the kidney.
> - The extracellular calcium receptor regulates release of PTH by a negative feedback mechanism whereby high calcium concentrations inhibit PTH release.
> - The CaR in the loop of Henle increases calcium, magnesium, sodium, and water loss from the kidney in response to high plasma calcium or magnesium concentrations.
> - Calcitriol is formed in the kidney from vitamin D under the influence of PTH and stimulates absorption of calcium from the gut.

magnesium, and potassium, and thus, potentially, acts as an antagonist of PTH. However, it does not appear to exert important physiological activity, except perhaps in pregnancy and neonatal life. A total absence of calcitonin appears to be without major physiological consequence.[8]

Physiological actions of calcium

Calcium ions function as a universal second-messenger system activating and regulating a wide range of cellular activity, the nature of which depends on the specialization of the individual cell. Not only does calcium trigger contraction in muscle cells but it also controls key metabolic enzymes, particularly those in the mitochondria, and stimulates hormone and neurotransmitter release. The mechanisms by which the calcium signal is generated are very diverse, ranging from brief, highly localized bursts of calcium release to long-acting global signals, which may even appear as repetitive waves of calcium throughout the cytosol. In order for calcium to function at peak efficiency, the intracellular concentration ($[Ca^{2+}]_i$) must be very tightly controlled. The mechanisms for regulating intracellular Ca^{2+} vary considerably between cell types and involve mechanisms to control Ca^{2+} entry, release, uptake, elimination, and protein binding. However, the sources of Ca^{2+} can essentially be divided into two: an infinite supply of extracellular calcium and a more limited internal store contained within the endoplasmic reticulum.

Cellular regulation

The $[Ca^{2+}]_i$ is extremely low, of the order of 100–200 nmol (1×10^{-7} molar), and consequently the Ca^{2+} gradient across the cell membrane is very large (10 000-fold)[10] compared with that of sodium, which is of the order of 10- to 20-fold. Furthermore, the gradient between the cytosol and the intracellular organelles, particularly the endoplasmic reticulum, is of a similar order of magnitude. The widespread role of $[Ca^{2+}]_i$ in ordering cell function demands that Ca^{2+} fluxes across cell membranes are tightly controlled, and this is achieved through a series of ion channels, pumps, calcium-binding proteins, and calcium exchangers.

The transcellular calcium gradient can be maintained because the cell membrane has a low natural permeability to divalent cations, and calcium entry into the cell can only occur through ion-specific channels. Nevertheless, the extreme transcellular gradient means that there is a constant trend for calcium influx into the cytosol, and thus the maintenance of the very low $[Ca^{2+}]_i$ is dependent on energy-requiring mechanisms that can extrude the ion against this large concentration gradient. There are at least two adenosine triphosphate (ATP)-dependent pumps, which remove calcium from the intracellular to the extracellular space. The first is a low-capacity, high-affinity Ca^{2+}/H^+ exchanger, which is directly dependent on ATP and which fine tunes the intracellular calcium concentration. The second mechanism is the Na^+/Ca^{2+} exchange pump, which is a high-capacity, low-affinity system that moves large quantities of calcium out of the cell, and is driven by the transmembrane sodium gradient ($[Na^+]_o/[Na^+]_i$). This pump exchanges three Na^+ ions for each Ca^{2+} ion removed from the intracellular space and the rate of removal of calcium is directly proportional to the $[Na^+]_o/[Na^+]_i$ ratio. Consequently, although this pump works independently of ATP, it is indirectly dependent on ATP as the sodium gradient across the cell membrane is maintained by the Na^+,K^+-ATPase mechanism. Both of these pump mechanisms have their capacity increased by increases in $[Ca^{2+}]_i$.[11] Increased calcium influx stimulates increasing calcium extrusion, mainly through an increase in the activity of various ATPases, thereby maintaining a dynamic balance within the cytosol provided that there are sufficient supplies of ATP to maintain the integrity of the pumps (Fig. 20.2).

There is an array of calcium-binding proteins both in the cytosol and in intracellular organelles. Some of these, such as calmodulin and troponin C, function as switches that activate cellular processes in response to changes in $[Ca^{2+}]_i$. The most important of these calcium-binding proteins, calmodulin, is found in virtually every eukaryotic cell type. It contains two pairs of Ca^{2+} binding sites that appear to bind Ca^{2+} cooperatively and sequentially. Calcium binding produces a conformational change that triggers the interaction of calcium–calmodulin complexes with a variety of effector molecules. Calcium–calmodulin complexes activate a number of protein kinases, notably myosin light chain kinase, which regulates smooth muscle contraction. Other calcium-binding proteins, such as the parvalbumins, act as Ca^{2+} buffers in the cytosol by taking free Ca^{2+} out of solution. A similar Ca^{2+}-buffering function is performed by other calcium-binding proteins such as calsequestrin, calreticulin, and the calbindins within cellular organelles, particularly the endoplasmic reticulum.[12]

The intracellular organelles also play a vital role in the maintenance of calcium homeostasis. Mitochondria have a high capacity for calcium but excess accumulation of calcium by the mitochondria binds phosphate, inhibiting ATP production, and also leads to mitochondrial damage.[13] Thus, this mechanism is, at best, a short-term safety valve and not part of the normal homeostatic mechanisms for calcium regulation. The major intracellular organelle involved in calcium regulation is the endoplasmic or, in the case of muscle, sarcoplasmic reticulum (ER/SR). In most cells this extensive labyrinth of membranous tubules provides not only the major storage site but also the chief source of calcium for rapid release in response to transient stimulation. The ER/SR structure contains ATP-driven Ca^{2+} pumps, intraluminal Ca^{2+}-binding proteins, and tightly regulated calcium release channels. A rise in $[Ca^{2+}]_i$ stimulates ATPases via, among other mechanisms, calcium–calmodulin complexes and this, in turn, activates ATP-dependent pumps that drive the Ca^{2+} into the ER. Within the lumen of the ER, calcium is stored both in the free ionized state and also complexed to calcium-binding proteins from which Ca^{2+} can be rapidly released in response to appropriate stimuli. The calcium-binding proteins thus decrease the effective concentration gradient of Ca^{2+} across the ER membrane, reducing the energy requirements for calcium uptake. Endoplasmic calcium release channels are regulated by an array of mechanisms that vary considerably between different cell types.

Calcium entry into cells of all types is also extremely tightly regulated (Fig. 20.3). Calcium entry into the cell normally occurs as a result of conformational changes in the proteins that constitute the calcium channels. Three main groups of calcium entry channels have been described which respond to different types of signals. Some channels open and admit calcium in response to depolarization and are termed voltage-operated calcium channels (VOCCs). The VOCCs are divided into four subtypes designated N, P, L, and T. The first two are found only

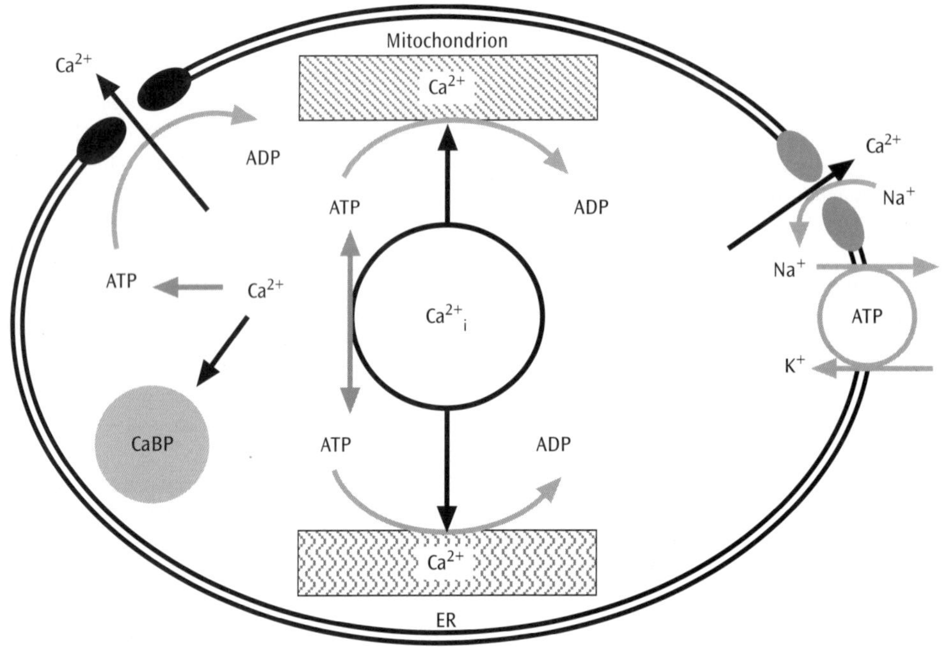

Figure 20.2 *Control of intracellular calcium. The intracellular* Ca^{2+} *is controlled at very low concentrations. A rise in intracellular calcium* (Ca^{2+}_i) *results in activation of ATPases, releasing energy to pump calcium out of the cell into the endoplasmic reticulum (ER) and the mitochondria. The main mechanism for calcium extrusion from the cell is the* Na^+/Ca^{2+} *antiporter that removes calcium in exchange for sodium. This pump is driven by the gradient for* Na^+ *across the cell membrane, and this is, in turn, maintained by the* Na^+,K^+*-ATPase pump.* Ca^{2+} *binds to calcium-binding proteins (CaBP), some of which (such as calmodulin) activate cellular processes, and others simply act as calcium buffers. Black arrows indicate movement of calcium; dark gray arrows indicate actions of calcium; light gray arrows indicate energy-requiring processes.*

in neuronal tissue. The L-type calcium channel is so named because it is long acting whereas the T-channel is more transient in its operation.[10] Others channels admit calcium as a result of changes produced in response to the binding of an appropriate ligand to its receptor and these are called receptor-operated calcium channels (ROCCs). These two channel types usually provide brief, high-intensity signals which produce rapid cellular responses. A third type of calcium entry channel, which appears to be regulated by the state of filling of calcium stores, has recently been described. These have been termed store-operated calcium channels (SOCCs) and appear to operate through a mechanism known as capacitative calcium entry, in which there is no calcium entry when the stores are filled but the channels are activated and permit calcium entry as the stores empty.[14] These channels apparently have a biphasic effect in which they are activated at low levels of calcium and inhibited at higher levels.[15] The importance of these SOCCs is that they provide a mechanism for the maintenance of the intracellular calcium stores necessary to sustain repetitive signaling in a wide range of cells.[14]

Release of calcium from internal stores, primarily the ER, is principally mediated by activation of either inositol triphosphate (IP_3) receptors or ryanodine receptors (RyRs). These massive, tetrameric proteins (> 1 MDa) function both as receptors and as calcium release channels. The RyRs are so named for their property of binding the plant alkaloid, ryanodine, which led to their discovery. Three different RyRs have now been identified: RyR_1, which is found predominantly in skeletal muscle, RyR_2, found mainly in the heart, and RyR_3, which occurs in the brain.[16] Both the IP_3 and the various RyR receptor types display the phenomenon of calcium-induced calcium release (CICR), in which a calcium signal stimulates either of the calcium release channels to release further calcium, thus providing amplification or gain of the initial signal. This mechanism accounts for the ability of calcium release channels to generate both brief, intense calcium signals – known as calcium spikes – and sustained calcium signals called calcium waves.[14] As a result, the calcium signal can vary from a localized increase in calcium in a limited area (called a microdomain) to a regenerative wave capable of sweeping through the cytoplasm, allowing for a slower, more sustained response.

The calcium signal

The response to alterations in cytosolic calcium concentrations is determined by the form of the calcium signal and the nature of the tissue involved.

Skeletal muscle

The SR is the structure mainly responsible for the regulation of $[Ca^{2+}]_i$ in all types of muscle. The SR in striated muscle has a longitudinal component and terminal cisterns.[12] The longitudinal SR is found mainly in the region of the A-band and is rich in a Ca^{2+}-ATPase known as sarcoplasmic–endoplasmic reticulum Ca^{2+}-ATPase (SERCA). The SERCA is responsible for the rapid reuptake of Ca^{2+} into the SR, and is thus largely responsible for termination of the contraction.[17] The terminal cisterns are tightly linked to the t-tubules. In striated muscle two of these cisterns are grouped around a single t-tubule in a structure known as a triad. Within this triad, the cisternal SR is linked to the t-tubule by a specific protein with junctional processes or "feet." These foot proteins have now been identified as RyRs, which are embedded in the SR membrane. The sarcolemma overlying the terminal cisterns contains a dihydropyridine receptor (DHPR) and this is tightly linked to the RyR. Stimulation of the RyR results in rapid release of calcium from the ER (Fig. 20.4). The calcium signaling system in skeletal muscle is designed to deliver a coordinated burst of calcium throughout the muscle fiber.[12] Depolarization of

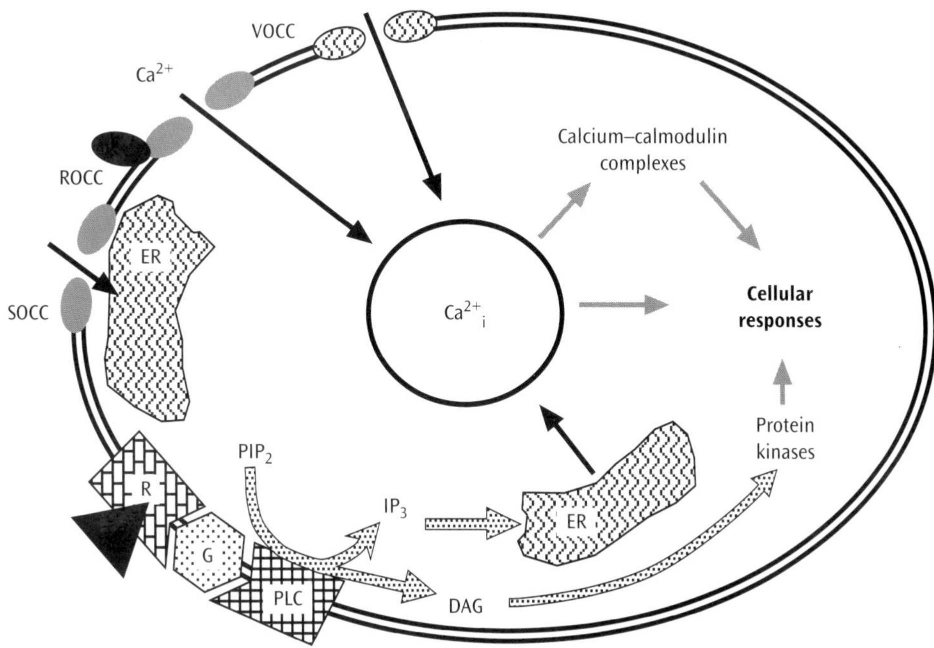

Figure 20.3 *Control of calcium entry. Calcium can enter the cell through voltage-operated calcium channels (VOCC) following depolarization in excitable tissue. Receptor-operated calcium channels (ROCC) open to admit calcium in response to the binding of an appropriate ligand to the receptor. Store-operated calcium channels (SOCC) are controlled by the calcium concentration within the endoplasmic reticulum (ER); when the ER Ca^{2+} is low, calcium enters the domain between the cell membrane and the ER apposed to the cell wall. Calcium release from the ER is controlled by Ca^{2+} itself (calcium-induced calcium release – CICR), and by the intracellular second messenger IP_3. IP_3 is generated from phosphatidylinositol bisphosphate (PIP_2) through activation of phospholipase C (PLC) by a G-protein (G)-coupled receptor. IP_3 binds to IP_3 receptors on the ER to release calcium when an appropriate ligand binds to the cell-surface receptor (R); the released calcium triggers a response that is specific to the cell type. PLC also releases diacylglycerol (DAG), which is also an intracellular second messenger. Black arrows indicate movement of calcium; dark gray arrows indicate actions of calcium; hatched arrows indicate second-messenger processes.*

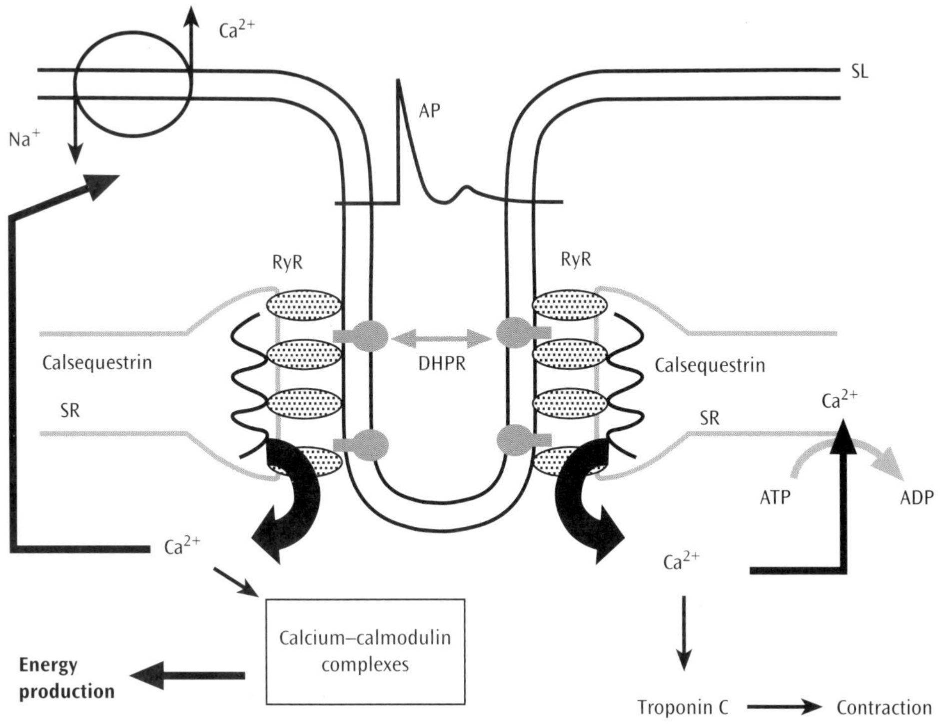

Figure 20.4 *Control of calcium in skeletal muscle. The excitation–contraction coupling unit is the triad consisting of the t-tubule and two terminal cisterns of the sarcoplasmic reticulum (SR). Depolarization of the sarcolemma (SL) by the action potential (AP) directly activates dihydropyridine receptors (DHPR), which in turn activate the underlying ryanodine receptors (RyR). The RyRs are also Ca^{2+} channels, and release Ca^{2+} from the SR into the cytosol to initiate contraction and energy production. The rise in Ca^{2+}_i activates ATPases, which pump the Ca^{2+} back into the SR, where it is bound by a calcium-binding protein, calsequestrin. Black arrows indicate movement of calcium; dark gray arrows indicate actions of calcium; light gray arrows indicate energy-requiring processes. ADP, adenosine diphosphate; ATP, adenosine triphosphate.*

the t-tubule is sensed by the sarcolemma-bound DHPR, which activates the RyR_1 receptor through a direct protein–protein interaction.[18,19] There are more RyR_1s than DHPRs, and this raises the possibility that either a DHPR may activate more than one RyR or that calcium release from one RyR may activate adjacent receptors. Until recently, it had been assumed that CICR did not occur in skeletal muscle, as the circumstances under which CICR had been observed in skeletal muscle did not exist under normal physiologic conditions. Furthermore, extracellular calcium is not essential for skeletal muscle contraction, unlike either cardiac or smooth muscle. However, recent research has suggested that a highly localized form of CICR may exist in skeletal muscle in which calcium released from either the DHPR or the RyR may induce further calcium release from adjacent RyRs.[20,21] This phenomenon may help to explain how graded responses can occur in a system that ought to be an all-or-none process. It is suggested that the elementary event is a calcium spark consisting of a brief pulse of calcium.[18] In a process analogous to synaptic transmission, spatial and temporal summation of these quantal calcium signals generates a global calcium signal.

The calcium released from the SR binds with troponin C, initiating muscular contraction. Simultaneously the rise in $[Ca^{2+}]_i$ causes the formation of calcium–calmodulin complexes, which in turn activate ATPases, increasing cellular metabolic rate and stimulating glycogenolysis, thus providing energy for muscle activity.[22]

Repolarization causes the DHPR to close the RyR_1, terminating the calcium signal. Studies have also suggested that, particularly in skeletal muscle, calcium-induced closure of calcium channels may also take place, increasing the speed of termination of the calcium signal.[20] The rise in calcium, and consequent activation of ATPases, stimulates SERCA pumps, which rapidly return the calcium to the sarcoplasmic reticulum, thus terminating the contraction. Within the lumen of the SR a protein known as calsequestrin has been proposed to act as a Ca^{2+}-binding agent, enhancing the ability of the SR to sequester calcium. This is a high-capacity, low-affinity calcium-binding agent, which can accumulate large amounts of calcium. Activation of the RyR_1 elicits a signal, which is transmitted to calsequestrin and appears to be important in the release of bound Ca^{2+} into the SR lumen, making it available for release into the cytosol.[19] A related isoform of this protein has been identified in cardiac muscle SR. There is a similar, but not identical, protein in the sarcoplasmic reticulum of smooth muscle called calreticulin.

In malignant hyperthermia (MH), the defect probably resides in the RYR_1. It is postulated that the abnormal RyR_1, in response to certain trigger substances, allows a continuous leak of calcium from the sarcoplasmic reticulum. After exposure of the muscle to triggering agents, the sustained release of calcium results in massive stimulation of aerobic and anaerobic metabolism. Creatine phosphate levels fall, followed by decreases in ATP. The drop in ATP results in a failure of SR uptake of calcium and produces muscle rigidity, lactic acidosis, hypercarbia, and, ultimately, hyperthermia, cardiac arrhythmias, and death.[19] The RyR has both high- and low-affinity binding sites for calcium, and it appears that the low-affinity site is responsible for the inhibition of Ca^{2+} release produced by dantrolene.[16]

Cardiac muscle

Although the basic structure of cardiac muscle is similar to that of skeletal muscle, there are essential structural and functional differences that affect the calcium signal. Unlike skeletal muscle, cardiac muscle is dependent on both extracellular and intracellular sources of calcium for myocardial contraction. This is reflected in the different shape of the myocardial action potential in which the plateau phase represents the inward calcium current. In cardiac muscle the relation between the terminal cisterns of the SR and the t-tubules is different from skeletal muscle in that there is usually only one terminal SR structure related to the t-tubule (a dyad). The RyR_2 in cardiac muscle is slightly, but significantly, different from the RyR_1 in skeletal muscle. Furthermore, there is no direct contact between the DHPRs and the RyR_2s.[18] When a voltage change is sensed by the DHPRs, these L-type calcium channels open to give a brief pulse of calcium into the underlying cleft between the sarcolemma and the SR.[14] This calcium signal then activates the adjacent RyR_2s.[23] Thus, electromechanical coupling in cardiac muscle is entirely dependent on CICR.[18] The DHPR-induced calcium release activates a small, localized group of RyR_2s (usually four), generating a quantal calcium spark.[18] The RyR_2 has fairly low calcium sensitivity, and thus neighboring units are functionally uncoupled from one another. Consequently, the magnitude of the calcium signal is determined by the number of DHPRs activated by the change in membrane voltage. Modulation of the magnitude of the Ca^{2+} influx by cAMP and β-adrenergic stimulation not only alters the size of the global Ca^{2+} signal, and hence the force of contraction, but also increases the rate of closure of the Ca^{2+} channels, resulting in accelerated relaxation (Fig. 20.5).

Calcium reuptake into the SR is also different from that in skeletal muscle. The SERCA in cardiac muscle SR is modulated by the activity of phospholamban. Phosphorylation of phospholamban by calcium–calmodulin-dependent cAMP increases the affinity of SERCA for Ca^{2+} and thus increases the rate of calcium transport back into the SR.[24] Increases in contractility, resulting from increased levels of cAMP are, thus, also accompanied by an increased rate of Ca^{2+} removal, and hence the increased force of contraction is also associated with a decreased duration contraction.

Alterations in contractility

All currently available inotropic agents exert their effects on contractility through alterations in intracellular calcium physiology, either directly or indirectly. They can essentially be divided into two groups: agents that increase $[Ca^{2+}]_i$ and those that alter the responsiveness of the muscle filaments to calcium. Adrenergic stimulation increases influx of calcium into the myocardial cell by increasing the probability of opening of the calcium channel, thus increasing the availability of $[Ca^{2+}]_i$. α-Adrenergic activity enhances the opening of the L-type calcium channel directly. β-Adrenergic stimulation exerts its far more pronounced effect, stimulating adenylate cyclase to activate cAMP with consequent phosphorylation of subunits of the L-type channel, which prolongs the opening of the channel.[10] Phosphodiesterase inhibitors, which decrease the rate of cAMP destruction, exert a similar effect in cardiac muscle. Increased concentration of cAMP not only increases $[Ca^{2+}]_i$ but also accelerates calcium reuptake into the SR by phosphorylation of phospholamban. Adrenergic stimulation also increases the rate of binding and dissociation of calcium with troponin C, and this accelerates the rate of both contraction and relaxation. However, the increasing calcium flux also increases the metabolic rate and consequent oxygen demand by myocardial cells that may predispose ischemic myocardium calcium overload. The cardiac glycosides inhibit the ATPase pump, causing the intracellular sodium concentration to rise. This decreases the efficiency of the sodium–calcium pump, causing an increase in resting $[Ca^{2+}]_i$. Although this will enhance contractility, it also diminishes diastolic relaxation.[25] The newer inotropic agents, pimobendan and levosimendan, are calcium sensitizers, which increase calcium sensitivity by binding to troponin C. It is thought that this may stabilize the calcium-induced conformational changes in troponin C, thus enhancing the effectiveness of calcium binding.[26]

The inositol triphosphate system

Inositol triphosphate (IP_3) is a phosphorylated hexose sugar that initiates the release of Ca^{2+} from ER. The IP_3 receptor (IP_3R)is also a calcium release channel and is found on the ER membranes of many cell types, including those that also carry RyRs. Most eukaryotic cells have some form of IP_3 receptor but the relative abundance and expression of these receptors is tissue specific and the system functions in both excitable

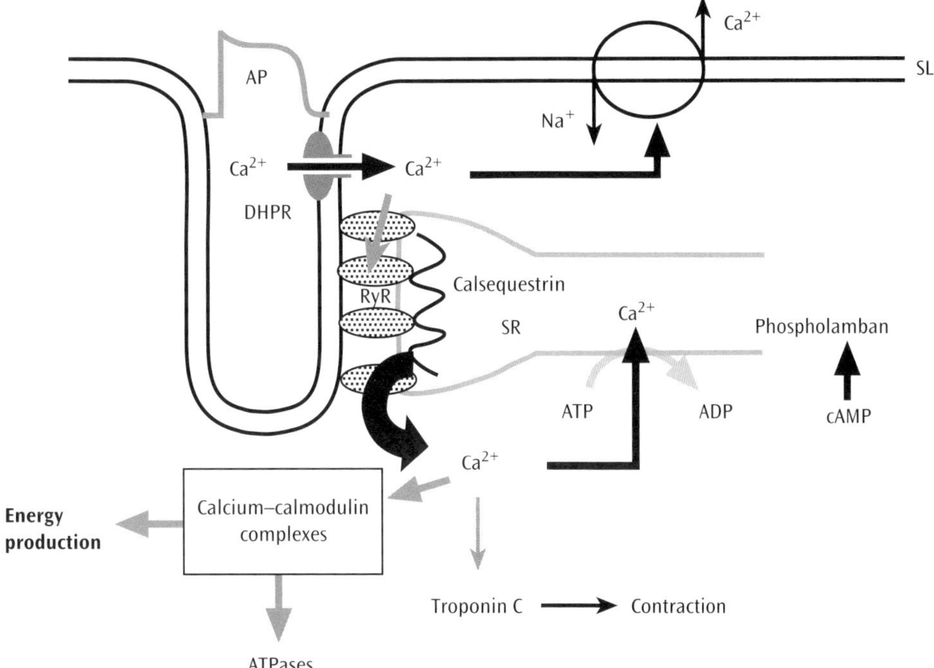

Figure 20.5 *Control of calcium in cardiac muscle. The excitation–contraction coupling unit consists of the t-tubule, an L-type calcium channel (DHPR), and one terminal cistern of the sarcoplasmic reticulum (SR). Depolarization of the sarcolemma (SL) by the action potential (AP) activates dihydropyridine receptors (DHPR), which open to admit calcium, resulting in the plateau phase of the AP. Calcium influx stimulates the underlying ryanodine receptors (RyR) to release Ca^{2+} from the SR (CICR) into the cytosol, thus initiating contraction and energy production. The rise in Ca^{2+}_i activates ATPases, which pump the Ca^{2+} back into the SR, where it is bound by a calcium-binding protein, calsequestrin. The relocation of Ca^{2+} into the SR is facilitated by the phosphorylation of phospholamban by cyclic adenosine monophosphate (cAMP). Black arrows indicate movement of calcium; dark gray arrows indicate actions of calcium; light gray arrows indicate energy-requiring processes. ADP, adenosine diphosphate; ATP, adenosine triphosphate.*

and nonexcitable cells.[14] IP_3 activation occurs when an appropriate ligand binds to its receptor and activates phospholipase C through a membrane-bound G-protein. The activated phospholipase C acts on a membrane-bound polyphosphoinositide – phosphatidylinositol 4,5-bisphosphate (PIP_2) – releasing two active components: IP_3 and diacylglycerol (DAG). The IP_3 then binds with its receptor on the ER, causing the calcium channel to open and resulting in the release of Ca^{2+} (Fig. 20.3). The time constant of the IP_3R channel is slow, and the channel itself shows a biphasic response to Ca^{2+}: an initial rise in calcium increases the sensitivity of the IP_3R but further increases in calcium diminish the responsiveness. These two factors may account for the generation of calcium waves in which successive IP_3Rs are stimulated creating a self-propagating wave of calcium through the cell. This wave of calcium and IP_3 may cross gap junctions and spread the signal to adjacent cells.[14] IP_3 itself is rapidly metabolized, limiting the extent and duration of the signal. Nonetheless, the system provides a more sustained response than RyR stimulation. DAG directly activates protein kinase C, creating a parallel limb of the signal transduction cascade, and this, too, creates a sustained response.

Smooth muscle

The molecular structure in smooth muscle is quite different from that in striated muscle and allows for the generation of greater tension, at lower energy expenditure, than that which occurs in striated muscle, but at the cost of a much slower shortening speed. The situation regarding calcium handling is also quite different. Some muscles, such as those in arteries and veins, display mechanisms similar to that in cardiac cells whereby calcium entry through VOCCs is further amplified by CICR from internal stores. However, the gain mechanism for Ca^{2+} release in smooth muscle cells is much less efficient than that in cardiac muscle and thus the entry of external calcium contributes a much larger portion of the global calcium signal.[14] This accounts for the greater sensitivity of vascular smooth muscle to calcium channel-blocking drugs. Depolarization of the plasma membrane need not take place in smooth muscle, as calcium may enter the smooth muscle cell through either VOCCs or ROCCs.[27] Smooth muscle also has the capacity for sustained response, and this depends on both the IP_3 and the DAG messenger systems. The IP_3 mechanism is primarily responsible for relatively rapid onset of effects. The protein kinase C mechanism maintains contraction, either by a direct effect through phosphorylation of myosin light chain kinase (MLCK) or via sustained calcium cycling across the cell membrane.[14] α-Adrenergic stimulation both increases transmembrane calcium flux and directly stimulates phospholipase C, thus increasing $[Ca^{2+}]_i$ by direct channel opening and through IP_3-mediated SR calcium release. There is also evidence that the reduction in membrane-bound PIP_2 may result in inhibition of the ATP-dependent calcium pump, thus decreasing calcium extrusion and effectively increasing $[Ca^{2+}]_i$. The action of calcium within smooth muscle is also quite different. It is hypothesized that calcium binds to calmodulin, and this complex then activates MLCK. The activated MLCK then catalyzes phosphorylation of the regulatory myosin light chain, resulting in actin–myosin interaction and hydrolysis of ATP.

Calcium-mediated cell death

There is now a large body of evidence that ischemia and hypoxia result in the accumulation of calcium in the intracellular space and that this is a major contributor to cell death.[28,29] Hypoxia results initially in a failure of the ATP-dependent Na^+,K^+-ATPase pump and as a consequence intracellular sodium concentrations rise. The increase in intracellular Na^+ impairs the Na^+/Ca^{2+} exchange mechanism, resulting in an increase in $[Ca^{2+}]_i$. In cardiac muscle, this accumulation of Ca^{2+} results initially in a failure of relaxation, and thus produces diastolic dysfunction as the earliest evidence of myocardial ischemia. Further accumulation of calcium results in uptake of calcium by the mitochondria, and this impairs the synthesis of ATP.[30] Mitochondrial dysfunction also leads to the genesis of oxygen free radicals, and this leads to disruption of cellular integrity.[13] Calcium-mediated activation of phospholipases results in the breakdown of membrane phospholipids and thus results in disruption of intracellular organelles and ultimately in destruction of the cell membrane and the triggering of the arachidonic acid cascade.[31] Calcium overload also stimulates glycogenolysis, which, in the face of hypoxia, results in accumulation of lactic acid.

In the brain, calcium accumulation is of special significance and the role of calcium in ischemic cell death has been extensively debated. Not only is the brain susceptible to calcium accumulation as a consequence of membrane energy failure, but, in addition, cerebral hypoxia triggers the release of excitotoxic neurotransmitters, notably glutamate. Glutamate activates further sodium influx through activation of AMPA and kainate receptor-gated Na^+ channels and also enhances Ca^{2+} influx through the *N*-methyl-D-aspartate (NMDA) receptor channel.[32] As a consequence, ischemia causes increases in $[Na^+]_i$ and $[Ca^{2+}]_i$ to nonphysiologic concentrations that are incompatible with cellular survival.[13] This process, however, does not adequately explain delayed neuronal cell death. It has been suggested that ongoing accumulation of calcium in the mitochondria may result in the impairment of ATP synthesis with resultant production of reactive oxygen species. However, recent research suggests that, while calcium influx may account for tissue necrosis, delayed cell death may involve additional mechanisms, including apoptosis. This process may be triggered by increasing extracellular potassium and, paradoxically, by a fall in $[Ca^{2+}]_o$ around the cells adjacent to the infarcted area. The decrease in the extracellular Ca^{2+} may be due to the rapid translocation of calcium to the intracellular spaces of dying cells, thus creating a penumbra in which there is a relative calcium deficit. This may be the trigger for the process of apoptosis in the cells within the penumbra, extending the area of cerebral damage.[33] Such a mechanism may help to explain the failure of the theoretically attractive NMDA antagonists to provide significant cerebral protection in the clinical situation.

Intracellular calcium

- Intracellular Ca^{2+} is extremely low and Ca^{2+} is rigorously extruded from the cytosol.
- Small increases in $[Ca^{2+}]_i$ cause powerful cellular responses, including muscle contraction, increases in metabolic rate, and increased protein turnover.
- Calcium enters the cytosol through Ca^{2+} channels, or is released from intracellular stores (mainly ER), by stimulation of the RyR or the IP_3 receptor. The calcium signal is amplified in many cells by calcium-induced calcium release.
- The mechanism of calcium release, and the response to it, is specific to each cell type.
- Excess calcium is very harmful to cells, and is a major mechanism of hypoxic cell damage.
- There is little place for pharmacological use of calcium salts other than for the correction of hypocalcemia.

Therapeutic use of calcium salts

Calcium salt solutions for intravenous administration are available as either the chloride or the gluconate. Calcium chloride contains 27.2 mg elemental calcium whereas the gluconate contains only 9.3 mg; apart from this, there is no evidence that one form is superior to another.[34] The chloride solution is very irritating to veins, and should not be administered through a peripheral line. Excessively rapid administration of either solution may induce arrhythmias. Neither solution should be given via a line through which blood or blood products are being administered, and calcium-containing solutions (such as Ringer's lactate) should be flushed out of an intravenous line before blood products are administered. The major use of injectable calcium solutions is the correction of hypocalcemia. The most common cause of hypocalcemia is an artifact of reduced plasma albumin; other causes include acute pancreatitis, hypoparathyroidism, malabsorption syndromes, and vitamin D deficiency. In anesthetic practice, acute hypocalcemia can arise from acute hemodilution and citrate loading as a result of rapid infusion of blood products. Alkalosis reduces the proportion of ionized calcium in the plasma and produces the typical symptoms of hypocalcemia including tetany, neuromuscular irritability, circumoral paraesthesia, laryngospasm, and seizures.

The use of calcium infusions in clinical practice has declined in recent years with the appreciation of the role that calcium may play in cell damage as a consequence of hypoxia. It is now widely recommended that calcium be excluded from most cardiopulmonary resuscitation regimens, as administering excess calcium may worsen reperfusion injury. Calcium is indicated in circumstances such as citrate toxicity in which calcium deficiency is the presumed cause of cardiac arrest, where potassium excess is suspected, or in cases of calcium antagonist toxicity. The use of calcium as a myocardial stimulant following cardiopulmonary bypass is controversial, as the improvement in contractility is brief but is associated with diastolic dysfunction[35,36] and coronary artery constriction.[37] Calcium probably should not be administered routinely upon emergence from cardiopulmonary bypass, but correction of significant hypocalcemia should be titrated against frequent estimations of ionized calcium in blood.[38]

Calcium supplementation during blood transfusion is also the matter of some debate. The effect of citrate on plasma Ca^{2+} is dependent on the rate of infusion and is negligible unless the infusion rate is at least $100\,mL\,min^{-1}$ in the average 70-kg adult.[39] The large stores of calcium and the rapid removal of citrate by the liver are usually sufficient to prevent depletion of Ca^{2+}. However, during massive blood transfusion,[40] or when liver function is impaired, the administration of calcium may be beneficial, especially during liver transplantation.[41] Again, calcium administration should be titrated against measurements of plasma Ca^{2+} wherever possible. Hypocalcemia is not usually a significant cause of coagulation difficulties, as the Ca^{2+} concentrations required to impair coagulation are low ($<0.6\,mmol\,L^{-1}$).[42]

Hypercalcemia

Hypercalcemia has many causes, which are summarized in Table 20.2. Patients should be evaluated for abnormalities of renal, cardiac, or central nervous systems. Mild hypercalcemia is seldom symptomatic and rarely warrants special treatment. Emergency treatment of hypercalcemia is indicated when the total serum calcium concentration exceeds $3.5\,mmol\,L^{-1}$. Rarely, emergency parathyroidectomy may be

Table 20.2 *Causes of hypercalcemia*

1	Common Artifactual – hyperalbuminemia, hypergammaglobulinemia Malignancy with skeletal metastases (e.g. breast, lung) Hematological malignancy (myeloma, lymphoma) Primary hyperparathyroidism
2	Uncommon Tertiary hyperparathyroidism – renal transplantation, chronic renal failure Vitamin D toxicity Increased responsiveness to vitamin D (e.g. sarcoidosis) Immobility – Paget's disease Milk alkali syndrome Thyrotoxicosis Thiazide diuretics Adrenal failure Pheochromocytoma Familial hypocalciuric hypercalcemia Hemodialysis – high dialysate calcium

required for very high levels of serum calcium (>5 mmol L^{-1}). The most crucial factor is the re-establishment of cardiovascular homeostasis and adequate renal function, rather than the reduction in the plasma Ca^{2+} to any predetermined value. Hypercalcemia induces a diuresis, due to the stimulation of the renal CaR (see above), and, consequently, patients with hypercalcemia are usually significantly fluid depleted. Fluid replacement should be with saline solutions and, once the plasma volume is re-expanded, the use of diuretics such as furosemide can assist in the reduction of serum calcium levels. Correction of the concomitant hypophosphatemia will inhibit the absorption of calcium from the gut, increase bone uptake of calcium, and correct the cardiac and skeletal muscle weakness that accompanies phosphate deficits. However, the use of sodium phosphate to lower calcium concentrations can no longer be recommended because of the risk of calcium phosphate deposition in the tissues. Other agents that will lower the plasma Ca^{2+} include the diphosphonates, plicamycin (mithramycin), calcitonin, and glucocorticoids. Plicamycin, a cytotoxic agent, impedes osteoclastic bone resorption, but may have renal, hepatic, and hematological toxic effects and must be used with caution. The diphosphonates also inhibit osteoplastic activity. Both of these agents will take several days to be effective, and their use to lower $[Ca^{2+}]_o$ prior to parathyroidectomy is seldom necessary. Saline diuresis may produce hypokalemia and hypomagnesemia, with a resultant increase in risk of cardiac dysrrhythmias, and potassium and magnesium supplementation should be considered. Once adequate fluid balance has been established, the management is that of the underlying condition. There is no literature to support any specific plasma calcium concentration as a cut-off value above which anesthesia becomes unacceptably hazardous.

MAGNESIUM

Magnesium (atomic weight 24.3) is the fourth most abundant cation in the body and the second most plentiful intracellular cation after potassium. The average adult male body contains approximately 24 g (1000 mmol) elemental magnesium; of this 50–60% is contained within bone and approximately 20% in skeletal muscle, with the remainder found in other body tissues, especially the liver and the heart. Only 1% of whole-body magnesium is in the extracellular fluid compartment including the plasma. In the plasma, approximately one-third of the total plasma magnesium is bound to protein and approximately 5.5% is complexed to phosphate, citrate, and other compounds. The normal plasma Mg^{2+} concentration is 0.75–1.1 mmol L^{-1} (1.5–2.2 mequiv L^{-1} or 1.8–2.5 mg dL^{-1}), of which 60–70% is ionized, 20–30% bound to protein, and the remainder (1–5%) complexed with other ions (Table 20.1).[43] As with calcium, the ionized Mg^{2+} fraction is believed to be the physiologically active form, and may be a more accurate reflector of total body magnesium stores,[44] but the relation between ionized measures of Mg^{2+} and the consequences of magnesium deficiency is not yet established.[45]

Regulation of magnesium homeostasis

In contrast to calcium, magnesium is predominantly an intracellular ion, and magnesium homeostasis is relatively poorly regulated by hormones, depending largely on absorption from the gut and excretion via the kidneys. The recommended dietary allowance for magnesium is 300–350 mg, with a higher requirement in pregnancy. Important dietary sources of magnesium include leafy vegetables, cereals, legumes, and nuts. Changes in diets and in food preparation have resulted in a marked decline in dietary magnesium content, and hypomagnesemia is becoming increasingly common. About 30% of ingested magnesium is absorbed from the gut through a poorly understood process that is a combination of passive diffusion and active transport.

The major regulatory system for absorbed magnesium is the kidney, which excretes between 120 and 150 mg Mg^{2+} per 24 h in an individual on a normal diet, although during periods of magnesium excess very much higher excretion rates can be achieved. About 70% of the total plasma Mg^{2+} is ultrafilterable through the glomerulus. In contrast with other ions, approximately 60% of the filtered magnesium is reabsorbed in the thick ascending limb of the loop of Henle, rather than the proximal tubule, mainly by passive mechanisms driven by the transepithelial voltage through paracellular pathways. The distal tubule also reabsorbs significant amounts of magnesium through a transcellular, active process.[46] A number of factors, including PTH, calcitonin, glucagon, vasopressin, and insulin, influence the reabsorption of magnesium, but the main regulator is the plasma concentration of the ion. The CaR (which also acts as a Mg^{2+} receptor) described above exerts considerable influence on renal magnesium clearance[1] and also accounts for the marked diuresis characteristic of the use of high-dose infusions of magnesium ions for therapeutic purposes. Insulin and PTH increase Mg^{2+} uptake in an additive fashion. Insulin acts in concert with other peptide and steroid hormones to control Mg^{2+} conservation in the distal convoluted tubule. Under conditions of reduced intake and normal renal function,[47] Mg^{2+} excretion can be limited to less than 1 mmol day^{-1}. Fluctuations in calcium, total inorganic phosphorus, potassium, parathyroid hormone, calcitonin, and aldosterone can influence magnesium turnover but, since magnesium itself can influence the turnover of most of these factors, the relation between them and control of total body magnesium is unclear.

Magnesium crosses the cell membrane only with difficulty, but the cytosolic concentration of Mg^{2+} is very much higher than that of calcium. The global $[Mg^{2+}]_i$ varies between 10 and 28 mmol L^{-1}, the vast majority of which is in the nucleus, the mitochondria, and the microsomes, while some is complexed with various lipid components of the cell. The free cytosolic $[Mg^{2+}]_i$ is in the range 1–3 mmol L^{-1}. Entry of Mg^{2+} into the cell occurs only during cell activity and requires active transport. It is stimulated by anabolic processes and insulin. Loss of Mg^{2+} from the cell occurs in response to catecholamine stimulation, potassium loss, catabolic processes, hypoxia, low-insulin states, and a fall in serum Mg^{2+}.

Physiological actions of magnesium

Magnesium is responsible for the activation of over 300 enzyme systems, including most of the enzymes involved in energy metabolism. It is an essential cofactor in energy production and utilization, being necessary for oxidative phosphorylation and the production and functioning of ATP. Other processes dependent on Mg^{2+} include the production of deoxyribonucleic acid (DNA) and ribonucleic acid (RNA) and protein synthesis.[48]

Magnesium is an important calcium regulator at both intracellular and extracellular sites, and has been described as the physiologic calcium antagonist.[49] Magnesium is essential for the release and action of PTH, and magnesium deficiency impairs the mobilization of calcium from bone. Magnesium exerts its calcium antagonist activity mainly by competing with calcium for entry through membrane channels in a variety of tissues. At an intracellular level, Mg^{2+} competes with calcium for binding sites on various calcium-binding proteins[50] and may thus act as a modulator of the effects of calcium as a second messenger. Magnesium also regulates the IP_3 receptor, where Mg^{2+} acts as a noncompetitive inhibitor, regulating CICR.[19] The uptake of calcium by the sarcoplasmic reticulum is highly Mg^{2+} dependent, and magnesium deficiency may thus predispose to intracellular calcium overload.

Magnesium is an essential cofactor for the Na^+,K^+-ATPase system and thus is an important regulator of transmembrane electrical potential. Magnesium blocks the efflux of potassium from the cell, possibly by closing a specific potassium channel. This may well be the mechanism by which magnesium counteracts hypokalemia. Consequently, disorders of magnesium metabolism, by altering the Na^+/K^+ gradients and transmembrane potentials, may result in irritability in various types of excitable tissues and thereby lead to conditions such as myocardial arrhythmias, tetany, and convulsions.

Skeletal muscle

Magnesium is necessary for normal energy metabolism, and in its absence muscle weakness occurs. Supplemental dietary magnesium and zinc apparently improve strength and muscle metabolism[51] and magnesium supplementation may enhance endurance and decrease the release of muscle enzymes during heavy exercise,[52] suggesting a protective role. Although Mg^{2+} is a major regulator of calcium release from the sarcoplasmic reticulum, it does not readily penetrate the intracellular space and, for this reason, magnesium is of limited value in the management of malignant hyperthermia, although the antagonism of catecholamine effects may offer some myocardial protection in a malignant hyperthermia episode.

Myocardium

Magnesium is essential for the regulation of calcium in the myocardium,[53] as well as for energy production and hence myocardial contractility. In addition to the magnesium dependence of ATP, it has been suggested that Mg^{2+} is necessary for the activation of cAMP and of SERCA, which may enhance diastolic relaxation.[54] In magnesium-deficient states, the myocardium is extremely sensitive to all types of arrhythmias, especially those associated with digitalis and catecholamines, probably through its actions in determining Na^+, K^+, and Ca^{2+} fluxes. Magnesium limits calcium influx in response to catecholamine stimulation and also minimizes the efflux of potassium and increase in lactate production that normally accompanies catecholamine stimulation. In smooth muscle, magnesium is a key modulator of blood vessel tone, acting at multiple sites, including transmembrane calcium channels and sarcoplasmic calcium release mechanisms.[55] Magnesium also acts as a direct α-adrenergic blocker.[56] It is, therefore, a major regulator of vascular tone, possibly also acting through an endothelium-dependent, nitric oxide-mediated mechanism,[57] and there is some evidence that magnesium deficiency may be important in certain forms of hypertension.

Metabolism

Magnesium is important in the release of neurotransmitters and certain hormones, notably thyroid-stimulating hormone and insulin, and in the degranulation of mast cells. It is crucial in protein synthesis and regulates, either directly or indirectly, most of the enzymes involved in the glycolytic pathway. Magnesium regulates the metabolic effects of $[Ca^{2+}]_i$ by competing for binding sites on protein kinases. Insulin also regulates $[Mg^{2+}]_i$ concentrations, and may enhance β-adrenergic stimulated increases in contractility in the myocardium through a Mg^{2+}-dependent mechanism.[58]

Magnesium deficiency

Hypomagnesemia exists when the serum concentration is less than $0.7\,mmol\,L^{-1}$. Patients are usually symptomatic at serum concentrations of $0.5\,mmol\,L^{-1}$, but symptoms may appear at higher concentrations than this.[59] However, since Mg^{2+} is primarily an intracellular ion, whole-body magnesium depletion may exist in the presence of normal serum Mg^{2+} concentrations. Consequently, detection of magnesium-deficient states may be very difficult. Whole-body magnesium deficiency can be safely assumed in the presence of hypomagnesemia, but the diagnosis of magnesium deficiency in the absence of a low plasma Mg^{2+} concentration is controversial. Various estimates of magnesium content have been recommended, including analysis of white cells and muscle or bone biopsies. No simple measurement of the real intracellular situation has emerged; measuring ionized magnesium in serum has little added value at present.[60] The magnesium load test, in which the 24-h excretion of magnesium is measured following an intravenous magnesium load of $0.1\,mmol\,kg^{-1}$ of a magnesium salt, may be useful in identifying hidden deficits.

Causes of magnesium deficiency

Magnesium deficiency occurs in a wide variety of conditions (Table 20.3). Despite this array of causes for hypomagnesemia, magnesium deficiency is seldom sought, and hypomagnesemia is frequently missed. Several drugs may contribute significantly to magnesium deficiency, particularly diuretics, and this is compounded by the concomitant use of cardiac glycosides. Infusions of epinephrine (adrenaline) and dopamine have been shown to produce significant reductions in serum magnesium concentration, although dobutamine and salbutamol apparently do not. Potassium and calcium abnormalities frequently accompany magnesium deficiency, particularly when the magnesium deficit is severe (total plasma $Mg^{2+} < 0.5\,mmol\,L^{-1}$), but neither can be used as an accurate pointer to the possibility of magnesium deficiency. Nevertheless, the occurrence of persistent hypokalemia or hypocalcemia should alert the clinician to the possibility of coexisting magnesium deficiency.

There are several groups of patients in whom magnesium deficiency is particularly likely to occur. Alcoholics are most at risk, and magnesium deficiency may occur in 30% of alcoholic patients, this being the most common electrolyte abnormality in these patients. Patients on diuretics are also a high-risk group, particularly if they are hypokalemic. As insulin is an important regulator of magnesium homeostasis, insulin-dependent diabetics are at significant risk of hypomagnesemia. The aminoglycosides and cisplatin and cyclosporine increase renal loss of magnesium. Stress hormones, particularly the catecholamines, also predispose to magnesium wasting and, consequently, there is a high

Table 20.3 *Causes of magnesium deficiency*

1	Decreased intake and absorption Poor diet Malnutrition Malabsorption syndromes Prolonged intravenous therapy Bowel dysfunction Pancreatic failure
2	Increased requirements Pregnancy Rapid growth and development Hungry bone syndrome
3	Gastrointestinal losses Prolonged diarrhea Small bowel fistulas Biliary fistulas Prolonged nasogastric suction Steatorrhea
4	Renal losses Primary renal tubular magnesium wasting Recovering ATN and renal transplantation Drugs: Thiazide diuretics, mannitol Aminoglycosides Cisplatin Digoxin Ethanol Stress aldosterone Catecholamines Hypokalemia Hypophosphatemia Hypercalcemia and hypercalciuria Diabetes

ATN, acute tubular necrosis.

incidence of magnesium deficiency among critically ill patients (up to 65%).[61] Citrate toxicity may also result in marked hypomagnesemia, and the deficit in magnesium induced by citrate overload may be even greater than the effect on calcium,[62] since the readily available stores of calcium are considerably greater than those of magnesium.

Consequences of magnesium deficiency

There is no clearly defined syndrome attributable to lack of magnesium, but rather a spectrum of nonspecific manifestations affecting various organ systems, which may be due to many factors of which magnesium deficiency is but one. This is probably because there is great variation in the individual response to magnesium deficiency and hypomagnesemia rarely occurs in isolation. However, magnesium deficiency almost certainly contributes to the impaired function of a number of organ systems, particularly in critically ill patients.

Magnesium deficiency results in increased potassium loss in the loop of Henle and the hypokalemia is refractory to potassium replacement unless the Mg^{2+} deficit is corrected first.[63] Magnesium replacement has a positive effect on potassium retention in potassium-deficient, critically ill patients.[64]

Cardiovascular manifestations

Electrocardiographic changes produced by magnesium deficiency are nonspecific and inconsistent, but there is usually an increase in heart rate. Severe magnesium deficiency results in prolongation of the PR and QT intervals, ST-segment depression, and T-wave flattening. The relevance of hypomagnesemia to the occurrence of both supraventricular and ventricular arrhythmias in magnesium-deficient patients has been reviewed recently.[65] It is not clear if magnesium deficiency is, in itself, arrhythmogenic, although magnesium deficiency is associated with increased incidence of arrhythmias after surgery.[66] Digoxin-induced arrhythmias may be refractory to conventional anti-arrhythmic agents but respond well to intravenous magnesium sulfate.[67]

Magnesium deficiency has been associated with increased levels of cholesterol, triglycerides, and low-density lipoproteins, and may be involved in the pathophysiology of cardiovascular complications from obesity.[68] Magnesium deficiency may also play some role in the development of hypertension,[69] and increased magnesium intake in the diet may improve hypertensive control.[70]

Magnesium deficiency appears to increase the risk of sudden death of patients suffering from myocardial infarction, and several studies have documented a loss of myocardial magnesium content following ischemic injury.[71] Hypomagnesemia may predispose to myocardial infarction, and may increase the risk of sudden death following an ischemic episode. In a recent epidemiological study, serum magnesium concentrations were inversely associated with mortality from ischemic heart disease and all-cause mortality.[72] Magnesium deficiency is associated with coronary artery vasospasm, and this, in turn, responds to magnesium replacement.[73]

Central nervous system manifestations

Personality changes and psychiatric manifestations have been described in association with magnesium deficiency and these may include depression, agitation, confusion, anxiety, and delirium. Seizures have also been described in association with magnesium deficiency but these are infrequent. Magnesium deficiency may contribute to the seizures associated with the alcohol withdrawal syndrome; it also interferes with thiamine utilization in the brain and may aggravate the Wernicke–Korsakoff encephalopathy. Disorders of Mg^{2+} metabolism in the brain occur in association with stroke and traumatic cerebral injury, and may contribute to cellular calcium overload.

Neuromuscular manifestations

Magnesium deficiency may produce frank tetany but this is uncommon. Of more importance, particularly in the intensive care unit, is that magnesium deficiency may result in weakness of the respiratory muscles and thus interfere with the weaning of patients from mechanical support. Correction of magnesium deficiency has been shown to improve respiratory muscle power.[74]

Magnesium replacement

Magnesium replenishment should be considered in all patients who are at risk (Table 20.3), particularly those who are persistently hypokalemic, hypocalcemic, or who have significant cardiac arrhythmias. The measurement of serum magnesium concentration, although limited, can act as a first-line guide to those needing magnesium replacement. Gambling *et al.*[75] considered that replacement of magnesium deficits should precede elective surgery in all patients at risk.

In the presence of normal renal function, Mg^{2+} replacement can be conducted very rapidly by the infusion of 40–50 mmol of Mg^{2+} (10–12 g $MgSO_4$) over 24 h; of this amount, up to 16 mmol can be infused rapidly over 5–10 min. During such replacement, routine monitoring of the tendon reflexes should be performed in spontaneously breathing patients and the infusion should be stopped and plasma concentration of Mg^{2+} checked if hypotension or bradycardia occurs, or renal output drops below 1 mL kg^{-1} h^{-1}. The aim should be to provide rapid restoration of whole-body stores without inducing excessive plasma concentrations of the ion (>2.5 mmol L^{-1}). This initial replacement can be followed by 24 mmol (6 g $MgSO_4$) for 2–5 days. Daily oral or slow intravenous administration of 4–8 mmol of Mg^{2+} can prevent further magnesium depletion once replacement is complete.

Pharmacology of hypermagnesemia

Accidental hypermagnesemia is rare in clinical medicine as absorption of the ion from the gastrointestinal tract is limited and the renal elimination of any excess Mg^{2+} is extremely rapid. Consequently, parenteral administration is the only way to achieve a significant increase in serum Mg^{2+} levels for therapeutic purposes. Increased concentration of Mg^{2+} in the plasma produces a wide variety of pharmacological responses of relevance to anesthesia. There has been growing interest in the use of magnesium as a pharmacological agent in a variety of situations, driven by an increasing awareness of the pharmacological effects of high concentrations of Mg^{2+} on the cardiovascular, respiratory, and nervous systems. In particular, the role of magnesium as a calcium antagonist with a short duration of action has suggested a number of possible applications.

Pharmacokinetics

The pharmacokinetic properties of magnesium salts have been relatively poorly studied, but the pharmacokinetics of magnesium infusions in pregnancy has been reviewed recently.[76] The distribution of magnesium to the intracellular space is at least partly determined by the initial level of magnesium stores, which can vary widely. This probably accounts for the wide variation in estimates of the volume of distribution of infused magnesium salts. Furthermore, the volume of distribution rapidly increases with a constant infusion, suggesting that active uptake of magnesium into the intracellular space is an important component of the redistribution process. A study using a rapid infusion followed by a slow infusion estimated a central compartment that approximated to the extracellular space ($0.25\,L\,kg^{-1}$) and a deep compartment that approximated to the intracellular space ($0.57\,L\,kg^{-1}$).[76] Thus, a loading dose of approximately 16 mmol (4 g $MgSO_4$) is required to raise the plasma magnesium concentration by $1\,mmol\,L^{-1}$. Absorption of magnesium following deep intramuscular injection is relatively slow, with a peak plasma concentration being achieved at around 60 min. For this reason, the initial loading dose of magnesium is usually given intravenously. A continuous intravenous infusion of $1\,g\,h^{-1}$ in the average adult will achieve a plasma concentration at steady state of around $1.7\,mmol\,L^{-1}$ and an infusion rate of $2\,g\,h^{-1}$ will produce a plasma concentration of the order of $2.2\,mmol\,L^{-1}$.

The sole route of elimination of magnesium is by renal clearance. Urinary excretion of magnesium is very rapid and is a roughly linear function of the plasma magnesium concentration.[77] However, once urinary output falls below about $0.4\,mL\,kg^{-1}\,h^{-1}$, it fails to match magnesium loading.[78] The α-elimination phase of a single bolus dose of $MgSO_4$ in sheep is of the order of 9 min (G L Ludbrook, R N Upton, and M F James, unpublished data) with a terminal elimination half-life of approximately 4 h. Urinary elimination of Mg^{2+} is accompanied by a brisk diuresis and a similar increase in the elimination of calcium, probably through activation of the renal CaR. In patients with normal renal function, the plasma concentration is dependent on the rate of infusion and renal clearance and not on the total dose administered. Continuous infusions (at an hourly rate of $15–30\,mg\,kg^{-1}$) or intramuscular injections are necessary to maintain serum Mg^{2+} levels in the generally accepted therapeutic range of $1.5–4.0\,mmol\,L^{-1}$.

Central nervous system

Magnesium inhibits calcium entry into neuronal cells at a variety of calcium channels, including acting as an NMDA antagonist. The ion penetrates the blood–brain barrier poorly and its level in the CSF is extremely tightly controlled. There is little evidence that parenterally administered magnesium salts have significant central nervous system (CNS) depressant effects. Provided ventilation is maintained, even very high levels of serum magnesium produce virtually no CNS depression.[79] The question therefore arises whether or not magnesium has major anticonvulsant properties, which would justify its use in obstetrics for the management of pre-eclampsia. Small but significant increases in CSF magnesium concentrations following magnesium treatment have been demonstrated but it is not clear whether or not this is sufficient to explain the anticonvulsant action. An alternative explanation for the anticonvulsant action of magnesium in gestational proteinuric hypertension is its cerebral vasodilator action, which reverses the cerebral vasospasm, now thought to be a principal cause of the convulsions.

Peripheral nervous system

Magnesium appears to have little axonal action on peripheral nerves, although it has been suggested that it may potentiate the action of local anesthetics. The major peripheral action of magnesium is by interfering with the release of neurotransmitter substances at all synaptic junctions.

Motor end plate

Magnesium produces a dose-dependent, presynaptic inhibition of neurotransmitter release in peripheral nerves by competing with calcium for membrane channels on the presynaptic terminal. At the neuromuscular junction, magnesium concentrations of $5\,mmol\,L^{-1}$ and above produce significant neuromuscular blockade, which is characterized by being reversed by increasing stimulus frequency, as opposed to fading. Magnesium potentiates the action and prolongs the duration of all nondepolarizing muscle relaxants,[80] and may precipitate severe muscular weakness in patients with the Lambert–Eaton syndrome or myasthenia gravis.[81] The combination of magnesium with aminoglycoside antibiotics has been reported to cause muscle weakness in a neonate,[82] but this complication has not been reported in adults. Nondepolarizing relaxants must be used with appropriate monitoring, in reduced doses, and at increased dosage intervals in patients who are significantly hypermagnesemic. Where difficulties in reversal of neuromuscular blockade occur, calcium may be of use in re-establishing normal motor function. Magnesium does not usefully shorten the onset time of nondepolarizing relaxants. There is no evidence that magnesium prolongs the action of depolarizing relaxants either in normal subjects[83] or in magnesium-treated pre-eclamptic mothers.[84] Patients treated with $MgSO_4$ do not demonstrate fasciculations, and acute administration of $MgSO_4$ prior to the use of succinylcholine (suxamethonium) appears to prevent the release of potassium provoked by the relaxant.[85] The possibility exists that magnesium may reduce the incidence and severity of succinylcholine-induced muscle pains, and may make succinylcholine usable in those circumstance in which the risks of excessive potassium release currently make the relaxant contraindicated, but, at the time of writing, no clinical use has been made of these interactions.

Autonomic nerve terminals

Magnesium exerts an effect, although less well known, on autonomic ganglia and on vagal nerve terminals similar to that demonstrated at the motor end plate. Serum Mg^{2+} concentrations exceeding $2.5\,mmol\,L^{-1}$ produce progressive inhibition of the release of catecholamines from both adrenergic nerve terminals and from the adrenal medulla, and higher levels produce ganglionic blockade.

Cardiovascular system

The early obstetric experience with magnesium showed minimal changes in the heart rate and blood pressure and created the incorrect impression that hypermagnesemia exerted no significant hemodynamic effects within the therapeutic range. On isolated heart preparations, hypermagnesemia is negatively inotropic, as would be expected from the calcium antagonistic action. However, in intact animals and humans, within the accepted therapeutic range, the dominant effect is one of a reduction in systemic vascular resistance with a compensatory increase in cardiac output, mainly mediated through an increase in stroke volume, and with only limited effects on blood pressure.[86,87] Within the range of 2–4 mmol L^{-1}, the reduction in systemic vascular resistance is of the order of 30%. Cardiac output, with improved lusitropy, is sustained up to plasma Mg^{2+} concentrations of 6.1 mmol L^{-1}.[88] At higher plasma concentrations, magnesium produces a bradycardia, resulting in a decrease in cardiac output and a fall in blood pressure but stroke volume is maintained above normal up to concentrations of 8 mmol L^{-1}.[86] The effect of magnesium on cardiac rhythm is complex; in isolated heart preparations, magnesium produces a slowing of the heart rate, but in intact animals and humans the vagolytic effect generally results in a small increase in heart rate. The effects of magnesium on the electrocardiogram (ECG) are minimal and inconsistent. The most common finding is a prolongation of atrioventricular conduction time and, in high doses, prolonged duration of the QRS complex.[65] Of particular importance is the fact that magnesium does not impair the cardiotonic action of epinephrine, even at plasma concentrations that reverse catecholamine-induced increases in blood pressure.[89]

Hypermagnesemia decreases peripheral vascular tone by a combination of mechanisms, which include calcium antagonism, antagonism of a range of hormonal vasoconstrictors, and interactions with prostacyclin and endothelium-dependent actions including nitric oxide. The interaction of magnesium with prostacyclin may also inhibit platelet function. Magnesium may also influence peripheral vascular tone by a number of other mechanisms including sympathetic blockade and inhibition of catecholamine release.

Respiratory system

Magnesium has no effect on central respiratory drive, and its only respiratory depressant effect is the result of respiratory muscle weakness. Because of its smooth muscle relaxant properties, magnesium is a bronchodilator and dilates the pulmonary vascular tree. Several studies have evaluated the use of magnesium infusions in asthma and meta-analysis suggests that the ion may be useful as an adjunct to standard therapy in severe asthma,[90] particularly for children,[91] but not as a sole agent or in mild asthma.

Genitourinary system

Magnesium has been widely used in obstetric practice, particularly in the USA, both as an anticonvulsant in eclampsia and as a tocolytic for the management of premature labor. It is also an effective renal vasodilator, and exerts a significant diuretic effect through its action on the CaR.[2] This mechanism is dose dependent, and increases the renal clearance of magnesium in proportion to the rate of rise of the plasma magnesium concentration, thus inducing elimination of the ion during periods of rapid administration.

Musculoskeletal system

Magnesium exerts its major effect on muscles at the motor end plate, although it does have minor calcium antagonist properties on the muscle itself. This may have some benefit in the management of malignant hyperpyrexia but the effect is small and probably not of great clinical significance.[92]

Therapeutic use of magnesium infusions

Magnesium salts have been used for hundreds of years for their aperient properties. For over 100 years, magnesium salts, particularly the sulfate, have been administered parenterally for a variety of clinical purposes, including anesthesia, the management of tetanus, the treatment of eclamptic convulsions, and the control of cardiac arrhythmias. Magnesium should be regarded first and foremost as a cardiovascular drug with the actions of both a calcium antagonist and an adrenergic antagonist with principally α-antagonistic actions. It is these actions of the ion that have led to considerable recent interest in the field of cardiology and cardiac anesthesia and surgery.

Obstetric use

By far the most established use of magnesium infusions has been in the control of eclampsia, an area of controversy until recently. In the last few years, several studies have established beyond doubt that magnesium sulfate is the agent of choice, at the present time, for the control of convulsions in the eclamptic patient.[93,94] The mechanism of action of the ion is unclear, although there are a number of possibilities. It is now well established that pre-eclampsia and eclampsia are characterized by intense vasospasm and increased sensitivity to pressor substances, particularly in the brain. Magnesium is a potent cerebral vasodilator[95] and reduces the cerebral arterial vasospasm in pre-eclamptic women.[96] Furthermore, magnesium is an effective antagonist at the NMDA receptor and intraperitoneal $MgSO_4$ has been shown to suppress convulsions induced by NMDA receptor activation.[97]

The role of magnesium in prophylactic management of the pre-eclamptic patient is far less certain as the incidence of eclamptic convulsions, even in severe pre-eclampsia, is very low. In a recent meta-analysis the authors concluded that there was insufficient evidence for the benefits and hazards to justify a clear recommendation on anticonvulsant prophylaxis at present, but that, if an anticonvulsant is to be used, $MgSO_4$ is the agent of choice.[98] Some studies have, however, suggested that severe pre-eclamptic patients may represent a subgroup in whom magnesium therapy may be beneficial.[99]

There are a number of considerations that the obstetric anesthesiologist, faced with a patient receiving a magnesium infusion, must bear in mind. The interaction of magnesium with muscle relaxants has been discussed, but it must be emphasized that the presence of significant hypermagnesemia in the pregnant patient makes the use of defasciculating doses of nondepolarizing relaxants prior to induction of anesthesia not only unnecessary but also potentially hazardous.

Magnesium may be of value in reducing the pressor response to intubation for patients with gestational proteinuric hypertension when general anesthesia is indicated. $MgSO_4$ (40 mg kg^{-1}) is superior to either lidocaine (lignocaine) (1.5 mg kg^{-1}) or alfentanil (10 mg kg^{-1}) for the control of the hypertensive response to intubation and produces less fetal depression than alfentanil.[100] A combination of 30 mg kg^{-1} $MgSO_4$ with 7.5 mg kg^{-1} alfentanil may be preferable to magnesium alone in severe pre-eclampsia.[101] Where general anesthesia is necessary for a patient with severe pre-eclampsia, it is our standard practice to administer 30 mg kg^{-1} $MgSO_4$ immediately after the induction agent to a patient who has received magnesium prior to surgery and 40mg kg^{-1} if she has not.

Potential interactions between magnesium and regional anesthesia are less well defined. Magnesium exerts a minor antiplatelet action, possibly similar to that produced by aspirin, but this should not pose a risk of intraspinal hemorrhage in a magnesium-treated patient requiring regional anesthesia. Magnesium increased the likelihood of modest hypotension during epidural anesthesia in normotensive ewes, but without increased risk to the fetus, probably because cardiac output was sustained.[102] A comparative study of the treatment of epidural hypotension in the presence of magnesium showed that, while ephedrine and phenylephrine were equally effective in correcting the hypotension, only ephedrine enhanced uterine blood flow, suggesting that this would be the vasopressor of choice.[103] A small human study suggested that epidural analgesia produced only small changes in hemodynamic status in pre-eclamptic patients receiving magnesium.[104] It appears, therefore, that regional blockade is safe in the presence of magnesium sulfate.

Cardiac applications

The value of hypermagnesemia in the treatment of arrhythmias is well established. The major role of magnesium in the management of rhythm disturbances is not primarily related to correction of magnesium deficiency but is because of the pharmacological actions of the ion, and its use has been advocated in the treatment of a wide range of cardiac rhythm disturbances. Magnesium supplementation has been shown to reduce the instance of atrial fibrillation following coronary artery surgery, but, overall, the evidence that magnesium salts are effective for control of supraventricular arrhythmias is weak. However, magnesium is now recommended for torsade de pointes, arrhythmias associated with digitalis toxicity, and ventricular arrhythmias refractory to other anti-arrhythmic agents such as lidocaine and bretylium. Baraka *et al.*[105] described a series of five patients with refractory ventricular fibrillation in whom a 2-g bolus of $MgSO_4$ was immediately effective in allowing successful defibrillation, and intra-aortic administration of 250 mg of $MgSO_4$ was effective in restoring the normal rhythm in a patient with intractable ventricular fibrillation during cardiac surgery.[106] Magnesium may also prevent bupivacaine-induced arrhythmias, possibly by controlling increases in intracellular potassium concentrations,[107] and has been useful in the treatment of bupivacaine-induced arrhythmias in the clinical situation (J M Thomas and A R Reed, personal communication). It would seem sensible to consider the early use of 2 g $MgSO_4$ in the management of persistent ventricular arrhythmias. Magnesium is particularly effective in controlling the arrhythmias associated with catecholamine administration,[108] being as effective as propranolol and more effective than verapamil.[109]

The place of magnesium in the management of acute myocardial ischemia is highly controversial. Several early studies suggested that magnesium might reduce both arrhythmias and mortality following myocardial infarction,[110] but the very large ISIS-4 (Fourth International Study of Infarct Survival) study failed to demonstrate any benefit.[111] Subsequent studies have suggested that the discrepancy may have been due to the fact that magnesium was administered after thrombolytic therapy in the ISIS-4 trial, and that early administration of magnesium sulfate either prior to, or at the time of, reperfusion may be beneficial in acute angina[112] and myocardial infarction by reducing infarct size, arrhythmia incidence, and even mortality.[113] However, all of these studies are relatively small, and a definitive answer on whether or not the early use of a magnesium infusion is valuable in the management of ischemic heart disease is still awaited.

Cardiovascular anesthesia

Magnesium depletion is common in patients undergoing cardiopulmonary bypass procedures and has been associated with postoperative arrhythmias, cardiogenic shock,[54] and coronary vasospasm.[114] Magnesium-containing cardioplegia is widely, but not universally, used and the inclusion of $MgSO_4$ in the pump prime and the cardioplegic solution has been shown to reduce the incidence of postoperative arrhythmias[115] and myocardial ischemia[116] and to improve myocardial performance.[117] It will not interfere with the inotropic action of epinephrine, even in the post-bypass patient.[89] Whatever the merits of the arguments around the use of pharmacologic doses of magnesium in cardiac surgical patients, it would seem logical, at the very least, to be scrupulous in avoiding magnesium depletion in the cardiac surgical patient.

The vasodilator and anti-arrhythmic properties of magnesium suggest that it may also be of use in the control of hypertension during aortic cross-clamping for major vascular surgery, and it has been used successfully when more conventional forms of treatment have been inadequate. The action of magnesium as an NMDA antagonist suggests that it may offer some protection against ischemia to the spinal cord during the surgical repair of suprarenal aortic aneurysms.[118–120] Similar neuronal protection may be offered by the infusion of magnesium during cerebrovascular surgery.[121]

Magnesium sulfate (40–60 $mg\,kg^{-1}$ intravenously) given prior to endotracheal intubation not only inhibits the rise in blood pressure but also prevents catecholamine release and is anti-arrhythmic.[122] Recent work has shown useful attenuation of the pressor response to intubation and a reduction in the incidence of myocardial ischemia in a group of patients with coronary artery disease.[123]

Pheochromocytoma

The anti-adrenergic, antihypertensive, and anti-arrhythmic actions of magnesium, together with its ability to inhibit the release of catecholamines, have been advanced as a rationale for the use of $MgSO_4$ infusions in the anesthetic management of patients undergoing resection of a pheochromocytoma. In a series of 17 anesthetics[124] and 43 subsequent cases it has been shown that magnesium effectively controls hemodynamic disturbances at induction of anesthesia, intubation of the trachea, and during surgical stimulation, and may also limit the release of catecholamines. A loading dose of 40–60 $mg\,kg^{-1}$, followed by an infusion of 2 $g\,h^{-1}$ together with 2-g incremental bolus doses, has been effective in controlling the cardiovascular responses. Very large doses are necessary to maintain therapeutic serum concentrations (which appear to be in the range of 2.5–4.0 $mmol\,L^{-1}$) and totals of up to 18 g of magnesium sulfate have been administered over a 2-h operation without subsequent neuromuscular difficulties. Additional sodium nitroprusside infusions may be needed on rare occasions during periods of tumor handling, although this has not been necessary for any of the most recent 50 of these cases. As the safety of magnesium in pregnant patients is so well established, $MgSO_4$ has obvious appeal in the pregnant patient who also happens to have a pheochromocytoma. The rationale for the use of magnesium in pheochromocytoma has been reviewed recently.[125]

Although magnesium does not inhibit the β_1-adrenergic actions of epinephrine, or diminish the effect of epinephrine on cardiac output, nevertheless, on present knowledge, caution must be advised when this agent is used for a patient with a pheochromocytoma complicated by impaired myocardial contractility. However, three patients who presented with cardiac failure due to catecholamine-induced cardiomyopathy have been successfully managed with $MgSO_4$ infusions, both in the intensive care unit and during surgery, with apparent benefit to myocardial performance. Calcium is useful in reversing the effects of magnesium when hypotension occurs following tumor excision and does not respond readily to fluid loading.

Intensive care

The deleterious effects of magnesium deficiency are now well recognized by those working in intensive care units, and most units now monitor magnesium levels in an effort to ensure that hypomagnesemia does not develop. Magnesium infusion, either on its own[126] or in conjunction with clonidine,[127] has been shown to reduce autonomic instability and to inhibit the release of catecholamines in patients with very severe tetanus. However, because magnesium lacks significant central sedative properties, it is inadequate as a sole agent, and should be used in conjunction with deep sedation regimes. Recently, the successful use of $MgSO_4$ infusions for tetanus and to avoid the need for controlled ventilation has been described[128] but caution must be used when using this form of therapy, as the combined effect of magnesium and tetanus toxin in inhibiting the release of acetylcholine may lead to respiratory muscle paralysis. Whether or not magnesium could be useful in controlling other types of autonomic instability, such as that associated with the Guillain–Barré syndrome, is unknown, but its successful use in a patient with paraplegia and autonomic instability during labor has recently been described.[129]

Other applications

Catecholamine antagonism, possible protection of ischemic cardiac tissue, and favorable pharmacokinetic properties suggest that magnesium salts may be useful in the management of perioperative hypertensive emergencies, particularly during anesthesia.[130] Magnesium modulation of NMDA-induced tissue damage, associated with neuronal injury, has led to the successful use of magnesium salts in ameliorating the outcome of brain injury[131] and cerebral ischemic events.[132]

Magnesium toxicity

Hypermagnesemia exerts its main toxic effects through respiratory paralysis, leading on to adverse hemodynamic events, including cardiac arrest. Some reports relating to massive, accidental overdose have highlighted this risk. Although fatalities have been reported,[133] the outcome generally seems to have been surprisingly good,[134] possibly because of the cerebral protective effect of magnesium. Treatment of such events requires routine resuscitative measures, possibly with the addition of calcium and support of ventilation until the excess magnesium is cleared. Unless the plasma concentration exceeds 12 mmol L^{-1}, cardiac decompensation (apart from the effects of hypoxia) should not present a major risk.[87,88] Should renal failure be part of the picture, dialysis may be required.

Magnesium

- Magnesium deficiency is one of the most common electrolyte disturbances, especially among critically ill patients, diabetics, alcoholics, and patients on diuretics.
- Magnesium deficiency may predispose to arrhythmias, may result in a deterioration in the control of hypertension, and may impair the control of diabetes.
- Magnesium infusion is the treatment of choice for control of eclamptic convulsions.
- Pharmacological doses of magnesium are highly effective against a wide range of ventricular arrhythmias, especially torsade de pointes, and should be considered in intractable ventricular fibrillation or tachycardia.
- Hypermagnesemia enhances the action of nondepolarizing muscle relaxants.
- Magnesium injections may be useful in controlling hypertensive emergencies, especially those related to catecholamine excess.
- Hypermagnesemia may offer some neuronal protection.

SUMMARY

Calcium

Calcium is both the most important structural mineral in the body and the most important cellular translator of biological signals. It is very tightly regulated at both extracellular and intracellular levels.

Extracellular calcium

The important points in relation to extracellular calcium are:

1. Plasma Ca^{2+} is regulated by the interaction of Ca^{2+} itself, PTH, calcitriol, and, to a lesser extent, calcitonin.
2. There is a unique, extracellular calcium-sensing receptor that regulates the release of PTH from the parathyroid gland.
3. The CaR also regulates renal excretion of sodium, magnesium, calcium, and water in the kidney and is responsible for the well-known diuretic effects of high plasma concentrations of calcium and magnesium.

Intracellular calcium

The important points relating to intracellular calcium are:

1. $[Ca^{2+}]_i$ is extremely tightly regulated and the free, cytosolic calcium concentration is of the order of 10^{-7} mol L^{-1}.
2. Ca^{2+} is the most important second-messenger system in the intracellular space, and small changes in $[Ca^{2+}]_i$ provoke many intracellular responses.
3. Ca^{2+} is extruded from the cytosol by energy-requiring pumps that transport Ca^{2+} either out of the cell or into intracellular organelles, mainly the ER and the mitochondria.
4. In skeletal muscle, extracellular Ca^{2+} is necessary for neuromuscular transmission, but within the myofibrils the Ca^{2+} required for contraction is entirely derived from the SR. Depolarization of the sarcolemma directly releases calcium from the SR by opening the RyR calcium channels. A genetic defect in the RyR_1 is the probable cause of malignant hyperthermia.
5. In cardiac muscle, Ca^{2+} release from the SR is dependent on an influx of Ca^{2+} through the L-type DHPR calcium channel. The Ca^{2+} signal induces opening of the RyR_2 with graded release of Ca^{2+} dependent on the magnitude of the initial Ca^{2+} signal (CICR). Smooth muscle is also dependent on this and other mechanisms (e.g. IP_3).
6. Calcium–calmodulin complexes activate a wide range of cellular functions.
7. Excess accumulation of intracellular Ca^{2+} is a critical part of the mechanism of hypoxic cell death.

The principal use of intravenous calcium administration is for the correction of hypocalcemia. Where calcium is given, dosage should be guided by regular measurement of ionized Ca^{2+} measurements. There is little place for calcium salts in cardiac resuscitation unless there is hyperkalemia or hypocalcemia.

Magnesium

Magnesium deficiency is common in hospital patients, especially the critically ill. Alcoholics, diabetics, and those on diuretics are at greatest risk. Hypomagnesemia predisposes to myocardial arrhythmias and should be corrected prior to surgery, especially cardiac surgery. Cardiac surgery and critical illness predispose to magnesium deficiency.

Therapeutic use of magnesium salts

The critical points in the therapeutic use of magnesium salts are as follows:

1 Magnesium is the first choice for control of eclamptic convulsions and may have other neuroprotective actions. It is usually administered as a loading dose of 4 g $MgSO_4$ (16 mmol) followed by an infusion of 1–2 g h^{-1}. Monitor tendon reflexes. Use with care if renal output is < 0.5 mL kg^{-1} h^{-1}.
2 Magnesium is the first choice as an anti-arrhythmic for torsade de pointes and catecholamine- or digitalis-associated arrhythmias. It may be life saving in intractable ventricular tachycardia or fibrillation. Dosage is a 2-g bolus repeated up to a maximum of 8 g in 1 h. The rôle of $MgSO_4$ for myocardial infarction is controversial.
3 Magnesium is excellent for controlling catecholamine-associated hypertension and is a valuable adjunct to the management of pheochromocytoma. In the absence of renal dysfunction, large doses of up to 20 g h^{-1} may be used intraoperatively for short periods, provided ventilation is maintained. Care with nondepolarizing relaxants is required.
4 Magnesium may be useful in the control of autonomic disturbances associated with tetanus or paraplegia.
5 Magnesium may have a place in assisting the management of poorly responsive asthma but not as a sole agent.
6 Magnesium may be regarded as a physiological calcium antagonist with a hemodynamic profile more resembling nifedipine than verapamil.

REFERENCES

1. Hebert SC. Extracellular calcium-sensing receptor: implications for calcium and magnesium handling in the kidney. *Kidney Int* 1996; **50:** 2129–39.
2. Hebert SC, Brown EM, Harris HW. Role of the Ca^{2+}-sensing receptor in divalent mineral ion homeostasis. *J Exp Biol* 1997; **200:** 295–302.
3. Hebert SC, Brown EM. The scent of an ion: calcium-sensing and its roles in health and disease. *Curr Opin Nephrol Hypertens* 1996; **5:** 45–53.
4. Pearce SH, Thakker RV. The calcium-sensing receptor: insights into extracellular calcium homeostasis in health and disease. *J Endocrinol* 1997; **154:** 371–8.
5. Silver J, Yalcindag C, Sela-Brown A, Kilav R, Naveh-Many T. Regulation of the parathyroid hormone gene by vitamin D, calcium and phosphate. *Kidney Int* 1999; **73:** S2–S7.
6. Coburn JW, Elangovan L, Goodman WG, Frazao JM. Calcium-sensing receptor and calcimimetic agents. *Kidney Int* 1999; **73:** S52–S58.
7. Wada M, Nagano N, Nemeth EF. The calcium receptor and calcimimetics. *Curr Opin Nephrol Hypertens* 1999; **8:** 429–33.
8. Mihai R, Farndon JR. Parathyroid disease and calcium metabolism. *Br J Anaesth* 2000; **85:** 29–43.
9. Marks KH, Kilav R, Naveh-Many T, Silver J. Calcium, phosphate, vitamin D, and the parathyroid. *Pediatr Nephrol* 1996; **10:** 364–7.
10. Mukherjee R, Spinale FG. L-type calcium channel abundance and function with cardiac hypertrophy and failure: a review. *J Mol Cell Cardiol* 1998; **30:** 1899–916.
11. Clark RB, Bouchard RA, Giles WR. Action potential duration modulates calcium influx, Na^+–Ca^{2+} exchange, and intracellular calcium release in rat ventricular myocytes. *Ann NY Acad Sci* 1996; **h**779: 417–29.
12. Lesh RE, Lynch C. Intracellular Ca^{2+} regulation. In: Yaksh TL (eds). *Anesthesia: Biologic Foundations.* Philadelphia: Lippincott-Raven Publishers, 1997: 105–129.
13. Kristian T, Siesjo BK. Calcium in ischemic cell death. *Stroke* 1998; **29:** 705–18.
14. Berridge MJ. Elementary and global aspects of calcium signalling. *J Physiol* 1997; **499:** 291–306.
15. Berridge MJ. Capacitative calcium entry. *Biochem J* 1995; **312:** 1–11.
16. Lunde PK, Sejersted OM. Intracellular calcium signalling in striated muscle cells. *Scand J Clin Lab Invest* 1997; **57:** 559–68.
17. Aubier M, Viires N. Calcium ATPase and respiratory muscle function. *Eur Respir J* 1998; **11:** 758–66.
18. Cheng H, Lederer MR, Xiao RP, *et al.* Excitation–contraction coupling in heart: new insights from Ca2+ sparks. *Cell Calcium* 1996; **20:** 129–40.
19. Mickelson JR, Louis CF. Malignant hyperthermia: excitation–contraction coupling, Ca^{2+} release channel, and cell Ca^{2+} regulation defects. *Physiol Rev* 1996; **76:** 537–92.
20. Rios E, Stern MD. Calcium in close quarters: microdomain feedback in excitation–contraction coupling and other cell biological phenomena. *Ann Rev Biophys Biomol Struct* 1997; **26:** 47–82.
21. Klein MG, Cheng H, Santana LF, *et al.* Two mechanisms of quantized calcium release in skeletal muscle. *Nature* 1996; **379:** 455–8.
22. Hayashi T, Wojtaszewski JF, Goodyear LJ. Exercise regulation of glucose transport in skeletal muscle. *Am J Physiol* 1997; **273:** E1039–E1051.
23. Wier WG, Lopez-Lopez JR, Shacklock PS, Balke CW. Calcium signalling in cardiac muscle cells. *Ciba Foundation Symposium* 1995; **188:** 146–60.
24. Koss KL, Kranias E.G.. Phospholamban: a prominent regulator of myocardial contractility. *Circ Res* 1996; **79:** 1059–63.
25. Brixius K, Pietsch M, Hoischen S, *et al.* Effect of inotropic interventions on contraction and Ca^{2+} transients in the human heart. *J Appl Physiol* 1997; **83:** 652–60.
26. Holubarsch C. New inotropic concepts: rationale for and differences between calcium sensitizers and phosphodiesterase inhibitors. *Cardiology* 1997; **88** (Suppl. 2): 12–20.
27. Somlyo AP, Somlyo AV. Signal transduction and regulation in smooth muscle. *Nature* 1994; **372:** 231–6.
28. Tymianski M. Cytosolic calcium concentrations and cell death in vitro. *Adv Neurol* 1996; **71:** 85–105.
29. Tymianski M, Tator CH. Normal and abnormal calcium homeostasis in neurons: a basis for the pathophysiology of traumatic and ischemic central nervous system injury. *NeuroSurg* 1996; **38:** 1176–95.
30. Nicholls DG, Budd SL. Mitochondria and neuronal survival. *Physiol Rev* 2000; **80:** 315–60.
31. Bagchi D, Wetscher GJ, Bagchi M, *et al.* Interrelationship between cellular calcium homeostasis and free radical generation in myocardial reperfusion injury. *Chem Biol Interact* 1997; **104:** 65–85.
32. Budd SL. Mechanisms of neuronal damage in brain hypoxia/ischemia: focus on the role of mitochondrial calcium accumulation. *Pharmaco Ther* 1998; **80:** 203–29.
33. Lee J-M, Zipfel GJ, Choi DW. The changing landscape of ischaemic brain injury mechanisms. *Nature* 1999; **399:** A7–A14.
34. Aguilera IM, Vaughan RS. Calcium and the anaesthetist. *Anaesthesia* 2000; **55:** 779–90.
35. DeHert SG, Ten Broecke PW, De Mulder PA, *et al.* Effects of calcium on left ventricular function early after cardiopulmonary bypass. *J Cardiothoracic Vasc Anesth* 1997; **11:** 864–9.
36. Virtanen VK, Saha HH, Groundstroem KW, *et al.* Calcium infusion and left ventricular diastolic function in patients with chronic renal failure. *Nephrol Dial Transplantation* 1998; **13:** 384–8.
37. Crystal GJ, Zhou X, Salem MR. Is calcium a coronary vasoconstrictor in vivo? *Anesthesiology* 1998; **88:** 735–43.
38. Robertie PG, Butterworth JF, Royster RL, *et al.* Normal parathyroid hormone responses to hypocalcemia during cardiopulmonary bypass. *Anesthesiology* 1991; **75:** 43–8.
39. Denlinger JK, Nahrwold ML, Gibbs PS, Lecky JH. Hypocalcaemia during rapid blood transfusion in anaesthetized man. *Br J Anaesth* 1976; **48:** 995–1000.
40. Linko K, Saxelin I. Electrolyte and acid–base disturbances caused by blood transfusions. *Acta Anaesthesiol Scand* 1986; **30:** 139–44.
41. Bertholf RL, Bertholf MF, Brown CM, Riley WJ. Ionized calcium buffering in the transfused anhepatic patient: Ab initio calculations of calcium ion concentrations. *Ann Clin Lab Sci* 1992; **22:** 40–50.
42. Ataullakhanov FI, Pohilko AV, Sinauridze EI, Volkova RI. Calcium threshold in human plasma clotting kinetics. *Thromb Res* 1994; **75:** 383–94.
43. Saris NE, Mervaala E, Karppanen H, *et al.* Magnesium. An update on physiological, clinical and analytical aspects. *Clin Chim Acta* 2000; **294:** 1–26.
44. Munoz R, Laussen PC, Palacio G, et al. Whole blood ionized magnesium: age-related differences in normal values and clinical implications of ionized hypomagnesemia in patients undergoing surgery for congenital cardiac disease. *J Thorac Cardiovasc Surg* 2000; **119:** 891–8.
45. Foley C, Zaritsky A. Should we measure ionized magnesium? *Crit Care Med* 1998; **26:** 1949–50.
46. Quamme GA, de-Rouffignac C. Epithelial magnesium transport and regulation by the kidney. *Frontiers Biosci* 2000; 5: D694–D711.

47. Burch GE, Giles TD. The importance of magnesium deficiency in cardiovascular disease. *Am Heart J* 1977; **94:** 649–57.
48. Weisinger JR, Bellorin-Font E. Magnesium and phosphorus. *Lancet* 1998; **352:** 391–6.
49. Iseri LT, French JH. Magnesium: Nature's physiologic calcium blocker. *Am Heart J* 1984; **108:** 188–93.
50. Malmendal A, Linse S, Evenas J, *et al.* Battle for the EF-hands: magnesium-calcium interference in calmodulin. *Biochemistry* 1999; **38:** 11844–50.
51. Lukaski HC. Magnesium, zinc, and chromium nutriture and physical activity. *Am J Clin Nutr* 2000; **72:** 585S–593S.
52. Golf SW, Bohmer D, Nowacki L. Is magnesium a limiting factor in competitive exercise? A summary of relevant scientific data. In: Golf SW, Dralle D, Vecchiet L (eds). *Magnesium*. London: John Libby, 2000: 209–20.
53. Griffiths EJ. Calcium handling and cell contraction in rat cardiomyocytes depleted of intracellular magnesium. *Cardiovasc Res* 2000; **47:** 116–23.
54. Storm W, Zimmerman JJ. Magnesium deficiency and cardiogenic shock after cardiopulmonary bypass. *Ann Thorac Surg* 1997; **64:** 572–7.
55. Karaki H. Magnesium as a modifier of smooth muscle contractility. *Microcirc Endothelium Lymphat* 1989; 5: 77–97.
56. James MF, Cork RC, Harlen GM, White JF. Interactions of adrenaline and magnesium on the cardiovascular system of the baboon. *Magnesium* 1988; 7: 37–43.
57. Yang ZW, Gebrewold A, Nowakowski M, *et al.* Mg^{2+}-induced endothelium-dependent relaxation of blood vessels and blood pressure lowering: role of NO. *Am J Physiol Regul Integr Comp Physiol* 2000; **278:** R628–R639.
58. Amano T, Matsubara T, Watanabe J, *et al.* Insulin modulation of intracellular free magnesium in heart: involvement of protein kinase C. *Br J Pharmacol* 2000; **130:** 731–8.
59. Tso EL, Barish MA. Magnesium: clinical considerations. *J Emerg Med* 1992; **10:** 735–45.
60. Sanders GT, Huijgen HJ, Sanders R. Magnesium in disease: a review with special emphasis on the serum ionized magnesium. *Clin Chem Lab Med* 1999; **37:** 1011–33.
61. Wong ET, Rude RK, Singer FR, Shaw ST. A high prevalence of hypomagnesemia and hypermagnesemia in hospitalized patients. *Am J Clin Pathol* 1983; **79:** 348–52.
62. Scott VL, De Wolf AM, Kang Y, *et al.* Ionized hypomagnesemia in patients undergoing orthotopic liver transplantation: a complication of citrate intoxication. *Liver Transplant Surg* 1996; 2: 343–7.
63. Ryan RP. Interrelationships of magnesium and potassium homeostasis. *Miner Electrolyte Metab* 1993; **19:** 290–5.
64. Hamill RR, McGory R. Magnesium repletion and its effect on potassium homeostasis in critically ill adults: results of a double-blind, randomized, controlled trial. *Crit Care Med* 1996; **24:** 38–45.
65. Arsenian MA. Magnesium and cardiovascular disease. *Prog Cardiovasc Dis* 1993; **35:** 271–310.
66. Aziz S, Haigh WG, Van Norman GA, *et al.* Blood ionized magnesium concentrations during cardiopulmonary bypass and their correlation with other circulating cations. *J Cardiac Surg* 1996; **11:** 341–7.
67. Tzivoni D, Keren A. Suppression of ventricular arrhythmias by magnesium. *Am J Cardiol* 1990; **65:** 1397–9.
68. Corica F, Corsonello A, Buemi M, *et al.* Platelet magnesium depletion in normotensive and hypertensive obese subjects: the role of salt-regulating hormones and catecholamines. *Magnesium Res* 1999; **12:** 287–96.
69. Peacock JM, Folsom AR, Arnett DK, *et al.* Relationship of serum and dietary magnesium to incident hypertension: the Atherosclerosis Risk in Communities (ARIC) Study. *Ann Epidemiol* 1999; 9: 159–65.
70. Katz A, Rosenthal T, Maoz C, *et al.* Effect of a mineral salt diet on 24-h blood pressure monitoring in elderly hypertensive patients. *J Hum Hypertens* 1999; **13:** 777–80.
71. Abraham AS. Potassium and magnesium status in ischaemic heart disease. *Magnesium Res* 1988; 1: 53–7.
72. Ford ES. Serum magnesium and ischaemic heart disease: findings from a national sample of US adults. *Int J Epidemiol* 1999; **28:** 645–51.
73. Douban S, Brodsky MA, Whang DD, *et al.* Significance of magnesium in congestive heart failure. *Am Heart J* 1996; **132:** 664–71.
74. Molloy DW, Dhingra S, Solven F, *et al.* Hypomagnesemia and respiratory muscle power. *Am Rev Respir Dis* 1984; **129:** 497–8.
75. Gambling DR, Birmingham CL, Jenkins LC. Magnesium and the anaesthetist. *Can J Anaesth* 1988; **35:** 644–54.
76. Lu JF, Nightingale CH. Magnesium sulfate in eclampsia and pre-eclampsia: pharmacokinetic principles. *Clin Pharmacokinet* 2000; **38:** 305–14.
77. Chesley LC. Parenteral magnesium sulfate and the distribution plasma levels, and excretion of magnesium. *Am J Obstet Gynecol* 1979; **133:** 1–7.
78. Pritchard JA. The use of the magnesium ion in the management of eclamptic toxemias. *Surg Gynecol Obstet* 1955; **100:** 131–40.
79. Somjen G, Hilmy M, Stephen CR. Failure to anesthetize human subjects by intravenous administration of magnesium sulfate. *J Pharmacol* 1966; **154:** 652–9.
80. Sinatra RS, Philip BK, Naulty JS, Ostheimer GW. Prolonged neuromuscular blockade with vecuronium in a patient treated with magnesium sulfate. *Anaesth Analg* 1985; **64:** 1220–2.
81. Bashuk RG, Krendel DA. Myasthenia gravis presenting as weakness after magnesium administration. *Muscle Nerve* 1990; **13:** 708–12.
82. L'Hommedieu CS, Huber PA, Rasch DK. Potentiation of magnesium-induced neuromuscular weakness by gentamicin. *Crit Care Med* 1983; **11:** 55–6.
83. James MF, Cork RC, Dennett JE. Succinylcholine pretreatment with magnesium sulfate. *Anesth Analg* 1986; **65:** 373–6.
84. Baraka A, Yazigi A. Neuromuscular interaction of magnesium with succinylcholine-vecuronium sequence in the eclamptic parturient. *Anesthesiology* 1987; **67:** 806–8.
85. James MF. Clinical use of magnesium infusions in anesthesia. *Anesth and Analg* 1992; **74:** 129–36.
86. James MF, Cork RC, Dennett JE. Cardiovascular effects of magnesium sulphate in the baboon. *Magnesium* 1987; 6: 314–24.
87. Nakaigawa Y, Akazawa S, Shimizu R, *et al.* Effects of magnesium sulphate on the cardiovascular system, coronary circulation and myocardial metabolism in anaesthetized dogs. *Br J Anaesth* 1997; **78:** 363–8.
88. Nakayama T, Nakayama H, Miyamoto M, Hamlin RL. Hemodynamic and electrocardiographic effects of magnesium sulfate in healthy dogs. *J Vet Int Med* 1999; **13:** 485–90.
89. Prielipp RC, Zaloga GP, Butterworth JF, *et al.* Magnesium inhibits the hypertensive but not the cardiotonic actions of low-dose epinephrine. *Anesthesiology* 1991; **74:** 973–9.
90. Rowe BH, Bretzlaff JA, Bourdon C, Bota GW, Camargo CAJ. Intravenous magnesium sulfate treatment for acute asthma in the emergency department: a systematic review of the literature. *Ann Emerg Med* 2000; **36:** 181–90.
91. Gurkan F, Haspolat K, Bosnak M, *et al.* Intravenous magnesium sulphate in the management of moderate to severe acute asthmatic children non-responding to conventional therapy. *Eur J Emerg Med* 1999; 6: 201–5.
92. Flewellen EH, Nelson TE. In vivo and in vitro responses to magnesium sulphate in porcine malignant hyperthermia. *Can Anaesthetists Soc J* 1980; **27:** 363–9.
93. Duley L, Henderson SD. Magnesium sulphate versus phenytoin for eclampsia. *The Cochrane Database of Systemic Reviews* 2000; CD000128.
94. Duley L, Henderson SD. Magnesium sulphate versus diazepam for eclampsia. *The Cochrane Database of Systemic Reviews* 2000; CD000127.
95. Ludbrook GL, James MF, Upton RN. The effect of magnesium sulfate on cerebral blood flow velocity, cardiovascular variables, and arterial carbon dioxide tension in awake sheep. *J Neurosurg Anesthesiol* 1999; **11:** 96–101.
96. Belfort MA, Moise KJJ. Effect of magnesium sulfate on maternal brain blood flow in preeclampsia: a randomized, placebo-controlled study. *Am J Obstet Gynecol* 1992; **167:** 661–6.
97. Hallak M, Berman RF, Irtenkauf SM, *et al.* Magnesium sulfate treatment decreases *N*-methyl-D-aspartate receptor binding in the rat brain: an autoradiographic study. *J Soc Gynecol Invest* 1994; 1: 25–30.
98. Duley L, Gulmezoglu AM, Henderson SD. Anticonvulsants for women with pre-eclampsia. *The Cochrane Database of Systemic Reviews* 2000; CD000025.
99. Coetzee EJ, Dommisse J, Anthony J. A randomised controlled trial of intravenous magnesium sulphate versus placebo in the management of women with severe pre-eclampsia. *Br J Obstet Gynaecol* 1998; **105:** 300–3.
100. Allen RW, James MF, Uys PC. Attenuation of the pressor response to tracheal intubation in hypertensive proteinuric pregnant patients by lignocaine, alfentanil and magnesium sulphate. *Br J Anaesth* 1991; **66:** 216–23.
101. Ashton WB, James MF, Janicki P, Uys PC. Attenuation of the pressor response to tracheal intubation by magnesium sulphate with and without alfentanil in hypertensive proteinuric patients undergoing caesarean section. *Br J Anaesth* 1991; **67:** 741–7.
102. Vincent RD, Chestnut DH, Sipes SL, *et al.* Magnesium sulfate decreases maternal blood pressure but not uterine blood flow during epidural anesthesia in gravid ewes. *Anesthesiology* 1991; **74:** 77–82.
103. Sipes SL, Chestnut DH, Vincent RDJ, *et al.* Which vasopressor should be used to treat hypotension during magnesium sulfate infusion and epidural anesthesia? *Anesthesiology* 1992; **77:** 101–8.
104. Newsome LR, Bramwell RS, Curling PE. Severe preeclampsia: hemody-

namic effects of lumbar epidural anesthesia. *Anesth Analg* 1986; **65:** 31–6.

105. Baraka A, Ayoub C, Kawkabani N. Magnesium therapy for refractory ventricular fibrillation. *J Cardiothor Vasc Anesth* 2000; **14:** 196–9.
106. Gopinath R, Reddy P, Rajagopal P. Intractable ventricular fibrillation after cross-clamp removal: intra -aortic magnesium a savior. *J Cardiothor Vasc Anesth* 1999; **13:** 801–2.
107. McCaslin PP, Butterworth J. Bupivacaine suppresses $[Ca^{2+}]_i$ oscillations in neonatal rat cardiomyocytes with increased extracellular K+ and is reversed with increased extracellular Mg^{2+}. *Anesth Analg* 2000; **91:** 82–8.
108. Zdanowicz MM, Barletta MA. Protective role of magnesium in catecholamine-induced arrhythmia and toxicity in vitro. *Magnesium Res* 1991; 4: 153–62.
109. Mayer DB, Miletich DJ, Feld JM, Albrecht RF. The effects of magnesium salts on the duration of epinephrine-induced ventricular tachyarrhythmias in anesthetized rats. *Anesthesiology* 1989; **71:** 923–8.
110. Woods KL, Fletcher S. Long-term outcome after intravenous magnesium sulphate in suspected acute myocardial infarction: the second Leicester Intravenous Magnesium Intervention Trial (LIMIT-2). *Lancet* 1994; **343:** 816–9.
111. The ISIS-4 Collaborative Group. A randomised factorial trial assessing early oral captopril, oral mononitrate, and intravenous magnesium sulphate in 58,050 patients with suspected acute myocardial infarction. ISIS-4 (Fourth International Study of Infarct Survival) Collaborative Group. *Lancet* 1995; **345:** 669–85.
112. Redwood SR, Bashir Y, Huang J, *et al.* Effect of magnesium sulphate in patients with unstable angina. A double blind, randomized, placebo-controlled study. *Eur Heart J* 1997; **18:** 1269–77.
113. Gyamlani G, Parikh C, Kulkarni AG. Benefits of magnesium in acute myocardial infarction: timing is crucial. *Am Heart J* 2000; **139:** 703.
114. Pearson PJ, Evora PR, Seccombe JF, Schaff HV. Hypomagnesemia inhibits nitric oxide release from coronary endothelium: protective role of magnesium infusion after cardiac operations. *Ann Tho Surg* 1998; **65:** 967–72.
115. Speziale G, Ruvolo G, Fattouch K, *et al.* Arrhythmia prophylaxis after coronary artery bypass grafting: regimens of magnesium sulfate administration. *Thorac Cardiovasc Surg* 2000; **48:** 22–6.
116. Shakerinia T, Ali IM, Sullivan JA. Magnesium in cardioplegia: is it necessary? *Can J Surg* 1996; **39:** 397–400.
117. Kronon MT, Allen BS, Hernan J, et al. Superiority of magnesium cardioplegia in neonatal myocardial protection. *Ann Thorac Surg* 1999; **68:** 2285–91.
118. Lang LL, Heurteaux C, Dupont H, *et al.* Prevention of ischemic spinal cord injury: comparative effects of magnesium sulfate and riluzole. *J Vasc Surg* 2000; **32:** 179–89.
119. Suzer T, Coskun E, Islekel H, Tahta K. Neuroprotective effect of magnesium on lipid peroxidation and axonal function after experimental spinal cord injury. *Spinal Cord* 1999; **37:** 480–4.
120. Simpson JI, Eide TR, Schiff GA, *et al.* Intrathecal magnesium sulfate protects the spinal cord from ischemic injury during thoracic aortic cross-clamping. *Anesthesiology* 1994; **81:** 1493–9.
121. Marinov MB, Harbaugh KS, Hoopes PJ, *et al.* Neuroprotective effects of preischemia intraarterial magnesium sulfate in reversible focal cerebral ischemia. *J NeuroSurg* 1996; **85:** 117–24.
122. James MF, Beer RE, Esser JD. Intravenous magnesium sulfate inhibits catecholamine release associated with tracheal intubation. *Anesth Analg* 1989; **68:** 772–6.
123. Puri GD, Marudhachalam KS, Chari P, Suri RK. The effect of magnesium sulphate on hemodynamics and its efficacy in attenuating the response to endotracheal intubation in patients with coronary artery disease. *Anesth Analg* 1998; **87:** 808–11.
124. James MF. The use of magnesium sulfate in the anesthetic management of pheochromocytoma. *Anesthesiology* 1985; **62:** 188–90.
125. O'Riordan JA. Pheochromocytomas and anesthesia. *Int Anesthesiol Clin* 1997; **35:** 99–127.
126. James MF, Manson ED. The use of magnesium sulphate infusions in the management of very severe tetanus. *Intensive Care Med* 1985; **11:** 5–12.
127. Sutton DN, Tremlett MR, Woodcock TE, Nielsen MS. Management of autonomic dysfunction in severe tetanus: the use of magnesium sulphate and clonidine. *Intensive Care Med* 1990; **16:** 75–80.
128. Attygalle D, Rodrigo N. Magnesium sulphate for control of spasms in severe tetanus. Can we avoid sedation and artificial ventilation? *Anaesthesia* 1997; **52:** 956–62.
129. Maehama T, Izena H, Kanazawa K. Management of autonomic hyperreflexia with magnesium sulfate during labor in a woman with spinal cord injury. *Am J Obstet Gynecol* 2000; **183:** 492–3.
130. Akazawa S, Shimizu R, Nakaigawa Y, Ishii R, Ikeno S, Yamato R. Effects of magnesium sulphate on atrioventricular conduction times and surface electrocardiogram in dogs anaesthetized with sevoflurane. *Br J Anaesth* 1997; **78:** 75–80.
131. Heath DL, Vink R. Neuroprotective effects of $MgSO_4$ and $MgCl_2$ in closed head injury: a comparative phosphorus NMR study. *J Neurotrauma* 1998; **15:** 183–9.
132. Muir KW. New experimental and clinical data on the efficacy of pharmacological magnesium infusions in cerebral infarcts. *Magnesium Res* 1998; **11:** 43–56.
133. Richards A, Stather DL, Moodley J. Cardiopulmonary arrest after the administration of magnesium sulphate. A case report. *S Afr Med J* 1985; **67:** 145.
134. Morisaki H, Yamamoto S, Morita Y, Kotake Y, Ochiai R, Takeda J. Hypermagnesemia-induced cardiopulmonary arrest before induction of anesthesia for emergency cesarean section. *J Clin Anesth* 2000; **12:** 224–6.

FURTHER READING

Berchtold MW, Brinkmeier H, Muntener M. Calcium ion in skeletal muscle: its crucial role for muscle function, plasticity, and disease. *Physiol Rev* 2000; **80:** 1215–65.

Stuyvers BD, Boyden PA, ter Keurs HE. Calcium waves: physiological relevance in cardiac function. *Circ Res* 2000; **86:** 1016–8.

Lamb GD. Excitation–contraction coupling in skeletal muscle: comparisons with cardiac muscle. *Clin Exp Pharmacol Physiol* 2000; **27:** 216–24.

Jackson WF. Ion channels and vascular tone. *Hypertension* 2000; **35:** 173–8.

Fawcett WJ, Haxby EJ, Male DA. Magnesium: physiology and pharmacology. *Br J Anaesth* 1999; **83:** 302–20.

21

Reproductive physiology

CAREN M STALBURG AND NORAH N NAUGHTON

Pregnancy is a unique physiologic condition that differs from the nonpregnant state. This chapter describes those differences from a systems-based perspective. Physical changes in the parturient lead to functional changes in many organ systems. The chin to chest ratio is shortened with elevation of the diaphragm. In addition, airway mucosa receives more blood flow and may be edematous. During pregnancy a woman's basal metabolic rate increases, as does her oxygen consumption. The elevation of the diaphragm leads to decreases in expiratory reserve volume, residual volume, and functional reserve capacity. As a result, the hemoglobin of the pregnant woman desaturates more quickly than that of the nonpregnant woman. However, both the minute ventilation and the tidal volume are increased. Therefore, pregnancy is a state of compensated respiratory alkalosis.

Cardiovascular changes are significant and occur by the eighth week of gestation. These include an increase in blood volume with resultant changes in cardiac output, left ventricular ejection fraction, stroke volume, and end-diastolic volume. The pregnant woman has lowered systemic vascular resistance because of the large vascular bed within the placenta. She also develops a physiologic anemia. The pregnant woman exhibits an increased glomerular filtration rate and the gravid uterus and progesterone combine to cause a physiologic hydronephrosis, usually right greater than left. The gravid uterus also acts as a mechanical obstruction to venous return and the pregnant woman can exhibit supine hypotension early in pregnancy. A shift to a left lateral decubitus position facilitates venous return and uterine perfusion.

Uterine blood flow is perfusion dependent. It is affected not only by maternal position and maternal perfusion pressure, but also by vascular resistance in the maternal and placental systems. The human placenta is hemochorial; there is no direct mixing of maternal and fetal blood. The maternal and fetal systems are separated by a thin chorionic membrane, however, allowing for transfer of oxygen and carbon dioxide via diffusion, glucose by facilitated diffusion and amino acids by active transport.

Pregnancy is a hypercoagulable state because of the increased production of numerous clotting factors. There is a decrease in factors XI and XIII. There is also increased fibrinolytic activity. All of this in combination leads to significant risk of thromboembolism and/or pulmonary embolism.

Hormonal changes also decrease gastric motility and place the pregnant woman at increased risk of hiatal hernia and aspiration. There is increased insulin resistance. Thus, pregnancy can be characterized as a diabetogenic state.

The pregnant woman undergoes a variety of physiologic changes throughout gestation. While these changes are normal and important for maternal and fetal well-being, many of the adaptations require anesthetic management that differs from that of the nonpregnant individual. This chapter reviews the physiologic changes associated with normal pregnancy and the pathophysiology of the more common disease states found in the parturient.

METABOLIC

The main metabolic differences during pregnancy are:

- The basal metabolic rate is raised 15% above the nonpregnant rate.
- Oxygen consumption is 35% above the nonpregnant level.

The basal metabolic rate is raised 15% above the nonpregnant rate at term. Oxygen consumption increases to 35% above the nonpregnant level primarily in response to the metabolic needs of the fetus, the uterus, and the placenta. Oxygen consumption increases further to 40% and 75% above the resting level during the first and second stages of labor respectively.[1] This progressive increase is secondary to the metabolic needs of the fetus, the uterus, and the placenta, and is secondarily related to the increase in cardiac and respiratory work.

RESPIRATORY

Anatomy

The main anatomical differences in the respiratory system during pregnancy are:

- The thoracic cage circumference increases by 5–7 cm.
- The diaphragm is elevated 4 cm.
- There is capillary engorgement of nasal, oral, pharyngeal, and laryngeal mucosa. Epistaxis may complicate instrumentation of the airway.
- The large airway resistance decreases.

The circumference of the thoracic cage increases by 5–7 cm during pregnancy due to an increase in both the anterior–posterior and transverse diameters.[1] The diaphragm is elevated 4 cm by the upward pressure exerted by the gravid uterus. These changes decrease the chin to chest distance and may impede access during laryngoscopy. There is progressive capillary engorgement of the nasal, oral, and pharyngeal mucosa, as well as the larynx. Nasal breathing becomes difficult and epistaxis can complicate nasal instrumentation. A voice change in the patient may result from edema involving the false cords and arytenoid region of the larynx.[2] Management of the airway may be difficult, with a reported 10-fold increase in difficult intubation in pregnancy compared with nonpregnant women.[3] The patient's airway examination, as assessed by Mallampati classification, can change as the patient progresses from the early phase of labor to the active phase.[4] An early airway assessment on admission to the labor and delivery suite may prove helpful; however, repeated airway assessment prior to the initiation of any major obstetric anesthetic is recommended.[5] Larger airways dilate because of the direct effects of progesterone, cortisone, and relaxin. This results in a decrease in airway resistance.[1]

Mechanics

The main differences in the mechanics of the respiratory system during pregnancy are:

- The closing volume, forced expiratory volume (FEV_1), FEV_1/FVC (forced vital capacity) ratio, and flow–volume loop are unchanged.
- Functional residual capacity (FRC) is decreased by 20%.
- Pregnant patients desaturate more quickly than nonpregnant patients following apnea due to decreased FRC, increased oxygen consumption, and unchanged closing volume.
- Tidal volume and minute ventilation increase by 45%.
- Pregnant patients maintain a primary respiratory alkalosis with compensatory metabolic acidosis.
- Extreme maternal hyperventilation may lead to uterine artery vasoconstriction.
- Arterial Po_2 and the P_{50} of the hemoglobin dissociation curve are increased in pregnancy.

Increased diaphragmatic excursion is made possible by diaphragmatic elevation in the resting state. Pregnant women demonstrate a 50% decrease in total pulmonary resistance, secondary to dilation of the large airways. This decrease compensates for the increased resistance that results from lower resting lung volumes and the decrease in the arterial pressure of carbon dioxide (P_aCO_2). The unaltered FEV_1, FEV_1/FVC ratio, and flow–volume loop are evidence for the normal functioning of the large airways.[1] The closing volume is normal in pregnancy; however, the elevated diaphragm results in a decrease in the expiratory reserve volume (ERV) and the residual volume (RV) by 25% and 15% respectively.[6] This results in an overall decrease in FRC of 20%. A reduction in FRC is of great importance to the obstetric anesthesiologist. The combination of an unchanged closing volume with a reduced FRC can lead to a tendency for small airway closure. Small airway closure is further aggravated in the supine position, in which FRC falls to 70% of its volume when compared with the sitting position.[6] Most patients in the supine position maintain normal oxygenation. However, the combination of reduced FRC and increased oxygen consumption can lead to a more rapid decline in oxygenation during periods of apnea. Pregnant patients have a twofold greater decrease in P_aO_2 during apnea compared with nonpregnant patients.[7] Minute ventilation increases by 45% over the prepregnant state.[8] The combination of decreased FRC and increased minute ventilation speeds nitrogen washout and oxygenation while breathing 100% oxygen. Two methods of preoxygenation and denitrogenation have been evaluated in the parturient: four-vital-capacity-breaths hyperventilation and 3-min tidal volume breathing. Norris and Dewan compared these two techniques in the pregnant patient.[9] Four-vital-capacity-breaths hyperventilation and 3-min tidal volume breathing produced similar levels of arterial oxygenation during rapid-sequence induction of general anesthesia. However, in a follow-up study, hyperventilation did not wash out nitrogen as effectively as the 3-min tidal volume breathing. However, it is debatable if the extra 10–15 additional seconds of apnea provided before hypoxemia is of clinical significance.[10]

Changes in lung volumes and capacities are listed in Table 21.1.[1] Tidal volume increases by 45% at term, accounting for the majority of the increase in minute ventilation. Inspiratory capacity increases 15% due to an increase in inspiratory reserve volume. This counterbalances the decrease in FRC, and, as a result, vital capacity and total lung capacity change very little, if at all.[1] Minute alveolar ventilation increases 45%.[1] Changes in ventilation are due to an increase in carbon dioxide production, the respiratory stimulant effects of progesterone and estrogen, and a progesterone-induced increase in the slope of the ventilatory response curve to arterial carbon dioxide. As a result, the pregnant patient maintains a partially compensated respiratory alkalosis. Pco_2 declines to 4 kPa (30 mmHg) by 12 weeks' gestation and does not change further in the second or third trimester. However, extreme maternal ventilation can increase uterine artery vascular resistance with a reduction in uterine blood flow and fetal oxygen delivery. In addition, hyperventilation may produce frank alkalemia with a leftward shift of the oxygen hemoglobin dissociation curve, resulting in reduced fetal oxygen delivery with the potential for fetal stress.

Pregnancy eliminates the gradient between the end-tidal and arterial carbon dioxide tension that begins early in pregnancy and persists through to term gestation. This is secondary to a reduction in alveolar dead space resulting from a marked increase in cardiac output.[1] The arterial Po_2 is increased significantly compared with values for nonpregnant subjects. This increase is due to the reduced arterial Pco_2, a decrease in the physiologic shunt, and a reduced arterial–venous oxygen difference. The latter increases in the third trimester and accounts for the slight decline in arterial Po_2 in late pregnancy, from 14.2 kPa (107 mmHg) in the first trimester to 13.7 kPa (103 mmHg) at term gestation.[1] Hemoglobin P_{50} is higher in pregnancy and allows for a greater volume of oxygen to be unloaded to the tissues at any given arterial Po_2. Of note, the increase in P_{50} is not observed in pre-eclampsia.[11]

The arterial Po_2 is influenced by the parturient's body position. Values after midgestation are frequently below 13.3 kPa (100 mmHg). Two factors are responsible for this decrease. First, a decrease in FRC without a corresponding change in the closing capacity can result in small airway closure. The second factor is reduced cardiac output secondary to aortocaval compression with an increase in the arterial–venous oxygen difference. Moving the pregnant woman from the supine to the erect or lateral decubitus position will improve arterial

Table 21.1 *Changes in respiratory physiology at term*

Parameter	Change[a]
Lung volumes	
Inspiratory reserve volume	+5%
Tidal volume	+45%
Expiratory reserve volume	–25%
Residual volume	–15%
Lung capacities	
Inspiratory capacity	+15%
Functional residual capacity	–20%
Vital capacity	No change
Total lung capacity	–5%
Dead space	+45%
Respiratory rate	No change
Ventilation	
Minute ventilation	+45%
Alveolar ventilation	+45%

a. Changes relative to values for nonpregnant women. From Conklin.[1]

oxygenation.[12,13] Maternal Pco_2 during mechanical ventilation should be maintained consistent with a normal pregnant state. Partial compensation for the respiratory alkalosis reduces serum bicarbonate concentration to approximately 20 mequiv L^{-1}, the base excess by 2–3 mequiv L^{-1}, and the total buffer base by approximately 5 mequiv L^{-1}.[14] This results in the patient's capacity to compensate for an acidosis.

The respiratory changes associated with pregnancy are exaggerated in the morbidly obese patient. Total respiratory compliance is decreased in association with the decreased chest wall compliance. Chest wall compliance is reduced by fat accumulated around the ribs and the diaphragm. The increased pulmonary blood volume can lead to a decrease in lung compliance. This decrease in total respiratory compliance is exacerbated further in the supine position. Ventilation-perfusion mismatch can easily occur in the morbidly obese patient as FRC falls within the closing volume and leads to airway closure. This can be exaggerated when the patient's position changes from standing to supine to the Trendelenburg position.[15]

CARDIOVASCULAR

Hemodynamics

The main differences in hemodynamics during pregnancy are:

- Total blood volume increases by 45%. Plasma and red blood cell volume increase by 50% and 30% respectively, which results in the physiologic anemia of pregnancy.
- Cardiac output increases by 45–50% and systemic vascular resistance decreases by 35%. The majority of these changes occur by 8 weeks' gestation.
- Central venous and pulmonary capillary wedge pressure (PCWP) are unchanged in pregnancy and left ventricular function is not hyperdynamic.
- Blood pressure decreases, reaching a nadir of 20% below baseline at 16–20 weeks.
- Aortocaval compression can occur as early as 13–16 weeks' gestation. Some degree of compression occurs in the majority of patients in the supine position and may compromise uterine blood flow.
- Aortocaval compression can be relieved with a 15° left uterine displacement.
- Parturients have decreased sensitivity to exogenous vasopressors.
- Patients with pre-eclampsia typically have low normal central venous pressure (CVP) and PCWP, elevated systemic vascular resistance (SVR), and hyperdynamic left ventricular function.

The cardiac examination in the pregnant patient differs from that in a nonpregnant person. The elevated diaphragm shifts the heart anteriorly and to the left with the apical impulse located in the fourth intercostal space, at least, and in the midclavicular line. The first heart sound is accentuated on auscultation with splitting of the mitral and tricuspid components as early as 12 weeks. The second heart sound varies little; however, a third heart sound is appreciated in the second half of pregnancy in up to 84% of parturients. A grade I–II early to midsystolic murmur, appreciated at the left sternal border, is secondary to cardiac enlargement with dilation of the tricuspid anulus leading to regurgitation. This sign is present in up to 96% of patients.[16] Also notable is a pericardial effusion, which is present in 9% of patients.[17]

Total blood volume increases by 45% in the third trimester. This is secondary to an increase in both the plasma (50%) and red blood cell (30%) volume (Table 21.2).[1] The hematocrit decreases by midgestation to approximately 34% because of the greater increase in plasma volume compared with red blood cell volume. However, by term the hematocrit has increased to 35.5% due to a greater increase in red blood cell mass.

Table 21.2 *Hematologic parameters at term*

Blood volume	+45%[a]
Plasma volume	+55%[a]
Red blood cell volume	+30%[a]
Hematocrit	35.5
Hemoglobin	11.6 g dL^{-1}
Cardiac output	+50%
Stroke volume	+25%
Heart rate	+20%

a. Changes relative to values for nonpregnant women. From Conklin.[1]

The increase in plasma volume is in response to a 100-fold increase in estrogen and progesterone. These hormones lead to increased renin activity and reabsorption of sodium and water by the renin–angiotensin–aldosterone system. Plasma protein concentrations decline, beginning in the first trimester.[18] Maternal colloid osmotic pressure decreases at term and this may predispose the pregnant patient to the development of pulmonary edema at hydrostatic pressures lower than those associated with volume overload. Plasma cholinesterase concentrations fall to approximately 25% during the first trimester and remain at this level.[19] However, this reduction usually has little clinical significance.

Significant cardiovascular hemodynamic changes occur throughout pregnancy. Capeless and Clapp evaluated cardiac output, ejection fraction, stroke volume, and end-diastolic volume using M-mode echocardiography in eight subjects before conception and at 8, 16, and 24 weeks' gestation.[20] The greater part of the total change in cardiac output and systemic vascular resistance occurs by 8 weeks' gestation. Cardiac output increases by 1 L min^{-1}, which represents greater than 50% of the total change. Systemic vascular resistance falls to 70% of its nonpregnant value. The increase in cardiac output is due primarily to an increase in stroke volume (Fig. 21.1).[20] Stroke volume and heart rate ultimately increase to 25% and 15% above prepregnant levels at term. The rise in stroke volume is due to an increase in left ventricular end-diastolic volume, which occurs without a change in end-systolic volume,[21,22] and results in an increase in the ejection fraction. Cardiac output peaks between 24 and 32 weeks' gestation at 45–50% greater than in the prepregnant state and generally does not increase further during the third trimester (Table 21.2).[1] Reports of a decrease in cardiac output as term approached were influenced by patient position and aortocaval

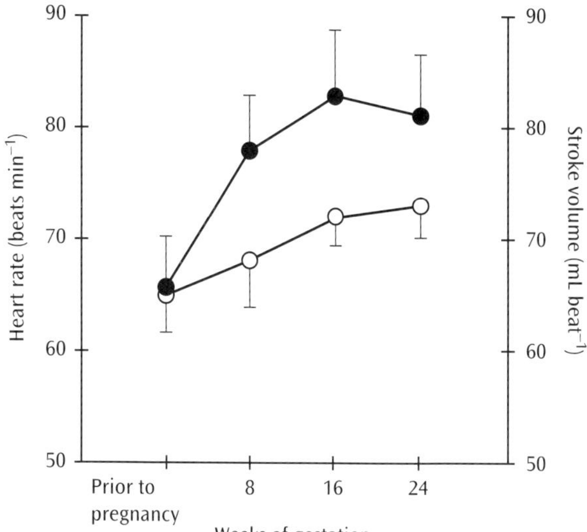

Figure 21.1 *The stroke volume (filled circles) and heart rate (open circles) components of cardiac output are presented for four study periods. (Reproduced with permission from Capeless and Clapp.[20])*

compression. Recently, measurements using pulse and continuous-wave Doppler demonstrated a further rise in cardiac output throughout the third trimester.[23]

Clark *et al.* assessed central hemodynamics in normal term pregnant patients (Table 21.3).[24] There is no significant change in the pulmonary capillary wedge pressure or central venous pressure despite the increase in left ventricular end-diastolic volume. This can be explained by ventricular dilation with the dilated left ventricle accommodating a greater volume without an increase in pressure. Additionally, the late phase of the third trimester is not associated with hyperdynamic left ventricular function as assessed by the left ventricular stroke work index/pulmonary capillary wedge pressure ratio.

Changes in regional blood flow accompany the changes in cardiac output. Blood flow to the uterus increases from 50–190 mL $min^{-1}$to 700–900 mL min^{-1} at term; 90% of this flow is to the intervillous space and the balance perfuses the myometrium. Renal plasma flow increases 50% at term and skin perfusion is 3–4 times greater than in the nonpregnant patient. Blood flow to other major organs is unchanged.

Cardiac output increases 11% in the late first stage of labor and increases an additional 30% during contractions.[25] Despite the increase in cardiac output, blood pressure decreases in midgestation because of a fall in systemic vascular resistance. This decrease in systemic vascular resistance reaches a nadir at 20 weeks' gestation approaching 35% below baseline and then rises toward term to 20% below baseline. Systolic blood pressure reaches the lowest levels at 16–20 weeks and returns to prepregnant levels at term gestation, whereas the diastolic blood pressure decreases by 20%, rebounds slightly, but remains below baseline at term.[1,24] These changes occur because of the presence of a low resistance vascular bed (intervillous space), as well as the vasodilative effects of prostacyclin, estrogens, and progesterone. The gradual increase in systemic vascular resistance as gestation progresses is due to compression of the aorta by the gravid uterus.

Patient position is a factor when measuring blood pressure in the parturient. Blood pressure decreases as the patient changes position from standing to sitting to left lateral position.[1] Aortocaval compression by the gravid uterus can have a significant impact on both the mother and the fetus. Patient position plays a significant role in its occurrence. Kerr *et al.* demonstrated complete obstruction of the inferior vena cava in 10 out of 12 subjects in the supine position.[26] Venous return to the heart occurs through collateral circulation comprising the intraosseous vertebral veins, paravertebral veins, and epidural venous plexus. The ovarian plexus also partially drains the uteroplacental vascular bed.[26] Caval compression can occur as early as 13–16 weeks gestation as evidenced by an elevated femoral venous pressure in the supine position.[27]

Central venous pressure is similar to that of a nonpregnant patient when the term parturient is in the lateral decubitus position.[24] This suggests that the collateral circulation maintains venous return. However, in the supine position right atrial pressure can fall significantly.[28] This can result in up to a 20% decrease in uterine blood flow with potential compromising of fetal oxygen delivery. These changes are evident by 20–28 weeks of gestation.[29]

Up to 8% of women will experience bradycardia and hypotension when supine. This is referred to as the supine hypotensive syndrome and occurs when the cardiovascular system is unable to compensate for a fall in venous return. These effects of the supine position on left ventricular filling pressure are reduced once the fetal head is engaged in the pelvis.[28] Hemodynamic changes can be minimized by a displacement of the uterus 15° to the left. Partial obstruction of the aorta can occur in the supine position between 27 weeks and term but does not occur in the lateral position.[30] A significant elevation of blood pressure can follow. This results from an increase in systemic vascular resistance, which is attributable to compression of the aorta by the gravid uterus and augmented sympathetic nervous system outflow.[31] It is important to note that a decrease in blood flow below the site of obstruction may not be reflected in the brachial blood pressure. Anesthetic techniques that result in a decrease in systemic vascular resistance may unmask compensated obstruction and endanger maternal cardiovascular homeostasis and organ blood flow.

The management of hypotension with vasoactive agents is influenced by the pregnant state. Sensitivity to exogenous vasopressors is decreased.[32] Vasopressors with pure α-adrenergic action have been shown to increase uterine vascular resistance and decrease uterine blood flow.[33] Ephedrine, a mixed α- and β-agonist, has been shown to not produce uterine artery vasoconstriction and has been the agent of choice to treat hypotension in the parturient. However, drugs such as phenylephrine, when administered in small doses (100-μg increments), have an action similar to that of ephedrine. Like ephedrine, α-agonists in small doses may increase perfusion pressure by increasing venous return without detrimental effect on uterine blood flow and neonatal status.[34] The decreased blood flow secondary to hypotension appears to be of greater concern than the choice of agent used for treatment.

In contrast, the hemodynamic characteristics associated with severe pre-eclampsia differ from those of the healthy parturient (Table 21.4).[35] The PCWP may be decreased, normal, or increased, but is typically low to low–normal, reflecting a decrease in intravascular volume. The average plasma volume in the pre-eclamptic patient has been reported to be 9% lower than that of normotensive parturients and 30–40% lower in patients with severe pre-eclampsia.[36] CVP is either decreased or normal and often does not correlate with the PCWP. This is thought to be secondary to the differences between the pulmonary and systemic vascular responses to pre-eclampsia. This may make CVP an unreliable indicator of volume status. SVR is usually elevated while pulmonary vascular resistance (PVR) is normal. The majority of patients with pre-eclampsia display hyperdynamic left ventricular function compared with nonpregnant patients. A small percentage have depressed left ventricular function, usually associated with markedly elevated

Table 21.3 *Central hemodynamic changes in pregnancy*

	Nonpregnant	Pregnant
Cardiac output (L min^{-1})	4.3 ± 0.9	6.2 ± 1.0
Heart rate (beats min^{-1})	71 ± 10	83 ± 10
Systemic vascular resistance (dyne s cm^{-5})	1530 ± 520	1210 ± 266
Pulmonary vascular resistance (dyne s cm^{-5})	119 ± 47	78 ± 22
Colloid oncotic pressure (mmHg)	20.8 ± 1.0	18.0 ± 1.5
Colloid oncotic pressure – pulmonary capillary wedge pressure (mmHg)	14.5 ± 2.5	10.5 ± 2.7
Mean arterial pressure (mmHg)	86.4 ± 7.5	90.3 ± 5.8
Pulmonary capillary wedge pressure (mmHg)	6.3 ± 2.1	7.5 ± 1.8
Central venous pressure (mmHg)	3.7 ± 2.6	3.6 ± 2.5
Left ventricular stroke work index (g m m^{-2})	41 ± 8	48 ± 6

Reproduced with permission from Clark *et al.*[24] 1 kPa = 7.5 mmHg.

Table 21.4 *Hemodynamic characteristics of severe pre-eclampsia*

Preload
Systemic (PCWP): variable but usually low
Pulmonary (CVP): low to normal
Afterload
Systemic (SVR): usually elevated
Pulmonary (PVR): normal
Contractility
Systemic (LVSWI): vast majority elevated
Heart rate: normal

Reproduced with permission from Fox *et al.*[35] CVP, central venous pressure; LVSWI, left ventricular stroke work index; PCWP, pulmonary capillary wedge pressure; PVR, pulmonary vascular resistance; SVR, systemic vascular resistance.

systemic vascular resistance. Heart rate is unchanged in pre-eclampsia compared with normal pregnant patients.[35] The use of central venous and pulmonary capillary pressure monitoring in the management of women with severe pre-eclampsia is controversial. Hypertension that is unresponsive to standard vasodilator therapy, pulmonary edema, and persistent oliguria that is unresponsive to a fluid challenge have been suggested as indications for use of a pulmonary artery catheter.[37]

Coagulation

The main differences in coagulation during pregnancy are:

- Pregnancy is a hypercoagulable state.
- Prothrombin time (PT) and partial thromboplastin time (PTT) are shortened by 20%.
- Fibrinolytic activity is increased.
- Platelet activation, consumption, and aggregation are increased and the platelet count is low–normal to normal.
- Significant thrombocytopenia (less than 100 000 mm^{-3}) occurs in 15% of patients with pre-eclampsia.
- Pregnant patients are predisposed to deep venous thrombosis and pulmonary embolism.

Pregnancy is considered to be a hypercoagulable state. There is an increase in the production of clotting factors I, VII, VIII, IX, X, and XII, while there is no change in the production of factors II and V. There is a decrease in factors XI and XIII. The PT and PTT are reduced by approximately 20%. There is also an increase in fibrin split products, suggesting an increase in fibrinolytic activity.[38] Twenty-one percent of patients have a significant increase in fibrin degradation products during labor, and 32% in the immediate postpartum period.[39] There is an increase in platelet activation, consumption, and aggregation and the platelet count may decrease slightly or show no change.[40,41] Interestingly, 7.6% of healthy parturients have a platelet count of less than 150 000 mm^{-3} and 0.9% have a platelet count of less than 100 000 mm^{-3}.[42] The bleeding time remains normal.

While platelet count is normal in the healthy parturient, thrombocytopenia should be investigated in the patient with pre-eclampsia. It is a common finding and occurs in one-third of all patients. Significant thrombocytopenia (less than 100 000 mm^{-3}) occurs in 15% of women with severe pre-eclampsia.[36] The mechanism of thrombocytopenia is multifactorial and includes increased platelet consumption, activation, and autoimmune mechanisms. The effect of thrombocytopenia on clinical bleeding is controversial. Bleeding times associated with thrombocytopenia in pre-eclampsia have been variable and the test itself is considered unreliable and difficult to reproduce.

The hypercoagulable state associated with pregnancy may predispose the patient to deep venous thrombosis and pulmonary embolism, the latter being the leading cause of maternal mortality in developed countries. Risk factors for the development of deep venous thrombosis include age greater than 35 years, operative delivery (particularly emergency cesarean section), obesity, and a personal or family history of thrombosis or thrombophilia.[43] There is a five- to sixfold increase in the risk of pulmonary embolism, in part because hypocoagulability, venous stasis, and vascular wall changes all occur in pregnancy. The incidence ranges between 1 per 1000 and 1 per 3000 deliveries, and 1 in 100 000 pregnant women die from pulmonary embolism.[44] There is an increase in clotting factors in pregnancy, while at the same time there is a decrease in natural anticoagulation. This includes an increased resistance to activated protein C and a decrease in protein S levels. In addition, fibrinolysis may be impaired because of an increase in plasminogen activator inhibitors 1 and 2 being produced by the placenta.[45]

The incidence of deep venous thrombosis on the left side is 90% in pregnant women compared with 55% in women who are not pregnant. The majority are iliofemoral rather than capillary venous thrombosis (72% vs. 9%).[45] Prophylaxis for, or management of, a deep venous thrombosis or pulmonary embolism in pregnancy involves primarily the use of anticoagulants, in particular heparin, low-molecular-weight heparins, and warfarin. Heparin or low-molecular-weight heparin are the preferred anticoagulants compared with warfarin as they do not cross the placenta. Warfarin crosses the placenta and poses a risk to the fetus. It is potentially teratogenic if administered in the first trimester. It can also result in abnormalities of cartilage and bone formation, known as chondrodysplasia punctata. It increases the risk of miscarriage and, when administered in the second or third trimester, has been associated with major fetal central nervous system abnormalities, in particular, microcephaly and optic atrophy. There is the potential to anticoagulate the fetus in the presence of a relatively immature clotting system with a risk of intracerebral bleed at the time of delivery.[44]

GASTROINTESTINAL

The main differences in the gastrointestinal system during pregnancy are:

- Pregnancy is associated with decreased gastric motility, lower esophageal sphincter (LES) tone, increased gastric pressure, and reduced esophageal barrier pressure gradient.
- Gastric emptying may be decreased in labor and is slowed further by opioid administration.
- Gastric emptying ante partum and 18 h post partum is not different from that in nonpregnant controls.
- The parturient is considered to be at risk of aspiration. However, it is not known at what gestational age or time interval post partum this risk is present.

Progesterone, a smooth muscle relaxant, decreases gastric motility during pregnancy. The LES tone decreases during pregnancy and reaches a nadir at 36 weeks.[46] At the same time, intragastric pressure rises during gestation because of the gravid uterus.[47] As a result, the esophageal barrier pressure gradient is reduced in the pregnant patient and is associated with the symptoms of heartburn. The altered position of the stomach and an increase in interabdominal pressure leads to a higher incidence of hiatal hernia in parturients. Up to 70% of gravidas complain of heartburn.[48,49] The effects of pregnancy on gastric emptying are controversial. This may in part reflect the variety of methods used to measure gastric emptying. Several studies have reported on gastric emptying using acetaminophen (paracetamol) absorption.

Using this technique, there is no significant difference in the gastric emptying times of women in the first, second, or third trimester of pregnancy compared with nonpregnant controls. In addition, there are no differences in gastric emptying compared with nonpregnant controls 18 h or more after delivery. There is, however, a delay in gastric emptying in patients within 2 h of delivery.[50] The influence of labor itself on gastric emptying has not been clearly defined; however, gastric emptying is markedly delayed when opioids are administered during labor.[51] Carp *et al.* reported a decrease in gastric emptying during labor.[52] Gastric volume is influenced by gastric secretion in addition to oral intake. Gastrin is secreted by the pyloric glands of the distal stomach and the proximal duodenum and induces copious gastric secretions. It also promotes an elevation in the LES tone and inhibits pyloric sphincter tone. A progressive increase in gastrin levels occurs as pregnancy advances and reaches mean peak levels during labor.[53] Historically, patients are considered to be at risk for the development of acid aspiration syndrome when gastric pH is equal to or less than 2.5 and gastric volume is greater than 25 mL. Despite the above findings, several investigators have reported no difference in the percentage of patients in the "at risk" category when comparing nonpregnant patients undergoing elective surgery with pregnant patients undergoing elective cesarean section or with women at a mean gestational age of 15 weeks.[54,55]

Clinicians are also not sure when to consider the postpartum patient no longer in the at risk category for acid aspiration. As mentioned previously, Whitehead *et al.* found no difference in gastric emptying between postpartum patients greater than 18 h after delivery and nonpregnant controls.[50] Gastric volumes in postpartum patients undergoing a postpartum tubal ligation at 1–8, 9–23, and 24–45 h following delivery are not different when compared with 15 women undergoing elective gynecologic surgery.[56] In addition, there is no difference between the two groups in the percentage at risk of acid aspiration syndrome. However, pregnant patients are considered to be at greater risk for aspiration despite the above findings. This may reflect the influence of pain, opioids, sedatives, and other drugs commonly administered during labor on gastric emptying. It still remains a clinical question as to the gestational age and postpartum interval at which intubation should be considered mandatory for the protection of the airway during general anesthesia.

RENAL

The main differences in the renal system during pregnancy are:

- Renal plasma flow and glomerular filtration rate increase by 75–85% and 50% respectively.
- Serum concentrations of blood urea nitrogen and creatinine are decreased.
- Glycosuria is common because of the decreased capacity of proximal tubules to reabsorb glucose.

Kidney size increases during pregnancy and the ureters and renal pelves dilate in response to hormonal changes as well the obstructive effect of the uterus as gestation advances. This may predispose the parturient to pyelonephritis. Renal plasma flow and glomerular filtration rate (GFR) increase by 75–85% and 50% respectively. Creatinine clearance increases to a maximum by the end of the first trimester and declines slightly near term.[57,58] Serum concentrations of blood urea nitrogen and creatinine are lower than in the nonpregnant state, approximately 8–9 $mg\,dL^{-1}$ and 0.5–0.6 $mg\,dL^{-1}$ by term respectively. Changes in tubular function affect glucose reabsorption. There is a decrease in the capacity of the proximal tubules to reabsorb glucose and as a result all pregnant patients exhibit some degree of glycosuria throughout pregnancy. The majority of parturients double or increase glucose excretion by 3–10 times the nonpregnant level.[59] Normal glucose excretion patterns return within 1 week of delivery.

ENDOCRINE

Glucose metabolism

The main differences in glucose metabolism during pregnancy are:

- Parturients have exaggerated responses to carbohydrate loading and starvation.
- Pregnancy is a diabetogenic state due to insulin resistance that is secondary to human placental lactogen.
- The diabetic parturient is at risk for hyperglycemia, diabetic ketoacidosis, pre-eclampsia, preterm labor, and hydramnios.
- Fetal mortality associated with diabetic ketoacidosis is a major threat. Additional fetal risks include macrosomia and other congenital anomalies, primarily cardiac and developmental respiratory distress syndrome.

Pregnancy is a diabetogenic state. There is an increase in insulin secretion throughout gestation; however, tissue sensitivity to insulin diminishes.[60,61] The insulin resistance is considered to be secondary to human placental lactogen (hPL), which has anti-insulin activity.[62] The blood glucose levels following a carbohydrate load are greater in the pregnant than in the nonpregnant woman, which favors a maternal–fetal glucose gradient. This is important because the fetus is dependent upon maternal glucose stores and placental passage of glucose is concentration dependent. Persistent hyperglycemia, however, is a sign of the development of excessive insulin resistance. Interestingly, fasting blood glucose levels are lower than in nonpregnant individuals.[63] This response is secondary to fetal–placental consumption of glucose. Pregnant women can experience a significant low blood glucose level, however symptomatic hypoglycemia is rare.

The diabetic parturient requires special consideration. She has exaggerated responses to both fasting as well as glucose loading. Typically, in early pregnancy, maternal hypoglycemia occurs frequently and requires a reduction in insulin dose. In the second half of pregnancy insulin resistance develops with a simultaneous requirement for an increase in insulin. Diabetic patients are at higher risk of developing additional obstetric complications including pre-eclampsia, preterm labor, and hydramnios. These parturients are more susceptible to developing diabetic ketoacidosis, and this occurs most commonly in the second and third trimesters. The changes are secondary to accelerated starvation, dehydration secondary to emesis, decreased buffering capacity (respiratory alkalosis of pregnancy), increased production of insulin antagonist, and stress.[64]

One of the most serious dangers facing the parturient with ketoacidosis is fetal mortality. The rate of fetal loss has been estimated at 9% in these patients over the past decade. Contributing factors include a massive osmotic diuresis, maternal intervascular volume depletion, and the potential for decreased uteroplacental blood flow. Maternal acidemia may also reduce uterine blood flow and predispose the fetus to hypoxemia. Additionally, maternal ketoacids cross the placenta, which can result in fetal acidosis. Maternal phosphate deficiency can lead to a reduction in red blood cell 2,3-diphosphoglycerate and an impaired delivery of oxygen to the fetus. A reduction in fetal myocardial contractility may occur in addition to cardiac arrhythmia secondary to profound hypokalemia.

Additional effects of diabetes on the fetus include an increase in the incidence of congenital anomalies, estimated to occur at a rate of 6–12%, which is 2–4 times that in the general population. The exact mechanism underlying these anomalies is not clear. Maternal hyperglycemia leads to fetal hyperglycemia, stimulating insulin production and anabolic metabolism. This results in an increase in fat deposition, hypertrophy of visceral organs, and increased skeletal growth. The incidence of macrosomia is estimated to be as high as 20–30%.[65]

Respiratory distress syndrome (RDS) is also a common cause of neonatal morbidity and mortality. Elevated fetal insulin may interfere with surfactant production and delay lung maturity. There is an estimated five- to sixfold greater risk of RDS in the premature fetus of the inadequately controlled diabetic parturient.[66]

Thyroid

The main differences in thyroid function during pregnancy are:

- There is an increase in thyroxine-binding globulin and total thyroid hormone concentrations.
- Free thyroid hormone levels are in the lower range of normal, resulting in a euthyroid state.

The thyroid gland may enlarge during pregnancy in response to an increase in human chorionic gonadotropin activity. This activity peaks in the first trimester with a corresponding transient decrease in thyroid-stimulating hormone (TSH). TSH returns to pregestation levels in the second and third trimester, and remains stable. Thyroxine-binding globulin (TBG) is increased in pregnancy as a result of an estrogen-induced increase in hepatic synthesis. It reaches a plateau in midpregnancy at two to three times pregestational levels. The increase in thyroid hormone-binding capacity favors a decrease in free thyroid hormone levels. This leads to TSH-mediated increases in thyroid hormone output. As a result, total thyroid hormone concentrations increase to approximately 50% greater than the pregestational levels and remain so throughout term. However, pregnancy is a euthyroid state as the free thyroid hormone levels tend to be at the lower end of the range seen in the nonpregnant patient.[67,68]

CENTRAL NERVOUS SYSTEM

The main differences in the central nervous system during pregnancy are:

- There is an increase in circulating endogenous analgesic neuropeptides.
- Less local anesthetic is required in pregnancy to give an equivalent cephalad level for spinal and epidural blockade.
- Less local anesthetic is required for peripheral nerve blockade.
- Minimum alveolar concentration (MAC) is decreased in pregnancy.
- There is increased sensitivity to the hypnotic effects of thiopental.

Pregnancy is associated with an increase in the circulating plasma concentrations of endogenous analgesic neuropeptides that further increase during labor.[69] Interestingly, pregnant women have an elevation in the pain threshold at term and during labor.[70] However, the explanation for these behavioral changes is controversial as cerebrospinal fluid (CSF) levels of β-endorphins do not change over the course of pregnancy or during labor.[69] Local anesthetic requirements are different in the pregnant patient as a result of both biochemical and mechanical factors.

There is a decrease in the volume of local anesthetic necessary for spinal and epidural local anesthesia per spinal segment blocked compared with the volume needed for nonpregnant controls. The gravid uterus obstructs the inferior vena cava, which results in a diversion of blood flow through the vertebral plexus with distension of the epidural veins. This increases epidural pressure, which in turn reduces CSF volume in the intrathecal space. CSF pressure remains unchanged. However, uterine contractions and maternal pushing increase CSF pressure. Because of the above changes, cephalad spread for a given volume of local anesthetic is higher in the pregnant patient than in the nonpregnant patient.[28,71,72] Biochemical factors also contribute to this increased sensitivity to local anesthetic drugs. Increased circulating levels of progesterone cause peripheral nerves to be more sensitive to the conduction blockade of local anesthetic drugs.[73]

Pregnancy also decreases the MAC in humans. Isoflurane MAC is 0.775% at 12 weeks' gestation versus 1.075% in nonpregnant patients.[74] Halothane and enflurane MAC values are decreased by 27% and 30% respectively.[75] Pregnant patients appear to be more sensitive to the hypnotic and anesthetic effects of thiopental. The dose of thiopental for hypnosis is 17% less and that for anesthesia 18% less in pregnant women at 7–13 weeks' gestation than in nonpregnant women.[76]

UTERINE AND PLACENTAL PHYSIOLOGY

Uterine vasculature

The main differences in the uterine vasculature during pregnancy are:

- The uterus receives perfusion from both the uterine and the ovarian arteries.
- The uterine and ovarian arteries anastomose within the uterus, allowing extensive collateral circulation.
- Stasis within this vascular cascade can lead to pelvic thrombus or septic pelvic thrombophlebitis.

The blood supply to the uterus arises from two primary sources: the uterine arteries and the ovarian arteries. The uterine artery arises from the internal iliac and runs medially and anteriorly along the pelvic sidewall, turning inward toward the uterus at the level of the internal cervical os. It then divides into the ascending and descending branches of the uterine artery. The descending branch supplies the cervical and vaginal arteries. The ascending branch is larger and traverses along the side of the uterus to supply the uterine body and fundus. It forms an anastomosis with the ovarian artery cascade from the cornual region of the uterus (Fig. 21.2).[77]

The ovarian artery is the most caudal branch arising from the aorta. The ovarian artery travels within the infundibulopelvic ligament into the pelvis to the ovary. The vessel then continues on toward the cornual region of the uterus to anastomose with the ascending branch of the uterine artery.

The uterine veins form a large plexus laterally within the broad ligament, which then drains into the internal iliac vein or the left renal vein. This enlarged venous plexus is often the site of thrombus or septic pelvic thrombophlebitis.

Innervation of the uterus

The main differences in the innervation of the uterus during pregnancy are:

- The sympathetic and afferent fibers from the uterus enter the spinal cord at the level of T10–L1.
- The lower portion of the vagina and perineum are innervated by S2–S4.

The nerves to the uterus and vagina form a dense plexus, called the uterovaginal plexus, and consist of a mixture of sympathetic and afferent fibers. There may also be parasympathetic fibers. The afferent supply from the uterine body and fundus travel with the hypogastric

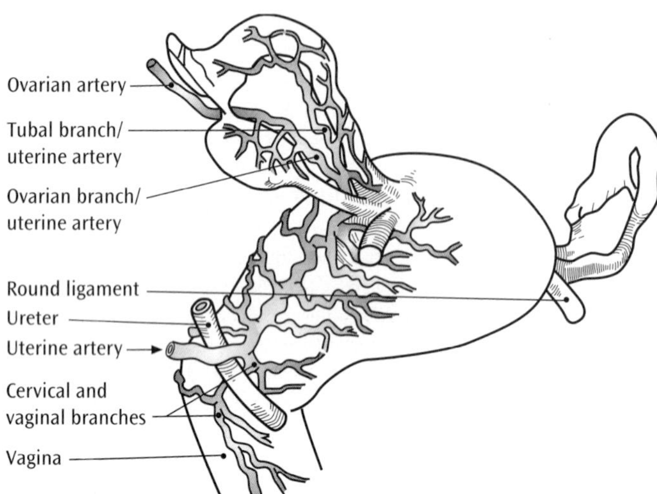

Figure 21.2 *Blood supply to the uterus, tube, and ovary. The vascular supply to the major organs is derived from the internal iliac (uterine) artery and the ovarian artery. Note the anastomotic plexuses of vessels along the lateral aspect of the uterus at the region of the cornu. Descending branches from the uterine artery supply the cervix and vagina. (From Gabbe* et al.[77]*)*

nerves and enter the spinal cord from T10 to L1. Pain fibers from the cervix run through the sacral nerves. The region of the vagina closer to the perineum sends afferent fibers to S2–4.

Uterine blood flow

The main differences in uterine blood flow during pregnancy are:

- Hypertrophy and hyperplasia of the myometrium lead to a 20-fold increase in uterine size at term.
- Uterine blood flow at term approximates to 700–900mL min^{-1}.
- During pregnancy, uterine blood flow is dependent on uterine artery perfusion pressure.
- Factors that decrease uterine artery perfusion pressure or increase uterine artery vascular resistance lead to decreased uteroplacental blood flow.
- While ephedrine produces a mild peripheral vasoconstriction, uterine blood flow is spared. Thus, ephedrine is the agent of choice for increasing the systemic blood pressure in the parturient.

Uterine blood flow changes dramatically during pregnancy. The nonpregnant uterus weighs approximately 50–70 g. Hypertrophy and hyperplasia of the myometrium leads to a 20-fold increase in uterine size, and at term the gravid uterus weighs approximately 1100 g. Uterine perfusion increases from 50–100 mL min^{-1} in the nonpregnant state to approximately 700–900 mL min^{-1} at term. At term uterine artery blood flow can account for almost 12% of maternal cardiac output, an increase from 5% before pregnancy. If one considers that maternal cardiac output increases to approximately 6 L min^{-1} at term, it would take a mere 6–9 min for a parturient to exsanguinate from an uncontrolled uterine artery hemorrhage.

Uterine blood flow is affected by many factors, including acute changes, local factors, and altered responses to vasoactive agents. Uterine blood flow is directly related to perfusion pressure and inversely related to uterine vascular resistance. Thus, uterine blood flow decreases with decreases in perfusion pressure. Decreased perfusion pressure can arise from a variety of scenarios including: (1) aortocaval compression and resultant supine hypotension syndrome; (2) maternal hemorrhage; (3) maternal hypovolemia; and (4) sympathetic blockade or high spinal or epidural blockade, with resultant maternal hypotension.

Increases in uterine vascular resistance will also decrease uterine blood flow. This can arise from: (1) vena caval compression; (2) uterine contractions; (3) performing the Valsalva maneuver while pushing; (4) drug-induced uterine hypertonus from agents such as oxytocin or cocaine; or (5) vasoactive agents.

The uterine artery response to vasoactive agents also changes during pregnancy. An increase in uterine artery vascular resistance may follow the use of some drugs and cause a decreased uterine artery blood flow. Such agents include catecholamines, vasopressin, epinephrine (adrenaline), and phenylephrine. In animal experiments (sheep), uterine vessels have been shown to be less sensitive to angiotensin II and endothelin than systemic vessels. However, the uterine arteries are more sensitive to the vasoconstrictive effects of α-adrenergic agonists than the systemic vessels.[78] Ephedrine normally causes constriction of the nonpregnant uterine artery; however, during pregnancy, the uterine artery has an increased diameter and an increased endothelial cell mass. The uterine artery synthesizes nitric oxide (NO) in larger quantities. This increase in nitric oxide is not apparent in peripheral vessels. Thus, in the parturient, ephedrine stimulates nitric oxide synthase in the uterine artery endothelium, preventing vasoconstriction. Conversely, ephedrine administration leads to vasoconstriction, as well as increased cardiac output, thereby increasing systemic blood pressure while sparing, or even improving, uteroplacental perfusion.[79]

Uterine blood flow and labor

The main points relating to uterine blood flow during labor are:

- The pain of labor increases systemic catecholamine release, leading to increased maternal cardiac output.
- While regional anesthetic-induced sympathetic blockade may improve blood flow to the placenta, maternal hypotension may decrease uteroplacental perfusion.

Cardiac adaptations to labor include increased cardiac output, from 12% to 34% by the second stage of labor, as documented by echocardiographic Doppler imaging.[80] Much of this rise is attributable to pain and apprehension, however, and can be minimized with effective analgesia and sedation. Shnider *et al.*[81] found that acute stress causes a 25% increase in plasma norepinephrine (noradrenaline) concentrations and a 50% reduction in uterine blood flow in pregnant ewes. Lederman *et al.*[82] showed that pain and stress are associated with increased plasma epinephrine concentrations and an increased incidence of abnormal fetal heart rate patterns in laboring women. Regional anesthesia may therefore increase uterine blood flow by decreasing circulating catecholamines and preventing periods of hyperventilation during contractions. Regional anesthesia may also decrease uterine blood flow as a result of maternal hypotension, unintentional intravenous injection of local anesthetic, and/or epinephrine.

Placental development

The main points relating to placental development are:

- Trophoblastic invasion of the endometrium leads to invasion and degradation of the maternal uterine spiral arterioles.
- Maternal blood enters the intervillous space, which surrounds the chorionic villi containing fetal vasculature.
- The human placenta is hemochorial. There is, overall, no direct mixing of maternal and fetal blood.

- Deoxygenated blood arrives at the placenta from the fetus via the two umbilical arteries.
- Oxygenated blood returns to the fetus via the single umbilical artery and bypasses the fetal lungs via the foramen ovale and ductus arteriosus.

Once blood has arrived at the uterus, the fetus receives oxygen and other crucial nutrients via the placenta. At term, the placenta receives approximately 90% of uterine blood flow. To understand placental function and its unique position between mother and fetus, one must start with its development. The mature ovum is fertilized within the fallopian tube, usually within 24–48 h of ovulation. The fertilized ovum now becomes a zygote (a diploid cell with 46 chromosomes) and cell division continues within the fallopian tube, leading to the formation of the morula. The morula enters the uterine cavity approximately 7 days after ovulation. The morula continues to divide, forming the blastocyst. The inner mass of cells of the blastocyst is destined to form the embryo, while the outer mass of cells goes on to form the trophoblasts. The blastocyst adheres to the endometrium and the trophoblasts burrow into the endometrium. Thus, the implanting blastocyst becomes completely covered by the endometrium. The trophoblastic cells continue to invade and intercalate between the endometrial epithelial cells. As the embryo enlarges, more maternal tissue is invaded, the walls of the superficial decidual capillaries erode, and maternal blood leaks out to form lacunae or lakes. The trophoblasts continue to invade into the arterioles and spiral arteries of the uterine wall and these vessels too are eroded.

Normal trophoblastic invasion of the spiral arterioles leads to a low-resistance, low-pressure, and high-flow system within the placental unit. In pre-eclampsia, these vascular changes do not occur because there is an abnormal response to placentation. The spiral arterioles maintain their responsiveness to vasoactive agents, thereby maintaining a high-resistance–low-capacitance profile.[83] Multiple studies now support the hypothesis that vascular endothelial abnormality is the critical factor in the development of pre-eclampsia.

On the fetal side, chorionic villi develop and fetal blood vessels invade the villi by about the 17th day of gestation. The villi in contact with the decidua basalis of the endometrium go on to form the fetal side of the placenta. Thus, the fetal component of the placenta arises from the chorionic villi that project into the intervillous space containing maternal blood. The fetal circulation is completed when the blood vessels of the embryo connect with the chorionic blood vessels via the umbilical cord. The maternal portion of the placenta is formed by the decidua basalis. Maternal blood enters the intervillous space from the spiral arterioles to bathe the chorionic villi containing fetal vessels. There is no direct mixing of maternal and fetal blood. The human placenta is, therefore, hemochorial (Fig. 21.3).[84] At term, the human placenta weighs approximately 450 g.

Placental circulation

Maternal blood circulates freely in the intervillous space but does not routinely mix with fetal blood.

Ramsey and colleagues have been instrumental in elucidating the mechanism of placental blood flow.[85,86] Blood leaves the maternal spiral arterioles and circulates freely in the intervillous space. Maternal blood flows in a pulsatile manner from the spiral arterioles and is propelled in a pulsating stream by the maternal blood pressure. The intervillous space contains approximately 350 mL of maternal blood.[87] The maternal blood then percolates slowly and under low pressure through the region

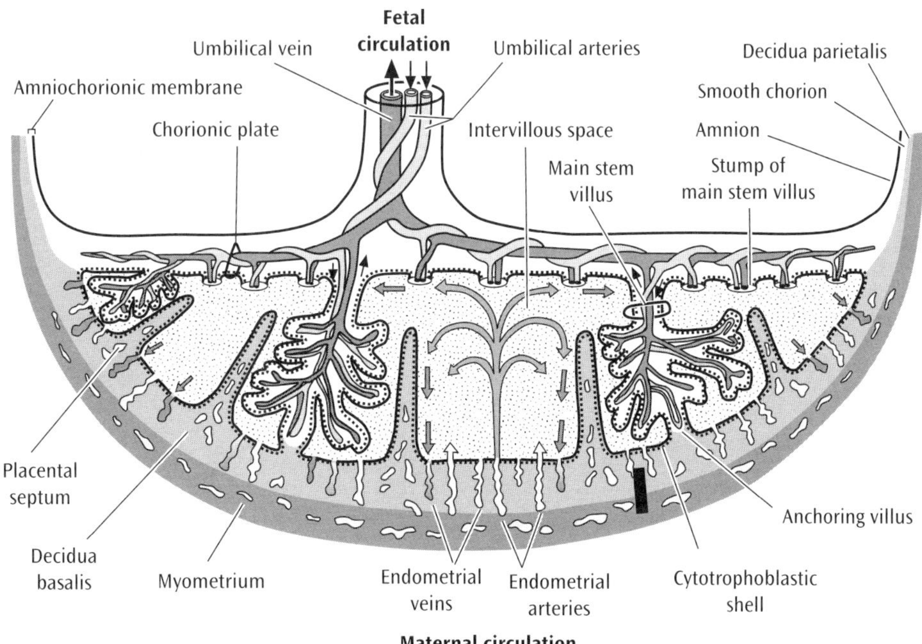

Figure 21.3 *Schematic drawing of a section through a full-term placenta, showing (1) the relation of the villous chorion (fetal part of the placenta); (2) the fetal placental circulation; and (3) the maternal placental circulation. Maternal blood flows into the intervillous spaces in funnel-shaped spurts and exchanges occur with the fetal blood as the maternal blood flows around the villi. The inflowing arterial blood pushes venous blood out into the endometrial veins, which are scattered over the entire surface of the decidua basalis. Note that the umbilical arteries carry deoxygenated fetal blood (shown in light shading) to the placenta and that the umbilical vein carries oxygenated blood (shown in dark shading) to the fetus. Note also that the cotyledons are separated from each other by the decidual septa of the maternal portion of the placenta. Each cotyledon consists of two or more main stem villi and their many branches. In this drawing, only one main stem villus is shown in each cotyledon, but the stumps of those that have been removed are indicated. (From Moore.[84])*

of densely packed terminal villi, where exchange occurs. Maternal blood then drains back through the basal plate and enters the uterine veins. These draining veins are affected by uterine muscular tone because they lie parallel to the uterine wall. Thus, during a contraction, maternal blood does not leave the intervillous space and can remain for continued transfer of nutrients.

Umbilical blood flow comprises deoxygenated blood from the fetus, which arrives via the two umbilical arteries. The arteries then travel along the chorionic surface and continue to subdivide into the multiple placental lobules and then enter into the chorionic villi to ultimately pass by the intervillous space for exchange of gases and nutrients. The venous tributaries, carrying oxygenated blood, return via the chorionic villi and along the chorionic surface to empty into one umbilical vein. This singular umbilical vein carries the blood back to the fetus and travels through the ductus venosus to the inferior vena cava (Fig. 21.4).[84] Blood flow through the ductus venosus is controlled by a sphincter, which is innervated by the fetal vagus nerve. The blood follows the path of least resistance in the fetus, flowing via the foramen ovale and ductus arteriosus and bypassing the fetal lungs.

Placental physiology

The main points relating to placental physiology are:

- Placental transport mechanisms include simple diffusion, facilitated transport, active transport, and pinocytosis.
- Oxygen is transferred via passive diffusion. The diffusion gradient is created by the different oxygen affinity between maternal and fetal blood.

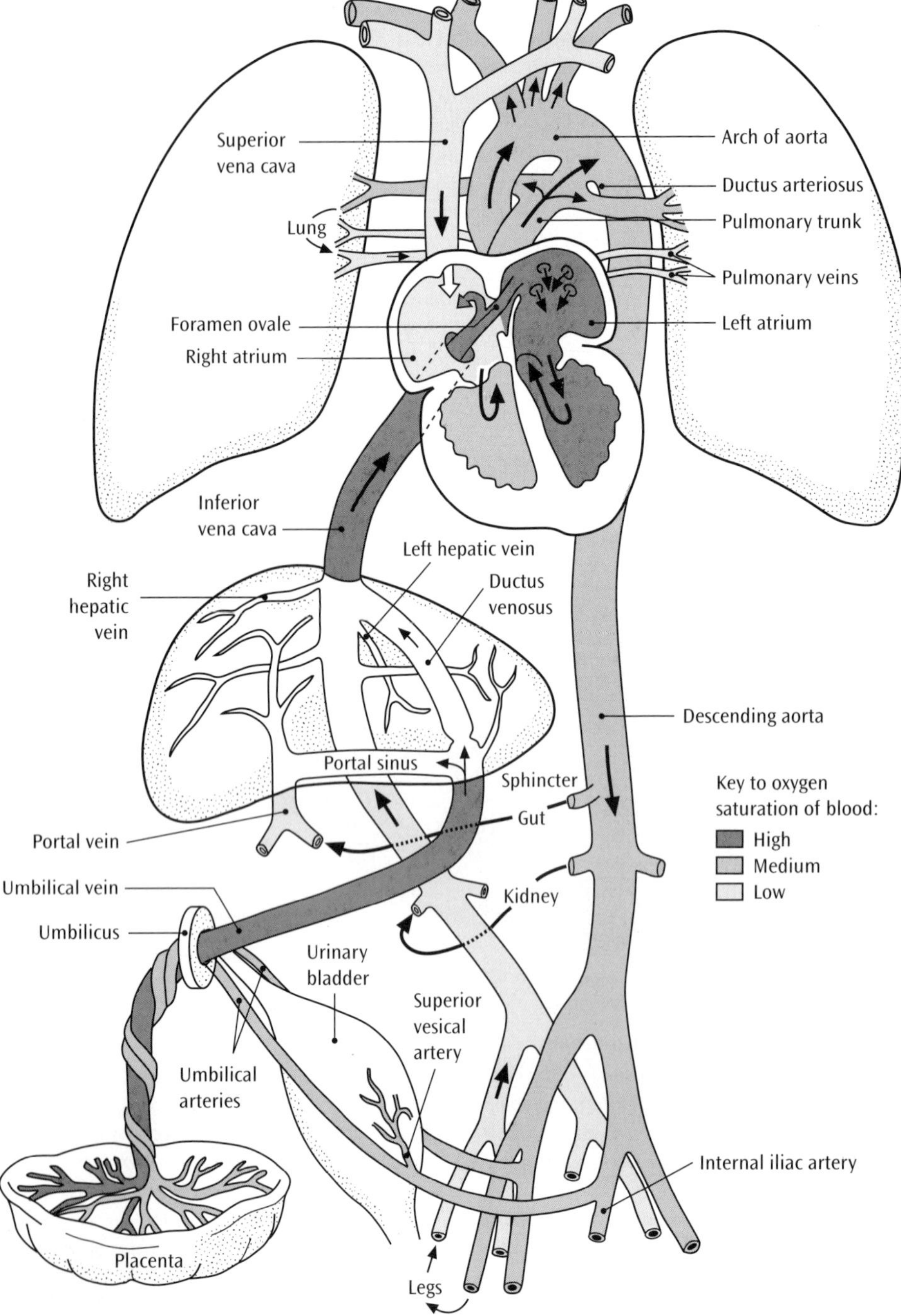

Figure 21.4 *A simplified scheme of the fetal circulation. The degree of shading indicates the oxygen saturation of the blood, and the arrows show the course of the fetal circulation. The organs are not drawn to scale. Note that three shunts permit most of the blood to bypass the liver and lungs: (1) the ductus venosus; (2) the foramen ovale; and (3) the ductus arteriosus. (From Moore.[84])*

- Carbon dioxide is transferred via simple diffusion. Maternal tachypnea decreases maternal $P\text{CO}_2$, thereby facilitating placental transfer.
- Glucose transfer occurs via carrier-mediated facilitated diffusion, while amino acids are actively transported across the placenta.

The placenta is mainly a transport and transfer organ. Transport can occur through a variety of mechanisms including: (1) simple diffusion; (2) facilitated transport; (3) active transport; and (4) pinocytosis. Multiple factors affect the ability of the placenta to transfer and transport substances as follows:

1 the concentration of the substance within the maternal plasma and its free vs. carrier-bound status;
2 the rate of maternal blood flow through the intervillous space;
3 the trophoblastic area available for exchange;
4 the physical characteristics of the substance undergoing transfer such as size, lipophilicity, and charge;
5 the kinetic limitations of the active transport mechanisms, both on the maternal and on the fetal side;
6 the amount of substance utilized and metabolized by the placenta itself;
7 the area available for exchange on the fetal side of the placenta;
8 the concentration of the substance in the fetal circulation and its bound vs. free status;
9 the rate of fetal blood flow through the villous capillaries.[88]

Placental transport of oxygen

Transfer of oxygen across the placenta is blood flow dependent and occurs by passive diffusion. The placenta must supply approximately $8\,\text{mL}\,\text{O}_2\,\text{min}^{-1}\,\text{kg}^{-1}$ fetal body weight.[89] Oxygen stores in the fetus are sufficient for only 1 to 2 min, thus an almost continuous blood flow is required. The average oxygen saturation in the intervillous space is about 65–75% with a partial pressure of oxygen of about 4–4.7 kPa (30–35 mmHg). The differences between the oxyhemoglobin dissociation curves of maternal and fetal blood may help to facilitate oxygen transport to the fetus. In addition, fetal hemoglobin has a higher affinity for oxygen because of the presence of hemoglobin F.

Placental transport of carbon dioxide

Carbon dioxide is also transferred across the placenta by simple diffusion. The partial pressure of carbon dioxide in the umbilical arteries is about 6.4 kPa (48 mmHg). This is higher than that in the maternal blood found in the intervillous space. Also, maternal blood has a higher affinity for carbon dioxide than does fetal blood, thereby facilitating transfer. Physiologic changes in maternal tidal volume leading to a slight tachypnea with hyperventilation also help to keep maternal $P\text{CO}_2$ lower than fetal $P\text{CO}_2$.

Placental transport of nutrients

The fetus is dependent on the transfer of glucose across the placenta, as it does not participate in gluconeogenesis. Glucose utilizes carrier-mediated, facilitated diffusion to cross the placenta. This process is not dependent on insulin, a sodium gradient, or cellular energy. The placenta also utilizes glucose for its own metabolic processes including oxidation, glycogen storage, and conversion to lactate.

Amino acids transfer is an active process involving the Na^+,K^+-ATPase pump. The fetus utilizes amino acids for protein synthesis, growth, and oxidation. The fetus also needs fatty acids for brain development, growth, and deposition of body fat. Fatty acids cross the placenta by simple diffusion. Ketones can be metabolized by the fetus in the brain tissue, kidney, heart, liver, and placenta. Most large molecules cannot cross the placenta. One important exception is IgG, which readily crosses the placenta and provides passive immunity to the fetus.

REFERENCES

1. Conklin KA. Maternal physiologic adaptations during gestation, labor, and the puerperium. *Semin Anesth* 1991; **10**: 221–34.
2. Leontic EA. Respiratory disease in pregnancy. *Med Clin North Am* 1977; **61**: 111–28.
3. Samsoon GL, Young JR. Difficult tracheal intubation: a retrospective study. *Anaesthesia* 1987; **42**: 487–90.
4. Mallampati SR, Gatt SP, Gugino LD, *et al.* A clinical sign to predict difficult tracheal intubation: a prospective study. *Can Anaesth Soc J* 1985; **32**: 429–34.
5. Farcon EL, Kim MH, Marx GF. Changing Mallampati score during labour. *Can J Anaesth* 1994; **41:** 50–1.
6. Russell IF, Chambers WA. Closing volume in normal pregnancy. *Br J Anaesth* 1981; **53**: 1043–7.
7. Archer Jr GW, Marx GF. Arterial oxygen tension during apnoea in parturient women. *Br J Anaesth* 1974; **46**: 358–60.
8. Byrne F, Oduro-Dominah A, Kipling R. The effect of pregnancy on pulmonary nitrogen washout. A study of preoxygenation. *Anaesthesia* 1987; **42**: 148–50.
9. Norris MC, Dewan DM. Preoxygenation for cesarean section: a comparison of two techniques. *Anesthesiology* 1985; **62**: 827–9.
10. Norris MC, Kirkland MR, Torjman MC, Goldberg ME. Denitrogenation in pregnancy. *Can J Anaesth* 1989; **36**: 523–5.
11. Kambam JR, Handte RE, Brown WU, Smith BE. Effect of normal and preeclamptic pregnancies on the oxyhemoglobin dissociation curve. *Anesthesiology* 1986; **65**: 426–7.
12. Ang CK, Tan TH, Walters WA, Wood C. Postural influence on maternal capillary oxygen and carbon dioxide tension. *Br Med J* 1969; **4**: 201–3.
13. Calvin S, Jones OW, 3rd, Knieriem K, Weinstein L. Oxygen saturation in the supine hypotensive syndrome. *Obstet Gynecol* 1988; **71**: 872–7.
14. Dayal P, Murata Y, Takamura H. Antepartum and postpartum acid–base changes in maternal blood in normal and complicated pregnancies. *J Obstet Gynaecol Br Commonw* 1972; **79**: 612–24.
15. Oberg B, Poulsen TD. Obesity: an anaesthetic challenge. *Acta Anaesthesiol Scand* 1996; **40**: 191–200.
16. Cutforth R, MacDonald CB. Heart sounds and murmurs in pregnancy. *Am Heart J* 1966; **71**: 741–7.
17. Enein M, Zina AA, Kassem M, el-Tabbakh G. Echocardiography of the pericardium in pregnancy. *Obstet Gynecol* 1987; **69**: 851–3.
18. Mendenhall HW. Serum protein concentrations in pregnancy. I. Concentrations in maternal serum. *Am J Obstet Gynecol* 1970; **106**: 388–99.
19. Leighton BL, Cheek TG, Gross JB, *et al.* Succinylcholine pharmacodynamics in peripartum patients. *Anesthesiology* 1986; **64**: 202–5.
20. Capeless EL, Clapp JF. Cardiovascular changes in early phase of pregnancy. *Am J Obstet Gynecol* 1989; **161**: 1449–53.
21. Laird-Meeter K, van de Ley G, Bom TH, *et al.* Cardiocirculatory adjustments during pregnancy: An echocardiographic study. *Clin Cardiol* 1979; **2**: 328–32.
22. Rubler S, Damani PM, Pinto ER. Cardiac size and performance during pregnancy estimated with echocardiography. *Am J Cardiol* 1977; **40**: 534–40.
23. Mabie WC, DiSessa TG, Crocker LG, *et al.* A longitudinal study of cardiac output in normal human pregnancy. *Am J Obstet Gynecol* 1994; **170**: 849–56.
24. Clark SL, Cotton DB, Lee W, *et al.* Central hemodynamic assessment of normal term pregnancy. *Am J Obstet Gynecol* 1989; **161**: 1439–42.
25. Robson SC, Dunlop W, Boys RJ, Hunter S. Cardiac output during labour. *Br Med J* (Clin Res Edn) 1987; **295**: 1169–72.
26. Kerr MG, Scott DB, Samuel E. Studies of the inferior vena cava in late pregnancy. Br Med J 1964; **1:** 532–3.
27. McLennan CE. Antecubital and femoral venous pressure in normal and toxemic pregnancy. *Am J Obstet Gynecol* 1943; **45:** 568–91.
28. Kerr MG. The mechanical effects of the gravid uterus in late pregnancy. *J Obstet Gynaecol Br Commonw* 1965; **72:** 513–29.
29. Ueland K, Novy MJ, Peterson EN, Metcalfe J. Maternal cardiovascular dynamics. IV. The influence of gestational age on the maternal cardiovascular response to posture and exercise. *Am J Obstet Gynecol* 1969; **104**: 856–64.

30. Abitbol MM. Aortic compression by pregnant uterus. *N Y State J Med* 1976; **76**: 1470–5.
31. Milsom I, Forssman L. Factors influencing aortocaval compression in late pregnancy. *Am J Obstet Gynecol* 1984; **148**: 764–71.
32. Hardebo JE, Edvinsson L. Reduced sensitivity to alpha- and beta-adrenergic receptor agonists of intra- and extracranial vessels during pregnancy. Relevance to migraine. *Acta Neurol Scand Suppl* 1977; **64:** 204–5.
33. Bonica JJ. *Principles and Practice of Obstetric Analgesia and Anesthesia*. Philadelphia: F A Davis Co., 1967.
34. Ramanathan S, Grant GJ. Vasopressor therapy for hypotension due to epidural anesthesia for cesarean section. *Acta Anaesthesiol Scand* 1988; **32**: 559–65.
35. Fox DB, Troiano NH, Graves CR. Use of the pulmonary artery catheter in severe preeclampsia: a review. *Obstet Gynecol Surv* 1996; **51**: 684–95.
36. Mushambi MC, Halligan AW, Williamson K. Recent developments in the pathophysiology and management of pre-eclampsia [see comments]. *Br J Anaesth* 1996; **76**: 133–48.
37. Clark SL, Cotton DB. Clin indications for pulmonary artery catheterization in the patient with severe preeclampsia [see comments]. *Am J Obstet Gynecol* 1988; **158**: 453–8.
38. Gerbasi FR, Bottoms S, Farag A, Mammen E. Increased intravascular coagulation associated with pregnancy. *Obstet Gynecol* 1990; **75**: 385–9.
39. Stiehm ER, Kennan AL, Schelble DT. Split products of fibrin in maternal serum in the perinatal period. *Am J Obstet Gynecol* 1970; **108**: 941–5.
40. Tygart SG, McRoyan DK, Spinnato JA, *et al.* Longitudinal study of platelet indices during normal pregnancy. *Am J Obstet Gynecol* 1986; **154**: 883–7.
41. Pitkin RM, Witte DL. Platelet and leukocyte counts in pregnancy. *JAMA* 1979; **242**: 2696–8.
42. Burrows RF, Kelton JG. Thrombocytopenia at delivery: a prospective survey of 6715 deliveries. *Am J Obstet Gynecol* 1990; **162**: 731–4.
43. Greer IA. The special case of venous thromboembolism in pregnancy. *Haemostasis* 1998; **28** (Suppl. 3): 22–34.
44. de Swiet M. Management of pulmonary embolus in pregnancy. *Eur Heart J* 1999; **20**: 1378–85.
45. Greer IA. Thrombosis in pregnancy: maternal and fetal issues [see comments]. *Lancet* 1999; **353**: 1258–65.
46. Van Thiel DH, Gavaler JS, Joshi SN, *et al.* Heartburn of pregnancy. *Gastroenterology* 1977; **72**: 666–8.
47. Lind JF, Smith AM, McIver DK, *et al.* Heartburn in pregnancy – a manometric study. *Can Med Assoc J* 1968; **98**: 571–4.
48. Ulmsten U, Sundstrom G. Esophageal manometry in pregnant and nonpregnant women. *Am J Obstet Gynecol* 1978; **132**: 260–4.
49. Hart DM. Heartburn in pregnancy. *J Int Med Res* 1978; **6** (Suppl. 1): 1–5.
50. Whitehead EM, Smith M, Dean Y, O'Sullivan G. An evaluation of gastric emptying times in pregnancy and the puerperium [see comments]. *Anaesthesia* 1993; **48**: 53–7.
51. Holdsworth JD. Relationship between stomach contents and analgesia in labour. *Br J Anaesth* 1978; **50**: 1145–8.
52. Carp H, Jayaram A, Stoll M. Ultrasound examination of the stomach contents of parturients. *Anesth Analg* 1992; **74**: 683–7.
53. Attia RR, Ebeid AM, Fischer JE, Goudsouzian NG. Maternal fetal and placental gastrin concentrations. *Anaesthesia* 1982; **37**: 18–21.
54. Roberts RB, Shirley MA. Reducing the risk of acid aspiration during cesarean section. *Anesth Analg* 1974; **53**: 859–68.
55. Wyner J, Cohen SE. Gastric volume in early pregnancy: effect of metoclopramide. *Anesthesiology* 1982; **57**: 209–12.
56. James CF, Gibbs CP, Banner T. Postpartum perioperative risk of aspiration pneumonia. *Anesthesiology* 1984; **61**: 756–9.
57. Dunlop W. Serial changes in renal haemodynamics during normal human pregnancy. *Br J Obstet Gynaecol* 1981; **88**: 1–9.
58. Davison JM, Hytten FE. Glomerular filtration during and after pregnancy. *J Obstet Gynaecol Br Commonw* 1974; **81**: 588–95.
59. Davison JM, Hytten FE. The effect of pregnancy on the renal handling of glucose. *Br J Obstet Gynaecol* 1975; **82**: 374–81.
60. Burt RL, Davidson IW. Insulin half-life and utilization in normal pregnancy. *Obstet Gynecol* 1974; **43**: 161–70.
61. Nordlander E, Hanson U, Persson B, Stangenberg M. Pancreatic B-cell function during normal pregnancy. *Diabetes Res* 1987; **6**: 133–6.
62. Fisher PM, Sutherland HW, Bewsher PD. The insulin response to glucose infusion in normal human pregnancy. *Diabetologia* 1980; **19**: 15–20.
63. Felig P, Lynch V. Starvation in human pregnancy: hypoglycemia, hypoinsulinemia, and hyperketonemia. *Science* 1970; **170**: 990–2.
64. Ramin KD. Diabetic ketoacidosis in pregnancy. *Obstet Gynecol Clin North Am* 1999; **26:** 481–8, viii.
65. Coustan DR. Management of gestational diabetes mellitus: a self-fulfilling prophecy? [editorial; comment]. *JAMA* 1996; **275**: 1199–200.
66. D'Alessio JG, Ramanathan J, Allen G, III. Diabetes mellitus in pregnancy: pathophysiology and obstetric management. In: Norris MC (ed.). *Obstetric Anesthesia*, 2nd edn. Philadelphia: Williams & Wilkins, 1999: 103–12.
67. Mortimer RH. Thyroid disease and pregnancy. *Aust NZ J Med* 1998; **28**: 647–53.
68. Glinoer D. The regulation of thyroid function in pregnancy: pathways of endocrine adaptation from physiology to pathology. *Endocr Rev* 1997; **18**: 404–33.
69. Steinbrook RA, Carr DB, Datta S, *et al.* Dissociation of plasma and cerebrospinal fluid beta-endorphin-like immunoactivity levels during pregnancy and parturition. *Anesth Analg* 1982; **61**: 893–7.
70. Cogan R, Spinnato JA. Pain and discomfort thresholds in late pregnancy. *Pain* 1986; **27**: 63–8.
71. Messih MN. Epidural space pressures during pregnancy. *Anaesthesia* 1981; **36**: 775–82.
72. Marx GF, Zemaitis MT, Orkin LR. Cerebrospinal fluid pressures during labor and obstetrical anesthesia. *Anesthesiology* 1961; **22:** 348–54.
73. Butterworth JF 4th, Walker FO, Lysak SZ. Pregnancy increases median nerve susceptibility to lidocaine. *Anesthesiology* 1990; **72**: 962–5.
74. Gin T, Chan MT. Decreased minimum alveolar concentration of isoflurane in pregnant humans. *Anesthesiology* 1994; **81**: 829–32.
75. Chan MT, Mainland P, Gin T. Minimum alveolar concentration of halothane and enflurane are decreased in early pregnancy. *Anesthesiology* 1996; **85**: 782–6.
76. Gin T, Mainland P, Chan MT, Short TG. Decreased thiopental requirements in early pregnancy. *Anesthesiology* 1997; **86**: 73–8.
77. Gabbe SG, Niebyl JR, Simpson JL. Anatomy of the pelvis. In: *Obstetrics Normal and Problem Pregnancies*, 3rd edn. New York: Churchill Livingstone, 1996: 3–30.
78. Magness RR, Rosenfeld CR. Systemic and uterine responses to alpha-adrenergic stimulation in pregnant and nonpregnant ewes. *Am J Obstet Gynecol* 1986; **155**: 897–904.
79. Weiner CP, Thompson LP. Nitric oxide and pregnancy. *Semin Perinatol* 1997; **21**: 367–80.
80. Hunter S, Robson SC. Adaptation of the maternal heart in pregnancy. *Br Heart J* 1992; **68**: 540–3.
81. Shnider SM, Wright RG, Levinson G, *et al.* Uterine blood flow and plasma norepinephrine changes during maternal stress in the pregnant ewe. *Anesthesiology* 1979; **50**: 524–7.
82. Lederman RP, Lederman E, Work Jr B, McCann DS. Anxiety and epinephrine in multiparous women in labor: relationship to duration of labor and fetal heart rate pattern. *Am J Obstet Gynecol* 1985; **153**: 870–7.
83. Khong TY, De Wolf F, Robertson WB, Brosens I. Inadequate maternal vascular response to placentation in pregnancies complicated by pre-eclampsia and by small-for-gestational age infants. *Br J Obstet Gynaecol* 1986; **93**: 1049–59.
84. Moore KL. *The Developing Human: Clinically Oriented Embryology*, 4th edn. Philadelphia: W B Saunders, 1988.
85. Ramsey EM, Davis RW. A composite drawing of the placenta to show its structure and circulation. *Anat Rec* 1963; **145:** 366.
86. Ramsey EM, Harris JWS. Comparison of uteroplacental vasculature and circulation in the rhesus monkey and man. *Contrib Embryol* 1966; **38:** 59.
87. Arey LB. *Developmental Anatomy: A Textbook and Laboratory Manual of Embryology*. Philadelphia: W B Saunders, 1974.
88. Cunningham FG, MacDonald PC, Gant NF, *et al. Williams Obstetrics*, 20th edn. Stamford, CT: Appleton & Lange, 1997.
89. Longo LD. Respiration in the fetal–placental unit. In: Cowett RM (ed.). *Principles of Perinatal–Neonatal Metabolism*. New York: Springer-Verlag, 1991: 304–15.

22

Inherited disease and anesthesia

P JANE HALSALL AND PHILIP M HOPKINS

In order to appreciate fully the significance of an inherited condition, having elicited a positive family history, the clinician must have a basic understanding of the genetic basis of the disease as well as its implications for anesthesia. Some important genetic concepts will therefore be briefly described.

The genetic code that determines the various characteristics of the individual is carried in the double helical structures of the deoxyribonucleic acid (DNA) that makes up the chromosomes of the nuclei of cells. The normal human chromosomal complement is 23 pairs, 22 of which are autosomes with one pair of sex chromosomes (XX in females, XY in males). Genes are regions of chromosomal DNA, which, by the nature of the order of the constituent nitrogenous bases, are responsible for the arrangement of the 20 different types of amino acids that form the various peptide chains, which are the building blocks of proteins. The site of a gene on its chromosome is termed the locus for that gene. As a result of a process of mutation over millions of years, each gene exists in one or more forms, or alleles. In many instances, different alleles of the same gene will produce a protein with identical function, but in others some alleles will produce proteins with altered function, which may give rise to pathology – an inherited disease. Whether the presence of a disease allele leads to the clinical expression of the condition (disease phenotype) is determined by the pattern of inheritance of the condition. A dominant condition is one that occurs when only one of the pair of alleles is the disease allele, that is the disease phenotype occurs with a heterozygous genotype. A recessive condition, however, requires two disease alleles or a homozygous genotype for the disease phenotype to be expressed. Inherited diseases are further classified according to whether the abnormal gene is present on the sex chromosomes (X-linked, as very little functioning genetic material is present on the Y chromosome) or absent (autosomal). Family pedigrees illustrating the three disorders (autosomal dominant, autosomal recessive, and X-linked recessive) are shown in Fig. 22.1. Table 22.1 lists the more common inherited disorders according to their mode of inheritance.

It can be seen in Table 22.1 that there are inherited diseases affecting each of the systems of the body, with many being multisystemic. The relevance of some of these to anesthesia is described in other chapters (Chapters 52 and 53). Many common disorders described in other sections of the book, such as diabetes mellitus and coronary heart disease, have a genetic component to a multifactorial etiology. Here we describe other inherited conditions that have a direct bearing on perioperative management. Two of these, malignant hyperthermia and plasma cholinesterase disorders, are discussed in greatest detail because their adverse effects are virtually confined to an abnormal response to certain drugs used in anesthesia. Also included in this chapter are the inherited myopathies and metabolic disorders.

MALIGNANT HYPERTHERMIA

There can be no doubt that malignant hyperthermia (malignant hyperpyrexia, MH) has been responsible for a proportion of anesthetic deaths almost since the introduction of ether and chloroform in the middle of the nineteenth century. However, it was not until 1960 that MH was first described in an Australian family by Denborough and Lovell.[1] This followed a clinical crisis in a patient with a family history of multiple anesthetic-related deaths. Thus, a very good description of the clinical reaction and its inheritance as an autosomal dominant characteristic was established. It was presumably because, until quite recently, death due to anesthesia was not uncommon that this relatively rare cause (the estimated incidence of MH in the UK population is 1 in 8000) was not recognized earlier. As anesthesia has become progressively safer, so morbidity and mortality due to MH have become relatively more significant. The original mortality rate from MH was 70–80%, so that MH was considered to be the commonest cause of anesthetic death in fit young patients. However, mortality has dropped significantly to 2–3% in recent years, mainly because of the improvements in monitoring and increased awareness of MH by anesthesiologists. The number of new MH cases identified each year remains fairly constant (~20 per annum in the UK) although the referral rate has increased. This suggests that the provisional clinical diagnosis is now being made more frequently. It is more commonly seen in the younger age groups (10- to 30-year-olds), with males predominating slightly. However, this may simply reflect the different lifestyles and therefore type of surgery and anesthesia required by males and females rather than a true gender difference. However, there is a slight preponderance of MH-positive fathers of probands compared with MH-positive mothers. One intriguing and unexplained fact is that 75% of UK probands have had at least one previous apparently uneventful anesthetic.[2,3]

Etiology of malignant hyperthermia

Although it was soon realized that MH was a muscle condition, which could be diagnosed from *in vitro* muscle studies (see later), it was not until 1985 that evidence of impaired Ca^{2+} homeostasis[4] during an MH reaction emerged.[5] This results in increased intracellular calcium, leading to intense muscle contractures and a marked increase in cell

A

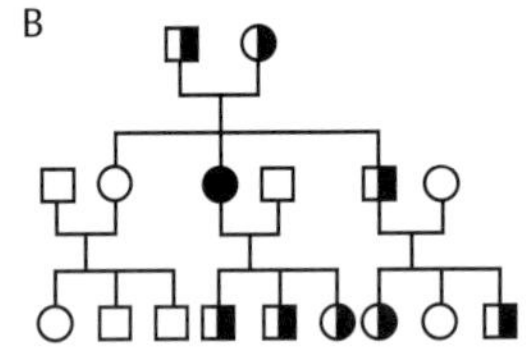

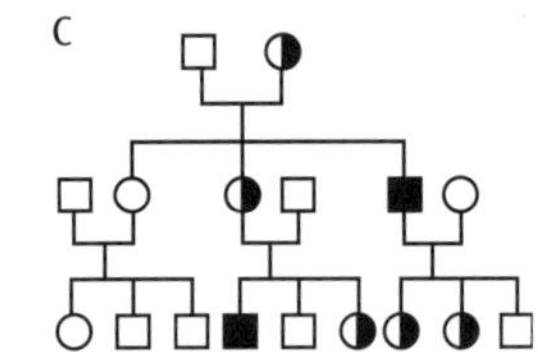

Figure 22.1 *The three most common patterns of inheritance. (A) Autosomal dominant. ◑, Affected female; ○, nonaffected female; ◨, affected male; □, nonaffected male. (B) Autosomal recessive. ●, Affected female; ○, nonaffected female; ◑, carrier female (nonaffected); ■, affected male; □, nonaffected male; ◨, carrier male (nonaffected). (C) X-linked recessive. ○, Nonaffected female; ◑, carrier female (nonaffected); ■, affected male; □, nonaffected male.*

metabolism. Ca^{2+} is a ubiquitous ion and loss of homeostasis could be caused by any molecular defect in any of the structures controlling Ca^{2+} movements along the excitation–contraction (E–C) coupling process.[6,7] This may explain why such chemically different agents as succinylcholine (suxamethonium) and halothane can trigger MH and why there is strong evidence of heterogeneity from DNA studies.

Interest has long been focused on the sarcoplasmic reticulum (SR) of the muscle as the site of the defect in MH. Caffeine is known to cause Ca^{2+} release from the SR, and MH muscle is more sensitive to caffeine. So, identification of the ryanodine receptor protein on the SR as a calcium efflux channel[8–10] and the subsequent identification of a link between the ryanodine receptor gene (*RYR1*) and MH[11,12] was of crucial importance, especially when it was shown that ryanodine could be used as an additional *in vitro* contracture test (IVCT) for MH.[13] Other potential sites of the MH defect in the E–C coupling process such as the sarcolemma and t-tubule have not been eliminated and may still be shown to have a significant role.

Genetics of malignant hyperthermia

Early family studies indicated an autosomal dominant inheritance for MH.[1] This mode of inheritance has been confirmed by the results of family screening using *in vitro* contracture tests. With the revolution in molecular biological techniques over the past 20 years, it has been possible to study MH susceptibility using DNA markers of known chromosomal location in individual MH families. Identification of the *Hal* gene in pigs, which suffer a similar but not identical MH syndrome, known as porcine stress syndrome, was the first lead.[14] There is a good preservation of groupings of loci across species and, as this area of the *Hal* gene transposed to human chromosome 19q12–13.2, intense research in this region was stimulated. Localization of the *RYR1* gene to this area (19q13–13.2) and subsequently two studies from North America and Ireland suggested a link between *RYR1* and MH.[11,12]

However, within the European populations *RYR1* accounts for around 50% of positive linkage findings in MH families. Furthermore, 23 mutations in *RYR1* cosegregating with MH have been identified.[15] Some occurred in isolated families and only 15 are reported to have functional properties.[16,17] There is evidence in some families of discordant data between the *in vitro* contracture tests and the genetic results. The incidence of the discordant data suggests that the inheritance of MH may be more complex than a straightforward autosomal dominant characteristic and could imply that additional genetic factors may influence the expression of MH.[22]

Other candidate genes have been detected on chromosomes 1 and 7, and possibly 3, 5, and 17. These genes involve the various subunits of the dihydropyridine receptor, which forms the triadic junction complex with the ryanodine receptor at the t-tubule/SR junction and also the adult muscle sodium channel. Consequently, the heterogeneity of MH is well established,[19] making the introduction of diagnostic DNA screening for MH complex (see later under diagnosis of MH).

Clinical presentation

When MH was first described, monitoring of the anesthetized patient was invariably purely clinical. Under these circumstances the most obvious abnormality of an MH reaction was a progressive rise in body temperature followed by death, hence the name malignant hyperthermia. With the description of further cases, however, it became apparent that hyperthermia is a relatively late manifestation of the reaction.

The clinical presentation of MH is very variable and therefore the recognition of a reaction and its treatment can also vary. In the UK, guidelines for the treatment of a crisis can be obtained from the Association of Anaesthetists and should be available in each operating room. MH patients are normal individuals; there is no way of identifying them prior to an MH event, other than by a personal or family history suggestive of MH, so preoperative assessment is important. The exception to this is central core disease (CCD), which is known to be associated with MH.[20] In the absence of a family history of MH, the first indication that an individual may be susceptible to the condition is the development of an exaggerated initial response to the depolarizing neuromuscular blocking drug succinylcholine (suxamethonium). It has been well demonstrated[21,22] that in most people, along with the more easily recognized fasciculations, succinylcholine causes an increase in tension of the jaw muscles. In some cases this is clinically apparent as resistance to opening of the mouth for laryngoscopy. When this jaw stiffness is severe, and especially when it is prolonged, the condition is

Table 22.1 *Mode of inheritance of some of the more common inherited disorders*

Autosomal dominant	Autosomal recessive	X-linked recessive
Huntington's chorea	Cystic fibrosis	Duchenne muscular dystrophy
Neurofibromatosis	Phenylketonuria	Hemophilia
Myotonic dystrophy	Sickle cell anemia	Fragile X syndrome
Malignant hyperthermia	Mucopolysaccharidoses	Childhood blindness
Polycystic kidneys	Friedreich's ataxia	
Polyposis coli	Cystinuria	
Hypercholesterolemia		
Acute intermittent porphyria		

called masseter muscle spasm (MMS). MMS may be accompanied by generalized muscular rigidity. MMS is associated with MH susceptibility, and after making this diagnosis the anesthesiologist must refer the patient for investigation of MH status (whether or not other signs of MH are detected). When MMS appears to occur alone, approximately 30% of cases are actually due to MH, and this rises to over 70% when there is evidence of muscle damage, such as a very high creatine kinase (CK) and myoglobinuria. MMS is difficult to interpret, not least because it is a subjective sign.[23]

The "true" MH response, as opposed to exaggerated succinylcholine-induced muscle rigidity, is characterized by metabolic stimulation, the consequences of the loss of sarcolemmal integrity (hyperkalemia and myoglobinemia), and a later-onset muscle rigidity. Such a response is very variable: it may have rapid and fulminant onset occurring soon after the introduction of one of the volatile anesthetic drugs, or it may be insidious, especially when inhalational agents have been used in low concentrations to prevent awareness during artificial ventilation. If the patient is carefully monitored, one or more abnormalities will always be detected during the course of the anesthetic. An MH reaction does not start after the discontinuation of the triggering drugs, although if it has progressed beyond the earliest stages it will not necessarily be stopped by the discontinuation of triggering drugs in the absence of other therapeutic measures. Consequently, a postoperative pyrexia occurring after a normal intraoperative and immediate recovery period is not an indicator of MH.[24]

The two early signs of hypermetabolism are a rising end-tidal CO_2 concentration (in the presence of appropriate ventilation and fresh gas flow for the particular circuit in use) and an inappropriate tachycardia. These signs may be accompanied, or followed, by hypertension, hypoxemia, tachypnea (in the spontaneously breathing patient), acidosis, early exhaustion of soda-lime in a circle system, and subsequently a rising body temperature. Hyperkalemia may lead to cardiac arrhythmias, including asystole, and myoglobinemia can cause acute renal failure. If the acute reaction is not terminated, the hypermetabolism and cellular destruction may lead to disseminated intravascular coagulation.

From this description it can be seen that the most essential monitoring devices for the early detection of an MH reaction are a capnograph, a pulse oximeter, and an electrocardiogram (ECG) monitor. A prerequisite for early diagnosis is, of course, an appropriate level of suspicion for the condition by the vigilant anesthesiologist. It is important that an early diagnosis is made because, as muscle rigidity develops, the blood supply to the muscle cells is restricted, thus impeding the supply of therapeutic agents to the muscle. It is also likely that a stage of the cellular pathological process is reached when the process, despite treatment, becomes irreversible.

Management of acute malignant hyperthermia reaction

The management of an acute MH reaction, as in the case of other medical emergencies, requires several therapeutic interventions to be employed as rapidly as possible: written descriptions of the appropriate actions cannot convey the urgency required. A poster entitled "Guidelines for the treatment of an MH crisis" can be obtained from the Association of Anaesthetists of Great Britain and Ireland.

Immediate measures

Stop the administration of trigger drugs

As well as actually turning off the vaporizer, the elimination of volatile drugs from the body can be enhanced by hyperventilation, and from the anesthetic breathing system by increasing fresh gas flow. If practicable, change the anesthetic circuit.

Dantrolene sodium

This drug was first used to reduce muscle spasms in those with neuromuscular disorders. It is effective in reducing muscle activity, resulting from an increase in intracellular calcium ion concentration from any cause, and is therefore efficacious in the treatment of MH. It acts at the site of E–C coupling, possibly at the sarcolemma, and is relatively sparing on cardiac and diaphragmatic muscle. Dantrolene for intravenous injection is prepared as an alkaline mixture with mannitol (3 mg per 20-mg vial) to increase its solubility; even so, its preparation for use is slow. The initial dose is 1–2 $mg\,kg^{-1}$, repeated until there is evidence that hypermetabolism is reversing, and further doses can be given if trends reverse. Up to 10 $mg\,kg^{-1}$ has been necessary.

Active body cooling

With better monitoring and the early diagnosis of MH, active cooling is now a less prominent feature. Cooling not only prevents the potentially harmful effects of hyperthermia on heat-labile cellular constituents but, if sufficiently effective, may also cool the body sufficiently to inhibit the MH response at the cellular level. Cooling can be achieved by converting warming blankets to cooling blankets, intravenous infusion of refrigerated crystalloid solutions, peritoneal lavage with cold saline, and applying icepacks to the axillae and groins, and in extreme cases (where facilities exist) a blood heat exchanger can be used. It is important to remember to try to prevent peripheral vasoconstriction as this will prevent heat loss. An adequate fluid load may be all that is required to do this, but, if not, methylprednisolone (10 $mg\,kg^{-1}$) is an effective vasodilator and has been shown to reduce halothane-induced muscle contracture *in vitro*.[25]

Intermediate treatment

Metabolic acidosis

The hyperventilation used to increase elimination of volatile drugs will partially compensate for the metabolic acidosis. Further correction can be achieved by titrating sodium bicarbonate against arterial pH and base excess.

Hypoxemia

Hyperventilation should initially be with 100% oxygen. This must be maintained until the reaction is controlled unless lower inspired oxygen fractions can be demonstrated to provide for adequate oxygen delivery in the face of the greatly increased oxygen consumption.

Hyperkalemia

Serum potassium concentrations must be measured frequently from the onset of an MH reaction. Intravenous calcium should be used only when life-threatening arrhythmias have occurred or are considered to be imminent, as it is possible that an influx of extracellular calcium is responsible for the generation of the MH response. Otherwise, hyperkalemia must be corrected with infusion of dextrose and insulin, ion exchange resins, or, if especially refractory, by hemodialysis.

Cardiac arrhythmias

These should be treated symptomatically along the usual lines. Antiarrhythmic drugs that may have an additional effect on reducing the MH response are verapamil and procainamide. However Ca^{2+} channel-blocking drugs must not be used if dantrolene has been administered, as the combination may have a profound negative inotropic effect on the heart.

Disseminated intravascular coagulation (DIC)

Disseminated intravascular coagulation (DIC) occurs rarely and only in very severe fulminating cases. Blood samples must be sent for clotting studies and analysis of fibrin degradation products. DIC should be managed along standard lines, with transfusion of platelets, fresh-frozen plasma, and cryoprecipitate. The use of tranexamic acid has not been reported in MH.

Myoglobinuria

Even before myoglobinuria is detected, significant myoglobinemia must be assumed to have occurred during an MH response. It is essential that urine output is monitored. The bladder should be catheterized and a diuresis established using fluids, mannitol, or furosemide. A high renal blood flow should be encouraged with dopamine during the acute phase of the illness. If myoglobinuria is severe it may block the renal tubules, leading to renal failure. Myoglobinuria is amenable to short-term dialysis over the acute period. Myoglobinuria can be detected in the first voided specimen of urine, whereas the highest CK associated with muscle damage will take approximately 24 h to develop.

Late treatment

Other conditions, such as thyrotoxic crisis, pheochromocytoma, and muscle diseases, may mimic MH. Therefore, appropriate investigations should be performed to exclude these potential diagnoses. All suspected MH reactions should be reported to an MH center for follow-up. Until the reaction has been confirmed, the proband and the whole family should be made aware of the potential implications of MH with regard to future anesthesia. MH is not a diagnosis to be made lightly without further referral to an MH center, otherwise the whole family may become erroneously labeled as being at risk of MH.

Laboratory diagnosis of malignant hyperthermia susceptibility

In 1970 and 1971 two *in vitro tests* for the diagnosis of MH susceptibility (MHS) were described by Kalow *et al.* (using caffeine)[26] and Ellis *et al.* (using halothane).[27] These tests still form the basis of current diagnostic methods, which involve open muscle biopsy and the exposure of live strips of muscle to halothane and to caffeine, following a set protocol. MHS muscle develops an abnormal contracture response to these agents. The results of the *in vitro* contracture test (IVCT), following the European MH Group (EMHG) protocol,[28] offers a 99% sensitivity and 93.6% specificity.[29] The IVCT is specifically designed to avoid dangerous false-negative diagnoses, but there is a consequent incidence of false-positive diagnoses. The responses of muscle bundles from MHS and normal individuals to halothane are shown in Fig. 22.2.

Diagnostic DNA testing for malignant hyperthermia

It can be appreciated from above that the use of DNA screening for MH will not be straightforward owing to the marked heterogeneity and the lack of identifiable functional mutations in many families (~75% in the UK). However, it is now recognized that DNA screening can be appropriate in a limited way, following the strict guidelines described by the European Malignant Hyperthermia Group.[30] These entail a careful analysis of both the IVCT and DNA results for a family. Only when the original proband (or the most appropriate relative when the proband has died) has proved to be susceptible to MH by muscle biopsy and also has a functional mutation can DNA analysis be offered to other family members as a screening test.

All patients who are suspected of developing an MH response should be referred to a recognized MH center to confirm (or refute) the clinical diagnosis and allow the follow-up of family members and also to offer support and advice to MH patients, their families, and medical attendants. Children (< 10–12 years old) are not offered IVCT screening as there are concerns that the contracture tests may yield negative results in young children. Such a diagnosis may have fatal consequences. Additionally, the amount of muscle tissue required might cause a functional deficit as well as being cosmetically unacceptable. In the case of young probands, the clinical MH diagnosis is confirmed indirectly by investigating the parents.

Anesthesia for the patient susceptible to malignant hyperthermia

The key to safe anesthesia for MHS individuals is to avoid the use of triggering drugs. Essentially, this now includes succinylcholine and *all* the anesthetic vapors. All local anesthetics are safe to use, as is ephedrine to control blood pressure during spinal/epidural anesthesia. Patients should not be denied surgery on the grounds of MH alone, but clearly MHS patients will be exposed to greater risk, especially when airway control is anticipated to be difficult, because either an inhalational technique or a rapid-sequence induction cannot be used, or in the prevention of awareness. Table 22.2 lists triggering drugs and those drugs known to be safe to use in MH; also listed are drugs that are thought to be safe but which should be used with caution. This last group mainly consist of drugs that have been implicated in early case reports as MH triggers. There must be doubts as to whether many of these cases were MH reactions. Furthermore, these drugs are in general use and therefore it could be expected that if they were MH triggers many "awake" MH reactions would have been reported following their use. Appropriate techniques are local anesthesia and intravenous general anesthesia. The routine use of total intravenous anesthesia (TIVA) over recent years has made anesthetizing MHS patients more straightforward. Many hospitals have dedicated "vapor-free" anesthetic machines for use with MHS patients. If such a machine is not available, both the machine and the ventilator can be prepared for use by removing the vaporizers and running maximum flows of oxygen through for at least 30 min. As volatile drugs are adsorbed on to plastics and rubber, new circuits and face masks should be used. If triggering drugs are meticulously avoided, the use of prophylactic dantrolene is neither required nor recommended. Although hepatitis, pleural effusion, pericarditis, and convulsions are associated only with chronic use of dantrolene, its short-term use does provoke nausea and vomiting and muscle weakness in a high proportion of recipients, thereby causing marked prolongation of the effects of muscle relaxants, as well as unpleasant central nervous system (CNS) effects. These include euphoria and disorientation. The relatively weak effects of dantrolene on cardiac and diaphragmatic muscle may also become significant for patients with pre-existing cardiac or respiratory disease.

OTHER INHERITED MUSCLE DISEASES

Anesthesia for patients with neuromuscular disease

Most anesthetic agents act directly or indirectly on muscle and nerve, so it is important to understand some general principles for anesthetizing any patient with a neuromuscular disease (NMD) as well as to have knowledge of the specific disorder in order to avoid any potential pitfalls. Occasionally the NMD only comes to light as a consequence of an unexpected abnormal reaction to anesthesia, another reason for the anesthesiologist to have an awareness of NMDs. Although individually rare, collectively NMDs are common, causing much morbidity and mortality. Patients may require surgery either because of their disease, e.g. correction of deformities, or because of a concurrent problem. Frequently patients have no specific diagnosis. The severity of the disease may vary, some patients posing little problem for anesthesia whereas others pose a severe risk. Many NMDs are progressive.

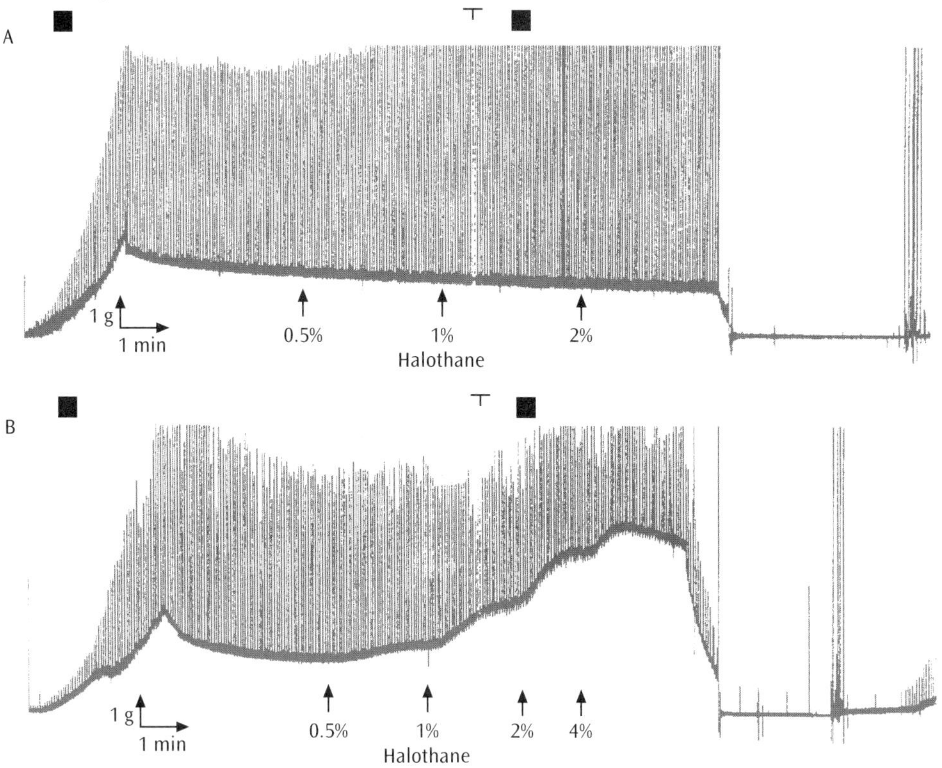

Figure 22.2 In vitro *responses to halothane of skeletal muscle bundles from (A) a normal individual and (B) a patient susceptible to malignant hyperthermia (MH). Freshly excised samples of vastus medialis muscle are mounted in a muscle bath and a baseline tension of 2g is applied. After a short stabilization period, incremental concentrations of halothane are vaporized into the gas mixture aerating the muscle bath. There is a dose-dependent increase in baseline tension (a contracture) in the specimen from the MH patient in response to halothane. This is not observed in normal muscle.*

There are several potential problems to consider: skeletal deformities, respiratory function, cardiomyopathy, myotonia, myoglobinuria, hyperkalemia, temperature regulation, and swallowing.

Skeletal deformities

These can cause technical difficulties, particularly when securing the airway, which may already be compromised. Decreased activity often makes adequate assessment of cardiorespiratory function impossible.

Respiratory function

Poor respiratory function is common and is due to weakness of the respiratory muscles, not of the lungs themselves, and leads to signs similar to those identified in restrictive lung disease. However, because of weakness of the oropharnyx, aspiration is common and frequent bouts of pneumonia, with consequent permanent lung damage, can occur. In some cases respiratory depression is of central origin because of increased somnolence, and these patients are particularly sensitive to respiratory depressant agents. It can be difficult to balance adequate pain relief with good respiratory function. Restoration of normal respiratory function is of prime concern and, although weaning from the ventilator can be difficult, there is no point in struggling to avoid postoperative controlled ventilation or even the use of a tracheostomy if the need for controlled ventilation becomes prolonged.

Cardiac problems

Cardiac problems in patients with NMD were recognized as far back as 1911. Conduction defects in muscular dystrophy are common, as

Table 22.2 *Classification of drugs according to their potential for triggering malignant hyperthermia*

Triggering drugs	Drugs that are probably safe	Safe drugs
Halothane	Phenothiazines	Benzodiazepines
Enflurane	Haloperidol	Thiopental
Isoflurane	Tricyclic antidepressants	Propofol
Desflurane	Monoamine oxidase inhibitors	Ketamine
Sevoflurane	Cyclopropane	Metoclopramide
Ether		Droperidol
Chloroform		Opioids
Succinylcholine		Nondepolarizing neuromuscular blocking drugs
		Atropine
		Neostigmine
		Nitrous oxide
		All local anesthetics

are increased P–R intervals, leading to heart block unresponsive to atropine. These may require pacing. Inhalational agents can predispose to arrhythmias, especially if CO_2 levels are raised due to inadequate respiration, although this is less likely to occur with the newer agents. There may be a cardiomyopathy with associated heart failure. The inhalational agents can have a significant adverse effect on cardiac contractility; there are several reports in the literature of cardiac arrest/failure due to halothane anesthesia. The newer agents are far better in this regard.

Hyperkalemia

Serum K^+ is often raised in muscle diseases, due to leakage through the damaged muscle membrane, and can cause cardiac arrhythmias, especially in an already abnormal heart. It is particularly important in the periodic paralyses. Careful monitoring and attention to fluid/blood replacement is important. In situations in which the serum K^+ is already high or leakage from damaged muscles is expected to be greater than normal, dangerous levels of hyperkalemia can be reached following the administration of succinylcholine.

Myotonia and myoglobinuria

Myotonia was first noticed in relation to anesthesia in 1915. It is solely a muscle problem and not affected by nondepolarizing or local anesthetic agents, in terms of either improving or worsening the myotonia. It can be attenuated by volatile agents, but this needs to be balanced against any cardiac complications. Myotonia was formerly thought to be solely a direct consequence of drug administration, but it can be precipitated by a variety of triggers such as surgical manipulation or the effect of cold. Succinylcholine will nearly always induce myotonia, most noticeably in the masseter muscles, causing difficulty with intubation. Myoglobinuria can be severe enough to induce renal failure. A high CK level (after 24 h) with severe and prolonged muscle stiffness can occur if muscle damage is severe enough for leakage to occur. Renal failure due to rhabdomyolysis may present 2–3 days after an anesthetic without apparent complications. Recovery is usually complete after hemodialysis. Myotonia congenita is often a mild condition, only coming to light after an abnormal response to succinylcholine and not always on the first exposure.

Other factors

Preoperative starvation is important especially in patients with some of the glycogen storage diseases as these patients are prone to hypoglycemia. Dehydration needs careful assessment and monitoring as it can prolong recovery. Inappropriate fluid or blood replacement can cause cardiac failure and hyperkalemia. Cooling and shivering may exaggerate muscle weakness and recovery from muscle relaxants and can precipitate myotonia. Finally, adequate pain relief may incur marked respiratory depression.

Preoperative assessment

This is clearly very important and needs the cooperation of many specialties if the patient is to be in optimal condition prior to surgery. Careful assessment of both cardiac and respiratory function is needed and CK and K^+ levels should be checked. The anesthetic regime needs careful consideration. Meticulous attention to detail is needed as the margins for error are very much reduced. Monitoring should continue well into the postoperative period and admission to a high dependency or intensive care unit may well be anticipated.

The X-linked muscular dystrophies

These are commonly known as the dystrophinopathies and include the two main types: Duchenne muscular dystrophy (DMD) and the milder Becker muscular dystrophy (BMD). Other examples include myotubular myopathy and Emery–Dreifuss muscular dystrophy. These diseases are caused by an absence of the structural protein dystrophin caused by various molecular defects in the gene *Xp21.2*. About 30% of cases are due to a new mutation rather than to inheritance.

Duchenne muscular dystrophy

DMD is the commonest of the muscular dystrophies, with an incidence of up to 35 per 10 000 live male births. The disease is characterized by rapidly progressive generalized muscle weakness with pseudohypertrophy of the calf muscles and occasionally of other muscle groups. Symptoms usually become apparent in the third year of life, progressing until around the age of 10, when the child requires a wheelchair. A wheelchair existence is often associated with kyphoscoliosis, fixed joint contractures, obesity, and impaired circulation to the legs and feet with dependent edema, along with psychological problems. The second decade of these boys' lives is punctuated by frequent chest infections due to impaired ventilatory effort. Death, due to pneumonia or cardiac disease, is usual by the age of 20. Symptoms of heart failure are deceivingly uncommon because of the enforced sedentary existence, but myocardial dysfunction is common, as is evident from echocardiographic studies.[31]

Anesthesia is rarely required in DMD patients for diagnostic muscle biopsy nowadays as a diagnosis can now be obtained by DNA analysis. Orthopedic procedures, for the release of fixed joint contractures to improve the duration of mobility, are becoming more common. Anesthetic problems are related to myocardial involvement, respiratory function, and the effects of drugs on the diseased skeletal muscles. Sethna *et al.*[32] reported their 5-year experience of anesthesia for 25 DMD patients, four of whom had complications, which, as it happens, typify most adverse events in other reports. In the first case, induction was followed within 10 min by cardiac arrest associated with acute hyperkalemia (8.9 mmol L^{-1}). The anesthetic in this case involved only halothane with nitrous oxide and oxygen. Even more dramatic hyperkalemic cardiac arrests have occurred when gaseous induction with halothane has been followed by administration of succinylcholine.[33] The second case[33] illustrates the need for awareness of cardiac involvement even in asymptomatic individuals. In this patient the echocardiogram was unremarkable but the boy died of cardiac failure during a prolonged procedure. The postmortem revealed biventricular dilation and hypertrophy with numerous fibrotic bands. An increased incidence of arrhythmias is another potential problem that can be exacerbated by hypercarbia secondary to depressant drugs at any stage during the perioperative period.[34] The last two cases of interest in their report both concern a rise in body temperature and a tachycardia that resolved when halothane was withdrawn. Tachycardia and hyperthermia are signs found during an MH reaction. These and other signs found in MH, such as hyperkalemia, acidosis, myoglobinuria, and raised creatine kinase (CK) levels, have been reported in DMD patients anesthetized with halothane and/or succinylcholine.[33] These authors incorrectly concluded, as did Sethna *et al.*, that their patients suffered MH. The possible responses of skeletal muscle to disease are limited in their expression, and the response of DMD muscle to halothane and succinylcholine in its similarity to MH is an example of this. The use of succinylcholine has also been implicated as the common factor in six DMD patients who required postoperative ventilation because of ventilatory insufficiency.[35]

The following approach to anesthetizing the patient with DMD seems appropriate:

- Use local/regional techniques when possible and acceptable to the patient (spinal anesthetic techniques that can cause sudden changes in afterload may not be appropriate for the patient with significant cardiac involvement).
- Avoid heavily depressant premedicants.
- Avoid succinylcholine.
- Consider carefully the choice of maintenance general anesthesia drugs for individual patients. Despite the reports of hypermetabolic reactions to volatile drugs, there is great experience in the safe use of inhalational agents in DMD patients: such reactions, if detected early in their course with the aid of appropriate monitoring, appear to be readily reversed by discontinuing the volatile drug. Of greater concern is the possibility of sudden massive rhabdomyolysis. These disadvantages of volatile drugs must be weighed against the detrimental cardiovascular effects of intravenous agents in patients with a cardiomyopathy.

Becker muscular dystrophy

BMD, in its clinical characteristics, closely resembles DMD but with a later onset (a mean of 11 years of age) and slower progression. Within a BMD family the clinical course of affected individuals is similar, but there is a wide spectrum of symptom onset and rate of disease progression between different BMD families.

There have been no recent reports of anesthetic problems in BMD. This probably reflects its rarity compared with DMD, the rarity of significant cardiac involvement despite ECG changes, and the milder nature of the skeletal muscle abnormality. However, the nature of this disease is so similar to that of DMD that there is potential for abnormal responses to succinylcholine, halothane, and related drugs. Indeed, muscle from a BMD patient has been shown to have an abnormal *in vitro* response to halothane.[36]

Other muscular dystrophies

These are generally less severe than the X-linked dystrophies discussed above and are given descriptive titles indicating the distribution of the muscle weakness and wasting, although other muscle groups may be involved as the disease progresses. Diseases with special anesthetic implications are listed below.

Humeroperoneal (Emery–Dreifuss) dystrophy

Early contractures involve the posterior cervical muscles. A consistent feature is atrioventricular block, which leads to recurrent episodes of syncope and embolic phenomena.

Oculopharyngeal dystrophy

Bulbar muscle involvement leads to a high risk of pulmonary aspiration.

Autosomal recessive diseases

Theses are usually severe with early onset and mortality. Examples include the distal hereditary motor neuropathies: spinal muscular atrophy, congenital muscular dystrophy, limb girdle dystrophy, and severe childhood muscular dystrophy. Charcot–Marie–Tooth disease is a heterogeneous condition occurring in childhood.

Autosomal dominant conditions

Facioscapulohumeral dystrophy

There is facial weakness but with sparing of bulbar muscles. Dresner and Ali[37] describe a patient who was successfully anesthetized using alfentanil, nitrous oxide, and atracurium. They observed a normal sensitivity to atracurium with a more rapid than usual recovery from neuromuscular blockade. This is difficult to attribute to the muscle pathology but perhaps reflects the contribution to neuromuscular blockade usually provided by a volatile anesthetic agent.

Other conditions in this group are the myotonic disorders, malignant hyperthermia, central core disease, and the periodic paralyses.

Myotonic disorders

There are two types of myotonic disorder, the dystrophic myotonias or multisystem diseases, such as myotonic dystrophy (dystrophia myotonica), and the nondystrophic myotonias, which are either Cl^- or Na^+ ion "channelopathies." Muscle biopsy is unhelpful in the myotonic disorders and should be avoided. The most important diagnosis is myotonic dystrophy, which requires genetic counseling.

Myotonic dystrophy (dystrophia myotonica)

This is a multisystem disease affecting the eyes (cataracts), hair (frontal baldness), bones (skull thickening), endocrine and metabolic function (hypogonadism, impaired glucose tolerance), immune system, and intelligence, as well as skeletal, cardiac, and smooth muscle. The skeletal muscle involvement is predominantly of the facial, oropharyngeal, and distal limb muscles. Muscle weakness is invariably the major symptom; myotonia is relatively mild in the early stages of the disease and becomes even less apparent as the dystrophic process progresses.

Aspiration pneumonia is a great hazard as the bulbar muscle weakness is compounded by esophageal dilation caused by smooth muscle involvement and by prolonged somnolence following the use of thiopental.[38,39] In one of these reports, etomidate was used in combination with thiopental.[39] This same patient had previously been anesthetized with propofol, which had resulted in prompt postoperative awakening. A normal recovery has also been reported following a 4-h infusion of propofol.[40] Postoperative respiratory problems may also be caused by respiratory muscle weakness.

Because of the muscle weakness, neuromuscular blocking drugs must be used with care. Vecuronium and atracurium have both been successfully used when the dose has been carefully titrated against response:[40,41] the doses used were about half the dose one would predict for a normal patient. Succinylcholine and other drugs that stimulate muscle (e.g. neostigmine) should be avoided in all myotonic disorders. Heart muscle involvement leads to dysrhythmias and/or conduction defects in about 60% of cases, and is progressive.

Local and regional anesthetic techniques overcome many of the problems of general anesthesia in myotonic dystrophy, with the notable exception of myotonia. Such a technique has been used for anesthesia for cesarean section.[42]

Safe anesthesia can usually be achieved for patients with myotonic dystrophy, but relies on the diagnosis having been made preoperatively. This is not always the case, as the number of typical features varies considerably, even between members of the same family, because of differences in gene expressivity. Therefore, to avoid unforeseen problems, the anesthesiologist should remember the features of this disease and, if any are present, a detailed family history should be taken.

Myotonic conditions due to ion "channelopathies"[43]

These conditions all result from autosomal inheritance.

Cl^- channel disorders

Myotonia congenita (Thomsen's disease) This rare condition causes weak but hypertrophied muscles with myotonia as a prominent symptom. The myotonia, described as muscle cramps or stiffness, is exacerbated by cold and inactivity. Muscle hypertrophy occurring within a limited fascial compartment may cause ischemic damage and intermittent claudication. Mild weakness may occur in the rarer autosomal recessive variety (Becker) but is usually confined to the limbs.

Na^+ channel disorders

There are three of these.

Paramytonia congenita Generalized myotonia is classically precipitated by cold and vigorous exercise. A flaccid paresis, most prominent in the feet and cranial musculature, may follow the myotonia and may persist for several hours, even after rapid rewarming.

Potassium-aggravated myotonia This is an allelic disorder characterized by severe permanent myotonia or fluctuating stiffness most prominent 20 min after exercise.

Streib[44] has reported two very interesting cases from the same paramyotonia family with known hyperkalemic-induced weakness, both of whom developed hypokalemic paralysis following general anesthesia, which required postoperative mechanical ventilation and large doses of potassium chloride by intravenous infusion. Unfortunately, knowledge of the details of the anesthetic agents used in each case is limited but our inference is that succinylcholine and a volatile agent were used in both.

Hyperkalemic periodic paralysis There are three types of the periodic paralyses but with differing etiology, the hyperkalemic type being caused by a Na^+ "channelopathy." The predominant symptom is episodic weakness, often after wakening, and which can become more progressive with age. Respiratory and cardiac muscles are usually unaffected. The paralysis is precipitated by changes in serum K^+, which can be induced by drugs, e.g. diuretics or insulin, or by fasting. Abnormal K^+ levels are found only during an attack and can cause T-wave changes on the ECG.

Anesthetic considerations include the administration of intravenous glucose (with no potassium!) during fasting, general measures for myotonic disorders (avoidance of succinylcholine, neostigmine, and cold; careful handling of muscles) and monitoring of the serum potassium concentration. Aarons *et al.*[45] have reported the successful use of vecuronium as part of a balanced anesthetic technique with fentanyl and isoflurane for a patient with hyperkalemic periodic paralysis. An attack can be treated with intravenous glucose and insulin.

Ca^{2+} channel disorders

Hypokalemic periodic paralysis This condition is caused by a defect in the α-subunit of the dihydropyridine receptor: the voltage sensor for E–C coupling in skeletal muscle. Attacks of flaccid paralysis of varying frequency, severity, and duration occur and are associated with a fall in the serum potassium concentration. A severe attack may render the patient quadriplegic but able to speak, swallow, and move the eyes, with minimal effect on respiratory function. The occurrence of most attacks is unpredictable, but they are commonly precipitated by heavy exercise, excessive carbohydrate intake, stress, trauma, and cold. The last three factors are obviously associated with anesthesia and surgery, and cannot always be avoided. Perioperatively, an acute episode may be prevented by maintaining normokalemia with the use of an infusion of potassium chloride and by monitoring the serum potassium level.

It should be noted that hypokalemic periodic paralysis can be an acquired condition, although this is a rare occurrence. It can occur in association with thyrotoxicosis, or secondary to renal or gastrointestinal potassium wasting.

Normokalemic periodic paralysis Episodic attacks, varying from mild extensor weakness to quadriplegic flaccid paralysis, lasting from minutes to days occur every few months. They occur usually during a period of rest following exertion but may also be precipitated by anxiety, ingestion of alcohol, and excessive sleep. General anesthesia must therefore be considered to be a potential precipitating factor. Attacks are not related to changes in the serum potassium concentration and myotonia is not a feature. Treatment is with intravenous sodium chloride.

Central core disease (CCD) CCD was first described by Shy and Magee[46] and is characterized by proximal weakness, which is usually nonprogressive. Sometimes it is associated with severe musculoskeletal deformities such as scoliosis and cardiomyopathy. Occasionally, it does not become clinically apparent until late adult life, and some patients who are known to have the morphological abnormality never develop symptoms. Diagnosis is by muscle biopsy revealing the characteristic central cores.

There is a strong association between CCD and malignant hyperthermia,[24] CCD being assigned to chromosome 19 in 1990.[47] Patients with CCD should be treated as potentially MHS, unless proved otherwise, and offered MH screening.[48,49] Mutations in the *RYR1* gene have been identified in some CCD patients,[50] although this is a very variable finding; for example at the time of writing no published mutations have been identified in any of the UK CCD families. Therefore, DNA screening is unsuitable for diagnosis of CCD at present.

Morphologically distinct myopathies

Rod (nemaline) myopathy

Rod myopathy exists as a familial congenital nonprogressive proximal weakness starting with a scapuloperoneal distribution. The more common congenital form is associated with secondary bony deformities such as pes cavus, kyphoscoliosis, and a high arched palate.

Specific anesthetic problems are related to the restrictive respiratory defect associated with scoliosis and the effects of drugs on postoperative muscle function. Cunliffe and Burrows[51] found the use of neuromuscular blocking agents unnecessary for establishing controlled ventilation, while Heard and Kaplan[52] used succinylcholine followed by pancuronium in their patient without untoward effect.

Type 1 fiber hypertrophy with central nuclei

This also known as centronuclear or myotubular myopathy. It covers a wide range of clinical presentations, from a fatal congenital form to a slowly progressive late-onset form. The predominant clinical feature is weakness.

Metabolic muscle diseases

The glycogenoses

The glyogenoses are a group of disorders characterized by defective glycogen and/or glucose metabolism. They can be classified as in Table 22.3.

Of the five glycogenoses that involve skeletal muscle, muscle symptoms predominate in three (types II, V, and VII), whereas in the other two (types III and IV) the dominant features are liver dysfunction and hypoglycemia.

McArdle's disease (type IV)

Myophosphorylase deficiency leads to an inability to utilize skeletal muscle glycogen stores. The muscle then becomes dependent on the entry of substrates such as glucose and fatty acids. Under conditions of increased energy requirement (exercise) or decreased substrate supply (fasting, ischemia) the muscle is liable to break down, releasing myoglobin, which can precipitate renal failure.

Table 22.3 *Classification of the glycogenoses*

Type	Name	Deficient enzyme	Skeletal muscle involvement	Liver involvement
I	von Gierke's disease	Glucose-6-phosphatase	No	Yes
II	Pompe's disease	Acid maltase	Yes	Yes
III	Forbes's disease, Cori's disease	Amylo-1,6-glucosidase (debranching enzyme)	Yes	Yes
IV	Andersen's disease	Amylo-1,4-1,6-transglucosidase (branching enzyme)	Yes	Yes
V	McArdle's disease	Myophosphorylase	Yes	No
VI	Hers's disease	Liver phosphorylase	No	Yes
VII	Tarui's disease	Phosphofructokinase	Yes	No

Perioperatively, an intravenous infusion of glucose should be maintained throughout, and the use of tourniquets avoided. If myoglobinuria occurs, a diuresis must be established.

Phosphofructokinase deficiency (type VII)

This presents a clinical picture similar to McArdle's disease. The principles of anesthetic management are also the same, with the exception that a fatty acid solution is required instead of the glucose in the Embden–Meyerhof pathway.

Acid maltase deficiency (type II)

The infantile variety (Pompe's disease) is associated with massive accumulation of glycogen in all tissues, death from cardiac failure usually occurring within the first year of life. The adult-onset form is restricted to skeletal muscle and eventually, in most cases, involves the respiratory muscles.

Disorders of muscle lipid metabolism

The energy for prolonged muscular effort is derived mainly from the oxidation of fatty acids in the mitochondria. The transport of long-chain fatty acids into the mitochondria depends on a carrier, carnitine, which is synthesized in the liver and actively taken up by muscle cells, and an enzyme, carnitine palmityl transferase 1.

Carnitine deficiency

Systemic

This is due to defective hepatic synthesis. Slowly progressing hepatorenal failure precedes a myopathy that produces a variable degree of weakness. Fasting may produce a fatal acidosis and therefore should be accompanied by an infusion of glucose.

Muscle

This type is due to a defective muscle uptake. It usually presents in childhood with proximal muscle weakness. A fatal cardiomyopathy may occur.

Carnitine palmityl transferase deficiency

Muscle cramping, pain, necrosis and myoglobinuria are associated with prolonged exercise. Anesthetic management includes constant provision of usable substrate (intravenous glucose).

Mitochondrial myopathies

Mitochondrial DNA is inherited from the mother. This is a group of rare, clinically heterogeneous conditions associated with many large and abnormal mitochondria in the skeletal muscle cells. In some patients a deficiency of one or more of the mitochondrial respiratory chain components has been demonstrated. Myopathic symptoms are usually weakness and excessive fatigue; other abnormalities may include central and peripheral nervous system problems, and cardiac conduction defects (these may be severe enough to warrant permanent cardiac pacing). Experimental mitochondrial myopathies have been produced by giving animals 2,4-dinitrophenol (2,4-DNP), which uncouples mitochondrial oxidative phosphorylation. 2,4-DNP has also been proposed as a tool for producing an animal model of malignant hyperthermia, as when it is administered with halothane animals become pyrexial, stiff, and then die. This implies that patients with defects of mitochondrial oxidative phosphorylation might exhibit a potentially dangerous response to the volatile anesthetic agents.

Inherited disorders of metabolism

The porphyrias

The porphyrias are a group of diseases that result from defects in the synthesis of heme. They are characterized by overproduction and excretion of heme precursors, including porphyrins, which are oxidized by ultraviolet light to form the purple-colored uroporphyrin and coproporphyrin. These can be detected easily in urine and feces. The rate-limiting step in the synthesis of heme is the formation of δ-aminolevulic acid (ALA) from succinyl-CoA and glycine – a reaction catalyzed by ALA synthetase (Fig. 22.3).

The significance of the porphyrias to anesthesiologists is that some of the hepatic porphyrias, acute intermittent and hereditary coproporphyria, are exacerbated by certain lipophilic drugs. Acute exacerbations produce acute neurologic disturbances involving central and peripheral sensory and motor nerves and the autonomic nervous system. The symptoms are dramatic and are as follows:

- *Central.* Agitation is a common early sign, but succeeding symptoms can mimic any psychotic illness.
- *Peripheral.* A progressive peripheral neuropathy may develop rapidly. Muscle weakness may be severe enough to necessitate artificial ventilation.
- *Autonomic.* Abdominal pain, vomiting, constipation, tachycardia, hypertension, postural hypotension, and urinary incontinence or retention may feature. The abdominal pain can mimic almost any acute surgical intra-abdominal emergency, and such a patient may therefore be presented to the anesthesiologist for laparotomy. Biochemical changes can result from vomiting and polyuria.

The key to uneventful anesthesia for porphyric patients is the avoidance of precipitating factors. It is important to remember those perioperative factors, other than drugs, that are imposed routinely, such as fasting. Infection is also a strong stimulus to increased porphyrin excretion; this may be a response to increased glucocorticoids or other

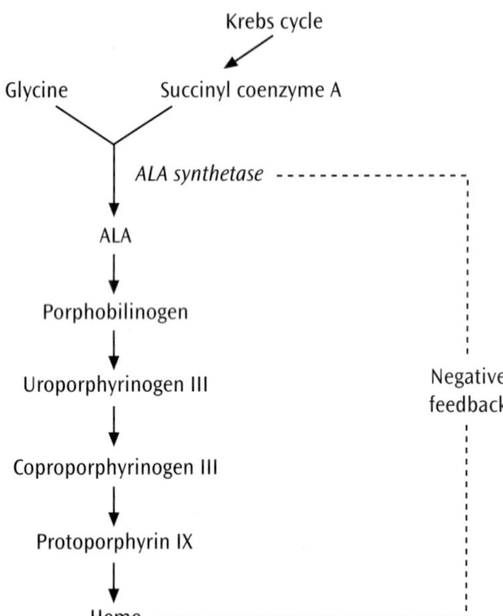

Figure 22.3 *The synthesis of heme.*

mediators of the "stress response." It would therefore seem logical to attempt to suppress the stress response associated with major surgery.

It is the lack of significant stress response with most elective surgical procedures that is perhaps the reason why drugs that are known to increase the activity of hepatic ALA synthetase, such as etomidate, have been used safely in porphyric patients undergoing such elective surgery.[53] The absence of an acute reaction in these circumstances means that safe use of potentially porphyrinogenic drugs may be reported. The duration of exposure may be important also. The reported safe use of propofol for induction may be an example of this,[54,55] as others have demonstrated increased excretion of porphyrins with its use by continuous infusion.[56,57] As barbiturates are strongly porhyrinogenic, the choice of intravenous induction agent is limited. In their recent review, James and Hift[58] recommend propofol as the induction agent of choice. In fact, there are many therapeutic groups of drugs, of which one or more members have been implicated (Table 22.4). Anesthesia can be safely given with halothane, nitrous oxide, opioids, and neuromuscular blocking drugs. Local anesthesia should be with bupivacaine or prilocaine, although lidocaine (lignocaine) is probably also safe.

The mucopolysaccharidoses

These are a group of disorders resulting from defects in the breakdown of proteomucopolysaccharides, which are structural components of cells in many tissues. All the disorders are inherited as autosomal recessive traits, other than Hunter syndrome, which is an X-linked recessive trait. The pathological findings are due to deposition of proteomucopolysaccharides in the tissues involved. They have in common a progressive course, skeletal and joint involvement, and coarse facial features. Other tissues involved in some are the brain (causing mental retardation), the heart and blood vessels, the liver, the spleen, and the cornea.

Anesthesia requires careful planning. Difficulties with airway control should be anticipated because of the large head, short neck, abnormal mandible, large tongue, hyperplastic lymphoid tissue, inelastic tissues, and abnormal laryngeal and tracheal cartilages. In addition, the cervical spine may be unstable in the Morquio and Maroteaux–Lamy syndromes. To add to these structural factors is an excessive production of viscid respiratory tract secretions. Other problems relate to potential failure of other organs involved in the disease.

The glycogenoses

These have been classified earlier in the section on muscle diseases (see Table 22.3). Types I, II, III, IV, and VI are characterized by liver failure and hypoglycemia because of affected individuals' inability to utilize glycogen. Type I (von Gierke's) patients also have a tendency to develop acidemia.

The anesthetic implications are those of liver failure, avoidance of excessive starvation, and administration of sufficient exogenous glucose to prevent hypoglycemia.

Hereditary fructose intolerance

Symptoms result acutely from hypoglycemia caused by the administration of fructose. Longer-term problems result from deposition of fructose 1-phosphate in the liver, kidneys, and intestinal mucosa. It is the failure of these organs that presents the only problem to the patient in whom the diagnosis has been made. Acute symptoms are completely controlled by diet.

Fructose-1,6-diphosphatase deficiency

Fructose-1,6-diphosphatase is essential for gluconeogenesis. Any stimulus to gluconeogenesis, such as starvation or surgery, will therefore result in hypoglycemia and lactic acidosis. Perioperatively, acid–base status and blood sugar should be monitored carefully and exogenous glucose supplied intravenously. Observing a fructose-free diet for 48 h prior to surgery also seems to limit the occurrence of hypoglycemia.

Disorders of amino acid metabolism

The most common is cystinuria, which is an epithelial amino acid transport defect leading eventually to chronic renal failure. While some renal function remains, it is important to maintain a high urine flow to prevent the formation of stones.

Perioperative problems common to disorders of amino acid degradation, such as homocystinuria, maple syrup urine disease, and phenylketonuria, include avoidance of an excessive breakdown of endogenous protein, which may accelerate progression of the disease. The increased levels of amino acids so produced may also cause hypoglycemia through several possible mechanisms. Periods of starvation should therefore be kept to a minimum, intravenous dextrose should be given, and measures to limit the catabolic response to surgery may be beneficial.

Homocystinuria is also associated with an increased tendency to form intravascular thromboses due to a platelet abnormality. Aspirin may be beneficial prophylactically. Circulatory stagnation should be prevented in both arterial and venous systems, and a degree of hemodilution is warranted. Low-dose subcutaneous heparin is advisable.

Familial dysautonomia

Otherwise known as Riley–Day syndrome, familial dysautonomia is an autosomal recessive condition with its highest incidence in ethnic Jews. It is a rare condition but one that presents major anesthetic problems. The disorder is thought to be due to a deficiency in dopamine-β-hydroxylase, which is responsible for the conversion of dopamine to norepinephrine (noradrenaline) in sympathetic (and probably central) nerve endings. This would explain why these patients display a "denervation hypersensitivity" to circulating catecholamines and only a limited sympathetic nervous system response to hypotensive stimuli such as inhalational anesthetic drugs.

The other features of the disease with implications for the anesthesiologist are not necessarily predictable from the term "dysautonomia." Respiratory secretions are excessive and thick, leading to recurrent chest infections. Respiratory drive is also abnormal and is reflected in reduced hypoxemic and hypercapnic responses, especially following opioid

Table 22.4 *Recommendations for the use of anesthetic drugs in the acute porphyrias*

Drugs	Recommendation
Inhalational agents	
Nitrous oxide, cyclopropane, halothane	Use
Enflurane, isoflurane, sevoflurane[a], desflurane[a]	UWC
Intravenous induction agents	
Propofol	Use
Ketamine	UWC
Barbiturates, etomidate	Avoid
Analgesics	
Acetaminophen (paracetamol), alfentanil, aspirin, buprenorphine, codeine, fentanyl, pethidine, morphine, naloxone, sufentanil	Use
Diclofenac, ketorolac,[a] phenacetin, tilidine	UWECO
Pentazocine	Avoid
Neuromuscular blocking drugs	
Tubocurarine, pancuronium, suxamethonium	Use
Alcuronium, atracurium, rocuronium,[a] mivacurium,[a] vecuronium	UWC
Neuromuscular block-reversing agents	
Atropine, glycopyrrolate, neostigmine	Use
Local anesthetic agents	
Bupivicaine, lidocaine, prilocaine, procaine, tetracaine	Use
Cocaine, mepivacaine	UWC
Ropivacaine	ND/avoid
Sedatives and antiemetics	
Droperidol, phenothiazines, temazepam, triazolam	Use
Benzodiazepines (other than listed), cimetidine, diazepam, lorazepam, metoclopramide, midazolam, ondansetron, oxazepam, ranitidine	UWC
Chlordiazepoxide, nitrazepam	UWECO
Cardiovascular drugs	
Epinephrine, magnesium, phentolamine, procainamide, α-agonists, β-blockers, β-agonists	Use
Diltiazem, disopyramide, sodium nitroprusside, verapamil	UWC
Hydralazine, nifedipine, phenoxybenzamine	UWECO

Adapted from James and Hift.[58] UWC, use with caution; UWECO, use with extreme caution only; ND, no data.
a. Based on comparisons with drugs in same class.

administration. The increased depressant effect of opioids may be exacerbated by the lower analgesic requirements of these patients, who are relatively insensitive to pain. Cyclical vomiting and fever are typical features of the disease and may be triggered by anesthesia and surgery.

Inherited abnormalities of plasma cholinesterase

Plasma cholinesterase (pseudocholinesterase) is an enzyme for which no physiologic role has been identified: those with no detectable enzyme activity have no disease or physiologic defect. However, reduced enzyme activity does occur in a number of conditions, e.g. pregnancy, hepatic failure, and uremia. Indeed, it was only following the introduction of succinylcholine, which depends on rapid destruction to succinic acid by plasma cholinesterase in a two-stage reaction for its short duration of action, that genetically inherited functional variants of the enzyme became apparent. This realization followed assessment of enzyme activity in the plasma of individuals (and their blood relatives) in whom succinylcholine had a prolonged action.

Characterization of allelic variants

The incidence of variants is 1 in 2500. Investigators have used percentage inhibition of enzyme activity by inhibitors to characterize variants rather than rely on plasma cholinesterase activity, which is a measure of the amount of enzyme present in a sample as well as the nature of the enzyme, cholinesterase. Kalow and Genest[59] first described such a method using the local anesthetic dibucaine (cinchocaine) and termed the percentage inhibition the dibucaine number (DN). They were thus able to identify patients homozygous for the usual allele (E_1^u,E_1^u) with a DN of ~80 (80% inhibition), patients homozygous for the atypical allele ($E_1^aE_1^a$) with a DN of ~20, and heterozygous patients with a DN of ~60. The atypical variant is the most common. Using analogous techniques with sodium fluoride, Harris and Whittaker[60] used the fluoride and dibucaine numbers to distinguish a fluoride-resistant allele, E_1^f. Family studies subsequently implicated a fourth allelic variant, which was termed the silent allele, E_1^s, because dibucaine and fluoride numbers in the heterozygous state were identical with those in the homozygote for the other allele.

There are families in whom the cholinesterase activities and inhibitor numbers cannot be explained by the alleles already described. Two of these have been called the "j" and "k" variants. If they are real entities, their occurrence is exceedingly rare.

More recently, pseudocholinesterase hyperactivity has been described.[61] This causes rapid inactivation of succinylcholine and apparent resistance to relaxation with resulting difficulties with intubation.

Table 22.5 *Noninherited causes of reduced plasma cholinesterase activity*

Physiological	Acquired	Iatrogenic
Peripartum women	Liver disease	Ecothiopate
Infants < 6 months of age	Collagen diseases	Chlorpromazine
	Cachexia	Pancuronium
	Chronic anemias	Procaine
	Uremia	Neostigmine
	Malnutrition	Oral contraceptives
	Hypothyroidism	Cancer chemotherapy
	Burns	Radiotherapy
		Organophosphorus insecticides

Succinylcholine apnea

This is the name of the condition exhibited by individuals who have a genetically determined reduction in plasma cholinesterase activity sufficient to produce a clinically apparent prolongation of the action of succinylcholine. Depending on the enzyme activity, the period of apnea may be anything from 10 min to 2 h. The condition is life-threatening only if not recognized. Treatment is artificial ventilation, with appropriate sedation until the return of spontaneous ventilation. Active enzyme is present in fresh-frozen plasma (unless the donor had abnormal cholinesterase activity), but spontaneous activity will often return before the plasma becomes available.

Investigation of succinylcholine apnea Noninherited causes of reduced cholinesterase activity should be excluded (Table 22.5) and plasma samples sent to a reference laboratory. If an inherited abnormality is confirmed, other family members should be similarly investigated.

Other drugs metabolized by plasma cholinesterase

Ester local anesthetics are now used infrequently, but repeated doses may cause unexpected toxicity in patients with low plasma cholinesterase levels.

Mivacurium, a relatively new nondepolarizing neuromuscular blocking drug, is metabolized primarily by plasma cholinesterase. Patients susceptible to succinylcholine apnea also have prolonged paralysis following administration of mivacurium.[62]

REFERENCES

1. Denborough MA, Lovell RRH. Anaesthetic deaths in a family. *Lancet* 1960; **2**: 15.
2. Ellis FR, Halsall PJ, Christian AS. Clinical presentation of suspected malignant hyperthermia during anaesthesia in 402 probands. *Anaesthesia* 1990; **45**: 838–41.
3. Ellis FR, Halsall PJ, Harriman DGF. The work of the Leeds Malignant Hyperthermia Investigation Unit 1971–84. *Anaesthesia* 1986; **46**: 806–15.
4. Lopez JR, Alamo L, Jones D, *et al.* Dantrolene reverses the syndrome of malignant hyperthermia by reducing the level of intracellular Ca^{2+}. *Biophys J* 1985; **47**: 313a.
5. Iaizzo PA, Klein W, Lehmann-Horn F. Fura-2 detected myoplasmic calcium and its correlation with contracture force in sleketal muscle from normal and malignant hyperthermia susceptible pigs. *Pflugers Arch* 1988; **411**: 648–53.
6. Stokes DL, Wagenknecht T. Calcium transport across the sarcoplasmic reticulum: structure and function of Ca^{2+}-ATPase and the ryanodine receptor. *Eur J Biochem* 2000; **267:** 5274–9.
7. Mickelson JR, Louis CF. Malignant hyperthermia: E-C coupling Ca^{2+} release channel and cell Ca^{2+} regulation defects. *Physiol Rev* 1996; **76** (2): 537–92.
8. Mickelson JR, Gallant EM, Litterer LA, *et al.* Abnormal sarcoplasmic reticulum ryanodine receptor in malignant hyperthermia. *J Biochem Chem* 1988; **263**: 9310–15.
9. Ervasti JM, Strand MA, Hanson TP, *et al.* Ryanodine receptor in different malignant hyperthermia susceptible porcine muscles. *Am J Physiol* 1991; **260**: C58–C66.
10. Fill M, Stefani E, Nelson ET. Abnormal sarcoplasmic reticulum Ca^{++} release channels in malignant hyperthermic skeletal muscle. *Biophys J* 1991; **59**: 1085–90.
11. MacLennan DH, Duff C, Zorato F, *et al.* Ryanodine receptor gene is a candidate for predisposition to malignant hyperthermia. *Nature* 1990; **343**: 559–601.
12. McCarthy TV, Healy JMS, Heffron JJA, *et al.* Localisation of the malignant hyperthermia susceptibility locus to human chromosome 19q12–13.2. *Nature* 1990; **343**: 562–4.
13. Hopkins PM, Ellis FR, Halsall PJ. Ryanodine contracture: a potentially specific *in vitro* diagnostic test for malignant hyperthermia. *Br J Anaesth* 1991; **66**: 611–13.
14. Harbitz I, Chowdray B, Thomsen PD, *et al.* Assignment of the Porcine Calcium Release Channel gene, a candidate for the malignant hyperthermia locus to the 6p11->q21 segment of chromosome 6. *Genomics* 1990; 8: 243–8.
15. Brandt A, Schleithoff L, Jurkat-Rott K, *et al.* Screening for the ryanodine receptor gene in 105 malignant hyperthermia families: novel mutations and concordance with the *in-vitro* contracture test. *Hum Mol Genet* 1999; 8: 2055–62.
16. Richter M. Schleithoff L, Deufel T, *et al.* Functional characterisation of a distinct ryanodine receptor mutation in human malignant hyperthermia-susceptible muscle. *J Biol Chem* 1997; **272**: 5256–60.
17. Tong J, Oyamada H, Demaurex N, *et al.* Caffeine and halothane sensitivity of intracellular Ca^{2+} relaese is altered by 15 calcium release channel (ryanodine receptor) mutations associated with malignant hyperthermia and/or central core disease. *J Biochem Chem* 1997; **272**: 26332–9.
18. Robinson RL, Curran JL, Ellis FR, *et al.* Multiple interacting gene products may influence susceptibility to malignant hyperthermia. *Ann Hum Genet* 2000; **64**: 307–320.
19. Deufel T, Golla A, Iles D, *et al.* Evidence for genetic heterogeneity of malignant hyperthermia susceptibility. *Am J Hum Genet* 1992; **50**: 1151–61.
20. Halsall PJ, Cain PA, Ellis FR. Retrospective analysis of anaesthetics received by patients before malignant hyperthermia was recognised. *Br J Anaesth* 1979; **51**: 949–54.
21. Van der Spek AFL, Fang WB, Ashton-Miller JA, *et al.* The effects of succinylcholine on mouth opening. *Anaesthesiology* 1987; **67**: 459–65.
22. Leary NP, Ellis FR. Masseteric spasm as a normal response to suxamethonium. *Br J Anaesth* 1990; **64**: 488–92.
23. Christian AS, Halsall PJ, Ellis FR. Is there a relationship between masseter muscle spasm and malignant hyperthermia? *Br J Anaesth* 1989; **65**: 540–4.
24. Halsall PJ, Ellis FR. Does post-operative pyrexia indicate malignant hyperthermia susceptibility? *Br J Anaesth* 1992; **68**: 209–10.
25. Cain PA, Ellis FR. Anaesthesia for patients susceptible to malignant hyperpyrexia: a study of pancuronium and methylprednisolone. *Br J Anaesth* 1977; **49**: 941–4.
26. Kalow K, Britt BA, Terreau ME, Haist C. Metabolic error of muscle metabolism after recovery from malignant hyperthermia. *Lancet* 1970; **2**: 895–8.
27. Ellis FR, Harriman DGF, Keaney NP, *et al.*. Halothane induced contracture as a cause of hyperpyrexia. *Br J Anaesth* 1971; **43**: 721–2.
28. European Malignant Hyperthermia Group. A protocol for the investigation of malignant hyperpyrexia (MH) susceptibility. *Br J Anaesth* 1984; **56**: 1267–9.
29. Ording H, for the European Malignant Hyperthermia Group. *In-vitro* contracture test for the diagnosis of malignant hyperthermia following the protocol of the European MH Group: results of testing patients surviving fulminant MH and unrelated low risk subjects. *Acta Anaesthesiol Scand* 1997; **41**: 955–66.
30. Urwyler A, Deufel T, McCarthy TV, West S, for the European Malignant

Hyperthermia Group. Guidelines for the molecular genetic testing of suceptibility to malignant hyperthermia. *Br J Anaesth* 2001; **86** (2): 283–7.

31. Goldberg S, Stern L, Feldman L. Serial two dimensional echocardiography in children with muscular dystrophy. *Neurology* 1982; **10**: 1101–5.
32. Sethna SF, Rockoff MA, Worthen HM, Rosnow JM. Anaesthesia-related complications in children with Duchenne muscular dystrophy. *Anaesthesiology* 1988; **68**: 462–5.
33. Wang JM, Stanley TH. Duchenne muscular dystrophy and malignant hyperthermia – two case reports. *Can Anaesth Soc J* 1986; **33:** 492–7.
34. Boba A. Fatal postanaesthetic complications in two muscular dystrophic patients. *J Paediatr Surg* 1970; **5**: 71–5.
35. Smith CL, Bush GH. Anaesthesia and progressive muscular dystrophy. *Br J Anaesth* 1985; **57**: 1113–8.
36. Heiman-Patterson TD, Natter HM, Rosenberg H, *et al.*. Malignant hyperthermia susceptibility in X-linked muscle dystrophies. *Paediatr Neuro* 1986; **2**: 356–8.
37. Dresner DL, Ali HH. Anaesthetic management of a patient with fascioscapulohumeral muscular dystrophy. *Br J Anaesth* 1989; **44**: 331–4.
38. Aldridge LM. Anaesthetic problems in myotonic dystrophy. *Br J Anaesth* 1985; **57**: 1119–30.
39. Pollard BJ, Young TM. *Anaesth* in myotonia dystrophica. *Anaesth* 1989; **44**: 699.
40. White DA, Smyth DG. Continuous infusion of propofol in dystrophica myotonica. *Can J Anaesthesiol* 1989; **36**: 200–3.
41. Wruck G, Tryba M. Vecuronium bei Dystrophia myotonica (Cursemann–Steinert). *Anaesthetist* 1989; **38**: 255–8.
42. Cope DK, Miller JN. Local and spinal anaesthesia for caesarian section in a patient with myotonic dystrophy. *Anaesth and Analg* 1986; **65**: 687–90.
43. Lehmann-Horn F, Rudel R. Molecular pathophysiology of voltage gated ion channels. *Rev Physiol Biochem Pharmacol* 1996; **128**: 195–268.
44. Streib EW. Hypokalaemic paralysis in two patients with paramyotonia congenita and known hyperkalaemic exercise-induced periodic paralysis. *Muscle Nerve* 1989; **12**: 936–7.
45. Aarons JJ, Moon RE, Camporesi MD. General anaesthesia and hyperkalaemic periodic paralysis. *Anaesthesiology* 1989; **71**: 303–4.
46. Shy GM, Magee KR. A new congenital non-progressive myopathy. *Brain* 1956; **79**: 610–9.
47. Haan EA, Freemantle, CH, McClure JA, Fiend KL, Mullery JC. Assignment of the gene for central core disease to human chromosome 19. *Hum Genet* 1990; **86**: 187–90.
48. Bridges LR, Halsall PJ, Hopkins PM, Ellis FR. Central Core Disease and malignant hyperthermia are not always associated. *J Neurol Neurosurg Psych* 1996; **61**: 119–21.
49. Curran JL, Hall WJ, Halsall PJ, *et al.* Segregation of malignant hyperthermia, central core disease and chromosome 19 markers. *Br J Anaesth* 1999; **83** (2): 217–22.
50. Quane KA, Healy JMS, Keating KE, *et al.* Mutations in the ryanodine receptor gene in central core disease and malignant hyperthermia. *Nature Genet* 1993; **5**: 51–5.
51. Cunliffe M, Burrows FA. Anaesthetic implications of nemaline rod myopathy. *Can Anaesth Soc J* 1985; **32**: 543–7.
52. Heard SO, Kaplan RF. Neuromuscular blockade in a patient with nemaline rod myopathy. *Anaesthesiology* 1983; **59**: 588–90.
53. Famewo CE. Induction of anaesthesia with etomidate in a patient with acute intermittent porphyria. *Can Anaesth Soc J* 1985; **32**: 171–3.
54. Meissner PN, Harrison GG, Hift RJ. Propofol as an i.v. anaesthetic induction agent in variegate porphyria. *Br J Anaesth* 1991; **66**: 60–5.
55. Mitterschiffthaler G, Theiner A, Hetzel H, Fuith LC. Safe use of propofol in a patient with acute intermittent porphyria. *Br J Anaesth* 1988; **60**: 109–11.
56. Kantor G, Rolbin SH. Acute intermittent porphyria and caesarian delivery. *Can J Anaesth* 1992; **39:** 282–5.
57. Weir PM Hodkinson BP. Is propofol a safe agent in porphyria? *Anaesthesia* 1988; **43**: 1022–3.
58. James MFM, Hift RJ. Porphyrias. *Br J Anaesth* 2000; **85**: 143–53.
59. Kalow W, Genest K. A method for the detection of atypical forms of human serum cholinesterase. Determination of dibucaine numbers. *Can J Biochem* 1957; **35**: 339.
60. Harris H, Whittaker M. Differential inhibition of human serum cholinesterase with fluoride: recognition of two new phenotypes. *Nature* 1961; **191**: 496.
61. Yao FS, Savarese JJ. Pseudocholinesterase hyperactivity with succinylcholine resistance: an unusual case of difficult intubation. *J Clin Anaesth* 1997; **9** (4): 328–30.
62. Ogunbigi OA, Branch KG. Mivacurium apnoea: a trap for the unwary. *Int J Clin Pract* 1999; **53** (2): 154–5.

23

The immune/inflammatory system

RENÉ ZELLWEGER, MARTIN G SCHWACHA, AND IRSHAD H CHAUDRY

INTRODUCTION

The primary function of the immune system is to protect the body from the deleterious effects of pathogenic organisms such as bacteria, viruses, fungi, and parasites and consequently from infection. This immune defensive activity is carried out primarily by leukocytes, which include lymphocytic cells (i.e. T and B cells and natural killer cells) and phagocytic cells (i.e. macrophages and neutrophils). Leukocytes are predominately found in the lymphoid organs [i.e. bone marrow, thymus, spleen, lymph nodes, and mucosa-associated lymphoid tissues (MALT)], but are also present in other tissues, such as the liver and lungs.

The primary subpopulations of lymphocytes are B and T cells. These immune cells, when functioning normally, specifically recognize "foreign" material (i.e. microorganisms) and distinguish it from the body's own components. The main function of B cells is to produce antibodies, whereas T cells have a number of functions, which include: (1) helping B cells make antibody; (2) controlling the immune response; (3) activating phagocytes (i.e. macrophages, neutrophils) to destroy pathogens and tumor cells; and (4) recognizing and destroying virally infected cells. Lymphocytes express antigen receptor molecules that recognize foreign material on their cell surface. Each lymphocyte expresses only one type of antigen receptor and can recognize only that antigen. However, since the antigen receptors differ on each lymphocyte clone, the lymphocyte population as a whole has the capacity to recognize a vast array of antigenic determinants.

Phagocytes include blood monocytes, macrophages, and neutrophils (Fig. 23.1). Their primary function is to phagocytose (i.e. ingest) and degrade pathogens, antigens, and cellular debris. However, they also possess the capacity to produce circulating factors (i.e. cytokines), which are central to the regulation of the immunoinflammatory response. Macrophages serve as antigen-presenting cells (APCs) along with other cell types such as dendritic and B cells. In general, the function of APCs is to present antigen to T cells in a form that can be recognized by the T cell. This interaction between APCs and T cells is critical to generation of an effective immune response as outlined in Fig. 23.2.

Additional immune accessory cells include the eosinophil, basophil, mast cell, and platelet. These accessory cells produce a variety of substances that mediate inflammation and thereby play a role in linking the immune system with inflammatory reactions.

LYMPHOCYTES

B cells are precursors to antibody-producing cells that are originally derived from hematopoietic stem cells. These lymphocytes initially develop in the fetal liver and subsequently mature in the bone marrow. Once mature, B cells express immunoglobulin on their surface, which acts as an antigen receptor. They respond to antigenic stimuli and T cell "help" by proliferating and differentiating into antibody-producing plasma cells. B cells also have the ability to function as APCs and, to a lesser degree, as cytokine-producing cells. They are found primarily in the red pulp of the spleen, the medulla of lymph nodes, MALT, and the circulation. To a lesser degree they are found at inflammatory sites, dependent upon the inflammatory stimuli.

T cells, like B cells, are derived from hematopoietic stem cells. Their development is thymic dependent. The maturation process in the thymus leads to the expression of specific antigen receptors on the cell surface. Within the thymus, critical events occur that determine the specificity of peripheral T cells and eliminate T cells that react with autologous (i.e. self) antigens. T cells further differentiate into the two major peripheral subsets, one of which expresses the CD4 surface marker (T helper cells) and the other of which expresses the CD8 surface marker (cytotoxic T cells). These lymphocytes play important roles in a range of immune responses including regulation of the immunoinflammatory response, antigen recognition, cytotoxicity, delayed-type hypersensitivity, and macrophage activation. *T helper* (TH) cells are mainly $CD4^+$ and they recognize antigen presented on the surface of APCs in association with class II major histocompatibility complex (MHC) molecules. They serve to help B cells divide and differentiate into antibody-producing plasma cells, they release cytokines that regulate the differentiation of various leukocytes from hematopoietic stem cells, they control the development of cytotoxic T cells, and they cause activation of macrophages, thus allowing them to destroy the ingested pathogens. *T cytotoxic* (Tc) cells are $CD8^+$ and they recognize antigen on the target cell surface associated with MHC class I molecules. They are capable of destroying virally infected target cells or allogenic cells.

Additional populations of lymphocytes include memory, null, suppressor, and natural killer cells. *T and B memory cells* are populations of long-lived lymphocytes that have been previously stimulated by antigen. These lymphocytes, when subsequently exposed to their specific

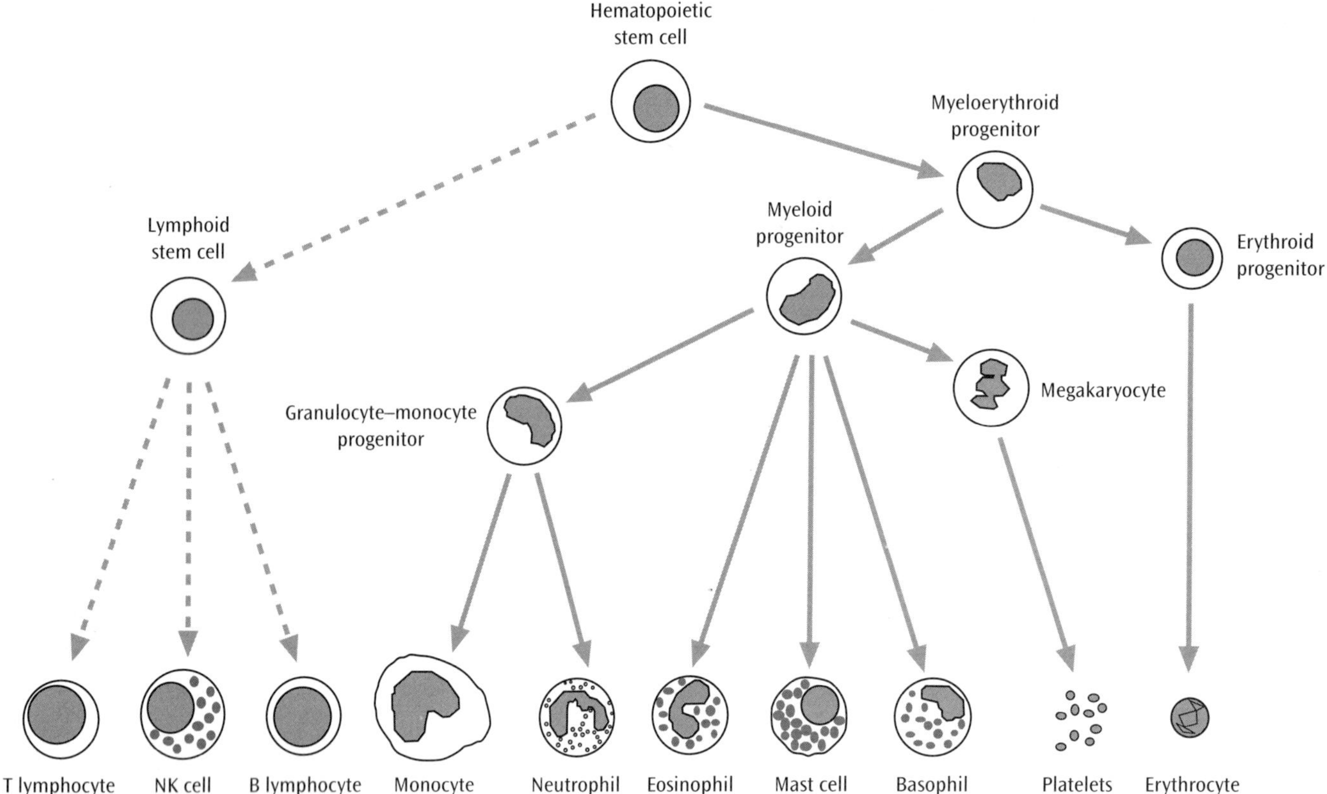

Figure 23.1 *Overview of hematopoiesis. - - -, a common lymphoid stem cell has not yet been isolated but is believed to exist; the histogenesis of natural killer (NK) cells is unknown.*

antigen, respond rapidly to initiate an immune response. *T suppressor* (Ts) cells downregulate the actions of other T and B cells, and thereby play an important role in controlling an immune response. *Null cells* are a distinct population of leukocytes that constitute approximately 14% of blood mononuclear cells. Although they lack conventional antigen receptors, they express surface markers of both the T-cell and mononuclear phagocyte lineages. The high density of Fc receptors on their surface permits them to recognize and kill antibody-sensitized target cells. *Natural killer* (NK) cells are another subset of cytotoxic immune cells that are capable of killing a variety of virally infected or tumor cells. The also serve as an important non-T-cell source of interferon-γ (IFN-γ), an important immunoregulatory cytokine.

PHAGOCYTES AND ANTIGEN-PRESENTING CELLS

Phagocytic cells are divided into two main populations, mononuclear cells (i.e. monocytes and macrophages) and granulocytes (i.e. neutrophils, eosinophils, and basophils). These cells originate from hematopoietic stem cells and their subsequent maturation is dependent on the growth factors to which they are exposed. Monocytes are the circulating form of macrophages. Tissue macrophages are found in all tissues and originate from the circulating monocyte. In addition to their capacity to ingest and degrade pathogens, macrophages also play a central role in the regulation of the immunoinflammatory response, having multiple capacities that can be modulated by inflammatory stimuli. Granulocytes are relatively short lived in the circulation, but are critical for the initial containment of an infection. This is due to their ability to phagocytose pathogens and produce various substances, such as reactive oxygen species and enzymes, that are cytotoxic. The response of granulocytes, however, is relatively nonspecific and the overproduction of these substances also contributes significantly to the inflammatory response and can cause tissue damage.

APCs are a group of functionally defined cells (i.e. dendritic cells and macrophages) which are capable of internalizing antigens and then presenting them on their cell surface to lymphocytes. B cells recognize antigen in its native form, whereas TH cells recognize antigenic peptides that are associated with MHC molecules on the surface of APCs. Consequently, in order to present antigen to a TH cell, an APC must internalize it, process it into small peptides, and re-express it at the cell surface in association with MHC class I or class II molecules.

Anesthetic agents

Studies on the effects of anesthetic agents on the immune function of animals were undertaken as long ago as 1904. Rubin[1] demonstrated that anesthetic inhalation agents, i.e. ether and chloroform, decreased the resistance of rabbits to infection. While most studies in animals have shown that some anesthetics have depressant effects on the immune response, caution should be used in directly extrapolating such results to humans. In attempting to control the nervous, respiratory, and circulatory systems, the anesthesiologist must use drugs that may have the potential of blocking, modifying, changing, and/or interacting with both the chemical messengers and the cell receptors of the immune system. Paradoxically, while trying to protect the patient from the effects of stress and trauma, the anesthesiologist deliberately chooses to use drugs that interfere with the activity of a variety of chemical messengers that mediate the immune response. There is an extensive literature dealing with the effect of the drugs used in anesthesia practice on immune function. Studies by Smith *et al.*[2] demonstrated significant depression of random leukocyte and lymphocyte migration by thiopen-

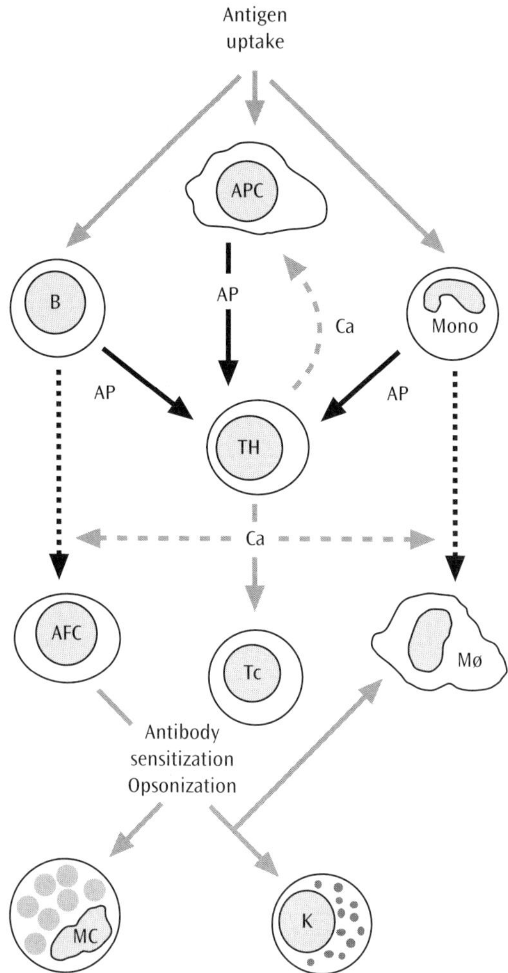

Figure 23.2 *Interaction between immune cells. AFC, antibody-forming cell; APC, antigen-presenting cell; B, B-cell; K, natural killer cell; Mø, macrophage; MC, mast cell; Tc, T cytotoxic cell; TH, T helper cell.*

tal at serum levels normally achieved following induction of anesthesia. Depression of leukocyte/lymphocyte migration by morphine occurred only at concentrations 1000-fold greater than normal serum analgesic levels. Nonetheless, such circulating levels of morphine are observed in opioid addicts, in whom there is evidence of immunosuppression and increased susceptibility to infection.[3]

Perioperative modulation of natural killer cell activity

NK-cell activity may be depressed for up to 3 days after hysterectomy under neuroleptic-induced anesthesia. This depression is not seen following epidural anesthesia. This difference may be partly due to the absence of a stress response [cortisol and norepinephrine (noradrenaline)] in the epidural group.[4] However, both *in vivo* and *in vitro* studies suggest that volatile anesthetic agents, nitrous oxide, halothane, and enflurane, have a transient dose-dependent depressive effect on interferon-stimulated NK-cell activity.[5,6] The effect of opiates on NK-cell activity is controversial, and appears to be dependent upon the experimental system employed. It has been postulated that NK cells have opioid receptors since β-endorphin can augment NK cytolytic activity *in vitro* through a naloxone-sensitive mechanism.[7] A preliminary report indicated that patients receiving high-dose fentanyl anesthesia had a depression in NK-cell activity that lasted for 3 days. This effect could, however, be reversed *in vitro* by the addition of interleukin 2 (IL-2).[8]

Catecholamines have been shown to influence NK-cell numbers and activity since it has been shown that an infusion of epinephrine (adrenaline) or dobutamine can increase NK-cell numbers.[9,10] Additionally, dobutamine infusion also increases lymphocyte numbers and NK-cell activity.[10]

Effect of anesthetic agents on neutrophil function

In view of the important role of neutrophils in the evolution of multiple organ failure, there has been much interest in the effects of anesthetic agents on various parameters of neutrophil function. The neutrophil activation process consists of polarization and locomotion, adherence, phagocytosis, and degranulation. *In vitro* studies have demonstrated that neutrophil polarization is reduced by clinical relevant concentrations of propofol and thiopental.[11] Propofol and intralipid also reduce neutrophil chemotaxis. The mechanism of action of propofol on chemotaxis appears to be dependent on lipid solubility, since lipid solubility in volatile anesthetic agents is correlated with reduction in granulocyte migration.[12] Neutrophils also display a naloxone-sensitive chemotactic response to endogenous opioids *in vitro*.[13,14]

Neutrophil phagocytosis is associated with increased oxygen consumption and the production of oxygen radicals, such as superoxide anion and hydrogen peroxide, and is termed "respiratory burst." Experimentally, volatile anesthetics can inhibit superoxide production and Ca^{2+} mobilization in neutrophils.[15] Propofol in clinical concentrations also inhibits the neutrophil "respiratory burst" as measured by chemiluminescence.[16] Barbiturates cause inhibition of neutrophil chemiluminescence as well as migration *in vitro*. This effect is 10–100 times greater for thiobarbiturates (i.e. thiopental) than for oxybarbiturates (i.e. methohexital). It is believed that the difference in inhibitory activity of the barbiturate depends on the presence of the sulfur atom.[17] Recent studies have shown that neutrophil respiratory burst and phagocytosis were reduced *in vitro* by thiopental and ketamine; however, this occurred only when these agents were employed at concentrations that were greater than that used in normal clinical practice.[18] Finally, neutrophils have opioid receptors and exposure to physiologic concentrations of opioid peptides rapidly induces naloxone-reversible superoxide production *in vitro*.[19]

Effect of anesthetic agents on lymphocytes

The proliferative response of lymphocytes is fundamental to the orchestration of an effective immune response. Lectins such as phytohemagglutinin (PHA), concanavalin A (ConA), and pokeweed mitogen (PWM) are often used selectively to induce B- and T-lymphocyte proliferation *in vitro*. Following anesthesia and surgery, decreased lymphocyte responsiveness to mitogens, decreased blastogenic responses to microbial antigens, decreased and delayed hypersensitivity reactions, and decreased mixed lymphocyte responses can be demonstrated. However, it is difficult to differentiate between the effects of anesthesia or surgery on the lymphocyte responsiveness. Anesthetic agents reduce some of the untoward responses of surgical stress, while producing direct and indirect effects on the function of lymphocytes. Experimentally, lymphocyte function, lymphocyte recirculation, cell-mediated cytotoxicity, and the ability of lymphocytes to kill tumor cells are depressed following anesthesia alone.[20–22] Thus, while operative trauma is considered to have a greater role in altering overall immune responses, the contribution of anesthetics may be more important than surgical stress in procedures that are less traumatic.

Clinical studies have attempted to differentiate the effects of volatile anesthetic agents on lymphocyte cytotoxicity from surgical trauma. Depression of lymphocyte function following inhalation anesthesia for tonsillectomy in otherwise healthy children has been reported.[23] Interestingly, washing the cells to remove traces of the anesthetic reversed the decrease in lymphocyte function. In one study comparing regional and general anesthesia, and surgical and nonsurgical procedures, the depression of lymphocyte function appeared to relate primarily to surgical trauma, and not to anesthetic technique or agent.[24] However, in another report comparing epidural with inhalation anesthesia a depression in lymphocyte (or monocyte) function was found only in the group that received general anesthesia.[25] Finally, in a study in which serum cortisol levels were assayed to control for the extent of surgical "stress," a depression in lymphocyte function occurred in the patients who received inhalation anesthesia but not spinal anesthesia.[26]

β-Endorphin is a potent inhibitor of PHA-induced human T-cell proliferation.[27] However, this effect is independent of opiate receptors, since it is insensitive to inhibition by naloxone.[27] It has also been postulated that increased levels of endogenous opioids contribute to the suppression of cell-mediated immune responses following major stress and trauma.[28]

The effects of propofol (Diprivan) and Intralipid on lymphocyte proliferation have also been examined.[28] The drugs had no effect on cells obtained from normal healthy volunteers, but in cells from the intensive care unit (ICU) patients propofol caused a reduction in the proliferative response to PWM. This suggests that B-lymphocyte proliferation in critically ill patients may be inhibited by propofol. Propofol or thiopental anesthesia followed by low-dose fentanyl induced a similar response in subpopulations of peripheral blood lymphocytes.[29] There is, however, an increase in the total number of T lymphocytes, as well as memory T and B lymphocytes, following administration of both drugs. In contrast, NK-cell numbers declined in both groups. However, there is one important difference between these anesthetics: propofol anesthesia increased helper T-cell numbers, whereas thiopental had no effect.

Studies have demonstrated a decrease in intra- and postoperative IgM, IgG, and IgA antibody levels.[30] Following regional or general anesthesia, a decline in antibody levels also occurs during the postinduction period, lasting briefly into the postoperative period. The mechanism responsible for this decline is not clear. The decline in antibody levels could be partly due to hemodilution or the formation of immune antigen–antibody complexes. The same mechanism(s) may also explain the decrease in complement levels observed intra- and postoperatively. Furthermore, experimental *in vitro* and animal data show little effect of anesthetic agents on T-cell-dependent antibody production by B cells if these agents are used at a therapeutic concentration.[31] Nonetheless, long-term use of high-dose thiopental infusions in the treatment of head injury and status epilepticus may produce increased susceptibility to bacterial pneumonia.[32]

Bupivacaine and lidocaine (lignocaine) inhibit immunoglobulin production only in *in vitro* systems in which B cells are exposed for prolonged period to concentrations of drugs that greatly exceed those occurring in plasma during regional anesthesia. Such *in vivo* concentrations of agents may be achieved after local infiltration of local anesthetics; however, the concentration of the anesthetics decreases rapidly, making it unlikely that there will be any detectable inhibitory effect. In fact, it has been reported that local anesthetics at high concentrations have antimicrobial activity.[33] Nonetheless, it should be recognized that concentrations of lidocaine and bupivacaine used for wound infiltration are bactericidal and toxic to immune cells.[34,35]

Perioperative immunomodulation of major histocompatibility complex class II molecules

A decrease in circulating monocyte (a major APC) numbers may lead to a depression in antigen presentation. This is known to occur during cardiopulmonary bypass, when monocytes adhere to the plastic tubing. In addition, a decrease in the relative number of TH cells should also have a similar effect. This has been reported following thiopental and vecuronium use during anesthesia, and to a lesser degree in patients receiving a dobutamine infusion.[10] The downregulation of MHC class II expression on monocytes or lymphocytes may lower immune responsiveness. In this regard, decreased expression of human MHC class II (HLA-DR) on lymphocytes and monocytes has been demonstrated as early as 10 min after high-dose fentanyl anesthesia for cardiac surgery.[36] At 2 h after the termination of cardiopulmonary bypass, monocyte HLA-DR expression was further decreased by 40%. At 24 h after surgery some recovery in monocyte HLA-DR expression was observed. In contrast to monocytes, lymphocyte HLA-DR expression was suppressed by 40% at 24 h postoperatively.[36] The perioperative immune response is, therefore, not attributable to surgery alone. Many drugs used by anesthesiologists have wide-ranging immunomodulatory properties. Clearly, more research is required to determine if the choice of anesthetic technique may have a clinically significant immunologic impact.

BLOOD TRANSFUSION AND INTRAVENOUS FLUIDS

Transfusion of blood from allogeneic donors has had a long and checkered history in the practice of medicine. Innovations in open-heart surgery, organ transplantation, treatment of leukemia and lymphoma, joint replacement surgery, and care of trauma patients were made possible by transfusion. The concept that transfusion-induced immunomodulation might be of broad clinical importance was not formulated until the 1980s. At that time the association between transfusion and increased cancer recurrence, postoperative infections, viral infection severity, and reduced severity of inflammatory diseases was reported in numerous epidemiological and animal studies.[37] Allogeneic blood transfusions generally cause upregulation of humoral immunity and downregulation of macrophage and T-cell immunity. Increased alloantibody formation to HLA-A,B (MHC class I) antigens and decreased cutaneous delayed-type hypersensitivity, T-cell proliferation, and NK-cell function were observed in transfused patients and experimental animals. These changes are hypothesized to be the mechanism underlying experimental and epidemiologic observations that allogeneic transfusions are strongly associated with prolonged survival of organ allografts, increased rates of cancer recurrence, and increased prevalence of postoperative bacterial and viral infections.[37] Nonetheless, major controversy exists over whether the association between allogeneic transfusion, immunomodulation, and increased postoperative infections and tumor recurrence are causal. There is now, however, a general consensus that transfusion downregulates APC and T-cell function. A variety of antigen-specific and nonspecific measures of immunity are also depressed following transfusion, including NK-cell function, macrophage chemotaxis, lymphocyte proliferation, and cutaneous delayed hypersensitivity responses.[37] These changes have been particularly prominent in the surgical setting, possibly because both anesthesia and surgery have immunomodulatory effects.

The prevailing hypothesis is that the stimulation of allogeneic transfusions drives the immune system toward what has been termed a T helper cell type 2 (TH2) response (e.g. IL-10, IL-4) with a concomitant downregulation of T helper cell type 1 (TH1)-dependent immune functions (e.g. IL-2, IL-12). TH2 responses support humoral immunity (i.e. antibody production), and TH1 responses support cellular immunity involving APC and T-cell function. The cytokines secreted in TH2-type responses have suppressive effects on antigen processing and presentation, and these functions are critical for many aspects of antibody formation. The concept that allogeneic transfusions generate a TH2-type immune response, and consequently impair TH1 responses, also provides a possible theoretical basis for understanding the beneficial effects of allogeneic transfusions in renal allotransplantation, Crohn's disease, and women with repetitive spontaneous abortions.[35] There are now approximately 100 epidemiologic studies that have examined the relation between transfusion and earlier cancer recurrence. Approximately two-thirds of these studies demonstrate a statistically significant deleterious effect on clinical outcome following transfusion. Approximately 40 epidemiologic studies have demonstrated that a dose-related increase in infections is seen in surgical patients who received allogeneic transfusions. The infections seen were predominantly bacterial and polymicrobial in nature. In contrast to allogeneic transfusions, autologous transfusions are not associated with an increased infection rate.[38]

The traditional belief that allogeneic blood is an effective and safe therapy with minimal risks has, however, been challenged by a heightened awareness of the problems of transfusion reactions, disease transmission, and immunomodulation. Surgeons have responded to these challenges by reassessing the reasons for transfusion, increasing use of autologous blood, modifying surgical techniques to reduce blood loss, and employing various drugs to reduce transfusion requirements. Blood should be transfused only when there is a documented need to increase O_2 delivery in those patients in whom O_2 demands exceed O_2 delivery. For more detail on this, refer to Chapter 9.

EFFECT OF GENDER, NUTRITION, AND AGE

Influence of gender on the immune system

Calzolari,[39] working in 1898, first demonstrated that sex hormones can affect the immune system by showing that castration of adult male rabbits resulted in an increase in thymic mass. More recently, gender differences in the susceptibility to, and morbidity from, sepsis have been observed in several clinical and epidemiologic studies.[40,41] Experimentally, the alterations in endocrine and immune functions have been investigated primarily using male laboratory animals. Nonetheless, immune function in normal males and females is influenced by sex steroids.[42,43] In this regard, it appears that better maintained immune functions in females are due not only to physiologic levels of female sex steroids, but also at least in part due to the lower levels of immunosuppressive androgenic hormones.[44,45]

The suppressive effects of androgens on immunity have been observed with regard to both *normal* and *abnormal* immune functions, such as the development of autoimmune disease.[46] In this regard, studies indicate a predominance of diverse autoimmune diseases in females, such as systemic lupus erythematosus, Hashimoto's thyroiditis, rheumatoid arthritis, and primary biliary cirrhosis.[47,48] Moreover, humoral and cell-mediated immune responses have been reported to be more vigorous in females than in males, suggesting a sexually dimorphic immune response.[49,50] With regard to humoral immunity, circulating concentrations of the major immunoglobulin classes (IgG, IgM, IgA) in females far exceed those found in males of the same species, age, and physiologic conditions when challenged with antigens such as polio virus, bovine serum albumin, or hemagglutinin.[51,52] This difference is reflected not only in higher titers of antibody but also in a more sustained primary and secondary response in females than in males.[53]

Increased plasma concentrations of prolactin in females are associated with increased TH and Tc lymphocyte activity.[54] The increased TH and Tc lymphocyte activity results in an increased cell-mediated immune response, accompanied by an increase in humoral immunity. Prolactin has been demonstrated to have stimulatory effects on the immune system, and may be a key hormone contributing to the dichotomy seen in the immune response between females and males.[55,56] Treatment of male septic mice with either prolactin or metoclopramide (which is known to elevate prolactin levels[57]) immediately after the onset of sepsis has been shown to result in significantly increased innate and inducible IL-1β, IL-6 and tumor necrosis factor (TNF)-α gene expression in both splenic and peritoneal macrophages.[58] Moreover, prolactin administration following hemorrhagic shock in male mice improved macrophage cytokine release capacity and decreased mortality from subsequent sepsis.[59] The physiologic release of prolactin from the pituitary fluctuates in a pulsatile circadian fashion, as do glucocorticoids, and is further modulated by behavioral and environmental stimuli, the reproductive cycle, steroid hormones, neurotransmitters, immunoregulatory cytokines, and various drugs. Additional studies also support the view that hormones of the endocrine system (i.e. prolactin, progesterone, the adrenal glucocorticoids, growth hormones, and endogenous opioids) are intimately involved in immunologic sexual dimorphism.[55,60,61]

Nutritional status and immune function

Nutrition is a critical determinant of immunocompetence and risk of illness. Young children with protein–energy malnutrition (PEM) exhibit increased mortality and morbidity, due largely to infectious disease. It has demonstrated that undernourished individuals have impaired immune responses. The most consistent abnormalities are in cell-mediated immunity, complement system activation, phagocyte function, mucosal secretory antibody responses, and antibody affinity. Malnutrition is associated with a number of acute and chronic sequelae, of which one of the most frequent complications is infection. Because of widespread occurrence of nutritional deficiency, it is the commonest cause of immunodeficiency worldwide. In this regard, epidemiologic studies have documented the adverse effect of PEM on morbidity and mortality.[62,63] Furthermore, several aspects of cell-mediated immunity are significantly altered by PEM. For example, delayed cutaneous hypersensitivity responses to both recall and new antigens are markedly depressed.

One plausible reason for reduced cell-mediated immunity in PEM is the reduction in the number of fully mature differentiated T lymphocytes. The number of $CD4^+$ TH cells is decreased markedly, often to values less than 50% of the controls, whereas the change in suppressor T cells ($CD8^+$) is less marked. Thus, the helper–suppressor ratio is significantly decreased. Lymphocyte proliferation is also reduced under such conditions. Antibody responses are among the first set of immune indices examined in PEM, and studies show that antibody affinity is decreased along with decreased secretory IgA antibody levels after immunization with viral antigens. The clinical implications of this immunodeficiency include an increased frequency of septicemia in undernourished patients.

The crucial role of several vitamins and trace elements in immunocompetence in patients with a given micronutrient deficiency has been established.[64] Deficiencies of pyridoxine, folic acid, vitamin A, vitamin C, and vitamin E result in impaired cell-mediated immunity and reduced antibody responses. Zinc deficiency, both acquired and inherited, is associated with lymphoid atrophy, decreased cutaneous delayed hypersensitivity responses and homograft rejection, and lower thymic hormone activity. Moreover, there are a reduced number of antibody-forming cells in the spleen and impaired T-killer cell activity. In addition, wound healing is impaired. Excessive dietary zinc can also depress neutrophil function and lymphocyte responses.[65] Deficiency of iron is the commonest nutritional problem worldwide, even in industrialized countries. Iron is critical for optimal neutrophil and lymphocyte activity. Responses to tetanus toxoid and herpes simplex antigens are low in iron-deficient subjects, but show significant improvement with iron therapy.[66]

In certain population segments (i.e. the elderly and smokers) immune activity can be increased by dietary supplementation of micronutrients, thus suggesting a rationale for increasing the recommended dietary allowances for these patients. In two separate studies the proliferation of peripheral blood lymphocytes to specific T- and B-cell mitogens increased significantly when the fat content of the diets was reduced from 30% or 40% of energy to 25% of energy.[67,68] An increase in lymphocyte proliferation and the secretion of IL-1 was also observed in a group of elderly subjects when fat intake was reduced from 36% to 27% of energy.[69] The lowering of fat intake from 32% to 22% of the total energy requirements also increased NK-cell activity in a group of healthy men.[70]

Animal studies have shown that *n*-6 polyunsaturated fatty acids (PUFAs) inhibit immune function to a greater extent than saturated fatty acids. Whether or not this is also the case in humans remains unclear. The available data suggest that a moderate increase in the intake of *n*-6 PUFAs in a diet containing >30% of energy from total fat and with adequate amounts of antioxidant nutrients should not have any adverse effects on immune response. However, such an increase may suppress immune response in individuals with low antioxidant-nutrient status who are consuming a high-fat diet.[71] Daly *et al.*[72] found that patients placed on enteral diets containing fish oil after major elective surgery demonstrated not only improved *in vitro* lymphocyte mitogenic responses but also fewer infection/wound complications and had a shorter hospital stay. Thus, the existing immunologic data support the current recommendations by the American Heart Association to decrease fat intake to 30% of energy, with 10% of energy from each of saturated, monounsaturated, and PUFAs. At the lower end ≥20% of energy from fat is needed for health maintenance and work efficiency in healthy adult populations.

Lifestyle and environmental factors can also adversely affect both nutritional status and immune responses. For example, tissue concentrations of vitamin C, vitamin E, β-carotene, vitamin B_6, and folate are lower in smokers than in nonsmokers. Smokers have elevated neutrophil oxidation activity, which may reduce antioxidant nutrient status. The elderly are another group at risk of decreased immune responsiveness. Chandra[73] showed a significant decrease in the number of sick days and in the use of antibiotics, as well as an increase in antibody response to the flu vaccine, in a group of healthy elderly subjects who supplemented their diets with a multivitamin. The multivitamin contained 100% of the recommended dietary allowance (RDA) of most vitamins and a moderately higher amount of vitamin C (80 mg day^{-1}), vitamin E (44 mg day^{-1}), and β-carotene (16 mg day^{-1}).

The numerous observations on the interactions between nutrition and immunity have led to several practical applications. For example, the outcome for surgical patients can be predicted on the basis of preoperative assessment of nutritional status and of immunocompetence. Severe malnutrition depresses immune responses which, in some patients, can be restored by nutritional support. Studies in which the effectiveness of enteral nutrition has been compared with total parenteral nutrition (TPN) have shown a higher incidence of septic complications in patients receiving TPN.[74] Furthermore, hepatobiliary abnormalities have also been reported following TPN.[75] Lipid-free parenteral nutrition, in contrast to standard parenteral nutrition given preoperatively, has been associated with improved outcome.[76] In addition, TPN leads to considerable mucosal atrophy by starvation of the gut mucosa. Meta-analysis of clinical studies[77] showed little, if any, clinically important benefit in surgical patients having received TPN.

Enteral feeding has been shown to be important in maintaining normal gut integrity and blood flow. Luminal nutrients are an essential source of nutrients for intestinal cells and for maintaining intestinal secretory IgA levels, thus limiting bacterial translocation. Traditionally, following surgery, surgeons have awaited the return of bowel sounds or the passage of flatus before commencing enteral feeding. However, "normal postoperative ileus" has been shown to affect only the stomach and colon, whereas small intestinal motility and function are maintained. Therefore, early feeding via a nasojejunal tube or a feeding jejunostomy can be employed.[78] The use of selective decontamination of the digestive tract, by administering nonabsorbable antibiotics, has not been proved to improve survival significantly in ICU patients, although the incidence of respiratory tract infections was reduced by 60%.[79] It should be recognized that certain amino acids, particularly glutamine and arginine, are important substrates for the maintenance of gastrointestinal integrity and function. Furthermore, these amino acids also play an important role in maintaining leukocyte activity and function.[80,81] Practicing anesthesiologists and surgeons should become knowledgeable about strategies involving the specialized nutritional regimens as potential new treatment options since such interventions may become an integral part in the care of critically ill surgical patients in the next decade.

THE EFFECT OF AGING ON THE IMMUNE SYSTEM

Optimal functioning of the immune system requires rapid proliferation of specific immune cells upon appropriate stimulation. Therefore, a decreased efficiency of protein metabolism, such as that which occurs during aging, might decrease the production of substances essential for normal functioning of the immune system. Conversely, activation of the immune system by illness may increase protein turnover in the elderly and place a higher demand on an already reduced lean body mass (LBM). Some of the primary hormones implicated in these changes associated with aging include growth hormone, prolactin, androgens, insulin, cortisol, and the thyroid hormones.

Growth hormones (GH) are potent anabolic agents that stimulate protein synthesis and cell growth and improve nitrogen balance, while reducing stored and circulating lipids.[82] Interestingly, increasing evidence suggests that lymphocytes also synthesize and secrete an immunoreactive GH that is similar, if not identical, in terms of bioactivity, antigenicity, and molecular weight, to that produced by cells of the anterior pituitary.[83] The production of GH is altered under various physiologic conditions. Exercise, for example, acts as a powerful stimulus to increase serum GH concentrations. In contrast, there is evidence that GH secretion declines with age after reaching maximal secretion at puberty.[84,85] Furthermore, it has been estimated that approximately 50% of individuals over 65 years of age are partially or totally deficient in GH.[86]

Testosterone is quantitatively the primary androgen. The difference in plasma testosterone levels between males and females (0.6 vs. 0.03 mg dL^{-1} respectively) seems to account for the fact that a female begins her adult life with a LBM only two-thirds that of a male.[86] Male testosterone secretion peaks at approximately 22 years of age and declines steadily thereafter, consistent with the decrease in LBM that occurs with advancing age.[87]

It has recently been reported that the well-recognized insulin resistance observed in the elderly is due to a variable decrease in pancreatic insulin output as well as a small decline in peripheral tissue responsiveness to insulin.[88] Given the known physiologic effects that insulin produces, a decrease in insulin bioactivity with aging would be consistent with the decrease in LBM and muscle activity observed in the elderly.

In addition to the influence of the classic neuroendocrine hormones on body composition, there is also considerable evidence supporting the notion that endogenous products of the immune system, the cytokines, also mediate LBM changes resulting from injury, inflammation, and perhaps aging. In recent years, increased attention has been paid to the effects of aging on the production of cytokines. It has been suggested that dysregulation of cytokine production may be in part responsible for the increased morbidity and mortality rates and the subtle presentation of infection in elderly patients.

Age itself, however, can no longer be considered a contraindication to well-managed anesthesia and surgery in any geriatric patient. Major neuroaxial conduction anesthesia and peripheral nerve and plexus blocks may not necessarily be preferable because they appear to be associated with an increased risk of nerve palsies, persistent numbness, and other neurologic complications in older patients.[89]

CYTOKINES IN ANESTHESIA

Cytokines are low-molecular-weight (< 80 kDa) secreted proteins, often glycosylated, and are extremely potent, generally acting at picomolar concentrations. They initiate their action by binding to specific receptors on the surface of the target cell. Cytokines tend to be paracrine (act on a nearby cell) or autocrine (act on the same cell), rather than endocrine (secreted into the circulation to act on a distant cell). Activation of surface receptors leads ultimately to a change in the pattern of cellular RNA and protein synthesis and to altered cell behavior. Cytokines act on many different cell types (pleiotropism) and often influence the synthesis and action of other cytokines. They are a heterogeneous group of proteins, variously termed lymphokines, monokines, interleukins, and interferons, which regulate a wide range of cellular functions, including cell growth, maturation, and repair (Tables 23.1 and 23.2). Cytokines are produced primarily by activated leukocytes; however, under certain conditions fibroblasts and endothelial cells can also produce cytokines. Activation of these cells is one of the earliest cellular responses to tissue injury from surgery or trauma and is associated with release of a variety of inflammatory mediators, which include arachidonic acid metabolites,

Table 23.1 *Overview of the interleukins*

Interleukin	Principal cell source	Principal effects
IL-1α and IL-1β	Macrophage Fibroblast Lymphocytes Other APCs Other somatic cells	Costimulation of APCs and T cells Phagocyte activation Inflammation and fever Hematopoiesis ↑ Prostaglandin synthesis Acute-phase response of liver
IL-2	T cells NK cells	T-cell growth and activation NK-cell function
IL-3	T cells Thymic epithelium	Growth of early hematopoietic progenitors
IL-4	Th2 cells Mast cells	TH2 cell proliferation and functions Inhibition of monokine production Eosinophil and mast cell growth and functions B-cell proliferation, IgE expression and class II MHC expression
IL-5	TH2 cells Mast cells	Eosinophil development and differentiation
IL-6	Macrophages TH2 cells APCs Other somatic cells	B-cell differentiation and growth Acute-phase response of liver Induces fever Synergistic effects with IL-1 or TNF
IL-7	Thymic and marrow stromal cells	T and B lymphopoiesis
IL-8	Monocytes/macrophages Fibroblast	Chemoattractant for neutrophils and T cells
IL-9	$CD4^+$ T cells	Hematopoietic and thymopoietic effects
IL-10	TH2 cells $CD8^+$ T cells B cells Macrophages	Inhibits cytokine production Promotion of B-cell proliferation and antibody responses Suppression of cellular immunity
IL-11	Stromal cells	Synergistic effects on hematopoiesis and thrombopoiesis
IL-12	Macrophages B cells	IFN-γ production Promotion of cell-mediated immune responses Activation of NK cells
IL-13	TH2 cells	↓ Cytokine production
IL-14	T cells B cells Tumor cells	Proliferation of activated B cells
IL-15	Monocytes/macrophages Nonlymphocytic cells Epithelial cells	Mimics IL-2 effects Synergistic effects with IL-12
IL-16	$CD8^+$ cells $CD4^+$ cells	Chemoattract for $CD4^+$ cells Comitogenic for $CD4^+$ T cells
IL-17	T cells	Proinflammatory

APCs, antigen-presenting cells; IFN, interferon; IL, interleukin; MHC, major histocompatibility complex; NK cell, natural killer cell; TH2, T helper cells type 2.

Table 23.2 *Immunoregulatory cytokines*

	Principal cell source	Principal effects
TNF-α (cachectin) TNF-β (lymphotoxin)	Activated macrophages Other somatic cells	Direct cytotoxicity IL-1-like effects Activates endothelial cells
IFN-α and -β	Macrophages	Activates macrophages Antiviral effects Antiproliferative effects
IFN-γ	Activated T cells Activated NK cells	Antiviral effects Activation of macrophages, neutrophils, and NK cells Promotion of cell-mediated immunity
TGF-β	Macrophages Activated T cells Platelets	Anti-inflammatory Antiproliferative for myelomonocytic cells and lymphocytes Promotion of fibroblast proliferation and wound healing

IFN, interferon; NK cell, natural killer cell; TGF, transforming growth factor; TNF, tumor necrosis factor.

complement products, lysosomal enzymes, and reactive oxygen and nitrogen molecules as well as cytokines.

The discovery of cytokines

Early studies of cytokines from 1950 to 1970 involved the description of numerous protein factors produced by a wide range of cells, which mediated specific cellular functions *in vitro.* The resulting evidence implicated thymus-derived T lymphocytes as the cells that specifically interacted with antigen to release these protein factors, which were termed lymphokines to indicate their origin and function. It was at this time that antiviral interferons, fever-producing pyrogens, and macrophage-activating factor were discovered. The second phase of cytokine research involved the purification and characterization of many of these secretory proteins. Somewhat surprisingly it was found that a single peptide (i.e. cytokine) could have a diverse range of cellular effects. Furthermore, it was realized that cytokines were synthesized principally by leukocytes to act primarily on other leukocyte populations, and because of this specific characteristic they were termed interleukins. In the past decade, molecular cloning and the production of highly specific neutralizing antibodies have resulted in the precise identification of the structure and properties of many of the individual cytokines.

The central role of cytokines in the immune response

When a foreign substance enters the body, the initial attempt to eliminate it comes from an inflammatory response led by neutrophils and macrophages. In engulfing the foreign molecules, some of these cells extrude foreign antigen on to the cell surface, thus becoming APCs. They are involved in the initial stages of specific immunity and also synthesize and release cytokines. In conjunction with other cells of the immune system, such as NK cells and TH lymphocytes, macrophage activation is critically dependent on cytokine production. Other cells involved in this nonspecific first line of defense are NK cells and lymphokine-activated cells (LAK cells). NK cells also release TNF and interferons.

Specific immune responses occur after exposure to antigens, following a chain of events that results in highly specific antibodies (humoral immunity) or production of a specific set of lymphocytes (cell-mediated immunity). Maturation of the TH subsets is cytokine dependent, TH1 is dependent on IFN-γ production, which is induced by IL-12, and predominantly produces further IFN-γ and IL-2. TH2 lymphocyte development is dependent on early IL-4 production and produces IL-4, IL-5, IL-10, and IL-13, and little or no IFN-γ.

Immunomodulation and the cytokine balance

For maintenance of health, pro- and anti-inflammatory cytokines need to be held in equilibrium. This equilibrium may be perturbed by the advent of trauma, sepsis, and neoplasia. Therapeutic interventions designed to manipulate the cytokine network and thus push the pathogenic process one way or the other are now emerging. For example, the clinical importance of the cytokine balance has been well illustrated in Lyme arthritis, in which it was shown that significant clinical improvement correlated with an elevation in plasma levels of IL-1 receptor antagonist in relation to IL-1β.[90]

Several investigators have observed the presence of a proinflammatory cytokine response during surgical procedures. For instance, during lung surgery a small increase has been observed in plasma IL-6, TNF-α, and IL-1α.[91] More dramatic and biologically relevant increases in these cytokines have been reported following cardiac surgery.[92,93] Recently, Hill *et al.*[94] showed that aprotinin, a serine protease inhibitor used primarily to reduce blood loss after cardiopulmonary bypass (CPB), reduces CPB-induced TNF-α in a similar way to glucocorticoids and enhances IL-10 release after cardiac operations. Furthermore, Latah *et al.*[92] first observed a significant elevation in TNF-α immediately after induction of anesthesia with high-dose fentanyl, even before surgery commenced. In addition to TNF-α, a significant rise in IL-8 occurs approximately 10 min after induction of anesthesia with high-dose fentanyl, independent of intubation and surgery.[36]

The important concept of perioperative cytokine modulation by anesthetic agents is exemplified by IL-6. This pro-inflammatory cytokine is released in response to major surgery[95] and is known to be directly correlated with postoperative morbidity.[96] Furthermore, a reduction in mortality of septic shock in response to treatment with monoclonal antibodies to IL-6 or IL-6 receptor has been reported.[97] Crozier *et al.*[98] have shown that propofol–alfentanil anesthesia delays the onset and reduces the magnitude of the IL-6 response during major abdominal surgery compared with isoflurane anesthesia. They suggest that this effect is mediated by alfentanil acting on opioid receptors, leading to a reduction in intracellular cyclic adenosine monophosphate (cAMP),[99] an important secondary messenger in triggering the release of IL-6.[100] Consequently a decrease in cAMP is associated with inhibition of IL-6 synthesis. In contrast to IL-6, a decrease in cAMP is associated with induction of TNF-α synthesis.

With regard to cyclic nucleotides, the balance of cAMP and cyclic guanosine monophosphate (cGMP) is controlled by seven phosphodiesterase isoenzymes that degrade these molecules to their noncyclic form. Phosphodiesterase (PDE) inhibitors are a diverse class of drugs with differing specificity for each of the isoenzymes. They include drugs such as methylxanthine, theophylline, milrinone, amrinone, petoxifylline, and dipyridamole. Pentoxifylline is in widespread use in the treatment of peripheral vascular disease. The use of this drug in experimental animal models of hemorrhage and endotoxic shock is associated with a marked improvement in survival rate.[101]

Dissection of the mechanisms whereby anesthetic agents modulate immune responses requires detailed *in vitro* analysis. For instance, intravenous induction agents have been reported to induce cytokine production by monocytes in culture.[102] Increased production of TNF-α occurred with propofol, thiopental, and ketamine, whereas IL-1α production was induced mainly by propofol and IL-6 was induced by ketamine. Furthermore, propofol has been shown to increase lymphocyte IFN-γ production *in vitro*.[103] Propofol and midazolam also reduce IL-8 release from lipopolysaccharide (LPS)-stimulated neutrophils *in vitro*.[95] *In vitro* studies suggest that the inhibitory effect of PGE_2 on TNF-α production may be attenuated by indomethacin. When this cyclo-oxygenase inhibitor was administered prior to cardiac surgery, TNF-α and IL-1β production by isolated peripheral blood mononuclear cells was enhanced *in vitro*.[104] Isoprenaline inhibits TNF-α production *in vitro* in a heparinized whole-blood model, while having no effect on IL-1β.[105] Furthermore, epinephrine inhibits human monocyte spreading and adherence *in vitro*, an effect that can be blocked by the β-adrenergic antagonist propranolol. Moreover, this effect is thought to be cAMP-mediated, since cAMP analogs induce similar results. In contrast to epinephrine, metenkephalin induced an increase in macrophage spreading and adherence. This effect was inhibited by concurrent treatment with epinephrine, suggesting that the two agents have opposite effects on cAMP levels.[106]

In addition to cytokines, cell adhesion molecules (CAM) function as a molecular mechanism by which cells of the immune system communicate with each other. These adhesion molecules appear on the surface of neutrophils and endothelial cells very early in an inflammatory response.[107] They are cell-surface proteins involved in the binding of cells either to each other, to endothelium, or to the extracellular matrix. Increased values of CAM may represent an earlier indicator of an activated immune response than an increase in cytokine secretion. The main groups of cell adhesion molecules are the selectins and immunoglobulin superfamily (IGSF). Selectins such as endothelial leukocyte adhesion molecule 1 (ELAM-1) act in the initial phases of cell adhesion to capture leukocytes from the circulation on to the vascular endothelium. Proinflammatory cytokines act on the endothelium to cause upregulation of a number of these CAMs. Cell adhesion molecules in the endothelium interact with complementary CAMs on neutrophils, leading to rolling of the neutrophil along the vascular endothelium, followed by activation (triggering) and more intense adherence, degranulation, or migration (Fig. 23.3). In addition, the cytokine cascade increases the prothrombotic potential of endothelium.

It has now been recognized that elevated IL-8, TNF-α, and IL-1β in the bronchoalveolar lavage fluid is predictive for the development of adult respiratory distress syndrome (ARDS) in patients in the ICU.[108,109] A decrease in the soluble form of the adhesion molecule L-selectin in plasma is also predictive of ARDS.[110] This may be related to a generalized endothelial activation occurring early in ARDS, which causes the upregulation of L-selectin ligands, which bind the soluble form of L-selectin, thereby decreasing plasma concentrations. It is possible that this phenomenon may prevent excessive neutrophil adhesion by blocking unoccupied ligands for L-selectin on the endothelium. With regard to neutrophil adhesion, adhesion to endothelium and other surfaces is enhanced by factors that decrease the negative charge of the endothelium. Cationic proteins, such as lactoferrin, are released by activated neutrophils and promote neutrophil adhesion.[111] In contrast, large anionic molecules such as heparin inhibit neutrophil adhesion in *in vitro* systems.[112] The highest *in vivo* concentrations of heparin occur during cardiac surgery and may be an important contributor to the lack of adverse clinical sequelae following cardiopulmonary bypass surgery, a period during which upregulation of neutrophil adhesion molecules occurs.[113]

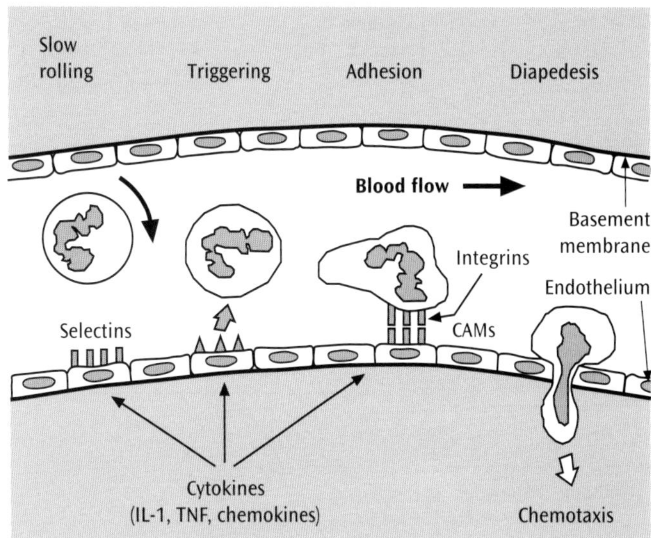

Figure 23.3 *Transendothelial leukocyte migration at site of infection. CAM, cell adhesion molecules; IL, interleukin; TNF, tumor necrosis factor.*

Our understanding of the importance of cytokine networks in health and disease is in its infancy. Further experimental analysis of the cytokine network should hopefully lead to the development of therapies or treatments to decrease many of the complications associated with anesthesia and surgery that are cytokine mediated.

IMMUNOLOGIC SEQUELAE OF SURGERY AND TRAUMA

Sepsis and the ensuing multiple organ failure cause 78% of late non-neurologic deaths associated with traumatic injury.[114] In this regard, trauma can be considered a multisystem disease. A great deal has been learned in the past 15 years about the role of the inflammatory and immunologic responses to traumatic injury. Recently, the relation between cellular inflammatory mediators, the neuroendocrine system, and nonspecific and specific immunity has further advanced the understanding of this complex area. Disruption of homeostasis following major elective surgery and major illness, as well as major traumatic injury, tends to produce a fairly similar pathologic response. Factors affecting the patient's premorbid host resistance and preinjury nutritional status are balanced against the extent of shock, tissue injury, and disruption of normal physiology that occurs with trauma. Following injury, various immune factors (i.e. cytokines, prostaglandins, coagulation factors, and toxic factors) affect the critical elements of gas exchange, energy metabolism, wound healing, and host resistance (Fig. 23.4).

A shock-producing insult results in a disruption of cellular potassium and sodium balance, leading to cell swelling.[115] The inflammatory

Trauma shock

Vasoactive factors
- Histamine
- Bradykinin
- C3a, C5a
- Prostanoids
- PAF
- Serotonin
- Leukotrienes
- Thromboxane A_2

Membrane dysfunction
↑ Capillary permeability

Chemotactic factors
- Cytokines
- LTB_4
- C5a

Recruitment and stimulation of inflammatory cells

Acute response
- PMNs
- Thrombocytes

Delayed response
- Macrophages
- Lymphocytes
- Plasma cells

Figure 23.4 *Trigger points of the inflammatory acute-phase response. LTB_4, leukotriene B_4; PMN, polymorphonuclear cell or neutrophil; PAF, platelet-activating factor.*

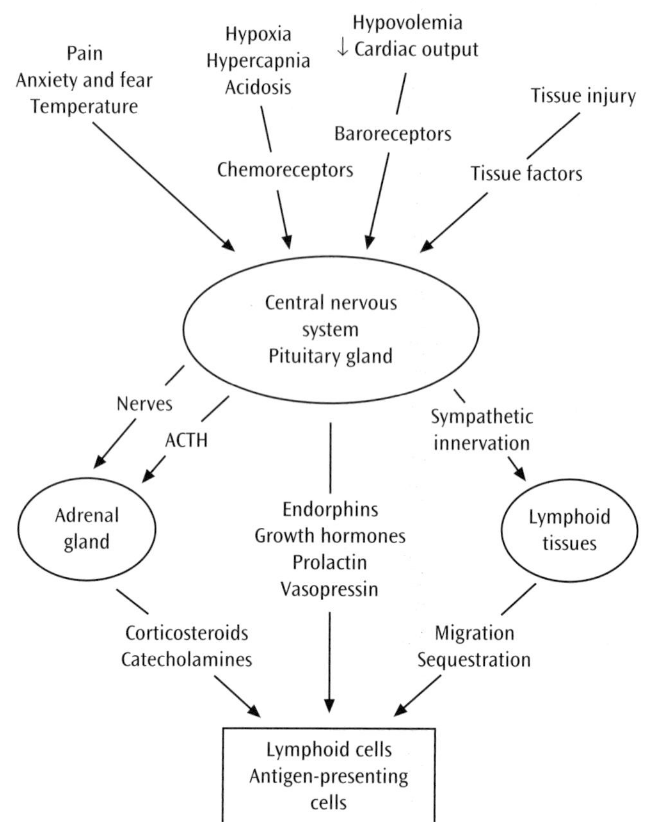

Figure 23.5 *The neuroendocrine response to injury. ACTH, adrenocorticotrophic hormone.*

mediators, such as TNF, platelet-activating factor (PAF), leukotrienes, and thromboxane A_2, have been implicated in the induction of this membrane dysfunction. In acute respiratory distress syndrome (ARDS) patients, O_2 consumption increases as O_2 delivery is augmented.[116] This increased O_2 consumption occurs despite the depression of peripheral O_2 extraction. Furthermore, O_2 demand and the arterial lactate concentration are both elevated. Injury also causes dramatic and complex changes in the neuroendocrine system, as shown in Fig. 23.5. For example, shock induces massive sympathetic output of norepinephrine (noradrenaline) and epinephrine (adrenaline) via the baroreceptor reflex. In turn, adrenocorticotropic hormone (ACTH) secreted from the pituitary promotes the release of glucocorticoids and, as a result, insulin levels fall and hyperglycemia is seen early after injury, in association with a relative "insulin resistance." There is extensive interaction between the hypothalamic–pituitary–adrenal axis (HPA) and the immune system, thus supporting the thesis that a two-way communication occurs between the site of injury and the central nervous system (CNS).[117]

Postinjury immune dysfunction

Various types of immune dysfunction have been identified following injury.[101] The hypothesis derived from these studies is that major trauma produces immunosuppression that can be further exacerbated by later-occurring sepsis. Faist *et al.*[118] demonstrated that T-cell numbers decreased in trauma patients; however, this reduction in T cells was primarily in the helper ($CD4^+$) rather than in the suppressor ($CD8^+$) cell population. In addition, IL-2 production and IL-2 receptor expression by TH cells was also decreased. These findings have been recently confirmed in other clinical[119] and experimental studies of shock and sepsis.[120] Interestingly, the production of IL-2 *in vitro* could be augmented by blocking PGE_2 production with the cyclo-oxygenase inhibitor indomethacin.

Severe head trauma carries a high risk of mortality and morbidity despite progress in its clinical management. In the USA, approximately 500 000 patients (median age 25 years) with traumatic brain injury (TBI) require hospitalization annually.[121] Moreover, patients surviving the initial insult have a mortality rate of greater than 30% during their intensive care period, and long-term survivors are confronted with neurobehavioral as well as socioeconomic consequences.[122] The high rate of secondary morbidity and mortality after TBI has been attributed to the post-traumatic inflammatory response within the intracranial compartment.[123] The resulting cerebral edema causes increased intracranial pressure (ICP) and loss of autoregulation of cerebral blood flow.[124] Post-traumatic cerebral ischemia and the intracranial release of neurotoxic mediators also contribute to delayed neuronal cell death.[125] Nonetheless, the inflammatory response of the injured brain also has beneficial effects, in terms of post-traumatic induction of neurotrophic factors, locally.[126] In this regard, clinical and experimental studies have shown that proinflammatory cytokines, such as IL-1β,[127] IL-6, and IL-8,[128] induce the production of the neurotrophin nerve growth factor within the injured CNS. The balance between the detrimental and the beneficial aspects of cerebral inflammation after TBI, however, remains to be determined.

Clinical impact and future directions

Inflammation and infection leading to organ dysfunction and failure continue to be the major problems after injury and operations, and in intensive care for many diseases and other conditions. When the systemic inflammatory response (SIRS) develops into multiple-organ distress syndrome (MODS) and multiple-organ failure (MOF), the mortality rate increases, ranging from 30% to 80%. Prospective, randomized, double-blind clinical trials are required to document the efficacy of various therapeutic agents. In this regard, many, if not all, such studies of single "magic bullets" have unfortunately not provided promising results.[129] Recent clinical studies are providing new insight into the treatment of severely injured patients. Prophylaxis with sucralfate or omeprazole is commonly used for the complication of gastrointestinal stress bleeding and it appears to be the best treatment in severely injured or ICU patients.[130] In contrast, treatment with ranitidine may increase infectious complications in trauma patients.[131] Patients with ARDS requiring ventilator support also benefit from rotational kinetic therapy.[132] With regard to head trauma, the use of hypertonic solutions appears to be of specific value as such solutions do not increase, and tend to decrease, intracranial pressure.[133]

The compensatory mechanisms of the body to survive overwhelming trauma are usually insufficient. The primary clinical goal of immunotherapy following trauma should, therefore, be to control the development of a SIRS and prevent subsequent sepsis. Ideally, the intervention employed needs to prevent SIRS from becoming a progressive nonreversible destructive inflammatory response (Fig. 23.6). Furthermore, the intervention/immunomodulation has to be employed in a calculated preventive fashion as early as possible following trauma and should encompass multiple cellular targets (e.g. lymphocytes, macrophages, granulocytes, and endothelial cells) to protect the host from cell hyperactivation and cell exhaustion. Crucial issues within the complex field of preventive immunotherapy for the control of SIRS and sepsis include patient selection, timing of administration of agents, controlled modulation of the inflammatory responses, and cost.

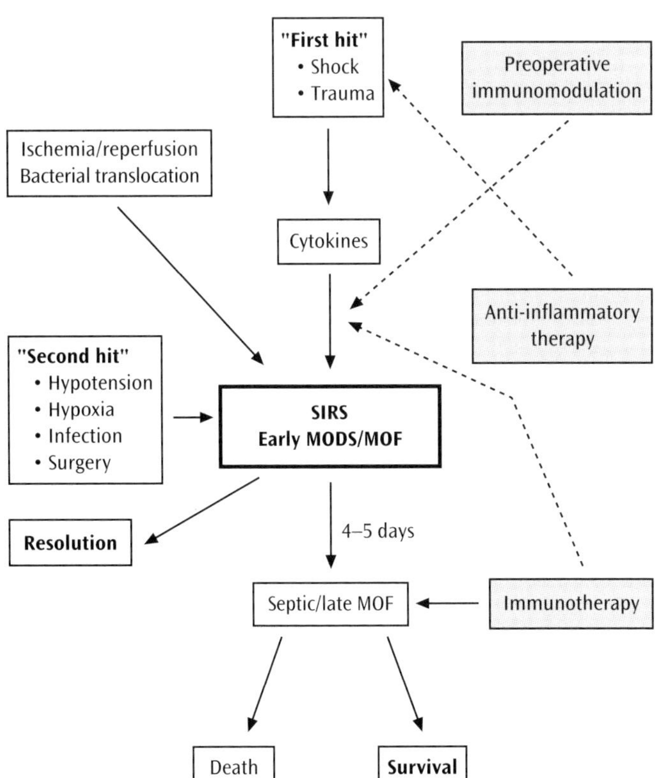

Figure 23.6 *Therapeutic strategies to prevent postinjury multiple-organ failure (MOF). MODS, multiple-organ dysfunction syndrome; SIRS, systemic inflammatory response syndrome.*

New surgical techniques and immune function

Open surgery has been recognized as causing a temporary impairment in cell-mediated immunity. Therefore, since immune function is greatly affected by the neuroendocrine response to trauma,[134] and laparoscopic surgery causes less tissue injury and pain than open surgery,[135] it is conceivable that laparoscopic surgery could result in a less pronounced stress-mediated effect on postoperative immune function. The success of laparoscopic cholecystectomy has encouraged surgeons to develop similar, alternative approaches to many operations that previously required incision into the chest or abdomen. In many cases, laparoscopic techniques are easier on patients because they produce smaller incisions and allow more rapid recovery and shorter hospital stays. Surgical laparoscopic techniques also minimize transfusion needs, thereby having less effect on immune responses. Improved operative field visualization, coupled with the knowledge that extra care must be taken in dissection through a minimal-access port, has resulted in reduced blood loss from laparoscopic procedures compared with open techniques.

Senagore *et al.*[136] compared 140 elective colonic resections for both benign and malignant disease; 102 patients underwent open procedures and 38 underwent laparoscopic procedures. Blood loss was significantly decreased with the laparoscopic approach compared with open surgery. In addition, Arbogast *et al.*[137] reported the successful use of laparoscopic-assisted hysterectomy as an alternative to open techniques. In this study, patients undergoing the laparoscopic-assisted procedure had significantly less blood loss than patients undergoing surgery using open techniques. Experimentally, Berguer *et al.*[138] compared laparoscopic fundoplication to open surgery in the rat and found lower adrenocortical hormone levels and better preserved TH-cell activation.

Recently developed laser techniques may either reduce or increase bleeding, depending on the disease treated and operation performed. Wyman and Rogers[139] performed a prospective, randomized trial comparing a neodymium yttrium–aluminum–garnet (YAG) laser scalpel with a conventional scalpel in 40 women undergoing modified radical mastectomy. Operative blood loss was significantly reduced with laser surgery. However, the mean operating time was approximately 25 min longer, thus leading the authors to question the use of the laser scalpel techniques for such surgery.

Although it appears that a systemic immune benefit exists for minimal invasive techniques, further clinical studies are needed to fully evaluate the regional immune responses to the new surgical procedures.

CONCLUSIONS

The prime function of the anesthesiologist remains the minimization and alleviation of pain and anxiety of patients undergoing surgical operations, with general or regional anesthesia, while maintaining physiologic homeostasis. Thus, during routine anesthetic and surgical practice, alterations in the immune response may pass unnoticed. An understanding of the immune system may not appear important on the surface; however, there is still an unacceptably high incidence of postoperative morbidity and mortality associated with infections and systemic activation of the inflammatory response. Numerous predisposing factors such as gender, age, pre-existing diseases, nutritional status, and socioeconomic background of the patient can influence the immunologic response and therefore outcome following anesthesia and surgery. Appropriate recognition and identification of those factors is likely to be helpful for the care and better management of patients. More attention needs to be directed toward understanding specific control and modulation of immune responses under such conditions. Clinical application of this new knowledge, as it is obtained, should provide improved outcomes following anesthesia and surgery.

A better knowledge of immunology will be helpful for anesthesiologists and particularly for those in the intensive care setting. Furthermore, the effect of current anesthetic agents on immune responses should continue to be systematically evaluated. Additionally, with the introduction of new anesthetic agents and surgical procedures, studies should be undertaken to determine the immunologic consequences of their use.

Acknowledgments

This work was supported by NIH grant GM 37127.

REFERENCES

1. Rubin G. The influence of alcohol, ether and chloroform on natural immunity in relation to leukocytosis and phagocytosis. *J Infect Dis* 1904; **1:** 425–44.
2. Smith CJ, Edwards AE, Gower, DE, *et al.* Leucocyte migration: effects of *in vitro* response to anesthetic agents: possible potentiation of effects by adrenaline. *Eur J Anesthesiol* 1992; **9:** 463–72.
3. Brown SM, Stimmel B, Taub RN, *et al.* Immunologic dysfunction in heroin addicts. *Arch Int Med* 1974; **134:** 1000–6.
4. Tonnesen E, Wahlgreen C. Influence of extradural and general anesthesia on natural killer cell activity and lymphocyte subpopulations in patients undergoing hysterectomy. *Br J Anesth* 1988; **60:** 500–7.
5. Woods GM, Griffiths DM. Reversible inhibition of natural killer cell activity by volatile anesthetic agents in vitro. *J Anesth* 1986; **58:** 535–9.
6. Markovic SN, Knight PR, Murasko, DM. Inhibition of interferon stimulation of natural killer cell activity in mice anesthetized with halothane or isoflurane (with an editorial). *Anesthesiology* 1993; **78:** 700–6.
7. Mandler RN, Biddison WE, Mandler R, Serrate SA. β-Endorphin augments the cytolytic activity and interferon production of natural killer cells. *J Immunol* 1986; **136:** 934–9.
8. Beilin B, Shavit Y, Hart J, *et al.* Effects of anesthesia based on large versus small doses of fentanyl on natural killer cell cytotoxicity in the perioperative period. *Anesth Analg* 1996; **82:** 492–7.
9. Crary B, Hauser SL, Borysenko M, *et al.* Epinephrine-induced changes in the distribution of lymphocyte subsets in peripheral blood of humans. *J Immunol* 1983; **131:** 1178–81.
10. Nomoto Y, Jhonokosi H, Karasawa S. Natural killer cell activity and lymphocyte subpopulations during dobutamine infusion in man. *Br J Anesth* 1993; **71:** 218–21.
11. O'Donnell NG, McSharry CP, Wilkinson PC, Asbury AJ. Comparison of the inhibitory effect of propofol, thiopentone and midazolam on neutrophil polarisation in vitro in the presence or absence of human serum albumin. *Br J Anesth* 1992; **69:** 70–4.
12. Jensen AG, Dahlgren C, Eintrei C. Propofol decreases random and chemotactic stimulated locomotion of human neutrophils *in vitro*. *Br J Anesth* 1993; **70:** 99–100.
13. Sharp BM, Keane WF, Suh HJ, *et al.* Opioid peptides rapidly stimulate superoxide production by human polymorphonuclear leukocytes and macrophages. *Endocrinology* 1985; **117:** 793–5.
14. Van Epps DE, Saland L. β-Endorphin and metenkephalin stimulate human peripheral blood mononuclear cell chemotaxis. *J Immunol* 1984; **132:** 3046–53.
15. Nakagawara M, Takeshijz K, Takamatsu J, *et al.* Inhibition of superoxide production and Ca^{2+} mobilization in human neutrophils by halothane, enflurane, and isoflurane. *Anesthesiology* 1986; **64:** 4–12.
16. Kellermann W, Rothe G, Briegel J, *et al.* Deterioration of respiratory burst of polymorphonuclear neutrophils by propofol. *Anesthesiology*, 1993; **79:** 430.
17. Kress HG, Eberlein T, Hörber B, Weis KH. Suppression of neutrophil migration and chemiluminescence is due to the sulphur atom in the thiobarbiturate molecule. *Acta Anaesthesiol Scand*, 1989; **33:** 122–8.
18. Davidson JAH, Boom SJ, Pearsall FJ, *et al.* Comparison of the effects of four iv anesthetic agents on polymorphonuclear leucocyte function. *Br J Anesth* 1995; **74:** 315–18.
19. Lopker A, Abood LG, Hoss W, Lionetti FJ. Stereoselective muscarinic acetylcholine and opiate receptors in human phagocytic leukocytes. *Biochem Pharmacol* 1980; **29:** 1361–5.
20. Lewis RE, Cruse JM, Hazelwood J. Halothane-induced suppression of cell-mediated immunity in normal and tumor-bearing $C3H_f$/He mice. *Anesth Analg* 1980; **59:** 666–71.
21. Vose BM, Moudgil GC. Effect of surgery on tumor-directed leukocyte responses. *Br Med J* 1975; **1:** 56–8.
22. Moore TC, Spruck CH, Leduc LE. Depression of lymphocyte traffic in sheep by anaesthesia and associated changes in efferent lymph PGE_2 and antibody levels. *Immunology* 1988; **63:** 139–43.
23. Espanol T, Todd GB, Soothill JF. The effect of anaesthesia on the lymphocyte response to phytohemagluttin. *Clin Exp Immunol* 1974; **18:** 73–9.
24. Cullen BF, Van Belle G. Lymphoctye transformation and and changes in leococyte count: effects of anesthesia and operation. *Anesthesiology* 1975; **43:** 563–9.
25. Hole A, Unsguard G, Breivik H. Monocyte function is depressed during and after surgery after general anaesthetia but not under epidural anaesthesia. *Acta Anaesthesiol Scand* 1982; **26:** 301–7.
26. Whelan P, Morris RJ. Immunological responsiveness after transurethral resection of the prostate *Clin Exp Immunol* 1982; **48:** 611–18.
27. McCain HW, Lamster IB, Bozzone JM, Grbic JT. β-Endorphin modulates human immune activity via non-opiate receptor mechanisms. *Life Sci* 1982; **31:** 1619–24.
28. Pirttikangas CO, Perttila J, Salo M. Propofol emulsion reduces proliferative responses of lymphocytes from intensive care patients. *Intensive Care Med* 1993; **19:** 299–302.
29. Pirttikangas CO, Perttila J, Salo M, *et al.* Propofol infusion anesthesia and immune response in minor surgery. *Anesthesia* 1994; **49:** 13–16.
30. Suttmann H, Doenicke A, Bretz C, *et al.* Einfluss der Narkose auf humorale Parameter. *Beitr Anaesthesiol Intensivmed* 1982; **1:** 39–65.
31. Koenig A, Koenig UD, Stoeckel H. Anesthesia and immunology. *Prakt Anaesth* 1978; **31:** 415–29.
32. Braun SR, Levin AB, Clark KL. Role of corticosteroids in the development of pneumonia in mechanically ventilated head-trauma victims. *Crit Care Med* 1986; **14:** 198–201.
33. Salo M. Effects of lignocaine and bubicavaine on immunoglobulin synthesis *in-vitro*. *Eur J Anesthesiol* 1990; **7:** 133–140.
34. Schmidt RM, Rosenkranz HS. Antimicrobial activity of local anesthetics: lidocaine and procaine. *J Infect Dis* 1970; **121:** 597–607.
35. Lowry, RP, Takeucki, T. *The Th1,Th2 Paradigm and Transplantation Tolerance*. Austin, TX: R G Landes, 1994.
36. McBride WT, Armstrong MA, Crockard AD, *et al.* Selective reduction in leukocyte antigen expression following high dose fentanyl administration at cardiac surgery. *Br J Anesth* 1994; **73:** 717P–718P.
37. Blumberg N, Heal JM. Effects of transfusion on immune function, cancer, recurrence and infection. *Arch Pathol Lab Med* 1994; **118:** 371–9.
38. Blumberg N, Heal JM. Immunomodulation by blood transfusion: an evolving scientific and clinical challenge. Am J Med 1996; **101:** 299–308.
39. Calzolari A. Recherches experimentales sur un rapport probable entre la function du thymus et celle des testicules. *Arch Ital Biol* 1898; **30:** 71–7.
40. Bone RC. Toward an epidemiology and natural history of SIRS (systemic inflammatory response syndrome). *JAMA* 1992; **268:** 3452–5.
41. McGowan JE, Barnes MW, Finland N. Bacteremia at Boston City Hospital: occurrence and mortality during 12 selected years (1935–1972) with special reference to hospital-acquired cases. *J Infect Dis* 1975; **132:** 316–35.
42. Homo-Delarche F, Fitzpatrick F, Christeff N, *et al.* Sex steroids, glucocorticoids, stress and autoimmunity. *J Steroid Biochem Mol Biol* 1991; **40:** 619–37.
43. Zellweger R, Ayala A, Stein S, *et al.* Females in proestrus state tolerate sepsis better than males. *Surg Forum* 1995; **46:** 65–7.
44. Wichmann MW, Ayala A, Chaudry IH. Male sex steroids are responsible for depressing macrophage immune function after trauma-hemorrhage. *Am J Physiol* 1997; **273:** C1335–C1340.
45. Luster MI, Pfeifer RW, Tucker AN. Influence of sex hormones on immunoregulation with specific reference to natural and environmental estrogens. In: Thomas JA, Korach KS, McLachlan JA (eds). *Endocrine Toxicology*. New York: Raven Press, 1985: 67–83.
46. Viselli SM, Stanziale S, Shults K, *et al.* Castration alters peripheral immune function in normal male mice. *Immunology* 1995; **84:** 337–42.
47. Olsen NJ, Kovacs WJ. Gonadal steroids and immunity. *Endocr Rev* 1996; **17:** 369–84.
48. Olsen NJ, Kovacs WJ. Case report: Testosterone treatment of systemic lupus erythematosus in a patient with Klinefelter's syndrome. *Am J Med Sci* 1995; **310:** 158–60.
49. Zellweger R, Wichmann MW, Ayala A, *et al.* Females in proestrus state maintain splenic immune functions and tolerate sepsis better than males. *Crit Care Med* 1997; **25** (1): 106–10.
50. Grossman CJ, Roselle GA. The control of immune response by endocrine

factors and the clinical significance of such regulation. *Proc Clin Biochem Med* 1986; **4:** 9–56.

51. Butterworth MB, McClellan B, Alansmith M. Influence of sex on immunoglobin levels. *Nature* 1967; **214:** 1224–5.
52. Ainbender E, Weisinger R, Hevizy M, Hodes HL. Difference in immunoglobulin class of polio antibody in the serum of men and women. *J Immunol* 1968; **101:** 92–8.
53. Terres G, Morrison SL, Habicht GS. A quantitative difference in the immune response between male and female mice. *Proc Soc Exp Biol Med* 1968; **127:** 664–7.
54. Grossman CJ. Possible underlying mechanisms of sexual dimorphism in the immune response, fact and hypothesis. *J Steroid Biochem* 1989; **34:** 241–51.
55. Shen GK, Montgomery DW, Ulrich ED, *et al.* Up-regulation of prolactin gene expression and feedback modulation of lymphocyte proliferation during acute allograft rejection. *Surgery* 1992; **112:** 387–94.
56. Athreya BH, Pletcher J, Zulian F, *et al.* Subset-specific effects of sex hormones and pituitary gonadotropins on human lymphocyte proliferation *in vitro. Clin Immunol Immunopathol* 1993; **66:** 201–11.
57. Brouwers JRBJ, Assies J, Wiersinga WM, *et al.* Plasma prolactin levels after acute and subchronic oral administration of domperidone and of metoclopramide: a cross-over study in healthy volunteers. *Clin Endocrinol* 1980; **12:** 435–40.
58. Zhu XH, Zellweger R, Wichmann MW, *et al.* Effects of prolactin and metoclopramide on macrophage cytokine gene expression in late sepsis. *Cytokine* 1997; **9:** 437–46.
59. Zellweger R, Zhu XH, Wichmann MW, *et al.* Prolactin administration following hemorrhagic shock improves macrophage cytokine release capacity and decreases mortality from subsequent sepsis. *J Immunol* 1996; **157:** 5748–54.
60. De M, Sanford TR, Wood GW. Interleukin-1, interleukin-6, and tumor necrosis factor α are produced in the mouse uterus during the estrous cycle and are induced by estrogen and progesterone. *Dev Biol* 1992; **151:** 297–305.
61. Ahmed SA, Penhale WJ, Talal N. Sex hormones, immune responses, and autoimmune diseases: review article. *Am J Pathol* 1985; **121:** 531–51.
62. Chandra RK. Nutrition, immunity, and infection: present knowledge and future directions. Lancet 1983: 688–91.
63. Chandra RK. Nutrition, immunity, and outcome. Past, present, and future. 11th Gopalan Gold Medal Oration. *Nutr Res* 1988; **8:** 132–46.
64. Bendich A, Chandra RK (eds). Micronutrient Effects on Immunologic Functions. New York: New York Academy of Sciences, 1990.
65. Chandra RK. Excess intake of zinc impairs immune responses JAMA, 1989 **252:** 1443–6.
66. Chandra RK. Immunocompetence is a sensitive and functional barometer of nutritional status. *Acta Paediatr Scand* 1991; **374** (Suppl.): 129–32.
67. Kelley DS, Branch, LB, Iacono, JM. Nutritional modulation of human immune system. *Nutr Res* 1989; **9:** 965–75.
68. Kelley DS, Dougherty, RM, Branch LB, *et al.* Concentration of dietary n-6 polyunsaturated fatty acids and the human immune status. *Clin Immunol Immunopathol* 1992; **62:** 240–4.
69. Meydani SN, Lichtenstein AH, Cornwall S, *et al.* Immunological effects of low fat high polyunsaturated fatty acid (NCEP – Step 2) diets on immune response of humans. *FASEB* 1992; **J**6: A1370.
70. Barone J, Hebert JR, Reddy MM. Dietary fat and natural-killer-cell activity. *Am J Clin Nutr* 1989; **50:** 861–7.
71. Rasmussen L B, Liens B, Pederson BD, Richer EA. Effect of diet and plasma fatty acid composition on immune status of elderly men. *Am J Clin Nutr* 1994; **59:** 572–7.
72. Daly JM, Lieberman MD, Goldfine J, *et al.* Enteral nutrition with supplemental arginine, RNA, and omega-3 fatty acids in patients after operation: immunologic, metabolic, and clinical outcome. *Surgery* 1992; **112:** 56–67.
73. Chandra RK. Effect of vitamin and trace-element supplementation on immune responses and infection in elderly subjects. *Lancet* 1992; **340:** 1124–7.
74. Moore F, Feliciano D, Andrassy R, *et al.* Enteral feeding reduces postoperative septic complications. *J Parenter Enteral Nutr* 1991; **15** (Suppl.): 225.
75. Clarke PJ, Ball MJ, Kettlewell MGW. Liver function tests in patients receiving parenteral nutrition. *J Parenter Enteral Nutr* 1991; **15:** 54–9.
76. Muller JM, Keller HW, Brenner V, *et al.* Indications and effects of preoperative parenteral nutrition. *World J Surg* 1986; **10:** 53–63.
77. Detsky AS, Baker JP, O'Rourke K, Goel V. Perioperative parenteral nutrition: a meta-analysis. *Ann Int Med* 1987; **107:** 195–203.
78. Maynard ND, Bihari DJ. Postoperative feeding. *Br Med J* 1991; **303:** 1007–8.
79. Meta-analysis of the Digestive Tract Trialists' Collaborative Group. Selective decontamination of the digestive tract. *Br Med J* 1993; **307:** 525–32.
80. Newsholme EA, Parry-Billings M. Properties of glutamine release from muscle and its importance for the immune system. *J Parenter Enteral Nutr* 1990; **14:** 635–75.
81. Kirk SJ, Barbul A. Role of arginine in trauma, sepsis and immunity. *J Parenter Enteral Nutr* 1990; **14:** 2265–95.
82. Crist DM, Peake GT, Loftfield RB, *et al.* Supplemental growth hormone alters body composition, muscle protein metabolism and serum lipids in fit adults: characterization of dose-dependent and response-recovery effect. *Mech Aging Dev* 1991; **58:** 191–205.
83. Weigent DA, Baxter JB, Wear WE, *et al.* Production of immunoreactive growth hormone by mononuclear leukocytes. *FASEB* 1988; **J**2: 2812–18.
84. Rudman D. Growth hormone, body composition, and aging. *J Am Geriatr Soc* 1985; **33:** 800–7.
85. Rudman D, Feller AG, Nagraj HS, *et al.* Effects on human growth hormone in men over 60 years old. *N Engl J Med* 1990; **323:** 1–6.
86. Forbes GB, Reina JC. Adult lean body mass declines with age: some longitudinal observations. *Metabolism* 1970; **19:** 653–63.
87. Roubenoff R, Rall LC. Humoral mediation of changing body composition during aging and chronic inflammation. *Nutr Rev* 1993; **51:** 1–11.
88. Broughton DL, James OFW, Alberti KGMM, Taylor R. Peripheral and hepatic insulin sensitivity in healthy elderly human subjects. *Eur J Clin Invest* 1991; **21:** 13–21.
89. Muravchik S. The aging process: anesthetic implications. *Acta Anaesthesiologica Belgica* 1998; **49** (2): 85–90.
90. Miller LC, Lynch EA, Isa S, *et al.* Balance of synovial fluid IL-1β and IL-1 receptor antagonist and recovery from Lyme arthritis. *Lancet* 1993; **341:** 146–8.
91. Tonnesen E, Wanscher M, Hohndorf K, *et al.* Effect of methylprednisolone on the cytokine response in patients undergoing lung surgery. *Acta Anaesthesiol Scand* 1993; **37:** 410–14.
92. Latah N, Zlotnick AY, Shtiller R, *et al.* Serum levels of IL-1, IL-6 and TNF in patients undergoing coronary artery bypass grafts of cholecystectomy. *Clin Exp Immunol* 1992; **89:** 255–60.
93. Kawamura T, Wakusawa R, Okada K, Inada S. Elevation of cytokines during open heart surgery with cardiopulmonary bypass: participation of interleukin 8 and 6 in reperfusion injury. *Can J Anesth* 1993; **40:** 1016–21.
94. Hill GE, Diego, RP, Stammers, AH, *et al.* Aprotinin enhances the endogenous release of Interleukin-10 after cardiac operations. *Ann Thorac Surg* 1998; **65:** 66–9.
95. Galley HF, Dubbels AM, Webster NR. The effect of midazolam and propofol on interleukin-8 from human polymorphonuclear leukocytes. *Anesth Analg* 1998; **86:** 1289–93.
96. Hall GM, Desborough JP. Interleukin-6 and the metabolic response to surgery. *Br J Anesth* 1992; **69:** 337–8.
97. Libert C, Vink A, Coulie P, Brouckaert P, *et al.* Limited involvement of interleukin-6 in the pathogenesis of lethal septic shock as revealed by the effect of monoclonal antibodies against interleukin-6 or its receptor in various murine models. *Eur J Immunol* 1992; **22:** 2625–30.
98. Crozier TA, Muller JE, Quittkat D, *et al.* Effect of anesthesia on the cytokine responses to abdominal surgery. *Br J Anesth* 1994; **72:** 280–5.
99. Kavelaars A, Ballieux, RE, Heijnen CJ. Differential effects of β-endorphin on cAMP levels in human peripheral blood mononuclear cells. *Brain Behav Immun* 1990; **4:** 171–9.
100. Zhang Y, Lin J-X, Vilcek J. Synthesis of interleukin-6 in human fibroblasts is triggered by an increase of intracellular cyclic AMP. *J Biol Chem* 1988; **263:** 6177–82.
101. Chaudry IH, Ayala A (eds). *Immunological Aspects of Hemorrhage: Medical Intelligence Unit*, Austin, TX: R G Landes Co, 1992: 1–132.
102. Rossano F, Tufano R, Cipollaro De L'Ero G, *et al.* Anesthetic agents induce human mononuclear leukocytes to release cytokines. *Immunopharmacol Immunotoxicol* 1992; **14:** 439–50.
103. Haeffner-Cavaillon N, Roussellier N, Ponzio O, *et al.* Induction of interleukin-1 production in patients undergoing cardiopulmonary bypass. *J Thor Cardiovasc Surg* 1989; **98:** 1100–6.
104. Markewitz A, Faist E, Lang S, *et al.* Regulation of acute phase response after cardiopulmonary bypass by immunomodulation. *Ann Thoracic Surg* 1993; **55:** 389–94.
105. Hartman DA, Ochalski SJ, Carlson RP. The effects of anti-inflammatory and antiallergic drugs on the release of IL-1β and TNF-α in the human whole blood assay. *Agents Actions* 1993; **39:** C70–C72.
106. Petty HR, Martin SM. Combinative ligand-receptor interactions: effects

of cAMP, epinephrine and met-enkephalin on RAW264 macrophage morphology, spreading, adherence and microfilaments. *J Cell Physiol* 1989; **138:** 247–56.

107. Shimizu Y, Newman W, Tanaka Y, Shaw S. Lymphocyte interactions with endothelial cells. *Immunol Today* 1992; **13:** 106–12.
108. Donnelly SC, Strieter RM, Kunkel SL, *et al.* Interleukin-8 and development of adult respiratory distress syndrome in at-risk groups. *Lancet* 1993; **341:** 643–7.
109. Suter PM, Suter S, Girardin E, *et al.* High bronchoalveolar lavage levels of tumor necrosis factor and its inhibitors, interleukin-1, interferon, and elastase in patients with adult respiratory distress syndrome after trauma, shock or sepsis. *Am Rev Respir Dis* 1992; **145:** 1016–22.
110. Donnelly SC, Haslett C, Dransfield I, *et al.* Role of selectins in development of adult respiratory distress syndrome. *Lancet* 1994; **344:** 215–19.
111. Boxer, L A, Bjorksten, B, Bjork, *et al.* Neutropenia induced by systemic infusion of lactoferrin. *J Lab Clin Med*, 1982; **99:** 886–872.
112. Bazzoni G, Beltran Nunez A, Mascellani G, *et al.* Effect of heparin, dermatan sulfate, and related oligo-derivatives on human polymorphonuclear leukocyte functions. *J Lab Clin Med* 1993; **121:** 268–75.
113. McBride WT, Armstrong MA, Crockard AD, *et al.* Selective reduction in leucocyte antigen expression following high dose fentanyl administration at cardiac surgery. *Br J Anesth* 1994; **73:** 717P–718P.
114. Baker CC, Oppenheimer L, Lewis FR, Trunkey DD. The epidemiology of trauma death. *Am J Surg* 1980; **140:** 144–50.
115. Sayeed MM, Adler, RJ, Chaudry, IH, Baue, AE. Effect of hemorrhagic shock on hepatic transmembrane potentials and intracellular electrolytes, in vivo. *Am J Physiol*, 1981; **240:** R211-R219.
116. Tuchschmidt J, Oblitas, D, Fried, JC, Oxygen consumption in sepsis and septic shock. *Crit Care Med*, 1991; **19:** 664–671.
117. Lilly MP, Gann, DS. The hypothalamic-pituitary-adrenal immune axis. *Arch Surg*, 1992; **127:** 1463.
118. Faist E, Ertel W, Salmen, B, *et al.* The immune-enhancing effect of perioperative thymopentin administration in elderly patients undergoing major surgery. *Arch* Surg, 1988; **123:** 1449–53.
119. McRitchie DI, Girotti MJ, Rotstein OD, Teodorczyk-Injeyan JA. Impaired antibody production in blunt trauma. *Arch Surg* 1990; **125:** 91–6.
120. Zellweger R, Ayala A, DeMaso CM, Chaudry IH. Trauma-hemorrhage causes prolonged depression in cellular immunity. *Shock* 1995; **4:** 149–53.
121. Jennett B. Epidemiology of head injury. *J Neurol Neurosurg Psychiatry* 1996; **60:** 362–9.
122. Ashley MJ, Persel CS, Clark MC, Krych DK. Long term follow-up of post acute traumatic brain injury rehabilitation: a statistical analysis to test for stability and predictability of outcome. *Brain Inj* 1997; **11:** 677–90.
123. Holmin S, Söderlund J, Biberfeld P, Mathisen T. Intracerebral inflammation after human brain contusion. *NeuroSurg* 1998; **42:** 291–9.
124. Regel G, Lehmann U, Rickels E, *et al.* Pathophysiology, management and outcome after multiple trauma. In: Schlag G, Redl H, Traber D (eds). *Brain Damage Secondary to Hemorrhagic-Traumatic Shock, Sepsis and Traumatic Brain Injury*. Berlin: Springer, 1996: 229–262.
125. Wieloch T. Mechanisms of neuronal death. In: von Wild KRH (ed.). *Pathophysiological Principles and Controversies in Neurointensive Care.* Munich: Zuckschwerdt, 1998: 3–14.
126. Meyer M. Neurotrophins: aspects of their in vivo action and physiology. In: Rothwell NJ (ed.). *Immune Responses in the Nervous System*. Oxford: Bios Scientific Publishers, 1995: 101–16.
127. DeKosky ST, Styren SD, O'Malley ME, *et al.* Interleukin-1 receptor antagonist suppresses neurotrophin response in injured rat brain. *Ann Neurol* 1996; **39:** 123–7.
128. Kossmann T, Stahel PF, Lenzlinger PM, *et al.* Interleukin-8 released into the cerebrospinal fluid after brain injury is associated with blood–brain barrier dysfunction and nerve growth factor production. *J Cerebral Blood Flow Metab* 1997; **17:** 280–9.
129. Baue AE. Multiple organ failure, multiple organ dysfunction syndrome, and the systemic inflammatory response syndrome: why no magic bullets? *Arch Surg* 1997; **132:** 703–7.
130. Phillips JO, Metzler MH, Palmieri MTL, *et al.* Prospective study of simplified omeprazole suspension for the prophylaxis of stress-related mucosal damage. *Crit Care Med* 1996; **24** (11): 1793–1800.
131. O'Keefe GE, Gentilello LM, Maier RV. Incidence of infectious complications associated with the use of histamine 2-receptor antagonists in critically ill trauma patients. *Ann Surg* 1998; **227** (1): 120–5.
132. Badia JR, Sala E, Rodriguez-Roisin R. Positional changes and drug interventions in acute respiratory failure. *Respirology* 1998; **3:** 103–6.
133. Shackford SR, Bourguignon R, Wald SL, *et al.* Hypertonic saline resuscitation of patients with head injury: a prospective, randomized clinical trial. *J Trauma* 1998; **44:** 50–8.
134. Cunnick JE, Lysle DT, Kucinski BJ, Rabin BS. Stress-induced alteration of immune function. Diversity of effects and mechanisms. *Ann NY Acad Sci* 1992; **650:** 283–7.
135. Troidl H, Spangenberger W, Langen R, *et al.* Laparoscopic cholecystectomy: technical performance safety and patient's benefit. *Endoscopy* 1992; **24:** 252–61.
136. Senagore AJ, Luchtefeld MA, Mackeigan JM, *et al.* Open colectomy versus laparoscopic colectomy: Are there differences? *Am Surg* 1993; **59:** 549–54.
137. Arbogast JD, Welch RA, Riza ED, *et al.* Laparoscopically assisted vaginal hysterectomy appears to be an alternative to total abdominal hysterectomy. *J Laparoendosc Surg* 1994; **4:** 185–90.
138. Berguer R, Dalton M, Ferrick D. Adrenocortical response and regional T-lymphocyte activation patterns following minimally invasive surgery in a rat model. *Surg Endosc* 1998; **12:** 236–40.
139. Wyman A, Rogers K. Randomized trial of laser scalpel for modified radical mastectomy. *Br J Surg* 1993; **80:** 871–3.

24

The endocrine system

ANTHONY WILTON

This chapter describes basic endocrine mechanisms at the cellular and subcellular levels. Building on these mechanisms, neuroendocrine control of the pituitary is then discussed. The hypothalamus–pituitary–adrenal and thyroid axes are emphasized, being of the most importance in anesthesia. Diseases of the adrenal and thyroid glands are reviewed. Finally, the rare disorders pheochromocytoma and carcinoid syndrome are summarized.

The prevalence of different endocrine disorders in a population is very variable. Aside from diabetes, the most common of the classical endocrine disorders are those of the thyroid gland. Thyroid disorders will be encountered by all anesthesiologists and the majority of cases will have been previously diagnosed and treated. Approximately 15% of cases of hyperthyroidism and 25% of hypothyroidism, however, remain undiagnosed and the majority of these are females.[1] Thyroid disorders, with the exception of the rare thyrotoxic crisis, are seldom life threatening during anesthesia. In contrast, the very rare disorder pheochromocytoma, which accounts for < 0.1% of all cases of hypertension, is diagnosed post mortem in 50% of cases.[2] A basic understanding of the normal function of the endocrine glands is essential for the diagnosis and management of their states of over- and underactivity and thus ensuring the safe anesthesia of patients with these disorders. This chapter summarizes selectively basic endocrine concepts and the components of the endocrine system of most relevance in anesthetic practice.

MECHANISM OF HORMONE ACTION

The action of a hormone on a target cell depends on the presence of specific receptors for that hormone. These receptors may be found on the cell membrane or intracellularly in the cytoplasmic or nuclear components. The chemical nature of individual hormones determines the type of receptors with which they interact. Peptide hormones and neurotransmitters, being lipid insoluble and hydrophobic, bind to cell membrane receptors. In contrast, the lipid-soluble thyroid hormones, steroid hormones, and vitamin D traverse the phospholipid plasma membrane and bind to intracellular receptors. This binding of the hormone to a receptor is the first event in the process by which an extracellular signal produces an intracellular response. This process, called signal transduction, differs between cell membrane receptor–hormone binding and intracellular receptor–hormone binding.[3]

CELL MEMBRANE RECEPTORS

Peptide hormones and neurotransmitters act via the generation of second messengers. These are generated when the first messenger, the hormone, interacts with membrane receptors on target cells and they mediate the effects of the hormone on gene expression.[4] Receptors play two roles in the transduction process. First, they bind with high affinity and specificity the extracellular signaling hormone molecule. Second, they relay the information inherent in the hormone to intracellular sites. The diversity of structure of hormones that bind to membrane receptors ranges from small molecules, such as catecholamines, to large glycoprotein hormones and is accommodated by variation in the binding domains of receptors. Complementary deoxyribonucleic acid (cDNA) studies have revealed four common motifs for the structure of membrane receptors – seven transmembrane G-protein-coupled receptors, receptor-type ion channels, single transmembrane receptors possessing intrinsic enzyme activities, and transmembrane receptors that interact with other cellular proteins with enzyme activity. Similarly, the signal produced by hormone binding is transduced intracellularly via multiple effector pathways. Cyclic adenosine monophosphate (cAMP) is the prototypical second messenger, intracellular levels of which are largely determined by ligand–receptor interactions. This process involves the interaction of three cellular components near the plasma membrane – the ligand receptor, a signal transducer (G-protein) and the effector enzyme (adenylate cyclase). Signal specificity and diversity is governed by the heterogeneity of each of the components, i.e the existence of multiple receptors, G-proteins, and effector adenylate cyclases. The G-proteins are the actual signal transducers between the receptor and effectors in the plasma membrane. The general mechanism of G-protein-linked hormone activation of adenylate cyclase is well understood. G-proteins exist as heterotrimers consisting of three different subunits: α, β, and γ. The α subunits have a single high-affinity binding site for guanine nucleotides and also intrinsic guanosine triphosphatase (GTPase) activity. Hormone binding to a G-protein-linked receptor results in increased exchange of GTP for guanosine diphosphate (GDP) on the α subunit. This results in decreased affinity between the α, β, and γ subunits, allowing the α subunit (the active form of the G-protein) to dissociate. This dissociated active subunit activates effector systems such as ion channels, or intracellular enzymes such as adenylate cyclase. After interaction with the effector systems, the intrinsic GTPase activity in the α subunit hydrolyzes GTP to GDP, returning the G-protein to its inactive form after reassociation with the β–γ complex. In the case of adenylate cyclase, its activation results in a transient increase in intracellular cAMP levels, which activate protein kinase A. The latter phosphorylates a variety of cellular substrates, including the nuclear transcription factors (TF), which mediate many of the known transcriptional responses to cAMP. Such phosphorylated transcription factors (TFP) bind to hormone response elements (HREs) in gene regulatory regions, leading to increased transcription and hence a change in cell function via protein synthesis (Fig. 24.1).

INTRACELLULAR RECEPTORS

The intracellular or nuclear receptors include those for steroid hormones, thyroid hormones, and vitamin D.[5] They are soluble receptors employing transcriptional regulation to mediate their hormone-binding effects. They can be divided into two major subgroups. The first, the steroid receptor family, includes the glucocorticoid (GR), mineralocorticoid (MR), androgen (AR), and progesterone (PR) receptors. The second, the thyroid receptor family, includes the thyroid hormone (TR), estrogen (ER), retinoic acid (RAR), and vitamin D (VDR) receptors. In the steroid receptor family, the hormone traverses the cell membrane and binds to specific receptors located in the cytoplasm. This binding of the hormone to the receptor results in dissociation of the receptor from a complex of proteins that includes the 90-kDa heat shock protein (hsp 90). The hormone–receptor complex is translocated to the nucleus, where it binds to a chromatin receptor consisting of a specific hormone receptor response DNA element (HRE), generally situated upstream of the transcription initiating site. Binding of the nuclear receptor molecule to the HRE sequence leads to stimulation of transcription of the specific genes involved in the particular hormone's actions. Protein synthesis ensues, mediating a change in cell function. Alternatively, inhibition of transcription may occur with decrease in a cell function. In the case of the thyroid receptor family, with the exception of estrogen, the receptor molecules are situated in the nucleus. The hormones diffuse through the cytoplasm into the nucleoplasm, where receptor binding occurs without the involvement of heat shock proteins (Fig. 24.2).

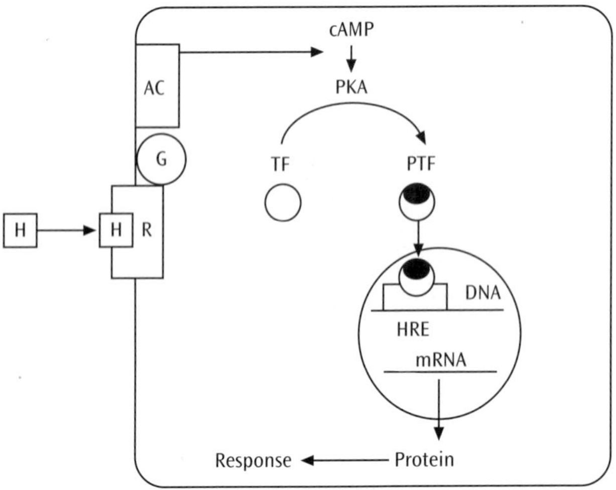

Figure 24.1 *Regulation of transcription by hormones acting on cell membrane receptors. AC, adenylate cyclase; G, G-protein; H, hormone; HRE, hormone response elements; PKA, protein kinase; PTF, phosphorylated TF; R, receptor; TF transcription factor.*

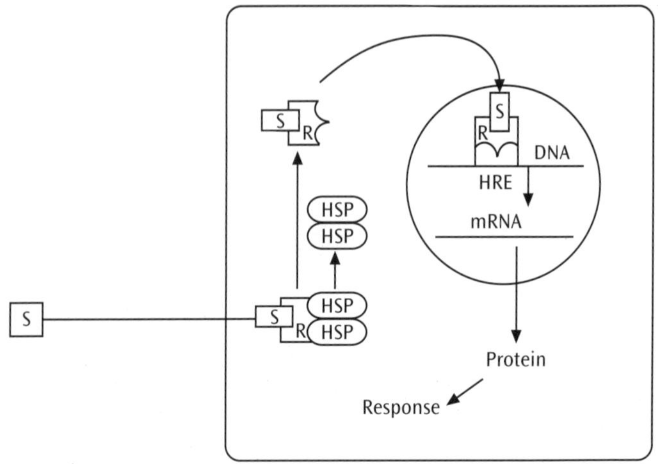

Figure 24.2 *Regulation of transcription by hormones acting on intracellular receptors. HSP, heat shock protein; HRE, hormone response elements; R, receptor; S, steroid.*

FEEDBACK MECHANISMS

Feedback control of hormone synthesis and release is characteristic of the endocrine system, with the interaction of the pituitary gland and peripheral endocrine organs furnishing classical examples.[6] Hormones produced in the peripheral target endocrine organs feed back via closed loops to the hypothalamus and pituitary, thus controlling the production of releasing or release-inhibiting hormones and trophic hormones respectively. The plasma level of the bioactive or unbound fraction of the peripherally produced hormone is the controlled variable and the set point is the normal resting plasma level of the hormone. This set point is determined by open-loop neural control by the central nervous system via modulation of hypothalamic releasing and release-inhibiting factors (Fig. 24.3). Physiological set point variation occurs over timescales ranging from minutes to hours to many years, with the greater timescale changes being superimposed on the shorter. These endogenous changes in set point can be further influenced by exogenous effects, such as environmental changes and stress, which may be physiologic (exercise, emotion) or pathological (trauma, disease states). The higher centers and hypothalamus are fundamental to set point regulation, which becomes abnormal if they are the subjects of disease states. Consideration of specific central nervous system – hypothalamopituitary – target organ systems will further elucidate these processes.

HYPOTHALAMOPITUITARY FUNCTION

Secretion of each of the six anterior pituitary hormones is controlled by one or more hypothalamic releasing or release-inhibiting hormones, interacting with feedback effects of target gland hormones.[7] Hypothalamic pituitary regulating hormones are synthesized in specialized neurons that represent the focal points at which neural information is converted into hormonal messages. These hypothalamic neurons can be considered to be a final common pathway by which signals from multiple systems reach the pituitary. These include nerve fibers from many parts of the brain concerned with homeostasis, stress responses, reproduction, etc. Cytokines, such as interleukins, that play a role in response to infection are also involved in regulation of hypothalamopituitary function. Hypothalamic neurohypophysial neurons secrete the posterior pituitary hormones antidiuretic hormone (ADH) and oxytocin into the general circulation, while hypotholamic hypophysiotrophic neurons secrete releasing and release-inhibiting

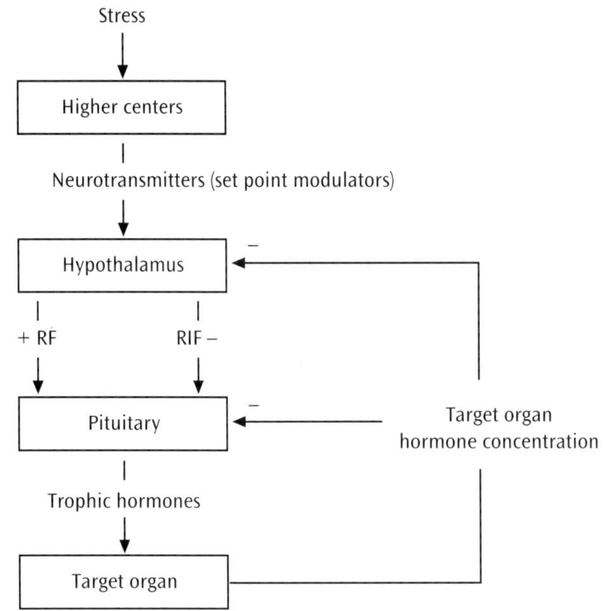

Figure 24.3 *Feedback loops of the hypothalamus–pituitary–adrenal axis.*

hormones into the blood supply in the anterior pituitary. In this account, of the six anterior pituitary hormones, adrenocorticotrophic hormone (ACTH) and thyroid-stimulating hormone (TSH) and their control of the adrenal and thyroid glands respectively will be described, these being of prime importance in anesthesia.

THE HYPOTHALAMUS–PITUITARY–ADRENAL AXIS

In this axis the level of biologically active or free cortisol in plasma is the controlled variable and the set point the normal resting cortisol level. The axis consists of open- and closed-loop components. Within the open-loop neural control component, the central nervous system controls the set point level of plasma cortisol through modulation of corticotrophin-releasing hormone (CRH) and ADH released by the hypothalamus. At the hypothalamus the secretion of CRH and ADH is regulated by both stimulatory and inhibitory neurotransmitters. Important stimulatory inputs come from the suprachiasmatic nuclei, which regulate the circadian rhythm of CRH and, in turn, ACTH and cortisol secretion. Within the circadian cycle there are 15–18 pulses of ACTH and cortisol secretion, the peaks of which vary with the time of day. The set point of feedback control of cortisol levels also varies in a circadian pattern. In the presence of high CRH levels, high concentrations of cortisol are required to inhibit ACTH secretion. Conversely, when CRH secretion is low, as at midnight, secretion is sensitive to cortisol suppression. This demonstrates that the episodic release of CRH and ACTH is independent of circulatory physiologic cortisol levels, the brain determining the set point. A variety of external stimuli or stressors, both physical and emotional, stimulate the axis, superseding the normal diurnal variation in axis activity. Typical physical stresses include pain, cold exposure, surgery, anesthesia, trauma, and shock, all of which activate the axis via higher center modulation or stimulatory neurotransmitter inputs to the CRH- and ADH-secreting hypothalamic neurons. The resulting high, but physiologic, levels of cortisol do not blunt the activation of the axis but high doses of exogenous glucocorticoids do. In some forms of stress, such as hypovolemic shock, ADH is the main stimulant of ACTH secretion. Similarly, emotional stresses such as failure of coping mechanisms, embarrassment, failure, and depression also activate the axis. An activating interaction with the immune system also exists, with circulatory cytokines released from activated lymphocytes, monocytes, and macrophages in response to antigens and toxins stimulating CRH and ADH release.[8] The axis is, however, also subject to inhibitory influences such as chronic morphine administration, which attenuates the activating affects of a variety of stresses. These inhibitory affects are via suppression of CRH and ADH secretion. The closed-loop components maintain the set point plasma cortisol level dictated by the neural open loop by means of a long negative feedback loop of cortisol at the pituitary and hypothalamus. At the hypothalamic level, cortisol inhibits secretion of CRH and ADH and also synthesis of their messenger ribonucleic acids (RNAs). It also acts directly on neuronal cell membranes to change CRH and ACTH secretion rapidly, but at the pituitary level cortisol inhibits secretion of ACTH and the synthesis of its pro-opiomelanocortin precursors.

Adrenocortical hormones

The adrenal cortex produces three main types of steroid hormones, glucocorticoids, androgens, and mineralocorticoids, zonally, depending on the presence of necessary synthesizing enzymes.[9,10] Glucocorticoid and androgen synthesis occurs in the inner zonae fasiculata and reticularis cells, which contain the enzyme, 17α-hydroxylase, necessary for the synthesis of their respective precursors 17α-hydroxyprogesterone and 17α-hydroxypregnenolone. The enzyme aldosterone synthetase is absent from these zones but is present in the outer zona glomerulosa, where synthesis of mineralocorticoids is sited. In contrast, 17α-hydroxylase is absent from the zona glomerulosa. The synthesis and release of cortisol, by far the major glucocorticoid, is controlled exclusively by ACTH. However, ACTH is only one of the factors involved in the synthesis and secretion of the adrenal androgens androstenedione, dehydroepiandrosterone (DHEA), and dehydroepiandrosterone sulfate (DHEAS). The synthesis and release of the major mineralocorticoid aldosterone by the cells of the zona glomerulosa is controlled predominantly by the renin–angiotensin system and plasma potassium concentration.[11] The aldosterone precursors, deoxycorticosterone, corticosterone, and 18-hydroxycorticosterone, which have some mineralocorticoid activity, are also synthesized in the fasciculata and reticularis zones under the control of ACTH. The enzyme renin is secreted by the juxtaglomerular cells of the afferent arterioles of the renal glomeruli. Secretion is stimulated by a fall in renal perfusing pressure, increased β_1-adrenergic stimulation, and decreased sodium concentration in the distal tubule. The last is sensed by the macula densa, a specialized group of distal convoluted tubule cells, which function as a chemoreceptor. Renin exerts its enzymatic effects on its substrate angiotensinogen, an α_2-globulin, to produce the inactive decapeptide angiotensin I. This is then converted by angiotensin-converting enzyme to the active octapeptide, angiotensin II. Further removal of the amino-terminal aspartate residue produces the heptapeptide angiotensin III. Angiotensins II and III are equipotent in stimulating aldosterone secretion, but angiotensin II is a far more potent vasoconstrictor. The actions of aldosterone and angiotensin II to raise plasma volume and blood pressure act as negative feedback effects on the secretion of renin.

Glucocorticoids exert effects on every body system and are essential to life. Their essential-to-life effects are predominantly on intermediary metabolism, increasing hepatic gluconeogenesis and glycogen deposition. Inhibition of glucose uptake in muscle and adipose tissue also occurs, in addition to stimulation of lipolysis in the latter. Their catabolic effects on peripheral tissue such as muscle cause the release of glucogenic amino acids for these processes. All these effects assume greater importance in the fasting state in order to maintain essential plasma glucose levels. Glucocorticoids exert a variety of effects on the immune and inflammatory responses including modulation and function of leukocytes, inhibition of prostaglandin synthesis, suppression of lymphokine release, and antibody production. The physiologic role of these effects in immune processes is not clearly understood. Adrenal androgens, although not potent androgens themselves, are converted to testosterone and dihydrotestosterone peripherally. In eugonadal males, adrenal androgens contribute only approximately 5% of total testosterone. In females the contribution is significant, with 60% of testosterone and 50% of dihydrotestosterone levels in the follicular phase of the menstrual cycle arising from conversion of adrenal androgen precursors. In midcycle the ovarian contribution increases and the adrenal contribution falls to 40% for testosterone. Mineralocorticoids regulate electrolyte transport across epithelial surfaces in the kidney, colon, and salivary glands via the effects on sodium potassium adenosine triphosphatase (ATPase). The result is maintenance of normal sodium and potassium concentrations and extracellular volume. These effects are mediated by activation of mineralocorticoid-responsive gene transcription with subsequent synthesis of proteins that regulate the Na^+, K^+-ATPase pump. Disease states involving hypo- and hyperfunction of the adrenal cortex illustrate the extremes of the effects of adrenocortical hormones.

DISEASES OF THE ADRENAL CORTEX

Hypofunction

Primary adrenal insufficiency, or Addison's disease, has an incidence of around 120 per million in Western countries.[12] Its early nonspecific symptoms can result in a delay in diagnosis, with eventual presentation as a life-threatening crisis an all too common occurrence. The etiologies of adrenal insufficiency have been grouped into three categories (Table 24.1): (1) adrenal dysgenesis; (2) adrenal destruction; and (3) impaired steroidogenesis.[13]

By far the commonest cause is autoimmune adrenalitis, which may occur in isolation or as part of the autoimmune polyglandular syndromes (APS). APS 1 is a rare recessive disease, associated with hypoparathyroidism, chronic mucocutaneous candidiasis, and gonadal failure. In APS 2 the associations are predominantly autoimmune thyroid disease and type 1 diabetes (Schmidt syndrome) or type 1 diabetes (Carpenter syndrome) and gonadal failure. Various modes of inheritance have been reported but both are more common in females. Circulating antibodies to the various endocrine organ autoantigens are present in both syndromes. Following the appearance of the adrenal autoantibodies, there is initially biochemical evidence of adrenal insufficiency. A rise in resting plasma renin activity, indicating zona glomerulosa failure, is followed months to years later by evidence of zona fasiculata dysfunction. Raised afternoon ACTH levels precede impaired cortisol responses to stimulation, and finally decreased basal plasma cortisol levels result in symptoms. Loss of more than 90% of the cortex occurs before symptoms ensue. The rate of cortical destruction is variable and so, therefore, is the clinical presentation (Table 24.2). In chronic adrenal insufficiency the early symptoms are nonspecific and can result in a delay in diagnosis, with an estimated 60% of patients having seen two or more physicians before the diagnosis is made.

Acute adrenal insufficiency, or adrenal crisis, in which the prime manifestation is shock, occurs in a patient previously undiagnosed with chronic insufficiency as a consequence of stress or in a previously diagnosed patient when glucocorticoid dose has not been increased to cover an intercurrent major illness. In the latter case, failure to retain medication due to vomiting or malabsorption may be responsible. The diagnosis of Addison's disease is confirmed by assessment of the pituitary–adrenal axis. Acutely ill patients should be stabilized prior to investigation. In such patients, a one-off cortisol level which is low or

Table 24.1 *Etiology of adrenal insufficiency*

Adrenal dysgenesis	
SF-1 gene mutation	
DAX-1 gene mutation	
ACTH resistance	
Adrenal destruction	
Autoimmune	Hemochromatosis
Infective	Amyloidosis
Hemorrhage	Adrenoleukodystrophy
Metastatic infiltration	Adrenomyeloneuropathy
Impaired steroidogenesis	
Congenital adrenal hyperplasia	
Drug effects	

ACTH, adrenocorticotrophic hormone.

Table 24.2 *Clinical features of adrenal insufficiency*

Chronic	
Weakness/fatigue	Hyperpigmentation
Anorexia	Gastroinestinal symptoms
Weight loss	Salt craving
Hypotension	Postural symptoms
Acute	
Shock	Hypoglycemia
Nausea/vomiting	Dehydration/volume depletion
Acute abdomen	Postural hypotension

inappropriately normal may be diagnostic. Simultaneous ACTH levels will distinguish between primary and secondary adrenal insufficiency. Replacement hydrocortisone should be administered if the diagnosis is considered a possibility as it is unlikely to cause any harm if the diagnosis is not subsequently confirmed.

In the chronic presentation, basal levels of cortisol in plasma and urine may be normal in unstressed patients and, although raised ACTH levels are helpful, conventional practice is to perform stimulatory testing. In the rapid, or short, tetracosactide (tetracosactrin; Synacthen) test, 250 μg of tetracosactide (ACTH 1–24) is administered intravenously or intramuscularly after taking a basal plasma cortisol sample. Further samples are drawn after 30 and 60 min. This test is best performed at 0900 h, when the basal level itself gives good evidence of the integrity of the axis if it is greater than 350 nmol L^{-1} in an unstressed patient. An impaired response in this test does not distinguish between primary or secondary adrenal insufficiency, or that due to suppression by previous glucocorticoid treatment. The long, or depot, tetracosactide test is then helpful. Depot tetracosactide (1 mg), which acts for approximately 24 h, is given intramuscularly. The 30- and 60-min cortisol levels are usually superimposable on those of the short tetracosactide test and, in both primary and secondary adrenal insufficiency, would be impaired. With secondary failure and adrenal suppression, cortisol levels continue to rise at 8 and 24 h, in contrast with the response in primary insufficiency. More recently, the low-dose tetracosactide test (1 μg intravenously) has been demonstrated to reveal partial adrenal insufficiency that may be missed by the short (250 μg) test.[14]

Treatment of primary adrenal insufficiency requires replacement glucocorticoid and mineralocorticoid. The latter is not usually required in secondary insufficiency, if the renin–angiotensin–aldosterone system is intact. There is no clear indication for replacement of adrenal androgen deficiency at present. It is not possible to mimic the natural circadian rhythm of cortisol secretion. Cortisol levels are undetectable during sleep at midnight and begin to rise coincidentally with the onset of rapid eye movement sleep in the early hours, reaching a peak at 08.00 to 09.00 h. Thereafter, there is a steady decline throughout the day with superimposed peaks in response to stress. Hydrocortisone replacement is therefore a compromise, with a view to achieving the well-being of the patient but avoiding overtreatment. The traditional dosage schedule of 20 mg on awakening in the morning and 10 mg in the evening has been shown to result in more cortisol levels above and below the normal population range than the now recommended 10 mg on rising, 5 mg at noon, and 5 mg at 16.00 h.[15] This schedule also produces a rise in osteocalcin, indicating increased bone formation, which may reduce the long-term risk of osteoporosis.

Mineralocorticoid is more easily replaced by the use of fludrocortisone at 0.05–0.20 mg day^{-1}. Adequacy of replacement can be monitored by measuring plasma renin activity, but in usual clinical practice assay of plasma electrolyte concentrations and supine and standing blood pressure levels suffice.[16] Dosage may need to be increased in summer to compensate for increased salt losses in sweat. In the treatment of the acute presentation, and similarly in the management of intercurrent illness and surgery, large multiple doses of intravenous or intramuscular hydrocortisone have traditionally been administered. This approach has no physiologic basis as normal and unstressed cortisol production is approximately 15 mg day^{-1}, rising to 45–60 mg in response to stresses such as pyrexia, anesthesia, and trauma. In these situations, plasma cortisol levels are in the range 600–1100 nmol L^{-1}, which is approximately the binding capacity of cortisol-binding globulin. Although the plasma half-life of cortisol is approximately 80 min, intracellular receptor occupancy is much longer, therefore multiple doses within 24 h are unnecessary. Doses of 300 mg day^{-1} or more are in the range of 24 times the basal production rate and also considerably exceed the physiologicly stressed maximum. Such doses may also result in hypokalemia, precipitation of diabetes (or exacerbation of existing diabetes), poor wound healing, immune suppression, myopathy (including that of respiratory muscles), and psychosis. It has been cogently argued that, for these reasons, hydrocortisone doses of > 150 mg in 24 h are unnecessary.[18]

Hyperfunction

Glucocorticoids

Chronic glucocorticoid excess leads to the group of symptoms and physical signs known as Cushing syndrome.[19] The commonest cause is iatrogenic, resulting from the therapeutic use of glucocorticoid, most commonly taken orally but also via the inhaled and topical routes. Noniatrogenic, or spontaneous, causes are conveniently classified as either ACTH dependent or independent (Table 24.3). Cushing's disease is defined as the specific type of Cushing syndrome that is caused by ACTH secretion by a pituitary adenoma and is eight times more common in women than in men. It occurs over an age range extending from childhood to the elderly. Ectopic ACTH secretion occurs from a variety of tumors of nonpituitary origin. The most common tumor type implicated is small-cell carcinoma of the bronchus. Other sources include carcinoid tumors of bronchial, thymic, gastrointestinal, and pancreatic origin.

That most body systems are susceptible to the effects of excess glucocorticoids is evident from the clinical features of Cushing syndrome (Table 24.4). The co-secretion of androgens explains other features. Although the presentation of ectopic ACTH-dependent Cushing syndrome may be indistinguishable from Cushing's disease, it should be suspected if onset is rapid or typical features are outweighed by marked weight loss, muscle wasting, weakness, and skin pigmentation. Adrenal adenomas typically present slowly with manifestations of mild glucocorticoid excess alone. In contrast, the presentation in carcinomas is of rapid onset with a combination of excess glucocorticoid and androgen manifestations. Androgen excess is usually greater than that of cortisol, resulting in signs of virilization. Food-dependent Cushing syndrome is due to the expression of ectopic gastric inhibitory peptide (GIP) receptors in the adrenal cortex.[20] Eating stimulates secretion of GIP, which binds to these receptors, inducing adrenal growth and cortisol synthesis.

Table 24.3 *Etiology of spontaneous Cushing syndrome*

Diagnosis	% of all causes
ACTH dependent	
Pituitary adenoma (Cushing's disease)	68
Ectopic ACTH	12
Macronodular hyperplasia	1
Ectopic CRH	< 1
ACTH independent	
Adrenal adenoma	10
Adrenal carcinoma	8
Food dependent	< 1

ACTH, adrenocorticotrophic hormone; CRH, corticotrophin-releasing hormone.

Table 24.4 *Clinical features of Cushing syndrome*

Weight gain/centripetal adiposity
Moon face/facial plethora
Hypertension
Glucose intolerance/diabetes
Weakness/proximal myopathy
Neuropsychiatric changes
Bruising/skin thinning
Hirsutism
Oligomenorrhea/amenorrhea
Decreased libido/impotence
Acne
Abdominal striae

The investigation of possible Cushing syndrome involves confirmation of the diagnosis followed by the differential diagnosis of the etiology. The two most commonly applied diagnostic tests are 24-h urinary free cortisol excretion and the low-dose dexamethasone suppression test. The former integrates the circulating plasma free cortisol over the 24-h period, and in the unstressed state levels > 280 nmol day^{-1} are diagnostic. The latter assesses the ability of dexamethasone (usually 1 mg orally at 23.00 h) to suppress the following morning's 09.00 h cortisol level. In normal individuals it will be suppressed to < 60 nmol L^{-1}. The differential diagnosis is then based on the simultaneous measurement of ACTH and cortisol levels. The finding of circulatory ACTH, coincidental with hypercortisolism, essentially excludes a primary autonomously secreting adrenocortical tumor. The finding of elevated ACTH levels is only the first step in the differential diagnosis of the ACTH-dependent syndrome. The exact siting of the source depends on sophisticated imaging and sampling techniques in specialist centers. The preferred treatment option is surgical removal of the CRH-, ACTH-, or cortisol-secreting lesion. Radiotherapy to the pituitary in Cushing's disease is an option for patients unfit or unwilling to undergo surgery and those not cured by surgery. The pharmacologic option is usually pursued in surgical failures and when awaiting the effects of radiotherapy. Metyrapone and ketoconazole inhibit steroidogenesis and opDD (mitotane) is adrenolytic, with a cytotoxic effect on adrenocortical cells.

Mineralocorticoids: hyperaldosteronism

Primary hyperaldosteronism, or Conn syndrome, is the commonest cause of mineralocorticoid hypertension, occurring in 0.5–3% of all hypertensive patients.[21] The diagnosis is important as it is a potentially reversible cause of hypertension. It is characterized by hypokalemia and suppressed plasma renin activity in the presence of elevated aldosterone levels. Symptoms attributable to hypokalemia include fatigue and proximal muscle weakness, with thirst, polyuria, and nocturia being secondary to hypokalemic nephropathy. It must be remembered, however, that approximately 30% of patients with primary hyperaldosteronism are normokalemic. The most common cause (in 65% of patients) is a solitary small (0.5–2.5 cm) adrenal adenoma. Bilateral adrenal hyperplasia is found in 30% of cases. Glucocorticoid-remediable aldosteronism (GRA), adrenal carcinoma, and renin-responsive aldosterone-producing adenomas constitute the remainder of cases. The diagnosis is confirmed by finding suppression of supine and standing plasma renin activity coincidental with elevation of plasma aldosterone levels. Ideally, investigations should be performed when patients have been off any antihypertensive therapy that has effects on the renin–angiotensin–aldosterone axis for 2 weeks. If hypertension is severe, prazosin may be used as it interferes the least. Once the diagnosis is confirmed, the etiology must be differentially diagnosed.[22] In adrenal hyperplasia, assuming an erect posture increases plasma aldosterone levels, but this is not the case with aldosterone-producing adenomas. Conversely, administration of captopril, which results in a fall in angiotensin II levels, produces a secondary fall in aldosterone levels in adrenal hyperplasia but not in the case of adenomas. The administration of ACTH has no effect on aldosterone secretion in adrenal hyperplasia and little effect in the presence of aldosterone-producing adenomas, which contrasts with a marked increase in GRA. Treatment of adenomas is by surgical removal, whereas in hyperplasia and GRA the treatment is pharmacologic. Amiloride or spironolactone is used in hyperplasia and dexamethasone in GRA.

THE HYPOTHALAMUS–PITUITARY–THYROID AXIS

In this axis, free thyroid hormones are the controlled variable and the set point their normal resting levels. As in the case of the adrenal gland, there are open- and closed-loop components to the axis.[23] The open-loop component determines the set point level via the effects of thyrotropin-releasing hormone (TRH) and somatostatin on thyroid-stimulating hormone (TSH) secretion by the thyrotroph cells of the anterior pituitary. The hypothalamic nuclei secreting the stimulatory TRH and inhibitory somatostatin receive neuroregulatory inputs from higher brain centers. Thus, the effects of stress in various forms, including psychological, starvation, temperature change, infection, and inflammation, on the set point, are mediated. Such influences are the basis of the euthyroid sick syndrome, in which low thyroid hormone levels are found without the normal compensatory rise in TSH secretion. The closed-loop component maintains precisely the set point determined by the opened-loop component via the negative feedback effects of thyroid hormones at both the pituitary and the hypothalamus.

In addition to the open- and closed-loop control mechanisms, the thyroid gland is capable of intrinsic autoregulation, which maintains euthyroidism despite wide variation in dietary iodide intake. Normally, the thyroid secretes T_4 and T_3 in a ratio of approximately 10:1. Most plasma T_3 is derived from peripheral metabolism by 5′-deiodination of T_4. The extent of T_4 conversion to T_3 raises the question of whether T_4 has any biological action itself or merely serves as a prohormone for T_3. A fall in dietary iodide causes a rapid decrease in T_4 concentration and a simultaneous rise in TSH. Circulatory T_3 levels are maintained as a consequence of preferential synthesis of T_3 rather than T_4, thereby preserving the metabolic effects of the secreted hormones.

In iodine deficiency, T_3 is mostly derived from thyroid synthesis rather than conversion from T_4. The deiodinase enzymes are intimately involved in this mechanism, as they are in the response to stress, in a complex and not fully understood manner. A rise in plasma iodide causes an acute inhibition of thyroidal iodide organification, called the Wolff–Chaikoff effect. As a consequence, the effects of TSH on the thyroid are decreased. If the increased plasma iodide level is maintained, the inhibitory effect disappears after 10–14 days and iodide organification increases. This escape from, or adaptation to, the Wolff–Chaikoff effect is due to the impairment of the ability of the thyroid to concentrate sufficient iodine to inhibit organification. High concentrations of plasma iodide can inhibit thyroid hormone secretion, but this effect may be incomplete or absent and, even if present initially, wanes with time. This phenomenon, known as iodine escape, is not to be confused with the escape from the Wolff–Chaikoff effect.

Thyroid hormones and the sympathoadrenal system

The sympathoadrenal system (the sympathetic nervous system and adrenal medulla) and thyroid hormones interact in a coordinated manner.[24] The former provides rapid adjustments to the environment and the latter affects the capacity of many tissues to respond to the actions of catecholamines. This synergistic interaction plays important adaptive roles, typified by the response to cold exposure, in which both systems interact to increase heat production. In other situations, such as starvation, both systems are decreased in activity to conserve energy, with sympathetic outflow decreasing along with decreased T_3 secretion and T_4 to T_3 conversion.

In hyper- or hypothyroidism the interaction between the two systems is disrupted as the activity of the thyroid is fixed at high or low levels respectively. In thyrotoxicosis, in which the effect of catecholamines is increased, as assessed by norepinephrine (noradrenaline) metabolism, sympathetic activity is diminished, and in hypothyroidism it is markedly increased. The sympathomimetic features of thyrotoxicosis cannot therefore be explained by enhanced sympathetic activity. These features are due to the similarity of the actions of the thyroid hormones and catecholamines, together with the synergistic action between them.

Thyroid hormones increase the number of β-adrenergic receptors on cells as well as decreasing the number of α-adrenergic receptors. This results in a rise in tissue cAMP levels, the effects of which are also potentiated. The postreceptor mechanisms, resulting in a rise in cAMP, are mediated by decreasing the cellular concentrations of certain G-protein subunits. T_3 downregulates some $G\alpha_i$ and $G\gamma$ subunits, the former leading to less G_i-mediated inhibition of adenylate cyclase whereas the latter makes more $G\alpha_s$ subunits available to mediate stimulation of adenylate cyclase. The effects of the disruption of the interaction between the sympathoadrenal system and thyroid in hypo- and hyperthyroidism are diverse, reflecting the widespread tissue actions of thyroid hormones.

Diseases of the thyroid

Hypothyroidism

This is the most common disorder of thyroid function with an incidence of 15 per 1000 females and 1 per 1000 males.[25] In cases in which iodine is replete, autoimmune thyroiditis followed by radiation-induced thyroid damage are the main causes (Table 24.5). The former is usually due to Hashimoto's thyroiditis and the latter therapeutic radioiodine treatment for thyrotoxicosis. In autoimmune thyroiditis, patients with thyroid autoantibodies may maintain normal thyroid function but approximately 50% have raised TSH levels. Patients in this state of subclinical hypothyroidism progress to overt hypothyroidism at the rate of 5% per annum.[26] Thyroxine replacement should be considered for patients with subclinical hypothyroidism.

Much less commonly, hypothyroidism is caused by decreased thyroid stimulation by TSH. This so-called central hypothyroidism is secondary if caused by TSH deficiency and tertiary if TRH is deficient. Although central hypothyroidism is more uncommon, its causes, which include pituitary tumor, hypothalamic tumors, and lymphocytic hypophysitis, may be life threatening due to coincidental ACTH deficiency.[27] The etiology of hypothyroidism therefore needs to be precisely determined, particularly when T_4 levels are low and TSH levels equivocal prior to instigating thyroxine replacement. A reduction in free or total T_4 coincidental with a rise in TSH indicates primary hypothyroidism. In central hypothyroidism, free or total T_4 is reduced coincidentally with a reduced or normal TSH level, indicating the need to assess hypothalamopituitary function. The biochemical changes of central hypothyroidism are also seen in nonthyroidal illness and in patients taking drugs such as glucocorticoids and anticonvulsants.

The clinical manifestations of hypothyroidism are influenced by the age of the patient, the presence of other diseases, and the rate at which it develops. The onset is usually insidious and the symptoms vague and nonspecific (Table 24.6). This is particularly the case in the elderly, in whom the diagnosis should be considered in the absence of other explanations for symptoms. Treatment of hypothyroidism is with sufficient oral thyroxine to restore patients to euthyroidism by normalizing T_4 and TSH concentrations.[28] T_4 levels above the normal range with suppressed TSH levels are no longer acceptable even if the patient is clinically euthyroid and well, particularly over the age of 60 because of the risk of atrial fibrillation.[29] The initial dose of thyroxine depends on the age of the patient, the severity and duration of the hypothyroidism, and the presence of other disorders. Previously healthy patients under 60 years of age and free of cardiac disease can be started on full replacement doses of thyroxine of 1.6–1.8 $\mu g\,kg^{-1}$. In females this usually translates to 75–125 $\mu g\,day^{-1}$ and in males 125–200 $\mu g\,day^{-1}$. Elderly patients and those with cardiac disease should be started on doses no higher than 50 $\mu g\,day^{-1}$ and those with long-standing severe hypothyroidism 25 $\mu g\,day^{-1}$. Patients who are unable to take oral preparations for 3–4 days do not require parenteral therapy because of the long half-life of thyroxine (approximately 7 days). When parenteral therapy is necessary, the required dose of thyroxine is 70–80% of the oral dose, based on the fraction of the oral dose absorbed. In the UK, triiodothyronine is the only preparation available for parenteral use. Thyroxine is available in the USA. It has recently been suggested that treatment with a combination of thyroxine and triiodothyronine may improve mood and neuropsychological function more effectively than an equivalent dose of thyroxine alone but this is not yet standard practice.[30]

Table 24.5 *Etiology of hypothyroidism*

Primary
Iodine deficiency (commonest cause worldwide)
Autoimmune thyroiditis (Hashimoto's disease)
Radioiodine/thyroidectomy
Antithyroid drugs
Lithium, amiodarone
Subacute/silent thyroiditis
Dyshormonogenesis/agenesis
Infiltrative disease (amyloid, hemochromatosis)
Central
Pituitary disease (secondary)
Hypothalamic disease (tertiary)

Table 24.6 *Clinical features of primary hypothyroidism*

Lethargy
Dry skin
Periorbital/facial edema
Cold intolerance
Weight gain
Impaired memory/mentation
Constipation
Hair loss
Hoarseness/aphonia
Menorrhagia

Thyrotoxicosis

Thyrotoxicosis is the clinical syndrome caused by excess circulating free thyroid hormones thyroxine (fT_4) and/or triiodothyronine (fT_3).[25] It has an incidence of 10 per 1000 females and 1 per 1000 males. Hyperthyroidism equates with thyroid gland overactivity, which results in thyrotoxicosis. Thyrotoxicosis can occur in the absence of hyperthyroidism, as in thyroiditis, in which stored thyroid hormones are released from the thyroid gland or when excess thyroid hormone is administered. The etiologies of thyrotoxicosis have been grouped into three categories (Table 24.7): (1) primary hyperthyroidism; (2) secondary hyperthyroidism; (3) thyrotoxicosis without hyperthyroidism.[31]

Graves' disease is the commonest cause of primary hyperthyroidism, accounting for 70–80% of cases, followed by toxic multinodular goiter and toxic adenoma (Plummer's disease). Graves' disease is caused by production of autoantibodies (TSH-RAb) that stimulate the TSH receptor. In addition to thyrotoxicosis, features exclusive to Graves' disease are ophthalmopathy, pretibial myxedema, and thyroid acropachy. These may occur coincidentally with the thyrotoxicosis, in combination or singly, but tend to run courses that are largely independent. In toxic multinodular goiter and toxic adenoma, thyroid hormone secretion is autonomous. Toxic multinodular goiter tends to occur after the age of 50 and is more common in women. Thyroid hormone levels are not as high as in Graves' disease but cardiovascular manifestation, such as atrial fibrillation and congestive cardiac failure, predominate because of the age of the patients. Ophthalmopathy and dermopathy are not present unless there is coincidental Graves' disease.

Toxic adenoma is less common, occurring most often between the ages of 30 and 50. The adenomas are usually solitary, the remainder of the gland being normal. Human chronic gonadotrophin (HCG) consists of α and β subunits, the α subunit being identical to TSH and the β subunit having considerable structural homology with those of TSH. The thyrotrophic activity of HCG is weak, but when levels are high, sufficient stimulation of thyroid TSH receptors may occur to cause hyperthyroidism. This situation occurs with trophoblastic tumors[32] and occasionally in the first trimester of pregnancy. In the latter case, the gestational thyrotoxicosis resolves spontaneously when HCG levels fall in the second trimester.[33] Amiodarone-induced thyrotoxicosis, which is becoming more common with increased use of the drug, is the result of two different mechanisms.[34] Type 1, or iodine-induced, is the more common, tending to occur in the presence of micro- or macronodular goiter. Such goiters are more likely to be present in the elderly, who are also more likely to be treated with the drug. Pre-existing autoimmune thyroid disease is also a predisposing factor. Type 2 is due to a destructive thyroiditis. Differentiation between the two is possible by radioiodine uptake studies and measurement of serum interleukin 6 (IL-6). In the destructive form, radioiodine uptake is always low and IL-6 levels tend to be markedly elevated. The situation is complicated, however, in that both types of thyrotoxicosis may be present simultaneously.

As in hypothyroidism, the clinical manifestations of thyrotoxicosis are influenced by the age of the patient, the rate of development and severity of the thyrotoxicosis, and the presence of other disease (Table 24.8). In children, rapid growth and accelerated bone maturation occurs. In older patients, weight loss (despite preservation of appetite), palpitations, anxiety, fatigue, and hyperkinesia are common. Over the age of 60, cardiovascular problems and myopathies predominate. TSH levels have been found to be suppressed in 28% of patients over the age of 65 presenting with atrial fibrillation.[29]

The diagnosis of thyrotoxicosis is confirmed by the finding of elevated thyroid hormone levels, and coincidental assay of TSH will

Table 24.7 *Etiology of thyrotoxicosis*

Primary thyrotoxicosis
Graves' disease
Toxic multinodular goiter
Toxic adenoma (Plummer's disease)
Thyroid carcinoma (follicular)
Iodine induced (Jod–Basedow phenomenon)
Secondary thyrotoxicosis
TSH-secreting pituitary adenoma
HCG dependent – trophoblastic tumor, gestational thyrotoxicosis
Thyrotoxicosis without hyperthyroidism
Destructive thyroiditis – post partum, subacute, amiodarone-induced
Excess thyroxine administration
Struma ovarii (ectopic autonomous thyroid tissue)

HCG, human chorionic gonadotrophin; TSH, thyroid-stimulating hormone.

Table 24.8 *Clinical features of thyrotoxicosis*

Weight loss
Fatigue/weakness
Heat intolerance/excess sweating
Increased appetite
Palpitations/tachycardia
Anxiety/irritability
Tremor
Diarrhea
Weight gain (2% of cases)
Pruritus

usually indicate the etiology. TSH levels are suppressed unless a very rare TSH secreted pituitary adenoma is present. Total thyroid hormone levels may be elevated in euthyroidism by the effects of estrogens (pregnancy or contraceptive pill), liver disease, and hereditary factors on thyroid hormone-binding proteins. Assay of free thyroid hormones is therefore preferable.

Treatment options are medical, surgical, or radioiodine. In Europe and Japan, patients below 50 years of age with Graves' disease tend to receive a course of antithyroid drugs. Carbimazole or propylthiouracil is used alone and dose titrated or continued at high dose with the addition of thyroxine in the block–replace regimen. In North America, radioiodine is more often the initial treatment. Over the age of 50, radioiodine is generally the preferred treatment option after initial control with antithyroid drugs. Surgical intervention is reserved for patients refusing other forms of treatment and for large nodular goiters, relapses, and in pregnancy if drugs cause unacceptable side-effects.

PHEOCHROMOCYTOMAS

Pheochromocytomas are rare catecholamine-secreting tumors of the adrenal medulla or paraganglia of the sympathetic nervous system, accounting for less than 0.1% of the causes of hypertension. They are of equal sex distribution and, although they occur from childhood to old age, they are more common in the third and fourth decades. In addition to the catecholamines [norepinephrine (noradrenaline), epinephrine (adrenaline), dopamine, and L-dopa], they may secrete a wide variety of neuropeptides. Secretion may be constant or episodic, which together with the protean manifestations of the disease, is responsible for its postmortem diagnosis in greater than 50% of cases.[2] Tumors are bilateral in 10%, malignant in 10%, and familial in 10% of cases. The inherited syndromes associated with pheochromocytoma include multiple endocrine neoplasia (MEN) types 2a and 2b, von Hippel–Lindau disease, and neurofibromatosis type 1.

In MEN type 2a the associates are medullary thyroid carcinoma, hyperparathyroidism, and pheochromocytoma. In MEN type 2b these are medullary carcinoma of the thyroid, multiple mucosal neuromas, marfanoid habitus, and pheochromocytoma. Mutational changes in the *RET* proto-oncogene are the genetic basis for MEN type 2. Von Hippel–Lindau is an autosomal dominant familial tumor syndrome with central nervous system and retinal hemangioblastomas, renal cysts and carcinomas, and associated pheochromocytomas. It is linked to chromosome 3p25. In neurofibromatosis type 1 (NF-1) there are *café-au-lait* spots, iris Lisch nodules, and multiple neurofibromas. Pheochromocytomas, most commonly involving the adrenal medulla, occur in 0.5% of such patients. The *NF-1* gene locus is on chromosome 17.

The commonest clinical feature in pheochromocytoma is hypertension which is resistant to treatment and may be sustained or paroxysmal. The wide variety of symptoms render pheochromocytoma a great mimic and it may present in a variety of ways to different specialties.[35] Crises or paroxysmal symptoms are typical and should lead to suspicion of the diagnosis. Distinctive features include postural hypotension (reduced plasma volume and downregulation of α-receptors), shock, myocardial ischemia, cardiac failure, pulmonary edema, hyperglycemia (increased glycogenesis and α-receptor-mediated inhibition of insulin secretion), hypercalcemia, increased hematocrit, and constipation (Table 24.9). Paroxysms may be precipitated by drugs, the commonest of which are propranolol, naloxone, metoclopramide, tricyclic antidepressants, phenothiazines, cytotoxins, and ACTH.[36] Diagnosis requires a high index of suspicion based on symptoms and signs. Biochemical confirmation is by measurement of free catecholamines in a 24-h urine specimen, this having superseded the older technique of measuring catecholamine metabolites in the form of vanillyl mandelic acid (VMA). Once the diagnosis is confirmed, localization of the tumor is by computed tomography (CT) scanning or, more commonly, magnetic resonance imaging (MRI). Tumors in unusual sites and metastases can be identified by [^{131}I]-metaiodobenzylguanidine (MIBG) scintigraphy. Treatment is primarily surgical resection after appropriate medical preparation with α- and β-blockade. Nonsurgical symptomatic treatment, particularly of metastases, is with the tyrosine hydroxylase (rate-limiting enzyme in catecholamine biosynthesis) inhibitor α-methyl paratyrosine. MIBG has also been used therapeutically.

CARCINOID SYNDROME

Approximately 85% of carcinoid tumors are found in the gastrointestinal tract. These gastrointestinal tract lesions are most commonly found in the appendix (1 in 300 appendicectomies) followed by the ileum (1 in 150 autopsies) and rectum (1 in 1500 proctoscopies). A further 10% are found in the lungs and the remainder in a variety of organs including the thymus, kidney, ovary, and prostate gland. Carcinoid tumors are the commonest small bowel neoplasms, contributing up to 35% of the total. Such tumors were previously classified, on the basis of their location,

Table 24.9 *Clinical features of pheochromocytoma*

Hypertension
Headache
Excess sweating
Palpitations
Anxiety
Tremulousness
Pallor
Chest/abdominal pain
Nausea/vomiting
Weight loss
Postural hypotension

into foregut, midgut, and hindgut tumors.[37] Foregut carcinoids include thymic, lung, stomach, duodenal, and pancreatic tumors. Midgut tumors arise in the duodenum, ileum, and descending colon, while hindgut tumors are confined to the colon and rectum. This classification has more recently been refined to include histological, functional, and biological characteristics in addition to the site of the tumor.[38]

Carcinoid syndrome describes the clinical manifestations caused by the secretory products of carcinoid tumors.[39] Most patients with carcinoid tumors do not develop carcinoid syndrome, which occurs only when the causative tumor products enter the systemic circulation. The syndrome is more common with tumors originating in the small bowel and proximal colon. Because the active substances released by these tumors pass via the portal vein and are inactivated by liver metabolism, the presence of the syndrome implies hepatic metastases with venous drainage into the systemic circulation. A small proportion of patients with tumors in these sites present with carcinoid syndrome in the absence of liver metastases. These patients may have retroperitoneal metastases, with drainage directly into the systemic circulation via the prevertebral veins. Substances released by carcinoid tumors include 5-hydroxytryptamine (serotonin), and tachykinins, such as substance P, neurokinin A, neuropeptide K, and bradykinin. Prostaglandins E and F and histamine are also secreted.

The clinical features of carcinoid syndrome are summarized in Table 24.10. Flushing takes the form of a paroxysmal diffuse erythematous phenomenon affecting the face, neck, and upper thorax and lasting 2–5 min. It occurs in up to 75% of patients and is associated with a feeling of warmth and palpitations. When the disease is long standing the flush is persistent and violaceous, with associated dilation of cutaneous veins and telangiectasia. Flushing usually occurs spontaneously, but recognized precipitants include eating, exercise, excitement, alcohol, and postural change. Mediating substances include the tachykinins neurokinin A, neuropeptide K, and substance P. A variant form occurs in gastric and bronchial carcinoids. The flush in this form is patchy and more erythematous, with serpiginous and sharply defined boundaries. This flush is typically precipitated by eating. It is associated with peptic ulceration rather than diarrhea and cardiac events, reflecting the predominant secretion of histamine. Bronchial carcinoids are sometimes associated with bluish-red flushes that persist for hours and are associated with facial edema, lacrimation, and hypotension. This severe type of flushing may be part of a carcinoid crisis. Pellagra-like skin lesions occur in a small number of patients with long-standing disease, in whom up to 60%, as opposed to the normal 1%, of available tryptophan is converted to 5-hydroxytryptamine. Diarrhea, taking the form of up to 30 watery stools per day, is almost as common as, but not always associated with, flushing. Colicky abdominal pain is an accompaniment and it is mediated by 5-hydroxytryptamine, which stimulates small bowel motility and secretion but not flushing. In contrast to this chemically mediated abdominal pain, approximately 40% of midgut carcinoids present with pain due to obstruction caused by the primary lesion. Bronchospasm occurs in up to 15% of cases and may be precipitated by anesthesia. It is associated with flushing and mediated by the same substances, the secretion of which may be increased by bronchodilatory drugs, thereby exacerbating the symptom.

Table 24.10 *Clinical features of carcinoid syndrome*

Flushing
Diarrhea
Abdominal pain/obstruction
Wheezing
Carcinoid heart disease
Pellagra

Aside from the blood pressure changes and palpitations, structural changes occur in carcinoid heart disease, caused by the same substances that mediate flushing and bronchospasm. These plaque-like lesions of mucopolysaccharide and collagen are found on the endocardium of valve leaflets, atria, and ventricles. They are predominantly right sided and cause tricuspid, and less frequently pulmonary, valve incompetence. The tumor growth factor (TGF)-β family of growth factors and 5-hydroxytryptamine have been implicated in their etiology.

The clinical diagnosis of carcinoid syndrome is confirmed by the finding of elevated levels of 5-hydroxyindoleacetic acid (5-HIAA) in urine. False positives occur if banana, avocado, pineapple, walnut, chocolate, and coffee are not excluded from the diet. Treatment with chlorpromazine, salicylates, L-dopa, imipramine, isoniazid, methyldopa, promethazine, and monoamine oxidase inhibitors cause false negatives. Localization of tumors is by CT and MRI scanning. The use of radionucleotide scanning with radiolabeled somatostatin analogs and metaiodobenzylguanidine (MIBG) has proved extremely helpful.

Treatment of carcinoid tumors and carcinoid syndrome aims to reduce tumor mass and control symptoms. Surgery to a primary tumor with only local metastases may be curative. Reduction of tumor mass may result in prolonged remissions, with improvement in symptoms, and enhance the chances of improvement with medical treatment. Previously, chemotherapy with a combination of streptozocin and 5-fluorouracil produced short responses in 10–30% of patients. More recently the use of α-interferon and somatostatin analogs, either alone or in combination, has produced responses in up to 70% of patients.[40]

REFERENCES

1. Tunbridge WMG, Evered DC, Haul R, *et al.* The spectrum of the thyroid disease in a community: the Whickham survey. *Clin Endocrinol* 1977; **7:** 481–93.
2. Stein PP, Black HR. A simplified approach to phaeochromocytoma. A review of the literature and report of one institution's experience. *Medicine (Baltimore)* 1991; **70:** 36–66.
3. Burrin JM. Molecular aspects of signal transduction in endocrine tissue. *Ann Clin Biochem* 1994; **31:** 205–14.
4. Kahn CR, Smith RJ, Chin WW. Mechanism of action of hormones that act at the cell surface. In: Wilson JD, Foster DW, Kronenberg HM, Reed Larsen P (eds). *Williams Text Book of Endocrinology,* 9th edn. Philadelphia: W B Saunders, 1998: 95–147.
5. Tsai M, Clark JH, Schrader WT, O'Malley BW. Mechanism of action of hormones that act as transcription – regulatory factors. In: Wilson JD, Foster DW, Kronenberg HM, Reed Larsen P (eds). *Williams Text Book of Endocrinology,* 9th edn. Philadelphia: W B Saunders 1998: 55–94.
6. Habener JF. Genetic control of hormone formation. In: Wilson JD, Foster DW, Kronenberg HM, Reed Larsen P (eds). *Williams Text Book of Endocrinology,* 9th edn. Philadelphia: W B Saunders 1998: 11–42.
7. Reichlin S. Neuroendocrinology. In: Wilson J D, Foster D N, Kronenberg H M, Reed Larsen P (eds) *Williams Text Book of Endocrinology,* 9th edn. Philadelphia: WB Saunders, 1998: 165–248.
8. Reichlin S .Neuroendocrine–immune interactions. *N Engl J Med* 1993: **329:** 1246–53.
9. Orth DN, Kovacs WJ. The adrenal cortex. In: Wilson JD, Foster DW, Kronenberg HM, Reed Larsen P (eds). *Williams Text Book of Endocrinology,* 9th edn. Philadelphia: W B Saunders 1998: 517–664.
10. Finding JW, Aron DC, Blake Tyrrel J. Glucocorticoids and adrenal androgens. In: Greenspan FS, Strewler GJ (eds). *Basic and Clinical Endocrinology*, 5th edn. Stamford, CT: Appleton and Lange, 1997: 317–58.
11. Valloton MB, Rossier MF, Capponi AM. Potassium–angiotensin interplay in the regulation of aldosterone biosynthesis *Clin Endocrinol* 1995; **42:** 111–20.
12. Oelkers W. Adrenal insufficiency. *N Engl J Med* 1996; **335:** 1206–12.
13. Ten S, New M, Maclaren N. Addison's disease 2001. *J Clin Endocrinol Metab* 2001; **86:** 2909–22.
14. Rasmusson S, Olsson T, Hagg E. A low dose ACTH test to assess the function of the hypothalamic–pituitary–adrenal axis. *Clin Endocrinol* 1996; **44:** 151–56.
15. Peacey SR, Guo C-Y, Robinson AM, *et al.* Glucocorticoid replacement

therapy: Are patients over treated and does it matter? *Clin Endocrinol* 1997; **46:** 255–2.62.

16. Fiad TM, Conwy JD, Cunningham SK, McKenna TJ. The role of plasma renin activity in evaluating the adequacy of mineralocorticoid replacement in primary adrenal insufficiency. *Clin Endocrinol* 1996; **45:** 529–34.
17. Esteban NV, Loughlin T, Yergey AL, *et al.* Daily cortisol production rate in man determined by stable isotope dilution/mass spectrometry. *J Clin Endocrinol Metab* 1991; **72:** 39–45.
18. Burke CN. Primary adrenocortical failure In: Grossman A (ed.). *Clinical Endocrinology,* 1st edn. Oxford: Blackwell Scientific Publications 1992: 393–404.
19. Trainer PJ, Besser GM. Cushing's syndrome. In: Besser GM, Thorner MO (eds). *Clinical Endocrinology,* 2nd edn. London: Mosby-Wolfe, 1994: 8.1–8.10.
20. Lacroix A, Bolté E, Tremblay J, *et al.* Gastric inhibitory polypeptide-dependent cortisol hypersecretion – a new cause of Cushing's syndrome. *N Engl J Med* 1992; **327:** 974–80.
21. Dluhy RG, Williams GH. Endocrine hypertension. In: Wilson JD, Foster DW, Kronenberg HM, Reed Larsen P (eds). *Williams Textbook of Endocrinology,* 9th edn. Philadelphia: WB Saunders 1998: 729–49.
22. Stewart PM, Dunne F. Primary hyperaldosteronism. In: Sheaves R, Jenkins PJ, Wass JAH (eds). *Clinical Endocrine Oncology.* Oxford: Blackwell Science 1997: 312–18.
23. Reed Larsen P, Davies TF, Hay ID. The thyroid gland. In: Wilson JD, Foster DW, Kronenberg HM, Reed Larsen P (eds). *Williams Textbook of Endocrinology,* 9th edn. Philadelphia: W B Saunders 1998: 389–515.
24. Enrique Silva J. Catecholamines and the sympathoadrenal system in thyrotoxicosis. In: Braverman LE, Utiger RD (eds). *Werner and Ingbar's The Thyroid,* 7th edn. Philadelphia: Lippincott-Raven, 1996: 661–70.
25. Vanderpump MPJ, Turnbridge WMG, French JM, *et al.* The incidence of thyroid disorders in the community: a twenty year follow up of the Whickam survey. *J Clin Endocrinol* 1995; **43:** 55–68.
26. Weetman AP. Hypothyroidism: screening and subclinical disease. *Br Med J* 1997; **314:** 1175–8.
27. Waise A, Belchetz PE. Unsuspected central hypothyroidism. *Br Med J* 2000; **321:** 1275–7.
28. Surks MI, Chopra IJ, Mariash CN, *et al.* American Thyroid Association guidelines for use of laboratory tests in thyroid disorders. *J Am Med Assoc* 1990; **263:** 1529–32.
29. Sawin CT, Geller A, Wolff PA, *et al.* Low serum thyrotrophin concentrations as a risk factor for atrial fibrillation in older persons. *N Engl J Med* 1994; **331:** 1249–52.
30. Bunevicius R, Kazanavicius G, Zalinkevicius R, Prange AJ. Effects of thyroxine as compared with thyroxine plus triiodothyronine in patients with hypothyroidism. *N Engl J Med* 1999; **340:** 424–9.
31. Weetman AP. Thyrotoxicosis. In: Wass JAH, Thakker RV (eds). *Endocrine Disorders. Medicine* 2001; **29:** 27–31.
32. Menimer JG, Hershman JM, Higgins HP. The thyrotrophin in hydatidiform moles is human chorionic gonadotrophin. *J Clin Endocrinol Metab* 1975; **40:** 482–91.
33. Tsuruta E, Tada H, Tamaki H, *et al.* Pathogenic role of asialo human chorionic gonadotrophin in gestational thyrotoxicosis. *J Clin Endocrinol Metab* 1995; **80:** 350–5.
34. Daniels GH. Amiodarone-induced thyrotoxicosis. *J Clin Endocrinol Metab* 2001; **86:** 3–8.
35 Prys-Roberts C. Phaeochromocytoma – recent progress in its management. *Br J Anaesth* 2000; **85:** 44–57.
36. Bouloux PG, Fakeeh M. Phaeochromocytoma. In: Sheaves R, Jenkins PJ, Wass JAH (eds). *Clininical Endocrine Oncology.* Oxford: Blackwell Science 1997: 299–305.
37. Williams ED, Sandler M. The classification of carcinoid tumours. *Lancet* 1963; **1:** 238–9.
38. Capella C, Heitz PU, Hofler H, *et al.* Revised classification of neuroendocrine tumours of the lungs, pancreas and gut *Virchows Arch Pathol Anat Histopathol* 1995; **425:** 547–60.
39. Oberg K. Carcinoid syndrome. In: Sheaves R, Jenkins PJ, Wass JAH (eds). *Clinical Endocrine Oncology.* Oxford: Blackwell Science 1997; 411–20.
40. Oberg K. Treatment of neuroendocrine tumours. *Cancer Treat Rev* 1994; **20:** 331–55.

25

Allergic reactions

MALCOLM FISHER AND DAVID SAGE

INTRODUCTION

In the professional lifetime of the average anesthesiologist, a life-threatening allergic reaction will happen only once or twice. Current peer and patient expectation is of a polished clinical performance: rapid diagnosis and treatment and full patient recovery. This chapter will provide the theoretical and practical framework for this perfect response to a rare emergency. While advances in molecular biology have greatly increased our knowledge of probable mechanisms, the best advice we have on treatment is very anecdotal, and diagnostic methods remain rudimentary.

Strictly defined, allergy implies a host immune mechanism, switching on in response to second or subsequent exposures to a specific antigen (allergen). This chapter will also consider clinically similar responses not involving immunoglobulin. It is also worthwhile remembering that the various mechanisms of mediator release described below do not happen in isolation, and that the coagulation, kallikrein and complement systems are often activated by the same stimulus.

ANAPHYLACTIC AND ANAPHYLACTOID MECHANISMS

Definitions

In practice, the four types of hypersensitivity described by Gell and Coombs are not completely separate entities, but the descriptive framework is useful. The mechanism of type 1 hypersensitivity summarized in Fig. 25.1 shows that exposure then re-exposure to antigen results (in a small minority of individuals) in IgE-mediated mast cell degranulation and release of mediators. It is not known why injected foreign material, such as drugs, can be innocuous on the vast majority of occasions but can also act as an antigen in certain rare individuals. Also, the concomitant occurrence of IgG antibodies to the same antigen, stimulating IgE production, is noted in insect venom and latex allergy, but the significance is unclear. The clinical appearances of asthma, eczema, hayfever, or urticaria, known collectively as atopy, result from localized mediator release, whereas anaphylaxis is the clinical picture of generalized (systemic) mediator release. The rapid generalized response of anaphylaxis, developing in minutes and seen as skin changes (erythema, urticaria, and angioedema), bronchospasm, and hypotension is clinically indistinguishable from mast cell degranulation caused by a variety of other mechanisms that do not require IgE. Thus, the term anaphylactoid is used to refer to these anaphylactic-like responses, or more loosely to describe all anaphylactic-like clinical pictures as they develop, since true type 1 hypersensitivity IgE-mediated anaphylaxis can be diagnosed only by investigation after the event.

Mast cell (basophil) mechanisms

Mast cells and basophils are functionally similar and derive from hemopoietic stem cells through the myeloid lineage (see Fig. 23.1). Basophils are found in small numbers in the bloodstream whereas mast cells are widely distributed in tissues adjacent to blood vessels, where their released mediators can act on vessel walls. Granules within both these cells contain heparin, slow reactive substance of anaphylaxis (SRS-A), eosinophil chemotactic factor of anaphylaxis (ECF-A), and histamine. They also contain several proteases, including tryptase and chymase, in contrast with basophils, which contain negligible amounts of these two enzymes. There are two subpopulations of mast cells distinguishable by their anatomical location and numerous differences in cell characteristics. The ubiquitous connective tissue mast cells (CTMCs) carry larger histamine and tryptase loads than mucosal mast cells (MMCs), which in turn are found in highest concentration in the midgut and the lung (Table 25.1). Further population differences include the relative amounts of arachidonic acid metabolites (prostaglandins and leukotrienes) produced, cell-surface Fc receptor numbers, and responsiveness to inhibitors of histamine release such as theophylline and disodium cromoglycate.

Mast cell degranulation is the rapid process of fusion of granules within the cell and expulsion of most or all granular contents. Mediators such as histamine thus released quickly reach the bloodstream and within minutes cause the signs and symptoms of an anaphylactoid reaction. In the type 1 mechanism (Fig. 25.1), in addition to release of preformed mediators, degranulating mast cells also release cytokines (low-molecular-weight secreted proteins), newly synthesized leukotrienes and prostaglandins, and proinflammatory factors such as the cytokine tumor necrosis factor (TNF-α) and platelet-activating factor (PAF), which all contribute to the inflammatory response. Cytokines (e.g. IL-4, -5, -13, -19) are also central to the control of IgE synthesis, and their overall importance in acute massive mediator release is becoming increasingly apparent with recent developments in identification and purification of individual cytokines.[1]

A scheme is shown in Fig. 25.2 of the processes thought to be involved in mast cell degranulation caused by various stimuli. Using the example of an individual sensitized to rocuronium, mast cells exist with previously manufactured rocuronium-specific IgE molecules adherent

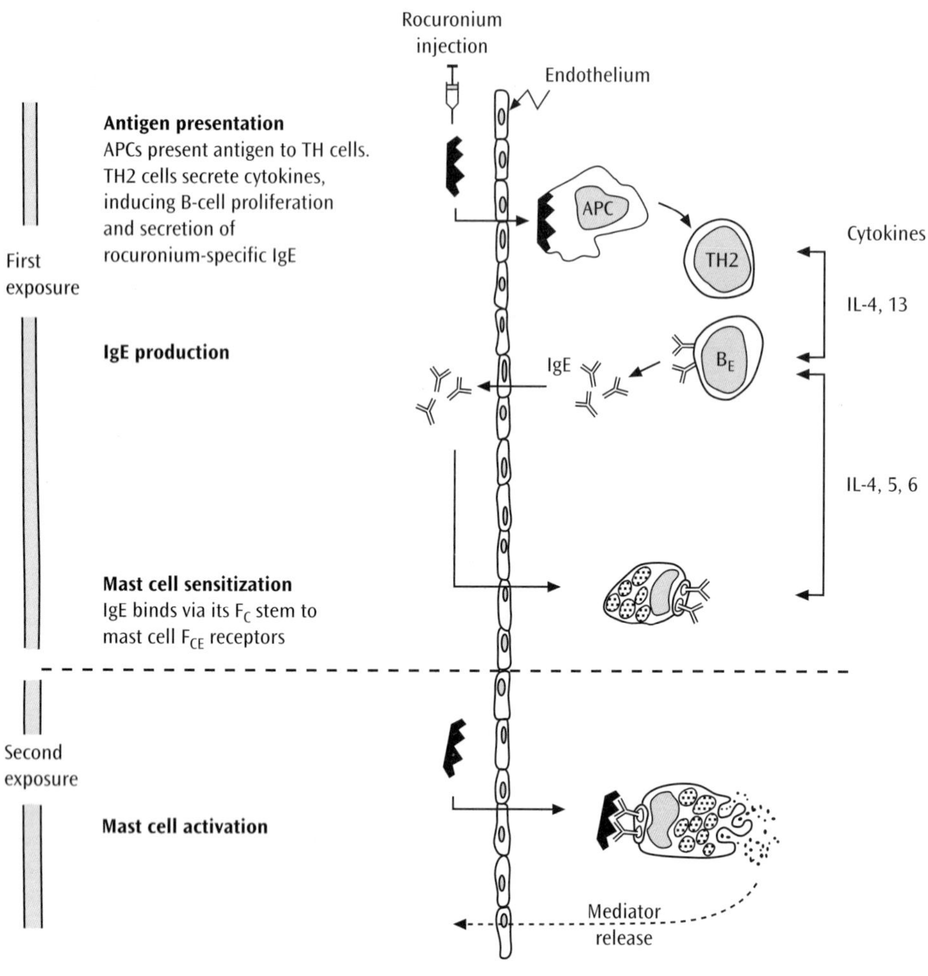

Figure 25.1 *Induction of type 1 hypersensitivtiy. APC, antigen-presenting cell; BE, B cell; IL, interleukin; TH2, T helper cell.*

Table 25.1 *Differences in the location and protease and histamine content of mast cells and basophils*

Cell type	Location	Protease content		Histamine content
		Tryptase	Chymase	
Mucosal mast cell	Intestine, lung, nose	+	–	+
Connective tissue mast cell	Skin, blood, vessels, intestine	+++	+	+++
Basophil	Bloodstream	–	–	–

to surface receptors. If this specific IgE is cross-linked by newly administered rocuronium, the surface receptors will aggregate to cause an influx of calcium ions into the cell. Various compounds are also known to actively cross-link IgE nonspecifically, for example across the Fc region (not the immune recognition Fab sites), such as lectins (carbohydrate-binding proteins found in foods), which is probably the explanation for some examples of food urticaria. The anaphylatoxins (complement fragments C3a and C5a) can trigger the degranulation of mast cells by binding to specific cell-surface receptors, and the structure of the C5a receptor in particular has been well delineated. These complement fragments are produced by activation of the complement cascade (by either classical or alternative pathways) by drugs such as protamine. However, any stimulus to mast cell degranulation produces tryptase, which directly cleaves C3, C4, and C5 to produce C3a and C5a, and thus the measurement of complement consumption following an anaphylactoid event is not helpful in elucidating the nature of the triggering stimulus.

The result of sudden calcium ion influx is twofold: exocytosis of granules containing preformed mediators (mainly histamine) and the induction of cell membrane synthesis of prostaglandins and leukotrienes from arachidonic acid, mediators with direct local histamine-like effects. The combined effect is the release of mediators that act systemically to constrict bronchial smooth muscle, vasodilate, and increase vascular permeability (plus a number of other systemic effects), and act locally to promote cellular inflammatory responses including activation of kinin and complement pathways (Fig. 25.2).

Low-grade histamine release

It is not clear whether the calcium influx and massive or low-grade degranulation produced by a long list of established mast-cell-triggering agents (e.g. compound 48/80, TNF-α, morphine, vancomycin, anesthetic drugs) operate through mast cell surface sites similar to the Fc receptors or through other individual mechanisms.

From a normal value of $<0.5\,ng\,mL^{-1}$, a very small transient rise in plasma histamine ($1–2\,ng\,mL^{-1}$) is measurable in most subjects after intravenous bolus injection of many drugs including opiates, anesthetic

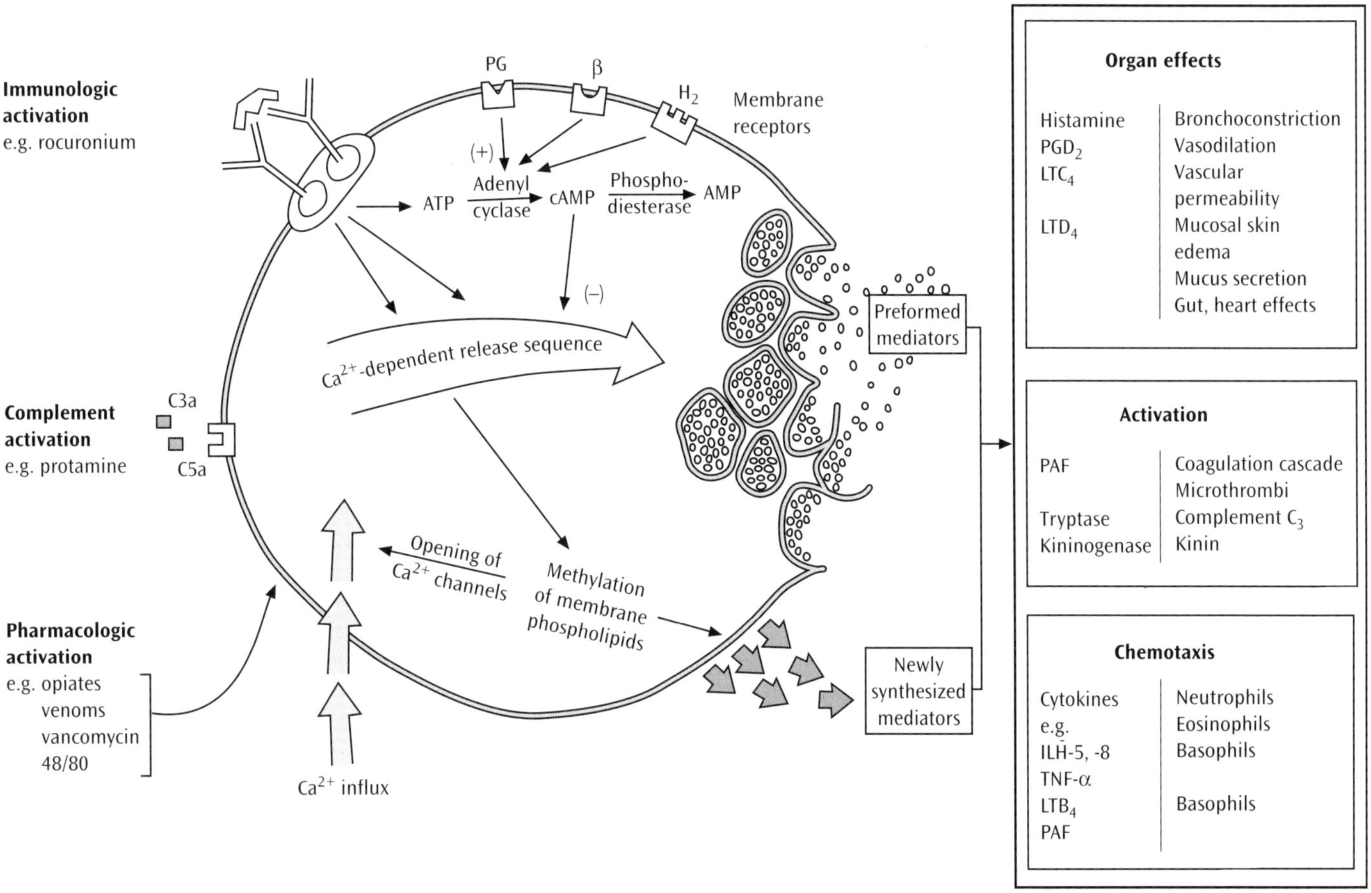

Figure 25.2 *Mast cell degranulation. ATP, adenosine triphosphate; cAMP, cyclic adenosine monophosphate; IL, interleukin; LT, leukotriene; PAF, platelet-activating factor; PG, prostaglandin; TNF, tumor necrosis factor.*

induction agents, and muscle relaxants. This is 10–100 times less than the levels common in anaphylaxis.[2] Fleeting erythema and minor heart rate and blood pressure changes are often noticed and ignored by anesthesiologists. The effects of these low levels of histamine release can be completely prevented by pretreatment with H_1 and H_2 receptor blockers.[3] Other stimuli such as surgery, trauma, and blood transfusion also cause low-grade histamine release, with marked variability between individuals in the extent of release. There is a correlation between low histamine blood levels, cardiovascular cutaneous signs, and subjective symptoms in volunteers, but blood levels do not correlate with bronchospasm.[4,5] Histamine-induced endogenous catecholamine release may explain this since histamine infusions produce bronchospasm only in the presence of β-blockade.[6] H_1 and H_2 blocking drugs effectively abolish histamine effects only at low plasma histamine levels ($<10\,ng\,mL^{-1}$) and, since blood levels in anaphylaxis are frequently greater than $50\,ng\,mL^{-1}$, these drugs are unsuitable for use in immediate resuscitation.

Potent low-grade histamine releasers such as morphine and *d*-tubocurarine show no increased propensity to produce massive degranulation; however, with all these drugs the histamine levels achieved are higher with multiple and rapid injection and higher doses. Mast cell populations from different parts of the body (skin, lung, heart, intestine, and also basophils), show different low-grade histamine release patterns with particular drugs. Morphine, for example, causes histamine release from skin mast cells only. Propofol, atracurium, and vecuronium release histamine from the lung mast cells, which may explain a number of referrals with nonimmunologic bronchospasm when these drugs are given together. In contrast, ketamine, a releaser of histamine from pulmonary mast cells, is effective in treating bronchospasm.[7–9]

Effects of histamine and other mediators

Although histamine as the dominant mediator explains most of the clinical anaphylactoid presentations, cases in which plasma histamine is normal have been recorded,[10] and the presence of other mediators explains this. Figure 25.2 lists mediators participating in the immediate circulatory–respiratory–inflammatory response and their three main areas of action. Other compounds detected are heparin, chondroitin sulfate, carboxypeptidese, peroxidase, chymase, and cathepsin G.

A summary of histamine pharmacology is given in Table 25.2. Arachidonic acid derivatives prostaglandin D_2 (PGD_2) and leukotrienes (LT) C_4 and D_4, which are newly synthesized in the mast cell membrane in response to exocytosis (Fig. 25.2), have histamine-like vascular and bronchial smooth muscle effects. Preformed and released by degranulation, cytokines induce chemotaxis of additional inflammatory cells. Activation of the kinin and complement system is achieved by preformed kininogen and tryptase.

Suppression of mediator release

Pretreatment with certain drugs effectively inhibits low-grade histamine release but cannot prevent anaphylaxis.

Table 25.2 *Histamine actions*

Organ/tissue	Receptor	Action
Heart	H_2	Positive inotropy
	H_2	Positive chronotropy
	H_1	AV conduction slowing
	H_3	Negative atrial chronotropy
Vascular smooth muscle	$H_1 + H_2$	Vasodilation
	H_3	?
Endothelium	H_1 (also H2?)	Increase permeability
bronchial smooth muscle	H_1	Bronchospasm
	H2	Bronchodilation – weak
Gastric mucosa	H_1	HCl secretion
Gut smooth muscle	H_1	Contraction
Skin peripheral neurons	H_1	Itch

AV, atrioventricular.

Adenyl cyclase activity in mast cells increases cyclic adenosine monophosphate (cAMP) synthesis, which has an inhibitory effect on the degranulation process (Fig. 25.2). Prostaglandins, β-agonists, and histamine itself stimulate adenyl cyclase activity via specific surface receptors. Thus, histamine appears to exert negative feedback on its own release, and the rationale for anaphylaxis resuscitation with epinephrine rather than α-agonists is based on β-receptor-mediated inhibition of further degranualation. Corticosteroids exert their anti-inflammatory action through cytokine effects on IgE synthesis and reduce mast cell excitability. Phosphodiesterase inhibitors increase intracellular cAMP by inhibiting its breakdown, and disodium cromoglycate probably inhibits calcium ion influx into the cell.

Risk factors for mediator release

There is poor understanding of why mast cells vary in sensitivity (their readiness to degranulate) both between and within individuals over time. Sensitivity for low-grade histamine release or massive degranulation appears to be unrelated. Anaphylaxis in neonates and the elderly is rare, perhaps reflecting their overall reduced immunocompetence. The catecholamine response to shock may provide protection since anaphylaxis is rare in shocked states.

Recent work has suggested that the clinical manifestations of anaphylaxis may be associated with impairment of the renin–angiotensin system. Hermann and Ring[11] described in 50 patients who had anaphylaxis to *Hymenoptera* venom significantly lower levels of renin, angiotensin I and II, and angiotensinogen compared with healthy controls. The levels were inversely correlated with the severity of symptoms and were returned to normal by immunotherapy. This failure of a protective mechanism is an attractive hypothesis to explain the lack of correlation between antibody levels and histamine responsiveness, and between histamine releasibility and the severity of reactions.[12]

Atopy and allergy

Although the literature reveals a three- to fivefold greater incidence of anaphylactoid reactions during anesthesia occurring in patients with allergy atopy or asthma compared with controls, this history as a predictor of anaphylactic reactions has a very low specificity and sensitivity.[13] A French study in which reactors were matched for age, gender, and social class and atopy was measured by antigen testing suggests that this increased incidence may be spurious.[14]

Overall, it must be realized that the majority of patients sustaining major anaphylactoid events are not atopic, and that the majority of atopic allergic or asthmatic patients do not sustain allergic reactions.

Gender

The female–male ratio for anaphylaxis to neuromuscular blocking drugs (NMBDs) is 4:1. This difference is somewhat less for colloids and thiopental (thiopentone). Sex differences in the age at which surgery is undertaken in men and women may partly explain this. A true difference might imply a gender difference in immune processing, or different environmental allergen exposure in women. For instance, sensitization to ammonium ion epitopes in cosmetics is a possible explanation.[15] For further discussion on immune differences between sexes, see Chapter 23.

Previous exposure

In anaphylaxis to thiopental, multiple uneventful exposures are not unusual, with up to 47 previous exposures in our series (M Fisher, unpublished data) and usually more than five.[16] A history of previous exposure is found in less than 50% of patients who are allergic to NMBDs, despite the demonstration of IgE antibodies that traditional wisdom suggests require previous exposure to be formed.[17] It is likely that the antibody that binds NMBDs has formed in response to exposure to some other antigen outside the field of anesthetic drugs. This is especially so of succinylcholine (suxamethonium), which is such a simple structure that it is unlikely that it could lead to antibody formation. It is also possible that even with previous exposure the antibody is formed not to the NMBDs themselves but to the outside antigens. Over 20 years of research has still not determined how people become sensitized to NMBDs.

Other allergic mechanisms

While the immediacy of type 1 hypersensitivity makes it of fundamental relevance to anesthesia practice, examples of type 2, type 3, and type 4 hypersensitivity may be encountered, and the reader is referred to any standard immunology text for a more detailed explanation.

Type 2 hypersensitivity reactions are caused by IgG or IgM antibodies against cell-surface antigens, such as occurs with incompatible blood transfusion.

Type 3 hypersensitivity produces immune complex disorders mediated by complement, which may include fixed drug skin disorders occurring days and weeks after exposure (as observed with barbiturates[18]).

Type 4 hypersensitivity has three variations, of which contact hypersensitivity is the most relevant to anesthesia practice. The reaction takes more than 12 h to develop and involves prior sensitization and memory T cells. Clinically, the reaction is characterized by an eczematous skin reaction at the point of contact with the allergen, for example latex gloves or, rarely, local anesthetics.

ANAPHYLAXIS DURING ANESTHESIA

Incidence

The incidence of anaphylaxis to a specific substance is a fraction in which the denominator is the number of cases in which the substance has been given and the numerator is the number of associated cases of anaphylaxis. These numbers are difficult to gather accurately. For anesthesia, the largest study is a multicenter French study, which found an incidence of anaphylaxis during anesthesia of 1:6000,[19] in agreement with a subsequent French pediatric survey.[20] The Boston Collaborative Drug Surveillance study[21] found an incidence of 1:900 to 1:20 000. At these rates, to establish an overall incidence of anaphylaxis during anesthesia with 5% confidence limits would require about 30 million patients.[22] On this basis, incidence data for specific drugs are likely to be even less meaningful.

Drugs producing anaphylaxis

The drugs producing anaphylaxis over a 25-year period of referrals to an Australian clinic (M Fisher, unpublished data) are shown in Table 25.3.

Neuromuscular blocking drugs

It can be seen from the table that NMBDs are the commonest cause of anaphylactic reactions, as in all large series. Succinylcholine is the most common culprit throughout the world. Pancuronium and vecuronium initially appeared safer than other NMBDs, suggesting that the steroid structure may be a safety factor. However, in France, changing patterns of usage have been associated with an increasing incidence of reactions to vecuronium.[19] In Australia and New Zealand, rocuronium appears to be fast becoming the commonest cause of anaphylaxis, which is almost certainly related to market share. Cross-sensitivity between NMBDs occurs in 60% of reactors.[23] Thus, the importance of skin testing for all NMBDs cannot be overemphasized. Cisatracurium and atracurium are antigenically identical.[24]

Thiopental

The use of propofol has led to the virtual disappearance of thiopental anaphylaxis. Two UK studies suggested the incidence was of the order of 1:20 000.[25,26] Multiple uneventful exposures usually occur before the abnormal reaction but, rarely, it may occur on the first exposure. There is variable cross-sensitivity with other barbiturates.[27]

Table 25.3 *Drugs producing life-threatening clinical anaphylaxis during anesthesia, 1974–98* (n = 666)[a]

Drug	No. of cases
Induction agents (*n* = 88)	
Thiopental	46
Alfathesin	29
Propanidid	6
Methohexitone	1
Propofol	5
Midazolam	1
Induction agent and NMBD (*n* = 3)	
Thiopental/succinylcholine	1
Thiopental/alcuronium	1
1-Thiopental/atracurium	1
NMBDs (n = 392)	
Reaction to single NMBD (*n* = 374)	
Alcuronium	125
Suxamethonium	127
Atracurium	38
d-Tubocurarine	23
Gallamine	16
Vecuronium	19
Mivacurium	1
Rocuronium	11
Cisatracurium	2
Pancuronium	12
Reaction to two NMBDs given on same occasion (*n* = 9)	
Succinylcholine/atracurium	1[b]
Succinylcholine/gallamine	2[b]
Succinylcholine/alcuronium	4[b]
Succinylcholine/vecuronium	1[b]
Succinylcholine/*d*-tubocurarine	1[b]
Reactions to two NMBDs on separate occasions (*n* = 9)	
d-Tubocurarine/alcuronium	3
Decamethonium/succinylcholine	1
Pancuronium/alcuronium	1
Gallamine/alcuronium	1
Succinylcholine/pancuronium	1
Alcuronium/vecuronium	1
Rocuronium/vecuronium	1
Colloid solutions (*n* = 37)	
Hemaccel	27
Dextran 70	6
Dextran 40	1
SPPS	1
NSA	1
Plasma	1
Local anesthetics (*n* = 6)	
Prilocaine/lidocaine	1[c]
Bupivacaine	2
Lignocaine	2
Ropivicaine/lidocaine	1
Opiates (*n* = 16)	
Morphine	8
Fentanyl	4
Omnopon	1
Meperidine	3
Antibiotics (*n* = 45)	
Ephalothin	12
Cephamandole	1
Cephazolin	10
Cefotaxime	3
Cefotetan	5
Penicillin	2
Ampicillin	4
Flucloxacillin	4
Vancomycin	2
Ampicillin/flucloxacillin	1[b]
Other drugs and agents (*n* = 29)	
Atropine	2
Blood	2
Contrast media	4
Ergometrine	1
Fragmin	1
Goretex	1
Latex	4
Neostigmine	1
Ondansetron	1
Patent blue	1
Platelets	2
Protamine	9
No drug determined	50

NMBD, neuromuscular block drug; NSA, normal soluble albumin; SPPS, stable plasma protein solution; lidocaine (lignocaine); meperidine (pethidine); succinylcholine (suxamethonium); thiopental (thiopentone).

a. Patients referred to M Fisher for investigation from Australia, New Zealand, and Europe.

b. Both drugs received prior to reaction and positive skin and/or radioallergosorbent tests.

c. Two reactions on separate occasions.

Cremophor-based drugs

Previously used anesthetic drugs althesin and propanidid, and initially propofol, were dissolved in Cremophor EL, which was associated with a very high incidence of anaphylaxis of up to 1:900. These allergic reactions were unusual in that they caused complement activation by the classical and alternative pathways. Skin testing produced positive results suggesting IgE involvement.[28,29] The precise roles in anaphylaxis of the active drug and the solvent were not elucidated.

Propofol

After changing the solvent from Cremophor to fat emulsion, life-threatening reactions to propofol still occurred to a lesser extent,[30] but the exact incidence is still unknown. Positive skin tests and propofol-specific IgE antibodies have been documented. There is no evidence in the literature to support the relation between allergy to eggs and allergy to the solvent causing anaphylaxis. Six patients have been referred to the Royal North Shore Hospital Clinic with late-onset (20 min) bronchospasm and rash but no elevation in mast cell tryptase levels after propofol and lidocaine (lignocaine) administered together.

Other induction agents

Reactions to ketamine, midazolam, etomidate, and methohexitone have been described but these reactions are extremely rare.

Opioids

Anaphylactic reactions to morphine, codeine phosphate, meperidine (pethidine), omnopon, and fentanyl have all been described but these are also rare. Fewer than 20 cases have been reported in the literature.[31]

Antibiotics

Antibiotics account for 2–6% of reported anaphylactic reactions, with cephalosporins being the most common culprit.[32] The incidence is increasing in Australia[33] and France (MC Laxenaire, personal communication). Cross-reactivity between cephalosporins is unusual because antigenicity is usually related to side chains rather than to the β-lactam group. Cross-sensitivity to penicillin through the β-lactam group is probably overestimated and there is no evidence of cross-sensitivity between penicillin and second, third, and fourth generation cephalosporins.[34] Cephalexin has a common side chain with ampicillin with some crossover in allergy while ceftazidine (without the common side chain) does not.[35] A recent study has shown that up to 25% of patients undergoing major surgery had nonimmune, nonhistamine-mediated reactions to antibiotics.[36]

Protamine

Reactions to protamine may involve a number of mechanisms including IgE, IgG, and complement.[37–39] Two different types of reaction may occur, a classical anaphylactic reaction or a syndrome producing pulmonary hypertension and right heart failure.[40,41] A prolonged and persistent capillary leak post bypass has been attributed to protamine and plasma products, although no direct cause and effect has been shown.[40] Protamine–insulin therapy, fish allergy, and vasectomy have been suggested as predisposing factors to protamine anaphylaxis, but there is no convincing association. Screening with skin testing or radioimmunoassay (RIA) tests is not useful.[42] Protamine anaphylaxis is less commonly reported today than in the past.

Colloids and blood products

All synthetic colloids have been shown to produce clinical anaphylaxis and their is no major evidence that one particular colloid has a higher incidence than another. As previously described, these reactions are rare during shock and there is little evidence that IgE is involved in the reactions. Pretreatment with high-molecular-weight dextrans (to cross-link any existing dextran-specific IgE) reduces the incidence of reactions to dextrans,[43] but anaphylaxis has occurred in response to the pretreatment and after the pretreatment. Reactions to blood products are well documented but are surprisingly infrequently reported to our unit in Australia.

Latex

Latex allergy is the IgE-mediated ocular, cutaneous, respiratory, or systemic allergic response to residual rubber-tree proteins in latex products. In some individuals, both IgG4 and IgE antibodies to the same rubber protein antigens have been detected, but the significance of this not known.[44]

The antigenicity of different rubber products is influenced by the manufacturing process. Tree sap from the rubber tree (*Hevea brasiliensis*) is collected into preservative (often ammonia). In the manufacturing process of latex rubber a number of chemicals are added. These include accelerators, curing agents, antioxidants, blowing compounds, the addition of sulfur in the vulcanization process, coloring agents, and corn starch powder. Latex rubber is about 30–40% *cis*-1,4-polyisoprene polymer, plus a mixture of some 200 latex peptides. Polyisoprene can also be manufactured synthetically from petrochemicals and itself has no allergic potential.

Latex allergy was first described in 1927. The next report appeared in 1979, the first perioperative case was reported in 1989, and between 1990 and 1994 the Food and Drug Administration (FDA) reported 1100 cases with 15 deaths, resulting in the recall of barium enema latex catheters. The multiple glove changes now required with the institution of universal precautions in hospitals and dental clinics has hugely increased the exposure to latex antigen of patients and healthcare workers.

In the general (nonatopic) population, the prevalence of latex allergy is $<1\%$; in healthcare workers regularly exposed to latex it is 7–10%, and in children with spina bifida 28–67%.[45–47] In a study in which the overall rate of anaphylaxis occurring during anesthesia was around 1: 7000 anesthetics, latex caused 76% of anaphylactic events in children, compared with 13% in adults.[20]

Clinical presentation

The commonest clinical presentation is hand dermatitis (type 4 delayed hypersensitivity). Far less common presentations are contact urticaria, rhinoconjunctivitis, wheeze, and anaphylaxis/death, which are all type 1 mechanisms. Although hand dermatitis may be a delayed type 4 response to latex proteins, nonlatex type 4 reactions to other chemicals in rubber (carbomates, thiazoles, etc.) may be the cause. Alternatively, these chemicals may be direct skin irritants (without an immune basis) and skin excoriation from these causes may predispose to latex allergy. With occupational exposure to latex there can be a progression from cutaneous symptoms to rhinoconjunctivitis, bronchospasm, and anaphylaxis over months or years, and detectable IgE may precede symptoms. The mode of exposure tends to influence the severity of the response: air particle exposure (glove powder) produces eye symptoms or itchy nose, cutaneous exposure induces urticaria and erythema locally, but mucosal or parenteral exposure induces anaphylaxis.

At-risk populations

Atopic individuals have an increased risk (fourfold). Repeated catherization and/or multiple surgery, such as occurs in children with spina bifida and congenital urogenital anomalies, creates the highest risk, followed by occupational exposure – in healthcare workers, usually as a result of wearing gloves or breathing latex-laden glove powder; among workers in the rubber industry or in greenhouses; and in employees in surgical glove and elastic textile factories, etc. Increased risk of latex allergy in those allergic to foods with similar antigens such as banana, kiwi, chestnut, avocado, potato, and tomato is alleged.

Diagnosis

This is essentially a clinical diagnosis made on the patient's history; however, detection of latex protein-specific IgE, usually by skin prick test (SPT) and RIA, is a useful adjunct. Questioning should explore:

1 atopy;
2 allergy – including banana, kiwi, chestnut, avocado, potato, and tomato;
3 multiple surgery, catheterization;
4 occupational exposure;
5 balloon, glove, and condom intolerance;
6 sequence of symptoms and signs, local and systemic urticaria, cutaneous, respiratory, generalized distribution.

History alone will not identify all latex-allergic subjects, but should be part of the anesthetic workup for high-risk patients. The accuracy of latex-specific IgE detection by SPT or RIA is extremely population dependent. For example, in the Toronto Sick Children's Hospital case series,[48] all 11 spina bifida children with clinically life-threatening anaphylaxis to rubber had positive latex prick tests. Prick testing is more sensitive and specific than RIA. Also, RIA-positive results occur in asymptomatic individuals and negative results occur in the presence of clinically unequivocal latex allergy.[47,49,50]

Clinical presentation perioperatively

Typically, the onset of allergic signs and symptoms is delayed 20–90 min from the onset of the procedure, sometimes with the gradual appearance of increased heart rate, decreased blood pressure, skin signs, and bronchospasm, and quite often with onset following skin closure. Plasma tryptase is typically elevated. Clinical management is identical for any anaphylactoid event occurring during anesthesia.

Management of a known case

Adopting a latex reduction protocol is probably more rational than extreme measures to eradicate all possible latex sources, since indirect evidence suggests that the latex antigen load required to induce anaphylaxis is quite variable and extreme measures are justified only if extreme sensitivity exists. Each operating room should have a protocol listing rubber-containing items that could come into contact with the patient, and their alternatives. Nonlatex gloves are the most important measure, and systematic elimination of rubber in contact with the patient (anesthetic equipment such as face mask, blood pressure (BP) cuff, pulse oximeter probe, syringes, and tape) and surgical equipment (Penrose drains, catheters, rubber-shod clamps, vascular tags, bulb syringes, rubber bands, and instrument mats) is logical.

In future, strict labeling regulations for latex content (introduced in 1998 in the USA) should reduce accidental exposure of latex-sensitive individuals. Isolation of the specific latex antigens causing allergy will allow the production of standardized antigen for testing and thus increased accuracy of IgE detection. Alternatives to latex gloves and the development of other latex-free products, and products with reduced latex protein levels (including powderless latex gloves), will undoubtedly become available in response to the high allergy incidence in the occupationally exposed.

Local anesthetics

Anaphylactic reactions to aminoamide local anesthetics (LAs) are extremely rare. A description of "collapse" from LA administration requires probing interrogation of the time sequence and whether there was loss of consciousness, seizures, or spontaneous recovery, bearing in mind that the diagnosis and treatment at the time may have been completely inappropriate. Inadvertent intravascular injection of epinephrine can cause extreme anxiety, a feeling of impending doom, and angina. Convulsions require a significant intravascular LA dose. The major cause of 'collapse" following LA injection is vasovagal, and hypoxic convulsions can occur as a result. Vasovagal unconsciousness can occur in the supine position and the reflex is particularly vigorous in young adults. Both these causes of "collapse" following LA are associated with rapid spontaneous recovery. In the absence of skin, respiratory, or cardiovascular signs of anaphylactoid reaction, evidence for profound bradycardia (associated with vasovagal causes but not anaphylaxis) and urticaria (the reverse) should be elicited. Of the possible adverse responses to LA injection, very few cannot be diagnosed from a detailed history.

Of the 264 patients referred to our unit in Australia, with a history of "allergy to local anesthetics" only six had severe anaphylaxis to local anesthetics, four reacted to additives and four had delayed reactions (probably a type 4 mechanism, as described above). The commonest "reactions" seen were psychological (mainly vasovagal) in 102 patients. In four other published studies only 11 of 468 patients with a history of local anesthetic allergy had positive skin tests to local anesthetics.[51,52] Although some of the reactions may be related to the additives in local anesthetics,[53] this is difficult to prove since the tests for preservatives are unreliable. Where additive(s) cannot be excluded as the cause, these solutions should be avoided.

Now used uncommonly, the aminoesters are inherently far more antigenic than the amides. They are structurally similar to *p*-aminobenzoic acid (PABA) and the sulfonamides and exhibit cross-sensitivity with these drugs (e.g. allergy to tetracaine and suntan cream).

A rare cause is aminoamide local anesthetic contact hypersensitivity. The "contact" may be cream applied directly to skin or via skin infiltration.[54,55] Patients with allergic contact dermatitis to topical lidocaine also develop severe localized reactions following injections of this drug, and similar reactions to injected prilocaine occur in those who exhibit contact dermatitis to EMLA® cream.

The phenomenon of transient patchy skin erythema and occasionally urticaria seen in the arm immediately following tourniquet release after intravenous regional anesthesia using prilocaine/methylparabens or 2-chloroprocaine is probably a direct histamine-releasing action of drug or preservative.[53]

Other perioperative causes

Injected radiocontrast material, syntocinon, heparin (contaminated with histamine during manufacture), chlorhexidine and povidone–iodine skin preparations, surgical fibrin glue, and surgical irrigation containing antibiotic should also be considered as causes for anaphylactoid responses in the operating room environment.

Clinical features of anaphylaxis

Reactions may occur at any time during anesthesia, but they are most common (90% of incidences) after induction. Reactions may be well established before they are noticed. Table 25.4 shows the first clinical feature noted in 646 patients, and the clinical features in 555 patients are shown in Table 25.5.

In the last few years, difficulty in lung inflation and pulse oximetry "desaturation", due to loss of plethysmographic waveform, have been the most common first features noted. Difficulty in inflation may lead the anesthesiologist to change the endotracheal tube, which has led to subsequent accusations in court that the reaction was due to esophageal intubation (although the manifestations of esophageal intubation usually appear later than those of anaphylaxis).

Cardiovascular signs are the most common feature. Cardiovascular collapse is associated with vasodilatation and supraventricular

Table 25.4 *First clinical feature noted by anesthesiologists reporting severe anaphylactoid reactions, 1974–98* ($n = 646$)[a]

Symptom	No. of cases
Subjective	12
Cough	43
No pulse	165
No bleeding	2
Swelling	8
Difficult to inflate	155
ECG abnormality	13
Rash	30
Flush	113
Urticaria	13
Other	20
Desaturation	74

ECG, electrocardiogram.
a. Patients referred to M Fisher for investigation.

tachycardia. As it is the only feature in approximately 10% of cases, there is a risk of the reaction being attributed to other causes.

Asthmatics invariably get bronchospasm during anaphylaxis. This is the most difficult feature to treat when severe. Pulmonary edema is a very rare component of acute anaphylaxis. On first principles, a low-pressure membrane edema due to leaky capillaries with an associated volume deficit would be expected. After the event, it may be impossible to distinguish between this picture and that of high-pressure pulmonary edema, secondary to epinephrine therapy, with acute heart failure. The factors that increase severity are a history of asthma, β-blockers, and epidural anesthesia. These states are all associated with reduced efficiency of the endogenous catecholamine response, which may make the reaction worse. Other presentations of mediator release occur. Delayed rashes (4 h to 2 weeks) and periorbital edema are not uncommon. These ("fixed drug") delayed reactions (type 3 and type 4) usually occur in relation to thiopental, occasionally with a spectacular exfoliative dermatitis that takes weeks to resolve.

Acute diagnosis and treatment

Understanding the differential diagnosis of bronchospasm and cardiovascular collapse following induction is a prerequisite for the rapid presumptive diagnosis of anaphylactoid reaction. The classical skin signs may never be seen or appear only following resuscitation and skin reperfusion. The following treatment algorithm can be applied to the wide spectrum of severity encountered:

1 Discontinue administration of all drugs, colloids, blood products, and skin preparations. Consider latex in the differential diagnosis.
2 Use 100% oxygen, intubate, ventilate, and start cardiopulmonary rescuscitation (CPR) if a pulse cannot be elicited.
3 Administer epinephrine intravenously (i.v.) at 100–1000 μg initially, titrated to blood pressure response.
4 Give rapid i.v. volume replacement with the most available crystalloid or colloid at 1–2 L initially but, if several liters are necessary, there may be a theoretical advantage in choosing colloid.[56,57]

German workers suggest that colloid fluid alone is preferable to using epinephrine because of the risk of adverse effects.[57] In our studies, sympathomimetic drugs appear to enable more rapid stabilization. Epinephrine usually stops the progression of angioedema.[58]

Once the blood pressure is adequate, its maintenance may be best achieved with an infusion of epinephrine. Intense bronchospasm responds well to the high doses of epinephrine needed to support the circulation but, if refractory, then salbutamol, aminophylline, ketamine, or isoflurane can be considered. Hand ventilation and manual lateral chest wall squeezing to aid expiration are life saving in this desperate situation. Again, anecdotal evidence supports the use of corticosteroid to reduce the extent of angioedema and using both H_1 and H_2 antagonists together to reduce the length and degree of adrenaline support required.[59]

Be prepared to use very high epinephrine doses in β-blocked patients. α-Agonists and glucagon may also be useful, as well as cardiopulmonary bypass in extreme situations. Pulmonary edema is very rare and best controlled by increasing the resistance to expiration (positive end-expiatory pressure or PEEP). Invasive monitoring is required to distinguish the expected low-pressure edema and probable volume deficit from acute left ventricular failure (LVF) secondary to the myocardial insult and epinephrine treatment. In rare reactions following cardiopulmonary bypass, large volumes of high-protein edema fluid may occur requiring pleural drainage to avoid cardiac and lung tamponade.[60]

It is appropriate to assess tryptase 1 h after the reaction. A decision to proceed with surgery must be based on urgency. A significant proportion of patients immediately after resuscitation have a coagulation screen abnormality (D Galletley, personal communication). Excessive gastric acid secretion and airway mucosal edema are factors to take into account when extubating after an anaphylactoid reaction.[61]

Definitive diagnosis

This is important not only to prevent subsequent reactions, but also for epidemiological and medicolegal reasons. The goals of diagnostic testing are to determine the cause of the event and the drug responsible, to

Table 25.5 *Clinical features of anesthetic anaphylaxis in 655 patients*

Clinical feature	No. of cases	Sole feature	Worst feature
Cardiovascular collapse	575	71	525
Bronchospasm	245	33	116
Transient	99		
Asthmatics	95		
Cutaneous			
Rash	89		
Erythema	297		
Urticaria	53		
More than one	32		
Angioedema	160	7	21
Generalized edema	41		
Pulmonary edema	17	2	3
Gastrointestinal disturbance	38		

detect other drugs that may produce a similar event (cross-reactivity), and to determine which drugs are safe to use in future anesthetics.

Patients should be referred for investigation when there is a high clinical index of suspicion. Reactions affecting only one system or those of intermediate severity may be overlooked. The history is very important. If, for example, a patient develops severe bronchospasm, erythema, and cardiovascular collapse after a single injection of propofol and all the investigations are negative, it is still important to give a written warning suggesting that the drug should not be administered subsequently and explain the seriousness of the situation to the patient.

Minor reactions restricted to the skin, reactions of short duration and intermediate severity, and delayed reactions are difficult to investigate and the available tests provide little help. We have not yet been able to document a case in which a minor reaction has led to or preceded a severe reaction.

Investigation of an anaphylactic reaction

Immediate investigations

The investigation during or shortly after the reaction must be designed to confirm the cause to have been massive mediator release. It is possible with RIA tests to detect specific drug antibodies immediately following a reaction.[62]

Histamine assays

Raised concentrations of plasma histamine implicate histamine in the reaction, but assay is not clinically practical. Because of histamine's brief plasma half-life (measured in minutes), sampling must occur within 10 min, at a time when resuscitation is a higher priority. Also, meticulous and complicated handling of the specimens is necessary.

Raised histamine levels do not establish the cause of the reaction, but concentrations above 20ng mL^{-1} suggest that histamine is involved and very high levels suggest that the reaction is anaphylactic.[2,63,64] The converse is, however, not true. No elevation in plasma histamine levels does not exclude histamine involvement because local release may be implicated.

Urinary methyl histamine

Urinary methyl histamine levels remain elevated for longer than plasma histamine and are simpler to assay. Unfortunately, the test is not very accurate and reached pathological levels in only 4 of 10 patients who had adverse reactions to anesthesia, with 10 of 10 having high plasma histamine and 9 of 10 an elevated mast cell tryptase level.[63]

IgE Levels

Alterations in total serum IgE levels after a reaction have been suggested as evidence that IgE is involved in such reactions. However, the IgE in these reactions is bound to cells and so serum level changes may not occur. Drug-specific IgE levels during the reaction usually (but not always) correlate with those on subsequent investigation.[62]

Complement levels

Changes in serum complement levels and activation of the classical and alternative pathways have been demonstrated after clinical anaphylaxis, particularly anaphylaxis due to althesin, contrast media, and protamine.[28,65,66] These changes have also been revealed in IgE-mediated reactions in which no complement activation is required and may represent activation secondary to shock or an independent process. Complement activation may occur without clinical manifestations, particularly those occurring after cardiopulmonary bypass due to heparin–protamine complexes.[67] The major limitation of complement activation measurement is that it determines neither mechanism nor cause.

Mast cell tryptase

Measurement of mast cell tryptase is the most reliable test for determining if an anaphylactoid reaction has occurred. It is also a marker for degranualtion in chronic proliferative conditions such as mastocytosis.

Tryptase is a neutral protease accounting for up to 25% of mast cell protein. Connective tissue mast cells have three times the mucosal mast cell content (Table 25.1) and there are negligible levels in circulating basophils. Thus, basophil degranulation is not detected by serum tryptase assay.

Tryptase has a plasma half-life of approximately 90 min.[68] In anaphylactic reactions, the levels are elevated for 1–5 h after the onset of the reaction,[69] enabling resuscitation to occur before the need for blood sampling. The assay is performed on serum separated from clotted blood and the specimens do not require preparation on site. Reliable samples can be obtained at postmortem in patients who survive an hour or longer after the reaction begins.[70] Conversely, postmortem tryptase can be elevated in the absence of anaphylaxis and thus elevated tryptase cannot be relied upon as a sole criterion for the postmortem diagnosis of anaphylaxis.[71] Nevertheless, in life, mast cell tryptase is highly specific and sensitive for anaphylaxis. Rarely, severe reactions may occur in which there is evidence of IgE involvement, either by skin testing or RIA, when serum taken at an appropriate time does not show elevated tryptase levels. Laroche *et al.*[63] postulate an allergic mechanism whereby the mediators of anaphylaxis are released from basophils which do not contain tryptase. Table 25.6 shows the incidence of positive skin and RIA tests associated with elevated tryptase. Although the association of elevated tryptase and positive skin tests is high, skin testing is still necessary when there is a strong history suggestive of anaphylaxis but normal tryptase.[72]

Investigations following recovery

Skin testing

Skin testing is performed 4–6 weeks after the reaction[73] to allow mast cell regeneration. Although such testing detects only reactions due to IgE, and possibly IgG, it gives a high yield of results reflecting the high incidence of IgE involvement in severe reactions. Two forms of skin testing are used – intradermal and prick testing. Intradermal tests involve diluting the drug and injecting it into the dermis; in prick testing, the undiluted drug is introduced into the dermis by pricking the patient's skin through a drop of the drug to be tested. It is usual to use controls such as histamine and/or high concentrations of an opioid to determine that histamine response and release are normal.[73,74] The great advantages of skin tests are that they have the highest yield of positive results, can be performed by anyone, and cross-sensitivity determined by skin testing usually enables safe subsequent anesthesia.[73,75–79] Prick testing has the advantages of reduced trauma and cost, safety, and ease of preparation. The two tests have a greater than 90% agreement in detecting the drug implicated[74,80] but less agreement in determining cross-sensitivity between NMBDs. There are no follow-up safety data published on subsequent anesthesia based on prick tests.

Skin tests are of little value for investigating reactions to colloids, contrast media, and blood products. Local anesthetic allergy is so rare

Table 25.6 *Incidence of IgE involvement in patients with elevated mast cell tryptase*

Group	No. of patients	IgE detected
Typtase not elevated	143	7/137
Elevated tryptase	158	125/158
P-value (χ^2)	< 0.0001	

Modified from Fisher and Baldo.[74]

that the aim is to exclude allergy. Skin testing with diluted drug will detect rare IgE-mediated allergy. If skin testing is negative, progressive challenge with up to 2 mL of undiluted drug should be performed. Before skin testing, the patient should be tested with 2 mL of saline, which may reproduce the symptoms when the cause is vasovagal. When delayed type 4 hypersensitivity is suspected, the skin testing sites must be reinspected at 12–24 h.

Deaths have occurred during skin testing (although not to anesthetic drugs). In over 2000 intradermal tests we have experienced two easily treatable reactions and one severe reaction.

Radioimmunoassay tests

This testing for circulating IgE is based on the assumption that it reflects IgE bound to mast cells. An antigen, which is either the drug or an analog, is coupled to a solid support. The antigen–support complex is then incubated with the patient's serum so that any antibodies will bind to the supported antigen. The serum is removed by rinsing and the residual complex is incubated with radiolabeled anti-IgE and the bound radioactivity assessed. This test is performed in only a few specialist laboratories.

Use of these tests in over 300 patients has shown the following:

1. RIA tests will detect the drug responsible for a reaction less often than skin tests, and drug-specific RIA is not available for all drugs.
2. A combination of RIA tests and skin tests will increase the detection of responsible drugs by about 5%.
3. RIA is more sensitive than skin testing for the detection of cross-sensitivity.
4. RIA tests identify significant *in vitro* cross-sensitivity between thiopental and NMBDs, which is not demonstrable clinically. Similarly, patients who react to NMBDs have a high incidence of positive RIAs to morphine, but this is not clinically significant and is probably related to the single quaternary group involved in morphine binding to the receptor on the antibody to NMBDs, which bind by their quaternary or tertiary groups.

In practice, if any one test is positive then the patient should avoid that drug.

Other tests

Leukocyte and basophil histamine release tests have been used in specialized laboratories and give results similar to RIA. When challenged *in vitro* by exposure to the drug causing the clinical event, significant histamine release from blood cells is highly suggestive of an immune mechanism.[9] The disadvantages of these tests are their limited availability, the relative lack of efficacy data, and the fact that the patient needs to travel to the laboratory. In four cases in which anaphylaxis was clinically highly likely and skin and RIA tests were negative, we have not found histamine-release tests to be able to determine the drug responsible.

In severe reactions, the current range of tests will find an identifying agent in 95% of patients. Clearly, for those patients in whom no causative agent is identified, other anesthesic agents should be considered.

Preoperative testing

Skin test screening of the general population for allergy to latex or NMBDs has no predictive value.[81] The value of screening high-risk subgroups is unclear. Some authors have advocated that for high risk patients there should be preoperative testing with RIA. The tests are limited, however, in both availability and predictive value.[22] The recent French studies showing a high incidence of positive skin tests in the surgical and allergic populations (see above) suggest that preoperative prick testing may be valid in high-risk patients and could be performed at virtually no cost. In 68 patients whom we tested preoperatively because of a family history of a reaction, multiple allergies, or alleged environmental chemical sensitivity syndrome we identified two weak positive skin tests.

Documentation

Allergic patients should be encouraged to wear a warning device, such as a Medic Alert bracelet. This is not sufficient on its own to ensure safe subsequent exposure. They should also carry a letter stating which drugs were given, what happened, which tests were performed, the results of those tests, and the conclusions. Details of subsequent anesthesia should be added to the letter. While a few patients lose their sensitivity over time, the majority do not, and anesthetic allergy has been shown to persist for up to 27 years.[82] We routinely add to warning devices the name of a drug shown by subsequent exposure or skin testing to be safe.

With this method of testing and follow-up we have seen six subsequent allergic reactions in 320 exposures.[83] Three were related to false-negative tests to alternative relaxants, two were related to using relaxants not tested, and one was probably due to latex allergy. Out of 69 patients who were diagnosed as not anaphylactic, 68 have had uneventful subsequent anesthesia and one had a second prolonged neuromuscular block.

Anaphylaxis and litigation

Anaphylaxis during anesthesia is associated with litigation. The anesthesiologist who was in charge when the reaction occurred has a clear duty to this patient to:

1. make the correct diagnosis and take corrective action;
2. investigate with skin testing as the minimum, appreciating that cross-sensitivity may exist;
3. communicate the results to the patient, update the hospital records, and equip the patient with a durable record/warning.

FUTURE DEVELOPMENTS

The search for suitable substitutes for unduly antigenic substances, such as latex and muscle relaxants, is unlikely to eliminate the problem of anaphylaxis; however, safer drug design is achievable. More efficient H-receptor antagonist drugs and blockers of the other mediators of anaphylaxis, particularly prostaglandins and cytokines, are promising areas of current research. Measurement of mast cell "triggeriness" in terms of circulating levels of IL-4, -5, and -13 is an interesting development but preoperative screening tests for susceptibility to individual agents look to be very distant possibilities.

REFERENCES

1. Sheeran P, Hall GM. Cytokines in anaesthesia. *Br J Anaesth* 1997; **78:** 201–19.
2. Laroche D, Vergnaud MC, Sillard B, *et al.* Biochemical markers of anaphylactoid reactions to drugs. Comparison of plasma histamine and tryptase. *Anesthesiology* 1991; **75:** 945–9.
3. Lorenz W, Duda D, Dick W, Sitter H, *et al.* Incidence and clinical importance of perioperative histamine release: randomised study of volume loading and antihistamines after induction of anaesthesia. *Lancet* 1994; **343:** 933–40.
4. Kaliner M, Sigler R, Summers R, *et al.* Effects of infused histamine: analysis of the effects of H-1 and H-2 histamine receptor antagonists on cardiovascular and pulmonary responses. *J Allerg Clin Immunol* 1981; **68:** 365–71.
5. Lorenz W, Doenicke A, Schoning B, *et al.* Definition and classification of the histamine-release response to drugs in anaesthesia and surgery: studies in the conscious human subject. *Klinische Wochenschrift* 1982; **60:** 896–913.
6. Ploy-Song-Sang Y, Corbin RF, Engel LA. Effects of intravenous histamine on lung mechanics in man after beta-blockade. *J Appl Physiol* 1978; **44** (5): 690–5.

7. Genovese A, Stellato, AC Marsella, CV, *et al.* Role of mast cells, basophils and their mediators in adverse reactions to general anesthetics and radiocontrast media. *Int Arch Allerg Appl Immunol* 1996; **110:** 13–22.
8. Stellato C, Casolaro V, Ciccarelli P, *et al.* General anaesthetics induce only histamine release selectively from mast cells. *Br J Anaesth* 1991; **67:** 751–8.
9. Stellato C, de Paulis A, Cirillo R, *et al.* Heterogeneity of human mast cells and basophils in response to muscle relaxants. *Anesthesiology* 1991; **74:** 1078–86.
10. Lorenz W, Doenicke A, Messmen K, Reimann J-J, *et al.* Histamine release in human subjects by modified gelatin (Haemaccel) and dextran: an explanation for anaphylactoid reactions observed under clinical conditions? *Br J Anaesth* 1976; **48:** 151–64.
11. Hermann K, Ring J. Association between the renin–angiotensin system and anaphylaxis. *Adv Exp Med Biol* 1995; **377:** 299–309.
12. Hermann K, von Eschenbach CE, von Tschirschnitz M, *et al.* Plasma concentrations of arginine vasopressin, oxytocin and angiotensin in patients with Hymenoptera venom anaphylaxis. *Regul Pept* 1993; **49:** 1–7.
13. Fisher MMcD, Outhred A, Bowey CJ. Can clinical anaphylaxis to anaesthetic drugs be predicted from allergic history? *Br J Anaesth* 1987; **59:** 690–2.
14. Charpin D, Benzarti M, Hemon Y, *et al.* Atopy and anaphylactic reactions to suxamethonium. *J Allerg Clin Immunol* 1988; **82:** 356–60.
15. Baldo BA, Fisher MM. Substituted ammonium ions as allergenic determinants in drug allergy. *Nature* 1983; **306:** 262–4.
16. Clark MM, Cockburn HA. Anaphylactoid response to thiopentone. Case report. *Br J Anaesth* 1971; **43:**185–9.
17. Fisher MM, Munro I. Life-threatening anaphylactoid reactions to muscle relaxants. *Anesth Analg* 1983; **62:** 559–64.
18. Bremang JA, Halasi S. Fixed drug eruption associated with anaesthesia. *Can J Anaesth* 1995; **42 (7):** 628–30.
19. Laxenaire MC, Moneret-Vautrin DA, Widmer S, *et al.* Substances anesthesiques responsables de chocs anaphylactiques. Enquete multicentrique francaise. [Anaesthetic drugs responsible for anaphylactic shock. French multi-center study] *Ann Fr Anesth Reanim* 1990; **9:** 501–6.
20. Murat I. Anaphylactic reactions during paediatric anaesthesia; results of the French Society of Paediatric Anaesthetists (ADARPEF) 1992–1992. *Paediatr Anaesth* 1993; **3:** 339–43.
21. Boston Collababorative Drug Surveillance Survey. Drug-induced anaphylaxis. *JAMA* 1973; **224:** 613–15.
22. Fisher M, Baldo BA. Anaphylaxis during anaesthesia: current aspects of diagnosis and prevention. *Eur J Anaesth* 1994; **11:** 263–84.
23. Fisher M, Munro I. Life threatening anaphylactoid reactions to muscle relaxants. *Anesth Analg* 1983; **62:** 559–64.
24. Fisher MM. Cisatracurium and atracurium as antigens. *Anesth Intensive Care* 1999; **27:** 369–70.
25. Beamish D, Brown DT. Adverse responses to IV anaesthetics. *Br J Anaesth* 1981; **53:** 55–7.
26. Evans JM, Keogh JAM. Adverse reactions to intravenous anaesthetic induction agents, *Br Med J* 1977; **ii:** 735–6.
27. Harle DG, Baldo BA, Fisher MM. The molecular basis of IgE antibody binding to thiopentone. Binding of IgE from thiopentone-allergic and nonallergic subjects. *Mol Immunol* 1990; **27:** 853–8.
28. Watkins J, Clark A, Appleyard TN, Padfield A. Immune mediated reactions to althesin (alphaxalone). *Br J Anaesth* 1976; **48:** 881–6.
29. Fisher M. Intradermal testing after anaphylactoid reaction to anaesthetic drugs: practical aspects of performance and interpretation. *Anaesth Intensive Care* 1984; **12:** 115–20.
30. Laxenaire MC, Mata Bermejo E, Moneret Vautrin DA, *et al.* Life-threatening anaphylactoid reactions to propofol (Diprivan) *Anesthesiology* 1992; **77:** 275–80.
31. Fisher MM, Harle DG, Baldo BA.Anaphylactoid reactions to analgesics. *Clin Rev Allerg* 1991; **9:** 309–18.
32. Fisher MM, Baldo BA. The incdence and clinical features of anaphalactic reactions during anesthesia in Australia. *Ann Fr Anesth Reanim* 1993; **12:** 97–104.
33. Fisher MM, Baldo BA. Mast cell tryptase in anaesthetic anaphylactoid reactions. *Br J Anaesth* 1998; **80:** 26–9.
34. Anne S, Reisman RE. risk of administering cephalosporimn antibiotics to patient with histories of penicillin allergy. *Ann Alerg Asthma Immunol* 1995; **74:** 167–70.
35. Audicana M, Bernaola I Urrutia S, *et al.* Allergic reactions to betalactans: studies in a group of patients allergic to penicillin and evaluation of cross-reactivity with cephalosporin. *Allergy* 1994; **49:** 108–13.
36. Kuenneke M, Celik I, Stinner B, *et al.* Cardiovascular adverse effects of antimicrobials in complex surgical cases. *Eur J Surg* 1996; **162:** 24–8.
37. Weiss ME, Nyhan D, Zhikang P, *et al.* Association of protamine IgE and IgG antibodies with life-threatening reactions to intravenous protamine. *N Engl J Med* 1989; **320:** 886–92.
38. Sharath MD, Metzger WJ, Richerson HB, *et al.* Protamine-induced fatal anaphylaxis. Prevalence of antiprotamine immunoglobulin E antibody. *J Thorac Cardiovasc Surg* 1985; **90:** 86–90.
39. Lakin J, Blocker T, Strong D, Yocum L. Anaphylaxis to protamine sulphate mediated by a complement dependent IgG antibody. *J Allerg Clin Immunol* 1978; **61:** 102–6.
40. Horrow JC. Protamine: a review of its toxicity. *Anesth Analg* 1985; **64:** 348–61.
41. Pharo GH, Harrow J, Van Riper DF, Levy JH. Suspected protamine allergy: diagnosis and management for coronary artery surgery. *Anesth Analg* 1994; **78:** 181–4.
42. Harrow JC, Pharo GH, Levit LS, Freeland C. Neither skin tests nor serum enzyme-linked immunosorbent assay tests provide specificity for protamine allergy. *Anaesth Analg* 1996; **82:** 386–9.
43. Messmer K, Ljungstrom KG, Gruber UF, *et al.* Prevention of dextran-induced anaphylactoid reactions by hapten inhibition [letter]. *Lancet* 1980; **1:** 975.
44. Alenius H, Reunala T, Turjanmaa K, Palosuo T Detection of IgG4 and IgE antibodies to rubber proteins by immunoblotting in latex allergy. *Allerg Proc* 1992; **13** (2): 75–7.
45. Sussman GL, Beezhold DH. Allergy to latex rubber. *Ann Intern Med* 1995; **122:** 43–6.
46. Mace SR, Sussman GL, Liss G, *et al.* Latex allergy in operating room nurses. *Ann Allerg Asthma Immun* 1998; **80:** 252–6.
47. Slater JE. Latex allergy. *J Allerg Clin Immunol* 1994; **94:** 139–49.
48. Swartz JS, Gold M, Braude BM, *et al.* Intraoperative anaphylaxis to latex: an identifiable population at risk. *Can J Anaesth* 1990; **37:** S131.
49. Moneret-Vautrin D-A, Beaudouin E, Widmer S, *et al.* Prospective study on risk factors in natural rubber latex hypersensitivity. *J Allerg Clin Immunol* 1993; **92:** 668–77.
50. Kelly KJ, Jurup V, Zacharisen M, *et al.* Skin and serologic testing in the diagnosis of latex allergy. *J Allerg Clin Immunol* 1993; **91:** 1140–5.
51. Fisher M, Bowey CJ. Alleged allergy to local anaesthetics. *Anaesth Intensive Care* 1997; **25:** 611–14.
52. Wildsmith JAW, Mason A, McKinnon RP, Rae SM. Alleged allergy to local anaesthetic drugs. *Br Dent J* 1998; **184:** 507–10.
53. Kajimoto Y, Rosenberg ME, Kytta J, *et al.* Anaphylactoid skin reactions after intravenous regional anaesthesia using 0.5% prilocaine with or without preservative – a double-blind study. *Acta Anaesthesiol Scand* 1995; **39**: 782–4.
54. Basset IB, Delaney TA, Freeman S. Can injected lignocaine cause allergic contact dermatitis? *Aust J Dermatol* 1996; **37:** 155–6.
55. Suhonen R, Kanerva L. Contact allergy and cross-reactions caused by prilocaine. *Am J Contact Dermatitis* 1997; **8:** 231–5.
56. Fisher M. Blood volume replacement in acute anaphylactic cardiovascular collapse related to anaesthesia. *Br. J Anaesth* 1977; 49: 1023–6.
57. Waldhausen E, Keser G, Marquardt B. Der Anaphlaktishe Schock [Anaphylactic shock]. *Anaesthetist* 1987; **36:** 150–8.
58. Fisher MM. Anaphylaxis to anaesthetic drugs: aetiology, recognition and management. *Curr Opin Anaesth Crit Care* 1991; **2:** 182–6.
59. De Soto H, Turk P. Cimetidine in anaphylactic shock refractory to standard therapy. *Anesth Analg* 1989; **69:** 260–9.
60. Olinger GN, Becker RM, Bonchek LI. Noncardiogenic pulmonary edema and peripheral vascular collapse following cardiopulmonary bypass: rare protamine reaction? *Ann Thorac Surg* 1980; **29:** 20–5.
61. Fisher MM, Raper RF. The cuff leak test for extubation. *Anaesthesia* 1992; **20:** 143–6.
62. Laroche D, Lefrancois C, Gerard JL, *et al.* Early diagnosis of anaphylactic reactions to neuromuscular blocking drugs. *Br J Anaesth* 1992; **69:** 611–14.
63. Laroche D, Dubois F, Lefrancois C, *et al.* Marquers biologiques precoces des reactions anaphylactoides peranesthesiques. *Ann Fr Anesth Reanim* 1992; **11:** 613–18.
64. Laroche D, Gallet E, Bricard H. Blood histamine and early retrospective diagnosis of anaphylactic shock. *Ann Fr Anesth Reanim* 1988; 7: 425–6.
65. Best N, Teisner B, Grudzinskas JG, *et al.* Classical pathway activation during an adverse response to protamine sulphate. *Br J Anaesth* 1983; **55:** 1149–53.
66. Cogen FC, Norman ME, Dunsky E, *et al.* Histamine release and complement changes following injection of contrast media in humans. *J Allerg Clin Immunol* 1979; **64:** 299–303.
67. Best N, Sinosich MJ, Teisner B, *et al.* Complement activation during cardiopulmonary bypass by heparin–protamine interaction. *Br J Anaesth* 1984; **56:** 339–41.
68. Enander I, Matsson P, Nystrand J, *et al.* A new radioimmunoassay for

human mast cell tryptase using monoclonal antibodies. *J Immunol Methods* 1991; **138:** 39–46.
69. Schwartz LB, Yunginger JW, Miller J, *et al.* Time course of appearance and disappearance of human mast cell tryptase in the circulation after anaphylaxis. *J Clin Invest* 1989; **83:** 1551–5.
70. Yunginger JW, Nelson DR, Squilace DL, *et al.* Laboratory investigation of deaths due to anaphylaxis. *J Forensic Sci* 1991; **36:** 857–65.
71. Randall B, Butts J, Halsey JF. Elevated post-mortem tryptase in the absence of anaphylaxis. *J Forensic Sci* 1994; **40:** 208–11.
72. Fisher MM, Baldo BA. Mast cell tryptase in anaesthetic anaphylactoid reactions. *Br J Anaesth* 1998; **80:** 26–9.
73. Fisher MM. Severe histamine mediated reactions to althesin. *Anaesth Intensive Care* 1976; **4:** 33–7.
74. Leynadier F, Sansarricq M, Didier JM, *et al.* Prick tests in the diagnosis of anaphylaxis to general anaesthetics. *Br J Anaesth* 1987; **59:** 683–9.
75. Leynadier F, Sansarricq M, Dry J. Reproducibility of intradermal tests after anaphylaxis caused by muscle relaxants. *Presse Med* 1987; **16:** 523–5.
76. Thacker MA and Gibbs JM. A hypersensitivity screening clinic following untoward reactions to anaesthesia. *N Z Med J* 1984; **97:** 232–4.
77. Moscicki RA, Sockin SM, Corsello BF, *et al.* Anaphylaxis during induction of general anaesthesia: subsequent evaluation and management. *J Allerg Clin Immunol* 1990; 86: 325–32.
78. Fisher MM, Baldo BA. Diagnosis and investigation of acute anaphylactoid reactions to anaesthetic drugs. *Int Anesthesiol Clin* 1985; **23:** 161–73.
79. Moneret-Vautrin DA, Laxenaire MC, Widmer S, Hummer M. [The value of prick tests in the detection of anaphylaxis caused by muscle relaxants]. *Ann Fr Anesth Reanim* 1987; **6:** 352–5.
80. Fisher MM, Bowey, CJ. Intradermal versus prick testing in the diagnosis of anaesthetic anaphylactic reactions. *Br J Anaesth* 1977; **79:** 59–63.
81. Porri F, Pradal M, Rud C, *et al.* Is systematic pre-operative screening for muscle relaxant and latex allergy advisable? *Allergy: Eur J Allerg Clin Immunol* 1995; **50**: 374–7.
82. Fisher MM, Baldo BA. Persistence of allergy to anaesthetic drugs. *Anaesth IntensiveCare* 1992; **20:** 143–6.
83. Fisher MM, Merefield D, Baldo B. Failure to prevent an anaphylactic reaction to a second anaesthetic drug during anaesthesia. *Br J Anaesth* 1999; **82:** 720–3.

FURTHER READING

Goss JE, Chambers CE, Heupler FA, *et al.* Systemic anaphylactoid reactions to iodinated contrast media during cardiac catheterization procedures: guidelines for prevention, diagnosis and treatment. *Cathet Cardiovasc Diagn* 1995; **35:** 99–104.

Jensen NF, Weiler JM, C1 esterase inhibitor deficiency, airway compromise and anesthesia. *Anesth Analg* 1998; **87**: 480–8.

Latex allergy on the internet: http://wwwlatexallergy/com/hhtp://moemedyaleedu/gta/latex.

Levy JH. *Anaphylactic Reactions in Anesthesia and Intensive Care*, 2nd edn. Boston, MA: Butterworth-Heinemann, 1994.

Roitt I, Brostoff J, Male D. *Immunology*, 4th edn. St Louis, MO: Mosby, 1996.

PART II

Anesthetic Considerations and Techniques

Perioperative Considerations

Clinical Pharmacology and Anesthetic Techniques

26

Preoperative assessment and premedication for adults

MICHAEL F ROIZEN AND J LANCE LICHTOR

The goals of preoperative medical assessment are to reduce anxiety by acquainting patients with their doctors and explaining procedures and protocol; to facilitate the return of patients to normal functioning; to improve outcome; to provide efficient and cost-effective care; and to obtain informed consent. Medical assessments enable physicians to reduce morbidity by optimizing health status and planning perioperative management. Because perioperative morbidity and mortality increase with the severity of pre-existing disease,[1-7] careful evaluation and treatment should reduce their occurrence. The preoperative evaluation is a time to ensure that the patient is in the best possible physical condition before surgery. Consequently, patients would benefit from a reliable method of preoperative assessment during which physicians examine them and order only the laboratory tests needed for perioperative care.[8,9]

From the 1940s to the 1960s, preoperative medical assessment relied primarily on accurate history-taking and physical examination. Then, in the late 1960s, multiphasic screening laboratory tests were introduced. The ease of ordering and low cost of obtaining many tests made this new mode of evaluation attractive. As a result, many hospitals, anesthetic departments, and outpatient surgery centers made rather arbitrary rules – recommendations that became requirements – regarding the tests that should be performed before elective surgery. When, with good intentions, anesthesiologists and surgeons tried to follow those rules, problems arose. Physicians believed that, by ordering inexpensive batteries of tests, they could efficiently screen for disease. Instead, because anesthesiologists were often still trying to determine which tests to order before surgery, what to do about an unexpectedly abnormal result on the morning of surgery, or how abnormal a result had to be before requesting a consultant opinion, the preoperative multiphasic screening with multiple tests became impracticable. Nonselective testing produced so many false-positive and false-negative results that the subsequent harm vastly outweighed any possible benefit. With the shift to outpatient surgery and same-day admissions, it became difficult to evaluate unexpected preoperative test abnormalities without creating inefficient operating room schedules.

Although laboratory screening tests can aid in optimizing a patient's preoperative condition once a disease is suspected or diagnosed, they have several shortcomings: they frequently fail to uncover pathological conditions; the abnormalities they detect do not necessarily affect patient care or outcome; and they are inefficient in screening for asymptomatic diseases. Finally, most abnormalities discovered on preoperative screening, or even on admission screening for non-surgical purposes, are not recorded (other than in the laboratory report) or appropriately pursued. Thus, preoperative testing should be used primarily to ensure the optimal preoperative condition of a patient who has not received healthcare recently. This conclusion can be drawn from a long series of epidemiologic studies and controlled trials.[10,11]

Even in the elderly, it appears that laboratory tests function to optimize care but are ineffective at screening for disease. Domoto *et al.*[12] examined the yield and effectiveness of a battery of 19 screening laboratory tests performed routinely in 70 functionally intact elderly patients (average age 82.6 years) who resided at a chronic care facility. The 70 patients underwent 3903 screening tests. "New abnormal" results occurred primarily in 5 of the 19 screening tests; most of these "new abnormalities" were only minimally outside the normal range. Only four (0.1% of all tests ordered) led to a change in patient management, none of which, Domoto and colleagues concluded, benefited any patient in an important way.

Wolf-Klein and colleagues[13] retrospectively studied the results of annual laboratory screening on a population of 500 institutionalized and ambulatory elderly patients (average age 80 years). From the 15 000 tests performed, 756 new abnormalities were discovered, 690 of which were ignored. Of those new abnormalities, 66 were evaluated; 20 new diagnoses resulted, 12 of which were treated. Two patients of the 500 ultimately may have benefited from eradication of asymptomatic bacteriuria (although eradication of asymptomatic bacteriuria has not been shown to improve the quality of life or extend the lifespan).

Studies show that the history and physical examination are the best measures for screening for disease. Delahunt and Turnbull[14] evaluated patients who were assessed preoperatively for varicose vein stripping or inguinal herniorrhaphy. Of 803 patients who underwent 1972 tests, only 63 abnormalities were uncovered in those patients whose history or physical findings had not indicated the need for tests; but in no instance did the discovery of these abnormalities influence patient management.

Narr and colleagues[15] discovered no benefit from screening tests for 3782 patients of American Society of Anesthesiologists (ASA) Physical Status I. After this study, the Mayo Clinic omitted laboratory tests for patients of ASA Physical Status I if, in the opinion of the physician who evaluated the patients, tests were not needed.[16] Lack of testing did not adversely affect any patient. Macpherson *et al.*[17] found that out of 3096 results of laboratory tests that had been normal within 1 year of surgery, upon repeat testing of patients, only 13 results had changed to a range unacceptable for surgery. These 13 were predictable from a change in patient history. Patient history was crucial in allowing 26 new diagnoses to be made by Mitchell *et al.*[18] for 550 patients on the general internal medicine ward of a university hospital.

Even in a referral population, history and physical examination determine more than 90% of the clinical course when a patient is referred for consultation for cardiovascular, neurological, or respiratory diseases.[19] Other studies have also demonstrated that the history and physical examination accurately indicate all areas in which subsequent laboratory testing proves beneficial for patients. For example, Rabkin and Horne[20,21] examined the records of 165 patients with "new" (i.e. a change from a previous tracing) abnormalities on the electrocardiogram (ECG) that were potentially "surgically significant" (i.e. that might affect perioperative management or outcome). In only two instances were the anesthetic or surgical plans altered by the discovery of new abnormalities on an ECG that were not indicated by history. Thus, for these 165 patients, for whom the benefits of a laboratory test should have been maximal because a new abnormality was detected preoperatively, the history or physical examination determined case management most of the time. Even in one of the two instances of altered case management – a patient with atrial fibrillation – the physical examination should have indicated that an ECG needed to be performed. A history or physical examination was not available for the other patient.

A randomized, controlled trial of laboratory tests before elective cataract removal in over 18 000 patients confirmed that if a patient does not need laboratory tests to facilitate return to daily activities, then extra testing is not needed before minimally invasive surgery.[8] In summary, the studies cited above point to the management of patient care, especially for minimally invasive surgery, and perhaps for all surgery. Data from the state of Maine (RM Flowerdew, personal communication) and the Mayo Clinic show that minimally invasive outpatient surgery is no more risky than daily living.[22] History and physical examination are the most effective ways to screen for disease.

Screening laboratory tests may even present extra risk to the patient. Unnecessary testing may lead physicians to pursue and treat abnormalities based on borderline positive and false-positive results. Few studies examine whether increased tests and the follow-up of false-positive tests adversely affect patients. In a retrospective examination of the adverse effects of chest radiographs on a population of 606 patients, 386 extra chest radiographs were ordered without being indicated.[23] In those 386 patients, one elevated hemidiaphragm and probable phrenic nerve palsy was found that may have resulted in improved care for that patient. In addition, three lung shadows were found that resulted in three sets of invasive tests, including one thoracotomy, without discovery of disease. These procedures caused considerable morbidity, including one pneumothorax and 4 months of disability.

In another study, Turnbull and Buck[24] examined the charts of 2570 patients undergoing cholecystectomy to determine the value of preoperative tests. The history and physical examinations successfully indicated all tests that ultimately benefited the patients, with four possible exceptions. But again, in those four patients it is doubtful if any benefit actually occurred. Among them was one patient whose emphysema was detected only by chest radiograph; he underwent preoperative physiotherapy without subsequent postoperative complications. Two patients had unsuspected hypokalemia (3.2 and 3.4 $mmol\,L^{-1}$ or $mequiv\,L^{-1}$) and received potassium treatment before surgery. No harm occurs to patients undergoing an operation with this degree of hypokalemia, and severe potential harm may be caused by treating such patients with oral or intravenous potassium. The fourth patient for whom possible benefit occurred received a blood transfusion before cholecystectomy for an asymptomatic hemoglobin concentration of 9.9 $g\,dL^{-1}$. Since cholecystectomy is not normally associated with major blood loss, it is concluded that this patient also received no benefit and only the risk of transfusion from that preoperative laboratory test. Thus, it is not clear that any patient in this study benefited from preoperative screening tests that were not indicated.

In another study, only two patients at most (whose asymptomatic bacteriuria was eradicated) benefited from the 9270 screening tests that were obtained.[25] At least one patient was seriously harmed from the pursuit of abnormalities on screening tests and her subsequent treatment; this woman developed atrial fibrillation and congestive heart failure after thyroid therapy was instituted for borderline low thyroxine and free thyroxine index tests. It is not clear if these investigators examined other patients for potential harm arising similarly from the pursuit and treatment of abnormalities.

More extensive screening tests are now being self-ordered and paid for by some patients. Whole-body computed tomography (CT) scans (about $400 in the USA) and magnetic resonance imaging (MRI) scans (about $500) result in sufficient false-positive results to generate a surgical schedule filled with patients who request removal of benign adrenal and other tumors. We also face the uncertain value of CT scans of lungs of former smokers. With the CT scans, the pursuit of new abnormalities with high-definition radiologic scans may cause undesirable radiation exposure. Thus, even in high-risk patients, some laboratory tests are beneficial only after the risk from the pursuit of uncertain abnormalities is reduced.[11]

When batteries of laboratory tests yield abnormal results that are neither pursued nor noted, medicolegal risk for physicians increases. Extra testing – testing that is not warranted by findings on a medical history – does not serve as medicolegal protection against liability. Roizen[26] reviewed a series of studies showing that 30–95% of all unexpected abnormalities found on preoperative laboratory tests are not noted on the chart preoperatively. Many reports of preoperative radiographs, for example, are not on the chart before anesthesia is administered. This lack of notation occurs not only at university medical centers but in community hospitals too. Failure to pursue an abnormality that has been detected poses a greater risk to medicolegal liability than does failure to detect that abnormality. In this way, extra testing can result in extra medicolegal risk to physicians.

Random preoperative testing is inefficient for operating room schedules. Surgeons say that they order preoperative tests to satisfy the anesthesiologist. They find it easier just to order all the tests and let the anesthesiologist sort them out. Surgeons also believe that it is much more efficient to order batteries of tests than for the anesthesiologist, who sees the patient the night before or the morning of surgery, to try to get the tests on an emergency basis. These surgeons apparently do not realize that the abnormalities detected are not discovered until the night before or the morning of surgery, if at all. Then, abnormal results on these tests delay or postpone schedules, as extra effort and time are wasted in obtaining consultant reviews of false-positive or slightly abnormal results.

Current guidelines separate surgery into different classes. No testing is indicated for minimally invasive surgery, and more testing is indicated to ensure the optimal condition of a patient before highly invasive surgery. One such system is described in Table 26.1.[11]

IMPLEMENTATION OF PREOPERATIVE EVALUATION

There are at least three methods for organizing preoperative evaluation efficiently. First, the surgeon, internist, family practitioner, or anesthesiologist who sees the patient before a scheduled procedure can obtain the history and perform the physical examination. Second, a clinic can be set up in an outpatient facility so that these two tasks are performed early enough to ensure that laboratory tests or consultations can be obtained without delaying schedules. Third, a questionnaire answered by the patient can be used to indicate likely disease processes and appropriate laboratory tests.

Of the first method one might ask: can the appropriate testing be easily generated from the surgeon's preoperative visit? One study found that it could. At the University of California, Kaplan *et al.*.[27] found that even a partial history conveyed enough information to indicate correctly all but

Table 26.1 *Types of surgical procedures*

Class A: minimally invasive Little potential to disrupt normal physiology Rarely associated with morbidity associated with the anesthetic Rarely require blood administration, invasive monitoring, or postoperative management in a critical care setting Examples: cataract removal, diagnostic arthroscopy, and postpartum interval tubal ligation
Class B: moderately invasive Modest potential to disrupt normal physiology *May* require blood administration, invasive monitoring, or postoperative management in a critical care setting Examples: carotid endarterectomy, transurethral resection of the prostate, and laparoscopic cholecystectomy
Class C: highly invasive Typically produce significant disruption of normal physiology Almost always require blood administration, invasive monitoring, and postoperative management in a critical care setting Examples: total hip replacement, open aortic aneurysm resection, aortic valve replacement, and posterior fossa craniotomy for aneurysm

22 abnormalities (none of which affected patient outcome) in more than 2785 preoperative blood tests obtained [counting the complete blood count and simultaneous multichannel analysis of six variables (SMA 6) as one test]. Knowing only the admission diagnosis, previous discharge diagnoses, and scheduled operation, and using previously determined indications for laboratory testing, enabled detection of virtually all abnormalities that would have been detected by routine screening.

As regards the patient questionnaire, several groups have tested the effects and sensitivity of orally administered or written questionnaires as a means of linking the selection of laboratory tests with a patient's medical history.[26,28] In 1987, McKee and Scott[29] used a verbally administered set of 17 questions and patient demographics to select preoperative tests for 400 patients. They found that age was the best predictor of abnormalities on preoperative tests. Complications occurred most commonly in patients who reported positive symptoms on the questionnaire and who were older.

A recent study determined that the responses of patients to written questions can be used to predict the laboratory tests that will yield abnormal results for those patients. After the patient answers the questionnaire, a plastic overlay reveals what tests are indicated. If the patient cannot answer the questions, a standard group of tests is ordered. Even in a tertiary care (specialist) hospital that admits very sick patients, more than 60% of those laboratory tests now routinely obtained could be eliminated.

The protocols outlined in Tables 26.1 and 26.2 are guidelines for using clinical judgment in ordering laboratory tests. A careful history and physical examination of the patient are required, with special attention to testing whenever indicators of disease entities listed in the tables are discovered. The protocol clearly places the burden on whoever takes the history to do so accurately.

OBTAINING A MEDICAL HISTORY

A medical history can be provided by a number of sources because patients undergoing surgery move through a continuum of medical care to which a primary care physician, an internist, an anesthesiologist, and a surgeon contribute. No aspect of medicine requires a greater degree of cooperation among physicians than does the performance of a surgical operation and the perioperative care of a patient. The importance of integrating practice is even greater in the context of the increasing lifespan of our population. As the number of the elderly and the very old (those older than 85 years of age) grows, so does the incidence among surgical patients of comorbidities and multiple drug regimens, knowledge of which is crucial to successful patient management. At a time when medical information is encyclopedic and medical subspecialization proliferates, it is difficult for even the most conscientious physician to keep abreast of the medical issues relevant to perioperative patient management. Thus, it is useful to coordinate care with the patient's general practitioner (primary care physician). Even when a good disease history is available, a screening review of these systems is beneficial: airway, chest, cardiovascular, renal, central nervous system, peripheral nervous system, gastrointestinal, musculoskeletal, and genitourinary. Questions should also be asked regarding medications, allergy, use of alcohol and drugs, smoking, family history of disease, activities, and exercise tolerance. Our patients take 25–35 min to respond to such questions on an automated questionnaire via telephone or on the Internet (www.healthquiz.com). Positive responses on the HealthQuiz to questions about an organ system elicit more questions about the system. Based on a patient's responses to the questions, certain laboratory tests are indicated. The rationale for the choice of tests relative to response is beyond the scope of this chapter, but some specific tests deserve comment.

HEMOGLOBIN, HEMATOCRIT, AND WHITE BLOOD CELL COUNTS

How many asymptomatic patients have a degree of abnormality on hematocrit (packed cell volume) or the white blood cell count (WBC) that alters perioperative management? The following values do not merit intervention perioperatively: a hematocrit of 27–54 for patients undergoing operations during which major blood loss is unlikely, and a WBC of 2400–16 000 mm^{-3} for individuals not undergoing insertion of a prosthesis. When values fall outside these ranges, we recommend seeking alternative diagnoses before anesthesia or surgery. Hematocrit or hemoglobin levels should be determined preoperatively for all surgical patients older than 60 years of age. Hematocrit or hemoglobin level and red blood cell antigen screenings (cross-matched blood) are warranted for all patients undergoing procedures involving possible loss of more than 2 units per 70 kg of body weight. WBCs appear to be rarely indicated in asymptomatic individuals but might be considered when a prosthesis is to be inserted.

BLOOD CHEMISTRY AND URINALYSIS

What blood chemistry would have to be abnormal, and how abnormal would the results have to be, to justify changing perioperative management? Abnormal hepatic or renal function might change the choice and dose of anesthetic or adjuvant drugs. About 1 in 700 supposedly healthy patients has subacute hepatitis, and 1 in 3 of these will become jaundiced. However, in our prospective study of the HealthQuiz involving 3500 patients, no asymptomatic patient who did not have risk factors for exposure to the hepatitis virus became jaundiced after uneventful surgery.[25] These data imply that either the screening history suffices or the incidence of asymptomatic hepatitis is decreasing. Unexpected abnormalities are reported for 2–10% of patients with multiphasic screening, and these abnormalities lead to many additional tests that usually (in approximately 80% of cases) have no significance for the patient. Unexpected abnormalities that are significant arise in 2–5% of patients studied. Of these abnormalities, approximately 70% are related to blood glucose and blood urea nitrogen (BUN) levels. The 4–19 additional tests on the screening SMAs 6–21 panels lead to very few important discoveries affecting anesthesia. In fact, the false-positive rate

Table 26.2 *Simplified strategy for preoperative testing for class B and C procedures*[a]

	HGB													
Preoperative condition	**M**	**F**	**WBC**	**PT/PTT**	**PLT/BT**	**Elect**	**Creat/BUN**	**Blood glu-cose**	**SGOT/ AlkPTAse**	**Radigraph**	**ECG**	**Prenancy test**	**Albumin**	**T/S**
Neonates	X	X												
Physiologic age ≥ 75	X	X					X	X		X	X		X	X
Class C procedure	X	X					X	X			X		X	X
Cardiovascular disease							X			X	X			
Pulmonary disease										X	X			
Malignancy	X	X	b	b						X				
Radiation therapy			X							X	X			
Hepatic disease				X					X					
Exposure to hepatitis									X					
Renal disease	X	X				X	X							
Bleeding disorder				X	X									
Diabetes						X	X	X			X			
Smoking ≥ 20 packs per year	X	X								X				
Possible pregnancy												X		
Diuretic use						X	X							
Digoxin use						X	X				X			
Steroid use						X		X						
Anticoagulant use	X	X		X										
CNS disease			X			X	X	X			X			

a. For minimally invasive class A procedures (cataracts, diagnostic arthroscopy), no tests are indicated. Not all diseases are included in this table. The anesthesiologist's own judgment is needed regarding patients with diseases not listed. For moderately invasive class B procedures (in which blood loss or hemodynamic changes are rare), use clinical judgment in test selection. Highly invasive class C procedures typically disrupt normal physiology (see Table 26.1).

b. Obtain for leukemias only. X, obtain in all cases.

BT, bleeding time; Creat/BUN, creatinine or blood urea nitrogen; ECG, electrocardiogram; Elect, electrolytes (i.e. sodium, potassium, chloride, carbon dioxide, and proteins); HGB, hemoglobin; PLT, platelet count; PT, prothrombin time; PTT, partial thromboplastin time; SGOT/AlkPTAse, serum glutamic oxaloacetic transaminase and alkaline phosphatase; T/S, blood typing and screen for unexpected antibodies; WBC, white blood cell count.
Modified from Roizen.[11]

is so high (96.5% for the test for calcium) that more harm than benefit is likely to result for asymptomatic patients who receive these tests.

If the data from our group on asymptomatic liver disease can be generalized, no blood chemistry tests are warranted for asymptomatic patients. One important exception is for patients undergoing major surgery (class C in Table 26.1), in whom albumin level has proved useful for prognosis. With or without surgery, prognosis is poor if a level below $2.0\,g\,dL^{-1}$ does not increase with enteral nutrition.[30]

Abnormalities are commonly found on urinalysis. The quality of urinalysis results obtained by dipstick technique has been variable at best. Abnormal results usually do not lead to beneficial changes in management. Most of those that do could have been obtained by history or determination of BUN and glucose levels, tests that are already recommended for routine care of all patients over 60 years of age. Thus, urinalysis, although initially inexpensive, becomes an expensive test to justify on a cost–benefit or benefit–risk basis.

CHEST RADIOGRAPHS

What abnormalities on chest radiographs would influence management of anesthesia? Certainly, it may be important to know about the existence of tracheal deviation; mediastinal masses; pulmonary nodules; a solitary lung mass; aortic aneurysm; pulmonary edema; pneumonia; atelectasis; new fractures of the vertebrae, ribs, or clavicles; dextrocardia; or cardiomegaly before proceeding to anesthesia and surgery. However, a chest radiograph probably would not detect the degree of chronic lung disease requiring a change in anesthetic technique any better than would the history and physical examination. Abnormalities are rare in the asymptomatic individual.[11] In fact, if a patient is asymptomatic and less than 74 years of age, the risks of chest radiograph examination probably exceed the possible benefits. This analysis is, of course, predicated on maximizing benefit to society in general, as one cannot predict in advance which patients will benefit or which will be harmed.

ELECTROCARDIOGRAPHY AND SCREENING FOR CARDIAC DISEASE

Although individual episodes of myocardial ischemia may not produce symptoms, almost all patients without diabetes or autonomic insufficiency have symptoms that lead one to screen for myocardial disease. An algorithm is presented in Fig. 26.1 for pursuing laboratory testing for cardiovascular disease.[11]

PULMONARY FUNCTION TESTING

These expensive tests are rarely needed but are useful for determining those who may benefit from bronchodilator therapy and for predicting the risk of thoracic operations before obtaining informed consent. The indications for pulmonary function tests in Table 26.3 seem justified by the data.[11] There is a debate about simple (FEV_1/FVC) spirometry for detection of asthma in the absence of wheezing in patients with dyspnea or those who do not exercise. This bedside test may be as good as the match test (blowing out a match burning 15 cm away from the lips) or a walking test, both of which serve clinicians well. Thus, like radiologic studies, lung function studies may not be needed before surgery if patients are in their optimal medical condition.

CLOTTING FUNCTION STUDIES

Virtually no asymptomatic patient in the literature has had unequivocal benefit from clotting function studies preoperatively. Most show symptoms or have a medication history suggesting that clotting function tests may be necessary. Aspirin at 325 mg per 70 kg of body weight per day does not seem to pose a risk for bleeding, but the data are not available for nonsteriodal anti-inflammatory drugs (NSAIDs) or cyclo-oxygenase (COX-2) inhibitors or for larger doses of aspirin taken within 12 h of surgery. Because the pharmacology of aspirin changes when more than 2 g per 70 kg body weight is consumed per day, patients should be

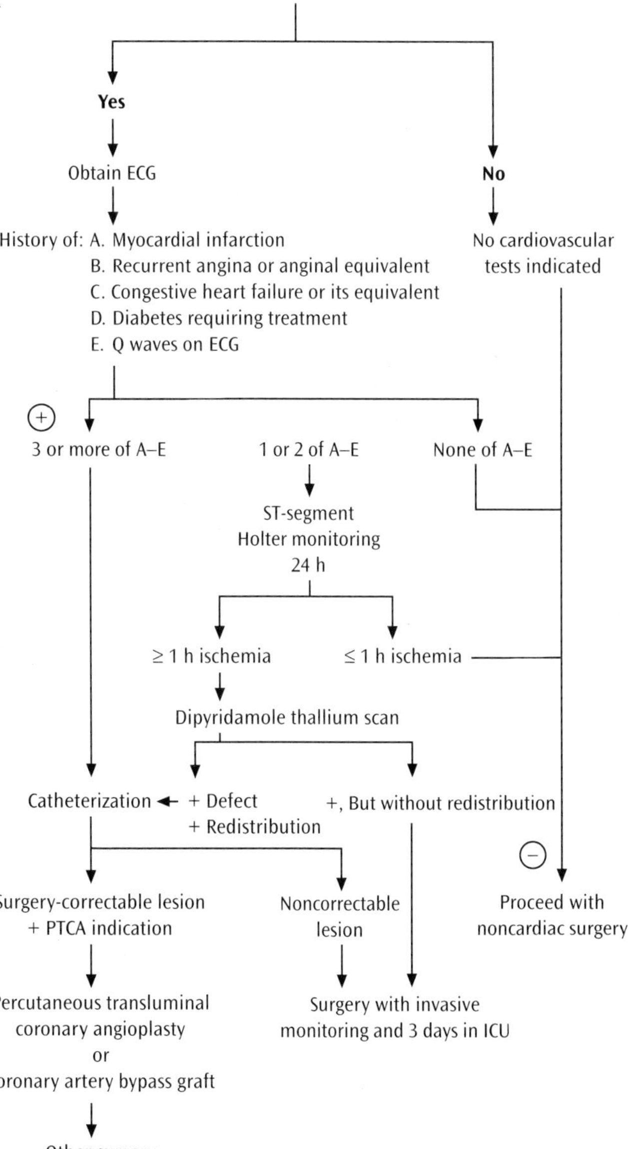

Figure 26.1 *How to decide which cardiovascular laboratory tests to obtain: use the history to segregate patients into groups to test and/or monitor invasively. PTCA, percutaneous transluminal coronary angioplasty.*

Table 26.3 *Indications for pulmonary function tests*

History of at least one of the following
1 Chronic obstructive pulmonary disease
2 Shortness of breath
3 Orthopnea
Also, at least one of the following needs to be determined
1 Reversibility of bronchospasm
2 Baseline condition if mechanical ventilation is expected preoperatively
3 Risk for lung resection (maximal midexpiratory flow rate, maximum breathing capacity, diffusing capacity for carbon monoxide)

evaluated if they cannot stop aspirin early enough to have undetectable acetylsalicylic acid or NSAID levels for 24 h before surgery (the period without acetylsalicylic acid necessary to generate the approximately 50 000 new platelets per mm^3 needed for normal platelet aggregation) or if surgical hemostasis cannot be assured or a regional anesthetic involving a closed space is planned.

PREGNANCY, HEMOGLOBINOPATHY, AND AIDS SCREENING

Tests for the acquired immunodeficiency syndrome (AIDS) and pregnancy, genetic testing, and screening for hemoglobinopathy and malignant hyperthermia raise ethical issues that may require close attention to institutional policy and the immediate availability of counseling services. Moreover, all of these tests have associated risks. The physician may therefore decide to limit testing to only at-risk populations (e.g. for pregnancy testing, only female patients who believe they may possibly be pregnant).

Testing of the asymptomatic population for AIDS is not likely to be the most effective way of uncovering the disease unless one or more risk factors are present. Few of the people in the USA who have had AIDS have not been gay, had sex with a prostitute or multiple partners, had unprotected sex (homo- or heterosexual), used intravenously administered drugs and shared needles, been stuck with a needle, cared for a family member with AIDS, been born of a woman with AIDS, or received a blood transfusion after 1979. One program, screening for human immunodeficiency virus (HIV) in asymptomatic individuals, was able to produce an "acceptably low false-positive rate" by diagnosing HIV infection only after one sample of blood produced positive results on four different tests and after a second sample of blood had been used for verification. Thus, for pregnancy, hemoglobinopathies, genetic testing, and AIDS, the history is still the best at identifying those at risk for a condition.

TOWARD A TECHNOLOGY FOR EFFICIENT, LESS EXPENSIVE, HIGH-QUALITY CARE

Even when anesthesiologists attempt to choose tests selectively, based on the history and physical examination of a patient, errors are made in ordering tests. When surgeons and anesthesiologists agreed on indications for testing, 30–40% of patients who should have had tests did not get them and 20–40% of patients who should not have had tests got them. For instance, Blery and coworkers[31] used a protocol based on suspected disease to order preoperative tests selectively for 3866 surgical patients in France, and found that, even after clinicians had been educated with regard to indications, 30% of tests ordered were not indicated and another 22% of tests that were indicated were not obtained. Thus, by ordering tests in the usual way, surgeons and anesthesiologists both increased costs and failed to obtain possibly valuable information. Blery *et al.* subsequently questioned anesthesiologists to assess whether management of the patient suffered from omission of one or more preoperative tests. Only 0.2% of omitted tests would have possibly been useful. They did not examine how many times such data might have led to pursuits that harmed patients.

Charpak *et al.*[32] examined the value of preoperative screening chest radiographs in 3849 patients. Surgeons and anesthesiologists agreed that any lung or cardiovascular disease, malignant disease, current smoking history in patients over 50 years of age, major surgical emergencies, immunodepression, or lack of prior health examination in immigrants were indications for ordering a chest radiograph. The surgeons ordered or did not order the chest radiograph after seeing the patient. Even with this agreement on indications, of a total of 1426 chest radiographs that should have been ordered in this group of 3849 patients, 271 were ordered although they were not recommended, and 596 were not ordered although they were recommended. Clinical judgments may account for some of these decisions, but it is presumed that many extra chest radiographs ordered or not ordered were simply errors. If so many errors occur in a single test trial, more laboratory tests are likely to generate more errors. The problem is how to order tests that are appropriate for each patient without decreasing efficiency. It appears that selective ordering strategies are better than nonselective methods for ordering tests, but an even easier, more efficient method exists.

At some institutions, a preoperative questionnaire is given to patients either by telephone or via the Internet in the surgeon's office or from home. This process can help segregate patients who need to be examined before surgery and can also suggest possible laboratory tests. The information is secure with an unattributable identifier known only to the patient and to the physician (see www.healthquiz.com). The Internet screen poses yes/no questions to patients about their health. Many practitioners think that questions about food supplements and vitamins which the patient may be taking are also important.[33] When the questions have been answered, the program generates a printout of the answers and a summary of symptoms. Reminders are given about items in the patient's history important to anesthetic care, such as allergies and capped teeth. Laboratory tests also are suggested based on the agreed indications and the patient's answers. The physician, surgeon, or anesthesiologist can override or add to the suggested tests to be ordered preoperatively. Other indications can be incorporated into this Internet technology, such as those developed by the National Health Studies Health Technology Program.[34] With the information from such a questionnaire, the anesthesiologist can spend quality time when meeting a patient preoperatively and have the time to emphasize the issues pertinent to his or her condition.

PREMEDICATION

Premedication controls anxiety, postoperative pain, nausea, and vomiting and reduces the risk of aspiration during induction of anesthesia. In the case of patients expected to go home on the day of surgery, the drugs given before anesthesia should not hinder recovery afterward. Given in appropriate doses for appropriate indications, most premedicants do not prolong recovery. For example, when patients who received 1 μg kg^{-1} fentanyl and 0.04 mg kg^{-1} midazolam before induction were compared with patients who received no premedication, maintenance requirements with desflurane, airway irritability, and blood pressure increases during induction were reduced by premedication, and discharge times were unaffected.[35]

Controlling anxiety

Patients scheduled to undergo surgery tend to be anxious long before they come to the hospital. In one study, the level of patient anxiety was measured daily from 4 days before hospital admission to several days after surgery.[36] Anxiety was high before admission, between admission and surgery, and 2 days after surgery (Fig. 26.2). There are subsets of patients, however, who are not anxious. For example, a study of the efficacy of drugs for relief of anxiety in outpatients before gynecologic surgery was unsuccessful simply because levels of preoperative anxiety were low.[37] Some operations certainly can generate more anxiety than others. Increased anxiety has been noted in women, young patients, in those accompanied by a friend or relative to the preoperative holding area, in those with a previous bad anesthetic experience, as well as before mutilating surgery, surgery for malignancy, or a first surgical experience. Something as simple as the need to remove dentures increases stress preoperatively. Worry about family more than about surgery stresses other patients. If in doubt about patient anxiety, ask: accuracy in predicting anxiety increases when patients are asked.[38]

As in the case of adults, children should have some idea of what to expect during a procedure. Even with this knowledge, a child may become anxious when separated from parent(s). But a child is less likely to cry or be uncooperative from the time of separation from parents to induction of anesthesia if a procedure has been explained preoperatively. A child who is overly anxious during the induction of anesthesia may wake up crying postoperatively, disobey parents, or have separation anxiety, bad dreams, or temper tantrums.[39] Both parents and children should be part of preoperative discussions so that the anxiety of the parents is not transmitted to the child. The transmission of anxiety is at least as problematic as is the separation itself, which for the child may recall being left with babysitters. If parents are calm and can effectively manage the physical transfer of their child to a warm and playful anesthesiologist or nurse, premedication is not necessary. Another option, semisedation, may be awkward or prolong recovery. Nonetheless, at least in one study, both parental and child anxiety around the time of induction was better managed with oral midazolam than with parental presence.[40]

Benzodiazepines

When medication is the treatment choice to reduce anxiety, midazolam is the benzodiazepine most commonly used preoperatively. It is water soluble and has an initial distribution half-life of 7.2 min and an elimination half-life of 2.5 h (range 2.1–3.4 h). Elimination half-life increases to 5.6 h in the elderly and to 8.4 h in obese patients.[41] Half of an orally administered dose undergoes first-pass metabolism in the liver, and extrahepatic metabolism may also occur. The metabolites of midazolam have negligible soporific effects. Although midazolam does not produce thrombosis or thrombophlebitis, it may cause nausea. The dose should be decreased for older patients (Fig. 26.3).[42] A dose of midazolam of 0.15 $mg\,kg^{-1}$ for a 20-year-old patient would be equivalent to a dose of 0.1 $mg\,kg^{-1}$ for a 60-year-old and to 0.03 $mg\,kg^{-1}$ for a 90-year-old. Midazolam at 0.07 $mg\,kg^{-1}$ given intravenously to 40 elderly patients for sedation before endoscopy of the esophagus, stomach, and duodenum was effective based on time to achieve sedation, adequacy of sedation, and absence of gagging during the procedure.[43]

Midazolam is a useful premedicant for children, especially in the oral formulation, which was approved by the US Food and Drug Administration in 1998. A dose of 0.5 $mg\,kg^{-1}$ produces sedation and reduces anxiety in 10 min so that children accept separation from their parents.[44] When midazolam is given before procedures lasting about 30 min with a halothane anesthetic, recovery is not prolonged[45] (Fig. 26.4). Although recovery after shorter-acting anesthetics such as sevoflurane or desflurane may be prolonged, discharge time is not affected. With the antifungal agents itraconazole or ketoconazole, serum concentrations of midazolam are increased, thereby increasing the potential for intense and prolonged sedation as well as respiratory depression. Cardiovascular, respiratory, and psychomotor depression are adverse effects of midazolam.

Another benzodiazepine, oral diazepam, is recommended for patients who are anxious before ambulatory surgery. Orally administered diazepam is well absorbed from the intestine. Plasma levels peak 60 min after ingestion, when anxiolytic effects are measurable; effectiveness lasts for several hours. Dose requirements decrease approximately 10% per decade of patient age. For adults, we prescribe diazepam in

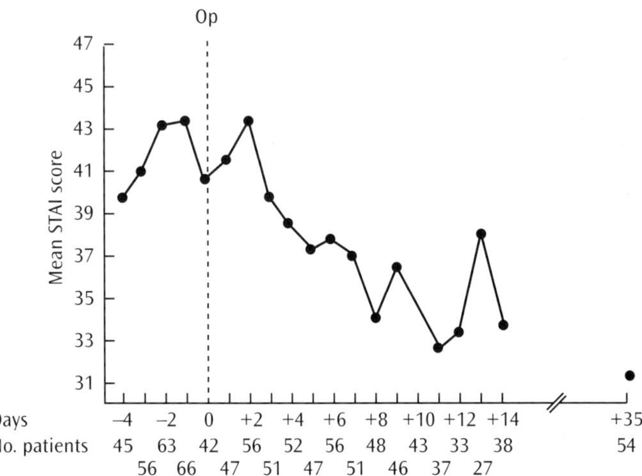

Figure 26.2 *Mean scores for the State-Trait Anxiety Inventory (STAI), which were obtained daily beginning 4 days before surgery, at home, at the time of admission to the hospital, and up to 35 days after surgery (when most patients had been discharged). "Op" indicates day of surgery. The level of anxiety was high not only before surgery but also at 2 days after surgery. (Reprinted with permission from Johnston.[36])*

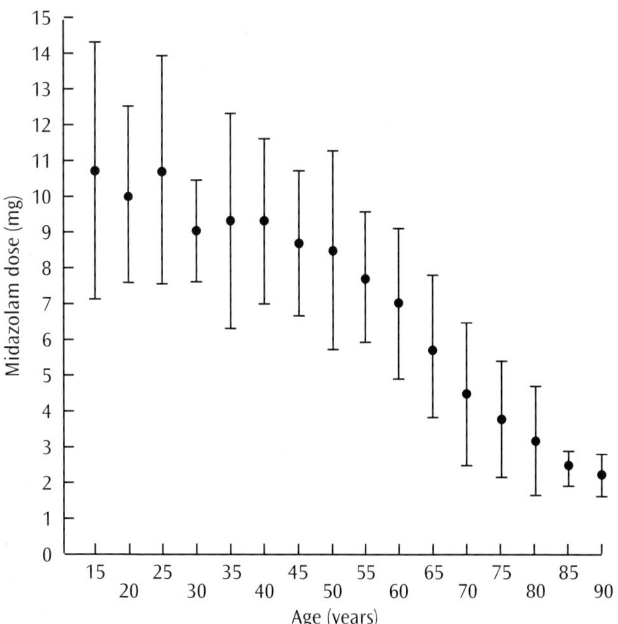

Figure 26.3 *The mean dose (± SD) of intravenous midazolam required to produce adequate sedation before upper gastrointestinal endoscopy decreases with age. (Reprinted with permission from Bell* et al.*[42])*

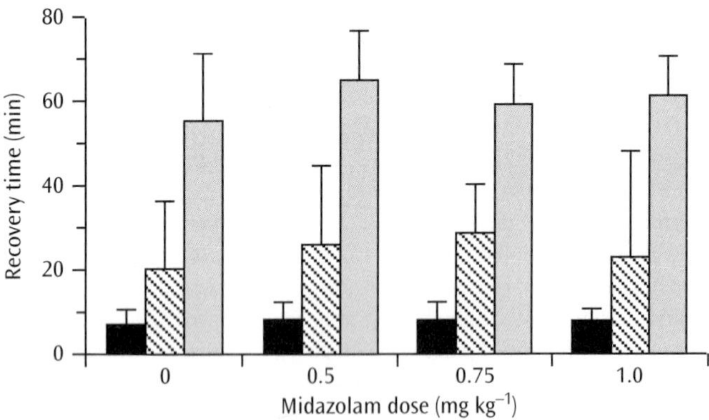

Figure 26.4 *Recovery is not affected by the preoperative use of midazolam. Black bars, surgery to PACU; stippled bars, PACU to eye opening; gray bars, PACU to discharge. PACU, postanesthesia care unit. (Reprinted with permission from McMillan* et al.*[45])*

a dose of 2–5 mg per 70 kg body weight. Its metabolite, desmethyldiazepam, has pharmacologic properties similar to those of the parent drug; concentrations can be detected after 2 h and decrease only after 36 h. The elimination half-lives of diazepam and desmethyldiazepam are longer in old subjects than in young ones. The activity of this drug, however, does not depend on plasma concentration alone. When young and old patients with equal plasma levels of diazepam are compared, the central nervous system of elderly patients is more sensitive to the depressant effects.

At proper doses, cardiovascular and respiratory depression are similar with diazepam and midazolam. A decrease in blood pressure in healthy individuals with the benzodiazepines is trivial (10%), but in old patients, particularly those with heart disease, decreases may range from 20% to 35% and may be associated with apnea.[46] The decrease in blood pressure is greater when other drugs, such as fentanyl, propofol, or thiopental, are coadministered. Oxygen saturation may decrease after injection of midazolam. In 100 patients, average baseline oxygen saturation of 95% decreased to 92% after intravenous (i.v.) administration of midazolam and to 89% during endoscopy (Fig. 26.5).[47] Oxygen saturation was below 80% in 7% of patients. Routine administration of supplemental oxygen, with or without continuous monitoring of arterial oxygenation, is recommended whenever benzodiazepines are given intravenously. This precaution is necessary not only when midazolam is the premedicant, but also when it is used alone or with other drugs for conscious sedation.

Fatigue associated with the effects of anxiolytics may delay or prevent the discharge of patients on the day of surgery, although more frequently discharge is delayed because of the effects of the operation. With regard to anesthesia effects, patients normally do not stay in the hospital because they are too sleepy but because they are nauseous.

The potential for amnesia after premedication is another concern, especially for patients undergoing ambulatory surgery. In one study, 42% of patients given a placebo, but only 2.8% of patients given midazolam (0.1 mg kg^{-1} intramuscularly), could remember induction of anesthesia for cervical dilation and uterine curettage ($P < 0.0001$).[48] It is noteworthy, however, that so many patients given placebo could not remember induction. No controlled studies have shown retrograde amnesia in patients after midazolam or diazepam.

Opioids and nonsteroidal analgesics

Opioids are administered preoperatively to sedate patients, to control hypertension during tracheal intubation, and to decrease pain. Meperidine (pethidine), but not morphine or fentanyl, is helpful for the control of shivering in the operating room, postanesthesia care unit (PACU), or recovery ward, although treatment is usually instituted at the time of shivering and not in anticipation of the event. The effectiveness of opioids in relieving anxiety in adults is controversial and probably nonexistent. A lozenge form of fentanyl (oral transmucosal fentanyl citrate) reduces children's anxiety, increases sedation, and improves the quality of induction.[49] In common with all opioids, fentanyl in lozenge form decreases respiratory rate and oxygen saturation,[50] an effect that is reversed with deep or big breaths. Oxygen saturation should be monitored. Pruritus, nausea, and vomiting are other undesirable effects. Droperidol, 50 μg kg^{-1}, given to 2- to 8-year-olds, did not reduce the incidence of vomiting.[50] With fentanyl, PACU stay is not prolonged and postoperative analgesia requirements are less, although if children are required to drink fluids before they can be discharged vomiting may delay their release. In adults, as in children, postoperative analgesic requirements are decreased, but nausea may be problematic with opioids.

Opioids are useful for the control of hypertension during tracheal intubation. Opioid premedication prevents increases in systolic pressure in a dose-dependent fashion. After tracheal intubation, however, systolic, diastolic, and mean arterial blood pressures sometimes decrease below baseline values.

Preoperative administration of opioids or nonsteroidal anti-inflammatory drugs controls pain in the early postoperative period. Among patients who received ketorolac (60 mg), dezocine (6 mg), or fentanyl (100 μg) before the start of laparoscopy,[51] 61% in the fentanyl group needed supplemental analgesia in the PACU compared with 34% in the ketorolac and 25% in the dezocine group. Less narcotic was required in the ketorolac and dezocine groups. Nausea was greatest after dezocine. In other studies, administration of diclofenac or naproxen before laparoscopy significantly reduced postoperative pain as well the need for supplemental analgesia. Ibuprofen, an anti-inflammatory drug with analgesic action, can be given rectally to children preoperatively.

Propofol

Propofol, which is used for sedation, induction, and maintenance of anesthesia, also reduces patient anxiety. When patients could self-administer propofol in 0.7-mg kg^{-1} boluses during an ambulatory surgical procedure, they described a feeling of well-being and relaxation.[52] Anxiety reduction and sedation were similar when propofol was compared with midazolam and methohexital for retrobulbar and peribulbar ocular block.[53] In one study in which patients were given either propofol or thiopental for induction and then enflurane, nitrous oxide, and oxygen for maintenance of anesthesia, anxiety increased postoperatively only in the thiopental group.[54]

Controlling the risk of aspiration

The risk for aspiration of gastric contents in ambulatory surgery patients is no greater than for inpatients. At greater risk for aspiration are pregnant or morbidly obese patients or those with a hiatal hernia. Preoperative anxiety probably has no effect on gastric acidity for individuals without a history of duodenal ulcer.

H_2-receptor antagonists

Cimetidine and ranitidine antagonize the action of histamine on H_2 receptors, reducing the concentration of hydrogen ions; they also decrease gastric volume. The effect of cimetidine begins 60–90 min after administration and lasts for at least 3 h. Ranitidine is four to six times as potent as cimetidine, yet the elimination half-lives, 2–3 h, are similar.[55] Famotidine and nizatidine, two new H_2-receptor antagonists, are similar

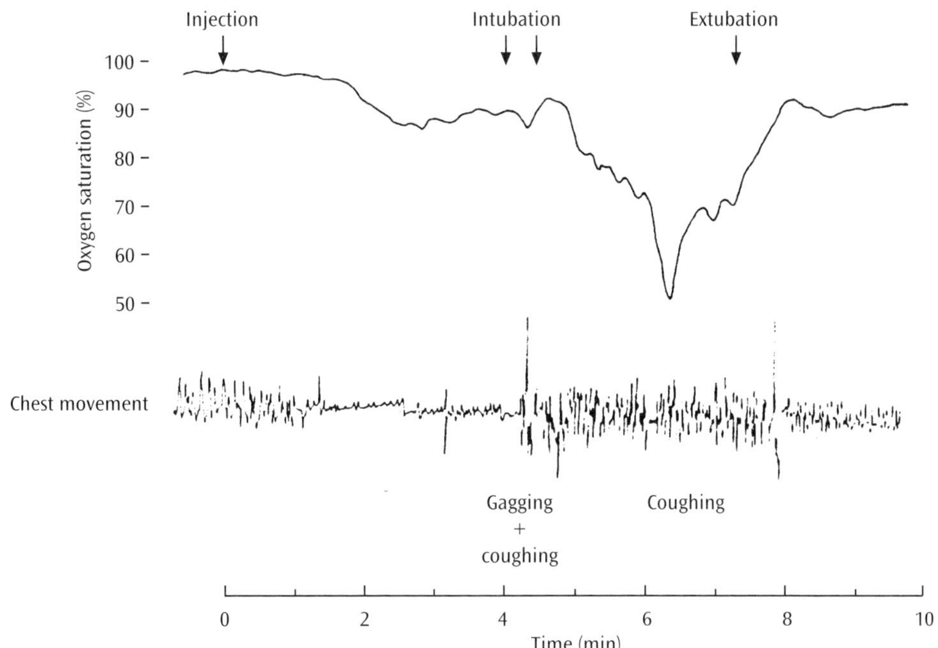

Figure 26.5 *Oxygen saturation and chest wall movements decreased in a patient after injection of midazolam during gastroscopy. After introduction of the gastroscope, the patient coughed and oxygen saturation decreased even more. (Reprinted with permission from Bell* et al.[47]*)*

to cimetidine and ranitidine. On an equimolar basis, famotidine is ~7.5 times more potent than ranitidine and 20 times more potent than cimetidine. Cimetidine inhibits the metabolism of drugs dependent on biotransformation by cytochrome P450. Cimetidine also decreases blood flow in the liver by 25% if administered acutely to a fasting patient and by 33% if administered slowly. When drugs such as propranolol, which depends on blood flow in the liver for hepatic elimination, are given in conjunction with cimetidine, they are eliminated from the body more slowly. Cimetidine sometimes causes mental confusion, particularly in elderly patients,[56] and usually within 48 h of the first dose. This syndrome is associated with drug concentrations of not lower than 1.25 $\mu g\,mL^{-1}$.

Omeprazole

Omeprazole is a substituted benzimidazole that inhibits the gastric enzyme, hydrogen–potassium adenosine triphosphatase (ATPase). This membrane transport protein is responsible for hydrogen ion secretion from the gastric parietal cell. The half-life of omeprazole ranges from 0.3 to 2.5 h.[57] Its metabolite is also active and binds irreversibly to gastric hydrogen–potassium ATPase. Omeprazole, like cimetidine, inhibits cytochrome P450 and, therefore, reduces the metabolism of drugs that depend on cytochrome P450 systems. When omeprazole (80 mg) was given to ambulatory patients the night before surgery, gastric volume was unchanged and gastric pH was increased.[58]

Sodium citrate

If aspirated, soluble antacids such as sodium citrate (Bicitra) produce less severe hypoxia and lung abnormalities than do nonabsorbable antacids, such as Mylanta (aluminum hydroxide, magnesium hydroxide, and simethicone). Customary doses (30 mL) of soluble antacids raise gastric pH but can also increase gastric volume. Very small doses of sodium bicarbonate (1.6 mL) increase gastric pH without affecting gastric volume.[59]

Metoclopramide

Metoclopramide is a dopamine antagonist that increases the pressure of the lower esophageal sphincter, speeds gastric emptying, and prevents or alleviates nausea and vomiting. To reduce gastric volume even more, metoclopramide is combined with other drugs. For example, the combination of cimetidine and metoclopramide during the preinduction phase was better than either drug alone before ambulatory surgery or increasing gastric pH and decreasing gastric volume.[60] Metoclopramide is also an effective antiemetic. Patients given metoclopramide before surgery may experience less nausea and vomiting not only during, but also after, surgery. However, the duration of action of metoclopramide is relatively brief, and its antiemetic effectiveness may be negligible at low doses. The typical oral doses of 0.15–0.3 $mg\,kg^{-1}$ before anesthesia did not prevent emesis induced by cisplatin, an antineoplastic drug given to cancer patients, whereas i.v. doses of 2 $mg\,kg^{-1}$ were effective.[61] These higher doses, however, have not been used perioperatively.

In our practice, sodium citrate and metoclopramide, or an H_2-receptor antagonist, are routinely administered to patients at risk for acid aspiration, particularly those with hiatal hernia, the morbidly obese, parturients, and those with a history of duodenal ulcer.

Controlling postoperative nausea preoperatively

More than any other factor, nausea, with or without vomiting, delays discharge of patients and increases unanticipated admissions of both children and adults after ambulatory surgery[62] (Fig. 26.6). Women, especially those who are pregnant, have a higher incidence of postoperative nausea and vomiting. Other risk factors include a previous history of motion sickness or postanesthetic emesis; surgery within 1–7 days of the menstrual cycle; and procedures such as laparoscopy, lithotripsy, and ear, nose, or throat surgery. Narcotics given for premedication may exacerbate the problem of postoperative nausea and vomiting. Other drugs such as metoclopramide may help alleviate this condition.

Droperidol

Droperidol has had variable success as an antiemetic. Lower doses (0.25–0.5 mg) seem to be more effective than higher doses, and recovery after anesthesia is not delayed.[63,64] Doses as low as 1.25 mg can produce restlessness in the postoperative period.[65] In children, 50–75 $\mu g\,kg^{-1}$ controls postoperative nausea, although this dose is also associated with

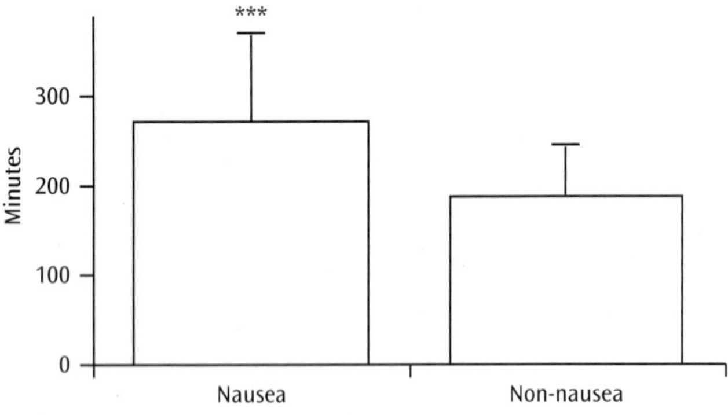

Figure 26.6 *Time to home-readiness (mean ± SD) in nauseated versus non-nauseated patients. Home-readiness is significantly delayed (***$P < 0.001$) if a patient is nauseous. (Reprinted with permission from Green and Jonsson.[62])*

a delay in discharge. When propofol and droperidol were compared, postoperative nausea in patients was similar, but fitness for discharge was1 h later after droperidol.[66] Droperidol has been withdrawn by the manufacturer from use in the UK.

Promethazine

Promethazine is the most common phenothiazine derivative used to control postoperative nausea and vomiting in children. The usual dose is 0.5–1.0 mg kg^{-1}. Promethazine, 0.5 mg kg^{-1} i.v. and intramuscularly (i.m.), was significantly more effective than droperidol in controlling overall postoperative vomiting, particularly vomiting after discharge from the hospital, when used for strabismus surgery in children.[67]

Serotonin antagonists

In the class of serotonin antagonists, the most studied is ondansetron. Its half-life is approximately 3.5 h in adults, shorter in children, and longer in the elderly (mean 7.9 h).[68] The primary adverse effect of ondansetron is headache; other effects are diarrhea, constipation, sedation, and transient minor elevations in liver function tests. The drug is not associated with extrapyramidal reactions. Doses of 4–8 mg were effective antiemetics, although 4 mg was not less effective than 8 mg[69] (Fig. 26.7). Ondansetron (4 mg) was superior to metoclopramide for control of postoperative nausea or vomiting.[70] An 8-mg dose was superior to droperidol (1.25 mg) and metoclopramide (10 mg).[71] In children, ondansetron (100 µg kg^{-1}), was more effective than droperidol (75 µg kg^{-1}) or placebo.[72] The reduction of postoperative nausea in patients was similar when ondansetron was compared with a placebo followed by a "rescue" antiemetic of 20 mg of i.v. metoclopramide and 25 mg of i.v. hydroxyzine.[73] Ondasetron is most effective when administered at the end of surgery.[74]

Acupressure

Acupressure may decrease postoperative nausea and vomiting. Acupressure bands that were placed preoperatively and removed 6 h postoperatively reduced nausea and vomiting by 50%[75] (Fig. 26.8). At the time of writing, the pressure bands cost only $15.00 and are reusable.

Recommendations

The routine use of antiemetics is controversial, given that a large percentage of patients do not experience postoperative nausea and vomiting. We consider drug treatment for nausea only when patients have a history of severe nausea and vomiting after anesthesia or when patients report a tendency to become nauseated easily (e.g. they become carsick easily). We use propofol for induction and then give metoclopramide early in the case. If, despite this regimen, patients are nauseous or vomiting in the PACU, we administer ondansetron. For children at risk for emesis, after an inhalation induction, we convert to an infusion of propofol.

Preoperative sedation is not needed for every patient. We use the following criteria for benzodiazepines. If a patient has been evaluated at least 24 h before a scheduled procedure and needs preoperative medication because of an expressed desire or anxiety that cannot be relieved with comforting, we prescribe oral diazepam, 2–5 mg per 70 kg body weight for the night before and 10 mg per 70 kg body weight for 6.00 a.m. on the day of surgery. If surgery is scheduled for 1.00 p.m. or later, the drug should be taken at 8.00 a.m. on the day of surgery. When patients are evaluated for the first time in the preoperative holding area and seem to need medication (again, because of an expressed desire, anxiety that cannot be relieved with assurances, or, on rare occasions, the ineffectiveness of a previously administered dose of diazepam), midazolam or propofol is administered intravenously with or without a narcotic. The initial dose of midazolam or propofol is 0.03 mg kg^{-1} or 0.7 mg kg^{-1} respectively. For children, when necessary, oral midazolam at 0.5 mg kg^{-1} is administered in the preoperative holding area.

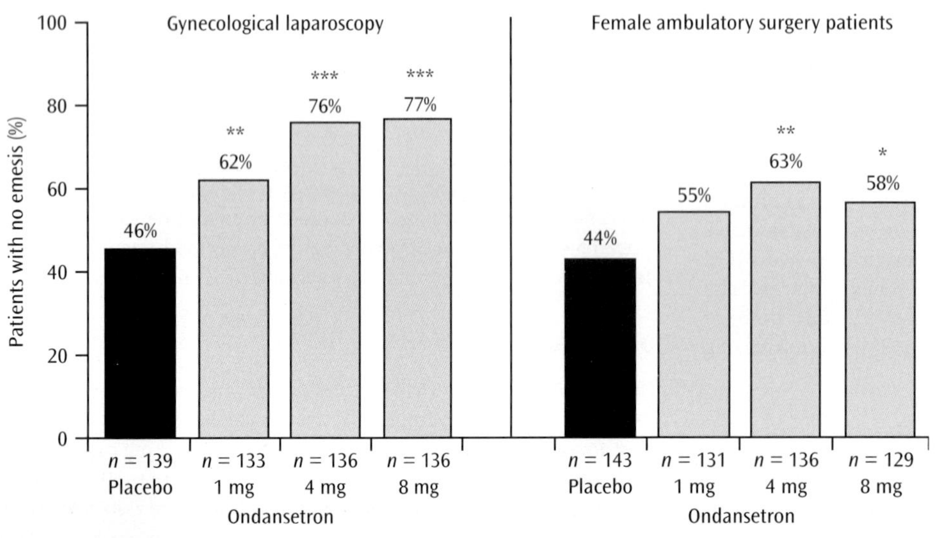

Figure 26.7 *Nausea and vomiting were significantly less in ambulatory surgery patients with 4 or 8 mg ondansetron given before induction of anesthesia compared with placebo or 1 mg ondansetron. *Significantly different from placebo at $P < 0.05$ level; **significantly different from placebo at $P < 0.02$ level; ***significantly different from placebo at $P < 0.01$ level. (Reprinted with permission from Pearman.[69])*

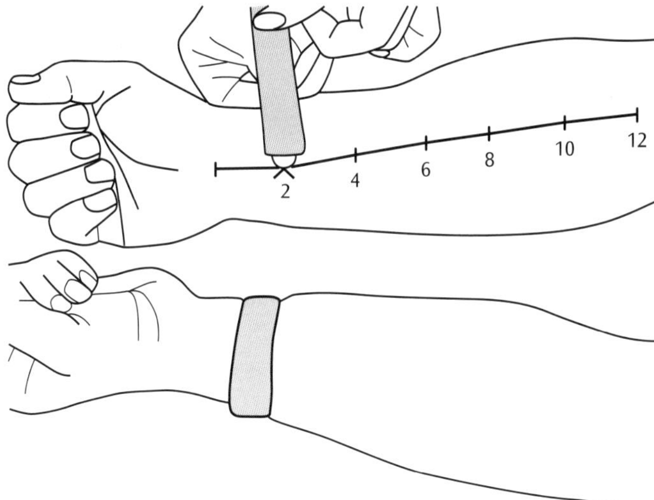

Figure 26.8 *The treatment point P.6 is located on the anterior surface of the forearm, 2 inches (5 cm) proximal to the distal wrist crease between the tendons of musculus flexor carpi radialis and musculus palmaris longus. The forearm of the patient from the transverse crease of the wrist to the cubital crease is measured as 12 inches (30 cm). (Reprinted with permission from Fan* et al.[75]*)*

In our practice, sodium citrate and metoclopramide or an H_2-receptor antagonist is routinely administered to patients at risk of acid aspiration, particularly those with hiatal hernia, the morbidly obese, and parturients. Although the idea of allowing patients to have clear liquids up to 2 h before surgery is attractive, this practice is not routinely recommended.

REFERENCES

1. Vacanti CJ, VanHouten RJ, Hill RC. A statistical analysis of the relationship of physical status to postoperative mortality in 68 388 cases. *Anesth Analg* 1970; **49:** 564–6.
2. Lewin I, Lerner AG, Green SH, *et al.*. Physical class and physiologic status in the prediction of operative mortality in the aged sick. *Ann Surg* 1971; **174**: 17–31.
3. Goldman L, Caldera DL, Nussbaum SR, *et al.* Multifactorial index of cardiac risk in noncardiac surgical procedures. *N Engl J Med* 1977; **297:** 845–50.
4. Keats AS. The ASA classification of physical status – a recapitulation. *Anesthesiology* 1978; **49:** 233–6.
5. Rehder K. Clinical evaluation of isoflurane: complications during and after anaesthesia. *Can Anaesth Soc J* 1982; **29** (Suppl.): S44–S48.
6. Cohen MM, Duncan PG. Physical status score and trends in anaesthetic complications. *J Clin Epidemiol* 1998; 41*:* 83–90.
7. Ziffren SE, Hartford CE. Comparative mortality for various surgical operations in older versus younger age groups. *J Am Geriatr Soc* 1972; **20:** 485–9.
8. Schein OD, Katz J, Bass EB, *et al.* The value of routine preoperative medical testing before cataract surgery. Study of Medical Testing for Cataract Surgery. *N Engl J Med* 2000; **342:** 168–75.
9. Eagle KA, Brundage BH, Chaitman BR, *et al.* Guidelines for perioperative cardiovascular evaluation for noncardiac surgery. Report of the American College of Cardiology/American Heart Association Task Force on Practice Guidelines (Committee on Perioperative Cardiovascular Evaluation for Noncardiac Surgery). *J Am Coll Cardiol* 1996; **27:** 910–48.
10. Roizen MF. More preoperative assessment by physicians and less by laboratory tests (editorial). *N Engl J Med* 2000; **342:** 204–5.
11. Roizen MF, Foss JF, Fischer SP. Preoperative evaluation. In: Miller RD (ed.). *Anesthesia*, 5th edn. Philadelphia: Churchill Livingstone, 2000: 824–83.
12. Domoto K, Ben R, Wei JY, *et al.* Yield of routine annual laboratory screening in the institutionalized elderly. *Am J Public Health* 1985; **75:** 243–5.
13. Wolf-Klein GP, Holt T, Silverstone FA, *et al.* Efficacy of routine annual studies in the care of elderly patients. *J Am Geriatr Soc* 1985; **33:** 325–9.
14. Delahunt B, Turnbull PRG. How cost effective are routine preoperative investigations? *N Z Med J* 1980; **92:** 431–2.
15. Narr BJ, Hansen TR, Warner MA. Preoperative laboratory screening in healthy Mayo patients: cost-effective elimination of tests and unchanged outcomes. *Mayo Clin Proc* 1991; **66:** 155–9.
16. Narr BJ, Warner ME, Schroeder DR, Warner MA. Outcomes of patients with no laboratory assessment before anesthesia and a surgical procedure. *Mayo Clin Proc* 1997; **72:** 505–9.
17. Macpherson DS, Snow R, Lofgren RP. Preoperative screening value of previous tests. *Ann Int Intern Med* 1990; **113:** 969–73.
18. Mitchell TL, Tornelli JL, Fisher TD, *et al.* Yield of the screening review of systems: a study on a general medical service. *J Gen Intern Med* 1992; **7:** 393–7.
19. Sandler G. Costs of unnecessary tests. *Br Med J* 1979; **2:** 21–4.
20. Rabkin SW, Horne JM. Preoperative electrocardiography: its cost-effectiveness in detecting abnormalities when a previous tracing exists. *Can Med Assoc J* 1979; **121:** 301–6.
21. Rabkin SW, Horne JM. Preoperative electrocardiography: effect of new abnormalities on clinical decisions. *Can Med Assoc J* 1983; **128:** 146–7.
22. Warner MA, Shields SE, Chute CG. Major morbidity and mortality within 1 month of ambulatory surgery and anesthesia. *JAMA* 1993; **270:** 1437–41.
23. Roizen MF, Kaplan EB, Schreider BD, *et al.* The relative roles of the history and physical examination, and laboratory testing in preoperative evaluation for outpatient surgery: the "Starling" curve of preoperative laboratory testing. *Anesthesiol Clin N Am* 1987; **5** (1): 15–34.
24. Turnbull JM, Buck C. The value of preoperative screening investigations in otherwise healthy individuals. *Arch Intern Med* 1987; **147:** 1101–5.
25. Levinstein MR, Ouslander JG, Rubenstein LZ, Forsythe SB. Yield of routine annual laboratory tests in a skilled nursing home population. *J Am Med Assoc* 1987; **258:** 1909–15.
26. Roizen MF. Preoperative evaluation. In: Miller RD (ed.). *Anesthesia*, 3rd edn. New York: Churchill Livingstone, 1990: 743–72.
27. Kaplan EB, Sheiner LB, Boeckmann AJ, *et al.* The usefulness of preoperative laboratory screening. *J Am Med Assoc* 1985; **253:** 3576–81.
28. Lutner RE, Roizen MF, Stocking CB, *et al.* The automated versus the personal interview. Do patient responses to preoperative health questions differ? *Anesthesiology* 1991; **75:** 394–400.
29. McKee RF, Scott EM. The value of routine preoperative investigations. *Ann Royal Coll Surg Engl* 1987; **69:** 160–2.
30. Khuri SF, Daley J, Henderson W, *et al.* Risk adjustment of the postoperative mortality rate for the comparative assessment of the quality of surgical care: results of the National Veterans Affairs Surgical Risk Study. *J Am Coll Surg* 1997; **185:** 315–27.
31. Blery C, Szatan M, Fourgeaux B, *et al.* Evaluation of a protocol for selective ordering of preoperative tests. *Lancet* 1986; **1:** 139–41.
32. Charpak Y, Blery C, Chastang C, *et al.* Prospective assessment of a protocol for selective ordering of preoperative chest X-rays *Can J Anaesth* 1988; **35:** 259–64.
33. Roizen MF. Is a patient's history of food supplement use simply supplementary? [editorial]. *J Clin Anesth* 1998; **10:** 89–90.
34. Munro J, Booth A, Nicholl J. Routine preoperative testing: a systematic review of the evidence. *Health Technol Assess* 1997; **1:** 1–62.
35. Kelly RE, Hartman GS, Embree PB, *et al.* Inhaled induction and emergence from desflurane anesthesia in the ambulatory surgical patient: The effect of premedication. *Anesth Analg* 1993; **77:** 540–3.
36. Johnston M. Anxiety in surgical patients. *Psychol Med* 1980; **10:** 145–52.
37. Aantaa R, Jaakola M-L, Kallio A, *et al.* A comparison of dexmedetomidine, an α_2-adrenoceptor agonist, and midazolam as i.m. premedication for minor gynaecological surgery. *Br J Anaesth* 1991; **67:** 402–9.
38. Badner NH, Nielson WR, Munk S, *et al.* Preoperative anxiety: detection and contributing factors. *Can J Anaesth* 1990; **37:** 444–7.
39. Kain ZN, Wang SM, Mayes LC, *et al.* Distress during the induction of anesthesia and postoperative behavioral outcomes. *Anesth Analg* 1999; **88:** 1042–7.
40. Kain ZN, Mayes LC, Wang SM, *et al.* Parental presence during induction of anesthesia versus sedative premedication: which intervention is more effective? *Anesthesiology* 1998; **89:** 1147–56.
41. Greenblatt DJ, Abernethy DR, Locniskar A, *et al.* Effect of age, gender, and obesity on midazolam kinetics. *Anesthesiology* 1984; **61:** 27–35.
42. Bell GD, Spickett GP, Reeve PA, *et al.* Intravenous midazolam for upper gastrointestinal endoscopy: A study of 800 consecutive cases relating dose to age and sex of patient. *Br J Clin Pharmacol* 1987; **23:** 241–3.

43. Brophy T, Dundee JW, Heazelwood V, *et al.* Midazolam, a water-soluble benzodiazepine, for gastroscopy. *Anaesth Intensive Care* 1982; **10:** 344–7.
44. Levine MF, Spahr-Schopfer IA, Hartley E, *et al.* Oral midazolam premedication in children: the minimum time interval for separation from parents. *Can J Anaesth* 1993; **40:** 726–9.
45. McMillan CO, Spahr-Schopfer IA, Sikich N, *et al.* Premedication of children with oral midazolam. *Can J Anaesth* 1992; **39:** 545–50.
46. Samuelson PN, Reves JG, Kouchoukos NT, *et al.* Hemodynamic responses to anesthetic induction with midazolam or diazepam in patients with ischemic heart disease. *Anesth Analg* 1981; **60:** 802–9.
47. Bell GD, Reeve PA, Moshiri M, *et al.* Intravenous midazolam: a study of the degree of oxygen desaturation occurring during upper gastrointestinal endoscopy. *Br J Clin Pharmacol* 1987; **23:** 703–8.
48. Raeder JC, Breivik H. Premedication with midazolam in out-patient general anaesthesia. A comparison with morphine-scopolamine and placebo. *Acta Anaesthesiol Scand* 1987; **31:** 509–14.
49. Feld LH, Champeau MW, van Steennis CA, Scott JC. Preanesthetic medication in children: a comparison of oral transmucosal fentanyl citrate versus placebo. *Anesthesiology* 1989; **71:** 374–7.
50. Friesen RH, Lockhart CH. Oral transmucosal fentanyl citrate for preanesthetic medication of pediatric day surgery patients with and without droperidol as a prophylactic anti-emetic. *Anesthesiology* 1992; **76:** 46–51.
51. Ding Y, White PF. Comparative effects of ketorolac, dezocine, and fentanyl as adjuvants during outpatient anesthesia. *Anesth Analg* 1992; **75:** 566–71.
52. Grattidge P. Patient-controlled sedation using propofol in day surgery. *Anaesthesia* 1992; **47:** 683–5.
53. Ferrari LR, Donlon JV. A comparison of propofol, midazolam, and methohexital for sedation during retrobulbar and peribulbar block. *J Clin Anesth*1992; **4:** 93–6.
54. Winwood MA, Jago RH. Anxiety levels following anaesthesia for day-case surgery: A comparison of state anxiety levels following induction of anaesthesia with propofol or thiopentone. *Anaesthesia* 1993; **48:** 581–4.
55. Douglass WW. Histamine and 5-hydroxytryptamine (serotonin) and their antagonists. In: Gilman AG, Goodman LS, Rall TW, Murad F (eds). *Goodman and Gilman's The Pharmacological Basis of Therapeutics*, 7th edn. New York: Macmillan, 1985: 605–38.
56. Schentag JJ, Cerra FB, Calleri G, *et al.* Pharmacokinetic and clinical studies in patients with cimetidine-associated mental confusion. *Lancet* 1979; **1:** 177–81.
57. Cederberg C, Andersson T, Skanberg I. Omeprazole: pharmacokinetics and metabolism in man. *Scand J Gastroenterol* 1989; **24** (Suppl.): 33–40.
58. Haskins DA, Jahr JS, Texidor M, Ramadhyani U. Single-dose oral omeprazole for reduction of gastric residual acidity in adults for outpatient surgery. *Acta Anaesthesiol Scand* 1992; **36:** 513–15.
59. Faure EA, Lim HS, Block BS, *et al.* Sodium bicarbonate buffers gastric acid during surgery in obstetric and gynecologic patients. *Anesthesiology* 1987; **67:** 274–7.
60. Dimich I, Katende R, Singh PP, *et al.* The effects of intravenous cimetidine and metoclopramide on gastric pH and volume in outpatients. *J Clin Anesth*1991; **3:** 40–4.
61. Gralla RJ. Metoclopramide: a review of antiemetic trials. Drugs 1983; **25** (Suppl.): 63–73.
62. Green G, Jonsson L. Nausea: the most important factor determining length of stay after ambulatory anaesthesia. A comparative study of isoflurane and/or propofol techniques. *Acta Anaesthesiol Scand* 1993; **37:** 742–6.
63. Millar JM, Hall PJ. Nausea and vomiting after prostaglandins in day case termination of pregnancy: the efficacy of low dose droperidol. *Anaesthesia* 1987; **42:** 613–18.
64. O'Donovan N, Shaw J. Nausea and vomiting in day-case dental anaesthesia: The use of low-dose droperidol. *Anaesthesia* 1984; **39:** 1172–6.
65. Melnick B, Sawyer R, Karambelkar D, *et al.* Delayed side effects of droperidol after ambulatory general anesthesia. *Anesth Analg* 1989; **69:** 748–51.
66. Watcha MF, Simeon RM, White PF, Stevens JL. Effect of propofol on the incidence of postoperative vomiting after strabismus surgery in pediatric outpatients. *Anesthesiology* 1991; **75:** 204–9.
67. Blanc VF, Ruest P, Milot J, *et al.* Antiemetic prophylaxis with promethazine or droperidol in paediatric outpatient strabismus surgery. *Can J Anaesth* 1991; **38:** 54–60.
68. Chaffee BJ, Tankanow RM. Ondansetron – the first of a new class of antiemetic agents. *Clin Pharm* 1991; **10:** 430–46.
69. Pearman MH. Single dose intravenous ondansetron in the prevention of postoperative nausea and vomiting. *Anaesthesia* 1994; **49** (Suppl.): 11–15.
70. Malins AF, Field JM, Nesling PM, Cooper GM. Nausea and vomiting after gynaecological laparoscopy: comparison of premedication with oral ondansetron, metoclopramide and placebo. *Br J Anaesth* 1994; **72:** 231–3.
71. Alon E, Himmelseher S. Ondansetron in the treatment of postoperative vomiting: a randomized, double-blind comparison with droperidol and metoclopramide. *Anesth Analg* 1992; **75:** 561–5.
72. Davis PJ, McGowan FX Jr, Landsman I, *et al.* Effect of antiemetic therapy on recovery and hospital discharge time. A double-blind assessment of ondansetron, droperidol, and placebo in pediatric patients undergoing ambulatory surgery. *Anesthesiology* 1995; **83:** 956–60.
73. Bodner M, White PF. Antiemetic efficacy of ondansetron after outpatient laparoscopy. *Anesth Analg* 1991; **73:** 250–4.
74. Tang J, Wang B, White PF, *et al.* The effect of timing of ondansetron administration on its efficacy, cost-effectiveness, and cost-benefit as a prophylactic antiemetic in the ambulatory setting. *Anesth Analg* 1998; **86:** 274–82.
75. Fan CF, Tanhui E, Joshi S, *et al.* Acupressure treatment for prevention of postoperative nausea and vomiting. *Anesth Analg* 1997; **84:** 821–5.

27

Essential monitoring

ANTHONY P ADAMS

Classically, information about a patient's progress was obtained by very simple clinical observations – a finger on the pulse, an ear to listen to breath and heart sounds (stethoscope), and an eye to see the chest movements and the patient's color. The value today of these kinds of clinical observations cannot be overemphasized despite the wonders of modern technology. It was always rightly emphasized that the finger needed to be glued, metaphorically, to the patient so that observations should be continuous and thus prevent any untoward events from being missed. It was common in the USA for a monaural esophageal stethoscope to be used in every case: a safety pin, to fix the tubing to the anesthesiologist's shirt, had the advantage of fixing him or her to the patient. Advances in anesthesia and surgery have demanded a better flow of continuous information (online) from the patient, and from the anesthetic and other equipment used, to the anesthesiologist. The anesthesiologist or the intensive care clinician has many tasks to perform simultaneously, and modern equipment can provide the necessary information continuously and immediately so that problems may be identified very early and corrected appropriately. Monitors are the "unsleeping eyes" that allow us to "see the invisible," especially early hypoxia. However, monitors are not likely to be of value unless the user can recognize and appropriately act on what he or she sees.

Hazards of equipment result not only from mechanical failure[1–4] but also from improper interaction between operator and machines. The most obvious dangers have largely long been eliminated from anesthetic machines and associated equipment in developed countries, but hazards of varying subtlety remain. Nevertheless, after human error (see below), equipment problems are the second most common cause of preventable critical incidents in anesthesia. A critical incident is defined as a human error or equipment failure that could have led (if not discovered or corrected in time), or did lead, to an undesirable outcome, ranging from increased length of hospital stay to death.[5] Included within this range of undesirable outcomes is an increased stay in a recovery room or intensive care unit. Disconnection of some part of the breathing system is very common: so common, in fact, that Cooper identified this general problem of disconnection [involving the breathing system, intravenous (i.v.) lines, monitoring apparatus] separately in his analysis of major errors and equipment failures in anesthesia management. A study commissioned jointly by the US and Canadian governments found that disconnections are so common that many anesthesiologists consider them routine.[6] Although this particular problem has been discussed by experts from the UK Department of Health (DoH),[7] the message appears not to have been persuasive. Indeed, important information, e.g. that male–female components of the breathing system should be mated by a "push and twist" technique (rather than by simply making the connection a push fit), so as to force a good connection,[8] appears to be often ignored, possibly because of a failure to convey and publicize the information sufficiently.

Monitoring systems in no way reduce the importance of training, continuing education, clinical skill, and vigilance in providing safe anesthesia and high-quality care.[9] Indeed, intense training is required in the correct use and interpretation of monitors. At what point do advanced safety features become positive hazards? And why, when manufacturers are trying to reduce cockpit clutter, are we prepared to put up with a plethora of different monitors or multifunction push buttons on the monitors? How can we prevent the brain being overloaded with too many good intentions? Litigation in the USA has forced hospitals into extensive monitoring of patients to protect themselves from multimillion dollar malpractice claims. In the UK, sums awarded in damages for medical negligence are rising: payments above £1 million are becoming commonplace, and there are cases in which brain-damaged patients are being awarded £2–4 million.

Monitoring in the operating room or in the intensive care unit may be considered from the viewpoint of: (1) monitoring the performance of the equipment (i.e. the supply of oxygen and the breathing system); and (2) monitoring the patient. The analysis of gases from the anesthetic machine must be established when the equipment is checked before anesthesia induction. The Association of Anaesthetists' *Checklist for Anaesthetic Apparatus*[10] is novel since it requires the use of an oxygen monitor, attached at the common gas outlet, to verify that, when the oxygen flow meter and emergency oxygen flush are opened, the gas issuing is indeed oxygen and that no "crossover" or contamination has occurred up to that point. This will also verify the correct operation of any antihypoxic device incorporated into the anesthetic machine.

The patient is monitored through clinical observations, continuous monitoring devices, and by intermittent monitoring devices. Additional specialized monitoring is required in certain instances: (1) where there is pre-existing medical disease; (2) when special techniques such as controlled hypotension are being used; (3) when surgery involves the lungs, cardiovascular, or central nervous systems; or (4) when major blood loss is expected. Furthermore, the same standards of monitoring should be applied when sedation or anesthesia is given for operations or procedures of brief duration, including those performed outside the conventional operating room. Monitoring should be continued during transfer of the patient and in the recovery room: a full range of monitoring devices as employed during anesthesia should be available. The *International Standards for a Safe Practice of Anaesthesia* – developed by The International Task Force on Anaesthesia Safety[11] – are recommended to anesthesiologists throughout the world. Their purpose is to provide guidance and assistance to anesthesiologists, professional societies, hospital administrators, and governments in improving the quality and safety of anesthesia. The World Federation of Societies of Anaesthesiologists in 1992 adopted these standards, which include standards of monitoring during anesthesia.

CLOSED CLAIM STUDY IN THE USA

A "closed claim"[12] for an adverse anesthetic outcome typically consists of relevant hospital and medical records, narrative statements from involved healthcare personnel, expert and peer reviews, deposition summaries, outcome reports, and the cost of settlement or jury award.[13] An anesthesiologist who has been specially trained for participation in the Closed Claim Study reviews each claim. Information from "closed claims" has been acquired from 20 insurance organizations involving a total of 1541 cases (dental damage – the most frequent injury in any surveys – is not considered). The most common cause of injury is difficulty in management of the respiratory system (34% of cases). This also represents the source of the most common result, namely death and brain damage. The three most common respiratory-related critical incidents are inadequate ventilation of the lungs, esophageal intubation, and difficult intubation. In an in-depth analysis of a sample of cases of inadequate ventilation, it was found that the majority of cases were due to poor monitoring of the respiratory system (42%) and personnel problems (13%), such as impaired vigilance of the anesthesiologist. Patient pathophysiology, such as obesity and impaired lung function, was noted in only 10% of cases. Esophageal intubation was the most frequent critical incident in the study – brain damage or death was the outcome in 94 such cases. It is notable that in 59 of the cases the person administering the anesthetic claimed to have auscultated both sides of the chest and thought that the tube was properly placed; this points to the unreliability of this sign alone.[14] The next most common respiratory emergency was difficult intubation, constituting 6% of the total cases. Detailed accounts of the closed-claim studies have been published as the information has been gathered.[15–17] Another conclusion from the American Society of Anesthesiologists (ASA) Closed Claims Study of data from 1079 analyzed claims "provides solid evidence" that the combination of pulse oximetry and capnometry can expect to help prevent anesthetic-related morbidity and mortality.[18]

MONITORING STANDARDS

The Health Council of the Netherlands, which is the main advisory council to the Ministry of Health, produced a pioneering advisory report on monitoring standards in 1978.[19] This was accepted and sent out to all hospitals with the requirement that they had to comply within 3 years; a team of inspectors under the Chief Inspector of Medical Affairs confirms compliance. In the Netherlands there has now been a reduction in the number of operating rooms covered by one anesthesiologist supervising nurse anesthesiologists (a 1:2 ratio).

In 1986, the ASA instituted minimal monitoring standards,[20] following the example of those promulgated by the Boston hospitals attached to Harvard Medical School.[21] Already, the effect of standards promulgated and laws enacted consequent upon the adoption of the Harvard standards by the ASA and other bodies has been to reduce the rate of the rise in premiums and now even to reduce premiums for malpractice insurance; it is becoming evident that this is a consequence of proper monitoring and not entirely due to greater awareness of the problem.[22,23] Advances in technology have played a very important part: although, for example, 10 different measurements were originally required in the Netherlands, this number has now been reduced by combination into fewer monitors, or even one. Technological advances have reduced the bulk and improved the reliability of monitors.[24]

Since 1986, the ASA standards have been upgraded several times. On 21 October 1998, two standards for basic anesthesia monitoring (these being in addition to other guidelines, statements, and protocols on related matters) were set. The standards apply to all anesthesia care although, in emergency circumstances, appropriate life-support measures take precedence. The basic standards may be exceeded at any time, based on the judgment of the responsible anesthesiologist. Moreover, the standards apply to all general anesthetics, regional anesthetics, and monitored anesthesia care. *Standard I* provides that qualified anesthesia personnel shall be present in the room throughout the conduct of all general anesthetics, regional anesthetics, and monitored anesthesia care. *Standard II* provides that during all anesthetics and the patient's oxygenation, circulation and temperature shall be continually evaluated. From 1 July 1999 further provisions came into effect. These comprise both objectives and methods (with the permission of the Association of Anaesthetists):

- *Objective (a): Oxygenation* To ensure adequate oxygen concentration in the inspired gas and the blood during all anesthetics.
  - *Methods (1): Inspired gas* During every administration of general anesthesia using an anesthesia machine, the concentrations of oxygen in the patient breathing system shall be measured by an oxygen analyzer with a low oxygen concentration limit alarm in use.
  - *Methods (2): Blood oxygenation* During all anesthetics, a quantitative method of assessing oxygenation, such as pulse oximetry, shall be employed. Adequate illumination and exposure of the patient are necessary to assess color.
- *Objective (b): Ventilation* To ensure adequate ventilation of the patient during all anesthetics.
  - *Methods (1)* Every patient receiving general anesthesia shall have the adequacy of ventilation evaluated continually. Qualitative clinical signs such as chest excursion, observation of the reservoir breathing bag, and auscultation of breath sounds are useful. Continual monitoring for the presence of expired CO_2 shall be performed unless invalidated by the nature of the patient, procedure, or equipment. Quantitative monitoring of the volume of expired gas is strongly encouraged.
  - *Methods (2)* When an endotracheal tube or laryngeal mask is inserted, its correct positioning must be verified by clinical assessment and by identification of CO_2 in the expired gas. Continual end-tidal CO_2 analysis, in use from the time of endotracheal tube/laryngeal mask placement until extubation/removal or initiating transfer to a postoperative care location, shall be performed using a quantitative method such as capnography, capnometry, or mass spectroscopy.
  - *Methods (3)* When ventilation is controlled by a mechanical ventilator, there shall be in continuous use a device that is capable of detecting disconnection of components of the breathing system. The device must give an audible signal when its alarm threshold is exceeded.
  - *Methods (4)* During regional anesthesia and monitored anesthesia care, the adequacy of ventilation shall be evaluated, at least, by continual observation of qualitative clinical signs.
- *Objective (c): Circulation* To ensure the adequacy of the patient's circulatory function during all anesthetics.
  - *Methods (1)* Every patient receiving anesthesia shall have the electrocardiogram (ECG) continuously displayed from the beginning of anesthesia until preparing to leave the anesthetizing location.
  - *Methods (2)* Every patient receiving general anesthesia shall have arterial blood pressure and heart rate determined and evaluated at least every 5 min.

- *Methods (3)* Every patient receiving general anesthesia shall have, in addition to the above, circulatory function continually evaluated by at least one of the following: palpation of a pulse, auscultation of heart sounds, monitoring of a tracing of intra-arterial pressure, ultrasound peripheral pulse monitoring, or pulse plethysmography or oximetry.
- *Objective (d): Body temperature* To aid in the maintenance of appropriate body temperature during all anesthetics.
  - *Methods* Every patient receiving anesthesia shall have temperature monitored when clinically significant changes in body temperature are intended, anticipated, or suspected.

The Association of Anaesthetists of Great Britain and Ireland (AAGBI) *Recommendations for Standards of Monitoring in Anaesthesia and Recovery* was published in 1988 and updated in 1994.[25] This also stresses the importance of the constant presence of the anesthesiologist and the absolutely fundamental tenets of clinical observation backed up by constant online information from monitors about the condition of the patient, the functioning of the apparatus, and the interactions between all of these. The document also addresses regional anesthesia, and the recovery and transport of patients. Half of the successful claims in the USA are due to failure to monitor, poor preoperative assessment, absence from the operating room, or inadequate recovery and follow-up. The first UK report of a confidential enquiry into perioperative deaths (CEPOD)[26] demonstrated that knowledge was not applied in 75% of anesthetic-related deaths. However, it is a fallacy to think that because equipment did not feature largely in this finding it is not important.

ALARMS

Importance of setting appropriate alarm limits

When a monitor is switched on, defaults for the thresholds of the various variables are automatically set. If any such threshold is violated, an alarm will be triggered. The default is a value(s) set up by the manufacturer in the expectation that it will be of use to the majority of users. Sometimes these settings are appropriate and sometimes not. For example, the default limit for low heart rate on one popular monitor is 40 beats per minute (b.p.m.) – hardly appropriate for an anesthetic conducted in a child, when the anesthesiologist would want to be alerted well before such a serious bradycardia developed. The alarm limits on anesthetic monitoring equipment rarely seem to be set up appropriately by the anesthesiologist before the anesthetic is started. There is a tendency to set such limits later on in the course of the anesthetic. There is too much reliance on the default values of individual monitors and an amazing lack of knowledge about the actual values involved. The presence of many similar and overobtrusive alarms in the operating room continues to confuse and irritate[27] and there is a need to rethink completely the characteristics of the different audible warnings. Intelligent alarm systems are being developed to organize these alarms, on the assumption that they will shorten the time that anesthesiologists need to detect and correct faults.[28] False positives often occur because the user does not fully understand the operation of the equipment and does not set appropriate alarm limits. False-positive alarms generate a sense of disregard and disbelief, yet modern equipment, correctly set up, is indicating that there really is something wrong. Errors of judgment by the anesthesiologist are a major problem, and this is usually a reflection of the anesthesiologist's inexperience, ignorance, or lack of skill.[29–31] A judgmental error occurs when the action taken is indeed the action intended, i.e. a bad judgment; these are errors based on faulty decisions, e.g. choice of face-mask anesthesia for a patient with a full stomach.

INVASIVE MONITORING

Invasive monitoring, used in the appropriate circumstances, provides vital information about a patient's current status and response to therapy. However, such monitoring techniques are not without risk. For example, the list of problems that may follow cannulation of the internal jugular vein is vast. Other techniques that pose risks are arterial cannulation and, particularly, pulmonary artery catheterization. Thus, it is essential that those who practice such techniques are correctly taught and are sufficiently exposed to them subsequently so that skills are maintained. The ASA first issued a guidance on invasive monitoring in 1984, which aims to reduce the risks to the patient by members of the anesthesia care team by stating that: (1) the decision to use invasive monitoring is a medical judgment and should, therefore, be made only by a qualified physician; (2) invasive monitoring techniques should be prescribed by a physician and, depending on their risk, should be applied only by a competent and trained physician, or under the immediate medical attention of such a person. The ASA statement provides for training and accrediting of nonphysician members of the team who may perform invasive monitoring [central venous pressure (CVP) catheterization via the upper extremity and arterial cannulation] if approved at local medical staff level by the anesthesia department and the active medical staff. Insertion of pulmonary artery catheters is a relatively hazardous procedure and should only be performed by an appropriately trained physician.

ARTERIAL (BLOOD) PRESSURE

When the American neurosurgeon Harvey Cushing was visiting Bern in Switzerland in 1901 he heard about Scipione Riva Rocci's method for measuring blood pressure, which had been described in 1896. Accordingly, he went to see him to learn more about this method, which was in continuous daily use by the bedside of every patient in the Ospedale di Matteo in Pavia near Milan. Cushing was so impressed that when he returned to the Johns Hopkins Hospital in the USA he insisted that those who anesthetized his patients used the technique during his operations. The method was later enhanced by listening to the Korotkoff sounds – described in 1905 – by auscultation over the brachial artery with a stethoscope. This is still a superb method for determining arterial pressure.

Indirect methods – intermittent noninvasive blood pressure

There have been many attempts to automate the measurement of arterial pressure using indirect methods. Most of the methods work satisfactorily in normal patients but are unreliable in hypotensive or restless patients. Systolic pressure can be detected more reliably than diastolic pressure. A number of physical principles have been used, such as electrical impedance changes, double- and triple-cuff pneumatic methods, using a microphone for detecting the Korotkoff sounds, and ultrasound sensing of movements of the arterial wall.

The technique of oscillotonometry was made popular by von Recklinhausen, who developed two instruments, the scala alternans and the scala altera. His technique was one that used two (double) cuffs that overlapped one another slightly. Both cuffs were inflated to above systolic pressure. The upper cuff was slowly deflated stepwise, thus eventually allowing jets of blood to pass under the upper cuff once its pressure had fallen below the systolic pressure. The lower cuff, which was still inflated, formed the sensing cuff and picked up the signals (systolic pressure) as the jets of blood impinged on it. At this point the lower cuff was slowly deflated, and the diastolic pressure was taken as the point at which the oscillations detected by this cuff died away.

The automated oscillotonometric technique uses a single cuff and a pressure transducer measures both the pressure and the oscillations. The onset of the oscillations and the point of maximum oscillation are sensed to give the systolic and mean pressures respectively.

Continuous noninvasive blood pressure

The best-known instrument is the Finapres. A small cuff is positioned over a finger and is attached to a transducer and an air pump. A light-emitting diode (LED) and a photocell are included in the cuff, so that the system is, in effect, a photoplethysmograph. The volume of blood in the arteries varies with the degree of distension during systole. The microprocessor senses this volume at a set point according to the mean arterial pressure and a servocontrol constantly adjusts the amount of air, and hence pressure, in the cuff in order to maintain a constant photoplethysmograph output. A continuous tracing of arterial pressure is obtained. The idea of measuring blood pressure accurately and noninvasively and in a finger is very alluring; unfortunately, it has been known for some time that finger blood flow and pulse pressure are regulated by sympathetic vasoconstriction.[32] Studies using finger and ear plethysmograms in anesthetized patients have shown that, whereas the pulse pressure in the pinna of the ear was minimally affected by sympathetic stimulation (laryngoscopy, surgical stimulation, etc.), pulse pressure in the finger is influenced greatly by such events.[33] Therefore, although the finger could be a good place to measure peripheral vascular response to sympathetic stimulation, it is not a good place to assess the general state of the circulation. Despite extensive trials the method is not thought to be sufficiently reliable.[34]

A new development is a method based upon the relations between pulse wave velocity (PWV) and blood pressure, which was initially described over 60 years ago. In any individual, changes in pulse wave velocity in the short term are due primarily to changes in blood pressure. Studies using two pressure transducers placed a known distance apart on a major artery identified a linear relation between PWV and mean blood pressure. Development of these concepts means that blood pressure may now be measured continuously and noninvasively. One pair of sensors measures blood pressure, heart rate, and arterial oxygen saturation by pulse oximetry. The system is based on photometric measurements that do not rely on compression or occlusion of arteries to track blood pressure (the Artrac system). The blood pressure cuff provides a calibration, or baseline, value. The sensors are placed on the forehead and a digit, and are used to measure changes in pulse transit time, microvascular volume, and other physiological values related to the blood pressure. Changes in these values are used in an empirically derived equation that calculates changes in blood pressure from the initial calibration value.

Invasive methods

In low cardiac output states, pulses may be poorly palpable and Korotkoff sounds difficult to hear, while the intra-arterial pressure may be only moderately reduced. This method is justified for difficult or major cases, as it is more reliable on a beat-to-beat basis than intermittent methods. In addition, blood samples can be obtained for analysis. Monitoring of intra-arterial pressure is easily accomplished by percutaneous insertion of a 20- or 22-gauge cannula into the radial, brachial, or dorsalis pedis artery. Occasionally, the femoral artery may be used but is best avoided in case of problems associated with any resulting infection or thrombosis. Long-term patency is assisted by intermittent or continuous flushing devices using heparinized saline (approximately 1 IU heparin per mL 0.9% NaCl solution). Miniature transducers can be attached to the arterial cannula, thus eliminating long fluid-filled catheters. Disposable transducers are now inexpensive.

CENTRAL VENOUS PRESSURE

Traditionally, CVP has been estimated using a catheter passed into the right atrium and connected to a saline manometer. Care must be taken that the reference zero of the system is in the phlebostatic axis of the patient. When the patient is supine the zero reference may be taken as level with the suprasternal notch. The small error should not pose a problem since the anesthesiologist is interested in trends and responses to therapy. Changes in CVP are also used to assist in the diagnosis of hypovolemia, cardiac failure, and tamponade. Sykes[35] has emphasized that the correct use of CVP is to assess the response to repeated small (200 mL) transfusions of fluid. In a patient with hypovolemia, CVP rises slightly after each such bolus and then rapidly falls to the preinfusion level. In a normovolemic patient the postinfusion fall in pressure is slower, taking about 3 min to return to the control value, while in a patient with fluid overload CVP will be high and the fall in pressure after infusion will be extremely slow.

ELECTROCARDIOGRAM

It is usual to use only a three-lead configuration during anesthesia. The best configuration is the CM5 lead in which the right electrode (negative) is positioned in the second or third intercostal space on the right side of the manubrium. The positive lead (left) is positioned in the fifth intercostal space in the anterior axillary line. The indifferent third lead may be positioned anywhere convenient. Since the mass of the heart lies between the positive and negative leads a good signal is obtained. Although information about heart rate and rhythm may be obtained by other leads, the value of the CM5 configuration for anesthesiologists is that signs of subendocardial ischemia are more readily detected. It should thus be regarded as the de facto method. The name CM5 (for central manubrium, fifth intercostal space) comes from the original position of the right electrode in the sternal notch, which is an uncomfortable location for an awake patient. Since it is important that the anesthesiologist can hear the sound of each heart beat, whether from the ECG signal or from the pulse oximeter, it is essential that the audible "bleep" of the monitor should be switched on; even small changes in heart rate will be instantly apparent.

CONTINUOUS INTRAVASCULAR BLOOD GAS ANALYSIS

The current standard[36] of Po_2, Pco_2, and pH, and derived variables, such as standard bicarbonate and base excess, involves procurement of an arterial blood sample that can be analyzed by a central laboratory or near to the bedside. The main problem with this approach is that sampling is intermittent and depends on the judgment of the person providing the care. Consequently, sampling may not be done when it is needed, or the timing of the sample may be inappropriate. Delays may occur between procurement of the sample and the report of the results. As a result, clinically important changes in blood gas status may go undetected or may occur after a sample has been drawn. Alternatively, excessive and unnecessary laboratory analyses may be performed. These problems should be overcome with the advent of indwelling, continuously monitoring arterial blood gas and pH sensors, but only recently, after three decades of research and development, have commercial systems become available.

The CIABA monitor

The CIABA system (3300 Intra-arterial Blood Gas Monitoring System, Puritan-Bennett, Carlsbad, CA, USA) is a continuous intra-arterial blood gas monitor with arterial values obtained periodically and analyzed by conventional equipment. The system consists of a sterile, disposable, fiberoptic sensor and a microprocessor-controlled monitor with a self-contained calibration unit and a detachable panel display. The sensor is inserted through a 20-gauge radial artery cannula. Light is transmitted from the monitor to the sensor tip, where it reacts with fluorescent dyes sensitive to oxygen or hydrogen ions (analytes). The change in the intensity of the photoluminescent radiation caused by the analytes is measured every 20 s and derived blood gas values are displayed. An assessment of the CIABA system concluded that it provides immediate blood gas results and trend information in sufficient agreement with *in vitro* results to be reliable for decision making in most clinical circumstances. Generally, the differences found in the values between the two methods of analysis resulted from the combination of the inherent errors of each method.[37]

The Paratrend 7

The accuracy and performance of a new intra-arterial blood gas sampling device, the Paratrend 7 [(PT7) Biomedical Sensors Ltd, Pfizer Hospital Products Group, High Wycombe, Bucks, UK], over a wide range of these variables during anesthesia with one-lung ventilation have been encouraging.[38–41] The PT7 is a multiparameter sensor system incorporating four different sensors: Po_2 is measured by a miniaturized Clark electrode; Pco_2 and pH are measured by optodes; and blood temperature is determined by a thermocouple. The four sensors are housed in a heparin-coated microporous polyethylene tube of about 0.5 mm diameter, suitable for insertion through a 20-gauge or larger catheter. The tip with the sensor elements, about 4 cm in length, must float freely within the arterial lumen. The element containing the blood gas sensor incorporates a tubing system that permits simultaneous and continuous measurement of intravascular arterial pressure, and intermittent aspiration via a side-port for repeated *in vitro* laboratory blood gas analysis. The disposable sensor is sealed during manufacture within a tonometer containing buffer solution that maintains hydration and serves as a calibration medium. Before insertion into the patient (e.g. into the radial artery), the sensor is calibrated under microprocessor control by the PT7 monitor using three precision gases bubbled through the tonometer. The calibration procedure takes 30 min. The manufacturer recommends that the sensor should be inserted into the artery before 8 h has elapsed. Recalibration of the system is not possible: instead values from *in vitro* laboratory blood gas analysis, as a reference every 12 h, are used to adjust the original calibration curve. The PT7 monitor displays the Po_2, Pco_2, and pH graphically and numerically. Temperature and calculated values for So_2, bicarbonate, and base excess are displayed numerically.

CARDIAC OUTPUT AND HEMODYNAMIC MONITORING

Pulmonary artery catheterization

The filling pressure of the left ventricle can be assessed as the pulmonary artery occlusion pressure after catheterization of the pulmonary artery with a balloon flotation catheter. Cardiac output is measured in most patients using these catheters. Correct interpretation requires assessment of the changes in pressure in response to therapeutic interventions. These catheters can assist in establishing the nature of the circulatory problem, optimize cardiac output while reducing the risk of pulmonary edema, and allow the rational use of inotropes and vasoactive drugs.[42] Diagnosis is often improved by the information gained. Pulmonary artery catheters are very invasive and should not be placed without due consideration of the risks and benefits.

Pulse dye densitometry

Pulse dye densitometry (PDD) belongs to the family of pulse spectrophotometry. It is a new method for monitoring cardiac output ($\dot{Q}$) and circulating blood volume (CBV). PDD detects arterial indocyanine green (ICG) dye concentration following its intravenous injection. The method relies on the measurement of ICG dye (cardio-green in the USA) in the arterial blood without the need for blood withdrawal; it has the potential to replace the thermodilution method.

The PDD system emits light at 805 nm and 900 nm and detects changes in absorption in accord with pulsation. In almost the same way as with pulse oximetry (see below), PDD detects the ratio of hemoglobin and ICG. The peak absorption of ICG is at 805 nm and the least absorption at 890 nm. The ratio between hemoglobin and ICG can be calculated using the absorption ratio between 805 nm and 940 nm. Manual input of the hemoglobin concentration – measured by an independent device – is required for the calculation of the ICG concentration. In essence, the PPD is a technique for depicting the dye densitogram of ICG. From this densitogram, several hemodynamic variables can be obtained.

PDD permits measurement of the cardiac output ($\dot{Q}$). The cuvette method was the gold standard for classic determination of $\dot{Q}$ using the Hamilton dye technique; it went out of favor following the introduction of the thermodilution method. In the classic method the concentration of ICG was measured in continuously drawn arterial blood. PDD measures the same concentration in arterial blood without the need for the withdrawal of blood. Comparisons of $\dot{Q}$ determination between PDD and thermodilution and cuvette, or PPD and thermodilution, show a bias of $0.15 \pm 0.72\ \text{L min}^{-1}$ (between PPD and cuvette), $0.50 \pm 0.92\ \text{L min}^{-1}$ (between PPD and thermodilution),[43] and $0.16 \pm 0.80\ \text{L min}^{-1}$ (between PPD and thermodilution)[44] – tolerable for clinical use.

Repeatability of measurement is important. ICG is excreted from the liver and therefore the residual ICG concentration depends on hepatic function. Arterial ICG concentration usually falls below 1% in 20 min. Thus, the PPD method can be used repeatedly during this time and over a longer interval in patients with liver dysfunction. However, for the measurement of cardiac output it is unnecessary to wait for ICG depletion in arterial blood – repeat measurements, up to five times, are possible. The residual concentration of ICG is subtracted automatically by the program. It is only necessary to wait for 20 min in order to measure circulating blood volume (CBV).

The PDD system permits quantitative assessment of the CBV and its accuracy has been compared with the gold standard labeled iodine method in healthy volunteers.[45,46] The mean bias between PDD and the radioisotope method was $3.99 \pm 10.54\%$; it may be acceptable for improving CBV measurement in a clinical setting. Examples include finding occult bleeding in emergency care patients or controlling blood volume in cases of pheochromocytoma. The CBV is not to be regarded as a static variable because it partly depends on cardiac output, which is dynamic.

Cardiac output monitoring by the NICO device

Another attractive new system for the measurement of $\dot{Q}$ is the noninvasive cardiac output (NICO) monitor (Novametrix Medical Systems Inc., Wallingford, CT, USA). The classical system used the rather laborious

Fick principle (dating from 1870), whereby oxygen content differences were found ($\dot{Q}$ = oxygen consumption/arteriovenous oxygen content difference). The NICO system permits the determination of $\dot{Q}$ from a Fick analysis of CO_2 differences using a partial rebreathing system fitted with a sophisticated sensor. The cardiac output is proportional to the change in CO_2 elimination, divided by the resulting change in arterial CO_2. This is accomplished by the NICO sensor after the periodic addition of a rebreathing volume. This sensor combines a rebreathing valve with the NICO loop (the rebreathing volume) and a CO_2 flow sensor. The change in arterial CO_2 is reflected by the change in end-tidal CO_2. Advantages claimed are that stroke volume and cardiac index can be computed at practically any time. Other variables including CO_2 elimination, alveolar ventilation, compliance, and resistance are also displayed.

The complete measurement cycles involve three phases over 3 min. After a baseline period (phase 1) of 60 s to gain stability, the patient rebreathes (phase 2), using the NICO loop (of rebreathing tubing) with the rebreathing valve turned on, for 50 s. During this time CO_2 output is reduced, P_aCO_2 and $ETCO_2$ (end-tidal CO_2) are elevated, but mixed venous CO_2 remains unchanged. Typically the rise in $ETCO_2$ is 0.4 kPa (3 mmHg). Phase 3 lasts 70 s and comprises a period of restabilization with the NICO valve turned off. During this period the three variables return to baseline values. Changes in $\dot{V}CO_2$ are measured by the integrated CO_2/flow sensor; changes in C_aCO_2 are measured by the mainstream CO_2 sensor (as reflected by a change in $ETCO_2$); a measurement of $C\bar{v}CO_2$ is not needed because it is eliminated from the Fick equation due to the differential method); finally, the measurement is corrected for pulmonary shunt based on F_iO_2 and S_pO_2. It is assumed that $\dot{Q}$, $C\bar{v}O_2$, and $V_D V_T$ do not change during the period of measurement.

Doppler systems for cardiac output measurement

Christian Doppler established in 1842 how the velocity of a moving object is proportional to the shift in reflected frequency of an optic wave of known frequency. Adaptation of this principle has led to the development of instruments that measure the velocity of blood flow and related variables in a continuous and relatively noninvasive manner. There were many difficulties: for instance, early machines could only evaluate patients who were not mechanically ventilated and whose $\dot{Q}$ values were close to normal limits. The most frequently used method was for aortic blood flow measurements to be made via the suprasternal notch: this required a well-trained operator and did not permit continuous monitoring.[47] The esophageal Doppler monitor (EDM)[48,49] is increasingly popular because it is the trend in cardiac output, rather than an absolute value, that is of particular interest in guiding therapy. The ODM provides an estimate of the cardiac output by using an estimated vessel diameter. This estimate is based on the curve of the diameter as it relates to body weight, height, and the age of the patient. Measurements can be made very easily and rapidly to provide beat-to-beat monitoring of $\dot{Q}$ and cardiac function. This device should reduce the use of more invasive methods but is not suitable for all patients. To use the technique of EDM also requires training.

VOLUMETRIC MEASUREMENTS OF VENTILATION

Monitoring respiration is often difficult unless the patient is receiving artificial ventilation. Leaks in the breathing system during spontaneous ventilation pose problems when a conventional anesthetic face mask is used. Measurement of minute volume and tidal volume may be made using simple devices such as the Wright respirometer (anemometer). However, delicate instruments such as this are easily damaged. Dry displacement gas meters are rugged, reliable, and quite accurate.[50] They are resistant to the effects of water vapor and can therefore be left in circuit continuously. Pneumotachographs have also been used but are difficult to use clinically, especially for long periods, because of water vapor condensation in the pressure lines and the calibration of the instrument changes during inspiration and expiration. Changes in the diameter of the chest and abdomen can be sensed in various ways. Impedance pneumography can be used to record changes in the electric impedance of the chest during respiration and a temperature sensor placed in the airway will record changes in air temperature during the phases of respiration and count the number of breaths per minute. Temperature probes may become displaced or covered with secretions and the impedance pneumogram may continue to record respiratory efforts made by the patient even though complete respiratory obstruction has occurred.

CAPNOGRAPHY

Capnography is the study of the shape or design of the changing concentrations of CO_2 in respired gas. A high-speed capnogram gives detailed information about each breath while overall changes in CO_2 may be followed at a slower paper speed. The capnograph is an excellent early-warning system. The association of certain patterns with specific circumstances is now recognized and the curves are often diagnostic; indeed, the effect of different breathing systems and malfunctions produce their own individual "signature" capnograms.

Luft developed the principle of capnography in 1943 from the fact that CO_2 is one of the gases that absorbs infrared (IR) radiation of a particular wavelength. Infrared radiation is absorbed by all gases with more than two atoms in the molecule. If there are only two atoms, absorption occurs only if the two atoms are dissimilar. A capnometer is an instrument that measures the concentration of CO_2 numerically. A device that continuously records and displays CO_2 concentration in the form of a tracing or waveform is called a capnograph and the tracing on recording paper is called a capnogram. The introduction of capnography into routine clinical practice was pioneered by Smalhout and Kalenda in the Netherlands.[51,52] The presentation of the CO_2 waveform obtained from breathing systems used in anesthesia and intensive care in the analog (waveform) format, i.e. the capnograph or capnogram, is vastly to be preferred to a meter or even a fast digital display. Indeed, the last two are useless in anesthetic practice, in which the breath-by-breath waveform needs to be displayed to permit continuous monitoring and analysis. This is essential where fractional rebreathing techniques are employed, such as with the Mapleson D/E/F and Bain breathing systems, because a meter or digital display cannot indicate the CO_2 concentration of the end-tidal CO_2 plateau in the face of CO_2 also appearing in the inspiratory part of the respiratory cycle. The measurement of changing CO_2 concentrations is of value in recognizing abnormalities of metabolism, ventilation, and circulation. In the normal state, alveolar CO_2 concentration is maintained within rather narrow limits independent of the metabolic state or the size of the physiological dead space. Thus, alveolar CO_2 concentration can serve as a valuable guide to CO_2 homeostasis during the prolonged periods of mechanical ventilation of the lungs required in anesthesia, intensive care, or other conditions associated with altered breathing.

Carbon dioxide in respired gas may be continuously measured by mass spectrometry, IR analysis, or photoacoustic spectrometry. Infrared rays are given off by all warm objects and are absorbed by nonelementary gases (i.e. those composed of dissimilar atoms); certain gases absorb particular wavelengths, producing absorption bands on the IR electromagnetic spectrum. The intensity of IR radiation projected through a gas mixture containing CO_2 is diminished by absorption, which allows the CO_2 absorption band to be identified and is proportional to the amount of CO_2 in the mixture.

Infrared rays have a wavelength greater than 1 µm and thus lie beyond the visible spectrum (0.4–0.8 µm); CO_2 shows strong absorption in the far IR at 43 µm and so this wavelength in the far IR range is used. A narrow-band IR filter prevents the passage of light that would otherwise be absorbed by gases other than CO_2. There is some overlap in the absorption bands of other gases (e.g. N_2O distorts the absorption bands for CO_2). Hence, due allowance must be made for any interfering gases; N_2O molecules also interact with CO_2 molecules to produce a collision broadening effect which affects the sensitivity of the IR CO_2 analyzer (see below).

An IR analyzer basically consists of a source of IR radiation, an analysis cell, a reference cell, and a detection cell. In the Luft system, rays of light from the source are filtered to obtain the required wavelengths and then pass through the analysis cell to fall on the detector, which contains pure CO_2. Any IR radiation that is not absorbed by the gases in the analysis cell is absorbed in the detector and heats the CO_2. The pressure in the detector (which is, in effect, a differential micromanometer as opposite sides are subjected to the light transmitted through the measuring and reference cells respectively) will vary according to the heating effect from the IR radiation. These alinear changes are suitably detected, amplified, and displayed; modern instruments use a linearizing circuit. Drift is reduced by interrupting or chopping the IR beam with a rotating shutter at 25–100 Hz; the pulses of IR radiation thus produce pulses of pressure in the detector cell.

The modern alternative to the classical Luft system uses an LED to produce light of the required wavelength. A solid-state photodetector (replacing the micromanometer) measures the amount of light reaching it alternately via the measuring and reference cells with the beam interrupted ("chopped") 4000 times per minute. In some designs, the chopper is omitted and the IR LED is switched on and off by a microprocessor. Some instruments dispense with the need for a reference cell and instead obtain a CO_2 zero for reference from the sample cell itself at a time when the cell is known not to contain CO_2. Thus, in both types of capnograph the electrical output consists of a series of pulses, the height of which varies with the CO_2 concentration in the analysis cell. The IR cell is the most critical part of the system and must be protected from contamination by liquids or particulate matter as these invariably cause erroneous high readings because of their high IR absorbance.

It has been common for capnographs to be provided with an automatic zeroing device that returns the trace to the baseline just as the next inspiration is sensed. This was of help in the past because of the drift experienced with electrical components. However, this facility is nowadays somewhat limiting because it does not permit the instrument to be used in the presence of breathing systems in which it may be normal to have some CO_2 in the inspired mixture, such as controlled fractional rebreathing during intermittent positive ventilation of the lungs with circuits such as the Bain breathing system.

Analysis of inspired oxygen, expired CO_2, and arterial oxygen saturation should be standard for every anesthetic. All patients, and certainly intubated patients, must be monitored by capnography to detect problems with the airway: systems that display the moving waveform of the capnogram are the best[53] although a chemical end-tidal CO_2 detector which uses a pH indicator is useful in many situations.[54]

There has been a growing awareness of the potential problems that may be induced by two-way radios and cellular telephones used in proximity to medical monitoring equipment. Disruptions of IR capnographs have been reported.[55] The problem mainly concerns the new digital mobile telephones using global positioning satellites (GPS). Within 2 m of the medical device, the electric fields from these telephones can exceed the immunity record of 7 V m^{-1} recommended by the US Food and Drug Administration (FDA) for medical electrical equipment. The electric fields produced by analog mobile telephones exceed the 7 V m^{-1} level only at relatively shorter distances.

Sidestream analyzers

These draw gas continuously from the sampling site via a small-bore tube of about 2 m in length to the measuring cell for analysis and display. The bore should be not greater than 1–2 mm to avoid mixing of gas, to resist the introduction of foreign matter, and to facilitate the withdrawal of small sample volumes. The length of the sampling tube should be kept as short as possible to obtain a fast response time for greatest accuracy. The sampling tube must be impermeable to CO_2 and so polyvinyl chloride (PVC) is often used, but because halogen hydrocarbons react with this material a tube made of Teflon is preferred in anesthetic practice. Several manufacturers provide sampling tubes and T-pieces that are hydrophobic, i.e. treated with a material that resists the entry of water. The sampling rate is of the order of 50–500 mL min^{-1} and can be varied either continuously or by preset steps. However, the flow control is often inconveniently positioned at the rear of some instruments so that the user may be unaware of the sampling rate. This may pose a hazard, for instance where excessive sampling rates are accidentally applied to children's breathing systems. Excessive sampling rates should generally be avoided in case loss of gas upsets the homeostasis of the breathing system. On the other hand, too low a sampling rate may produce a capnogram in which the curves are raised above the baseline and are sinusoidal in form without a plateau. A poor connection at some point along the sampling tube can cause the entrainment of air, thus producing an abnormal capnogram. Gas that has been sampled by the analyzer is usually discarded and not returned to the breathing circuit because of the inconvenience involved as well as the possibility of interfering with the gaseous homogeneity of the breathing system. However, the loss of gas through sampling may pose a problem in pediatric practice or with the use of closed or low-flow circle breathing systems. In such circumstances gas may be returned to the breathing system or an extra equivalent fresh gas inflow provided to compensate.

Sampling sites

It used to be common for the tip of the sampling catheter to be positioned just above the carina to obtain a good sample of alveolar gas. However, this is inconvenient and the risk of aspiration of secretions and water into the apparatus is considerable. It is now usual to position the end of the sampling tube at the proximal end of the endotracheal tube using a T-piece adapter; this is also analogous with the position of the IR measuring cell in mainstream analyzers (see below). Care must be taken in obtaining the correct sampling position when T-piece breathing systems on the Ayre principle are used lest fresh gas from the anesthetic machine is drawn into the sampling tube along with the expired gas sample to produce, because of the dilution, an erroneous low value for the end-tidal sample. The same problem occurs with the use of lung ventilators that produce a constant flow. The problem can be prevented by interposing a right-angle adapter (such as that used with a facepiece) between the breathing system (Ayre's T-piece or Bain system) and the endotracheal tube and interposing the sampling tube on the patient's side of the angle piece. Where conventional twin breathing hoses are used with a Y-piece, the sampling site should be as close to the patient's mouth as possible. When a catheter mount is used, care must be taken to ensure that the sampling site is not at the junction of the Y-piece with the catheter mount because of the extra dead space introduced by the mount. The same consideration obtains with the use of bacterial filters and condenser humidifiers despite the increased risk of water getting into the sampling tube. Manufacturers produce a wide variety of adapters for sampling and their use is recommended; special adapters to cope with the special problems of small children are also available. The use of a hypodermic needle inserted through breathing tubes to achieve access to the respired gas is to be deplored.

Mainstream analyzers

These do not draw gas but incorporate the analysis cell with IR source, detector, and associated electronics into a specially designed airway adapter, which is interposed into the breathing system. There is no specific reference cell. This form of "no loss" system offers the advantages of a very fast response. The risk of condensation of water vapor is minimized by heating the measurement chamber to about 40°C but there remains the possibility of contamination from secretions, which absorb IR radiation and lead to a spurious high value for CO_2 concentration. The added dead space is a serious disadvantage in infants. In clinical practice, the sidestream system is often to be preferred if only because of the expense involved in the repair of accidental damage sustained to the delicate components in the mainstream adapter.

Calibration

Problems occur because CO_2 and N_2O share the same mass number of 44. Unfortunately, N_2O absorbs some light at the most convenient CO_2 wavelength of 4.3 µm. Furthermore, the absorbance properties of CO_2 molecules are affected by the presence of N_2O molecules that collide with them. The effect is to cause the absorption spectrum to become broader with the result that the degree of overlap in the absorption bands of different gases varies according to the gas concentrations. This collision broadening effect (sometimes also called pressure broadening) results from the fact that the IR absorption of CO_2 is based on the vibrational motion of the molecules. When the CO_2 molecule vibrates in a crowd of other molecules, the collisions affect their vibrational energy states and thus the absorption of IR light. The degree of interaction depends on the ambient pressure and on the mass and nature of the neighboring molecules. The overall effect when CO_2 is measured in gas mixtures containing N_2O is an overestimate by an amount of about 10% for a mixture containing 50% N_2O, 45% O_2, and 5% CO_2. This is overcome commercially by introducing an electronic bias to the results through compensation buttons for N_2O, and often for O_2 as well; sophisticated instruments also monitor N_2O (by another IR LED) and O_2 concentrations simultaneously to provide a continuous and varying compensation according to the changing concentration of the interfering gases.

Other considerations include the influence of water vapor, atmospheric pressure, and calibration procedures. Erroneous results will occur if water or particulate matter, which have high IR absorbance, enter the cell. An effective water separation system is required for continuous use but a filter may produce an undesirable sinusoidal curve because of a mixing effect. A water trap is used in sidestream analyzers to remove water in particulate form before it can enter the analysis cell. The design of the trap relies on gravitational forces to separate drops of water from the gas stream and the trap must be frequently dried out and attention directed to preventing water accumulating.

Because the principle of capnography is based on the measurement of partial pressure of CO_2 the method is somewhat affected by changes in the barometric pressure. It is for this reason that calibration procedures with gaseous mixtures must be performed using the same type of sampling tube as will be used when the analyzer is connected to the patient system. Omission of the standard, long, narrow 2-m sampling tube during such calibration procedures will thus fail to take account of the large pressure drop across the ends of the tube and a measuring error will therefore result during subsequent clinical use. Equipment suppliers now provide canisters of gas mixtures containing known amounts of CO_2 in a mixture of anesthetic gases and vapors. Although modern instruments provide means for electronic calibration, regular checks using such gaseous calibration are recommended. Some modern capnometers sense changes in barometric pressure and automatically correct the CO_2 reading. In cases of doubt, a rough check may be made by a healthy individual making a forced vital capacity breath into the sampling tube and observing the peak CO_2 reading, which should be about 50–55% (mean 5.3 kPa, 40 mmHg). The presence of water vapor also affects the reading because the temperature of the patient is usually 37 °C whereas that of the instrument cell is, say, 25 °C, i.e. a difference of 3 kPa (23 mmHg) in $P\text{H}_2\text{O}$, resulting in an overestimate of $P\text{CO}_2$ by 0.15% (0.15 kPa, 1.13 mmHg).

The normal capnogram

In conditions of cardiovascular stability, the end-tidal CO_2 concentration ($P_{ET}\text{CO}_2$) bears a constant relation to $P_a\text{CO}_2$ and the normal $P_{ET}\text{CO}_2$–$P_a\text{CO}_2$ difference is 0.7 kPa (5 mmHg). If the alveoli from all areas of the lung are emptying synchronously, $P_{ET}\text{CO}_2$ will be synonymous with $P_a\text{CO}_2$. The normal capnogram is shown in Fig. 27.1. The fast speed (12.5 mm s^{-1}) is essential to detect changes in individual respiratory cycles. When expiration begins, the first part of the gas passing out of the patient's mouth is composed of gas from the mechanical and anatomical dead space and since this normally contains no CO_2 the capnograph registers zero. Next, a sharply rising front is seen, which represents the mixing of dead-space gas with alveolar gas. It is important to note that the end-expiratory plateau that follows is not an isocapnic trace but that there is a very slight and steady increase in the end-tidal CO_2 concentration as the alveolar fraction is expelled from the lungs. This effect is exaggerated in patients with chronic bronchitis and emphysema. There then follows a sharp downward return of the trace towards zero as gas flow ceases during the expiratory pause until the next inspiration begins. It is common to see a ripple effect superimposed on this downward part of the trace, the so-called cardiac oscillations, although this is now thought to be due to small gas movements created largely by the pulsations of the aorta. These oscillations are especially noticeable at slow respiratory rates and when opioids such as fentanyl have been given. It is claimed that

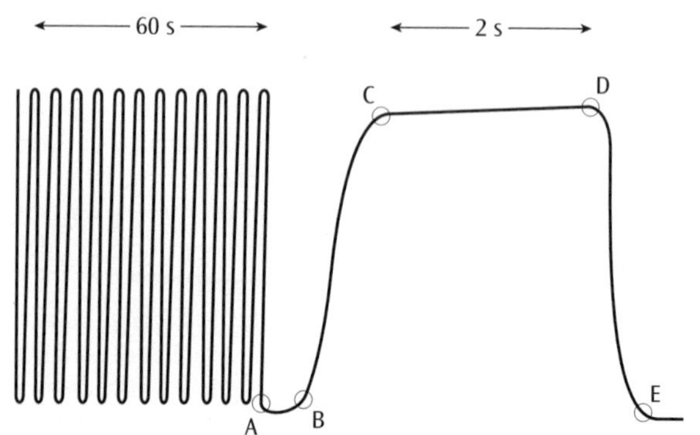

Figure 27.1 *The normal capnogram at slow and fast recording speeds. A–D denotes the expiration of gas from the anatomical dead space (containing no O_2); A–B denotes the exhalation of mixed expired gas; C–D is the alveolar or end-tidal "plateau;" D denotes the onset of inspiration and D–E denotes the return of the CO_2 tracing to the baseline as fresh gas is inspired.*

individual drugs produce their own characteristic shapes or signatures, and observation of this part of the capnogram is helpful in this respect.

The normal capnogram seen at low (trend) speed recording (25 mm s^{-1}) is rather like looking at an open box of matches and observing the striped effect of the heads of the matches all lined up next to one another. Trends are best observed at this recording speed. Reference has already been made to the often distinctive "fingerprint" or "signature" shapes produced in the capnogram in special circumstances. Such pattern recognition (as with the electrocardiogram) enables instant detection of problems with the patient or breathing apparatus. Figure 27.2 shows the normal characteristic capnogram "signature" of a healthy patient undergoing uneventful intermittent positive-pressure ventilation (IPPV) of the lungs with a Bain breathing system. The small amount of CO_2 appearing during inspiration (the rebreathing wave) represents the controlled fractional rebreathing, which enables a predetermined P_aCO_2 to be achieved in the face of large tidal volumes (thus avoiding excessive hypocapnia with all its attendant disadvantages) and hence the maintenance of good oxygenation. The exact position and shape of this rebreathing wave depend on the magnitude of the fresh gas flow from the anesthetic machine.

The abnormal capnogram

Abnormalities should be sought by analyzing the various phases of the capnogram for individual breaths as well as observing the trends occurring over a period of time. Five characteristics should be inspected: height, frequency, rhythm, baseline, and shape. Rebreathing may be observed by the appearance of CO_2 in the inspired gas; this may or may not be abnormal depending on the type of breathing system used. Blunting of the normal sharp upward deflection as expiration proceeds (mixed alveolar gas) occurs with atelectasis or with a leak in the breathing circuit. A second alveolar plateau superimposed on the first (the so-called "camel" capnogram) represents one lung emptying slightly before the other and may be seen in patients in the lateral position. Small indentations or dips in the final portion of the alveolar plateau may represent gas movement due to someone leaning on the chest or the patient making a very small movement of the diaphragm as a muscle relaxant is wearing off (the so-called "curare cleft"). Complete disconnection or total obstruction of the breathing system results in a sudden return to a zero trace, but torsion or kinking of the endotracheal tube or breathing circuit with some gas passage remaining shows as a peaked effect in place of the normal end-tidal plateau. Disconnection alarms are not infallible. The commonest types monitor the pressure in the airway and the thresholds for "high" and "low" must be set carefully

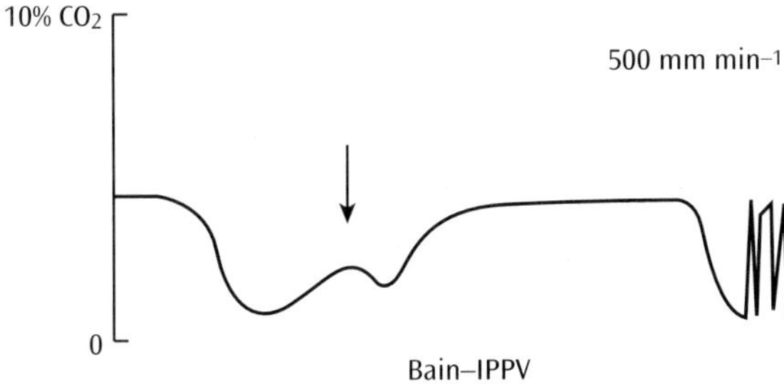

Figure 27.2 *The normal "signature" capnogram of a patient anesthetized using intermittent positive-pressure ventilation with the Bain breathing system. Note the rebreathing wave (arrow) during inspiration.*

and closely according to the prevailing circumstances. The "high" and "low" alarm limits form a pressure "window" which just spans the peak pressure observed when the system is set up on the patient. A window of about 10 cmH_2O (1 kPa) correctly set (with the peak pressure reaching its center) will permit a change of 5 cmH_2O (0.5 kPa) on either side of the high and low-threshold values before the alarm is sounded. A window of a lesser span is even better. Under some circumstances partial or even complete disconnections of some part of the breathing system may go undetected should cyclic pressure changes prevent the alarm from operating. Hence, continuous capnography is valuable.

Unrecognized intubation of the esophagus instead of the trachea is a common problem in anesthetic practice and accounts for many medicolegal actions. It is often thought that intubation of the esophagus by mistaking it for the trachea is associated with a zero CO_2 signal. However, this is not necessarily the case because previous attempts to inflate the lungs by face mask drive some expired gas into the esophagus and stomach so that when esophageal intubation unknowingly occurs some of this CO_2 returns to the breathing system to appear on the capnograph when IPPV is attempted. Such a tracing has a peaked effect and does not resemble the normal end-tidal plateau; the concentration of CO_2 is low and gastric CO_2 decreases to zero after about 1 min (five "breaths"). A spin-off from this work is the observation that intubation of the esophagus followed by intermittent compression of the reservoir breathing bag, or use of a ventilator, ventilates the esophagus and stomach to an extent that produces some gas movement in and out of the lungs as they are compressed by the movements of the mediastinum. This accounts for the fact that accidental esophageal intubation often goes undetected for a considerable period of time when valiant attempts have previously been made at preoxygenation by face mask. The golden rule to remember with capnography is that any trace other than the normal pattern with a smooth distinct end-tidal plateau should immediately suggest that something is wrong somewhere.

In a few countries, CO_2 is still used by some anesthesiologists as part of the anesthetic technique to stimulate breathing, to aid blind nasal intubation, or to prevent hypocapnia in pediatric anesthesia. In such circumstances the capnograph should be mandatory to warn of an excess in $P\text{CO}_2$ or its continued accidental administration. In the UK, such incidents of inadvertent CO_2 administration continue to occur with tragic results. In the Netherlands, capnography in anesthetic practice has been mandatory by law since 1978. It should be borne in mind that during spontaneous breathing return of the CO_2 tracing to the zero level between each breath does not necessarily imply that rebreathing is not occurring because the retention of CO_2 stimulates breathing; simultaneous measurement of expired volume should indicate whether or not this is the case. However, failure of the CO_2 trace to return to zero during spontaneous breathing with any breathing system indicates the presence of gross rebreathing of CO_2.

The measurement of the CO_2 fraction of mixed expired gas ($F_E\text{CO}_2$) to permit the calculation of physiological dead space and the rate of elimination of CO_2 ($\dot{V}\text{CO}_2$) is classically performed by analyzing mixed expired gas over a period of time by collection into a Douglas bag. However, a more convenient method for obtaining $F_E\text{CO}_2$ is to measure the instantaneous expiratory flow ($\dot{V}_E$) and expiratory CO_2 fraction ($F_E'\text{CO}_2$ or ETCO_2). The product of these two signals gives CO_2 flux, and integration with time yields expiratory CO_2 volume. Processing of these signals is achieved online electronically and provides particularly useful information for patients in intensive care who are receiving IPPV. Because it is not practicable for commercial systems to measure both flow and ETCO_2 at the same point in the system, the CO_2 production is overestimated. The error occurs in the measurement of the instantaneous flow of CO_2 to and from the patient as a result of rebreathing, which corresponds to about 24 mL of end-expiratory gas per breath using the standard Y-piece and tubing of the Siemens-Elema Servo ventilator with the Siemens-Elema CO_2 analyzer. This problem can be largely decreased by the use of nonreturn valves in the Y-piece.

Continuous monitoring of $ETCO_2$ is of value for the early detection of the malignant hyperthermia syndrome (MHS), and dramatic rises in P_aCO_2 occur before body temperature has much increased. Continuous CO_2 monitoring is also useful in other conditions associated with increases in metabolism such as shivering, pain, and seizures.

Reductions in cardiac output are accompanied by reductions in CO_2 output, and $ETCO_2$ monitoring is quite a useful adjunct in monitoring cardiogenic or hypovolemic shock. A gradually diminishing $ETCO_2$ concentration should alert the anesthesiologist to the possibility that blood loss has been more than is realized. When a sudden interruption in pulmonary perfusion occurs, as it does with cardiac arrest (or cardiac failure or gross arrhythmias), the transport of CO_2 to the lungs ceases and the capnograph tracing quickly and exponentially decays toward zero. The capnograph is also a very sensitive monitor of venous air embolism and is second only in sensitivity to the Doppler ultrasonic technique, without having the disadvantage of interference by surgical diathermy. The blockage in the lung capillaries caused by emboli disturbs the existing ventilation–perfusion ratio so that gas exchange in affected units either is grossly impaired or ceases. The overall effect is thus one of an increased physiological dead space, with gas returning from affected alveolar units (having the same composition of fresh gas, i.e. not containing CO_2), hence diluting the mixed expired gas containing CO_2 from unaffected regions of the lung to produce a lowering of the $ETCO_2$ concentration. This monitor is of particular value in neurosurgical operations, and continuous monitoring of the CO_2 tracing is important. In such circumstances even the slightest reduction in the $ETCO_2$ concentration should raise the possibility that an air embolus has occurred. However, the more expensive nitrogen meter is a far better monitor of air embolus because, once denitrogenation has been achieved as part of the anesthetic process, any ingress of air (whether as an air embolus or as an air leak into the breathing system) will produce a strong positive signal.

Carbon dioxide measurements are not accurate, especially in children, if the response time of the CO_2 analyzer is too slow and its output fails to reach the actual carbon dioxide concentration at the end of each breath. An accurate high-frequency response is essential when end-tidal PCO_2 is monitored during pediatric anesthesia. Six IR capnometers and one multiplexed mass spectrometer were assessed in a laboratory study in the face of increasing respiratory rates from 8 to 101 cycles min^{-1}.[56] At or below frequencies of 31 cycles min^{-1}, four capnometers overestimated and three underestimated the true $P_{ET}CO_2$. At frequencies above 31 cycles min^{-1}, six capnometers underestimated and one overestimated $P_{ET}CO_2$. The differences in displayed CO_2 from known CO_2 over the entire range of frequencies studied was between –2.19 kPa and +0.88 kPa (–16.4 mmHg and +6.6 mmHg), although if two suspect values obtained from one capnograph are removed from the reported results the range narrows to between–1.52 kPa and +0.88 kPa (–11.4 mmHg and +6.6 mmHg), and is–0.99 kPa to +0.88 kPa (–7.4 mmHg to +6.6 mmHg) if the mass spectrometer results are also discarded (see below). The cause of the underestimation in $P_{ET}CO_2$ is thought to be the mixing of adjacent breaths during transport down the sampling catheters and in the analysis chamber; the long sampling line (50 m) of the multiplexed mass spectrometer system presumably contributes to this error. The Hewlett-Packard 47210A capnometer was the instrument least affected, presumably because of its mainstream analysis cell, thus no sampling tube.

The rise time of a capnograph is the time taken for the analyzer output to respond to a sudden step change in CO_2 concentration, i.e. the time (T_{90}) it takes for the analyzer to change from 10% of the final value to 90% of the final value. Alternatively, the response time, T_{70}, is used in place of T_{90} because the 70% point is a steeper part of the response curve; for all practical purposes, T_{90} is twice the value of T_{70}. The rise times of capnographs for clinical use range from 50 to 600 ms. The distortion of the CO_2 waveform is a function of the rise time of the analyzer. The rise times of 11 commercially available CO_2 analyzers were measured in a laboratory study: only six instruments responded quickly to be accurate for rates up to 100 breaths min^{-1}. All 11 responded rapidly enough to measure end-tidal CO_2 concentration with 5% accuracy when ventilatory rates were less than 30 breaths min^{-1}. To measure CO_2 output ($\dot{V}CO_2$) with 5% accuracy an analyzer should have a rise time of 20 ms; the analyzer rise time (for analyzers with T_{70} rise times < 200 ms) can be estimated clinically to within 10 ms (±8 ms SD) by a simple breath hold and forced exhalation, thus providing an estimate of the accuracy of CO_2 measurements in adults or children. Hence, the limitations of capnography should be appreciated in special situations, such as in pediatric anesthesia, as some capnographs show a better performance than others. It has been recommended that a CO_2 analyzer should have a T_{90} of less than 100 ms to measure $ETCO_2$ accurately in adults; when the ventilatory rate is high, as in children, even faster rise times are recommended. A sidestream capnometer should be considered reliable only if the total delay time is less than the respiratory cycle time; total delay time can be reduced by increasing the rate of gas sampling, or by reducing the length of the sampling tube, or both, although other factors are involved.

Capnography is not a measurement solely of respiratory function, and capnograms must be interpreted in conjunction with other clinical findings. The capnogram, like the ECG, requires systematic analysis to obtain the best information (namely baseline, height, frequency, rhythm, and shape). Various monographs detail numerous such examples.

PHOTOACOUSTIC SPECTROSCOPY

Monitors for analysis of anesthetic vapors are becoming more widespread. They have a special value in low-flow and closed-circle techniques since overdosage and insufficient anesthesia (awareness) should be apparent at an early stage. The eavesdropping microphones used in World War II, and even today in some businesses as bugging devices, can be put to good use in medicine. Such instruments (Brüel and Kjær Ltd, BK-2850, Naerum, Denmark) use the principle of photoacoustic spectroscopy (PAS):[57] with the exception of oxygen, all gas and vapor concentrations are determined by this technique (Fig. 27.3). Much the same basic principles are used as found in the IR monitor, namely the ability of CO_2 and N_2O and anesthetic agents to absorb IR light. However, the measurement techniques differ. Infrared spectroscopy uses the optical method whereas PAS uses the acoustic technique. This is based on the fact that, if IR energy is applied to a gas, the gas will expand, leading to an increase in pressure. If the applied energy is delivered in pulses, the pressure will be intermittent, thus resulting in a fluctuating pressure. If the pulsation lies within the audible range, an acoustic signal is produced that can be detected by a microphone. The advantages claimed for PAS over the basic IR method are high accuracy, increased reliability, reduced preventive maintenance, and the need for less frequent calibration. Moreover, as the amount of IR light absorbed is measured directly without use of a reference cell, zero drift is nonexistent with PAS. If there is no gas in the chamber, there can be no acoustic signal. A magnetoacoustic technique is used to measure gaseous oxygen concentrations. In some instruments the same microphone is used for both measurement methods. This means that the rise time is the same for all gases and gives a true real-time relation between all the gas waveforms.

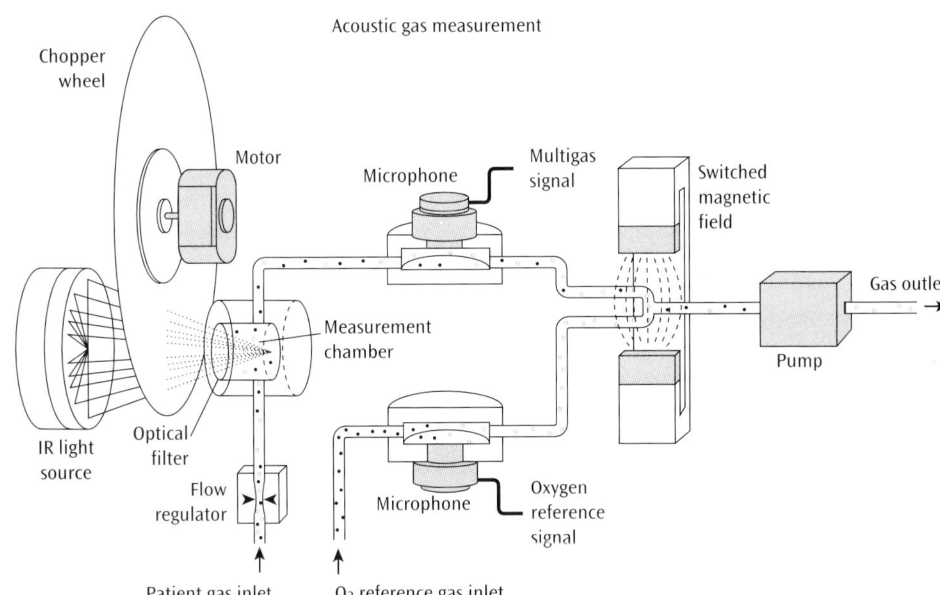

Figure 27.3 *The principle of photoacoustic spectroscopy.*

RAMAN SCATTERING

Raman scattering, a powerful and widely used laboratory spectroscopic technique, was discovered in 1928. Accurate high-speed analysis of gases requires an intense monochromatic light source such as a laser. Raman scattering of light provides continuous and trend measurement of anesthetic and respiratory gases. A precisely regulated laser beam (helium–neon laser) is recirculated hundreds of times through a gas cell. During each pass through the cell the laser beam interacts with a flowing sample of gas being continuously withdrawn from the anesthesia breathing system. When a photon from the laser beam collides with a gas molecule in the cell, its energy excites the vibrational and rotational modes of the molecule. As the molecule loses energy after the collision, it re-emits scattered light at a lower energy and consequently at greater wavelength. The amount of wavelength "shift" corresponds to characteristic vibrational and rotational energies of the gas molecule. Because these shifts are different for each gas, the wavelength components present in Raman-scattered light provide specific chemical identification of the gases present. The quantities of scattered photons produced at each wavelength are directly proportional to the concentration of a particular gas within the cell. Proprietary filters and photon-counting circuits are used to measure simultaneously the scattered light at multiple wavelengths. The molecules of each respiratory and anesthetic gas in the sample give out distinct Raman-scattered light with characteristic wavelengths when irradiated by the laser beam. The number of scattered photons for each wavelength is directly proportional to the concentration of a particular gas present in the mixture. The RASCAL (*Ra*man *sc*attering *a*na*l*ysis) is one such instrument.

OXIMETRY

Transient hypoxemia is common during anesthesia, often resulting from hypoventilation during induction and recovery or from minor degrees of obstruction. Measures can be taken to avoid its occurrence when hypoxia may be anticipated such as during endoscopy, one-lung anesthesia, or possible difficult intubation. At other times it is unexpected, and may be unrecognized and lethal. For decades, attempts have been made to find a convenient and reliable means of monitoring the delivery of oxygen to the tissues. Matthes published at least 20 papers on oximetry between 1934 and 1944 and may safely be regarded as the father of oximetry. In the mid-1930s, Professor Robert Brinkman used the newly invented barrier layer photocell to measure oxygen saturation of blood. During World War II, noninvasive ear oximeters were developed for use in aviation research; this led to the introduction of the classic Atlas and Cyclops oximeters, but although the benefits of continuous oximetry were appreciated, technical problems prevented their routine clinical use. In 1948 Brinkman substituted the conventional technique of light transmission for a reflection measurement. In the late 1960s, Shaw developed a self-calibrating eight-wavelength ear oximeter, which eventually became the Hewlett-Packard ear oximeter. However, the introduction of the Clark oxygen electrode in 1956 directed clinical thinking and technology for the ensuing 30 years away from the concept of saturation and focused instead upon the tension of oxygen in the blood. Hence the concept of tension as the driving gradient for oxygen between the inspired air and the mitochondria of tissue cells, through the various intermediate steps of alveolar gas, pulmonary capillary blood, etc., dominated thinking.

General principles of pulse oximetry

Many devices have been used as pulse meters, e.g. mercury-in-rubber strain gauges, microphones, piezoelectric crystals, Doppler devices, and photoelectric cells. Although Hertzman reported the use of photoelectric finger plethysmography in 1937, it was not until 1975 that the concept of pulse oximetry was reported from Japan, developed by Minolta, and tested by other Japanese researchers. The introduction into clinical practice of the Nellcor pulse oximeter, by Yelderman and New[58] in 1983, enabled arterial oxygen saturation to be measured easily by noninvasive means and revolutionized continuous monitoring of oxygen saturation, producing reliable results in every patient. Pulse oximetry is the most useful method as it is simple, noninvasive, and accurate under most circumstances.[53,59] Cyanosis is notoriously difficult to detect clinically because of variation in lighting conditions and variability among individual observers; it is even more difficult to detect where the epidermis is thickened, the skin is pigmented, or there is pigment associated with jaundice or Addison's disease. Cyanosis and bradycardia are late signs of hypoxemia, and pulse oximetry represents a very significant advance in patient safety because even astute clinicians fail to detect cases of severe arterial desaturation. It is worth remembering that $S_{a}O_2$ will not decrease until the $P_{a}O_2$ is below 11.3 kPa (85 mmHg) because of the shape of the oxyhemoglobin dissociation curve. Furthermore, when the low-threshold alarm sounds as saturation falls below the default setting of 90%, the corresponding PO_2 is 7.7 kPa (57.8 mmHg) on the standard oxygen dissociation curve.

The basis of oximetry is to shine light of known intensity and given wavelength through a substance in solution and to measure the amount of light that is transmitted through it. The chosen wavelength depends on the absorption spectrum of the substance under investigation. The fundamental law (the Lambert–Beer law) governing the transmission, or the absorption, of the light is $I_t = I_0 e^{-Ecd}$ (where I_0 is the intensity of the incident light, and I_t is the intensity of the light after transmission through a solution of a substance of concentration, c; d is the distance that the light has to travel through the substance, e is the base of natural logarithms, and E is a proportionality constant known as the extinction coefficient). The term Ecd is called the absorbance or optical density, D, of the solution. It can be shown that $D = 2.303 \log_{10}(I_0/I_t)$. In the red region of the spectrum, at a wavelength of 650 nm, there is a large difference in optical absorption between reduced hemoglobin and oxyhemoglobin (Fig. 27.4). When hemoglobin is oxygenated, the transmission of light is increased. In the near-IR region of the spectrum, at 805 nm, there is an isobestic point. There are several of these points and they represent wavelengths at which the optical absorption of fully reduced and fully oxygenated hemoglobin are equal. Hence, a measurement at this wavelength determines the total amount of hemoglobin present, and the difference in output between the measurements at the two wavelengths (650 nm and 805 nm) is an index of the oxygen saturation of the blood. However, when light is shone through a substance or tissue it is reflected and scattered as well as being transmitted, and so the Lambert–Beer law is to be regarded as entirely empirical.

A pulse oximeter analyzes the changes in the transmission of light through any pulsating arterial vascular bed. The amount of light transmitted, such as through the nail bed of the finger or the lobe or pinna of the ear, depends on the amount absorbed by the various structures present, such as skin, muscle, bone, venous, and capillary blood, etc. The path length that the light has to travel through the finger is constant until it is changed (increased and decreased) because of expansion and relaxation from the entry and exit of pulsing arterial blood into the system to produce the familiar plethysmographic waveform. The amount of light absorbed and transmitted will then alter. This "pulse added" signal (Fig. 27.5) is subtracted from the background transmission signal by a microprocessor-controlled empirical algorithm computed hundreds of times per second; the saturation is averaged over a short time interval of 3–6 s to produce a rapid response. The algorithm is created by measuring pulse-added absorbances in healthy, awake volunteers breathing various gas mixtures. These absorbances are then correlated with actual oxygen saturations obtained by arterial sampling and a CO oximeter. The differing light absorption characteristics of oxygenated and nonoxygenated blood are thus used to compute continuously the oxygen saturation of the arterial blood.

Two narrow band LEDs are used at wavelengths of 660 nm in the red and 910 nm in the IR part of the spectrum. Some manufacturers use an LED at 940 nm instead of 910 nm but, as either value corresponds to a plateau on the curve, the isobestic point of 810 nm is in effect mimicked (it is not technically possible to produce a reliable LED for 810 nm). Because only two wavelengths are used, the pulse oximeter cannot distinguish between more than two forms of pigment, i.e. reduced and oxyhemoglobin. If a third form is present, such as carboxyhemoglobin (COHb), it is not clear what the pulse oximeter will actually measure. Each LED switches on and off at about 720 Hz (red on, red off, and IR on, both off, etc.) and a single broad-band photodiode detects the amount of light transmitted. The photodetector produces outputs for the transmitted light from each of the diodes and also for any ambient light detected during the off periods in the 720-Hz cycle. The LEDs and photodetector are housed in a probe, which is attached to a digit,

Figure 27.4 *Absorption spectrum of reduced (Hb) hemoglobin (solid line) and oxygenated (HbO_2) hemoglobin (dashed line). D is the optical density (an index of the opaqueness of the medium) and λ is the wavelength in nanometers. 810 nm is one of the isobestic points at which the absorbance of the two forms of hemoglobin is the same. The two vertical lines denote wavelengths in the red and infrared parts of the spectrum used by the light-emitting diodes of pulse oximeters.*

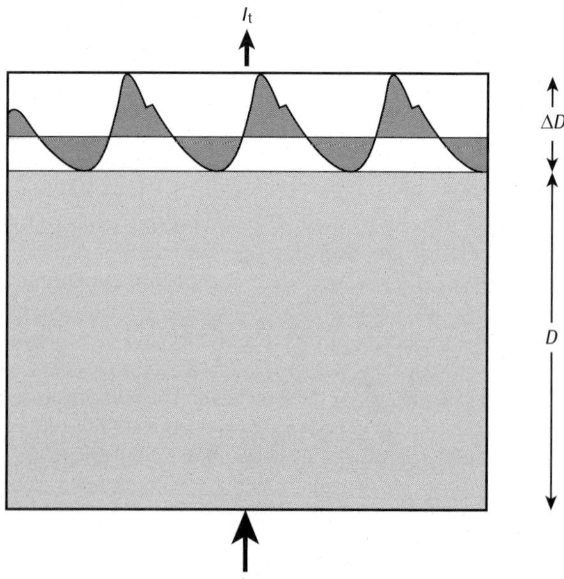

Figure 27.5 *The principle of pulse oximetry. D is the fixed absorbance of light shone through the nonpulsating structures (e.g. bone, muscle, skin, veins) of a tissue; ΔD is the "pulse added" component, or variable absorbance, of light as a result of the pulsating arterial system in the tissue. I_0 is the intensity of the incident light and I_t is the intensity of the transmitted light emerging from the tissue.*

the pinna or lobe of the ear, or across the foot, heel, or hand in the case of infants. Skin, flesh, bone, and venous blood reflect and absorb a constant amount of light; arterial blood, by contrast, absorbs varying amounts of light because of the pulsatile blood flow. Until recently, all commercially available LEDs were homostructures, i.e. they consisted of pn junctions formed in one type of material. Over the past few years new types of LEDs (heterostructures) such as those based on the aluminum–gallium–arsenide (AlGaAs) system have appeared with significant improvements in light output efficiency, and even further advancements in LED technology are due to appear.

Calibration and performance

The calibration of the instrument is preset during manufacture and cannot be altered by the user; it is unfortunate that no external standards have so far been developed. Most instruments are programmed to check their internal calibration and sensor function when switched on and intermittently thereafter. The majority of pulse oximeters are tested down to saturation values of 70%, the lower limit of tolerable hypoxemia; the error above this value is about ±2 %, and ±3% in the range 70–50% saturation. The $P_{a}O_2$ corresponding to a saturation of 70% on the standard oxygen dissociation curve is 5 kPa (37 mmHg). Below this point on the dissociation curve the calibration is generally achieved by extrapolation. In this region the detection of very small optical signals together with the need to reject artifacts requires the averaging of the data over several seconds, and this procedure can affect the response to rapid changes in saturation. In a study of six different models of pulse oximeter, it was found that some instruments continued to show nearly normal saturation when the true saturation was down to 40–70%, and some routinely failed to indicate any saturation at all during the critical period of falling saturation. Response times tend to be longer for desaturation than for increasing saturation, perhaps as a result of an increase in finger and ear blood flow when hypoxic blood reaches the tissue. Other studies have explored the range of saturation from 95.5% down to 56% and have found good correlation with arterial blood samples. Studies of oxygen saturation in volunteers submitted to hypoxic gas mixtures have shown a number of differences between the various instruments available; however, improved models are continually appearing. The arterial oxygen saturation is usually displayed digitally with the provision of an audible tone accompanying each pulse so that the pitch falls as saturation falls. The magnitude of the pulse waveform is indicated either by a bar graph or else by display of the pulse waveform; however, in some instruments this method of waveform presentation can be rather misleading because decreases in the signal produced, e.g. by vasoconstriction, are compensated by an increase in gain of the amplifier.

The pulse oximeter is designed to be insensitive to changes in hemodynamics, although situations in which the pulse is diminished, such as in peripheral vascular disease, hypothermia, extreme hypotension, or vasoconstriction, may produce too weak a signal. However, from Lawson and his colleagues' study[60] it appears that a pulse oximeter is able to estimate saturation even in states of severely reduced peripheral blood flow. They found that when the arm was progressively occluded using a blood pressure cuff the flow rate, which was measured with a laser Doppler flow probe, decreased to approximately 9% of the control value before the pulse oximeter (Nellcor N-100) was unable to estimate the saturation. When the cuff was released from total occlusion, the pulse oximeter regained a measured pulse and an estimation of saturation at only 4% of the original blood flow. No attempt was made in that study[60] to compare the saturations obtained with an independent method, but another study addressed the problem that venous congestion may cause low readings of saturation. In this study on the effect of venous congestion,[61] the average value of $S_{a}O_2$ measured by pulse oximetry in the finger tip and finger base was found to be between 1.5% and 7.8% lower than when the digit was elevated. This effect is thought to be a result of venous pulsations effected through shunting of arterial blood through open arteriovenous anastomoses in the cutaneous circulation. Desaturation and resaturation are best determined by centrally placed sensors, e.g. tongue, cheek, or ear, in preference to fingers or toes. Movement artifacts are a nuisance but only a problem in nonanesthetized patients. The Nellcor N-200 model has the facility to synchronize the determinations of arterial saturation with the patient's ECG and thus is particularly useful for monitoring awake patients.

Forms of hemoglobin such as methemoglobin (metHb) and carboxyhemoglobin (COHb) cannot be distinguished from oxyhemoglobin by pulse oximetry. Because COHb is red it is "seen" by the pulse oximeter as oxyhemoglobin, therefore in the presence of COHb the oximeter reads the sum of the oxyhemoglobin and the COHb. In heavy smokers, in whom 10% of hemoglobin may be combined with CO as COHb, hemoglobin saturation may be overestimated by 2–3% when in fact only 90% of the available hemoglobin is saturated. On the other hand, transcutaneous PO_2 falls as COHb increases. The effective acute "anemia" of CO poisoning does not alter the oximeter reading and thus the instrument does not alert the clinician to the low arterial oxygen content under these circumstances. It appears that a pulse oximeter "sees" COHb as 90% oxyhemoglobin and 10% reduced Hb.

Methemoglobinemia has a more complex effect because the ability of the pulse oximeter to register desaturation is impaired and no indication of the functional hemoglobin is given. Methemoglobin is seen as a large absorbance in both the red and IR wavelengths of the pulse oximeter. The large pulsatile absorbance seen in both these wavelengths forces the ratio of the added pulse absorbance toward unity, which is interpreted by the pulse oximeter as a saturation of 85% oxyhemoglobin and 15% reduced Hb. Therefore, in the presence of significant amounts of metHb the pulse oximeter will tend toward a reading of 85% regardless of the saturation. The Radiometer "OXImeter" has provision for adjusting the readout from the instrument according to known amounts of abnormal forms of hemoglobin, determined separately from the Radiometer OSM3 hemoximeter. This approach has obvious value when dealing with victims of smoke inhalation, in whom high concentration of COHb are common.

Dyes that absorb light in the region of 660 nm, such as indocyanine green, indigo carmine, and especially methylene blue, may also cause sudden false low readings for a time after intravenous injection. The time-course for these changes is about 1–2 circulation times and recovery to baseline values occurs within 3 min of bolus dye injection in young healthy subjects breathing room air.

Artifacts may result from interference from radiofrequency diathermy apparatus, light of high intensity, and some IR heat lamps. Because the photodetector can measure weak signals, oximeters are designed to reject ambient light. When the intensity of ambient light is high the photodetector cannot sense light transmitted through tissue or calculate $S_{a}O_2$. Certain operating room lights may cause interference and cause erroneous high saturation readings. It is recommended that the probe be shielded by wrapping it in a thin opaque metal foil. One study considered the effects of nail polishes of different colors; black, blue, and green nail polish lower pulse oximeter readings of $S_{a}O_2$. Blue and green produced greater decreases than purple and red; black produced an intermediate decrease. Nail polish should therefore be routinely removed before pulse oximetry. The probe should always be carefully placed so that no undue pressure or torque is applied and careful inspection made of both site of application and probe. Other problems appear to be few, such as minor burns, abrasions and a suntanning effect.

Clinical applications of pulse oximetry

Pulse oximetry is now a valuable routine monitor in anesthesia and is especially valuable for patients with skin pigmentation and those with poor physical status with a low arterial oxygen tension, i.e. below 13 kPa (95 mmHg). Pulse oximetry is also of value for patients undergoing regional anesthesia, sedation, endoscopies, and procedures of brief duration as severe hypoxemia is far commoner than hitherto realized. The clinical use of pulse oximetry has led to many interesting observations such as the high incidence of hypoxemia during manual ventilation (compared with ventilator-controlled or spontaneous ventilation) and in patients in the lithotomy position. It also reveals the hypoxemia of inadvertent bronchial intubation. Although pulse oximetry provides rapid noninvasive evaluation of total blood oxygenation and displays information about pulse amplitude, conclusions that pulse oximeters monitor tissue perfusion and tissue oxygen delivery must be approached with caution.

Pulse oximetry is a useful monitor in the preparation of patients before anesthesia (e.g. while intravascular lines are being inserted), during one-lung ventilation, and as a valuable tool during surgical manipulation of the pulmonary artery, such as banding or clamping where pulmonary artery flow is reduced. It is a valuable monitor of oxygenation in the recovery room, intensive care unit, and ward; also during transfer of patients. Hypoxemia [defined as an $S_{a}O_2$ of 90% or less (= $P_{a}O_2$ of 7.7 kPa or 58 mmHg)] occurred in 35% and severe hypoxemia [defined as an $S_{a}O_2$ of 85% or less (= $P_{a}O_2$ of 6.7 kPa or 50 mmHg)] occurred in 12% of ASA class 1 or 2 patients breathing room air during their transfer from the operating room to the recovery room.[62] Postoperative hypoxemia did not correlate with anesthetic agent, age, duration of anesthesia, or level of consciousness. Smith and Crul[63] have demonstrated early profound decreases in $S_{a}O_2$ in healthy patients during transfer to the recovery room, in spite of the administration of 100% O_2 for 5 min at the end of the anesthetic. They suggest that ventilation–perfusion mismatch is most likely to be responsible; no patient given 2 L min^{-1} by nasopharyngeal catheter during transport had an $S_{a}O_2$ below 90%. Children are potentially more susceptible than adults to airway closure and disturbances in pulmonary gas exchange. In children, 21% oxygen (room air) is a potentially hypoxic mixture in the early recovery period. Substantial desaturation has been observed in patients receiving either traditional parenteral analgesia or epidural morphine following cesarean section. Because oxygen is innocuous under most circumstances, the safe course is to provide air enriched with oxygen during postoperative transfer and in the early recovery period. In the intensive care unit, pulse oximetry is also valuable as an online noninvasive indicator of the benefits or otherwise of therapy; it is a particularly useful monitor during chest physiotherapy and suctioning procedures.

A Danish group[64,65] published a large, multicenter, prospective controlled study of the value of pulse oximetry on the outcome of anesthetic care. Of the participating anesthesiologists, 80% felt more secure with pulse oximetry. Despite the enormous effort involved and over 20 000 patients studied, the sample was too small to conclude that pulse oximetry had any effect on patient outcome. However, intuitively it is believed that brief exposure to mild levels of hypoxemia may be harmful to severely ill patients, whereas healthy patients probably tolerate longer periods of more severe hypoxia. The technology provides for early warning and enables earlier intervention; additional time is available to resolve a problem.[66]

TEMPERATURE

Temperature measurement is useful for the prevention of hypothermia during long operations and as a monitor of the methods used to keep patients warm. In some institutions a single disposable esophageal probe, which incorporates a unipolar ECG, a thermistor, and a hollow tube connecting to a monaural stethoscope, is routine for every case. The nasopharynx is another popular site for temperature measurement. For major operations, and especially in children, the use of a second more peripheral temperature sensor (e.g. on a digit) is used to allow measurement of the temperature gradient and hence provides an index of cardiac output and peripheral perfusion. In 1994 the *ASA Standards for Postoperative Care* (1988) were supplemented by a new reference to the monitoring of temperature. The relevant section now reads "particular attention should be given to monitoring oxygenation, ventilation, circulation and temperature."

INTRACRANIAL PRESSURE

The measurement of intracranial pressure (ICP) is a useful adjunct to the management of patients with neurological disease in the intensive care unit. ICP measurement is valuable in cases of trauma for the indication of the onset of cerebral edema or hemorrhage. The most accurate method relies on ventricular puncture. Extradural sensors are less reliable but may be left *in situ* for longer periods. The technique demands electronic systems for the best results. Absolute sterility and an aseptic technique are vital. Monitoring of the EEG or its derivatives, and the problem of monitoring the depth of anesthesia, is discussed in Chapter 32.

COMPUTER-ASSISTED MONITORING

The advent of the microprocessor has resulted in the automation of clinical monitoring and the collection of many data that can be used as a permanent record and for the purposes of audit and research. However, early enthusiasm often produced instruments that were difficult to use and presented far too much information without much attempt to present it in order of priority. A common difficulty is the requirement for the anesthesiologist to have to scroll through pages of menus on the screen in order to get the information sought. Automatically generated records of the anesthetic process are now being introduced.[67]

CONCLUSIONS

Continuous observation of anesthetized patients has been considered vital for patient safety since the earliest days of anesthesia. There are now sufficient reports that indicate that dedicated monitoring instruments can benefit the patient as an extension of the anesthesiologist's human senses. Indeed, in several countries standards of monitoring have now been laid down by professional anesthetic organizations or even by law. To a great extent this has come about because of the escalating rise in medical malpractice insurance premiums. Monitoring instruments are not a substitute for careful clinical observation. However, good monitoring benefits not only the patient by constant and close presentation of many vital signs and other parameters but also the anesthesiologist by freeing him or her from many manual tasks, thus helping to relieve fatigue and tension and so concentrating attention better on the overall care of the patient. Capnography and pulse oximetry can noninvasively provide continuous information that would not otherwise be available and the use of reliable, audible, and visual alarms increases patient safety, particularly when access is restricted or room lighting is reduced. There is a strong analogy between the anesthesiologist and the civil airline pilot. Both must rely heavily on instruments for information and the fallacies of human error are well known to both professions. In some operations the anesthesiologist cannot get near to the patient – rather like flying in cloud; however, with the use of adequate instruments (monitors) everything should be perfectly safe. Cooper and his colleagues[29,30] have shown that human error, rather than equipment failure, is overwhelmingly responsible for anesthetic mishaps. Attention must nevertheless be directed toward combining the various monitors used in anesthesia into a common system to simplify and reduce the number of controls and switches. It is imperative that sufficient reliable equipment is purchased and great attention must paid to the training of anesthesiologists in its use and to proper maintenance and checking. There is a powerful argument for the use of routine capnography and pulse oximetry in all patients, in addition to traditional monitors such as the ECG, blood pressure, etc., which may be expected to make a considerable contribution to patient safety.

REFERENCES

1. Eger EI II, Epstein RM. Hazards of anesthesia equipment. *Anesthesiology* 1964; **25:** 490–504.
2. Rendell-Baker L. Problems with anesthetic gas machines and their solutions. In: Rendell-Baker (ed.). Problems with Anesthetic and Respiratory Equipment. *Int Anesthesiol Clin* 1982; **20** (3): 1–82.
3. Schreiber P. *Anaesthesia Equipment Performance, Classification and Safety* Berlin: Springer-Verlag, 1972.
4. Schreiber P. *Safety Guidelines for Anesthesia Systems.* Philadelphia: The North American Dräger Company, 1985.
5. Cooper JB, Newbower RS, Kitz RJ. An analysis of major errors and equipment failures in anesthesia management: considerations for prevention and detection. *Anesthesiology* 1984; **60:** 34–42.
6. Interim report available from study of accidental breathing system disconnections. *Med Devices Bull* 1984; **2:** 1–2.
7. Spurring PW, Small LFG. Breathing system disconnexions and misconnexions. A review of some common causes and some suggestions for safety. *Anaesthesia* 1983; **38:** 683–8.
8. Health Equipment Information, No. 150. *Evaluation of Breathing attachments for Anaesthetic Apparatus to BS 3849.* London: Department of Health and Social Security, 1965.
9. Wood MD. Monitoring equipment and loss reduction: an insurer's view. In: Gravenstein JS, Holtzer JF (eds). *Safety and Cost Containment in Anesthesia.* London: Butterworth, 1988: 47–54.
10. *Checklist for Anaesthetic Apparatus – 2.* London: Association of Anaesthetists of Great Britain and Ireland, 1997.
11. International Standards for a Safe Practice of Anaesthesia. *Eur J Anaesthesiol* 1993; **10** (Suppl. 7): 12–15.
12. Cheney FW. ASA closed claims study. *Am Soc Anesthesiol Newsletter* 1989; **53** (11): 8–9.
13. Caplan RA, Posner KL, Ward RJ, Cheney FW. Adverse respiratory events in anesthesia: a closed claims analysis. *Anesthesiology* 1990; **72:** 828–33.
14. Birmingham PK, Cheney FW, Ward RJ. Esophageal intubation. A review of detection techniques. *Anesth Analg* 1986; **65:** 886–91.
15. Caplan RA, Ward RJ, Posner KL, Cheney FW. Unexpected cardiac arrest during spinal anesthesia: a closed claims analysis of predisposing factors. *Anesthesiology* 1988; **68:** 5–11.
16. Caplan RA, Posner KL, Ward RJ, Cheney FW. Peer review agreement for major anesthetic mishaps. *Qual Rev Bull* 1989; **14:** 363–8.
17. Cheney FW, Posner KL, Caplan RA, Ward RJ. Standard of care and anesthesia liability. *J Am Med Assoc* 1989; **261**: 1599–603.
18. Dull DL, Tinker JH, Caplan RA, Ward FW. ASA closed claims study: can pulse oximetry and capnography prevent anesthesia mishaps? *Anesth Analg* 1989; **68:** S74.
19. Committee of the Health Council of The Netherlands. *Advisory Report on Anaesthesiology,* Part I: *Recent Developments in Anaesthesiology*, 1978.
20. American Society of Anesthesiologists. Standards of basic intraoperative monitoring. *Am Soc Anesthesiol Newsletter* 1986; **50:** 9.
21. Eichhorn JH, Cooper JB, Cullen DJ, *et al.* Standards of patient monitoring during anesthesia at Harvard Medical School. *J Am Med Assoc* 1986; **256:** 1017–20.
22. Moss E. New Jersey continues as a center of anesthesia regulatory activity. *Anesth Patient Safety Found Newsletter* 1990; **5** (1): 4–5.
23. Moss E. Insurance premiums cut in New Jersey. *Anesth Patient Safety Found Newsletter* 1990; **5** (1): 1–2.
24. Sykes MK. Essential monitoring. *Br J Anaesth* 1987; **59:** 901–12.
25. Association of Anaesthetists of Great Britain and Ireland. *Recommendations for Standards of Monitoring during Anaesthesia and Recovery, – 1994,* rev. edn. London: Association of Anaesthetists of Great Britain and Ireland, 1994.
26. Buck N, Devlin H, Lunn JN. *The Report of A Confidential Enquiry into Perioperative Deaths.* London: The Nuffield Provincial Hospitals Trust, 1987.
27. Hedley-Whyte J. Monitoring and alarms – philosophy and practice. In: Dinnick OP, Thompson PW (eds). Some Aspects of Anaesthetic Safety. *Baillière's Clin Anaesthesiol* 1988; **2:** 379–89.
28. Westenskow DR, Orr JA, Simon FH, *et al.* Intelligent alarms reduce anesthesiologist's response time to critical faults. *Anesthesiology* 1992; **77:** 1074–9.
29. Cooper JB, Newbower RS, Kitz RJ. An analysis of major errors and equipment failures in anesthesia management: considerations for prevention and detection. *Anesthesiology* 1984; **60:** 34–42.
30. Cooper JB, Newbower RS, Long CD, McPeek B. Preventable anesthesia mishaps: a study of human factors. *Anesthesiology* 1978; **49:** 399–406.
31. Gaba DM, Maxwell M, DeAanda A. Anesthesia mishaps: breaking the chain of accident evolution. *Anesthesiology* 1987; **66:** 670–6.
32. Shepherd JT. *Physiology of the Circulation in Human Limbs in Health and Disease.* Philadelphia: Saunders, 1963: 9–17.
33. Nijboer JA, Dorias JC. Comparison of plethysmograms taken from finger and pinna during anaesthesia. *Br J Anaesth* 1985; **57:** 531–4.
34. Imholz BPM, van Montfrans GA, Settels JJ, *et al.* Continuous non-invasive blood pressure monitoring: reliability of the Finapres device during the Valsalva manouvre. *Cardiovasc Res* 1988; **22:** 390–7.
35. Sykes MK. Central venous pressure as a guide to the adequacy of transfusion. *Ann R Coll Surg Engl* 1963; **33:** 185.
36. Adams AP, Hahn CEW. *Principles and Practice of Blood Gas Analysis,* 2nd edn. London: Churchill Livingstone, 1982.
37. Larson CP Jr, Vender J, Seiver A. Multisite evaluation of a continuous intraarterial blood gas monitoring system. *Anesthesiology* 1994; **81:** 543–52.
38. Zollinger A, Spahn DR, Singer T, *et al.* Accuracy and clinical performance of a continuous intra-arterial blood-gas monitoring system during thoracoscopic surgery. *Br J Anaesth* 1997; **79:** 47–52.
39. Adams AP. Blood-gases and acid–base balance. In: Nimmo WS, Rowbotham DJ, Smith G (eds). *Anaesthesia,* 2nd edn. Oxford: Blackwell Scientific Publications, 1994, 291–307.
40. Venkatesh B, Clutton-Brock TH, Hendry SP. Evaluation of the Paratrend 7 intravascular blood gas monitor during cardiac surgery: comparison with the C4000 in line blood gas monitor during cardiopulmonary bypass. *J Cardiothorac Vasc Anaesth* 1995; **9:** 412–19.
41. Abraham E, Gallagher TJ, Fink S. Clinical evaluation of a multi-parameter intra-arterial blood-gas sensor. *Intensive Care Med* 1996; 22: 507–513.
42. Hinds CJ, Watson D. ABC of intensive care. Circulatory support. *Br Med J* 1999; **318:** 1749–52.
43. Iijima T, Aoyagi T, Iwao Y, *et al.* Cardiac output and circulating blood volume analysis by pulse dye-densitometry. *J Clin Monitoring* 1997; 13: 81–9.
44. Imai T, Takahashi K, Fukura H, Morishita Y. Measurement of cardiac output by pulse dye densitometry using indocyanine green; a comparison with the thermodilution method. *Anesthesiology* 1997; **87:** 816–22.
45. Iijima T, Iwao Y, Sankawa H. Circulating blood volume measured by pulse dye-densitometry: comparison with 131I-HAS analysis. *Anesthesiology* 1998; **89:** 1329–35.
46. Haruna M, Kumon K, Yahagi N, *et al.* Blood volume measurement at the bedside using ICG pulse spectrophotometry. *Anesthesiology* 1998; **89:** 1322–8.
47. Malagon I, Karalliedde L, Adams AP. Non invasive cardiac output measurement by suprasternal Doppler: its clinical applications. *Med Sci Monitoring* 1996; **2:** 514–19.
48. Mark JB, Steinbrook RA, Gugino LD, *et al.* Continuous noninvasive monitoring of cardiac output with esophageal Doppler ultrasound during cardiac surgery. *Anesth Analg* 1986; **65:** 1013–20.
49. Singer M, Clarke D, Bennett D. Continuous hemodynamic monitoring by esophageal Doppler. *Crit Care Med* 1989; **17:** 447–52.
50. Adams AP, Vickers MDA, Munroe JP, Parker CW. Dry displacement gas meters. *Br J Anaesth* 1967; 39: 174–83.
51. Smalhout B, Kalenda Z. *An Atlas of Capnography,* 2nd edn. The Netherlands: Kerckebosch, Zeist, 1981.
52. Swedlow DB. Capnometry and capnography: the anesthesia early disaster warning system. In: Katz, RL (ed.). *Semin Anesth* 1986; **5:** 194–205.
53. Adams AP. Capnography and pulse oximetry. In: Atkinson RS, Adams AP (eds). *Recent Advances in Anaesthesia and Analgesia,* 16th edn. London: Churchill Livingstone, 1989: 155–75.
54. O'Flaherty D, Adams AP. The end-tidal carbon dioxide detector. *Anaesthesia* 1990; **45:** 653–5.

55. Sprung J, Siker D, Koch R, Beaudin P. Disruption of an infra-red capnograph monitor by hand-held radio receivers. *Anesthesiology* 1995; **83:** 1352.
56. From RP, Scamman FL. Ventilatory frequency influences accuracy of end-tidal CO_2 measurements: analysis of seven capnometers. *Anesth Analg* 1988; **67:** 884–6.
57. Møllgaard K. Acoustic gas measurement. *Biol Instrum Technol* 1989; **23:** 495–7.
58. Yelderman M, New W Jr. Evaluation of pulse oximetry. *Anesthesiology* 1983; **59:** 349–52.
59. Payne J P, Severinghaus JW. *Pulse Oximetry.* London: Springer-Verlag, 1986.
60. Lawson D, Norley I, Korbon G, *et al.* Blood flow limits and pulse oximeter signal detection. *Anesthesiology* 1987; **67:** 599–603.
61. Kim J-M, Arakawa K, Benson KT, Fox DK. Pulse oximetry and circulatory kinetics associated with pulse volume amplitude measured by photoelectric plethysmography. *Anesth Analg* 1986; **65:** 1333–9.
62. Hanning CD. "He looks a little blue down this end." Monitoring oxygenation during anaesthesia. *Br J Anaesth* 1985; **57:** 359–60.
63. Smith DC, Crul J. Early postoperative hypoxaemia during transport. *Br J Anaesth* 1988; **61:** 625–7.
64. Moller JT, Pedersen T, Rasmussen LS, *et al.* Randomized evaluation of pulse oximetry in 20802 patients. I. Design, demography, pulse oximetry failure rate and overall complication rate. *Anesthesiology* 1993; **78:** 436–44.
65. Moller JT, Johannessen NW, Espersen K, *et al.* Randomized evaluation of pulse oximetry in 20802 patients. II. Perioperative events and postoperative complications. *Anesthesiology* 1993; 7**8:** 445–53.
66. Orkin FK, Cohen MM, Duncan PG. The quest for meaningful outcomes. *Anesthesiology* 1993; 7**8:** 417–22.
67. De Mello WF, Adams AP. Record keeping in anaesthesia. In: Adams AP, Cashman JC (eds). *Recent Advances in Anaesthesia and Analgesia,* 19th edn. London: Churchill Livingstone, 1995: 17–31.

28

Principles of airway management

BRIAN J POLLARD AND MARTIN L NORTON

Management of the airway is central to the practice of anesthesia. It is not simply confined to proficiency with techniques for intubation of the trachea, but encompasses the whole range of airway manipulations that may be required during the course of anesthesia. Airway control is also central to other spheres of the anesthesiologist's work, e.g. in the critical care unit.

In order to understand airway management fully, the anesthesiologist must be fully conversant with the anatomy of the region and its variants, with its innervation, its possible pathological conditions, and its physiology, and with the consequences and complications of airway maneuvers. The anesthesiologist must have the ability to recognize those patients who may present with a difficult airway and must be able to formulate a plan of action to deal with any such problem.

The history of airway control and the importance of breathing for the maintenance of life dates back many thousands of years (Genesis; Second Kings, iv, 34–35). Tracheal insufflation in animals was first described in the 1600s, although the development of tracheal intubation as we know it today dates from about 1900. The history can be found in a number of published texts.[1]

THE AIRWAY

The airway commences at the nose or mouth and extends to the terminal bronchioles. For the purposes of this chapter, however, only the upper airway will be considered. This consists of the nose, mouth, pharynx, larynx, trachea, and main bronchi.

The nose

This may be divided anatomically into two parts: the external nose and the internal nasal cavity. The former has an upper bony part and a cartilaginous lower part. The nasal septum divides it into two. The nasal cavity is also separated into two parts by the backward continuation of the nasal septum. Each side has a roof, a floor, a medial wall (the nasal septum), and a lateral wall, and each side opens anteriorly by the external nares and posteriorly into the nasopharynx. The majority of adults have a deviated nasal septum, which may be important in the context of airway management because air flow through one side (nostril) will be better than through the other. The function of the nose is to warm, filter, and humidify incoming gases as well as to subserve the function of smell. There are three turbinates on each side that increase the mucosal surface area. Innervation comes mainly from the nasociliary and maxillary branches of the trigeminal nerve, with olfactory fibers derived directly from the first cranial nerve. Openings exist from the various ethmoid and maxillary air cells and the paranasal sinuses into the nasal cavity, and tears drain into the nose via the nasolacrimal duct.

The mouth

The mouth opens via the lips, and just within lie the gums and teeth with the cheeks at the sides. The upper boundary is the alveolar arch, the hard palate, and the soft palate, with the anterior two-thirds of the tongue forming the floor of the mouth. The hard palate separates the mouth below from the nasal cavity above. The mouth is opened by movement of the mandible, which pivots on the temporomandibular joints. These joints are unusual in that they permit movement in a number of different directions, namely rotation (mouth opening), sliding forwards and backwards (protrusion of the jaw), and sliding side to side (necessary for mastication of food). The tongue is almost entirely muscle and can be moved in all directions. Its bulk prevents direct vision of the larynx, which is why it has to be displaced or depressed in order to perform a direct laryngoscopy. Protrusion of the tongue is required in some assessments of airway patency and ease of access. The motor supply to the tongue is derived from the hypoglossal nerves (cranial nerve XII). Sensation on the anterior two-thirds of the tongue is from the facial nerves (cranial nerve VII), whereas sensation on the posterior one-third is supplied by the glossopharyngeal nerves (cranial nerve IX).

The pharynx

This wide fibromuscular tube joins the nasal cavity and oral cavity in the front to the larynx below (Fig. 28.1). The nasopharynx closes off during swallowing by elevation of the soft palate. The Eustachian tubes enter at the rear of the nasopharynx. The adenoids lie on the roof and posterior wall of the nasopharynx, and the tonsils lie one on each side of the pharynx between the pillars of the fauces. There are three muscles within the pharynx, termed the superior, middle, and inferior constrictors. These partially encircle the pharynx, being attached to the base of the skull above and to the mandible, hyoid bone, and cricoid cartilage, respectively, below. These are essential to the act of swallowing, in which food is pushed to the back of the mouth by the tongue and the bolus of food is propelled into the esophagus. It is prevented from entering the larynx by a complex mechanism, which includes closure of the sphincter system of the larynx, pulling the larynx upwards and forwards behind the base of the tongue. The epiglottis is used to guide the bolus of food

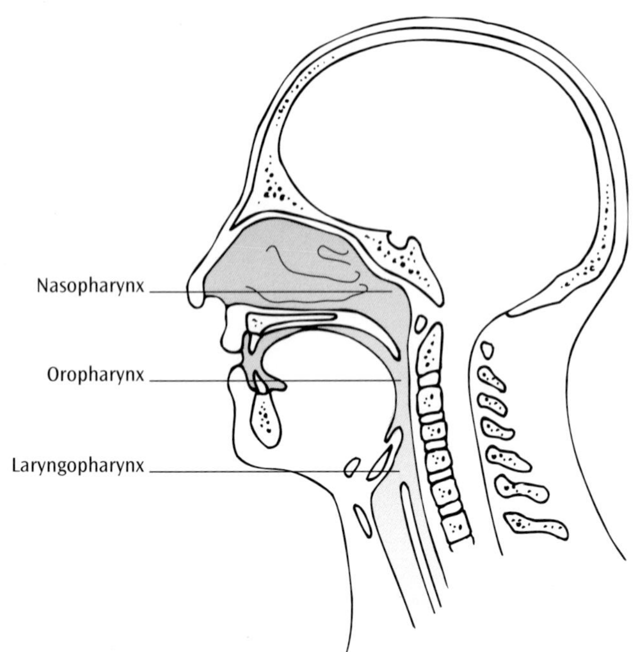

Figure 28.1 *Sagittal section of the pharynx. (Reproduced with permission from Hwang NC.* Fiberoptic Guided Tracheal Intubation. *Singapore: McGraw Hill, 1995.)*

away from the laryngeal entrance. Initiation of swallowing is under voluntary control, but the act of swallowing is an involuntary reflex.

The larynx

Every anesthesiologist should have a comprehensive knowledge and understanding of the larynx (Fig. 28.2). Partly for this reason, it is a common question in professional examinations in the specialty. The larynx subserves two main functions. First, it is a protective valve at the upper end of the trachea; second, it is the organ of speech. It lies at the level of the 4th to 6th cervical vertebrae and is composed of a framework of cartilages interconnected by muscles and ligaments. The cartilages can move in relation to each other. It is "slung" from the underside of the hyoid bone and can easily be palpated through the skin. It is covered superficially by the skin, deep fascia, and the thin strap muscles of the neck. The principal cartilages are the thyroid cartilage, the cricoid cartilage, and the two arytenoid cartilages, although there are a number of other small cartilaginous structures within the larynx.

The thyroid cartilage is often described as "shield shaped" and consists of two laminae that are joined in the midline. The cartilaginous protrusion known as the Adam's apple at the front of the neck is produced mainly by the thyroid cartilage. The cricoid cartilage lies immediately below the thyroid cartilage and is a complete cartilaginous ring. It articulates with the thyroid cartilage and the arytenoids. The arytenoid cartilages are pyramidal in shape, and one sits on each side of the upper lateral border of the cricoid. The vocal folds are attached to the anterior surfaces of the arytenoids. The posterior and lateral cricoarytenoid muscles are inserted onto the lateral sides of the arytenoids. The epiglottis is attached to the back of the thyroid cartilage on its lower side and to the back of the hyoid bone on its upper side. It projects backwards and upwards behind the base of the tongue, partially covering the inlet of the larynx.

The muscles of the larynx may be divided into two types: the external muscles and the internal muscles. There are a number of extrinsic muscles, including the sternothyroid and thyrohyoid muscles. From their position between the larynx and the surrounding structures, these are responsible for moving the larynx. The omohyoid elevates the hyoid, thereby raising the larynx. The intrinsic muscles include the cricoarytenoid muscles, the interarytenoid muscle, the thyroarytenoid muscle, and the cricothyroid muscle. Their role is to move the cartilages within the larynx. The results of these movements are principally to adduct, abduct, and adjust the tension in the vocal folds. The nerve supply to the larynx travels through the right and left superior and recurrent laryngeal nerves, all of which are branches of the vagus nerves. The nerves to the larynx pass very close to the thyroid gland and its vascular supply. These may be damaged during surgery to the anterior neck or involved in pathology of this region, e.g. tumors of the neck and thyroid gland. Damage to these nerves causes specific patterns of voice changes and may result in stridor.

The trachea

The trachea begins at the level of C6, where it is attached to the lower side of the cricoid cartilage. It is about 10 cm long in the adult and ends at the carina. The position of the carina alters with posture and respiration, but is usually regarded as being at about the T6 level on a chest radiograph. The diameter of the trachea depends on the physical stature of the patient, but a rule of thumb is that its diameter is similar to that of the patient's index finger. Its patency is maintained by a series of C-shaped cartilaginous rings. The anterior aspect of the trachea is covered with skin, pretracheal fascia, the thyroid isthmus, and the thin strap muscles of the neck until it passes behind the sternum. The carotid sheaths lie laterally, and the posterior relation is the esophagus. The innominate artery, the left common carotid artery, and the arch of the aorta cross the trachea within the thorax.

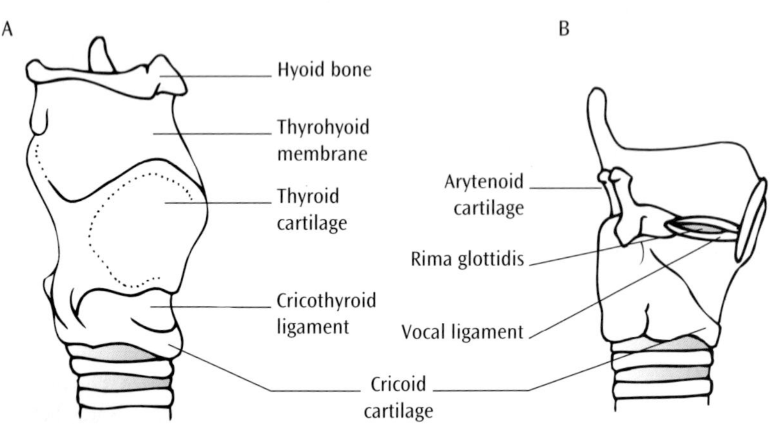

Figure 28.2 *The larynx. (A) Side view; (B) sagittal section. (Reproduced with permission from Hwang NC.* Fiberoptic Guided Tracheal Intubation. *Singapore: McGraw Hill, 1995.)*

The main bronchi

The trachea bifurcates at the carina to form the right and left main bronchi. The right main bronchus is shorter and wider than the left and descends at a steeper angle (about 25° to the vertical compared with 45° on the left side). The branch to the right upper lobe arises after about 2–3 cm. This more vertical angle of the right main bronchus is important in that inhaled foreign bodies are more likely to pass down the right side than the left.

MANAGEMENT OF THE AIRWAY

In the awake patient, the airway is maintained by the tone in the muscles of the neck, pharynx, and tongue. Loss of consciousness results in loss of this muscular tone and the tongue falls back to obstruct the airway. If the patient is supine, this obstruction can be complete and, without intervention, potentially fatal hypoxia will ensue. If the patient is in the lateral position, the tongue should fall to the side and the airway is not completely obstructed. This is a part of the rationale behind the use of the lateral position for resuscitation and during unconsciousness. The supine position is commonly used during anesthesia, and one of the anesthesiologist's fundamental roles is to maintain a patent airway at all times. Airway control is therefore one of the most basic skills taught to trainee anesthesiologists.

Basic principles

The simple expedient of elevating the chin and extending the head on the neck may be all that is required to produce a patent airway. Placing a small pillow behind the occiput and/or a roll under the shoulders may also help. Overextension of the neck may, however, make matters worse. If these simple movements are not effective, an upward thrust on the jaw should be attempted. This is effected by placing the fingers or thumbs behind the angle of the mandible and lifting it forwards. Anterior dislocation of the mandible may be the result, but this is not a problem as it can be returned to the normal position without difficulty. The mechanism by which this maneuver clears the airway is by displacing the tongue in an anterior direction and pulling it away from the posterior pharyngeal wall. It is tiring to maintain this position and so the use of an artificial airway is commonplace.

The face mask

The face mask is designed to fit the face of the ideal patient, and the usual pattern fits over the mouth and nose with the lower part between the lower lip and chin. There is a range of sizes. Many anesthesiologists believe that edentulous patients should be encouraged to continue to wear their dentures because a better fit can be obtained on the face with the mask than can be achieved if they are removed. This must be balanced against the risk of obstruction from the dentures themselves should they become displaced. The old style black rubber masks have been largely superseded by clear plastic disposable ones which are more pleasant for the patient. Furthermore, any secretions on the lips can be easily seen through the clear plastic variety. These masks can even be made to taste or smell sweet and pleasant for children and anxious patients.

The airway

The oral airway is a curved rigid plastic tube, which was originally described by Guedel. It is usually inserted into the mouth with the concavity of the curve pointing upwards and then rotated through 180° as it is advanced into the mouth. It may also be inserted directly with the concavity pointing downwards and the airway slid in over the tongue until the flange touches the lips. The timing of airway insertion is very important. It is generally inserted in order to relieve an obstruction. However, if the patient is too lightly anesthetized, coughing, breath-holding, and laryngospasm may result, leading to a further deterioration in airway control.

A nasal airway may be used instead of an oral airway. This is indicated for patients with fragile teeth, crowns, or bridges, or when an oral airway cannot be inserted. Nasal airways are better tolerated than oral airways at light levels of sedation and even in the awake patient. Mucosal damage is relatively common, and trauma to the posterior pharyngeal wall can result in the development of a pharyngeal abscess. Damage to the turbinates within the nose may occur and polyps have been avulsed, and these can block the tube. It is advisable to avoid using a nasal airway for patients or those with bleeding disorders or with a base-of-skull fracture.

The laryngeal mask

The laryngeal mask (LM) is a relatively new airway device that is inserted through the mouth and comes to lie at the back of the pharynx with its opening sitting anteriorly over the entrance to the larynx.[2,3] Inflation of its cuff then seals the airway around the laryngeal opening (Fig. 28.3). Air should be inserted into the cuff of the LM slowly to reduce the likelihood of coughing and the cuff must not be overinflated. Easy insertion requires the patient to be deeply anesthetized with a relaxed mouth and pharyngeal muscles. Propofol is the induction agent which currently provides the best conditions for insertion of the LM. There is a small failure rate of insertion, and if in doubt the LM should be deflated, removed, and reinserted. A bite block is recommended to prevent patients closing their teeth on the tube part of the LM. It is common practice to leave an LM in position until the patient is awake. The LM can be removed in the recovery room.

The LM has proved to be a very useful aid to tracheal intubation. The position of the LM over the larynx allows a smaller tube or a guide passed through the lumen of the LM tube to be very likely to enter the larynx. Some small adjustment of the position of the LM might

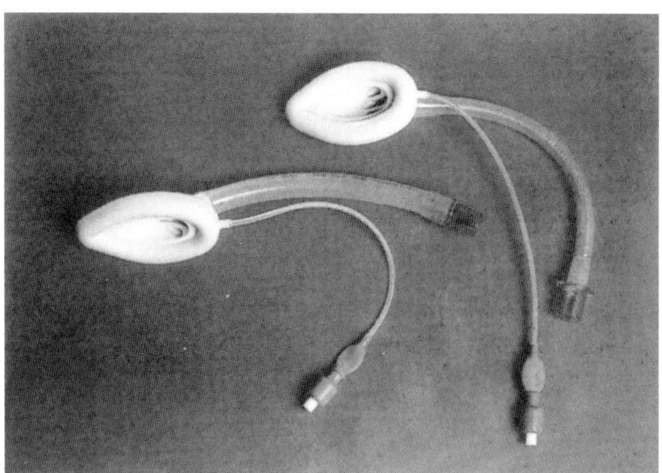

Figure 28.3 *Laryngeal masks. Two examples illustrating the design of the laryngeal mask. The cuff is inflated in the hypopharynx so the lumen is held over the laryngeal inlet. The lower mask is the original design for routine use when intubation is not indicated, but has proved life saving with failed intubation. The upper mask is a more recent refinement, with a flexible armored tube extension, which is more suited to head and neck surgery. (Reproduced with permission from Brown ACD. Anesthetic principles of airway management. In: Ferlito A (ed.).* Diseases of the Larynx. *London: Arnold, 2000.)*

be required in individual cases. The intubating laryngeal mask was developed to exploit this further and to permit more easy blind placement of a tracheal tube.[4] A smaller diameter tracheal tube may have to be used than would be ideal for the patient in order for it to pass through the lumen of the LM. This does not usually present a problem. The LM can also be used as an aid to fiberoptic-guided intubation by inserting the fiberoptic scope through the LM and directing it into the larynx and down the trachea.

Although originally developed as an airway aid for spontaneous ventilation, it is possible to perform positive-pressure ventilation through an LM. However, there is a serious risk of gastric dilation owing to anesthetic gases entering the esophagus, and this can lead to regurgitation of gastric contents. Care should therefore be taken to keep inflation pressures as low as possible, and patients must be selected carefully for this procedure. The LM does not offer the same protection to the airway as a tracheal tube.[5,6]

The LM has also found a place in the resuscitation room. With a little practice, many healthcare professionals find a laryngeal mask to be just as satisfactory as, and sometimes easier to use than, a tracheal tube in cardiac arrest management.

The Combitube

The Combitube is a device with two lumens and two inflatable cuffs (Fig. 28.4). It is easier to insert if a laryngoscope is used. One cuff will seal within the esophagus and the other within the pharynx. It is possible to isolate the esophagus from the trachea using this device, and any regurgitated gastric material is vented to the exterior through the esophageal lumen. It owes its origin to the earlier esophageal obturator devices that were designed for use by paramedical staff and others not skilled in tracheal intubation. It may be more traumatic than the LM. It does, however, allow higher inflation pressures to be used for controlled ventilation. This device has also found some use in the resuscitation situation.[7]

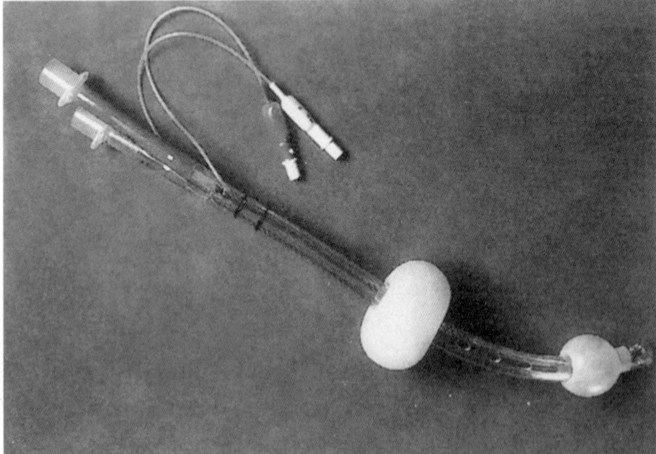

Figure 28.4 *The Combitube™. This device is a double-lumen tube with two cuffs. It is placed with its tip in the esophagus and the lower small cuff is inflated. The upper larger cuff is then inflated behind the base of the tongue. One tube lumen passes through the lower cuff and provides a route for regurgitation; the other lumen ends blindly above the lower cuff, but has side holes between the two cuffs that permit ventilation through the second lumen by virtue of the cuff seals above and below the hypopharynx. (Reproduced with permission from Brown ACD. Anesthetic principles of airway management. In: Ferlito A (ed.).* Diseases of the Larynx. *London: Arnold, 2000.)*

The tracheal tube

There are a number of indications for a tracheal tube, including the following situations:

- when the airway needs to be protected from the possible entry of foreign material, e.g. gastric contents, blood, irrigation fluid;
- to maintain the airway during operative procedures on the head and/or neck;
- when the patient is to be placed in the prone or sitting positions and sometimes the lateral position;
- in patients with airway abnormalities;
- for prolonged periods of airway control, e.g. the critical care unit;
- when repeated tracheal suction is required for secretion control;
- most intracranial, intrathoracic, and intra-abdominal operations.

Intubation of the trachea is unnecessary for many general anesthetics and carries with it a number of hazards – damage to the vocal folds probably being the most serious. The complications of tracheal intubation are listed in Table 28.1.

Orotracheal intubation is performed far more commonly than nasotracheal intubation. Indications for nasotracheal intubation include intraoral surgery and inability to open the mouth. Contraindications include nasal abnormalities or trauma, base-of-skull fracture, and a coagulopathy. A tube that is of a smaller diameter and longer than that which would be used for the oral route should be selected. A

Table 28.1 *Complications of tracheal intubation*

Damage to teeth, lips, tongue, gums, larynx
Perforation of pharynx, esophagus, trachea
Fracture or dislocation of the cervical spine
Endobronchial intubation
Esophageal intubation
Increased intracranial pressure
Increased intraocular pressure
Kinking or obstruction of tube
Hemorrhage, infection
Aspiration of gastric contents or foreign material
Fire from laser beam hitting tube
Bronchospasm
Accidental extubation
Hypoxia, hypercarbia, hypertension
Increased work of breathing

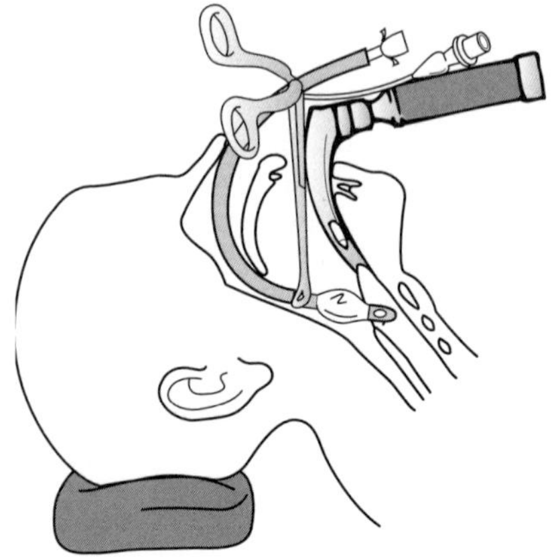

Figure 28.5 *Magill forceps are used to grasp and direct the endotracheal tube during nasotracheal intubation. (Reproduced with permission from Barash PG, Cullen BF, Stoetling RK (eds).* Clinical Anesthesia, *2nd edn. Philadelphia: J B Lippincott, 1992.)*

topical vasoconstrictor is recommended before passing a tube through the nose, and the nostril through which it is easier for the patient to breathe should be chosen if possible. Nasotracheal intubation is usually performed under direct vision using Magill forceps (Fig. 28.5), but may be performed "blind" by an experienced operator. The prior passage of a well-lubricated soft nasal airway to dilate the nasal passage is recommended by some anesthesiologists.

Severe nasal bleeding (from Kiesselbach's plexus in Little's area), amputation of the ethmoid or inferior turbinate, and impaction of foreign material into the orifice of the Eustachian tube have occurred. The reason for choosing the nasal route is the relatively gradual curve through which the tracheal tube passes to the glottic opening compared with the oral route.

Intubation of the trachea following the induction of general anesthesia is the normal procedure, although awake intubation under local analgesia is possible (see below). Following the induction dose of general anesthetic, airway control must be verified to ensure that ventilation is possible using a face mask before administering a muscle relaxant (with the exception of rapid-sequence induction). Following the muscle relaxant, intubation can take place once relaxation is adequate. If the anesthesiologist cannot guarantee that ventilation of the lungs is possible using a face mask, then a muscle relaxant must not be given.

Technique of tracheal intubation

Once the muscle relaxant has taken effect, the tube can be inserted into the trachea. The operating table or trolley on which the patient is lying should already have been adjusted so that it is at a comfortable height for the anesthesiologist. A pillow is placed beneath the patient's head to move it into the "sniffing" position. The patient's mouth is opened as wide as possible and the head extended on the neck (but not overextended). The laryngoscope blade is inserted into the right-hand side of the mouth and advanced using a lifting motion (Fig. 28.6). The tongue should slide to the left in the groove of the laryngoscope. The tip of the blade is advanced into the vallecula if using a standard curved (Macintosh) blade. If using a straight blade, the tip is advanced so as to elevate the epiglottis directly. The handle of the blade is then lifted upwards and forwards until the glottic opening is exposed (Fig. 28.7). Levering on the handle should be avoided because the upper incisor teeth may be damaged. Once the glottic opening can be seen, the tracheal tube is advanced through the vocal folds until the cuff lies beyond the vocal folds. The laryngoscope can then be carefully removed, taking care not to damage the teeth or withdraw the tube in the process.

The tracheal tube size should be carefully selected. For a man, an 8.5-mm tube is usually adequate, and a 7.5-mm tube is adequate for a woman. For a child, the correct formula should be consulted. The tube should be cut to length such that the connector is just beyond the teeth. If the tube is too long, migration of the tube tip can occur, resulting in endobronchial intubation (usually of the right side). The average man requires a tube cut to about 23 cm at the teeth, and the average woman about 21 cm at the teeth.

Once inserted, the position must be verified. Seeing the tube enter the trachea is important, but this must not be relied upon entirely. Auscultation of both sides of the chest should be performed to ensure that there is air entry to both sides. It is also advisable to listen over the stomach to ensure that no air is passing down the esophagus. The operator should also look for chest movements. None of these tests is 100% reliable, and so other tests should be performed. The presence of carbon dioxide in the exhaled gas from the tracheal tube is an essential test. Small detectors have been developed in the event that a properly calibrated capnograph is unavailable.[8] The presence of condensing water vapor in the lumen of the connecting tube is a useful sign, as is the return of gas into an expansible reservoir.[9]

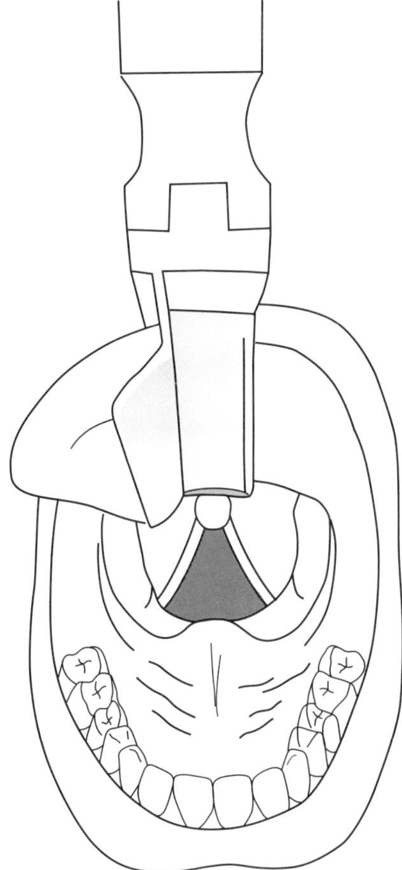

Figure 28.6 *The laryngoscope blade is inserted along the side of the tongue so that the tip is directed toward the epiglottis. The blade handle is then lifted upward and simulataneously rotated to the left side of the mouth. These movements are designed to lift the tongue and expose the glottic opening.*

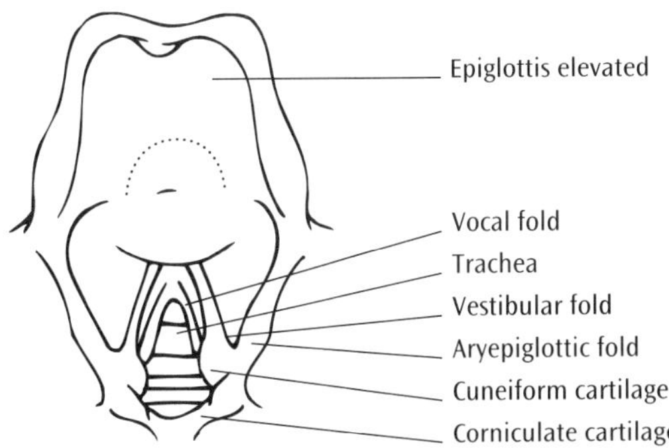

Figure 28.7 *The larynx as seen on direct laryngoscopy. (Reproduced with permission from Hwang NC.* Fiberoptic Guided Tracheal Intubation. *Singapore: McGraw Hill, 1995.)*

Endobronchial intubation

Endobronchial intubation may be required to control or isolate intrapulmonary bleeding or lower endobronchial bleeding, to permit one-lung anesthesia, and for pulmonary lavage in cases of alveolar proteinosis (Fig. 28.8). A number of double-lumen tubes have been described, of which the Robertshaw pattern is commonly used. A single-use version is available in a range of sizes. A double-lumen tube must be positioned

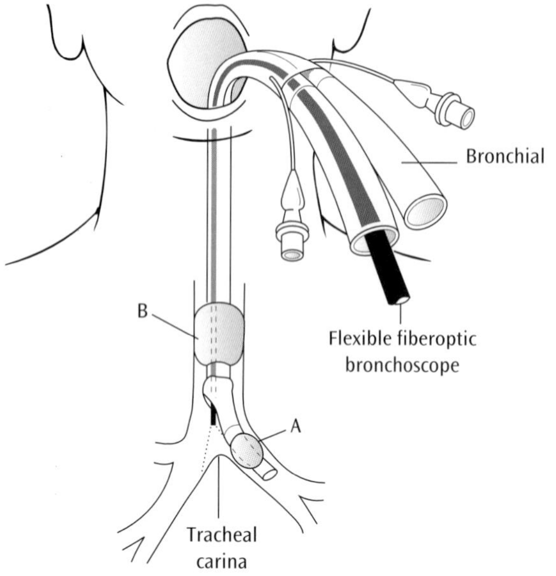

Figure 28.8 *Double-lumen endobronchial tubes permit one or both lungs to be ventilated. The left endobronchial tube is positioned with the distal cuff (A) in the left bronchus and the proximal cuff (B) in the trachea. A fiberoptic bronchoscope can be used to confirm proper tube placement. (Reproduced with permission from Barash PG, Cullen BF, Stoetling RK (eds).* Clinical Anesthesia, *2nd edn. Philadelphia: J B Lippincott, 1992.)*

with great care and accuracy to be used safely. A left-sided tube is used when possible owing to the proximity of the right upper lobe bronchus to the carina. It is essential to be certain that the two sides can be satisfactorily isolated before surgery begins. Many anesthesiologists prefer to check the position by direct vision using a fiberoptic bronchoscope. Dependency on visualization through the endoscope will obviate its use in the bleeding patient. In this circumstance, the Fogarty embolectomy catheter is of value if properly placed via a rigid bronchoscope. Vigorous suction may be required.

Tracheostomy

The airway may be managed following the direct insertion of a tube into the trachea, bypassing the mouth and larynx. This is usually a surgical procedure, although, presently, the percutaneous technique has found much favor, particularly on intensive care units and in out-of-hospital situations. Indications for a tracheostomy include major head and neck surgery, malignant tumors of the head or neck, long-term ventilation, and secretion control. Complications include hemorrhage, infection, damage to structures in the anterior neck, damage to the larynx, and erosion of major blood vessels.

PHYSIOLOGIC RESPONSES TO TRACHEAL INTUBATION

A number of responses to tracheal intubation occur, including hypertension, tachycardia, raised intraocular pressure, and raised intracranial pressure.[10] The magnitude of these responses depends in some part on the individual patient, but it may also be influenced by the depth of anesthesia and the presence or absence of other adjuvant drugs, e.g. analgesics. Fentanyl and alfentanil are effective in attenuating the hypertension and tachycardia associated with laryngoscopy and intubation and are often used for this purpose.[11] Intravenous lidocaine (lignocaine),[12] esmolol,[13] sodium nitroprusside,[14] and glyceryl trinitrate[15] may also be effective. The cardiovascular responses may have serious consequences, including myocardial ischemia, cerebrovascular hemorrhage, and cardiac arrest.

The rises in intracranial pressure with laryngoscopy and intubation are not usually significant unless a raised intracranial pressure is already present or intracranial compliance is severely impaired. Similarly, the rises in intraocular pressure are of little consequence unless the patient already has a pathologically high pressure or an open eye injury.

STARVATION PERIOD

When the patient is anesthetized, the airway protective reflexes are lost. Any foreign material gaining access to the pharynx can then pass down the larynx and enter the airways. This material might include blood, tooth particles, irrigation fluids from trauma or surgery, upper airway secretions, or gastric contents. It is important to prevent access of foreign material to the lower airway, and this is often achieved by the use of a tracheal tube. There are at-risk times when a tracheal tube is not within the airway, i.e. in the time between the onset of anesthesia and isolation of the airway or when reflexes are obtunded at recovery.

The substances that cause most damage to the lower airway are gastric acid and gastric contents. It is, therefore, essential to prevent aspiration of gastric contents. Vomiting can occur at induction and during recovery. The most dangerous, however, is probably the "silent regurgitation," which can take place at almost any time. Some patients are at a greater risk of regurgitation than are others. These include those patients with known gastroesophageal reflux, pre-existing hiatus hernia, and obesity. Particular precautions need to be taken for these patients with respect to isolating the airway, in particular the use of the rapid-sequence induction technique (see below).

Minimizing the risk by trying to ensure that the stomach is empty is important, and the universally accepted rule is that there should have been no food intake for the previous 6 h at a minimum. This equates to starvation from midnight for operations in the morning, although patients having surgery in the afternoon are permitted a light, very early breakfast. This rule used to apply to fluids also, but evidence has suggested that clear fluids (water or dilute juice but not milky drinks) are cleared from the stomach fairly quickly, assuming no gastric outlet pathology.[16] Reasonable intake of clear fluids is permitted up to 2 h before surgery in many institutions. The patient's normal routine medications should be taken together with a sip of water.

In patients at risk, the use of agents to reduce gastric acidity and resting volume, and possibly promote gastric emptying, has been recommended. Administration of 30 mL of 0.3 M sodium citrate will rapidly neutralize much of the gastric acid and raise the pH. Preoperative administration of a histamine H_2 blocker (e.g. ranitidine) has achieved general acceptance in a number of countries.[17] Metoclopramide has been used in an attempt to promote gastric emptying, but its efficacy is not guaranteed. Physical emptying of the stomach with a wide-bore tube or inducing vomiting have been used in the past, but are not currently recommended except in unusual circumstances.

Patients with particular needs, such as the frail elderly patient or the neonate, constitute a special case and prolonged starvation is unwise. A preoperative intravenous infusion may be necessary together with careful timing of the surgery.

Figure 28.9 *The ASA difficult airway algorithm. This is a useful consensus attempt to offer guidance to a rational sequence of management techniques for dealing with a difficult airway. It is not a protocol, but it helps to establish a sequence of care to be used by anesthesiologists.(Reproduced from* Anesthesiology *1993;* **78:** *597–602, with the permission of Lippincott-Raven.)*

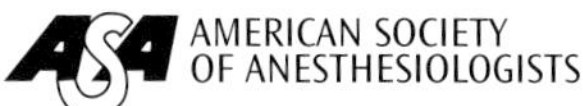

DIFFICULT AIRWAY ALGORITHM

1. Assess the likelihood and clinical impact of basic management problems:

A. Difficult Intubation
B. Difficult Ventilation
C. Difficulty with Patient Cooperation or Consent

2. Consider the relative merits and feasibility of basic management choices:

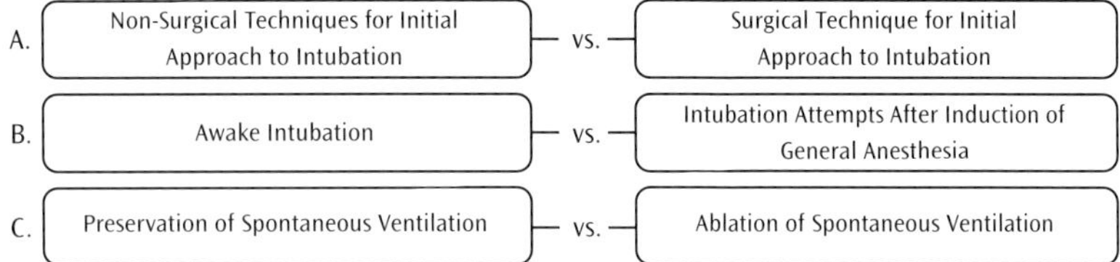

3. Develop primary and alternative strategies:

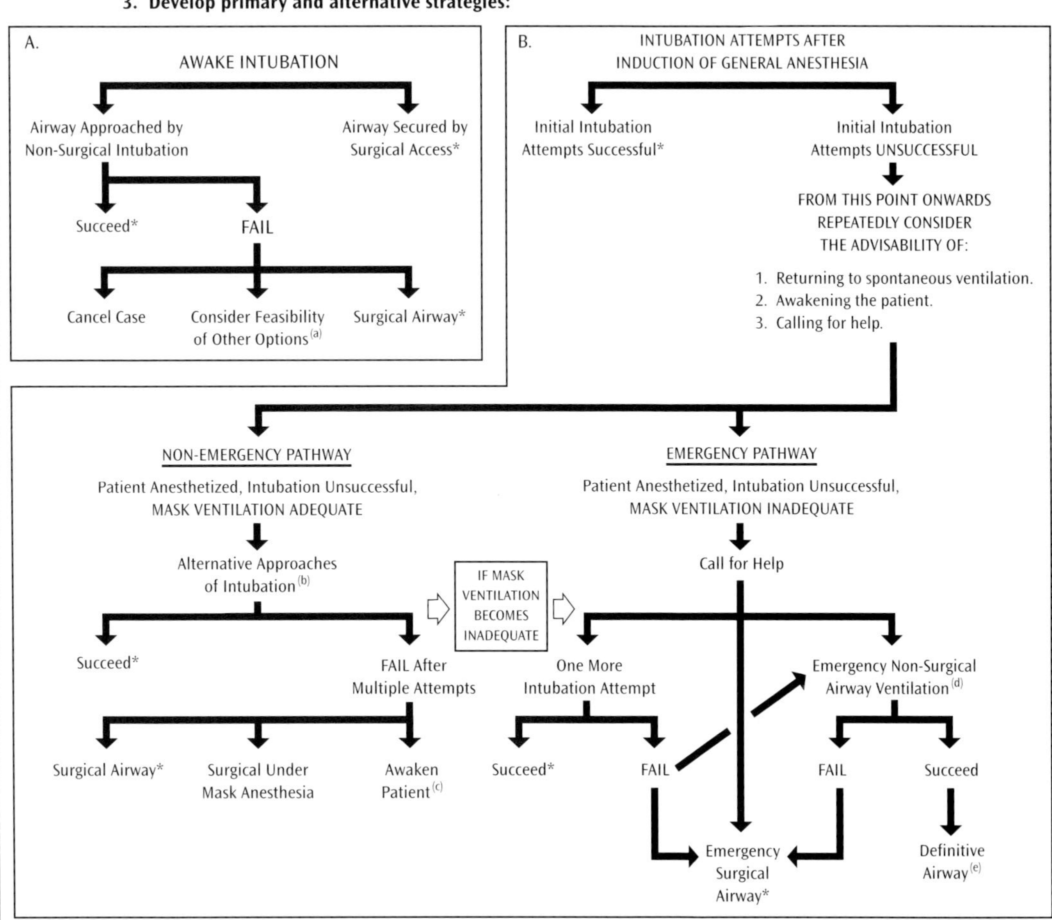

* CONFIRM INTUBATION WITH EXHALED CO_2

(a) Other options include (but are not limited to): surgery under mask anesthesia, surgery under local anesthesia infiltration or regional nerve blockade, or intubation attempts after induction of general anesthesia.

(b) Alternative approaches to difficult intubation include (but are not limited to): use of different laryngoscope blades, awake intubation, blind oral or nasal intubation, fiberoptic intubation, intubating stylet or tube changer, light wand, retrograde intubation, and surgical airway access.

(c) See awake intubation.

(d) Options for emergency non-surgical airway ventilation include (but are not limited to): transtracheal jet ventilation, laryngeal mask ventilation, or esophageal–tracheal Combitube ventilation.

(e) Options for establishing a definitive airway include (but are not limited to): returning to awake state with spontaneous ventilation, tracheotomy, or endotracheal intubation.

THE DIFFICULT AIRWAY

The difficult airway continues to be a problem for anesthesiologists. If a difficult airway can be anticipated, then appropriate preparations can be made (Fig. 28.9). It is the unanticipated difficult airway which is every anesthesiologist's worst nightmare. Studies in the UK, Australia, and the USA have shown that significant anesthetic-related mortality and morbidity are related to airway management.[18–22] The report of the Confidential Enquiry into Maternal Deaths published for England and Wales, 1986,[22] revealed that a difficult or failed intubation contributed to 6 of the 4034 deaths reported. Indeed, as many as 600 deaths may occur each year as a result of a difficult intubation.[23]

Simple tests exist that may be able to identify many patients who are apparently normal but who will prove difficult to intubate. These should be available for all patients. There are a number of complex tests described later in this chapter which cannot be applied as a routine to all surgical patients but which may be appropriate for use in specific situations.

The simple action of asking patients to open their mouth widely and protrude the tongue may identify the occasional patient with restricted mouth opening. This test was refined by Mallampati[24] when he divided the view on visual examination of the posterior wall of the pharynx into four grades (Fig. 28.10). In class I, the soft palate, uvula, faucial pillars, and posterior pharyngeal wall are visible; in class II, the upper part of the faucial pillars and the soft palate are visible; in class III, only the soft palate is visible; and in class IV, none of these structures is visible. In patients who are classified as Mallampati class I, there should be no difficulty with direct laryngoscopy and tracheal intubation. The anticipated difficulty increases as the class increases, and difficulty in tracheal intubation can be expected with those patients who are classified as III or IV.

A number of additional bedside tests have been proposed. Patil and colleagues[25] examined the thyromental distance and showed that if it was less than 7 cm there was an increased likelihood of a difficult intubation (Fig. 28.11). Frerk[26] combined these tests and showed that, when the posterior pharyngeal wall can be seen below the soft palate with the patient's mouth open wide, intubation should be straightforward (class I or II). On the other hand, if the posterior pharnygeal wall cannot be seen, the patient should be classed as III or IV and may be difficult to intubate, particularly if the thyromental distance is short (i.e. less than 7 cm). Fortunately, when an unexpected difficulty arises, flexible fiberoptic endoscopy may often provide a solution.

No problem is more frustrating than the anesthetic management of a patient of apparently normal appearance in whom it is impossible to visualize the glottis and insert a tracheal tube.

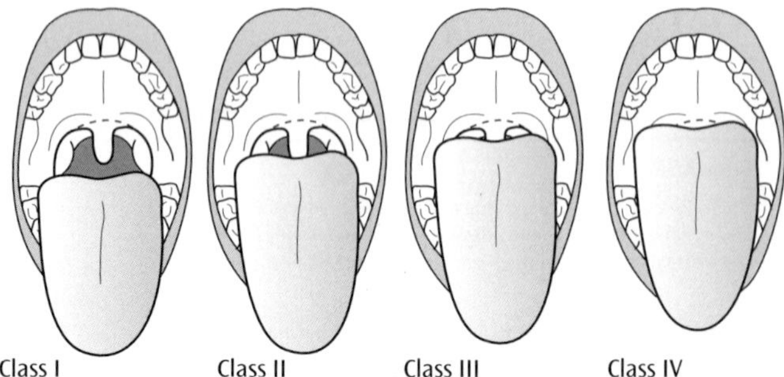

Figure 28.10 *Mallampati oropharyngeal scale. (Reproduced with permission from Mallampati SR, Galt SP, Gugino LD,* et al. *A clinical sign to predict difficult intubation: a prospective study.* Can Anaesth Soc J *1985;* **32:** *429–34.)*

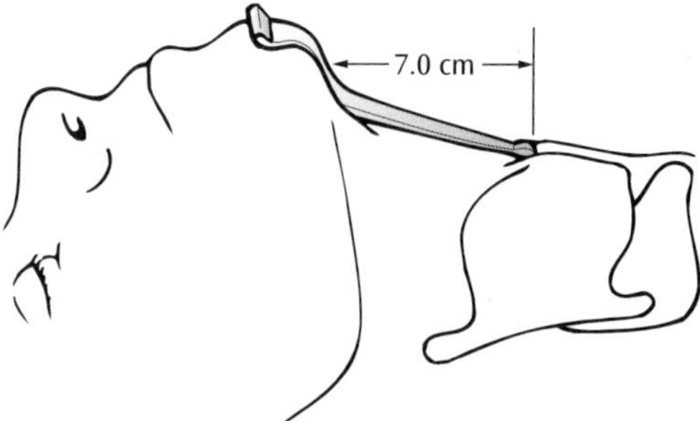

Figure 28.11 *An intubation gauge can be used to estimate the degree of difficulty with endotracheal intubation. (Modified with permission from Barash PG, Cullen BF, Stoetling RK (eds).* Clinical Anesthesia, *2nd edn. Philadelphia: J B Lippincott, 1992.)*

Defining the difficult airway

Definition of the "difficult airway" is usually related solely to tracheal intubation or problems with mask ventilation. Central to management must be an understanding of the anatomical, biomechanical, or pathophysiologic mechanisms responsible for airway complications. For example, an understanding of the disease processes mucopolysaccharidosis or fibrofascial myositis ossificans can warn of potential airway disaster just as much as retrognathia or micrognathia (separate but overlapping entities).

In approaching the difficult airway, it is useful to consider the following broad categories:

1 Previous history of difficulty or failure in establishing control and access to the patient's airway.
2 Presence of anatomical or physiologic pathology that might predictably be associated with difficulty in airway management. Although previous documented success in such a patient may put the practitioner at ease, it does not necessarily guarantee that the planned anesthetic will be uneventful.
3 Limited experience in evaluating, planning, and managing the difficult airway.

Various reports to date have attempted to focus on single, and sometimes simplistic, factors such as macroglossia or micrognathia.[27] These studies have all been based on a search for prospective reproducible criteria of value to the clinical practitioner. Another suggestion (Table

Table 28.2 *Signs suggesting difficult laryngoscopy*

Sign	Score
Micrognathia with acute mandibular angles	5
Glossoptosis or basal macroglossia	4
Difficulty with prior laryngoscopy	3
Long, high-arched palate associated with long, narrow dental arch	2
Temporomandibular joint limitation	4
Short muscular neck with full dentition	2
Protruding maxillary dentition with premaxillary overgrowth	2
Increased alveolomental depth	1
Limited extension of the upper cervical vertebrae	2
Limited motion of lower cervical vertebrae	3
Pathological signs of airway obstruction	3
Decreased distance between hyoid and thyroid cartilages	2
Decreased distance of epiglottis from posterior wall of pharynx	3
Skill of the anesthesiologist	1–5
Planning for endoscopy	1–5
Miller's sign (3–4)[a]	3

a. Scale ranges from 1 to 5, with 1 being best and 5 being worst. (Reproduced, with permission, from Norton ML, Brown ACD (eds). *Atlas of the Difficult Airway*. St Louis: Mosby Year Book, 1991: 8.)

28.2) is to score a number of criteria in attempting to predict whether there will be difficulty with airway management. This approach has yet to be fully validated, but it must not be forgotten that the best of predictive methods may fail to draw attention to the patient for whom difficulties become obvious only after the induction of anesthesia. Thus, as in all aspects of practice, the anesthesiologist must continually be prepared to manage unexpected and potentially life-threatening loss of control of an airway. It is tempting to believe that the use of a regional anesthetic technique for surgery will obviate such problems. This may, unfortunately, not be the case. Inadequate regional anesthesia, too high a spinal level, a sudden unexpected event, or a toxic reaction may all require emergency airway management. Failure to guarantee an airway can risk a patient's life. It always has been – and remains – the anesthesiologist's obligation to be certain that he/she can control the patient's airway.

The skilled clinician may have justifiable pride in his or her abilities, but a degree of objectivity is essential for optimum patient management. Thus, whenever a difficult intubation is anticipated, the presence of another skilled practitioner may be invaluable in providing intelligent and definitive assistance. Furthermore, there will be occasions when consultation with colleagues, referral of patients to others with more experience in a particular aspect of airway abnormality, or even deferral of surgery for additional planning will be in the patient's best interest. The anesthesiologist may face situations involving various external pressures; these should be recognized and dealt with maturely. There is no shame in being unable to solve a problem at the specific moment; there must be no reluctance to step back in order to rethink and plan. The safety of the patient is the first priority.

When it is judged necessary to intubate a patient while awake and under local analgesia, a thorough explanation of the reasons as well as the process is part of the anesthesiologist's responsibility. Explanations must not be rushed. Just as topical anesthesia requires meticulous time and effort, so too does gaining the patient's confidence. Once trust has been established, patient cooperation will be enhanced, leading to a smoother procedure with a greater chance of success.

Responsibility does not end with placement and ultimate removal of the tracheal tube. Remember that a patient will probably come to surgery again. Consideration must be given to the fact that the patient may have a future need for tracheal intubation. The patient, as well as the referring practitioner, must be fully informed about the problem airway. A written report must be provided because, with the passage of time, memory becomes inaccurate.[28]

Preoperative assessment of the airway should minimize the occurrence of pathology presenting unexpectedly during a "routine" general anesthetic. Schemata for the expected and the unexpected problem airway range from the complex[29] to the simple.[30] Algorithms represent a valid training aid but do not completely satisfy the needs of the situation in that they do not provide the rationale. It is necessary to constantly seek those factors that can be recognized, are reproducible, and can be solved. Similarly, technology may provide a tool, but an understanding of the essentials of medicine and knowledge of the anatomy, physiology, pharmacology, biomechanics, and pathology are required. The flexible fiberoptic endoscope has made it possible for visual approaches to be the norm for these patients, reducing but not obviating the need for "blind" techniques. Finally, the skilled clinician must be familiar with all approaches to the difficult airway and must, therefore, develop skills that do not depend only on the most advanced technology.

The difficult airway clinic

The difficult airway clinic[31] has developed in order to concentrate experience in complex examinations and to provide clinical management advice for the solution of demonstrated or potential upper airway problems. Planning the best first approach, with back-up options, can eliminate the need for tracheostomy or can reduce the incidence of anesthetic induction trauma as well as operating room delays or case cancellations.

Premedication

Ideally, the patient should be brought to the operating room without any premedication that can suppress ventilation. Even small doses of narcotic, tranquilizer, or barbiturate can turn a partial obstruction into a complete obstruction with alarming rapidity. The use of an antisialogogue (e.g. glycopyrollate or hyoscine) is controversial. A reduction in secretions, which may obstruct the view, is desirable. However, the resulting increase in viscosity of secretions following an antisialogogue may make it more difficult to suction away mucoid collections. Furthermore, those very secretions may serve as a lubricant and facilitate the passage of instruments. Perhaps of greater importance is the decision to continue or discontinue the patient's usual medication. Unless it presents a significant risk in the presence of anesthetic agents or procedures that is greater than the underlying pathophysiology for which these drugs were prescribed, the patient's usual medication should be continued.

Monitoring

All patients being evaluated for, or undergoing, control of the airway require routine anesthesia monitoring. The pulse oximeter provides the most useful information. The effects of the Valsalva maneuver, increase in airway obstruction, and changes in cardiac rate are rapidly identified by this device. The continuous electrocardiogram display should also be used, and, for patients with a history of cardiac disease or arrhythmias, online ST segment analysis may be valuable. The blood pressure can usually be measured using a noninvasive automated cuff system; a direct arterial line is required only if indicated by other clinical demand. Facilities for measuring the end-tidal P_{CO_2} assist in confirming correct intubation and are considered mandatory for patients with a history of bronchospastic disease.[32]

Conduct of the anesthetic

Anesthetic techniques designed solely for efficiency are inappropriate in the management of a difficult airway. Rapid induction of anesthesia by administration of a precalculated dose of barbiturate followed by a rapidly acting muscle relaxant is likely to be devastating for patients with a difficult airway, and may require urgent or emergency action. When airway difficulties are anticipated, the selection of a technique should include consideration and anticipation of all potential complications (Tables 28.3 and 28.4). Muscle relaxants must be withheld until the anesthesiologist is certain that the airway can be controlled.

Opening the mouth

The mechanics of normal mouth opening involve both muscular and bony components. The principal bony component to be considered is the temporomandibular joint. The contour of the zygomatic arch and temporal bone is that of an elongated "S" lying on its side. The joint is located between the mandibular (glenoid) fossa of the inferior surface of the temporal bone and the condylar process of the mandibular bone. The condyloid process of the mandible seats into the glenoid sulcus and a bursa lies within the joint. The mechanical pattern of mouth opening involves a hinge motion accompanied by rotation and translocation forwards. This joint can be temporarily dislocated, allowing the mouth

Table 28.3 *Complications and constraints of some airway devices*

Technique	Complications
Jet (Venturi)	Pneumolarynx and trachea, pneumomediastinum, pneumothorax, infection
Retrograde	Trauma to vocal folds, infection, laryngeal and tracheal trauma
Light wand	Tissue burn from heat of bulb
Fiberoptic (nasal)	Hemorrhage, nasal trauma
Fiberoptic (oral)	Trauma to mouth or teeth from intubation airway
Intubation guide	Trauma to mouth or teeth from intubation airway
Tracheostomy	Tracheal infection, stenosis, loss of Valsalva mechanism, communication problems, cicatrix, stenosis, hemorrhage
Nasal airway	Hemorrhage
Laryngeal mask	Gastric acid reflux, disruption of esophagopharyngeal introitus

The above list does not include reactions to topical anesthetics and adjuvants required for "shrinking" the mucosae, reduction of sensation to passage of instruments, depression of gag reflex, and psychotropic effects.

Table 28.4 *Examples of soft-tissue conditions causing airway difficulty*

Congenital
Glottic webs
Hemangiomas
Hypoplastic mandible
Laryngomalacia
Infection and progressive airway obstruction
Epiglottis
Croup
Ludwig's angina
Retropharyngeal abscess
Diphtheria
Sudden
Foreign body aspiration
Trauma
Retropharyngeal hematoma
Large neck hematoma
Tumors
Tongue
Epiglottis
Larynx

to be opened further with the use of muscle relaxants. A common error when learning airway control is to attempt opening the patient's mouth by simply pushing downward on the lower jaw with the patient supine. This maneuver impacts the coronoid process into the sulcus, limiting the translocation motion of the joint, and inhibits mouth opening. The required movement is downward, then outward, lifting both the mandible and base of the tongue in a C-shaped motion. This can be accomplished by the following maneuvers:

1 Place the thumb over the index finger in a scissor position. The index finger should then be placed as far posteriorly on the occlusal surface of the upper dentition as possible and the thumb on the lower dentition. A scissor motion with the thumb extending downward, outward, and upward should then achieve mouth opening.
2 Insert the thumb over the tongue base as far posteriorly as possible, and then grasp the tongue base and mandible below the chin with the remaining fingers. A motion lifting downward, outward, and upward should then achieve mouth opening. This maneuver is better suited to the edentulous patient and is useful for those with unstable cervical vertebrae.

Trismus, a pathological muscle spasm secondary to pain, limits mouth opening. It usually responds to local anesthetic infiltration, analgesia, or general anesthesia. However, what appears to be trismus may not necessarily result from muscular spasm. Thus, if difficulty in opening the mouth is caused by bony pathology or soft-tissue disease, local or general anesthesia may not be effective. This can result in a potentially hazardous situation if the assumption is made that the mouth will open after the induction of anesthesia and is proved wrong.

Extending the head

Standard teaching has been that the best position for airway control and for intubation of the trachea is the "sniffing the morning air" position.[33] The rationale behind this is based on better alignment of the oral, pharyngeal, and tracheal axes.[34] Unfortunately, this has been overemphasized to the point of resultant neck flexion (by too many blankets or pillows behind the head), which also stresses the restraining ligaments of the ventrally placed odontoid process (C1–C2 complex), most important in atlantoaxial stability and instability. Another mistake is to place one hand on the chin with the other on the occipitoparietal area of the cranium and push the head into extreme extension. This not only distorts the airway axis by artificially displacing the tracheal cartilage ventrally, but also forces the odontoid process against the body of the C1 vertebra. This is particularly hazardous for patients with osteoporosis, Paget's disease, or achondroplasia, in whom there is a risk of odontoid fracture and displacement against the spinal cord. Thus, extension of the head into the correct position is of paramount importance.

Placement of the laryngoscope blade

Difficulty in direct laryngoscopy may be the problem because of, for example, pathology within the airway. It is possible, however, for an airway that is not difficult to be labeled as difficult owing to inexperience of the operator or to faulty technique. Visual obstruction can readily occur because of improper placement of a laryngoscope blade. The lateral flange of the blade was designed to deflect the bulk of the tongue to the side (normally the left). Placement of the blade directly in the midline induces the tongue on the opposite side to curl around into the channel of the blade, thus obstructing vision. Proper placement requires that the instrument is placed in the right lateral part of the mouth (left hand holding the laryngoscope) and then moved toward the midline as necessary, deflecting the tongue by the flange of the laryngoscope to the left paramedian position. (A left-handed anesthesiologist may choose to use a laryngoscope that is designed to be held in the right hand, in which case the side of placements and direction of movement are reversed.)

The view of the larynx may vary from all to none. The classification proposed by Cormack and Lehane[35] is commonly adopted for grading the view on direct laryngoscopy and correlates with the difficulty in intubation of the trachea (Fig. 28.12). Most anesthesiologists note the Cormack and Lehane grading on the anesthesia record for the benefit of future anesthesiologists.

Rapid-sequence induction

This is the universally accepted way of securing the airway for a patient who has (or who might have) a full stomach. It must be emphasized that, first and foremost, delaying the induction of anesthesia until the stomach has had time to empty is the most important consideration. There are times, however, when it is necessary to proceed, e.g. in an emergency for the patient with gastric outlet obstruction, or for the obstetric case. In these cases, precautions to minimize (you can never

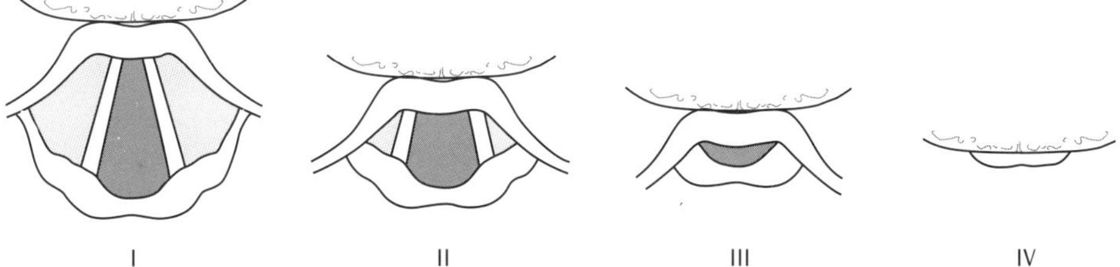

Figure 28.12 *Laryngoscopy grading. Grade I: the full glottis and both commissures are visible. Grade II: most of the glottis and the posterior commissure are visible. Grade III: only the posterior rim of larynx is visible but arytenoids indicate the location of the midline. Grade IV: the tip of the epiglottis or only the base of the tongue is visible. (Reproduced with permission from Cormack RS, Lehane J. Difficult tracheal intubation in obstetrics.* Anaesthesia *1984;* **39:** *1105–11.)*

completely prevent) regurgitation and aspiration of gastric contents are of paramount importance. Strict adherence to all details of the induction technique are essential. All equipment must be checked and available to hand before starting, and the assistant must be competent to help and know exactly what to do. The supine position is the most commonly used and is probably the most reliable, although head-up and head-down tilt have both also been advocated. If there is a nasogastric tube *in situ*, some recommend its removal before induction in case its presence compromises the integrity of the lower esophageal sphincter, although others do not consider that there is a problem.[36]

The patient should be preoxygenated for a minimum of 3 min using a tight-fitting anesthetic face mask and 100% oxygen. The calculated intravenous induction dose is administered into the fast-running intravenous infusion followed immediately by succinylcholine (suxamethonium) 1.5 mg kg^{-1}. Cricoid pressure (Sellick's maneuver) is applied (Fig. 28.13). The fasciculations from the succinylcholine are awaited and, as soon as muscular relaxation of the jaw is adequate, direct laryngoscopy and tracheal intubation are performed. The lungs should not be inflated if possible, although evidence suggests that this may not present a problem provided that the inflation pressure is kept low and care is taken not to inflate the stomach. The suction apparatus should be connected, working, and immediately to hand, e.g. underneath the pillow. A wide-bore, rigid-type sucker is recommended, e.g. the Yankaur type. Cricoid pressure is not released until the anesthesiologist is completely convinced that the tracheal tube is correctly inserted into the trachea and the cuff inflated.

The Sellick maneuver[37] is not an absolute assurance against the aspiration of liquids. It may also make intubation more difficult by distorting the anatomy (Fig. 28.14). The hyoid bone is prevented from moving forward with the tongue during laryngoscopy, misplaced pressure can drive the thyroid up under the wings of the hyoid cartilage so reducing the visualization available for insertion of the tracheal tube, and, rarely,

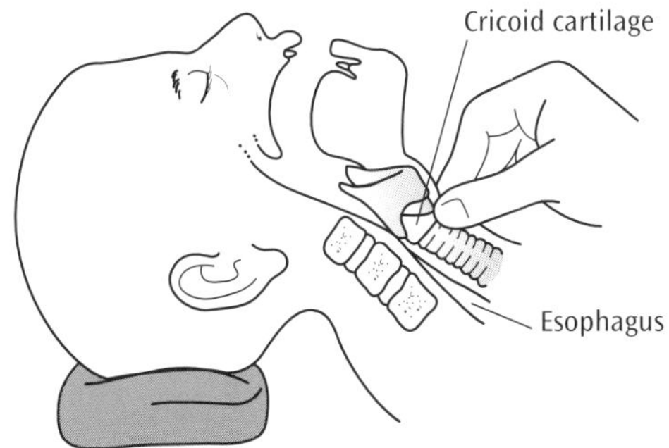

Figure 28.13 *Cricoid pressure (Sellick's maneuver) is applied to occlude the esophagus and prevent aspiration of gastric contents. (Reproduced with permission from Barash PG, Cullen BF, Stoetling RK (eds).* Clinical Anesthesia, *2nd edn. Philadelphia: J B Lippincott, 1992.)*

lingual nerve damage can be caused by stretching the nerve as it crosses the hyoglossus,[38] which leads to hyperesthesia of the tongue.[39] This technique has, however, reduced morbidity and mortality.

Unexpected airway problems in the operating room

An unexpected problem is quite different from that faced by the anesthesiologist with a patient whose airway pathology has been diagnosed before anesthesia is commenced. Most anesthesiologists have, however, been confronted with an apparently normal patient who proves difficult to intubate. Such an eventuality should always be borne in mind when planning the induction and intraoperative anesthetic management of all patients.

The first rule is to plan for all eventualities in airway management. This includes having readily available the equipment that might be needed if a problem arises. This need not be complex, and one method is to have a number of pre-prepared boxes or trolleys within the operating suite. The "kit" should include intubation guides (e.g. Norton, Eschmann, Sheridan), light wand, gum-elastic bougie, a range of laryngoscope blades, and a selection of small tubes. To this is often added a large-bore cannula and connector or a proprietary minitracheostomy set for emergency ventilation directly into the trachea. A prepared "airway trolley" for specialized techniques (e.g. fiberoptic laryngoscope, Bullard laryngoscope, jet ventilation set) should also be available at short notice. It must be remembered that one should always look through the lumen of the chosen tracheal tubes for obstructive blebs or membranes produced during manufacture or a constricted lumen on inflation of the cuff.

During operation, other factors may be important. The tubes, or tracheal tube cuffs, may be cut if the surgeon is operating in that vicinity. Plugs of mucus or blood may collect in the lumen of the tube or even in the tracheobronchial tree, especially when using dry, cold gases. Kinking, torsion, and compression of the airways can occur, as can kinking, torsion, or compression of the tracheal tube. Improper placement or migration of the tube may occur so that the distal tip becomes occluded by soft tissue. The distal tip may also become occluded against the wall of the trachea or bronchus. A tube that is too long may inadvertently enter the right main bronchus either at the time of intubation or following movement during surgery. Auscultation of both sides of the chest should be intermittently performed to rule out this possibility. If obstruction, or partial obstruction, of a tube is suspected, merely passing a suction catheter through the lumen may be insufficient because of a ball-valve or trap-door action of some mucus plugs. In these cases, it is necessary to pass a fiberoptic flexible endoscope to locate and determine the nature of the plug and remove it. It may require special forceps (for highly viscous or solid materials), changing the airway device, or, in very rare instances, rigid bronchoscopy for removal. If in doubt, never be afraid to change the tracheal tube for a new one or resort to a new and different airway device.

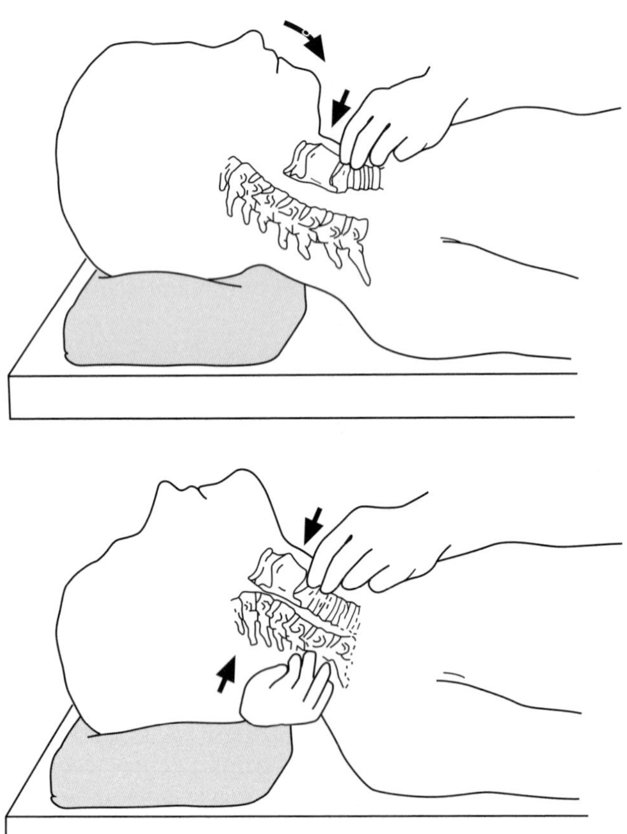

Figure 28.14 *In order to apply cricoid pressure, the anesthesiologist's assistant must carefully place his/her index fingure and thumb over the cricoid cartiledge immediately below the prominent thyroid cartilage. Pressure is then applied downward in order to compress the esophagus. Unopposed pressure on the cricoid may cause flexion of the neck, thus distorting the anatomy and making visualization of the larynx more difficult. This can be easily corrected by repositioning the pillows or by the assistant placing a hand behind the neck. (Modified with permission from Barash PG, Cullen BF, Stoetling RK (eds).* Clinical Anesthesia, *2nd edn. Philadelphia: J B Lippincott, 1992.)*

Positioning for endoscopy

The standard position for rigid endoscopy is with the patient supine and the anesthesiologist above the head of the patient. Flexible fiberoptic intubation can be performed in the same way but may not be the ideal position, particularly for the patient with a difficult airway.[40] Many operators find that the optimum position is with the patient sitting, and the endoscopist standing or sitting beside and facing the patient. The advantages of this position are:

1 The patient's face and facial reaction can be observed.
2 The light reflection (nasal or cervical), which indicates the position of the fiberscope, can be seen.
3 Awake patients do not feel disoriented and remote as they are face to face with the endoscopist.
4 Blood or secretions draining from the pharynx can be swallowed.

The normal larynx is protected from above by the base of the tongue, the epiglottis, and the funnel action of the pharyngeal muscles. When the patient is supine, the suspensory structures tend to relax, decreasing the airway channel to one-half to one-third of its erect diameter. This reduction has been demonstrated with radiological views using C-arm dynamic fluoroscopy (the "image intensifier"), even in the awake subject. However, when the patient sits up, the larynx tends to uncoil[41,42] as the suspensory structure becomes functional. The hyoid separates further from the tracheal cartilage, permitting the normal adult tracheal cartilage to open up and become more heart shaped.

The chin and the base of the tongue should be brought forward. This motion, via the pulley of the hyoid (anterior and posterior digastric and omohyoid muscles), pulls the hyoid wings cephalad, away from the thyroid cartilage, further opening the airway.

The phrase "anterior larynx" is often used to describe patients in whom the larynx cannot be easily visualized on direct laryngoscopy. In reality, it would be hard to find anything more anteriorly placed than the thyroid prominence just under the skin and a better description would be "superiorly shifted larynx" with a relative posterior displacement (glossoptosis) of the tongue base and epiglottis. In the supine position, there is a cephalad displacement of the tracheal cartilage wings such that the larynx rises within the limits of the hyoid, narrowing the aperture. The sitting position, which reduces biomechanical obstruction, is therefore more appropriate than the supine for opening up the airway for endoscopy. Whereas the flexible fiberoptic endoscope is very useful for safe airway management, in the unexpected emergency it may be helpful only in the hands of the expert. The presence of blood, viscous mucus, or massive tissue edema will lead to failed airway visualization. Furthermore, the supine position, with its reduced airway support, will contribute to the difficulty.

Use of the fiberscope

The flexible fiberoptic endoscope is an extremely useful aid to intubation. Key factors include knowledge of the anatomy, the use of the sitting position, and repeated practice to develop and maintain adequate skill. The position of maximum airway opening has been reviewed by Fink.[41,42] It can be used to guide the tracheal tube through either the oral or nasal passages having previously loaded the chosen tube onto the endoscope. There are times when advancing the endoscope is not possible, however, in spite of the laryngeal opening being in view. In these circumstances, a guide wire may prove useful. The wire should have a flexible tip which can be guided, either by direct vision or by radiological assistance, through the larynx. The flexible endoscope tip can be used to direct the wire through the laryngeal aperture. The wire is then advanced into the lower trachea to reduce the chance of its being pulled out of the trachea by a "whipping" action as the endoscope is advanced over the wire guide down to the carina under wire guide and direct vision control. Finally, the previously placed warm-water-softened tracheal tube can be advanced over the endoscope into the trachea. The fiberscope should then be withdrawn to allow a period of oxygenation through the tracheal tube. The fiberscope may then be reinserted, via a fiberoptic bronchoscope swivel adapter, down to the carina to enable the anesthesiologist to count four or five rings up from the carina to ensure that the tracheal tube can be sited correctly so that it will not inadvertently advance into the right main bronchus. It is appropriate to auscultate over both sides of the chest to ensure that air or anesthetic gases are entering throughout both lungs.

Local analgesia of the airway

Topical analgesia may be combined with a regional nerve block for airway analgesia, especially of the larynx (Fig. 28.15). Use of the Jackson (Krause) right-angle toothed forceps with cocaine-impregnated packing of the pyriform fossae is the usual approach. Superior laryngeal nerve block and transtracheal instillation of local anesthetic agent through the cricothyroid membrane are also used.[43] Another technique is to ask a sitting patient to inhale deeply and slowly while the "spray" from a local anesthetic nebulizer, with a variable direction tip and oxygen as the carrier, is activated.[44] It is important to spray both transnasally and orally in order to anesthetize the dorsal surface of the uvula. This is equally important for both nasal and oral intubation using fiberoptic endoscopy. In the case of fiberoptic oral intubation, it is necessary to spray the hard and soft palate to prevent stimulation by the oral intubation airway.

Once the fiberoptic scope has been placed just above the larynx, the larynx and trachea may be anesthetized using local analgesic solution instilled through a suitable thin catheter (Fig. 28.16).

The agents suitable for topical analgesia are 4% lidocaine and 2% cocaine in a 10:2 ratio. If there is a history of thyrotoxicosis, hypertension, or other contraindication, cocaine should be omitted. There are other local analgesics which may also be suitable. For nasal intubation, the nasal route may be packed with anesthetic-soaked nasal packs using

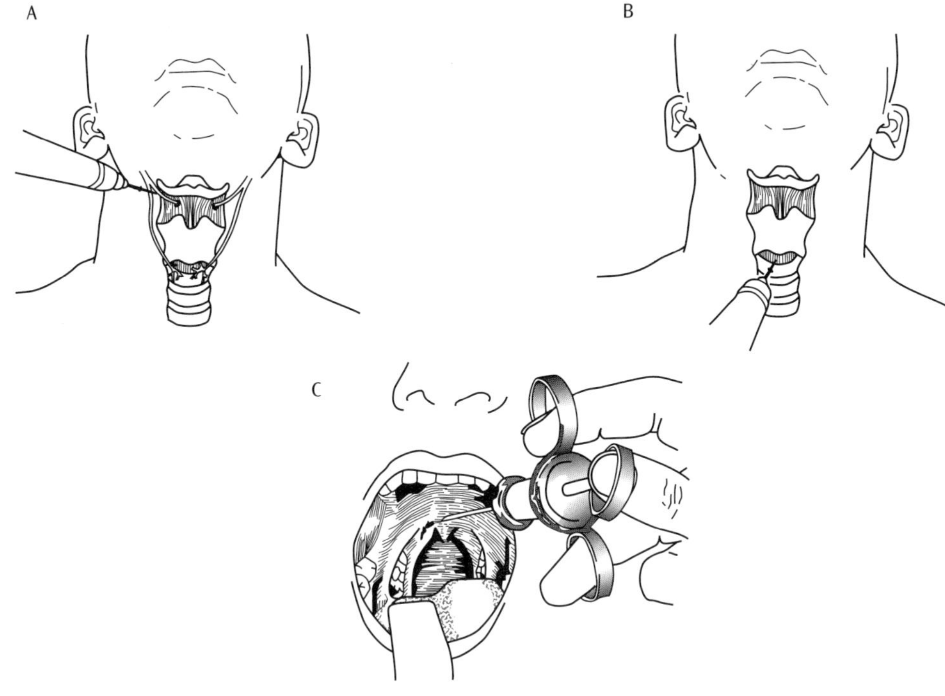

Figure 28.15 *Conduction blockage of the airway. The three illustrations in this figure show the common percutaneous/conduction blocks of the airway. (A) The block of the superior laryngeal nerve where it divides into its internal and external branches adjacent to the posteroinferior aspect of the hyoid cornu major. This is to achieve anesthesia of the mucous membrane of the hypopharynx. (B) The percutaneous instillation of local anesthetic through the cricothyroid membrane to achieve tracheal anesthesia and laryngeal intrinsic muscle relaxation. (C) The use of a guarded needle and dental syringe to block the branch of the glossopharyngeal that enters the pillar of the fauces in order to anesthetize the base of the tongue and block the afferent arc of the gag reflex. (Reproduced with permission from Brown ACD. Anesthetic principles of airway management. In: Ferlito A (ed.).* Diseases of the Larynx. *London: Arnold, 2000.)*

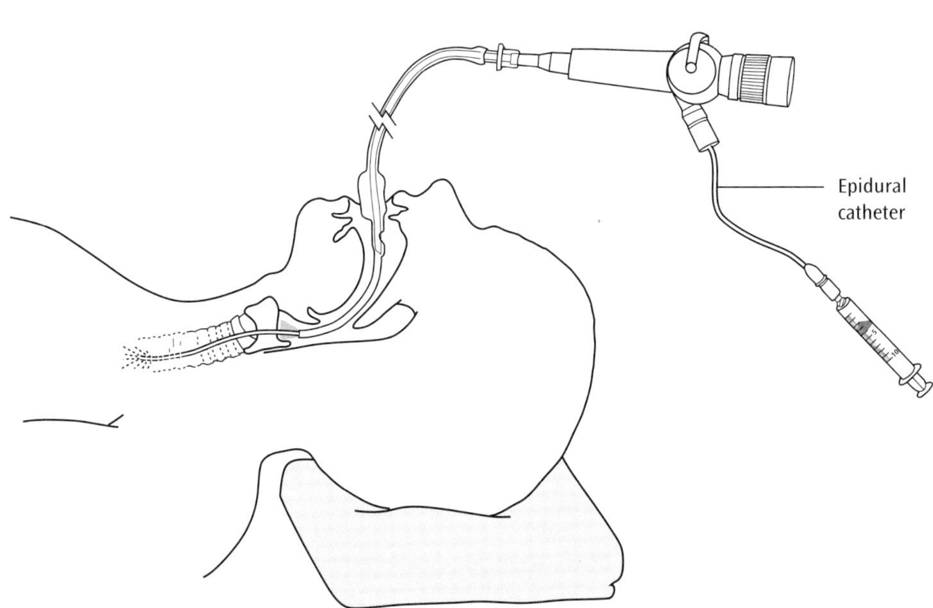

Figure 28.16 *Epidural catheter trachea instillation technique, rather than a percutaneous block of tracheal sensation. This method, utilizing direct vision of the glottis through a fiberoptic endoscope to pass an epidural catheter from the suction channel into the trachea, has been found particularly useful, as careful positioning of the catheter causes little stimulation. Directly injecting local anesthetic through the suction or biopsy port of the endoscope is equally efffective. (Reproduced with permission from Brown ACD. Anesthetic principles of airway management. In: Ferlito A (ed.).* Diseases of the Larynx. *London: Arnold, 2000.)*

Magill, Cohen, or Hartman forceps. On occasion, it may be necessary to dilate the nasal passage using progressively increased sizes of nasal trumpet.

When there is excessive mucoid secretion, this may be reduced by intravenous glycopyrollate or hyoscine. These drugs may, however, increase the viscosity of the secretions, making it harder to suction them effectively through the small fiberoptic endoscope suction channel. This problem can often be resolved by passing a suction catheter through the contralateral nasal passage and down to the larynx. Intermittent suction can then be used as required.

Local anesthesia for nasal intubation

The nasal airway should first be examined to determine whether there is an anterior obstruction due to septal deviation, anomaly of the inferior turbinates or floor of nasal passage, or the presence of polyps. Asking the patient to sniff with each nostril occluded in turn can be used as an initial guide, although one cannot rely on the patient's account of the ease of breathing through either side unless there is an almost total obstruction. An otic speculum of appropriate size with otoscope can be used for a more accurate assessment. A deeper examination requires a nasopharyngoscope or the fiberoptic endoscope.

A long, moistened cottonwool bud may then be inserted to obtain the tactile sense of any posterior obstruction as well as the direction and depth of the inferior ethmoid passage. If the depth (from maxillary entrance to posterior pharyngeal wall) is much less than 9–9.5 cm in the normal adult, suspect a posterior passage abnormality. As the cottonwool bud is withdrawn, it should be swept in a circular motion to get a tactile sense of the canal diameter. Note that the size of the nares contributes nothing to this evaluation.

Finally, the nasopharynx should be included in the examination as the flexible fiberoptic endoscope is inserted. Unsuspected polyps or other pathology may be revealed. Mirror nasopharyngoscopy can readily reveal posterior canal polyps and adenoidal masses, as well as lesions on the base of the tongue.

Following local anesthetic preparation mentioned above, a Codman pack (2.5 × 10 cm) soaked in 2% cocaine may be inserted for anesthesia, vasoconstriction, and canal dilation, after which nasal trumpets, thoroughly lubricated with an anesthetic gel, may be inserted to dilate and lubricate the canal. At this stage, a previously prepared tracheal tube that has been softened in a warmed solution of saline or water may be inserted. If flexible fiberoptic intubation is to be used, it is imperative not to insert the tracheal tube too far because it may limit movement of the tip of the endoscope to be passed through it or, more frequently, it may impact against the posterior pharynx. Some anesthesiologists feel that, although this is time-consuming and requires meticulous attention, the result is a more comfortable patient, almost complete elimination of bleeding, and improved intubation success. The need for nasal intubation is not without other complications (e.g. maxillary sinusitis). It must not be undertaken lightly. Studies indicate that bacterial maxillary sinusitis is found in more than 60% of recently intubated patients.[45–47]

Oral intubation guides

The oral route is usually used for fiberoptic intubation when the supine position is chosen. However, this approach does require that the mouth can open sufficiently to insert an intubating oral airway. Thus, it is not possible when the mouth cannot be opened, as in temporomandibular joint ankylosis.

A typical oral intubation airway is the Berman intubation airway, which has a side slit so that it can be removed. Another guide is the Williams airway, which has the disadvantage of not being similarly slotted and removable. A third frequently used approach is the Ovassapian airway, which is particularly useful for a patient with a large, broad tongue; its disadvantage is the open top (proximal to the hard and soft palate). When using oral intubation airways, the tracheal tube should be preplaced in the airway lumen, but not beyond the distal opening analogous with the transnasal technique.

The laryngeal mask has also made possible airway access for either the intubation guide or the flexible fiberoptic endoscope (see above).[48]

Sublaryngeal difficult airways

Other important uses of the fiberoptic endoscope include (1) positioning of tracheal and endobronchial tubes and (2) placement of tracheal tubes below areas of tracheal compression.

Tracheal tube positioning

The value of the fiberoptic endoscope for the insertion of tracheal tubes through the airway has been discussed elsewhere. It is often forgotten that the usual techniques for checking tube placement are fraught with error. Auscultation does not guarantee proper placement. However, direct visualization via a tracheal fiberoptic swivel adapter can readily be accomplished, visualizing the carina and then counting the number of rings up to the tip of the tracheal tube, and is an absolute assurance of the tube position.

Similarly, the fiberoptic techniques taught by Ovassapian[49] for placement of endobronchial double-lumen tubes and blockers provide absolute assurance of proper placement.

The compressed trachea

The usual cause of a compressed trachea is a massively enlarged thyroid. The most frequent effects may be lateral displacement, significant compression of the trachea, and, less often, compression of the main stem bronchi (substernal goiter). An obvious concern is tracheal torsion or further obstruction during surgical manipulation, and possible tracheal collapse after the tracheal tube is removed. Tracheomalacia is a problem that must be considered following all long-term tracheal compression. It is relatively rare. Its effects are not usually obvious until the supportive tumor structure is removed, at which time the weathered tracheal cartilages collapse. These possibilities must be anticipated and the tracheal tube must be placed beyond the point of compression or potential collapse. This can best be achieved using fiberoptic evaluation. Other examples include mucopolysaccharidoses infiltrating the trachea and post-traumatic tracheal disruption. For these conditions, visual extubation of the trachea is of value in determining whether tracheal collapse will make extubation inadvisable at this time, while providing a visual guide for immediate reintubation.

Aids to intubation

Many devices have been described over the years as aids to tracheal intubation for the patient in whom direct laryngoscopy and intubation are not straightforward. There are many different types and modifications to the simple laryngoscope blade, although they tend to fall into two broad categories: straight blade, for example Miller (Fig. 28.17), and curved blades, e.g. the Macintosh (Fig. 28.18). Most anesthesiologists find the Macintosh blade (which is available in several sizes) the easiest to use. The technique is slightly different in that, when using a straight blade, the tip of the laryngoscope is advanced beneath the epiglottis in order to lift up the epiglottis directly (Fig. 28.19). There are occasions when obstruction prevents the normal positioning of the handle, for example

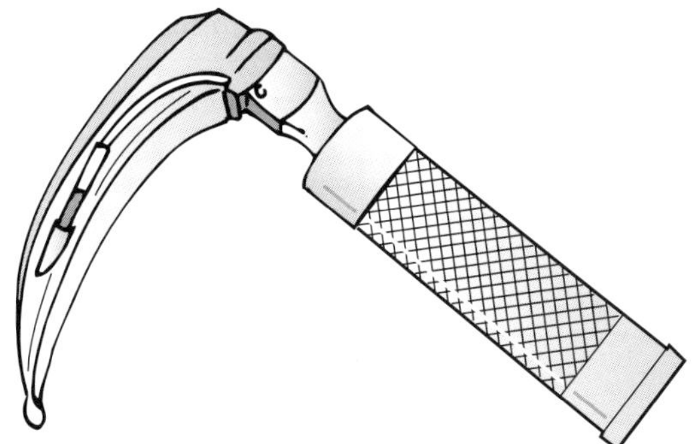

Figure 28.17 *Macintosh curved blade. (Reproduced from Vukmir RB.* Airway Management in the Critically Ill. *Carnforth, Lancs: Parthenon Publishing Group, 2001.)*

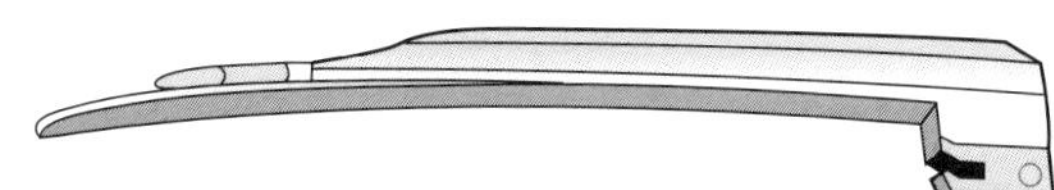

Figure 28.18 *Miller modified straight blade. (Reproduced from Vukmir RB.* Airway Management in the Critically Ill. *Carnforth, Lancs: Parthenon Publishing Group, 2001.)*

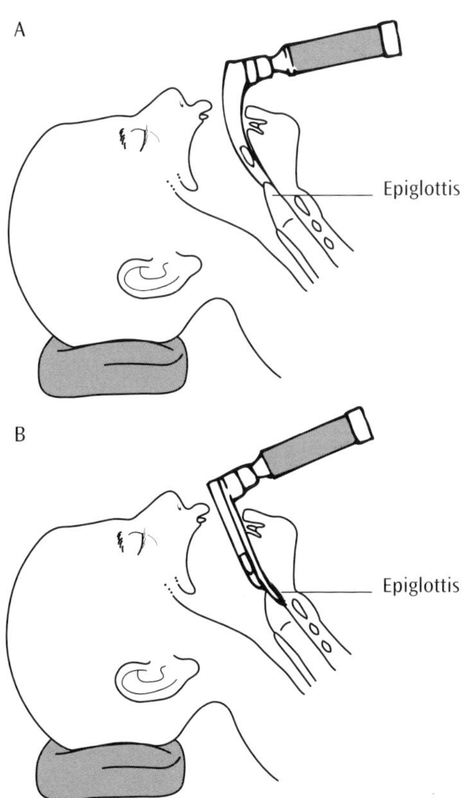

Figure 28.19 *(A) When a curved laryngoscope blade is used, the tip of the blade is placed in the vallecula – the space between the base of the tongue and the pharyngeal surface of the epiglottis. (B) The tip of a straight blade is advanced beneath the epiglottis. (Reproduced with permission from Barash PG, Cullen BF, Stoetling RK (eds).* Clinical Anesthesia, *2nd edn. Philadelphia: J B Lippincott, 1992.)*

a rigid neck collar, and for these situations different handle–blade angles are available, e.g. the Polio laryngoscope.

Even if laryngoscopy is possible, the larynx may not be seen, and a number of different devices have been described to enable better vision "around the corner." Plastic prisms were popular at one time, and some laryngoscopes have a small mirror built into their blade. The McCoy blade (Fig. 28.20), with its mobile tip, is very helpful for cases in which vision is impaired. Many different types of guide have been described with fixed and movable ends to facilitate the location of the laryngeal inlet. The majority of these are now redundant or are used only on rare occasions since the widespread availability of the fiberoptic laryngoscope.

INTUBATION GUIDES

Intubation guides include the Sheridan TXX (hollow tubing), Eschmann woven, and Norton Teflon rod. These are commonly, but incorrectly, called bougies. A bougie is actually a tapered instrument for introduction into tubular structures for dilation and diagnosis of strictures. On the other hand, a guide is just that – an instrument to guide or direct another instrument along a particular pathway. In the context of intubation, guides are long instruments that are passed through a tracheal tube over which the tube is passed through the oropharynx and larynx into the trachea (Fig. 28.21). They are often used at time of extubation in reverse manner. The guide is gently inserted through the tracheal tube and the tube is then carefully removed, leaving the guide in place (Fig. 28.22). This is very important because it ensures that reintubation can be accomplished if a patient with a difficult airway develops postextubation edema or other complications, some of which require reintubation (Table 28.5). It is possible to adapt a hollow flexible tube to act as a stylet and also permit ventilation of the lungs.[50]

Light wand

Light wand techniques (Fig. 28.23) involve inserting a light bulb on the tip of a long flexible wand through the tracheal tube.[51] The bulb of the wand is illuminated. It may be advantageous for the room to be partly darkened and the reflection of light sought in the patient's neck. When the reflection is noted superficially in the midline, the tube is advanced into the trachea.[52]

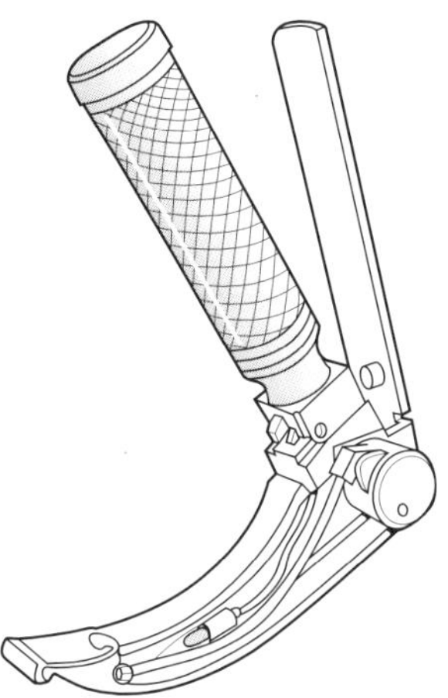

Figure 28.20 *McCoy laryngoscope blade. (Reproduced with permission from Penlon, Abingdon, UK.)*

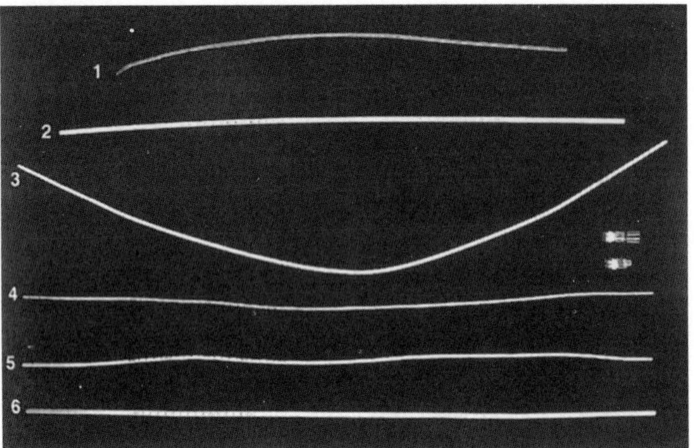

Figure 28.21 *Examples of tube guides. 1, The gum-elastic bougie with its "ski-tip" to the left is a long-established aid to intubation. 2, The original hollow "Tube-hanger™," first introduced for managing tube changes in the ICU environment. 3, A home-made device comprising a solid Teflon rod in different diameters developed for use with double-lumen tubes and laser tubes. 4–6, Examples of the different diameters of "Cook Airway Exchange Catheters™" that are now available for use even in pediatric situations. The catheters are hollow and, by use of the attachments, may be used for both low-pressure gas insufflation and jet ventilation in situations other than just tube changes. (Reproduced with permission from Brown ACD. Anesthetic principles of airway management. In: Ferlito A (ed.).* Diseases of the Larynx. *London: Arnold, 2000.)*

Intubation with radiographic assistance

Many techniques, ranging from simple to computer assisted, are now available for radiological examination of the neck and airway. The traditional upper airway film, a lateral view of the soft tissue of the neck, is useful for a quick limited review of the upper airway. Computer-driven technology such as computed tomography (CT) or magnetic resonance imaging (MRI) can provide a valuable insight in the imaging of both the cervical spine and soft tissues of the neck. Digitized CT scans make it possible to study tongue volume.[53] The combination of cineradiographic observation with simultaneous polysomnography (somnofluoroscopy) provides a relatively new technique for the diagnosis of sleep apnea,[54] and this also permits observation of the changes occurring during general anesthesia.

C-head dynamic fluoroscopy (the "image intensifier"), although not itself a new technique, offers a flexible, expeditious technique for assessment of the upper airway and for assisting tracheal intubation. This enables airway configuration, over a wide range of patient motion, to be quickly determined. The C-arm is a fixed radiographic tube that is aimed at a phosphorus image receptor. The image receptor is then photographed using a small camera within the C-arm head. The photograph is displayed by the monitor. The final image can be adjusted by changing radiation factors or standard brightness/contrast controls on the monitor itself.

The patient is placed on the table in the sitting position for intubation. The radiologist and the anesthesiologist determine the placement of the C-arm so as to insure that lateral and anterior/posterior radiographic positions are available and that the appropriate operating room table or patient position is used. Occasionally, the neurosurgical

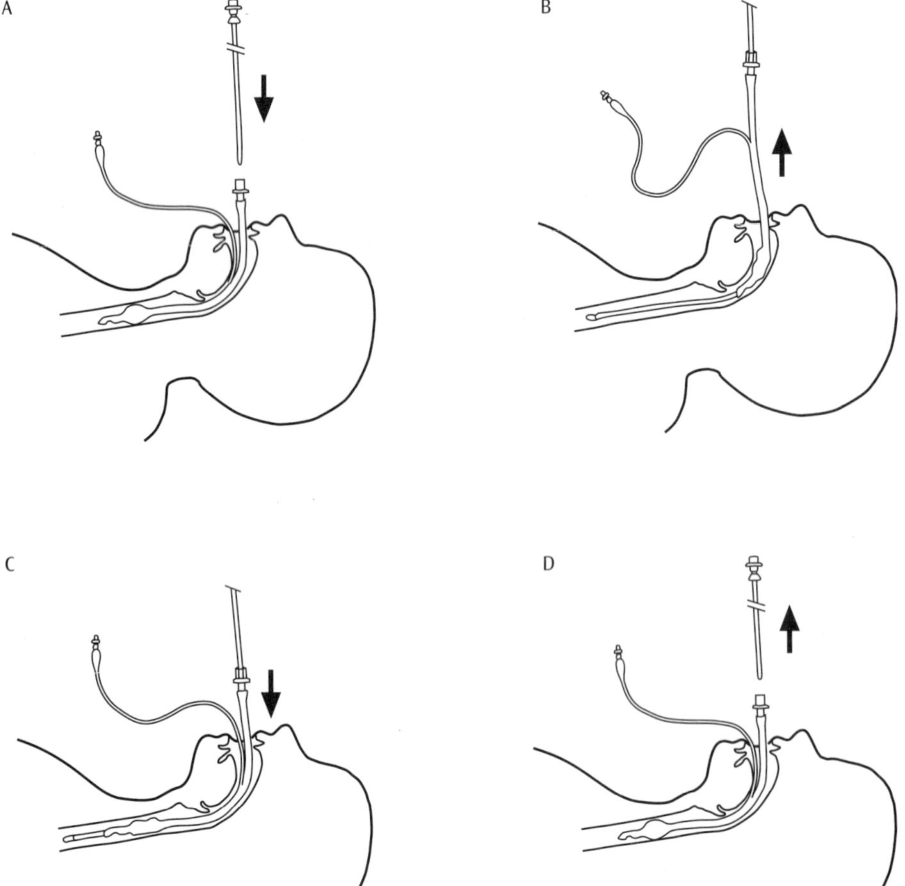

Figure 28.22 *Technique for tube guide use in extubation protocol. The choice of a hollow tube guide permits the insufflation of oxygen during the following maneuvers. (A) After preparation of the patient, the tube guide is inserted into the original endotracheal tube, so that its tip protrudes a centimeter beyond its bevel in the trachea. (B) The tube is then withdrawn over the guide, leaving the guide in place, ensuring that the guide's extent of insertion relative to the teeth is not changed. The patient is then observed for a period with the guide taped in place. (C) If spontaneous ventilation deteriorates and reintubation is necessary, a new tube is "railroaded" over the guide into the trachea. If the new tube will not pass the larynx, the guide permits the continuation of oxygen by insufflation until a smaller tube can be placed. (D) Once the patient is safely reintubated the guide is removed and the tube secured. (Reproduced with permission from Brown ACD. Anesthetic principles of airway management. In: Ferlito A (ed.).* Diseases of the Larynx. *London: Arnold, 2000.)*

Table 28.5 *Complications following extubation*

Laryngospasm
Edema of airway
Sore throat
Hoarse voice or loss of voice
Aspiration of gastric contents or foreign material
Vocal fold paralysis (nerve damage)
Vocal fold granulomata
Tracheomalacia
Noncardiogenic pulmonary edema
Tracheal stenosis
Incompetence of the larynx

Mayfield Swivel Horseshoe Head Rest may be very useful. The radiological monitor is placed so that it can be seen by both the radiologist and the anesthesiologist.

During the intubation, the anesthesiologist will view through the fiberoptic scope. The radiologist will provide a report of the image on the C-arm monitor screen. Using this method, it has been possible to guide the fiberoptic scope when blood, mucus, redundant tissue, etc. have temporarily obscured direct fiberoptic visualization. The use of the C-arm for patients who have suffered trauma enables the airway to be visualized with the fiberoptic scope within it.

The use of the C-arm enables the anesthesiologist or radiologist to know when the fiberoptic scope is being misdirected. Anterior/posterior (A/P) positioning of the fiberscope can be seen using the lateral view. The lateral view also identifies when the fiberscope is being directed to the left/right midline. Assuming that the image is a true lateral of the airway, the image of the scope, if in midline, should have a flat tip. Therefore, the first indication of a rounded appearance of the tip of the scope will alert the operator to the fact that the scope is moving away from the midline. Confirmation of left/right positioning can be made with the A/P view.

The most difficult intubations can often be performed with wire-guided intubation. Under C-arm guidance, a tracheal tube is positioned in the nasal or oral passage, although not too deeply. The fiberscope is then passed through the tracheal tube and guided by direct vision and/or with the C-arm so as to be pointed at the tip of the epiglottis and in view of the glottic opening. A flexible-tip guide wire is passed through the fiberscope suction channel and, under real-time fluorographic vision, advanced along the posterior surface of the epiglottis, through the vocal folds, and into the trachea to the carina. The fiberscope is then advanced (using the wire as a guide) into the trachea down to the point of the carina. The wire is then removed and the tracheal tube is advanced over the fiberscope. The fiberscope is used to confirm positioning of the tracheal tube tip at approximately four or five rings above the carina. The use of the C-arm need not be confined to those patients whose airway is known to be difficult; it may be used when no difficulty has been foreseen but when the intubation proves unexpectedly impossible.

Attention must be paid to radiation exposure dosage to both patients and staff. Patient exposure dosages average 300–450 mrad min^{-1}. This is very much in line with, or below, other ionizing imaging modalities. The average examination exposure time should be under 2 min actual fluorographic time for diagnosis.

Jet ventilation

The term "jet ventilation" has been used for different forms and means of introducing gas (oxygen) into the tracheobronchial tree. The technique may be used for laser surgery.[55] Another use has been advocated, i.e. for airway management of the difficult airway.[56] The latter involves the introduction of large-bore needles into the tracheal lumen. It is essentially a blind technique and incorrect placement or excessive pressure can produce a pneumothorax, pneumomediastinum, pneumotrachea, pneumolarynx, or pneumopericardium. However, in extreme situations when time is crucial, the technique can buy time. In

A

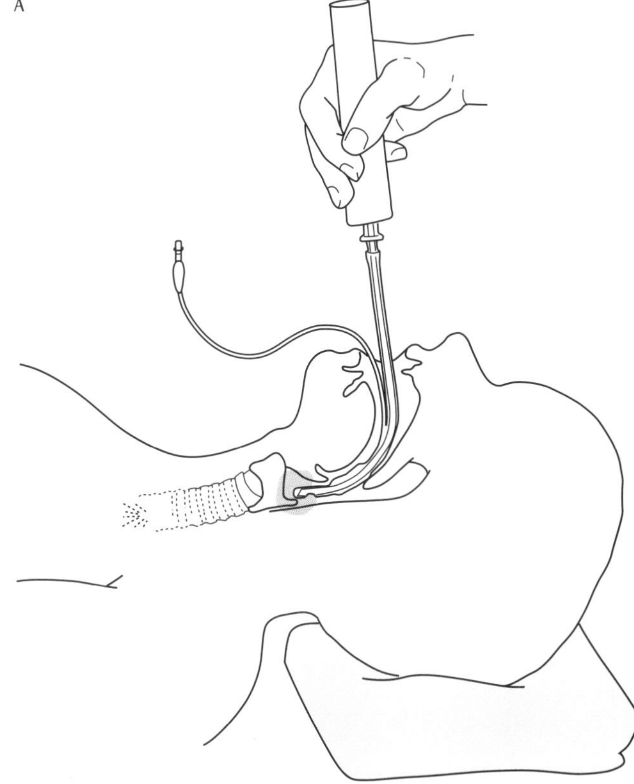

B

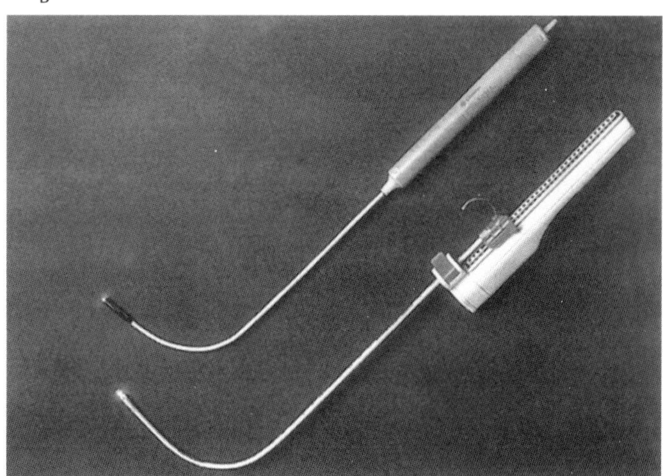

Figure 28.23 *Light-wand intubation. (A) The light wand in use. The tube is placed over the wand, which is then introduced to the midline hypopharynx with the patient in the standard "sniffing position." The wand is then manipulated until a "flare" of light down the trachea is seen transilluminating the neck. The tube is then slid off the wand into the trachea. (B) Two examples of proprietary light wands. The upper wand (Flexilum™) is cheap and robust but its use requires the tube to be cut to length, so it is better suited to planned use with standard tubes. The lower wand (Trachlight™) is more expensive but it permits the rapid use of uncut or preformed tubes by virtue of its adjustable wand section. (Reproduced with permission from Brown ACD. Anesthetic principles of airway management. In: Ferlito A (ed.).* Diseases of the Larynx. *London: Arnold, 2000.)*

this era of technological advances, flexible fiberoptic endoscopes, the Bullard laryngoscope, the Bellhouse laryngoscope, the noninvasive light wand, and intubation guides are recommended.

Jet ventilation via a "needle" placed within the lumen of an otolaryngological laryngoscope may permit laser surgery without a tracheal tube.[57] This is particularly suitable for patients with glottic, subglottic, and tracheal stenosis or other obstruction.

Retrograde intubation

This approach, originally suggested by Waters,[58] involves passing a needle via the cricothyroid membrane. A long, flexible catheter is advanced cephalad through the needle, the larynx, and out of the mouth (Fig. 28.24). The tracheal tube is either passed over this guide or tied to it via the Murphy eye. The major difficulty is guiding the tracheal tube past the epiglottis and vestibular/vocal folds. Suitable catheters include an epidural catheter and a fine ureteric stent.

There are many variations on this theme. Unfortunately, there are also a number of complications to be considered, including infection, needle laceration of the posterior tracheal wall, needle trauma to the vocal folds, amputation of a vocal fold by a sawing motion when attempting to pull the tethered tracheal tube past the epiglottis, and hemorrhage. This technique, as in the case of the transtracheal jet needle, should be used only as a last resort.

The Bullard laryngoscope

The Bullard laryngoscope (Fig. 28.25) has an associated stylet/guide which has greatly increased its application. The main advantage of the Bullard laryngoscope is that visualization of the upper airway is permitted, although there may be limited views of the orolaryngeal structures. The Bullard laryngoscope is an excellent aid for diagnostic evaluation of glottic/supraglottic airway obstruction or other malfunction, post-thyroidectomy evaluation of the vocal folds, and problems involving glossoptosis and basal macroglossia. However, it is inadequate for infraglottic diagnoses, placement of double-lumen tubes, or determining the position of the distal tip of a tracheal tube. In practiced hands, it can be used to introduce tracheal tubes through the glottic aperture.

The patient with facial trauma may present problems of distorted anatomy, massive edema, hemorrhage, urgency of management, shock, and air hunger. These pathologies are seen primarily following automobile accidents and gunshot (especially shotgun) wounds. Facial trauma is often accompanied by patient restlessness and inability to cooperate. The surgical option of tracheostomy may be limited by massive trauma of soft tissue in the neck. In this circumstance, the Bullard laryngoscope can be a useful aid to intubation.

The rigid bronchoscope

Foreign bodies in the airway as well as "clothes line" and "handle bar" (motorcycle, bicycle) injuries to the trachea represent a specific indication for use of the rigid bronchoscope. The terms "handle bar" and "clothes line" refer to trauma to the neck involving tracheal ring dislocation and, in rare cases, disruption. The injury is seen most frequently after motorcycle, bicycle, or snow-mobile accidents during which the rider is propelled toward the handle bar. Similar trauma is seen in touring car (convertible, cabriolet) accidents in which the top of the automobile is retracted, leaving a windshield extending upwards. The

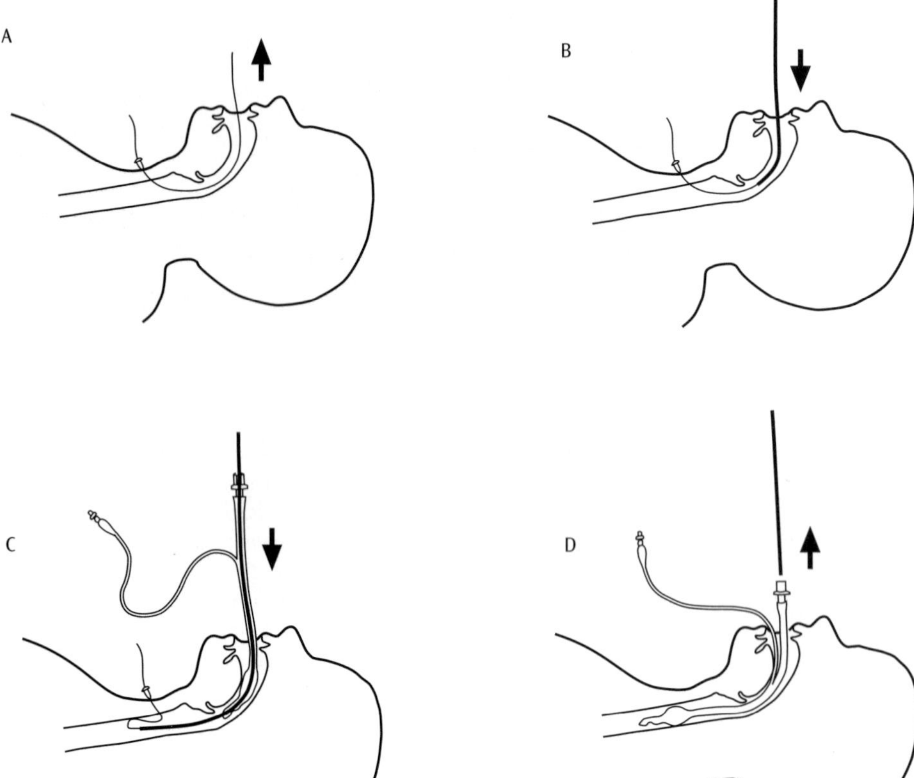

Figure 28.24 *Retrograde intubation. This illustration shows the principle of the technique using a proprietary retrograde intubation kit. (A) A soft wire is introduced via a cricothyroid needle puncture of the trachea, after instillation of local anesthetic, and passed gently cephalad until the end can be retrieved through the mouth. (B) A hollow tube guide is threaded over the wire which guides it into the trachea. (C) The guide is pushed below the point of insertion of the wire, and an endotracheal tube is "railroaded" over the guide into the trachea. (D) The wire is then cut at the point of insertion, to prevent contamination of the airway, and the guide and the wire are withdrawn from the airway. (Reproduced with permission from Brown ACD. Anesthetic principles of airway management. In: Ferlito A (ed.).* Diseases of the Larynx. *London: Arnold, 2000.)*

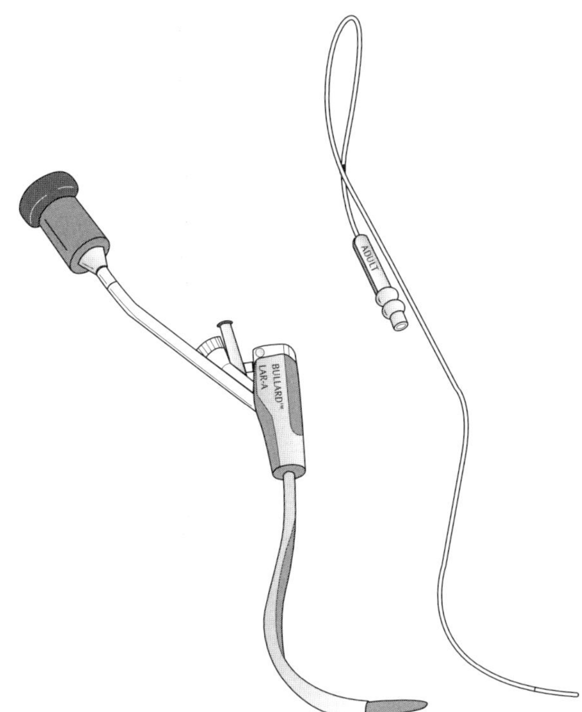

Figure 28.25 *The Bullard laryngoscope. (Reproduced with permission from Norton ML. The difficult airway. In: Healy TEJ, Cohen PJ (eds).* Wylie and Churchill-Davidson's A Practice of Anaesthesia, *6th edn. London: Edward Arnold, 1995.)*

"clothes line" description refers to runners or cyclists who literally run into a clothes line, producing a transection-like injury. The important factor to keep in mind is that there may be little external sign of trauma, but the injury must be suspected from the history of the accident. The patient usually has discomfort on swallowing and breathing. There is often minimal stridor or fremitus. On looking into the larynx and trachea, one may see arytenoid displacement (high injury) with skewing of the horizontal axis of the arytenoid/interarytenoideus complex. More often, the appearance of a cricoid shelf is noted below the level of the cricoid, which is a manifestation of tracheal ring dislocation. If the mucosa is swollen and discolored, disruption with hemorrhage and edema is evident. In this circumstance, immediate intubation and internal stenting are required to prevent near-total airway occlusion. Note particularly that these patients rarely tolerate the supine position. This is explained by the biomechanics of airway support.[42]

This situation is encountered primarily in the emergency room or in the patient rushed to the operating room. The techniques for management are as follows:

1 Foreign bodies in the upper airway can usually be visualized using a nasal speculum or nasopharyngeal mirror (nasal foreign bodies), or by indirect and direct laryngoscopy. In these situations, the prime loci are tonsillar fauces, vallecula of the epiglottis, pyriform sinuses, vestibule of the larynx (between vestibular and vocal folds), and at the level of the cricoid ring.
2 Foreign bodies in the trachea (including cricoid ring and extending into the main stem and lower bronchi) are most frequently found on the right side because of the angulation of the bronchi. These require a rigid bronchoscope for removal. In the anesthetic setting, the problem commonly occurs in the obstetric delivery room following aspiration of solid matter.

The bronchoscope should be inserted using direct laryngoscopy to rule out upper airway obstruction. The bevel of the bronchoscope should initially be facing posteriorly, visualizing any potential cricopharyngeal lesion (e.g. Zenker's pouch or diverticulum). When entering the larynx, the bevel should be directed laterally to approximate the long axis of the rima glottidis and vocal folds. On passage, the level should again be directed posteriorly, watching for pulsations suggestive of aneurysmal encroachment on the soft wall of the trachea (especially in the elderly patient).

When the foreign body is visualized, it should be impacted into the distal end of the bronchoscope (by grasping forceps or use of a Fogarty catheter vascular balloon). Then both the object and the bronchoscope are removed as one unit. No attempt should be made to pull the object through the bronchoscope.

"Clothes line" or "handle bar" injuries present a very different problem. There may or may not be a true "fracture" of the tracheal cartilages. Usually, there is more of a disruption of continuity of the trachea with dislocations of the "rings." This then presents a figure-of-eight configuration with some overlapping. The mucosae may not be disrupted, but may have an internal shelf-like configuration. The objective then is to restore the anatomic pattern of the rings and splint them for optimum channel integrity. A bronchoscopic telescope (0° or 180°) is of great value in delineating the lumen. The bronchoscope itself can be used as a tracheal stent or passed through a tracheal tube. Once in place, the bronchoscope can be removed, leaving the tracheal tube in the tracheal lumen as a stent. An alternative approach is rigid bronchoscopy, followed by insertion of an intubation guide to assist the passage of a tracheal tube. This technique must be used with extreme caution because the tip of the tracheal tube may impinge on the dislocated tracheal ring, causing further disruption of the channel.

The essential warning in these situations is never to advance an instrument without visualizing the distal pathway, and certainly never against resistance.

Transmission of infection

Some patients with upper airway problems have chronic infection, particularly in the nasal passages and paranasal sinuses. Patients with relatively flat facies, a depressed nasal bridge, and a deviated nasal septum or post-traumatic obstruction fall into this category, as do those with herpetic lesions.

The problem that arises is the transmission of infection via the endoscopes or tracheal tubes during the process of "controlling" the airway. Concern should be directed toward disinfection or sterilization of the instruments.[59] Instruments, including suction channels, should be flushed with cold water as soon as possible after use to wash away blood and other debris before it dries. Insertion of a fresh channel brush in fiberoptic suction channels to remove particulate matter is also advised.

Postoperative management

A patient who has been very difficult to intubate may be exceedingly difficult to extubate safely or to reintubate should this become necessary. Serious consideration should be given to placing an intubation guide before extubation. This will facilitate reintubation during the immediate postoperative period and until the airway is considered safe. This can be carried out with ease in adults, and the option is now readily available for children.

When the decision is made to extubate the patient, the tracheal tube connector (proximal end) should be removed. Then, the guide is passed intraluminally to a depth below the distal end of the tracheal tube. The tube is removed, leaving the guide in place for 1.5–2 h. Experience has confirmed that situations requiring reintubation occur well within this period. Simultaneously, the larynx and trachea should be moisturized with appropriate nebulization, e.g. racemic epinephrine (adrenaline) in saline and dexamethasone may be administered to counteract edema development. Patients may be given 4 mg dexamethasone before intubation, 4 mg more during surgery, and 4 mg in the recovery room.

An ice collar is often applied, although this may have more psychologic effect than physical value.

Perhaps the most useful ancillary aid is the sitting position. This promotes venous drainage and biomechanically opens up the airway.

Pediatrics

There are fundamental differences between the airway of the adult and that of the small child, and airway management for pediatric patients requires an understanding of developmental anatomy linked with an understanding of the mechanics of the airway function of the tongue, pharynx, epiglottis, larynx, and subglottic tissues (cricoid ring). The bony configurations of the mandible, temporomandibular joints, palate, nose, and dentition must also be considered. Routine airway maintenance requires a different approach, not just a different size of the equipment. The child's head is larger in relation to the body than that of the adult. Positioning a roll under the shoulders may therefore be rather more helpful for the child than for the adult (Fig. 28.26). When a face mask is used, it must be remembered that dead space in relation to the patient's airway is relatively larger than that in an adult. When a tracheal tube is selected, it is necessary to consider the use of an uncuffed tube. The correct size can be determined from the commonly used formula (Chapter 59). The narrowest part of a child's upper airway is at the level of the cricoid and not at the laryngeal aperture.

Children may present with morphologic abnormalities or abnormal function due to a variety of disease processes. The most common morphologic anomalies involve mandibular dysostoses such as the Pierre Robin anomaly as well as associated macroglossia (Beckwith–Wiedemann syndrome and cystic hygroma, among others). Careful assessment is crucial, as many of these syndromes have coexistent midfacial hypoplasia (Stickler, Treacher Collins, Goldenhar syndromes) or velocardiofacial syndromes with pharyngeal hypotonia. The mucopolysaccharidoses (Hurler and Hunter syndromes) represent aberrations of both structure and function. A combination of facial, upper airway, and cervical spine (often with thoracic components) anomalies produces major difficulties in airway management in these patients.

Apart from the above, airway obstruction may occur for a variety of reasons, even in morphologically normal patients. The anteroposterior diameters of head and thorax which influence neck extension, as well as relative macroglossia and glossoptosis, contribute to our concerns. Thus, variation in the patient's oxygenation and ventilation requirements will also affect flow patterns across the site of a relative obstruction. Management of these patients is superficially analogous to that of the adult. However, the margin of safety and tendency to convert from urgent to emergency airway conditions are increased. For a detailed discussion, the reader is referred to Chapters 58 and 59 on pediatric and neonatal anesthesia.

The bleeding tonsil

The patient with a bleeding tonsil bed represents a frightening situation for any anesthesiologist, however experienced. It demands a particular care in its management. The patient with a bleeding tonsil should be placed on the operating table in the lateral position on his/her left or right side depending on whether the anesthesiologist holds the laryngoscope in his/her left or right hand respectively, i.e. the patient lies left side down for an anesthesiologist who is holding the laryngoscope in his/her left hand. The reason for this is to avoid the need to perform a laryngoscopy while at the same time struggling to prevent a slippery tongue falling under gravity into the field of vision, i.e. gravity is used to help rather than hinder laryngoscopy. Additionally, the need to rotate the head to obtain a satisfactory view under the hand and the laryngoscope handle is obviated. Some anesthesiologists remove the pillow support for the head. The absence of a pillow facilitates gravity drainage of blood away from the larynx. Alternatively, the pillow may be left *in situ* to stabilize the head and the table adjusted to provide a few degrees of head-down tilt. The assistant or assistants support the patient in the lateral position during the laryngoscopy. An appropriate induction technique using 100% oxygen is used. A variety of tracheal tube sizes and laryngoscope blades must be instantly available. When an adequate depth of anesthesia for laryngoscopy is achieved, the table may be raised to the appropriate height for the anesthesiologist. The laryngoscope may then be introduced. The absence of a pillow or the use of a pillow with a slight head-down tilt ensures that the bleeding points are below the larynx. After intubation, any blood or other debris may be removed from the mouth and pharynx, the table lowered, and the patient turned to the supine position (Fig. 28.27).

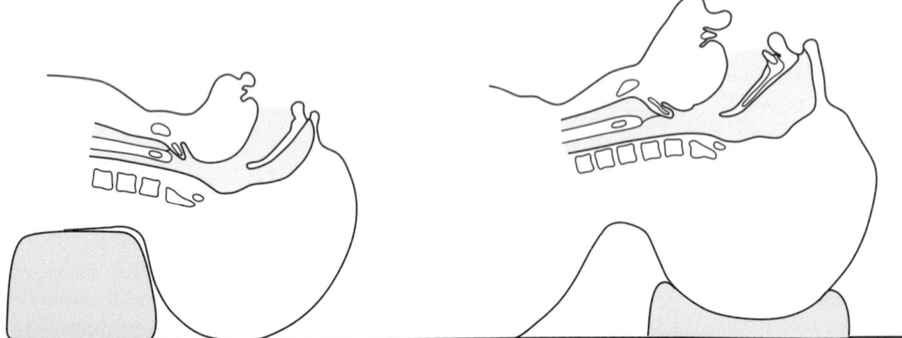

Figure 28.26 *When positioning the head for intubation in the young infant, the use of a smaller pillow together with a roll under the shoulders is recommended because a child (left) has a larger head compared with the body than does an adult (right).*

A

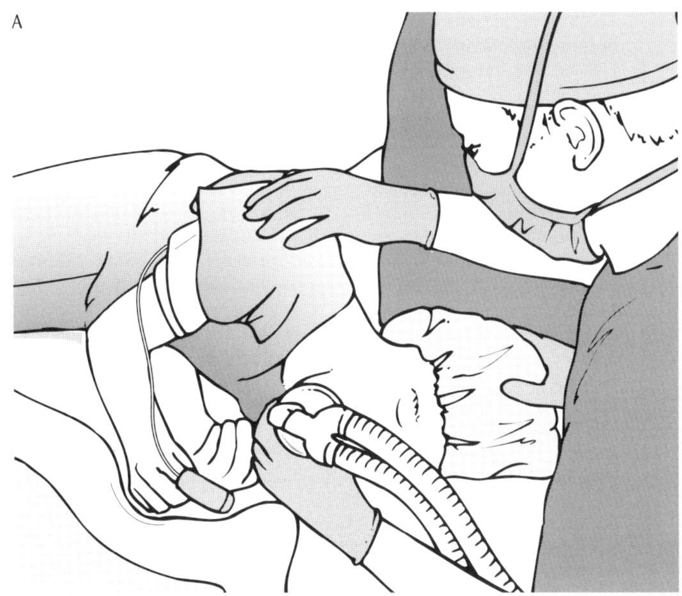

B

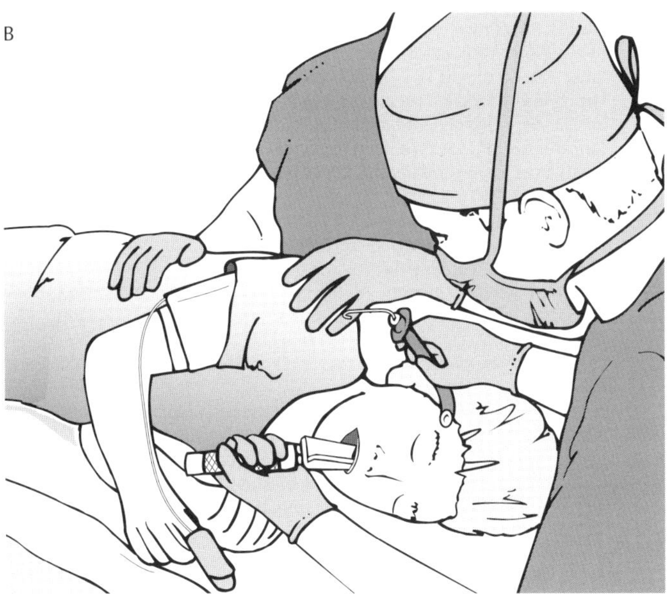

C

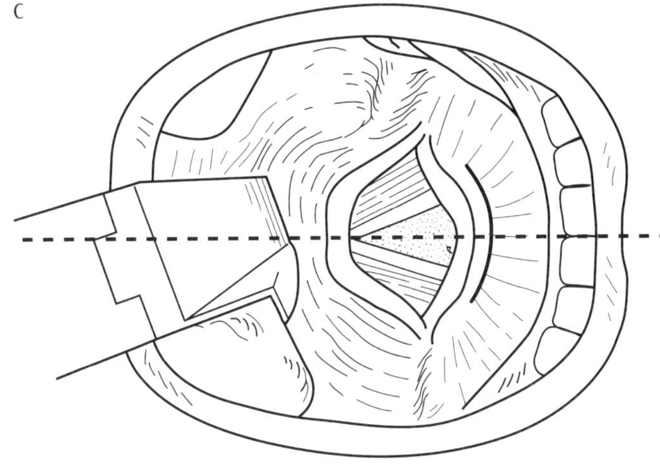

Figure 28.27 *(A) The patient is placed on the operating table in the "tonsil position" on the left side with an assistant to steady the patient during inhalation induction. (B) When stable third-stage anesthesia is achieved, the patient is rolled into the full lateral position with minimal support under the head to facilitate gravity drainage of blood or secretions from the mouth. (C) The laryngoscope blade is now introduced, but instead of lifting in the usual sagittal plane, the tongue and mandible are lifted at a 45° angle to the plane. This permits the pooling of contaminants inside the left cheek and drainage from the mouth.*

REFERENCES

1. Atkinson RS, Rushman GB, Lee JA. Tracheal intubation. In: Atkinson RS, Rushman GB, Lee JA (eds). *A Synopsis of Anaesthesia*, 8th edn. Bristol: John Wright and Sons, 1977: 237–59.
2. Brain AI, McGhee TD, McAteer EJ, *et al*. The laryngeal mask airway. Development and preliminary trials of a new type of airway. *Anaesthesia* 1985; **40:** 356–61.
3. Brain AI. The laryngeal mask: a new concept in airway management. *Br J Anaesth* 1983; **55:** 801–5.
4. Kapila A, Addy EV, Verghese C, Brain AIJ. The intubating laryngeal mask airway: an initial assessment of performance *Br J Anaesth*, 1997; **79:** 710–13.
5. Sidaras G, Hunter JM. Is it safe to artificially ventilate a paralysed patient through the laryngeal mask? The jury is still out. *Br J Anaesth* 2001; **86:** 749–53.
6. McCrory C, McShane AJ. Laryngeal mask airway is associated with reflux in the lithotomy position. *Br J Anaesth* 1996; **77:** 693.
7. Agro F, Frass M, Benumof JL, Krafft P. Current status of the Combitube: a review of the literature. *J Clin Anesth* 2002; **14:** 307–14.
8. O'Flaherty D, Adams AP. The end-tidal carbon dioxide detector: assessment of a new method to distinguish oesophageal from tracheal intubation. *Anaesthesia* 1990; **45:** 653–5.
9. Williams KN, Nunn JF. The oesophageal detector device. A prospective trial on 100 patients. *Anaesthesia* 1989; **44:** 412–14.
10. Shribman AJ, Smith G, Achola KJ. Cardiovascular and catecholamine responses to laryngoscopy with and without tracheal intubation. *Br J Anaesth* 1987; **59:** 295–9.
11. Kautto UM. Attenuation of the circulatory response to laryngoscopy and intubation by fentanyl. *Acta Anaesth Scand* 1982; **26:** 217–21.
12. Tam S, Chung F, Campbell M. Intravenous lidocaine: optimal time of injection before tracheal intubation. *Anesth Analg* 1987; **66:** 1036–8.
13. Sheppard S, Eagle CJ, Strunin L. A bolus dose of esmolol attenuates tachycardia and hypertension after tracheal intubation. *Can J Anaesth* 1990; **37:** 202–5.
14. Stoelting RK. Attenuation of blood pressure responses to laryngoscopy and tracheal intubation with sodium nitroprusside. *Anesth Analg* 1979; **58:** 116–19.
15. Grover VK, Sharma S, Mahajan RP, Singh H. Effect of intranasal nitro-

glycerine on circulatory responses to laryngoscopy and endotracheal intubation. *Indian J Med Res* 1987; **86:** 629–34.

16. Scarlett M, Crawford-Sykes A, Nelson M. Preoperative starvation and pulmonary aspiration. New perspectives and guidelines. *West Indian Med J* 2002; **51:** 241–5.
17. Kallar SK, Everett LL. Potential risks and preventive measures for pulmonary aspiration: new concepts in preoperative fasting guidelines. *Anesth Analg* 1993; **77:** 171–82.
18. American Society of Anesthesiologists, Committee on Professional Liability. Preliminary study of closed claims. *ASA Newsletter* 1988; 4, **52:** 8–10.
19. Caplan RA, Ward RJ, Posner K, *et al.* Unexpected cardiac arrest during spinal anesthesia: closed claims analysis of pre-disposing factors. *Anesthesiology* 1988; **68:** 5–11.
20. Caplan RA, Posner K, Ward RJ, *et al.* Adverse respiratory events in anesthesia: a closed claims analysis. *Anesthesiology* 1990; **72:** 828–33.
21. Holland R. Anesthesia related mortality in Australia. In: Pierce EC, Cooper JB (eds). *Instructional Anesthesia Clinics.* Boston: Little, Brown, 1984: 61–71.
22. Department of Health and Social Security. Report on Confidential Enquiries into Maternal Deaths in England and Wales, 1979–1981. *Report on Health and Social Security Subjects, 29.* London: HMSO, 1986.
23. King TA, Adams AP. Failed tracheal intubation. *Br J Anaesth* 1990; **65:** 400–14.
24. Mallampati SR, Gatt SP, Gugino LD, *et al.* A clinical sign to predict difficult tracheal intubation: a prospective study. *Can Anaesth Soc J* 1985; **32:** 429–34.
25. Patil VU, Stehling LC, Zaunder HL. *Fiberoptic Endoscopy in Anesthesia.* Chicago: Year Book Medical, 1983.
26. Frerk CM Predicting difficult intubation. *Anaesthesia* 1991; **46:** 1005–8.
27. White A, Kander PL. Anatomical factors in difficult direct laryngoscopy. *Br J Anaesth* 1975; **47:** 468.
28. Mark LJ, Beattie C, Ferrell CL, *et al.* The difficult airway: mechanisms for effective dissemination of critical information. *J Clin Anesth* 1992; 4, **3:** 247–51.
29. Latto IP, Rosen M. Management of difficult intubation. In: Latto IP, Rosen M (eds). *Difficulties in Tracheal Intubation.* Eastbourne: Bailliere Tindall, 1985: Ch. 7.
30. Norton ML, Brown ACD. The difficult airway clinic. In: Norton ML, Brown ACD (eds). *Atlas of the Difficult Airway.* St Louis: Mosby Year Book, 1991: Ch. 4.
31. Norton ML, Wilton N, Brown AC. The difficult airway clinic. *Anesthesiol Rev* 1988; **15:** 25–8.
32. Smalhout BA. *Quick Guide to Capnography and its Use in Differential Diagnosis.* Boblingen: Hewlett Packard Medical Products Group, 1983.
33. Elze CJ. Anatomie des Kehlkopfes. In: Denker A (ed.). *Handbuch des Halo, Nasen Ohrenteilkunde.* Berlin: Springer, c. 1868.
34. Dripps RD, Eckenhoff E, Vandam LD. *Introduction to Anaesthesia*, 6th edn. Philadelphia: WB Saunders, 1982.
35. Cormack RS, Lehane J. Difficult tracheal intubation in obstetrics. *Anaesthesia* 1984; **39:** 1105–11.
36. Salem MR, Joseph NJ, Heyman HJ, *et al.* Cricoid compression is effective in obliterating the esophageal lumen in the presence of a nasogastric tube. *Anesthesiology* 1985; **63:** 443–6.
37. Sellick BA. Cricoid pressure to control regurgitation of stomach contents during induction of anaesthesia. *Lancet* 1961; **2:** 404.
38. Jones BC. Lingual nerve injury: a complication of intubation. *Br J Anaesth* 1971; **43:** 730.
39. Terchner RL. Lingual nerve injury: a complication of orotracheal intubation. *Br J Anaesth* 1971; **43:** 413–44.
40. Brock-Utney JG, Jaffo RA. Tracheal intubation with the patient in a sitting position. *Br J Anaesth* 1991; **67:** 225–6.
41. Fink BR. *The Human Larynx: a Functional Study.* New York: Raven Press, 1975: 42.
42. Fink BR, Demarest RJ. *Laryngeal Biomechanics.* Cambridge, MA: Harvard University Press, 1978.
43. Norton ML, Brown ACD. Fig. 15–4. In: Norton ML, Brown ACD (eds). *Atlas of the Difficult Airway.* St Louis: Mosby Year Book, 1991: 184.
44. Norton ML, Brown ACD. Fig. 15–3. In: Norton ML, Brown ACD (eds). *Atlas of the Difficult Airway.* St Louis: Mosby Year Book, 1991: 184.
45. Gosgnach M, Ghedira S, Xiang J, *et al.* Incidence of maxillary sinusitis in recently intubated critically ill patients. *Anesthesiology* 1990; **73:** A1224.
46. Leguillou JL, Rouby JJ, Xiang J, *et al.* Endotracheal intubation induced sinusitis and nosocomial pneumonia in critically ill patients. *Anesthesiology* 1991; **75:** A1019; and Endotracheal intubation induced maxillary sinusitis: a prospective randomized study. *Anesthesiology* 1991; **75:** 1020.
47. Rouby JJ, Rossignon MD, Nicolas MH, *et al.* A prospective study of protected bronchoalveolar lavage in the diagnosis of nosocomial pneumonia. *Anesthesiology* 1989; **71:** 679–85.
48. Allison A, McCrory J. Tracheal placement of a gum elastic bougie using the laryngeal mask. *Anaesthesia* 1990; **45:** 419–20.
49. Ovassapian A, Schrader SC. Fiber-optic-aided bronchial intubation. *Semin Anesth* 1987; **7:** 133–42.
50. Benger RC, Chang J-L. A jet-stylet endotracheal catheter for difficult airway management. *Anesthesiology* 1987; **66:** 221–3.
51. Ducrow M Throwing light on blind intubation. *Anesthesia* 1978; **33:** 827–9.
52. Norton ML, Brown ACD. Fig. 15–11. In: Norton M, Brown ACD (eds). *Atlas of the Difficult Airway.* St Louis: Mosby Year Book, 1991: 193.
53. Lowe AA, Gionhaku N, Takeuchi K, *et al.* Three-dimensional CT reconstructions of tongue and airway in adult subjects with obstructive sleep apnea. *Am J Orthod Dentofacial Orthop* 1986; **90:** 364–73.
54. Katsantonis GP, Walsh JK. Somnofluoroscopy: its role in the selection of candidates for uvulopalatopharyngoplasty. *Orolaryngol Head Neck Surg* 1966; **94:** 1.
55. Norton ML, Strong S, Vaughan C. Endotracheal intubation and Venturi (jet) ventilation for laser microsurgery of the larynx. *Ann Otol Rhinol Laryngol* 1976; **85:** 656–64.
56. Benumof JL. Management of the difficult adult airway. With special emphasis on awake tracheal intubation. *Anesthesiology* 1991; **75:** 1087–110.
57. Spink LK. *Principles and Practice of Flow Meter Engineering*, 8th edn. Foxboro, MA: Foxboro Co., 1958.
58. Waters DJ. Guided blind endotracheal intubation. *Anaesthesia* 1963; **18:** 158–62.
59. Centers for Disease Control. Nosocomial infections and pseudoinfection from contaminated endoscopes and bronchoscopes. *Wisconsin Missouri MMWR* 1991; **40:** 675–8. Reprinted in *JAMA* 1991; **266:** 2197–8.

FURTHER READING

Fried MP. *The Larynx.* Boston: Little Brown, 1988.

Latto IP, Rosen M (eds). *Difficulties in Tracheal Intubation.* Eastbourne: Bailliere Tindall, 1985.

Norton ML (ed.). *Atlas of the Difficult Airway*, 2nd edn. St Louis: Mosby Year Book, 1996.

29

The anesthetic machine and breathing systems

CHRISTOPHER J VALLIS, PETER HUTTON, THOMAS H CLUTTON-BROCK, AND ROGER STEDMAN

UNITS AND SYSTEMS OF MEASUREMENT

There is a profusion of different systems of units in use across the world. Traditional units tended to be defined in terms of a convenient quantity, e.g. a foot (of length), an atmosphere (of pressure), a knot (of velocity), or a horsepower (of power). To provide a common set of internationally agreed units, the Système International d'Unités (or SI units; see also Chapter 3) was agreed by most countries at a conference in Paris in 1960. However, many units outside this system remain in common use.

The advantages of SI units are:

- It is a decimal system based on unchanging, fundamental, and reproducible units.
- Derived units are built up from fundamental units.
- All units and derived units mean the same in all branches of science. Thus a joule, a unit of energy that combines dimensions of mass, time, and length, is the same whether it refers to a unit of electrical, mechanical, or heat energy.

The SI practice is to use the basic unit or multiples of 10^3 or 10^{-3} in expressing numerical values. Thus, length is expressed in meters (10^1), millimeters (10^{-3}), and kilometers (10^3). Other examples are given in Table 29.1.

To prevent errors in clinical practice, the particular multiple chosen should avoid decimals wherever possible. There is then less likely to be confusion when, for example, the dose of a drug is expressed as 50 μg rather than 0.05 mg, or worse still 0.00005 g.

Derived units

Area, volume, and flow

Area is expressed in square meters (m^2), or in convenient multiples, e.g. mm^2. Other common units are square feet and square miles. Volume is in cubic meters or m^3. The liter (1000 mL) is a special name for the cubic decimeter and is not an SI unit but is retained for general use. $1\ m^3 = 10^3$ L.

Flow is the measure of volume per unit time. In anesthesia, the common units are liters per minute ($L\,min^{-1}$). If it is a gas that is flowing, then it is usually referred to a given temperature and pressure.

Velocity and acceleration

Velocity (v) is the rate of change of distance with time (meters per second or $m\,s^{-1}$) and acceleration (a) is the rate of change of velocity with time (meters per second, per second or $m\,s^{-2}$). The constant acceleration known as the *acceleration due to gravity* is $9.81\ m\,s^{-2}$, although it varies slightly at different latitudes. It is given the symbol g.

Force and pressure

Force (F) is that property which when applied to a mass causes acceleration, or a change in the direction of motion. The SI unit of force is the newton (N), which is defined as that force which, if applied to mass of 1 kg, gives it an acceleration of 1 meter per s per s ($1\ m\,s^{-2}$) along the line of the applied force (i.e. $F = ma$). A newton, in gravitational terms, exerts the same force as the gravitational pull on 102 g (i.e. a small apple). Commonly used traditional units of force, the kg weight or lb weight, are equal to the force of gravitational attraction on a mass of 1 kilogram or 1 pound respectively.

Pressure is the intensity of force over a defined area such that:

$$\text{Pressure} = \text{total force } (F)/\text{total area } (A) = \text{force per unit area}$$

Force is measured in newtons and area in m^2. The force of 1 N applied uniformly over an area of $1\ m^2$ produces a pressure of 1 pascal (Pa). This is such a small pressure that kilopascals (kPa) are used in

Table 29.1 *Multipliers used in the SI system*

Multiplier	Power of 10	Symbol	Example
Pico	10^{-12}	(p)	Picofarads, a measurement of capacitance
Nano	10^{-9}	(n)	Nanomoles, a number of hydrogen ions
Micro	10^{-6}	(μ)	Micrograms, drug dosage
Milli	10^{-3}	(m)	Milliamps, current to cause ventricular fibrillation
Kilo	10^3	(k)	Kilopascals, pressure
Mega	10^6	(M)	Megawatts, the power from an electricity generator
Giga	10^9	(G)	Gigabytes, as in computer memory

medicine. The principle of pressure being a distribution of force over area is immediately understood if one imagines a person wearing skis or stiletto heels. The dangers of localized pressure damage to skin or nerves during anesthesia are well recognized by anesthesiologists.

Pressure retains some traditional units in common use such as pounds per square inch (p.s.i.), millimeters of mercury (mmHg), centimeters of water (cmH_2O), and atmospheres. All traditional units of pressure involve the use of the force of gravity or the height of a liquid column supported by the atmosphere. The bar, although not an SI unit, is an approved unit of pressure, equal to 100 kPa. It is approximately equal to the atmospheric pressure at sea level:

1 bar = 100 kPa = approximately 760 mmHg = approximately 1000 cmH_2O = approximately 14.7 p.s.i.

Figure 29.1 shows practical examples of the relation between pressures, forces, and areas.

The type of device used to measure pressure depends upon the magnitude of the pressure under consideration. For clinical use in anesthesia, electronic transducers, Bourdon gauges, aneroid gauges, and liquid columns can all be used.

Gauge pressure describes the pressure *above* atmospheric pressure. Absolute pressure *includes* atmospheric pressure. The pressure in a full oxygen cylinder can be quoted as 137 bar gauge pressure or 138 bar absolute pressure. Negative pressure (properly called subatmospheric pressure) always refers to gauge pressure as negative absolute pressures do not exist.

Energy, work, and power

Energy and work are closely inter-related but not identical: when work is done, in essence it is the manifestation of energy being released in a useful and controlled fashion, e.g. the burning of petrol in a car engine. If energy is released in an uncontrolled manner, e.g. when a volcano erupts, no useful work results. Heat is also a form of stored energy. Because of this link, energy, work, and heat are measured in the same units. The SI unit is the joule (J) and 1 joule is the work done when a force of 1 newton moves through 1 meter in the direction of the force. One joule therefore is synonymous with 1 newton meter (N m). The most common non-SI unit of heat is the calorie, which is defined as the amount of heat needed to raise 1 g of water through 1 °C.

Energy exists in two main forms, kinetic and potential. Kinetic energy is a property of a moving body and the energy it possesses is released as it slows down. The formula for kinetic energy is $\frac{1}{2}mv^2$ (m = mass; v = velocity). By virtue of the form of this equation, at low speed, kinetic energy depends principally on the mass of the body, whereas at high speed the velocity becomes the dominant term. This is why an object of low mass, e.g. a bullet, can be so destructive.

A body has potential energy because of its position or state: there is no visual expression of its presence. Potential energy can exist in many forms, e.g.:

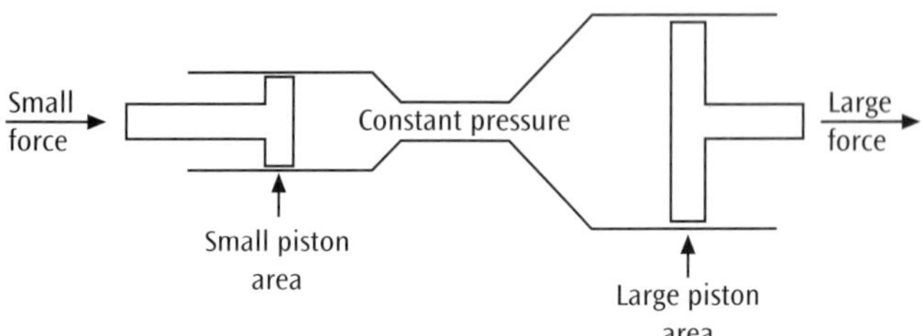

Figure 29.1 *Relation between pressure, forces, and area (see also Fig. 29.8).*

- compression, extension, or deformation of elastic materials, e.g. a wound-up spring;
- chemical bonds, e.g. energy stores such as oil, carbohydrates, or fats;
- compression of gases, e.g. air hoses, rockets;
- high-temperature fluids, e.g. heat exchangers;
- stored charge in an electrical capacitor;
- height above surroundings, e.g. weight at the top of a slope, a pile-driver hammer; under these conditions, the potential energy of a mass m which falls through a height h under gravity releases $m \times g \times h$ joules, where g is the acceleration due to gravity.

The principle of conservation of energy states that a given amount of energy in one form can be converted into a variety of other forms of energy, or converted into work, but the sum total of the energy expressed in each form is always equal to the original amount. This is the first law of thermodynamics. Work is, however, a more valuable form of energy than heat: although work can always be totally transformed into heat, heat can never be completely transformed into work. This is a consequence of the second law of thermodynamics. No process converting heat to work can run at 100% efficiency: most engines run at well below 50% efficiency and steam engines often struggle to reach 3%. When mechanical energy is turned into heat, because the conversion is 100%, there is a fixed relation between the work done and the heat generated. This ratio is called the mechanical equivalent of heat and is approximately 0.24 calories to 1 joule (more frequently written as 4.2 joules to 1 calorie).

Power is the rate at which energy is expended, often in doing work. It is measured in watts, which are equal to joules per second or newton meters per second ($N\,m\,s^{-1}$). Step aerobics provides a familiar idea of the difference between work and power. The same work (increase in potential energy) is done by getting up on to the step no matter how long it takes. The power expended depends on the number of steps made in a unit of time. In a similar manner, the work done by electricity is the energy needed to move a charge against a potential difference [voltage (V)]. Current (I) is charge being moved per second, so electrical power is ($V \times I$) measured in joules per second or watts.

SOLIDS, LIQUIDS, AND GASES

Changes of state

Given the correct conditions of temperature and pressure, most substances can exist as either a solid, a liquid, or a gas. Solids are held together by three-dimensional intermolecular bonds, which hold the molecules in a fixed position relative to each other. When subject to stress, solids deform and the amount of deformation is measured by a property known as their elasticity. The commonest expression of this is Hooke's law, which states that, within the elastic limit, the extension of a metal bar is proportional to the load. The elastic limit is the load that is sufficient to seriously disrupt the internal molecular structure and cause permanent damage to it.

Liquids do not have such strong intermolecular forces as solids and hence deform easily and are capable of flowing. All the molecules are, however, closely packed together so applied forces result in a change of shape but not in a change in volume: because of this, liquids are often termed "incompressible." The "stickiness" (or viscosity) of liquids, which determines how easily their adjacent layers slide over one another, is measured by the coefficient of viscosity. The higher the coefficient, the more difficult it is to produce flow. The hematocrit is the main determinant of the viscosity of the blood. With a normal hematocrit, the viscosity of blood is more than twice that of the plasma alone.

Gases have weak intermolecular forces that allow individual molecules to flow freely in random directions. Most of the volume of a gas is in fact empty space, the total volume of the molecules occupying only a minute fraction of the gas volume. This allows gases to be compressed and their volume reduced. The pressure exerted by a gas results from the momentum change of all its molecules hitting the wall of the container and bouncing back into the body of the gas. The magnitude of the momentum change, which determines the pressure, depends upon the velocity of the individual molecules. This velocity, in turn, depends on the temperature of the gas. Kinetic theory predicts that the average kinetic energy of a molecule is directly proportional to the absolute temperature of the gas. Hence, as the temperature of the gas in a closed container rises, so does the pressure exerted on the walls of the container.

It could be assumed from the above that if the compression of a gas continued inexorably, it would eventually be liquefied. In the majority of instances, this is true. If, however, the temperature is high enough, such is the momentum of the individual molecules that, however much the pressure is increased, liquefaction remains impossible. This temperature, above which a gas cannot be liquefied, is known as its critical temperature. It varies enormously depending on the gas, being 36.5 °C for nitrous oxide and –118 °C for oxygen. Because of their importance in anesthesia, the properties of gases are considered in more detail later.

Latent heat

Water is a good example of a common substance that can exist as a solid, liquid, or gas. If a beaker of water in a standard atmosphere has a steady flow of heat applied to it, the graph of temperature against time will be as shown in Fig. 29.2. It can be seen from this that there are two plateaux at 0 °C and 100 °C on an otherwise steadily rising slope. From A to B, ice is being turned into water at 0 °C, and from C to D water is being turned into steam at 100 °C. The energy required to change from a solid at A to a liquid at B is known as the latent heat of fusion and has a value of 19 J g^{-1} (80 cal g^{-1}). Hence, it takes as much energy to melt 1 g of ice as it does to then raise its temperature to 80 °C. It can be seen from Fig. 29.2 that the ratio of AB:CD is equal to 80:540 because the latent heat of vaporization (or evaporation) is 128.6 J g^{-1} (540 cal g^{-1}). The energy required to convert from liquid to gas is therefore much more than that required to convert from solid to liquid.

Vaporization

As is known from everyday experience, a pool of water does not have to be at 100 °C for it to evaporate by converting from a gas to a liquid. So, how can the experiment defining latent heat (as described above) be reconciled with this? The explanation lies in the link between temperature (which reflects the average molecular kinetic energy) and the kinetic energy of individual molecules as shown in Fig. 29.3. It can be seen that there is a wide range of individual kinetic energies and that the higher-energy molecules have sufficient energy to leave the liquid. As they do, the average kinetic energy of those remaining falls, and with it the temperature of the remaining liquid.

Now consider an open dish containing liquid in a closed container. Under these conditions, if there is sufficient liquid, the liquid will evaporate until the number of molecules leaving the liquid is equal to those returning by random motion. Then, if the temperature remains constant, a form of equilibrium will be established between the liquid and the vapor. Under these conditions, the partial pressure exerted by the vapor is termed the saturated vapor pressure (SVP) at that temperature. As the temperature rises, the average and individual kinetic energies of the molecules increases because the SVP depends only on the temperature. A demonstration of this and a comparison of isoflurane with water is shown in Fig. 29.4. Gases close to saturation conditions do not behave as perfect gases because of intermolecular forces; this is described later in the section on nitrous oxide.

In order for a vaporizer to be useful in clinical practice, it must give a constant concentration of vapor over a wide range of flows and settings. Their design therefore employs wicks (to increase the evaporative area), thermal buffering, and temperature-sensitive control mechanisms. For details of these factors, specialized texts should be consulted.

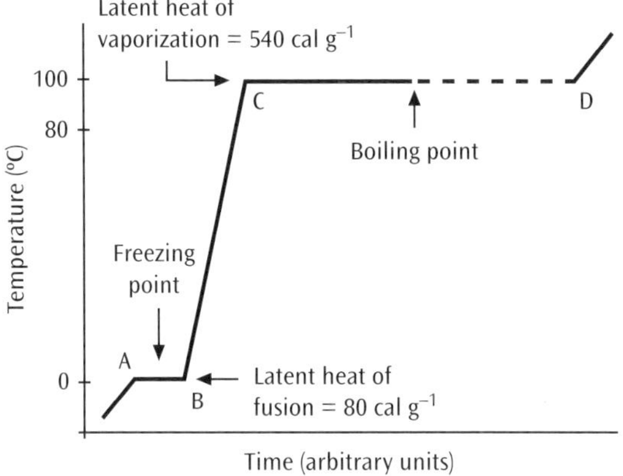

Figure 29.2 *Behavior of ice when heated steadily. Figure not to scale.*

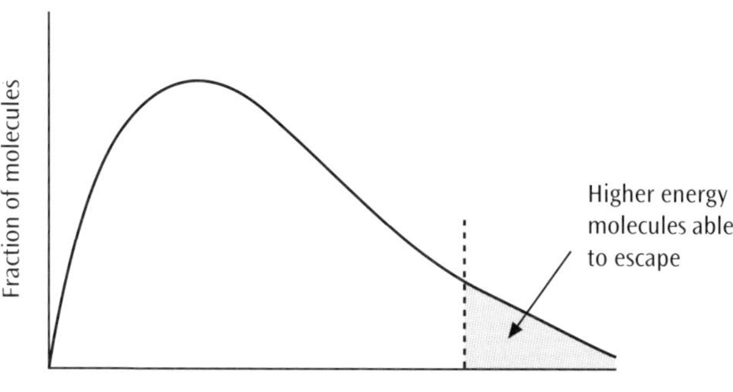

Figure 29.3 *Reduction in a liquid's mean molecular energy by evaporation.*

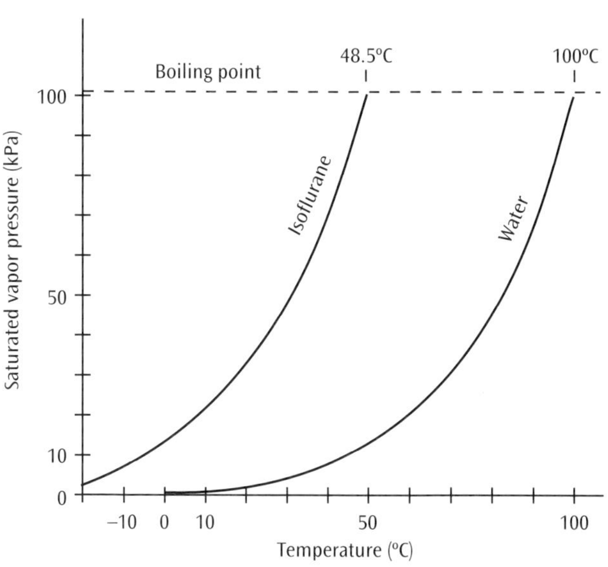

Figure 29.4 *Saturated vapor pressures of isoflurane and water.*

THE BEHAVIOR OF GASES

The component molecules

Because the actual volume of a gas is dependent upon the movement of molecules rather than the volume of the molecules per se, it is the number of molecules in a gas that determines its behavior rather than the specific molecular structure. This concept is contained in Avogadro's hypothesis, which states that :

> Equal volumes of all gases under the same conditions of temperature and pressure contain equal numbers of molecules: it therefore follows that masses of gases in proportion to their molecular weights also have the same number of molecules.

The gram molecular weight of a gas is its molecular weight expressed in grams. At 0 °C and 1 atmosphere pressure (101 kPa, 760 mmHg), all gases contain 6.023×10^{23} molecules (Avogadro's number). The quantity of a substance that contains Avogadro's number of molecules is termed a mole and the universal gas constant (R) (see later), is the same for 1 mole of any perfect gas.

The gas laws

The relations between the pressure, volume, and temperature of a fixed mass of gas are inextricably associated with the names of Boyle, Charles, and Gay-Lussac. Boyle examined gases held at a constant temperature, Charles those at a constant pressure, and Gay-Lussac those at a constant volume. The results for constant temperature and constant pressure are shown in Fig. 29.5. The great importance of Charles's work was that it led to the development of the constant-pressure gas thermometer and the concept of absolute zero (−273.2 °C). Whatever gas was under consideration, the back-extrapolation of the volume–temperature graph demonstrated zero volume at the same temperature. Absolute zero is now the zero point for the kelvin scale of temperature, which has unitary divisions equal to those of the Celsius scale. 0 °C is therefore 273.2 K.

Summarizing these relations mathematically, we get:

Boyle's law: Pressure (P) × Volume (V) = Constant [at fixed temperature (T)]

Charles's law:
Volume (V)/Temperature (T) = Constant [at fixed pressure (P)]

Gay-Lussac's law: Pressure (P)/Temperature (T) = Constant (at fixed volume (V))

Combining these three relations together results in the universal gas equation, which is usually written $PV = nRT$, where n is the number of moles (see below) of a gas and R is the universal gas constant, which is the same for all gases.

These relations all depend upon the gas behaving as a "perfect gas." This, in turn, requires the molecules of the gas to be sufficiently separated that they will not interfere with each other, no chemical reactions will occur, and no changes of state will be imminent. In anesthesia practice this implies that oxygen and medical air approximate to perfect gas behavior but that nitrous oxide does not.

The behavior of nitrous oxide

Nitrous oxide (N_2O) has a critical temperature of 36.5 °C and is supplied in cylinders that are 90–95% full of liquefied N_2O. Consequently, it does not behave like a perfect gas: the phase relations of N_2O are shown in Fig. 29.6. Although a vapor and a gas are essentially indistinguishable, it is conventional to refer to a vapor below the critical temperature and a gas above it, hence the expression "nitrous oxide is inhaled as a vapor and exhaled as a gas."

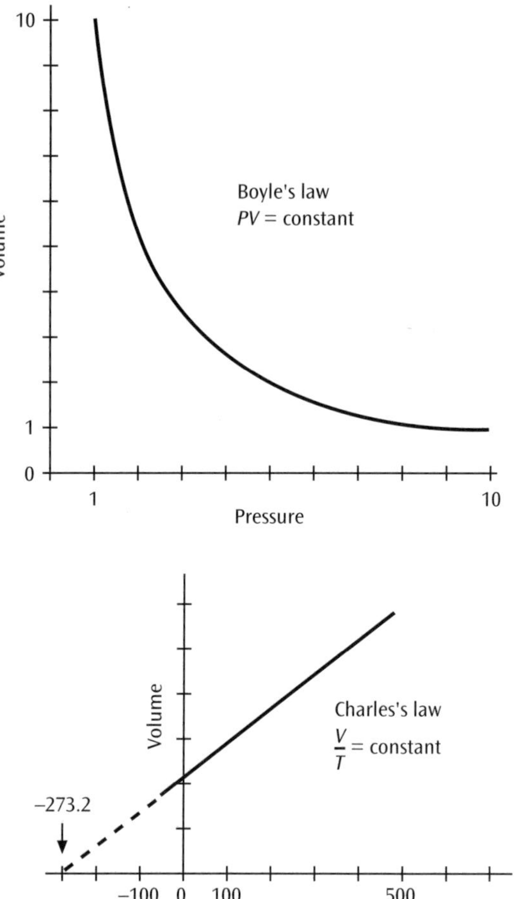

Figure 29.5 *Boyle's law and Charles's law plotted graphically.*

The pressure recorded on a gauge attached to a nitrous oxide cylinder will, if there is liquid present and the cylinder is in thermal equilibrium with its surroundings, record the SVP of nitrous oxide at ambient temperature. There is a common misconception that as N_2O is delivered the cylinder pressure will remain constant at this level until all the liquid has been used up and then fall as if it were an ideal gas. This assumption is, however, untrue because the rate of supply of heat from the surroundings is too slow to maintain isothermal conditions.

As gas is drawn off, the higher-energy molecules leave the liquid and the temperature of the liquid falls, and together with it the SVP and the recorded cylinder pressure. The rate of temperature fall depends upon the rate of gas usage, and under high-flow conditions ice can form on the outside of the cylinder. This process is shown in Fig. 29.7, which also demonstrates that if there is sufficient content left in the cylinder to maintain the liquid phase, as it warms up back to ambient temperature, the pressure will recover to equal that in the original full cylinder. Consequently, the pressure in a nitrous oxide cylinder bears little relation to its content until it is largely exhausted and the contents are entirely gaseous; this occurs at the point at which the cylinder is about five-sixths depleted. Only those cylinders being used to supply low-flow systems at below 2 L min^{-1} will empty without undue cooling and approximate to isothermal behavior.

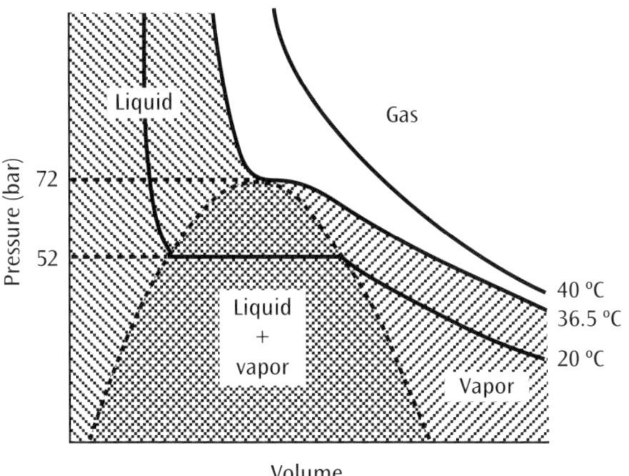

Figure 29.6 *Phase diagram of nitrous oxide.*

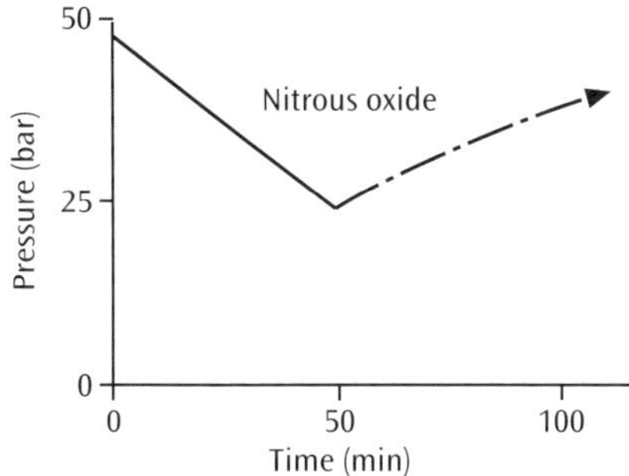

Figure 29.7 *Pressure changes accompanying incomplete emptying of a nitrous oxide cylinder.*

FLUID FLOW

Laminar flow

Molecules of a fluid passing along a tube are subject to drag from the walls of the tube. Molecules close to the wall are affected most, and these in turn affect adjacent molecules to a lesser extent, and so on until those in the center of the flow are least affected. This leads to a velocity profile that is parabolic in shape, so that in a given time the central molecules have traveled furthest, and those near the wall have not moved very far. Factors affecting flow include the pressure on the fluid, the radius and length of the tube, and the viscosity of the fluid. These are combined in the Hagen–Poiseuille equation:

$$\text{Flow} = \frac{\text{pressure gradient} \times \pi \times (\text{tube radius})^4}{8 \times \text{viscosity} \times \text{tube length}}$$

Turbulent flow

As flow becomes faster, or fluid passes a constriction or orifice, flow becomes less ordered. Rather than flowing in layers, the molecules collide with one another, and move in eddies. The molecules are accelerated and decelerated, and hence flow depends on their mass or inertia, reflected by the density of the gas, rather than its viscosity, as described by the Reynolds number:

$$\text{Reynolds number} = \text{Mean velocity} \times \text{density} \times \text{diameter/viscosity}$$

This has practical application in the design of flowmeters (see below). A Reynolds number of 2000–2500 predicts the point at which laminar flow breaks down and the transition to turbulent flow occurs.

THE ANESTHETIC MACHINE

As anesthesia machines have become more complex, understanding of their function has become more necessary as malfunctions, should they occur, may not be obvious. Time spent diagnosing and resolving machine or breathing system malfunction is time spent away from concentrating directly on patient care. Gaining a general understanding of the principles of anesthesia machines, plus a detailed knowledge of the actual models being used, should result in improved patient care.

Contemporary machines increasingly incorporate modular monitoring systems and ventilators. The latest standards refer extensively to the provision of a minimal level of monitoring for every use of the machine. It is useful to look at the development and function of the gas delivery and vaporization sections of the machine in some detail.

Historical development

In the early 1800s, Sir Humphry Davy used the "mercurial air-holder and breathing machine" to deliver undiluted nitrous oxide from a mercury-sealed bell spirometer. In 1846, Morton used a glass draw-over vaporizer for his public demonstration of general anesthesia. By 1880, both oxygen and nitrous oxide were available as compressed gases in iron bottles and the development of the basic anesthetic machine had begun.

In the late nineteenth century, Sir Frederick Hewitt described a machine in which oxygen and nitrous oxide from cylinders was stored in two rubber bags and delivered in a variable concentration via a stopcock that he designed. In 1912, Cotton and Boothby developed the nitrous oxide–oxygen–ether "perfected apparatus," with compressed gas cylinders, reducing valves, bubble flowmeters and a flow-through ether vaporizer.

World War I stimulated major developments. In the USA James Gwathmey developed practical anesthesia machines, but it is Dr Henry Edmund Gaskin Boyle whose name has become almost synonymous with the anesthetic machine. In 1917, Geoffrey Marshall designed a machine while serving in the Royal Army Medical Corps in France and had it made by the apparatus manufacturer Coxeter in London. Illustrations of the machine were borrowed by Boyle and used by him in a presentation to the Anaesthetics Section of the Royal Society of Medicine in 1918. A major advantage of the Marshall/Boyle design over Gwathmey's was the use of the Hewitt stopcock to prevent rebreathing.

The developments continued between the wars, with Jackson in the UK introducing a circle system in 1915 and Waters in the USA for carbon dioxide absorption in 1924 (using granular sodium and calcium hydrate). At this time, water sight-feed meters or bubble-bottles indicated gas flows. In the early 1930s, Coxeter introduced the dry gas meter. The rotameter still used today had been designed by Küppers in 1908 and was widely used in industry for gas and fluid flow measurements. It was not until 1937 that it was introduced into anesthetic machines.

During the next 50 or so years much of the development was focused on safety and standardization of design. However, since the early 1990s the introduction of sophisticated monitoring has placed a new set of demands on machine design.

Standards and anesthetic machines

To date (2003), anesthesia machines are not covered by a single International Standards Organization (ISO) standard. The current standards in force, EN740: 1999 in Europe and ASTM F1850-00 in the USA (BS EN 740:1999, BS 5724-2204:1999 in the UK), are available over the Internet. Both refer extensively to other standards governing the design of many of the anesthetic machine's components. ASTM F1850-00 recognizes that the anesthetic machine (anesthesia work station) will be part of a larger system incorporating decision support, central monitoring, and automated anesthetic record keeping (AARK). Extensive reference is made to IEEE 1073, governing communication between medical devices (medical information bus).

Gas supply

Pipelines

Hospital medical gas pipelines are now the primary source of gas supply to the machine. Oxygen produced by the fractional distillation of liquid air is stored at −150 to −175 °C as a pale blue liquid in a large vacuum flask (vacuum insulated evaporator, VIE). Liquid oxygen occupies 1/860 of the space the gas would occupy, compared with 1/142 for oxygen in a cylinder. Oxygen from the flask is warmed to ambient temperature and is regulated to a pressure of 4 atmospheres (approximately 404 kPa; 58.8 p.s.i.; 3030 mmHg), or 330 kPa (3.3 atmospheres; 50 p.s.i.; 2475 mmHg) in the USA, before entering the hospital medical gas pipeline system. A backup system of oxygen cylinders, or a second VIE, is provided, with an automated and alarmed switching system.

Nitrous oxide is stored at ambient temperature in a bank of cylinders, the pressure again being reduced to about 404 kPa (3030 mmHg) before entering the pipeline system. There are strict controls on the labeling of medical gas pipelines within the hospital and central and local monitoring panels give visual and audible indication of gas supply problems. Emergency shut-off valves are fitted outside each main clinical area.

Operating departments may have medical air from compressors delivered at two pressures, 404 kPa (3030 mmHg) and a higher pressure of 707 kPa(5400 mmHg) for powered surgical instruments.

Pipelines are color coded corresponding to cylinder coding and cannot be incorrectly connected. The pipe is connected to the machine by a noninterchangeable screw thread (NIST), which is specific for each gas. (In the USA, the DISS system – diameter index safety system). The Schrader probe, which connects the machine to the gas outlet, is of the same diameter for all gases but misconnection is prevented by a collar, specific for each gas. The collars are both internally and externally indexed and the collar must fit into the socket before gas is released.

Gas pipelines are provided with pressure gauges at the machine end and these should be clearly visible. Flow restrictors operating at 300–400 kPa (2250–3000 mmHg) are placed in the machine to protect the flowmeters when the pipelines are first connected.

Gas cylinders

Modern anesthetic machines primarily use the cylinders on the machine itself for emergency backup use. It is therefore unusual for the cylinders to be used at all, and few trainees have experience of the use of machine-mounted cylinders and their potential hazards.

To identify the contents, gas cylinders are both color coded and labeled (Table 29.2). Historically, different countries developed their own methods of distinguishing cylinder contents by color. During World War II confusion was caused by the lack of standard cylinder coloring. Eventually international agreement was reached and cylinder colors are covered by ISO 32 (1977). Not all countries conform, notably the USA, which relies on the Compressed Gas Association (CGA) standard.

Cylinders are manufactured from lightweight chrome molybdenum steel, for portable cylinders, or from heavier high-carbon or low-carbon and manganese steel, for hospital use. Some portable cylinders, or those designed for magnetic resonance imaging units, are made of aluminum.

Cylinders are made individually identifiable by a stamp on the shoulder, or by a fitted plastic collar. Cylinders are tested following manufacture and at regular intervals according to the country. Testing includes exterior and endoscopic visual inspection and a hydraulic test to a pressure 50% greater than the normal maximum working pressure.

Filling ratio

To prevent cylinders, the contents of which are normally in liquid form, from being overfilled, a filling ratio (or filling density) is specified. This is the ratio of the total weight of gas in a cylinder to the weight of water that the cylinder would hold at 16 °C. For nitrous oxide (and carbon dioxide) it is 0.67 for tropical climates and 0.75 for temperate areas in which the temperature is not expected to exceed 25 °C (Table 29.3). (Note that the filling ratio is not the proportion of the cylinder occupied by liquid. A full nitrous oxide cylinder, filling ratio 0.75, would be over 90% full of liquid.)

Safe handling of cylinders

Oxygen, nitrous oxide, and mixtures containing these gases, such as entonox, support combustion, particularly at high concentrations and pressures. In the presence of oxygen at high partial pressures, many substances such as oil may ignite spontaneously. Cylinders are stored in cool, well-ventilated areas, away from fire. Storage areas must be free of flammable materials.

Valves, regulators, and gauges should be kept free of oil and grease. A seal should protect cylinders. Before connecting a cylinder to the anesthetic machine, the seal is removed and the valve opened briefly to blow away any dust. Cylinders should be opened slowly when attached to the anesthetic machine – rapid compression of the small volume of the yoke will generate heat, which cannot dissipate quickly (i.e. an adiabatic process). This may ignite any dust or grease present. In any case it is advisable to avoid rapid rises in pressure in the pipes and pressure gauges of the machine.

ANESTHESIA MACHINE COMPONENTS

The pneumatic part of anesthesia machines is conveniently divided into three parts. The high-pressure part receives high-pressure gas from the cylinder and reduces the pressure. It consists of the yoke block, and the cylinder pressure regulators and gauges (Fig. 29.8). The intermediate part receives gases from the high-pressure part, or from the pipelines, and delivers them to flowmeters, or to the oxygen flush. It includes the pipeline inlets and pressure gauges and an oxygen pressure-failure safety device. The low-pressure part delivers the gases to the common gas outlet, and includes valves, flowmeters, and vaporizers.

Yoke

The yoke supports the gas cylinder in the correct orientation. It includes a valve allowing one-way passage of gas from the cylinder into the anesthetic machine, but preventing gas from leaving the machine when there is temporarily no cylinder in place. The valve minimizes trans-filling between cylinders if two are opened at once, allows an empty cylinder to be changed while the machine is in use, and reduces the risk of gas leak to the atmosphere from an empty yoke. The yoke also contains a filter to remove any particulate material. Cylinders should be turned off after use. Yokes that are not in use should be blocked with a sealing plug in place of the cylinder.

A gas-tight seal between the cylinder and the yoke is achieved using a Bodock seal with a maximum thickness of 2.4 mm before compression. The Neoprene gasket expands when pressurized in the center and as it is restrained externally by the metal ring must increase in thickness. The

Table 29.2 *Color coding of medical gas cylinders*

Gas	UK color	Australian color	US color	Pin index position
Oxygen	Black body, white shoulder	Black body, white shoulder	Green	2,5
Carbon dioxide	Gray	Gray-green	Gray	1,6
Nitrous oxide	Blue	Blue	Blue	3,5
Entonox (N_2O/O_2 = 50:50)	Blue body, shoulder blue/white quartered	Blue body, shoulder blue/white quartered	N/A	Single central hole
Air	Gray body, shoulder black/white quartered	Gray body, shoulder black/white quartered	Yellow	1,5
Helium	Brown	Brown	Brown	–
Vacuum (pipeline)	Yellow	Yellow	White	–

Table 29.3 *Contents of medical gas cylinders*

Cylinder size and volume		C (1.2 L)	D (2.3 L)	E (4.7 L)	F (9.4 L)	G (23.6 L)
Gas	**Pressure when full (kPa at 15 °C)**	**Liters of gas available**				
Oxygen	13 650	170	340	680	1360	3400
Carbon dioxide	5000	450		1800		
Nitrous oxide	4400	450	900	1800	3600	9000
Entonox (N_2O/O_2 = 50:50)	13 650	500			2000	5000
Air	13 650			640	1280	3200

Note that when running on two equal-sized cylinders of oxygen and nitrous oxide at an F_IO_2 of 0.33, the oxygen cylinder will run out first.

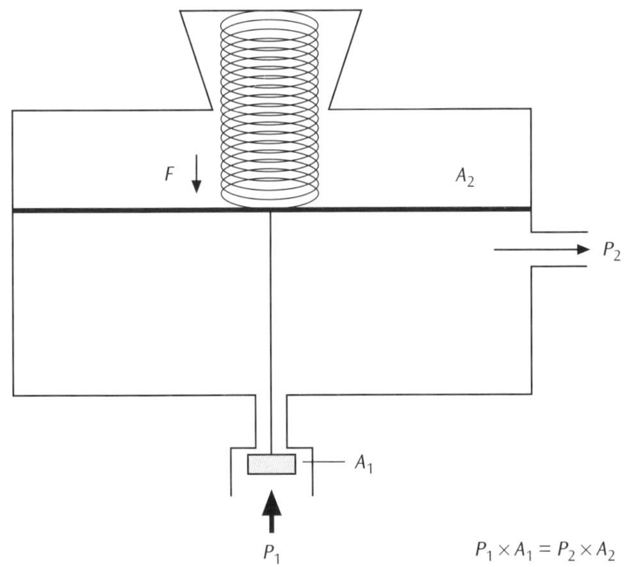

Figure 29.8 *High-pressure gas from the cylinder at pressure P_1 tends to keep the small valve seat of area A_1 closed. Opening a flowmeter and drawing gas off reduces the pressure in the main chamber, so that the spring pushing down on the diaphragm now opens the valve, allowing gas to flow into the chamber. Reducing valves used in anesthesia machines are located under the surface of the machine, and pressure P_2 is factory preset by adjusting the spring tension. The outlet pressure varies little over a wide range of cylinder pressures.*

effect is that a small amount of gas escapes under pressure before the ring expands enough to seal. Once turned on, the Bodock seal should prevent leakage. An audible leak indicates a missing or worn seal.

Pin index system

To prevent misconnection, gas cylinder valve blocks have holes drilled in two of six positions (a single hole in the case of entonox). The system may be defeated by removing the pins, using extra sealing washers, or by inverting the gas cylinder! Recently, in the UK cylinders of oxygen with a built-in finger-operated valve have been introduced, the shortened shoulder below the valve knob allowing pin-indexed regulators to be attached upside down.

Cylinder gauges

Cylinder gauges are usually of the Bourdon type – i.e. a hollow metal tube, flattened in cross-section, bent into a curve, and sealed at one end. It is linked to an indicator needle passing over a dial identified by the standard color for the gas. The tube is fixed at the open end. As gas pressure increases, the tube straightens and the closed end moves, causing the indicator to move across the scale. Cylinder pressure gauges indicate gauge pressure, i.e. pressure above atmospheric pressure. The back of the gauge body is vented to prevent damage to personnel in the event of a high-pressure leak inside the gauge.

With small variations due to temperature fluctuation, the pressure in a cylinder, the contents of which are gaseous such as oxygen, will reflect its remaining content, showing a steady decline until the cylinder is empty. As already discussed, gases stored partially in liquid form do not show such a relation. If desired, the gas remaining in the cylinder can be estimated by weighing.

Pressure regulators

The pressure regulators convert a high, variable cylinder pressure to a lower constant pressure downstream of the regulator. Designs vary, but the underlying principle is the same (Fig. 29.8). The total force exerted by a gas is the pressure multiplied by the area on which it is exerted. Thus, a large pressure over a small area produces the same force as a small pressure over a larger area. The high pressure of the cylinder gas on a small valve seat produces the same force as the gas pressure in a low-pressure chamber on a larger diaphragm. The outlet pressure of the gas leaving the regulator is determined by a spring pressing on the diaphragm, and is slightly less than pipeline pressure to prevent slow depletion of the cylinder if it is left open while the pipeline is also in use.

Pipeline supply pressures may vary somewhat depending on demand around the hospital. Some anesthesia machines have a second pressure regulator to regulate the pipeline oxygen supply. This ensures a constant oxygen flowmeter input until the supply pressure falls below 82–110 kPa (615–825 mmHg).

Flowmeters

The most commonly used gas flow measuring devices in anesthesia machines are flowmeters. These are often referred to by an original commercial name, rotameter, or occasionally as Thorpe tubes. A needle valve controls gas flow through a conical transparent tube, tapered, with the smallest diameter at the bottom, and with an indicator float or bobbin. At zero flow, the bobbin rests at the bottom of the tube. When gas flows, the indicator floats in the tube at a position at which the downward force on the float (gravity) is balanced by the pressure drop of the gas flowing past. Since the weight of the float is constant, the gas pressure drop must be constant at all gas flows and all bobbin positions. Because the tube is tapered, the orifice around the float varies according to its position in the tube. Thus, the flowmeter is a variable orifice, constant-pressure device.

At low gas flows, the float is low in the tube. The gap between float and tube is small, so gas flow is largely laminar and dependent on the viscosity of the gas, as described in the Hagen–Poiseuille equation. At higher flows the bobbin moves up the tubing, so that the annular area around the float is greater to permit the higher gas flow. The annular area around the bobbin is now larger in comparison with the length of the float, and gas flow is more turbulent and hence depends on the gas density. Thus float height and indicated flow depend on the physical properties of the gas, so each flowmeter is specific for one gas. Typically, accuracies of ± 2.5% of reading over a 10:1 ratio of flows are achieved

Most anesthesia flowmeters have a bobbin-shaped float with an upper rim. The bobbin is sighted along its upper, flat surface and the flow read from a scale on the tubing. A stuck bobbin would give erroneous readings. Grooves cut into its surface cause the bobbin to spin, preventing it from sticking, and there is a stop to prevent the bobbin sticking at the top of the tube. The tubing is made of a conducting material or incorporates a conductive strip to prevent the build-up of static electricity, and the needle valves that regulate gas flow include a dust filter. Some flowmeters have a spherical float, which is read from its center.

The flow of gas through a flowmeter is controlled by a needle valve, operated by a knob of a color appropriate to the gas. The control knob moves a long, narrow spindle in and out of the gas flow. Gas flow around the spindle or needle is very fast. The flow of gas in such a valve, in terms of mass flow (i.e. mass per unit time, rather than volume per unit time), is relatively unaffected by small changes in downstream pressure.

Flowmeters are calibrated at room temperature (20 °C) and 101 kPa (760 mmHg). Temperature variations will affect the density of the gas and produce a small, clinically insignificant change in the flowmeter reading. However, pressure changes will produce visible alterations in the indicated gas flow. If the downstream pressure rises, there will be a reduction in the indicated flow even though the actual mass gas flow is almost unchanged.

The flowmeter tube may be double or single tapered. A double taper has a lower taper to make measurement of low flows easier, while the tapering increases higher up the tube for high flows. An increasingly common practice, however, is for two tubes in series, each with a single taper, to be used for low and high flows. Where both bobbins have risen up their tubes, the total flow is that shown by the bobbin in the high-flow tube. (In the past, separate low- and high-flow oxygen rotameters were provided, which led to a number of accidents.) On some machines the oxygen control valve has a minimum flow rate of about 200 mL min^{-1}, enough to provide basal oxygen flow in a closed circuit.

It is standard practice in the UK for the oxygen control knob to be situated at the left of the flowmeter assembly, whereas in the USA it is normally on the right. In most countries it is both color coded and touch coded, being larger than the other knobs. For safety, in the event of a leak from the top of the rotameter block, oxygen should be the last gas added to the mixture. This is achieved easily in the US arrangement of rotameters with oxygen on the right. The UK persists with the oxygen rotameter on the left, however, and an internal sleeve is used to ensure that oxygen is the last gas added to the mixture.

In some modern machines a separate auxiliary oxygen flowmeter is provided, which allows nasal cannulae, variable performance oxygen masks, etc. to be supplied with oxygen without dismantling the ventilator breathing circuit. Although useful as a supply for a self-inflating bag in the event of a ventilator failure, they are supplied from the same oxygen supply as the rest of the anesthetic machine and so are of no use in a pipeline failure.

The latest generation of anesthetic machines makes extensive use of electronic flowmeters that are digitally controlled. Digital flowmeters can achieve a precision some 5–10 times greater than the rotameter and allow automated anesthesia record systems to chart the fresh gas flow rates.

Emergency oxygen flush

Anesthetic machines incorporate an emergency oxygen flush valve, which connects a supply of oxygen directly from the first part of the regulated supply to the common gas outlet, bypassing all flowmeters, vaporizers, etc. The flow rate should be between 35 and 75 L min^{-1} and it should not be possible either to activate the valve by accident or to lock the valve in the "on" position. Older designs have led to barotrauma and awareness.

Antihypoxia devices (proportioning systems)

Prior to the 1980s it was possible to deliver 100% nitrous oxide through the machine. New anesthesia machines are required to have some means of preventing the delivery of a hypoxic gas mixture.

The Ohmeda Link 25 system uses a chain to connect the oxygen and nitrous oxide flow control knobs. Either gas can be adjusted independently but the mechanical link maintains a minimum ration of 1:3 of oxygen to nitrous oxide. The nitrous oxide is also reduced in a second-stage regulator to 173 kPa (1298 mmHg). Dräger use a pneumatic interlock (ORMC) that maintains fresh gas oxygen concentrations at 25 ± 3% by limiting nitrous oxide flow, the system also activating electronic alarms as required. Both systems assume that oxygen and nitrous oxide are the only gases in use – if a third inert gas is introduced, such as carbon dioxide or helium, then hypoxic mixtures can still be produced. A calibrated oxygen analyzer should therefore always be used at the common gas outlet; modern machines incorporate this into the machine itself.

It should be remembered that compliance with standards does not necessarily mean that the patient cannot be administered a hypoxic mixture of gases. For example, the administration of the lowest permissible F_IO_2 at low flow into a circle system will still potentially allow the development of a hypoxic mix of gases, even though the machine is not delivering one to the breathing system. It is still *essential* to monitor the concentration of oxygen received by the patient.

Oxygen failure safety device and alarm

Should an oxygen cylinder become fully depleted, or the oxygen pipeline fail, there is a potential danger to the patient. Oxygen failure safety devices are located upstream of the flowmeter. ASTM F1850–00 (51.12.1) states that:

> The anesthesia gas supply device shall be designed so that whenever the oxygen supply pressure is reduced to below the manufacturer-specified minimum the delivered oxygen concentration shall not decrease below 19% at the common gas outlet. The performance of the anesthesia gas supply device under these conditions shall be stated in the accompanying documents.

And (51.12.2) states that:

> Whenever the oxygen supply pressure falls below the manufacturer-specified threshold, at least a medium priority alarm shall be activated within 5 s. This alarm shall not be capable of being disabled.

The level at which the system is activated is usually set at 200 kPa (1500 mmHg). Historically, both battery- and nitrous oxide-driven systems have been described. These required a second system to be operational for the alarm to work and have been replaced by oxygen-powered devices. In the simpler systems, a small cylinder is pressurized by oxygen from the internal intermediate-pressure system in the machine; if the pressure falls below the preset level, then a valve is triggered and the cylinder discharges through a whistle. The common gas outlet may also be opened, so allowing entrainment of room air. More sophisticated machines use combined audible and visual alarms triggered by a low oxygen pressure. Datex-Ohmeda use a "pressure-sensor shut-off valve," whereby at 133 kPa (998 mmHg) the flow of all other gases is shut off, whereas Dräger's "oxygen failure protection device" is a proportional system with complete shut-off of nitrous oxide occurring when the oxygen pressure falls below 67 kPa (502 mmHg). Ohmeda also includes a second-stage oxygen regulator in its machines, ensuring a constant pressure of oxygen at the flowmeter until pressures fall below 80–107 kPa (600–802 mmHg).

Vaporizers

Vaporizers may be low-efficiency draw-over vaporizers or high-efficiency plenum vaporizers in which a separate measured gas flow is saturated with vapor by bubbling through the agent and then mixed back into the main fresh gas flow.

Plenum vaporizers

Nearly all vaporizers attached to the anesthesia machine are of the plenum type – variable-bypass, flow-over, temperature-compensated, agent-specific, out-of-circuit vaporizers; the Dräger Vapor 19.1, Penlon Sigma, Datex-Ohmeda AS/3 ADU Aladin (see below), and Datex-Ohmeda Tec 4 and 5 are all examples of this type of device. Modern anesthesia machines that allow for more than one vaporizer to be fitted at a time incorporate a vaporizer interlock ensuring that only one vaporizer can be switched on at a time. Vaporizers need to be securely fitted and locked in place if leaks from the fresh gas supply are to be avoided

Gas flowing into variable-bypass vaporizers is split into carrier gas (< 20% of flow) that is saturated with vapor and then mixed back into the bypass gas at the outlet of the vaporizer. The ratio, the splitting ratio, is controlled by the dial and by the internal automatic temperature compensation valve. The output of current variable-bypass vaporizers is reasonably constant over a range of flows, from 250 mL min^{-1} to 15 L min^{-1}, because of the extensive internal wick and baffle systems, which increase the surface area available for vaporization.

Effect of temperature

Without temperature compensation, the effect of the loss of the latent heat of vaporization as the volatile liquid evaporated would be to rapidly reduce the temperature in the vaporization chamber, accompanied by a drop in the evaporation rate and a fall in the delivered vapor concentration. This occurs to only a minor extent in modern vaporizers because of two mechanisms: (1) the vaporizer itself is constructed of a large mass of metal, which acts as a heat reservoir; (2) in addition, a temperature compensation mechanism varies the splitting ratio, increasing the proportion of gas flowing through the vaporization chamber as the temperature falls. The mechanism achieving this is either an aneroid bellows or a bimetallic strip. A bimetallic strip consists of two metals bonded together. The differing rates of thermal expansion of the two metals change the curvature of the strip as temperature changes (a mechanism first developed by clock makers).

Sevoflurane vaporizers are less accurate due to the low vapor pressure of the agent (Table 29.4); at high fresh gas flow rates and high concentration settings (e.g. after induction) they deliver significantly less than the dial setting. Modern vaporizers also incorporate a check valve at the vaporizer outlet to reduce the "pumping effect" of intermittent back-pressure from the breathing system, a common problem when older style minute-volume divider ventilators are used. Vaporizers and flowmeters are also protected by a safety blow-off valve from a prolonged rise in gas pressure caused by the occlusion of the common gas outlet. This valve typically opens at 35–40 kPa (158–300 mmHg) and plays no role in protecting the patient from high breathing system pressures.

The Datex-Ohmeda Aladin vaporizer consists of an agent-specific cassette that is inserted into a port on the AS/3 anesthetic machine. The electronic control system recognizes the cassette type and dispenses agent into the fresh gas stream. As there is no bypass channel in the cassettes, they can be tipped without danger, and will not discharge agent without electrical power and adequate oxygen pressure in the system.

Modern vaporizers also make use of keyed filling systems in which a specially designed adapter connects a keyed bottle to the vaporizer filling port. It is important not to overfill or tip vaporizers as very small amounts of liquid agent produce large volumes of concentrated agent (typically 1 mL of liquid yields about 200 mL of vapor!)

The Datex-Ohmeda Tec 6 is a specialized vaporizer designed for use with desflurane only; the vaporizer is heated internally to a thermostatically controlled temperature of 39 °C and is a gas–vapor blender rather than a variable-bypass system. It is filled using a specially designed gas-tight adapter and incorporates a low-level alarm. The Aladin desflurane vaporizer works without being heated.

The common gas outlet

This is the exit point for gases leaving the machine. It has a 22-mm-diameter outer male–15-mm-diameter inner female connection. It may be situated on either side of the machine.

Humidification

Humidifiers compensate for the loss of the heat and moisture exchange function of the upper respiratory tract when it is bypassed. The absolute humidity of tracheal gas is 44 mg L^{-1} at the carina, i.e. 100% relative humidity at 37 °C. The ideal situation is to reproduce this and to humidify and warm anesthetic gases, which leave the machine at virtually zero humidity, to body temperature and 100% relative humidity. For anesthesia use, the most common methods are hot water baths and heat and moisture exchangers. Other methods of humidification are available, such as ultrasonic nebulizers, but are less commonly used, partly because of the risk to the patient of water overload.

Agent	SVP (kPa) at 20 °C	SVP (mmHg) at 20 °C	Boiling point °C (1 atm)
Desflurane	89.2	669	23.0
Enflurane	23.3	175	56.5
Halothane	32.4	243	50.2
Isoflurane	31.7	238	48.5
Sevoflurane	21.6	163	58.5

Table 29.4 *Properties of volatile anesthetic agents*

Hot water baths

These are mainly used in intensive care units but have some use in the operating room, particularly for pediatric cases. The dry anesthetic gases are passed over a heated bath of sterile water. Condensation on cooling in the tubing is a problem, dealt with in some systems by moisture traps, and by a heating wire in the breathing system. Should the water bath humidifier be insecurely fixed, there is a risk of water tipping into the breathing system.

Heat and moisture exchangers

The principle of operation is that exhaled gas passes through the heat and moisture exchanger (HME), water vapor condenses out, and the HME is warmed. During inspiration, the dry gases are humidified by the condensed water and warmed. Unlike water baths, HMEs do not add heat or water to the system but are 60–70% efficient at returning the patient's own water vapor and heat. HMEs are more efficient with longer cases as, during the first minutes of an operation, efficiency is low. The elements of an HME can be either hygrosopic (the element becomes wet) or hydrophobic (water droplets sit on the surface of the membrane). Hydrophobic HMEs with small pore sizes (200 nm or 0.2 µm) can act as protective filters.

Protective filters

For many years filters have been available, which, when inserted in the breathing system at the patient's end, will protect the patient from viral and bacterial contamination. As a cost-saving measure it has become common to reuse anesthesia breathing systems, with a fresh filter used for each patient.

Protective filters may be placed at various positions relative to the breathing system and patient, but protective filters placed at the patient's end of the breathing system will protect the patient from contamination from the breathing system, and will also protect the breathing system from contamination by the patient. Potential problems with this siting of the filter include increased dead space, increased potential for disconnections, and increased resistance to gas flow, particularly if the filter becomes obstructed with secretions.

Modern filters have a relatively low volume, typically 35 mL, so increased dead space is only a problem with small children. Typical retention efficiency for small (0.30 µm) airborne viral and bacterial contaminants is 99.999%, while that for larger (0.45 µm or above) particles is 99.9999%. The hydrophobic nature of the membrane also prevents the passage of hepatitis C. An added advantage of breathing system filters is the ability to trap latex particles generated in the anesthetic equipment, which may prevent allergic reactions.

CHECKING THE ANESTHESIA MACHINE

From what has gone before, it is apparent there are many potential hazards within the anesthesia machine, many of which can be detected by a careful preuse check. The Food and Drug Administration (FDA) in the USA and the Association of Anaesthetists (AAGBI) in the UK have issued recommended checklists. There is, however, a trade-off between the complexity of the test and the way in which it is likely to be performed on regular basis. Occluding the common gas outlet in an attempt to detect leaks in the internal workings of the machine is ineffective as the one-way and blow-off valves described above prevent the pressure being applied to the vaporizers and flowmeters. Step 5 in the current (1993) FDA checkout recommendations requires a deflated suction bulb to be attached to the common gas outlet with the master switch, the flowmeters, and the vaporizers switched off. The bulb should not reinflate in less than 10 s and the test is repeated with each vaporizer switched on in turn. The AAGBI have also issued a checklist that makes use of an oxygen analyzer at the common gas outlet, so allowing detection of internal pipeline cross-connections. The latest generation of machines such as the Datex-Ohmeda AS3 ADU and the Dräger Julian incorporate an automated, electronic system checkout. The operator follows a series of "on-screen" instructions, activating gas flows and occluding the breathing system as required. The checkout covers all the requirements of the FDA checklist and takes 3–6 min to complete.

Conclusion

The design of anesthesia machines has changed much since their introduction at the turn of the last century. The modern machine is a highly sophisticated piece of mechanical, pneumatic, and electronic engineering, built to strict safety standards and incorporating state-of-the-art monitoring and ventilator systems. The absolute requirement for electrical power is now a reality and the use of integrated digital gas and agent control allows a truly comprehensive automated anesthetic record to be kept. Gas delivery equipment accounted for only 2% of claims in the American Society of Anesthesiologists Closed Claims Project, most of these being due to breathing system problems.

The most dangerous part of an anesthetic machine remains the operator! It is incumbent on the manufacturer to make the new machines implicitly easy to use and the anesthesiologist to understand how to use them safely.

BREATHING SYSTEMS

The term "breathing system" is nowadays the preferred term rather than the former term "circuit" as the flow of gases is not necessarily circular. A breathing system is the conduit between an already pressure-reduced and flow-restricted gas source (e.g. the common gas outlet of an anesthetic machine) and the patient's airway.

A breathing system has three main functions to achieve:

- the supply of oxygen to the patient;
- the elimination of carbon dioxide;
- the supply of anesthetic gases and vapors.

Many breathing systems also incorporate the facility to artificially ventilate the patient, a system of humidification, and also a facility to connect to a scavenging system.

Carbon dioxide removal

If the breathing system is such that the patients expired gases are not reinspired, carbon dioxide will be eliminated. This is the situation in a nonrebreathing system. Alternatively, in systems in which rebreathing occurs to a significant degree, i.e. the expired gases are not removed from the system, the carbon dioxide must be absorbed.

Classification of breathing systems

There has been much contention over the classification of breathing systems and different approaches of varying complexity have been made.

According to the ISO,[1] breathing systems are classified as nonrebreathing, partial rebreathing, and complete rebreathing. Semiopen and semiclosed are terms that are not used. Others who have proposed functional classifications of anesthesia breathing systems include Dripps *et al.*,[2] McMahon,[3] and Baraka.[4] Some classifications include newer breathing systems such as the enclosed Mapleson A.[5] Hamilton[6] has proposed a descriptive classification system based on the fresh gas flow and the equipment used. A simple approach by Conway was to divide systems into the two categories of absorber and nonabsorber systems (Fig. 29.9).

The approach to be taken here is that most breathing systems fall within in the three categories (with some overlap) of open systems, semiopen or semiclosed systems, and closed systems. There are subclassifications within each of these categories.

Open systems

These are valveless systems without boundaries and include the early methods of anesthesia administration by soaking a cloth in a volatile agent held away from the patient's face. A modern example is a fixed flow of gas being delivered to the patient via a loose-fitting mask or other device such as nasal prongs. There is no restriction to the patient's gas flow. They are suitable for providing oxygen support therapy to spontaneously breathing patients. The clinician has only limited control over the inspired gas mixture, as in open systems the patient will entrain air during inspiration. The degree of entrainment will depend on the patient's peak inspiratory flow, which in turn depends on respiratory rate and minute volume.

High-air-flow oxygen enrichment (HAFOE) systems use a fixed ratio air entrainment device. These devices work on the Venturi principle, using the high flow of oxygen through a constriction in the delivery system to entrain a known proportion of room air. In this way the device can deliver a known concentration of oxygen at a flow approaching that of the patient's peak inspiratory flow (about 30 L min^{-1}). The principle limitation of these devices is that the maximum deliverable oxygen concentration is probably about 60%. Attempts at higher concentrations result in a lower total flow and thus greater air entrainment around the mask.

Semiopen and semiclosed systems

The distinction between these two categories is somewhat blurred and laboring the differences between them is not helpful in practical terms. Both types fall within the Mapleson classification of anesthetic breathing systems and they have been combined here. It should be noted that the function of these systems depends not only on the arrangements of the components making up the breathing system but also on the level of fresh gas flow and whether the ventilation is spontaneous or controlled.

The main difference is that semiopen systems are valveless and entrainment of room air can still occur (although in normal modern use this should not happen). A semiclosed system cannot entrain room air because it uses an expiratory adjustable pressure-limiting (APL) valve. These systems are distinguished from open systems by the fact that there is a seal between the breathing system and the patient's airway, either through a tight-fitting mask or by connection to an airway device such as an endotracheal tube or laryngeal mask airway. The problem of coping with peak inspiratory flow is overcome by the incorporation of a reservoir bag. The bag collapses during inspiration sufficiently to compensate for the difference between fresh gas flow and peak inspiratory flow. As long as the fresh gas flow is sufficient to replace losses from the system via the expiratory APL valve, the bag will return to its original full state during expiration.

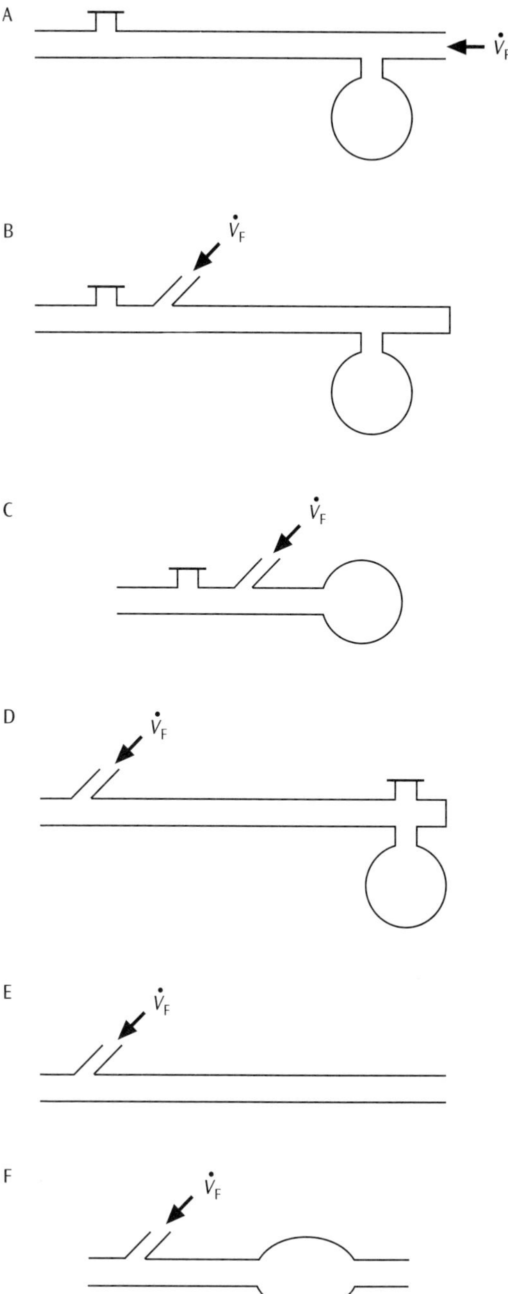

Figure 29.9 *The Mapleson classification of nonabsorber breathing systems.*

Mapleson classification

Mapleson, at Mushin's suggestion, classified anesthetic breathing systems according to the possible physical configurations of the components of a basic breathing system, namely fresh gas flow, APL valve, reservoir bag, and corrugated tubing.[7] He pointed out that if, as an exercise, these components are drawn on separate pieces of paper and then assembled in every way possible, only five practical breathing systems can be assembled. Mapleson examined the conditions necessary to eliminate rebreathing in each of these.

Mapleson A

Mapleson A systems include the Magill attachment and the Lack systems (parallel and coaxial). The essential features of these systems are that the reservoir bag is attached to the same limb of the system as that into which the fresh gas flow is introduced and that the APL valve is part of the expiratory limb or directly over the patient's airway. These systems are particularly efficient when used on spontaneously breathing patients. The fresh gas flow need be no higher than the patient's alveolar ventilation because the anatomical dead space is rebreathed whereas alveolar gas that has taken part in gas exchange is vented through the APL valve. Note again the function of the reservoir bag in reducing the necessary fresh gas flow – without a reservoir the fresh gas flow would have to be sufficient to cope with the maximum inspiratory flow rate, which may be 30 L min^{-1}.

The degree of rebreathing is determined by the pressure-limiting valve. If a patient requires manual ventilation while attached to a Mapleson A system, the pressure on the APL valve has to be increased in order to generate sufficient pressure to positively pressure ventilate the patient. This makes the system very inefficient as extensive mixing of fresh gas and alveolar gas will take place in the inspiratory limb of the system unless the fresh gas flows are high (2–3 times minute volume).

Mapleson C

This system is often found in recovery areas, and may be used for manual ventilation for short-distance patient transfers. It is not used for maintenance of anesthesia. For both spontaneous ventilation and controlled ventilation, there is a degree of rebreathing and the fresh gas flow should be at least 2–3 times minute ventilation. When used for manual ventilation, expansion of the reservoir bag depends on the fresh gas flow, so failure of the gas supply renders the system useless (in comparison with self-inflating resuscitation bags, which will still ventilate the patient with air in this situation).

Mapleson D

The Bain system is an example of a Mapleson D system. This system is configured such that the reservoir bag and APL valve are on the expiratory limb and fresh gas is introduced as close to the airway as possible. The Bain achieves this using a coaxial system with the fresh gas flow forming the core of the coaxial tube. These systems are most efficient when used for positive-pressure ventilation of the patient. Fresh gas fills the expiratory limb of the system, pushing expired gases further up the expiratory limb as the reservoir bag fills. When the bag is squeezed the fresh gas in the expiratory limb enters the patient. When the APL valve opens, it is the gas mixture in the reservoir bag that is vented, which is mostly expired gases, although some fresh gas is also lost. Rebreathing occurs if fresh gas flow is insufficient (under 1.5–2 times minute volume when spontaneously breathing) or if the volume of the expiratory limb is too small (a length of 1.8 m of 22-mm tubing is recommended for adults). During mechanical ventilation the fresh gas flow can be used as a means of controlling the patient's arterial P_{CO_2} using the algorithm described by Henville and Adams.[8] A potential problem with the Bain circuit is disconnection or kinking of the inner fresh gas tube. The Pethick test is designed to detect this hazard (Table 29.5).

Mapleson E

The Ayre's T-piece is a Mapleson E type breathing system. Philip Ayre introduced the T-piece system in 1937.[9] Ayre was principally an adult neuroanesthesiologist, and it was thought that cerebral congestion was made worse by the presence of the valves in the existing breathing systems, which increased expiratory resistance. His breathing system, which is a valveless arrangement of tubes connected in a T configuration, corresponds with Mapleson's E classification. Ayre also gave anesthetics to children for cleft lip and cleft palate surgery (Ayre himself had this condition), and adopted the system for pediatric anesthesia.[10] It was designed for use in spontaneously breathing patients as it presents almost no resistance to expiration. It is a semiopen system, as there are no valves in the system, and the expiratory limb of the system is open to room air. Table 29.6 summarizes the advantages and disadvantages of the T-piece and Table 29.7 the desirable characteristics of breathing systems for pediatric use.

Mapleson F

The Jackson Rees modification of Ayre's T-piece (Mapleson F) incorporates a reservoir bag attached to the expiratory limb of the T-piece. Movements of the bag allow the patient's breathing to be observed. (Previously a strand of cotton wool would be placed over the end of the expired limb and observed swaying as the patient breathed.) The reservoir bag has a small outlet. This remains open throughout the respiratory cycle for spontaneous ventilation. The partial occlusion of the open end of the bag and the manual squeezing of the bag can achieve more satisfactory ventilation, with more optimal inspiratory flow, than simple occlusion of the open end of a T-piece.

As modified by Rees, the T-piece is sometimes described as a Mapleson F, though with the open end of the bag partially occluded for controlled ventilation it also resembles a Mapleson D. It has many advantages for pediatric and in particular neonatal anesthesia, and some drawbacks. These are summarized in Table 29.6.

Function of the T-piece

Fresh gas flows continuously into the T-piece system. The fresh gas flow rate is lower than the patient's peak inspiratory flow rate, in the case of both spontaneously breathing patients and those ventilated with bag-squeezing ventilators. Therefore, inspired gases are a mix of the fresh gas flowing into the T-piece and gas from the "expiratory" limb, which is thus better called the reservoir limb.

The fresh gas flow pushes expired gas away down the reservoir limb, so that when inspiration commences the reservoir limb holds fresh gas. An inadequate fresh gas flow will result in reinspiration of alveolar gas from the reservoir tube. A short reservoir tube may result in the inspiration of room air drawn into the tube.

Ayre described different sizes of expiratory or reservoir limb for effective ventilation of patients of differing sizes. This is now known to be unnecessary, as the effective ventilation of the patient depends on the fresh gas flow washing out expired gas, not the dimensions of the T-piece. The early T-pieces were made with the fresh gas inflow extending down the lumen of the wide-bore tube, with the fresh gas flow directed toward the patient. This is also not necessary, and modern T-pieces are a simple T arrangement with no inner continuation of the fresh gas tube.

Rees[11] has pointed out that in Ayre's original T-pieces, by virtue of the inner concentric fresh gas tube causing a Venturi effect, continuous positive pressure would exist in the system. Thus, Ayre was, inadvertently, the first user of continuous positive airway pressure (CPAP) in anesthesia. Because of the longer expiratory limb in modern T-pieces, a

Table 29.5 *The Pethick test for testing a Bain breathing system*

1	Occlude the distal (patient) end of the circuit
2	Close the APL valve
3	Fill the system using the oxygen flush
4	Release the occlusion of the system and flush it
5	If the inner tube is patent, the reservoir bag will flatten due to the Venturi effect

APL valve, adjustable pressure-limiting valve.

Table 29.6 *Advantages and disadvantages of the T-piece*

Advantages
Lightweight
Minimal resistance to flow
Can be used for both spontaneous and controlled ventilation
Simple design with no valves
Disadvantages
Exhaust gases not easy to scavenge
Obstruction of expiratory limb exposes patient to high pressures if APL valve not used

APL valve, adjustable pressure-limiting valve.

Table 29.7 *Desirable characteristics of breathing systems for pediatric use*

1	Light in weight
2	As few connections as possible making assembly and use easy
3	Dead space should be minimized
4	Delivery of anesthetic vapors and gases must be reliable
5	Reliable removal of carbon dioxide
6	Moisture and heat retention
7	Disposal of expired gases to reduce pollution of the operating environment
8	Ease of cleaning/sterilization
9	Economy of use

constant expiratory pressure is necessary to expel gases from the system. Thus, for a different reason, a degree of CPAP or positive end-expiratory pressure (PEEP) is still applied to patients using modern T-pieces.

A disadvantage of the Ayre's T-piece is that it does not incorporate any means for artificially ventilating the patient. At the time of its introduction, most patients were anesthetized breathing spontaneously. With the introduction of relaxant drugs, it was easy to use the T-piece by simple occlusion of the gas outflow. While the outflow was occluded, the fresh gas flowed into the patient. Removal of the occlusion allowed expiration. This is the principle of T-piece occlusion, a mode of ventilation suitable for intensive care rather than anesthesia. Only in the case of T-piece occluding ventilators, in which the expiratory limb is simply occluded, does inspired gas consist entirely of the fresh gas flow. In this case, it can be seen that high fresh gas flows are necessary to give an adequate inspiratory flow.

Factors affecting rebreathing with the T-piece

The following factors will affect rebreathing, and hence CO_2 elimination, with the T-piece.

Fresh gas flow

Increasing fresh gas flow (FGF) causes expired alveolar gas to be expelled further down the reservoir tube, reducing the rebreathing of exhaled gases. This applies equally to both spontaneously breathing patients and those ventilated with a bag-squeezing anesthesia ventilator. Above a certain FGF there is no rebreathing, assuming tidal volume remains constant. Increasing FGF beyond this level has no point and is wasteful as it does not further reduce inspired CO_2. Conversely, reducing FGF below the critical level increases the reinhalation of expired gases, so inspired CO_2 rises. Thus, manipulation of FGF controls the elimination of CO_2, regardless of other ventilatory parameters.

Tidal volume

Should end-tidal CO_2 rise, it is a natural response to increase the tidal volume. However, an increase in tidal volume at a low FGF may have no effect on CO_2 elimination. Additional rebreathing may occur due to the failure of the FGF to fully wash out the increased volume of expired gases. This in fact may be useful as it allows the anesthesiologist to set high tidal volumes, adequate to prevent basal atelectasis, without necessarily producing hypocapnia. If a fall in the patient's $P_{a}CO_2$ is desired it is necessary to increase the FGF as well as increasing tidal volume.

Rate of ventilation

In a manner analogous to the situation in which tidal volume is increased, an increase in rate may not produce an increase in CO_2 elimination unless FGF is also increased. At higher ventilatory rates, there is a shortened expiratory phase and pause, in which there is less time for washout by the fresh gas to occur, and hence more rebreathing. An increase in rate without adjustment of FGF may produce a paradoxical reduction in CO_2 elimination, and the patient's $P_{a}CO_2$ rises.

Spontaneous ventilation with the T-piece

Spontaneous ventilation without rebreathing requires a FGF of 2.5–3 times the patient's minute ventilation to prevent rebreathing. Practically, the anesthetized patient's minute ventilation will not be known so this is not a very helpful statement. Neonates are usually anesthetized using controlled ventilation, so the problem rarely arises. Formulae were once employed to relate FGF requirements to body weight. An FGF of at least $3\,L\,min^{-1}$ is usually recommended even for neonates.

It is easier to calculate FGF from the patient's body weight (BW). For an intubated patient spontaneously breathing:

$$FGF = 3 \times (1000 + 100\,mL\,kg^{-1})$$

For patients breathing spontaneously with a mask, allowing for the greater dead space:

$$FGF = 4 \times (1000 + 100\,mL\,kg^{-1})$$

Alternative formulae are:

$$FGF = 2 \times \sqrt{BW} \text{ (spontaneous respiration)}$$

$$FGF = \sqrt{BW} \text{ (controlled ventilation)}$$

With the general availability of capnometry, these formulae have limited modern application.

However, capnometry may not be entirely reliable with a T-piece. A sampling port placed in the usual position near the breathing system–endotracheal tube connection may under-report the end-tidal carbon dioxide because of dilution of the expired gases by the FGF.

Controlled ventilation with the T-piece

This is the normal situation with neonates. An FGF of between 2 and $3\,L\,min^{-1}$ is normally sufficient to prevent hypercapnia. Even lower FGFs may be used if end-tidal CO_2 is reliably measured.

Humphry ADE system

This system incorporates a flow switch to allow a breathing system to be rapidly reconfigured from a Mapleson type A to D or E.[12] This allows the anesthesiologist to maximize the efficiency of the system during the different phases of the anesthetic when the patient may be spontaneously breathing or artificially ventilated.

Summary of Mapleson breathing system performances

Spontaneously breathing patient

The Mapleson A is the most efficient. It approaches the ideal, in that FGF may be set to equal alveolar ventilation. There is virtually no rebreathing, and no fresh gas is wasted – it all reaches the patient's alveoli. This performance is achieved regardless of the breathing pattern (Fig. 29.10).

In comparison, there is some wastage of fresh gas with systems B, C, D, and E. Performance is to some degree dependent on the pattern or waveform of breathing

Controlled ventilation

The Mapleson A is much less efficient. The performances of the other systems are still ventilation waveform dependent and are still not efficient.

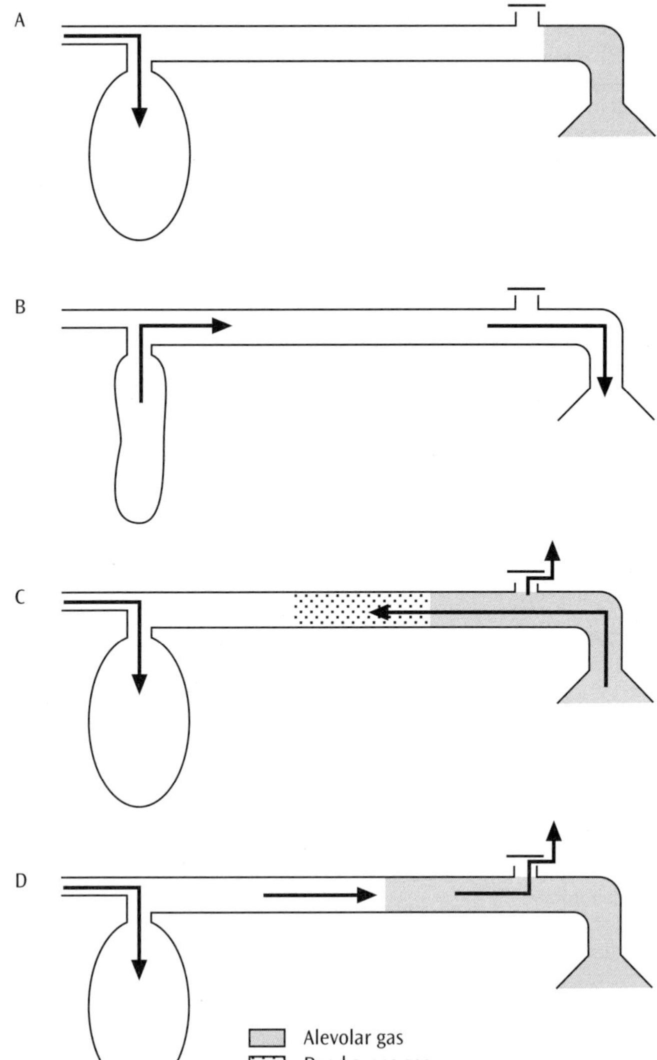

Figure 29.10 *The Mapleson A breathing system during spontaneous ventilation. (A) Reservoir bag filled with fresh gas at end of expiratory phase; (B) inspiration – the patient draws gas from fresh gas flow and from reservoir bag; (C) expiration – dead space gas enters breathing system, followed by alveolar gas, and passes expiratory valve – reservoir bag filled by fresh gas flow; (D) reservoir bag full – pressure in system rises, expiratory valve opens, and system tubing swept by fresh gas flow prior to inspiration.*

Closed systems

The strict definition of a closed system is one in which no communication between the system and the outside takes place (i.e. there is no entrainment of room air and no venting of expired gases). However, in practice it has come to mean any system in which deliberate rebreathing takes place. Such systems must incorporate a mechanism for removing CO_2 from the expired gases before they are rebreathed and this usually takes the form of a canister of soda-lime. These systems allow the use of much reduced FGF, to the extent that in some circumstances the system can be closed completely, with the FGF replacing only the patient's oxygen and anesthetic consumption. The advantage of these systems is that they conserve expensive and environmentally harmful anesthetic agents, they provide a means of monitoring the patient's metabolic status, and the soda-lime provides warming and humidification of the gases. The principal disadvantage is that the systems are more complex and closer attention must be paid to the patient's oxygen and anesthetic requirements if hypoxic gas mixtures and awareness are to be avoided. This makes the use of oxygen, nitrous oxide, and volatile agent monitoring mandatory.

The classic rebreathing system is the Water's to-and-fro system. This is essentially a Mapleson C system with a canister of soda-lime placed in line between the patient's airway and the reservoir bag. Although it works well, the proximity of the soda-lime canister to the airway makes it cumbersome and also there is the danger that particles of the highly caustic soda-lime may be aspirated.

Circle breathing systems

The circle breathing system is by far the most commonly used closed breathing system. The circle system has an expiratory and inspiratory limb, and in each are valves that ensure the circular flow of gas through the system. It also incorporates a soda-lime canister and an APL valve in the expiratory limb and a reservoir bag (or ventilator bellows) that can be placed at any point in the circle. The earlier circle systems also incorporated the anesthetic vaporizer within the circle. These were of the type that present only a low resistance to the flow of gas through them (e.g. the Goldman draw-over vaporizer). The vaporizer in circle (VIC) systems were necessary because the high blood–gas solubility and relatively low potency of the older inhalational agents meant that insufficient amounts of vapor could be carried into the circle by the low FGFs if the vaporizer was outside the circle. The danger with the VIC system is that the concentration of anesthetic agent leaving the vaporizer increases as FGF into the circle decreases. The vaporizer also adds to the concentration already present in the rebreathed fraction of gas allowing very high concentrations to develop.

The introduction of the modern inhalation agents with high potency and low blood–gas solubility has meant that circle systems are now almost universally "vaporizer outside the circle" (VOC) systems. This, however, has not eliminated the problem of carrying sufficient agent into the circle on low flows of fresh gas. During the early stages of the anesthetic, the absorption of the inhalational agent by the patient is at its greatest and often exceeds the rate at which it is carried into the circle by the FGF. For example, in a 70-kg adult an inspired concentration of isoflurane of 2% results in an initial uptake of approximately 100 mL per minute (of vapor). In order to carry this into the circle, if the vaporizer is set at 2%, an FGF of $5\,L\,min^{-1}$ is required in order to maintain the concentration of isoflurane in the system. Even if the anesthesiologist turns the vaporizer up to the maximum setting of 8%, an FGF of $1.25\,L\,min^{-1}$ is still required. These figures assume that the breathing system is already primed with the desired concentration of anesthetic agent, which in practice is rarely the case, and thus a period of washin of the system itself must also be allowed for. The internal volume of most circle breathing systems is between 6 and 10 L, which makes this consideration an important one.

The actual inspired concentration of volatile agent in a circle breathing system is the product of the complex interaction between the patient (size, cardiac output, minute volume, and oxygen consumption), the anesthetic vapor used (blood gas solubility), the system (the internal volume, the concentration of anesthetic and oxygen in the prime, and the configuration of the system), and the FGFs. The relation between these must be understood if a circle breathing system is to be used safely at low flows. Lowe and Ernst produced a set of tables to assist the anesthesiologist in administering low-flow anesthesia.[13] They based their uptake model for volatile agents on the single-compartment square root of time model developed by Severinghaus for nitrous oxide. The model states that if alveolar concentration of anesthetic is constant, then uptake can be approximated by the formula:

$$\dot{V}an = F_{A}an \times \lambda_{b/g} \times \dot{Q} \times \sqrt{t}$$

where $\dot{V}an$ is anesthetic uptake ($mL\,min^{-1}$), $F_{A}an$ is alveolar concentration of anesthetic, $\lambda_{b/g}$ is blood–gas partition coefficient, $\dot{Q}$ is cardiac output ($mL\,min^{-1}$), and t is time from the start of the anesthetic.

This model has been incorporated into a computer simulation for circle breathing systems called PsiGas, which is available for the Psion 3 series pocket computer. This simulator allows the anesthesiologist to experiment with different sizes of patient under differing physiologic conditions, various configurations of the circle, its size and how it is primed, different anesthetic agents with or without nitrous oxide, even allowing for the invention of fictitious agents, and different FGFs. It demonstrates how it is possible to both under- and overdose the volatile agent within a closed circle, how it is possible to deliver a hypoxic gas mixture, and under what circumstances these might occur.

The square root of time model has been criticized for overestimating the uptake of volatile agents, and other models exist, including the Westkensow model and the Lin model. Both of these, as in the case of the Lowe and Ernst model, are based on experimental data and differ mainly in their interpretation of whether washin of the alveolar compartment constitutes uptake. Multicompartmental pharmacokinetic modeling can be achieved using the Zuntz equation, which because of its complexity is of little practical assistance unless incorporated in a computer simulation.

The circle breathing system has become popular again because of its versatility. It can be used safely at a variety of flows, from very high flows (greater than minute volume), at which it is effectively a Mapleson D system and carbon dioxide absorption is not required, down to basal flows at which FGFs are no greater than the patient's oxygen and anesthetic uptake. Table 29.8 summarizes the advantages and disadvantages of low-flow circle absorber systems.

A recent development in the field of closed system anesthesia is the high-flow closed system. An example of this is the Physioflex anesthetic machine. In these systems, a blower is incorporated into the system which circulates the gases in the circle at around $70\,L\,min^{-1}$. This results in complete mixing of all the gases within the system and completely eliminates the problem of the long time constant of traditional low-flow systems. This means that any drop in concentration of volatile agent due to absorption is immediately detected and compensated for by computer-controlled injection of agent. This is done in the form of liquid anesthetic, which is instantly and reliably vaporized by the high flow of gases within the system. The system has, as well as a soda-lime canister, a charcoal absorber, which can be switched in and out of the system. This allows for rapid recovery at the end of anesthesia as volatile agent is scrubbed from the system very rapidly, preventing the rebreathing of expired inhalational agent, which in normal circumstances delays its elimination. These systems are extremely efficient at conserving anesthetic agent and are useful when expensive agents are being used such as desflurane and xenon. They are also a very good way of monitoring the patient's metabolic status as oxygen consumption can be very closely followed. The control of these highly engineered systems is via a computer interface, which is considered by some to be a disadvantage as it completely divorces the anesthesiologist from the mechanics of delivering the anesthetic.

Use of low-flow circle systems in pediatric anesthesia

Although the first circle system was developed and used in Germany as long ago as 1924,[14] pediatric anesthesiologists have long been reluctant to adopt their use on account of various concerns, particularly excessive dead space and resistance in the system.[15] There have also been concerns over safety because of the greater complexity and potential for incorrect assembly.[16] However, there is now more interest in the use of circle systems in pediatrics, particularly with the increased awareness of pollution and for reasons of cost associated with the use of newer, more expensive, volatile agents.

There is no generally accepted definition of "low flow." Meakin[17] has suggested that low-flow anesthesia should be defined as the use of a flow rate less than the patient's alveolar ventilation. This is a low rate, less than that required with a Mapleson A system, the most efficient system not using an absorber.[18] Note that low-flow and closed system are not necessarily synonymous terms. Closed systems, as mentioned above, have no or minimal overflow, and gas replacement into the system is limited to that necessary to replace that taken up by the patient.

Safety aspects of the breathing system

The breathing system can present a safety hazard to the patient through disconnection, leakage, and transmission of infection, or by excessive airway pressure.

There are many connections between the various components in most systems. Each connection may fail and result in disconnection of the patient from the ventilator and oxygen supply. Anesthetic breathing system connectors have been standardized to a system of conical male/female push-fit connectors with diameters of 22 mm and 15 mm for adult systems and 15 mm and 8.5 mm for pediatric systems. In pediatrics, endotracheal tube connectors of 8.5 mm are now sometimes used as an alternative to the more bulky 15-mm connectors (which remain the ISO standard). There is a risk of incompatible connections, however, if both 15-mm and 8.5-mm sizes are allowed to coexist in the same area.

Both the connectors and the tubing of the breathing system can crack and leak as a result of wear and tear, especially through repeated autoclaving. The plastic corrugated construction of the tubing confers a degree of flexibility, which helps to prevent cracking. The problems of wear and tear have largely been eliminated by the introduction of modern systems designed for single use. These systems, however, are often used on more than one patient, which means they may potentially act as a source for transmission of infection between patients. Bacterial filters are almost always incorporated into the system at the point of

Table 29.8 *Advantages and disadvantages of a low-flow circle absorber system*

Advantages	Disadvantages
Low FGFs	Slow changes in volatile agent concentration
Reduction of room pollution	Gas monitor essential otherwise delivered agent and oxygen concentrations not known
	Potential CO_2 accumulation in event of absorber exhaustion
Reduced patient heat loss	Possible toxicity problems
Reduced patient evaporative water loss	More bulky
More difficult technique? – more vigilance required	Higher compressible gas volume
	More difficult technique?
	Infection risk ? – more difficult to sterilize
	Potential for gas leaks

FGFs, fresh gas flows.

connection with the airway device. These often function as devices for the conservation of heat and moisture (see below).

The first line of defense against excessive airway pressure is the APL valve. This is described below. If the APL valve happens to be closed, or the system does not incorporate one, the next line of defense would be the reservoir bag. Under pressure, this will normally distend and will continue to do so, maintaining a more or less constant pressure of approximately 40 cmH_2O. If this fails or happens to be switched out of the system, as happens in some systems when a ventilator is on, then the only remaining defense will be the pressure limiters within the anesthetic machine itself. These pressure limiters are designed for the protection of the machine and not the patient and will not prevent the patient from coming to harm as a result of barotrauma.

Other components of the breathing system

The adjustable pressure-limiting valve

The APL valve is a common feature of all semiclosed and closed breathing systems. Its function is to vent gas from the otherwise sealed breathing system when a certain pressure is reached. The pressure at which this occurs is adjusted by changing the tension in a spring, which holds the valve closed. The valve itself is a metal disk, which is seated on an upfacing aperture in the system. The rim of the aperture is knife edged to minimize the contact area of the disk and reduce the risk of sticking. A safety mechanism incorporated into most APL valves prevents the tension rising above 60 cmH_2O, which prevents barotrauma to the patient. During spontaneous breathing the tension is reduced to a minimum, allowing the venting of expired gases and providing as little resistance to expiration as possible. During artificial ventilation the tension in the valve is increased to around the peak inspiratory pressure of the ventilation cycle. This provides a controlled leak of gas (usually a mixture of fresh gas and expired gases) from the system. During closed-system anesthesia the valve is shut completely so that the only gas to leave the system is that absorbed by the patient, however it continues to provide a pressure-limiting safety mechanism in these circumstances. Most APL valves are incorporated into a plastic sleeve, which allows connection to the anesthetic gas scavenging system.

The soda-lime canister

Soda-lime is used for the absorption of CO_2 in rebreathing systems. Its composition when dry is as follows:

- calcium hydroxide (94%);
- sodium hydroxide (5%);
- potassium hydroxide (1%);
- silicates, kieselguhr, and indicator dye (< 1%).

In use it is hydrated with 15–20% water. The chemical reaction that takes place when CO_2 is absorbed is as follows:

$$CO_2 + 2NaOH \rightarrow Na_2CO_3 + H_2O$$

$$Na_2CO_3 + Ca(OH)_2 \rightarrow 2NaOH + CaCO_3$$

The reactions are exothermic and result in the production of water as well as a drop in pH as the calcium hydroxide is converted to calcium carbonate. (If the canister does not feel warm to touch, the soda-lime may not be functioning and CO_2 absorption may not be taking place.) The water is present as a thin film over the granules. Water is essential, as the chemical reactions only take place between ions in the presence of water. The efficiency of the soda-lime depends on its physical structure. A sufficient surface area is required to maximize the use of the chemicals, however smaller granules pack too tightly and provide excessive resistance to the flow of gas. Granules that are too large result in the channeling of gas, so that some fails to come into contact with the soda-lime at all. The silica is used to structure the granules to their optimal size and reduce dust formation. Most canisters will hold 1 kg, which is sufficient, when used at low flows, for about 5 h use. In normal use when higher flows are used, this life can be extended. Some systems have two canisters or jumbo canisters holding up to 2 kg of soda-lime.

Soda-lime has been associated with a number of adverse events. The heat generated and the highly caustic environment inside the soda-lime has resulted in the chemical breakdown of some of the volatile anesthetic agents. The classic example is trichloroethylene, which breaks down to dichloroacetylene, which is a potent neurotoxin. More modern agents have also been shown to decompose in soda-lime, including sevoflurane, however this has not proved to be of clinical significance. It is recommended, however, that sevoflurane is not used for periods longer than 3 h in a closed system without flushing the system. If soda-lime is allowed to dry out, for example by leaving fresh gas flowing through the canister while the machine is not in use, then its subsequent use with certain agents has been associated with the production of carbon monoxide. These agents include isoflurane, enflurane, and desflurane. Carbon monoxide is not detected by gas monitors routinely used in clinical anesthesia.

Baralyme

Baralyme is a mixture of 80% calcium hydroxide and 20% barium hydroxide, plus indicator. Potassium hydroxide may also be present. It is the barium hydroxide that is the active component, reacting in a similar manner to the sodium hydroxide in soda-lime.

VENTILATORS

A ventilator is a machine that provides ventilation or supplements the patient's own ventilation. Most adults receiving artificial ventilation for anesthesia do so from a ventilator rather than manually. In anesthesia, a ventilator, in conjunction with the breathing system, must perform three functions:

1 supply oxygen to the patients;
2 eliminate carbon dioxide;
3 supply gaseous or volatile anesthetic agents.

Artificial ventilation has a long history – Robert Hooke ventilated a dog manually in the seventeenth century using a pair of bellows.[19] This section describes some of the principles of ventilators. It is not possible to describe in detail all the individual ventilators available. Whichever ventilator is in use, the anesthesiologist should be familiar with its working principles and controls. Table 29.9 outlines the classification of positive pressure ventilators.

Advantages of using a ventilator for anesthesia

The advantages can be summarized as follows:

1 A ventilator may produce more consistent ventilation than manual ventilation.
2 Anesthesia personnel can concentrate on other tasks.
3 There is less fatigue experienced by anesthesia personnel.
4 Monitoring and recording of some ventilation parameters is easier.

Possible disadvantages of using a ventilator for anesthesia

Some of the potential disadvantages of using a ventilator are:

1 There is a loss of contact between the anesthesiologist and the patient. Many publications, over 300 years after Hooke's publication, describe neonates and infants in particular as being better ventilated with manual rather than mechanical ventilation. It is the view of many pediatric anesthesiologists that this allows detection of breathing system problems, such as disconnection or airway obstruction, and allows the anesthesiologist to compensate for changes in compliance caused by surgical manipulations.[20] However, at least one study[21] found that even experienced anesthesiologists were not always able to detect these changes.
2 Some older ventilators may lack adequate monitoring and alarm functions, and may continue to make the appropriate sounds even if the patient is not being ventilated, giving the anesthesiologist a false sense of security.
3 Compared with intensive care ventilators, anesthesia ventilators are relatively simple in design, and have fewer controls. While this may be an advantage, some newer modes of ventilation may not be possible. Conversely, more complex ventilators may not be as user-friendly in the rapidly changing environment of an operating room when the anesthesiologist has other matters on which to concentrate.
4 High flows of fresh gas or driving gas may be needed, a drawback in situations in which supplies of gas may be limited.
5 Sterilization of components may not be easy, with a risk of cross-infection if this is not performed adequately.

With the above points in mind, the properties required of a ventilator suitable for anesthesia are summarized in Table 29.10.

Table 29.9 *Classification of positive-pressure ventilators*

Power source
1 Electricity
2 Gas (high pressure)
3 Gas (low-pressure anesthetic gas)

Mechanism of action
1 Minute volume divider
2 Mechanical thumb
3 Bag squeezer
4 Intermittent blower
5 High-frequency oscillator
6 Jet ventilator

A functional classification of ventilators
1 The method of cycling (the separation of inspiration from expiration)
2 The method whereby gas flow is generated in the ventilator
3 The method of producing a pulmonary pressure gradient

Classification of ventilators

There is more than one way of classifying ventilators, and some ventilators may fall into more than one category according to the mode of use.

Negative- vs. positive-pressure ventilation

A fundamental classification is into negative- and positive-pressure ventilators. Negative-pressure ventilators, though they have a role for long-term ventilatory support, are not routinely used for anesthesia, although they were originally conceived for such use.

Cycling between phases of ventilation

Time cycling

The point at which inspiration ends and expiration is allowed to commence is usually determined by a fixed time, which is set by the anesthesiologist, either directly or indirectly. This is called time cycling and is the most common arrangement.

Pressure cycling

The ventilator cycles when a preset pressure has been reached. In this case, a change in compliance may affect the volume of gas delivered. For example, a surgeon leaning on the patient's chest may reduce tidal gas flow.

Volume cycling

It is also possible to cycle when a given volume of gas has been delivered. The ventilatory pressures necessary to deliver this may vary. The pressure may become high if the patient's compliance is reduced, unless a limit is put on it (Fig. 29.11).

Characteristics of ventilators

Ventilators may be described in various ways (see Table 29.9). In broad terms, anesthesia ventilators may be divided into constant-flow generators and constant-pressure generators. A major functional classification

Table 29.10 *Desirable properties of an anesthesia ventilator*

1 Easy to use
2 Difficult to misconnect or misuse
3 Easy to sterilize
4 Reliable
5 Easy conversion to manual ventilation
6 Differing ventilation modes available, e.g. pressure or flow generation
7 Ventilation parameters adjustable over a wide range
8 Economical over its lifetime
  a Cost of purchase
  b Running costs

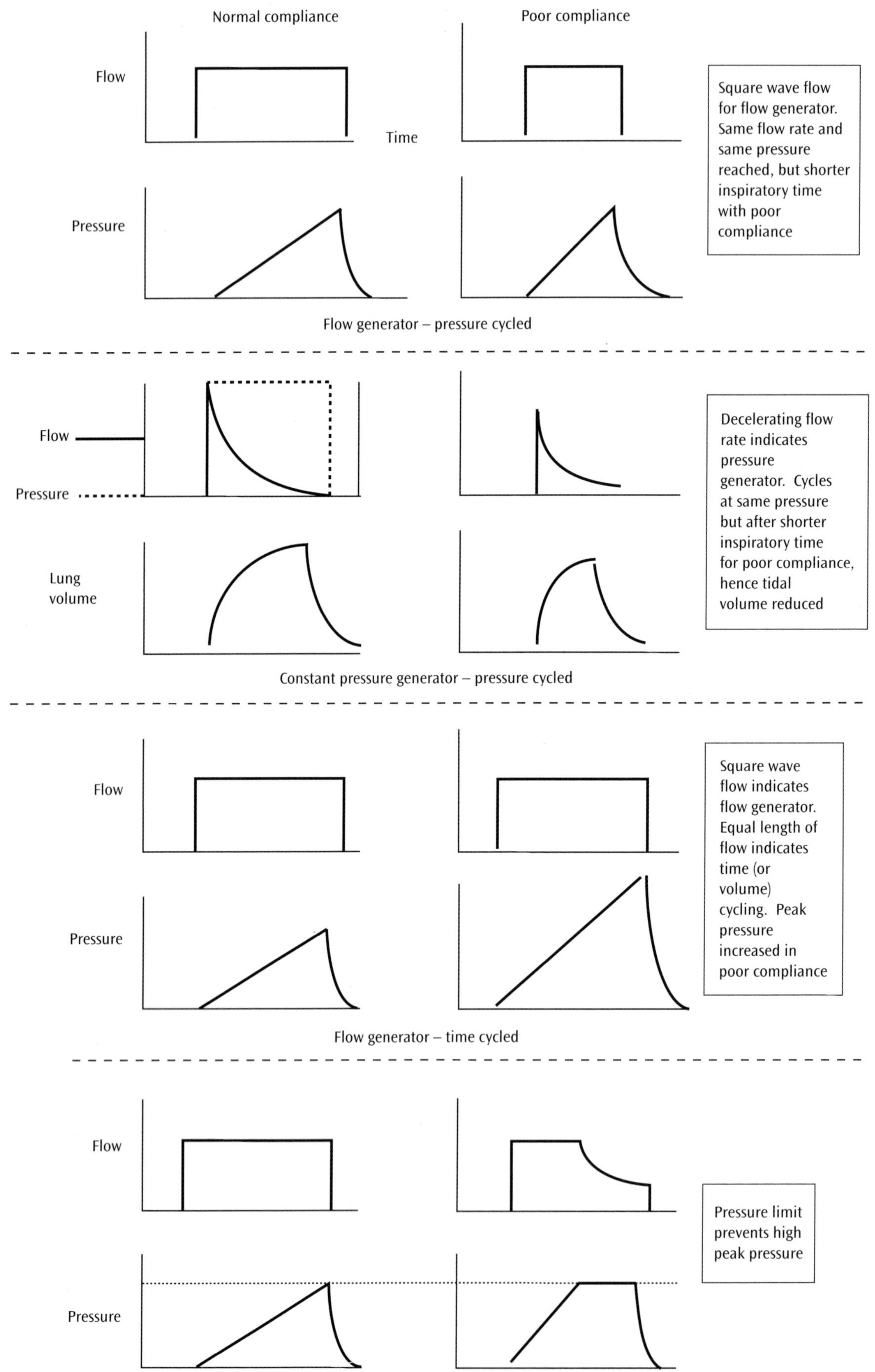

Figure 29.11 *The diagram shows simplified inspiratory flows and pressures for ventilators in a patient with normal compliance and one with reduced compliance.*

is the manner in which a pressure gradient is produced, driving gas into the patient during inspiration.

It should be remembered that this division is not rigid, and that with the appropriate circumstances, a given ventilator may operate as either type, or may only approximately function in one of these categories.

Constant-pressure generators

A preset increase in pressure in the breathing system is developed, producing an inspiratory flow. The flow rate of gases into the patient will depend on the characteristics of the whole system, i.e. the resistance and compliance of the breathing system as well as that of the patient's airways and lungs. The mean flow rate and the inspiratory time will determine the tidal volume of gas delivered to the system. In some situations, the tidal volume may be measured, but in other cases the tidal volume is not known.

The initial flow rate is high, falling away as the pressure gradient diminishes. The decelerating flow rate is characteristic of constant pressure generators.

Note that if overall compliance changes, for example by surgical retraction on a lung during a thorocotomy, or by partial obstruction of an airway or the endotracheal tube by a plug of mucus, there is a danger that the resulting reduction of tidal flow may not be noticed, unless flow to the patient is monitored.

The advantages of this approach include automatic compensation for small leaks in the system or around an uncuffed endotracheal tube. Hence, pressure generators have remained popular in pediatric anesthesia. Also, as the pressure is preset, barotrauma is avoided.

Constant-flow generators

A constant flow in the system is produced, the tidal volume depending on the magnitude of the flow and the duration of inspiration. The driving force producing the constant flow is very high in relation to the resistance to flow in the system. Although the pressure in the lungs rises during inspiration, this is small in proportion to that of the driving gas. Thus, for practical purposes the flow remains constant throughout inspiration. In the presence of increased airway resistance or of reduced lung compliance, the airway pressure will rise to maintain a constant flow. In practice, a blow-off valve limits the rise in pressure to prevent barotrauma. A leak in the breathing system will reduce patient tidal volume, as the flow remains constant in comparison with constant-pressure generators.

Control of ventilation variables

Tidal volume

Tidal volume is the volume of gas entering or leaving the patient with inspiration or expiration. Note that the two are not necessarily exactly the same because of the respiratory quotient (or respiratory exchange ratio), the effect of warming the gas, and the presence of water vapor. Some of the tidal volume leaving the ventilator may be absorbed by the compliance of the breathing system, and a mechanism to compensate for this may be present. This involves checking the system compliance before connecting the patient to the system. In addition, if there is a leak around the endotracheal tube, the volume of gas leaving the breathing system may not be the same as that entering the patient's airway.

Tidal volume is directly set on most ventilators used for adults. On other ventilators, tidal volume is set indirectly by adjusting minute ventilation and rate or by varying flow rate and inspiratory time.

Minute volume

This is either directly set or is the product of tidal volume and rate.

Maximum pressure

It is usually possible to limit the pressure attainable during the inspiratory phase. If this pressure is reached as a result of low lung compliance, the volume of gas delivered may be limited.

Frequency

This is directly or indirectly set. Indirect control involves setting the total cycle time by controlling inspiratory and expiratory times.

Inspiratory–expiratory ratio

The inspiratory–expiratory (I/E) ratio may be adjusted directly on some ventilators, particularly those used in pediatrics. However, it is more common for it to be determined indirectly by the setting of other variables.

Expiration

In most anesthesia ventilators, expiration is a passive process and relies on the elastic recoil of the patient's chest and lungs. In patients, such as asthmatics, in whom there is resistance to gas flow, it is not possible to assist expiration. It is therefore necessary to have an expiratory time prolonged sufficiently to allow passive expiration to occur. If expiration does not fully occur it may lead to hyperinflation, decreased cardiac output, barotrauma, and even pneumothorax.

The ventilator and the patient breathing system – the mechanism of action of ventilators

Functionally, ventilators my be divided into three types:

- intermittent gas flow occluders ("mechanical thumbs");
- minute volume dividers;
- intermittent tidal volume generators.

Gas flow occluders

The gas in the Mapleson E breathing system flows constantly into the T-system. Intermittent occlusion of the reservoir tube will force the gas to flow into the patient, followed by expiration as the occlusion is released. Tidal volume into the patient depends on gas flow and duration of inspiration, as will peak inspiratory pressure (unless this is limited by a pressure-limiting valve). There are dangers inherent in such a system, in that failure of the ventilator in the occlusion position potentially exposes the patient to a continuous inspiratory flow of gas and resulting high pressures.

Minute volume dividers

The total minute volume of gas delivered from the anesthetic machine is divided into tidal volumes, of a size determined by the anesthesiologist, which are all delivered to the patient. The smaller the set tidal volumes, the greater will be the frequency of breathing. During expiration the FGF runs into a bellows. The bellows expands to reach the set tidal volume, the time taken to do this depending on the FGF. At this point the gas is driven into the patient by a weight acting on the bellows. The effect is to produce a time-cycled constant-pressure generating ventilator. The ventilator is powered by the pressure of the fresh gas.

Bag in bottle ventilators

During manual ventilation, the anesthesiologist's hand squeezes the reservoir bag of the breathing system to drive gas into the patient. The bag in bottle ventilator replaces the anesthesiologist's hand.

Most modern ventilators are of the "bag in bottle" type. The bag, or concertina bellows, is inside a transparent chamber. The inside of the bellows is connected to the patient's breathing system and contains anesthetic gases. There is often a scale on the chamber, so that the tidal excursions of the bag can be judged.

During inspiration, the bellows is compressed by driving gas flowing into the chamber and compressing the bellows, in the same way that the anesthesiologist's hand would squeeze the bag. The driving gas, usually oxygen, cannot leave the chamber as an exhaust valve is closed, so the pressure in the chamber rises, the bellows are compressed, and the gas inside the bellows is driven toward the patient.

At the end of inspiration, the chamber exhaust valve is opened, allowing the driving gas to escape from the chamber. The bellows is no longer compressed, allowing it to fill again with anesthetic gases. Once the bag is full, toward the end of the patient's expiratory phase, an overspill valve in the bellows opens and any excess anesthetic gas is vented into the exhaust system. This valve closes again when inspiration commences. This dumping of excess anesthetic gas in the expiratory phase contrasts with manual ventilation, in which excess anesthetic gases are vented during inspiration. Furthermore, during mechanical ventilation, the APL valve is either fully closed manually or, more commonly, is automatically isolated and thus rendered inoperative.

Ascending versus descending bellows

Bellows may function in two ways. In expiration, when the bellows are filling, they may either rise from the base of the chamber, and then be compressed downward during inspiration, or they may be attached to the top of the chamber and descend during expiration (filling) and then be compressed upwards during inspiration. Most ventilators designed during the 1990s are of the ascending type. There are safety arguments in favor of this arrangement – if a major leak develops in the system, the ascending bellows will usually collapse. However a descending bellows may still descend, sucking room air into the system. Thus, ventilation with room air may continue to a degree, and alarms may not be activated, giving rise to potential problems both of awareness and reduced F_IO_2.

The ventilator controls the flow of driving gas, and the timing of operation of the valves. Controls are either pneumatic (fluidic) or electronic. Pneumatically controlled ventilators do not require electrical power, whereas the more common electronic ventilators require both electrical power to operate the valves and a source of driving gas to power the bellows. The operation of valves does not require much power, and it is usual for electronic anesthesia ventilators to have a reserve battery, in case of power failure, which is usually capable of running the ventilator for at least an hour.

General problems associated with ventilator use

Most anesthesia ventilators perform reliably for long periods. In the unlikely event of failure, a system to hand-ventilate the patient should always be present, giving time for the anesthesiologist to consider the cause of the failure. A procedure for checking ventilators, recommended by the AAGBI, is outlined in Table 29.11.

Disconnection

This may occur anywhere in the breathing system, and is a common and preventable anesthetic problem.

Ventilator failure

Causes of failure include disconnection of the power source and internal mechanical dysfunction. Many electrically powered ventilators incorporate a battery in case of power failure, but this must be kept charged. Apparent ventilator failure may result from faults in the monitoring of ventilatory variables, e.g. a pneumotachograph at the patient's end of the breathing system may become clogged with mucoid secretions.

Leak of driving gas

A leak around the bellows housing may result in a loss of driving gas and a consequent loss of tidal volume.

Leak of gas from the breathing system

Flow generators which are time or volume cycled do not compensate for loss of gas from the breathing system. A descending bellows system may descend normally despite loss of breathing system gas, and sufficient pressure may still be developed such that a low-pressure alarm may not signal.

Occlusion of the breathing system

This may be an equipment- or patient-related problem.

Ventilation alarms

Disconnect/apnea alarms may be triggered by monitoring end-tidal carbon dioxide, or by monitoring pressure cycling failure. Other ventilator alarms commonly found include high pressure, low tidal volume, low (subatmospheric) pressure, and reverse flow in a circle system.

OTHER MODES OF VENTILATION

High-frequency ventilation

There are three modes of high-frequency ventilation (HFV): high-frequency positive-pressure ventilation, high-frequency jet ventilation, and high-frequency oscillation.

High-frequency positive-pressure ventilation

High-frequency positive-pressure ventilation (HFPPV) is possible via an endotracheal tube using a conventional ventilator. Ventilators using pneumatic (fluidic) valves are often used, though many conventional pediatric ventilators are capable of delivering the frequencies required without modification. Typical rates of ventilation for adults are 1–2.5 Hz (60–150 cycles min^{-1}). Other modes of delivery include endotracheal catheters via bronchoscopes.

Table 29.11 *Recommended procedure for checking a ventilator*

1. Check that the ventilator is configured correctly for its intended use. Ensure that the ventilator tubing is securely attached. Set the controls for use and ensure that adequate pressure is generated during the inspiratory phase.
2. Check that a disconnect alarm is present and functions correctly.
3. Check that the pressure relief valve functions correctly at the set pressure.
4. Ensure that there is an alternative means to ventilate the patient's lungs in the event of ventilator malfunction.

Recommended by the Association of Anaesthetists of Great Britain and Ireland.

High-frequency jet ventilation

High-frequency jet ventilation (HFJV)may be delivered via a catheter placed in a bronchoscope, via a modified double- or treble-lumen endotracheal tube, or through a cricothyroid catheter. Low tidal volumes (up to 150 mL) are utilized at rates of between 1 and 10 Hz (60–600 cycles min^{-1}), and airway pressures are low at about 0.5 kPa (5 cmH_2O). Ventilation with a conventional ventilator and a HFJV in tandem is sometimes used for patients with severe barotrauma or a bronchopleural fistula.

All the above types of high-frequency ventilators have active inspiration only. Expiration occurs passively as in conventional ventilation.

High-frequency oscillation

The feature of high-frequency oscillation (HFO), defined as 3–15 Hz (180–900 cycles min^{-1}), which distinguishes it from other forms of high-frequency ventilation, is that both inspiration and expiration are active. Active inspiration and expiration produce a sinusoidal pressure waveform that oscillates above and below the baseline continuous positive airway pressure. Either a piston- or a loudspeaker-type diaphragm is used to create the oscillations, which have an amplitude of 1–3 mL kg^{-1} (i.e. less than dead space). Short, noncompliant tubing is necessary to prevent the oscillations being absorbed by the tubing. Oxygen is added via a side arm.

Clinical matters are outside the scope of this chapter, but, broadly speaking, two modes of HFO are utilized. In general, for diffuse alveolar disease, the mean airway pressure on the oscillator should be 3–4 cmH_2O higher than on a conventional ventilator. For unilateral or nonhomogeneous lung disease, or air leak, the mean airway pressure should be equal to or less than that of the conventional ventilator. Should the ventilator and patient become disconnected, for example during transfers, alveoli will collapse, and a sustained inflation will be necessary to re-establish the patient's functional residual capacity. The mechanism of gas exchange is not clear. However, in patients with restrictive lung disease such as adult respiratory distress syndrome (ARDS), oxygenation is related to mean airway pressure, and ventilation (i.e. CO_2 removal) is related to FGF and the magnitude of the oscillations, and is inversely related to the oscillation frequency. HFO ventilation may be combined with conventional ventilation.

Injector ventilation

The Saunders injector uses manually controlled jets of air or, more usually, oxygen, delivered by a needle injector down a rigid bronchoscope or similar tube. Room air is entrained via the open end of the bronchoscope. Expiration is via the open end of the bronchoscope and is passive. Different sizes of needle are used according to patient size.

Noninvasive ventilation

Brief mention is made of this here as, although not primarily intended as a mode of ventilation for operating room use, the anesthesiologist may encounter patients with this form of ventilation in other settings.

The chief aims of noninvasive ventilation are to reduce the work of breathing, improve gas exchange, and minimize risk, partly by the avoidance of intubation or tracheostomy. Home ventilation is possible for many patients. Ventilation may be on a 24-h basis or nocturnal only to give respite to weak respiratory muscles.

Noninvasive intermittent positive-pressure ventilation

The use of noninvasive ventilation has increased in the past decade, partly because of the greater use of nasal ventilation, often achieved by a nasal mask. The ventilation modes of conventional ventilators may be used by noninvasive ventilators. In addition, it is possible to arrange for spontaneous patient triggering of the inspiratory cycle, which improves patient comfort. Leakage around the mask may be a problem, particularly for patients with incomplete dentition.

Intermittent negative pressure ventilation

The whole of the patient, apart from the head ("iron lung" ventilator), is surrounded by a rigid container. A flexible seal around the neck is necessary. Cuirass ventilators operate similarly, but are more convenient as only the thorax is enclosed. The pressure within the container is cycled between atmospheric and subatmospheric pressures, causing respiratory excursions. An important benefit is that the patient does not require intubation to achieve ventilation.

Transport ventilators

The requirements of a transport ventilator vary from those used in the operating room environment. Anesthesiologists are frequently called upon to accompany ventilated patients, and familiarity with the particular ventilator being used is essential, as is some additional means of ventilation should power supplies or compressed gas supplies fail.

The general requirements include:

- portability – relatively low weight and small overall volume;
- reliability – during patient transport, a back-up mechanical ventilator is unlikely to be present;
- ability to withstand knocks and even being dropped;
- tolerance of wide range of ambient temperature;
- tolerance of variation in ambient atmospheric pressure (e.g. if the ventilator is to be used in unpressurized aircraft cabins or in hyperbaric conditions undersea);
- power supply self-contained, i.e. from compressed gas or battery – in either case, battery usage or compressed gas use should be as low as possible to give adequate endurance;
- if electrically powered, no broadcast radio interference or interference with nearby navigational instruments (particularly important for airborne use).

As a minimum set of requirements, a transport ventilator should have the following capabilities:

- have independent control of tidal volume and frequency;
- be able to monitor airway pressure and have a high-pressure alarm;
- have a disconnect alarm;
- be capable of providing PEEP;
- be capable of providing a wide range of $F_{I}O_2$.

Some modern transport ventilators have more sophisticated ventilation modes incorporated such as assisted spontaneous breathing (ASB), pressure control ventilation, and flow triggering.

SCAVENGING SYSTEMS

Occupational anesthetic agent exposure has been implicated in spontaneous abortion, malformation, cancer, polyneuropathy, and behavioral malformation. Numerous studies have suggested, but have not proved, that exposure to anesthetic agents may be hazardous. Despite this lack of hard evidence, maximum exposure levels were decreed and incorporated into recommendations by the National Institute for Occupational Safety and Health (NIOSH) in the USA and the equivalent regulations for the Control of Substances Hazardous to Health (COSHH), issued by the Health and Safety Executive (HSE) in the UK. These levels are set at 2 p.p.m. for any halogenated agent and 25 p.p.m. for nitrous oxide.

Unscavenged operating rooms have had measured levels as high as 70 p.p.m. for halogenated agents and 3000 p.p.m. for nitrous oxide; meticulous scavenging can reduce these levels to 0.005 and 1 p.p.m. respectively.

The scavenging system performs the important function of carrying exhausted gases from the breathing system away from the operating area and preventing contamination of the operating room environment with potentially toxic anesthetic gases.

A scavenging system consists of:

- a collecting system, often leading from the ventilator expiratory port or a breathing system APL valve;
- a receiving interface or reservoir to protect the breathing system from back-pressure, should the system become occluded, and also to protect from excessive negative pressure;
- further tubing leading to the gas dispersal point at which gases are vented to the atmosphere.

For breathing systems with an APL valve the collecting system is a plastic sleeve with a 30-mm connector to the transfer system. For open and semiopen systems the collecting system may have a funnel or similar device, which is held close to the area where anesthetic gases are exhausted from the breathing system. The transfer system has to be wide bore so as to have low resistance to the flow of gas. Usually this is 30-mm corrugated tubing. The patient must be protected from both excessive positive and negative pressures, and this can be achieved either by using an "open" system with a high-flow air brake or by using a "closed" system with a reservoir bag and carefully adjusted valves. The open-type receiving system is a reservoir, often an open-ended cylinder, hence preventing any positive or negative pressure being transmitted to the patient.

The disposal system can be active or passive though active scavenging is more common.

Passive systems

In passive systems, the gas is driven along wide-bore tubing by the patient's own expiratory flow. Thus, low resistance to flow is essential. The drawback of passive systems is vulnerability to external factors, mainly at the point at which gases are vented to the atmosphere. Changes in wind direction may lead to reversal of flow in the scavenging system, and even to pollution of one operating area with gases from another if the venting points are close together.

Active systems

Gas is actively pumped to the external site, sometimes via a pipeline from the gas pendant. The negative pressure is usually provided either by a Venturi system or from the main vacuum system. The reservoir assembly may have an indicator float that rises to indicate that the negative system pressure is turned on and the system is operational. An active scavenging system typically generates a flow of 30–80 L min^{-1} without producing a negative pressure more than 50 Pa (0.5 cmH_2O).

Other methods of reducing pollution

Activated charcoal canisters can be used if a fixed active or passive system is unavailable. However, there may be variations in efficiency with changes in gas flow through the canister. Also, activated charcoal does not adsorb nitrous oxide so pollution from this source is not removed.

A poor mask fit, filling vaporizers in the operating room, and failing to scavenge the exhaust from gas analyzers can easily defeat effective scavenging. Efficient room ventilation is also essential in the recovery area, where significant pollution may otherwise occur.

Monitoring of pollution

Portable infrared analyzers are available to monitor atmospheric pollution levels. In addition, personal monitoring systems are available. These consist of badges worn by individuals in a manner akin to the radiation exposure badges worn by radiology personnel.

REFERENCES

1. International Standards Organization. *Anaesthesiology Vocabulary (ISO 4135: 1995)*. Geneva: ISO, 1995.
2. Longnecker DE, Murphy FL. *Dripps Echenofff Vadam Introduction to Anesthesiology*, 9th edn. Philadelphia: WB Saunders, 1997.
3. McMahon J. Rebreathing as a basis for classification of anaesthesia circuits. *J Am Assoc Nurse Anesthetists* 1951; **19:** 133–58.
4. Baraka A. A functional classification of anaesthesia circuits. *Anaesth Intensive Care* 1977; **5:**172–8.
5. Miller D. Breathing systems reclassified. *Anaesth Intensive Care* 1995; **23:** 281–3.
6. Hamilton WK. Nomenclature of inhalation anaesthetic systems. *Anesthesiology* 1964; **25:** 3–5.
7. Mapleson WW. The elimination of rebreathing in various semi-closed anaesthetic systems. *Br J Anaesth* 1954; **26:** 323–32; *Br J Anaesth* "Citation Classic" 1998; **80:** 263–4.
8. Henville JD Adams AP. The Bain anaesthetic system. An assessment during controlled ventilation. *Anaesthesia* 1976; **31:** 247–56.
9. Ayre P. Anaesthesia for intra-cranial operations. *Lancet* 1937; **1:** 561–3.
10. Ayre P. Anaesthesia for hare-lip and cleft palate operation. *Br J Surg* 1937; **25:** 131.
11. Rees GJ. An early history of paediatric anaesthesia. *Paediatr Anaesth* 1991; **1:** 3–11.
12. Humphrey D. A new anaesthetic breathing system combining Mapleson A, D and E principles. A simple apparatus for low flow universal use without carbon dioxide absorption. *Anaesthesia* 1983; **38:**361–72.
13. Ernst EA, Lowe HJ. *The Quantitative Practice of Anaesthesia*. Baltimore, MD: Wiliams and Wilkins, 1981.
14. Baum JA. *Low Flow Anaesthesia. The Theory and Practice of Low Flow, Minimal Flow and Closed System Anaesthesia*, 2nd Engl. edn. London: Butterworth-Heinemann, 2001.
15. Peters JWB, Bezstarosti-Van Ereden J, Erdmann W, Meursing AEE. Safety and efficacy of semi-closed circle ventilation in small infants. *Paediatr Anaesth* 1998; **8:** 299–304.
16. Hughes DG. Paediatric anaesthesia equipment. In: Hughes DG, Mather SJ (eds). *Handbook of Paediatric Anaesthesia*. Oxford: Oxford University Press, 1991.
17. Meakin GH. Low-flow anaesthesia in infants and children. *Br J Anaesth* 1999; **83:** 50–7.
18. Meakin GH, Jennings AD, Beatty PCW, Healy TEJ. Fresh gas requirements of an enclosed afferent reservoir breathing system in anaesthetized spontaneously breathing children. *Br J Anaesth* 1992; **68:**333–337.
19. Hook R. An account of the experiment made by Mr Hook, of preserving animals alive by blowing through their lungs with bellows. *Phil Trans Royal Soc* 1667; **2:** 539–540.
20. Coté CJ. Paediatric breathing circuits and anesthesia machines. *Int Anesthesiol Clin* 1992; **30** (3): 51–61.
21. Spears Jr RS, Yeh A, Fischer DM, Zwass MS. The "educated hand." Can anesthesiologists assess changes in neonatal pulmonary compliance manually? *Anesthesiology* 1991; **75:** 693–6.

FURTHER READING

Dorsch JA, Dorsch SE. *Understanding Anaesthesia Equipment*, 4th edn. Baltimore, MD: Williams and Wilkins, 1999.

The Virtual Anesthesia Machine (interactive website) http://www.anest.ufl.edu/~eduweb/vam/

30

Computers and simulators in anesthesia

JAMES G BOVILL

As in virtually every other field of modern society, computers and computer technology have made significant inroads into anesthetic practice. Every new physiologic monitor and most of the newer generation of ventilators rely on this technology. The generation of graphical trends, simultaneous graphical and alphanumerical displays, arrhythmia detection, and S–T segment analysis would not be possible without the dedicated processors present in these devices. Often the presence of computers is transparent to the user. Many anesthesiologists also use a personal computer for word processing and administrative and statistical purposes. The modern anesthesiologist needs to be computer literate.

HISTORICAL BACKGROUND

Mechanical counting machines had been devised in the seventeenth century. The French scientist Blaise Pascal invented a digital adding machine in 1642, using a mechanical gear system, for the computations for his father's business accounts. The English mathematician and inventor Charles Babbage (1791–1871) conceived the first automatic digital computer in the 1830s. He produced plans for a Difference Engine that would automatically construct mathematical, nautical, and astronomical tables. In 1991, to celebrate the 200th anniversary of Babbage's birth, a team at the Science Museum in London constructed a complete Difference Engine from his original drawings. It worked exactly as Babbage had predicted. His greatest achievement, however, was a detailed plan for an Analytical Engine. This embodied many features found in later computers, including internal registers and a range of peripherals. It could make decisions based on previous calculations, and included features such as sequential control, branching, and looping. Babbage never constructed his Analytical Engine, largely because he was unable to raise the necessary financial support.

The first all-purpose, modern electronic computer was the ENIAC (Electronic Numerical Integrator and Calculator), completed in 1946 at the University of Pennsylvania. ENIAC was 1000 times faster than its electromechanical predecessors and could execute 5000 basic arithmetical operations per second (a modern computer can execute many million instructions per second). ENIAC was an externally programmed machine in which the sequence of operations required to solve any particular problem was wired on plugboards by hand. Each new problem required the wiring to be manually altered, a process taking days. The first stored-program electronic digital computer was the "Small Scale Experimental Machine" developed in the UK at the University of Manchester in 1948. A successor of this computer, the Ferranti Mark 1, was the first commercially available computer, production starting in February 1951. Another pioneering computer was the EDSAC (Electronic Delay Storage Automatic Calculator), developed in the UK at the University of Cambridge in 1959. These first-generation computers were massive machines and needed a small army of technicians to maintain them. They used valve technology and had a power consumption equivalent to that of a small town. The Ferranti Mark 1 contained about 4000 valves and 6 miles of wiring, and occupied two bays each 16 feet long, 8 feet high, and 4 feet wide (approximately 4.8 × 2.4 × 1.2 m). It had a power consumption of 27 kW. The successor to ENIAC, UNIVAC, contained 18 000 valves.

The real breakthrough in computer technology came with the discovery of the transistor in the 1950s. Its small size, much greater reliability, and its relatively low power consumption made it far superior to the valve. During the 1960s and 1970s electronic components were further miniaturized, resulting in dramatic improvements in computer technology. Today's computers use very large-scale integration (VSLI) technology, in which several million electronic components can be contained on a silicon chip (integrated circuit) less than 5 mm^2.

COMPUTER BASICS

Computers can be divided into two broad types, analog and digital. Analog computers solve problems by operating on continuous variables whereas digital computers operate on discontinuous or discrete values. Today, analog computers are only used for highly specialized tasks, e.g. by engineers for complex simulations. In general, in speaking about computers one is referring to digital computers.

The fundamental "language" of all digital computers is written in binary numbers (base 2). Information is stored as groups of binary digits called bits. Each bit can be in one of only two possible states, "on" or "off." These states are more often represented logically by the symbols "1" and "0", and internally as + 5 volts and 0 volts respectively. A pattern of eight bits is called a byte, and a number of bytes, the actual number varying between computers, is referred to as a word. Although modern computers can work with up to 8-byte (64-bit) words, the byte remains the basic unit in computer technology. In computer terminology one kilobyte (1 kB) represents 1024 (2^{10}) bytes, not 1000 bytes, and one megabyte (1 MB) represents 1024 kB. A binary number of even modest size is very long and difficult for humans to manipulate easily (365 decimal = 101 101 101 binary). Therefore, computer programmers often use another means of representation, the hexadecimal (base 16) number system, in which a group of 4 bits (a nibble) is encoded as one hexadecimal digit. Using 4 bits, it is possible to count from zero up to 15 (2^4–1) by extending the decimal number system using the letters A, B, C, D, E, and F (Table 30.1). The decimal number 365 is represented in hexadecimal as 16D. Occasionally, the octal system is used. This has its origin in the time when some mainframe computers had an internal organization based on 6-bit units rather than 8-bit bytes. The octal digit requires 3 bits ($2^3 = 8$, hence octal) and a 6-bit unit could be made up of two octal digits.

Every digital computer performs five basic functions: input, storage, control, processing, and output. The most common input sources are the keyboard and magnetic disk units, but input can also be via a parallel or serial port from a peripheral device such as a scanner or even from an electrocardiogram (ECG) monitor. Input data are stored in various internal storage devices, referred to as memory, until needed. Also held in memory are the instructions that govern the functioning of the computer and the program that will operate on the input data. The primary internal storage device is a high-speed random-access memory (RAM). The central processing unit (CPU) can both read from and write to RAM, and external programs and the data on which they operate must be read into RAM, e.g. from the hard disk, before execution. RAM is, however, volatile, and all stored information is lost when power is turned off. The second type of internal memory is ROM (read-only memory), which, in contrast to RAM, is permanent. ROM stores the programs the computer needs to function, such as the BIOS (basic input–output system). BIOS contains one of the most vital programs for the computer, the operating system software that handles the input and output functions and various routines that test and report errors in the components of the computer when power is switched on.

The control function involves retrieval of instructions from storage in the appropriate sequence and relaying the proper command to the arithmetic/logic unit (ALU), which is the part of the CPU where information processing takes place. It is this control function that distinguishes a computer from a calculator. The "brain" of a computer is the CPU, an integrated circuit that contains all the arithmetic, logic, and control circuitry needed for the computer to function. It is the CPU that interprets and executes instructions. In addition to the CPU, a computer will contain several other microprocessors dedicated to specific tasks such as control of the keyboard and disk drives or required for creating the video signals needed to put images on the monitor. Communication between the various parts of the computer, and with external devices, is by means of three special communication lines called buses (Fig. 30.1). The address bus enables communication between the CPU and memory. The data bus passes the actual information to and from the CPU, and the control bus defines the type of communication, e.g. read or write. For

Table 30.1 *Computer number systems*

Decimal	Binary	Octal	Hexadecimal
0	0	0	0
1	1	1	1
2	10	2	2
3	11	3	3
4	100	4	4
5	101	5	5
6	110	6	6
7	111	7	7
8	1000	10	8
9	1001	11	9
10	1010	12	A
11	1011	13	B
12	1100	14	C
13	1101	15	D
14	1110	16	E
15	1111	17	F

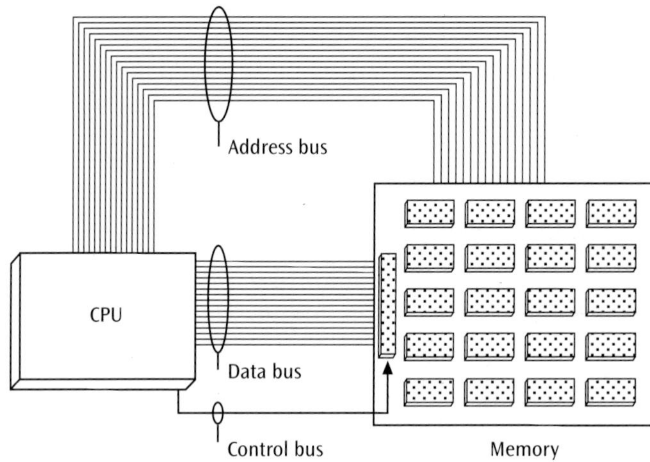

Figure 30.1 *A schematic representation of the connections between memory and the central processing unit (CPU) of a microprocessor.*

reliable data transfer, all the bus signals are accurately synchronized by an internal clock. Because each instruction takes at least one clock tick, the speed of the computer is a function of the clock speed.

Nowadays it is standard to have several internal clocks, each one dedicated to a different purpose. The fastest clock is the one controlling the CPU, which can run at a frequency of 400 MHz or higher. This is the clock speed usually quoted in computer advertisements. For most computers the CPU is the only part that runs at this speed. Main memory cannot operate at this high speed and the main memory clock typically runs at a fraction of the CPU frequency, e.g. at 100 MHz for a 400-MHz CPU. Indeed, it is the main memory clock that drives the CPU clock. Other clocks are used for the video monitor, hard disk drive, modem, etc. Because the CPU works much faster than memory, it contains a specialized high-speed memory, the cache, into which instructions and data can be fetched in advance of their being needed by the CPU. The cache acts as a temporary holding place for information on its way to or from the CPU, avoiding long CPU-idle periods.

The output device that receives processed data from the computer can take many forms, such as the video screen, printer, or mass-storage systems such as magnetic disk. Another form of storing large amounts of information is the CD-ROM, developed from audio compact disk (CD) technology. A CD-ROM disk can store about 650 MB information (the standard 3.5-inch floppy disk has a capacity of 1.4 MB). Many current software programs require 50 MB or more storage space and are usually delivered on a CD-ROM. Initially, CD-ROMs were read-only devices, but more recently recordable CDs (CD-R) have become widely available. There are also CDs (CD-RW) on which information can be written and erased many thousands of times, like magnetic disks. The latest development in mass-storage devices is the digital versatile disk or DVD. Unlike CDs, which use infrared lasers, DVDs use a laser tuned to the red band of the visible spectrum (635 or 650 nm), similar to a laser pointer. The much shorter wavelength makes it possible to pack data more densely. Some DVD systems employ two lasers, one infrared and one red, allowing them to read both conventional CDs and DVDs. DVD disks can be double sided, and some have double layers accessed by focusing the laser beam, effectively making them four-sided. DVD disks can have a storage capacity of 12–17 GB (1 GB = 1024 MB).

Digital information can be transmitted between the computer and external devices in either serial or parallel format. With serial transmission, digital data are sent in sequence on a single wire, whereas with parallel transmission all 8 bits of a byte are sent simultaneously on eight separate wires. Parallel transmission is generally much faster than serial but, to avoid problems with synchronization, is restricted to cable distances of about 3 m. For longer distances, serial transmission must be used. Transmission speed is indicated in bauds (one baud equals 1 bit per second). Because each transmitted byte requires at least 2 extra bits to indicate the beginning and end of the byte, a transmission rate of 9600 bauds, represents the transmission of only about 960 rather than 1200 bytes or characters per second. There are many different types of serial interfaces, the most popular being the RS-232C and the newer RS-422. The newest form of serial transmission uses the universal serial bus (USB), which can transmit information over 10 times faster than conventional serial lines. Networks use a special kind of serial transmission in which the information is modulated so that transmission rates of 10 megabit per second are possible.

The power of the digital computer rests not only on its speed and capacity for manipulating large quantities of data but also on its ability to perform complicated sequences of actions under control of a stored program. The first step in programming should be to express the solution of the problem to be solved as a series of step-by-step procedures – such a solution is called an algorithm. The next step is to translate the algorithm into a language that is understood by the computer. Early-generation computers required that the individual steps of the algorithm were entered, in the correct sequence, in binary or hexadecimal format, a task that was tedious and very prone to errors. Subsequently, a programming language close to machine language, called assembly language, was created. Each step of the algorithm was represented by a mnemonic code designed to assist the memory of the programmer. For example, the assembly language instruction "ADD AX, ADR" (add the contents of memory address "ADR" to register AX) is much easier to remember than the hexadecimal equivalent "132 7D3". Having coded the complete algorithm in assembly language, a translator program or assembler translates the mnemonic into a form ready for execution. Assembly language programming is still used when high-speed processing is needed. However, most programming today is done using high-level languages such as C, Pascal, or Fortran, which are much easier to use than assembly language.

NETWORKS

The enormous increase in the computing power and storage capacity of the modern personal computer (PC) in recent years has been paralleled by an even greater increase in the size and complexity of the programs that are available, and in the data files that are sometimes generated. The original IBM PC had as little as 16 kB memory and one or two 128 kB floppy disks. Today, many commercial programs occupy 50–60 MB or more of storage capacity and require several MB of internal memory. These large programs can often be most appropriately installed on a central computer in a local area network (LAN), where they can be shared by several users concurrently. In simplest terms, a LAN is a high-speed communication link, allowing personal computers to communicate with each other and with other electronic devices. One of the major reasons for using a network includes sharing programs, data files, and resources such as printers and mass-storage systems that need to be accessed by many people.

The computers and devices in a LAN are connected using a system of cables, network interfaces, and appropriate communication software. The network interface is the physical connection between the computers or other devices and the network cabling system. Its function is to organize and control the transmission of data. Most PC-based LANs operate in a client–server environment in which some or all of the application processing is done on the client computer, while a dedicated computer called a file server is used to provide controlled access to files and access to network printers or mass-storage facilities. The particular computer that is used as a file server might be a standard PC or a specialized machine designed specifically for that purpose. It is the software running in that machine that defines it as a file server.

COMPUTER-CONTROLLED INFUSIONS

The increasing interest in total intravenous anesthesia (TIVA; see Chapter 39) has focused attention on the role of computers for this application. TIVA makes use of a continuous intravenous infusion of hypnotics, analgesics, and muscle relaxants at a variable rate determined by the patient's response to surgical or anesthetic stimuli. With manually adjusted infusions, frequent adjustments to the infusion rate are usually required to achieve stable anesthesia. To rapidly achieve and maintain a constant plasma concentration over a period of time requires a combination of a bolus dose to fill the central compartment, a constant-rate infusion to replace drug lost by elimination, and an exponentially decreasing infusion to replace drug lost from the plasma by transfer or distribution to peripheral tissues. The complexity of the mathematics involved in calculating a constantly changing exponential rate is considerable. This, together with the manual dexterity required to transfer the calculated rates to an infusion pump, makes the task impossible to perform without a computer. Target-controlled infusion (TCI) is a method for administering intravenous drugs whereby a set drug concentration (or target concentration) in the blood, or occasionally at some other site, can rapidly be reached, maintained and, when needed, changed. This is achieved by using a computer running a program based on standard pharmacokinetic principles and supplied with appropriate pharmacokinetic parameters for the drug being used to control an infusion pump.

When first developed, TCI systems used standard desktop PCs. These are large, bulky, and not very suited for use in a crowded operating room. More recent innovations in TCI technology integrate the computer within the housing of the infusion pump. Such a system is incorporated in the Diprifusor, a commercial TCI device for administering propofol.[1,2] The computer program sends information to the pump about infusion rates, but must also receive information from the pump to confirm that the infusion rate being delivered matches that requested. Information from the pump is also needed about any pump alarms, e.g. syringe empty, line occlusion, etc. When an empty syringe is changed, the program automatically compensates for the time during which no drug is being infused to restore the plasma concentration to the set target.

MONITORING DEPTH OF ANESTHESIA

There is an increasing interest in methods for monitoring the depth of anesthesia, and especially an emphasis on detecting intraoperative awareness. There is no universally reliable monitor of the depth of anesthesia, although several have been investigated, with varying success. The most successful have used either a parameter derived from the electroencephalogram (EEG) or sensory-evoked responses. EEG analysis, evoked response monitoring, and changes in respiratory sinus arrhythmia rely on computer technology (see Chapter 32).

Most anesthetic drugs cause slowing of the EEG in a dose-related fashion, the exception being the benzodiazepines, which shift the EEG frequency distribution towards higher frequencies. The most widely used technique for EEG frequency analysis uses the fast Fourier transform (FFT). This is a mathematical technique that transforms successive epochs of a signal in the time domain, i.e. a voltage that varies with time, into one in the frequency domain in which the signal is represented in terms of amplitude, phase, and frequency. Modern computers allow FFT analysis to be carried out in real time. Changes in EEG frequency are frequently presented as a single parameter derived from the frequency spectrum, such as the median frequency or spectral edge frequency. The median frequency is the 50th percentile of the cumulative power distribution and the spectral edge frequency is the 95th percentile.

A more recent approach to EEG analysis during anesthesia is bispectral analysis. This is an advanced signal processing technique that provides a more comprehensive description of the information available from Fourier analysis. Bispectral analysis has been in use since the 1960s by physicists and geologists but until recently has found little application in medicine, mainly because of the heavy computational requirements. With the increased computing power available with current computers, the technique has become more widely available. Bispectral analysis, as implemented on the Aspect A-1000 EEG monitor, generates a variable, the bispectral index (BIS), computed by applying a multivariate discriminant analysis algorithm to parameters generated by the bispectral analysis and a variety of clinical signs.[3] BIS appears to be especially sensitive to the hypnotic component of anesthesia.[4,5]

An evoked response is the change in the EEG in response to a specific stimulus. The amplitude of the response to a single stimulus is very low, a few microvolts, whereas the EEG, electromyogram (EMG), and other extraneous electrical activity may be 50 to several hundred microvolts. Fortunately, the evoked response is time-locked to the originating stimulus, whereas the EEG and other electrical signals are essentially random, so that if repeated stimuli at 5–10 Hz are presented the response can be extracted using computer-averaging techniques. Of the three commonly used stimulus modalities (visual, somatosensory, and auditory), the auditory-evoked response (AER) appears to be promising as a possible predictor of anesthetic depth. A disadvantage of the AER is that as many as 1024 averages may be required to reliably acquire a valid response. This would give a response time much too slow to provide a reliable real-time index of anesthetic depth. However, using a moving average of the incoming responses it is possible to obtain a reasonable approximation to a real-time display of the AER. It is also possible to derive a numerical index giving an indication of anesthetic depth.[6]

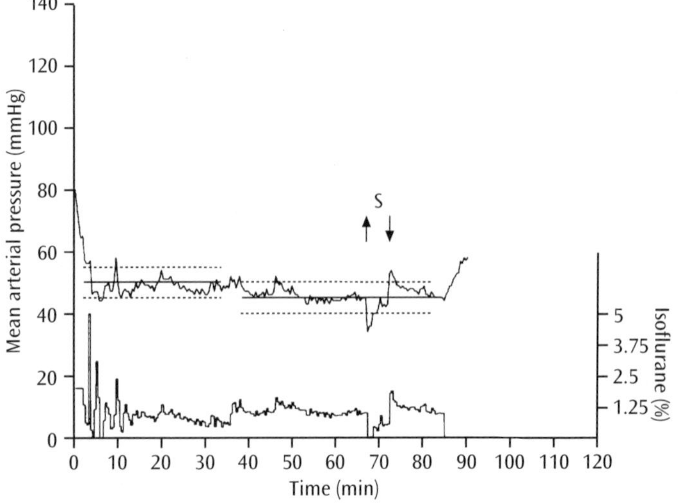

Figure 30.2 *Mean arterial blood pressure and isoflurane inspired concentration in a patient during controlled hypotension, in whom regulation of blood pressure was achieved by means of automatic closed-loop control of isoflurane inspired concentration. Initial control to 50 mmHg target pressure (——) is followed by a period of 45 mmHg (------ = ± 5 mmHg control band). Two perturbations in MAP (mean arterial pressure), mimicked by transducer shifts at the points indicated by S, resulted in changes in the isoflurane inspired concentration to regain regulation. The controller was switched off at the end of surgery to allow the MAP to return towards normal. (From Monk* et al.[12] *with permission.)*

CLOSED-LOOP CONTROL IN ANESTHESIA

Closed-loop control systems are widely used in industry and engineers have extensively studied system control theory. They have a long history in anesthesia. In 1937 Gibbs *et al.*[7] suggested the possibility of employing the EEG for controlling the depth of anesthesia. In the 1950s and early 1960s several systems were developed whereby the integrated output from EEG amplifiers was used to drive electromechanical devices controlling the delivery of drugs.[8] More recently, a variety of parameters derived from the EEG have been used as control variables to control automatically the depth of anesthesia.[9–11] Monk *et al.*[12] described an adaptive feedback, or self-tuning, controller to regulate the inspired concentration of isoflurane to achieve controlled hypotension in patients undergoing ear, nose, and throat (ENT) surgery (Fig. 30.2). Computer-controlled feedback has been applied to postoperative hypertension, and its superiority over manual control has been demonstrated.[13,14]

Closed-loop control also has a role in closed-circuit anesthesia. Both for economic reasons, in particular the high cost of the newer volatile anesthetic agents, and to reduce the risk of polluting the environment, there has been a movement toward the use of low-flow or totally closed-circuit anesthesia. When using a closed circuit the uptake of nitrous oxide and the volatile agents constantly changes, so that their administration needs to be precisely controlled to maintain a constant alveolar partial pressure. Another problem is that at very low flow rates conventional vaporizers are inaccurate and sluggish in their response. The solution is, first, to incorporate the monitoring of the anesthetic concentration into an automatic closed-loop control system, and, second, to replace the conventional vaporizer by a system whereby the liquid anesthetic is injected directly into the circuit – the exact amount to be injected being calculated and delivered using computer control. This approach has been incorporated into one commercially available closed-loop anesthesia machine (Physioflex).

Methods for closed-loop control

Closed-loop feedback control systems accept an input control variable, compare its value with a predetermined set point, and use the difference (the error parameter) to determine the amount by which the controlled process must be modified to reduce the error signal to zero and achieve the set point. The output feeds back its information to modify the input to the system. A physiologic example of closed-loop feedback control is the baroreceptor system. Changes in blood pressure alter the firing frequency of the baroreceptors. This information is processed in the central nervous system (CNS), which then adjusts heart rate and peripheral resistance to return the blood pressure to its previous level.

The simplest form of closed-loop control is one in which the error signal is multiplied by a constant, K_p, to yield a signal that is the input to the process, e.g. pump infusion rate. This arrangement is called proportional control. The numerical value of the constant K_p determines the amount of corrective effort that is applied for a given magnitude of error. By varying the value of K_p the dynamic behavior of the system can be altered. For low values of K_p the corrective effort is small and the response likely to be sluggish, and the set point may never be reached (Fig. 30.3). If K_p is very large, significant oscillation or instability is likely to result. For this reason, one or more additional control actions are usually added to proportional control. Proportional plus integral (or PI) control involves adding to the proportional term a signal proportional

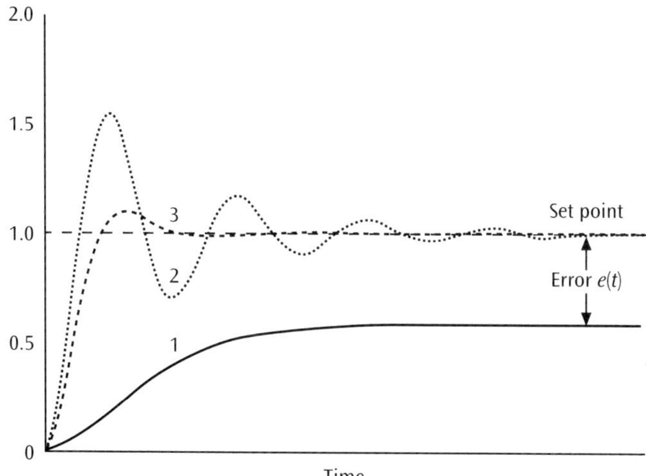

Figure 30.3 *Response of a closed-loop feedback control system to a unit step input. Curve 1 – the response of a proportional controller with a control constant (K_p) of low value. The response is sluggish and the set point is never reached. Curve 2 – the response of a proportional controller with a control constant (K_p) of high value. There is a rapid response but the system exhibits instability with marked oscillation about the set point. Curve 3 – the response of a PID (proportional–integral–derivative) controller. The set point is quickly reached with minimum overshoot.*

to the time integral of the error. Thus, the controller output (C_s) may be represented by the equation:

$$C_s(t) = K_p \cdot e(t) + K_I \int dt\, e(t)$$

where $e(t)$ is the error signal at time t and K_I is the integral control constant. PI controllers have the advantage that even the smallest error eventually produces a corrective signal of sufficient magnitude to ensure that the error signal is reduced to zero, i.e. the set point is always reached. In addition, by careful selection of the control constants, K_p and K_I, it is possible to achieve a rapid response without excessive overshoot or oscillation. Adding a derivative feedback loop to the control action can increase damping. The derivative signal responds to the rate of change, or derivative, of the error signal. Controllers that incorporate all three control actions are known as proportional–integral–derivative (PID) controllers (Fig. 30.4). The equation for a PID controller is:

$$C_s(t) = K_p \cdot e(t) + K_I \int dt\, e(t) + K_D \frac{de(t)}{dt}$$

In general, controllers can be tuned to provide the best possible combination of accuracy, response time, and damping by adjusting the value of the control constants. Increasing the integral constant increases the accuracy of the system and increasing the derivative component reduces oscillations and improves the response time.[8] A common example of the use of a PID control system is the computer disk drive. When the head is required to read information from a distant track it initially moves toward that track at maximum speed, slowing as it approaches the designated track under the influence of the PID algorithm, and eventually stopping without overshooting.

Fuzzy logic

In recent years, engineers have increasingly moved from PID control to fuzzy logic control. A fuzzy controller uses variables that have fuzzy rather than crisp values. These terms are best described by reference to set theory. A set is a group of distinguishable items, e.g. blood pressure can be classified into sets containing, for example, low, normal, or high values. In classical set theory, membership of a set is mutually exclusive. Thus, if we define low systolic blood pressure as a pressure less than 100 mmHg, normal as 100–140 mmHg (13.3–18.7 kPa), and high as a pressure greater than 140 mmHg, then a pressure of 101 mmHg (13.5 kPa) is normal while one of 99 mmHg (13.2 kPa) is low. Such sets are described as "crisp," and the type of logic associated with them is termed crisp, or binary, logic. This is the type of logic used by computers. The drawing of such rigid boundaries is obviously arbitrary, and an anesthesiologist would be more likely to say that a blood pressure of 99 mmHg is "a little low but essentially normal." This is an example of an imprecise, or fuzzy, definition. Humans, but not computers, are happy dealing with this sort of imprecision.

Fuzzy logic was introduced to deal with sets in which the boundaries are fuzzy rather than crisp. It is an appropriate, simple, and effective technique for controlling nonlinear and imprecise processes dealing with "fuzzy" terms such as low, normal, or high. In fuzzy set theory, elements can simultaneously belong to several sets, the degree of membership being defined by membership functions, which take values between 0 and 1. This is illustrated in Fig. 30.5 for systolic blood pressure, where the ordinate indicates the extent of membership and the boundaries of

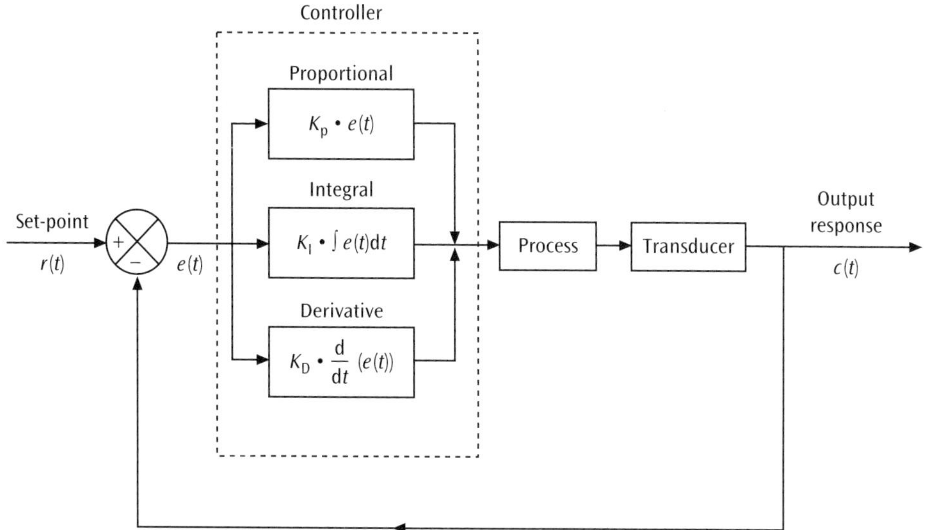

Figure 30.4 *Block diagram of a closed-loop feedback system with PID (proportional–integral–derivative) control.*

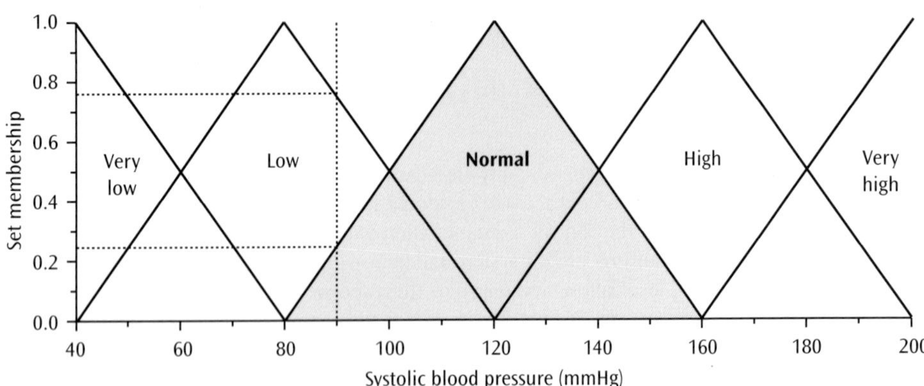

Figure 30.5 *Classification of systolic blood pressure using fuzzy sets. The boundaries of each set form a triangle and overlap with neighboring sets. The shaded area represents the extent of the "normal" set. The membership for a blood pressure of 90 mmHg is indicated by the dotted lines.*

each set form a triangle and overlap with neighboring sets. A pressure of 90 mmHg (12 kPa) would have membership functions of 0.25 for normal pressure and 0.75 for low pressure. A fuzzy controller applies membership functions to a set of fuzzy rules to produce a fuzzy control output based on control inputs. A defuzzification module then converts this fuzzy output to a "crisp" control value that can be used by the computer (Fig. 30.6). Fuzzy logic control has found many applications in anesthesia.[15] The technique has been applied to the automatic control of arterial blood pressure,[16–18] neuromuscular block during surgery,[19,20] control of mechanical ventilation during anesthesia,[21] and the control of inspired isoflurane and oxygen concentrations using minimal-flow anesthesia.[22]

Neural networks

Artificial neural networks consist of many nonlinear computational elements (nodes) linked by weighted interconnections. They are analogous to the networks of neurons and axons in animal neurological systems. Each node in a neural network performs a simple computation independently of the other nodes. This parallel structure allows neural networks to explore competing hypotheses simultaneously, and makes them especially suitable for implementation on parallel processing computers. They can also run on conventional computers, although these are slower. The weights on the internode connections, together with the overall topology of the neural network, define the output for a given input. Many network topologies are possible, from single-layer configurations such as the Hopfield net to complex multilayer ones such as the Kohonen self-organizing net. The weights need not be known in advance but can be learned automatically by training the network with exemplars (Fig. 30.7). Even when subsequently presented with noisy or incomplete data, they will produce an approximate answer rather than one that is incorrect. Neural networks are particularly useful for classification of data. A common application is in optical character readers. Neural networks and fuzzy logic often represent alternative solutions to problems, and increasingly the two technologies are being applied together.

SIMULATORS AND TRAINING DEVICES

The use of simulation has gained wide acceptance in many branches of those industries that involve complex processes, such as civil and military aviation, the merchant navy, the nuclear industry, and railway systems. There is currently considerable interest in the use of simulators in anesthesia. Traditionally, anesthetic skills have been acquired by anesthesiologists-in-training by hands-on experience with real patients under the supervision of a senior colleague. Quite rightly, that colleague will intervene when a situation threatens the well-being of the patient but, of course, the learning process for the trainee is compromised. In a simulated situation the instructor can let a potentially critical situation develop to its natural conclusion. We all learn from our mistakes – in a simulator trainees can even be encouraged to make mistakes and by observing the consequences the learning process is enhanced. Most humans learn best by active rather than by passive learning. Simulators are also ideally suited to maintaining the competence and skills of qualified anesthesiologists, however long they have been in the specialty, and are particularly useful for upgrading competence in handling those uncommon but potentially fatal problems that require a rapid and correct response.

A distinction is usually made between simulators and training devices. A simulator is a machine that attempts to reproduce or represent the exact or nearly exact phenomena likely to occur in the real world, e.g. a complex operating room environment. Training devices often concentrate on specific aspects of anesthetic knowledge such as pharmacology or physiology, using computer-screen-based simulation rather than reproducing the real operating room environment. A sophisticated training device is the Anesthesia Simulator Consultant (ASC, University of Washington, Seattle, WA), which creates the workspace of the anesthesiologist on the screen of a personal computer and simulates the patient's responses to a wide variety of interventions. Its case library contains a wide variety of critical incidents, emergency situations, and difficult clinical problems. ASC is an expanded version of a system described by Schwid and O'Donnell.[23] Both full-scale simulators and training devices such the ASC have proved their value in the education of trainees and in improving the performance of qualified anesthesiologists.[24,25] A heart/lung bypass simulator has been described that can be used to teach perfusionists, anesthesiologists, and surgeons the principles of cardiopulmonary bypass and allow them to gain experience with conducting bypass in both routine and complex cases.[26]

Anesthesia simulators are not new; the first anesthesia simulator was developed by Denson and Abrahamson in 1969.[27] However, the technology needed to develop true highly realistic or high-fidelity anesthesia simulators has only became available in the past two decades. Since the late 1980s, several high-fidelity anesthesia simulators have been developed. Two are commercially available, the CAE-Link "Eagle" simulator, based on the system developed at the University of Stanford in California,[28] and the Loral system developed by the University of Florida.[29] Full-scale simulators have also been developed at the University of Leiden in the Netherlands,[30] and by groups in Copenhagen in Denmark[31] and Cambridge in the UK.[32] Full-scale simulators are expensive to develop and maintain. The commercial versions cost in the region of US$200 000. In addition, adequate space and manpower are required to operate simulators effectively. In particular, it is essential to have a well-trained team of instructors if the maximum benefit of simulator training is to be achieved. Technical support is also essential. Several anesthesia simulator centers have been established in Europe,

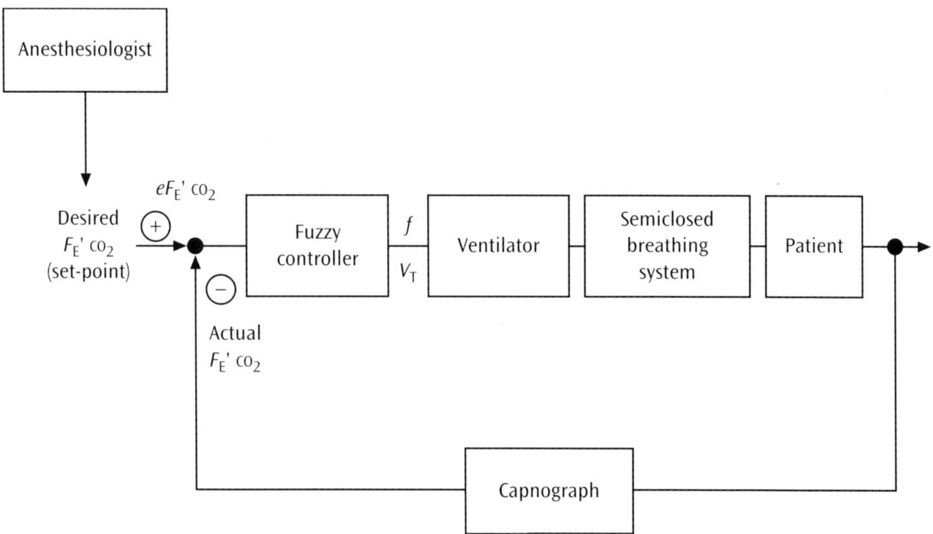

Figure 30.6 *Block diagram of a fuzzy logic control loop used to for the control of mechanical ventilation. Deviations of the actual end-tidal CO_2 from the desired end-tidal CO_2 set point are compensated by changes in ventilatory frequency (f) or tidal volume (V_T) or both, computed by the fuzzy controller. (From Schäublin* et al.[21] *with permission.)*

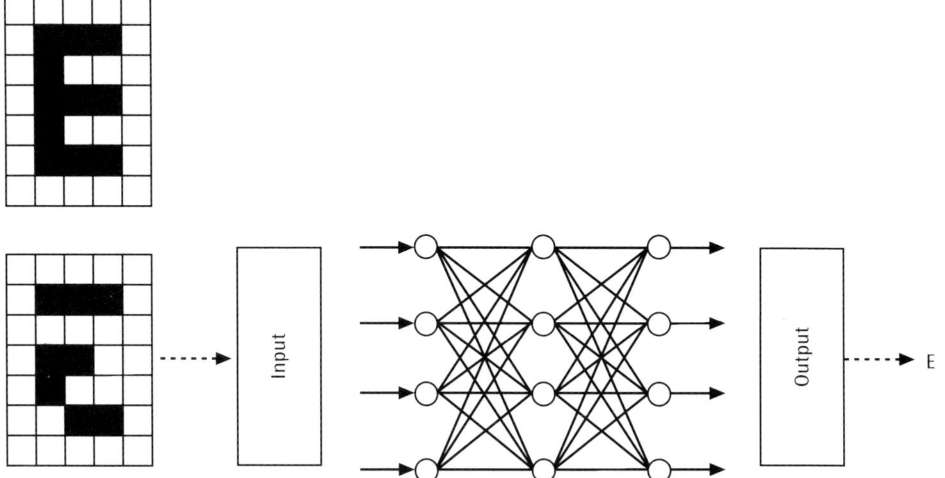

Figure 30.7 *Schematic diagram of a neural network with one input layer, one hidden layer, and one output layer. Input and output are usually in the form of vectors. In this example the input vector would be derived from the individual cells of the matrix representing the letter "E." An open cell would be represented by "0" and a filled cell by "1." After appropriate learning the network would be able to correctly identify the letter even when the information is incomplete, as shown here.*

the USA, and Australia, and more are being planned. It is obvious that the anesthetic community recognizes the educational potential of this technology.

The Leiden Anaesthesia Simulator is representative of most full-scale anesthesia simulators. It can simulate, in a highly realistic manner, almost all aspects of anesthesia. A modified manikin attached to an electromechanical lung represents the simulated patient. The lung allows both spontaneous and mechanical ventilation. The movement of the right and left halves of the thorax can be differentially controlled to allow simulation of bronchial intubation or pneumothorax. The tidal volume and breathing frequency during spontaneous ventilation can be varied under computer control, as can lung compliance and resistance. Carbon dioxide production and oxygen uptake are simulated. Breath sounds, generated by specially developed software, are transmitted to microphones incorporated in the thoracic walls of the manikin and can be externally auscultated. Carotid pulses can be felt. Laryngospasm and gastric regurgitation can be electromechanically simulated. Computer-generated physiologic signals provide input to the monitors. There are also facilities for simulating noninvasive blood pressure measurement and pulse oximetry.

Fifteen different parameters can be simulated and adjusted independently to generate a variety of clinical scenarios. Mathematical models of cardiovascular and respiratory physiology, pharmacokinetics, and pharmacodynamics are used to predict the simulated patient's responses to anesthetic and other drugs and to pathologic changes. In addition to providing scenarios that simulate both common and extremely rare situations (e.g. malignant hyperthermia, anaphylaxis), it allows personnel to be trained with new apparatus and working methods, the use of new drugs such as remifentanil, and crisis resource management. The last has become one of the most important applications of simulators in addition to more routine training. Human factors are a major cause of critical incidents in anesthesia. Many of these result from failure in teamwork and communication at the interface between different groups, e.g. consultant/trainee, anesthesiologist/surgeon.[33–35] The anesthetic simulator can be a powerful tool in a comprehensive human factors program designed to increase awareness of this type of problem.

AUTOMATED ANESTHETIC RECORDS

Anesthesia records fulfill several functions. A properly prepared record, accurately documenting the progress of anesthesia, is of value not only to the anesthesiologist in detecting untoward trends during the case but also to staff involved in the postoperative care of the patient. It is an essential source of information for those who may be responsible for providing subsequent anesthetics to that patient. Anesthetic records are also a valuable source of information for education and research purposes, and these are required for medicolegal purposes in most countries. In a court of law the medical record is considered the primary source of facts, and juries tend to believe what is written over what is said – "if it isn't documented, it wasn't done." A full and accurate record may make the vital difference between the defensible and the indefensible in a claim for damages in which professional negligence is alleged. Unfortunately, it is probably true that the majority of anesthetic records do not reflect a "full and accurate record" of what happened to the patient during anesthesia. Even with the best will in the world, it is virtually impossible to record accurately all events, vital signs, drug and fluid or blood administration, etc., as these occur, especially during induction, recovery, or critical incidents. At these times the anesthesiologist is, quite rightly, concerned with more important aspects of patient care and data must be recorded retrospectively. Even during times of relative stability, it is probably not possible to record data manually more often than every 5 minutes, while adequately performing the other clinical tasks and demands on the anesthesiologist's time. To enter data more frequently than this requires some form of automated record keeping if the anesthesiologist is to cope with the growing complexity of pharmacological intervention and physiological monitoring.

An automated anesthetic record system is a computer-based device that acquires data from physiological monitors, ventilators, etc., as well as data entered directly by the anesthesiologist, and displays these, in a suitable format online, to the anesthesiologist. In addition, the acquired data will be stored to enable the automatic generation and printing of the anesthetic record at the end of the case, as well as allowing subsequent retrieval for clinical, administrative, or research purposes. The core of such a system is data acquisition. Most modern equipment used in anesthesia and intensive care has the facility to output data in digital form, allowing relatively straightforward connection to a computer. It is this ability to exchange information between medical devices that forms the foundation of modern data management in anesthesia.

In addition to automatic data capture, there is also a need for manual input, for example to enter drug or intravenous fluid administration, events, etc. The most common method of input is via the computer keyboard but other possibilities include touch-screen, mouse or trackerball driven menus, light pen, or voice recognition.[36] The use of bar codes on ampules and prefilled syringes and infusion bags not only simplifies drug and fluid administration input but also reduces the risk of input errors.

An important aspect of automated record systems is validation of data input. Concern is often expressed that erroneous or artifactual values of physiologic parameters might be incorporated into an automated record with possible medicolegal consequences. The automated record system will, and should, faithfully record the information presented to it. In contrast, the anesthesiologist keeping a handwritten record is unlikely to record readings that are considered artifactual or unexpectedly out of range. There is also a tendency to record high values a bit lower and low values a bit higher, a phenomenon known as "smoothing."[37] It is possible to incorporate artifact detection algorithms in the automated record system software that would allow "flags" to be attached to those stored items considered to be artifacts. In many cases the artifactual data may be physiologically unrealistic or even impossible. Blood pressures of 300/300 mmHg (40/40 kPa), negative pressures, or a zero pressure recorded within 1 second of a normal blood pressure, such as might occur during a catheter flush or transducer zeroing, are obvious artifacts that would be of no clinical or medicolegal significance.

Another aspect that must be considered is the security of the database containing the automated records. It must not be possible to edit data once they are stored in the database, although errors may be corrected at the time of entry. While an alteration to a handwritten record can easily be detected, this is much more difficult, if not impossible, to detect with an electronic record. The security of the database becomes even more important if it is maintained on a central computer serving a LAN. It is then vitally important that adequate safeguards are built into the system to prevent unauthorized access, and to preserve patient confidentiality.

The use of automated record systems in a LAN rather than as stand-alone devices offers many advantages. The ability to link into the hospital information computer system can give immediate, online access to laboratory data and other information of importance to the clinical management of the patient. Storage of data centrally on a file server is also more economical and improves data security. It is possible for the complete anesthetic records of upward of 15 000 patients to be stored on one optical storage device, and details of any patient recalled within a few seconds. One of the fears concerning automated records is loss of information due to computer failure. This risk can be reduced to a minimum when an LAN is used. All data are transmitted as they are entered down the network for storage on the central storage facility; they can also be stored on hard disk in the local computer in the operating room during a case. Should the local computer fail, then all information up to that moment is safely stored centrally. Conversely, should either the network or the file server fail, the anesthesiologist can confidently continue with local storage. The chance of both the network and the local computer going down simultaneously is extremely remote. With a network, intraoperative data can also be immediately available to medical and nursing staff responsible for the patient in the recovery room or intensive care. And, of course, using a network offers administrative advantages. Having virtually instantaneous access to a database containing detailed information about all patients anesthetized by the department in the past makes evaluation of trends in drug usage etc. and preparation of statistical reports very easy.

Several investigators have compared handwritten and automated anesthetic records. Lerou *et al.*[38] quantified the differences in the documented values of eight physiological variables recorded online by a commercially available automated system with the values from the same patients recorded on handwritten anesthesia records. The incidence of erroneous data in the handwritten record was between 1% and 11% while the incidence of missing data varied from 8% to 31%. Most missing or erroneous data occurred during the period of induction and at the end of the case, when the anesthesiologist often records from memory after-the-event data. Erroneous data were most frequently observed for the recorded blood pressures, with 57% more erroneous data for diastolic than for systolic pressure. Similar discrepancies between handwritten and automated blood pressure records were noted by Cook *et al.*[39] and explained by faulty reconstruction of handwritten records from memory, and bias in favor of less controversial values. No handwritten record contained a diastolic pressure above 110 mmHg (14.7 kPa) whereas the automated system recorded diastolic pressure over 110 mmHg 33 times in 15 of the 46 patients, including eight measurements greater than 125 mmHg (16.7 kPa). Those factors that lead to significant inaccuracy in the handwritten record, including observer bias, missed readings, and errors of memory, may be avoided by using automated data management systems.[40]

It is often claimed that these systems, by accurately recording what is happening to the patient, and by freeing the anesthesiologist from the drudgery of maintaining a handwritten record, allow more time to be devoted to direct patient care, and that they thereby contribute to an improvement in patient safety. An argument used by opponents of these systems is that they might reduce, rather than increase, the attention that the anesthesiologist pays to the patient. The discipline of having to note mentally and record manually a value for physiological parameters at regular intervals may, in fact, enhance patient contact and increase the vigilance of the anesthesiologist. Removing the anesthesiologist from the information feedback loop could have an adverse effect on vigilance. Current evidence, however, is that automatic record keeping allows the anesthesiologist to deal more effectively with other intraoperative problems.[41]

THE INTERNET AND ANESTHESIA

The Internet has resulted in a revolution of truly global proportions in information exchange. It developed from networks designed in the mid-1960s by the US Department of Defense to control ballistic missiles and other weapons.[42] A network is a group of computers connected so that information can be shared between them. Today the Internet is a network of networks of worldwide dimensions, giving users access to information stored on many million computers across the globe. Information is transferred using a standard format that is independent of the type of computer. Individual computers are connected to local networks, which are in turn connected to regional ones, and from those to national and international networks. Each computer connected to the Internet has an individual "host name." These form part of a system of uniform resource locators (URLs), a standardized syntax describing the location and method of accessing Internet resources.

URLs were developed for the World Wide Web (WWW) but are now almost universally in use throughout the Internet. They consist of three parts, a code identifying the transfer protocol to be used, the host name of the computer being accessed. and the path and file to be retrieved. As an example, the URL for accessing information from the medical library (the Walaeus Library) of the University of Leiden is http://www.medfac.leidenuniv.nl/walaeus/online.html. The first part (in this case *http*) is the protocol name and indicates the type of Internet service. HTTP (hypertext transfer protocol) is the protocol used by the WWW. Other protocols that might be used are FTP (file transfer protocol) and Telnet. A colon and two forward slashes always follow the protocol. The next part is the domain name of the computer: *www* indicates that it is a WWW site in a subnetwork of the Faculty of Medicine (*medfac*) of the University of Leiden (*leidenuniv*); finally *nl* indicates that the computer is located in the Netherlands. Each country, except the USA, has a unique country identifier. In the USA locations are frequently identified by endings such as *edu* (educational institution), *org* (organization, e.g. the American Society of Anesthesiology) or *com* (commercial institution). The final part of the URL is the directory (*walaeus*) and the name of the file to be retrieved (*online.html*). This file has been created using hypertext markup language (HTML), which creates hypertext documents that can be used on any computer. In a hypertext document one can jump from one document to another, which may be located anywhere on the Internet, simply by clicking with a mouse on a highlighted word (a hyperlink). By this means information can be downloaded without knowing from which computer, country, or continent it originated.

The World Wide Web

The World Wide Web or WWW was developed at the CERN Institute for Particle Physics at Geneva in 1992 as a means of disseminating information about the physical sciences. It presents information using a graphical user interface known as a page. Since 1992 it has grown from a few thousand to more than 21 million pages of information. In addition to printed and graphical information, audio and video material can be downloaded. Indeed, it is possible via the WWW to follow online international conferences from any continent in the privacy of one's office. Another use of these facilities is teleconferencing. The WWW has allowed the transfer of information virtually without limitation, almost instantly and at a low price. There is a vast amount of medical information available, for both the layman and the professional. Some Internet sites relevant to anesthesia are listed in Table 30.2. However, while the Internet has obvious benefits in providing for widespread dissemination of information, there is growing concern within the medical community about the quality of this information.[43,44] The Internet provides absolute literary freedom, without the requirement for peer review or any other form of quality control.

Table 30.2 *Websites relevant to computing and to anesthesia*

History of computers

http://www.ex.ac.uk/babbage/
Biographical information about Charles Babbage, details about his Difference and Analytical Engines, and much more

http://www.computer50.org/mark1/new.baby.html
Background history and specifications about the Manchester "Small Scale Experimental Machine," nicknamed the "Baby." There are links to the Ferranti Mark 1 and other sites of historical interest

http://ei.cs.vt.edu/~history/UNIVAC.Weston.html
History of the development of the ENIAC and UNIVAC computers

http://www.maa.org/mathland/mathland_7_1.html
Details of the EDSAC computer. An EDSAC simulator can be downloaded

General sites

http://www.usyd.edu.au/su/anaes/VAT/VAT.html
The *Virtual Anesthesia Textbook* uses a familiar "textbook" style to present a comprehensive set of links to anesthesia-related Internet information

http://www.hsc.missouri.edu/~msa/palmtop/palmtop.html
Many useful links to sites from which programs for a variety of palmtop computers with applications in anesthesia and critical care can be downloaded

http://groucho.med.yale.edu/
Gasnet, a globally distributed anesthesia server network. There are mirror sites in Europe (http://gasnet.eur.nl), Australia (http://gasbone.herston.uq.edu.au:8000), and the UK (http://gasnet.dundee.ac.uk)

Societies and Associations

http://www.ncl.ac.uk/~nassoca/
The Association of Anaesthetists of Great Britain and Ireland (AAGBI)

http://www.asahq.org/
American Society of Anesthesiologists (ASA)

http://units.ox.ac.uk/departments/anaesthetics/wfsa/index.htm
World Federation of Societies of Anaesthesiologists (WFSA)

http://www.iars.org/
The International Anesthesia Research Society (IARS)

http://www.halcyon.com/iasp/
International Association for the Study of Pain (IASP)

http://www.oaa-anaes.ac.uk/
Obstetric Anaesthetists' Association

Electronic mail

Electronic mail (email) is one of the most frequently used services provided by the Internet. In addition to plain text messages, documents and graphical and audio files can be sent to recipients anywhere in the world. Email addresses consist of two parts, the user name and the host name, separated by the "@" (at) symbol. The author's email address is j.g.bovill@lumc.nl; *j.g.bovill* is the user name and *lumc.nl* the host name.

REFERENCES

1. Gray JM, Kenny GN. Development of the technology for 'Diprifusor' TCI systems. *Anaesthesia* 1998; **53** (Suppl. 1): 22–7.
2. Glen JB. The development of 'Diprifusor': a TCI system for propofol. *Anaesthesia* 1998; **53** (Suppl. 1): 13–21.
3. Rampil IJ. A primer for EEG signal processing in anesthesia. *Anesthesiology* 1998; **89:** 980–1002.
4. Liu J, Singh H, White PF. Electroencephalographic bispectral index correlates with intraoperative recall and depth of propofol-induced sedation. *Anesth Analg* 1997; **84:**185–9.
5. Liu J, Singh H, White PF. Electroencephalographic bispectral index predicts the depth of midazolam-induced sedation. *Anesthesiology* 1996; **84:**64–9.
6. Mantzaridis H, Kenny GN. Auditory evoked potential index: a quantitative measure of changes in auditory evoked potentials during general anaesthesia. *Anaesthesia* 1997; **52:** 1030–6.
7. Gibbs FA, Gibbs EL, Lennox WG. Effect on the electroencephalogram of certain drugs which influence nervous activity. *Arch Intern Med* 1937; **60:** 154–66.
8. O'Hara DA, Bogen DK, Noordergraaf A. The use of computers for controlling the delivery of anesthesia. *Anesthesiology* 1992; **77:** 563–81.
9. Schwilden H, Schüttler J, Stoeckel H. Closed-loop feedback control of methohexitone anesthesia by quantative EEG analysis in humans. *Anesthesiology* 1987; **67:** 341–7.
10. Schwilden H, Stoeckel H, Schüttler J. Closed-loop feedback control of propofol anaesthesia by quantitative EEG analysis in humans. *Br J Anaesth* 1989; **62:** 290–6.
11. Mortier E, Struys M, De Smet T, *et al.* Closed-loop controlled administration of propofol using bispectral analysis. *Anaesthesia* 1998; **53:** 749–54.
12. Monk CR, Millard RK, Hutton P, Prys-Roberts C. Automatic arterial pressure regulation using isoflurane: comparison with manual control. *Br J Anaesth* 1989; **63:** 22–30.
13. Reid JA, Kenny GNC. Evaluation of closed-loop control of arterial pressure after cardiopulmonary bypass. *Br J Anaesth* 1987; **59:** 247–55.
14. Murchie CJ, Kenny GN. Comparison among manual, computer-assisted, and closed-loop control of blood pressure after cardiac surgery. *J Cardiothorac Anesth* 1989; **3:** 16–19.
15. Asbury AJ, Tzabar Y. Fuzzy logic: new ways of thinking for anaesthesia. *Br J Anaesth* 1995; **75:** 1–2.
16. Ying H, McEachern M, Eddleman DW, Sheppard LC. Fuzzy control of mean arterial pressure in postsurgical patients with sodium nitroprusside infusion. *IEEE Trans Biomed Eng* 1992; **39:** 1060–70.
17. Zbinden AM, Feigenwinter P, Petersen Felix S, Hacisalihzade S. Arterial pressure control with isoflurane using fuzzy logic. *Br J Anaesth* 1995; **74:** 66–72.
18. Tsutsui T, Arita S. Fuzzy logic control of blood pressure through enflurane anesthesia. *J Clin Monit* 1994; **10:** 110–7.
19. Mason DG, Ross JJ, Edwards ND, *et al.* Self learning fuzzy control of atracurium induced neuromuscular block during surgery. *Med Biol Eng Comput* 1997; **35:** 498–503.
20. Ross JJ, Mason DG, Linkens DA, Edwards ND. Self learning fuzzy logic control of neuromuscular block. *Br J Anaesth* 1997; **78:** 412–5.
21. Schaublin J, Derighetti M, Feigenwinter P, *et al.*. Fuzzy logic control of mechanical ventilation during anaesthesia. *Br J Anaesth* 1996; **77:** 636–41.
22. Curatolo M, Derighetti M, Petersen Felix S, *et al.* Fuzzy logic control of inspired isoflurane and oxygen concentrations using minimal flow anaesthesia. *Br J Anaesth* 1996; **76:** 245–50.
23. Schwid HA, O'Donnell D. The Anesthesia Simulator-Recorder: a device to train and evaluate anesthesiologists' responses to critical incidents. *Anesthesiology* 1990; **72:** 191–7.
24. Gaba DM. Improving anesthesiologists' performance by simulating reality. *Anesthesiology* 1992; **76:** 491–4.
25. Schwid HA, O'Donnell D. Anesthesiologists' management of simulated critical incidents. *Anesthesiology* 1992; **76:** 495–501.
26. Leonard RJ. A total heart/lung bypass simulator. *ASAIO Trans* 1988; **34:** 739–42.
27. Denson JS, Abrahamson S. A computer-controlled patient simulator. *JAMA* 1969; **208:** 504–8.
28. Gaba DM, DeAnda A. A comprehensive anesthesia simulation environment: re-creating the operating room for research and training. *Anesthesiology* 1988; **69:** 387–94.
29. Euliano T, Good ML. Simulator training in anesthesia growing rapidly; LORAL model born in Florida. *J Clin Monit* 1997; **13:** 53–7.
30. Chopra V, Engbers FHM, Geerts MJ, *et al.* The Leiden anaesthesia simulator. *Br J Anaesth* 1994; **73:** 287–92.
31. Christensen UJ, Andersen SF, Jacobsen J, *et al.* The Sophus anaesthesia simulator v 20. A Windows 95 control-center of a full-scale simulator. *Int J Clin Monit Comp* 1997; **14:**11–6.
32. Byrne AJ, Hilton PJ, Lunn JN. Basic simulations for anaesthetists. A pilot study of the ACCESS system. *Anaesthesia* 1994; **49:** 376–81.
33. Howard SK, Gaba DM, Fish KJ, *et al.* Anesthesia crisis resource management: teaching anesthesiologists to handle critical incidents. *Aviat Space Environ Med* 1992; **63:** 763–70.
34. Davies JM. Simulation: it's a start. *Can J Anaesth* 1996; **43:** 425–9.
35. Kurrek MM, Fish KJ. Anaesthesia crisis resource management training: an intimidating concept, a rewarding experience. *Can J Anaesth* 1996; **43:** 430–4.
36. Murchie CJ, Kenny GN. Comparison of keyboard, light pen and voice recognition as methods of data input. *Int J Clin Monit Comput* 1998; **5:** 243–6.
37. Block FE Jr. Normal fluctuation of physiologic cardiovascular variables during anesthesia and the phenomenon of "smoothing." *J Clin Monit* 1991; **7:** 141–5.
38. Lerou JGC, Dirksen R, van Daele M, *et al.* Automated charting of physiological variables in anesthesia: a quantitative comparison of automated versus handwritten anesthesia records. *J Clin Monit* 1988; **4:** 37–47.
39. Cook RI, McDonald JS, Nunziata E. Differences between handwritten and automatic blood pressure records. *Anesthesiology* 1989; **71:** 385–90.
40. Thrush DN. Are automated anesthesia records better? *J Clin Anesth* 1992; **4:** 386–9.
41. Allard J, Dzwonczyk R, Yablok D, *et al.* Effect of automatic record keeping on vigilance and record keeping time. *Br J Anaesth* 1995; **74:** 619–26.
42. Ruskin KJ. The Internet. A practical guide for anesthesiologists. *Anesthesiology* 1998; **89:** 1003–14.
43. Rampil IJ. Medical information on the Internet. *Anesthesiology* 1998; **89:** 1233–45.
44. Tramèr MR. How can we cope with the Internet? *Anesth Analg* 1999; **89:** 271–2.

31

Operating room safety

DAVID H MORISON, HOMER YANG, AND PETER T-L CHOI

INTRODUCTION

Safety in the operating room is of paramount importance in the practice of anesthesia. This chapter considers the hazards to both patients and staff presented by electrical faults, explosions, and fires, as well as by the gases that continue to be a mainstay of anesthetic practice.

ELECTRICAL SAFETY

Basic principles

Electrical charge is measured in coulombs; 1 coulomb (C) is the charge carried by 6.2418×10^{18} electrons. Current through an electrical circuit is measured in amperes; 1 ampere (A) is the flow of 1 coulomb through a circuit in 1 second. The electrical difference required to force current through a circuit is measured in volts. One volt equals 1 joule per coulomb. One volt-coulomb is therefore a unit of energy (1 joule). The law that governs the flow of current through a circuit is Ohm's law:

$$R = V/I \text{ or } V = I \times R$$

where I is current, V is voltage, and R is the proportionality constant, or resistance through the circuit. Resistance is measured in ohms (W).

In measuring hemodynamics, the systemic vascular resistance (SVR) is governed by a similar equation:

$$\text{SVR} = (\text{MAP} - \text{CVP})/\text{CO} \text{ or } (\text{MAP} - \text{CVP}) = \text{CO} \times \text{SV}R$$

where CO is MAP is mean arterial pressure, CVP is central venous pressure, and CO is cardiac output. SVR is analogous to the resistance in an electrical circuit; the pressure difference between MAP and CVP is analogous to the electrical potential difference; and CO is analogous to current through the electrical circuit.

Electrical power system

Electric power companies supply electricity as an alternating current (a.c.), and the polarity of the current reverses itself at a set frequency, measured in cycles per second or hertz (Hz). In North America, electricity is supplied as 120 V at 60 Hz; in the UK, it is 240 V at 50 Hz. With a.c., resistance is expressed as impedance, Z:

$$Z = V/I \text{ and } Z = 1/f$$

where f is cycles per second. Impedance therefore drops as frequency increases, and current increases as impedance decreases.

Alternating current gives rise to two electromagnetic properties: inductance and capacitance. These properties are central to the operating room line isolation and current leakage. In the case of inductance, the arrangement of two coils of wire wound around a common iron core allows an electrical current to be induced in one coil when an alternating current is passed through the other (Fig. 31.1). This property is used in power transformers to step up or step down power line voltage by changing the ratio of turns between the coils around the core. In the operating room, power can be induced and yet isolated from the utility plant power supply as, using electromagnetic inductance, the two coils are not in contact, hence line isolation.

Electromagnetic capacitance is the storage of electrical charge between two conducting surfaces with an insulation in between (Fig. 31.2). When electricity is applied, a transient current is seen in the circuit until the two surfaces are saturated with positive and negative charges. In the a.c. circuit, the constant reversal of polarity allows the

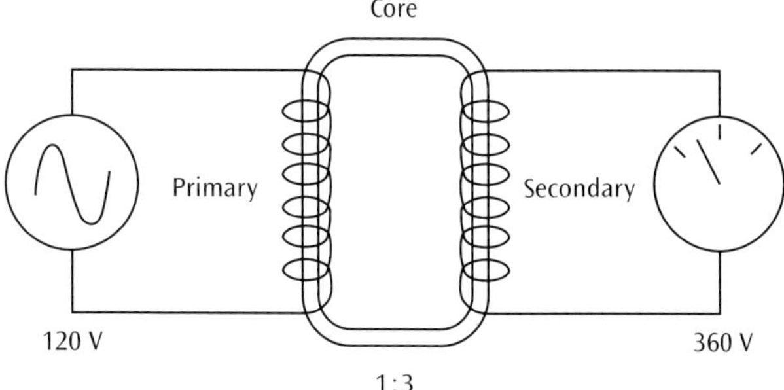

Figure 31.1 *Two electrically insulated coils of wire wound around a single iron "core'" to form a transformer. Alternating current flowing through the primary coil produces a varying magnetic field, which generates or "induces" an alternating current in the secondary coil. The primary/secondary voltage ratio is the same as the ratio of turns in the primary and secondary coils.*

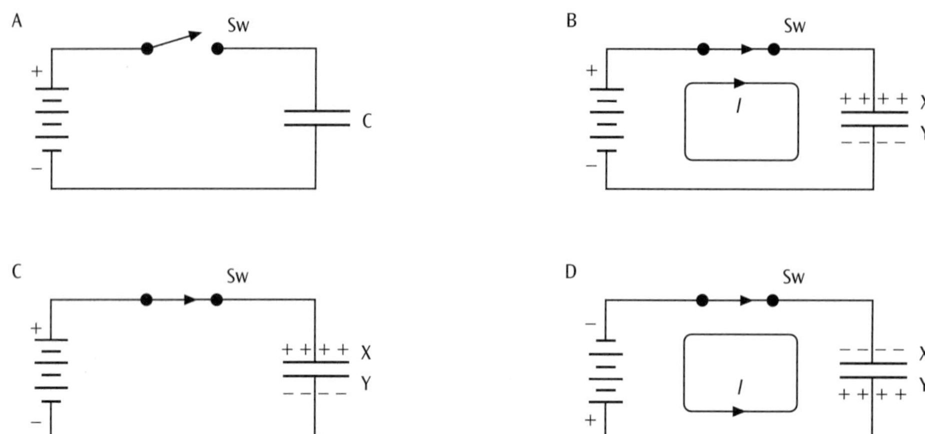

Figure 31.2 *(A) Electrical circuit consisting of a battery (source of unidirectional or d.c. voltage), two closely spaced but insulated conductors forming a capacitor (C), and a switch (Sw). (B) When the switch is closed, the battery causes electrons to accumulate on plate Y. These repel electrons from plate X, leaving it positively charged. The net effect is a transient flow of current (I). (C) Within a short time, plate Y can accept no more electrons, and plate X has no more electrons to be repelled. At this time, the flow of current ceases. (D) By reversing the battery, the electrons on plate X are replenished, while those on plate Y are repelled, leaving X negatively charged and Y positively charged. In the process, there is a transient flow of current (I) in the opposite direction.*

conducting surfaces to alternate between being positively and negatively charged. This results in a constant current through the rest of the circuit, even though the circuit is interrupted by the insulation. Capacitance is used in many electrical applications; however, capacitative coupling, seen in household appliances and operating room electrical equipment, is an unwanted effect. Two wires in a power cord, although insulated, may generate capacitative coupling merely by their proximity to each other and being plugged into an a.c. supply. An electric motor in a refrigerator compressor may also generate capacitative coupling between the motor's circuit wiring and the refrigerator metal casing. The result is a small current, a type of leakage current, where there should be none (Fig. 31.3).

Leakage current may result from capacitative coupling but also from faults in the equipment circuit such that a current actually flows onto other conductive surfaces, typically the equipment casing. This may result from worn insulation, component failures, or moisture, especially in equipment not designed for but exposed to liquid spills.

Grounding

Household electrical appliances should be grounded to provide an electrical path between the appliance casing and earth. If a fault in the appliance circuitry develops, and if the appliance is not grounded, the appliance casing may become electrically charged. In this situation, touching the casing would create an electrical path through the user and could result in electrocution. Earth is a better conductor than the human body, so if an appliance is grounded touching it would result in the current preferentially flowing to earth, leaving the user unharmed. Should the fault be large, the current would be large and trip the fuse.

Electrical equipment in the operating room is grounded for the same reason. In addition, line isolation, a common feature in the operating room, requires the electrical equipment to be grounded for its proper use. Using the property of inductance, operating room power supply may be isolated from the utility power supply (Fig. 31.4). In Fig. 31.4, neither line 1 nor 2 has a path to ground. Should an equipment fault develop, i.e. the first fault, current may leak to the casing and then to ground. With line isolation, the user who touches the casing is exposed only to one power line and will not experience an electrical shock as there is no electrical path to the second power line. For an electrical hazard to occur, a second fault in the system, i.e. another piece of faulty equipment, is necessary, along with the user simultaneously touching both pieces of equipment. The initial loss of line isolation, i.e. the first fault, may be noted by monitoring the amount of leakage current, using a line isolation monitor (see below). The user is then alerted before harm can result. Without grounding, leakage in the equipment is otherwise undetectable until harm results.

Ground fault circuit interrupter (GFCI)

This device monitors the current in the hot and neutral side of a circuit. If any difference is detected, it is assumed that current leakage outside the circuit is occurring and power is immediately interrupted. The device works well in certain hazardous areas such as bathrooms or kitchens. In the operating room, an uncontrolled and unanticipated power interruption may be hazardous, especially if the equipment affected is essential to patient well-being.

Line isolation monitor (LIM)

This device monitors the current leakage to ground and alarms when the leakage is greater than 2 or 5 mA, depending on the age of the LIM. The alarm indicates the occurrence of a first fault prior to the occurrence of macroshock. As alluded to above, the proper use of LIM requires the electrical equipment to be grounded. With line isolation, macroshock, in theory, would not occur unless there are two faults in the electrical system. The user then may respond by removing the responsible equipment at an opportune moment before the second fault occurs. It must be emphasized that line isolation is not designed to prevent microshocks.

Line isolation is required as a standard only where flammable anesthetic agents are used.[1] With the disappearance of explosive anesthetic agents, operating room line isolation has been claimed by some to be anachronistic.[2] Most electrical equipment in the operating room nowadays incorporates a power transformer in its design and isolates itself from the operating room power supply. The use of line isolation in the operating room power supply therefore gives rise to double isolation and may be redundant.[3] The low incidence of electrical accidents over a 42-month period in a 1100-bed hospital provides further support for the use of line isolation being unnecessary.[3] The largest single cause of

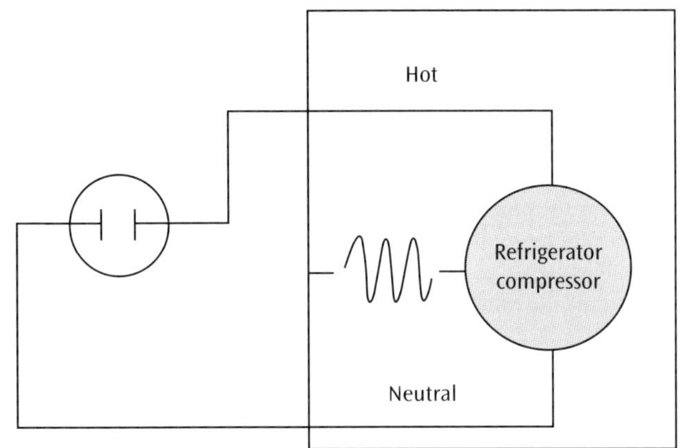

Figure 31.3 *Capacitative coupling and leakage (wavy line) between a refrigerator's compressor and casing.*

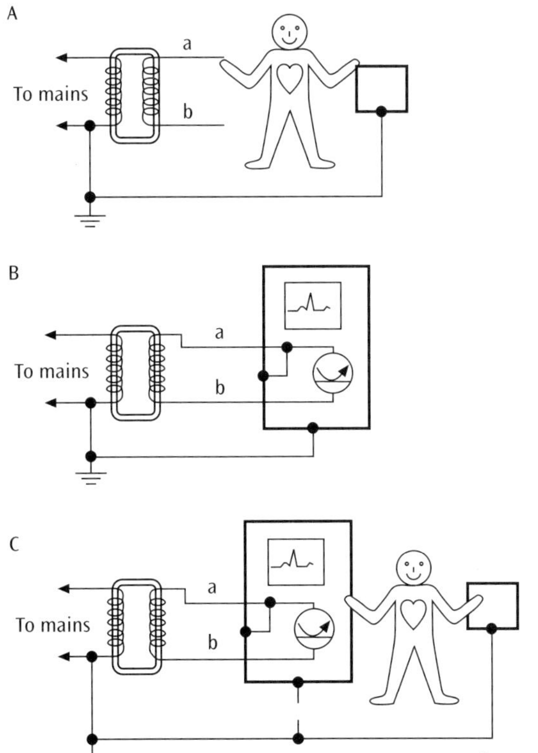

Figure 31.4 *(A) In an isolation transformer, the primary and secondary coils are coupled magnetically but not electrically; note that neither conductor of the secondary coil is attached to ground. Thus, an individual can simultaneously contact either one of the secondary lines and ground without completing a circuit. (B) A defect has caused a direct connection between one side of the isolated power system and the case of the electrocardioscope. The electrocardioscope continues to function normally (line voltage continues to be present between conductors A and B). However, the power system is no longer isolated from ground. A second defective unit could create a hazard by bringing a patient into simultaneous contact with conductor B and ground. (C) Even in the presence of a direct connection from one side of the line to the equipment case and a simultaneous faulty ground connection, an individual can safely contact the electrocardioscope and a grounded object without completing a circuit.*

electrical accidents is equipment ground faults. As LIM works only if the faulty equipment is grounded, its use to reduce electrical hazards seems dubious. Finally, a survey showed that routine equipment checks for ground faults are not adopted by many hospitals.[4] Opponents of LIM argue that resources would be better spent in ensuring that equipment is properly grounded.[5]

Line isolation does give operating room personnel and patients a theoretical advantage compared with conventional grounded power supply against macroshock. Its ability to alert the user and the fact that equipment can continue to be used under first fault conditions is also attractive. In spite of improved plugs and rugged power cords, the operating room is still a location "normally subject to wet conditions while patients are present."[6,7] The potential for line-to-ground faults under wet conditions remains a concern in the operating room. The costs versus benefits of line isolation have not been clearly resolved. Nevertheless, when a significant amount of fluid or drenching may occur during surgery, such as in the arthroscopy or urology suite, it would seem to be prudent to consider the use of line isolation and an LIM.

Macroshock

This is an electrical shock at high current, i.e. 1 mA or greater. The resistance of skin to electrical current is approximately 100 000 Ω, and the resistance of tissue is 1000 Ω; thus, the current through intact skin must be high before an electrical shock is hazardous. The factors governing the development of macroshock include the size of the current, the contact area (current density), the pathway through the body, the duration of exposure, and the current frequency. In the operating room, macroshock is usually due to leakage current and equipment ground faults.

In the case of finger contact, the effects of various currents at 60 Hz are well documented.[8] Current usually becomes perceptible at 0.3 mA, unpleasant at around 1 mA, results in "letting go" between 10 and 20 mA, and is likely to result in ventricular fibrillation at approximately 100 mA or greater; severe shock or burns will occur at currents between 10 and 100 A. In the case of ECG electrodes applied to skin, current sensations at 60 Hz were documented in volunteers.[9] The mean current for threshold sensation was 83 μA, while there was definite sensation at 107 μA, strong sensation at 298 μA, and painful sensation at 401 μA. In that study, there was no difference in the sensing currents between pediatric and adult patients.

Current density influences the shock hazard: a pinprick sensation is felt if a current of 100 μA is concentrated close to a nerve, whereas 100 μA spread over the fingers is hardly felt. If a large enough current enters the body but exits through a path that includes the heart, cardiac dysrhythmias or ventricular fibrillation may result. If the pathway bypasses the heart, serious shock and burn may result, but not necessarily resulting in any cardiac dysrhythmias. If the duration of current exposure is 10 ms or less, ventricular fibrillation is not expected unless a large amount of energy is applied,[10] or at a critical point in the cardiac cycle, i.e. upstroke of the T wave.[11]

The current frequency and the current at which one could let go have been studied.[12] In the case of direct current, the let-go current generally results from fear due to the shock rather than the ability to move one's muscles. Interestingly, 60 Hz a.c. is probably the most dangerous frequency when considering the ability to let go.

Microshock

This refers to electrical shock at low current, i.e. in the microamp range. For microshock to be hazardous requires a conduit that bypasses the intact skin, such as a saline-filled cardiac catheter. At such low currents, the only body system that is affected in a significant way is the heart, resulting in ventricular fibrillation or pump failure.

Leakage current, as alluded to earlier, may lead to microshocks in the presence of pacemaker wires or pulmonary arterial catheters. An additional possible source of leakage current is from a patient contacting two separate pieces of equipment with a common ground, one piece of equipment having a significant leakage current to ground, while the second piece of equipment is connected to the patient through a heart catheter. If the second piece of equipment has a fault in its circuits and therefore a pathway to ground, leakage current from the first piece of equipment may travel via the ground to the second piece of equipment and enter the patient's heart, causing microshocks and cardiac dysrhythmias. Nowadays, equipment directly connected to a patient's heart must contain a low-leakage power transformer in its design. In essence, the equipment isolates itself from other equipment and thereby prevents such an occurrence.

It has been found that the minimum current necessary to induce ventricular fibrillation in dogs ranges from 20 to 35 μA.[13,14] The threshold for the human heart seems to differ between the atrium and ventricle. In a study conducted in eight patients about to undergo cardiopulmonary bypass, a bipolar right atrial pacemaker catheter was unable to induce sustained cardiac dysrhythmias even at currents of up to 3 mA.[15] In the same study, in nine patients, the smallest current produced by a bipolar right ventricular pacemaker catheter that could cause a rhythm disturbance was 80 μA.[15] In another study of 58 human subjects undergoing cardiopulmonary bypass, epicardial disk electrodes, intramyocardial needles, and endocardial electrodes were compared.[16] Epicardial disk electrodes were the least likely to induce dysrhythmias, with the predicted minimum fibrillating current being 735 μA. Intramyocardial needles were more likely to induce dysrhythmias, with the predicted minimum fibrillating current being 199 μA. The predicted minimum fibrillating current for endocardial electrodes was 67 μA. Using probit analysis, an estimated 50% of the patients would experience ventricular fibrillation with a right ventricular pacemaker catheter and a current of 200 μA, 1% with a current of 64 μA, and 0.1% with a current of 44 μA.[17]

Prevention of microshock depends on all endocardial monitoring lines being electrically isolated. As explained above, electrical grounding is not a substitute for electrical isolation as grounding may provide a return path for leakage current from another piece of equipment. North American standards allow a maximum of 20 μA, whereas the European standards allow 50 mA of leakage current to pass through the isolated equipment connected to the patient. The maintenance of the isolation limits is essential if microshock is to be avoided.

Electrocautery

The use of electrocautery is commonplace in modern surgery. The early development of electrosurgery in the 1890s was principally achieved by numerous French investigators, including D'Arsonval, Nagelschmidt, and Revière. Revière was the first to successfully remove an indolent ulcer (on a musician's hand) using diathermy.[18] In North America, William L Clark was the first to remove benign growths using electrosurgery. William Bovie, a physicist, faced significant resistance in his early attempts to develop electrosurgery, mostly due to the prevailing prejudice against electrotherapy. Harvey Cushing in 1926 was impressed by Bovie's electrified loop to "scoop" out malignant tissue without bleeding.[19] With Cushing's encouragement, significant strides were made in developing the electrosurgical unit, subsequently known as the Bovie unit.

In 1891, D'Arsonval noted that when an alternating current at a frequency above 10 000 Hz is passed through the human body it causes no pain or muscle contractions but a rise in body temperature.[18] The amount of heat generated is proportional to the square of the current density. The modern electrosurgical unit (ESU) uses a high-voltage radiofrequency between 500 and 3000 kHz. The principle is still the same as Bovie described in the early days, "In electrosurgery, a high current density is obtained by making the active ('operating') electrode small, whereas the inactive ('indifferent') electrode, through which the electrical circuit between the patient and machine is completed, is made large so that the current density in its immediate vicinity will be sufficiently low to permit the small amount of heat developed to be readily dissipated by the blood stream."[19]

In the past, the return electrode, or grounding pad, was connected to earth. Modern ESUs contain a capacitor to isolate the return plate from ground to reduce the risk of electrical shock. Thus, the term "grounding" seems less appropriate nowadays. The key feature of the return electrode or dispersive pad is to create a large area so that the current density and therefore the underlying tissue temperature remains low. The pad should have an area of at least 0.66 cm^2 per watt of ESU output.[20] The contact between the return electrode and the patient should also be uniform so that the current density is uniformly distributed, thereby preventing a "hotspot" from developing and leading to burns. The heat generated in the tissues is dissipated by the underlying blood flow. Placing the pad over muscular tissue usually ensures adequate perfusion for heat dissipation; a pad over a bony prominence may result in nonuniform current density but also inadequate perfusion for heat dissipation. Similarly, placing the pad over a prosthetic implant that is electrically conductive, e.g. an artificial hip joint, may result in a nonuniform current density. In both cases, a burn may result.

When electrosurgery is applied to tissues close to the body surface, the current generally flows evenly toward the returning electrode, following the path of least resistance. When electrosurgery is applied endoscopically or during brain surgery, the current path may be confined at certain points and result in thermal burns. The use of a bipolar ESU ensures that the electrical field is confined between the tips of the forceps and that the risk of tissue damage beyond the field is minimized.

Burns from electrical devices in the operating room

Malfunction of an ESU usually results in a thermal burn. Nonuniform current density and inadequate blood flow to dissipate the underlying tissue temperature have already been discussed. Burns resulting from an improperly applied dispersive pad, such as occurs when part of the pad lifts off, are well known. Numerous other causes of a burn during the use of an ESU have been reported: a breakdown of the ESU capacitor used for isolating the return electrode from ground,[21] e.g. capacitative coupling between the ESU and a flow-directed pulmonary artery catheter,[22] an esophageal temperature probe,[23] or a faulty battery-operated Doppler monitor.[24] A fault in the spark gap in a bipolar ESU leading to a macroshock has also been reported, illustrating that bipolar ESU is not immune to equipment malfunction.[2]

Burns may also result from battery-operated equipment. Inadvertent application of direct current (d.c.) to the electrodes of a neuromuscular stimulator has been reported.[25] The result is an electrolysis of the electrode gel, with the generation of sodium hydroxide and a chemical burn to the patient. Voltage as low as 3 V has been implicated.[26]

The proper use of an ESU is obviously extremely important in modern-day surgery. The reported malfunctions illustrate the need for all personnel in the operating room to be vigilant, as well as to exercise proper care of all electrical devices, cords, and plugs. Breaks in equipment wiring and plugs due to rough handling may lead to a breakdown in electrical isolation, creating opportunities for ESU burns. The requirement of inordinately high wattage from the ESU or significant interference with monitoring devices such as the ECG may also indicate an undesirable current path, which might potentially result in a thermal burn, although abnormalities in the ECG are not always noted. A tingling sensation when touching the patient or the operating table with an ungloved hand should also alert the anesthesiologist to the possibility of an unacceptable current path.

When a burn has been noted, a critical incident investigation should follow. All electrical equipment used in the case should be removed for subsequent inspection and testing.[25] Disposable components should not be discarded, including the stimulating electrode, dispersive pad, and ECG and neuromuscular stimulator electrodes. Equipment mounted on an ad hoc basis should not be removed as the critical incident may be the result of such ad hoc tampering.[25]

Electromagnetic interference

Radiofrequency (RF) is generated from most electrical and telecommunication devices. Electromagnetic interference (EMI) refers to interference in the operation of electrical devices, including medical devices, due to RF. Although EMI has received much publicity, the true scope of the problem and the setting of appropriate standards remain elusive. Analog cellular phones have probably received the most publicity, but other sources of RF may potentially affect the operation of electrical medical devices in the operating room. These include sources within the operating room, such as ESUs and electrical warming blankets, or outside the operating room, such as two-way radios, transmission towers, etc. Interference can cause an extra ventilator breath, turn on the neuromuscular stimulator, or change volumetric pump settings.

The problem of EMI may be approached from the point of view of limiting RF emission by electrical devices or by instituting electromagnetic immunity standards. An electrical device may be designed to withstand a certain amount of RF and therefore confer "immunity" against EMI. There are existing standards adopted from the International Electrotechnical Commission (IEC), and the current immunity standard is $3\,V\,m^{-1}$.[27] Generally, the immunity level is deemed not appropriate for all medical equipment in all environments.[28] Higher immunity levels may be required for some healthcare environments, whereas immunity levels may not be as critical in other environments. The cost of implementing the IEC standard 601.1.2 ranges from C$5000 to C$30 000[28] per piece of equipment. Surveys by Industry Canada and others have found that 10% of electromagnetic field measurements around urban homes are above $3\,V\,m^{-1}$, and, in some areas, may be as high as $20\,V\,m^{-1}$. In the operating room environment, several pieces of equipment in addition to the ESU may emit RF. The total field strengths may therefore be much higher than $3\,V\,m^{-1}$, and higher immunity levels would seem prudent.

Electromagnetic field strength is directly proportional to the square root of a source's power and inversely proportional to the distance. Analog cellular phones are, in fact, less problematic than two-way radios in that regard: 0.6 W versus 2–5 W. Some cellular phones now operate at 10 mW (0.01 W). The separation distance to prevent EMI between a device emitting RF and a susceptible device has been determined: 6 m for 4 W two-radios, 2 m for 0.6-W cellular phones, and 0.3 m for 10-mW cellular phones.[29] In view of the transmitting power of cellular phones, it is not surprising that, of the 34 reported incidents of EMI in Canada between 1984 and 1995, only one involved an analog cellular phone.[30] This was confirmed in a national survey by the Committee on Technology of the Canadian Anesthesiologists' Society in 1996: one reported incident of EMI due to an analog cellular phone.

Many hospitals have now banned cellular phones in critical care areas, including the operating room environment. Some have completely banned cellular phones in the hospital environment. The position adopted by most biomedical engineers is to develop an individual hospital-based electromagnetic compatibility policy (Table 31.1).

FIRE SAFETY IN THE OPERATING ROOM

Since the first report of an operating room fire caused by ether in Boston in 1850,[31] fire safety has been an important issue for anesthesiologists and operating room staff. Reliable estimates of incidence are scant and difficult to find as most fires are small, quickly controlled, and often not reported. Although the use of flammable anesthetics has decreased, operating room fire remains a concern with the increasing number of potential ignition sources, such as lasers, ESUs, and fiberoptic light devices. Statistically, the incidence of operating room fires declined from 1 in 80 000 anesthetic procedures in 1955 to 1 in 150 000 in 1963.[32] Based on estimates of 20–30 operating room fires per year in an estimated 27 million surgical procedures,[33] the incidence in the 1990s could be as low as 1 in 900 000. Despite such a low incidence, vigilance is still required. This section will focus on the etiology of operating room fires, the issues related to prevention and management, and the fire regulations and policies pertinent to the operating room environment.

Etiology

Three elements, the so-called fire triad, must be present for a fire to occur: an oxidizing agent, a flammable substrate, and an ignition source. Removal of one of the three elements will extinguish a fire. Table 31.2 categorizes the possible sources of each element.

Oxidizing agents

Although oxygen supplementation is desirable to oxygenate patients adequately, care must be taken, especially during procedures around the head, neck, and thoracic cavity. A number of case reports have described fires resulting from leakage of high oxygen concentrations from nasal cannulae[34,35] or face masks,[36] or through lung tissue during lung resection.[37,38] Epstein and Halmi[36] measured the maximum percent oxygen leakage during 100% oxygen delivery to children undergoing general anesthesia with spontaneous ventilation via face mask and spontaneous or controlled ventilation via a laryngeal mask airway (LMA). They

Table 31.1 *Hospital-based electromagnetic compatibility policy (adapted from Canadian Bio-Medical Engineering Society[28])*

1 Encourage biomedical engineers to learn how to assess the electromagnetic environment of their hospitals
2 Take action on:
  a managing (increasing) distance between sources of electromagnetic interferences and susceptible devices
  b managing (removing or relocating) devices that are highly susceptible to electromagnetic interference
  c lowering power from internal electromagnetic interference sources under hospital control
  d labeling devices susceptible to electromagnetic interference
  e educating staff (including nurses and physicians) to be aware of, and to recognize, electromagnetic interference-related problems
  f conducting technical remedial action to eliminate electromagnetic interference, such as shielding, using ferrite cones, or optical coupling, if possible
  g sharing relevant electromagnetic-interference electromagnetic-compatibility information with others
  h considering electromagnetic interference when planning hospital layouts
3 Consider electromagnetic compatibility when purchasing new medical equipment (e.g. acquiring devices that have met the safety and performance requirements of the International Electrotechnical Commission standard 601 and its collateral standards)
4 Educate patients, especially those using medical devices in a home care setting

Table 31.2 *List of common fire hazards found in the operating room*

Oxidizing agents	Flammable substrates	Ignition sources
Oxygen	Inhalational anesthetics	Lasers
Nitrous oxide	Endotracheal tubes	Electrosurgical units
	Surgical drapes and swabs	Fiberoptic equipment
	Warming blankets	Defibrillators
	Gastrointestinal gas	Electrical short-circuit
	Skin cleansing agents	

found that use of a face mask resulted in leakage of high concentrations (63%) of oxygen, whereas the LMA resulted in a leak of 22% and 31% oxygen with spontaneous and controlled ventilation respectively. Given the risk of combustion, the lowest inspired oxygen concentration that ensures adequate oxygenation should be used to minimize oxygen accumulation.

Combination of oxygen with other gases has also been used to minimize the risk of combustion. The addition of inert gases such as helium and nitrogen to oxygen decreases the probability of causing a fire.[39] The exception is nitrous oxide, which supports combustion and does not minimize the risk associated with oxygen.[40,41]

Flammable substrates

Historically, inhalational anesthetic agents have been the main cause of operating room fires. Diethyl ether, ethylene, acetylene, ethyl chloride, and cyclopropane have all been implicated in explosions and fires.[42] With the current volatile agents, the risk is negligible. Halothane, isoflurane, and enflurane support combustion even in an oxygen–nitrous oxide environment. However, they do so only at extremely high concentrations, which are not used in the clinical environment.[31,43,44] Sevoflurane and desflurane have not been evaluated with respect to flammability.

Endotracheal tubes are a common fire hazard during airway surgery with ESUs and lasers, as evidenced by the 15 case reports reviewed by Chee and Benumof.[45] Suggested preventive measures have included the use of a helium–oxygen mixture,[39] jet ventilation without tracheal intubation,[46] laser-resistant endotracheal tubes, positive end-expiratory pressure,[47] and the use of harmonic scalpels.[48] Further details can be found in Chapter 50.

Materials applied near or onto the patient are also potential fuel sources. Surgical drapes, especially disposable ones, and swabs have become important fire hazards with the increasing number of ignition sources. Disposable paper drapes are treated with flame-retardant chemicals, but once ignition occurs combustion is extremely rapid and severe.[49,50] The potential for ignition is increased when oxygen accumulation occurs under the drapes. Forced air warming blankets may also be a potential fire hazard.

Flammable or explosive agents are other potential fire hazards in the operating room. Alcohol solutions are found in skin cleansing agents and in catgut suture conditioning fluids. These have all been implicated in operating room fires.[42,51,52] Although alcohol-based antiseptics (povidone–iodine, chlorhexidine, methanol, ethanol) are not recommended for use in the presence of ignition sources, they continue to be used in the operative setting. Nitroglycerin patches, like alcohol, also serve as a potential fire hazard.[53]

Gastrointestinal gas has also been the cause of explosions and fires in the operating room. Human bowels contain both hydrogen and methane, both of which are flammable.[42] Hydrogen production is dependent on bacterial metabolism of ingested food; methane production is not.[42] A low-residue diet, preoperative fasting for 12 h, and preoperative bowel preparations will reduce the amount of flammable gas to 5% of normal levels.[54] However, the use of mannitol as a bowel preparation will increase hydrogen production.[55] Both hydrogen and methane require an oxygen concentration over 5% for combustion to occur. Unfortunately, normal oxygen concentrations are 10% and 5% in the stomach and colon respectively.[42] In addition, oxygen concentrations in these areas increase during anesthesia with oxygen supplementation. The risk of combustion is further increased if nitrous oxide is used, owing to accumulation of this gas in the bowel. Carbon dioxide insufflation into the bowel has been shown to decrease the risk of combustion but is not commonly performed.[42] The majority of explosions and fires from gastrointestinal gas occur during either laparoscopy or colonoscopy. Most incidents during laparoscopy occur in the presence of intra-abdominal insufflation with air or nitrous oxide.[42] The current practice of insufflation with nonflammable carbon dioxide is safer from a combustion perspective.

Ignition sources

With advances in technology, the number of ignition sources in the operating room has increased. These include ESUs, lasers, fiberoptic light sources, defibrillators, and electrical short circuits. Laser safety is discussed further in Chapter 50. Electrocautery has been described earlier in this chapter. As well as being a potential electrical hazard, electrocautery is a common ignition source. In some devices, temperatures can reach up to 1200 °C.[56] Common surgical materials such as gauze and drapes will ignite at these temperatures even in the absence of supplemental oxygen.[56] The use of an electrically insulated, nonflammable holster to reduce accidental arcing or direct contact, cleaning the cautery tip to prevent accumulation of debris, and allowing the cautery tip to cool at the operative site before moving the cautery are all measures which can reduce accidental ignition of flammable materials. Similar care should be taken with fiberoptic light sources, which can also generate sufficient heat at their distal ends to start a fire.[33]

With the relaxation of electrical safety codes in operating rooms so that isolated power sources and line isolation monitors are no longer required, electrical short circuits may become another potential ignition source. Electrical fires in anesthetic monitors have been described. Sodium chloride contamination of the interior of monitors has been reported in three cases and has resulted in electrical short circuits, which have led to overheating and ignition of the monitors.[57]

Prevention

The easiest way to reduce the incidence of fires is to prevent them. Prevention of operating room fires consist of three components: national and regional legislation, hospital administrative policies (emergency planning), and operating room engineering controls. All are necessary to ensure the success of any fire safety program.

Legislation

Operating room and hospital fire safety is encompassed within legislation for building fire codes, occupational health, and workplace safety. Most of this information is difficult to access by conventional information retrieval methods used for medical literature; however, some information can be found on the Internet. In Canada, each province has its own fire legislation. The entire text of each province's legislation can be searched and viewed via the Canadian Centre for Occupational Health and Safety (CCOHS) website: www.ccohs.ca/products/legislation/legislation.html. In the UK, fire prevention is legally enforced by the 1997 Fire Precautions (Workplace) Regulations. Copies of the Regulations are available from Her Majesty's Stationery Office in London. Details of the Regulations can be found at www.safetyshop.com/legislation/legislation/2.html. In the USA, standards for workplace safety are outlined by the National Institute for Occupational Safety and Health (NIOSH) and the US Department of Labor Occupational Safety and Health Administration (OSHA). The OSHA publishes fact sheets on fire safety and workplace emergencies that are meant to be educational and not legally binding.[58,59] As one can see from these examples, legislation varies from country to country.

Hospital emergency plans

Emergency plans serve a number of functions, which are highlighted in Table 31.3. In the UK, emergency planning for fires is required by the Department of Health and Social Security. In the USA, development of hospital disaster plans is required by the Joint Commission on Accreditation of Healthcare Organizations (JCAHO).[60] Details of the elements of an emergency plan are described at the website www.ccohs.ca/oshanswers/hsprograms/planning.html and by Aghababian *et al.*[60]

One of the functions of emergency plans is to promote safety awareness and education. Fire drills are useful exercises to practice critical elements of a fire plan (such as evacuation) and to review fire safety.[61,62] Problems that were not predicted may also be identified during drills and allow revisions to be made to the plan. Similarly, review after an actual fire is invaluable for highlighting strengths and weaknesses of an existent fire plan. This proved to be the case after a major fire in the hospital of one of the authors.[63]

Operating room engineering controls

Operating room engineering controls deal with the physical layout of the surgical suite as well as the policies and procedures employed to prevent fires. Although the physical environment and regulations may differ between hospitals, the key features are the avoidance or minimization of all three elements of the fire triad at a given site and routine safety checks of potential ignition sources.

Management

The principles of fire-fighting and fire prevention are similar: removal of one or more of the elements of the fire triad will extinguish the fire. In practical terms, fire-fighting entails interruption of the oxidizing source (usually oxygen), removal of the flammable substrate, and extinguishing the ignition source.

In combating small fires, removal of the oxidizing agent is usually the most efficient method. This is especially important for fires around or in the patient's airway. Respiratory gases should be discontinued immediately as further interventions are initiated. Although this maneuver appears counterintuitive, there are three reasons to stop gas flow to the patient during an airway fire. First, most patients will tolerate momentary interruptions of oxygen. Second, most of the delivered oxygen will actually be consumed by the combustion process before reaching the alveoli. Third, the gas flow can potentially spread the fire further into the respiratory tract and lead to greater injury.

Table 31.3 *Functions of a hospital emergency plan*

Prevent fatalities and injuries
Reduce damage and loss of building and material
Accelerate resumption of normal operations
Highlight past and potential hazards (risk assessment)
Define resources (equipment, personnel) needed in the event of an emergency
Promote safety awareness

Discontinuation of the oxidizing agent should be quickly followed by removal of any flammable material from the combustion site. Removal of the ignition source or removal of the heat by cooling agents such as water should be performed concurrently. Following these maneuvers, oxygenation, ventilation, and circulatory support of the patient can be resumed.

The equipment required to achieve the above objectives will depend upon the magnitude of the fire. In the case of small fires, a wet towel or a fire blanket may be the only equipment needed. In the case of moderate or large fires, fire extinguishers may be employed. Fire extinguishers are classified according to their ability to extinguish three classes of fires: class A (wood, paper, cloth, most plastics), class B (flammable liquids), and class C (electrical fires). Table 31.4 outlines the details of the different types of fire extinguishers available. To extinguish large fires, fire hoses and other specialized equipment may be necessary. In those cases, the fire-fighting is best left to trained personnel while the operating room staff care for the patient.

If efforts to extinguish the fire with fire extinguishers are unsuccessful, evacuation of the operating room and activation of the fire alarm should be considered. As products of combustion will float near the ceiling (because their density is lower than air) and fresh air tends to layer near the floor, personnel should remain as low as possible. The patient should be evacuated with manual ventilation. Gas lines, electrical equipment, and the room ventilation system should be shut down and the doors should be closed to contain the fire.

Three important points of the successful management of an operating room fire should be highlighted. First, speed is of essence. Rapid recognition and quick action to control a fire will reduce the magnitude of the disaster. Second, patient safety should take precedence over any fire-fighting strategies. Third, communication between members of the operating team (and other hospital or fire-fighting personnel) is essential to avoid chaos, to initiate successful fire-fighting measures, and to undertake (if necessary) a safe evacuation of the patient and staff. As mentioned previously, fire drills to practice these elements are invaluable in ensuring a successful outcome.

GAS SAFETY

The basis for most general anesthetics is still supplied from compressed gas sources. Therefore, it is very important that these gases be supplied in a safe manner.

Identification

The anesthesiologist must be able to recognize the cylinders and pipelines from which these gases are derived.

Cylinders filled with medical gases are controlled by a number of safety regulations, which are determined by the authorities – in the USA these include the Code of Federal Regulations, Department of Transport, and the Compressed Air Association (CGA).[64] In Canada, the Canadian Standards Association (CSA) has published a number of standards.

Identification of cylinder is by color, pin indexing of the cylinder yoke, and labels. Unfortunately, the colors of gas cylinders are not the same in

Table 31.4 *Description of available fire extinguishers*

	Fire blanket	Water	Carbon dioxide	Dry chemical	Halon
Type of fire	Small class A	Class A Some class B	Small class A Class B and C	Class A, B, and C	Class A, B, and C
Mechanism	Interrupts oxidizers	Interrupts oxidizers Disperses heat	Interrupts oxidizers Disperses heat	Interrupts oxidizers Disperses heat	Interrupts oxidizers Disperses heat
Notes	Inexpensive Non-toxic	Heavy, bulky devices Risk of electric shock	Heavy, bulky devices	Leaves residue Damages equipment Potential toxicity?	Small, light devices Leaves no residue Low toxicity

every country. Oxygen cylinders in the USA are green, whereas in the UK they are black with a white collar and in Canada they are white. Table 31.5 shows the colors of common gas cylinders. The pin index safety system is designed to avoid connecting the wrong cylinder to a port on an anesthetic gas machine. However, this system is not foolproof as the pins can be knocked off, washers placed between the cylinder yoke port, or the cylinder connected in a crooked fashion.[65] The cylinder may also be filled with the wrong gas. It is important, therefore, that gas analyzers and close patient monitoring be used to avoid mishaps.

Figure 31.5 and Table 31.6 show the pin indexes for common gases used.

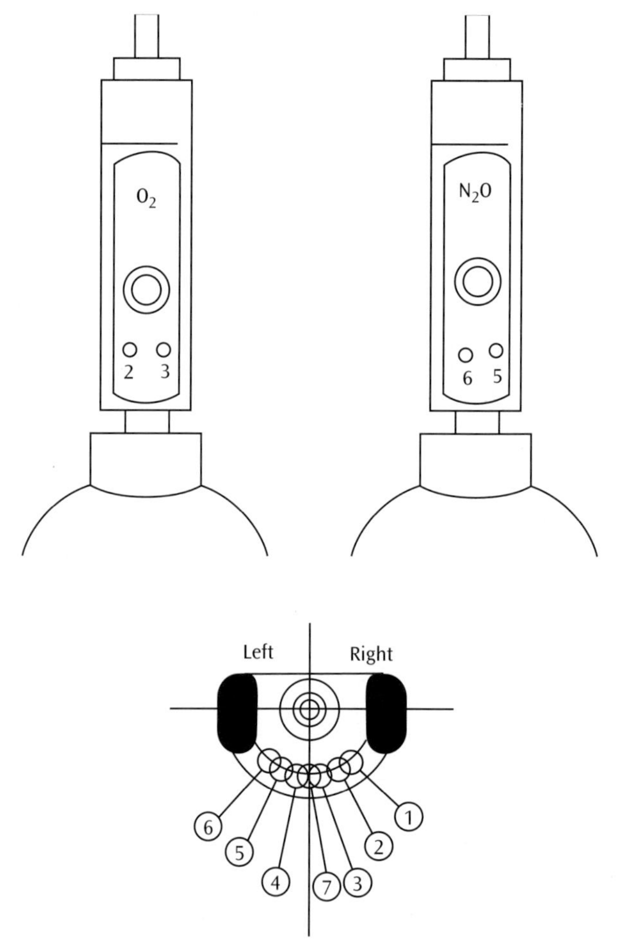

Figure 31.5 *Pin index safety system. (Reproduced with permission from Dorsch and Dorsch.[66])*

Distribution systems

Though cylinders are still in use in every system, usually they are a back-up supply to a central source.

Central supplies

Most hospitals supply oxygen, medical air, and nitrous oxide from a central source via pipelines. Standards for these systems are set by regulatory agencies in each country, including the National Fire Protection Association (NFPA)[67] in the USA and the CSA in Canada, as well as the International Standards Organization (ISO).

Storage requirements

The central gas source must be stored in an appropriate manner, usually with a primary and secondary (back-up) source. Oxygen (O_2) can only be stored in cylinders, to a maximum of 20 000 cubic feet. If larger supplies are needed, oxygen can be stored in a liquid form, in insulated vessels, so that the boiling point of liquid O_2 is not reached (2148 °C). These vessels are stored outside and can be filled or exchanged without disruption of supply.

Oxygen concentrators provide an alternative source of O_2. This source of oxygen has been developed for situations in which conventional supplies, i.e. cylinders, are impossible or too expensive. Concentrated O_2 is produced from air by absorption of nitrogen (N_2) onto a molecular sieve. O_2 and trace gases are allowed to pass through, resulting in an O_2 concentration of 90–98% with an argon concentration in the range of 5%.[68] The product gas from the concentrator is referred to as oxygen 93% USP or oxygen 90.[69]

Table 31.5 *Color code*

Cylinder contents	Europe, Canada	USA
Air	Black, white	Yellow
Carbon dioxide	Gray	Gray
Helium	Brown	Brown
Nitrogen	Black	Black
Nitrous oxide	Blue	Blue
Oxygen	White[a]	Green

[a]In UK, black with white collar.

Pipelines

The distribution of medical gases from the central source to the user outlet is via pipelines. The pipelines are classified into three general types:

1 main lines – connecting the central source to the other line;
2 risers – vertical pipes connecting the main sources to different floor levels of the institution;
3 branch or lateral lines – go to the user outlets in a room or group of rooms.

Table 31.6 *Pin index system*

Gas	Index pins
Air	1,5
Carbon dioxide (<7.5% in oxygen)	2,6
Helium (>80.5% in oxygen)	4,6
Nitrogen	1,4
Nitrous oxide	3,5
Nitrous oxide (47.5% in oxygen)	7
Oxygen	2,5

A typical layout is shown in Fig. 31.6. Pressure relief and shut-off valves must be incorporated into the system. Emergency shut-off valves must be readily accessible to the users so that they can be quickly turned off in an emergency. In addition, alarm systems are incorporated to signal to users when the pressure differs from the normal operating pressure by 20%. It is important that users are aware of the significance of these alarms and notify the responsible personnel when the alarm(s) sounds.[70]

Terminal units

The terminal unit is the site in a medical gas distribution system at which the user makes connections and disconnections. Equipment is connected directly or via a flexible hose. This unit incorporates a primary valve, which allows flow of gas only when the equipment is attached. Two main types of connections are used:

1. Diameter index safety system (DISS). This was designed so that only the correct flexible hose could be connected to the outlet of the pipeline. For each gas connection, i.e. air, oxygen ,and nitrous oxide, there is a unique fitting. This connector consists of an inner nipple and an outer screw nut, which are specific to the particular gas.
2. Quick connectors. These are designed to allow for easy one-handed connections of medical gas equipment, e.g. an O_2 flowmeter. Each connector consists of gas-specific male and female components, with a releasable spring mechanism to hold the two parts together.

Testing, regulations, and monitoring

There is a potential for problems and errors at all levels of a central storage and pipeline system. A number of reports of such problems have been published. These can range from a wrong gas supplied at the source,[71] crossed pipelines[72,73] or fitting equipment to an incorrect gas

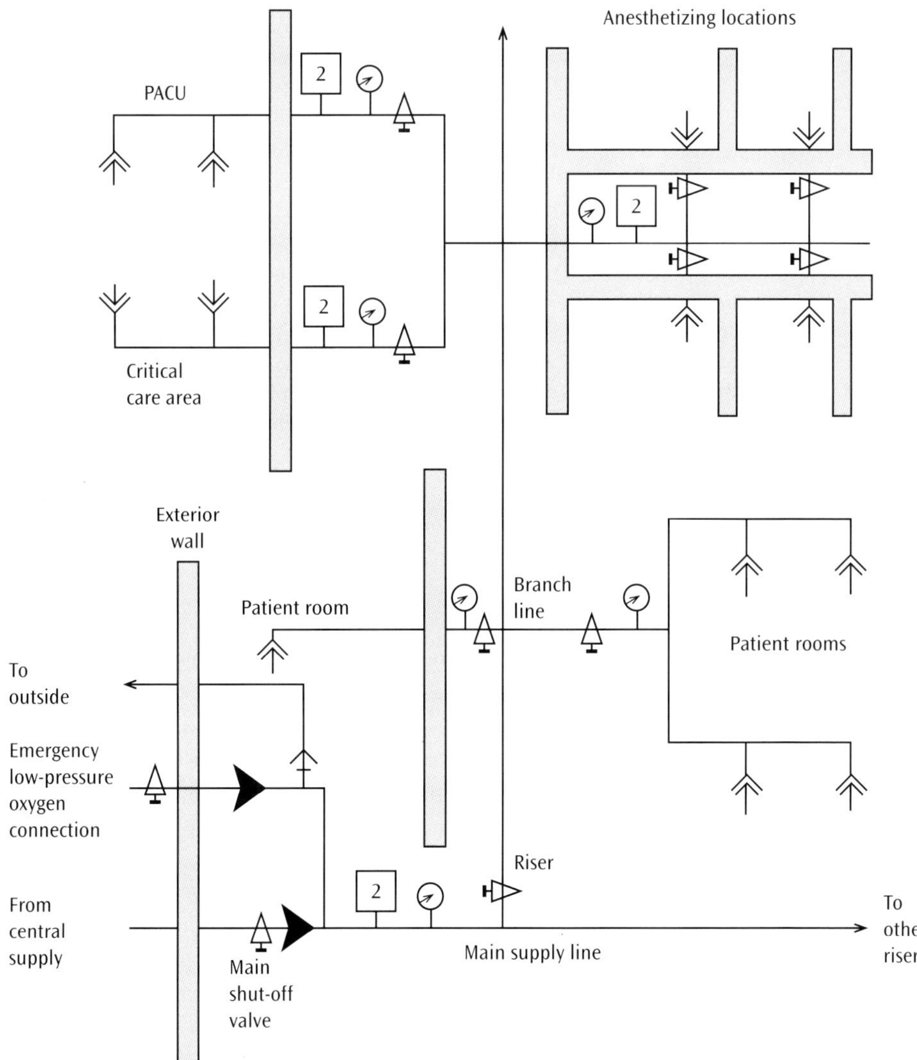

Figure 31.6 *Typical medical gas piped distribution system. (Reproduced with permission from Dorsch and Dorsch.[66])*

source.[74] Regulations are present in many countries or states that require appropriate testing of supply and pipeline systems at initial installation and after any maintenance or repair work. The Canadian standard requires independent testing to be performed at time of installation or repair, and it also requires that a member of staff and representative of the installer be present at the time of testing.[75] Problems can obviously also occur at times not related to installation or repair. These can include contamination and failure of the gas supply.[71] Most incidents reported relate to hypoxia from either failure of or incorrect oxygen supply. However, decreased nitrous oxide supply could lead to inadequate anesthesia.

Contamination from water and bacteria has also been reported.[76] It is important that the anesthesiologist be alert to these possible problems at all times. In-line monitoring of gas concentrations, particularly oxygen, is essential and may be a required regulation.[77] Vigilance for such occurrences as odors in pipelines is important as medical gases should be odor free.

Local supplies

Cylinders remain a vital part of medical gas supply. They provide a back-up to a pipeline system – anesthetic machines should all carry yokes for at least O_2 and N_2O cylinders. In addition, cylinders may be necessary to supply gas to places where a pipeline is not installed or for gases, e.g. carbon dioxide, that is not often supplied from a central system (Table 31.7 shows the characteristics of typical medical gas cylinders).

Storage

Cylinders all carry specific requirements for storage to meet safety standards. Cylinders contain gases under pressure in a gas or liquid phase depending on the gas concerned. Thus, the cylinder has to be able to withstand high pressures, which will increase as the ambient temperature increases. Cylinders can be refilled for up to 10 years, but only if they pass test requirements by pressuring them above their service pressure.[64] The test date (month and year) must be stamped on the cylinder. Cylinders should be stored in a cool, clear room constructed of fire-resistant material with adequate ventilation. Signs should be placed to warn that they should be moved in the event of a fire, and that there should be no open flames, sparks, or smoking in the storage room. Temperature should be maintained above freezing (0 °C) and below 52 °C. Cold temperatures are especially hazardous for N_2O–O_2 cylinders as the two gases may separate, with the potential to deliver a hypoxic mixture.

The tap on a cylinder should never be opened without a pressure-reducing valve being in place. Otherwise, gas under high pressure is released, which could lead to injury of personnel or patients. The tap should always be opened slowly to check for leaks – its important that a sealing washer be in place over the gas port. Valves should be closed before a cylinder is removed from its yoke to avoid release of gas under pressure. The portion of the label should be removed so as to read empty. Nitrous oxide cylinders should be stored in a secure place to avoid the potential for theft and abuse, and their use should be monitored.[78]

Monitoring of gas supply, as was described for pipelines, must be used for cylinders as cylinders can be contaminated or filled incorrectly.[79]

Trace gas exposure

Waste anesthetic gases during at least the first 100 years of anesthesia were exhausted directly into the operating environment. Initial attempts to reduce waste gases were designed to reduce the concentrations of flammable exhaust gases such as ether to reduce the risk of an explosion.

Modern interest in reducing exposure to waste gases came about because of reports of hazards resulting from such exposure.[80] Initial reports focused on increased abortion rates among female operating room personnel, including nurses and anesthesiologists. However, many other possible hazards have been studied, including rates of cancer, infertility, and mortality, among anesthesia personnel.[81,82]

The evidence that trace anesthetic gases are harmful is not strong, and any hazard is not great. These studies, however, have led to an awareness of the existence of these trace gases with resultant regulations for exposure and equipment to reduce their level.

Regulations

Agencies in many countries have set standards for exposure to trace anesthetic gases. A trace level of gas is far below anesthetic levels, cannot be detected by smell, and is usually measured in parts per million (ppm). This is expressed as volume/volume (1% gas is 10 000 ppm). Levels set by regulation relate to averaged measurements over a period of time.

The UK Committee for Occupational safety and Health has set threshold levels of 100 ppm for N_2O, 50 ppm for isoflurane, and 10 ppm for halothane. Other jurisdictions,[1] including Canada and the USA, have set acceptable levels as low as 25 ppm for N_2O and 2 ppm for halogenated agents.[1]

Table 31.7 *Typical medical gas cylinders, volumes, weights, and pressures*

Cylinder size	Dimensions: outer diameter × length in cm	Capacities and pressures at 21 °C	Air	CO_2	Helium	N_2O	Nitrogen	Oxygen
B	8.85×414	Liters	–	370	–	–	–	200
		kPa × 100	–	838	–	–	–	1900
D	11×41.5	Liters	375	940	300	940	370	400
		kPa × 100	1900	838	1600	745	1900	1900
E	10.5×63.5	Liters	625	1590	500	1590	610	660
		kPa × 100	1900	838	1600	745	1900	1900
M	17×105.5	Liters	2850	7570	2260	7570	3200	3450
		kPa × 100	1900	838	1600	745	2200	2200
G	21×125	Liters	5050	12300	4000	13800	–	–
		kPa × 100	1900	838	1600	745	–	–
H	22.5×125	Liters	6550	–	6000	15800	6400	6900
		kPa × 100	2200	–	2200	745	2200	2200

Monitoring

Only regular monitoring can ensure that trace gas concentrations are at an appropriately low level. This should form part of a routine protocol for any environment using anesthetic gases. A high level of gas can exist without being noticed as, for example, nitrous oxide is odorless and halothane may not be detected by smell at levels below 300 ppm.[83]

Monitoring can be performed by either hospital-based personnel or commercial laboratories. In-house analysis can be performed using moderately priced equipment with the advantage of an immediate report. Such equipment can, if necessary, be shared by a group of hospitals.

There are a number of choices for the monitoring equipment. Infrared analyzers are best at measuring nonhalogenated agents, e.g.N_2O, but the presence of CO_2 or water vapor can interfere with the analysis. This problem is reduced by sampling at least 6–10 inches from personnel. Passive dosimeters measure the amount of N_2O that diffuses into a molecular sieve. Analysis is usually carried out by the manufacturer. Passive dosimeters are a good method for obtaining a sample for a time-weighted average. Other equipment available for monitoring include the ionizing leak detector (suitable for halogenated agents) and the thermocamera.

Several options are available for sampling air samples for detection of trace gas levels. The simplest method, in which a sample of air is drawn into a container which is then sent for testing, is instantaneous. This method only represents the level of gas(es) in a small area of a room at one point in time. Time-weighted average sampling probably better reflects the time exposure of personnel to trace gases.[84] This approach can be used to monitor personnel or room exposure. Both nitrous oxide and halogenated gases can be measured, but different containers are necessary. Continuous monitoring is useful for the detection of leaks from equipment. In addition, end-tidal, blood, and urine sampling have been used to monitor individuals but, while accurately reflecting exposure, samples are more tedious to collect.

Monitoring is achieved by attaching a dosimeter to the clothing of personnel (not directly in the line of expired air). In addition, room levels can be measured by attaching a sampling device to the exhaust grille of the air exchange system or at an open door. If there are at least 15 air exchanges per hour, then homogeneous levels in a room can be expected except close to the gas leak.[85]

Control of waste gases

Scavenging systems are designed to exhaust waste anesthetic gases from the working environment to a discharge site, usually in the outside air. This is necessary because most anesthetic systems allow for leaks of gases, and also flowmeters are usually set to deliver a gas flow in excess of the patients' requirement.

A scavenger system consists of up to five basic parts:

1 a gas-collecting assembly at the site of emission;
2 a means of transfer to
3 an interface (providing a positive or negative pressure relief);
4 gas disposal tubing, which connects to the
5 gas disposal assembly.

Standards have been set for these components both internationally and in the USA.[86,87] Standards now require that the fitting at the outlet gas-collecting assembly be a 30-mm fitting. Previously, 14- and 22-mm fillings had been used, which allowed for possible misconnection. Most anesthetic circuits allow for easy connection to a gas-collecting device, however T-piece circuits require special adaption to allow such a fitting.[88] It is also possible to collect waste gases from other equipment such as ventilators, resuscitation equipment, or masks and nasal cannulae (by means of a hood).

Interfaces also require special connections, usually 30 or 19 mm, and if the direction of flow is specific then the inlet and outlet connectors should be different. Interfaces are open or closed depending on whether positive or negative pressure relief is used. In an open system, the collection reservoir must be large enough to avoid spillage. A closed system does not need a reservoir and can be used only with an active disposal system. Figure 31.7 shows samples of open interfaces and Fig. 31.8 shows closed interfaces.

The final gas disposal is achieved using either a passive or an active system. Passive systems include the room ventilation, piping directly to the outside air, and an adsorption device. As the room ventilation system requires circulation of air, it may be termed an assisted-passive system and the room air should be exhausted directly to the outside atmosphere.

Active systems usually work through a connection to the piped vacuums or an active duct system. If the piped vacuum is used, there must be a high-volume flow (30 L min^{-1}) and sufficient outlets and the system must not be easily overloaded.[89]

The anesthetic technique used can determine the likelihood of gases being exhausted into air. The least likely situation is with a closed circuit in an intubated patient. Common sources of gas leakage include poorly fitting anesthetic masks, leaks around endotracheal cuffs, and open circuits.[90] In this regard, laryngeal mask airways are associated with less leakage than anesthetic masks. The difficulty in exhausting gases from T-piece systems has already been mentioned. In addition, other

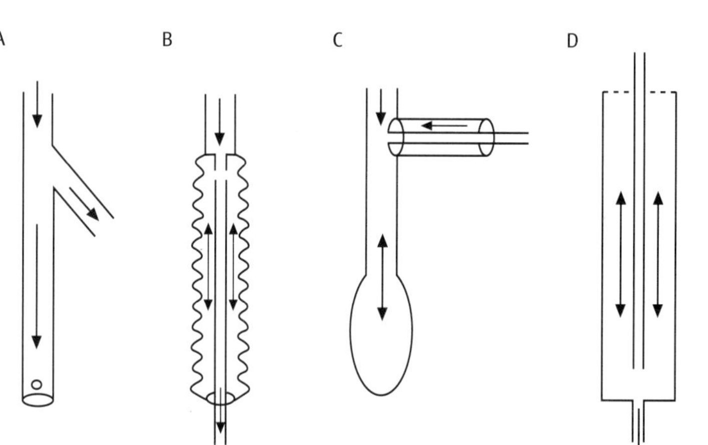

Figure 31.7 *Open interfaces. (Reproduced with permission from Dorsch and Dorsch.[66])*

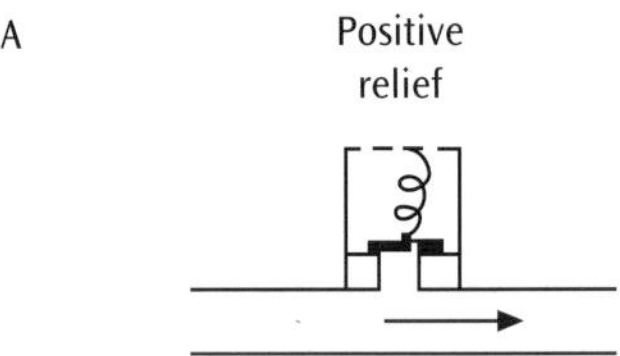

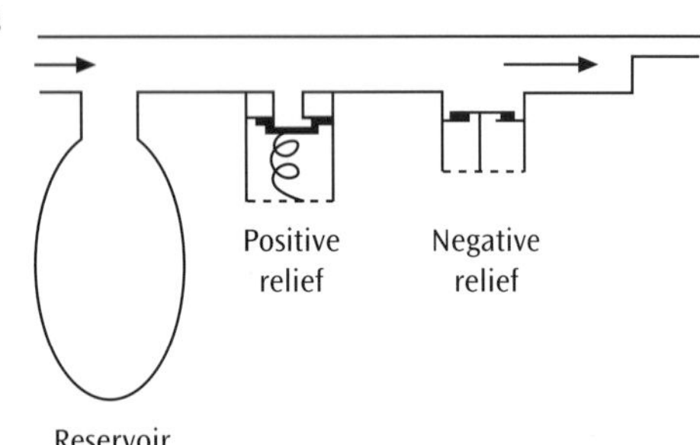

Figure 31.8 *Closed interfaces. (Reproduced with permission from Dorsch and Dorsch.[66])*

work practices can lead to gas pollution, such as leaving flowmeters and vaporizers on between and at the end of cases and spilling inhalational agents when filling vaporizers (more likely if keyed fillers are not used).

Room ventilation is also an important factor in controlling waste gases, and at least fifteen air exchanges per hour are recommended for nonrecirculating systems. Ideally, the potential source of leaks, i.e. the anesthetic machine, should be placed close to the exhaust air grille.

SUMMARY

Despite advances in equipment and monitoring, safety continues to be an important consideration for the practice of anesthesia.

Explosions are unlikely to occur with the disappearance of flammable gases, but electrical hazards can cause injury to patients and staff. Each new piece of equipment brings its own problems, i.e. the possible interference from cellular phones.

Gases may be a source of injury to patients and exposure is of concern for all staff.

Anesthesiologists must be knowledgeable about these possible hazards and be alert at all times in the operating room to ensure a safe environment.

REFERENCES

1. Klein BR. *Health Care Facilities Handbook*, 4th edn. Quincy, MA: National Fire Protection Association, 1993.
2. Gilbert TB, Shaffer M, Matthews M. Electrical shock by dislodged spark gap in bipolar electrosurgical device. *Anesth Analg* 1991; **73:** 355–7.
3. Bruner JMR, Aronow S, Cavicchi V. Electrical incidents in a large hospital: a 42 month register. *J Assoc Adv Med Instrument* 1972; **6:** 222–30.
4. Spalding CK, Klein BR. A survey of 20 Massachusetts hospitals' approach to the micro–macro shock hazard problems and their programs of corrective measures. In: *7th Annual Meeting of the Association of Advancement of Medical Instrumentation*, Las Vegas, 1972.
5. Bruner JMR. Common abuses and failures of electrical equipment. *Anesth Analg* 1972; **51:** 810–20.
6. Day FJ. Electrical safety revisited: a new wrinkle. *Anesthesiology* 1994; **80:** 220–1.
7. Lennon RL, Leonard PF. A hitherto unreported virtue of the isolated power system. *Anesth Analg* 1987; **66:** 1056–7.
8. Dalziel CF, Massoglia FP. Let-go currents and voltages. *AIEE Trans* 1956; **75**(Pt II, May): 49–56.
9. Tan KS, Johnson DL. Threshold of sensation for 60 Hz leakage current: results of a survey. *Biomed Inst Tech* 1990; **24:** 207–11.
10. Bruner JMR. Hazards of electrical apparatus. *Anesthesiology.* 1967; **28:** 396–425.
11. Wegria R, Wiggers CJ. Production of ventricular fibrillation by alternating currents. *Am J Physiol* 1940; **131:** 119.
12. Kouwenhoven WB, Hooker DR, Lotz EL. Electrical shock: effects of frequency. *Elect Eng* 1936; April.
13. Weinberg D, Artley JL, Whalen RE, McIntosh HD. Electric shock hazards in cardiac catheterization. *Circ Res* 1962; **11:** 1004–9.
14. Weinberg D. Grounding for electrical safety. *Med Elect Bio Eng* 1964; **2:** 435.
15. Raftery EB, Green HL, Yacoub MH. Disturbances of heart rhythm produced by 50 Hz leakage currents in human subjects. *Cardiovasc Res* 1975; **9:** 263–5.
16. Loughman J. Electrical thresholds for ventricular fibrillation in man. *Med J Aust* 1973; **1:** 1179–82.
17. Hull CJ. Electrocution hazards in the operating theatre. *Br J Anaesth* 1978; **50:** 647–57.
18. Goldwyn RM. Bovie: the man and the machine. *Ann Plast Surg* 1979; **2:** 135–53.
19. Cushing H. Electrosurgery as an aid to the removal of intracranial tumours. *Surg Gynecol Obstet* 1928; **47:** 751–84.
20. Battig, CG. Electrosurgical burn injuries and their prevention. *JAMA* 1968; **204:** 1025–9.
21. Schneider AL, Apple HP, Braun RT. Electrosurgical burns at skin temperature probes. *Anesthesiology* 1977; **47:** 72–74.
22. McNulty SE, Cooper M, Staudt S. Transmitted radiofrequency current through a flow directed pulmonary artery catheter. *Anesth Analg* 1994; **78:** 587–9.
23. Parker EO. Electrosurgical burn at the site of an esophageal temperature probe. *Anesthesiology* 1984; **61:** 93–5.
24. Bloch EC, Burton LW. Electrosurgical burn while using a battery-operated Doppler monitor. *Anesth Analg* 1979; **58:** 339–42.
25. Cooper JB, DeCesare R, Ambra MN. An engineering critical incident: direct current burn from a neuromuscular stimulator. *Anesthesiology* 1990; **73:** 168–72.
26. Leeming MN, Ray C Jr, Howland WS. Low voltage direct current burns. *JAMA* 1970; **214:** 1681–4.
27. Canadian Standards Association. *C22.2 Canadian Electrical Code, No. 601.1.2 Medical Electrical Equipment. Part 1: General Requirements for Safety – 2. Collateral Standard: Electromagnetic Compatibility Requirements and Tests.* Toronto: Canadian Standards Association, 1999.
28. Canadian Bio-Medical Engineering Society. Round table on EMC in health care. CMBES Conference Charlottetown, 1996.
29. Segal B, Retfalvi S, Townsend, Pavlesek T. Recommendations for electromagnetic compatibility in health care. CMBES Conference, Charlottetown, 1996.
30. Tan KS Himberg I. Investigation of electromagnetic interference with medical devices in Canadian hospitals. *Proceedings of a Workshop on Electromagnetics, Health Care and Health.* Montreal, 1995: 20–2.
31. MacDonald AG. A short history of fires and explosions caused by anaesthetic agents. *Br J Anaesth* 1994; **72:** 710–22.
32. Nicholson MJ, Crehan JP. Fire and explosion hazards in the operating room. *Anesth Analg* 1967; **46:** 412–24.
33. Podnas YD, Williams RA. Fires in the operating room. *Bull Am Coll Surg* 1997; **82:** 14–17.
34. Howard BK, Leach JL. Prevention of flash fires during facial surgery performed under local anesthesia. *Ann Otol Rhinol Laryngol* 1997; **106:** 248–51.
35. Eade GG. Hazard of nasal oxygen during aesthetic facial operations. *Plast Reconstr Surg* 1986; **78:** 539.
36. Epstein RH, Halmi BH. Oxygen leakage around the laryngeal mask airway during laser treatment of port-wine stains in children. *Anesth Analg* 1994; **78:** 486–9.
37. Bennett JA, Agree M. Fire in the chest. *Anesth Analg* 1994; 1994; **78:**406.
38. Ortega RA. A rare cause of fire in the operating room. *Anesthesiology* 1998; **89:** 1608.
39. Pashayan AG, Gravenstein JS. Helium retards endotracheal tube fires from carbon dioxide lasers. *Anesthesiology* 1985; **65:** 274–7.
40. Wolf GL, Simpson JI. Flammability of endotracheal tubes in oxygen and nitrous oxide enriched atmosphere. *Anesthesiology* 1987; **67:** 236–9.
41. Simpson JI, Wolf GL. Flammability of esophageal stethoscopes, nasogastric tubes, feeding tubes, and nasopharyngeal airways in oxygen-and nitrous oxide-enriched atmospheres. *Anesth Analg* 1988; **67:** 1093–5.
42. MacDonald AG. A brief historical review of nonanaesthetic causes of fires and explosions in the operating room. *Br J Anaesth* 1994; **73:** 847–56.

43. Brown TA, Morris G. The ignition risk with mixtures of oxygen and nitrous oxide with halothane. *Br J Anaesth* 1966; **38:** 164–73.
44. Leonard PF. The lower limits of flammability of halothane, enflurane, and isoflurane. *Anesth Analg* 1975; **54:** 238–40.
45. Chee WK, Benumof JL. Airway fire during tracheostomy: extubation may be contraindicated. *Anesthesiology* 1998; **89:** 1576–8.
46. Koufman JA, Little WB, Weeks DB. Proximal large-bore jet ventilation for laryngeal laser *Surg. Arch Otolaryngol* 1987; **113:** 314–20.
47. Pashayan AG, SanGiovanni C, Davis LE. Positive end-expiratory pressure lowers the risk of laser-induced polyvinylchloride tracheal-tube fires. *Anesthesiology* 1993; **79:** 83–7.
48. Coulson AS, Bakhshay SA. Harmonic scalpel prevents tracheotomy fires. *Chest* 1998; **114:** 349.
49. Milliken RA, Bizzarri DV. Flammable surgical drapes – a patient and personnel hazard. *Anesth Analg* 1985; **64:** 54–7.
50. Stouffer DJ. Fires during surgery: two fatal incidents in Los Angeles. *J Burn Care Rehab* 1992; **13:** 114–7.
51. Briscoe CE, Hill DW, Payne JP. Inflammable antiseptics and theatre fires. *Br J Surg* 1976; **63:** 981–3.
52. Buyers RA. Fire in the operating room caused by fluid from suture package. *JAMA* 1977; **237:** 531.
53. Wrenn K. The hazards of defibrillating through nitroglycerin patches. *Ann Emerg Med* 1990; **19:** 1327–8.
54. Bond JH, Levitt MD. Factors affecting the concentration of combustible gases in the colon during colonoscopy. *Gastroenterology* 1975; **68:** 1445–8.
55. Avgerinos A, Kalantzis N, Rekoumis G, *et al.* Preparation and risk of explosion during colonoscopic polypectomy. *Gut* 1984; **25:** 361–4.
56. Axelrod EH, Kusnetz AB, Rosenberg MK. Operating room fires initiated by hot wire cautery. *Anesthesiology* 1993; **79:** 1123–6.
57. Reynolds DS, Plant E, Bancroft L, *et al.* Electrical fires in Hewlett-Packard monitors due to saline contamination. *Anesthesiology* 1998; **89:** 521–4.
58. US Department of Labor. Workplace fire safety. Fact Sheet [serial online] No. OSHA 91–41 [cited 1999 April 19; 3 screens]. Available from: www.ccohs.ca/othersinfo/alerts/osha-41.txt
59. US Department of Labor. Responding to workplace emergencies. Fact Sheet [serial online] No. OSHA 92–19 [cited 1999 April 19; 3 screens]. Available from: www.ccohs.ca/othersinfo/alerts/osha-19.txt
60. Aghababian R, Lewis CP, Gans L, Curley FJ. Disasters within hospitals. *Ann Emerg Med* 1994; **23:** 771–7.
61. Vidor KK, Puterbaugh S, Willis CJ. Fire safety training: A program for the operating room. *AORN J* 1989; **49:** 1045–9.
62. Nagel EL, Perdue M, Hayes JD, Kennedy W. Drill prepares O.R. for fire emergency. *J Am Hosp Assoc* 1973; **47:** 99–105.
63. Scanlon J. F-I-R-E! Evacuating St. Joseph's. *Dimensions in Health Service* 1983; **60:** 18–19.
64. Compressed Gas Association. *Handbook of Compressed Gases*, 3rd edn. New York, NY: Van Nostrand, Reinhold, 1990.
65. Sosis MB (ed.) *Anesthesia Equipment Manual*. Philadelphia: Lippincott, 1997.
66. Dorsch JA, Dorsch S.E. *Understanding Anesthesia Equipment.* Philadelphia: Wilkins and Wilkins.
67. National Fire Protection Association. *Standards for Health Care Facilities* (NFPA '99). Quincy, MA: NFPA, 1996.
68. Carter BA, Baskett PJ, Simpson PJ. The 'Pennox' oxygen concentrator. *Anesthesia* 1985; **40:** 560–5.
69. Friesen RM. Oxygen concentration and the practice of anesthesia. *Can J Anesth* 1992; **39:** R80–4.
70. Feeley TW, Hedley-Whyte J. Bulk oxygen and nitrous oxide delivery systems: designs and dangers. *Anaesthesiology* 1976; **44:** 301–5.
71. Sprague DH, Archer EW. Intraoperative hypoxia from an erroneously filled liquid oxygen reservoir. *Anaesthesiology* 1975; **4:** 360–2.
72. Lebourdais E. Nine deaths linked to cross-contamination: Sudbury General inquest makes hospital history. *Dimens Hlth Services* 1974, **51:** 10–12.
73. Scammas FL. An analysis of the factors leading to crossed gas lines causing profound hypercardia during general anesthesia. *J Clin Anesth* 1993; **5:** 439–41.
74. Lane GA. Medical gas outlets – a hazard from interchangeable "Quick-connect" couples. *Anesthesiology* 1980; **32:** 86–7.
75. Canadian Standards Association. *Qualification Requirements for Agencies Testing Non-flammable Medical Gas Piping Systems* (CSA 2305.4 – M85). Toronto: CSA, 1985.
76. Bjerning P, Oberg B. Bacterial contamination of compressed air for medical use. *Anesthesia* 1986; **41:** 148–50.
77. CAS Monitoring Standards. *CAS Guidelines to the Practice of Anesthesia*. Toronto: CAS, 2002.
78. Rowbottom SJ. Nitrous oxide abuse. *Anesth Intensive Care* 1988; **16:** 241–2.
79. Menon MRB. Incorrectly filled cylinders. *Anesthesia* 1991; **46:** 155–6.
80. Cohen EN, Bellville JW, Brown BW. Anesthesia, pregnancy and miscarriage: a study of operating room nurses and anesthetists. *Anesthesiology* 1971; **35:** 343–7.
81. Knill-Jones RP, Rodriques LV, Morr DD, Spence AA. Anesthetic practice and pregnancy. *Lancet* 1972; **1:** 1326–8.
82. Ad Hoc Committee on the Effects of Trace Anesthetics in the Health of Operating Room Personnel, American Society of Anesthesiologists. *Occupational Disease Among Operating Room Personnel: a National Study*. Park Ridge, IL: ASA.
83. Halsey MJ, Chard S, Diurzewski, AR, *et al.* Olfactory thresholds: detection of operating room contamination. *Br J Anaesth* 1977; **49:** 510–11.
84. Campbell D, Danis PD, Halliday MM, *et al.* Comparison of personnel pollution monitoring techniques for use in the operating room. *Br J Anaesth* 1980; **521:** 885–92.
85. *Draft Report on Anesthetic Waste Gas: Scavenging*. Ontario: Ministry of Health, 1977.
86. *Inhalational Gas Systems – Part 3: Anesthetic gas scavenging systems transfer and receiving systems – transfer and receiving systems* (ISO8835). Geneva: International Standards Organization. 1997.
87. American Society for Testing and Materials. *Standard Specification for Anesthetic Equipment-scavenging Systems for Anesthetic Gases.*(ASTMFI 343-91). West Conshohocken, PA: ASTM, 1991.
88. Van Hasselt G, Phillips J. T-piece scavenging: simple alternatives. *Anesthesia* 1994; **49:** 263–4.
89. Enderly DH, Booth AM, Churchill-Davidson HC. Removal of anesthetic waste gases. An inexpensive antipollution system for use with pipeline suction. *Anesthesia* 1978; **33:** 820–6.
90. Barnett R, Gallant B, Forsey S, *et al.* Nitrous oxide environmental pollution. A comparison between face mask, laryngeal mask and endotracheal intubation. *Can J Anesth* 1992; **9:** A151.

32

Measurement of the depth of anesthesia

GAVIN N C KENNY AND THOMAS E J HEALY

Anesthesiologists have sometimes been complacent about the possibility of awareness during anesthesia. However, patients who have been aware and can explicitly recall the event in detail, especially the horrifying experience of pain, may suffer post-traumatic stress syndrome. Awareness, in the absence of pain or fear or recall, may have no untoward sequelae. Awareness occurs most frequently in the paralyzed patient and most anesthesiologists have heard about patients who, paralyzed on the operating table, attempt to cry, move, or shout out. The spontaneously breathing patient may also suffer awareness, but such a patient can make purposeful movements to alert the anesthesiologist to the problem.

The use of minimal doses of neuromuscular blocking agents can reduce the frequency of patients experiencing awareness during anesthesia. However, in a recent study Sandin *et al.*[1] reported results from almost 12 000 patients. Eighteen patients had experienced awareness, of whom four had not received neuromuscular blocking agents.

The percentage of patients who suffer awareness during general anesthesia is small. However, even a fraction as low as 0.2%, i.e. 1 in 500, can, taking into account the many clinical situations in which general anesthesia is used, result in many patients being conscious during their operation. It is therefore very important that anesthesiologists are able to identify changes in the depth of anesthesia that can threaten conscious awareness.

The development of monitors to assess the depth of anesthesia has been the subject of much study. The introduction of appropriate measurement techniques can be expected to reduce the incidence of awareness during general anesthesia but allow anesthesia to be light enough to facilitate rapid recovery and reduce both the human and the financial costs. However, the use of a monitor does not necessarily guarantee that it will be used appropriately. It would be expected that the use of end-tidal agent monitoring would decrease the frequency of awareness during anesthesia. However, in the study by Sandin there was no difference in the frequency of awareness in patients who had end-tidal monitoring of their inhalational anesthetic agents and those who had no monitoring.[1]

A depth of anesthesia monitor would indicate the possibility that a patient might be aware and give an anesthesiologist the opportunity to increase the amount of anesthetic drug and thereby protect the patient from suffering. The provision of an effective monitor would be a considerable advance but in addition would lend itself to the possibility of combining the electronic measurement of depth of anesthesia, via a feedback link, with an injector or flow controller. Such a development could further improve the dosing accuracy but might allow the anesthesiologist to concentrate attention on the other aspects of anesthetic care.

Awareness results from the failure to deliver an adequate dose of the hypnotic component of anesthesia. Deeply anesthetized patients do not report that they were aware during their surgery but, on the other hand, awareness is not an inevitable consequence of light anesthesia. Light anesthesia may, under certain conditions, pass into awareness and yet still disrupt the mechanism underlying the formation of memory, thereby limiting the chance of recall. Nonetheless, light anesthesia must be monitored very carefully.

General anesthesia is a dynamic balance between the level of hypnosis, analgesia, and stimulation (Fig. 32.1).[2] Painful surgical stimulation can alter the level of anesthesia, and therefore appropriately secure levels of anesthesia are required to ensure unconsciousness. Unless nerve blockade has been introduced, nocioceptive pathways remain intact during general anesthesia. It is important, therefore, to combine adequate dosing with the anesthetic drug and appropriate analgesia.

Anesthesiologists should consider the level of anesthetic depth that they wish to achieve. A patient given an appropriate dose of hypnotic drug will have loss of cognitive ability and be unaware of self and surroundings, be unable to form an emotional response to stimuli, and will not recognize pain. However, the afferent stimulation of the brain, by the painful stimulus, may well reduce the level of sedation, making increased hypnotic dosing essential if awareness is to be avoided.

The development of new anesthetic drugs is generally a response to the need for, or the advantages of, a faster recovery. Xenon anesthesia, in particular, offers the likelihood of a complete recovery of cognitive function, including awareness of self, emotion, and recall within minutes of the cessation of anesthesia. Agents used previously that had a slower offset provided a greater opportunity for the anesthesiologist to identify and correct problems such as disconnection of the anesthetic circuit. New agents with very short offset times will increase the need for improved and dependable depth of anesthesia monitoring technology.

AWARENESS

There are different levels of awareness that can occur, ranging from complete recall to no evidence of awareness.

- conscious awareness with spontaneous or prompted recall (explicit recall);
- conscious awareness with amnesia;
- dreaming;
- unconscious awareness with amnesia (implicit recall);
- no evidence of awareness.

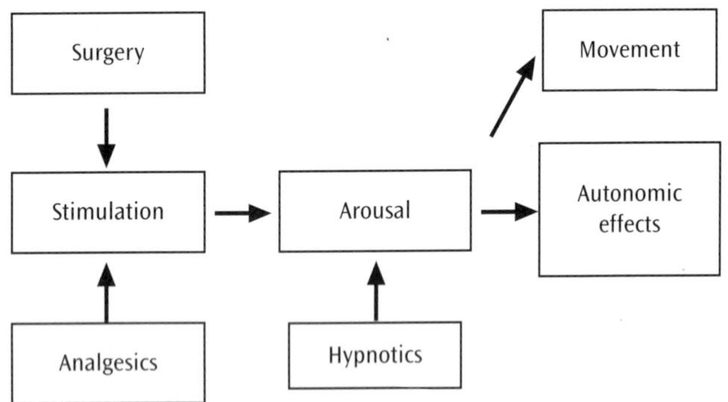

Figure 32.1 *Schematic diagram of the interaction between surgical stimulation, analgesia, and hypnosis. Analgesic agents decrease the stimulating effects of surgery and reduce the requirements for hypnotic agents.*[2]

Conscious awareness with recall describes the normal awake patient who is fully able to describe explicit memories of events during surgery. Conscious awareness with amnesia describes patients who are able to respond during surgery but have no recollection of their experience. In a study by Russell,[3] using the isolated forearm technique, 72% of patients responded to command during major surgery but none had spontaneous, unprompted recall. Almost two-thirds of the patients indicated that they had experienced pain at some point during their surgery. Patients who report dreaming present a difficult group to classify since the dreams may have occurred during anesthesia or in the immediate postoperative period. Unconscious awareness with amnesia describes the patient who has implicit expression of memory. The patient has no voluntary recall but events such as morbid conversations by the surgical team are memorized subliminally and may be recalled later by patients presenting with adverse behavioral reactions.[4]

It has been reported by the Medical Defence Union in the UK that, of its total claims during 1 year, amounting to £50 million, 12.2% were related to awareness during general anesthesia.[5] This exceeded the claims involving perioperative death (11.6%). A faulty technique was accepted as the cause for 70% of the complaints of awareness and 20% were due to a failure by the anesthesiologist to check the equipment. Only 2.5% of the claims for awareness were attributed to apparatus failure, spurious claims, unknown causes, or justified risks.

Careful experimental design is required to identify the incidence of explicit recall. Public awareness of the possibility of conscious awareness has been raised in recent years, and it is important to discriminate awareness from dreams, hallucinations, or even false claims. The results of correctly planned and conducted trials, including structured interviews with the subjects, have revealed that the incidence of awareness ranges from 0.2% to 1.6%.[6] The levels of dreaming were reported to range from 0.9 to 26% in the same study. Other studies without structured interviews conclude that the incidence of awareness is around 8% for cesarean section.[7] The incidence extends to 45% during accident and emergency surgery, during which there were periods of inadequate level of anesthetic depth.[8] It has been estimated that approximately 10% of patients who suffer from awareness experience pain.[4]

There have been attempts using benzodiazepines to convert conscious awareness with recall into awareness with amnesia. The prevention of memory is not the same as the prevention of awareness. Implicit recall of events may still be possible even following the retrograde disruption of explicit memory by an amnesic drug.

All anesthesiologists should design their anesthetic techniques to obviate awareness. In one study of 68 patients undergoing cesarean section, morphine and diazepam were shown to reduce significantly the incidence of awareness and unpleasant dreams.[9] The combination of diazepam and morphine was shown to cause both anterograde and retrograde amnesia and, interestingly, in two of the patients (3.8%) who were aware during their anesthesia, neither the pupil size nor the blood pressure changed. It seems likely that the absence of pupil reactivity was due to the morphine, which quickly decreases pupil diameter.[10]

Explicit awareness is linked with, though not caused by, the use of muscle relaxant drugs. The spontaneously breathing unparalyzed patient moves when too lightly anesthetized. Only one case of a spontaneously breathing patient who experienced awareness during anesthesia had been reported before the recent study of Sandin *et al.*[1] in which four patients were aware in the absence of paralyzing drugs.[11,12]

Subconscious awareness with amnesia can be demonstrated by testing for a behavioral response to an intraoperative suggestion. A group of 33 patients in whom anesthesia was induced with thiopental and maintained with nitrous oxide/oxygen and halothane or enflurane was studied.[13] A significant number (9 out of 11) exhibited postoperative ear-touching behavior in response to intraoperative verbal suggestions. No patient was able to recall the suggestions during subsequent hypnosis and no patient complained that he or she had been aware during anesthesia. Word sequences presented during anesthesia may be recalled postoperatively.[14] Detection of 10 keywords out of a 40-word sequence was significantly better in those patients who listened to a tape of the keywords intraoperatively rather than a tape of radio static.[14] The authors recommended the use of ear plugs to prevent the recall of words heard during anesthesia. The use of ear plugs, while inappropriate as a way of preventing awareness under anesthesia, does remove the likelihood that a patient who is aware might recognize key phrases spoken by the surgical team.

It has been suggested that positive verbal comments presented intraoperatively, and subject to implicit recall, might shorten the duration of postoperative recovery. In one study, positive intraoperative comments were made to 91 patients and it was reported that these comments resulted in a reduction in the time that elderly patients remained in hospital.[15] No patient was shown to have explicit recall of the verbal stimuli following anesthesia. These findings were not confirmed in a later study in which positive verbal suggestions were given to patients undergoing total abdominal hysterectomy.[5] There was no evidence of a reduction in hospital stay or of an improved postoperative outcome. Decreased requirements for morphine, delivered by patient-controlled analgesia, have been reported following positive intraoperative suggestions.[16]

Good clinical practice requires that an anesthesiologist visits each patient following general anesthesia. One study has noted the benefit of the postoperative visit to calm and reassure patients who had suffered from awareness.[17] A postoperative review of even good clinical records may not always reveal an obvious cause for awareness, as was the case in that study in which the anesthetic notes of patients who had been aware were concealed among the records of those who had not. The clinical records were examined by a panel of experienced anesthesiologists but they were unable to identify from the notes those patients who had experienced awareness. Similar results have been reported by Domino and colleagues,[18] who found that awareness was associated with hypertension in only 15% of cases and with tachycardia in 7%.

There have been few reports of awareness in the literature following the use of total intravenous anesthesia (TIVA). In a study in which 2500 patients received propofol with alfentanil, five (~2%) reported awareness.[19] Two of these patients recalled some pain. The authors, however, asked the patients only if they had slept well, and this question did not form part of a correctly structured interview. Sandin and his colleagues[1] reported zero incidence of awareness during intravenous anesthesia in their study of almost 12 000 patients, in which the overall frequency of awareness was 0.15%. There is a need for more studies, including correctly structured postoperative interviews, to identify the incidence of awareness during the use of different anesthetic drugs and drug combinations.

The incidence and the implications of implicit awareness of subliminal suggestions will be more difficult to assess. It must concern anesthesiologists that a negative health suggestion may be subconsciously remembered by the patient and be implicitly recalled and affect the prognosis. In one study in which 10 patients were anesthetized with thiopental, nitrous oxide, and ether, the anesthesiologist was required to make negative statements during the surgery such as, "Stop the operation. I don't like the patient's color. His/her lips are too blue. I am going to give a little oxygen." These negative suggestions were followed by reassuring positive comments such as, "There, that's better now. You can carry on with the operation."[20] No patient exhibited explicit recall of the comments. However, at interview 1 month later, under hypnosis four patients recalled the comments exactly, four had partial recall, and two had no recall. All the patients during anesthesia exhibited irregular slow electroencephalogram (EEG) waves monitored using a six-channel scalp recording. The EEG evidence of "adequate anesthesia" did not prevent implicit recall.

Levinson described a patient who was anesthetized with thiopental, nitrous oxide, oxygen, and halothane during the removal of a cyst from the mouth. A surgical colleague exclaimed, "Good gracious! This may not be a simple cyst, it may be cancer." After the surgeon had removed the cyst he said, "On second thoughts, it was only a simple cyst." Following recovery, the patient, who was shown the laboratory report confirming that the cyst was not malignant but who under hypnosis had recalled the surgeon's words, remarked that she had not believed the surgeon's reassurances. This patient died 2 years later with cancer of the uterus. The fact that this patient could recall a negative comment and fail to believe the positive assurance suggests that operating room staff should be most careful in their discussions in the presence of an anesthetized patient.

HISTORY

Anesthesia, if deepened to its ultimate conclusion, leads to death. John Snow described "five stages of narcotism." These were later refined by Guedel.[21] Guedel's sleep stages form the basis of assessment during anesthesia with most modern volatile anesthetics, even though the method was developed with ether and before the introduction of muscle relaxants. It must be remembered that staging anesthetic depth is not the same as staging for possible levels of awareness. The first stage of Guedel's classification was analgesia. The second was the stage of excitement. Stage 3 was named the stage of surgical anesthesia. This originally consisted of four sequential planes: plane 1, extending from the onset of automatic respiration or regular breathing to the cessation of eye movements; plane 2, extending from the onset of intercostal paralysis; plane 3, extending to complete intercostal muscle paralysis; and plane 4, extending to diaphragmatic paralysis. Guedel's stage 4 therefore extended from the onset of diaphragmatic paralysis to apnea and death and represented overdosage. As ether anesthesia is deepened there is progressive dilation of the pupil from stage 3, plane 1, through to death. There is loss of the pupillary light reflex during stage 3, plane 3. White[22] expressed the process of deepening anesthesia in terms of a continuum, in which as anesthesia deepens there is a progressive loss of physiological control. Sedation is an intermediate state between consciousness and unconsciousness in which the patient remains arousable at all times.

Muscle relaxants do not alter the depth of anesthesia but have decreased the need for deep anesthesia to reduce muscle tone. Concern about inadequate anesthesia and the use of muscle relaxants as adjuncts to anesthesia has resulted in a legal requirement to ensure adequate depth of anesthesia during animal experimentation in the UK.[23]

MEASUREMENT OF ANESTHETIC DEPTH

Dose-related estimates of anesthetic depth and adequacy are empirical and require the correct functioning of the anesthetic equipment used to deliver the hypnotic agent. Vaporizers, even when correctly calibrated, do not measure the amount of anesthetic present in the patient. Mechanical failure, airway obstruction, or abnormal metabolism can all conspire to reduce the hypnotic effect of anesthesia. End-tidal gas analyzers may provide useful information concerning the amount of anesthetic being given and indeed even brain concentration, but they do not provide a complete answer to the problem of depth measurement. These monitors measure gas or vapor concentration but do not measure the hypnotic state. No monitor based on anesthetic concentrations can anticipate the physiologic responses of a patient during anesthesia or detect the effects of surgical stimulation on anesthetic depth.

Subjective methods have been applied to the assessment of anesthetic depth but these rely on the experience and opinion of the anesthesiologist that the patient is adequately anesthetized. Until a reliable monitor of anesthetic depth is available, the anesthesiologist must rely on easily detectable presentations of changes in brain function, such as the pupillary light reflex, and, more importantly, on the hemodynamic changes, in blood pressure and pulse rate, which occur in response to surgery.

Subjective measurement

Autonomic changes

Changes in blood pressure or heart rate may indicate lightening of anesthesia to levels at which awareness may occur.[19] Unfortunately, changes in blood pressure and pulse rate may be responses to other events and the time taken to exclude these may permit awareness, if light anesthesia is the cause. A study in which patients were repeatedly taken from consciousness to unconsciousness and back to consciousness showed no correlation between cardiovascular responses and the conscious level of the patients.[24] Russell[3] has also reported that cardiovascular measurements could not detect conscious awareness.

Pupil diameter

The classical staging of ether anesthesia describes the initial contraction of the pupil followed by progressive dilation as anesthesia becomes deeper.[21] Changes in pupil size are unreliable. Pupil dilation is affected by circulating catecholamines; atropine and hyoscine induce mydriasis whereas opiates induce miosis. The pupillary light reflex may also be affected by intraoperative opioid analgesics[14] and by anoxia and therefore an unresponsive pupil does not confirm that a patient is deeply anesthetized (Fig. 32.2).

Isolated forearm technique

The isolated forearm technique[25] is based on the isolation of an arm from intravenously administered muscle relaxants. A tourniquet is placed on an arm and inflated before the muscle relaxant is given. The arm can therefore be expected to remain unparalyzed and free to move. The patient is able therefore to respond to commands by the anesthesiologist or to alert the anesthesiologist to the fact that he or she has regained consciousness. Ischemia may be a problem, though it can be avoided by periodically releasing the tourniquet. This is usually done before topping up the neuromuscular blockade, i.e. at a time when circulating levels of neuromuscular blocking agent are at their lowest.

In spite of the ease of this technique very few anesthesiologists use it. The possibility of patient movement is an anathema to them and to surgeons. Furthermore, patients have reported that they have heard commands to move their arm but have been unable to do so, even

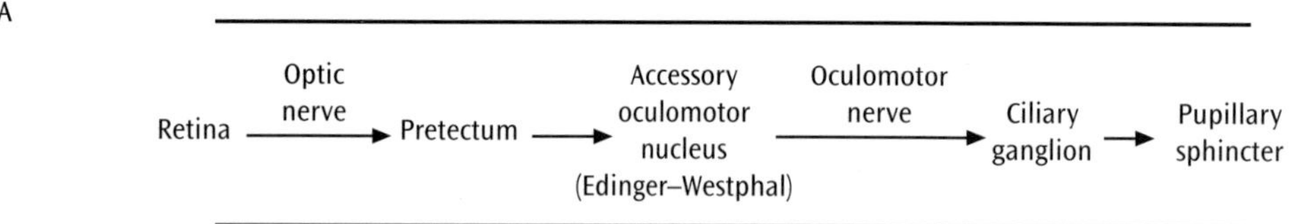

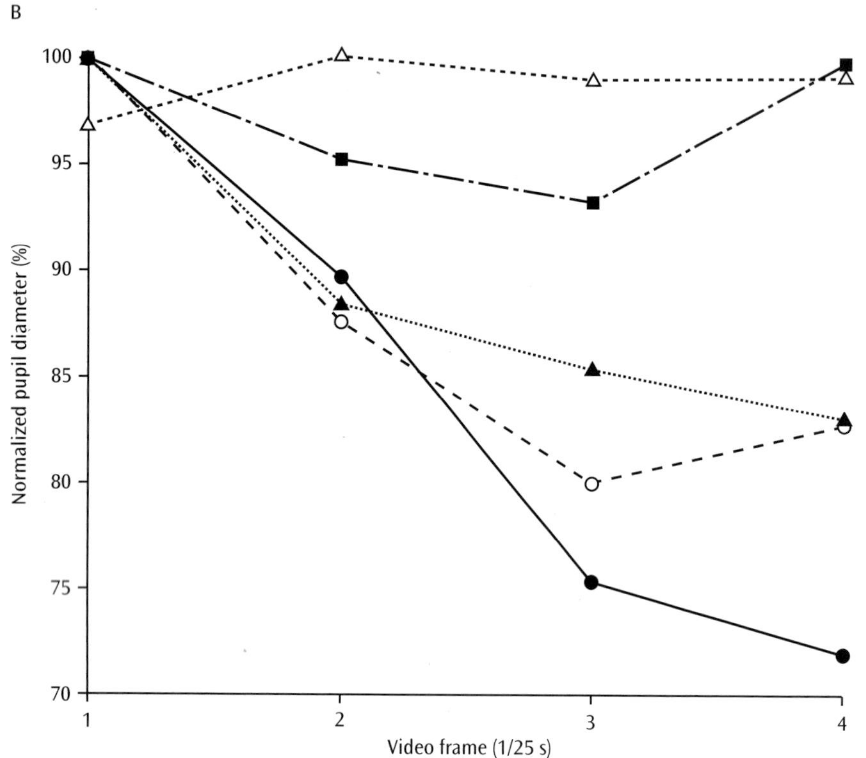

Figure 32.2 *Simplified derivation of the bispectral index. (A) Pupil light reflex: neural pathway. (B) The pupil reaction velocity. Following a bolus dose of propofol the pupil reaction to light slowed but then recovery started as the effect of this dose began to wane. The pupil response to a steady-state propofol infusion is shown. Fentanyl disrupted the light reflex and recovery was only marginal 5 min after anesthesia ceased.* ●, *Preinduction;* ▲, *propofol (2.5 mg kg^{-1}) induction;* ○, *propofol (10 mg kg^{-1} h^{-1}) infusion;* Δ, *fentanyl;* ■, *postfentanyl recovery.*

though electrical nerve stimulation suggested that their arm was not paralyzed.[26]

Objective measurement

An objective monitor of anesthetic depth should meet certain requirements in order to be of clinical use:

- adequate cardiovascular and respiratory stability;
- ideally no, or at least only minimal, patient movement;
- no awareness or recall of events during the procedure;
- similar values for different types of anesthetic agents at equipotent doses;
- values at recovery from anesthesia similar to those obtained before induction;
- appropriate change during surgical stimulation;
- unaffected by alterations in the cardiovascular system or by cardioactive drugs;
- marked difference in the signal between consciousness and unconsciousness.

An objective measurement should indicate the stage during light anesthesia that precedes conscious awareness; it should reflect changing concentrations of anesthetic agents and be sensitive to stimuli of different modalities, especially surgical stimulation; the monitor should have a high temporal resolution and should be able to stage the depth of anesthesia. It should also be quick and easy to set up and work for all modern anesthetic drugs, and the characteristics of the response should be the same with the separate anesthetic agents at equivalent levels of anesthesia.

It must be remembered that the minimum alveolar concentration (MAC) is not a measurement of anesthetic depth. MAC is the concentration of anesthetic at which 50% of subjects respond to an unpleasant stimulus, such as a skin incision in humans or tail clamping in rats. MAC is just one point on the dose–response curve for an anesthetic and does not require cortical or forebrain structure.[27] While MAC does not measure or indicate anesthetic depth, it provides an opportunity for the anesthesiologist, measuring expired vapor concentrations, to set a level of anesthetic at which noxious stimuli are very unlikely to cause conscious awareness. The concept of MAC therefore makes the use of a vapor concentration monitor essential during general anesthesia.

Electroencephalogram and derived indices

Electroencephalogram

The raw EEG is a small (1–500 μV) voltage deflection recorded from silver/silver chloride electrodes fixed to the scalp. An active electrode is positioned over a site of neuronal activity and an indifferent electrode is positioned at a site on the scalp some distance away. The EEG is the sum of ionic currents from thousands of neurons around the site of the active electrode. The spatial organization of pyramidal neurons, with dendrites perpendicular to the surface of the cerebral cortex, results in these contributing the most to the EEG. In addition, slow-wave synaptic potentials, rather than action potentials, contribute more to the EEG as these, being slower potentials, summate more readily at the scalp. The nature of the deflection in the EEG waveform may differ according to the site of the neuronal event in the cerebral cortex. Excitatory postsynaptic potentials cause an upward deflection in the scalp-recorded EEG if the synapse is in the superficial layers of the cerebral cortex but a downward deflection if it originates in the deeper layers. Conversely, inhibitory postsynaptic potentials cause a downward deflection if they originate in the superficial layers and an upward deflection if present in the deeper layers.[28]

EEG recording is noninvasive. It is important that the recording electrodes are attached to the scalp carefully in order to limit impedance to the lowest possible level and to obtain the greatest possible EEG wave amplitude. This is usually achieved by sequential application of an abrasive paste and adhesive gel combined with the use of an electrode impedance meter to confirm good connections. Making these attachments increases the time spent in the anesthetic room but, in spite of great care with the attachment of electrodes, poorly screened electrical equipment and diathermy contribute to interference in the EEG, which can make the waveform difficult to interpret or damage sensitive recording amplifiers. Care should be taken in the selection of amplifiers. Amplifiers designed for research purposes may be unsuitable for use in operating rooms.

Visual inspection of the EEG shows it to be a rapidly fluctuating waveform, varying from periods of intense high-frequency fluctuations to an almost flat line (Fig. 32.3). Identification of the components in the EEG requires classification into its component frequencies: α (8–13 Hz), β (13–30 Hz), δ (0.5–4.5 Hz), and θ (4–7 Hz).[28] The EEG in the conscious patient with eyes closed generally shows a predominance of α frequencies and contrasts with sleep and general anesthesia, which are associated with more low-frequency activity, including δ and θ frequencies.

Spectral analysis

The raw EEG waveform is complex and changes in rhythm during anesthesia are due not only to the level of anesthesia but also to the type of anesthetic and to other factors such as the hemodynamic state of the patient. Interpretation of the EEG requires much experience, and studies have been directed to develop an automatic interpretation of the EEG. Early studies employed an electronic filtering of the EEG with the integrated amplitude of the EEG waveform used to indicate the level of brain activity (Fig. 32.4).

The introduction of affordable microcomputers in the 1980s resulted in an increase in research using algorithms rather than electronic components to digitally filter the EEG waveform into spectral components. The most common algorithm is the fast Fourier transform (FFT). By squaring the results of the FFT, the power spectrum of the EEG may be obtained. This may be plotted as power against frequency to give the frequency distribution in the EEG recording. The individual distributions may be considered to be "time slices" and joined together into a 3D plot generally called the compressed spectral array (CSA). Several commercial versions of the CSA have been incorporated into monitors designed to determine the level of brain function during procedures such as carotid clamping, when the intention is to detect ischemia and prevent damage. A number of limitations have to be placed on the nature of the signal. The FFT algorithm assumes that the data sample, interval, or epoch of the EEG data is stationary, i.e. there is no change in the characteristics of the waveform during the epoch. This requires a reliable indicator during changing levels of anesthesia. Epochs should therefore be as brief as possible, but see below. However, artifacts within the EEG may affect the FFT analysis and appear as erroneous and potentially misleading peaks in the power spectrum. This is especially true within short epochs. Ideally, the raw EEG should be inspected for artifacts before spectral analysis but this cannot be achieved by a real-time system. Appropriate filtering must also be performed on any waveform to be analyzed using FFT-based techniques. Unless low-pass filtering is applied to the data at half the original sampling frequency of the waveform (Nyquist frequency), false aliasing and harmonics may appear in the data. For example, if the highest frequency of interest is 40 Hz, the sampling frequency must be at least 80 Hz and a low 40-Hz

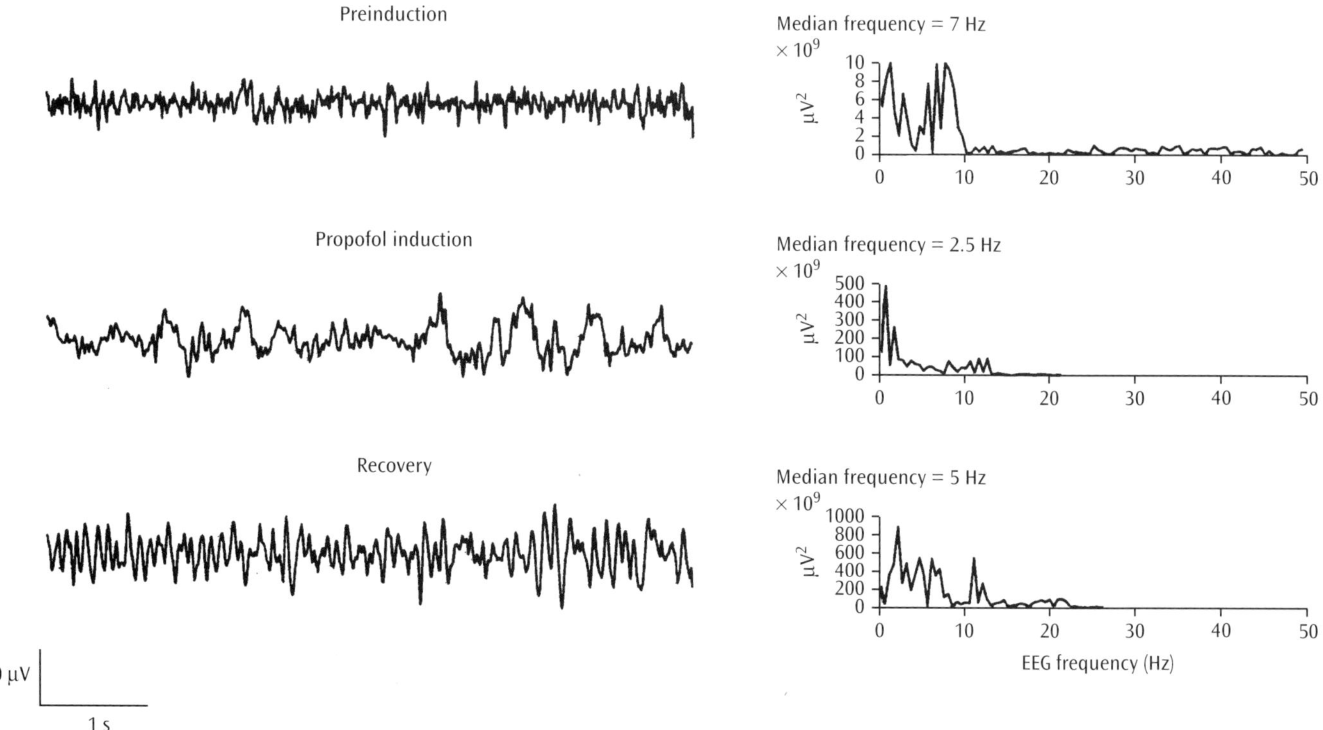

Figure 32.3 *Changes in the amplitude and frequency of the raw EEG and the spectral derivatives of the EEG during anesthesia. An increase in low-frequency activity followed induction with propofol (2.5 mg kg⁻¹). This was reflected in a reduction in the median frequency from 7 to 2.5 Hz. The median frequency had increased from 2.5 Hz to 5 Hz 5 min following recovery as some high-frequency activity returned.*

pass filter must be applied to the data. Substantially higher sampling frequencies allow detection and rejection of artifacts, such as electrical spikes, in the data. Other artifacts, such as EEG complexes appearing on the EEG, may also adversely affect an automated EEG spectral frequency analysis and must be excluded from the analysis.

Characteristic changes in the CSA have been documented during anesthesia.[29] The characteristics of the CSA vary depending on the type of anesthesia used, but the general trend is for deeper anesthesia to result in low-frequency activity, shifting the peaks of the CSA from higher frequencies. At recovery, there is a progressive increase in the amount of high-frequency activity, with a corresponding decrease in low-frequency activity. However, the spectral components of the EEG do not return quickly to exactly the same characteristics seen before exposure to the anesthetic. Nitrous oxide provides a good example of this phenomenon, changing characteristics of the EEG at recovery and giving a different EEG response on subsequent exposure within 30 min of the initial exposure. This has led authors to suggest that patients may develop a measurable tolerance to N_2O.[30] It has, in addition, been suggested that atropine may affect the EEG frequency distribution.[31] This effect appears to be independent of the EEG frequency changes observed with changes in anesthetic depth.[32]

Although the CSA is considerably more compact than the raw EEG, it is still a complex display that takes time to interpret, and changes within it are difficult to quantify. Several single-figure numeric indices have been derived from power spectral analysis of the EEG. These include mathematical expressions of the spectral distribution (mean,[33] median,[33] and spectral edge[34] frequencies) and analyses of coincident spectral frequencies e.g. the bispectral index.[35] Initial studies using the spectral edge frequency[34] described the use of a pattern-matching technique to detect the highest frequency at which significant levels of power were present in the EEG. Most researchers have now simplified the methods and describe the spectral edge frequency as that below which 95% of the EEG power is contained. The mean frequency describes the arithmetic mean of the power distribution. However, the mean frequency tends not to accurately represent high-frequency (β) outliers in the power distribution. The median frequency, above and below which 50% of the power spectrum is distributed, is generally accepted as a good indicator of changing distributions of EEG power during anesthesia. The median frequency has been studied using different anesthetic drugs. In the case of intravenous propofol anesthesia, a frequency of 5 Hz has been suggested as an empirical guideline for adequate surgical anesthesia. Higher frequencies suggest that anesthesia is too light.[33]

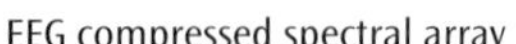

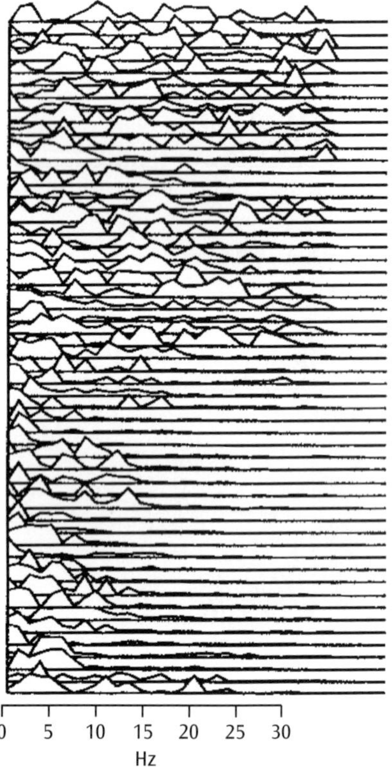

Figure 32.4 *The EEG compressed spectral array during cesarean section following induction of anesthesia with thiopental. The reduction in the high-frequency components can be seen.*

The bispectral index

Bispectral analysis is a more recent method of EEG analysis based on the interfrequency phase relations of the EEG.[36] The bispectral index (BIS) is the weighted average of three subparameters that analyze the phase and frequency relations among the component frequencies in the EEG (Fig. 32.5).

This has proved more reliable than other types of analysis, such as the compressed spectral array, but may still suffer from some degree of interagent variability.[37,38] In addition, patients who have been rendered unconscious following administration of nitrous oxide[39] or fentanyl[40] may exhibit no change in the BIS value during the transition from awake to unconscious. Furthermore, *increasing* doses of isoflurane have been shown to cause the expected decrease in the BIS in some patients, no effect in others, and an *increase* in the BIS in yet others.[41]

As is the case for all proposed monitors for depth of anesthesia, BIS does not warn of impending awareness but does indicate that awareness has occurred and may therefore reduce the stress suffered by those who are aware, by alerting the anesthesiologist, who can then quickly deepen anesthesia.

Evoked potentials

Analysis of the EEG incorporates the responses of many thousands of neurons in the cerebral cortex. Evoked potentials (EP) display the responses of more localized areas of the brainstem, midbrain, and cerebral cortex to specific stimuli. Most research has explored the use of evoked potentials in the elucidation of the integrity of functional pathways, but it is also possible to examine changes in the activity of these pathways related to the effects of anesthesia. EP studies rely on time-locking the stimulus relative to small changes in the raw EEG in response to the stimulus. The time-locked signals are then averaged in order to minimize the effects of other EEG components such as random noise, which are canceled out as these are not time-locked to the stimulus. The duration of the sampling epoch is a major drawback of any EP-based technique for use as a depth of anesthesia monitor. Stimulus presentation rates of up to 10 Hz and averaging over 1024 samples require a sampling epoch of at least 102 s. The adoption of advanced signal processing techniques will undoubtedly produce displays of evoked potential that can be used to assess the depth of anesthesia. One

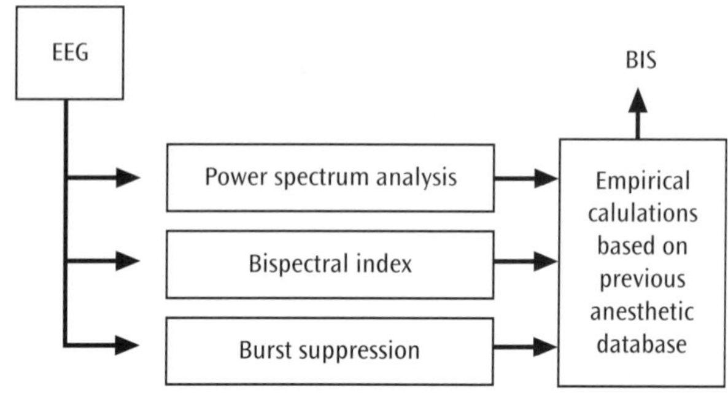

Figure 32.5 *Simplified derivation of bispectral index.*

such approach monitors the coherent frequency of the EEG to a high-frequency auditory stimulus (10–46 Hz; Fig. 32.6).[42]

Standard silver chloride EEG scalp electrodes are used to obtain the EP. The position of these electrodes depends on the type of EP to be recorded. The EP signals are small and therefore are easily swamped by electrical interference in the operating room such as the surgical diathermy. The need for filtering, isolation, low-noise, and high-gain EEG amplifiers has made the technology expensive. More recent EEG amplifiers employ digitization of the EEG signal in a computer-controlled amplifier close to the patient's head, and this technology may make EP recordings more accessible in the electronically hostile environment of the operating room.

Auditory-evoked potentials

Much research has been directed to determine the changes in the characteristics of auditory-evoked potentials (AEP) during anesthesia. Newton and others have demonstrated the changes in specific components of the AEP during anesthesia and recovery from anesthesia.[43] Halothane, isoflurane, and enflurane tend to increase the latencies of the brainstem AEP waves III and V as anesthesia is deepened. Furthermore, increases in the depth of anesthesia also increase the latency and decrease the amplitude of the early cortical AEP components P_a and N_b (Fig. 32.7).

The changes were similar for the volatile agents and were present across a range of inspired concentrations appropriate for general anesthesia. However, intravenous barbiturates also increased the latency of brainstem components III and V. Other intravenous anesthetics (i.e. etomidate, althesin, and propofol) did not affect the brainstem response, but did change cortical P_a and N_b latency and amplitudes in a manner comparable to that observed for the volatile anesthetic agents. The brainstem response did not change with some intravenous agents and, therefore, it has been dismissed as a putative method for determining the depth of anesthesia. The early cortical AEP remains a useful method for determining the depth of anesthesia, especially because surgical stimulation has been shown to affect the amplitude of the early cortical wave N_b during light halothane anesthesia (0.3% end-tidal, in 67% N_2O).[43]

A single derivative of the auditory-evoked response (AER), the AEP_{ex}, has been shown to correlate well with the clinical condition of the patient during studies in which patients were repeatedly taken from being unconscious to conscious[44–46] and to display less variability and overlap between awake and unconscious states than the BIS.[46,47] Similarly, during cold cardiopulmonary bypass, the AEP_{ex} provided consistent values of around 30–40 while the BIS ranged between values of 10 and 90.[48] The BIS has been considered to be a monitor of the level of hypnosis and does not predict response to noxious stimulation. In contrast, the AEP_{ex} has been shown to be able to predict movement during insertion of the laryngeal mask in patients receiving propofol[49] and movement after incision in patients receiving sevoflurane.[50]

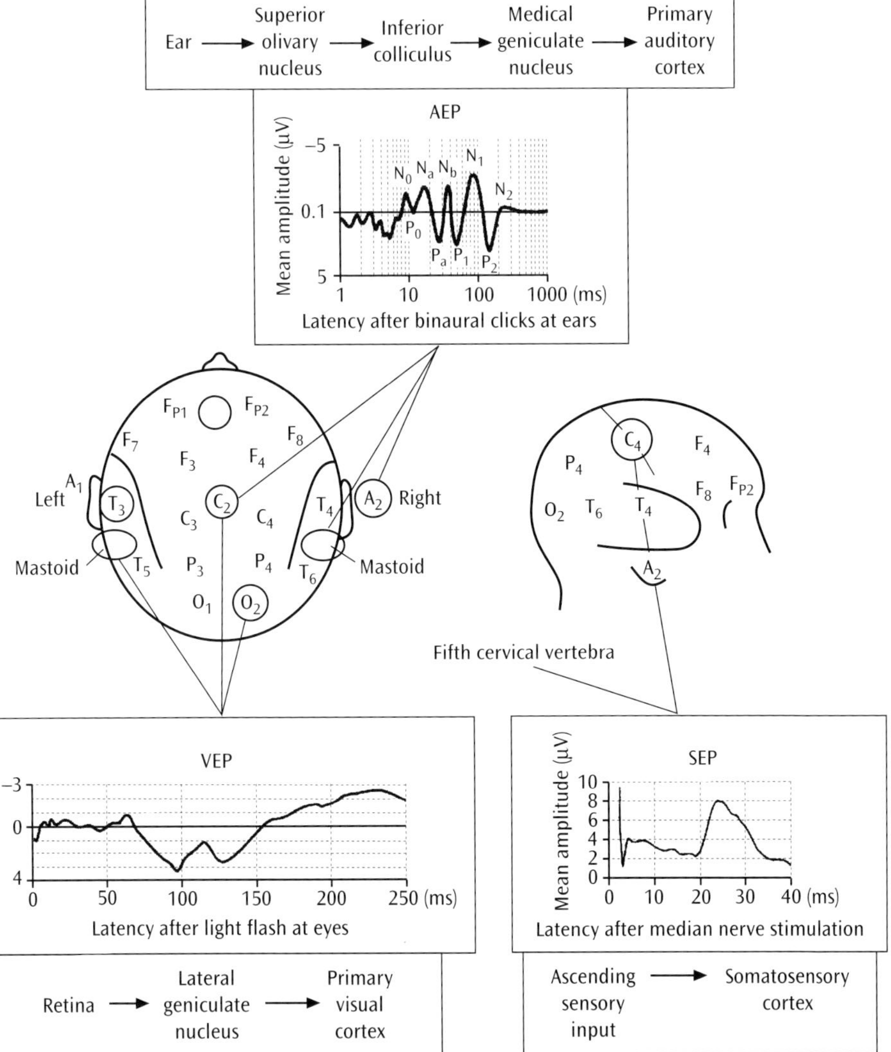

Figure 32.6 *The sensory pathway leading to the evoked responses are shown. Anesthesia results in a progressive increase in latency and a reduction in amplitude of the components of each response.*

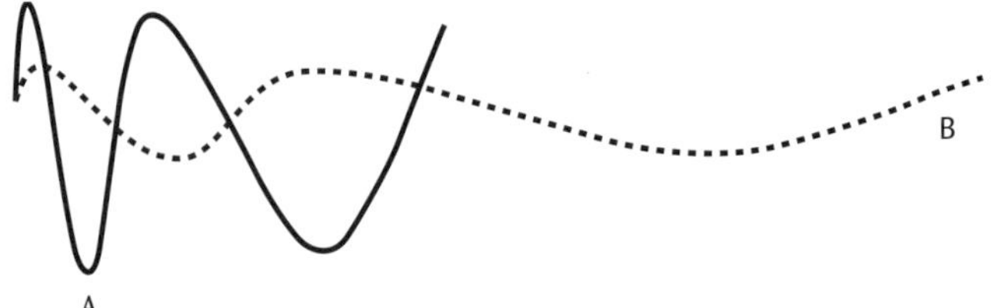

Figure 32.7 *Typical auditory-evoked potential waveform recorded from a conscious (A) and an anesthetized patient (B) (latencies of the wave peak are increased and amplitudes are decreased).*

Closed-loop control of anesthesia

The ultimate proof for a measurement of anesthetic depth is that the signal should be able to control automatically the delivery of an anesthetic agent to produce satisfactory anesthesia in a patient breathing spontaneously during surgery. Any closed-loop control system must be reliable, robust, and rapid in response. It must be able to respond with sufficient speed to a change in the input signal.

A closed-loop anesthesia (CLAN) system using systolic arterial pressure as the input signal has been described.[51] This system altered administration of a volatile agent during surgery and advised on the need for supplementary morphine. However, the system was used only when satisfactory anesthesia had already been established and in patients who were paralyzed during surgery. Three patients could not be controlled satisfactorily. The median frequency of the compressed spectral array has also been used to control the administration of intravenous anesthetics but not in patients breathing spontaneously during surgery.[33]

A closed-loop control system based on the AEP has been used to control the delivery of propofol in 100 patients breathing spontaneously during surgery.[45] The derivative, the AEP_{ex}, was extracted from the signal every 3 s and the quality of anesthesia was controlled within acceptable limits as assessed by a satisfactory "PRST" score (a common measure derived from pulse rate, systolic blood pressure, and lacrimation[52]) and the occurrence of minimal movement during surgery. A closed-loop control system for altering the degree of propofol sedation and for general anesthesia has been developed using the BIS as the input signal.[53–55] The AEP system has been used to demonstrate the pharmacodynamic requirements for propofol[56] and to provide an unbiased assessment of the propofol-sparing effects of remifentanil.[57]

Hypnosis and analgesia

The study of the propofol-sparing effects of remifentanil demonstrated the interdependence of hypnosis, analgesia, and stimulation and illustrated that there is no single concentration of an anesthesia agent that results in satisfactory anesthesia for all patients. Indeed, within individual patients, the requirements for anesthetic vary considerably depending on the degree of surgical stimulation and the quality of analgesia provided at any point in time. The AEP_{ex} appears able to provide information that incorporates the level of hypnosis, the quality of analgesia, and the stimulation from surgery (Fig. 32.1).

Relatively high concentrations of a hypnotic agent are required when a low-dose analgesic technique is used. When a high concentration of analgesic is administered, smaller doses of hypnotic are then required to maintain satisfactory anesthesia. This is shown most clearly when patients have good premedication and a fully functioning local block in place. In this situation, the requirements for anesthetic can be reduced to very low values.

However, there are still a number of problems which need to be addressed before the AEP can be used routinely. One of these is the significant change in evoked potentials observed during mild hypoglycemia,[58] and its use in those patients with a nerve deafness.

Visual-evoked potentials

Visual-evoked potentials (VEP) have been studied during anesthesia with isoflurane, enflurane, and thiopental.[59] The VEP is commonly generated by the presentation of bright flashes through the closed eyelid using light-emitting diodes mounted within goggles. Since the eyelids are commonly taped shut during anesthesia, the VEP is an attractive putative method for measuring the depth of anesthesia. Three components of the VEP waveform have been studied: P60, N70, and P100. The origin of P100 has been described as the primary visual cortex, but the origin of the earlier waves has not been characterized. Since the earlier components have a shorter latency than the P100, it is logical to assume that they originate from earlier stages in the visual pathway such as the lateral geniculate nucleus. Single-neuron recordings in the visual cortex of cats have shown that a range of velocity and spatial frequency coding properties, including the identification of textured visual stimuli, still occur in the primary visual cortex during light halothane anesthesia.[60] The primary visual cortex is, therefore, well able to process simple flash stimuli during anesthesia. However, the P60 and N70 components of the human VEP are not reliably reproduced in all subjects under anesthesia, and the P100 component does not change in latency or amplitude through the range of volatile anesthetic concentrations used for deep surgical anesthesia. In spite of this, the VEP shows real promise as a technique for use in assessing the level of sedation in patients in the intensive care unit,[61] and could be used to warn of excessively light anesthesia.

Somatosensory-evoked potentials (SEP)

Relatively few studies have considered the SEP as a putative method of determining anesthetic depth. The SEP takes some 80 s to calculate and requires time-locked averaging of responses to stimuli presented to sites such as the median nerve. Typical recording sites are the fifth cervical vertebra and the scalp above the contralateral somatosensory cortex. One carefully designed study described a small increase in latency (21.1 ms ± 1.8 SD to 21.9 ms ± 1.8 SD) and a reduction in amplitude (4.6 μV ± 2.5 SD to 2.9 μV ± 1.5 SD) following induction of anesthesia with thiopental.[62] However, this trend was not observed in all patients from the group ($n=22$). In two patients there was an increase in SEP latency, and in one patient there was no change in latency with anesthesia. No correlation could be determined between changes in SEP and either heart rate or blood pressure, although these autonomic indices are by no means "gold standards" for determining anesthetic depth. Unfortunately, SEPs were not recorded during recovery of the patient because of contamination of the recordings by muscle artifacts. The results do not discount SEPs as a putative index of anesthetic depth, but, as with all evoked potentials, considerable progress needs to be made in the subject before a commercial depth of anesthesia monitor employing the techniques could be made available for use in everyday clinical anesthetic practice.

Heart rate variability

Changes in autonomic tone are the basis of most subjective estimates of anesthetic depth, e.g. changes in heart rate and blood pressure. Ideally, one needs a measurement of autonomic tone that is not affected by factors other than anesthetic depth and is easy to measure.

Recent research using animal models has cast doubt on the value of the measurements of cerebral cortical activity, such as the EEG, when estimating the efficacy of anesthesia. In particular, in rats, MAC has been shown to depend on neural circuitry within the brainstem and not higher cortical influences.[63]

Analysis of specific components of the rat electromyogram has revealed that MAC equivalent responses to noxious stimuli can be explained by the effect of anesthetic agents either directly or indirectly on motor neurons, and not on higher regions of the central nervous system.[64] If anesthesia does originate in the brainstem, and then subsequently affects higher cortical centers, it seems logical to propose that the first signs of wakening due to light anesthesia or inadvertent recovery will be determined by opening a window not just on the cerebral cortex but also on the brainstem. Such a window should include areas of the brainstem responsible for mediating both afferent and efferent information, rather than primarily afferent sensory pathways via regions such as the auditory nuclei.

A possible explanation for the anesthetic effects on the brainstem is provided by activation of inhibitory glycine synapses, which play a major role, in contrast with γ-aminobutyric acid (GABA), the main inhibitory neurotransmitter in the brain.[65] Anesthetic drugs appear to act on the brainstem by enhancing inhibitory glycine-mediated activity. Anesthesia that originates in the brainstem probably inhibits the cerebral cortex via ascending, efferent projections from the midbrain.[66]

Objective measurement of brainstem-mediated autonomic tone has been an area of particular interest for those screening for autonomic neuropathy, especially in the study of diabetes. The heart rate is not constant from beat to beat in subjects with a healthy autonomic nervous system; there is a balance between sympathetic excitation and parasympathetic inhibition of the sinoatrial and atrioventricular nodes in the heart, leading to heart rate variability (HRV). Subjects exhibiting autonomic neuropathy show a reduction, and eventual loss, of HRV. Spectral analysis of HRV has revealed three components: a low-frequency fluctuation, which is generally believed to be circadian; a medium-frequency variation, which is attributed to the baroreceptor reflex; and a high-frequency component, which coincides with breathing. The high-frequency variation is respiratory sinus arrhythmia (RSA), and is typically characterized as a greater that 10% variation in the electrocardiogram (ECG) P-wave interval over 5 min. RSA is easily visible on an ECG monitor that is time-locked to an ECG R-wave peak, but it is difficult to distinguish using modern monitors with a rolling display. During RSA, heart rate increases during inspiration and decreases during expiration are under the control of a predominantly parasympathetic reflex in the supine subject.

Since 1985, there have been a number of reports that the level of RSA changes during anesthesia. One study, using offline analysis of 10-min epochs of ECG, suggested that the RSA diminished during isoflurane anesthesia and then increased again at recovery.[67] The authors suggested that a real-time system could form the basis of a monitor for measuring the level of anesthesia. A later study also suggested that the technique could be used for anesthetic agents other than isoflurane.[68] A dose–response relation between RSA and the level of isoflurane anesthesia measured at different MAC levels has been demonstrated (Fig. 32.8).[32]

Methods for measuring heart rate variability

Various techniques have been used to screen for autonomic neuropathy based on measurements of HRV. The simplest is by determining the mean heart rate and the standard deviation from the mean. The standard deviation provides an estimate of the HRV. Unfortunately, the mean heart rate and ectopic contractions have a direct effect on the standard deviation so that it cannot be used in isolation as a measurement of HRV. Spectral analysis of HRV has been used. However, epochs of at least 5 min are required in order to resolve the low-frequency components. FFT-based spectral analysis requires that data are stationary during an epoch, and it is difficult to guarantee that the ECG will not change during the course of an epoch during surgery, when surgical stimulation with hemodynamic changes may impose a change in heart rate (Fig. 32.9).

A circular statistical technique has been used to quantify the level of uncontaminated RSA using ECG R-wave times correlated against respiratory cycles. This has the advantage that, when compared with other techniques which use the standard deviation or power spectrum of ECG R–R intervals, ectopic beats and other irregularities not related to breathing are separated from those variations caused by breathing.

The results obtained using this technique have been reported following studies performed during anesthesia with total intravenous propofol[69] (Fig. 32.10) and isoflurane maintenance,[32] as well as during propofol sedation in the intensive care unit,[70] for cesarean section,[71] and as a result of other surgical stimulation during light enflurane anesthe-

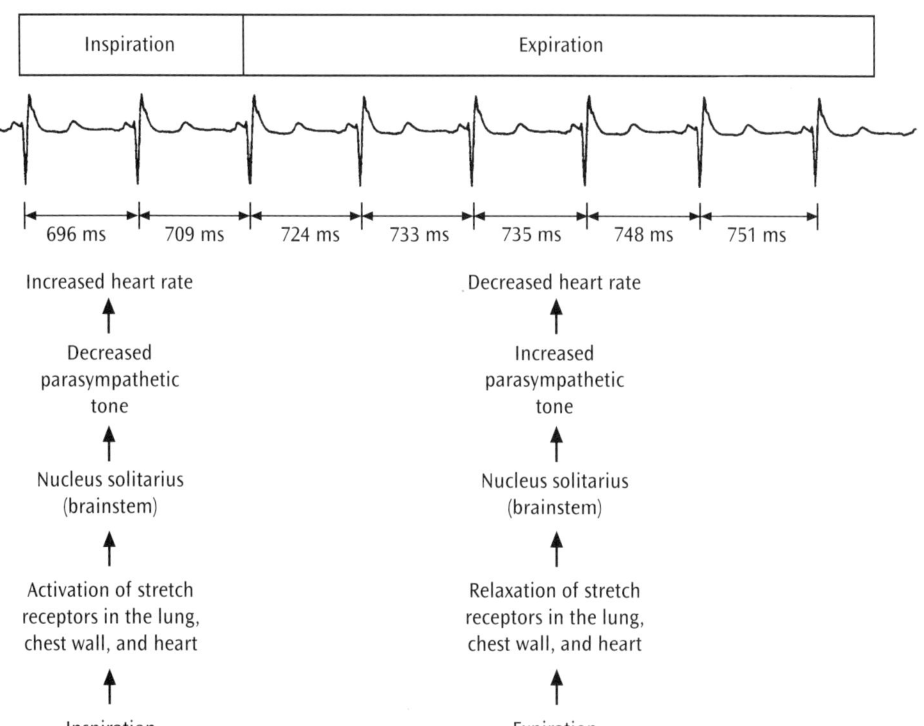

Figure 32.8 *There is a cyclic variation in heart rate coincident with respiration, known as respiratory sinus arrhythmia.*

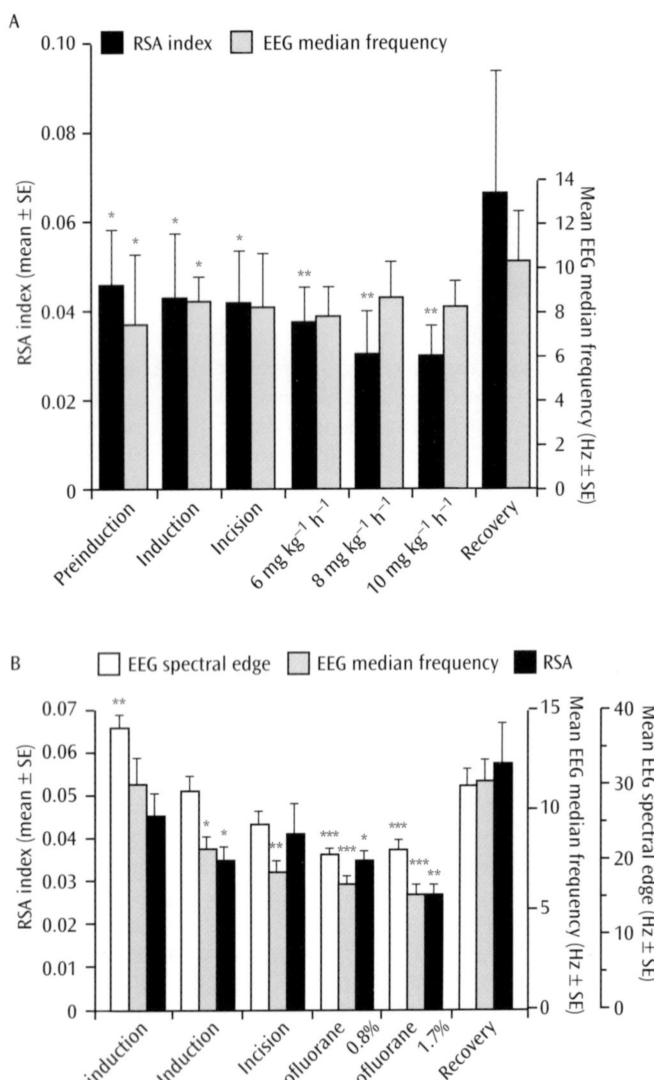

Figure 32.9 *Respiratory sinus arrhythmia (RSA) results. Reduction in RSA and derived indices of the electroencephalogram (EEG) during anesthesia. The differences between the values obtained during anesthesia and at recovery were significant (*P < 0.05, **P < 0.01, ***P < 0.001). (A) RSA and the median frequency of the EEG were reduced in 10 patients during total intravenous anesthesia with propofol. (B) RSA, median, and spectral edge frequencies were reduced as the concentrations of isoflurane were increased. (Redrawn from data in references 32 and 68.)*

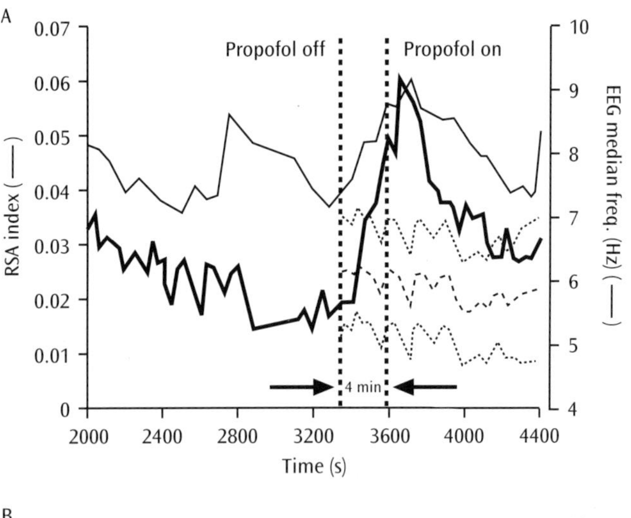

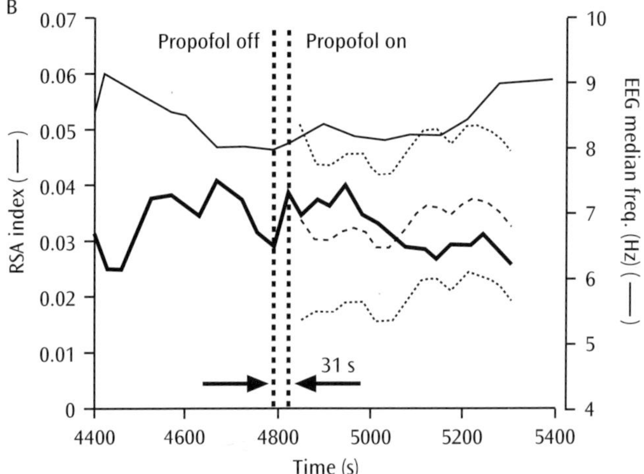

Figure 32.10 *Time-course of changing respiratory sinus arrhythmia (RSA index, ——) and median EEG frequency (——) during an interruption of the infusion of propofol.[69] - - - - -, Predicted. (A) Effect of a 4-min interruption in the propofol infusion. The increase in RSA index exceeds the 99% confidence limits (·····) predicted from the RSA index based on the previous 15 min data. (B) Nonsignificant change in RSA index following a 31-s interruption in the propofol infusion.*

sia.[72] It appears likely that the level of RSA reflects the level of anesthetic depth. Deeper anesthesia elicits a greater increase in RSA than that seen during light anesthesia alone. RSA is a convenient window on the brainstem, which needs only standard ECG and respiratory signals.

THE FUTURE

It may be that no single method will be found to measure the depth of anesthesia reliably for all patients and all anesthetic agents. The different molecular structure of anesthetic drugs suggests the possibility that they will elicit responses in different populations of neuronal membrane receptors and must therefore act in subtly different ways on different regions of the brain.[44] In addition, all the methods proposed for determining the depth of anesthesia have some potential exclusion criteria. For example, evoked potentials depend on an intact neural pathway from which to obtain the response to stimulation. Any break in the pathway, such as visual impairment with VEPs or loss of hearing in AEPs, will change the response characteristics before an anesthetic is given. Similarly, techniques based on monitoring the autonomic nervous system, such as monitoring HRV, will be impaired in the event of autonomic neuropathy. The only reliable way of determining the depth of anesthesia will require a real-time noninvasive measure of cerebral activity and a localization of the activity to specific cortical regions and areas of the brainstem.

Positron emission tomography (PET) has been used in a limited number of studies to monitor brain function during anesthesia. However, the technique is invasive to the extent that isotopes of glucose with a short half-life are used and these have to be prepared with the cyclotron close to the recording site, and cannot, therefore, form the basis of a cheap operating room monitor for use by the anesthesiologist. However, PET scanning has revealed that propofol anesthesia has a widespread suppressive effect on cerebral metabolism, and it is probable that future research will allow the localization of specific regions in the brain that are affected by anesthesia.[73] Ultimately, this approach may lead to the adoption of a standard, absolute scale of anesthetic depth, against which future clinicians may calibrate their putative tests of anesthetic depth.

Ultra-sensitive superconducting quantum interference devices (SQUIDS) have been used to provide a new insight into cerebral function by noninvasively measuring not only structures, as resolved with more conventional magnetic resonance imaging, but also functional activity in the brain. Although prohibitively expensive, new technology may lead to the provision of relatively cheap, direct imaging brain function monitors based on SQUID technology. This will provide the anesthesiologist with the ultimate monitor, being capable of determining not just anesthetic depth, but also awareness, anoxia, ischemia, and unusual pathology. Although the routine use of such devices seems unlikely in the very near future, one has only to appreciate the rapid adoption of microcomputer technology over the past 10 years to realize that new monitoring technologies may be available in the relatively near future.

REFERENCES

1. Sandin RH, Enlund G, Samuelsson P, Lennmarken C. Awareness during anesthesia: a prospective case study. *Lancet* 2000; **355:** 707–11.
2. Gajraj RJ, Doi M, Mantzaridis H, Kenny GN. Comparison of bispectral EEG analysis and auditory evoked potentials for monitoring depth of anaesthesia during propofol anaesthesia. *Br J Anaesth* 1999; **82** (5): 672–8.
3. Russell IF.Midazolam–Alfentanil: an anaesthetic? An investigation using the isolated forearm technique. *Br J Anaesth* 1993; **70:** 42–6.
4. Dixon NF. Unconscious perception and general anaesthesia. *Baillière's Clin Anaesthesiol* 1989; **3** (3): 473–85.
5. Aitkenhead AR. Awareness during anaesthesia: what should the patient be told? *Anaesthesia* 1990; **45:** 351–2.
6. Liu WHD, Thorp TAS, Graham SG, Aitkenhead AR. Incidence of awareness with recall during general anaesthesia. *Anaesthesia* 1991; **46:** 435–7.
7. Schultetus RR, Hill CR, Dharamraj CM, Banner TE, Berman LS. Wakefulness during caesarean section after anesthetic induction with ketamine, thiopental, or ketamine and thiopental combined. *Anesth Analg* 1986; **65:** 723–8.
8. Bogetz MS, Katz JA. Recall of surgery for major trauma. *Anesthesiology* 1984; **61:** 6–9.
9. Abouleish E, Taylor FH. Effect of morphine–diazepam on signs of anaesthesia, dreams of patients under N_2O for caesarean section. *Anesth Analg* 1976; **55:** 702–5.
10. Miller CD, Asbury AJ, Brown JH. Pupillary effects of alfentanil and morphine. *Br J Anaesth* 1990; **65:** 415–17.
11. Saucier N, Walts LF, Moreland JR. Patient awareness during nitrous oxide, oxygen and halothane anaesthesia. *Anesth Analg* 1983; **362:** 239–40.
12. Aitkenhead A. Awareness: incidence and medico-legal implications. In: *Awareness in Anaesthesia and Awareness of Current Issues*, Report of a Symposium held at Queens College, Cambridge, UK, 28–29 June 1993. Oxford: Oxford Clinical Communications, 1993.
13. Bennett HL, Davis HS, Giannini JA. Non-verbal response to intraoperative conversation. *Br J Anaesth* 1985; **57:** 174–9.
14. Millar K, Watkinson N. Recognition of words presented during general anaesthesia. *Ergonomics* 1983; **26:** 585–94.
15. Bonke B, Schmitz PIM, Verhage F, Zwaveling A. A clinical study of so-called unconscious perception during general anaesthesia. *Br J Anaesth* 1986; **58:** 957–64.
16. McLintock TT, Aitken H, Downie CF, Genny GNC. Postoperative analgesic requirements in patients exposed to positive intraoperative suggestions. *Br Med J* 1990; **301:** 788–90.
17. Moerman N, Bonke B, Oosting J. Awareness and recall during general anaesthesia. Facts and feelings. *Anesthesiology* 1993; **79:** 454–64.
18. Domino KB, Posner KL, Caplan RA, Cheyney FW. Awareness during anesthesia: a closed claims analysis. *Anesthesiology* 1999; **90:** 1053–61.
19. Sandin R, Norstrom O. Awareness during total IV anaesthesia. *Br J Anaesth* 1993; **71:** 782–7.
20. Levinson B. The states of awareness in anaesthesia in 1965. In: Bonke B, Fitch W, Millar K (eds). *Memory and Awareness in Anaesthesia.* Amsterdam: Swetz and Zeitlinger, 1990: 11–18.
21. Guedel A. Third stage ether anesthesia: a sublassification regarding the significance of the position and movements of the eyeball. *Am J Surg* 1920; **34** (Quarterly Suppl. in Anesthesia): 53–7.
22. White DC. Anaesthesia: a privation of the senses. An historical introduction and some definitions. In: Rosen M, Lunn JN (eds). *Conscious Awareness and Pain in General Anaesthesia*. London: Butterworth, 1987: 1–9.
23. Flecknell PA. Anaesthesia of animals for biochemical research. *Br J Anaesth* 1993; **71:** 885–94.
24. Davies FW, Mantzaridis H, Fisher AC, Kenny GN. Middle latency auditory evoked potentials during repeated transitions from consciousness to unconsciousness. *Anaesthesia* 1996; **51:** 107–13.
25. Tunstall ME. Detecting wakefulness during general anaesthesia for caesarean section. *Br Med J* 1977; **1:** 1321.
26. Russell IF. Auditory perception under anaesthesia. *Anaesthesia* 1979; **34:** 211.
27. Rampil IJ, Mason P, Singh H. Anesthetic potency (MAC) is independent of forebrain structures in the rat. *Anesthesiology* 1993; **78:** 707–12.
28. Kandel ER, Schwartz JH, Jessell TM. *Principles of Neural Science*, 3rd edn. New York: Elsevier, 1991.
29. Pichmayer I. *EEG Atlas for Anaesthesiologists*. Berlin: Springer-Verlag, 1987.
30. Avramov MN, Shingu K, Mori K. Progressive changes in electrencephalographic responses to nitrous oxide in humans: a possible drug tolerance. *Anesth Analg* 1990; **70:** 369–374.
31. Pickworth WB, Herning RI, Koeppl B, Henningfield JE. Dose-dependent atropine-induced changes in spontaneous electroencephalogram in human volunteers. *Milit Med* 1990; **155:** 166–170.
32. Pomfrett CJD, Sneyd JR, Barrie JR, Healy TEJ. Respiratory sinus arrhythmia: comparison with EEG indices during isoflurane anaesthesia at 0.65 and 1.2 MAC. *Br J Anaesth* 1994; **72:** 397–402.
33. Schwilden H. Use of median frequency and pharmacokinetics in determining depth of anaesthesia. *Balliere's Clin Anaesthesiol* 1989; **3** (3): 601–21.
34. Rampil IJ, Sasse FJ, Smith NT, *et al.* Spectral edge frequency – a new correlate of anesthetic depth. *Anesthesiology* 1980; **53:** S12.
35. Vernon J, Bowles S, Sebel PS, Chamoun N. EEG bispectrum predicts movement at incision during isoflurane anesthesia. *Anesthesiology* 1992; **77:** A502.
36. Rampil IJ. A primer for EEG signal processing in anesthesia. *Anesthesiology* 1998; **89:** 980–1002.
37. Vernon JM, Lang E, Sebel PS, Manberg P. Prediction of movement using bispectral electroencephalographic analysis during propofol/alfentanil or isoflurane/alfentanil anesthesia. *Anesth Analg* 1995; **80:** 780–5.
38. Gajraj RJ, Doi M, Kenny GNC. A comparison of auditory evoked potentials and bispectral EEG analysis in spontaneously breathing anesthetized patients. *Anesthesiology* 1996; **85:** A462.
39. Barr G, Jakobsson JG, Owall A, Anderson RE. Nitrous oxide does not alter bispectral index: study with nitrous oxide as sole agent and as an adjunct to i.v. anaesthesia. *Br J Anaesth* 1999; **82:** 827–30.
40. Barr G, Anderson RE, Owall A, Jakobsson JG. Effects on the bispectral index during medium–high dose fentanyl induction with or without propofol supplement. *Acta Anaesthesiol Scand* 2000; **47** (7): 807–11.
41. Detsch O, Schneider G, Kochs E, *et al.* Increasing isoflurane concentration may cause paradoxical increases in the EEG bispectral index in surgical patients. *Br J Anaesth* 2000; **84:** 33–7.
42. Munglani R, Andrade J, Sapsford DJ, *et al.* A measure of consciousness and memory during isoflurane administration: the coherent frequency. *Br J Anaesth* 1993; **71:** 633–41.
43. Thornton C, Newton DEF. The auditory evoked response: a measure of depth of anaesthesia. *Balliere's Clin Anaesthesiol* 1989; **3** (3): 559–585.
44. Davies FW, Mantzaridis H, Kenny GNC, Fisher AC. Middle latency auditory evoked potentials during repeated transitions from consciousness to unconsciousness. *Anaesthesia* 1996; **51:** 107–13.
45. Kenny GN, Mantzaridis H. Closed-loop control of propofol anaesthesia. *Br J Anaesth* 1999; **83:** 223–8.
46. Gajraj RJ, Doi M, Mantzaridis H, Kenny GN. Analysis of the EEG bispectrum, auditory evoked potentials and the EEG power spectrum during repeated transitions from consciousness to unconsciousness. *Br J Anaesth* 1998; **80:** 46–52.
47. Doi M, Gajraj RJ, Mantzaridis H, Kenny GNC. Relationship between calculated blood concentration of propofol and electrophysiological variables during emergence from anaesthesia: a comparison of bispectral index, spectral edge frequency, median frequency and auditory evoked potential index. *Br J Anaesth* 1997; **78:** 180–4.
48. Doi M, Mantzaridis H, Kenny GN. Effects of cardiopulmonary bypass and hypothermia on electroencephalographic variables. *Anaesthesia* 1997; **52:** 1048–55.
49. Doi M, Gajraj RJ, Mantzaridis H, Kenny GN. Prediction of movement at laryngeal mask airway insertion: comparison of auditory evoked response index, bispectral index, spectral edge frequency and median frequency. *Br J Anaesth* 1999; **82:** 203–7.

50. Kurita T, Doi M, Katoh T, *et al.* Auditory evoked potential index predicts the depth of sedation and movement in response to skin incision during sevoflurane anesthesia. *Anesthesiology* 2001; **95:** 364–70.
51. Robb HM, Asbury AJ, Gray WM, Linkens DA. Towards a standardized anaesthetic state using isoflurane and morphine. *Br J Anaesth* 1993; **71:** 366–9.
52. Evans JM, Davies WL, Wise CC. Lower oesophageal contractility: a new monitor of anaesthesia. *Lancet* 1984; **1:** 1151–4.
53. Mortier E, Struys M, De ST, *et al.* Closed loop controlled administration of propofol using bispectral analysis. *Anaesthesia* 1998; 366–9.
54. Absalom A, Kenny GN. Closed loop control of anaesthesia using bispectral index. Performance assessment of patients undergoing major orthopedic surgery under combined general and regional anesthesia. *Anesthesiology* 2002; **96:** 67–73.
55. Leslie K, Absalom A, Kenny GN. Closed loop control of sedation for colonoscopy using the Bispectral Index. *Anaesthesia* 2002; **57:** 693–7.
56. Kenny GN, McFadzean WA, Mantzaridis H, Fisher AC. Propofol requirements during closed loop anesthesia. *Anesthesiology* 1993; **79:** A329.
57. Milne SE, Kenny GN. Increasing the remifentanil target blood concentration reduces closed-loop propofol administration. *Br J Anaesth* 1999; **82** (Suppl.): 119.
58. Jones TW, McCarthy G, Tamborlane WV, *et al.* Mild hypoglycemia and impairment of brainstem and cortical evoked potentials in healthy subjects. *Diabetes* 1990; **39:**1550–5.
59. Chi OZ, Field C. Effects of enflurane on visual evoked potentials in humans. *Br J Anaesth* 1990; **64:** 163–6.
60. Hammond P, Pomfrett CJD. Direction and orientational tuning of feline striate cortical neurones: correlation with neuronal class. *Vision Res* 1989; **29:** 653–62.
61. Wang DY. Indices of sedation in the intensive care unit. PhD thesis. University of Manchester, 1994.
62. Sebel PS. Somatosensory, visual and motor evoked potentials in anaesthetized patients. *Balliere's Clin Anaesthesiol* 1989; **3** (3): 587–602.
63. Rampil IJ, Mason P, Singh H. Anesthetic potency is independent of forebrain structures in the rat. *Anesthesiology* 1993; **78:** 707–12.
64. Rampil IJ. "F-waves" – a nonsynaptic, but sensitive indicator of anaesthetic effect in rats. *Anesth Analg* 1994; **78:** S350.
65. Franks NP, Lieb WR. Molecular and cellular mechanisms of general anaesthesia. *Nature* 1994; **367:** 607–14.
66. Donchin Y, Feld JM, Porges SW. Respiratory sinus arrhythmia during recovery from isoflurane–nitrous oxide anesthesia. *Anesth Analg* 1985; **64:** 811–15.
67. Porges SW. Vagal mediation of respiratory sinus arrhythmia. Implications for drug delivery. *Ann NY Acad Sci* 1991; **618:** 57–66.
68. Kato M, Komatsu T, Kimura T, *et al.* Spectral analysis of heart rate variability during isoflurane anesthesia. *Anesthesiology* 1992; **77:** 669–74.
69. Pomfrett CJD, Barrie JA, Healy TEJ. Respiratory sinus arrhythmia: an index of light anaesthesia. *Br J Anaesth* 1993; **71:** 212–17.
70. Wang DY, Pomfrett CJD, Healy TEJ. Respiratory sinus arrhythmia: a new objective score. *Br J Anaesth* 1993; **71:** 354–8.
71. Healy TEJ, Bellman MH, Pomfrett CJD. Respiratory sinus arrhythmia indicates light anesthesia during caesarean section. *Anesth Analg* 1994; **78:** S156.
72. Pomfrett CJD, Barrie JR, Healy TEJ. Respiratory sinus arrhythmia reflects surgical stimulation during light enflurane anesthesia. *Anesth Analg* 1994; **78:** S344.
73. Alkire MT, Barker SJ, Haier RJ, *et al.* A positron emission tomography study of cerebral metabolism in a volunteer during propofol anesthesia. *Anesth Analg* 1994; **78:** S5.

33

Volatile anesthetics

NIALL O'KEEFFE

INTRODUCTION

Inhalational anesthetics date back to the dawn of anesthesia. Humphry Davy first observed the analgesic effects of nitrous oxide as long ago as 1800, and called it "laughing gas." He was at that time the superintendent of the Pneumatic Institute in Bristol, where different gases were used in the treatment of pulmonary tuberculosis. However, it was not until 1844 that Horace Wells described the use of nitrous oxide to facilitate the extraction of a tooth. Unfortunately, the first public demonstration of his technique ended in failure. Despite this, he continued to use the gas, and eventually the qualities of nitrous oxide were recognized; it is still in use today.

In 1824, Henry Hill Hickman, who received his medical education in Edinburgh, then worked in general practice in Ludlow in Shropshire, demonstrated in animals that anesthesia could be induced and surgical procedures carried out using carbon dioxide. Thus, it was he who introduced the concept of anesthesia using an inhaled substance. The first recorded general anesthetic administered in humans was in 1842, when both C W Long and W Clarke successfully induced anesthesia using diethyl ether. Unfortunately, they did not publicize their work until a much later date. The first successful public demonstration of anesthesia was in 1846, when W T G Morton successfully induced anesthesia using ether on 16 October at Massachusetts General Hospital. Following this, the word spread rapidly around the world.

The first general anesthetic in the UK was administered in December 1846, and again ether was used. In November of the following year, chloroform was introduced by James Young Simpson, professor of midwifery at Edinburgh University, to control pain in labor.

The first deaths associated with ether occurred in 1847, less than a year after its introduction, and the first death associated with chloroform was in 1848 (11 weeks after its introduction). It therefore became apparent quite quickly that, although these agents provided vastly improved conditions for surgery for both patient and surgeon, their use was not without risk. Most deaths associated with chloroform were probably cardiac in origin, most likely due to arrhythmia leading to ventricular fibrillation. These deaths usually occurred during light anesthesia, often shortly after the commencement of the induction. In the case of chloroform, there was also the additional problem of hepatotoxicity, which could result in hepatic necrosis in the postoperative period. The principal advantage of chloroform over ether was that it was relatively nonirritant to inhale. Ether, however, was much safer to use than chloroform. The main problems associated with the use of ether were that it is extremely irritating to the airway, induction and recovery are slow because of its pharmacokinetic properties, and it is explosive when mixed with oxygen.

These two agents, along with nitrous oxide, remained the mainstays of anesthesia for the next 80 years, until the introduction of cyclopropane in 1930 by Lucas and Henderson in Toronto. A significant advantage of cyclopropane over the previously used agents was its ability to provide a rapid, smooth induction. However, as in the case of ether, it is explosive in oxygen, and it can also cause ventricular ectopic contractions and ventricular fibrillation. Cyclopropane is also associated with a syndrome of circulatory collapse and bradycardia, often referred to as cyclopropane shock. This occurred in the postoperative period following deep cyclopropane anesthesia. The mechanism of cyclopropane shock is uncertain.

Other agents used around this time included divinyl ether, trichlorethylene, and ethyl chloride. The general anesthetic properties of ethyl chloride were discovered during its use as a local anesthetic spray for dental extractions. Trichlorethylene was initially used as a fat solvent in industry, and Lehmann first described its general anesthetic effects in 1911. Trichlorethylene was used both to produce general anesthesia, usually in combination with nitrous oxide, and also on its own as an inhalational analgesic. It was used for many years, with specially designed inhalers, for controlling labor pain.

In 1932, Booth and Bixby observed that the greatest potential for new noncombustible anesthetic agents lay with organic fluoride compounds, because the substitution of fluoride for other halogens reduces the boiling point, increases the stability, and generally reduces the toxicity of gases.[1] A large number of fluorinated compounds were produced over the next 20 years, culminating in 1950 with the development of fluroxene, and then in 1952 with the synthesis of halothane, the first of the truly modern anesthetics. Although halothane lacked many of the qualities of an ideal anesthetic, it represented a significant advantage over previously available agents. Research into fluorinated compounds continued and has led to the production of all the modern anesthetic agents. Fluroxene, the first fluorine-containing anesthetic agent, introduced in 1950, and methoxyflurane, introduced in 1960, have since been superseded by the newer agents. Fluroxene is explosive in concentrations greater than 3%, and methoxyflurane is associated with high-output renal failure, caused by fluoride toxicity resulting from metabolism.

The introduction of halothane, and subsequently enflurane and isoflurane, and the research that followed has identified which properties are desirable in a volatile anesthetic agent (Table 33.1).

No agent currently available meets all the criteria, although several of the modern agents do combine many of them.

Table 33.1 *Properties of an ideal inhalational anesthetic agent*

It should be cheap and easy to produce
It should be chemically stable and not decompose on exposure to light or interact with anesthetic circuits or soda-lime. It should have a long shelf-life without the addition of preservatives
It should be nonflammable and nonexplosive
It should have a low blood–gas solubility, thereby allowing rapid induction, rapid recovery, and rapid alteration of depth of anesthesia
It should have a pleasant odor and not irritate the airway to facilitate inhalational induction
It should be sufficiently potent to allow administration in conjunction with high concentrations of oxygen if necessary
It should produce unconsciousness with some degree of analgesia and muscle relaxation
It should cause no cardiovascular or respiratory depression and no central nervous system excitation
It should have no organ toxicity and should not undergo any metabolism, being excreted completely unchanged by the lungs
It should not cause histamine release or cause allergic reactions
It should not trigger malignant hyperpyrexia
It should not interact with other drugs

HALOTHANE

Halothane was synthesized in the laboratories of Imperial Chemical Industries in 1951 by C W Suckling and was first introduced into clinical practice by Michael Johnstone in Manchester in 1956.[2]

Physical properties

Halothane (2-bromo-2-chloro-1,1,1-trifluoroethane) is a clear colorless liquid with an acceptable, nonirritating odor. Its physical properties are summarized in Table 33.2 and its structure shown in Fig 33.1. It has a low boiling point, 50 °C, and a saturated vapor pressure of 32.4 kPa (243 mmHg) at 20 °C, which makes it amenable to administration through a standard temperature- and flow-controlled vaporizer. It has a blood–gas solubility coefficient of 2.3.

Halothane is relatively stable, although it decomposes on exposure to light, with the formation of volatile acids. For this reason, it is stored in amber bottles, and 0.01% (w/w) thymol is added to retard decomposition. It is noninflammable and nonexplosive in all concentrations of oxygen, and it does not interact with soda-lime.[3] It is soluble in rubber and the plastics commonly found in anesthetic circuits.[4] This has obvious implications for patients with halothane sensitivity or who are at risk from malignant hyperthermia, in whom an "anesthetic-free" circuit should be used.

In 1963, the term minimum alveolar concentration (MAC) was introduced as an index of comparison in order to allow the potency of the different inhalational anesthetics to be compared.[5] The MAC was further defined in 1964 as the minimum alveolar concentration of inhaled anesthetic, at steady state, required to prevent movement in 50% of patients exposed to a painful stimulus.[6] The MAC is useful both as a guide for the administration of inhalational anesthetics and as an index for comparing the potency of different inhalational anesthetic agents. Alveolar concentration is used as an approximation of brain anesthetic tension. Various factors have been found to affect the MAC. If ambient pressure is doubled, then the MAC is halved, the blood concentration remaining more or less the same. The MAC of halothane falls with increasing age. It varies from 1.08 in neonates to 0.64 in the elderly. The MAC of halothane in adults aged 31–55 was found to be 0.76%.[7] The addition of 70% nitrous oxide to halothane has been shown to reduce MAC by 61%[6]. MAC in dogs has been shown to vary linearly with temperature, increasing up to 40.7 °C at a rate of 8% per degree.[8] Anesthetic requirements are reduced by hypothermia, and it has been observed that humans enter into a "narcotic state" at temperatures below 30 °C.[9] The administration of narcotics, sedatives, or tranquilizers also reduces the MAC.[9]

Pharmacokinetics

Halothane has a lower blood–gas solubility than agents that had previously been available, which means that both induction and recovery are quicker. The blood–gas solubility coefficient of a substance refers to the relative solubility of that substance in the two different media. The more soluble an agent is in blood, the greater the quantity that is required to achieve a given tension. The minute ventilation of the lungs and the inspired concentration of the agent determine the quantity entering the bloodstream. It follows, therefore, that the greater the solubility of the agent in blood, the longer it will take for sufficient agent be taken up to achieve a given blood tension. Although the potency of an agent is commonly referred to in terms of its MAC, depth of anesthesia is determined by the brain (and indirectly blood) partial pressure. Therefore, the higher the blood–gas solubility, the longer it takes to achieve the desired partial pressure and the slower induction will be. Similarly, at the end of a procedure, the greater the blood–gas solubility of an agent, the greater will be the amount of the agent that has to be cleared from the system, and therefore the longer it will take and the slower recovery will be. The blood–gas solubility of halothane varies from 2.14 in neonates to a peak of 2.65 in adults (20–40 years old). It falls to 2.41 in the elderly (75–85 years old).[10] It is not clear why the blood–gas solubility varies with age in this way, but it may be related to differences in the serum albumin, cholesterol, or triglyceride levels between the different age groups.

A five-compartment model best describes the distribution of halothane.[11] It has been postulated that these may be the lungs, the vessel-rich group of organs, muscle, fat around the vessel-rich organs, and, finally, peripheral fat.

Ether has a blood–gas solubility of 12.1 and chloroform has a blood–gas solubility of 10.3, so halothane represented a significant

Table 33.2 *Properties of volatile anaesthetic agents*

Agent	Formula	Molecular weight (Da)	Boiling point (°C)	SVP at 20 °C		Blood–gas solubility	MAC (in O_2) (%)	Metabolism (%)
				kPa	mmHg			
Halothane	$C_2HBrClF_3$	197.39	50.2	32.4	243.3	2.5	0.75	20
Enflurane	$C_3H_2CF_5O$	184.5	56.5	22.9	172	1.91	1.68	2.4
Isoflurane	$C_3H_2CF_5O$	184.5	48.5	33.2	250	1.4	1.15	0.2
Sevoflurane	$C_4H_3F_7O$	200.5	58.5	21.3	160	1.69	2	4
Desflurane	$C_3H_2F_6O$	168.04	22.8	88.3	664	0.42	6	0.02
Nitrous oxide	N_2O	44	−88	–	–	0.42	105	0
Xenon	Xe	131.3	−107.1	–	–	0.115	71	0

Halogenated hydrocarbon

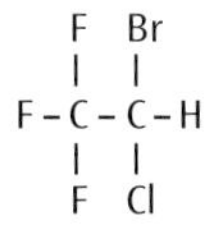

```
  F  Br
  |  |
F-C- C-H
  |  |
  F  Cl
```

Halothane

Ethers

```
  F    H  F           F    F  H           F    F  F
  |    |  |           |    |  |           |    |  |
H-C-O-C - C-F       H-C-O-C - C-F       H-C-O - C - C-H
  |    |  |           |    |  |           |    |  |
  F    Cl F           F    F  Cl          F    H  F
```

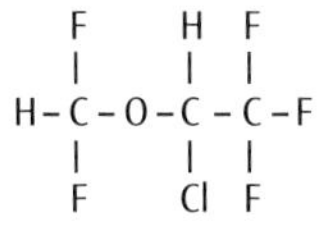

Isoflurane 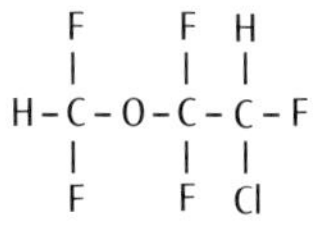   Enflurane 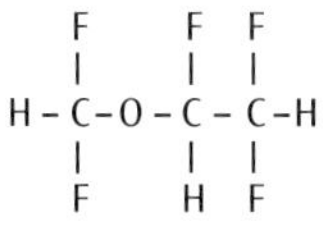   Desflurane

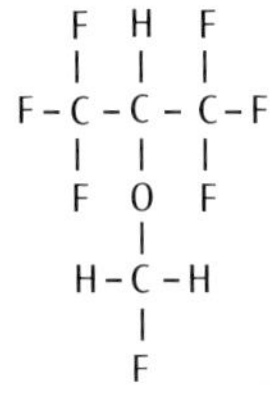

```
  F  H  F
  |  |  |
F-C- C- C-F
  |  |  |
  F  O  F
     |
   H-C-H
     |
     F
```

Sevoflurane

Figure 33.1 *Structural formulae of inhalational anesthetic agents.*

improvement on these agents. Uptake and elimination through the lungs is also quicker when ventilation is controlled because halothane is a respiratory depressant (see Respiratory effects below), and in spontaneously breathing patients this will have the effect of slowing any changes in the alveolar concentration. Although halothane is excreted through the lung, up to 46% may be metabolized, mainly by the liver.[12] It undergoes primarily oxidative metabolism, and the major metabolites are chlorine, bromine, and trifluoroacetic acid. Trifluoroacetic acid has been implicated in the etiology of the fulminant hepatitis, which occasionally occurs after halothane anesthesia (see Toxicity below). Halothane can also undergo reductive metabolism, and this is thought to be favored at low oxygen tension. The reductive pathway is associated with the production of fluoride ions, although not at the concentrations associated with renal toxicity. It may also be reactive metabolites, produced by the reductive pathway, which are responsible for the transient liver damage commonly seen after halothane anesthesia. Metabolism of halothane is catalyzed by cytochrome P450. Drugs acting on cytochrome P450, such as alcohol or isoniazid, which induce this enzyme system, or cimetidine and disulfiram, which inhibit it, may alter halothane metabolism.

Pharmacodynamics

Central nervous system effects

Halothane causes cerebral vasodilation and increases cerebral blood flow (CBF), provided systemic blood pressure is maintained. A concentration of 1 MAC halothane doubles CBF, and 1.6 MAC halothane almost quadruples it.[13] CBF is further increased by the addition of nitrous oxide. Halothane also abolishes CBF autoregulation and reduces cerebrospinal fluid (CSF) production by up to 30%.[14,15] The net effect on intracranial pressure and cerebral perfusion pressure (CPP) depends on systemic pressure and brain compliance. The increase in CBF induced by halothane may be prevented or reversed by hypocapnia.[16] In patients with intracranial disease resulting in raised intracranial pressure (ICP), the addition of halothane to a nitrous oxide–oxygen mixture resulted in a further increase [mean 1 kPa (7.6 mmHg)] in ICP despite hyperventilation.[17]

Halothane reduces cerebral oxygen consumption by up to 25%. The greatest reduction in oxygen consumption occurs at an inhaled concentration of halothane of between 0.5% and 0.8%. The reduction in oxygen consumption corresponds with a change in the electroencephalograph (EEG).[18] There is little further change in cerebral oxygen consumption with further increases in halothane until toxic levels are reached. EEG monitoring has not revealed epileptiform activity during halothane anesthesia. There have been reports of seizures following halothane anesthesia, but all these patients had also received other drugs, which may possibly be implicated. It is not a widely used anticonvulsant, although it has been successfully used in the treatment of status epilepticus in children.[19]

Halothane influences sensory evoked potentials, reducing the amplitude and increasing the latency, but this effect is not sufficiently pronounced to allow the depth of anesthesia to be monitored, and it does not interfere with the use of sensory evoked potentials used to evaluate CNS function.[20,21]

Respiratory effects

Halothane is very well tolerated in the concentrations used for induction and maintenance of anesthesia, and it causes very little airway irritation. For many years now it has been the agent of choice for inhalational induction of anesthesia, although with the recent introduction of sevoflurane this position is now changing.[22]

Halothane is a potent respiratory depressant. Although it increases respiratory rate, it also reduces tidal volume, and the overall effect is a reduction in alveolar minute ventilation and a rise in the arterial CO_2 (P_aCO_2) concentration.[23] The ventilatory response to a raised P_aCO_2 is also reduced.[24]

Similarly, the ventilatory response to hypoxemia is impaired, with concentrations as low as 0.1 MAC significantly reducing it and concentrations of 1.1 MAC abolishing it completely.[24] The site of action is probably the peripheral chemoreceptors of the carotid bodies.[25]

In addition to impairing the response to hypoxemia, halothane anesthesia is also associated with the development of atelectasis in dependent lung regions and an increase in shunt both in patients breathing spontaneously and in ventilated patients.[26] This is increased by muscle paralysis. The atelectasis is diminished by the use of positive end-expiratory pressure (PEEP).

A large number of studies have been directed to look at the effect of halothane on hypoxic pulmonary vasoconstriction (HPV), which has implications both for patients with lung disease resulting in ventilation–perfusion mismatch and in patients undergoing one-lung anesthesia. Although halothane has been shown to reverse HPV in isolated lung preparations, *in vivo* studies suggest that HPV is not likely to be a problem clinically.[27,28]

Halothane is also a potent bronchodilator. It has been shown to inhibit or reverse the bronchoconstriction caused by histamine and a variety of other mediators, and it reverses bronchoconstriction in subjects with asthma.[29,30] It is the most potent bronchodilator of the available anesthetic agents.[30] However, its use in asthmatics may be limited because it sensitizes the heart to cathecholamines, and as a result can cause ventricular arrhythmia, particularly in the presence of hypercapnia and raised catecholamine levels (see Cardiovascular effects). There is also evidence that it can interact with aminophylline, again resulting in an increased incidence of ventricular arrhythmia.[31]

Cardiovascular effects

There have been many studies into the effect of halothane on the circulation, with conflicting results. There are a number of possible reasons for this, including the use of different drugs for premedication, differing depths of anesthesia, differing P_aCO_2 levels, different degrees of surgical stimulation, and the simultaneous use of nitrous oxide and other drugs.

However, a number of properties have been identified. Halothane produces little change in the total systemic vascular resistance and, although skin vasodilation does occur, this is probably at the expense of other organ perfusion. There is a significant reduction in renal and splanchnic blood flow.[32–34] Coronary blood flow is reduced, probably as a result of reduced perfusion pressure and a reduction in myocardial oxygen consumption secondary to reduced contractility. Animal studies suggest that coronary blood flow autoregulation is slightly impaired, but this has the effect of increasing blood flow relative to demand.[35] The main hemodynamic effect of halothane is a reduction in blood pressure secondary to a fall in cardiac output.[36] There is a reduction in contractility manifested by a rise in right atrial pressure and a reduction in stroke volume. This reduction in contractility is due to alterations in calcium metabolism. There is a reduction in the influx of calcium through slow channels, and the binding of calcium by the plasma membrane is increased.[37] The uptake and release of calcium by the sarcoplasmic reticulum is also impaired.[38] The overall effect of this is a reduction in intracellular calcium and therefore a reduction in contractility.

There is no evidence for an increase in heart rate; indeed, heart rate often falls during halothane anesthesia. This may be due to a reduction in sympathetic activity or a direct effect on the rate of discharge of the sinoatrial node.[39] The reflex tachycardia one would normally expect in response to the hypotension that occurs, mediated by the baroreceptors, is depressed with increasing doses of halothane, and at 1.1% end-tidal concentration of halothane, the baroreceptor reflex is completely inhibited.[40]

An increased incidence of arrhythmia is associated with halothane anesthesia, which may result from three different mechanisms. First, halothane can decrease the automaticity of the sinoatrial node, thereby favoring the emergence of alternative pacemakers in the atrium or the atrioventricular node.[39,41] Second, halothane also slows myocardial conduction.[42] This favors the development of re-entry of the cardiac impulse, which results in either atrial or ventricular arrhythmia, depending on where the re-entry occurs. Finally, halothane interacts with epinephrine (adrenaline), increasing the incidence of cardiac arrhythmia.[43] This effect is potentiated in the presence of hypercapnia.[44] Johnston *et al.*[45] calculated the ED_{50} (the dose producing a positive response in 50% of patients) of epinephrine that produces arrhythmia during halothane anesthesia to be 2.1 μg kg^{-1}, and Katz and Katz[43] considered that a maximum dose of 10 mL of 1:100 000 epinephrine in any 10-min period, up to a maximum of 30 mL, was safe.

It appears that the incidence of cardiac arrhythmia associated with the use of halothane is particularly high for dental anesthesia.[46] Hutchison *et al.*[47] found that in the vast majority of patients, arrhythmia diminished when isoflurane was substituted for halothane.

There is recent evidence to suggests that the action of general anesthetics is mediated by ligand-gated ion channels, which includes calcium channels (See Mechanism of action of inhalational anesthetics). Halothane may also interact with calcium channel blockers, which is not surprising given that they both alter calcium metabolism and have similar effects on the heart. Both are negative inotropes and slow conduction, and there is evidence that these effects may be additive.[48] Studies in dogs have shown that verapamil reduces the MAC of halothane.[49] Although long-term use of oral calcium channel blockers is unlikely to cause problems, intravenous calcium channel blockers should be used with caution in patients receiving halothane.[50]

There is recent evidence to suggest that halothane, in common with isoflurane, enflurane, and sevoflurane, protects against the effects of myocardial ischemia if it is commenced before the ischemia occurs, and it may also improve recovery post ischemia.[51] This effect was greater than any seen with propofol.[51] The mechanism of this myocardial-protective effect of halothane has not been fully elucidated.

Neuromuscular effects

Halothane, used on its own, produces moderate muscle relaxation with increasing depth of anesthesia, although it is not as potent in this respect as are the other volatile agents. Gissen *et al.*[52] showed, using a frog sciatic nerve–sartorius muscle preparation, that the postjunctional membrane is the structure most sensitive to the neuromuscular blocking effects of halothane. Halothane also increases the duration and degree of block produced by nondepolarizing muscle relaxants. The mechanism of this interaction with nondepolarizing muscle relaxants is again mainly through its effect on the postjunctional membrane.[53] It also relaxes uterine muscle. Although the use of halothane has been associated with an increased incidence of bleeding following obstetric procedures, low concentrations have been used to prevent awareness during cesarean section without problems.[54]

There is a significant incidence of shivering and muscle spasticity during emergence from anesthesia, and particularly emergence from halothane anesthesia– so much so that the effect is often referred to as the "halothane shakes." Oxygen consumption is significantly increased and hypoxemia can result.[55] The incidence with halothane has been reported to be as high as 80%.[56] There is significant heat loss during anesthesia as a result of exposure to the operating room environment and the cutaneous vasodilation that occurs. The thermoregulatory response is also impaired during halothane anesthesia.[57] Patients are therefore commonly hypothermic during recovery, and shivering is a normal physiological response to this.[58] However, this is not the complete explanation. There is evidence for a central or spinal effect of halothane, which results in altered muscle activity during emergence from anesthesia.[56] A wide selection of agents have been used successfully to reduce this shivering, including opiates, magnesium sulfate, muscle relaxants, and clonidine. The drug found to be most effective in reducing the shivering is meperidine (pethidine).[59]

Toxicity

A major problem associated with the use of halothane is hepatotoxicity. This was recognized shortly after its introduction and manifests itself in two forms. The first occurs in about one in three patients exposed to halothane and manifests as a subclinical transient increase in liver enzymes shortly after exposure.[60] The etiology is not known and previous exposure is not a prerequisite. Halothane does cause a reduction in hepatic blood flow, and this, combined with the unique dual blood supply of the liver (hepatic artery and portal vein), may produce areas of reduced oxygen tension around the central vein. There are two possible pathways of halothane metabolism, an oxidative pathway and a reductive pathway. The reductive pathway, which is favored under conditions of low oxygen tension, may result in the production of toxic metabolites, thereby causing a rise in liver enzymes.[61]

The second form of halothane hepatotoxicity results in hepatic necrosis. This is a rare but often fatal complication. The incidence is estimated at between 1 in 6000 and 1 in 35 000 administrations, and is most likely immune mediated.[61] The risk is increased with repeat exposure. Although it has been recommended that halothane administration should not be repeated within 3 months, hepatic necrosis can occur irrespective of when halothane was previously administered. Any patient who has a history of liver dysfunction following exposure to any of the halogenated anesthetic agents should not subsequently be exposed to any of these agents because there is some evidence of cross-sensitization.[62] As discussed above (see Pharmacokinetics), metabolism of halothane results in the production of a trifluoroacetyl (TFA) halide, which binds covalently to liver microsomal proteins. It has been demonstrated that exposure to halothane, isoflurane, enflurane, and desflurane results in the production of TFA-labeled proteins, and that serum from patients with a history of halothane hepatitis reacts with acylated liver proteins from rats exposed to halothane.[63]

This suggests that the TFA halide may bind to hepatocytes, creating neoantigens and thereby exciting an autoimmune response against the hepatocyte. The first signs of liver damage may be delayed for up to a month after exposure to halothane, and are often preceded by pyrexia, rash, or arthralgia.[60] Two different tests have been described for the detection of antibodies: the immunoblotting assay, which is the less sensitive and more time-consuming; and the enzyme-linked immunosorbent assay (ELISA), which was reported as being positive in 72% of one group of patients diagnosed clinically as having halothane hepatitis.[62]

Although fluoride ions are also be produced by the reductive metabolism of halothane, this is a minor pathway, and significant amounts are not produced. Halothane decomposes on contact with soda-lime to CF_2CClBr, which is nephrotoxic. However, only small amounts accumulate, and it does not appear to be a clinical problem. There is no evidence of nephrotoxicity associated with the use of halothane.

Halothane is also a trigger for malignant hyperthermia (MH). Malignant hyperthermia is an autosomal dominant inherited condition. Affected individuals have a defect in their skeletal muscle that makes them susceptible to massive release of intracellular calcium from the sarcoplasmic reticulum of skeletal muscle on exposure to certain trigger agents. It results in an uncontrolled increase in metabolism in the muscle, leading to a rise in temperature of over 2 °C per hour and serious biochemical derangement.

Rhabdomyolysis can occur with associated hyperkalemia. In the absence of appropriate management, mortality can be as high as 70%; however, with early intervention this can be reduced significantly. Management includes supportive measures, active cooling, and the use of the muscle relaxant dantrolene, which inhibits the release of calcium from the sarcoplasmic reticulum. All the volatile agents and the muscle relaxant succinylcholine (suxamethonium) are trigger agents. Halothane may be a more potent trigger than the fluorinated ethers.[60] The incidence of MH is estimated at between 1:15 000 and 1:50 000.

Clinical use

Halothane has been available for over 40 years and is still widely used despite the introduction of newer agents. The major advantage of halothane over the other modern inhalational anesthetics, with the exception of sevoflurane, is that it is very well tolerated during inhalation induction. This has sustained its use, particularly in pediatric practice. Until the advent of sevoflurane it was the agent of choice for an inhalation induction. However, the use of halothane has been declining, fueled mainly by concerns about toxicity, and with the wider availability of sevoflurane it now looks set to disappear almost completely from clinical practice.

ENFLURANE

Enflurane is one of the 700 compounds produced by R C Terrell of Ohio Medical Products. It was first tested in animals in 1963, and in man in 1966.[64] Interest in new anesthetic agents was driven mainly by concerns about the toxicity of the metabolites of halothane and methoxyflurane. A major potential advantage of enflurane is that it is much more stable in the body than are these other agents.

Physical properties

Enflurane is a halogenated methyl ethyl ether. As illustrated in Fig. 33.1, it is a structural isomer of isoflurane, which was produced a little later. It is noncorrosive, nonflammable, and stable in light, so it can be stored in glass bottles without any chemical stabilizer. It is not as pleasant to inhale as halothane, and is therefore less useful for inhalation induction. Although enflurane is quite stable, under certain conditions it may interact with soda-lime and Baralyme® with degradation of the enflurane, resulting in the production of carbon monoxide (CO) (see Toxicity below).

The boiling point of enflurane is 56.5 °C, and its saturated vapor pressure is 22.9 kPa (172 mmHg) at 20 °C. Its blood–gas solubility is 1.91 at 37°C, slightly less than that of halothane but greater than isoflurane and the newer agents desflurane and sevoflurane.

It has a MAC of 1.68 in young adults when used in oxygen, which is greater than that of isoflurane, and almost double the MAC of halothane.[64] When 70% nitrous oxide is introduced, the MAC is reduced to 0.6%.[64] As with the other agents, the MAC is higher in children and lower in the elderly.

Pharmacokinetics

Enflurane has a lower blood–gas solubility than halothane, which suggests that the equilibration of alveolar and blood concentrations should be quicker. This is indeed the case, although enflurane is significantly less potent than halothane, and therefore higher partial pressures are required. Airway irritation will limit the rate at which the inspired concentrations may be increased during induction in the spontaneously breathing patient.

Enflurane is metabolized to organic and inorganic fluoride ions. The degree of biotransformation is much less than that of halothane, and has been estimated to be about 2.4%. A major problem with methoxyflurane is the high levels of fluoride ions resulting from its metabolism, which can result in high-output renal failure. Fluoride concentrations greater than 100 $\mu mol\,L^{-1}$ have been reported in patients treated with an enzyme-inducing agent following exposure to enflurane, particularly patients taking isoniazid who are "fast acetylators."[65] However, even in these patients renal dysfunction has not proved to be a clinical problem (see Toxicity below).

Pharmacodynamics

Central nervous system effects

A significant problem associated with the use of enflurane is that its use in humans may be associated with convulsions. These can occur in patients with no previous history of epilepsy. Initial studies with rats showed that, at a concentration of 1.5%, spontaneous spike wave complexes were displayed on the EEG, and repetitive auditory stimulation often precipitated seizures.[64] In humans, the likelihood of EEG changes and of seizures is increased at increasing concentrations of enflurane.[64] Cerebral irritability is also increased by hypocapnia, and can be reduced by hypercapnia.[64,66] This increase in cerebral irritability associated with reduced arterial CO_2 levels is greatest at inspired enflurane concentrations above 2.5%.[66] The addition of nitrous oxide does not alter the EEG patterns.

The effect of enflurane on evoked potentials is similar to that of halothane: the amplitude is reduced and the latency is increased.[21]

Enflurane produces a slight increase in CBF, significantly less than that of halothane but greater than that of isoflurane.[67] Autoregulation of CBF is absent during 1 MAC enflurane anesthesia, although it may be partially restored by hypocapnia.[14] It also results in a reduction in cerebral oxygen consumption, most marked at concentrations up to 1 MAC.[18]

Respiratory effects

Of the currently available volatile agents, enflurane is the most potent respiratory depressant.[68,69] Although it is associated with a smaller reduction in tidal volume than halothane and isoflurane, enflurane does not increase the respiratory rate to the same extent as do these agents, and the overall result is a greater reduction in minute ventilation.[64,69] As with halothane, 0.1 MAC significantly reduces the ventilatory response to hypoxia and 1.1 MAC abolishes it almost completely. The slope of the CO_2 response curve is also significantly reduced.[70] Concentrations of 2 MAC have been shown to result in apnea in some subjects.[71] Some adaptation to the respiratory depressant effect of enflurane does occur over time, and after 7 h of enflurane anesthesia there is no difference in the degree of respiratory depression from that seen with either isoflurane or halothane.[71] Enflurane is somewhat irritating to the airway, and that, combined with respiratory depression, may limit the ability to achieve adequate levels of anesthesia quickly when using enflurane for inhalational induction.

Enflurane and halothane have been shown to be equally effective for the attenuation of experimentally induced bronchoconstriction in dogs, although enflurane is not quite as effective in attenuating the response to intravenous histamine.[72,73]

In vitro studies show that enflurane inhibits hypoxic pulmonary vasoconstriction in a dose-dependent manner to the same degree as halothane and insoflurane.[74] Enflurane has been used successfully for one-lung anesthesia, and a comparison with intravenous anesthesia using ketamine for patients undergoing lung resection found no difference between the two drugs in the $P_{a}O_2$ and right to left shunt.[75]

Cardiovascular effects

Enflurane increases heart rate, reduces blood pressure, and reduces cardiac output.[64] Although it has a dose-dependent negative inotropic effect, there is little impairment in left ventricular diastolic performance.[76] At low doses, the increase in heart rate partially compensates for the reduction in contractility. Low concentrations of enflurane have less effect than similar concentrations of halothane, but the cardiovascular dose–response curve is much steeper than that of halothane.[77] Animal studies have shown that concentrations of 1 MAC may disrupt coronary autoregulation to a similar degree as halothane and isoflurane, producing coronary vasodilation and slightly increasing coronary blood flow out of proportion to demand, and human studies have shown that the two vapors have a similar effect on systemic vascular resistance (SVR).[35,78] Deeper levels of anesthesia (2 MAC) have been associated with profound cardiovascular depression, although some recovery may occur if anesthesia is maintained for several hours.[78]

Enflurane does not sensitize the heart to catecholamines, either endogenous or exogenous, to the same extent as halothane. Although the threshold for arrhythmia with enflurane is higher than with either isoflurane or halothane, the variation in patient response is more variable, so that arrhythmia can occur at relatively low concentrations.[45,77] Enflurane has less effect on myocardial conduction than halothane.[54] Like halothane, it interacts with calcium channel blockers. Intravenous verapamil causes significantly more hemodynamic depression with enflurane than with either halothane or isoflurane.[48]

There is evidence that enflurane offers the heart some protection against the effects of myocardial ischemia.[51] The mechanism of this is likely to be similar to that associated with isoflurane (see under Cardiovascular effects).

Neuromuscular effects

Enflurane causes a dose-dependent depression of neuromuscular function. A concentration of 1 MAC causes no depression of single-twitch response but does cause fade and post-tetanic facilitation.[64] The effect is more pronounced than that seen with halothane.[77] It is possible to produce sufficient relaxation to allow abdominal surgery without neuromuscular blocking drugs, although hypotension can be a limiting factor. It also relaxes uterine muscle, the effect being slight at 0.5 MAC but pronounced at 1.5 MAC. The response of the uterus to oxytocin is retained at concentrations less than 1.75 MAC.[77]

Enflurane augments the effect of neuromuscular blocking agents to a greater degree than either halothane or isoflurane.[79] There is some evidence that this effect is time dependent, increasing with longer duration of anesthesia.[80]

Shivering does occur during emergence from enflurane anesthesia, and, as with halothane, it can be suppressed with meperidine.[59]

Toxicity

Enflurane metabolism results in the production of TFA, which has been implicated in hepatotoxicity (see above). Liver damage can occur with enflurane anesthesia, and the incidence has been estimated at 1 in 800 000.[60]

Experience with methoxyflurane suggested that concentrations of fluoride greater than 50 μmol L^{-1} are associated with renal impairment, characterized by serum hyperosmolarity, hypernatremia, urinary hypo-osmolarity and vasopressin-resistant polyuria.[81] Fluoride levels of over 100 μmol L^{-1} have been detected after enflurane anesthesia in patients treated with isoniazid, which is a specific inducer of cytochrome P450 2E1, but there was no evidence of impaired renal function.[65] There are several possible explanations for this. First, methoxyflurane has much higher tissue solubility than enflurane, and therefore it is likely that high serum levels will be more prolonged following methoxyflurane anesthesia than after enflurane. Second, more recent work suggests that with methoxyflurane there is intrarenal production of fluoride ions, perhaps resulting in high intrarenal concentrations of fluoride ions, and that this in fact may be more important in the etiology of the fluoride toxicity seen with methoxyflurane than the serum fluoride concentration.[82]

A potential problem that was mentioned above (see Physical properties) is production of carbon monoxide when enflurane is exposed to either soda-lime or Baralyme®.[83] This appears to occur only if the soda-lime or Baralyme® is allowed to dry out. Their normal water content is about 15%, and carbon monoxide production is negligible above 4.8%, which appears to be the critical level. Under laboratory conditions, concentrations of carbon monoxide as high as 5000 p.p.m. have been generated from enflurane exposed to completely dry Baralyme® at 45 °C.[83] Carbon monoxide production is greater with Baralyme® than with soda-lime. This phenomenon can also occur with desflurane and isoflurane (all of which contain a CHF_2 moiety), with carbon monoxide production being greater with desflurane and less with isoflurane.[83] Carbon monoxide production increases with higher temperatures and higher anesthetic concentrations. There have been no reports of patient injury as a result of this problem, and drying of the absorbers can be minimized by avoiding fresh gas flow through absorbers when they are not in use, and simply by adding a little water if drying is suspected to be a problem. Alternatively, it has been demonstrated, at least in the case of desflurane, that removal of sodium hydroxide and potassium hydroxide from soda-lime may significantly decrease carbon monoxide production without impairing CO_2 absorption.[84]

As with the other halogenated anesthetics, enflurane is a trigger agent for malignant hyperthermia in susceptible patients.[60]

Clinical use

Enflurane was introduced in response to concerns about the side-effects of the older agents. However, enflurane is not without problems itself. Compared with the recently introduced volatile agents, it is a more potent cardiac and respiratory depressant, and it also causes cerebral irritation, all of which effects preclude its use in high concentrations and make it particularly unsuitable for neurosurgical patients. The incidence of cardiac arrhythmia with enflurane is lower than with halothane, as is the incidence of hepatotoxicity, so its initial reception was favorable. Its use declined following the introduction of isoflurane, which has significant clinical advantages over enflurane.

ISOFLURANE

Isoflurane was first produced in 1968 by Dr R C Terrell as one of the series of 700 compounds that he produced. Although early work suggested that it might have significant advantages over the then available agents, the introduction of isoflurane was delayed because synthesis and purification were more difficult than in the case of the earlier agents. A pilot study published in 1976, which suggested that administration during gestation and early life in mice caused hepatic neoplasia, further delayed its introduction into clinical practice.[85] This work was subsequently repeated using a larger number of mice, and no increased incidence of neoplasia was found – it was subsequently realized the increase found in the earlier study was probably related to contaminated feed that had been eaten by the mice.[86]

Isoflurane was approved for clinical use in the USA in 1979, and introduced into clinical practice in the UK in 1983.

Physical properties

Isoflurane is a structural isomer of enflurane, a halogenated methyl ethyl ether (Fig. 33.1). It has a pungent ethereal odor, which is moderately irritating. The three fluorine atoms on the terminal ethyl carbon make it resistant to chemical or biological degradation.[87] It is nonflammable, stable in ultraviolet light, and noncorrosive, and can be stored without a preservative at room temperature.[88] Like enflurane and desflurane, it contains a CHF_3 moiety and may undergo some degradation when exposed to dried soda-lime or Baralyme®, resulting in the production of carbon monoxide, although not to the same degree as with enflurane or desflurane.

The boiling point of isoflurane is 48.5 °C and its blood–gas solubility is 1.4 (Table 33.2). The saturated vapor pressure is 33.2 kPa (250 mmHg) at 20 °C, which is almost the same as that of halothane [32.4 kPa (243mmHg)]. This means that halothane and isoflurane vaporizers could be used interchangeably with little loss in accuracy in the delivered concentration. For obvious reasons, this practice is not encouraged. Isoflurane is absorbed by the plastics and rubber found in anesthetic circuits, although not to the same extent as halothane.[4] The MAC of isoflurane is intermediate between that of halothane and enflurane. It decreases with increasing age, ranging from 1.28% in young adults down to 1.05% in patients over the age of 55 years.[89] However, the MAC of isoflurane in a premature or newborn infant is less than the MAC for a 6-month-old.[90] The MAC in middle-aged patients is 1.15%. The addition of 70% nitrous oxide roughly halves the MAC, which is also reduced by lidocaine (lignocaine), alcohol, and narcotic analgesics.[68,89] The MAC is also reduced by hypothermia, with animal studies showing a 5.3% fall for every degree drop in temperature.[91] The MAC is not influenced by the duration of anesthesia.

Pharmacokinetics

Isoflurane has a lower blood–gas solubility than either halothane or isoflurane, which means that the inspired concentration and the alveolar concentration equilibrate more quickly. It takes only 4 min to reach an F_A/F_I (ratio of the alveolar concentration to the inspired concentration) of 0.5 with isoflurane, compared with 5 min for enflurane and 30 min with halothane.[92,93] The use of higher initial concentrations to achieve a given alveolar concentration can compensate for the slow equilibration. However, because of its pungency, rapidly increasing the inspired concentration of isoflurane during induction may induce coughing and breath-holding. This limits the rate of induction in patients breathing spontaneously. Pungency does not limit the rate at which anesthetic depth is changed, and is not a problem during recovery, both of which should be quicker with isoflurane than with either enflurane or halothane. As with the other modern agents, a five-compartment model best describes the distribution of isoflurane.[94]

Isoflurane undergoes minimal metabolism in man, with less than 0.2% being recovered as urinary metabolites.[95] Excretion is primarily through the lungs. Metabolism is by oxidation by hepatic cytochrome P450 2E1 with the production of inorganic fluoride and trifluoroacetic acid.[68] Although enzyme induction with drugs such as isoniazid may increase metabolism, the absolute increase is small and unlikely to be clinically significant.[88]

Pharmacodynamics

Central nervous system effects

Isoflurane produces a dose-dependent depression of CNS activity. Concentrations above 0.25 MAC produce amnesia.[96] Animal studies have shown a nonlinear reduction in cerebral oxygen consumption, with the greatest reduction occurring at concentrations below 1 MAC. In dogs, cerebral oxygen consumption is reduced by 23% at 1 MAC and 30% at 2 MAC.

Unlike its isomer enflurane, isoflurane is not associated with epileptiform activity, even at deeper levels of anesthesia with profound hypocapnia.[87] As the concentration of isoflurane increases toward 1 MAC there is an increase in the voltage amplitude and the frequency of the EEG.[68] As the concentration increases above 0.4 MAC, the higher voltage shifts from the posterior part of the brain to the anterior part of the brain. At concentrations up to around 1 MAC, the voltage amplitude of the EEG continues to increase, but the frequency starts to decrease. As anesthesia deepens further, both frequency and amplitude start to decrease. At 1.5 MAC, burst suppression occurs, and at 2 MAC an isoelectric pattern appears.[97] Concentrations of 1 MAC isoflurane also increase the latency of auditory evoked brainstem potentials.[98]

Isoflurane does not increase CBF in normocapnic, normotensive patients in concentrations up to 1.1 MAC, but 1.6 MAC is associated with a doubling of CBF if blood pressure is maintained.[68] If mean arterial pressure (MAP) is allowed to fall, CPP and cerebral blood flow are both reduced.[99] Cerebral autoregulation is also impaired by isoflurane compared with propofol.[100] In normocapnic patients without an intracranial mass lesion, isoflurane, sevoflurane, and desflurane slightly increase lumbar CSF pressure compared with propofol.[101,102] The increase in intracranial pressure that occurs with isoflurane is easier to reverse with hypocapnia than the increase that occurs with halothane.[103] In hypocapnic neurosurgical patients with supratentorial mass lesions [end-tidal CO_2 2.4–2.9 kPa (18–22 mmHg)], concentrations of 1 MAC isoflurane were associated with no change in ICP.[104]

Respiratory effects

Isoflurane is quite irritating to the airway, and is not particularly well suited for inhalational induction. It causes slightly greater dose-related respiratory depression than halothane, but less than enflurane.[69,105] Respiratory rate is increased and tidal volume is reduced, with a net reduction in minute ventilation. The ventilatory response to increasing P_aCO_2 is decreased with increasing concentrations, and approaches zero at 2 MAC.[106] The ventilatory response to hypoxemia is also impaired by isoflurane. Concentrations as low as 0.1 MAC can reduce it by up to 70%, and concentrations above 1.1 MAC abolish it completely.[107] Isoflurane seems particularly to depress the ventilatory responses mediated by peripheral chemoreceptors.[107]

Isoflurane reduces functional residual capacity and pulmonary compliance at concentrations of 1 MAC, with no further decrease at 2 MAC, and airways resistance is increased.[108] While studies with isolated lungs have shown that isoflurane reduces hypoxic pulmonary vasoconstriction, in the clinical situation this is not a significant problem.[27,109]

Isoflurane does not increase airways resistance, and its use in patients with chronic asthma does not seem to cause any particular problems.[88] It is as effective as halothane in preventing the bronchoconstriction produced by inhalation of the *Ascaris* antigen by dogs that were allergic to this antigen.[88]

Cardiovascular effects

Although *in vitro* studies have shown that isoflurane depresses the contractility of an isolated heart, clinically it is associated with minimal apparent myocardial depression at concentrations of up to 2 MAC, partly because of a fall in peripheral vascular resistance. Heart rate increases, stroke volume decreases, and cardiac output remains at awake levels.[110] Animal studies suggest that there is a wider margin of cardiovascular safety with isoflurane than with enflurane or halothane.[68] Sudden exposure to high concentrations of isoflurane may be associated with tachycardia and a rise in blood pressure similar to that seen with desflurane (see Cardiovascular effects of desflurane). Isoflurane causes a significant drop in peripheral vascular resistance, and hence blood pressure, although this can be reversed by surgical stimulation. While there is a reduction in tone in all vascular beds, there is a proportionally greater reduction in the vascular tone of the skin and muscle beds, and therefore an increase in blood flow to these areas. As a result of the fall in perfusion pressure, blood flow to the splanchnic area may fall.[88] There is a reduction in renal blood flow, glomerular filtration rate, and urine production.[88]

Ventricular work and myocardial oxygen consumption are reduced, thereby improving the oxygen supply–demand ratio of the heart. In addition, isoflurane is also a coronary vasodilator. Indeed, there is evidence in dogs that it may cause coronary steal, and this has been a cause of some concern.[111] Coronary steal occurs when blood is directed away from collateral-dependent myocardium to areas of normal flow as a result of coronary vasodilation. This can result in ischemia in the collateral-dependent area. However, the coronary steal phenomenon has been demonstrated only in animal models and has not been confirmed in human studies. The use of isoflurane in patients with steal-prone anatomy has been compared with the use of halothane, enflurane, or high-dose sufentanil; no difference in the incidence of myocardial ischemia was found to be associated with any of the four agents.[112,113]

The coronary vasodilation produced by isoflurane is mediated through adenosine triphosphate (ATP)-gated potassium channels (K_{ATP}).[114] These channels are generally inhibited in the presence of normal intracellular ATP levels. When ATP levels fall, as they will during ischemia, these channels open. This causes hyperpolarization and a reduction in cellular activity. In vascular smooth muscle, muscle tone is reduced and blood flow is therefore increased. This contributes to the regulation of blood flow. These channels are distributed throughout the cardiovascular system, including the heart. In myocardial cells, activation of these channels results in reduced action potential duration, reduced calcium entry, and a reduction in contractility. This helps to protect the cell from the effects of ischemia. Nicorandil is a K_{ATP} agonist that is licensed for use in the management of angina. In addition to producing coronary vasodilation, K_{ATP} agonists have been shown to protect against the effects of myocardial ischemia and enhance recovery post ischemia.[115] There is now evidence that isoflurane may protect the myocardium from ischemia by a similar effect on K_{ATP} channels.[115] The sulfonylurea oral hypoglycemic drug glibenclamide blocks the effect of K_{ATP} agonists.[114]

Although recent research has focused on the potential protective effect of isoflurane on the heart during and after myocardial ischemia, all the currently used agents may offer protection against myocardial ischaemia.[51] It is likely that this protection is multifactorial and includes free radical inhibition (enflurane > halothane > isoflurane), preservation of myocardial ATP concentrations, opening of K_{ATP} channels, and alteration in calcium flux.

Although isoflurane does cause some slowing of myocardial conduction, this is less than occurs with either enflurane or halothane, and the cardiac rhythm is more stable.[54] The doses of epinephrine required to produce arrhythmia in 50% of patients receiving 1.25 MAC isoflurane is three times the dose required in patients receiving 1.25 MAC halothane.[88] There is some evidence for an interaction with calcium channel blockers, although the hemodynamic depression produced with intravenous verapamil is not as significant as that seen with enflurane.[48]

Neuromuscular effects

The effect of isoflurane on neuromuscular function is similar to that of enflurane. It has no effect on twitch height, but does cause fade with repeated stimulation. The neuromuscular effect is dose related and roughly equivalent to that seen with enflurane, but more pronounced than that observed with halothane.[87] Isoflurane also augments the effect of muscle relaxants. In this it is more potent than halothane but less potent than enflurane.[79]

Shivering also occurs during emergence from isoflurane anesthesia, and can be suppressed with meperidine.[59] Although this is often a thermoregulatory response to hypothermia, as with halothane (see Neuromuscular effects) isoflurane may also cause clonus and tonic stiffening despite normal temperatures.[58]

Toxicity

Hepatotoxicity has been reported following isoflurane anesthesia, although not as frequently as with halothane or enflurane, despite isoflurane now being used more frequently.[60] This may be because isoflurane undergoes significantly less metabolism. The mechanism of the hepatotoxicity is probably a result of the TFA metabolite forming neoantigens, as occurs with halothane and enflurane, and possibly desflurane (see Toxicity of desflurane).

Fluoride ions are also produced by isoflurane metabolism, but only in clinically insignificant amounts because of the low rate of metabolism. Although renal blood flow, glomerular filtration rate, and urine flow are all reduced during isoflurane anesthesia, this does not appear to cause any long-term adverse effects. There is no evidence for nephrotoxicity associated with isoflurane anesthesia. Isoflurane is degraded by desiccated CO_2 absorbers to produce carbon monoxide, although not to the same degree as enflurane or desflurane.

Isoflurane is a trigger agent for malignant hyperthermia in susceptible patients.[60]

Clinical use

Isoflurane has several advantages over both enflurane and halothane. It has a lower blood–gas solubility, which results in a more rapid induction and recovery. Although it is a potent respiratory depressant, it is still less so than enflurane. It is a coronary vasodilator. Initial concerns about its use in patients with ischemic heart disease as a result of "coronary steal syndrome" have proved to be unfounded. Indeed, more recent research shows isoflurane to be protective against myocardial ischemia through several different mechanisms. Its use in neurosurgical patients is discussed in Chapter 44. A major drawback with isoflurane is that it is not suitable for inhalation induction. Like halothane and enflurane, it contributes to the depletion of the ozone layer, and it may be this factor that ultimately results in its withdrawal from clinical practice.

SEVOFLURANE

Sevoflurane was first synthesized in the late 1960s at Baxter-Travenol laboratories by R F Wallin and coworkers. The first published record of its use in humans was in 1981, when the results of a phase I trial of the drug in six healthy adults were published, and it was found then to be worthy of further study.[116] It has two drawbacks: metabolism results in the production of potentially significant levels of fluoride ions and it has also been found to be chemically unstable in the presence of soda-lime. Baxter-Travenol decided not to develop this drug commercially. It contracted with a Japanese firm, Maruishi Pharmaceuticals (Osaka), and following further research it was approved for clinical use in Japan in 1990, where it eventually became the most popular inhalational anesthetic agent.[117] Its success in Japan was subsequently followed by its introduction into practice in the USA and Europe.

Physical properties

Sevoflurane contains no chlorine or bromine ions, and therefore, unlike other volatile agents, with the exception of desflurane, it should have no effect on the ozone layer (Fig. 33.1). It is colorless, nonflammable, and a liquid at room temperature. In contrast to isoflurane, it is not unpleasant to inhale. It has a boiling point of 58.5 °C and a saturated vapor pressure (SVP) of 21.3 kPa (160 mmHg) at 20 °C and can therefore be administered using a conventional temperature-compensated vaporizer. It has a blood–gas solubility coefficient of 0.69, which is more or less half that of isoflurane and quarter that of halothane.[118] Induction and recovery should therefore be more rapid, and this does appear to be the case (see Physical properties of halothane). Sevoflurane blood–gas solubility, unlike that of halothane and isoflurane, does not alter with age.[119] It is also less soluble in the rubber and plastic of anesthetic circuits than halothane or isoflurane.[4]

As with the other inhalational agents, the MAC of sevoflurane decreases with age from 3.3. in neonates to 1.48 in the elderly.[120] The MAC in adults has been variously estimated at 1.7–2.1.[121,122] The MAC is reduced by nitrous oxide, opioid drugs, and hypnotics.[123]

Pharmacokinetics

The low blood–gas partition coefficient of sevoflurane should mean that anesthetic concentrations are rapidly achieved. The F_A/F_I ratio of sevoflurane has been compared with that of isoflurane. At 30 min after the start of anesthesia, the F_A/F_I for sevoflurane was 0.85 compared with 0.73 for isoflurane. When the elimination of sevoflurane was also compared with that of isoflurane, the elimination F_A/F_{AO} ratios (F_{AO} being the F_A when administration of the agents ceases) 5 min after ceasing administration were 0.157 for sevoflurane and 0.23 for isoflurane.[94] This confirmed that set concentrations are achieved more quickly and elimination is also quicker, as predicted. A five-compartment model best describes the distribution of sevoflurane.[94] Sevoflurane is primarily excreted through the lung, although a small amount is metabolized. The proportion metabolized has been estimated at between 1.6% and 4.9%.[82,116]

Metabolism occurs in the liver, catalyzed by the cytochrome P450 2E1 enzyme.[124] Sevoflurane is broken down into inorganic fluoride ions and the organic fluoride metabolite hexafluoroisopropanol (HFIP).[116] HFIP is conjugated with glucuronic acid to form HFIP glucuronide, which is excreted by the kidneys (Fig. 33.2).[125] There is no evidence of toxicity associated with HFIP.

Pharmacodynamics

Central nervous system effects

Sevoflurane and isoflurane cause similar dose-dependent changes in the EEG.[126] However, there is some evidence that sevoflurane may also have neuroexcitatory properties. There has been a case report of EEG changes consistent with seizure activity in a nonepileptic patient under deep sevoflurane anesthesia, and also a report of tonic–clonic seizure-like movements in a patient recovering from sevoflurane anesthesia.[127,128] There is evidence that the neuroexcitatory properties of sevoflurane are greater than those of isoflurane, and that they are not altered by hypocapnia.[129] Nevertheless, there are still only isolated case reports of convulsions following sevoflurane anesthesia despite widespread use for several years.

Animal studies suggest that sevoflurane has an effect on CBF similar to that isoflurane, with minimal increase at normocapnia, and that both agents significantly reduce the cerebral metabolic rate for oxygen.[130] Observations in humans have confirmed this, although MAP and CPP are better maintained with sevoflurane than with isoflurane.[99] The cerebrovascular response to carbon dioxide and cerebrovascular autoregulation are both preserved under sevoflurane anesthesia.[131] Sevoflurane causes a slight increase in ICP in normocapnic patients, similar to that seen with desflurane and isoflurane.[102]

Respiratory effects

Sevoflurane is quite pleasant to inhale and has virtually no irritant effect on the airway. This, combined with its low blood–gas solubility, makes it very suitable for inhalational induction. It may, in fact, be the least irritant of the currently available anesthetic agents.[132] It is a less potent agent than halothane, but this can be overcome by using higher inspired concentrations, which are generally well tolerated. As in the case of halothane, it is a respiratory depressant, causing a reduction in minute ventilation. Tidal volume is reduced, and, although respiratory rate is increased, this does not compensate for the reduction in tidal volume.[133] The ventilatory response to carbon dioxide is depressed to a slightly

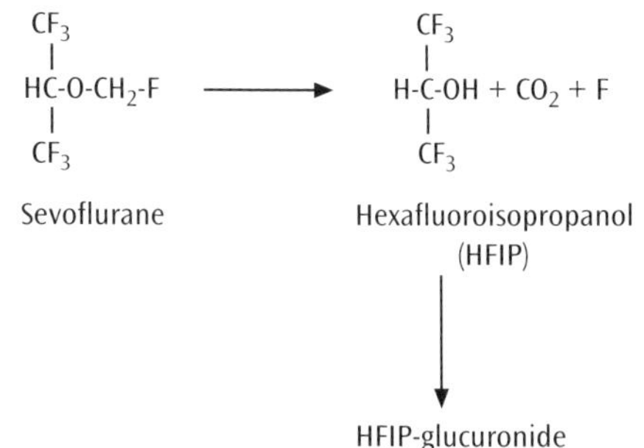

Figure 33.2 *Metabolism of sevoflurane.*

greater degree than with halothane, and 0.1 MAC causes a 30–40% depression of the ventilatory response to hypoxia[25,134]

Sevoflurane also abolishes hypoxic pulmonary vasoconstriction in a dose-dependent manner in isolated perfused rabbit lungs.[135] However, in a randomized crossover study, there was no difference in arterial oxygenation between isoflurane and sevoflurane when used to maintain anesthesia during one-lung ventilation, so in most cases it is unlikely to cause significant clinical problems.[136]

Sevoflurane is also effective as a bronchodilator. It has been shown to be as effective as isoflurane in attenuating bronchospasm in antigen-induced anaphylaxis in dogs, although other studies in dogs have shown that it is not as effective as halothane in attenuating changes in airway resistance after intravenous histamine.[30,137]

Cardiovascular effects

Sevoflurane has a number of different hemodynamic effects. Unlike isoflurane and desflurane, both of which can cause tachycardia, sevoflurane has a minimal effect on heart rate.[138,139] Animal studies have suggested that sevoflurane can produce direct myocardial depression through an effect on calcium channels.[140,141] It causes a dose-dependent depression of cardiac output and a reduction in systemic vascular resistance that is similar to that seen with isoflurane and which results in a fall in systemic blood pressure.[139,142] It also causes a reduction in pulmonary arterial pressure that is not dose dependent.[139] Hepatic and renal blood flows are well preserved, at least with concentrations up to 1 MAC.[123]

Sevoflurane does not sensitize the myocardium to epinephrine.[143] Although it is a coronary vasodilator, it is less potent in this regard than isoflurane, and in canine models this does not lead to coronary steal.[144,145] In a study of patients with cardiac disease undergoing noncardiac surgery, there was no difference in the incidence of myocardial ischemia or of adverse cardiac events between sevoflurane and isoflurane.[146]

Sevoflurane does not cause the sympathetic-mediated cardiovascular stimulation associated with rapid increases in end-tidal concentration that is seen with desflurane and isoflurane.[123,147,148] It also protects against some of the metabolic changes associated with myocardial ischemia.[149]

Neuromuscular effects

Sevoflurane produces dose-dependent muscle relaxation. At deeper levels of anesthesia, it provides sufficient relaxation to allow tracheal intubation.[122] In common with the other volatile agents in current use, sevoflurane potentiates the action of neuromuscular blocking agents.[150] It prolongs the train-of-four recovery by 15–20% when compared with a droperidol/fentanyl combination and with halothane.[53] The rate of train-of-four recovery is very similar to that seen with isoflurane.[151] It has no effect on recovery of post-tetanic twitch, which suggests that, as with other agents, its action is mainly on the postjunctional region of the neuromuscular junction.[53]

Toxicity

Although *in vitro* experiments suggested that sevoflurane would be metabolized extensively, *in vivo* metabolism is less significant because its tissue solubility is so low.[152] Metabolism of sevoflurane results in the production of inorganic fluoride ions and HFIP, as discussed above (see Pharmacokinetics). Although serum inorganic fluoride levels greater than 50 μmol L^{-1} have been recorded in humans following administration of sevoflurane, as in the case of enflurane (see Toxicity of enflurane) there have been no reports of renal failure.

Another possible mechanism by which sevoflurane anesthesia could cause nephrotoxicity in humans involves a degradation product called compound A. When sevoflurane is exposed to soda-lime or Baralyme®, it is absorbed and degraded to a variety of compounds (compounds A–E), of which two are produced in significant amounts (Fig 33.3), fluoromethyl-2,2-difluoro-1-(trifluoromethyl) vinyl ether (compound A) and fluoromethyl-2-methoxy-2,2-difluoro-l-(trifluoromethyl) ethyl ether (compound B).[153] Compound A has been shown to be toxic in rats (LD_{50} 1000 ppm after 1 h exposure), causing lung and renal damage, and there are fears it may also be toxic to humans. The lower the flow in a circle system, the higher will be the concentration of compound A. The addition of water to soda-lime and the use of partially exhausted soda-lime seem to reduce the production of compound A during low-flow anesthesia.[154,155] Although the addition of water reduces the carbon dioxide-absorbing capacity of the soda-lime, in practice this is not a problem.

The significance of the risk from compound A has yet to be established. One study, in which eight volunteers were given 1.25 MAC sevoflurane for 4h at a flow rate of 1 L min^{-1}, found an average maximum concentration of compound A of 39 ppm, and no significant increase in sensitive markers of renal function (proteinuria, albuminuria, glucosuria, and urinary a- and p-glutathione-S-transferase).[156] In contrast, other studies have found that exposure to 1.25 MAC at a flow rate of 2 L min^{-1} for both 4 h or 8 h was associated with transient renal injury (albuminuria, glucosuria, and raised levels of urinary a- and p-glutathione-S-transferase).[157,158] There was no evidence of renal injury following 2 h exposure.[157] While there is no evidence to date of serious long-term renal injury associated with the use of sevoflurane, it would seem prudent to avoid prolonged exposure to sevoflurane with fresh gas flows of less than 2 L min^{-1}.

Despite its relatively high metabolism, sevoflurane does not appear to be hepatotoxic. Several studies have found no change in transaminases in patients given sevoflurane for up to 4 h.[156,159] Of the halogenated anesthetic agents currently in widespread use, sevoflurane is the only one not metabolized to trifluoroacetic acid, which has been implicated in hepatotoxicity.

As with other volatile agents, sevoflurane should be avoided in patients susceptible to malignant hyperthermia. Sevoflurane triggers malignant hyperthermia in susceptible pigs, and there have also been several reports of malignant hyperthermia in humans following sevoflurane anesthesia.[123]

Clinical use

Sevoflurane compares quite favorably with isoflurane in most aspects, and it also has a number of significant advantages. It has a lower blood–gas solubility, so induction and recovery are slightly quicker. It offers good hemodynamic stability. It contains no chlorine ions and therefore it is environmentally friendly. However, the major advantage of sevoflurane over the currently used agents, with the exception of halothane, is that it is pleasant to inhale, and therefore it is suitable for inhalational induction. It has fewer side-effects than halothane, and there are the same concerns about toxicity as with halothane. Although there is some concern about renal toxicity from compound A as a result of degradation of sevoflurane by desiccated CO_2 absorbers, this has not proved to be a clinical problem even with low flows for prolonged periods.

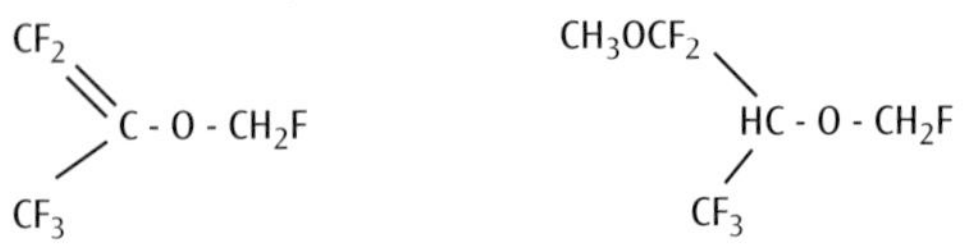

CF_2=C(CF₃)-O-CH_2F — Compound A

CH_3OCF_2-CH(CF_3)-O-CH_2F — Compound B

Figure 33.3 *Compounds A and B.*

DESFLURANE

Desflurane was another one in the series of 700 compounds produced by Dr Ross Terrell, which also included isoflurane and enflurane. Several factors delayed the development of desflurane. Initial production involved a potentially hazardous process utilizing elemental fluorine. Another disadvantage was that its SVP is very close to 1 atmosphere at room temperature. This precludes the use of conventional vaporizers for its administration. However, the structure of desflurane suggested that it may have very low blood–gas solubility, and the increasing frequency of day-case surgery and a desire for rapid recovery rekindled interest in desflurane. A safer process for synthesizing it was developed, and the results of the phase I evaluation were published in 1990.[1] Desflurane was subsequently approved for clinical use in the USA in 1992.

Physical properties

Desflurane is a fluorinated methyl ethyl ether. Like sevoflurane, it contains no chlorine or bromine ions and therefore should not deplete the ozone layer (Fig. 33.1). It is otherwise very similar to isoflurane, the only difference being the substitution of fluorine for the chlorine on the a-ethyl carbon (Fig. 33.1). As with enflurane, both soda-lime and Baralyme® can degrade it with the production of carbon monoxide (see Toxicity of enflurane).

Desflurane has a pungent odor, which makes it irritating and unpleasant to inhale. Where it differs significantly from the other modern volatile agents is in its boiling point of 22.8 °C, which is just above room temperature, and its SVP of 88.3 kPa (664 mmHg) at 20 °C. This means that it cannot be administered using a standard vaporizer. To facilitate the accurate delivery of desflurane, a new vaporizer has been developed in which the anesthetic agent is converted to a gas by heating it to a constant temperature and maintaining it at a constant pressure [about 200 kPa (1500 mmHg)]. It is then mixed in a controlled fashion with the carrier gas. The user interface is similar to that of the standard vaporizers, a dial that alters the resistance to outflow from the heated desflurane container, thereby altering the concentration delivered. Unlike other vaporizers, this vaporizer needs an external power source.

Desflurane has a blood–gas solubility coefficient of 0.42, the lowest of all the inhalational agents available with the exception of xenon, which means equilibration and recovery should occur quickly.[160] It has a lower solubility in rubber and plastic than halothane, isoflurane, or sevoflurane[4]. The MAC of desflurane varies from 4.58% to 7.25% depending on the stimulus used, and as with the other agents the MAC decreases with increasing age.[1,161,162] The MAC is reduced by nitrous oxide.[163]

Pharmacokinetics

Desflurane has the lowest blood–gas solubility of all the volatile anesthetic agents, and thus should result in the fastest induction and recovery. Yasuda *et al.*[11] have shown that equilibration of the F_A/F_I ratio of desflurane is higher than that of either isoflurane or halothane. At 30 min the F_A/F_I ratio of desflurane was 0.9 compared with 0.73 for isoflurane and 0.58 for halothane. The elimination of desflurane is also faster.[11]

The distribution of desflurane is similar to that of sevoflurane, isoflurane, and halothane, following a five-compartment model which, it has been postulated, may be as follows – the lungs, the vessel-rich group of organs, muscle, fat around the vessel-rich organs, and, finally, peripheral fat.[11]

The elimination of desflurane is almost exclusively through the lungs, with metabolism by the liver estimated to be less than 0.02%.[164] Increased levels of trifluoroacetic acid, a breakdown product of the halogenated ethers, have been found in the urine of patients given desflurane, but the levels were only about one-tenth of the levels seen after exposure to isoflurane.[165] However, this does suggest that there is a possibility of hepatotoxicity associated with desflurane (see Toxicity). Increased serum or urine fluoride levels have not been reported after exposure to desflurane.[166]

Pharmacodynamics

Central nervous system effects

The effects of desflurane on the EEG have been shown to be similar to those of isoflurane.[167] Both produce a dose-dependent suppression of the EEG. Desflurane produces burst suppression at concentrations greater than 1.24 MAC, and at a MAC of greater than 1.66 the EEG becomes isoelectric.[167] As in the case of isoflurane, there is no evidence of epileptiform activity. Desflurane does depress somatosensory evoked potentials in patients, with the amplitude but not latency decreasing with increasing doses.[168]

Studies in dogs have demonstrated that desflurane causes dose-dependent cerebral vasodilation and a dose-dependent reduction in cerebral metabolism.[169,170] It also impairs cerebral autoregulation to the same extent as isoflurane.[100]

Desflurane, like isoflurane, increases lumbar CSF pressure in normocapnic patients without an intracranial mass lesion.[101] In a comparative study carried out on patients with a supratentorial mass lesion given 1 MAC desflurane or isoflurane, ICP increased progressively in the desflurane group, even with hypocapnia, whereas there was no increase in the isoflurane group.[104]

To date, no clear advantage has been shown for any given inhalation agent over another in neurosurgical anesthesia. The more rapid recovery associated with desflurane anesthesia may offer a small advantage in patients undergoing prolonged neurosurgical procedures.

Respiratory effects

Desflurane is unsuitable for an inhalation induction because it is extremely irritating to the airway. Concentrations of 6% or more have been shown to cause coughing, breath-holding, and laryngospasm in both children and adults.[171,172]

In common with the other volatile agents, desflurane is a potent respiratory depressant. It causes a dose-dependent decrease in tidal volume and an increase in respiratory rate, with an overall reduction in minute alveolar ventilation.[1,173] $P_{a}CO_2$ increases and the ventilatory response to carbon dioxide is reduced. The intrapulmonary shunt fraction and the physiological dead space are also increased.[173] Despite the fact that desflurane is a potent airway irritant, the incidence of bronchospasm in asthmatics is not increased during the induction of anesthesia with desflurane, and *in vitro* studies suggest that, like other inhalation agents, desflurane causes concentration-dependent bronchodilation.[174–176]

Cardiovascular effects

Desflurane causes a dose-dependent tachycardia in humans that is associated with a depression in myocardial contractility and a decrease in the SVR resulting from peripheral vasodilation.[1,177] These changes occur at concentrations ranging from 0.83–1.66 MAC.[177] In ventilated patients, the cardiac index remains unchanged, and thus systemic blood pressure falls. In spontaneously breathing patients, the cardiac index is increased.[178] The administration of equivalent MAC doses in 60% nitrous oxide results in higher central venous and systemic pressures and higher left ventricular stroke work index than when desflurane alone is used.[179] Studies in dogs suggest that splanchnic blood flow is well preserved. Although there may be a slight fall in portal blood flow, hepatic artery blood flow is maintained and there is no change in renal blood flow at concentrations up to 2 MAC.[163] Desflurane is a direct coronary vasodilator and produces an overall reduction in cardiac work.[180,181] The potential improvement in coronary blood flow due to coronary vasodilation is offset by the tachycardia and fall in coronary perfusion pressure resulting from peripheral vasodilation. Although this also raises the potential for coronary steal, research using a canine model of coronary artery disease failed to find any evidence for this.[182] There is some evidence however that the use of desflurane is associated with an increased incidence of myocardial ischemia in patients with ischemic heart disease, at least when compared with a sufentanil-based technique.[183]

A rapid increase in the concentration of desflurane to greater than 1 MAC will cause an increase in heart rate and blood pressure similar to that seen with isoflurane.[148] This transient cardiovascular stimulation is greater with desflurane than with isoflurane, and it is reduced by nitrous oxide.[179,184,185] Although the mechanism of this reaction is not fully understood, there is evidence that it is mediated by receptors at multiple sites, which include the upper airway, the lungs, and systemic receptors.[186] It can be significantly attenuated by small doses of opioids, clonidine, or esmolol.[187] Desflurane does not sensitize the myocardium to epinephrine, although it may slow atrioventricular conduction or induce a junctional bradycardia.[181,188,189]

Neuromuscular effects

Desflurane significantly depresses neuromuscular function. It reduces the force of contraction of the adductor pollicis muscle and increases the degree of tetanic fade.[190] It can provide sufficient relaxation to allow tracheal intubation. This effect is independent of the duration of anesthesia. It also potentiates the action of nondepolarizing muscle relaxants to the same degree as isoflurane.[190]

Toxicity

Desflurane has very low blood–gas and blood–tissue solubility, is very stable and undergoes minimal metabolism. These are properties that should favor low toxicity, and this does appear to be the case.

However, a very small amount of desflurane is metabolized with the production of trifluoroacetic acid, which, as discussed above, may interact with hepatic proteins and induce an immune response in susceptible patients.[63] Sera from patients with a diagnosis of halothane hepatitis have been shown to contain circulating antibodies to liver microsomal proteins modified by trifluoroacetic acid.[191] Although the risk with desflurane is likely to be very low because of its extremely low metabolism, there has, nonetheless, been a case of nonfatal hepatitis associated with desflurane.[192] It is possible that this particular patient had previously been sensitized by exposure to halothane.

There is no evidence of renal toxicity with desflurane, even after prolonged exposure. Markers of renal function (albuminuria, urinary a-glutathione-transferase, and serum creatinine and blood urea nitrogen) were measured before and for up to 7 days after exposure to 8 h of MAC 1.25% desflurane, and no evidence of renal injury was found.[158]

Desflurane, like enflurane and isoflurane, is degraded under certain conditions by CO_2 absorbers, and carbon monoxide is produced. In common with the other halogenated anesthetic agents, desflurane is a trigger agent for malignant hyperthermia. There have been several reports of this occurring following desflurane anesthesia.[193]

Clinical use

Desflurane has the lowest blood–gas solubility of the halogenated anesthetic agents, and therefore provides the most rapid induction and recovery. It undergoes minimal metabolism, and thus the risk of toxicity from metabolites is expected to be very low, although it is metabolized to TFA, which has been implicated in hepatotoxicity. Desflurane does also have some significant disadvantages, however. It is quite irritating to the airway and therefore it is not suitable for an inhalation induction. Rapid changes in the inspired concentration are associated with sympathetic stimulation, resulting in hypertension and tachycardia, and there are also some concerns about its use in patients with ischemic heart disease. It offers no advantage over sevoflurane except for a lower blood–gas solubility coefficient, a property that may have no significant clinical impact.

NITROUS OXIDE (N_2O)

The use of nitrous oxide dates back to the earliest days of anesthesia, and it is a reflection of its safety and versatility that it is still being used today. However, nitrous oxide is a potent greenhouse gas, and environmental considerations will probably result in a reduction in its use in the future.

Physical properties

Nitrous oxide has a molecular weight of 44 and its boiling point is −88 °C. It is a colorless, sweet-smelling, and nonirritant gas, slightly heavier than air. It is nonflammable, although it does support combustion, even in the absence of oxygen. It is stable in the presence of soda-lime.

Nitrous oxide is supplied in two different ways, as pure nitrous oxide and as a mixture of equal parts nitrous oxide and oxygen (Entonox). Nitrous oxide alone is supplied and stored in cylinders, under pressure of 5000 kPa at 20 °C. A full cylinder at room temperature contains liquid, not vapor. For this reason, the cylinder should be kept upright when in use. As the gas is used, the cylinder will cool because energy is required to convert the liquid inside the cylinder to gas. The pressure in a nitrous oxide cylinder will not reflect how much nitrous oxide is in the cylinder as long as there is liquid nitrous oxide in the cylinder. The contents of a nitrous oxide cylinder can only be ascertained by weighing until it is nearly empty and contains only gas. At this stage the pressure inside the cylinder begins to fall, and the pressure gauge will then give some indication of contents of the cylinder. The critical temperature of nitrous oxide is 36.5 °C. If it is stored at temperatures above this it can only exist in gaseous form.

As mentioned above, nitrous oxide is also available as a 50:50 mixture with oxygen. Nitrous oxide–oxygen mixture is supplied in cylinders pressurized to 15 000 kPa at 20 °C. Contrary to what might be expected, both gases are in gaseous form. The oxygen alters the behavior of the nitrous oxide so that it does not liquefy at this pressure unless the temperature drops to below −7 °C. Below −7 °C the nitrous oxide will liquefy and, as the oxygen remains in gaseous form, the two gases separate out. This will result in high-concentration oxygen gas over nitrous oxide liquid. If the cylinder is used at this time in the upright position, high concentration oxygen will be released first, leaving ultimately a hypoxic mixture of oxygen in nitrous oxide behind. Where there is a possibility of a cylinder of nitrous oxide in oxygen having been exposed to a temperature of −7 °C or below, thorough mixing of the gases is necessary before the cylinder is used.

The MAC of nitrous oxide is 105%. This was established experimentally by putting volunteers in a pressure chamber and subjecting them to a pressure of 2 atmospheres. The MAC required at 2 atmospheres (55%) is half that which is required at atmospheric pressure.

The blood–gas solubility coefficient of nitrous oxide is 0.42, which is less than that of any of the other available inhalational agents with the exception of xenon. Nitrous oxide does not undergo any metabolism.

It is eliminated unchanged from the body, predominantly through the lungs.

Pharmacokinetics

Nitrous oxide has a low blood–gas solubility compared with most other volatile agents. This ensures rapid equilibration of the F_A/F_I ratio. However, it is still much more soluble in blood than nitrogen, and because of the concentrations generally used this has several implications, especially during induction and recovery. When a patient changes from breathing a high concentration of nitrogen to breathing a high concentration of nitrous oxide, the concentration of nitrous oxide in the alveoli rises rapidly. Because nitrous oxide is more soluble in blood than nitrogen, the volume of nitrous oxide taken up by the blood is greater than the volume of nitrogen entering the alveoli from the blood. The alveoli therefore get smaller, and the fractional concentration of the remaining gases in the alveoli increases. Although the volume of nitrous oxide has decreased, the concentration does not diminish to the same degree because the volume of the alveoli has also decreased. The relative concentrations of other gases in the alveoli are also increased, including CO_2. If another anesthetic agent is given with nitrous oxide, the relative concentration of this will also increase. This phenomenon is referred to as the "second gas effect." During the early part of induction, using high concentrations of nitrous oxide, gas volumes of the order of 1 L min^{-1} may be transferred from the lungs to blood.[194] It has been demonstrated that the higher the inspired concentration of nitrous oxide, the more rapidly the alveolar concentration approaches the inspired concentration. This has been referred to as the "concentration effect."[194]

At the end of anesthesia, the opposite occurs. If the patient is allowed to breathe air, nitrous oxide will diffuse into the alveoli faster than the blood can take up nitrogen. The volume of the alveoli will increase as the nitrous oxide diffuses into the lung, and the concentration of all the other gases in the alveoli, including oxygen, will fall. This could result in hypoxia, and is generally referred to as "diffusion hypoxia" or the Fink effect.

The other consideration in relation to this is that, if there is an enclosed gas-filled cavity within the body, then when nitrous oxide is given it may also diffuse into this more quickly than the gas that it originally contained can diffuse out. This can cause the gas-filled area to expand significantly, often with serious consequences. Examples are a pneumothorax, bullae within the lung, gas-filled bowel, gas bubbles in the eye following retinal surgery or in the middle ear in the case of Eustachian tube blockage. Similarly, in patients at risk from gas embolism, the presence of nitrous oxide in the blood would increase the size of any gas embolus that might occur.

Pharmacodynamics

Central nervous system effects

Evidence to date suggests that, when nitrous oxide is administered as the sole agent, it will produce significant increases in CBF and ICP. The addition of nitrous oxide to patients already anesthetized with halothane has been associated with significant increases in CBF.[195] The replacement of isoflurane with an equipotent concentration of nitrous oxide in patients with brain tumors has also resulted in a significant increase in ICP.[196] The administration of 50% nitrous oxide in oxygen to patients with severe head injuries has resulted in a significant increase in ICP.[197] When intravenous anesthetic agents are administered in conjunction with nitrous oxide, these effects on ICP may be greatly attenuated.[17] The other possibility to consider when nitrous oxide is used for neurosurgery is that it may diffuse into air pockets left within the skull following closure of the wound.

The recorded effect of nitrous oxide on cerebral metabolism is variable, probably because in many cases the data have been collected from patients already anesthetized with agents that themselves have an impact on cerebral metabolism. On balance, if it has any significant effect, nitrous oxide probably results in a slight increase in cerebral metabolism.[19] Despite these potential disadvantages, the use of nitrous oxide in patients undergoing neurosurgery and at risk from raised ICP remains an established and accepted practice.

While there is some evidence that epileptic activity is associated with nitrous oxide administration in animals, EEG studies have not demonstrated any evidence of seizure activity in humans.[19] Increasing concentrations of nitrous oxide have been shown to reduce the amplitude of visual and somatosensory evoked potentials, and to increase the latency of visual evoked potentials.[198]

Respiratory effects

Nitrous oxide is pleasant to inhale and not irritating to the airway. Its pharmacokinetic characteristics make it very useful as a supplement to volatile agents, particularly for inhalational induction. It increases the uptake of the accompanying agent in addition to reducing the MAC.

Nitrous oxide should be used with caution in patients with respiratory disease. It diffuses into closed air spaces, causing significant expansion of lung bullae with prolonged time constants, producing a clinical condition that can mimic a tension pneumothorax. When given alone, nitrous oxide has a minimal effect on ventilation. It does not alter the ventilatory response to changes in CO_2, although it does significantly reduce the ventilatory response to hypoxia.[199] As discussed above, when nitrous oxide is discontinued at the end of anesthesia, supplementary oxygen should be given because of the risk of diffusion hypoxia.

Nitrous oxide produces a small reduction in hypoxic pulmonary vasoconstriction. This may increase the right to left shunt in one-lung ventilation.[200] However, a higher inspired oxygen requirement during one-lung anesthesia very often precludes the administration of high concentrations of nitrous oxide.

Cardiovascular effects

Nitrous oxide is a direct myocardial depressant and causes a reduction in cardiac output. However, myocardial depression is offset by increased sympathetic nerve activity, resulting in peripheral vasoconstriction, so that overall there is minimal change in blood pressure.[201,202] Urinary catecholamines, plasma norepinephrine (noradrenaline), and peripheral vascular resistance have all been shown to increase during the administration of nitrous oxide. Although nitrous oxide diminishes the baroreceptor-mediated tachycardia that normally occurs in response to hypotension, it does not affect the baroreceptor-mediated increase in sympathetic nerve activity.

Toxicity

Although nitrous oxide is metabolized minimally, it does interact with vitamin B_{12}. It converts the cobalt in vitamin B_{12} from the monovalent form to the bivalent form. In the bivalent form, vitamin B_{12} can no longer carry out its function as a methyl carrier. This oxidation is irreversible, and recovery depends on the absorption of replacement vitamin B_{12}. Vitamin B_{12} is a cofactor for methionine synthase and is involved in the production of 5,10-methylene tetrahydrofolate, which is essential to DNA synthesis. Chronic exposure to high concentrations of nitrous oxide could result in a condition resembling subacute combined degeneration of the cord. Shorter term exposure results in megaloblastic anemia and agranulocytosis.[203] There is considerable interspecies variation. In humans, exposure for less than 30 min will not cause any measurable change in methionine synthase activity; exposure for more than 2h will probably interfere with methionine synthase activity, this effect increasing with increasing duration of exposure. There is likely to be considerable interindividual variability. Patients have received nitrous oxide for up to 24 h without coming to any harm, although it is likely that after this degree of exposure there would be megaloblastic marrow changes, and there has been a report of reduced neutrophil counts.[203] The inhibition of methionine synthase will take some time to recover – this should be considered if exposure to nitrous oxide is likely to be repeated within 3 days. The administration of folic acid 30 mg twice a day may prevent the development of the megaloblastic changes associated with nitrous oxide.[203]

Nitrous oxide is not thought to be a trigger agent for malignant hyperthermia.[60]

Clinical use

Nitrous oxide is a good analgesic, and the 50:50 nitrous oxide–oxygen mixture is widely used to alleviate pain in labor and to facilitate minor surgical procedures. It is a very weak anesthetic and is likely to be inadequate as a sole anesthetic agent. When used for anesthesia, it is generally used in combination with a second agent. It reduces the MAC of the second agent, reducing the amount required for effect, and it also increases the uptake (and elimination) of the other agent by the second gas effect, increasing the rate of induction and recovery.

XENON

The anesthetic properties of xenon were first recognized more than 50 years ago. Cullen and Groaa[204] first used it as an anesthetic in 1951, in an 81-year-old man undergoing orchidectomy. They administered xenon at a concentration of 80%, which appears to have been sufficient for anesthesia. Following the procedure, the patient was conscious at 2 min and fully oriented 5 min after xenon administration was stopped.

The main factor limiting the use of xenon is availability. Although it is an atmospheric gas, it only constitutes 0.0000087% of the atmosphere.[205] It is produced by fractional distillation of air, often as a byproduct of oxygen production. It has found a variety of applications in the modern world, from X-ray tubes to high-intensity lights. Radioactive xenon has been used for many years in cerebral blood flow studies, in the measurement of lung volume, and for some time for routine anesthesia in Germany, The Netherlands, Sweden, and Russia.

Physical properties

Xenon is one of the noble gases. Its atomic number is 54 and its molecular weight is 131.3. It is colorless, odorless, nonirritating, and is four times heavier than air. It also has a higher viscosity than nitrogen. It freezes at −111.9 °C and boils at −107.1 °C. It is nonflammable and does not support combustion. Being extremely unreactive, it does not interact with soda-lime, but it will diffuse readily through rubber.[205] In view of its limited availability, this has significant implications.

Xenon is more potent than nitrous oxide with a MAC of 71%, and therefore it should be possible, at least in some patients, to use it as the sole anesthetic agent. At 0.115, its blood–gas partition coefficient is the lowest coefficient of all the available agents.[206]

Pharmacokinetics

Xenon is a more potent anesthetic gas than nitrous oxide and, even when it cannot be used as the sole agent, it should need less supplementing than nitrous oxide.

Although xenon has a blood–gas solubility coefficient of less than one-third of that of nitrous oxide, there is still the potential for diffusion hypoxia during recovery, and it should also offer the benefit of the concentration effect and the second gas effect during induction, as discussed for nitrous oxide (see Pharmacokinetics of nitrous oxide). Similar considerations would apply as with nitrous oxide regarding diffusion into gas-filled cavities within the body. However, the lower blood–gas partition coefficient of xenon should result in rapid induction and recovery, and this indeed does appear to be the case.[206] Xenon is a noble gas, which implies that it is extremely unlikely to be involved in any biochemical reactions. The elimination of xenon is mainly through the lungs.[205]

Pharmacodynamics

Central nervous system effects

Studies carried out to date suggest that, although the effect is variable, in most cases xenon causes an increase in CBF.[207] In patients undergoing abdominal surgery with no intracranial pathology, it was found using transcranial Doppler that the administration of 65% xenon increased CBF.[208] Independent of its anesthetic effect, xenon is radiodense, and inhaled stable xenon has been used for a number of years to enhance computed tomography images and thereby facilitate measurement of CBF and its regional distribution in patients with severe head injury. However, a number of studies have demonstrated clearly that xenon can increase ICP. A study of 13 patients 3 days after severe head injury and sedated with barbiturates found that inhalation of 33% xenon increased ICP in all patients, despite moderate hyperventilation.[207] Of these 13 patients, the raised ICP was associated with a reduction in CPP in 11. Although hyperventilation reduced ICP, it did not attenuate the effect of xenon on the ICP. On the basis of these data, xenon should be used with caution in patients at risk from raised ICP.

Respiratory effects

Xenon is colorless and odorless, and therefore, like nitrous oxide, it should be useful for inhalational induction. However, the density of xenon is four times greater than that of nitrogen and three times greater than that of nitrous oxide, and it also has a higher viscosity than both nitrogen and nitrous oxide. Gas density and viscosity both have a significant effect on pulmonary mechanics, with higher values increasing airway resistance. Animal studies have confirmed that ventilation with 70% xenon is associated with moderately increased airway resistance, and under conditions of induced bronchoconstriction airway pressures were also significantly higher with xenon than with equivalent concentrations of nitrous oxide or nitrogen.[209] Caution should therefore be exercised when administering xenon to patients with respiratory disease, and it probably should not be used for patients in whom inhalation induction is indicated because of a narrowing or an obstruction of the airway. Similar considerations also apply in terms of expansion of emphysematous bullae and diffusion hypoxia with xenon as with nitrous oxide, although because of the lower solubility of xenon the effect will not be as great (see Pharmacokinetics of nitrous oxide).

Central control of ventilation is altered by xenon. Respiratory rate is slowed and there is a compensatory increase in tidal volume, with little change in minute ventilation.[205]

Cardiovascular effects

The evidence currently available indicates that xenon provides good hemodynamic stability with little change in blood pressure. An assessment of left ventricular function using transesophageal echocardiography found no change during administration of 65% xenon.[208] Xenon has also been shown to cause a slight reduction in heart rate, but otherwise it has no effect on the heart.[205]

Toxicity

There are limited data on the effects of long-term exposure to xenon, but it is chemically unreactive. It does not undergo any metabolism in the body, and therefore it is likely to have very low, if any, toxicity. There is some evidence that it may potentiate platelet aggregation at pressures greater than 2 atmospheres.[205]

Current available evidence suggests that xenon is not a trigger for malignant hyperthermia.[205]

Clinical use

Xenon, like nitrous oxide, appears to be quite a good analgesic and has been shown to reduce opiate requirements.[205,210]

It has many of the properties of nitrous oxide, with the added advantages that it is more potent and is environmentally friendly. The main problem with xenon is availability – it is very expensive to produce. Future use of xenon is likely to involve the use of very low-flow systems and may involve reclamation of the xenon. A number of completely closed systems have been designed, which aim to match gas flow with patient uptake. However, even these systems will require a flush from time to time to prevent the build-up of other gases. The other option which is also being considered is to reclaim xenon from the waste gases. Two different systems for recycling xenon have been described.[205]

Xenon has many of the properties of an ideal anesthetic. It also has the advantage that it is an atmospheric gas, so that its use is not associated with the same environmental concerns as with some of the other inhalational agents. It seems likely that technological developments will soon make delivery and recovery of xenon both feasible and economical, thereby facilitating more widespread use of xenon as an anesthetic agent.

MECHANISM OF ACTION OF INHALATIONAL ANESTHETICS

The variability in the structure and physical properties of currently identified agents that produce anesthesia in humans is such that it seems unlikely that there is a common mode of action. However, what is striking is the link between lipid solubility and potency. This was first recognized by Meyer and Overton at the turn of the last century. They demonstrated that the potency of an anesthetic agent is directly related to its lipid solubility, which raised the possibility that all inhalational anesthetic agents may have a common site of action. Early studies of the mechanism of anesthetics were based around this theory, with the presumption being that the mechanism of action must be lipid based. It was suggested that anesthetic agents might interrupt lipid interactions in cell membranes, or cause an expansion of the cell membrane, resulting in the closure of channels across it. A variety of solvents were tested in the hope of finding a correlation between lipid solubility and anesthetic potency, thus identifying the site of action, but without much success. The other factor that influenced the development of theories of how anesthetic agents exerted their effect was the observation that the action of anesthetics can be reversed by the application of high pressures.

It has recently been realized that a major problem with the early search for the mechanism of action of anesthetic agents was that the experiments were carried out at room temperature based on gas phase concentrations rather than aqueous phase concentrations. The gas phase potency of anesthetic agents is much greater at room temperature than at body temperature, which means that the actual concentrations being used were much higher than would be found clinically.[211] The aqueous phase potency does not vary with temperature to the same degree.

However, it was the development of agents that did not follow the Meyer–Overton rule, and particularly the isolation of optical isomers of anesthetic agents, which finally undermined these early theories on the mechanism of action of inhalation anesthetics, and subsequent research has focused on other possible mechanisms. Many volatile anesthetic agents have an asymmetric carbon atom and can therefore exist as optically active isomers. The general anesthetic effect of many optical agents including etomidate, ketamine, barbiturates, and isoflurane, is stereoselective to a variable degree.[212] These agents are generally supplied as racemic mixtures. Recently, isolation of the two enantiomers of isoflurane has allowed their individual potencies to be assessed. The dextrorotatory (+) enantiomer was found to be 53% more potent than the levorotatory (–) enantiomer, with a MAC of 1.06% compared with a MAC of 1.62%.[212] By comparing the relative effect of optical isomers on various receptors *in vitro* with their clinical effect *in vivo*, it should be possible to start to identify their sites of action. The fact that both the enantiomers of isoflurane have similar lipid solubility is an argument against a lipid site of action. In addition, studies have shown that the concentrations of general anesthetics used to produce anesthesia have a minimal effect on lipid bilayers, and a lipid-free protein that is inhibited by the concentrations of volatile agents that are normally used for anesthesia has been discovered. The effects of clinical concentrations of anesthetics on lipid bilayers are so small that they can be mimicked by a 1 °C rise in temperature.[211]

It is now apparent that anesthetic agents exert an effect at a variety of sites throughout the CNS, at both central and spinal level. It has long been apparent that anesthetic agents modify calcium flux. More recently, it has become apparent that they also modify potassium flux. It is significant that, although they may have some effect on impulse conduction through axons, their main effect seems to be the inhibition of synaptic transmission. Axonal conduction is less sensitive to anesthetics than synaptic transmission.[212] There is now evidence that anesthetics may exert their effect through neurotransmitter-gated ion channels, which tend to be concentrated at synapses.[211] While these ligand-gated ion channels are sensitive to anesthetic agents, the voltage-gated ion channels that are responsible for impulse propagation seem to be quite resistant, with the exception of some calcium channels.[211]

A number of neurotransmitter-gated receptor channels have been shown to be sensitive to modulation by general anesthetics.[213] They are the neuronal and muscle nicotinic acetylcholine receptor channels, serotonin 5-HT_3 receptor channels, the inhibitory gamma-aminobutyric acid type A ($GABA_A$) receptor channel, and the glycine receptor channel. These channels are all structurally quite similar, having homologous amino acid sequences and a pentameric structure. Each channel is made up of five subunits (Fig. 33.4). The subunits have four membrane-spanning regions (M1–M4), an extracellular amino terminus, and a small extracellular carboxy-terminal region. The five subunits come together at the M2 region, forming an aqueous pore through which the ions move. The agonist binds at the extracellular amino-terminal domain and initiates small rotations in these domains, changing the conformation of the M2 α-helices, which in turn results in opening of the channel.

GABA receptors are influenced by a wide variety of CNS depressants, including benzodiazepines and barbiturates. There are at least two different types of GABA receptors. GABA appears to be the most significant inhibitory neurotransmitter in the mammalian brain. Binding of GABA enhances the inward movement of chloride ions, resulting in hyperpolarization. It is likely that anesthetics increase the affinity of the receptors for GABA. At levels of GABA too low to produce an effect, the addition of halothane increases GABA-induced currents.[211]

Anesthetic agents appear to inhibit nicotinic receptors. This may also explain their effect on the neuromuscular junction. Neuronal nicotinic

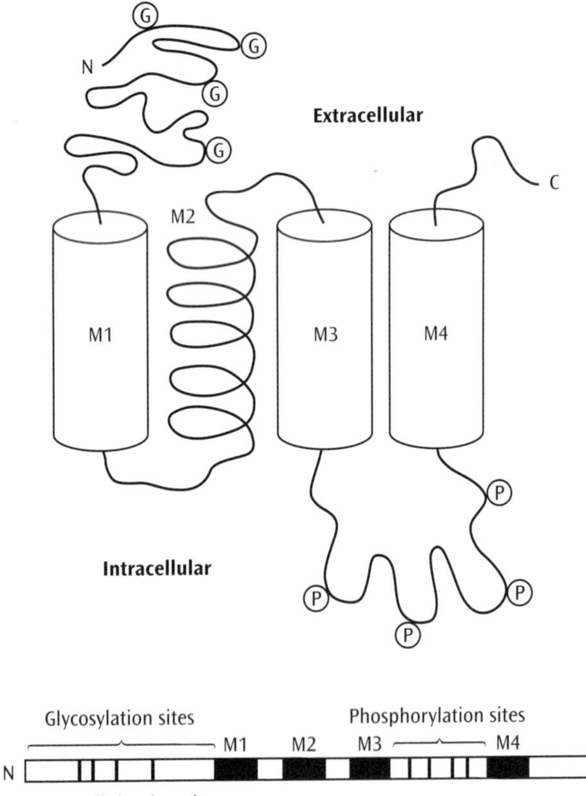

Figure 33.4 *Diagrammatic representation of a subunit of a neurotransmitter-gated ion channel, with four membrane-spanning regions (M1–4). Each channel is made up of five of these subunits. (Reproduced with permission from Franks and Lieb.[213])*

receptors are much more sensitive to general anesthetics than are muscle nicotinic acetylcholine receptors.[212] Much less is known about the effects of anesthetics on glycine and 5-HT_3 receptor channels.

OCCUPATIONAL EXPOSURE

The use of inhalational anesthetics in enclosed areas without any system to prevent their release into the local environment is undesirable and may be potentially hazardous to personnel working in that area. With the earlier anesthetic agents, the major worry was the risk of fire and explosion. This is no longer such a problem, and the major concern now is the effect of long-term exposure to the agents themselves, both because of their potential effect on performance and because of the possible deleterious effect of chronic exposure to trace levels. To date there is no evidence that any of the inhalational agents are carcinogenic. There was some concern that female operating room personnel exposed to trace levels of anesthetic agents were more at risk of spontaneous abortion or giving birth to a child with congenital abnormalities. Nitrous oxide was thought to be the most likely cause. Whether this is indeed the case has never been conclusively established.

Common sense dictates, however, that, where possible, unnecessary exposure should be avoided. Most modern operating rooms are fitted with scavenging systems or absorbers that, for the most part, prevent anesthetic agents polluting the environment. In addition, the increasing use of low fresh gas flows and closed breathing systems also reduces the pollution risk.

REFERENCES

1. Jones RM. Desflurane and sevoflurane: inhalation anaesthetics for this decade. *Br J Anaesth* 1990; **65:** 527–36.
2. Johnstone M. The human cardiovascular response to Fluothane anaesthesia. *Br J Anaesth* 1956; **28:** 392–6.
3. Seiflow GHF. The non-inflammability of Fluothane. *Br J Anaesth* 1957; **29:** 438.
4. Targ AG, Yasuda N, Eger EI II. Solubility of I-653, sevoflurane, isoflurane, and halothane in plastics and rubber composing a conventional anesthetic circuit. *Anesth Analg* 1989; **69:** 218–25.
5. Merkel G, Eger EI II. A comparative study of halothane and halopropane anesthesia. Including method for determining equipotency. *Anesthesiology* 1963; **24:** 346–57.
6. Saidman LJ, Eger EI 2nd. Effect of nitrous oxide and narcotic premedication on the alveolar concentration of halothane required for anesthesia. *Anesthesiology* 1964; **25:** 302–6.
7. Gregory GA, Eger EI 2nd, Munson ES. The relationship between age and halothane requirements in man. *Anesthesiology* 1969; **30:** 488–91.
8. Steffey EP, Eger EI II. Hyperthermia and halothane MAC in the dog. *Anesthesiology* 1974; **14:** 392–6.
9. Quasha AL, Eger EI II, Tinker JH. Determination and applications of MAC. *Anesthesiology* 1980; **53:** 315–34.
10. Lerman J, Gregory GA, Willis MM, Eger EI. Age and solubility of volatile anesthetics in blood. *Anesthesiology* 1984; **61:** 139–43.
11. Yasuda N, Lockhart SH, Eger EI, *et al.* Kinetics of desflurane, isoflurane and halothane in humans. *Anesthesiology* 1991; **74:** 489–98.
12. Carpenter RL, Eger EI 2nd, Johnson BH, *et al.* The extent of metabolism of inhaled anesthetics in humans. *Anesthesiology* 1986; **65:** 201–5.
13. Frost EAM. Inhalational anaesthetic agents in neurosurgery. *Br J Anaesth* 1984; **56:** 47S–56S.
14. Miletich DJ, Ivankovich AD, Albrecht RF, *et al.* Absence of autoregulation of cerebral blood flow during halothane and enflurane anesthesia. *Anesth Analg* 1976 **55:** 100–6.
15. Artru AA. Effects of halothane and fentanyl on the rate of CSF production in dogs. *Anesth Analg* 1983; **62:** 581–5.
16. Adams RW, Gronert GA, Sundt TM, Michenfelder JD. Halothane, hypocapnia and cerebrospinal fluid pressure in neurosurgery. *Anesthesiology* 1972; **37:** 510–57.
17. Misfeldt BB, Jorgensen PB, Rishoj M. The effect of nitrous oxide and halothane upon the intracranial pressure in hypocapnic patients with intracranial disorders. *Br J Anaesth* 1974; **46:** 853–8.
18. Stullken EH, Milde JH, Michenfelder JD, Tinker JH. The nonlinear responses of cerebral metabolism to low concentrations of halothane, enflurane, isoflurane and thiopental. *Anesthesiology* 1977; **46:** 28–34.
19. Modica PA, Tempelhoff R, White PF. Pro- and anticonvulsant effects of anaesthetics (Part 1). *Anesth Analg* 1990; **70:** 303–15.
20. Uhl RR, Squires KC, Bruce DL, Starr A. Effect of halothane anaesthesia on the human cortical visual evoked response. *Anesthesiology* 1980; **53:** 273–6.
21. Thornton C, Heneghan CPH, James MFM, Jones JG. Effects of halothane or enflurane with controlled ventilation on auditory evoked potentials. *Br J Anaesth* 1984; **56:** 315–23.
22. Inomata S, Yamashita S, Toyooka H, *et al.* Anaesthetic induction time for tracheal intubation using sevoflurane or halothane in children. *Anaesthesia* 1998; **53:** 440–5.
23. Black GW. A review of the pharmacology of halothane. *Br J Anaesth* 1965; **37:** 688–705.
24. Knill RL, Gelb AW. Ventilatory responses to hypoxia and hypercapnia during halothane sedation and anaesthesia in man. *Anesthesiology* 1978; **49:** 244–51.
25. Dahan A, Teppema L. Influence of low-dose anaesthetic agents on ventilatory control: where do we stand? *Br J Anaesth* 1999; **83:** 199–201.
26. Tokics L, Hedenstierna G, Strandberg A, Brismar B, Lundquist H. Lung collapse and gas exchange during general anesthesia: effects of spontaneous breathing, muscle paralysis, and positive end-expiratory pressure. *Anesthesiology* 1987; **66:** 157–67.
27. Rogers DN, Benumof JL. Halothane and isoflurane do not decrease PaO2 during one-lung ventilation in intravenously anesthetised patients. *Anesth Analg* 1985; **64:** 946–54.
28. Johnson D, Mayers I. The effects of halothane in hypoxic pulmonary vasoconstriction. *Anesthesiology* 1990; **72:** 125–33.
29. Hirshman CA, Edelstein G, Peetz S, *et al.* Mechanism of action of inhalational anesthesia on airways. *Anesthesiology* 1982; **56:** 107–11.

30. Katoh T, Ikeda K. A comparison of sevoflurane with halothane, enflurane and isoflurane on bronchoconstriction caused by histamine. *Can J Anesth* 1994; **41:** 1214–19.
31. Roizen MF, Stevens WC. Multiform ventricular tachycardia due to the interaction of aminophylline and halothane. *Anesth Analg* 1978; **57:** 738–41.
32. Epstein RM, Deutsch S, Cooperman LH, *et al.* Splanchnic circulation during halothane anesthesia in normal man. *Anesthesiology* 1966; **27:** 654–61.
33. Deutsch S, Goldberg M, Stephen GW, Wu WH. Effects of halothane anesthesia on renal function in normal man. *Anesthesiology* 1966; **27:** 793–804.
34. Gelman S, Fowler KC, Smith LR. Regional blood flow during isoflurane and halothane anaesthesia. *Anesth Analg* 1984; **63:** 557–65.
35. Hickey RF, Sybert SE, Verrier ED, Casong BA. Effects of halothane, enflurane, and isoflurane on coronary blood flow autoregulation and coronary vascular reserve in the canine heart. *Anesthesiology* 1988; **68:** 21–30.
36. Eger EI II, Smith NT, Stoelting RK, *et al.* Cardiovascular effects of halothane in man. *Anesthesiology* 1970; **32:** 396–409.
37. Rusy BF, Komai H. Anesthetic depression of myocardial contractility: a review of possible mechanisms. *Anesthesiology* 1987; **67:** 45–66.
38. Housmans PR, Murat I. Comparative effects of halothane, enflurane and isoflurane at equipotent anesthetic concentrations on isolated ventricular myocardium of the ferret. *Anesthesiology* 1988; **69:** 451–63.
39. Atlee JL, Bosjnak ZJ. Mechanisms for cardiac dysrhythmias during anesthesia. *Anesthesiology* 1990; **72:** 347–74.
40. Duke PC, Fownes D, Wade JG. Halothane depresses baroreflex contro1 of heart rate in man. *Anesthesiology* 1977; **46:** 184–7.
41. Merlos JR, Bosnjak ZJ, Purtock RV, *et al.* Halothane and enflurane effects on SA node cells. *Anesthesiology* 1980; **53:** S143.
42. Atlee JL III, Peterson ML. Halothane, isoflurane, enflurane and A-V conduction: awake vs. anesthesia. *Anesthesiology* 1982; **57:**A15.
43. Katz RL, Katz GJ. Surgical infiltration of pressor drugs and their interaction with volatile anaesthetics. *Br J Anaesth* 1966; **38:**712–718.
44. Black GW, Linde HW, Dripps RD, Price HL. Circulatory changes accompanying respiratory acidosis during halothane (Fluothane) anaesthesia in man. *Br J Anaesth* 1959; **31:** 238–46.
45. Johnston RR, Eger EI, Wilson C. A comparative interaction of epinephrine with enflurane, isoflurane and halothane in man. *Anesth Analg* 1976; **55:** 709–12.
46. Willatts DG, Harrison AR, Groom JF, Crowther A. Cardiac arrhythmias during outpatient dental anaesthesia: comparison of halothane with enflurane. *Br J Anaesth* 1983; **55:** 399–403.
47. Hutchison GL, Davies CA, Main G, Gray IG. Incidence of arrhythmias in dental anaesthesia: a crossover comparison of halothane and isoflurane. *Br J Anaesth* 1989; **62:** 518–521.
48. Kapur PA, Bloor BC, Flacke WE, Olewine SK. Comparison of cardiovascular responses to verapamil during enflurane, isoflurane, or halothane anesthesia in the dog. *Anesthesiology* 1984; **61:**156–60.
49. Maze M, Mason DM, Kates K. Verapamil decreases MAC for halothane in dogs. *Anesthesiology* 1983; **59:** 327–9.
50. Durand PG, Lehot JJ, Foëx P. Calcium-channel blockers and anaesthesia. *Can J Anesth* 1991; **38:** 75–89.
51. Ross S, Foëx P. Protective effects of anaesthetics in reversible and irreversible ischaemia–reperfusion injury. *Br J Anaesth* 1999; **82:** 622–32.
52. Gissen AJ, Karis JH, Nastuk WL. Effect of halothane on neuromuscular transmission. *JAMA* 1966; **197:** 116–20.
53. Saitoh Y, Toyooka H, Amaha K. Recoveries of post-tetanic twitch and train-of-four responses after administration of vecuronium with different inhalation anaesthetics and neurolept-anaesthesia. *Brit J Anaesth* 1993; **70:** 402–4.
54. Jones RM. Clinical comparison of inhalation anaesthetic agents. *Br J Anaesth* 1984; **56:** 57S–60S.
55. Bay J, Nunn JF, Prys-Roberts C. Factors influencing arterial PO_2 during recovery from anaesthesia. *Br J Anaesth* 1968; **40:** 398–407.
56. Soliman MG, Gillies DMM. Muscular hyperactivity after general anaesthesia. *Can Anesth Soc J* 1972; **19:** 529–35.
57. Sessler DI, Olofsson CI, Rubinstein EH, Beebe JJ. The thermoregulatory threshold in humans during halothane anesthesia. *Anesthesiology* 1988; **68:** 836–42.
58. Sessler DI, Rubinstein EH, Moayeri A. Physiologic response to mild perianesthetic hypothermia in humans. *Anesthesiology* 1991; **75:** 594–610.
59. Macintyre PE, Pavlin EG, Dwersteg JF. Effect of meperidine on oxygen consumption, carbon dioxide production and respiratory gas exchange in post-anesthesia shivering. *Anesth Analg* 1987; **66:** 751–5.
60. Fee JPH, Thompson GH. Comparative tolerability profiles of the inhaled anaesthetics. *Drug Safety* 1997; **16:** 157–70.
61. Ray DC, Drummond GB. Halothane hepatitis. *Br J Anaesth* 1991; **67:** 84–99.
62. El Mikatti N, Healy TEJ. Hepatic injury associated with halogenated anaesthetics: cross sensitisation and its clinical implications. *Eur J Anaesth* 1997; **14:** 7–14.
63. Njoku D, Laster MJ, Gong DH, *et al.* Biotransformation of halothane, enflurane, isoflurane, and desflurane to trifluoroacetylated liver proteins: association between protein acylation and hepatic injury. *Anesth Analg* 1997; **84:** 173–8.
64. Adams AP. Enflurane in clinical practice. *Br J Anaesth* 1981; **53:** 27S–41S.
65. Mazze RI, Woodruff RE, Heerdt ME. Isoniazid-induced enflurane defluorination in humans. *Anesthesiology* 1982; **57:** 5–8.
66. Persson A, Peterson E, Wahlin A. EEG changes during general anaesthesia with enflurane (Efrane) in comparison with ether. *Acta Anaesthesiol Scand* 1978; **22:** 339–48.
67. Eintrei C, Leszniewski W, Carisson C. Local application of 133Xenon for measurement of regional cerebral blood flow (rCBF) during halothane, enflurane, and isoflurane anesthesia in humans. *Anesthesiology* 1985; **63:** 391–4.
68. Eger EI II. Isoflurane: a review. *Anesthesiology* 1981; **55:** 559–76.
69. Wren WS, Allen P, Synnott A, *et al.* Effects of halothane, isoflurane and enflurane on ventilation in children. *Br J Anaesth* 1987; **59:** 399–409.
70. Knill RL, Manninen PH, Clement L. Ventilation and chemoreflexes during enflurane sedation and anaesthesia in man. *Can Anesth Soc J* 1979; **26:** 353–60.
71. Calverley RK, Smith NT, Jones CW, *et al.* Ventilatory and cardiovascular effects of enflurane anaesthesia during spontaneous ventilation in man. *Anesth Analg* 1978; **57:** 610–18.
72. Hirshman CA, Bergman NA. Halothane and enflurane protect against bronchospasm in an asthma dog model. *Anesth Analg* 1978; **57:** 619–28.
73. Katoh T, Ikeda K. A comparison of sevoflurane with halothane, enflurane and isoflurane on bronchoconstriction caused by histamine. *Can J Anesth* 1994; **41:** 1214–19.
74. Marshall C, Lindgren L, Marshall BE. Effects of halothane, enflurane, and isoflurane on hypoxic pulmonary vasoconstriction in rat lungs in vitro. *Anesthesiology* 1984; **60:** 304–8.
75. Rees DI, Gaines GY. One-lung anaesthesia – a comparison of pulmonary gas exchange during anaesthesia with ketamine or enflurane. *Anesth Analg* 1984; **63:** 521–5.
76. Zimpfer M, Gilly H, Krosl P, *et al.* Importance of myocardial loading conditions in determining the effects of enflurane on left ventricular function in the intact and isolated canine heart. *Anesthesiology* 1983; **58:** 159–69.
77. Black GW. Enflurane. *Br J Anaesth* 1979; **51:** 627–39.
78. Calverley RK, Smith NT, Prys-Roberts C, *et al.* Cardiovascular effects of enflurane anesthesia during controlled ventilation in man. *Anesth Analg* 1978; **57:** 619–28.
79. Rupp SM, Miller RD, Gencarelli PJ. Vecuronium-induced neuromuscular blockade during enflurane, isoflurane, and halothane anesthesia in humans. *Anesthesiology* 1984; **60:**102–5.
80. Withington DE, Donati F, Bevan DR, Varin F. Potentiation of atracurium neuromuscular blockade by enflurane: time-course of effect. *Anesth Analg* 1991 **72:** 469–73.
81. Cousins MJ, Mazze RI. Methoxyflurane toxicity: a study of dose response in man. *JAMA* 1973; **225:** 1611–16.
82. Kharasch ED, Hankins DC, Thummel KE. Human kidney methoxyflurane and sevoflurane metabolism. Intrarenal fluoride production as a possible mechanism of methoxyflurane toxicity. *Anesthesiology* 1995; **82:** 689–99.
83. Fang ZX, Eger EI II, Laster MJ, et al. Carbon monoxide production from degradation of desflurane, enflurane, isoflurane, halothane, and sevoflurane by soda lime and Baralyme.® *Anesth Analg* 1995; **80:** 1187–93.
84. Neumann MA, Laster MJ, Weiskopf RB, *et al.* The elimination of sodium and potassium hydroxides from desiccated soda lime diminishes degradation of desflurane to carbon monoxide and sevoflurane to compound A but does not compromise carbon dioxide absorption. *Anesth Analg* 1999; **89:** 768–73.
85. Corbett TH. Cancer and congenital anomalies associated with anesthetics. *Ann NY Acad Sci* 1976; **271:** 58–66.
86. Eger EI II, White AE, Brown CL, *et al.* A test of the carcinogenicity of enflurane, isoflurane, halothane, methoxyflurane, and nitrous oxide in mice. *Anesth Analg* 1978; **57:**678–694.

87. Wade JG, Stevens WC. Isoflurane: an anesthetic for the eighties. *Anesth Analg* 1981; **6:** 666–82.
88. Eger EI II. The pharmacology of isoflurane. *Br J Anaesth* 1984; **56:** 71S–99S.
89. Stevens WC, Dolan WM, Gibbons RT, *et al.* Minimum alveolar concentrations (MAC) of isoflurane with and without nitrous oxide in patients of various ages. *Anesthesiology* 1975; **42:** 197–200.
90. Cameron CB, Robinson S, Gregory GA. The minimum anesthetic concentration of isoflurane in children. *Anesth Analg* 1984; **63:** 418–40.
91. Vitez TS, White PF, Eger EI II. Effects of hypothermia on halothane MAC and isoflurane MAC in the rat. *Anesthesiology* 1974; **41:** 80–1.
92. Cromwell TH, Eger EI II, Stevens WC, Dolan WM. Forane uptake, excretion, and blood solubility in man. *Anesthesiology* 1971; **35:** 401–8.
93. Munson ES, Eger EI II, Tham MK, Embro WJ. Increase in anesthetic uptake, excretion, and blood solubility in man after eating. *Anesth Analg* 1978; **57:** 224–31.
94. Yasuda N, Lockhardt SH, Eger EI. Comparison of kinetics of sevoflurane and isoflurane in humans. *Anesth Analg* 1991; **72:** 316–24.
95. Holaday DA, Fiserova-Bergerova V, Latto IP, Zumbiel MA. Resistance of isoflurane to biotransformation in man. *Anesthesiology* 1975; **43:** 325–32.
96. Adam N. Effects of general anesthetics on memory functions in man. *J Comp Physiol Psychol* 1973; **83:** 294–305.
97. Eger EI II, Stevens WC, Cromwell TH. The electroencephalogram in man anesthetized with Forane. *Anesthesiology* 1971 **35:** 504–8.
98. Manninen PH, Nicholas JF, Lam AM. Effects of isoflurane and isoflurane-nitrous oxide anesthesia on brain stem auditory evoked potentials in man. *Anesth Analg* 1984; **63:** 245.
99. Artru AA, Lam AM, Johnson JO, Sperry RJ. Intracranial pressure, middle cerebral artery flow velocity, and plasma inorganic fluoride concentrations in neurosurgical patients receiving sevoflurane or isoflurane. *Anesth Analg* 1997; **85:** 587–92.
100. Strebel S, Lam AM, Matta B, *et al.* Dynamic and static cerebral autoregulation during isoflurane, desflurane, and propofol anesthesia. *Anesthesiology* 1995; **83:** 66–76.
101. Talke P, Caldwell J, Dodsont B, Richardson CA. Desflurane and isoflurane increase lumbar cerebrospinal fluid pressure in normocapnic patients undergoing transphenoidal hypophysectomy. *Anesthesiology* 1996; **85:** 999–1004.
102. Talke P, Caldwell JE, Richardson CA. Sevoflurane increases lumbar cerebrospinal fluid pressure in normocapnic patients undergoing transsphenoidal hypophysectomy. *Anesthesiology* 1999; **91:** 127–30.
103. Adams RW, Cucchiara RF, Gronert GA, *et al.* Isoflurane and cerebrospinal fluid pressure in neurosurgical patients. *Anesthesiology* 1981; **54:** 97–9.
104. Muzzi DA, Losasso TJ, Dietz NM, *et al.* The effect of desflurane and isoflurane on cerebrospinal fluid pressure in humans with supratentorial mass lesions. *Anesthesiology* 1992; **76:** 720–4.
105. Eger EI II. Isoflurane: a review. *Anesthesiology* 1981; **55:** 559–76.
106. Fourcade HE, Stevens WC, Larson CP, *et al.* The ventilatory effects of Forane, a new inhaled anaesthetic. *Anesthesiology* 1971; **35:** 26–31.
107. Knill RL, Kieraszewicz HT, Dodgson BG, Clement JL. Chemical regulation of ventilation during isoflurane sedation and anaesthesia in humans. *Can Anesth Soc J* 1983; **30:** 607.
108. Rehder K, Mallow JE, Fibuch EE, *et al.* Effects of isoflurane anesthesia and muscle paralysis on respiratory mechanics in normal man. *Anesthesiology* 1974; **41:** 477–85.
109. Carlsson AJ, Bindslev L, Hedenstierna G. Hypoxia-induced pulmonary vasoconstriction in the human lung. The effect of isoflurane anesthesia. *Anesthesiology* 1987; **66:** 312–16.
110. Stevens WC, Cromwell TH, Halsey MJ, *et al.* The cardiovascular effects of a new inhalation anesthetic, Forane, in human volunteers at constant arterial carbon dioxide tension. *Anesthesiology* 1971; **35:** 8–16.
111. Priebe HJ. Isoflurane causes more severe regional myocardial dysfunction than halothane in dogs with a critical coronary artery stenosis. *Anesthesiology* 1988; **69:** 72–83.
112. Slogoff S, Keats A, Dear WE, *et al.* Steal prone coronary anatomy and myocardial ischemia associated with four primary anesthetic agents in humans. *Anesth Analg* 1991; **72:** 22–7.
113. Leung JM, Hollenberg M, O'Kelly BF, *et al.* and the SPI Research Group. Effects of steal-prone anatomy on intraoperative myocardial ischemia. *J Am Coll Cardiol* 1992; **20:** 1205–12.
114. Cason BA, Shubayev I, Hickey RF. Blockade of adenosine-triphosphate sensitive potassium channels eliminates isoflurane-induced coronary artery vasodilatation. *Anesthesiology* 1994; **81:** 1245–55.
115. Kersten JR, Schmeling TJ, Hettrick DA, *et al.* Mechanism of myocardial protection by isoflurane. Role of adenosine triphosphate potassium (KATP) channels. *Anesthesiology* 1996; **85:** 794–807.
116. Holaday DA, Smith FR. Clinical characteristics and biotransformation of sevoflurane in healthy human volunteers. *Anesthesiology* 1981; **54:** 100–6.
117. Brown B Jr. Sevoflurane: introduction and overview. *Anesth Analg* 1995; **81:** S1–3.
118. Strum DP, Eger EI. Partition coefficients for sevoflurane in human blood, saline and olive oil. *Anesth Analg* 1987; **66:** 654–6.
119. Malviya S, Lerman J. The blood/gas solubility of sevoflurane, isoflurane, halothane and serum constituent concentrations in neonates and adults. *Anesthesiology* 1990; **80:** 814–24.
120. Nakajima R, Nakajima Y, Ikeda K. Minimum alveolar concentrations of sevoflurane in elderly patients. *Br J Anaesth* 1993; **70:** 273–5.
121. Katoh T, Ikeda K. The minimum alveolar concentration (MAC) of sevoflurane in humans. *Anesthesiology* 1987; **66:** 301–3.
122. Kimura T, Watanabe S, Asakura N, *et al.* Determination of end tidal sevoflurane concentration for tracheal intubation and minimum alveolar concentration in adults. *Anesth Analg* 1994; **79:** 378–81.
123. Patel SS, Goa KL. Sevoflurane: a review of its pharmacodynamic and pharmacokinetic properties and its clinical use in general anaesthesia. *Drugs* 1996; **51:** 658–99.
124. Kharasch ED, Thummel KE. Identification of cytochrome P450 2E1 as the predominant enzyme catalyzing human liver microsomal defluorination of sevoflurane. *Anesthesiology* 1993; **79:** 795–807.
125. Jiaxiang N, Sato N, Fojii K, Yuge O. Urinary excretion of hexafluoroisopropanol glucuronide and fluoride in the urine in patients after sevoflurane anesthesia. *J Pharm Pharmacol* 1993; **45:** 67–9.
126. Kameyama Y. Effect of isoflurane and sevoflurane on evoked potentials and EEG. *Masui* 1994; **43:** 657–64.
127. Woodforth IJ, Hicks RG, Crawford MR, *et al.* Electroencephalographic evidence of seizure activity under deep sevoflurane anesthesia in a non-epileptic patient. *Anesthesiology* 1997; **87:** 1579–82.
128. Terasako K, Ishii S. Postoperative seizure-like activity following sevoflurane anesthesia. *Acta Anaesthesiol Scand* 1996; **40:** 953–4.
129. Watts ADJ, Herrick IA, McLachlan RS, *et al.* The effect of sevoflurane and isoflurane anesthesia in interictal spike activity among patients with refractory epilepsy. *Anesth Analg* 1999; **89:** 1275–81.
130. Scheller MS, Nakakimura K, Fleischer JE, Zornow MH. Cerebral effects of sevoflurane in the dog: comparison with isoflurane and enflurane. *Br J Anaesth* 1990; **65:** 388–92.
131. Kitaguchi K, Ohsumi H, Kuro M, *et al.* Effects of sevoflurane on cerebral circulation and metabolism in patients with ischemic cerebrovascular disease. *Anesthesiology* 1993; **79:** 704–9.
132. Doi M, Ikeda K. Airway irritation produced by volatile anaesthetics during brief inhalation: comparison of halothane, enflurane, isoflurane and sevoflurane. *Can J Anesth* 1993; **40:** 122–6.
133. Doi M, Takahashi T, Ikeda K. Respiratory effects of sevoflurane used in combination with nitrous oxide and surgical stimulation. *J Clin Anesth* 1994; **6:** 1–4.
134. Doi M, Ikeda K. Respiratory effects of sevoflurane. *Anesth Analg* 1987; **66:** 241–4.
135. Ishibe Y, Gui X, Uno H, *et al.* Effect of sevoflurane on hypoxic pulmonary vasoconstriction in the perfused rabbit lung. *Anesthesiology* 1993; **79:** 1348–53.
136. Shimizu T, Abe K, Kinouchi K, Yoshiya I. Arterial oxygenation during one lung ventilation. *Can J Anesth* 1997; **44:** 1162–6.
137. Mitsuhata H, Saitoh J, Shimizu R, *et al.* Sevoflurane and isoflurane protect against bronchospasm in dogs. *Anesthesiology* 1994; **81:**1230–4.
138. Frink EJ, Malan TP Jr, Atlas M, *et al.* Clinical comparison of sevoflurane and isoflurane in healthy patients. *Anesth Analg* 1992; **74:** 241–5.
139. Malan T, DiNardo J, Isner R, *et al.* Cardiovascular effects of sevoflurane compared with those of isoflurane in volunteers. *Anesthesiology* 1995; **83:** 918–28.
140. Hatakeyama N, Ito Y, Momose Y. Effects of sevoflurane, isoflurane and halothane on mechanical and electro-physiological properties of canine myocardium. *Anesth Analg* 1993; **76:** 1327–32.
141. Park WK, Pancrazio JJ, Suh CK, Lynch C. Myocardial depressant effects of sevoflurane. Mechanical and electrophysiologic actions in vitro. *Anesthesiology* 1996; **84:** 1166–76.
142. Ebert TJ, Muzi M, Lopatka CW. Neurocirculatory responses to sevoflurane in humans. A comparison to desflurane. *Anesthesiology* 1995; **83:** 88–95.
143. Navarro R, Weiskopf R, Moore M, *et al.* Humans anesthetized with sevoflurane or isoflurane have similar arrhythmic response to epinephrine. *Anesthesiology* 1994; **80:** 545–9.
144. Larach DR, Schuler HG. Direct vasodilatation by sevoflurane, isoflurane and halothane alters coronary flow reserve in the isolated rat heart. *Anesthesiology* 1991; **75:** 268–78.

145. Kersten JR, Brayer AP, Pagel PS, *et al.* Perfusion of ischemic myocardium during anesthesia with sevoflurane. *Anesthesiology* 1994; **81:** 995–1004.
146. Ebert TJ, Kharasch ED, Rooke GA, *et al.* Myocardial ischemia and adverse cardiac outcomes in cardiac patients undergoing non cardiac surgery with sevoflurane and isoflurane. Sevoflurane Ischemia Study Group. *Anesth Analg* 1997; **85:** 993–9.
147. Yli-Hankala A, Randell T, Seppälä T, Lindgren L. Increases in hemodynamic variables and catecholamine levels after rapid increase in isoflurane concentration. *Anesthesiology* 1993; **78:** 266–71.
148. Moore MA, Weiskopf RB, Eger EI 2nd, *et al.* Rapid 1% increases of end-tidal desflurane concentration to greater than 5% transiently increases heart rate and blood pressure in humans. *Anesthesiology* 1994; **81:** 94–8.
149. Takahata O, Ichihara K, Ogawa H. Effects of sevoflurane on ischaemic myocardium in dogs. *Acta Anaesthesiol Scand* 1995; **39:** 449–56.
150. Izawa H, Takeda J, Fukushima K. The interaction between vecuronium and sevoflurane and its reversibility by neostigmine in man. *Anesthesiology* 1992; **77:** A960.
151. Morita T, Tsukagoshi H, Sugaya T, *et al.* The effects of sevoflurane are similar to those of isoflurane on the neuromuscular block produced by vecuronium. *Br J Anaesth* 1994; **72:** 465–7.
152. Kenna JG and Jones MJ. The organ toxicity of inhaled anesthetics. *Anesth Analg* 1995; **81:** 551–66.
153. Wallin RF, Regan BM, Napoli M, Stern IJ. Sevoflurane: A new inhalational agent. *Anesth Analg* 1975; **54:** 758–66.
154. Moriwaki G, Bito H, Ikeda K. Partly exhausted soda lime or soda lime with water added inhibits the increase in compound A concentration in the circle system during low flow sevoflurane anesthesia. *Br J Anaesth* 1997; **79:** 782–6.
155. Bito H, Ikeuchi Y, Ikeda K. Effects of the water content of soda lime on compound A concentration in the anesthesia circuit in sevoflurane anesthesia. *Anesthesiology* 1998; **88:** 66–71.
156. Ebert TJ, Messana LD, Uhrich TD, Staacke TS. Absence of renal and hepatic toxicity after 4 hours of 1.25 minimum alveolar concentration sevoflurane anesthesia in volunteers. *Anesth Analg* 1998; **86:** 662–7.
157. Eger EI, Gong D, Koblin DD, *et al.* Dose related biochemical markers of renal injury after sevoflurane versus desflurane anesthesia in volunteers. *Anesth Analg* 1997; **85:** 1154–63.
158. Eger EI, Koblin DD, Bowland T, *et al.* Nephrotoxicity of sevoflurane versus desflurane anesthesia in volunteers. *Anesth Analg* 1997; **84:** 160–8.
159. Frink Jr EJ, Ghantous H, Malan TP. Plasma inorganic fluoride with sevoflurane anesthesia: correlation with indices of renal and hepatic function. *Anesth Analg* 1992; **74:** 231–5.
160. Eger EI. Partition coefficients of I-653 in human blood, saline, and olive oil. *Anesth Analg* 1987; **66:** 971–3.
161. Rampil IJ, Lockhart SH, Zwass MS, *et al.* Clinical characteristics of desflurane in surgical patients: minimum alveolar concentration. *Anesthesiology* 1991; **74:** 429–33.
162. Taylor RH, Lerman J. Minimum alveolar concentration of desflurane and hemodynamic responses in neonates, infants and children. *Anesthesiology* 1991; **76:** 975–9.
163. Patel SS, Goa KL. Desflurane: a review of its pharmacodynamic and pharmacokinetic properties and its efficacy in general anaesthesia. *Drugs* 1995; **50:** 742–67.
164. Koblin DD, Weiskopf RB, Holmes MA, *et al.* Metabolism of I-653 and isoflurane in swine. *Anesth Analg* 1989; **68:** 147–9.
165. Sutton TS, Koblin DD, Gruenke, *et al.* Fluoride metabolites after prolonged exposure of volunteers and patients to desflurane. *Anesth Analg* 1991; **73:** 180–5.
166. Smiley RM, Ornstein E, Pantuck EJ, *et al.* Metabolism of desflurane and isoflurane to fluoride ion in surgical patients. *Can J Anesth* 1991; **38:** 965–8.
167. Rampil IJ, Lockhart SH, Eger EI 2nd, *et al.* The electroencephalographic effects of desflurane in humans. *Anesthesiology* 1991; **74:** 434–9.
168. Black S, Konstadt SN, Sami H, Rao TK. Effect of I-653(desflurane) on somatosensory evoked potentials. *Anesthesiology* 1990; **73:** A181.
169. Newberg LA, Milde JH, Michelfelder JD. The cerebral metabolic effects of isoflurane at and above concentrations that suppress cortical electrical activity. *Anesthesiology* 1983; **59:** 23–8.
170. Lutz LJ, Milde JH, Milde LN. The cerebral functional, metabolic and haemodynamic effects of desflurane in dogs. *Anesthesiology* 1990; **73:** 125–31.
171. Zwass MS, Fisher DM, Welborn LG, *et al.* Induction and maintenance characteristics of anesthesia with desflurane and nitrous oxide in infants and children. *Anesthesiology* 1992; **76:** 373–8.
172. Bunting HE, Kelly MC, Milligan KR. Effects of nebulized lignocaine on airway irritation and haemodynamic changes during induction of anesthesia with desflurane. *Br J Anaesth* 1995; **75:** 631–3.
173. Lockhart SH, Rampil IJ, Yasuda N, *et al.* Depression of ventilation by desflurane in humans. *Anesthesiology* 1991; **74:** 484–8.
174. Eger EI II. New inhaled anesthetics. *Anesth Analg* 1994; **80:** 906–22.
175. Mazzeo AJ, Cheng EY, Stadnicka A, *et al.* Topographical differences in the direct effects of desflurane and halothane on canine airway smooth muscle. *Anesth Analg* 1994; **78:** S274.
176. Park KW. Dai HB. Lowenstein E. Sellke FW. Epithelial dependence of the bronchodilatory effect of sevoflurane and desflurane in rat distal bronchi. *Anesth Analg* 1998; **86:** 646–51.
177. Weiskopf RB, Cahalan MK, Eger EI 2nd, *et al.* Cardiovascular actions of desflurane in normocarbic volunteers. *Anesth Analg* 1991; **73:** 143–56.
178. Weiskopf RB, Cahalan MK, Ionescu P, *et al.* Cardiovascular actions of desflurane with and without nitrous oxide during spontaneous ventilation in humans. *Anesth Analg* 1991; **73:** 165–74.
179. Cahalan MK, Weiskopf RB, Eger EI, *et al.* Hemodynamic effects of desflurane/nitrous oxide anesthesia in volunteers. *Anesth Analg* 1991; **73:** 143–56.
180. Merin RG, Bernard JM, Cohen M, Chelly JE. Comparison of the effects of isoflurane and desflurane on cardiovascular dynamics and regional blood flow in the chronically instrumented dog. *Anesthesiology* 1991; **74:** 568–74.
181. Boban M, Stowe DF, Buljabasic N, *et al.* Direct comparative effects of isoflurane and desflurane in isolated guinea pig hearts. *Anesthesiology* 1992; **76:** 775–80.
182. Hartmann JC, Pagel PS, Kampine JP, Warltier DC. Influence of desflurane on regional blood flow in a chronically instrumented canine model of multi vessel coronary artery obstruction. *Anesth Analg* 1991; **72:** 289–99.
183. Helman JD, Leung JM, Bellows WH, *et al.*, The SPI Research Group. The risk of myocardial ischemia in patients receiving desflurane versus sufentanil anesthesia for coronary artery bypass graft surgery. *Anesthesiology* 1992; **77:** 47–62.
184. Ebert TJ, Muzi M. Sympathetic hyperactivity during desflurane anesthesia in healthy volunteers. *Anesthesiology* 1993; **79:** 444–53.
185. Weiskopf RB, Moore MA, Eger EI II, *et al.* Rapid increases in desflurane concentration is associated with greater transient cardiovascular stimulation than with rapid increase in isoflurane concentration in humans. *Anesthesiology* 1994; **80:** 1035–45.
186. Muzi M, Ebert TJ, Hope WG, Robinson BJ, Bell LB. Site(s) mediating sympathetic activation with desflurane. *Anesthesiology* 1996; **85:** 737–47.
187. Weiskopf RB, Eger EI II, Noorani M, Daniel M. Fentanyl, esmolol and clonidine blunt the transient cardiovascular stimulation induced by desflurane in humans. *Anesthesiology* 1994; **81:** 1350–5.
188. Moore MA, Weiskopf RB, Eger EI, *et al.* Arrhythmogenic doses of epinephrine are similar during desflurane or sevoflurane anesthesia in humans. *Anesthesiology* 1993; **79:** 943–7.
189. Rampil IJ, Zwass M, Lockhart SH, *et al.* Hemodynamics of I-653 in patients. *Anesthesiology* 1989; **71:** A25.
190. Caldwell JE, Laster MJ, Magorian T, *et al.* The neuromuscular effects of desflurane, alone and combined with pancuronium or succinylcholine in humans. *Anesthesiology* 1991; **74:** 412–18.
191. Kenna JG, Satoh H, Christ DD, Pohl LR. Metabolic basis for drug hypersensitivity: antibodies in sera from patients with halothane hepatitis recognize liver neoantigens that contain the trifluoracetyl group derive. *J Pharmacol Exp Ther* 1988; **245:** 1103–9.
192. Martin JL, Plevak DJ, Flannery KD, *et al.* Hepatotoxicity after desflurane anesthesia. *Anesthesiology* 1995 **83:** 1125–9.
193. O'Keeffe NJ, Healy TEJ. The role of new anaesthetic agents. *Pharmacol and Therapeutics* 1999; **84:** 233–48.
194. Korman B, Mapleson WW. Concentration and second gas effect: can the accepted explanation be improved? *Br J Anaesth* 1997; **78:** 618–25.
195. Sakabe T, Kuramoto T, Kumagae S, Takeshita H. Cerebral responses to the addition of nitrous oxide to halothane in man. *Br J Anaesth* 1976; **48:** 957–62.
196. Jung R, Reinsel R, Marx W, *et al.* Isoflurane and nitrous oxide: comparative impact on cerebrospinal fluid pressure in patients with brain tumors. *Anesth Analg* 1992; **75:** 724–8.
197. Moss E, McDowall DG. ICP increases with 50% nitrous oxide in oxygen in severe head injuries during controlled ventilation. *Br J Anaesth* 1979; **51:** 757–61.
198. Sebel PS, Flynn PJ, Ingram DA. Effect of nitrous oxide on visual, auditory and somatosensory evoked potentials. *Br J Anaesth* 1984; **56:** 1403–7.
199. Yacoub O, Doell D, Kryger MH, Anthonisen NR. Depression of hypoxic ventilatory response by nitrous oxide. *Anesthesiology* 1976; **45:** 385–9.

200. Benumof JL, Wahrenbrock EA. Local effects of anesthetics on regional hypoxic pulmonary vasoconstriction. *Anesthesiology* 1975; **43:** 525–32.
201. Eisle JH, Smith NT. Cardiovascular effects of 40 percent nitrous oxide in man. *Anesth Analg* 1972; **51:** 956–62.
202. Ebert TJ. Differential effects of nitrous oxide on baroreflex control of heart rate and peripheral sympathetic nerve activity in humans. *Anesthesiology* 1990; **72:** 16–22.
203. Nunn JF. Clinical aspects of the interaction between nitrous oxide and vitamin B_{12}. *Br J Anaesth* 1987; **59:** 3–13.
204. Cullen SC, Groaa EG. The anaesthetic properties of xenon in animals and human beings, with additional observations on krypton. *Science* 1951; **113:** 580–2.
205. Dingley J, Ivanova-Stoilova TM, Grundler S, Walln T. Xenon: recent developments. *Anaesthesia* 1999; **54:** 335–46.
206. Goto T, Saito H, Shinkai M, *et al.* Xenon provides faster emergence from anaesthesia than does nitrous oxide-sevoflurane or nitrous oxide-isoflurane. *Anesthesiology* 1997; **86:** 1273–8.
207. Ploughmann J, Astrup J, Pedersen J, Glydensted C. Effect of stable xenon inhalation on intracranial pressure during measurement of cerebral blood flow in head injury. *J Neurosurg* 1994; **81:** 822–8.
208. Luttrop HH, Romner B, Perhag L, *et al.* Left ventricular performance and cerebral haemodynamics during xenon anaesthesia. A transoesophageal echocardiography and transcranial Doppler study. *Anaesthesia* 1993; **48:** 1045–9.
209. Calzia E, Stahl W, Handschuh T, *et al.* Respiratory mechanics during xenon anesthesia in pigs. *Anesthesiology* 1999; **91:** 1378–86.
210. Boomsma R, Ruprecht J, Man in't Veld AJ, *et al.* Haemodynamic and neurohumoral effects of xenon anaesthesia. A comparison with nitrous oxide. *Anaesthesia* 1990; **45:** 273–8.
211. Franks NP, Lieb WR. Selective actions of volatile general anaesthetics at molecular and cellular level. *Br J Anaesth* 1993; **71:** 65–76.
212. Sidebotham DA, Schug SA. Stereochemistry in anaesthesia. *Clin Exp Pharm Phys* 1997; **24:** 126–30.
213. Franks NP, Lieb WR. An anesthetic-sensitive super family of neurotransmitter-gated ion channels. *J Soc Clin Anesth* 1996; **8:** 3S–7S.

34

Pharmacology of analgesia

T ANDREW BOWDLE

> Among the remedies which it has pleased Almighty God to give to man to relieve his sufferings, none is so universal and so efficacious as opium.
>
> Sydenham (1680)

INTRODUCTION

The neurophysiology of nociception is complicated. Many neuronal pathways and different neurotransmitters are involved (see Chapter 12). Despite this, a single large class of drugs, opioid analgesics, have been the mainstay of pain therapy since ancient physicians discovered the useful effects of the alkaloids derived from the opium poppy, *Papaver somniferum*. A specific opium alkaloid was first isolated from crude opium in 1806 and named morphine, after Morpheus, the Greek god of dreams. A major breakthrough in the understanding of opioid pharmacology occurred in 1973 with the simultaneous announcement from several laboratories of the discovery of stereospecific binding sites for opioids. Endogenous opioid receptor ligands (neurotransmitters), the pentapeptides, met- and leu-enkephalin, were identified in 1975. Subsequently, three families of endogenous opioid peptides have been identified (enkephalins, endorphins, dynorphins), and three distinct types of opioid receptors, designated mu (μ), kappa (κ), and delta (δ); there is also evidence for subtypes of these receptors. Thus, our understanding of opioid drugs and the manner in which they affect the nervous system has grown tremendously in recent years. On the other hand, the molecular structure and function of the opioid receptors is not nearly as well understood as some other receptors in the central nervous system (CNS). A more detailed molecular biology of opioid receptors is currently emerging as the receptors are cloned and additional receptors are discovered. This will undoubtedly result in modification of some of the current concepts about opioid receptors and their ligands.

The main purpose of this chapter is to present the clinical pharmacology of opioid drugs. While opioids are by far the most important analgesic drugs used in surgical patients, other classes of drugs are used adjunctively, particularly the nonsteroidal anti-inflammatory drugs (NSAIDs). Therefore, the pharmacology of NSAIDs will also be included in this chapter. Alpha-2 (α_2) agonists (e.g. clonidine, dexmeditomidine) and novel agents such as the N-type calcium-channel antagonist ziconotide may gain importance in the future, and these will also be covered briefly.

There is some confusion of terminology with regard to drugs with morphine-like actions. The older term, "opiate," continues to be used occasionally. However, the predominant practice is to use the term "opioid" to refer to all drugs with morphine-like effects. The term "narcotic" has no specific pharmacologic meaning and should be avoided; derived from the Greek word for stupor, it has been applied to any drug that produces sleep. The term opioid will be used in this chapter.

OPIOID RECEPTOR PHARMACOLOGY

In order to understand opioid receptor pharmacology and particularly to understand partial agonist and agonist–antagonist opioids it is necessary to first define certain terminology and review relevant aspects of drug receptor theory.

"Potency" refers to the quantity of drug required to produce a particular degree of receptor occupancy and is related to the affinity of the drug for the receptor. In clinical pharmacology, potency is usually expressed in terms of the dose administered, often in mg or $mg\,kg^{-1}$; in molecular pharmacology, potency is considered in terms of concentration. A reduction in potency shifts the dose–response curve (to the right) but does not change its shape.

"Efficacy" or "intrinsic activity" refers to the shape of the dose–response curve and is related to the consequences of the molecular interaction between the drug and the receptor. There is a spectrum of intrinsic activity ranging from a maximum (full agonist) to zero (antagonist). Agonists are capable of producing the maximum effect possible by binding to the receptor. Antagonists bind to the receptor but cause no direct effects. Between these two extremes are partial agonist drugs with intermediate activity that produce some effect but are incapable of producing the maximum effect of the full agonist.

Partial agonists produce a dose–effect curve that is less steep and has a lower maximum effect. A lower maximum response does not necessarily imply a lack of potency; hypothetically, partial agonists may be quite potent, such that very small quantities of drug may produce a significant (albeit submaximal) effect.

An interesting and somewhat complicated phenomenon occurs when a full agonist and a partial agonist are applied together. If the concentration of the full agonist is low, introduction of the partial agonist results in an additive effect. However, if the concentration of the full agonist is relatively high, introduction of the partial agonist results in a net reduction in the effect. The opioid nalorphine (*N*-allylnormorphine), an *N*-allyl substituted derivative of morphine, is an example of a partial agonist drug. It is a potent analgesic, yet it is capable of antagonizing morphine.

When nalorphine was evaluated as a possible therapeutic agent, investigators realized that its pharmacologic properties could not be explained entirely on the premise that it was a partial agonist of the morphine receptor. The subjective effects of nalorphine in human subjects differed from morphine, and the abstinence syndrome associated with nalorphine dependence was qualitatively different from the morphine abstinence syndrome. W R Martin proposed in 1967 that there must be multiple opioid receptors.[1] Subsequently, Martin postulated a family of opioid receptors consisting of three members: μ, standing for the prototype agonist, morphine; κ, from the prototype agonist ketocyclazocine; and sigma (σ), for the prototype agonist SKF 10 047 (*N*-allylnormetazocine). All opioid drugs were thought to have a variable degree of activity at one or more of these receptors.

Since 1967 much research has resulted in many changes to Martin's original proposal. However, the postulated existence of multiple opioid receptors has been confirmed. The opioid receptor family is now recognized as being extremely complex. Research in this area proceeds rapidly and opioid receptor pharmacology undergoes frequent revision. Thus, the presentation below is somewhat simplified and very much subject to modification.

Opioid receptors are currently classified into three major types based upon bioassays and binding studies: μ, κ, and δ. These receptors appear to exert inhibitory actions primarily by presynaptic modulation of the release of excitatory neurotransmitters. Their molecular mechanism of action is by coupling to G-proteins (guanine nucleotide-binding proteins) that ultimately affect the activity of various ion channels. All three types of receptors are involved in regulating nociception through extremely complex inter-relations that are not well understood.

The μ receptor

μ receptors appear to mediate many of the clinical effects of morphine-like drugs. Two subtypes of the μ receptor have been identified in rodents, μ_1 and μ_2.[2] μ_1 receptors appear to mediate supraspinal analgesic effects of morphine-like opioids. The endogenous ligands (i.e. neurotransmitters) of μ_1 receptors appear to be opioid peptides. μ_2 receptors appear to mediate respiratory depression and spinal analgesia. Significant species differences exist, but, assuming that different μ-receptor subtypes mediate analgesia and respiratory depression in humans as well as in rodents, there would be a hypothetical possibility of specific μ-receptor subtype agonists that would produce analgesia without respiratory depression.

The κ receptor

κ receptors were named for the agonist–antagonist drug ketocyclazocine. The endogenous ligands of this receptor are probably the opioid peptides known as dynorphins. The traditional concept was that κ receptors mediated analgesia in the spinal cord but not in the brain. Currently it is believed that both spinal and supraspinal κ receptors are involved in antinociception. There appear to be three major κ receptor subtypes, designated κ_1, κ_2, and κ_3. κ_1 receptors appear to mediate spinal analgesia in rodents. κ_3 receptors are found in the rodent brain with a density twice that of μ or δ receptors.[3] The agonist–antagonist drug nalorphine has been shown to produce analgesia mediated by κ_3 receptors, and this receptor has been regarded as the "original" κ receptor proposed by Martin.[3]

Although μ and κ agonists both produce analgesia, the subjective effects of κ agonists are distinct from μ agonists. While μ agonists tend to produce euphoria, κ agonists tend to produce sedation and dysphoria (the opposite of euphoria). Perhaps because of these differences, experimental animals and human subjects tend to prefer self-administration of μ agonists to κ agonists. This implies that κ agonists should produce a lower potential for abuse and dependence.

κ receptors appear to mediate the psychotomimetic (hallucinosis, delirium) effects[4] that are prominent with certain opioids, especially benzomorphan derivatives; highly selective κ agonists produce naloxone-sensitive dysphoria and psychotomimetic effects in humans.

An interesting neuroendocrine role of κ receptors involves the regulation of vasopressin release from the posterior pituitary.[2] The κ receptor peptide ligand dynorphin is contained with vasopressin in the neurosecretory vesicles of the neuron terminals in the posterior pituitary. Dynorphin appears to mediate an inhibitory feedback loop in which dynorphin released with vasopressin activates κ receptors, inhibiting further release. Thus κ agonist drugs tend to produce a diuresis by inhibiting release of vasopressin. This is an example of a bioassay that can be used to detect the κ agonist properties of an opioid drug.

Highly selective κ agonists have not produced respiratory depression in animals.[5,6]

The δ receptor

δ refers to the opioid receptors with greatest selectivity for the endogenous opioid peptides known as enkephalins. There is evidence for two δ receptor subtypes, designated δ_1 and δ_2.[3] Because of their relative selectivity for enkephalins, δ receptors may be somewhat less important for the effects of exogenously administered opioids. On the other hand, many opioid drugs bind δ receptors to some degree, thus δ receptors may have some part in mediating the effects of opioid drugs. δ receptors may be involved in opioid-induced respiratory depression.[7]

The σ receptor

The σ receptor was one of the original triad of opioid receptors proposed by W R Martin in 1976.[1] Martin postulated such a receptor to explain the psychotomimetic and cardiovascular effects of *N*-allylnormetazocine (SKF 10 047), and related agonist–antagonist opioids. Opioids with such properties were regarded as "σ opioids." Subsequently, an enormous effort was made to identify and characterize the σ receptor, an effort that continues to the present. While the σ receptor is not entirely understood, the results of many studies now suggest that actually it does not mediate the psychotomimetic effects of agonist–antagonist opioids, as originally proposed. Natural opioids (such as morphine) are levorotatory (−) isomers. Dextrorotatory (+) enantiomers do not have opioid activity. Many synthetic opioids are racemic mixtures (others are nonchiral). (±)SKF 10 047 (as originally used by Martin[1]) is a racemic mixture which is now recognized as binding (at least) three types of receptors: (−)SKF 10 047 binds mainly to μ and κ opioid receptors; (+)SKF 10 047 binds to phencyclidine (PCP) receptors (ketamine also acts at this receptor) and to another receptor currently designated as σ.[8] The σ receptor shows a preference for dextrorotatory compounds and is not sensitive to naloxone (which is levoratatory). Because the psychotomimetic effects of agonist–antagonist opioids are mediated by levorotatory enantiomers and can be antagonized by naloxone, it appears that neither PCP nor σ receptors are involved, contrary to Martin's original scheme.[9] Presumably, opioid psychotomimetic effects are mediated by κ receptors or by some unknown receptors.[4] The physiologic significance, if any, of actions by dextrorotatory opioids on σ or PCP receptors is unknown.

Other opioid receptors

Recently, several putative opioid receptors have been identified that do not fit the simple scheme of μ, κ, and δ. This is perhaps not surprising, and undoubtedly there will be additional opioid receptors discovered in the future. Pasternak and Standifer[10] have identified a receptor for the morphine metabolite morphine 6-glucuronide. The physiologic role of this receptor is unknown. Interestingly, morphine, thebaine, and codeine have been identified in mammalian tissues and mammalian cytochrome P450 enzymes are able to catalyze the transformation of thebaine to codeine and morphine, suggesting that morphine and, presumably, morphine 6-glucuronide may be endogenous ligands. Another recently discovered opioid receptor is known as opioid-receptor-like 1 (ORL1). This receptor has been cloned and has a high degree of homology to μ and κ receptors. An endogenous peptide ligand known as nociceptin (or orphanin FQ) has been associated with this receptor.[11] Interestingly, the opioid agonists etorphine and lofentanil bind the receptor, but naloxone does not.

Opioid receptors have been identified in mammalian lung.[12] Sapru *et al.*[13] found that administration of a stable enkephalin analog into the right atrium of rats produced apnea that was prevented by vagotomy or naloxone. They hypothesized that opioid-induced apnea was mediated by pulmonary J-receptor stimulation. Yeadon and Kitchen[14] reported that respiratory depression in rats given fentanyl analogs was mediated through peripheral μ–receptors and centrally through μ and non-μ receptors. The apneic response was abolished by either bilateral vagotomy or the quaternary opioid antagonist *N*-methyl levallorphan (which acts peripherally).

Ohtani *et al.*[15] reported that buprenorphine effects on breathing involve peripheral opioid receptors. They found that the buprenorphine metabolite, norbuprenorphine, was a much more potent respiratory depressant in rats than the parent drug. The respiratory effects of norbuprenorphine were antagonized by the specific μ-receptor antagonist β-funaltrexamine (FNA). Interestingly, norbuprenorphine penetrated the blood–brain barrier poorly, and the respiratory depression resulting from norbuprenorphine was much greater after intravenous administration than after central intra-arterial administration (bypassing the lungs), suggesting a peripheral rather than a central respiratory depressant effect.

RELATIONS BETWEEN STRUCTURE AND ACTIVITY

The structures of the opioid drugs discussed in this chapter are shown in Fig. 34.1. Morphine, a naturally occurring opium alkaloid, is the prototype compound. Many clinically useful opioid drugs are semisynthetic derivatives of morphine or thebaine, another natural opium alkaloid. Some other opioid drugs, including the fentanyl analogs, are synthetic. Opioids can be classified by examining their derivation from a basic parent structure. The major structural classes include: opium alkaloids (or their derivatives), morphinans, benzomorphans, methadones, and phenylpiperidines. Semisynthetic derivatives of morphine or thebaine of interest in anesthesiology include nalorphine (obsolete, but of great historical significance), nalbuphine, buprenorphine, naloxone, and naltrexone. Butorphanol is a morphinan and pentazocine is a benzomorphan. Methadone is a unique structure, thus it constitutes a class of its own. Meperidine (pethidine) and the fentanyl analogs are phenylpiperidines.

Opioid receptors are stereoselective. The levorotatory (−) isomer is the active enantiomer at opioid receptors. Dextrorotatory (+) enantiomers may have pharmacological effects (see the section The σ receptor above), but they are not reversible by naloxone (not opioid receptor mediated).

Modifications corresponding to positions 3, 6, and 17 of morphine (see Fig. 34.1) are particularly important for relations between structure and activity. Particular substituents on the tertiary amine (position 17) result in antagonist activity. The first opioid with significant antagonist activity was nalorphine (*N*-allylnormorphine), the *N*-allyl analog of morphine. Incorporation of *N*-allyl substituents in almost all series of synthetic opioids that contain three of the five rings present in morphine results in antagonist activity. *N*-cyclopropylmethyl (naltrexone, buprenorphine) and *N*-cyclobutylmethyl (butorphanol, nalbuphine) subtituents have also resulted in clinically useful compounds with agonist–antagonist or pure antagonist activity.

In general, the opioids in clinical use do not have an extremely high degree of receptor specificity. However, morphine, meperidine (pethidine), methadone, and the fentanyl analogs probably interact primarily with μ receptors. Sufentanil is a particularly potent μ-receptor agonist. Nalorphine, pentazocine, nalbuphine, and butorphanol are probably partial μ agonists and partial κ agonists (see sections Partial agonists and Agonist–antagonists, below). Buprenorphine is a partial μ agonist; it has activity at κ receptors as well. Naloxone is a pure antagonist at μ, κ, and δ receptors, although it is most potent at μ receptors.

THERAPEUTIC DRUG EFFECTS

Endogenous opioid peptide neurotransmitters appear to exert subtle modulatory effects on the CNS under normal conditions. The administration of naloxone to normal subjects produces remarkably few noticeable effects. This is in dramatic contrast to the effects of administering therapeutic doses of opioid agonists. Opioid agonists produce analgesia, sedation, and, in large doses, unconsciousness and anesthesia.

The capability of opioids to produce general anesthesia has been debated. It is useful to consider general anesthesia in terms of its component parts: amnesia, analgesia, unconsciousness, immobility, muscle relaxation, and control of autonomic and endocrine responses to surgery. No currently existing intravenous anesthetic agent provides all of these features in every situation. Therefore, it would be inappropriate to recommend the routine use of any particular drug as a sole anesthetic agent. However, opioids are capable of producing many of the features of general anesthesia, especially analgesia, unconsciousness, and control of autonomic and endocrine responses to surgery; from this perspective it is reasonable to regard opioids as anesthetic agents.

There is clear evidence that opioids alone are capable of producing unconsciousness in humans (see section Dose–effect relations). In rats, sufentanil virtually replaced halothane for preventing movement in response to a tail clamp.[16]

The capability of opioids to produce amnesia in conscious subjects has not been well studied. Generally, it has been assumed that smaller doses of opioids do not effectively produce amnesia. It is interesting that butorphanol has been reported to have a small but significant anterograde amnesic effect.[17]

High doses of opioids blunt the neuroendocrine stress response to surgery; plasma concentrations of catecholamines, cortisol, antidiuretic hormone (ADH), glucose, insulin, and growth hormone can be maintained at normal levels. However, the endocrine stress response to cardiopulmonary bypass is not completely controlled by opioids. Opioids are useful for reducing the hyperdynamic cardiovascular response to a surgical stimulus (see the section Cardiovascular effects, below). Many anesthesiologists use opioids in large doses as primary anesthetic agents, in combination with other intravenous agents or inhaled agents. The term "balanced anesthesia" (as currently used) refers to the combination of substantial doses of opioids with inhaled anesthetics.

Electroencephalographic effects

Opioids produce high-voltage slow (δ) waves. Higher doses of opioids do not produce a progression to burst suppression and a flat electroencephalogram (EEG) as with volatile anesthetics. The EEG effects of opioids provide a convenient, continuous measurement of drug effect that has been exploited for numerous pharmacodynamic studies. When monitoring cerebral function with the EEG (e.g. during carotid

Morphine or thebaine derivatives

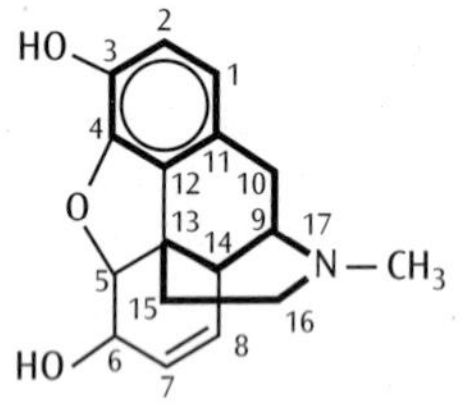

Morphine
(Ag)

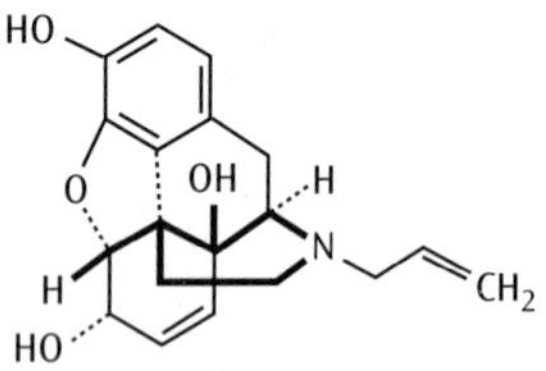

Nalorphine
(Ag–ant)

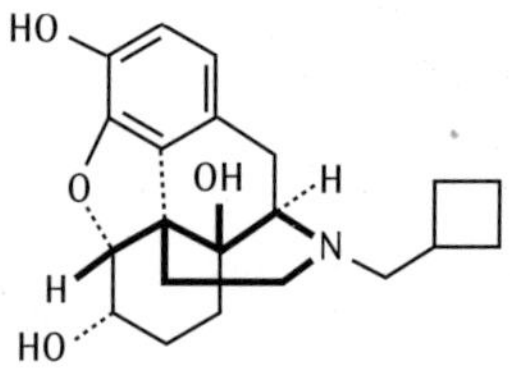

Nalbuphine
(Ag–ant)

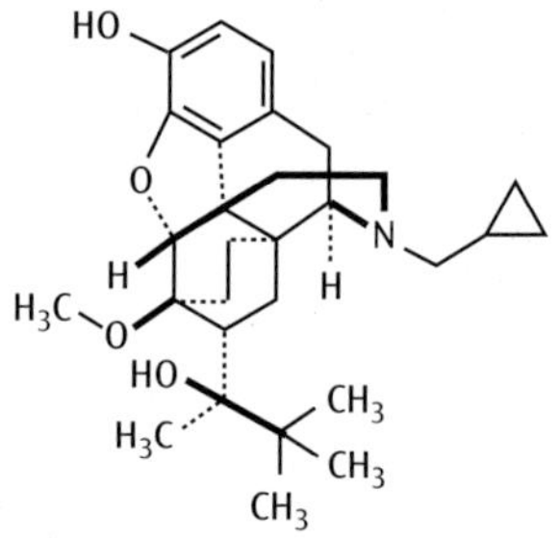

Buprenorphine
(Ag–ant)

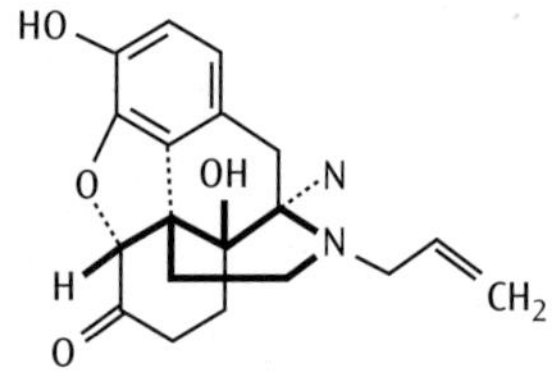

Naloxone
(Ant)

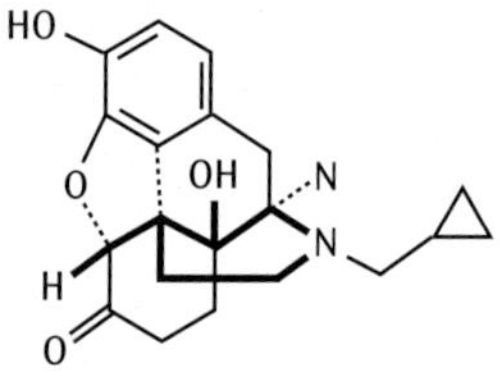

Naltrexone
(Ant)

Phenylpiperidines

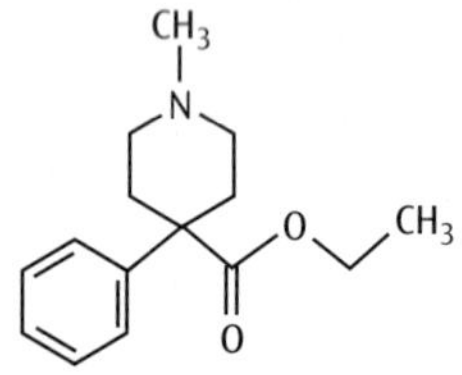

Meperidine
(pethidine)
(Ag)

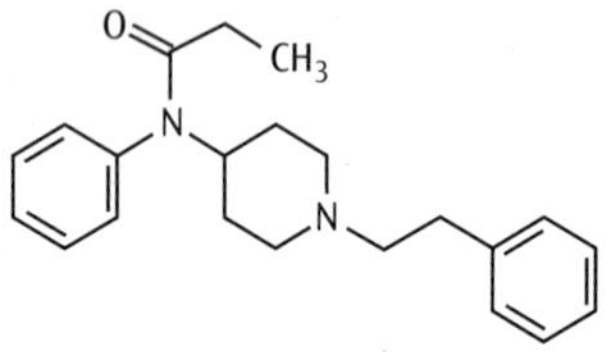

Fentanyl
(Ag)

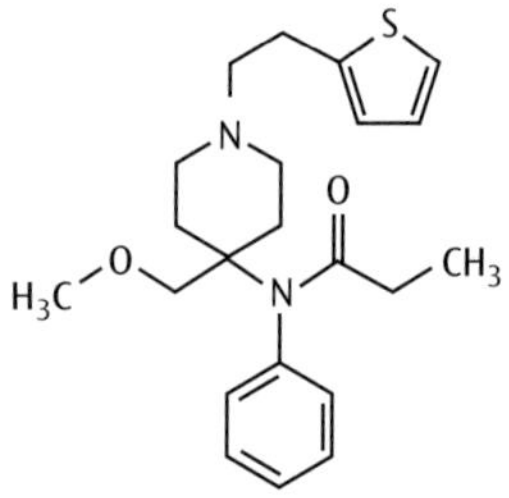

Sufentanil
(Ag)

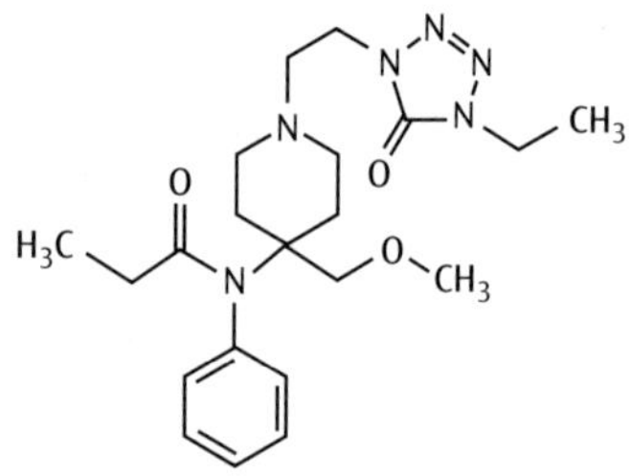

Alfentanil
(Ag)

Morphinan

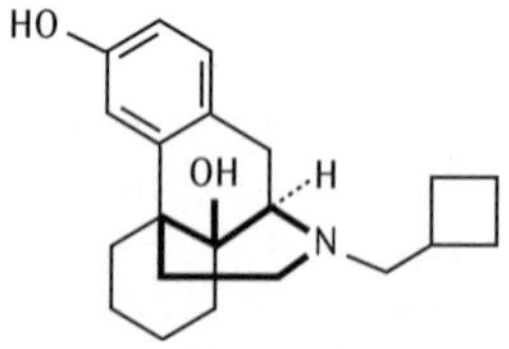

Butorphanol
(Ag–ant)

Methadone

Methadone
(Ag)

Benzomorphan

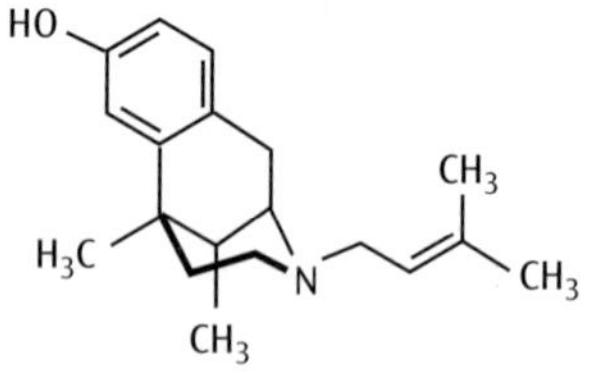

Pentazocine
(Ag–ant)

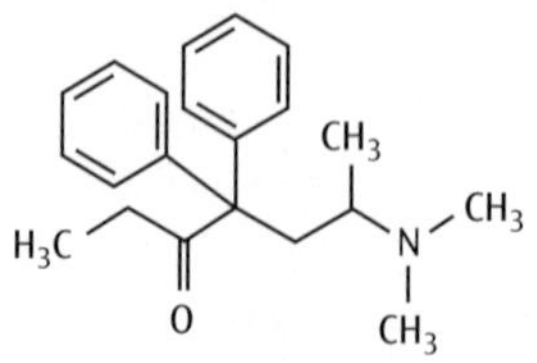

Figure 34.1 *Chemical structures of opioids. Ag, agonist; Ag–ant, agonist–antagonist; Ant, antagonist.*

endarterectomy) it is important to realize that the appearance of slow waves produced by opioids may be indistinguishable from slowing produced by cerebral ischemia; therefore it is advisable to avoid bolus doses of opioid at critical times (such as carotid cross-clamping) when confusion with cerebral ischemia could arise.

Shivering

Postanesthetic shaking or shivering that is not related to hypothermia can be effectively abolished by certain opioids. Meperidine is effective for this purpose.[18] Morphine is not effective. There is evidence that butorphanol[19] and tramadol[20] are also effective. The reason why some opioids are effective while others are ineffective is not known.

RELATIONS BETWEEN DOSE AND EFFECT

Data describing relations between dose and effect are extremely valuable for answering an important practical question in therapeutics: "How much drug should be given in order to obtain a particular, desired effect?" Unfortunately, high-quality dose–effect data for humans are relatively scarce, probably because of the difficulty in performing clinical studies that typically require large numbers of patients and data "points."

There is a large amount of variability in response to opioids between patients. The important clinical implication is that the dose of opioid must always be individualized. Information from the literature can be a useful guide to dosing, however there is no substitute for a thoughtful and observant anesthesiologist. Figure 34.2 provides an example of the large variation in individual responsiveness.[21]

McDonnell *et al.*[22] and Vinik *et al.*[23] have reported dose–effect studies of alfentanil for induction of anesthesia. McDonnell *et al.* determined the ED_{50} and ED_{90} for unconsciousness in unpremedicated young adults using both loss of response to verbal commands and loss of response to a nasopharyngeal airway as endpoints to identify unconsciousness (Fig. 34.3). The ED_{50} and ED_{90} were 92 and 111 μg kg^{-1} respectively for loss of response to verbal stimulus and 111 and 169 μg kg^{-1} respectively for loss of response to a nasopharyngeal airway. Several practical aspects of opioid clinical pharmacology are made evident by this study. An opioid in sufficient dose can produce unconsciousness when used as the sole agent for induction of anesthesia. However, the clinical endpoint to identify unconsciousness during induction is not entirely clear. It is the author's experience that the loss of the "eyelash reflex," commonly used to confirm unconsciousness during induction with barbiturates, is not a useful endpoint during induction with opioids. The data of McDonnell *et al.*[22] demonstrate that responsiveness to a verbal stimulus may not be an adequate endpoint during opioid induction and some more intense test stimulus may be necessary. The author has occasionally seen patients who did not respond to verbal or gentle tactile stimuli during opioid induction, but opened their eyes when an oral airway was inserted; the practice of inserting an airway (or providing some other comparable stimulus) prior to the administration of an intubating dose of neuromuscular blocker may be advisable when opioids are used as the primary induction agent. Vinik *et al.*[23] reported an ED_{50} for induction of anesthesia with alfentanil of 130 μg kg^{-1} (Fig. 34.4), remarkably similar to that found by McDonnell *et al.*[22]

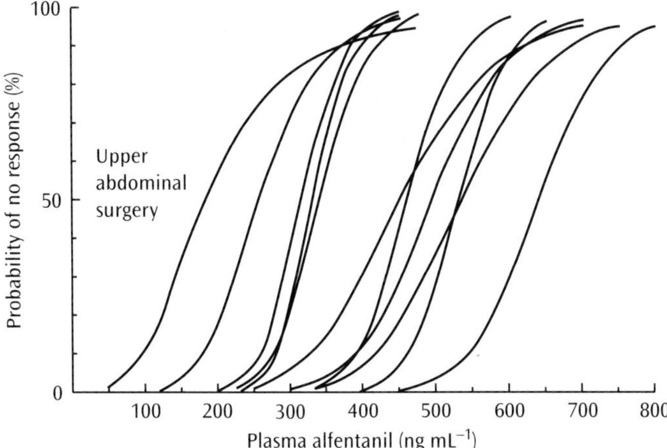

Figure 34.2 *Alfentanil plasma concentration vs. effect curves for probability of not responding to a surgical stimulus during upper abdominal surgery. Anesthesia consisted of alfentanil and 66% nitrous oxide. Each curve represents one patient. The tremendous variation in plasma concentration required to prevent response to a surgical stimulus is evident. (From Ausems* et al.,[21] *with permission.)*

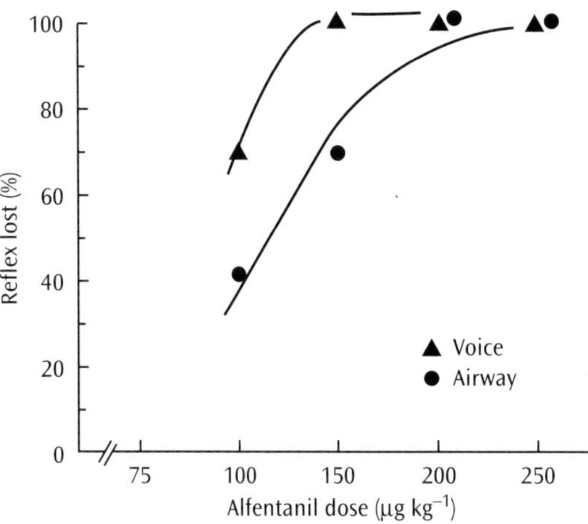

Figure 34.3 *Dose–effect curves for induction of anesthesia with alfentanil in unpremedicated young adults. Alfentanil alone, in sufficient dose, produced unconsciousness. Absence of response to placement of a nasopharyngeal airway was a more reliable sign of unconsciousness than a verbal stimulus. (From McDonnell* et al.,[22] *with permission.)*

Ausems *et al.*[21] have determined alfentanil plasma concentration–effect curves for patients anesthetized with alfentanil–nitrous oxide undergoing lower abdominal gynecologic, upper abdominal, or breast surgery (Fig. 34.2).

The ED_{50} for remifentanil in combination with 67% nitrous oxide for preventing response to surgical stimulation was 0.52 μg kg^{-1} min^{-1}.[24] This figure is remarkably close to the infusion rate reported to produce 50% of the maximum EEG effect, 0.56 μg kg^{-1} min^{-1}, at the age of 50 years; the same study found that dose requirement decreased with age due to both pharmacokinetic and pharmacodynamic influences.[25]

NONTHERAPEUTIC DRUG EFFECTS

The side-effects of opioids drugs have been recently reviewed.[26] While opioids have proved to be relatively safe drugs, management of side-effects is critical to successful application in clinical practice.

Depression of breathing

μ agonist opioids produce dose-related depression of breathing. Resting minute ventilation and tidal volume are decreased. Respiratory rate was found to be decreased in some studies but not in others; slow breathing

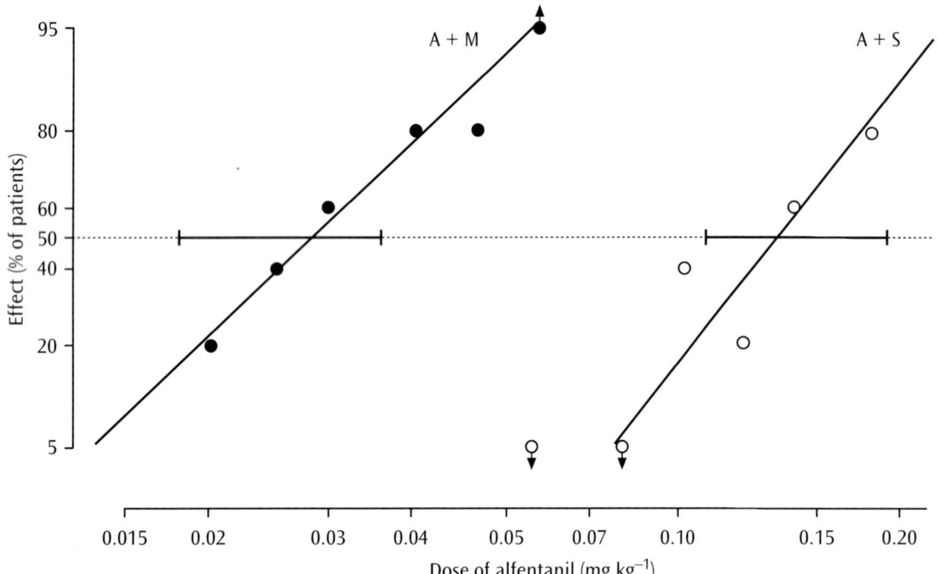

Figure 34.4 *Dose–effect curves for induction of anesthesia with alfentanil (right-hand side) or alfentanil plus midazolam (left-hand side) in unpremedicated patients. Data are plotted on a log–log scale. Midazolam, 0.07 mg kg^{-1}, reduced the alfentanil ED_{50} for unconsciousness by about 80%. (From* Vinik et al.,[23] *with permission.)*

certainly may occur, but a normal rate of breathing does not ensure the absence of opioid-induced depression of breathing. The ventilatory responses to hypercarbia and hypoxia are blunted. Opioids may also alter the normal rhythm of breathing, resulting in irregular breathing and apneic intervals. Sufficient doses of opioids produce complete apnea, although apneic patients who remain conscious may continue to breathe on command.

Analgesic effects and depression of breathing from μ agonists are generally assumed to be proportional. However, Bailey *et al.*[27] have suggested that sufentanil produces less depression of breathing than fentanyl, relative to analgesia. The existence of μ receptor subtypes provides a hypothetical explanation: μ agonists, having relatively less effect on μ receptor subtype(s) involved with breathing, could produce less depression of breathing relative to analgesia. This hypothesis remains to be tested.

The agonist–antagonist opioids are probably partial μ agonists, therefore the maximum effects on breathing are expected to be less than those of full μ agonists such as morphine. Nalorphine,[28], nalbuphine,[29] and dezocine[30] were found to have a "ceiling" for depression of breathing equivalent to about 30 mg of morphine per 70 kg of body weight. At lower doses, the depression of breathing was dose related. Higher doses produced no additional depression of CO_2 response. The pentazocine dose–effect curve was flatter than for morphine, but a plateau could not be demonstrated because intense dysphoria in the volunteers limited the maximum dose.[28] The dose–effect curve for butorphanol was flatter than for morphine, but doses large enough to establish a true ceiling were not studied.[31] The effects of buprenorphine on breathing have not been fully characterized. An important clinical observation is that the depression of breathing caused by buprenorphine cannot always be antagonized by naloxone (see sections Partial agonists and Agonist–antagonists); doxapram, an analeptic drug that stimulates ventilation, has been suggested as an alternative antidote for buprenorphine-induced depression of breathing.[32] Very large doses of naloxone (5–10 mg) can also be tried and may be effective.[33]

There are a number of case reports of severe, delayed depression of breathing following balanced anesthesia with fentanyl analogs.[34] In most cases neuromuscular blockers were adequately reversed and patients were awake and breathing spontaneously on arrival in the recovery room. After an interval of apparently adequate ventilation, ranging from minutes to about an hour, severe respiratory depression supervened. Prompt response to naloxone has confirmed the suspected relation to opioids in many cases. Because these events followed an interval of apparently adequate ventilation, the depression of breathing has often been described as delayed or recurrent. The mechanism is not known with certainty. Enterohepatic circulation of opioids sequestered in the stomach by acid trapping has been postulated to cause fluctuating plasma concentrations in the postoperative setting. However, studies of fentanyl and alfentanil distribution in rats suggest that this is an unlikely mechanism. An appealing alternative is the possibility that opioids stored in "peripheral compartments" such as muscle are mobilized as patients begin to move about, resulting in transient increases in plasma concentrations and drug effects. Delayed depression of breathing may not be the result of a single pharmacokinetic phenomenon, but rather the common endpoint of several possible etiologies, including excessive opioid plasma concentrations at the time of extubation, the relatively short duration of action of naloxone (given to some patients at the time of extubation), drug interactions (e.g. benzodiazepines), or the onset of sleep (adding to the depression of breathing caused by opioids). Whatever the etiology may be, recovery room personnel should be well aware of the possibility for severe depression of breathing in patients that initially appear to be breathing adequately.

Patients receiving opioids for postoperative analgesia on the surgical wards may also undergo episodes of depressed breathing and hypoxemia. This problem has not been thoroughly studied, but some studies suggest that postoperative hypoxemia related to opioids is remarkably common.[35]

Cardiovascular effects

The cardiovascular system is extraordinarily complex. While it is relatively simple to measure drug effects on vital signs, such as blood pressure and heart rate, determination of the mechanism of drug action can be very difficult. The effects of opioids on the cardiovascular system are not completely understood. Nevertheless, certain basic aspects of opioid cardiovascular pharmacology are understood well enough to be clinically useful.

Stimulation of histamine release by morphine or meperidine, but not by fentanyl analogs, can provoke significant hypotension and tachycardia.[36] Flacke *et al.*[36] administered incremental equipotent doses of meperidine (4.3 ± 0.1 mg kg^{-1}), morphine (0.6 ± 0.02 mg kg^{-1}), fentanyl (7.0 ± 0.4 μg kg^{-1}), or sufentanil (1.3 ± 0.1 μg kg^{-1}) for induction of anesthesia. Subsequent plasma histamine levels were elevated in 31% of patients receiving meperidine, 10% of patients receiving morphine, and in none of the patients receiving fentanyl or sufentanil. Elevations of plasma histamine were significantly correlated with reduction of mean blood pressure, elevation of heart rate, and elevation of circulating epinephrine (adrenaline) (Fig. 34.5). The relation between dose and effect for histamine release by meperidine or morphine are unknown, but slow administration of morphine (<5 mg min⁻¹) appears to minimize histamine release.

Opioids depress contractility of isolated heart muscle. However, the concentrations of morphine or fentanyl analogs necessary to produce myocardial depression are greatly in excess of concentrations achieved in patients. Thus, morphine and fentanyl are believed not to produce significant myocardial depression in the clinical setting. On the other hand, meperidine produces substantial myocardial depression at clinically relevant concentrations; meperidine was estimated to be 200 times more potent as a myocardial depressant than morphine or fentanyl.[37] Severe hypotension limits the usefulness of meperidine as a primary anesthetic agent. Meperidine (2.5 mg kg⁻¹) produced severe cardiovascular depression in dogs; higher doses (e.g. 35 mg kg⁻¹) quickly produced cardiac arrest.[38]

Morphine and the fentanyl analogs typically reduce heart rate by a vagomimetic action that is antagonized by atropine. The reduction in heart rate is variable, but severe bradycardia or even asystole are possible, especially with the fentanyl analogs (see section Drug interactions). Reduction of heart rate induced by opioids may have a desirable therapeutic effect on the balance between coronary oxygen supply and demand in patients with coronary disease,[39] provided that bradycardia does not result in severe hypotension; it is this author's opinion that the heart rate-lowering effects of the fentanyl analogs are among their most useful properties. Meperidine, which was originally investigated for its anticholinergic properties, tends to increase heart rate.

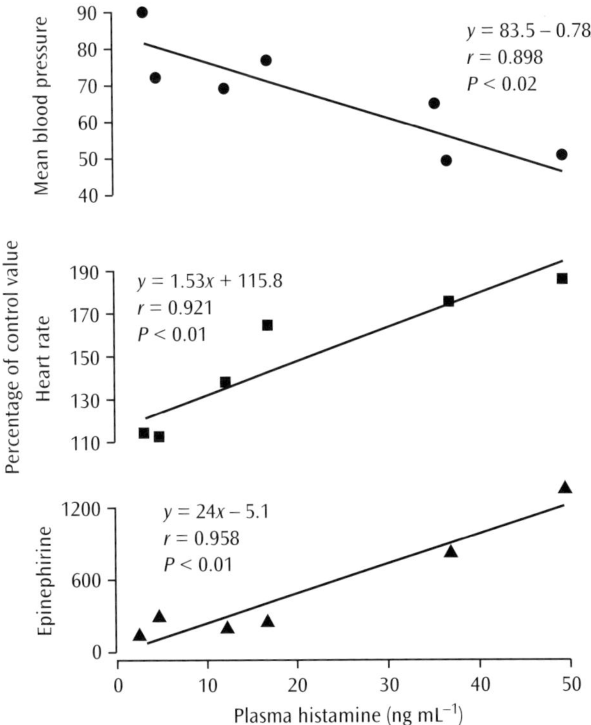

Figure 34.5 *Histamine release was stimulated by administration of morphine or meperidine (pethidine), resulting in reduction of blood pressure and elevation of heart rate and plasma epinephrine (adrenaline). The changes in vital signs and epinephrine levels were significantly correlated to plasma histamine concentration. (From Flacke* et al.*,[36] with permission.)*

Fentanyl analogs often produce minor reductions in blood pressure and occasionally are associated with severe hypotension. In the absence of histamine release or significant myocardial depression, a reduction in systemic vascular resistance is implicated. Flacke *et al.*[40] have suggested that the mechanism may involve a centrally mediated reduction in sympathetic tone. They showed that fentanyl (100 μg kg⁻¹) produced no cardiovascular depression in dogs previously deprived of autonomic tone by a combination of vagal transection and subarachnoid block. They also showed that the cardiovascular depressant effects of fentanyl in dogs were antagonized by naloxone and that clonidine prevented naloxone from reversing fentanyl's cardiovascular effects, presumably by decreasing sympathetic outflow from the CNS.[41] Severe hypotension following administration of fentanyl analogs can probably be avoided by paying close attention to the patient's volume status (opioids may be hazardous in hypovolemic patients) and by avoiding certain drug interactions that exacerbate hemodynamic effects (see section Drug interactions). Opioid-induced hypotension can usually be treated effectively by intravenous fluid and/or an α–adrenergic agonist drug (e.g. phenylephrine) to restore vascular tone.

While discussions of cardiovascular effects usually emphasize cardiovascular depression, there is evidence of cardiovascular stimulation in some cases. Thomson *et al.*[42] reported that induction of anesthesia with fentanyl, 50 μg kg⁻¹, resulted in substantial increases in heart rate, blood pressure, pulmonary artery pressure, and cardiac index in some patients. It is interesting that certain agonist–antagonist opioids, notably pentazocine, produce cardiovascular stimulation more often than not (see below). The incidence of cardiovascular stimulation and the mechanism are unknown; the author has certainly observed such responses by patients in his own practice.

It is evident from the foregoing discussion that morphine and meperidine are more likely to produce cardiovascular problems than the fentanyl analogs. Meperidine, in particular, has potentially hazardous cardiovascular effects. It is interesting that the proclivity for cardiovascular effects is inversely related to both the potency and the therapeutic index of opioids. The therapeutic indices (LD_{50}/ED_{50}, the ratio of lethal dose to effective dose) in rats are 4.8 for meperidine, 70 for morphine, 277 for fentanyl, and 26 700 for sufentanil; potency is in the same rank order (sufentanil is most potent).[43]

Cardiovascular effects of agonist–antagonist opioids

The cardiovascular effects of the agonist–antagonist opioids have not been studied nearly as extensively as the full μ agonists discussed above. The older agonist–antagonist drugs, nalbuphine and pentazocine, have considerable cardiovascular stimulating effects; pentazocine produces increases in blood pressure, heart rate, systemic vascular resistance, pulmonary artery pressure and left ventricular end-diastolic pressure. Butorphanol has been shown in some studies to cause a small increase in pulmonary artery pressure (reminiscent of pentazocine),[44] however other studies find no change in pulmonary pressures. The newer agents generally appear to have relatively minor cardiovascular effects (except meptazinol and dezocine; see below).

Meptazinol appeared to produce only minor hemodynamic effects when given in analgesic doses. Larger doses of meptazinol, 2, 3, or 4 mg kg⁻¹, given to a small number of patients anesthetized with etomidate, produced substantial reductions in heart rate and blood pressure.[45] Pulmonary artery pressures were unaffected. These results suggest that the hemodynamic effects of meptazinol may be of clinical importance. Additional studies are warranted.

Dezocine is capable of producing serious cardiovascular depression in dogs.[46] Marked cardiovascular effects are not generally found in humans given analgesic doses of dezocine. Additional studies are needed to elucidate the mechanism of cardiovascular depression in dogs and to determine if similar effects are possible in humans.

Rigidity and other neuroexcitatory effects

Muscle rigidity is seen commonly during induction of anesthesia with larger doses of opioids. A simple experiment convincingly demonstrated that opioid rigidity is central in origin. After a tourniquet was applied to the arm, preventing the entry of drugs, administration of alfentanil produced rigidity in the entire body, including the isolated extremity. Studies in rodents suggest that opioid rigidity is mediated by μ receptors in brainstem midline nuclei; a naloxone analog applied by microinjection to these brain areas antagonized alfentanil-induced rigidity.[47] The basal ganglia have also been implicated in opioid rigidity.

Because opioid rigidity frequently prevents ventilation of the lungs with a bag and mask, it has been often associated in the first instance with the chest wall muscles. Benthuysen *et al.*[48] have shown that opioid rigidity affects not only the chest muscles, but virtually all of the major muscle groups in the body. They quantified rigidity during induction of anesthesia with alfentanil, 175 μg kg^{-1}, by recording electromyograms (EMG) from sternocleidomastoid, deltoid, biceps, forearm flexors, intercostal, rectus abdominus, vastus medialis/lateralis, and gastrocnemius muscles. Rigidity occurred in all of the muscles, beginning first in the upper body (sternocleidomastoid, deltoid, biceps, forearm). Ridigity was often sudden in onset and could be provoked by stimulation such as passive movement of an extremity, manipulation of the anesthesia mask, or a loud sound. Stereotyped postures were noted: flexion of the upper extremity, extension of the lower extremity, rigid immobility of the head, flexion of the neck with chin on chest, and severe rigidity of the abdomen and chest wall.

Opioid-induced rigidity is usually observed during induction of anesthesia; however, there are case reports of rigidity occurring either immediately upon emergence from anesthesia,[49] or up to 3–5 h postoperatively.[50] Naloxone administration has dramatically relieved the rigidity in cases in which it was tried, implicating an opioid mechanism. The explanation for delayed rigidity is unknown, much as the explanation for delayed depression of breathing from opioids is unknown.

Currently, the only reliable treatment for opioid-induced rigidity is the administration of neuromuscular blocking drugs, in doses large enough to facilitate intubation. A very small dose of pancuronium, 1.5 mg per 70 kg body weight (e.g. for defasciculation) was reported to attenuate rigidity;[51] however, it is difficult to explain how a dose of neuromuscular blocker that is generally too small to prevent voluntary movement could significantly affect the considerable motor activity necessary to produce rigidity. Another study using electromyography to quantify rigidity found that small doses of neuromuscular blockers did not significantly attenuate rigidity.[52] Considering the neuroanatomical basis of opioid rigidity, drugs that act on GABA-ergic, serotonergic or adrenergic pathways might be expected to affect rigidity. The serotonin receptor antagonist ketanserin and the α_2-adrenergic agonist dexmedetomidine prevented opioid-induced rigidity in rats.[53,54] Benzodiazepines and thiopental (GABA-ergic mechanisms of action) have also been reported to attenuate rigidity in rats and humans, although this finding has not been consistent.[55]

In addition to tonic rigidity, opioids have been associated with tonic–clonic movement, or myoclonus. Opioid-induced myclonus may be quite dramatic, resembling generalized epileptic convulsions. Opioids in very large doses have produced seizure activity in laboratory animals. However, there appears not to be any EEG evidence that opioids produce generalized, cortical seizure activity in humans, despite many studies of opioids in which EEG recordings have been made [with the exception of normeperidine (norpethidine), see below].[56] To the contrary, myoclonus has been observed during simultaneous EEG recording, in the absence of EEG evidence of seizure activity.[57] Fentanyl (mean dose 25 μg kg^{-1})[58] and alfentanil (50 μg kg^{-1})[59] have been reported to produce localized temporal lobe electrical seizure activity in patients with complex partial epilepsy, but this was not accompanied by motor activity. Thus, it is tempting to speculate that the mechanism of opioid-induced myoclonus may be closely related to opioid-induced tonic rigidity.

The N-demethylated metabolite of meperidine (normeperidine) is capable of producing CNS excitation and generalized seizures that are not antagonized by naloxone.[60] Normeperidine is eliminated by the kidney and by hydrolysis to normeperidinic acid. The half-life of normeperidine is 15–40 h, thus it may accumulate with prolonged meperidine administration. Patients with impaired renal function are probably at increased risk for normeperidine toxicity.

Cerebral blood flow and intracranial pressure

Opioids were once considered to produce no change, or only modest reductions, in cerebral blood flow and cerebral metabolic oxygen consumption. However, Milde *et al.*[61] reported that sufentanil caused substantial increases in cerebral blood flow in normocapnic dogs anesthetized with small doses of halothane; for the most part the increase in cerebral blood flow was not explained by concomitant changes in cerebral oxygen consumption, implying that sufentanil was dilating cerebral vessels directly.

Sperry *et al.*[62] studied intracranial pressure in patients with severe head trauma. The patients were paralyzed with vecuronium and their intracranial pressure was controlled using standard clinical procedures, including hyperventilation, elevation of the head, sedation with midazolam, and osmotic agents. Intracranial pressure was monitored by a subarachnoid bolt device. Administration of fentanyl (3.0 μg kg^{-1}) or sufentanil (0.6 μg kg^{-1}) resulted in a mean increase in intracranial pressure of about 10 mmHg (1.33 kPa) (Fig. 34.6). Mean blood pressure declined by about 10 mmHg. The maximum increase in intracranial pressure occurred about 5 min after opioid administration and persisted for about 20 min.

The explanation for the apparent increase in cerebral blood flow or intracranial pressure in these studies is unknown. Because of cerebral autoregulation of blood flow, alterations in blood pressure caused by opioids may indirectly result in changes in cerebrovascular tone. It is interesting that feline cerebrovascular smooth muscle is reported to dilate in response to direct microapplication of μ or δ agonists.[63] There is also some evidence for neuroexcitatory effects of opioids, including localized electrical (but not motor) seizure activity in neurosurgical patients (see Rigidity and other neuroexcitatory effects, above)[58] that could be associated with increases in regional cerebral blood flow.

The subject of opioid effects on the cerebral circulation has become very complex and somewhat controversial because of unexplained discrepancies between studies. These issues were recently reviewed.[64] Some studies have found increased cerebral blood flow or increased intracranial pressure following opioid administration, and some have not. The effects of opioids on the cerebral circulation may be variable depending upon the circumstances. These issues should be considered when opioids are used in patients with critically reduced intracranial compliance.

Gastrointestinal effects

Potency varies between particular drugs, but virtually all commonly used opioids produce gastrointestinal side-effects, by a combination of central and peripheral actions. Intestinal motility is generally reduced and constipation can be a problem. Increased tone in the sphincter of

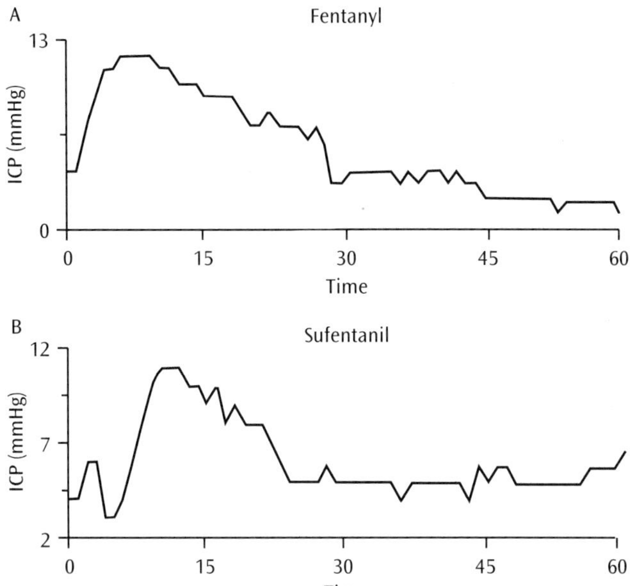

Figure 34.6 *Intracranial pressure was elevated significantly within minutes of administration of (A) fentanyl (3 µg kg^{-1}) or (B) sufentanil (0.6 µg kg^{-1}) to patients with severe head trauma. Each plot represents a single patient. (From Sperry* et al.,[62] *with permission.)*

Oddi can produce increased pressure in the biliary ducts, occasionally producing pain. Opioid-induced spasm of the sphincter may prevent radiographic dye from entering the duodenum during intraoperative cholangiography, simulating the presence of a common bile duct gallstone. Some anesthesiologists prefer to avoid opioid-balanced anesthesia for cholecyctectomy because of the possibility of interfering with the cholangiogram. However, this is a relatively uncommon problem,[65] and may be resolved by administering glucagon (or naloxone or nalbuphine), which relaxes the sphincter of Oddi. Obstruction of the common bile duct persisting after glucagon administration is unlikely to be related to opioid effects.

Nausea and vomiting

Opioids commonly produce nausea and vomiting. The neurophysiology and pharmacology of nausea and vomiting are complex. The vomiting center in the medulla receives input from the cerebral cortex, the gut, the vestibular system, and the chemoreceptor trigger zone. The chemoreceptor trigger zone is located in the floor of the fourth ventricle, outside the blood–brain barrier. The chemoreceptor trigger zone contains many types of receptors, including opioid receptors, that promote vomiting. Experiments in cats have suggested that opioids actually have an antiemetic effect on the vomiting center that can be reversed by naloxone. Thus, opioids appear to have opposite effects on emesis in the vomiting center and the chemoreceptor trigger zone. Intracerebroventricular injection of naloxone prevented opioid-induced emesis, but intravenous administration of naloxone did not, suggesting that the vomiting center was much more sensitive to naloxone than the chemoreceptor trigger zone. Intravenous naloxone appeared to reverse the antiemetic effects of opioids on the vomiting center selectively, promoting emesis; for example, fentanyl did not produce emesis in cats until they were pretreated with naloxone.[66] This is consistent with observations by Longnecker *et al.*[67] that administration of naloxone to antagonize morphine-induced depression of breathing frequently produced vomiting in patients.

Some patients may experience significant differences between particular opioid drugs in the severity of nausea and vomiting; it is reasonable to switch to an alternative opioid if nausea and vomiting are particularly troublesome.

Pruritus

Pruritus is a common opioid side-effect, especially with neuraxial opioid administration. Pruritus is generally quite sensitive to very small doses of µ antagonists (either naloxone or agonist–antagonist drugs such as nalbuphine); it may be possible to antagonize the pruritus selectively while preserving analgesia in many patients.

DRUG INTERACTIONS

There are several drug interactions between opioids and other anesthetic agents of vital significance in clinical practice. The interactions of greatest interest include those with intravenous induction agents, benzodiazepines, and neuromuscular blocking drugs.

Although most of the clinically significant opioid drug interactions apply broadly to all opioids, there appears to be a unique interaction between opioids that block reuptake of serotonin (e.g. meperidine, dextromethorphan, pentazocine, and tramadol) and monoamine oxidase inhibitor antidepressants (MAOIs), which block the enzymatic degradation of serotonin in the synaptic cleft, and selective serotonin reuptake inhibitors (SSRIs), which block the reuptake of serotonin into nerve terminals.[68,69] This interaction has been called the serotonin syndrome.[70] The syndrome was first described in animals, which became hypermetabolic, with fever, myoclonus, stiffness in the hindlimbs, tremor, stereotyped movements, and autonomic instability. The first clinical case was reported in 1955, in a patient treated with iproniazid (an MAOI) and meperidine.[71] Subsequently, there were a number of case reports describing a syndrome of hyperpyrexia, hypotension, and coma following administration of meperidine to patients taking MAOIs; some fatalities were recorded. The apparent rarity of this syndrome, in the face of widespread use of both meperidine, MAOIs, and SSRIs, suggests an idiosyncratic mechanism (i.e. affecting only uniquely susceptible patients). However, avoidance of drug combinations that may produce the serotonin syndrome is advisable.

Concomitant use of opioids generally reduces the dose of intravenous induction agent (e.g. thiopental, etomidate, propofol) or benzodiazepine required to induce anesthesia (produce unconsciousness). Bowdle and Ward[72] studied induction of anesthesia with a moderate dose of sufentanil or fentanyl followed by incremental doses of thiopental. They found an inverse relation between the dose of opioid and the dose of thiopental required to produce unconsciousness (Fig. 34.7). The mean thiopental requirement following sufentanil at 0.5 µg kg^{-1} was 100 mg, but following sufentanil at 1.3 µg kg^{-1} the mean thiopental requirement was only 5 mg (9 out of 10 subjects required no thiopental; one subject required 50 mg).

Fentanyl appears to attenuate the usual sympathomimetic effects of ketamine. Ketamine, 1.5 µg kg^{-1}, following fentanyl, 50 µg kg^{-1}, administered to patients undergoing coronary artery bypass surgery, produced no significant hemodynamic changes.

Vinik *et al.*[23] determined dose–effect curves for the combination of midazolam and alfentanil for induction of anesthesia and found a synergistic interaction (Fig. 34.4). Midazolam, 0.07 mg kg^{-1}, reduced the ED_{50} (for unconsciousness) for alfentanil from 0.13 mg kg^{-1} to 0.028 mg kg^{-1}, an 80% reduction in dose requirement for alfentanil.

The interaction of opioids and benzodiazepines may also produce significant hemodynamic effects. Tomicheck *et al.*[73] studied the hemodynamic consequences of administration of diazepam, 0.125–0.5 mg kg^{-1}, followed by fentanyl, 50 µg kg^{-1}, to patients undergoing coronary artery surgery. They found a dramatic reduction in mean blood pressure due entirely to reduction in systemic vascular resistance in patients receiving diazepam and fentanyl (Fig. 34.8). Hemodynamic changes were insignificant in control patients receiving fentanyl alone or diazepam alone. Flacke *et al.*[40] have suggested that this interaction occurs as a consequence of reduction of sympathetic tone; they found

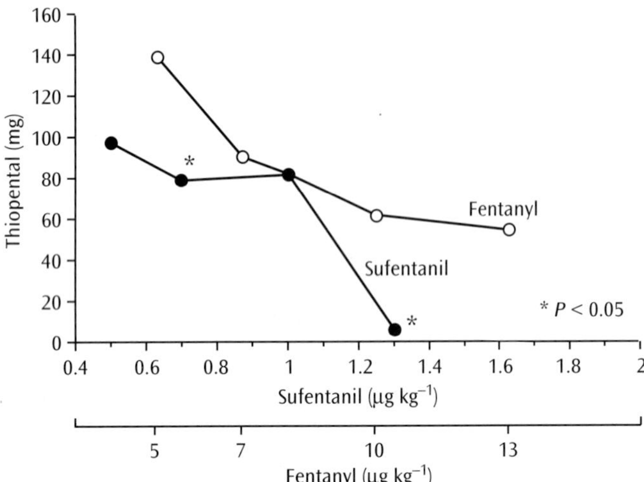

Figure 34.7 *Sufentanil or fentanyl boluses were administered over 1 min. Three minutes later, thiopental was administered in 25-mg increments every 30 s until the patient was unconscious. Sufentanil and fentanyl doses were plotted on an equipotent scale [potency ratio of 1:8, based on the electroencephalogram (EEG) effects]. There was an inverse relation between opioid dose and thiopental requirement. (From Bowdle and Ward,*[72] *with permission.)*

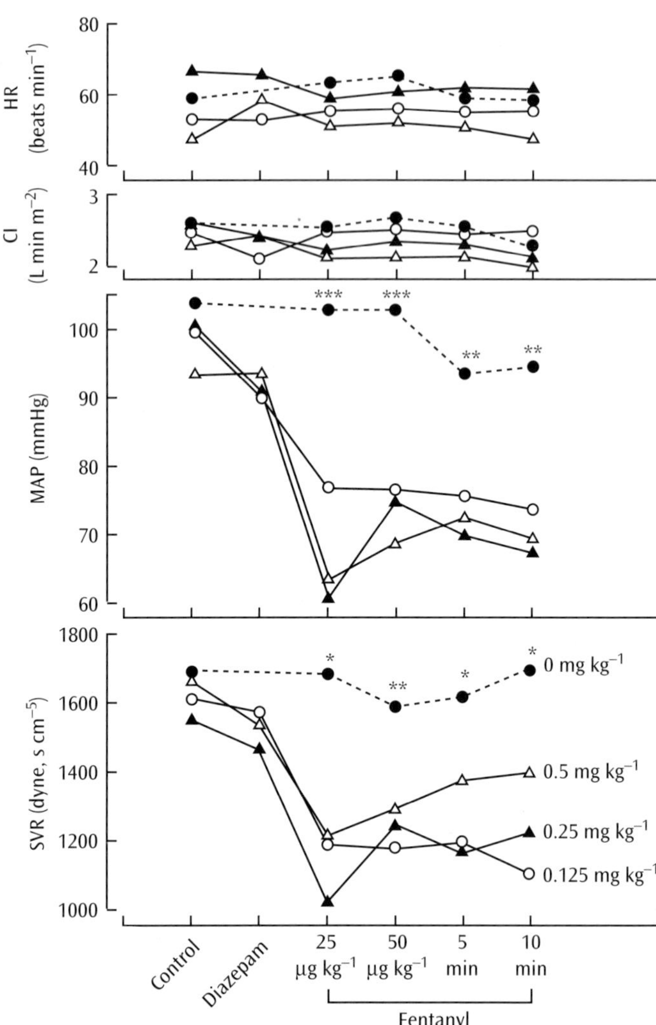

Figure 34.8 *Fentanyl or diazepam separately produced no significant changes in (from top of figure) heart rate (HR), cardiac index (CI), mean arterial pressure (MAP), or systemic vascular resistance (SVR) when administered to cardiac surgery patients for induction of anesthesia. The combination of fentanyl and diazepam (0.5, 0.25, or 0.125 mg kg*$^{-1}$*) resulted in substantial reductions in MAP and SVR. (From Tomicheck* et al.,[73] *with permission.)*

that fentanyl and diazepam did not produce cardiovascular depression in dogs previously deprived of autonomic tone. Some investigators have suggested that the interaction of benzodiazepines and opioids may produce myocardial depression, however this has not been found consistently.

Interaction between opioids and benzodiazepines may also affect ventilation. Bailey *et al.*[74] administered midazolam (0.05 mg kg^{-1}) and fentanyl (2.0 µg kg^{-1}) to healthy, young volunteers, measured CO_2 responsiveness and oxygen saturation by pulse oximetry, and observed the pattern of breathing. They found that fentanyl alone produced hypoxemia in 6 out of 12 of the subjects (breathing room air) and apnea in none. Midazolam alone did not produce hypoxemia or apnea. The addition of midazolam to fentanyl produced hypoxemia in 11 out of 12 subjects and apnea in six, suggesting a synergistic interaction.

The interaction between opioids and neuromuscular blockers has received considerable attention because of the effects on heart rate. The fentanyl analogs often produce reductions in heart rate, occasionally resulting in severe bradycardia or even asystole. Some anesthesiologists favor the concomitant use of pancuronium to facilitate intubation, based on the premise that pancuronium tends to elevate heart rate, thereby opposing the heart rate-lowering effect of the opioid. However, the combination of fentanyl, 100 µg kg^{-1}, and pancuronium, 0.1 mg kg^{-1}, produced S–T segment depression in some patients undergoing coronary artery surgery, associated with significant increases in heart rate; no S–T segment changes occurred in control groups receiving metocurine or a metocurine–pancuronium combination.[75] In the opinion of the author the choice of a combination of opioid and muscle relaxant depends upon the clinical priority. If the priority is to avoid bradycardia, pancuronium is a reasonable choice. On the other hand, if the priority is to avoid increases in heart rate, an alternative muscle relaxant devoid of cardiac stimulating properties may be preferable.

An interesting interaction has been reported between epidural morphine and the local anesthetic 2-chloroprocaine. A test dose of either lidocaine (lignocaine) or 2-chloroprocaine was administered to confirm the proper placement of epidural catheters, prior to bupivacaine epidural anesthesia for cesarean section. The duration of action of epidural morphine, given for postoperative pain control, was significantly shorter in patients receiving the 2-chloroprocaine test dose (16 h in the 2-chloroprocaine group vs. 24 h in the lidocaine group; $P < 0.05$).[76] Based upon these results, the authors recommended avoiding 2-chloroprocaine when epidural opioid analgesia is contemplated. The mechanism of this interaction is not entirely understood.[77]

PHARMACOKINETICS AND PHARMACODYNAMICS

Pharmacokinetics and pharmacodynamics constitute the study of the time-course of drug disposition and the time-course of drug effects respectively. Clinicians are ultimately most interested in pharmacodynamics; however, pharmacokinetic events often have significant impact on the time-course of drug effects. Therefore, opioid pharmacokinetics and pharmacodynamics must be considered together.

The two pharmacokinetic/pharmacodynamic questions of greatest importance for clinicians are: (1) what is the time interval between drug administration and onset of effects? and (2) what is the duration of the effects?

Speed of onset

The precise explanation for the time-course of onset of effects of an intravenously administered drug is unknown. There are several factors that could be important, including molecular size, lipid solubility, plasma protein binding, tissue binding, and distributional phenomena, such as first-pass tissue binding by the lung. Lipid solubility is probably quite important for drugs that traverse lipid membranes to gain entry to the site of action; the blood–brain barrier incorporates the lipid membranes of significance for opioids. The degree of ionization is an important determinant of lipid solubility. The opioids are weak bases with pK_a ranging from 6.5 (alfentanil) to 9.3 (methadone) (see Table 34.1). Based on the pK_a, and assuming a blood pH of 7.4, the percentage of uncharged opioid molecules (percentage "free base") can be calculated, ranging from 1.4% (methadone) to 89% (alfentanil). Overall lipid solubility has often been determined from the distribution of a drug between a mixture of octanol (an organic solvent) and water. The ratio of drug in octanol to drug in water at equilibrium is the octanol–water partition coefficient; this coefficient is usually adjusted to reflect the degree of ionization at pH 7.4. The apparent octanol–water partition coefficient at pH 7.4 ranges from 1757 (sufentanil; most lipid soluble) to 1.4 (morphine; least lipid soluble). The propensity to cross lipid barriers and enter the CNS has been estimated by combining the lipid solubility with the effect of plasma protein binding by multiplying the octanol–water partition coefficient by the free fraction in plasma; this hybrid parameter ranges from 0.91 for morphine (less likely to penetrate CNS) to 130 and 123 for fentanyl and sufentanil respectively (more likely to penetrate CNS). Based solely upon pH-adjusted lipid solubility and plasma protein binding, morphine should have the slowest onset of action and fentanyl and sufentanil the fastest. Indeed, morphine has a very slow onset (see below); however, alfentanil and remifentanil, with intermediate lipid solubility, are considerably faster in onset than fentanyl and sufentanil. The explanation for this is not known with certainty, but several factors may be involved.

The lungs temporarily take up significant amounts of lipophilic, basic drugs on the "first pass" through the pulmonary arterial circulation, and then release them back into the pulmonary venous circulation. The first-pass retention of fentanyl and sufentanil is in the order of 60–75% of the administered dose, while the first-pass retention of alfentanil is much smaller, about 10%. Alfentanil has also been shown to be released back into the circulation more quickly than sufentanil. Thus, Boer *et al.*[78] suggested that the lung may act as a "capacitor," tending to reduce the peak arterial concentration of fentanyl and sufentanil, but not alfentanil. This may explain the faster speed of onset of alfentanil; further study is needed to understand the pharmacodynamic significance of first-pass lung uptake.

After penetration of the blood–brain barrier, drugs must diffuse through a partially aqueous extracellular environment to gain access to receptor sites. Lipid solubility may be relatively disadvantageous at this point. Bernards and Hill[79] studied diffusion of drugs through spinal meninges that contain both lipophilic and lipophobic regions, and found that very lipophilic or very lipophobic drugs penetrated less well than drugs with intermediate lipid solubility. Interestingly, alfentanil penetrated much better than either fentanyl or sufentanil. A hypothetical explanation for this would be that the highly lipid-soluble drugs are bound to many nonspecific lipid sites in tissues, reducing the availability of free drug at the receptor site.

Morphine has a very slow onset of action, probably because of poor lipid solubility. Hug *et al.*[80] administered an intravenous bolus of morphine to dogs and showed that the peak concentration in cerebrospinal fluid (CSF) did not occur for approximately 15–30 min (Fig. 34.9). By comparison, more lipid-soluble drugs, such as lidocaine and fentanyl, attain peak CSF concentrations within a few minutes of an intravenous bolus. They also measured end-tidal CO_2 as a measure of morphine-induced ventilatory depression. End-tidal CO_2 did not peak until about 60 min following drug administration, a remarkably delayed onset of action.

The fentanyl analogs are much faster in onset than morphine. The EEG effects of the fentanyl analogs have been used to quantify their action in the brain. Scott *et al.*[81] fitted EEG data to a pharmacodynamic model and reported a half-time of equilibration between the central compartment and the effect compartment ($t_{1/2Keo}$) of 6.4 min for fentanyl and 1.1 min for alfentanil; as mentioned, alfentanil is remarkably faster in onset than fentanyl or sufentanil, perhaps because of its intermediate lipid solubility. The speed of onset of remifentanil is similar to that of alfentanil, while the speed of onset of sufentanil closely resembles that of fentanyl. Bowdle and Ward[72] reported that peak EEG effects of fentanyl or sufentanil occurred less than 2 min after an intravenous bolus, the 2 min including 1 min taken to administer the drug. They also observed that speed of onset was dose related: larger doses had earlier peak effects.

Duration of action

Plasma concentrations of morphine may not correspond closely with morphine effects. The lipid insolubility that retards penetration of morphine into the brain also tends to prevent it from leaving the brain once it has arrived. In addition, the morphine metabolite morphine 6-glucuronide is pharmacologically active and probably contributes substantially to the effects of morphine. Within 6 min of intravenous administration of morphine to human volunteers, the concentration of morphine 6-glucuronide in plasma exceeded that of morphine.[82]

Table 34.1 *Physical properties of and pharmacokinetic data for opioids*

Variable	Morphine	Meperidine	Fentanyl	Sufentanil	Alfentanil	Methadone
pK_a	8.0	8.5	8.4	8.0	6.5	9.3
% unionized, pH 7.4	23	7	8.5	20	90	1.4
Octanol–water partition coefficient (pH 7.4)	1.4	39	813	1778	145	116
% bound to plasma protein	35	70	84	93	92	89
$V_{d(ss)}$ (L kg^{-1})	3–5	3–5	3–5	2.5–3.0	0.4–1.0	6.1
Clearance (mL min^{-1} kg^{-1})	15–30	8–18	10–20	10–15	4–9	2.7
$t_{1/2\beta}$ (h)	2–4	3–5	2–4	2–3	1–2	35
Hepatic extraction ratio (*E*)	0.8–1.0	0.7–0.9	0.8–1.0	0.7–0.9	0.3–0.5	<0.2
Potency (mg, relative to morphine, 10 mg)	10	75	0.10	0.010	1.0	10

$V_{d(ss)}$, volume of distribution at steady state; $t_{1/2\beta}$, elimination half-life; meperidine (pethidine).
Numbers in this table are rough estimates, intended to facilitate comparisons between drugs. Actual values may vary considerably in specific situations. Relative potency is for parenteral administration.

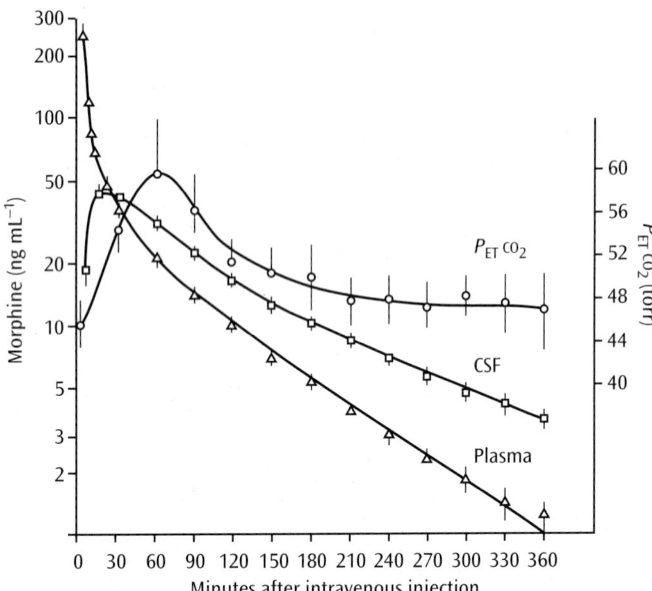

Figure 34.9 *An intravenous bolus of morphine was administered to dogs. Plasma and cerebrospinal fluid (CSF) morphine concentrations and end-tidal CO_2 were measured. Peak morphine concentrations did not occur in CSF until 15–30 min after morphine administration. End-tidal CO_2 did not reach a peak until about 60 min. The delay in the peak effect is probably related to the low lipid solubility of morphine and possibly to the active metabolite, morphine 6-glucuronide. (From Hug* et al.,[80] *with permission.)*

Morphine 6-glucuronide had a potency 45 times greater than morphine when administered intracerebrally to mice, and its ventilatory depressant effects in dogs were 5–10 times more potent than morphine itself. However, the potency in humans appears to be in the order of 2–2.5 times the potency of morphine (interspecies differences in opioid effects are expected).[83] Morphine 6-glucuronide crosses the blood–brain barrier (albeit slowly because of its polarity), and is eliminated more slowly from the CSF than morphine. Lotsch *et al.*[84] showed that morphine 6-glucuronide contributed little to the effect of morphine following a single intravenous bolus, probably because of the slowness of morphine 6-glucuronide in crossing the blood–brain barrier, but had a substantial effect during chronic administration of morphine.[85] Pharmacokinetic simulation indicated that, at steady state, morphine 6-glucuronide concentration at the effect site would be twice the concentration of morphine. Because morphine 6-glucuronide is cleared by the kidney, renal failure is expected to promote accumulation and prolong its action.

There is a close correspondence between plasma concentrations of the lipid-soluble opioids, such as the fentanyl analogs, and pharmacologic effects. Therefore, pharmacokinetic data are useful for predicting duration of action. These drugs all have relatively large volumes of distribution. Because of this, plasma concentrations fall rapidly following an intravenous bolus as drug moves from the circulation into tissues. When distribution has reached pseudoequilibrium, plasma concentrations continue to decline because of metabolic clearance, but more slowly than during the initial distribution phase.

The duration of action of drugs that undergo extensive tissue distribution is dose related in the following manner. If plasma concentrations fall below the threshold for significant pharmacologic effects during the distribution phase, as with a relatively small dose, the duration of action is short because distribution takes place rapidly. This is the reason why thiopental has a short duration of action when given as a bolus for induction of anesthesia, despite having an elimination half-life of many hours; this principle applies to almost all intravenous anesthetic agents, as well as to thiopental. On the other hand, if the plasma concentrations do not fall below the effect threshold after distribution is completed, as with a relatively large dose, the duration of action is longer, because clearance takes place less rapidly than distribution (Fig. 34.10).

Following repeated doses or continuous infusions, predicting duration of action becomes considerably more complicated because the tissue compartments begin to "fill up," altering the kinetic profile. Hughes *et al.*[86] have simulated the relation between duration of a continuous infusion and the time required for drug concentrations to fall by 50% after the infusion is turned off. They have referred to this as the "context-sensitive half-time," not to be confused with elimination half-life; the context refers to the duration of the infusion (Fig. 34.11). One of the interesting results of these simulations was that sufentanil had a shorter context-sensitive half-time than alfentanil or fentanyl, following infusions less than about 10 h long, despite having a substantially longer elimination half-life than alfentanil. This occurs because sufentanil has a much larger volume of distribution than alfentanil. Even after a prolonged infusion, this large volume of distribution acts as a "sink" for sufentanil, causing plasma concentrations to fall relatively rapidly, due to continued distribution. By contrast, the smaller volume of distribution for alfentanil is relatively "filled up," and reduction in alfentanil plasma concentration depends more heavily on metabolic clearance. Remifentanil has by far the shortest context-sensitive half-time of the fentanyl analogs (see Pharmacokinetics of remifentanil, below) at about 5 min, which does not vary with the duration of infusion. Remifentanil is a true "ultrashort-acting" drug.

The concept of context-sensitive half-time demonstrates the importance of distribution on the duration of action of drugs with

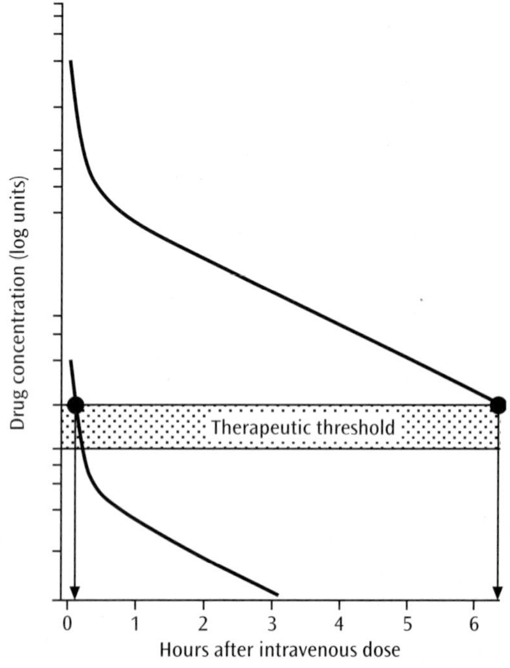

Figure 34.10 *The plasma concentrations of a large and a small intravenous bolus dose of a hypothetical anesthetic drug are shown. After the smaller dose, distribution causes plasma concentrations to fall below the therapeutic threshold within minutes. After the larger dose, plasma concentrations are well above the therapeutic threshold after distribution pseudoequilibrium is reached. Eventually (after many hours), clearance lowers plasma concentrations below the therapeutic threshold. Thus, the duration of action of this drug is dose dependent. Most intravenous anesthetics agents are subject to this effect.*

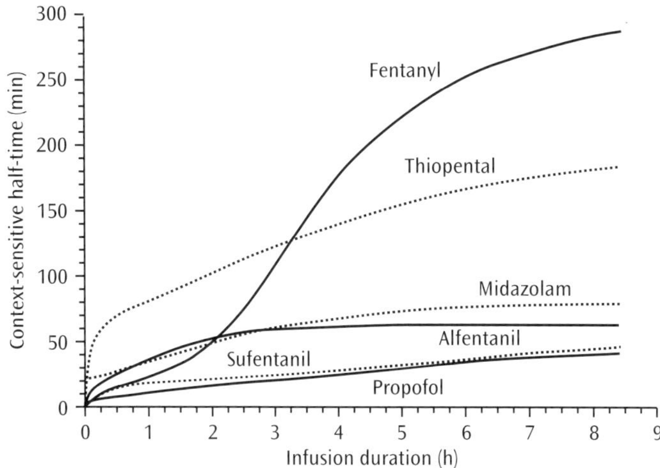

Figure 34.11 *The time required for plasma concentration to fall by 50% after stopping an infusion (context-sensitive half-time) is plotted against the duration of the infusion by computer simulation. The context-sensitive half-times are heavily influenced by the distribution kinetics of the drugs. See text for details. (From Hughes* et al.*,[86] with permission.)*

large volumes of distribution. Predicting the duration of action under conditions of continuous infusion or multiple bolus doses is complex, and not necessarily intuitive.

PHARMACOKINETIC PROPERTIES OF PARTICULAR AGENTS

A summary of pharmacokinetic parameters is provided in Table 34.1. The values in the table are averages from representative studies. There is enormous variation in pharmacokinetic parameters between patients due to normal biologic diversity and disease processes. Further comments on the pharmacokinetic properties of particular agents follows.

Morphine: unique pharmacokinetics for spinal analgesia

The pharmacokinetics and pharmacodynamics of morphine have been described extensively above. Distinguishing characteristics of morphine include poor lipid solubility and conversion to a pharmacologically active metabolite, morphine 6-glucuronide. The slow onset and prolonged duration of action of morphine may be disadvantageous when attempting to titrate the analgesic effects of intravenous morphine. However, these same properties confer on morphine a unique role in spinal analgesia (the term spinal analgesia, as used here, includes intrathecal and epidural administration). The systemic absorption of morphine after intrathecal or epidural administration is very slow, resulting in long duration of analgesia and low plasma concentrations. Intrathecal morphine, 0.3 mg, produced a peak plasma concentration of 4.5 ng mL^{-1} (minimum analgesic concentration in plasma, 20–40 ng mL^{-1}), while concentration in CSF was 6410 ng mL^{-1}.[87] Thus, the effects of spinal morphine are mediated by direct penetration into the CNS, not absorption into the circulation and subsequent redistribution to the CNS. Therapeutic effects of spinal morphine probably occur mainly within the spinal cord, although larger doses of morphine may reach the brain by cephalad spread of morphine in CSF. If sufficient spinal morphine reaches brainstem respiratory centers, depression of breathing may result. Respiratory depression from spinal morphine tends to occur after a number of hours (the precise timing being highly variable), reflecting the time required for morphine-containing CSF to migrate to the brainstem.

Highly lipid-soluble opioids, such as the fentanyl analogs, are much more rapidly absorbed into the circulation after neuraxial administration, resulting in relatively short duration of action and clinically significant plasma concentrations. When systemic absorption of an opioid from the neuraxis becomes sufficiently rapid, the plasma concentrations and concomitant effects resemble intravenous administration; under these circumstances, the effective spinal dose is similar in size to the intravenous or intramuscular dose, and neuraxial opioid administration may not be advantageous. For example, epidural infusion and intravenous infusion of fentanyl following knee surgery produced similar plasma fentanyl concentrations and comparable analgesia. Camman *et al.*[88] have reviewed the literature and concluded that the effects of lipophilic opioids in general are substantially the same whether given intravenously or spinally. On the other hand, single bolus doses (as opposed to continuous infusions) of lipid-soluble opioids probably produce selective spinal analgesia for brief periods of time and may be advantageous under particular circumstances. Epidural analgesia for labor with combinations of dilute local anesthetics and opioids produces less motor block than local anesthetics alone.

Many drugs, including some opioids, have been administered by the spinal route in the absence of adequate preclinical animal toxicology to determine whether or not the drugs or their vehicles produce direct spinal cord irritation or injury. Such practices may be unwise.

Fentanyl and sufentanil: high-extraction drugs

Fentanyl and sufentanil have hepatic extraction ratios approaching unity. The intrinsic capacity of the liver to metabolize these drugs (intrinsic clearance) is so great that the blood passing through the liver is virtually completely cleared of drug. Plasma protein binding does not affect clearance in this situation because the liver virtually "strips" the drug from plasma protein. Clearance of fentanyl or sufentanil will be nearly identical to liver blood flow, and consequently clearance will be diminished if liver blood flow is reduced. Clearance of these drugs is relatively insensitive to changes in activity of liver enzymes (because there is a substantial excess), unless they are extreme. Interestingly, the clearance of sufentanil was not altered in one study of patients with hepatic cirrhosis.[89]

Alfentanil: an intermediate-extraction drug

The hepatic extraction ratio of alfentanil was estimated to be 0.3–0.5. This intermediate extraction ratio corresponds to a relatively low intrinsic capacity of the liver to metabolize alfentanil and also reflects the high degree of alfentanil plasma protein binding; under these circumstances clearance of bound drug tends to be "restricted." Thus, clearance of alfentanil is determined by a complex relation between intrinsic clearance, plasma protein binding, and liver blood flow. Reductions in plasma protein binding will increase clearance, while reductions of liver enzyme activity or liver blood flow will decrease clearance. The clearance of alfentanil was reduced substantially in hepatic cirrhosis, and even mild hepatic dysfunction may have a significant effect. Shafer *et al.*[90] found that patients without a clinical history of liver disease but with mild abnormalities in liver function tests had alfentanil clearance 50% lower than patients without liver function test abnormalities. Patients with liver function test abnormalities frequently required naloxone to restore spontaneous ventilation at the conclusion of balanced anesthesia with alfentanil.

Pharmacokinetics of remifentanil

Remifentanil, the newest fentanyl analog, was developed deliberately to have an ultrashort duration of action. Previous experience in medicinal chemistry had identified a strategy for incorporating an ester moiety into a drug molecule that could be inactivated by ester hydrolysis, resulting in a drug with very rapid clearance. The best-known example of this approach is the ultrashort-acting β-adrenoceptor blocking drug esmolol. This strategy was applied to the 4-anilidopiperidine structure of fentanyl. A series of 26 compounds was synthesized and one of these was remifentanil.[91] The ultrashort duration of action of remifentanil distinguishes it from all other currently available opioids. Aside from the pharmacokinetic properties, remifentanil appears to be a conventional μ-receptor agonist with a pharmacologic profile similar to that of fentanyl.

Ester hydrolysis of remifentanil results in the major metabolite known as GR90291, which retains a minor amount of opioid agonist activity. The effects of GR90291 in dogs suggest that it is about 4600 times less potent than remifentanil. GR90291 is cleared by the kidney with a terminal elimination half-life in the range of 88–137 min (compared with less than 10 min for remifentanil).[92] When remifentanil is administered to patients with renal failure, clearance of GR90291 is reduced, but substantial opioid effect due to accumulated GR90291 does not appear to be clinically significant.[93]

The esterase enzymes responsible for metabolizing remifentanil have not been identified. Remifentanil is not metabolized by pseudocholinesterase,[94] acetylcholinesterase, or carbonic anhydrase. Remifentanil esterase activity is present in red cells but not in plasma. Red cell esterase activity probably does not account for the rapidity of remifentanil clearance, suggesting that tissue esterase is significantly involved. Interestingly, remifentanil elimination did not change during the anhepatic phase of liver transplantation, suggesting that liver esterase is relatively unimportant.

The very large clearance of remifentanil, of the order of 3–5 L min^{-1}, results in rapid decrement of blood levels following discontinuation of a remifentanil infusion. The elimination half-life is less than 10 min, and the context-sensitive half-time is about 5 min. The context-sensitive half-time does not increase during an infusion.[95,96]

Effect of aging on the pharmacokinetics of fentanyl analogs

Numerous studies have documented alteration in pharmacokinetics or pharmacodynamics of fentanyl analogs in elderly patients. Taken as a whole, these studies suggest that the elderly will be more sensitive to opioids. However, it is difficult to be specific because the results of several studies are in conflict. An interesting study by Lemmens *et al.*[97]showed that there was a negative correlation between alfentanil clearance in female surgical patients but not in males, a reminder that gender can make a significant difference in the disposition of certain drugs. Recent studies of remifentanil suggested that brain sensitivity increases with aging, and plasma clearance decreases, resulting in a substantially reduced dose requirement in older patients, with a typical 80-year-old requiring one-third of the infusion rate of a typical 20-year-old to attain the same effect.[25]

Methadone

Methadone has an unusual pharmacokinetic profile because of its relatively low clearance and large volume of distribution, resulting in a very long elimination half-life averaging 35 h in surgical patients.[98] Gourlay *et al.*[98] reported that methadone, 20 mg intravenously, produced a median duration of analgesia of 27 h in surgical patients. The speed of onset of methadone is similar to that of fentanyl.[99]

TARGET-CONTROLLED INFUSION OF OPIOIDS

Target-controlled infusion

Target-controlled infusion (TCI) is a system for delivering anesthetic drugs by a pump, usually a syringe pump, which is controlled by a computer. These systems are also known by other jargon, including CACI (computer-assisted continuous infusion). The computer is programmed with pharmacokinetic algorithms and parameters that are used to achieve rapidly and maintain an approximation (see below) of the target plasma concentration "dialed in" by the anesthesiologist. Alternatively, the biophase concentration or "effect site" concentration may be targeted instead of the plasma concentration; in this case the computer takes into account the time required for the drug to diffuse from the plasma to the effect site, and attempts to attain a steady effect site concentration. The pharmacokinetic, computer, and pump technology for TCI is readily available for investigational purposes, and commercially available for clinical use in Europe (Diprifusor, for the administration of propofol); TCI is not commercially available in the USA at the time of writing. The necessary computing power can be miniaturized sufficiently to be incorporated directly into a syringe pump. The pharmacokinetic technique usually employed for TCI is known as BET, which stands for bolus, elimination, and transfer. When a new target is entered that is higher than the current target, the computer calculates and instructs the pump to deliver a loading *bolus*, a maintenance infusion to compensate for *elimination* of drug out of the body, and an exponentially decreasing infusion to compensate for intercompartmental *transfer* (distribution). Hypothetically, the result of this technique is that the blood concentration moves very rapidly to the new target, with minimal undershooting or overshooting of the target, as occurs commonly with empirical bolus and infusion administration. Importantly, TCI does not alter the offset of drug action, which depends upon discontinuing the infusion and waiting for drug distribution and clearance to take place.

Accuracy of target-controlled infusion

The pharmacokinetic parameters used to calculate the instructions for the pump are mean values derived from studies of patients or normal volunteers, which almost certainly do not accurately reflect the pharmacokinetic properties of the individual patient who will receive the drug, since there is substantial pharmacokinetic variability between individuals. A mean variation of actual (measured) concentrations from target concentrations of 20–30% is expected with TCI.[100,101] The problem of individual pharmacokinetic variability could hypothetically be solved by online plasma concentration measurement, perhaps with some sort of biosensor technology. Information about plasma concentration would be fed back to the pump controller, resulting in adjustments to the pharmacokinetic algorithm and greatly improved accuracy. Unfortunately, online measurement of plasma concentration is probably many years away.

Clinical outcome and target-controlled infusion

There is only very limited information about the clinical utility of TCI. Alvis *et al.*[102] used fentanyl TCI compared with manual fentanyl bolus administration for cardiac anesthesia. The TCI group had greater hemodynamic stability and required fewer adjuvant drug interventions. Ausems *et al.*[103] compared alfentanil TCI plus nitrous oxide with manual bolus alfentanil plus nitrous oxide for lower abdominal surgery. The TCI group had greater hemodynamic stability and a lower incidence of responsiveness. These studies suggest that TCI may be associated with an improved quality of anesthetic care, however additional well-controlled studies would certainly be desirable to further explore these issues.

TCI vs. ultrashort-acting drugs

With a constant rate infusion, five half-lives are required to achieve 97% of steady state. Constant infusion of drugs with relatively small volumes of distribution and rapid clearance (and therefore short half-lives) results in steady-state plasma concentrations within a relatively short time. Arguably, TCI has less potential value for these drugs than for drugs with longer half-lives. The only current example of an ultrashort-acting intravenous anesthetic drug is remifentanil, which has a half-life of less than 10 min. A constant infusion of remifentanil reaches roughly 50–75% of steady state in 5 min or less. Remifentanil can be administered very effectively without using bolus doses, because changes in infusion rate are translated very rapidly into changes in plasma concentration and drug effect, even without TCI.

Target plasma and effect site concentrations for opioids

When using TCI the clinician must think about target plasma or effect site concentration rather than dose. There will be a range of target concentrations for any drug, depending on the intensity of surgical stimulation, the effects of other anesthetic drugs, variability between patients, and other factors. Titration of drug effect for each individual patient is just as important with TCI as with any other method of drug administration. Table 34.2 provides the steady-state plasma concentrations of the fentanyl analogs that produced half-maximal slowing of the EEG in volunteers.[104,105] These are particularly useful plasma concentration targets for comparison of one drug with another because they are determined under standardized conditions, in the absence of other anesthetic drugs or surgical stimulation.

Table 34.2 *Steady-state plasma target concentrations for opioids*

Opioid	Reference	EEG IC_{50} (ng mL^{-1})[a]
Fentanyl	Scott *et al.*[104]	8.1
Sufentanil	Scott *et al.*[104]	0.7
Alfentanil	Egan *et al.*[105]	376
Remifentanil	Egan *et al.*[105]	19.9

a. Steady-state concentration in plasma causing half-maximal slowing of the electroencephalogram (EEG) in human volunteers.

PARTIAL AGONISTS AND AGONIST–ANTAGONISTS

The pharmacology of partial agonists and agonist–antagonists has been previously reviewed.[106] While not as important as full agonist drugs in anesthetic practice, these drugs are nevertheless commonly used, and are sometimes the source of confusion because of their complexity.

Nalorphine-like drugs

The so-called nalorphine-like drugs, including nalorphine, pentazocine, nalbuphine, and butorphanol, were originally believed to be μ antagonists and κ agonists. These drugs are probably more accurately described as partial agonists at both μ and κ receptors, with the intensity of agonist activity varying somewhat from one drug to another. Some of the reasons for classifying nalorphine-like drugs as partial μ and partial κ agonists are interesting to examine. While nalorphine-like drugs uniformly depress breathing (see Depression of breathing section above), selective κ agonists do not; the selective κ agonist bremazocine did not produce depression of breathing in dogs or rats[5] and the highly selective prototype κ agonist drug U-50 488 did not depress breathing when given by intrathecal or intracerebroventricular routes to rats.[6] These results imply that κ receptors do not mediate the respiratory effects of opioids and suggest that nalorphine-like drugs mediate depression of breathing through μ receptors. β-FNA is a highly selective μ receptor antagonist. β-FNA markedly shifts to the right, in a nonparallel fashion, the dose–response curves of nalorphine, nalbuphine, and butorphanol in the mouse abdominal constriction assay, a bioassay that reflects opioid-mediated analgesia. This further supports the notion that nalorphine-like drugs are partial μ agonists.[107] Thus, the ability of nalorphine-like drugs to antagonize morphine-like μ agonists is probably because of μ partial agonist activity.

Suppression of vasopressin levels and resulting diuresis has been a useful bioassay for classifying κ agonist activity. Results of such studies suggest that nalorphine-like drugs are partial κ agonists; nalorphine and butorphanol suppress vasopressin levels but do not have the full efficacy of prototype κ agonists such as U-50 488.

Although nalorphine-like drugs share many similarities, there are significant differences between the particular drugs. Nalorphine and pentazocine produce more intense dysphoria and psychotomimetic effects than nalbuphine or butorphanol and have cardiovascular stimulating properties. Butorphanol and nalbuphine do not tend to produce as much dysphoria or cardiovascular stimulation, however they do produce sedation. Butorphanol, in particular, appears to have a marked sedative effect.[17] All of the nalorphine-like drugs have antagonist activity toward full μ agonists, but nalbuphine appears to have the most prominent antagonist properties (see below).

Buprenorphine

Buprenorphine appears to be a partial agonist at μ and κ receptors; to this extent it resembles the nalorphine-like drugs. However, slow dissociation from μ receptors and an unusual "bell-shaped" dose–response curve give buprenorphine a unique pharmacologic profile.

Several studies have demonstrated that buprenorphine dissociates very slowly from opioid receptors in rat brain and guinea pig ileum.[108] Clinical reports suggest an analogous phenomenon in humans; naloxone does not always effectively reverse buprenorphine adverse effects, such as depression of breathing.

Dum and Herz[109] examined the antinociceptive effects of buprenorphine in rats and found that doses of buprenorphine up to about 0.5 mg kg^{-1} produced the expected dose-related analgesia but doses greater than 0.5 mg kg^{-1} resulted in a paradoxical reduction in antinociception (Fig. 34.12). The opioid antagonist naltrexone shifted the buprenorphine dose response curve symmetrically to the right, suggesting that the bell shape is related to opioid receptor activity. The explanation for the unusual buprenorphine dose–response curve is unknown.

Comparable dose–response studies in humans are not available, however it is interesting to consider a case report of two patients with severe postoperative pain after balanced anesthesia with buprenorphine and nitrous oxide.[110] The anesthesiologists were aware of the bell-shaped dose–response curve and reasoned that the patients had received too much buprenorphine, placing them on the downsloping side of the curve (dose-related reduction in analgesia). Administration of naloxone to these patients resulted in "total pain relief," consistent with a shift to the right of a bell-shaped dose–response curve.

Buprenorphine binds κ receptors in rat brain and it antagonizes the diuretic effects of the κ agonist bremazocine in morphine-tolerant rats, suggesting antagonist or partial agonist activity at κ receptors. Buprenorphine pharmacology is complicated and not completely understood. Under some circumstances naloxone may not completely antagonize buprenorphine agonist effects or naloxone may actually cause a paradoxical increase in buprenorphine agonist effects.

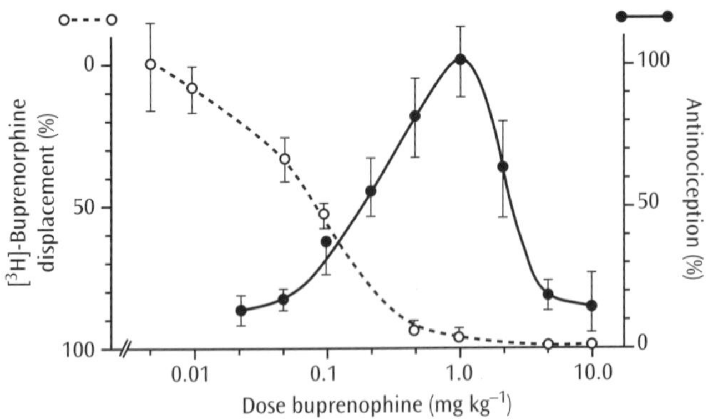

Figure 34.12 *Buprenorphine dose–effect curve for antinociception in rats (right-hand side). The curve is "bell shaped." The extent of buprenorphine binding to receptors in rat brain is also shown for the same range of buprenorphine doses (left-hand side). (From Dum and Herz,[109] with permission.)*

There is considerable interest in the use of buprenorphine as an alternative to methadone in substitution therapy for heroin addiction. Buprenorphine is probably less prone to abuse than methadone, and concomitant use of heroin is discouraged by the antagonist effects of buprenorphine.

Dezocine

Dezocine is a partial μ agonist. Subjective effects (sedation or dysphoria) in humans suggest κ activity and dezocine binds κ receptors *in vitro*.[111] Dezocine antagonized morphine effects and produced an abstinence syndrome in morphine-dependent animals. Dezocine appeared to be a more efficacious μ agonist than other agonist–antagonist drugs, judging from its analgesic and respiratory effects in animals and humans. A plateau of analgesic activity and depression of breathing could be demonstrated in humans, but the level of the plateau appeared higher than for butorphanol or nalbuphine.[112] The anesthetic-sparing effect [reduction of enflurane minimum alveolar concentration (MAC); see below] of dezocine in dogs was similar to morphine, and much greater than that of nalbuphine or butorphanol.[46]

Meptazinol

Meptazinol binds μ receptors in rat brain with moderate affinity and behaves clinically as a partial μ agonist; it is moderately selective for μ_1 receptors.[113] It has very low affinity for rat brain κ receptors, and therefore may not have appreciable κ effects. The antinociceptive effects of meptazinol in animals appear to be mediated in part by a cholinergic mechanism.[114]

Tramadol

Tramadol has a complicated mechanism of action that involves weak partial μ agonist effects combined with blockade of monoamine reuptake.[115] Analgesia is only partially reversed with naloxone but almost completely abolished by the α_2-adrenoceptor antagonist yohimbine. Thus, tramadol shares the analgesic mechanisms of opioids and α_2-agonists. Houmes *et al.*[116] performed a blinded, randomized comparison of tramadol and morphine for postoperative pain control following gynecologic surgery. Under the conditions of their study, analgesia was clinically acceptable with either drug, although there was a trend for morphine to be more effective in patients with severe pain. Oxygen saturation was measured by pulse oximetry as a measure of respiratory depression; supplemental oxygen was not given during the study. In the morphine group, 13% of patients had oxygen saturation less than 86%, compared with 0% in the tramadol group. The authors suggested that tramadol was preferable to morphine because of this apparent difference in respiratory effects. Concomitant use with MAOIs or SSRIs should be avoided, as discussed above (see Drug interactions).

Agonist–antagonists as anesthetic agents

There is an interesting literature describing the use of agonist–antagonist opioids as analgesic supplements in various regimens of balanced anesthesia. Murphy and Hug[117] studied the enflurane-sparing effect (MAC reduction) of morphine, fentanyl, butorphanol, and nalbuphine in dogs. Morphine or fentanyl reduced enflurane MAC by about 65%, while butorphanol or nalbuphine reduced enflurane MAC by only 11% or 8% respectively. The authors suggested that the smaller MAC reduction with the agonist–antagonists was the result of a "ceiling" for analgesia. Hall *et al.*[46] studied dezocine in the same dog model and found a 58% reduction in enflurane MAC; the maximum dose of dezocine was limited by cardiovascular depression. These studies could be interpreted as suggesting that butorphanol and nalbuphine would not be efficacious as analgesic supplements to general anesthesia. However, this conclusion may not be warranted. There are substantial differences in opioid pharmacology between various species; experiments in dogs may not apply directly to humans. The contribution of "analgesia" to general anesthesia is unclear, and many drugs that produce general anesthesia (e.g. most of the intravenous induction agents and potent volatile anesthetics) do not produce analgesia in conscious subjects. Even with a "ceiling" for antinociceptive effects, other opioid effects, such as the sedation mediated by κ receptors, might contribute to the anesthetic state.

"MAC reduction" studies with agonist–antagonists have not been performed in humans. However, a substantial number of clinical studies of agonist–antagonist opioids, including blinded, randomized comparisons with full μ agonists, suggest that agonist–antagonists can be efficacious as the opioid component of "balanced" anesthesia. For example, Aldrete *et al.*[118] compared butorphanol with morphine, combining either opioid with diazepam, pancuronium, and nitrous oxide in a randomized, blinded study of anesthesia for coronary artery bypass surgery. The average dose of butorphanol was 25 mg compared with 127 mg of morphine. The average dose of diazepam was 22 mg in both groups. The two opioids were equally satisfactory and there were no significant differences in hemodynamic changes during surgery. The "blinded" anesthesiologists were unable to discern which drug they were using. In three out of four cases of patient movement, intraoperative awareness, or hemodynamic instability in which the anesthesiologist was convinced the opioid was butorphanol when it was in fact morphine.

The use of agonist–antagonists to antagonize full agonists

The agonist–antagonist opioids can antagonize full agonists under certain conditions. The antagonist properties of nalbuphine have been studied most often. Nalbuphine (15 mg per 70 kg body weight) actually increased depression of breathing produced by a small dose of morphine (15 mg per 70 kg body weight), as predicted by theory.[119] However, several studies have shown that nalbuphine is effective for antagonizing the respiratory depressant effects of large doses of μ agonists.[120–122] The dose–response for nalbuphine antagonist effects has not been rigorously determined and a wide range of doses have been used, from about 1–20 mg per 70 kg intravenously; 2.5–5.0 mg is probably a reasonable starting dose.

There is considerable interest in opioid antagonists that would preserve analgesia and not elevate sympathetic tone, because of the clinical problems associated with naloxone. Nalbuphine did not elevate circulating catecholamines in dogs anesthetized with fentanyl and enflurane, in contrast with naloxone. Bailey *et al.*[120] suggested that nalbuphine preserved analgesia better than naloxone. On the other hand, the use of nalbuphine as an antagonist has been associated with a spectrum of naloxone-like adverse effects, including pulmonary edema.[123] Nalbuphine is an interesting alternative to naloxone in the clinical setting; whether it is superior to naloxone is not clear.

Butorphanol[124] and buprenorphine[125] have also been used experimentally to antagonize respiratory depression caused by fentanyl, however insufficient information is available to recommend their use for this purpose in clinical practice.

Pharmacokinetics of partial agonist and agonist–antagonist opioids

The pharmacokinetic properties of partial agonist and agonist–antagonist opioids have not been studied nearly as extensively as for full agonist drugs. Pharmacokinetic data for agonist–antagonist opioids are summarized in Table 34.3.

ANTAGONISTS

Naloxone is a pure antagonist of all three types of opioid receptors, although higher doses are required to antagonize κ and δ receptors than μ receptors. Naloxone has a relatively short duration of action compared with many of the opioid agonists; the terminal half-life is about 1–1.5 h. Thus, there may be a risk of recurrence of opioid agonist effects when naloxone is given in small bolus doses. Longnecker *et al.*[67] were able to prolong the action of naloxone by giving it intramuscularly; from 80 min (0.35 mg per 70 kg body weight, intravenously) to 6 h (0.7 mg per 70 kg body weight, intramuscularly).

Naloxone has been given by intravenous infusion in attempts to antagonize opioid side-effects such as pruritus and ventilatory depression while preserving analgesia. Some authors have reported successful results. However, interference with analgesia is always a possibility when naloxone is used.

The use of naloxone to antagonize opioid agonist overdosage can be associated with serious cardiovascular problems. Severe hypertension, cardiac arrhythmias (including ventricular fibrillation), and pulmonary edema have been reported. A few deaths have been attributed to naloxone administration. These adverse effects may not be dose related; pulmonary edema has been reported following a small dose (0.1 mg). The mechanism of cardiovascular side-effects is believed to be a sudden increase in sympathetic tone, as demonstrated in dogs by Flacke *et al.*[41] The mechanism of pulmonary edema is presumed to be similar to neurogenic pulmonary edema.

Naloxone has been used to treat cardiovascular shock states, stroke, spinal cord injury, and a variety of miscellaneous conditions. There is also evidence that naloxone may antagonize some anesthetic drugs that are not opioids, such as nitrous oxide, benzodiazepines, and barbiturates. However, these miscellaneous uses of naloxone are not firmly established.

There are remarkably few pure opioid antagonists, compared with the number of opioid agonists that are available. Naltrexone and nalmefene are pure opioid antagonists that are analogs of naloxone. Naltrexone is the *N*-cyclopropylmethyl analog of oxymorphone, whereas naloxone is the *N*-allyl analog. Several antagonists have resulted from modificaton of the C_6 keto group of naltrexone, including nalmefene, naltrindole, and norbinaltorphimine (nor-BNI). Naltrindole and norbinaltorphimine are selective antagonists at δ and κ receptors respectively (not available for clinical use). Naltrexone and nalmefene, like naloxone, are most potent at μ receptors but have significant activity at all three types of opioid receptor. They are both much longer acting than naloxone (terminal half-life in excess of 8 h) and have significant oral bioavailability. Joshi *et al.*[126] found that administration of nalmefene reduced side-effects (nausea, itching) associated with patient-controlled analgesia with morphine, without altering morphine requirements.

PERIPHERAL MECHANISMS OF ANALGESIA: OPIOIDS AND NONSTEROIDAL ANTI-INFLAMMATORY DRUGS

Traditional pharmacologic strategies for producing analgesia are largely concerned with blunting nociceptive afferent stimuli inside the CNS. An alternative strategy is to prevent the afferent stimulus from ever reaching the CNS. Sensory nerve conduction block by local anesthetics is an example of this approach. Recently, there has been considerable interest in methods of blocking nociception at the most peripheral possible site, the afferent nerve ending. Two classes of drugs have been tried with some success, the opioids and the nonsteroidal anti-inflammatory agents; these drugs have significant peripheral, as well as central, effects on nociception.

Nonsteroidal anti-inflammatory drugs

Nonsteroidal anti-inflammatory drugs (NSAIDs) are a heterogeneous group of agents that mediate anti-inflammatory, analgesic, antipyretic, and platelet-inhibitory effects. There are over 100 NSAIDs marketed around the world. NSAIDs are also referred to as "aspirin-like," after the prototype drug of the class, acetylsalicylic acid (aspirin), which was introduced into clinical use in 1899. The term "nonsteroidal anti-inflammatory" is probably preferable to "aspirin-like" because many of the drugs are chemically unrelated to aspirin. The anti-inflammatory, analgesic, antipyretic, and platelet-inhibitory effects vary between specific NSAIDs. For example, acetaminophen (paracetamol) is antipyretic and analgesic but lacks significant anti-inflammatory activity.

Table 34.3 *Pharmacokinetic data for partial agonists and agonist–antagonists*

Variable	Pentazocine	Nalbuphine	Butorphanol	Buprenorphine	Dezocine	Meptazinol
Clearance (L min^{-1})	1.38	1.5	2.7	1.3	3.0 L h^{-1} kg^{-1}	1.3
$V_{d(ss)}$ (L) or *$V_{d\beta}$ (L kg^{-1})	396	315	350	188	11 L kg^{-1}*	5.0 L kg^{-1}*
$t_{1/2\beta}$ (min)	203	222	160	184	156	120
Potency (mg, relative to morphine, 10 mg	30	10	2	0.2	10	100

$V_{d(ss)}$, volume of distribution at steady state; $V_{d\beta}$, volume of distribution during terminal elimination ($V_{d\beta} > V_{d(ss)}$); $t_{1/2\beta}$, elimination half-life. Numbers in this table are rough estimates, intended to facilitate comparisons between drugs. Actual values may vary considerably in specific situations. Relative potency is for parenteral administration.

NSAIDs are particularly effective for producing analgesia in settings in which inflammatory mediators, such as prostaglandins, have sensitized afferent sensory nerve endings. NSAIDs interfere with protaglandin biosynthesis by inhibition of the enzyme prostaglandin synthase also known as cyclo-oxygenase (COX). NSAID inhibition of COX is highly stereospecific; the (+) isomer is more potent. There are two forms of COX: COX-1, which has a role in the normal physiologic regulation of renal parenchyma, gastric mucosa, platelets, and other tissues; and COX-2, which is involved in inflammation. Many adverse effects of NSAIDs are mediated by COX-1, while the therapeutic effects are mediated by COX-2. Thus, agents that affect COX-2 selectively might be predicted to have relatively fewer adverse effects. Available NSAIDs have a wide range of COX-1 vs. COX-2 activity, and toxicity, especially gastrointestinal ulceration, does in general correspond with COX-1 action. However, toxicity is not entirely explained by COX activity; for example, the non-COX selective NSAID nabumetone has a relatively low incidence of gastrointestinal side-effects.[127]

The mechanism of inhibition of COX varies with different agents. Some are competitive inhibitors, while others irreversibly block the enzyme; for example, aspirin inhibits COX by irreversible acetylation of a serine associated with the active site. Platelets are particularly vulnerable to irreversible inhibition of COX because they have no cellular apparatus for producing new enzyme. Thus, a single dose of aspirin will inhibit platelet aggregation and prolong bleeding time until sufficient numbers of normal platelets enter the circulation to restore normal platelet function; this process typically requires 3 or 4 days.

COX inhibition explains many of the anti-inflammatory effects of NSAIDs. Adverse effects of NSAIDs, including platelet dysfunction, gastrointestinal ulceration, and decreased renal function, are also related to inhibition of COX. However, other mechanisms of action are probably important. The potency of NSAIDs to inhibit prostaglandin synthesis is not well correlated with anti-inflammatory activity, and a number of other NSAID effects on the inflammatory process have been identified. There is also evidence that NSAID actions in the CNS may affect peripheral inflammation. Catania *et al.*[128] found that lysine acetylsalicylate and sodium salicylate injected into the lateral cerebral ventricle of mice inhibited inflammatory edema in the mouse ear. Indomethacin did not have this effect; the lack of anti-inflammatory activity with indomethacin implied that prostaglandins were not involved in the central anti-inflammatory activity of salicylates, because both indomethacin and salicylates inhibit prostaglandin synthesis.

NSAIDs can produce serious side-effects. They decrease renal blood flow, normally a harmless effect. However, renal failure can be precipitated in patients with impaired renal circulation from low cardiac output, chronic renal disease, or hypovolemia. Gastric and intestinal ulceration is a common side-effect, mediated both by local irritation (with oral administration) and by systemic action. Platelet inhibition and prolongation of bleeding time has been mentioned; whether this results in clinically significant hemorrhage depends upon specific circumstances, including the type of surgery and the status of other aspects of the patient's hemostatic system.

An idiosyncratic reaction to NSAIDs occurs in perhaps 20–25% of patients with asthma, nasal polyps, or chronic urticaria. These patients may respond to NSAIDs with a potentially life-threatening syndrome resembling anaphylaxis. Although this syndrome is often associated with aspirin, it may occur with any NSAID. The mechanism is unknown. Treatment is the same as for anaphylaxis; epinephrine is the drug of choice.

NSAIDs appear to be moderately effective for the treatment of postoperative pain. Interest in the use of these drugs exploded in the USA following the marketing of ketorolac, an NSAID that has been promoted specifically for postoperative pain. However, ketorolac is not the only NSAID available for parenteral use, and whether it has any advantages over other NSAIDs (even including aspirin) is unknown. Ketorolac or other NSAIDs are often used in combination with opioids. The required dose of opioids may be reduced in this circumstance.[129] Such "opioid sparing" may be beneficial by virtue of minimizing opioid side-effects, such as respiratory depression; on the other hand, NSAIDs also have their own side-effects. Additional clinical research is needed to clearly establish the role of NSAIDs in the therapy of postoperative pain.

Recently, NSAIDs that are highly selective for COX-2, such as rofecoxib and celecoxib, have become available,. Early experience suggests that gastrointestinal toxicity is reduced with these drugs, although further experience will be required to fully understand their side-effect profiles.[130]

PERIPHERAL OPIOIDS

Until recently, opioid-mediated analgesia was thought to occur entirely within the CNS. Now there is evidence that opioid receptors on peripheral afferent neurons may mediate analgesia, especially in the setting of inflammation.[131, 132] Opioid peptides produced by immune cells in the vicinity of the neurons may be the source of endogenous ligands for these receptors. Exogenous opioid agonist drugs can also mediate peripheral antinociceptive effects; there is evidence for peripheral analgesic activity of μ, δ, and κ agonists, suggesting that all three known opioid receptors may be involved. Results from the few available clinical studies of the peripheral administration of opioid drugs are inconclusive but positive results from some studies are encouraging. For example, Khoury *et al.*[133] instilled morphine, 1 mg, into the knee joint at the conclusion of arthroscopic surgical procedures and compared the resulting analgesia with intra-articular bupivacaine. The onset of analgesia after morphine was delayed compared with bupivacaine, but the duration of analgesia was substantially longer; from the fourth postoperative hour until 2 days later (the end of the study period), analgesia was superior with morphine. A combination of bupivacaine and morphine produced rapid onset and prolonged analgesia.

THE α_2-AGONISTS

α_2-Adrenoceptor agonists produce sedative–hypnotic, anesthetic-sparing, analgesic, and sympatholytic effects, and attenuate opioid-induced muscle rigidity. While very promising as anesthetic and/or analgesic agents, clinical application of these drugs has been hampered by side-effects, mainly bradycardia and hypotension.[134] The effects of α_2-agonists on blood pressure are biphasic. Smaller doses tend to produce hypotension by central reduction of sympathetic tone, while larger doses induce peripheral vasoconstriction by activation of postsynaptic α_2-adrenoceptors on vascular smooth muscle. Currently available α_2-adrenoceptor agonists do not distinguish between the several α_2-adrenoceptor subtypes and they contain an imidazole ring that causes binding to the imidazoline receptor. Improvement in the side-effect profile in this drug class will probably depend upon elimination of imidazoline-mediated effects and greater α_2-receptor subtype specificity. Clonidine, the best-described α_2-adrenoceptor agonist, has been administered orally, intravenously, and epidurally in the treatment of acute and chronic pain, and as an anesthetic adjunct.[135] Dexmedetomidine, which has about a 10-fold greater α_2- vs. α_1-adreneceptor selectivity than clonidine, has recently been licensed in the USA. The place of dexmedetomidine in anesthetic practice has yet to be established.[136] A specific α_2-adrenoceptor antagonist has been investigated.[134, 137]

CONOPEPTIDES

Ziconotide (formerly SNX-11) is derived from a conopeptide, MVIIA, from the venom of fish-hunting marine snails. Following intrathecal or epidural administration ziconotide produces analgesia by blockade of N-type calcium channels, interrupting primary afferent transmission in the spinal cord, and antagonizing central sensitization. The spinal route of administration minimizes potential adverse effects that would otherwise occur with systemic administration, including hypotension. Ziconotide appears not to produce typical opioid side-effects, such as respiratory depression and bowel dysfunction. Tolerance to the analgesic effects of ziconotide has not been observed, and ziconotide has been effective for treating pain refractory to opioids. The results of clinical trials suggest that spinally administered ziconotide is effective for both acute and chronic pain.[138] Although the clinical utility of this drug remains to be established, future prospects appear bright.[139]

REFERENCES

1. Martin WR. History and devlopment of mixed opioid agonists, partial agonists, and antagonists. *Br J Clin Pharmacol* 1979; **7:** 273S–279S
2. Cox BM. Peripheral actions mediated by opioid receptors In: Pasternak GW (ed.). *The Opiate Receptors*. Clifton, NJ: The Humana Press, 1988.
3. Pasternak GW. Pharmacological mechanisms of opioid analgesics. *Clin Neuropharmacol* 1993; **16:** 1–18.
4. Millan MJ. Kappa-opioid receptors and analgesia. *Trends Pharmacol Sci* 1990; **11:** 70–6.
5. Freye E, Hartung E, Schenk GK. Bremazocine: an opiate that induces sedation and analgesia without respiratory depression. *Anesth Analg* 1983; **62:** 483–8.
6. Castillo R, Kissin I, Bradley E. Selective kappa opioid agonist for spinal analgesia without the risk of respiratory depression. *Anesth Analg* 1986; **65:** 350–4.
7. Pazos A, Florez J. Interaction of naloxone with mu and delta opioid agonists on the respiration of rats. *Eur J Pharmacol* 1983; **87:** 309–14.
8. Walker JM, Bowen WD, Walker FO, *et al.* Sigma receptors: biology and function. *Pharmacol Rev* 1990; **42:**355–402.
9. Musacchio J. The psychotomimetic effects of opiates and the sigma receptor. *Neuropsychopharmacology* 1990; **3:** 191–200.
10. Pasternak GW, Standifer KM. Mapping of opioid receptors using antisense oligodeoxynucleotides: correlating their molecular biology and pharmacology. *Trends Pharmacol Sci* 1995; **16:** 344–50.
11. Henderson G, McKnight AT. The orphan opioid receptor and its endogenous ligand-nociceptin/orphanin FQ. *Trends Pharmacol Sci* 1997; **18:** 293–300.
12. Hughes J, Kosterlitz AW, Smith TW. The distribution of methionine-enkephalin and leucine-enkephalin in the brain and peripheral tissues. *Br J Pharmacol* 1977; **61:** 639–47.
13. Sapru HN, Willette RN, Krieger AJ. Stimulation of pulmonary J receptors by an enkaphalin-analog. *J Pharmacol Exp Ther* 1981; **217:** 228–34.
14. Yeadon M, Kitchen I. Multiple opioid receptors mediate the respiratory depressant effects of fentanyl-like drugs in the rat. *Gen Pharmacol* 1990; **21:** 655–64.
15. Ohtani M, Kotaki H, Nishitateno K, *et al.* Kinetics of respiratory depression in rats induced by buprenorphine and its metabolite, norbuprenorphine. *J Pharmacol Exp Ther* 1997; **281:** 428–33.
16. Hecker BR, Lake CL, DiFazio CA, *et al.* The decrease in the minimum alveolar anesthetic concentration produced by sufentanil in rats. *Anesth Analg* 1983; **62:** 987–90.
17. Dershwitz M, Rosow CE, DiBiase PM, Zaslavsky A. Comparison of the sedative effects of butorphanol and midazolam. *Anesthesiology* 1991; **74:** 717–24.
18. Macintyre PE, Pavlin EG, Dwersteg JF. Effect of meperidine on oxygen consumption, carbon dioxide production and respiratory gas exchange in postanesthesia shivering. *Anesth Analg* 1987; **66:** 751–5.
19. Vogelsang J, Hayes SR. Stadol attenuates postanesthesia shivering. *J Post Anesth Nurs* 1989; **4:** 222–7.
20. Pausawasdi S, Jirasirithum S, Phanarai C. The use of tramadol hydrochloride in the treatment of post-anesthetic shivering. *J Med Assoc Thai* 1990; **73:** 16–20.
21. Ausems ME, Hug CC, Stanski DR, Burm AGL. Plasma concentrations of alfentanil required to supplement nitrous oxide anesthesia for general surgery. *Anesthesiology* 1986; **65:** 362–73.
22. McDonnell TE, Bartowski RR, Williams JJ. ED_{50} of alfentanil for induction of anesthesia in unpremedicated young adults. *Anesthesiology* 1984; **60:** 136–40.
23. Vinik HR, Bradley EL, Kissin I. Midazolam–alfentanil synergism for anesthetic induction in patients. *Anesth Analg* 1989; **69:** 213–17.
24. Dershwitz M, Randel GI, Rosow CE, *et al.* Initial clinical experience with remifentanil, a new opioid metabolized by esterases. *Anesth Analg* 1995; **81:** 619–23.
25. Minto CF, Schnider TW, Shafer SL. Pharmacokinetics and pharmacodynamics of remifentanil. II. Model application. *Anesthesiology* 1997; **86:** 24–33.
26. Bowdle TA. The comparative tolerability of opioid agonists. *Drug Safety* 1998; **19:** 173–89.
27. Bailey PL, Streisand JB, East KA, *et al.* Differences in magnitude and duration of opioid-induced respiratory depression and analgesia with fentanyl and sufentanil. *Anesth Analg* 1990; **70:** 8–15.
28. Keats AS, Telford T. Studies of analgesic drugs. X. Respiratory effects of narcotic antagonists. *J Pharmacol Exp Ther* 1966; **112:** 126–132.
29. Romagnoli A, Keats AS. Ceiling effect for respiratory depression by nalbuphine. *Clin Pharmacol Ther* 1980; **27:** 478–85.
30. Romagnoli A, Keats AS. Ceiling respiratory depression by dezocine. *Clin Pharmacol Ther* 1984; **35:** 367–73.
31. Nagashima H, Karamanian A, Malovany R, *et al.* Respiratory and circulatory effects of intravenous butorphanol and morphine. *Clin Pharmacol Ther* 1976; **19:** 738–45.
32. Orwin JM. The effect of doxapram on buprenorphine induced respiratory depression. *Acta Anaesth Belg* 1977; **2:** 93–105.
33. Gal TJ. Naloxone reversal of buprenorphine-induced respiratory depression. *Clin Pharmacol Ther* 1989; **45:** 66–71.
34. Krane BD, Kreutz JM, Johnson DL, Mazuzan JE. Alfentanil and delayed respiratory depression: case studies and review. *Anesth Analg* 1990; **70:** 557–61.
35. Catley DM, Thornton C, Jordan C, *et al.* Pronounced, episodic oxygen desaturation in the postoperative period: its association with ventilatory pattern and analgesic regimen. *Anesthesiology* 1985; **63:** 20–8.
36. Flacke JW, Flacke WE, Bloor BC, *et al.* Histamine release by four narcotics: a double-blind study in humans. *Anesth Analg* 1987; **66:** 723–30.
37. Strauer BE. Contractile responses to morphine, piritramide, meperidine, and fentanyl: a comparative study of effects on the isolated ventricular myocardium. *Anesthesiology* 1972; **37:** 304–10.
38. Freye E. Cardiovascular effects of high dosages of fentanyl, meperidine, and naloxone in dogs. *Anesth Analg* 1974; **53:** 40–7.
39. Buffington CW. Hemodynamic determinants of ischemic myocardial dysfunction in the presence of coronary stenosis in dogs. *Anesthesiology* 1985; **63:** 651–62.
40. Flacke JW, Davis LJ, Flacke WE, *et al.* Effects of fentanyl and diazepam in dogs deprived of autonomic tone. *Anesth Analg* 1985; **64:**1053–9.
41. Flacke JW, Flacke WE, Bloor BC, Olewine S. Effects of fentanyl, naloxone and clonidine on hemodynamics and plasma catecholamine levels in dogs. *Anesth Analg* 1983; **62:** 305–13.
42. Thomson IR, Putnins CL, Friesen RM. Hyperdynamic cardiovascular responses to anesthetic induction with high-dose fentanyl. *Anesth Analg* 1986; **65:** 91–5.
43. Janssen PAJ. The past, present and future of opioid analgesics in anesthesia. In: Estafanous F (ed.). *Opioids in Anesthesia II*. Boston: Butterworth-Heinemann, 1991: xvi.
44. Popio KA, Jackson DH, Ross AM, *et al.* Hemodynamic and respiratory effects of morphine and butorphanol. *Clin Pharmacol Ther* 1978; **23:** 281–7.
45. Camu F, Rucquoi M. Cardiac and circulatory effects of high-dose meptazinol in anaesthetized patients. *Postgrad Med* J 1983; **59** (Suppl. 1): 60–3.
46. Hall RI, Murphy MR, Szlam F, Hug CC. Dezocine-MAC reduction and evidence for myocardial depression in the presence of enflurane. *Anesth Analg* 1987; **66:** 1169–74.
47. Weinger MB, Smith NT, Blasco TA, Koob GF. Brain sites mediating opiate-induced muscle rigidity in the rat: methylnaloxonium mapping study. *Brain Res* 1991; **544:** 181–90.
48. Benthuysen JL, Smith NT, Sanford TJ, *et al.* Physiology of alfentanil-induced rigidity. *Anesthesiology* 1986; **64:** 440–6.
49. Bowdle TA, Rook GA. Postoperative myoclonus and rigidity after anesthesia with opioids. *Anesth Analg* 1994; **78:** 783–6.
50. Klausner JM, Caspi J, Lelcuk S, *et al.* Delayed muscular rigidity and respiratory depression following fentanyl anesthesia. *Arch Surg* 1988; **123:** 66–7.

51. Bailey PL, Wilbrink J, Zwanikken P, *et al*. Anesthetic induction with fentanyl. *Anesth Analg* 1985; **64:** 48–53.
52. Blasco TA, Smith NT, Sanford TJ, *et al*. A clinical study of the effects of various pretreatment agents on alfentanil-induced rigidity: EMG data. *Anesthesiology* 1985; **63:** A380.
53. Weinger MB, Segal IS, Maze M. Dexmedetomidine, acting through central alpha-2 adrenoceptors, prevents opiate-induced muscle rigidity in the rat. *Anesthesiology* 1989; **71:** 242–9.
54. Weinger MG, Cline EJ, Smith NT, Koob GF. Ketanserin pretreatment reverses alfentanil-induced muscle rigidity. *Anesthesiology* 1987; **67:** 348–54.
55. Vacanti CA, Silbert BS, Vacanti FX. The effects of thiopental sodium on fentanyl-induced muscle rigidity in a human model. *J Clin Anesth* 1991; **3:** 395–8.
56. Smith NT, Benthuysen JL, Bickford RG, *et al*. Seizures during opioid anesthetic induction – are they opioid-induced rigidity? *Anesthesiology* 1989; **71:** 852–62.
57. Bowdle TA. Myoclonus following sufentanil without EEG seizure activity. *Anesthesiology* 1987; **67:** 593–5.
58. Tempelhoff R, Modica PA, Bernardo KL, Edwards I. Fentanyl-induced electrocorticographic seizures in patients with complex partial epilepsy. *J Neurosurg* 1992; **77:** 201–8.
59. Cascino GD, So EL, Sharbrough FW, Al E. Alfentanil-induced epileptiform activity in patients with partial epilepsy. *J Clin Neurophysiol* 1993; **10:** 520–5.
60. Armstrong PJ, Bersten A. Normeperidine toxicity. *Anesth Analg* 1986; **65:** 536–8.
61. Milde LN, Milde JH, Gallagher WJ. Effects of sufentanil on cerebral circulation and metabolism in dogs. *Anesth Analg* 1990; **70:** 138–46.
62. Sperry RJ, Bailey PL, Reichman MV, *et al*. Fentanyl and sufentanil increase intracranial pressure in head trauma patients. *Anesthesiology* 1992; **77:** 416–20.
63. Wahl M. Effects of enkephalins, morphine and naloxone on pial arteries during perivascular microapplication. *J Cereb Blood Flow Metab* 1985; 5: 451–7.
64. Artru AA. Effects of fentanyl, sufentanil, and alfentanil on epileptiform EEG activity, cerebral blood flow, and intracranial pressure. In: Hines R, Bowdle TA (eds). *Anesthesiology Clinics of North America Annual of Anesthetic Pharmacology*. Philadelphia: WB Saunders, 1997: 117–54.
65. Jones RM, Detmer M, Hill AB, *et al*. Incidence of choledochoduodenal sphincter spasm during fentanyl-supplemented anesthesia. *Anesth Analg* 1981; **60:** 638–40.
66. Costello DJ, Borison HL. Naloxone antagonizes narcotic self-blockade of emesis in the cat. *J Pharmacol Exp Ther* 1977; **203:** 222–30.
67. Longnecker DE, Grazis P, Eggers GWN. Naloxone antagonism of morphine induced respiratory depression. *Anesth Analg* 1973; **52:** 447–52.
68. Bodner RA, Lynch T, Lewis L, Kahn D. Serotonin syndrome. *Neurology* 1995; **45:** 219–23.
69. Kam PCA, Chang GWM. Selective serotonin reuptake inhibitors: pharmacology and clinical implications in anaesthesia and critical care medicine. *Anaesthesia* 1997; **52:** 982–8.
70. Sternbach H. The serotonin syndrome. *Am J Psychiatry* 1991; **148:** 705–13.
71. Mitchell RS. Fatal toxic encephalitis occurring during iproniazid therapy in pulmonary tuberculosis. *Ann Intern Med* 1955; **42:** 417–24.
72. Bowdle TA, Ward RJ. Induction of anesthesia with small doses of sufentanil or fentanyl: dose versus EEG response, speed of onset and thiopental requirement. *Anesthesiology* 1989; **70:** 26–30.
73. Tomicheck RC, Rosow CE, Philbin DM, *et al*. Diazepam–fentanyl interaction – hemodynamic and hormonal effects in coronary artery surgery. *Anesth Analg* 1983; **62:** 881–4.
74. Bailey PL, Pace NL, Ashburn MA, *et al*. Frequent hypoxemia and apnea after sedation with midazolam and fentanyl. *Anesthesiology* 1990; **73:** 826–30.
75. Thompson IR, Putnins CL. Adverse effects of pancuronium during high-dose fentanyl anesthesia for coronary artery bypass grafting. *Anesthesiology* 1985; **62:** 708–13.
76. Eisenach JC, Schlairet TJ, Dobson CE, Hood DH. Effect of prior anesthetic solution on epidural morphine analgesia. *Anesth Analg* 1991; **73:** 112–18.
77. Coda B, Bausch S, Haas M, Chavkin C. The hypothesis that antagonism of fentanyl analgesia by 2-chloroprocaine is mediated by direct aciton on opioid receptors. *Reg Anesth* 1997; **22:** 43–52.
78. Boer F, Bovill JG, Burm AGL, Mooren RAG. Uptake of sufentanil, alfentanil and morphine in the lungs of patients about to undergo coronary artery surgery. *Br J Anaesth* 1992; **68:** 370–5.
79. Bernards C, Hill HF. Physical and chemical properties of drug molecules governing their diffusion through the spinal meninges. *Anesthesiology* 1992; **77:** 750–6.
80. Hug CC, Morphy MR, Rigel EP, Olson WA. Pharmacokinetics of morphine injected intravenously into anesthetized dog. *Anesthesiology* 1981; **54:** 38–47.
81. Scott JC, Ponganis KV, Stanski DR. EEG quantitation of narcotic effect: the comparative pharmacodynamics of fentanyl and alfentanil. *Anesthesiology* 1985; **62:** 234–41.
82. Osborne R, Joel S, Trew D, Slevin M. Morphine and metabolite behavior after different routes of morphine administration: demonstration of the importance of the active metabolite morphine 6-glucuronide. *Clin Pharmcol Ther* 1990; **47:** 12–19.
83. Hanna MH, Peat SJ, Woodham M, *et al*. Analgesic efficacy and CSF pharmacokinetics of intrathecal morphine 6-glucuronide: comparison with morphine. *Br J Anaesth* 1990; **64:** 547–50.
84. Lotsch J, Kobal G, Stockmann A, *et al*. Lack of analgesic activity of morphine 6-glucuronide after short-term intravenous administration in healthy volunteers. *Anesthesiology* 1997; **87:** 1348–58.
85. Lotsch J, Weiss M, Ahne G, *et al*. Pharmacokinetic modeling of M6G formation after oral administration of morphine in healthy volunteers. *Anesthesiology* 1999; **90:** 1026–38.
86. Hughes AH, Glass PSA, Jacobs JR. Context-sensitive half-time in multicompartment pharmacokinetic models for intravenous anesthetic drugs. *Anesthesiology* 1992; **76:** 334–41.
87. Sjostrom S, Tamsen A, Persson MP, Hartvig P. Pharmacokinetics of intrathecal morphine and meperidine in humans. *Anesthesiology* 1987; **67:** 889–95.
88. Camann WR, Loferski BL, Fanciullo GJ, *et al*. Does epidural administration of butorphanol offer any clinical advantage over the intravenous route? *Anesthesiology* 1992; **76:** 216–20.
89. Chauvin M, Ferrier C, Haberer JP, *et al*. Sufentanil pharmacokinetics in patients with cirrhosis. *Anesth Analg* 1989; **68:**1–4.
90. Shafer A, Sung M-L, White PF. Pharmacokinetics and pharmacodynamics of alfentanil infusions during general anesthesia. *Anesth Analg* 1986; **65:** 1021–8.
91. Feldman PL, James MK, Brackeen MF, *et al*. Design, synthesis, and pharmacological evaluation of ultrashort- to long-acting opioid analgetics. *J Med Chem* 1991; **34:** 2202–8.
92. Westmoreland CL, Hoke JF, Sebel PS, *et al*. Pharmacokinetics of remifentanil (GI87084B) and its major metabolite (GI90291) in patients undergoing elective inpatient surgery. *Anesthesiology* 1993; **79:** 893–903.
93. Hoke JF, Shlugman D, Dershwitz M, *et al*. Pharmacokinetics and pharmacodynamics of remifentanil in persons with renal failure compared with healthy volunteers. *Anesthesiology* 1997; **87:** 533–41.
94. Manullang J, Egan T. Remifentanil's effect is not prolonged in a patient with pseudocholinesterase deficiency. *Anesth Analg* 1999; **89:** 529–30.
95. Egan TD, Lemmens HJM, Fiset P, *et al*. The pharmacokinetics of the new short-acting opioid remifentanil (GI897084B) in healthy adult male volunteers. *Anesthesiology* 1993; **79:** 881–92.
96. Glass PSA, Hardman D, Kamiyama Y, *et al*. Preliminary pharmacokinetics and pharmacodynamics of an ultra-short-acting opioid: remifentanil (GI87084B). *Anesth Analg* 1993; **77:** 1031–40.
97. Lemmens HJM, Burm GL, Hennis PJ, *et al*. Influence of age on the pharmacokinetics of alfentanil. *Clin Pharmacokinet* 1990; **19:** 416–22.
98. Gourlay GK, Wilson PR, Glynn CJ. Pharmacodynamics and pharmacokinetics of methadone during the postoperative period. *Anesthesiology* 1982; **57:** 458–67.
99. Inturrisi CE, Colburn WA, Kaiko RF, *et al*. Pharmacokinetics and pharmacodynamics of methadone in patients with chronic pain. *Clin Pharmacol Ther* 1987; **41:** 392–401.
100. Glass PSA, Jacobs JR, Smith RL, *et al*. Pharmacokinetic model-driven infusion of fentanyl: assessment of accuracy. *Anesthesiology* 1990; **73:** 1082–90.
101. Maitre PO, Ausems ME, Vozeh S, Stanski DR. Evaluating the accuracy of using population pharmacokinetic data to predict plasma concentrations of alfentanil. *Anesthesiology* 1988; **68:** 59–67.
102. Alvis JM, Reves JG, Govier AV, *et al*. Computer-assisted continuous infusions of fentanyl during cardiac anesthesia: comparison with a manual method. *Anesthesiology* 1985; **63:** 41–9.
103. Ausems ME, Vuyk J, Hug CCJ, Stanski DR. Comparison of a computer-assisted infusion verssus intermittent bolus administration of alfentanil as a supplement to nitrous oxide for lower abdominal surgery. *Anesthesiology* 1988; **68:** 851–61.
104. Scott JC, Cooke JE, Stanski DR. Electroencephalographic quantitation of opioid effect: comparative pharmacodynamics of fentanyl and sufentanil. *Anesthesiology* 1991; **74:** 34–42.
105. Egan TD, Minto CF, Hermann DJ, *et al*. Remifentanil versus alfentanil:

comparative pharmacokinetics and pharmacodynamics in healthy adult male volunteers. *Anesthesiology* 1996; **84:** 821–33.

106. Bowdle TA, Galer BS. Agonist–antagonist and partial agonist opioids: pharmacologic mechanisms and clinical application in the treatment of headache. *Headache Q* 1993; 4: 322–36.
107. Zimmerman DM, Leander JD, Reel JK, Hynes MD. Use of β-funaltrexamine to determine mu opioid receptor involvement in the analgesic activity of various opioid ligands. *J Pharmacol Exp Ther* 1987; **241:** 374–8.
108. Schulz R, Hertz A. The guinea pig ileum as an *in vitro* model to analyse dependence liability of narcotic drugs. In: Kosterlitz HW (ed.). *Opioids and Endogenous Opioid Peptides*. Amsterdam: North-Holland, 1976: 319–26.
109. Dum JE, Herz A. *In vivo* receptor binding of the opiate partial agonist, buprenorphine, correlated with its agonistic and antagonistic actions. *Br J Pharmacol* 1981; **74:** 627–33.
110. Pedersen JE, Chraemmer-Jorgensen B, Schmidt JF, Risbo A. Naloxone – a strong analgesic in combination with high-dose buprenorphine? *Br J Anaesth* 1985; **57:** 1045–6.
111. O'Brien JJ, Benfield P. Dezocine: a preliminary review of its pharmacodynamic and pharmacokinetic properties, and therapeutic efficacy. *Drugs* 1989; **38:** 226–48.
112. Gal TJ, DiFazio CA. Ventilatory and analgesic effects of dezocine in humans. *Anesthesiology* 1984; **61:** 716–22.
113. Spiegel K, Pasternak GW. Meptazinol: a novel mu-1 selective opioid analgesic. *J Pharmacol Exp Ther* 1984; **228:** 414–19.
114. Bill DJ, Hartley JE, Stephens RJ, Thompson AM. The antinociceptive activity of meptazinol depends on both opiate and cholinergic mechanisms. *Br J Pharmacol* 1983; **79:** 191–9.
115. Raffa RB, Friderichs E, Reimann W, *et al.* Opioid and nonopioid components independently contribute to the mechanism of action of tramadol, an "atypical" opioid analgesic. *J Pharmacol Exp Ther* 1992; **260:** 275–85.
116. Houmes RM, Voets MA, Verkaaik A, *et al.* Efficacy and safety of tramadol versus morphine for moderate and severe postoperative pain with special regard to respiratory depression. *Anesth Analg* 1992; **74:** 510–14.
117. Murphy MR, Hug CC. The enflurane sparing effect of morphine, butorphanol and nalbuphine. *Anesthesiology* 1982; **57:** 489–92.
118. Aldrete JA, de Campo T, Usubiaga LE, *et al.* Comparison of butorphanol and morphine as analgesics for coronary bypass surgery: a double-blind, randomized study. *Anesth Analg* 1983; **62:** 78–83.
119. Bailey PL, Clark NJ, Pace NL, *et al.* Failure of nalbuphine to antagonize morphine: a double-blind comparison with naloxone. *Anesth Analg* 1986; **65:** 605–11.
120. Bailey PL, Clark NJ, Pace NL, *et al.* Antagonism of postoperative opioid-induced respiratory depression: nalbuphine versus naloxone. *Anesth Analg* 1987; **66:** 1109–14.
121. Freye E, Azevedo L, Hartung E. Reversal of fentanyl related respiratory depression with nalbuphine. *Acta Anaesthesiol Belg* 1985; 4: 365–74.
122. Latasch L, Teichmuller T, Dudziak R, Probst S. Antagonisation of fentanyl-induced respiratory depression by nalbuphine. *Acta Anaesth Belg* 1989; **40:** 35–40.
123. DesMarteau JK, Cassot AL. Acute pulmonary edema resulting from nalbuphine reversal of fentanyl-induced respiratory depression. *Anesthesiology* 1986; **65:** 237.
124. Bowdle TA, Greichen SL, Bjurstrom RL, Schoene TB. Butorphanol improves CO_2 response and ventilation after fentanyl anesthesia. *Anesth Analg* 1987; **66:** 517–22.
125. Boysen K, Hertel S, Chraemmer-Jorgensen B, *et al.* Buprenorphine antagonism of ventilatory depression following fentanyl anaesthesia. *Acta Anaesthesiol Scand* 1988; **32:** 490–2.
126. Joshi GP, Duffy L, Chehade J, *et al.* Effects of prophylactic nalmefene on the incidence of morphine-related side effects in patients receiving intravenous patient-controlled analgesia. *Anesthesiology* 1999; **90:** 1007–11.
127. Freston JW. Rationalizing cyclooxygenase (COX) inhibition for maximal efficacy and minimal adverse events. *Am J Med* 1999; **107:** 78S–89S.
128. Catania A, Arnold J, Macaluso A, *et al.* Inhibition of acute inflammation in the periphery by central action of salicylates. *Proc Natl Acad Sci USA* 1991; **88:** 8544–7.
129. Gillies GWA, Kenny GNC, Bullingham RES, McArdle CS. The morphine sparing effects of ketorolac tromethamine. *Anaesthesia* 1987; **42:** 727–31.
130. Richardson C, Emery P. The clinical implications of inhibition of the inducible form of cyclo-oxygenase. *Drug Safety* 1996; **15:** 249–60.
131. Stein C. Peripheral mechanisms of opioid analgesia. *Anesth Analg* 1993; **76:** 182–91.
132. Kolesnikov YA, Jain S, Wilson R, Pasternak GW. Peripheral morphine analgesia: synergy with central sites and a target of morphine tolerance. *J Pharmacol Exp Ther* 1996; **279:** 502–6.
133. Khoury GF, Chen ACN, Garland DE, Stein C. Intraarticular morphine, bupivacaine, and morphine/bupivacaine for pain control after knee videoarthroscopy. *Anesthesiology* 1992; **77:** 263–6.
134. Khan ZP, Ferguson CN, Jones RM. Alpha-2 and imidazoline receptor agonists: their pharmacology and therapeutic role. *Anaesthesia* 1999; **54:** 146–65.
135. Eisenach JC, De Kock M, Klimscha W. Alpha-2 adrenergic agonists for regional anesthesia: a clinical review of clonidine (1984–1995). *Anesthesiology* 1996; **85:** 655–74.
136. Venn RM, Bradshaw CJ, Spencer R, *et al.* Preliminary UK experience of dexmedetomidine, a novel agent for postoperative sedation in the intensive care unit. *Anaesthesia* 1999; **54:** 1136–42.
137. Scheinin H, Aantaa R, Anttila M, *et al.* Reversal of the sedative and sympatholytic effects of dexmedetomidine with a specific alpha-2 adrenoceptor antagonist atipamezole: a pharmacodynamic and kinetic study in healthy volunteers. *Anesthesiology* 1998; **89:** 574–84.
138. Brose WG, Gutlove DP, Luther RR, *et al.* Use of intrathecal SNX-111, a novel, N-type, voltage-sensitive, calcium channel blocker, in the management of intractable brachial plexus avulsion pain. *Clin J Pain* 1997; **13:** 256–9.
139. Bowersox SS, Luther R. Pharmacotherapeutic potential of omega-conotoxin MVIIA (SNX-111), an N-type neuronal calcium channel blocker found in the venom of *Conus magus*. *Toxicon* 1998: **36:** 1651–8.

35

Clinical pharmacology and anesthetic techniques

ANDREW R A RUSHTON AND J ROBERT SNEYD

INTRODUCTION

The administration of an appropriate dose of an intravenous anesthetic results in the pleasant, rapid, and reliable induction of general anesthesia. This fact is taken for granted by patients, and those anesthesiologists who adopt a "cookbook" approach to clinical pharmacology. However, the optimal choice and safe use of intravenous anesthetics, particularly for the maintenance of anesthesia, requires a deeper understanding of the pharmacologic properties that characterize this group of drugs, and the specific peculiarities which differentiate them. The pharmacologic issues are:

- pharmaceutics, including the formulation, stability, and solubilizing agents and preservatives;
- pharmacokinetics, drug distribution, metabolism and elimination over time, and the variability in drug concentrations that occur between individuals and in disease states;
- pharmacodynamics, defining the range of effective drug concentrations for sedation and anesthesia, and noting the wide range of additional drug effects, synergism with other drugs, and adverse effects.

This theoretical framework for practice is grounded in experimental evidence and will enhance the satisfaction and safety of intravenous anesthesia, tailored to the needs of individual patients. It will also promote the understanding and introduction into practice of new intravenous anesthetics and techniques.

Maintenance of anesthesia with intravenous anesthetic drugs is becoming increasingly popular. The favorable pharmacologic profile of modern agents and technological developments for safe and predictable continuous drug infusion have made intravenous anesthesia no more difficult than using volatile anesthetic agents from a vaporizer. The advantages of intravenous anesthesia are particularly evident when volatile anesthetics are contraindicated, and in some specialist anesthetic practice, for example neurosurgical and day-stay anesthesia.

Intravenous anesthetic drugs specifically produce unconsciousness. Large doses, which prolong recovery and increase unwanted side-effects, are required to suppress reflex autonomic and muscular movements in response to surgery. This problem is mitigated by using a combination of drugs to achieve desired clinical endpoints in a balanced anesthetic technique: an intravenous anesthetic produces hypnosis and opiate analgesic drugs or local anesthetic blockade suppress motor and autonomic reflex responses to noxious stimuli. Additional muscle relaxation, which may be required for intubation or surgery within body cavities, can be achieved with neuromuscular blocking drugs.

Intravenous anesthetics are dangerous drugs. Unconsciousness threatens the security and protection of the airway with the attendant risks of airway obstruction or aspiration. Intravenous anesthetics produce a variable degree of respiratory or cardiovascular depression, with reduced tone and coordination of pharyngeal and respiratory muscles, and an impaired response to hypoxia. Safe administration requires the skills, staff, and equipment to administer oxygen, ensure an open airway with appropriate protection, support ventilation and cardiovascular depression, and cope with rare, severe adverse reactions. These essential requirements may not be appreciated by personnel without anesthetic training.

PHARMACOLOGIC PRINCIPLES

Pharmaceutical issues

All intravenous anesthetics are lipid soluble, with a significant nonionized fraction at blood pH 7.4. These are essential requirements for easy passage across the blood–brain barrier to the sites of action in the brain. However, poor water solubility hampers the formulation of a stable intravenous preparation. The method of formulation of an intravenous drug has no therapeutic value but a disproportionate impact on both drug costs and adverse reactions. There are three general approaches to solubilizing poorly water-soluble drugs for intravenous use: pH adjustment, a lipophilic carrier, and a lipid emulsion.

pH adjustment

The barbiturate anesthetics, thiopental and methohexital, are weakly acidic. Their sodium salts are stable in a strongly alkaline aqueous solution. Both drugs are presented as a crystalline powder, to be reconstituted with water before use. They are incompatible with the majority of drugs used during anesthesia, and precipitation occurs with acidic solutions, including muscle relaxants. These formulations are extremely irritant, and severe tissue damage has followed extravasation or inadvertent intra-arterial injection.

Lipophilic carrier

Lipophilic carriers are more problematic. Rare but serious anaphylactoid reactions to the solvent Cremaphor EL, mediated by complement activation,[1] caused the withdrawal of two clinically useful intravenous anesthetic drugs, althesin and propanidid, and the reformulation of etomidate in propylene glycol, and propofol in a lipid emulsion.

Cremaphor EL is still used as the solubilizing agent in a number of unrelated parenteral drug preparations including vitamin K.

Etomidate and diazepam are dissolved in a solution containing 35% propylene glycol. The extreme hyperosmolarity of this formulation is associated with pain on injection and thrombophlebitis. Clinically significant hemolysis can occur with large cumulative doses.

Lipid emulsion

Propofol, and a new formulation of etomidate, are presented in an aqueous and isotonic emulsion of tiny lipid droplets, with a mean diameter of 0.2 µm. An important determinant of emulsion stability is the zeta potential. This negative electrostatic charge creates a repulsive force which opposes coalescence of emulsion droplets.[2] The addition of other drugs can reduce the magnitude of the zeta potential and jeopardize the stability of the emulsion; for example, the addition of 10–20 mg lidocaine (lignocaine) solution to 200 mg propofol causes an immediate fall in electrostatic charge and within 90 min coalesced droplets of 2–3 µm appear in the emulsion.[2] This is not clinically important provided that the resultant mixture is used immediately. The emulsion contains no antimicrobial preservatives and supports microbial growth. It should be administered in an aseptic manner, and without delay once the sealed container is opened.[3] A new formulation containing disodium edetate has been introduced in the USA. This significantly reduces bacterial growth without affecting the pharmacokinetic profile.[4]

A number of measures may reduce the risks of these complications associated with using intravenous anesthetics. A fresh preparation or sealed ampule should be drawn up immediately prior to administration into a secure and patent cannula, preferably in a large vein. Slow injection, observation of the site of injection, and questioning for any discomfort minimizes the risk of serious extravasation. Mixing of drugs is avoided by flushing the cannula following injection or delivery through a running intravenous infusion.

Pharmacokinetics and pharmacodynamics

Intravenous bolus injection of anesthetic drugs causes a short period of unconsciousness with rapid onset following an intravenous bolus. Pharmacokinetic studies describe the time-course and factors governing drug concentration at the site of action following drug administration. Pharmacodynamic studies describe the relation between concentration of drug at the molecular sites of action (the biophase) and the consequent responses. Both are required to understand and predict the relation between the administration of drugs and their effects; this important point is illustrated by plotting propofol concentrations following a bolus dose in relation to the ranges of therapeutic action (Fig. 35.1).

Pharmacokinetics

The pharmacokinetic profile of an intravenous anesthetic is described by the time-course of drug concentrations in the blood following intravenous administration (Fig. 35.1). Drugs are distributed to all tissues including, but not limited to, their sites of action. Other tissues may provide passive storage and removal from the body by metabolism or elimination.

Distribution of intravenous anesthetics

Distribution is an important pharmacologic concept. It represents the dynamic and reversible process of transfer of drug between organs and tissues via the blood. In contrast, metabolism and elimination are irreversible processes that occur in specific organs and tissues.

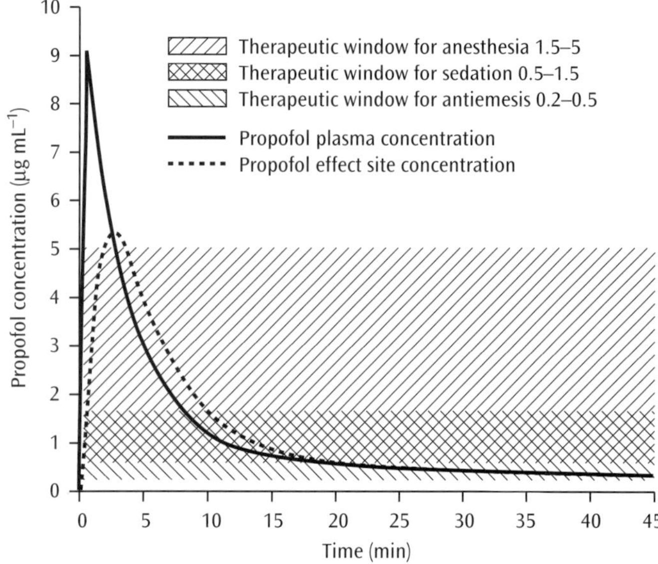

Figure 35.1 *Pharmacokinetic simulations of the plasma and effect site concentrations produced by an intravenous bolus of propofol, 2 mg kg^{-1}. The pharmacodynamic significance is indicated by therapeutic windows for anesthesia, sedation, and antiemesis.*

The major factors that affect the distribution of intravenous anesthetic drugs include:

- blood flow to tissues;
- the concentration gradient between blood and tissues;
- tissue mass;
- the blood–tissue partition coefficient;
- differential protein binding or pH-dependent nonionized fraction.

Organs and body tissues have been assigned to three physiological compartments according to their drug solubility and perfusion characteristics:[5]

1. *The vessel-rich group.* The brain, heart, liver, and kidneys account for only 9% of body weight but are perfused by 75% of cardiac output.
2. *The muscle group.* Muscle tissue accounts for at least 50% of body mass but receives 18% of cardiac output.
3. *The fat group.* Fat tissue represents a significant 19% of body mass, but is poorly perfused with 5.4% of cardiac output.

Following an intravenous bolus, the drug mixes with the blood. This process is rapid, but not instantaneous. Arterial concentrations of intravenous anesthetic drugs are many times greater than peripheral venous concentrations during the first 2 min following a bolus dose, with an average difference of 10% in most subjects persisting for up to 9 min.[6] The drug is distributed by blood flow and molecular diffusion throughout body tissues according to the rate of perfusion, tissue affinity for the drug, and relative concentrations in tissue and blood. Differential perfusion between these physiologic compartments profoundly influences the dynamic distribution of intravenous drugs.

After bolus administration, lipid-soluble drug rapidly equilibrates with the vessel-rich group of tissues: high blood flow delivers a large proportion of drug to a small mass of tissue with modest partition coefficients. This includes the brain and results in rapid loss of consciousness.

As the drug is more slowly distributed to other tissues, plasma concentration falls, and equilibration with the vessel-rich group is reversed. The drug leaves the vessel-rich group, which includes the site of drug action, and is redistributed via the blood to a large reservoir of less well-perfused lean tissue, primarily muscle. This redistribution accounts for the rapid initial recovery following administration (Fig. 35.1). Irreversible removal of intravenous anesthetic drugs through clearance by metabolism in the liver or elimination is slow relative to the process of redistribution to lean tissue. Despite a high affinity for lipid-soluble anesthetic drugs, fat takes up drug slowly because of poor perfusion.

Metabolism and elimination of intravenous anesthetics

Most intravenous anesthetic drugs are metabolized in the liver. The hepatic extraction ratio describes the arteriovenous drug concentration gradient across the liver. It is influenced by liver blood flow, intrinsic enzyme activity, and protein binding. Drugs with a high extraction ratio, including propofol and methohexital, are readily extracted from blood passing through the liver. Clearance from the blood is high and very sensitive to changes in liver blood flow. In contrast, metabolism of drugs such as thiopental, which has a low extraction ratio, is strongly influenced by changes in intrinsic hepatic enzyme activity and protein binding. Midazolam shares characteristics of both patterns of hepatic metabolism. The contribution of metabolism to the termination of anesthetic effect of a bolus induction dose is modest for drugs such as propofol, which has a high metabolic clearance, and insignificant for drugs such as thiopental, which are slowly metabolized.

Physiological factors influencing the bolus induction dose

Lean body weight Both blood volume and the distribution volume are related to lean body weight. Obesity has little effect on the early distribution kinetics and anesthetic effect of a bolus induction dose, although accumulation in the poorly perfused fat stores following repeated or continuous infusion may prolong the elimination half-life and recovery. Bolus dosing regimens based on a dose per kilogram will be excessive in obese patients, risking dose-related side-effects, and should be adjusted to lean body weight and titrated to response.

Cardiac output Physiologic pharmacokinetic models emphasize the role of perfusion in the distribution of lipid-soluble drugs to all tissues, including the site of action. A sophisticated model of the distribution, recirculation, and metabolism of propofol and thiopental in sheep has been constructed from measurements against time of: propofol or thiopental concentration in pulmonary arterial, arterial, and sagittal venous sinus blood; cerebral blood flow and previous studies of cardiac output; and depth of anesthesia based on response to a painful stimulus.[7,8] The model was used to analyze the determinants of induction of anesthesia with propofol, and their implications for dose requirements.[9] Cardiac output was identified as the most important physiologic factor that influenced the induction dose (Fig. 35.2).[8,9]

In the face of reduced cardiac output, whether caused by hypovolemia or heart failure, anesthetic drug concentrations in blood perfusing the brain are higher and more sustained, producing a greater and more prolonged drug effect.[9,10] Physiologic mechanisms of compensation maximize perfusion to the essential organs of the vessel-rich group, through vasoconstriction and reduced blood flow to the muscle and fat groups. Cerebral blood flow is maintained at the expense of perfusion of other organs, especially muscle. Consequently, drug concentrations in blood perfusing the brain and other tissues of the vessel-rich group are increased and remain elevated for a longer period because early redistribution from the brain is curtailed. This is directly reflected in the intensity and duration of drug effect. Dependence on cardiac output may be responsible for much of the variability in induction dose requirement that is associated with increasing age, disease states, and concurrent cardiodepressant medication.[8,9]

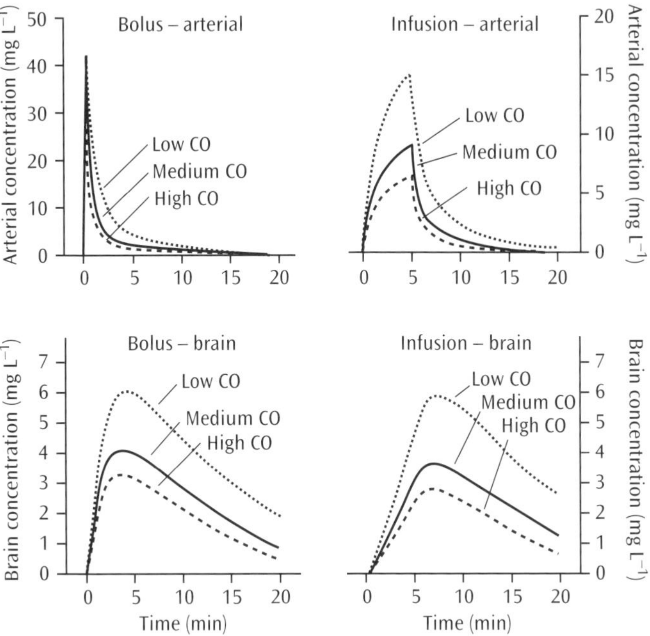

Figure 35.2 *Physiologic modeling of the effect of changes in cardiac output (CO), 50% lower and 50% higher than normal on arterial and brain concentrations of propofol. (From Ludbrook and Upton.[9])*

Dose and injection rate The dose and rate of injection profoundly influence the speed of onset, depth, and duration of anesthesia produced by an intravenous bolus.[7,9] Predictions from the sheep model correlate closely with clinical studies of the effects of infusion rates on the dose and time for anesthetic effect.[11,12] Brain concentration lags behind changes in arterial concentration. The sheep model predicted that fast injection does not substantially increase the depth of anesthesia. The onset of anesthesia was faster, but at the expense of markedly increased peak concentrations in the arterial system (Fig. 35.3). This reflects the finite time required for distribution from blood to the biophase and depends on cerebral blood flow and the partitioning characteristics of the particular drug in the brain. Hypotension during induction with propofol may be related to the direct exposure of vascular smooth muscle to very high initial blood concentrations.

Very rapid injections of propofol produced a sharp peak in arterial concentrations that were too transient to load the brain, whereas for very slow injections the peak brain concentration was attenuated by redistribution and metabolism of drug before the time of the peak (Fig. 35.3). Between these extremes was an optimal duration of injection of 2 min. The predicted benefits of slower injection over 2 min rather than a rapid bolus included a direct dose-sparing effect and reduced peak arterial blood concentrations with potential hemodynamic advantage. Fast induction of anesthesia can be achieved with a rapid bolus injection of propofol, but with a higher dose and inevitable overshoot in blood concentrations, depth of anesthesia, and attendant side-effects.

The blood–brain equilibration time of thiopental was significantly faster than that of propofol and a dose-sparing effect of slower injection was not seen with thiopental. Blood–brain equilibration was sufficiently rapid for fast injections over 10 s to maximally load the brain.[8] Equianesthetic doses of thiopental produced a more rapid onset of anesthesia than propofol, at all rates of administration.

Freely diffusible, unbound, nonionized drug Only unbound and nonionized drug can freely cross lipid membranes into tissues. Absolute

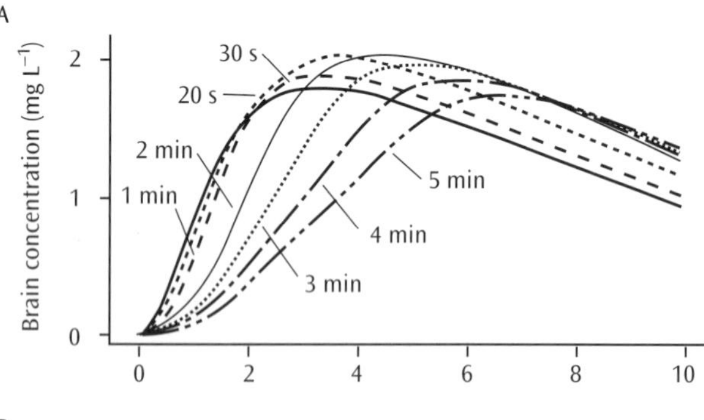

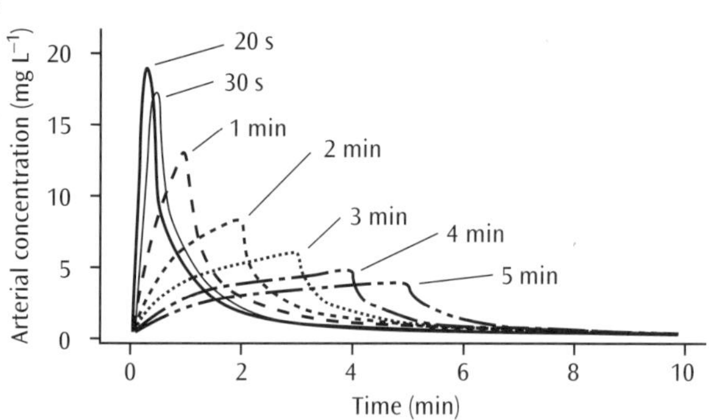

Figure 35.3 *Physiological modeling of administration of propofol, 100 mg, at different rates of injection on the time course of brain and arterial concentrations. (From Ludbrook and Upton.[9])*

decreases in protein binding with increased free fraction are seen in disease states including hypovolemia and renal and liver disease. The desired drug effects following an intravenous bolus are achieved with a smaller dose injected more slowly. The proportion of nonionized drug depends on the drug pK_a and blood pH. For weakly acidic intravenous anesthetic drugs, notably the barbiturates, acidemia favors the nonionized fraction, which is free to cross lipid barriers with increased drug effect. The influence of changes in the free fraction and drug partitioning on the effects of a bolus dose of intravenous anesthetic is probably much less important compared with the three major factors: lean body weight, cerebral perfusion as a proportion of cardiac output, and the dose and injection rate, which are described above.[7,13]

Population pharmacokinetics and factors influencing the bolus induction dose

Mathematical compartment modeling of the changes in plasma concentration provides a different quality of evidence concerning the pharmacokinetic behavior of intravenous anesthetic drugs.[14] Hypothetical mathematical compartments, characterized by an imaginary distribution volume and equilibration rate constant, cannot be directly equated with the physiologic parameters, blood flow, tissue volume, and partition coefficient. However, compartment modeling has proved enormously useful for defining and comparing the pharmacokinetic properties of different drugs, including variability, in many diverse populations.

One application has been to identify and quantify sources of variability in drug response. Aging patients have reduced induction dose requirements. For intravenous anesthetic drugs, the explanation is not an age-related increase in pharmacodynamic brain sensitivity or equilibration rate between plasma and the brain, but pharmacokinetic differences in the early distribution volumes and rates. This has been demonstrated for thiopental and etomidate,[15,16] and is probably true for propofol. The predicted effect site concentration at the time of onset of anesthesia produced by different rates of propofol infusion does not vary with age (A R A Rushton and J R Sneyd, unpublished observations). Population-based pharmacokinetic studies cannot define the underlying physiologic mechanisms. However, the primacy of lean body weight and cardiac output in physiologic models of induction dose requirements has been described above and both decrease with age.

The interface between drug kinetics and dynamics is the drug concentration in the biophase. This cannot be measured directly, but the relation between blood concentration and a continuous measure of drug effect can be modeled as the "effect site" (Fig. 35.1).[17] The temporal dissociation or hysteresis between blood concentration and drug effect for each drug is evident in Fig. 35.1 and can be quantified by a rate constant, K_{eo} (see Chapter 2). Interpatient variability in the hypothetical effect site equilibration time accounts for much of the variability in required thiopental induction doses.[18] Effect site equilibration time reflects a complex composite of physiologic variables, including perfusion as a proportion of cardiac output and partitioning.[8] It is, however, a convenient unitary index of a real clinical phenomenon that is an important consideration in modeling dosing regimens and comparing intravenous anesthetic drugs.[18]

Relation between distribution, elimination, and duration of drug action

The effects of a bolus dose of intravenous anesthetic are short lived because of rapid clearance from the blood by distribution to well-perfused tissues. Following repeated doses or continuous infusion, tissue drug concentrations rise. Ongoing redistribution occurs to tissues and the gradient between blood and tissues falls. Total clearance from blood is substantially reduced and clearance by elimination becomes increasingly important with time. The rate of decline of plasma concentration, and therefore clinical effect, depends on the prior dose and duration of administration. This is illustrated by a simple simulation of the predicted plasma concentrations of propofol following cessation of a target-controlled infusion at 15, 60, 180, and 360 min (Fig. 35.4). This pharmacokinetic phenomenon has been defined for many intravenous anesthetic drugs by this process of simulation and described by the term "context-sensitive half-time" (Fig. 35.5).[19] The fact that the decline in blood concentration and clinical effect are dependent on the dose and duration of drug administration profoundly influences the choice and use of intravenous anesthetic drugs for repeated or continuous administration.

The pharmacokinetic profile of a drug does not by itself predict clinical effects. This depends on the pharmacodynamic relation between blood concentration and drug effect at any moment. Intravenous anesthetic drugs produce a rapid onset and recovery from anesthesia because the clinically effective concentrations coincide with the steep initial distribution phase (Fig. 35.1). However, the lower drug concentrations during the elimination phase are still high enough to produce a detectable hangover with sedation and impairment of higher cerebral processing for many hours, particularly for drugs such as thiopental and diazepam, which are slowly metabolized to active metabolites. The much higher metabolic clearance of propofol contributes to the decline in plasma concentration during the initial distribution phase and the proportionately lower plasma concentrations during the elimination phase.

Pharmacodynamics

By definition, all intravenous anesthetic drugs produce unconsciousness following an intravenous bolus. Clinically effective concentrations have been established, and for some drugs, notably barbiturates and benzodiazepines, the effects of highly specific drug–receptor interactions have been characterized.[20] Lower drug concentrations produce drug and dose-dependent amnesia, sedation, and impairment of higher cerebral

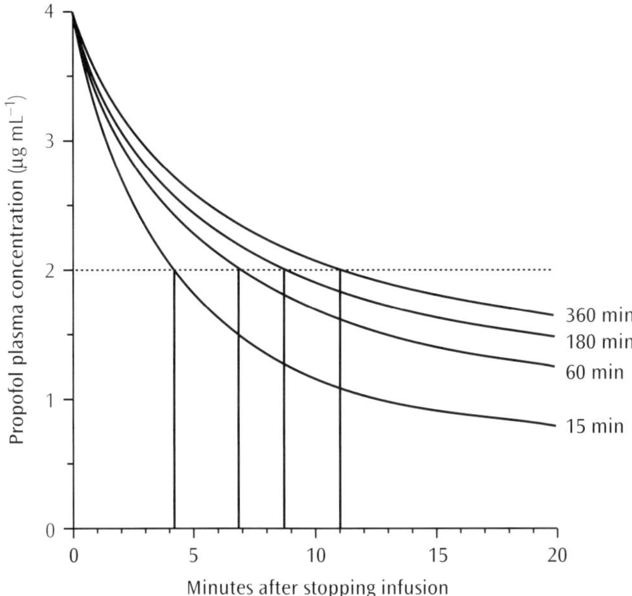

Figure 35.4 *Simulations of declining plasma propofol concentrations following cessation of 4 μg mL^{-1} target-controlled infusions (TCIs) of 15, 60, 180, and 360 min duration. Drop lines at 2 μg mL^{-1} demonstrate the context-sensitive dependence of half-time on duration of infusion.*

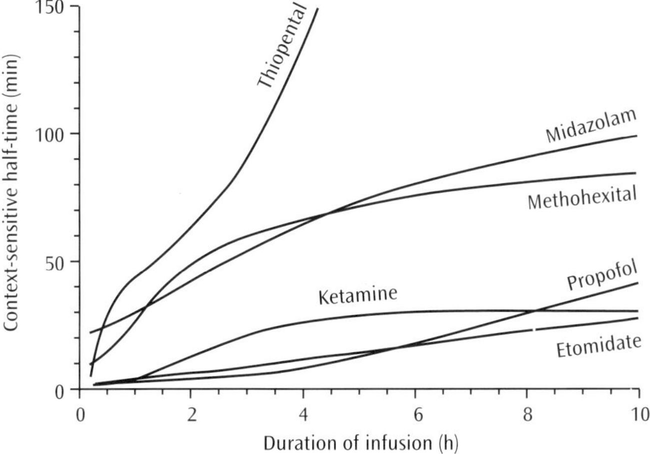

Figure 35.5 *Simulations of the context-sensitive half-times of intravenous anesthetic drugs plotted against the prior duration of infusion.*

processing, motor performance, and coordination. Other patterns of neurologic effects are common and specific to each anesthetic drug: excitatory phenomena, including myoclonus and dyskinetic movements; pro- or antiepileptic activity; altered respiration, cardiovascular reflexes, and sympathetic vasomotor tone; and different effects on analgesia and postoperative nausea and vomiting.

Studies of the relation between blood concentration and anesthetic effect require a clear, measurable endpoint for anesthesia. This may be a discrete clinical observation, for example cessation of counting, loss of response to verbal command, loss of eyelash reflex, or loss of manual grip. Prevention of movement to increasingly strong surgical stimuli is clinically relevant and requires greater blood concentration and depth of anesthesia. Such discrete measurements are clinically useful but cannot provide a continuous measure of drug effect. Concentration-dependent changes in measures of the electroencephalogram (EEG) have been widely used as a continuous surrogate measure of drug effect for the experimental definition of the effect site kinetic parameters of intravenous anesthetics and opioids.[21]

Optimal dosing of intravenous anesthetics

The optimal use of intravenous anesthetic drugs in a particular patient is achieved by combining a priori dosing regimens that have been shown to achieve therapeutic concentrations of drug in defined populations of patients with a posteriori adjustment to the observed drug responses.

Population pharmacokinetic approach

The pharmacokinetic properties of any drug can be defined experimentally and used in computer simulations and empirical clinical studies to develop dosing regimens that produce therapeutic concentrations and drug effects in defined populations of patients. The therapeutic window is a useful concept that describes the clinically effective range of concentrations that lie between low subtherapeutic concentrations and high, toxic concentrations associated with unwanted side-effects (Fig. 35.1).

In practice, the therapeutic window required to achieve the desired clinical effect varies widely depending upon:

- dynamic need, the intensity of the noxious stimulus;[22]
- dynamic interactions, profound synergism between hypnotics and opiates;
- dynamic variability, particularly age, comorbidity, and receptor sensitivity.

Therapeutic windows of effective blood concentrations can be defined for populations of patients which incorporate variability in dynamic need and interactions (Fig. 35.6).[23]

A recipe-based anesthetic technique will aim to achieve a target blood concentration that produces the desired degree of effect in the most patients, for example 95% of the study population sample. However, excessive amounts of drug will be administered to patients who are sensitive, in whom the effective concentrations are relatively low. This is safe for drugs with a wide therapeutic index but otherwise risks drug toxicity and prolonged recovery.

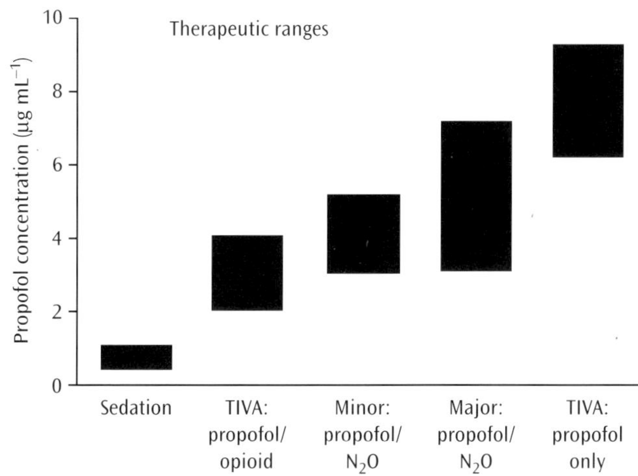

Figure 35.6 *Therapeutic windows of propofol concentration incorporating dynamic need, drug interactions, and variability in response. TIVA, total intravenous anesthesia. (From Shafer.[23])*

The application of dosing regimens derived from population pharmacokinetic studies to an individual patient is limited by the variability of response in the population and the host of confounding factors, including concurrent diseases and medications, which make individual patients unrepresentative of a selected study population. The administration of intravenous anesthetics must be fine-tuned to achieve and maintain the desired response.

Titration to effect

Feedback from accurate, precise, and continuous measurement of the desired therapeutic effect would be the most reliable mechanism for titrating drug delivery to achieve the desired effects in individual patients. Concentration-dependent changes in indices derived from the EEG or evoked responses have been used as a continuous but surrogate measure of the depth of anesthetic effect.[24,25] Although useful in research, the commercial development of a reliable, automated, continuous monitor of depth of anesthesia has been limited by technical difficulties, especially the poor signal-to-noise ratio and complex interpretation of recordings. Unlike pulse oximetry and capnography, anesthesiologists have not readily accepted that information about depth of anesthesia is worth the time and trouble of making the recordings using expensive equipment that is difficult to understand.

Clinical endpoints of unconsciousness during induction include loss of verbal contact, or purposeful grip, or the eyelash reflex. Adequate anesthesia is defined by the absence of response to surgical stimulus. In clinical practice, establishing the depth of anesthesia can be very difficult, particularly when neuromuscular blockade abolishes reflex motor responses. The natural tendency is for generous dosing of anesthetics, which safeguards against inadequate anesthesia but slows recovery and increases dose-related side-effects.

PHARMACOLOGY OF INDIVIDUAL DRUGS

Propofol

Propofol (Diprivan) is the most recent intravenous anesthetic to be marketed for clinical use. The favorable pharmacokinetic profile makes it suitable for both induction and extension, by repeated bolus or infusion, to the maintenance of anesthesia with easy and responsive titration to effect and rapid recovery. The pharmacodynamic profile includes pleasant sedation and onset of anesthesia and a demonstrable antiemetic effect with few side-effects or adverse reactions.

For over 50 years, thiopental was the standard anesthetic drug used to induce anesthesia. Study of the structure–activity relations of barbiturate derivatives[26,27] and the physiologic modeling of the disposition of thiopental and methohexital[28,29] profoundly influenced understanding of the pharmacology of fast-acting intravenous drugs. However, propofol now holds this pivotal position, with a kinetic and dynamic profile closer to the ideal – suitable for short and prolonged use for both anesthesia and sedation – and a good vehicle for bringing to a wide audience new thinking about intravenous anesthesia and new techniques, notably target-controlled infusion.

Pharmaceutics

Propofol is an alkylphenol, 2,6-disopropylphenol. It is highly soluble in lipid but not water and is formulated as an aqueous emulsion with Intralipid, specifically an isotonic 1% solution with 10% soya bean oil, 2.25% glycerol, and 1.2% purified egg phosphatide. This is stable at room temperature and not light sensitive. The addition of disodium edetate 0.005% (w/v) suppresses bacterial growth without compromising the clinical safety, efficacy, and stability of propofol. This modified formulation has been approved for clinical use and marketed in the USA since 1996, but is not yet licensed in Europe.

Dilution or the addition of drugs to the propofol emulsion, to reduce the pain on injection or provide systemic analgesia, can destabilize the emulsion.[2] The drug license specifies acceptable combinations and conditions of use: for example, propofol may be mixed with preservative-free lidocaine, 0.5% or 1%, in a ratio up to 20:1 with aseptic precautions and immediate administration, and with alfentanil, 500 μg mL^{-1}, in a ratio from 20:1 to 50:1 for use within 6 h of preparation.

Pharmacokinetics

The decline in propofol plasma concentration that follows an intravenous bolus can be fitted to a typical three-compartment model (Fig. 35.1). The initial volume of distribution is 20–40 L and the initial distribution half-life 1–8 min.

Following an intravenous bolus, plasma levels initially decline rapidly (Fig. 35.1), due to redistribution of propofol from highly perfused, low-capacity tissues, including the brain, to high-capacity sites with lower perfusion. This initial distribution clearance of propofol from the central compartment is rapid (3–4 L kg^{-1} min^{-1}), but no faster than other intravenous anesthetic drugs. Effect site equilibration is fairly rapid (K_{eo} = 0.291 min^{-1}), although not as fast as the barbiturate anesthetics. This reflects modest hysteresis between changes in plasma concentration and the depth of propofol anesthesia.

Subsequent metabolic clearance is extremely large (1.5–2.2 L min^{-1}) and in some studies exceeds hepatic blood flow. However, the large volume of distribution at steady state (400–700 L or 2–12 L kg^{-1}) results in a long elimination half-life estimated to be between 4 and 23.5 h, but with low, subtherapeutic plasma concentrations during the long elimination phase (Fig. 35.1). In practice, extensive redistribution to poorly perfused tissues that equilibrate slowly, but are lipophilic with a large capacity for propofol, results in a context-sensitive half-time for infusions up to 8 h of less than 40 min (Figs 35.4 and 35.5).[19] Clinical recovery from propofol sedation or anesthesia that has been titrated to therapeutic effect is relatively fast, even following prolonged infusions.

Propofol is rapidly metabolized in the liver by conjugation, to produce inactive water-soluble glucuronide and sulfate compounds, which are excreted by the kidneys. The hepatic extraction ratio is high: propofol degradation is more dependent on liver blood flow than on metabolism. Additional extrahepatic metabolism has been demonstrated during the anhepatic phase of liver transplantation.[30]

Pharmacodynamics

A commercial system for the target-controlled infusion of propofol has been marketed (Diprifusor; see Chapter 39). This delivers a predicted plasma propofol concentration and not the desired drug effect. No pharmacodynamic data are included in the three-compartment pharmacokinetic model, and the operating anesthesiologist must estimate the target plasma concentration required to achieve the desired effect. This depends upon the extent of surgical stimulation, the synergistic effects of analgesic and sedative drugs, and population variability. The therapeutic plasma propofol concentrations required for a variety of anesthetic applications have been estimated (Fig. 35.6).[23]

Effects on the central nervous system

Propofol causes dose-dependent sedation and hypnosis. However, amnesia is poor compared with barbiturates and benzodiazepines and very high infusion rates may be required to prevent awareness if propofol is used as the sole anesthetic.[31] Propofol is associated with an elevation of mood and a general state of well-being.[32] Hallucinations and sexual fantasies have been reported:[33] unimpeachable standards of conduct and care are essential, and the presence at induction of a chaperone for female patients is sensible.

The EEG effects of increasing propofol concentration include a transient β-excitation at low doses followed by a concentration-dependent decrease in median EEG frequency and an increase in EEG amplitude, leading to burst suppression at high blood concentrations greater than 8 μg mL^{-1}. Propofol also causes a dose-dependent increase in latency and decrease in the amplitude of cortical middle-latency auditory-evoked potentials.[25]

The excitatory effects of propofol include occasional involuntary movements, myoclonus, dystonic posturing, and opisthotonus.[34] These are less frequent than with etomidate, thiopental, or methohexital.[35] They are subcortical in origin and not associated with epileptiform EEG activity. Propofol demonstrates dose-dependent anticonvulsant properties in animal models, reduces the motor and EEG seizure activity during electroconvulsive therapy (ECT), and has been successfully used to control status epilepticus. However, occasional case reports have described grand mal seizures up to 6 days following propofol administration, with the majority, but not all cases, in patients with a history of previous convulsions. Grand mal seizures are sufficiently rare that administration of propofol to patients with a history of seizures, whether or not taking prophylactic antiepileptic medication, may be justified in situations in which propofol offers other clear advantages, for example anesthesia for neurosurgery, previous postoperative nausea and vomiting, or sedation during intensive care. Propofol would be sensibly avoided in patients with a history of seizures for whom an unexpected grand mal seizure could have devastating consequences, for example injury while operating machinery or the mandatory loss of a driving license.[36]

Propofol reduces cerebral oxygen consumption ($CMRO_2$) and cerebral blood flow (CBF).[37] This is associated with decreased intracranial pressure (ICP) in patients with normal or elevated ICP. Cerebrovascular autoregulation and reactivity to carbon dioxide are maintained. However, a greater fall in mean arterial pressure can reduce cerebral perfusion pressure (CPP).[38]

Effects on the cardiovascular system

Propofol causes a significant and concentration-dependent decrease in arterial blood pressure during induction of anesthesia. This is more marked than other intravenous induction agents. A fall in cardiac output is caused by myocardial depression and reduced ventricular filling pressures, and a decrease in systemic vascular resistance is associated with reduced sympathetic activity and a direct effect of propofol on vascular smooth muscle tone.[39] Heart rate does not change significantly despite the fall in aortic pressure.

Although coronary perfusion pressure is reduced, the global myocardial oxygen supply–demand ratio is preserved by a parallel decrease in left ventricular stroke work and preservation of the diastolic perfusion period.[40] Perioperative ischemia and myocardial contractility following cardiac surgery are no worse with propofol than with alternative hypnotics.

The relative fall in systemic blood pressure is not a significant problem in healthy patients. It can be minimized by adequate preoperative hydration and the slow, controlled titration of propofol dose to achieve the desired effect. However, patients with limited cardiovascular reserve, whether caused by hypovolemia, concurrent myocardial depressant or vasodilating drugs, or cardiac disease with reduced cardiac output may demonstrate exaggerated hypotension requiring immediate recognition and treatment.

Effects on the respiratory system

Propofol causes respiratory depression with a rise in arterial carbon dioxide tension and a reduced ventilatory response to both carbon dioxide and hypoxia. The effects of barbiturate or volatile anesthetics are similar. Apnea is common following an induction dose of propofol: the incidence and duration depend upon the dose and rate of administration of propofol and synergistic effects of opiates or sedative premedication.

Miscellaneous effects

Pain on injection into small peripheral veins occurs in many patients, although it is not associated with phlebitis. This can be distressing and radiates proximally above the elbow. It can be substantially reduced by delivery into large veins, pretreatment with alfentanil or lidocaine, or mixing alfentanil or lidocaine with the lipid emulsion of propofol immediately before administration.

Propofol produces a greater degree of relaxation of laryngeal muscles and better conditions for airway instrumentation than an equihypnotic dose of thiopental.[41] This is sufficiently pronounced for propofol to be used in combination with alfentanil or remifentanil to achieve tracheal intubation without neuromuscular block. Neither drug potentiates neuromuscular blockade nor affects the evoked electromyogram or twitch tension. Propofol does not trigger malignant hyperpyrexia and has been used to provide safe anesthesia for muscle biopsy. It is also considered safe to use in patients with porphyria.

Subhypnotic doses of propofol reduce nausea and vomiting postoperatively and following chemotherapy. The median plasma concentration associated with an antiemetic response is 0.343 μg mL^{-1}.[42] Similar doses also relieve the pruritus associated with cholestasis and spinal opiates.[43]

Rare anaphylactoid reactions due to propofol, and not the lipid emulsion, have been reported.[44] Most have occurred in patients with a history of allergic responses.

Clinical uses

Propofol is a commonly used induction agent and hypnotic component of a balanced anesthetic technique. Smooth induction of anesthesia, easy titration to effect for sedation or anesthesia, short clinical duration of action, and a demonstrable antiemetic effect represent the most balanced clinical profile of the available intravenous hypnotics. The advantages of propofol are particularly evident in day-case anesthesia, neuroanesthesia, cardiac anesthesia, especially during cardiopulmonary bypass, sedation for intensive care, or comfort during radiologic interventions, endoscopy, or minor surgery with local anesthesia. It is extremely useful in situations in which volatile anesthetic agents are not available or applicable and an intravenous anesthetic technique must be employed, for example rigid laryngoscopy and bronchoscopy, tracheobronchial surgery with apneic oxygenation or ventilation, transfer of anesthetized patients, high risk of postoperative nausea and vomiting, and susceptibility to malignant hyperpyrexia. Propofol has now become the intravenous induction agent of choice in the majority of patients for many anesthesiologists, with alternative agents reserved for specific clinical indications.

Day-case patients

The clinical and pharmacoeconomic benefits of propofol have been well documented in the field of day-case anesthesia. Rapid recovery with minimal side-effects is as important as smooth induction of anesthesia and optimum intraoperative conditions. Propofol offers many advantages, particularly when used for maintenance of anesthesia in addition to induction: more rapid recovery and improved early psychomotor performance compared with barbiturates and benzodiazepines; similar recovery times following etomidate but fewer side-effects; and substantially lower incidence of postoperative nausea and vomiting compared with barbiturates and etomidate. The greater degree of hypotension with propofol is less problematic in fit day-case patients, and pain on injection is easily controlled with lidocaine or alfentanil or by injection into a large vein.

The benefits of propofol compared with volatile agents for day-case anesthesia are more controversial. Difficulties in standardizing depth of anesthesia, synergistic use of opioids and midazolam, and variable criteria for discharge have led to studies with conflicting results and conclusions. In general, the recovery time to wakefulness is quicker with modern volatile anesthetics. This is particularly true for sevoflurane when used for both induction and maintenance of anesthesia. However, this early recovery is not reflected in a reduced time to discharge because of an excess of postoperative vomiting in patients receiving volatile anesthetics.[4,45,46] Studies comparing anesthetic techniques in terms of drug costs, incidence of side-effects, or recovery times can miss important human costs.[47] Postoperative nausea and vomiting (PONV) is an unpleasant experience for patients and their carers and the antiemetic effects of propofol are most clearly evident in this patient population.

Children

The role of propofol in pediatric anesthesia is more controversial. It is not approved by the manufacturer for anesthesia in children less than 3 years old or for sedation for intensive care or surgical and diagnostic procedures. Propofol sedation was blamed for the deaths of several children with respiratory tract infections, who developed severe acidosis, lipemia, and multiple organ failure. A causal mechanism has not been established and extremely high doses of propofol were used in these children.[48]

The volume of distribution and the clearance of propofol in children are larger as a proportion of body weight compared with adults and higher doses are required. In addition, children may be more resistant to the pharmacodynamic effects. In practice, induction doses of 2.5–3.5 $mg\,kg^{-1}$ followed by infusion rates of 100–300 $\mu g\,kg^{-1}min^{-1}$ are satisfactory. Specific indications are similar to those for adults.[49] This includes the beneficial reduction in PONV,[50] perhaps in part related to the avoidance of nitrous oxide.

Summary

In summary, the advantages of propofol are:

- pleasant sedation and recovery;
- rapid onset and easy titration to effect;
- suitable for both induction and maintenance of anesthesia;
- suppression of airway reflexes;
- antiemetic effects;
- safe in porphyria.

The disadvantages are:

- pain on injection;
- lipid emulsion carrier, which supports bacterial growth;
- vasodilation causes hypotension, especially with limited cardiovascular reserve;
- expensive.

Barbiturates: thiopental and methohexital

Thiopental and methohexital are the only barbiturates still in common use as intravenous hypnotic agents. Both produce very rapid induction of anesthesia, which is short lived following a single bolus because of redistribution into lean tissue. Both are also tried and tested and cost-effective. Accumulation following repeated or continuous dosing is particularly marked with thiopental. Blood concentrations sufficient to cause prolonged hangover effects during the elimination phase reflect a relatively small volume of distribution and slow metabolic clearance.

Pharmaceutics and physicochemical properties

Both thiopental and methohexital are weak acids with slightly alkaline pK_a values (thiopental 7.6, methohexital 7.9), and are highly lipid soluble. Their sodium salts are dissolved in a strongly alkaline aqueous solution ($pH > 10$). This can cause serious tissue damage if injected subcutaneously or intra-arterially. Precipitation when mixed with many other preparations, especially acidic solutions of muscle relaxants, can block a fine cannula. The solutions are bacteriostatic and stable if cooled, although the manufacturers recommend that solutions are freshly prepared and used within 24 h.

Pharmacokinetics

High lipid solubility results in very fast effect site equilibration (thiopental $K_{eo} = 0.3\,min^{-1}$ and methohexital $K_{eo} = 0.6\,min^{-1}$) and a clinically rapid induction of anesthesia. The initial and steady-state volumes of distribution are smaller than those of propofol and reflect the very high binding to plasma albumin. Reduction in the albumin concentration or binding increases the unbound fraction in blood, consequent drug effect, and metabolic clearance.

Metabolism

Both barbiturates are metabolized and eliminated via the liver with very little renal involvement. Pentobarbital is a major and pharmacologically active metabolite of thiopental and contributes to the prolonged effects of large or repeated doses.

Thiopental metabolism is slow and depends on liver enzyme activity and, to a lesser extent, changes in protein binding. The hepatic extraction ratio is less than 20% and the clearance during the elimination phase is modest (250 $mL\,min^{-1}$). The slow metabolic clearance of thiopental produces a long and context-dependent elimination half-life (Fig. 35.5). It is not suited to the maintenance of anesthesia.

High thiopental blood concentrations saturate the capacity of the hepatic P450 cytochromes and metabolism reaches a ceiling "zero order" fixed rate. This occurs at concentrations required for EEG burst suppression (50–60 $\mu g\,mL^{-1}$), which have been used in clinical practice in uncontrolled status epilepticus and for putative cerebral protection, but are much greater than required for anesthesia. In the face of unknown and unpredictable metabolism, prolonged thiopental infusions must be titrated against measured blood concentration and EEG effects.

In contrast, methohexital has a much higher hepatic extraction ratio (50–80%) and a greater clearance during the elimination phase (690 $mL\,min^{-1}$). The context-sensitive half-time is much shorter than for thiopental (Fig. 35.5) and methohexital has been used for maintenance of anesthesia.

Pharmacodynamics

Barbiturates affect many central neurotransmitter systems, although interactions with the γ-aminobutyric acid-A ($GABA_A$) receptor are stereospecific and correlate with anesthetic potency. The mechanisms by which potentiation of the inhibitory effects of GABA and hyperpolarization of pre- and postsynaptic membranes are translated into loss of consciousness and the clinical state of anesthesia are not understood. The barbiturates have no analgesic effects and thiopental may be hyperalgesic at subanesthetic concentrations, exaggerating responses to pain.

Central nervous system

Thiopental and methohexital both cause depression of cerebral electrical activity and cerebral metabolism.[37] Thiopental depresses $CMRO_2$, in a dose-dependent manner, to a maximum of 55% of conscious levels when the EEG becomes flat. Reduced $CMRO_2$ causes cerebral vasoconstriction, reducing cerebral blood flow and intracranial pressure. Cerebral perfusion pressure is usually maintained or slightly elevated. This is beneficial for patients with raised intracranial pressure.

EEG depression is dose dependent. The awake α pattern progresses to higher amplitude and slower frequency δ and θ waves until burst suppression precedes a flat EEG. The excitatory movements commonly seen with methohexital and occasionally seen with thiopental are not accompanied by EEG changes.[35] Thiopental is a potent anticonvulsant. However, methohexital has proconvulsant properties, with an increased incidence of postoperative seizures following neurosurgery and precipitation of seizures in previously undiagnosed epileptics.

Cardiovascular system

Thiopental causes venodilation, reducing preload, and direct myocardial depression at high concentrations. Systemic vascular resistance and arterial blood pressure remain relatively unaltered following a normal induction dose in healthy patients. Both thiopental and methohexital cause an increase in heart rate, which increases myocardial oxygen consumption. Provided aortic root pressure remains unchanged, this is more than compensated for by a proportional decrease in coronary artery resistance and increased myocardial blood flow. However, in the presence of fixed, severe coronary obstruction or low diastolic arterial pressure, coronary blood flow may be severely compromised. Hence, barbiturates must be used cautiously in patients for whom an increase in heart rate or a decrease in preload might be detrimental, for example those with hypovolemia, critical coronary artery disease, ventricular hypertrophy, or heart failure.

Respiratory system

Thiopental and methohexital produce dose-dependent ventilatory depression, and apnea usually follows an induction dose. Responses to hypoxia and hypercapnia are also depressed for a prolonged period. Laryngeal and tracheal reflexes are depressed to a lesser degree than by equipotent anesthetic doses of propofol.[51] Laryngospasm and bronchospasm may be related to insertion of artificial airways, laryngeal masks, or tracheal tubes in lightly anesthetized patients. Although safe in asthmatic patients, neither drug causes bronchodilation.

Adverse effects

Thiopental, but not methohexital, produces dose-dependent histamine release. Rarely, IgE-mediated anaphylaxis is reported.

Pain on injection into small veins and local thrombophlebitis is well recognized with methohexital (5%) but less common with thiopental, unless extravasation occurs. Subcutaneous injection of thiopental causes pain and inflammation, which depends on the dose; severe tissue necrosis has been reported. Accidental intra-arterial injection can be much more serious. Intense and painful arterial spasm and chemical arteritis can lead to irreversible thrombosis. Immediate treatment with saline is necessary to dilute the barbiturate with local anesthetic block of somatic and sympathetic innervation, to relieve vascular spasm and pain, and with heparin anticoagulation to inhibit thrombosis.

Barbiturates can cause involuntary excitatory movements, hypertonus, coughing, and hiccuping. The incidence and severity are dose dependent and much greater following methohexital than thiopental.

The incidence of nausea and vomiting after barbiturate anesthesia is less than after inhaled anesthetics, or after ketamine or etomidate, but is even less following propofol or midazolam anesthesia.

Barbiturates are contraindicated in patients with porphyria. They are potent inducers of δ-aminolevulinic acid synthetase and can precipitate attacks of acute intermittent or variegate porphyria in susceptible patients.

Clinical uses

Suitable induction doses for healthy adults would be thiopental at 2.5–4.5 mg kg^{-1} and methohexital at 1.5 mg kg^{-1}, adjusted for comorbidity and synergistic sedative premedication or opioids, and titrated to response.

Thiopental is cheap, effective, tried, and trusted, and still used as an induction agent in situations in which rapid recovery for neurologic assessment or early "street fitness" is not important. Prolonged recovery makes it unsuitable for maintenance of anesthesia for all but the shortest of procedures. Thiopental remains the most effective drug for controlling status epilepticus refractory to benzodiazepines and specialized anticonvulsant drugs. As a consequence of interactions with these drugs and prolonged seizure activity, airway protection, assistance of ventilation, support of the circulation, and transfer to an intensive care unit are usually necessary.

Methohexital is most commonly used as a single bolus dose for ECT because of its well-established effects on the convulsive response. Infusions of methohexital have been used for maintenance of anesthesia. However, pain on injection, a longer context-sensitive half-life and recovery, frequent excitatory phenomena, and higher incidence of nausea and vomiting are disadvantages relative to propofol.

Summary

Thiopental

The advantages of thiopental are:

- very rapid onset of anesthesia;
- potent anticonvulsant;
- tried and tested and cheap.

The disadvantages are:

- unsuitable for maintenance of anesthesia: slow metabolism prolongs recovery from cumulative doses;
- contraindicated in patients with porphyria.

Methohexital

The advantages of methohexital are:

- rapid onset of anesthesia;
- cheap.

The disadvantages are:

- pain on injection;
- involuntary movements;
- proconvulsant properties;
- contraindicated in patients with porphyria.

Etomidate

Etomidate is a potent, short-acting intravenous anesthetic, characterized by hemodynamic stability, minimal respiratory depression, and cerebral protective effects. Concerns about the potential consequences of inhibition of steroid synthesis and troublesome side-effects, including a relatively high incidence of nausea and vomiting, excitatory events, and myoclonus on induction, pain on injection, and superficial thrombophlebitis related to the propylene glycol carrier, have limited its widespread use.

Pharmaceutics and physicochemical properties

Etomidate is an imidazole derivative. Although presented as a racemic mixture, only the (+) isomer is an active hypnotic. It is insoluble in water and formulated in 35% propylene glycol as a 2 mg mL^{-1} solution. This mixture has a low pH (5.6) and high osmolality (4600 mosmol kg^{-1}), which is responsible for the frequent occurrence of pain on injection (30%) and superficial thrombophlebitis (20%), particularly when injected into small peripheral veins. The extremely hyperosmolar solvent also causes transient hemolysis. Although not a problem in healthy patients, significant hemolysis may occur in patients with fragile red cells, for example spherocytosis or post transfusion, or by interaction with other drugs or diseases causing hemolysis. Hemoglobinuria is undesirable with pre-existing renal disease. The total dose must not exceed 30 mL. Reformulation in Lipofundin, a lipid emulsion (Etomidate Lipuro), has solved both of these problems.

Pharmacokinetics

Etomidate rapidly crosses the blood–brain barrier, producing peak effect site concentrations within 1 min of administration, and a similarly fast onset of hypnosis. Plasma concentration and the related hypnotic effect of an intravenous bolus of etomidate decline rapidly. Moderate initial and steady-state volumes of distribution and high redistribution clearance and metabolic clearance (18–25 mL kg^{-1} min^{-1}) both contribute to exceptionally short half-lives for redistribution (2.7 min) and elimination (2.9–5.3 h). This pharmacokinetic profile is ideally suited for rapid recovery following single or repeated doses or a continuous infusion (Fig. 35.5).

Metabolism

Etomidate is rapidly metabolized in the liver, primarily by ester hydrolysis, to the carboxylic acid derivative, which is inactive. The extraction ratio is high (0.5–0.9) and metabolic clearance is therefore dependent on liver blood flow, but relatively unaffected by hepatic dysfunction.

Pharmacodynamics

Etomidate has hypnotic but not analgesic activity. The main sites of action appears to lie within the neocortex and its primary effects involve inhibition of the GABA-ergic system.[52]

Effects on the central nervous system

A high incidence of myoclonus (50–80%) is observed during induction of anesthesia with etomidate in the absence of premedication. Although usually self-limiting and of short duration, it can persist beyond recovery of consciousness. This is a subcortical effect, associated with depressed slow δ-wave EEG activity indicating deep anesthesia and no epileptiform EEG activity. Myoclonus can be reduced by pretreatment with low-dose etomidate, opioids, or benzodiazepines. The incidence is also lower with etomidate reformulated in Lipofundin.

Rare case reports associate etomidate with epileptic attacks in at-risk patients. Increased EEG activity in epileptogenic foci has been used during intraoperative mapping prior to surgical ablation. No clinical or EEG signs of epileptic seizures have been observed in patients receiving etomidate who have no previous history of epilepsy. Etomidate demonstrates potent anticonvulsant properties in experimental animals and humans.[53,54]

Etomidate lowers cerebral blood flow (36%) and cerebral oxygen consumption (45%). Cerebral perfusion pressure is well maintained.[37] Intracranial and intraocular pressure are both substantially reduced. Cerebrovascular reactivity is maintained and hyperventilation further reduces intracranial pressure. In rat models, neuroprotective properties prior to ischemia are equivalent to thiopental. However, decreases in cerebral blood flow precede the decrease in cerebral oxygen consumption, raising concerns about potential cerebral ischemia in areas of critical perfusion. It has been postulated that free hemoglobin produced by hemolysis secondary to the propylene glycol may be scavenging local vasodilating nitric oxide.

Effects on the cardiovascular system

Etomidate minimally affects hemodynamic stability and myocardial function in healthy patients. This contrasts with other fast-acting intravenous induction agents, and may be related to a unique lack of effect on the sympathetic nervous system and baroreceptor function. Even in patients with moderate cardiac dysfunction, etomidate (0.3 mg kg^{-1}) produces only minor cardiovascular changes, typically less than a 10% decrease in cardiac index. Coronary vascular resistance falls, increasing coronary perfusion, and the myocardial oxygen supply–demand ratio is well maintained. Control of the sympathetic and hemodynamic responses to laryngoscopy requires large doses of etomidate or synergistic doses of intravenous opiate. Compared with alternative currently available intravenous induction agents, etomidate may be the drug of choice in patients with pre-existing cardiovascular disease.

Effects on the respiratory system

Etomidate has fewer ventilatory depressant properties than propofol, thiopental, and methohexital. Apnea occurs less frequently and an increase in minute ventilation is sometimes seen. Hiccups and coughing are noted with an incidence comparable to that of methohexital.

Endocrine effects

Increased mortality in a group of patients sedated with etomidate infusions in an intensive care unit was associated with low cortisol levels and attributed to etomidate-induced suppression of adrenal cortisol synthesis.[55] Etomidate is a dose-dependent but reversible inhibitor of 11β-hydroxylase in the adrenal cortex, and is more potent than metyrapone. This enzyme is required for both mineralocorticoid and corticosteroid production. Minor adrenocortical suppressive effects [impaired response to adrenocorticotrophic hormone (ACTH) stimulation] follow induction doses or short infusions, although in many studies the mean cortisol levels in the etomidate group remain within the normal range. The effect of a single bolus is short lived (6–8 h) and the clinical significance is uncertain. Other drugs and anesthetic techniques can depress plasma cortisol levels, for example high-dose opioids. No studies have reported adverse outcomes secondary to short-term adrenocortical suppression. Enthusiasts argue that the many benefits of etomidate outweigh this theoretical disadvantage and that etomidate is safe to use for induction and for short-term maintenance of anesthesia as part of a total intravenous anesthesia (TIVA) technique.

Adverse effects

Nausea and vomiting is common following etomidate, with an incidence of 30–40% (compared with 20 –30% for barbiturates). This has severely limited the use of etomidate for day-case surgery, and it should be avoided in patients with increased risk of PONV. This side-effect may, however, have been reduced by reformulation in lipid.

No histamine release is produced by etomidate and hypersensitivity reactions are extremely unusual. Etomidate inhibits aminolevulinic acid synthetase and it has been administered to patients with porphyria without precipitating a clinical crisis.

Clinical use

An induction dose of 0.3 mg kg^{-1} produces sleep lasting 6–10 min in healthy adults. In other patient groups, this dose should be reduced and titrated to effect.

Etomidate is suitable for patients who will benefit from specific desirable properties, including hemodynamic stability, minimal respiratory depression, cerebral protection, and rapid recovery, following either a single dose or a short-term continuous infusion. In practice, these are patients compromised by trauma, serious illness, shock, or cardiovascular comorbidity. The fast onset of anesthesia and high therapeutic index for cardiovascular side-effects are helpful during a rapid-sequence induction.

However, widespread use is limited by several prominent adverse effects: pain on injection, thrombophlebitis, myoclonus, a relatively high incidence of nausea and vomiting, hemolysis, and concerns about the disputed significance of transient adrenal suppression. Reformulation in lipofundin has improved the side-effect profile. The availability of Etomidate Lipuro in Europe may herald its more widespread use.

Summary

Etomidate

The advantages of etomidate are:

- hemodynamic stability;
- reduction in $CMRO_2$, CBF, and ICP, with maintenance of CPP;
- very rapid onset of hypnosis and recovery.

The disadvantages are:

- hyperosmolar propylene glycol carrier causes pain on injection, thrombophlebitis, and hemolysis;
- profound but transient inhibition of steroidogenesis;
- excitatory effects and myoclonus common;
- postoperative nausea and vomiting.

Ketamine

Ketamine is the only clinically useful phencyclidine derivative marketed for clinical use. This group of drugs is characterized by an unusual "dissociative" anesthetic state, profound analgesia, cardiorespiratory stability, and troublesome psychomimetic effects during recovery.

Pharmaceutics

Ketamine is presented as a racemic mixture of two optically active isomers, *S*[+] and *R*[−], in equal amounts. It is a clear colorless solution containing 1%, 5%, or 10% ketamine hydrochloride with a pH of 3.5–5.5. These aqueous solutions are not irritant and ketamine can be administered by the intramuscular, extradural, and intrathecal routes.

Pharmacokinetics

Low molecular weight, low protein binding, a pK_a close to the physiologic pH, and high lipid solubility all contribute to very rapid penetration of the blood–brain barrier and onset of effect. The duration of anesthesia following a typical intravenous anesthetic dose of $2\,mg\,kg^{-1}$ in an adult is 10–15 min, with recovery to full orientation in 15–30 min. This is produced by rapid early redistribution ($t_{1/2\alpha}$ = 11–16 min) into a large central compartment (20–100 L). The high lipid solubility of ketamine and low degree of protein binding are also reflected in the extensive steady-state volume of distribution (100–400 L). Terminal clearance is also high ($1.4\,L\,min^{-1}$) and approaches liver blood flow. The dependence of recovery time on the dose and duration of infusion is relatively small and similar to that of propofol and etomidate (Fig. 25.5).

Ketamine can be administered intravenously, intramuscularly, orally, and rectally. Following intramuscular administration, onset of sedation occurs within 5 min and peak effect within about 20 min. Topical anesthetic creams and modern volatile agents have reduced the trauma of induction of anesthesia for children and their parents. Oral or intramuscular ketamine is now rarely used in children.

The principal metabolite of N-demethylation by hepatic microsomal enzymes is norketamine. This is pharmacologically active but with less than 30% of the potency of ketamine. Diazepam competitively inhibits N-demethylation of ketamine, decreasing its hepatic clearance. High hepatic extraction means that clearance is dependent on liver blood flow and therefore reduced by drugs or comorbidity that impair cardiac output and visceral perfusion.

Pharmacodynamics

Effects on the central nervous system

Ketamine produces an unusual cataleptic state with profound analgesia described as "dissociative anesthesia." The endpoint of induction of anesthesia may be unclear. Eyes may remain open, and corneal, gag, and swallowing reflexes are well preserved, although not necessarily protective. Analgesia is produced by considerably lower blood levels than loss of consciousness, providing considerable postoperative analgesia following anesthesia maintained with ketamine.

The neuropharmacology of ketamine is complex and quite distinct from that of other intravenous anesthetics.[56] Noncompetitive antagonism of glutamate at *N*-methyl-D-aspartate (NMDA) ligand-gated calcium channels accounts for most of the anesthetic, analgesic, amnestic, and psychotomimetic effects.[56] Ketamine also interacts with non-NMDA glutamate receptors, nicotinic and muscarinic cholinergic, and monoaminergic and opioid receptors. Inhibition of neuronal voltage-dependent sodium channels provides a modest local anesthetic effect.

Ketamine increases cerebral metabolism, cerebral oxygen consumption, and cerebral blood flow. The consequent rise in intracranial pressure is particularly marked in the presence of intracranial pathology, and may exceed sympathetically mediated increases in mean arterial pressure with a reduction in cerebral perfusion pressure.[57] Ketamine is contraindicated by raised intracranial pressure or intracranial pathology with a mass effect. Cerebrovascular responsiveness to ketamine is preserved, and reducing the arterial carbon dioxide tension by hyperventilation and the depressant effects of other intravenous anesthetic drugs attenuates the ketamine-induced rise in intracranial pressure. A parallel increase in intraocular pressure may be detrimental in patients with open eye injuries or glaucoma, or during vitreoretinal surgery.

Emergence reactions include vivid dreams, surreal experiences, and illusions during the first hour of recovery. These can be emotionally intense, with excitement and euphoria or unpleasant confusion and fear. At least one-third of adults will be affected following a ketamine-based anesthetic. The incidence is higher in adults than in children, in women compared with men, and in patients with a previous history of psychological problems. Psychomimetic side-effects are aggravated by centrally active anticholinergic drugs, including atropine, and can be successfully minimized or treated with benzodiazepines.

Effects on the cardiovascular system

In contrast with other intravenous anesthetic agents, ketamine stimulates the cardiovascular system, with increases in heart rate, arterial pressure, and cardiac output. The mechanism is a centrally mediated increase in sympathetic tone and circulating catecholamines, further potentiated by inhibition of neuronal catecholamine reuptake. This sympathetic stimulation is not dose dependent and overrides the direct myocardial depressant effects of ketamine except at high concentrations. Pulmonary vascular resistance is also increased. Undesirable tachycardia and hypertension can be effectively attenuated by prior administration of benzodiazepines, other intravenous or inhalational anesthetics, or adrenergic antagonists. The propensity to tachycardia and hypertension means that ketamine must be used extremely carefully in patients with ischemic heart disease or vascular aneurysms. Resistance to the adrenergic effects of ketamine in shocked and critically ill patients can unmask marked direct myocardial depression and peripheral vasodilation.

Effects on the respiratory system

Ketamine produces minimal respiratory depression and an unaltered response to carbon dioxide at clinically useful concentrations. Functional residual capacity, minute volume, tidal volume, and the coordinated contribution of intercostal muscle function to inspiration are maintained. However, synergistic respiratory depression occurs with concurrent use of sedatives and other anesthetic drugs.

Ketamine has a clinically useful bronchodilating effect and has been used in life-threatening and unresponsive status asthmaticus. It has also been used during one-lung anesthesia in patients with severe pulmonary disease. Hypoxic pulmonary vasoconstriction is unaffected and effective intravenous ketamine anesthesia permits high inspired oxygen concentrations.

Increased salivary and tracheobronchial secretions can be troublesome, particularly in children. This may promote laryngospasm or airway obstruction but can be minimized by antisialagogues, for example glycopyrollium.

Other clinical effects

Anesthetic doses of ketamine increase uterine tone and the intensity of uterine contraction. Sympathetic stimulation and maintenance of cardiovascular tone make ketamine a potentially life-saving anesthetic for parturients with exsanguinating obstetric hemorrhage and a flaccid uterus.

Ketamine has been safely used for patients with malignant hyperthermia and acute intermittent and variegate porphyria.

Clinical uses

There are no widespread or consistent clinical indications for the use of ketamine, but it is promoted by enthusiasts in special clinical situations, particularly anesthesia for patients with severe shock or who are cardiovascularly compromised.

War and civilian disasters often coexist with limited medical resources for anesthesia and postoperative care. Ketamine may be the anesthetic agent of choice when supplies of oxygen and monitoring and disposable equipment are limited and anesthesia is administered by inexperienced anesthesiologists or paramedical personnel. It is cheap, stable, and undemanding to store and transport. The relative preservation of airway control and respiration, maintenance of cardiac output and arterial pressure, and provision of analgesia can deliver remarkably safe and effective anesthesia in difficult circumstances.

The profound analgesia of subanesthetic doses of ketamine has been used during painful minor procedures, for example changing of burns dressings. Such use of ketamine is not a substitute for appropriate local anesthetic infiltration or blockade or for modern standards of monitoring and anesthesia.

Case reports support the use of ketamine in ventilated patients with severe asthma who are unresponsive to other bronchodilator and anti-inflammatory therapy.

Summary

The advantages of ketamine are:

- dissociative anesthesia and marked analgesia;
- very rapid onset of effects;
- cardiorespiratory stability;
- relative preservation of airway reflexes;
- safe in patients with porphyria.

The disadvantages are:

- unpleasant and troublesome psychotomimetic emergence reactions;
- tachycardia and hypertension, undesirable with ischemic heart disease;
- contraindicated by raised intracranial pressure.

Benzodiazepines

Benzodiazepines are important drugs in anesthetic practice. They are characterized by potent amnestic, sedative, and anticonvulsant effects and the availability of a pure competitive antagonist. Solo administration provides a slow onset of poor-quality anesthesia with little suppression of motor and autonomic responses to surgery. The main role for benzodiazepines in anesthesia is sedation and supplementation of opioids and other intravenous anesthetic drugs.

Pharmaceutics and physicochemical properties

Benzodiazepines are small molecules and lipid soluble at physiologic pH. Parenteral diazepam and lorazepam are formulated in propylene glycol. Midazolam incorporates an imidazole ring, which is ionized and water soluble in an acidified aqueous solution of pH 3.5. Following injection, the ring closes at physiologic pH. This nonionized form of midazolam is the most lipid soluble of the three benzodiazepines.

Pharmacokinetics

High lipophilicity contributes to rapid central nervous system effects, although the onset of action is slower than that of other intravenous anesthetics. Recovery from a bolus dose is dependent on redistribution. The very slow metabolism of diazepam and lorazepam causes accumulation and prolonged clinical effects with large or repeated doses. Recirculation of diazepam and its metabolites may also slow recovery.[58] The metabolic clearance of midazolam is much greater ($6–11\,mL\,kg^{-1}\,min^{-1}$). This contributes to the relatively short duration of clinical effect by bolus. The rise in context-sensitive half-time with duration of infusion is substantially lower for midazolam than for diazepam and thiopental, but twice as long as for propofol, etomidate, and ketamine (Fig. 35.5).

Metabolism

Biotransformation in the liver is dependent on phase I enzyme activity. This is susceptible to outside influences, for example impaired metabolism with age, diseases including cirrhosis, or enzyme induction. Unlike midazolam, diazepam is very slowly metabolized to active metabolites, desmethyl diazepam and oxazepam, which enhance and prolong its effects and contribute to a particularly wide population variability in response.

Pharmacodynamics

Benzodiazepines facilitate inhibitory actions of GABA on central neuronal transmission. Allosteric modulation of a binding site on the $GABA_A$ receptor increases chloride ion influx, causing hyperpolarization and resistance to excitation.[59] All benzodiazepines share this common action but with variable receptor affinity and intrinsic activity.

Effects on central nervous system

The wide range of central effects include hypnosis, sedation, anxiolysis, prominent amnesia, anticonvulsant action, and centrally mediated muscle relaxation – but no useful analgesia.

Benzodiazepines produce a dose-related reduction in cerebral metabolism and blood flow and intracranial pressure, provided that other influences are controlled. Hypercarbia and possibly hypoxia secondary to benzodiazepine sedation may cause a dangerous rise in intracranial pressure in patients with poor intracranial compliance. Nevertheless, potent anticonvulsant activity, a high therapeutic ratio for adverse cardiorespiratory responses relative to other anesthetics, and a rapid onset relative to other anticonvulsants make diazepam and midazolam the first-line intravenous anticonvulsant drugs on general hospital wards.

The effects of benzodiazepines depend on the dose: low plasma concentrations are anxiolytic and anticonvulsant, increasing doses cause sedation and amnesia, and a high concentration causes hypnosis, but with no analgesia and strong reactions to stimulation. A wide variation in the degree and duration of response is common, especially in young unpremedicated patients. Marked synergistic interactions with other central nervous depressants are dangerous if unrecognized but have become a useful part of balanced anesthesia.

Effects on cardiovascular system

When used alone, benzodiazepines produce modest and dose-related hemodynamic effects. Homeostatic mechanisms are relatively well preserved. However, the mild, transient, dose-related fall in arterial pressure associated with reduced catecholamine concentrations and sympathetic tone can be dangerously exaggerated by hypovolemia and coadministered opioids or intravenous anesthetics.

Effects on respiratory system

Reduced phasic and tonic contraction of airway muscles causes a tendency to airway obstruction. The ventilatory responses to hypoxia are also depressed, particularly in hypercarbic patients. Supplemental oxygen may be needed to prevent hypoxia, with continuous observation of airway patency and respiration.

Minor respiratory depression is more profound in the presence of limited respiratory reserve and increasing age. Synergistic interaction with other respiratory depressant drugs, notably opioids, can produce severe respiratory depression and apnea.

Hypersensitivity reactions are extremely uncommon.

Clinical uses

Benzodiazepines are not suitable for use as the sole hypnotic. The unconscious state is not profound and, if noxious procedures are intended, lower doses should be combined with opiates and other intravenous or volatile anesthetics.

Oral benzodiazepines are commonly used for preoperative sedation. Midazolam is useful in children: rapid absorption produces a short period of sedation, within 20 min of administration. In the absence of an oral preparation, the bitter intravenous solution has been mixed with a more palatable syrup. The low bioavailability requires an oral dose of 0.5 mg kg^{-1}.

Dosage guidelines

The response to benzodiazepines is highly variable, especially when combined with opioids or other anesthetic drugs and in elderly patients with exaggerated pharmacodynamic responses and slower distribution and metabolism. The profound synergistic interaction with intravenous anesthetics and opioids is used to advantage in a technique of "coinduction," which significantly reduces required drug doses. The dose must be tailored to the needs and response of the individual patient. Midazolam has the fastest onset of action of the benzodiazepines, but the peak effect of a bolus dose occurs several minutes after bolus injection and small incremental doses should be administered with patience.

Titratable sedation, reliable amnesia, and reasonable preservation of respiratory and hemodynamic reflexes make benzodiazepines suitable for conscious sedation for procedures and sedation for intensive care. However, two problems are common. Despite the wide margin of safety, continuous observation is required to ensure airway patency and adequate oxygenation and respiration. Amnesia is prominent and may appear out of proportion to the degree of sedation: memory for both instructions and events is impaired. Short-term recall is unaffected and patients appear awake and engage in conversation, but without recall. *Consent cannot be reliable or informed following even small doses of benzodiazepines.* Important postoperative instructions are likely to be forgotten and are usefully reinforced by a written reminder.

Midazolam is the only benzodiazepine suitable for induction of anesthesia. Onset is slow but accompanied by reliable amnesia. Midazolam 0.2 mg kg^{-1} will induce anesthesia in less than 2 min in healthy unpremedicated patients. Substantially reduced doses are required in the elderly and unfit [American Association of Anesthesiologists (ASA) class III patients], and there is synergistic interaction with other intravenous anesthetics and opiates. Awakening from a bolus dose depends on redistribution of drug from the brain to other well-perfused tissues and is slower than with other intravenous anesthetics. This is not significant following long operations. Accumulation may delay recovery following repeated doses or prolonged infusions, for example following conscious sedation, maintenance of anesthesia, and especially following sedation in intensive care units.

Summary

The advantages of midazolam are:

- potent amnestic, sedative, and anticonvulsant effects;
- competitive antagonist available;
- relatively high therapeutic ratio for cardiorespiratory depression.

The disadvantages are:

- profound, useful, but potentially dangerous synergism with opioids;
- slow onset of action and peak effect;
- poor quality of anesthesia.

Flumazenil

Flumazenil is a highly selective, intravenous, competitive benzodiazepine antagonist which produces immediate recovery from the depressant effects of benzodiazepine agonists.[60] Unlike naloxone reversal of opioids, administration of flumazenil is remarkably free of cardiovascular effects. Careful titration of the dose of flumazenil reduces the potential for unpleasant withdrawal effects from the abrupt termination of the benzodiazepine effect.

The high clearance and small volume of distribution of flumazenil produces a short elimination half-life of less than 1 h but carries the risk of the reappearance of sedation and amnesia. This is not a clinical problem with the short periods of sedation with midazolam. Flumazenil does not reduce the need for postoperative surveillance but it does facilitate nursing. Patients are more responsive and mobile and there is a reduced risk of loss of airway control or aspiration.

INTRAVENOUS ANESTHETICS AND SEDATION

A very large number of minimally invasive diagnostic and therapeutic procedures are performed on patients by a wide range of specialists, particularly in the fields of endoscopy, endoscopic surgery, and interventional radiology. Sedative drugs address three specific issues: fear and feelings of panic, with associated sympathetic responses; discomfort and restlessness following periods of immobility on hard surfaces; and amnesia, which reduces anxiety about repeated procedures.

Sedation is not a substitute for general anesthesia in situations in which anesthesia services are not provided, basic resucitation equipment is not to hand, or the patient is considered unfit for general anesthesia. During appropriately controlled sedation, verbal communication is maintained with a comfortable, relaxed, and cooperative patient, with patently well-maintained protective reflexes.

Sedation is not a substitute for adequate analgesia. Discomfort or pain associated with the procedure must be properly controlled, with sedative drugs used to provide appropriate relaxation and relief of anxiety. Local anesthetic techniques including topical preparations, local infiltration, or nerve blocks provide both effective analgesia and control of autonomic and motor reflex responses. This is particularly successful in dentistry and urology.[61] Centrally acting analgesic drugs, commonly opioids, are less satisfactory, but must be used for some procedures for which local anesthesia is not feasible, for example colonoscopy. Marked synergism can rapidly and unpredictably produce dangerously deep sedation or anesthesia, with compromise of the airway and respiratory and cardiovascular control.

Intravenous drugs used in sedation

Propofol and midazolam are the most commonly used intravenous sedatives, with ketamine reserved for special situations.

Propofol produces a pleasant sedation, which is easily controlled with experience. The responsive pharmacokinetic profile results in easy titration and rapid recovery following repeated doses or infusion. However, the therapeutic window is narrow (Fig. 35.1), with easy and rapid progression from sedation to anesthesia with cardiorespiratory depression or apnea. Injection pain is common. Propofol must be restricted to monitored anesthesia care and administered by a vigilant anesthesiologist with the equipment and trained support to manage the dangerous consequences of inadvertent anesthesia. Continuous infusion provides a more consistent degree of sedation than repeated dosing for prolonged periods. Typical doses in a fit adult are in the range of 30–50 mg for a loading dose to establish sedation and a continuous infusion of 100–600 mg h^{-1} to maintain sedation. Transient increases in requirement are easily treated with a further bolus of 10–30 mg.

Midazolam exhibits a much greater margin of safety and is regularly used for sedation, not only by anesthesiologists but by a wide range of practitioners with minimal or no training in anesthesia and airway management. Safe sedation still requires careful patient selection, reduction in dose to compensate for the effects of age, comorbidity, or synergistic drug interactions, and continuous monitoring of the degree of sedation. The peak sedative effect of a bolus dose will not be attained for several minutes. If the impatient desire for a more rapid onset leads to the use of a large or repeated bolus dose, then excessive sedation several minutes later is inevitable. Midazolam and opioid analgesics act synergistically, and substantially reduced doses are required. An acceptable margin of safety is provided by the specific competitive antagonists flumazenil and naloxone and both drugs should be available. For fit patients, a suitable range for a sedation dose is 0.04–0.07 mg kg^{-1} but this must be substantially reduced in elderly or unfit patients.

The sympathetic and unpleasant psychotropic effects of ketamine preclude its use in routine clinical practice. However, its wide therapeutic index, good analgesic properties, relative preservation of airway reflexes, and minimal cardiorespiratory depression make it invaluable in difficult environments or emergency situations, particularly for the management of trauma victims.

Techniques of administration

In practice, an anticipated bolus dose to achieve the desired degree of sedation is estimated from a range of recommended doses and adjusted according to personal experience and the age and physical condition of the patient. Small bolus doses may be safely administered to prolong sedation after the induction bolus has achieved peak effect. The slower onset and recovery profile of midazolam is suited to a regimen of bolus doses titrated to sedative effect. Rapid effect site equilibration, distribution, and hepatic metabolism of propofol mean that continuous infusion produces more stable sedation.

Patient-controlled sedation allows patients to control their own sedation.[62] This results in high levels of patient satisfaction and is appropriate for longer procedures. The dosing regimen and control system for patient demands must deliver a dose sufficient for the patient to experience the effect quickly and gain confidence in the system but have restrictions on the size and maximum frequency of the bolus to avoid oversedation.[62] Either propofol or midazolam is satisfactory for patient-controlled sedation.[63] Propofol is associated with rapid early recovery but pain at the injection site can be troublesome. Recovery with midazolam is marginally slower but balanced by the greater therapeutic ratio and the availability of the specific antagonist flumazenil to reverse unwanted effects.

DRUG INTERACTIONS

The spectrum of effects that constitute general anesthesia, including analgesia, amnesia, unconsciousness, and suppression of reflex motor, autonomic, and hormonal responses to surgery, should not be regarded as several components of anesthesia resulting from one anesthetic action; rather, they represent separate pharmacologic actions, even if anesthesia is produced by one drug.[64,65] In clinical practice with currently available drugs, at least two drugs are used to achieve the clinical goals of adequate anesthesia.[66,67] Complex and profound drug interactions are inevitable and are dangerous traps for the inexperienced anesthesiologist but have also been studied and incorporated into the development of improved dosing schedules for intravenous anesthetic drugs.[68]

Types of drug interaction

Drug interactions can be quantified by comparing the relation between the dose and response of each individual drug with the combination using the technique of isobolographic analysis. The plasma concentrations of two different drugs that produce the same net effect are measured and plotted: the resulting line of equivalent effect is called the isobole (Fig. 35.7). Three types of interaction define the combined effects of different drugs. Volatile anesthetics demonstrate additive effects, that is the sum of their individual effects. The interaction of ketamine with thiopental, propofol, or midazolam is simply additive.[69–71] A reduced drug effect defines an antagonistic interaction, for example the clinically useful antagonism of the depressant effects of benzodiazepines by flumazenil. However, the most common and important interaction involving intravenous anesthetics is synergism, whereby the combined effect is greater than the sum of the individual drug effects. This is most prominent with the combined use of intravenous anesthetic drugs and opioids.

Altered pharmacokinetic distribution and metabolism, particularly caused by changes in cardiac output and the pattern of tissue blood flow, may explain some of the synergistic effects. The observed plasma concentrations of propofol are elevated by approximately 10% by the

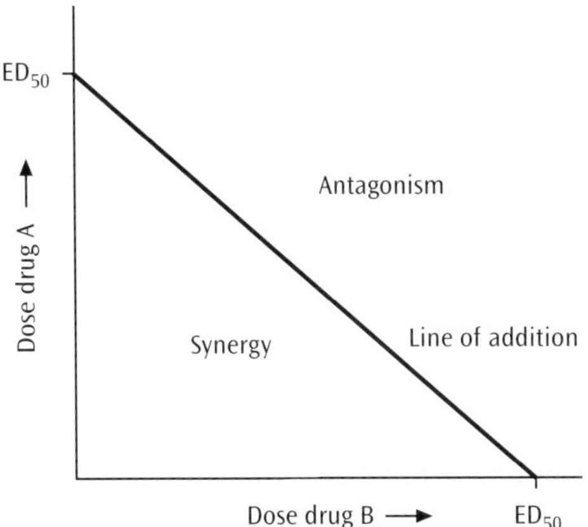

Figure 35.7 *An isobologram: the effects of doses of two drugs A and B that produce the same response are plotted. Independent actions produce a simple additive effect, illustrated by the straight line of addition. Observations above this line represent an antagonism and below this line a supra-additive, synergistic effect. ED_{50}, effective dose of drug in 50% of patients.*

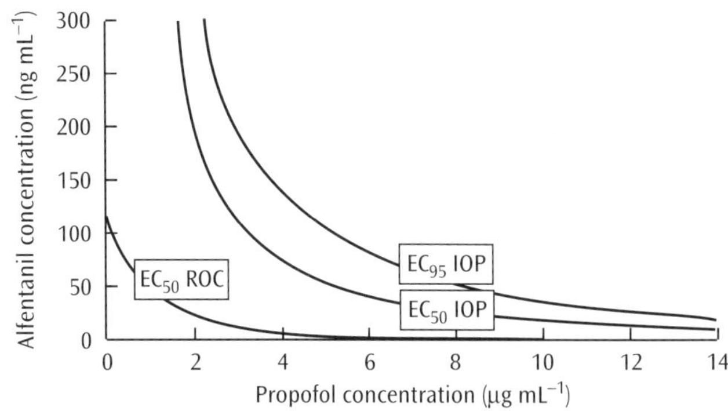

Figure 35.8 *Interaction curves (isobolograms) of propofol and alfentanil associated with the 95% (EC_{95} IOP) and 50% (EC_{50} IOP) probability of no response to surgical stimuli intraoperatively and a 50% probability of return of consciousness (EC_{50} ROC) demonstrate profound synergism. (From Vuyk* et al.[68]*)*

simultaneous administration of alfentanil.[72] This contribution to the supra-additive effects of the drug combination is modest in comparison with pharmacodynamic interaction. The combined effect of drugs that have different, complementary mechanisms of action can demonstrate profound synergism.

Supra-additive interactions include adverse effects. The synergistic interaction between intravenous opioids and all intravenous anesthetic drugs substantially increases the incidence and duration of apnea and hypotension. This is potentially dangerous if the intended effect was sedation and respiratory depression was not anticipated, recognized, or appropriately managed. Deaths have been reported involving a combination of opioid and benzodiazepine for sedation.

Propofol and synthetic opioids

The interaction between synthetic opioids and propofol for prevention of purposeful movement at skin incision has been quantified.[68,73,74] The isobolograms of propofol and alfentanil for three different drug effects are shown in Fig. 35.8: the 95% and 50% probability of no response to surgical stimuli intraoperatively and the 50% probability of return of consciousness demonstrate a profound synergistic interaction.[68] Low analgesic concentrations of alfentanil produce a steep decrease of approximately 50% in the propofol concentrations required to prevent purposeful movement at skin incision. However, the further reduction in propofol requirements becomes much less marked with increasing opioid concentration and approximates toward a minimum propofol concentration required to maintain anesthesia. Furthermore, this minimum plateau concentration is the same magnitude as the concentration required for unconsciousness in the absence of surgical stimulus.[75] The interaction between other lipid-soluble opioids, including fentanyl, sufentanil, and remifentanil, and both propofol and the volatile anesthetics is remarkably similar.

Analgesic concentrations of opioids suppress the noxious stimulation of surgery and reduce the concentration of propofol needed for anesthesia in a strongly synergistic manner down to the minimum plateau required for unconsciousness. Most of this synergistic effect occurs within the analgesic concentration range of the opiate.[76] A number of practical conclusions can be drawn. The concentration of anesthetic agent should not be titrated much below the effective concentration for awakening because of the risk of awareness and recall. When low, analgesic, concentrations of opioid are used, deeper anesthesia can be achieved by increasing either the opioid or the hypnotic concentration. At high opioid concentrations, a further increase in concentration achieves little; increasing the concentration of hypnotic is more appropriate.[76]

Coinduction

The appropriate use of intravenous anesthetics and opioid drugs to achieve the smooth induction of anesthesia while avoiding adverse cardiovascular side-effects requires understanding of both the early pharmacokinetics of bolus doses and the synergistic pharmacodynamic drug interactions. This has been successfully exploited in the technique of coinduction, in which a small dose of midazolam, up to 2.5 mg, produces amnesia for the induction process, a substantial reduction in the requirement for the induction agent, and a more stable hemodynamic profile, without substantially compromising recovery.[77,78] Predosing with propofol at $0.4\,mg\,kg^{-1}$ produces a similar reduction in the induction dose,[79] although it is not clear whether this is more effective than a single induction dose of propofol administered over the optimum period of approximately 2 min in achieving the maximum dose-sparing effect.[9] Even more profound synergism is found with the triple combination of propofol with midazolam and alfentanil (Fig. 35.9).[80,81]

Rational use

The rational use of intravenous anesthetics to maintain anesthesia must also take account of the context-dependent recovery (that is dependence on dose and duration of infusion) that follows the distribution and accumulation of drug in peripheral tissues (Fig. 35.8). This issue has been comprehensively addressed by integrating pharmacokinetic models of the plasma concentrations of propofol and synthetic opioids, following variable duration infusions, with the pharmacodynamically synergistic drug concentrations required to achieve adequate anesthesia with no response to surgery and awakening in 50% and 95% of patients and the time to recovery.[68] The nadir of optimal drug concentrations for the shortest time to awakening was primarily dependent on the pharmacokinetic profile of the opioid and to a lesser extent on the duration of infusion.

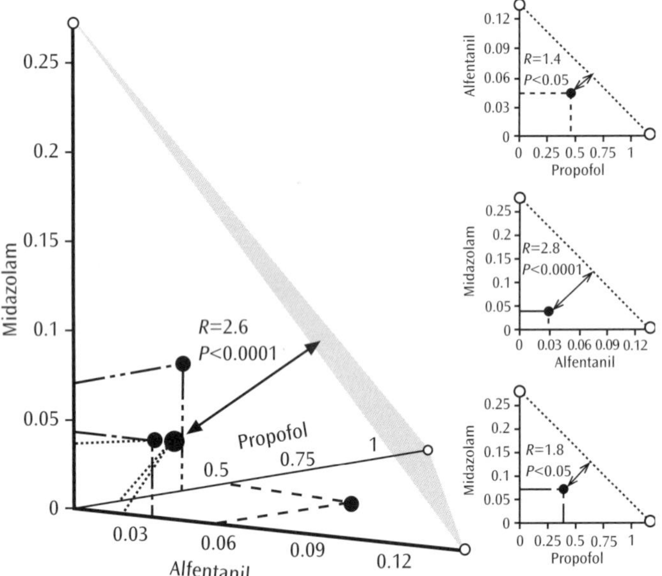

Figure 35.9 *Isobolograms for the hypnotic interactions of propofol, midazolam, and alfentanil are on the right. All combinations fall below the line of additive effect representing synergism, but midazolam and alfentanil produce the greatest synergism. The triple interaction, on the left, demonstrates that the combination of all three drugs is also synergistic. (From Vinik* et al.[81]*)*

FUTURE PROSPECTS

New intravenous anesthetic drugs

Molecular biological research has made enormous progress in the identification, sequencing, and cloning of ligand-gated ion channels in the central nervous system.[20] The future promise is that an understanding of drug–receptor interactions at a molecular level might lead to the engineering of new intravenous anesthetic drugs with greater specificity and fewer unwanted side-effects.

New uses for established classes of drugs

Established classes of drugs have been evaluated for suitability in anesthesia. Derivatives of 5α- and 5β-reduced progesterone have anesthetic properties, although none is currently marketed.[82] These drugs are characterized by a short duration of action and a high therapeutic ratio for cardiorespiratory depression but are limited by excitatory effects and difficulties in formulation. Eltanolone, also called pregnanolone, was formulated as an emulsion in Intralipid and demonstrated an excellent kinetic profile with a modest volume of distribution and very high clearance.[83] A low incidence of nausea and vomiting, good cardiovascular stability, and minimal respiratory depression were attractive features. However, involuntary movements and hypertonus, slow effect site equilibration and onset of action, and a higher than expected incidence of urticaria were problematic and the manufacturer has discontinued further evaluation.

Amino-ester derivatives of 21-hydroxypregnanedione are water-soluble anesthetics without accompanying cardiovascular or respiratory depression. Water solubility solves the problems of formulation but is inevitably associated with a slow effect site kinetic profile. Recent human volunteer studies of the experimental, water-soluble Org 21465 showed a slow onset of anesthesia caused by restricted access to the effect site and an unacceptably high incidence of excitatory side-effects.[84]

Two water-soluble, experimental imidazobenzodiazepines (Ro 48-6791 and Ro 48-8684) have been evaluated.[85] Compared with midazolam, both drugs showed a higher clearance, a larger volume of distribution, and a faster effect site equilibration. This was reflected in quicker onset and recovery.

Racemic intravenous anesthetics: exploitation of drug chirality

Enantiomers may share similar chemical properties but the specificity of their interactions with the chiral centers of receptors and enzymes produces pharmacokinetic and pharmacodynamic differences. *S*-ketamine (+) is a more potent anesthetic and analgesic and produces fewer psychotomimetic emergence reactions than racemic ketamine.[56] Other benefits include a greater clearance and a steeper concentration effect response, resulting in more rapid recovery and easier titration to desired clinical effect. *R*-ketamine (−) acts as a competitive partial agonist at the effect site and competitively inhibits the metabolism of *S*-ketamine (+). The cardiovascular stimulation produced by equipotent doses is similar. Separation of pure enantiomers from a racemic mixture is an expensive manufacturing process and *S*-ketamine (+) is not commercially viable at present.

New formulations of existing intravenous anesthetics

Reformulation of etomidate in a lipid emulsion reduced the incidence of pain on injection and myoclonus. No venous thrombosis or hemolysis were evident. Potency, pharmacokinetic profile, and the inhibition of adrenal steroidogenesis were unchanged.

The development of new intravenous anesthetics is limited by the enormous cost of development, manufacturing difficulties, protracted animal and human studies, and stringent licensing requirements. Successful marketing of a new intravenous anesthetic appears increasingly unlikely in a competitive market that requires demonstrable clinical and cost benefits over the current market leader, propofol.

Optimal use of current intravenous anesthetic drugs

The prospects for improving the ways in which existing drugs are used are more promising. Synergism between drugs can be quantified and applied in clinical practice for the benefit of patients.[86] The commercial target-controlled infusion of propofol (Diprifusor) uses a pharmacokinetic model to achieve a selected plasma concentration. Computer-controlled infusion systems, which incorporate mathematical models of effect site kinetics, are widely used in research. The incorporation of a pharmacodynamic model of the relation between effect site concentration and drug effect could permit the user-friendly selection of a desired clinical drug effect, rather than a drug concentration, incorporating physiologic sources of variability and with optimal recovery time whatever the duration of infusion.[87] The application of pharmacologic models to individual patients will always be limited by the wide interindividual variation in response to anesthetic drugs, which is greatly exaggerated by comorbidity, particularly cardiovascular compromise, which affects the differential distribution and elimination of drugs, and synergistic drug interactions.

The alternative engineering solution to this problem involves titration of drug delivery according to feedback from an accurate, real-time, continuous monitor of cerebral response. This has been achieved in the laboratory and clinical research using derived indices from the EEG.[88] However, technical difficulties and the poor signal-to-noise ratio have limited commercial development. In the absence of a reliable monitor of depth of anesthesia, guidelines for drug administration, whether presented as dosage and infusion rates or target drug concentrations, must be tailored to the anticipated needs of the patient and adjusted according to clinical response.

Acknowledgments

Pharmacokinetic simulations of propofol following an intravenous bolus (Fig. 35.1) and recovery from propofol infusions (Fig. 35.4) were calculated using Stanpump pharmacokinetic software. The simulations of the context-sensitive half-times of intravenous anesthetics (Fig. 35.5) were calculated using Recov software. Both Stanpump and Recov software are freely available, courtesy of Dr S L Shafer, from the Pharmacokinetics and Pharmacodynamics Software Server at the VA Palo Alto Health Care System (http://anesthesia.stanford.edu/pkpd).

REFERENCES

1. Moneret-Vautrin DA, Laxenaire MC, Viry-Babel F. Anaphylaxis caused by anti-Cremophor EL IgG STS antibodies in a case of reaction to althesin. *Br J Anaesth* 1983; **55:** 469–71.
2. Lilley EM, Isert PR, Carasso ML, Kennedy RA. The effect of the addition of lignocaine on propofol emulsion stability. *Anaesthesia* 1996; **51:** 815–8.
3. Sklar GE. Propofol and postoperative infections. *Ann Pharmacother* 1997; **31:** 1521–3.
4. Schnider TW, Minto CF, Gambus PL, *et al.* The influence of method of administration and covariates on the pharmacokinetics of propofol in adult volunteers. *Anesthesiology* 1998; **88:** 1170–82.
5. Mapleson WW. An electrical analogue for uptake and exchange of inert gases and other agents. *J Appl Physiol* 1963; 18: 197.
6. Barratt RL, Graham GG, Torda TA. Kinetics of thiopentone in relation to the site of sampling. *Br J Anaesth* 1984; **56:** 1385–91.
7. Upton RN, Ludbrook GL. A physiological model of induction of anaesthesia with propofol in sheep. 1. Structure and estimation of variables. *Br J Anaesth* 1997; **79:** 497–504.
8. Upton RN, Ludbrook GL. A model of the kinetics and dynamics of induction of anaesthesia in sheep: variable estimation for thiopental and comparison with propofol. *Br J Anaesth* 1999; **82:** 890–9.
9. Ludbrook GL, Upton RN. A physiological model of induction of anaesthesia with propofol in sheep. 2. Model analysis and implications for dose requirements. *Br J Anaesth* 1997; **79:** 505–13.
10. Wada DR, Björkman S, Ebling WF, *et al.* Computer simulation of the effects of alterations in blood flows and body composition on thiopental pharmacokinetics in humans. *Anesthesiology* 1997; **87:** 884–99.
11. Peacock JE, Spiers SP, McLauchlan GA, *et al.* Infusion of propofol to identify smallest effective doses for induction of anaesthesia in young and elderly patients. *Br J Anaesth* 1992; **69:** 363–7.
12. Stokes DN, Hutton P. Rate-dependent induction phenomena with propofol: implications for the relative potency of intravenous anesthetics. *Anesth Analg* 1991; **72:** 578–83.
13. Burch PG, Stanski DR. Decreased protein binding and thiopental kinetics. *Clin Pharmacol Ther* 1982; **32:** 212–17.
14. Wright PM. Population based pharmacokinetic analysis: why do we need it; what is it; and what has it told us about anaesthetics? *Br J Anaesth* 1998; **80:** 488–501.
15. Stanski DR, Maitre PO. Population pharmacokinetics and pharmacodynamics of thiopental: the effect of age revisited. *Anesthesiology* 1990; **72:** 412–22.
16. Arden JR, Holley FO, Stanski DR. Increased sensitivity to etomidate in the elderly: initial distribution versus altered brain response. *Anesthesiology* 1986; **65:** 19–27.
17. Shafer SL, Stanski DR. Improving the clinical utility of anesthetic drug pharmacokinetics. *Anesthesiology* 1992; **76:** 327–30.
18. Jacobs JR, Reves JG. Effect site equilibration time is a determinant of induction dose requirement. *Anesth Analg* 1993; **76:** 1–6.
19. Hughes MA, Glass PS, Jacobs JR. Context-sensitive half-time in multicompartment pharmacokinetic models for intravenous anesthetic drugs. *Anesthesiology* 1992; **76:** 334–41.
20. Lees G. Molecular mechanisms of anaesthesia: light at the end of the channel?. *Br J Anaesth* 1998; **81:** 491–3.
21. Gregg KM, Varvel JR, Shafer SL. Application of semilinear canonical correlation to the measurement of opioid drug effect. *J Pharmacokinet Biopharmaceut* 1992; **20:** 611–35.
22. Shafer SL. Constant versus optimal plasma concentrations. *Anesth Analg* 1993; **76:** 467–9.
23. Shafer SL. Advances in propofol pharmacokinetics and pharmacodynamics. *J Clin Anesth* 1993; **5** (Suppl. 1): 14S–21S.
24. Glass PS, Bloom M, Kearse L, *et al.* Bispectral analysis measures sedation and memory effects of propofol, midazolam, isoflurane, and alfentanil in healthy volunteers. *Anesthesiology* 1997; **86:** 836–47.
25. Thornton C, Barrowcliffe MP, Konieczko KM, *et al.* The auditory evoked response as an indicator of awareness. *Br J Anaesth* 1989; **63:** 113–15.
26. Andrews PR, Mark LC. Structural specificity of barbiturates and related drugs. *Anesthesiology* 1982; **57:** 314–20.
27. Dundee JW. Clinical pharmacology of general anesthetics. *Clin Pharmacol Ther* 1967; **8:** 91–123.
28. Price HL, Kovnat PJ, Safer JN, *et al.* The uptake of thiopental by body tissues and its relation to duration of narcosis. *Clin Pharmacol Ther* 1960; **43:** 324–31.
29. Gillis PP, DeAngelis RJ, Wynn RL. Nonlinear pharmacokinetic model of intravenous anesthesia. *J Pharmaceut Sci* 1976; **65:** 1001–6.
30. Veroli P, O'Kelly B, Bertrand F, *et al.* Extrahepatic metabolism of propofol in man during the anhepatic phase of orthotopic liver transplantation. *Br J Anaesth* 1992; **68:** 183–6.
31. Glass PS. Prevention of awareness during total intravenous anesthesia. *Anesthesiology* 1993; **78:** 399–400.
32. McDonald NJ, Mannion D, Lee P, *et al.* Mood evaluation and outpatient anaesthesia. A comparison between propofol and thiopentone. *Anaesthesia* 1988; **43** (Suppl.):68–9.
33. Hocking G. Propofol – an interesting new side effect? *Anaesthesia* 1996; **51:** 101.
34. Sneyd JR. Excitatory events associated with propofol anaesthesia: a review. *J R Soc Med* 1992; **85:** 288–91.
35. Reddy RV, Moorthy SS, Dierdorf SF, *et al.* Excitatory effects and electroencephalographic correlation of etomidate, thiopental, methohexital, and propofol. *Anesth Analg* 1993; **77:** 1008–11.
36. Sneyd J. Propofol and epilepsy. *Br J Anaesth* 1999; **82:** 168–9.
37. Cheng MA, Theard MA, Tempelhoff R. Intravenous agents and intraoperative neuroprotection. Beyond barbiturates. *Crit Care Clin* 1997; **13:** 185–99.
38. Herregods L, Verbeke J, Rolly G, Colardyn F. Effect of propofol on elevated intracranial pressure. Preliminary results. *Anaesthesia* 1988; **43** (Suppl.): 107–9.
39. Goodchild CS, Serrao JM. Cardiovascular effects of propofol in the anaesthetized dog. *Br J Anaesth* 1989; **63:** 87–92.
40. Stephan H, Sonntag H, Schenk HD, *et al.* Effects of propofol on cardiovascular dynamics, myocardial blood flow and myocardial metabolism in patients with coronary artery disease. *Br J Anaesth* 1986; **58:** 969–75.
41. McKeating K, Bali IM, Dundee JW. The effects of thiopentone and propofol on upper airway integrity. *Anaesthesia* 1988; **43:** 638–40.
42. Gan TJ, Glass PS, Howell ST, *et al.* Determination of plasma concentrations of propofol associated with 50% reduction in postoperative nausea. *Anesthesiology* 1997; **87:** 779–84.
43. Borgeat A, Wilder-Smith OH, Suter PM. The nonhypnotic therapeutic applications of propofol. *Anesthesiology* 1994; **80:** 642–56.
44. Laxenaire MC, Mata-Bermejo E, Moneret-Vautrin DA, Gueant JL. Life-threatening anaphylactoid reactions to propofol (Diprivan). *Anesthesiology* 1992; **77:** 275–80.
45. White PF, Song D. New criteria for fast-tracking after outpatient anesthesia: a comparison with the modified Aldrete's scoring system. *Anesth Analg* 1999; **88:** 1069–72.
46. Dashfield AK, Birt DJ, Thurlow J, *et al.* Recovery characteristics using single-breath 8% sevoflurane or propofol for induction of anaesthesia in day-case arthroscopy patients. *Anaesthesia* 1998; **53:** 1062–6.
47. Macario A, Weinger M, Truong P, Lee M. Which clinical anaesthesia outcomes are both common and important to avoid? The perspective of a panel of expert anesthesiologists. *Anesth Analg* 1999; **74:** S225.
48. Susla GM. Propofol toxicity in critically ill pediatric patients: show us the proof [editorial; comment]. *Crit Care Med* 1998; **26:** 1959–60.
49. Smith I, White PF, Nathanson M, Gouldson R. Propofol. An update on its clinical use. *Anesthesiology* 1994; **81:** 1005–43.
50. Woodward WM, Barker I, John RE, Peacock JE. Propofol infusion vs thiopentone/isoflurane anaesthesia for prominent ear correction in children. *Paediatr Anaesth* 1997; **7:** 379–83.
51. Brown GW, Patel N, Ellis FR. Comparison of propofol and thiopentone for laryngeal mask insertion. *Anaesthesia* 1991; **46:** 771–2.
52. Ostwald P, Doenicke A. Etomidate revisited. *Curr Opin Anaesthesiol* 1998; **11:** 391–8.
53. Modica PA, Tempelhoff R, White PF. Pro- and anticonvulsant effects of anesthetics (Part I). *Anesth Analg* 1990; **70:** 303–15.

54. Modica PA, Tempelhoff R, White PF. Pro- and anticonvulsant effects of anesthetics (Part II). *Anesth Analg* 1990; **70:** 433–44.
55. Ledingham IM, Watt I. Influence of sedation on mortality in critically ill multiple trauma patients. *Lancet* 1983;**1** (8336): 1270.
56. Kohrs R, Durieux ME. Ketamine: teaching an old drug new tricks. *Anesth Analg* 1998; **87:** 1186–93.
57. Wyte SR, Shapiro HM, Turner P, Harris AB. Ketamine-induced intracranial hypertension. *Anesthesiology* 1972; **36:** 174–6.
58. Baird ES, Hailey DM. Delayed recovery from a sedative: correlation of the plasma levels of diazepam with clinical effects after oral and intravenous administration. *Br J Anaesth* 1972; **44:** 803–8.
59. Möhler H, Richards JG. The benzodiazepine receptor: a pharmacological control element of brain function. *Eur J Anaesthesiol* (Suppl.) 1988; **2:** 15–24.
60. Whitwam JG, Amrein R. Pharmacology of flumazenil. *Acta Anaesthesiol Scand* (Suppl.) 1995; **108:** 3–14.
61. Birch BR, Anson KM, Miller RA. Sedoanalgesia in urology: a safe, cost-effective alternative to general anaesthesia. A review of 1020 cases. *Br J Urol* 1990; **66:** 342–50.
62. Cook LB, Lockwood GG, Moore CM, Whitwam JG. True patient-controlled sedation. *Anaesthesia* 1993; **48:** 1039–44.
63. Rudkin GE, Osborne GA, Finn BP, *et al.* Intra-operative patient-controlled sedation. Comparison of patient-controlled propofol with patient-controlled midazolam. *Anaesthesia* 1992; **47:** 376–81.
64. Kissin I. General anesthetic action: an obsolete notion? *Anesth Analg* 1993; **76:** 215–18.
65. Collins JG, Kendig JJ, Mason P. Anesthetic actions within the spinal cord: contributions to the state of general anesthesia. *Trends Neurosci* 1995;**18:** 549–53.
66. Stanski DR, Shafer SL. Quantifying anesthetic drug interaction. Implications for drug dosing. *Anesthesiology* 1995; **83:** 1–5.
67. Glass PS, Howell S, Gan TJ, Ginsberg B. How to manage drug interactions. *Eur J Anaesthesiol* 1997; **15** (Suppl.): 33–9.
68. Vuyk J, Mertens MJ, Olofsen E, *et al.* Propofol anesthesia and rational opioid selection: determination of optimal EC_{50}–EC_{95} propofol–opioid concentrations that assure adequate anesthesia and a rapid return of consciousness. *Anesthesiology* 1997; **87:** 1549–62.
69. Roytblat L, Katz J, Rozentsveig V, *et al.* Anaesthetic interaction between thiopentone and ketamine. *Eur J Anaesthesiol* 1992; **9:** 307–12.
70. Hui TW, Short TG, Hong W, *et al.* Additive interactions between propofol and ketamine when used for anesthesia induction in female patients. *Anesthesiology* 1995; **82:** 641–8.
71. Hong W, Short TG, Hui TW. Hypnotic and anesthetic interactions between ketamine and midazolam in female patients. *Anesthesiology* 1993; **79:** 1227–32.
72. Vuyk J. TCI: supplementation and drug interactions. *Anaesthesia* 1998; **53** (Suppl.): 35–41.
73. Smith C, McEwan AI, Jhaveri R, *et al.* The interaction of fentanyl on the CP_{50} of propofol for loss of consciousness and skin incision. *Anesthesiology* 1994; **81:** 820–8.
74. Vuyk J, Lim T, Engbers FH, *et al.* The pharmacodynamic interaction of propofol and alfentanil during lower abdominal surgery in women. *Anesthesiology* 1995; **83:** 8–22.
75. Glass PS. Anesthetic drug interactions: an insight into general anesthesia – its mechanism and dosing strategies. *Anesthesiology* 1998; **88:** 5–6.
76. Lang E, Flaishon R, Sebel P. Monitoring the adequacy of intravenous anaesthesia. *Anaesth Pharmacol Rev* 1995; 3: 37–45.
77. Whitwam JG. Co-induction of anaesthesia: day-case surgery. *Eur J Anaesthesiol* 1995; **12** (Suppl.):25–34.
78. Amrein R, Hetzel W, Allen SR. Co-induction of anaesthesia: the rationale. *Eur J Anaesthesiol* 1995; **12** (Suppl.): 5–11.
79. Djaiani G, Ribes-Pastor MP. Propofol auto-co-induction as an alternative to midazolam co-induction for ambulatory surgery. *Anaesthesia* 1999; **54:** 63–7.
80. Vinik HR, Bradley EL Jr, Kissin I. Triple anesthetic combination: propofol–midazolam–alfentanil. *Anesth Analg* 1994; **78:** 354–8.
81. Vinik HR, Bradley EL Jr, Kissin I. Propofol–midazolam–alfentanil combination: is hypnotic synergism present? *Anesth Analg* 1993; **76:** S450.
82. Sear JW. Eltanolone: 50 years on and still looking for steroid hypnotic agents! [editorial]. *Eur J Anaesthesiol* 1998; **15:** 129–32.
83. Hering WJ, Ihmsen H, Langer H, *et al.* Pharmacokinetic–pharmacodynamic modeling of the new steroid hypnotic eltanolone in healthy volunteers. *Anesthesiology* 1996; **85:** 1290–9.
84. Sneyd JR, Wright PM, Harris D, *et al.* Computer-controlled infusion of ORG 21465, a water soluble steroid i.v. anaesthetic agent, into human volunteers. *Br J Anaesth* 1997; **79:** 433–9.
85. Dingemanse J, Häussler J, Hering W, *et al.* Pharmacokinetic–pharmacodynamic modelling of the EEG effects of Ro 48–6791, a new short-acting benzodiazepine, in young and elderly subjects. *Br J Anaesth* 1997; **79:** 567–74.
86. Vinik HR. Intravenous anaesthetic drug interactions: practical applications. *Eur J Anaesthesiol* 1995; **12** (Suppl.): 13–9.
87. Egan TD. Intravenous drug delivery systems: toward an intravenous vaporizer. *J Clin Anesth* 1996; **8** (Suppl. 3): 8S–14S
88. Huang JW, Lu YY, Nayak A, Roy RJ. Depth of anesthesia estimation and control. *IEEE Trans Biomed Eng* 1999; **46:** 71–81.

36

Neuromuscular blocking agents and their antagonists

RAJINDER K MIRAKHUR AND FRANÇOIS DONATI

Neuromuscular blocking agents have been an essential part of the anesthetists' armamentarium for more than 50 years. The first relaxant used in clinical practice, *d*-tubocurarine, is rarely used now and is not available in many areas of the world, partly because of its unacceptable side-effects and partly because of the development of much safer and more predictable newer agents. The general principles supporting the use of muscle relaxants and the commonly used individual agents are described in this chapter.

PHARMACODYNAMIC CONCEPTS

Potency and dose–response curves

The potency of neuromuscular blocking agents, like that of any other drugs, is estimated by constructing dose–response curves. This was traditionally achieved using incremental doses of the relaxant in the same patient when the block had stabilized after the previous increment until 95% block developed.[1] Another method is to give single doses of different concentrations (at least three but usually 4–6) to separate groups of patients, each patient receiving only a single dose of the relaxant. Whereas the cumulative method has been shown to yield the same results as the single-dose method for long-acting relaxants, it underestimates the potency of intermediate and short-acting relaxants.[2–5] The main disadvantage of the single-dose method is the large number of subjects needed to establish dose–response curves. The data are subjected to some type of transformation to produce straight lines from sigmoid-shaped curves. The effective dose that results in 50%, 90%, or 95% block is termed the ED_{50}, ED_{90}, or ED_{95} respectively. Potency is also influenced by the mode of stimulation used.[6] Recently, some investigators have determined potency using only two doses.[7] The ED_{95} values of commonly used relaxants are given in Table 36.1. Roughly the same order of relative potency was found when potency was assessed *in vitro* using recombinant muscle-type acetylcholine receptors.[8] In general, a dose that is 2–3 times the ED_{95} is administered for facilitating tracheal intubation.

Stimulating the ulnar nerve at the wrist and measuring the resultant responses of the adductor pollicis muscle is the most convenient method for determining response to neuromuscular blocking agents, but it is well established that other important muscles, such as the diaphragm and the laryngeal muscles, have different sensitivities.[9]

Onset and duration of action

The onset of neuromuscular block in clinical terms is the time it takes for the drug to effect depression of measurable responses, although by that time nearly 70% of the receptors will be occupied by the drug. The speed of onset of action depends upon cardiac output, muscle blood flow, the potency and dose of the relaxant used, and some kinetic characteristics (e.g. clearance).[10] The passage of the relaxant into the effect compartment is dependent upon the rate constant, k_{eo},[11] which is influenced by the above factors. The influence of cardiac output and blood flow is apparent from the observations of a rapid onset of effect of muscle relaxants in children and a slower onset in the elderly. High blood flow is probably also the reason for a faster onset of action in muscles such as the diaphragm and the larynx and when repeated nerve stimulation or stimulation at high rates is applied to the muscle being studied. Onset time is also rapid for drugs whose redistribution is rapid or which are rapidly cleared from the plasma into the effect compartment.

It is now established that drugs with a low potency have a more rapid onset of action.[12–14] Potent drugs are expected to be slow acting as fewer molecules are injected and the concentration gradient into the receptor is low. The most potent muscle relaxant used in man, doxacurium, also has the slowest onset of action. Potent relaxants also have a high affinity for the receptor and their effects therefore wear off slowly (Fig. 36.1).

The size of the dose administered also influences the onset time of relaxants, within limits. A large dose acts more rapidly but is also associated with slower recovery. The reason for the quick onset is principally the rapid development of high concentrations of the drug at the neuromuscular junction. One of the other ways in which onset of neuromuscular block can be accelerated is by the use of the "priming" technique. In this technique, an initial small dose is followed by the main dose, the effect of which becomes apparent more quickly. However, rapid onset is not consistently observed with this technique, which also has the disadvantage that many patients experience symptoms of muscle weakness before they are anesthetized.

The duration of action of neuromuscular blocking agents depends upon their redistribution and rate of clearance, the size of the dose, and the mode and site of metabolism. Some of these factors are described with individual agents.

Pharmacokinetic considerations

Muscle relaxants are quaternary ammonium compounds and thus are highly ionized and water soluble. Their absorption from intramuscular

Table 36.1 *ED_{95} values and intubating doses for commonly used muscle relaxants*

	ED_{95} (mg kg^{-1})	Usual intubating dose (mg kg^{-1})
d-Tubocurarine	0.45	0.5
Pancuronium	0.06	0.1
Doxacurium	0.03	0.03–0.04
Pipecuronium	0.045	0.06–0.08
Vecuronium	0.04	0.08–0.1
Atracurium	0.25	0.5–0.6
Rocuronium	0.3	0.6–1.0
Cisatracurium	0.05	0.1–0.15
Mivacurium	0.08	0.15–0.2
Rapacuronium	0.75	1.5–2.0
Succinylcholine	0.3	1.0–1.5

Succinylcholine (suxamethonium).

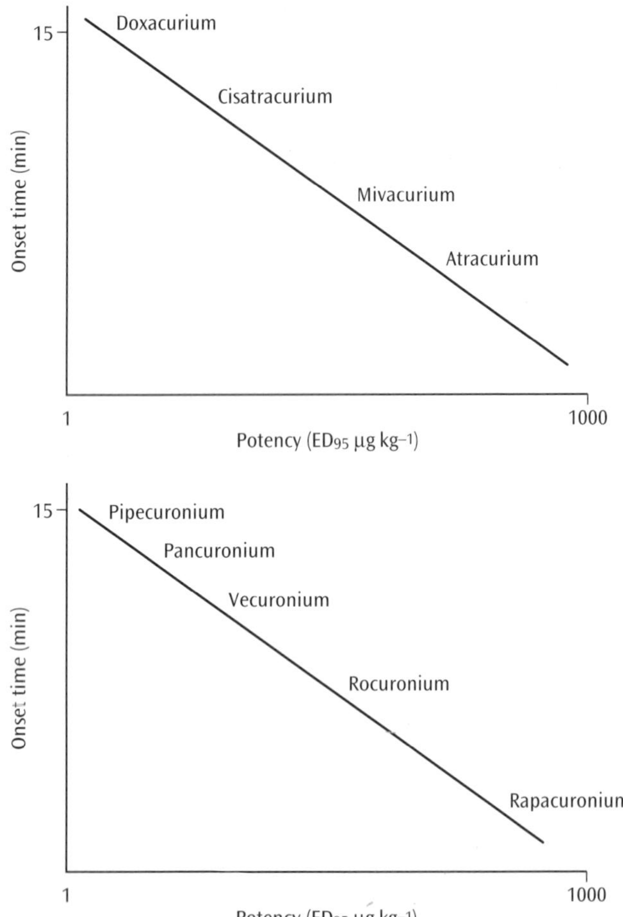

Figure 36.1 *Schematic diagrams showing inverse relation between potency and onset time for benzylisoquinolinium (top) and aminosteroid (bottom) relaxants.*

sites is therefore relatively slow. The distribution of currently used relaxants can be described by two- or three-compartment models. They are distributed from a central compartment into a peripheral compartment followed by one or two elimination phases, when the drugs are metabolized and excreted. Most muscle relaxants have both a distribution half-life ($t_{1/2\alpha}$) and an elimination half-life ($t_{1/2\beta}$).

The volume of distribution of relaxants is low owing to their poor lipid solubility. The initial volume of distribution usually varies between 80 and 150 mL kg^{-1}, and the volume of distribution at steady state varies between 200 and 500 mL kg^{-1}. The initial volume of distribution determines the peak plasma concentration after injection of a rapid bolus. The volume of distribution and the clearance of relaxants is influenced by age, pregnancy, and diseases of the liver and kidney. Cardiac output also influences the kinetics of relaxants because it influences drug distribution.

Protein binding of muscle relaxants is relatively low, varying between 30% and 80%. Changes in plasma proteins in disease states influence the volume of distribution, metabolism, and excretion of drugs including relaxants.[15] The pharmacokinetic data for commonly used relaxants are given in Table 36.2.

DEPOLARIZING NEUROMUSCULAR BLOCKING AGENTS

Succinylcholine (suxamethonium)

Succinylcholine is the only depolarizing muscle relaxant still in clinical use, although its demise has been forecast many times. It is still widely employed in clinical practice because of its unique properties of a short onset time and a short duration of action. It resembles acetylcholine (Fig. 36.2) and, like acetylcholine, depolarizes the postsynaptic membrane although its effect is more persistent[16–18] than that of acetylcholine, as the latter is metabolized much more rapidly by acetylcholinesterase. Succinylcholine produces a characteristic depolarizing block that is associated with the absence of fade in response to train-of-four and tetanic stimulations, the absence of post-tetanic facilitation, and increased block in the presence of anticholinesterase drugs. The type of block may change into a nondepolarizing type following prolonged administration of the drug (phase II block). The transition from a depolarizing to a phase II block is gradual and usually occurs after administration of 7–10 mg kg^{-1} of succinylcholine. The recovery from a phase II block is much slower.

It is difficult to estimate the pharmacokinetic parameters for succinylcholine because of its rapid degradation. Its half-life has been indirectly estimated by some to be between 16 and 47 s, the short half life being considered to be due to its rapid hydrolysis by plasma cholinesterase.[19,20] However, others have estimated the half-life to be 2–4 min.[21]

The onset of block following administration of succinylcholine is heralded by fasciculations, which represent this agent's acetylcholine-like agonist activity.[22] This usually happens in 30–40 s, with maximum block occurring in 1–1.5 min following a dose of 1 mg kg^{-1} (representing approximately three times the ED_{95}.)[23] The doses required for diaphragmatic paralysis are greater than those required for paralysis of the adductor pollicis muscle; however, the doses required for paralysis of the vocal cords are lower.[24] The onset times are shorter in children than in adults. The duration of action of a dose of succinylcholine of 1 mg kg^{-1} is 5–10 min. Increasing the dose does not result in prolongation of effect of the same magnitude as with nondepolarizing relaxants. Succinylcholine provides near ideal intubating conditions within 60–90 s following a dose of 1 mg kg^{-1}.[25,26]

Table 36.2 *Pharmacokinetic parameters for muscle relaxants*

	$V_{d(ss)}$ (mg kg^{-1})	Cl (mL kg^{-1} min^{-1})	Elimination half-life (min)
d-Tubocurarine[56]	425	1.71	173
Pancuronium[69]	212	1.5	130
Doxacurium[75]	150	2.22	86
Pipecuronium[82]	353	1.8	161
Vecuronium[92]	246	4.26	58
Atracurium[105]	182	6.1	20.6
Rocuronium[136]	207	3.7	97.2
Cisatracurium[153]	175	5.09	24.8
Mivacurium[158]	210	95	1.53 (cis–trans isomer)
	200	70	2.32 (trans–trans isomer)
	266	5.2	50.3 (cis–cis isomer)
Rapacuronium[181]	220	5.3	88
Succinylcholine[19]	16.4	40.5 L min^{-1}	16.6 s

$V_{d(ss)}$, volume of distribution at steady state; Cl, clearance; succinylcholine (suxamethonium).

$(CH_3)_3N^+—CH_2—CH_2—O—C(=O)—CH_3$

Acetylcholine

$(CH_3)_3N^+—CH_2—CH_2—O—C(=O)—CH_2—CH_2—C(=O)—O—CH_2—CH_2—N^+(CH_3)_3$

Succinylcholine

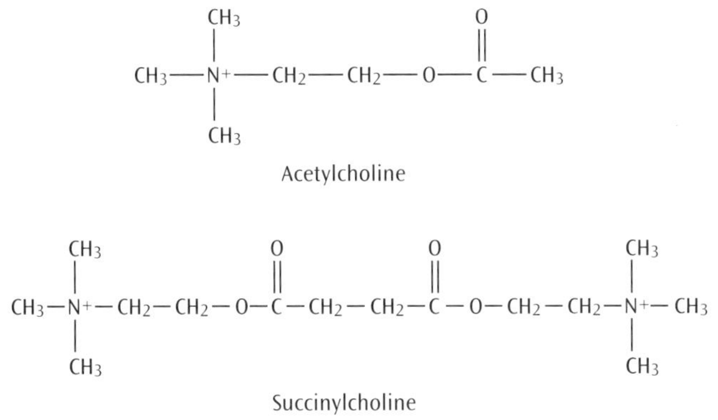

Figure 36.2 *Acetylcholine and succinylcholine (suxamethonium).*

Depolarizing drugs such as succinylcholine show significant interactions during anesthesia. Administration of a nondepolarizing agent tends to antagonize the effects of succinylcholine. This is characteristically seen when succinylcholine is preceded by a small dose of a nondepolarizing relaxant.[23] Neostigmine, a potent anticholinesterase drug, may prolong the effects of succinylcholine whereas edrophonium, a drug with only minimal anticholinesterase activity, may not.[27–29] There is conflicting evidence as to whether the dosage of nondepolarizing relaxants following succinylcholine administration should or should not be increased.

The effects of succinylcholine are potentiated in the presence of isoflurane anesthesia, although not in the presence of other volatile agents unless administered over a long period.[30,31]

Although succinylcholine does have the advantages of a rapid onset and a short duration of action, its use is associated with a wide spectrum of side-effects, some of which are very serious, and it is contraindicated in some patients. Muscle pains are probably the most commonly observed side-effect and have been reported in 25–80% of patients.[32] These are more common in young and fit patients and those who are mobilized early. Various strategies have been used to prevent these pains, but administration of small doses of nondepolarizing relaxants remains the most commonly used technique.[32,33] These reduce but do not completely abolish the pains. It remains unclear whether there is a direct correlation between the observation of muscle fasciculations and the occurrence of muscle pains.

Cardiovascular effects following succinylcholine are unpredictable. It can produce vagally mediated severe bradycardia, particularly in children and after a second dose; this can be prevented by administration of an anticholinergic agent. Succinylcholine may also give rise to hypertension and tachycardia as a result of an increase in circulating catecholamines.[34] This latter effect may counteract the bradycardic effect.

Succinylcholine produces an increase in serum potassium[33] of about 0.5 mmol L^{-1} that is of little consequence in normal patients. This is believed to originate from the depolarization of skeletal muscle, increasing the potassium efflux from muscle cells.[35] The increase can be marked and may have adverse consequences for patients with lesions of the spinal cord, extensive burns, skeletal muscle diseases, or renal failure, and in immobile subjects. Pretreatments given to attenuate the muscle pains also attenuate the increase in plasma potassium to a certain extent. Marked hyperkalemia may also give rise to cardiovascular effects.

Of all the drugs used by anesthetists, the frequency of allergic and/or anaphylactic reactions is probably highest with succinylcholine.[36] The likelihood of a reaction is high if there is a history of previous reaction. As is the case with all muscle relaxants, succinylcholine may give rise to cross-sensitivity. The management of such reactions should be on standard lines.

Administration of succinylcholine is associated with an increase in intraocular, intragastric, and intracranial pressures. Most of these effects are believed to be based on the depolarizing mode of action of succinylcholine. Although they are of minimal importance in normal patients, they may have adverse consequences for patients with pre-existing disease or a perforated eye. The increase in intragastric pressure is not important as the opening pressure of the lower esophageal sphincter also increases. These effects may be partly attenuated by pretreatment with a small dose of a nondepolarizing relaxant.

Administration of succinylcholine has been observed to give rise to masseter muscle spasm. This may be severe in some patients, making laryngoscopy and intubation difficult. In such cases the smaller doses of nondepolarizing relaxants are not of much benefit. This may be due to inadequate dosage of succinylcholine or may simply represent an exaggerated form of normal response. It has been suggested that this is an early warning sign of the development of malignant hyperthermia,[37] but it is not invariably associated with the syndrome. Succinylcholine administration has been associated with occurrence of malignant hyperthermia in susceptible individuals. This condition is characterized by rapidly increasing temperature, metabolic acidosis, hypercapnia, and an increase in serum potassium, and is associated with considerable mortality.

Succinylcholine shows a prolonged response when the plasma cholinesterase activity is low (less than 40% of normal) or the patient has genetically atypical plasma cholinesterase. The enzyme activity is low in patients with liver disease or cancer as well as in elderly, pregnant, or malnourished patients and following anticholinesterase drugs. The prolongation of block in these conditions is not very long. Very prolonged block is, however, associated with the presence of silent or atypical genes in homozygous individuals.[38] The block in these cases lasts several hours until succinylcholine is broken down and eliminated very slowly.

NONDEPOLARIZING (COMPETITIVE) NEUROMUSCULAR BLOCKING AGENTS

Long-acting agents

d-Tubocurarine

The use of *d*-tubocurarine (Fig. 36.3) as a neuromuscular blocking agent in clinical practice was first described in 1942 and heralded the era of the use of such agents, which have revolutionized the practice of anesthesia during the last 60 years. This agent is used very rarely now and in fact is no longer included in many pharmacopeias.

Tubocurarine is a member of the benzylisoquinolinium group of compounds and was originally thought to be a bisquaternary compound. This categorization was however, revised in 1970, when it was found that it is actually a monoquaternary compound, although it becomes a bisquaternary compound at body pH.[39]

The main site of action of tubocurarine is at the postjunctional membrane, where it competes with acetylcholine molecules. It also has some prejunctional effect, reducing the liberation of acetylcholine. This has been demonstrated indirectly also by observation that fade in response to tetanic and train-of four stimulations is greater than with agents such as pancuronium and vecuronium.[40–44]

The ED_{95} of *d*-tubocurarine is approximately 0.5 mg kg^{-1}, and this is the dose commonly employed to facilitate tracheal intubation and abdominal muscle relaxation (in contrast to other relaxants, for which the most commonly used dose is 2–3 times the ED_{95}). The onset of block with this dose is quite slow, more than 5 min being required to produce maximum block.[45] *d*-Tubocurarine is justifiably classified as a long-acting agent – 25% recovery of the twitch (duration of clinical relaxation) occurs in 60–100 min. The time to recovery after additional doses is prolonged.[46]

The pharmacological antagonism of *d*-tubocurarine depends upon the depth of block at which antagonism is carried out.[47] Commonly used anticholinesterase agents, e.g. neostigmine, pyridostigmine, and edrophonium, have all been evaluated as antagonists of *d*-tubocurarine block. Edrophonium is faster in its onset of action than equipotent doses of neostigmine.[48] Whereas Morris *et al.*[49] reported adequate antagonism of block with edrophonium, others have observed it not to be reliable, particularly if the block is relatively deep.[50]

d-Tubocurarine produces cutaneous flushing and a significant reduction in arterial pressure in doses that are commonly used clinically. This is mostly due to histamine liberation and ganglionic blockade.[51–54] A direct myocardial depressant effect has also been reported.[55] It is excreted mostly unchanged in urine, and, to some extent via the liver, and has a long elimination half-life.[56]

Dimethyltubocurarine

Dimethyltubocurarine is a methylated derivative of *d*-tubocurarine, being nearly twice as potent as *d*-tubocurarine with an ED_{95} of 0.28 mg kg^{-1}.[45] Its speed of onset is only marginally faster than equipotent doses of *d*-tubocurarine, duration of clinical relaxation also being similar. Its main advantage over *d*-tubocurarine appears to be that it is associated with fewer cardiovascular effects, although some histamine liberation has been reported.[45,57,58] The drug has never been popular in clinical use.

Pancuronium

Pancuronium is a synthetic bisquaternary aminosteroidal muscle relaxant (Fig. 36.4) introduced into clinical practice in 1967.[59] It is 8–10 times as potent as *d*-tubocurarine, with an ED_{95} of about 0.06 mg kg^{-1}; commonly administered doses are in the range 0.07–0.1 mg kg^{-1}.

Pancuronium has a relatively slow onset of action, producing maximum block at the adductor pollicis muscle in about 3–4 min at a dose of 1–1.5 times the ED_{95},[60] and intubating conditions are acceptable only after 3–4 min of administration of this dose. The clinical duration of this dose of pancuronium is about an hour, with full recovery taking up to 2 h. Higher doses have a faster onset but are associated with a much longer duration of action. A progressive increase in the duration of action occurs with repeated administration.[61] Recovery can be accelerated by administration of anticholinesterase drugs, but recovery from deeper levels of block takes longer.[62] Although edrophonium in equipotent doses can also reverse the block, and perhaps at a faster rate, it is not as effective as neostigmine if the block is relatively deep.[50]

Pancuronium tends to increase the heart rate, arterial pressure, and cardiac output in clinically used doses.[63] Although this may be advantageous in some situations, such as when using high-dose opiate anesthesia during cardiac surgery, it may be associated with arrhythmias and cardiac ischemia in susceptible individuals.[64,65] The postulated mechanisms for the occurrence of these cardiovascular changes include muscarinic receptor blockade, increased release and decreased reuptake of catecholamines, and possibly direct myocardial stimulation.[66–68]

Elimination of pancuronium is mostly via the kidney, about half of it in an unchanged form. As in the case of *d*-tubocurarine, it has a relatively long elimination half-life.[69] Its clinical duration and elimination half-life are markedly increased in patients with renal failure. It also undergoes some hepatic metabolism, producing the 3-hydroxy metabolite, which has neuromuscular blocking properties, the elimination of which is reduced in patients with liver disease.[70]

Although the use of pancuronium has decreased markedly following the introduction of intermediate-acting agents, it was the first relaxant introduced into clinical practice which did not have the ganglion-blocking or histamine-releasing properties of *d*-tubocurarine. It is still a popular choice with many for use during cardiac surgery as it tends to counteract the vagal effects of high-dose opiate anesthesia.

Doxacurium

Doxacurium (Fig. 36.3) is the most potent relaxant presently available, with an ED_{95} of 25–30 μg kg^{-1}.[71] It is the first benzylisoquinolinium compound not to have the propensity to release histamine. A striking feature of doxacurium is its clean cardiovascular profile; it has no significant effects on heart rate, blood pressure, or cardiac output.[72] The drug has a slow onset of action, which may exceed 10 min, and a very variable and prolonged duration of effect (duration of clinical relaxation of 1–2 h following doses of 1–2 × ED_{95}).[73,74] It is mainly excreted unchanged in the urine, with less than 10% being metabolized. It has an elimination

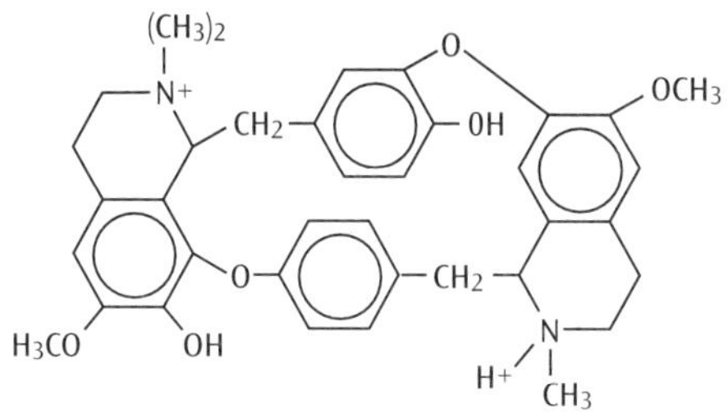

Tubocurarine

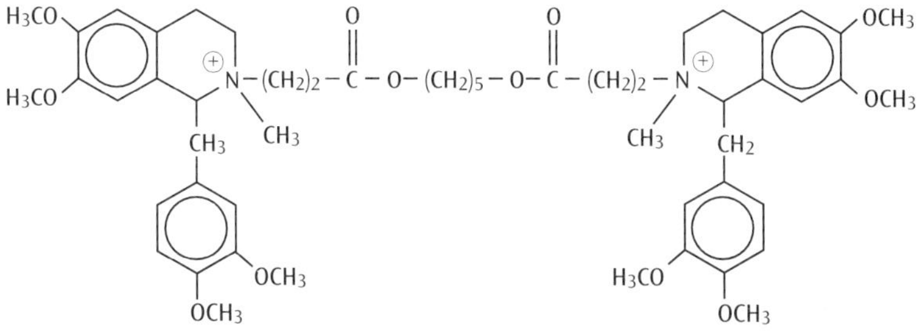

Atracurium

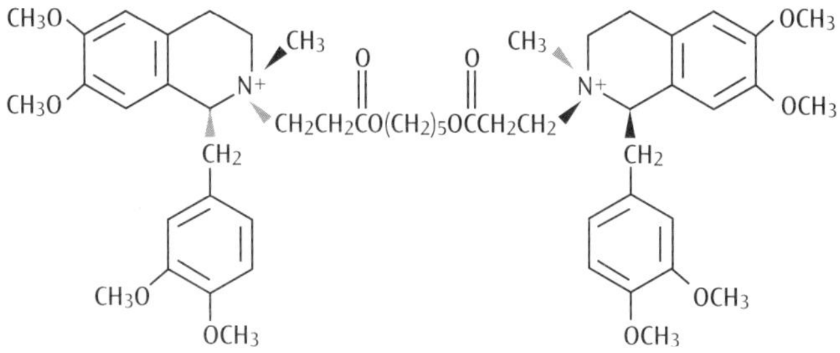

Cisatracurium

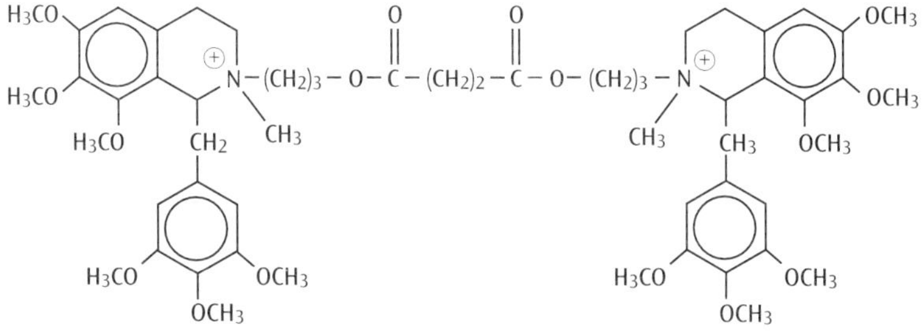

Doxacurium

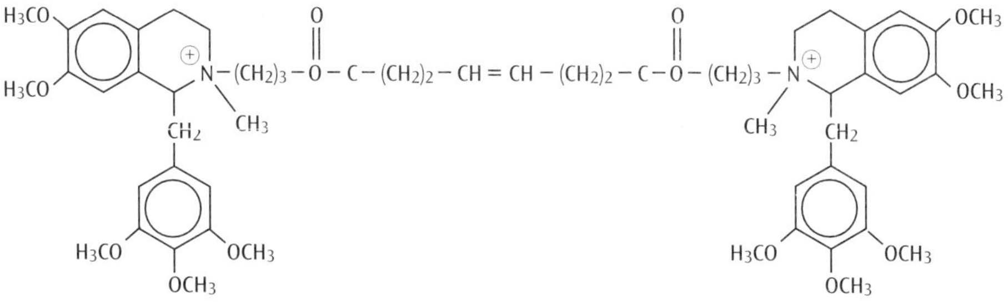

Mivacurium

Figure 36.3 *Benzylisoquinolinium relaxants.*

half-life which is shorter than that of the other long-acting relaxants but it has a similarly long duration of action.[75] Recovery is prolonged in patients with renal failure, and in the elderly.[74] It is recommended that doxacurium block should always be reversed. Doxacurium is available only in the USA, and the use there is limited. It is unlikely to become available in the UK or elsewhere.

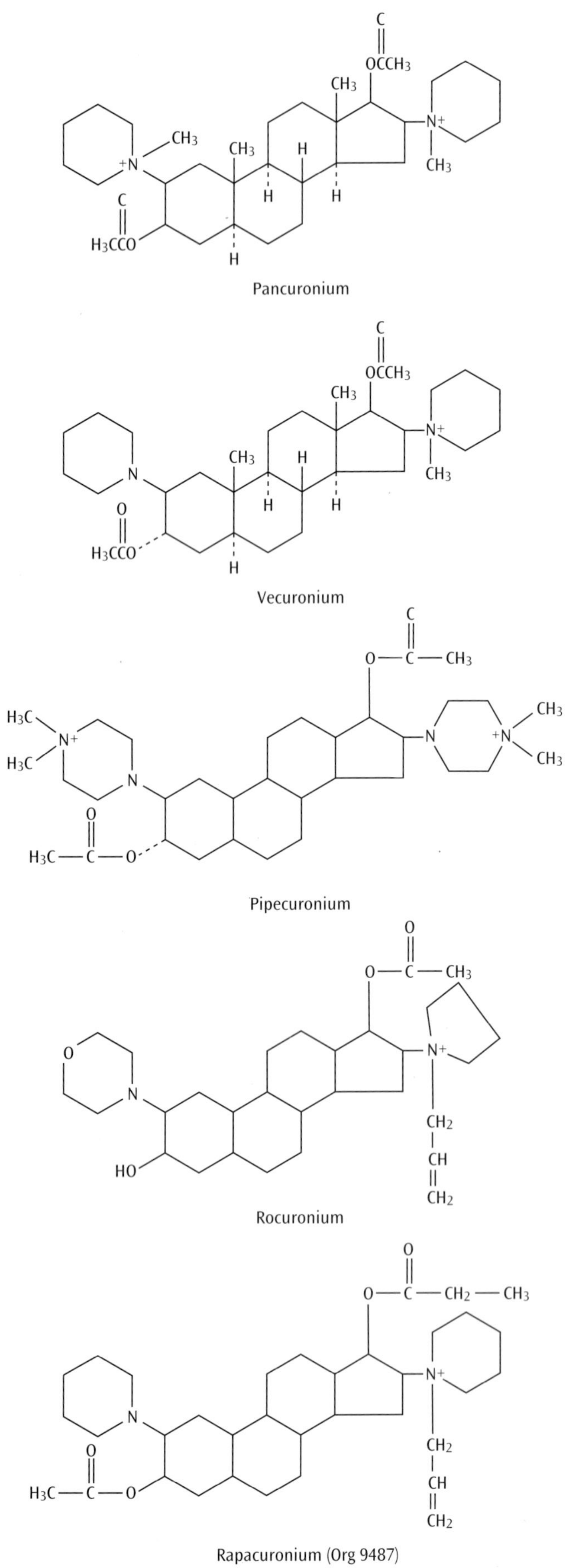

Pancuronium

Vecuronium

Pipecuronium

Rocuronium

Rapacuronium (Org 9487)

Figure 36.4 *Aminosteroid relaxants.*

Pipecuronium

Pipecuronium was available in Eastern Europe for many years and it became available in the West in 1992. Its onset and duration of action are similar to those of pancuronium in equipotent doses, but it is free from the cardiovascular side-effects of the latter. It is also a bisquaternary compound (Fig. 36.4).

The ED_{95} of pipecuronium during balanced anesthesia is about 45 μg kg^{-1}.[76] The time to onset of neuromuscular block decreases in a dose-dependent fashion. The onset time has been reported to be between 2.5 and 4.5 min with doses of 1–2 × ED_{95}.[77,78] Pipecuronium has a long duration of action, which is influenced by the size of the dose and the anesthetic technique used. The clinical duration of action at doses of 1–2 × ED_{95} varies from 50 to 100 min. The spontaneous recovery from a pipecuronium block is slow;[77] antagonism using neostigmine at the end of surgery is therefore recommended. Reversal of neuromuscular block can be successfully achieved with neostigmine administration provided twitch height has already recovered spontaneously to between 10% and 25% of control but may still take up to 10 min.[79] The principal feature of pipecuronium is its almost complete lack of cardiovascular side-effects.[80,81] Histamine release does not appear to be a problem. The drug is eliminated slowly and mainly through the kidney.[82]

Owing to its relatively slow onset of action and minimum advantages over more recently introduced agents, the use of pipecuronium is limited and it is unlikely to become available in those parts of the world where it is not available now.

Other long-acting agents

Gallamine was the first synthetic nondepolarizing agent to be introduced into clinical practice. It is a drug with a low potency (ED_{95} approximately 2.5 mg kg^{-1}). It is a relatively long-acting agent and its action is slow to reverse following administration of neostigmine. Gallamine suffers from two major disadvantages, namely a highly potent vagolytic effect and almost total dependence upon the kidneys for its elimination. These have rendered it of mainly historical interest.

Alcuronium is a semisynthetic compound (with an ED_{95} of approximately 150 μg kg^{-1}) originally introduced in the belief that it would have a short duration of action; however, in clinical practice it has not proved to be any different from *d*-tubocurarine. It is excreted almost entirely unchanged through the kidneys and has a moderate vagolytic effect. Alcuronium has no particular advantage over other similar nondepolarizing relaxants and has been largely withdrawn from clinical practice owing to the occurrence of anaphylactic reactions.

Fazadinium was introduced into clinical practice in the UK in the 1970s in an attempt to provide an agent with a rapid onset and a short duration of action. However, it soon became apparent that it was neither rapid in onset of effect nor short acting and was associated with a marked tachycardia. This drug has also been withdrawn from clinical use.

Intermediate-acting agents

The introduction of intermediate-acting agents vecuronium and atracurium revolutionized the use of muscle relaxants. For the first time anesthetists had nondepolarizing relaxants with much shorter durations of action than *d*-tubocurarine or pancuronium and with durations of action that were much more predictable.

Vecuronium

Vecuronium is the 16-monoquaternary derivative of pancuronium (Fig. 36.4) with an ED_{95} of 0.04–0.05 mg kg^{-1}.[4,83] A dose of 0.1–0.15 mg kg^{-1} provides acceptable intubating conditions within 90–120 s and surgical muscle relaxation for 25–40 min.[84] The onset of action of a standard intubating dose of 0.1 mg kg^{-1} occurs in about 3 min. Both the onset and duration of action are dose related. The onset of action can also be accelerated by inducing anesthesia with a potent volatile agent such as sevoflurane.[85] The onset of vecuronium block is slightly faster in children, in whom it also has a shorter duration of action. The drug has a longer duration of action in the elderly and in the obese if dosed on actual body weight. Both neostigmine and edrophonium, in equipotent doses, are effective antagonists of a vecuronium block, although the latter is slow and somewhat ineffective if the block at the time of reversal is deep.[50]

The use of vecuronium is associated with extremely good cardiovascular stability even when used in large doses.[49,86,87] There is a wide separation between vagal and neuromuscular blocking doses (68:1) and it has little ganglion-blocking or sympathetic activity. As a result, large doses (3–4 × ED_{95}) can be administered to achieve a faster onset of action and good intubating conditions at an earlier time. Although vecuronium does not cause tachycardia or hypotension, its use may be associated with bradycardia as a result of vagal stimulation or when administered along with other drugs. Vecuronium can be administered in repeated doses of 1–2 mg or by a continuous infusion for maintenance of block.[88] A general rule of thumb for administration by infusion is to use 0.1 mg kg^{-1} h^{-1} following some recovery from a bolus dose of 0.1 mg kg^{-1}. The dose requirements diminish after some time as peripheral storage sites become saturated. It is strongly advocated that neuromuscular block be routinely monitored during prolonged administration.

Although initial studies showed little evidence of cumulation with vecuronium,[61] subsequent work has demonstrated that it does occur to some degree.[89] This is partly because recovery is shifted from the rapid distribution to the less rapid elimination phase and partly because of the formation of the metabolite 3-desacetylvecuronium, particularly when vecuronium is administered in larger doses. Despite this, vecuronium has been used safely by infusion in individuals with normal organ function over considerable periods of time.[90]

Vecuronium is metabolized to 3-, 17-, and 3,17-dihydroxy metabolites, the main route of elimination being hepatic, with about 40% being excreted in the bile.[91] The 3-hydroxy metabolite, 3-desacetylvecuronium, has 40–80% of the potency of the parent compound and is eliminated by the kidneys. For these reasons, the effects of vecuronium are prolonged in patients with hepatic or renal failure.[92,93] This metabolite may be responsible for cases of prolonged paralysis seen after long-term administration of vecuronium to patients in intensive care units.[94] Hypothermia and hypothermic cardiopulmonary bypass also produce a prolongation of effect and reduced vecuronium requirements.[95] This may be due to a reduction in the uptake in the liver and reduced metabolism and clearance of the drug itself or its active metabolites.[96,97] The dosage of vecuronium should therefore be reduced in such circumstances and the block monitored.

Atracurium

Atracurium is a synthetic bisquaternary benzylisoquinolinium compound (Fig. 36.3) developed because of its novel method of metabolism by the Hofmann elimination reaction.[98] This reaction takes place at a pH of 7.4 and a temperature of 37 °C. It is, thus, metabolized at body temperature and pH, and is stored at 4 °C and buffered to a pH of 3.

The ED_{95} of atracurium, calculated using the single-dose technique under balanced anesthesia,[3] is approximately 0.22 mg kg^{-1} and the onset of action of an ED_{95} dose approximately 3–5 min. This can be reduced by increasing the intubating dose. Spontaneous recovery occurs reliably from an atracurium neuromuscular block, such that an intubating dose of about 0.5 mg kg^{-1} can be expected to provide surgical muscle relaxation for 25–40 min in the normal healthy patient.[99] Repeated administration of atracurium does not lead to an increase in the duration of action.[100] Satisfactory neuromuscular block can be maintained with an atracurium bolus of 0.6 mg kg^{-1} followed by an infusion at a rate of 0.6 mg kg^{-1} h^{-1}; the requirement is less in the presence of potent volatile agents. The unique metabolism of atracurium makes it suitable for use in the critically ill patient as it is associated with a rapid recovery. This is true even in patients with renal failure, in whom rapid recovery has been reported (as rapid as after a bolus dose) after infusions lasting up to 37 h.[101] The reversal of an atracurium block can be easily accomplished by neostigmine or edrophonium; however, the latter is not reliable if the block is relatively deep.[50]

The pharmacodynamics of atracurium are unchanged with advancing age.[102] There is, however, some evidence for a reduction in clearance and an increase in elimination half-life.[103] No statistically significant differences have been observed in the recovery characteristics between healthy patients and those with chronic renal failure with unchanged pharmacokinetics.[104,105] The pharmacodynamics of atracurium are little changed in the presence of hepatic cirrhosis; resistance to onset of block may occur, but, if anything, recovery is faster than in healthy patients as the result of an increased rate of clearance.[106,107]

At physiological pH and temperature, atracurium is eliminated by spontaneous degradation through Hofmann elimination and ester hydrolysis.[108] Fisher *et al.* [109] have estimated that 60% of the total clearance of atracurium occurs via pathways other than Hofmann elimination and ester hydrolysis, presumably by metabolism or excretion by the liver and/or the kidney.

Hofmann degradation of atracurium produces the tertiary compound laudanosine, which in animal studies at concentrations above 17 μg mL^{-1} is known to produce epileptiform fits.[110] Ester hydrolysis of atracurium produces a monoquaternary alcohol, which also undergoes Hofmann degradation to laudanosine. Thus, two molecules of laudanosine are produced from the breakdown of each molecule of atracurium. Laudanosine is more lipid soluble than atracurium; it is metabolized in the liver, and also excreted unchanged in the urine. In humans, the highest plasma laudanosine concentrations of about 5 μg mL^{-1} have been recorded after 5 days of atracurium administration in critically ill patients.[111] There have been no reported adverse effects attributable to laudanosine. The highest reported laudanosine concentration of 8.6 μg mL^{-1} in man was in a neurosurgical patient with normal renal and hepatic function and produced no adverse effects.[112]

Atracurium gives rise to minimal cardiovascular effects except for some histamine liberation if the drug is given rapidly or in high doses.[113] It does not produce a tachycardia, and the patient may even show a bradycardia in its presence, owing to the effects of other agents such as the opiates or as a result of vagal stimulation. The histamine release is about one-third of that observed after *d*-tubocurarine administration.[114]

Rocuronium

Rocuronium, a low-potency drug (Fig. 36.1) was developed as a relaxant with a fast onset of effect in an attempt to develop a nondepolarizing agent that would have an onset of action closer to that of succinylcholine. The basis for this development was the observation that potency and the speed of onset of action were inversely related.[12]

Rocuronium is a desacetoxy analog of vecuronium (Fig. 36.4) that is stable in solution and formulated as an aqueous ready to use solution. The potency of rocuronium is between one-sixth and one-eighth that of vecuronium with an estimated ED_{95} of approximately 0.3 mg kg^{-1}.[6,115] This value is slightly lower in the presence of potent volatile anesthetics.

Early animal and subsequent human studies have shown the onset of action of rocuronium to be faster than that of other nondepolarizing relaxants.[116–118] The onset of maximum block following an intubating dose of 0.6 mg kg^{-1} occurs in about 2 min, which is slightly slower than after succinylcholine 1.0 mg kg^{-1}.[26,119,120] Larger doses have a more rapid onset of effect. The duration of action of rocuronium is similar to that of vecuronium and atracurium in comparable doses and is dose related, with a clinical duration of about 30 min with a 0.6 mg kg^{-1} dose, full spontaneous recovery taking about an hour.[115,120] Even in lower doses such as 0.45 mg kg^{-1}, particularly during anesthesia with desflurane, the onset of action of rocuronium is faster than after a standard dose of atracurium but with a shorter duration of action than the latter.[121] The effects can be readily antagonized by neostigmine or edrophonium on similar lines as after atracurium and vecuronium. The duration of action is prolonged by potent volatile agents, and in particular by sevoflurane, which may also slow the antagonism by neostigmine.[122–124] Repeat administration does not usually result in a prolonged effect.

Intubating conditions with a 0.6 mg kg^{-1} dose during normal induction of anesthesia are similar to those after succinylcholine within about 90 s.[26,125] However, a dose of about 1.0 mg kg^{-1} is required to obtain good intubating conditions during a rapid-sequence induction.[126,127] Intubating conditions at the lower dose may be improved by the addition of opiates, by using ketamine or etomidate as the induction agent, or by the administration of a small dose of ephedrine, these measures maintain a better cardiac output, which facilitates a rapid delivery of the relaxant to the neuromuscular junction.[128–130]

Commonly used doses of rocuronium are associated with cardiovascular stability and only a small increase in heart rate.[131,132] Higher doses may give rise to some increase in heart rate as a result of a lower vagal to neuromuscular blocking ratio than with vecuronium.[116,133]

While more than half of an administered dose of rocuronium is taken up by the liver and excreted unchanged in the bile, about a third of the dose is eliminated in the urine.[134] Of the possible metabolites, only very small amounts of 17-desacetylrocuronium have been found. Recent studies have shown that fecal and urinary excretion of unchanged rocuronium are the major routes of rocuronium elimination.[135] Clearance is reduced in patients with significant renal and hepatic disease with a possible prolongation of effect.[136,137] Both the onset and recovery are slower in the elderly.

Rocuronium is administered in an initial bolus dose of 0.6–1.0 mg kg^{-1} depending upon the anticipated duration of surgery. The block can be maintained by repeated administration of about 10 mg or by a continuous infusion in a dose of 0.5–0.6 mg kg^{-1} h^{-1} for a 90% block. The dosage requirements are lower in the presence of anesthetics such as isoflurane, enflurane, or sevoflurane. The dosage in obese and postpartum patients should be based on the lean body mass to avoid overdose and prolongation of effect.[138,139] Recovery after prolonged infusion may be somewhat slower than after cisatracurium.[140] Maintenance dosage during hypothermia is lower.[141] While the use of intermediate-acting agents such as rocuronium may not help with the early discharge of patients undergoing relatively prolonged cardiac surgery, it facilitates early extubation and is associated with a lower incidence of residual curarization in such patients.[142,143]

With its rapid onset of action, rocuronium may be useful for facilitating tracheal intubation during rapid-sequence induction of anesthesia in place of succinylcholine or when the latter is contraindicated. A useful dose in this situation is 1.0 mg kg^{-1}, although it must be realized that this dose will have a clinical duration of about an hour. It is also important to assess the airway carefully if the use of rocuronium is contemplated in this setting.

Cisatracurium

Cisatracurium (Fig. 36.3) is one of the 10 stereoisomers of atracurium. Previously known as 51W89, it is the 1*R* cis-1′*R* cis isomer of atracurium and has been used in clinical practice now for about 6 years. It constitutes about 15% of commercially available atracurium.[144] It differs from atracurium in being more potent, liberating histamine only minimally, and being predominantly metabolized via the Hofmann elimination pathway.

The ED_{95} of cisatracurium is about 0.05 mg kg^{-1}, making it about four times as potent as atracurium.[145] The estimated potency is not markedly different in infants and children.[146] Being more potent, the drug has a slower onset of action than atracurium, taking 3–5 min for maximum block with a dose of 0.1 mg kg^{-1}.[145,147] Although increasing the dose to 0.15 mg kg^{-1} accelerates the onset, it is still slower than that of atracurium 0.5 mg kg^{-1}.[147] The intubating conditions 2 min after relaxant administration are somewhat better with atracurium 0.5 mg kg^{-1} than 0.1 or 0.15 mg kg^{-1} cisatracurium.[147,148] Both the onset and the intubating conditions may be improved by prior administration of a small dose of ephedrine.[149]

The duration of clinical relaxation following cisatracurium is dose dependent and ranges from about 35 to 65 min at doses of 0.1–0.15 mg kg^{-1}.[147,150] This is similar to or slightly longer than the duration of neuromuscular block after an equipotent dose of atracurium. The rate of recovery from a cisatracurium block appears to be independent of the dose. The maintenance dose by infusion is reduced in the presence of potent volatile anesthetics and hypothermia.[141] Administration of neostigmine accelerates the recovery significantly, but it makes little difference whether the block is reversed from a 10% or a 25% recovery of twitch height.[147] Cisatracurium can be administered either by repeat dosing (25 μg kg^{-1} increments lasting for 18–20 min each) or by a continuous infusion (about 1.5 μg kg^{-1} min^{-1} for a 90% block) for procedures of long duration.

Minimal cardiovascular effect is an important attribute of cisatracurium. When administered in doses up to and including eight times the ED_{95}, cisatracurium does not give rise to any significant changes in arterial pressure or heart rate.[151] Cisatracurium in these doses does not cause any significant changes in median plasma histamine levels, although there is great inter-patient variation.[150,151] Similarly, there are no significant changes in intracranial pressure with its use.

Hofmann clearance accounts for about 75% of total body clearance, with organ clearance accounting for the remainder; renal clearance, a component of organ clearance, is about 16% of total body clearance.[152] Lien *et al.*[153] showed that the pharmacokinetics of cisatracurium are independent of dose in healthy adult patients after 0.1 and 0.2 mg kg^{-1} doses. The recovery profile is not altered in patients with liver failure, but the clearance is slightly reduced and recovery slightly slower in patients with renal failure.[154–156] This is in contrast with atracurium, which exhibits little change in pharmacokinetics or duration of action in the presence of renal disease; the difference in real terms is small. Compared with atracurium, much less laudanosine is produced by metabolism of cisatracurium, even when the drug is given by continuous infusion over a prolonged period of time.[157]

Short-acting agents

Mivacurium

Mivacurium chloride is a bisbenzylisoquinolinium diester (Fig. 36.3) that is hydrolyzed by plasma cholinesterase at about 80% of the rate of succinylcholine. Enzymatic hydrolysis gives the drug its short duration of action. The length of paralysis is approximately 2–2.5 times that of succinylcholine and one-half to one-third that of the intermediate-acting relaxants. Mivacurium is a mixture of three stereoisomers: the two short-acting cis–trans and trans–trans isomers, which constitute about 94% of the mixture, have very short half-lives of about 2 min, while the much less potent cis–cis isomer, which has about one-tenth the neuromuscular blocking potency of the other two isomers, undergoes some renal excretion as well as being broken down by plasma cholinesterase, with a half-life of about 50 min.[158] The short-acting isomers are broken down almost entirely by plasma cholinesterase, with a high rate of clearance and a short duration of action (Table 36.2).

The ED_{95} of mivacurium is about 80 μg kg^{-1}.[159,160] As with other nondepolarizing muscle relaxants, the time to onset of neuromuscular block is dose dependent. Savarese *et al.*[159] reported onset times ranging from 3.8 to 1.9 min with 0.1–0.3 mg kg^{-1} doses of mivacurium. It is currently the shortest acting nondepolarizing relaxant available, with a duration of clinical relaxation of about 15 min following a dose of 0.15 mg kg^{-1} (2×ED_{95}) with complete spontaneous recovery in under half an hour.[159,161] Its duration of action is 2–3 times that of succinylcholine.[162] The increase in the duration of action with increasing doses is not as marked as with other nondepolarizing relaxants. As in the case of other relaxants, spontaneous recovery of the effect is slower in the presence of potent volatile anesthetics such as isoflurane and sevoflurane.[163,164]

Mivacurium is a very suitable agent for maintaining relaxation by infusion; in fact, this is the preferred method for mivacurium administration for anything but brief procedures. The average dose required to maintain approximately 90–95% block is 6–8 μg kg^{-1} min^{-1}.[165,166] The recovery profile does not vary significantly following administration by repeat bolus doses or infusion of varying duration, suggesting minimal cumulation.[165] The reduction in the duration of action by administering anticholinesterase agents is relatively small, perhaps because of the inherently short duration of action of the drug.[161,167] Theoretically, neostigmine, which is a potent anticholinesterase agent, may prolong the action of mivacurium, but this has not been found to occur when neostigmine has been administered to antagonize a mivacurium block. However, previous administration of neostigmine prolongs the effects of subsequently administered mivacurium.[168]

Mivacurium has a propensity for histamine release even in clinically useful doses of 0.15–0.20 mg kg^{-1}. This may be the reason for the reduction in the arterial pressure and systemic vascular resistance reported by Loan *et al.*[169]

The duration of action of mivacurium is increased when there is a reduction in plasma cholinesterase activity, as in patients with marked renal and hepatic disease.[170,171] The same is true for elderly patients.[166] The prolongation is significant and marked in those with inherited homozygous silent or atypical plasma cholinesterase variants.[172] The effect of a single dose may last several hours in such patients. Heterozygotes show only moderate prolongation of effect.[173]

Rapacuronium

The introduction of rocuronium provided a neuromuscular blocking agent with a rapid onset of effect but lacking a short duration of action. The development of rapacuronium was an attempt to achieve this objective. Rapacuronium is the 16-*N*-allyl-17-β-propionate analog of vecuronium (Fig. 36.4) and is a low-potency compound with an ED_{95} of about 0.75 mg kg^{-1}.[174] Wierda *et al.*[175] reported its first use in humans and reported that a dose of 1.5 mg kg^{-1} produced complete block in 83 s compared with 67 s for succinylcholine 1.0 mg kg^{-1} and that the effect could be reversed by neostigmine within 2 min of relaxant administration. The rapid onset has been confirmed in recent studies, which have also shown it to be faster acting than mivacurium and vecuronium.[176,177] The onset of action is dose dependent.[176,178] The rapid onset is due to a high k_{eo} value, possibly related to its low potency, indicating a rapid access to the site of action.[179]

Although the initial study of Wierda *et al.*[175] found the clinical duration of rapacuronium 1.5 mg kg^{-1} to be 8–9 min, recent studies have reported this value to be 14–20 min.[176–178,180–182] The drug has also been shown to have cumulative properties after repeated administration or administration by infusion, even for only 30 min,[177,183,184] possibly as a result of the accumulation of its metabolite Org 9488.

Initial enthusiasm for rapacuronium was also based on its early reversibility with neostigmine, giving an overall duration of action similar to that of succinylcholine, about 11 min.[175] However, later studies found the duration to be longer, 15–20 min with reversal and about 35 min spontaneously at a dose of 1.5 mg kg^{-1}.[177,180,182] Nevertheless, the drug has a short duration of action similar to that of mivacurium but with a rapid and predictable onset.

Intubating conditions at 60 s with rapacuronium 1.5 mg kg^{-1} during stable anesthesia were reported to be similar to those of succinylcholine 1.0 mg kg^{-1}.[175,177] A more recent large study, however, showed that the conditions after succinylcholine 1.0 mg kg^{-1} were significantly better than after rapacuronium 1.5 mg kg^{-1}.[185] Higher doses are required during a rapid-sequence induction. A study employing a dose of 2.5 mg kg^{-1} showed that the conditions were not as good as after succinylcholine at 60 s.[186]

The principal route of elimination of rapacuronium is hepatic uptake and biliary excretion with a half-life of 88 min.[181] In addition to Org 9488 (3-hydroxy derivative), the other predicted metabolites of rapacuronium are Org 9502 (17-hydroxy derivative) and Org 9504 (3,17-dihydroxy derivative), but these have low neuromuscular blocking potency.

Rapacuronium administration leads to a dose-related increase in heart rate, which may be greater than 30% with a dose of 2.5 mg kg^{-1}.[176] In addition, a decrease in arterial pressure and systemic vascular resistance and an increase in cardiac output have been reported.[187] Although these results suggest the possibility of histamine release, which can occur with higher doses,[188] vasodilation may be due to inhibition of receptor and voltage-activated Ca^{2+} channels.[189]

The use of rapacuronium has been associated with a high frequency of respiratory side-effects, principally bronchospasm. This has been reported in both adults and children,[185,186,190,191] and many patients have required bronchodilators. Bronchospasm has been reported to be particularly severe in children in whom ventilation was occasionally difficult. In comparative trials and case-control studies, respiratory side-effects were observed more commonly with the administration of rapacuronium than with the comparators.[185,186,192] The identified risk factors are an irritable upper airway, a history of smoking, and use of the drug during a rapid-sequence induction.[186,192] The exact cause of bronchospasm with rapacuronium has not been determined. Histamine release probably plays a minor role, and muscarinic receptor stimulation in the airways may be responsible.

The drug was withdrawn from clinical use in March 2001 because of the much greater risk of occurrence of bronchospasm with this agent.

New agents undergoing investigation

Several drug series are being investigated currently for their potential use as rapid and short-acting nondepolarizing relaxants.

GW280430A

This agent, an asymmetrical mixed-onium chlorofumarate, has been tested in some animal species and in a few human volunteers. It is rapidly degraded in plasma and has a rapid onset and a very short duration of effect. The ED_{95} in humans is about 0.18 mg kg^{-1}, and a 2×ED_{95} dose has an onset time at the larynx of about 1.1 min and clinical duration of about 7 min.[193] The onset and recovery times following GW280430A 0.36 mg kg^{-1} and succinylcholine 1.0 mg kg^{-1} are similar.[194] Recovery can be shortened further by the administration of edrophonium.[194] Further investigation of its neuromuscular and cardiovascular effects is required before determining its place in clinical practice.

Tropinyl diesters

The rigid structure of tropane alkaloids has prompted research in stereochemistry to develop compounds with a variety of properties, including that of nondepolarizing neuromuscular blockade. These are low potency compounds shown to have an ultrashort duration of action in rats and pigs;[195] however, there is no human experience with these compounds as yet. Other tropinyl diester derivatives, such as TAAC3, have undergone animal investigation, and early results suggest that these compounds also have a rapid onset and ultrashort duration of action with minimal cumulative effects.[196]

PROBLEMS WITH THE USE OF MUSCLE RELAXANTS

Drug interactions

Muscle relaxants interact with a large variety of agents used in the perioperative period. The potentiation of their effect by volatile agents such as isoflurane, enflurane, and sevoflurane is well known. In general, intravenous anesthetics do not cause significant potentiation. Aminoglycoside antibiotics such as neomycin and gentamicin potentiate the effects of the relaxants and make antagonism difficult. This is particularly true of long-acting relaxants. The effect may be due to increased sensitivity of the postjunctional membrane and a presynaptic component. Verapamil has been shown in animal models to potentiate a nondepolarizing block, but studies in human patients on chronic nifedipine therapy have shown no such effect. Steroids may show a biphasic effect. The effects of some nondepolarizing relaxants may be potentiated by simultaneous or prior administration of other nondepolarizing agents; this usually happens if combinations of aminosteroid and benzylisoquinolinium relaxants are used. If two nondepolarizing relaxants with different durations of action are administered sequentially, the second relaxant may show a pattern of duration of action of the one given first.

Anticonvulsant agents such as carbamazepine and phenytoin produce resistance to the effects of relaxants.

Residual paralysis

It is more than 20 years since the first prospective study of residual paralysis in patients arriving in the recovery ward after routine anesthesia and surgery.[197] It was noticed that 42% of patients given pancuronium arrived in the recovery ward with train-of four ratios of <0.7 even though, in the vast majority, the block had been reversed. It has now been shown that this may be associated with a high frequency of postoperative pulmonary complications.[198] There have been several other reports since then. Although the vast majority have shown that the frequency of residual paralysis is lower with intermediate- and short-acting agents, a recent study showed that, using the newer standard of train-of four ratio of at least 0.8 to denote adequate recovery, the incidence was still high.[199] The incidence is high if reversal of block is not routinely carried out. The advantage of using intermediate- and short-acting agents is that any residual paralysis will be of short duration. It is advocated that monitoring, with proper attention to detail and interpretation, particularly to ascertain recovery, should be routinely employed.

Use of relaxants in the intensive therapy unit

Although the use of muscle relaxants in patients in the intensive therapy unit (ITU) has reduced considerably, these agents may still need to be used to facilitate tracheal intubation, and to facilitate ventilation and gas exchange in some situations, and in neurosurgical patients and those with tetanus. Multiple organ disease may alter the pharmacokinetics of relaxants, particularly when these are used over a prolonged period. There have been many reports of prolonged weakness in patients in the ITU, many of which are associated with the use of muscle relaxants.[94] This may be due to development of myopathy or neuropathy.[200] The link is not always clear, but steroidal relaxants have been implicated most often. Metabolites of pancuronium and vecuronium may accumulate in patients with renal dysfunction and lead to prolonged paralysis. There are occasional reports of this developing even when no relaxant has been used. The presence of sepsis and concomitant use of corticosteroids have also been implicated. It is not clear if monitoring the block is sufficient to prevent this developing, but it should help to tailor the dose of the relaxants and avoid overdosing patients. The use of atracurium or cisatracurium is preferable for patients in the ITU as these agents undergo considerable nonorgan-dependent elimination.

Allergic/anaphylactic reactions

Muscle relaxants are the most commonly implicated drugs in allergic/anaphylactic reactions occurring during anesthesia.[201] This is considered to be due to their quaternary structure and previous natural sensitization to such molecules. Allergic/anaphylactic reactions present themselves almost immediately after drug administration. Manifestations include cutaneous flushing, tachycardia, and hypotension, which may be severe enough to lead to cardiac arrest. Severe bronchospasm occurs in a proportion of patients. The reactions may be genuinely immune drug-specific hypersensitivity or nonimmune. Succinylcholine is the most commonly implicated agent, but increasingly other agents have been implicated as their use has increased, and cross-reactivity may be present.[202] Recently, rocuronium and cisatracurium have been implicated in several reactions,[203–205] although this probably reflects their increasing use.[206]

Occasionally, the reaction may simply be a pharmacological (chemical) histamine release characteristically seen with *d*-tubocurarine; this is usually dose related. Measurement of histamine levels may not be feasible when a reaction takes place, but measurement of serum tryptase and urinary methylhistamine are helpful in diagnosis. Determination of the actual causative agent involves demonstration of specific antibodies and skin testing. Management consists of the administration of oxygen and epinephrine, ventilation, volume expansion, and treatment of bronchospasm.

REVERSAL OF NEUROMUSCULAR BLOCK

Recovery from the effects of nondepolarizing relaxants can occur by elimination of the agent either unchanged or after metabolism. However, except for short-acting relaxants such as mivacurium, this may take a considerable time and cannot be reliably predicted and may result in residual curarization. In addition, surgical procedures can be of unpredictable duration and may require intense relaxation until near the completion of surgery. Pharmacological antagonism of neuromuscular block is therefore indicated in clinical practice and is accomplished by the administration of anticholinesterase drugs.

Anticholinesterase agents

The anticholinesterase agents in common use are neostigmine, pyridostigmine, and edrophonium, neostigmine being the most commonly used (Fig. 36.5).

The main mechanism of action of anticholinesterase agents is the inhibition of acetylcholinesterase, which results in an increased concentration of acetylcholine, thereby increasing the likelihood of acetylcholine occupying an unblocked receptor. Acetylcholinesterase has an anionic and an esteric site of action. The acid-transferring inhibi-

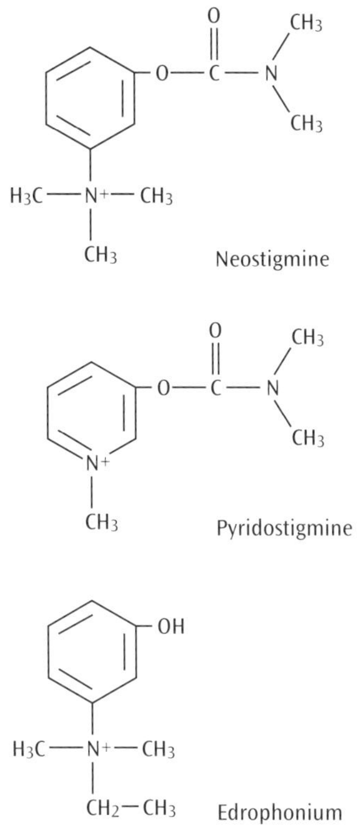

Neostigmine

Pyridostigmine

Edrophonium

Figure 36.5 *Anticholinesterase drugs.*

tors, neostigmine and pyridostigmine, are carbamated compounds which combine at both sites in almost the same way as acetylcholine but with a longer dissociation half-life of about 7 min.[207] These agents are hydrolyzed at a slower rate and the breakdown products also have weak anticholinesterase actions. The prosthetic inhibitor edrophonium attaches mainly to the anionic site and dissociates more readily from the enzyme with a much shorter dissociation half-life of about 20 s.

Anticholinesterase drugs may also have a direct stimulating effect on the receptor, facilitating neuromuscular transmission.[208] Another effect of these drugs is their presynaptic action, involving enhanced liberation of acetylcholine. This effect is particularly marked with edrophonium, which is thought to act mostly by increasing liberation of acetylcholine rather than by inhibition of acetylcholinesterase.[209,210] This hypothesis is indirectly supported by the observation that the antifade properties of edrophonium are greater than those of other drugs.

Anticholinesterase drugs, if administered in large doses or in the absence of muscle relaxants, may produce fasciculations and even a depolarizing type of block, similar to that produced by succinylcholine. However, this is unlikely to occur if a nondepolarizing relaxant has been given, even if almost complete recovery appears to have occurred; it is likely that the explanation is that a large proportion of receptors are still occupied by the muscle relaxant.

Pharmacokinetic studies of neostigmine have estimated its half-life to be about 80 min (Table 36.3).[50] About half of an administered dose of neostigmine is renally excreted, the rest being metabolized. The clearance is markedly reduced in the presence of significant renal disease; this may be a safety factor when using muscle relaxants in such patients.

The kinetics of pyridostigmine follow a similar pattern. The elimination half-life of edrophonium when given in a dose of 0.5–1.0 mg kg^{-1} is similar to that of neostigmine and pyridostigmine (Table 36.3). Elderly patients show a reduced rate of clearance for all three agents.

Dose–response studies carried out in the presence of a constant *d*-tubocurarine block have shown pyridostigmine to be about five times less potent and edrophonium about 10 times less potent than neostigmine.[48] Others have shown edrophonium to be much less potent.[211,212] This variation in findings may be due to use of different muscle relaxants or different methods of stimulation and to estimating potency at different stages of spontaneous recovery. It has also been shown that the dose–response curves for neostigmine and edrophonium are not parallel, indicating that edrophonium probably has a different mode of action. The elderly require a larger dose of neostigmine to attain the same rate of recovery[213] while the dose of reversal agents should be reduced in children.[214]

The commonly recommended doses of anticholinesterase agents are given in Table 36.4. Edrophonium is the most rapid acting of the three, with peak effect apparent in 1–2 min, while the effect of neostigmine may take up to 10 min and pyridostigmine even longer. Pyridostigmine is therefore too slow for routine use. On the other hand, although edrophonium is faster acting, it is not always effective in antagonizing a relatively deep block.

Anticholinesterase drugs exert effects at sites other than the neuromuscular junction. The most prominent of these are at the muscarinic receptors, resulting in bradycardia, increased secretions, and an increase in the activity of smooth muscles. These effects are prevented by the simultaneous or prior administration of antimuscarinic (anticholinergic) agents such as atropine (20–30 μg kg^{-1}) or glycopyrrolate (10 μg kg^{-1}). The use of glycopyrrolate is associated with greater stability of the heart rate when neostigmine is used, although atropine is the preferred agent with edrophonium because of their similar speed of onset of effect.[50] Glycopyrrolate may have other advantages as it does not cross the blood–brain barrier. Edrophonium requires a lower dose of the anticholinergics as its muscarinic effects are less. Contraction of smooth muscles of the bowel, in particular, could theoretically lead to the breakdown of bowel anastomosis, but in practice this is not a problem. Administration of neostigmine has also been thought to increase the incidence of postoperative emetic symptoms, but critical assessment of the evidence shows this not to be the case.[215] Neostigmine and pyridostigmine, but not edrophonium, produce marked inhibition of plasma cholinesterase activity, which may result in the prolongation of the effect of subsequently administered succinylcholine or mivacurium.

Other agents for reversal of neuromuscular block

4-Aminopyridine

This is a tertiary compound that acts predominantly by increasing the release of acetylcholine.[216] 4-Aminopyridine may be useful in combination with an anticholinesterase drug for reversing block in the presence of antibiotics. However, apart from its inability to antagonize block consistently, it produces marked central and autonomic effects that limit its usefulness. It may be useful in the treatment of Eaton–Lambert syndrome.[217]

Table 36.3 *Pharmacokinetics of anticholinesterase agents*

	$V_{d(ss)}$ (mg kg^{-1})	Cl (mL kg^{-1} min^{-1})	Elimination half-life (min)
Neostigmine	700	9	80
Pyridostigmine	1100	8.6	112
Edrophonium	1100	9.6	110

$V_{d(ss)}$, volume of distribution at steady state; Cl, clearance.

Table 36.4 *Dosage of anticholinesterase agents*

	Dose ($mg\,kg^{-1}$)	Peak effect (min)
Neostigmine	0.035–0.05	4–10
Pyridostigmine	0.20–0.25	10–15
Edrophonium	0.5–1.0	2–4

Galanthamine

Galanthamine, like 4-aminipyridine, is a tertiary amine with anticholinesterase effects.[217] Central excitatory actions in addition to its inconsistent reversal effect have limited its clinical usefulness. Both galanthamine and 4-aminopyridine may be useful as analeptics.

Org 25969

This is new class of drugs which is agent specific. This novel compound uses the principle of chemical chelation, forming complexes with the aminosteroid relaxant molecule, resulting in the reversal of the relaxant effect.[218] Animal studies have shown a rapid reversal of rocuronium-induced block even from a very deep level of block without the need for concomitant anticholinergic drugs, as the mechanism of action does not involve cholinergic systems.[219] This potentially exciting agent along with a rapid-acting relaxant such as rocuronium may form an alternative to succinylcholine. Clinical studies will, however, be needed to assess its potential.

Factors affecting reversal

Depth of block is an important determinant of the speed and efficacy of reversal. This also is true for intermediate-acting relaxants, although the underlying rate of recovery with such agents is faster. Neostigmine has been found to be a more reliable antagonist than edrophonium for antagonism of deep blocks. The advantages of edrophonium overall are perhaps small, and neostigmine should be considered a more universal antagonist. It is recommended that reversal is not attempted in the presence of a complete block.

The speed of reversal is related to the inherent duration of action and the rate of spontaneous recovery from the effects of the relaxant. Intermediate-acting drugs are therefore easier and faster to reverse than are long-acting relaxants. It has also been observed that reversal following single bolus doses of the relaxant is easier than after relaxant infusion.[214,220] It is the slower rate of spontaneous recovery that leads to slow reversal of block in the elderly.

Potent volatile agents result in slower recovery following pharmacologic muscle relaxant reversal; however this is so only if the use of volatile agents is continued during the reversal.[124,214] This effect is particularly marked with sevoflurane. Reversal may also be impaired in the presence of aminoglycoside antibiotics.

Acidosis has also been believed to delay reversal of neuromuscular block. The impairment of the ability of neostigmine to antagonize a pancuronium block in the presence of acidosis has been shown in animal studies. Hypokalemia may also impair antagonism of block.

It is safer to administer a reversal agent even if only minimal degrees of block are present; reversal should be omitted only when absence of any residual block has been definitely demonstrated.

REFERENCES

1. Donlon JV, Ali HH, Savarese JJ. A new approach to the study of four nondepolarizing relaxants in man. *Anesth Analg* 1974; **53:** 934–9.
2. Donlon JV, Savarese JJ, Ali HH, *et al.* Human dose–response curves for neuromuscular blocking drugs: a comparison of two methods of construction and analysis. *Anesthesiology* 1980; **53:** 161–6.
3. Gibson FM, Mirakhur RK, Lavery GG, Clarke RSJ. Potency of atracurium: a comparison of single dose and cumulative dose techniques. *Anesthesiology* 1985; **62:** 657–9.
4. Gibson FM, Mirakhur RK, Clarke RSJ, Lavery GG. Comparison of cumulative and single bolus dose techniques for determining potency of vecuronium. *Br J Anaesth* 1985; **57:** 1060–2.
5. Gibson FM, Mirakhur RK. Dose response curves for pancuronium and tubocurarine: comparison of single and cumulative dose techniques. *Eur J Anaesthesiol* 1987; **4:** 143–7.
6. Cooper RA, Mirakhur RK, Elliott P, McCarthy GJ. Estimation of the potency of Org 9426 using two different modes of nerve stimulation. *Can J Anesth* 1992; **39:** 139–42.
7. Kopman AF, Klewicka MM, Neuman GG. An alternate method for estimating the dose–response relationships of neuromuscular blocking drugs. *Anesth Analg* 2000; **90:** 1191–7.
8. Paul M, Kindler CH, Fokt RM, *et al.* The potency of new muscle relaxants on recombinant muscle-type acetylcholine receptors. *Anesth Analg* 2002; **94:** 597–603.
9. Ibebunjo C, Donati F. Sensitivities of different muscles to relaxant drugs. *Bailliere's Clin Anaesthesiol* 1994; **8:** 369–94.
10. Donati F. Onset of action of relaxants. *Can J Anaesth* 1988; **35** (Suppl.): S52–S58.
11. Sheiner LB, Stanski DR, Vozeh S, *et al.* Simultaneous modelling of pharmacokinetics and pharmacodynamics: application of d-tubocurarine. *Clin Pharmacol Ther* 1979; **25:** 358–71.
12. Bowman WC, Rodger IW, Houston J, *et al.* Structure: action relationships among some desacetoxy analogs of pancuronium and vecuronium in the anesthetized cat. *Anesthesiology* 1988; **69:** 57–62.
13. Kopman AF. Pancuronium, gallamine and d-tubocurarine compared: is speed of onset inversely related to drug potency? *Anesthesiology* 1989; **70:** 915–20.
14. Kopman AF, Klewicka MM, Kopman DJ, Neuman GG. Molar potency is predictive of the speed of onset of neuromuscular block for agents of intermediate, short, and ultrashort duration. *Anesthesiology* 1999; **90:** 425–31.
15. Wood M. Plasma drug binding: implications for anesthesiologists. *Anesth Analg* 1986; **65:** 786–804.
16. Browne JG, Collier HOJ, Somers GF. Succinylcholine (succinoxylcholine): muscle relaxant of short duration. *Lancet* 1952; **1:** 1225–8.
17. Waud DR. The nature of depolarization block. *Anesthesiology* 1968; **29:** 1014–24.
18. Waud DR, Waud BE. Depolarisation block and phase II block at the neuromuscular junction. *Anesthesiology* 1975; **43:** 10–20.
19. Hoshi K, Hashimoto Y, Matsukawa S. Pharmacokinetics of succinylcholine in man. *Tohoku J Exp Med* 1993; **170:** 245–50.
20. Torda TA, Graham GG, Warwick NR, Donohue P. Pharmacokinetics and pharmacodynamics of suxamethonium. *Anaesth Intens Care* 1997; **25:** 272–8.
21. Cook DR, Wingard LB, Taylor FH. Pharmacokinetics of succinylcholine in infants, children, and adults. *Clin Pharmacol Ther* 1976; **20:** 493–8.
22. Hartman GS, Flamengo SA, Riker WF. Succinylcholine: mechanism of fasciculations and their prevention by d-tubocurarine or diphenylhydantoin. *Anesthesiology* 1986; **65:** 405–13.
23. Szalados JE, Donati F, Bevan DR. Effect of d-tubocurarine pretreatment on succinylcholine twitch augmentation and neuromuscular blockade. *Anesth Analg* 1990; **71:** 55–9.
24. Meistelman C, Plaud B, Donati F. Neuromuscular effects of succinylcholine on the vocal cords and adductor pollicis muscles. *Anesth Analg* 1991; **73:** 278–82.
25. Blitt CD, Carlson GL, Rolling GD, *et al.* A comparative evaluation of pretreatment with nondepolarizing blockers prior to the administration of succinylcholine. *Anesthesiology* 1981; **55:** 687–9.
26. Cooper R, Mirakhur RK, Clarke RSJ, Boules Z. Comparison of intubating conditions after administration of Org 9426 (rocuronium) and suxamethonium. *Br J Anaesth* 1992; **69:** 269–73.
27. McCoy EP, Mirakhur RK. Comparison of the effects of neostigmine and edrophonium on the duration of action of suxamethonium. *Acta Anaesthesiol Scand* 1995; **39:** 744–7.
28. Mirakhur RK. Edrophonium and plasma cholinesterase activity. *Can Anesthesiol Soc J* 1986; **33:** 588–90.
29. Mirakhur RK, Clarke RSJ, Collier PS. Effects of neostigmine and pyridostigmine on serum cholinesterase activity. *Can Anesthesiol Soc J* 1982; **29:** 287.
30. Miller RD, Way WL, Dolan WM, *et al.* Comparative neuromuscular effects

of pancuronium, gallamine and succinylcholine during forane and halothane anesthesia in man. *Anesthesiology* 1971; **35:** 509–14.

31. Futter ME, Donati F, Bevan DR. Prolonged suxamethonium infusion during nitrous oxide anaesthesia supplemented with halothane or fentanyl. *Br J Anaesth* 1983; **55:** 947–53.
32. Pace NL. Prevention of succinylcholine myalgias; a meta-analysis. *Anesth Analg* 1990; **70:** 477–43.
33. McLoughlin C, Elliott P, McCarthy G, Mirakhur RK. Muscle pains and biochemical changes following suxamethonium administration after six pre-treatment regimens. *Anaesthesia* 1992; **47:** 202–6.
34. Nigrovic V. Succinylcholine, cholinoceptors and catecholamines: proposed mechanism of early adverse haemodynamic reactions. *Can Anesthiol Soc J* 1984; **31:** 382–94.
35. Gronert GA, Theye RA. Pathophysiology of hyperkalaemia induced by succinylcholine. *Anesthesiology* 1975; **43:** 89–99.
36. Watkins J. Second report from an anaesthetic reactions advisory service. *Anaesthesia* 1989; **44:** 157–9.
37. Donlon JV, Newfield P, Streter F, *et al.* Implications of masseter spasm after succinylcholine. *Anesthesiology* 1978; **49:** 298.
38. Whittaker M. Plasma cholinesterase variants and the anaesthetist. *Anaesthesia* 1980; **35:** 174–97.
39. Everrett AJ, Lowe LA, Wilkinson S. Revision of the structures of (+)-tubocurarine chloride and (+)-chondrocurine. *J Chem Soc* 1970; **10:** 1020–1.
40. Hubbard JI, Wilson DF, Miyamoto M. Reduction of transmitter release by d-tubocurarine. *Nature* 1969; **223:** 531–3.
41. Blaber LC. The prejunctional actions of some non-depolarizing blocking agents. *Br J Pharmacol* 1973; **47:** 109–16.
42. Williams NE, Webb SN, Calvey TN. Differential effects of myoneural blocking drugs on neuromuscular transmission. *Br J Anaesth* 1980; **52:** 1111–15.
43. Bowman WC. Prejunctional and postjunctional cholinoceptors at the neuromuscular junction. *Anesth Analg* 1980; **59:** 935–43.
44. Gibson FM, Mirakhur RK. Train-of-four fade during onset of neuromuscular block with nondepolarising neuromuscular blocking agents. *Acta Anaesthesiol Scand* 1989; **33:** 204–6.
45. Savarese JJ, Ali HH, Antonio RP. The clinical pharmacology of metocurine: dimethyltubocurarine revisited. *Anesthesiology* 1977; **47:** 277–85.
46. Walts LF, Dillon JB. d-Tubocurarine cumulation studies. *Anesth Analg* 1968; **47:** 696–701.
47. Katz RL. Neuromuscular effects of d-tubocurarine, edrophonium and neostigmine in man. *Anesthesiology* 1967; **28:** 327–36.
48. Cronnelly R, Morris RB, Miller RD. Edrophonium: duration of action and atropine requirement in humans during halothane anesthesia. *Anesthesiology* 1982; **57:** 261–6.
49. Morris RB, Cahalan MK, Miller RD, *et al.* The cardiovascular effects of vecuronium (ORG NC45) and pancuronium in patients undergoing coronary artery bypass grafting. *Anesthesiology* 1983; **58:** 438–40.
50. Mirakhur RK. Antagonism of neuromuscular block. *Bailliere's Clin Anesthesiol* 1994; **8:** 461–81.
51. McCullough LS, Reier CE, Delaunois AL, *et al.* The effects of d-tubocurarine on spontaneous post-ganglionic sympathetic activity and histamine release. *Anesthesiology* 1970; **33:** 328–34.
52. Hughes R, Chapple DJ. Effects of non-depolarizing neuromuscular blocking agents on peripheral autonomic mechanisms in cats. *Br J Anaesth* 1976; **48:** 59–68.
53. Stoelting RK, McCammon RL, Hilgenberg JC. Changes in blood pressure with varying rates of administration of d-tubocurarine. *Anesth Analg* 1980; **59:** 697–9.
54. Moss J, Roscow CE, Savarese JJ, *et al.* Role of histamine in the hypotensive action of d-tubocurarine in humans. *Anesthesiology* 1981; **55:** 19–25.
55. Johnstone M, Mahmoud AA, Mrozinski RA. Cardiovascular effects of tubocurarine in man. *Anaesthesia* 1978; **33:** 587–93.
56. Matteo RS, Backus WW, McDaniel DD, *et al.* Pharmacokinetics and pharmacodynamics of d-tubocurarine and metocurine in the elderly. *Anesth Analg* 1985; **64:** 23–9.
57. Stoelting RK. Hemodynamic effects of dimethyltubocurarine during nitrous oxide–halothane anesthesia. *Anesth Analg* 1974; **55:** 513–15.
58. Hughes R, Chapple DJ. Cardiovascular and neuromuscular effects of dimethyl tubocurarine in anaesthetized cats and rhesus monkeys. *Br J Anaesth* 1976; **48:** 847–52.
59. Baird WLM, Reid AM. The neuromuscular blocking properties of a new steroid compound, pancuronium bromide. *Br J Anaesth* 1967; **39:** 775–80.
60. Norman J, Katz RL, Seed RF. The neuromuscular blocking action of pancuronium in man during anaesthesia. *Br J Anaesth* 1970; **42:** 702–9.
61. Fahey MR, Morris RB, Miller RD, *et al.* Clinical pharmacology of ORG NC45 (Norcuron): a new nondepolarizing muscle relaxant. *Anesthesiology* 1981; **55:** 6–11.
62. Katz RL. Clinical neuromuscular pharmacology of pancuronium. *Anesthesiology* 1971; **34:** 550–6.
63. Kelman GR, Kennedy BR. Cardiovascular effects of pancuronium in man. *Br J Anaesth* 1971; **43:** 335–8.
64. Saemund O, Dalenius E. Pancuronium and nodal rhythm. *Br J Anaesth* 1981; **53:** 780.
65. Thomson IR, Putnins CL. Adverse effects of pancuronium during high-dose fentanyl anesthesia for coronary artery bypass grafting. *Anesthesiology* 1985; **62:** 708–13.
66. Docherty JR, McGrath JC. Sympathomimetic effects of pancuronium bromide on the cardiovascular system of the pithed rat: a comparison with the effects of drugs blocking the neural uptake of noradrenaline. *Br J Pharmacol* 1978; **64:** 589–99.
67. Iwatsuki N, Hashimoto Y, Amaha K, *et al.* Inotropic effects of non-depolarizing muscle relaxants in isolated canine heart muscle. *Anesth Analg* 1980; **59:** 717–21.
68. Appadu BL, Lambert DG. Studies on the interaction of steroidal neuromuscular blocking drugs with cardiac muscarinic receptors. *Br J Anaesth* 1994; **72:** 86–8.
69. Rupp SM, Castagnoli KP, Fisher DM, Miller RD. Pancuronium and vecuronium pharmacokinetics and pharmacodynamics in younger and elderly adults. *Anesthesiology* 1987; **67:** 45–9.
70. Duvaldestin P, Agoston S, Henzel D, *et al.* Pancuronium pharmacokinetics in patients with liver cirrhosis. *Br J Anaesth* 1978; **50:** 1131–6.
71. Basta SJ, Savarese JJ, Ali HH, *et al.* Clinical pharmacology of doxacurium chloride, a new long-acting nondepolarizing muscle relaxant. *Anesthesiology* 1988; **69:** 478–486.
72. Emmott RS, Bracey BJ, Goldhill DR, *et al.* Cardiovascular effects of doxacurium, pancuronium and vecuronium in anaesthetized patients presenting for coronary artery bypass surgery. *Br J Anaesth* 1990; **65:** 480–6.
73. Maddineni VR, Cooper R, Stanley JC, *et al.* Clinical evaluation of doxacurium chloride. *Anaesthesia* 1992; **47:** 554–7.
74. Martlew RA, Harper NJ. The clinical pharmacology of doxacurium in young adults and in elderly patients. *Anaesthesia* 1995; **50:** 779–82.
75. Dresner DL, Basta SJ, Ali HH, *et al.* Pharmacokinetics and pharmacodynamics of doxacurium in young and elderly patients during isoflurane anesthesia. *Anesth Analg* 1990; **71:** 498–502.
76. Stanley JC, Mirakhur RK. Comparative potency of pipecuronium bromide and pancuronium bromide. *Br J Anaesth* 1989; **63:** 754–5.
77. Stanley JC, Mirakhur RK, Bell PF, *et al.* Neuromuscular effects of pipecuronium bromide. *Eur J Anaesthesiol* 1991; **8:** 151–6.
78. Sanfilippo M, Fierro G, Vilardi V, *et al.* Clinical evaluation of different doses of pipecuronium bromide during nitrous oxide–fentanyl anaesthesia in adult surgical patients. *Eur J Anaesthesiol* 1992; **9:** 49–53.
79. Foldes FF, Nagashima H, Nguyen HD, *et al.* Neuromuscular and cardiovascular effects of pipecuronium. *Can J Anesth* 1990; **37:** 549–55.
80. Tassonyi E, Neidhart P, Pittet JF, *et al.* Cardiovascular effects of pipecuronium and pancuronium in patients undergoing coronary artery bypass grafting. *Anesthesiology* 1988; **69:** 793–6.
81. Stanley JC, Carson IW, Gibson FM, *et al.* Comparison of the haemodynamic effects of pipecuronium and pancuronium during fentanyl anaesthesia. *Acta Anaesthesiol Scand* 1991; **35:** 262–6.
82. Wierda JMKH, Karliczek GF, Vandenbrom RHG, *et al.* Pharmacokinetics and cardiovascular dynamics of pipecuronium bromide during coronary artery surgery. *Can J Anesth* 1990; **37:** 183–91.
83. Agoston S, Salt P, Newton D, *et al.* The neuromuscular blocking action of ORG NC 45, a new pancuronium derivative, in anaesthetized patients. A pilot study. *Br J Anaesth* 1980; **52** (Suppl. 1): 53S–59S.
84. Mirakhur RK, Ferres CJ, Clarke RSJ, *et al.* Clinical evaluation of Org NC45. *Br J Anaesth* 1983; **55:** 119–24.
85. Yamaguchi S. Egawa H. Okuda K, *et al.* High concentration sevoflurane induction of anesthesia accelerates onset of vecuronium neuromuscular blockade. *Can J Anesth* 2001; **48:** 34–7.
86. Rorvik K, Husby P, Gramstad L, *et al.* Comparison of large dose of vecuronium with pancuronium for prolonged neuromuscular blockade. *Br J Anaesth* 1988; **61:** 180–5.
87. Wierda JM, Maestrone E, Bencini AF, *et al.* Haemodynamic effects of vecuronium. *Br J Anaesth* 1989; **62:** 194–8.
88. Mirakhur RK, Ferres CJ. Muscle relaxation with an infusion of vecuronium. *Eur J Anaesthesiol* 1984; **1:** 353–9.
89. Wright PMC, Hart P, Lau M, *et al.* Cumulative characteristics of atracurium and vecuronium. *Anesthesiology* 1994; **81:** 59–68.
90. Darrah WC, Johnston JR, Mirakhur RK. Vecuronium infusions for pro-

longed muscle relaxation in the intensive care unit. *Crit Care Med* 1989; **17:** 1297–300.

91. Bencini AF, Scaf AH, Sohn YJ, *et al.* Hepatobiliary disposition of vecuronium bromide in man. *Br J Anaesth* 1986; **58:** 988–95.
92. Lebrault C, Berger JL, D'Hollander AA, *et al.* Pharmacokinetics and pharmacodynamics of vecuronium (ORG NC 45) in patients with cirrhosis. *Anesthesiology* 1985; **62:** 601–5.
93. Lepage JY, Malinge M, Cozian A, *et al.* Vecuronium and atracurium in patients with end-stage renal failure. A comparative study. *Br J Anaesth* 1987; **59:** 1004–10.
94. Segredo V, Matthay MA, Sharma ML, *et al.* Prolonged neuromuscular blockade after long-term administration of vecuronium in two critically ill patients. *Anesthesiology* 1990; **72:** 566–570.
95. Withington D, Menard G, Harris J, *et al.* Vecuronium pharmacokinetics and pharmacodynamics during hypothermic cardiopulmonary bypass in infants and children. *Can J Anesth* 2000; **47:** 1188–95.
96. Caldwell JE, Heier T, Wright PM, *et al.* Temperature-dependent pharmacokinetics and pharmacodynamics of vecuronium. *Anesthesiology* 2000; **92:** 84–93.
97. Beaufort TM, Proost JH, Maring J, *et al.* Effect of hypothermia on the hepatic uptake and biliary excretion of vecuronium in the isolated perfused rat liver. *Anesthesiology* 2001; **94:** 270–9.
98. Stenlake JB, Waigh RD, Urwin J, *et al.* Atracurium: conception and inception. *Br J Anaesth* 1983; **55:** 3S–10S.
99. Katz RL, Stirt J, Murray AL, Lee C. Neuromuscular effects of atracurium in man. *Anesth Analg* 1982; **61:** 730–4.
100. Mirakhur RK, Lavery GG, Clarke RSJ, *et al.* Atracurium in clinical anaesthesia: effect of dosage on onset, duration and intubating conditions. *Anaesthesia* 1985; **40:** 801–5.
101. Griffiths RB, Hunter JM, Jones RS. Atracurium infusions in patients with renal failure on an ITU. *Anaesthesia* 1986; **41:** 375–81.
102. d'Hollander AA, Luyckx C, Barvais L, De Ville A. Clinical evaluation of atracurium besylate requirement for a stable muscle relaxation during surgery: lack of age-related effects. *Anesthesiology* 1983; **59:** 237–40.
103. Kent AP, Parker CJR, Hunter JM. Pharmacokinetics of atracurium and laudanosine in the elderly. *Br J Anaesth* 1989; **63:** 661–6.
104. Hunter JM, Jones RS, Utting JE. Use of atracurium in patients with no renal function. *Br J Anaesth* 1982; **54:** 1251–8.
105. Fahey MR, Rupp SM, Fisher DM, *et al.* The pharmacokinetics and pharmacodynamics of atracurium in patients with and without renal failure. *Anesthesiology* 1984; **61:** 699–702.
106. Bell CF, Hunter JM, Jones RS, Utting JE. Use of atracurium and vecuronium in patients with oesophageal varices. *Br J Anaesth* 1985; **57:** 160–8.
107. Parker CJR, Hunter JM. Pharmacokinetics of atracurium and laudanosine in patients with hepatic cirrhosis. *Br J Anaesth* 1989; **62:** 177–83.
108. Hughes R, Chapple DJ. The pharmacology of atracurium: a new competitive neuromuscular blocking agent. *Br J Anaesth* 1981; **53:** 31–44.
109. Fisher DM, Canfell PC, Fahey MR, *et al.* Elimination of atracurium in humans: contribution of Hofmann elimination and ester hydrolysis versus organ-based elimination. *Anesthesiology* 1986; **65:** 6–12.
110. Chapple DJ, Miller AA, Ward JB, Wheatley PL. Cardiovascular and neurological effects of laudanosine: studies in mice and rats, and in conscious and anaesthetized dogs. *Br J Anaesth* 1987; **59:** 218–25.
111. Yate PM, Flynn PJ, Arnold RW, *et al.* Clinical experience and plasma laudanosine concentrations during the infusion of atracurium in the intensive therapy unit. *Br J Anaesth* 1987; **59:** 211–17.
112. Gwinnutt CL, Eddleston JM, Edwards D, Pollard BJ. Concentrations of atracurium and laudanosine in cerebrospinal fluid and plasma in three intensive care patients. *Br J Anaesth* 1990; **65:** 829–32.
113. Scott RPF, Savarese JJ, Basta SJ, *et al.* Atracurium: clinical strategies for preventing histamine release and attenuating the haemodynamic response. *Br J Anaesth* 1985; **57:** 550–3.
114. Naguib M, Samarkandi AH, Bakhamees HS, *et al.* Histamine-release haemodynamic changes produced by rocuronium, vecuronium, mivacurium, atracurium and tubocurarine. *Br J Anaesth* 1995; **75:** 588–92.
115. Wierda JM, de Wit AP, Kuizenga K, Agoston S. Clinical observations on the neuromuscular blocking action of Org 9426, a new steroidal non-depolarizing agent. *Br J Anaesth* 1990; **64:** 521–3.
116. Muir AW, Houston J, Green KL, *et al.* Effects of a new neuromuscular blocking agent (Org 9426) in anaesthetized cats and pigs and in isolated nerve-muscle preparations. *Br J Anaesth* 1989; **63:** 400–10.
117. Mayer M, Doenicke A, Hofmann A, Peter K. Onset and recovery of rocuronium (Org-9426) and vecuronium under enflurane anesthesia. *Br J Anaesth* 1992; **69:** 511–12.
118. Bartkowski RR, Witkowski TA, Azad S, *et al.* Rocuronium onset of action: a comparison with atracurium and vecuronium. *Anesth Analg* 1993; **77:** 574–8.
119. Foldes FF, Nagashima H, Nguyen HD, *et al.* The neuromuscular effects of ORG 9426 in patients receiving balanced anesthesia. *Anesthesiology* 1991; **75:** 191–6.
120. Cooper RA, Mirakhur RK, Maddineni VR. Neuromuscular effects of rocuronium bromide (Org 9426) during fentanyl and halothane anaesthesia. *Anaesthesia* 1993; **48:** 103–5.
121. Miguel RV, Soto R, Dyches P. A double-blind, randomized comparison of low-dose rocuronium and atracurium in a desflurane anesthetic. *J Clin Anesth* 2001; **13:** 325–9.
122. Oris B, Crul JF, Vandermeersch E, *et al.* Muscle paralysis by rocuronium during halothane, enflurane, isoflurane, and total intravenous anesthesia. *Anesth Analg* 1993; **77:** 570–3.
123. Lowry DW, Mirakhur RK, McCarthy GJ, *et al.* Neuromuscular effects of rocuronium during sevoflurane, isoflurane and intravenous anesthesia. *Anesth Analg* 1998; **87:** 936–40.
124. Reid JE, Breslin DS, Mirakhur RK, Hayes AH. Neostigmine antagonism of rocuronium block during anesthesia with sevoflurane, isoflurane or propofol. *Can J Anesthesiol* 2001; **48:** 351–5.
125. Huizinga AC, Vandenbrom RH, Wierda JM, *et al.* Intubating conditions and onset of neuromuscular block of rocuronium (Org 9426); a comparison with suxamethonium. *Acta Anaesthesiol Scand* 1992; **36:** 463–8.
126. McCourt KC, Salmela L, Mirakhur RK, *et al.* Comparison of rocuronium and suxamethonium for use during rapid sequence induction of anaesthesia. *Anaesthesia* 1998; **53:** 867–71.
127. Andrews JI, Kumar N, van den Brom RH, *et al.* A large simple randomized trial of rocuronium versus succinylcholine in rapid-sequence induction of anaesthesia along with propofol. *Acta Anaesthesiol Scand* 1999; **43:** 4–8.
128. Fuchs-Buder T, Sparr HJ, Zeigenfu BT. Thiopental or etomidate for rapid sequence induction with rocuronium? *Br J Anaesth* 1998; **80:** 504–6.
129. Hans P, Brichant JF, Hubert B, *et al.* Influence of induction of anaesthesia on intubating conditions one minute after rocuronium administration: comparison of ketamine and thiopentone. *Anaesthesia* 1999; **54:** 276–9.
130. Tan CH, Onisong MK, Chiu WKY. The influence of induction technique on intubating conditions 1 min after rocuronium administration: a comparison of a propofol–ephedrine combination and propofol. *Anaesthesia* 2002; **57:** 223–6.
131. McCoy EP, Maddineni VR, Elliott P, *et al.* Haemodynamic effects of rocuronium during fentanyl anaesthesia: comparison with vecuronium. *Can J Anesth* 1993; **40:** 703–8.
132. Levy JH, Davis GK, Duggan J, Szlam F. Determination of the hemodynamics and histamine release of rocuronium (Org 9426) when administered in increased doses under N_2O/O_2–sufentanil anesthesia. *Anesth Analg* 1994; **78:** 318–21.
133. Cason B, Baker DG, Hickey RF, *et al.* Cardiovascular and neuromuscular effects of three steroidal neuromuscular blocking drugs in dogs (ORG 9616, ORG 9426, ORG 9991). *Anesth Analg* 1990; **70:** 382–8.
134. Wierda JM, Kleef UW, Lambalk LM, *et al.* The pharmacodynamics and pharmacokinetics of Org 9426, a new non-depolarizing neuromuscular blocking agent, in patients anaesthetized with nitrous oxide, halothane and fentanyl. *Can J Anesth* 1991; **38:** 430–5.
135. Proost JH, Eriksson LI, Mirakhur RK, *et al.* Urinary, biliary and faecal excretion of rocuronium in humans. *Br J Anaesth* 2000; **85:** 717–23.
136. Cooper RA, Maddineni VR, Mirakhur RK, *et al.* Time course of neuromuscular effects and pharmacokinetics of rocuronium bromide (Org 9426) during isoflurane anaesthesia in patients with and without renal failure. *Br J Anaesth* 1993; **71:** 222–6.
137. van Miert MM, Eastwood NB, Boyd AH, *et al.* The pharmacokinetics and pharmacodynamics of rocuronium in patients with hepatic cirrhosis. *Br J Clin Pharmacol* 1997; **44:** 139–44.
138. Pühringer FK, Khuenl-Brady KS, Mitterschiffthaler G. Rocuronium bromide: time course of action in underweight, normal weight, overweight, and obese patients. *Eur J Anaesthesiol* 1995; **12** (Suppl. 11); 107–10.
139. Gin T, Chan MTV, Chan KL, Yuen PM. Prolonged neuromuscular block after rocuronium in postpartum patients. *Anesth Analg* 2002; **94:** 686–9.
140. Jellish WS, Brody M, Sawicki K, Slogoff S. Recovery from neuromuscular blockade after either bolus and prolonged infusions of cisatracurium or rocuronium using either isoflurane or propofol-based anesthetics. *Anesth Analg* 2000; **91:** 1250–5.
141. Cammu G, Codens J, Hendrickx J, Deloof T. Dose requirements of infusions of cisatracurium or rocuronium during hypothermic cardiopulmonary bypass. *Br J Anaesth* 2000; **84:** 587–90.
142. McEwan L, Merrick PM, Bevan DR. Residual neuromuscular blockade after cardiac surgery: pancuronium vs rocuronium. *Can J Anesth* 1997; **44:** 891–5.

143. Murphy GS, Szokol JW, Marymont JH, *et al.* Impact of shorter-acting neuromuscular blocking agents on fast-track recovery of cardiac surgical patient. *Anesthesiology* 2002; **96:** 600–6.
144. Wastila WB, Maehr RB, Turner GL, *et al.* Comparative pharmacology of cisatracurium (51W89), atracurium, and five isomers in cats. *Anesthesiology* 1996; **85:** 169–77.
145. Belmont MR, Lien CA, Quessy S, *et al.* The clinical neuromuscular pharmacology of 51W89 in patients receiving nitrous oxide/opioid/ barbiturate anesthesia. *Anesthesiology* 1995; **82:** 1139–45.
146. De Ruiter J, Crawford MW. Dose–response relationship and infusion requirement of cisatracurium besylate in infants and children during nitrous oxide-narcotic anesthesia. *Anesthesiology* 2001; **94:** 790–2.
147. Carroll MT, Mirakhur RK, Lowry D, *et al.* A comparison of the neuromuscular blocking effects and reversibility of cisatracurium and atracurium. *Anaesthesia* 1998; **53:** 744–8.
148. Littlejohn IH, Abhay K, E1 Sayed A, *et al.* Intubating conditions following 1R CIS, 1R′ CIS atracurium (51W89): a comparison with atracurium. *Anaesthesia* 1995; **50:** 499–502.
149. Albert F, Hans P, Bitar Y, *et al.* Effects of ephedrine on the onset time of neuromuscular block and intubating conditions after cisatracurium: preliminary results. *Acta Anaesthesiol Belg* 2000; **51:** 167–71.
150. Lepage JY, Malinovsky JM, Malinge M, *et al.* Pharmacodynamic dose–response and safety study of cisatracurium (51W89) in adult surgical patients during N_2O–O_2–opioid anesthesia. *Anesth Analg* 1996; **83:** 823–9.
151. Lien CA, Belmont MR, Abalos A, *et al.* The cardiovascular effects and histamine-releasing properties of 51W89 in patients receiving nitrous oxide/opioid/barbiturate anesthesia. *Anesthesiology* 1995; **82:** 1131–8.
152. Kisor DF, Schmith VD, Wargin WA, *et al.* Importance of organ-independent elimination of cisatracurium. *Anesth Analg* 1996; **83:** 1065–71.
153. Lien CA, Schmith VD, Belmont MR, *et al.* Pharmacokinetics of cisatracurium in patients receiving nitrous oxide/opioid/barbiturate anesthesia. *Anesthesiology* 1996; **84:** 300–8.
154. De Wolf AM, Freeman JA, Scott VL, *et al.* Pharmacokinetics and pharmacodynamics of cisatracurium in patients with end-stage liver disease undergoing liver transplantation. *Br J Anaesth* 1996; **76:** 624–8.
155. Eastwood NB, Boyd AH, Parker CJR, Hunter JM. Pharmacokinetics of 1R-*cis* 1′R-*cis* atracurium besylate (51W89) and plasma laudanosine concentrations in health and chronic renal failure. *Br J Anaesth* 1995; **75:** 431–5.
156. Boyd AH, Eastwood NB, Parker CJR, Hunter JM. Pharmacodynamics of the 1R *cis*-1′R *cis* isomer of atracurium (51W89) in health and chronic renal failure. *Br J Anaesth* 1995; **74:** 400–4.
157. Boyd AH, Eastwood NB, Parker CJR, Hunter JM. Comparison of the pharmacodynamics and pharmacokinetics of an infusion of *cis*-atracurium (51W89) or atracurium in critically ill patients undergoing mechanical ventilation in an intensive therapy unit. *Br J Anaesth* 1996; **76:** 382–8.
158. Head-Rapson AG, Devlin JC, Parker CJR, Hunter JM. Pharmacokinetics of the three isomers of mivacurium and pharmacodynamics of the chiral mixture in hepatic cirrhosis. *Br J Anaesth* 1994; **73:** 613–18.
159. Savarese JJ, Ali HH, Basta SJ, *et al.* The clinical neuromuscular pharmacology of mivacurium chloride (BW B1090U) a short-acting nondepolarizing ester neuromuscular blocking drug. *Anesthesiology* 1988; **68:** 723–32.
160. Maddineni VR, Mirakhur RK, Cooper R, McCoy E. Potency estimation of mivacurium: comparison of two different modes of nerve stimulation. *Br J Anaesth* 1993; **70:** 694–5.
161. Connolly FM, Mirakhur RK, Loan PB, *et al.* Antagonism of mivacurium block with edrophonium from various degrees of spontaneous recovery. *Br J Anaesth* 1995; **74:** 229–30.
162. Brandom BW, Woelfel SK, Cook DR, *et al.* Comparison of mivacurium and suxamethonium administered by bolus and infusion. *Br J Anaesth* 1989; **62:** 488–93.
163. Weber S, Brandom BW, Powers DM. Mivacurium chloride (BW B1090U) induced neuromuscular blockade during nitrous oxide-isoflurane and nitrous oxide-narcotic anaesthesia in adult surgical patients. *Anesth Analg* 1988; **67:** 495–9.
164. Lowry DW, Mirakhur RK, Carroll MT, *et al.* Potency and time course of mivacurium block during sevoflurane, isoflurane and intravenous anesthesia. *Can J Anesthesiol* 1999; **46:** 29–33.
165. Diefenbach C, Mellinghoff H, Lynch J, Buzello W. Mivacurium: dose–response relationship and administration by repeated injection or infusion. *Anesth Analg* 1992; **74:** 420–3.
166. Maddineni VR, Mirakhur RK, McCoy EP, Sharpe TDE. Neuromuscular and haemodynamic effects of mivacurium in elderly and young adult patients. *Br J Anaesth* 1994; **73:** 608–12.
167. Goldhill DR, Whitehead JP, Emmott RS, *et al.* Neuromuscular and clinical effects of mivacurium chloride in healthy adult patients during nitrous oxide–enflurane anaesthesia. *Br J Anaesth* 1991; **67:** 289–95.
168. Symington MJ, Mirakhur RK, Kumar N. Neostigmine but not edrophonium prolongs the action of mivacurium. *Can J Anesth* 1996; **43:** 1220–3.
169. Loan PB, Elliot P, Mirakhur RK, *et al.* Comparison of the haemodynamic effects of mivacurium and atracurium during fentanyl anaesthesia. *Br J Anaesth* 1995; **74:** 330–2.
170. Phillips BJ, Hunter JM. Use of mivacurium chloride by constant infusion in the anephric patient. *Br J Anaesth* 1992; **68:** 492–8.
171. Devlin JC, Head-Rapson AG, Parker CJR, Hunter JM. Pharmacodynamics of mivacurium chloride in patients with hepatic cirrhosis. *Br J Anaesth* 1993; **71:** 227–31.
172. Maddineni VR, Mirakhur RK. Prolonged neuromuscular block following mivacurium. *Anesthesiology* 1993; **78:** 1181–4.
173. Ostergaard D, Jensen FS, Jensen E, *et al.* Mivacurium-induced neuromuscular blockade in patients with atypical plasma cholinesterase. *Acta Anaesthesiol Scand* 1993; **37:** 314–18.
174. Kopman AF, Klewicka MM, Ghori K, *et al.* Dose–response and onset/offset characteristics of rapacuronium. *Anesthesiology* 2000; **93:** 1017–21.
175. Wierda JM, van den Broek L, Proost JH, *et al.* Time course of action and endotracheal intubating conditions of Org 9487, a new short-acting steroidal muscle relaxant; a comparison with succinylcholine. *Anesth Analg* 1993; **77:** 579–84.
176. Miguel R, Witkowski T, Nagashima H, *et al.* Evaluation of neuromuscular and cardiovascular effects of two doses of rapacuronium (ORG 9487) versus mivacurium and succinylcholine. *Anesthesiology* 1999; **91:** 1648–54.
177. Hayes A, Breslin D, Reid J, Mirakhur RK. Comparison of recovery following rapacuronium, with and without neostigmine, and suxamethonium. *Anaesthesia* 2000; **55:** 859–63.
178. Kahwaji R, Bevan DR, Bikhazi G, *et al.* Dose-ranging study in younger adult and elderly patients of ORG 9487, a new, rapid-onset, short-duration muscle relaxant. *Anesth Analg* 1997; **84:** 1011–18.
179. Proost JH, Wright PMC. A pharmacokinetic–dynamic explanation of the rapid onset-offset of rapacuronium. *Eur J Anaesthesiol* 2001; **18** (Suppl. 23): 83–9.
180. Connolly FM, Mirakhur RK, Loan PB, *et al.* Time course of action of Org 9487 with or without reversal: comparison with suxamethonium. *Br J Anaesth* 1995; **74:** 473P.
181. Duvaldestin P, Slavov V, Rebufat Y. Pharmacokinetics and pharmacodynamics of rapacuronium in patients with cirrhosis. *Anesthesiology* 1999; **91:** 1305–10.
182. Purdy R, Bevan DR, Donati F, Lichtor JL. Early reversal of rapacuronium with neostigmine. *Anesthesiology* 1999; **91:** 51–7.
183. van den Broek L, Wierda JM, Smeulers NJ, Proost JH. Pharmacodynamics and pharmacokinetics of an infusion of Org 9487, a new short-acting steroidal neuromuscular blocking agent. *Br J Anaesth* 1994; **73:** 331–5.
184. McCourt KC, Mirakhur RK, Lowry DW, *et al.* Spontaneous or neostigmine-induced recovery after maintenance of neuromuscular block with Org 9487 (rapacuronium) or rocuronium following an initial dose of Org 9487. *Br J Anaesth* 1999; **82:** 755–6.
185. Fleming NW, Chung F, Glass PS, *et al.* Comparison of the intubation conditions provided by rapacuronium (ORG 9487) or succinylcholine in humans during anesthesia with fentanyl and propofol. *Anesthesiology* 1999; **91:** 1311–17.
186. Blobner M, Mirakhur RK, Wierda JMKH, *et al.* Rapacuronium 2.0 or 2.5 mg kg^{-1} for rapid sequence induction: comparison with succinylcholine 1.0 mg kg^{-1}. *Br J Anaesth* 2000; **85:** 724–31.
187. McCourt KC, Elliott P, Mirakhur RK, *et al.* Haemodynamic effects of rapacuronium in adults with coronary artery or valvular disease. *Br J Anaesth* 1999; **83:** 721–6.
188. Levy JH, Pitts M, Thanopoulos A, *et al.* The effects of rapacuronium on histamine release and hemodynamics in adult patients undergoing general anesthesia. *Anesth Analg* 1999; **89:** 290–5.
189. Yamaguchi K, Huraux C, Szlam F, Levy JH. Vascular effects of Org 9487 in human mammary arteries, a new short acting muscle relaxant. *Anesth Analg* 1998; **86:** SCA109.
190. Meakin GH, Pronske EH, Lerman J, *et al.* Bronchospasm after rapacuronium in infants and children. *Anesthesiology* 2001; **94:** 926–7.
191. Onrust SV, Foster RH. Rapacuronium bromide: a review of its use in anaesthetic practice. *Drugs* 1999; **58:** 887–918.
192. Rajchert DM, Pasquariello CA, Watcha MF, Schreiner MS. Rapacuronium and the risk of bronchospasm in pediatric patients. *Anesth Analg* 2002; **94:** 488–93.
193. Belmont MR, Lien CA, Savarese JJ, *et al.* Neuromuscular blocking effects

of GW280430A at the adductor pollicis and larynx in human volunteers. *Br J Anaesth* 1999; **82** (Suppl. 1): A.419.

194. Lien CA, Belmont MR, Gurvitch DL, *et al.* Spontaneous and edrophonium augmented recovery from GW280430A-induced neuromuscular block. *Anesthesiology* 1999; **91:** A1017.
195. Gyermek L, Lee C, Cho Y-M, Nguyen N. Alkoxy-acetoxy benzyl quaternary derivatives of tropinyl diesters. Ultrashort acting non-depolarizing muscle relaxants. *Eur J Anaesthesiol* 2001; **18** (Suppl. 23): 104.
196. van Egmond J, van de Pol F, Booij L, Muir A, Bom A. New fast neuromuscular blocking agent, TAAC3, in the anaesthetized dog. *Eur J Anaesthesiol* 2001; **18** (Suppl. 23): 94.
197. Viby-Mogensen J, Jorgensen BC, Ording H. Residual curarization in the recovery room. *Anesthesiology* 1979; **50:** 539–41.
198. Berg H, Viby-Mogensen J, Roed J, *et al.* Residual neuromuscular block is a risk factor for postoperative pulmonary complications. A prospective, randomised and blinded study of postoperative pulmonary complications after atracurium, vecuronium and pancuronium. *Acta Anaesthesiol Scand* 1997; **41:** 1095–103.
199. Hayes AH, Mirakhur RK, Breslin DS, *et al.* Postoperative residual block after intermediate-acting neuromuscular blocking drugs. *Anaesthesia* 2001; **56:** 312–18.
200. Coakley JH. Muscle relaxants and neuromuscular disorders in the intensive care unit. *Bailliere's Clin Anesthesiol* 1994; **8:** 483–99.
201. Tamayo E, Perez M, Gomez JI, Alvarez FJ. Allergy of anaesthetizing agents in Spain. *Br J Anaesth* 1999; **83:** 336–7.
202. Matthey P, Wang P, Finegan BA, Donnelly M. Rocuronium anaphylaxis and multiple neuromuscular blocking drug sensitivities. *Can J Anesth* 2000; **47:** 890–3.
203. Neal SM, Manthri PR, Gadiyar V, Wildsmith JAW. Histaminoid reactions associated with rocuronium. *Br J Anaesth* 2000; **84:** 108–11.
204. Toh KW, Deacock SJ, Fawcett WJ. Severe anaphylactic reaction to cisatracurium. *Anesth Analg* 1999; **88:** 462–4.
205. Legros CB, Orliaguet GA, Mayer MN, *et al.* Severe anaphylactic reaction to cisatracurium in a child. *Anesth Analg* 2001; **92:** 648–9.
206. Rose M, Fisher M. Rocuronium: high risk for anaphylaxis? *Br J Anaesth* 2001; **86:** 678–82.
207. Wilson IB. The interaction of tensilon and neostigmine with acetylcholinesterase. *Arch Int Pharmacodynam Ther* 1955; **54:** 204–13.
208. Deana A, Scuka N. Time course of neostigmine; action on the endplate response. *Neurosciences* 1990; **118:** 82–4.
209. Blaber LC. The mechanism of the facilitatory actions of edrophonium in the cat skeletal muscle. *Br J Pharmacol* 1972; **46:** 498–507.
210. Sakuma N, Hasimoto Y, Iwatsuki N. Effects of neostigmine and edrophonium on human erythrocyte acetylcholinesterase activity. *Br J Anaesth* 1992; **68:** 316–17.
211. Breen PJ, Doherty WG, Donati F, Bevan DR. The potencies of edrophonium and neostigmine as antagonists of pancuronium. *Anaesthesia* 1985; **40:** 844–7.
212. Smith CE, Donati F, Bevan DR. Dose–response relationship for edrophonium and neostigmine as antagonists of atracurium and vecuronium neuromuscular blockade. *Anesthesiology* 1989; **71:** 37–43.
213. McCarthy GJ, Cooper AR, Stanley JC, Mirakhur RK. Dose–response relationships for neostigmine antagonism of vecuronium-induced neuromuscular block in adults and the elderly. *Br J Anaesth* 1992; **69:** 281–3.
214. Bevan DR, Donati F, Kopman AF. Reversal of neuromuscular blockade. *Anesthesiology* 1992; **77:** 785–805.
215. Tramèr MR, Fuchs-Buder T. Omitting antagonism of neuromuscular block: effect on postoperative nausea and vomiting and risk of residual paralysis. A systematic review. *Br J Anaesth* 1999; **82:** 379–86.
216. Soni N, Kam P. 4-Aminopyridine, a review. *Anaesth Intens Care* 1982; **10:** 120–6.
217. Bowman WC. *Pharmacology of Neuromuscular Function*, 2nd edn, London: Wright, 1990: 196–202.
218. Bom A, Cameron K, Clark JK, *et al.* Chemical chelation as novel method of NMB reversal – discovery of Org 25969. *Eur J Anaesthesiol* 2001; **18** (Suppl. 23): 99
219. Hope F, Bom A. Org 25969 reverses rocuronium-induced neuromuscular blockade in the cat without important haemodynamic effects. *Eur J Anaesthesiol* 2001; **18** (Suppl. 23): 99
220. Kopman AF. Recovery times following edrophonium and neostigmine reversal of pancuronium, atracurium and vecuronium steady-state infusions. *Anesthesiology* 1986; **65:** 572–8.

37

Regional anesthetic techniques

IAN McCONACHIE, JOHN McGEACHIE, AND JANET BARRIE

The purpose of this chapter is to provide an overview of the principles of safe practice of regional anesthesia, emphasizing patient preparation, the importance of a thorough knowledge of relevant anatomy, and intra-operative management. Clinical pharmacology of the local anesthetic drugs will be briefly discussed where it is relevant to clinical practice. The usefulness of regional anesthetic techniques as a component of balanced anesthesia and the ongoing controversy regarding potential improvements in outcome, especially with central neural blocks, is discussed in some detail. The technical aspects of performing the blocks will be only briefly described for two reasons. First, learning the blocks is best achieved in the operating room, preferably by demonstration. Second, a complete description of all aspects of all available techniques is outside the scope of one chapter. Hence, only the most common and most important techniques for the practicing anesthesiologist will be included. However, the study of this and other chapters in this book that describe regional anesthetic techniques is not a substitute for a thorough study of the relevant anatomy or practical teaching in the operating room.

FACILITIES REQUIRED

The most important prerequisite is a thorough knowledge of anatomy. The facilities required for successful and safe performance of regional anesthesia depend on whether regional anesthesia is to be provided in isolation or in combination with general anesthesia. Similar standards of monitoring apply for regional anesthesia as for general anesthesia. Full resuscitation facilities must be immediately available. The requirements for the safe performance of regional anesthesia are shown in Table 37.1. Also shown are the "optional extras" for which the need may be a matter of personal preference. Certain aspects are controversial, for example routine monitoring during the injection of the block, although this can be useful – particularly for central neural blockade.[1]

Many anesthesiologists do not routinely wear a sterile gown or face mask for all regional techniques. However, the majority of anesthesiologists wear a gown and mask for catheter techniques and central neural blockade.

Good-quality disposable "kits" are widely available from different manufacturers, containing all the equipment required for performing the block, and are preferred by some practitioners.

Table 37.1 *Facilities required*

Essentials
Gloves, cleaning fluid, towels, gowns, masks, dressings, etc.
Resuscitation drugs
Appropriate needles, syringes, labels, and catheters
Tipping trolley
Access to circulation
Thiopental, succinylcholine, and other drugs
Intravenous fluids
Trained assistance (e.g. for positioning)
Oxygen and means of administering under pressure
Means of assisted ventilation
Laryngoscopes and tracheal tubes
Suction
Monitoring
All facilities for general anesthesia
Appropriate local anesthetic drugs, including lidocaine for skin infiltration
Adjuncts to local anesthesia e.g. α_2-agonists if required
Sharps container
Optional extras
Peripheral nerve stimulator
Music and headphones
Screen to prevent patient viewing operation
Sedation drugs if used
Oxygen face mask if sedating
Skin marker
Tourniquets if required

Lidocaine (lignocaine); succinylcholine (suxamethonium).

Needles

There is controversy over the most suitable type of needle for performing regional anesthesia. Standard sharp-pointed, long-beveled needles are suitable for many blocks and may permit smoother needle passage through the tissues, enabling fine control of the needle tip. However short-beveled "blunt" needles, e.g. Sprotte needles, may enable tissue planes to be identified more easily.

Nerve damage related to needle type is controversial. It is logical to assume that standard needles will cause less damage if the nerve is pierced. This would presumably be due to the fibers being separated rather than torn. Animal studies have shown that sharp needles penetrate nerves less commonly with less damage and quicker recovery.[2] Unfortunately, convincing patient studies are not available to resolve this issue.

Unless otherwise stated, all blocks described here are performed with a 23-s.w.g. (standard wire gauge) needle.

Peripheral nerve stimulators

Nerve stimulators can be used to identify nerves with a motor component. Eliciting paresthesiae may be unpleasant for an awake patient and may result in an increased incidence of neurologic complications.[3] Nerve stimulators may not solve all the problems, and are not helpful if an anesthetized patient has received muscle relaxants. Care must be taken to ensure that the response observed with stimulation is not a result of direct muscle stimulation. The response should be sought in an area where direct local stimulation cannot occur. The value of electrical stimulators is confirmed by evidence that their use increases the success rate for some blocks.[4] Contrary to some reports, special sheathed needles that are electrically insulated apart from the tip are not required; the point of maximum current density lies just in front of the tip of the needle. Nerve stimulation should occur before the nerve is touched by the needle, as the point of the needle is behind the point of maximum stimulation.

CLINICAL PHARMACOLOGY

Factors influencing the choice of local anesthetic drug

In general, a highly lipid-soluble drug will have a prolonged duration of action; for example, bupivacaine is more lipid soluble than lidocaine (lignocaine). The degree of ionization is inversely related to the lipid solubility: poorly ionized drugs will be present in a higher free form and will therefore exhibit a rapid onset of anesthesia. Lowering the pH in the tissues (as with local infection) will increase the amount of ionized drug and reduce the amount of free lipophilic drug present and retard the development of anesthesia. Conversely, if the pH of the drug is increased (e.g. by adding sodium bicarbonate), the free portion of drug should increase (all local anesthetic drugs have a pK_a greater than 7) and hasten the onset of anesthesia.[5] Not all the results of various studies are convincing,[6] and the additional effect is of doubtful practical significance. The degree of protein binding also influences the duration of action; for example, tetracaine and bupivacaine are highly protein bound and produce prolonged blockade compared with procaine, which is weakly protein bound.

From a practical point of view, the greater the concentration of anesthetic used, the shorter the duration of onset, the more prolonged the duration of action, and the more profound the block (i.e. motor as well as sensory). The duration of blockade is increased if the local anesthetic remains at the required site, i.e. if vascular uptake is inhibited, by the addition of epinephrine (adrenaline) to the anesthetic solution. The reduced rate of absorption and consequent lowering of blood concentration by the addition of adrenaline raises the "quoted" maximum safe dose of lidocaine from 3 to 7 mg kg^{-1}. However, there are factors involved in systemic toxicity other than the relation between the amount of drug and the patient's weight.[7]

Practical points in the use of nerve stimulators

- A low current of approximately 0.5 mA should be selected, or stimulation may occur when the needle tip is still some distance away from the nerve.
- The negative electrode or cathode must be attached to the stimulating needle.
- The positive electrode or anode must be attached to a site distant to the block site.
- The first 1–2 mL of anesthetic should abolish evoked contraction immediately if a safe block is to be ensured. This implies that the needle is immediately adjacent to the nerve fibers. This mechanism is not due to a pharmacological action of the local anesthetic but is probably due to physical deformation of the nerve fibers by the small volume injected (saline will have the same effect). If injection cannot be easily performed, the needle should be withdrawn to avoid a possible intraneural injection.
- Stimulators that permit battery reserve to be checked are best lest unrecognized battery failure leads to failure to identify the site of block. In some machines, completion of the electrical circuit is heralded by a change in tone of the signal confirming circuit integrity.

Adjuncts to local anesthetic drugs

Adjuncts are often given with local anesthetics in regional blocks, particularly central blocks, to which most of the published data refer. The aim of using adjuncts is to improve analgesic intensity, to increase duration of action, to achieve faster onset, or to achieve acceptable analgesia with lower drug doses and thus reduced risks of side-effects.

There are many studies with various combinations of agents in varying doses. These studies often contain small groups and use different methodologies. Many studies show theoretical or statistical benefits that are of dubious clinical relevance.

Opioids

Centrally administered opioids result in vascular levels that are too low for systemic analgesic effects. It is thought therefore that analgesia results from activation of opioid receptors located in laminae I and II of the dorsal horn. Uptake of opioid by the spinal cord is proportional to lipid solubility; lipophilic drugs therefore show faster onset and elimination than hydrophilic agents. Conversely, hydrophilic drugs are taken up by the spinal cord to a lesser extent and therefore show greater cephalad spread than lipophilic opioids. Elimination from the subarachnoid or extradural spaces is by vascular uptake.

Centrally administered opioids are synergistic with concomitantly administered local anesthetics, particularly lidocaine. This synergy is best seen at low doses of both opiate and local anesthetic. They are also synergistic with centrally administered clonidine and other α_2-agonists.

Neurotoxicity is not a feature of opioids given via the extradural space but has been reported with high-dose sufentanil given intrathecally. Side-effects include:

1 nausea;
2 pruritus, particularly of the face and upper trunk;
3 respiratory depression – the incidence of respiratory depression is about 0.3% at low doses of opioid and results from migration of the agent to the brain and is therefore seen most frequently with the more hydrophilic compounds;
4 vertigo, particularly with morphine;
5 urinary retention.

Numerous dose–agent combinations have been published, with little obvious advantage to any. Despite widespread clinical experience,[8] opioids remain unlicensed for administration via the spinal or extradural routes in the UK.

Clonidine

α_2-Receptors are present both pre- and postsynaptically in the primary afferents of the dorsal horn and are part of the descending noradrenergic pathways. Their stimulation inhibits firing of nociceptively driven cells. α_2-Agonists at this site reduce the activity of wide-dynamic-range neurons in the dorsal horn and reduce the release of substance P and other neurotransmitters in response to noxious stimuli.[9] Animal studies suggest that clonidine is not neurotoxic even during chronic administration[10] and does not reduce neuronal blood flow.[11]

Postoperatively, 3–10 μg kg^{-1} extradural clonidine as the sole agent results in 4–6 h analgesia but at the expense of bradycardia, hypotension, and sedation.[12] Likewise, 150 μg clonidine prolongs the action and increases the effect of extradural fentanyl[13] or bupivacaine.[14] Respiratory depression and urinary retention after intrathecal clonidine are mild. Clonidine is not licensed in the UK for spinal or extradural use but has recently been licensed by the Food and Drug Administration (FDA) in the USA for extradural use for chronic pain management.

Studies in sheep indicate that clonidine does not alter uterine blood flow.[12] There is evidence that central clonidine is associated with an increased incidence of suspicious fetal cardiotochographs but not necessarily with worse fetal condition.[15]

The addition of clonidine to lidocaine for brachial plexus block results in reduced onset time, greater extent of block, and increased duration of action at the expense of sedation and reduced systolic blood pressure.[16]

Steroids

Steroids have been used extensively in the extradural space and are regarded as safe for use by this route. The extradural injection of steroids for their anti-inflammatory effects in chronic pain is discussed further in Chapter 75. There is less experience with the use of steroid injected into the subarachnoid space. There is, however, some evidence of adhesive arachnoiditis or aseptic meningitis after repeated injection of intrathecal methylprednisolone. There are also anecdotal reports of cauda equina syndrome or cerebral vein thrombosis following intrathecal steroid use.[17]

Epinephrine

Centrally administered epinephrine may potentiate local anesthetic action in two ways:

1. The vasoconstrictor properties of epinephrine may reduce vascular uptake of local anesthetic and therefore help to maintain the concentration at the site of injection. Some local anesthetics are vasoconstrictors in low concentrations, and this may explain why epinephrine has little effect on duration of action of potent drugs.
2. Low doses of extradural epinephrine may have direct α_2 activity in the dorsal horn and potentiate other centrally acting drugs.

Concurrent benzodiazepines

These may remove the signs of central nervous system (CNS) toxicity but do not raise the threshold for cardiovascular collapse. The usefulness of "warning signs" of CNS toxicity before impending cardiovascular collapse is therefore removed. They may also make resuscitation less successful.[18]

There are benzodiazepine binding sites in substantia gelatinosa and intrathecal midazolam may potentiate intrathecal morphine.

Dextrose

Dextrose is often added to bupivacaine to render it hyperbaric. This solution is often used for subarachnoid anesthesia, the hyperbaric solution being felt to act in a more predictable manner than hypobaric plain bupivacaine. The peripheral nerve toxicity of local anesthetics is increased in the presence of 7.5% dextrose. It is uncertain whether this is a direct effect of the dextrose or whether the presence of dextrose enhances the toxic effect of the local anesthetic.[19]

Future possibilities

The complex neurophysiology of the dorsal horn involves many neurotransmitters and intermediate substances. This leads to many possible therapeutic options. Animal studies suggest that the following may have antinociceptive properties when administered intrathecally:

1. *Adenosine agonists.* These probably act via A_1 adenosine receptors. They are said to produce analgesia with little motor block.[20]
2. *Somatostatin.* Somatostatin is a neurotransmitter within the spinal cord. Central administration of somatostatin has potent analgesic effects but its clinical use may be limited by neurotoxicity secondary to vasoconstriction.[21] Octreotide, a somatostatin analog, may be less neurotoxic.
3. *Neostigmine.* Neostigmine probably acts via M_1 muscarinic receptors to produce analgesia when given intrathecally.[22] Neostigmine may act synergystically with clonidine or morphine. Its use is associated with motor dysfunction, nausea, vomiting, and sedation.[23]
4. *Ouabain.* This Na^+/K^+ pump inhibitor, when administered intrathecally, results in a dose-dependent increase in tail flick latency in rats. It is active alone and is synergistic with morphine but not lidocaine. The effect of ouabain is inhibited by atropine and is therefore possibly mediated via muscarinic receptors. Neural Na^+/K^+ pump inhibition can increase acetlycholine release from nerve endings.[24]
5. N-*Methyl-*D-*aspartate (NMDA)* is thought to be involved in the development of chronic pain via increased nitric oxide synthesis. Antagonists of either NMDA or nitric oxide synthesis potentially limit or even reverse this response.

CLINICAL ASPECTS OF TOXICITY

"Toxic dose" is a misnomer as the development of toxicity correlates poorly with dose or total plasma levels. Peak total plasma concentration achieved after stellate[25] or interscalene[26] blocks and time to peak concentration both show wide interindividual variation. Peak plasma concentration is related to the vascularity of the injection site and inversely to the weight of the patient.

Local anesthetics bind to both albumin and, predominantly, α_1-acid glycoprotein. The latter is an acute-phase protein and its plasma concentration is variable, rising secondary to trauma, inflammatory processes, and other stimuli. The free serum concentration of local anesthetic agent resulting from a given bolus dose is therefore also variable, decreasing as the plasma α_1-acid glycoprotein concentration rises.

As the uptake of local anesthetic agents into the brain and cerebrospinal fluid (CSF) is related to the free serum concentration, the effects of a given bolus dose of local anesthetic on the CNS decrease with increasing α_1-acid glycoprotein concentration in plasma. Cardiotoxicity may similarly be related to free, rather than total, drug concentration.

Despite these observations, the manufacturers suggest that the maximum safe dose of local anesthetic should not be exceeded. Drugs of low toxicity (e.g. prilocaine) should be used for intravenous regional anesthesia or when the risk of intravascular injection is high. Toxicity is further minimized by scrupulous attention to technique, aspiration prior to injection, use of incremental doses, and maintenance of verbal contact with the patient.

The toxic effects of local anesthetic agents are described below and the management of local anesthetic toxicity is summarized.

Central nervous system

Initial toxic effects of local anesthetic agents on the CNS are stimulatory, due to depression of inhibition mechanisms by the local anesthetic. Local anesthetic CNS toxicity is made worse by hypoxia or acidosis. The CNS symptoms related to plasma levels are listed below, in order of increasing plasma levels:

- numbness of mouth and tongue;
- light headache;
- tinnitus;
- visual disturbance;
- irrational speech and behavior;
- muscle twitching;
- convulsions;
- coma;
- apnea.

Cardiovascular system

Cardiovascular system (CVS) toxicity occurs at higher plasma levels than CNS toxicity for all agents except bupivacaine, for which CVS and CNS reactions occur at similar plasma levels.

The CVS effects of local anesthetics are due to the membrane-stabilizing effect of the agent on the conducting and myocardial tissue, rendering these membranes resistant to depolarization. All agents reduce cardiac conductance of Na^+, leading to a reduction in the maximum upstroke velocity (V_{max}) of the action potential. With most agents, therefore, patients develop loss of contractility, hypotension bradycardia, and asystole, with this trend being exacerbated by hypoxia. Asystole may require prolonged cardiopulmonary resuscitation (CPR) and be resistant to pacing.

Bupivacaine differs from the above pattern in its tendency to induce arrhythmias because ionized bupivacaine may locate within the phospholipid bilayer of cell membranes at physiologic intracellular pH to a greater extent than the other agents.[27] Bupivacaine reduces V_{max} to a greater extent than other agents. This leads to prolongation of the P–R and QRS intervals of the electrocardiogram (ECG) and predisposes to re-entrant arrhythmias. Bupivacaine cardiotoxicity may therefore present as ventricular tachycardia/ventricular fibrillation (VT/VF) or the induction of heart blocks or loss of contractility with cardiac failure.

The Na^+ ions are blocked in a "fast in, slow out" manner, therefore recovery is slow but bupivacaine may "wash out" if coronary circulation is maintained.[28] There is some suggestion that this washout may be enhanced by treatment with a lipid infusion in which the lipophilic bupivacaine is thought to dissolve.[29] It also appears that *R*-bupivacaine is more cardiotoxic than *S*-bupivacaine and that *R*-bupivacaine may dissociate more slowly from ion channels than the *S*-form.[30]

Ropivacaine cardiotoxicity presents in a similar manner to lidocaine cardiotoxicity and its effect on V_{max} is intermediate between that of lidocaine and bupivacaine.[31] It is less arrhythmogenic than bupivacaine.

The management of toxic reactions includes:

- Stop further injection.
- Provide oxygen.
- Secure airway and ventilation if necessary.
- Stop convulsions – these may be resistant to treatment and may require intravenous thiopental.
- Treat hypotension with inotropes.
- CPR – asystole may be resistant to pacing and bupivacaine-induced VF may be resistant to defibrillation.

Toxic effects on peripheral nerves

Neuropathy following regional anesthesia may be due to direct nerve trauma, hemorrhage with nerve compression, infection, or neurotoxic effects of local anesthetic agents.

Local anesthetic agents are vasoactive, being constrictor in low concentrations and dilator in high concentrations. This may potentially lead to demyelination or local neuronal damage due to ischemia secondary to constriction of the nerve's blood supply. The addition of epinephrine will enhance this effect.[32]

There may also be a direct relation between local toxicity and concentration of agent, possibly due to inhibition of mitochondrial respiration. This phenomenon may have been involved in the development of the cauda equina syndrome after high concentrations of local anesthetic were administered via microspinal catheters.[33] The use of hyperbaric solutions may have exacerbated this complication. The role of specific local anesthetic agents in the development of cauda equina syndrome has been questioned.[34]

Muscle

Local anesthetic agents are directly myotoxic.[35] This effect is dose dependent and exacerbated by repeated injections, increased concentration of agent, and the concomitant use of steroids and epinephrine. Although rare in clinical practice, it presents with muscle tenderness exacerbated by stretching of the muscle involved. Recovery within 3–4 weeks is usual, but occasionally muscle atrophy persists. This myotoxicity is possibly secondary to calcium release from the sarcoplasmic reticulum.

Allergy

True allergy to local anesthetics is very rare. Less than 4% of people claiming local anesthetic allergy show true allergic reaction, and these reactions are divided approximately equally between anaphylaxis and delayed hypersensitivity. Over 90% of allergic individuals were found not to react to other local anesthetics.[36] Approximately 15% of people describing allergy may react to the preservative – usually methylparaben or sodium bisulphate. No true allergic reaction was noted in any patient describing allergy after dental block or who presented with collapse or hypotension and recovered without treatment.

REGIONAL ANESTHESIA AND THE STRESS RESPONSE TO SURGERY

The effect of regional anesthesia, and central neural blockade in particular, on the stress response has been a subject of much research. The concept that the stress response in some patients may have an adverse effect on patient morbidity and that this morbidity may be lessened by blunting the stress response is, at least, intriguing.

Although discussed elsewhere in detail, a brief summary of the stress response is given in Table 37.2. As can be seen, the triggers could not all be amenable to regional anesthesia, e.g. the role of wound chemicals and hemorrhage, but afferent stimuli via both the peripheral and the central nervous systems could be open to modification with regional anesthesia.

There are several important points regarding regional anesthesia and the stress response :

1 The intensity of the stress response is related to the degree of tissue trauma, i.e. minor surgery stimulates a minor, transient response whereas major abdominal surgery may stimulate a stress response persisting for days or even weeks.
2 The desirability of totally abolishing the stress response, as opposed to modifying its excessive effects, is questionable.
3 Intraoperative regional anesthesia may only delay the development of the stress response. The optimum duration of blockade is not known.
4 If modification of the response into the postoperative period is desired, a continuous regional technique is required – continuous extradural analgesia has been most studied.
5 Extradural analgesia has significant modifying effects on the hormonal and catecholamine responses to surgery of the lower half of the body.
6 The effects of extradural anesthesia on the stress response following upper abdominal and thoracic surgery are less impressive. This could be due to failure to adequately block all afferent stimulation. For example, continuous spinal anesthesia, with its denser block, is more effective at blocking the hormonal stress response than is extradural anesthesia.

Many anesthesiologists believe that the increase in patient well-being following major surgery in those in whom a regional technique has been successfully employed is, in part, due to the suppression of this response. However, objective proof that morbidity or mortality from surgery is improved because of suppression of the hormonal and metabolic stress response is not available.

The influence of anesthetic technique on the immune function after surgery has been less well studied than the effects on the metabolic response. In general, any modification of the immune response to surgery by regional compared with general anesthesia is probably of less clinical importance than the different effects on the hormonal and metabolic changes.

Table 37.2 *Summary of stress response*

Triggers of stress response
Neural pathways
Wound chemicals
Sympathetic nervous system, e.g. from gut
Cytokines
Hemorrhage
Infection
Starvation
Function of stress response
Generates substrate
Synthesizes acute-phase proteins
Mobilizes protein for wound healing
Effects of stress response
Increased catabolic hormones
Negative nitrogen balance
Increased release of catecholamines
Water and sodium retention
Increased coagulability
Decreased fibrinolysis
Decreased immune competence
Possible detrimental effects of stress response
Increased demands on organs, possibly with reduced reserve
Muscle wasting
Fatigue
Thromboembolism
Possible increase in cardiac and respiratory complications

REGIONAL ANESTHESIA AND PERIOPERATIVE MORBIDITY

The possible effects of regional blockade on perioperative outcome are of major interest. These include effects on coagulability and fibrinolyis, with their impact on blood loss and thrombotic complications, which are part of the effect on the stress response. In addition, the role of regional anesthesia and postoperative analgesia on overall morbidity and cardiac and respiratory complications has been increasingly investigated.

There is no consensus on whether certain types of patient undergoing certain types of surgery benefit more from a regional anesthetic, a general anesthetic, or a mixture of the two. Obvious indicators such as mortality have not proved to be helpful.

In truth, there may not be a significant difference for all patients. Much will depend on how a technique is performed rather than on which technique is performed, the skill of the practitioner, patient factors such as cardiac or respiratory disease, and the occurrence of side-effects or complications. The practitioner should attempt to weigh up risks versus benefits for each patient even though it may not be certain what these are.

Different generations of anesthesiologists may have different priorities and preferences; an example is the fall in popularity of intrathecal anesthesia in the UK in the 1950s and 1960s following the Woolley and Roe court case.[37] For many anesthesiologists the benefits of regional anesthesia appear to be self-evident and worth attaining. Others perform virtually no regional techniques throughout their entire practice.

Despite the lack of consensus, there are certain advantages and disadvantages of the two main forms of anesthesia that are generally accepted universally, and these are outlined in Table 37.3. Some of these are expanded upon below and in relevant chapters elsewhere in this volume. Combinations of regional and general techniques or regional techniques with accompanying sedation will tend to blur these advantages and disadvantages.

Blood loss and central neural blockade

Reduced blood loss following central block, especially during hip arthroplasty surgery[38] and transurethral prostatectomy,[39] is well established. There seems to be little reduction in bleeding associated with upper abdominal and thoracic surgery. The mechanism is a reduction in venous pressure, leading to reduced venous oozing, and a reduction in arteriolar bleeding from relaxation of capillary sphincters, with added contribution from a reduced mean blood pressure, if present.

An alternative point of view is that extradural anesthesia is not associated with reduced bleeding but that general anesthesia is associated with *increased* bleeding,[40] i.e. any benefits of reduced blood loss from the use of an extradural technique are lost if a general anesthetic is given as well.

Thrombotic complications and central neural blockade

A considerable body of evidence supports the concept of reduced thrombotic complications [deep venous thrombosis (DVT) and pulmonary embolism]. The effect in hip surgery may be as great as a 50% reduction.[41] However, most of the older studies included no

Table 37.3 *Regional vs. general anesthesia*

Advantages of regional anesthesia	Advantages of general anesthesia
Decreased blood loss for certain surgery	Patent airway may be assured
Decreased DVT rate for certain surgery	Adequate oxygenation may be assured
Decrease in metabolic changes following surgery	Cardiovascular effects usually titratable
Better for severe respiratory impairment	Familiarity for most anesthetists
Preserves airway (if no sedation)	Patient preference
Cardiovascular stability (if no sympathetic blockade)	
Residual postoperative analgesia	
Allows verbal communication: warning of, for example, hypoglycemia	
Better recovery with less risk of airway obstruction, aspiration, etc.	
Excellent muscle relaxation	
No atmospheric pollution	
Less expensive than many GA techniques	
Avoids rare complications of GA, e.g. malignant hyperthermia	
Patient can drink and/or eat immediately after surgery (depending on type of operation)	
Disadvantages of regional anesthesia	**Disadvantages of general anesthesia**
Discomfort, especially for prolonged operations	Cardiovascular depression
Discomfort eliciting paresthesiae	Decreased protective reflexes
Contraindicated in confused patients	Prolonged psychomotor impairment
Potential for nerve damage (rare)	Nausea, vomiting, headache, etc.
Profound cardiovascular effect with central neural blockade	Possibility of inadvertent awareness
Leg weakness and urinary retention with central neural blockade	
Toxic doses for some combinations of blocks	
Toxicity with high serum levels of anesthetic or accidental i.v. injection	
Poor communication of intentions if patient deaf	
Patient preference to be asleep	
Certain positions are embarrassing for awake (and especially elderly) patients, e.g. lithotomy	

DVT, deep venous thrombosis; GA, general anesthetic; i.v., intravenous.

antithrombotic prophylaxis in the control group. There has been little evaluation of the effect of combining central neural block with other methods of prophylaxis or even comparing central neural block with such a common technique as subcutaneous heparin prophylaxis.

Whether extradural anesthesia continued into the postoperative period is superior to single-shot intrathecal anesthesia is unknown, although a consideration of the theories of the mechanisms of actions would suggest that it should be.

Suggested mechanisms include increased leg blood flow, maintenance of muscle temperature, and inhibition of coagulation and stimulation of fibrinolysis.[42] There may also be a direct pharmacologic effect related to blood levels of local anesthetic following vascular uptake. Certainly, *in vitro*, one can see inhibition of platelet aggregation from local anesthetic drugs.[43] In the postoperative period extradural anesthesia limits the increase in factor VIII and von Willebrand factor.

Gastrointestinal function and surgery

Postoperative ileus involves sympathetic and parasympathetic pathways. These can be blocked by extradural anesthesia, leading to a reduction in the incidence of ileus following abdominal surgery.[44] Surgeons are often concerned that the increase in intestinal motility may increase the incidence of anastomotic breakdown. However, any anesthetic influences are probably less important than the quality of the surgical technique. Controlled trials of intrathecal or extradural anesthesia show no increase in the rate of bowel anastomotic breakdown. In fact, by increasing intestinal blood flow one might expect extradural anesthesia to have a favorable effect on a bowel anastomosis.

Postoperative nitrogen balance after bowel surgery is improved by extradural anesthesia.[45]

Postoperative mental disturbances

One might expect the use of a regional anesthetic technique to reduce the incidence of postoperative confusion, either by reducing the "toxic" effects of general anesthesia and/or by less reduction in cerebral blood flow, combined with a reduced stress response. However, studies suggest no significant difference between regional and general anesthesia in terms of postoperative confusion in the elderly patient.[46]

Milder forms of postoperative mental disturbance, such as subtle degrees of cognitive dysfunction leading to loss of memory and psychomotor impairment, are common (5.5% at 6 months), with no difference between extradural anesthesia and general anesthesia.[47] A reduction in postoperative fatigue related to a reduced stress response has been suggested as a benefit of extradural anesthesia but results are conflicting.

The general high-risk patient

Owing to the generally low mortality rate after major surgery, the beneficial effects on complication rates and morbidity detailed above may ultimately be more persuasive than any uncertain benefit on mortality when deciding to choose a regional technique. However, extradural anesthesia and postoperative analgesia is not a panacea for the high-risk patient and carries its own morbidity, e.g.:

- respiratory depression with spinal opioids;
- cardiovascular problems;
- difficulty in identifying the etiology of hypotension and the possibility of unsuspected bleeding;
- inappropriate use of vasopressors in some patients;
- conversely, excessive use of fluids in the elderly patient;
- urinary retention.

The effect of extradural and intrathecal opioids on morbidity and mortality in high-risk surgical patients is less well studied but is likely to be less significant than following central neural block with local anesthetics. However, the use of opioids in this manner as opposed to local anesthetic drugs avoids the complications associated with sympathetic block.

The patient with respiratory disease

If the proposed surgery is suitable, a form of regional anesthesia is superior to general anesthesia for the patient with severe respiratory disease.

There is evidence that the excellent postoperative analgesia with continuous extradural analgesia leads to a reduction in respiratory complications.[48] The impairment in pulmonary function following abdominal surgery is reduced (in particular, diaphragmatic dysfunction is less[49]), but pulmonary function is still reduced compared with preoperative values. Thoracic surgery patients benefit from thoracic extradural analgesia, but this is discussed elsewhere.

It is possible that high-quality analgesia from other methods (e.g. patient-controlled analgesia) may also lead to a reduction in complications. The provision of adequate analgesia may be more important than the method of analgesia employed.

The patient with cardiac disease

Peripheral regional blocks (e.g. brachial plexus block) are probably safer than general anesthesia for patients with severe cardiac disease. However, central blocks, following which hypotension may not always be preventable, e.g. intrathecal anesthesia, are not necessarily a safer alternative to careful general anesthesia, particularly in inexperienced hands.[50] Central neural blocks are particularly hazardous for patients who require well-maintained preload, e.g. patients with aortic stenosis. Conversely, a small degree of afterload reduction from central neural blockade may be beneficial for patients with regurgitant valves. However, even with such seemingly clear-cut issues, there is controversy. An extradural block that is carefully titrated and planned to avoid sudden falls in preload and allows judicious, simultaneous use of fluids and vasoconstrictors may be no more hazardous in a patient with mild to moderate aortic stenosis than the tachycardia associated with inadequate pain relief. Appropriate invasive monitoring of filling pressures, cardiac output, and systemic vascular resistance may be indicated in such patients and may lessen the potential problems.

It is crucial in many cardiac patients to avoid sudden falls in diastolic blood pressure with resultant falls in coronary perfusion. Several studies have examined whether extradural anesthesia in association with general anesthesia, or, more commonly, on its own, results in less cardiac morbidity. This might be related to a reduction in thrombotic tendency, a reduction in catecholamine levels, and avoidance of cardiac depression. The original prospective randomized trial to address this issue reported beneficial effects from extradural anesthesia in high-risk surgical patients in the intensive care unit (ICU).[51] Unfortunately, later studies have shown conflicting results, with interpretation of these studies hampered by their lack of statistical power and poor control of other management protocols. The largest trial to examine this issue in lower limb vascular surgery patients found no significant reduction in cardiac morbidity from the use of extradural anesthesia.[52]

Indeed, the majority of patients may not expect an improvement in their overall prognosis when extradural anesthesia is provided. However, many practitioners argue that individual subgroups of patients should benefit and, therefore, continue to offer extradural anesthesia to their high-risk patients (if only to improve the quality of their postoperative analgesia).

Aortic and peripheral vascular surgery

Several important studies have been designed to examine aortic surgery specifically because of the high incidence of morbidity, especially cardiac morbidity. Claimed advantages for an extradural-based technique are reduced cardiovascular morbidity[53] (but see above), improved graft patency (related to reduced thrombotic tendency as well as improved graft blood flow), and better quality of postoperative analgesia with less sedation. Unfortunately, the studies to date are modest in size[54,55] and definitive studies are still awaited. Nevertheless, the majority of practitioners consider an extradural catheter combined with general anesthesia to be the method of choice for anesthesia for elective aortic surgery. Few patients presenting for emergency surgery are stable enough to permit insertion of an extradural catheter.

Peripheral leg blocks are not widely performed for peripheral vascular surgery, whereas central blocks are widely used. The perceived benefits are as already described but there is still active debate.

Carotid surgery

Carotid artery surgery can be performed under either general anesthesia or a regional technique.[56] The chief advantage of a regional technique is that one can easily monitor the patient's mental and neurological status; disadvantages include the unfamiliarity for many practitioners, the perceived difficulties of performing the blocks, and the lack of access for interventions, especially airway control. The chief advantage of a general anesthetic technique is the ability to manipulate variables of cerebral blood flow and intracranial pressure, especially arterial $P\text{CO}_2$. General anesthesia has the disadvantages of drowsiness afterwards and difficulty in monitoring the patient's neurologic state.

If a regional technique is preferred, the easiest method is to perform superior and deep cervical plexus blocks. Cervical extradural is another potential technique, but many are discouraged from this technique by the potential for severe complications.

Femur fracture surgery

In the special circumstance of fractured hips in the elderly, meta-analysis of 15 randomized trials shows that intrathecal anesthesia is associated with a reduced incidence of early mortality and a reduced incidence of DVT[57] compared with general anesthesia but no significant difference in late mortality (for which other factors, including pre-existing medical disease, quality of postoperative care including nutrition, and aggressive mobilization, have the major influence).

PREPARATION AND MANAGEMENT OF THE PATIENT

The patient should be prepared exactly as one would prepare a patient who is to have a general anesthetic, especially with regard to fasting. Some aspects involved in preparation are presented in Table 37.4.

All regional techniques have a small failure rate, and the patient who is to have a regional anesthetic may require general anesthesia. Indeed, all patients who are to have a regional anesthetic should be forewarned of this possibility. However, despite this pessimistic counsel, it is important to project an air of confidence to the patient. Many patients will prefer to "go to sleep." These patients should be reassured that sedation will be available if required. Other patients have fears of permanent neurologic complications (particularly paralysis following extradural or intrathecal anesthesia). These patients should be reassured of the safety of regional anesthesia. Appropriate sedative premedication may be used.

Finally, many techniques, especially extradural and brachial plexus

Table 37.4 *Preparation for regional anesthesia*

Patient
Preoperative visit
Previous anesthetics, problems
Cardiovascular and respiratory status
Medication
Allergies
Is surgery suitable?
Is regional anesthesia/analgesia indicated?
Examination of CVS/RS
Site of block
Discussion with patient
Advantages/disadvantages/risks
Informed consent
Document in case notes/anesthetic chart
Explanation of what to expect (especially if block performed awake)
Sedation, nerve stimulator, etc.
Anesthetic room
Planning
Anticipate problems
Do not be rushed or pressurized
Acceptance of failure
Alternative(s)

CVS, cardiovascular system; RS, respiratory system.

blockade, require up to 20 min after their completion for surgical anesthesia to be achieved. Thus, the operating schedule must be carefully planned to prevent delays. Impatience and/or pressure from the surgeons may result in too early testing of the quality of the block, which may lead to loss of confidence by the patient.

Arguably, the time spent performing a regional technique may be more than compensated for by the improved quality of postoperative analgesia. In addition, time spent at the beginning of the case may lead to time saved at the end, e.g. by avoiding the time required for reversal of neuromuscular blockade, awakening, and extubation. Time in the recovery room may also be reduced. Many blocks can be performed more efficiently and quickly once staff are familiar with the technique, e.g. positioning the patient, setting up trays and drugs, etc. An efficient team that is familiar with regional anesthesia can avoid significantly delayed operating schedules.

There are several cardinal rules to follow when preparing the patient and performing the block:

1 The risks and benefits of the proposed technique should be discussed in advance with the patient. This discussion should be recorded in the patient's charts. Current advice in the UK from the Association of Anaesthetists of Great Britain and Ireland is that verbal consent is sufficient if this is recorded in the charts. Specific written consent is considered unnecessary but different institutions may have different policies and rules regarding consent. Suggestions for appropriated documentation of regional techniques are made in Table 37.5.
2 Many practitioners use a skin marker pen to delineate the anatomy prior to performing the block. This helps ensure that no injection sites are missed when multiple injections are performed, e.g. intercostal blocks.
3 The site of injection of the block must be cleaned with an appropriate agent according to local policy. After skin cleansing, either the skin must not be touched again during the injection ("no touch" technique) or sterile gloves must be worn. Gown and face mask may be advisable for catheter techniques and central neural blockade.
4 Prior to injection, aspiration must be performed to detect blood and/or CSF depending on the site. This minimizes the risk of inadvertent intravascular or intrathecal injection of local anesthetic and is therefore essential. Aspiration should be repeated when large-volume injections are used. The only exception is the "fanwise" infiltration of local anesthetic into the tissues. On these occasions it is sufficient to aspirate as injection commences and then to continually move the needle point during injection to ensure that, even if a small vessel is entered, only a very small portion of anesthetic will be injected intravascularly.
5 If the patient is awake, the procedure is made more tolerable by subcutaneous infiltration with lidocaine, 1%, and then by allowing several minutes for its action to take effect.
6 Care must be taken to avoid inadvertent intravenous injection of local anesthetic drugs. This may be achieved by appropriate labeling of syringes and by not preparing drugs in advance of need. Many practitioners also physically separate the areas for preparation of local anesthetic drugs from other drugs to avoid potential confusion.
7 Local anesthetics containing vasoconstrictors must never be injected around digits or the penis.

Table 37.5 *Documentation of regional block technique*

Skin preparation/"sterility"
Awake or asleep?
Position of patient
Block and anatomical approach
Local infiltration?
Needle type and size
Number of attempts
Paresthesia/use of nerve stimulator
Aspiration before/during/after injection
Concentration/volume/additives
Method of injection
Manufacturer's name and lot number
Level of block (intrathecal/extradural)
Record of all problems/complications
Record of preoperative discussion and explanation

Some keys to successful regional anesthesia are presented in Table 37.6.

Awake versus asleep

There has been recent controversy regarding the performance of regional anesthesia (particularly central neural blockade) in the anesthetized patient.[58,59]

There is no published evidence to support the view that all regional anesthesia should be performed with the patient awake. Although there is a theoretical argument that suggests that the awake patient will tell the anesthesiologist when neural tissue is threatened by a needle or catheter or injection, there have been cases reported when damage has followed and the patient did not complain at the time of the institution of the regional anesthetic technique.

It is easier to perform regional anesthesia in a patient who is asleep, (particularly in children), but there is no doubt that the warning signs, paresthesia and pain, associated with impending nerve damage will be masked. The careful use of nerve stimulators when a nerve with motor function is to be blocked is imperative during regional anesthesia in the anesthetized patient. Blocks of purely sensory nerves cannot be performed using a nerve stimulator in the anesthetized patient.

Central neural blockade in the anesthetized patient is potentially the most hazardous. Intrathecal anesthesia with lumbar puncture carried out below the level of the termination of the spinal cord will avoid damage to the spinal cord but does not rule out the possibility of nerve root

Table 37.6 *Keys to success*

Careful selection of patients
Preoperative visit
Meticulous attention to detail
Dialogue/explanation
Careful considered use of supplementation
Anticipation and prompt treatment of complications

damage. One can argue that a patient having an intrathecal block should not also need to have a general anesthetic.

Extradural anesthesia, and particularly thoracic extradural injections or catheters for postoperative analgesia, are arguably the most difficult situation to resolve. The technique of thoracic extradural anesthesia is often technically challenging, and it can be argued that success is more likely when the patient is asleep. However, if epidural or intrathecal injections are undertaken in the anesthetized patient and damage, motor or sensory, occurs, it may be difficult to defend the technique in court, even though others use the same practice.

Choice of suitable patients

Despite the use of sedation there are some patients who are unsuitable for a regional technique alone. These include the extremely anxious patient, the psychotic patient, or the confused and uncooperative patient. However, they may still be suitable for a combined regional and general technique. Patients who cannot tolerate the positioning or injection of an essential block because of pain are also unsuitable for a regional technique without general anesthesia. The systemic or local contraindications to regional anesthesia described below should be noted.

Contraindications to regional anesthesia

As for any technique or therapy, there are both relative and absolute contraindications to regional techniques. Relative contraindications may on occasion be outweighed if the technique proposed carries appropriate benefits. However, it must be emphasized that none of the contraindications should be taken lightly. There are also contraindications that are specific for the central neural blocks.

Absolute contraindications are as follows:

1 patient refusal or lack of cooperation or understanding;
2 proved allergy to the local anesthetic drugs;
3 absence of resuscitation equipment;
4 no intravenous access for resuscitation;
5 coagulopathy;
6 local sepsis at the point of injection.

The following are the relative contraindications:

1 *Neurological disease.*
2 *Orthopedic disorder.* This is especially the case for patients with backache for whom a central block is proposed. There is no confirmed scientific evidence that performing a block will exacerbate a neurologic or orthopedic disorder, but coincidental exacerbation of the condition may be attributed to the block. Certainly, if a neurological impairment is present, the nature and extent of the disease must be documented before performing any regional anesthetic technique.
3 *Performing blocks on awake children.* Young patients may not understand or be able to cooperate with the procedure. The occasional pediatric anesthesiologist should not perform intrathecal or lumbar extradural anesthesia on small children and infants. Specialized centers, however, report the value of intrathecal anesthesia in neonates.[60]

Additional relative contraindications to central neural blocks are also recognized:

1 Severe cardiac disease, when cardiac output depends on either vascular tone or an adequate preload, is a contraindication. A sympathetic block could lead to a marked fall in cardiac output. This may be particularly relevant in pregnant women with heart disease. Careful titration of anesthetic to achieve a controlled extradural block using a catheter is safer than single-shot intrathecal anesthesia, after which the extent of sympathetic block may be rapid and unpredictable.
2 High abdominal surgery is a contraindication. The difficulty here is in achieving an adequate height of block with adequate muscle relaxation but without extensive sympathetic block.
3 Increased intracranial pressure is a contraindication, because deliberate or inadvertent intrathecal puncture may result in a sudden fall in CSF pressure, with herniation of the brainstem through the foramen magnum.
4 Hypovolemia or continuing rapid blood loss is an absolute contraindication for a central block. The induced sympathetic block may cause rapid and catastrophic cardiovascular collapse.
5 General sepsis is a contraindication for central neural blocks, as an infection may become seeded in an extradural hematoma.

INTRAOPERATIVE MANAGEMENT OF A REGIONAL TECHNIQUE

Most patients, except those undergoing very minor surgery, expect to be rendered unconscious for their surgical procedures. A notable exception is the obstetric patient.

A common problem may relate to patients' previous experiences of regional anesthesia in the dental chair – painful during the injection and providing unsatisfactory analgesia in many instances. This leads to low expectations of regional anesthesia. Patients' fears and misconceptions need to be addressed.

Aspects other than the block must be considered to ensure that the overall experience for the patient is as pleasant as possible. For example, attention must be paid to the patient's overall comfort and warmth while lying on a hard table and the provision of a relaxed environment. The patient should be protected from viewing the operation by the use of screens and towels.

In some operations the position of the patient may itself give rise to some discomfort, exposure, and embarrassment. Sedation may make such a procedure more tolerable. Supplementation of a regional anesthetic technique may be by one of several methods.

Distraction therapy

The simple action of diverting the patient's attention from his or her concerns may be of great benefit during surgery performed under regional anesthesia. The use of personal stereos is a particularly good method,[61] as it should be possible to accommodate the musical taste of most patients. Alternatively, a member of the operating room staff may offer reassurance and encouragement when required.

General anesthesia

While it may seem perverse to deliberately render a patient insensible when the regional anesthetic is providing perfect operating conditions, any anxiety or doubt concerning the efficacy of the anesthesia provided will be removed. Only a very light general anesthetic may be needed.

The combination of general anesthesia and extradural blockade will give excellent operating conditions as well as prolonged postoperative analgesia. However, caution is required, especially in the elderly, because of the potential combined hemodynamic effects. This is even more of a potential problem with combined general and intrathecal anesthesia, in which the sudden onset of sympathetic block from the intrathecal component and the cardiac depression of general anesthesia can cause considerable hemodynamic compromise but without any potential benefit of significant postoperative analgesia.

Relative analgesia

Patients' anxiety can be reduced and cooperation increased and additional analgesia be provided by the use of mixtures of nitrous oxide and oxygen, with the concentration titrated to the patient's response. Although this technique is particularly popular with dental surgeons, it has yet to become commonplace in the hospital environment.

Intravenous supplementation

There is no doubt that advances in pharmacology have provided anesthesiologists with safer and more predictable sedative agents that can be used to supplement regional anesthesia. However, the extensive use of sedation in conjunction with regional anesthesia is illogical at best and dangerous at worst, and the anesthesiologist must be able to justify the use of sedative drugs. There is no doubt, however, that the provision of amnesia for the events surrounding the time spent in the operating room can be an advantage for many patients. However, some patients find this loss of memory disturbing.

The choice of sedative drugs appears to be wide in theory, but in practice only a few drugs are used. The water-soluble benzodiazepine midazolam offers considerable advantages over its predecessor diazepam and may be administered by intravenous bolus ($0.07–0.15\,mg\,kg^{-1}$) or by continuous infusion ($0.25\,mg\,kg^{-1}\,h^{-1}$). Care and caution are required with midazolam as there is a wide variation in dose response; these doses are for guidance only.

The newer anesthetic agent propofol can also be administered by increment, although a continuous infusion is probably the best method of administration for sedation throughout the whole of the surgical procedure.[62] An infusion of propofol of $2–4\,mg\,kg^{-1}\,h^{-1}$ will provide sedation with a rapid recovery. Newer methods of administration of propofol are of interest. Software algorithms within the infusion pump aim to maintain blood levels of propofol at the selected level (target-controlled infusion). Precise degrees of sedation may be maintained.[63] Another method worthy of consideration is to allow the patient to self-administer propofol at anxiolytic doses (patient-controlled sedation) in a manner analogous to patient-controlled analgesia.[64] This method of supplementation is still under evaluation.

The advantages of propofol over midazolam are that the drug is easier to titrate, oversedation is probably less common, and recovery is more rapid. Care with regard to the cardiorespiratory systems is required with this drug and the amnesic effect of propofol is not as powerful as that provided by midazolam.

Small doses of short-acting opioid drugs such as alfentanil (0.25–0.5 mg) and fentanyl (50–100 μg) can be used for analgesia in addition to or instead of sedative drugs. Supplementary analgesia may help with discomfort relating to position and may help reduce the pain of the local anesthetic injection or the pain from the tourniquet used for intravenous regional anesthesia.

Combinations of sedative and analgesic drugs are not without their dangers,[65] and it is mandatory that supplemental oxygen is administered and oxyhemoglobin saturation is monitored continuously whenever sedative and/or analgesic drugs are administered to supplement any regional anesthetic, especially extradural and intrathecal anesthesia.

The anesthesiologist should be present throughout for monitoring and appropriate care of the patient.

The inadequate block

If the resultant block is clearly inadequate for the proposed surgery, it can occasionally be supplemented more peripherally, for example a wrist block to supplement a brachial plexus block or local infiltration by the surgeon. Care must be taken with the total dose of anesthetic. Systemic opioids may on occasion be useful but their overenthusiastic use can be dangerous. It is probably wiser to admit defeat and convert to controlled general anesthesia than to administer excessive amounts of "sedation." The "failed" block may still provide residual postoperative analgesia. Persistence with surgery in the face of a clearly inadequate block has led to litigation.

CENTRAL NEURAL BLOCKADE

There are essentially two forms of central neural blockade: intrathecal (spinal or subarachnoid) anesthesia and extradural (epidural) anesthesia. Caudal anesthesia is a variant of extradural anesthesia. Contraindications have already been discussed.

The spinal cord and its associated structures are enclosed within the bones of the vertebral column. Knowledge of the anatomy and physiology of the spinal canal is the foundation of successful central neural blockade. The clearly defined endpoint (CSF dripping from the hub of the spinal needle) confirms that there is likely to be a high level of success in establishing intrathecal anesthesia. However, failure to achieve a satisfactory block is not unknown despite CSF visualization. Worldwide, intrathecal anesthesia is the most commonly performed regional anesthetic technique. Extradural blockade is used to provide analgesia for labor and postoperative analgesia in addition to surgical anesthesia.

Some of the differences between intrathecal and extradural anesthesia are shown in Table 37.7.

Intrathecal anesthesia

Subarachnoid block can be used to provide surgical anesthesia for all procedures carried out on the lower half of the body. Indications include surgery on the lower limb, pelvis, genitals, and perineum, and most urological procedures. Recently, the technique has found favor in obstetric practice in providing anesthesia for both elective and emergency procedures. While patients with respiratory disease may benefit from the avoidance of general anesthesia, caution should be exercised in patients with severe cardiac disease.

The concept of spinal anesthesia is simple enough. The injection of a local anesthetic drug into the cerebrospinal fluid produces anesthesia/analgesia of the lower extremities and torso. In recent years, many other drugs (opioids and α-agonists for example) have also been injected to modify the modulation of noxious stimuli as they are transmitted to the brain via the spinal cord.

This simple concept can become complex when all the complications,

Table 37.7 *Some of the differences between extradural and intrathecal anesthesia.*

	Extradural		**Intrathecal**
	Caudal	**Lumbar/thoracic**	
Technique	Single injection; catheter not common	Single injection; catheter common	Single injection; catheter out of favor
Onset[a]	5–20 min	5–20 min	5 min
Duration[a]	Single shot: 120–240 min	Single shot: 120–240 min Catheter: potentially many days	Single shot: 120–180 min
Volume Dose (bupivacaine)	10–20 mL 25–150 mg	10–20 mL 25–150 mg	1.0–4.0 mL 5–20 mg
Cardiovascular effects	Area of block will influence Generally any fall in blood pressure is slower than with intrathecal, but can be profound with large doses of local anesthetics Bradycardia with high block/thoracic blocks		Can be a problem Fall can be sudden and profound Bradycardia with high blocks
Headache	Unlikely unless accidental dural tap. Then likely and may require aggressive treatment		Low incidence with modern needles (< 2%)

a. Choice of local anesthetic may influence.

side-effects, and variety of factors affecting the spread, duration, and predictability of a spinal anesthetic are considered.

Dural puncture is usually performed below the level of the first lumbar vertebra to avoid damage to the spinal cord, which terminates about this level. The final choice of which interspace to use for the lumbar puncture must depend on the anatomy of the particular patient.[66]

Technique

Figure 37.1 displays the relevant anatomy of the vertebral bodies.

Before positioning the patient, it is mandatory that reliable intravenous access be secured with a large-bore indwelling cannula and monitoring commenced. The administration of a bolus of 0.5–1.0 L of intravenous fluid to limit the hypotension that may be precipitated by the sympathetic blockade associated with intrathecal anesthesia is considered standard practice but care may be required for those patients with severe heart disease. Treatment with vasoactive drugs is an alternative approach. Controversy surrounds this topic.[67,68] Standard monitoring of the patient should also have started before the patient is positioned for the lumbar puncture.

The choice of position of the patient will be dictated by a number of factors. The patient can be placed in one of two positions, the sitting or the lateral position. (The prone position has also been described, but is not used in modern anesthesia.) The sitting position has the advantage that generally the vertebrae remain in a line and the identification of the interspinous spaces and the block is easier to perform. Some patients may find it difficult to sit for the lumbar puncture (fractured neck of femur, for example) and the lateral position will be more appropriate. In the lateral position the vertebrae may not be in a straight line with a slight curve developing because of the position. Lumbar puncture may therefore be less straightforward. The lateral position may offer an advantage when the proposed surgery is unilateral (joint replacement in the lower limb, for example).

Sitting position

The patient should be asked to swing his or her legs over the edge of the trolley or operating table. Care may be required if premedication has been administered and there should be assistance with the positioning of the patient. The patient's feet may be allowed to rest on a stool or chair to encourage the legs to flex and the patient then asked to bend over to help in flexing the lumbar spine. The assistant can provide support. The lower back should then be examined by the anesthesiologist and if necessary the patient's position can be altered. A few moments spent on careful consideration of the most appropriate interspinous space to use for the lumbar puncture may save much time, increases the chances of successful lumbar puncture, and will ensure that the procedure is as speedy and comfortable as possible for the patient.

Lateral position

The patient should be asked to turn, or be assisted in turning, on to the side. If a unilateral procedure (for example a total hip replacement) is to be performed, the operative side can be dependent if the patient will tolerate this position. The patient is then asked to bring the knees up toward the chest to encourage flexion of the lumbar spine. A pillow or blanket can be placed between the patient's knees to try and maintain the horizontal relation of the vertebral bodies. As with the sitting position, careful consideration of the bony landmarks and choice of interspace will increase the chances of a successful lumbar puncture.

Lumbar puncture and injection of local anesthetic

The lumbar puncture must be conducted with a strict aseptic technique and all the equipment required should be placed on a sterile towel, preferably on a trolley. Once the anesthesiologist is happy with the patient's position, the skin of the lower back should be cleaned with an antiseptic solution or spray and allowed to dry. A sterile towel should be placed at the base of the spine when the patient is sitting and a towel placed over the dependent aspect of the flank when the patient is in the lateral position. When in the lateral position use of an O towel is an alternative method of draping the skin favored by some anesthesiologists. The skin and deeper structures can be infiltrated with local anesthetic prior to insertion of the spinal needle.

The anesthesiologist has a choice of several needle types for lumbar puncture, from the traditional Quincke point to the more recently introduced pencil-pointed Whitacre and Sprotte needles (Fig. 37.2). The pencil-pointed needles have been shown to be associated with a reduced incidence of postdural puncture headache and are now the first choice of many anesthesiologists for intrathecal anesthesia.[69]

Most anesthesiologists perform lumbar puncture in the midline. The space between the third and fourth or second and third lumbar vertebral spinous processes is usually selected. The spinal needle is inserted

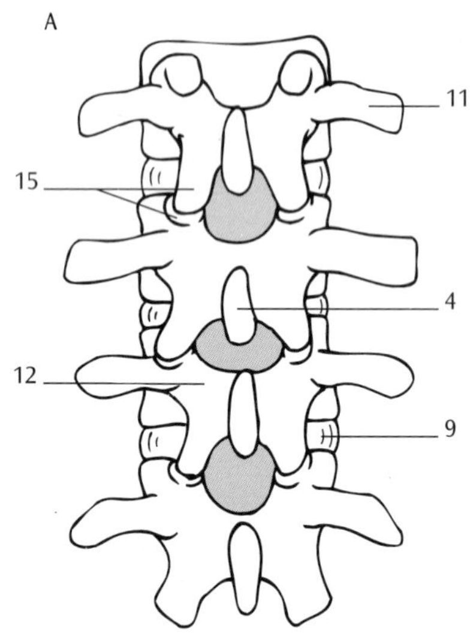

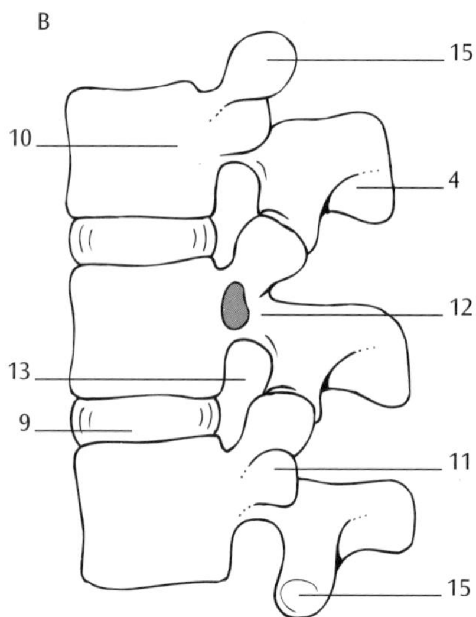

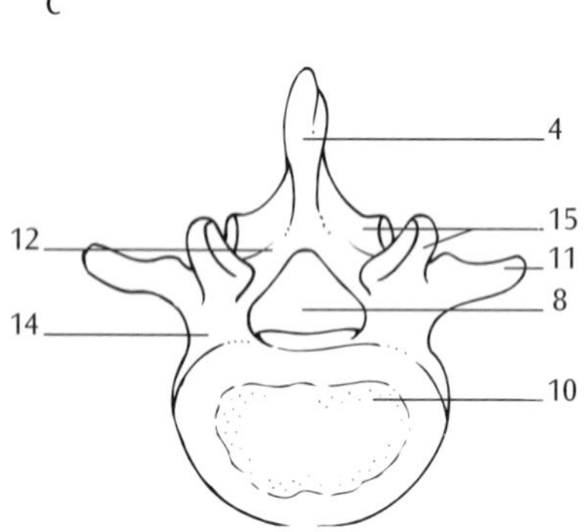

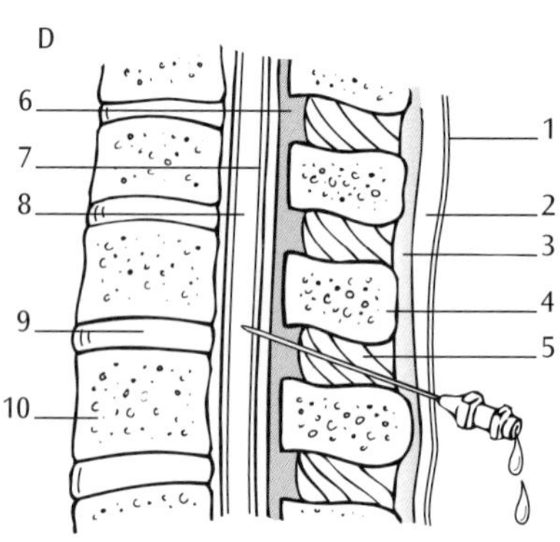

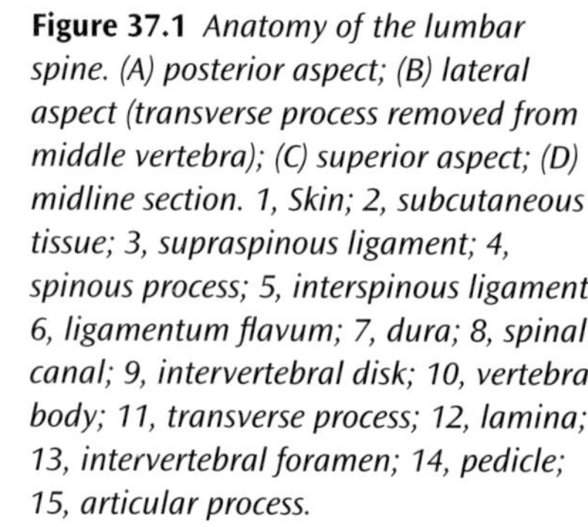
Figure 37.1 *Anatomy of the lumbar spine. (A) posterior aspect; (B) lateral aspect (transverse process removed from middle vertebra); (C) superior aspect; (D) midline section. 1, Skin; 2, subcutaneous tissue; 3, supraspinous ligament; 4, spinous process; 5, interspinous ligament; 6, ligamentum flavum; 7, dura; 8, spinal canal; 9, intervertebral disk; 10, vertebral body; 11, transverse process; 12, lamina; 13, intervertebral foramen; 14, pedicle; 15, articular process.*

through the area of anesthetized skin with the needle angled cranially to compensate for the angle of the spinous processes. The needle will pass through the skin, subcutaneous tissue, the supraspinous ligament, the interspinous ligament, the ligamentum flavum, and finally the dura before entering the subarachnoid space. There is often a characteristic "give" when the tip of the needle passes through the dura. Successful lumbar puncture is confirmed when removal of the stylet of the spinal needle is followed by the appearance of cerebrospinal fluid at the hub of the needle. This may take some time if a very fine needle is used. If there is doubt regarding the authenticity of the fluid, the use of a bedside glucose testing strip may be helpful. Passage of the spinal needle (particularly smaller needles and the pencil-pointed needles) is assisted by the use of an introducer needle, which aids passage through the tougher ligamentous structures of the vertebral column. In the older patient (in whom the ligamentous structures of the back may become calcified) it may be impossible to insert a fine pencil-pointed needle without use of an introducing needle. If a beveled needle is used it is recommended that the needle is inserted with the bevel parallel to the fibers of ligamentum flavum and dura so that the fibers are parted rather than cut by the needle tip as it is advanced. Inserting the needle in this fashion also reduces the chances of postdural puncture headache.[70]

The lateral approach to the subarachnoid space is useful when the midline approach is difficult (because of scar tissue or arthritic changes, for example).

Once the tip of the needle is confirmed to be lying in the subarachnoid space, the local anesthetic solution is injected. It is good practice to confirm that the tip of the needle has not moved by aspirating cerebrospinal fluid at some point during the injection. Once the block has become established, the area of anesthesia produced should be identified, with loss of sensation to pinprick a common measurement, although some would suggest that touch is a more reliable method of blockade assessment. It is worthwhile remembering that the sympathetic block produced may extend for several dermatomes above that of the sensory block.

Factors influencing the spread of subarachnoid block

Dose of local anesthetic drug

Logically, the larger the dose of local anesthetic that is injected into the cerebrospinal fluid, the more extensive the intrathecal block will be. The same dose injected in different volumes has been shown to produce similar levels of block. However, the relation between dose and extent of block is not linear, and studies with 0.5% bupivacaine in dextrose have shown that, although below 3 mL of injectate there is predictability, above this volume there are proportionally smaller increases in the extent of the block.[71,72]

Gravity/position/baricity

These three factors are related when considering the extent of the block that is produced. Gravity and the position of the patient are closely related in the spread of the local anesthetic, particularly when using hyperbaric solutions. If unilateral surgery is proposed, then the patient should ideally be placed on the operative side when the injection is made. This may not be possible or fair to the patient if there is pain

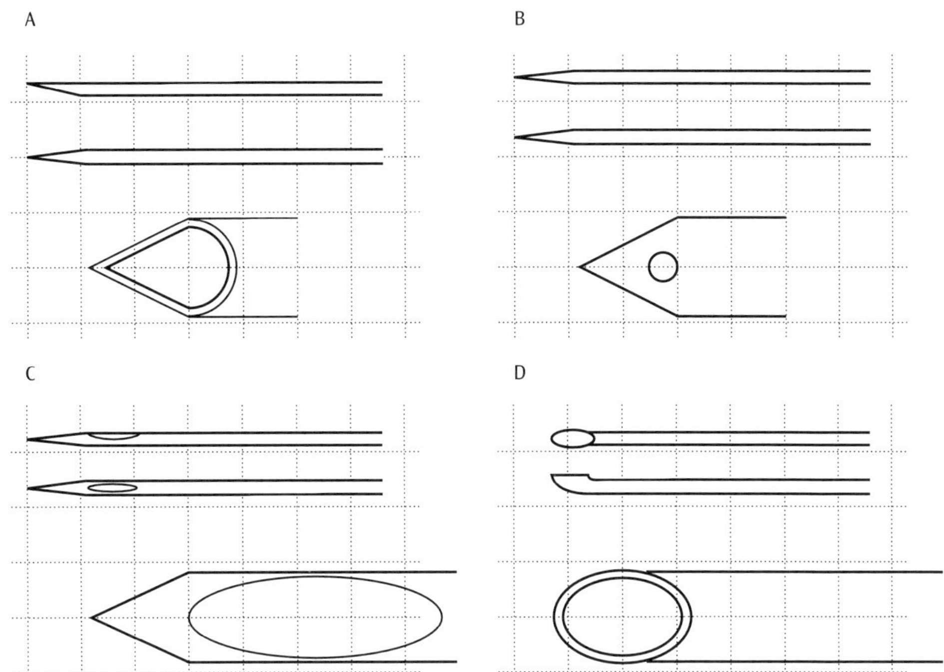

Figure 37.2 *Needles for central neural blockade (not to scale). (A) Quincke-type needle; (B) Whitacre-type needle; (C) Sprotte-type needle; (D) Tuohy needle.*

associated with this, e.g. fractured neck of femur, and injection with the operative side uppermost followed by a swift return to the supine position usually produces a bilateral block to the same level. Leaving the patient on his or her side for 5–10 min after the injection is more likely to produce a unilateral block on the dependent side. The use of hyperbaric solutions is preferred by most clinicians as it is felt that these solutions are more predictable in terms of the resulting block. However, there is considerable variation between patients. Baricity can influence the duration of blockade.[73]

Duration of blockade

Choice of local anesthetic solution

Comparisons of different studies (different drugs, volumes, doses, etc.) is difficult as often different measurements of duration have been used. The most important factor in duration of action is the local anesthetic drug that is used by the anesthesiologist. Many different drugs have been used, but only a few drugs remain in current use, and in recent years the choice of drugs available to anesthesiologists has been reduced, (particularly in the UK), with the most commonly used drug being 0.5% bupivacaine in 8% dextrose. Other drugs that are available include procaine, lidocaine, mepivacaine, and tetracaine. The duration of action of each of these drugs varies, with a range quoted for each, but, in general, procaine has a short duration of action, with lidocaine and mepivacaine having a moderate duration and tetracaine and bupivacaine a longer duration of action. The action of hypobaric solutions persists for longer than that of isobaric solutions, which in turn have a more prolonged action than have hyperbaric solutions. The addition of epinephrine is advocated by some clinicians to extend the duration of action of the block, with a doubling of the length of duration of the block being possible. The epinephrine may also have a direct antinociceptive effect on the spinal cord by a direct activation of descending inhibitory systems that modulate dorsal horn neural activity. The addition of clonidine and opioid drugs to the local anesthetic solution may have benefits by providing postoperative analgesia well after the effects of the local anesthetic drug have ceased.[74,75]

Problems with lumbar puncture

Unfortunately, not all attempts at lumbar puncture will be successful and there are several problems that may be encountered.

Incorrect direction of the needle is a common cause of failure. The needle can pass in the wrong direction and either miss the spinal canal or be stopped by one of several bony parts of the vertebral body. Withdrawal of the needle, reappraisal of the anatomy, and a change of direction (sometimes surprisingly small) may be all that is required. Repositioning of the patient and change to another interspace may be needed in other cases. Occasionally, it can be impossible to locate the intrathecal space. The anesthesiologist should be wary of making frequent attempts at different interspaces. The patient's comfort and dignity must be respected at all times.

Continuous spinal anesthesia

Very small spinal needles (27 s.w.g. and 29 s.w.g.) and very small catheters (30 s.w.g. and 32 s.w.g.) have made it possible to consider this technique without the risks of severe postdural puncture headache (PDPH) which resulted from the use of 16-s.w.g. and 18-s.w.g. Tuohy needles. The intrathecal catheters are inserted through the spinal needles and small doses of local anesthetic drugs are administered to establish an intrathecal block, which can be maintained postoperatively with the introduction of additional intrathecal local anesthetic. However, reports of cauda equina syndrome[76] associated with the technique led to the FDA in the USA banning the sale of the needles and catheters. Further debate on the safety of local anesthetic drugs has also followed.[34,77] Although there is still some interest in the technique, it is generally not widely practiced at present. In addition, the size of the needle and catheters makes successful lumbar puncture more difficult.

Complications of intrathecal anesthesia

Hypotension[78]

Approximately one-third of patients will suffer from hypotension following an intrathecal anesthetic.[79] Hypotension is more likely in the older patient, in patients with higher blocks (T5 and above), and in cases in which a high lumbar puncture site is used. The definition of hypotension varies, but a systolic blood pressure of less than 12 kPa (90 mmHg) is clearly challengeable and it is more appropriate to consider a fall of 25–30% from the preoperative blood pressure as a more practical level at which to consider treatment. A fall in blood pressure may be of benefit, for example, in patients with ischemic heart disease, and may lead to reduced blood loss, for example in a total hip replacement. The fall in blood pressure is due to the thoracolumbar sympathectomy produced by the local anesthetic solution, which produces a decrease in systemic vascular resistance and an increase in venous pooling. While the optimal treatment of intrathecal anesthesia-induced hypotension remains unresolved, a correction of the fall in systemic vascular resistance will generally include treatment with α-adrenergic agonists. These drugs may produce or extend a bradycardia. Venous pooling may be corrected with intravenous fluids, elevation of the legs, or with β-adrenergic agonists. A slight head-down tilt will encourage venous return in patients undergoing intrathecal anesthesia.

While the management of hypotension will depend on whether a bradycardia is present (treatment of the bradycardia may restore blood pressure to an acceptable level), the initial management should be along the lines of:

1 Increase the inspired oxygen concentration.
2 Increase the rate of administration of the intravenous fluids. Often a bolus of 0.5–1.0 L will restore the blood pressure. Debate continues over the choice of crystalloid or colloid solution.[80,81] Caution may be required for the patient with cardiac disease, and smaller volumes of intravenous fluids, plus earlier use of vasopressors, may be advisable. The administration of large volumes of intravenous fluids as the only treatment for persistent hypotension associated with a central neural block is potentially dangerous and is not recommended.
3 Search for the cause of the fall in blood pressure, e.g. blood loss, packs, and retractors in abdominal surgery.
4 Consider a change in the patient's position, e.g. raise the legs. Caution may be required with head-down tilt as this may encourage further cranial spread of the local anesthetic block if this is undertaken in the early stages of intrathecal anesthesia (see also Chapter 40). Changes in the patient's position may also not be possible if surgery has started.
5 Consider administration of vasoactive drugs. This should not be delayed.

Ephedrine is often the first choice of vasopressor. Administered intravenously in a bolus dose of 3–6 mg this drug has a predominantly β-adrenergic agonist effect and produces an increase in heart rate, with some effect on the venous pooling but little direct effect on peripheral resistance. This is advantageous in pregnancy, when preservation of uterine blood flow in the presence of hypotension is important. Methoxamine is an α-adrenergic agonist and increases peripheral resistance. It will restore pressure, perhaps at the expense of blood flow, but is preferable to ephedrine when a tachycardia is present. Caution should be exercised when there is a normal or lower than normal heart rate as a reflex bradycardia may follow the administration of methoxamine. The initial intravenous bolus dose should be 2 mg.

Bradycardia

Bradycardia is more likely with a high block (T5 and above), in patients with a normal heart rate of less than 60 beats per minute, American Society of Anesthesiologists (ASA) class I patients, and patients prescribed β-adrenergic antagonists. If the heart rate falls below 60 beats per minute and the blood pressure is not adversely affected, careful monitoring is all that is required. However, if hypotension or other cardiovascular events present then treatment is indicated. If the heart rate drops to 50 beats per minute or less then treatment will be necessary for the older patient and the patient with heart disease. Intravenous glycopyrrolate, 0.2 mg, or atropine, 0.3 mg, should be administered. The circulation time may be much prolonged by the bradycardia and patience may be required to avoid administration of further, unnecessary doses of the drugs. Should the hypotension and bradycardia prove resistant to treatment, administration of intravenous epinephrine should be considered.[79,82,83]

Nausea and vomiting

Nausea and vomiting are commonly associated with hypotension, bradycardia, and a high block. Treatment of the cardiovascular problem(s) often relieves these symptoms, but not in every case. The use of conventional antiemetics can be beneficial but not in every case.

Postdural puncture headache

Headache has always been recognized as a side-effect of dural puncture and therefore of intrathecal anesthesia. The headache is believed to be the result of CSF leak, both at the time of the dural puncture and, more importantly, continuing afterward. Factors known to increase the likelihood of PDPH include the size of the needle used for the dural puncture (the larger the needle, the higher the incidence), the age of the patient (younger patients are more likely to have a headache than older patients) and early ambulation[70,84] Newer needle designs (Sprotte and Whitacre) are associated with a significantly lower incidence of PDPH, especially in higher risk groups. Needles of very small diameter (27–32 s.w.g.) are available, but practical difficulties have limited their widespread use.

PDPH is characteristically throbbing in nature, is eased by lying down, and returns on standing. It is unusual for the headache to present more than 48 h after lumbar puncture.

The conservative management of PDPH (bedrest, simple analgesia, and good fluid intake) is not successful in all cases. Severe PDPH will render the patient bedbound and merits more aggressive treatment if conservative management is ineffective after 24 h. The most reliable and effective method of treatment is the autologous extradural blood patch: 20–30 mL of blood is removed aseptically from the patient and injected into the extradural space. It is usual for two doctors to be involved in this procedure, one to remove the blood and one to perform the extradural injection. The headache usually disappears within minutes of the injection with a good long-term safety record. If the patient is pyrexial it is not advisable to use this technique.[70]

High block (total spinal)

While the injection of local anesthetic into the subarachnoid space usually provides a predictable regional anesthetic block, there are occasions when the resulting block is much higher than that anticipated or planned. Should the block extend above the T4 level, then severe cardiovascular problems may develop, with bradycardia and hypotension. These should be managed with appropriate aggressive intravenous therapy and the administration of chronotropic and vasoconstrictor drugs. Very rarely with subarachnoid anesthesia the block may extend higher and the patient may develop respiratory difficulties if the phrenic nerves (C3, C4, and C5) are affected. There may be warning of this developing if the patient complains of tingling or numbness in the hand(s). If respiratory difficulties are reported then the anesthesiologist should be prepared to intubate and ventilate the patient. It is important to remember that, although the patient may be unable to breathe, he or she may still be conscious, and a small dose of an intravenous induction agent is indicated to render the patient unconscious. Upper airway reflexes may also still be active and muscle relaxants may be needed to facilitate intubation. The patient may require some form of general anesthesia to maintain unconsciousness until the block wanes and spontaneous respiration returns. If the block is high enough then unconsciousness will occur, but consciousness may return before the patient can breathe spontaneously. The accidental injection of a large dose/volume of local anesthetic into the subarachnoid space can be a complication of extradural blockade and may result in a total spinal anesthetic.

Failure of block

Complete failure to produce any block when cerebrospinal fluid has been identified at the hub of the needle is very unusual. A problem with the local anesthetic solution may be responsible, but it is more likely that the tip of the needle has moved and the local anesthetic has not been injected into the subarachnoid space. Rarely, fluid-filled cysts in the subarachnoid space may be responsible, with membranes in the subarachnoid space limiting the spread of the local anesthetic.

Partial failure is a more common problem than complete failure and is usually due to insufficient dose of local anesthetic rather than the result of individual variation. The block can be repeated, but often a general anesthetic technique is more appropriate.

Urinary retention

Although the neural block provided by subarachnoid anesthesia usually only lasts for a few hours, urinary retention can sometimes be a problem even after the block has regressed. Some anesthesiologists routinely catheterize the bladder in patients having intrathecal anesthesia, either before or after the block has been instituted. If intravenous fluids have been administered as part of the management of the block, then this fluid may cause problems as it is excreted by the kidneys. Retention is a particular problem in the older male patients, who may have pre-existing problems related to prostatatic enlargement. Bladder catheterization is often associated with a transient bacteremia. This in itself does not usually cause problems, but there are groups of patients in whom the administration of prophylactic intravenous antibiotics (such as gentamicin) is advisable. These groups of patients include those having prosthetic joint replacements and those with valvular heart disease.

Extradural anesthesia

The techniques of extradural anesthesia and analgesia have become common in surgical patients following their introduction in the labor ward and obstetric operating room. Although extradural anesthesia for obstetric surgery has been superseded by spinal anesthetic techniques, extradural analgesia following major surgery is now commonplace in modern postoperative care.

The anatomical considerations for extradural anesthesia are similar to those for intrathecal anesthesia, although there are some important differences between the thoracic and lumbar vertebral bodies. Caudal anesthesia is a form of extradural anesthesia but the anatomical considerations are different and are described later. Anesthesia is provided by the effect of the local anesthetic drugs on the spinal nerve roots as they pass from the spinal cord to the periphery through the extradural space. Analgesia can be provided by the same mechanism, although the addition of other drugs (such as opioids) introduces other mechanisms of action such as effect(s) on receptors in the spinal cord.

Indications for extradural anesthesia

The indications for extradural anesthesia are similar to those for intrathecal anesthesia. As mentioned above, postoperative analgesia (of a high quality) can be provided either by intermittent injections or by continuous infusion using an extradural catheter, and this is probably the commonest indication for the technique.

Technique

Success is dependent upon the tip of the needle being accurately placed in the extradural space. As with intrathecal anesthesia, care with the positioning of the patient is vital. The awake patient can be placed in either the sitting or the lateral position. If the patient is anesthetized, then the lateral position is adopted. The choice of side that the patient lies on is not important. Reliable large-bore intravenous access should be established before extradural anesthesia is attempted. The practice of intravenous preloading with 500–1000 mL of intravenous fluid is common. The controversy surrounding the use of crystalloid/colloid vasopressors in the prevention of hypotension during extradural anesthesia is similar to that in intrathecal anesthesia. Strict asepsis is essential when extradural techniques are employed. If the patient is awake, the skin and subcutaneous tissues should be infiltrated with a local anesthetic solution (such as lidocaine) before the needle is inserted. It is common practice to use a Tuohy needle (see Fig. 37.2) for the identification of the extradural space. Awake patients should be reassured that the procedure should be painless though they may be aware of the needle insertion despite the generous use of local anesthesia.

The extradural space is usually identified by the use of the loss of resistance technique, which relies upon the inability to inject (either air or saline) through the Tuohy needle while the tip of the needle lies in the ligamentum flavum. Once the tip of the needle passes through the ligamentum flavum it should lie in the extradural space and injection should become possible. In practice, this can be difficult. The potential difficulties with extradural anesthesia are similar to those encountered with intrathecal anesthesia. The midline approach is the easier technique to adopt (see below for thoracic extradural anesthesia), but it is important to keep the needle in the correct position as even small angulations from the midline can cause problems.

The choice of site of introduction of the Tuohy needle is determined by the surgical incision. The insertion should be at the level of the middle of the dermatomes that innervate the area of the skin in which the incision will lie. However, once the patient is positioned it may be that the best interspinous space is one above or below the ideal level. Clearly, the anesthesiologist should balance the practical problems of a potentially difficult space against the benefits of a successful first-time identification of the extradural space.

Above the level of the first lumbar vertebral body there is a danger of direct damage to the spinal cord should accidental dural puncture occur. In general, the higher up the vertebral column, the larger the cord becomes and there is also relatively less cerebrospinal fluid surrounding the cord. In theory, thoracic extradural anesthesia and analgesia presents greater risk than the lumbar technique and serious controversy surrounds the placement of the extradural needle in the anesthetized patient. (See below for neurologic complications of central neural blockade.)

Lumbar extradural technique

Once a sterile field has been established (and local anesthetic infiltrated if appropriate), the Tuohy needle should be inserted in the midline of the chosen interspinous space. The lateral approach (described in the section on thoracic extradural technique) can be adopted if problems are encountered with the midline approach. A small incision in the skin will ease insertion. The needle passes through the subcutaneous tissues, the supraspinous ligament, the interspinous ligament, and then reaches the ligamentum flavum. There is often a characteristic feel to the needle at this point as it reaches the tough fibers of the ligamentum flavum, although this is not universal. Once the ligamentum flavum has been reached, the stylet should be removed from the needle and a syringe containing either air or saline attached to the needle. At this point it is (almost) impossible to inject into the ligamentum flavum and this is central to the loss of resistance technique for identification of the extradural space. Some anesthesiologists recommend the use of a well-lubricated glass syringe, others an ordinary plastic syringe, and yet others the use of a specially designed loss of resistance syringe.

Saline 0.9% or air can be used for the loss of resistance technique. Saline, being a liquid, is less compressible than air, and this is one reason advocated for the use of saline, as the identification of the extradural space is said to be more convincing. However, saline may flow from the end of the needle when the syringe is removed and this may mimic a dural tap. The flow of saline, however, is usually transient and saline will feel cold on the back of an ungloved hand, whereas CSF will feel warm. There should be no difficulty in correctly identifying a dural tap, particularly when this occurs in the sitting position, as the flow of CSF that results is usually obvious and continuous. If there is still doubt, a bedside glucose analysis strip will change color if the liquid is CSF. Obviously, if air is used, then fluid appearing at the end of the needle is likely to be CSF.[85]

Once attached, the needle is advanced very carefully through the ligamentum flavum until the extradural space is reached. The passage through the ligamentum flavum can be either a series of very small advances of the needle, with an attempt at injection after each advancement, or a very slow, controlled continuous movement forward with continuous pressure on the syringe plunger. Once the tip of the needle enters the extradural space, injection will become possible. The syringe is then removed from the needle and either an injection of local anesthetic solution given or a plastic catheter introduced into the extradural space.

If an injection of local anesthetic is planned, the injection should be made very slowly or in the form of 5-mL bolus injections.

If a catheter is to be placed in the extradural space, then it should pass easily through the needle. If difficulty is encountered in passing the catheter, a number of maneuvers can be employed to facilitate its passage into the extradural space. It is important to exercise great caution, as accidental dural puncture should be avoided because of the problems of postdural puncture headache that the large Tuohy needle will cause. First, one can reattach the syringe and attempt to inject again. It may be that the tip of the needle has come back into the ligamentum flavum and injection is not possible. Careful advancement of the needle should re-establish the position of the needle tip in the extradural space. If injection remains easy, the additional volume of air/saline may assist the passage of the catheter. If this is not successful, then careful advancement of the needle a very short distance may overcome the problem. If these maneuvers are unsuccessful at resolving the problem, the needle should be removed and another attempt made at finding the extradural space. One reason for difficulty in passing the catheter may be that the needle tip is not lying in the extradural space. If any length of catheter has already passed the tip of the Tuohy needle and resistance is encountered, the temptation to withdraw the catheter should be resisted as there is a small chance that this will lead to the end of the catheter being sheared off and left in the extradural space. The needle and catheter should be removed together.

In adult patients there are no advantages in passing the catheter more than 4 or 5 cm into the extradural space.

Before securing the catheter to the patient's skin with a plastic waterproof transparent dressing and waterproof adhesive tape, the anesthesiologist must aspirate the catheter to ensure that no blood or CSF is obtained. If blood is aspirated, then no local anesthetic drugs should be injected through the catheter. Pulling the catheter back 1 cm may remove the tip from the lumen of the blood vessel, but occasionally removal and replacement may be required. If CSF is aspirated, then the planned use of the catheter should be reassessed. The catheter could still be used to provide a spinal anesthetic but its use for continuous postoperative analgesia would have to be abandoned. Many anesthesiologists prefer to abandon their plans to use the catheter, remove it, and resite at a different level. Caution will be required with use of a new catheter and plans to deal with a dural headache may be needed.

After securing the catheter to the skin, the first dose of local anesthetic may be injected into the extradural space. Controversy surrounds the use of a "test dose," i.e. a small dose of local anesthetic with or without epinephrine to determine that the catheter is not in the subarachnoid space or in the lumen of a blood vessel. In theory, if the catheter is in a blood vessel, the injection of a small volume of an epinephrine solution will result in a tachycardia. This is not without risk in the patient with severe heart disease. If the catheter lies in the subarachnoid space, then the injection of a dose of local anesthetic similar to that used in intrathecal anesthesia should result in a sudden onset of loss of sensation and weakness in the legs in the awake patient. Hypotension may also develop swiftly. It is important that a false sense of security does not develop if a test dose has no adverse effects. Although it is rare, it is not unknown for extradural catheters to migrate into blood vessels or into the subarachnoid space after satisfactory test doses. The anesthesiologist must be vigilant at all times.

Selection of the therapeutic dose and choice of local anesthetic will be influenced by a number of factors, including the proposed use of the technique: is it for intraoperative anesthesia only, or will the catheter be used for postoperative analgesia as well? The use of a high concentration of the local anesthetic may be indicated to provide muscle relaxation intraoperatively but a dense motor block is not desirable once the patient has returned to the ward and a lower concentration (perhaps with the addition of an opioid) may be chosen. How large is the proposed incision? Larger incisions across more dermatomes will require larger volumes/doses of local anesthetic agents. The spread of the local anesthetic is variable and additional injections may be required to establish the desired level of sensory blockade.[86]

Thoracic extradural technique

For upper abdominal and thoracic surgery the extradural injection should be made in the thoracic part of the vertebral column as the dermatomal innervation for the surgery is located in this part of the spinal column. However, the incidence of cardiovascular side-effects may be increased (sympathetic innervation of the heart) and placement of the catheter can be technically more difficult than in the lumbar region because of the different structure of the vertebral bodies, in particular the angulation of the spinous processes.

Technique

Patient positioning and preparation are as for the lumbar approach. The patient can be sitting if the procedure is to be carried out with the patient awake. Accurate identification of the interspinous spaces can be difficult and it may be easier to count down from the prominent seventh cervical spinous process. When the midline approach is used, the needle will have to be directed far more in the cranial direction than for the lumbar approach. The loss of resistance technique is used but great care must be taken to avoid dural puncture as the ligamentum flavum is thinner in the thoracic region. There is also relatively less distance between the dura and the spinal cord in the thoracic region of the spinal column as the cord is relatively larger than in the lumbar region. Theoretically, this makes direct damage to the spinal cord more likely should an accidental dural puncture be performed. Many clinicians strongly advocate that this is a powerful indication for performing thoracic extradural anesthesia only in awake patients, even though it is easier for the anesthesiologist as a patient who is anesthetized will remain still.

If the midline approach is unsuccessful, the lateral or paramedian approach should be considered, and some experienced anesthesiologists use the lateral approach to the extradural space routinely in the thoracic region. The difficulties presented by the angles of the thoracic spinous processes and calcified interspinous ligaments are avoided by this approach. The needle is introduced about 1 cm from the midline and deliberately directed into the lamina of the thoracic vertebra. The depth at which this occurs should be noted. The needle is then withdrawn about 1 cm and redirected in a cranial and medial direction until the ligamentum flavum and the extradural space are identified in the usual fashion. It is important that the needle is not allowed to be introduced more than 1 cm beyond the depth at which the lamina was encountered if damage to the spinal cord is to be prevented. Once the catheter is in place, injection of local anesthetic drugs may then be performed after aspiration of the catheter etc., as for the lumbar extradural technique. Smaller volumes/doses of local anesthetics are required for a similar dermatomal spread when compared with the lumbar region.

Complications of extradural anesthesia

Dural puncture

An unrecognized dural puncture can place the patient at great risk, particularly when an extradural catheter technique is used. Large doses of local anesthetic drugs injected intrathecally can have rapid and dramatic effects on the cardiovascular and respiratory systems. The risk of developing a postdural puncture headache is high because of the large bore of the Tuohy needle, which leads to CSF leak. Aggressive management, as outlined above in the section on intrathecal block, should be considered.

Total spinal

Please refer to the section above on intrathecal block.

Blood vessel damage

It is unusual for the Tuohy needle to damage blood vessels in the extradural space, but damage is more likely when a catheter is introduced into the extradural space. Damage is more likely when intra-abdominal pressure is raised (ascites, large tumors, and patients in the later stages of pregnancy). If blood flows back through the catheter or is aspirated through the catheter it should be pulled back 1 cm and reaspirated. After withdrawing the catheter about 3 cm it is probably advisable to remove the catheter and introduce a new catheter in a different interspace. In a patient with normal coagulation the chances of serious sequelae are very small.

Hypotension

The sympathetic blockade provided by the extradural blockade can produce hypotension in the same fashion as during intrathecal anesthesia. Its management should be on the same lines, with the use of intravenous fluids and vasoactive drugs.

Urinary retention

Retention of urine is a common problem with extradural anesthesia, particularly when a catheter technique is adopted. Management is discussed in the section on subarachnoid anesthesia. It should be remembered that there is a significant incidence of urinary retention in patients who receive parenteral opioid analgesia, so the problem may still occur if extradural analgesia is avoided.

Neurological sequelae

See below.

Catheter problems

Occasionally, an extradural catheter may be difficult to remove. Catheters may be damaged on removal, and there have been cases in which several centimeters of catheter has been left in a patient's back. If difficulty is encountered, despite flexion of the spine, extension of the spine may make removal easier. If a piece of catheter is accidentally left behind, there has been debate over whether the patient should be informed. It is probably best to be honest, explain what has happened, and reassure the patient that the chances of adverse long-term sequelae are remote.

Local anesthetic toxicity

Adverse reactions to the injection of a large dose of local anesthetic drug into the extradural space may occur. There may be a number of reasons for such a reaction. Toxicity may result if the maximum recommended dose of the local anesthetic has been exceeded. Such a reaction is usually delayed for some minutes until the plasma level rises above that which will lead to signs and symptoms of toxicity (see earlier). If the reaction occurs soon after the injection, then the possibility of accidental intravascular injection must be considered. Such a reaction may occur with even a small dose of the local anesthetic drug.

Failure of block

Complete failure to produce any block at all, despite a convincing loss of resistance (and easy introduction of the extradural catheter), is not uncommon and suggests that the needle was not in the extradural space when the injection was made (or the catheter was passed). The procedure must be repeated to establish a block, but remember that, if large doses of local anesthetic drugs have already been administered, then further doses risk a toxic reaction.

Partial failure is a more common problem than complete failure and is usually due to insufficient dose of local anesthetic rather than the result of individual variation. Additional dose(s) of the local anesthetic usually resolves this problem.

Differential block

A common feature of extradural block, indeed a desirable feature when extradural analgesia is employed for obstetric analgesia, is differential block, in which different sensory modalities are blocked to different extents. Various mechanisms have been suggested to explain the phenomenon of differential block. These mechanisms include:

1. Blockade depends on the diameter of the axon.
2. Differential block is related to the time available for the drug to diffuse into nerves of different thickness – thus blockade of thicker motor nerves takes longer to achieve .
3. Blockade relates to the number of nodes blocked. The blockade of three consecutive nodes is required to prevent transmission of the action potential. This is particularly relevant when small lengths of nerve are exposed in areas limited by anatomical constraints. For example, during extradural anesthesia, blockade of three nodes is less likely to be achieved in motor fibers that have a greater internodal distance than in pain-carrying fibers.
4. There is a reduction in the induced current in successive nodes that are bathed in a weak solution of local anesthetic that is not in itself strong enough to abolish electrical activity completely. Conduction may therefore cease even if no individual node is blocked completely. This phenomenon is known as decremental conduction. In these circumstances the concentration of local anesthetic required to induce blockade is related inversely to the number of nodes exposed and therefore to the length of the exposed segment. Thus, C fibers, with their short internodal distances, are blocked by lower concentrations of local anesthetic than are A fibers, with their long internodal distances.
5. Alternatively, blockade of A fibers requires that a longer segment of nerve is exposed to local anesthetic of a given concentration. The length of nerves in the subarachnoid space is less for cervical than for sacral roots and, during subarachnoid block, the concentration of local anesthetic in the cerebrospinal fluid decreases with cephalad spread. Thus, at the upper extent of a subarachnoid block the combination of length of nerve exposed to anesthetic and the concentration of anesthetic to which it is exposed may be inadequate for blockade of A fibers while inducing near total blockade of C fibers. This is manifest clinically by sympathetic block extending roughly four segments higher than motor block.
6. Different agents have different ED_{50} values for different axon types and also for vagal or sympathetic axons. Drugs of low pK_a and high lipid solubility preferentially block A fibers rather than C fibers – thus ropivacaine, with low lipid solubility, preferentially blocks C fibers to a greater extent than does bupivacaine.

Caudal anesthesia and analgesia

Any surgical procedure performed on the perineum, anus, genitalia, and lower urinary tract can be performed under caudal anesthesia and the patient will benefit from the postoperative analgesia that a caudal block may provide. The anatomy is outlined in Fig. 37.3.

A needle inserted through the sacrococcygeal membrane will lie in the most distal part of the extradural space, and injection of local anesthetic will provide anesthesia and analgesia, as would an injection in the lumbar or thoracic extradural space. It is unusual for a catheter technique to be used because the lumbar region is a more convenient and easier site in which to secure a catheter and nurse postoperatively. Unfortunately, there is more variety in the normal anatomy than in other parts of the spinal column and therefore insertion of the needle is not always easy.

Technique

The patient can be placed in the prone or, more usually, the lateral position for the injection. The patient is placed in a lateral position with the knees drawn up to the chest. In the obese patient the uppermost buttock can overlie the midline and this may make palpation of the coccyx difficult. The usual conditions of sterility must be adopted with thorough skin cleaning and the use of sterile towels and gloves. The sacral hiatus is located by palpating the coccyx at the base of the spine and then moving the finger cranially. The sacral cornuae lie on either side of the hiatus and the finger will identify the hiatus as a hollow between the cornuae. If the patient is awake, the skin and subcutaneous tissues can be infiltrated with local anesthetic, although large volumes should be avoided as the landmarks may be obscured. The needle should be inserted at right angles through the skin and advanced into the sacral hiatus. Once the sacrococcygeal ligament is penetrated by the needle (a slight "give" or "pop" may be felt at this point), the needle direction should be changed to angle it up into the sacral canal. Once in place, the local anesthetic solution may be injected after careful aspiration. If blood is aspirated, a slight withdrawal of the needle usually rectifies the problem. The needle may be placed subcutaneously, in which case a swelling will be noted as the injection is started. Periosteal injection should be easily recognized as the injection will be very difficult. Repositioning of the needle usually corrects these problems. The local anesthetic injection should be made either very slowly or in 5-mL boluses. Attempted aspiration during the course of the injection is prudent. In the adult patient, 20 mL of the local anesthetic solution should produce a reliable anesthetic block of the sacral and most of the lumbar nerve roots. On occasions the block may extend higher.

Complications

Dural puncture Very rarely, CSF may be aspirated from the needle, as the subarachnoid space may descend into the sacral area in some individuals. Should this occur, injection of a large volume/dose of a local anesthetic into the subarachnoid space is clearly undesirable and the needle should be withdrawn and reaspiration attempted. If there is any doubt about the position of the needle then the procedure should be abandoned. A PDPH may occur.

Hypotension and urinary retention Management of these problems is discussed in the section on extradural blockade.

Neurologic complications of central neural blockade

Neurologic complications following central neural blockade fall into one of two categories: first, those that occur by coincidence with the central blockade; and, second, those that are directly related to the regional anesthetic procedure.

Central neural blockade is a safe anesthetic technique with a very low incidence of permanent neurological damage related directly to the procedures. There is much published work to support this.[87–91] However, there is no doubt that there are some factors that appear to increase the risk of neurologic damage following central blockade and, clearly, the anesthesiologist should be aware of these before considering the use of extradural or intrathecal anesthesia.

Such factors include:[92]

- physical trauma: injury from needle and catheter placement;
- chemical trauma: local anesthetic toxicity, wrong drug injected;
- ischemia following severe, prolonged hypotension: related to technique, unrelated to technique (anterior spinal artery syndrome);
- spinal hematoma: pathological and pharmacologic clotting problems;[93]
- systemic infection.[94]

While there are no large controlled studies and no incidence figures to support the logical fears that some of the above situations may generate, the final decision lies with the anesthesiologist, who may wish to discuss these with the patient. The true incidence of problems developing is probably small and the benefit to the individual patient may be great.

Anticoagulation and central neural blockade

Hemorrhagic complications can follow most regional anesthetic techniques. However, bleeding within the spinal canal may be unrecognized at the time of the placement of the block (intrathecal or extradural)[95] and may continue unrecognized, and, as the spinal canal is a confined space, an expanding space-occupying lesion may develop which may compress the contents of the spinal canal and can lead to catastrophic permanent neurologic damage. These lesions can remain masked by, or interpreted as, the effects of the central neural blockade, delaying prompt diagnosis and treatment. Spinal hematoma may be spontaneous, with no prior instrumentation in the region, or in association with therapeutic anticoagulant treatment, or with the pathology of the clotting mechanisms.

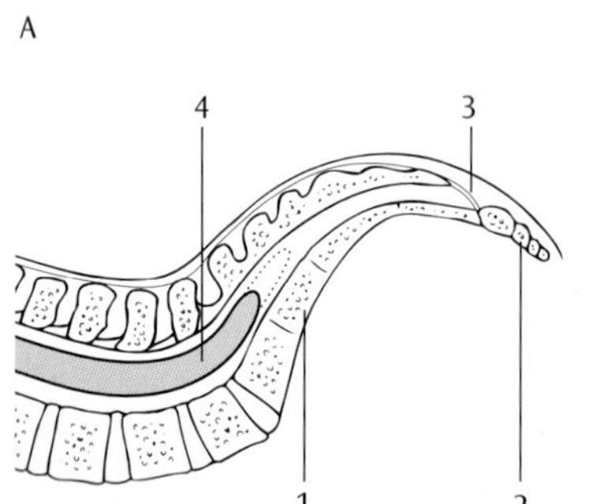

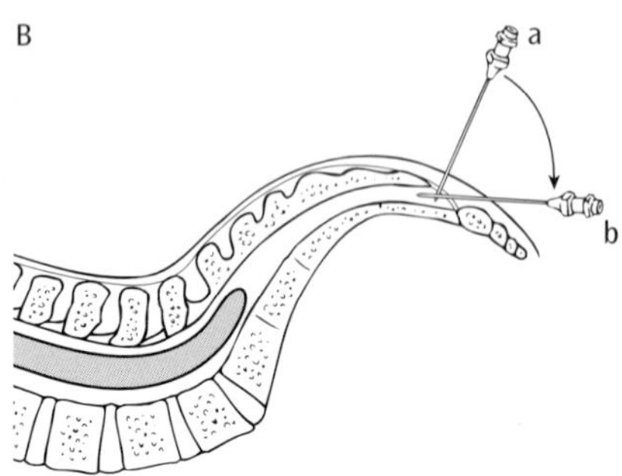

Figure 37.3 *Caudal extradural technique. (A) Anatomy: 1, sacrum; 2, coccyx; 3, sacrococcygeal membrane; 4, dural sac. (B) Technique: a, initial angle of needle for entry; b, position of needle for injection of anesthetic.*

There is no doubt that some therapeutic situations and illnesses affecting hemostasis clearly present risks. However, there has been much debate surrounding some of the therapeutic strategies designed to minimize the development of postoperative deep venous thrombosis and central neural blockade, particularly those involving the use of so-called low-dose anticoagulation. This debate led to the publication of *Recommendations for Neuraxial Anesthesia and Anticoagulation* following a consensus conference of the American Society of Regional Anesthesia in May 1998.[96] A summary of this document is contained in Table 37.8.

Every central neural block carries a risk.[92] While any increase in this small risk in the presence of pharmacologic attempts to minimize postoperative thrombosis may be difficult to quantify, the benefits of central neural blockade must not be overlooked. Postoperative extradural analgesia is now accepted. It has been recommended for high-risk surgical patients and shown to increase blood flow and contribute to fibrinolysis in the postoperative patient.[97]

When it is felt that there may be a slightly increased risk of hematoma development in the spinal canal, then a rigorous postoperative observation regime should be followed so that, if problems do develop, then these are detected quickly. The avoidance of higher concentrations of local anesthetic drugs, together with the careful use of adjuvant drugs such as low-dose opioids, will mimimize the chances of the development of motor block in the lower limbs and facilitate early diagnosis.

Consultation and cooperation between the clinicians involved in patient care will lead to optimal management with the maximum benefit provided to the patient from the anticoagulant drugs and the regional anesthetic technique.

Table 37.8 *Anticoagulation and central neural blockade*

Oral anticoagulants
Long-term therapy
Stop drug
? Convert to i.v. heparin and stop 4 h preoperatively
Restart postoperatively when hemostasis secure
Beware of interaction with other drugs affecting clotting

Low-dose DVT prophylaxis
If administered >24 h before surgery check INR before block
If administered after catheter insertion and >36 h since first dose check INR before removal
Routine neurological testing should be performed and continued after catheter removal
Use low concentrations of LA to minimize motor block

Antiplatelet drugs
There are no specific concerns regarding the use of antiplatelet drugs. Significance of interaction with other anticoagulant drugs is uncertain.

Fibrinolytic/thrombolytic drugs
Patients receiving or who have recently received or who may receive these drugs are at high risk of adverse bleeding. Great caution should be exercised if block used and routine neurologic testing should be performed.

Heparin
s.c. DVT prophylaxis
Avoid before block; avoid until 60 min after block; remove catheter 60 min before next dose.

i.v. therapeutic
Blocks should be avoided once established. If heparin started after catheter insertion, delay removal until heparin has been stopped for >4 h.

LMWH
Preoperative treatment
Block/catheter should be done 12 h after last dose

Postoperative treatment
Delay start 24 h postoperatively
? Remove catheters first
? Leave catheter and remove 2 h before next dose (10 h after last)
Use low concentrations of LA to minimize motor block

DVT, deep venous thrombosis; INR, international normalized ratio; i.v., intravenous; LA, local anesthetic; LMWH, low-molecular-weight heparin; s.c., subcutaneous. (From reference 96.)

PERIPHERAL REGIONAL BLOCKS

Wound infiltration

Simple infiltration along the wound margins is remarkably effective in promoting postoperative analgesia after minor surgery.[98] A prolonged effect may be obtained from local anesthetic irrigation via a catheter twice a day.[99]

Whether infiltration performed prior to incision reduces the total amount of pain compared with infiltration after skin suture (the concept of pre-emptive analgesia) is not clear.

Wound infiltration may not be as useful following abdominal surgery (in which much of the pain comes from deeper structures). For example, pain scores and morphine requirements following abdominal hysterectomy are not altered by wound infiltration,[100] nor is wound infiltration effective in reducing pain following open cholecystectomy.[101]

Many anesthesiologists routinely infiltrate lidocaine prior to venous cannulation with large cannula, an approach that significantly reduces in pain scores.[102]

To achieve analgesia for suturing lacerations, injection of local anesthetic from within the wound, as compared with through the intact skin, is less painful.[103] Local anesthetic infiltration of fracture sites is commonly performed in the emergency room for fracture manipulation, with acceptable results. Strict asepsis is crucial. Lidocaine, 1%, 10–15 mL, is injected into the periosteum around the fracture. Blood levels may rise rapidly, and therefore, for this and other blocks in the emergency room, resuscitation skills and equipment must be available.

BLOCKS ON THE TRUNK

Intercostal blocks

The three sensory branches of each intercostal nerve are:

1 a posterior cutaneous branch supplying skin and muscle in the paravertebral region;
2 a lateral cutaneous branch, arising anterior to the midaxillary line, supplying the skin over most of the thorax and abdominal wall;
3 an anterior cutaneous branch, supplying the front of the thorax, the sternum, and the front of the abdominal wall.

The areas of innervation of each nerve undergo significant overlap both vertically and across the midline. One must remember that the neuromuscular bundle lies in the costal groove behind the inferior margin of the rib. The nerve lies below the artery and vein.

Intercostal blocks are generally performed either at the angle of the rib or in the anterior axillary line. For blockade at the angle of the rib, just lateral to the sacrospinalis muscle, the patient is turned either three-quarters or fully prone. At the anterior axillary line the block can be performed with the patient supine or on the opposite side. There is evidence that distal spread along the rib may occur whichever site of injection is chosen.[104] Adjacent ribs may also be blocked by one large injection,[105] implying perhaps subpleural spread. At the angle of the rib there may also be spread into the extradural space via the paravertebral gutter.

For both approaches, the cardinal rule when performing an intercostal block is that one must be able to palpate the rib; otherwise, the chance of a successful block is low but the chance of pneumothorax is high. However, if the rib is palpated and the technique is sound, the success rate is very high. When blocking multiple ribs, most practitioners start with the most inferior rib and work upward. The safest technique which allows full control of the point of the needle at all times is as follows (see also Fig. 37.4):

1 Standing alongside the patient, the uppermost hand (for most people the left hand, while standing to the patient's right) firmly retracts the skin superiorly. The other (right) hand then places the point of the needle with attached syringe directly on to the rib.
2 As the skin retraction is slackened, the needle "walks" off the rib. As the needle slides off the rib, the point is advanced 2–3 mm only and 3–5 mL of anesthetic is injected. The aspiration test must be scrupulous in this very vascular area. Many practitioners use local anesthetic and vasoconstrictor to reduce the vascular uptake from this area, which would reduce the plasma anesthetic levels.
3 After injection, the needle is placed back on the rib just blocked while the upper hand palpates the next rib. This is necessary as otherwise it is surprisingly easy to block some ribs twice and others not at all.
4 The procedure is repeated as often as desired. For the upper ribs the point of injection should be more medial, with the shoulder abducted in order to avoid the scapula.
5 There is no need to change sides when performing bilateral blocks.

Intercostal blocks are indicated for pain relief following fractured ribs and for intra- and postoperative analgesia for operations on the abdominal wall (e.g. cholecystectomy) and chest wall (e.g. mastectomy). For prolonged analgesia after rib fractures, a catheter may be inserted.[106] For an indication of the extent of block required, a dermatome chart should be consulted. Bilateral blocks are required for abdominal surgery. (Performing bilateral blocks is considered controversial in view of the potential for causing bilateral pneumothoraces.) Less commonly considered, but very effective, is the use of intercostal blocks for lower abdominal surgery (e.g. appendicectomy).[107] However, intercostal nerve blocks following renal transplant surgery are associated with improved analgesia only in the first 4 h after surgery[108]

Some practitioners combine bilateral intercostal blocks with celiac plexus blocks for complete analgesia for intra-abdominal surgery. The role of the T12 block for analgesia after hip surgery is discussed below.

Pneumothorax is not as common a complication as one might expect (as long as the technique is sound) – the reported incidence is 0.073%.[109]

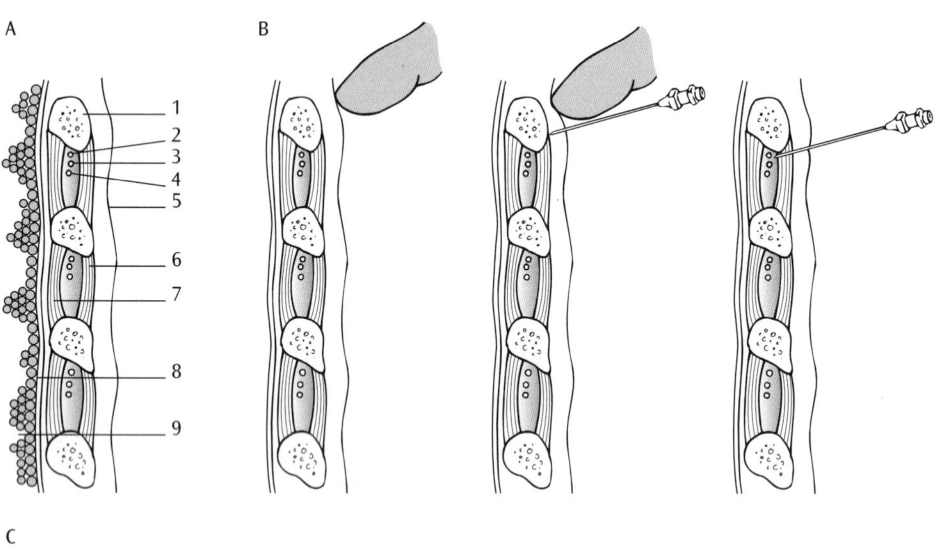

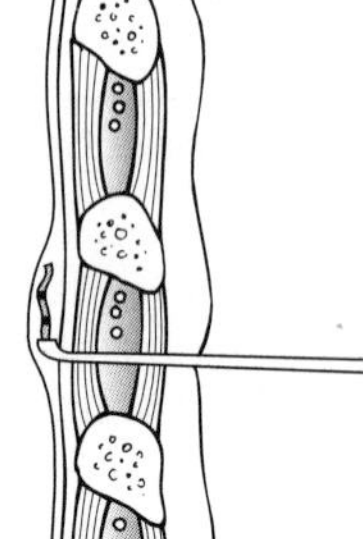

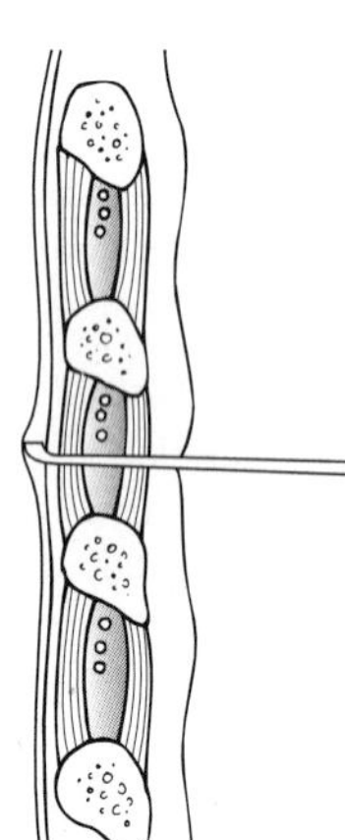

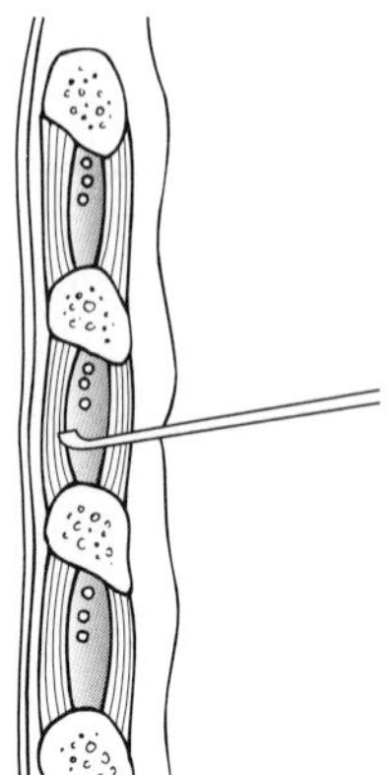

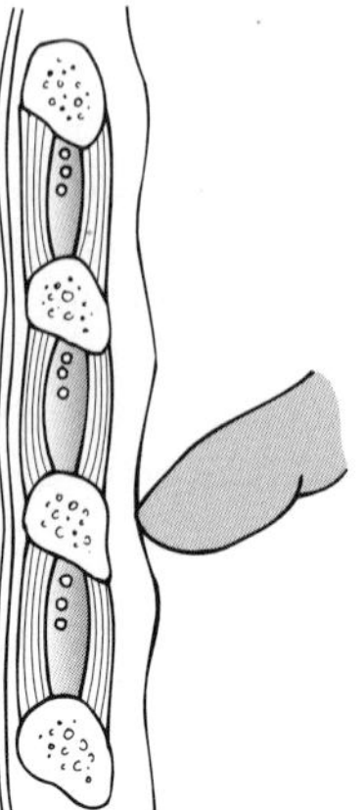

Figure 37.4 *Intercostal and intrapleural techniques. (A) Intercostal space in the midaxillary line: 1, rib; 2, intercostal vein; 3, intercostal artery; 4, intercostal nerve; 5, skin; 6, external intercostal muscle; 7, internal intercostal muscle; 8, parietal pleura; 9, lung. (B) Intercostal nerve block (see text for details). (C) Intrapleural catheter technique (see text for details).*

Intrapleural catheter block

This technique was first reported in 1984 for management of postoperative pain and has been used successfully for post-traumatic pain, especially in the management of fractured ribs.[110] The expected pain should be in the distribution of the intercostal nerves that will be bathed by the local anesthetic agent once it has been injected into the pleural cavity. This effectively means that the area from the second to the tenth intercostal nerves can be reliably blocked. As bilateral block is not recommended, midline incisions will require alternative methods of pain relief.

Special contraindications include obesity, which renders palpation of the ribs difficult or impossible, and previous lung disease, which increases the likelihood of pleural adhesions.

When the technique is to be used for postoperative pain management, the catheter may be inserted once the patient is anesthetized but generous local infiltration with lidocaine may be needed if the patient is awake while the catheter is inserted.

Technique

The patient should be positioned in the lateral position with the affected side uppermost. As with the intercostal block, it is mandatory that the ribs are palpable for this technique. Aseptic technique is also mandatory. In the anterior axillary line at the level of the third to the sixth ribs, depending upon which is most easily palpated, a Tuohy needle is inserted superior to the rib with the needle angle slightly upward (Fig. 37.4). A small incision with a scalpel blade will make insertion of the needle easier and offer better control of the needle as it passes through the chest wall, The negative pressure that exists inside the pleural space can be utilized to safely identify the endpoint in the insertion of the needle (the loss of resistance technique is not recommended).

Once the needle tip has passed into the subcutaneous tissues, a well-lubricated 10-mL glass syringe filled with sterile saline solution is attached to the needle. The two are then advanced slowly through the remaining chest wall. Artificial ventilation should be suspended at this point until the catheter has been inserted, to minimize the chances of damage to the visceral pleura. If the patient is awake and is able to do so, he or she should be asked to breathe out and remain in expiration until the needle is in the correct position. Once the posterior intercostal membrane is punctured (often with a "click") the parietal pleural membrane will be punctured shortly afterward and the barrel of the syringe pulled down by the negative intrathoracic pressure.

The syringe should be removed and, as quickly as possible, an extradural catheter inserted into the pleural space. At least 10 cm of catheter should be inserted before removing the Tuohy needle over the catheter. The catheter should then be covered with a sterile swab and waterproof tape dressing. After negative aspiration of the catheter for air or blood, 15–20 mL of 0.5% bupivacaine with epinephrine can be injected slowly over 5 min. Pain relief from a single injection can last for 6–9 h. A continuous infusion of local anesthetic, at a rate of 5–10 mL an hour, can provide longer-lasting pain relief, which is particularly effective with unilateral fractured ribs. When used for postoperative analgesia the catheter can be left in place for 48 h, but longer periods may be considered if required.

The catheter can also be placed in the thorax and passed out from the inside of the chest at thoracotomy by the surgeon.

Complications and side-effects

Rapid injection of local anesthetic may lead to high or toxic plasma levels of the local anesthetic. Lack of attention to detail may permit air to enter the pleural cavity during insertion of the catheter. Certainly, small amounts may be introduced if air is used instead of saline in the glass syringe. These small pneumothoraces can be demonstrated radiologically but, provided there has been no damage to the lung or visceral pleura, they will resolve spontaneously.

The significance of the introduction of a small amount of air at the beginning of a general anesthetic that features nitrous oxide is also a matter of debate and techniques have been described to minimize its occurrence.[111] The visceral pleura may be damaged by the Tuohy needle, and a pneumothorax requiring underwater seal drainage may be required.

Paravertebral block

As spinal nerves pass through the intervertebral foramina, they can be blocked with local anesthetic injections. Several adjacent nerves can be blocked by the injection of a large volume of local anesthetic into the paraverebral space, especially in the thoracic region. Catheter techniques have been described to permit prolonged analgesia.

Thoracic paravertebral block

The key anatomical landmark is the spinous process of the vertebral body. It is important to appreciate the relation between the spinous process and the transverse process of the vertebral body as this has its own characteristics in the thoracic region. The angle of the spinous process is greatest in the mid-thoracic region and the tip of the spinous process is at the level of the transverse process of the vertebra immediately below. Where the angulation is less severe (above T4 and below T9), the tip of the spinous process is approximately opposite the transverse process of the same vertebra. The midpoint of the desired area of block should be chosen as the point of injection. When several roots are to be blocked a volume of 10–20 mL of anesthetic solution may be required (approximately 5 mL per root).

Strict asepsis should be adopted for the procedure and, if the patient is awake, local anesthetic should be injected before the needle is inserted. Some workers recommend that the prone position be adopted, but the block can be performed with the patient in the lateral position with the block side uppermost. A 10-cm needle should be used. Once the appropriate level for the injection has been identified, a point 3–4 cm from the midline is chosen to introduce the needle and the needle is advanced until the transverse process is struck. The needle is then withdrawn slightly and redirected caudally to pass below the transverse process. Advancement of the needle 2–2.5 cm further should place the needle tip adjacent to the spinal nerve. Paresthesia may be produced in the awake patient. In the unconscious patient the use of a nerve stimulator may be helpful in placing the needle tip close to the nerve, but as the motor function of some of the thoracic nerves is small and may be difficult to observe, this technique may be of limited value. The injection of the local anesthetic should be made slowly in 5-mL boluses after careful aspiration.

Lumbar paravertebral block

The key anatomical landmark is the spinous process of the vertebral body, which in the thoracic region is opposite the corresponding transverse process. The midpoint of the desired area of block should be chosen as the point of injection, and when several roots are to be blocked a volume of 10–20 mL of anesthetic solution may be required. The technique is similar to thoracic paravertebral block, with the needle "walked off" the transverse process.

There has been some debate concerning the psoas sheath block and whether in some cases it is actually a lumbar paravertebral block that is produced.[112]

Complications

While the incidence of complications compares favorably with alternative techniques for unilateral analgesia,[113] the anesthesiologist should be aware of problems that can occur.

Toxicity

When large doses or volumes of local anesthetic are injected, there is always the possibility of toxicity.

Pneumothorax

Thoracic paravertebral block is associated with this complication. Management is by the standard method. An intercostal drain may be required.

Damage to individual spinal nerves

When this block is performed "blind" (i.e. without a peripheral nerve stimulator) in an anesthetized patient, there is always the risk of nerve damage. When performed in an awake patient, the patient will complain of severe pain should an injection be made into a nerve root, and paresthesia may be a symptom should the needle tip touch a nerve root in the awake patient.

Subarachnoid or extradural injection of local anesthetic

As the spinal nerve leaves the spinal cord, it is enveloped by tissue associated with the membranes that surround the spinal cord. Thus, it is possible for the local anesthetic injection to be placed in a tissue plane that may lead to the development of an extradural anesthetic and rarely an intrathecal anesthetic. Clearly, the inadvertent injection of a large volume of local anesthetic into the extradural or intrathecal space will lead to unexpected effects on the patient. If the patient is awake, then symptoms of an extradural block or total spinal block will be expressed and appropriate treatment should be instituted. In the anesthetized patient the only sign may be that of hypotension, which may be sudden and severe, requiring aggressive treatment with intravenous fluids and vasopressors.

Inguinal block

Traditionally employed for postoperative analgesia following surgery for an inguinal hernia,[114] this block may be useful for other operations for which the incision lies along the L1 dermatome (e.g. lower segment cesarean section[115]and hysterectomy).[116]

The inguinal region is supplied by the ilioinguinal and iliohypogastric nerves arising from T12, LI, and L2. The medial end of the lower part of the inguinal canal is supplied by the genital branch of the genitofemoral nerve arising from the same spinal levels. The ilioinguinal and iliohypogastric nerves may easily be blocked by generously instilling up to 20 mL of anesthetic between the external and internal oblique abdominal muscles. The point of injection is approximately 2 cm medial and 2 cm inferior to the anterior superior iliac spine. When a short-beveled needle is used, a definite "click" will be felt as the appropriate tissue plane is identified. If no click is identified, the solution should be infiltrated in a "fanwise" manner through the abdominal layers in several directions from the point of entry.

Some specialists routinely block the genital branch of the genitofemoral nerve for hernia surgery by a similar fanwise infiltration of 10 mL of anesthetic at the inferior end of the inguinal canal. However, others do not, as postoperative analgesia seems effective in its absence. Midline infiltration of local anesthetic may be required if an overenthusiastic surgeon has extended the incision across the midline.

Penile blocks

In many centers penile blocks are increasingly employed for intraoperative and postoperative analgesia for surgery of the penis. The technique is simple and may be preferred to caudal analgesia owing to the lack of effect on motor power and avoidance of urinary retention. The dorsal nerve of the penis is a terminal branch of the pudendal nerve and passes under the symphysis pubis to pass along the penis on the dorsal surface of the corpora cavernosa. At the symphysis pubis a branch is given off to supply the ventral surface and frenulum. A commonly used technique is to "walk off" the symphysis pubis with a fine, short needle and deposit 5–10 mL of 0.25% bupivacaine (less in infants and children) approximately 5 mm below the bone.[117] Occasionally, a click will be felt as Buck's fascia is penetrated. Other practitioners inject half the total dose on each side of the midline at an angle of approximately 15°. A third technique is to perform a superficial "ring" block around the base of the penis. However, in a recent study the use of a ring block produced inferior analgesia and more frequent problems from tissue swelling and edema than did penile block.[118]

Complications mainly arise if the dorsal vessels are punctured or the corpora cavernosum entered, leading to failed block, intravascular injection, or hematoma formation. Hematoma or excessive volumes of anesthetic can result in compression ischemia. A total dose of 10 mL in adults should not be exceeded to minimize the risk of compression whichever technique is employed. The use of vasoconstrictor-containing anesthetics at the base of the penis must be avoided because spasm of the vessels and profound ischemia may ensue. Performing a caudal block, if such accidents occur, has been recommended to promote sympathetic block and vasodilation.[118]

UPPER LIMB BLOCKS

Cervical plexus block

This is included here for convenience although not strictly an upper limb block. The anterior primary rami of C2, C3, and C4 unite to form the cervical plexus as they leave the intervertebral foramina and pass between the anterior and medial scalene muscles posterior to the sternocleidomastoid muscle, approximately halfway down its length. The superficial plexus is easily blocked by a fanwise injection of 10 mL of anesthetic at the point at which the external jugular vein crosses the posterior edge of the sternocleidomastoid muscle. This will provide surface analgesia in the distribution of the C2–C4 nerve roots – that is the neck above the clavicle, the upper shoulder area, and a lateral area of the cranium around the ear.

Both the superficial and deep plexuses may be blocked by injecting 2–3 mL of anesthetic at each transverse process of the cervical vertebra or, less reliably, by injecting a larger volume of 6–10 mL at just one site. (Anesthetics containing vasoconstrictors should not be used because of the proximity of the vertebral artery and other vessels.) This will provide deeper analgesia, for example for thyroid surgery or tracheostomy. Deep cervical plexus block will also cover the posterior rami, providing analgesia around the back of the neck and occiput. However, extreme caution must be exercised because of the risk of both vascular and dural puncture. Convulsions will result from injection of even very low doses of local anesthetic into the vertebral artery.

Bilateral blocks may be complicated by respiratory distress as the stellate ganglion, recurrent laryngeal nerve, and phrenic nerve can all be affected during deep cervical plexus block. Cervical plexus block is a recognized "complication" of the interscalene approach to the brachial plexus.

Brachial plexus block

Brachial plexus block is a valuable addition to a general anesthetic for surgery of the upper limb or a suitable alternative to general anesthesia in certain patients. Brachial plexus blocks are among the most commonly performed, and most commonly studied, peripheral blocks owing to their high success rate and their ability to provide prolonged postoperative analgesia. In addition, the sympathetic block produced is of value for arm or hand reimplantation surgery or to establish a vascular shunt for dialysis.

The anatomy of the brachial plexus is complex and should be studied in a standard anatomy textbook for detailed description. Successful blockade of the branches of the plexus relies on the fact that these branches are enveloped in a tubular sheath of fascia. Thus, if one branch is identified by eliciting paresthesiae or by using a nerve stimulator, and a reasonably large volume of anesthetic is injected, blockade of the entire plexus may be predicted. Only the three main approaches to the plexus are discussed here: interscalene, supraclavicular, and axillary. For a more complete discussion, see the Further reading section.

Note: owing to the large volumes of anesthetic required, many anesthesiologists attach an extension set to the needle so that the needle point may be held immobile during injection, syringe removal, and syringe reattachment.

Interscalene approach

The roots of the plexus exit from their intervertebral foramina and pass laterally and inferiorly between the anterior and middle scalene muscles, uniting to form three main trunks. The interscalene groove can usually be palpated posterior to the sternocleidomastoid muscle. With the patients head turned to the opposite side, the needle tip should be inserted at the level of the transverse process of the sixth cervical vertebra (the level of the cricoid cartilage - often the level where the sternocleidomastoid is crossed by the external jugular vein) in a slightly posterocaudal direction until paresthesiae or muscle contractions with the nerve stimulator are elicited. The transverse process is often only about 2 cm below the skin, and care should be taken to prevent damage to deeper structures. A large volume of up to 40 mL of anesthetic is required to ensure blockade of the entire plexus.[119] Lower volumes may result in sparing of the lower trunk (i.e. chiefly the ulnar nerve). Cervical plexus block is also achieved, resulting in analgesia of the shoulder region. Indeed, interscalene brachial plexus block is the analgesic technique of choice for shoulder surgery and may reduce intraoperative blood loss.[120]

Of all the approaches to the brachial plexus, the interscalene approach is most commonly associated with blockade of the following:

1 the phrenic nerve, resulting in unilateral diaphragmatic paresis, reducing pulmonary function by up to 25%;
2 the sympathetic chain, resulting in Horner syndrome;
3 the recurrent laryngeal nerve, resulting in hoarseness; and, more rarely
4 accidental intrathecal or extradural injection;
5 direct injection into the vertebral artery, causing convulsions.

Supraclavicular block

Of the three common approaches to brachial plexus block, this is the most hazardous owing to the risk of pneumothorax. This is not to discourage practitioners, but this approach may be relatively contraindicated for the obese patient or for any patient in whom the landmarks are difficult to palpate.

However, at the level of the supraclavicular approach the brachial plexus is arranged in a very compact space as the plexus crosses the first rib, and thus inclusion of all three trunks in the block may be predicted. If surgical conditions permit, one may ask the awake patient to try to stretch the arm on the side to be blocked down toward the patient's foot. With the patient's head turned to the opposite side, the subclavian artery may be palpated about 1 cm posterolateral to the midpoint of the clavicle. If this is so, the point of insertion of the needle is immediately lateral to this point at about 80° to the skin. If paresthesiae are not obtained, the needle is advanced until the first rib is contacted. The needle is then "walked" in the longitudinal direction of the rib until paresthesiae or evoked muscle contractions with the nerve stimulator are obtained, at which stage the needle point is assumed to lie within the sheath. If the artery is not palpated, the first rib should be sought approximately 1 cm posterolateral to the midpoint of the clavicle.

When the needle point is thought to be within the sheath, 30 mL of anesthetic should be injected after aspiration. Up to 30 min may he required for complete anesthesia to be obtained.

With careful technique, the incidence of pneumothorax is probably as low as 0.5 %. Horner syndrome and phrenic nerve palsy may also develop. Bilateral supraclavicular blocks are contraindicated by the risks of bilateral pneumothoraces and phrenic nerve paralysis (and by the toxic doses of local anesthetic that would be required). Damage to the lung or pleura may provoke a cough at the time of injection. A chest radiograph should be performed if the patient complains of cough, pleuritic pain, or dyspnea at or after performance of the block. However, it should be remembered that a small leak may take some time to result in a pneumothorax large enough to cause symptoms or show on a radiograph. Thus, if the radiograph is performed immediately, a false sense of security may ensue. Many specialists do not routinely obtain screening chest radiographs in asymptomatic patients.

Axillary block

Owing to the lack of risk of pneumothorax and the ease of execution, this is the favored approach to the brachial plexus for many anesthesiologists. There is a high success rate - up to 92% in some series.[121] This block is performed most easily when the head is turned to face the opposite direction and the arm abducted to 90°. The axillary artery is palpated as proximal as possible in the axilla. A short-beveled needle inserted over the pulse toward the axilla will result in a characteristic "click" as it penetrates the sheath (often surprisingly superficial). The needle should then oscillate with the pulse beat. If blood is aspirated, this is good evidence that the needle tip is within the sheath and the needle should be withdrawn until the needle tip is no longer within the vessel. Deliberate puncture of the artery is a feature of this approach to axillary block. Despite concerns regarding vascular damage and hematoma formation it seems that this approach to axillary block is safe.[122]

Using a nerve stimulator, it is possible to confuse the endpoint of axillary brachial plexus blockade if one causes direct stimulation of the head of biceps muscle. Evoked muscle contraction below the elbow should be sought as no muscle crosses the elbow joint, thus avoiding potential direct muscle stimulation.

Up to 40 mL of anesthetic is required, especially if spread to the more proximal parts of the plexus is desired. This may be encouraged by applying digital pressure over the sheath distal to the point of injection, both during and after the injection. A tourniquet should not be used during needle placement as this may cause collapse of the vessels, a false-negative aspiration test, and inadvertent intravascular injection of anesthetic. A catheter may be placed in the sheath for prolonged analgesia. Intermittent bolus injections through the catheter result in lower plasma levels compared with continuous infusion for equivalent analgesia.[123]

Axillary block is very safe but there is no room for complacency. A recent report demonstrated that if injection is made outside the sheath, i.e. a failed block, the resulting plasma levels will be higher than if the block is successful.[124]

Note that with the axillary approach, the musculocutaneous nerve may not be blocked as it leaves the sheath proximal to the site of axillary block, so an area on the radial side of the forearm may not be covered by axillary block unless this nerve is blocked separately. As the nerve passes through the coracobrachialis muscle, it can be infiltrated with anesthetic at the level of the needle insertion for the axillary block. With a large volume of local anesthetic injected by the axillary approach and massaged proximally up the sheath, this separate injection may not be necessary.

Some advantages and disadvantages of the three main approaches to brachial plexus blockade are shown in Table 37.9.

DISTAL ARM BLOCKS

Blockade of the more distal nerves of the arm may be useful as a supplement to an inadequate brachial plexus block or for surgery when a brachial plexus blockade is inappropriate (e.g. difficult anatomy, bilateral surgery). Because the origins of the innervation of the forearm are proximal to the elbow, the functional result in the hand will be similar if the nerves are blocked at either the wrist or elbow. Paresthesiae or evoked muscular contractions with the nerve stimulator may be used. Alternatively, fanwise infiltration in the appropriate areas will usually suffice.

Ulnar nerve

An injection of 5 mL of anesthetic can be made between the olecranon and medial epicondyle of the elbow along the ulnar groove. The nerve is very superficial at this point, and care should be taken to avoid intraneural injection. At the wrist, 5 mL of anesthetic can be infiltrated from the deep fascia and bone to the subcutaneous tissues between the ulnar side of the ulnar artery and the radial side of the flexor carpi ulnaris.

Median nerve

An infiltration of 5–10 mL of anesthetic can be made in fanwise manner at several levels just medial to the brachial artery in the antecubital fossa. At the wrist, 5 mL of anesthetic is infiltrated in a similar fashion to ulnar nerve block at the wrist, between the palmaris longus and the flexor carpi radialis.

Radial nerve

It is uncommon to block this nerve at the level of the elbow. At the wrist, 5–10mL of anesthetic solution can be infiltrated subcutaneously along the radial border of the wrist for a simple and effective block.

Note that for all wrist blocks, care must be taken to prevent damage to, or accidental injection into, the arteries and numerous small veins in this area.

Digital nerve block

Simple surgery on the digits can be performed under "ring" block of the digital nerves or the block can be performed for postoperative analgesia. Each digit is supplied by two dorsal and two palmar or plantar nerves running along the digit. All four branches need to be blocked for successful analgesia. Small digits will probably be blocked by instilling 2 mL of anesthetic containing no vasoconstrictor on each side of the base of the digit using a fine, short needle. Larger digits will benefit from 1–2 mL injected both superficially and deeply on both sides of the digits to ensure that all four branches are reached. Care should be taken and smaller volumes used if the digit is already traumatized, as the circulation may be more readily compromised.

Intravenous regional anesthesia (Bier's block)

Intravenous regional anesthesia (IVRA or Bier's block) has a long history and is an accepted part of anesthetic and emergency department practice.[125] It is a safe technique with a long and proved track record, but care and attention to detail are the best protection against complications. Technical or operator error is responsible for most failures or adverse effects.

Table 37.9 *Comparison of different approaches to brachial plexus blocks*

	Interscalene	Supraclavicular	Axillary
Advantages	Landmarks usually easy to identify, even in obese patients	Reliable complete block of all three trunks	No risk of pneumothorax
	Does not require change in patient position Shoulder analgesia included Minimal risk of pneumothorax Rapid onset (usually in 15 min)	No movement of arm for performance	Suitable for most hand surgery Catheters may be inserted Paresthesiae not essential
Disadvantages	Ulnar nerve may be missed Potential rare but serious complications	Slow onset without paresthesiae Risk of pneumothorax	Arm abducted for performance Usually inadequate for upper arm surgery
		May be contraindicated in respiratory cripples as risk of pneumothorax and phrenic nerve paralysis	Circumflex nerve and musculocutaneous nerve often missed as left sheath more proximal Area at base of thumb (radial) may be missed
Special complications	Intrathecal/extradural Vertebral artery injection Phrenic nerve paralysis Horner syndrome Recurrent laryngeal nerve paralysis	Phrenic nerve paralysis Horner syndrome	Intravascular injection Hematoma due to artery puncture

There is some controversy over whether IVRA works via the nerve trunks or the peripheral nerve endings. Radiographic studies[126] have shown that the local anesthetic accumulates around the antecubital fossa and so blocks the vascular nerve trunks of the median and ulnar nerves prior to blocking the less vascular radial nerve. Because the anesthetic is carried into the vascular core of the nerve trunks, the block starts distally (innervated by the more central fibers of the nerve at the vascular core) and progresses proximally to the elbow. This is an interesting contrast with, for example, brachial plexus blockade, in which the anesthetic diffuses inwards through the nerve trunk. Thus, the inner fibers supplying the distal part of the arm are affected last and the block progresses distally.

IVRA can be used for manipulations of fractures of the forearm and minor surgery of the hand and forearm. A peripheral cannula is inserted as distal as possible in the forearm to be operated upon. A second cannula must be inserted in the opposite arm to permit access to the circulation if required. A double pneumatic tourniquet cuff is applied to the upper arm and then an exsanguinator is used to exsanguinate the arm below. If the arm is too painful to permit exsanguination, the arm may be elevated for 2 min.

Ideally, the pulse occlusion pressure should be measured using the operative tourniquet and a pulse oximeter or by manually palpating the radial artery. The tourniquet should then be inflated to 13.3 kPa (100 mmHg) above the pulse occlusion pressure. The use of pulse occlusion pressure is the safest method, particularly when the patient has a large arm. However, systolic blood pressure plus 13.3 kPa (100 mmHg) is widely used and it has been demonstrated over time to be safe. The tourniquet should remain connected to the pressure gauge at all times: cross-clamping is dangerous.

Up to 40 mL of anesthetic is then injected into the vein in the exsanguinated arm. A characteristic mottling of the skin will be seen. It is generally recommended that a distal vein is used. Radioisotope studies have shown that proximal injection is associated with raised venous pressures, leading to increased leak under the tourniquet. The same study showed that rapid injection was also associated with venous pressures of up to 33.3 kPa (250 mmHg) and recommended an injection time of at least 90 s. Leakage of local anesthetic via intraosseous veins has been postulated, but there is no conclusive evidence for its occurrence.

In the UK and Europe, prilocaine, 0.5%, 3 mg kg^{-1} (preservative-free), is the standard agent, giving a normal dose of around 40 mL. This is not the case in the USA, where prilocaine is not licensed by the Food and Drug Administration (FDA) for use in IVRA. In the USA, preservative-free lidocaine, 0.5%, 3 mg kg^{-1}, is standard practice. The great advantage of prilocaine over lidocaine is that the peak plasma concentrations are never as high for the same dose administered.[127] One concern in the USA is that prilocaine can cause methemoglobinemia, leading to a cyanotic color. For this to be clinically significant, levels of methemoglobin must be greater than 10%, and it has been shown that following IVRA with prilocaine methemoglobin levels are never greater than 3%.[127] Bupivacaine has been widely used in the past but is no longer approved for this purpose owing to deaths from cardiac toxicity.[128]

Once anesthesia is obtained after 10–15 min, the proximal cuff can be inflated on the anesthetic upper arm and the distal cuff then deflated. This will tend to ameliorate "tourniquet pain."

Anesthesia is limited by the allowable duration of occlusion of circulation to the arm, but in any case the distal cuff should not be deflated for at least 20 min. By this time, most of the anesthetic will have "fixed" to the tissues and there should be no overt toxicity. Intermittent deflation followed by full reinflation of the cuff to limit washout of anesthetic into the circulation has also been advocated. Once the circulation is restored, residual analgesia is short lived (which tends to contradict the assumption that the anesthetic is fixed to the tissues). The use of anesthetic solutions containing epinephrine in an attempt to prolong the block is dangerous. IVRA is contraindicated in situations in which tourniquets are contraindicated (e.g. sickle cell or Raynaud's disease). Although theoretically possible, lower limb IVRA is not often performed owing to the large volumes (60–80 mL) of anesthetic required.

Although it is a very simple technique, many surgeons find the relaxation obtained to be poor, with better conditions the more distal the procedure. Other limitations include inadequate duration of anesthesia, wet tissue planes for delicate hand surgery, and the short duration of analgesia after tourniquet deflation. Different drugs have been investigated as additions to the standard technique in an attempt to resolve some of these problems. Opioids are probably not helpful. Ketamine[129] used alone will provide anesthesia but is not recommended perhaps because of the obvious side-effects when the cuff is deflated. The addition of nonsteroidal anti-inflammatory drugs (NSAIDs) is well supported by studies. For example, Ketorolac, 20 mg, has been shown to provide improved postoperative analgesia[130] when added to lidocaine, compared with systemic ketorolac at the same dose. A more controversial additive is a muscle relaxant. The addition of 2 mg of atracurium provides improved muscle relaxation.[131] However, the use of muscle relaxants could produce a clinical effect in a small group of patients who are sensitive to small amounts of nondepolarizing muscle relaxants, and therefore one cannot recommend this practice. The addition of sodium bicarbonate to prilocaine is useful and produces a block of faster onset and more intense anesthesia.[132]

Many doctors in the UK, particularly in the emergency department, perform IVRA without the assistance of anesthesiologists. However, there is always the potential for severe toxic reactions, especially if there is sudden, early, or unexpected cuff deflation. The double tourniquet must be checked regularly and shortcuts in technique avoided. Therefore, any practitioner performing IVRA must be skilled in airway management, resuscitation, and recognition of signs of local anesthetic toxicity. Even if such skills are possessed, the use of IVRA by a single operator/anesthesiologist is to be deprecated.

BLOCKS FOR LOWER LIMB SURGERY

Lower limb surgery is easily performed under central neural block. Many practitioners have in the past, because of the availability of central neural blocks, neglected lower limb peripheral block (unlike upper limb surgery, for which central neural blocks have never been an alternative).

However, on occasion, central neural block may be contraindicated, even if only by patient refusal or preference for general anesthesia. On such occasions, the ability to perform lower limb peripheral blocks for postoperative analgesia is important.

Lumbar plexus or psoas sheath block

The lumbar plexus forms within the psoas sheath and, as such, can be blocked if a large volume of anesthetic (up to 40 mL) is deposited after loss of resistance or a "pop" is felt on entering the compartment. The patient is positioned fully or three-quarters prone and the tip of a Tuohy needle is "walked off" the transverse process of the L3 vertebra.

The correct compartment is usually reached approximately 1–3 cm beneath the transverse process. A nerve stimulator may be used to produce evoked contractions of the quadriceps muscles. In view of the large volume required, the variability found for the site of injection, and the resulting potential for complications, some practitioners do not advocate the block.[133] However, others report success in providing analgesia for hip surgery.[134] The requirements for turning the patient and the large volumes required have led to the development of an inguinal approach to the main components of the lumbar plexus – the so-called "3-in-1" block.

Femoral and "3-in-1" blocks

Femoral nerve block

The femoral nerve is the main product of the lumbar plexus and runs into the leg deep to the inguinal ligament in the groove between the psoas major and iliac muscles. In the inguinal region it lies approximately 1 cm lateral to the femoral artery, which is the main landmark sought for its effective blockade. The femoral nerve divides into a superficial branch supplying the anterior surface of the thigh and sartorius and pectineus muscles and a deep branch supplying the quadriceps muscles, articular branches to the hip and knee joints, and terminating as the saphenous nerve. This division is variable and may occur above the inguinal ligament. It is important to realize that the femoral nerve is deep to both fascia lata and fascia iliaca while the artery and vein are only deep to fascia lata; that is, they are not all in the same neurovascular compartment.

Blockade is achieved by injection of 10 mL of local anesthetic with one of two techniques. Using a nerve stimulator, the nerve may be located lateral to the artery in anesthetized or sedated patients. Alternatively, if two "pops" are felt using a short-beveled needle just lateral to the artery, blockade can be predicted with or without eliciting paresthesiae.

Blockade of the femoral nerve provides analgesia for knee surgery, relieves muscle spasm and pain from fractures off the femur,[135] and can be used as the sole anesthetic for muscle biopsy as an investigation into malignant hyperthermia susceptibility or for the donor site for skin grafts. Classic teaching is that complete analgesia is not achieved unless the other nerves supplying the knee, especially the sciatic nerve, are blocked. However, a recent study found that the addition of a sciatic block did not add to the analgesia following femoral nerve block.[136] Another study demonstrated excellent analgesia for anterior cruciate ligament reconstruction from femoral nerve block.[137]

Complications (e.g. intravascular injection, hematoma, and nerve damage) are uncommon with careful technique. Femoral nerve block is contraindicated in the presence of artificial grafts to the femoral artery.

"3-in-1" block

Winnie described the "3-in-1" block, whereby injection of up to 30 mL of local anesthetic by one of the above methods enables blockade of the other two main components of the lumbar plexus, namely the lateral cutaneous nerve of the thigh (supplying the skin on the lateral aspect of the thigh) and the obturator nerve (supplying the adductor muscles of the thigh and articular branches to both the hip and knee joints). This technique relies on the large volume of anesthetic filling up the fascial canal and traveling upward toward the lumbar plexus (cf. the brachial plexus block). However, either lateral cutaneous nerve block or obturator nerve block may not be achieved, and this block has been described as "femoral block with overdosage."[133] In view of the importance of blocking both the femoral and the lateral cutaneous nerve for hip surgery, specific blockade of each with 10 mL of anesthetic may be preferred, although single "3-in-1" block can be effective in producing analgesia following surgery for a fractured neck of femur.

Continuous low-dose "3-in-1" block has been shown to significantly improve postoperative pain relief following knee[138] and hip[139] replacement.

Lateral cutaneous nerve of thigh block

This nerve enters the thigh by passing under the lateral attachment of the inguinal ligament 1–2 cm medial to the anterior superior iliac spine. The anterior superior iliac spine thus acts as the chief landmark for individual blockade of this nerve. Using a short-beveled needle, 10 mL of anesthetic can be deposited under the fascia lata 1–2 cm both inferior and medial to the anterior superior iliac spine. A "pop" and loss of resistance indicate puncture of the fascia. The success rate can be improved by employing a fanwise injection of a larger volume of anesthetic around this point. A nerve stimulator is of no help for performing this block in the anesthetized patient because the nerve is purely sensory. In addition to surgery for fractures of the femur, this block is also useful for analgesia of skin graft donor sites.

T12 or the subcostal nerve supplies fibers to the ilioinguinal and iliohypogastric nerves and also supplies a small area of skin laterally at the extreme top of the thigh. It has been shown that analgesia following hip surgery is improved by blocking T12 by subcutaneously infiltrating anesthetic across the top of the iliac crest.[140]

Obturator block

Blockade of the obturator nerve is rarely performed in isolation but is required, along with femoral and sciatic nerve block, for complete anesthesia of the knee. However, postoperative analgesia following knee surgery seems adequate if only the others are blocked. The obturator nerve may be included in the femoral "3-in-1" technique but this is controversial. Occasionally blockade of the obturator nerve is helpful in cases of spasm of the adductor muscle of the hip, e.g. following cerebrovascular accident.

The easiest method of blocking the obturator nerve is to abduct the upper leg and insert a needle between the adductor tendons inserting into the pubis. If this needle is advanced toward the ipsilateral anterior superior iliac spine, either the obturator foramen or the bony margins of this foramen will be encountered. In either event, manipulation of the needle tip and the use of a nerve stimulator should enable identification of the obturator nerve by producing contraction of the adductor muscles. A dose of 10 mL of local anesthetic should be sufficient.

Sciatic nerve block

The sciatic nerve arises from the sacral plexus and is the largest peripheral nerve in the body. The nerve leaves the pelvis through the sciatic notch or foramen, and passes through the saddle area beneath the gluteus maximus to enter the thigh approximately equidistant between the ischial tuberosity and the greater trochanter of the femur. There are three main approaches:[141]

1 The posterior approach historically has been the most popular. A needle at least 10 cm in length will be needed even in thin patients, owing to the distance from skin to the nerve. The patient is placed on the opposite side from that to be blocked, with the uppermost leg flexed at the hip and knee joints (i.e. the recovery position). A line may be drawn or imagined between the greater trochanter of the femur and the posterior superior ischial spine. The point of skin entry is approximately 4 cm caudally from the midpoint of this line and the nerve is usually found at 8–10 cm of depth. The needle point may have to be "walked" until paresthesiae or evoked muscular contractions are elicited (movements of the foot should be sought to avoid confusion with direct muscle stimulation).

2 Possibly the easiest is the lithotomy approach, performed with the patient lying supine with one leg supported with both the hip and the knee flexed to 90° – similar to being in lithotomy position. Here the nerve is relatively superficial and held taut like a bowstring. The needle is inserted perpendicular to the skin midway between the greater trochanter of the femur and the ischial tuberosity. If the leg muscles are well defined this is through the groove between the biceps femoris and semitendinosus muscles. The nerve may be as little as 4 cm below the surface using this technique.
3 The anterior approach has the advantage that it can be performed with the patient supine without painful movements. A line is visualized or drawn from the greater trochanter to the lesser trochanter, parallel to the inguinal ligament. A 10-cm needle should be inserted at this level such that it can be "walked" off the medial border of the femur. Paresthesiae or evoked muscular contractions should be sought approximately 5 cm beyond the femur. Unfortunately, owing to variations in anatomy, the success rate is lower with this approach.

Paresthesiae or evoked muscular contractions with the nerve stimulator should be sought. A recent study suggests that a higher success rate will be achieved by using a nerve stimulator than by eliciting parasthesiae.[4]

For all approaches, 20 mL of anesthetic should be injected. With such a volume the posterior cutaneous nerve of the thigh is also usually blocked. Owing to the size of the sciatic nerve, up to 30 min may be required to achieve full analgesia.

BLOCKS AROUND THE KNEE

Intra-articular local anesthetic for arthroscopy

Arthroscopy of the knee is a common surgical procedure, often performed as a "day-case" procedure. Effective analgesia, therefore, must not restrict the potential for discharge, thus limiting the role of, for example, femoral nerve block. Useful analgesia is achieved by injecting 10–20 mL of local anesthetic into the joint cavity at the end of the procedure. Infiltration of anesthetic around the instrument entry ports is also recommended. The addition of 1 mg of morphine to the anesthetic solution injected into the joint cavity may improve analgesia by an effect on peripheral opioid receptors, though not all studies have shown a convincing effect.[142]

Popliteal fossa block

A simple approach to the sciatic nerve for surgery below the knee is to perform the block at the level of the popliteal fossa behind the knee. The sciatic nerve usually bifurcates at the popliteal fossa into the tibial and common peroneal nerves, although it may bifurcate higher up the thigh. With the patient in the prone or lateral position, the popliteal fossa can be thought of as a diamond-shaped, fat-filled space with the popliteal vessels and the above-mentioned nerves contained within it. The tibial nerve will usually be found with the aid of the nerve stimulator at the apex of the fossa. in the midline, lateral to the popliteal artery The common peroneal nerve lies slightly more lateral, the nerve eventually winding round the head of the fibula. A "pop" may be felt as the fascia is punctured. Results are better if both nerves are located, either by paresthesiae or with the nerve stimulator, but even if only one is found injection of 30 mL of anesthetic will usually produce a satisfactory block. The success rate for this block is high, especially with a nerve stimulator. The combination of a popliteal fossa block and a femoral/saphenous nerve block will provide complete analgesia of the lower leg. The need to turn the patient prone is a drawback of this technique.

Common peroneal nerve block

As a partial alternative to popliteal fossa block, the common peroneal nerve may be blocked as it winds round the head of the fibula with the patient remaining supine. A dose of 5 mL of anesthetic may be deposited just posterolateral to the head of the fibula or a nerve stimulator may be used.

Saphenous nerve

As an alternative to blocking the whole nerve in the inguinal region, saphenous nerve blockade can be achieved at the level of the knee. The nerve is quite superficial, and 10–15 mL of anesthetic solution can be deposited along the medial epicondyle of the tibia.

These blocks are ideal for surgery of the lower leg and ankle.

BLOCKS FOR FOOT SURGERY

Ankle block

Five main nerves supply the foot, and all can be easily blocked by appropriate injections around the ankle. Apart from the saphenous nerve, which is the terminal branch of the femoral nerve, it should be noted that these nerves are all branches of the sciatic nerve.

Tibial nerve

The anesthetic (5 mL) is injected just anterolateral to the posterior tibial artery, if this is palpable, at the level of the upper border of the medial malleolus. If the artery is not palpable, 10 mL of anesthetic should be injected at the same level medial to the Achilles tendon. Branches of the tibial nerve supply the majority of the sole of the foot.

Saphenous nerve

The anesthetic (5 mL) is injected subcutaneously around the saphenous vein anterior to the medial malleolus. The saphenous nerve supplies the medial malleolus and the medial edge and dorsum of the foot.

Deep peroneal nerve

The anesthetic (5 mL) should be injected lateral and slightly beneath the dorsalis pedis artery. If the artery is not palpable, the injection should be given about 1 cm lateral to the extensor hallucis longus tendon. This block is necessary only if anesthesia of the first two toes is required.

Superficial peroneal nerve

This nerve branches higher up the leg and must therefore be blocked by subcutaneously infiltrating up to 10 mL of anesthetic along the area between the anterior border of the tibia and the lateral malleolus. The nerve supplies the majority of the dorsal aspect of the foot.

Sural nerve

The anesthetic (5 mL) is injected between the lateral malleolus and the border of the Achilles tendon. The sural nerve supplies the heel, lateral malleolus, and lateral edge of foot and the posterolateral part of the sole of the foot. Alternatively, this block can be usefully combined with a superficial peroneal nerve block by infiltrating subcutaneously down the entire lateral border of the ankle.

These blocks are easily performed after general anesthesia has been induced (eliciting paresthesiae is difficult and may be painful for the patient – but will hasten the onset of analgesia). It seems wise to avoid epinephrine-containing solutions for blocks around the two major arteries in the presence of peripheral vascular disease.

In addition, analgesia for foot surgery can be provided by injecting local anesthetic as either a digital block or a metatarsal block, depending on the site of surgery. Metatarsal block involves injecting 6 mL of anesthetic into the dorsum of the foot on both sides of the appropriate metatarsal bones, filling the space above the plantar fascia (taking care not to penetrate the plantar fascia or the sole of the foot !). Metatarsal block is preferred to digital block for surgery at the base of the toes.

TEACHING AND TRAINING

There are many excellent textbooks covering the subject of regional anesthesia and recently a number of interactive CD-ROMs have been made available.

Regional anesthesia is a practical field and, as such, training needs to be conducted with an experienced practitioner demonstrating and assisting the trainee through the range of techniques available. As the techniques are demonstrated and practiced the theoretical knowledge should be discussed, with the anatomy and complications of the techniques emphasized. Extra time may be needed to allow trainees to gain the confidence to perform regional anesthesia without direct supervision.[143]

The American Society of Regional Anesthesia (ASRA) published guidelines[144] listing the knowledge base and technical skills that residents involved in the practice of regional anesthesia should be expected to have. These include acquiring a working knowledge base of anatomy, physiology, and pharmacology and being able to acquire the technical skill and practical experience in a wide range of regional anesthetic techniques. Experience should have been gained in a minimum number of cases (e.g. 50 subarachnoid and 50 extradural blocks) and, if possible, specific attachments for training should be completed with an emphasis on the intensive exposure of the resident to the performance of regional anesthesia under supervision in a wide range of different clinical situations in a range of patients from the fit ASA class I patient to the critically ill. Once acquired, these skills require regular updating, in the form of reviews of the published literature (original research and review articles) and attendance at meetings both small and large.

REFERENCES

1. McConachie I. Vasovagal asystole after spinal anaesthesia. *Anaesthesia* 1991; **46:** 281–2.
2. Rice AS; McMahon SB. Peripheral nerve injury caused by injection needles used in regional anaesthesia: influence of bevel configuration, studied in a rat model. *Br J Anaesth* 1992; **69:** 433–8.
3. Selander D, Edshage S, Wolff T. Paraesthesiae or no paraesthesiae? Nerve lesions after axillary block. *Acta Anaesthesiol Scand* 1979; **23:** 27–33.
4. Davies MJ, McGlade DP. One hundred sciatic nerve blocks: a comparison of localisation techniques. *Anaesth Intens Care* 1993; **21:** 76–8.
5. DiFazio CA, Carron R Grosslight KR. Comparison of pH adjusted lidocaine solutions for epidural anesthesia. *Anesth Analg* 1986; **65:** 760–4.
6. Bedder MD, Kozody R, Craig DB. Comparison of bupivacaine and alkalinized bupivacaine in brachial plexus anesthesia. *Anesth Analg* 1988; **67:** 49–52.
7. Scott DB. "Maximum recommended doses" of local anaesthetic drugs. *Br J Anaesth* 1989; **63:** 373–4.
8. Hamber EA, Viscomi CM. Intrathecal lipophilic opioids as adjuncts to surgical spinal anesthesia. *Reg Anesth Pain Med* 1999; **24:** 255–63.
9. Eisenach JC, De Kock M, Klimscha W. Alpha(2)-adrenergic agonists for regional anesthesia. A clinical review of clonidine (1984–1995). *Anesthesiology* 1996; **85:** 655–74.
10. Gordh Jr T, Post C, Olsson Y. Evaluation of the toxicity of subarachnoid clonidine, guanfacine and a substance P-antagonist on rat spinal cord and nerve roots Light and electron microscopic observations after chronic intrathecal administration. *Anesth Analg* 1986; **65:** 1303–18.
11. Eisenach JC, Castro ML, Dewan DM, Rose JC. Epidural clonidine analgesia in obstetrics: sheep studies. *Anesthesiology* 1989; **70:** 51–6.
12. Eisenach JC, Lysak S, Viscomi C. Epidural clonidine analgesia following surgery: Phase 1. *Anesthesiology* 1989; **71:** 640–6.
13. Rostaing S, Bonnet F, Levron JC, *et al.* Effect of epidural clonidine on analgesia and pharmacokinetics of epidural fentanyl in postoperative patients. *Anesthesiology* 1991; **75:** 420–5.
14. Carabine UA, Milligan KR, Moore J. Extradural clonidine and bupivacaine for postoperative analgesia. *Br J Anaesth* 1992; **68:** 132–5.
15. Tremlett MR, Kelly J, Parkins J, *et al.* Low dose clonidine infusion in labour. *Br J Anaesth* 1999; **83:** 257–61.
16. Bernard JM, Macaire P. Dose-range effects of clonidine added to lidocaine for brachial plexus block. *Anesthesiology* 1997; **87:** 277–84.
17. Abram SE. Intrathecal steroid injection for postherpetic neuralgia: what are the risks? *Reg Anesth Pain Med* 1999; **24:** 283–5.
18. Bernards CM, Carpenter RL, Rupp SM, *et al.* Effect of midazolam and diazepam premedications on central nervous system and cardiovascular toxicity of bupivacaine in pigs. *Anesthesiology* 1989; **70:** 318–23.
19. Lambert LA, Lambert DH, Strichartz GR. Irreversible conduction block in isolated nerve by high concentrations of local anesthetics. *Anesthesiology* 1994; **80:** 1082–93.
20. Karlsten R, Gordh T Jr, Hartvig P, Post C. Effects of intrathecal injection of the adenosine receptor agonists *R*-phenylisopropyl-adenosine and *N*-ethylcarboxamide-adenosine on nociception and motor function in the rat. *Anesth Analg* 1990; **71:** 60–4.
21. Taura P, Planella V, Balust J, *et al.* Epidural somatostatin as an analgesic in upper abdominal surgery: a double-blind study. *Pain* 1994; **59:** 135–40.
22. Hwang JH, Hwang KS, Leem JK, *et al.*. The antiallodynic effects of intrathecal cholinesterase inhibitors in a rat model of neuropathic pain. *Anesthesiology* 1999; **90:** 492–9.
23. Liu SS, Hodgson PS, Moore JM, *et al.* Dose–response effects of spinal neostigmine added to bupivacaine spinal anesthesia in volunteers. *Anesthesiology* 1999; **90:** 710–7.
24. Zeng W, Dohi S, Shimonaka H, Asano T. Spinal antinociceptive action of Na+-K+ pump inhibitor ouabain and its interaction with morphine and lidocaine in rats. *Anesthesiology* 1999; **90:** 500–8.
25. Wulf H, Maier C, Schele HA, Wabbel W. Plasma concentration of bupivacaine after stellate ganglion blockade. *Anesth Analg* 1991; **72:** 546–8.
26. Pihlajamaki KK. Inverse correlation between the peak venous serum concentration of bupivacaine and the weight of the patient during interscalene brachial plexus block. *Br J Anaesth* 1991; **67:** 621–2.
27. Butterworth JF 4th, Strichartz GR. Molecular mechanisms of local anesthesia: a review. *Anesthesiology* 1990; **72:** 711–34.
28. Mazoit JX, Orhant EE, Boico O, *et al.* Myocardial uptake of bupivacaine. I Pharmacokinetics and pharmacodynamics of lidocaine and bupivacaine in the isolated perfused rabbit heart. *Anesth Analg* 1993; **77:** 469–76.
29. Weinberg GL, Vade Boncouer T, Ramaraju GA, *et al.* Pretreatment or resuscitation with a lipid infusion shifts the dose–response to bupivacaine-induced asystole in rats. *Anesthesiology* 1998; **88:** 1071–5.
30. Cox CR, Checketts MR, Mackenzie N, *et al.*. Comparison of *S*-bupivacaine with racemic *R*-bupivacaine in supraclavicular brachial plexus block. *Br J Anaesth* 1998: **80:** 594–8.
31. McClure JH. Ropivacaine. *Br J Anaesth* 1996; **76:** 300–7.
32. Johns R. Local anesthetics inhibit endothelium-dependent vasodilation. *Anesthesiology* 1989; **70:** 805–11.
33. Rigler ML, Drasner K, Krejcie TC, *et al.* Cauda equina syndrome after continuous spinal anesthesia. *Anesth Analg* 1991; **72:** 275–81.
34. Moore DC, Thompson GE. Commentary: neurotoxicity of local anesthetics – an issue or a scapegoat? *Reg Anesth Pain Med* 1998; **23:** 605–10.
35. Hogan Q, Dotson R, Erickson S, *et al.* Local anesthetic myotoxicity: a case and review. *Anesthesiology* 1994; **80:** 942–7.
36. Fisher MM, Bowey CJ. Alleged allergy to local anaesthetics. *Anaesth Intens Care* 1997; **25:** 611–4.
37. Hutter CD. The Woolley and Roe case. A reassessment. *Anaesthesia* 1990; **45:** 859–64.
38. Modig J. Beneficial effects on intraoperative and postoperative blood loss in total hip replacement when performed under lumbar epidural anaesthesia. *Acta Chir Scand* (Suppl.) 1988; **550:** 95–103.
39. Peters CA, Walsh PC. Blood transfusion and anesthetic practices in radical retropubic prostatectomy. *J Urol* 1985; **134:** 81–3.
40. Shir Y, Raja SN, Frank SM, Brendler CB. Intraoperative blood loss during radical retropubic prostatectomy: epidural versus general anesthesia. *Urology* 1995; **45:** 993–9.

41. Prins MH, Hirsh J. A comparison of general anesthesia and regional anesthesia as a risk factor for deep vein thrombosis following hip surgery: a critical review. *Thromb Hemost* 1990; **64:** 497–500.
42. Donadoni R, Baele G, Devulder J, Rolly G. Coagulation and fibrinolytic parameters in patients undergoing hip replaceinent: influence of the anaesthesia technique. *Acta Anesthesol Scand* 1989; **33:** 588–92.
43. Cooke ED, Bowcock SA, Lloyd MJ, Pilcher NF. Intravenous lignocaine in prevention of deep venous thrombosis after elective hip surgery. *Lancet* 1977; **2:** 797–9.
44. Liu SS, Carpenter RL, Mackey DC, *et al.* Effects of perioperative analgesic technique on rate of recovery after colon surgery. *Anesthesiology* 1995; **83:** 757–65.
45. Vedrinne C, Vedrinne JM, Guirard M, *et al.*. Nitrogen sparing effect of epidural administration of local anaesthetics in colon surgery *Anesth Analg* 1989; **60:** 354–9.
46. Crul BJ, Hulstijn W, Burger IC. Influence of the type of anaesthesia on post-operative subjective physical well-being and mental function in elderly patients. *Acta Anaesthesiol Scand* 1992; **36:** 615–20.
47. Williams-Russo P, Sharrock NE, Mattis S, *et al.* Cognitive effects after epidural vs. general anesthesia in older adults. A randomized trial. *JAMA* 1995; **274:** 44–50.
48. Ballantyne JC, Carr DB, de Ferranti S, *et al.* The comparative effects of postoperative analgesic therapies on pulmonary outcome: cumulative meta-analyses of randomized, controlled trials. *Anesth Analg* 1998; **86:** 598–612.
49. Manikian B, Cantineau JP, Bertrand M, *et al.* Improvement of diaphragmatic function by a thoracic extradural block after upper abdominal surgery. *Anesthesiology* 1988; **68:** 379–86.
50. Holland R. Trends recognised in cases reported to the New South Wales special committee investigating deaths under anaesthesia. *Anaesth Intens Care* 1987; **15:** 97–8.
51. Yeager MP, Glass DD, Neff RK Brinck-Johnsen T. Epidural anesthesia and analgesia in high risk surgical patients. *Anesth Analg* 1987; **66:** 729–36.
52. Bode RH Jr, Lewis KP, Zarich SW, *et al.* Cardiac outcome after peripheral vascular surgery. Comparison of general and regional anesthesia. *Anesthesiology* 1996; **84:** 3–13.
53. Tuman KJ, McCarthy RJ, March RJ, *et al.* Effects of epidural anesthesia and analgesia on coagulation and outcome after major vascular surgery. *Anesth Analg* 1991; **73:** 696–704.
54. Naesh O, Haljamae H, Hindberg I, *et al.* Epidural anaesthesia prolonged into the postoperative period prevents stress response and platelet hyperaggregability after peripheral vascular surgery. *Eur J Vasc Surg* 1994; **8:** 395–400.
55. Christopherson R, Beattie C, Frank SM, *et al.* Perioperative morbidity in patients randomized to epidural or general anesthesia for lower extremity vascular surgery. Perioperative Ischemia Randomized Anesthesia Trial Study Group. *Anesthesiology* 1993; **79:** 422–34.
56. Hannallah MS. Management of patients undergoing carotid endarterectomy. *Anesthesiol Clin N Am* 1995; **13:** 154–6.
57. Urwin SC, Parker MJ, Griffiths R. General versus regional anaesthesia: a meta-analysis of randomized trials. *Br J Anaesth* 2000; **84:** 450–5.
58. Fischer HBJ. Regional anaesthesia – before or after general anaesthesia? *Anaesthesia* 1998; **53:** 727–9.
59. Krane EJ, Dalens BJ, Murat IM, Murell D. The safety of epidurals placed during general anaesthesia. *Reg Anaesth Pain Med* 1998; **23:** 433–8.
60. Abajian JC, Mellish PWP, Browne AE, *et al.* Spinal anesthesia for surgery in the high risk infant. *Anesth Analg* 1984; **63:** 359–62.
61. Van Nest RL. Radio headset for use with regional anaesthesia. *Anesthesiology* 1979; **50:** 275.
62. Mackenzie N, Grant IS. Propofol for intravenous sedation. *Anaesthesia* 1987; **42:** 3–6.
63. Thorpe SJ, Balakrishnan VR, Cook LB. The safety of patient-controlled sedation. *Anaesthesia* 1997; **52:** 1144–50.
64. Skipsey IG, Colvin JR, Mackenzie N, Kenny GN. Sedation with propofol during surgery under local blockade. Assessment of a target-controlled infusion system. *Anaesthesia* 1993; **48:** 210–3.
65. Smith DC, Crul JF. Oxygen desaturation following sedation for regional anaesthesia. *Br J Anaesth* 1989; **62:** 206–9.
66. Vandam LD. Anatomy of spinal anaesthesia: some old and new findings. *Reg Anaesth Pain Med* 1998; **23: 4:** 340–3.
67. Venn PJ, Simpson DA, Rubin AP, Edstrom HH. Effect of fluid preloading on cardiovascular variables after spinal anaesthesia with glucose free bupivacaine. *Br J Anaesth* 1989; **63:** 682–7.
68. Arndt JO, Borner W, Krauth J, Marquardt B. Incidence and time course of cardiovascular side effects during spinal anaesthesia after prophylactic administration of intravenous fluids or vasoconstrictors. *Anaesth Analg* 1998; **87:** 347–54.
69. Rosenberg PH. Novel technology: needles, microcatheters and combined techniques. *Reg Anaesth Pain Med* 1998; **23:** 363–9.
70. Spencer HC. Postdural puncture headache: what matters in technique. *Reg Anaesth Pain Med* 1998; **23:** 374–9.
71. Liu SS. Drugs for spinal anaesthesia: past, present and future. *Reg Anaesth Pain Med* 1998; **23:** 344–6.
72. Chiari A, Eisenach JC. Spinal anaesthesia: mechanisms, agents, methods and safety. *Reg Anaesth Pain Med* 1998; **23:** 357–62.
73. Stienstra R, Veering BT. Intrathecal drug spread: is it controllable? *Reg Anaesth Pain Med* 1998; **23:** 347–51.
74. Veering BT, Stienstra R. Duration of block: drug, dose and additives. *Reg Anaesth Pain Med* 1998: **23:** 352–6.
75. Frey K, Holman S, Mikat-Stevens M, *et al.* The recovery profile of hyperbaric spinal anaesthesia with lidocaine, tetracaine and bupivacaine. *Reg Anaesth Pain Med* 1998; **23:** 156–63.
76. Lambert DH, Hurley RJ. Cauda equina syndrome and continuous spinal anaesthesia. *Anaesth Analg* 1991; **72:** 817–19.
77. Neal JM, Pollock JE. Can scapegoats stand on shifting sands? *Reg Anaesth Pain Med* 1998; **23:** 533–7.
78. McCrae AF, Wildsmith JAW. Prevention and treatment of hypotension during central neural blockade. *Br J Anaesth* 1993; **70:** 672–80.
79. Butterworth J. Physiology of spinal anaesthesia : what are the implications for management? *Reg Anaesth Pain Med* 1998; **23:** 370–3.
80. Marhofer P, Faryniak B, Oismuller C, *et al.* Cardiovascular effects of 6% hetasterch and lactated ringer's solution during spinal anaesthesia. *Reg Anaesth Pain Med* 1999; **24:** 399–404.
81. Critchley LA, Short TG, Gin T. Hypotension during subarachnoid anaesthesia: haemodynamic analysis of three treatments. *Br J Anaesth* 1994; **72:** 151–5.
82. Geffin B, Shapiro L. Sinus bradycardia and asystole during spinal and epidural anaesthesia: a report of 13 cases. *J Clin Anaesthesiol* 1998; **10:** 278–85.
83. Caplan RA, Ward RJ, Posner K, Cheney FW. Unexpected cardiac arrest during spinal anaesthesia: a closed claims analysis of predisposing factors. *Anaesthesiology* 1988; **68:** 5–11.
84. Reid JA. Thorburn J. Headache after spinal anaesthesia. *Br J Anaesth* 1991; **67:** 674–7.
85. Saberski LR, Kondomamuri S, Osinubi UB. Identification of the epidural space: is loss of resistance to air a safe technique? A review of the complications related to the use of air. *Reg Anaesth* 1997: **22:** 3–15.
86. Kaneko T, Iwama H. : The association between injected volume of local anaesthetic and spread of epidural analgesia: a hypothesis. *Reg Anaesth Pain Med* 1999: **24:** 153–7.
87. Wildsmith JAW. Problems with combined spinal and epidural anaesthesia. *Reg Anaesth Pain Med* 1998; **23:** 388–9.
88. Dahlgren N, Tornebrandt K. Neurological complications after anaesthesia. A follow up of 18000 spinal and epidural anaesthetics performed over three years. *Acta Anaesthesiol Scand* 1995; **39:** 872–80.
89. Aromaa U, Lahdensuu M, Cozanitis DA. Severe complications associated with epidural and spinal anaesthesia in Finland 1987–1993. A study based on insurance claims. *Acta Anaesthesiol Scand* 1997; **41:** 439–44.
90. Dripps RD, Vandam LD. The long term follow up of patients who received 10,098 spinal analgesics: failure to discover major neurological sequelae. *JAMA* 1954; **156:** 1486–91.
91. Wang LP, Hauerberg J, Schmidt JF. Incidence of spinal epidural abscess after epidural analgesia: A national 1 year survey. *Anaesthesiology* 1999; **91:** 1928–36.
92. Horlocker TT, Wedel DJ. Neurological complications of spinal and epidural anaesthesia. *Reg Anaesth Pain Med* 2000; **25:** 83–98.
93. Rosenquist RW, Brown DL. Neuraxial bleeding: fibrinolytics/thrombolytics. *Reg Anesth Pain Med* 1998; **23** (Suppl. 2): 152–6.
94. Wedel DJ, Horlocker TT. Regional anaesthesia and infection. In: Finucane BT (ed.). *Complications of Regional Anaesthesia*. Philadelphia, PA: Saunders, 1999: 170–83.
95. Knowles PR, Randall NPC, Lockhart AS. Vascular trauma associated with routine spinal anaesthesia. *Anaesthesia* 1999; **54:** 647–50.
96. Neuroaxial anaesthesia and anticoagulation. *Reg Anaesth Pain Med* 1998; **23** (Suppl.): 6.
97. Rosenfield BA. Benefits of regional anaesthesia on thromboembolic complications following surgery. *Reg Anaesth* 1996; **21:** 6 (Suppl.): 9–12.
98. Owen R, Galloway DJ, Mitchell KG. Analgesia by wound infiltration after surgical excision of benign breast lumps. *Ann Royal Coll Surg Engl* 1985; **67:** 114–15.
99. Thomas DFX, Lambert WG, Lloyd-Williams K. The direct perfusion of surgical wounds with local anaesthetic solutions. An approach to postoperative pain. *Ann Royal Coll Surg Engl* 1983; **65:** 226–9.

100. Cobby TF, Reid MF. Wound infiltration with local anaesthetic after abdominal hysterectomy. *Br J Anaesth* 1997; **78:** 431–2.
101. van Raay JJ, Roukema JA, Lenderink BW. Intraoperative wound infiltration with bupivacaine in patients undergoing elective cholecystectomy. *Arch Surg* 1992; **127:** 457–9.
102. Harrison N, Langham BT, Bogod DG. The appropriate use of local anaesthesia for venous cannulation. *Anaesthesia* 1992; **47:** 210–12.
103. Bartfield JM, Sokaris SJ, Raccio-Robak N. Local anesthesia for lacerations: pain of infiltration inside vs. outside the wound. *Acad Emerg Med* 1998; **5:** 100–4.
104. Moore DC. Intercostal nerve block: spread of India ink injected to the rib's costal groove. *Br J Anaesth* 1981; **53:** 325–9.
105. Kirno K, Lindell K. Intercostal nerve blockade. *Br J Anaesth* 1986; **58:** 246.
106. O'Kelly E, Garry B. Continuous pain relief for multiple rib fractures. *Br J Anaesth* 1981; **53:** 989–91.
107. Bunting P, McGeachie JF. Intercostal nerve blockade producing analgesia after appendicectomy. *Br J Anaesth* 1988; **61:** 169–72.
108. Knowles P, Hancox D, Letheren M, Eddleston J. An evaluation of intercostal nerve blockade for analgesia following renal transplantation. *Eur J Anaesthesiol* 1998; **15:** 457–61.
109. Moore DC. Intercostal nerve block for postoperative somatic pain following surgery of thorax and upper abdomen. *Br J Anaesth* 1975; **47:** 284–6.
110. Rocco A, Reiestad F, Gudman J, McKay W. Intrapleural administration of local anaesthetics for pain relief in patients with multiple rib fractures. Reg Anesth 1986; **12:** 12–14.
111. Scott PV. Interpleural regional analgesia: detection of the interpleural space by saline infusion. *Br J Anaesth* 1991; **66:** 131–3.
112. Pinnock CA, Fischer HBJ, Jones RP. *Peripheral Nerve Blockade*. Edinburgh: Churchill Livingstone, 1996: 90.
113. Lonnqvist PA, Mackenzie J, Soni A, Conacher ID. Paravertebral blockade, failure rate and complications. *Anaesthesia* : 1995; **50:** 813–15.
114. Bugedo GJ, Carcamo CR, Mertens RA, *et al.* Preoperative percutaneous ilioinguinal and iliohypogastric nerve block with 0.5% bupivacaine for post-herniorrhaphy pain management in adults. *Reg Anesth* 1990; **15:** 130–3.
115. Bunting P, McConachie L. Ilioinguinal block for analgesia after lower segment caesarean section. *Br J Anaesth* 1988; **61:** 773–5.
116. Kelly MC, Beers HT, Huss BK, Gilliland HM. Bilateral ilioinguinal nerve blocks for analgesia after total abdominal hysterectomy. *Anaesthesia* 1996; **51:** 406.
117. Bacon AK. An alternative block for post circumcision analgesia. *Anaesth Intens Care* 1977; **5:** 63–4.
118. Berens R, Pontus SP. A complication associated with dorsal penile nerve block. *Reg Anaesth* 1990; **15:** 309–10.
119. Winnie AP. Interscalene brachial plexus block. *Anesth Analg* 1970; **49:** 455–66.
120. Tetzlaff JE, Yoon HJ, Brems J. Interscalene brachial plexus block for shoulder surgery. *Reg Anesth* 1994; **19:** 339–43.
121. Pearce H, Lindsay D, Leslie K. Axillary brachial plexus block in two hundred consecutive patients. *Anaesth Intens Care* 1996; **24:** 453–8.
122. Stan TC, Krantz MA, Solomon DL, *et al.* The incidence of neurovascular complications following axillary brachial plexus block using a transarterial approach. A prospective study of 1000 consecutive patients. *Reg Anesth* 1995; **20:** 486–92.
123. Mezzatesta JP, Scott DA, Schweitzer SA, Selander DE. Continuous axillary brachial plexus block for postoperative pain relief. Intermittent bolus versus continuous infusion. *Reg Anesth* 1997; **22:** 357–62.
124. Yamamoto K, Nomura T, Shibata K, Ohmura S. Failed axillary brachial plexus block techniques result in high plasma concentrations of mepivacaine. *Reg Anesth* 1997; **22:** 557–61.
125. Davis KJ, McConachie I. Intravenous regional anaesthesia. *Curr Anaesth Crit Care* 1998; **9:** 261–4.
126. Sorbie C, Chacha P. Regional anaesthesia by the intravenous route. *Br Med J* 1965; **1:** 957–61.
127. Bader A, Concepcion M, Hurley R, Arthur GR. Comparison of lignocaine and prilocaine for intravenous regional anaesthesia. *Anesthesiology* 1988; **69:** 409–12.
128. Heath MC. Deaths after intravenous regional anaesthesia. *Br Med J* 1982; **285:** 913–14.
129. Durrani Z, Winnie AP, Zsigmond EK, Burnett MC. Ketamine for IVRA. *Anesth Analg* 1989; **68:** 328–32.
130. Reuben SS, Steinberg RB, Kreitzer JM, Duprat KM. IVRA using lignocaine and ketorolac. *Anesth Analg* 1995; **81:** 110–13.
131. McGlone R, Heyes F, Harris P. The use of muscle relaxant to supplement local anaesthetics for Bier's blocks. *Arch Emerg Med* 1988; **5:** 79–85.
132. Solak M, Arthur G, Erciyes N, *et al.* The addition of sodium bicarbonate to prilocaine solution during IVRA. *Acta Anaesthesiol Scand* 1991; **35:** 572–4.
133. Smith BE, Haydock JC. Local anaesthesia for surgery of the lower limb. *Curr Anaesth Crit Care* 1992; **3:** 37–41.
134. Ben-David B, Lee E, Croitoru M. Psoas block for surgical repair of hip fracture: a case report and description of a catheter technique. *Anesth Analg* 1990; **71:** 298–301.
135. Haddad FS, Williams RL. Femoral nerve block in extracapsular femoral neck fractures. *J Bone Joint Surg Br* 1995; **77:** 922–3.
136. Allen HW, Liu SS, Ware PD, *et al.* Peripheral nerve blocks improve analgesia after total knee replacement surgery. *Anesth Analg* 1998; **87:** 93–7.
137. Edkin BS, Spindler KP, Flanagan JF. Femoral nerve block as an alternative to parenteral narcotics for pain control after anterior cruciate ligament reconstruction. *Arthroscopy* 1995; **11:** 404–9.
138. Fournier R, Van Gessel E, Gaggero G, *et al.* Postoperative analgesia with "3-in-1" femoral nerve block after prosthetic hip surgery. *Can J Anaesth* 1998, **45:** 34–8.
139. Edwards ND, Wright EM. Continuous low-dose 3-in-1 nerve blockade for postoperative pain relief after total knee replacement. *Anesth Analg* 1992; **75:** 265–7.
140. Smith BE, Allison A. Nerve block for hip surgery. *Anaesthesia* 1987; **42:** 1916–17.
141. Tagariello V. Sciatic nerve blocks: approaches, techniques, local anaesthetics and manipulations. *Anaesthesia* 1998; **53** (Suppl. 2): 15–17.
142. Kalso E, Tramer M, Carrol D, *et al.* Pain relief from intra-articular morphine after knee surgery: a qualitative systematic review. *Pain* 1997; **71:** 64–51.
143. Kopacz DJ. Regional anaesthesia training: do we have the confidence to go on? *Reg Anaesth Pain Med* 1999; **24:** 1–4.
144. Educational guidelines for subspecialty training in regional anesthesia. *American Society for Regional Anesthesia News* 1995; November: 10–11.

FURTHER READING

Cousins MJ, Bridenbaugh PO. *Neural Blockade Pain Management*, 3rd edn. Philadelphia: Lippincott, 1998.

Finucane BT (ed.) *Complications of Regional Anaesthesia*. Philadelphia, PA: Saunders, 1999.

Pinnock CA, Fischer HBJ, Jones RP. *Peripheral Nerve Blockade*. Edinburgh: Churchill Livingstone, 1996

Raj P, Nolte H, Stanton-Hicks M. *Illustrated Manual of Regional Anaesthesia*. Berlin: Springer-Verlag, 1988.

Scott DB. *Techniques of Regional Anaesthesia*. Fribourg, Switzerland: Mediglobe SA, 1995.

Winnie AP. *Plexus Anaesthesia*, Vol 1, *Perivascular Techniques of Brachial Plexus Block*. Edinburgh: Churchill Livingstone, 1983.

38

Other drugs used in anesthesia

BARBARA J PLEUVRY

In this chapter, a collection of unrelated drugs that may be used in patients undergoing anesthesia is considered. The largest group is the antiemetic drugs, which will be discussed in some detail. Included in the antiemetic drugs are the dopamine antagonists, which have also been used as neuroleptics in techniques such as neuroleptanalgesia and neuroleptanesthesia. The use of neuroleptics in anesthesia for this purpose is gradually dying out, with only a few papers being published in recent years (mainly in the Russian language). Consequently, this section will be relatively brief. Heparin, protamine, and the intravenous contrast media and dyes will be considered mainly in relation to adverse effects that must concern the anesthesiologist.

ANTIEMETIC DRUGS

Anatomy and physiology of vomiting

When the unpleasantness of nausea and vomiting is considered, it is perhaps surprising that the mechanisms by which they occur have been studied relatively little.

The major physiologic reason for the vomiting reflex is to protect the body from toxins ingested in food that have not been detected by sight, taste, or smell. As such, it is a second line of defense.[1] Nausea and vomiting may also be induced by irritation or distension of the upper gastrointestinal tract (GIT), distension of the duodenum being a particularly strong stimulus. In view of this it is not surprising that vagal and sympathetic afferent impulses from the GIT to the vomiting or emetic center can induce vomiting. Of the two, the vagal afferents are the most important. These afferent impulses are initiated by either mechanoreceptors, which detect distension, or mucosal chemoreceptors, which detect acids, alkalis, irritants, and probably bacterial toxins. Induction of vomiting, for example with cytotoxic drugs, is associated with mucosal damage and the liberation of 5-hydoxytryptamine (5-HT) from the enterochromaffin cells.[2] The released 5-HT probably stimulates the vagal afferent nerves by interaction with a 5-HT_3 receptor. There is recent evidence that mucosally released substance P acting on tachykinin NK_1 receptors may act cooperatively with 5-HT (acting on 5-HT_3 receptors) in the upper GIT to induce vomiting.[3]

Vomiting can also be induced by chemicals carried in the blood that are detected by the chemosensitive trigger zone (CTZ) in the area

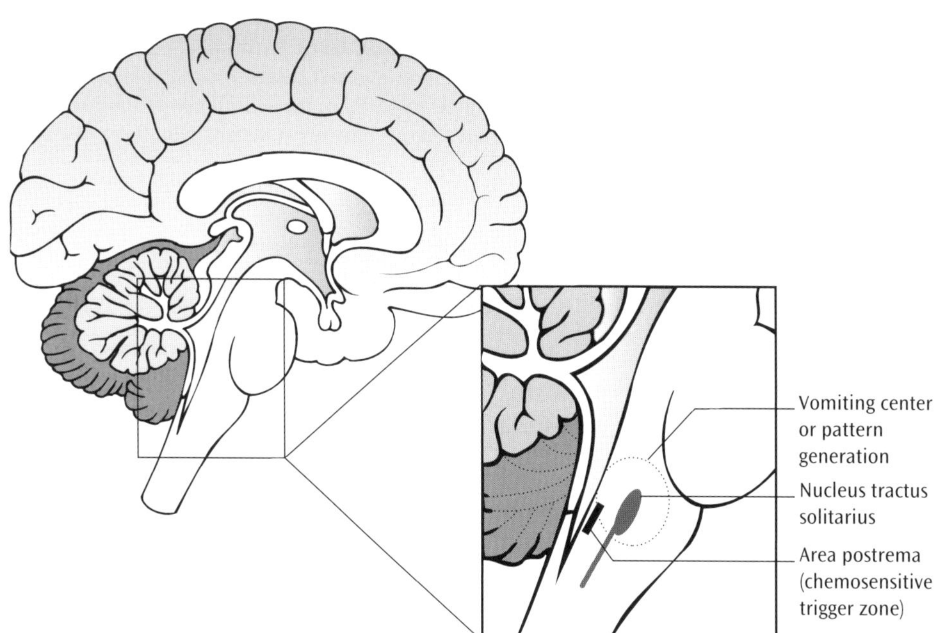

Figure 38.1 *Areas of the brain associated with nausea and vomiting.*

postrema on the caudal floor of the fourth ventricle (Fig. 38.1).[4] From a pharmacologic point of view, it is interesting and exploitable that the CTZ is functionally outside the blood–brain barrier.[5] Animal studies have shown that the area postrema contains high concentrations of 5-HT_3,[6] dopamine (D_2),[7] and opioid receptors.[8] In the human, agonists at these receptors cause nausea and vomiting and, whereas antagonists at 5-HT_3 and D_2 receptors are effective antiemetic agents (see later), to my knowledge opioid antagonists are not useful in this respect.

Motion sickness requires the vestibular system to be present and labyrinthine stimulation enhances the emetic effects of many other vomiting triggers.[9] The receptors present in the vestibular nuclei are muscarinic cholinergic and histamine H_1 receptors.[10]

Both the vestibular system and the CTZ send impulses to the vomiting center, which initiates the sequence of smooth and skeletal muscle contraction associated with vomiting. The vomiting center is a physiologic rather than an anatomical structure and is found in the area of the brain that includes the nucleus tractus solitarius (Fig. 38.1), close to the area postrema. Both muscarinic cholinergic and histamine H_1 receptors are found in this area.[10] In addition, [^{3}H]-substance P binds with high density in the nucleus tractus solitarius and is displaced by the NK_1 receptor antagonist CP-99994.[11] CP-99994 has broad-spectrum antiemetic effects and the main site of action appears to be the nucleus tractus solitarius, although an action on the area postrema cannot be ruled out.[11] Vomiting can also occur due to inputs from higher centers such as the limbic system, although the mechanisms underlying these are as yet unexplained.

The receptors involved in emesis and useful antiemetic drugs are summarized in Table 38.1.

Use of antiemetic drugs in anesthesia

The mechanism by which postoperative nausea and vomiting (PONV) occurs is unclear and almost certainly multifactorial. The percentage of patients exhibiting PONV varies with type of surgery. A particularly high incidence occurs with strabismus and ovum retrieval.[12] PONV increases with age up to 10 years old and adult female patients are more likely to experience PONV than males, a fact that appears to be related to female sex hormone concentrations, as fluctuations in the incidence of PONV occur during the menstrual cycle.[12] Anesthetic factors, including the drugs used and anesthetic technique selected, can also influence PONV, although many clinical studies have given contradictory results.[9,13] Although the incidence of PONV is highly variable, it can be reduced significantly by the corporate acceptance of departmental protocols designed to reduce this adverse effect.[14]

Unfortunately, animal models of PONV did not exist until recently (a house musk shrew model of PONV was described by Gardner and Perrin in 1998[15]) and PONV is not a common veterinary problem, even in species that respond to other emetic stimuli in a manner similar to man. In view of this, drug treatment has been restricted to trials of agents that are effective antiemetics in other emetogenic situations, rather than a rational design of drugs based on an understanding of the condition.

Dopamine receptor antagonists

The three main neuronal tracts utilizing dopamine as a neurotransmitter are shown in Fig. 38.2.

The nigrostriatal pathway from the substantia nigra to the corpus striatum is involved in motor control, and a deficit in dopamine in this pathway is associated with Parkinson's disease. Emotion and stereotypical behavior are linked to the mesolimbic/mesocortical pathway, and this is believed to be the site of the beneficial effects of antipsychotic drugs. All the currently useful antipsychotic drugs are dopamine antagonists, although many have affinity for other receptors, especially the 5-HT_3 receptor in respect of the atypical agents.[16] Hormone secretion from the pituitary gland is regulated by the tuberohypophyseal dopaminergic neurons running from the hypothalamus to the pituitary gland. Dopamine agonists are used to treat hyperprolactinemia, which is a cause of infertility.

As mentioned earlier, dopamine is also involved in the production of emesis, and dopamine antagonists are effective antiemetics. Unfortunately, most dopamine antagonists, such as droperidol, have no selectivity for the dopamine receptors in the CTZ so they also produce neurolepsis (see below), hyperprolactinemia, and extrapyramidal motor disturbances similar to Parkinson's disease. An exception is domperidone, a drug that is less likely to cross the blood–brain barrier than other agents[17] and thus is less prone to, but not free from, extrapyramidal actions. There is some debate concerning the effectiveness of domperidone in PONV. In addition, there have been reports of severe cardiac arrhyhthmias after large doses, which resulted in the withdrawal of the parenteral preparation. These last three factors have caused a loss of interest in domperidone from an anesthetic point of view.[18] Interestingly, despite the drug's adverse effects, droperidol is still the standard antiemetic with which others are compared.

Dopamine receptors were originally divided into two groups depending on their ability either to stimulate adenylyl cyclase (D_1) or to inhibit or have no effect on adenylyl cyclase (D_2). Subsequently, cloning techniques revealed subgroups D_1 to D_5, of which the D_2 has two splice variants (long and short) and the D_4 is subject to genetic polymorphism.[19] Both D_1 and D_5 are of the original D_1 type while D_2, D_3, and D_4, which are more important from the therapeutic point of view, are of the original D_2 type. Since the distribution of these receptor subtypes differs in the central nervous system (CNS), there has been

Table 38.1 *Neurotransmitters involved in nausea and vomiting*

Detectors of emetic stimuli	Stimulus	Neurotransmitter	Receptors involved	Antiemetic drugs
Afferent input from the GIT	Irritation and distension	5-HT	5-HT_3	Ondansetron, granisetron
		Substance P	NK_1	Sendide (not clinically available)
Area postrema (CTZ)	Toxins and chemicals	Dopamine	D_2	Droperidol, prochlorperazine, perphenazine, domperidone, metoclopramide
		5-HT	5-HT_3	Ondansetron, granisetron
Vestibular nuclei	Motion	Acetylcholine	Muscarinic	Hyoscine, atropine
		Histamine	H_1	Cyclizine, promethazine
Vomiting or emetic center	Inputs from other areas (above)	Acetylcholine	Muscarinic	Hyoscine, atropine
		Histamine	H_1	Cyclizine, promethazine
		Substance P	NK_1	CP-99994

CTZ, chemosensitive trigger zone; GIT, gastrointestinal tract.

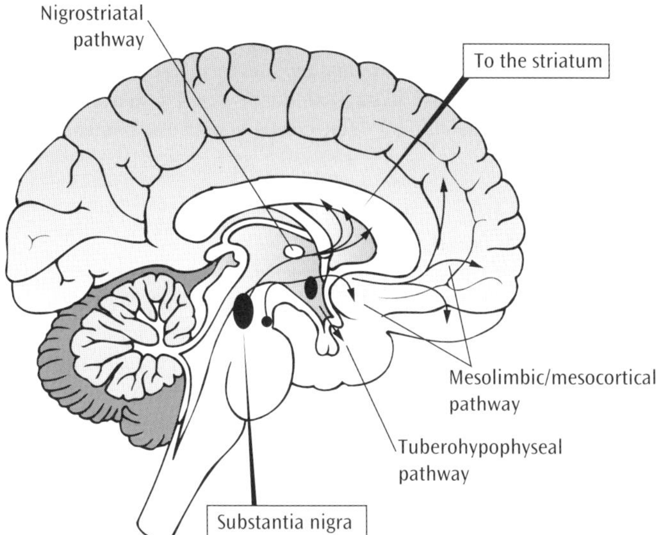

Figure 38.2 *Main dopaminergic pathways in the brain.*

considerable interest in developing selective compounds that might possess fewer side-effects. For example, the receptors in the basal ganglia, which mediate the extrapyramidal side-effects of dopamine antagonists, are mainly of the D_2 subtype, thus drugs selective for D_3 or D_4 receptors may not posses this side-effect. Clozapine and other newer atypical antipsychotic drugs have some selectivity for D_4 receptors and have a much better side-effect profile when used as antipsychotic agents than the traditional dopamine antagonists. However, they also bind to several other nondopaminergic receptors, which may explain this phenomenon.[16] The application of this approach to the reduction of adverse effects associated with dopamine antagonists used as antiemetic agents seems to have been ignored, probably because alternatives (see below) have now been introduced.

Individual dopamine antagonists that have been used as antiemetic agents are summarized in Table 38.2.

Metoclopramide and domperidone have additional prokinetic activity (enhanced gastric and upper intestinal motility), which may contribute to their antiemetic action. Metoclopramide also has some 5-HT_3 antagonistic effects at higher doses.[20] Although not of particular interest for anesthetic purposes, dopamine antagonists are not useful for motion sickness unless they have coincident muscarinic cholinoceptor antagonist properties.

Muscarinic cholinoceptor antagonists

In the treatment of PONV, the muscarinic receptors present in the vomiting center itself are a more important target than those in the vestibular nuclei, which are involved in motion sickness. Some differences in the muscarinic receptors in the cortex and pons have been described in man, and these could lead to a more selective antimuscarinic antiemetic drug in the future, at least with respect to motion sickness.[22] At present, three muscarinic antagonists are used in anesthesia – hyoscine, atropine, and glycopyrrolate – but of these only the first two penetrate the CNS and have useful antiemetic activity. A recent study in children found that the use of atropine with neostigmine for reversal of neuromuscular blockade was associated with significantly less postoperative emesis than reversal with glycopyrrolate and neostigmine.[23]

Hyoscine, used intramuscularly, has been found to be generally more effective as an antiemetic than atropine, but it was associated with increased drowsiness and delayed recovery from anesthesia.[18] In order to increase its duration of action, hyoscine has also been used as a transdermal preparation for the control of both motion sickness and PONV. The patch needs to be applied several hours before the emetic stimulus to enable an adequate plasma concentration to be obtained. While several authors have demonstrated the efficacy of transdermal hyoscine in PONV, others have failed to detect a significant difference from the placebo. Negative results were more likely when the prior duration of patch application was brief or additional premedication drug administration was uncontrolled.[18] A typical adverse effect of muscarinic antagonists, dry mouth, was a frequent, but not serious, observation.

Histamine H_1-receptor antagonists

Many examples of antihistamine drugs are used to treat motion sickness, but most have additional antimuscarinic activity. It is not clear which property is more important with respect to their antiemetic action,

Table 38.2 *Dopamine antagonists used as antiemetics in postoperative nausea and vomiting (PONV)*

Drug	Route	Elimination half-life	Adverse effects	Comments
Droperidol[a]	i.v. and i.m.	2 h	Extrapyramidal disorders Delayed recovery Hypotension Anxiety	Some studies have shown negative effects when the drug is administered prior to surgery. Most anesthesiologists are reluctant to use it for day-cases. More adverse effects than metoclopramide and domperidone for major gynecologic surgery[21]
Perphenazine	i.v.	9.4 h	Extrapyramidal disorders Delayed recovery	Not recommended for children
Prochlorperazine	i.v. and i.m.	6.8 h	Extrapyramidal disorders Delayed recovery	Fewer adverse effects than perphenazine?
Metoclopramide	Oral, i.v., i.m.	4 h	Extrapyramidal disorders Restlessness	Poor brain penetration so fewer adverse effects than others except domperidone. Still preferred over droperidol by many European anesthesiologists despite perceived lower efficacy than droperidol
Domperidone	Oral and rectal?		Cardiac dysrhythmias	Few trials demonstrate efficacy when compared with placebo

a. Now withdrawn.

i.m., intramuscular; i.v., intravenous.

although both receptors are present in both the vomiting center and the vestibular nucleus. Cyclizine has been used extensively to treat PONV and most reports demonstrate efficacy with few side-effects such as sedation.[18] Promethazine is a markedly sedative drug and has been used by anesthesiologists to premedicate children, but whether this is for its sedative effect or its antiemetic effect is debatable. Oral dimenhydrinate, given at least 1 h before surgery, has also been used to prevent PONV. Second-generation antihistamines, such as terfenadine and astemizole, are not effective antiemetic drugs as they do not cross the blood–brain barrier. Neither muscarinic antagonist nor antihistaminic drugs are particularly useful in treating the emesis due to chemotherapy.

5-HT$_3$-receptor antagonists

The relative lack of effectiveness of dopamine antagonists in severe chemotherapy-induced emesis suggested that no dopaminergic emetic mechanisms were involved. The observations with respect to 5-HT release by these cytotoxic agents (see above) prompted the successful trial of 5-HT$_3$ antagonists such as ondansetron. Subsequently, oral ondansetron was found to be effective in PONV,[24] a finding that has been confirmed, using both the oral and the intravenous route, in many postoperative situations.[25] Generally, the adverse effects of ondansetron were mild and no signs of the extrapyramidal symptoms or dry mouth seen with alternative antiemetics were reported. Another 5HT$_3$-receptor antagonist that has successfully extended its indications from cytotoxic drug-induced emesis to PONV is granisetron. It has been shown to be useful by the oral route in children[26] and by both the oral and the intravenous route in adults.[27, 28] The antiemetic activity of other 5-HT$_3$ antagonists, such as dolasetron and tropisetron, has been reported only in the treatment of patients given emetogenic chemotherapy.

Comparative studies between individual 5-HT$_3$ antagonists in PONV have not been carried out, but there are some reports of comparisons with other antiemetic drugs. The more recent examples are summarized in Table 38.3.

It must be appreciated that most of the trials involved single doses and the equivalence of the dose of comparitor may be questioned. However, in general the 5-HT$_3$ antagonists appear to be more effective and to exhibit fewer adverse effects than alternative antiemetics used for PONV. However, the cost implications of treating all patients at risk of PONV with these relatively new agents must be considered.

Other antiemetics

Although the cannabinoid nabilone and glucocorticosteroids have been used as antiemetic drugs for emotogenic chemotherapy, they have not been used extensively for emesis associated with anesthesia. The intravenous anesthetic propofol has also been used to treat PONV in a patient-controlled antiemetic therapy.[34] Although sedation could be a problem if the dose was too high, moderate doses were effective and, when compared with placebo, reduced the stay in the postanesthetic care unit.

NEUROLEPTIC DRUGS

A neurolept is a drug that causes neurolepsis – a state of altered consciousness characterized by quiescence, reduced motor activity, and indifference to the surroundings. Although he or she may sleep, the patient remains conscious and is able to respond to commands. These drugs find their chief use as antipsychotic agents and all are antagonists at dopamine receptors (described under Antiemetic drugs above). Blockade of the mesolimbic/mesocortical pathway (Fig. 38.2) is believed to lead to the state of neurolepsis. Neuroleptic drugs were first described by Campan and Lazothes in 1954[35] as part of an anesthetic technique that aimed to reduce the perception of pain without affecting cognition. Combinations of analgesics, such as meperidine (pethidine), and neuroleptics, such as chlorpromazine, were subsequently used under a number of guises such as "ataraxy," a state of calmness and freedom from pain, or as a "lytic cocktail" with the addition of promethazine. Neuroleptanalgesia with haloperidol (neurolept) and phenoperidine (potent opioid analgesic) was first described in 1959, and the addition of nitrous oxide or a hypnotic drug to render the patient unconscious was known as neuroleptanesthesia.[36] The development of drugs with shorter durations of action, such as droperidol and fentanyl, led to the increased use of the technique and a fixed-dose combination of the two drugs was introduced into the anesthetic market, despite the fact that the two drugs had completely different durations of action. Over the next few years, neuroleptanalgesia was tried as an alternative to general anesthesia in all types of surgery, resulting in numerous reports of postoperative ventilatory depression. After this, the application of neuroleptanalgesia was limited to minor surgical procedures, often as an adjunct to local anesthesia.[37] Neuroleptanalgesia has also been used as preanesthetic medication, although a minority of patients suffered from dysphoria, restlessness, and dyskinesia. These side-effects are also seen when the neuroleptic component is used strictly as an antiemetic. However, in combination with light general anesthesia the droperidol and fentanyl combination proved better in some circumstances than any previous anesthetic protocol, especially when cardiovascular stability was required.[37]

Table 38.3 *Comparisons between 5-HT$_3$ antagonists and other antiemetics for postoperative nausea and vomiting (PONV)*

5-HT$_3$ antagonist	Comparator	Surgery	Result	Reference
Granisetron (oral)	Domperidone (oral)	Major gynecological	Patients with no PONV 88% granisetron, 48% domperidone	27
Ondansetron (i.v.)	Metoclopramide (i.v.)	Laparoscopic cholecystectomy	Ondansetron superior to metoclopramide in females (males showed little PONV)	29
Granisetron (i.v.)	Droperidol (i.v.) Metoclopramide (i.v.)	Cesarean section (spinal anesthesia)	Granisetron was effective in preventing nausea and emesis during and after spinal anesthesia. Droperidol and metaclopramide were ineffective for PONV	28
Ondansetron (i.v.)	Dimenhydrinate (i.v.)	Adenotonsillectomy	42% of children vomited with ondansetron compared with 79% vomiting with dimenhydrinate	30
Ondansetron (i.v.)	Droperidol (i.v.)	Laparoscopy	Both drugs equally effective in preventing nausea, although ondansetron was slightly superior in preventing vomiting	31
Ondansetron (i.v.)	Droperidol (i.v.) Metoclopramide (i.v.)	Strabismus surgery	Ondansetron and droperidol were equally effective and better than metoclopramide in decreasing predischarge vomiting but none were effective in decreasing postdischarge vomiting	32
Ondansetron (oral)	Metoclopramide (oral)	Major orthopedic	Ondansetron was significantly better than metoclopramide for reducing PONV	33

A rare complication of neuroleptic drug administration is the neuroleptic malignant syndrome (NMS), characterized by rigidity, tremor, autonomic dysfunction, and fever, coupled with an increase in serum creatinine phosphokinase and white blood cell count. It is more likely to occur when high parenteral doses are used and there is appreciable mortality (over 10%). Treatment involves removal of the drug and supportive therapy. Unlike the malignant hyperthermia induced by general anesthetics, the use of drugs such as dantrolene does not appear to be helpful, and a disorder of Ca^{2+} metabolism in skeletal muscle is probably not the cause. However, there has been a report of both syndromes occurring in the same patient.[38] Recovery from NMS occurs in about 14 days without any cognitive impairment induced by the syndrome itself, although impairment may be caused by high fever, hypoxia, or other complications of the syndrome.[39]

As new drugs were introduced, particularly propofol, alfentanil, and midazolam, it became clear that conscious sedation could be produced without the risk of the serious side-effects posed by the neurolept-opioid combination.[40] Despite the occasional report that there were no advantages to the use of total intravenous anesthesia with midazolam and alfentanil over neuroleptanalgesia,[41] the publication of papers describing neuroleptanalgesia has gradually ceased.

HEPARIN AND PROTAMINE

Heparin is present, together with histamine, in mast cells and is extracted from animal tissue such as cattle lung. It is a family of sulfated glycosaminoglycans with a range of molecular weights and, as its constitution is variable, it is bioassayed against an international standard and is measured in units of activity rather than mass. Heparin is an anticoagulant with a rapid onset and a short duration of action after intravenous or subcutaneous administration. It may be referred to as standard or unfractionated heparin to distinguish it from the low-molecular-weight heparins, such as dalteparin, which have a longer duration of action and are administered subcutaneously. Heparin is used in the treatment of deep venous thrombosis and pulmonary embolism, and low doses may be used in anesthesia to prevent the development of these two conditions in high-risk patients undergoing general surgery. The low-molecular-weight heparins are being increasingly used for this purpose.[42, 43] In cardiopulmonary bypass surgery and hemodialysis, heparin is used to maintain the extracorporeal circuits.

Heparin is an effective anticoagulant both *in vivo* and *in vitro*. It activates a protease inhibitor, antithrombin III, which inhibits many of the active forms of the coagulation factors (Fig. 38.3). Thrombin is particularly sensitive to standard heparin, which provides a catalytic template to which both antithrombin III and thrombin bind. The low-molecular-weight heparins are not long enough to bind to both antithrombin and thrombin and have their major anticoagulant action via inhibition of activated factor X (Fig. 38.3). They have very limited effects on clotting *in vitro*.

Heparin exhibits saturation kinetics, with the apparent half-life increasing with dose. In contrast, while they have a longer half-life than standard heparin, the low-molecular-weight heparins follow first-order kinetics and the half-life does not depend upon dose. This simplifies dose regimens.

The principal unwanted effect of heparin is hemorrhage. This can be controlled by stopping drug administration or, if more active treatment is required, by administering the antagonist. Protamine sulfate is a strongly basic protein that forms an inactive complex with the acidic heparin molecule. It is important that the patients should not be overdosed with this heparin antagonist as it can prolong bleeding time in its own right. Protamine can, as in the case of most strong bases, release histamine, and rapid intravenous injections can result in hypotension. It also activates the immune system, and IgG- and IgE-mediated allergic responses have been described, particularly in patients with a history of fish allergy (protamine is derived from fish) or in the case of neutral protamine Hagedorn (NPH) in patients with insulin-dependent diabetes. Catastrophic pulmonary vasoconstriction is a rare but may be a fatal consequence of the use of protamine to neutralize heparin.[44] A recent paper suggests that inhaled nitric oxide, a potent pulmonary vasodilator, is an effective treatment for this condition.[45] Thrombocytopenia can be linked to the use of standard heparin, but this is unlikely to be a serious problem in anesthetic use unless therapy is prolonged.

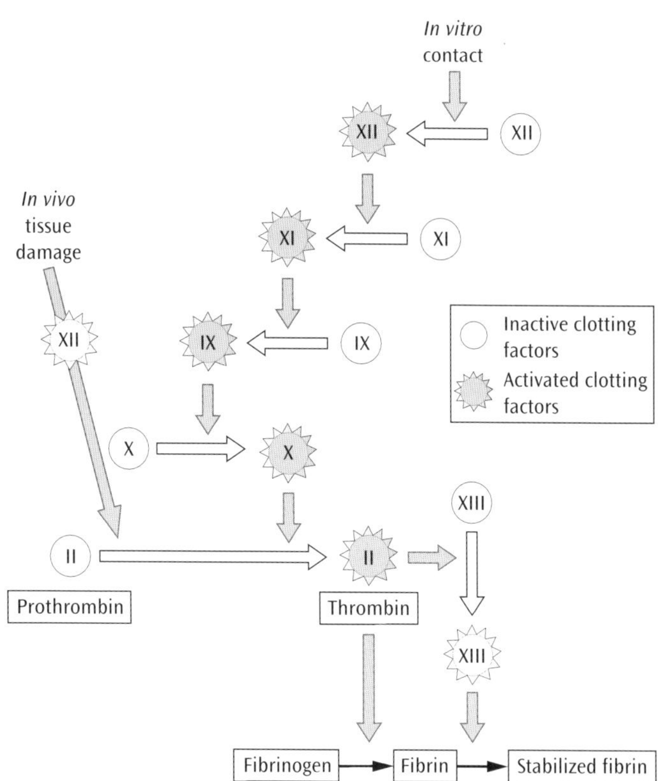

Figure 38.3 *Blood coagulation cascade showing clotting factors (shaded symbols) inhibited by heparin-activated antithrombin factor III. Note that low-molecular-weight heparins only inhibit activated factor X.*

INTRAVENOUS DYES

The intravenous dyes probably include the radiographic contrast media used to delineate blood vessels or other organs by increasing the absorption of X-rays as they pass through the body. Substances containing heavy metals are the most suitable for this purpose, and many contrast media contain iodinated organic compounds, which have a degree of radiodensity proportional to their iodine content. Iodinated contrast media may be divided into ionic, in which the compound is dissociated into cations and anions, and nonionic, in which no dissociation has occurred. In addition, the compounds may be monomeric, usually containing three iodine atoms per molecule, or dimeric, containing six iodine atoms per molecule. The ionic monomeric compounds have the highest osmolality when given in effective concentrations, and their hypertonicity results in a high incidence of adverse effects (Table 38.4).

The lowest osmolality is achieved with the dimeric nonionic compounds, with a consequent reduction in adverse effects. Adverse reactions requiring medical attention occurred in 29% of patients receiving ionic agents, but only 9% had adverse reactions to the nonionic compounds.[46] However, the increased cost of these compounds

Table 38.4 *Adverse effects seen with iodinated contrast media*

Hypersensitivity reactions (about 12% incidence)
Mild
Nausea and vomiting
Taste disturbances
Mild urticaria
Sensations of heat or cold
Pain on injection (not life-threatening, but may necessitate anesthesia)
Intermediate
Hypotension
Widespread urticaria
Bronchospasm and laryngospasm
Angioneurotic edema
Serious (potentially fatal)
Cardiovascular and pulmonary collapse
Refractory bronchospasm and laryngospasm
Other adverse effects
Diuresis leading to hypovolemia
Nephrotoxicity
Salivary gland enlargement
Hyperthyroidism

Table 38.5 *Some examples of contrast media*

Ionic		Nonionic	
Monomeric	Dimeric	Monomeric	Dimeric
Diaztrizoic acid	Ioxaglic acid	Iohexol	Iotrolan
Iothalamic acid	Iomeprol	Iodixanol	
Metrizoic acid			

Some may be given as sodium or meglutamine salts.

may make the choice less clear cut.[47] Some examples of the iodinated compounds are shown in Table 38.5.

The intravenous route is commonly used for radio-opaques, compounds designed to allow the visualization of the kidney and urinary tract. The molecule must be small and water soluble with very low protein binding to encourage glomerular filtration and passage through the urinary tract. The ionic compounds, such as metrizoic acid, have a high side-effect profile and newer drugs such as iohexol are preferred. Similar drug characteristics are required for angiography and the lower osmolality compounds are much less painful on injection and may be used without general anesthesia. Despite the general reduction in adverse effects with the low-osmolality drugs, visual hallucinations have been reported even when the drug has not been directly infused into the CNS.[48] A noniodinated compound used in retinal angiography is fluorescein, which can be described as a dye with more confidence than the contrast media mentioned above. The commonest adverse effect of fluorescein is nausea and vomiting, which may be reduced by oral granisetron.[49] Hypersensitivity reactions have also been described.

In order to enhance contrast in magnetic resonance imaging (MRI), newer (noniodine-containing) compounds based on gadolinium are used. Adverse effects include headache, nausea, and vomiting, together with transient taste disturbances or sensations of heat.

A number of other dyes are used as diagnostic agents and are listed in Table 38.6. As can be seen from the table, the major adverse effects seen with most of these are hypersensitivity reactions. The use of these agents is becoming less common, but there is still an extensive literature concerning the use of indocyanine green to measure blood volume and cardiac output. The development of pulse dye densitometry, in which indocyanine green-sensitive optical probes are attached to a finger rather than necessitating the insertion of a pulmonary catheter to obtain samples for cuvette densitometry, has simplified the procedure without sacrificing accuracy.[50, 51] As with other dyes, hypersensitivity reactions can occur.[52]

The use of crystal violet (gentian violet) and potassium permanganate as cleansers and disinfectants is of limited interest to the anesthesiologist.

Table 38.6 *Dyes used in diagnostic procedures*

Dye	Diagnostic use	Comments
Methylene blue	Fistula detection	Mild antiseptic; may cause methemoglobinemia
Indocyanine green	Cardiac output and blood volume	Occasional anaphylactoid reactions
Patent blue V (sulfan blue)	Coloring lymph vessels	Hypersensitivity reactions
Congo red	Detection of amyloid disease	
Indigo carmine	Renal function	Better agents available; may cause hypersensitivity reactions and hypertension
Phenolsulfonphthalein	Renal function and drug absorption studies	Hypersensitivity reactions
Rose Bengal	Determination of hepatobiliary function; staining nonviable tissue	May be painful on injection

Table 38.7 *Therapeutic uses of methylene blue*

Therapeutic use	Comment
Methemoglobinemia	Particularly useful in nitrite poisoning
Refractory septic shock	Acute vasopressor action with no deleterious effect on respiratory function
Targeting melanoma cells	High affinity for melanin; α-particle-emitting derivative
Antimalarial activity	Inhibits *Plasmodium falciparum* glutathione reductase
Adjuvant therapy for schizophrenia	Significant but modest decrease in psychopathology score
Antiviral	Mainly *in vitro* studies
Anxiolytic and antidepressant activity	Intermittent use in manic–depressive illness over the past century

The last dye that deserves a more detailed mention is methylene blue. I first came across methylene blue at school, where we used it to stain the nephridia of earthworms. Since then the reports of its use both as a stain and as a therapeutic agent have grown exponentially. Table 38.7 lists just some of the therapeutic applications that have been described in recent years. Although the major use of methylene blue is to treat methemoglobinemia, it can precipitate this condition at higher doses or in patients with glucose-6-phosphate dehydrogenase deficiency.[53] These patients are unable to reduce the methylene blue to leucomethylene blue, which, in turn, reduces methemoglobin to hemoglobin. Methylene blue is a messy drug. It is known to be an inhibitor of soluble guanyl cyclase and an inhibitor of iron-containing enzymes such as NO synthase. In addition it has anticholinesterase activity and an affinity for the muscarinic receptors for acetylcholine.[54] It has also been reported to reduce the minimum alveolar anesthetic concentration of sevoflurane in the rat.[55]

REFERENCES

1. Davis CJ, Harding RK, Leslie RA, Andrews PLR. The organisation of vomiting as a protective reflex. In: Davis CJ, Lake-Bakaar GV, Grahame-Smith DG (eds). *Nausea and Vomiting: Mechanisms and Treatment.* Berlin: Springer-Verlag, 1986: 65–75.
2. Hawthorn J, Ostler KJ, Andrews PLR. The role of abdominal visceral innervation and 5-hydroxytryptamine M receptors in vomiting induced by cytotoxic drugs cyclophosphamide and cis-platin in the ferret. *Q J Exp Physiol* 1988; **73:** 7–21.
3. Minami M, Endo T, Kikuchi K, *et al.* Antiemetic effects of sendide, a peptide tachykinin NK_1 receptor antagonist, in the ferret. *Eur J Pharmacol* 1998; **363:** 49–55.
4. Wang SC, Borison HL. A new concept of organisation of the central emetic mechanism: recent studies on the sites of action of apomorphine, copper sulfate and cardiac glycosides. *Gastroenterology*, 1952; **22:** 1–12.
5. Leslie RA. Comparative aspects of the area postrema: fine structural considerations help to determine its function. *Cell Mol Neurobiol* 1986; **6:** 95–120.
6. Waeber C, Dixon K, Hoyer D Palacios JM. Localisation by autoradiography of neuronal 5-HT_3 receptors in the mouse. *Eur J Pharmacol* 1988; **151:** 351–2.
7. Stefanini E, Clement-Cormier Y. Detection of receptors in the area postrema. *Eur J Pharmacol* 1981; **74:** 257–60.
8. Atweh SF, Kuhar MJ. Autoradiographic localisation of opiate receptors in the rat brain: II The brain stem. *Brain Res* 1977; **129:** 1–12.
9. Andrew PLR. Physiology of nausea and vomiting. *Br J Anaesth* 1992; **69** (Suppl. 1): 2S–19S.
10. Peroutka SJ, Snyder SH. Antiemetic: neurotransmitter receptor binding predicts therapeutic actions. *Lancet* 1982; **1:** 658–9.
11. Watson JW, Gonsalvas SF, Fossa AA, *et al.* The antiemetic effects of CP-99 994 in the ferret and the dog: role of the NK_1 receptor. *Br J Pharmacol* 1995; **115:** 84–94.
12. Lerman J. Surgical and patient factors involved in postoperative nausea and vomiting. *Br J Anaesth* 1992; **69** (Suppl. 1): 24S–32S.
13. Rabey PG, Smith G. Anaesthetic factors contributing to postoperative nausea and vomiting. *Br J Anaesth* 1992; **69** (Suppl. 1): 40S–45S.
14. Hadji F, Eastwood D, Fear S, Corfield HJ. The impact of audit in a district general hospital on post-operative nausea and vomiting after major gynaecological surgery. *Eur J Anaesthesiol* 1998; **15:** 595–9.
15. Gardner C, Perrin M. Inhibiton of anaesthetic-induced emesis by NK_1 or 5-HT_3 receptor antagonist in the house musk shrew, *Suncus murinus. Neuropharmacology* 1998; **37:** 1643–4.
16. Rang HP, Dale MM, Ritter JM. Antipsychotic drugs. In: Rang HP, Dale MM, Ritter JM (eds). *Pharmacology*, 4th edn. Edinburgh: Churchill Livingstone, 1999: 539–49.
17. Brogden RN, Carmine AA, Heel RC, *et al.* Domperidone. A review of its pharmacological activity, pharmacokinetics and therapeutic efficacy in the symptomatic treatment of chronic dyspesia and as an antiemetic. *Drugs* 1982; **24:** 360–400.
18. Rowbotham DJ. Current management of post operative nausea and vomiting. *Br J Anaesth* 1992; **69** (Suppl. 1): 46S–59S
19. Jaber M, Robinson SW, Missale C, Caron MG. Dopamine receptors and brain function. *Neuropharmacology* 1996; **35:** 1503–19.
20. Fozard JR. Neuronal 5-HT receptors in the periphery. *Neuropharmacology* 1984; **23:** 1473–86.
21. Madej TH, Simpson KH. Comparison of the use of doperidone, droperidol and metoclopramide in the prevention of nausea and vomiting following major gynaecological surgery. *Br J Anaesth* 1986; **58:** 884–7.
22. McCarthy BG, Peroutka SJ. Differentiation of the cholinoreceptor subtypes in human cortex and pons: implications for antiemetic therapy. *Aviat Space Environ Med* 1988; **59:** 63–6.
23. Chhibber AK, Lustik SJ, Thakur R, *et al.* Effects of anticholinergics on postoperative vomiting, recovery, and hospital stay in children undergoing tonsillectomy with or without adenoidectomy. *Anesthesiology* 1999; **90:** 697–700.
24. Leeser J, Lip H. Prevention of postoperative nausea and vomiting using ondansetron, a new, selective 5-HT3 receptor antagonist. *Anesth Analg* 1991; **72:** 751–5.
25. Russell D, Kenny GNS. 5-HT_3 antagonists in postoperative nausea and vomiting. *Br J Anaesth* 1992; **69** (Suppl. 1): 63S–68S
26. Fujii Y, Toyooka H, Tanaka H. Oral granisetron prevents postoperative vomiting in children. *Br J Anaesth* 1998; **81:** 390–2.
27. Fujii Y, Saitoh Y, Tanaka H, Toyooka H. Prophylactic oral antiemetics for preventing postoperative nausea and vomiting: granisetron versus domperidone. *Anesth Analg* 1998; **87:** 1404–7.
28. Fujii Y, Tanaka H, Toyooka H. Prevention of nausea and vomiting with granisetron, droperidol and metoclopramide during and after spinal anaesthesia for ceasarean section: a randomized, double-blind, placebo-controlled trial. *Acta Anaesthesiol Scand* 1998; **42:** 921–5.
29. Dabbous A, Itani M, Kawas N, *et al.* Post-laparoscopic vomiting in females versus males: comparison of prophylactic antiemetic action of ondansetron versus metoclopramide. *J Soc Laparoendoscop Surg* 1998; **2:** 273–6.
30. Hamid SK, Selby IR, Sikich N, Lerman J. Vomiting after adenotonsillectomy in children: a coparison of ondansetron, dimenhydrinate, and placebo. *Anesth Analg* 1998; **86:** 496–500.
31. Koivuranta M, Laara E, Ranta P, *et al.* Comparison of ondansetron and droperidol in the prevention of postoperative nausea and vomiting after laparoscopic surgery in women. A randomised, double-blind, placebo-controlled trial. *Acta Anaesthesiol Scand* 1997; **41:** 1273–9.
32. Scuderi PE, Weaver RG, James RL, *et al.*. A randomized, double-blind, placebo-controlled comparison of droperidol, ondansetron, and metoclopramide for the prevention of vomiting following outpatient strabismus surgery in children. *J Clin Anesth* 1997; **9:** 551–8.
33. Alexander R, Fennelly M. Comparison of ondansetron, metaclopramide and placebo as premedicants to reduce nausea and vomiting after major surgery. *Anaesth* 1997; **52:** 695–8.
34. Gan TJ, El-Molem H, Ray J, Glass PSA. Patient controlled antiemesis. *Anesthesiology* 1999; **90:** 1564–70.
35. Campan L, Lazothes G. L'hibernotherapie en chirurgie cerebrale, sa justification clinique et pathologenique. In: Laborit H, Huguenard P (eds). *Practique de l'hibernotherapie en Chirurgie et en medicine.* Paris: Masson et Cie, 1954: 137–80.
36. De Castro J, Mundeleer P. Anesthesie sans sommeil: "neuroleptanalgesie." *Acta Chir Belg* 1959; **58:** 689–93.
37. Edmonds-Seal J, Prys-Roberts C. Pharmacology of drugs used in neuroleptanalgesia. *Br J Anaesth* 1970; **42:** 207–16.
38. Portel L, Hilbert G, Gruson D, *et al.* Malignant hyperthermia and neuroleptic malignant syndrome in a patient during treatment for acute asthma. *Acta Anaesthesiol Scand* 1999; **43:** 107–10.
39. Pelonero AL, Levensen JL, Pandurangi AK. Neurolepic malignant syndrome: a review. *Psychiatr Serv* 1998; **49:** 1163–72.
40. Bissonnette B, Swan H, Raussin P, Un V. Neuroleptanesthesia: current status. *Can J Anesth* 1999; **46:** 154–68.
41. Jensen AG, Moller JT, Lybecker H, Hansen PA. A random trial comparing recover after midazolam–alfentanil anaesthesia, with and without reversal with flumazenil, and standard neurolept anaesthesia for major gynecologic surgery. *J Clin Anesth* 1995; **7:** 63–70.
42. The European Fraxiparin Study (EFS) Group. Comparison of a low molecular weight heparin and unfractionated heparin for the prevention of deep vein thrombosis in patients undergoing abdominal surgery. *Br J Surg* 1988; **75:** 1058–63.
43. Lepaux T, Charpentier C, Pertek JP, *et al.* Assessment of deep vein thrombosis prophylaxis in surgical patients: a study conducted at Nancy University Hospital, France. *Eur J Clin Pharmacol* 1998; **54:** 671–6.
44. Lowenstein E, Johnston WE, Lappas DG, *et al.* Catastrophic pulmonary vasoconstriction associated with protamine reversal of heparin *Anesthesiology* 1983; **59:** 470–3.
45. Ralley FE. The use of nitric oxide for managing catstrophic pulmonary vasoconstriction arising from protamine administration. *Anesth Analg* 1999; **88:** 505–7.
46. Barrett BJ,Parfley PS, Vavasour HM, *et al.* A comparison of non ionic

low osmolality radiocontrast agents during catheterization. *N Engl J Med* 1992; **326:** 431–6.

47. Henry DA, Evans RB, Robertson J. The safety and cost effectiveness of low osmolar contrast media. Can economic analysis determine the real worth of new technology? *Med J Aust* 1991; **154:** 766–72.
48. Iliopoulou A, Giannakopoulos G, Goutou P, *et al.* Visual hallucinations due to radiocontrast media. Report of two cases and review of the literature. *Br J Clin Pharmacol* 1999; **47:** 223–30.
49. Mattioli V, Calo A, Pisoni G, *et al.* Oral granisetron as prophylaxis for nausea and vomiting during fluorescein angiography. A multicentre, double blind, randomised, parallel group, placebo-controlled study. *Minerva Anestesiol* 1998; **64:** 553–61.
50. Iijima T, Aoyagi T, Iwao Y, Masuda J, *et al.* Cardiac output and circulating blood volume analysis by pulse dye-densitometry. *J Clin Monit* 1997; **13:** 81–9.
51. He YL, Tanigami H, Ueyama H, *et al.* Measurement of blood volume using indocyanine green measured with pulse-spectrophotometry: its reproducibility and reliability. *Crit Care Med* 1998; **26:** 1446–51.
52. Speich R, Saesseli B, Hoffman U, *et al.* Anaphylactoid reactions after indocyanine green administration. *Ann Int Med* 1988; **109:** 345–6.
53. Bilgin H, Ozcan B, Bilgin T. Methemoglobinaemia induced by methylene blue pertubation during laparoscopy. *Acta Anaesthesiol Scand* 1998; **42:** 594–5.
54. Pfaffendorf M, Bruning TA, Batink HD, van Zwieten PA. The interaction between methylene blue and the cholinergic system. *Br J Pharmacol* 1997; **122:** 95–8.
55. Masaki E, Kondo I. Methylene blue, a soluble guanylyl cyclase inhibitor, reduces the sevoflurane minimum alveolar anaesthetic concentration and decreases the brain cyclic guanosine monophosphate content in rats. *Anesth Analg* 1999; **89:** 484–9.

39

Total intravenous anesthesia

MICHAEL B HOWIE

Early anesthesia in the mid- and late nineteenth century was based almost totally on the use of inhalational agents. During the last 150 years, anesthesiologists have acquired vast experience and expertise in the administration of these types of drugs.

The use of intravenous anesthesia has been plagued by two parallel problems, the unavailability of satisfactory drugs and inadequate methods of administration, resulting in either underdosage or overdosage and almost invariably in excessively long recovery times. Today, both of these problems have been addressed. More favorable drugs and more appropriate means of delivering them have been developed, and enthusiasm for total intravenous anesthesia (TIVA) has markedly increased. Nevertheless, TIVA is currently used in only approximately 25% of cases where general anesthesia is administered.

PROBLEMS ASSOCIATED WITH INHALATION ANESTHESIA

Inhalation anesthetics provide the anesthesiologist with only two options: either to change the anesthetic state over time or to set a higher inspiratory concentration. Many aspects of the transfer process to the brain of inhalational anesthetics have an adverse effect on cardiac output, respiratory rate, total volume, and respiratory dead space.

Possible environmental damage caused by nitrous oxide and halogenated volatile anesthetics (e.g. depletion of the ozone layer) is also a concern. Nitrous oxide is a significant "greenhouse gas." It reacts with oxygen to produce nitric oxide, which affects the ozone layer, and has an atmospheric lifetime of 150 years. The anesthetic hydrochlorofluorocarbons such as isoflurane are less stable than chlorofluorocarbons and can undergo photolysis in the upper atmosphere, with the release of free chlorine atoms. Free chlorine atoms act as catalysts for ozone destruction, with an estimated loss of 100 000 ozone molecules per atom of chlorine released.[1,2]

For many years, anesthesiologists have been aware of the need for an intravenous line by which to inject an intravenous agent such as thiopental to deepen the level of anesthesia either for induction or as a rapid response to inadequately maintained anesthesia that would have had to be treated with inhalational agents using inhalational agents in an increased vaporizer setting. Thus, the intravenous injection of hypnotics, analgesics, and muscle relaxants has long blurred the distinction of purist methods.

BENEFITS OF TIVA

TIVA has multiple effects, including sleep hypnosis, analgesia, suppression of autonomic and somatic reflexes response, and muscle relaxation. With TIVA it is possible to provide truly "balanced" anesthesia by selecting a pure hypnotic such as propofol and an opioid together with a muscle relaxant. By independently titrating each of these different drugs to provide the desired levels of hypnosis, analgesia, and relaxation, it is possible to adjust anesthesia to the needs of the individual patient according to the surgical situation.[3]

The development in recent years of new hypnotic and analgesic drugs (e.g. propofol, remifentanil) with pharmacokinetic and pharmacodynamic profiles that are more suitable for TIVA than those offered by their predecessors has renewed interest in this type of anesthesia. Newer muscle relaxants are also more suitable for administration by continuous infusion.

Many anesthetic techniques now dispense with the use of nitrous oxide. Successful provision of solely intravenous agents has improved appreciation of intravenous methods and has shown that TIVA has the potential to provide anesthesia with equal or greater flexibility and control than has hitherto been possible with the use of inhalational agents. Because the onset and offset times of these drugs are known, intravenous anesthesia enables the anesthesiologist to obtain a specific desired effect (e.g. quick induction, rapid response to increased analgesia or hypnosis, convenient and stress-free emergence) within a specific time frame.

MODELS OF THE PHARMACOKINETICS AND PHARMOCODYNAMICS OF TIVA

For an in-depth discussion, see Chapter 2.

Physiologic models

Physiologic models may be divided into flow and recirculatory types. Flow models are complex but offer the most realistic representation of drug kinetics because they define these processes in terms of parameters that relate to the underlying physiology, anatomy, and biochemistry. The events occurring in each organ, tissue, or groups of tissues are described with respect to tissue size, vascular perfusion, binding or partitioning of drug between blood and tissue components, and any elimination processes that occur.

Unlike empirical and compartmental models, which are fitted to experimental data, complex physiologic models are developed a priori in that previous independent measurements are combined to predict pharmacokinetic behavior. In practice, however, the models are not mutually exclusive.

CLINICAL APPLICATION OF PHARMACOKINETIC THEORY

The clinical application of pharmacokinetic theory is concerned primarily with the design of dosage regimens. This requires some target profile of the plasma drug concentration–time relation that is consistent with optimum pharmacologic effect.

The simplest application assumes a threshold range of plasma drug concentrations that is safe and effective. The challenge is to reach this range and maintain it as long as desired. If this were a simple one-compartment problem, we could say that the loading dose is the product of the volume of distribution and the target concentration and the maintenance or infusion rate is the product of clearance and target level.

To achieve and maintain a constant plasma concentration over a period of time requires a combination of three processes:

1 a bolus dose calculated to fill the central compartment (which includes blood) to the required concentration;
2 a constant-rate infusion to replace drug lost by elimination; and
3 an exponentially decreasing infusion that will replace drug lost from the plasma by transfer or distribution to peripheral issues.[4,5]

The infusion of a bolus at a constant rate poses no great technical problems, but the administration of an infusion at a rate that must change according to predetermined exponential function is obviously much more demanding. To accurately achieve such an infusion scheme requires the use of an infusion pump controlled by a computer that is programmed with appropriate pharmacokinetic data of the drug to be infused. This simplistic approach is not sufficient, however, and has been replaced by the bolus elimination transfer (BET) infusion scheme. It is possible to approximate an exponentially decreasing infusion by a series of stepwise constant rate infusions (Fig. 39.1).

Roberts *et al.*[6] described a three-stage infusion regimen designed to achieve a steady-state propofol concentration of 3 μg mL^{-1}. This scheme can be used to derive a pharmacokinetic model or, more practically, by reading dependable known literature and then using an empirical approach, which Crankshaw *et al.*[7] called the *plasma drug efflux method*.

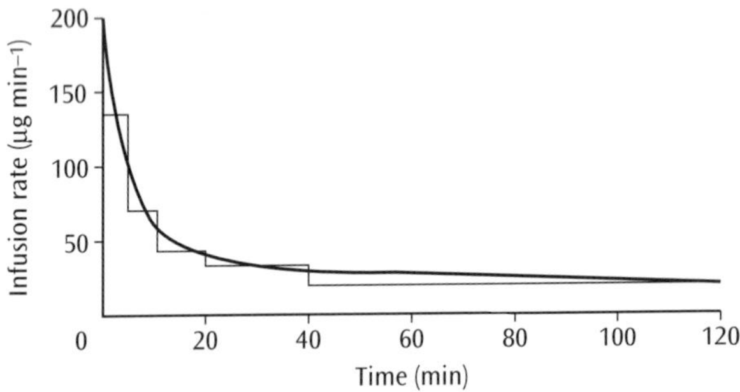

Figure 39.1 *The smooth curve shows how an intravenous infusion must change exponentially to achieve rapidly and maintain a constant plasma drug concentration. This example represents the infusion required to achieve an alfentanil concentration of 100 ng mL^{-1}.[21] The stepped curve shows how the exponentially decreasing infusion rate can be approximated by a series of constant-rate infusions.*

An initial group of patients received a series of changing drug infusion schemes. Plasma concentrations were measured, and a relation between infusion over time was constructed. They used these infusion sequences at different time points, first to ensure an adequate anesthesia level and then to predict recovery from the infused drug. The duration of effect after stopping a BET infusion was incorporated into the index of recovery, called the *context-sensitive half-time*. and defined as the time for the plasma drug concentration to decrease by 50% after the end of a BET input given over a specific time.

DESIRED PHARMACOLOGIC EFFECT

The desired effect is an ideal pharmacologic effect, which is not necessarily synonymous with the optimal plasma drug concentration. Anesthetic agents seldom produce immediate effects; their physiochemical characteristics and molecular structure determine the time to enter biophase. In fact, the concentration at the effect site – the biosphere concentration – and not the plasma concentration governs the drug effect. However, the actual anatomic site of the biophase may be difficult to identify, and direct physical measurements of drug concentrations in the biophase is impossible.

By measuring the drug effect and blood concentrations accurately and frequently, one can characterize the time for equalization of drug concentrations in the biophase with that in the blood. A significant lag between the time of drug effect and the plasma concentration gives rise to a hysteresis loop in the effect–concentration plot. This can be used to describe the rate of drug movement into a distinct effect compartment of negligible volume, hence the term *effect compartment models*. We assume that the effect compartment is so small that it has no effect on pharmacokinetics. We also assume that the effect site is connected linearly to the plasma compartment in the simplest case by a mathematical first-order rate constant derived, k_{eo}, which determines the time delay between changes in drug concentration in the blood and measured changes in drug effect. The k_{eo} combines access to receptor from plasma with on/off rates at the receptor and any postreceptor events that might contribute to time delays in response.

The k_{eo} and half-life k_{eo} have been characterized for many drugs used in anesthesia. Equilibration between the plasma and the effect site is rapid for thiopental, propofol, alfentanil, and remifentanil; intermediate for fentanyl and perhaps sufentanil and the nondepolarizing muscle relaxants; and slow for morphine and ketorolac.

The logical extension of pharmacokinetic and dynamic models in anesthesia is to apply them to the automatic control of pharmacologic effect. Thus, when a value and continuous measure of desired response is available, we can use a desired loop. At the present time we use neuromuscular stimulation and bispectral analysis, but both of these methods are controlled by a loose loop control in which the anesthesiologist controls the clinical response; this could become a tight loop with automatic control.

COMPUTER-CONTROLLED INFUSION OF TIVA

The true benefit of TIVA has not yet been realized. Many clinicians prefer inhalational agents because they are more familiar and less complicated to use. Some believe that TIVA has doubtful benefits and is more expensive to use.

When a bolus is given, TIVA can be administered by a manual infusion pump to maintain anesthesia, but this approach can be used to deliver only a zero-order infusion. A steady-state concentration of drug in the blood cannot be obtained until four to five times the distribution half-life has elapsed. Intuitively, we have used bolus plus zero-order infusions and have used multiple changes at the time of perceived stress or lack of it.

The ability of the anesthesiologist to respond to changes in anesthetic and surgical conditions in a predictable manner without the need to perform calculations that are mathematically complex requires the use of computers. Programs are available that will calculate predictable blood concentrations of anesthesia-related drugs in response to any given input regimen. An even more sophisticated approach is to have the computer directly control the syringe pump in such a way that the device achieves and maintains predicted target concentrations. By using such a target control infusion, concentrations can be manipulated in any direction with the same ease as a vaporizer, permitting delivery of anesthesia according to the surgical conditions and the individual patient's requirements.

When the infusion stops, drug concentrations fall at a rate that is dependent on the duration of infusion. Some agents, such as thiopental, slow recovery because of their relatively low clearance rate. These poor recovery characteristics ensured that TIVA remained an unpopular technique. The introduction of newer intravenous anesthetic drugs with more favorable pharmacokinetic profiles that permit faster recovery after infusion has improved the performance of TIVA. These new agents include muscle relaxants, remifentanil, and propofol.

The advent of these new agents made a different approach to computer-controlled infusions necessary. Work began at a number of academic centers, including the University of Glasgow, Scotland, on the use of computer-controlled infusions of propofol and the concept of target-controlled infusions (TCI) systems that would maintain the desired blood propofol concentration.[8,9] One of these systems, the Diprofuser, has been shown to be the most versatile, and thus is preferred by anesthesiologists.

The European anesthesiologist using intravenous anesthesia with propofol or remifentanil now changes the target concentration, and the Diprofusor system automatically adjusts the rate of infusion to achieve the required blood concentration. When the anesthesiologist wants to change the depth of anesthesia, either to respond to surgical stimulation or to pre-empt a response to it (e.g. sternotomy), the pharmacokinetic variables built into the system ensure that the patient receives an appropriate bolus dose followed by an increased rate of infusion when the target concentration needs to be increased. The system also works when the concentration needs to be lowered, in which case the pump stops the infusion until the system predicts that the required blood concentration has been reached and then restarts the infusion at a lower rate.[10]

The Diprofusor system does not determine how much anesthesia a patient needs. It is not a monitor of the depth of anesthesia, and control still rests with the anesthesiologist, who should be using clinical signs or more sophisticated means of monitoring the depth of anesthesia. Thus, the Diprofuser system provides flexibility in manipulating plasma concentrations similar to that offered by calibrated vaporizers for the volatile anesthetic agents.

Propofol has been used successfully to maintain anesthesia by either a stepped manual infusion or a TCI system. The extensive and rapid distribution of the drug to peripheral compartments, combined with a high central clearance rate, ensures that blood concentrations decrease rapidly after the infusion is stopped.

Opiate drugs can also be administered as continuous infusions. An ideal opioid has rapid transfer between blood and the effect compartment and a rapid decrease in concentration on cessation of infusion to levels that permit rapid recovery from effects. Alfentanil, sufentanil, and remifentanil are all ideal opioids. Remifentanil is an exciting opioid. Alfentanil, as in the case of remifentanil, produces rapid onset of intense analgesia, but its recovery profile is unaffected by duration of infusion.

Target-controlled infusion devices automatically implement pharmacokinetic principles to produce reasonably predictable results. The models for such systems, however, are grossly oversimplified. Even with efforts to make them more sophisticated, they remain inadequate and fail to deal with either the homogeneity of pharmacokinetic handling among individuals or the physiologic changes that occur during anesthesia delivery and surgery. It is unreasonable to expect that a precise concentration of drug can be predicted at all times. There is considerable pharmacokinetic and pharmocodynamic variability even in matched patient populations. This variability is also seen with inhalation agents. Fortunately, the target concentration does not have to be completely accurate. A system bias of 10% and a precision of 30–50% seem to be adequate for routine clinical practice.

Successful use of a computer-controlled infusion requires knowledge of the therapeutic concentrations appropriate for the specific anesthetic technique and the prevailing surgical stimulus. The anesthesiologist must determine the adequacy of the patient response and must change the target concentration as necessary. The control system must be surprisingly complex. It must provide acceptable performance with regard to the time to induction (i.e. reaching the target, the degree of overshoot, the time to stability, the extent of oscillation at a steady state, and the maximum deviation from the target). Pumps should be programmed to use the effect phase or site as a more logical target. Targeting the plasma results in a significant delay; targeting the effect site instead allows faster attainment of therapeutic concentration in the biosphere.

DOSE INTERACTIONS OF TIVA

The last area of inquiry is clinical pharmacology, in particular the interactions of different doses of intravenous agents.

In 1997, Vuyk *et al.*[11] analyzed the use of propofol and opioids in combination. They stated that the clinical concentration range of propofol is substantial. The combination of distinct propofol and alfentanil concentrations has been defined and was associated with a 50% probability of no response to surgical stimuli.[12] The study indicated that the speed of recovery varies with intraoperative propofol and alfentanil concentrations, even when they were equivalent. Stanski and Shafer[13] determined the infusion rates to maintain optimal propofol concentrations when combined with alfentanil or remifentanil. Because the pharmacokinetics of propofol and the various opioids vary, the optimal intraoperative propofol concentration varies with the selected opioid and duration of infusion.

Return of consciousness is governed not only by the decrease in the effect site propofol concentration relative to the effect site opioid concentration, but also by pharmacodynamic interaction between these two agents intraoperatively, relative to that for return of consciousness postoperatively. The optimal combination of propofol and opioid in both 50% and 95% of patients (EC_{95}) has been evaluated, with the shortest time to return of consciousness in 50% of patients. This optimal concentration was found with a variety of infusion times.

Compared with other opioids, for all durations of infusion, the effect site propofol concentration decreases much less (25%) in the time to return to consciousness than the effect site remifentanil concentration (>60%). For this reason, remifentanil is called a "forgiving" drug. For all concentration combinations of propofol and remifentanil associated with adequate intraoperative anesthesia in 50% and 95% of patients for all durations of infusion, recovery after propofol–remifentanil anesthesia is much faster than after anesthesia with propofol combined with alfentanil, fentanyl, or sufentanil at equivalent concentrations. For infusion durations of 15–600 min, the context-sensitive half-times of the opioids decrease in the following order: fentanyl > alfentanil > sufentanil > remifentanil.[11]

Concentrations do not need to decrease by as much as 50% to achieve return of consciousness or spontaneous breathing. The other factor that determines the values of the optimal propofol–opioid concentrations is the position of the interaction curve associated with a 50% or 95% probability of no response to surgical stimuli relative to the return of consciousness. At intraoperative effect site EC_{95} concentrations, return of consciousness is postponed less by relatively high propofol concentrations than by high alfentanil, fentanyl, or sufentanil concentrations because the decay in the propofol concentration is steeper than that for these three opioids. In contrast, combined with remifentanil, return of consciousness is postponed less by high remifentanil concentrations because remifentanil concentrations decrease more rapidly than concentrations of propofol. These characteristics of drug interactions can be used specifically with intravenous anesthetics to produce the overall anesthetic state.

The role of specificity of action in the combined effect of intravenous anesthetics can be illustrated by a number of synergistic reactions. One impressive synergistic reaction was reported with a midazolam–thiopental combination for the loss of ability to open eyes in patients. Dose–response curves for thiopental, midazolam, and their combination were determined and compared with isobolographic analysis [a statistical assessment of drug–drug interactions (additivity, synergy, or antagonism)]. The combined midazolam–thiopental fractional dose was only half of the single drug fractional dose. In other words, the hypnotic potency was twice that of midazolam. This result has been noted with many hypnotic combinations. The role of the physiologic mechanisms of actions of intravenous drugs in anesthetic interactions is especially evident in combinations that include an opioid component.

Opioids, however, have a ceiling effect; Smith *et al.*[14] observed this effect with a fentanyl–propofol interaction. The interaction was studied with steady biophase concentrations of both agents. A plasma fentanyl concentration of $3\,ng\,mL^{-1}$ resulted in an 89% reduction in the propofol EC_{50} value for blockage of motor response to skin incision. Fentanyl concentrations above $3\,ng\,mL^{-1}$ provided very little further reduction in propofol requirements, suggesting that the extent of interaction with opioids is limited. However, other effects (respiratory depression) that are often detrimental may continue to increase beyond such limits.

Sophisticated analysis of a decrease in the requirement of one drug by another can show a synergistic, additive, or even antagonistic interaction, depending on the extent of the decrease. Philip and colleagues[15] compared the use of remifentanil–propofol with alfentanil–propofol administered in TIVA regimens in patients undergoing ambulatory laparoscopic procedures scheduled to last more than 30 min. As indicated by fewer hemodynamic responses to intubation and trocar insertion and fewer dose adjustments during maintenance, remifentanil provided better intraoperative stability than alfentanil because it could be administered in a relatively larger dose owing to the decreased risk of delayed recovery and prolonged respiratory depression associated with higher infusion doses of remifentanil. Additionally, as the dose of remifentanil increased, the propofol dose decreased. As remifentanil can be administered right up until the end of surgery, it was considered useful for procedures in which high levels of surgical stimulation persist until the end of surgery or in which the duration is uncertain. Many more patients in the remifentanil group required fentanyl in the postanesthetic care unit, or required it earlier than patients in the alfentanil group, because of the short-acting nature of remifentanil due to metabolism.

INDIVIDUAL VARIABILITY

Many studies have indicated that TIVA is equivalent to standard inhalation methods. Some questions with regard to individual variability must be answered to realize the full potential of TIVA.

The choice of an appropriate pharmacokinetic model has been the concern of many investigators.[16] When individuals are given identical doses of a drug or even identical doses per kilogram of body weight, vast differences in pharmacologic response may be seen. Also, the dose required to produce a specific response may vary between individuals. Two sources contribute to this variability: differences in plasma or blood concentrations (pharmacokinetic variability) and differences in effect produced by a given drug concentration (pharmacodynamic variability).

Body weight

In adults with normal fat content, the volumes of both total body water and extracellular fluid are directly proportional to body weight. Most anesthesiologists believe that obese patients may be at risk of overdose when weight-normalized infusions are administered. A lean body mass correction is made to account of this, but it has not been universally used. The Diprofuser TCI system considers body weight when determining the central volume of distribution. This approach is appropriate for patients with normal fat content, but for markedly obese patients a modification of ideal weight plus 0.4 times excess weight has been suggested.[17] With propofol, this modification may not be necessary; Servin *et al.*[18] showed that the pharmacokinetics of propofol in obese patients are unaltered, and clearance values and volumes of distribution correlate well with body weight.

Age

Children require and tolerate larger weight-adjusted doses of drugs than do adults. However, the lean body mass per unit surface decreases as a function of age from 21 to 81 years and is probably responsible for decreasing volumes of distribution in elderly patients.

Disease

Pharmacokinetic variability is much greater in ill than in healthy patients. Disease affects various organ functions and the way in which drugs are distributed, metabolized, and excreted. For example, renal disease directly affects drug excretion, but it also alters drug binding to plasma proteins. Hepatic disease has an effect on drug metabolism, with some drugs being more sensitive to these changes than others. Cardiovascular disease can substantially interfere with the transport of drugs to eliminating organs by perfusion alterations but also influences the rate of distribution and redistribution to various compartments.

CONCLUSION

Several factors have contributed to renewed interest in total intravenous anesthesia (TIVA). The trend toward outpatient surgery has made speed and completeness of recovery from anesthesia important considerations. New intravenous drugs with desirable properties have been developed. The availability of reliable and accurate infusion pumps has improved delivery and made TIVA a more popular option. Finally, better understanding of the pharmacokinetic and pharmacodynamic characteristics has made it possible to use TIVA successfully as an option to inhalation drugs.

REFERENCES

1. Logan M, Farmer SG. Anesthesia and the ozone layer. *Br J Anaesth* 1989; **63:** 645–7.
2. Westthorpe R, Blustein H. Anesthetic agents and the ozone layer. *Anaesth Intens Care* 1990; **18:** 102–9.

3. Bovill JG. Total intravenous anesthesia – a pharmacokinetic approach. *Middle East J Anesthesiol* 1995; **13:** 37–60.
4. Vaughn DP, Tucker GT. General derivation of the ideal intravenous drug input required to achieve and maintain a constant plasma drug concentration. Theoretical application to lignocaine therapy. *Eur J Clin Pharmacol* 1976; **10:** 433–40.
5. McMurray TJ, Robinson FP, Dunes SW, *et al.* A method for producing constant plasma concentration of drugs. Application to methohexitone. *Br J Anaesth* 1986; **58:** 1085–90.
6. Roberts FL, Discan J, Lewis GT, *et al.* Induction and maintenance of propofol anesthesia. A mammalian infusion scheme. *Anesthesia* 1988; **43** (Suppl.): 14–17.
7. Crankshaw DP, Boyd MD, Bjorkston AR. Plasma drug efflux: a new approach to optimization of drug infusion for constant and blood concentration of thiopental and methohexital. *Anesthesiology* 1987; **67:** 32–41.
8. Schuttler J, Kloes S, Schwilden H, Stoeckel H. Total intravenous infusion with propofol and alfentanil by computer assisted infusion. *Anaesthesia* 1988; **43** (Suppl.): 2–7.
9. Kenny GNC, White M. A portable target controlled propofol infusion system. *Int J Clin Monitoring Computing* 1999; **9:** 179–92.
10. Gray JM, Kenny GNC. Development of the technology for "Diprofusor" TCI systems. *Anaesthesia* 1998; **53** (Suppl. 1): 22–7.
11. Vuyk J, Mertens MJ, Olofsen E, *et al.* Propofol anesthesia and rational opioid selection: determination of optimal EC50–EC95 propofol–opioid concentrations that assure adeaquate anesthesia and a rapid return of consciousness. *Anesthesiology* 1997; **89:** 1549–62.
12. Vuyk J, Lim T, Engbers FHM, *et al.* The pharmacodynamic interaction of propofol and alfentanil during lower abdominal surgery in female patients. *Anesthesiology* 1995; **83:** 8–22.
13. Stanski DR, Shafer SL. Quantifying anesthetic drug interaction: Implications for drug dosing. *Anesthesiology* 1997; **83:** 1–5.
14. Smith C, McEwan A, Jhaveri R, *et al.* The interaction of fentanyl on the CP_{50} of propofol for loss of consciousness and skin incision. *Anesthesiology* 1994; **81:** 820–8.
15. Philip BK, Philip ES, Chung F, *et al.* Remifentanil compared with alfentanil for ambulatory surgery using total intravenous anesthesia. *Anesth Analg* 1997; **84:** 515–51.
16. Coetzee SF, Glen JB, Wium CC, Boshoff L. Pharmacokinetic model selection for target controlled infusions of propofol. Assessment of three parameter sets. *Anesthesiology* **82:** 1995; 1328–45.
17. Gepts E. Pharmacokinetic concepts for TCI anesthesia. *Anesthesia* 1998; **53** (Suppl. 1): 4–12.
18. Servin F, Fannotti R, Haberer SP, Desmonts SM. Propofol infusion for maintenance of anesthesia in markedly obese patients receiving nitrous oxide. A clinical and pharmacokinetic study. *Anesthesiology* 1993; **78:** 657–65.

40

Trauma and physiologic dangers associated with patient transfer and the positioning process

JOHN M ANDERTON

TRAUMA RESULTING FROM THE TRANSFER AND POSITIONING PROCESS

Accidents in the operating and recovery rooms can never be totally prevented. Inadequate staffing, fatigue, and relative inexperience are undoubtedly contributing factors. A patient may fall from the operating table or be dropped by attendants involved in either positioning or transfer duties at any stage of the positioning process. Anecdotal reports of such mishaps undoubtedly occur from time to time. The potential for serious harm is considerable and fractured ribs have been reported.[1] It is not unreasonable to anticipate that long bones or hips could also be fractured, or that spinal or intracranial damage could ensue. Such an accident is likely to happen in the following circumstances.

Inadequate patient supervision

This can occur at any time after the administration of premedicant drugs. In pediatric anesthetic practice the problem is well recognized and assistance by attendant parents a useful safety factor. Adult patients, who may also be confused by unfamiliar surroundings in the immediate preinduction period, may make the presence of more than one attendant essential prior to induction of anesthesia. Narrow operating tables or transfer trolleys without side guard rails further increase the hazard.

If the early recovery phase is complicated by restlessness it must be the primary duty of all available operating room staff to assist in the management of the patient until safety can be ensured. The first and most important step in this process is undoubtedly transfer off the operating table either to the patient's bed or to a safe transfer trolley. Washing the surgical instruments or recounting the swabs is not a priority for operating room staff when such a crisis occurs. The presence of an anesthesiologist in the recovery room, as recently advocated by Vaughan,[2] albeit primarily for problems of airway management, would be a help in the later management of the restless patient.

Faulty patient transfer procedures

Although patient transfer systems that reduce direct handling to the minimum have been devised, there is almost always one stage at which the patient must be moved manually. Commonly, a stretcher canvas and poles are used or, alternatively, a "slide" may be employed. The first step is to ensure that the brakes are applied to any potentially mobile part of the system. Second, the task must be easily within the capabilities of the staff involved. Inadequacy in either of these prerequisites can result in problems; inadequacy in both is courting disaster.

There are two major hazards associated with the use of stretcher canvases. Repeated use can leave a weakness in the sleeves, which may cause one pole to tear out under the weight of the patient. With luck, the patient may fall only a few centimeters to the surface of the trolley or table. In less fortunate circumstances, a fall between the two could occur. A second hazard is the accidental placement of two canvases beneath the patient. The inefficiency of placing a pole in one sleeve of each canvas is revealed only on attempting to lift the patient. Unfortunately, some movement can be generated but ultimately the patient will fall between the poles; again the patient may end up on the operating room floor if there is a gap, or potential gap, between table and trolley.

Unhurried, gentle handling of the patient by an *adequate number* of operating room attendants at all stages of patient transfer is essential to avoid both minor injuries and the occasional catastrophe. Unfortunately, a recent survey has shown that we are some way off obtaining these ideals.[3] Difficulty in transferring patients occurred in one-third of cases. All the anesthesiologists questioned had scanty knowledge of the relevant handling regulations and, despite the fact that five or more staff were available to assist in 95% of transfers, 96% of patient transfers were performed by two staff alone and often by the anesthesiologists themselves. Operating room practice in the UK seems to have altered little since some of the legal aspects of lifting patients were addressed in 1970.[4] In that editorial it was stated that "it is not considered that the lifting of a patient can form part of the normal duties of medical or nursing staff in the operating theatre."

Badly designed operating tables

Operating tables designed using the principles of a separate operating room-sited pedestal with mobile "transfer tops" are hazardous if the locking mechanism for the two parts fails. The author has seen such a table top fall off the pedestal after the transfer vehicle had been removed. Fortunately for the patient, the foot end fell first and the table top remained propped against the pedestal at an angle of approximately 60°. The patient was able to be retained in place and was unharmed. The foot end of the transfer top made a 0.5-cm groove in the antistatic tiled flooring and could certainly have amputated part of an attendant's foot. A similar case has been described in which total collapse of the operating room table occurred just as the patient was being transferred to the transport trolley[5] (Fig. 40.1). Subsequent examination showed that the table top had been on the pedestal in the reverse position.

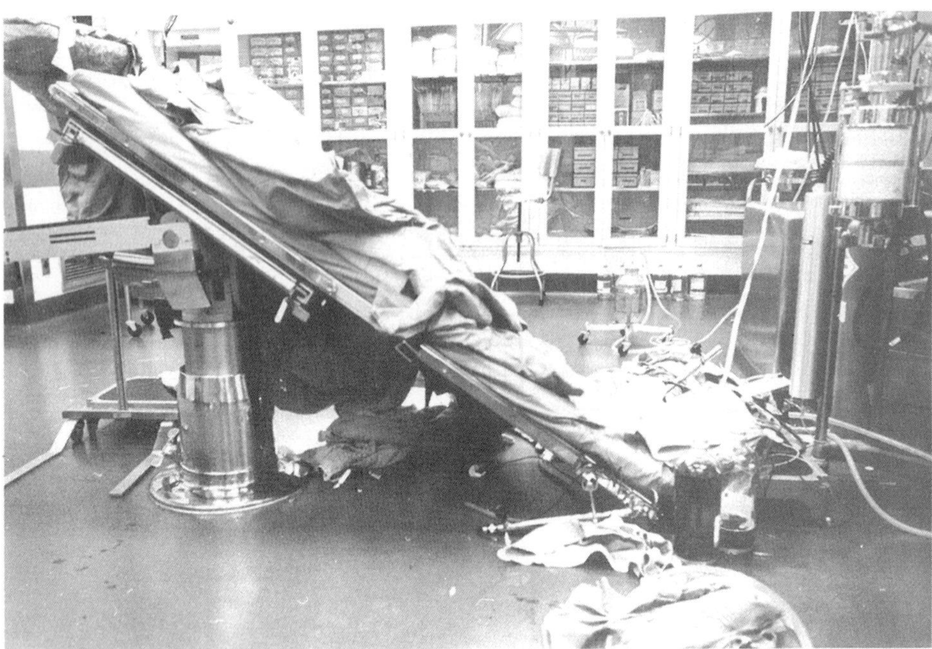

Figure 40.1 *The use of colored arrows to designate proper alignment of the table top on the pedestal might have prevented this mishap.*[5]

A note of caution should also be added concerning the use of "home-made" additions to the operating table, particularly those described to facilitate prone positioning. The wooden blocks used to support the pelvis were a significant advance in their day but were often not stable.[6] Modern operating tables with properly engineered accessories are now much safer and have rendered earlier methods obsolete (Fig. 40.2).

As far as the future is concerned, it is worth noting that some of the new electrically controlled operating tables do not have any means of manually changing their tipping function or any of their positional maneuvers should the electrical supply be compromised or any other fault render them "fixed." The facility to achieve rapid head-down tilt for the management of regurgitation or airway-threatening hemorrhage is undoubtedly of value but is uncatered for in these circumstances.

Use of the prone and other specialized positions

For maximum safety, employing the prone position requires skill, experience, and a team with an adequate number of assistants. The larger the patient, the greater the importance of this last requirement. The use of a "frame" or other more sophisticated propping system will further increase the risks. Methods of turning the patient vary. The change from supine to prone can be achieved after transfer to the operating table; alternatively, the patient can be turned in the process of transfer from the trolley to the operating table. The former is probably the safer method. Having achieved the prone position, stability must be ensured. This is not a problem with the simple horizontal position supported by pillows, but when more complex methods are required the choice should certainly be made with this in mind. The Tarlov[7] knee–chest (Fig. 40.3) or seated prone position is both reliable and applicable to a wide range of body shapes and sizes.[6]

At the completion of surgery, returning the patient to the supine position again requires the help and coordination of trained attendants. It is a wise precaution to maintain a good depth of anesthesia until the

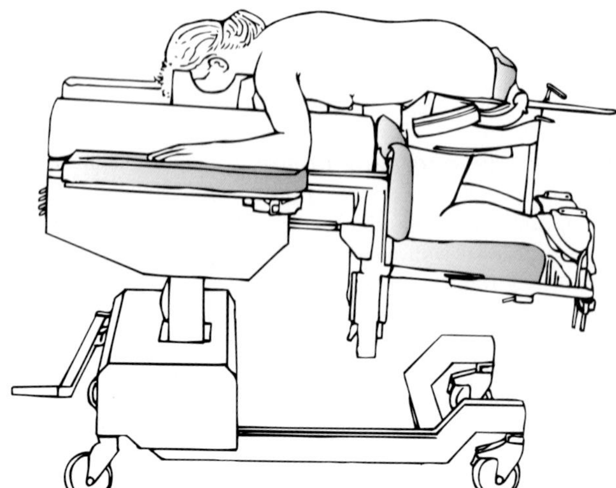

Figure 40.2 *Once the patient has been placed in the prone horizontal position other positions can be achieved by manipulation of the table controls. No physical lifting of the patient is required.*

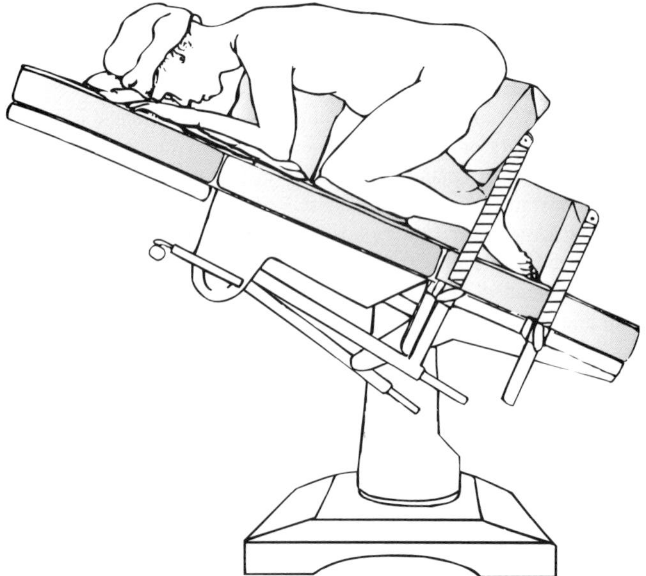

Figure 40.3 *Tarlov*[7] *described this as the "knee–chest" position. However, the use of the term "seated prone" distinguishes it from similar but less satisfactory positions.*[6]

patient is safely in the supine position. The situation can rapidly become out of control if a lightly anesthetized patient, still intubated and in the prone position, moves spontaneously on a narrow operating table.

The lateral decubitus position is probably the next most potentially unstable position although the use of evacuation mattresses has considerably increased the safety factor here. I have known a surgeon unhappy with either the view of, or access to, a difficult intrathoracic operating site almost dislodge the patient from the operating table in his attempts to improve these.

Fortunately, nowadays, the sitting position is rarely used except in neurosurgical operating rooms. Great skill is necessary to achieve safety for these patients and, although the risks are self-evident, a specialized text should be consulted.

Localized trauma due to the positioning process

The joints

During the positioning of patients under anesthesia joints may be subjected to a range of passive movements that would not be tolerated if conscious. Patients with any history of congenital or degenerative joint disease or who have had a prosthetic joint replacement should have their normal range of movement elicited prior to anesthesia. This range of movement should not be exceeded in the positioning process. The lithotomy position is particularly hazardous, and associated sacroiliac strain is a well-recognized sequela of failure to coordinate movement of the legs. To my knowledge a patient with a prosthetic hip replacement suffered such severe postoperative pain following stretching of the capsular ligaments that radiographic investigations were necessary to rule out dislocation. In other positions, the knees, shoulders, and elbows should be protected. Problems encountered with the spinal axis are dealt with later in this chapter.

Muscular trauma

Serious damage to muscle groups can occur, either because of direct external pressure or as a result of interference with venous drainage. The simplest example of the former is a case of deltoid muscle necrosis encountered in the underlying arm of a laterally positioned patient.[8] The presence or absence of a supporting axillary pad is not clear in the original article. Cases of "crush syndrome" following thigh and calf muscle compression in the Mohammedan prayer position, at one time advocated for use in lumbar intervertebral disk surgery, are of much greater importance[9] (Fig. 40.4). A death from acute renal failure was reported in 1952,[10] and a similar but nonfatal case in 1970.[11] The use of the exaggerated lithotomy position, now being used for radical perineal prostatectomy, resulted in ischemic compression of the lower back and pelvic muscles.[12] Surgery took 6 h and renal failure ensued. Technetium scanning on the third postoperative day demonstrated intense uptake in the posterior spinal, psoas, and gluteal muscles. This appears to be a useful investigation when the source of the rhabdomyolysis is not clinically obvious. Direct external pressure on muscles of the anterolateral aspect of the leg can lead to edema and swelling, and is one of the causes of acute "compartment syndrome."[13] This condition has been reported following surgery in the lithotomy position[14–16] and the Lloyd Davies position,[17] and the risk may be increased in these positions if intermittent pneumatic compression apparatus is used.[18] Support systems that place direct pressure on the popliteal fossa or the calf itself seem to pose greater risk than a simple sling encircling the heel and foot. Postoperative renal failure and permanent loss of function in the muscles affected result from failure to diagnose the condition quickly. As the muscles concerned are enclosed within a well-defined fascial sheath, capillary blood perfusion is reduced below a level necessary for

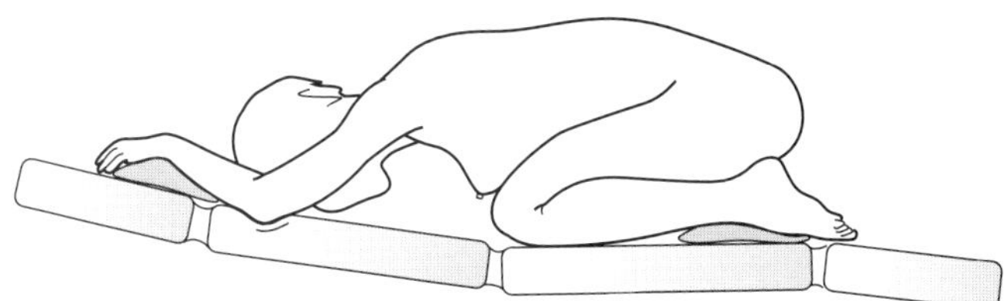

Figure 40.4 *The "Mohammedan prayer" position described by Lipton.[9] There is obvious potential for serious congestion and muscle damage in the lower limbs.*

tissue viability. This in turn will lead to edema and further ischemia. Experimental evidence shows that, as the pressure increases, different components of the compartment are affected. Muscle damage with a rise in creatine phosphokinase occurs at an early stage, as does damage to the nerve; damage to the latter becomes irreversible after 12 h. The period that the legs are held elevated in lithotomy appears to be a crucial factor. It rarely occurs in cases of less than 4–5 h duration.[16,19,20] In animal studies irreversible damage to muscle and nerve occurs between 3 and 4 h. The best way to reduce the perfusion problems in potentially long surgical procedures is to limit the use of lithotomy to the stages necessary for surgical access. Postoperatively, the legs will be very painful (out of proportion to the physical signs), tender, and somewhat swollen; there may also be numbness and tingling in the distribution of the nerve to the compartment. Confirmation of the diagnosis can be assisted by direct pressure measurements using a side port needle and may have the further advantage of limiting the extent of surgery to those compartments that require fasciotomy.[21,22] This is the only reliable method for terminating the ischemic cycle. The onset of acute renal failure may occur before the swelling and pain are clinically obvious, and the use of postoperative epidural analgesia may be a cause of delayed diagnosis,[23] but there are reports of cases in which this has not occurred.[16,24]

Trauma to internal organs

Patients who have been admitted to hospital for treatment of multiple injuries may be at further risk of trauma to internal organs at any time from the commencement of their transfer from the scene of the accident.

Great care must be taken to ensure the integrity of the spinal cord when injury to the cervical spinal vertebrae is suspected or diagnosed. Both positioning the patient for airway management and the method of achieving this can increase the risks of exacerbating the damage. Various methods of performing laryngoscopy and intubation have been investigated from the point of view of avoiding cervical spine movement but the most appropriate technique in this situation remains debatable.[25]

Heath[26] assessed ease of laryngoscopy in uninjured volunteer patients using two different cervical spine immobilization techniques. The use of a rigid collar with tape across the forehead and sandbags on either side of the neck were compared with an assistant providing manual in-line immobilization. Finally, laryngoscopy in the routine intubating position was also assessed. It was concluded that the use of a rigid collar and sandbags impedes laryngoscopy significantly, resulting in difficult intubation, which may be dangerously prolonged. Manual in-line immobilization was therefore recommended as the method of choice, provided that the collar and sandbags could be used once the airway had been secured. Data from the Maryland Shock Trauma Center in the USA would appear to support this view.[27] A retrospective analysis showed that over a 2-year period 73 patients with traumatic cervical spine injuries intubated within 24 h of admission showed no secondary neurologic injury associated with the procedure. A conventional rapid-sequence induction with the application of cricoid pressure and manual in-line stabilization of the head and neck was routinely used.

The above advice has, however, been challenged by Morley *et al.*,[28] commenting that, although it may be acceptable for patient management within the hospital environment, it may not be ideal in the prehospital situation. Here the practical difficulties of extricating trapped patients with multiple injuries may make uninterrupted manual support not always possible and so a collar affords at least some protection. Any need to remove and reapply the collar may also increase the risk of cord damage. Their preference for roadside tracheal intubation (when necessary) is for manual in-line stabilization with the collar in place. Preoxygenation and a rapid-sequence intravenous technique is used. They agree that mouth opening is indeed reduced by the presence of a cervical collar but that intubation assisted by the use of a gum elastic bougie invariably overcomes the difficulty. This technique has been successfully used in 307 out of 310 patients. It seems likely that the key to successful management of this potentially dangerous anesthetic situation lies more in the availability of an experienced team than in the method used.

Unstable rib and long bone fractures can also be a source of trauma following multiple injury. Perforation of the internal organs of the chest and abdomen when patients are transferred to and positioned on the operating table is always a possibility and should be considered in any acute deterioration of the patient's general condition. Tension pneumothorax, cardiac tamponade, or hypovolemic hypotension may occur. Manipulation of fractured long bones may cause fat embolism.

Skin trauma

Skin trauma can arise from pressure, heat, chemical, or electrical sources, either singly or in combination. Weight-bearing surfaces are particularly susceptible and of course vary with the intraoperative position used. There is a greater susceptibility to skin trauma in patients on steroid medication and in the elderly, who have lost supportive subcutaneous tissues.

In the *supine position*, pressure necrosis over the sacrum, heels, and occiput may easily occur unless effective support is provided. With advances in the safety of anesthesia this has become more of a problem as complex surgery extends operating times beyond previous expectations. At the end of a lengthy operation for hypospadias in a boy aged 4 years, the child's buttocks were discovered to have prolapsed into the triangular hole that is found in the mattress of many operating tables. Once his bottom had been extracted some skin necrosis was evident, but healing was uneventful.[29] The use of warming blankets to maintain body temperature, though necessary, adds a further risk to the sacral area. The use of a "fleece" or silicone-gel padding between skin and warming blanket is strongly recommended. The more widespread use of forced-air active heating devices should be strongly encouraged. Not only are they more efficient but they also considerably reduce the risk of thermal damage to the sacral area.

Diabetic patients, especially those with neuropathy or absent foot pulses, are particularly prone to develop ulcers on the heels if there has been inadequate protection during their time on the operating table. Connor[30] states quite categorically that these ulcers are not due to misfortune or misadventure but are preventable. Foam leg-troughs or ample padding with cotton wool are recommended but sheepskin heel-muffs do not appear to be of value. External pneumatic compression apparatus on the legs will prevent calf muscle compression and stasis, and certainly in nondiabetic patients protects the skin of the heels.

Postoperative pressure alopecia has been reported following prolonged surgery in which deliberate hypotensive techniques were employed.[31,32] Cardiopulmonary bypass surgery in particular has been implicated in this problem by Lawson and colleagues.[33] Follicular ischemia is clearly an important factor in most cases. Hair loss may be delayed for some days or weeks after the operation. It would seem prudent during long surgical procedures to ensure that the area of scalp under pressure is adequately supported with soft padding or pillows and to release pressure occasionally by readjusting the position of the head. However, this may not always prevent the problem, and alternative causes such as alopecia areata and damage by chemicals, drugs, or infection may have to be considered.

Skin damage caused by pneumatic tourniquets applied to the limbs is said to be uncommon. Pressure necrosis or shearing due to inadequate padding or poor application in patients with loose or thin skin is an obvious cause. Perhaps less well known is the danger of chemical burns occurring when spirit solutions commonly used in skin preparations are allowed to seep beneath the tourniquet and are held tightly against the skin.[34] Both full- and partial-thickness skin loss in the areas concerned have been described. It would seem a sensible precaution to use a self-adhesive surgical drape to seal off the tourniquet from the operative field before skin preparation commences.

With the patient in the *prone position*, damage to the skin of the malar region is a risk if the horseshoe headrest is used. Blistering and even full-thickness skin loss may result from excessive pressure, abrasive forces, or both. Craniotomy involving the use of the Gigli saw is a particular risk, as the reciprocating movement inevitably rubs the malar skin against the headrest. In cases not involving cranial surgery the skin at the tip of the nose can be very sore postoperatively if the head was placed face down on a pillow. Special props or frames occasionally cause superficial skin blistering in the areas of bony contact, particularly the iliac crests. In contrast, the seated knee–chest prone position very rarely causes anything more than a slight erythematous reaction to the skin of the knees.

Trauma to appendages

The fingers can be crushed or even amputated in accidents involving the moving sections of the operating table. Courington and Little[32] graphically described such an incident in which the arms of a patient in the lithotomy position were at her sides. Fingers were amputated as the foot section of the table was raised. Similar accidents occurring at the side of the table are possible with operating tables designed on the "pedestal" and "transfer top" principle. Probably the safest place for the patient's hands is across the chest; they should most certainly not be "tucked under the buttocks" to prevent the arm from falling off the sides of the operating table! (Unfortunately, elbow flexion may put the ulnar nerve at risk; see The ulnar nerve, below.) The longer and more complex the operation, the more important it is that the hands are within the view of the anesthesiologist. In this way, problems associated with arterial cannulation or failure of intravenous lines will be immediately apparent. A considerable volume of blood can be pumped subcutaneously if an intravenous cannula becomes dislodged. Splinting the hand and wrist using 2-cm Velcro tapes in order to maintain an extended position following radial artery cannulation has caused intensely painful wounds where the tapes cut into the flesh below the index and little fingers. It was thought that the prolonged period of hypotension that was necessary during cardiopulmonary bypass, and postoperatively for 12 h, may have exacerbated the ischemic effect of external pressure.[35]

Courington and Little[32] drew attention to the possibility of an ear becoming necrosed if caught up and folded either by a face mask harness or between the head and a supporting head ring.[32] The dangers to the genitalia and pudendal nerves in contact with the vertical post of the fracture table are dealt with fully elsewhere in this chapter.

Potential damage to breast tissue may be a problem in the prone position. The first priority must always be the prevention of any traumatic damage due to pressure. If the breasts are so large as to cause any instability of the patient as a whole on the operating table or supporting frame, it would be wise to opt for the lateral position. Patients who have had a mastectomy present a different problem, and prolonged pressure on a tender scar may result in postoperative pain or even ischemic damage. Care must also be taken with patients who have had an augmentation mammoplasty using pliable silicone breast implants. The latter could rupture if subjected to pressure or stretching and leaking contents may damage the surrounding tissues.

Smith and colleagues,[36] after discussion with conscious volunteer subjects, advised attempting where possible to displace the breasts laterally during the positioning process. Martin and Warner,[37] following a similar but unpublished review, disagree and state that "medial placement seems more satisfactory than lateral placement for most breast sizes during surgical procedures in the prone position." This view is also supported by senior surgical colleagues of Martin and Warner who have extensive experience in specialized breast surgery.

Backache following anesthesia and surgery

Attention has sporadically been drawn to backache for at least half a century.[32,38–40] The commonly perceived explanation is that anesthesia, general or regional, relaxes paraspinal muscles, allowing the supine position to flatten the convexity of the lumbar spine. This stresses the interlumbar and lumbosacral ligaments. In the lithotomy position, backward rotation of the pelvis flattens the convexity of the lumbar spine to an even greater extent than does the supine position.

Unfortunately, it is still very common for anesthesiologists to ignore recommendations that have been made to reduce the incidence of these problems. Courington and Little[32] first described modifying the operating table so that the patient "no longer lies to attention supine," and Martin and Warner[37] have both renamed it the "lawn-chair" position and quite rightly attempted to popularize it (Fig. 40.5). It may be of benefit to a great many patients.

Alternatively, simply supporting the lumbar spine has been suggested by other authors. An inflatable 3-L urologic irrigation bag linked via a three-way tap connector to a sphygmomanometer bulb and aneroid pressure gauge can easily be assembled for such use. O'Donavan *et al.*[41] assessed comfort levels on conscious volunteers and found that the most satisfactory pressures were 3.33 kPa (25 mmHg) for supine and 4 kPa (30 mmHg) for lithotomy patients. One hundred and fifty-five patients were divided into study and control groups; the incidence of postoperative backache was 8.5% and 38% respectively ($P < 0.001$). A further more complex analysis from the same department showed a reduction in first-day back pain from 46% in the unsupported group to 21% in the supported group.[42] Patients were also shown to have benefited if they had a previous history of backache or if they were anesthetized for more than 40 min. The incidence and severity of the backache was, not surprisingly, also shown to be greater if the surgery was performed on a very firm operating table surface compared with a softer one.

In practice, a fixed contour support would probably be more convenient to use and would not be prone to accidental deflation. However, the normal variation in degree of lumbar lordosis might require that a range of differently shaped supports would need to be available. More widespread use of the lawn-chair position or lumbar supports is to be recommended. Postoperative backache is a largely unrecognized form of trauma caused by failure to support the spine in the supine or the lithotomy position and results from a serious error of omission. The figures from the above studies speak for themselves.

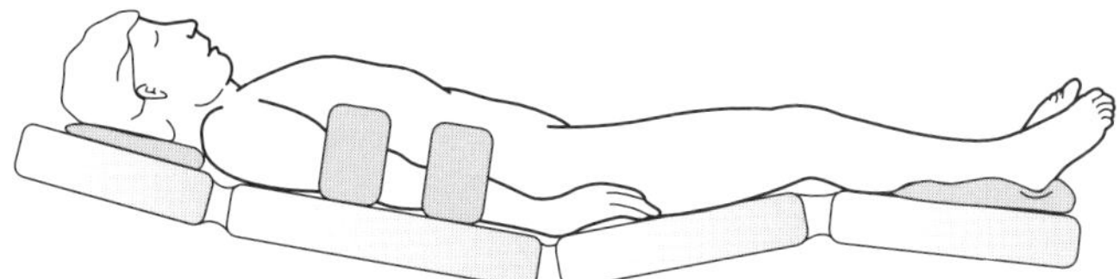

Figure 40.5 *The lawn-chair position. (After Martin,[37] with permission from the publishers.)*

HEAD AND NECK: SOME SPECIFIC PROBLEMS

Care of the patient's eyes

Probably every textbook of practical anesthesia contains some advice on this subject. Whatever the position of the head during surgery, the eyelids should be closed and taped down so that they stay closed. The routine installation of aqueous solutions, viscous gels, and ointments is not recommended. They do not offer sufficient additional protection, and ointments in particular contribute to ocular morbidity.[43] Additional cover of the orbit with an occlusive dressing is a sensible extra safeguard in most cases. Failure to tape the eyelids together beneath such an occlusive dressing can result in corneal trauma. Any temptation to omit these precautions in minor surgical cases should be resisted. The risks to the corneal epithelium are ever present, irrespective of the length of surgery. Contamination with acid- or bile-containing vomit can cause corneal ulceration and easily occurs with the lateral decubitus position for tracheal extubation. Any head-down tilt applied in these circumstances to prevent aspiration into the trachea virtually guarantees contamination of one or even both eyes. Aerosol-sprayed wound dressings and skin antiseptics may also gain access to an unprotected cornea and conjunctiva.

A further danger, often unappreciated by anesthesiologists, is that approximately 10 min of corneal exposure without eyelid movement is sufficient to start the process of surface dehydration. This is an important precursor of corneal abrasion. Studies involving the continuous monitoring of the exposed corneas of patients undergoing elective general anesthesia have shown that corneal changes start to occur after 100 min, always in the lower half of the cornea, and that the peak incidence of corneal abrasions is between 90 and 150 min of anesthesia.[43] Central corneal oxygenation is dependent on atmospheric oxygen dissolved in tears. General anesthesia itself is responsible for a significant reduction in tear production and further surface drying completes the destructive scenario. An analysis of closed insurance claims in the USA has shown that abrasions constitute 35% of postoperative eye injuries associated with anesthesia (Table 40.1). On balance it seems likely that corneal drying is largely responsible for the majority of the cases.[44] Approximately 20% of cases result either from chemical injury or from inadvertent direct trauma. Face masks, the anesthesiologists' and other attendants' hands, surgical drapes, and instruments have all been implicated. Symptomatically there is considerable pain and distress and permanent scarring can result from epithelial breakdown and infection. Permanent ocular damage was found in 16% of patients in the series quoted above.[44] A secondary iridocyclitis may also develop. Immunosuppressed patients from special care units in which virulent organisms are frequently encountered are at particular risk from these complications.

External pressure on the eye can result from a variety of causes. A badly fitting face mask that extends too high up the bridge of the nose and presses into the medial aspect of the orbits is a recognized hazard. The obvious danger is that intraocular pressures will be raised. Four cases of central retinal artery occlusion resulting from this have been reported.[45] Hypovolemic hypotension was thought to have been a contributory factor.

Tipping the patient head-down also has adverse effects on intraocular pressure. This was reported by Tarkannen and Leikola in 1967.[46] Significant elevations in intraocular pressure were shown in tilts of up to 70° from the horizontal. Fortunately, this is rarely necessary in modern surgery. Friberg and Şanborn[47] investigated optic nerve function in subjects volunteering to be completely inverted, and concluded that the direct effects on intraocular pressure were of primary importance. It can be concluded that steep head-down tilting for any length of time

Table 40.1 *Mechanisms of eye injury*[44]

Mechanism of injury	Eye injury (total) ($n = 71$)	Corneal abrasions ($n = 25$)
Patient movement	21 (30%)	0
Chemical injury	9 (13%)	1 (4%)
Direct trauma	6 (8%)	4 (16%)
Pressure on eye	2 (3%)	0
Other	3 (4%)	0
Unknown	30 (42%)	20 (80%)

is undesirable and may cause optic nerve dysfunction. Even a 6° head-down tilt maintained for 20 min will produce significant effects.[48]

The incidence of acute glaucoma following nonophthalmic surgery is probably only in the order of 1 in 12 000 and appears to have decreased markedly in the last 20 years. Two cases are described that have no predisposing factors caused by positioning or direct pressure.[49] However, as this condition has catastrophic ocular effects if not diagnosed and treated promptly, all postoperative cases of acute, painful red-eye require ophthalmologic assessment.

The avoidance of external pressure on the eyeballs is of particular importance in patients with an intraocular lens implant of the older type that clips on to the iris. Displacement of the lens can cause intraocular hemorrhage, or damage to the generative epithelium on the posterior corneal surface. The newer posterior chamber intraocular lenses are much more stable and are unlikely to be dislodged, though interactions with the coats of the eye remain a possibility. Significant external pressure on the eye is most likely to occur when the patient is placed in the prone position. It is less common, but has been recorded, with lateral positioning. Walkup and colleagues[50] first described two cases of retinal ischemia with resulting unilateral blindness occurring during thoracotomy carried out in the prone position. Undetected rotation of the head on a "horseshoe" support resulted in protracted direct pressure on the globe. Eight similar cases were later reported from the Mayo Clinic.[51] Animal studies by the same authors suggested that induced hypotension and hypovolemia were necessary in addition to the external pressure, in order to produce findings similar to those observed in humans. A modification in the design of the headrest was also suggested and initial experience of its use was encouraging, but further reports have not been found. It has, of course, been largely superseded by the use of a skull clamp. The horseshoe headrest was implicated as a factor in a case of postoperative blindness described by Jampol and colleagues[52] and in another case described by A. Cooper and S. Ingham (personal communication) at a National Neurosurgical Anesthesiologists Meeting in 1989.

Edema of the periorbital tissues is occasionally seen following prone positioning. It does not appear to be of any importance. Periorbital bruising is a fairly common complication following the removal of eyelid tapes from fragile skin, especially in patients taking high-dose steroids.

Finally, it is worth noting that should postoperative blindness or even a deterioration in visual acuity ensue unexpectedly and for no obvious external reason (e.g. pressure), other causes should be considered. An embolic episode affecting the retinal artery may have occurred: fat in particular has been implicated and paradoxical air embolism is a rarer possibility. Alternatively, the condition of postoperative ischemic optic neuropathy may be associated with such perioperative factors as anemia, hypotension, blood loss, venous obstruction, and vascular anomalies. This subject has been extensively reviewed by Williams *et al.*[53]

Damage to the cervical spine and consequences of head rotation

An unconscious patient loses the protection of the tone in the musculature supporting the cervical vertebrae. Damage is therefore easily produced by passive movements, especially if they are poorly controlled. It can range from a simple musculotendinous "strain" to intervertebral disk herniation or even facet joint fracture and dislocation. Within the spinal canal itself the delicate structure of the spinal cord, nerve roots, and, most importantly, its blood supply may also be compromised. Even the young patient with a spacious spinal canal (Fig. 40.6) may suffer from the effects of muscle or ligamentous damage, or even a traction injury to the nerve roots. The more elderly patient, who may have a spinal canal narrowed by osteophytes and degenerated intervertebral disk hernation, is at much greater risk from mishandling of the neck (Fig. 40.7). Patients with rheumatoid arthritis are well known to have serious weakness of the cervical spine ligaments and degeneration of the associated joints. The atlantoaxial region is at particular risk of subluxation. Patients with Down syndrome are similarly at risk of spinal cord compression. However, in this group, research has shown that neck radiology will not reliably identify those susceptible and is therefore no longer recommended.[54]

In positioning the patient, neck injury can be produced in a variety of ways. Probably the best known is "whiplash" injury, which occurs when support for the head is suddenly withdrawn. The classic example of this may be produced by lifting a patient with poles and stretcher canvas where the latter has been incorrectly placed and does not support the patient's pillow. Lifting the patient allows the pillow to drop swiftly away and the head to swing violently downwards (Fig. 40.8). Turning the patient into the prone or lateral positions also carries similar risks unless the person supporting the head makes a positive effort to avoid hyperextension of the neck.

A "Lesson of the Week" article in the *British Medical Journal* entitled "Don't twist my child's head off" graphically describes the risk of iatrogenic cervical dislocation.[55] Excessive rotation of the necks of two children whilst they were undergoing cervical lymph node biopsy probably resulted in C1–C2 dislocation (Figs 40.9 and 40.10).The most likely mechanism was that the children were placed supine on the operating table and, to gain access, the head was rotated and held to one side to expose the posterior triangle of the neck. If diagnosed and dealt with at an early stage, conservative management with traction, manipulation, and immobilization with a collar is often successful. The delayed diagnosis in these cases necessitated complex spinal surgery to correct the deformity. Surgeons and anesthesiologists must ensure that overvigorous positioning of the child's head and neck does not occur.[55]

Head and neck rotation with the neck in forward flexion is particularly dangerous with respect to the integrity of the facet joints. These are not easily disrupted in the neutral or extended position but can readily

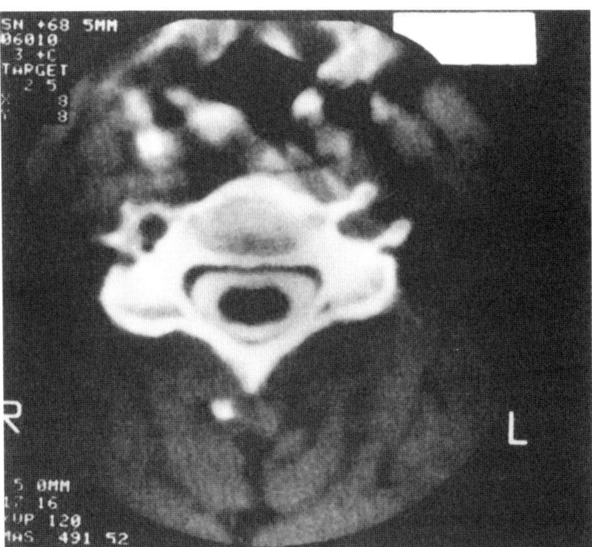

Figure 40.6 *A normal cervical spinal canal with no compression of the cerebrospinal fluid and spinal cord.*

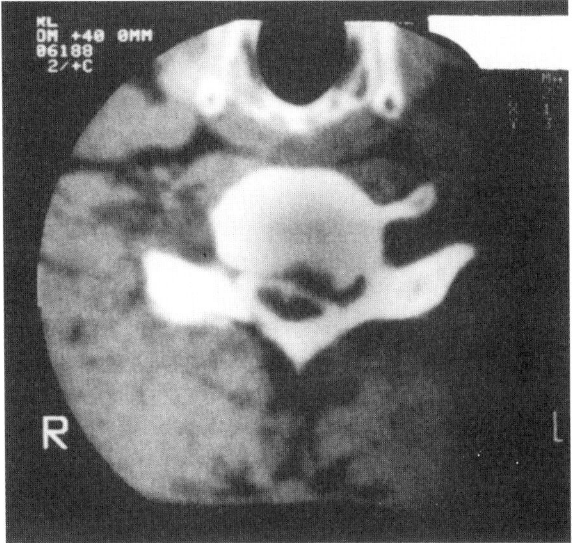

Figure 40.7 *The spinal cord is displaced and compressed by a bulging cervical intervertebral disk and large osteophyte. The rim of cerebrospinal fluid is considerably narrowed.*

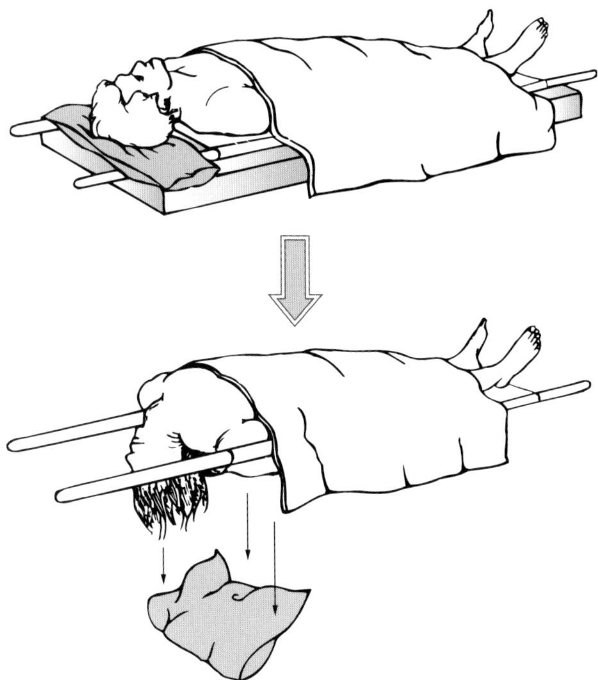

Figure 40.8 *It is essential that the stretcher canvas supports the head and neck.*

become dislocated, with fracture of the delicate articulating surfaces, by such a maneuver. The adjacent vertebral arteries running through their bony canals can easily become damaged or occluded by such injury. Any method of lifting or turning the unconscious patient can result in damage to the structures of the neck; responsibility for "holding the head" should not therefore be taken lightly.

Excessive head rotation can compromise the circulation to the spinal cord and brainstem even in the *unanesthetized patient*. Cerebrovascular accidents secondary to obstruction of the vertebral artery have been reported following swimming,[56] ceiling painting,[57] and yoga exercises.[58] Chiropractic manipulation of the neck has a particularly bad record in this respect.[59,60] Radiologic studies in healthy men have shown that complete occlusion of the contralateral vertebral artery can occur when the head is turned to one side.[61] Abrupt changes in the head position, whether active or passive, may injure the intima of the vertebral artery at the level of the atlanto-occipital joint, giving rise to thromboembolism and progressive brainstem infarction.[62] Kim *et al.*[63] monitored electroencephalogram (EEG) changes in anesthetized patients having an internal jugular vein catheter inserted with approximately 70° of head rotation. This demonstrated adverse effects in 15 out of 28 patients studied, and these were bilateral in five of the affected patients. McPherson *et al.*[64] noted complete disappearance of cortical somatosensory-evoked potential recordings in a patient positioned with the head flexed and laterally rotated in the "park-bench" position. The tracings returned on restoration of the head to the neutral position.

Patients with cervical spondylosis are obviously going to be at increased risk of postoperative deterioration of neurologic function, particularly after neurosurgical procedures. Such damage appears to take one of two forms.

The *central cord syndrome* originally described by Scheider *et al.*[65] in 1954 occurs most commonly in patients having had severe *hyperextension* of the neck but has also been noted to be due to minor hyperextension injury.[66] It is a known complication of decompressive cervical laminectomy, with an incidence of 1.6%.[67] The essential clinical features are arm weakness, leg spasticity, and diminished perception of pain and temperature in the upper half of the body. It has been suggested that the mechanism of the injury may involve buckling of the ligamentum flavum and direct spinal cord compression, or a "pincher effect" between the posterior elements of the vertebral body below and the laminae above. Limiting neck movement by fitting a firm cervical collar before awakening and very careful patient movement in the immediate postoperative period may give some protection.

Alternatively, cases of postoperative *midcervical tetraplegia* have mainly been reported in patients operated on with the *neck flexed and the head laterally rotated,* in either the park-bench or sitting position.[68] Although still a relatively rare condition a considerable bibliography is accruing. Some 30 cases have now been reported.[69] The syndrome has also been described in a patient with severe cervical spondylosis having thoracolumbar surgery in the prone position,[70] in an infant positioned supine with the neck in extreme hyperflexion,[71] and in a victim tied up by bandits in a position of extreme cervical flexion for several hours.[72]

The etiology of injury is probably different to central cord syndrome in that pressure is unlikely to be involved and that stretching of the spinal

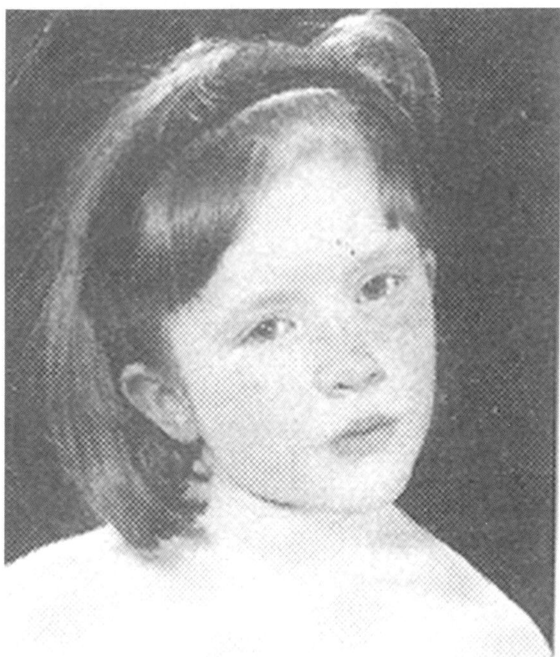

Figure 40.9 *Child with a wry neck showing the typical "Cock Robin" position. Prompt evaluation by detailed cervical spine radiography is indicated.*[55]

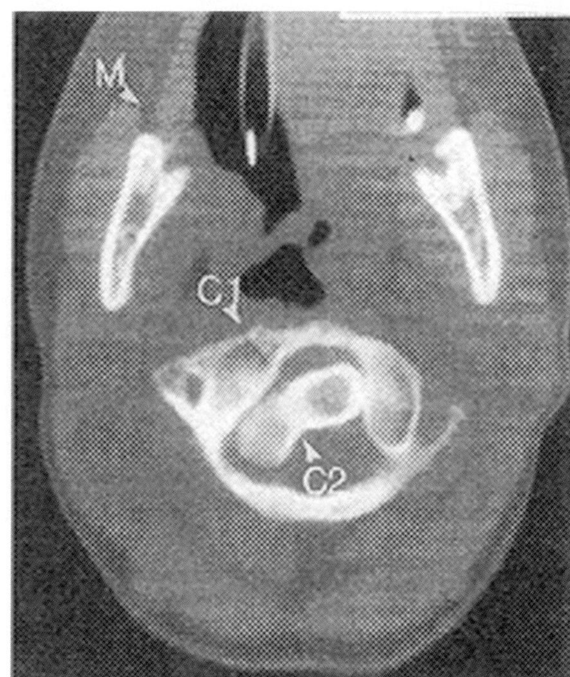

Figure 40.10 *Axial computed tomogram showing rotary atlantoaxial dislocation C1 and C2, indicated by arrows.*

cord with compromise of its vascular supply could be of importance. Somatosensory-evoked potentials can be used to assist monitoring but animal experiments have shown that they are not always sufficiently sensitive to be reliable.[73] Motor-evoked potentials may be shown to have value in the future. Maintenance of adequate perfusion pressures and meticulous attention to maintaining a neutral neck position remain the mainstay of management, although these precautions alone will not always guarantee success.[70] Limiting the degree of neck flexion so that two fingers can be placed between the chin and the sternum or clavicle and having the head as near as possible to the sagittal plane remain sound advice. Short periods of head and neck rotation may have an adverse effect on cerebral blood flow and, until monitoring of the latter is commonplace practice in the operating room, these positions should be avoided whenever possible.

Serious airway complications have also been reported and attributed to extremes of head flexion with or without cervical spine rotation.[74,75] They have occurred in patients operated on in the sitting position, and it is thought that impaired venous and lymphatic drainage occurs and is responsible for the gross edema of the face, soft palate, and tongue. Some cases have required tracheostomy. However, positioning alone is not always responsible for this alarming complication. Sublingual hematoma, angioedema, and sialadenitis can all result in a similar clinical picture.[76]

Dangers of some special head supports

The horseshoe headrest

Surgical procedures on the head and neck may require the head to be supported so that pressure can be applied without the danger of any movement occurring. This is particularly important in some of the intracranial microsurgical procedures that have become more common in recent years. Probably one of the earliest such devices was the "horseshoe headrest." It must be stressed that there is no longer any justification for using this device as a head support for patients in either the lateral or the prone position when the head or neck is *not* the site of the surgical operation. The risks of the head becoming displaced and blindness ensuing are too great. Safer methods such as silicone-filled "rings," foam padding, or pillows are available. Extreme care must be exercised in their use when the face is in the prone position for operative procedures on the cervical spine or posterior cranial fossae. The eyes in particular and the skin of the malar areas are vulnerable and have already been discussed.

Skull clamps

Alternatively, a three-pin neurosurgical skull clamp may be used for accurate and very stable fixation of the head (Fig. 40.11).[77] Although it is an instrument of barbaric appearance, it virtually eliminates the risk of pressure-related complications involving the face. It is essential for operations in the sitting position and highly desirable for cervical or intracranial procedures in the prone or lateral position. It appears to have had a very good overall safety record apart from two cases of intracranial hemorrhage (see below).

Disadvantages of the skull clamp

Its application is associated with a quite severe surge of systemic and intracranial hypertension. This is undesirable for any patient, but particularly so in those presenting for intracranial aneurysm surgery or with raised intracranial pressure. The use of local anesthetic at the pin sites or intravenous lidocaine (lignocaine) or thiopental has been advocated to attenuate the response.[78,79]

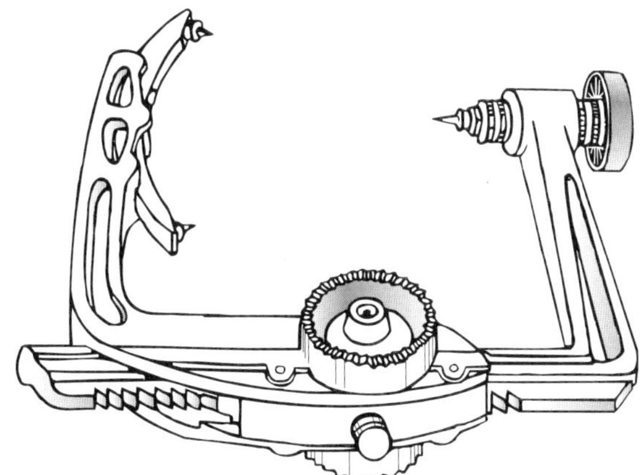

Figure 40.11 *The Mayfield modification of Gardner's headrest.*

The second physiologic risk is that of venous air embolism. Because the pins are designed to pierce the outer table of the skull, diploic veins are likely to be damaged by their insertion. Air can enter these veins when the pins are removed if the head is at a higher level than the heart. It is important, when applying the clamp, to do so with the patient horizontal and to obtain the correct siting of the headrest at the first attempt. Multiple unsuccessful attempts to do so increase the risk of venous air embolism. At the termination of the case, especially if the sitting position has been used, the clamp should not be removed until the patient has been placed supine. The use of an antibacterial ointment around the entry points of the pins may help to seal these. Hemorrhage from the site of skin puncture can occasionally be a problem and may require suturing. Skin necrosis can occur if a small area of skin is trapped between the bone and the shoulder of the pin. This is likely if pediatric size pins are used for an adult, or if the correct size pins are applied at an angle rather than at 90° to the skin surface. If, on application, this occurs and there is "blanching" of an area of skin around the puncture site, the clamp should be reapplied correctly.

Scalp laceration can occur as a result of inadequate bony penetration and subsequent head movement. The most serious danger associated with the use of this skull clamp concerns the use of too great a pressure in its application, with resulting puncture of both the outer and the inner tables of the skull. This can lead to loosening of the remaining pins, which may allow the head to slip out of the clamp. Other potential complications relate to the depth of the penetration of intracranial structures. Epidural hematoma, meningitis, cerebrospinal fluid fistula, and cortical brain injury are possible. A fatality from serious intracranial hemorrhage occurred and resulted in a UK Department of Health "Hazard Warning Notice 46" being issued. The Gardner models 19–1020 and 19–1026 of this headrest were withdrawn from clinical use.[80] A case of epidural hematoma that did not present until 10 days postoperatively has also been reported.[81]

The Boyle–Davis gag

The Boyle–Davis combined mouth gag and tongue depressor is widely used for intraoral access, especially by ear, nose, and throat (ENT) surgeons (Fig. 40.12). There are some obvious dangers inherent in its use, such as damage to the teeth and bruising of the lips, dislocation of the mandible, and tracheal tube occlusion or disconnection. Hyperextension of the cervical vertebrae must be prevented. Failure to pay attention to the latter during the course of curetting adenoid tissue may result in damage to the ligaments overlying the anterior surface of the vertebral bodies. For this reason, some surgeons prefer to hold the gag by hand rather than use the supporting rods for this procedure.

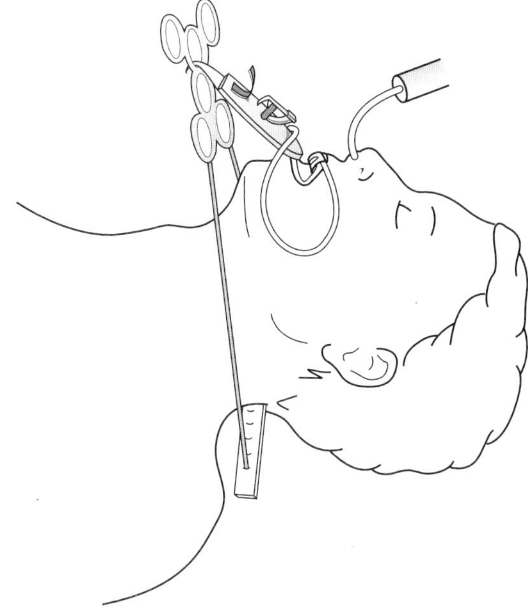

Figure 40.12 *The Boyle–Davis gag, commonly used for tonsillectomy.*

Nerve lesions of the head and neck

There are several reports of damage to nerves in the head and neck region resulting from problems in positioning the patient or maintenance of the patient's airway. Superficial branches of the trigeminal nerve are vulnerable at two sites.

Compression of the supraorbital nerve as it emerges around the supraorbital ridge by the metallic end of an endotracheal tube connector held in place by a Hudson's harness, even though protected by a layer of gamgee, was sufficient to produce a neurapraxia persisting for 3 weeks.[82] The patient complained of pain in the right eye, headache, photophobia, and numbness over the right side of the forehead and scalp. There was impaired sensation to touch, heat, cold, and pain in the distribution of the nerve, but no impairment of corneal sensation. A right-sided conjunctivitis also ensued, but this may have been coincidental and it resolved quickly.

The mental branch of the inferior dental nerve exits from its foramen on the anterior surface of the mandible in a position that is susceptible to pressure from the lower rim of a tightly fitting face mask.[83] Two cases of lower lip numbness with loss of touch and temperature sensation have been described.[83] The patients were at risk from inadvertent self-induced thermal injury and experienced the distressing inability to drink fluids without spillage from both corners of the mouth. The condition resolved within 5–6 weeks.

Deeper branches of the trigeminal nerve are susceptible to external pressure, which affects the position of the mandible. This may be due to efforts to maintain a patent airway[84] or from prone positioning.[85] In the first of these cases hyperesthesia of the tongue, with numbness and loss of taste sensation, followed a 3-h anesthetic administered via a face mask necessitating continuous bilateral anterior pressure at the mandibular angles. The cause of the problem was thought to be trapping of the lingual and chorda tympani nerves between the lateral and medial pterygoid muscles (Fig. 40.13). Anterior displacement of the mandible could be responsible, especially if the muscles became edematous. A combined lingual and buccal neuropathy has been documented in a patient placed prone for lumbar laminectomy. The lesion was unilateral and after a lengthy dissertation it was concluded that positioning the

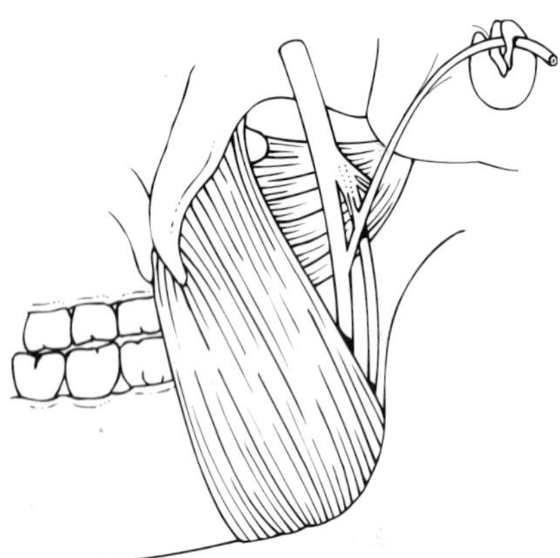

Figure 40.13 *The relation of the chorda tympani and lingual nerves to the pterygoid muscles.*

patient's head with some slight rotation caused an asymmetric retraction of the mandible. This in turn had caused passive tension of the lateral and medial pterygoid muscles on the side of the lesion, thereby trapping both buccal and lingual nerves. The patient complained of numbness and parasthesiae on the right side of the face and tongue, which resolved over 4 weeks.

Branches of the facial nerve are well known to be at risk from face masks, harnesses, or tapes used to secure the endotracheal tube; however there are few reported cases. The buccal branch has been reported to be susceptible to injury, particularly if it has an unusually superficial relation to the parotid gland and can thus be compressed against the body of the mandible.[86] The early cases described by Fuller and Thomas[87] involved the marginal mandibular branch and occurred after application of pressure behind the mandible for only 10–30 min. A similar case, but of a unilateral presentation, has been reported following 40 min of anesthesia.[88] Airway control was moderately difficult and required an oral airway with firm facial and submandibular pressure applied bilaterally to the body and angles of the mandible. The patient complained of increasing difficulty in talking, dribbled food, and was unable to move the left lower lip. Taste sensation to the anterior two-thirds of the tongue was intact, as was motor function in the remaining distribution of the facial nerve. Anatomical studies have shown that in 19% of cases this branch of the nerve lies up to 1 cm below the inferior border of the mandible and that after crossing the facial artery it lies above the inferior border in all cases.[89] At the angle of the jaw, therefore, upward pressure may well compress the nerve against bone. A case of similar etiology but with bilateral nerve damage has also been described.[90] In this instance, a difficult airway was successfully managed for 75 min using a mask and bilateral digital pressure behind the angle of the mandible in order to spare a medical colleague the risks of endotracheal intubation. Unfortunately, the ensuing and striking weakness of the lower facial muscles, poor control of saliva, and parotid tenderness took 5 weeks to resolve.

On the posterior surface of the neck, the C1–C3 nerve roots, which constitute the greater and lesser occipital nerves, may be damaged by any hyperextension of the occiput against the atlantoaxial region. These nerve roots are not protected by bony foraminae and are at risk as they emerge through the muscular and ligamentous attachments between skull and spine. Parasthesiae or pain may result in their area of distribution and may be mistakenly diagnosed and treated as postoperative headache. In the neck region, stretching of the cervical sympathetic chain can result in unilateral Horner syndrome.[91] This has been described in a patient maintained in the full lateral position for renal surgery in which the head had probably been positioned with insufficient support to ensure that cervical and thoracic spines remained level. The symptoms resolved over 3 days.

POSTOPERATIVE PERIPHERAL NERVE LESIONS

The brachial plexus

Probably the best-known and most feared nerve injury associated with surgery or anesthesia is damage to the brachial plexus. It is highly susceptible to damage associated with poor positioning during anesthesia. Its anatomical fixation in the neck and axilla and its close proximity to the bony structures of the clavicle, first rib, and head of the humerus are well-known predisposing factors to traction injury. In recent years this has been almost entirely associated with the practice of having one arm abducted on an arm-board for ease of access to intravenous infusion sites and blood pressure measurements. Limiting the abduction to approximately 80°, pronating the hand, and turning the head toward the abducted arm will considerably reduce the risks (Fig. 40.14). Surgical assistants can inadvertently increase the degree of abduction unless the arm-board has a locking device to maintain its position. Failing to pronate the forearm has been associated with brachial plexus damage when the arm was abducted to only 60°. Changing practices associated with the availability of more sophisticated and reliable monitoring techniques appear to be leading to arm positioning either fully adducted (Fig. 40.15) or adducted with the forearm across the chest. It is to be anticipated that this will result in a reduced incidence of brachial plexus injury. The clinical presentation of a traction injury is of a motor deficit, usually painless, affecting the C5–C7 roots. This physiologic deficit is suggestive of a focal conduction block, and a case described by Trojaborg,[92] in which nerve conduction tests were performed, confirmed this hypothesis. Most patients recover within 3 months, although some prolonged recoveries requiring up to 1 year after injury have been recorded. Surgical exploration of the plexus is not indicated. It is to be hoped that such possible causes of brachial plexus injury as restraining "Trendelenburg" patients by the wrists or

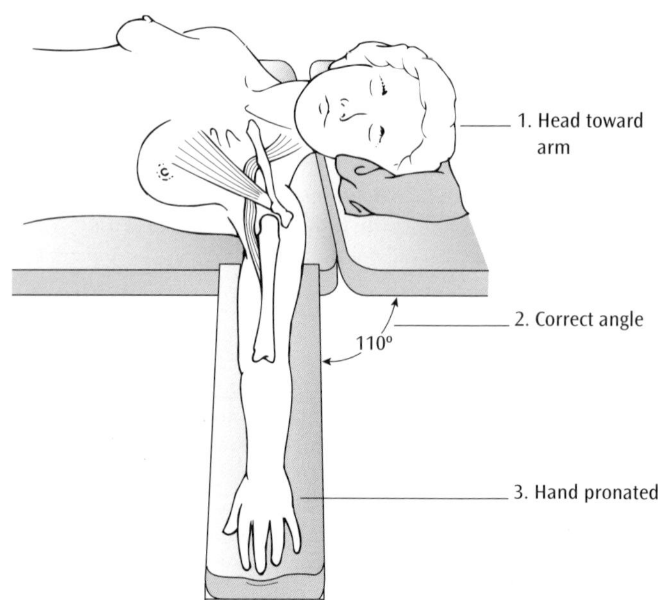

Figure 40.14 *The correct position for the head, arm, and hand when an arm-board is used.*

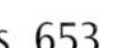

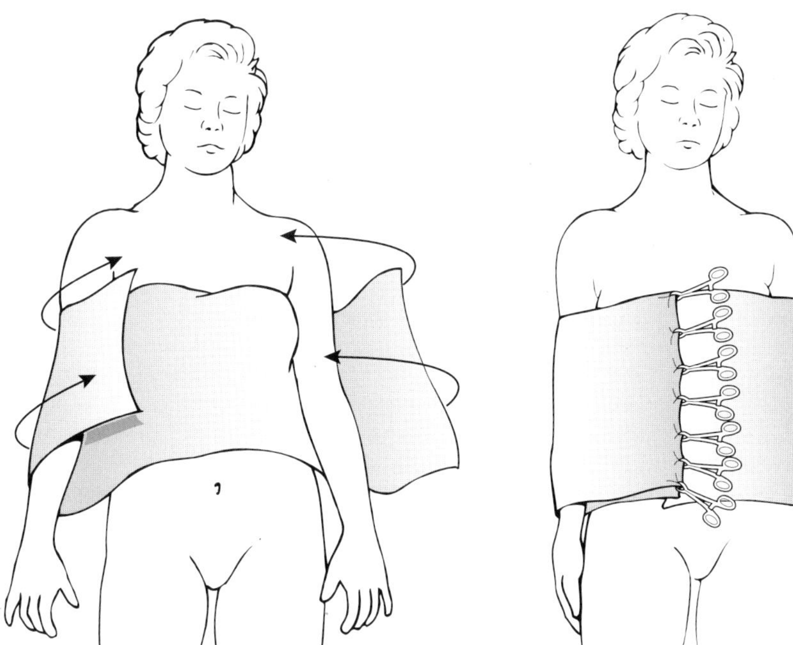

Figure 40.15 *A useful method of supporting the arms using a length of toweling. The same principle can be used in either the supine or the prone patient. Damage to main nerve trunks from external pressure by arm retainers or the surface of the table is prevented.*

preventing them slipping off the operating table head first by the use of shoulder retainers has been long abandoned. *Direct compression* of the plexus is probably a very rare cause of brachial plexus injury. It may be the culprit when patients are placed in the full lateral position without a protective air cushion or "foam cylinder" supporting the rib cage adjacent to the axilla. Failure to provide this support can result in compression of the axillary neurovascular bundle between the head of the humerus and the lateral aspect of adjacent ribs. This support also has another important function, i.e. to prevent deltoid muscle necrosis, and may have been omitted in the case described earlier.[8,32] An inadequate axillary roll support was one possible factor in the etiology of a complex case of postoperative brachial plexus neurapraxia described as "axillary compression syndrome." Extensive swelling of the shoulder area necessitated an emergency decompression procedure by dividing the pectoral and anterior scalene muscles.[93]

Some surgical procedures carried out in the *prone position*, particularly those on the dorsal or lumbar spine, allow for either the arms to be fully adducted or the shoulders to be extended so that the arms lie above the head resting on the operating table (Fig. 40.16). The former position is clearly quite safe for the brachial plexus, provided that the security of the retaining system is reliable. The extended position was thought to be safe, having been advocated following investigations on conscious volunteers.[36] The illustrations in that article show the upper arms to be in close proximity to the sides of the face. Recent experience has shown that this can be associated with isolated axillary nerve damage and brachial plexus neurapraxia.[94,95] This position should be avoided if preoperative questioning reveals any symptoms of cervical spondylosis, or parasthesia when the arms are held above the head. Even when no such symptoms are present, it would be wise to avoid excessive arm abduction. There are reports of brachial plexus lesions in patients operated on in the sitting position through failure to support adequately the weight of the arm[96,97] (Fig. 40.17).

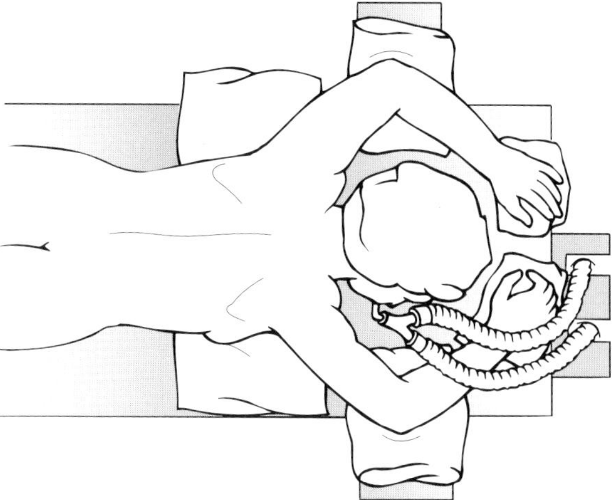

Figure 40.16 *Avoid having the hands any further forward than this. It is unwise to have the upper arms abducted against the sides of the head.*[94,95]

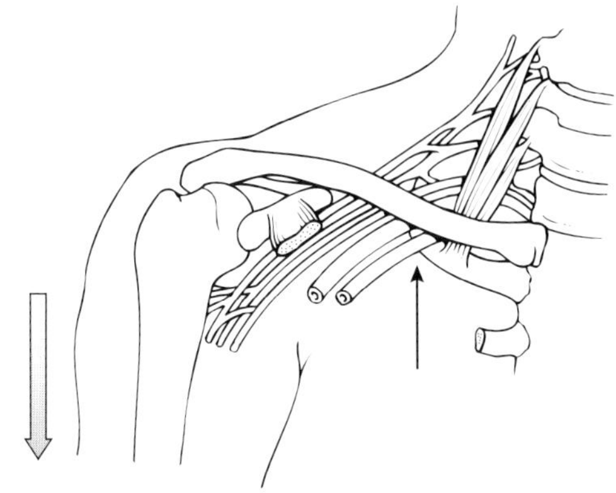

Figure 40.17 *In the sitting position the weight of the arm, if inadequately supported, can cause compression of the neurovascular bundle between the clavicle and the first rib.*

Brachial plexus injury due to open heart surgery

Although this is not a positioning problem for which, at first sight, the anesthesiologist can be held responsible, awareness of its occurrence and possible etiology is important. The brachial plexus injury is related to the median sternotomy approach and occurs without arm abduction or any of the other potential causes of stretch injury. It differs from arm abduction injury in that the lower (C8–T1) roots of the plexus are most affected and it may be bilateral, although not necessarily symmetrical. Pain is a prominent feature of some cases and, although recovery may be protracted and incomplete,[98] the majority of cases have a good prognosis with rapid return of nerve function within days or weeks. The two most common causes are thought to be stretching of the nerve fibers, secondary to an increased distance between the axillary fascia and the insertion of the plexus, and direct trauma to the plexus from fracture of the first rib. The same mechanical forces can be responsible for both categories and placing the sternal retractor too high up is especially harmful in respect of first rib fractures.

A possible cause of damage by attempts at internal jugular vein cannulation has been suggested in a large prospective study from the Cleveland Clinic in which the overall incidence was 5%.[99] In 19 of the 26 patients with brachial plexopathies the plexus lesion occurred on the same side as the cannulation of the internal jugular vein. In all instances arms were positioned at the patient's sides throughout the surgical procedure. Direct needle trauma is the obvious inference, but compression by anticoagulant-induced hematomas is another possible causative factor. It is not a report that has been universally accepted.

Idiopathic brachial neuritis

Anesthesiologists should be aware that this rare condition can also present following surgery. The features are acute onset of severe pain along the shoulder, followed by a patchy amyotrophy of the associated muscles. The condition can be distinguished from intraoperative causes by the delayed onset of the presenting symptoms and the results of electromyographic investigations.[100] This underlines the importance of always obtaining skilled neurologic assistance in any such event at the earliest possible opportunity.

The ulnar nerve

Within the last decade evidence has become available to the effect that postoperative malfunction of the ulnar nerve has become the most frequent peripheral neuropathy encountered in litigation claims in the USA. It is now therefore a serious medicolegal problem.[101–103] At the same time, studies have shown that the etiology is potentially much more complex than was previously thought and, furthermore, that the condition can appear even when precautions for its avoidance have indisputably been taken.

The ulnar nerve is vulnerable to both external and internal compressive forces. The former is well recognized and occurs where the nerve lies superficially in the groove behind the medial epicondyle of the humerus. The edge of the operating table mattress has been a frequently quoted culprit. Pronation of the extended forearm leaves the nerve more vulnerable at this site than does supination.[104] Internal compression can occur as the nerve then passes distally between the two heads of the flexor carpi ulnaris muscle (Fig. 40.18). Full flexion of the elbow alone can cause entrapment here as it enters this cubital tunnel. As the elbow is flexed from zero to 45° the arcuate ligament tightens because the distance between its points of attachment increases by 5 mm.[105] A combination of both external and internal compressive forces may occur. It is not possible to differentiate either clinically or by electophysiologic testing between damage occurring at these two sites.

Three criteria for the diagnosis have been postulated: onset after general anesthesia, persistent neural deficit, and clinical and electrophysiologic evidence of a pure ulnar neuropathy. The symptoms may consist of numbness, tingling, or pain in the fourth and fifth fingers. It is unusual for all three symptoms to be present. On physical examination sensory deficit may be elicited and there may be weakness of the interosseous muscles. Onset ranges from immediate to 3 days but may initially be unreported owing to preoccupation with the primary illness.

Careful follow-up of the condition is important. Only half the patients can be expected to show improvement or complete resolution at 6 months, and further exacerbation with development of motor nerve signs affecting the intrinsic muscles of the hand will occur in some. Surgical decompression of the nerve may be required.

In recent years there has been a striking increase in the incidence of litigation associated with its occurrence. Analysis of 227 anesthesia-related nerve injuries involved in litigation claims showed that ulnar neuropathy accounted for one-third of the total.[101] But, since the population of anesthetized patients from which these events were drawn is unknown, the actual incidence cannot be deduced. A very large consecutive series of just over one million patients analyzed retrospectively showed an incidence of one case per 2729 patients.[103] No association was found either with anesthetic technique or with patient position.

In a situation in which the patient appears to have been previously symptom-free, it is easy to suggest that negligent practice in positioning the limb is a clear and obvious cause. Alvine and Schurrer,[106] in an extensive prospective study, demonstrated that this is most certainly not the case. A total of 6538 patients were followed through convalescence, and 17 (0.26%) developed an ulnar nerve palsy during the postoperative period. When investigated at 6 months the most important finding was that the nerve conduction was abnormal not only on the affected side *but also on the opposite side*. The authors concluded "that many patients may have a subclinical ulnar neuropathy that may become symptomatic as a result of the many maneuvers and manipulations that are associated with surgical procedures." This is supported by evidence from examination of ulnar nerves obtained during routine autopsy of 12 subjects without known disease of the peripheral nervous system.[107] Localized histolologic changes were found in five, indicating subclinical entrapment.

Alvine and Schurrer[106] also showed that preventive measures have only a limited degree of success. Preoperative screening for symptoms of neuropathy, the use of elbow pads during the procedure, and careful positioning of the arms were all strictly adhered to during the subsequent 4 years. Nevertheless, a further 11 patients with postoperative ulnar nerve lesions were identified. The authors stress the importance of eliciting a preoperative history of nocturnal neuropathy in surgical patients. When found, the patients should be warned of the risks that the surgical procedure may aggravate this condition.

It is not within the scope of this text to discuss the various anatomical and congenital causes of ulnar nerve entrapment: recurrent dislocation of the ulnar nerve at the elbow, "double crush" syndrome, or inherited peripheral neuropathies, all of which are now thought to be possible etiologic precursors of the postoperative syndrome. Common sense care in positioning the arm and supporting the elbow remains standard management but cannot be regarded as wholly effective.

The axillary nerve

The axillary nerve is derived from the fifth and sixth cervical nerve roots and is a branch of the posterior cord of the brachial plexus. Anatomically it is closely related to the lowest part of the articular capsule of the shoulder joint and then runs below the surgical neck of the humerus. Anterior and posterior branches supply the deltoid and teres minor muscles and an area of the skin on the lateral surface of the arm.

Isolated lesions are usually the result of either inferior dislocation of the shoulder joint or adjacent fracture of the humerus. Pollock and Davis[108] first observed that stretching during prolonged sleep or anesthesia could also be a cause. Gwinnutt[94] has described a case resulting from prone positioning of the patient for revision spinal surgery, in whom the shoulders were extended and the arms placed above the head,

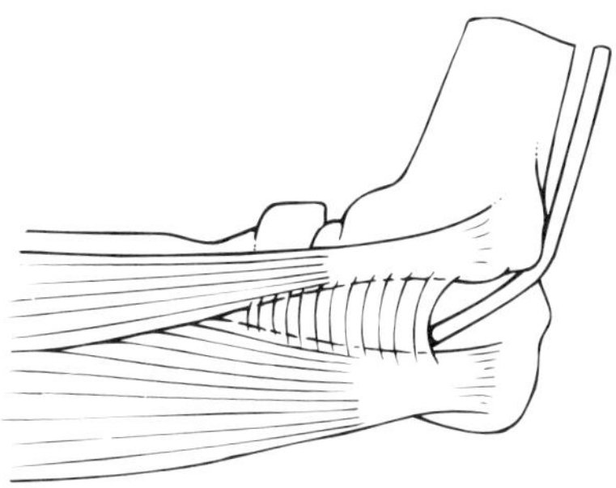
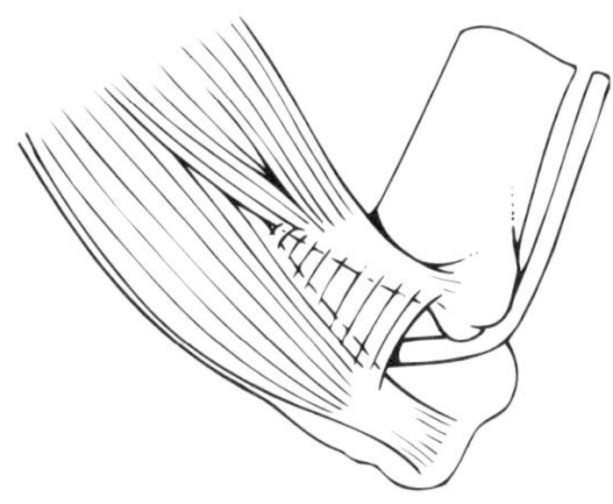

Figure 40.18 *The ulnar nerve can be trapped both at the level of the medial epicondyl and at the entrance of the muscle, especially with elbow flexion.*[105]

resting on the operating table. Postoperatively the patient complained of weakness and numbness in her left arm. Examination revealed an inability to abduct the arm more than 50° against gravity, and an area of decreased skin sensation affecting the lateral aspect of the upper arm. Despite the fact that both arms were placed similarly, the lesion was unilateral and had also occurred some 15 years previously at her first operation. Both incidents resolved uneventfully within 2 months. Although this is a rare nerve injury, the increased incidence of surgical treatment for spinal column problems may result in further cases being recognized. Hyperabduction of the arms should be avoided when patients are positioned for surgery, either prone or supine.

The radial nerve

Arising from cervical segments 6, 7, and 8 and leaving the brachial plexus at its posterior cord, the radial nerve runs through the axilla before winding round the lateral aspect of the mid-third of the humerus in the spiral groove. Proximally, it is at risk from external pressure in the axilla if the arm is permitted to "overhang" the side of the operating table. The posterior cord of the plexus then rubs against the table edge.[109] The classic operating room injury is that of a misplaced "ether screen" pressing against the lateral mid-third of the arm. With a neurosurgical patient in the sitting position a similar injury can occur if the arm rests against the support bars of the three-pin headrest. The result is wrist drop due to paralysis of the extensor muscles of the forearm and loss of sensation in the posterior surface of the forearm and posterolateral aspect of the hand.

Damage to the nerve from misplaced intramuscular injections into the lower part of the deltoid muscle has resulted in this practice being discontinued.

The suprascapular nerve

This large motor nerve arises from the posterior border of the upper trunk of the brachial plexus and is derived from the fifth and sixth cervical nerves. On its route to supply the posterior muscles arising from the scapula it passes through the suprascapular notch and is tethered to adjacent structures at this position. Forced passive adduction of an extended arm across the midline may result in traction injury (in the proximal segment between its origin from the plexus and the suprascapular notch). Alternatively, marked lateral tilt of the head toward the contralateral shoulder would have the same effect. Laterally positioned patients who become unstable and roll away from the vertical to either semiprone or semisupine may also be at a similar risk. Entrapment neuropathies of this nerve can also occur and may be unrecognized as a source of upper extremity pain. The pain is of a deep, poorly localized nature and is accentuated by shoulder movement involving the scapula. There may be secondary pain radiation in the distribution of the radial nerve.[110] Surgical division of the transverse scapular ligament may be necessary to resolve the entrapment neuropathy. Medicolegally it may be important to differentiate between the naturally occurring neuropathy and claims for traumatic damage due to faulty positioning technique.

The median nerve

Postoperative median nerve neuropathy resulting from faulty positioning of the arm is extremely uncommon. Parks,[111] reviewing 50 000 operative procedures over a 13-year period, discovered only two cases of paresis. Both patients were in the supine position; one had the arms abducted and the other had both arms at the sides. Traumatic damage during venipuncture attempts in the antecubital fossa or brachial artery catheterization is well recognized, as is severance of the palmar cutaneous branch of the median nerve during carpal tunnel compression surgery.

The long thoracic nerve

This nerve arises from the anterior branches of the C5, C6, and C7 spinal roots that form the brachial plexus. After entering the neck on the surface of the scalenus posterior muscle it descends down the anterolateral aspect of the chest wall for some 24–30 cm, exclusively supplying motor branches to the serratus anterior muscle. Dysfunction of the nerve produces the classical "winged scapula." On rare occasions this has presented in the postoperative period and unaccountably has been associated with shoulder pain. Malpractice in the positioning or transport of the patient is almost certain to be leveled at the anesthesiologists and ancillary staff. Medical personnel unfortunate enough to find themselves in this predicament should consult Martin's[112] well-balanced review. He could come to no firm conclusion regarding etiology. There was a loose association with the lateral decubitus position and the palsy was nearly always right sided. An independent neuropathy could not be ruled out in many cases.

The lower spinal cord and cauda equina

Unexpected paraplegia or symptoms of cauda equina compression that follow unrelated surgery are rare but are an extremely distressing occurrence. In 1969 Ehni[113] published four cases of paraplegia secondary to operating table position (lordosis) in patients with spinal stenosis. He believed that this was a poorly understood phenomenon and that it was frequently blamed on spinal anesthesia or vascular complications. A further case report also implicated the operating table position as a causative factor.[114] A 61-year-old patient with a pre-existing but asymptomatic spinal canal stenosis was placed in the lateral position with some spinal extension and lateral bend for hip surgery. This position, combined with severe spinal stenosis (proved later at operation), caused enough compression on the neural elements to produce permanent irreversible paraplegia. It is well known in patients with symptomatic spinal stenosis that flexion gives relief, and that extension exacerbates the symptoms. The implications for surgical positioning of elderly patients are therefore clear. The supine position, with the spine at least straight if not moderately flexed, would be the safest. This is a group of patients in whom it might be unwise to provide lumbar support in order to prevent postoperative backache.

In 1968 Moiel and Ehni[115] described a case of postoperative cauda equina syndrome that was due to compression of the structure between intact fifth lumbar vertebral laminae and the upper sacral centrum in which spondylolisthesis had occurred. The etiology of the neurologic sequelae was almost certainly associated with the lithotomy position. Decompressive laminectomy produced considerable improvement in the neurologic deficit.

The cases described above occurred before sophisticated electrophysiological and magnetic resonance imagining (MRI) was available. Amoiridis *et al.*[116] have recently reported a similar case for which these investigations could be utilized to make a definitive diagnosis for the postoperatic paraplegia. The patient had undergone a 10-h radical surgical procedure for bladder carcinoma. This was performed in the hyperlordotic supine position with a 17° head- and trunk-down tilt and the legs extended 17° at the hips to raise the pubis. Serial MRI scanning over the first postoperative month gradually revealed findings that were consistent with ischemic infarction of the spinal cord, dura mater, and the posterior part of the vertebral bodies at the L2–L3 level. Electrophysiologic testing proved an anterior horn or root lesion and, concerning the sensory pathways, a supraganglionic site of the lesion. Consideration of these findings and three other cases cited in their references led to the conclusion that a prolonged hyperlordotic supine position for surgery, which could promote an inferior vena cava compression and aggravate lumbar canal stenosis, should be avoided when possible.

Acute lumbar intervertebral disk disruption and even sequestration of a fragment within the spinal canal do not appear to have been reported as a cause of postoperative pain or neurological deficit. It is, however, easy to see that this might well occur as a result of positioning, turning, or recovery room transfer procedures. Indeed, the ease with which this seems to occur in the conscious subject makes the absence of such reports all the more remarkable. In any case of unexpected postoperative spinal neurologic deficit, urgent surgical exploration and decompression of the spinal canal may offer the only hope of alleviating the condition. The appropriate advice for this problem should be sought quickly.

The sciatic nerve

This main branch of the lumbosacral plexus exits from the pelvis via the greater sciatic notch. From this point onward it is vulnerable to damage by pressure, trauma, or stretching. Very rarely, placing an emaciated patient in the lateral position with insufficient soft padding beneath the buttock can result in damage to the underlying sciatic nerve.[111] The main source of direct trauma is from needlestick injury and disruption by misplaced intramuscular injections. In this context it is worth mentioning that flexion of the thigh to 90° or more alters the course of the nerve through the gluteal region to a more lateral and superficial position. This renders the conventional "upper outer quadrant" advice less reliable and it would be safer to avoid this area altogether unless the hip is in the neutral position. The pneumatic tourniquet is a well-recognized potential cause of damage to the sciatic nerve. Pressures of more than 40–46.7 kPa (300–350 mmHg) are rarely required in the thigh and the duration of application should be carefully monitored.[117]

Stretching of the main length of the nerve can easily occur with the thigh flexed as in the lithotomy position. Anatomical studies have drawn attention to the fact that it is relatively fixed to underlying structures both at the sciatic notch and where its common perineal branch passes around the neck of fibula (Fig. 40.19).[118] It is therefore important to minimize flexion of the thighs to reduce tension on the nerve between these two points. Variations in the lithotomy position in which the legs were held fully extended and almost vertical to the body have been associated with (reversible) sciatic nerve damage.[119,120] External rotation of the hip with the legs in the more conventional position again puts the sciatic nerve "on the stretch." Surgical assistants should be discouraged from leaning against the knees or lower legs with the patient in lithotomy as this might exacerbate the hip rotation and thus stretch the nerve. In 1972 a review of 1000 consecutive vaginal hysterectomy cases carried out in the lithotomy position showed a 0.4% incidence of postoperative sciatic nerve neuropathy.[120] A recent (1994) very much more extensive retrospective review found it to be 0.03%.[121] A very thin body habitus, recent cigarette smoking, and surgery in excess of 4 h appear to be predisposing factors.

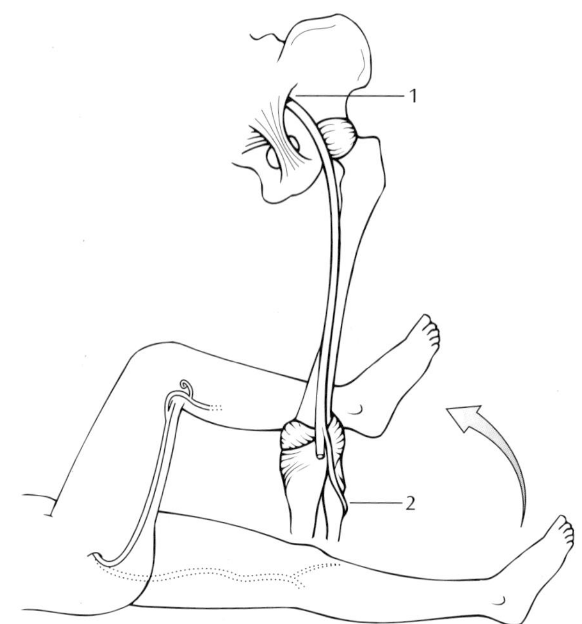

Figure 40.19 *Anatomical fixation of the sciatic nerve at the sciatic notch (1) and the head of the fibula (2) may predispose to damage from tension.[118] Hip flexion makes the nerve more taut.*

With the patient in full lateral position it is occasionally necessary to increase stability by using a broad leather or canvas strap running beneath the table top and over the patient's gluteal region. Sciatic nerve damage can ensue if insufficient padding is used or the strap is too tight. Patients having surgery in the sitting position can also have sciatic nerve damage if there is insufficient appropriate padding beneath the ischial tuberosities.[122]

The sciatic nerve in the thigh gives off branches to the hamstring muscles. Ability to flex the knee joint confirms that the nerve is intact at this level. Division into its two main terminal branches occurs at the level of the knee joint. The tibial branch takes a deep course through the popliteal fossa and lower leg and there are no recorded dangers to it from positioning. The common perineal branch extends laterally around the head of the fibula, where it is extremely superficial and vulnerable to the external pressure (Table 40.2). Foot drop and loss of cutaneous sensation on the lateral aspect of the leg and dorsum of the foot are the consequences of damage. This may be seen in the underlying limb when the patient has been in the lateral decubitus position and after use of some of the less common methods of lithotomy positioning. In the study of exaggerated lithotomy position by Angermeier and Jordan[123] it was the most common (15.8%) complication noted. In those cases it was probably related to prolonged stretching of the nerve due to flexion of both the hip and the knee, with a component of internal compression as it is stretched over the fibular head. The method of leg positioning for surgical exposure of the saphenous veins in patients who undergo coronary artery bypass graft surgery has resulted in two case reports of the complication.[124] The use of external pneumatic compression apparatus has been considered to be a factor in the development of bilateral peroneal neuropathies in a cachectic patient during pancreatic surgery.[18]

Table 40.2 *Incidence of postlithotomy lower extremity motor neuropathy persisting for more than 3 months[121] (retrospective review of 198461 procedures)*

Common peroneal nerve	43
Sciatic nerve	8
Femoral nerve	4
Obturator nerve	0
Total	55

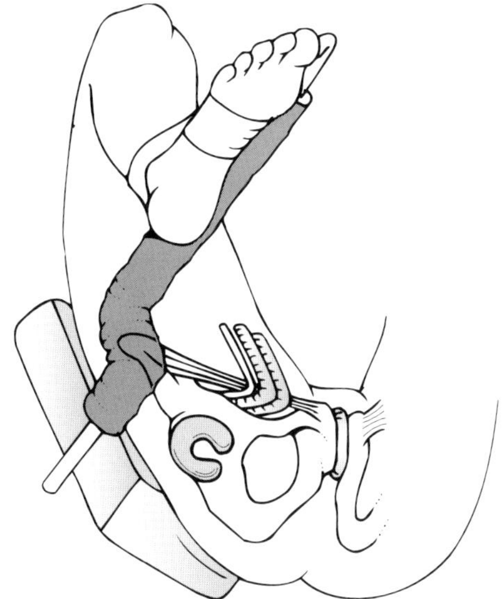

Figure 40.20 *The femoral neurovascular bundle may be damaged by kinking around the inguinal ligament when there is extreme flexion of the thigh.[125] Excessive hip abduction and external rotation can also stretch the nerve.[126]*

The femoral nerve

The femoral nerve arises from L2, L3, and L4 nerve roots, and is susceptible to damage from positioning only as it passes beneath the tough inguinal ligament. It can become kinked around the latter when the patient is placed in some forms of lithotomy position (Fig. 40.20). It becomes a problem either when there is excessive flexion of the thighs or when extremes of abduction and external rotation of the hip are permitted. The use of straight-leg sling systems has been implicated as one cause of the latter.[125]

Branches of the femoral nerve trunk arising above the pelvic bones supply the psoas muscle and are intact if the thigh can be flexed toward the trunk. Damage occurring at or below the inguinal ligament affects the quadreceps femoris muscle, and its ability to extend the knee joint, and the integrity of the knee jerk reflex. Sensory impairment or parasthesiae are localized to the anterior surface of the thigh. Over the years there have been many reports of femoral neuropathy in the literature and there are a great many causes other than simple positioning. Hakim and Katirji[126] have recently reported a further five cases in young women who underwent either uncomplicated vaginal delivery or laparoscopy in the lithotomy position. Sophisticated nerve conduction studies and compound muscle action potentials were used to assess the neurologic deficit. They concluded that use of the lithotomy position alone can cause femoral nerve neuropathy, regardless of its indication for use and without the involvement of other risk factors.

It is worth noting that the self-retaining abdominal retractors commonly used in pelvic surgery have been incriminated as a cause of femoral nerve damage,[127] as has retroperitoneal hematoma and compression by the fetal head.

The lateral femoral cutaneous nerve of the thigh

This nerve arises from the L2 and L3 roots and after running retroperitoneally enters the thigh either through the substance of, or deep to the lateral end of, the inguinal ligament. Anterior and posterior branches are distributed to skin of the lateral lower gluteal region and the anterolateral surface of the thigh extending distally as far as the knee.

Damage to this nerve can result in the condition of meralgia parasthetica; there is numbness and an annoying hyperalgesia of the upper lateral thigh. When patients are positioned prone using any of the frames that support the anterior superior iliac spines there is theoretically the risk of compression or stretching of this nerve. A prospective study of postpartum patients (managed in the lithotomy position) revealed neuropathies in 21% of cases overall, and 38% of these involved the lateral femoral cutaneous nerve. Cesarean delivery and a prolonged duration of pushing during vaginal delivery were factors correlating with parasthesiae.[128] Surgical causes of this condition include iliac bone procurement for grafting and groin-flap procedures.[98]

The saphenous nerve

With the patient in the lithotomy position the saphenous nerve may be compressed against the medial tibial condyle if the legs are placed outside the vertical stirrup support.[109] Usually, however, the stirrup is positioned more distally. Numbness or parasthesiae of the medial side of the leg may occur.

The pudenal nerves

The pudenal nerves emerge from the pelvis into the ischiorectal fossae passing round the spine of the ischium (the classic site for infiltration of local anesthetic nerve blockade). Each divides into branches supplying the skin of the external genitalia. A smaller posterior branch becomes the inferior hemorrhoidal nerve, with the very important function of external anal sphincter control. Sexual impotence and dysfunction following fractures of the pelvis have been well documented but it is probably not widely appreciated that pudendal nerve neurapraxia can occur as a complication of traction against the perineal post on the fracture table.[129] Hoffman and colleagues[130] described two patients operated on in the *prone position* for pin fixation of subcapital femoral fractures and muscle pedicle grafting. These patients developed numbness of the shaft and bulb of the penis and inability to obtain an erection for 3–4 months following surgery. In the prone position the genitalia hang dependently across the symphysis pubis, and both dorsal nerves of the penis are vulnerable to compression between the bone and the perineal post.

They also describe two patients operated on in the *supine position* for simple pinning of a fractured neck of the femur, who developed unilateral anesthesia of the penis and scrotum. The anesthetic area in each case was on the same side as the fracture. In one of these cases the perineal post had been positioned against the ipsilateral pubic ramus. Cadaver dissections have shown that the nerve is skeletally protected from the fracture table post by the ischial tuberosity and the inferior pubic ramus but it becomes vulnerable distally after trifurcation. Pudendal nerve neurapraxia may be more common than the literature indicates. Hoffman *et al.*[130] cited five other cases in the orthopedic literature. A case of inferior hemorrhoidal nerve damage resulting in incontinence of feces has also been reported. The sensitive nature of the symptoms may inhibit patients from disclosing the occurrence of these complications. Prevention is clearly very important. The perineal post must be wide and well padded to distribute the traction pressure evenly. It should be placed between the genitalia and the uninjured limb when the patient is in the supine position, and should not be in the exact midline of the symphysis or in contact with the genitalia when the patient is in the prone position. Patients can be reassured that sensation will return but complete return of sexual function seems to be more prolonged.

Etiology of perioperative nerve lesions

Accidental surgical damage, from either direct trauma or compression by a hematoma, occasionally occurs and is a recognized hazard of some operations. In other cases the precise mechanism of nerve injury is often unclear. When these lesions occur and are a result of faulty positioning, the three most likely causes are compression, traction, or ischemia. In the case of the brachial plexus, traction seems to be the most probable explanation. Once the natural laxity of the nerves has been taken up, rupture of the epineurium occurs and, although this may result in some axonal degeneration, providing that the internal neural architecture is not completely destroyed a good recovery can be anticipated (neurapraxia). Mild stretching effects have been studied experimentally in the cat and it was found that epineural hemorrhage occurred. The resulting ischemia was thought to be the most likely explanation of the ensuing transient muscle weakness. Other workers found signs of myelin disruption at moderate degrees of nerve stretch. An increase of 15% in the resting length of the nerve stops blood flow completely. Conduction failure and even nerve degeneration may result if stretching is maintained for long periods. If the stretching injury is significant enough to produce a separation of the related parts of the ruptured axons (neurotmesis), recovery will be poor. This type of injury can occur even if the nerve appears to be anatomically intact. With very severe traction injuries of the brachial plexus, Wallerian degeneration occurs with the inevitable pain, long-standing paralysis, and sensory changes.

With lesions of the ulnar, peroneal, and pudendal nerves, compression between bone and a hard surface is usually the cause, although in the case of the ulnar nerve it may not be quite as simple as this. Duration of the pressure is more important than the compressive force and local asphixia is the predominant causative factor. This type of injury is not dissimilar from the effects of pneumatic tourniquets applied to the limbs for surgical hemostasis.[131]

Peripheral nerve injuries may also aggravate pre-existing nerve damage, or a combination of the two may unmask a subclinical problem. The patient with diabetes mellitus is a good example of this. Ischemic changes already present in the nerves make them more susceptible to the effects of the injury. In the acute situation, there is displacement of the nodal myelin followed by paranodal demyelination and conduction block. Recovery can take 2 months following remyelination. A much longer period for recovery was described in a case in which edema between the axon and the myelin was a prominent feature. In the most serious compression injuries, Wallerian degeneration is found.[98] Patients with inherited primary peripheral neuropathies may have a susceptibility to intraoperative nerve damage.[132] It is also possible for normal peripheral nerves to have two separate and unrelated sites of entrapment, one of which may occur as a result of patient positioning. This "double crush" syndrome, first described by Upton, postulates that either lesion can potentiate the severity of the other irrespective of their site on the nerve. Changes in axoplasmic flow are thought to be responsible for the nerve dysfunction. The association of abnormalities of the brachial or cervical plexus with carpal tunnel syndrome is often quoted.[133]

Etiology is important because the prognosis for recovery depends on the nature of the neurologic deficit. It is necessary to know whether there is functional disturbance of nerve fibers that remain in continuity, or complete axonal loss. In the early postoperative period this may be difficult to assess clinically, but an expert in electrophysiologic testing should be able to elucidate this as well as the exact localization of the nerve lesion. The functional integrity of both *motor* and *sensory* fibers must be assessed and the test repeated at appropriate intervals to monitor progress. The diagnosis is more difficult if evaluation by conduction studies and electromyography is delayed until concern is expressed over the lack of spontaneous recovery. After many weeks the electrophysiologic changes of chronic denervation differ from those seen in the acute stages. The opportunity for early surgical exploration and possible reconstruction will have been missed if complete denervation has occurred.

Despite the extensive reporting of cases and an undoubted increase in awareness of potential problems among operating room teams, incidents still occur.[101] This happens even when it appears that all the necessary "accepted" precautions for prevention have been taken. It is clear that 100% safety for the patient in respect of nerve "injuries" may never be attainable, but only by attempting to achieve this will avoidable accidents be minimized.

SOME PHYSIOLOGIC DANGERS OF POSITIONING THE SURGICAL PATIENT

The main dangers can be divided into those affecting the respiratory system and those affecting the cardiovascular system. There may be secondary effects involving other systems.

The respiratory system

Diagnosis and management impeded by difficult access to the patient

Any position that seriously limits the anesthesiologist's access to the patient's head and thorax is undoubtedly a source of potential danger. Neurosurgical procedures, in which the anesthesiologist is confined to the foot of the operating table, are classic examples. Simple complications, such as the migration of a tracheal tube into the right main bronchus, can be difficult to assess and correct. Serious situations, such as acute tension pneumothorax or the life-threatening onset of severe bronchospasm, are challenging enough crises without the extra complication of impeded access. Positioning the patient should always be carried out so that such dangers, though admittedly rare, can be dealt with expeditiously; delay can be fatal.

Position-related changes in respiratory function

Altered lung mechanics and changes in blood flow in both the systemic and the pulmonary circulations have been studied in patients under general and regional anesthesia and have been well reviewed.[134] These may be either improved or made worse by positioning the patient for surgery. This is particularly the case if extremes of positioning (e.g. Trendelenburg or sitting position) are employed.[135,136] Dangers resulting from such changes inevitably stem from hypoxia or hypercarbia. Areas of atelectasis are almost certainly the commonest cause, but fluid transudation into the alveoli is another possibility when left atrial pressures exceed alveolar pressure, e.g. in a prolonged head-down position. In the lateral position pulmonary edema may be unilateral (down lung syndrome), especially if fluid volume overload has occurred.[137]

Taken in isolation, changes in respiratory function are almost always in practice corrected by anesthesia with tracheal intubation and intermittent positive-pressure ventilation. Indeed, blood gas analysis figures that improve on the patient's preoperative status are often produced.

In terms of patient management, it may sometimes be difficult to separate the dangers arising from changes to the respiratory or the cardiovascular systems. A recent case anesthetized by the author illustrates the point. General anesthesia was induced and tracheal intubation performed uneventfully. The patient was turned to the "Tarlov" prone position and within 3 min the end-tidal CO_2 alarm was activated, indicating "apnea." This was perplexing because the tracheal tube was clearly still in place and both sides of the chest were unmistakably expanding in time with the ventilator. However, the next automatic indirect blood pressure recording revealed a catastrophic fall in arterial blood pressure. Both the hypotension and the low CO_2 output responded to immediate treatment with a small dose of vasopressor and intravenous fluids.

Tipping the patient into the Trendelenburg position has been shown radiologically to cause upward displacement of the carina in 40% of patients. In half of these this will be sufficient to cause a tracheal tube previously in position with the tip just above the carina to enter the right main bronchus. It is wise therefore to recheck for adequate aeration of both sides of the chest after the patient has been positioned in this way.[138] Laparoscopic tension pneumoperitoneum can produce a similar carinal shift even if the patient is tilted head up.[139] Toung *et al.*[140] have shown by computed tomography scans that neck flexion also risks endobronchial intubation if the endotracheal tube is already too low in the trachea. Conversely, neck extension may risk accidental extubation of the patient if the endotracheal tube tip is too high (Figs. 40.21 and 40.22). This is the opposite of what may previously have been taught: confusion has probably arisen from the mistaken concept that the oropharynx moves "upward" with flexion, thereby extracting the endotracheal tube with it. The head and neck flexion and extension that take place when surgical drapes are being applied or adjusted, particularly in the pediatric patient, may produce either of these scenarios. There is a chance that endobronchial intubation may correct itself on repositioning; extubation clearly will not, and its identification is an urgent priority.

The recovery period

This is probably the most dangerous in respect of risk of pulmonary complications. Two investigations have shown that about 20% of all cases of death and serious neurologic damage occur at this time.[141,142] The danger of aspiration can be minimized by correct lateral positioning, which would almost certainly have prevented some of these tragedies. Nurses in the recovery room should accept patients into their care in the supine position only if these are already fully conscious or if there is some overriding surgical or medical reason for avoiding the lateral position. Even after recovery of consciousness, there is evidence that the glottic reflexes can be obtunded for up to 2 h.[143]

Once consciousness has been regained and vital functions are stable, a change in posture may be thought to be appropriate, particularly as ventilatory excursion is impaired by narcotics and pain. However, placing the patient supine with a backrest raised to approximately 45° has been shown by Russell[144] to have no advantage, despite previous work by Hsu and Hickey,[145] which demonstrated that functional residual capacity of the lungs is increased. Russell studied 19 patients at approximately 30–60 min following the completion of surgery. There was a statistically significant deterioration in arterial oxygenation in most.

The cardiovascular system

The patient's position may result in occlusion of major arteries

Occlusion of a major artery is a considerable danger with many of the positions used for surgery. With the patient placed supine or prone, cervical spine rotation can result in occlusion of the contralateral vertebral artery (dealt with elsewhere in this chapter). It is quite remarkable that many long ENT procedures carried out with the head at almost 90° to the spinal axis appear to cause no neurological sequelae.

The arterial supply to the lower limbs can be compromised in several different positions. The femoral neurovascular bundle can become kinked around the inguinal ligament in the lithotomy position if too great a degree of flexion, abduction, and lateral rotation of the thighs is allowed. In the prone position when props or "frames" for the iliac crests are used they must be carefully adjusted to ensure that they are directly beneath the bone and that no lateral movement is possible. Stability throughout the whole surgical procedure must be guaranteed. Any lateral movement of either the support or the patient's body will result in direct pressure on the patient's groin and occlusion of the femoral artery. Even with the degree of adjustment afforded by the Relton and Hall "four-poster frame"[146] it is still possible for the patient's pelvis to slip sideways on the pelvic supports, so that pressure can come to bear on the femoral vessels. In the prone "Mohammedan prayer" position,[9] occlusion of the femoral and popliteal arteries is a near certainty, but this is only one of the reasons for declaring the position to be totally unacceptable.

Nowadays it is unusual for there to be any postoperative sequelae that suggest that the blood supply to the upper limbs has been compromised by the position of the patient's arms. Perhaps it is the well-known concern for protecting the brachial plexus that inadvertently serves the same function. In 1945 Wright,[147] a US Army physician, described several unusual cases (one of which even had superficial gangrene of the finger tips) associated with patients who habitually slept with their hands and arms in a hyperabducted position. As a result of this he studied 150 fit, normal, adult army personnel, observing the effects on the radial pulses as the arms were raised above their heads into the hyperabducted position. The frequency of obliteration of the pulse was much higher than he anticipated – around 80% of subjects. One of his conclusions was that "special attention be paid to the state of the pulse and to complaints of parasthesiae and numbness from patients whose arms are in hyperabduction on operating tables or in splints or casts, in order to avoid neurovascular complications which occasionally occur as a result of neglect of this principle."

The position of the arms when the patient is placed in the prone position was studied by Smith,[36] who, contrary to the advice of the previous author, concluded that the arms should be resting on the operating table above the head (see Fig. 40.16). However, this author has heard of one anecdotal report in which bilateral loss of the peripheral pulses occurred after such positioning of the arms and was followed by severe postoperative upper limb weakness for 48 h. As the symptoms resolved quite rapidly, it is unlikely that this was due to brachial plexus damage. This position for the arms can occasionally result in neurological sequelae and has already been discussed. It is not therefore as safe for the neurovasculature as was previously thought. The degree of abduction should not be extreme and peripheral pulses should be checked when it is used. It may be safer, if surgically acceptable, to position the arms at the sides of the body. This can be achieved as illustrated in Fig. 40.15. Unfortunately, this method has the disadvantage of making access to monitoring probes and intravenous infusion more difficult. A case can be made for the use of adjustable arm supports that attach to the side rails of the operating table.

Patients who have previously had coronary artery bypass surgery may be at some risk if positioned prone. A case has been reported of a patient in whom pressure under the sternum resulted in intraoperative electrocardiogram (ECG) evidence of myocardial ischemia.[148] In the recovery room massive anterolateral ischemia was diagnosed and emergency coronary revascularization was undertaken. During the operation, both saphenous vein bypass grafts were found to be patent and pulsatile. A further graft was inserted and a good recovery was obtained. It would appear that the thin-walled veins used as coronary grafts easily become compressed by pressure on the anterior chest wall. Since this report in 1985 many similar patients have undoubtedly required lumbar disk surgery in the prone position but similar sequelae do not appear to have been reported. However, it would be wise to

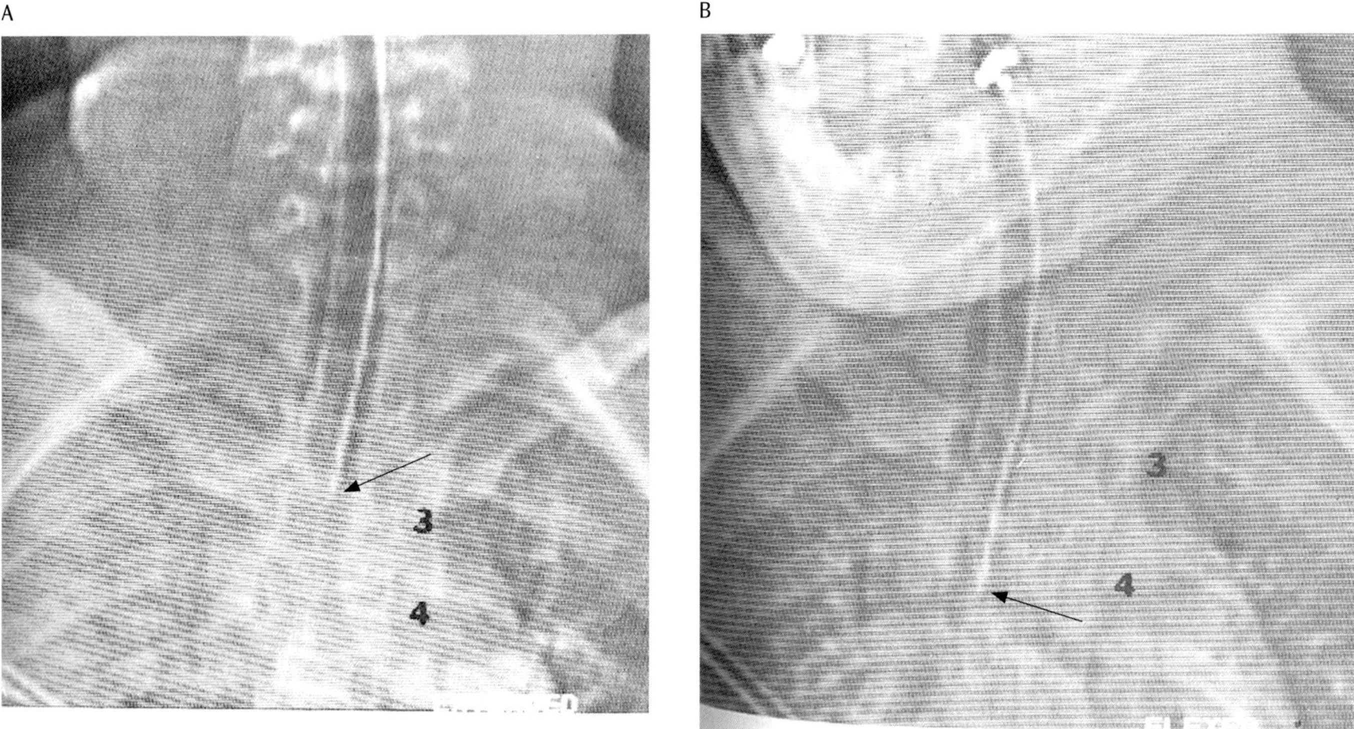

Figure 40.21 *With the neck in the extended position, the ETT tip lies above the carina (A), but during flexion (B), the tip moves down the right main bronchus. Note the minimal movement of the carina relative to the third and fourth thoracic vertebrae. Arrow, ETT tip.*

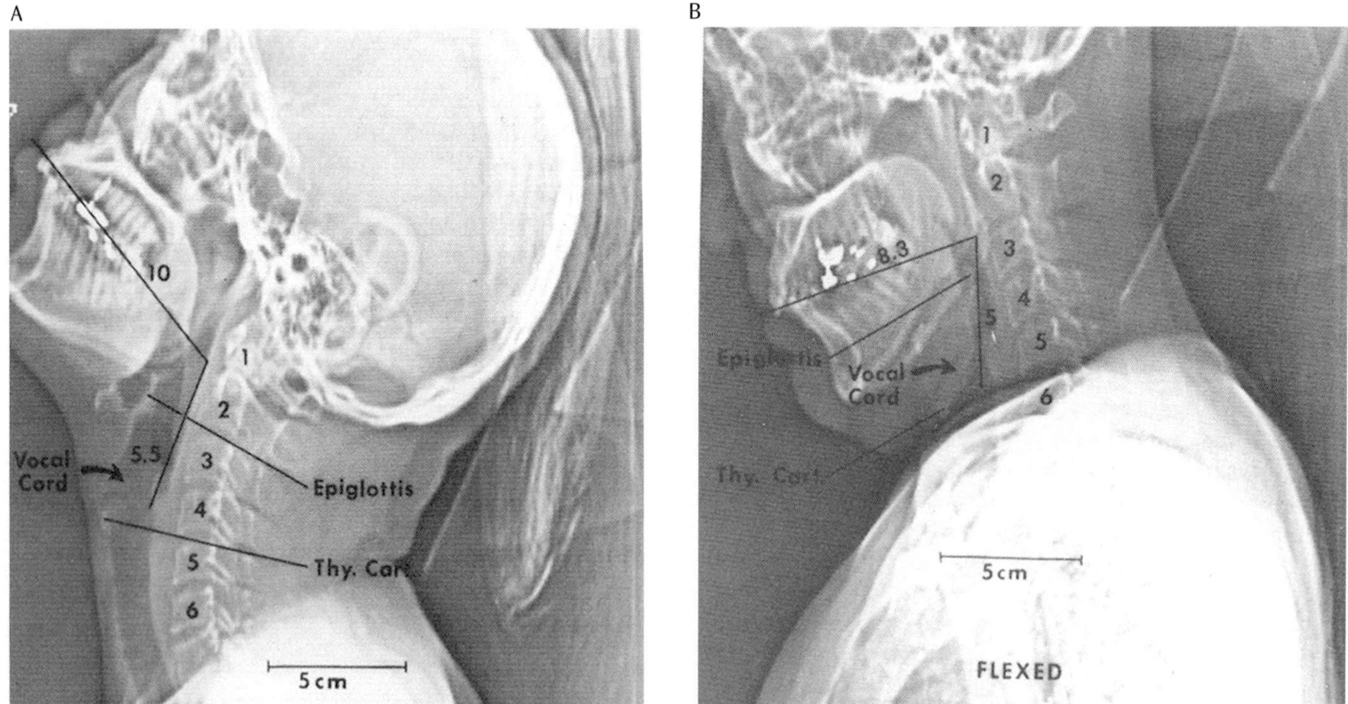

Figure 40.22 *Cervical vertebrae 1–6, upper, and middle airways taken from computed tomography scans of an adult with the neck extended (A) and flexed (B). Note some upward displacement of the cords and a result of head and neck extension (C5 to C4). Also note the larger increase in distance from incisors to oropharynx to vocal cords during extension. Distances are in centimeters.*

give careful thought to the positioning process and to use appropriate monitoring for such cases. A case of ventricular fibrillation was reported during back stabilization surgery in a 15-year-old boy with Duchenne's muscular dystrophy.[149] The patient was successfully resuscitated *in situ* (i.e. still prone) by internal cardiac massage and cardioversion via a left posterior thoracotomy. This case suggests the need for careful preoperative assessment of the likely responses of the cardiovascular system to major surgery and position.

The abdominal aorta and its branches are compressed by the pregnant uterus in the supine position.[150] During the last trimester both its course and its size are disrupted as it is pushed posteriorly, narrowed, and applied closely to the vertebral column. It is usually displaced to the left below the origin of the renal arteries. Compression takes place at the first lumbar vertebra, being most marked at the level of the third and extending to the bifurcation. Systemic hypotension exaggerates these phenomena. The dangerous effect on placental blood flow is discussed further in the section on venous obstruction. Other large intra-abdominal tumors can of course cause a similar clinical outcome.[151,152]

Obstruction of venous return to the heart

Venous return at a high superior vena caval level can be compromised when the anesthetized patient is turned from the supine to the lateral position. The mediastinum shifts toward the down side and rotates the heart on its axis. Monitoring of arterial blood pressure at this time is therefore essential so that measures to restore cardiac output can be taken.

Obstruction of the inferior vena cava from any cause will impede filling of the right ventricle and may seriously reduce cardiac output. Zuck[153] has traced the earliest known description of this phenomenon to the *Tractus de C'orde* [*Treatise on the Heart*] of 1669 by Richard Lower (1631–1691). Credit for more recently recognizing the association between arterial hypotension and the supine position in late pregnancy is due to Hansen.[154] Recognition for investigation and further publicizing the problem must go to McRoberts[155] and Howard *et al.*,[156] who described "postural shock in pregnancy" and "supine hypotensive syndrome" respectively. An excellent review of the 50-year history of aortocaval compression syndrome has recently been published by Marx.[157] In the UK, Holmes' 1960 study of 500 patients was an important contribution and has recently been republished in *Anaesthesia* as a "classic" paper.[158]

The important physiologic sequelae of inferior vena caval compression depend on whether blood can bypass the obstruction, via enlarged paravertebral venous pathways, and on the capacity of the systemic vascular resistance to maintain arterial blood pressure. From the anesthesiologist's point of view all near-term pregnant patients are at risk from the dangers of this problem. However, they fall into two distinct groups. First, there are the majority who are symptom-free and appear to have no obvious discomfort or adverse effects when they lie in the supine position. This can lead to a false sense of security and a very serious fall in arterial blood pressure following induction of general or regional anesthesia, the sympathetic blockade induced by either method abolishing the ability to compensate by vasoconstriction. Routine use of the "obstetric wedge" beneath the right buttock has become standard practice and is of undoubted value. However, it has recently been shown that the standard 15° of tilt usually used in the UK is insufficient to relieve aortocaval compression completely. Both left and right pelvic tilt failed to reverse the decreased blood flow in the leg associated with the supine position.[159] Other workers have demonstrated that at cesarean section cardiac output increased toward the value found in the left lateral position when left-sided table tilt was supplemented with uterine displacement.[160] In the author's experience, simple "wedging" can delay, by a few minutes, the onset of serious hypotension. When such a dramatic fall in blood pressure occurs, it is vital that there are an adequate number of operating room assistants available to reposition the patient fully lateral. If the obstetrician has already opened the peritoneum the crisis can be resolved either by the very rapid delivery of the infant or by the surgeon holding the gravid uterus forward off the underlying great vessels until adequate cardiac output has been restored.

A second group of patients complain of feeling faint when supine, and indeed cannot usually be persuaded to stay in this position. Acute hypotension, pallor, and sweating rapidly ensue and tachycardia gives way to a marked bradycardia. Complete relief occurs after these women turn fully lateral. At first sight it appears that a vasovagal or emotional fainting attack is superimposed in some patients who have aortocaval compression syndrome. The rational explanation for this seemed obscure for many years. More recent studies into circulatory collapse and acute blood loss offer an explanation. In any situation in which blood is lost to the circulation, whether externally, by obstruction, or by extreme peripheral vasodilation (as in "emotional" fainting), there is an initial increase in vasoconstrictor drive. This can be measured directly by both microneurography and estimation of plasma norepinephrine (noradrenaline) concentration. When the volume of blood loss, either true or simulated, exceeds approximately 25% of the circulating volume, peripheral resistance, arterial pressure, and heart rate fall profoundly. The light-headedness or loss of consciousness that follows is secondary to cerebral hypoxia. Sympathetic vasoconstrictor drive has stopped abruptly and the cardiovascular reflexes that maintained constant blood pressure suddenly seem to have been "switched off." At the same time, another vasoconstrictor mechanism is "switched on." There is a massive outpouring of antidiuretic hormone into the bloodstream; this is responsible for the nausea and skin pallor that persist for some 30–40 min after cardiovascular hemodynamics have been restored. This dramatic change in physiologic response probably acts in a protective role. The initial increased sympathetic drive and falling venous return will induce powerful, rapid myocardial contractions around small volumes of blood. The supervening bradycardia may prevent myocardial damage and allow improved ventricular filling during a falling preload.[161,162]

The small number of antenatal patients who exhibit these serious symptoms of "supine hypotensive syndrome" should not present too great a management problem to an experienced obstetric anesthesiologist, especially when diagnosed preoperatively. A regional anesthetic technique for cesarean section, performed with the patient tipped as far lateral as practicable, is probably the management of choice. At the other end of the scale, general anesthesia with the patient in the lithotomy position, even with a "wedged" pelvis, is likely to be extremely hazardous. Without a "wedge" it could rapidly result in a maternal fatality.

If, for any reason, cardiopulmonary resuscitation is required in a pregnant patient near to term, it will be obvious from the foregoing discussion that a successful outcome will be very unlikely if the patient is left in the standard supine position. In such circumstances, it has been shown that an assistant kneeling on the floor and sitting on his or her heels can provide support for the patient's back. This "human wedge" then uses one arm to stabilize the patient's shoulder and the other to stabilize the pelvis. Performance assessed using resuscitation mannikins has been favorable.[163] Dark and Engelhart, in a letter entitled "Are you alright Mrs Tilt?", have pointed out that tilting the patient should be carried out by the rescuer right at the start of the obstetric resuscitation. Their experience in the instruction of basic obstetric life support was that many candidates failed to accord it correct priority.[164]

Marx[165] has advocated that if manual displacement of the uterus to the left and slightly cephalad does not achieve hemodynamic stability within a few minutes, immediate abdominal delivery of the infant must be performed to give the mother any chance of surviving without brain damage, and this is supported by the International Liaison Committee on Resuscitation.[166] Two cases managed in this way have reported successful outcomes.[167,168]

Dangers to the fetus of the maternal supine position

The fact that the majority of mothers appear superficially to show no adverse effects from the unsupported supine position, and indeed often produce apparently healthy babies, has made gaining acceptance of "lateral tilt" in the labor room an uphill struggle over the past 30 years. The evidence now accumulated leaves no room for doubt that the fetus is at risk, and the only correct management is to treat all mothers with this in mind. One of the earliest investigations reviewing placentograms showed diminution of placental perfusion with the mother in the unsupported supine position. Direct catheter studies showed reduced arterial pressure measurements in the different branches of the aorta distal to its obstruction by the gravid uterus.[169] Simultaneous brachial and femoral blood pressure measurements have shown that 60% of women had significant femoral hypotension whereas only 18% had similar brachial hypotension.[170] Studies by Kauppila *et al.*[171] suggest that the autoregulation system for uteroplacental circulation is operative only in the nonplacental component of the pregnant uterus. Evidence from the examination of the fetus during labor and both its physiologic and its physical status at birth further condemn failure to ensure prevention of aortocaval compression. It has been demonstrated that deceleration of the fetal heart rate occurring while the mother was lying on her back could be reversed by turning her into the lateral position, regardless of whether or not there was maternal hypotension. Umbilical blood gas and acid–base studies in patients having vaginal deliveries in either the supine or the supine/tilted position demonstrated that in the offspring of the supine mothers there was a time-related decrease in pH, whereas acid–base status was maintained within the normal range in the tilted group.[172] Evidence seems to be accumulating that, wherever possible, the full lateral position is to be preferred.[173]

In contrast, the use of lateral tilt at cesarean section became well established much earlier. Ansari and colleagues,[174] measuring umbilical venous and arterial oxygen saturations, demonstrated statistically significant advantages. The work of Crawford *et al.*[175] on Agpar scores at 1 and 5 min showed the cardiorespiratory status in infants of tilted mothers to be less depressed. Although it is more inconvenient to the obstetrician, the superiority of left lateral tilt as opposed to right tilt has been demonstrated by Buley *et al.*[176] on the basis of pH and blood gas values. This is to be expected because, anatomically, the inferior vena cava lies marginally to the right of the vertebral column. Elevation of the hip with a foam rubber wedge or similar device seems to have become the method of choice over mechanical devices designed to attach to the operating table and displace the uterus to the left.

Position for lumbar regional anesthetic techniques

The ideal hemodynamic position for the insertion of a lumbar epidural catheter in the obstetric patient has, until recently, received little consideration. Individual preference usually determines the choice of lateral or sitting position.

The danger of an emotional vasovagal syncopy is present in *both* positions.[177] In the former, the patient is at least already horizontal and will probably require a only short period of head-down tilt to refill the heart for resuscitation (provided that she has not been so tightly "curled up" with "knees to chest" that aortocaval compression is not itself the cause of the syncope). In the sitting position the danger depends on the speed with which the syncopal reaction supervenes and whether there is adequate support to prevent her falling forward. Fortunately, there is usually time to take action and allow the patient to adjust into the lateral decubitus position.

Noninvasive assessment of cardiac output using the principle of thoracic bioimpedance (BOMED NCCOM3 monitor; Bomed Medical Manufacturing, Irvine, CA, USA) has provided a method for comparison of sitting and lateral positions. Chadwick and colleagues[178] studied 20 healthy patients at term and 20 controls who were placed sequentially in four positions: supine; 15° wedge position; left lateral with hips and spine flexed; and sitting with the spine and neck flexed. The "wedge" position was taken as the baseline. The most striking change in the pregnant population occurred in the left lateral position, in which stroke index and consequently cardiac index were reduced by 21.8% and 23.4% respectively. In comparison, in the sitting position, stroke index and cardiac index were reduced by 13.1% and 8.5% respectively (Figs 40.23 and 40.24). Systolic blood pressure was significantly reduced in the lateral position, by 8.6% (Fig. 40.25). The study demonstrated that, of the two positions chosen by anesthesiologists for the insertion of the epidural, the flexed left lateral position has significantly more adverse effects on maternal cardiac output. Therefore, in the already compromised patient it may be preferable to perform the regional block in the sitting position.

Elstein and colleagues[179] have reported the use of similar noninvasive methods of cardiac output measurement to determine the optimal posture during cesarean section for a patient with triplet gestation complicated by severe "supine hypotensive syndrome." With more widespread availability of such apparatus it may, in the future, be possible to alleviate scientifically the dangers in positioning obstetric patients.

Peripheral venous obstruction or stasis and the danger of postoperative deep vein thrombosis

Deep vein thrombosis (DVT) remains a common event in hospital patients and carries the serious risk of pulmonary embolism. Although its etiology is multifactorial, it is not difficult to argue that positioning for surgery and the lack of muscular activity while under anesthesia will make a significant contribution. Intermittent pneumatic compression of the legs in general surgical patients has been shown to reduce the incidence of DVT from 27%, with no prophylaxis, to 18%. When combined with graduated compression stockings, there is further reduction to 4.5%.[180]

Vasovagal or emotional fainting

Although fainting is often regarded as a trivial, well-known, self-correcting curiosity, it has over the years had serious and sometimes lethal consequences when not recognized. Induction of general anesthesia for dental surgery in the sitting position is of course the classic example. Studies of the physiologic process have shown that the changes that take place are extremely complex and it would be inappropriate to discuss them in detail here. Relevant current knowledge is mainly based on the 1968 article by Epstein *et al.*,[181] "The role of the capacitance and resistance vessels in vasovagal syncope." Physiologically, the changes of syncopy can be summarized as a serious fall in venous return to the heart, which triggers reflex cardiovascular and endocrine compensating mechanisms. Unlike the previous discussion on aortocaval compression there is, however, no mechanical pressure on the great vessels to initiate this.

In the management of patients the anesthesiologist should have the following important points in mind:

1 Anybody can faint, but some faint more easily than others. Unfortunately, patients often forget to mention this at preoperative assessment. Such a history should be actively sought out.
2 Fainting is not at all uncommon in patients having regional anesthetics performed in the sitting position, particularly spinal or epidural procedures.[182] In addition to the prior placement of ECG electrodes and automated blood pressure and $S_{p}o_2$ monitoring, it is essential that an attendant is positioned in front of, and facing, the patient throughout the procedure so that easy transfer to the lateral position can be effected if symptoms ensue. Do not do as I once did in a very busy labor ward and ask the patient's husband to take on this role. He fainted, a midwife nearby failed to prevent him falling, and he had to be sent for a skull radiograph, thereby missing the birth of his son. Fortunately, there were no problems.
3 Fainting can occur *even when the patient is supine*[177] or in the lateral

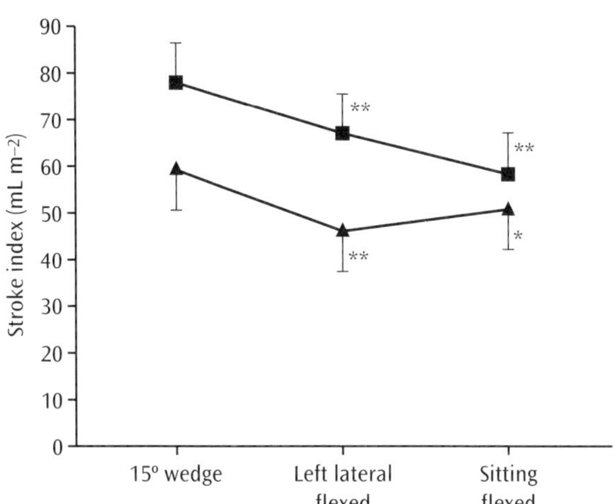

Figure 40.23 *Effect of posture on the stroke index. Mean with 95% confidence limits (mL m⁻²). ■, Control group; ▲, pregnant group; *P < 0.05 compared with 15° wedge position; ** P < 0.01 compared with 15° wedge position. (Reproduced, with permission, from Chadwick* et al.[178]*)*

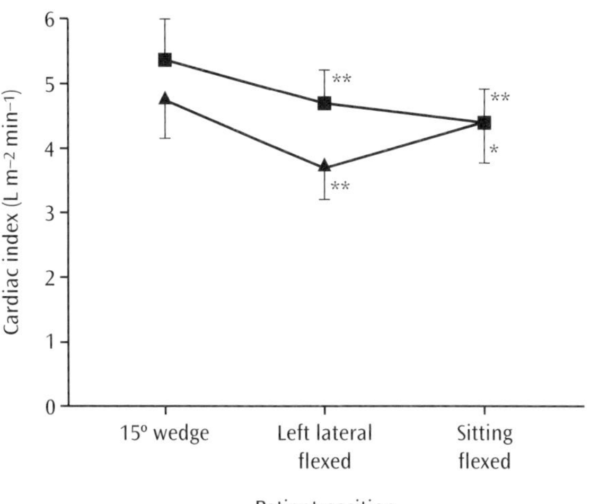

Figure 40.24 *Effect of posture on cardiac index. Mean with 95% confidence limits (L m⁻² min⁻¹). ■, control group; ▲, pregnant group; * P < 0.05 compared with 15° wedge position; ** P < 0.01 compared with 15° wedge position. (Reproduced, with permission, from Chadwick* et al.[178]*)*

decubitus position. It is not very common: I have seen it twice. At first sight this may seem a contrary state of affairs, as patients who faint in the upright position usually respond to repositioning supine. Possibly the onset period is longer in those already supine but there is no doubt that the full scenario does occur. Diagnosis is not difficult if the patient is sufficiently awake to make a warning comment. The more difficult cases occur when the patient has a syncopal reaction coincident with induction of general anesthesia. The routine application of cardiovascular monitoring prior to induction of anesthesia should immediately alert the anesthesiologist to a problem. However, if the possible diagnosis of vasovagal attack is not considered by the anesthesiologist, inappropriate and possibly dangerous management may ensue. Two recently reported cases of cardiovascular collapse at induction, one implicating drug reactions and one vasovagal attacks, occurred with the patient supine.[183,184]

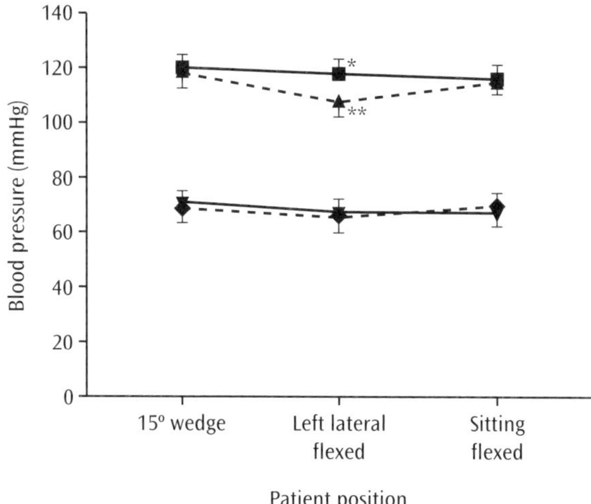

Figure 40.25 *Effect of posture on systolic (■, ▲) and diastolic (▼, ◆) blood pressure. Mean with 95% confidence limits (mmHg; 60 mmHg = 8 kPa). ■, ▼, Control group; ▲, ◆, pregnant group; *P < 0.05 control group (left lateral position) compared with pregnant group; ** P < 0.01 pregnant group (left lateral position) compared with baseline 15° wedge position. (Reproduced, with permission, from Chadwick* et al.[178]*)*

4 Even though emotional factors may initiate the cardiovascular events of vasovagal syncope, the loss of consciousness is always secondary to poor cerebral perfusion. Time is therefore at a premium in the management of the patient if brain damage is to be avoided, and it is especially important if the syncopal attack occurs coincidentally with induction of anesthesia.

5 The triggering mechanisms at cerebral level for vasovagal syncopy are not understood and the exact sequence of physiologic changes is complex. In summary there is:

   a A preliminary phase in which arterial blood pressure declines gradually and it is likely that blood is being lost to the circulation by pooling in the lower limb musculature. This phase may be extremely brief. From a clinical point of view it may be missed and is probably of less significance than the following more dramatic, clinically obvious phase.

   b The onset of this phase is characterized by a sudden precipitous fall in blood pressure, heart rate, and vascular resistance. As previously explained in the discussion on aortocaval compression of pregnancy, sympathetic vasoconstrictor reflexes that tend to maintain constant blood pressure in phase 1 have been "switched off." At the same time, another vasoconstrictor mechanism has been "switched on," i.e. there is a massive outpouring of antidiuretic hormone into the bloodstream. This is responsible for the nausea and skin pallor that persists for some 30–40 min after cardiovascular hemodynamic performance has been restored. This physiologic response probably acts in a protective role. The raised initial sympathetic drive and falling venous return of phase 1 will have induced rapid powerful myocardial contractions around small volumes of blood. The supervening bradycardia may prevent myocardial damage and allow improved ventricular filling during a fall in preload.[161,162] This physiologic response is thought to take place whenever blood volume loss to the circulation exceeds approximately 25% of circulating volume. (NB Bradycardia, as opposed to tachycardia, is also seen in severe, external and occult, internal hemorrhage.[185])

The message from this discussion is that syncope does not need electrical or chemical cardioversion! What is required is that blood sequestered in peripheral locations should be shunted back into the chambers of the heart. Positioning the patient to achieve this is the key first-aid measure and the simple expedient of raising the patient's legs to 90°, with some slight head-down tilt to empty the pelvic vessels, will immediately achieve this. Baroreceptor reflexes that have switched off the sympathetic drive are reactivated and quickly restore pulse rate and blood pressure. The temptation to reach for atropine to reverse the bradycardia is understandable, but as early as 1931 Sir Thomas Lewis, presenting the prestigious eponymous lecture in Philadelphia at which he coined the phrase "vasovagal," drew attention to the fact that, when the bradycardia associated with fainting was reversed by atropine, the arterial pressure did not return to normal, nor did the patients regain full consciousness.[186] However, both atropine and small doses of vasopressor could be a beneficial second-line management depending on the clinical and ECG response to refilling the heart. Some patients with recurrent syncope that may progress to asystole are now placed in the category of "cardioinhibitory malignant vasovagal syndrome," for which pacemaker insertion may become advocated.[187] Tilt-table testing has been shown to be of value in elucidating this condition.[188] Hart and Yanny[189] have recently described the management of a patient with "needle phobia and malignant vasovagal syndrome."

Vasovagal syncope induced by fear is probably still the commonest initial cause of acute cardiovascular collapse in patients awaiting induction of anesthesia. Day-case anesthesia without premedication and the replacement of potent opiates with short-acting benzodiazepine drugs of doubtful tranquilizing value will ensure that the problem persists. The fact that patients can faint in the supine or lateral decubitus position needs to be more widely appreciated. The value of patient monitoring prior to induction of anesthesia is self-evident, although a vasovagal attack can start even before there is time to do this. Incorrect management may, especially in the presence of coronary hypoxia, volatile anesthetic agents, and high epinephrine levels, culminate in ventricular fibrillation.[190]

The dangers of augmenting venous return to the heart

Tipping patients head-down, either to facilitate pelvic surgery or as a first-aid management of all forms of "shock," could be described as one of the 10 commandments of medical practice in the first half of the twentieth century. Despite considerable accumulated evidence of its dangers, it may well still have some adherents to this day. Old practices, well entrenched, die hard. The original hypothesis anticipated that improved venous return to the heart would increase atrial filling pressures, stimulate cardiac output, and support the blood pressure. As early as 1918 it was demonstrated that 45° of head-down tilt did not result in any significant change in blood pressure,[191] but much more sophisticated investigations were required before any impact could be made on the popularity of the practice. Between 1950 and 1970 various authors demonstrated no specific beneficial effect for patients.[192–194] Other workers demonstrated that in animal models all forms of shock were made worse by head-down tilt.[195,196] In the clinical field, two important papers concluded that the use of muscle relaxants had rendered the use of the Trendelenburg position for surgery "obsolete."[197,198] The report of Sibbald and his colleagues[199] in 1979 was probably (or should have been!) the investigative *coup de grâce* for the use of head-down tilt in the management of the hypotensive patient. It demonstrated convincing data for both cardiovascular and intracranial dangers. Seventy-six intensive care patients were divided into normotensive (61) and hypotensive (15) groups. The underlying pathology was either sepsis, acute cardiac dysfunction, or miscellaneous acute conditions. Each patient was placed into 15–20° of head-down tilt. In the normotensive group, invasive monitoring showed that the preload to the right and left ventricles was increased with a slight increase in cardiac output, systemic vascular resistance (SVR) decreased and mean arterial pressure (MAP) was therefore unchanged. In the hypotensive patients there was no increase in preload, a slightly increased afterload, and a fall in cardiac output. The very patients it was supposed to help were disadvantaged. A more recent study published the results of head-down tilt on oxygen transport in eight hypovolemic postoperative adults in an intensive care unit.[200] All subjects had an initial pulmonary artery wedge pressure of 0.8 kPa (6 mmHg) or less. Measurements were recorded with the patient in the supine position and again 10 min after instituting head-down tilt. Pulmonary artery wedge pressure, SVR, and MAP all rose but cardiac index oxygen delivery and consumption and extraction ratios were all unchanged. It was concluded that, although the blood pressure may have increased, it was not matched by any improvement in blood flow or tissue oxygenation.

There are several other factors that also have to be taken into consideration when head-down tilt is requested nowadays to facilitate an operative procedure. Probably the most important of these is the state of the patient's cardiovascular system. Two studies have measured the hemodynamic effects of the head-down position on anesthetized and awake patients with coronary artery disease.[201,202] Both found similar adverse effects. Some patients with low ejection fractions were unable to adjust to the increased filling pressures and had significant decreases in cardiac output, and half the patients in one study had elevations of pulmonary capillary wedge pressures above 2.4 kPa (18 mmHg) consistent with the onset of pulmonary congestion. This, therefore, is a very serious risk factor for the use of head-down tilt, whatever the indication.

The second disease state that is an absolute contraindication to head-down tilt is the patient with diagnosed or suspected raised intracranial pressure. Shenkin and colleagues[203] did the first important work on this topic in 1949. Five awake, physiologically normal adult volunteers showed no change in cerebral blood flow (CBF) when placed in a 20° head-up position. Four similar normal adults were then tipped 20° head down and a 14% decrease in CBF occurred despite a 10% increase in mean carotid artery blood pressure. Intracranial pressure rose from 13.7 to 29 cmH_2O (it had fallen to −0.9 cmH_2O in the head-up series). Changes in position are therefore able to alter cerebrovascular resistance. It is also likely that the effects may not be uniform throughout the brain. Single-photon emission computed tomography measurements of regional cerebral blood flow in normal male subjects during a brief period of 6° head-down tilt demonstrated significantly increased blood flow in the basal ganglia and cerebellum.[204] These variables, together with the effects of the anesthetic technique chosen, add to the complexity of the physiologic outcome. It seems fairly certain that head-down tilt is one adverse factor that should be avoided in the patient with intracranial pathology.

The combination of head-down tilt with or without lithotomy and the intra-abdominal insufflation of gases for laparoscopic surgery is likely to stress the cardiovascular system of even the most robust patient. Tilt of between 30° and 45° is not uncommonly requested with obvious potential for enhanced venous return to the heart. One study has shown that, at the time of maximum hemodynamic stress, stroke index and cardiac index are reduced by approximately 40% with no significant changes in either heart rate or MAP. In one group in the study, receiving halothane, SVR increased by 50%, and in the second group, receiving balanced anesthesia, there was a 100% increase in SVR. The authors concluded that positional factors and abdominal insufflation were much more important than the anesthetic technique.[205]

In summary, tipping a normovolemic patient head down increases central blood volume and central venous pressure. Central baroreceptors interpret this as being generally representative of the situation throughout the body and the response is an inappropriate fall in SVR. The MAP does not rise and there may be a decrease in cardiac output.

Despite the fact that over the years countless patients have survived the Trendelenburg position, its use at the current time should always be questioned, particularly in the less healthy individual.

Apart from the purely physiologic response to tipping, it must always be remembered that blood loss can be masked by the autotransfusion that continually takes place, particularly when the legs are in the lithotomy position. This can suddenly become very apparent when the supine position is reattained. Lowering the legs can require some 500–800 mL of blood to refill the vascular space depending on the depth of anesthesia and the degree of vasodilation.[206] Both anticipation and caution are needed at this time.

The position of the patient and the risk of venous air embolism

In 1983 *Anesthesiology* carried an editorial by Maurice Albin[207] in which he wrote: "It is to be remembered that venous air embolism [VAE] was a much feared complication during the nineteenth century in the spontaneously ventilating (anesthetized or nonanesthetized) patient, with many procedures carried out in the sitting or semi-sitting position. In fact, more than 150 articles, reviews, and books were published on air embolism in the 1800s." By this time, a great deal of the pathophysiology of the condition had been elucidated. More recent advances in the knowledge of the subject include bubble detection by the use of ultrasonics and end-tidal CO_2 monitoring, an understanding of the enhancement of bubble size by nitrous oxide, and management of VAE via the use of a right-sided catheter. More recently, transesophageal Doppler ultrasound and echocardiography have presented further potential for monitoring and investigating this condition.

Although no-one could maintain that the risks are as prevalent as they were, VAE can still cause a crisis in the operating room, severe morbidity, and the occasional fatality. Although most anesthesiologists are familiar with its classic association with the posterior cranial fossa surgery in the sitting position, technology is revealing the presence of air emboli in less familiar situations. To some extent it is unfortunate that VAE has been associated with such a specific surgical operation, as this may have hindered the formulation of a correct diagnosis in less likely situations. Quite simply, VAE can occur whenever the patient is positioned so that open veins or a traumatized venous sinus are situated at a site above that of the right atrium of the heart. Other factors are described below.

The first is the inability of a venous channel to collapse under the influence of gravity or pressure of adjacent tissues. Venous sinuses and diploic or emissary veins, the adventitious coat of which is fused to adjacent periosteum, are the classic examples. Self-retaining surgical retractors may have a similar effect, and a less widely appreciated example is the risk that is incurred with both removal and insertion of central venous catheters. Although predicable with their insertion, it has only recently been appreciated that fibrin tracks form consistently around catheters, *sometimes within 24 h of insertion*, creating a potential portal for VAE after catheter removal.[208] It is therefore important to remove the catheter with the patient slightly head down and to ensure immediate, complete cover of the wound with an air-occlusive dressing. Over a 20-year period, Peters[209] has collected data in which VAE associated with central venous catheterization has been responsible for 50 fatalities and 151 cases of cardiorespiratory distress or considerable neurologic morbidity.

The second most important factor is the level of venous pressure present in the veins concerned. For air to enter, this must be low or even negative. The effects of *posture* on the pressure within the venous sinuses of the skull was measured by Iwabuchi *et al.*[210] They found that, when the upper half of the body was raised, the confluens sinuum pressure decreased to reach zero at +22°. When the angle was +90°, a marked negative pressure of 12.7 ± 3.0 cmH_2O was observed in adults. To obtain a confluens sinuum pressure of zero or a little higher the most favorable position is with the sinus 15 cm higher than the right atrium. In children under 6 years of age, however, such negative pressure was not observed even at an angle of +90°. A low venous pressure at the operation site may be potentiated by negative intrathoracic pressures generated by spontaneous ventilation. Albin *et al.*[211] drew attention to the fact that in the prone knee–chest position a pendulous, free-moving abdomen could also exert a suction effect on veins opened during the course of spinal axis surgery. Gradients as low as 5 cmH_2O have been shown to allow large amounts of air, up to 200 mL, to become entrained.

The widespread use of muscle relaxants and intermittent positive-pressure ventilation (IPPV) during anesthesia may have reduced the incidence of VAE, and this may have made anesthesiologists less likely to suspect its occurrence. It is a risk that may not have been appreciated in the UK where there has been a resurgence of regional anesthesia for the conscious patient. Manual removal of a morbidly adherent placenta under spinal anesthesia recently resulted in rapidly fatal air embolism. This could have been due to a combination of deep inspiratory efforts, a low inferior vena caval pressure due to hemorrhage, and repeated introduction of air into the uterus by the hand of the obstetrician.

Apart from the well-known VAE problems of neurosurgery performed in the sitting position, some recent reports have drawn attention to similar dangers in the following procedures.

Cesarean section

During cesarean section carried out under regional anesthesia, patients not uncommonly complain of quite severe chest pain after delivery of the baby. On occasion the symptomatology is indistinguishable from angina. The ECG may appear quite unaltered. $S_{p}O_2$ monitoring may show coincident falls in saturation to around 90% but equally may not be associated with any symptoms. Vartikar and colleagues[212] prospectively investigated 78 patients with precordial Doppler ultrasound, ECG, and peripheral pulse oximetry. Both elective and emergency cases were studied, and anesthesia was either regional or general. Sixty-five percent had Doppler changes consistent with a diagnosis of VAE, and three-quarters of these had a decrease in $S_{p}O_2$ averaging 5.2% (range 3–20%). Chest pain or ECG changes were not seen unless both abnormal Doppler recordings and $S_{p}O_2$ depression were present simultaneously. Both the $S_{p}O_2$ and ECG changes resolved within the following 3 h. Rather unexpectedly, most of the Doppler changes were seen during the repair of the hysterotomy wound. Exteriorization of the uterus and traction on the wound edges increase the risks. The Trendelenburg position should now most certainly be avoided for cesarean section or any form of uterine manipulation, and patient positioning should be adopted that ensures that abdominal and uterine incision is always below heart level. Slight breaking of the table with head-up tilt to increase inferior vena cava pressure should theoretically confer some protection. One Doppler ultrasound study has, however, shown the incidence of VAE is unchanged by the use of 5–10° head-up tilt.[213] Two groups of 50 patients were studied and VAE was identified 15 times in 11 patients – seven in supine and four in head-up patients (no statistically significant difference). There were no clinically important sequelae from these events in either group. Perhaps the highest degree of head-up tilt compatible with surgical technique should be advocated, along with other measures, e.g. generous volume preloading where appropriate, to ensure central venous pressure is not low. Younker *et al.*[214] reported a case of massive air embolism during cesarean section performed under general anesthesia; resuscitation was successful.

The dangers of air embolism in posterior spinal surgery

Almost all of these procedures are carried out in the prone position and the risks of VAE occurring are extremely small when routine, uncomplicated lumbar disk surgery is being performed. This type of operation is currently the most commonly encountered reason for spinal axis surgery. Reconstructive orthopedic procedures on the thoracic spine and posterior fossa exploration, also carried out in the prone position, obviously carry a great potential for all manner of operative complications.

The necessity for a high level of complex patient monitoring is self-evident in these last procedures, and may well include a facility for detecting and managing VAE. There are lessons to be learnt from looking at the development of techniques for prone positioning for lumbar disk surgery.[6] Some methods advocated in the period between 1945 and 1965 took no account of the already well-documented anatomical connection between the vena cava and the extradural veins via the lumbar plexus. Inevitably, back-pressure from compression by pillows in the epigastrium or misplaced props in the groins could cause so much hemorrhage at the site of operation that VAE was clearly no risk whatsoever. In fact, excessive bleeding could result in premature termination of the surgery.[215] With greater recognition of the etiology of this problem, positioning with well-designed frames or props to support the iliac crests was advocated. Probably the most significant advance was in the method of propping the "knee–chest" positioned patient with a "seat" under the ischial tuberosities (Fig. 40.3). With the back horizontal in this position it has been shown that venous pressure is usually small – approximately 0–2 cmH_2O (Table 40.3).[216] Inferior vena cava pressures measured in different positions by DiStefano and colleagues[217] confirmed these findings (Table 40.4). It seems, therefore, that the search for more satisfactory surgical operating conditions and greater patient safety may theoretically set the stage for the development of VAE. In 1969 the first report of a fatality from air embolism in the prone position described a case in which surgery was being performed for a large arteriovenous malformation in the posterior cranial fossa.[218] In 1977 the "questions and answers" section of the *Journal of the American Medical Association* posed the question: "is right atrial catheterization a prerequisite for lumbar disk surgery in the knee–chest position?"[219] Tarlov,[220] replying, stated that in his experience of several hundred patients it was not necessary for lumbar surgery. He made the point that spinal veins, unlike the large intracranial veins and dural sinuses, are not kept open by bony and fascial attachments. In further correspondence, Albin *et al.*[211] disagreed and advocated the use of both right atrial catheters and Doppler ultrasonic transducers even for lumbar surgery. They quoted detection of VAE in the lateral, supine, and prone positions, with gradients between the wound and the heart as small as 5 cm. At that time, therefore, it appeared that, at least in the USA, there were two dramatically opposed schools of thought. In the UK there was no evidence of the routine use of atrial catheters for uncomplicated lumbar disk surgery, and it can be assumed that the morbidity from jugular or supraclavicular vein puncture for monitoring central venous pressure (CVP) on a routine basis would almost certainly have been expected to outweigh the advantages.

Since this early correspondence, Albin and colleagues[221] have described two fatalities in three case reports of VAE occurring during lumbar laminectomy in the prone position. Both fatalities occurred in patients positioned on the "four-poster" Relton and Hall frame. The surviving patient had been positioned in the seated knee–chest position (Tarlov). The cases described were, however, at the extreme end of the spectrum of surgical and anesthetic difficulty. All were revision procedures requiring fusion and all three weighed over 100 kg. Blood loss was excessive in all cases, and the operation times when the incidents occurred were 5 h in two cases and 3.5 h in the third. On the basis of these three cases, it would be unwise to make general recommendations regarding invasive CVP monitoring, with multiorificed catheters sited in the right atrium for all routine lumbar laminectomies. The great majority of these cases are primary procedures, blood loss should not exceed 150–200 mL, and an operating time of 1.5–2 h suffices.

As always, more complex cases will justify more complex monitoring, which could well include a thermodilution catheter as advocated by Backofen and Schauble.[222] These workers pointed out that the value of a right atrial catheter lies more in its propensity as a route of aspiration than for the information it may provide. They recommend that poor-risk patients who would be unlikely to tolerate a reduction in cardiac index of around 20% should have arterial and thermodilution catheters inserted if they are to be positioned prone.

Table 40.3 *Effects of position on central venous pressure in patients undergoing laminectomy*[216]

		Central venous pressure (cmH_2O)		
Patient's weight (kg) (lb)	**Operation**	**Supine under general anesthesia**	**Prone on laminectomy frame**	**Sitting prone position**
91.7 (200)	Thoracic	1	14	1
49.9 (110)	Lumbar	3	10	2
68.0 (150)	Thoracic	10	16	2
91.7 (200)	Lumbar	5–6	8–10	1
77.1 (170)	Thoracic	3–4	12–14	0–1
113.4 (250)	Lumbar	1	16	1
79.4 (175)	Lumbar	2	13	0
68.0 (150)	Lumbar	6	7.5	0
91.7 (200)	Lumbar	4	6	0
81.6 (180)	Lumbar	6–7	10–12	0–1
77.1 (170)	Lumbar	4	8	0
81.6 (180)	Lumbar	3–4	8	0

1 kPa = 10 cmH_2O.

Table 40.4 *Central venous pressure values in a variety of positions*[217]

Arrangements	Average central venous pressure (cmH_2O)
Georgia prone	20.7
Prone chest rolls	15.9
Lateral decubitus	11.1
Wilson frame	10.1
Tuck position	9.4
Hastings frame	1.4

1 kPa = 10 cmH_2O.

Air embolism and newly introduced surgical procedures

Radical retropubic prostatectomy and orthotopic liver transplantation have both been the subject of VAE case reports.[223,224]. The former certainly had a significant gravitational gradient between operative site and the right atrium.

CONCLUSION

Most episodes resulting in avoidable harm to the patient in the operating room are due to human error and repetition of these errors is all too common. Responsibility for the mishap that so dramatically resulted in the patient's finger ends being amputated (see under Trauma to appendages, above) was summarized by the Court Recorder: "During general anesthesia, the patient is unconscious ... and ... is no longer able to protect himself against injury. Responsibility for the prevention of such injuries then falls solely upon the anesthesiologist."[32] Nowadays this may be regarded as too sweeping a verdict and obvious negligence by other members of the operating team may mean that the blame would be, at least, shared. However, the underlying principle is clear.

Taylor[102] has pointed out that "the surgeon is ultimately responsible for the patient's position, although the duty is usually shared with the theatre nursing team and the anaesthetist." If any difference between the best choice of position from a surgical standpoint conflicts with the anesthesiologist's consideration of patient safety it is to be hoped that a sensible compromise can be achieved. Preoperative dilemmas of this type should always be recorded in the patient's records. Taylor[225] has also stressed that the anesthesiologist's responsibility "extends from the induction of anaesthesia to full recovery" and therefore encompasses both postoperative patient transfer and recovery room management.

Aitkenhead,[1] discussing risk management in anesthesia, makes it clear that Health Service managers and doctors may in the UK find that they are held accountable if the Crown Prosecution Service believes that the death of a patient was the result of a predictably preventable occurrence. The dangers of failing to position the surgical patient safely may result in greater morbidity than that due to the condition for which the patient is receiving surgery. A fatality is not unknown as the ultimate complication of this process. An appreciation of the potential problems, constant vigilance, and a high standard of patient monitoring are all necessary to minimize the risks.

REFERENCES

1. Aitkenhead AR. Risk management in anaesthesia. *J Med Defence Union* 1991; **4:** 86–90.
2. Vaughan RS. Airway management in the recovery room. *Anaesthesia* 1997; **52:** 617–18.
3. Luntley JB, Ross J, Pearce J. Lifting and handling of patients by anaesthetists. *Anaesthesia* 1995; **50:** 729–32.
4. Editorial. *Anaesthesia* 1970; **25:** 1–2.
5. Birch AA. Collapse of an operating room table. *Anaesthesiology* 1978; **49:** 62.
6. Anderton JM. The prone position for the surgical patient: a historical review of the principles and hazards. *Br J Anaesth* 1991; **67:** 452–63.
7. Tarlov IM. The knee–chest position for lower spinal operations. *J Bone Joint Surg (Am)* 1967; **49:** 1193–4.
8. Betlach DW. Wisconsin Anesthesia Study Commission of the Wisconsin Society of Anesthesiologists. *Wisconsin Med J* 1958; **57:** 185–6.
9. Lipton S. Anaesthesia in the surgery of retropulsed vertebral discs. *Anaesthesia* 1950; **5:** 208–12.
10. Gordon BS, Newman W. Lower nephron syndrome following prolonged knee–chest position. *J Bone Joint Surg (Am)* 1952; **35:** 764–8.
11. Keim HA, Weinstein JD. Acute renal failure. A complication of spine fusion in the tuck position. *J Bone Joint Surg (Am)* 1970; **52:** 1248–50.
12. Ali H, Nieto JG, Rhamyh RK, *et al.* Acute renal failure due to rhabdomyolysis associated with extreme lithotomy position. *Am J Kidney Dis* 1993; **22:** 865–9.
13. Julian D, Scott A, Allen MJ. Acute and chronic compartment syndromes. *Surgery* 1987; **46:** 1088–93.
14. Leff RG, Shapiro SR. Lower extremity complications of the lithotomy position: prevention and management. *J Urol* 1979; **122:** 138–9.
15. Lydon JC, Spielman FJ. Bilateral compartment syndrome following prolonged surgery in the lithotomy position. *Anesthesiology* 1984; **60:** 236–8.
16. MacIntyre PA. Compartment syndrome following prolonged positioning in the lithotomy position. *Anaesthesia* 1996; **51:** 511.
17. Stoodley NG, Thomson WHF. Compartment syndrome: a cautionary tale. *Br J Surg* 1989; **76:** 1297.
18. Lachman EA, Rook JL, Tunkel R, *et al.* Complications associated with intermittent pneumatic compression. *Arch Phys Med Rehab* 1992; **73:** 482–5.
19. Neagle CE, Schaffer JL, Heppenstall RB. Compartment syndrome complicating prolonged use of the lithotomy position. *Surgery* 1991; **110:** 566–9.
20. Martin JT. Compartment syndromes: concepts and perspectives for the anaesthesiologist. *Anaesth Analg* 1992; **75:** 275–83.
21. Scott DJA, Allen MJ, Barnes MR. Compartment syndromes in unconscious patients. *Br Med J* 1987; **295:** 330.
22. Moed BR, Thorderson PK. Measurement of intra-compartment pressure: a comparison of the slit catheter, side-ported needle and simple needle. *J Bone Joint Surg (Am)* 1993; **75:** 231–5.
23. Strecker WB, Wood MB, Bieber EJ. Compartment syndrome masked by epidural analgesia for postoperative pain. *J Bone Joint Surg (Am)* 1986; **68:** 1447–8.
24. Montgomery CJ, Ready LB. Epidural opioid analgesia does not obscure diagnosis of compartment syndrome resulting from prolonged lithotomy position. *Anaesthesiology* 1991; **75:** 541–3.
25. Fitzgerald RD, Kraft P, Skrbensky T, *et al.* Excursions of the cervical spine during tracheal intubation: blind oral intubation compared with direct laryngoscopy. *Anaesthesia* 1994; **49:** 111–15.
26. Heath KJ. The effect on laryngoscopy of different cervical spine immobilization techniques. *Anaesthesia* 1994; **49:** 843–5.
27. Criswell JC, Parr MJA, Nolan JP. Emergency airway management in patients with cervical spine injuries. *Anaesthesia* 1994; **49:** 900–3.
28. Morley A, Haji-Michael PG, Mahoney P. Cervical spine control during pre-hospital tracheal intubation of trauma victims. *Anaesthesia* 1995; **50:** 661–662.
29. Kay AR, Dickson MG. In "MINERVA." *Br Med J* 1992; **305:** 660.
30. Connor H. Iatrogenic injuries in theatre. *Br Med J* 1992; **305:** 956.
31. Abel RR, Lewis GM. Postoperative (pressure) alopecia. *Arch Dermatol* 1960; **81:** 34–42.
32. Courington FW, Little DM. Clinical anaesthesia 3. The role of posture in anaesthesia. In: Jenlans MT (ed.). *Common and Uncommon Problems in Anaesthesia.* Philadelphia: FA Davis, 1968: 24–54.
33. Lawson NW, Mills NL, Ochsner JL. Occipital alopecia following cardiopulmonary bypass. *J Thor Cardiovasc Surg* 1976; **71:** 342.
34. Dickenson JC, Bailey BN. Chemical burns beneath tourniquets. *Br Med J* 1988; **297:** 1513.
35. Luscombe F, Teasdale A, Powell J. Ischaemic lesions related to pressure from the bindings of a wrist splint and cardiopulmonary bypass. *Anaesthesia* 1989; **44:** 610–11.
36. Smith RH, Gramling ZW, Volpitto PP. Problems related to the prone position for surgical operations. *Anaesthesiology* 1961; **22:** 189–93.

37. Martin JT, Warner MA (eds). *Positioning in Anaesthesia and Surgery,* 3rd edn. Philadelphia: WB Saunders, 1997.
38. Magill IW. Postoperative care: anaesthetic prospects. *Practitioner* 1937; **138:** 247.
39. Schleyer-Sanders E. Prevention of backache in women. *Br Med J* 1954; **1:** 28.
40. Brown EM, Elman DS. Postoperative backache. *Anesth Analg – Curr Res* 1961; **40:** 683–5.
41. O'Donovan N, Healy TEJ, Faragher EB, *et al.* Postoperative backache: the use of an inflatable wedge. *Br J Anaesth* 1986; **58:** 280–3.
42. Hickmott KC, Healy TEJ, Roberts P, Faragher EB. Back pain following general anaesthesia and surgery. *Br J Surg* 1990; **77:** 571–5.
43. White E, Crosse MM. The aetiology and prevention of perioperative corneal abrasions. *Anaesthesia* 1998; **53:** 157–61.
44. Gild WM, Posner KL, Caplan RA, Cheney FW. Eye injuries associated with anaesthesia. *Anaesthesiology* 1992; **76:** 204–8.
45. Givner I, Jaffe N. Occlusion of the central retinal artery following anaesthesia. *Arch Ophthalmol* 1950; **43:** 197–201.
46. Tarkannen A, Leikola J. Postural variations of the intraocular pressure as measured with the Mackay–Marg Tonometer. *Acta Ophthalmol* 1967; **45:** 569–75.
47. Friberg TR, Sanborn G. Optic nerve dysfunction during gravity inversion; pattern reversal evoked potentials. *Arch Ophthalmol* 1980; **103:** 1687–9.
48. Linder BJ, Trick GL, Wolf ML. Altering body position effects intraocular pressure and visual function. *Invest Opthalmol Vis Sci* 1988; **29:** 1492.
49. Eldor J, Admoni M. Acute glaucoma following non-ophthalmic surgery. *Israel J Med Sci* 1989; **25:** 652–4.
50. Walkup HE, Murphy JD, Oteen NC. Retinal ischaemia with unilateral blindness – complications during pulmonary resection in prone position: two cases. *J Thoracic Surg* 1952; **23:** 174–5.
51. Hollenhorst RW, Svien HJ, Benoit CF. Unilateral blindness occurring during anaesthesia for neurosurgical operations. *Arch Ophthalmol* 1954; **52:** 819.
52. Jampol LM, Goldbaum M, Rosenberg M, Bahr R. Ischaemia of ciliary arterial circulation from ocular compression. *Arch Ophthalmol* 1975; **93:** 1311–17.
53. Williams EL, Hart WM, Tempelhoft R. Postoperative ischaemic neuropathy. *Anaesth Analg* 1995; **80:** 1018–29.
54. Cervical spine instability in people with Down Syndrome. *Chief Medical Officer's Update 7.* London: Department of Health, 1995: 4.
55. Casey ATH, O'Brien M, Kumar V, *et al.* Don't twist my child's head off: iatrogenic cervical dislocation. *Br Med J* 1995; **311:** 1212–13.
56. Tramo MJ, Hainline B, Petito F, *et al.* Vertebral artery injury and cerebella stroke while swimming. Case report. *Stroke* 1985; **16:** 1039–42.
57. Okawara S, Nibbelink D. Vertebral artery occlusion following hyperextension and rotation of the head. *Stroke* 1974; **5:** 640–2.
58. Hanus SH, Homer TD, Harter DH. Vertebral artery occlusion following yoga exercises. *Arch Neurol* 1977; **34:** 574–5.
59. Krueger BR, Okazaki H. Vertebral–basilar distribution infarction following chiropractic cervical manipulation. *Mayo Clin Proc* 1980; **55:** 322–32.
60. Schmidley JW, Koch T. The noncerebrovascular complications of chiropractic manipulation. *Neurology* 1984; **34:** 684–5.
61. Faris AA, Poser CM, Wilmore DW, Agnew CH. Radiologic visualization of neck vessels in healthy men. *Neurology* 1963; **13:** 386–96.
62. Sherman DG, Hart RG, Easton JD. Abrupt change in head position and cerebral infarction. *Stroke* 1981; **12:** 2–6.
63. Kim BY, Ngeow JYF, Kitahata LM, Swift CA. EEG changes with lateral rotation of the head. *Anesthesiol Rev* 1985; **12:** 36–7.
64. McPherson RW, Szymanski J, Rogers MC. Somatosensory evoked potential changes in position-related brain stem ischaemia. *Anesthesiology* 1984; **61:** 88–90.
65. Schneider RC, Cherry G, Pantek H. The syndrome of acute central cervical cord injury. *J Neurosurg* 1954; **11:** 546–77.
66. Peterson EI, Altman K. Central cervical spinal cord syndrome due to minor hyperextension injury. *Western J Med* 1989; **150:** 691–4.
67. Levy WJ, Dohn DF, Hardy RW. Central cord syndrome as a delayed postoperative complication of decompressive laminectomy. *Neurosurgery* 1982; **11:** 491–5.
68. Hitselberger WE, House WF. A warning regarding the sitting position for acoustic tumour surgery. *Arch of Otolaryngol* 1980; **106:** 69.
69. Black S, Ockert DB, Oliver WC, Cucchiara RF. Outcome following posterior fossa craniectomy in patients in the sitting or horizontal positions. *Anaesthesiol* 1988; **69:** 49–56.
70. Deem S, Shapiro HM, Marshall LF. Quadriplegia in a patient with cervical spondylosis after thoracolumbar surgery in the prone position. *Anesthesiology* 1991; **75:** 527–528.
71. Grundy B, Gravenstein N, Reid SA. The central nervous system complications of positioning. In: Martin JT (ed.). *Positioning in Anaesthesia and Surgery.* Philadelphia: WB Saunders 1987: 297.
72. Levy LM. An unusual case of flexion injury of the cervical spine. *Surg Neurol* 1982; **17:** 255–9.
73. Cottrell JF, Hassan NF, Hartung J, *et al.* Hyperflexion and quadriplegia in the seated position. *Anaesthesiol Rev* 1985; **12:** 34.
74. Tattersall MP. Massive swelling of the face and tongue. A complication of posterior fossa surgery in the sitting position. *Anaesthesia* 1984; **39:** 1015–17.
75. Munshi CA, Dhamee MS, Ghandi SK. Postoperative unilateral facial oedema: a complication of acute flexion of the neck. *Can Anaesth Soc J* 1984; **31:** 197–9.
76. Huehns TY, Yentis SM, Cumberworth V. Apparent massive tongue swelling. *Anaesthesia* 1994; **49:** 414–16.
77. Gardner WJ. Intracranial operations in the sitting position. *Ann Surg* 1935; **101:** 138–46.
78. Colley PS, Dunn R. Prevention of blood pressure response to skull-pin holder by local anesthesia. *Anaesth Analg* 1979; **58:** 241.
79. Bedford RF, Marshall WK, Persing JS. Rapid reduction of intracranial pressure: thiopentone versus lidocaine *Anesth Analg* 1980; **59:** 528.
80. Hazard warning notice. *HC (Hazard) (91) 15.* London: Department of Health, 16 July 1991.
81. Baerts WDM, De Lange JJ, Leo HD. Complications of the Mayfield skull clamp. *Anaesthesiology* 1984; **61:** 460–1.
82. Barron DW. Suprorbital neurapraxia. *Anaesthesia* 1955; **10:** 374.
83. Azar I, Lear E. Lower lip numbness following general anaesthesia. *Anaesthesiology* 1986; **65:** 450–1.
84. James FM. Hypesthesia of the tongue *Anaesthesiology* 1975; **42:** 359.
85. Winter R, Munroe M. Lingual and buccal nerve neuropathy in a patient in the prone position: a case report. *Anaesthesiology* 1989; **71:** 452–4.
86. Churchill-Davidson HC. *A Practice of Anaesthesia,* 3rd edn. London: Lloyd-Luke, 1972: 1263.
87. Fuller JE, Thomas DV. Facial nerve paralysis after general anaesthesia, *JAMA* 1956; **162:** 645.
88. Nightingale PJ, Løngren A. Iatrogenic facial nerve paresis. *Anaesthesia* 1982; **37:** 322–3.
89. Dingman RO, Grabb WC. Surgical anatomy of the mandibular ramus of the facial nerve based on the dissection of 100 facial halves. *Plas Reconstruct Surg* 1962; **29:** 266–72.
90. Glauber DT. Facial paralysis after general anaesthesia. *Anaesthesiology* 1986; **65:** 516–17.
91. Jaffe TB, McLeskey CH. Position induced Horner's syndrome. *Anaesthesiology* 1982; **56:** 49–50.
92. Trojaborg W. Electrophysiologic findings in pressure palsy of the brachial plexus. *J Neurol Neurosurg Psychiatry* 1977; **40:** 1160–7.
93. Nambisan RN, Karakousis CP. Axillary compression syndrome with neurapraxia due to operative positioning. *Surgery* 1989; **105:** 449–54.
94. Gwinnutt CL. Injury to the axillary nerve. *Anaesthesia* 1988; **43:** 205–6.
95. Anderton JM, Schady W, Markham DE. An unusual case of postoperative brachial plexus palsy. *Br J Anaesth* 1994; **72:** 605–7.
96. Patel RI, Thein RMH, Epstein BS. Costoclavicular syndrome and the sitting position during anesthesia. *Anaesthesiology* 1980; **53:** 341–2.
97. Saady A. Brachial plexus palsy after anaesthesia in the sitting position. *Anesthesiology* 1981; **36:** 194.
98. Dawson DM, Krarup C. Perioperative nerve lesions. *Arch Neurol* 1989; **46:** 1355–60.
99. Hanson MR, Breuer AC, Furlan AJ, *et al.* Mechanism and frequency of brachial plexus injury in open heart surgery: a prospective analysis. *Ann Thorac Surg* 1983; **36:** 675–9.
100. Malamut RI, Wilson M, England JD, *et al.* Post surgical idiopathic brachial neuritis. *Muscle Nerve* 1994; **17:** 320–24.
101. Kroll DA, Caplan RA, Posner K, *et al.* Nerve injury associated with anaesthesia. *Anaesthesiology* 1990; **73:** 202–7.
102. Taylor TH. Avoiding iatrogenic injuries in theatre. *Br Med J* 1992; **305:** 595–6.
103. Warner MA, Warner ME, Martin JT. Ulnar neuropathy Incidence outcome and risk factors in sedated or anaesthetised patients. *Anaesthesiology* 1994; **81:** 1332–40.
104. Wadsworth TG, Williams JR. Cubital tunnel external compression syndrome. *Br Med J* 1973; **1:** 662–6.
105. Wadsworth TG. The external compression syndrome of the ulnar nerve at the cubital tunnel. *Clin Orthop* 1977; **124:** 189–204.

106. Alvine GF, Schurrer ME. Postoperative ulnar nerve palsy. Are there predisposing factors? *J Bone Joint Surg (Am)* 1987; **69:** 255–9.
107. Neary D, Ochoa J, Giliatt RW. Sub-clinical entrapment neuropathy in man. *J Neurol Sci* 1975; **24:** 283–98.
108. Pollock LJ, Davis L. Peripheral nerve injuries. *Am J Surg* 1932; **17:** 461–71.
109. Britt BA, Gordon RA. Peripheral nerve injuries associated with anaesthesia. *Can Anaesth Soc J* 1964; **11:** 514–36.
110. Kopell HP, Thompson WAL. *Peripheral Entrapment Neuropathies.* New York: Robert E Krieger, 1976.
111. Parks BJ. Postoperative peripheral neuropathies. *Surgery* 1973; **74:** 348–57.
112. Martin JT. Postoperative isolated dysfunction of the long thoracic nerve: a rare entity of uncertain etiology. *Anaesth Analg* 1989; **69:** 614–19.
113. Ehni G. Significance of the small lumbar spinal canal. Cauda equina compression syndromes due to spondylosis. 4. Acute compression artificially induced during operation. *J Neurosurg* 1969; **31:** 507–12.
114. Wilkes LL. Paraplegia from operating position and spinal stenosis in non-spinal surgery. *Clin Orthopaed* 1980; **146:** 148–9.
115. Moiel R, Ehni G. Cauda equinal compression due to spondylolisthesis with intact neural arch. Report of two cases. *J Neurosurg* 1968; **28:** 262–5.
116. Amoiridis G, Wöhrle JC, Langkafer M, *et al.* Spinal cord infarction after surgery in a patient in the hyperlordotic position. *Anaesthesiology* 1996; **84:** 228–30.
117. Shaw JA, Murray DG. The relationship between tourniquet pressure and underlying soft tissue pressure in the thigh. *J Bone Joint Surg* 1981; **64A:** 1148–52.
118. Sunderland S. Relative susceptibility to injury of the medial and lateral division of the sciatic nerve. *Br J Surg* 1953; **41:** 300–2.
119 Burkhart FL, Daly JW. Sciatic and peroneal nerve injury. A complication of the vaginal operations. *Obstet Gynaecol* 1966; **28:** 99–102.
120. McQarrie HG, Harris SW, Elsworth HS, *et al.* Sciatic neuropathy complicating vaginal hysterectomy. *Am J Obstet Gynaecol* 1972; **113:** 223–32.
121. Warner MA, Martin JT, Schroeder DR, *et al.* Lower extremity motor neuropathy associated with surgery performed on patients in a lithotomy position. *Anaesthesiology* 1994; **81:** 6–12.
122. Gozal Y, Pomeranz S. Sciatic nerve palsey as a complication after acoustic neuromas resection in the sitting position. *J Neurosurg Anaesth* 1994; **6:** 6–40.
123. Angermeier KW, Jordan GH. Complications of the exaggerated lithotomy position: a review of 177 cases. *J Urol (USA)* 1994; **151:** 866–8.
124. Hatono Y, Arai T, Iida H, Soneda J. Common peroneal nerve palsy. A complication of coronary artery bypass grafting surgery. *Anaesthesia* 1988; **43:** 568–9.
125. Roblee MA. Femoral neuropathy from the lithotomy position. Case report and a new leg holder for prevention. *Am J Obstet Gynaecol* 1967; **97:** 871–2.
126. Hakim M-AL, Katirji MB. Femoral mononeuropathy induced by the lithotomy position: a report of 5 cases with a review of the literature. *Muscle Nerve* 1993; **16:** 891–5.
127. Kinges KG, Wilbanks GD, Cole GR. Injury to the femoral nerve during pelvic operations. *Obstet Gynaecol* 1965; **25:** 619–23.
128. O'Donnell D, Rottman R, Kotelko D, *et al.* Incidence of maternal post-partum neurological dysfunction [abstract]. *Anaesthesiology* 1994; **81:** A1127.
129. Lembecke W. [Rare nerve paralysis due to pressure while lying on an extension table. Two cases.] *Chirugie* 1947; **264:** 17–18.
130. Hoffman A, Jones RE, Schoenvogel R. Pudendal nerve neurapraxia as a result of traction on the fracture table. A report of 4 cases. *J Bone Joint Surg (Am)* 1982; **64:** 136–8.
131. Ochoa J, Fowler TJ, Gilliath RW. Anatomical changes in peripheral nerves compressed by a pneumatic tourniquet. *J Anat* 1972; **113:** 433–55.
132. Lupinski JR, Chance PF, Garcia CA. Inherited primary peripheral neuropathies: molecular genetics and clinical implications. *JAMA* 1993; **270:** 2326–30.
133. Upton ATM, McComas AJ. The double crush in nerve entrapment syndromes. *Lancet* 1973; **2:** 359–61.
134. Corvino BG, Fossard HA, Relider K, *et al.* (eds). *Effects of Anaesthesia.* Bethesda, MD: Americal Physiological Society, 1985.
135. Coonan TJ, Hope CE. Cardiorespiratory effects of change in body position *Canadian Anaesthetists' Society J* 1983; **30:** 424–37.
136. Marshall WK, Bedford RF, Miller ED. Cardiovascular responses in the seated position – impact of four anesthetic techniques. *Anaesth Analg* 1983; **62:** 648–53.
137. Snoy FJ, Woodside JR. Unilateral pulmonary oedema (down lung syndrome) following a urological operation. *J Urol* 1984; **132:** 776–7.
138. Heinonen J, Takki S, Tammisto T. The effect of Trendelenburg tilt and other procedures on the position of endotracheal tubes. *Lancet* 1968; **1:** 850–3.
139. Morimura N, Inour K, Miwa T. Chest roentgenogram demonstrates cephalad movement of the carina during laparoscopic cholecystectomy [correspondence]. *Anaesthesiology* 1994; **81:** 1301.
140. Toung TJK, Grayson R, Saklad J, Wang H. Movement of the distal end of the endotracheal tube during flexion and extension of the neck. *Anaesth Analg* 1985; **64:** 1029–32.
141. Green RA. A matter of vigilance. *Anaesthesia* 1986; **41:** 129–30.
142. Lunn JN, Mushin WW. *Mortality Associated with Anaesthesia.* London: Nuffield Provincial Hospitals Trust, 1982: 21–2.
143. Tomlin PJ, Howarth FH, Robinson JS. Postoperative atelactasis and laryngeal incompetence. *Lancet* 1968; **1:**1402–5.
144. Russell WJ. Position of the patient and respiratory function in the immediately postoperative period. *Br Med J* 1981; **283:** 1079–80.
145. Hsu H, Hickey RF. Effect of posture on the functional residual capacity postoperatively. *Anesthesiology* 1976; **44:** 520–1.
146. Relton JES, Hall JE. An operation frame for spinal fusion – a new apparatus designed to reduce haemorrhage during operation. *J Bone Joint Surg (Br)* 1967; **49:** 327–32.
147. Wright IS. The neurovascular syndrome produced by hyperabduction of the arms. *Am Heart J* 1945; **29:** 1–19.
148. Weinlander CM, Coombs DW, Plume SK. Myocardial ischemia due to obstruction of an aortocoronary bypass graft by intra-operative positioning. *Anaesth Analg* 1985; **64:** 933–6.
149. Reid JH, Appleton PJ. A case of ventricular fibrillation in the prone position during back stabilisation surgery in a boy with Duchenne's muscular dystrophy. *Anaesthesia* 1999; **54:** 364–71.
150. Bieniarz J, Crottogini JJ, Curuchet E, *et al.* Aortocaval compression by the uterus in late human pregnancy. *Am J Obstet Gynecol* 1968; **100:** 203–17.
151. Matalinski J, Kadlic T. Inferior vena cava occlusion in the left lateral position. *Br J Anaesth* 1974; **46:** 165–7.
152. Schroeder EM, Jebson PJ. The supine hypotensive syndrome in a young boy. *Anaesthesiology* 1986; **64:** 377–8.
153. Zuck D. Caval compression. *Anaesthesia News* July 1999: 12, or the home page of the Association of Anaesthetists of Great Britain and Ireland, www.aagbi.org.
154. Hansen R. Ohnmacht und schwangerschaft. *Klinische Wochenschrift* 1942; **21:** 241–5.
155. McRoberts WA. Postural shock in pregnancy. *Am J Obstetrics and Gynecology* 1951; **62:** 627–32.
156. Howard RK, Goodson JH, Mengert WF. Supine hypotensive syndrome in late pregnancy. *Obstetrics and Gynecology* 1953; **1:** 371–377.
157. Marx GF. Aortocaval compression syndrome: its 50 year history. *Int J Obstetric Anaesth* 1992; **1:** 60–4.
158. Holmes F. The Supine Hypotensive Syndrome Its importance to the Anaesthetist. *Anaesthesia* 1995; **50:** 972–7.
159. Kinsella SM, Lee A, Spencer JAD. Maternal and foetal effects of the supine and pelvic tilt positions in late pregnancy. *Eur J Obstetrics, Gynecology Reproductive Biol* 1990; **36:** 11–17.
160. Secher NJ, Arnsbo P, Heslet Anderson L, Thomson A. Measurement of cardiac stroke volume in various body positions in pregnancy and during caesarean section: a comparison between thermodilution and impedance cardiography. *Scandinavian J Clin and Lab Invest* 1979; **39:** 569–76.
161. Ludbrook J. Faint heart. Opioids have a role in circulatory collapse due to acute blood loss. *Br Med J* 1989; **298:** 1053–4.
162. Anderson ID. Faint heart [letter]. *Br Med J* 1989; **298:** 1449–50.
163. Goodwin APL, Pearce AJ. The human wedge: a manoeuvre to relieve aortocaval compression during resuscitation in late pregnancy. *Anaesthesia* 1992; **47:** 433–4.
164. Dark A, Engelhardt T. "Are you alright Mrs Tilt"? *Anaesthesia* 1998; **53:** 927.
165. Marx GF. Cardiopulmonary resuscitation of late pregnant women. *Anesthesiology* 1982; **56:** 156.
166. International Liaison Committee on Resuscitation. Special resuscitation situations. 1997; **34:** 129–49.
167. McIndoe AK, Hammond EJ, Babington PCB. Peripartum cardiomyopathy presenting as cardiac arrest at induction of anaesthesia for emergency caesarean section. *Br J Anaesth* 1995; **75:** 97–101.

168. McCartney CJL, Dark A. Caesarean delivery during cardiac arrest in late pregnancy. *Anaesthesia* 1998; **53:** 310–11.
169. Abitol MM. Aortic compression by pregnant uterus. *N Y J Med* 1976; **76:** 1470–5.
170. Eckstein KL, Marx GF. Aortocaval compression and uterine displacement. *Anesthesiology* 1974; **40:** 92–6.
171. Kauppila A, Koskinin M, Puolokka J, *et al.* Decreased intervillous and unchanged myometrial blood flow in supine recumbency. *Obstetrics and Gynecology* 1980; **55:** 203–5.
172. Humphrey MD, Chang A, Wood EC, *et al.* A decrease in foetal pH during the second stage of labour when conducted in the dorsal position. *J Obstet Gynaecol Br Commonwealth* 1974; **81:** 600–2.
173. Kinsella SM, Whitwam JG, Spencer JAD. Reducing aortocaval compression: how much tilt is enough? Do as much as possible in the lateral position. *Br Med J* 1992; **305:** 539–40.
174. Ansari I, Wallace G, Clemetson CAB, *et al.* Tilt caesarean section. *J Obstet Gynaecol Br Commonwealth* 1970; **77:** 713–21.
175. Crawford JS, Burton M, Davies P. Time and lateral tilt at caesarean section. *Br J Anaesth* 1972; **44:** 477–84.
176. Buley RJR, Downing JW, Brock-Utne JG, *et al.* Right versus left lateral tilt for caesarean section. *Br J Anaesth* 1977; **49:** 1009–15.
177. Verrill PJ, Aellig WH. Vasovagal faint in the supine position. *Br Med J* 1970; **4:** 348.
178. Chadwick IS, Eddleston JM, Candelier CK, Pollard BJ. Haemodynamic effects of the position chosen for the insertion of an extradural catheter. *Int J Obstet Anaesth* 1993; **2:** 197–201.
179. Elstein ID, Schwalbe SS, Marx GF. Cardiac output measurements during and after triplet gestation. *Obstet Gynecol*1989; **74:** 452–3.
180. Colditz GA, Tuden RL, Oster G. Rates of venous thrombosis after general surgery; combined results of clinical trials. *Lancet* 1986; **2:** 143–6.
181. Epstein SE, Stampfer M, Beiser GD. Role of the capacitance and resistance vessels in vasovagal syncope. *Circulation* 1968; **37:** 524–33.
182. McConachie I. Vasovagal asystole during spinal anaesthesia. *Anaesth* 1991; **46:** 281–2.
183. Dorrington KL. Asystole with convulsion following sub anaesthetic dose of propofol plus fentanyl. *Anaesthesia* 1989; **44:** 658–9.
184. McCoy EP, Wilson CM. Cardiac arrest before induction of anaesthesia. *Today's Anaesth* 1989; **4:** 260.
185. Sander-Jensen K, Secher NH, Bie P, *et al.* Vagal slowing of the heart during haemorrhage, observations from 20 consequative hypotensive patients. *Br Med J* 1986; **292:** 364–6.
186. Lewis T. Vasovagal syncope and the carotid sinus mechanism with comments on Gower's and Nothnagal's syndrome. *Br Med J* 1932; 873–6.
187. Petersen MEV, Chamberlain-Webber R, Fitzpatrick AP, *et al.* Permanent pacing for cardio-inhibitory malignant vaso-vagal syndrome. *Br Heart J* 1994; **71:** 274–81.
188. Kenny RA, Ingram A, Bayliss J, Sutton R. Head-up tilt a useful test for investigating unexplained syncope. *Lancet* 1986; **2:** 1352–5.
189. Hart PS, Yanny W. Needle phobia and malignant vasovagal syndrome. *Anaesthesia* 1998; **53:** 1002–4.
190. Bourne JG. Cardiac arrest – a personal view. *Proc Assoc Dent Anaesth* 1989; **7:** 22.
191. Henderson Y, Haggard HW. The circulation in man in the head-down position and a method of measuring the venous return to the heart. *J Pharmacol Exp Ther* 1918; **11:** 189–201.
192. Cole F. Head lowering in the treatment of hypotension. *JAMA* 1952; **150:** 273–4.
193. Taylor J, Weil MH. Failure of the Trendelenburg position to improve circulation during clinical shock. *Surg Gynaecol Obstet* 1967; **124:** 1005–10.
194. Wilkins RW, Bradley ES, Friedland CK. The acute circulatory effects of the head down position (negative G) in normal man with a note on some measures to relieve cranial congestion in this position. *J Clin Invest* 1950; **29:** 940–9.
195. Weil MH, Whigham H. Head down (Trendelenburg) position for treatment of irreversible haemorrhagic shock. Experimental study on rats. *Ann Surg* 1965; **162:** 905–9.
196. Guntheroth WG, Abel FL, Mullins GL. The effect of Trendelenburg's position on blood pressure and carotid flow. *Surg Gynaecol Obstet* 1964; **119:** 345–8.
197. Inglis JM, Brook BN. Trendelenburg tilt: obsolete position. *Br Med J* 1956; **2:** 343–4.
198. Swain J. The case for abandoning the Trendelenburg position in pelvic surgery. *Med J Aust* 1960; **ii:** 536–7.
199. Sibbald WJ, Patterson NAM, Holliday RL, Baskeville J. The Trendelenburg potion: hemodynamic effects in hypotensive and normotensive patients. *Crit Care Med* 1979; 7: 218–24.
200. Sing FR, O'Hara D, Sawyer MA, *et al.* Trendelenburg position and oxygen transport in hypovolaemic adults. *Ann Emerg Med* 1994; **23:** 564–7.
201. Kopman EA, Sandza Jr JG . Hemodynamic effects of head-down lithotomy position in patients with coronary artery disease. *Obstetrics and Gynaecology* 1979; **53:** 273.
202. Kubal K, Komatsu T, Sanchala V, *et al.* Trendelenburg position used during venous cannulation increases myocardial oxygen demand [abstract]. *Anaesth Analg* 1984; **63:** 239.
203. Shenkin HA, Scheuerman EB, Spitz EB, *et al.* Effects of change of posture upon cerebral circulation of man. *J Appl Physiol* 1949; **2:** 317–26.
204. Satake H, Konishi T, Kawashima T, *et al.* Intra-cranial blood flow measured with single photon emission computer tomography (SPECT) during transient –6 degrees head down tilt. *Aviat Space Environ Med* 1994; **65:** 117.
205. Johannsen G, Andersen M, Juhl B. The effects of general anaesthesia on the haemodynamic events during laparoscopy with CO_2 insufflation. *Acta Anaesthesiol Scand* 1989; **33:** 132–6.
206. Little DM Jr. Posture and anaesthesia. *Can Anaesth Soc J* 1960; **7:** 2–15.
207. Albin MS. The sights and sounds of air. *Anesthesiology* 1983; **58:** 113–14.
208. Meninim P, Coyle CF, Taylor JD. Venous air embolism associated with removal of central venous catheter. *Br Med J* 1992; **305:** 171–2.
209. Peters JL. Removal of central venous catheter and venous air embolism. *Br Med J* 1992; **305:** 524–5.
210. Iwabuchi T, Sobata E, Susuki M, *et al.* Dural sinus pressure is related to neurosurgical positions. *Neurosurgery* 1983; **12:** 203–7.
211. Albin MS, Newfield P, Paulter S, *et al.* Atrial catheter and lumbar disc surgery [correspondence]. *J Am Med Assoc* 1978; **239:** 496.
212. Vartikar JV, Johnson MD, Datta S. Precordial doppler monitoring and pulse oximetry during caesarean section delivery; detection of venous air embolism. *Regional Anaesth* 1989; **14:** 145–8.
213. Karuparthy YR, Downing JW, Husain FJ, *et al.* Incidence of venous air embolism during caesarean section is unchanged by the use of 5–10° head-up tilt. *Anaesth Analg* 1989; **69:** 620–3.
214. Younker D, Rodriguez V, Kavanagh J. Massive air embolism during caesarean section. *Anesthesiology* 1986; **65:** 77–9.
215. Hunter AR. Anesthesia for operations in the vertebral canal. *Anesthesia* 1950; **12:** 367–73.
216. Cook AW, Siddiqui TS, Nidzgorski R, *et al.* Sitting prone position for the posterior surgical approach to the spine and posterior fossa. *Neurosurgery* 1982; **10:** 232–5.
217. DiStefano VJ, Klein KS, Nixon JE, Andrews TE. Intraoperative analysis of position and body habitus on surgery of the low back. *Clin Orthopaed* 1974; **99:** 51–6.
218. Shenkin HN, Goldfedder P. Air embolism from exposure of posterior cranial fossa in prone position. *J Am Med Assoc* 1969; **210:** 726.
219. Goldberg D. Lumbar disc surgery in the knee–chest position: preanaesthetic atrial catheter unnecessary. Questions and Answers. *J Am Med Assoc* 1977; **238:** 253.
220. Tarlov I. Lumbar disc surgery in knee–chest position. Pre-anaesthetic atrial catheter unnecessary. Questions and Answers. *J Am Med Assoc* 1977; **238:** 253.
221. Albin MS, Ritter RR, Pruett CE, Kalff K. Venous air embolism during lumbar laminectomy in the prone position: a report of three cases. *Anesth Analg* 1992; **73:** 346–9.
222. Backofen JE, Schauble JF. Hemodynamic changes with prone position during general anaesthesia [abstract]. *Anesth Analg* 1985; **64:** 194.
223. Albin MS, Ritter RR, Reinhart R, *et al.* Venous air embolism during radical retropubic prostatectomy. *Anesth Analg* 1992; **74:** 151–3.
224. Prager MC, Gregory GA, Ascher NL, *et al.* Massive venous air embolism during orthotopic liver transplantation. *Anesthesiology* 1990; **72:** 198–200.
225. Taylor T. Postoperative recovery. *Med Protection Soc Casebook* 1996; **7:** 4–7.

41

Incident monitoring in anesthesia

MICHAL T KLUGER AND WILLIAM B RUNCIMAN

INTRODUCTION

Although adverse events in medical practice are not a new phenomenon, their impact on the care of patients in our hospitals is becoming, increasingly, a source of public concern. Incident monitoring, as a tool for managing organizational error, has been used for many years in nonmedical areas such aviation, engineering, and the space and nuclear industries. Over the past 50 years, healthcare workers have slowly embraced this concept and developed applications mirroring those in industry to identify and manage problems in their own areas. Despite being a relatively new medical specialty, anesthesia is acknowledged as one of the leaders in addressing patient safety and error reduction in clinical medicine.[1]

The aim of this chapter is to develop a conceptual framework for error and how it impacts on our understanding of incidents and accidents in anesthetic practice. The role of incident monitoring is discussed in association with other methods of data acquisition. Finally, the place of incident monitoring as a component of a risk management program is reviewed with particular reference to the Australian Incident Monitoring Study (AIMS).

Although we are focusing on incident monitoring as a valuable tool for improving patient safety and reducing error, it should not be seen as a single solution – there is no "magic bullet' for this problem. Rather, it is one component of a multifaceted approach to patient safety.

ERROR AND RISK IN MEDICINE

> Cure the disease and kill the patient.
>
> Francis Bacon 1561–1626[2]

> I do not want two diseases – one nature made – one doctor made.
>
> Napoleon Bonaparte (1769–1821)[3]

> Cur'd yesterday of my disease, I died last night of my physician.
>
> Matthew Prior (1664–1721)[3]

Adverse events in health care

The concept of medical error and iatrogenic injury is not new. It has been recognized for thousands of years that attempts to improve health and reduce suffering could themselves be associated with harmful effects to the patient. It constitutes the basis of the Hippocratic Oath – *primum non nocere* – or "first do no harm," first enunciated over 2000 years ago. Patient safety has been highlighted more recently by widely publicized investigations at local, national, and international levels. Unprecedented attention from both the media and the public over such cases as the Bristol Inquiry (pediatric cardiac surgery, UK) and the Gisborne cervical screening disaster (missed cervical cancer smears, New Zealand) has focused attention on professional bodies. It is now obvious that doctors will be held much more accountable for their actions in the future than they have been to date.

United States

The importance of this issue was recently demonstrated by the huge public outcry and comments made by Congress and the President of the United States in response to the Institute of Medicine of the National Academy of Science's publication, *To Err is Human*.[4] This governmental committee recognized the active role played by anesthesia, with particular reference to the Anesthesia Patient Safety Foundation (APSF) as the only named specialty-affiliated body that was actively addressing patient safety within the USA. This committee issued several recommendations as a result of its studies. These included: the creation by Congress of a Center for Patient Safety within the Agency for Healthcare Research and Quality; the creation of a national integrated mandatory incident reporting system; increased legal protection for reports that were filed; encouraging professional groups to address safety issues; improving drug surveillance; and, finally, implementing safety programs within healthcare institutions with documented executive responsibility for safety.

The committee commented unfavorably on the safety profile and culture (or lack of it) in the healthcare industry compared with aviation. The airline fatality rate between 1990 and 1994 was one-third that of the rate experienced in the 1950s despite a greatly increased number of flights. There were no deaths on a commercial aircraft in 1998 in the USA. When this is contrasted with the 0.3–0.5% of admissions being associated with deaths attributable to iatrogenic injury (up to 100 000 per annum in the USA), it is not surprising that this committee stated: "Given current knowledge about the magnitude of the problem, the committee believes it would be irresponsible to expect anything less than 50 percent reduction in error [in healthcare] over five years."

The forerunner to many of the recent studies examining medical negligence and iatrogenic injury was based in California in the 1970s. Escalating malpractice claims led to an exponential rise in medical insurance premiums, which in turn led to a litigation crisis. A major study was commissioned by the California Medical Association, which identified that 4.6% of all hospital admissions were associated with a "potentially compensatable event."[5] However only 1 in 5 negligent injuries actually led to a malpractice claim.

This study was followed by the widely cited Harvard Medical Practice Study (HMPS) in which Brennan and colleagues[6,7] reviewed the medical records of 30 121 patients admitted to 51 acute care institutions in New York State in 1984. In addition, over 60 000 malpractice claims were reviewed and interviews were conducted with 2400 patients. Adverse events (injuries caused by medical management that led to or prolonged hospitalization or resulted in disability at the time of discharge or death) were identified in 3.7% of all admissions; in two-thirds of these human error was deemed to have caused the injury. This was extrapolated to 13 000 deaths resulting from negligence and almost 100 000 people suffering from adverse events in New York State each year.[8]

The Utah–Colorado Study (UTCOS)[9] reviewed the records of 14 700 patients randomly selected from 28 hospitals using the HMPS methodologies. Adverse events were identified in 2.9% of all hospitalizations, with death occurring in 0.3% of these adverse events. Operative procedures accounted for 45% of all events, 1% of which were deemed negligent and 17% of which led to permanent disability.

Australia

The Quality in Australian Health Care Study (QAHCS), released in 1995, reviewed 14 179 randomly selected admissions to 28 hospitals in New South Wales and South Australia.[10] The results of this study indicated that 16.6% of all admissions were associated with an "adverse event" caused by healthcare management rather than a disease process. Of significance, half of all adverse events were considered preventable, 13.7% led to permanent disability, and in 4.9% of cases the patient died. Anesthesia contributed to only 47 (2%) of all adverse events, with one-third of these cases deemed preventable The main anesthesia-related categories were relatively minor in comparison with some other clinical areas Over one-third comprised hospitalization for postoperative nausea and vomiting or postdural puncture headache; the remainder were made up of well-recognized anesthesia-related complications such as aspiration and dental, eye, and neurologic damage.

Although there initially appeared to be fewer adverse events in the USA than in Australia (2.9% vs. 16.6% of admissions), when methodologic differences were corrected for,[11] the overall rates for major disability (1.7%) and death (0.3%) were virtually identical in both studies.[12] The discrepancy was accounted for, after correcting for some methodological differences, by there being seven times more minor adverse events in the Australian study than in the US one. The authors concluded that differences in the thresholds for "calling" an adverse event were mainly responsible for the apparent differences in the rates of adverse events and that there was no evidence for a difference in quality of healthcare delivery in the two countries.[11,12]

United Kingdom

The Department of Health commissioned an expert group to examine the impact of adverse events within the National Health Service (NHS). This report, *An Organisation with a Memory*,[13] mirrored many of the comments made by the US and Australian reports. The committee reported that there were an estimated 850 000 adverse events per year in the NHS hospital sector, and 38 000 complaints in primary care. In addition, 600 reports had been filed with the Medical Devices Agency, which included 87 deaths and at least 13 patients who had been paralyzed since 1985 due to a wrong drug being injected into the subarachnoid space. This report identified four processes that needed to occur in order to improve safety. These were: a unified incident reporting mechanism; the development of a more open safety-oriented reporting culture; the implementation of corrective strategies; and a wider appreciation of the systems approach in measuring, analyzing, and learning from human error.

Reports from the USA, Australia, and the UK, therefore, highlighted the need for a single, unified incident monitoring system as an essential component of the foundation on which could be built future improvements in healthcare safety.[4,13,14]

Financial implications

The cost of medical error is high. In the USA, medical error may contribute to up to 98 000 unnecessary deaths per annum and in excess of 1 million injuries, with a projected annual cost of as much as US$30 billion.[4] In comparison, the QAHCS predicted 18 000 deaths per annum in Australia and more than 50 000 permanent disabilities, with 10% of hospital admissions being associated with a preventable adverse event.[12] The NHS report also estimated that 10% of hospitalized patients had been subject to an adverse event with a direct cost of £250 000 per 1011 admissions, projected to 850 000 admissions and a cost of £2 billion for the NHS in the UK per annum.[13] Overall, the direct medical costs of iatrogenic injury may be estimated to account for 5% of the total amount spent on health care.[4,14,15,16]

Whereas some countries such as New Zealand and Sweden have no-fault compensation schemes, others such as the USA, Australia, and the UK rely on the tort system for compensation. With increasing public concern about iatrogenic injury, it is not surprising that no-fault compensation schemes are being considered in a number of countries. Clearly, this would benefit the consumer and, given the high administration costs of the tort system, would probably cost little more than the present system.[17] Indeed, the data from the NHS study indicate that the £2 billion spent on treating adverse events is five times the cost of clinical negligence litigation in the UK.[13]

Health care – a risky business

Risk can be compared between medical specialties and with other activities by using an easily measurable end-point. Death is such an end-point. The fatal accident frequency rate (FAFR) is defined as: "the number of fatal accidents in a certain place during a certain activity that occur over 100 million hours of activity." The UK chemical industry uses an FAFR of 4 as an acceptable rate, above which steps will be actively taken to reduce it.[18] Table 41.1 shows calculated FAFRs for a combination of medical and nonmedical activities. It should be noted that being an inpatient in an Australian acute care hospital is 40 times more dangerous that being in traffic, and only 10 times safer than jumping out of an aircraft with a parachute![14] The relative safety profile of anesthesia is emphasized by the fact that having an hour under anesthesia is no more risky than simply being in hospital for an hour!

There remains no good estimate of anesthesia-related mortality and morbidity. The 1992 Confidential Enquiry into Perioperative Death (CEPOD) Study, conducted in the UK, concluded that anesthesia as the *sole* cause of mortality, *directly caused* one death per 150 000 procedures, but *contributed to* one death per 1300 procedures. Current annual figures suggest an estimated 20 000 deaths within 30 days of surgery per year in the UK.[13] In the most recent review of anesthesia-related mortality in Australia (1994–1996), 7% of all perioperative deaths were attributed to some degree to anesthesia.[20] This represents one death per 63 000 procedures in which anesthesia contributed to the death, and one in over 150 000 in which anesthesia was the definite cause of death.

Table 41.1 *Average fatal accident rates (per 100 million hours of exposure) for various activities. Data taken from Runciman and Moller[14] and Zelders[19]*

Being pregnant[a]	1
Train travel[b]	5
Working at home[b]	8
Working in agriculture[b]	10
Having a unit of blood and developing HIV infection[c]	10
Being in traffic[b]	50
Flying in commercial aircraft[b]	100
Being a patient in an Australian hospital[d]	2000
Being anesthetized[e]	2000
Parachute jumping[f]	20 000
Elective abdominal aneurysm operation[g]	200 000
Emergency abdominal aneurysm operation[g]	2 000 000

a. Calculated from Dutch health statistics.
b. References are *c*. 20 years old but give an idea of magnitude.
c. Assuming 1 h to transfuse one unit and one case of human immunodeficiency virus per 10 million transfused units.
d. Calculated from number of deaths in the Quality in Australian Health Care Study.
e. Calculated from number of deaths directly attributable to anesthesia in Australia.
f. Calculated from Dutch figures.
g. Assuming a 5% mortality for elective procedures and 50% for emergency procedures.

THE CAUSATION OF INCIDENTS AND ACCIDENTS

The delivery of health care takes place in a complex environment, with rapidly evolving technology and high consumer expectations, all set against a backdrop of cost containment and fiscal accountability. Although safety should be paramount in medicine, cost issues can and do impact on the commitment of resources for safety efforts. The medical environment is constantly changing and is subject to dynamic interactions between patients, their disease processes, medical and nursing staff, system processes, societal mores, cultural issues, and hospital and government policies. It should not be surprising that this sets the stage for the development of a wide range of individual and organizational problems.

The model depicted in Fig. 41.1 forms the theoretical basis for modern risk management programs.[21,22] Incident and accident causation can be seen to arise from complex, dynamic interactions between organizational, workplace, and human factors (errors and violations), all of which may contribute to the accident pathway.

Reason's[22] "Swiss cheese" model envisages the system defenses as a series of barriers (Fig. 41.2). Inevitably, "holes" appear in these defenses (like those in Swiss cheese!) Usually we have a multilayered series of defenses, one or more of which will usually act as a barrier to a problem progressing. However, on occasions these holes (deficiencies) can align, allowing the now successful accident trajectory to pass through and damage the system. It is critical to understand that these defense lapses or "holes" are not static. They are constantly changing in size and position. This has important implications when we are trying to address the issues of how to prevent them from occurring in our own system.

The latent failure pathway (Fig. 41.1) comprises the "resident pathogens" in the system. They lie dormant before combining with active (human) failures or local workplace factors to assist in bypassing the host's defenses. Latent conditions are always present, but may never surface. However, because of this they can be systematically eradicated (if identified). This is in contrast to active failures (errors and violations), which, by their very nature, are more difficult to identify and predict. The example below illustrates a latent failure in our own system.

A surgical service manager decides that it is too expensive to run a resident anesthetic assistant (anesthetic technician/anesthetic nurse) at night and initiates an on-call roster. An obstetric patient is rushed to the operating room with a prolapsed umbilical cord requiring immediate cesarean section. The anesthesiologist has to perform a rapid-sequence induction using an operating room nurse with no anesthetic training. The intubation proves difficult, and the patient aspirates gastric contents, which results in an intensive care admission.

It is possible that this latent error (i.e. on-call anesthetic assistant) might never have surfaced but, because of a specific combination of factors, it did and subsequently caused harm. Both the head of anesthetic services and the surgical services manager who made this decision could have predicted this event, yet it is not always possible to convince a manager to go against his or her dominant management paradigm, which may be to maintain elective surgery in the face of a shrinking budget, leading to reducing the resources available for an emergency service.

Organizational factors

Organizational processes include management decisions, workplace arrangements, and corporate culture. The organization may be limited in its ability to fund adequately the introduction of new services because of budgetary constraints. Hence its ability to cover operating lists with adequate numbers of trained anesthesiologists or to have sufficient numbers of trained anesthetic assistants may be compromised. This may be illustrated by the example in Box 41.1.

A hospital refused to increase specialist numbers and took on even more work to increase funding. Morale quickly dropped among those

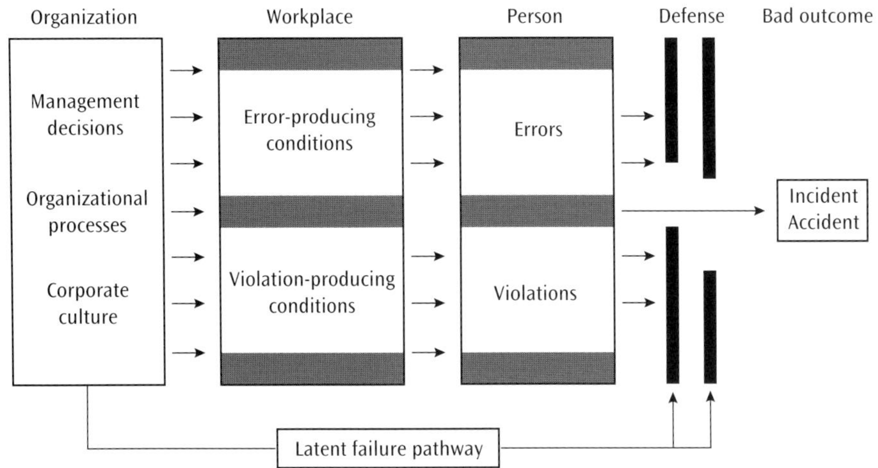

Figure 41.1 *Stages in the development of an accident or incident. (Adapted from Reason,[21,22] with permission.)*

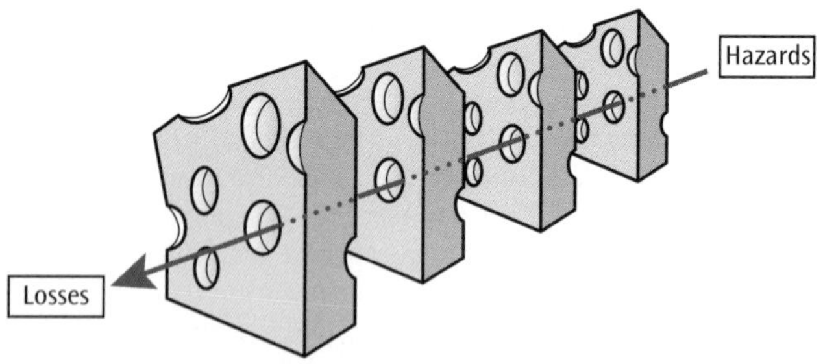

Figure 41.2 *Reason's "Swiss cheese" model of accident causation (with permission).*[22] *Note that the breaches in the defenses are constantly changing in both position and time.*

> **Box 41.1** *Case history taken from the Australian Incident Monitoring Study (AIMS) database*
>
> A 35-year-old woman, American Association of Anesthesiologists (ASA) class III, with insulin-dependent diabetes, hypertension, and morbid obesity, presented as a day-of-surgery admission for an elective, nonurgent, general surgical procedure. She had undergone no preoperative assessment by an anesthesiologist, and was poorly informed about her pending anesthetic. As she had arrived at the hospital, some distance from her home, considerable pressure was put on the anesthesiologist (junior) by the surgeon (senior) and patient to proceed. A cursory history and rushed examination was followed by induction of anesthesia. No preoperative investigations were performed. The patient developed intraoperative bronchospasm, probably from aspiration, and had to be intubated. She continued to have problems in recovery, but was sent to the ward prior to review by the anesthesiologist. She sustained a cardiac arrest soon after arriving in the ward and resuscitation was unsuccessful.

anesthesiologists left, which resulted in mass resignations of anesthesiologists and an absolute reduction in operating lists.

The corporate culture of some hospitals is to "press on regardless." Anesthesiologists are frequently at the end of a long process that involves recruiting patients, investigating them, and finally getting them ready for surgery. The anesthesiologist is subject to pressure to proceed from various sectors with vested interests. The patient wants the operation carried out with minimal fuss and delay, relatives may have canceled work to be available for support, the surgeon is there and ready to go, and the institution has already paid for the operating room time and staff salaries. The pressure to "carry on regardless" is very high. This pattern of management has been shown to create the conditions in which procedures may take place in a setting of inadequate perioperative patient preparation and care.

Workplace factors

Error-producing conditions

Operating room design and position can lead to potential problems (e.g. with the operating room on a different floor or building from a labor and delivery ward, with reliance on lifts for transferring emergency patients). A poor or nonexistent equipment maintenance program can result in equipment failure or in the use of poorly functioning equipment. Staffing problems may contribute to errors. This may be due to dysfunctional individual staff members – such as a specialist who refuses to come in at the request of a junior staff member, or dysfunctional teams – such as one with ongoing conflict between anesthesiologists, surgeons, or other staff.

Violation-producing conditions

The scene may be set for violation in a system by the existence of "bad" rules, checklists, or protocols. For example, new monitors may be purchased because they were the cheapest available. However, the alarm settings may prove to be very difficult to customize. If not correctly set, "false" alarms will occur frequently, and the anesthesiologists' automatic response may be to cancel the alarm before reviewing the problem that led to the alarm being activated. Alternatively, many anesthesiologists may disable the alarms. An inadvertent breathing circuit disconnection with resulting apnea may not therefore be detected for several minutes until the surgeon notices that the patient's blood is blue or, worse, until the patient becomes bradycardic.

Human factors

It is well recognized that human error contributes to adverse events in up to 80% of all incidents and accidents.[21,22,23] However, a certain level of human error is inevitable, quite usual, and is necessary for learning.[24] In addition, the various types of error described below often occur in association with a combination of factors that involves fatigue, cognitive overload, poor interpersonal communication, inadequate critical decision making, and impaired central processing.

In order to address the issue of human factors it is necessary to understand the various types of errors and violations. A classification of human error is given in Fig. 41.3.[25]

Knowledge-based errors

These were thought to have been involved in 35% of Australian Incident Monitoring Study (AIMS) incidents. They are the result of forming either the wrong intention or making the wrong plan and are based on inadequate knowledge and/or experience. Anesthetizing a patient with known aortic stenosis (valve area 0.2 cm^2) and poor left ventricular function using a high spinal anesthetic would be an example of a plan based on flawed knowledge.

Rule-based errors

These were thought to have been involved in 33% of AIMS incidents and include failure to apply or misapplying a good rule or applying a "bad" rule. Examples of these include:

1 *The failure to apply a rule designed to avoid an error.* A patient undergoing major revision joint surgery does not get a preoperative assessment, no blood tests are ordered, and no blood cross-matching is carried out. This patient's operation is canceled on the day of surgery due to the discovery of biventricular failure. The written preoperative guidelines were not followed, which led to a process problem and hence failure of the intended outcome.
2 *Applying a "bad," inadequate, or outdated rule.* A patient is transfused 1 unit of blood preoperatively, initiated by a junior trainee anesthesiologist. The patient's hemoglobin was 99 g L^{-1}. A departmental protocol dated 1985 had indicated that all anemic patients should have a hemoglobin greater than 100 g L^{-1} before elective surgery. This rule was based on an old attitude to perioperative anemia management that is not considered appropriate today.
3 *Misapplying a "good" rule in some problem-solving situation.* An anesthesiologist initiates a cardiac arrest protocol for a "cardiac arrest" without realizing that the electrocardiogram (ECG) picture

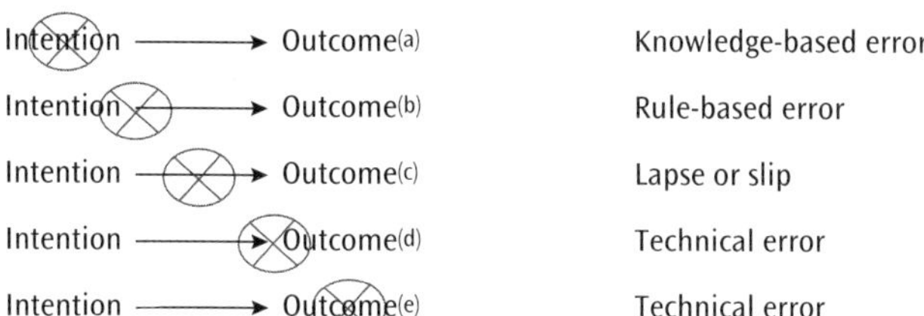

Figure 41.3 *A classification of human error. (From Runciman,[25] with permission.) The X represents where an error occurs in the chain between intention and planning, action (arrow) and outcome. (a) The administration of succinylcholine (suxamethonium) to a patient with malignant hyperthermia. (b) Cardiopulmonary resuscitation is commenced for asystole, but the electrocardiograph leads have in fact come off the patient, who is hemodynamically stable. (c) Succinylcholine is injected instead of fentanyl prior to induction of anesthesia. Technical errors occur when the outcome fails, or the wrong outcome occurs. This may not be an error in the true sense as there has been no breach of rule, slip/lapse, or knowledge problem. Some workers have suggested they are classified differently. (d) An epidural is inserted but there is no block. (e) An epidural is inserted and it becomes a subarachnoid placement.*

of ventricular fibrillation was in fact due to the surgeon dabbing dry the patient's abdomen during skin preparation.

Skill-based errors

These are so called because skilled people who are "multitasking" are most likely to commit them, and they include *slips* and *lapses*. Slips and lapses occur when an action deviates from that intended due to an execution failure and/or a storage failure. They can be understood by the result of the temporary dissociation of automatic and conscious processing. The automatic process consists of stored-action templates, which can be accessed with little attention. It is fast and efficient but rigid and does not require active environmental monitoring

Slips and lapses are not uncommon in anesthetic practice and have been noted to contribute to at least 10% of anesthetic incidents. An example of a slip would be the reconstitution of an antibiotic powder with lidocaine (lignocaine) instead of sterile water. A lapse would be the drawing up of heparin prior to cardiopulmonary bypass but forgetting to administer this as a result of taking a phone call.

Violations

A violation is a deliberate, but not necessarily a reprehensible, deviation from those practices appreciated by the individual as being required by regulation or necessary or advisable to achieve an appropriate objective while maintaining the safety of people and equipment and the ongoing operation of a device or system (A F Merry, personal communication, adapted from Reason[21]). In the majority of cases there is intention involved in this process, although usually there is no intention to damage the system or patient. In anesthetic practice this may take the form of intentional breaches of college, society, or other professional standards. Wider ethical, societal, and cultural standards may also be breached.

It is difficult to assess how common violating behavior is in medicine. As a follow-on from an AIMS analysis of the factors involved in inadequate preoperative preparation and management,[26] clear violations (reports that clearly demonstrated intention plus obvious rule breaking) could be identified in 6% of all reports. This is undoubtedly an underestimation due to reporting bias and the subjective processes involved in this type of data interpretation. This figure is consistent with the 5% suggested by the QAHCS for adverse events produced by violations,[10] which is also likely to be an underestimate because of the limitations of what is recorded in, and may therefore be extracted from, the medical record.

Violations are frequently inherited or "knocked on" from other areas and/or people. The final common pathway in the surgical process tends to involve the anesthesiologist; hence anesthesiologists are among those who are most interested in reducing such problems. Patients can breach preoperative fasting rules and medication management. Surgical colleagues may, for a variety of reasons, fail to follow normal preoperative evaluation or investigation processes. Our own anesthetic colleagues may violate standards on monitoring and investigation and then expect others to manage an anesthetic after such a flawed perioperative process.

Although the classification of violations is difficult, three major categories are described. These are routine, optimizing, and necessary violations.[21]

Routine violations

Routine violations involve the bypassing of necessary procedures, which by themselves may be perceived as making the process inefficient or cumbersome. If the system tolerates these violations, they tend to recur with no corrections. One of the most common routine violations in anesthetic practice is failing to do a complete anesthetic machine check. Despite attempts by colleges and societies to provide clear checklists, the time, complexity, and ease of starting a case without the performance of a comprehensive machine check means this "rule" is frequently breached intentionally and routinely.

Optimizing violations

Optimizing violations involve the avoidance of following specific rules for the benefit of the individual performing the task. These are uncommon in medical practice. An example might be an anesthesiologist who wishes to be perceived as someone who can do anything at any time and never cancels a case. He performs an anesthetic on a footballer who has eaten within 2 h of proposed surgery. He also wants to avoid any complications on emergence and so uses a laryngeal mask airway. The private surgeon and patient thank him profusely for not delaying surgery! The anesthesiologist feels highly pleased and is offered further work by the surgeon in private practice. In this case, violating safe rules has given the individual the positive feedback that may encourage recurrence of this pattern of action.

Necessary violations

These can also be known as system "double-binds." In this situation a violation must occur for a process to take place successfully. Another example from the AIMS database illustrates this type of violation (Box 41.2).

ADDRESSING THE PROBLEM

The factors contributing to an incident or accident can be interpreted and managed in two ways, either by the "person approach" or by the "system approach."[27] Most incidents and accidents usually have a number of antecedent contributing factors, each necessary but none sufficient to cause the problem on its own. Box 41.3 gives an account of an incident report with a number of contributing factors to illustrate how several lateral errors may combine with several human errors to breach a number of defenses and result in an incident or accident.

The person approach is what is commonly seen when the media portray major mishaps and disasters. Individuals (anesthesiologists, surgeons, pathologists) involved in the case are portrayed as having perpetrated an unsafe act mediated by innate "weaknesses" within

Box 41.2 *Case history from the Australian Incident Monitoring Study (AIMS) database*

A patient with a platelet disorder had received a platelet transfusion prior to his scheduled elective abdominal aneurysm repair. Unfortunately, he had already eaten something 1 h prior to his planned start of surgery. An intensive care unit bed had been specially reserved for him and additional staff called in. The anesthesiologist decided to go ahead despite the fasting protocol violation. There were no adverse sequelae.

themselves. These might include: forgetfulness, inattention, poor motivation, low professional standards, chemical dependence, negligence, and possibly overt violations. Errors are thus treated as moral issues, and are designated by the "just world hypothesis," which intimates that "bad things happen to bad people."[28] Corrective strategies used in this person approach attempt to address human variability. Thus, emphasis is placed on correcting personal deficiencies by improving knowledge and training, emphasizing sequelae of error (e.g. litigation, loss of income, loss of prestige) and attempting to write detailed policies and guidelines for every eventuality. In essence, this can be summarized as the "name, blame, and shame" approach.

This approach has several limitations. The requirement to allocate blame is seriously flawed, as certain types of error are inevitable. The creation of a culture that reports incidents to develop a database and history on which to formulate quality improvements cannot be achieved in such a tort-based system. Additionally, the unsafe acts are frequently considered in isolation from the system and circumstances in which they occur. As Reason stated, "the best people make the worst mistakes; error is not the monopoly of the unfortunate few. [In addition,] mishaps tend to fall into recurrent patterns."[27]

The system approach looks "upstream" from the incident and attempts to identify precursors to the problem. It assumes that humans can and do make mistakes. Most systems have barriers and defenses that need to be breached before an error can occur or result in harm. Therefore, when something does go wrong, rather than focusing on the individual at the end of the line, the entire chain of problems and the reasons for the failure of defenses should be investigated. Incident monitoring is one of the ways in which the details about the "things that go wrong" may be collected.

Incident monitoring

General principles

The terms "incident reporting" and "incident monitoring" are often used interchangeably, but in reality they arose from two different concepts.[29]

Incident reporting is a process whereby an identifiable person completes a form as a result of patient harm, potential harm, departure from documented policy or protocol, complaint, equipment failure, laboratory error, or medication mishap.[29] It is usually targeted to one specific incident and area and emphasizes the precise nature of the incident. Although incident reports can account for several thousands of forms per annum, their ability to create change "system wide" has been

Box 41.3 *A case based on an Australian Incident Monitoring Study report illustrating events that led to the development of an anesthetic incident*

Clinical scenario	Causative factor
A 14-year-old boy presented for an elective tonsillectomy. He was Vietnamese and spoke no English. He had not attended a preadmission clinic.	*Violation:* preadmission criteria: the patient's medical condition cannot be assessed if it is not possible to communicate with the patient. *Latent failure:* pressure from management to reduce interpreter services meant that this was not organized by nurses.
He had suffered from sleep apnea in past but this was not identified.	*Inadequate communication*
The boy was anesthetized and operated upon. He re-bled on emergence and was therefore reanesthetized.	*Technical error:* the surgeon failed to get hemostasis. He had been partially distracted by a telephone call during diathermy and ongoing hemostasis (*lapse*). A junior anesthesiologist was assigned to the list with minimal supervision. The patient awoke after the first case straining and coughing on the endotracheal tube (knowledge-based error). *Latent failure:* the surgeon was on acute call while performing elective surgery.
The patient was given a large dose of morphine prior to extubation. Following extubation in the recovery unit, he became hypoxic and desaturated to 50%, requiring continuous positive airway pressure via a T-piece. Naloxone, 40 μg, was administered.	*Rule-based error and knowledge-based error:* given the initial problem, the patient should have been extubated in the operating room. In addition, the patient received a relative overdose of morphine
The next patient was being anesthetized by another senior anesthesiologist to help catch up and avoid delaying the surgeon who had to be perform a private case in the next 20 min.	*Organizational problem:* culture of pressure to proceed and conflict of interest (*violation-producing conditions)*
The boy was eventually extubated and spent the night in the high-dependency unit. It was eventually recognized that the boy had evidence of sleep apnea and was probably susceptible to the central nervous system depressant effects of opioids.	

successful in only a handful of institutions. This is mainly due to the piecemeal nature of the collection, classification, and analysis of these reports, which tend to be handled individually, preventing patterns of incidents and their causation from being identified.

Incident monitoring is based on the critical incident technique, as described by Flanagan,[30] and was developed during World War II and subsequently refined for nonmedical, and more recently medical, applications. The early studies analyzed the reasons behind candidate pilots being eliminated from flying school and studied the critical requirements needed for combat troops to be successful in the field. The principal objective was to determine the "critical requirement demonstrated to have made the difference between success and failure" from "first hand [subjective] reports" or "objective reports." [30] This qualitative approach was, and still is, relatively new to medical science, which has espoused an evidence-based approach, based on quantitative data gathered, ideally, from randomized controlled trials. Qualitative research reveals how people actually behave and think in common everyday situations. This validity contrasts with quantitative research methodology, which, although supported for its reliability and objectivity, takes place in a highly controlled, contrived, and often unrealistic environment.[31,32]

Although initially developed to identify and modify human behavior in these military applications, it soon became evident that system factors were also being addressed.[29,30] Thus, improvements in job design, operating procedures, and equipment also resulted from these studies, although this was not intended from the original study design. The medical applications of incident monitoring have been remarkably consistent with Flanagan's original methods. What has altered over the past 10 years is the increasing realization of the importance of these system-based problems and of taking a proactive approach to formally integrate evaluation of both human error and systems failure into risk management.

Incident reporting in nonmedical areas

Several sources of data are used to assess aviation safety. Confidential pilot surveys provide some insight into personal approaches, relationships, attitudes, and commitment to various safety regimens. Attitude surveys define pilots' professional culture. Although aviation in general, and pilots in particular, has been held up as a role model for medicine to follow, it is of interest that a recent study showed some similarities between pilots and medical staff. A survey of 30 000 pilots and 1033 doctors and nurses showed that pilots were less likely to deny the effects of fatigue on performance than were consultant anesthesiologists and consultant surgeons – however around one-quarter (26%) of pilots denied that fatigue had any effect on their performance. Of note in this survey, 47% of anesthesiologists denied the effects of fatigue on their performance compared with 70% of consultant surgeons.[33]

A continuum can be seen between minimal, trivial events and full-blown disasters; it is of interest that similar factors may be involved in the generation of both extremes of outcome. Adequacy (or failure) of defense mechanisms may account for the differences in final outcome. Schemes for reporting "near misses" and "close calls" are well established in the fields of aviation, the petrochemical industry, the nuclear power industry, heavy industry, the space industry, and the military.

The Aviation Safety Reporting System now has over 500 000 incident reports on file.[34] This is a US federally funded project, which relies on voluntary reporting but offers anonymity and immunity from prosecution. This provides a strong incentive to report all incidents without fear of legal consequences. Importantly, a weekly newsletter, *Callback*, gives detailed accounts of actions and events leading to incidents, thus providing two-way communication pathways between respondents and investigators. Hence, the aviation industry has been able to provide a wealth of information from these incidents, allowing improvements in aircraft design, pilot training, and air traffic control to take place. Not all aviation systems are the same. Some make reporting mandatory (e.g. British Airways' *Air Safety Report*) and many are not anonymous (e.g. the Airline Pilots Association Aviation Safety Airways Program, *Air Safety Report*, and Confidential Human Factors Reporting System) but all are confidential and all give feedback. Only two systems confer legal immunity (the Aviation Safety Reporting System and the Special Event Search and Master Analysis), although even this has been challenged in some countries recently.[35]

Medical applications of incident monitoring

Cooper *et al.*[36] were the first to apply the critical incident technique to anesthesia in 1978. Prior to this there had been isolated studies evaluating drug errors by nurses[37] and the effects of doctors' performance on patient management.[38] Cooper and colleagues' original definition of a critical incident was an occurrence that could have led (if not discovered or corrected in time) or did lead to an undesirable outcome, ranging from increased hospital stay to death and permanent disability. As a trained interviewer collected these data, as opposed to the respondent, the inclusion criteria were very specific. In addition, in order to be included each incident had to have the following characteristics: it had to involve an error by a member of the anesthesia team; it had to involve a failure of anesthesia equipment; it had to occur when the patient was under the care of the anesthesiologist; it had to be described in clear detail by a person who either observed or was involved in the incident; and it had to be clearly preventable.

Two groups working independently in Australia were the first to use a written, anonymous reporting system on a structured form based on Cooper and colleagues' methods.[39,40] A third group recorded details of any event that could have affected patients adversely.[41]

Australian Incident Monitoring Study

Soon afterwards, these groups collaborated and combined under the auspices of the then newly formed Australian Patient Safety Foundation (APSF) and set up the Australian Incident Monitoring Study (AIMS).[42] The initial study was set up in 1988 to investigate incidents related to anesthetic practice, and in 1993 a symposium issue in *Anaesthesia and Intensive Care* published 30 papers relating to the first 2000 AIMS reports.[43] This mass of data produced invaluable information on a wide variety of subjects including: monitoring (capnograph, oximeter, ECG, blood pressure, oxygen analyzer, stethoscope), crisis management, drug error, difficult intubation, ventilation problems, anaphylaxis, cardiac arrest, pneumothorax, regional anesthesia problems, recovery room incidents, awareness, pediatric incidents, equipment failure, and human failure. Over the next 7 years, the AIMS–Anesthesia project collated over 7000 reports. These have been used to generate reports, crisis management algorithms, and review papers and to provide data to support new safety initiatives. Ongoing studies have addressed evolving areas of concern and interest including: fatigue in anesthesiologists,[44] obstetric issues,[45] aspiration during anesthesia,[46] assistance for the anesthesiologist,[47] and preoperative management.[26] Furthermore, the original database has been used to develop a series of crisis management algorithms to assist with the treatment and management of conditions such as laryngospasm, airway obstruction, aspiration, bronchospasm, pulmonary edema, desaturation, arrythmias, hypotension, hypertension, myocardial ischemia, cardiac arrest, anaphylaxis, pneumothorax, embolism, sepsis, awareness, and water intoxication.[14]

The success of the AIMS–Anesthesia project led to further funding to coordinate pilot incident monitoring schemes in other medical areas (general practice,[48] psychiatry,[49] emergency medicine,[50] intensive care,[51] pathology, gastroenterology, obstetrics, and gynecology). As a natural progression, the AIMS concept developed into a system-wide approach.

This was intended to cover the whole range of health care and allowed incidents or issues relating to staff, visitors, nonclinical areas, personal property, and equipment to be reported. Thus, for this wider context, an incident was described as "any event which could have or did harm anyone or which could result in a complaint, loss or damage."[14] Any staff member could complete the form. Importantly, there did not have to be any evidence of error, equipment failure, or preventability.

The spread of incident monitoring

Studies using similar reporting and collecting formats were reported from the Netherlands[52] and Hong Kong,[53] leading to improved quality assurance activities and documented error reduction as a direct result of implementing quality initiatives, while other groups developed their own individually formatted incident monitoring systems.[54]

The Royal College of Anaesthetists in the UK piloted a critical incident program in 1995.[55] They defined a critical incident as one that led to harm or could have caused harm if it had been allowed to progress. In addition, the critical incident should be preventable by a change in practice.

The results of this pilot study were disseminated to all anesthetic departments within the UK in 1999 via College tutors. The Royal College has continued to support such a scheme, and the form can be easily accessed from the College website (www.rcoa.ac.uk). In a recent publication, *Raising the Standard*,[56] the Royal College of Anaesthetists has suggested that the above form should be used to allow collection of data arising from adverse events. This form includes a minimum data set and suggests a critical incident reporting rate of about 6.7% or 1 in 15 procedures.[57]

Rationale for using incidents/near misses as a measurement tool

Although detecting adverse events is a key element in reducing future problems, it is important to realize that not all unsafe systems frequently produce bad outcomes. In reality latent failures in systems may never surface, despite their potential to do harm. In addition, in a specialty such as anesthesia, in which major morbidity and mortality are now rare, learning only from events with bad outcomes would significantly restrict progress. As a consequence, these systems need to collect, analyze, and promulgate information for both adverse events and near misses. It has been known for years that minor sequelae from accidents occur with a much higher frequency than major problems. For every major injury there are 30 minor injuries and 300 no-injury accidents.[58]

Limitations of incident monitoring

There are, of course, limitations to all systems, and incident monitoring is no exception.[14] Potential barriers and problems with incident monitoring programs have been highlighted in both medical and nonmedical systems. These can have implications at various levels (individual, organizational, or societal) and be influenced by factors such as legal, cultural (values, attitudes, and beliefs), regulatory, and financial constraints.

Corporate culture

This is probably the greatest single barrier to overcome in the healthcare system. Inertia combined with skepticism, fear of the unknown, and comfort with the *status quo*, are all contributory factors. Developing a "safety culture" is a new concept to most specialties, although less so in anesthesia.[1]

Medicolegal implications

For any system to be truly workable, anonymity along with freedom from any legal consequences of reporting are prerequisites, although they have been claimed in some quarters to represent another ploy by doctors to "keep things in house." Improved communication about critical incident techniques is essential to educate both the public and the media about their importance in protecting patients and staff from stress and harm.

Increasing exposure to adverse events

There is no doubt that a reporting system does force individuals, groups, and institutions to confront previously unrecognized or acknowledged deficiencies in their care processes and interactions with patients, relatives, and other staff. This can reduce morale, and on occasion lead to a false impression of increased medicolegal risk.

Expense

There is some cost to setting up and running a comprehensive incident monitoring system. Although this expenditure is often seen as a wasted resource and not cost-effective, this perception is usually based on experience of the historical piecemeal collection of information, without any systematic collation and analysis and without introducing measures to control the problems identified.

Poor feedback

For any incident reporting system to work, there needs to be regular feedback to promote continued reporting. Frequently processes are started but rapidly fall by the wayside because of low reporting levels. It is usually necessary for there to be a "champion" of any incident reporting system, ideally supported by senior administration and at least one clinical "opinion leader."

Prevention and management of incidents and accidents – a risk management framework

The previous sections have given an overview of the epidemiology of error in medicine, with particular emphasis on anesthesia. Simple classifications for errors and violations have been presented. The attributes of a successful incident monitoring system, such as that set up by the APSF in Australia, have been outlined. All of this now needs to be set in the context of a comprehensive approach to the problem of iatrogenic injury. A risk management framework, such as the new Australian and New Zealand standard AS/NZS 4390, provides such an approach;[59] one advantage of using it as a basis for discussion is that it has been adopted as the basis for a risk management framework within the UK NHS. This framework, with multiple feedback loops, provides an approach to the ongoing management of any risk at any level within a system (departmental, hospital, regional, or national). The key components are shown in Fig. 41.4; incident monitoring can play an important role in the risk identification, evaluation, and analysis components of this framework. Indeed, incident monitoring may be the only feasible approach to gaining an understanding of the low-frequency events that make up more than three-quarters of all adverse events.[14]

Understanding the context

Health care occurs in a complex environment, subject to the vagaries of human error and systems failure. Further work is needed to define these problems, to determine their relative importance, and to subsequently alter clinical practice. This will have important implications for the frequency, pattern, cost, and impact of error within medicine. There are several areas that need addressing. Healthcare professionals and consumers alike need to be informed about expected risks in relation to benefits of specific health delivery services and/or procedures. Along with standard written and verbal communication channels, innovative media such as videotapes and web-based information systems need to be considered. As has been seen with the larger aviation safety agencies,

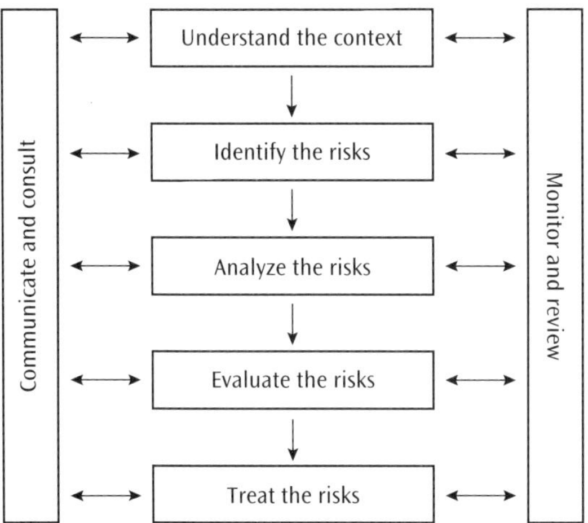

Figure 41.4 *Overview of the risk management process using AS/NZS 4360.*[59]

Table 41.2 *Methods for identifying problems*

Incident monitoring
Incident reporting
Case note/chart reviews
Mortality committee reports
Morbidity committee reports
Departmental mortality and morbidity meetings
Medical defense reports
Closed claims studies
Medical record review
Hazard alerts
Observation studies
Simulation studies
Case reports/anecdotes
Clinical indicators/sentinel event recording

legal privilege and, where necessary, anonymity for risk management and quality improvement activities need to be granted to those workers actively involved with frontline patient management. This does not, however, lead to the minimization of accountability. In truth, it forces the organization to move toward greater accountability at a system level for iatrogenic injury and its sequelae. Finally, it is hoped that, as a consequence of the above, the expensive, inefficient tort system will be replaced by some form of blameless but rapidly responsive and efficient no-blame compensation scheme. In order for this process to have any chance of success, all major stakeholders - government, professional bodies, health insurers, industry, healthcare facilities, and consumers - need to be actively involved in the various levels of each process.

Identifying the risks

The initial step is to define both what is going to be reported and what will be the general aim of the whole process. Flanagan[30] stated that "considerable effort is required to avoid defeating the purpose of the general aim by cluttering up the statement with specific details and qualifying conditions." Although incident monitoring is the major model we are reviewing, there are other valuable sources of information that can and should be used, if applicable and feasible (Table 41.2).

Although Flanagan used a structured interview, later groups realized that it was more cost-effective to have respondents complete a written form as soon after the incident as possible. A basic requirement for any collection system is that it has to be immediately available and quick and easy to complete. The AIMS-Anesthesia form consisted of four pages and had sections for free narrative as well as detailed tick boxes. Page 1 provided instructions for the respondent; page 2 consisted of a blank page for free narrative along with a keyword section; page 3 was allocated to the completion of tick boxes on "what happened" and "why it happened;" and page 4 consisted of demographic information regarding procedure, monitoring, time of incident, and outcome. Other specialist groups used their own forms.[51]

Feedback from most pilot sites indicated that a single form that could be used across all specialties within a hospital would be advantageous. At the same time, incident reports continued to be completed on different forms. Hence, a decision was made to incorporate both incident reporting and incident monitoring on the same form. This became the generic AIMS form. It also became very clear that the most important information came from the "free narrative" section. Therefore, subsequent forms relied on questions such as "Where did the incident take place?" rather than having 20 tick boxes.

A new generic "AIMS+" form has now been introduced,[14] which can be tailored to the needs of special groups, but which has a standardized "core" structure. This is suitable for use across the entire spectrum of health care.

Mortality and morbidity committee reports

These are an extremely useful form of review for specific areas or geographical regions. Examples of successful reporting systems include the triennial reports looking at maternal mortality and morbidity in the UK, Confidential Enquiry - Stillbirths and Deaths in Infancy, the Confidential Enquiry into Perioperative Deaths (CEPOD), and the triennial mortality reports from Australia. These reports, which require review by committee after dissemination, are often produced some years after the actual date of the incidents. Also, some systems such as CEPOD require considerable infrastructure, are moderately expensive, and have, to date, no consistent format or classification system. Hence, international comparisons are difficult.

Mortality and morbidity/meetings

Mortality and morbidity (M&M) meetings have limited scope in areas, such as anesthesia, with low complication rates. Although they are important to retain, they are prone to peer group pressure and biased presentation of information. They can, however, be used in conjunction with an incident monitoring scheme. Indeed, some institutions base their M&M meetings on regular reviews of incident reports.

Medical defense unions/closed claim studies

Medicolegal information in claims files can be collated and analyzed and the findings disseminated to assist in improving patient safety. Like M&M committee reports, there is often a considerable time delay between the incident and the presentation of data in a formalized report. Although this has proved very successful in the USA, where a closed claims study group provides regular feedback on issues such as nerve injury, cardiac arrest under spinal anesthesia, liability, monitoring, respiratory complications, and obstetric issues,[60,61] this valuable source of information has not been systematically exploited in most countries. Reports from medical defense organization and closed claims-type sources are, by their nature, tort or blame oriented and hence tend to provide information of relevance mainly to problems likely to be subject to litigation, but they are nevertheless most valuable. The NHS has reports on NHS Litigation Authority claims data (810 cases per annum, settled by the authority above local excess levels) and complaints data both from hospitals (27 949) and from primary care (38 857).[13]

Medical record reviews

These provide cross-sectional "snapshots" of adverse events in selected hospitals. This method was the basis of the HMPS, the QAHS, and the Utah-Colorado studies. Although effective, they are subject to observer bias and interobserver variability and are very expensive and time consuming. Despite using seemingly similar methodologies, comparisons are not reliable.[11,12] At a local level they can be of value for reviewing individual cases and have been used to good effect in some institutions.[14,62]

Regulatory agencies

Hazard alerts from agencies, such as the Therapeutic Device Evaluation Committee (Australia), Pharmac (New Zealand), the Emergency Care Research Institute (USA), the Medical Devices Agency, and the Medicines Control Agency, produce regular up-to-date reports. However, these are often solely equipment or drug related and may not always be easily accessible to practicing clinicians.

Observational studies

Personal observation has been used in studies to observe deviations from normal procedure in anesthesia and aviation. An ongoing study in the aviation field using observational methodology, the line operation safety audit (LOSA), in over 3500 domestic and international flights has revealed interesting comparisons for anesthesia.[63] There were, on average, two threats and two errors observed by a trained cabin observer on each flight. Moreover, half the errors were violations of established practice. Examples of violations included performing a preflight checklist from memory, whereas errors included entering incorrect data into a flight computer, misunderstanding altitude clearances, and unnecessary navigation through adverse weather. Very similar results have been obtained from a study in clinical anesthesia. An analysis of anesthesia system errors reported that there were on average 8.1 factors identified that were considered to have significantly contributed to the development and evolution of each reported error.[64] The importance of recovery pathways was also highlighted, which influenced the outcome of the error as much as those factors involved with its causation. The same group evaluated the accuracy of data entered on to anesthesia records using trained observers, much like the aviation studies above. Omissions of data occurred in 35%, incorrect entries in 3.4%, and unwarranted entries in 1% of all records.[65] Thus, the largest number of errors related to omitting, rather than falsifying, data. Falsification of data is not uncommon. Using a survey technique this group evaluated the frequency of data omission or modification in anesthesia records: 55% of respondents indicated that they had on occasion deliberately omitted or recorded false information.[66] Although such observational studies as described above in both aviation and medicine are labor intensive and expensive, they do provide an indication of how anesthesiologists work in an error-prone domain.

Simulation studies

Anesthesiologists have pioneered the development of computer-screen- and mannequin-based interactive simulators. These systems offer the advantages of standardization of scenario, comparison of practitioners and systems, and ability to get immediate feedback.[67] In addition, there is no risk to patients and rare but critical conditions can be presented and allowed to proceed as far as the scenario dictates. However, they are expensive and labor intensive and require considerable infrastructure and commitment of personnel and resources. Some workers also question their validity, despite their widespread use in the aviation industry.

Case reports/anecdotes

Much of medical practice is based on noncorroborated anecdote and experience. However, this is an inefficient method of acquiring knowledge and again can be biased by local factors and the threat of censure or litigation.

Clinical indicators

Prespecified markers of quality can be determined and subsequently audited. This limits the scope of information that is collected. It is also necessary to ensure that the data that are collected are uniform in quality; this has not been the case so far in countries such as Australia and New Zealand, which precludes comparisons between departments and hospitals. In Australia, the indicators that are collected include: unanticipated admission to the intensive care unit, uncontrolled pain in recovery, cardiac arrest in the operating room, hypothermia, and airway incidents. At a local level, hospital health information units may be able to "tag" specified cases for regular audit (e.g. postoperative myocardial infarction or unanticipated day surgery admission).

Sentinel event monitoring

This involves the "root-cause analysis" of specified types of problems with poor outcomes. These are generally so rare that this process is not useful for improving safety or quality across the system.[14] However, it does serve a political purpose, as an extensive investigation is seen to have been done when there has been a nasty event (e.g. a baby being stolen).

Evaluating and analyzing the risks

Once data from incident monitoring and other sources have been collated, review and analysis are required. In early studies, details of the incident gained from the trained interviewer were transcribed and coded into branching summaries..[23] Basically, these were coded by the respondent according to his or her own evaluation of the failure. These summaries could be retrieved using codes for looking at various subgroups.

The AIMS–Anesthesia study entered both the free narrative (with identifiers removed) and the tick box section on to an interactive database. Keywords were added to assist with subsequent coding. Groups of analysts (primarily specialist anesthesiologists and hospital scientists) would then review particular topics of interest. This formed the basis for the symposium issue of *Anaesthesia and Intensive Care*.[43] These analysts typically would review all the tagged reports using either keywords, phrases from the narrative, or specified demographic information. In many cases combinations would be analyzed. Reports that were not associated with the specified problem were discarded and an appropriate classification system created by an iterative review process. Depending on the size of the dataset, all reports would be read by all analysts or else subsets of the entire database would be classified by all to ensure the reliability, reproducibility, and validity of the classification. This system was not without limitations; it relied heavily on keywords and was labor intensive in producing the *post hoc* categorizations.

Analysts who were working on the "Which monitor?" and "Crisis management" papers in the original AIMS study described commonly arising situations, which they called "clinical situations" or, later, "natural categories."[43] A natural category is a descriptor (usually a short phrase) that is succinct and understandable and encapsulates the essence of an event.[68] The term "natural mapping" refers to connecting the groups in an intuitively reasonable way.[68]

Webb and Runciman identified 60 "natural categories" in their papers on monitoring and crisis management in the analysis of the first 2000 AIMS incident reports.[43] Forty percent of incidents were accounted for by only five natural categories or clinical situations, 60% by 10, and nearly 80% by 20, while 98% were accounted for by 60 situations.

The recognition of "natural categories" and of the limitations of using keywords and free text analysis led to the development of the generic occurrence classification system (GOC).[68] Existing classifications at the time of GOC development, such as ICD-9-AM[69] and the Read system,[70] were found to be unsuitable for classifying "things that go wrong" in medicine. Initially, 1000 AIMS reports from teaching hospitals were collected and grouped into natural categories connected by natural mapping. Branching, tree-like structures were created and, using group discussion techniques, it was decided how these should be categorized. Relevant upstream factors were grouped under "intuitive" headings, while those downstream had their details grouped. This process was modified, computerized, and expanded using a further 2000 AIMS reports plus 800 reports from the Quality in Australian Health Care Study. This allowed incidents and accidents to be analyzed down to a level of detail that provides sufficient information to enable clinical problems to be identified and correction strategies developed.[68] The GOC also proved to be a flexible tool that could be used to explain differences and/or similarities in patterns of data from different sources and/or different instruments.

The GOC has now been expanded and redesigned to facilitate accurate coding, easier analysis, and better reporting, based on experience from over 50 000 incidents and adverse events. The new system, GOC+, was released in 2002.[14] It has subsequently been further refined to code for different healthcare incident types (HITs), and a more streamlined classification will be released in 2003.

Treating the risks

Once the reports have been collated, analyzed, and evaluated, the final step is to devise and implement some strategies to minimize the risk. These can be targeted at several levels. The most important factor in achieving ongoing support for such a continuous quality management process is regular feedback. As a system such as AIMS is anonymous and voluntary, it is heavily reliant on regular input from respondents. Without such feedback, responses wane and the value of the process is reduced.

Feedback about implementation of risk-reducing strategies can be initiated and carried out at different levels. These levels are not independent but tend to complement each other, thus simultaneously strengthening the risk management processes at a number of levels.

Individual anesthesiologists

An anesthesiologist reported a case of awareness during a routine general anesthetic for a hip replacement. There had been no recognized problem intraoperatively. The anesthesiologist reviewed the data for awareness from the AIMS database.[71] There were 16 cases of awareness in the first 2000 reports. In seven cases there had been no obvious reason for the problem; in three cases there was a documented low concentration of volatile anesthetic; in six cases there had been a syringe swap prior to induction leading to paralysis before hypnosis. These facts were incorporated into his report following a complaint.

Until recently most anesthesiologists were unaware of modern management techniques such as quality assurance, continuous quality improvement, and total quality improvement. Despite the facts that "doctors are only human" and technology has increased exponentially over the past 10 years, the overall expectation of society is one of medical perfection. Anesthesiologists, being facilitators and offering no primary therapeutic intervention, can be placed in an invidious position. They get no recognition when things go well but are placed at the forefront when something goes wrong. As has been stated by Wu,[72] "confession is often discouraged, passively by the lack of appropriate forums for discussion, and sometimes (actively) by risk mangers and hospital lawyers."

The "second victim" in any adverse event is often forgotten, namely the doctor or nurse. The ability to be able to document the problem in an anonymous manner goes some way toward alleviating the distress of this second victim and making him or her at least feel that they have made a contribution to a process for reducing the chance of a similar problem causing harm in the future. In addition, completion of a specific report form empowers the individual to a greater extent than simply documenting the problem in the notes and encourages further reporting. This has obvious benefits for the anesthesiologist, improves job satisfaction, and improves patient safety. Moreover, the ease of obtaining relevant knowledge from the whole AIMS database provides a valuable back-up for individuals.

Hospital, group, or practice level

The AIMS process involves the collation of incident reports at the local level by a designated "person on the spot," who is responsible for reviewing the local reports, disseminating the relevant information, removing identifiers, and forwarding the reports to the central collection center.[73] This process area can provide the agenda for M&M meetings at a local level. Forms can also be completed retrospectively as a result of these meetings. Local quality improvement projects can then provide the basis for corrective strategy development and implementation, followed in turn by ongoing incident monitoring. Two examples are described:

1 Several forms appeared that indicated potential and actual adverse events resulting from the emergency booking of acute obstetric cases by midwives instead of the obstetrician concerned. Lack of detail about medical comorbidities, status of the patient, degree of urgency, and patient prioritization were cited as problems. As a result of this, a policy was instituted that all obstetric cases requiring an operative procedure were to be discussed directly by the obstetrician and the anesthesiologist.
2 One hospital reported a higher incidence of malfunctioning unidirectional valves than would have been expected. Investigation revealed that this hospital had changed to a new, cheaper type of valve prone to sticking and malfunction, without the knowledge of the practicing clinicians. This was rectified and the problem eliminated.

The coordinating body level

At the level of the coordinating body, e.g. the APSF, the Royal College of Anaesthetists, a tool to supplement and/or complement the monitoring process is sometimes produced. These tools include checklists (e.g. an anesthetic machine checklist), crisis management algorithm cards, booklets of forms, instructional videos, and specific classifications.[74]

A crisis management handbook has been developed based on real-life reported incidents.[14] This mnemonic-based crisis resource-management tool assists with the diagnosis and management of acute emergencies. It is based on the mnemonic COVER ABCD – A SWIFT CHECK, which leads from a "core" algorithm (COVER ABCD)[75] into over 20 subalgorithms. These have been validated against 4000 real incidents and ensure that a logical process is followed for any emergency.

Although this is presented in a handbook format at present, it is envisioned that it will become incorporated into the software of anesthetic monitors so that a split-screen format will allow crisis algorithms to be viewed at the same time as physiological data. An example of a page of the handbook is shown in Figs 41.5 and 41.6. Each emergency has an easily identifiable tag. Simple, clear, and succinct instructions are given on one side, with annotated comments on the reverse. These give back-up information, which can be read after correcting the initial problem. In the example quoted for anaphylaxis, the common notion that anaphylaxis presents with tachycardia was found to be incorrect, with 50% of respondents noting a bradyarrythmia as the presenting ECG abnormality. Validation and rationale for the algorithm is provided. Finally, as this is a dynamic, living database, new changes in presentation of disease states, or new information can be incorporated, such as an updated incidence of anaphylaxis to newer muscle relaxants.

There has been concern about the active reduction in recruitment and retention of trained anesthetic assistants in hospitals in Australia and New Zealand. A study was conducted to evaluate the role of assistants in anesthetic practice in this area.[47] Skilled assistance was deemed to have actively minimized the consequences of the incident in 808 of

ANAPHYLAXIS

LOOK FOR
Cardiovascular changes **(1)**
Hypotension ⟶ collapse
Tachy- OR bradycardia **(2)**
Respiratory changes
Bronchospasm **(3)**
Pulmonary oedema
Skin rash/pruritus
Oedema of the face and lips
Nausea and vomiting in awake patients **(5)**

PRECIPITATING FACTORS (6)
Reaction to drugs
Colloids
Blood products
Latex allergy

EMERGENCY MANAGEMENT
Complete COVER ABDC–A SWIFT CHECK
Inform the surgeon
Request immediate assistance
Cease all drugs/plasma expanders/blood products
Immediate volume expansion **(7)**
Maintain ventilation with 100% oxygen
Give adrenaline bolus IV 0.001 mg/kg/min
If pulseless treat as cardiac arrest ⟶ page 38
Adrenaline; for easy adult dosing **(4)**, page 71
Titrate against heart rate and blood pressure

FURTHER CARE
The patient may relapse
Continue the adrenaline infusion, if necessary
Consider other drugs **(9)**
Admit to ICU/HDU
Take blood for testing as soon as possible **(10)**
Counsel the patient/relatives as soon as possible See page **(9)** page 15.
Arrange for allergy testing (skin) at 1 month
Adrenaline bolus
Adrenaline infusion

ANAPHYLAXIS

Figure 41.5 *Crisis management algorithm for anaphylaxis. (From the Australian Patient Safety Foundation Crisis Management Manual.) Adrenaline (epinephrine).*

5837 AIMS reports. Of note, however, was that untrained assistants actually contributed to the generation of an incident in 147 cases. This resulted from inadequate equipment preparation (misconnection of circuits and intravenous lines), communication problems, and inadequate staffing levels (number and/or skill mix). This report is the only one available to support ongoing training for assistants and quantify (albeit qualitatively) their impact on patient safety. Clinical directors faced with budget restraints and national technical organizations have used this data to enhance their ability to provide support for the recruitment and retention of assistants for anesthesiologists.

National and international levels

As part of the risk management program, there is ongoing feedback to governmental agencies, regulatory authorities, the medical profession, and industry.

Fifteen of the current AIMS projects require systematic interaction between clinicians, distributors, and manufacturers in order to solve current problems. These include: that all monitors default to a standard setting when initially switched on; that Seldinger wires should have soft-tipped ends to prevent vessel and heart puncture; that all relaxant syringes (the most common group of drugs implicated in syringe errors) be color coded red; and that endotracheal tubes should have designated marking to minimize the potential for endobronchial intubation.

It has been recognized for some time that inadequate preoperative preparation and investigation of the patient can contribute to adverse events. The most recent mortality report from Australia indicated that, of the 135 deaths attributable to anesthesia, inadequate preoperative assessment contributed to 40 cases, just over 33%.[20] The report concluded that "increased emphasis should be given during training and continuing medical education to the importance of preoperative assessment and management."

Data were extracted from the AIMS database to further investigate this problem; 197 cases out of 6271 reports made to AIMS were attributable to inadequate preoperative assessment and planning.[26] In 10% of reports the patient had received no preoperative assessment by any anesthesiologist, while in 23% the assessing anesthesiologist was not the person administering the anesthetic. As a result of inadequate preoperative assessment, seven patients died, 17 patients were admitted to intensive care/high-dependency care, 23 suffered major morbidity, and surgery was canceled in nine cases. The principal areas causing problems were poor airway assessment, communication problems, and inadequate medical evaluation of patients. The reporters considered that the incident would have been preventable in 57% of cases. Partly as a result of this study, an national initiative, sponsored by the Australian and New Zealand College of Anaesthetists, has been embarked upon to

ANAPHYLAXIS

Notes: The earliest signs of anaphylaxis are hypotension, bronchospasm and integumentary signs. At least one of these manifested in 55% of cases, and two in 44%. 65% of patients were ASA grades 1–2. It was judged that correct use of the algorithm would have led to earlier recognition of the problem and/or better management in 25% of 148 relevant incidents reported to AIMS. **For the basis of the figures reported here see (11) below**

(1) Half of all reactions were judged as severe, and 55% of these involved circulatory collapse. There was hypotension in 68% of all cases.
(2) Heart rate changes were documented in 28% of reports, being equally split between tachy- and bradycardias. Bradycardia heralded circulatory collapse.
(3) Bronchospasm was documented in 42% of cases.
(4) Erythema/urticaria/rash was documented in 44% of cases. Facial oedema was an uncommon sign.
(5) Nausea and vomiting occurred in 45% of awake patients.
(6) 35% of cases involved polydrug therapy at induction. Drugs or agents commonly implicated were:
Cephalosporins–24%
Non depolarising muscle relaxants–9%
Haemaccel–8%
Penicillin–5%
Thiopentone–5%
Blood products–2%
Other drugs implicated included: suxamethonium, propofol, protamine, amide type local anaesthetics.
(7) Immediate crystalloid bolus of 10 mL/kg. Review and repeat as necessary. Haemaccel and blood products should be avoided as necessary.
(8) For easy adult dosing see (4) page 71.
(9) Consider hydrocortisone IV 5 mg/kg.
(10) In the course of an allergic response to a foreign antigen(s), consumption of IgG and IgE occurs. Comparison of IgAM/IgGE ratios before and after the event will detect consumption of IgG and IgE (most patients will have a preoperative blood screen). If there is no preoperative sample, a blood test at six weeks post incident will allow a similar ratio to be calculated. Mast cell tryptase is a specific test, which, due to expense is performed as a batch at intervals. It is an absolute level. Normal range < 2, equivocal 2–10, unequivocal anaphylactic reactions give results > 10. The test can be performed post mortem.
(11) Anaesthesia and Intensive Care 1996, Vol 24, No X.

Figure 41.6 *The reverse side of the crisis management algorithm. This allows cross-reference to other related areas. (From the Australian Patient Safety Foundation Crisis Management Manual.)*

develop evidenced-based decision-support systems designed to clarify, simplify, and unify the preoperative assessment process.

The results of large ongoing databases such as AIMS–Anesthesia need to be fed back to international organizations. Issues such as endotracheal tube design and the labeling and color coding of syringes have been forwarded to the International Standards Organization (ISO). The World Federation of Societies of Anesthesiologists has been proactive in adopting this project as part of the activities of its Safety and Quality of Practice Committee, and has disseminated AIMS "starter kits" to over 30 countries world wide.

Incident monitoring, anesthesia, and the future

Developments in incident monitoring reporting systems

Comprehensive systems for incident reporting have now been established. Doctors other than anesthesiologists have been slow to participate, although successful pilot projects have been carried out in 12 medical specialties.[14]

Paper-based reports are subject to damage and misinterpretation due to poor writing and require some method of transcription to digital format. Moreover, the dissemination of collated and analyzed reports takes time and is itself subject to the vagaries of paper-based information. Staender *et al*,[75] stimulated by the Aviation Safety Reporting System (ASRS), attempted to set up an Internet-based HTML (hypertext mark-up language) reporting form for use in critical incidents. This was directly linked to the University of Basle Department of Anaesthesia. The reports were subsequently converted, using templates, to anecdotal text and stored to create a teaching database. This type of system has the potential for unlimited flexibility, not only for collecting data but also for transferring, analyzing, and interpreting large numbers of reports from many countries.

The new AIMS+ system, likewise, has the facility for "web-based" reporting, and plans are under way for establishing an "e-warning" system for rapid dissemination of new information.[14]

Improvements in the generic occurrence classification

Further developments in the APSF generic occurrence classification (GOC) incident monitoring system are continuously being made. The GOC+ is an upgraded system that allows for a greater number of natural categories and for cross-linking with the ICD-10 and other coding systems. This will allow not only anesthesia but the entire healthcare system to come under the one unified reporting umbrella, a concept actively sought by national reports from the USA, Australia, and the UK.

Implications for anesthetic practice

Once we have derived national and international databases with a sufficient number of natural categories, we may then proceed to re-engineer our systems to avoid potential problems in the future. Various methods have already been described. Work is already under way to generate software-driven systems for prompting, history taking, examination, and investigation of preoperative patients. This explicit process will then feed into computer-based decision-support systems tailored to local conditions and individual patient profiles with respect to pre-existing disease, correct problem, and type of surgery and anesthetic plans. At the end of the preoperative consultation, protocols will automatically be printed on to order forms for thromboembolism, nausea and vomiting, pain, and nosocomial infection prophylaxis, as well as for problems such as asthma and diabetes.

Future interest will also be drawn to areas previously in the domain of engineering systems, such as that of probabilistic risk analysis (PRA).

This technique has been utilized in offshore drilling operations and the space shuttle program. Paté-Cornell *et al.*[76] have applied this model to anesthesia by addressing four main areas: first, the probability of an initiating event; second, the probability of an accident occurring conditional on a particular initiating event; third, the effects of the state of the anesthesiologist; and, finally, the effects of organizational policy. Using complex mathematical modeling, outcomes can be determined along with factors that may limit system damage. Of interest from this early pilot study was the potential benefit derived from increased trainee supervision, anesthesia simulators, periodic recertification, and regular medical examinations for all anesthesiologists. These are potentially valuable tools, which with refinement and validation may offer answers to the perpetual problem of managing resource constraints while maintaining productivity and ensuring adequate safety.

Integration of human factor concepts to reduce system-based problems

There is no doubt that the aim of incident monitoring should be to assist in the reduction of errors to as close to zero as possible. Further collaboration between human factors experts and reliability engineers may lead us some way down the path to offer zero risk to patients under our anesthetic care. Tactics fall into five mandates: reduce the complexity of procedures; optimize information processing; automate wisely; use constraints; and, finally, mitigate against the unwanted side-effects of change.

SUMMARY

Adverse events in the healthcare sectors are increasingly becoming a cause for concern. Estimates derived from UK, US, and Australian studies indicate that adverse events are associated with about 10% of all hospital admissions, and account in direct medical costs for 5% of the total health budget. Most accidents are caused by a combination of organizational, workplace, and personal factors. Personal factors include errors (slips/lapses and rule- and knowledge-based mistakes) and violations. Latent failures in the system also contribute to the generation of organizational and individual accidents.

Incident monitoring is a valuable risk management tool, with a long history in engineering and aviation, which has been introduced into medical practice over the past 20 years. It allows the reporting, analysis, evaluation, and treatment of risk in an organization by analyzing near misses, incidents, and accidents. The AIMS project has been at the forefront of developing this process and has contributed to an anesthesia database that spans over 7000 reports and has promulgated over 70 scientific papers, crisis management algorithms, protocols, videos, and improvements in equipment. The subsequent development of a GOC has allowed AIMS to develop into a health-system-wide incident monitoring tool with potential international applications.

Incident monitoring as a component of risk management in the healthcare industry has great potential and, with ongoing interaction with human factors experts, will progress the goal of reducing risk for the health sector overall as well as for the discipline of anesthesia.

REFERENCES

1. Leape L. Error in medicine. J Am Med Assoc 1994; **272:** 1851–7.
2. *The Concise Oxford Dictionary of Quotations.* London: Oxford University Press, 1964: 14.
3. Cited in Laurence DR, Bennett PN (eds). *Clinical Pharmacology*, London: Churchill Livingstone, 1995.
4. Kohn LT, Corrigan JM, Donaldson MS (eds). *To Err is Human. Building a Safer Health System.* Washington, DC: National Academy Press, 1999.
5. Mills DH. *Report on the Medical Insurance Feasibility Study*, San Francisco: Sutter Publications, 1977.
6. Brennan TA, Leape LL, Laird N, et al. Incidents of adverse events and negligence in hospitalized patients. Results of the Harvard Medical Practice Study I. N Engl J Med 1991; **324:** 370–6.
7. Leape LL, Brennan TA, Laird N, et al. The nature of adverse events in hospitalized patients. Results of the Harvard Medical Practice Study II. N Engl J Med 1991; **324:** 377–84.
8. Leape LL, Lawthers AG, Brennan TA, Johnson WG. Preventing medical injury. Qual Rev Bull 1993; **19:** 144–9.
9. Thomas MJ, Studdert DM, Burstin HR, *et al.* Incidences and types of adverse events and negligent care in Utah and Colorado. *Med Care* 2000; **38:** 261–71.
10. Wilson RM, Runciman WB, Gibberd RW, *et al.* The Quality in Australian Health Care Study. *Med J Aust* 1995; **163:** 458–71.
11. Thomas EJ, Studdert D, Runciman WB, *et al.* A comparison of iatrogenic injury studies in Australia and the USA. I: Context, methods, casemix, population, patient and hospital characteristics. *Int J Qual Health Care* 2000; **12:** 371–378.
12. Runciman WB, Webb RK, Helps SC, *et al.* A comparison of iatrogenic injury studies in Australia and the USA. II Reviewer behaviour and quality of care. *Int J Qual Health Care* 2000; **12:** 379–88.
13. *An Organisation with a Memory. Report of an Expert Group on Learning from Adverse Events in the NHS.* Department of Health, London: The Stationery Office, 2000.
14. Runciman WB, Moller JJ. *Iatrogenic Injury in Australia.* Adelaide: Australian Patient Safety Foundation, 2001.
15. Rigby KD, Litt JC. Errors in health management: what do they cost? *Qual Health Care* 2000; **9:** 216–21.
16. Vincent CA. Presentation at *British Medical Journal Conference "Reducing Error in Medicine,"* London, March 2000.
17. Studdert DM, Thomas EJ, Burstin HR, *et al.* Negligent care and malpractice claiming behavior in Utah and Colorado. *Med Care* 2000; **38:** 250–60.
18. Kasperson RE. Acceptability of human risk. Environ Health Perspect 1983; **52:** 15–20.
19. Zelders T. Patient risks: an underdeveloped area. J Clin Monit 1996; **12:** 237–41.
20. Davis NJ (ed.). *Anaesthesia Related Mortality in Australia 1994–1996.* Melbourne: Australian and New Zealand College of Anaesthetists, 1999.
21. Reason J. *Human Error.* New York: Cambridge University Press, 1990.
22. Reason J. *Managing the Risks of Organizational Accidents.* Aldershot: Ashgate Publishing Limited, 1997.
23. Runciman WB, Webb RK, Lee R, Holland R. System failure: an analysis of 2000 incident reports. Anaesth Intens Care 1993; **21:** 684–95.

24. Allnutt MF. Human factors in accidents. *Br J Anaesth* 1987; **59:** 856–64.
25. Runciman WB, Sellen A, Webb RK, et al. Errors, incidents and accident in anaesthetic practice. Anaesth Intens Care 1993; **21:** 506–19.
26. Kluger MT, Tham EJ, Coleman NA, *et al.* Inadequate pre-operative evaluation and preparation: a review of 197 reports from the Australian incident monitoring study. *Anaesthesia* 2000; **55:** 1173–8.
27. Reason J. Human error: models and management. Br Med J 2000; **320:** 768–70.
28. Lerner MJ. The desire for justice and reactions to victims. In: McCauley J, Berkowitz L (eds). *Altruism and Helping Behavior.* New York: Academic Press, 1970.
29. Runciman WB. Incident monitoring. *Baillière's Clin Anaesth* 1996; **10:** 333–56.
30. Flanagan JC. The critical incident technique. Psychol Bull 1954; **51:** 327–58.
31. Merry AF, Davies JM, Maltby JR. Qualitative research in health care. *Br J Anaesth* 2000; **84:** 552–5.
32. Runciman WB. Qualitative versus quantitative research – balancing cost, yield and feasibility. Anaesth Intens Care 1993; **21:** 502–5.
33. Sexton JB, Thomas EJ, Helmreich RL. Error, stress, and teamwork in medicine and aviation: cross sectional surveys. Br Med J 2000; **320:** 745–9.
34. Federal Aviation Administration. *Aviation Safety Action Programs. Advisory Circular 120–66A.* Washington, DC: FAA, 1999.
35. Barach P, Small SD. Reporting and preventing medical mishaps: lessons from non-medical near miss reporting systems. Br Med J 2000; **320:** 759–63.
36. Cooper JB, Newblower RS, Long CD, McPeek B. Preventable anesthesia mishaps: a study of human factors. Anesthesiology 1978; **49:** 399–406.
37. Safren MA, Chapanis A. A critical incident study of hospital medication errors. Hospitals 1960; **34:** 32–66.
38. Sanazaro PJ, Williamson JW. Physician performance and its effects on patients: a classification based on reports by internists, surgeons, paediatricians and obstetricians. *Med Care* 1970; 8: 299–308.
39. Currie M, Pybus DA, Torda TA. A prospective survey of anaesthetic critical events. A report on a pilot study of 88 cases. Anaesth Intens Care 1988; **16:** 103–7.
40. Williamson JA, Webb RK, Pryor GL. Anaesthesia safety and the "critical incident" technique. *Aust Clin Review* 1985; 5: 57–61.
41. Morgan C. Incident reporting in anaesthesia. Anaesth Intens Care 1988; **16:** 98–100.
42. Runciman WB. The Australian Patient Safety Foundation. *Anaesth Intens Care* 1988, **18:** 114–16.
43. Symposium. The Australian Incident Monitoring Study. Anaesth Intens Care 1993; **21:** 501–684.
44. Morris GP, Morris RW. Anaesthesia and fatigue: an analysis of the first 10 years of the Australian Incident Monitoring Study 1987–1997. *Anaesth Intens Care* 2000; **28:** 300–4.
45. Sinclair M, Simmons S, Cyna A. Incidents in obstetric anaesthesia and analgesia: an analysis of 5000 AIMS reports. Anaesth Intens Care 1999; **27:** 275–81.
46. Kluger MT, Short TG. Aspiration during anaesthesia: a review of 133 cases from the Australian Anaesthetic Incident Monitoring Study (AIMS). Anaesthesia 1999; **54:** 19–26.
47. Kluger MT, Bukofzer M, Bullock M. Anaesthetic assistants: their role in the development and resolution of anaesthetic incidents. Anaesth Intens Care 1999; **27:** 269–74.
48. Steven ID, Malpass A, Moller J, *et al.* Towards safer drug use in general practice. *J Qual Clin Pract* 1999, **19:** 47–50.
49. Wright M, Parker G. Incident monitoring in psychiatry. J Qual Clin Pract 1998; **18:** 249–61.
50. Vinen J. Incident monitoring in Emergency Departments: an Australian Model. *Acad Emerg Med* 2000, **7:** 1290–7.
51. Beckmann U, Baldwin I, Hart GK, Runciman WB. The Australian Incident Monitoring Study in Intensive Care: AIMS–ICU. An analysis of the first year of reporting. *Anaesth Intens Care* 1996; **24:** 320–29.
52. Chopra V, Bovill JG, Spierdijk J, Koorneef F. Reported significant observations during anaesthesia; a prospective analysis over an 18-month period. Br J Anaesth 1992; **68:** 13–17.
53. Short TG, O'Regan A, Lew J, Oh T. Critical incident reporting in an anaesthetic department quality assurance programme. Anaesthesia 1993; **48:** 3–7.
54. Kumar V, Barcellos WA, Hehta MP, Carter JG. An analysis of critical incidents in a teaching department for quality assurance. A survey of mishaps during anaesthesia. Anaesthesia 1988; **43:** 879–83.
55. Critical Incident Reporting Scheme. The Royal College of Anaesthetists, London (www.rcoa.ac.uk).
56. Lack JA, White LA, Thoms GM, Rollin A-M (eds). *Raising the Standard.* London: Royal College of Anaesthetists, 2000.
57. Spittal MJ, Findlay GP, Spencer I. A prospective analysis of critical incidents attributable to anaesthesia. *Int J Qual Health Care* 1995; **7:** 363–71.
58. Heinrich HW. *Industrial Accident Prevention: A Scientific Approach.* New York, 1941.
59. The Australian Standard AS/NZS 4360 – Risk Management (www.standards.com.au).
60. Caplan RA, Posner KL, Ward RJ, Cheney FW. Adverse respiratory events in anaesthesia: a closed claims analysis. Anesthesiology 1990; **72:** 828–33.
61. Tinker JH, Dull DL, Caplan RA, et al. Role of monitoring devices in prevention of anaesthetic mishaps: a closed claims analysis. Anesthesiology 1989; **71:** 541–6.
62. Wolff A. Limited adverse occurrence screening: an effective and efficient method of medical quality control. J Qual Clin Pract 1995; **15:** 221–33.
63. Klinect JR, Wilhelm JA, Helmreich RL. Threat and error management: data from line operations safety audits. In: *Proceedings of the Tenth International Symposium on Aviation Psychology*, Ohio State University, Columbus, 1999: 683–8.
64. Galletly DC, Mushet NN. Anaesthesia system errors. Anaesth Intens Care 1991; **19:** 66–73.
65. Rowe L, Galletly DC, Henderson RS. Accuracy of text entries within a manually compiled anaesthetic record. Br J Anaesth 1992; **68:** 381–7.
66. Galletly DC, Rowe WL, Henderson RS. The anaesthetic record: a confidential survey on data omission or modification. Anaesth Intens Care 1991; **19:** 74–8.
67. Gaba DM. Anaesthesiology as a model for patient safety in health care. Br Med J 2000; **320:** 785–8.
68. Runciman WB, Helps SC, Sexton EJ, Malpass A. A classification for incidents and accidents in the health care system. J Qual Clin Pract 1998; **18:** 199–211.
69. *ICD-9-AM. Australian Version of the International Classification of Diseases*, 9th rev, Clinical modification. National Coding Centre, Faculty of Health Sciences, University of Sydney, Sydney, 1996.
70. Stannard.CF. Clinical terms project: a coding system for clinicians. Br J Hosp Med 1994; **52:** 46–8.
71. Osborne GA, Webb RK, Runciman WB. Patient awareness during anaesthesia: an analysis of 2000 incident reports. Anaesth and Intens Care 1993; **21:** 653–4.
72. Wu AW. Medical error: the second victim. Br Med J 2000; **320:** 726–7.
73. Webb RK, Currie M, Morgan CA, et al. The Australian Incident Monitoring Study. Anaesth Intens Care 1993; **21:** 520–8.
74. Runciman WB, Webb RK, Klepper ID, et al. Crisis management: validation of an algorithm by analysis of 2000 incident reports. Anaesth Intens Care 1993; **21:** 579–92.
75. Staender S, Davies J, Helmreich B, Kaufmann M. The anaesthesia critical incident reporting system: an experience based database. Int J Med Informatics 1997; **47:** 87–90.
76. Paté-Cornell ME, Lakats LM, Murphy DM, Gaba DM. Anesthesia patient risk: a quantitative approach to organizational factors and risk management options. *Risk Anal* 1997; **17:** 511–23.

FURTHER READING

Reason J. *Human Error.* New York: Cambridge University Press, 1990.

Reason J. *Managing the Risks of Organizational Accidents.* Aldershot: Ashgate Publishing Limited, 1997.

The Australian Incident Monitoring Study Symposium. *Anaesth Intensive Care* 1993; **21:** 501–684.

Medical error. Special issue. *Br Med J* 2000; **320**.

Kohn LT, Corrigan JM, Donaldson MS (eds). *To Err is Human. Building a Safer Health System.* Washington, DC: National Academy Press, 1999.

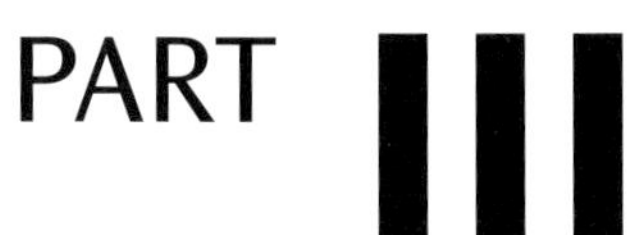

PART III

Subspecialty-oriented Management of Anesthesia

42

Trauma anesthesia

CARL L GWINNUTT AND JERRY P NOLAN

Each year, many people die or are seriously disabled as a result of trauma. In the UK, there are approximately 19 000 trauma deaths per annum, and it is the leading cause of death among people aged 1–34 years. In the USA, trauma is the leading cause of death in people aged 1–38 years and accounts for over 150 000 injury-related deaths annually. In comparison with the UK, the availability of firearms in the USA results in significantly more patients with penetrating injuries.[1] Mortality is only the tip of the trauma "iceberg;" it is estimated that, for each death, three people are rendered permanently disabled. In the USA, this results in 300 000 permanent and 8.7 million disabled temporarily each year.[2] It is not surprising, therefore, that anesthesiologists encounter large numbers of trauma patients in all aspects of their work.

The local organization of trauma care will determine the role of the anesthesiologist in caring for the trauma patient.[3] The spectrum of responsibilities is shown in Table 42.1. The USA has developed a system of care based around regionalized "trauma centers" in order to concentrate the necessary expertise and provide an adequate case load to allow teaching and to maintain skills. The role of the anesthesiologist in the majority of these institutions is to establish a secure airway, ensure adequate ventilation, and provide anesthesia for surgery. In the UK, anesthesiologists undertake much wider roles, ranging from prehospital care, resuscitation, and anesthesia to postoperative care in an intensive care or high-dependency unit. In other parts of Europe, ambulance technicians are frequently supported by physicians, often anesthesiologists, in hospital mobile units, e.g. those used by the Service D'Aide Medical Urgente (SAMU) in France. Within whichever system anesthesiologists work, the skills of airway and ventilatory management, vascular access and fluid resuscitation, analgesia and the ability to monitor the effectiveness of such interventions are among the essential prerequisites for the initial management of the patient following trauma.

This chapter will concentrate on the role of the anesthesiologist in the prehospital environment, the emergency department and operating room.

Table 42.1 *Anesthesiologists' responsibilities in trauma care*

Prehospital care
Emergency department
Trauma team leader
Trauma team member
Anesthesiologist
Operating room
Anesthesia
Postoperative care
Intensive care unit
High-dependency unit
Acute pain team
Transportation
Major incident/disaster management

PREHOSPITAL CARE AND THE ANESTHESIOLOGIST

Any anesthesiologist providing care for patients after trauma in the prehospital environment must be adequately trained, clothed, and equipped.[4] Anesthesiologists possess many skills, which can be used at the scene of an accident to complement those of a paramedic in managing victims of trauma (Table 42.2). However, despite providing an enhanced level of care, there is no overwhelming evidence that the patient's outcome is improved. Published studies reveal conflicting results that continue to fuel the debate between policies of "scoop and run" and "stay and play."[5–10] Even when the patient's physiological status is improved, this does not automatically translate into an improved outcome.[11]

Ultimately, the most effective prehospital care will probably depend on the treatment delivered being tailored to the type of injuries sustained, rather than trying to treat all patients following major trauma as a homogeneous group.[12] Currently, therefore, an anesthesiologist attending the scene of an accident as part of the emergency medical team should limit initial interventions to securing a patent airway, ensuring effective ventilation, controlling external hemorrhage, and expediting transfer of the patient to a center capable of dealing with the injuries.[13] The only acceptable exceptions to this are those who have suffered prolonged entrapment or head injuries when, in addition to the above, intravenous fluids or analgesia may be required.

Table 42.2 *Anesthetic skills which can be used before arrival at a hospital*

The use of neuromuscular blocking drugs to facilitate tracheal intubation
Analgesia
Anesthesia
The use of a greater range or volume of intravenous fluids
Insertion of chest drain (tube thoracostomy)
Cricothyroidotomy
Triage of patients to the most appropriate hospital

Prehospital general anesthesia

Occasionally the anesthesiologist may be called to the scene of an accident to administer a general anesthetic, e.g. to facilitate extrication or the amputation of a nonviable limb. The administration of a general anesthetic in such circumstances must be a planned event – it must not be the accidental result of injudicious administration of sedatives and analgesics.

Prior to inducing anesthesia, all physical dangers to the anesthesiologist and patient must have been eliminated as far as possible, and access to the patient maximized. All immediately life-threatening injuries must be identified first and dealt with using the ABC principles (see Table 42.5), and the equipment to be used must have been fully checked. An assistant should be designated to help the anesthesiologist and, if unfamiliar with the equipment, they must be fully briefed beforehand. Monitoring of the patient should be established using an electrocardiogram (ECG), noninvasive blood pressure device, and pulse oximeter.[14] If access is limited, a pulse oximeter can be used alone to assess oxygenation, heart rate, and rhythm and to give an indication of perfusion.

Induction of anesthesia is not without risk. It may result in loss of airway patency and the protective reflexes, resulting in an increased risk of the patient aspirating gastric contents. Shock may be exacerbated by both decreased ventilation and reduced cardiac output. Consideration should be given to the effects of anesthesia on injuries to the central nervous system and loss of muscle tone reducing support for the spinal column.

Choice of anesthetic agent

The ideal anesthetic agent for use prehospital in trauma patients should possess the features shown in Table 42.3.

Ketamine

Ketamine is the agent which comes closest to the ideal for the prehospital general anesthetic (Ketalar, Ketaject). Following intravenous administration of 0.75–1 mg kg^{-1}, anesthesia is induced over 30–60 s. Anesthesia can also be induced by intramuscular administration, but erratic uptake makes this inadvisable in the shocked patient. Airway patency and respiratory function are generally well preserved. Pharyngeal reflexes are depressed less than with other agents, but silent aspiration may occur.[15] An increase in jaw muscle tone and salivary and tracheobronchial secretions may compromise the airway. Secretions may be reduced by the prior administration of glycopyrrolate (0.2 mg intravenously). Respiratory depression is dose related; the carbon dioxide response curve is shifted to the right, but the slope is maintained. The functional residual capacity (FRC) is maintained along with the pulmonary hypoxic vasoconstriction response, both of which help to maintain oxygenation.[16] Ketamine antagonizes the action of histamine on bronchial smooth muscle and can be used safely for asthmatics. In contrast with the other currently available induction agents, ketamine causes a tachycardia and an increase in systemic blood pressure, secondary to central sympathetic stimulation and inhibition of catecholamine reuptake.[17,18] However, in the shocked trauma patient, in whom sympathetic stimulation is already maximal, cardiac output and blood pressure may fall as a vasodilatory effect is unmasked. The main concern with the use of ketamine is in its use for patients with head injuries in whom a rise in cerebral blood flow and intracranial pressure (ICP) may compromise cerebral perfusion in patients whose ICP is already raised – a view which has recently been challenged.[19] Furthermore, *N*-methyl-D-aspartate (NMDA) receptor antagonists, of which ketamine is one, have been shown to improve neurological outcome in experimental models of brain injury.[20] These observations, coupled with current investigations into the use of the S(+) enantiomer of ketamine, may change the future role of ketamine for these patients.[21]

Table 42.3 *Properties of an ideal anesthetic agent for use in the prehospital environment*

Rapid onset
Preserve laryngeal reflexes
No respiratory depression
No cardiovascular depression
No increase in intracranial pressure
Provide good analgesia
No histamine release
Short duration of action with rapid recovery

Following induction, anesthesia may be maintained by an infusion or repeat boluses of ketamine according to clinical need. Recovery may be accompanied by a variety of emergence phenomena including hallucinations and delirium, the incidence of which can be significantly decreased by the concurrent administration of midazolam.[22]

Much of the evidence for the use of ketamine in difficult circumstances remains either anecdotal or in the form of uncontrolled clinical reports. However, the consensus is that, overall, it offers a greater margin of safety than many other anesthetics in these circumstances.[23–25]

Alternatives to ketamine

Etomidate causes less cardiovascular and respiratory depression than do other agents in healthy adults; however, for the hypovolemic patient, it should be used following adequate fluid resuscitation and in a reduced dose. It may be useful for patients with isolated head injuries as it reduces cerebral blood flow, cerebral oxygen consumption, and intracranial pressure while maintaining cerebral perfusion pressure.[26,27] Unfortunately, administration of etomidate is frequently accompanied by myoclonus, which may be potentially hazardous in the prehospital environment.

Propofol causes a significant decrease in systemic blood pressure secondary to reduced peripheral resistance and a fall in cardiac output. It has effects on cerebral blood flow that are similar to etomidate and it has been used successfully for patients with head injuries after volume resuscitation.[28] A major advantage of propofol use is that it can be administered subsequently as a continuous infusion to maintain anesthesia without the risk of accumulation or delayed recovery. Neither etomidate nor propofol possesses analgesic properties and, therefore, appropriate doses of opioids must be administered concurrently.

Neuromuscular blocking drugs

Succinylcholine (suxamethonium) remains the agent of choice when muscle relaxation is required to facilitate tracheal intubation. However, in the prehospital environment, the associated side-effects must not be ignored (see Table 42.14). The administration of succinylcholine commits the anesthesiologist to maintaining the patient's ventilation, a situation which may be made more difficult in these circumstances by limited access to the patient. Even intubating a patient lying supine on the ground is more difficult, and may be facilitated by the anesthesiologist adopting the left lateral decubitus position.[29]

The administration of an anesthetic in the difficult circumstances of the prehospital environment should not be seen as an excuse to operate at a reduced standard of care. Whether the anesthetic lasts only a few minutes or for a prolonged period, the patient must be adequately monitored. Once the patient has been extricated, and during transportation, one should aim for a standard of care commensurate with that provided in hospital. In addition to being monitored, the patient's vital signs should be recorded frequently along with the details of dose and timing of all drugs administered.

THE ANESTHESIOLOGIST IN THE EMERGENCY DEPARTMENT

In most hospitals, the emergency department is the first contact between the anesthesiologist and the trauma patient. It is essential that any anesthesiologist, working as either a member of the trauma team or providing analgesia or anesthesia as part of the care of the trauma patient, fully understands the currently accepted system of managing this group of patients so as not to jeopardize their treatment.

Communication and preparation

Time is absolutely crucial to the successful resuscitation of a severely injured patient. Ideally, ambulance personnel or a doctor at the scene should be able to communicate directly with the emergency department staff.[30] Concise and essential information on the patient's condition and estimated time of arrival must be given. The receiving department staff can then decide whether to alert individual specialists, or if available, the trauma team. With advance warning, the medical and nursing staff can prepare the resuscitation area with the appropriate equipment based on the information received. The relevant nurses and doctors should be assigned tasks before the patient arrives. The primary responsibilities of the anesthesiologist are shown in Table 42.4.

RESUSCITATION OF THE PATIENT FOLLOWING TRAUMA

Deaths following trauma are generally considered to occur with a trimodal distribution.[31] The first peak in deaths is within seconds to minutes of injury, as a result of major neurological or vascular injury. This can currently be reduced only by preventative measures. The second peak, the early deaths, occurs in patients dying from airway, breathing, or circulatory problems. This period has been called "the golden hour"[32] to emphasize the importance of rapid and timely resuscitation to reduce mortality. The third peak in the number of deaths occurs in days to a few weeks later, as a result of sepsis and multiple organ failure. Appropriate management of the patient in the resuscitation phase, with rapid restoration of cellular oxygenation, should not only reduce deaths in the golden hour but also those that occur in this third peak. This classic trimodal distribution of deaths in patients following trauma has been challenged recently, but this should not detract from the philosophy of rapid, systematic, and appropriate management.[33,34]

The traditional medical practice, which is the taking of a history from the patient, performing a full examination, and ordering diagnostic investigations in order to construct a differential diagnosis before commencing treatment, is not appropriate for the severely injured patient. Instead, assessment and resuscitation take place simultaneously, with the aim being to identify and treat first the greatest threats to life. The lack of a *definitive* diagnosis should not impede the start of appropriate treatment, and furthermore a detailed history is not a prerequisite before starting to assess the patient. These are the fundamental principles taught in the Advanced Trauma Life Support (ATLS) course, developed by the Committee on Trauma of the American College of Surgeons.[35] Although aimed at the single-handed physician working in a rural hospital, the ATLS protocols can be easily adapted for a team approach and provide a useful framework on which resuscitation efforts in any environment can be based. The focus of ATLS is the management of patients with major injuries during the golden hour and is considered in four phases: primary survey, resuscitation, secondary survey, and definitive care. Although the first two phases are listed consecutively, they are performed simultaneously. The aim of the primary survey can be summed up as "to look for and treat, any immediately life-threatening injuries as soon as they are identified."

The primary survey is conducted using the ABCDE mnemonic to ensure that the most time-critical conditions are dealt with first. The correct sequence is summarized in Table 42.5.

Any life-threatening problem detected is treated immediately (resuscitation) before proceeding to the next step of the primary survey, even if on occasion this requires emergency surgery, e.g. to arrest uncontrollable hemorrhage. Once the primary survey and resuscitation have been completed, the secondary survey, a detailed head-to-toe examination of the patient, must be performed. The aim is to identify all other injuries and concurrent medical problems. Clearly, on some occasions, this may be delayed by several hours, but it must not be omitted. Finally, definitive care of each condition can commence, depending on its priority.

Resuscitation of the trauma patient using this approach is most efficient if undertaken by a team of appropriately trained doctors and nurses.[36] This enables a variety of tasks to be undertaken simultaneously, a process known as "horizontal organization." The most difficult problem that some hospitals may face is the lack of experienced doctors who are immediately available, and the precise composition of those tasked with caring for the traumatized patient will inevitably vary between hospitals. When trauma teams are established, the role of the team leader is particularly important, and in the UK this has been defined comprehensively by a British Trauma Society Standards Working Party.[37]

The primary survey and resuscitation

Airway with control of the cervical spine

During the resuscitation of any severely injured patient, the initial priorities are to ensure a clear, secure airway and to maintain adequate oxygenation. If the airway is obstructed, immediate basic maneuvers such as chin lift or jaw thrust along with suction may temporarily relieve the obstruction. In the semiconscious patient, an oropharyngeal (Guedel) airway or a nasopharyngeal airway may help to maintain patency while preparation is made for more definitive management (see below). Every patient with multiple injuries should receive a high inspired oxygen concentration. In those who are not intubated but are breathing

Table 42.4 *The responsibilities of the anesthesiologist in preparing for a patient following trauma*

Prior to the arrival of the trauma patient, the anesthesiologist must check:
- The range of basic airway equipment – oropharyngeal, nasopharyngeal airways
- The equipment for tracheal intubation, in particular laryngoscopes and tracheal tubes
- The suction apparatus
- The equipment for ventilation, both manual and mechanical
- The drugs available, correctly labeled with name and concentration
- That equipment for monitoring is functioning and calibrated correctly
- The abilities of an assistant

Table 42.5 *The primary survey*

Airway with control of the cervical spine
Breathing and ventilation
Circulation and hemorrhage control
Disability – a rapid assessment of neurological function
Exposure with environmental control

spontaneously, a face mask and reservoir bag with a high flow of oxygen ($15\,L\,min^{-1}$) will increase the inspired concentration to approximately 85%. A pulse oximeter may give valuable information about the patient's oxygen saturation, but frequently peripheral vasoconstriction makes it difficult to obtain a reliable reading.

The cervical spine cannot be deemed undamaged until the patient has been examined by an experienced clinician and appropriate radiological procedures have been completed.[38] Clearly, a reliable clinical examination cannot be obtained if the patient has sustained a significant head injury, is intoxicated, or has a reduced conscious level from any other cause. Therefore, every patient sustaining significant blunt trauma, particularly above the clavicles or if unconscious, should be assumed to have a cervical spine injury until it is proved otherwise.[39] The most effective method for achieving this comprises a combination of an appropriately sized semirigid cervical collar (e.g. Stiffneck or Philadelphia) and bilateral sandbags or blocks, joined with tape or straps across the forehead (Fig. 42.1).[40] This combination will virtually eliminate neck flexion, although 30% of normal extension is still possible. The only acceptable alternative to this is manual inline stabilization.

If the patient has an unstable cervical spine injury, further movement may result in permanent injury to the spinal cord. In fresh cadavers with unstable cervical injuries, basic and advanced airway maneuvers caused significant subluxation of the cervical spine during aggressive chin lift or jaw thrust despite the presence of a Philadelphia collar.[41] Mask ventilation can also produce a similar degree of displacement of the cervical spine to that produced by oral intubation.[42] Thus, all airway maneuvers must be performed carefully, and without moving the neck (Fig. 42.2).

Advanced airway management

Intubation of the trachea with a cuffed tube remains the gold standard. The indications for performing tracheal intubation are given in Table 42.6.

The choice of technique to use when intubating a patient will depend on the indication, the skill and experience of the clinician, and whether there is a suspected or confirmed cervical spine injury. Blind nasotracheal intubation has been advocated for clinicians not experienced in the use of neuromuscular blocking drugs and laryngoscopy, thereby avoiding the potential scenario of "can't intubate, can't ventilate." However, this method is not as successful as direct laryngoscopy and

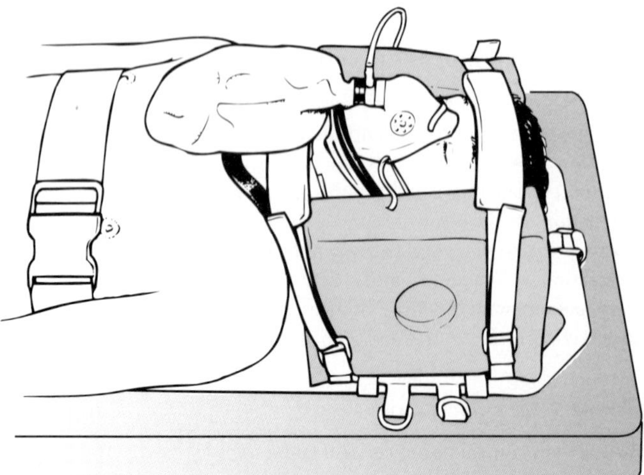

Figure 42.1 *Cervical spine immobilization in a patient on a long spine board with rigid collar, lateral blocks and straps. (Reproduced with permission from Nolan and Parr.[30])*

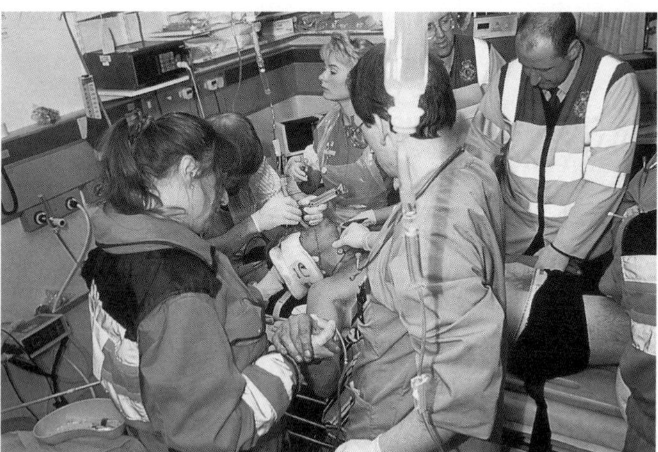

Figure 42.2 *Tracheal intubation in the emergency department. The head and neck are immobilized manually and cricoid pressure is applied as the anesthesiologist attempts intubation.*

oral intubation and has a higher risk of aspiration.[43] Other associated problems include profuse bleeding, coughing, laryngospasm, and unrecognized esophageal intubation. It has been suggested that awake tracheal intubation via either the nasal or oral route is safe and effective and allows the patient to act as their own "spinal cord monitor."[44] These techniques have been criticized by anesthesiologists in the UK,[45] who are more likely to follow the approach used for intubation at the Maryland Institute for Emergency Medical Services Systems Shock Trauma Center.[46] This consists of:

- manual inline stabilization of the cervical spine by an assistant;
- preoxygenation for 2–3 min;
- administration of an intravenous anesthetic induction agent;
- application of cricoid pressure by a separate assistant;
- administration of a rapidly acting neuromuscular blocking drug;
- intubation of the trachea;
- check the position of the tracheal tube;
- release of cricoid pressure.

It is the continuous immobilization of the neck during tracheal intubation that is the important factor for reducing the incidence of secondary spinal cord injury, rather than the technique used to achieve intubation.[47,48] Manual inline stabilization (MILS) reduces neck movement during intubation,[49,50] but care must be taken to avoid excessive axial traction, which may distract a cervical fracture.[51,52] By placing the patient's head and neck in neutral alignment and applying MILS, one can expect the view of the larynx to be grade 3[53] or worse in approximately 20% of patients, compared with 64% when immobilization is achieved using a rigid collar, sandbags, and tape.[54] Intubation will be aided greatly by the use of a gum-elastic bougie[55] and a McCoy levering

Table 42.6 *Indications for tracheal intubation in the trauma patient*

Coma – Glasgow coma scale (GCS) ≤8
Loss of protective airway reflexes
Hemorrhage into the airway
Ventilatory insufficiency
$P_{a}O_2$ <8 kPa (60 mmHg) breathing air
$P_{a}CO_2$ >6 kPa (45 mmHg)
Seizures
Combative patient requiring investigations
General anesthesia
Cardiac arrest

laryngoscope, use of which reduces the effective incidence of grade 3 or worse views to 5%.[56] If intubation of the patient proves impossible and the patient cannot be adequately ventilated using a face mask, there are a number of options. Needle cricothyroidotomy with a 14G cannula followed by jet insufflation of oxygen from a high-pressure source (400 kPa; 3000 mmHg) will usually provide satisfactory oxygenation, but hypercarbia is likely. Alternatives are to use a laryngeal mask airway (LMA), intubating laryngeal mask (ILM), or esophageal tracheal combitube (see below).

Breathing and ventilation

Once the airway is clear and secure, attention is turned to ensuring adequate alveolar ventilation and identifying life-threatening chest injuries (Table 42.7). Most of these can be dealt with initially without the need for surgery.

There are three major chest injuries that may rapidly impair ventilation and therefore need to be excluded: a tension pneumothorax, an open pneumothorax, and a flail chest.

The presence of a tension pneumothorax is a clinical diagnosis. The patient will be in respiratory distress and, on examination, there will be reduced chest movement, reduced breath sounds, a hyper-resonant percussion note on the affected side, hypotension, and a tachycardia. Deviation of the trachea to the opposite side is a late sign, and neck veins may not be distended in the presence of hypovolemia. Treatment is immediate decompression with a large (14G, 2.0 mm) cannula. This is inserted into the second intercostal space, in the midclavicular line on the affected side, and has the effect of converting a tension to a simple pneumothorax. Once intravenous access has been obtained, a large chest drain (36FG) should be inserted into the fifth intercostal space in the anterior axillary line and connected to an underwater seal drain.

In the presence of an open pneumothorax that is greater than two-thirds the tracheal diameter, air will preferentially enter the pleural cavity via the defect. Pulmonary ventilation is impaired, resulting in hypoxia and hypercarbia. The defect should be covered and a chest drain inserted to prevent the risk of a tension pneumothorax developing. Alternatively, an Ashermann seal can be applied, which acts as a one-way valve allowing escape, but not entrainment, of air into the pleural cavity.

Table 42.7 *Assessment of breathing and ventilation*

Speech
- Sentences or odd words

Look at the chest
- Excursion
- Symmetry of movement
- Rate of breathing
- Use of accessory muscles
- Supraclavicular, intercostal recession
- Wounds

Auscultate the chest
- Reduced breath sounds
- Wheeze
- Stridor

Percuss the chest
- Hyper-resonance
- Dullness

Feel for surgical emphysema

Check the neck
- Tracheal position
- Veins
- Wounds

A flail chest is an indication of a severe chest injury; the underlying pulmonary contusion may cause life-threatening hypoxia, requiring intubation and mechanical ventilation. The classic description of paradoxical movement at the site of the flail may not be seen in younger patients, as fractured ribs will be splinted by the muscles of the chest wall. It is only in the elderly or exhausted patient that this clinical sign will be obvious.

Two further problems can be conveniently excluded at this stage. A massive hemothorax (more than 1500 mL blood in a hemithorax) will result in reduced chest movement, a dull percussion note, hypoxemia, and hypovolemia. Once volume resuscitation has commenced, a chest drain should be inserted. This will allow re-expansion of compressed lung and improve oxygenation. Insertion of a chest drain does not increase blood loss.[57] Finally, cardiac tamponade should be considered while examining the chest, particularly if the patient has sustained a penetrating injury to the chest or upper abdomen. The diagnosis should be considered in a patient with distended neck veins in the presence of hypotension, after rapid volume resuscitation. The classic description of muffled heart sounds may not be distinguishable in the midst of a busy resuscitation room. If the diagnosis is suspected, and the patient is deteriorating despite all resuscitative efforts, pericardiocentesis should be performed. In the presence of a suitably experienced surgeon, open pericardiotomy is the more effective procedure. A myocardial contusion may also present with similar signs.

Circulation and control of hemorrhage

The patient's hemodynamic status must be assessed rapidly and an ECG attached. Until proved otherwise, assume hypotension is the result of hypovolemia. Less likely causes include myocardial contusion, neurogenic shock, or cardiogenic shock. In the young trauma patient, loss of 15–30% of the total blood volume will typically be associated with a tachycardia and, as a result of peripheral vasoconstriction, a rise in diastolic pressure, which reduces the pulse pressure. A fall in systolic pressure suggests a loss of more than 30% of total blood volume – approximately 1500 mL in a 70-kg adult.

Intravenous access

Two short, large-bore, intravenous cannulae (14G, 2.0 mm or larger) should be inserted rapidly. The easiest site is usually the antecubital fossa, but anywhere on the upper limb is acceptable. In the lower limb, the femoral or long saphenous veins can be used but are not ideal if the patient has pelvic or intra-abdominal injuries. Blood samples for baseline investigations and cross-match can be taken from the first successfully inserted cannula.

Any major external hemorrhage should be controlled with direct pressure, or in the case of a major pelvic fracture causing exsanguinating hemorrhage (Fig. 42.3), the application of an external fixator.

If peripheral access is impossible percutaneously, other options include cut-down onto a peripheral vein, central venous cannulation, or the intraosseous route. Cut-downs have few complications, can be performed quickly with minimal training, and allow standard large-bore cannulae to be inserted into the antecubital fossa and the saphenous vein. Anesthesiologists are more familiar with the use of the Seldinger technique to allow insertion of catheters into central veins. Using this technique to cannulate the femoral vein may also be a quicker option than performing a cut-down onto the saphenous vein.[58] Inserting a central line may not be easy in the hypovolemic patient, and there is a risk of creating a pneumothorax. If the central route is to be used for rapid fluid resuscitation, a relatively short, large-bore catheter (e.g. 8.5FG pulmonary artery catheter introducer sheath) should be used. The intraosseous route,[59] usually via the proximal tibia, is useful in children but will not allow high enough flow rates for effective fluid resuscitation in adults.

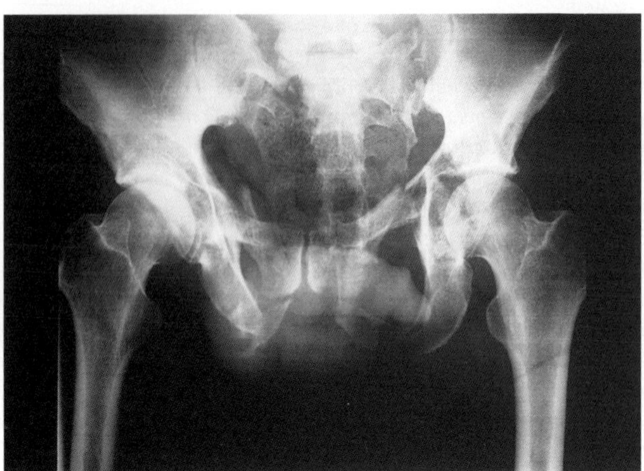

Figure 42.3 *Multiple pelvic fractures causing life-threatening hemorrhage.*

Fluids

Once intravenous access has been achieved, an initial fluid challenge of either crystalloid (2 L) or colloid (1 L) is administered[60] (Table 42.8). There is a wealth of literature describing the most appropriate of the many fluids available for resuscitation.[61–63]

Edwards and colleagues[64] have described the "ideal" solution (Table 42.9), but for the majority of hypovolemic patients in the emergency department the initial choice is less important than speed and adequacy of replacement.

A transient response to this fluid challenge suggests ongoing bleeding and, in addition to fluid resuscitation, these patients require immediate surgical assessment. A sustained reduction in heart rate and increase in blood pressure suggests only moderate blood loss (<20% blood volume).

Table 42.8 *Fluids used for resuscitation*

Isotonic crystalloids
Physiologic (0.9%) saline
Hartmann's solution
Lactated Ringer's
Plasmalyte 148
Hypertonic crystalloid
7.5% saline
Gelatin solutions
Gelofusine
Haemaccel
Hydroxyethyl starches
Medium molecular weight
Low molecular weight
Dextrans
Blood

Table 42.9 *The ideal solution for volume resuscitation in the trauma patient*

Molecular weight (weight and number average) 35 000 Da
Increases plasma volume, cardiac index, and oxygen delivery
No organ toxicity
No effect on coagulation or cross-matching
Nonallergenic
Complete and predictable elimination
Cheap
Long shelf-life

Colloids are more efficient than crystalloids in that equivalent intravascular volume expansion will be achieved with less colloid. Colloid oncotic pressure is better maintained with colloid. Colloids are more expensive than crystalloids. Fluid overload is bad for the patient regardless of the type of fluid used. Two recent meta-analyses purport to show increased mortality with colloids in patients following trauma, but they are based on very small studies that used a variety of fluids.[65,66] There are no prospective, randomized trials that clearly demonstrate the superiority of either colloids or crystalloids for resuscitation following trauma. Double-blind studies with the power to define any advantages are unlikely given the complexity of trauma cases and the difficulty in establishing matched controls.

Crystalloids The American College of Surgeons' Committee on Trauma recommends the use of Hartmann's solution for the initial resuscitation of severely injured patients.[2] Part of the rationale for using crystalloids is that trauma patients will have sustained considerable interstitial fluid losses as well as intravascular loss. Replacement volumes should be three to four times the estimated intravascular loss.

Gelatin solutions In comparison with other colloids, gelatin solutions are cheap and they can be infused in relatively unrestricted volumes. They have no effects on the cross-matching of blood and act as an osmotic diuretic. *In vitro* studies suggest that gelatins may reduce the quality of clot formation,[67] but in the clinical setting they do not appear to have a significant effect on bleeding. In comparison with other colloids, the intravascular half-life of gelatins is relatively short (approximately 2 h).

Hydroxyethyl starch (HES) solutions HES solutions are synthetic polymers derived from amylopectin. Different degrees of substitution of hydroxyethyl groups for glucose result in solutions of varying properties.[68] The high molecular weight starches with high degrees of substitution (e.g. HES 450/0.7) have a very long half-life (over 24 h) and tend to increase bleeding by reducing factor VIII and von Willebrand factor. Thus, the maximum dose of high molecular weight HES is restricted to 20 $mL\,kg^{-1}\,day^{-1}$. The medium molecular weight starches (e.g. HES 200/0.5) have an intravascular half-life of approximately 6 h and, in doses less than 33 $mL\,kg^{-1}\,day^{-1}$, will not impair coagulation. Use of these medium molecular weight starches may reduce post-traumatic capillary leak.[69]

Hypertonic saline solutions Hypertonic crystalloid solutions provide small-volume resuscitation and rapid restoration of hemodynamic stability. The reduction in edema may improve microcirculatory hemodynamic function. They exert their effect by recruitment of interstitial volume, thus increasing circulating volume and increasing blood pressure. However, a rise in the blood pressure may not always be an ideal goal, and their role in resuscitation following trauma has yet to be defined. Head-injured patients with a Glasgow Coma Scale (GCS) score of <9 may benefit from hypertonic saline,[70] but this has yet to be proved conclusively.

Hemoglobin solutions Once a patient has lost more than 30–40% of the blood volume, a resuscitation fluid with good oxygen-carrying capability will become necessary. Currently, this implies the need for a blood transfusion.

Having overcome a number of problems related to toxic stroma, short intravascular half-life, and high colloid osmotic pressure, a number of hemoglobin solutions are now undergoing phase III clinical trials.[71] An increase in mean arterial pressure (resulting partly from nitric oxide binding), in conjunction with a reduction in viscosity, may result in significantly better oxygen delivery to vital organs. The long-term safety of massive transfusion with hemoglobin solutions in humans has yet to be demonstrated.

Blood When resuscitating a patient in hemorrhagic shock following trauma, the time taken to complete a full cross-match (45–60 min) is too long. Type-specific blood can be issued by the blood bank within approximately 10 min, and is acceptable and preferable to prolonged delay in the resuscitation setting. Significant incompatibility reactions to type-specific blood are rare. The exsanguinating patient may require group O blood, which will be available immediately.

Hemoglobin targets in trauma

Hypovolemia is tolerated considerably less well than anemia. Normovolemic patients with good cardiopulmonary function will tolerate hemoglobin levels[72] as low as $<7\,g\,dL^{-1}$. Recent evidence suggests that even critically ill patients may fare better when managed with a restrictive strategy of red cell transfusion.[73] As long as normovolemia is achieved, a reduction in viscosity results in a significant increases in cardiac output and tends to improve tissue oxygenation. One problem facing the clinician when resuscitating a patient immediately after trauma is that a history of ischemic heart disease or significant respiratory disease may not be available. Furthermore, the hemoglobin concentration of a hemorrhaging patient undergoing resuscitation will be changing rapidly. Under these conditions, the margin of safety is very small when the hemoglobin concentration is reduced as low as $7\,g\,dL^{-1}$. Thus, until more data are available, the hemoglobin concentration of the severely injured patient should be targeted at around $10\,g\,dL^{-1}$.

Fluid warming

Hypothermia (a core temperature less than 35 °C) is a serious complication of severe trauma and hemorrhage.[74] The etiology of hypothermia in these patients is multifactorial and includes exposure, tissue hypoperfusion, and infusion of inadequately warmed fluids. All intravenous fluids should be warmed properly as prevention is better than cure. A high-capacity fluid warmer, such as the Level 1 (Fig. 42.4),[75] will be required to cope with the rapid infusion rates used during resuscitation of a patient with multiple injuries. Following severe trauma, survival correlates with the degree of hypothermia: those with a core temperature dropping below 34 °C have a 40% mortality compared with 7% for those whose lowest recorded core temperature is 34 °C or above.[76] Hypothermia also increases fluid requirements and independently increases acute mortality after trauma.[77]

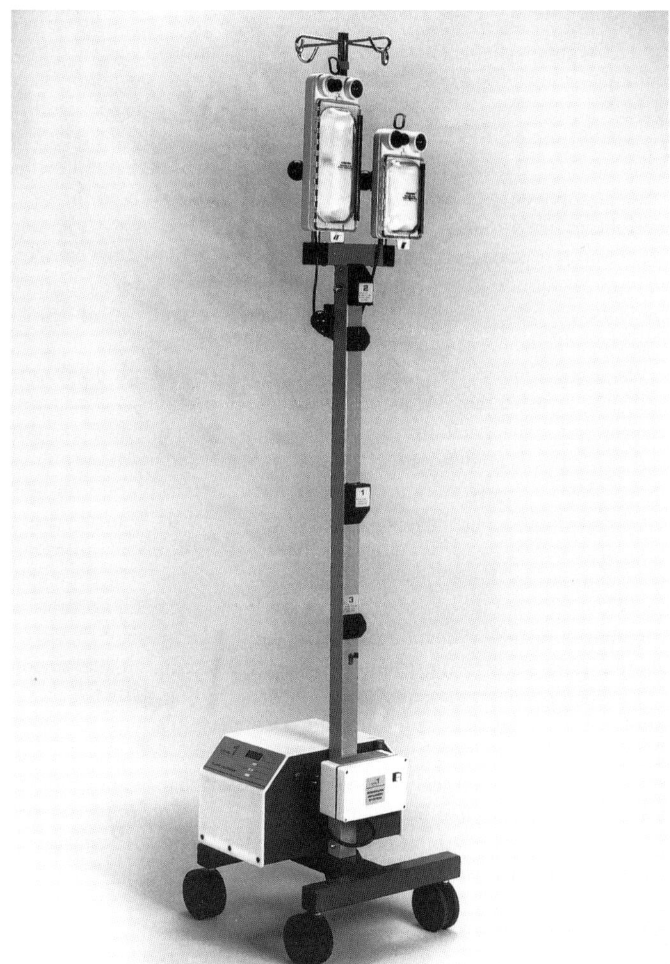

Figure 42.4 *A high-capacity, Level 1 fluid warmer.*

Disability: a rapid assessment of neurological function

The patient's conscious level is assessed at this stage to ensure that any possible compromise owing to hypoxia or hypotension has been eliminated. The size of the pupils and their reaction to light should be checked. This is particularly important at this stage if the patient requires urgent induction of anesthesia and intubation. Conscious level must be assessed rapidly using the GCS to record the patient's verbal response, eye-opening response, and best motor response. Clearly, problems can arise when assessing the verbal response in the intubated patient and eye opening may be impeded by the presence of bilateral periorbital edema. In such cases, this should be recorded rather than omitting the assessment. Motor assessment is made bilaterally and the best response recorded to ensure that limb injuries or focal brain lesions, both of which may restrict movement unilaterally, do not artificially lower the score achieved. The most appropriate painful stimulus is pressure on the supratrochlear nerve rather than on a nail bed, as the latter may not be sensed in the presence of a spinal cord lesion. Localizing to pain is defined as the patient's hand reaching above the level of the clavicle.

The GCS is a reliable, reproducible, and dynamic measurement; the trend in the conscious level is more important than one static reading. Although alcohol and other drugs can affect the level of consciousness, these must never be assumed to be the sole cause. Hypoxia and hypotension must be excluded and any persisting changes must be considered to be indicative of intracranial pathology until proved otherwise.

The pupillary response and the presence of any lateralizing signs must be recorded. A dilated pupil in a patient in coma can be due to pressure on the occulomotor nerve from a displaced medial temporal lobe, and is therefore a sign of ipsilateral hematoma or brain injury. A hematoma pressing on the motor cortex usually causes contralateral motor weakness. However, it may be of such magnitude that the whole hemisphere is shifted, pressing the opposite cerebral peduncle against the edge of the tentorium. This will cause ipsilateral weakness, although its clinical detection will be masked in what will probably be a deeply comatose patient.

Exposure with environmental control

In the patient with multiple injuries, it is essential that all clothing be removed to allow examination of the entire body surface. The patient's injuries and the possibility of spinal instability preclude removing clothes in the normal way and these are best removed by cutting along the seams. The conscious patient should always be given an explanation and permission sought! Once this has been achieved, it is essential to protect the patient from hypothermia with warm blankets and by keeping the room temperature adequate.

Monitoring

During the primary survey, the adequacy of resuscitation is best guided by quantitative assessment of the patient's physiological status. The

ECG will provide the heart rate while, at the same time, arrhythmias and ST segment changes may also give early indication of cardiac injury. Initially, blood pressure is measured using an automated noninvasive device. A pulse oximeter gives useful information about the hemoglobin oxygen saturation, but does not give information about the adequacy of ventilation. In the cold, shocked, and vasoconstricted patient following trauma, these devices often fail to give information owing to the poor peripheral perfusion. An arterial blood sample for gas analysis should be obtained as soon as practical, usually toward the end of the primary survey or sooner if there are sufficient personnel. Severely injured patients will have a marked base deficit, and its correction will help to confirm adequate resuscitation.

By any definition, the patient with major injuries is critically ill, and warrants invasive monitoring at the earliest opportunity.[78] The anesthesiologist is the usual member of the trauma team to undertake this task. An arterial cannula (radial, brachial, or femoral) allows continuous direct blood pressure monitoring and frequent arterial blood sampling for the assessment of gas exchange and acid–base status. Central venous pressure monitoring gives useful information after the initial fluid challenge and is also best displayed continuously. In the ventilated patient, end-tidal CO_2 should be monitored to guide the adequacy of ventilation, but it must be remembered that in the shocked patient there is a significant increase in the arterial to alveolar gradient. Catheterization of the bladder allows measurement of the urine output, a further useful indicator of the adequacy of resuscitation of the circulation, albeit over a slightly longer period. The patient's temperature should be monitored, rather than relying on feeling the skin, to ensure that hypothermia is avoided. A nasogastric tube will allow stomach contents to be drained and reduce the risk of aspiration. If there is any suspicion of a basal skull fracture, the orogastric route should be used.

Resuscitation endpoints

Some investigators have questioned whether simply returning the heart rate, blood pressure, and urine output to normal represents a suitable resuscitation endpoint for the traumatized patient. Once bleeding has been controlled, goal-directed therapy, with the aim of increasing oxygen delivery and oxygen consumption, may increase survival following severe trauma.[79] This approach requires the early insertion of a pulmonary artery floatation catheter (see Chapter 67).

Hypotensive resuscitation

Recent evidence from a number of animal studies and one human study has suggested that, in some circumstances, aggressive fluid resuscitation before surgical control of bleeding may be detrimental.[80–83] Simplistically, increasing the blood pressure with fluid in the presence of active bleeding merely accelerates the loss of red blood cells and may hamper clotting mechanisms. However, it must be emphasized that the evidence supporting a "delayed" fluid resuscitation strategy relates only to young adults with penetrating torso injuries occurring in an urban environment where there is rapid transport to hospital. Until further evidence is available, it would be inappropriate to extrapolate these findings to all traumatized patients, particularly those following blunt trauma, those with head injuries, the older population, or those who may be some distance from hospital.

Radiographs

All patients sustaining significant blunt trauma need their chest and pelvis to be radiographed. These films must be taken in the resuscitation room and must be obtained as soon as possible, but without interrupting the resuscitation process. The cervical spine is usually radiographed during the secondary survey.

The secondary survey

The objectives of the secondary survey are shown in Table 42.10. The secondary survey should not begin until the immediately life-threatening conditions have been identified and treated and the patient is stable. For those patients who require urgent surgical intervention, usually as a result of either exsanguinating or intracranial hemorrhage, the secondary survey will be postponed, but must take place later on the intensive care unit.

The following is intended as a brief outline of the conditions identified in the secondary survey that are of immediate relevance to the anesthesiologist. For greater detail, the reader is advised to see the current edition of the ATLS manual.[2]

Head

The scalp must be inspected and palpated for lacerations, hematomas, or depressed fractures. These may signify underlying brain injury and an increased risk of intracranial hematoma. Signs of a basal skull fracture include raccoon eyes, cerebral spinal fluid (CSF) rhinorrhea and otorrhea, and hemotympanum. If suspected, pass an oral tube but avoid passing a nasogastric tube. Inspect the mouth for loose or missing teeth, particularly prior to laryngoscopy and intubation. The airway may be compromised by middle third facial fractures which can bleed profusely, whereas mandibular fractures may result in posterior displacement of the tongue. Neurological status is reassessed using the GCS, pupillary response, and symmetry of motor response. This must always be performed and documented before the administration of anesthetic drugs. With any deterioration from a previous assessment, it is essential to exclude hypoxia and hypotension, following which further investigation, usually a computed tomography (CT) scan, will be required. Indications for an urgent CT scan will vary according to local policy. The indications used in the UK[84] are shown in Table 42.11.

Table 42.10 *The objectives of the secondary survey*

Examine the patient
- Head to toe
- Front to back

Obtain a complete medical history
Obtain all clinical, laboratory, and radiological information
Formulate a management plan

Table 42.11 *Indications used in the UK for urgent computed tomography (CT) scanning*

Coma persisting after resuscitation
Deteriorating conscious level or progressive neurological signs
Skull fracture with any of the following:
- Confusion or worsening impairment of consciousness
- Epileptic seizure
- Neurological signs or symptoms

Open injury:
- Depressed compound skull vault fracture
- Fracture of skull base
- Penetrating injury

Confusion or neurological signs persisting after resuscitation
Uncertain diagnosis:
- Drugs or alcohol complicating assessment
- Patients with a history of a loss of consciousness requiring prolonged anesthesia for other injuries

Unstable state precluding safe transfer to neurosurgical center

Neck

With an assistant providing MILS, the cervical spine is palpated for deformity, muscle spasm, and, in the case of a conscious patient, tenderness and pain. The neck must be inspected anteriorly for wounds, crepitus, and surgical emphysema. Injuries in this region may hinder laryngoscopy, tracheal intubation, and the insertion of central venous catheters.

Lateral, anteroposterior (AP), and odontoid radiographs are taken of the cervical spine. The craniocervical junction to the junction of the seventh cervical (C7) and first thoracic (T1) vertebrae must be clearly visible in the lateral view. This may entail careful caudal traction of the patient's arms to pull the shoulders out of the field (Fig. 42.5) or, alternatively, a swimmer's view (lateral oblique with one arm raised).

If these fail to show the C7–T1 junction, a CT scan will be required.[38] Interpretation of cervical spine radiographs is notoriously difficult. Alignment can be checked by identifying the four lordotic curves on the lateral radiograph: the anterior vertebral line, the anterior spinal canal, the posterior spinal canal, and the spinous process tips (Fig. 42.6). Widening of the prevertebral space may be another indication of cervical spine injury. It is important to be aware that radiographs show only the resting position and not the dynamics of the injury; apparently normal cervical radiographs alone do not exclude injury to the cervical spine or spinal cord at this level – they must be accompanied by a reliable clinical examination. Thus, a sensible approach to the resuscitation of traumatized patients with known mechanisms of injury is to initially treat all of them as if they have an unstable cervical spine injury, even if the initial plain films are normal.[85] The use of appropriate radiographs, targeted CT scanning, and, if necessary, dynamic fluoroscopy will allow possible damage to the cervical spine to be excluded in due course.[86,87]

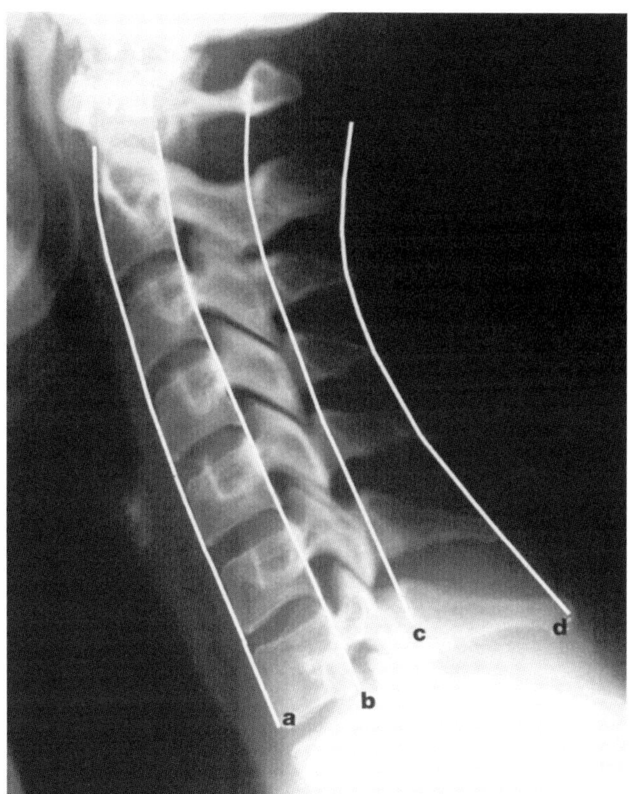

Figure 42.6 *Lateral radiograph of the cervical spine showing (a) the anterior vertebral line; (b) the anterior spinal canal; (c) the posterior spinal canal; and (d) the tips of the spinous processes. Note: taken in a patient following a whiplash injury with resultant loss of the normal cervical lordosis.*

Chest

A thorough examination is mandatory for all patients presenting for anesthesia and surgery following severe trauma (Table 42.7). Do not forget the back! Fractured ribs may indicate underlying pulmonary contusions, the commonest potentially lethal chest injury. Fractures also predispose to a pneumothorax if mechanical ventilation is required.

Myocardial contusion

Cardiac contusion must be considered in any patient with severe blunt chest trauma, particularly those with sternal fractures. An elevated central venous pressure (CVP) in the presence of hypotension may be the earliest indication of myocardial dysfunction secondary to severe cardiac contusion, but cardiac tamponade must be excluded. The right ventricle is the most frequently injured as it is predominantly an anterior structure. Cardiac arrhythmias and ST changes on the ECG may indicate contusion, but these signs are very nonspecific.[88,89] A rise in serum creatine kinase MB (CK-MB) is very nonspecific after trauma as it can be elevated as a result of injury to skeletal muscle alone. Rises in cardiac troponin I may be more specific for the detection of cardiac contusion.[90] The severely contused myocardium is likely to require inotropic support in conjunction with invasive hemodynamic monitoring.

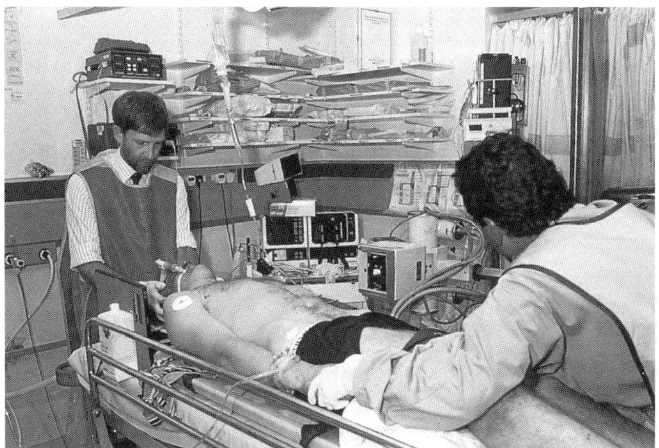

Figure 42.5 *Caudal traction on the patient's arms while taking a lateral radiograph of the cervical spine to ensure an adequate film is obtained (to C7–T1 junction).*

Blunt aortic injury

Blunt aortic injury (Fig. 42.7) should be suspected in any patient with a history of a significant decelerating force (e.g. fall from a height or high-speed road traffic accident). The commonest site of injury is the aortic isthmus, just distal to the origin of the left subclavian artery at the level of the ligamentum arteriosum. Although patients sustaining traumatic aortic rupture usually have multiple injuries and are therefore hypotensive at presentation, upper extremity hypertension is present in 40% of cases as the hematoma compresses the true lumen, causing a "pseudo-coarctation." In 85% of cases, a supine chest radiograph will show a widened mediastinum and possibly other features,[91] which are listed in Table 42.12. Although a widened mediastinum is a sensitive sign of aortic rupture, it is not very specific: 90% of cases are due to venous bleeding.

Although arteriography is traditionally the definitive investigation for blunt aortic injury,[92] it is increasingly being superseded by

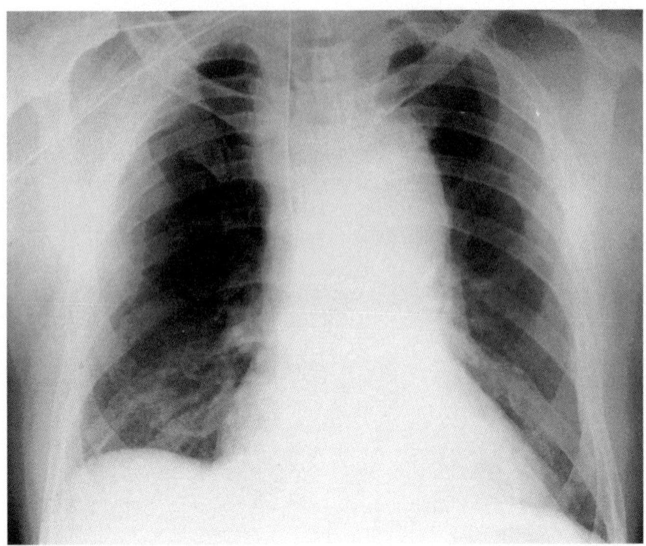

Figure 42.7 *Chest radiograph of a patient with blunt aortic injury. Note the widened mediastinum and deviation of the trachea and nasogastric tube to the right.*

Table 42.12 *Chest radiograph appearances suggesting aortic injury*

Pleural capping
Left hemothorax
Deviation of the trachea to the right
Depression of the left mainstem bronchus
Loss of the aortic knob
Deviation of the nasogastric tube to the right
Fracture of the thoracic spine

transesophageal echocardiography[93,94] along with helical CT scanning.[95] Arteriography is more prolonged, invasive, and requires a relatively stable patient. Once a rupture of the thoracic aorta is suspected, the patient's blood pressure should be stabilized at 12–13.3 kPa (90–100 mmHg) systolic[95,96] in an effort to reduce the risk of complete rupture and the patient transferred immediately to the nearest cardiothoracic unit. Short-acting beta-blocking drugs, for example esmolol, will reduce dP/dt and are the preferred agents for reducing the blood pressure. In a recent study in the USA, the mortality of 274 patients with blunt aortic injury reaching hospital alive was 31%, with 63% of deaths being attributable to aortic rupture.[97]

Diaphragmatic rupture

Rupture of the diaphragm occurs in about 5% of patients who sustain severe blunt trauma to the trunk, with 75% occurring on the left side. Signs and symptoms may include diminished breath sounds on the ipsilateral side, pain in the chest and abdomen, and respiratory distress.

Diagnosis can be made on a plain radiograph. Signs include an elevated hemidiaphragm, gas bubbles above the diaphragm, shift of the mediastinum to the opposite side, and presence of the gastric tube in the chest. Despite this, the diagnosis is initially commonly missed. Instilling contrast media through the gastric tube and repeating the radiograph makes the definitive diagnosis.

Injury to the major airways

Transections of the trachea or bronchi proximal to the pleural reflection cause massive mediastinal and cervical emphysema. Injuries distal to the pleural sheath lead to pneumothoraces, which do not resolve after chest drainage because the bronchopleural fistula causes a large air leak. Most bronchial injuries occur within 2.5 cm of the carina and the diagnosis is confirmed by bronchoscopy.

Abdomen

The priority is to determine the need for laparotomy rather than attempting to define precisely which viscus is injured.[98] Diagnostic peritoneal lavage, ultrasound, or CT is indicated whenever abdominal examination is unreliable. This will include patients:

- with a depressed level of consciousness (head injury, drugs, or alcohol);
- with fractures of the lower ribs or pelvis;
- in whom examination is equivocal, particularly if prolonged general anesthesia for other injuries will make reassessment impossible.

Ultrasound is being used increasingly to allow rapid identification of pericardial and peritoneal blood. The technique of "focused assessment with sonography for trauma" (FAST) can be undertaken by appropriately trained members of the trauma team.[99] The procedure can be learnt after 8 h of training and 200 supervised patient examinations.

Extremities

All limbs must be inspected for bruising, wounds, and deformities, and examined for vascular and neurological defects. Appropriate reduction of any deformity and splinting of the limb reduces blood loss, neurovascular impairment, pain, and the risk of fat emboli. All these factors must be taken into account before attempting to achieve vascular access or positioning a patient before surgery.

Spinal column

A detailed neurological examination for signs of spinal cord injury must be performed, particularly in the unconscious patient. Simply leaving a patient on a long spine board "just in case" is unacceptable because of the risk of developing decubitus ulcers. Patients in whom clinical examination is unreliable (distracting injuries, reduced level of consciousness) will require AP and lateral radiographs of the entire thoracolumbar spine. However, if the urgency of surgery prevents this, it is mandatory to assume injury to the spinal column or cord and to ensure that the patient is turned only using a log-roll technique, with an appropriate number of people, to maintain spinal alignment.

Medical history

During the secondary survey, or sooner if urgent surgery is required, a medical history must be obtained as this may affect subsequent management. Ideally, this may be obtained from the patient, but, if this is impossible, relatives, paramedics, hospital, and general practitioner records can be useful sources of information. Essential details can be obtained using the "AMPLE" mnemonic (Table 42.13).

A large proportion of the population take medication and the incidence increases with age.[100] Cardiac drugs may modify the response to both the initial injury and the resuscitation. The link between alcohol consumption and trauma is well recognized, but it is important to remember the potential for complications arising from chronic use.

Table 42.13 *Essential medical details*

Allergies
Medications
Past medical history
Last food or fluid
Events of the incident and the environment

The use of recreational drugs will also modify the patient's response to trauma.[101] The patient's past medical history is a very relevant factor as this has a profound influence on eventual outcome. In the USA, the incidence of premorbid conditions ranges from 5% to 16%, whereas in the UK it has been reported as being as high as 39%.[102] All age groups are affected, the elderly being most at risk, with cardiovascular and respiratory diseases being the most common. Although the timing of last intake of food or fluid is useful, patients following trauma are treated in the acute phase as having a full stomach.

Details of the events and environment relating to the incident are important, in particular the mechanism of injury because this may give clues to the presence of undiagnosed injuries.

Analgesia

Effective analgesia should be given to the patient as soon as practically possible. If the patient needs surgery imminently, then immediate induction of general anesthesia is a logical and very effective solution to the patient's pain. If not, an intravenous opioid (e.g. fentanyl or morphine) should be titrated to the desired affect. Head-injured patients will require adequate pain relief for any other injuries. Careful titration of intravenous morphine or fentanyl will provide effective pain relief without serious respiratory depression. The popular use of intramuscular codeine in head-injured patients is illogical. It is a weak opioid with the same side-effects as morphine, and in equianalgesic doses it is a more potent releaser of histamine. Intravenous administration of codeine is never clinically indicated and may be associated with a significant risk of severe hypotension.

Nonsteroidal anti-inflammatory drugs (NSAIDs) alone provide moderate analgesia but are relatively contraindicated in hypovolemia as these patients depend on prostaglandins to maintain renal blood flow. The new, highly selective cyclo-oxygenase 2 (COX-2) inhibitors may prove to be useful in the treatment of moderate pain after trauma.[103] In normovolemic patients following trauma, NSAIDs are synergistic with, and may reduce the dose of, opioids required for analgesia.

Local anesthetic blocks would have many advantages for the traumatized patient. Unfortunately, there are relatively few of these that are both simple and effective. One example is the femoral nerve block for patients with a fracture of the femoral shaft. Central neural blockade may have a role in some acute traumatized patients, but it is essential that hypovolemia and coagulopathy be first excluded. In patients with multiple ribs fractures, including flail segments, an appropriately placed thoracic epidural provides excellent analgesia.[104] This is usually instituted in an intensive therapy unit (ITU)/high-dependency unit (HDU) setting where it will help the patient to tolerate aggressive physiotherapy and maintain adequate ventilation, which may reduce the requirement for intubation and mechanical ventilation. A lumbar epidural will benefit those patients with lower limb injuries and, assuming there are no contraindications, this can be placed either preoperatively or postoperatively.

THE ANESTHESIOLOGIST IN THE OPERATING ROOM

For the majority of anesthesiologists, most of their contact with patients following severe trauma will be in the operating room; in the UK, this will constitute as much as 30–40% of their emergency workload. There are four main categories of severely injured patients requiring anesthesia for surgery:

1 patients requiring emergency surgery, who are transferred directly from the emergency department, with ongoing resuscitation;
2 patients who require limb-saving surgery after resuscitation;
3 patients who require major reconstructive surgery;
4 patients requiring follow-up surgery, e.g. repeat laparotomy, multiple orthopedic procedures.

It is the first group who provide the major challenge for the anesthesiologist in terms of continuing resuscitation while having to provide safe and effective anesthesia for surgery. The following guidance focuses on this group of patients.

Preparation for anesthesia

A full check of all drugs and equipment before use is a well-established principle in anesthesia. However, nowhere is this more important than when awaiting the arrival of a seriously injured patient, as the injuries that may have been sustained and the type and length of surgery likely to be required are varied. The following should be regarded as the minimum preparation for such a case:

1 Assemble adequate numbers of trained anesthetic assistants. At least two will be required to assist with emergency tracheal intubation (see below) and a third to administer drugs and fluids and to monitor the patient. The latter may be another anesthesiologist.
2 A full check of the anesthesia machine and ventilator must be performed. It may be necessary to change the ventilator to one capable of providing a variety of ventilatory modes to effectively ventilate lungs with poor compliance or high resistance. In particular, it must be capable of providing positive end-expiratory pressure (PEEP).
3 Assemble the equipment for ventilation. In addition to the usual range of tracheal tubes, laryngoscopes, bougies, and introducers, include double-lumen tubes for potential thoracotomy. The equipment for needle and surgical cricothyroidotomy should be immediately available, and either a fiberoptic laryngoscope or bronchoscope sterilized and assembled ready for immediate use.
4 A variety of different size and length venous cannulae/catheters, with and without guidewires, should be prepared, along with devices that allow rapid infusion of warmed intravenous fluids (e.g. a Level 1 fluid warmer).
5 Anesthetic and resuscitation drugs should be drawn up in syringes labeled to show contents and concentration.
6 All monitoring equipment should be checked for function and calibrated ready for immediate use. The seriously injured patient will require invasive monitoring.
7 Patient-warming devices, for example warming blankets, should be on and at operating temperature. A forced air warming system is the most efficient method of preventing hypothermia.
8 All the appropriate equipment for the safe positioning of the patient should be ready, with sterile padding.
9 Check that there is the equipment available to insert or change chest drains.

Anesthesia

Regional techniques

Central neural blockade and other regional anesthetic techniques are associated with a number of potential problems in the acute situation:

- sympathetic block may precipitate or increase hypotension;
- it may prove difficult to adequately or comfortably position a patient to institute the block;
- there may be unacceptable delays in achieving adequate surgical anesthesia;

- the technique may prove inadequate when there are injuries in different body areas that require surgery;
- the patient may find it difficult to be comfortable and to remain still during long surgical procedures.

The main role for regional techniques is to provide anesthesia for surgery in patients with an isolated skeletal injury, after they have been fully resuscitated. Consequently, general anesthesia with tracheal intubation is the most commonly used technique for the seriously injured patient who requires emergency surgery. The technique will be determined by a number of factors that include the physiological status of the patient, the surgery planned, the availability of drugs and equipment, and the skill and experience of the anesthesiologist.

Induction of anesthesia and intubation of the trachea

The patient must be regarded as having a full stomach and a possible injury to the cervical spine unless proved otherwise. The technique of choice is the same as that used in the emergency department, namely rapid sequence induction with manual inline stabilization of the head and neck (Fig. 42.8).[105,106] Stene and colleagues[107] have described a variation on this, which consists of gentle manual ventilation with 100% oxygen via a face mask prior to attempting intubation. This has two effects: (1) it improves oxygenation before intubation and (2) it indicates the ability to support ventilation of the patient in the event of a failed intubation.

All intravenous anesthetic agents depress both the cardiovascular and the respiratory systems to a varying degree; to date, there is no evidence that the choice of agent affects survival. The appropriate use of these agents in the seriously injured patient involves a careful assessment of the patient's clinical condition and a thorough knowledge of the pharmacology of the agents used. The safest course of action is for the anesthesiologist to use drugs with which he/she is most familiar. The patient who has sustained major trauma is not a suitable candidate for the evaluation of new techniques. Severely injured patients requiring anesthesia and intubation can be divided into three main groups:

1. Those who are severely hypotensive (systolic blood pressure < 10.6 kPa; < 80 mmHg), with ongoing resuscitation, and are severely neurologically obtunded. Induction agents are not usually required, but a neuromuscular blocking drug is used to facilitate tracheal intubation.
2. Those who are hypotensive (systolic blood pressure 10.6–13.3 kPa; 80–100 mmHg), hemodynamically unstable, or inadequately resuscitated. A reduced dose of intravenous induction agent is used. A neuromuscular blocking drug is used to facilitate intubation, along with a reduced dose of an analgesic.
3. Patients with an isolated head injury, with signs of raised intracranial pressure (bradycardia, hypertension, and irregular respiration). Normal doses of an induction agent, neuromuscular blocking drug, and analgesic are administered. Intubation may also be preceded by an intravenous bolus of lidocaine (lignocaine) intravenously.

Succinylcholine (suxamethonium) remains the neuromuscular blocking drug that provides optimal conditions for tracheal intubation in the shortest time and remains the first choice for the seriously injured patient. Despite this advantage, there are a number of important side-effects associated with the use of this drug, many of which are pertinent to these patients (Table 42.14). Previous concerns of an increase in intracranial pressure (ICP) in patients with a severe head injury are unfounded, provided that adequate anesthesia is provided.[108,109] The exaggerated release of potassium seen after the administration of succinylcholine in patients following severe burns does not occur within the first 48 h after the burn. A large dose of vecuronium has been a popular alternative in the USA,[110] but this has now been superseded by rocuronium.

Difficult intubation

Some seriously injured patients will be difficult to intubate as a result of:

- trauma to the soft tissues of the face and neck;
- midface fractures with significant hemorrhage;
- burns to the upper airway;
- a pre-existing anatomic difficulty combined with maintaining the neck in a neutral position.

In such circumstances, the immediate aim is to maintain adequate oxygenation using whatever method is available. This may include:

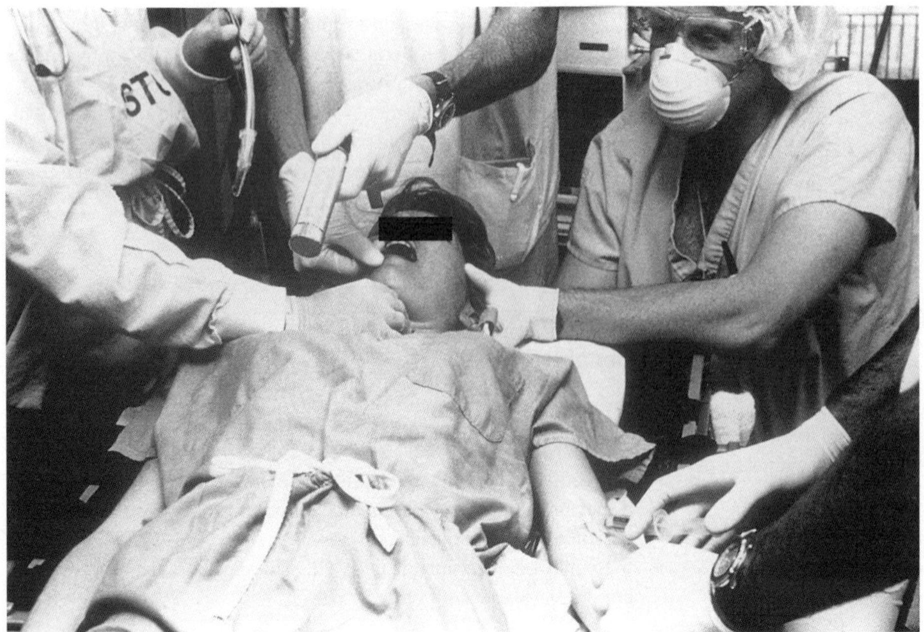

Figure 42.8 *Rapid-sequence induction of anesthesia prior to surgery. Note the similarity between this and Fig. 42.2.*

Table 42.14 *Potential adverse side-effects of succinylcholine (suxamethonium)*

Hyperkalemia
Worse after burns, denervation injury, major trauma with crush injuries
Trigger malignant hyperpyrexia
Increases intraocular pressure
Histamine release
Bradycardia – worse after large or repeat doses
Prolonged paralysis in atypical cholinesterase
Muscle pains

- bag–mask ventilation with an oro/nasopharyngeal airway and maintenance of cricoid pressure;
- insertion of a laryngeal mask airway, intubating laryngeal mask, or Combitube;
- needle or surgical cricothyroidotomy.

An algorithm to direct the management of such patients has been published by the American Society of Anesthesiologists' Task Force on Difficult Airway Management and has been modified to include the laryngeal mask airway (LMA) and Combitube (Fig. 42.9).[111] An LMA may provide a temporary airway and allow effective ventilation.[112,113] The use of this device does not guarantee protection against aspiration, but the risks are significantly reduced. It does protect against soiling of the airway from above,[114] which may be more relevant in the seriously injured patient with facial injuries in whom blood is more likely to be aspirated than gastric contents. A correctly positioned LMA may also be used as a conduit to pass a tracheal tube either blindly[115] or with the aid of an intubating bronchoscope. More recently, an intubating LMA (ILM) has been described to facilitate blind tracheal intubation[116] and has been used successfully following failed orotracheal intubation.[117] The Combitube[118] is a double-lumen tube which is inserted blindly and has been designed to allow ventilation of the patient's lungs irrespective of whether it enters the esophagus (over 90% of placements) or the trachea. It offers protection against aspiration from any direction, but to avoid inflation of the stomach, care must be taken to ensure that ventilation is via the correct lumen. The Combitube has been used successfully following failed intubation in seriously injured patients[119,120] and after cardiac arrest.[121]

Awake fiberoptic intubation is frequently proposed as the solution to difficult intubation, but this may prove difficult in a patient who is uncooperative or where significant hemorrhage into the upper airway reduces visibility.

The traditional solution to many cases of difficult intubation would have been inhalational induction of anesthesia, direct laryngoscopy, and attempted intubation, while maintaining spontaneous ventilation. This is inappropriate in the acute trauma patient because of the combination of the time taken, risk of aspiration, cardiovascular depression, breath-holding, and coughing. The recent introduction of sevoflurane may offer a solution to some of these problems. Sevoflurane is relatively insoluble and nonirritant, allowing rapid induction of anesthesia with minimal cardiovascular effects.[122] To date, there are only anecdotal reports of its use in emergency situations to induce anesthesia and allow intubation,[123,124] and further clinical evidence is required before this technique can be advocated in the seriously injured patient.

Once the patient has been intubated, or arrives in the anesthetic room already intubated, it is essential to confirm correct placement of the tube and to ensure adequacy of ventilation. End-tidal CO_2, oxygen saturation, expired tidal and minute volumes, ventilatory rate, and inspiratory pressure should be monitored. Ventilation should be achieved with the lowest peak and mean intrathoracic pressures to reduce the risk of barotrauma and to minimize the impediment to venous return.

A

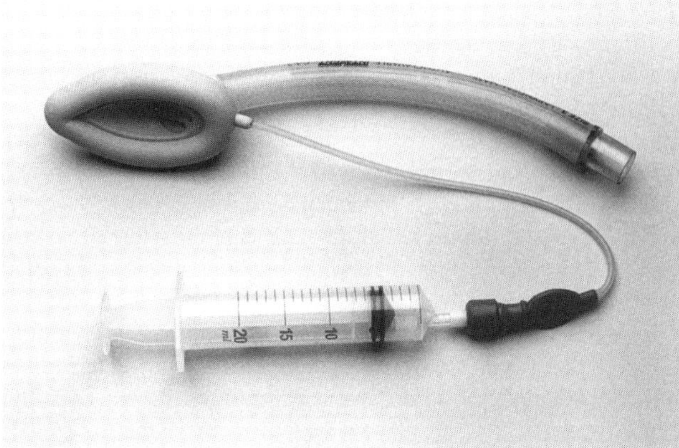

B

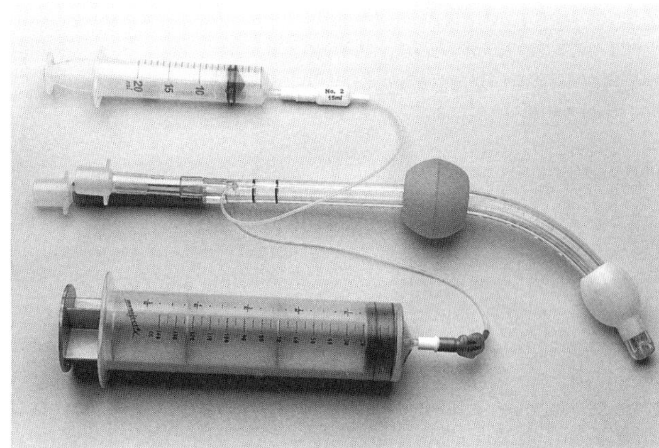

Figure 42.9 *(A) A laryngeal mask airway (LMA) with the cuff inflated. (B) A Combitube with both the proximal (oropharyngeal) and distal cuffs inflated.*

Oxygenation should be optimized by adjusting the inspiratory to expiratory ratio and PEEP. The final arbiter of adequacy of oxygenation and ventilation is arterial blood gas analysis. Normocarbia should be the aim unless the patient has a severe head injury, when mild hypocarbia is permissible (4.6 kPa; 35 mmHg), or in order to avoid barotrauma in the presence of severe pulmonary contusions, when a degree of hypercarbia is acceptable. If there are persistent difficulties with ventilation, there are a number of conditions that should be eliminated (Table 42.15).

Maintenance of anesthesia

The main aim is to provide an adequate flow of oxygenated blood to the vital organs, and to keep the patient unaware of the surgical procedure.

Table 42.15 *Common causes of impaired ventilation in the trauma patient*

Gastric dilation – pass an oro/nasogastric tube
Pneumothorax – insert a chest drain
Hemothorax – insert a chest drain
Ruptured diaphragm – surgical intervention
Pulmonary hemorrhage – endoscopy, consider double-lumen tube if unilateral
Bronchopleural fistula – double-lumen tube

Seriously injured patients are known to be at risk of awareness,[125] and anesthetic requirements will need to be judged on an individual basis. Patients who are initially profoundly shocked but in need of urgent surgery will usually tolerate the hemodynamic effects of anesthetic agents only when hemorrhage is under control and the mean arterial pressure (MAP) is adequate to ensure cerebral perfusion. Anesthesia is most commonly maintained by titrating inhalational agents, remembering that hypotension significantly reduces the minimum alveolar concentration (MAC). In addition, a potent analgesic, for example fentanyl or sufentanil, is usually administered. The effects of inhalational agents on the cerebral vasculature and intracranial pressure must also be considered in those patients with head injuries.

The use of nitrous oxide is controversial; however, it should be avoided in those patients whose injuries result in air entering body cavities, for example pneumocephalus and pneumothorax, or in those patients requiring a laparotomy where there are loops of gas-filled bowel. During prolonged surgery, there is the potential for interference with methionine synthesis. In those patients with pre-existing myocardial disease or myocardial injury, it can cause profound depression. Relying on nitrous oxide also limits the inspired oxygen concentration that can be administered. It is perhaps therefore more appropriate to identify those patients for whom nitrous oxide is specifically indicated, rather than using it routinely.

Monitoring

The choice of monitoring will depend upon the physiological status of the patient and the extent of surgery. All patients should be monitored in accordance with the local minimal standards, e.g. those of the Association of Anaesthetists of Great Britain and Ireland[126] or the American Society of Anesthesiologists.[127] Such recommendations apply in all areas where seriously injured patients are anesthetized. The more seriously injured will require more invasive monitoring. An intra-arterial cannula allows direct blood pressure measurement and frequent sampling of arterial blood for analysis of blood gases and metabolic status. Central venous and urinary catheters help to assess fluid balance. A pulmonary artery catheter may be required in patients who have suffered massive hemorrhage, either preoperatively or during surgery, in patients with extensive burns, and in patients with pre-existing heart disease or myocardial injury. An esophageal Doppler device is an alternative to the pulmonary artery catheter for the estimation of cardiac output. A Doppler probe positioned in the esophagus provides a beat-by-beat estimate of blood traveling through the descending aorta. This technique shows good correlation with the thermodilution techniques,[128] and has been widely evaluated in healthy and critically ill patients.[129] Hemodynamic deterioration can be detected by alterations in the waveform displayed, often earlier than changes in either arterial pressure or heart rate (Fig. 42.10).

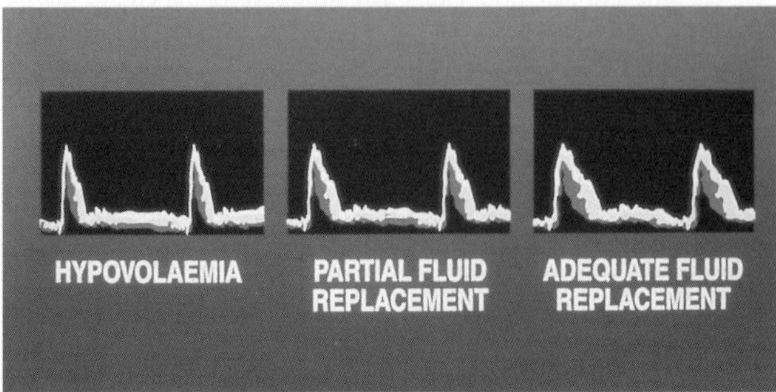

Figure 42.10 *Typical esophageal Doppler traces seen during the correction of hypovolemia. (Illustration courtesy of Medicina Ltd.)*

Specific problems during anesthesia for the seriously injured patient

Hypothermia

The majority of seriously injured patients will arrive in the operating room already hypothermic as a result of a prolonged time at the scene of the accident, exposure in the emergency department, and the administration of large volumes of cold intravenous fluids during resuscitation. In the operating room, further heat loss occurs as a result of evaporation of fluids from the surgical site and the respiratory tract, convection and radiation of heat from exposed body surfaces, and the continued administration of cold fluids, especially blood. These patients will need to be rewarmed and kept warm (Table 42.16). Hypothermia increases mortality after major trauma[77] through a number of mechanisms:

- It causes a gradual decline in cardiac output while increasing the propensity for myocardial dysrhythmias.[130] During surgery, there is an increase in the incidence of morbid cardiac events, even in mildly hypothermic patients.[131,132]
- The oxyhemoglobin dissociation curve is shifted to the left, impairing peripheral oxygen delivery at a time when it is most needed.
- Shivering may compound the lactic acidosis that typically accompanies hypovolemia, and this may be further aggravated by a decreased metabolic clearance of lactic acid by the liver.
- It contributes to the coagulopathy accompanying massive transfusion.[133] The likely mechanisms involved include retarding the function of enzymes in the clotting cascade,[134] enhanced plasma fibrinolytic activity,[135] reduced platelet aggregation,[136] and prolongation of the bleeding and prothrombin times.[137,138] Even mild hypothermia has been shown to increase blood loss during hip arthroplasty.[139]
- In the perioperative period, it increases the incidence of wound infection.[140]

Massive blood loss

Surgery for major trauma is frequently prolonged and is associated with the loss of large volumes of blood from intra-abdominal, intrathoracic, and vascular injuries and bone fractures. In addition, soft-tissue injuries will result in large "third-space" losses of fluid, all of which will be exacerbated by losses due to evaporation from wounds and open body cavities and insensible losses. The anesthesiologist may therefore be faced with replacing the equivalent of the patient's blood volume several times, along with large volumes of crystalloid and colloid solutions. Stored blood is usually supplied as plasma reduced and lacking clotting factors and platelets. Consequently, a coagulopathy and dilutional thrombocytopenia are common and will need to be treated. Although there are many "rules of thumb" for the administration of clotting fac-

Table 42.16 *Prevention of hypothermia in seriously injured patients during surgery*

Use a forced air-warming device
Use a heat and moisture exchanger (HME) between the tracheal tube and breathing system; actively warm and humidify anesthetic gases
Cover all body surfaces when exposure is not required for surgery, including the head
Maintain the operating room temperature as warm as possible (but still tolerable for the clinical staff)
Warm all fluids, both intravenous and those used for lavage by the surgeons
Place the patient on a warming blanket

tors and platelets, it is preferable to monitor the patient's coagulation status objectively and provide replacement therapy based upon the findings. Maintenance of the circulating volume is of greater importance than a normal hemoglobin, and a degree of hemodilution is acceptable. The concentration to which the hemoglobin can be allowed to fall will depend upon the presence of myocardial disease or injury, which limits the ability to increase cardiac output and maintain oxygen flux in the presence of anemia. Adequacy of volume replacement should be guided using the monitoring techniques already described. A metabolic acidosis is not uncommon in patients with major injuries. Frequent monitoring of base deficit and/or lactate along with invasive hemodynamic monitoring will guide therapy with fluids and inotropic agents.

Early compared with delayed stabilization of long-bone fractures

There is a sound theoretical and practical rationale for the primary internal or external fixation of long-bone fractures:[141,142]

- to reduce the incidence of acute respiratory distress syndrome;
- to allow upright or prone positioning of the patient and reduce the risk of atelectasis;
- to reduce the need for analgesia, which may impair ventilation;
- there is some evidence that it reduces the length of hospitalization and possibly mortality.

Recently, experimental data from animal models have shown that early intramedullary nailing of femoral fractures causes fat embolism and a systemic inflammatory response. Although some degree of microembolization undoubtedly occurs during reaming and intramedullary nailing of human femoral fractures, clinical studies of patients with or without primary chest injury have failed to show conclusively that this increases the incidence or severity of acute lung injury. Nonetheless, it would seem sensible to minimize the amount of reaming in patients with serious thoracic trauma.[143] In patients with head injuries, early fixation of long-bone fractures does not increase the incidence of adverse cerebral events, as long as hypoxia and hypotension are avoided. However, where possible, extensive surgery should be avoided and intracranial pressure should be monitored.

On the basis of current data, the general concept that early stabilization of long-bone fractures in multiply injured patients is beneficial remains valid.

SUMMARY

Following severe injury, patients will continue to make a significant contribution to the anesthesiologists' workload. The anesthesiologists' skills are relevant at almost every stage of the patient's management. Those involved in prehospital care must be properly trained and equipped. Accurate and precise communication from prehospital personnel will provide the opportunity for the anesthesiologist and other trauma team members to prepare for the patient's arrival in the resuscitation room. The management of the severely injured is divided into four phases: the primary survey, resuscitation, secondary survey, and definitive care. The primary survey and resuscitation are undertaken simultaneously. Those injuries that pose the greatest threat to life are dealt with first. Lack of a definitive diagnosis does not retard the start of appropriate treatment. The standard approach to advanced airway management for the acute trauma patient is preoxygenation, manual inline stabilization of the cervical spine, rapid sequence induction, the application of cricoid pressure, and oral intubation. The precise combination and doses of drugs used for the induction of anesthesia should be tailored to the hemodynamic and neurological state of the patient. Initial fluid resuscitation may be undertaken with crystalloid or colloid; there are no robust data to support a better outcome with one or the other. Hemoglobin solutions may become a useful option in the near future. Specific problems encountered in the operating room include hypothermia, massive blood loss, prolonged surgical time, and multiple surgical teams. In the patient with multiple injuries, early stabilization of long-bone fractures allows subsequent management of the patient to be optimized and improves outcome.

REFERENCES

1. Gupta KJ, Parr MJA, Nolan JP. Epidemiology of trauma. The role of the anesthesiologist. *Anesthesiol Clin North Am* 1999; **17:** 17–32.
2. The American College of Surgeons Committee on Trauma. *Advanced Trauma Life Support Program For Physicians: Instructor Manual*. Chicago: American College of Surgeons, 1997.
3. Parr MJA, Nolan JP, Desjardins G. Creating a trauma anaesthetic service. In: Berlot G, Delooz H, Gullo A (eds). *Trauma Operative Procedures*. Milan: Springer Verlag, 1999: 127–43.
4. Gwinnutt CL, Wilson AW, Driscoll P. Prehospital Care. In: Skinner D, Driscoll P, Earlam R (eds). *ABC of Major Trauma*, 3rd edn. London: BMJ Publishing Group, 2000: 129–33.
5. Potter D, Goldstein G, Fung SC, Selig M. A controlled trial of prehospital advanced life support in trauma. *Ann Emerg Med* 1988; **17:** 582–8.
6. Reines HD, Bartlett RL, Chudy NE, *et al.* Is advanced life support appropriate for victims of motor vehicle accidents? The South Carolina Highway Trauma Project. *J Trauma* 1988; **28:** 563–570.
7. Schmidt U, Frame SB, Nerlich ML, *et al.* On-scene helicopter transport of patients with multiple injuries – comparison of a German and an American system. *J Trauma* 1992; **33:** 548–55.
8. Sampalis JS, Lavoie A, Williams JI, *et al.* Impact of on-site care, prehospital time, and level of in hospital care on survival in severely injured patients. *J Trauma* 1993; **34:** 252–61.
9. Sampalis JS, Boukas S, Lavoie A, *et al.* Preventable death evaluation of the appropriateness of the on-site trauma care provided by Urgences-Sante physicians. *J Trauma* 1995; **39:** 1029–35.
10. Nicholl J, Hughes S, Dixon S, *et al.* The costs and benefits of paramedic skills in prehospital trauma care. *Health Technol Assess* 1988; **2** (17).
11. Cayten CG, Murphy JG, Stahl WM. Basic life support versus advanced life support for injured patients with an injury severity score of 10 or more. *J Trauma* 1993; **35:** 460–7.
12. Deakin CD. Strategies in the prehospital management of major trauma. *JEUR* 1995; **8:** 140–6.
13. Sampalis JS, Dennis R, Frechette P, *et al.* Direct transport to tertiary trauma centres versus transfer from lower level facilities: impact on mortality and morbidity among patients with major trauma. *J Trauma* 1997; **43:** 288–95.
14. Morley AP. Prehospital monitoring of trauma patients: experience of a hospital emergency medical service. *Br J Anaesth* 1996; **76:** 726–30.
15. Taylor PA, Towey RM. Depression of laryngeal reflexes during ketamine anaesthesia. *Br Med J* 1971; **2:** 688–9.
16. Reich DL, Silvay G. Ketamine: an update on the first twenty-five years of clinical experience. *Can J Anaesth* 1989; **36:** 186–97.
17. White PF, Way WL, Trevor AJ. Ketamine – its pharmacology and therapeutic uses. *Anesthesiology* 1982; **56:** 119–36.
18. Lundy PM, Lockwood PA, Thompson G, Frew R. Differential effects of ketamine isomers on neuronal and extraneuronal catecholamine uptake mechanisms. *Anesthesiology* 1986; **64:** 359–63.
19. Albanese J, Arnode S, Rey M, *et al.* Ketamine decreases intracranial pressure and electroencephalographic activity in traumatic brain injury patients during propofol sedation. *Anesthesiology* 1997; **87:** 1328–34.
20. Shapira Y, Lam AM, Eng CC, *et al.* Therapeutic time window and dose response of the beneficial effects of ketamine in experimental head injury. *Stroke* 1994; **25:** 1637–43.
21. Pfenninger E, Himmelseher S. Anesthesia with S(+)-ketamine. *Acta Anaesthesiol Scand* 1998; **112** (Suppl.): 213–15.
22. Cartwright PD, Pingel SM. Midazolam and diazepam in ketamine anaesthesia. *Anaesthesia* 1984; **39:** 439–42.
23. Szappanyos G, Gemperle M, Rifat K. Selective indications for ketamine anaesthesia. *Proc R Soc Med* 1971; **64:** 1156–9.
24. Bond AC, Davies CK. Ketamine and pancuronium for the shocked patients. *Anaesthesia* 1974; **29:** 59–62.
25. Bull PT, Merrill SB, Moody RA, *et al.* Anaesthesia during the Falklands campaign. The experience of the Royal Navy. *Anaesthesia* 1983; **38:** 770–5.

26. Cold GE, Eskesen V, Eriksen H, *et al.* CBF and $CMRO_2$ during continuous etomidate infusion supplemented with N_2O and fentanyl in patients with supratentorial cerebral tumour. A dose response study. *Acta Anaesthesiol Scand* 1985; **29:** 490–4.
27. Modica PA, Tempeloff R. Intracranial pressure during induction of anaesthesia and tracheal intubation with etomidate – induced EEG burst suppression. *Can J Anaesth* 1992; **39:** 236–41.
28. Heath KJ, Samra JS, Davis GE, *et al.* Blood pressure changes in head-injury patients during pre-hospital anaesthesia with propofol. *Injury* 1994; **25** (Suppl. 2): B7–B8.
29. Adnet F, Sydulka RK, Lapandry C. Emergency tracheal intubation of patients lying supine on the ground: Influence of operator body position. *Can J Anaesth* 1998; **45:** 266–9.
30. Nolan JP, Parr MJA. Aspects of resuscitation in trauma. *Br J Anaesth* 1997; **79:** 226–40.
31. Trunkey DD. Trauma. *Sci Am* 1993; **249:** 28–35.
32. Cowley R, Scanlan E. University Trauma Centre: operation, design and staffing. *Am Surg* 1979; **45:** 79–85.
33. Sauaia A, Moore FA, Moore EE, *et al.* Epidemiology of trauma deaths: a reassessment. *J Trauma* 1995; **38:** 185–93.
34. Wyatt J, Beard D, Gray A, *et al.* The time of death after trauma. *Br Med J* 1995; **310:** 1502.
35. Gwinnutt CL, Driscoll PA. Advanced trauma life support. *Eur J Anaesthesiol* 1996; **13:** 95–101.
36. Driscoll PA. Trauma: today's problems, tomorrow's answers. *Injury* 1992; **23:** 151–8.
37. Oakley PA. Setting and living up to national standards for the care of the injured. *Injury* 1994; **25:** 595–604.
38. Woodring JH, Lee C. Limitations of cervical radiography in the evaluation of acute cervical trauma. *J Trauma* 1993; **34:** 32–9.
39. Hills MW, Deane SA. Head injury and facial injury: Is there an increased risk of cervical spine injury? *J Trauma* 1993; **34:** 549–54.
40. Podolsky S, Baraff LJ, Simon RR, *et al.* Efficacy of cervical spine immobilisation methods. *J Trauma* 1983; **23:** 461–5.
41. Aprahamian C, Thompson BM, Finger WA, Darin JC. Experimental cervical spine injury model: Evaluation of airway management and splinting techniques. *Ann Emerg Med* 1984; **13:** 584–7.
42. Hauswald M, Sklar DP, Tandberg D, Garcia JF. Cervical spine movement during airway management: cinefluroscopic appraisal in human cadavers. *Am J Emerg Med* 1991; **9:** 535–8.
43. Dronen SC, Merigian KS, Hedges KR, *et al.* A comparison of blind nasotracheal and succinylcholine assisted intubation in the poisoned patient. *Ann Emerg Med* 1987; **16:** 650–2.
44. Meschino A, Devitt JH, Koch JP, *et al.* The safety of awake tracheal intubation in cervical spine injury. *Can J Anaesth* 1992; **39:** 114–17.
45. Wood PR, Lawler PGP. Managing the airway in cervical spine injury. A review of the Advanced Trauma Life Support protocol. *Anaesthesia* 1992; **47:** 792–7.
46. Criswell JC, Parr MJA, Nolan JP. Emergency airway management in patients with cervical spine injury. *Anaesthesia* 1994; **49:** 900–3.
47. Crosby ET. Tracheal intubation in the cervical spine-injured patient. *Can J Anaesth* 1992; **39:** 105–9.
48. Hastings RH, Kelley SD. Neurologic deterioration associated with airway management in a cervical spine-injured patient. *Anesthesiology* 1993; **78:** 580–3.
49. Majernick TG, Bieniek R, Houston JB, Hughes HG. Cervical spine movement during orotracheal intubation. *Ann Emerg Med* 1986; **15:** 417–20.
50. Hastings RH, Wood PR. Head extension and laryngeal view during laryngoscopy with cervical spine stabilization manoeuvres. *Anesthesiology* 1994; **80:** 825–31.
51. Bivins HG, Ford S, Bezmalinovic Z, *et al.* The effect of axial traction during orotracheal intubation of the trauma victim with an unstable cervical spine. *Ann Emerg Med* 1988; **17:** 25–9.
52. Turner LM. Cervical spine immobilization with axial traction: a practice to be discouraged. *J Emerg Med* 1989; **7:** 385–6.
53. Cormack RS, Lehane J. Difficult tracheal intubation in obstetrics. *Anaesthesia* 1984; **39:** 1105–11.
54. Heath KJ. The effect on laryngoscopy of different cervical spine immobilisation techniques. *Anaesthesia* 1994; **49:** 843–5.
55. Nolan JP, Wilson ME. Orotracheal intubation in patients with potential cervical spine injuries. An indication for the gum elastic bougie. *Anaesthesia* 1993; **48:** 630–3.
56. Laurent SC, de Melo AE, Alexander-Williams JM. The McCoy laryngoscope is superior to the Macintosh laryngoscope for laryngoscopy in patients with potential cervical spine injuries. *Anaesthesia* 1996; **51:** 74–5.
57. Ali J, Qi W. Effectiveness of chest tube clamping in massive hemothorax. *J Trauma* 1995; **38:** 59–63.
58. Westfall MD, Ray Price K, Lambert M, *et al.* Intravenous access in the critically ill trauma patient: a multicentered, prospective, randomised trial of saphenous cutdown and percutaneous femoral access. *Ann Emerg Med* 1994; **23:** 541–5.
59. Kruse JA, Vyskocil JJ, Haupt MT. Intraosseous infusions: a flexible option for the adult or child with delayed, difficult, or impossible conventional access. *Crit Care Med* 1994; **22:** 728–9.
60. Baskett PJF, Nolan JP. Hypovolaemic shock. In: Skinner D, Driscoll P, Earlam R (eds). *ABC of Major Trauma*, 3rd edn. London: BMJ Publishing Group, 2000: 27–33.
61. Ducey JP, Mozingo DW, Lamiell M, *et al.* A comparison of the cerebral and cardiovascular effects of complete resuscitation with isotonic and hypertonic saline, hetastarch, and whole blood following hemorrhage. *Crit Care Med* 1989; **17:** 1510–18.
62. Sutcliffe AJ. Crystalloid and colloids for volume replacement. *Trauma* 1999; **1:** 115–23.
63. Nolan JP. Fluid replacement. In: Yates DW (ed.). *Trauma: The Science of Success. Br Med Bull* 1999; **4:** 821–43.
64. Edwards JD, Nightingale P, Wilkins RG, Faragher EB. Hemodynamic and oxygen transport response to modified fluid gelatin in critically ill patients. *Crit Care Med* 1989; **17:** 996–8.
65. Schierhout G, Roberts I. Fluid resuscitation with colloid or crystalloid solutions in critically ill patients: a systematic review of randomised trials. *Br Med J* 1998; **316:** 961–4.
66. Choi PTL, Yip G, Quinonez LG, Cook DJ. Crystalloids vs. colloids in fluid resuscitation: a systematic review. *Crit Care Med* 1999; **27:** 200–10.
67. Mardel SN, Saunders FM, Allen H, *et al.* Reduced quality of clot formation with gelatin-based plasma substitutes. *Br J Anaesth* 1998; **80:** 204–7.
68. Treib J, Baron JF, Grauer MT, Strauss RG. An international view of hydroxyethyl starches. *Intensive Care Med* 1999; **25:** 258–68.
69. Gosling P. Prevention of post-traumatic capillary leak syndrome. *Trauma* 1999; **1:** 91–103.
70. Wade CE, Kramer GC, Grady JJ, *et al.* Efficacy of hypertonic 7.5% saline and 6% dextran-70 in treating trauma: a meta-analysis of controlled clinical studies. *Surgery* 1997; **122:** 609–16.
71. Conhaim RL, Harms BA. Hemoglobin therapeutics in hemorrhagic shock. *Curr Opin Crit Care* 1998; **4:** 442–6.
72. Weiskopf RB, Viele MK, Feiner J, *et al.* Human cardiovascular and metabolic response to acute severe isovolemic anemia. *JAMA* 1998; **279:** 217–21.
73. Hebert PC, Wells G, Blajchman MA, *et al.* A multicenter, randomized, controlled clinical trial of transfusion requirements in critical care. Transfusion requirements in Critical Care Investigators, Canadian Critical Care Trials Group. *N Engl J Med* 1999; **340:** 409–17.
74. Luna GK, Maier RV, Pavlin EG, *et al.* Incidence and effect of hypothermia in seriously injured patients. *J Trauma* 1987; **27:** 1014–18.
75. Browne DA, De Boeck R, Morgan M. An evaluation of the Level 1 blood warmer series. *Anaesthesia* 1990; **45:** 960–3.
76. Jurkovich GJ, Greiser WB, Luterman A, Curreri PW. Hypothermia in trauma victims: an ominous predictor of survival. *J Trauma* 1987; **27:** 1019–24.
77. Gentilello LM, Jurkovich GJ, Stark MS, *et al.* Is hypothermia in the victim of major trauma protective or harmful? A randomized, prospective study. *Ann Surg* 1997; **226:** 439–49.
78. Abou-Khalil B, Scalea TM, Trooskin SZ, *et al.* Hemodynamic responses to shock in young trauma patients: need for invasive monitoring. *Crit Care Med* 1994; **22:** 633–9.
79. Bishop MH, Shoemaker WC, Appel PL, *et al.* Prospective, randomized trial of survivor values of cardiac index, oxygen delivery, and oxygen consumption as resuscitation endpoints in severe trauma. *J Trauma* 1995; **38:** 780–7.
80. Stern SA, Dronen SC, Birrer P, Wang X. Effect of blood pressure on hemorrhage volume and survival in a near fatal model incorporating a vascular injury. *Ann Emerg Med* 1993; **22:** 155–63.
81. Kowalenko T, Stern SA, Dronen SC, Wang X. Improved outcome with hypotensive resuscitation of uncontrolled haemorrhagic shock in a swine model. *J Trauma* 1992; **33:** 349–53.
82. Capone AC, Safar P, Stezoski W, *et al.* Improved outcome with fluid restriction in treatment of uncontrolled hemorrhagic shock. *J Am Coll Surg* 1995; **180:** 49–56.
83. Bickell WH, Wall MJ, Pepe PE, *et al.* Immediate versus delayed fluid resuscitation for hypotensive patients with penetrating torso injuries. *N Engl J Med* 1994; **331:** 1105–9.
84. Bartlett J, Kett-White R, Mendlow AD, *et al.* Guidelines for the initial management of head injuries. *Br J Neurosurg* 1998; **12:** 349–52.
85. Stemp LI. A normal cervical spine X-ray does not "clear" the patient with suspected cervical spine injury. *Anesthesiology* 1993; **79:** 619–20.

86. Gupta KJ, Clancy M. Discontinuation of cervical spine immobilisation in unconscious patients with trauma in intensive care units – telephone survey of practice in South and West region. *Br Med J* 1997; **314:** 1652–5.
87. Lochey AS, Handley R, Willett K. Clearance of cervical spine injury in the obtunded patient. *Injury* 1998; **29:** 493–7.
88. Roxburgh JC. Myocardial contusion. *Injury* 1996; **27:** 603–5.
89. Petre R, Chilcott M. Blunt trauma to the heart and great vessels. *N Engl J Med* 1997; **336:** 626–32.
90. Adams JE, Davila-Roman VG, Bessey PQ, *et al.* Improved detection of cardiac contusion with cardiac troponin I. *Am Heart J* 1996; **131:** 308–12.
91. Mattox KL. Red River anthology. *J Trauma* 1997; **42:** 353–67.
92. Ahrar K, Smith DC, Bansal RC, *et al.* Angiography in blunt thoracic aortic injury. *J Trauma* 1997; **42:** 665–9.
93. Vignon P, Lagrange P, Boncoeur MP, *et al.* Routine transesophageal echocardiography for the diagnosis of aortic disruption in trauma patients without enlarged mediastinum. *J Trauma* 1996; **40:** 422–7.
94. Smith MD, Cassidy JM, Souther S, *et al.* Transesophageal echocardiography in the diagnosis of traumatic rupture of the aorta. *N Engl J Med* 1995; **332:** 356–62.
95. Fabian TC, Davis KA, Gavant ML, *et al.* Prospective study of blunt aortic injury. Helical CT is diagnostic and antihyperversive therapy reduces rupture. *Ann Surg* 1998; **227:** 666–77.
96. Frick EJ, Cipolle MD, Pasquale MD, *et al.* Outcome of blunt thoracic aortic injury in a level 1 trauma center: an 8 year review. *J Trauma* 1997; **43:** 844–51.
97. Fabian TC, Richardson D, Croce MA, *et al.* Prospective study of blunt aortic injury: multicenter trial of the American Association for the Surgery of Trauma. *J Trauma* 1997; **42:** 374–83.
98. Schuster-Bruce M, Nolan JP. Priorities in the management of blunt trauma. *Curr Opin Crit Care* 1999; **5:** 500–5.
99. Scalea TM, Rodriguez A. Focused assessment with sonography for trauma (FAST): results of an international consensus conference. *J Trauma* 1999; **46:** 466–72.
100. Walley T, Scott AK. Prescribing in the elderly. *Postgrad Med J* 1995; **71:** 466–71.
101. Soderstrom CA, Smith GS, Dischinger PC, *et al.* Psychoactive substance use disorder among seriously injured trauma centre patients. *JAMA* 1997; **277:** 1769–74.
102. Wardle TD. Medical problems in major trauma patients. In: Driscoll P, Skinner D (eds). *Trauma Care: Beyond the Resuscitation Room.* London: BMJ Publishing Group, 1998: 295–302.
103. Hawkey CJ. Cox-2 inhibitors. *Lancet* 1999; **353:** 307–14.
104. Moon MR, Luchette FA, Gibson SW, *et al.* Prospective, randomised comparison of epidural versus parenteral opioid analgesia in thoracic trauma. *Ann Surg* 1999; **229:** 684–92.
105. Suderman VS, Crosby ET, Lui A. Elective oral tracheal intubation in cervical spine-injured adults. *Can J Anaesth* 1991; **38:** 785–9.
106. Shatney CH, Brunner RD, Nguyen TQ. The safety of orotracheal intubation in patients with unstable cervical spine fracture or high spinal cord injury. *Am J Surg* 1995; **170:** 676–9.
107. Stene JK, Grande CM, Barton CR. Airway management for the trauma patient. In: Stene JK, Grande CM (eds). *Trauma Anesthesia.* Baltimore, MD: Williams & Wilkins, 1991: 64.
108. Brown MM, Parr MJA, Manara AR. The effects of suxamethonium on intracranial pressure and cerebral perfusion pressure in patients with severe head injuries following blunt trauma. *Eur J Anaesthiol* 1996; **13:** 474–7.
109. Kovarik WD, Mayberg TS, Lam AM, *et al.* Succinylcholine does not change intracranial pressure, cerebral blood flow velocity or the electroencephalogram in patients with neurologic injury. *Anesth Analg* 1994; **78:** 469–73.
110. Norwood S, Myers MB, Butler TJ. The safety of emergency neuromuscular blockade and orotracheal intubation in the acutely injured trauma patient. *J Am Coll Surg* 1994; **179:** 646–52.
111. Benumof JL. Laryngeal mask airway and the ASA difficult airway algorithm. *Anesthesiology* 1996; **84:** 686–99.
112. Greene MK, Roden R, Hinchley G. The laryngeal mask airway. Two cases of pre-hospital trauma care. *Anaesthesia* 1992; **47:** 688–9.
113. Pennant JH, Pace NA, Gajraj NM. Role of the laryngeal mask airway in the immobile cervical spine. *J Clin Anesthesiol* 1993; **5:** 226–30.
114. John RE, Hill S, Hughes TJ. Airway protection by the laryngeal mask: a barrier to die placed in the pharynx. *Anaesthesia* 1991; **46:** 366–7.
115. Heath ML, Allagain J. Intubation through the laryngeal mask. A technique for unexpected difficult intubation. *Anaesthesia* 1991; **46:** 545–8.
116. Baskett PJF, Parr MJA, Nolan JP. The intubating laryngeal mask. Results of a multi-centre trial with experience of 500 cases. *Anaesthesia* 1998; **53:** 1174–9.
117. Parr MJA, Gregory M, Baskett PJF. The intubating laryngeal mask. Use in failed and difficult intubation. *Anaesthesia* 1998; **53:** 343–8.
118. Frass M, Frenzer R, Zhadral F, *et al.* The oesophageal tracheal Combitube: preliminary results with a new airway for CPR. *Ann Emerg Med* 1987; **16:** 768–72.
119. Eichinger S, Schreiber W, Heinz T, *et al.* Airway management in a case of neck impalement: use of the oesophageal tracheal combitube airway. *Br J Anaesth* 1992; **68:** 534–5.
120. Blowstein PA, Koestner AJ, Hoak S. Failed rapid sequence intubation in trauma patients: esophageal tracheal combitube is a useful adjunct. *J Trauma* 1998; **44:** 534–7.
121. Lefrancois D. Use of the esophageal–tracheal combitube (ETC) in pre-hospital cardiorespiratory arrest (CRA) in a EMT-D level EMS system. *Resuscitation* 1998; **37:** S44.
122. Smith I, Nathanson M, White PF. Sevoflurane – a long awaited volatile anaesthetic. *Br J Anaesth* 1996; **76:** 435–45.
123. Mostafa SM, Atherton AMJ. Sevoflurane for difficult tracheal intubation. *Br J Anaesth* 1997; **79:** 392–3.
124. Ip-Yam PC. Sevoflurane in acute airway obstruction. *Br J Anaesth* 1998; **80:** 272–3.
125. Bogetz MS, Katz JA. Recall of surgery for major trauma. *Anesthesiology* 1984; **61:**6–9.
126. Association of Anaesthetists of Great Britain and Ireland. *Recommendations for Standards of Monitoring during Anaesthesia and Recovery.* London: The Association of Anaesthetists of Great Britain and Ireland, 1998.
127. Cass NM, Rosby WM, Holland RB. Minimal monitoring standards. *Anesth Intensive Care* 1988; **16:** 110–13.
128. Singer M, Clarke J, Bennett ED. Continuous hemodynamic monitoring by esophageal Doppler. *Crit Care Med* 1989; **17:** 447–52.
129. Singer M. Esophageal Doppler monitoring of aortic blood flow: beat by beat cardiac output monitoring. In: Royston D, Feely TW (eds). *International Anesthesiology Clinics, Monitoring in Anesthesiology: Current Standards and Newer Techniques.* 1993; **3:** 3.
130. Paton BC. Cardiac function during accidental hypothermia. In: Pozos RE, Wittmer LE (eds). *The Nature and Treatment of Hypothermia.* Minneapolis: University of Minnesota Press, 1983: 133–42.
131. Frank SM, Fleisher LA, Breslow MJ, *et al.* Perioperative maintenance of normothermia reduces the incidence of morbid cardiac events. *JAMA* 1997; **277:** 1127–34.
132. Sessler DI. Mild perioperative hypothermia. *N Engl J Med* 1997; **336:** 1730–6.
133. Patt A, McCroskey BL, Moore EE. Hypothermia-induced coagulopathies in trauma. *Surg Clin North Am* 1988; **68:** 775–85.
134. Reed II RL, Bracey AW, Hudson JD, *et al.* Hypothermia and blood coagulation: dissociation between enzyme activity and clotting factor levels. *Circ Shock* 1990; **32:** 141–52.
135. Paul J, Cornillon B, Baguet J, *et al.* In vivo release of a heparin-like factor in dogs during profound hypothermia. *J Thorac Cardiovasc Surg* 1981; **82:** 45–8.
136. Valeri CR, Feingold H, Cassidy G, *et al.* Hypothermia-induced reversible platelet dysfunction. *Ann Surg* 1987; **205:** 175–81.
137. Staab DB, Sorensen J, Fath JJ, *et al.* Coagulation defects resulting from ambient temperature induced hypothermia. *J Trauma* 1994; **36:** 634–8.
138. Valeri CR, MacGregor H, Cassidy G, *et al.* Effects of temperature on bleeding time and clotting time in normal male and female volunteers. *Crit Care Med* 1995; **23:** 698–704.
139. Scmied H, Kurz A, Sessler DI, *et al.* Mild hypothermia increases blood loss and transfusion requirements during hip arthroplasty. *Lancet* 1996; **347:** 289–92.
140. Kurz A, Sessler DI, Lenhardt R. Perioperative normothermia to reduce the incidence of surgical-wound infection and shorten hospitalization. *N Engl J Med* 1996; **334:** 1209–15.
141. Rommens PM, Hessmann M. Early versus delayed surgery for musculoskeletal trauma in polytraumatized patients. *Curr Opin Crit Care.* 1998; **4:** 424–8.
142. Philips TF, Contreras DM. Timing of operative treatment of fractures in patients who have multiple injuries. *J Bone Joint Surg* 1990; **72-A:** 784–8.
143. Bosse MJ, Mackenzie EJ, Riemer BL, *et al.* Adult respiratory distress syndrome, pneumonia, and mortality following thoracic injury and a femoral fracture treated either with intramedullary nailing with reaming or with a plate. *J Bone Joint Surg* 1997; **79-A:** 799–809.

FURTHER READING

Dutton RP, Mackenzie CF, Scalea TM. Hypotensive resuscitation during active hemorrhage: impact on in-hospital mortality. *J Trauma* 2002; **52:** 1141–6.

Eastern Association for the Surgery of Trauma (EAST). Determination of cervical spine stability in trauma patients (update of the 1997 EAST cervical spine clearance document), www.east.org.

Ford P, Nolan JP. Cervical spine injury and airway management. *Curr Opin Anaesthesiol* 2002; **15:** 193–201.

Gestring ML, Gracias VH, Feliciano MA, *et al.* Evaluation of the lower spine after blunt trauma using abdominal computed tomographic scanning supplemented with lateral scanograms. *J Trauma* 2002; **53:** 9–14.

McLeod ADM, Calder I. Spinal cord injury and direct laryngoscopy – the legend lives on. *Br J Anaesth* 2000; **84:** 705–8.

Nolan J. Fluid resuscitation for the trauma patient. *Resuscitation* 2001; **48:** 57–70.

Pasquale MD, Nagy K, Clarke J. EAST Practice Parameter Workgroup for Screening Blunt Cardiac Injury. Practice management guidelines for screening of blunt cardiac injury, www.east.org.

43

Anesthesia for orthopedic surgery

HEIDI V GORDON AND FRANK L MURPHY

INTRODUCTION

Orthopedic operations rarely compromise the function of major organ systems in the same way that invasive neurosurgical, abdominal, cardiac, or thoracic procedures may. Therefore, relatively few patients die as an immediate result of orthopedic surgery, provided that they receive competent care. Nevertheless, these patients gain much from skillful management of their anesthetics. Enhanced patient comfort, fewer transfusions, a reduced rate of nerve damage, fewer infections, fewer and less severe episodes of hypotension and hypertension, lessened risk of thromboemboli, and even a reduced death rate may all be achieved by sophisticated anesthesia management directed at the special needs of orthopedic patients.

Such management calls on information found elsewhere in this book. Orthopedic patients may be taking steroids or suffer from endocrine diseases associated with osteoporosis (Chapter 24). With increasing frequency, they are elderly (Chapter 60); children also require special techniques (Chapter 59). Orthopedic procedures frequently require positions more hazardous than the supine (Chapter 40). Patients who undergo minor orthopedic procedures often return home on the day of operation (Chapter 62). This chapter addresses issues specific for patients requiring anesthesia for orthopedic procedures.

ISSUES COMMON TO PATIENTS REQUIRING ORTHOPEDIC PROCEDURES

Preoperative evaluation

Preoperative evaluation of patients scheduled for orthopedic procedures requires special attention to a number of matters. Difficulties in positioning arise, owing to arthritis, fractures, joint deformities, or unstable vertebrae; sometimes it is profitable to rehearse the surgical position while the patient is awake. Patients with aseptic necrosis of the femoral or humeral head may abuse alcohol, take steroids, or have suffered from barotrauma. If the patient has donated autologous blood in anticipation of a major operation, it is prudent to assure the availability of these units before inducing anesthesia.

Rheumatoid arthritis and ankylosing spondylitis

Patients suffering from rheumatoid arthritis and ankylosing spondylitis present for a wide variety of orthopedic procedures, ranging from spine surgery to prosthetic replacement of hip, knee, and hand joints. Patients with rheumatoid arthritis are more likely to be women. Peripheral joints are more severely affected with sparing of the thoracic and lumbar spines, making spinal and epidural anesthesia practical choices. The most common locus for instability of the cervical spine is at C1–C2; the cervical spine is usually stable in extension, but not in flexion. Cervical spine disease may progress in the absence of symptoms. Arthritis affecting the temporomandibular joints may also restrict opening of the mouth, while cricoarytenoid joint disease may leave the patient hoarse, with limited vocal cord mobility, and with a restricted glottic opening.[1]

Ankylosing spondylitis occurs more often in men, is more likely to be confined to the spine, and affects the entire spine, making spinal and epidural anesthesia often impractical and leaving the spine unusually brittle. However, Schelew and Vaghadia[2] showed spinal anesthesia to have been successful in 76% of patients with ankylosing spondylitis for whom it was planned. The cervical spine is especially susceptible to fracture and dislocation at the C5–C7 level.[3]

These diseases introduce difficulties for the management of anesthesia. Immobility and fragility of the cervical spine result from either. Spinal cord or cervical root damage may already be present despite the absence of symptoms. Cervical spine films in flexion and extension should be obtained for patients with neck symptoms or long-standing erosive disease who will require general anesthesia. Careful radiologic evaluation of the cervical spine allows a specific approach to positioning for intubation.[4] Airway abnormalities often require techniques such as blind nasal intubation, fiberoptic intubation, or lighted stylet intubation (see Chapter 28).

Both rheumatoid arthritis and ankylosing spondylitis may affect organ systems other than bones and joints, but remaining function is almost always sufficient to permit orthopedic procedures. Restrictive pulmonary disease results from fibrosis and limitation of chest wall movement. Atherosclerosis following chronic steroid use, and coronary arteritis, may cause ischemic heart disease. Pericarditis, conduction defects, valvular disease, and renal damage may all be present.

Corticosteroid therapy

Many patients admitted for orthopedic procedures use or have used corticosteroids in the past. It has become routine for many surgeons and anesthesiologists to treat these patients with large doses of corticosteroids on the day of operation to avoid the risk of acute adrenal insufficiency. This practice is open to question. The rare harmful effect of corticosteroid deficiency, unwanted hypotension, may be treated after it occurs. Also, large doses of steroids can impair wound healing and immune function. Thus, it is possible that prophylactic corticosteroids do more harm than good; large-scale outcome studies are lacking. Furthermore, the dose or duration of previous steroid therapy does not predict the occurrence of adrenocortical deficiency. This makes it impossible to select those patients who should receive prophylactic treatment without formal testing of adrenal responses.[5] The patient's daily dose of corticosteroids should suffice unless the magnitude of the operative stress warrants larger doses of corticosteroids.[6]

Sickle cell disease

Patients with sickle cell disease are prone to ischemic necrosis of the femoral head and may require total hip arthroplasty, as well as other orthopedic procedures. It is logical to fear that the cooling, hypoxemia, and acidosis that occur distal to the tourniquet may provoke sickling. However, experience suggests that the use of a tourniquet does not increase the risk of sickle crisis in these patients.[7]

Patients suffering multiple trauma

Some victims of multiple trauma require immediate orthopedic surgery to treat an open bone or joint injury (6 h is a recommended maximum delay) or to relieve neurovascular compromise. There are a number of special concerns for the patient with fractures.

Cervical spine injury occurs in 1–3% of patients suffering major trauma, and the anesthesiologist should have an airway management plan for patients with neck injuries.[8] Blood loss from pelvic and femoral fractures, or from multiple fractures of smaller bones, can amount to many liters, and is difficult to estimate. Those caring for these patients must be prepared to deal with massive blood loss. In many cases, unreplaced blood loss and the difficulties in positioning the patient with multiple injuries make spinal or epidural anesthesia impractical. Inducing general anesthesia before transferring the patient from the stretcher or bed can provide welcome relief from the pain involved in movement. Respiratory distress unexplained by chest trauma may be due to pulmonary embolism from fat or thrombus, which is prevalent in these patients. If hypocapnia is needed to control increased intracranial pressure, arterial blood gas determination must be used to supplement measurement of end-tidal carbon dioxide as pulmonary injury widens the disparity between the two values by increasing functional dead space. Furthermore, augmented ventilation is also needed to treat the transient hypercapnia that follows deflation of the pneumatic tourniquet.[9]

Other injuries do not require immediate operation; the visit to the operating room can be delayed for days or weeks, so that acute problems of cardiovascular instability or respiratory insufficiency may resolve. However, the patient's injuries or the use of skeletal traction may still limit positioning for spinal or epidural anesthesia. If there has been extensive muscle injury, succinylcholine (suxamethonium) may provoke dangerous hyperkalemia. Thrombi that have accumulated in an injured leg may be mobilized during positioning, with skin preparation, during wrapping with an elastic bandage to express blood, or even with simple tourniquet inflation.[10] In such cases, it is best to avoid using the elastic bandage and simply elevate the leg to allow blood to drain before inflating the tourniquet.

Blood loss

Expected blood loss

During orthopedic procedures blood is lost from raw bone and muscle surfaces, rather than from identifiable blood vessels. This limits the surgeon's ability to control bleeding directly, allows much of the shed blood to escape collection by suction wands or gauze sponges, and insures that bleeding continues after the wound is closed. Surgeons and anesthesiologists almost always underestimate blood losses. A radioisotope study of blood lost in major orthopedic procedures showed that estimates of loss were, on average, 50% of the true measured losses.[11]

So many factors affect the volume of blood lost that tables of expected losses for various procedures are of little use. However, under the following circumstances blood losses will be greater than usual during orthopedic procedures:

1 proximal site of operation, without a tourniquet;
2 large areas of raw bone;
3 previous surgery at operative site;
4 radiation therapy at operative site;
5 infection at operative site;
6 tumor at operative site;
7 proliferative bone disease (e.g. Paget's disease);
8 the surgeon's technique.

Benefits of reduced blood loss

When blood loss is kept to a minimum, patients benefit because their exposure to blood donated by others is reduced. The two major viruses transmitted through blood transfusion are human immunodeficiency virus (HIV) and hepatitis viruses, the latter being by far the more common. Present screening methods reduce the risk of hepatitis transmission to three cases per 10 000 units transfused, making bank blood a relatively safe product if only the risk of viral infection is considered.[12]

The use of banked blood may have other harmful effects on patients undergoing orthopedic operations. A study of 84 patients undergoing hip replacement surgery found that 16 of the 50 patients who received homologous blood suffered various postoperative infections, including wound infections, compared with 1 of the 34 patients who received only autologous blood.[13] This increased rate of infection raises the fear of bacterial infections of implanted prostheses. A more recent study of patients undergoing hip replacement failed to confirm these findings.[14] Further studies are required before concluding that homologous transfusion increases the postoperative infection rate, but this complication may become a contraindication to the use of bank blood.

Reduced bleeding in the operative field not only facilitates surgery, but might also improve surgical results. Radiographic assessment (without long-term follow-up) of the cement–bone interface in the acetabular component of cemented total hip arthroplasties showed that patients managed with deliberate hypotension and who had operative blood losses less than 300 mL exhibited improved penetration of the cement into the bone.[15]

Methods of limiting blood loss

A pneumatic tourniquet placed proximal to the site of a peripheral procedure and inflated to occlude arterial flow eliminates blood loss during surgery. However, significant losses still occur postoperatively, when the tourniquet is removed. Some surgeons routinely deflate the tourniquet before closing the wound to control bleeding. While this may be of use in some procedures on the hand or other areas where hematomas compromise the surgical result, it was shown in one study not to reduce overall blood loss during total knee arthroplasty.[16] Avoiding hypothermia will also help to minimize blood loss. Mild hypothermia (35.0 °C) has been associated with an average increase of 500 mL of blood loss during total hip arthroplasty.[17]

Hemodilution, maintaining the patient's blood volume with cell-free fluids such as saline, pasteurized albumin, or starch, is the most common method of managing blood loss without resorting to bank blood. When the patient's hemoglobin concentration is between 6 and $10\,g\,dL^{-1}$ the anesthesiologist must determine whether the patient's risk for complications of inadequate oxygenation justify transfusion.[18]

Autologous blood, collected from the surgical field or donated before operation by the patient, is safer than banked blood. It is difficult to justify proceeding with an elective orthopedic operation that entails significant blood loss until adequate supplies of the patient's own blood have been collected, unless the patient cannot provide blood. Much attention has been directed at using synthetic erythropoietin (epoetin alpha) to increase red cell mass preoperatively. Epoetin alpha increased the number of autologous units deposited and reduced the amount of homologous blood transfused in anemic patients undergoing orthopedic surgery.[19]

Bleeding during major orthopedic procedures occurs by oozing from large surfaces; induced hypotension reduces blood losses.[20] During total hip arthroplasty or other hip operations, spinal or epidural anesthesia reduces blood losses significantly. When high levels of epidural anesthesia (T4) are combined with general anesthesia, and mean arterial pressure is allowed to decrease to about 7.3 kPa (55 mmHg), total hip arthroplasty can be performed with intraoperative blood losses of 300 mL or less.[21] Many patients scheduled for such operations are old and may present relative contraindications to hypotensive anesthesia. Nevertheless, Sharrock *et al.*[21] reported a series of 1016 consecutive patients who underwent total hip arthroplasty, 987 of whom were managed with combined epidural and general anesthesia, using epinephrine (adrenaline) infusions to produce mean arterial blood pressures of 6.9–7.3 kPa (52–55 mmHg). One-third of these patients were suffering preoperatively from hypertension; postoperatively there were no strokes, no renal failure, two myocardial infarctions, and three deaths, one due to myocardial infarction, one to aspiration, and one to pulmonary embolism. These results suggest that the combination of high levels of epidural anesthesia with general anesthesia may be safer than one would predict and deserves wider application as a means of reducing blood loss during orthopedic surgery.

Although early studies suggested that desmopressin (DDAVP) might reduce blood loss during Harrington rod surgery, a recent controlled study revealed no reduction in blood loss in healthy patients in the absence of preoperative blood coagulopathies.[22] Tranexamic acid and aprotinin have been shown in several studies to reduce blood loss and the need for homologous transfusion during orthopedic surgery. Fortunately, the antifibrinolytic properties of these agents did not lead to an increase in thromboembolism in these preliminary studies.[23,24]

Management of blood loss (see also Chapter 9)

The proper management of blood loss during major orthopedic procedures begins with maintaining normothermia, recommending regional anesthesia when other factors permit, and using autologous blood or blood salvaged from the operative field whenever possible. Giving cell-free fluids to prevent hypovolemia, rather than basing fluid therapy on unreliable estimates of blood loss, ensures that patients do not suffer from hypovolemia and low cardiac output. Hemodilution and moderate reductions in blood pressure are almost sure to be safe and useful.

Tourniquets

Orthopedic surgeons place occlusive pneumatic tourniquets about patients' arms and legs, usually after expressing the blood from the limb with a tightly wrapped elastic bandage. This may reduce total blood loss (see above), and it provides a dry field, making exposure and dissection more precise.

Effects of inflating tourniquets

The tourniquet must be placed over smoothly applied padding to prevent skin damage; antiseptic solutions used to prepare the skin must not be allowed under the tourniquet, otherwise chemical burns may occur. The width of the cuff should be more than half the diameter of the limb in order to improve transmission of cuff pressures to the deeper tissues.[25] Overinflation may increase tissue damage. Inflation pressure should be limited to that needed to block arterial flow, usually 6.7–13.3 kPa (50–100 mmHg) above the patient's systolic pressure. The patient's blood pressure may increase after incision, so that blood pressure measured during the surgical preparation is not always a reliable guide to setting the pressure of the tourniquet. The time at which the cuff is inflated and deflated, as well as the pressure, must be recorded on the anesthesia record. The pneumatic tourniquet, as in the case of all medical devices, requires periodic inspection and calibration.

The immediate effect of applying the tourniquet is to increase the central blood volume; if both legs are exsanguinated at once, marked increases in central venous pressure may occur, which may not be tolerated by patients with heart disease. Within 10–20 min, conduction fails in nerves underlying the tourniquet, contributing to anesthesia at the surgical field. The isolation of the limb from the central circulation allows it to cool, which also reduces sensation.

Intense aching pain at the site of the tourniquet rules out use of this device for more than brief periods, if local anesthesia alone is to be used. Unmedicated volunteers tolerated thigh tourniquets for 30 min, reporting pain not only under the tourniquet but elsewhere in the leg, suggesting that "tourniquet pain" is a complex entity.[26]

In some but not all patients undergoing general anesthesia, there occurs within the first hour a progressive increase in blood pressure that may reflect the pain inflicted by the tourniquet. This hypertension is difficult to treat with the usual doses of narcotic or inhaled anesthetics, considering that the operation is likely to end immediately after deflation of the tourniquet. Delayed occurrence is likely if large doses of these drugs are used. If the patient is otherwise well anesthetized, a vasodilator such as nitroprusside or nicardipine may be the best choice for the treatment of hypertension induced by a pneumatic tourniquet.

In patients under intravenous regional, spinal, or epidural anesthesia (but usually not brachial plexus block), tourniquet pain sometimes appears before anesthesia fails, or before the level assessed by pinprick has receded to the level of the tourniquet. This pain occurs inconsistently, coming on at various intervals after the inflation of the tourniquet.

Sympathetic nerve fibers, once cited as pathways for tourniquet pain, are not the sole mediators of this discomfort, as tourniquet pain is experienced despite blockade up to T4 spinal levels. Similarly, stellate ganglion block does not ameliorate tourniquet pain experienced during intravenous regional anesthesia of the arm.[27]

Administering greater doses of drug for spinal anesthesia decreases the incidence of tourniquet pain.[28] Hypobaric and isobaric spinal techniques result in a lower incidence of pain than do hyperbaric techniques, even when the drugs, dose, and dermatome levels are the same.[29] A given dose of near isobaric spinal bupivacaine provides better freedom from tourniquet pain than does the same dose of tetracaine, despite identical levels of anesthesia.[30] This may be related to the fact that, in isolated rabbit C-fiber preparations, bupivacaine is the more potent drug in blocking higher-frequency repeated impulses.[31] Intrathecal narcotics reduce the severity of tourniquet pain.[32]

Taken together, these observations are best explained by assuming that tourniquet pain represents a maximal pain stimulus, perhaps carried by C-fibers. Its appearance during spinal or epidural anesthesia represents an inadequate or dissipating block. The fact that tourniquet pain can be relieved during continuous spinal or epidural anesthesia by adding additional drug is consistent with this hypothesis. This explanation suggests that to reduce the incidence of tourniquet pain for patients undergoing spinal or epidural anesthesia, one can use larger doses and higher concentrations of local anesthetics, add opioids, and supplement the anesthetic through an indwelling catheter. The addition of bicarbonate to local anesthetic solutions speeds the onset of epidural anesthesia, by increasing the fraction of the drug present as the free base. It seems likely that this technique might also reduce the incidence of tourniquet pain.

Neuropraxia sometimes follows the use of a pneumatic tourniquet. Electrophysiologic testing and a thorough neurologic examination serve to distinguish these injuries from more proximal injuries that might be attributed to spinal or epidural anesthesia. Pneumatic tourniquets produce tissue ischemia, with cell damage and death inevitably following if ischemia is prolonged. Though changes may be seen after inflation times of only a few minutes, and limbs have survived complete occlusion of flow lasting many hours, some guidelines as to safe limits can be offered, based on electron microscopic evidence of cell disruption, and depletion of high-energy phosphate stores. Between 90 and 120 min seems to be an appropriate interval, with reperfusion periods of 5–10 min allowed between episodes of tourniquet inflation.[33]

Effects of deflating tourniquets

When the pneumatic tourniquet is deflated, the resulting effects depend on the volume of ischemic tissue and the duration of the ischemia. Sequelae are usually negligible when a single arm tourniquet is deflated after a brief procedure and are unmistakable when double leg tourniquets are deflated after an operation lasting more than 2 h.

Products of anaerobic metabolism are released; the venous blood coming from the leg demonstrates mixed respiratory and metabolic acidosis. For about 5 min after deflation of a single leg tourniquet, the patient's CO_2 excretion is increased by about 50%.[34] The patient's core temperature decreases as the limb is rewarmed. Hypotension results, probably from a combination of the abrupt decrease in peripheral resistance, the increase in venous capacitance, the release of vasoactive and myocardial depressant mediators derived from ischemic vascular endothelium and tissue, and the onset of bleeding. Hypoxemia may be caused by showers of platelet aggregates, thromboemboli, air emboli, or fat and other marrow emboli. Recent echocardiographic evidence shows that pulmonary embolism is actually common after tourniquet release, and there are case reports of severe cardiac instability and death following tourniquet release.[35]

Usually, these effects are transient and well tolerated. However, patients must be monitored closely in the minutes following deflation of a pneumatic tourniquet. Oxygen and vasopressors usually suffice to treat any severe responses, but staged or intermittent deflation can spread these effects out over time and moderate their severity.

Methacrylate cement

Methyl methacrylate cement is used as a space filler (not an adhesive) to improve the fit of implanted orthopedic prostheses to bone. The vapors given off by the curing cement are pungent and have raised some concern about operating room air pollution. The polymerizing reaction is exothermic, suggesting that there may be some risk of thermal injury to patients' tissues. However, the major problem arising from the use of cement is the cardiovascular response.

When the cement is placed, some patients develop hypotension and hypoxemia of varying severity, including cardiac arrest. These reactions are not as common or as severe with uncemented prostheses. These responses to the use of cement are poorly understood and are probably mediated by several complex mechanisms. The direct effect of the liquid monomer itself is to produce vasodilation, but the concentrations required in blood in animal models to produce these effects are greater than those typically measured after their clinical use. A secondary effect of cement may be more important than its direct effects: by improving the seal between the prosthesis and the walls of the marrow cavity, the cement acts to increase intramedullary pressures as the prosthesis is inserted, thereby forcing marrow contents into the bloodstream. This may explain why inserting the stem of a femoral prosthesis, which can produce intraluminal pressure exceeding 1 atmosphere, produces much more severe effects than does the cementing of an acetabular prosthesis, when no such piston and cylinder effect is present. A recent study using transesophageal echocardiography revealed showers of echogenic material in the right heart in almost all of 48 patients studied during total hip arthroplasty. The emboli were seen during acetabular and femoral cementing, but the largest emboli (in size and total amount) occurred during the placement of the femoral component.[36] In patients undergoing total knee replacement, the reaction is delayed until deflation of the tourniquet. Reactions do not seem to be as severe when prostheses are cemented at other sites, such as in the proximal humerus.

As most of the hypotension after cementing results from impaired left ventricular filling due to an increase in pulmonary vascular resistance, hypovolemia will further impair filling. Management includes insuring that the patient's blood volume is well replaced before the cement is applied, as hypovolemia increases the hypotension. Close monitoring of the blood pressure and treatment with vasopressors and oxygen usually suffice to treat the reaction.

Fat embolism

Fat embolism, the appearance of fat globules in the bloodstream, occurs in as many as 90% of the victims of major trauma. Fat embolism syndrome (FES) is rarer, with a recent study reporting an incidence of 11% following long bone or pelvic fractures.[37]

The clinical diagnosis of FES (Table 43.1) is based on criteria described by Gurd.[38] Numerous tests have been proposed to aid in the diagnosis of FES, including serum lipase and triglyceride levels, staining for fat after bronchoalveolar lavage, and evaluation of blood obtained from a pulmonary artery catheter. None has been shown to be specific.

Two mechanisms may explain the appearance of fat droplets in the blood in FES. Fat from the bone marrow may enter torn medullary veins. Fat droplets may then pass through the pulmonary blood vessels or an intracardiac shunt to become arterial emboli.[39] Evidence supporting this mechanical theory includes the absence of lung embolism during bone manipulations if the femoral vein is first cross-clamped and the postmortem finding of histologically recognizable bone marrow elements in the lungs. Alternatively, fat may agglutinate in the plasma, due to the release of enzymes that affect lipid solubility.[40] This biochemical theory explains FES seen with inflammatory conditions such as pancreatitis, alcohol-related hepatic failure, and sickle cell disease.

When blood-borne fat globules reach the lung, with the platelets and fibrin that adhere to them, they occlude blood vessels less then 20 μm in diameter. This neutral fat is hydrolyzed to toxic free fatty acids, which can induce acute respiratory distress syndrome. In addition, these fat and platelet aggregates lodged in the lung can cause the release of numerous vasoactive, bronchoconstricting, inflammatory modulating substances, including serotonin, histamine, products of arachidonic acid metabolism, and proinflammatory cytokines. Patients' reactions to fat embolism range from imperceptible minor effects, to FES, to death. The gravity of the illness may depend on the dose of fat and on concurrent medical problems, in particular reduced cardiopulmonary reserve and hypovolemia.

Table 43.1 *Criteria for diagnosis of fat embolism syndrome*

Major criteria	Minor criteria
Petechiae: conjunctiva, axilla	Tachycardia >110
$P_{a}O_2$ <8 kPa (60 mmHg), $F_{I}O_2$ >0.4	Fever (temperature >38.5 °C)
CNS depression	Emboli on fundoscopic examination
Pulmonary edema	Fat in urine
	Fat in sputum
	Unexpected anemia
	Increased sedimentation rate
	Unexpected thrombocytopenia

Surgical risk factors for FES include intramedullary nailing, especially of the femur and tibia, and joint replacements of the hip or knee with prostheses that displace large volumes of marrow. Fat embolization occurs regularly during placement of cemented femoral prostheses in dogs unless the medullary cavity is vented.[41] As discussed above, during total hip arthroplasty and total knee arthroplasty, transesophageal echocardiography reveals emboli of unknown nature in the right heart. Among patients who came to autopsy shortly after operative repair of fractured hips, fat emboli were found in the lungs of 7% of those treated with cemented femoral components and in none of those treated with uncemented prostheses. This suggests that the cement increased the level of fat embolism.[42] Any instrumentation of the marrow cavities of long bones may produce fat emboli. In sheep undergoing intramedullary nailing, echocardiography demonstrated that the maximum number of emboli appeared during insertion of the nail despite only minimal increases in intramedullary pressure.[43]

The respiratory distress of FES is treated with the usual supportive care. If possible, it is best to delay all but emergency surgery until patients with FES improve or at least are no longer deteriorating. An exception is the patient who requires fixation of fractures to halt continuing fat embolization. In studies in dogs, steroids and nonsteroidal anti-inflammatory agents have not been found to ameliorate the hemodynamic instability or prostanoid response to fat embolism.[44,45] Several small studies suggest a decrease in the incidence and severity of hypoxemia when prophylactic steroids are given at the time of injury. No human studies support the use of steroids for established FES.[46]

Neurologic symptoms of FES usually consist of dementia or disturbances in consciousness. Only rarely does FES present as a neurologic disorder without accompanying respiratory symptoms. The characteristic appearance of cerebral fat embolism on T2-weighted magnetic resonance images make this the best method for confirming the diagnosis.[47] The cerebral edema that may accompany cerebral fat embolism is treated with the usual supportive therapy for increased intracranial pressure. The role that subclinical fat embolism plays in causing the postoperative hypoxemia and deteriorated mental function, so often seen in patients undergoing intramedullary procedures, is yet to be determined.

Venous thrombosis and thromboembolism

Deep venous thrombosis (DVT), with the associated risk of pulmonary embolism, occurs in 45–70% of patients who undergo orthopedic procedures on the lower extremities.[48] The factors responsible for this include postoperative immobilization, intraoperative limb blood flow reduction (tourniquets or kinking of femoral vessels from dislocation and flexion of the hip during total hip arthroplasty), and the hypercoagulable state seen after surgery.

Many measures have been employed to prevent this complication; none is fully effective. Early mobilization, elevation of the foot of the bed, and pneumatic compression stockings seem safe. After total knee arthroplasty, a device that compresses only the foot, combined with aspirin, reduced the incidence of DVT to half, compared with aspirin alone.[49] Many anticoagulation regimens employing varying doses of coumarin, heparin, low-molecular-weight heparin (LMWH), recombinant hirudin, aspirin, or dextran have been investigated. These therapies typically reduce the rate of DVT by 50–70% compared with placebo, but hematomas are more frequent and the induced coagulopathy may discourage the use of spinal or epidural anesthesia, for fear of producing an epidural hematoma.[50,51] Indeed, 40 cases of spinal hematoma in patients undergoing spinal or epidural anesthesia while receiving LMWH perioperatively were reported between 1993 and 1997 in the USA. The majority of these patients were elderly women receiving their first dose of LMWH while an epidural catheter was present. This may indicate the need to avoid concomitant epidural analgesia and LMWH therapy.[52,53]

Spinal or epidural anesthesia has been shown in numerous trials to reduce the rate of DVT and thromboembolism by about one-half for patients undergoing total hip prosthesis surgery.[54,55] For patients undergoing total knee arthroplasty, the beneficial effect of regional anesthesia is less marked. In one study, the use of epidural anesthesia served to decrease the incidence of DVT after total knee arthroplasty to only 48%, as compared with 64% with general anesthesia.[56]

Two mechanisms have been proposed for this beneficial effect of regional anesthesia. First, spinal and epidural anesthesia increase blood flow to the lower extremities, which would be expected to decrease clot formation. In particular, during total hip arthroplasty, epidural anesthesia is associated with better flow in the operative limb than is general anesthesia.[57] Second, regional anesthesia seems to alter the overall stress response to surgical trauma, including the generalized activation of clotting mechanisms and inhibition of fibrinolysis. This effect has been clearly demonstrated in patients undergoing lower limb revascularization procedures, for whom epidural anesthesia has been shown to reduce the rate of thrombotic complications and to moderate the hypercoagulable state seen in patients receiving a general anesthetic.[58] The reduced effectiveness of regional anesthesia against DVT during total knee arthroplasty may be due to the overwhelming effect of the mechanical obstruction to blood flow produced by the tourniquet, unaltered by the effects of regional anesthesia.

Although regional anesthesia does reduce the rate of DVT and thromboemboli, especially for patients undergoing major hip surgery, it is inappropriate to recommend the technique universally to everyone who is to undergo orthopedic surgery below the waist. First, regional anesthesia does not reduce the rate of DVT to zero, and other methods of prophylaxis, listed above, are likely to be as effective as regional anesthesia. Second, the optimum combination of prophylactic techniques has yet to be defined; it seems likely that some combination of postoperative mechanical enhancement of lower limb flow, regional anesthesia, and a postoperative anticoagulation regimen will offer the greatest protection with the fewest complications. Third, the anticoagulative effect, if any, of extending regional anesthesia or analgesia into the postoperative period for orthopedic patients remains undetermined. Last, it is not certain that reducing the rate of DVT using these various prophylactic measures will decrease the mortality from thromboemboli.

Air and gas embolism

Fatal air or gas embolism has been reported in patients undergoing a wide variety of orthopedic operations, including procedures on the humerus, shoulder, spine, pelvis, and femur. Minor air embolism is common during total hip arthroplasty, and may play a part in the cardiovascular reaction that follows placement of cement into the femoral marrow cavity (see above). Air trapping beneath the cement and the extent of air embolism are reduced by using a long nozzle to introduce cement into the bottom of the femoral canal.[59] Air embolism has been reported during the use of a pulse irrigation device during extensive debridement.[60] Liquid nitrogen used to ablate bone tumors has produced gas emboli, as has nitrogen escaping from gas-powered tools.[61,62]

Except for surgery in which the operative field is elevated above the heart, so that local venous pressures are subatmospheric, air embolism is rare enough that special precautions such as prophylactic placement of a right heart catheter are not warranted. Nevertheless, gas embolism must be included among the possible diagnoses when patients undergoing orthopedic operations suffer intraoperative cardiovascular distress.

Measures to prevent infection

Wound infections are so catastrophic for patients, especially those with implanted prostheses, that orthopedic surgeons omit no measure that might prevent infection. Some of these measures affect anesthetic practice.

Laminar flow air filtration systems reduce the bacterial count in the air in the operating room but increase surface cooling of the patient. This makes patients vulnerable to inadvertent hypothermia, especially when large areas of skin are covered with antiseptic solutions. In addition to the usual risks of increased oxygen consumption, tachycardia, and hypertension produced as the patient's temperature returns to normal, hypothermia interferes with coagulation mechanisms and increases blood loss. Mild hypothermia (34.7 °C) alone has been shown to triple the incidence of wound infection.[63] To minimize this effect, as much of the patient as possible must be kept covered at all times. Usually some form of active warming is required to prevent intraoperative hypothermia; forced air warming is the most effective method. Patients exposed on fracture tables are especially vulnerable and require aggressive measures to prevent hypothermia.

Prophylactic antibiotics are most effective when given shortly before the skin incision and are ineffective if given later.[64] In some cases, surgeons may withhold antibiotics until specimens can be obtained from the wound for culture. The anesthesiologist can, after discussion with the surgeon, give the appropriate drug at the right time. Antibiotics such as gentamicin may reduce the required dose of nondepolarizing neuromuscular blockers. Another popular drug, vancomycin, produces hypotension and flushing if administered too quickly.

The possibility of HIV infection has become a cause for concern for orthopedic surgeons. This has led to adoption of reinforced gloves, clear face shields, and even other protective garments. When blood and bone chips fly from the operative field throughout the room, anesthesiologists must also give thought to protecting themselves.

Postoperative pain relief

The general principles of managing postoperative pain are given in Chapter 74. The physiologic benefits of postoperative analgesia are not as striking in patients who have undergone orthopedic operations as they are in patients who have undergone operations on the chest or abdomen, because pain relief does not result in the same dramatic improvement in diaphragmatic mobility. Patient-controlled analgesia, epidural or subarachnoid opioids, and other conventional measures all have been applied successfully to orthopedic patients. Some techniques have special application.

Continuous (via an indwelling catheter) or intermittent blockade of the brachial plexus or the femoral nerve provides good postoperative pain relief without the drawbacks of epidural or spinal narcotics. A study on postoperative knee rehabilitation after total knee arthroplasty found continuous femoral nerve blockade to be identical to epidural blockade for the provision of pain relief and rapid postoperative rehabilitation.[65] Intra-articular bupivacaine or morphine, which has a less intense but longer lasting effect, or a combination of the two, is effective after arthroscopic surgery of the knee.[66] Analgesia is improved by maintaining tourniquet inflation for 10 min after intra-articular morphine, to allow an increase in local tissue binding prior to the postischemic hyperemic response.[67] Intra-articular local anesthetics have also been used after arthroscopic surgery for other joints. The severe pain often experienced by patients at the donor site of iliac crest bone grafts can be relieved temporarily by infiltration of local anesthetic solution, or by longer term infusions administered through a catheter placed in the wound.[68] Ketorolac is a useful analgesic adjunct for orthopedic procedures, though it may increase bleeding, especially if administered to patients already receiving anticoagulants for DVT prophylaxis.[69] Patients who are to be placed in passive motion devices to maintain joint mobility after surgery benefit especially from postoperative analgesia.

After some operations, patients require repeat evaluation to detect neurovascular compromise. Inappropriately prolonged anesthesia can hinder the prompt detection of nerve injury, compartment syndromes, or tight casts. In such cases, confining analgesia to opioids or low doses of local anesthetics may be the most appropriate choice.

SPECIFIC ORTHOPEDIC PROCEDURES

Joint manipulation, reduction of dislocations

Patients with scars or adhesions limiting motion of a joint may require anesthesia so that the surgeon can put the joint through a range of motion that otherwise would be too painful to bear. Dislocations not managed successfully in the office or emergency room may also require reduction under general anesthesia. The management of these two groups of patients is similar.

Because the procedures are so brief, general anesthesia is often preferred to regional techniques. Profound muscle relaxation allows the surgeon to distinguish anatomical limitations of joint motion, as opposed to guarding. Thus, short-acting intravenous anesthetics and succinylcholine are effective. If the surgical lesion permits, the injection of intra-articular local anesthetic may provide some postoperative analgesia.

Closed treatment of fractures

Patients with closed fractures who require anesthesia may already have undergone a trial of reduction with sedation or with the injection of a local anesthetic into the hematoma. These procedures can be lengthy, with fluoroscopy, radiographs, casts, and sometimes percutaneous pins, making regional anesthesia more appropriate than in the case of dislocations. Colles' fracture is common in the elderly; intravenous regional anesthesia or brachial plexus block can provide an appropriate means of anesthetizing an elderly patient with multiple medical problems and a full stomach. If general anesthesia is chosen, it may be important to avoid violent fasciculations caused by succinylcholine, which may disturb some fractures.

Injuries that do not involve the spine or cranium present less of an immediate threat to life than does trauma to the chest or abdomen.

However, fractures of the femur or pelvis or multiple fractures of other bones are major injuries. The problems that result are the same as those resulting after other forms of severe trauma and include life-threatening blood loss, coagulopathy, shock, hypothermia, and complications due to other injuries. The specific sequelae of massive bone and muscle injury include myoglobinemia, bleeding, third-space fluid losses, shock, fat embolism, and hyperkalemic responses to succinylcholine. In the more severe cases, renal failure and pulmonary injury can result.

Fractures of the hip

In the USA alone, approximately 250 000 patients suffer hip fractures each year. In a prospective study, mortality 6 months after subcapital hip fracture was 23%. Among the 534 patients who died, significant predictors of death included the following factors:[70]

- depressed mental function preoperatively;
- postoperative chest infection;
- neoplasia;
- old age, > 85 years;
- deep wound infections.

Other predictors of 1-year mortality, which ranges in studies from 14% to 36%, include institutionalization, psychiatric illness, and operative management before stabilization of coexisting illness.[71] Operative repair of proximal femoral fractures is undertaken in the hope of getting elderly patients out of bed quickly in order reduce the harmful effects of prolonged bed rest, which include pneumonia, skin deterioration, and pulmonary thromboemboli. Although immediate surgery is not required, the operation is usually performed within a day or two of the accident, allowing time for medical evaluation and treatment of intercurrent disease. In a survey of 468 patients with hip fracture, delaying operation beyond 48 h did not result in an increased mortality, but did increase the incidence of complications, most of which were bed sores.[72] A prospective study of 367 elderly patients with hip fractures who were able to walk and who were not demented before the fracture found that an operative delay of more than 2 days doubled the mortality at 1 year.[73] The disagreement between these two studies may lie in the fact that the second studied a population of hip fracture patients who normally do well after surgery.

Preoperative evaluation includes attention to several special issues. First, the use of psychotropic drugs is associated with falls and fractures in the elderly,[74] and dementia is associated with delayed recovery and increased mortality in those with fractured hips. A mental status examination is an important part of the preanesthetic examination. Mentally impaired patients who cannot communicate may not be suitable for regional anesthesia. Second, it can be illuminating to ask why the patient fell to determine whether this followed a stroke, a myocardial infarction, or a cardiac arrhythmia. Third, these patients are often severely dehydrated secondary to diuretic use, impaired thirst recognition, delay before rescue, and blood loss into the fracture site (400 mL for intracapsular neck fractures and 800 mL for trochanteric fractures). Correction may require vigorous intravenous therapy and even invasive cardiovascular monitoring in some cases. Fourth, these patients may be more hypoxemic than one would expect for their age, possibly as a result of fat embolism.[75]

Controlled prospective studies have demonstrated 1-month mortality rates of 6–8% with both spinal and general anesthesia.[76,77] A recent meta-analysis of 13 randomized controlled trials of anesthetic techniques for surgical repair of femoral neck fractures has found no important differences in mortality between regional and general anesthesia.[78] There has been an impression that patients given regional anesthesia are less likely to be confused and mentally impaired after surgical repair of hip fractures. However, a randomized controlled study, in which epidural anesthesia was compared with halothane general anesthesia for patients with fractured femoral necks, found that postoperative confusion correlated with preoperative confusion, the use of drugs with anticholinergic effect, and with early postoperative hypoxemia, but not with the choice of anesthesia.[79] Another prospective study showed that general and regional anesthesia produced the same minimal postoperative mental impairment in patients undergoing elective hip or knee replacement.[80]

The outcome of an operation to repair a fractured hip in an elderly patient depends not only on the anesthesiologist and surgeon, but also on nurses, other physicians, and intensive care specialists. Regional anesthesia can be expected to confer benefits of reduced blood loss, a reduction in DVT and thromboemboli (see above), and perhaps a more prompt return to the preoperative mental state. However, many of these benefits are lost if patients are oversedated, especially with long-acting agents, or allowed to become hypoxemic. If regional anesthesia is entertained, using a continuous spinal or epidural technique may allow for better control of the level of anesthesia, limiting hypotension and bradycardia.

If practical considerations such as difficulties in positioning or dementia make regional anesthesia impracticable, general anesthesia can be recommended with confidence, because bank blood is relatively safe and because DVTs can be prevented by means other than the use of regional anesthesia. A well-conducted general anesthetic for these patients resembles a well-conducted regional anesthetic in that it is planned to avoid postoperative sedation, hypoxemia, and hypothermia. For the frailer patients, this goal can be achieved with small (seemingly homeopathic) doses of the shortest acting drugs and the least soluble inhaled anesthetics.

Total hip arthroplasty

The considerations described above for managing patients with fractured hips apply to patients who undergo total hip arthroplasty, except that these elective patients are usually younger and healthier with greater muscle mass and less osteoporosis. The lateral position is often used. In addition to the usual precautions, the anesthesiologist must collaborate with the surgeon to assure proper placement of an anterior pelvic brace used to hold these patients in the lateral position. If it is placed too far caudally and exerts too much pressure on the femoral triangle of the dependent leg, venous or arterial obstruction can result. If it is placed too far cephalad and pressed into the patient's abdomen too forcefully, it can limit motion of the diaphragm and compress the vena cava.

Transesophageal echocardiography reveals emboli (fat, marrow, or air) in patients undergoing hip arthroplasty. Measures taken to avoid emboli include drilling a venting hole in the distal femur, washing out the femoral canal, and omitting cement. As judged by transesophageal echocardiography, more emboli occurred in patients who have cement rather than uncemented total hip arthroplasty.[81] Uncemented total hip arthroplasty may be the preferred procedure for patients at higher risk for FES.

Emboli produce recognizable clinical problems in a minority of patients undergoing total hip arthroplasty. Increased pulmonary artery pressure at the time of cementing the femoral prosthesis is the usual finding. This reaction may occur at the end of the operation when the hip is relocated and emboli are dislodged from the previously obstructed femoral vein.[82] Careful maintenance of blood volume and increasing the inspired oxygen concentration at the time of prosthesis placement and hip relocation attenuates the decreases in arterial blood pressure and oxygenation.[83] Severe hypotension reflects large increases in pulmonary vascular resistance and resultant right heart failure. Immediate inotropic support is the recommended management.

Because DVT and thromboembolism are so prevalent after this procedure, the measures described above to prevent these complications have all been used when managing total hip arthroplasty. All offer some benefit, but none has emerged as the best prophylaxis.

Blood loss in patients managed without special precautions is expected to be about 1500 mL for primary total hip arthroplasty and 2000 mL for a revision. These losses can be reduced substantially by deliberately inducing hypotension (see Chapter 11). For example, a combination of light general anesthesia and continuous lumbar epidural anesthesia, with anesthetic levels up to T4, could be employed. With mean arterial pressures maintained at 6.7–8 kPa (50–60 mmHg), blood losses can amount to less than 300 mL. Autologous blood transfusion and moderate degrees of deliberate hemodilution are safe techniques that allow these patients to be managed without bank blood when total blood losses are limited to 1500–2000 mL. It should be possible to keep blood losses below these values without very high epidural anesthesia, invasive cardiovascular monitoring, or extremes of hypotension.

In the recovery room, bleeding and third-space losses continue and require treatment with appropriate fluids. Unexpected hypoxemia, especially if accompanied by deteriorating mental status, must raise the question of FES.

In the absence of contraindications and with the patient's permission, the best anesthesia plan seems to be a spinal or epidural anesthetic with supplemental general anesthesia if the duration of the operation or the patient's comfort requires it. There is not enough proved benefit from regional anesthesia to require the patient's compliance with this form of anesthesia. Moderate depression of arterial blood pressure can be obtained with low thoracic levels of spinal or epidural anesthesia, or with adequate depths of supplemental general anesthesia. Unless the patient is at particular risk of myocardial ischemia or failure, or of pulmonary hypertension, measuring blood pressure by an arm cuff and measuring urine output with a bladder catheter usually suffice for monitoring the cardiovascular system.

Total knee arthroplasty

The considerations involved in managing patients for total knee arthroplasty are similar to those for total hip arthroplasty. The supine position makes it easier to manage patients under regional anesthesia alone. DVT and thromboemboli are prevalent, but prophylactic measures do not seem to reduce the incidence of these problems as much as with total hip arthroplasty. This may be because of the outright obstruction of blood flow produced by the tourniquet usually employed to prevent bleeding.

When cemented total knee arthroplasty is performed without a tourniquet, a progressive syndrome of systemic hypotension and pulmonary vascular obstruction may begin immediately upon insertion of the prosthesis.[84] When a tourniquet is used, the onset of this syndrome is delayed until deflation of the tourniquet at the end of the operation. At this time, patients can suffer from the combined effects of tourniquet deflation, blood loss, and embolization of cement, thrombi, fat, and other marrow contents. As with total hip arthroplasty, the use of cement aggravates the severity of the effect.[85] Emboli may be identified in the right heart on echocardiography, and arterial hypoxemia is sometimes seen. Large emboli (greater than 0.5 cm) in the right heart at the time of tourniquet deflation are associated with a marked increase in pulmonary vascular resistance, and these large emboli are more likely when a tourniquet is used during total knee arthroplasty.[86,87]

A study of 80 patients found that the complication rate and initial recovery of knee movement was improved when knee arthroplasty was performed without a tourniquet. Overall blood loss was similar regardless of tourniquet use.[88] Larger clinical trials of total knee arthroplasty with and without tourniquet are required to establish the safest technique. During the period after tourniquet deflation, vital signs must be measured frequently and the patient treated with fluids, pressors, and oxygen as required. Patients with cardiovascular disease who might not be able to compensate adequately for these events may require invasive cardiovascular monitoring.

About 1500 mL of blood is lost into the knee after total knee arthroplasty, much of it in the first minutes after the tourniquet is deflated. Techniques of deliberate hypotension, to decrease these losses, are inappropriate because of the simultaneous problem with pulmonary embolism.

The physiologic insult that occurs at the end of a single total knee arthroplasty is usually tolerated well by patients who do not suffer severe cardiovascular disease. Simultaneous bilateral total knee arthroplasty has been accomplished safely, but doubling the dose of bleeding and embolization has also resulted in more blood transfusions, postoperative confusion, and cardiopulmonary complications.[89] Outcome may be improved by selection of healthier patients, monitoring pulmonary vascular resistance, and staging the two procedures so that the second does not begin until it is seen that the patient has weathered the first successfully.

Patients benefit from a period of close monitoring in the operating room (usually less than 5 min) after deflation of the tourniquet. Treatment includes fluids, pressors, and oxygen. Transfer to the recovery suite is delayed until heart rate, blood pressure, and peripheral oxygen saturation have recovered. In the recovery room, any unexplained hypoxemia or deterioration in mental status provides warning of possible FES and demands evaluation and treatment.

Spinal or epidural anesthesia offers several advantages to patients undergoing total knee arthroplasty. Hypertensive reactions to prolonged tourniquet inflation are rare and postoperative pain relief can be provided. Epidural anesthesia is associated with more rapid achievement of postoperative in-hospital rehabilitation goals than general anesthesia.[90] However, given careful attention to details, general anesthesia can also provide satisfactory anesthesia.

Arthroscopic surgery of the knee

The majority of knee operations once requiring arthrotomy are now done through the arthroscope, including ligament repairs, meniscectomy, removal of loose bodies, and replacement of the anterior cruciate ligament. All forms of anesthesia are suitable, but the less invasive and least prolonged of these procedures can be performed with the intra-articular injection of local anesthetic solutions. Absorption of local anesthetic is not rapid, although the addition of epinephrine decreases the maximum blood concentrations; 30 mL of bupivacaine 0.5%, with or without epinephrine, is a safe dose.[91] Femoral nerve block also provides good analgesia. DVT may occur after knee arthroscopy; a recent study demonstrated an incidence of 18% within 1 week. Tourniquet duration of more than 60 min was the only variable associated with an increased risk of DVT. Short-term prophylaxis may prove beneficial for these patients.[92]

Operations on the foot and the lower extremity

Operations on the lower leg can be accomplished with peripheral nerve blocks, either at the level of the femoral and sciatic nerves or by individual nerve blocks at the level of the knee. If a thigh tourniquet is not used, operations on the foot are amenable to ankle block. Instead of a thigh tourniquet, a tightly wrapped rubber bandage at the ankle is a safe and effective method for the occlusion of arterial inflow.[93]

Operations on the hand and distal arm

Operations on the hand and arm are well suited to regional anesthesia. If the operation is limited in extent, a distal block of a specific nerve, such as the ulnar nerve at the elbow, may suffice. Intravenous regional anesthesia is widely applicable, but does not allow for deflation of the tourniquet to obtain hemostasis and is limited in the duration of anesthesia it can provide. Tourniquet pain does not usually occur with brachial plexus block if care is taken to anesthetize the intercostobrachial nerve as it enters the upper arm superficial to the fascia overlying the axillary artery.

Procedures about the elbow can usually be accomplished under axillary block, but more proximal procedures require an approach to the brachial plexus above the level of the clavicle, such as an interscalene block. This is especially advantageous in elderly patients who suffer fractures of the proximal humerus.

Operations on the shoulder

The deep structures of the shoulder are innervated by C5–C6, so that interscalene and other supraclavicular approaches to the brachial plexus provide good regional anesthesia. Anesthesia of the skin over the anterior shoulder may require infiltration of local anesthetics because of innervation from thoracic dermatomes. As a rule, regional anesthesia is more successful for anterior than posterior approaches to the shoulder.

Patients, surgeons, and anesthesiologists often prefer general anesthesia for shoulder procedures because of the proximity of the surgical field to the patient's face. The combination of light general anesthesia and a brachial plexus block may provide good postoperative pain relief along with intraoperative comfort for the patient. Intra-articular local anesthetic solutions can be used alone for anesthesia for arthroscopy and for postoperative pain relief after more extensive procedures performed under general anesthesia. Whether regional anesthesia alone or in combination with general anesthesia provides any special health benefits analogous to those seen with surgery on the lower extremity has not been investigated.

Regardless of the anesthetic technique, three relatively infrequent complications require vigilance during these operations. Shoulder procedures are often carried out with the patient in a semisitting position, increasing the possibility of venous air embolism. When dissection is carried to deep levels, pneumothorax is possible. Operations on the clavicle can result in injury to the underlying subclavian vessels with abrupt, massive blood loss.

Operations on the spine

Operations on the spine carried out by orthopedic surgeons are divided into several categories. Laminectomy and spinal fusions of limited extent, which are usually on the lumbar spine, present challenges, mostly because of the position required. More extensive operations, such as instrumented fusions such as the Harrington procedure, raise the possibility of significant blood loss or damage to the spinal cord. Such patients may also suffer from kyphoscoliosis with attendant restrictive lung disease and even right heart failure from cor pulmonale. In the sitting position, approaches to the cervical spine create the risk of air embolism. Anterior approaches to the spine require incision in the anterior neck, thorax, or abdomen.

Positioning

Patients in the prone position suffer pressure on the abdomen; in all but the slimmest of individuals, this elevates the diaphragm, interferes with diaphragmatic motion, and obstructs the vena cava. Obstruction to the vena cava, in turn, increases flow and pressure in the veins of the epidural venous plexus, thereby increasing operative blood loss and making many spinal operations technically more difficult. Devices such as the Andrews frame position the patient so that the abdomen is free, thereby ameliorating this problem. The efficacy of these positions in decreasing venous pressures may explain why air embolism has now been reported during lumbar spine surgery.[94] It is fortunate that serious air embolism due to this mechanism is rare. Studies in a dog model with the abdomen hanging freely suggest that it is difficult to retrieve significant quantities of air from the right heart under these circumstances.[95]

Blood loss

Controlled hypotension reduces blood loss in patients undergoing extensive spine surgery and has become a popular technique for these patients (see Chapter 11). Blood recovery, autologous blood transfusion, and deliberate hemodilution also reduce the need for bank blood in these patients.

Spinal cord injury

Intraoperative spinal cord ischemia may produce neurologic damage in patients in whom extensive surgery is carried out or in whom a marked kyphoscoliosis is to be corrected. To prevent this, patients are monitored during the operation to detect spinal cord damage. Somatosensory evoked potentials (SSEPs), produced by stimulating the lower extremities and monitoring the cerebral cortex or the spinal cord above the level of the operation, are ablated when ischemia affects the sensory tracts in the spinal cord. When this technique is in use, a constant level of anesthesia helps to avoid confusing anesthetic effects with ischemia.

An alternative is the "wake-up test," which assesses the integrity of motor tracts. As the spine is straightened or distracted, the patient is awakened partially and asked to move toes or fingers. If the patient moves his or her hands but not the feet, it is presumed that there is spinal cord compromise. In order to accomplish this test, the anesthesiologist must coach and reassure the patient carefully beforehand. An analgesic and an amnesic sedative administered as part of the anesthetic mixture allows the patient to participate without discomfort or distressing memories. Spontaneous recovery of neuromuscular function to the level of one or two responses to a train of four stimuli enables the patient to execute commands but not to move violently and disrupt the operation. Rapid lightening and deepening of the anesthetic are easily accomplished by employing nitrous oxide, desflurane, sevoflurane, isoflurane, or propofol.

Choice of anesthesia

More extensive surgery on the spine requires general anesthesia, but simple excision of a lumbar intervertebral disk or a limited laminectomy may also be performed under spinal or epidural anesthesia. The usual advantages of regional anesthesia obtain, but several unique dangers have limited the popularity of the technique. First, in the prone patient heavy sedation may produce apnea and airway obstruction that are difficult to manage. Second, obese patients, patients with respiratory disease, or those at special risk of hypotension from the prone position, who would otherwise be appropriate candidates for regional anesthesia, may require support of ventilation or circulation using intubation, controlled ventilation, and high concentrations of inspired oxygen. Third, postoperative neural deficits due to surgical trauma may be blamed inappropriately on the anesthetic technique.

Epidural or spinal anesthesia can be advantageous techniques for lumbar spine surgery, but their safe application requires care, skill, and discretion by both surgeon and anesthesiologist. If the duration of the operation exceeds the duration of the block, the surgeon can easily give a supplemental subarachnoid injection via the surgical field.

Amputation

Amputation of a limb represents two special problems for anesthesia management. First, the psychologic trauma to the patient of losing a major part of the body may require that general anesthesia or heavy sedation be employed. Second, many patients suffer phantom limb sensations or pain for months or years after the operation. The pain, which may occur during complete neural block, can be treated with spinal narcotics.[96] One controlled study in elderly patients receiving leg amputations for painful ischemia demonstrated that 3 days of preoperative epidural blockade with local anesthetics and opioids markedly reduced the incidence of postoperative phantom limb pain.[97] This was confirmed in a similar study of patients receiving epidural local anesthetic, clonidine, and opioid prior to and for at least 3 days after lower limb amputation.[98] Clearly, regional anesthesia offers special benefits to patients undergoing limb amputation.

Reimplantation and free microvascular grafts

Reimplantation of severed parts and the *en bloc* grafting of bone and soft tissue with vascular anastomoses are lengthy operations that present several special challenges to anesthesia management. Care that is important for less prolonged procedures becomes crucial when surgery extends over an entire day. Meticulous positioning and padding reduce the risks of neuropathies and skin damage. Repeated testing to ensure that the endotracheal tube cuff is not overinflated may lessen damage to the tracheal mucosa. The patient must be kept at a normal body temperature.

Because of the duration of the procedure, patient comfort virtually demands general anesthesia. One case report described prolonged emergence from general anesthesia after such a procedure, but this can be avoided by careful management of anesthetic depth to avoid relative overdoses.[99]

Regional anesthesia offers advantages of increased blood flow to the limb secondary to sympathectomy and can be employed with general anesthesia. Repeated blocks with prolonged acting local anesthetics or indwelling catheters can extend these benefits to the postoperative period. Other measures directed to maintain adequate perfusion include maintaining an optimal hematocrit (probably 30%), keeping the patient warm, and administering heparin or dextran.

REFERENCES

1. Matti MV, Sharrock NE. Anesthesia on the rheumatoid patient. *Rheum Dis Clin N Am* 1998; **24**: 19–34.
2. Schelew BL, Vaghadia H. Ankylosing spondylitis and neuraxial anaesthesia – a 10 year review. *Can J Anaesth* 1996; **43:** 65–8.
3. Salathé M, Jöhr M. Unsuspected cervical fractures: a common problem in ankylosing spondylitis. *Anesthesiology* 1989; **70:** 869–870.
4. Macarthur A, Kleiman S. Rheumatoid cervical joint disease – a challenge to the anaesthetist. *Can J Anaesth* 1993; **40:** 154–9.
5. Schlaghecke R, Kornely E, Santen R Th, Ridderskamp P. The effect of long-term glucocorticoid therapy on pituitary–adrenal responses to exogenous corticotropin-releasing hormone. *N Engl J Med* 1992; **326:** 226–30.
6. Salem M, Tainsh RE, Bromberg J, *et al.* Perioperative glucocorticoid coverage. A reassessment 42 years after emergence of a problem. *Ann Surg* 1994; **219:** 416–25.
7. Stein RE, Urbaniak J. Use of the tourniquet during surgery in patients with sickle cell hemoglobinopathies. *Clin Orthop Rel Res* 1980; **151:** 231–3.
8. Hastings RH, Marks JD. Airway management for trauma patients with potential cervical injuries. *Anesth Analg* 1991; **73:** 471–82.
9. Conaty KR, Klemm MS. Severe increase of intracranial pressure after deflation of a pneumatic tourniquet. *Anesthesiology* 1989; **71:** 294–5.
10. Hofman AA, Wyatt RWB. Fatal pulmonary embolism following tourniquet inflation. *J Bone Joint Surg* 1985; **67A:** 633–4.
11. Gardner RC. Blood loss in orthopedic operations: comparative studies in 19 major orthopedic procedures utilizing radioisotope labeling and an automatic blood volume computer. *Surgery* 1970; **68:** 489–91.
12. Donahue JG, Munoz A, Ness PM, *et al.* The declining risk of post-transfusion hepatitis C virus infection. *N Engl J Med* 1992; **327:** 369–73.
13. Murphy P, Heal JM, Blumberg N. Infection or suspected infection after hip replacement surgery with autologous or homologous blood transfusions. *Transfusion* 1991; **31:** 212–17.
14. Vamvakas EC, Moore SB, Cabanela M. Blood transfusion and septic complications after hip replacement *Surg Trans* 1995; **35:** 150–6.
15. Ranawat CS, Beaver WB, Sharrock NE, *et al.* Effect of hypotensive epidural anaesthesia on acetabular cement-bone fixation in total hip arthroplasty. *J Bone Joint Surg* 1991; **73B:** 779–82.
16. Lotke PA, Faralli VJ, Orenstein EM, Ecker ML. Blood loss after total knee replacement. *J Bone Joint Surg* 1992; **73A:** 1037–40.
17. Schmied H, Kurz A, Sessler DI, *et al.* Mild hypothermia increases blood loss and transfusion requirements during total hip arthroplasty. *Lancet* 1996; **347:** 289–92.
18. American Society of Anesthesiologists. Practice guidelines for blood component therapy. *Anesthesiology* 1996; **84:** 732–47.
19. Price TH, Goodnough LT, Vogler W, *et al.* The impact of recombinant erythropoietin administration on the efficacy of autologous blood strategies in patients with low hematocrits. *Blood* 1992; **80:** 219a (Suppl. 1, abstract 867).
20. Rosberg B, Fredin H, Gustafson C. Anesthetic techniques and surgical blood loss in total hip arthroplasty. *Acta Anaesthesiol Scand* 1982; **26:** 189–93.
21. Sharrock NE, Mineo R, Urquhart B. Haemodynamic effects and outcome analysis of hypotensive extradural anaesthesia in controlled hypertensive patients undergoing total hip arthroplasty. *Br J Anaesth* 1991; **67:** 17–25.
22. Guay J, Reinberg C, Poitras B, *et al.* A trial of desmopressin to reduce blood loss in patients undergoing spinal fusion for idiopathic scoliosis. *Anesth Analg* 1992; **75:** 405–10.
23. Hiippala ST, Strid LJ, Wennerstrand MI, *et al.* Tranexamic acid radically decreases blood loss and transfusions associated with total knee arthroplasty. *Anesth Analg* 1997; **84:** 839–44.
24. Murkin JM, Shannon NA, Bourne RB, *et al.* Aprotinin decreases blood loss in patients undergoing revision or bilateral total hip arthroplasty. *Anesth Analg* 1995; **80:** 343–8.
25. Hargens AR, McClure AG, Skyhar MJ, *et al.* Local compression patterns beneath pneumatic tourniquets applied to arms and thighs of human cadavera. *J Orthop Res* 1987; **5:** 247–52.
26. Hagenouw RRPM, Bridenbaugh PO, van Egmond J, Stuebing R. Tourniquet pain: a volunteer study. *Anesth Analg* 1986; **65:** 1175–80.
27. Farah R-S, Thomas PS. Sympathetic blockade and tourniquet pain in surgery of the upper extremity. *Anesth Analg* 1987; **66:** 1033–5.
28. Egbert LD, Deas TC. Cause of pain from a pneumatic tourniquet during spinal anesthesia. *Anesthesiology* 1962; **23:** 287–90.
29. Bridenbaugh PO, Hagenouw RR, Gielen MJ, Edstrom HH. Addition of glucose to bupivacaine in spinal anesthesia increases incidence of tourniquet pain. *Anesth Analg* 1986; **65:** 1181–5.
30. Concepcion MA, Lambert DH, Welch KA, Covino BG. Tourniquet pain during spinal anesthesia: a comparison of plain solutions of tetracaine and bupivacaine. *Anesth Analg* 1988; **67:** 828–32.
31. Stewart A, Lambert DH, Concepcion MA, *et al.* Decreased incidence of tourniquet pain during spinal anesthesia with bupivacaine. *Anesth Analg* 1988; **67:** 833–7.
32. Touminen M, Valli H, Kalso E, Rosenberg PH. Efficacy of 0.3 mg morphine intrathecally in preventing tourniquet pain during spinal anaesthesia with hyperbaric bupivacaine. *Acta Anaesthesiol Scand* 1988; **32:** 113–16.
33. Sapega AA, Heppenstall RB, Chance B, *et al.* Optimizing tourniquet application and release times in extremity surgery. *J Bone Joint Surg* 1985; **67A:** 303–14.
34. Bourke DL, Silberberg MS, Ortega R, Willock MM. Respiratory responses associated with release of intraoperative tourniquets. *Anesth Analg* 1989; **69:** 541–14.

35. Cohen JD, Keslin JS, Nili M, *et al.* Massive pulmonary embolism and tourniquet deflation. *Anesth Analg* 1994; **79:** 583–5.
36. Lafont ND, Kalonji MK, Barre J, *et al.* Clinical features and echocardiography of embolism during cemented hip arthroplasty. *Can J Anaesth* 1997; **44:** 112–17.
37. Fabian TC, Hoots AV, Stanford DS, *et al.* Fat embolism syndrome: prospective evaluation in 92 fracture patients. *Crit Care Med* 1990; **18:** 42–6.
38. Gurd AR. Fat embolism: an aid to diagnosis. *J Bone Joint Surg* 1970; **52B:** 732–7.
39. Byrick RJ, Mullen JB, Mazer CD, Guest CB. Transpulmonary systemic fat embolism. Studies in mongrel dogs after cemented arthroplasty. *Am J Respir Crit Care Med* 1994; **150:** 1416–22.
40. Hulman G. The pathogenesis of fat embolism. *J Pathol* 1995; **176:** 3–9.
41. Kallos T, Enis JE, Gollan F, Davis JH. Intramedullary pressure and pulmonary embolism of femoral medullary contents in dogs during insertion of bone cement and a prosthesis. *J Bone Joint Surg* 1974; **56A:** 1363–7.
42. Sevitt S. Fat embolism in patients with fractured hips. *Br Med J* 1972; **2:** 257–62.
43. Wozasek GE, Simon P, Redl H, Schlag G. Intramedullary pressure changes and fat intravasation during intramedullary nailing: an experimental study in sheep. *J Trauma* 1994; **36:** 202–7.
44. Byrick RJ, Mullen JB, Wong PY, *et al.* Prostanoid production and pulmonary hypertension after fat embolism are not modified by methylprednisolone. *Can J Anaesth* 1991; **38:** 660–7.
45. Byrick RJ, Wong PY, Mullen JB, Wigglesworth DF. Ibuprofen pretreatment does not prevent hemodynamic instability after cemented arthroplasty in dogs. *Anesth Analg* 1992; **75:** 515–22.
46. King MB, Harmon KR. Unusual forms of pulmonary embolism. *Clin Chest Med* 1994; **15:**561–580.
47. Yoshida A, Okada Y, Nagata Y, *et al.* Assessment of cerebral fat embolism by magnetic resonance imaging in the acute stage. *J Trauma* 1996; **40:** 437–40.
48. Consensus Conference. Prevention of venous thrombosis and pulmonary embolism. *JAMA* 1986; **256:** 744–9.
49. Westrich GH, Sculco TP. Prophylaxis against deep venous thrombosis after total knee arthroplasty. *J Bone Joint Surg* 1996; **78A:** 826–34.
50. Lieberman JR, Geerts WH. Prevention of venous thromboembolism after total hip and knee arthroplasty. *J Bone Joint Surg* 1994; **76A:** 1239–50.
51. Eriksson BI, Wille-Jorgensen P, Kälebo P, *et al.* A comparison of recombinant hirudin with a low-molecular-weight heparin to prevent thromboembolic complications after total hip replacement. *N Engl J Med* 1997; **337:** 1329–35.
52. Horlocker T, Wedel D. Spinal and epidural blockade and perioperative low molecular weight heparin: smooth sailing on the Titanic. *Anesth Analg* 1998; **86:** 1153–5.
53. Hynson JM, Katz JA, Bueff HU. Epidural hematoma associated with Enoxaparin. *Anesth Analg* 1996; **82:** 1072–5.
54. Thorburn J, Louden JR, Vallance R. Spinal and general anaesthesia in total hip replacement: frequency of deep vein thrombosis. *Br J Anaesth* 1980; **52:** 1117–21.
55. Modig J, Borg T, Karlström G, *et al.* Thromboembolism after total hip replacement: role of epidural and general anesthesia. *Anesth Analg* 1983; **62:** 174–80.
56. Sharrock NE, Haas SB, Hargett MJ, *et al.* Effects of epidural anesthesia on the incidence of deep-vein thrombosis after total knee arthroplasty. *J Bone Joint Surg* 1992; **73A:** 502–6.
57. Davis FM, Laurenson VG, Gillespie WJ, *et al.* Leg blood flow during total hip replacement under spinal or general anaesthesia. *Anaesth Intens Care* 1989; **17:** 136–43.
58. Rosenfeld BA, Beattie C, Christopherson R, *et al.* The effects of different anesthetic regimens on fibrinolysis and the development of postoperative arterial thrombosis. Perioperative ischemia randomized anesthesia trial study group. *Anesthesiology* 1993; **79:** 435–43.
59. Evans RD, Palazzo MGA, Ackers JWL. Air embolism during total hip replacement: comparison of two surgical techniques. *Br J Anaesth* 1989; **62:** 243–7.
60. Buxbaum JL, Muravchick S, Chen L. Intraoperative air embolism with pulse irrigation device. *J Clin Anesth* 1996; **8:** 519–21.
61. Dwyer DM, Thorne AC, Healey JH, Bedford RF. Liquid nitrogen instillation can cause venous gas embolism. *Anesthesiology* 1990; **73:** 179–81.
62. Whitehill R, Moskal JT, Scully KS, *et al.* Nitrogen-gas injection from a power reamer: a complication of closed intramedullary nailing of the femur. *J Bone Joint Surg* 1983; **65A:** 860–1.
63. Kurz A, Sessler DI, Lenhardt R. Perioperative normothermia to reduce the incidence of surgical-wound infection and shorten hospitalization. *N Engl J Med* 1996; **334:** 1209–15.
64. Classen DC, Evans RS, Pestotnik SL, *et al.* The timing or prophylactic administration of antibiotics and the risk of surgical-wound infection. *N Engl J Med* 1992; **326:** 281–6.
65. Singelyn FJ, Deyaert M, Joris D, *et al.* Effects of intravenous patient-controlled analgesia with morphine, continuous epidural analgesia, and continuous three-in-one block on postoperative pain and knee rehabilitation after unilateral total knee arthroplasty. *Anesth Analg* 1998; **87:** 88–92.
66. Khoury GF, Chen ACN, Garlad DE, Stein C. Intraarticular morphine, bupivacaine, and morphine/bupivacaine for pain control after knee videoarthroscopy. *Anesthesiology* 1992; **77:** 263–6.
67. Healy WA, Joshi GP, McCarroll SM, O'Brien TM. The effect of tourniquet release time on the analgesic efficacy of intraarticular morphine after arthroscopic knee. *Surg Anesth Analg* 1997; **84:** 791–3.
68. Brull SJ, Lieponis JV, Murphy MJ, *et al.* Acute and long-term benefits of iliac crest donor site perfusion with local anesthetics. *Anesth Analg* 1992; **74:** 145–7.
69. Delaporte-Cerceau S, Samama C-M, Riou B, *et al.* Ketorolac and Enoxaparin affect arterial thrombosis and bleeding in the rabbit. *Anesthesiology* 1998; **88:** 1310–17.
70. Wood DJ, Ions GR, Quinby JM, *et al.* Factors which influence mortality after subcapital hip fracture. *J Bone Joint Surg* 1992; **74A:** 199–202.
71. Zuckerman JD. Hip fracture. *N Engl J Med* 1996; **334:** 1519–25.
72. Parker MJ, Pryor GA. Timing of surgery for proximal femoral fractures. *J Bone Joint Surg* 1992; **74B:** 203–5.
73. Zuckerkman JD, Skovron ML, Koval KJ, *et al.* Postoperative complications and mortality associated with operative delay in older patients who have a fracture of the hip. *J Bone Joint Surg* 1995; **77A:** 1551–6.
74. Ray WA, Griffin MR, Schaffner W, *et al.* Psychotropic drug use and the risk of hip fracture. *N Engl J Med* 1987; **316:** 363–9.
75. Sari A, Miyauchi Y, Yamashita S, *et al.* The magnitude of hypoxemia in elderly patients with fractures of the femoral neck. *Anesth Analg* 1986; **65:** 892–4.
76. Valentin N, Lomholt B, Jensen JS, *et al.* Spinal or general anaesthesia for surgery of the fractured hip. *Br J Anaesth* 1986; **58:** 284–91.
77. Davis FM, Woolner DF, Frampton C, *et al.* Prospective, multi-centre trial of mortality following general or spinal anaesthesia for hip fracture surgery in the elderly. *Br J Anaesth* 1987; **59:** 1080–8.
78. Sorenson RM, Pace NL. Anesthetic techniques during surgical repair of femoral neck fractures. *Anesthesiology* 1992; **77:** 1095–104.
79. Berggren D, Gustafsorl Y, Eriksson B, *et al.* Postoperative confusion after anesthesia in elderly patients with femoral neck fractures. *Anesth Analg* 1987; **66:** 497–504.
80. Jones MJT, Piggott SE, Vaughan RS, et al. Cognitive and functional competence after anaesthesia in patients aged over 60: controlled trial of general and regional anaesthesia for elective hip or knee replacement. Br Med J 1990; **300:** 1683–7.
81. Ereth MH, Weber JG, Abel MD, *et al.* Cemented versus noncemented total hip arthroplasty. – embolism, hemo-dynamics, and intrapulmonary shunting. *Mayo Clin Proc* 1992; **67:** 1066–74.
82. Urban MK, Sheppard R, Gordon MA, Urquhart BL. Right ventricular function during revision total hip arthroplasty. *Anesth Analg* 1996; **82:** 1225–9.
83. Al-Shaikh B. Effect of inspired oxygen concentration on the incidence of desaturation in patients undergoing total hip replacement. *Br J Anaesth* 1991; **66:** 580–2.
84. Samil K, Elmelik E, Goutalier D, Viars P. Hemodynamic effects of prosthesis insertion during knee replacement without tourniquet. *Anesthesiology* 1980; **52:** 271–3.
85. Samil K, Elmelik E, Mourtada MB, *et al.* Intraoperative hemodynamic changes during total knee replacement. *Anesthesiology* 1979; **50:** 239–42.
86. Berman AT, Parmet JL, Harding SP, *et al.* Emboli observed with use of transesophageal echocardiography immediately after tourniquet release during total knee arthroplasty with cement. *J Bone Joint Surg* 1998; **80A:** 389–96.
87. Parmet JL, Horrow JC, Berman AT, *et al.* The incidence of large venous emboli during total knee arthroplasty without pneumatic tourniquet use. *Anesth Analg* 1998; **87:** 439–44.
88. Abdel-Salam A, Eyres KS. Effects of tourniquet during total knee arthroplasty. *J Bone Joint Surg* 1995; **77B:** 250–3.
89. Lane GJ, Hozack WJ, Shah S, *et al.* Simultaneous bilateral versus unilateral total knee arthroplasty. *Clin Orthop Res* 1997; **345:** 106–12.
90. Williams-Russo P, Sharrock NE, Haas SB, *et al.* Randomized trial of epidural versus general anesthesia. Outcomes after primary total knee replacement. *Clin Orthop Res* 1996; **331:** 199–208.
91. Carnes RS, Butterworth JF, Poehling GS, Samuels MP. Safety and efficacy

of intra-articular bupivacaine and epinephrine anesthesia for knee arthroscopy. *Anesthesiology* 1989; **71:** A729.

92. Demers C, Marcoux S, Ginsberg J, *et al.* Incidence of venographically proved deep vein thrombosis after knee arthroscopy. *Arch Intern Med* 1998; **158:** 47–50.
93. Biehl WC, Morgan JM, Wagner FW, Gabriel RA. The safety of the Esmarch tourniquet. *Foot Ankle* 1993; **14:** 278–83.
94. Albin MS, Ritter RR, Pruett CE, Kalff K. Venous air embolism during lumbar laminectomy in the prone position: report of three cases. *Anesth Analg* 1991; **73:** 346–9.
95. Artru AA. Venous air embolism in prone dogs positioned with the abdomen hanging freely: percentage of gas retrieved and success rate of resuscitation. *Anesth Analg* 1992; **75:** 715–19.
96. Jacobson L, Chabal C. Prolonged relief of acute postamputation phantom limb pain with intrathecal fentanyl and epidural morphine. *Anesthesiology* 1989; **71:** 984–5.
97. Bach S, Noreng MF, Tjéllden NU. Phantom limb pain in amputees during the first 12 months following limb amputation, after preoperative lumbar epidural blockade. *Pain* 1988; **33:** 297–301.
98. Jahangiri M, Bradley JWP, Jayatunga AP, Dark CH. Prevention of phantom pain after major lower limb amputation by epidural infusion of diamorphine, clonidine, and bupivacaine. *Ann R Coll Surg Engl* 1994; **76:** 324–6.
99. Caplan RA, Long MC. Prolonged anesthesia – management and sequelae of a two day general anesthetic. *Anesth Analg* 1984; **63:** 353–8.

44

Anesthesia for neurosurgery

JOHN M TURNER

THE PATIENT

The patient who requires neurosurgery sets many problems for the anesthesiologist. Some of these relate to the disordered physiology caused by neurosurgical disease and some to the special requirements of neurosurgery. The brain is in a unique position, being confined within a rigid closed box (the skull), and its function depends on the maintenance of the cerebral circulation within that restricted space. Disease and injury interfere with the control of the cerebral circulation in ways that predispose to cerebral ischemia and therefore cerebral damage.

Anesthetic drugs have powerful effects on the brain. The alterations they produce in cerebral function can be used to ensure good operating conditions for neurosurgery and to limit the extent of any neuronal damage that may occur.[1,2] They may, however, have side-effects that interfere with the production of good operating conditions. Modern drugs allow the anesthesiologist considerable control over cerebral and cerebrovascular function and new monitoring techniques have enabled a re-evaluation of some traditional drugs and techniques.

Neurosurgical operations are relatively high-risk procedures. The patient with intracranial space occupation is at risk from the development of high intracranial pressure, and as the space-occupying lesion (SOL) grows the danger increases. The patient who has suffered a subarachnoid hemorrhage (SAH) is at further risk from repeated bleeds and may suffer from vascular spasm and cerebral infarction. Patients with pituitary disease suffer from endocrine disturbances that affect their fitness for surgery.

Intracranial space occupation

The skull is essentially a closed box, containing the brain (about 1400 g in the adult) and about 140 mL of cerebrospinal fluid (CSF), of which half is in the cranial space and half in the spinal CSF space and arterial and venous blood. Cerebral blood flow (CBF) is controlled by cerebral metabolic requirements and is about 50 mL per 100 g brain per min. A distinct pressure, the intracranial pressure (ICP), exists in the skull and is considered normal up to about 2 kPa (15 mmHg). The pressure is the result of many forces, including CSF production and reabsorption and the arterial pressure forcing blood into the skull. Other factors such as the "stiffness" of the brain modify the ICP.[3]

Once intracranial space occupation begins, surgery becomes relatively urgent. Intracranial tumors may be benign or malignant, primary or secondary. An abscess or a hematoma can also cause space occupation. The clinical course of space occupation depends on the area in which the SOL is developing and the speed at which it increases in size. Thus, the brain is less able to compensate for the rapid development of a hematoma following injury than for the slower development of a tumor.[4] A tumor developing in an "eloquent" area of the brain will present earlier by producing neurologic symptoms and signs. A tumor developing in a "silent" area of the brain, such as the frontal lobe, may become large before presenting, and, indeed, may present with the general signs of high intracranial pressure (Fig. 44.1).

The four intracranial constituents (brain, CSF, arterial blood, and venous blood), being essentially liquid, are incompressible, but two of them (CSF and venous blood) are connected to low-pressure systems outside the skull. The mechanisms that compensate for the presence of an SOL rely on these extracranial connections. As the SOL develops, intracranial CSF is lost to the spinal CSF space and venous blood from the thin-walled cerebral veins to the great veins in the chest. The ICP does not therefore rise in the early stages of intracranial space occupation. There is, of course, a limit to the amount of space occupation that can be accommodated in this way. Once that limit has been reached, the ICP will quickly rise to very high levels. The relation between the ICP and the volume of any SOL is expressed as the volume–pressure curve (Fig. 44.2).

The volume of the posterior fossa of the skull is much less than the supratentorial space. An SOL developing in the posterior fossa will tend to produce a rise in ICP relatively early, partly because of the small volume of the posterior fossa and partly because it may produce hydrocephalus by obstructing the flow of CSF. Infratentorial tumors also produce symptoms and signs related to the lower cranial nerves and to cerebellar compression and distortion (Fig. 44.3).

Cerebrospinal fluid and extracellular fluid

CSF is formed in the choroid plexus of the lateral ventricles by an active process. The rate of production[5] is about 0.4 mL min^{-1} and requires carbonic anhydrase and a sodium/potassium-activated ATPase. The CSF circulates through the third ventricle, aqueduct, and fourth ventricle. It reaches the subarachnoid space through the exit foramina in the fourth ventricle and is eventually reabsorbed through the arachnoid villi, which are in contact with the blood in the sagittal sinus. The composition of the CSF in the lateral ventricles resembles that of an ultrafiltrate of plasma,[6] but its composition is gradually modified as it circulates by the addition of brain extracellular fluid moving across the ependyma.

Obstruction to the flow of CSF can occur in a number of ways. Aqueduct blockage may follow SAH or head injury (HI), so that hydrocephalus results as a complication. Tumors and other mass lesions

Figure 44.1 *Computed tomography scan showing a large bifrontal meningioma.*

also distort or compress the CSF pathways, and by causing ventricular dilation will accentuate the effects of any SOL.

The rate of CSF production can be markedly modified. Alkalosis,[7] acetazolomide, furosemide, spironolactone,[8] and cardiac glycosides[9] all reduce the rate of CSF production. Enflurane[10] and desflurane[11] produce an increase in CSF production, presumably as a result of vasodilation of the choroid plexus. Isoflurane and sevoflurane do not show that effect.[11,12]

The interstitial fluid of the brain is limited by the blood–brain barrier (BBB), and any fluid forms, as elsewhere in the body, under the influence of the Starling balance at the capillary. Cerebral edema occurs under many clinical conditions and can affect brain bulk to a great extent. A simple classification of edema into vasogenic or cytotoxic was described by Klatzo,[13] although, as he points out, it is only rarely that one of the two mechanisms would be operating without some elements of the other. In vasogenic brain edema, there is an increase in vascular permeability in the cerebral capillaries, and edema associated with leakage of serum proteins into the brain parenchyma occurs. The edema fluid spreads through the brain by bulk flow; the white matter, which has a less dense structure than the gray, offers less resistance to such flow. Cytotoxic brain edema may exist after ischemia or hypoxia and may also be a feature of Reye syndrome.[14]

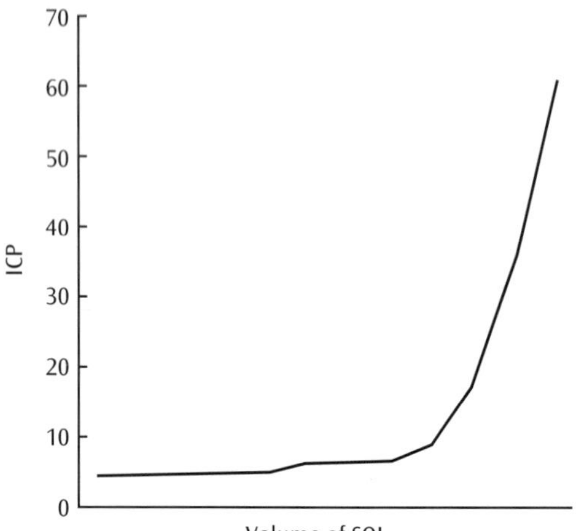

Figure 44.2 *Graph representing the change in ICP as intracranial space occupation develops.*

Tumors may be associated with the production of cerebral edema; therefore, the mass effect of the tumor is added to by the increase in brain bulk caused by the edema. Thus, the edema associated with a small SOL may result in a clinically insignificant degree of intracranial space occupation becoming a more serious clinical problem (Fig. 44.4).

Symptoms and signs of raised intracranial pressure

Raised ICP, whether existing preoperatively or caused during anesthesia, constitutes a significant risk to the patient. In the preoperative assessment of a patient for neuroanesthesia, the possibility of raised ICP needs to be considered. The symptoms and signs of raised ICP need to be distinguished from those due to the lesion producing the raised ICP. Miller[15] suggested that headache, vomiting, papilledema, and drowsiness are the symptoms and signs likely to be due to raised ICP alone, whereas bradycardia, arterial hypertension, and pupillary changes, although often occurring together with raised ICP, may arise from brainstem distortion or ischemia.

When the mechanisms that compensate for intracranial space occupation are exhausted, the ICP can rise to high levels. The medulla and cerebellar tonsils may be forced from the posterior fossa into the narrow confines of the foramen magnum so that the vital centers in the medulla are compressed, producing the syndrome described by Cushing[16] of bradycardia, hypertension, and ventilatory irregularity (Table 44.1).

Cerebral blood flow

The blood supply to the brain is about 15% of the cardiac output. It is provided mainly by the two internal carotid arteries, which together provide two-thirds of the CBF, and the vertebral arteries, which provide one-third. The basilar artery, formed from the two vertebral arteries, and the two internal carotid arteries join to form the circle of Willis

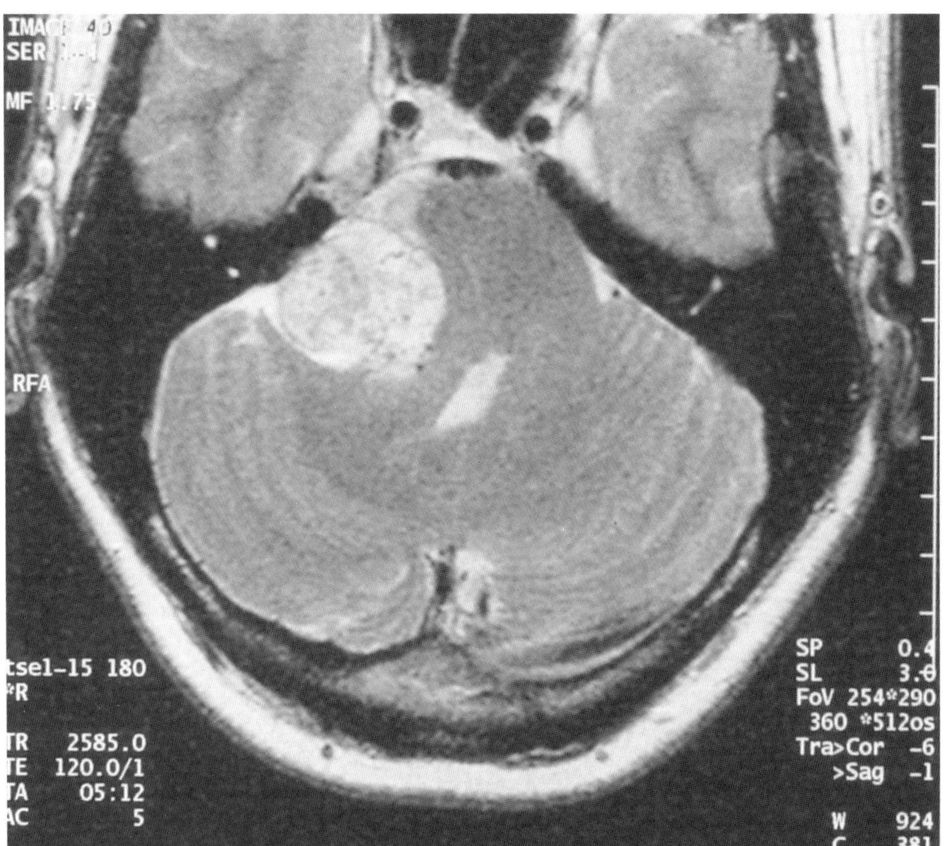

Figure 44.3 *Acoustic neuroma showing distortion of the cerebellum and fourth ventricle.*

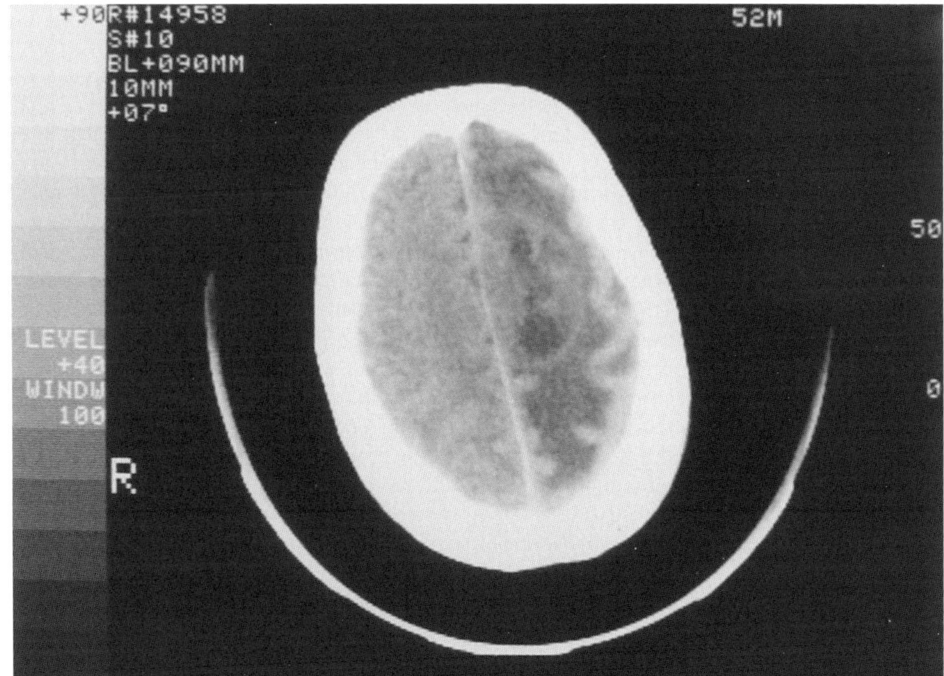

Figure 44.4 *Computed tomography scan showing a glioma surrounded by extensive edema.*

at the base of the skull. The morphology of the circle of Willis is quite variable, but from it arise the cerebral arteries.

The cerebral veins are thin walled and contain no valves. Being thin walled, they are exposed to the ICP. They drain into the cerebral venous sinuses, which, being contained within two layers of dura, are somewhat protected from the pressure changes in the skull. CSF drainage takes place along a pressure gradient through the arachnoid villi into the dural sinuses. Venous drainage takes place either through the internal jugular veins or through the vertebral venous plexus.

Control of cerebral blood flow

Metabolism

The dominant factor controlling CBF is cerebral metabolism. Cerebral metabolism, as revealed by oxygen utilization ($CMRO_2$), is normally about 3.0–3.5 mL per 100 g per minute, although regional differences exist. If metabolism increases, a cerebral vasodilation produces a rise in CBF to meet the increased need for oxygen; if metabolism falls, as for example with thiopental (thiopentone), CBF also falls.

Table 44.1 *Assessment of intracranial space occupation*

Clinical
Papilledema? Vomiting?
Level of response
Neurologic deficit
Computed tomography scan and angiography
Size and position of space-occupying lesion
Midline distortion
Cerebrospinal fluid obstruction
Edema
Vascularity; feeding vessels
Proximity to venous sinus

The normal cerebral circulation responds to changes in carbon dioxide (CO_2), but some situations, such as injury or SAH, and some drugs or techniques modify the relation. Normally, there is a sigmoid relation between P_aCO_2 and CBF. Between 2.7 kPa (20 mmHg) and 10.7 kPa (80 mmHg) the CBF increases fourfold. At lower levels of P_aCO_2, cerebral vasoconstriction does not continue to increase and CBF does not fall away to any great extent. Similarly, at high values of P_aCO_2, maximum cerebral vasodilation appears to occur. Intracranial disease and injury may reduce the reactivity of the cerebral circulation to P_aCO_2, especially when local cerebral ischemia produces a local acidosis.

Autoregulation

Autoregulation maintains the CBF at a remarkably constant value between 6.66 kPa (50 mmHg) and 20 kPa (150 mmHg) mean arterial pressure (MAP) by cerebral vasodilation when the MAP falls and by vasoconstriction when it rises. Outside these limits, the CBF passively follows the MAP. When intracranial disease or injury abolishes or impairs autoregulation, the CBF may be pressure passive even at normal MAP values, so that there is a danger of significant cerebral ischemia at relatively small reductions of MAP. At high levels of MAP, there is a danger of BBB damage and, therefore, cerebral edema formation. Cerebral perfusion pressure (CPP) is normally defined as the difference between MAP and mean ICP; this appears to be the source of the autoregulatory response rather than the MAP. There is evidence that, when the CPP is reduced by a rise in ICP, the CBF is maintained to a lower CPP level than when the CPP is reduced by lowering the MAP.[17,18] As the CPP falls with increasing ICP, the brain is less compliant and the ICP pulse pressure increases, so that the volume of blood forced into the skull with each cardiac stroke provokes a greater pressure response.

The autoregulatory response is relatively slow to act in response to a change in the CPP and may take up to 2 min. Autoregulation can be affected by intracranial disease, such as SAH, or by space occupation, trauma, or anesthesia.[19] Isoflurane and desflurane [at 1.5 MAC (minimum alveolar concentration)] impaired autoregulation, whereas propofol (200 $\mu g\,kg^{-1}\,min^{-1}$) preserved it.

Neurogenic control

CBF falls with increasing sympathetic stimulation, although the maximum change of CBF is about 10%. Although this change is not large, it is of some clinical significance. If blood loss occurs during surgery so that the MAP is reduced, it is likely that a degree of sympathetic stimulation will exist as a result of the hemorrhage. The sympathetic-induced vasoconstriction will add to the effects of the MAP reduction on the CBF, producing a further reduction in regional CBF and increasing the ischemia.

Aneurysm and arteriovenous malformations

Aneurysms may develop in the cerebral circulation in the young adult, but most patients are aged 40–60 years. An aneurysm usually develops where an artery branches. Cerebral aneurysms present by causing a SAH, which may be confined to a minimal leakage into the subarachnoid space or may involve massive bleeding with extensive cerebral disruption and death. The initial bleed carries a distinct mortality (about 30% of patients die in the early stages after the SAH) and subsequent bleeds demonstrate an increasing mortality if not treated.

SAH presents with sudden-onset severe headache, perhaps with loss of consciousness. Nausea and vomiting, photophobia, and neck stiffness may be part of the presentation. During the bleed, the ICP is thought to rise to the level of the arterial pressure, and this may be involved in preventing continued bleeding from the arterial weakness. The SAH sets in train various complications (hypertension, unconsciousness, high ICP, neurologic deficits) that affect the status of surviving patients. The patient's condition can be assessed by scales such as that produced by the World Federation of Neurological Surgeons[20] (Table 44.2).

SAH may produce other systemic effects that affect the patient's fitness for anesthesia. Bed rest is a central part of the management of the patient after SAH, and therefore dehydration, decubitus pneumonia, and deep vein thrombosis may occur. Fluids should be prescribed to keep the hematocrit at about 30%. Patients who are comatose need to be intubated and ventilated. Hypoxia and hypercarbia must be avoided.

Hypertension may be noted and is difficult to evaluate because it may have been present before the SAH and may have been a contributory factor. In other patients, the sympathetic overactivity that not infrequently follows SAH may be responsible. Electrocardiogram (ECG) abnormalities are present in 60% of patients, including changes suggestive of ischemia with ST segment depression or elevation, T-wave inversion, or QT prolongation. Unless supported by other evidence of myocardial disease, these changes do not constitute a contraindication to surgery. Computed tomography (CT) scan, lumbar puncture, and angiography will establish the diagnosis and the vessel affected.

A major cause of morbidity after SAH is cerebral vasospasm. Neurologic signs developing after an initially good recovery from SAH suggest the development of vasospasm, which occurs in 30% of SAH patients.[21] Once cerebral vasospasm has developed, blood supply to an area of the brain may be inadequate and the neurologic deficit may develop into a completed stroke. The commonest time when signs referable to vasospasm develop is the eighth day following the initial bleed.

Much work has been carried out to understand the etiology and management of cerebral vasospasm, and the British Aneurysm Nimodipine Trial[22] demonstrated the dramatic effects of nimodipine. If administration of nimodipine was begun soon after the SAH and continued through the operative period, there was a 34% reduction in completed stroke and a 40% reduction in poor outcome. The mechanism driving the improvement is not fully understood. Calcium entry blocking drugs are associated with the production of cerebral vasodilation, but nimodipine appears not to reverse the angiographically demonstrated vasospasm. Following subarachnoid hemorrhage, cerebral vasospasm occurs in the majority of patients, and is accompanied by cerebral ischemia in 30%. Cerebral vasospasm may decrease cerebral blood flow, disturb autoregulation, and place the patient at risk for delayed cerebral

Table 44.2 *Grading of patients with subarachnoid hemorrhage*

Grade	Glasgow coma score	Neurologic deficit (aphasia, hemiparesis, or hemiplegia)
0	15	Absent
I	15	Absent
II	13–14	Absent
III	13–14	Present
IV	7–12	Present or absent
V	3–6	Present or absent

ischemia. Intraoperatively induced hypotension and hypocapnia can decrease the CBF further, although the effects of either on outcome have not been evaluated. SAH (especially in the worse grades) reduces the reactivity of the cerebral circulation to changes in P_aCO_2 and impairs autoregulation.

Surgery to clip the aneurysm may be performed in the first few days after the SAH, or 10–14 days after it. Delaying the surgery exposes the patient to the danger of rebleeding. Early surgery may be complicated by the presence of cerebral edema and a hyperemic cerebral circulation, which make the surgical approach more difficult.[23]

Pituitary tumors

Patients presenting for pituitary surgery may show evidence of endocrine deficiency and require replacement therapy before surgery. If bleeding takes place into a pituitary tumor, the sudden increase in size may cause compression of the optic chiasm and sudden blindness. Urgent operation to decompress the optic chiasm is required to prevent permanent blindness. Such patients are likely to show an acute endocrine deficiency.

Patients may also suffer from hypersecreting tumors. Those with Cushing's disease may have been accustomed to high plasma cortisol levels and require higher postoperative doses of steroids. Acromegalic patients are traditionally said to be difficult to intubate as a result of the large tongue and reduplication of the oropharyngeal mucosa. The earlier diagnosis with improved imaging of the pituitary may mean that this problem will become less serious. Acromegalic patients often suffer from compartment syndromes such as carpal tunnel syndrome. Evidence suggests that, in such patients, it may be wise to avoid placement of a cannula in the radial artery.[24]

Patients with pituitary disease may also develop hypertension, diabetes mellitus, and thyroid and adrenal insufficiency.

DRUG EFFECTS

Intravenous anesthetic agents

Thiopental, propofol, and etomidate all produce a fall in the $CMRO_2$ and a concomitant fall in the CBF. When sufficient thiopental has been given to produce an isoelectric electroencephalogram, the $CMRO_2$ is about half the awake value. No further fall in the $CMRO_2$ occurs if more thiopental is given.[25] The decrease in the CBF produces a fall in the ICP, and there is some evidence that the fall is greater when the ICP is high.[26]

Propofol (1.5 mg kg^{-1}) produces a fall in the CSF pressure of 32% after 2 min.[27] The reduction in the MAP produced by propofol may be greater than that produced by thiopental, and there is evidence that propofol protects more effectively against the pressor response to intubation than thiopental.[28] Propofol has been implicated in inducing seizure activity.[29,30] These authors demonstrated an activation of the electrocortigram in 17 out of 20 epileptic patients; the mean dose of propofol required for burst suppression was 88.2 mg, with a range of 25–175 mg.

In contrast, etomidate has a minimal effect on the cardiovascular system, although Renou *et al.*[31] found a 45% reduction in the $CMRO_2$ and a 34% reduction in the CBF. Milde *et al.*[32] also demonstrated a reduction in the $CMRO_2$ and the CBF and showed that the reduction was proportional to the dose of etomidate. The lack of any major cardiovascular depression ensures that the CPP is well preserved with etomidate.

Volatile anesthetic agents

Volatile anesthetic agents tend to uncouple the relation between $CMRO_2$ and CBF. The effect is well demonstrated by the action of *halothane*: 1% halothane causes a decrease in the $CMRO_2$ of 26% but an increase in the CBF of 27%, and therefore a considerable rise in the ICP.[33] Low concentrations of halothane (0.6 MAC) have relatively little effect on the CBF, but 1.1 MAC may triple it.

Isoflurane produces a reduction in the $CMRO_2$ that is greater than that produced by equivalent MAC values of halothane, but the CBF increase with isoflurane is minimal below 1.1 MAC.[34] Isoflurane (2.5 MAC) produces an isoelectric electroencephalogram (EEG), and increasing the concentration of isoflurane will not cause a further lowering of the $CMRO_2$. Some early studies showed that ICP can be increased significantly with isoflurane, especially if there is an already existing high ICP, if the patient is normocapnic, or if a mass lesion has produced a marked shift of the midline structures as revealed by CT or magnetic resonance imaging (MRI).[35,36]

Several groups have studied the cerebral effects of *sevoflurane*.[37,38] It seems that, as in the case of other volatile anesthetic agents, sevoflurane has an intrinsic dose-dependent cerebral vasodilator effect. However, this effect is less than that of isoflurane. In one study in neurosurgical patients,[39] sevoflurane has been shown to decrease middle cerebral artery flow velocity and not to cause an increase in ICP. On the other hand, Talke *et al.*[40] studied 20 patients, without evidence of mass effect, undergoing transsphenoidal hypophysectomy and requiring lumbar drains. Lumbar CSF pressure increased with sevoflurane (both 0.5 and 1.0 MAC) compared with a control group of patients receiving a propofol infusion. Half of the patients receiving sevoflurane required phenylephrine to support the blood pressure. Lumbar CSF pressure, cerebral perfusion pressure, and systolic blood pressure did not change in the propofol group. Sevoflurane may be of considerable value in neurosurgery because of its low blood gas solubility that allows rapid induction of anesthesia and prompt recovery.

Muzzi *et al.*[41] compared a single dose (1 MAC) of *desflurane* with a single dose of *isoflurane* during operation in hypocapnic patients with supratentorial mass lesions. They reported a gradual increase in lumbar CSF pressure [from 1.47 ± 0.53 kPa (11 ± 4 mmHg) to 2.4 ± 0.8 kPa (18 ± 6 mmHg)] during administration of desflurane but not isoflurane. Beginning 20 min after the institution of desflurane, lumbar CSF pressure was significantly greater than baseline. The continued increase in CSF pressure is attributed to an increase in CSF production due to choroid plexus vasodilation. The same effect appears to apply to enflurane. Although enflurane is associated with seizure-like activity on the EEG, the incidence of postoperative convulsions is no greater than that following isoflurane.

Nitrous oxide

Nitrous oxide has been used as part of an anesthetic sequence for neurosurgery for many years, but it has considerable cerebral effects. The main advantage of its use is that, by combining the effects of different anesthetic agents, a lower dose of each agent is given, so that recovery may be faster.

Early work showed that nitrous oxide increased the $CMRO_2$. It has also been shown to increase ICP.[42,43] In a study in patients with intracranial pathology,[43] it was shown that hyperventilation was able to prevent the rise in ICP. In 1988, Hansen *et al.*[44] showed that adding 0.5 MAC nitrous oxide to a background anesthetic of 0.5 MAC halothane or enflurane produced a greater increase in CBF than would have been expected by doubling the concentration of the background agent. Measuring cerebral blood flow velocity in volunteers has shown that the increase in CBF was prevented by hyperventilation.[45] In order for this to be relevant during neuroanesthesia, we need to be sure that vascular reactivity to CO_2 is maintained.[46]

Therefore, the question of whether it is safe to use nitrous oxide in neuroanesthesia depends, first, on the immediate response of the patient with intracranial disease to the drug and, second, whether the outcome of surgery is affected. This was the aim of a study in animals[47] in which nitrous oxide seemed to be associated with the worst outcomes. There are no clinical studies relating outcome to nitrous oxide usage.

Muscle relaxants

Being highly charged molecules, muscle relaxants do not pass the blood–brain barrier. Therefore, they ought to have no direct effect on the brain, and their use in neurosurgery depends more on their systemic effects than on any cerebral effects.

The choice and use of muscle relaxants should be compatible with the rapid and complete recovery required after neurosurgery. Any tendency to prolonged muscle weakness needs to be avoided in the postoperative neurosurgical patient, who is, of course, especially sensitive to the accompanying dangers of hypoxia or hypercarbia. Ballantyne and Chang[48] have calculated the mean recovery time associated with various muscle relaxants in a retrospective study of 270 patients. The difference in mean recovery time between patients receiving vecuronium and those receiving pancuronium (the two most commonly used drugs) was 33 min.

Pancuronium

Pancuronium causes an increase in heart rate and blood pressure.[49] This should have no discernible cerebral effect in patients with normal intracranial dynamics. There is, however, a possibility that the pressor response to laryngoscopy and intubation will be greater with pancuronium than with other relaxants, so particular care must be taken to prevent the pressor response when pancuronium is used.

Atracurium

Atracurium has some potential for histamine release. The question of histamine causing central nervous system (CNS) effects was investigated when tubocurarine was in frequent use. Some studies in animals and humans showed an increase in ICP and CSF production with histamine,[50,51] but with atracurium this is unlikely to have significant cerebral effects.[52] The metabolite of atracurium, laudanosine, is well known as a convulsant, but plasma levels do not seem to reach dangerous levels.

Vecuronium and rocuronium

Vecuronium would seem to have many of the properties of the ideal relaxant as it has no cerebral and few systemic side-effects. Rocuronium[53] has also been recommended.

Succinylcholine (suxamethonium)

The use of succinylcholine (suxamethonium) has been said to raise ICP. One explanation for this is that the fasciculations cause an increase in intra-abdominal pressure and therefore an increase in central venous pressure (CVP). This may not be the entire story. Minton *et al.*[54] gave succinylcholine to patients with intracranial space occupation both before and after muscle paralysis had been established with vecuronium. When given before the patient was paralyzed, succinylcholine caused a consistent rise in ICP from a mean of 2 kPa (15 mmHg) to 2.66 kPa (20 mmHg). After vecuronium had been given, the increase generated by succinylcholine was still present, but much smaller – the maximum increase being only 0.4 kPa (3 mmHg). The evidence suggests that increased muscle spindle activity generating afferent neuronal traffic produces an increase in cerebral activity, and therefore in regional CBF (rCBF). Lanier and colleagues confirmed the observations.[55]

Analgesics

The synthetic opioids are a valuable part of modern neuroanesthesia. Investigation of their actions on the brain and cerebral circulation has been complicated by their systemic actions. It is important when assessing the action of analgesics (as, indeed, for any drug) to ensure that they are not generating an effect, such as respiratory depression or hypotension, which has its own action on the cerebral circulation. For example, sufentanil[56] and alfentanil[57] may be associated with significant increases in CBF and/or ICP. Another study of fentanyl, alfentanil, and sufentanil using brain retractor pressure (BRP)[58] demonstrated no general tendency for the BRP to rise. When the MAP decreases after drug administration, it is likely that a compensatory cerebral vasodilation will occur; this produces a rise in ICP, which may be erroneously attributed to the drug action. Remifentanil[59] has many advantages compared with fentanyl, including better control of the pressor response to intubation and faster recovery.

ANESTHESIA

Anesthesia may be required in the operating room and also in the imaging departments for radiographs, CT scans, or MRI. The patient should be assessed in the usual way for fitness for anesthesia and surgery, but in addition the various risk factors arising from the neurosurgical disease must be evaluated so that the appropriate anesthetic can be chosen.

Premedication

Heavy premedication, particularly with narcotic analgesics, is inappropriate for neurosurgical patients, especially if there is a critical degree of space occupation. Any depression of conscious level may lead to an increase in $P_{a}CO_2$ from respiratory depression and therefore cerebral vasodilation and increased ICP.

Careful premedication is, however, of considerable value. Many people will be apprehensive at the thought of having to undergo neurosurgery and the resulting high levels of circulating catecholamines may produce cardiovascular instability in the early stages of anesthesia. Undue hypertension is obviously dangerous in the presence of an unclipped aneurysm. The use of oral benzodiazepines (10–30 mg temazepam or 10–20 mg diazepam) has proved effective in providing an acceptable degree of sedation.[60]

Patients presenting for spinal surgery with an acute disk prolapse may be in severe pain preoperatively, and the use of analgesic drugs in the premedication is valuable. Nonsteroidal anti-inflammatory drugs such as diclofenac can be used with diazepam and the modified release preparations provide a useful degree of analgesia into the postoperative period.

Induction

At all stages of the anesthetic, cerebral vasodilation produced by hypoxia or hypercarbia, or by the injudicious use of vasodilating anesthetic agents, must be avoided. It is important to produce a low CVP. This means ensuring profound muscle relaxation, with no tendency to cough or strain. A sudden increase in blood pressure is potentially dangerous and should be prevented. Some neurosurgical conditions, including subarachnoid hemorrhage and head injury, produce local cerebral ischemia, so hypotension needs to be avoided in case it increases the extent of the ischemia. The patient's position should be such that the drainage from the cerebral veins is unobstructed.

Intravenous induction of anesthesia is preferred; both thiopental and propofol[61] may be used. The reduction in $CMRO_2$ produced by both drugs and the resultant reduction in CBF and ICP are of particular value when an SOL is present. Etomidate can be used: the depression of $CMRO_2$ is about the same, but the greater cardiovascular stability characteristic of the drug is associated with a greater rise in MAP on laryngoscopy and intubation than with thiopental or propofol. The use of a bolus injection of induction agent has been commonplace; however, if propofol infusion is being used for the maintenance of anesthesia, the infusion may be usefully started at induction. Techniques such as target-controlled infusion (TCI) or total intravenous anesthesia (TIVA) have been well studied and are appropriate for induction and maintenance of neuroanesthesia.[62]

The induction technique needs to abolish the hypertension that results from laryngoscopy and intubation. Although a problem for many patients,[63–65] the pressor response to intubation presents an obvious extra risk to neurosurgical patients with an arterial weakness, such as an aneurysm or arteriovenous malformation (AVM), of further hemorrhage. There is also a significant danger for patients with a vascular tumor because, as the blood pressure rises with intubation, the bulk of the tumor will increase, causing a rise in ICP. Indeed, there is likely to be a rise in the ICP in patients without a vascular tumor because the rapidity of the pressor response will outstrip the ability of the cerebral circulation to autoregulate.

If intubation is being effected using a nondepolarizing relaxant, a second, partial dose of the induction agent just before intubation is sensible. An infusion of the induction agent is an effective way of preventing the pressor response. Many other maneuvers have been suggested. The difference between thiopental and propofol is intriguing.[66] Propofol tends to depress the blood pressure more than thiopental and the blood pressure rise on intubation is greater with thiopental. Fentanyl (200–300 μg) at induction is only a partial protection. Use of beta-blockers has been recommended; calcium entry blockers (particularly verapamil, given 1 min before intubation) have been found to attenuate the blood pressure response without reducing the increase in circulating catecholamines.[67] Lidocaine (lignocaine) given intravenously 90 s before intubation is valuable in patients with cardiovascular instability.[68] Remifentanil[69] (1 $\mu g\,kg^{-1}$ bolus given over 30 s, followed by an infusion of 0.5 $\mu g\,kg^{-1}\,min^{-1}$) was effective in attenuating the pressor response in one study, although this study and another[70] point to the high incidence of hypotension or bradycardia with this dose of remifentanil. Sufentanil has also been recommended.

Intubation should only be performed when muscle relaxation is complete. The coughing and straining that result from premature attempts at intubation will produce a rise in intrathoracic pressure, so there will be not only a marked pressor response but also an increase in central and, therefore, cerebral venous pressure. ICP is certain to rise. The introduction of the laryngoscope and the traction necessary to view the vocal folds may be associated with jugular venous distortion, so that venous blood flow out of the skull is impaired.

Maintenance of anesthesia

Neurosurgical operations may last several hours. The airway, venous access, and monitoring must be instituted and secured in such a way as to be completely reliable for the whole of the operating period.[71] In particular, the airway needs to be secure because access to the head may be impossible. Normally, an armored tube should be used and fixed in such a way as to leave cerebral venous drainage free. Some anesthesiologists also support the tracheal tube with an oropharyngeal pack, especially if the patient is prone or sitting. Placement of the tracheal tube should be carried out carefully; if the neurosurgeon flexes the patient's head and neck to facilitate surgery, the tracheal tube will be advanced along the trachea. It is possible therefore that a tube placed too close to the carina will be advanced into the right main bronchus.

Throughout the surgery, the anesthesiologist should choose drugs and techniques with the provision of good intracranial operating conditions in mind. There are many facets to this, including:

1. maintaining adequate cerebral perfusion pressure;
2. maintaining stable MAP;
3. avoiding factors leading to increased ICP
   a. hypoxia
   b. hypercarbia
   c. vasodilating drugs
   d. cerebral venous obstruction
   e. incomplete muscle relaxation;
4. reducing brain bulk;
5. protecting against the sudden development of cerebral ischemia.

At the end of surgery, a rapid recovery of consciousness is essential so that the level of response can be assessed. Other techniques such as hypothermia or hypotension may be required.

The head is often held in a head clamp in which pins mounted in a frame are fixed into the outer table of the skull; this is a painful procedure. The increase in blood pressure caused by this procedure needs to be prevented by appropriate analgesia given just before the pins are applied. A sudden rise in the MAP owing to a painful stimulus needs to be prevented. A sustained hypertension may lead to the acceleration of edema formation. Some groups[72] perform a local anesthetic skull block to avoid the painful stimulation, which they say allows the surgeon to review the placement of the pins. Others[73] infiltrate the scalp with local anesthetic just where the pins will be placed.

Sneyd *et al.*[74] studied three opioid regimens. The first was 50 $\mu g\,kg^{-1}$ alfentanil followed by 0.833 $\mu g\,kg^{-1}\,min^{-1}$ until dural closure. The second was alfentanil followed by remifentanil: 50 $\mu g\,kg^{-1}$ alfentanil followed by 0.833 $\mu g\,kg^{-1}\,min^{-1}$ for 2 h, then 0.25 $\mu g\,kg^{-1}\,min^{-1}$ remifentanil. The third treatment was 1 $\mu g\,kg^{-1}$ remifentanil followed by 0.5 $\mu g\,kg^{-1}\,min^{-1}$, reducing to 0.25 $\mu g\,kg^{-1}\,min^{-1}$ after craniotomy. Anesthesia was maintained with an infusion of propofol and 66% nitrous oxide in oxygen. The patients receiving remifentanil had the least intraoperative hemodynamic responses and those receiving alfentanil the most.

The initial part of the craniotomy is also painful, particularly cutting the skin and reflecting the galea. As the burr holes are drilled, there may be pressure on the skull, raising ICP. Further, if the dura has to be stripped away from the inner table of the skull (most likely if the surgeon is using a saw guide and Gigli saw), an intensely painful stimulus is produced as the periosteum is removed from the bone. At the same time, there may be marked sympathetic stimulation.[75] Both factors (pain and sympathetic stimulation) tend to raise blood pressure. Surgery inside the skull is not markedly painful unless the surgeon stretches the dura, which is most likely to happen near the points of dural attachment.

Once the bone flap is cut, any brain swelling will produce the risk of brain herniation through the bone defect; if that occurs, the herniated brain will infarct, so the anesthesiologist must attempt to reduce the brain bulk. Reducing brain bulk will also aid the surgeon, who may need to retract the brain to give access to deeper structures. An increase in brain bulk will lead to greater pressure on the brain retractors, leading to an increased amount of neuronal damage. The significance of retractor pressure can be assessed by using retractors capable of measuring the pressure applied to the brain.[76]

Blood loss in a craniotomy is usually less than 500 mL, but may be marked in special circumstances. Some tumors, such as meningiomas, are vascular, and surgery can produce fast and extensive blood loss. A vascular tumor, having a low vascular resistance, may generate relatively high pressure in draining veins. Rapid blood loss may therefore occur if they are damaged. This may happen particularly while the bone flap is removed when a meningioma on the convexity of the brain is being excised. The ability to replace blood that is lost and to control blood pressure is essential.

Urethral catheterization is essential, particularly if osmotic diuretics are to be used. Urine flow should be noted regularly to check that a diuresis has developed after the use of osmotic diuretics.

The agents used during maintenance of anesthesia have been subject to controversy for some time. All the volatile agents increase cerebral blood flow, to differing extents, and this may mean that the bulk of the brain will increase.

Some authors have pointed out that volatile agents may be used quite successfully as long as hyperventilation is employed at the same time, when the increase in the CBF generated by the agent is to a certain extent overcome by the reduction in CBF produced by the hyperventilation. Others have suggested that this may not be so, especially if the mechanisms compensating for intracranial space occupation are near exhaustion, when a further, even small, addition of space occupation to the intracranial volume may be critical. Studies have suggested, particularly in relation to isoflurane, that ICP can be increased, especially if the patient is normocapnic or if a preoperative CT scan shows that a mass lesion has produced shift of the midline structures.[36,77] Volatile anesthetics may also affect the reactivity of the cerebral circulation to changes in $P_{a}CO_2$.[78] It appears that changes in the CBF caused by alteration of the $P_{a}CO_2$ are greater with isoflurane anesthesia than with sevoflurane anesthesia. The authors suggest that attempting to decrease intracranial pressure by decreasing $P_{a}CO_2$ may be more successful during isoflurane anesthesia than during sevoflurane anesthesia.

Ravussin *et al.*[79] and Todd *et al.*[80] reviewed several anesthetic techniques. The latter group studied patients undergoing supratentorial craniotomy for tumor. Their patients were carefully assessed. The ICP was measured and the extent of brain swelling noted. The speed of emergence from anesthesia was also recorded. The group also measured total stay and hospital costs. Patients were assigned to one of three groups. The first group received propofol induction and maintenance of anesthesia with 10 μg kg^{-1} fentanyl load followed by 2–3 μg kg^{-1} h^{-1}. The propofol infusion was set between 50 and 300 μg kg^{-1} min^{-1}. In the second group, anesthesia was induced with thiopental and maintained with nitrous oxide (N_2O), oxygen, and isoflurane; up to 2 μg kg^{-1} fentanyl was given only after bone flap replacement. The third group also had thiopental induction of anesthesia, but with fentanyl as in group one and "low-dose" isoflurane. It was reported that the ICP before craniotomy was 1.6 ± 0.93 kPa (12 ± 7 mmHg) in group 1; 2 ± 1.6 kPa (15 ± 12 mmHg) in group 2; and 1.47 ± 1.07 kPa (11 ± 8 mmHg) in group 3. The authors suggest that all three anesthetic regimens were acceptable, pointing out that there were only small differences in ICP among the three groups. In assessing such a complex study, it is worth noting that only two patients in groups 1 and 3 had ICP levels greater than 3.2 kPa (24 mmHg), but that nine patients in group 2 had ICP levels greater than this.

The position of N_2O as part of the anesthetic technique is controversial. The main advantage is that, by combining nitrous oxide with other anesthetics and analgesics, the dose of each drug may be minimized so that recovery is likely to be faster.[81]

Propofol infusion, whether in combination with N_2O[82] or as TCI, is a valuable technique and avoids the need for vasodilating anesthetic agents. Ravussin *et al.*[79] considered that, in their study, propofol gave better control of responses to painful stimuli and faster recovery than thiopental/isoflurane, whereas Todd *et al.*[80] thought the differences in their patients were minimal. One group[81] used 2.0–2.5 mg kg^{-1} propofol for induction of anesthesia followed by 12 mg kg^{-1} h^{-1} for 10 min, then 9 mg kg^{-1} h^{-1} for another 10 min, and then 3–6 mg kg^{-1} h^{-1} for the rest of the study. They showed that with this dosage the responsiveness of the cerebral circulation to $P_{a}CO_2$ change was well maintained – the slope of the CBF vs. $P_{a}CO_2$ being 1.56 mL per 100 g per min per mmHg.

Hyperventilation

Hyperventilation[83] has been an important part of neuroanesthesia for many years because of its ability to reduce ICP by producing cerebral vasoconstriction. The vasoconstriction also reduces the intracapillary hydrostatic pressure and therefore shifts the Starling balance at the capillary in favor of fluid reabsorption from the brain extracellular space. Consequently, hyperventilation helps to provide improved operating conditions. Intraoperative surgical requirements (reduction of brain bulk) may necessitate hyperventilation but risks increasing cerebral ischemia.

Concern about the fact that hyperventilation "uncoupled" the link between the $CMRO_2$ and the CBF, reducing oxygen supply without reducing metabolism, has led to a re-evaluation of the technique. The CBF changes 4% for every mmHg change in $P_{a}CO_2$; thus, at high values of $P_{a}CO_2$ (10.6 kPa; 80 mmHg) the CBF is twice that at normocapnia. Any further rise in $P_{a}CO_2$ is not associated with a further rise in CBF. Maximum vasoconstriction occurs below 2.6 kPa (20 mmHg), at which level the CBF is reduced by 40%.[84] Hyperventilation is also associated with a slowing of the EEG consistent with cerebral ischemia and an increase in brain tissue and cerebrospinal fluid lactate concentrations.[85] Concern about the effect of ischemia worsened by hyperventilation has been voiced in head injury care.[86] The availability of easy jugular venous oxygen content measurement has allowed the study of the effects of hyperventilation.[87] Using jugular venous catheters, Matta *et al.*[88] studied the effects of varying the $F_{I}O_2$ on jugular bulb venous oxygen tension ($P_{jv}O_2$), saturation ($S_{jv}O_2$), and content ($C_{jv}O_2$) in hyperventilated patients. They showed that an increased $F_{I}O_2$ during acute hyperventilation in the anesthetized patient improves oxygen delivery to the cerebral circulation, as measured by a higher cerebral venous oxygen content and saturation. They recommended that "An increased $P_{a}O_2$ should be considered for those patients in whom aggressive hyperventilation is contemplated."

Muscle relaxants

The use of muscle relaxants in doses adequate for the provision of profound muscle relaxation is important for producing good intracranial operating conditions. It is important to remember that, as recovery from muscle relaxants begins, abdominal and thoracic muscle tone will recover faster than neuromuscular function tested by a nerve stimulator on the arm or leg. The recovery of muscle tone produces a rise in intra-abdominal and intrathoracic pressures and therefore in CVP. The increased CVP is transmitted to the cerebral veins, thereby raising ICP. If the brain is found to be tight at surgery, checking that the venous drainage from the head is clear and unimpeded is one of the first checks that should be performed; part of that check is to confirm adequate muscle relaxation.

Reversal of muscle relaxation and extubation

Care should be taken with the management at the end of the anesthetic.[89] The aim must be to ensure that the patient makes as full a recovery as possible, but without periods of coughing and straining or inadequate breathing. Coughing and straining, through the associated increase in intrathoracic pressure, expose the patient to the possibility of intracranial venous bleeding. Reversal of muscle relaxation must wait until after the head dressing or bandages have been applied, so that there is no chance of the patient coughing as the head is moved. A practical routine is to reverse the muscle relaxant, and immediately to remove any oropharyngeal pack that has been used. When the reversal is judged complete, so that the patient is able to breathe, a gentle laryngoscopy should be carried out and the pharynx cleared quickly. If breathing starts, the tracheal tube can be removed. Any hypertension at the time of extubation can be attenuated by the use of intravenous (i.v.) lidocaine ($1.5\,mg\,kg^{-1}$) 90 s before laryngoscopy (A Cooper and JM Turner, unpublished observations). Esmolol has also been recommended.[90,91] Others have used verapamil and i.v. lidocaine 2 min before extubation, either alone or in combination ($0.1\,mg\,kg^{-1}$ verapamil and $1\,mg\,kg^{-1}$ lidocaine).[92] Remifentanil ($1\,\mu g\,kg^{-1}$) has also been used to attenuate the cardiovascular response to extubation.[93]

Postoperative pain after neurosurgery has been shown to be less severe than after other forms of surgery,[94] although some patients do experience severe pain, especially those having had a frontal craniotomy.

Air is frequently left in the cranial cavity when surgery is finished and the craniotomy closed.[95] In a study,[95] air was seen in all scans obtained in the first 2 postoperative days, and in two-thirds of the patients the collection was judged to be moderate or large. At the end of the first week following surgery, the incidence decreased to 75%. Of the scans obtained during the second postoperative week, 11.8% had collections of air that were judged to be moderate or large. Another study[96] evaluated the changes in ICP at closure of the craniotomy cavity, relating ICP to whether N_2O was continued. The latter study demonstrated that ICP was reduced significantly in the N_2O group as the gas washed out of the entrapped air. Clearly, however, the high incidence of air in the skull means that nitrous oxide should be avoided if repeated anesthesia is required in the few weeks after a craniotomy.

SPECIAL PROBLEMS

Aneurysm surgery

In surgery for clipping an aneurysm, the anesthesiologist has to protect against a rise in blood pressure that may burst the unprotected aneurysm. Subarachnoid hemorrhage may be instrumental in causing vascular spasm, so that cerebral ischemia is a danger; the anesthesiologist must therefore avoid significant hypotension that will further reduce rCBF. The cerebrovascular reactivity to CO_2 and autoregulation are likely to be impaired after SAH in the worst affected patients. The surgeon needs to be able to retract the brain to approach the aneurysm site, so the anesthesiologist has to be careful to provide good operating conditions.

If the aneurysm bursts during the surgical dissection, control of the bleeding is a priority. The best outcome is achieved by a surgical clip placed across the feeding vessel[97] rather than inducing hypotension to reduce blood flow. Covering this period with thiopental or propofol may be of value,[98] although the greatest evidence for cerebral protection is demonstrated with barbiturates in the treatment of focal cerebral ischemia.[99]

If surgical control of the bleeding aneurysm is not immediately possible, the anesthesiologist should be prepared to lower the MAP to reduce the rate of bleeding, bearing in mind that this is associated with a high morbidity. Thiopental, propofol, labetalol, or isoflurane may be used.

Treatment of high intracranial pressure

Intracranial pressure falls to atmospheric pressure when the skull is open, as at craniotomy. If any processes that increase brain bulk are active, the brain will be difficult for the surgeon to retract and the operation may become impossible; or at least increased pressure on the brain retractors may be required, producing neuronal damage. More seriously, if the brain swelling is marked, part of the brain will be pushed out through the dural incision and the tight edges of the dura will interfere with rCBF, thus producing infarction of the herniated brain.

Intraoperatively, therefore, it is important to avoid factors that may increase brain bulk. Such factors may include faulty technique, the choice of drugs, and positioning. Although there are many agents that can be used to lower high ICP, the avoidable factors that raise ICP need to be identified and corrected first (Table 44.3).

Hyperosmolar diuretics

Mannitol, the standard agent to treat raised ICP, should be given as a 20% solution. It has many systemic and cerebral effects. When given in doses of $0.5–1.0\,g\,kg^{-1}$, it raises serum osmotic pressure so that water is drawn from the tissues into the vascular system. Therefore, initially, the circulating blood volume rises and the hematocrit falls.[100] The blood volume remains elevated for about 15–20 min and, during this time, blood pressure and CVP may also be elevated. The diuresis that occurs limits the extent of the rise in blood volume. The increased plasma oncotic pressure draws water from the brain and therefore reduces brain bulk. Mannitol, in addition to reducing ICP, also reduces the volume pressure response (VPR).[101] As a result of decreased blood viscosity, the decreased hematocrit also allows a greater CBF; in patients with intact autoregulation, this leads to a cerebral vasoconstriction (oxygen supply being kept in balance with demand), which lowers ICP. This effect is not seen in patients in whom autoregulation is impaired and in whom the increased CBF persists.[102]

Loop diuretics

Some diuretics have actions on the brain that may be useful when combined with other drugs. Acetazolamide, furosemide, and spironolactone decrease the rate of CSF production.[103]

Furosemide, given in doses of $1.0\,mg\,kg^{-1}$, produces a fall in ICP similar to that produced by $1\,g\,kg^{-1}$ of mannitol, but without the electrolyte changes that result from mannitol.[104] It acts by the inhibition of sodium and chloride reabsorption in the ascending limb of the loop of Henle and has a separate action in reducing CSF production by suppressing sodium transport. It is able to lower ICP by mobilizing normal brain extracellular fluid and cerebral edema.

The reduction in blood volume that occurs following the diuresis also contributes to the reduction in ICP because the genesis of a low CVP promotes, through the related low dural sinus venous pressure, resorption of CSF. Furosemide appears not to reduce the VPR.

Spironolactone reduces the rate of CSF secretion, and may therefore be of value when combined with other drugs. Ethacrynic acid, alone or in combination with mannitol, decreased ICP in experimental studies.[105]

Table 44.3 *Faults in technique*

- Inadequate muscle relaxation
- Poor cerebral venous drainage
  - Jugular venous obstruction
    - Neck rotation
    - Tapes round neck
    - Raised mean intrathoracic pressure
    - Poorly adjusted ventilator
  - Positive end-expired pressure
  - Inadequate head-up position
- Hypercapnia
- Hypoxia
- Overtransfusion
- Hypertension; increasing cerebral edema

Corticosteroids

Steroids have a marked effect in reducing cerebral edema. This is most dramatically seen in patients who have a focal lesion around which there is extensive edema. Steroids are much less effective when there is widespread brain injury. Following the administration of steroids to patients with edema surrounding a tumor, there is often a rapid improvement in conscious level and neurologic state. The mechanism of action is not clear, but stabilization of the cell membranes so that intracellular–extracellular gradients for water and electrolytes are preserved is one possible explanation. Steroids also reduce the extrachoroidal production of CSF.[106]

Steroids have little place in the acute control of intraoperative raised ICP, but may be given intraoperatively to reduce edema postoperatively. Dexamethasone (8 mg i.v.) as a single dose, followed by 4 mg 6-hourly, is an appropriate regime.

Cerebrospinal fluid removal

CSF removal may be achieved in a number of ways. The surgeon may choose to cannulate the cerebral ventricles, either through the incision or through a separate burr hole. Placement of a supratentorial burr hole used to be routine before starting posterior fossa surgery, so that if pressure rose in the posterior fossa during surgery the general ICP could be lowered without delay by tapping the ventricles.

In selected patients, without significant intracranial space occupation, a lumbar subarachnoid catheter may be placed in the CSF at the start of the anesthetic. Drainage of CSF to give better surgical access should not begin until after the dura is opened.

Metabolic suppression

Cerebral metabolic suppression has been used during neurosurgery. This was initially produced by hypothermia used as part of an operative technique during circulatory arrest to enable cerebral aneurysms to be clipped,[111] but is also of value in reducing brain swelling.

Shapiro[107] described the use of barbiturates, which depressed $CMRo_2$ and therefore lowered ICP as a result of the associated vasoconstriction. Other agents used in a similar way are propofol and etomidate. Thiopental and propofol lower ICP, but may also depress cardiovascular function. Lidocaine ($1.5\,mg\,kg^{-1}$) also lowers ICP and is valuable in the patient with cardiovascular instability.[68] It has been suggested that $1.5\,mg\,kg^{-1}$ lidocaine is as effective in reducing ICP as $3\,mg\,kg^{-1}$ thiopental.

Cerebral protection

Limiting the damage caused by cerebral ischemia has provoked much work of interest to anesthesiologists.[108,109] Some work has related to anesthetic drugs, some to nonanesthetic drugs, and some to hypothermia.[110] Hypothermia has been used during neurosurgery for many years.[111,112] The effects of drugs and techniques depend on whether focal or global ischemia is present, the duration and severity of the ischemia, and the blood glucose values.

Michenfelder[108,109] indicated that there is a difference between the effects of hypothermia and barbiturates on the brain. He suggested that hypothermia acted by decreasing the rates of all intracellular biochemical reactions, a function of temperature, rather than just the electrical activity of the brain. Barbiturates (and other anesthetic agents) stabilize electrically active membranes, thus decreasing the work of the brain and, therefore, its energy requirements. They appear to be particularly protective in focal ischemia.[113] Propofol has been less well studied in humans, but some animal studies suggest that it may provide some neuroprotection,[114] particularly when burst suppression is induced. It is worth noting that, while the reduction in $CMRo_2$ is undoubtedly the mechanism for much of the protective effect, propofol is well known as a free radical scavenger.

Todd and Warner,[115] reviewing the mechanisms of cerebral protection, suggested that the simple idea that metabolic depression will protect the brain needs modification. They point out that the ability of agents to protect the brain does not parallel their ability to suppress the EEG or the $CMRo_2$, and that the protective effects of hypothermia may not be related to the degree of cerebral metabolic depression.

Focal ischemia in the operating room is most likely to occur when a main artery feeding an aneurysm is clipped to gain control of that aneurysm. Pretreating that event with thiopental or propofol to produce burst suppression may be of value.

Other nonanesthetic drugs such as calcium channel blockers may provide some cerebral protection. Nimodipine, used to protect against the development of a completed stroke after SAH, is one such drug. Sodium channel blockers are under investigation. The action of lidocaine in reducing $CMRo_2$ has been known for some time, and its potential protective effects have been studied.[116] Excitatory amino acid antagonists such as the *N*-methyl-D-aspartate (NMDA) antagonists phencyclidine and MK-801 (dixocilpine) have been extensively investigated in an attempt to control the glutamate levels after cerebral ischemia.[117] They are also effective in focal ischemia, but have not been introduced widely into clinical practice. Many other drugs, including ketamine and dextromethorphan, free radical scavengers, and free fatty acid inhibitors, are being studied.

Pituitary surgery

The surgical approach may be transcranial or trans-sphenoidal. The advantages of the transsphenoidal route are that, because it minimizes direct neuronal damage, the postoperative morbidity and the incidence of seizures are low. The disadvantages of the transsphenoidal route center around surgical difficulties if the tumor extends outside the sella. Transsphenoidal hypophysectomy is quite a painful procedure[118] and the use of TIVA with remifentanil is valuable. Steroid replacement therapy and thyroid therapy may be required. Diabetes insipidus may follow, so hourly urine output needs to be observed carefully. It may persist for 7–10 days and should be treated with desmopressin (DDAVP), up to 2 μg initially.

Placement of a lumbar subarachnoid catheter is common because it allows the addition of saline to the CSF, raising ICP so that the pituitary tumor is made more accessible to the surgeon. Care is needed to identify the CSF catheter so that inadvertent administration of intravenous drugs is avoided. A bacterial filter in the catheter is a valuable safeguard against CSF infection.

Postoperatively, there may be bleeding into the airway and the blood may be swallowed. The surgeon may use nasal packs to control bleeding.

Posterior fossa surgery

Most operations in the posterior fossa are for space-occupying lesions. The relatively small capacity of the posterior fossa and the ease with which these tumors may cause hydrocephalus means that surgery should not be unduly delayed once space occupation has been diagnosed. Ventriculoperitoneal shunting may be required urgently to reduce ICP. There may be a generally raised ICP, and the lower cranial nerves need to be examined for signs of bulbar palsy. Any patient who presents with laryngeal incompetence or difficulty in swallowing will need specific airway care in the postoperative period.

It is also important to assess the proximity of the tumor to the vital centers in the floor of the fourth ventricle and to look for signs of cardiovascular disturbance during surgery. The older approach of maintaining spontaneous ventilation with a midline fourth ventricular tumor has been replaced by the near universal use of controlled ventilation of the lungs in such cases. If cardiovascular disturbance occurs during surgery, the surgeon should be told and the patient considered for pressure ventilation of the lungs in the postoperative period.

Some aneurysms present in the posterior fossa, particularly the posterior inferior cerebellar artery aneurysms and aneurysms on the basilar artery.

POSITIONING

Supine

Much neurosurgery is performed with the patient supine. All patients undergoing intracranial surgery should be positioned slightly head up (about 10° is usually enough) so that cerebral venous drainage is free. Frequently, the head will be turned to one or other side and it is important to ensure that the degree of neck rotation is not excessive, usually by raising the shoulder on a support. Excessive rotation of the head is well known as a cause of jugular vein obstruction.[119] Pressure points need particular care because of the length of the neurosurgical procedures. The eyes should be closed and covered, especially for a frontal operation because of the possibility of the surgical skin preparation fluids entering the eye.

Prone

Spinal surgery and posterior fossa surgery may be carried out with the patient prone. The airway must be carefully secured; the difficulties of reintubation should the tracheal tube fall out during a prone procedure are daunting to consider. Positive pressure ventilation is required and great care needs to be taken to ensure that no undue increase in CVP results from an inappropriate setting of the ventilator. There are many ways of supporting the patient in the prone position, so the method chosen needs to be related to the needs of the operation planned. Sometimes, firm supports under chest and pelvis, which leave the abdomen clear, are all that is required. On other occasions, such as for lumbar spine surgery, the surgeon needs the vertebral column flexed and supports such as the Wilson frame are required. Compression of the abdomen by faulty positioning will result in an increase in central venous pressure and, in the case of spinal surgery, engorged epidural veins. The eyes need to be closed and covered and the arms padded, either by the patient's side or on arm boards by the head, as appropriate for the surgery. Care should be taken to avoid pressure on the femoral neurovascular bundle.

Sitting

The use of the sitting position for surgery of the posterior fossa or posterior cervical spine has been reducing,[120–122] but it is still used in some centers and new procedures are finding it useful.[123] The disadvantages of the position include difficulties in maintaining the blood pressure and venous air embolism. The advantages include a low venous pressure, unrestricted chest movement, and, facilitating surgery, the fact that the blood flows away from the surgical field rather than collecting at the base of the incision.

As an anesthetized patient is placed in the sitting position, blood tends to pool in the lower extremities, so that venous return and therefore cardiac output are reduced; the peripheral vascular resistance rises to maintain blood pressure.[124,125] Anesthesia therefore needs to maintain the integrity of the baroreceptor arc. Hypotension should not be tolerated. The reported incidence of hypotension is variable: 10% in one series[126] and 30% in another.[127] High-risk patients should not be exposed to the sitting position. If hypotension is found on moving the patient into the sitting position, the patient should be returned to the supine position and the cause for the hypotension identified and treated. Light anesthesia, with muscle relaxants and opioid analgesics, is a good basis for the technique. Pancuronium is a particularly valuable relaxant. A fluid load is helpful and hyperventilation should be avoided. Many maneuvers have been described to avoid hypotension. These range from simply wrapping the legs in a firm bandage and flexion of the thighs and knees so that the legs are not dependent, to the use of a G-suit.[128]

Venous air embolism

The reported incidence from many centers of venous air embolism is variable, but, in the case of sitting patients, figures up to 50% have been reported[129,130] and a common saying is that the incidence is proportional to the degree of monitoring. The incidence is high and the dangers of venous air embolism (VAE) can be reduced to an acceptable degree only with good monitoring, a careful anesthetic and surgical technique, and good communication between the anesthesiologist and the surgeon. The use of specific methods to detect *early* embolism is essential.

When the patient is sitting, the hydrostatic level of the central venous pressure is likely to be considerably lower than the operation site, so the pressure in the veins in the area of the operation will be subatmospheric. In that situation, if a vein is opened by the surgeon, air will be drawn into the vascular system and passed on to the heart and lungs.

A method that is effective in detecting air embolism involves using a Doppler flow probe[131] with the crystal positioned at the right sternal edge between the third and fourth costal interspace. The signal from the probe is audio modulated, and air bubbles as small as 0.5 mL can be heard passing the probe. The major limitation of the Doppler method is that the radiofrequency signal of the surgical diathermy may interfere with the Doppler signal and, as the greatest danger from VAE is during the muscle dissection and bone work, the diathermy may be in use for quite long periods of time. Modern equipment should provide for rejection of the diathermy signal. The precordial probe must be positioned with care, and checked once the patient is sitting.

End-tidal CO_2 measurement must also be used. If the air enters the circulation gradually and passes on to embolize the pulmonary circulation, the peak value of end-tidal CO_2 reduces gradually. If a large volume of air enters the circulation quickly, the fall in observed end-tidal CO_2 may be rapid. The measurement is not as sensitive as the Doppler technique, but is quite adequate for clinical purposes. A disadvantage is that, if the cardiac output falls for any reason, the CO_2 level will also fall.

Both methods of air detection require that, as soon as a positive signal is obtained, the surgeon is informed and neck compression started so as to occlude the neck veins. The surgeon should if possible flood the operation site with saline. These measures prevent further embolism and the neck compression causes venous bleeding from the site at which the vein was opened, thus allowing the surgeon to seal the point at which air was entering. There is some value in pressing on the neck at agreed times during the operation to detect any veins opened inadvertently. This is most logically carried out during the periods of greatest risk for VAE, while the muscle is being dissected and during the bone work. Transesophageal echocardiography has also been used for air-bubble detection.[132]

A central venous catheter should always be placed in sitting patients so that air can be aspirated easily if the simple methods for preventing large amounts of air entering the vascular system fail. Bunegin *et al.*[133] showed that more air can be aspirated from a catheter placed in the superior vena cava than from one placed in the right atrium. The use of a flow-directed pulmonary artery (PA) catheter is advocated by some because it helps to identify patients at risk of hypotension as they are moved into the sitting position. It is possible that use of these catheters may also identify patients at risk from paradoxical VAE from probe-patent foramen ovale; such patients should not be in the sitting position for surgery. The PA catheter can also be used to aspirate air.

Auscultation of the heart sounds will demonstrate the classic mill wheel murmur only after a large VAE has taken place.

Positioning the sitting patient

The sitting patient should be positioned with care. The arms need to be supported to avoid traction injury to the brachial plexus. The back should be supported in the lumbar area with the hips and knees flexed so that no undue strain is placed on the back or the sciatic nerve in a paralyzed patient. In an operation on the cervical spine, the presence of cervical spondylosis or a central prolapsed intervertebral disk may lead to spinal cord damage if the head and neck are flexed as the patient is put into the head support.

MONITORING

Neurosurgery is likely at times to produce considerable and rapid blood loss. Some operations, especially those in the posterior fossa, may involve cardiovascular disturbance. Hypotension may be required on occasions. It seems obvious therefore that patients undergoing neurosurgery require a large-bore intravenous cannula capable of rapid blood transfusion, arterial cannulation, and central venous cannulation and CVP measurement for all operations inside the dura. The transducers should be positioned so that CPP can be derived, which means referencing the zero adjustment to the level of the base of skull. The ICP can be measured during the procedure from the intact side and allows the derivation of the CPP. In the case of sitting patients, positioning the transducer at the level of the base of the skull ensures that the arterial pressure forcing blood into the head is accurately known.

Core temperature, preferably nasopharyngeal or esophageal, must be measured. The length of neurosurgical operations may produce quite large falls in temperature, and the dangers of postoperative shivering, producing hypoxemia, ventilatory impairment, and increased intrathoracic pressure are well known.

Oximetry

Oxygen saturation measurements have been accepted as routine in all forms of anesthesia. The neurosurgical patient is especially sensitive to arterial hypoxemia, which causes brain swelling from the hypoxemia-induced hyperemia and the edema it is likely to cause. Many of the conditions for which neurosurgery is required involve some degree of local cerebral ischemia, to which the addition of hypoxemia is obviously dangerous.

End-tidal CO_2

End-tidal CO_2 ($P_{ET}CO_2$) measurements are essential to neuroanesthesia to set accurate levels of ventilation and, in relevant patients, as part of the monitoring for VAE. The value of the $P_{ET}CO_2$ should be compared with arterial blood gas sampling at the start of surgery and repeated through the procedure. In normal individuals, the difference between the P_aCO_2 and the $P_{ET}CO_2$ may vary by 0.27–0.67 kPa (2–5 mmHg), and the relation is not reliable through a prolonged procedure.[134]

Transcranial Doppler flow analysis

The ability of Doppler flow probes to pick up flow in the arteries of the circle of Willis, usually the middle cerebral artery, has permitted the noninvasive measurement of flow velocity.[135] Measurements of CBF, as distinct from flow velocity, are difficult in the operating room, but recent use of near-infrared analysis for patients undergoing craniotomy[136] suggests that measurements of CBF may be available in the near future.

Jugular venous oxygen sampling

Measurement of oxygen saturation in the jugular bulb ($S_{jv}O_2$) provides a useful measure of global cerebral oxygenation,[85] with the normal range being 55–85%. Values below that range suggest that oxygen demand is exceeding supply, and high values indicate a relative hyperemia.

Hypotension

The use of induced hypotension for neurosurgery has changed significantly over recent years.[137] It has been used extensively for surgery on vascular tumors, such as meningiomas, and for aneurysm surgery. Although inherently risky, because of the danger of cerebral ischemia, the technique has proved valuable and there are large series showing its freedom from major morbidity.[138]

NEURORADIOLOGY

Interventional neuroradiology is most commonly used for obliterating an aneurysm, for treating an arteriovenous malformation (AVM), or for reducing the blood flow to a vascular tumor before surgery. In most cases, a large vascular sheath (7.5Fr) is placed in the femoral artery and a catheter passed through the sheath to one of the major cerebral vessels. Finer catheters and guidewires are passed through this catheter into the cerebral vessels and up to the lesion. Angiography is performed at all stages of the procedure to delineate the anatomy. The radiograph is processed to "subtract out" radio-opaque structures such as bone, so that the vascular anatomy is clearer. A "road map" image is available, in which an angiogram view is retained on the radiologist's monitor screen with the current screening view superimposed on top.

Anesthesia should be set up as for similar patients in the operating room. The vasodilation produced by some anesthetic agents may mean that the angiographic images are less clear because the bolus of contrast cannot fill the vascular lumen.[139] Conversely, vasoconstriction, such as that produced by hyperventilation, not only improves the quality of the images but also allows more images to be taken because the cerebral circulation is slowed.[140]

The treatment of intracerebral aneurysms has been advanced by the development of the Guglielmi detachable coils,[141,142] i.e. platinum coils attached to a stainless-steel guidewire. The coil is passed through a fine catheter and in the aneurysmal sac opens to hold itself in position. Angiography is performed to check that the position of the coil is satisfactory. The connection between the guidewire and coil is fused by passing an electrical current through the system. The guidewire is then removed, leaving the coil in place. Several coils may be required for an aneurysm (Figs 44.5 and 44.6).

AVMs present a dramatic picture on angiography, with many feeding vessels and large, arterialized draining veins produced by the fistulae (Fig. 44.7A and B). Flow through the AVM is extremely rapid and not under autoregulatory control. Embolization is frequently performed in several stages, and in some centers conscious sedation is preferred.[143,144] The main advantage of conscious sedation is that, when a microcatheter

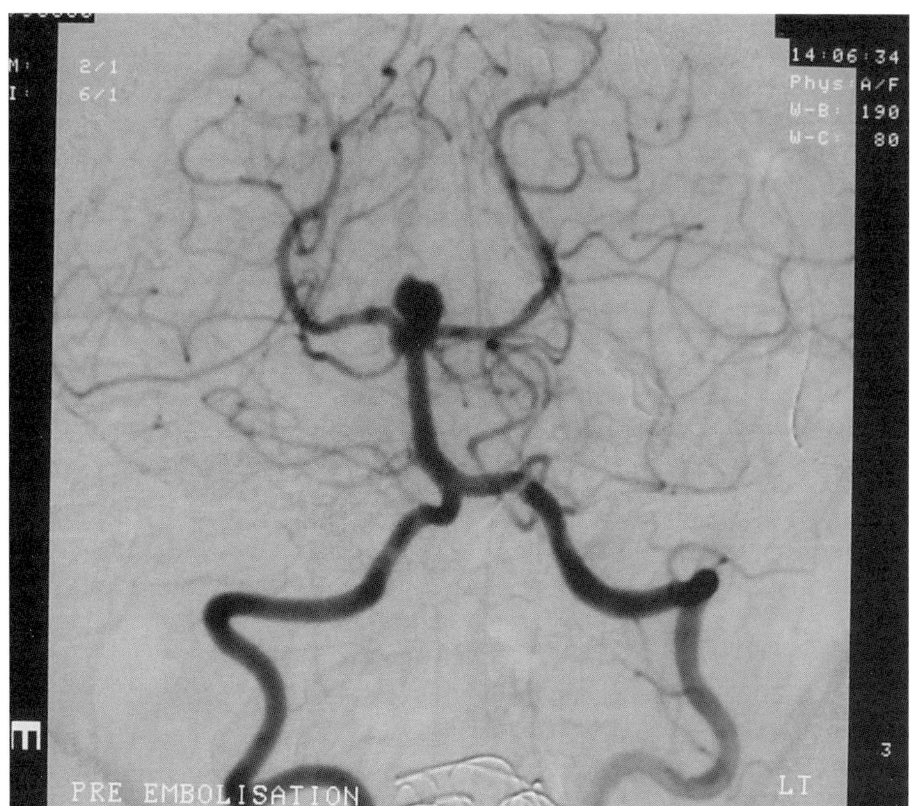

Figure 44.5 *Vertebral angiogram showing basilar tip aneurysm.*

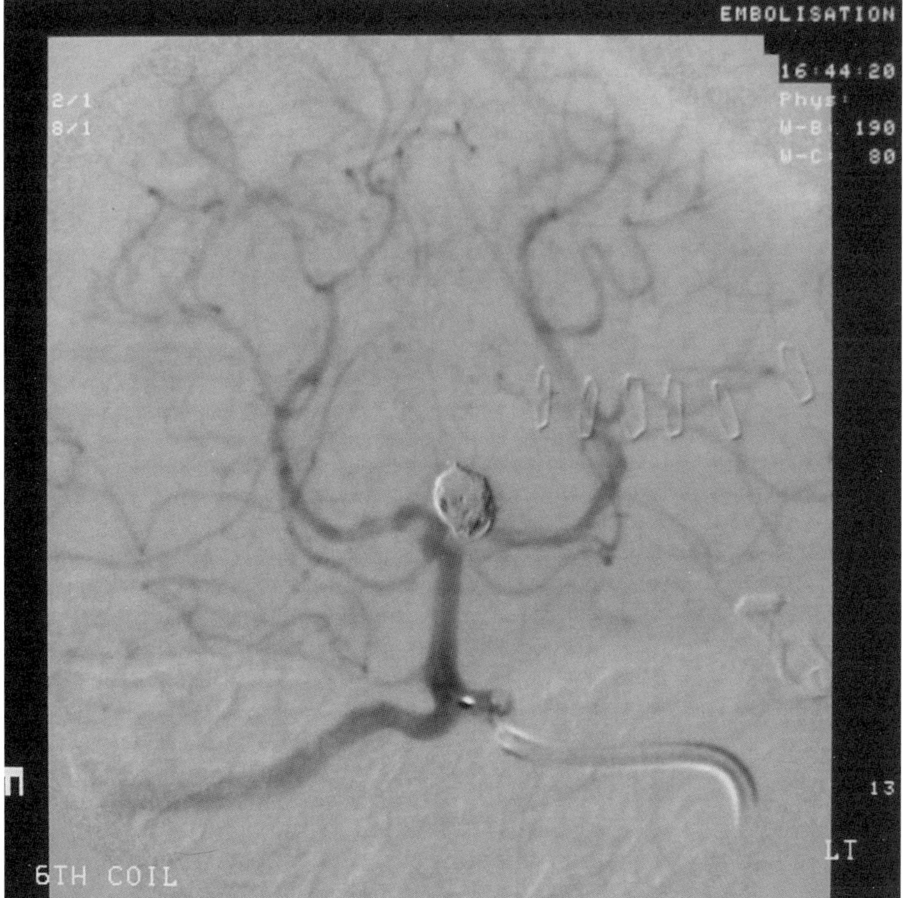

Figure 44.6 *Vertebral angiogram showing the appearance of the aneurysm shown in Fig. 44.5 after six coils have been inserted.*

A

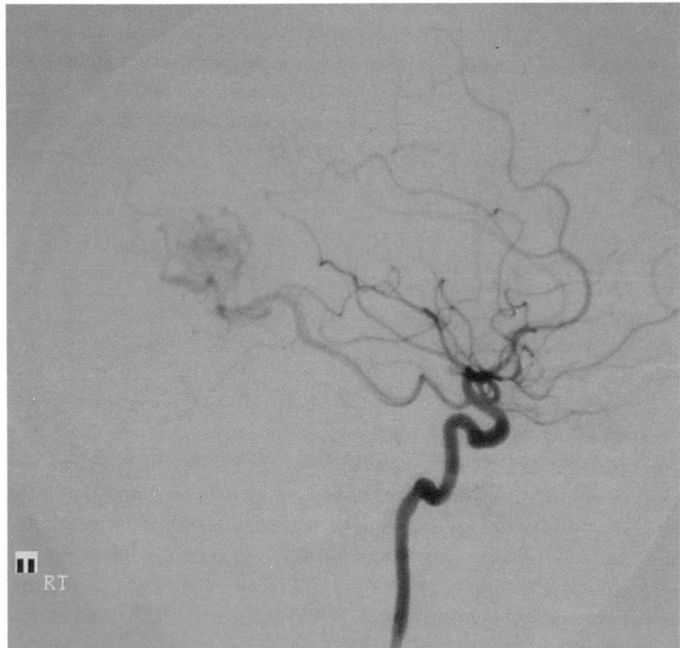

B

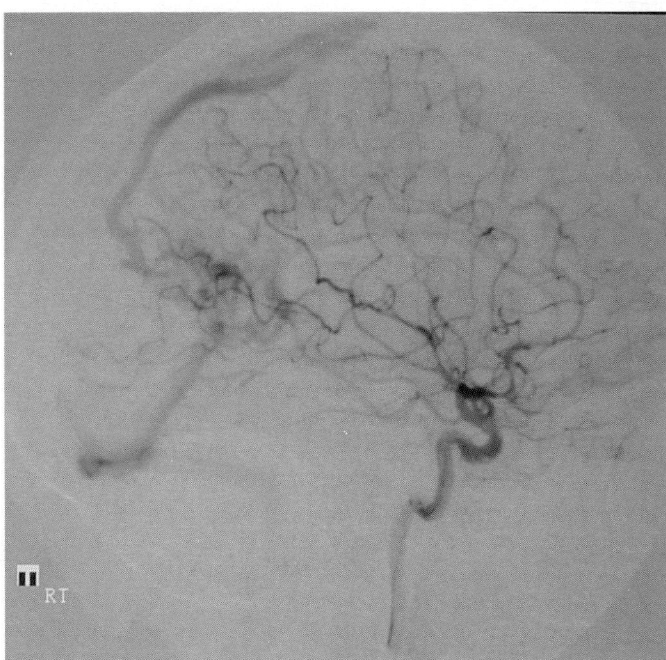

Figure 44.7 *Carotid angiogram lateral view showing AVM with (A) fast flow and (B) early filling vein.*

is placed ready for the embolization, the safety of the placement can be checked by injection of sodium amytal (30 mg) or lidocaine (30 mg)[1]45 with subsequent neurologic assessment.[146] General anesthesia does not easily allow for such an examination, but does allow the manipulation of the $P_{a}CO_2$ as well as the production of hypo- or hypertension as required. Many materials have been used for embolization, including contact adhesive (*N*-butyl-cyanoacrylate), coils, and pellets of silastic. More recently, the use of an ethylenevinylalcohol copolymer in dimethyl sulfoxide (DMSO) solvent has been recommended.

The successful placement of the embolic material within the AVM, avoiding it passing through to the venous circulation, may be quite difficult, and the ability of the anesthesiologist to modify blood flow to the AVM is valuable. Many techniques can be used, but this author's group uses a combination of hypotension produced by labetalol and sodium nitroprusside.[147,148] Once a stable level of hypotension has been produced, positive end-expiratory pressure (PEEP) is applied to the airway as the radiologist injects the embolic material to reduce, temporarily, the venous outflow. Anticoagulation is required and should be closely monitored with hourly measurements of activated partial thromboplastin time (APTT) and prothrombin time (PT).

Complications of interventional neuroradiology

Neuroradiology has a significant morbidity.[149,150] The two most serious complications of interventional radiology are hemorrhage and vascular occlusion. Hemorrhage takes place into the intact skull, so cardiovascular disturbance is noticeable. Control of any undue hypertension with thiopental or propofol will help to minimize the extent of the intracranial bleeding. Young and Pile-Spellman[146] are insistent on the necessity for the immediate reversal of the heparinization.

Vascular occlusion may lead to cerebral infarction if it is untreated. It may be due to thrombosis, to the malpositioning of catheters or coils, or to other embolic material. Vascular spasm may also be induced and may be treated by phentolamine or rogitine. Thrombolysis may be required. Induced hypertension may be required to maintain cerebral perfusion.

POSTOPERATIVE CARE

Good postoperative care is essential for the neurosurgical patient. Many of the disease processes, such as cerebral edema or local cerebral ischemia, that were present before the operation or that started during the operation persist and even develop further in the postoperative period. Additional complications may arise after surgery and the recovery room should be so organized that these can be recognized early and treated.

Hematoma formation

The incidence of postoperative hematoma formation should be low because of the care taken to achieve hemostasis before closure of the dura. The surgeon should always be aware when hypotension has been used so that he/she may be meticulous in securing hemostasis. Following hypotension, the systolic blood pressure should be at least 13.3 kPa (100 mmHg) before closure.

Cerebral edema

Edema is often present before surgery. A certain amount of edema formation always follows intracranial surgery and may continue to increase in extent for 24–36 h postoperatively. Extensive edema may affect conscious level.

Edema in the vicinity of the vital centers in the brainstem may lead to respiratory irregularity or apnea in the postoperative period.[151] The impairment of breathing may be recognized immediately on recovery from anesthesia or it may be delayed by several hours. Such patients require elective postoperative positive pressure ventilation of the lungs.

Respiratory failure

The indications for postoperative pressure ventilation are as follows:

- long operation;
- high intraoperative ICP;
- surgery close to vital centers;
- intraoperative vasomotor instability;
- midbrain edema;
- major blood loss;
- temporary clipping of a major artery.

Vasospasm

If vasospasm exists after surgery for clipping an aneurysm, fluid balance should be controlled carefully so that hypotension does not occur. Nifedipine infusion should be continued and therapy to raise the blood pressure, such as dopamine infusion, started if there are neurologic signs suggesting the existence of vasospasm.

Seizures

Seizures constitute a major emergency because they cause increased cerebral activity and metabolism at a time when the oxygen supply may be reduced by airway obstruction or respiratory insufficiency. Use of appropriate anticonvulsants such as phenytoin is usual.

Postoperative monitoring

The level of response, as indicated in an objective, repeatable way by such scales as the Glasgow coma scale,[152] is central to the detection of postoperative complications. It is essential, therefore, that the neurosurgical patient recovers rapidly and quickly from anesthesia and that observations made in the recovery room are comparable with those made later, when the patient has returned to the ward.

There must be regular assessment of localizing signs. Many neurologic signs can be attributable to supratentorial lesions, but the detection of muscle weakness on one side is the most valuable. Pupillary examination will reveal unilateral dilation. Measurement of heart rate, blood pressure, central venous pressure, and intracranial pressure as appropriate are important to ensure the maintenance of CPP.

Pain after craniotomy is not normally considered severe,[153] although some patients do experience severe pain. Codeine phosphate has traditionally been used to control the pain. Attempts to reduce postoperative pain by performing scalp blocks have not been successful.[154]

SUMMARY

The neuroanesthesiologist has always had to relate the anesthetic to the outcome of neurosurgery knowing that a badly judged anesthetic may make surgery difficult. The neuroanesthesiologist, therefore, has used a detailed knowledge of the disordered physiology of neurosurgical disease and of the effects of anesthetic drugs to ensure the best outcome for the patient. Currently, new measurement techniques are extending our knowledge of neurophysiology, sometimes confirming old ideas, sometimes contradicting favorite dogma. As these ideas work through into clinical practice, neuroanesthesia will continue to change and improve, possibly quite quickly.

REFERENCES

1. Polis TZ, Lanier WL. An evaluation of cerebral protection by anesthetics, with special reference to metabolic depression. In: Heyer EJ, Young WL (eds). *Anesthesiology Clinics of North America: Anesthesia for the Patient with Neurologic Disease.* Philadelphia: W.B. Saunders Co., 1997: 691–717.
2. Doyle PW, Matta BF. Burst suppression or isoelectric encephalogram for cerebral protection: evidence from metabolic suppression studies. *Br J Anaesth* 1999; **83:** 580–4.
3. Pickard JD, Czosnyka M. Management of raised intracranial pressure. *J Neurol Neurosurg Psychiatry* 1993; **56:** 845–58.
4. Fitch W, McDowall DG. Gradients of intracranial pressure produced by halothane in experimental space-occupying lesions. *Br J Anaesth* 1971; **43:** 704.
5. Plum F, Siesjö BK. Formation of cerebrospinal fluid. Recent advances in CSF physiology. *Anesthesiology* 1975; **42:** 708.
6. Ames A, Sakanoue M, Endo S. Sodium, potassium, calcium, magnesium and chloride concentrations in choroid plexus fluid and cisternal fluid compared with plasma ultrafiltrate. *J Neurophysiol* 1964; **27:** 672.
7. Oppelt WW, Maren TH, Ownes ED. Effects of acid–base alterations on cerebrospinal fluid production. *Proc Soc Exp Biol Med* 1963; **114:** 86.
8. Plum F, Siesjö BK. Formation of cerebrospinal fluid. Recent advances in CSF physiology. *Anesthesiology* 1975; **42:** 708.
9. Ames A, Higashi K, Nesbett FB. Effects of P_aCO_2, acetazolamide and ouabain on volume and composition of choroid plexus fluid. *J Physiol* 1965; **181:** 516.
10. Artru AA, Nugent M, Michenfelder JD. Enflurane causes a prolonged and reversible increase in the rate of CSF production in the dog. *Anesthesiology* 1982; **57:** 225.
11. Muzzi DA, Losasso TJ, Dietz NM, *et al.* The effect of desflurane and isoflurane on cerebrospinal fluid pressure in humans with mass lesions. *Anesthesiology* 1992; **76:** 720–4.
12. Scheller MS, Teteishi A, Drummond JC, Zornow MH. The effects of sevoflurane on cerebral blood flow, cerebral metabolic rate for oxygen, intracranial pressure, and the electroencephalogram are similar to those of isoflurane in the rabbit. *Anesthesiology* 1988; **68:** 548–51.
13. Klatzo I. Brain oedema following brain ischaemia and the influence of therapy. *Br J Anaesth* 1985; **57:** 18.
14. De Vivo DC. Reye syndrome: a metabolic response to an acute mitochondrial insult? *Neurology* 1978; **28:** 105.
15. Miller JD Intracranial pressure monitoring. *Br J Hosp Med* 1978; **19:** 497.
16. Cushing H. The blood pressure reaction of acute cerebral compression, illustrated by cases of intracranial haemorrhage. *Am J Med Sci* 1903; **125:** 1017.
17. Miller JD, Stanek AE, Langfitt TW. Concepts of cerebral perfusion pressure and vascular compression during intracranial hypertension. *Prog Brain Res* 1972; **35:** 411.
18. Grubb RL, Raichle ME, Eichling JD. The effects of changes in P_aCO_2 on cerebral blood volume, blood flow and vascular mean transit time. *Stroke* 1974; **5:** 630.
19. Strebel SM, Lam AM, Matta B, *et al.* Dynamic and static cerebral autoregulation during isoflurane, desflurane, and propofol anesthesia. *Anesthesiology* 1995; **83:** 66–76.
20. Drake CC, Hunt WE, Sano K, *et al.* Report of a World Federation of Neurological Surgeons Committee on a Universal Subarachnoid Haemorrhage Grading Scale. *J Neurosurg* 1988; **68:** 985–6.
21. Archer DP, Shaw DA, Leblanc RL, Tranmer BI. Haemodynamic considerations in the management of patients subarachnoid haemorrhage. *Can J Anaesth* 1991; **38:** 454.
22. Pickard JD, Murray GD, Illingworth R, *et al.* Effect of oral nimodipine on cerebral infarction and outcome after subarachnoid haemorrhage: British Aneurysm Nimodipine Trial. *Br Med J* 1989; **298:** 636.
23. Ohman J, Heiskanen O. Timing of operation for ruptured supratentorial aneurysms; a prospective randomised study. *J Neurosurg* 1989; **70:** 55–60.
24. Campkin TV. Radial artery cannulation: potential hazard in patients with acromegaly. *Anaesthesia* 1980; **35:** 1008.
25. Michenfelder JD. The interdependency of cerebral function and metabolic effects following maximum doses of thiopentone in the dog. *Anesthesiology* 1974; **41:** 231.
26. Turner JM, Coroneos NJ, Gibson RM, *et al.* The effect of Althesin on intracranial pressure in man. *Br J Anaesth* 1973; **45:** 168.
27. Ravussin P, Guinard JP, Ralley F, Thorin D. Effect of propofol in cerebrospinal fluid pressure and cerebral perfusion pressure in patients undergoing craniotomy. *Anaesthesia* 1988; **43** (Suppl.): 37.
28. Harris CE, Murray M, Anderson JM, *et al.* Effects of thiopentone, etomidate and propofol on the haemodynamic response to tracheal intubation. *Anaesthesia* 1988; **43** (Suppl.): 32.

29. Hodkinson BP, Frith RW, Mee EW. Propofol and the electroencephalogram. *Lancet* 1987; **2:** 1518.
30. Smith M, Smith SJ, Scott CA, Harkness WFJ. Activation of the electrocorticogram by propofol during surgery for epilepsy. *Br J Anaesth* 1996; **76:** 499–502.
31. Renou AM, Vernhiet J, Macraz P, *et al.* Cerebral blood flow and metabolism during etomidate anaesthesia in man, *Br J Anaesth* 1978; **50:** 1047.
32. Milde LN, Milde JH, Michenfelder JD. Cerebral functional, metabolic and hemodynamic effects of etomidate in dogs. *Anesthesiology* 1985; **63:** 371.
33. Christensen MS, Høedt-Rasmussen K, Lassen NA. Cerebral vasodilation by halothane anaesthesia in man and its potentiation by hypotension and hypocapnia. *Br J Anaesth* 1967; **39:** 927.
34. Eger EI. *Isoflurane (Forane). A Compendium and Reference*. Madison, WI: Anaquest, a Division of BOC Inc., 1986: 1.
35. Campkin TV, Flinn RM. Isoflurane and cerebrospinal fluid pressure – a study in neurosurgical patients undergoing intracranial shunt procedures. *Anaesthesia* 1989; **44:** 50.
36. Grosslight K, Foster R, Colohan AR, Bedford RF. Isoflurane for neuroanesthesia; risk factors for increases in intracranial pressure. *Anesthesiology* 1985; **63:** 533.
37. Matta BF, Heath KJ, Tipping K, Summors AC. Direct cerebral vasodilatory effects of sevoflurane and isoflurane. *Anesthesiology* 1999; **91:** 677–80.
38. Kuroda Y, Murakami M, Tsuruta J, *et al.* Blood flow velocity of middle cerebral artery during prolonged anesthesia with halothane, isoflurane, and sevoflurane in humans. *Anesthesiology* 1997; **87:** 527–32.
39. Artru AA, Lam AM, Johnson JO, Sperry RJ. Intracranial pressure, middle cerebral artery flow velocity, and plasma inorganic fluoride concentrations in neurosurgical patients receiving sevoflurane or isoflurane. *Anesth Analg* 1997; **85:** 587.
40. Talke P, Caldwell JA, Richardson CA. Sevoflurane increases lumbar cerebrospinal fluid pressure in normocapnic patients undergoing transsphenoidal hypophysectomy. *Anesthesiology* 1999; **91:** 127.
41. Muzzi DA, Losasso TJ, Dietz NM, *et al.* The effect of desflurane and isoflurane on cerebrospinal fluid pressure in humans with supratentorial mass lesions. *Anesthesiology* 1992; **76:** 720–4.
42. Greenbaum R, Cooper R, Hulme A, Macintosh IP. The effects of the induction of anaesthesia on intracranial pressure. In: Arias A (ed.). *Recent Progress in Anesthesiology and Resuscitation.* Amsterdam: Excerpta Medica, 1975: 794.
43. Hendrik HT, Jorgensen PB. The effect of nitrous oxide on intracranial pressure in patients with intracranial disorders. *Br J Anaesth* 1973; **45:** 486.
44. Hansen TD, Warner DS, Todd MM. Nitrous oxide is a more potent vasodilator than either halothane or isoflurane. *Anesthesiology* 1988; **69:** A537.
45. Hörmann C, Schmidauer C, Haring, HP, *et al.* Hyperventilation reverses the nitrous oxide-induced increase in cerebral blood flow velocity in human volunteers. *Br J Anaesth* 1995; **74:** 616.
46. Misfeldt BB, Jorgensen PB, Rishoj M. The effect of nitrous oxide and halothane upon intracranial pressure in hypocapnic patients with intracranial disorders. *Br J Anaesth* 1974; **46:** 853–68.
47. Baughman VL, Hoffman WE, Thomas C, *et al.* The interaction of nitrous oxide and isoflurane with incomplete cerebral ischemia in the rat. *Anesthesiology* 1989; **70:** 767–74.
48. Ballantyne JC, Chang Y. The impact of choice of muscle relaxant on postoperative recovery time: a retrospective study. *Anesth Analg* 1997; **85:** 476–82.
49. Coleman AJ, Downing JW, Leary WP, *et al.* The immediate cardiovascular effects of pancuronium, alcuronium and tubocurarine in man. *Anaesthesia* 1972; **27:** 415.
50. Weiss MH, Kurze T, Apuzzo ML, Heiden JS. Effect of curare in intracranial dynamics. *Surg Forum* 1974; **25:** 458.
51. Tarkkanen L, Laitinen L, Johansen G. Effects of *d*-tubocurarine on intracranial pressure and thalamic electrical impedance. *Anesthesiology* 1974; **40:** 247.
52. Minton MD, Stirt JA, Bedford RF, Haworth C. Intracranial pressure after atracurium in neurosurgical patients. *Anesth Analg* 1985; **64:** 1113.
53. Schramm WM, Strasser K, Bartunek A, *et al.* Effects of rocuronium and vecuronium on intracranial pressure, mean arterial pressure and heart rate in neurosurgical patients. *Br J Anaesth* 1996; **77:** 607–11.
54. Minton MD, Grosslight K, Stirt JA, Bedford RF. Increases in intracranial pressure from succinylcholine. Prevention by prior non-depolarising blockade. *Anesthesiology* 1986; **65:** 165.
55. Lanier WW, Milde JH, Michenfelder JD. Cerebral stimulation following suxamethonium in dogs. *Anesthesiology* 1986; **65:** 165.
56. Milde LN, Milde JH, Gallagher WJ. Effects of sufentanil on cerebral circulation and metabolism in dogs. *Anesth Analg* 1990; **70:**138–46.
57. Marx W, Shah N, Long C. Sufentanil, alfentanil and fentanyl: impact on cerebrospinal fluid pressure in patients with brain tumors. *J Neurosurg Anesthesiol* 1989; **1:** 3–7.
58. Herrick IA, Gelb AW, Manninen PH, *et al.* Effects of fentanyl, alfentanil and sufentanil on brain retractor pressure. *Anesth Analg* 1991; **72:** 359.
59. Guy J, Hindman BJ, Baker KZ, *et al.* Comparison of remifentanil and fentanyl in patients undergoing craniotomy for supratentorial space-occupying lesions. *Anesthesiology* 1997; **86:** 514–24.
60. Lodge D. *Therapy*. London: Penguin Books, 1995: 68.
61. Hoffman WE, Kochs E. Propofol: an intravenous anesthetic for neuroanesthetic practice? *J Neurosurg Anesthesiol* 1992; **4:** 75–7.
62. Gouldson R, Nathanson M, White PF, Smith I. Propofol: an update on its clinical use. *Anesthesiology* 1994; **81:** 1005.
63. Prys-Robert C, Foëx P, Biro GP, Roberts JG. Studies of anaesthesia in relation to hypertension. V. Adrenergic betareceptor blockade. *Br J Anaesth* 1973; **45:** 671–80.
64. Edwards DN, Alford AM, Dobson PMS, *et al.* Myocardial ischaemia during tracheal intubation and extubation. *Br J Anaesth* 1994; **72:** 537–9.
65. Roy WL, Edelist G, Gilbert B. Myocardial ischemia during noncardiac surgical procedures in patients with coronary-artery disease. *Anesthesiology* 1979; **51:** 393–7.
66. Lindgren L, Yli-Hankala A, Randell T, *et al.* Haemodynamic and catecholamine responses to induction of anaesthesia and tracheal intubation: comparison between thiopentone and propofol. *Br J Anaesth* 1993; **70:** 306–10.
67. Mikawa K, Nishina K, Maekawa N, Obara H. Comparison of nicardipine, diltiazem and verapamil for controlling the cardiovascular responses to tracheal intubation. *Br J Anaesth* 1996; **76:** 221–6.
68. Bedford RF, Persing JA, Pobereskin L, Butler A. Lidocaine or thiopental for rapid control of intracranial hypertension? *Anesth Analg* 1980; **58:** 435.
69. Thompson JP, Hall AP, Russell J, *et al.* Effect of remifentanil on the haemodynamic response to orotracheal intubation. *Br J Anaesth* 1998; **80:** 467–9.
70. O'Hare R, McAtamney D, Mirakhur RK, *et al.* Bolus dose remifentanil for control of haemodynamic response to tracheal intubation during rapid sequence induction of anaesthesia. *Br J Anaesth* 1999; **82:** 283–5.
71. Spiekermann BF, Stone DJ, Bogdonoff DL, Yemen T. Airway management in neuroanaesthesia. *Can J Anaesth* 1996; **43:** 820–34.
72. Pinosky ML, Fishman RL, Reeves ST. The effect of bupivicaine skull block on the hemodynamic response to craniotomy. *Anesth Analg* 1996; **83:** 1256.
73. Colley PS. Blunting the hemodynamic response to skull-pin placement. *Anesth Analg* 1997; **84:** 942.
74. Sneyd JR, Whaley A, Dimpel HL, Andrews CJH. An open, randomized comparison of alfentanil, remifentanil and alfentanil followed by remifentanil in anaesthesia for craniotomy. *Br J Anaesth* 1998; **81:** 361–4.
75. Shapiro HM, Wyte SR, Harris AB, Galindo A. Acute intraoperative intracranial hypertension in neurosurgical patients: mechanical and pharmacological factors. *Anesthesiology* 1972; **37:** 399–405.
76. Rosenorn J, Diemer NH. Reduction in regional cerebral blood flow during brain retraction pressure in the rat. *J Neurosurg* 1982; **56:** 826–9.
77. Campkin TV, Flinn RM. Isoflurane and cerebrospinal fluid pressure – a study in neurosurgical patients undergoing intracranial shunt procedures. *Anaesthesia* 1985; **63:** 533.
78. Nishiyama T, Matsukawa T, Yokoyama T, Hanaoka K. Cerebrovascular carbon dioxide reactivity during general anesthesia: a comparison between sevoflurane and isoflurane. *Anesth Analg* 1999; **89:** 1437–41.
79. Ravussin P, Tempelhoff R, Modica PA, Bayer-Merger M-M. Propofol vs thiopental-isoflurane for neurosurgical anesthesia: comparison of hemodynamics, CSF pressure and recovery. *J Neurosurg Anesthesiol* 1991; **3:** 85.
80. Todd MM, Warner DS, Sokoll MD. A prospective comparative trial of three anesthetics for elective supratentorial craniotomy. Propofol/fentanyl, isoflurane/nitrous oxide and fentanyl/nitrous oxide. *Anesthesiology* 1993; **78:** 1005.
81. Samra SK. Place of nitrous oxide in neuroanesthesia: still a valuable drug. *J Neurosurg Anesthesiol* 1992; **4:** 290–4.
82. Fox J, Gelb AW, Enns J, *et al.* The responsiveness of cerebral blood flow to changes in arterial carbon dioxide is maintained during propofol–nitrous oxide anesthesia in humans. *Anesthesiology* 1992; **77:** 453.
83. Brian JE. Carbon dioxide and the cerebral circulation. *Anesthesiology* 1998; **88:** 1365.
84. Harper AM, Glass HI. Effect of alterations in arterial carbon dioxide ten-

sion on the blood flow through the cerebral cortex at low and normal arterial blood pressures. *J Neurol Neurosurg Psychiatry* 1965; **28:** 449.
85. Plum F, Posner JB. Blood and cerebrospinal fluid lactate during hyperventilation. *Am J Physiol* 1967; **212:** 864–70.
86. Chesnut RM. Hyperventilation in traumatic brain injury: friend or foe? *Crit Care Med* 1997; **25:** 1275–8.
87. Matta BF, Lam AM, Mayberg TS, *et al.* A critique of the intraoperative use of jugular venous bulb catheters during neurosurgical procedures. *Anesth Analg* 1994; **79:** 745–50.
88. Matta BF, Lam AM, Mayberg TS. The influence of arterial oxygenation on cerebral venous oxygen saturation during hyperventilation. *Can J Anaesth* 1994; **41:** 1041.
89. Lowrie A, Johnston PL, Fell D, Robinson SL. Cardiovascular and plasma catecholamine responses at tracheal extubation. *Br J Anaesth* 1992; **68:** 261–3.
90. Spiekermann, BF, Stone DJ, Bogdonoff DL, Yemen TA. Airway management in neuroanaesthesia. *Can J Anaesth* 1996; **43:** 820–34.
91. Dyson A, Isaac PA, Pennant JH, *et al.* Esmolol attenuates cardiovascular responses to extubation. *Anesth Analg* 1990; **71:** 675–6.
92. Mikawa K, Nishina K, Takao Y, *et al.* Attenuation of cardiovascular responses to tracheal extubation: comparison of verapamil, lidocaine, and verapamil–lidocaine combination. *Anesth Analg* 1997; **85:** 1005–10.
93. Shajar MA, Thompson JP, Hall AP, *et al.* Effect of a remifentanil bolus on the cardiovascular response to emergence from anaesthesia and tracheal extubation. *Br J Anaesth* 1999; **83:** 654–6.
94. Dunbar PJ, Visco E, Lam AM. Craniotomy procedures are associated with less analgesic requirements than other surgical procedures. *Anesth Analg* 1999; **88:** 335–40.
95. Reasoner DK, Todd M, Scamman FL, Warner DS. The incidence of pneumocephalus after supratentorial craniotomy. Observations on the disappearance of intracranial air. *Anesthesiology* 1994; **80:** 1008.
96. Domino KB, Hemstad JR, Lam AM, *et al.* Effect of nitrous oxide on intracranial pressure after cranialdural closure in patients undergoing craniotomy. *Anesthesiology* 1992; **77:** 421.
97. Gianotta SL, Oppenheimer JH, Levy MI, Zelman V. Management of intraoperative rupture of aneurysm without hypotension. *Neurosurgery* 1989; **25:** 54.
98. McDermott MW, Durity FA, Borozny M, Mountain MA. Temporary vessel occlusion and barbiturate protection in cerebral aneurysm surgery. *Neurosurgery* 1989; **25:** 54.
99. Polis TZ, Lanier WL. An evaluation of cerebral protection by anesthetics, with special reference to metabolic depression. In: Heyer EJ, Young WL (eds). *Anesthesiology Clinics of North America: Anesthesia for the Patient with Neurologic Disease.* Philadelphia: W.B. Saunders Co., 1997: 691–717.
100. Muizelaar JP, Wei EP, Kontos HA, Becker DP. Mannitol causes compensatory cerebral vasoconstriction and vasodilatation in response to blood viscosity changes. *J Neurosurg* 1983; **59:** 822.
101. Miller JD, Leech PJ. Effects of mannitol and steroid therapy on intracranial volume pressure relationships in patients. *J Neurosurg* 1975; **42:** 274.
102. Muizelaar JP, Lutz HA, Becker DP. Effect of mannitol on ICP and CBF and correlation with pressure autoregulation in severely head injured patients. *J Neurosurg* 1984; **61:** 700.
103. Plum F, Siesjo BK. Recent advances in CSF physiology. *Anesthesiology* 1975; **42:** 708.
104. Cottrell JE, Robustelli A, Post K, Turndorf H. Furosemide and mannitol induced changes in ICP and serum osmolality and electrolytes. *Anesthesiology* 1977; **47:** 28.
105. Wilkinson HA, Wepsie JG, Austin G. Diuretic synergy in the treatment of acute experimental cerebral oedema. *J Neurosurg* 1971; **34:** 203.
106. Martins AM, Ramirez A, Soloman LS, Weise GM. The effect of dexamethasone on the rate of formation of cerebrospinal fluid in the monkey. *J Neurosurg* 1974; **41:** 550.
107. Shapiro HM. Intracranial hypertension: therapeutic and anesthetic considerations. *Anesthesiology* 1975; **43:** 445.
108. Michenfelder JD. Cerebral protection with barbiturates: relation to anesthetic effect. *Stroke* 1978; **9:** 140.
109. Michenfelder JD. Hypothermia plus barbiturates: apples plus oranges? *Anesthesiology* 1978; **49:** 157.
110. Sano T, Drummon J, Patel P, *et al.* A comparison of the cerebral protective effects of isoflurane and mild hypothermia in a model of incomplete forebrain ischaemia in the rat. *Anesthesiology* 1992; **76:** 221.
111. Campkin TV, McNeil WT. Hypothermia for neurosurgery. *Br J Anaesth* 1964; **36:** 77.
112. Solomon RA, Smith CR, Raps EC, *et al.* Deep hyothermic circulatory arrest for the management of complex anterior and posterior circulation aneurysms. *Neurosurgery* 1991; **29:** 732.
113. Cottrell JE. Possible mechanisms of pharmacological neuroprotection. *J Neurosurg Anesthesiol* 1995; **7:** 31.
114. Young Y, Menon DK, Tisavipat N. Propofol neuroprotection in a rat model of ischaemia reperfusion injury. *Eur J Anesthesiol* 1997; **14:** 320.
115. Todd MM, Warner, DS. A comfortable hypothesis reevaluated. Cerebral metabolic depression and brain protection during ischemia. *Anesthesiology* 1992; **76:** 161.
116. Astrap J, Sorensen PM, Sorensen HR. Inhibition of cerebral oxygen and glucose consumption in the dog by hypothermia, pentobarbital and lidocaine. *Anesthesiology* 1981; **55:** 263.
117. Hudspith MJ. Glutamate: a role in normal brain function, anaesthesia, analgesia and CNS injury. *Br J Anaesth* 1997; **78:** 731.
118. Klimek M, Ammann J, Weigand C, *et al.* Pain after TIVA with remifentanil vs. fentanyl in patients undergoing transsphenoidal hypophysectomy. *Br J Anaesth* 1999; **82:** 192–3.
119. Turner JM, McDowall DG. The measurement of intracranial pressure. *Br J Anaesth* 1976; **48:** 735.
120. Campkin TV. Posture and ventilation during posterior fossa and cervical operations. *Br J Anaesth* 1981; **53:** 881–3.
121. Elton RJ, Howell SC. The sitting position in neurosurgical anaesthesia: a survey of British practice in 1991. *Br J Anaesth* 1994; **73:** 247–8.
122. Porter JM, Pidgeon C, Cunningham AJ. The sitting position in neurosurgery: a critical appraisal. *Br J Anaesth* 1999; **82:** 117–28.
123. Kahn RL, Hargett MJ. β-Adrenergic blockers and vasovagal episodes during shoulder surgery in the sitting position under interscalene block. *Anesth Analg* 1999; **88:** 378–81.
124. Albin MS, Babinski M, Maroon JC, Janetta PJ. Anaesthetic management of posterior fossa surgery in the sitting position. *Acta Anaesthesiol Scand* 1976; **20:** 117.
125. Dalrymple DG, MacGowan SW, Macleod GF. Cardiorespiratory effects of the sitting position in neurosurgery. *Br J Anaesth* 1979; **51:** 1079.
126. Young ML, Smith DS, Murtagh F, *et al.* Comparison of surgical and anesthetic complications in neurosurgical patients experiencing venous air embolism in the sitting position. *Neurosurgery* 1986; **18:**157–61.
127. Albin MS, Babinski M, Maroon JC, Jannetta PJ. Anaesthetic management of posterior fossa surgery in the sitting position. *Acta Anaesthesiol Scand* 1976; **20:** 117–28.
128. Martin JT. Neuroanesthetic adjuncts for surgery in the sitting position. II. The anti-gravity suit. *Anesth Analg* 1970; **49:** 588.
129. Michenfelder JD, Miller RH, Gronert GD. Evaluation of an ultrasonic device (Doppler) for the diagnosis of venous air embolism. *Anesthesiology* 1972; **36:** 164.
130. Voorhies RM, Fraser AR, Van Poznak A. Prevention of air embolism with positive end expiratory pressure. *Neurosurgery* 1983; **12:** 503–6.
131. Gildenberg PL, O'Brien P, Brett WJ, Frost EA. The efficacy of Doppler monitoring for the detection of venous air embolism. *J Neurosurg* 1981; **54:** 75–8.
132. Cucchiara RF, Nugent M, Seward JB, Messick JM. Air embolism in upright neurosurgical patients: detection and localization by two-dimensional transoesophageal echocardiography. *Anesthesiology* 1984; **60:** 353.
133. Bunegin L, Albin MS, Helsel PE, *et al.* Positioning the right atrial catheter. *Anesthesiology* 1991; **55:** 343.
134. Russell GB, Graybeal JM. The arterial to end-tidal carbon dioxide difference in neurosurgical patients during craniotomy. *Anesth Analg* 1995; **81:** 806.
135. Aaslid R, Markwalder T-M, Nornes H. Non-invasive transcranial Doppler ultrasound recording of flow velocity in basal cerebral arteries. *J Neurosurg* 1982; **57:** 769.
136. Owen-Reece H, Elwell CE, Harkness W, *et al.* Use of near infra-red spectroscopy to estimate cerebral blood flow in conscious and anaesthetized adult subjects. *Br J Anaesth* 1996; **76:** 43.
137. Moss E. Cerebral blood flow during induced hypotension. *Br J Anaesth* 1995; **74:** 635–7.
138. Kerr AR. Anaesthesia with profound hypotension for middle ear surgery. *Br J Anaesth* 1977; **49:** 447–52.
139. Dallas SH, Moxon CP. Controlled ventilation for cerebral angiography. *Br J Anaesth* 1969; **41:** 597.
140. Samuel JR, Grange RA, Hawkins TD. Anaesthetic technique for carotid angiography. *Anaesthesia* 1968; **23:** 543.
141. Guglielmi G, Vinuela F, Dion J, Duckwiler G. Electrothrombosis of saccular aneurysms via endovascular approach. *J Neurosurg* 1991; **75:** 8–14.
142. Guglielmi G, Vinuela F, Duckwiler G, *et al.* Endovascular treatment of posterior circulation aneurysms by electrothrombosis using electrically detachable coils. *J Neurosurg* 1992; **77:** 515–24.
143. Manninen PH, Chan ASH, Papworth D. Conscious sedation for inter-

ventional neuroradiology: a comparison of midazolam and propofol infusion. *Can J Anaesth* 1997; **44:** 26–30.
144. Menon DK, Gupta AK. Anaesthesia and sedation for diagnostic procedures. *Curr Opin Anesthiol* 1994; **7:** 495–9.
145. Rauch RA, Vinuela F, Dion J, *et al.* Preembolization functional evaluation in brain arteriovenous malformations: the ability of superselective amytal test to predict neurological dysfunction before embolization. *Am J Neuroradiol* 1992; **13:** 303–8.
146. Young WL, Pile-Spellman J. Anesthetic considerations for interventional neuroradiology. *Anesthesiology* 1994; **80:** 427–56.
147. Turner JM, Powell D, Gibson RM, McDowall DG. Intracranial pressure changes in neurosurgical patients during hypotension induced with sodium nitroprusside or trimetaphan. *Br J Anaesth* 1977; **49:** 419.
148. O'Mahony BJ, Bolsin SNC. Anaesthesia for closed embolisation of cerebral arterial malformations. *Anaesth Intensive Care* 1988; **16:** 318–23.
149. Earnest 4th F, Forbes G, Sandok BA, *et al.* Complications of cerebral angiography: prospective assessment of risk. *Am J Roentgenol* 1984; **142:** 247–53.
150. Purdy PD, Batjer HH, Samson D. Management of hemorrhagic complications from preoperative embolization of arteriovenous malformations. *J Neurosurg* 1991; **3:** 101–6.
151. Artru AA, Cucchiara RF, Messick JM. Cardiorespiratory and cranial nerve sequelae of surgical procedures involving the posterior fossa. *Anesthesiology* 1980; **52:** 83.
152. Teasdale G, Jennett WB. Assessment of coma and impaired consciousness. A practical scale. *Lancet* 1974; **2:** 81.
153. Jeffrey HM, Charlton P, Mellor DJ, *et al.* Analgesia after intracranial surgery: a double blind prospective comparison of codeine and tramadol. *Br J Anaesth* 1999; **83:** 245.
154. Bloomfield EL, Schubert A, Secic M, *et al.* The influence of scalp infiltration with bupivicaine on hemodynamics and postoperative pain in adult patients undergoing craniotomy. *Anesth Analg* 1998; **87:** 579.

45

Surgery of the heart and thoracic aorta

CHARLES HANTLER AND MARK PATRICK

INTRODUCTION

Heart disease is the commonest cause of death in the Western world. Approximately 40 000 open heart procedures are performed annually in the UK,[1] and worldwide the figure is closer to 1 000 000.[2] About 85% of adult cardiac surgery in the UK is performed for ischemic heart disease, and 15% for valvular heart disease, with aortic valve surgery about twice as common as mitral.[1] The fact that the anesthesiologist contributes to the outcome of heart surgery is accepted. This chapter deals with the preparation of patients for heart surgery, the conduct of anesthesia, cardiopulmonary bypass, and postoperative care.

PREOPERATIVE MANAGEMENT OF ADULTS

The purpose of preoperative workup is to establish the type and severity of cardiac disease, the presence of other pathology, and the need for further investigation and treatment, and to inform the patient. Operative risk can be quantified using risk stratification methodology based on preoperative findings.

Assessment of cardiac disease

Diagnostic methods

Diagnostic methods are clinical (history and examination), electrical (resting and exercise ECG), and imaging (plain radiography, echocardiography, nuclear imaging, cardiac catheterization, and angiography).

Pathophysiology and assessment of ischemic heart disease (IHD)

The important features in the history of patients with IHD are prior myocardial infarction (including when it occurred) and severity of functional limitation due to angina, breathlessness, or both. The severity of symptoms reflects the reduction in coronary flow reserve. Angina may be classified as stable, of which there are four grades (see Classification of symptoms), or unstable. The latter is characterized by a deterioration of symptoms over a few days or weeks. It almost always indicates intracoronary thrombosis without infarction, serial cardiac enzymes being normal. Unstable angina is an indication for hospitalization and usually requires parenteral therapy with nitrates and low-molecular-weight heparin, antiplatelet therapy, and early revascularization.

Breathlessness is due to pulmonary venous hypertension, which, in IHD, is due to left ventricular (LV) dysfunction. This may be irreversible, in which case it is usually associated with prior "Q"-wave myocardial infarction, or reversible, when due to either "hibernating" myocardium[3] or transient myocardial ischemia. The latter can occur in the presence of otherwise normal LV function. Hibernating myocardium is a condition in which regions of LV muscle are chronically too underperfused to contract, but are still potentially viable. In both cases, revascularization can lead to return of function. The prognosis in patients with either hibernating myocardium or transient ischemia (LV function recoverable) is different from that of patients with prior infarction (LV function irrecoverable).

Physical examination is usually normal but may reveal signs of left ventricular failure (LVF) and occasionally congestive cardiac failure (CCF). Other evidence of occlusive vascular disease may be found.

The ECG may be normal at rest. The most important ECG abnormality is "Q"-wave myocardial infarction, and this is indicative of myocardial damage. Exercise ECG, which is frequently performed when IHD is suspected, aids the assessment of functional limitation. The chest radiograph is normal unless LVF is present. Detailed evaluation is obtained by cardiac catheterization, LV cineangiography, and coronary angiography.

Only in two circumstances does coronary revascularization improve survival: triple-vessel disease with poor LV function and left main stem disease.[4] Otherwise, the procedure is performed to relieve symptoms.

Assessment of valvular heart disease (VHD)

Aortic valve disease (AVD)

In aortic stenosis (AS), the obstruction may be valvular, supravalvular, or subvalvular, the first being most common. AS usually occurs in a valve without any obvious underlying structural abnormality, but sometimes the valve is bicuspid or rheumatic. Obstruction occurs as a result of progressive calcification, leaflet thickening, and fusion.

In AS, a systolic pressure gradient exists between the left ventricle and the aorta. Thus, systolic tissue pressure in the left ventricle is much higher than coronary perfusion pressure, and this compresses the coronary circulation in systole. The combination of hypertrophy and high tissue pressure means that myocardial oxygen consumption is high. Thus, myocardial oxygenation is at risk, and one-third of patients with AS experience angina, although only 50% of these have significant coronary disease. The pressure-overloaded left ventricle undergoes progressive concentric hypertrophy. However, dilation of the ventricle only occurs once left ventricular failure supervenes. Late in the disease, cardiac output falls and the pressure gradient across the valve decreases.

Patients become symptomatic late in AS. Symptoms are breathlessness, angina, and syncope. Symptoms are indicative of advanced disease, and such patients have a life expectancy of, at best, 5 years. Syncope and pulmonary edema are ominous signs. Patients with these symptoms require early surgery.

Aortic regurgitation (AR) arises either from abnormality of the valve or from dilation of the aortic root leading to functional AR. Rheumatic fever and endocarditis affect the valve; ascending aortic dissection and Marfan syndrome affect the root. Chronic AR often produces no symptoms until late in the disease. Although dilation of the LV occurs early due to volume overload, the LV is capable of withstanding chronic AR very well for long periods. Usually, it is the onset of failure that initiates symptoms. By contrast, acute AR due to endocarditis, aortic dissection, or trauma precipitates LVF rapidly.

Physical examination in aortic valve disease usually reveals the typical pulse characteristics. Arterial pressure measurement may reveal a narrow pulse pressure in AS and a wide pulse pressure in AR. Cardiac enlargement is common, particularly in AR, but not invariable. Typical murmurs are present, and in isolated AR these can include a systolic aortic flow murmur. Signs of LVF may be present.

The ECG varies from normal to a pattern indicating left ventricular hypertrophy (LVH) with repolarization abnormalities. The rhythm is usually sinus but occasionally atrial fibrillation (AF). The chest radiograph may be normal, especially in AS, but cardiac enlargement is common.

Aortic valve replacement is almost always indicated for patients with symptomatic aortic valve disease of either type. Without surgery, these patients are likely to develop LVF, or, in the presence of AS, die suddenly within a few years. The advisability of surgery for patients with asymptomatic disease is less clear, as the risk of sudden deterioration is small and has to be balanced against the risk of surgery and complications of prosthetic valves. Echocardiographic follow-up should be performed at least annually in patients with asymptomatic AVD.

Mitral valve disease (MVD)

In adults, virtually all mitral stenosis (MS) is rheumatic. Mitral regurgitation (MR) may be rheumatic, congenital, degenerative, or ischemic. In ischemic MR, it is papillary muscle dysfunction or tethering that causes the valve to leak, rather than failure of the valve itself. All MS is chronic, but MR may occur acutely, as a result of either papillary muscle rupture following myocardial infarction or chordal rupture.

Symptoms occur far earlier in patients with MVD than in those with AVD. The only common symptoms of chronic MVD are breathlessness, fatigue, and palpitations. LVF may occur in MR, but almost never in isolated MS, although the LV is frequently abnormal. Possible reasons for the LV abnormality in MS are calcification and fibrosis of the mitral apparatus and adjacent myocardium, and the after-effects of rheumatic carditis. The occurrence of LVF in MR is important. Normally, retrograde flow into the low-pressure left atrium (LA) reduces ventricular afterload. This tends to maximize the ejection fraction (EF). Thus, the finding of a low EF in MR is indicative of severe LV dysfunction.

Fatigue is caused by chronic low cardiac output. Palpitations indicate tachyarrhythmias, and in mitral valve disease this is almost always AF. The physical examination may reveal AF, signs of LVF or CCF, and typical murmurs. ECG abnormalities include AF, digoxin effects, and, in MR, LV hypertrophy.

The chest radiograph may show an abnormal cardiac outline, with enlargement of the LA, but the actual size of the LA can only be seen with a penetrated film. Overall cardiac enlargement is common in MR (but not invariable) and less common in MS. Massive cardiac enlargement occurs only if there is associated tricuspid regurgitation (TR). TR is more commonly functional regurgitation secondary to chronic pulmonary hypertension than the result of rheumatic tricuspid disease. Mitral valvular calcification may be seen on a lateral chest radiograph, the valve being posteroinferior to the center of the cardiac shadow.

Rheumatic mitral disease is usually irreparable and valve replacement is required. The only exception is that valvotomy can be performed in cases of simple commissure fusion. Mitral regurgitation due to degenerative disease is usually suitable for repair.[5]

Special diagnostic methods

Echocardiography

Echocardiography is used to assess both structure and function. It may be performed by transthoracic (TTE) or transesophageal (TEE) routes, and may be done at rest or using a myocardial stressor (stress echocardiography). Echocardiography has four main modes: "M" mode (M = motion) shows movement in one dimension; two-dimensional echo shows the moving heart in one plane; Doppler color flow mapping shows patterns of flow; and spectral Doppler techniques measure velocities. TTE is used in adults to assess structural abnormalities of valves and cardiac chambers, to quantify LV function, and to show pericardial fluid. The systolic aortic valve gradient in AS can be calculated from measurement of velocity of blood through the valve. Stress echocardiography, usually with an infusion of dobutamine as the stressor, is used to show reversible LV segmental wall motion abnormalities due to ischemia provoked by the stress. Preoperative TEE is used principally for the detailed assessment of mitral valve structure and function with regard to suitability for valve repair.

Nuclear cardiology

Nuclear imaging is used to assess LV function (using technetium) and myocardial perfusion (using thallium). As with echocardiography, imaging can be performed during a stress test to reveal reversible defects of myocardial blood flow. The stressor is usually dipyridamole.

Cardiac catheterization and angiography

Echocardiography and nuclear imaging are not always mandatory prior to cardiac surgery, but cardiac catheterization and angiography almost always are. Catheterization measures pressures and oxygen saturations within the heart. Angiography shows LV function, aortic and mitral valve abnormalities, and the coronary circulation. Although most valvular and other structural abnormalities can be demonstrated very well using echocardiography, only angiography can give detailed information about the coronary circulation. Given the high prevalence of IHD, most clinicians prefer to have this information before undertaking valve surgery.

Arrhythmias: pacemakers

The only common tachyarrhythmia seen preoperatively is AF. The commonest cause of AF is MVD, but it may occur in association with other types of VHD and IHD. Most patients in AF require drugs to control ventricular rate, and almost all are anticoagulated to reduce the risk of embolization of left atrial thrombus. It is usual to withhold coumarin anticoagulants for about 3 days prior to surgery. Subcutaneous heparin or low-molecular-weight heparin may be used instead.

Most patients with symptomatic bradyarrhythmias (blackouts or dizziness) are permanently paced. If not, they require preoperative temporary pacing, and will ultimately require permanent pacing. Permanent pacemakers must be electrically checked prior to surgery to verify normal box and lead function. Some pacemakers are inhibited by diathermy and the usual precautions – pacemaker reprogramming and/or bipolar diathermy – must be taken to avoid inhibition in a pacemaker-dependent patient.

Classification of symptoms

Symptoms causing functional limitation are classified according to the protocols of the Canadian Cardiovascular Society (CCS) and the New York Heart Association (NYHA). Details are shown in Table 45.1.

Drugs in heart disease

Classes and uses of drugs

The main classes of drugs used in the treatment of heart disease are listed in Table 45.2.

Interactions with anesthesia and bypass; discontinuing drugs

There are no interactions between drugs used to treat heart disease and anesthesia of such severity that the drug must be stopped before surgery. However, caution is required with the agents listed in Table 45.3.

It is generally recommended that drugs be continued up to surgery. Overwhelming evidence exists that beta-blockers should always be continued. Some prefer to omit ACE inhibitors for a few days, but there is no evidence that these drugs are associated with adverse outcome, at least in patients with normal LV function.[6] To avoid embarrassing the patient, diuretics are best avoided with sedative premedication. Aspirin and other inhibitors of platelet function such as clopidogrel are usually discontinued 1 week preoperatively. Discontinuation of aspirin is controversial as it is sometimes associated with increased symptoms of myocardial ischemia.

Evaluation of other relevant conditions

Table 45.4 lists the investigations required before surgery. History, examination, and the results of investigations may indicate the need for further evaluation of the conditions listed below.

Cerebral vascular disease

Stroke is a feared complication of open-heart surgery. Its incidence varies from 1% to over 10% and it is commoner in older patients. Prior neurologic event, aortic atheroma, and long bypass time are all risk factors for perioperative stroke during open-heart surgery. Patients with

Table 45.1 *Abbreviated functional classification of the severity of heart disease*

Class	New York Heart Association	Canadian Cardiovascular Society
I	Patients with cardiac disease without resulting limitations of physical activity. Ordinary physical activity does not cause undue fatigue, palpitation, dyspnea, or anginal pain	Ordinary physical activity such as walking or climbing stairs does not cause angina. Angina occurs during strenuous or rapid or prolonged exertion at work or recreation
II	Patients with cardiac disease resulting in slight limitation of physical activity. They are comfortable at rest. Ordinary physical activity results in fatigue, palpitation, dyspnea, or anginal pain	Slight limitation of ordinary activity. Walking or climbing stairs rapidly, walking uphill, or walking or stair climbing after meals, in cold or windy weather, or when under emotional stress induces anginal pain, or pain occurs only during the first few minutes after awakening. Walking more than two blocks on the level and climbing more than one flight of ordinary stairs at normal pace and in normal conditions induces anginal pain
III	Patients with cardiac disease resulting in marked limitation of physical activity. They are comfortable at rest. Less than ordinary physical activity results in fatigue, dyspnea, palpitation, or anginal pain	Marked limitation of ordinary physical activity. Walking one to two blocks on the level or climbing one flight in normal conditions induces anginal pain
IV	Patients with cardiac disease resulting in inability to carry on any physical activity without discomfort. Symptoms may be present at rest. If any physical activity is undertaken, discomfort is increased	Inability to carry on any physical activity without discomfort. Angina may be present at rest

Table 45.2 *Classes of drugs in heart disease and their principal uses*

Class of drugs	Principal uses
Diuretics	Preload reduction in heart failure Hypertension
Beta-blockers	Angina Hypertension Control of ventricular rate in AF
Calcium antagonists	Angina Hypertension
Nitrates	Angina Preload reduction in heart failure
ACE inhibitors	Preload and afterload reduction in heart failure
Potassium channel activators	Angina
Antiplatelet drugs	Inhibition of platelet function in IHD
Coumarin anticoagulants	Prevention of atrial thrombus formation in AF Inhibition of thrombosis on prosthetic valves
Unfractionated heparin and low-molecular-weight heparin	Prevention of coronary thrombosis in unstable angina
Antiarrhythmic drugs	Atrial and ventricular tachyarrhythmias

Table 45.3 *Interactions between anesthesia and drugs used to treat heart disease*

Drugs	Interaction	Solution
Diuretics	Hypokalemia leading to arrhythmias	Potassium administration
Beta-blockers	Extreme bradycardia in combination with opioids	Anticholinergic drugs
Nitrates	Venodilation leading to hypovolemia at induction of anesthesia	Fluid therapy prior to induction of anesthesia
ACE inhibitors	Venodilation leading to hypovolemia at induction of anesthesia	Fluid therapy prior to induction of anesthesia
	Hypotension during cardiopulmonary bypass	Vasopressors during cardiopulmonary bypass
Antiplatelet drugs	Increased bleeding	Aprotinin
Coumarin anticoagulants	Increased bleeding	Fresh-frozen plasma

Table 45.4 *Preoperative investigation of patients on admission for open-heart surgery. Italics indicate need in special circumstances only*

Classes of investigation					
Clinical	**Cardiologic**	**Radiologic**	**Hematologic**	**Biochemical**	**Microbiologic**
Temperature	Twelve-lead ECG	Posteroanterior chest radiograph	Full blood count	Urea	Nasal swab
Pulse		*Lateral chest radiograph (mitral valve disease)*	Coagulation screen	Creatinine	Throat swab
Arterial pressure			*Sickle test*	Electrolytes	Urine culture
Weight				Liver function	
Height				Cardiac enzymes	
				Blood glucose	–

a recent history of transient ischemic attacks or who have abnormal carotid pulses or bruits should undergo duplex ultrasonic imaging of the carotid arteries. Although many studies have been conducted, there is no consensus as to whether coronary and cerebral revascularization should be undertaken separately or simultaneously.

Pulmonary disease

Pulmonary disease is accepted as a risk factor for open-heart surgery. Preoperative management of patients with pulmonary disease should be as follows:

- A plain posteroanterior chest radiograph must be obtained for all patients preoperatively. Important radiographic features are those of chronic obstructive pulmonary disease or neoplasia.
- Routine heart surgery should not be undertaken in the presence of an undiagnosed lesion on chest radiograph.
- Pulmonary function testing is required for patients with a history of symptomatic chronic pulmonary disease, or for patients with unexplained breathlessness.
- Optimization of pulmonary status must be achieved by treating infection or bronchospasm.
- Nasal carriage of *Staphylococcus aureus* should be treated, as its presence is a risk factor for sternal infection.[7]

Renal disease

Abnormalities of renal function are common in this patient group, and may be due to heart failure, renovascular disease, or intrinsic renal disease. Preoperative chronic renal failure increases the mortality and morbidity of cardiac surgery.[8] The following steps should be taken:

- In patients requiring dialysis, the interval between the last dialysis and surgery should be less than 24 h.
- Radial arteries and forearm veins should not be cannulated.
- Anemia, if severe, will necessitate using blood as part of the bypass priming fluid. Potassium in cardioplegia should be used sparingly and avoided altogether in other fluids. Ultrafiltration during bypass is easily performed and can be used to remove fluid.
- Early postoperative dialysis may be needed to correct volume overload, hyperkalemia, or acidosis.
- The development of postoperative renal failure in patients with previously normal renal function carries a poor prognosis and is associated with persistent low cardiac output and multiple organ failure.

Diabetes mellitus

The rules for managing diabetes mellitus during open-heart surgery are similar to those for other major surgery. The neuroendocrine stress of cardiopulmonary bypass is so great that virtually all diabetic patients will need insulin perioperatively, and the dose of insulin required is significantly greater than for noncardiac surgery. Management should be as follows:

- Diabetes must be well controlled preoperatively. Blood glucose must be consistently below 14 mmol L^{-1}. On admission, glucose measurements should be performed before meals and at bedtime. Biguanides must be stopped.
- If glucose control is inadequate, it must be improved, and this may require insulin. Insulin should be given in soluble form before meals and a long-acting preparation at bedtime. Alternatively, an intravenous glucose–insulin–potassium regime may be used on a sliding

scale. Blood glucose should be measured 2-hourly until stability is achieved.

- On the day of surgery, sulfonylureas must be omitted. Two-hourly glucose estimations must be started. For morning surgery, the morning insulin dose should be omitted and an insulin regime instituted at the start of anesthesia. For afternoon surgery, insulin-dependent diabetic patients should be given breakfast along with one-quarter of their normal total daily dose of insulin as soluble insulin. Thereafter, an intravenous glucose–insulin–potassium regime should be started on a sliding scale. Noninsulin-dependent diabetic patients should be given breakfast, and an intravenous regime similar to that above should be started.
- During surgery, the aim is to maintain blood glucose at 5–10 mmol L^{-1}. The catabolic effects of the stress response mobilize glucose stores, and it is virtually never necessary to administer exogenous glucose intraoperatively. During bypass, large amounts of insulin may be needed, especially if glucose-containing cardioplegic solutions are used.
- Postoperatively, the sliding scale regime should be continued until the patient is eating reasonably. This usually takes about 3 days. A four times daily subcutaneous insulin regime similar to that described above for stabilization can then be recommenced. About 25% more insulin is usually required to be given than preoperatively. Conversion back to the patient's usual regime can be achieved by about day 5 postoperatively.

Hypertension

Preoperative arterial hypertension greater than 18.7/12 kPa (140/90 mmHg) is a risk factor for adverse outcome following open heart surgery.[9] Control of arterial pressure must therefore be achieved preoperatively, the aim being to maintain arterial pressure consistently below this value.

Premedication

All sources advocate premedication, its purpose being to achieve anxiolysis, and there is evidence that omission of premedication is associated with anxiety. Opinions differ as to the precise content. Most use either a benzodiazepine, an opioid–antiemetic mixture, or a combination of both. The dose used must reflect the size and fitness of the patient. Heavy premedication, for example benzodiazepine plus opioid–antiemetic combinations, produces significant hypoxemia, and oxygen should be administered, although the evidence that hypoxemia is associated with myocardial ischemia is weak. The incidence of deep venous thrombosis is sufficiently high during open-heart surgery that thromboprophylaxis is advisable. Pulmonary embolism occurs in about 0.5% of patients.

INTRAOPERATIVE MANAGEMENT OF ADULTS

Equipment

Monitoring

Surgeon, anesthesiologist, and perfusionist all require information from the monitors. The location and size of monitor displays must allow unobstructed vision of screens by all parties, and at least two displays are needed. Displays must be large and clear, and color is better than monochrome. Individual configuration of screens allows unnecessary information to be removed. Recording facilities must be available to allow printing of waveforms and derived hemodynamic parameters. An arrhythmia computer is optional.

Electrocardiographic monitoring (ECG)

Five-lead ECG is a minimum requirement. This allows recording of all six limb leads and one chest lead. For practical reasons, the latter is usually positioned at V6. Two leads must be displayed, one anterior lead and one inferior lead, to show both anterior and inferior ischemia. Usually, leads II and V are chosen.

Hemodynamic monitoring

Display of three pressure channels is essential. Display configuration must allow easy interpretation of waveforms and rapid recognition of changes. In particular, the pulmonary artery pressure (PAP) and pulmonary capillary wedge pressure (PCWP) must be easily distinguishable. Derived hemodynamic parameters obtained from cardiac output measurement must be available. Transducer systems must be zero stable over long periods, and accurate calibration must be verified.

Temperature monitoring

Core temperature can be measured from the nasopharynx (the commonest method), the tympanic membrane, the bladder, or the rectum (the least satisfactory site due to slow response). Heart temperature can be indirectly measured via the esophagus, although this is rarely used. Peripheral temperature can be measured on a finger or toe, but the latter is unsatisfactory in the presence of peripheral vascular disease.

Selection of monitoring

Physiologic monitoring for straightforward cases consists of five-lead ECG with S–T segment analysis, arterial and central venous pressures, core and peripheral temperature, metered urine output, pulse oximetry, and analysis of blood gases, acid–base status, electrolytes, glucose, hematocrit, and coagulation. More complex cases require additional monitoring consisting of the above plus one or more of pulmonary vascular pressures, cardiac output with derived parameters, mixed venous oxygen saturation ($S_{\bar{v}}O_2$),[10] TEE,[11,12] and cerebral monitoring. Indications for additional monitoring are shown in Table 45.5. Contraindications to the use of a pulmonary artery catheter are shown in Table 45.6.

Management of anesthesia

Anesthetic techniques

Techniques vary considerably between anesthesiologists. Whatever method is used, there are always two essential aims. The first is adequate anesthesia and the second is good hemodynamic stability. The actual drug combination used does not appear to affect outcome.[13]

The commonest approach is balanced anesthesia using a large dose of opioid. Muscle relaxation is universal, and most use a nondepolarizing agent from the outset. Techniques ranging from inhalational anesthesia using halothane, enflurane, isoflurane, desflurane, or sevoflurane to pure high-dose opioid anesthesia have been described. High thoracic epidural or spinal analgesia combined with general anesthesia has been advocated.[14] This has advantages, notably reduced opioid requirements, allowing more rapid awakening and inhibition of the stress response to bypass. Its use is, however, still limited by fears about the combination of neuraxial blockade and full anticoagulation. With large trials of thoracic epidural analgesia under way, this controversy is likely to be resolved soon.

Antibiotic prophylaxis is routine. Endocarditis and mediastinitis are very serious complications with high mortality. Endocarditis on a new prosthetic valve carries a mortality of more than 60%. The most important organisms to cover are *Staphylococcus aureus* and Gram-negative bacilli. Precise drug regimes vary, but most include an antistaphylococcal penicillin plus Gram-negative cover, usually an aminoglycoside.

Table 45.5 *Indications for additional monitoring. CABG, coronary artery bypass grafting; OPCAB, off-pump coronary artery bypass surgery*

Type of monitoring	Indications
Pulmonary vascular pressures	Left ventricular ejection fraction (LVEF) less than 40% Mitral valve disease Left, right, or congestive heart failure CCS class III or IV, or unstable angina Heart transplants Lung transplants (but not heart–lung transplants)
Cardiac output and derived parameters	Left, right, or congestive heart failure Any patient who is hypotensive after cardiopulmonary bypass despite adequate filling and inotrope therapy
Continuous mixed venous oxygen saturation	Single and bilateral sequential lung transplants
Transesophageal echocardiography (TEE)	Mitral repair, valvotomy, and homograft replacement Stentless and homograft aortic valve replacement Congenital heart defect repairs Ross procedure and aortic root replacement Dissection involving aortic valve Pericardial window for loculated effusion Monitoring LV function in high-risk OPCAB and CABG
Cerebral monitoring (oximetry, EEG, Doppler)	Symptomatic carotid disease and other high-risk scenarios such as carotid surgery with CABG

Table 45.6 *Contraindications to the use of a pulmonary artery catheter*

Contraindication	Clinical setting	Reason
Absolute contraindications	Mechanical prosthesis in tricuspid or pulmonary position	Interference with valve function
Relative contraindications	Aortic stenosis	Arrhythmias (AF and rarely VF) during insertion
	Left bundle branch block	Complete heart block during insertion

Management of hemodynamics during anesthesia

Except in certain conditions (described below), hemodynamics should be maintained to meet two conditions. The first is to prevent myocardial ischemia by maintaining global and regional myocardial oxygen supply in excess of demand. The second is to ensure adequate oxygen delivery to vital organs. These two aims may conflict and a balance has to be struck. The maintenance of myocardial oxygen supply in excess of demand is most crucial during coronary artery bypass grafting (CABG) (see Anesthesia for specific procedures: CABG).

Heart rate should be kept between 55 and 75 beats min^{-1}. It may be increased using anticholinergic agents and reduced using intravenous beta-blockade, for which esmolol is ideal. Mean arterial pressure should be maintained up to about 20% below awake levels. Thus, depending on the preoperative level, mean arterial pressure during anesthesia should usually be between 9.3 and 13.3 kPa (70 and 100 mmHg). It may be increased using vasoconstrictors and reduced either by deepening anesthesia or with nitroglycerine.

According to the law of Laplace, filling the heart increases left ventricular wall tension, and this increases myocardial oxygen consumption. Adequate filling is mandatory but unnecessary overfilling should be avoided. Ventilation should aim to maintain normocarbia and avoid hypoxemia, hyperoxemia, and overdistension of the lungs. The use of positive end-expiratory pressure (PEEP) is acceptable but sometimes hinders surgical access.

Anesthetic procedures

Arterial cannulation

The radial artery is the preferred site in most cases. Radial pulses may be absent, and alternative sites, including brachial, axillary, femoral, and pedal, may be used. The radial artery can sometimes give misleading information, especially immediately after bypass and in patients with low cardiac output, and cannulation of the femoral or axillary artery is preferable for patients with low-output states such as congestive heart failure.

Venous cannulation

Peripheral venous cannulation must be with a 14-gauge cannula. Central venous catheterization is usually performed via the right internal jugular vein, although occasionally the superior or infraclavicular subclavian routes are used. The use of ultrasound to locate the internal jugular or subclavian vein is associated with fewer failures and greater safety. If more than one catheter is to be placed in the same central vein, a Seldinger technique must be used and both needles must be in position before either catheter is placed. Mitral valve and right heart surgery require bicaval cannulation for bypass, and central lines must be no longer than 15 cm so as not to interfere with the superior caval cannula. Pulmonary artery catheters must be withdrawn 5–10 cm during bypass to prevent perforation of the pulmonary artery during surgical manipulation.

Preparation prior to induction of anesthesia

Before induction of anesthesia, an anticholinergic agent, a vasoconstrictor, heparin, and antibiotics must be ready. If antifibrinolytic agents or inotropes are needed, these should also be ready.

Surgery may be long and associated with reduced skin perfusion. Thus, the patient must be placed on a soft surface on the operating table to prevent pressure sores.

It is usual to attach the ECG and pulse oximeter and to insert peripheral venous and arterial lines before induction. This is the minimum monitoring required. Some anesthesiologists also insert the central line(s) at this time. This gives more information during induction. Volume may be required prior to induction.

Induction of anesthesia

Preoxygenation is mandatory. A suitable induction sequence is midazolam 0.15 $mg\,kg^{-1}$, fentanyl 15 $\mu g\,kg^{-1}$ (although there are alternatives to both of these), and a muscle relaxant. Before intubation, gentle ventilation through an absolutely clear airway is essential. Dynamic hyperinflation must be avoided as this reduces right heart filling and decreases cardiac output. Hypotension following anesthetic induction is treated using small doses of vasoconstrictors, such as metaraminol 0.25 mg. Hemodynamic stability during intubation is achieved by ensuring that all the induction drugs have time to be effective, and intubation should not be attempted for 2 min after induction. After intubation, anesthesia can be maintained with either an inhalational or intravenous anesthesia of choice. The central line(s), temperature probe(s), urinary catheter, TEE probe, and CNS monitoring should now be placed. A nasogastric tube may be passed, but there is no evidence that this is necessary.

Maintenance of anesthesia

The prebypass period

Hypotension secondary to decreased sympathetic tone is common before surgery starts and may need treating. Ventilation is usually discontinued during sternotomy to help prevent entering one or both pleural cavities, although there is little evidence that this is effective.[15] Blood gases, electrolytes, glucose, and hematocrit estimations must be performed at least once before bypass. A baseline activated clotting time (ACT) is measured or, if a heparin management system is used, a heparin dose–response calculation is performed. The heparin dose can be derived empirically, in which case 3–4 $mg\,kg^{-1}$ is given, or calculated from the dose–response curve. Heparin is administered and ACT must be greater than 300 s before cannulation of the aorta (see Cardiopulmonary bypass).

Arrhythmias are common. Surgical manipulation of the heart causes ectopic beats or AF. This may be treated with synchronized internal cardioversion using 10–20 J, although correction is not necessary if hemodynamics are satisfactory and there is no ECG evidence of myocardial ischemia. Very occasionally, ventricular fibrillation occurs. It is almost always indicative of myocardial ischemia. It requires either defibrillation or rapid institution of bypass.

The postbypass period

After bypass, the cardiac pathology should have been corrected, and a raised level of cardiac performance is needed compared with that before surgery. However, the heart has inevitably endured a period of hypoxia/ischemia and manipulation, which may have reduced cardiac performance.

During CABG, full revascularization cannot be assumed to have occurred, and it is still necessary to avoid gross tachycardia. A heart rate of 70–90 beats min^{-1} is usually ideal, with mean arterial pressure maintained at 9.3–13.3 kPa (70–100 mmHg). Hypertension can disrupt arterial anastomoses, and mean arterial pressure should not exceed this figure. Venous pressures should be sufficient to ensure adequate filling, but overfilling the heart may stretch a short bypass graft to the point of occlusion. Inotropic agents are preferable to overfilling. However, these drugs must never be used to boost arterial pressure in the presence of hypovolemia.

Choice of inotrope varies and is often influenced by local practice. No strong evidence supports the use of any one particular agent. In theory, vasodilator inotropes such as dobutamine and the phosphodiesterase inhibitors are preferable when the systemic vascular resistance (SVR), prior to weaning from bypass, is high. Conversely, norepinephrine (noradrenaline) may be preferable in the patient with a low SVR. Sometimes a combination of inotrope and vasoconstrictor is required. Unlike the catecholamines, the phosphodiesterase inhibitors can be administered either by infusion or bolus, and they produce tachycardia less commonly, but when failure is severe they are rarely adequate alone.

The circulatory and biochemical parameters that were corrected prior to discontinuation of bypass must be maintained in their normalized state. If inotropic and/or mechanical agents have been required to wean from bypass, they should usually be maintained at least until the end of surgery, although the dose may need modification. Inotropic agents may be needed for a prolonged period. Occasionally, the agent chosen may have undesirable effects, such as excessive tachycardia or vasodilation, and may need changing.

Before discontinuation of bypass, the lungs should be inflated manually to re-expand collapsed areas, particularly if either pleural cavity has been opened, but overinflation can disrupt an internal mammary graft. It is usually necessary to use a higher inspired oxygen concentration (F_IO_2) to maintain adequate arterial oxygenation after bypass. In about 1% of patients, bypass has profound adverse effects on pulmonary function and an F_IO_2 of 1.0 with PEEP may be required. Anesthesia may be maintained inhalationally or intravenously.

Once the bypass cannulae have been removed and sources of obvious surgical bleeding corrected, anticoagulation is reversed with protamine (see Cardiopulmonary bypass). Protamine may cause profound hypotension, and some anesthesiologists administer it while the arterial cannula is still *in situ* in order to allow rapid reinstitution of bypass after further heparin administration. Blood gases, electrolytes, glucose, and hematocrit estimations must be performed in the operating room at least once after discontinuation of bypass.

ANESTHESIA FOR SPECIFIC PROCEDURES

Coronary artery bypass grafting (CABG)

This is by far the most common procedure and will be considered in some detail. It is usually conducted through a median sternotomy and with the use of cardiopulmonary bypass. However, alternative techniques include surgery on the beating heart without bypass, through either a median sternotomy or left anterolateral thoracotomy, and laser revascularization.

Anesthetic considerations

Prevention of myocardial ischemia in the period between premedication and the initiation of bypass is the single most important aim. Evidence exists that the incidence of perioperative myocardial infarction (PMI) is increased if the heart is ischemic during this period.[16] PMI is associated with an increase in operative mortality and reduced long-term survival.

Induction and maintenance of anesthesia must achieve the desired aim of maintaining global and regional myocardial oxygen supply in excess of demand. This is achieved by paying very close attention to the control of arterial oxygenation, heart rate, arterial pressure, and filling pressures.

In order to prevent myocardial ischemia one must be able to detect it. Various methods exist to do this, and these are shown in Table 45.7. Most sensitive is TEE. If this is not available, ECG and PCWP are used to detect ischemia. PCWP measurement should be used for all patients with impaired left ventricular function, or unstable angina. However, among patients with stable class II angina and normal left ventricular function, there is no evidence that the use of PCWP measurement improves outcome.

If myocardial ischemia is detected at any stage in the prebypass period, it must be treated by reducing myocardial oxygen demand without reducing myocardial oxygen supply, or by increasing supply without increasing demand. Thus, tachycardia is treated with esmolol. Hypotension is treated with a vasoconstrictor. High PCWP is treated with glyceryl trinitrate infusion, with concomitant arterial vasoconstriction if needed to maintain arterial pressure. If myocardial ischemia cannot be rapidly reversed, early initiation of bypass is advisable.

Special situations

Some conditions present additional difficulty during CABG. These are repeat operations, unstable angina, and heart failure. Repeat surgery is complicated by adhesions between the heart and pericardium. These require careful dissection. Occasionally, adhesions may result in the sternal saw entering the right ventricle. For this reason, blood must be available in the operating room and checked prior to sternotomy. Blood loss after bypass is also usually increased.

Unstable angina implies the presence of intracoronary thrombosis and coronary flow is critically compromised. Prebypass management of hemodynamic performance to prevent myocardial ischemia is especially difficult. The combination of all three or any two of unstable angina, poor left ventricular function (EF < 25%), or redo surgery is an indication for insertion of an intra-aortic balloon pump (IABP) before or immediately after induction of anesthesia. Patients with the complications of myocardial infarction, namely papillary muscle rupture or post-infarction ventricular septal defect, are invariably in severe heart failure.

Surgery for aortic valve disease

Aortic valve replacement is the only common procedure used for aortic valve disease. Attempts to avoid some of the disadvantages of standard valve replacement with a mechanical or stented bioprosthesis (anticoagulation or repeat surgery) have led to the development of alternative procedures. These include stentless bioprostheses, homograft valves, and the Ross operation, in which the pulmonary valve is excised and relocated in the aortic position with a homograft replacement of the pulmonary valve. All these alternative procedures mandate the use of intraoperative TEE to confirm correct alignment and function of the prosthesis. The mortality for isolated first-time aortic valve surgery is 3%.[1] With concomitant CABG, the mortality rises to 7%.[1]

Aortic stenosis: anesthetic considerations

Patients with AS are at greater risk than others during induction of anesthesia, and those with LVF are at greatest risk. Hypotension must be prevented at all costs, as this reduces the coronary blood flow to the myocardium with a high oxygen consumption. Thus, myocardial depression and vasodilation must be avoided. A low heart rate and high SVR are desirable except in patients with LVF, who frequently have a resting tachycardia to compensate for reduced stroke volume. In this subgroup, bradycardia may cause an unacceptable reduction in cardiac output. The loss of atrial "kick" that may occur during anesthesia may also result in an unacceptable decrease in cardiac output.

Although CVP is inaccurate as a measure of left atrial pressure in AS, the dangers of inserting a pulmonary artery catheter are slightly greater than in other conditions. This is because the catheter may induce AF (and rarely VF) during insertion.

Aortic regurgitation: anesthetic considerations

A degree of vasodilation is desirable to offload the LV, but hypotension will compromise coronary blood flow. Conversely, a high "afterload" must be avoided. Because the LV volume overload in AR occurs in diastole, a low heart rate can cause excessive ventricular distension, particularly in acute AR. This is avoided by maintaining heart rate at 75–90 beats min^{-1} before bypass.

Surgery for mitral valve disease

This includes mitral valvotomy (for MS), mitral valve repair (for MR), and mitral valve replacement. In the first two cases, the use of intraoperative TEE to quantify valve gradient and regurgitation before completion of surgery is mandatory. This allows corrective further surgery if needed. The mortality of first-time mitral valve repair is 2.8%, and for replacement with a mechanical prosthesis 4.9%.[1] With concomitant CABG, the mortality rises to 8.6%.[1]

Mitral valve disease: anesthetic considerations

Many of these patients, and in particular those with rheumatic heart disease, will have pulmonary hypertension. This can lead to tricuspid regurgitation and/or right heart failure, which in turn can result in hepatic congestion and hyperbilirubinemia. Large doses of those drugs that are metabolized in the liver appear to have prolonged sedative effects in these patients. Doses of such drugs need to be reduced and, for example, 7.5 $\mu g\,kg^{-1}$ fentanyl is adequate.

The presence of chronic heart failure with low cardiac output and

Table 45.7 *Methods for the detection of intraoperative myocardial ischemia in decreasing order of sensitivity*

Method	Information obtained	Sensitivity
Transesophageal echocardiography	New segmental wall motion abnormality (SWMA)	Highest
Coronary sinus lactate estimation	Myocardial lactate production	↑
Pulmonary capillary wedge pressure measurement	Rise in PCWP accompanied by "a" and "v" waves	↕
ECG S–T segment monitoring	S–T segment changes (usually depression)	↓
Systemic pressures	Fall in arterial pressure and rise in CVP	Lowest

pulmonary hypertension makes pulmonary artery catheterization particularly useful. Mitral surgery is well known to adversely affect ventricular performance after bypass. It results in increased preload (in MS) and afterload (in MR).[17] Thus, patients are more difficult to wean from bypass than are those with other conditions, and hypotension despite adequate filling is common. Inotropes are often required, and cardiac output measurement is very useful when hemodynamic responses are unsatisfactory.

Surgery for diseases of the tricuspid and pulmonary valves

Surgery on the valves of the right heart is uncommon in adults. It is almost entirely confined to surgery to correct functional tricuspid regurgitation (TR) in patients with pulmonary hypertensive mitral valve disease. It is not always necessary to treat TR in this setting as the degree of regurgitation may reduce or it may disappear completely following treatment of the left heart lesion. Functional TR is usually treated by annuloplasty to reduce the valve area rather than by replacement. Organic causes of TR are rare and include endocarditis, carcinoid syndrome, and Ebstein's anomaly.

Anesthetic considerations

The management of patients with TR is determined by the underlying left heart pathology. Specific measures are sometimes required when TR is present. The pressure- and volume-overloaded right heart may become massively enlarged. This can cause deviation of the interatrial and interventricular septa, thus reducing left heart volume and performance. This can only be evaluated using TEE. A pulmonary artery catheter will have to be removed if tricuspid valve replacement rather than annuloplasty is performed. Increased pulmonary vascular resistance (PVR) during anesthesia must be avoided, as an elevation of PVR impairs the ejection of an already compromised right ventricle. Avoidable causes include nitrous oxide, alveolar hypoxia, acidosis, hypoventilation, extreme hyperventilation, inadequate anesthetic depth, and α-adrenergic agonists.

Surgery for congenital heart disease in adults

Congenital anomalies of the cardiovascular system occur in about 1% of newborn infants. The majority of conditions are operated on in infancy and childhood. However, an estimated 10–15% of patients with congenital heart disease may survive untreated to adulthood. Owing to calcification of abnormal valves, progressive ventricular dysfunction, onset of arrhythmias, pulmonary hypertension, or infective endocarditis, these patients often have irreversible myocardial damage at the time of initial presentation for surgery.

Atrial septal defect

Of the common congenital heart defects, atrial septal defect (ASD) is the most important lesion in adults. ASDs may not be detected until adulthood because they rarely produce symptoms in children and may be confused with normal physical findings at younger ages. However, if left untreated, the risks of death are 25% by 27 years, 50% by 36 years, 75% by 50 years, and 90% by 60 years.[18] ASDs are classified on an anatomic basis: ostium secondum, ostium primum, and sinus venosus. All are associated with a left to right shunt at the atrial level and volume overload of the right ventricle. The two major complications of ASD are pulmonary arterial hypertension and right ventricular failure. In about 15% of cases, elevated pulmonary vascular resistance develops after adolescence. As a result of the chronic volume overload, patients older than 40 years may develop right ventricular failure leading to atrial dysrhythmias, tricuspid regurgitation, and eventual congestive heart failure. In the most severe of cases, an Eisenmenger-like syndrome may occur, resulting in a cyanotic patient.

Surgery for ASD closure is indicated for any patient in whom the ratio of pulmonary blood flow to systemic blood flow is 2:1 or greater. ASD repair is contraindicated when pulmonary hypertension approaches or exceeds systemic pressures. In such patients, the pulmonary vascular resistance does not decrease after surgery and the operative mortality is high. The ostium primum type of ASD often poses a greater degree of difficulty for surgical repair as this is often associated with cleft mitral and tricuspid valves and the defect may extend down to, or even into, the ventricular septum.

Nonsurgical closure of ASDs via cardiac catheterization with a clamshell- or umbrella-like device is utilized in selective patients with favorable anatomical features, such as an adequate rim of septal tissue. This technique avoids the need for sternotomy and cardiopulmonary bypass. However, no data comparing the two procedures are currently available.

Coarctation of the aorta

Coarctation of the aorta results in some degree of blood flow obstruction, from insignificant obstruction (termed pseudocoarctation) to complete obstruction. The basic anatomical abnormality in coarctation of the aorta is a localized deformity of the media resulting in an infolding that narrows concentrically the aortic lumen. The area of coarctation is usually located in proximity to the origin of the left subclavian artery and may actually extend proximally as a narrowed segment of aorta to just distal to the innominate artery. The coincidence of a bicuspid aortic valve is approximately 20–40%. Reduced, delayed, or absent femoral pulses points to a diagnosis of coarctation. A 4.7 kPa (35 mmHg) pressure gradient between the arm and the ankle in a patient at rest signifies that the lumen of the coarctation is less than 50% of normal.

In the absence of surgical correction, 90% of patients with coarctation die before the age of 50 from cardiovascular and cerebrovascular disease. Treatment by surgical resection is generally very successful, with a survival rate of 70% at 40 years after surgery.[19] However, despite the early success of coarctation repair, there remains an increased risk of premature death in these patients from hypertension, premature coronary heart disease, re-coarctation, and aortic valve disease. Coarctation repair in adolescence or adulthood has resulted in more late problems with hypertension.

Other conditions

The commonest congenital cardiac malformation is ventricular septal defect (VSD). It is rarely seen in adults because the incidence of spontaneous closure of VSDs is high, and those that persist are usually associated with high mortality in childhood. Isolated VSDs that are diagnosed in adulthood are usually less than 1 cm in diameter and tend not to result in elevated right ventricular and pulmonary arterial pressures. Surgical closure is usually performed to prevent infective endocarditis and paradoxical embolism. However, the risk of developing conduction abnormalities as a result of the right atrial or right ventricular surgical approach may outweigh the risk of leaving the defect uncorrected.

Patent ductus arteriosus left untreated has a mortality rate of 40% by the age of 50 years and leaves the patient prone to infective endocarditis. Increased pulmonary vascular resistance and volume overload of the left ventricle may occur if the duct is large. Even after ligation of the ductus, these changes may not entirely regress, resulting in a state of chronic pulmonary hypertension.

Patent foramen ovale causes no detectable hemodynamic abnormalities. However, it may be found in patients who have suffered a stroke or transient ischemic attack as a result of paradoxical embolization. No specific guidelines for treatment have been established for this defect, but closure may be indicated in some instances.

Patients with tetralogy of Fallot which has been palliated with a systemic to pulmonary shunt, or is entirely uncorrected, are occasionally seen in adulthood. These patients have chronic hypoxemia and polycythemia, but may display fairly good effort tolerance and show little or no cyanosis. However, they may become disabled due to gradual shunt closure or infundibular pulmonary stenosis. Complications include infective endocarditis, cerebral thromboembolism, and brain abscess if the anomaly is not repaired. Sudden cardiac death caused by arrhythmia is the most common cause of late mortality. The mortality risk for total surgical correction is less than 5%, with late results remaining generally good.

Heart transplantation

This is performed for end-stage cardiac failure from any cause. Postoperative care is lifelong, arduous, and expensive, and recipients will have received full psychologic and physical evaluation.

Donor considerations

Heart donors must have good hemodynamic function on minimal inotropic support. The condition of donor hearts can be improved by appropriate donor management. The maximal permissible ischemic time for a heart is 4 h.

Preoperative preparation; recipient exclusion criteria

Essential in the recipient are freedom from malignancy, infection, and any other organ failure. The only absolute circulatory requirement is a low pulmonary vascular resistance index (PVRI) or transpulmonary pressure gradient (TPG). PVRI must be below 640 dyne s cm^{-5}, or TPG less than 1.9 kPa (14 mmHg). Values higher than these are associated with severe right heart failure after bypass. If PVRI is elevated, the patient may receive a "conditioned" heart, i.e. one that is accustomed to an elevated PVR, or a heart–lung transplant must be performed. Donor weight must be matched to within 20% of recipient weight.

Anesthetic and prebypass considerations

Anesthesia is similar to that for any patient with severe heart failure, but some aspects of management are different. The patient will be receiving immunosuppressive therapy. Very careful attention must be directed to prevention of infection by administration of appropriate antibiotic therapy and scrupulous aseptic care with invasive procedures. Monitoring is the same as in other open-heart procedures, but a profusion of drugs is often required, therefore plentiful central venous access is essential. Anesthetics must be titrated carefully to myocardial performance. Inotropic agents will frequently be required before bypass. Pulmonary artery catheterization is useful for postbypass care, but the catheter must be withdrawn during bypass.

Postbypass considerations

Arrhythmias and right heart failure are common. Antiarrhythmic agents (usually amiodarone) and pulmonary vasodilators (nitroglycerine, isoprenaline, prostaglandin I_2, nitric oxide, phosphodiesterase inhibitors) are often required. Heart rate should be kept high (over 100 beats min^{-1}) to avoid myocardial distension. This requires β-adrenergic agonists or pacing, as anticholinergic agents have no effect in the denervated heart. Hemorrhage is common and full measures to prevent it must be taken. TEE is very helpful in the assessment of biventricular function in the transplanted heart.

Surgery for miscellaneous conditions

Hypertrophic cardiomyopathy

Hypertrophic cardiomyopathy (HCM) is a heterogeneous genetic disease of the myocardial contractile apparatus.[20–22] Multiple gene mutations at multiple locations are responsible for encoding production of cardiac sarcomere contractile proteins that give rise to abnormalities in myocardial morphology and function. The incidence of the disease may be as high as 1 in 500. Most individuals with HCM remain asymptomatic, although a minority require multiple medical interventions and infrequently cardiac surgery to improve symptoms of LVF.

In HCM, there is asymmetric hypertrophy primarily involving the interventricular septum. This is coupled with systolic anterior motion (SAM) of the anterior mitral valve leaflet toward the septum. The combination causes dynamic left ventricular outflow tract (LVOT) obstruction. Obstruction is made worse by stress or exercise, and by preload or afterload reduction. Echocardiography can detect both septal hypertrophy and SAM, either at rest or following catecholamine stimulation, and provide a gradient across the outflow tract. Symptoms of LVF are related to the degree of LVOT obstruction, diastolic dysfunction due to LV hypertrophy, and, late in the disease, abnormal systolic function. Medical therapy for patients with normal systolic function is designed to reduce contractile function and heart rate. Beta-blockers, calcium channel blockers, and ventricular pacing have been used alone or in combination to improve symptoms. When medical therapy fails, surgical intervention is indicated.

Anesthetic considerations include maintenance of preload and afterload, slow heart rate, and reduced inotropic state. Thus, adequate anesthesia, a well-filled circulation, and beta-blockers are all indicated. Surgical repair is performed during cardiopulmonary bypass through an aortotomy, to expose the interventricular septum. The septum is incised below the annulus and septal muscle removed (myectomy). Following resection, TEE is used to assess residual SAM and the LVOT pressure gradient. Surgery results in dramatic symptomatic improvement and has a mortality less than 5% in centers familiar with the procedure. Recently, nonsurgical procedures to reduce intraventricular septal thickness have been described with good initial outcomes.[23,24]

Less invasive forms of cardiac surgery

Off-pump bypass (OPCAB) surgery is a procedure in which coronary revascularization is achieved without the use of cardiopulmonary bypass.[25] Single or multiple vessels may be bypassed. This can be accomplished via small left anterior thoracotomy (minimally invasive direct coronary artery bypass or MIDCAB), usually involving the left anterior descending coronary artery only, or through a standard median sternotomy for multivessel operations. Possible advantages of OPCAB surgery include avoiding the inflammatory response to bypass and less manipulation of the ascending aorta with the expectation of decreased postoperative neurologic dysfunction. However, this has not yet been established.

Both arterial and venous conduits may be used. When the ascending aorta is used for proximal anastomoses, partial cross-clamping of the aorta is required. However, it is possible to perform the surgery without any manipulation of the aorta. This is achieved by using the left and/or right internal mammary arteries, which are left attached proximally to the subclavian arteries. Additional conduits using vein or radial artery can be attached to the internal mammary artery. Avoiding manipulation of the aorta may be an advantage for patients with known aortic atheromatous disease.

Prior to the introduction of coronary stabilizers, formation of distal anastamoses required low heart rates. There is less movement of the coronary arteries and less bleeding with stabilizers, and therefore a low heart rate and blood pressure are usually not necessary. The need for a double-lumen endotracheal tube depends upon the approach and requirements of the surgeon. During distal anastomosis of the right, circumflex, and posterior descending coronary arteries, the apex of the heart has to be lifted. This impedes venous return, reducing cardiac output and arterial pressure. The hemodynamic impairment can be minimized by careful dislocation of the heart, use of the Trendelenburg position, and administration of α-agonists. Although TEE is frequently employed during this procedure, the echo image may be lost when the heart is lifted out of the pericardial sac. Placement of a pulmonary artery catheter is warranted in patients with depressed LV function. The usual dose of heparin prior to coronary occlusion is 1–1.5 $mg\,kg^{-1}$. The heparin is not routinely reversed with protamine.

Another type of "minimal access" cardiac surgery uses endovascular catheters and balloons to perform cardiopulmonary bypass and apply cardioplegia using percutaneous vascular access. Positioning of an aortic "balloon" clamp, retrograde cardioplegia catheter, and other venous catheters is performed with the aid of TEE. Small thoracotomy incisions are typically used for cardiac exposure. This technique has been extensively used for mitral valve replacement/repair, and has been used for coronary revascularization and aortic valve replacement in patients without evidence of aortic regurgitation. The advantage of this technique over standard bypass is the avoidance of median sternotomy.

These new approaches continue to be refined and data are being collected on outcomes. The major unanswered question is the rate of graft patency and need for repeat procedures.

ANESTHESIA FOR CARDIAC PROCEDURES IN CHILDREN

Two principles apply universally to the proper care of children with congenital heart defects. First and foremost, the goal of the anesthetic plan should be to maintain or improve existing circulatory homeostasis. Once cardiovascular collapse occurs, resuscitation may be very difficult in these patients. Second, careful attention to details and anticipation of potential problems will not only prevent avoidable catastrophes, but will also maximize the chances of getting even the sickest children through surgery.

Investigative procedures

A thorough history and physical examination may detect the presence of congenital heart disease in children. Analysis of the electrocardiogram can give evidence of chamber enlargement, axis deviation, or conduction defects. The chest radiograph provides data regarding the shape and size of the heart and the prominence of pulmonary vascularity. Often with the above information one can accurately make a preliminary diagnosis, which can then be confirmed with further selective use of noninvasive and invasive diagnostic studies.

Echocardiography, both transthoracic (TTE) and transesophageal (TEE), has great value in the diagnosis and management of congenital heart defects. With echocardiography, one can assess the size of the cardiac chambers, abnormalities of the valves, subvalvular obstruction, and the connections of the great vessels. Visualization of the size of a shunt or the direction of flow through a septal defect or valvular lesion can be assessed with the addition of Doppler ultrasonography and color flow imaging techniques.

Magnetic resonance imaging (MRI) provides another means of evaluating cardiac anatomy. Like echocardiography, MRI can provide information regarding valvular gradients and blood flow velocities, and may offer advantages over echocardiography in the demonstration of anomalies involving the great vessels. When TTE in adults is unsatisfactory because of interference from the chest wall and lungs, MRI may be superior. However, in children, confinement in an MRI scanner is not well tolerated and examination by echocardiography is usually adequate because of their smaller chest and lung size.

Cardiac catheterization and selective angiocardiography remain the gold standard for definitive diagnosis of congenital heart defects. Hemodynamic data of pressures and oxygen saturations in each chamber and great vessel can be collected using this technique. The use of contrast agents allows for a definitive radiographic image of the congenital lesion. Cardiac catheterization almost always requires general anesthesia for the pediatric patient. It is recommended that a pediatric cardiac surgeon and operating room be on standby during catheterization because of the many potential complications that can occur during the procedure.

Open heart surgery

Preoperative evaluation and preparation

It must be emphasized that the preoperative evaluation of a patient with congenital heart disease is anything but routine. It is imperative that the anesthesiologist thoroughly understands the child's cardiac anatomy and pathophysiology. Additional systemic disease and coexisting noncardiac anomalies should be well delineated. Consultation with the patient's pediatrician or cardiologist may assist the anesthesiologist in better assessing the potential complications of the case. Review of the patient's medical records can be useful for obtaining information regarding previous anesthetics, cardiac investigative procedures, and laboratory results. A careful history and physical examination, with particular attention to examination of the airway, and a detailed review of medications, allergies, and nutritional status are important so that any problems can be addressed prior to surgery. The presence of even a mild upper respiratory tract infection, especially during the winter months, when respiratory syncytial virus abounds, can result in significant morbidity for children with congenital heart disease and cancellation of elective surgery for these patients is prudent. One should document preoperative vital signs, including room air oxyhemoglobin saturation, to help assess and manage intraoperative care.

There are no specific laboratory tests or diagnostic procedures that are always indicated in patients with congenital heart defects. Each patient is individually evaluated and the appropriate tests ordered, with the hematocrit level obtained most commonly. If a change in the child's clinical condition has occurred, an electrocardiogram or echocardiogram may provide valuable information.

The choice of premedication for children with congenital heart disease can be difficult. On the one hand, preoperative sedation may produce less crying during separation from the parents, resulting in decreased oxygen consumption and decreased requirement for anesthetic agents. However, some anesthesiologists believe that even minimal respiratory depression often associated with the premedicants may result in significant oxyhemoglobin desaturation in children with cyanotic congenital heart defects. Oral midazolam (0.75 $mg\,kg^{-1}$) appears to be safe and efficacious for this group of patients.

Anesthetic considerations

Classification of congenital heart defects is based on whether there is increased pulmonary blood flow (left to right shunts), decreased pulmonary blood flow (right to left shunts), a mixing of pulmonary and systemic circulation (complex shunt), or an obstruction to flow.

The basic tenet of anesthetic management during surgery for congenital heart defects is the ability to alter the relation between flow, pressure, and resistance:

$$\dot{Q} = P/R$$

where $\dot{Q}$ is blood flow (cardiac output), P is pressure within a chamber or vessel, and R is vascular resistance of the pulmonary or systemic bed. Pressure (P) within a given intracardiac chamber may be altered with positive and negative inotropic agents. Flow ($\dot{Q}$) can be improved by maximizing preload. Manipulating resistance (R) is accomplished by the use of various dilators and constrictors. The decision to manipulate one or more of the variables during anesthesia is based on the specific pathophysiology of the lesion.

Postoperative management

The postoperative care of the patient with congenital heart disease should be individualized based on the type of repair and its physiologic effects. However, several considerations can be universally applied. Patients with congenital heart disease are (1) prone to arrhythmias in the postoperative period, (2) particularly susceptible to the deleterious effects of hypoventilation and decreases in oxyhemoglobin saturation, and (3) dependent on vasoactive and inotropic pharmacological support, which should not be discontinued abruptly. It is very important that these patients are followed closely in the postoperative period by an anesthesiologist, pediatric intensivist, and/or cardiologist familiar with their specific cardiac disease.

ANESTHESIA FOR SURGERY ON THE THORACIC AORTA

Surgery on the thoracic aorta may be required for aneurysm, aortic dissection, pseudoaneurysm, or other consequences of atherosclerosis that increase the risk of aortic rupture and/or lead to embolus formation with consequent end-organ damage.

The prevalence of thoracic aortic disease is poorly described. Postmortem reports suggest that the incidence of aneurysm may be as high as 3–5 per 1000, while the incidence of aortic dissection is probably higher. The etiologies of disease of the thoracic aorta are varied and are listed in Table 45.8.

Thoracic aortic aneurysm

Aneurysmal dilation of the aorta is the most common condition requiring surgical intervention. Aneurysmal dilation is defined as a localized increase in aortic diameter of greater than 50% of normal. Atherosclerosis is the most common cause of a thoracic aortic aneurysm; cystic medial necrosis may occur with connective tissue diseases such as Marfan syndrome and Ehlers–Danlos syndrome.

Trauma resulting from deceleration injury usually affects the descending thoracic aorta because this is the least mobile portion. Blunt chest trauma is more likely to cause proximal aortic disruption as a result of either inferior displacement of the heart, or aortic compression between the manubrium and the spine. These traumatic causes of thoracic aortic disease may present as surgical emergencies requiring prompt diagnosis and operative intervention.

Aortic dissection causes aortic dilation as blood flow traverses into the aortic media via a tear in the intima. Medial degeneration is thought to be the cause of most nontraumatic aortic dissections. Risk factors include hypertension, advanced age, bicuspid aortic valve, pregnancy, and Marfan syndrome. Chronic dissection is a common cause of thoracic aortic aneurysm. Infection is a rare cause of aortic aneurysm.

The natural progression of thoracic aortic aneurysm is not as well described as that for abdominal aortic aneurysm. There is no consensus about the optimal time to perform elective surgery. Aneurysm size and rate of expansion, the presence of chronic dissection, and Marfan syndrome seem to be important predictors of the risk of rupture.

Table 45.8 *Diseases of the thoracic aorta*

Type	Causes
Aneurysm	Atherosclerosis
	Hypertension
	Poststenotic dilation
	Trauma
	Cystic medial necrosis
	Ehlers–Danlos syndrome
	Infection (mycotic aneurysm)
	Takayasu's disease
Pseudoaneurysm	Prior surgery
	Trauma
Dissection	Hypertension
	Aortic stenosis
	Aortic coarctation
	Age
	Marfan syndrome
	Trauma
	Prior surgery

Aortic dissection

There are two systems for classification of thoracic aortic dissections, the DeBakey and Stanford classifications, which depend upon the location and extent of the dissection (Fig. 45.1). In these systems, the important distinctions between the types of dissection are location, either proximal or distal to the arch, and extent, involving the arch and/or abdominal visceral organs. More than 50% of dissections occur in the proximal ascending aorta, distal to the aortic sinuses. Approximately 10% involve a tear in the arch itself, and 30% arise in the descending thoracic aorta distal to the left subclavian artery.

Proximal thoracic aortic dissection is a surgical urgency. The majority of patients with proximal dissection who do not undergo surgical correction will die. Death is due to rupture, cardiac tamponade, or obstruction of coronary or cerebral arteries. The operative mortality for acute proximal dissection is 10–20%. Surgery on distal dissection (Stanford B or DeBakey III) carries far higher mortality and significant morbidity from paraplegia. These patients are managed medically by reducing aortic stress (dP/dt) with beta-blockers and arterial vasodilators as needed. Long-term management of these patients remains controversial. In the absence of end-organ involvement such as renal insufficiency, pleural hematoma, or symptoms of rapid expansion, long-term medical management is preferred to elective surgical repair provided that regular follow-up is maintained.

Diagnosis of thoracic aortic disease

Accurate diagnosis is required for management of all diseases of the thoracic aorta. This is particularly true in acute dissection and in asymptomatic patients, in whom delay in diagnosis may cause death. Chest radiography may show aortic dilation, but up to 20% of cases may be missed. Computed tomographic (CT) scanning is the most widely used screening and follow-up test for disease of the thoracic aorta. Although CT scanning with contrast and three-dimensional reconstruction is useful for the diagnosis of dissection, magnetic resonance imaging (MRI) has superior sensitivity and specificity. When rapid intraoperative diagnosis of acute aortic dissection is required, the use

DeBakey classification

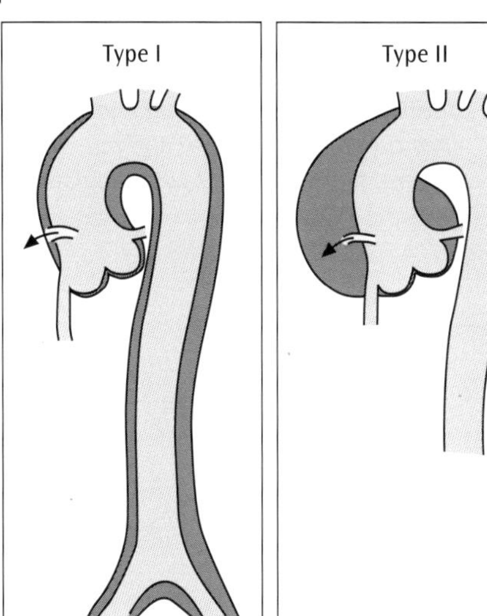

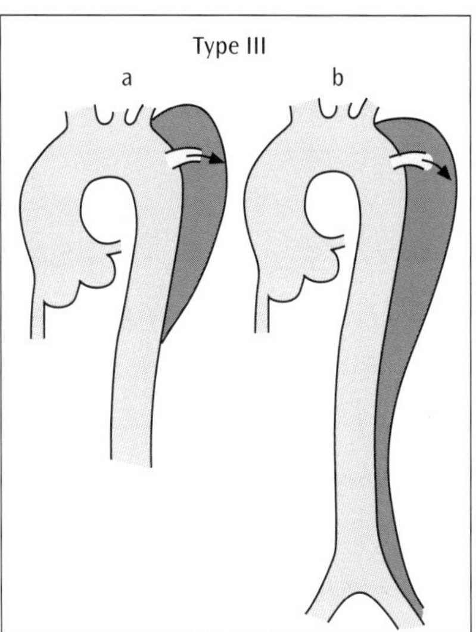

Stanford classification

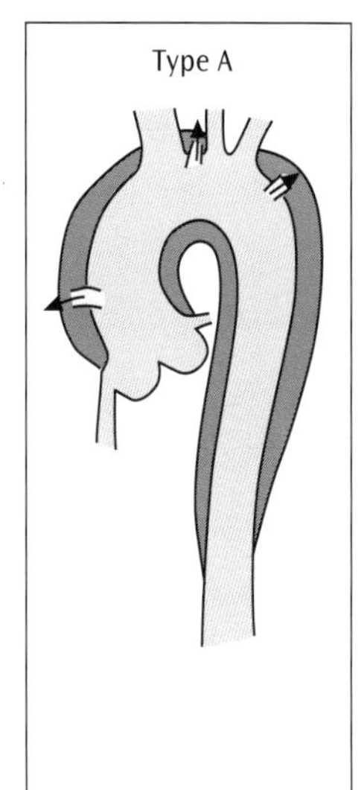

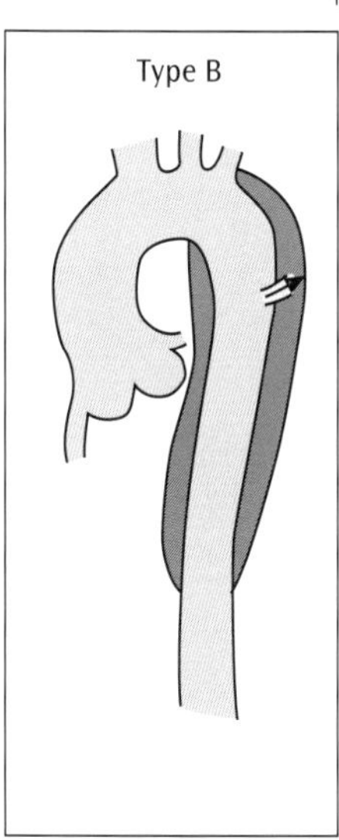

Figure 45.1 *The two most commonly used classifications for aortic dissection. The DeBakey classification defines three types of dissection depending on the location of the intimal tear and the extent of the dissection. Type I refers to a proximal tear with extension to the descending thoracic aorta. Type II is also a proximal tear but the dissection is confined to the ascending aorta. Type III refers to a dissection that originates distal to the aortic arch. The Stanford classification uses two categories, either proximal or distal dissection, depending on whether the proximal is involved or spared. Reproduced with permission from Kouchoukos and Dougenis.*[21]

of transesophageal echocardiography (TEE) with color flow mapping is useful. Aortography remains the standard for diagnosis of thoracic aortic disease in elective cases. This technique allows examination of aortic valve competency and the coronary arterial system as well as the precise location of the aneurysm or point of aortic dissection.

Surgical correction

General recommendations are to repair an ascending aneurysm when its diameter exceeds 5–5.5 cm, arch aneurysm when it exceeds 5.5–6 cm, and descending aneurysm when it exceeds 5–6 cm.[26–28] Preoperative preparation of all patients with nonemergent thoracic aortic disease must include evaluation for pulmonary disease, renal insufficiency, coronary artery disease, and cerebrovascular disease. Thus, coronary angiography and duplex carotid scans will be required.

Operations on the thoracic aorta are often attended by major blood loss. Blood and blood products are usually required and the use of cell salvage is universal. Aprotinin use has gained in popularity. However, there is concern, though little systematic evidence, that aprotinin might cause disseminated intravascular coagulation during circulatory arrest.

Repair of the ascending aorta

It is usually necessary to replace the aortic valve during repair of the aortic root. This is usually accomplished with a composite aortic graft that includes an aortic valve incorporated into the aortic graft. When the most proximal aorta is replaced, the coronary arteries can be reimplanted with graft material or directly by using the coronary ostia from the replaced aorta sewn to the new graft. Sparing of the aortic valve may be beneficial for patients in whom the proximal ascending aorta is dilated but the aortic leaflets and annulus are normal.

Bypass is usually performed using right atrial and femoral arterial cannulation. For surgery not involving circulatory arrest, routine anesthetic considerations include the possibilities of aortic perforation and large blood loss during sternotomy. Left radial artery pressure monitoring is preferred because the right innominate artery may be compressed during repair. EEG monitoring can provide information about regional cerebral ischemia, which may be treated by adjusting the aortic clamp or by increasing blood pressure. One must be prepared for circulatory arrest should arch vessels be involved. Hospital mortality is below 5% but increases with age.

Repair of the aortic arch

Repair of an aortic arch aneurysm requires interruption of cerebral blood flow. The use of deep hypothermic circulatory arrest (DHCA) reduces neurologic injury and allows a bloodless field. The "safe" time for circulatory arrest when the temperature is 15–20 °C is thought to be 30–40 min. Some have recommended cooling until the EEG is silent and then further cooling by 3 °C prior to initiating total circulatory arrest. Steroids, mannitol, barbiturates, avoidance of hyperglycemia, and packing the head in ice to prolong cerebral cooling have all been advocated.

Methods aimed at reducing cerebral injury during DHCA include antegrade and retrograde cerebral perfusion (ACP and RCP), the latter being in wider use. The use of ACP in conditions of moderate total body hypothermia at 28 °C and cold perfusion of the cerebral and coronary vessels has been described with an overall mortality of 17% and a stroke rate of 12%.[29] More commonly, RCP is used with the aim of prolonging ischemic time, enhancing brain cooling, and reducing embolic episodes (Fig. 45.2). Cold blood at less than 10 °C is pumped in a retrograde direction through the superior vena cava cannula at a rate of 250–400 mL min^{-1}. The retrograde perfusion pressure is maintained at less than 3.3 kPa (25 mmHg) by adjustment of flow.

Although there are no randomized, prospective trials comparing DHCA with or without cerebral perfusion, historical data suggest that retrograde perfusion extends the safe DHCA duration. In a large series of surgical operations performed under DHCA, Svensson *et al.*[30] found that the safe time of arrest while avoiding neurologic injury was increased by 40 min. After the aortic arch is repaired and air is removed from the operative field, perfusion to the arch vessels is reinstituted.

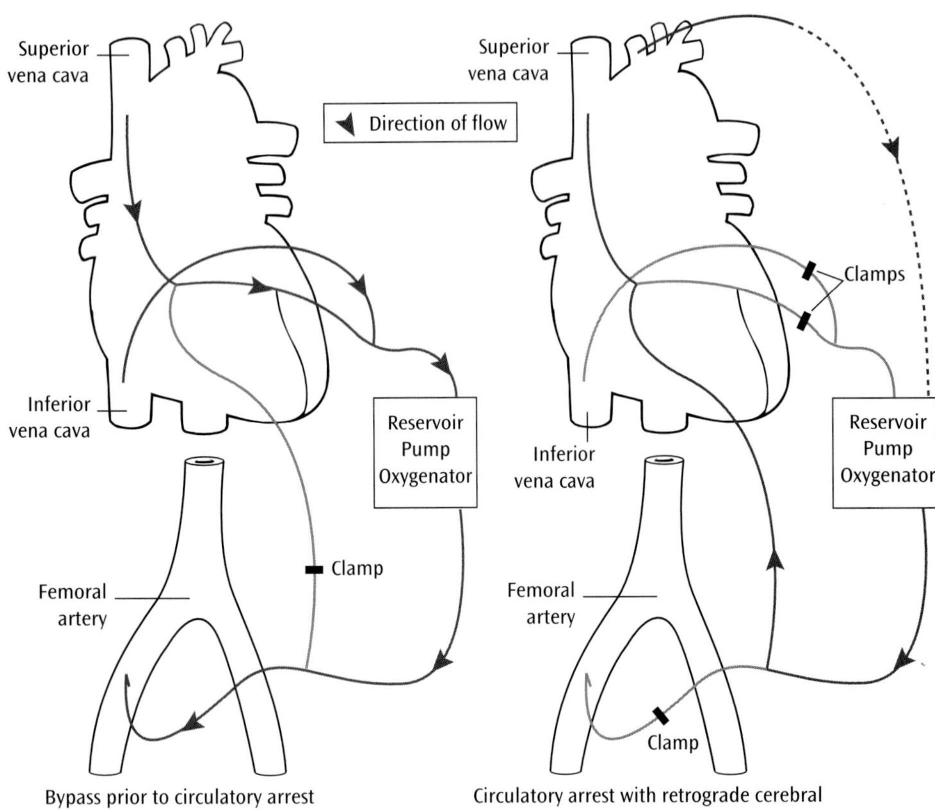

Figure 45.2 *Example of circuits used for retrograde cerebral perfusion. Normal bypass configuration is depicted on the left. With the changing of clamps, flow is directed only through the superior vena cava cannula on the right and retrograde cerebral flow is initiated with circulatory arrest.*

Repair of the descending thoracic and thoracoabdominal aorta

A useful classification of descending thoracic aortic aneurysm based on location and extent has been established by Crawford *et al.*[31]

There are several techniques for surgery on the descending aorta. These have been developed to attempt to reduce the high incidence of perioperative paraplegia (see below). Simplest is the "clamp and sew" technique, in which the aorta is cross-clamped with no attempt being made to perfuse the lower body. Alternatively, distal perfusion can be provided passively using a "Gott" shunt. This is a plastic heparin-bonded shunt, which is placed from the ascending aorta (or occasionally the left ventricle) to the distal abdominal aorta. It provides limited distal perfusion. Much better is left heart bypass, in which blood is pumped using a centrifugal pump from left atrium to femoral artery (Fig. 45.3). During left heart bypass, left atrial blood is divided. Some passes through the mitral valve into the LV and provides cardiac output to the body above the level of the cross-clamp. The remainder is pumped via the bypass from left atrium to femoral artery. Upper body and distal pressures are manipulated by changing pump flow, with distal pressure being raised by increasing flow through the pump. This reduces left ventricular filling, cardiac output, and arterial pressure above the clamp. Arterial pressure below the clamp should be measured via the femoral or a more distal artery. Distal mean arterial pressure (MAP) should exceed 8 kPa (60 mmHg). To guarantee adequate pressure and flow above and below the pump, adequate intravascular volume must be maintained. Vasoconstrictors are rarely required.

When the clamps are removed, circulatory support is weaned and the entire cardiac output reverts back to the left ventricle. For left heart bypass, low levels of systemic heparinization can be employed or heparin-bonded circuits used. Full femoral vein to femoral artery bypass using an oxygenator is occasionally used for lower body perfusion. It requires full heparinization, is associated with more bleeding, and may also increase the risk of using cerebrospinal fluid (CSF) drainage (see below).

The most feared complication during repair of the descending thoracic or thoracoabdominal aorta is postoperative paraplegia, which has an incidence of 10–30%. It has been reported to occur up to 8 days postoperatively. Paraplegia is caused by interruption of blood flow through the artery of Adamkiewicz. This artery, which provides most of the blood flow to the anterior spinal cord, is a confluence of spinal arteries that arises from the aorta between T9 and L2. More than 85% of the time it arises between T10 and T12 (Fig. 45.4). The absence of blood flow leads to spinal cord infarction. The incidence of paraplegia is markedly reduced with the use of bypass to provide distal perfusion, as described above, particularly in complex cases involving the abdominal aorta.

CSF drainage with a continuous spinal catheter to maintain a CSF pressure of 1.3–2 kPa (10–15 mmHg) has been shown to reduce the incidence of perioperative paraplegia. CSF pressure monitoring is required and is commenced at the time of surgery. CSF is removed 10–30 mL at a time. CSF drainage has been successful in reversing delayed paraplegia, and it is usually continued for several days postoperatively. Systemic or local cooling may help protect the cord. Active cord cooling may be implemented by infusion of iced saline into an epidural catheter. Agents that alter nerve transmission, such as barbiturates and magnesium, free radical scavengers, steroids, and other pharmacologic adjuncts, have been examined for their possible protective effect on spinal cord ischemia.[33]

Motor-evoked potentials are used in some centers to detect anterior spinal cord ischemia. Reimplantation of some or all of the intercostal arteries involved in the aneurysm has been attempted. However, this increases cross-clamp time, which may itself increase the risk of paraplegia, and the practice is not widespread.

Without the use of distal perfusion, cross-clamping the proximal descending aorta causes severe hypertension. This places significant

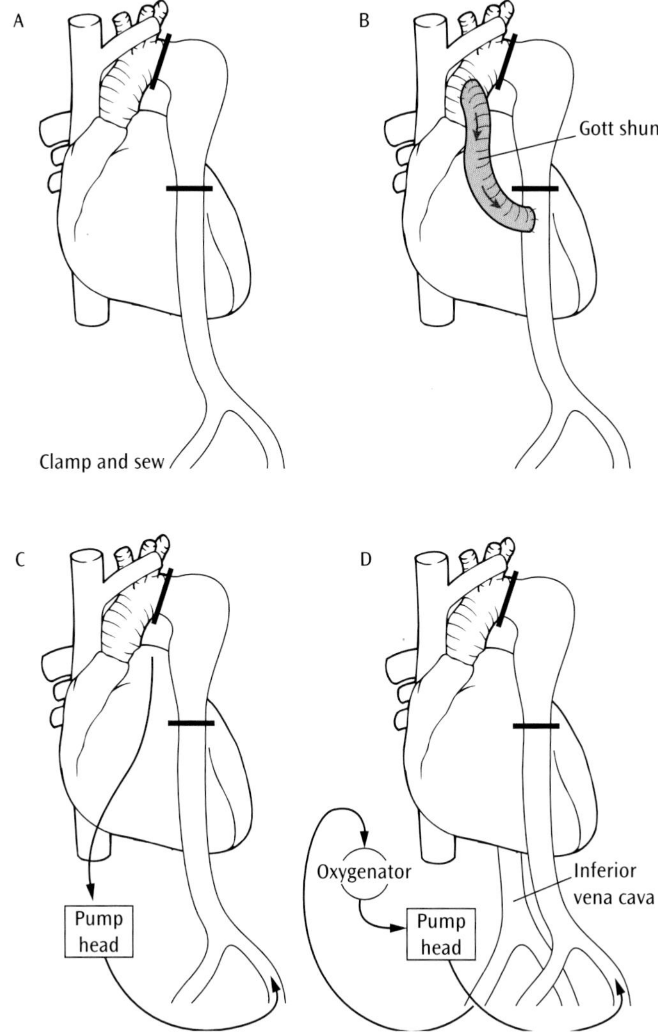

Figure 45.3 *Drawings of techniques for repairing descending thoracic aorta. (A) No bypass, "clamp and sew." (B) Heparinized Gott shunt. (C) Left heart bypass, from left atrium via pump head (roller or centrifugal). (D) Full cardiopulmonary bypass, with an oxygenator, using femoral artery and femoral vein.*

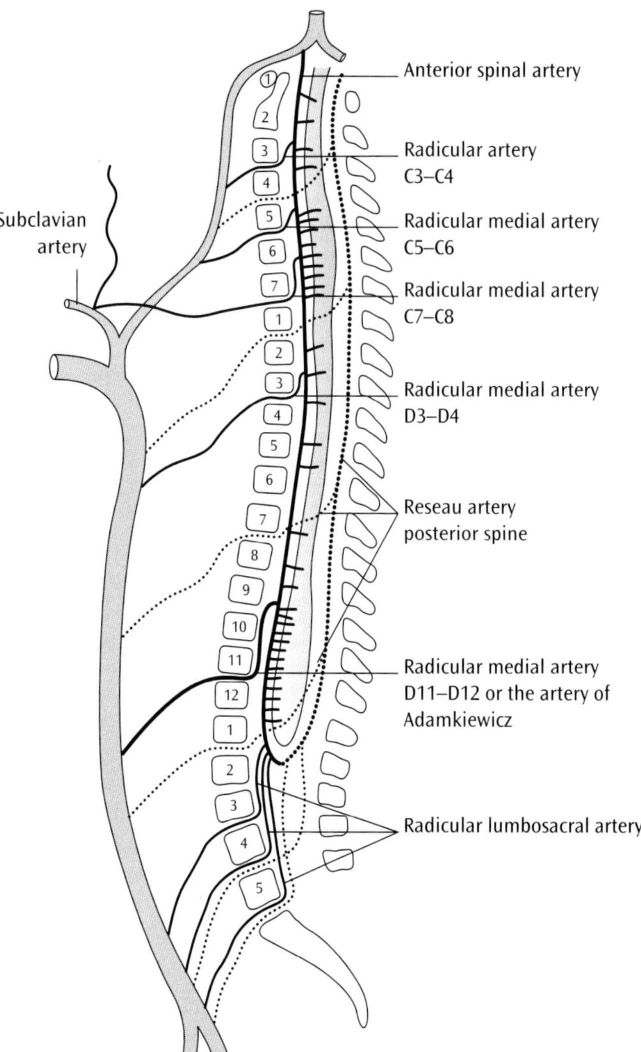

Figure 45.4 *Thoracic and lumbar contributions to the arterial supply of the spinal cord. See text. (Reproduced with permission from Djindjian et al.[32])*

stress on the left ventricle, and a Swan–Ganz catheter is advisable to measure PCWP and help detect impending LVF. If the LV is able to sustain the high pressure without decompensation, the hypertension is probably best left untreated. However, vasodilators are often needed to control arterial pressure. The abdominal viscera, lower extremities, and the artery of Adamkiewicz all depend on collateral flow. Lowering the proximal aortic pressure with vasodilators causes reduced collateral flow, and the use of vasodilators has been associated with increased neurologic deficits in experimental trials.[34–37]

Whichever technique is used, there are some anesthetic considerations that should be applied. The surgical approach requires placement of a left-sided double-lumen endotracheal tube (DLT) to facilitate collapse of the left lung. Uncommonly, there may be compression of the left mainstem bronchus by the aneurysm, increasing the risk of aneurysm rupture during intubation or leading to difficulty in placing the DLT. In these rare instances, a right-sided DLT or bronchial blocker should be considered. Arterial monitoring must include pressures proximal and distal to the aortic cross-clamp. Some passive cooling is recommended to reduce the risk of paraplegia. Rewarming must be conducted so as to avoid hyperthermia. Prior to cross-clamping, furosemide or mannitol is usually administered to help preserve renal function, although evidence for this is weak. If no form of bypass is used, there is typically a severe metabolic acidosis after release of the cross-clamp, which may need correcting. It is recommended that mean arterial pressure be maintained at 10.7–13.3 kPa (80–100 mmHg) postoperatively to enhance cord blood flow, despite the potential risk of bleeding.

Anesthesia for patients with pericardial disease

Acute pericarditis

Acute pericarditis is an inflammatory process usually due to a viral infection. Other causes include uremia, acute myocardial infarction (Dressler syndrome), bacterial infection, tuberculosis, trauma, and neoplastic invasion of the pericardium. The clinical diagnosis of acute pericarditis is suggested by the onset of severe chest pain that is exacerbated by lying supine, coughing, deep inspiration, or swallowing. The presence of a pericardial friction rub on auscultation is pathognomonic for acute pericarditis. S–T segment elevation present in all leads except aVR and V_1 with upright T-waves is the most common electrocardiographic change and is diagnostic for pericarditis. Sinus tachycardia and a low-grade fever may also be present. Treatment of acute pericarditis is symptomatic with the administration of nonsteroidal anti-inflammatory drugs (NSAIDs) and corticosteroids. In the absence of an associated pericardial effusion, acute pericarditis does not alter cardiac function.

Pericardial effusion

The pericardial space normally contains approximately 25 mL of pericardial fluid and has a subatmospheric pressure, which decreases on inspiration and increases on expiration. If an effusion develops gradually, the pericardium can stretch to accommodate a fairly large amount of fluid without a significant increase in pressure. However, the rapid accumulation of even a small amount of fluid (100–200 mL) can result in acute cardiac tamponade. Elevation of intrapericardial pressure above that of right atrial or right ventricular diastolic pressure results in a decrease in transmural filling pressure and cardiac output. Reduction in stroke volume is compensated initially by increases in heart rate and adrenergic tone. However, as these compensatory mechanisms fail, severe circulatory compromise becomes evident.

The definitive treatment of cardiac tamponade is relief of the cardiac compression. The goal of anesthetic management is the preservation of cardiac compensatory mechanisms until surgical drainage is accomplished. The cornerstones of hemodynamic stability are adequate intravascular volume, tachycardia, and peripheral vasoconstriction ("full, fast, and tight"). Adequate intravenous access for volume resuscitation, central venous access for infusion of vasoactive medications, and arterial cannulation for systemic blood pressure monitoring are required. "Prepping" and "draping" of the patient prior to induction are suggested in the event of rapid hemodynamic deterioration. The induction technique should avoid drugs with significant vasodilator properties. Low tidal volumes and rapid respirations are also recommended in order to prevent compromise of venous return.

Constrictive pericarditis

Constrictive pericarditis, like cardiac tamponade, restricts ventricular filling, resulting in hemodynamic changes. Diastolic filling is restricted by a stiff, fibrosed, adherent pericardium rather than accumulation of fluid within the pericardial sac. Most cases of constrictive pericarditis are of unknown etiology.

The symptoms of constrictive pericarditis include weakness and progressive dyspnea and fatigue. Syncope is occasionally seen. Patients may develop ascites with or without peripheral edema, as well as other signs associated with increased venous pressure. Pericardial "knock" is a classic sign on auscultation.

Unlike cardiac tamponade, filling is unimpeded in early diastole in constrictive pericarditis. As a result, stroke volume is maintained because left ventricular end-diastolic pressure is preserved by rapid ventricular filling in early diastole. Systolic contraction of the ventricles is usually normal, although in chronic cases myocardial atrophy may occur. Atrial fibrillation may be present in 25% of patients. Pulsus paradoxus is unusual as the stiff pericardium shields the heart from intrathoracic pressure changes.

Acute hemodynamic decompensation is not the predominant problem in constrictive pericarditis, and hence the choice of anesthetic drugs is less critical. However, the anesthesiologist must choose a technique that maintains heart rate, adequate vascular volume, and contractility. Use of positive-pressure ventilation usually poses little problem. On the other hand, surgical manipulation required to excise the adherent pericardium can cause arrhythmias, hypotension, and bleeding. Most arrhythmias respond to the cessation of manipulation and antiarrhythmics are seldom necessary. Occasionally, cardiopulmonary bypass may be required to control bleeding from friable areas of the heart.

POSTOPERATIVE MANAGEMENT OF ADULTS

Early postoperative care

Continuous monitoring of ECG, arterial pressure, and oxygen saturation must be performed during return of the patient to the postoperative care area. Handover to postoperative care staff must include full details of the operation performed, the condition of the heart, circulation, ventilation and blood gas values, blood chemistry, hemoglobin, blood loss, blood and blood product replacement, and information about untoward events.

Rate and rhythm: arrhythmias

Heart rate should ideally be 70–100 beats min^{-1}. Sinus bradycardia is treated using anticholinergic agents or α-adrenergic agonists. Bradycardia unresponsive to the above treatments requires temporary pacing, either using the leads placed at the time of surgery or by the transvenous route. Sinus tachycardia is almost always a physiologic response to a low stroke volume secondary to either hypovolemia or poor ventricular function; thus, reduction in heart rate in sinus rhythm may be inappropriate. The common causes of pathological tachyarrhythmias are perioperative myocardial infarction and electrolyte disturbances, notably hypokalemia and hypomagnesemia. With the exception of chronic atrial fibrillation, tachyarrhythmias need to be treated. Electrolyte disturbances must be corrected, and magnesium sulfate up to 5 g may be given without prior measurement. Intravenous lidocaine (lignocaine) or amiodarone may be used to treat ventricular arrhythmias.

Assessment of circulatory filling

Correct filling of the circulation is essential. An assessment of filling is usually made by the anesthesiolgist after bypass and used postoperatively. In many patients, measurement of CVP may be adequate as a guide to filling postoperatively. However, if more than minimal doses of inotropic agents are needed to produce satisfactory cardiovascular performance in the presence of a CVP of 1.3 kPa (10 mmHg), it is sensible to insert a pulmonary artery catheter to measure pulmonary vascular pressures and cardiac output. This allows a better-targeted approach to improving cardiovascular performance. Measurement of venous pressure (including PCWP) gives no information about circulating volume, and can be misleading, especially in obese patients, in patients who are inadequately settled during ventilation, and during cardiac tamponade. In these three situations, venous pressures are high when circulating volume is low. In uncertain cases, TEE is invaluable, providing information about intracardiac volume, biventricular systolic and diastolic performance, valve function, and cardiac tamponade.

Inotropic agents, vasodilators, and vasoconstrictors

Pharmacologic cardiovascular support must be targeted to the underlying abnormality. The systemic vascular resistance index should be in the normal range, and cardiac index should be at least 2.4 L min m^{-2}. More than one drug may be required to achieve this, but therapy should be kept as simple as possible. Such support, if needed at all, can usually be withdrawn within a few hours to 1 day. Occasionally, support may be required for several days.

Postoperative care of heart transplant patients is the same as for other open-heart procedures except for the need for immunosuppression and the requirement to keep pulmonary vascular resistance (PVR) low. Pulmonary vasodilators are often continued for several days.

Hemorrhage

Overt blood loss should never be greater than 200 mL h^{-1}, and never be more than 1000 mL total in adults. If loss is greater and there is no treatable coagulopathy, the sternotomy should be re-explored. Hemorrhage does not always occur through the drains: blood may collect in the pericardium or pleura. The former results in cardiac tamponade; the latter in unexplained hypovolemia. Suspicion of either should lead to the immediate performance of a chest radiograph and/or TEE to confirm the diagnosis.

The treatment of coagulopathy depends on the cause. Persistence of heparin is reversed with further protamine. Deficiency of coagulation factors due to hemodilution is common and is treated with fresh-frozen plasma. Although severe thrombocytopenia is rare, platelet dysfunction is invariable and platelets may be required. Antifibrinolytic agents, Cyclokapron (tranexamic acid), or aprotinin, may be needed.

Ventilation

There is no set time period for postoperative ventilation. Some prefer to extubate within a few minutes of completion of surgery. The concept of early extubation is generally taken to mean extubation within 4 h of surgery. Most patients can be extubated within this time, and evidence supports such a policy. Extubation should only be undertaken when certain conditions have been met (Table 45.9). Extubation on the operating table is associated with a requirement to reintubate some patients to treat either hemorrhage or failure of cardiovascular, neurologic, or respiratory function. The presence of an IABP is not a contraindication to extubation provided the other criteria have been met and the IABP has been inserted percutaneously. Extubation may be associated with myocardial ischemia in patients following CABG.

Impairment of gas exchange occurs in all patients during and after cardiac surgery. Its etiology is multifactorial and includes atelectasis, increased extravascular lung water, and altered chest wall mechanics. The impairment is greater if either pleural cavity is opened. The resulting hypoxemia can be overcome with oxygen therapy and physiotherapy in most patients. Phrenic nerve injury is a rare complication of heart surgery. It is commoner following internal mammary artery dissection.

One percent of patients develop the adult respiratory distress syndrome (ARDS) and severe hypoxemia. Risk factors include current smoking, hypertension, emergency surgery, NYHA disease classes III and IV, low preoperative cardiac output, and ejection fraction < 40%.[38] Furthermore, bypass is known to activate the complement cascade. Soluble human complement type 1 receptor blockade reduces pulmonary dysfunction after bypass in pigs; complement activation is, thus, implicated.[39]

Analgesia

There are various approaches to analgesia. These include intermittent intramuscular opioids, nurse-controlled intravenous infusions, patient-controlled analgesia, and spinal and thoracic epidural analgesia.

Later postoperative care

Arrhythmias

Atrial fibrillation during the first few days postoperatively is very common after heart surgery of any type. Possible causes are hypovolemia, hypokalemia, hypomagnesemia, withdrawal of beta-blockade, and surgical trauma. Hypovolemia and electrolyte disturbances should be corrected. Unless sinus rhythm returns spontaneously, AF usually requires treatment to reverse it or control ventricular rate. Evidence exists that postoperative beta-blockade significantly reduces the incidence of AF. Other arrhythmias are uncommon at this stage.

Analgesia

Median sternotomy is not as painful as some other surgical wounds, but analgesia must be adequate to allow the patient to cooperate effectively with chest physiotherapy. Strong analgesics are not often required after the first postoperative day. Combinations of weak opiates and NSAIDs provide highly satisfactory analgesia at this stage.

CARDIOPULMONARY BYPASS

History

The first cardiopulmonary bypass (CPB), performed by Gibbon in 1953, utilized the four basic components of bypass machinery: (1) a pump to create forward flow; (2) an oxygenator (i.e. artificial lung) for exchange of oxygen and carbon dioxide; (3) a blood reservoir to preserve forward

Table 45.9 *Criteria for postoperative extubation after open-heart surgery in adults*

System	Criteria
Cardiovascular	Good cardiovascular performance on no more than moderate inotropic or vasoactive support Presence of percutaneous intra-aortic balloon pump acceptable Absence of arrhythmias requiring cardioversion
Respiratory	Normal respiratory pattern Tidal volume > 5 mL kg^{-1} No residual neuromuscular blockade Respiratory rate > 8 and < 20 min^{-1} P_{aO_2} > 13 kPa (100 mmHg) and P_{aCO_2} < 7.3 kPa (55 mmHg) with F_{IO_2} < 0.6 and PEEP < 0.5 kPa (5 cmH_2O)
Neurologic	Awake, alert, and cooperative No evidence of major neurologic damage (fitting or paresis)
Hemorrhage	Consistently less than 50 mL h^{-1}
Thermoregulation	Normothermia (core temperature at least 36 °C)

flow; and (4) cannulae for gravity-driven venous return and pump-driven arterial flow. This simple design allowed surgery on an empty, fibrillating heart.

Mechanics of bypass

Cardiopulmonary bypass (Fig. 45.5) requires drainage of venous blood from either the right atrium or vena cavae. This is usually accomplished by gravity, but it may be augmented by pump- or vacuum-assisted venous return, and this allows use of smaller venous cannulae. The drained blood is actively pumped through either a membrane or a hollow fiber oxygenator. Bubble oxygenators are no longer used because membrane and hollow fiber oxygenators cause less trauma to red blood cells, introduce fewer gaseous emboli, probably induce less inflammatory response, and result in better outcomes. The membrane or fiber bundle, through which oxygen and carbon dioxide diffuse, is made of Teflon, silicone, or similar materials (Fig. 45.6). The rate of CO_2 removal depends on the gas flow, whereas oxygenation depends on the oxygen concentration in the fresh gas. A heat exchanger allows rapid cooling and warming of blood. After gas exchange, blood passes through an arterial filter with a bubble trap into the arterial cannula and then into the upper ascending aorta or, occasionally, the femoral artery.

The entire bypass circuit is primed with fluid. Contents vary, but most centers use a mixture of crystalloid and colloid. To this may be added a small amount of bicarbonate as buffer, 2 g of magnesium to prevent hypomagnesemia, and mannitol as a diuretic and free radical scavenger. Blood is occasionally required in the priming fluid to prevent excessive hemodilution in small (< 45 kg) or anemic patients.

Pumps are of two types, roller or centrifugal (Fig. 45.7). Roller pumps work by occlusion and therefore must be carefully set to avoid excessive trauma to red cells. Centrifugal pumps cause less red cell trauma. Mean arterial pressure is usually reduced to about 9.3 kPa (70 mmHg) during placement of the arterial cannula in the aorta to reduce wall tension. Arterial and venous cannulae are shown in Fig. 45.8. Incorrect positioning of the cannula in the aorta can occur, with the tip either passing into one of the arch branches or (very rarely) causing a dissection. Both of these manifest after initiation of CPB as a high driving pressure measured proximal to the aortic cannula. A checklist prior to initiation of bypass is shown in Table 45.10, and a checklist after commencement of bypass is shown in Table 45.11.

Cardioplegia

Except during OPCAB procedures, the heart is arrested in either VF or asystole. This renders it still and allows it to be opened or surface coronary arteries to be bypassed. Prior to the introduction of cardioplegia, cardiac arrest was achieved by cross-clamping the ascending aorta proximal to the arterial cannula and inducing VF. This was accompanied by mild to moderate systemic hypothermia. Such a technique without coronary perfusion allows for only a short ischemic time, which should be no longer than 10 min. If the ischemic time is much longer than this, severe and persistent myocardial dysfunction occurs when the heart is restarted. Cardioplegic solutions containing K^+ arrest the heart in asystole. This allows a far longer ischemic time and has become the mainstay for electromechanical arrest during cardiac surgery. The goals of cardioplegia are (1) a quiet, bloodless field; (2) limitation of myocardial damage by reduction of intracellular acidosis, edema, and depletion of ATP stores; (3) preservation of coronary endothelial function and myocardial flow; and (4) reduced injury during reperfusion. There are several strategies for delivering cardioplegia. It may be antegrade

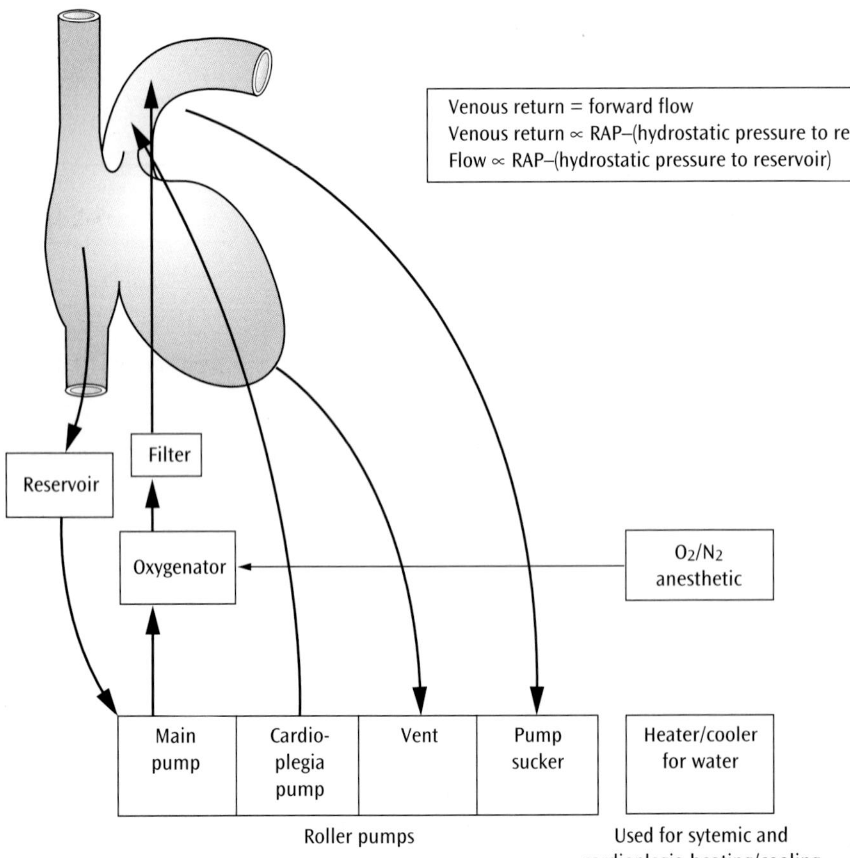

Figure 45.5 *Simplified depiction of the mechanics of CPB. Arrows show direction of blood flow. The reservoir is above the oxygenator (in this configuration); heating and cooling take place at the oxygenator and in the cardioplegia circuit (not shown). Venous return is passive in this configuration and obeys the formulae shown in equations above. See text.*

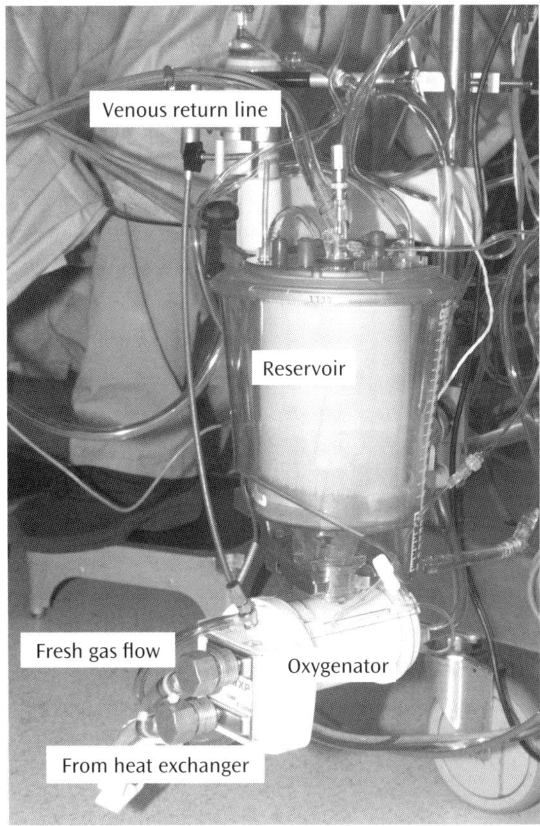

Figure 45.6 *Clean venous return line connected to reservoir above the oxygenator with lines from heater–cooler and fresh gas flow. See text.*

or retrograde, warm or cold, crystalloid or blood, and continuous or intermittent.

Antegrade cardioplegia is delivered into the aortic root; retrograde into the coronary sinus. Retrograde cardioplegia may lead to better distribution of cardioplegia when significant coronary artery disease is present, but adequate delivery to the right ventricular myocardium is difficult. This is because the posterior interventricular vein (which drains right ventricular myocardium) enters the coronary sinus very close to its entry into the right atrium, and the cannula is usually beyond the vein. Optimal preservation probably requires combined cold and warm cardioplegia with antegrade and retrograde perfusion, especially for patients with acute ischemia or infarction, left ventricular hypertrophy, severely impaired left ventricular function, or cardiac surgery requiring long periods of aortic cross-clamping.

Cold cardioplegia is delivered at or below 10 °C with the use of a heat exchanger. Warm cardioplegia is administered at 37 °C. The purpose of cold cardioplegia is to decrease oxygen demand and ischemic damage. However, electromechanical work constitutes the major component of myocardial oxygen consumption, and asystole can also be produced with warm cardioplegia. There is some evidence that this may have advantages, including reduced reperfusion injury, preserved coronary endothelial function, rapid re-establishment of myocardial energy stores, reduced calcium influx, and less activation of leukocytes and platelets. Warm cardioplegia may also upregulate protective heatshock proteins.

Blood cardioplegia provides a source of oxygen to the heart and has buffering and antioxidant properties, which are absent in crystalloid solutions. Intermittent cardioplegia is delivered at high flow at intervals of not more than 20 min in volumes of a few hundred milliliters to 1 L. Continuous cardioplegia is delivered at lower flow. It is difficult to provide homogeneous distribution of flow using continuous techniques, and there is concern about protection of the right ventricle and posterior septum. Nonetheless, studies of continuous warm cardioplegia have reported excellent myocardial protection and outcomes, and it has been advocated for better myocardial protection during prolonged cross-clamp periods. Single "hot shots" of warm cardioplegia at the initiation and termination of asystolic arrest have also been advocated for restoring ATP levels and reducing subsequent injury. The final "hot shot" can be enriched with the amino acids glutamate and aspartate to replenish depleted Krebs cycle intermediates and enhance aerobic metabolism, decreasing lactate production and increasing ATP.

The K^+ concentration of cardioplegia is usually about 20 mmol L^{-1}. Calcium-free solutions are never used because they lead to massive influx of calcium into myocardial cells on reperfusion, a phenomenon known as "calcium paradox." Mannitol may be added to reduce edema formation, glucose for myocardial substrate, and bicarbonate to buffer

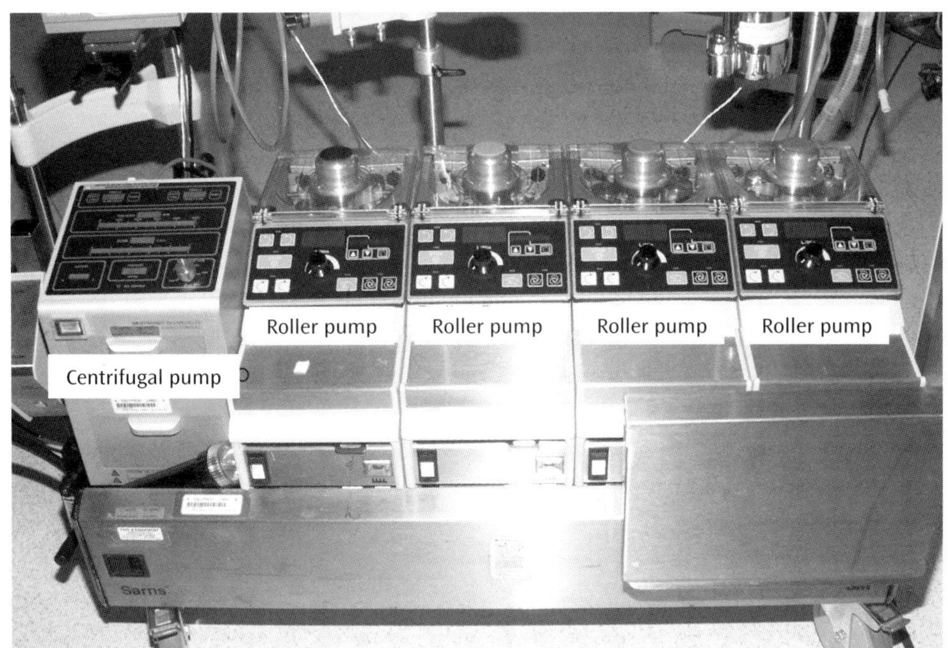

Figure 45.7 *Standard Sarns pump with four roller heads and a Medtronic centrifugal pump used for systemic flow. Additional roller pumps are used for blood recovery, cardioplegia, and ventricular sumps as needed. See text.*

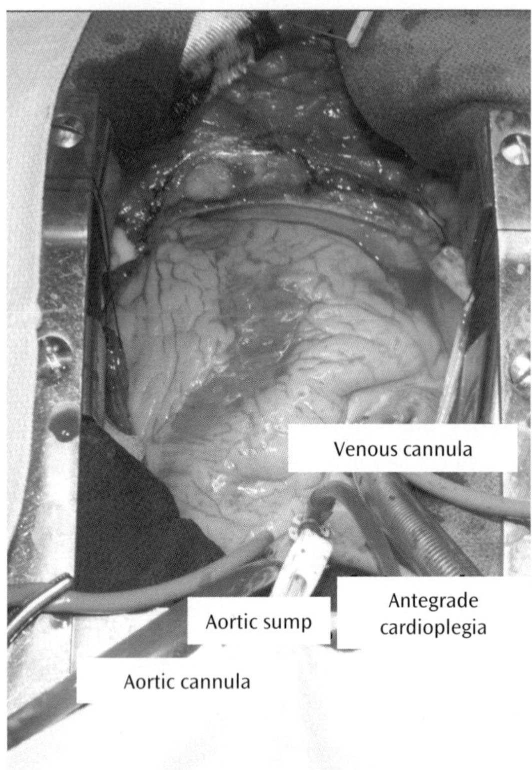

Figure 45.8 *Actual venous and arterial cannulation along with the cardioplegia line (with additional aortic sump line). This is taken from the head of the table looking over the field.*

intracellular acidosis. There is little experimental support or consensus for the use of other additives including beta-blockers, calcium channel blockers, steroids, free radical scavengers, and adenosine.

Anesthetic management

Both inhalational and intravenous techniques are used to maintain anesthesia during CPB. Inhalational agents are vaporized into the fresh gas flow to the pump. The concentration of, for example, isoflurane, is usually in the range of 0.5–1%. When inhalational agents are administered, effluent gas should be scavenged. Propofol is widely used by infusion, usually at a dose of 3 mg kg^{-1} h^{-1}. Other adjuncts, such as opioids, benzodiazepines, and muscle relaxants, may also be used. Hypothermia reduces anesthetic requirements for all agents, although implicit memory, unconscious memory, and awareness may occur during hypothermic CPB.

Blood gas management

There are two methods for managing blood gases during hypothermic CPB. These are called pH-stat and alpha-stat. pH-stat methodology entails maintaining arterial P_{CO_2} at 5.3 kPa (40 mmHg) during hypothermia, based on blood gas results corrected to actual patient temperature. The correction is performed by the blood gas analyzer, which always performs the analysis at 37 °C and then calculates values for pH, P_{O_2}, and P_{CO_2} at the patient temperature. Alpha-stat methodology entails maintaining arterial P_{CO_2} at 5.3 kPa (40 mmHg) during hypothermia, based on blood gas results uncorrected for patient temperature. Actual pH is higher, but actual P_{O_2} and P_{CO_2} are both lower during alpha-stat management.

Autoregulation of cerebral flow is preserved during hypothermia only with alpha-stat management, whereas cerebral blood flow is increased with pH-stat management. Postoperative neuropsychological outcomes are better when alpha-stat management is used.[40–42] This is almost certainly because the total quantity of microemboli to the cerebral circulation, which arise from the pump during bypass, is increased with pH-stat management. However, when DHCA is used, studies support the use of pH-stat management because increased cerebral perfusion may promote more complete cooling of the brain.[43,44]

Arterial pressure

During normothermic CPB, relatively small changes in cerebral blood flow occur when MAP is in the range 5.3–13.3 kPa (40–100 mmHg).[45] With alpha-stat management, cerebral autoregulation is preserved during hypothermia with MAP between 4 and 13.3 kPa (30 and 100 mmHg).[46] However, patients with diabetes, hypertension, and significant cerebral vascular disease may have impaired autoregulation. Although there is no absolute consensus, a reasonable lower MAP during moderate hypothermia (28–32 °C) is 5.3–6.7 kPa (40–50 mmHg). During normothermia (above 36 °C), this should be increased to 6.7–8 kPa (50–60 mmHg). It is usually accepted that these values should be higher in hypertensive patients. During CPB, MAP is controlled by changing pump flow rates and administering vasoactive drugs.

Pump flow

Flow should be set at a level high enough that total oxygen consumption is not flow dependent. Signs of inadequate flow include decreased mixed venous oxygen saturation, acidosis, and reduced urine output. A flow

Table 45.10 *Anesthetic checklist prior to CPB*

Item	Anesthetic checklist
Anesthetic level	Narcotics, benzodiazepine, muscle relaxant by infusion or additional dose, or volatile anesthetic available on pump
Anticoagulation	Heparin given centrally; ACT adequate for bypass
Monitors	Visible to anesthesiologist and perfusionist, retrograde pressure monitored (if used); Swan–Ganz pulled back 5–10 cm prior to bypass
Arterial line	Check for air
Venous line	Check fluid filled; minimal air to prevent air lock
Retrograde cardioplegia line	Pressure displayed (usually RV trace); position confirmed by echocardiography (if available)

Table 45.11 *Checklist after CPB initiated*

Item	Objectives	Problems	Solutions
Arterial blood flow	Adequate pump flow, normal pump pressure, adequate MAP [>4 kPa (30 mmHg)]	High pump pressure with low flow and low MAP	Check for line closed or kinked; aortic dissection; innominate cannulation
Arterial blood color	Arterial blood bright	Arterial blood dark	Check oxygen supply to oxygenator
Venous return	Good venous return; low venous pressure	Poor venous return; high venous pressure	Check venous line for air or kinking; if bicaval cannulae check head color and IVC cannula; check table height above reservoir adequate
Ventilation	Cessation with deflated lungs	Ventilator on; lungs inflated	Turn ventilator off unless partial bypass; check PEEP valve
Fluids	Off	Still running	Stop
Heart filling	Empty	Distended ventricles	Check venous return; vent heart; if aortic regurgitation present, reduce flow or cross-clamp aorta
Anesthesia	Adequate depth	Anesthesia too light	Check infusions running; add vapor to pump gas supply

of 2.4 $L\,min^{-1}\,m^{-2}$ at normothermia is widely accepted as satisfactory. Lower flows are acceptable during hypothermia but only for short periods during normothermia.

Anticoagulation and hemostasis

Anticoagulation with heparin is required during CPB to prevent platelet activation and clot formation when blood comes into contact with the plastic surfaces of the bypass circuit. The primary action of heparin is to enhance binding of thrombin with antithrombin III (ATIII).[47] Factor Xa and other factors are also inhibited by heparin, but to a lesser extent.

Adequacy of heparinization is usually monitored using activated clotting time (ACT). Blood is added to a tube containing activator (celite or kaolin) and the time for clot formation at 37 °C is measured. The normal value is 100–140 s. The usual dose of heparin is 3–4 $mg\,kg^{-1}$ and the desired ACT is at least 300 s, although many believe that it should be over 480 s. Visible clot forms below 250 s.[48] Higher levels of heparin result in less fibrin formation and plasmin activation, with better preserved platelet function. However, lower levels of heparin require less protamine for neutralization after CPB, protamine itself being an inhibitor of platelet function. Although there is some controversy about the optimum dose of heparin and ACT, there is no doubt that the greatest danger is a clotted pump, which is almost universally fatal. For this reason most err on the side of generosity with heparin.

An alternative to empirical dosing of heparin is the use of a heparin management system. A heparin dose–response curve is performed by titrating blood against varying levels of heparin and measuring the time for clot formation to occur. This permits calculation of the level of heparin needed to produce the required ACT, in units of heparin per mL of blood. The dose of heparin is then calculated from this value and the patient's projected blood volume. The use of this system has been shown to result in the administration of more heparin (and less protamine), and is associated with reduced postoperative bleeding.[49] In heparin-resistant patients with low levels of antithrombin III (ATIII), such as those with active endocarditis, administration of ATIII is required ,and this is usually achieved by giving fresh-frozen plasma.

Heparin is neutralized with protamine after termination of CPB. In the absence of a heparin management system, the initial dose of protamine is at best an estimate. In theory, each milligram of heparin requires 1 mg of protamine for reversal, but the heparin dose–response curve and the rate of heparin metabolism are both unknown. Excess protamine should be avoided, as it inhibits ADP-induced platelet aggregation *in vitro*, thus impairing platelet function, and prolongs the ACT. A reasonable approach is to give an initial dose of protamine equal to about half the total heparin. Five minutes later an ACT can be performed and correction made. If a heparin management system is used, the dose of protamine is derived from a heparin–protamine titration. Reversal is verified by performing another titration after protamine administration.

Protamine has important hemodynamic effects. It causes vasodilation via nitric oxide release, increases pulmonary vascular resistance (sometimes drastically) as a result of thromboxane A_2 production in the lung, and reduces arterial pressure. These effects are related to rate of administration, and protamine should be given over at least 5 min. A high F_IO_2 also augments the hemodynamic changes and should be avoided if possible. Allergy to protamine is occasionally encountered.

Most nonsurgical bleeding after CPB is related to abnormalities in platelet function,[50] although reduced levels of coagulation factors are also found. This is independent of heparin or protamine, and other tests of coagulation may be useful if there is excess nonsurgical bleeding. These include prothrombin time (PT), activated partial thromboplastin time (aPTT), thromboelastography, and platelet function analysis. The thromboelastograph is a device in which the rate of clot formation, clot strength, and the rate of clot lysis are measured in a kaolin-activated sample of blood. The rate of clot formation ("R time") is related to coagulation factor activity, clot strength (maximum amplitude or MA) is related to platelet function, and rate of clot lysis relates to fibrinolytic activity. Results allow targeted therapy, and the thromboelastograph is gaining widespread acceptance.

Partial reactivation of heparin may occur postoperatively, and additional protamine may be needed. Some patients will arrive in the operating room direct from the catheter laboratory, having received antibodies to the platelet GPIIb/IIIa receptor such as abciximab and tirofiban. Ultrafiltration during CPB can remove these antibodies.[51]

Antifibrinolytic agents are used in a majority of patients. These are ε-aminocaproic acid (EACA), tranexamic acid, and aprotinin (a serine protease inhibitor). All are effective in reducing bleeding, aprotinin being the most effective. With aprotinin, the reduction in bleeding is proportional to the complexity of surgery and amount of anticipated blood loss. Although there have been concerns that these agents (especially aprotinin) may be associated with coronary graft failure, there is no evidence that this occurs. The dose of tranexamic acid is at least 1 g and of aprotinin at least 4 million kallikrein-inhibiting units (KIU). Both are given either before CPB or in the pump priming fluid.

Heparin-induced thrombocytopenia (HIT) is occasionally seen in patients scheduled for CPB, usually as a result of prior heparin therapy. There are two types. Type I occurs within 4 days of exposure to heparin. It is nonimmune mediated and benign. Type II is much more serious with a mortality of 20–30%. It occurs 1–2 weeks after exposure to heparin and is immune mediated through interactions between IgG platelet factor 4 (PF4) and heparin. It is associated with arterial and venous thrombosis.[52] Heparin must be discontinued. Should a patient with HIT type II require CPB, other methods of anticoagulation are required. These include ancrod to reduce fibrinogen level, hirudin to inhibit thrombin, danaparoid (a synthetic, low-molecular-weight heparinoid), and prostaglandin I_2. ACT monitoring of anticoagulation is not useful with these techniques and no reversal agents exist.

Patients undergoing procedures involving CPB receive 10–20% of all blood transfusions in the USA.[53–56] Decisions to transfuse should be based upon laboratory evidence and consistent with recommendations of the ASA.[57] An algorithm for the management of postbypass bleeding is provided in Fig. 45.9.

Neurologic and neuropsychological dysfunction

As mortality rates from cardiac surgery continue to fall, attention has focused on neurologic and cognitive deficits following CPB. All cohort-controlled trials have demonstrated higher neurologic and cognitive deficits following cardiac surgery with CPB than after noncardiac surgery or cardiac surgery without CPB.[58,59] The major cause of post-CPB neurologic dysfunction is cerebral emboli. These occur in two forms. Macroemboli arise from the aorta when there is unstable atheroma and from particulate matter in the heart, particularly calcific debris, which has been loosened during valve surgery. These emboli cause stroke. Microemboli arise from the bypass circuit itself and from cardiotomy suction. They may be solid or gaseous and are associated with postoperative diffuse neuropsychologic dysfunction. Other factors, such as an imbalance in cerebral oxygen demand and supply during CPB, may also be important contributors to overall neurologic dysfunction. Preventive measures remain elusive. The risk for postoperative adverse neurologic outcome is influenced by age, diabetes, atherosclerotic disease of the aorta, carotid bruit, prior neurologic event, cardiac reoperation, CCF, and hypertension. Delayed strokes occurring more than 24 h after surgery may result from postoperative hypotension, hypercoagulability, or AF, as well as intraoperative events with delayed clinical manifestation.

Global cerebral edema has been shown to occur within 24–48 h of CPB with MRI.[60] Regional abnormalities in glucose uptake detectable by positron emission tomography (PET) imaging occur within 2 weeks of CPB.[61] A recent trial[62] showed that burst suppression of the EEG with propofol during CPB did not reduce neuropsychologic dysfunction after CPB. Blood pressure management remains a dilemma. Most try to avoid hypotension during CPB in patients with a high-grade carotid lesion or chronically elevated blood pressure. The stress response to CPB increases blood glucose. Hyperglycemia is known to be deleterious to the injured brain. Maintenance of normoglycemia is widely advocated. A recent report suggests that the renal reabsorption of glucose is increased during CPB.[63] There may be genetic predisposition to increased neurologic injury.[64]

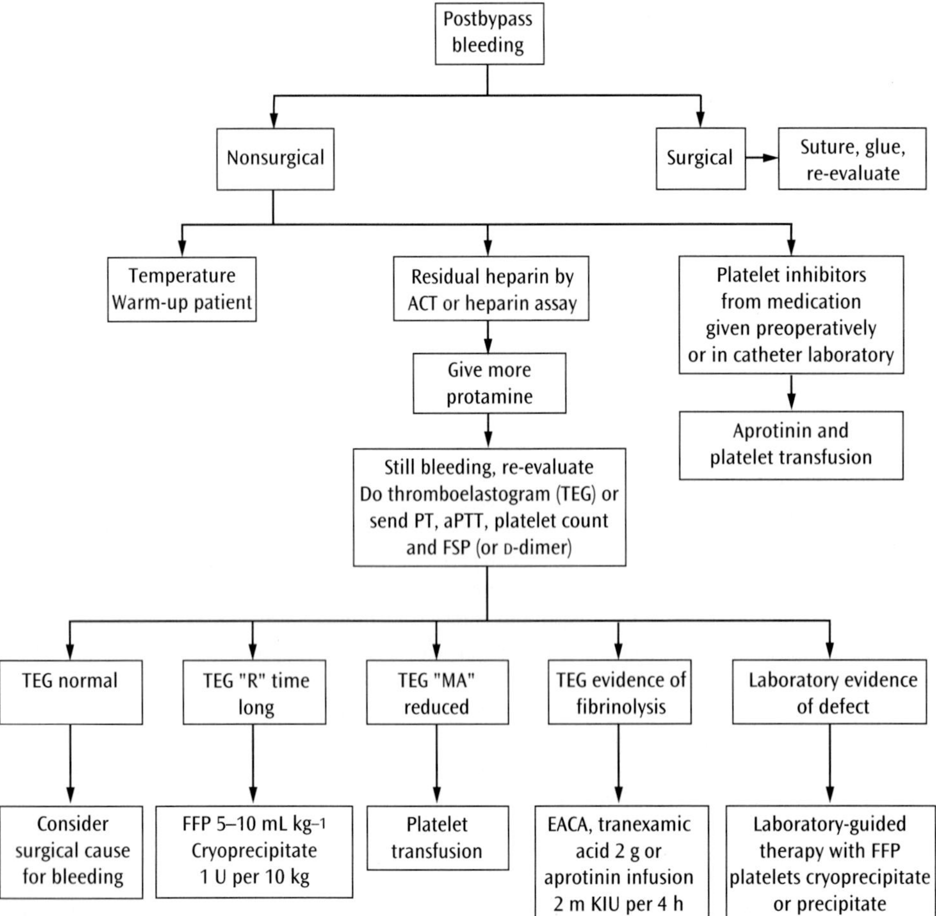

Figure 45.9 *Management of postbypass bleeding. See text.*

The inflammatory response

CPB is associated with a generalized inflammatory response. Blood components contacting artificial surfaces, ischemia–reperfusion injury to heart, brain, and gastrointestinal tract, heparin, protamine, and surgical trauma may all contribute to it. It manifests as complement activation, production and release of cytokines and leukotrienes, and subsequent activation of polymorphonuclear cells (PMNs), lymphocytes, monocytes, platelets, and endothelial cells.

There is evidence that endotoxin is released into the circulation during CPB. This may be the result of mesenteric ischemia, and it is associated with decreased gastric mucosal pH. The ischemic myocardium can produce proinflammatory cytokines and platelet-activating factor, leading to leukocyte and endothelial adhesive interaction. The outcome depends on the extent of the inflammatory response, anti-inflammatory cytokine production, and end-organ injury. Any organ with an ischemia–reperfusion injury is further damaged by leukocyte activation with the release of toxic products.

Many interventions have been attempted to reduce the inflammatory response, with some success in clinical trials. These include biocompatible circuits, steroids, aprotinin, complement antibody, antibody to PMN adhesive receptors, and hemofiltration.

Failure to wean from CPB

A mental checklist is performed before weaning from CPB (Table 45.12), and an algorithm for preparation to wean is shown in Fig. 45.10. Algorithms for managing weaning and difficulty with weaning are shown in Figs. 45.11 and 45.12. It is important that the cardiac repair is optimal, with no valvular dysfunction or kinking or vasospasm of coronary bypass grafts. Blood gases and electrolytes must be normalized. Core temperature must be at least 36 °C. Heart rate and rhythm must be optimized. When hypotension is present, rational decisions regarding manipulation of heart rate, preload, contractility, and afterload can be made with the help of arterial and venous pressure measurements, thermodilution cardiac output, and TEE.

The most commonly used inotropic agents are the adrenergic agonists epinephrine (adrenaline), dobutamine, dopamine, and isoproterenol. The side-effects of these agents include tachycardia and tachyarrhythmias. The phosphodiesterase III inhibitors work by a mechanism independent of β-adrenergic stimulation, and the combination of these two classes of drug has been shown to enhance left ventricular performance with fewer side-effects. Phosphodiesterase III inhibitors enhance calcium entry into myocardial cells, enhance reuptake of calcium in the sarcoplasmic reticulum (SR), increasing diastolic relaxation, and do not reduce myofibril sensitivity to calcium (as do β-agonists). As these compounds inhibit cyclic 3,5-AMP degradation in vascular smooth muscle as well as the myocardium, they are potent vasodilators as well as inotropes. The most commonly used phosphodiesterase inhibitors are milrinone and enoximone. Calcium "sensitizers" are a recent and promising development. Levosimendan is the prototype agent. It increases the affinity of the myofilament for free calcium by binding and stabilizing troponin C and opens K^+ channels in vascular smooth muscle. The result is increased contractile function and vasodilation. There is little experience in cardiac surgery and levosimendan is not yet in general use.[65]

Placement of an IABP should be considered when there is failure to wean from CPB despite therapy with the above agents.

Right ventricular (RV) failure is more difficult to treat. The normal right ventricle is anatomically and physiologically unsuited to increases in afterload. When RV dysfunction is present due to injury or infarction, any left ventricular (LV) failure will also worsen RV performance by increasing RV afterload and reducing the LV augmentation of RV systolic pressure generation known as systolic interaction or interdependence.[66] When vasodilators are used to reduce pulmonary artery pressure, systemic pressure is also reduced. In the presence of severe pulmonary hypertension, the right ventricle becomes more dependent on systemic pressure for perfusion. Therefore, administration of vasodilators may increase RV dysfunction by decreasing systemic pressure.

Table 45.12 *Checklist for weaning from CPB*

Item	Objectives	Problems	Solutions
Transducers	Zeros correct	Zero drift	Re-zero
Temperature	Core 36 °C; peripheral 33 °C	Inadequate rewarming	Continue rewarming
Acid–base status	Normal acid–base status	Base deficit > 5 mmol L^{-1} ECF	Correct with bicarbonate unless minor abnormality in otherwise fit patient
Electrolytes	Normal K^+, Ca^{2+}, Mg^{2+}	Low or high K^+, low Ca^{2+} or Mg^{2+}	Correct as appropriate; use insulin only if K^+ very high
Glucose	< 15 mmol L^{-1}	Hyperglycemia	Treat with insulin
Hematocrit	> 20%	Anemia	Transfuse into pump
Inotropes	Ready if needed	Not ready	Prepare and administer
Protamine	Ready	Not ready	Prepare
Heart rate	> 70 min^{-1}	Bradycardia	Treat with anticholinergic drug
Heart rhythm	Sinus or other appropriate rhythm	Heart block, AF, VF, multiple VEs	Pace (preferably DDD), cardiovert, or defibrillate; lidocaine or amiodarone if unstable ventricular rhythm
SVR	Normal	Inappropriate vasodilatation or vasoconstriction	Calculate SVR from pump flow and MAP; normalize SVR with vasopressor or vasodilator
Anesthesia	Adequate depth	Anesthesia too light	Check infusions running or turn on vapor
Intravenous fluid	Ready to run	Not ready	Prepare i.v. fluid
Ventilation	Ventilator on; F_{IO_2} > 50%	Ventilator off; F_{IO_2} < 50%	Turn ventilator on; increase F_{IO_2}

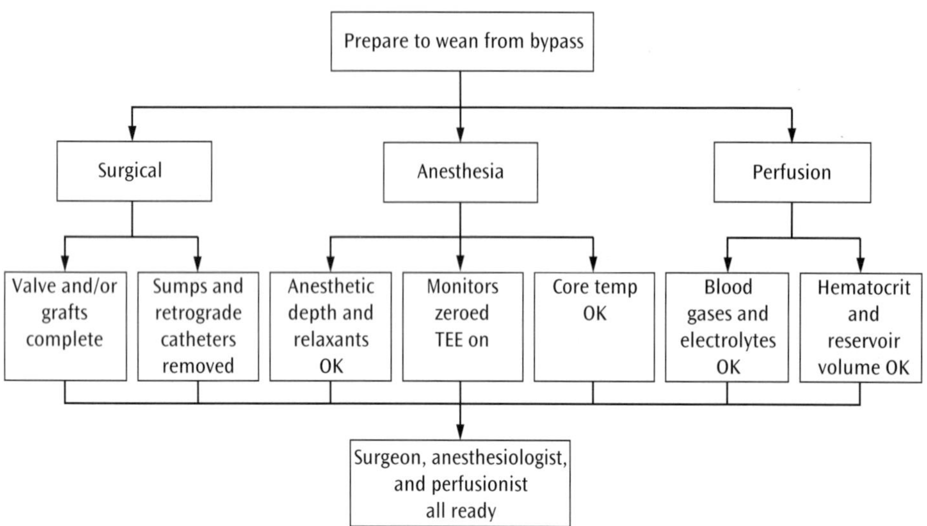

Figure 45.10 *Preparation for weaning from bypass. See text.*

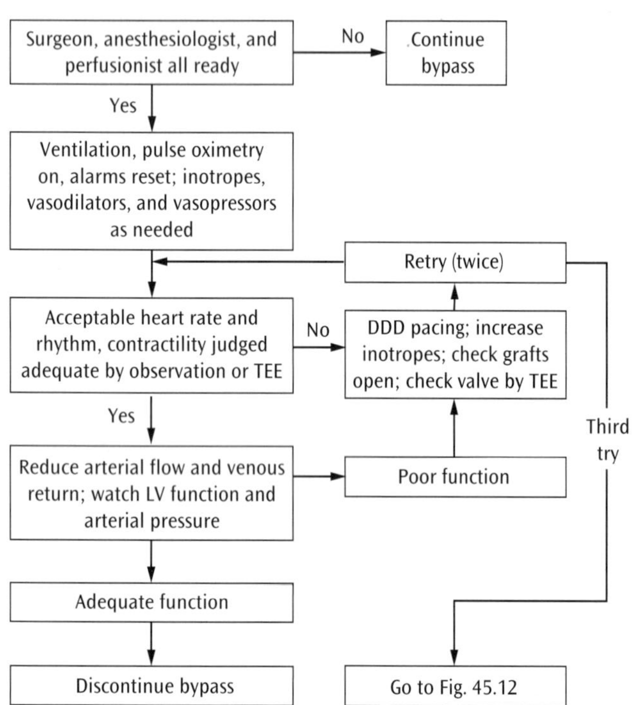

Figure 45.11 *Weaning from bypass. DDD, dual chamber demand pacing. See text.*

Nitric oxide can be useful in this situation. Use of an IABP may aid RV function and improve RV diastolic coronary blood flow.

There is evidence that circulating levels of thyroid hormones are reduced following CPB. Tri-iodothyronine (T_3) is the active compound, potentiating β-agonism, increasing myofibril activity, and having beneficial effects on intracellular and intraorganelle ATPase. Administration of $0.8\,\mu g\,kg^{-1}$ T_3, with or without infusion ($0.1–0.2\,\mu g\,kg^{-1}\,h^{-1}$),[67,68] has been advocated for patients proving difficult to wean from CPB, although support for this practice is not uniform. Prospective trials have failed to support important differences in outcome between patients receiving infusions of T_3 and those receiving placebo.[69] Other alternative approaches have included administration of glucose, insulin, and potassium, as well as rearrest of the ischemic, failing heart with warm, substrate-rich cardioplegia, a technique that may represent an alternative before mechanical assist.

Very low systemic vascular resistance is not uncommon after CPB. When cardiac function and output are adequate but the blood pressure is too low for weaning from CPB, administration of α-agonists should be considered. Vasoconstrictors, usually norepinephrine (noradrenaline), are used to treat hypotension due to low systemic vascular resistance. Artificially low radial artery pressures compared with central aortic pressure sometimes occur and appear to be related to forearm vasodilation and reduced radial artery diameter. Accurate blood pressure may be obtained directly from the ascending aorta or femoral artery. Usually, differences between radial and central aortic pressure after CPB are short-lived.

Recent reports suggest that the frequent occurrence of hypomagnesemia after CPB causes dysrhythmias. Administration of 2 g of magnesium during CPB has been recommended despite a potential depressant effect on platelet function.[70]

Intra-aortic balloon pumps (IABPs)

IABPs are usually placed percutaneously and then advanced into the descending aorta. The balloon tip should lie 3–5 cm distal to the left subclavian artery. The position of the tip must be assessed daily by chest radiography. Proximal migration into either left common carotid or subclavian arteries can cause damage or dissection, and distal migration can lead to obstruction and possible embolization of the mesenteric or renal vessels. Helium, 30–50 mL, is used to inflate the balloon. The device is triggered to inflate shortly after aortic valve closure and deflate just prior to ventricular contraction. The timing of inflation and deflation is adjusted to allow maximal diastolic coronary perfusion with maximal ventricular systolic unloading. This is best appreciated by observation of the arterial pressure trace. Use of an IABP improves coronary perfusion and cardiac output and reduces pulmonary artery pressure. Regular rhythm is desirable to allow proper timing of inflation, and deflation and control of tachyarrhythmias should be attempted.

Contraindications are severe aortic regurgitation, mobile atheroma of the descending aorta, aortic dissection, and dynamic left ventricular outflow tract obstruction. Evidence of limb ischemia requires balloon removal or replacement either in the contralateral limb or directly into the descending thoracic aorta via sternotomy. Anticoagulation may be achieved with heparin or low-molecular-weight dextran. The most common complications relate to vascular damage, including hematoma, lower extremity ischemia, and aortic dissection.

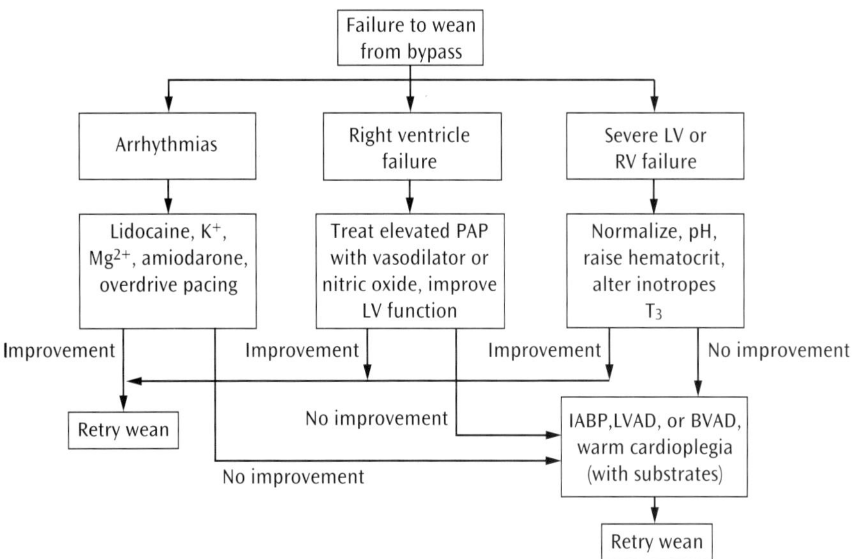

Figure 45.12 *Failure to wean. BVAD, biventricular assist device; IABP, intra-aortic balloon pump; LVAD, left ventricular assist device. See text.*

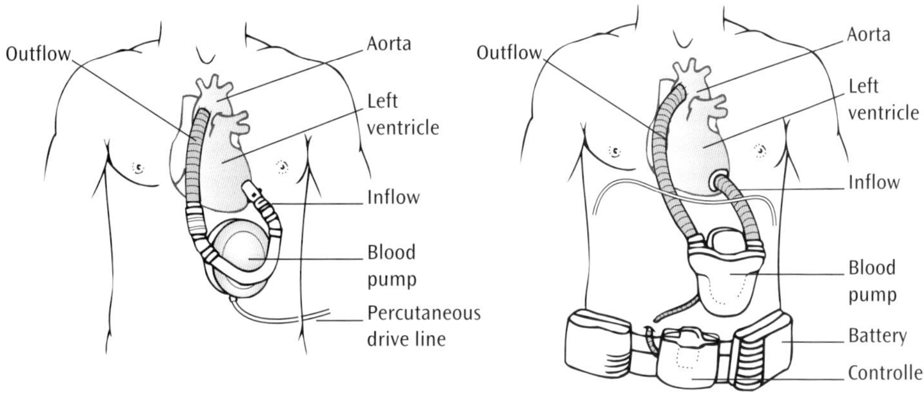

Figure 45.13 *The Heartmate implantable device on the left and the Novacor LVAD on the right.*

Assist devices and artificial hearts

Cardiac assist devices include centrifugal pumps, left and right ventricular assist devices (LVAD and RVAD), and total artificial hearts (TAH). These devices are used to support the circulation in severe low-output failure. They allow time for myocardial recovery or may be used as a bridge to transplantation. Cannulae for centrifugal pumps (which are the pumps used for normal bypass) are easy to insert and the pumps are familiar to perfusionists, but they can only be used for a few days. They may be used to support either ventricle and are connected with an inflow cannula in the relevant atrium and outflow in the pulmonary artery or ascending aorta.

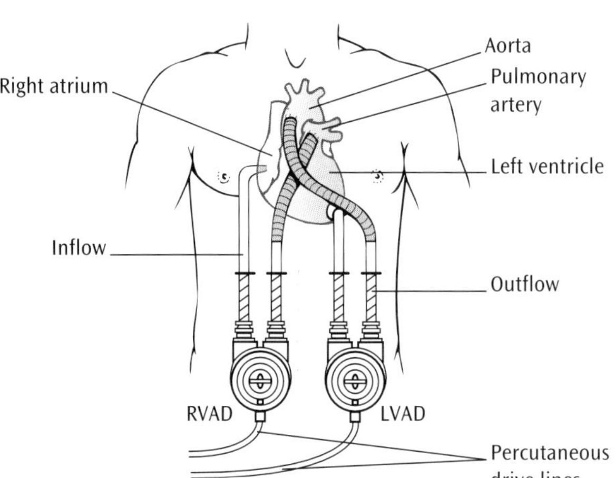

Figure 45.14 *Thoratec extracorporeal left and right ventricular devices.*

There are two LVADs, the Heartmate (Themo Cardiosystems) and the Novacor (Baxter Healthcare Corporation) (Fig. 45.13). These are placed intra-abdominally with the inflow cannula in the left ventricle and the outflow cannula in the ascending aorta. When an LVAD is used, tissue perfusion is dependent on right ventricular function. This requires adequate right ventricular filling and possibly inotropes and/or nitric oxide. Severe mitral stenosis or aortic regurgitation and intracardiac shunts are all contraindications to an LVAD and must be corrected at the time of device insertion.

Bridging to transplant is performed with the Thoratec paracorporal device or the TAH. The Thoratec is a biventricular assist device. It is pneumatically powered with the assist chambers placed outside on the surface of the abdomen (Fig. 45.14). At present, one total artificial heart, the Cardio West TAH, is undergoing clinical trials. This device is fully internal except for the percutaneous drive lines (Fig. 45.15).

Placement of all devices is associated with major bleeding, but reports suggest that aprotinin reduces this significantly.[71] The rate of infection is high at 25%. Thromboembolism has been reduced with the use of newer biocompatible materials. The Heartmate requires minimal or no anticoagulation because of specialized lining of blood-contacting surfaces. The other devices require anticoagulation with heparin and/or coumarin.

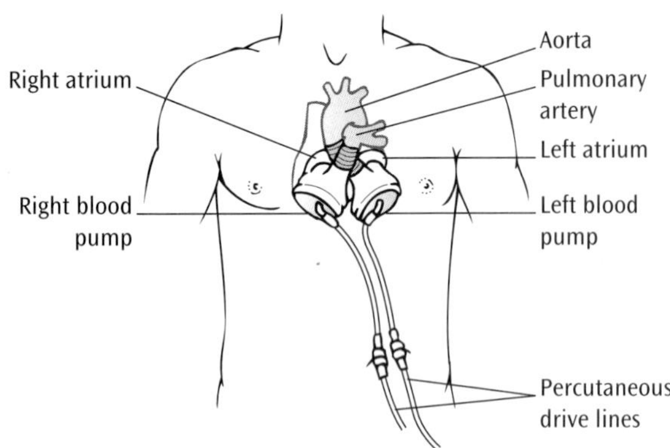

Figure 45.15 *The CardioWest total artificial heart.*

REFERENCES

1. The United Kingdom Cardiac Surgical Register. In: Keogh BE, Kinsman R. *The United Kingdom National Adult Cardiac Surgical Database Report.* 1999–2000. Reading: Dendrite Clinical Systems Ltd.
2. Ferguson TB Jr, Dziuban SW Jr, Edwards FH, *et al.* The STS National Database: current changes and challenges for the new millennium. Committee to establish a National Database in Cardiothoracic Surgery, The Society of Thoracic Surgeons. *Annals of Thoracic Surgery* 2000; **69:** 680–91.
3. Heusch G, Schulz R. Hibernating myocardium: a review. *J Mol Cell Cardiol* 1996; **28:** 2359–72.
4. Coles JC, Goldbach MM, Ahmed SN, *et al.* Left main-stem coronary artery disease: surgical versus medical management. *Can J Surg* 1984; **27:** 571–3.
5. Lawrie GM. Mitral valve repair vs replacement. Current recommendations and long-term results. *Cardiol Clin* 1998; **16:** 437–48.
6. Pigott DW, Nagle C, Allman K, *et al.* Effect of omitting regular ACE inhibitor medication before cardiac surgery on haemodynamic variables and vasoactive drug requirements. *Br J Anaesth* 1999; **83:** 715–20.
7. Kluytmans JA, Mouton JW, Ijzerman EP, *et al.* Nasal carriage of *Staphylococcus aureus* as a major risk factor for would infections after cardiac surgery. *J Infect Dis* 1995; **171:** 216–19.
8. Durmaz I, Buket S, Atay Y, *et al.* Cardiac surgery with cardiopulmonary bypass in patients with chronic renal failure. *J Thorac Cardiovasc Surg* 1999; 118.
9. Parsonnet V, Dean D, Bernstein AD. A method of uniform stratification of risk for evaluating the results of surgery in acquired adult heart disease. *Circulation* 1989; **79:** I3–I12.
10. Vedrinne BO, De Varax R, Blanc P, *et al.* Predictive factors for usefulness of fiberoptic pulmonary artery catheter for continuous oxygen saturation in mixed venous blood monitoring in cardiac surgery. *Anesth Analg* 1997; **85:** 2–10.
11. Grimm RA, Stewart WJ. The role of intraoperative echocardiography in valve surgery. *Cardiol Clin* 1998; **16:** 477–89.
12. Bergquist BD, Bellows WH, Leung JM. Transesophageal echocardiography in myocardial revascularisation. II. Influence on intraoperative decision making. *Anesth Analg* 1996; **82:** 1139–45.
13. Tuman KJ, McCarthy RJ, Spiess BD, *et al.* Does choice of anesthetic agent significantly affect outcome after coronary artery surgery? *Anesthesiology* 1989; **70:** 189–98.
14. Desborough JP. Thoracic epidural analgesia in cardiac surgery. *Anaesthesia* 1996; **51:** 805–7.
15. Ronday M, Damen J, van der Tweel I. Disconnection of the ventilatory system does not prevent pleural lesions during sternotomy. *J Thorac Cardiovasc Anesth* 1993; **7:** 535–7.
16. Slogoff S, Keats AS. Does perioperative myocardial ischemia lead to postoperative myocardial infarction? *Anesthesiology* 1985; 107–14.
17. Ross J, Jr. Afterload mismatch in aortic and mitral valve disease: implications for surgical therapy. *J Am Coll Cardiol* 1985; **5:** 811–26.
18. Campbell M. Natural history of atrial septal defect. *Br Heart J* 1970; **32:** 820–6.
19. Brouwer RM, Erasmus ME, Ebels T, *et al.* Influence of age on survival, late hypertension, and recoarctation in elective aortic coarctation repair. Including long-term results after elective aortic coarctation repair with a follow-up from 25 to 44 years. *J Thorac Cardiovasc Surg* 1994; **108:** 525–31.
20. Spirito P, Seidman CE, McKenna WJ, *et al.* The management of hypertrophic cardiomyopathy. *N Engl J Med* 1997; **336:** 775–85.
21. St John Sutton M, Epstein JA. Hypertrophic cardiomyopathy – beyond the sarcomere. *N Engl J Med* 1998; **338:** 1303–4.
22. Kai H, Muraishi A, Sugiu Y, *et al.* Expression of proto-oncogenes and gene mutation of sarcomeric proteins in patients with hypertrophic cardiomyopathy. *Circ Res* 1998; **83:** 594–601.
23. Faber LH, Seggewiss H, Gleichmann U. Percutaneous transluminal septal myocardial ablation in hypertrophic obstructive cardiomyopathy: results with respect to intraprocedural myocardial contrast echocardiography. *Circulation* 1998; **98:** 2415–21.
24. Nagueh SF, Kakkis NM, Middleton KJ, *et al.* Changes in left ventricular diastolic function 6 months after nonsurgical septal reduction therapy for hypertrophic obstructive cardiomyopathy. *Circulation* 1999; **99:** 344–7.
25. Cohn LH, Chitwood WR, Dralle JG, *et al.* Policy statement: minimally invasive coronary artery bypass surgery. STS/AATS Ad Hoc Committee on New Technology Assessment. American Association for Thoracic Surgery. *J Thorac Cardiovasc Surg* 1998; **116:** 887–8.
26. Kouchoukos NT, Dougenis D. Surgery of the thoracic aorta. *N Engl J Med* 1997; **336:** 1876–88.
27. Greenberg R, Risher W. Clinical decision making and operative approaches to thoracic aortic aneurysms. *Surg Clin N Am* 1998; **78:** 805–26.
28. Coady MA, Rizzo JA, Hammond GL, *et al.* What is the appropriate size criterion for resection of thoracic aortic aneurysms? *J Thorac Cardiovasc Surg* 1997; **113:** 476–91.
29. Bachet J, Guilmet D, Goudot B, *et al.* Antegrade cerebral perfusion with cold blood: a 13-year experience. *Ann Thorac Surg* 1999; **67:** 1874–8.
30. Svensson LG, Crawford ES, Hess KR, *et al.* Deep hypothermia with circulatory arrest. Determinants of stroke and early mortality in 656 patients. *J Thorac Cardiovasc Surg* 1993; **106:** 19–28.
31. Crawford ES, Crawford JL, Safi HJ, *et al.* Thoracoabdominal aortic aneurysms: preoperative and intraoperative factors determining immediate and long-term results of operations in 605 patients. *J Vasc Surg* 1986; **3:** 389–404.
32. Djindjian R, Hurth RM, Houdart M, *et al.* Arterial supply of the spinal cord. In: *Angiography of the Spinal Cord.* Baltimore: University Park Press, 1970: 3–13.
33. Lintott P, Hafez HM, Stansby G. Spinal cord complications of thoracoabdominal aneurysm surgery. *Br J Surg* 1998; **85:** 5–15.
34. Simpson JI, Eide TR, Newman SB, *et al.* Trimetaphan versus sodium nitroprusside for the control of proximal hypertension during thoracic aortic cross-clamping: the effects on spinal cord ischemia. *Anesth Analg* 1996; **82:** 68–74.
35. Simpson JI, Eide TR, Schiff GA, *et al.* Isoflurane versus sodium nitroprusside for the control of proximal hypertension during thoracic aortic cross-clamping: effects on spinal cord ischemia. *J Cardiothorac Vasc Anesth* 1995; **9:** 491–6.
36. Marini CP, Nathan IM, Efron J, *et al.* Effect of nitroglycerin and cerebrospinal fluid drainage on spinal cord perfusion pressure and paraplegia during aortic cross-clamping. *J Surg Res* 1997; **70:** 61–5.
37. Gelman S, Reves JG, Fowler K, *et al.* Regional blood flow during cross-clamping of the thoracic aorta and infusion of sodium nitroprusside. *J Thorac Cardiovasc Surg* 1983; **85:** 287–91.
38. Christenson JT, Aeberhard JM, Badel P, *et al.* Adult respiratory distress syndrome after cardiac surgery. *Cardiovasc Surg* 1996; **4:** 15–21.
39. Gillinov AM, DeValeria PA, Winkelstein JA, *et al.* Complement inhibition with soluble complement receptor type 1 in cardiopulmonary bypass. *Ann Thorac Surg* 1993; **55:** 619–24.
40. Murkin JM, Martzke JS, Buchan AM, *et al.* A randomized study of the influence of perfusion technique and pH management strategy in 316 patients undergoing coronary artery bypass surgery. I. Mortality and cardiovascular morbidity. *J Thorac Cardiovasc Surg* 1995; **110:** 340–8.
41. Murkin JM, Martzke JS, Buchan AM, *et al.* A randomized study of the influence of perfusion technique and pH management strategy in 316 patients undergoing coronary artery bypass surgery. II. Neurologic and cognitive outcomes. *J Thorac Cardiovasc Surg* 1995; **110:** 349–62.
42. Patel RL, Turtle MR, Chambers DJ, *et al.* Alpha-stat acid–base regulation during cardiopulmonary bypass improves neuropsychologic outcome in patients undergoing coronary artery bypass grafting. *J Thorac Cardiovasc Surg* 1996; **111:** 1267–79.
43. Jonas RA, Bellinger DC, Rappaport LA, *et al.* Relation of pH strategy and

developmental outcome after hypothermic circulatory arrest. *J Thorac Cardiovasc Surg* 1993; **106:** 362–8.

44. du Plessis AJ, Jonas RA, Wypij D, *et al.* Perioperative effects of alpha-stat versus pH-stat strategies for deep hypothermic cardiopulmonary bypass in infants. *J Thorac Cardiovasc Surg* 1997; **114:** 991–1000.
45. Govier AV, Reves JG, McKay RD, *et al.* Factors and their influence on regional cerebral blood flow during nonpulsatile cardiopulmonary bypass. *Ann Thorac Surg* 1984; **38:** 592–600.
46. Murkin JM, Farrar JK, Tweed WA, *et al.* Cerebral autoregulation and flow/metabolism coupling during cardiopulmonary bypass: the influence of PaCO2. *Anesth Analg* 1987; **66:** 825–32.
47. Despotis GJ, Gravlee G, Filos K, *et al.* Anticoagulation monitoring during cardiac surgery: a review of current and emerging techniques. *Anesthesiology* 1999; **91:** 1122–51.
48. Bull BS, Huse WM, Brauer FS, Korpman RA. Heparin therapy during extracorporeal circulation. II. The use of a dose–response curve to individualize heparin and protamine dosage. *J Thorac Cardiovasc Surg* 1975; **69:** 685–9.
49. Despotis GJ, Joist JH, Hogue Jr CW, *et al.* The impact of heparin concentration and activated clotting time monitoring on blood conservation. A prospective, randomized evaluation in patients undergoing cardiac operation. *J Thorac Cardiovasc Surg* 1995; **110:** 46–54.
50. Despotis GJ, Skubas NJ, Goodnough LT. Optimal management of bleeding and transfusion in patients undergoing cardiac surgery. *Semin Thorac Cardiovasc Surg* 1999; **11:** 84–104.
51. Poullis M, Manning R, Haskard T, *et al.* Reopro removal during cardiopulmonary bypass using a hemoconcentrator. *J Thorac Cardiovasc Surg* 1999; **117:** 1032–4.
52. Pravinkumar E, Webster NR. HIT/HITT and alternative anticoagulation: current concepts. *Br J Anaesth* 2003; **90:** 676–85.
53. Goodnough LT, Soegiarso RW, Birkmeyer JD, Welch HG. Economic impact of inappropriate blood transfusions in coronary artery bypass graft surgery. *Am J Med* 1993; **94**: 509–14.
54. Goodnough LT, Johnston MF, Toy PT. The variability of transfusion practice in coronary artery bypass surgery. Transfusion Medicine Academic Award Group. *JAMA* 1991; **265:** 86–90.
55. Goodnough LT, Johnson MF, Ramsey G, et al. Guidelines for transfusion support in patients undergoing coronary artery bypass grafting. Transfusion Practices Committee of the American Association of Blood Banks. Ann Thorac Surg 1990; **50:** 675–83.
56. Stover EP, Siegel LC, Parks R, *et al.* Variability in transfusion practice for coronary artery bypass surgery persists despite national consensus guidelines: a 24-institution study. Institutions of the Multicenter Study of Perioperative Ischemia Research Group. *Anesthesiology* 1998; **88:** 327–33.
57. Praseedom RK. Perioperative blood transfusion: a plea for guidelines. *Ann Roy Coll Surg Engl* 1997; **79:** 469.
58. Vanninen R, Aikia M, Kononem M, *et al.* Subclinical cerebral complications after coronary artery bypass grafting: prospective analysis with magnetic resonance imaging, quantitative electroencephalography, and neuropsychological assessment. *Arch Neurol* 1998; **55:** 618–27.
59. Libman RB, Wirkowski E, Neystat M, *et al.* Stroke associated with cardiac surgery. Determinants, timing, and stroke subtypes. *Arch Neurol* 1997; **54:** 83–7.
60. Sellman M, Hindmarsh T, Ivert T, *et al.* Magnetic resonance imaging of the brain before and after open heart operations. *Ann Thorac Surg* 1992; **53:** 807–12.
61. Jacobs A, Neveling M, Horst M, *et al.* Alterations of neuropsychological function and cerebral glucose metabolism after cardiac surgery are not related only to intraoperative microembolic events. *Stroke* 1998; **29:** 660–7.
62. Roach GW, Newman MF, Murkin JM, *et al.* Ineffectiveness of burst suppression therapy in mitigating perioperative cerebrovascular dysfunction. Multicenter Study of Perioperative Ischemia (McSPI) Research Group. *Anesthesiology* 1999; **90:** 1255–64.
63. Braden H, Cheema-Dhadli S, Mazer CD, *et al.* Hyperglycemia during normothermic cardiopulmonary bypass: the role of the kidney. *Ann Thorac Surg* 1998; **65:** 1588–93.
64. Tardiff BE, Newman MF, Saunders AM, *et al.* Preliminary report of a genetic basis for cognitive decline after cardiac operations. The Neurologic Outcome Research Group of the Duke Heart Center. *Ann Thorac Surg* 1997; **64:** 715–20.
65. Cleland JG, McGowan J. Levosimendan: a new era for inodilator therapy for heart failure? *Curr Opin Cardiol* 2002; **17:** 257–65.
66. Farrar DJ, Woodard JC, Chow E. Pacing-induced dilated cardiomyopathy increases left-to-right ventricular systolic interaction. *Circulation* 1993; **88:** 720–5.
67. Broderick TJ, Wechsler AS. Triiodothyronine in cardiac surgery. *Thyroid* 1997; **7:** 133–7.
68. Bennett-Guerrero E, Jimenez JL, White WD, *et al.* Cardiovascular effects of intravenous triiodothyronine in patients undergoing coronary artery bypass graft surgery. A randomized, double-blind, placebo-controlled trial. Duke T3 study group. *JAMA* 1996; **6: 275:** 687–92.
69. Teiger E, Menasche P, Mansier P, *et al.* Triiodothyronine therapy in open-heart surgery: from hope to disappointment. *Eur Heart J* 199; **14:** 629–33.
70. Storm W, Zimmerman JJ. Magnesium deficiency and cardiogenic shock after cardiopulmonary bypass. *Ann Thorac Surg* 1997; **64:** 572–7 [Published erratum appears in *Ann Thorac Surg* 1997; **64:** 1878].
71. Goldstein DJ, Oz MC, Smith CR, *et al.* Safety of repeat aprotinin administration for LVAD recipients undergoing cardiac transplantation. *Ann Thorac Surg* 1996; **61:** 692–5.

46

Anesthesia for vascular surgery

BRUCE A CRIDER AND ANDREW J MORTIMER

Elective vascular surgical procedures are mostly performed for the relief of ischemic symptoms resulting from atherosclerotic occlusive disease of the internal carotid, aortoiliac, and femoropopliteal arteries. Emergency vascular surgery, on the other hand, is most commonly concerned with repair of an acutely ruptured aorta that has as its cause atherosclerotic aneurysmal disease or the acutely thrombosed mesenteric or femoral arterial trees.

Elective and emergency surgical intervention within this patient population carries with it a significantly increased intraoperative as well as perioperative morbidity and mortality compared with the general surgical population.[1] The increased morbidity and mortality is due to the comorbid conditions present in the patients, rather than the primary vascular lesion requiring repair. In general, vascular disease is not isolated to one vascular bed but is a generalized condition affecting all the vascular beds supplying the various organ systems. The major cause of perioperative morbidity and mortality in this patient population is cardiac related.[2] Repair of the primary arterial lesion, which improves or restores blood flow, may also lead to the complication of ischemia–reperfusion injury, which may result in local cellular hypoxia and tissue necrosis plus multisystem organ failure. Surgically induced blood loss, fluid shifts, and the overall effects of activation of the stress response exacerbate these factors.

Anesthesia for vascular surgical procedures is therefore a high-risk subspecialty of anesthesia. This is reflected in the higher level of premiums required from anesthesiologists, vascular surgeons, and intensive care physicians for the provision of medical indemnity insurance (Medical Defence Union Limited, London).

Before considering the perioperative anesthetic considerations surrounding the care of patients presenting for vascular surgery, the disease process of atherosclerosis will be discussed.

EPIDEMIOLOGY OF ATHEROSCLEROSIS AND PERIPHERAL VASCULAR OCCLUSIVE DISEASE

Atherosclerosis is the most common cause of death and morbidity in the well-developed nations of the world. Deaths in the USA from cardiovascular disease have risen dramatically over the last 50–60 years, with the primary cause being atherosclerosis. Peripheral vascular occlusive disease (PVOD) affects up to 12% of the general population and 20% of people over the age of 70.[3-5] PVOD is associated with a markedly increased risk of cardiovascular events.[3] On average, an age-matched control group has an all-cause mortality rate of 1.6% per year. This rate increases to 4.8% per year for patients with PVOD. Cardiovascular mortality rates have an overall event rate of 0.5% per year in controls and 2.5% per year in PVOD patients. This represents a 3.4-fold increase in relative risk (Table 46.1).[6-10] It is also remarkable that asymptomatic individuals have a markedly greater risk of cardiovascular events. The presence of PVOD is now known as an independent risk factor for mortality, even when other known risk factors are controlled for.

RISK FACTORS

Risk factors for the development and progression of PVOD include age, diabetes mellitus, smoking, lipid metabolic abnormalities, hypertension, and elevated blood concentration of homocysteine or fibrinogen (Table 46.2).[5,11-22]

Active cigarette smoking almost doubles the risk of progression of PVOD (Table 46.3).

PATHOGENESIS OF ATHEROSCLEROSIS

The term atherosclerosis is formed from the Greek words *athere*, meaning porridge, and *scler*, meaning hard. This describes well the fatty deposits seen in the arterial wall at surgery. These hard fatty deposits are the final result of the response to injury of the vascular endothelium. Whether it is hypertension, hypercholesterolemia, diabetes mellitus, or tobacco use, there appears to be a final common pathway that leads to endothelial injury. Common endothelial abnormalities include increased generation of superoxide anion and reduced bioactivity or production of nitric oxide (Fig. 46.1).[23-26] Any one of these risk factors for atherosclerosis-associated conditions may have as its initial endothelial injury that of an intracellular oxidative stress.[27] This elicits the release of vascular adhesion molecules and chemokines, which with other factors attract monocytes that will ultimately adhere to and infiltrate the vascular subendothelium. As the monocytes accumulate lipids, they become foam cells, which will ultimately develop into a *fatty streak*. As more macrophages and smooth muscle cells are incorporated, more oxidation of low-density lipoprotein cholesterol occurs within the subintimal space. These "fatty" macrophages continue to take up LDL until they take on the appearance of *"foam" cells*. With the expansion of the subintimal space, the endothelial surface becomes irregular, and attracts platelets, which adhere to it. The platelets then release growth factors that will induce smooth muscle proliferation in the area of the lesion, forming an extracellular matrix and ultimately developing into a *fibrous plaque*. With even more lipid accumulation, the plaque becomes

Table 46.1 *Mortality risk in peripheral arterial occlusive disease*

			All mortality (event rate per year)			CVD mortality (event rate per year)		
Author (year)	**No.**	**Group**	**Control**	**PAOD**	**RR (95% CI)**	**Control**	**PAOD**	**RR (95% CI)**
Criqui *et al.* (1992)[6]	565	Men	1.7	6.2	3.1 (1.9–4.9)	0.8	4.2	5.9 (3.0–11.4)
		Women	1.2	3.3		0.4	1.8	
Vogt *et al.* (1993)[10]	1492	Women	1.1	5.4	3.1 (1.7–5.5)	0.4	3.0	4.0 (1.7–9.1)
Leng *et al.* (1996)[8]	1498	Symptomatic	2.0	3.8	1.6 (0.9–2.8)	0.7	2.7	2.7 (1.3–5.3)
		Asymptomatic	2.0	6.1	2.4 (1.6–3.7)	0.7	2.3	2.1 (1.1–3.8)
	1582	All patients	2.1	4.4	1.8 (1.3–2.4)	0.1	2.4	2.3 (1.5–3.6)
Newman *et al.* (1997)[9]	1537	Men	1.5	5.3	3.0 (2.8–5.3)	0.3	2.2	3.4 (1.3–8.9)
		Women	1.3	3.8	2.7 (1.6–4.6)	0.4	1.6	3.3 (1.3–8.6)
Total/average	6674		1.6	4.8	2.5	0.5	2.5	3.4

CI, confidence interval; CVD, cardiovascular disease; PAOD, peripheral arterial occlusive disease; RR, relative risk.

more complex and develops a necrotic core that contains the cellular debris and thrombogenic tissue factor secreted by the macrophages. Calcification of the necrotic core may occur late in the process.

PATHOPHYSIOLOGY OF ATHEROSCLEROSIS

The responses to the usual hemodynamic stresses on the arterial wall include a compensatory increase in wall thickness, thereby reducing the diameter of the lumen. Arterial wall thickness is directly proportional to tangential tension, whereas lumen diameter is directly related to shear stress. Abnormal responses include significant plaque formation that ultimately results in lumen stenosis; weakening of the vascular wall leading to aneurysm formation; and intimal hyperplasia, which may result in complete arterial occlusion.

Plaque formation is considered to play a major role in cardiovascular disease, with rupture being the predominant cause of acute coronary syndromes.[28] Plaque rupture has also been observed at the site of coronary thrombosis in two-thirds of cases investigated.[28] Plaque characteristics that predispose it to rupture include thinning of the overlying fibrous plaque, a large necrotic core, intraplaque and intraluminal thrombosis, and an overwhelming invasion of the plaque with macrophages.[27] There is evidence that many of the above characteristics that lead to rupture result from the role of the macrophages in this process.[29–31] There is also speculation that infectious agents such as cytomegalovirus, herpesviruses, and *Chlamydia pneumoniae* play a role in atherosclerotic-related events such as plaque rupture and the furthering of local inflammation.[32–36]

Angiographically, most plaques appear as projections into the arterial lumen. This is because angiography depicts contour in a longitudinal or axial projection. *In vivo*, the distending intraluminal pressure causes the cross-sectional lumen contour to be regular and round despite being significantly atherosclerotic.[37] Perfusion cross-sections of fixed arteries that appear irregular with intraluminal protrusions may indicate that the plaque has been subject to ulceration, hemorrhage, dissection, or thrombosis. An increase in artery size may also accompany an increase in plaque volume.[38–41]

Although the majority of vascular beds are usually affected by atherosclerosis, there are factors such as hemodynamic variables and arterial wall properties that may cause certain areas of a vascular bed to be free of atherosclerosis. Hemodynamic variables that may influence plaque distribution include shear stress, flow separation, stasis, turbulence, and hypertension.[42]

Distribution of plaque

Specific areas that are vulnerable to plaque formation include the carotid arteries, the coronary arteries, the abdominal aorta, and the superficial femoral artery. At the carotid artery bifurcation, plaque formation occurs predominantly at the origin of the internal carotid artery. The proximal common carotid artery and the distal internal carotid artery are usually spared. The tortuous nature and the mechanical stress of the pumping myocardium lead to dramatic fluctuations in flow rate in these vessels. These factors may explain why the coronary arteries are particularly susceptible to plaque formation. The thoracic aorta rarely has significant plaque formation whereas the infrarenal aorta is especially prone to plaques, ulceration, thrombi, and aneurysmal degeneration. Factors that may help to explain this distribution include flow conditions, mural architecture, and vasovasorum blood supply.[43] It seems that diabetes mellitus and tobacco use are likely to be the primary predisposing influences on atherosclerosis in the lower extremities, of which the superficial femoral artery is most commonly affected.[44]

Table 46.2 *Major peripheral vascular occlusive disease (PVOD) risk factors and associated increases in risk*

Major risk factors	
Age	Risk ↑ 1.5–2-fold every 10 years ↑ in age[5,11,12]
Diabetes	Risk ↑ four to five times; blood glucose control (HbA_{1C}) not associated with PVOD severity[7–9]
Cigarette smoking	Threefold ↑ in risk[5,11,12]
Hyperlipidemia	↑Total cholesterol, ↑LDL, triglycerides, ↑lipoprotein (a); 10% ↑ in PVOD risk for every 10 mg dL^{-1} ↑ total cholesterol[5,12,13]
Hypertension	↑ Risk of PVOD two to three times[5,11,13–15]
Homocysteinemia	↑ Risk twofold[16–21]
Fibrinogenemia	↑ Fibrinogen associated with claudication symptoms[22]
Minor risk factors	
Include male gender, nonwhite race, high-fat diet, hypercoagulable states, excessive alcohol, asymmetric dimethylarginine, C-reactive protein[3]	

Table 46.3 *Effects of tobacco on outcomes of peripheral arterial occlusive disease (PAOD)*

Clinical event	Tobacco use (%)	Abstinence (%)
PAOD clinical progression		
Claudication to rest pain: 5-year progression	18	0
Revascularization procedure success rates		
Vein graft patency at 1 year	70	90
"Reconstruction success"	19	81
Vein graft patency at 3 years	50	90
Patency rate at 3 years	78	94
Prosthetic bypass patency rate at 1 year	65	85
Cumulative patency rate		
1–12 months	66.7	75.4
1–2 years	55.2	65.5
2–3 years	52.6	63.6
3–4 years	48.6	60.8
4–5 years	48.6	55.7
Secondary graft patency		
1 month	70	91
12 months	40	75
Vein graft patency (femoropopliteal at 2 years)	60	90
Vein/Dacron graft patency (aortofemoral) at 4 years	75	90
Vein graft patency at 1 year	63	84
Amputation rates		
Amputation rate	23	10
Cumulative limb loss rate		
1–12 months	2.7	2.0
1–2 years	14.9	3.3
2–3 years	22.8	6.5
3–4 years	28.1	6.5
4–5 years	28.1	10.9
Patient survival		
1 year	85	100
3 years	40	67
5 years	36	66

Adapted from Hirsch AT, Treat-Jacobsen D, Lando HA, *et al*. The role of tobacco cessation, antiplatelet and lipid-lowering therapies in the treatment of peripheral arterial disease. *Vasc Med* 1997; **2:** 243–51 (summarizes literature).

Clinical manifestations of plaque

The clinical manifestations of atherosclerosis are usually the result of complications caused by plaque disintegration, fragment formation following plaque fracture, or fissuring. The symptoms are related to the region or organ system that is rendered ischemic by the thrombosis or embolism of plaques or plaque fragments. Plaques may have various characteristics. They may be calcific, sclerotic, friable, cohesive, or pliable. Hemodynamic stress or direct mechanical stress in the form of movement or torsion may result in plaque disruption. Alteration in the vessel configuration by plaque development might also create hemodynamic forces that result in plaque fracture or rupture. The acute complications of plaque are superimposed on the chronic symptoms arising from the arterial stenosis. There are usually no symptoms arising from chronic arterial occlusion until the diameter is reduced by 50%. This corresponds to a reduction in cross-sectional area of 75%. Symptoms of angina and claudication intensify as the diameter is reduced to 70% (area reduction of 90%). These symptoms occur only during exertion, when oxygen consumption in the tissues distal to the obstruction is temporarily increased and oxygen delivery is limited by the stenosis. Above 70% reduction in diameter (90% area reduction), oxygen delivery is inadequate to match oxygen consumption and rest pain results.

The relation between atherosclerosis and aneurysm formation is not yet fully understood. Evidence suggests that aneurysm formation is genetically linked and may have no direct causal link with atherosclerosis.[45–48] On the other hand, aneurysm formation has been associated with plaque regression leading to a deterioration in the medial layer of the arterial wall.[49,50] The thinning and destruction of the arterial medial wall caused by plaque degeneration make it unable to withstand the hemodynamic shear stresses to which it is exposed. This can result in a progressive arterial enlargement and aneurysm formation. The results of this process are embolization and thrombosis of the contents of the aneurysm as well as the actual dissection or rupture of the aneurysm wall.

MECHANISMS OF CELLULAR INJURY

Ischemia leading to cellular hypoxia and cellular injury and ultimately cell death occurs when the blood supply or oxygen delivery is insufficient to support aerobic metabolism. Regardless of the cause of cellular injury, there are four basic intracellular homeostatic systems that are especially sensitive to injury. These include (1) maintenance of cell membrane integrity, (2) aerobic respiration, (3) synthesis of enzymatic and structural proteins, and (4) preservation of genetic integrity.[51] The manifestations and degree of injury to the cell are directly related to the type of cell injured, its ability to adapt, and the type and duration of system failure. Regardless of whether the damage is due to ischemia or to other mechanisms, there are four common biochemical changes that play integral roles in cell injury or cell death. These are (1) oxygen

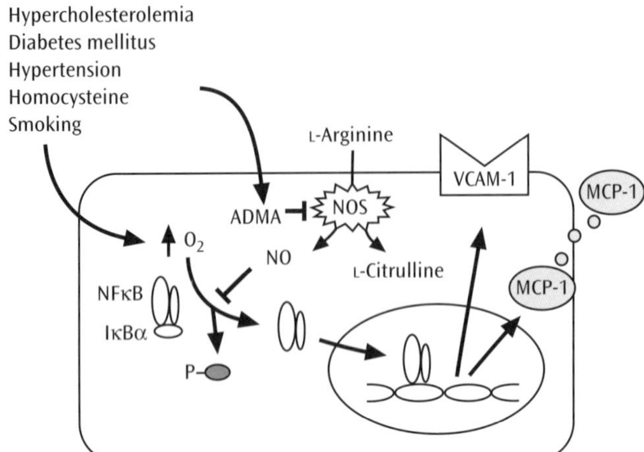

Figure 46.1 *Atherosclerotic risk factors such as hypercholesterolemia, hypertension, tobacco use, and diabetes mellitus lead to increased free radical production and decreased nitric oxide (NO) activity in endothelial cells. This endothelial dysfunction has not only acute effects on vascular tone but also chronic effects on vessel structure. Increased superoxide anion leads to activation of nuclear factor κB (NFκB) via phosphorylation and degradation of the inhibitor protein (IκBα). NFκB is then free to translocate into the nucleus to initiate transcription of proatherogenic genes such as vascular cell adhesion molecule (VCAM-1) and monocyte chemoattractant peptide (MCP-1). NO can inhibit these processes by inhibiting superoxide production, directly scavenging superoxide anions, and increasing the transcription and activity of IκBα. Moreover, since NO is a paracrine factor, it can have important inhibitory effects on circulating leukocytes and underlying smooth muscle cells. NOS, nitric oxide synthase; ADMA, asymmetric dimethylarginine.*

and oxygen-derived free radicals, (2) intracellular calcium and loss of calcium homeostasis, (3) adenosine triphosphate (ATP) depletion, and (4) breakdown in cell membrane permeability.[51]

Free radicals

The three most notorious free radicals are the superoxide (O_2^-), hydrogen peroxide (H_2O_2), and hydroxyl ions (OH). Superoxide is the product of mitochondrial auto-oxidation or enzymatic generation by cytoplasmic enzymes such as xanthine oxidase, cytochrome P450, and others. Hydrogen peroxide is generated in peroxisomes or the dismutation of superoxides. Hydroxyl radicals are produced by the hydrolysis of water initiated by ionizing radiation. Nitric oxide (NO) is another species that can act as a free radical. These radicals are both unstable and reactive. They play a central role in the mechanisms of cell injury and cell death. These mechanisms include lipid peroxidation of plasma and organellar membranes, oxidative alteration of proteins, and alterations in deoxyribonucleic acid integrity.

Loss of calcium homeostasis

Ischemic or other damaging factors cause an increase in the cytoplasmic calcium concentration, which is due primarily to the breakdown of both cellular or organ membrane structure and membrane calcium pump function. The increase in cytoplasmic calcium results in an accelerated structural breakdown by activation of various enzymes such as phospholipases, proteases, ATPases, and endonucleases.

ATP depletion

ATP depletion results from the loss of mitochondrial pyridine nucleotides and decreased ATP synthesis. The relative lack of this primary energy substrate causes the failure of membrane pumps that maintain membrane permeability and ultimately leads to membrane disintegration.

Cell membrane breakdown

At some point in the process of cellular injury, reversible cell membrane breakdown becomes irreversible (Fig. 46.2). Injury to lysosomal membranes seems to play a predominant role in this transition. The release of lysosomal enzymes such as RNAases, DNAases, proteases, phosphatases, glucosidases, and cathepsins may result in an inability to reverse mitochondrial dysfunction and in irreversible deleterious alterations in membrane function. Associated with these changes, a progressive loss of phospholipids, cytoskeletal abnormalities, the production of reactive oxygen species, and an accumulation of lipid breakdown products occur (Fig. 46.3).

An interesting paradox occurs when blood flow and an adequate oxygen supply to ischemic tissue is restored, namely the concentration of free radicals increases rather than decreases. This is thought to be primarily due to oxygen free radicals produced by polymorphonuclear leukocytes infiltrating the ischemic area.[52] This phenomenon is known as reperfusion injury.

PATIENT PROFILE

There is an increased incidence of concomitant cardiovascular disease in this patient population, such as hypertension, ischemic coronary artery disease including congestive heart failure, chronic obstructive airways disease (COAD), and renal insufficiency.[1,53–59] As might be expected, disease in one vascular bed is not usually an isolated event. The disease processes that result in the need for reconstructive surgical procedures also affect other vascular beds even though these may be asymptomatic.

COEXISTING DISEASE

The morbidity and mortality of vascular surgery are determined not only by factors related to the site of the operation but also by the performance of the heart, lungs, and kidneys. Coronary artery disease and hypertension are very common (Table 46.4).[60,61] The incidence of fatal and nonfatal cardiovascular complications appears to be similar in patients undergoing carotid or aortic surgery. However, in the case of patients undergoing revascularization procedures for lower limb ischemia, the cardiac morbidity and mortality are higher than in the other two groups.[58] This does not appear to be widely appreciated, but it does need to be taken into consideration when plans are made for the perioperative care of patients in this higher risk group.

Coronary artery disease

Radiologically significant atherosclerotic disease of the coronary arteries is present in almost two-thirds of all patients with peripheral vascular disease.[62] In the majority of these, it is clinically significant, having resulted in previous myocardial infarction (50%) or the symptoms of angina (15%). Many of these patients are asymptomatic with silent myocardial ischemia, which is associated with a poor prognosis. Thus, around 50% of all patients have had a major myocardial complica-

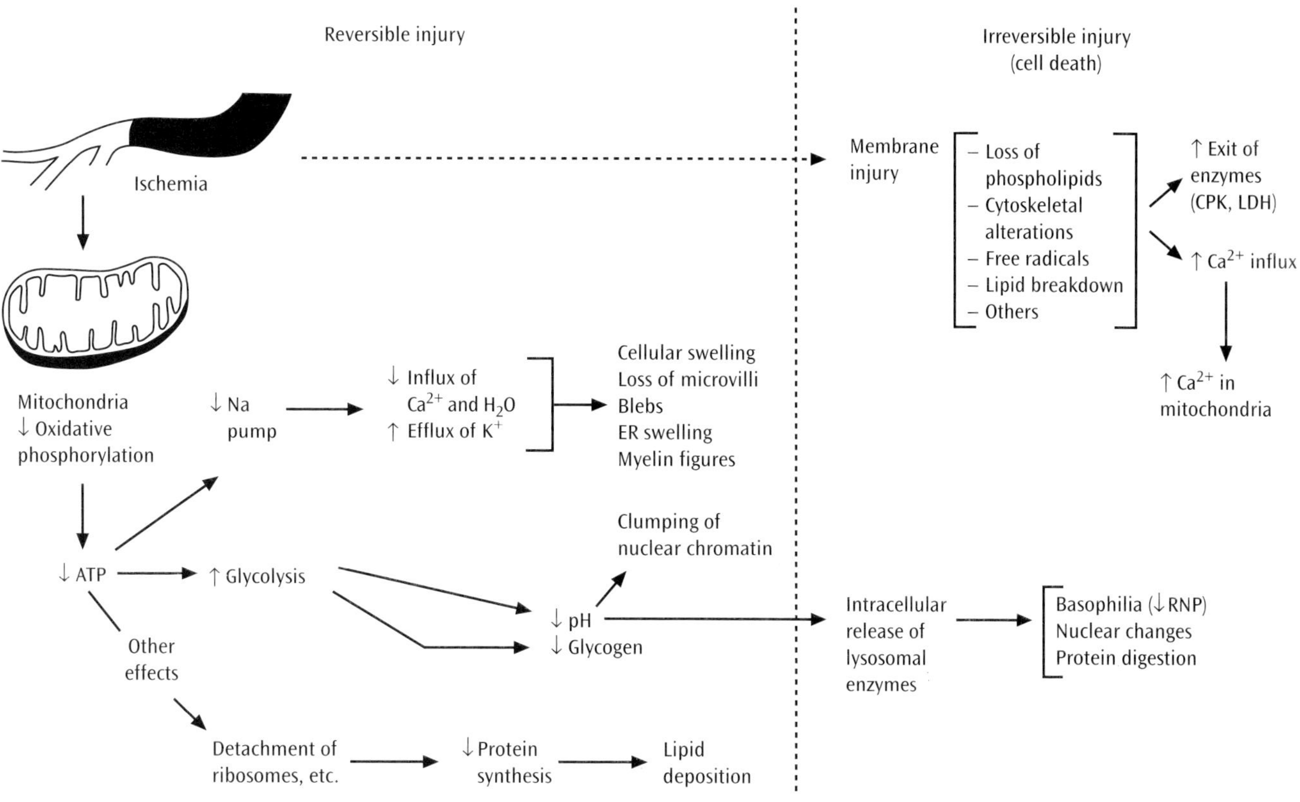

Figure 46.2 *Postulated sequence of events in ischemic injury. Note that, although reduced oxidative phosphorylation and ATP levels have a central role, ischemia can cause direct membrane damage.*

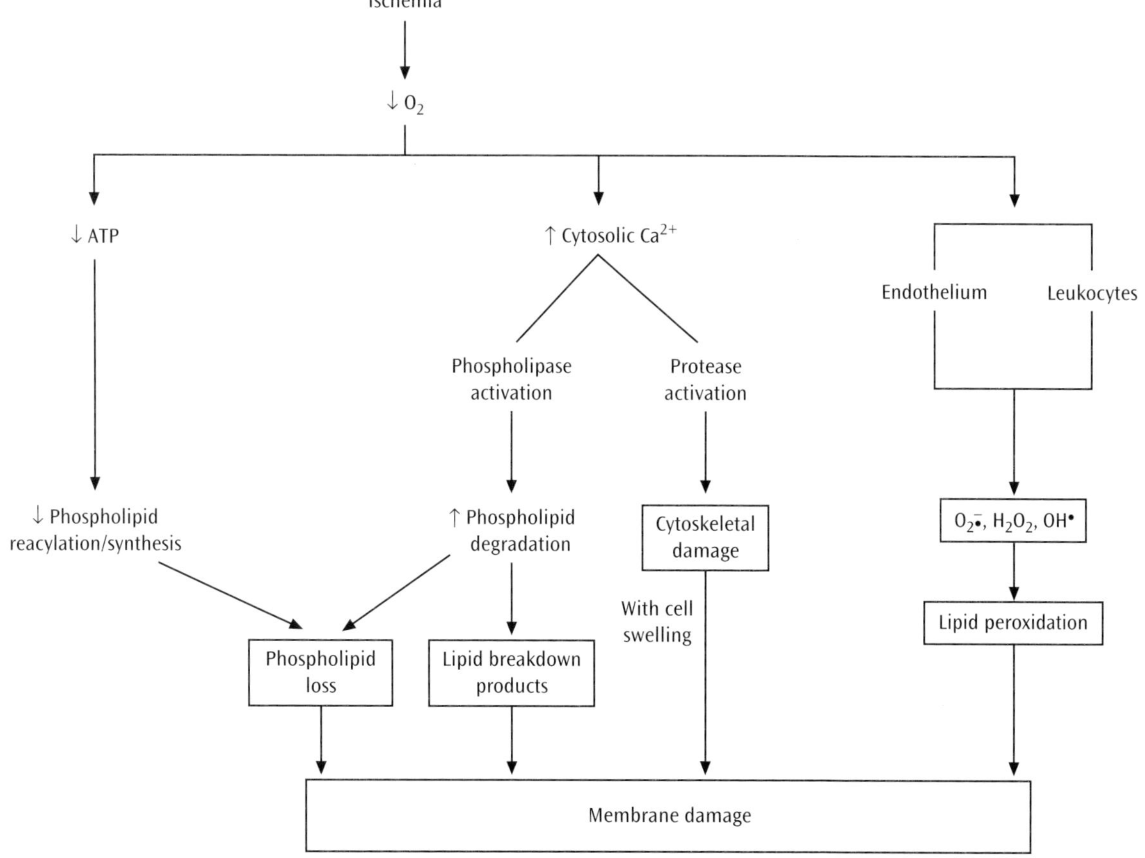

Figure 46.3 *Mechanisms of membrane damage in ischemia.*

Table 46.4 *Incidence of coexisting disease in vascular surgical patients*

Condition	Incidence (%)
Coronary artery disease	65
Angina	15
Previous myocardial infarction	50
Hypertension	50
Chronic obstructive airways disease	35
Congestive cardiac failure	15
Renal disease	10
Diabetes mellitus	10

Compiled from data in Hessel[60] and Cunningham.[61]

tion before surgery is undertaken! This is especially important because myocardial infarction is the principal cause of death in the perioperative period and accounts for 50% of all early postoperative deaths. Consequently, determination of the functional severity of coronary artery disease is an essential part of the preoperative assessment.

The significance of previous myocardial infarction is emphasized by the high incidence of perioperative reinfarction in such patients, which ranges from 6% to 13%.[63,64] The peak incidence is on the third postoperative day, possibly associated with nocturnal hypoxia and intravascular hypovolemia. Its occurrence may be reduced by intensive perioperative cardiovascular monitoring and by avoiding surgery when possible within 6 weeks of a myocardial infarction, as by that time the myocardium will have developed adequate scar tissue.[65]

Hypertension

Fifty percent of all patients have hypertension as defined by the World Health Organization and the International Hypertension Society.[66] The high incidence of hypertension is to be expected in an elderly patient population and is also a major factor in the pathogenesis of atherosclerotic disease.

Hypertension is important because of its pathophysiological effects. The increase in peripheral (arteriolar) resistance increases the afterload on the left ventricle for a given cardiac output. Consequently, myocardial work and therefore oxygen demand are increased, necessitating greater oxygen delivery via the coronary arteries. Since these are partially occluded in the majority of patients, it is not surprising that the incidence of perioperative myocardial infarction is high. Untreated hypertension results in left ventricular hypertrophy and, eventually, dilation as the heart fails. The hypertrophied left ventricle requires higher filling pressures because of the decrease in the ventricular compliance. The practical consequences of these compensatory changes is labile blood pressure, especially during induction of anesthesia or hypovolemia (exaggerated hypotension), and surgical stimulation (exaggerated hypertension). Frequent noninvasive (every 3 min) or invasive (continuous) blood pressure monitoring, provision of adequate intravascular volume, and slow administration of intravenous anesthetic drugs are essential during anesthesia for any vascular operation, or indeed for any patient with coronary artery disease or hypertension.

Another major effect of chronic hypertension is the shift to the right of blood flow autoregulation in the cerebral and renal circulations (Fig. 46.4). The significance of this rightward shift is that ischemia of the brain or kidneys may occur at apparently normal blood pressures, hence the importance of frequent or continuous blood pressure monitoring.

Because the majority of patients with hypertensive disease are taking medication, it is essential that this is continued right up to the operation and afterwards if possible. In a patient with untreated hypertension in whom surgery is urgent, a single dose of β-adrenoceptor blocker given with the premedication has been shown to reduce the incidence of intraoperative myocardial ischemia from 28% to 2%.[67]

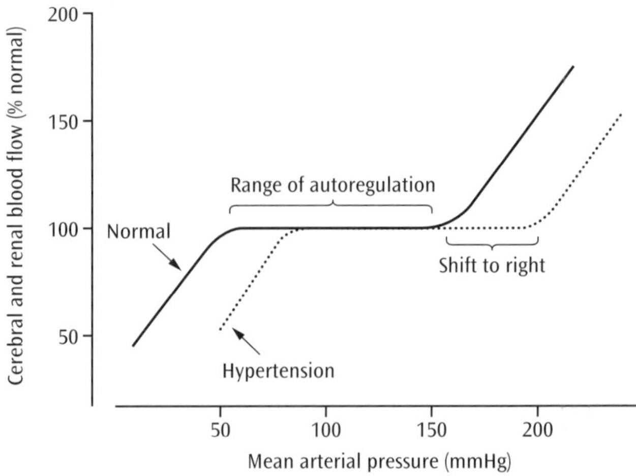

Figure 46.4 *The relation between cerebral and renal blood flow (% normal) and mean arterial pressure (MAP). In health (solid line), normal blood flow is maintained when the MAP is approximately 6.7–20 kPa (50–150 mmHg). In hypertension (dotted line), the curve is shifted to the right. Consequently, an apparently normal MAP may result in reduced organ blood flow.*

Congestive heart failure

Cardiac failure is present in 10–15% of patients preoperatively and in up to 30% of patients postoperatively.[68] Left ventricular failure resulting from hypertension and coronary artery disease usually precedes right ventricular failure, which occurs in response to persistently elevated left ventricular end-diastolic pressures. Ultimately, biventricular or congestive cardiac failure is present with signs of pulmonary and peripheral edema.

The presence of decompensated heart failure implies very severe cardiovascular disease, which is associated with a perioperative mortality of 15–20% Consequently, *all* patients with heart failure must be treated vigorously with diuretics, inotropes, and vasodilators prior to surgery.

Dysrhythmias

Atrial fibrillation is the dysrhythmia most frequently encountered, usually in association with coronary artery disease and hypertension. It may also arise *de novo* in the postoperative period in association with hypokalemia, hypovolemia, or an intra-abdominal procedure. The goal of treatment is to reduce the ventricular rate to between 70 and 90 beats per minute by increasing atrioventricular conduction blockade. The significance of atrial fibrillation is that, if left uncontrolled, cardiac output is invariably reduced in the absence of the 30% atrial contribution to ventricular filling. The resultant hypotension impairs coronary, cerebral, and renal perfusion, with all the associated complications.

Pulmonary disease

Chronic obstructive airway disease (COAD) is present in around one-third of patients. The high incidence reflects the high frequency of previous and present cigarette smokers in this patient population. The problems resulting from COAD are twofold. First, there is the potential for the development of right-heart failure due to the increased afterload caused by chronic elevation of pulmonary artery pressures. Second is the increased production of mucus, which leads to small airway closure especially prevalent in the early postoperative period. Decreased mobility of the chest wall because of pain plus splinting of the diaphragm due to swelling after intra-abdominal surgery may aggravate this.

Basal atelectasis leading to bronchopneumonia and hypoxemic respiratory failure are frequent complications of aortic surgery. When the airways are also filled with fluid in addition to mucus, as may occur in aortic rupture leading to pulmonary reperfusion injury, the hypoxemic respiratory failure is especially severe.

Renal disease

Renal function is vulnerable in patients with hypertension or heart failure, and is manifest in 10–15% of patients as elevated blood concentrations of urea and creatinine. Hypertensive patients have a marked increase in total body sodium and water retention, possibly mediated via aldosterone and atrial natriuretic peptide together with a rightward shift of blood flow autoregulation. The low perfusion pressure in patients with cardiac failure decreases glomerular filtration. The impaired blood flow autoregulation may lead to renal ischemia. For these reasons, and the presence of atherosclerotic plaques that are found in the renal arteries in two-thirds of patients, the kidneys are especially vulnerable to hypotension that occurs during myocardial ischemia, dysrhythmias, or the rapid blood loss following aortic rupture.

Diabetes mellitus

Patients with diabetes mellitus constitute about 10% of all patients with vascular disease and a proportion of those with peripheral vascular disease.[61] They have not only premature atherosclerotic occlusive disease of the large conducting arteries but also small-vessel (arteriolar) occlusive disease. Consequently, their feet and toes are underperfused and often develop infection and gangrene. Diabetic patients are therefore frequently scheduled for femoropopliteal reconstructive surgery and, when that fails, progressive proximal amputation of the toes, feet, and lower leg.

Points to be considered during anesthesia are the likelihood of coronary artery disease,[69] awkward venous access because of obesity, maintenance of steady blood glucose concentrations by appropriate intravenous insulin treatment (between 6 and 10 mmol L^{-1}), and adequate intravascular hydration to optimize tissue perfusion.

CHRONIC MEDICATION

Almost every patient scheduled for vascular surgery is receiving regular oral medication from one or more of the drug groups discussed below. The significance of these drugs, apart from the antithromboembolic and hypoglycemic agents, is that they may interact with intravenous and volatile anesthetics, causing undue hypotension. All cardiovascular drugs should be continued up to the day of surgery. Otherwise, the blood pressure may be more labile than expected. Antithromboembolic drugs, although they may not directly interact with anesthetics, can significantly alter anesthetic choice. Over the past decade or so, there has been a significant increase in the various types of antihypertensive medications that patients might be taking long term. Also, with the introduction of so-called "mini-dose" heparin and low molecular weight heparins, anesthetic considerations for the conduct of regional anesthesia in this patient population have changed.

Digitalis glycosides

Digitalis glycosides increase myocardial contractility and conduction blockade between the atria and ventricles. Digoxin is used for patients with atrial fibrillation to reduce the ventricular rate and as an inotrope in heart failure. The previous practice of routine administration of digoxin to elderly patients who may be at risk of developing heart failure or atrial fibrillation is no longer indicated.

Diuretics

Diuretics can be divided into five categories. These include thiazide-type diuretics (e.g. hydrochlorothiazide), indoline derivatives (e.g. indapamide), loop diuretics (e.g. furosemide), potassium-sparing diuretics (e.g. spironolactone), and osmotic diuretics (e.g. mannitol). The mechanism of action of diuretics is not precisely known; however, there is an acute decrease in plasma volume. This effect lessens over time but plasma volume does not usually return to pretherapy levels. Systemic blood pressure is lowered via an initial lowering of cardiac output (cardiac output eventually returns to baseline) and a lowering of systemic vascular resistance. Fewer than one-third of the patients on nonpotassium-sparing diuretics experience hypokalemia, and this should be avoided especially by the elderly, diabetic patients, and patients taking digitalis. Frequently, thiazide diuretics are used in combination with other antihypertensives. Examples include the combination of captopril or bisoprolol with hydrochlorothiazide. This combination lowers the thiazide dose necessary and reduces the need for close monitoring of serum potassium and the potential need for potassium supplementation. Other possible side-effects of diuretics include insulin resistance and hypercalcemia.[70]

β-Adrenergic receptor blockers

Nonspecific β-adrenoreceptor blockade may result in vasoconstriction, bronchospasm, decreased heart rate, decreased cardiac output, and a decrease in systemic blood pressure. Beta-blockers are classed as nonselective, blocking both β_1 and β_2-adrenergic receptors, or as selective β-adrenergic blockers, blocking either β_1 or β_2 receptors. Examples of the so-called "cardioselective" or β_1-blockers include atenolol, acebutolol, bisoprolol, and metoprolol. It should be noted that, even though these agents work primarily by blocking β_1 receptors, they also possess slight β_2-blocking activity. Their avoidance should be considered for patients with asthma, severe peripheral vascular occlusive disease, Raynaud's disease, and insulin-dependent diabetes.

Other effects of beta-blockers include bradycardia, decreased atrioventricular conduction, prolonged hypoglycemia in insulin-dependent diabetics, and the masking of symptoms of insulin-induced hypoglycemia such as tachycardia and tremors.[71]

Combined α- and β-blockers

Examples of the combination of these two classes of antihypertensives include labetalol and carvedilol. Labetalol combines nonspecific β-blocking activity with some α_1-blocking activity. Carvedilol is a combination of drugs with similar blocking activity. These agents decrease peripheral vascular resistance with relatively fewer cardiac effects than the pure β-blockers. Heart rate decreases slightly and there are only slight changes in renin and catecholamine levels. Side-effects include postural hypotension and dizziness.[72]

Peripheral adrenergic inhibitors

This class of medication includes such drugs as guanethidine and guanadrel, which inhibit sympathetic activity by preventing the release of norepinephrine (noradrenaline) from storage granules.

Reserpine, on the other hand, acts to prevent or inhibit the transport of norepinephrine into storage granules. This eventually leads to depletion of norepinephrine stores. While in both of these examples catechol-induced hypertension is reduced by different mechanisms, they are effective in reducing blood pressure. They are, however, rarely used in current medical practice.[73]

Central α_2-agonists

Central agonists act on central α_2-receptors, thereby increasing inhibitory activity and decreasing central nervous system sympathetic outflow. The end result of this action is a decrease in systemic vascular resistance, cardiac output, and systemic blood pressure. Examples of medications in this category are α-methyldopa, clonidine, and guanabenz. Acute withdrawal of clonidine treatment should be avoided as this may cause severe rebound hypertension.[74]

α_1-Adrenergic inhibitors

This class of antihypertensives acts by blocking postsynaptic α_1-receptors on vascular smooth muscle, thereby reducing the uptake of catecholamines. This results in vasodilation. Examples of this class of antihypertensives include doxazosin, prazosin, and terazosin. Relatives of this category are the nonselective α-inhibitors. They are nonselective in the sense that they block both α_1-receptors and presynaptic α_2-receptors. Phentolamine and phenoxybenzamine are examples of these medications. This action on these presynaptic receptors blocks the inhibiting effect on norepinephrine release, causing a depletion of norepinephrine stores. Tachycardia, postural hypotension, and dizziness are frequent side-effects of these drugs, thus their use is limited.[75]

Direct vasodilators

These drugs act by directly dilating arterioles, with the result being a reduction in systemic vascular resistance and systemic blood pressure. A baroreceptor-mediated reflex tachycardia may occur as well as catecholamine release, resulting in sodium retention and consequent fluid accumulation. Consequently, these drugs are often used in combination with β-blockers or diuretics. Tachyphylaxis develops frequently. Examples of medications in this class are hydralazine and minoxidil.[76]

Angiotensin-converting enzyme (ACE) inhibitors

These agents prevent the conversion of angiotensin I to angiotensin II, which is a potent vasoconstrictor. They also inhibit the breakdown of bradykinin – a potent vasodilator – by blocking kininase II, the enzyme responsible for the degradation of bradykinin. There is no increase in aldosterone secretion and vasoconstriction does not occur. As a result, systemic vascular resistance is decreased, as is systemic blood pressure. There is only a slight increase in heart rate along with natriuresis and retention of potassium. Elanapril, lisinopril, and captopril are examples of drugs in this category. Anesthetic interactions include the compounding of their hypotensive effects with those of the volatile anesthetics.[77] Because of the potent hypotensive effect of ACE inhibitors, some authorities recommend that they be withheld on the day of surgery.

Angiotensin II receptor blockers

Systemic vascular resistance is reduced by blockade of the peripheral effects of angiotensin II on blood vessels. Unlike the angiotensin-converting enzyme inhibitors, there is no effect on the bradykinin system. Serum potassium increases are uncommon. These medications can be combined with other lines of antihypertensive therapy such as diuretics. Losartan, valsartan, irbesartan, candesartan, and eprosartan are members of this new class of medication.[78]

Calcium channel blockers

Calcium channel blockers reduce blood pressure by blocking the calcium influx into vascular smooth muscle cells. This, in turn, causes a reduction in systemic vascular resistance by reducing vascular tone leading to vasodilation. Diltiazem and verapamil also act on cardiac muscle cells and will also cause partial blockade of both the atrioventricular and sinoatrial nodes, possibly slowing heart rate and prolonging any atrioventricular heart block. The major anesthetic consideration with this class of drugs is that the hypotension that sometimes accompanies these drugs may exacerbate the hypotensive effect of the volatile anesthetics.[79]

Nitrates

Nitroglycerin (glyceryl trinitrate, GTN) and isosorbide mononitrate are vasodilators used in the treatment of myocardial ischemia. They act directly on the coronary vasculature, improving subendocardial perfusion as well as reducing ventricular preload through dilation of venous capacitance vessels. Glyceryl trinitrate given intravenously is very useful for the intraoperative treatment of acute myocardial ischemia. It may also be administered by cutaneous patches to minimize the likelihood of myocardial ischemia during induction of anesthesia and tracheal intubation. The major drawback to this group of drugs is tachyphylaxis. Consequently, they should be used only intermittently in order to maintain their pharmacological effect.

ANTITHROMBOEMBOLIC DRUGS

Anticoagulants

Patients on full anticoagulation with oral vitamin K antagonists such as warfarin should have their treatment changed to a continuous intravenous infusion of 1000 units of heparin per hour 48–72 h prior to surgery. The dose is then adjusted to maintain either the activated partial thromboplastin time (APTT) or activated clotting time (ACT) at about twice normal. In an emergency, coagulation factors will need to be administered in the form of fresh-frozen plasma and possibly factor concentrates, the quantity required being monitored by measurement of the prothrombin time (PT). Full anticoagulation is an *absolute* contraindication to regional anesthetic techniques.

Low-molecular-weight heparin

Perhaps the easiest way to discuss low-molecular-weight heparins is to compare and contrast them with the properties of standard heparin. Standard heparin has as its mechanism of action the binding of a high-affinity sequence to antithrombin III, which then interacts or inhibits the action of anti-IIa or anti-Xa.[80] In the case of standard heparin, there is a significant degree of protein binding that reduces both its bioavailability and its ability to anticoagulate. Standard heparin has a relatively short half-life of approximately 0.5–1.0 h. These factors result in there being a significant patient-to-patient variability. It is therefore necessary for close laboratory monitoring of the activated partial thromboplastin time (APTT) as well as frequent dose adjustments to achieve the targeted level of anticoagulation. Another characteristic of standard heparin is that it is known to have adverse effects on platelet aggregation.[81]

In contrast, the low molecular weight heparins have a longer plasma half-life of 4–6 h and little protein binding.[81] It should also be noted that this class of anticoagulants has fewer platelet effects, especially when compared with standard heparin. As a consequence, there is no need in most cases for dose adjustment or laboratory monitoring. Clinical uses of low molecular weight heparins include prophylaxis against venous thromboembolism, treatment of acute pulmonary embolism, and venous thrombosis prophylaxis in the pregnant population.[81]

Antiplatelet drugs

The principal antiplatelet drug is aspirin, which reduces the aggregation of platelets (and therefore the formation of platelet emboli) by irreversible inhibition of platelet cyclo-oxygenase, the enzyme responsible for thromboxane A_2 (TXA_2) synthesis. Thromboxane A_2 is the substance that normally initiates and promotes platelet aggregation. A single dose of aspirin is effective as a cyclo-oxygenase inhibitor for the 7- to 10-day lifespan of a platelet.[83] Aspirin is now given to patients with symptoms of atherosclerotic occlusive disease such as angina, previous myocardial infarction, transient ischemic attack (TIA), and stroke. Indeed, the majority of patients scheduled for surgery in the authors' practice are now taking this drug. The recently reported results of a meta-analysis of 300 controlled trials prepared by the Anti-Platelet Triallists Collaboration[82] revealed a 25% reduction in vascular events in these high-risk patients. Significant improvements were also observed in postoperative coronary and peripheral arterial vein grafts. As a result, all or most vascular surgical patients will probably be taking aspirin for the duration of their lives.

The anesthetic implications of aspirin include the possibility of increased intraoperative blood loss and the logical attendant risk of a spinal or epidural hematoma. However, this risk has not been confirmed by published trials (see Chapter 74). Control of the blood loss is achieved by meticulous attention to hemostasis given by the surgical team. However, there appears to be no consensus of opinion regarding regional neural blockade in aspirin-treated patients. The safest answer is to regard aspirin as a *relative* contraindication and to consider the risks and benefits for each individual patient.

OTHER SIGNIFICANT MEDICATION

Steroids

Patients with an inflammatory condition such as Takayasu's arteritis or severe COAD may be taking oral prednisolone. This should be changed to intravenous hydrocortisone in increased dosage during the perioperative period.

Hypoglycemic drugs

The oral hypoglycemic drugs must be stopped preoperatively. Long-acting insulin preparations should be changed to short-acting soluble insulin. In all diabetic patients, the blood glucose concentration should be measured hourly and appropriate doses of insulin given with the goal of avoiding hypo- and hyperglycemia (aim for a blood glucose concentration of 6–10 $mmol\,L^{-1}$).

PREOPERATIVE ASSESSMENT

The cornerstones of preoperative assessment are the medical history, clinical examination, routine laboratory tests, and special investigations. The last are focused on providing a detailed assessment of cardiovascular function. Only a brief survey of preoperative assessment will be given here because the topic is considered fully elsewhere in this book.

History and physical examination

In addition to documenting the symptoms caused by the particular surgical lesion, questions must be asked about cerebral, cardiac, pulmonary, and renal function.

Loss of cerebral function may have occurred following stroke or TIA. Details of any residual neurological deficits must be recorded prior to carotid endarterectomy. Otherwise, it may be difficult to determine whether an apparently new deficit was present preoperatively or occurred intraoperatively. Similarly, it is important to note crude spinal cord function prior to abdominal aortic surgery and is absolutely essential with thoracic aortic procedures.

Symptoms of coronary artery disease and heart failure should be sought. Coronary artery disease manifests (after 75–90% arterial lumen occlusion) as angina, arrhythmias, heart failure, or infarction. Anginal pain is typically crushing in nature with or without radiation to the left arm, lower jaw, back, and right arm. In the case of stable angina, the pain is elicited by activity and is predictable. In unstable angina, there is no discernable pattern and may even occur at rest. This may be the result, all or in part, of coronary artery spasm. Myocardial ischemia may even be totally silent, as is the case in some diabetic patients. Myocardial infarction may be transmural (main coronary artery) or subendocardial, and is characterized by persistent pain usually necessitating emergency medical treatment and admission to hospital.

Assessment of ventricular function will be straightforward for a patient with frank congestive cardiac failure with ankle or sacral edema and shortness of breath due to increased pulmonary extravascular fluid. Early left ventricular failure may be indicated by orthopnea. This results from the chronically raised left ventricular end-diastolic pressure.

All patients must be questioned about their present and former smoking habits. Signs and symptoms of chronic obstructive pulmonary disease should be sought. Shortness of breath, wheeziness, and recurrent episodes of excessive production of mucus that readily becomes infected will be evident in one-third of all patients.

Mild-to-moderate renal impairment is usually asymptomatic, but should be considered in any patient with diabetes mellitus, atrial fibrillation, or heart failure. Severe renal impairment manifests as oliguria or anuria and is usually associated with shock resulting from a ruptured aortic aneurysm.

The patient's weight should be recorded for use as a guide when planning intravenous anesthetic drug dose requirements and when estimating circulating blood volume for operations in which blood loss is anticipated (estimated blood volume = weight in $kg \times 70\,mL\,kg^{-1}$). Additionally, the patient's height should be measured. This, together with the weight, can be used to estimate the body surface area for those in whom a pulmonary artery catheter (PAC) may be used and cardiac index derived from measurements of cardiac output.

Laboratory investigations

A full blood count (hemoglobin, white blood cells, and platelets) plus biochemical profile (calcium, potassium, and creatinine in particular) should be performed for every patient. Mild-to-moderate anemia is frequently discovered, whereas polycythemia usually indicates severe COAD.

Hypokalemia (<3.5 mmol L^{-1}) is occasionally observed in patients taking diuretics. Some believe that it is best corrected by intensive oral potassium replacement over 3–4 days. In emergencies, surgery should proceed because it is the ratio of extracellular to intracellular potassium that is physiologically important and not the absolute concentration.

Hepatocellular enzymes and plasma proteins should be measured in patients with heart failure as an index of liver congestion. When coagulation disorders arise either by dilution due to anticipated blood loss or by factor XII activation during tissue ischemia, a coagulation screen to establish baseline values should be carried out.

A single measurement of the arterial blood gases with the patient breathing air is a useful guide to the management of oxygenation and pulmonary ventilation in the perioperative period for those with dyspnea at rest or abnormal findings on spirometry. For example, a lowered P_{aO_2} [<9 kPa (<67.5 mmHg)] indicates the optimum that patients may achieve 1 week postoperatively without supplemental oxygen, whereas a raised P_{aCO_2} [>7 kPa (>52.5 mmHg)] indicates the likelihood of the need for postoperative ventilation.

Finally, the patient's blood group must be determined. For operations in which blood loss is inevitable, such as arterial trauma or aortic reconstruction, 4–6 units of fresh whole blood should be cross-matched in accordance with hospital transfusion policy. Blood transfusion is rarely required for other operations. The potential need for platelets should be considered especially for those patients that may require massive transfusion. This potential need can be increased if the patient in question has been on nonsteroidal anti-inflammatory medication, which could very well render the patient's native platelets dysfunctional.

SPECIAL INVESTIGATIONS AND ASSESSMENTS

Since coronary artery disease is the most common cause of death after major vascular procedures,[84–87] it follows that extreme care and vigilance should be taken when evaluating a patient's cardiac status preoperatively. Several special screening tests are available to assist in this investigation. These include electrocardiogram (ECG) treadmill testing (ETT), Holter monitoring (ambulatory ECG), radionuclide ventriculography, dipyridamole thallium scintigraphy (DTS), dobutamine stress echocardiography, and coronary angiography. The routine preoperative resting ECG is not a reliable predictor of perioperative cardiac risk. This has led investigators to use the investigations listed above.

Identifying those patients at risk for perioperative ischemia can assist with their management and may lead to surgical intervention or percutaneous angioplasty for those patients found to have surgically amenable coronary lesions. For example, in one study[85] of 216 patients there was a 72% 5-year survival among those who underwent surgery for correctable coronary lesions. For the 35 patients who had surgically correctable disease and refused surgical intervention, the 5-year survival was 43%. These data must be assessed in the context that there is a definite morbidity and mortality associated with surgical intervention for demonstrable coronary disease as well as the risks of the prospective major vascular procedure being considered. Patients should be considered on a case-by-case basis, weighing risk versus benefit for each. It is not clear that surgical intervention is always in the patient's best interest.

ECG exercise treadmill testing (ETT)

This testing modality is usually used for patients that have the ability to exercise. Unfortunately, the patients who present for major vascular procedures are frequently limited in their ability to exercise because of claudication in their ischemic lower extremities. These patients are therefore unable to generate the heart rates necessary to evaluate them for the presence of ischemic coronary artery disease. Attempts at conducting exercise stress testing via upper extremity ergometry usually fall short of the level of exercise needed for standard assessment ETT protocols. It has been found in at least one study[88] that normal ETT values were present in two-thirds of men and one-third of women with angiographically documented significant CAD. Other studies have found significant false positives and false negatives associated with this testing technique. A positive ETT only slightly increases the likelihood of CAD and a negative ETT poorly correlates with the absence of CAD.[89]

Holter monitoring (ambulatory ECG)

Prospective studies[90–92] have supported the use of ambulatory ECG as a predictor of perioperative cardiac events. Characteristics of these studies are of interest. Twenty-eight percent of patients having noncardiac operations had significant preoperative ischemia detected by Holter, and the incidence of postoperative ischemia in these patients was nearly doubled. Also of interest is the fact that nearly all of these documented ischemic episodes were silent (94%). The use of this method of assessment is also supported by Raby *et al.*,[93] who found that in their study of the patients who demonstrated significant ischemia by Holter preoperatively just under one-third went on to experience postoperative cardiac events. Fewer than 1% of the patients who tested negative preoperatively went on to have a cardiac event postoperatively. This positive predictive reliability of Holter monitoring sets it apart from many of the other modalities discussed in that it is easily available and is inexpensive.

Radionuclide ventriculography (RNVG)

RNVG is a nuclear cardiographic technique that is typically used to assess ejection fraction (EF) and to demonstrate left ventricular dysfunction. It has been used for several years to assess and identify those patients at greatest risk for perioperative cardiac events surrounding major vascular procedures. Pasternack *et al.*[94,95] found that, of those patients undergoing vascular surgery who had an EF of greater than 56%, none went on to suffer a perioperative myocardial infarction. In contrast, of those patients who had an EF under 30%, 70–80% went on to experience adverse cardiac events. Although the predictive value of this technique is not universally accepted, it is nonetheless frequently used.

Dipyridamole–thallium scintigraphy (DTS)

When there is a demand for increased coronary blood flow either by exercise or by injection of dipyridamole, the usual response of normal coronary arterioles is to dilate. When arterioles are diseased and are either stenosed or unable to dilate normally in response to these demands, blood flow is preferentially diverted away from the diseased arterial beds in favor of the normally responding coronary vascular beds. This phenomenon is known as coronary artery "*steal*" syndrome. Once the demand for increased coronary blood flow has ceased, the normal vessels constrict, returning blood flow once again to those areas supplied by the diseased vessels. This process is referred to as redistribution. These shifts in blood flow patterns can be monitored by the injection of radioactive tracers such as thallium-201. The shifts in the tracer molecules are then translated into a picture by the use of photon emission computed tomographic imaging techniques. Areas that *redistribute* after exercise or after dipyridamole-induced coronary vasodilation has ceased are identified as areas at risk of ischemia. Areas that never appear under scintigraphy are called *fixed defects* and, in essence, receive no detectable blood flow. These include areas that are essentially "dead" as the result of previous ischemic damage usually in the form of myocardial infarction.

The ability of DTS to be used as a tool for predicting perioperative adverse cardiac events is controversial. In one study,[96] 54% of known ischemic cardiac events occurred in those patients who did not show reversible defects on DTS. This study found both poor positive and negative predictive value with this technique. In another study,[97] there appeared to be an improved predictive correlation when the number of defects on DTS was taken into account. This implies that the predictive ability of the study increases as the number of defects that are detected by DTS increases. Another perceived disadvantage of this technique is the high cost. In the USA, the cost of this screening procedure per patient is of the order of $3000.

Dobutamine stress echocardiography

This test couples the ability of echocardiography to detect wall motion abnormalities with the effects of the β_1-agonist dobutamine, which increases myocardial oxygen demand. Any wall motion abnormalities elicited by ischemic areas of the myocardium can then be picked up by two-dimensional echocardiography. Sensitivity and specificity of this modality for detecting coronary artery disease varies widely between different studies. Sensitivity can range from 54% to 96% and specificity from 57% to 95% compared with the angiographic results.[98]

Coronary angiography

The Coronary Artery Surgery Study[88] concluded that left main or multivessel coronary artery disease correlates well with early and late mortality. Coronary artery disease that was amenable to surgery was present in 34% of those patients who had clinical evidence of coronary artery disease. Surgically amenable coronary lesions were also found in 14% of patients who had no clinical signs of coronary artery disease. The presence of significant coronary artery lesions does not mean that intervention is necessary. In many cases, adequate collateral blood flow will have been established.

RISK ASSESSMENT

In the process of performing a thorough history and physical examination together with all the indicated laboratory and special investigations, a patient profile is generated. Each patient will present with his or her own constellation of clinical findings.

Several risk factors have already been identified in the vascular surgery population. This implies that these factors appear often enough in this patient population to be associated with certain adverse outcomes. These factors are identified in Table 46.5. Risk factors for vascular surgery include angina pectoris,[57,58] previous myocardial infarction,[56,58] congestive heart failure,[1,57] diabetes mellitus,[58,59] ventricular ectopy and/or cardiac arrhythmias,[56,58] abnormal ECG,[56,57] and previous cerebrovascular accident.[56] In many cases, these findings will help to determine a patient's surgical risk for the procedure in question, and assist in intra- and postoperative management.

Table 46.5 *Risk factors for major vascular surgery*

Clinical assessment
Previous myocardial infarction
Angina pectoris
Silent myocardial ischemia
Congestive heart failure
Age > 70 years
Significant aortic valvular stenosis
Cardiac arrhythmias
Renal insufficiency or failure
Pulmonary insufficiency
Diabetes mellitus
Laboratory investigations
Abonormal ECG (at rest or during exercise)
Thallium redistribution on dipyridamole–thallium myocardial perfusion imaging
Radionuclide ejection fraction < 0.35
Elevated serum creatinine
Intraoperative (or procedure related)
Type of operation (i.e. major vascular surgery itself)
Intraoperative hypotension or shock
Intraoperative myocardial ischemia
Oliguric/anuric renal insufficiency

ANESTHESIA FOR SPECIFIC PROCEDURES

It will by now be recognized by the reader that anesthesia for vascular surgery is high risk because of the significant cardiac mortality even for elective surgery. Local anesthetic methods with the patient awake and general anesthetic techniques with spontaneous or controlled ventilation have all been employed for the various operations. Furthermore, all the different intravenous induction agents, analgesics, muscle relaxants, and volatile anesthetics have been used. As the advantages and disadvantages of the different techniques and drugs have been discussed in other chapters, what follows is a synopsis of the current anesthetic techniques that are most widely used in the UK and the USA for carotid artery and aortic surgery. What matters most is the way the various drugs are used rather than which drugs are chosen.

Carotid endarterectomy

Carotid endarterectomy (CEA) was first described in 1954 as a procedure for the prevention of ischemic stroke in a patient with atherosclerotic stenosis at the origin of the internal carotid artery.[99] The operation has since been performed 19–27 times more frequently in the USA than in the UK.[100] This huge difference is likely to decrease now that the benefits of the operation have been proved in the North American[101] and European[102] carotid artery surgery trials. The operation is superior to medical treatment for patients with TIA or stroke when there is greater than 70% internal carotid artery stenosis on the relevant side. This defect is the current indication for surgery.

Cerebral circulation

Anatomy

The brain is supplied with blood from the two internal carotid and two vertebral arteries, which anastomose at the base of the brain to form the circle of Willis. Minor extracranial to intracranial anastomoses via the ophthalmic, trigeminal, intrapetrosal, and intracavernous arteries also contribute to the cerebral blood supply. This collateral circulation of blood via the communicating arteries ensures that the cerebral hemispheres remain perfused despite a reduction of blood flow associated with an atherosclerotic plaque in one or both carotid arteries.

Pathophysiology

Cerebral blood flow (CBF) amounts to 50 mL per 100 g brain per min and accounts for 15% of the resting cardiac output. Cerebral oxygen consumption ($CMRo_2$) is 3–5 mL per 100 g of brain per min, being higher in the gray matter than in the white matter. Cerebral perfusion pressure (CPP) is determined by the difference between mean arterial pressure (MAP) and intracranial pressure (ICP). It is important to emphasize that up to two-thirds of patients undergoing CEA are hypertensive and therefore subject to loss of autoregulation during anesthesia, thereby further reducing a blood flow that is already reduced by plaque. Consequently, hypotensive episodes must be avoided at all times.

Cerebral blood flow is affected by two other factors which may change during anesthesia. The arterial Po_2 and Pco_2 have independent and profound effects. A reduction in P_ao_2 below 7 kPa (52.5 mmHg) causes a massive increase in CBF by vasodilation, whereas the CBF varies directly with the P_aco_2. Clinically, although hypoxia must be avoided for obvious reasons, so too must hypocapnia resulting from hyperventilation because this will also impair cerebral perfusion.

Surgical principles

The cutaneous incision is made along the anterior border of the sternomastoid muscle. Subcutaneous fat, the platysma muscle, and the facial vein are divided. The sternomastoid muscle is retracted laterally, and the internal jugular vein and vagus nerve are separated from the common carotid artery. The fascia around the carotid bifurcation is then dissected, avoiding damage to the hypoglossal nerve. Clamps are then placed on the external, internal, and common carotid arteries, thereby isolating the stenotic plaque from the circulation. An incision extending above and below the plaques is then made in the internal and common carotid arteries. The intimal plaque is then dissected, as are the plaques in the origin of the external carotid artery. The arteriotomy is then closed and the arteries unclamped following saline flushing to remove air and debris.[103] When the residual internal diameter of the internal carotid artery is 5 mm or less, many surgeons now perform a Dacron patch angioplasty to widen the artery.

Although the operation is intended to prevent future TIA and stroke, it may be complicated by stroke. This currently occurs in around 2% of operations. Of these strokes, 80% are mechanical and are due to plaque emboli arising from clamping procedures whereas the remaining 20% are hemodynamic and are due to inadequate cerebral blood flow while the carotid arteries are clamped.[104]

Carotid shunting

To minimize the likelihood of cerebral ischemia intraoperatively, some surgeons insert an intraluminal carotid shunt or bypass to maintain cerebral perfusion during the cross-clamping period. The decision to shunt is surgical and appears to be based on personal preference as there are no precisely defined criteria. Measurement of the stump pressure[105] (internal carotid artery back pressure when the external and common carotids are clamped) and the reduction in blood velocity in the middle cerebral artery (MCA) during cross-clamping measured by transcranial Doppler ultrasonography[106] have both been recommended, but the safe lower limits of pressure and blood velocity are not known.

Techniques of anesthesia

Because of the superficial location of the carotid bifurcation, CEA is a suitable operation for regional as well as general anesthetic techniques.

Regional anesthesia

Regional anesthesia by local infiltration or by superficial and deep cervical plexus block are methods favored by some surgeons. The major advantage claimed is a lower incidence of cerebral and myocardial complications (approximately 2% for each), but these do not appear to be significantly different from those occurring when general anesthesia is used.[107] Proponents of regional anesthesia claim a better ability to monitor the patient's neurological status. Some investigators have shown a reduction in both intensive care unit and general ward stays, thereby reducing overall cost.[108] The controversy over which anesthetic technique is superior for these procedures will undoubtedly continue. Until there are compelling data favoring one technique over another, the choice of technique is a matter of personal preference. History and the varieties of practice show that both methods when performed competently are more than satisfactory.

Disadvantages of regional techniques are, first, failure of the anesthetic block and, second, the need for prolonged immobility required of an elderly patient while the operation is performed. Because of this and the likely need for intravenous sedation, proponents of general anesthesia will espouse a greater degree of control over physiological variables. Although not previously popular in the UK, the use of regional anesthesia is increasing, just as it is in the USA. However, there are proponents of both anesthetic techniques (regional and general) in both countries. The use of regional anesthesia for CEA in the USA has grown significantly over the past decade.

General anesthesia

General anesthesia has the advantages that the patient is unaware of the procedure and is in the ideal position to facilitate surgery and it enables some degree of control over cardiovascular and respiratory variables. The major anesthetic considerations are summarized in Table 46.6.

Premedication Light sedation is desirable to decrease the likelihood of tachycardia and aggravated hypertension. Antisialogogue agents are not required with modern anesthetic agents. Sedation can be achieved with a short to medium duration benzodiazepine (e.g. midazolam or temazepam). Prolonged, deep central nervous system (CNS) depression should be avoided because this delays recovery and may make postoperative evaluation of CNS function difficult.

Induction With the patient awake, five-lead ECG and fingertip or earlobe oxygen saturation (S_ao_2) monitoring are attached. A five-lead ECG permits ST-segment monitoring (acute myocardial ischemia) in leads II and V_5. When this is not possible, a three-lead recording should be made using the CM_5 configuration.

Table 46.6 *Anesthetic considerations for carotid endarterectomy*

Preoperative	
Coexisting conditions	Hypertension Coronary artery disease TIAs and stroke
Cardiovascular drugs	Continue
Light premedication	
Perioperative	
Goals	Normotension Normocapnia Normovolemia Optimize cerebral perfusion Maintain high arterial Po_2
Monitoring	ECG (five lead) S_ao_2 BP (direct radial) End-tidal Pco_2 Transcranial Doppler ultrasonography
Complications	Hypotension (carotid sinus dissection) Hypertension (cross-clamping)
Postoperative	
Assessment of neurological function	Stroke
Blood pressure instability	Monitor and treat
Hemorrhage with hematoma	Airway obstruction

A crystalloid intravenous infusion is set up and a radial arterial cannula inserted following cutaneous anesthesia with lidocaine (lignocaine). If this proves technically very difficult, it can be deferred until after induction of anesthesia in order to reduce the patient's stress. In this situation, blood pressure should be measured temporarily with a noninvasive cuff method at frequent intervals (3 min).

Following preoxygenation, anesthesia is slowly induced with intravenous thiopentone, etomidate, or propofol. All these agents reduce $CMRO_2$ and therefore the demand for cerebral perfusion; thiopentone and propofol also reduce systemic blood pressure and must be administered with care, hence the merit of arterial cannulation before induction of anesthesia while the radial pulse is easily palpable.

Intubation of the trachea is essential to safeguard the airway and ensure adequate pulmonary gas exchange. Either depolarizing [succinylcholine (suxamethonium)] or nondepolarizing muscle relaxants may be used. Of the latter, the agents of choice are pancuronium, atracurium, and vecuronium. Pancuronium has the advantage of causing mild tachycardia, which antagonizes vagal stimulation which may occur during dissection of the carotid bifurcation. The other two drugs have no significant cardiovascular effects but need to be given in repeated doses because of their short duration of action. Venous engorgement during coughing and straining is a possibility when these drugs wear off unexpectedly.

The sympathetic stress response to laryngoscopy and intubation may be obtunded in four ways. First, intubation should proceed rapidly and smoothly only after full muscle relaxation is achieved. Second, the vocal cords and trachea may be sprayed with lidocaine. Intravenous lidocaine 2–3 min prior to intubation can also obtund the responses to laryngoscopy. Third, an intravenous opioid such as fentanyl or alfentanil may be administered. Fourth, a short-acting β-adrenoceptor blocker such as esmolol may be given intravenously.[109]

The tracheal tube selected (e.g. cuffed oral RAE) should be positioned to leave the mouth on the side opposite that of the operation and fixed in place using adhesive tape. Tying the tube in place would interfere with the surgical incision. The eyes should be protected in the usual way. The patient should then be positioned for surgery. This usually entails a small pad being placed between the shoulder blades to produce moderate cervical extension with the head facing away from the operation site. The operating table is adjusted to head-up tilt to optimize venous drainage and minimize venous pooling at the operation site.

Maintenance Anesthesia is maintained with a volatile agent using spontaneous or controlled ventilation. Spontaneous ventilation has a theoretical advantage that it provides both a continuous monitor of brainstem perfusion intraoperatively and moderate to high arterial $P\text{CO}_2$ tensions. Its disadvantage is the need for moderate to high concentrations of volatile agent, and therefore myocardial depression, for the duration of the surgery. It is a technique best reserved for procedures of short duration.

Volatile agents Controlled ventilation is the most widely used method with isoflurane or sevoflurane in an air–oxygen or oxygen nitrous oxide mixture. The volatile anesthetics, like the intravenous induction agents, all depress cerebral blood flow and $CMRO_2$, but isoflurane is the agent of choice because of its cerebral protective effects.[110,111] With isoflurane, cerebral ischemia develops only when cerebral blood flow reaches 10 mL per 100 g brain tissue per min compared with 15–18 mL min^{-1} with enflurane and 20 mL min^{-1} with halothane. Against this must be considered the coronary vasodilator effects of isoflurane, which are more potent than those of enflurane and halothane and may cause the coronary artery steal syndrome. However, this appears to be a theoretical problem and not clinically important.[112]

Ventilation is adjusted to achieve an end-tidal $P_{ET}\text{CO}_2$ of 4.5–5.5 kPa (34–41 mmHg). This ensures an arterial $P\text{CO}_2$ of 5–6 kPa (37–45 mmHg) when the alveolar–arterial $P\text{CO}_2$ difference is taken into account.

Intravenous analgesia is usually achieved with incremental fentanyl or an alfentanil infusion. The concentration of volatile agent may be reduced by using an analgesic, so that the cardiovascular hypotensive effects may be minimized.

A practical goal for the intraoperative management of blood pressure is to maintain the systolic pressure within ± 5.3 kPa (40 mmHg) of the preoperative values. This usually means keeping it between 16 and 26.7 kPa (120 and 200 mmHg).

Fluids Crystalloid intravenous fluids, avoiding dextrose-containing solutions except in diabetic patients, are administered at a moderate rate (100–200 mL h^{-1}) following an initial 500- to 1000-mL bolus to counteract preoperative dehydration. It is essential to be wary of fluid overload in these elderly patients, many of whom have decreased left ventricular compliance owing to hypertension or scarring from previous myocardial infarction. Dextrose-containing solutions should be avoided because hyperglycemia has been shown to aggravate ischemic brain damage.[113] Two liters of balanced crystalloid solution is usually sufficient fluid to be given intraoperatively.

Heparin Intravenous heparin is usually requested by the surgeon prior to cross-clamping the internal carotid artery. Up to 5000 units may be given. It is usual to allow the anticoagulant effect to decay spontaneously and not to use protamine for reversal.

Cerebral monitoring Although the adequacy of cerebral perfusion is uncertain intraoperatively and the safe lower limits of blood flow are not yet defined, it is usual for some form of cerebral function monitoring to be used. This is most valuable during carotid cross-clamping, which is when plaque embolization and resultant cerebral ischemia are most likely to occur. Cerebral blood flow has been assessed indirectly from global hemisphere function in the awake patient, and from stump pressure measurements in the unconscious patient. Other forms of monitoring that have been used are the electroencephalograph (EEG), somatosensory-evoked potentials (SSEP), transcranial Doppler ultrasonography (TCD), and, more recently, near infrared cerebral spectroscopy (NIRS).[114] The last provides a continuous display of cerebral oxygen saturation ($C\text{SO}_2$) and, when combined with TCD, gives simultaneous measurements of ipsilateral global blood flow [middle cerebral artery (MCA) blood velocity] and cerebral perfusion. Both of these methods are noninvasive, requiring only an ultrasound probe in a headband (TCD) and a flexible plate electrode (NIRS) to be attached to the skull. These techniques are used in the authors' hospital.

The principle of $C\text{SO}_2$ measurement is to beam light of wavelengths between 650 and 1100 nm from an emitting electrode through the skull into the brain. The light may be transmitted, absorbed, or reflected. The reflected light is detected by two detectors – one near and one more distant from the emitter. Light detected by the near detector represents light transmitted through the scalp and skull, whereas that detected by the far detector represents light transmitted through the scalp, skull, and brain (Fig. 46.5).

Subtraction of the near signal from the far signal gives a value for the brain which is normally between 65% and 75%. This value is lower than noncerebral tissue because about 70% of blood within the skull is venous. Typical signals for $C\text{SO}_2$ observed perioperatively are shown in Fig. 46.6. Carotid cross-clamping usually results in a fall in TCD peak blood flow velocity and $C\text{SO}_2$ because the ipsilateral hemisphere is entirely dependent on collateral blood flow. When the cross-clamp is removed following closure of the arteriotomy, the TCD peak velocity and $C\text{SO}_2$ signals increase owing to the large increase in blood flow resulting from the patent artery and reactive hyperemia.

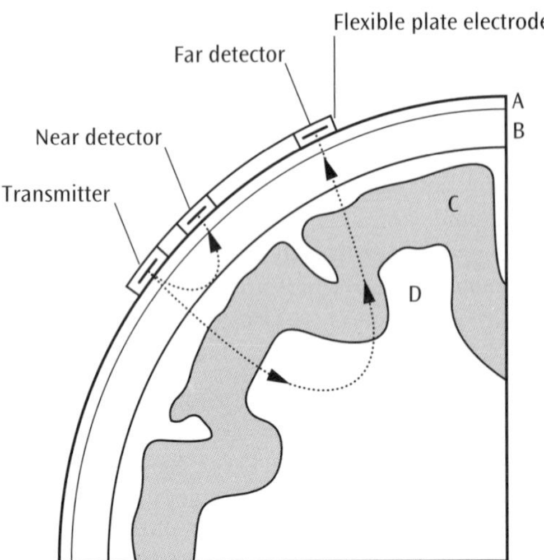

Figure 46.5 *The principle of near infrared cerebral spectroscopy. A flexible plate electrode is fixed to the scalp over the hemisphere to be monitored. Light between 650 and 1100 nm in wavelength is directed through the scalp (A), skull (B), gray matter (C), and white matter (D) from the transmitting electrode. Reflected light is detected by both near (A and B) and far (A, B, C, and D) electrodes, subtraction of the former from the latter providing a value for cerebral oxygen saturation (65–75%).*

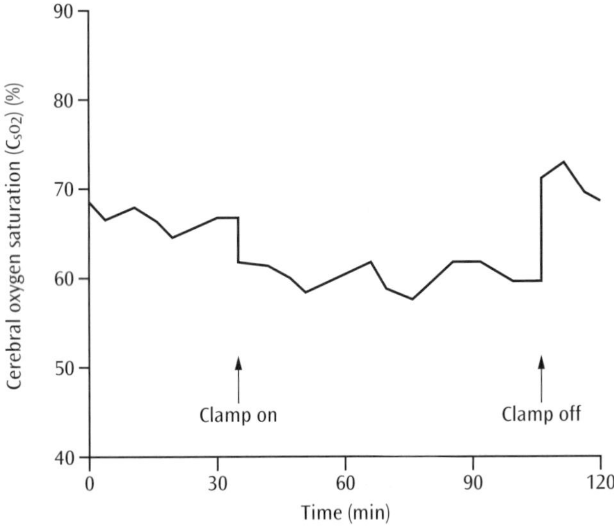

Figure 46.6 *Typical changes in cerebral oxygen saturation (Cso_2) during carotid endarterectomy in a patient with a poor collateral circulation. When the internal carotid artery is cross-clamped, Cso_2 falls by approximately 5% and remains unchanged during the endarterectomy procedure. Following unclamping, Cso_2 increases and exceeds precross-clamp values initially, indicating hyperemic reperfusion of the ischemic brain. In patients with a good collateral circulation, no significant change in Cso_2 is observed following application of the cross-clamp.*

Reversal and recovery Following skin closure, the muscle relaxants are reversed in the standard way and the patient is given 100% oxygen. Once spontaneous ventilation is established, the patient is transferred to the recovery room for postoperative ECG, S_aO_2, and radial arterial pressure monitoring for up to 2 h. When appropriate, the tracheal tube is removed after tracheal and oropharyngeal suction have been performed. A simple clinical assessment is made of the patient's neurological state by asking him to move each arm and leg in turn. Occasionally (1 patient in 50) an intraoperative stroke will have occurred, causing hemiplegia. This should be recorded in the clinical notes. Patients should be monitored for 24 h in a high-dependency area.

Postoperative pain is not a major concern because the surgery is superficial. Infiltration of the wound with long-acting local anesthetic (bupivacaine) followed by simple oral analgesics are usually sufficient.

Complications

Intraoperative

Intraoperative anesthetic complications are either hypotension or hypertension.

Hypotension Intraoperative hypotension may develop gradually or suddenly. Gradual hypotension usually results from the combined effects of hypovolemia and the vasodilator and cardiac depressant effects of volatile anesthetic agents. Sudden hypotension usually follows baroreceptor stimulation.

The baroreceptors are located in the carotid sinus in the wall of the internal carotid artery just above the bifurcation. During manipulation and dissection of this area, the carotid sinus nerve (a branch of the glossopharyngeal nerve) transmits impulses to the vasomotor center in the brainstem with resultant vagal efferent activity which causes vasodilation plus bradycardia. When this occurs, the surgeon should be asked to stop operating momentarily, the concentration of volatile anesthetic should be reduced and ephedrine (α- and β-adrenoceptor activity) given intravenously in 3-mg doses until the previous blood pressure reading is restored. If a continuous infusion of vasoconstrictor is required, dopamine, which is a mixed agonist, may be given in low dosage. At higher dosages, dopamine becomes predominantly an α-adrenergic agonist. Phenylephrine can also be used as a continuous infusion to maintain blood pressure. Its disadvantage is that it is virtually all α-adrenergic and therefore increases cardiac afterload and may cause vasoconstriction in all vascular beds including the coronary vascular bed. Other α-adrenoceptor agonists such as methoxamine or metaraminol may also be given. If bradycardia and hypotension persist, the carotid sinus nerve should be infiltrated with up to 3 mL of lidocaine. Surgery may proceed when the blood pressure has recovered.

Hypertension Apart from light anesthesia (empty vaporizer, etc.) hypertension may follow cross-clamping of the internal carotid artery.[115] Just as with hypotension, this is also presumed to be a baroreceptor-mediated reflex, but on occasion the absence of blood flow in the ipsilateral carotid artery causes vasoconstriction and inhibition of vagal activity via the brainstem. The systolic pressure may rise rapidly and reach 40 kPa (300 mmHg) within 5 min. Such a hypertensive response may be beneficial in terms of cerebral perfusion but is dangerous and life-threatening because of the cardiac complications. Increased afterload on the left ventricle and the high intraventricular pressure result in the conflicting conditions of increased myocardial demand for oxygen in the face of reduced myocardial perfusion. Profound myocardial ischemia is likely to occur (ST-segment depression), leading to subendocardial infarction. Prompt treatment is therefore essential. Immediate intravenous glyceryl trinitrate to augment subendocardial perfusion and offload the left ventricle is the initial treatment, followed by intravenous labetalol (combined α- and β-adrenoceptor blockade) given in 25-mg boluses until the pressure is controlled. The response to treatment is rapid and usually permanent.

Postoperative

Postoperative complications are either surgical or medical.

Surgical The principal surgical complications are hemorrhage with hematoma formation, and stroke. The hemorrhage may be acute, arising directly from a flaw in closure of the arteriotomy in the carotid artery, or subacute, arising from all the wound surface as may occur in patients taking aspirin preoperatively. If a substantial hematoma develops within the first hour postoperatively, the wound should be re-explored. Deviation and compression of the trachea with partial airway obstruction should be taken into account in planning induction of anesthesia.

Stroke should be considered in any patient who is hemiplegic or remains sleepy and uncoordinated 30 min after reversal of anesthesia (using the anesthetic technique described). Assessment of cerebral blood flow with TCD or carotid angiography should be considered. Re-exploration of the carotid artery may be necessary to exclude an intimal flap, stenosis, or kinking as a cause of the stroke.

Medical Derangement of blood pressure is common in the early postoperative period, affecting between 19% and 68% of all patients.[107] Hypertension [>26.7 kPa (200 mmHg)] is more common than hypotension [<16 kPa (120 mmHg)]. These disorders are attributed to resetting of the baroreceptors, which may take up to 6 months to return to normal.[116]

In the recovery room, specific treatment may need to be given once adequacy of analgesia and circulating volume are confirmed. Systolic pressures greater than 26.7 kPa (200 mmHg) usually settle spontaneously but may need to be reduced with hydralazine or sublingual nifedipine.

Low blood pressure, although less common, may need pharmacological treatment *having first excluded a myocardial cause*. Modest intravenous doses of a α-adrenoceptor agonist such as phenylephrine, metaraminol, or methoxamine may be used. Methoxamine is probably the drug of choice since an increased incidence of myocardial infarction has been observed with metaraminol,[117] and the duration of action of phenylephrine is very brief. The authors' practice is to avoid intravenous hypertensive drugs in the postoperative period, if possible, by ensuring minimal cerebral depression by use of light premedication and anesthetic agents that permit rapid recovery. Methoxamine has now been withdrawn from clinical use in the UK.

ABDOMINAL AORTIC RESECTION

Resection and grafting of the abdominal aorta is performed for the treatment of aneurysms and stenosing occlusive disease. These two conditions occur together in about 25% of patients.[118] The goals of surgery are avoidance of rupture and relief of symptoms with restoration and maintenance of blood flow to the viscera and legs.

The operation requires temporary cross-clamping of the aorta, which may cause indirect impairment of cardiac function owing to the potential massive increase in left ventricular afterload. Direct impairment of blood flow to the intestines and lower limbs causes ischemic reperfusion injury, the magnitude of which varies with the collateral circulation. Renal and spinal cord perfusion may also be impaired. These pathophysiological effects are severely exacerbated by the acute blood loss associated with aortic rupture.

In addition to enabling surgery to be performed, the goals of anesthesia are maintenance of cardiopulmonary function, preservation of renal and spinal cord perfusion, and minimizing the effects of ischemia–reperfusion injury during and following aortic cross-clamping.

Regional, general, and combined anesthetic techniques have all been employed successfully. A balanced general anesthetic with tracheal intubation, muscle relaxation, and controlled ventilation combined with postoperative epidural infusion analgesia is widely used and enables the anesthetic objectives to be met.

The goals are similar in emergency anesthesia for a ruptured aorta, but organ function is usually severely impaired owing to acute profound hypovolemia. Only a light general anesthetic technique is appropriate, with special emphasis on rapid correction of the intravascular volume deficit to minimize the tissue ischemia.

Indications for surgery

Aneurysms

The majority of abdominal aortic aneurysms are asymptomatic, the pulsatile swelling being detected only incidentally during abdominal examination, radiography, or ultrasonography. Symptomatic aneurysms manifest either as thromboembolic disease of the leg or severe pain and shock associated with rupture.

The natural history of an aneurysm is expansion at an average rate of 0.4 cm per annum with ultimate rupture. The mortality from rupture is 100% unless surgically treated.[119] In the UK, only 40–50% of all patients with a ruptured aorta reach hospital alive, and of those who undergo surgery the overall mortality may reach 75%.[120] Thus, the total survival rate of 10–15% for surgical repair of the ruptured aorta compares very unfavorably with the 90–95% survival following elective aortic repair. Surgery is therefore indicated to prevent inevitable rupture occurring.

Aneurysms are mostly fusiform or occasionally saccular in shape, and infrarenal in origin in about 90% of patients and juxtarenal or suprarenal in the remainder.[121] Preoperative definition of the upper and lower limits of the aneurysm is performed by computed tomographic scanning. The upper limit determines the location of aortic cross-clamp application, i.e. whether it is above or below the origin of the renal arteries, whereas the lower limit, which may involve the iliac arteries, determines whether a tube or bifurcation graft is required.

The indications for operating on patients with small asymptomatic aneurysms await clarification following large-scale ultrasound screening programmes.[122] Currently, most surgeons would offer surgery to patients with a 4.5-cm-diameter aneurysm because, when the ultrasound measurement error of ± 0.5 cm is taken into account, the aneurysm could be larger. Furthermore, since surgery will inevitably be required, the sooner it is performed, the lower the morbidity and mortality are likely to be because the coexisting cardiac, pulmonary, and renal disease will be less advanced.

Occlusive disease

Atherosclerotic occlusive disease of the aorta and its branches tends to be progressive and results from chronic exposure to the risk factors previously discussed. Unlike the majority of patients with aneurysms who are asymptomatic, all patients with occlusive disease have symptoms. Approximately two-thirds have intermittent claudication, and the other one-third have either ischemic rest pain or gangrene.[62] The other major differences from aneurysmal disease are (1) the peak incidence of surgery which is performed in patients 10 years younger, (2) a decreased incidence of coexisting disease (because the patients are younger), and (3) a decreased requirement for blood transfusion.[123] Otherwise, the two groups are similar, with myocardial infarction being the major perioperative complication.

Abdominal and lower limb circulation

The intestines and lower limbs are supplied with blood from the abdominal aorta, which is a tapering, smooth-walled tube extending from the aortic hiatus in the diaphragm to the bifurcation into the left and right common iliac arteries (segmental level L4). Each common iliac artery divides into internal and external iliac arteries anterior to the upper end of the sacroiliac joint. The internal iliac supplies the pelvic organs, perineum, and buttocks, whereas the external iliac runs round the pelvic brim and, after emerging under the inguinal ligament, becomes the common femoral artery which supplies the leg.

The blood supply of the intestines follows the embryological origins of the fore-, mid-, and hindgut. The foregut, comprising the stomach and duodenum as far as the entry of the bile duct, is supplied from the celiac artery (T12). The midgut, comprising the duodenum, ileum, and ascending and transverse colon as far as the splenic flexure, is supplied from the superior mesenteric artery (L1), whereas the hindgut, comprising the descending and sigmoid colon and first part of the rectum, is supplied by the inferior mesenteric artery (L3). There are anastomoses between the branches of these arteries which maintain continuity of blood supply to the intestinal mucosa when blood flow is compromised. This is especially significant for the hindgut because the inferior mesenteric artery is invariably totally or partially occluded in both aneurysmal and occlusive disease.

The renal arteries (L2) supplying the kidneys are the largest branches of the abdominal aorta (25% cardiac output). Other branches of significance in vascular disease are the four pairs of lumbar arteries that supply the back and anterior abdominal wall plus the anterior spinal artery (artery of Adamkiewicz), which is a small branch of an intercostal or lumbar artery which may originate anywhere between T8 and L2.[124]

Awareness of the origin of these various arteries from the aorta enables the anesthesiologist to consider the ischemic consequences of aortic cross-clamping and to plan to minimize the effects. For example, suprarenal cross-clamp application renders not only the kidneys ischemic but also most of the intestines in addition to the legs. This is a far greater pathophysiological insult than infrarenal aortic cross-clamping, in which only the legs may be ischemic.

Surgical principles

Successful repair of an abdominal aortic aneurysm using preserved human artery (homograft) was first described in 1952[125] and subsequently in the same year using a textile prosthesis.[126] Currently available prostheses are made either from knitted or woven Dacron or polytetrafluoroethylene (PTFE).

The abdominal aorta is retroperitoneal and is most often approached through the peritoneal cavity via either a vertical midline or transverse supraumbilical incision. The transperitoneal approach is favored by most surgeons because it facilitates access to the aorta and its branches in addition to the abdominal organs. The disadvantages of this technique are (1) the severe postoperative pain which may limit chest movement and lung expansion, (2) the loss of heat and fluid from the intestines, and (3) the paralytic ileus which may persist for several days. To minimize these complications, which contribute significantly to the postoperative morbidity of the operation, a retroperitoneal approach is used by some surgeons.[127]

The abdominal contents are thoroughly explored, following which the transverse colon, greater omentum, and small intestine are lifted superiorly and placed outside the abdomen between moist packs.[128] The posterior peritoneum is incised and dissected to expose the aorta from the left renal vein superiorly to the common iliac arteries inferiorly. Dissection near the aneurysm is kept to a minimum to prevent bleeding.

Systemic heparin (5000–10 000 units) is given to prevent distal thrombus formation during the cross-clamp period. Vascular clamps are then applied, first to both common iliac arteries to prevent embolization of thrombus and debris into the legs, and then to the aorta, which is incised longitudinally. All atherosclerotic debris and thrombus are removed from the aortic lumen and the paired ostia of the lumbar arteries is oversewn. The inferior mesenteric artery is dealt with similarly if it is still patent.

The chosen graft is sutured into the infrarenal aorta at its proximal end and the anastomosis tested by brief unclamping of the aorta. If necessary, repairs are made to the suture line. The distal anastomosis is then sutured (aorta–tube graft or iliac arteries–bifurcation graft) and, before completion, the distal vascular clamps are released to permit backbleeding and the vessel is flushed to remove any residual intraluminal debris. Restoration of blood flow to the lower limbs should be permitted to occur in a controlled fashion one leg at a time, to minimize unclamping hypotension. The original aortic wall is then wrapped round the graft and sutured, the peritoneum is closed, the intestines are returned to the abdominal cavity, and the abdominal wall is repaired.[129]

Anesthetic technique

The anesthetic technique is similar for all types of abdominal aortic disease. A controlled airway with tracheal intubation and ventilation is essential because of the huge abdominal incision. This may be supplemented with epidural analgesia, which is especially advantageous postoperatively. A regional anesthetic technique alone is inappropriate for such major body cavity surgery.

The choice to include regional anesthesia as part of the anesthetic plan may offer some advantages. With respect to perioperative cardiac morbidity and mortality, the response to surgery is thought to include sympathetic nervous system activation through which either coronary vasoconstriction or the impedance of coronary blood flow via a hypercoagulable state may occur.[130–133] Regional anesthesia may play a role in blunting sympathetic outflow and therefore reduce cardiac morbidity. In some investigations, the combination of thoracic epidural anesthesia with general anesthesia is thought to reduce the hemodynamic correlates of myocardial oxygen consumption,[134] improve intraoperative hemodynamic stability,[135] and reduce postoperative cardiac morbidity and mortality especially when epidural analgesia is extended well into the postoperative period. Using epidural anesthesia as a component of the anesthetic plan in these patients has also been correlated with reduced postoperative pulmonary complications.[136,137] Any advantages of using regional anesthesia to reduce perioperative morbidity and mortality are most significant for patient populations in which high-risk patients present for major surgery.[138]

Surgical anesthesia

Premedication Anxiolytic premedication is desirable to minimize the release of endogenous catecholamines and decrease sympathetic nervous system stimulation that result from stress in the preoperative period. Oral benzodiazepines (temazepam, diazepam, or lorazepam) given 60–90 min preoperatively are effective in maintaining stable cardiovascular conditions. Another approach is to include either α- or β-adrenoceptor blockade with the premedication using drugs such as clonidine[139] or atenolol.[67] These drugs blunt the heart rate and hypertensive responses to the emotional stress of waiting for surgery and the physical stress of induction of anesthesia. Beta-blockers have the additional benefit of significantly reducing postoperative mortality.[67]

Monitoring Cardiorespiratory monitoring must be established prior to induction of anesthesia. This includes EGG (five-lead for ST-segment monitoring), peripheral S_aO_2, and direct measurement of blood pressure through a radial arterial cannula. A peripheral intravenous infusion of crystalloid is started. It is convenient if both arterial and venous cannulae are placed in the same arm to facilitate connections with the monitoring equipment. In the mid- to late 1980s, it was the common practice to place both the arterial cannulae and a pulmonary artery catheter in almost all patients, especially those with known coronary artery disease and/or left ventricular dysfunction. Over the past decade, there has been a change, limiting the use of pulmonary artery catheters to those patients who present with most limited cardiac reserve. Usually, this invasive monitoring is delayed until after induction of anesthesia. Certainly, in the case of the isolated infrarenal aneurysm with no other clinical indication of disease elsewhere, the placement of invasive monitoring can be delayed until induction of anesthesia without compromising hemodynamic control.

Induction and maintenance Preoxygenation is performed for 3–5 min, after which anesthesia is induced intravenously. The choice of induction agent is less critical than the way in which the drug is administered. The goal is to prevent hypotension followed by tachycardia and hypertension during laryngoscopy and intubation. Etomidate, thiopentone, and propofol are equally suitable provided that they are given slowly to minimize cardiovascular changes. Fentanyl is the most widely used analgesic, given as an initial bolus to minimize the stress response to intubation, with further increments to minimize the responses to skin incision and aortic cross-clamping.

As with carotid artery surgery, either depolarizing (succinylcholine) or nondepolarizing (pancuronium, atracurium, or vecuronium) muscle relaxants may be used to facilitate tracheal intubation. Pancuronium has the advantage that a single dose may provide muscle relaxation for the duration of the operation whereas atracurium and vecuronium, which have a more brief duration of action, are suitable for a total intravenous anesthetic technique (TIVA). When considering pancuronium, it should be remembered that renal excretion is part of its pharmacodynamics. TIVA may be used for those patients with pre-existing renal insufficiency (elevated blood urea and creatinine) or with intraoperative signs of developing renal failure (oliguria or anuria). TIVA using a combination of the shorter-acting agents propofol, atracurium, alfentanil, or remifemtamil avoids the need to use a volatile anesthetic agent to maintain anesthesia. When a volatile anesthetic is required, isoflurane or sevflurane appears to be the agent of choice. Although it is a more potent coronary artery vasodilator than either halothane or enflurane and causes a greater incidence of coronary artery steal syndrome, as demonstrated in laboratory animals,[112] the incidence of myocardial ischemia in patients is no higher with isoflurane than with the other options.[140] Furthermore, this volatile agent provides the greatest cerebral protection (as previously discussed) and causes far less impairment of renal function than halothane during aortic cross-clamping.[141]

After intubation and the placement of a nasogastric tube, the lungs are ventilated with an air–oxygen or oxygen–nitrous oxide mixture. The former mixture is preferable to the latter as there is no intestinal distention, which facilitates wound closure for the surgeon. Ventilation is adjusted to achieve normal values of arterial $P\text{CO}_2$ for each patient (usually 5.0–5.5 kPa; 37.5–41.3 mmHg), allowing for the alveolar–arterial $P\text{CO}_2$ difference. Maintenance of normocapnia throughout the operation contributes to the global cardiovascular stability. End-tidal $P\text{CO}_2$ monitoring is continued throughout the operation with this objective in mind.

After the patient is anesthetized, central venous pressure (CVP) monitoring is established. A useful technique is to insert a large-bore (8.5 French gauge) percutaneous sheath in the right internal jugular (RIJ) vein. Identification of the vein is facilitated by the rapid infusion of crystalloid and tilting the patient 20–30° head down. Using a wide-bore sheath permits use of this alone for CVP monitoring and the rapid infusion of fluids, or it enables a triple-lumen catheter or pulmonary artery flotation catheter (PAFC) to be inserted at any time. Use of a portable ultrasound scanning device further facilitates identification of the RIJ. This vein is absent in 2.5% of the population. A PAFC is indicated when the ejection fraction is less than 30% or there is any major disorder of myocardial function detected on preoperative echocardiography.

At some stage, a lumbar epidural catheter is inserted and taped into position. In the USA, the more common practice is for epidural placement to take place prior to induction so that the patient can relate any paresthesiae that might occur. This practice is becoming more common in the UK, although some anesthesiologists still insert the epidural in the unconscious patient. Placing the epidural preinduction also has the advantage that the effect of a test dose [lidocaine 5% with epinephrine (adrenaline)] may be assessed. This helps to rule out intrathecal placement. Placement of the catheter at this stage ensures that any bleeding will have stopped before heparinization. There is no advantage in thoracic epidural catheter placement over lumbar when only epidural opioids are used in the case of infraumbilical surgery.[142] However, there are advantages in placing a thoracic epidural as opposed to a lumbar epidural when a local anesthetic agent is used, either alone or in combination with opioids.

In the USA, the decision to proceed with surgery in spite of the occurrence of a "bloody" tap in the process of epidural placement remains controversial. Practice varies from canceling the case for up to 24 h to going ahead with the operation and maintaining a high index of suspicion concerning the possibility of epidural hematoma.

A member of the surgical team catheterizes the bladder at this stage. The hourly urine production can then be monitored. Surgery proceeds as outlined previously. The interval up to aortic cross-clamping provides the anesthetic team with plenty of time to establish and control the normal values of cardiorespiratory variables for the patient. When a PAFC is used, measurements of pulmonary artery occlusion pressure (PAOP) and cardiac output (CO) are made and the derived variables of cardiac index (CI) and systemic vascular resistance (SVR) calculated. The relation of CVP to PAOP is observed and recorded since there is a poor correlation between the two when one ventricle is diseased and the other is not.[143] Arterial blood gases should be measured to enable pulmonary gas exchange to be optimized.

Body temperature Core temperature is measured either by the thermistor on a PAFC or by an esophageal temperature probe. Because the operation involves a large abdominal incision with evisceration of the intestines, the core temperature may decline by up to 3–4 °C.

Heat loss by conduction and radiation is reduced by ensuring that the operating room temperature is kept at 20 °C minimum and the patient is lying on a heated mattress. In the USA and UK, more centers are favoring the use of forced-air warming devices that involve covering exposed areas of the patient with warmed air mattresses that are constantly exchanging large volumes of warmed air. All intravenous fluids are also heated. Loss of heat from the patient's head can be minimized by enclosing it in a heat-reflective cap. Heat loss by evaporation is minimized by thorough wrapping of the intestines in moist gauze packs and use of a condenser humidifier in the patient's airway. If the patient is cold at the end of the operation, this may be an indication for postoperative ventilation to permit normal body temperature to recover gradually. This ensures that there are no sudden massive increases in oxygen consumption due to shivering, and minimal risk of hypoxia which may aggravate myocardial ischemia.

Circulating volume Adequacy of circulating volume is judged from measurements of the CVP and PAOP. The values of these measurements are similar in a healthy heart, but are often different in patients undergoing aortic surgery because two-thirds have significant coronary artery disease. Previous myocardial infarction, which affects 50% of patients, results in some degree of ventricular wall scarring and higher values of PAOP than CVP, hence the importance of monitoring both pressures. By using PAOP as the guide to filling pressures, hydrostatic pulmonary edema is likely to be prevented if PAOP is kept below 2.4 kPa (18 mmHg). Suitable intraoperative goals for PAOP and CVP are 2 kPa (15 mmHg) and 1.3 kPa (10 mmHg) respectively. In the absence of the facility to measure PAOP, the CVP should be maintained between 0.67 kPa (5 mmHg) and 1.3 kPa (10 mmHg) throughout the operation to ensure near optimal ventricular function with no significant risk of pulmonary edema developing.

Fluid and blood losses are large compared with abdominal surgery. Extracellular fluid is lost by evaporation, sequestration into the lumen of the intestines, and the development of interstitial edema (third-space effect) due to handling and mobilization of a large mass of tissue. These losses, which are superimposed on preoperative dehydration and relative hypovolemia as a result of the vasodilation caused by anesthetic agents (propofol or isoflurane), should be replaced with a continuous infusion of a balanced electrolyte solution (Hartmann's solution, UK; Ringer's lactate, USA). The infusion rate ranges from 6 to 16 $mL\,kg^{-1}\,h^{-1}$ (average about 10 $mL\,kg^{-1}\,h^{-1}$) to maintain a stable circulation and prevent oliguria.[60] Some 3–6 L of crystalloid may thus be required in the perioperative period, and occasionally more.

Blood loss averages 2.15 ± 1.15 L during aneurysm surgery, with an average transfusion requirement of 4.5 ± 2.4 units of blood.[60] However, blood transfusion with homologous blood is potentially dangerous. In the past, up to 10% of patients have experienced either immunological red and white cell incompatibility or infectious – hepatitis B or C or human immunodeficiency virus (HIV) – complications. In recent years, routine screening of blood products for these infectious agents has reduced this possibility greatly. In many institutions, homologous blood transfusions are now avoided unless necessary.

Until recently, it has been customary to transfuse blood when the loss exceeds 20% of the predicted circulating blood volume, but there is no evidence to support a single criterion for transfusion. Although no major complications appear to result when the hemoglobin concentration is allowed to fall to 7 $g\,dL^{-1}$, it is recommended to aim for 10 $g\,dL^{-1}$ in patients with CAD.[144]

The hazards of blood transfusion can be avoided by meticulous surgical techniques and the use of autologous blood, and minimized by using as little homologous blood as necessary. Autologous blood can be removed from the patient preoperatively (predonation) or intraoperatively (normovolemic hemodilution). When combined with intraoperative red cell autotransfusion, homologous transfusion is avoided in around two-thirds of patients.

Cardiovascular stability

Cardiovascular stability is achieved by minimizing heat loss, maintaining normocapnia and adequate volume loading [CVP of 1.3 kPa (10 mmHg)], and ensuring an appropriate depth of anesthesia in relation to surgical stimulation (e.g. deepening anesthesia prior to skin incision). Major disturbances in the circulation may arise at three points in the operation: in association with placement of intra-abdominal retraction and clamping and unclamping of the aorta.

Abdominal retraction

Removal of the intestines from the abdominal cavity followed by placement of large retractors to enable the aorta to be exposed may result in mechanical obstruction of venous return via the inferior vena cava. If hypotension develops rapidly in association with a low CVP, the retractors should be repositioned to correct the disturbance.

Another cause of hypotension in association with sudden tachycardia and facial flushing is the mesenteric traction syndrome described by Selzer *et al.*[145] in 1985. This syndrome occurs following mesenteric traction, lasts less than 30 min, and is associated with an increased plasma prostacyclin concentration. Prostacyclin is a prostaglandin derived from arachidonic acid in vascular endothelium. It may be synthesized in response to intestinal ischemia resulting from displacement of the intestines from the abdominal cavity. When cyclo-oxygenase, an enzyme involved in the synthesis of prostacyclin, is inhibited by preoperative treatment with either aspirin[146] or ibuprofen[147] the syndrome does not occur.

Aortic cross-clamping

The consequences of cross-clamping are similar regardless of the level at which the aorta is occluded, but the magnitudes of the changes are greater the higher the level. Infrarenal cross-clamping is the norm (90% of patients), with mechanical effects on the circulation and ischemic consequences for the pelvis and lower limbs.

The circulatory effects result from the abrupt increase in left ventricular afterload, which leads to increased PAOP, SVR, and mean arterial pressure with decreases in cardiac output and preload. When coronary artery disease is present, these changes may result in the occurrence of subendocardial ischemia (ST-segment depression) and arrhythmias.[61] These complications may need rapid intravenous treatment with coronary vasodilators such as GTN.

The ischemic consequences for the pelvis and lower limb result from the interruption to the arterial blood supply, which renders the tissues ischemic during the cross-clamping period. Anaerobic metabolism occurs with accumulation of lactic acid initially and subsequent production of reactive oxygen species, as outlined previously. In patients with a well-developed collateral circulation via the abdominal wall and back, ischemia may be minimal. A good collateral circulation is more likely in patients with occlusive disease.[148]

Suprarenal and supraceliac cross-clamping impose a much greater afterload on the left ventricle, resulting in cardiovascular changes of greater magnitude. A continuous intravenous infusion of vasodilator such as GTN or nitroprusside may be required to control blood pressure. The kidneys are rendered ischemic and so too are the intestines, which appear to be especially sensitive to deprivation of their blood supply. For example, in laboratory animals, superficial mucosal acidosis from anaerobic metabolism develops within minutes of occlusion of the mesenteric artery.[149] Disruption of the mucosal barrier has been proposed as the mechanism for development of septicemia with intestinal organisms and death from multiple organ failure following abdominal aortic surgery.[150]

Aortic unclamping

Aortic unclamping results in restoration of blood flow to the ischemic tissues and vasodilated blood vessels of the lower torso. The cardiovascular changes are broadly the opposite of those occurring during cross-clamping. Thus, the blood pressure and SVR decrease (unclamping shock). The cardiac output, however, may decrease further owing to decreased preload from pooling of blood in the hyperemic lower extremities before returning to previous levels. There may also be acute blood loss from the graft anastomosis site.

Unclamping shock is usually of short duration (< 10 min) and its magnitude can be reduced in several ways. First, the surgeon can release the clamp slowly (over 2–3 min), thereby minimizing the rate at which the stagnant blood in the lower torso is washed into the trunk. Second, when a bifurcation graft is used, blood flow can be restored to one leg at a time, again reducing the rate at which acidic blood mixes with the circulation. Third, the anesthesiologist can prepare for unclamping by stopping any infusion of vasodilator and reducing the concentration of volatile anesthetic agent 5–10 min before the anticipated release of the clamp. Simultaneously with these maneuvers, if the ventricular preload (CVP or PAOP) has not been rigorously maintained at the values suggested, it is raised rapidly by 0.67 kPa (5 mmHg) or so by rapid infusion of fluid. These measures, when applied together, will usually minimize the complications of unclamping.

Renal and spinal cord perfusion

Renal Renal function is impaired preoperatively in about 10% of patients and this may be aggravated by hypovolemia and hypotension intraoperatively. Despite infrarenal application of the aortic cross-clamp, renal blood flow may be reduced by about 40% with an increase of up to 75% in renal vascular resistance which is not affected by sympathetic blockade.[151] The reduction in blood flow reduces the glomerular filtration rate and urine formation. The mechanism for the reduction in blood flow is uncertain but may be related in part to the reduction in cardiac output during cross-clamping and possibly also a humoral mechanism because concentrations of renin are increased following cross-clamping.

Provided that cardiovascular function is optimized with maintenance of cardiac filling pressure, renal function is usually adequately maintained with the production of 40–60 mL h^{-1} of urine. Some authorities consider that pharmacological support of the kidney is essential and routinely administer intravenous mannitol (25–50 g), furosemide, or dopamine by infusion (1–3 μg kg^{-1} h^{-1}).

Mannitol acts in two ways. First, as an osmotic diuretic it is a renal vasodilator and promotes renal tubular urine flow, and, second, it is a hydroxyl radical scavenger and thereby lessens the effects of ischemia–reperfusion injury. To be most effective, the mannitol must be administered before the ischemic episode.[152] Mannitol is essential whenever one or both kidneys are likely to be ischemic, as in suprarenal cross-clamping. Furosemide is also a renal vasodilator that may be used to augment urine flow.

Dopamine is very effective in increasing sodium, potassium, urine output, and creatinine clearance during cross-clamping.[153] Its use may be considered when renal impairment already exists.

Spinal cord Complete flaccid paraplegia may follow aortic cross-clamping. It is attributed to spinal cord ischemia due to interruption of flow in the anterior spinal artery; the segmental origin of this is not known to the surgeon before the clamp is applied.

The incidence of paraplegia is about 0.25% in patients undergoing elective abdominal aneurysm surgery and about 2.5% when the aorta has ruptured. The incidence is also higher during surgery on thoracic and thoracoabdominal aneurysms because of the higher segmental level of cross-clamp application.[154] Various methods have been utilized with varying success to reduce the incidence of paraplegia from spinal cord ischemia. This is especially true in the case of thoracoabdominal procedures. These methods include spinal cord cooling, hypothermia, aortic and left-heart bypass with retrograde perfusion, and lumbar intrathecal drainage. The success or failure of each one of these techniques is a subject of ongoing debate.

Ischemia–reperfusion injury

Primary ischemic injury occurs in the muscles of the pelvis and lower limbs during infrarenal aortic cross-clamping, with the addition of the kidneys and intestines during suprarenal cross-clamping. The same sites are also exposed to reperfusion injury, which follows restoration of blood flow together with systemic reperfusion injury in the lungs in particular.

Advances in the management of patients undergoing surgery for advanced atherosclerotic disease are likely to occur through attempts to minimize by pharmacologic blockade the toxic effects of oxygen-derived free radicals. The role of mannitol in the prevention of ischemic reperfusion injury of the kidney has already been discussed. The same drug in doses of 0.2 g kg^{-1} just before cross-clamp application also limits the acute lung injury and pulmonary edema which follow aortic unclamping.[155,156] The systemic effects of reperfusion injury are much more severe following aortic rupture. Therefore, mannitol should be administered to every patient undergoing aortic surgery and should always be given before the onset of ischemia to be most effective. Allopurinol, which inhibits the action of xanthine oxidase, has been studied in animals. Treatment of rabbits prior to hindlimb ischemia reduced the skeletal muscle reperfusion injury.[157]

POSTOPERATIVE MANAGEMENT

The goals of postoperative management are similar to those pertaining intraoperatively. Good analgesia is essential to enable adequate pulmonary ventilation to occur, and this can be better achieved with epidural infusion analgesia using a combination of dilute local anesthetic and opioid than intramuscular or intravenous opioids alone.[142]

Maintenance of adequate circulating volume must be continued to optimize cardiac output and mean arterial pressure, and this requires continued monitoring of CVP ± PAOP for approximately 24 h. A postoperative ileus will be present in most patients, which prevents oral fluid intake usually until the second postoperative day.

Cardiovascular stability is achieved by attention to pulmonary gas exchange, body temperature, pain relief, and adequate circulating volume. Renal function is monitored by observation of the hourly urine output and creatinine clearance.

All these objectives can be met only if the patient is transferred postoperatively to a high-dependency or intensive care unit where cardiorespiratory monitoring and intensive nursing care can be given. Many patients are suitable for reversal of anesthesia and extubation at the end of surgery. However, when the operation is complicated or prolonged, postoperative ventilation should be considered and carried out until complete physiological stability has been achieved. Only then is extubation performed. By following these guidelines the potential cardiac,[158] pulmonary,[159] and renal[160] complications can be prevented or minimized.

Ruptured aortic aneurysm

Leakage or rupture of an abdominal aortic aneurysm is fatal unless surgical treatment is attempted. Rupture is retroperitoneal in 75% of patients and intraperitoneal in the remainder.[161] The latter is associated with more severe hypotension from blood loss because of the lack of tamponade effect which contains the hemorrhage when it is retroperitoneal. The outcome of surgery is determined by the interval between the onset of symptoms (abdominal or back pain plus collapse due to shock) and control of the hemorrhage by cross-clamping, plus the severity of the patient's coexisting cardiac, pulmonary, and renal disease.

The goal of hospital management is resuscitation, rapid diagnosis, immediate laparotomy, and control of the hemorrhage. All patients need massive volume replacement using crystalloids and colloids initially while a minimum of 10 blood group-specific units of blood are cross-matched. Time should not be wasted on elaborate laboratory investigations in any patient with shock, back pain, and a pulsatile abdominal mass. The principles of anesthetic management are dealing with the exaggerated cardiovascular responses to induction of anesthesia, skin incision, cross-clamping and unclamping, plus the major blood loss. The major anesthetic considerations are summarized in Table 46.7.

Anesthesia must be induced in the operating room with the surgeon ready to make the incision. Two wide-bore intravenous infusions are established, the ECG and peripheral $S_{a}O_2$ are monitored, and the blood pressure is measured by a noninvasive cuff. Two or more anesthesiologists are essential. The patient is given 100% oxygen while basic

Table 46.7 *Anesthetic considerations in ruptured aortic aneurysm*

Preoperative
Coexisting cardiac, pulmonary, and renal disease
Pain and shock
Fluid resuscitation – two large-bore intravenous cannulae
Mannitol

Intraoperative
Preoxygenation – monitor ECG, $S_{a}O_2$, noninvasive BP
Rapid-sequence induction
Light anesthesia
Cross-clamping hypertension – vasodilators
Unclamping hypotension – vasopressors
Massive blood transfusion – coagulopathy

Postoperative
Ventilate until physiologically stable
Death
  Early – cardiac failure
  Late – multiple organ failure (ischemia–reperfusion injury)

monitoring is established, following which anesthesia is induced with a rapid-sequence induction technique using drugs such as etomidate and succinylcholine. Once the trachea is intubated, surgery may begin. Anesthesia is continued with ventilation of the lungs using 100% oxygen, intravenous opioid, and a muscle relaxant such as atracurium until the patient's response to stress indicates the need for deeper anesthesia, when a volatile agent such as isoflurane may be added. Mannitol is given (50 g) intravenously in an attempt to minimize the systemic ischemia–reperfusion injury and augment urine production. A dopamine infusion is set up in an attempt to preserve renal function.

The main complication following induction is undue hypotension, which may be resistant to fluid and blood administration. Muscle relaxation and opening of the abdomen may also contribute to the hypotension by removal of the tamponade which has previously contained the hemorrhage. Once the aorta is cross-clamped, undue hypertension may be the next complication necessitating deepening of anesthesia and a GTN infusion. When the primary hemorrhage is surgically controlled, the anesthetic team can concentrate on establishing arterial, CVP, and PAOP monitoring to attempt to optimize cardiac filling pressures, cardiac output, and renal perfusion.

Anesthesia and surgery then proceed in accordance with the descriptions given for an elective operation. During the operation a massive blood transfusion may be required and may also be associated with a dilutional coagulopathy. This is treated with fresh-frozen plasma and platelets based on the results of laboratory tests. The final intraoperative problem is persistent unclamping hypotension, which may occur despite adequate cardiac filling pressures. In this situation, intravenous vasopressors, either as a single dose (metaraminol) or by infusion (norepinephrine or phenylephrine), are administered.

Postoperatively, the patient is ventilated in intensive care until physiological stabilization is achieved and then extubation is attempted. Epidural analgesia is inappropriate because of the likely coagulation disorder. Analgesia is therefore administered using traditional techniques. Of the patients who survive surgery, there are very few who do not have major complications affecting the heart, lungs, or kidney, resulting from precross-clamp ischemia (shock) and postcross-clamp reperfusion injury. Cardiac ischemia is the usual cause of perioperative death whereas multiple organ dysfunction syndrome is the usual cause of late death.

REFERENCES

1. Gersh BJ, Rihal CS, Rooke TW, Ballard DJ. Evaluation and management of patients with both peripheral vascular and coronary artery disease. *J Am Coll Cardiol* 1991; **18:** 203–14.
2. Mangano DT. Perioperative cardiac morbidity. *Anesthesiology* 1990; **72:** 153–84.
3. Hiatt WR, Cooke JP. Atherogenesis and the medical management of atherosclerosis. In: Rutherford RB (ed.). *Vascular Surgery*, 5th edn. Philadelphia: WB Saunders, 2000: 333.
4. Criqui MH, Fronek A, Barrett-Connor E, *et al.* The prevalence of peripheral arterial disease in a defined population. *Circulation* 1985; **71:** 510–15.
5. Hiatt WR, Hoag S, Hamman RF. Effect of diagnostic criteria on the prevalence of peripheral arterial disease. The San Luis Valley Diabetes Study. *Circulation* 1995; **91:** 1472–9.
6. Criqui MH, Langer RD, Fronek A, *et al.* Mortality over a period of 10 years in patients with peripheral arterial disease. *N Engl J Med* 1992; **326:** 381–6.
7. Leng GC, Fowkes FG, Lee AJ, *et al.* Use of ankle brachial pressure index to predict cardiovascular events and death: a cohort study [comment]. *Br Med J* 1996; **313:** 1440–4.
8. Leng GC, Lee AJ, Fowkes FG, *et al.* Incidence, natural history and cardiovascular events in symptomatic and asymptomatic peripheral arterial disease in the general population. *Int J Epidemiol* 1996; **25:** 1172–81.
9. Newman AB, Tyrrell KS, Kuller LH. Mortality over four years in SHEP participants with a low ankle–arm index. *J Am Geriatr Soc* 1997; **45:** 1472–8.
10. Vogt MT, Cauley JA, Newman AB, *et al.* Decreased ankle/arm blood pressure index and mortality in elderly women. *JAMA* 1993; **270:** 465–9.
11. Vogt MT, Cauley JA, Kuller LH, Hulley SB. Prevalence and correlates of lower extremity arterial disease in elderly women. *Am J Epidemiol* 1993; **137:** 558–68.
12. Murabito JM, D'Agostino RB, Silbershatz H, Wilson WF. Intermittent ckaudication. A risk profile from The Framingham Heart Study. *Circulation* 1997; 96: 44–9.
13. Johansson J, Egberg N, Johnsson H, Carlson LA. Serum lipoproteins and hemostatic function in intermittent claudication. *Arterioscler Thromb* 1993; **13:** 1441–8.
14. Safar ME, Laurent S, Asmar RE, *et al.* Systolic hypertension in patients with arteriosclerosis obliterans of the lower limbs. *Angiology* 1987; **38:** 287–95.
15. Sutton KC, Wolfson Jr SK, Kuller LH. Carotid and lower extremity arterial disease in elderly adults with isolated systolic hypertension. *Stroke* 1987; **18:** 817–22.
16. Brattstrom L, Israelsson B, Norrving B, *et al.* Impaired homocysteine metabolism in early-onset cerebral and peripheral occlusive arterial disease. Effects of pyridoxine and folic acid treatment. *Atherosclerosis* 1990; **81:** 51–60.
17. Clarke R, Daly L, Robinson K, *et al.* Hyperhomocysteinemia: an independent risk factor for vascular disease. *N Engl J Med* 1991; **324:** 1149–55.
18. Hoogeveen EK, Kostense PJ, Beks PJ, *et al.* Hyperhomocysteinemia is associated with an increased risk of cardiovascular disease, especially in non-insulin-dependent diabetes mellitus: a population-based study. *Arterioscler Thromb Vasc Biol* 1998; **18:** 133–8.
19. Malinow MR, Kang SS, Taylor LM, *et al.* Prevalence of hyperhomocyst(e)inemia in patients with peripheral arterial occlusive disease. *Circulation* 1989; **79:** 1180–8.
20. Molgaard J, Malinow MR, Lassvik C, *et al.* Hyperhomocyst(e)inaemia: an independent risk factor for intermittent claudication. *J Intern Med* 1992; **231:** 273–9.
21. Taylor Jr LM, DeFrang RD, Harris Jr EJ, Porter JM. The association of elevated plasma homocyst(e)ine with progression of symptomatic peripheral arterial disease. *J Vasc Surg* 1991; **13:** 128–36.
22. Lowe GD, Fowkes FG, Dawes J, *et al.* Blood viscosity, fibrinogen, and activation of coagulation and leukocytes in peripheral arterial disease and the normal population in the Edinburgh Artery Study. *Circulation* 1993; **87:** 1915–20.
23. Ohara Y, Peterson TE, Harrison DG. Hypercholesterolemia increases endothelial superoxide anion production. *J Clin Invest* 1993; **91:** 2546–51.
24. Rajagopalan S, Kurz S, Munzel T, *et al.* Angiotensin II-mediated hypertension in the rat increases vascular superoxide production via membrane NADH/NADPH oxidase activation. Contribution to alterations of vasomotor tone. *J Clin Invest* 1996; **97:** 1916–23.
25. Tesfamariam B, Cohen RA. Free radicals mediate endothelial cell dysfunction caused by elevated glucose. *Am J Physiol* 1992; **263:** H321–6.
26. Tsao PS, Lewis NP, Alpert S, Cooke JP. Exposure to shear stress alters endothelial adhesiveness. Role of nitric oxide. *Circulation* 1995; **92:** 3513–9.
27. van der Wal AC, Becker AE, van der Loos CM, Das PK. Site of intimal rupture or erosion of thrombosed coronary atherosclerotic plaques is characterized by an inflammatory process irrespective of the dominant plaque morphology. *Circulation* 1994; **89:** 36–44.
28. Fuster V, Lewis A. Conner Memorial Lecture. Mechanisms leading to myocardial infarction: insights from studies of vascular biology. *Circulation* 1994; **90**: 2126–46 [published erratum appears in *Circulation* 1995; **91:** 256.
29. Galis ZS, Sukhova GK, Libby P. Microscopic localization of active proteases by in situ zymography: detection of matrix metalloproteinase activity in vascular tissue. *FASEB J* 1995; **9:** 974–80.
30. Lendon CL, Davies MJ, Born GV, Richardson PD. Atherosclerotic plaque caps are locally weakened when macrophages density is increased. *Atherosclerosis* 1991; **87:** 87–90.
31. Shah PK, Falk E, Badimon JJ, *et al.* Human monocyte-derived macrophages induce collagen breakdown in fibrous caps of atherosclerotic plaques. Potential role of matrix-degrading metalloproteinases and implications for plaque rupture. *Circulation* 1995; **92:** 1565–9.
32. Grattan MT, Moreno-Cabral CE, Starnes VA, *et al.* Cytomegalovirus infection is associated with cardiac allograft rejection and atherosclerosis. *JAMA* 1989; **261:** 3561–6.
33. Melnick JL, Adam E, DeBakey ME. Possible role of cytomegalovirus in atherogenesis. *JAMA* 1990; **263:** 2204–7.

34. Minick CR, Fabricant CG, Fabricant J, Litrenta MM. Atheroarteriosclerosis induced by infection with a herpesvirus. *Am J Pathol* 1979; **96:** 673–706.
35. Saikku P, Leinonen M, Mattila K, *et al*. Serological evidence of an association of a novel Chlamydia, TWAR, with chronic coronary heart disease and acute myocardial infarction. *Lancet* 1988; **2:** 983–6.
36. Libby P, Egan D, Skarlatos S. Roles of infectious agents in atherosclerosis and restenosis: an assessment of the evidence and need for future research. *Circulation* 1997; **96:** 4095–103.
37. Zarins CK, Zatina MA, Glagov S. Correlation of postmortem angiography with pathologic anatomy: quantitation of atherosclerotic lesions. In: Bond MG, Insull Jr W, Glagov S, *et al* (eds). *Clinical Diagnosis of Atherosclerosis*. New York, NY: Springer-Verlag, 1983: 283–303.
38. Bond MG, Adams MR, Bullock BC. Complicating factors in evaluating coronary artery atherosclerosis. *Artery* 1981; **9:** 21–9.
39. Beere PA, Glagov S, Zarins CK. Experimental atherosclerosis at the carotid bifurcation of the cynomolgus monkey. Localization, compensatory enlargement, and the sparing effect of lowered heart rate. *Arterioscler Thromb* 1992; **12:** 1245–53.
40. Armstrong ML, Heistad DD, Marcus ML, *et al*. Structural and hemodynamic response of peripheral arteries of macaque monkeys to atherogenic diet. *Arteriosclerosis* 1985; **5:** 336–46.
41. Holvoet P, Theilmeier G, Shivalkar B, *et al*. LDL hypercholesterolemia is associated with accumulation of oxidized LDL, atherosclerotic plaque growth, and compensatory vessel enlargement in coronary arteries of miniature pigs. *Arterioscler Thromb Vasc Biol* 1998; **18:** 415–22.
42. Zarins CK, Glagov S. Atherogenesis and the medical management of atherosclerosis. In: Rutherford RB (ed.). *Vascular Surgery*, 5th edn. Philadelphia: WB Saunders, 2000: 333.
43. Wolinsky H, Glagov S. Comparison of abdominal and thoracic aortic medial structure in mammals. Deviation of man from the usual pattern. *Circ Res* 1969; **25:** 677–86.
44. Gordon T, Kannel WB. Predisposition to atherosclerosis in the head, heart, and legs. The Framingham study. *JAMA* 1972; **221:** 661–6.
45. Campa JS, Greenhalgh RM, Powell JT. Elastin degradation in abdominal aortic aneurysms. *Atherosclerosis* 1987; **65:** 13–21.
46. Dobrin PB, Baker WH, Gley WC. Elastolytic and collagenolytic studies of arteries. Implications for the mechanical properties of aneurysms. *Arch Surg* 1984; **119:** 405–9.
47. Menashi S, Campa JS, Greenhalgh RM, Powell JT. Collagen in abdominal aortic aneurysm: typing, content, and degradation. *J Vasc Surg* 1987; **6:** 578–82.
48. Johansen K, Koepsell T. Familial tendency for abdominal aortic aneurysms. *JAMA* 1986; **256:** 1934–6.
49. Glagov S, Grande JP, Xu CP, *et al*. Limited effects of hyperlipidemia on the arterial smooth muscle response to mechanical stress. *J Cardiovasc Pharmacol* 1989; **14** (Suppl. 6): S90–7.
50. Zatina MA, Zarins CK, Gewertz BL, Glagov S. Role of medial lamellar architecture in the pathogenesis of aortic aneurysms. *J Vasc Surg* 1984; **1:** 442–8.
51. Cotran RS, Kumar V, Robbins SL. Cellular injury and cellular death. In: Schoen FJ (ed.). *Pathologic Basis of Disease*, 5th edn. Philadelphia: WB Saunders, 1994: 4–10.
52. Menger MD, Pelikan S, Steiner D, Messmer K. Microvascular ischemia–reperfusion injury in striated muscle: significance of "reflow paradox." *Am J Physiol* 1992; **263:** H1901–6.
53. McGill Jr HC. George Lyman Duff memorial lecture. Persistent problems in the pathogenesis of atherosclerosis. *Arteriosclerosis* 1984; **4:** 443–51.
54. Diehl JT, Cali RF, Hertzer NR, Beven EG. Complications of abdominal aortic reconstruction. An analysis of perioperative risk factors in 557 patients. *Ann Surg* 1983; **197:** 49–56.
55. Towne JB, Weiss DG, Hobson 2nd RW. First phase report of cooperative veterans administration asymptomatic carotid stenosis study – operative morbidity and mortality. *J Vasc Surg* 1990; **11:** 252–8; discussion 258–9.
56. Cooperman M, Pflug B, Martin Jr EW, Evans WE. Cardiovascular risk factors in patients with peripheral vascular disease. *Surgery* 1978; **84:** 505–9.
57. Yeager RA, Weigel RM, Murphy ES, *et al*. Application of clinically valid cardiac risk factors to aortic aneurysm surgery. *Arch Surg* 1986; **121:** 278–81.
58. Eagle KA, Coley CM, Newell JB, *et al*. Combining clinical and thallium data optimizes preoperative assessment of cardiac risk before major vascular surgery. *Ann Intern Med* 1989; **110:** 859–66.
59. Yeager RA, Moneta GL, McConnell DB, *et al*. Analysis of risk factors for myocardial infarction following carotid endarterectomy. *Arch Surg* 1989; **124:** 1142–5.
60. Hessel 2nd EA. Intraoperative management of abdominal aortic aneurysms. The anesthesiologist's viewpoint. *Surg Clin North Am* 1989; **69:** 775–93.
61. Cunningham AJ. Anaesthesia for repair of abdominal aortic aneurysms. In: Atkinson RS, Adams AP (eds). *Recent Advances in Anaesthesia and Analgesia*. Edinburgh: Churchill Livingstone, 1992: 49–69.
62. Szilagyi DE, Elliott Jr JP, Smith RF, *et al*. A thirty-year survey of the reconstructive surgical treatment of aortoiliac occlusive disease. *J Vasc Surg* 1986; **3:** 421–36..
63. Rao TL, Jacobs KH, El-Etr AA. Reinfarction following anesthesia in patients with myocardial infarction. *Anesthesiology* 1983; **59:** 499–505.
64. Ennix Jr CL, Lawrie GM, Morris Jr GC, *et al*. Improved results of carotid endarterectomy in patients with symptomatic coronary disease: an analysis of 1,546 consecutive carotid operations. *Stroke* 1979; **10:** 122–5.
65. Goldman L. Assessment of the patient with known or suspected ischaemic heart disease for non-cardiac surgery. *Br J Anaesth* 1988; **61:** 38–43.
66. Summary of 1993 World Health Organization. International Society of Hypertension guidelines for the management of mild hypertension. Subcommittee of WHO/ISH Mild Hypertension Liaison committee. *Br Med J* 1993; 307: 1541–6 [published erratum appears in *Br Med J* 1994; **308:** 45.
67. Stone JG, Foex P, Sear JW, *et al*. Myocardial ischemia in untreated hypertensive patients: effect of a single small oral dose of a beta-adrenergic blocking agent. *Anesthesiology* 1988; **68:** 495–500.
68. Young AE, Sandberg GW, Couch NP. The reduction of mortality of abdominal aortic aneurysm resection. *Am J Surg* 1977; **134:** 585–90.69.
69. Mangano DT. Pre-operative assessment of the patient with cardiac disease. *Balliere's Clin Anesthesiol* 1989; **3:** 47–102.
70. Moser M. *Clinical Management of Hypertension*. Caddo, OK: Professional Communications, 1998: 63.
71. Moser M. Beta-adrenergic receptor blockers. In: *Clinical Management of Hypertension*. Caddo, OK: Professional Communications, 1998: 91.
72. Moser M. Combined alpha and beta blockers. In: *Clinical Management of Hypertension*. Caddo, OK: Professional Communications, 1998: 105.
73. Moser M. Peripheral adrenergic inhibitors. In: *Clinical Management of Hypertension*. Caddo, OK: Professional Communications, 1998: 109.
74. Moser M. Central agonists. In: *Clinical Management of Hypertension*. Caddo, OK: Professional Communications, 1998: 113.
75. Moser M. Alpha-1 adrenergic inhibitors. In: *Clinical Management of Hypertension*. Caddo, OK: Professional Communications, 1998: 119.
76. Moser M. Direct vasodilators. In: *Clinical Management of Hypertension*. Caddo, OK: Professional Communications, 1998: 125.
77. Moser M. ACE inhibitors. In: *Clinical Management of Hypertension*. Caddo, OK: Professional Communications, 1998: 129.
78. Moser M. Angiotensin II receptor blockers. In: *Clinical Management of Hypertension*. Caddo, OK: Professional Communications, 1998: 145.
79. Moser M. Calcium channel blockers. In: *Clinical Management of Hypertension*. Caddo, OK: Professional Communications, 1998: 151.
80. Heit JA. Low-molecular-weight heparin: biochemistry, pharmacology, and concurrent drug precautions. *Reg Anesth Pain Med* 1998; **23** (6 Suppl. 2): 135–9.
81. Horlocker TT, Heit JA. Low molecular weight heparin: biochemistry, pharmacology, perioperative prophylaxis regimens, and guidelines for regional anesthetic management. *Anesth Analg* 1997; **85:** 874–85.
82. Vandermeulen EPE, Vermylen J, Van Aken H. Epidural and spinal anesthesia in patients receiving antioagulant therapy. *Baillière's Clin Anesthesiol* 1993; **7:** 663–89.
83. Underwood MJ, More RS. The aspirin papers. *Br Med J* 1994; **308:** 71–2.
84. Hertzer NR. The natural history of peripheral vascular disease. Implications for its management. *Circulation* 1991; **83** (Suppl. 2): I12–19.
85. Hertzer NR, Beven EG, Young JR, *et al*. Coronary artery disease in peripheral vascular patients. A classification of 1000 coronary angiograms and results of surgical management. *Ann Surg* 1984; **199:** 223–33.
86. Hollier LH, Plate G, O'Brien PC, *et al*. Late survival after abdominal aortic aneurysm repair: influence of coronary artery disease. *J Vasc Surg* 1984; **1:** 290–9.
87. Criqui MH, Coughlin SS, Fronek A. Noninvasively diagnosed peripheral aortic aneurysm repair: influence of coronary artery disease. *J Vasc Surg* 1984; **1:** 290–9.
88. Foster ED, Davis KB, Carpenter JA, *et al*. Risk of noncardiac operation in patients with defined coronary disease: The Coronary Artery Surgery Study (CASS) registry experience. *Ann Thorac Surg* 1986; **41:** 42–50.
89. Krupski WC, Bensard DD. Preoperative cardiac risk management. *Surg Clin North Am* 1995; **75:** 647–63.
90. Krupski WC, Layug EL, Reilly LM, *et al*. Comparison of cardiac morbidity

between aortic and infrainguinal operations. Study of Perioperative Ischemia (SPI) Research Group. *J Vasc Surg* 1992; **15:** 354–63; discussion 364–5.

91. Mangano DT, Hollenberg M, Fegert G, *et al.* Perioperative myocardial ischemia in patients undergoing noncardiac surgery. I. Incidence and severity during the 4 day perioperative period. The Study of Perioperative Ischemia (SPI) Research Group. *J Am Coll Cardiol* 1991; **17:** 843–50.
92. Mangano DT, Wang MG, London MJ, *et al.* Perioperative myocardial ischemia in patients undergoing noncardiac surgery. II. Incidence and severity during the 1st week after surgery. The Study of Perioperative Ischemia (SPI) Research Group. *J Am Coll Cardiol* 1991; **17:** 851–7.
93. Raby KE, Goldman L, Creager MA, *et al.* Correlation between preoperative ischemia and major cardiac events after peripheral vascular surgery. *N Engl J Med* 1989; **321:** 1296–330 [comment: *N Engl J Med* 1990; **322:** 931–2].
94. Pasternack PF, Imparato AM, Bear G, *et al.* The value of radionuclide angiography as a predictor of perioperative myocardial infarction in patients undergoing abdominal aortic aneurysm resection. *J Vasc Surg* 1984; **1:** 320–5.
95. Pasternack PF, Imparato AM, Riles TS, *et al.* The value of the radionuclide angiogram in the prediction of perioperative myocardial infarction in patients undergoing lower extremity revascularization procedures. *Circulation* 1985; **72** (3 Pt 2): II13–17.
96. Mangano DT, London MJ, Tubau JF, *et al.* Dipyridamole thallium-201 scintigraphy as a preoperative screening test. A reexamination of its predictive potential. Study of Perioperative Ischemia Research Group. *Circulation* 1991; **84:** 493–502.
97. Bry JD, Belkin M, O'Donnell Jr TF, *et al.* An assessment of the positive predictive value and cost-effectiveness of dipyridamole myocardial scintigraphy in patients undergoing vascular surgery. *J Vasc Surg* 1994; **19:** 112–21; discussion 121–4.
98. Krupski WC, Bensard DD. Preoperative cardiac risk management. *Surg Clin North Am* 1995; **75:** 647–63.
99. Eastcott HHG, Pickering GW, Robb CG. Reconstruction of internal carotid artery in a patient with intermittent attacks of hemiplegia. *Lancet* 1954; **2:** 994–6.
100. Garrioch MA, Fitch W. Anaesthesia for carotid artery surgery. *Br J Anaesth* 1993; **71:** 569–79.
101. Barnett HJ, Taylor DW, Eliasziw M, *et al.* Benefit of carotid endarterectomy in patients with symptomatic moderate or severe stenosis. North American Symptomatic Carotid Endarterectomy Trial Collaborators. *N Engl J Med* 1998; **339:** 1415–25.
102. European Carotid Surgery Trialists' Collaborative Group. MRC European Carotid Surgery Trials: interim results for symptomatic patients with severe (70–99%) or with mild (0–29%) carotid stenosis. *Lancet* 1991; **337:** 1235–43.
103. Sandmann W. Carotid endarterectomy. In: Bell PFR, Jamieson CCV, Ruckley CV (eds). *Surgical Management of Vascular Disease.* London: WB Saunders, 1992: 671–81.
104. Naylor AR, Bell PR, Ruckley CV. Monitoring and cerebral protection during carotid endarterectomy. *Br J Surg* 1992; **79:** 735–41.
105. Archie Jr JP. Technique and clinical results of carotid stump back-pressure to determine selective shunting during carotid endarterectomy. *J Vasc Surg* 1991; **13:** 319–26; discussion 326–7.
106. Bishop CC, Powell S, Rutt D, Browse NL. Transcranial Doppler measurement of middle cerebral artery blood flow velocity: a validation study. *Stroke* 1986; **17:** 913–15.
107. Youngberg JA, Gold MD. Carotid artery surgery: perioperative anaesthetic considerations. In: Kaplan JA (ed.). *Vascular Anesthesia.* New York: Churchill Livingstone, 1991: 333–61.
108. Godin MS, Bell 3rd WH, Schwedler M, Kerstein MD. Cost effectiveness of regional anesthesia in carotid endarterectomy. *Am Surg* 1989; **55:** 656–9.
109. Cucchiara RF, Benefiel DJ, Matteo RS, *et al.* Evaluation of esmolol in controlling increases in heart rate and blood pressure during endotracheal intubation in patients undergoing carotid endarterectomy. *Anesthesiology* 1986; **65:** 528–31.
110. Michenfelder JD, Sundt TM, Fode N, Sharbrough FW. Isoflurane when compared to enflurane and halothane decreases the frequency of cerebral ischemia during carotid endarterectomy. *Anesthesiology* 1987; **67:** 336–40.
111. Messick Jr JM, Casement B, Sharbrough FW, *et al.* Correlation of regional cerebral blood flow (rCBF) with EEG changes during isoflurane anesthesia for carotid endarterectomy: critical rCBF. *Anesthesiology* 1987; **66:** 344–9.
112. Hobbhahn J, Hansen E, Keyi C. Volatile anaesthetics in patients with coronary artery disease and with heart failure. *Bailliere's Clin Anesthesiol* 1993; **7:** 1057–77.
113. Pulsinelli WA, Levy DE, Sigsbee B, *et al.* Increased damage after ischemic stroke in patients with hyperglycemia with or without established diabetes mellitus. *Am J Med* 1983 **74:** 540–4.
114. Harris DN, Bailey SM. Near infrared spectroscopy in adults. Does the Invos 3100 really measure intracerebral oxygenation? *Anaesthesia* 1993; **48:** 694–6.
115. Kane CM, Le Cheminant D, Horan BF. Acute cardiovascular responses to internal carotid artery occlusion during carotid endarterectomy and to the restoration of internal carotid flow. *Anaesth Intensive Care* 1987; **15:** 289–95.
116. Dehn TC, Angell-James JE. Long-term effect of carotid endarterectomy on carotid sinus baroreceptor function and blood pressure control. *Br J Surg* 1987; **74:** 997–1000.
117. Riles TS, Kopelman I, Imparato AM. Myocardial infarction following carotid endarterectomy: a review of 683 operations. *Surgery* 1979; **85:** 249–52.
118. Johnston KW, Scobie TK. Multicenter prospective study of nonruptured abdominal aortic aneurysms. I. Population and operative management. *J Vasc Surg* 1988; **7:** 69–81.
119. Reid DB, Welch GH, Pollock JG. Abdominal aortic aneurysm: a preventable cause of death? *J R Coll Surg (Edinburgh)* 1990; **35:** 284–8.
120. Lambert ME, Baguley P, Charlesworth D. Ruptured abdominal aortic aneurysms. *J Cardiovasc Surg* 1986; **27:** 256–61.
121. Kwitka G, Kidney SA, Nugent M. Thoracic and abdominal aortic aneurysm resections. In: Kaplan JA (ed.). *Vascular Anesthesia.* New York: Churchill Livingstone, 1991: 363–94.
122. Greenhalgh RM. Prognosis of abdominal aortic aneurysm. *Br Med J* 1990; **301:** 136.
123. Sumpio BE, Traquina DN, Gusberg RJ. Results of aortic grafting in occlusive vs aneurysmal disease. *Arch Surg* 1985; **120:** 817–19.
124. Picone AL, Green RM, Ricotta JR, *et al.* Spinal cord ischemia following operations on the abdominal aorta. *J Vasc Surg* 1986; **3:** 94–103.
125. Dubhost C, Allary M, Oeconomos N. Resection of an aneurysm of the abdominal aorta. Reestablishment of continuity by a preserved human arterial graft, with result after five months. *Arch Surg* 1952; **64:** 405–8.
126. Vorhees AB, Joretzki A, Blasmore AH. The use of tubes constructed from Vinyon 'N' cloth in bridging arterial defects. *Ann Surg* 1952; **135:** 332–6.
127. Sicard GA, Allen BT, Munn JS, Anderson CB. Retroperitoneal versus transperitoneal approach for repair of abdominal aortic aneurysms. *Surg Clin North Am* 1989; **69:** 795–806.
128. Imparato AM. Surgical management of abdominal aortic aneurysms. In: Bell PFR, Jamieson CCV, Ruckley CV (eds). *Surgical Management of Vascular Disease.* London: WB Saunders, 1992: 843–57.
129. Mannick JA, Whittemore AD, Couch NP. Abdominal aortic aneurysms. In: Greenhalgh RM (ed.). *Vascular Surgical Techniques.* London: Butterworth, 1984: 107–16.
130. Anonymous. A randomized trial of propranolol in patients with acute myocardial infarction. II. Morbidity results. *JAMA* 1983; **250:** 2814–19.
131. Anonymous. Reduction of infarct size with the early use of timolol in acute myocardial infarction. *N Engl J Med* 1984; **310:** 9–15.
132. Tofler GH, Brezinski D, Schafer AI, *et al.* Concurrent morning increase in platelet aggregability and the risk of myocardial infarction and sudden cardiac death. *N Engl J Med* 1987; **316:** 1514–8.
133. Brezinski DA, Tofler GH, Muller JE, *et al.* Morning increase in platelet aggregability. Association with assumption of the upright posture. *Circulation* 1988; **78:** 35–40.
134. Kataja J. Thoracolumbar epidural anaesthesia and isoflurane to prevent hypertension and tachycardia in patients undergoing abdominal aortic surgery. *Eur J Anaesthiol* 1991; **8:** 427–36.
135. Baron JF, Coriat P, Mundler O, *et al.* Left ventricular global and regional function during lumbar epidural anesthesia in patients with and without angina pectoris. Influence of volume loading. *Anesthesiology* 1987; **66:** 621–7.
136. Diebel LN, Lange MP, Schneider F, *et al.* Cardiopulmonary complications after major surgery: a role for epidural analgesia? *Surgery* 1987; **102:** 660–6.
137. Yeager MP, Glass DD, Neff RK, Brinck-Johnsen T. Epidural anesthesia and analgesia in high-risk surgical patients. *Anesthesiology* 1987; **66:** 729–36.
138. Liu S, Carpenter RL, Neal JM. Epidural anesthesia and analgesia. Their role in postoperative outcome. *Anesthesiology* 1995; **82:** 1474–506.
139. Ghignone M, Calvillo O, Quintin L. Anesthesia and hypertension: the effect of clonidine on perioperative hemodynamics and isoflurane requirements. *Anesthesiology* 1987; **67:** 3–10.
140. Slogoff S, Keats AS. Randomized trial of primary anesthetic agents on

outcome of coronary artery bypass operations. *Anesthesiology* 1989; **70:** 179–88.

141. Colson P, Capdevilla X, Cuchet D, *et al*. Does choice of the anesthetic influence renal function during infrarenal aortic surgery? *Anesth Analg* 1992; **74:** 481–5.
142. Vercauteren MP. The role of the perispinal route for postsurgical pain relief. *Baillière's Clin Anesthesiol* 1993; **7:** 769–92.
143. Ansley DM, Ramsay JG, Whalley DG, *et al*. The relationship between central venous pressure and pulmonary capillary wedge pressure during aortic surgery. *Can J Anaesth* 1987; **34:** 594–600.
144. Carson JL, Willett LR. Is a hemoglobin of 10 g/dL required for surgery? *Med Clin North Am* 1993; **77:** 335–47.
145. Seltzer JL, Ritter DE, Starsnic MA, Marr AT. The hemodynamic response to traction on the abdominal mesentery. *Anesthesiology* 1985; **63:** 96–9.
146. Gottlieb A, Skrinska VA, O'Hara P, *et al*. The role of prostacyclin in the mesenteric traction syndrome during anesthesia for abdominal aortic reconstructive surgery. *Ann Surg* 1989; **209:** 363–7.
147. Hudson JC, Wurm WH, O'Donnel Jr TF, *et al*. Ibuprofen pretreatment inhibits prostacyclin release during abdominal exploration in aortic surgery. *Anesthesiology* 1990; **72:** 443–9.
148. Cunningham AJ. Anaesthesia for repair of abdominal aortic aneurysms. In: Atkinson RS, Adams AP (eds). *Recent Advances in Anaesthesia and Analgesia*. Edinburgh: Churchill Livingstone, 1992: 49–69.
149. Fiddian-Green RG, Gantz NM. Transient episodes of sigmoid ischemia and their relation to infection from intestinal organisms after abdominal aortic operations. *Crit Care Med* 1987; **15:** 835–9.
150. Fiddian-Green RG. Splanchnic ischaemia and multiple organ failure in the critically ill. *Ann R Coll Surg Engl* 1988; **70:** 128–34.
151. Gamulin Z, Forster A, Simonet F, *et al*. Effects of renal sympathetic blockade on renal hemodynamics in patients undergoing major aortic abdominal surgery. *Anesthesiology* 1986; **65:** 688–92.
152. Ouriel K, Smedira NG, Ricotta JJ. Protection of the kidney after temporary ischemia: free radical scavengers. *J Vasc Surg* 1985; **2:** 49–53.
153. Salem MG, Crooke JW, McLoughlin GA, *et al*. The effect of dopamine on renal function during aortic cross clamping. *Ann R Coll Surg Engl* 1988; **70:** 9–12.
154. Szilagyi DE, Hageman JH, Smith RF, Elliott JP. Spinal cord damage in surgery of the abdominal aorta. *Surgery* 1978; **83:** 38–56.
155. Paterson IS, Klausner JM, Pugatch R, *et al*. Noncardiogenic pulmonary edema after abdominal aortic aneurysm surgery. *Ann Surg* 1989; **209:** 231–6.
156. Paterson IS, Klausner JM, Goldman G, *et al*. Pulmonary edema after aneurysm surgery is modified by mannitol. *Ann Surg* 1989; **210:** 796–801.
157. Oredsson S, Plate G, Qvarfordt P. Allopurinol – a free radical scavenger – reduces reperfusion injury in skeletal muscle. *Eur J Vasc Surg* 1991; **5:** 47–52.
158. Heagerty AM, Barnett DB. Postoperative cardiac complications following vascular surgery. In: Bell PFR, Jamieson CCV, Ruckley CV (eds). *Surgical Management of Vascular Disease*. London: WB Saunders, 1992: 999–1011.
159. Coley S, Smith G. Respiratory problems in the postoperative period. In: Bell PFR, Jamieson CCV, Ruckley CV (eds). *Surgical Management of Vascular Disease*. London: WB Saunders, 1992: 1013–25.
160. Smithies M, Cameron JS. Renal failure following reconstructive arterial surgery. In: Bell PFR, Jamieson CCV, Ruckley CV (eds). *Surgical Management of Vascular Disease*. London: WB Saunders, 1992: 1027–48.
161. Roizen MF. Anesthesia for emergence surgery for abdominal aortic reconstruction. In: Roizen MF (ed.). *Anesthesia for Vascular Surgery*. New York, NY: Churchill Livingstone, 1990: 311–16.

47

Anesthesia for thoracic surgery

JAY B BRODSKY

PREOPERATIVE ASSESSMENT

All patients undergoing thoracic surgery must give a complete medical history and have a complete physical examination prior to surgery. The physical examination is directed primarily to the cardiovascular and pulmonary systems. The presence of wheezing, rales, rhonchi, or other abnormal breath sounds suggests the need for further medical intervention. Any deviation of the trachea from the midline should alert the anesthesiologist to a potentially difficult intubation or to the possibility of airway obstruction during induction of anesthesia.

The electrocardiogram (ECG) of the patient with chronic obstructive pulmonary disease may reveal right atrial or ventricular hypertrophy. An enlarged P-wave in lead II ("P" pulmonale) indicates right atrial enlargement. A low-voltage QRS complex may be due to lung hyperinflation.

Many patients undergoing thoracic surgery have pre-existing pulmonary problems, and alterations in pulmonary function are to be expected in every patient after thoracotomy. Pulmonary function tests and an arterial blood gas sample are usually indicated to establish baseline values before major surgery.[1]

Bedside spirometric tests for forced vital capacity (FVC) and forced expiratory volume (FEV) are usually adequate (see Chapter 5).[2] FVC can be compared with normal values based on sex, height, and age and then expressed as a percentage of the predicted vital capacity (%FVC). A %FVC greater than 80 is considered normal, 70–80 is borderline normal, 60–70 suggests pulmonary disease, and less than 60 indicates significant restriction of pulmonary function.

The FEV_1 is the volume of air forcefully expired in the first second of an FVC maneuver. FEV_1 can be compared with the actual measured FVC (ratio $FEV_1/FVC = \%FEV_1$) to differentiate between restrictive and obstructive pulmonary disease. The $\%FEV_1$ is normally greater than 70. In restrictive disease, both FEV_1 and FVC decrease, so $\%FEV_1$ remains normal.

In obstructive disease, only FEV_1 is reduced, so $\%FEV_1$ is lowered. A $\%FEV_1$ less than 70 suggests significant airway resistance, which increases the work of breathing during stress. A 15% improvement in $\%FEV_1$ after bronchodilator therapy indicates some reversibility of airway obstruction, and in these patients bronchodilators should be administered preoperatively.

Pulmonary function tests are used to predict the degree to which the pre-existing obstructive and restrictive components of pulmonary function may compromise the ability to ventilate adequately and to maintain clear lungs after thoracic surgery.

An FVC that is at least three times greater than tidal volume is necessary for an effective cough. A preoperative FVC of less than $20\,mL\,kg^{-1}$, a FEV_1 of less than 1.2 L, and a $\%FEV_1$ of less than 35 are each associated with postoperative respiratory problems. Improvements in operative and postoperative management of high-risk surgical patients have rendered these absolute measurements invalid. Thoracotomy and video-assisted thoracoscopic surgery are now safely performed in patients who were not previously considered surgical candidates based on the above spirometric criteria.[3]

Flow–volume loop measurements are another means of assessing airway status. The shape and peak air flow rates during expiration at high lung volumes are effort dependent and indicate the patency of the larger airways. Expiration at low lung volumes is effort independent and reflects resistance in smaller airways.

Split-lung ventilation/perfusion studies predict the amount of functional lung tissue remaining after pulmonary resection. These tests are especially useful before pneumonectomy. Radioactive xenon is injected intravenously, and the radioactivity subsequently measured in each lung is proportional to regional perfusion. Ventilation is measured by the inhalation of radioactive gas. The radioactivity measured in each lung area is proportional to the degree of regional ventilation.

Diffusing capacity is another sensitive measure of pulmonary function. Abnormal diffusing capacity measurements may reveal the existence of emphysematous changes in the lung, even when spirometric values are considered acceptable. Decreased diffusing capacity is a strong predictor of both pulmonary and cardiac complications following lung resection.[4]

Pulmonary and cardiac complications continue to present major sources of morbidity and mortality for patients undergoing thoracic operations. Determination of the specific factors associated with increased risk is therefore important so that those patients who might be predisposed to develop serious complications can be identified.[5]

Such factors include carbon monoxide diffusion capacity, peak oxygen (O_2) uptake, pulmonary artery pressure, oxygen tension (P_aO_2) during pulmonary artery occlusion, and presurgical exercise testing. Patient age, the site and extent of the operative procedure, duration of anesthesia, pre-existing cardiovascular or neurologic dysfunction, obesity, the degree of postoperative pain expected, and the interval between surgery and ambulation affect postoperative outcome.[6–9]

Patients with respiratory muscle weakness have a high incidence of postoperative pulmonary complications. Preoperative respiratory muscle testing and then training can reduce complications by increasing both inspiratory and expiratory muscle strength in patients undergoing thoracic surgery.[10]

A cardiopulmonary risk index (CPRI) has been used to predict postoperative outcome following thoracotomy (Table 47.1).[11] This system assigns numerical values to certain cardiac factors (congestive heart failure, recent myocardial infarction, arrhythmia, aortic stenosis) and to pulmonary factors [obesity, cough, elevated carbon dioxide ($P_{a}CO_2$), poor spirometric performance, cigarette smoking, and diffuse wheezing].

A CPRI score of 4 or higher is associated with a 22-fold increase in post-thoracotomy complications compared with patients with a score of less than 4. Other studies have failed to correlate a high CPRI score with an adverse outcome.[12,13]

For patients with significant chronic pulmonary disease or retained secretions, a significant improvement in vital capacity (VC) and FEV_1 can be obtained preoperatively with appropriate bronchial hygiene therapy (aerosol therapy with or without bronchodilator, chest physiotherapy, intermittent positive-pressure breathing).[14] Every patient should be encouraged to cough, breathe deeply, and sit up and ambulate as soon as possible after surgery.

Preoperative spirometry used to predict postoperative FEV_1 is probably the best predictor of outcome.[15] However, no index or comorbidity is completely accurate. With appropriate perioperative management, even patients with severely compromised pulmonary function, such as those undergoing lung volume reduction surgery or pulmonary transplantation, can be safely anesthetized for pulmonary resection.[16]

CHOICE OF ANESTHETIC AGENT

General anesthesia normally increases airway resistance by reducing functional residual capacity (FRC). Airway resistance may be further increased during thoracic surgery by obstruction with secretions or tumor and from surgical trauma that can cause hemorrhage and bronchospasm. Associated medical conditions [chronic obstructive pulmonary disease (COPD), asthma, cystic fibrosis, or other lung diseases] can also affect airway caliber and reactivity. Intentional intubation of a bronchus with a double-lumen tube (DLT) or bronchial blocker can produce bronchospasm from direct mucosal stimulation.

These effects can be partially alleviated by using an inhalational anesthetic agent (Table 47.2). Halothane, enflurane, isoflurane, desflurane, and sevoflurane have direct bronchodilator properties. They also obtund bronchoconstrictive airway reflexes in patients with reactive airways.

Isoflurane, sevoflurane, or desflurane, which allow rapid changes in depth of anesthesia with fewer ventilatory arrhythmias, is preferred for thoracic surgery. No differences in oxygenation, shunt fraction, or hemodynamic stability result from the use of isoflurane or sevoflurane[17,18] or from isoflurane or desflurane[19] during selective one-lung ventilation.

Drugs that release histamine (thiopental, thiamylal, propanidid) can produce bronchospasm. These agents must be used with caution in patients with reactive airway disease. Methohexital, etomidate, and propofol do not cause histamine release and should be considered for anesthetic induction of the patient with asthma.[20]

Some muscle relaxants (vecuronium, mivacurium, curare) also cause histamine release. Pancuronium and cisatracurium are completely devoid of any chemically mediated histamine release and can be used for patients with reactive airways.[21]

Ketamine has direct bronchodilatory effects and antagonizes bronchoconstriction from histamine without depressing respiration. It also maintains the hypoxic pulmonary vasoconstrictive (HPV) response.[22] It has a rapid onset of action while tending to maintain cardiovascular stability. Ketamine is a particularly useful agent for induction of anesthesia in unstable patients undergoing emergency thoracotomy.[23] Ketamine offers no advantages for routine thoracic surgery.[24]

In the lungs, regional hypoxia causes arteriolar constriction with diversion of blood flow away from a hypoxic segment to areas that are better oxygenated. The HPV response improves gas exchange by matching perfusion to ventilation. The primary stimuli for HPV are alveolar oxygen tension ($P_{A}O_2$) and mixed venous oxygen tension ($P_{v}O_2$).[25]

The overall effects of anesthetics on HPV are complex.[26] In both *in vitro* and *in vivo* animal studies, all intravenous drugs (barbiturates, hypnotics, droperidol, ketamine, opioids) do not depress HPV. In experimental models, all inhalational anesthetics, including the newer agents sevoflurane and desflurane, directly inhibit HPV.[27–30]

The direct depression of HPV by the inhalational anesthetics is believed to be due to release of endogenous nitric oxide (NO).[31] Conversely, inhibition of NO production results in an increased HPV response, even in the presence of an inhalational anesthetic agent.[32]

Although in experiments the inhalational agents all inhibit HPV, clinically a wide range of effects are seen with those same agents. This may be due in part to their effects on cardiac output, oxygen consumption, regional wasted perfusion of the collapsed lung during one-lung ventilation ("shunt"), and $P_{v}O_2$, and to mechanical factors such as

Table 47.1 *Cardiopulmonary risk index (CPRI) for lung resection*

CRI		PRI	
Variable	**Points**	**Variable**	**Points**
Congestive heart failure	11	Obesity	1
Myocardial infarction (within 6 months of surgery)	10	Cigarette smoking (within 8 weeks of surgery)	1
>5 PVCs min^{-1}	7	Productive cough (within 5 days of surgery)	1
Other arrhythmia	7	Diffuse wheezing or rhonchi (within 5 days or surgery)	1
Age >70 years	5	FEV_1/FVC <70%	1
Aortic stenosis	3	$P_{a}CO_2$ >45 mmHg	1
Poor general medical condition	3		
Thoracic operation	3		

Score = 1 (0–5 CRI points)
2 (6–12 CRI points)
3 (12–25 CRI points)
4 (>25 CRI points)

CRI, cardiac risk index; PRI, pulmonary risk index; PVCs, premature ventricular contractions; FEV, forced expiratory volume; FVC, forced vital capacity. CPRI score is obtained by adding the CRI and PRI scores. A minimum CRI score of 3 is assigned to each patient because they are undergoing a thoracic operation. A CPRI score ≥4 was associated with a 22-fold increase in postoperative complications.

Table 47.2 *Properties of anesthetic agents used for thoracic surgery*

Agent	Desirable	Undesirable
Inhalational anesthetics	Permit high $F_{I}O_2$	Inhibit HPV
	Bronchodilator properties	Myocardial depression
	Diminished airway reflexes	
	Rapidly eliminated	
Opioids	Do not inhibit HPV	May depress ventilation
	Postoperative analgesia	
	No myocardial depression	
Nitrous oxide	Rapidly eliminated	Reduces $F_{I}O_2$
	No effect on HPV	May expand blebs, tube cuffs
Ketamine	Diminishes airway irritability	Emergence delirium
	Does not inhibit HPV	
	Cardiovascular stability during hypovolemia	
Thiopental	Does not inhibit HPV	Releases histamine
Propofol	Does not inhibit HPV	
	Rapid emergence	
Muscle relaxants	Facilitate mechanical ventilation	Potential postoperative weakness
	Improve surgical exposure	Release histamine
	Reduced dose of anesthetic	Requires reversal agent

HPV, hypoxic pulmonary vasoconstriction.

manipulation of the lung and the use of positive end-expiratory pressure (PEEP) during thoracic surgery.

By directly increasing the shunt by depression of HPV, inhalational agents produce modest reductions in P_aO_2. However, if the anesthetic lowers cardiac output more than it decreases oxygen consumption, P_vO_2 will drop. This is a potent stimulus for HPV. Therefore, the effectiveness of the HPV response varies inversely with cardiac output. A myocardial depressant such as halothane, which decreases cardiac output, reduces blood flow to the collapsed lung, thereby neutralizing any direct depression of HPV during one-lung ventilation.[33]

In clinical practice, the overall effects by inhalational and intravenous anesthetic agents on HPV during thoracotomy are small.[34,35] Intravenous propofol did not increase shunt fraction during one-lung ventilation, whereas shunt did increase threefold in patients receiving isoflurane.[36] However, there is no difference in oxygenation between a total intravenous (propofol–alfentanil) anesthetic which spares the HPV response, and an inhalational anesthetic (isoflurane) which depresses HPV during one-lung ventilation.[37]

Vasoconstrictive drugs [dopamine, epinephrine (adrenaline), phenylephrine] preferentially constrict pulmonary vessels perfusing normoxic or hyperoxic lung segments during one-lung ventilation. This increases pulmonary vascular resistance in the ventilated lung, causing redistribution of blood flow to the collapsed lung, lowering P_aO_2, and possibly increasing the shunt.

Vasodilator drugs (nitroprusside, nitroglycerin) blunt HPV in the atelectactic lung during one-lung ventilation. This increases blood flow to that lung, thereby lowering P_aO_2. Similarly, manipulation of the collapsed lung during surgery causes endogenous thromboxane and prostaglandin I_2-mediated local vasodilation, which may blunt HPV.[38]

Nitrous oxide (N_2O) expands air-containing spaces (such as a pneumothorax, lung cyst, or an air bleb) and dilutes the amount of oxygen that can be delivered during one-lung ventilation. There is no reason to use N_2O during thoracic surgery. If exposure to high oxygen concentration is undesirable, as in the patient receiving bleomycin,[39] then air should be substituted for N_2O. There may even be a lower incidence of postoperative atelectasis in the ventilated lung after pulmonary surgery when air is substituted for N_2O during one-lung ventilation.[40]

INTRAOPERATIVE MONITORING

Routine monitoring during thoracic operations should include noninvasive blood pressure, pulse oximetry, end-tidal capnography, ECG, and temperature. A urinary catheter should also be placed before long procedures and/or when epidural opioids are planned.

During one-lung ventilation, monitoring oxygenation by oxygen saturation (S_pO_2) is usually adequate.[41] However, in the presence of prolonged hypotension, pulse oximetry may be inaccurate. An indwelling arterial line allows intermittent sampling of arterial blood to monitor oxygenation, ventilation, and acid–base status. It is also useful for beat-to-beat hemodynamic monitoring, especially in situations in which surgical retraction on the heart or great vessels can cause hypotension and arrhythymias.

Continuous intra-arterial blood gas monitoring (CIABG) is now feasible.[42,43] This technology has been used successfully during thoracic surgery,[44] although PO_2 values are relatively inaccurate during one-lung ventilation.[45]

Since intermittent arterial blood gas sampling may fail to detect transient arterial hypoxemia during one-lung ventilation, the application of CIABG as a trend monitor in critical situations such as lung transplantation, lung volume reduction surgery, and pulmonary alveolar lavage seems reasonable.[46] Because of the high cost of the intra-arterial probes, at present there is no role for CIABG during routine thoracotomy or video-assisted thoracoscopic surgery.

Fluid status monitoring with a central venous pressure (CVP) or pulmonary artery (PA) line is not routinely needed during thoracotomy because volume changes are not large. Fluid restriction is indicated for most pulmonary resections.[47] Less than 20 mL kg^{-1} of crystalloid solution over 24 h is recommended, and increasing fluid input to achieve a urine output of 0.5 mL kg^{-1} h^{-1} is not necessary.[48]

Pulmonary edema can occur following any thoracotomy from a variety of causes, including fluid overload, cardiac failure, and aspiration. For procedures with large volume shifts (esophageal resection, pneumonectomy), postoperative volume monitoring with a central catheter is normally indicated.

Open thoracotomy in the lateral decubitus position limits the usefulness of information derived from CVP or PA catheters during surgery. Normally, the CVP reflects blood volume, venous tone, and right ventricular performance. During thoracotomy, the CVP may be altered by surgical retraction, mediastinal and diaphragmatic shifts, and the application of PEEP, which changes intrathoracic pressure. With advanced pulmonary disease and/or left ventricular dysfunction, the CVP may not reflect left-sided filling pressures.

A PA catheter for monitoring hemodynamic function (preload, afterload, and cardiac output) may be useful in patients with pre-existing myocardial dysfunction, ischemia, and valvular heart disease (see Chapter 27). A PA catheter can also be used to follow $S_{\bar{v}}O_2$, which is a reflection of oxygen supply and demand. $S_{\bar{v}}O_2$ gives indirect information of end-organ perfusion and may reflect decreases in cardiac output, decreased arterial oxygen content, anemia, or increased oxygen consumption.[49]

When a PA catheter is used, its position should be documented radiographically before surgery since catheters enter the right pulmonary artery 85% of the time. Therefore, during right thoracotomy the catheter tip will be in the nondependent pulmonary artery, and during left thoracotomy the catheter tip will be in the vessel of the nonoperated, dependent lung. In both situations, the data obtained may be inaccurate. Hemodynamic and $S_{\bar{v}}O_2$ measurements are lower during right thoracotomy than during left thoracotomy because both are affected by reduced blood flow to the nonventilated right lung.

Transesophageal echocardiography (TEE) has been used during pulmonary surgery. Clamping the pulmonary artery during pneumonectomy was associated with transient left ventricular dysfunction and mild mitral regurgitation from acute right ventricular dilation.[50] TEE monitoring of high-risk patients with associated cardiac disease during pneumonectomy may help to identify those patients who will go on to develop right ventricular failure and/or hypoxemia in the postoperative period. There were no TEE changes during pulmonary lobectomy. During thoracotomy, TEE can also identify tumor in pulmonary veins, tumor embolism, and tumor invasion into the atrium.[51,52]

ISOLATION OF THE LUNGS

During intrathoracic procedures in which the operated lung is selectively collapsed, hemodynamic stability and oxygenation must be maintained while ventilating only one lung. Isolation of the lungs is essential when it is necessary to protect the dependent lung from contamination while the patient is in the lateral decubitus position.[53,54] Collapsing the operated lung provides optimal operative exposure.

Although selective one-lung ventilation is required for many procedures (e.g. repair of a bronchopleural fistula, lung transplantation, and video-assisted and lung volume reduction surgery), any thoracic surgery will benefit from selective lung collapse. A completely atelectactic lung eliminates the need for vigorous retraction during surgery, so there is less intraoperative lung trauma. Improved exposure shortens the duration of the procedure, therefore total operative costs are also reduced. Isolation and selective collapse of a lung can be achieved by either bronchial blockade or with a double-cuffed DLT.

Bronchial blockade

Lung tissue distal to any obstruction will collapse from absorption atelectasis. Historically, bronchial blockade has been achieved with a variety of different devices, including gauze tampons, special cuffed rubber blockers, and with the inflated balloons used for embolectomy, pulmonary artery, and even urinary catheters.[55,56] Bronchial blockade with a Fogarty embolectomy or some other small (4–6Fr) balloon-tipped catheter is the only practical method for lung separation in small children.[57] Larger (8–12Fr) embolectomy catheters are occasionally used for adults.[58,59] In patients with a restricted mouth opening, a nasal intubation with an endotracheal tube followed by bronchial blockade with a Fogarty catheter may be the only practical means of achieving one-lung ventilation.[60] Bronchial blockade should also be considered for patients with a previous laryngectomy and permanent tracheostomy when the stoma is too small to accommodate a DLT.[61]

In adults, the blocker catheter is passed, using a flexible fiberoptic bronchoscope, through an endotracheal tube, whereas in children it is passed alongside the endotracheal tube. Once the catheter is in position in the bronchus, its balloon is inflated until it completely obstructs the airway.

Blockers have several disadvantages. They can be easily displaced when changing the position of the patient or during surgical manipulation. If the blocker slips into the trachea, it may obstruct ventilation to the nonoperated lung and/or fail to isolate the healthy lung from contamination. Another disadvantage is that lung tissue distal to the obstruction cannot be suctioned or re-expanded during the procedure. Continuous positive airway pressure (CPAP) cannot be applied if the patient becomes hypoxemic during one-lung ventilation.

All catheters currently used for bronchial blockade are manufactured for other uses and have low-volume balloons that generate very high pressures when inflated. Tracheobronchial rupture can occur if the balloon is overinflated or if it becomes overdistended with N_2O during the anesthetic.[62] The largest balloon whose catheter will fit the endotracheal tube should be used. The balloon should be inflated with the smallest volume of air that seals the bronchus while under direct observation.

The Univent tube (Fuji Systems, Tokyo, Japan) is designed for bronchial blockade in adults and larger children.[63–65] The tube is a conventional endotracheal tube with an additional small lumen. This lumen contains another smaller tube that can be advanced up to 8 cm past the tip of the larger tube into either bronchus. A balloon located near the tip of the smaller tube, when inflated, serves as the airway blocker while the nonoperated lung is ventilated through the larger endotracheal tube. Bronchoscopy is required for accurate placement of Univent tubes.[66,67]

The operated lung can be suctioned or lavaged, and supplemental oxygen can be insufflated through the lumen of the blocker tube.[68,69] High-frequency jet ventilation can also be used through this lumen.[70] Ventilation to both lungs can be reinstituted at any time by deflating the blocker balloon and withdrawing the blocker back into the body of the main tube. A major advantage of the Univent tube is that the airway need not be reintubated with another endotracheal tube at the completion of surgery if postoperative ventilation is planned.

Although some consider a Univent tube is easier to use than a DLT,[71,72] the time required to position both tubes, the number of tube malpositions, and the surgical exposure provided by each did not differ when the Univent tube was compared with a DLT.[73] Since the blocker tube is so small, its balloon must be inflated with 2–10 times as much air as the bronchial cuff of a DLT in order for it to obstruct the bronchus.[74] This generates high, potentially dangerous pressures that predispose the balloon to carinal herniation or can damage the airway.[75]

Several unique complications have been reported with the Univent tube.[76] A tension pneumothorax can occur when the rigid blocker tube is advanced into the airway wall.[77] Failure to withdraw the blocker completely at the time of airway resection can result in inclusion of the blocker in the staple line.[78] Obstruction of ventilation to both lungs may result if the cuff on the blocker balloon is retracted completely back into the main tube without deflation. This complication is more likely to occur postoperatively in the critical care setting with personnel who are not familiar with the properties of the Univent tube.[79] Removal of the pilot balloon to the blocker will eliminate the risk of this complication.

Double-lumen tubes

The major advantage of a DLT is that either or both lungs can be deflated, re-expanded, or suctioned at any time during the procedure. In addition, CPAP can be administered to the collapsed lung during one-lung ventilation without interrupting ventilation to the nonoperated lung.

Properties

All DLTs are constructed of two tubes of unequal length. The shorter tube ends in the trachea, whereas the longer tube reaches into a bronchus. A cuff placed above the distal opening of the tracheal tube prevents gas leaks during positive-pressure ventilation. Inspired gas can be diverted into either or both lungs by a second cuff on the longer tube in the bronchial lumen. The inflated bronchial cuff isolates and protects each lung. In tubes designed for the right bronchus, the lateral aspect of the bronchial cuff or bronchial lumen itself is fenestrated to allow gas exchange with the right upper-lobe bronchus.

The proximal end of each lumen is fitted to a special connector that allows ventilation to be distributed to either or both lungs. Each tube can be independently opened to the atmosphere, thereby allowing the lung on that side to collapse while ventilation to the other lung can continue. A suction catheter or bronchoscope can be passed down either lumen while ventilating the other lung.

The original rubber Carlens's and White's DLTs had a hook to engage the carina to help position the tube. Carinal hooks make passage through the glottis difficult and often injure the airway. The rubber Robertshaw's DLT has no hook and has larger internal lumens than either the Carlens's or the White's tube. DLTs are now made of polyvinylchloride plastic material and resemble Robertshaw's design.

Because of their numerous advantages, disposable plastic DLTs have now almost universally replaced reusable rubber tubes.[80] Plastic DLTs are sold by several manufacturers in a range of sizes (26, 28, 32, 35, 37, 39, and 41Fr). An even smaller, uncuffed DLT is available for very small children.[81] Each tube differs slightly in bronchial cuff design[74] and in the length of the endobronchial segment distal to the bronchial cuff.[82] The relatively large lumens in all plastic tubes allow easy passage of a suction catheter or bronchoscope to either lung while presenting less resistance to airflow during one-lung ventilation.[83,84] The transparent plastic makes continuous observation of moisture during ventilation and the presence of secretions or blood in either lumen possible. Each bronchial cuff is dyed blue and is easily visualized during fiberoptic bronchoscopy.

In contrast with the low-volume/high-pressure cuffs of rubber DLTs, the bronchial cuff of plastic tubes have high-volume/low-pressure characteristics. This reduces the danger of ischemic pressure damage to the respiratory mucosa.[85,86] Since cuff shape differs among the different DLTs, each tube exerts a different degree of pressure on the airway wall when its bronchial cuff is inflated. As a general rule, less than 2–3 mL of air should be all that is needed for the bronchial cuff of any adult DLT.[87] As cuffs are extremely fragile, care must be taken when intubating the airway (see below).[88]

Choice of double-lumen tube

A malpositioned DLT will usually obstruct the upper-lobe bronchus. Therefore, the rationale for intubating the bronchus of the operative lung (right or left) is that the intubated lung is always visible during surgery. If the tube is not in a satisfactory position, the upper lobe will either be atelectactic when the chest is opened or the lung will fail to collapse when the appropriate lumen is clamped.[89,90] Bronchoscopy is not needed to confirm tube placement or to aid in repositioning.[91] The surgeon can manually help guide the tube if repositioning does become necessary.[92]

The potential disadvantage of placing the DLT in the bronchus of the operated lung is that there is a risk of displacing the tube with surgical manipulation. A DLT in the operated bronchus may also complicate the resection of that bronchus.[93] A DLT in the nonoperated bronchus (right or left) will stent the airway, thereby decreasing the chance that a sagging mediastinum will obstruct ventilation. However, lung distal to the tube tip can still be compressed.[94]

The human airway is asymmetrical. The average length of the adult left bronchus is about 5.0 cm, whereas the right bronchus is less than 2.0 cm long. Many anesthesiologists prefer a left DLT for both right and left operations in order to reduce the chance of obstructing the upper-lobe bronchus.[95]

A right DLT must be used if there is an intrinsic (tumor, stenosis) or extrinsic (tumor, aortic aneurysm) obstruction of the left bronchus. A right DLT is also used for sleeve resections of the left bronchus and during left single-lung transplants. If a right bronchial intubation is planned, a right rubber Robertshaw's tube may be a better choice. Rubber DLTs have a right upper-lobe ventilation slot that is approximately twice as long as the slot on a right plastic tube. A rubber right DLT therefore has less chance of obstructing the right-upper lobe.[93] The rubber Robersthaw's DLT is also shorter and has a larger external circumference than a plastic tube, so it is unlikely that it will be advanced too far into the right bronchus.

Size selection

The largest DLT with a bronchial lumen that fits the desired bronchus should be used.[96] Many of the problems with DLTs result from using a tube that is too small. Small tubes are often advanced too far into the bronchus, where they are more likely to obstruct the upper-lobe bronchus.[97] Since the bronchial cuff of a smaller tube must be inflated with a larger volume of air to seal the bronchus, the risk of airway injury is increased. During one-lung ventilation, there is more resistance to airflow through the lumen of a smaller tube and this generates higher levels of "auto-PEEP" in patients with COPD.[98]

Direct measurement of bronchial width from a chest radiograph has been tried as a means of selecting DLT size,[96] but the bronchus is not always visible on the chest radiograph. Measurement of the bronchus on the chest computed tomography (CT) scan is accurate, but may be impractical since it requires the assistance of a radiologist.[99,100]

The width of the left bronchus is directly proportional to the size of the trachea.[101] Since the trachea is visible and easily measured from a chest radiograph, tracheal width can be used to predict the size of the left bronchus. This allows selection of the appropriate size left DLT[102] (Table 47.3). The airway of most men will accept a 39Fr or 41Fr DLT, and for most women a 37Fr or 39Fr tube is indicated.[103]

A smaller tube may be needed if there is an intrinsic or extrinsic obstruction of the mainstem bronchus to be intubated.[104] Following a lung transplant, patients may have a bronchus that is significantly smaller than predicted from measurements of the native trachea.[105] For adult patients with very small bronchi relative to tracheal size owing to airway pathology, a bronchial blocker may be indicated.[106]

Placement

An appropriate size left DLT is selected using tracheal width guidelines.[107] Following preoxygenation, general anesthesia is induced and the patient is paralyzed for airway intubation. A Macintosh laryngoscope blade provides the largest area in which to pass a DLT. The improved vision (IV-MAC) laryngoscope blade is particularly useful for DLTs.[108] Extra care must be taken with plastic DLTs since their cuffs are fragile and easily torn by the patient's teeth. The tracheal cuff is usually the cuff that is damaged.[88,109]

The distal tip of the tube is advanced just past the vocal cords. The

Table 47.3 *Guidelines for left BronchoCath double-lumen tubes (DLTs)*

Measured tracheal width (mm)	Predicted left bronchus width (mm)	Recommended DLT size	OD (mm)	
			Main body	Left lumen
≥18	≥12.2	41Fr	14–15	10.6
≥16	≥10.9	39Fr	13–14	10.1
≥15	≥10.2	37Fr	13–14	10.0
≥14	≥9.5	35Fr	12–13	9.5
≥12.5	≥8.5	32Fr	10–11	8.3
≥11	≥7.5	28Fr	9.4	7.4

Tracheal width (mm) as measured from the chest radiograph.
Predicted size of left bronchus = tracheal width (mm) × 0.68
DLT, left-sided BronchoCath (Mallinckrodt Medical, St Louis, MO, USA); OD, outside diameter (mm) for main body and for left lumen of the BronchoCath DLT. Size specifications provided by the manufacturer.

stylet in the bronchial lumen is then removed. It has been recommended that the stylet be kept in place during the entire placement sequence to increase the success rate of entering the left bronchus.[110] The safety of this maneuver has not been demonstrated.

The tube is rotated 90–120° counterclockwise (toward the left bronchus) and is only then advanced down the trachea. The recommended endpoint of advancing the tube until a moderate resistance is encountered will often result in a DLT that is too deep in the bronchus, especially when a small tube is used. In both men and women, depth of placement is directly proportional to height.[111] For a man or woman of height 170 cm, the DLT should be advanced into the airway 29 cm, and for each ± 10-cm change in height the tube should be advanced or withdrawn ± 1 cm.

Several variations have been described for "blindly" positioning a DLT. The bronchial cuff can be partially inflated while the tube is in the trachea. Then the tube is advanced. When the bronchial lumen enters a bronchus, a marked rise in the tension in the bronchial cuff's pilot balloon will be noted and breath sounds will be heard only over the intubated lung.[112–114] Another method is to intentionally advance the tube deep into the bronchus until resistance is encountered. The bronchial cuff is inflated and the tube is withdrawn until the tension in the bronchial cuff's pilot balloon suddenly drops as the cuff enters the trachea. The tube is then readvanced back into the bronchus.[115] Both these methods involve moving the DLT while its bronchial cuff is inflated. This has the potential for damaging the airway. The following sequence of steps for safe "blind" placement of a left DLT is recommended.[116]

The tube is advanced into the bronchus to a depth based on the patient's height and both cuffs are inflated. When an appropriate size (large) tube is used, only 1–2 mL of air should be needed for the bronchial cuff. The patient is then ventilated through both lumens. Moisture should appear in each, indicating that both lumens are open to the lungs. Both sides of the chest should move with ventilation and bilateral breath sounds should be present.

Initially, the tracheal lumen is clamped. If the tube is in the left bronchus, breath sounds should now be heard only over the intubated left lung. If breath sounds are present bilaterally, the tube is probably not deep enough and should be advanced still further into the bronchus.

If at this point breath sounds are heard only over the right lung, the tube is in the right bronchus. In this situation, both cuffs should be deflated and the tube withdrawn several centimeters until it is in the trachea. Turning the patient's head and neck to the right while bending the head down will help direct the tube into the left bronchus.[117] The tube is rotated to the left and readvanced. Once the tube is in the left bronchus, the left lumen is clamped and the patient is ventilated through the tracheal lumen. Breath sounds should now be heard over the right lung. If the tube is not in a satisfactory position, there will be difficulty ventilating the patient since the inflated tracheal and bronchial cuffs will be obstructing gas flow from the tracheal opening. In this situation, by deflating the bronchial cuff and continuing to ventilate through the tracheal lumen one can accurately determine tube position. If the tube is not deep enough breath sounds will now be present bilaterally. If the tube is too deep, breath sounds will now be present only over the left lung. Both cuffs should be deflated and the tube should be advanced or withdrawn in 0.5-cm increments until it is in a satisfactory position.

Confirmation of double-lumen tube placement

DLT position must always be reconfirmed before surgery since tubes are easily displaced while moving the patient to the lateral decubitus position.[118] The tension in the pilot balloon to the bronchial cuff should be noted after first inflating that cuff.[119] DLTs are often displaced proximally with lateral positioning.[120] Therefore, after turning the patient or at any time during the procedure if the pilot balloon becomes softer the bronchial cuff is no longer completely in the bronchus. The tube should be advanced further into the bronchus until the initial tension in the pilot balloon returns. Confirmation of tube position is accomplished by physical examination of the chest, including auscultation and observation of chest wall movement and measurement of peak inspiratory pressures during independent ventilation of each lung. Water vapor in both lumens usually indicates that both lumens are open to gas-exchanging areas.

Controversy exists as to whether a bronchoscope should[121,122] or should not[91,123,124] be used *routinely* for DLT placement. A bronchoscope is often used to visually confirm DLT position.[125] Looking down the tracheal lumen, there should be an unobstructed view of the blue bronchial cuff below the carina in the appropriate bronchus.[126] Several studies have reported that DLTs placed "blindly," i.e. without bronchoscope confirmation, are frequently not in an "ideal" position.[127–130] A tube is considered to be in an ideal position when the proximal edge of its bronchial cuff is immediately below the carina in the appropriate bronchus.[126] Most "malpositioned" tubes are actually only slightly deeper in the bronchus and will function without problems.[107] Since most tubes will be displaced proximally when turning the patient,[120] bronchoscopic visualization in the supine position is really only useful to determine whether the endobronchial lumen has been placed on the appropriate side.[131] A bronchial cuff 0.5–1.0 cm inside the left bronchus initially will avoid cuff displacement into the trachea when the patient is turned to the decubitus position.

The bronchoscope should also be passed down the bronchial lumen to insure patency of that lumen and to confirm that the upper-lobe orifice is not obstructed. A 4.9-mm-diameter bronchoscope will pass down larger DLTs, but a 3.6-mm-diameter bronchoscope is needed if smaller (35Fr, 37Fr) tubes are used.[132] Very thin pediatric bronchoscopes are needed for smaller (28Fr or 32Fr) tubes. Capnography,[133,134] continuous monitoring by spirometry with flow–volume or pressure–volume loops,[135] and even chest radiographs and fluoroscopy have been used to determine the correct DLT position. If visualization of the glottis by direct laryngoscopy is not possible, a DLT can be advanced over a bronchoscope. Likewise, a bronchoscope in the bronchial lumen can be used as a stylet to advance the DLT into the bronchus if "blind" intubation of that bronchus fails.[136]

If continued ventilatory support is required at the completion of thoracotomy, the DLT may need to be replaced with a conventional endotracheal tube. This can be challenging if the initial intubation was difficult, or even hazardous if airway edema has developed during the procedure. A variety of stylets and tracheal tube exchangers can be used to more safely change from a DLT to an endotracheal tube.[137,138]

Complications

Although DLTs are generally safe and easy to use, complications do occur (Table 47.4). The most frequent problems relate to DLT position. A misplaced DLT can result in airway damage and hypoxemia or compromise any procedure if the operated lung fails to collapse.

DLT position can change at any time during surgery, so constant vigilance is important. Ventilation of the dependent lung, through either the tracheal or bronchial lumen, is never directly visualized. The patient must be monitored by observing changes in the peak inspiratory pressure to the dependent lung, end-tidal CO_2 levels, S_{pO_2}, and most importantly mediastinal movement during inspiration. If in doubt, a bronchoscope should be used to confirm tube position.

The airway can be traumatized during intubation and extubation. Most injuries are clinically insignificant – usually asymptomatic ecchymosis of the mucous membranes.[110] More serious problems (arytenoid dislocation, torn vocal cords) occur, but have become relatively uncommon since plastic DLTs replaced the more rigid rubber DLTs.

When the softer plastic DLTs were introduced in the early 1980s, it was thought that they were safer than rubber tubes.[86,139] However, airway rupture has been reported with both rubber[140–145] and plastic DLTs.[146–151] The factors that increase the risk of airway rupture are listed in Table 47.5. Airway damage can present with air leak, subcutaneous surgical emphysema, airway hemorrhage, and cardiovascular instability due to tension pneumothorax. With incomplete laceration, air may dissect into the adventitia, producing an aneurysmal dilation of the membranous wall. If N_2O is used, it will further distend this air collection. The signs of injury may not be evident for many hours after the initial injury, when rupture into the mediastinum or pleural space occurs.[152]

Both cuffs should be deflated when moving the patient or changing the position of the DLT. It is safer to keep the bronchial cuff deflated whenever lung isolation or selective ventilation is not required.

A fiberoptic bronchoscope should be available to inspect the airway if mediastinal emphysema or loss of tidal volume occurs at any time during the surgery. Bronchoscopy should be performed before extubation to identify evidence of trauma if an airway disruption is suspected as this requires immediate surgical intervention for a favorable prognosis.[153] At the completion of every thoracotomy, the integrity of the intubated bronchus should be tested with manual ventilation for leaks with only the tracheal cuff inflated. Table 47.6 lists recommendations to reduce the incidence of major airway injury from a DLT.

A DLT should never be forcibly advanced. One should be even more cautious in patients who have airway pathology such as tracheomalacia or tumor infiltration, and for patients who are immunosuppressed or who are receiving steroids.

Both the bronchial and tracheal cuffs must be inflated with air slowly. It is extremely important not to overinflate the bronchial cuff. A 3-mL syringe can be used for the bronchial cuff as a reminder that 2–3 mL of air is usually the volume needed if an appropriate size (large) tube has been selected.

Table 47.4 *Complications of double-lumen tubes (DLTs)*

Intubation
Carinal hook unable to pass by glottis (Carlens's or White's DLT)
Unable to advance bronchial limb into bronchus
Tube too large
Airway obstruction (intrinsic or extrinsic)
Trauma
Dental trauma
Airway injury
Laryngitis, mucosal ecchymosis, arytenoid dislocation, tracheobronchial rupture
Ruptured thoracic aneurysm
Position
Not far enough into bronchus
Bronchial cuff in carina
Unable to ventilate nonintubated lung with both cuffs inflated or unable to deflate intubated lung
Failure to seal airway – contamination of healthy lung
Down wrong bronchus
Too deep in correct bronchus
Obstruction of upper lobe causing hypoxemia
Failure to collapse upper lobe
Changes during surgery
Surgical manipulation
Movement of patient to decubitus position
Head flexion or extension
Tube inadequately taped or secured
Hypoxemia
Malpositioned DLT
Collapse upper lobe of nonoperated lung
Obstruction by bronchial cuff in trachea
Torsion of tube or bronchial lumen opening against bronchial wall
Carinal hook bent back, obstructing tracheal lumen
Miscellaneous
Bronchial lumen interferes with surgical procedures
Pneumonectomy, carinal or sleeve resection, lung transplant
Displacement of mediastinal mass
Bronchial lumen sutured to pulmonary vessel

Nitrous oxide should avoided.[154] When N_2O is used, both cuffs should be inflated with either saline or an O_2/N_2O mixture to prevent cuff distention during the procedure. The bronchial and tracheal cuffs should be deflated periodically to avoid build-up of excessive pressure on the mucosa.

Underinflation of the bronchial cuff can result in a cross-leak with failure to collapse the lung undergoing surgery and contamination of the dependent lung. Overinflation of the bronchial cuff can damage the airway or obstruct the trachea. Several techniques have been described to determine the exact endpoint for cuff inflation.[155,156]

OPTIMIZING OXYGENATION DURING ONE-LUNG VENTILATION

In the lateral decubitus position, approximately 40% of the cardiac output flows to the nondependent lung and 60% goes to the dependent lung. There is normally perfusion of nongas-exchanging areas in each

Table 47.5 *Risk factors associated with airway rupture*

Direct trauma
Forceful insertion
Frayed tube tip (rubber DLTs only)
Too large DLT – bronchial lumen too large for bronchus
Tube advanced with stylet in place (?)
Movement of tube with cuffs inflated
Carinal hook damages upper airway (Carlens's and White's DLTs)
Cuff overinflation
Too rapid inflation
Too large a volume
Too small DLT (requires larger volume to seal the bronchus)
Overdistention from N_2O
Asymmetric cuff distension – pushes tip into airway wall (rubber DLTs)
Pre-existing airway pathology
Congenital airway wall abnormalities
Airway wall weakness from tumor infiltration or infection
Airway distortion from lymph nodes, intra- and extrabronchial tumors
Patients receiving steroids
Patients with leukemia and lymphoma
Hypotension with hypoperfusion to the airway

DLTs, double-lumen tubes.

Table 47.6 *Recommendations for DLT placement*

1	Select the largest plastic DLT that will safely fit the airway
2	Remove the bronchial stylet as soon as the tube is past the vocal cords
3	Be extra cautious with patients who have tracheobronchial wall pathology, leukemia, steroids, hypoperfusion
4	Advance the DLT into the bronchus to a depth based on the patient's height
5	Inflate both cuffs slowly – never overinflate either cuff
6	Use a 3-mL syringe to inflate bronchial cuff – usually < 3 mL air is adequate if an appropriate size (large) DLT is selected. If more air is needed, reassess tube position by auscultation or by bronchoscopy
7	If you use N_2O, inflate both cuffs with saline or an O_2/N_2O mixture rather than air alone – measure cuff pressures intermittently and periodically relieve pressure (if necessary) by partially deflating the cuff to the original inflation volume. Keep bronchial cuff pressure < 30 cmH_2O
8	Deflate both cuffs before moving the patient, deflate the bronchial cuff when lung isolation or selective ventilation is not needed
9	During esophageal procedures, consider partial deflation of the cuff when surgical dissection is near either cuff
10	Test the integrity of the intubated bronchus at the completion of surgery, use fiberoptic bronchoscopy to determine site and extent of injury

DLT, double-lumen tube.

lung, so during two-lung ventilation with the patient in the lateral position approximately 35% of the cardiac output participates in gas exchange in the nondependent lung.

Following selective lung collapse, the lung undergoing surgery continues to be perfused but is not ventilated. Several factors influence the magnitude of this "shunt." Blood flow to the dependent, ventilated lung is increased by the effects of gravity and by the increased vascular resistance in the lung undergoing surgery from surgical retraction and the effects of total atelectasis. Other factors that influence the degree of arterial hypoxemia during one-lung ventilation include inadequate inspired oxygen concentration ($F_{I}O_2$) and alveolar hypoventilation. Additionally, the right lung has more gas-exchanging areas than the left, and there is a greater drop in $P_{a}O_2$ with one-lung ventilation during right-sided operations than during similar procedures on the left side.[157]

Systemic vasopressors (dopamine, epinephrine, phenylephrine) preferentially constrict vessels perfusing normoxic or hyperoxic lung segments, resulting in redistribution of blood flow to the collapsed lung. Vasodilators (nitroprusside, nitroglycerin) relax vascular smooth muscle in the collapsed lung by releasing NO. This increases blood flow to the operated lung, thereby lowering $P_{a}O_2$. Drugs that inhibit NO release maintain the HPV response.[158] Surgical manipulation of the lung releases vasoactive substances that blunt HPV.[38] During video-assisted thoracoscopic surgery there is less direct trauma to the lung, so HPV may play a more important role during this type of surgery than during open thoracotomy. Increased pulmonary vascular resistance may be present preoperatively in a chronically diseased lung, so blood flow may already be preferentially diverted to the healthy lung.

When changing from two- to one-lung ventilation, tidal volume should be continued unchanged. The ventilator rate should be adjusted to keep $P_{a}CO_2$ at 4.8–5.33 kPa (36–40 mmHg). If end-tidal CO_2 measurements are used, it must be realized that, in the lateral decubitus position, these values during one-lung ventilation may be as much as 1.33 kPa (10 mmHg) lower than actual $P_{a}CO_2$. Hypocarbia should be avoided because it will increase pulmonary vascular resistance in the ventilated lung and redirect blood flow to the nonventilated lung. Hypercarbia is usually not a problem if minute ventilation is maintained.

The position of the DLT or bronchial blocker should be immediately reconfirmed if hypoxemia occurs. Other mechanical problems (tube obstruction, bronchospasm) should be considered. Clinically significant hypoxemia usually does not occur immediately after initiation of one-lung ventilation, but after 10–15 min because it takes that long for the nonventilated lung to completely collapse and for any remaining O_2 in that lung to be absorbed.

The largest proportion of the cardiac output is directed to the ventilated lung, therefore matching ventilation to perfusion is important. In the lateral decubitus position, the intra-abdominal contents shift the diaphragm cephalad, thus reducing the FRC of the dependent lung. General anesthesia further decreases FRC. Therefore, during lateral thoracotomy, the dependent lung may have areas of low ventilation to perfusion ratios and areas that are completely atelectactic. To maximize $P_{a}O_2$ the dependent lung should be ventilated with 100% O_2 with a large tidal volume.[159]

Relatively large tidal volumes (10–14 mL kg^{-1}) are needed to recruit dependent lung alveoli. Tidal volumes of less than 8 mL kg^{-1} result in a further decrease in FRC, which leads to increased areas of dependent lung atelectasis. Larger tidal volumes (> 15 mL kg^{-1}) overdistend the alveoli and increase pulmonary vascular resistance, thereby causing redistribution of blood flow to the nondependent lung.

Even with a shunt of 25% to the nonventilated lung, an $F_{I}O_2$ of 1.0 and large tidal volume ventilation will usually produce a $P_{a}O_2$ > 20 kPa (150 mmHg).[160] At this oxygen tension, arterial hemoglobin is 100% saturated. A high $F_{I}O_2$ causes vasodilation of the vessels in the dependent lung, increasing perfusion of that lung and further decreasing shunt.

A theoretical concern is that an $F_{I}O_2$ of 1.0 can lead to absorption atelectasis of the dependent lung. Although the addition of 10–20% nitrogen to the inspired gas mixture will decrease the propensity for the dependent lung to collapse, clinically this maneuver is unnecessary. Concerns about pulmonary damage from hyperoxia are only relevant for patients with histories of certain drugs (bleomycin, nitrofurantoin, amiodarone, mitomycin C) or acute inflammatory lung diseases. These have been associated with postoperative pulmonary oxygen toxicity.[161–163]

During one-lung ventilation, peak inspiratory pressure will be high because the dependent lung will have decreased compliance while being inflated with a relatively large tidal volume.[164] In addition, airway resistance will be increased through the single lumen of the DLT. Since airway pressure changes may be great, continuous monitoring of ventilatory mechanics during one-lung ventilation has been recommended.[165] Special ventilators employing instantaneous breath-to-breath analysis to adjust ventilatory patterns (adaptive lung ventilation) have been used during one-lung ventilation.[166]

The traditional practice of using large tidal ventilation during one-lung ventilation is now questioned. Barotrauma, presumably from high peak pressures during one-lung ventilation, has been associated with pulmonary complications following thoracotomy. Pressure-controlled ventilation has been suggested as an alternative to volume-controlled ventilation during one-lung ventilation. Pressure-controlled ventilation is associated with lower peak airway pressures, lower shunt, and higher oxygen levels than conventional volume-controlled ventilation.[167]

If hypoxemia occurs during one-lung ventilation, PEEP can be applied to the ventilated lung. Many factors cause a reduction in FRC during one-lung ventilation, including the effects of general anesthesia, the pressure of the abdominal contents on the diaphragm, the weight of the sagging mediastinum, and incorrect positioning of the patient on the operating room table. In the presence of decreased FRC, PEEP [10 cmH_2O (1.0 kPa)] will recruit collapsed and underinflated alveoli and improve oxygenation. However, with normal or increased FRC, PEEP will decrease cardiac output, increase alveolar airway pressure, and increase dependent lung pulmonary vascular resistance, which in turn will divert blood flow to the nonventilated lung, thereby increasing hypoxemia.[168]

During one-lung ventilation, if alveolar pressure fails to fall to atmospheric pressure at the end of expiration, "intrinsic" or auto-PEEP will be generated.[169,170] The degree of auto-PEEP that develops is determined by several factors, including the extent of preoperative pulmonary disease, the time allowed for expiration, and airflow resistance through the single lumen of the DLT. Auto-PEEP also increases with age, perhaps because of loss of lung elastic recoil.

Although some patients do benefit from the addition of external PEEP during one-lung ventilation, at present it is not possible to predict who those patients are.[171] External PEEP may be therapeutic during one-lung ventilation in patients who do not generate significant levels of auto-PEEP.[172]

The collapsed lung can be partially re-expanded to treat severe hypoxemia. A single breath to the operated lung will temporarily correct the ventilation–perfusion imbalance.[173] The lung will slowly recollapse, so it must be re-expanded about every 5 min. This maneuver cannot be used during video-assisted thoracoscopic surgery as it will interfere with operative exposure.

Insufflation with 100% O_2 to the nonventilated lung is inadequate treatment for hypoxemia because the O_2 will fail to reach and recruit collapsed alveoli. However, insufflation by CPAP with 100% O_2 to the nonventilated lung is a very effective means of correcting hypoxemia.[174–176]

CPAP maintains the patency of the operated alveoli with O_2, so unsaturated mixed venous blood perfusing that lung becomes oxygenated. Any increased airway pressure from the CPAP may further increase pulmonary vascular resistance, which will divert blood flow to the dependent, ventilated lung. The nonventilated lung remains partially distended but "quiet" with CPAP.

Initially, relatively high pressures are required when applying CPAP to an atelectatic lung in order to open the collapsed alveoli. CPAP should be applied during the deflation phase of a full breath to the nondependent lung.[177] Once distended, relatively small levels of CPAP [5–10 cmH_2O (0.5–1.0 kPa)] are all that is required to maintain satisfactory oxygenation. Higher levels of CPAP overdistend the lung and interfere with surgical exposure.

CPAP is effective only when there are no major disruptions in the airway because a nonintact bronchus will not allow distending pressures to be maintained. CPAP is therefore not helpful with a bronchopleural fistula, during sleeve resection of the airway, or during massive pulmonary hemorrhage or bronchopleural lavage. Any airway obstruction by mucus, blood, or tumor may not permit adequate airway pressures to reach the lung. CPAP is not normally used for treating hypoxemia during video-assisted thoracoscopic surgery since any distention of the lung undergoing surgery will compromise the surgical exposure.

The combination of PEEP (5–10 cmH_2O) applied to the ventilated lung and CPAP (5–10 cmH_2O) to the nonventilated lung has been used to treat severe hypoxemia, but is seldom necessary when upper-lung CPAP is used alone.[178]

In animal models, inflation of a nonocclusive pulmonary artery catheter balloon located in the main pulmonary artery of the lung undergoing surgery can redistribute blood flow to the lung not undergoing surgery. However, if the pulmonary artery catheter were to shift to the dependent lung, inflation of the balloon could potentially increase hypoxemia by redirecting blood to the upper lung.

During a pneumonectomy, ligation of the pulmonary artery completely eliminates shunt, thus maximizing the relation between ventilation and perfusion. Clamping the lobar pulmonary artery during lobectomy should increase vascular resistance in that lung segment, directing more blood to the ventilated lung. Occlusion of the main pulmonary artery during limited pulmonary resection is not advised as this maneuver will alter the activity of the alveolar lining material (surfactant) and will deleteriously affect lung re-expansion following surgery, i.e. it will potentially induce an ischemia–reperfusion injury.

Pharmacologic manipulation of the pulmonary blood flow is another approach to matching perfusion with ventilation. It has been suggested that, since some endogenous prostaglandins inhibit HPV, prostaglandin inhibitors might potentiate the HPV response and improve oxygenation during one-lung ventilation. In an *in vitro* study, ibuprofen, a cyclo-oxygenase inhibitor, did reverse the depression of HPV by halothane.[179]

Direct infusion of prostaglandin F_{2a}, a potent pulmonary vasoconstrictor, into the pulmonary artery of the nonventilated lung during one-lung ventilation results in a significant decrease in shunt and an increase in $P_{a}O_2$.[180] The continuous infusion of a vasodilator, prostaglandin E_1, into the pulmonary artery of the ventilated lung improved both arterial oxygenation and venous admixture during one-lung ventilation.[181,182]

Nitric oxide has an important physiologic role in the modulation of vascular tone. The vasodilator properties of inhaled NO (NO_i) are restricted to the pulmonary circulation.[183] NO_i (5–80 p.p.m.) decreases pulmonary vascular resistance in animal models.[184] NO_i also decreased pulmonary vascular resistance during one-lung ventilation in supine patients.[185] However, during one-lung ventilation in the lateral position, NO_i (40 p.p.m.) did not decrease mean pulmonary artery pressure in patients with normal pulmonary vascular resistance and the shunt remained unchanged.[186]

The use of NO_i to improve oxygenation during one-lung ventilation has been disappointing. This may be because the effects of NO_i are directly proportional to the degree of pulmonary vascular resistance present in the ventilated lung before NO administration and most patients undergoing pulmonary resection have normal or only slightly elevated pulmonary artery pressures.

During one-lung ventilation, the combination of NO_i to the ventilated lung and a potent pulmonary vasoconstrictor (almitrine) decreased perfusion to lung undergoing surgery and markedly improved oxygenation.[187] NO_i and other pulmonary vasoconstrictors may prove helpful for hypoxemia during video-assisted thoracoscopic surgery when application of CPAP is not practical.[188]

VENTILATION AT THE COMPLETION OF THORACOTOMY

Prior to reinflating the collapsed lung, both lumens of the DLT should be suctioned to remove any mucus, blood, or debris from each lung. Both lungs must be fully re-expanded and the mediastinum must be midline at the completion of one-lung ventilation. Following total collapse, the operated lung will re-expand unevenly during inflation. Lung volume increases as collapsed alveoli are recruited. Alterations in pulmonary surfactant occur during one-lung ventilation and this necessitates the application of high-sustained pressures in order to reopen the atelectactic lung. Once the lung has been fully reinflated and deflates to residual volume, subsequent inflation will require lower pressures consistent with normal surfactant activity.

Following any pulmonary resection, the integrity of the bronchial repair or the bronchial stump must be tested before the chest is closed. The surgeon pours warm saline into the pleural cavity while the anesthesiologist applies increasing levels of inflation pressures [up to 30–40 cmH_2O (3–4 kPa)] by manually compressing the reservoir bag. This maneuver demonstrates air leaks and, when repeated several times, allows the previously collapsed lung to fully re-expand. Although a lung that has been collapsed for several days can develop unilateral ("re-expansion") pulmonary edema if inflated too rapidly, this is extremely uncommon following one-lung ventilation.

Immediately after most thoracic procedures (including pneumonectomy), patients should be extubated and allowed to breathe spontaneously. After any pulmonary resection, positive-pressure ventilation places stress on the bronchial suture line and exacerbates air leakage and formation of a bronchopleural fistula.

POST-THORACOTOMY PAIN MANAGEMENT

The decrease in FRC and the ability to cough and breathe deeply following thoracotomy are influenced by pain. The patient who experiences pain may be unable or unwilling to clear secretions. This in turn can lead to atelectasis and eventually pneumonia. Besides improved pulmonary function, comfortable patients have a lower incidence of cardiac complications after thoracic procedures.[189]

Analgesic regimens associated with the best post-thoracotomy pulmonary function are generally felt to be superior. In addition to spirometry and arterial blood gas values, post-thoracotomy pain is also assessed by visual analog pain scores (at rest and with cough and movement), the amount of additional opioid requested, the length of hospital stay, and overall patient satisfaction.

The lateral thoracotomy incision is very painful.[190] The site and extent of the incision influences the degree of pain. Disruption of intercostal nerves and inflammation of the chest wall and pleura all contribute to the discomfort. The number and the sites of the chest drainage tubes also influence pain. Some patients also experience shoulder pain of unknown etiology following thoracotomy.[191]

Systemic opioids

Systemic opioids have a very narrow therapeutic window. With inadequate pain relief, the patient will be unwilling to cough and clear secretions while the overmedicated patient will be oversedated and unable to cough and breathe deeply.

Intermittent opioid administration may be associated with a significant time lag between the request for medication, the actual administration of the medication, and the onset of action. When systemic opioids are used, patient-controlled analgesia (PCA) or continuous intravenous infusion are preferred.[192,193]

Neuraxial opioids

Neuraxial (epidural, intrathecal) analgesia can reduce pain and improve pulmonary function following thoracotomy.[194]

The current practice is to combine epidural local anesthetics with epidural opioids.[195] However, the addition of a local anesthetic may not significantly improve the analgesia achieved by epidural opioids alone.[196,197] The addition of bupivacaine (0.1%) does not affect epidural meperidine (pethidine) requirements, but does reduce pruritus after thoracotomy.[198] Hypotension or motor blockade from the local anesthetic may limit the patient's ability to ambulate. The addition of epinephrine, even in concentrations as low as 1:300 000, does decrease the amount of opioid needed for effective analgesia.[199]

Post-thoracotomy opioid neuraxial analgesia, when compared with parenterally administered opioids, improves pulmonary function and oxygenation and reduces postoperative complications.[200–203] This has been demonstrated with every opioid that has been given either intrathecally or epidurally following thoracic surgery.[204–206]

Unlike local anesthetics, neuraxial opioids are "selective." Other than potentiation of analgesia, they have no known hemodynamic or motor effects. Opioids work by binding to opiate receptors in the spinal cord. There is some evidence that pre-emptive administration of epidural opioids before surgical incision can reduce pain following thoracotomy.[207] Single-shot intrathecal morphine produces analgesia for up to 24 h, but the intrathecal route is limited by the need for repeated injections unless a catheter is placed.[208]

The epidural route is generally preferred since the incidence of respiratory depression is less than with intrathecal opioids and the presence of a catheter allows for continuous, prolonged drug administration in the postoperative period. Patient-controlled epidural opioid analgesia is also possible if a catheter is present.[209] Depending on the agent selected, a catheter placed at either the lumbar or the thoracic epidural level is effective for post-thoracotomy analgesia.[210]

Lipophilic agents rapidly diffuse across the dura into the cerebral spinal fluid, bind to the spinal opiate receptors, and produce a rapid onset of action. The more lipid soluble the agent, the more potent it is. Lipophilic agents such as fentanyl and sufentanil are better suited for epidural administration at the thoracic level.[211] These drugs provide satisfactory analgesia following thoracotomy, but because of their relatively short duration of action they should be administered by constant infusion.

Lipophilic opioids are rapidly absorbed into the systemic and cerebral circulation, and severe acute postoperative respiratory depression may occur with even small doses of epidural sufentanil.[212] Hydrophilic agents (morphine, hydromorphone) diffuse more slowly into the cerebral spinal fluid.[213] Their onset of action is delayed, but the length of action is longer than with the lipophilic agents. These agents are preferred when a continuous infusion is not possible.

Hydrophilic opioids can also be safely administered by constant infusion. Their low lipid solubility allows these drugs to be given either at the thoracic or at the lumbar level for post-thoracotomy pain relief without any difference in analgesic efficacy.

The complications of epidural opioids administered during surgery occur in the postoperative period. All epidural opioids decrease the ventilatory response to CO_2, but significant respiratory depression and apnea are rare. The lipophilic drugs cause *acute* respiratory depression owing to central effects from systemic absorption. The hydrophilic opioids are associated with *delayed* respiratory depression occurring hours after administration, presumably as a result of the rostral spread of the drug in the cerebrospinal fluid to the brain.

The factors predisposing to delayed respiratory depression include: concomitant administration of opioids or sedatives by other routes prior to or during surgery; high doses; the hydrophilicity of the agent;

advanced age; and the site of administration (intrathecal > thoracic epidural > lumbar epidural). With appropriate dosing and selection of patients, serious respiratory depression is uncommon. The frequency and occurrence of minor complications (pruritus, urinary retention, nausea, and vomiting) varies with the specific opioid used and should not be a contraindication for their use following thoracotomy.

Adjuncts

Cryoanalgesia, the freezing of intercostal nerves, can reduce incisional pain following thoracotomy. The nerve at the incision space and the two intercostal nerves above and below are frozen. The loss of sensory and motor function that follows cryoanalgesia usually lasts 1–6 months. However, many patients experience painful neuralgias at the treatment sites.[214] Cryoanalgesia may reduce, but does not eliminate, post-thoracotomy pain and is useful only as a supplement to other forms of pain control.[215]

Electrodes can be placed on either side of the thoracic incision and electrical stimulation applied (transcutaneous electric nerve stimulation; TENS). TENS does not reduce opioid requirements or improve pulmonary function following thoracotomy, but is effective in treating pain after video-assisted thoracoscopic surgery.[216]

Intercostal nerve blocks can be performed directly intraoperatively with the lung collapsed or percutaneously following surgery. These blocks reduce opioid requirements following thoracotomy. Continuous blocks are more practical than repeated individual blocks owing to the relatively short action of the local anesthetics.[217,218] Continuous intercostal blockade can be achieved by placing several catheters in the intercostal grooves during surgery. Systemic toxicity from intravascular absorption or from direct injection and unrecognized dural puncture resulting in marked hypotension are major complications of intercostal nerve blocks.

Interpleural blockade can be performed by injecting local anesthetics into the thoracic cavity between the visceral and parietal pleura.[219] One approach is to place an epidural catheter directly through the chest wall. Local anesthetics can also be given directly into the chest drainage tube after the lung has been re-expanded. Because a significant loss of local anesthetic can occur with an open chest drainage tube, clamping the chest tube following anesthetic administration increases the success rate.[220] Pain relief following thoracotomy is incomplete when the interpleural technique is used alone.[221,222] Local anesthetic on the diaphragm may actually impair respiratory function.[223] Interpleural analgesia is useful for analgesia following video-assisted thoracoscopic surgery.[224]

Ipsilateral stellate ganglion block is also effective for treating shoulder pain after thoracotomy.[225] Nonsteroidal anti-inflammatory drugs (NSAIDs) are also effective for shoulder pain resistant to epidural analgesia. When used in combination with other analgesics, NSAIDs improve pain relief and postoperative pulmonary function following thoracotomy.[226,227] Ketorolac supplementation of hydromorphone epidural analgesia reduced total opioid requirement and was associated with better postoperative pulmonary function than the combination of epidural hydromorphone and bupivacaine.[228]

NSAIDs have a peripheral site of action, have anti-inflammatory and antipyretic activity, and can be conveniently administered intravenously or by rectal suppository. One advantage after thoracotomy is that they are not respiratory depressants. Side-effects, including increased bleeding time, gastrointestinal and central nervous system symptoms, and a deterioration of renal function, may limit their use in some at-risk patients.

Low-dose intramuscular or intravenous ketamine is another useful adjunct for post-thoracotomy analgesia.[229,230] Intravenous tramadol, an analgesic with mixed μ-opioid and nonopioid activity, is also effective in the treatment of post-thoracotomy pain.[231]

POST-THORACOTOMY COMPLICATIONS

Atelectasis

The most common pulmonary complication following thoracotomy is atelectasis. Significant atelectasis will cause a mismatch of ventilation with perfusion and result in hypoxemia.

Atelectasis may develop from pulmonary injury during surgery, incomplete lung re-expansion following one-lung ventilation, or from bronchial obstruction by mucus as a result of inadequate clearance of secretions. Deep breathing, coughing, pulmonary toilet with suctioning, and clearance of secretions with incentive spirometry, aerosolized bronchodilators, and early postoperative ambulation are important. Effective pain relief is essential.

For lobar or whole lung atelectasis due to mucus plugging, the patient should be placed in the lateral position with the healthy lung dependent. This position improves ventilation/perfusion and promotes mucus drainage from the operated lung. If oxygenation does not improve with lateral positioning and chest physiotherapy, fiberoptic or rigid bronchoscopy and lavage may be required.

Unresolved atelectasis can proceed to pneumonia, a potentially fatal condition following pneumonectomy and in patients with borderline pulmonary reserve. Associated respiratory failure may require reintubation of the airway and mechanical ventilation.[232] This increases the risk of stump disruption and formation of a bronchopleural fistula. Empyema (pus in the pleural space) may result from pneumonia.

Airway trauma

Injury to the airway can occur at any time during surgery and may go unrecognized intraoperatively. A damaged airway can present postoperatively with respiratory distress, an air leak, subcutaneous emphysema, hemorrhage, or cardiovascular instability owing to tension pneumothorax.

Immediate surgical intervention is essential. Any positive-pressure ventilation, even mask-assisted ventilation, will cause gas to enter either subcutaneous tissue or the chest, further exacerbating the situation. An awake bronchoscope-guided intubation of the airway is recommended, followed by spontaneous ventilation with an inhalational anesthetic agent. For a tracheal injury, the endotracheal tube should be carefully advanced past the defect. For a bronchial injury, the tube should be placed in the intact bronchus and the injured lung isolated.

Pneumothorax

In the presence of a bronchopleural communication, the volume of air in the pleural space will increase. A tension pneumothorax will develop if air continues to enter the chest and is not effectively decompressed. The risk of pneumothorax following pulmonary resection is reduced by placement of a pleural drainage tube. However, a pneumothorax can still develop if the chest tube or suction apparatus malfunctions, or if the tube is occluded. The tube must have access to the air leak. Positive-pressure ventilation, especially with PEEP, increases the risk of developing a pneumothorax.

If the pneumothorax continues to enlarge it will displace mediastinal structures and compress the great vessels, leading to cardiovascular collapse. Signs of a tension pneumothorax include decreased chest movement and diminished breath sounds, a unilateral wheeze, and hyper-resonance to percussion on the affected side. The peak inspiratory pressure during mechanical ventilation will increase and may reach very high levels. A chest radiograph is diagnostic. The patient may experience increasing respiratory distress, tachypnea, tachycardia, and hypotension. A decrease in S_pO_2 may occur before other signs become obvious. Immediate decompression with a large intravenous catheter or new chest tube may be lifesaving.

Cardiac herniation

Cardiac herniation can occur after pneumonectomy if the adjacent pericardium has been disrupted.[233] If the pericardial defect is repaired intraoperatively, the risk of herniation is low. Herniation is more common following right pneumonectomy. After left pneumonectomy, the great vessels and mediastinal structures provide more of a barrier to herniation. Factors that contribute to cardiac herniation include suction applied to the side of pneumonectomy, positioning the patient with the operated side dependent, positive-pressure ventilation, coughing, and vomiting.

The signs of cardiac herniation occur following surgery and may include radiographic abnormalities, atrial and ventricular dysrhythmias, sudden hypotension, and superior vena caval syndrome.[234] Cardiovascular collapse occurs as a result of acute angulation of the heart and great vessels.

Hemodynamic stability can only return following surgical replacement of the heart to its normal position. If not immediately diagnosed and promptly treated, cardiac herniation is almost uniformly fatal. Even with aggressive treatment the mortality rate is 50%.[235] Until the chest is reopened, the patient should be positioned on the side with the remaining lung dependent.

Hemorrhage

The clinical signs of major hemorrhage (tachycardia, hypotension, oliguria) are usually obvious in hypovolemic patients. Excessive chest tube drainage and a falling hematocrit are indications for surgical reexploration.

Structural injuries

Structural injuries following thoracotomy occur from intraoperative surgical trauma or from malpositioning. The phrenic nerve is often injured, especially during extensive mediastinal dissection or if the nerve is embedded in tumor. The patient may experience some distress during spontaneous breathing. For the patient with limited pulmonary reserve, this complication can be devastating. The chest radiograph will reveal an elevated hemidiaphragm.

The left recurrent laryngeal nerve can be injured during hilar dissection. A unilateral injury usually results in hoarseness, but is otherwise asymptomatic.

Damage to the thoracic duct can occur from surgery or from central venous cannulation on the left side. Surgical intervention may be necessary to stop the resulting chylothorax.[236]

Dysrhythmias

Supraventricular dysrhythmias (atrial tachycardia, atrial flutter, and atrial fibrillation) occur in as many as 20% of patients following pneumonectomy.[237] Arrhythmias can occur after any thoracotomy or video-assisted thoracoscopic procedure.[238] Advanced age and pre-existing cardiac disease are important risk factors.

Any resulting impaired cardiac output may require fluid loading to enhance preload, which in turn can adversely affect pulmonary function. Prophylactic digitalization has long been recommended, especially following pneumonectomy, but recent studies have reported either no difference[239] or a higher incidence[189] of arrhythmias in thoracic surgical patients receiving digoxin. Prophylactic metoprolol can decrease the incidence of atrial fibrillation after pulmonary resection.[240]

Arrhythmias associated with profound hypotension require immediate cardioversion. Verapamil has been reported to be effective for atrial flutter or multifocal atrial tachycardia after lung resection.[241] Verapamil can cause hypotension from vasodilatory and negative inotropic effects and significant bradycardia occurs in as many as 25% of patients.[242] The administration of phenylephrine will support cardiac output. Beta-blockade may be necessary for rapid supraventricular dysrhythmias associated with hypertension and myocardial ischemia, but beta-blockers may cause bronchospasm. Esmolol is effective but short acting, so a continuous intravenous infusion may be needed.

Postpneumonectomy pulmonary edema

Pulmonary edema after pneumonectomy, an often fatal complication, is relatively common. Postpneumonectomy pulmonary edema occurs in as many as 5% of patients.[243] Some studies have associated positive fluid balance,[244,245] while others find no clear-cut relation between intraoperative fluid load and the development of pulmonary edema.[246] Postpneumonectomy pulmonary edema may be the result of increased pulmonary endothelial permeability after pneumonectomy[247] or impaired lymphatic drainage following radical lymph node dissection.

Cardiac output and right-heart filling pressures should be monitored following pneumonectomy if there is evidence of tissue hypoperfusion, especially when epidural-administered local anesthesia has caused vasodilation and hypotension. In most situations, small amounts of a vasopressor (ephedrine or neosynephrine) rather than intravenous fluid should be used to improve cardiac performance.

Right-heart failure

Extensive lung resection decreases pulmonary vascular cross-sectional area, resulting in increased pulmonary vascular resistance, which may lead to acute right-heart failure with or without pulmonary edema. Prior to pneumonectomy, if temporary unilateral occlusion of the main pulmonary artery to the operated lung by a PA catheter increases mean PA pressure more than 4–5.33 kPa (30–40 mmHg), the risk for postoperative right-heart failure is high. Even when predicted right-heart function is adequate, postoperative hypoxemia can precipitate right-heart failure.

Clinical signs of right-heart failure include supraventricular dysrhythmias, distended neck veins, hepatomegaly, and peripheral edema. The electrocardiogram may demonstrate left and right ventricular strain, and a chest radiograph may reveal right atrial and ventricular enlargement. Echocardiography will confirm the diagnosis.

The therapeutic goal is to support right ventricular preload and decrease pulmonary vascular resistance without lowering systemic blood pressure. Ventilatory support may be needed to correct reversible causes of increased pulmonary vascular resistance (hypoxemia, hypercarbia, and respiratory acidosis). Volume loading supports right ventricular preload. Pharmacologic treatment includes dobutamine, an inotrope whose vasodilatory action decreases pulmonary vascular resistance. Amrinone, which has less chronotropic effect than dobutamine, is an alternate choice, especially in the presence of myocardial ischemia, but systemic hypotension may limit its usefulness.

For pulmonary vasodilation and right ventricular afterload reduction, nitroglycerin is superior to nitroprusside. Both agents cause systemic hypotension and blunt HPV. The potential use of inhaled NO during and following pulmonary resection has been investigated.[248]

SPECIAL PROCEDURES

Fiberoptic bronchoscopy

Fiberoptic bronchoscopy can be performed under local or general anesthesia. If local anesthesia is chosen, sedatives should be used with caution since they may not be well tolerated by patients with pulmonary disease, particularly those that retain CO_2.

An anticholinergic agent is given to dry the airway and to blunt irritative reflexes. Glycopyrrolate is preferred to atropine or scopolamine. The upper airway is first anesthetized with local anesthetic solution delivered by nebulizer or with viscous lidocaine (lignocaine) gargle. Tracheal anesthesia is achieved by transtracheal injection of local anesthetic.[249] Superior laryngeal and glossopharyngeal nerve blocks can also be performed. These blocks depress airway reflexes so the patient should be told to take nothing by mouth for several hours following bronchoscopy.

During awake bronchoscopy, the patient should receive supplemental O_2. This is achieved using mouth-held nasal prongs or with a special face mask (Patil-Syracuse mask) which has a diaphragm through which the bronchoscope is passed.

Any general anesthetic (inhalational or intravenous) technique is acceptable for fiberoptic bronchoscopy, but N_2O is usually avoided to allow a higher F_{IO_2}.[250] A bronchoscope passed through an endotracheal tube produces a significant PEEP effect. Barotrauma can result if ventilation is attempted through a small tube obstructed by the bronchoscope. An endotracheal tube with an internal diameter of 8.0 mm or larger should be used. Suctioning through the bronchoscope decreases alveolar O_2, reduces FRC, and can cause significant hypoxemia.

The laryngeal mask airway (LMA) may be used instead of an endotracheal tube for therapeutic or diagnostic bronchoscopy under local or general anesthesia.[251] There is a larger internal diameter for easy passage of the bronchoscope. There may be less discomfort and trauma with an LMA, and capnographic and volume monitoring of respiration is also possible during the procedure. The endoscopist will also have access to the vocal cords and upper trachea

Rigid bronchoscopy

During rigid bronchoscopy, the patient should be paralyzed and ventilation controlled in order to minimize the risk of trauma from movement. Patients with suspected malignancy may have an increased sensitivity to nondepolarizing muscle relaxants (myasthenic or Eaton–Lambert syndrome), so short-acting relaxants should be given in small incremental doses or a continuous intravenous infusion of succinylcholine (suxamethonium) used and effects should be titrated using a blockade monitor.

A variety of ventilatory techniques can be used during rigid bronchoscopy.[252] Following hyperventilation with 100% O_2 to denitrogenate the lungs and to lower $P_{a}CO_2$, O_2 can be delivered by insufflation at a high flow (10–15 L min^{-1}) ("apneic oxygenation") without actually ventilating the patient. Although satisfactory oxygenation can be achieved for long periods, apnea should not extend beyond 5 min because of CO_2 accumulation.

Oxygen and anesthetic gases can also be delivered through the side arm of the bronchoscope by intermittent ventilation. Ventilation is possible as long as the eyepiece is in place, but must be interrupted whenever biopsy or suctioning is performed. An intravenous anesthetic technique with a short-acting agent such as propofol, alfentanil, or remifentanil allows continuous administration of anesthetic, which may not be possible with an inhalational anesthetic technique.[253]

During long procedures, CO_2 accumulates, thereby predisposing the patient to dysrhythmias, particularly in the presence of light anesthesia. Intermittent hyperventilation lowers $P_{a}CO_2$ and deepens the anesthetic. High fresh gas flows are needed to compensate for the leak around the bronchoscope. Oxygen can also be delivered by a Sanders system, which uses the Venturi principle to deliver O_2 by jet ventilation. The presence of an eyepiece is not necessary with this technique.

The complications of bronchoscopy include damage to the teeth, hemorrhage, broncho- and laryngospasm, subglottic edema, and airway perforation. A chest radiograph should be obtained following bronchoscopy to exclude the presence of pneumothorax or mediastinal emphysema from barotrauma.

Mediastinoscopy

Transcervical mediastinoscopy is usually performed on the right side of the chest with the patient in the reverse Trendelenburg position. For left mediastinal pathology, an open Chamberlain procedure is performed. The mediastinoscope is advanced following the anterior aspect of the trachea, passing close to the innominate vessels and the aortic arch.

Mediastinoscopy can be performed under local anesthesia. However, with the patient breathing spontaneously, the risk of venous air embolism and mediastinal injury from movement are greatly increased. General anesthesia, muscle paralysis, and controlled positive-pressure ventilation is preferred. An anticholinergic agent should be given to blunt the autonomic reflexes (bradycardia) that result from compression or stretching of the trachea, vagus nerve, or great vessels.

The mediastinoscope may compress the innominate artery, causing a loss of the right radial pulse in the presence of a normal ECG. This may be misinterpreted as "hypotension" and lead to inappropriate aggressive treatment. During mediastinoscopy, blood pressure measurements should be obtained from the left arm, and the right radial pulse should be continuously monitored by plethysmography or by pulse oximetry. A decrease in the right radial pulse with normal left arm blood pressure indicates that the mediastinoscope needs to be repositioned. This is especially important if the patient has a history of impaired cerebral vascular circulation since carotid artery perfusion can be compromised by vascular compression by the mediastinoscope.

The major complications of mediastinoscopy include pneumothorax, recurrent laryngeal nerve damage, air embolism, and hemorrhage. If a large mediastinal blood vessel is torn, fluids given through an intravenous line in the arm may enter the mediastinum through the tear in the vein. In this situation, a large-bore catheter should be placed in a lower extremity vein. Although blood loss is usually quite small, blood should always be available since an emergency thoracotomy or sternotomy may be required to control bleeding. Other complications of mediastinoscopy include acute tracheal collapse, tension pneumomediastinum, hemothorax, and chylothorax. All patients must have a chest radiograph in the immediate postoperative period.

Mediastinal mass

Anterior mediastinal masses may compress the superior vena cava, the major airways, and even the heart. Complete or partial airway obstruction from an anterior mediastinal mass can occur following patient positioning and/or with relaxation of the muscles maintaining airway patency.[254] Preoperatively, it is important to ask whether the patient has experienced dyspnea in the supine position. A chest CT scan and other radiologic studies should be obtained to determine the extent of the tumor mass and any involvement with surrounding structures. Flow–volume loops are needed in both the upright and supine positions. A marked decrease in FEV_1 and peak expiratory flow rate in the supine position suggests the potential for airway obstruction with anesthesia. In this situation, it is appropriate to consider radiotherapy to the mass prior to surgery.

A rigid bronchoscope may be needed to bypass an obstruction occurring in the trachea during induction of anesthesia and to allow the patient to be ventilated. The patient's position may need to be changed from supine to lateral or even prone to relieve the compression.

If biopsy of the mediastinal mass cannot be performed under local anesthesia, an awake fiberoptic bronchoscopy-assisted airway intubation followed by induction of general anesthesia is usually recommended. Spontaneous ventilation helps to maintain airway patency. The Trendelenburg position and positive-pressure ventilation should be avoided if superior vena caval obstruction is present.

Bronchial obstruction

Secretions, blood, anatomic distortion, tumor, or foreign bodies can each cause bronchial obstruction. Retention of secretions can occur distal to the obstruction. A preoperative chest radiograph or CT scan may reveal consolidation or an abscess cavity beyond the airway obstruction.

Isolation of the lungs is critically important since pus can flood the airway as the obstruction is relieved. Manipulation of the lung or simply turning the patient to the lateral decubitus position can dislodge a foreign body or secretions into the trachea or dependent lung. Therefore, the lungs should be isolated before turning the patient. A DLT is preferred to a bronchial blocker as this provides protection to the dependent lung while allowing the involved lung to be suctioned. Only the dependent lung is ventilated while the lumen to the nondependent lung is left open for drainage or suction.

The obstruction, in some instances, can behave as a ball valve. Positive-pressure ventilation distends the bronchus and allows gas to pass the obstruction during inflation, but then the gas is trapped during deflation. A progressive rise in peak inspiratory pressure and a decrease in expired volume compared with inspired volume may indicate gas trapping. Ventilation of only the dependent lung is extremely important in this situation.

Nd-YAG laser

The neodymium–yttrium–aluminum–garnet (Nd-YAG) laser is used to debulk tumors and to tunnel through or widen obstructed airways.[255] The Nd-YAG laser beam can be transmitted through a flexible quartz monofilament, so it can be used with either rigid or flexible bronchoscopes. Although the procedure can be performed under local anesthesia, general anesthesia with muscle relaxants is preferred as any movement could result in a misfired laser causing damage to healthy tissue. There is improved airway control with general anesthesia, and debris and blood are more easily removed so that aspiration is avoided.

The patient should not be premedicated with a sedative or opioid. Atropine or glycopyrrolate can be used as a drying agent. After intravenous induction and muscle relaxation, an inhalational anesthetic agent is used. Patients should be ventilated with an F_{IO_2} of 0.4 or less and 60% or more nitrogen (from inspired air) to reduce the chance of an airway fire. Nitrous oxide, which is combustible, should be avoided. No special endotracheal tube is needed since the laser is only fired beyond the tip of the tube. However, if misfired, tube ignition is possible. The laser should only be fired deep in the airway, but damage to the anesthesiologist's eyes is possible from a misfired laser, so goggles or glasses are recommended.

In an alternative technique, with total intravenous anesthesia (TIVA) with propofol or remifentanil, laser surgery may be performed through a rigid bronchoscope.[256] This technique requires a high concentration of O_2 delivered through jet system, so combustion is a possibility.

Only the surface of the treated tissue is visible. Any underlying damage and edema will not be apparent, and airway obstruction and hemorrhage can develop as late as 48 h after the procedure. Hypoxemia, perforation of the tracheobronchial tree, and airway hemorrhage are major complications of Nd-YAG procedures. The surgeon may need to apply epinephrine-soaked pledgets directly if bleeding is profuse.

Airway stenting

Placement of a tracheal or bronchial stent will maintain patency of airways with stenosis and malacia. Stenting is particularly useful following pulmonary transplantation. Either silicone stents or self-expanding stainless-steel stents are used.

For general anesthesia, a fiberoptic bronchoscope-assisted airway intubation of an awake, cooperative, spontaneously breathing patient allows visualization while minimizing the risk of airway obstruction. An inhalational anesthetic induction is an alternative choice. Once the trachea is intubated, there is still the possibility that the airway distal to the endotracheal tube can collapse so a rigid bronchoscope should be available to re-establish a patent airway if necessary.

The stenting procedure requires an immobile field for accurate airway length measurements and for positioning of the stents, therefore muscle relaxants may be needed. Associated bronchial balloon dilation of the airway can be extremely stimulating, so a rapid-acting intravenous anesthetic agent should be available and given if the patient moves.

All inhalational anesthetic agents have bronchodilatory effects which are useful because of the frequent presence of reactive airway disease in patients undergoing stenting procedures. Intravenous agents such as propofol or remifentanil can maintain anesthesia during the periods of bronchial dilation and stenting when ventilation with an inhalational agent is not possible.

Stenting procedures are usually performed in the confined, unfamiliar, environment of the radiology suite. One must always be prepared for complications. Common problems can include marked resistance to ventilation from a misplaced or dislodged stent or even airway rupture. Emergence from anesthesia can also be challenging. The anesthesiologist must have all the necessary airway equipment available in order to re-establish a patent airway, including tracheostomy.

Pulmonary hemorrhage

Protecting the noninvolved airway is the first priority in the management of massive pulmonary hemorrhage. Death usually results from drowning in blood, rather than from hypovolemia or exsanguination. The methods used for isolating the lung during pulmonary hemorrhage include a DLT, bronchial blockade with the Univent tube, or placement of a single-lumen endotracheal tube into the bronchus of the nonbleeding lung. If bleeding is massive and visualization of the larynx is difficult, awake laryngoscopy and intubation is recommended.

Advancing an uncut endotracheal tube to its full length will usually intubate the right main bronchus. If bleeding is coming from the right lung, the tube may have to be passed over a fiberoptic bronchoscope into the left lung. If the left lung is bleeding, an endotracheal tube inserted into the right main bronchus will probably obstruct the right upper lobe as well as isolating the entire left lung, so hypoxemia may occur.[257] Confirmation of lung isolation by bronchoscopy is necessary before the patient is turned to the lateral decubitus position.

Once the airway is established and the contralateral lung is protected, attention is directed toward detecting and controlling the site of bleeding while maintaining adequate gas exchange. The site of hemorrhage is determined by bronchoscopy. The larger lumen of a rigid bronchoscope makes the suctioning of greater volumes of blood easier, but fiberoptic bronchoscopy through a tube in the airway is safer.

Video-assisted thoracoscopic surgery

Insertion of an endoscope into the thoracic cavity is an accurate, safe, and reliable alternative to open thoracotomy for a broad spectrum of intrathoracic procedures. Video-assisted thoracoscopic surgery is used to obtain pulmonary and pleural biopsies and for limited lung resection, laser treatment of tumors, lung volume reduction surgery (LVRS), treating spontaneous and traumatic pneumothoraces, sympathectomies, chest wall resections, and limited cardiac, orthopedic, and many other intrathoracic operations.[258,259]

Patients undergoing video-assisted thoracoscopic surgery procedures range from healthy, low-risk (e.g. bilateral sympathectomies) patients to those with very severe pulmonary disease (e.g. LVRS).[260] Therefore, each anesthetic will vary depending on the patient, and the choice of monitors will depend on the overall status of the patient and not necessarily on the procedure alone. The benefits of video-assisted thoracoscopic surgery include less pain, better postoperative pulmonary function, and more rapid recovery with a shortened hospital stay.

Video-assisted thoracoscopic surgery can be performed under local, regional, or general anesthesia, the choice depending on the duration and extent of the operative procedure.

When the incision is made, air enters the pleural cavity, causing a partial pneumothorax. If the procedure is performed using local anesthetics with the patient awake, the pneumothorax is usually well tolerated because the skin and chest wall form a seal around the thoracoscope, thus limiting the degree of atelectasis.

Several rules apply for all video-assisted thoracoscopic procedures. When general anesthesia is indicated, a DLT or bronchial blocker must be used because collapse of the operated lung is essential. DLTs offer the advantage of allowing passage of a fiberoptic bronchoscope or suction catheter to aid lung collapse and for pulmonary toilet.

Ventilation to the lung undergoing surgery is discontinued by opening the lumen of the DLT to air. Collapse of the lung undergoing surgery occurs when air enters the pleural cavity. Intermittent suction down the lumen of the DLT may help to hasten collapse. To augment selective collapse, CO_2 has been insufflated into the pleural space. This maneuver should be avoided because it can cause marked hemodynamic instability owing to a response similar to that of a tension pneumothorax.[261,262]

If the patient undergoing video-assisted thoracoscopic surgery becomes hypoxemic, the application of CPAP is not practical as even a modest distention of the lung undergoing surgery will compromise surgical exposure. The combined use of NO and a pulmonary vasoconstrictor to correct hypoxemia during video-assisted thoracoscopic surgery may be beneficial.[188]

Pain after video-assisted thoracoscopic surgery is unpredictable and analgesic requirements vary greatly between individual patients. Systemic opioids remain the analgesic regimen of choice. NSAIDs, intercostal nerve blocks, and even epidural opioids have been used. TENS has been used with some success in patients undergoing video-assisted thoracoscopic surgery.[216]

Local anesthesia (0.25% bupivacaine plus $0.5\,\text{mL}\,\text{kg}^{-1}$ epinephrine) administered through the chest drainage tube at the completion of surgery after the lung has been reinflated also works well. The local anesthetic solution must be given before the drainage tube is placed on suction.

Bronchopleural fistula

A bronchopleural fistula is a pathologic communication between the airway and the pleural cavity. The fistula may extend to the skin (bronchopleural–cutaneous fistula). Bronchopleural fistulae occur following pulmonary resections (most common after pneumonectomy), from rupture of a bullae, bleb, or cyst into the pleural space, from erosion of a carcinoma, and from trauma.

If an empyema is present, it should be drained prior to surgery on the fistula. The safest means is to drain the empyema under local anesthesia with the patient sitting up and leaning toward the affected side. A drain, connected to an underwater seal, should be left in the cavity. The empyema may be loculated, so complete drainage of the empyema is not always possible.

The most important anesthetic concerns when managing a bronchopleural fistula are separation and isolation of the lungs to avoid contamination and selective ventilation of the healthy lung. These goals are best achieved with a DLT.

Prior to intubation, the chest drainage tube should be left unclamped for continued drainage of pus and to avoid a tension pneumothorax. Intubation can be performed in an awake patient or under general anesthesia provided the patient breathes spontaneously. Controlled ventilation must be avoided until the lungs are completely separated, i.e. until the DLT is in place, to prevent a tension pneumothorax.

The bronchus of the healthy lung should be intubated. Because a tube "blindly" advanced can pass through the fistula, a fiberoptic bronchoscope is used to direct the DLT into the noninvolved bronchus. Once in position, the bronchial cuff should be inflated immediately to separate the lungs. Only the healthy lung is ventilated. In the presence of an empyema, there may be a massive outpouring of pus through the tracheal lumen immediately after intubation.

Bronchopleural fistulae can be treated without surgery using a DLT to independently ventilate each lung ("split-lung" ventilation). The healthy lung is ventilated with a normal tidal volume while the affected lung is ventilated with a smaller volume or is left unventilated. CPAP can also be applied at pressures below the opening pressure of the fistula. The critical opening pressure is found by adding small increments of CPAP to the affected bronchus until continuous bubbling appears in the underwater sealed chest drain. High-frequency jet ventilation is ineffective and may make the bronchopleural fistula worse.[263]

Lung cysts and bullae

Thin-walled, air-filled cavities in the lungs (cysts and bullae) may represent end-stage emphysematous lung changes or may be congenital and isolated findings. Repeated pneumothoraces from spontaneous rupture, infection, and/or dyspnea are the usual indications for surgery. The degree of functional impairment depends on the condition of the remaining lung, the size of the airspace, and the amount of compression of the surrounding healthy lung tissue by the cyst.

Patients with spontaneous pneumothoraces can be divided into two clinical groups. The first have apical blebs and are usually young with excellent pulmonary reserve. The second group have emphysematous blebs, are older, and have advanced COPD often with CO_2 retention. These latter patients would benefit by avoiding thoracotomy. Video-assisted thoracoscopic resection of bullae and blebs is usually attempted in both groups, although those in the emphysematous group frequently requires open thoracotomy.

If the bulla is very compliant, during controlled ventilation a large portion of the applied tidal volume will be wasted in this additional dead space. Positive-pressure ventilation should be used with caution in case the bulla ruptures, leading to a tension pneumothorax. Nitrous oxide must always be avoided. Once the chest is opened, the risk of a tension pneumothorax disappears.

Intubation with a DLT in a spontaneously breathing awake or anesthetized patient is recommended. Positive-pressure ventilation with rapid small tidal volumes at pressures less than $15\,\text{cmH}_2\text{O}$ (1.5 kPa) can be used during induction and maintenance of anesthesia. Once the DLT is in place, the nonaffected lung (if free of bullae) is ventilated with a normal tidal volume. After resection of each bulla, the operated lung should be re-expanded and checked for air leaks and for the presence of additional bullae. Most patients can be extubated at the completion of surgery, but if postoperative controlled ventilation is needed, low positive pressures should be used to reduce the chance of developing a tension lung cyst or pneumothorax.

Bronchopleural lavage

The whole lung may be irrigated in the treatment of alveolar proteinosis, bronchiectasis, refractory asthma, inhalation of radioactive dust, and cystic fibrosis.[264] When bilateral lung disease is present, ventilation–perfusion scans should be obtained preoperatively so that lavage can be performed first on the more severely affected lung.

With the patient under general anesthesia, a DLT is used to isolate the lungs. The bronchial lumen should enter the bronchus on the side to be lavaged. An $F_{I}O_2$ of 1.0 is used throughout the procedure. The cuff of the bronchial lumen should maintain separation of the lungs at pressures as high as 50 cmH$_2$O (5 kPa) in order to prevent the leak of lavage fluid into the healthy, ventilated lung. Some anesthesiologists prefer the lavaged lung to be dependent so that the risk of leakage to the healthy (nondependent) lung is reduced. Others prefer the lavaged lung to be nondependent as in this position perfusion will more closely match ventilation in the dependent lung. As a compromise, lavage may be performed in the supine position.

Warm, heparinized, isotonic saline is infused by gravity down the bronchial lumen from a height of 30–40 cm above the chest while the patient is in a head-up position. When the lavage fluid ceases to flow, the patient is placed in a head-down position, and chest percussion and vibration are applied for 1 min to loosen material. The infused fluid is then allowed to drain passively in to a collecting system. As many as 20 repetitions of this procedure may be required before the drained lavage fluid becomes clear. Accurate measurement of inflow and outflow volumes is important. Following the last passive drainage, the lung is suctioned and then re-expanded using large tidal volumes and high pressures. Most patients can be extubated in the operating room.

The most serious complication of this procedure is aspiration of the lavage fluid into the ventilated lung. This may result in a marked decrease in oxygenation requiring immediate reinstitution of two-lung ventilation with PEEP.

Lung volume reduction surgery

Lung volume reduction is the only surgical treatment for emphysema. It is performed using either video-assisted thoracoscopic surgery with laser ablation of the lung[265] or sternotomy with surgical excision of lung tissue.[266] Not all patients with advanced emphysema are candidates for LVRS.[267] Table 47.7 lists the selection criteria.

The aim of either LVRS operation is to reduce the lung volume by 20–30%. The mechanism of benefit by reducing nonfunctioning lung tissue is to enhance elastic recoil of the remaining lung and to improve the efficiency of the diaphragm.[268] This in turn leads to better matching of ventilation to perfusion and improved right ventricular filling.

The lungs must be isolated and ventilated with a DLT or bronchial blocker. Higher levels of potentially dangerous auto-PEEP are produced if a small DLT is used in patients with advanced COPD.[98] Therefore, it is very important to use a large DLT. Because of significant obstruction to expiratory flow, the ventilator tidal volume, rate, and inspiratory–expiratory ratio must be adjusted for the individual patient to avoid air trapping. Unlike the usual practice of ventilating the nonoperated lung with large tidal volumes, smaller tidal volumes are used because of the presence of bullous emphysema in the ventilated lung. The ventilator must be adjusted to provide a long expiratory–inspiratory ratio (1:4 or 1:5), and maximum peak inspiratory pressure during one-lung ventilation should be limited to 35 cmH$_2$O (3.5 kPa).

A contralateral tension pneumothorax should be considered if $S_{p}O_2$ drops and peak inspiratory pressure rises during one-lung ventilation. Air trapping with hyperinflation of the ventilated lung is another potential cause of increased airway pressures. Transient hypoxemia can result from mucus plugging, so frequent suctioning for pulmonary toilet is indicated. Significant parenchymal air leaks are present in almost every patient following LVRS.

An arterial line is mandatory for continuous pressure monitoring and for frequent blood gas analysis. A pulmonary artery catheter may be helpful for patients with pulmonary hypertension especially in the presence of right ventricular hypertrophy.[269]

Permissive hypercapnia must also be accepted since these patients are intentionally hypoventilated. End-tidal CO$_2$ levels may not reflect the higher arterial $P_{a}CO_2$ because of significant dead space wasted ventilation. Despite very high $P_{a}CO_2$ levels at the completion of surgery, most patients have their airway extubated in the operating room. After surgery, the patient must be continuously monitored and the anesthesiologist must be available.

Assisted ventilation by mask may be needed in the immediate postextubation period. Equipment must be available should reintubation and mechanical ventilatory support become necessary.

The key to the anesthetic management of patients undergoing LVRS, whether performed through a sternotomy incision or by video-assisted thoracoscopic surgery, is satisfactory postoperative analgesia. Epidural analgesia with smaller amounts of opioids should be used even when LVRS is performed by the video-assisted thoracoscopic surgery approach. If the epidural ceases to function, it should be replaced. Parenteral opioid analgesia should be avoided if possible.

Lung transplantation

Indications for lung transplantation include infectious (cystic fibrosis, bronchiectasis), obstructive (COPD, α_1-antitrypsin deficiency), restrictive (idiopathic pulmonary fibrosis), or severe pulmonary hypertension.

Table 47.7 *Selection criteria for lung volume reduction surgery (LVRS) patients*

Medical history
Severe COPD (emphysema rather than chronic bronchitis)
Age < 75 years
No cigarette smoking for 6 months
"Lowest" effective prednisone dose
No previous chest surgery
Pulmonary function
FEV$_1$ > 15% but < 30–35% of predicted
TLC > 120% of predicted
$P_{a}CO_2$ < 50 mmHg
Cardiac function
If suspect PA hypertension, measure PA pressure (< 35 mmHg)
No evidence of LV dysfunction (normal dobutamine stress test)
Radiographic
$\dot{V}/\dot{Q}$ scan with predominantly upper lobe disease – decreased upper lobe perfusion
CT scan with heterogeneous distribution of air trapping – emphysema with upper lobe predominance
Hyperinflation, flattened diaphragm (chest radiograph)

COPD, chronic obstructive pulmonary disease; FEV, forced expiratory volume; TLC, total lung capacity; PA, pulmonary artery; LV, left ventricular; CT, computed tomography.

In some instances, patients with COPD may undergo LVRS as a "bridge" or as an alternative to transplantation. Patients with cystic fibrosis, bullous emphysema, or vascular diseases may require double-lung transplantation, whereas patients with Eisenmenger syndrome may require combined heart–lung transplantation.

Patients are usually dyspneic at rest. Many are hypoxemic, and CO_2 retention is not uncommon. Most procedures are performed on an emergency basis to minimize ischemia time, but donor lobectomy for lung transplantation in children can be scheduled on an elective basis.

Transplant recipients are usually started on cyclosporine (cyclosporin) preoperatively, and intravenous azathioprine is also administered before the start of anesthesia. Premedication with opioids or sedatives is avoided because of the tenuous respiratory status of these patients.

Many patients do not tolerate the supine position and must have their backs elevated during induction. Cricoid pressure is needed for those at risk for aspiration. Induction usually consists of etomidate, ketamine, and/or high doses of opioid to avoid hypotension.

Hypoxemia and hypercarbia must be avoided to prevent further increases in pulmonary artery pressure. Hypotension is treated with vasopressors. Large fluid boluses are avoided. An anesthetic technique combining opioids with an inhalational agent and 100% O_2 and muscle relaxants is recommended. Nitrous oxide is not used since it exacerbates pulmonary hypertension, reduces the concentration of inspired O_2, and expands intravascular air bubbles. Arterial blood gases are followed so that acid–base balance can be maintained. A pulmonary artery catheter is also required, but may have to be withdrawn into its sterile sheath if the pulmonary artery on the side of transplantation has been catheterized.

A DLT, Univent tube, or bronchial blocker is required for single-lung transplantation through a lateral thoracotomy incision. Cardiopulmonary bypass should also be available. Hypoxemia during lung collapse or marked pulmonary hypertension when the pulmonary artery is clamped may necessitate the need for cardiopulmonary bypass. Prostaglandin E_1, amrinone or milrinone, nitroglycerin, and dobutamine may be required to control pulmonary hypertension and prevent right ventricular failure. More recently, NO has been used to treat pulmonary hypertension during pulmonary transplantation.[270,271]

Most patients require ventilatory support for 24–48 h after transplantation. If cardiopulmonary bypass is not used, or once coagulation studies return to normal, a thoracic or lumbar epidural catheter should be placed for administration of neuraxial opioids.

Cyclosporine may exacerbate renal dysfunction. Mannitol and furosemide may be required postoperatively to induce diuresis. Inotropic support with dopamine, isoproterenol, and epinephrine may be necessary, especially if pulmonary hypertension and right ventricular failure are present. TEE is helpful in differentiating between right ventricular and left ventricular dysfunction and for evaluating pulmonary blood flow after transplantation.

Transplantation disrupts neural innervation of the transplanted lung. Although the respiratory pattern is not affected, the cough reflex is abolished below the carina and there is bronchial hyperactivity in some patients. Loss of lymphatic drainage increases extravascular lung water, predisposing the transplanted lung to pulmonary edema. Intraoperative fluid replacement should be kept to a minimum.

Atelectasis and retained secretions require frequent postoperative bronchoscopy. Other surgical complications include damage to the phrenic, vagus, and recurrent laryngeal nerves.

REFERENCES

1. Slinger PD. Perioperative respiratory assessment and management. *Can J Anaesth* 1992; **39:** 115–31.
2. Zeiher BG, Gross TJ, Kern JA, *et al.* Predicting postoperative pulmonary function in patients undergoing lung resection. *Chest* 1995; **108:** 68–72.
3. Cottrell JJ, Ferson PF. Preoperative assessment of the thoracic surgical patient. *Clin Chest Med* 1992; **13:** 47–53.
4. Ferguson MK, Little L, Rizzo L, *et al.* Diffusing capacity predicts morbidity and mortality after pulmonary resection. *J Thorac Cardiovasc Surg* 1988 **96:** 894–900.
5. Busch E, Verazin G, Antkowiak JG, *et al.* Pulmonary complications in patients undergoing thoracotomy for lung carcinoma. *Chest* 1994; **105:** 760–6.
6. Gerson MC, Hurst JM, Hertzberg VS, *et al.* Prediction of cardiac and pulmonary complications related to elective abdominal and noncardiac thoracic surgery in geriatric patients. *Am J Med* 1990; **88:** 101–7.
7. Morice RC, Peters EJ, Ryan MB, *et al.* Exercise testing in the evaluation of patients at high risk for complications from lung resection. *Chest* 1992; **101:** 356–61.
8. Bollinger CT, Soler M, Stulz P, *et al.* Evaluation of high-risk lung resection candidates: pulmonary haemodynamics versus exercise testing. A series of five patients. *Respiration* 1994; **61:** 181–6.
9. Ferguson MK, Reeder LB, Mick R. Optimizing selection of patients for major lung resection. *J Thorac Cardiovasc Surg* 1995; **109:** 275–81.
10. Nomori H, Kobayashi R, Fuyuno G, *et al.* Preoperative respiratory muscle training. Assessment in thoracic surgery patients with special reference to postoperative pulmonary complications. *Chest* 1994; **105:** 1782–99.
11. Epstein SK, Faling LJ, Daly BD, Celli BR. Predicting complications after pulmonary resection: preoperative exercise testing vs multifactorial cardiopulmonary index. *Chest* 1993; **104:** 694–700.
12. Melendez JA, Carlon VA. Cardiopulmonary risk index does not predict complications after thoracic surgery. *Chest* 1998; **114:** 69–75.
13. Prause G, Offner A, Ratzenhofer-Komenda B, *et al.* Comparison of two preoperative indices to predict perioperative mortality in non-cardiac thoracic surgery. *Eur J Cardiothorac Surg* 1997; **11:** 670–5.
14. Gass GD, Olsen GN. Clinical significance of pulmonary function tests. Preoperative pulmonary function testing to predict postoperative morbidity and mortality. *Chest* 1986; **89:** 127–35.
15. Kearney DJ, Lee TH, Reilly JJ, *et al.* Assessment of operative risk in patients undergoing lung resection. Importance of predicted pulmonary function. *Chest* 1994; **105:** 753–9.
16. Cerfolio RJ, Allen MS, Trastek VF, *et al.* Lung resection in patients with compromised pulmonary function. *Ann Thorac Surg* 1996; **62:** 348–51.
17. Shimizu T, Abe K, Kinouchi K, Yoshiya I. Arterial oxygenation during one lung ventilation. *Can J Anaesth* 1997; **44:** 1162–6.
18. Abe K, Mashimo T, Yoshiya I. Arterial oxygenation and shunt fraction during one-lung ventilation: a comparison of isoflurane and sevoflurane. *Anesth Analg* 1998; **86:** 1266–70.
19. Pagel PS, Fu JL, Damask MC, *et al.* Desflurane and isoflurane produce similar alterations in systemic and pulmonary hemodynamics and arterial oxygenation in patients undergoing one-lung ventilation during thoracotomy. *Anesth Analg* 1998; **87:** 800–7.
20. Eisenkraft JB. Effects of anaesthetics on the pulmonary circulation. *Br J Anaesth* 1990; **65:** 63–78.
21. Doenicke AW, Czeslick E, Moss J, Hoernecke R. Onset time, endotracheal intubating conditions, and plasma histamine release after cisatracurium and vecuronium administration. *Anesth Analg* 1998; **87:** 434–8.
22. Lumb PD, Silvay G, Weinreich Ai, Shiang H. A comparison of the effects of continuous ketamine infusion and halothane on oxygenation during one-lung anaesthesia in dogs. *Can Anaesth Soc J* 1979; **26:** 394–401.
23. Weinreich AI, Silvay G, Lumb PD. Continuous ketamine infusion for one-lung anaesthesia. *Can Anaesth Soc J* 1980; **27:** 485–90.
24. Rees DI, Gaines III GY. One-lung anesthesia – a comparison of pulmonary gas exchange during anesthesia with ketamine or enflurane. *Anesth Analg* 1984; **63:** 521–5.
25. Domino KB, Wetstein L, Glasser SA, *et al.* Influence of mixed venous oxygen tension (PvO_2) on blood flow to atelectatic lung. *Anesthesiology* 1983; **59:** 428–34.
26. Benumof JL. One-lung ventilation and hypoxic pulmonary vasoconstriction. Implications for anesthetic management. *Anesth Analg* 1985; **64:** 821–33.
27. Marshall C, Lindgren L, Marshall BE. Effects of halothane, enflurane, and isoflurane on hypoxic pulmonary vasoconstriction in rat lungs in vitro. *Anesthesiology* 1984; **60:** 304–8.
28. Ishibe Y, Gui X, Uno H, *et al.* Effect of sevoflurane on hypoxic pulmonary vasoconstriction in the perfused rabbit lung. *Anesthesiology* 1993; **79:** 1348–53.
29. Loer SA, Scheeren TW, Tarnow J. Desflurane inhibits hypoxic pulmonary vasoconstriction in isolated rabbit lungs. *Anesthesiology* 1995; **83:** 552–6.

30. Karzai W, Haberstroh J, Priebe HJ. Effects of desflurane and propofol on arterial oxygenation during one-lung ventilation in the pig. *Acta Anaesthesiol Scand* 1998; **42:** 648–52.
31. Lennon PF, Murray PA. Attenuated hypoxic pulmonary vasoconstriction during isoflurane anesthesia is abolished by cyclooxygenase inhibition in chronically instrument dogs. *Anesthesiology* 1996; **84:** 404–14.
32. Moore PG, Nguyen DK, Reitan JA. Inhibition of nitric oxide synthesis causes systemic and pulmonary vasoconstriction in isoflurane-anesthetized dogs. *J Cardiothorac Vasc Anesth* 1994 **8:** 310–16.
33. Benumof JL, Augustine SD, Gibbons JA. Halothane and isoflurane only slightly impair arterial oxygenation during one-lung ventilation in patients undergoing thoracotomy. *Anesthesiology* 1987; **67:** 910–15.
34. Satoh D, Sato M, Kaise A, *et al.* Effects of isoflurane on oxygenation during one-lung ventilation in pulmonary emphysema patients. *Acta Anaesthesiol Scand* 1998; **42:** 1145–8.
35. Slinger P, Scott WA. Arterial oxygenation during one-lung ventilation: a comparison of enflurane and isoflurane. *Anesthesiology* 1995; **82:** 940–6.
36. Kellow NH, Scott AD, White SA, Feneck RO. Comparison of the effects of propofol and isoflurane anaesthesia on right ventricular function and shunt fraction during thoracic surgery. *Br J Anaesth* 1995; **75:** 578–82.
37. Reid CW, Slinger PD, Lenis S. A comparison of the effects of propofol-alfentanil versus isoflurane anesthesia on arterial oxygenation during one-lung ventilation. *J Cardiothorac Vasc Anesth* 1996; **10:** 860–3.
38. Arima T, Matsuura M, Shiramatsu T, *et al.* Synthesis of prostaglandins TXA_2 and PGI_2 during one lung anesthesia. *Prostaglandins* 1987; **34:** 668–78.
39. Brodsky JB, Shulman MS. Oxygen monitoring of bleomycin-treated patients. *Can Anaesth Soc J* 1984; **31:** 488–9.
40. Browne DR, Rochford J, O'Connell U, Jones JG. The incidence of post-operative atelectasis in the dependent lung following thoracotomy: the value of added nitrogen. *Br J Anaesth* 1970; **42:** 340–6.
41. Brodsky JB, Shulman MS, Swan M, Mark JBD. Pulse oximetry during one-lung ventilation. *Anesthesiology* 1985; **63:** 212–14.
42. Larson Jr CP, Vender J, Seiver A. Multisite evaluation of a continuous intraarterial blood gas monitoring system. *Anesthesiology* 1994; **81:** 543–52.
43. Uchida T, Makita K, Tsunoda Y, *et al.* Clinical assessment of a continuous intraarterial blood gas monitoring system. *Can J Anaesth* 1994; **41:** 64–70.
44. Zollinger A, Spahn DR, Singer T, *et al.* Accuracy and clinical performance of a continuous intra-arterial blood-gas monitoring system during thoracoscopic surgery. *Br J Anaesth* 1997; **79:** 57–2.
45. Ishikawa S, Makita K, Nakazawa K, Amaha K. Continuous intra-arterial blood gas monitoring during oesophagectomy. *Can J Anaesth* 1998; **45:** 273–6.
46. Zaugg M, Luccinetti E, Zalunardo MP, *et al.* Substantial changes in arterial blood gases during thoracoscopic surgery can be missed by conventional intermittent laboratory blood gas analyses. *Anesth Analg* 1998; **87:** 647–53.
47. Mathru M, Blakeman BP. Don't drown the "down lung." *Chest* 1993; **103:** 1644–5.
48. Slinger PD. Perioperative fluid management for thoracic surgery: the puzzle of postpneumonectomy pulmonary edema. *J Cardiothorac Vasc Anesth* 1995; **9:** 442–51.
49. Herrera A, Pajeulo A, Morano MJ, *et al.* Continuous monitoring of hemoglobin oxygen saturation in mixed venous blood during thoracic anesthesia with selective single-lung ventilation. *Rev Esp Anesthesiol Reanim* 1993; **40:** 258–67.
50. Barletta G, Del Bene MR, Palminiello A, Fantini F. Left-ventricular diastolic dysfunction during pneumonectomy – a transesophageal electrocardiographic study. *Thorac Cardiovasc Surg* 1996; **44:** 92–6.
51. Neustein SM, Cohen E, Reich D, Kirschner P. Transoesophageal echocardiography and the intraoperative diagnosis of left atrial invasion by carcinoid tumor. *Can J Anaesth* 1993; **40:** 664–6.
52. Wang KY, Lin CY, Kuo-Tai J, *et al.* Use of transesophageal electrocardiography for evaluation of resectability of lung cancer. *Acta Anaesthesiol Sin* 1994; **32:** 255–60.
53. Brodsky JB. Clinical separation of the lungs. *Ann Fr Anesth Reanim* 1992; **11:** 178–92.
54. Inoue H, Shohtsua A, Ogawa J, *et al.* Endotracheal tube with movable blocker to prevent aspiration of intratracheal bleeding. *Ann Thorac Surg* 1984; **37:** 497–9.
55. Conacher ID. The urinary catheter as a bronchial blocker. *Anaesthesia* 1983; **38:** 475–7.
56. Dalens B, Labbe A, Haberer JP. Selective endobronchial blocking vs selective intubation. *Anesthesiology* 1982; **57:** 555–6.
57. Hammer GB, Manos SJ, Smith BM, *et al.* Single-lung ventilation in pediatric patients. *Anesthesiology* 1996; **84:** 1503–6.
58. Ginsberg RJ. New technique for one-lung anesthesia using an endobronchial blocker. *J Cardiovasc Surg* 1981; **82:** 542–6.
59. Oxorn D. Use of fiberoptic bronchoscope to assist placement of a Fogarty catheter as a bronchial blocker. *Can J Anaesth* 1987; **34:** 427–8.
60. Harvey SC, Alpert CC, Fishman RL. Independent placement of a bronchial blocker for single-lung ventilation: an alternative method for the difficult airway. *Anesth Analg* 1996; **83:** 1330–1.
61. Kraenzler EJ, Rice TW, Stein SL, Insler SR. Bilateral bronchial blockers for bilateral pulmonary resections in a patient with a previous laryngectomy. *J Cardiothorac Vasc Anesth* 1997; **11:** 201–2.
62. Borchardt RA, LaQuaglia MP, McDowall RH, Wilson RS. Bronchial injury during lung isolation in a pediatric patient. *Anesth Analg* 1998; **87:** 324–5.
63. Kamaya H, Krishna PR. New endotracheal tube (Univent tube) for selective blockade of one lung. *Anesthesiology* 1985; **63:** 342–3.
64. Karwande SV. A new tube for single lung ventilation. *Chest* 1987; **92:** 761–3.
65. Hammer GB, Brodsky JB, Redpath JH, Cannon WB. The Univent tube for single-lung ventilation in paediatric patients. *Paediatr Anaesth* 1998; **8:** 55–7.
66. MacGillivray RG. Evaluation of a new tracheal tube with a movable bronchus blocker. *Anaesthesia* 1988; **43:** 687–9.
67. Doi Y, Uda R, Akatsuka M, *et al.* Damaged Univent tube. *Anesth Analg* 1998; **87:** 732–733.
68. Benumof JL, Gaughan S, Ozaki GT. Operative lung constant positive airway pressure with the Univent bronchial blocker tube. *Anesth Analg* 1992; **74:** 406–10.
69. Foroughi V, Krucylak PE, Wyatt J, Bowen C. A technically simple means for administration of continuous positive airway pressure during one-lung ventilation using a Univent tube. *Anesth Analg* 1995; **81:** 656.
70. Ransom E, Detterbeck F, Klein JI, Norfleet EA. Univent tube provides a new technique for jet ventilation. *Anesthesiology* 1996; **84:** 724–6.
71. Ransom ES, Carter L, Mund GD. Univent tube: a useful device in patients with difficult airways. *J Cardiothorac Vasc Anesth* 1995; **9:** 725–7.
72. Garcia-Aquado R, Mateo EM, Onrubia VJ, Bolinches R. Use of the Univent System tube for difficult intubation and for achieving one-lung anaesthesia. *Acta Anaesthesiol Scand* 1996; **40:** 765–7.
73. Campos JH, Massa FC. Is there a better right-sided tube for one-lung ventilation? A comparison of the right-sided double-lumen tube with the single-lumen tube with right-sided enclosed bronchial blocker. *Anesth Analg* 1998; **86:** 696–700.
74. Guyton DC, Besselievre TR, Devidas M, *et al.* A comparison of two different bronchial cuff designs and four different bronchial cuff inflation methods. *J Cardiothorac Vasc Anesth* 1997; **11:** 599–603.
75. Kelley JG, Gaba DM, Brodsky JB. Bronchial cuff pressures of two tubes used in thoracic surgery. *J Cardiothorac Vasc Anesth* 1992; **6:** 190–2.
76. Arai T, Hatano Y. Yet another reason to use a fiberoptic bronchoscope to properly site a double lumen tube. *Anesthesiology* 1987; **66:** 581–2.
77. Schwartz DE, Yost CS, Larson MD. Pneumothorax complicating the use of a Univent endotracheal tube. *Anesth Analg* 1993; **76:** 443–5.
78. Thielmeier KA, Anwar M. Complication of the Univent tube. *Anesthesiology* 1996; **84:** 491.
79. Dougherty P, Hannallah M. A potentially serious complication that resulted from improper use of the Univent tube. *Anesthesiology* 1992; **77:** 835–6.
80. Burton NA, Watson DC, Brodsky JB, Mark JBD. Advantages of a new polyvinyl chloride double-lumen tube in thoracic surgery. *Ann Thorac Surg* 1983; **36:** 78–84.
81. Marraro G. Selective endobronchial intubation in paediatrics: the Marraro paediatric bilumen tube. *Paediatr Anaesth* 1994; **4:** 255–8.
82. Watterson LM, Harrison GA. A comparison of the endobronchial segment of modern left-sided double-lumen tubes in anesthesia for bilateral sequential lung transplantation. *J Cardiothorac Vasc Anesth* 1996; **10:** 583–5.
83. Hannallah MS, Miller SC, Kurzer SI, Tefft MC. The effective diameter and airflow resistance of the individual lumens of left polyvinyl chloride double-lumen endobronchial tubes. *Anesth Analg* 1996; **82:** 867–9.
84. Slinger PD, Lesiuk L. Flow resistances of disposable double-lumen, single-lumen, and Univent tubes. *J Cardiothorac Vasc Anesth* 1998; **12:** 142–4.
85. Brodsky JB, Adkins MO, Gaba D. Bronchial cuff pressures of double-lumen tubes. *Anesth Analg* 1989; **69:** 608–10.
86. Slinger PD, Chripko D. A clinical comparison of bronchial cuff pressures in three different designs of left double-lumen tubes. *Anesth Analg* 1993; **77:** 305–8.

87. Hannallah MS, Benumof JL, Bachenheimer LC, Mundt DJ. The resting volume and compliance characteristics of the bronchial cuff of left polyvinyl chloride double-lumen endobronchial tubes. *Anesth Analg* 1993; **77:** 1222–6.
88. Coppa GP, Brodsky JB. A simple method to protect the tracheal cuff of a double-lumen tube. *Anesth Analg* 1998; **86:** 675.
89. Gibbs N, Giles K. Malposition of left-sided PVC double-lumen endobronchial tubes. *Anaesth Intensive Care* 1986; **14:** 92.
90. Greene Jr ER, Gutierrez FA. Tip of polyvinyl chloride double-lumen endotracheal tube inadvertently wedged in lower lobe bronchus. *Anesthesiology* 1986; **64:** 406.
91. Burke III WJ. Should a fiberoptic bronchoscope be routinely used to position a double-lumen tube? *Anesthesiology* 1988; **66:** 826.
92. Cohen E, Kirschner PA, Goldofsky S. Intraoperative manipulation for positioning of double-lumen tubes. *Anesthesiology* 1988; **68:** 170.
93. McKenna MJ, Wilson RS, Botelho RJ. Right upper lobe obstruction with right-sided double-lumen endobronchial tubes: A comparison of two tube types. *J Cardiothorac Anesth* 1988; **6:** 734–40.
94. Desai FM, Rocke DA. Double-lumen tube fault. *Anesthesiology* 1990; **73:** 575–6.
95. Benumof JL, Partridge BL, Salvatierra C, Keating J. Margin of safety in positioning modern double-lumen endotracheal tubes. *Anesthesiology* 1987; **67:** 729–38.
96. Hannallah MS, Benumof JL, Ruttimann UE. The relationship between left mainstem bronchial diameter and patient size. *J Cardiothorac Vasc Anesth* 1995; **9:** 119–21.
97. Brodsky JB, Shulman MS, Mark JBD. Malposition of left-sided double-lumen tubes. *Anesthesiology* 1985; **62:** 667–9.
98. Bardockzy G, d'Hollander A, Yernault JC, *et al.* On-line expiratory flow-volume curves during thoracic surgery: occurrence of auto-PEEP. *Br J Anaesth* 1994; **72:** 25–8.
99. Hannallah M, Benumof JL, Silverman PM, *et al.* Evaluation of an approach to choosing a left double-lumen tube size based on chest computed tomographic scan measurement of left mainstem bronchial diameter. *J Cardiothorac Vasc Anesth* 1997; **11:** 168–71.
100. Chow MYH, Liam BL, Lew TWK, *et al.* Predicting the size of a double-lumen endobronchial tube based on tracheal diameter. *Anesth Analg* 1998; **87:** 158–60.
101. Jesseph JE, Merendino KA. The dimensional relationships of the major components of the human tracheobronchial tree. *Surg Gynecol Obstet* 1957; **105:** 210–14.
102. Brodsky JB, Macario A, Mark JBD. Tracheal diameter predicts double-lumen tube size: a method for selecting left double-lumen tubes. *Anesth Analg* 1996; **82:** 861–4.
103. Brodsky JB, Mackey S, Cannon WB. Selecting the correct size left double-lumen tube. *J Cardiothorac Vasc Anesth* 1997; **11:** 924–5.
104. Saito S, Dohi S, Tajima K. Failure of double-lumen endobronchial tube placement: congenital tracheal stenosis in an adult. *Anesthesiology* 1987; **66:** 83–5.
105. Habibi A, Mackey S, Brodsky JB. Selecting a double-lumen tube after lung transplantation. *Anesth Analg* 1997; **84:** 938–9.
106. Capdeville M, Hall D, Koch CG. Practical use of a bronchial blocker in combination with a double-lumen endotracheal tube. *Anesth Analg* 1998; **87:** 1239–41.
107. Brodsky JB, Macario A, Cannon WB, Mark JBD. "Blind" placement of plastic double-lumen tubes. *Anaesth Intensive Care* 1995; **23:** 583–6.
108. Gaeta RG, Brodsky JB. A new laryngoscopy blade to facilitate double-lumen tube placement. *J Cardiothorac Anesth* 1991; **5:** 418–19.
109. Erb JM. A less difficult method to protect the tracheal cuff of a double-lumen tube. *Anesth Analg* 1998; **87:** 1217.
110. Lieberman D, Littleford J, Horaan T, Unruh H. Placement of left double-lumen endobronchial tubes with or without a stylet. *Can J Anaesth* 1996; **43:** 238–42.
111. Brodsky JB, Benumof JL, Ehrenwerth J, Ozaki GT. Depth of placement of left double-lumen endobronchial tubes. *Anesth Analg* 1991; **73:** 570–2.
112. Russell WJ. A blind guided technique for placing double-lumen endobronchial tubes. *Anaesth Intensive Care* 1992; **20:** 71–4.
113. Russell WJ. Further reflections on a "blind guided technique for endobronchial intubation." *Anaesth Intensive Care* 1996; **24:** 123.
114. Panadero A, Iribarren MJ, Fernandez-Liesa I, Monedero P. A simple method to decrease malposition of Robertshaw-type tubes. *Can J Anaesth* 1996; **43:** 984.
115. Bahk J-H, Oh Y-S. A new and simple maneuver to position left-sided double-lumen tube without the aid of fiberoptic bronchoscopy. *Anesth Analg* 1998; **86:** 1271–5.
116. Brodsky JB, Mark JBD. A simple technique for accurate placement of double-lumen endobronchial tubes. *Anesth Rev* 1983; **10:** 26–30.
117. Neustein SM, Eisenkraft JB. Proper lateralization of left-sided double-lumen tubes. *Anesthesiology* 1989; **71:** 996.
118. Saito S, Dohi S, Naito H. Alteration of double-lumen endobronchial tube position by flexion and extension of the neck. *Anesthesiology* 1985; **62:** 696–7.
119. Araki K, Nomura R, Urushibara R, *et al.* Displacement of the double-lumen endobronchial tube can be detected by bronchial cuff pressure change. *Anesth Analg* 1997; **84:** 1349–53.
120. Cheng KS, Wu RSC. Displacement of double-lumen tubes after patient positioning. *Anesthesiology* 1998; **89:** 1282–3.
121. Ehrenwerth J. Pro: proper positioning of a double-lumen endobronchial tube can only be accomplished with endoscopy. *J Cardiothorac Anesth* 1988; **2:** 101–4.
122. Benumof JL. The position of a double-lumen tube should be routinely determined by fibreoptic bronchoscopy. *J Cardiothorac Vasc Anesth* 1993; **7:** 513–14.
123. Grum DF, Porembka D. Misconceptions regarding double-lumen tubes and bronchoscopy. *Anesthesiology* 1988; **68:** 826–7.
124. Brodsky JB. Con: proper positioning of a double-lumen endobronchial tube can only be accomplished with endoscopy. *J Cardiothorac Anesth* 1988; **2:** 105–9.
125. Hurford WE. Fiberoptic endobronchial intubation. *Anesth Clin North Am* 1991; **9:** 97–109.
126. Smith GB, Hirsch NP, Ehrenwerth J. Placement of double-lumen endobronchial tubes. Correlation between clinical impressions and bronchoscopic findings. *Br J Anaesth* 1986; **58:** 1317–20.
127. Alliaume B, Coddens J, DeLoof T. Reliability of auscultation in positioning of double-lumen endobronchial tubes. *Can J Anaesth* 1992; **39:** 687–90.
128. Hurford WE, Alfille PH. A quality improvement study of the placement and complications of double-lumen endobronchial tubes. *J Cardiothorac Vasc Anesth* 1993; **7:** 517–20.
129. Cohen E, Neustein SM, Goldofsky S, Camunas JL. Incidence of malposition of polyvinylchloride and red rubber left-sided double-lumen tubes and clinical sequelae. *J Cardiothorac Vasc Anesth* 1995; **9:** 122–7.
130. Klein U, Karzai W, Bloos F, *et al.* Role of fiberoptic bronchoscopy in conjunction with the use of double-lumen tubes for thoracic anesthesia. A prospective study. *Anesthesiology* 1998; **88:** 346–50.
131. Desiderio DP, Burt M, Kolker AC, *et al.* The effects if endobronchial cuff inflation on double-lumen endobronchial tube movement after lateral decubitus positioning. *J Cardiothorac Vasc Anesth* 1997; **11:** 595–8.
132. Slinger PD. Fiberoptic bronchoscopic positioning of double-lumen tubes. *J Cardiothorac Anesth* 1989; **3:** 486–96.
133. Shafieha MJ, Sit J, Kartha R, *et al.* End-tidal CO_2 analyzers in proper positioning of the double-lumen tubes. *Anesthesiology* 1986; **64:** 844–5.
134. Shankar KB, Moseley HSL, Kumar AY. Dual end-tidal CO_2 monitoring and double-lumen tubes. *Can J Anaesth* 1992; **39:** 100.
135. Bardoczky GI, Levarlet M, Engelman E, Defrancquen P. Continuous spirometry for detection of double-lumen endobronchial tube displacement. *Br J Anaesth* 1993; **70:** 499–502.
136. Shulman MS, Brodsky JB, Levesque PR. Fiberoptic bronchoscopy for tracheal and endobronchial intubation with a double-lumen tube. *Can J Anaesth* 1987; **34:** 172–3.
137. Rusch VW, Freund PR, Bowdle TA. Exchanging double-lumen for single-lumen endotracheal tubes after thoracotomy. *Ann Thorac Surg* 1991; **51:** 323–4.
138. Hannallah M. Evaluation of tracheal tube exchangers for replacement of double-lumen endobronchial tubes. *Anesthesiology* 1992; **77:** 609–10.
139. Clapham MCC, Vaughan RS. Bronchial intubation. A comparison between polyvinyl chloride and red rubber double lumen tubes. *Anaesthesia* 1985; **40:** 1111–14.
140. Holden MP, Jones WM, Bekassy SM, *et al.* Ruptured left main bronchus during a right lung resection. *Anaesthesia* 1972; **27:** 204–8.
141. Guernelli N, Bragaglia RB, Bricolli A, *et al.* Tracheobronchial ruptures due to cuffed Carlens tubes. *Ann Thorac Surg* 1979; **28:** 66–8.
142. Heiser M, Steinberg JJ, MacVaugh H, Klineberg PL. Bronchial rupture, a complication of use of the Robertshaw double-lumen tube. *Anesthesiology* 1979; **51:** 88.
143. Foster JMG, Lau J, Alimo EB. Ruptured bronchus following endobronchial intubation. *Br J Anaesth* 1983; **55:** 687–8.
144. Roxburgh JC. Rupture of the tracheobronchial tree. *Thorax* 1987; **42:** 681–8.
145. Kaloud H, Smolle-Juttner F-M, Prause G, List WF. Iatrogenic ruptures of the tracheobronchial tree. *Chest* 1997; **112:** 774–8.
146. Burton NA, Fall SM, Lyons T, Graeber GM. Rupture of the left main-stem bronchus with a polyvinylchloride double-lumen tube. *Chest* 1983; **6:** 928–9.

147. Wagner DL, Gammage GW, Wong ML. Tracheal rupture following the insertion of a disposable double-lumen endotracheal tube. *Anesthesiology* 1985; **63:** 698–700.
148. Hannallah M, Gomes M. Bronchial rupture associated with the use of a double-lumen tube in a small adult. *Anesthesiology* 1989; **71:** 457–9.
149. Peden J, Galiza EJ, Smith B. Bronchial trauma secondary to intubation with a PVC double-lumen tube. *J R Soc Med* 1992; **85:** 705–6.
150. Hasan A, Low DE, Ganado AL, Norton R, *et al.* Tracheal rupture with disposable polyvinylchloride double-lumen endotracheal tubes. *J Cardiovasc Anesth* 1992; **6:** 208–11.
151. Sakuragi T, Kumano K, Yasumoto M, Dan K. Rupture of the left mainstem bronchus by the tracheal portion of a double-lumen endotracheal tube. *Acta Anaesthesiol Scand* 1997; **41:** 1218–20.
152. Marty-Ane CH, Picard E, Jonquet O, Mary H. Membranous tracheal rupture after endotracheal intubation. *Ann Thorac Surg* 1995; **60:** 1367–71.
153. MacGillivay RG, Rockne DA, Mahomedy AE. Endobronchial tube placement in repair of ruptured bronchus. *Anaesth Intensive Care* 1987; **15:** 459–62.
154. Brodsky JB, Shulman MS, Mark JBD. Airway rupture with a disposable double-lumen tube. *Anesthesiology* 1986; **64:** 415.
155. Hannallah MS, Benumof JL, McCarthy PO, Liang M. Comparison of three techniques to inflate the bronchial cuff of left polyvinylchloride double-lumen tubes. *Anesth Analg* 1993; **77:** 990–4.
156. Hannallah MS, Gharagozloo F, Gomes MN, Chase GA. A comparison of the reliability of two techniques of left double-lumen tube bronchial cuff inflation in producing water-tight seal of the left mainstem bronchus. *Anesth Analg* 1998; **24:** 1027–31.
157. Lewis JW, Servin JP, Gabriel FS, *et al.* The utility of a double-lumen tube for one-lung ventilation in a variety of noncardiac thoracic surgical procedures. *J Cardiothorac Vasc Anesth* 1992; **6:** 705–10.
158. Fischer SR, Deyo DJ, Bone HG, *et al.* Nitric oxide synthesis inhibition restores hypoxic pulmonary vasoconstriction in sepsis. *Respir Crit Care Med* 1997; **156:** 833–9.
159. Kerr JH, Smith AC, Prys-Roberts C, *et al.* Observations during endobronchial anaesthesia. II. Oxygenation. *Br J Anaesth* 1974; **46:** 84–92.
160. El-Baz N, Jensik R, Faber LP, Faro RS. One-lung high-frequency ventilation for tracheoplasty and bronchoplasty: a new technique. *Ann Thorac Surg* 1982; **34:** 564–70.
161. Jackson RM. Pulmonary oxygen toxicity. *Chest* 1985; **88:** 900–5.
162. Nalos PC, Kass RM, Gang ES, *et al.* Life-threatening postoperative pulmonary complications in patients with previous amiodarone pulmonary toxicity undergoing cardiothoracic operations. *J Thorac Cardiovasc Surg* 1987; **93:** 904–12.
163. Thompson CC, Bailey MK, Conroy JM, Bromley HR. Postoperative pulmonary toxicity associated with mitomycin-C therapy. *South Med J* 1992; **85:** 1257–9.
164. Szegedi LL, Bardiczky GI, Engelman EE, d'Hollander AA. Airway pressure changes during one-lung ventilation. *Anesthesiology* 1997; **84:** 1034–7.
165. Iwasaka H, Itoh K, Miyakaw H, *et al.* Continuous monitoring of ventilatory mechanics during one-lung ventilation. *J Clin Monit* 1996; **12:** 161–4.
166. Weiler N, Eberle B, Heinrichs W. Adaptive lung ventilation (ALV) during anesthesia for pulmonary surgery. automatic response to transitions to and from one-lung ventilation. *J Clin Monit Comput* 1998; **14:** 245–52.
167. Tugrul M, Camci E, Karadeniz H, *et al.* Comparison of volume controlled with pressure controlled ventilation during one-lung anaesthesia. *Br J Anaesth* 1997; **79:** 306–10.
168. Katz JA, Laverne RG, Fairley HB, Thomas AN. Pulmonary oxygen exchange during endobronchial anesthesia: effects of tidal volume and PEEP. *Anesthesiology* 1982; **56:** 164–71.
169. Yokota K, Toriumi T, Sari A, *et al.* Auto-positive-end-expiratory pressure during one-lung ventilation using a double-lumen endobronchial tube. *Anesth Analg* 1996; **82:** 1007–10.
170. Bardoczky GI, d'Hollander AA, Cappello M, Yernault JC. Interrupted expiratory flow on automatically constructed flow-volume curves may determine the presence of intrinsic positive end-expiratory pressure during one-lung ventilation. *Anesth Analg* 1998; **86:** 880–4.
171. Slinger PD, Hickey DR. The interaction between applied PEEP and auto-PEEP during one-lung ventilation. *J Cardiothorac Vasc Anesth* 1998; **12:** 133–6.
172. Inomata S, Nishikawa T, Saito S, Kihara S. "Best" PEEP during one-lung ventilation. *Br J Anaesth* 1997; **78:** 754–6.
173. Malmkvist G. Maintenance of oxygenation during one-lung ventilation. Effect of intermittent reinflation of the collapse lung with oxygen. *Anesth Analg* 1989; **68:** 763–6.
174. Capan LM, Turndorf H, Chandrakant P, *et al.* Optimization of arterial oxygenation during one-lung anesthesia. *Anesth Analg* 1980; **59:** 847–51.
175. Hogue Jr CW. Effectiveness of low levels of nonventilated lung continuous positive airway pressure in improving arterial oxygenation during one-lung ventilation. *Anesth Analg* 1994; **79:** 364–7.
176. Cohen E, Eisenkraft JB. Positive end-expiratory pressure during one-lung ventilation improves oxygenation in patients with low arterial oxygen tensions. *J Cardiothorac Vasc Anesth* 1996; **10:** 578–82.
177. Slinger P, Triolet W, Wilson J. Improving arterial oxygenation during one-lung ventilation. *Anesthesiology* 1988; **68:** 291–5.
178. Cohen E, Eisenkraft JB, Thys DM, *et al.* Oxygenation and hemodynamic changes during one-lung ventilation: effects of $CPAP_{10}$, $PEEP_{10}$, and $CPAP_{10}/PEEP_{10}$. *J Cardiothorac Anesth* 1988; **2:** 34–40.
179. Marshall C, Kim SD, Marshall BE. The actions of halothane, ibuprofen and BW755C on hypoxic pulmonary vasoconstriction. *Anesthesiology* 1987; **66:** 537–42.
180. Scherer RW, Vigfusson G, Hultsch E, *et al.* Prostaglandin F_{2a} improves oxygen tension and reduces venous admixture during one-lung ventilation in anesthetized paralyzed dogs. *Anesthesiology* 1985; **62:** 23–8.
181. Chen TI, Ueng TH, Huang CH, *et al.* Improvement of arterial oxygenation by selective infusion of prostaglandin E1 to ventilated lung during one-lung ventilation. *Acta Anaesthesiol Scand* 1996; **40:** 7–13.
182. Chen TL, Lee YT, Wang MJ, *et al.* Endothelin-1 concentrations and optimisation of arterial oxygenation and venous admixture by selective artery infusion of prostaglandin E1 during thoracotomy. *Anaesthesia* 1996; **51:** 422–6.
183. Carmona MJC, Auler Jr JOC. Effects of inhaled nitric oxide on respiratory system mechanics, hemodynamics, and gas exchange after cardiac surgery. *J Cardiothorac Vasc Anesth* 1998; **12:** 157–61.
184. Pison U, Lopez FA, Heidelmeyer CF, *et al.* Inhaled nitric oxide reverses hypoxic pulmonary vasoconstriction without impairing gas exchange. *J Appl Physiol* 1993; **74:** 1287–92.
185. Rich GF, Lowson SM, Johns RA, *et al.* Inhaled nitric oxide selectively decreases pulmonary vascular resistance without impairing oxygenation during one-lung ventilation in patients undergoing cardiac surgery. *Anesthesiology* 1994; **80:** 57–62.
186. Wilson WC, Kapelanski DP, Benumof JL, *et al.* Inhaled nitric oxide (40 ppm) during one-lung ventilation, in the lateral decubitus position, does not decrease pulmonary vascular resistance or improve oxygenation in normal patients. *J Cardiothorac Vasc Anesth* 1997; **22:** 172–6.
187. Moutafis M, Liu N, Dalibon N, *et al.* The effects of inhaled nitric oxide and its combination with intravenous almitrine on PaO_2 during one-lung ventilation in patients undergoing thoracoscopy procedures. *Anesth Analg* 1997; **85:** 1130–5.
188. Pearl RG. Phenylephrine and inhaled nitric oxide in adult respiratory distress syndrome. When are two better than one? *Anesthesiology* 1997; **87:** 1–3.
189. Neustein SM, Kahn P, Kreellenstein DJ, Cohen E. Incidence of arrhythmias after thoracic surgery: thoracotomy versus video-assisted thoracoscopy. *J Cardiovasc Thorac Anesth* 1998; **12:** 659–61.
190. Kavanagh BP, Katz J, Sandler AN. Pain control after thoracotomy: a review of current techniques. *Anesthesiology* 1994; **81:** 737–59.
191. Burgess FW, Anderson M, Colonna D, *et al.* Ipsilateral shoulder pain following thoracic surgery. *Anesthesiology* 1993; **78:** 365–8.
192. Furrer M, Rechsteiner R, Eigenmann V, *et al.* Thoracotomy and thoracoscopy: postoperative pulmonary function, pain and chest wall complaints. *Eur J Cardiothorac Surg* 1997; **12:** 82–7.
193. Salzer GM, Klingler P, Klingler A, Unger A. Pain treatment after thoracotomy: is it a special problem? *Ann Thorac Surg* 1997; **63:** 1411–14.
194. Lubenow TR, Faber LP, McCarthy RJ, *et al.* Postthoracotomy pain management using continuous epidural analgesia in 1,324 patients. *Ann Thor Surg* 1994; **58:** 924–9.
195. George KA, Wright PMC, Chisakuta A. Continuous thoracic epidural fentanyl for post-thoracotomy pain relief: with or without bupivacaine? *Anaesthesia* 1991; **46:** 732–6.
196. Badner NH, Komar WE. Bupivacaine 0.1% does not improve post-operative epidural fentanyl analgesia after abdominal or thoracic surgery *Can J Anaesth* 1992; **39:** 330–6.
197. Aguilar JL, Rincon R, Domingo V, *et al.* Absence of an early pre-emptive effect after thoracic extradural bupivacaine in thoracic surgery. *Br J Anaesth* 1996; **76:** 72–6.
198. Etches RC, Gammer T-L, Cornish R. Patient-controlled epidural analgesia after thoracotomy: a comparison of meperidine with and without bupivacaine. *Anesth Analg* 1996; **83:** 81–6.
199. Baron CM, Kowalski SE, Greengrass R, *et al.* Epinephrine decreases postoperative requirements for continuous thoracic epidural fentanyl infusions. *Anesth Analg* 1996; **82:** 760–5.
200. Shulman M, Sandler AN, Bradley JW, *et al.* Postthoracotomy pain and pulmonary function following epidural and systemic morphine. *Anesthesiology* 1984; **61:** 569–75.

201. Guinard J-P, Mavrocordatos P, Chiolero R, Carpenter RL. A randomized comparison of intravenous versus lumbar and thoracic epidural fentanyl for analgesia after thoracotomy. *Anesthesiology* 1992; **77:** 1108–15.
202. Warner DO, Warner MA, Ritman EL. Human chest wall function during epidural anesthesia. *Anesthesiology* 1997; **85:** 761–73.
203. Logas WG, El-Baz N, El-Ganzouri A, *et al.* Continuous thoracic epidural analgesia for postoperative pain relief following thoracotomy. A randomized prospective study. *Anesthesiology* 1987; **67:** 787–91.
204. Patrick JA, Meyer-Witting M, Reynolds F. Lumbar epidural diamorphine following thoracic surgery. A comparison of infusion and bolus administration. *Anaesthesia* 1991; **46:** 85–9.
205. Rosseel PMJ, van den Broek WGM, Boer EC, Prakash O. Epidural sufentanil for intra- and postoperative analgesia in thoracic surgery: a comparative study with intravenous sufentanil. *Acta Anaesthesiol Scand* 1988; **32:** 193–8.
206. Brodsky JB, Chaplan SR, Brose WG, Mark JBD. Continuous epidural hydromorphone for postthoracotomy pain relief. *Ann Thorac Surg* 1990; **50:** 888–93.
207. Katz J, Kavanagh BP, Sandler AN, *et al.* Preemptive analgesia: clinical evidence of neuroplasticity contributing to postoperative pain. *Anesthesiology* 1992; **77:** 439–46.
208. Gray JR, Fromme GA, Nauss LA, *et al.* Intrathecal morphine for post-thoracotomy pain. *Anesth Analg* 1986; **65:** 873–6.
209. Grant RP, Dolman JF, Harper JA, *et al.* Patient-controlled lumbar epidural fentanyl compared with patient controlled intravenous fentanyl for post-thoracotomy pain. *Can J Anaesth* 1992; **39:** 214–19.
210. Coe A, Sarginson R, Smith MW, *et al.* Pain following thoracotomy: a randomized, double-blind comparison of lumbar versus thoracic epidural fentanyl. *Anaesthesia* 1991; **46:** 918–21.
211. Hansdottir V, Bake B, Nordberg G. The analgesic efficacy and adverse effects of continuous epidural sufentanil and bupivacaine infusion after thoracotomy. *Anesth Analg* 1996; **83:** 394–400.
212. Whiting WC, Sandler AN, Lau LC, *et al.* Analgesic and respiratory effects of epidural sufentanil in patients following thoracotomy. *Anesthesiology* 1988; **69:** 36–43.
213. Brose WG, Tanelian DL, Brodsky JB, Mark JBD. CSF and blood pharmacokinetics of hydromorphone and morphine following lumbar epidural administration. *Pain* 1991; **45:** 11–15.
214. Roxburgh JC, Markland CG, Ross BA, Kerr WF. Role of cryoanalgesia in the control of pain after thoracotomy. *Thorax* 1987; **42:** 292–5.
215. Gough JD, Williams AB, Vaughan RS, Khalil JF. The control of post-thoracotomy pain. A comparative evaluation of thoracic epidural fentanyl infusions and cryo-analgesia. *Anaesthesia* 1988; **43:** 780–3.
216. Benedetti F, Amanzanio M, Casadio C, *et al.* Control of postoperative pain by transcutaneous electrical nerve stimulation after thoracic operations. *Ann Thorac Surg* 1997; **63:** 773–6.
217. Sabanathan S, Smith PJB, Pradhan GN, *et al.* Continuous intercostal nerve block for pain relief after thoracotomy. *Ann Thorac Surg* 1988; **46:** 425–6.
218. Kaiser AM, Zollinger A, De Lorenzi D, *et al.* Prospective, randomized comparison of extrapleural versus epidural analgesia for posthoracotomy pain. *Ann Thorac Surg* 1998; **66:** 367–72.
219. Mann LJ, Young GR, Williams JK, *et al.* Intrapleural bupivacaine in the control of postthoracotomy pain. *Ann Thorac Surg* 1992; **53:** 449–54.
220. Ferrante FM, Chan VWS, Arthur GR, Rocco AG. Intrapleural analgesia after thoracotomy. *Anesth Analg* 1991; **72:** 105–9.
221. Schneider RF, Villamena PC, Harvey J, *et al.* Lack of efficacy of intrapleural bupivacaine for postoperative analgesia following thoracotomy. *Chest* 1993; **103:** 414–16.
222. Gaeta RR, Macario A, Brodsky JB, *et al.* Pain outcomes after thoracotomy: Lumbar epidural hydromorphone versus intrapleural bupivacaine. *J Cardiothorac Vasc Anesth* 1995; **9:** 534–7.
223. Richardson J, Sabanathan S, Shah RD, *et al.* Pleural bupivacaine placement for optimal postthoracotomy pulmonary function: a prospective, randomized study. *J Cardiothorac Vasc Anesth* 1998; **12:** 166–9.
224. Brodsky JB, Eggen M, Cannon WB. Spontaneous pneumothorax in early pregnancy: successful management by thoracoscopy. *J Cardiothorac Vasc Anesth* 1993; **7:** 585–7.
225. Garner L, Coats RR. Ipsilateral stellate ganglion block effective for treating shoulder pain after thoracotomy. *Anesth Analg* 1994; **78:** 1195–6.
226. Perttunen K, Kalso E, Heinonen J, Salo J. I.V. diclofenac in post-thoracotomy pain. *Br J Anaesth* 1992; **68:** 474–80.
227. Rhodes M, Conacher I, Morritt G, Hilton C. Nonsteroidal antiinflammatory drugs for postthoracotomy pain. A prospective controlled trial after lateral thoracotomy. *J Thorac Cardiovasc Surg* 1992; **103:** 17–20.
228. Singh H, Bossard RF, White PF, Yeatts RW. Effects of ketorolac versus bupivacaine coadministration during patient-controlled hydromorphone epidural analgesia after thoracotomy procedures. *Anesth Analg* 1997; **84:** 564–9.
229. Dich-Nielsen JO, Svendsen LB, Berthelsen P. Intramuscular low-dose ketamine versus pethidine for postoperative pain treatment after thoracic surgery. *Acta Anaesthesiol Scand* 1992; **36:** 583–7.
230. Chou TKF, Penberthy AJ, Goodchild CS. Ketamine as adjunct to morphine in postthoracotomy analgesia: an unintended N-of-1 study. *Anesth Analg* **87:** 1372–4.
231. James MFM, Heijke SAM, Gordon PC. Intravenous tramadol versus epidural morphine for postthoracotomy pain relief: a placebo-controlled double-blind trial. *Anesth Analg* 1996; **83:** 87–91.
232. D'Arsiny C, Goldberg P. Mechanical ventilation for respiratory failure postthoracotomy. *Chest Surg Clin North AM* 1998; **8:** 585–610.
233. Weinlander CM, Abel MD, Piehler JM. Spontaneous cardiac herniation after pneumonectomy. *Anesth Analg* 1986; **65:** 1085–8.
234. Baaijens PF, Hasenbos MA, Lacquet LK, Dekhuijzen PN. Cardiac herniation after pneumonectomy. *Acta Anaesthesiol Scand* 1992; **36:** 842–5.
235. Cassorla L, Katz JA. Management of cardiac herniation after intrapericardial pneumonectomy. *Anesthesiology* 1984; **60:** 362–4.
236. Robinson CL. The management of chylothorax. *Ann Thorac Surg* 1985; **39:** 90–5.
237. Mitsudimi T, Mizoue T, Yoshimatsu T, *et al.* Postoperative complications after pneumonectomy for treatment of lung cancer: multivariate analysis. *J Surg Oncol* 1996; **61:** 218–22.
238. Jaklitsch MT, DeCamp MM, Liptay MJ, *et al.* Video-assisted thoracic surgery in the elderly. *Chest* 1996; **110:** 751–8.
239. Ritchie AJ, Tolan M, Whiteside M, *et al.* Prophylactic digitalization fails to control dysrhythmia in thoracic esophageal operations. *Ann Thorac Surg* 1993; **55:** 86–8.
240. Jakobsen CJ, Bille S, Ahlburg P, *et al.* Perioperative metoprolol reduces the frequency of atrial fibrillation after thoracotomy for lung resection. *J Cardiothorac Vasc Anesth* 1997; **11:** 746–51.
241. Lindgren L, Lepantalo M, Von Knorring J, *et al.* Effect of verapamil on right ventricular pressure and atrial tachyarrhythmia after thoracotomy. *Br J Anaesth* 1991; **66:** 205–11.
242. Van Mieghem W, Tits G, Demuynck K, *et al.* Verapamil as prophylactic treatment for atrial fibrillation after lung operations. *Ann Thorac Surg* 1996; **61:** 1083–6.
243. van der Werff YD, van der Houwen HK, Heijmans PJ, *et al.* Postpneumonectomy pulmonary edema. A retrospective analysis of incidence and possible risk factors. *Chest* 1997; **111:** 1278–84.
244. Shapira OM, Shahian DM. Postpneumonectomy pulmonary edema. *Ann Thorac Surg* 1993; **56:** 190–5.
245. Parquin F, Marchal M, Mehiri S, *et al.* Post-pneumonectomy pulmonary edema: analysis and risk factors. *Eur J Cardiothorac Surg* 1996; **10:** 929–32.
246. Turnage WS, Lunn JL. Postpneumonectomy pulmonary edema. A retrospective analysis of associated variables. *Chest* 1993; **103:** 1646–50.
247. Waller DA, Keavey P, Woodfine L, Dark JH. Pulmonary endothelial permeability changes after major lung resection. *Ann Thorac Surg* 1996; **61:** 1435–40.
248. Cohen E. Physiology of the lateral position and one-lung ventilation. *Chest Surg Clin North Am* 1997; **7:** 753–71.
249. Isaac PA, Barry JE, Vaughan RS, *et al.* A jet nebuliser for delivery of topical anaesthesia to the respiratory tract. A comparison with cricothyroid puncture and direct spraying for fibreoptic bronchoscopy. *Anaesthesia* 1990; **45:** 46–8.
250. Crawford M, Pollock J, Anderson K, *et al.* Comparison of midazolam with propofol for sedation in outpatient bronchoscopy. *Br J Anaesth* 1993; **70:** 418–22.
251. Birmingham B, Mentzer SJ, Body SC. Laryngeal mask airway for therapeutic fiberoptic bronchoscopic procedures. *J Cardiothorac Vasc Anesth* 1996; **10:** 519–20.
252. Plummer S, Hartley M, Vaughan RS. Anaesthesia for telescopic procedures in the thorax. *Br J Anaesth* 1998; **80:** 223–34.
253. Kestin IG, Chapman JM, Coates MB. Alfentanil used to supplement propofol infusions for oesophagoscopy and bronchoscopy. *Anaesthesia* 1989; **44:** 994–6.
254. Neuman GG, Weingarten AE, Abramowitz RM, *et al.* The anesthetic management of the patient with an anterior mediastinal mass. *Anesthesiology* 1984; **60:** 144–7.
255. Hanowell LH, Martin WR, Savelle J, Foppiano LE. Complications of general anesthesia for Nd:YAG resection of endobronchial tumors. *Chest* 1991; **99:** 72–6.
256. Conacher ID, Paes LL, McMahon CC, Morritt GN. Anesthetic management of laser surgery for central airway obstruction: a 12-year case series. *J Cardiothorac Vasc Anesth* 1998; **12:** 153–6.

257. Lammers CR, Hammer GB, Brodsky JB, Cannon WB. Failure to separate and isolate the lungs with an endotracheal tube positioned in the bronchus. *Anesth Analg* 1997; **85:** 946–7.
258. Wakabayashi A. Expanded applications of diagnostic and therapeutic thoracoscopy. *J Thorac Cardiovasc Surg* 1991; **102:** 721–3.
259. Carillo EH, Schmact DC, Gable DR, *et al.* Thoracoscopy in the management of posttraumatic persistent pneumothorax. *J Am Coll Surg* 1998; **186:** 636–9.
260. Fredman B, Olsfanger D, Jedeikin R. Thoracoscopic sympathectomy in the treatment of palmar hyperhidrosis: anaesthetic implications. *Br J Anaesth* 1997; **79:** 113–99.
261. Baraka A. Hazards of carbon dioxide insufflation during thoracoscopy. *Br J Anaesth* 1998; **81:** 100.
262. Peden CJ, Prys-Roberts C. Capnothorax: implications for the anaesthetist. *Anaesthesia*1993; **48:** 664–6.
263. Bishop MJ, Benson MS, Sato P, Pierson DJ. Comparison of high-frequency jet ventilation with conventional mechanical ventilation for bronchopleural fistula. *Anesth Analg* 1987; **66:** 833–8.
264. Cohen E, Eisenkraft JB. Bronchopulmonary lavage. effects on oxygenation and hemodynamics. *J Cardiothorac Anesth* 1990; **4:** 609–15.
265. Wakabayashi A, Brenner M, Kayaleh RA, *et al.* Thoracoscopic carbon dioxide laser treatment of bullous emphysema. *Lancet* 1991; **337:** 881–3.
266. Cooper JD, Trulock EP, Triantafillou AN, *et al.* Bilateral pneumonectomy (volume reduction) for chronic obstructive pulmonary disease. *J Thorac Cardiovasc Surg* 1995; **109:** 106–19.
267. Doyle RL, Brodsky JB. Lung volume reduction surgery. An option for your COPD patient? *J Crit Illness* 1997; **12:** 666–71.
268. Fein AM. Lung volume reduction surgery: answering the crucial questions. *Chest* 1998; **113:** 277S–282S.
269. Kruculak PE, Naunheim KS, Keller CA, Baudendistel LJ. Anesthetic management of patients undergoing unilateral video-assisted lung reduction for treatment of end-stage emphysema. *J Cardiothorac Vasc Anesth* 1996; **10:** 850–3.
270. Mylles PS, Venema HR. Avoidance of cardiopulmonary bypass during bilateral sequential lung transplantation using inhaled nitric oxide. *J Cardiothorac Vasc Anesth* 1995; **9:** 571–4.
271. Bacha EA, Head CA. Use of inhaled nitric oxide for lung transplantation and cardiac surgery. *Respir Care Clin North Am* 1997; **3:** 521–36.

48

Anesthetic management of patients with endocrine disease

CHRISTOPHER J HULL AND ANNA M BATCHELOR

The anesthetic management of a variety of endocrine disorders will be discussed. Some, such as diabetes mellitus, are included because they occur so frequently. Others, such as pheochromocytoma, despite relative rarity, are discussed because they present severe problems to the anesthesiologist. The underlying endocrine disorders are described in detail in Chapter 24.

DIABETES MELLITUS

Diabetes mellitus is a common condition characterized by inappropriate hyperglycemia and is associated with a wide range of complications. Most of these are of direct significance to the anesthesiologist.

Problems associated with the diabetic patient

It is widely held that diabetic patients are at greater perioperative risk than the general population. The high incidence of coronary and cerebral atherosclerosis, hypertension, and peripheral vascular and renal disease is of major importance.[1] Diabetic patients may also suffer from somatic or autonomic neuropathy. Furthermore, animal studies have suggested that uncorrected hyperglycemia may be associated with poor wound healing and impaired resistance to infection.[2,3]

In a 1982 analysis of 2300 surgical deaths, Fowkes *et al.*[4] found that patients with diabetes were 11 times more likely to succumb than patients with no preoperative abnormality. However, it appears that the diabetic patient is at risk not so much from acute metabolic derangement as from comorbidity such as ischemic or valvular heart disease, nephropathy, and peripheral vascular disease with sepsis.[5]

The metabolic problem

In uncontrolled type 1 diabetes, there is a generalized catabolic state. Lipids are mobilized with release of fatty acids. Ketogenesis increases, leading to acidosis and loss of cellular potassium. Protein breakdown exceeds protein synthesis. Gluconeogenesis and glycogenolysis, combined with reduced tissue utilization of glucose, lead to hyperglycemia. When the renal threshold for glucose (10–11 mmol L^{-1}) is exceeded, glycosuria leads to osmotic polyuria and dehydration. Plasma hyperosmolarity, acidosis, and hyperkalemia lead to coma and then death.

Patients with type 2 diabetes may also present in hyperosmolar coma requiring urgent stabilization.

Unless managed appropriately, most diabetic patients undergoing surgery will become hyperglycemic during the operation and severely catabolic afterwards.

Increased catecholamine, adrenocorticotropic hormone (ACTH), and cortisol production commences before surgery and is probably caused by emotional factors. The surgical stress response then causes further increases in cortisol, growth hormone, and glucagon with inhibition of insulin secretion, leading to hyperglycemia, increased metabolic rate, and increased nitrogen excretion.

Postoperatively, there is increased lactate and pyruvate formation, with increased gluconeogenesis, probably driven by increased secretion of insulin-opposing mediators such as glucagon and catecholamines. A negative protein balance develops as part of the overall catabolic state.

These changes apply equally to type 1 patients with no insulin secretion and to type 2 patients who, although capable of secreting enough insulin for daily life, may fail to increase insulin secretion after surgery so that gluconeogenesis and fat and protein breakdown, combined with impaired glucose tissue uptake, may lead to severe hyperglycemia and hyperosmolar coma.

All the above changes can be prevented by the appropriate administration of insulin and glucose, demand for which increases with the severity of surgery.[6]

"Stiff joint" syndrome

Some 30% of insulin-dependent diabetes mellitus (IDDM) patients develop "stiff joint" syndrome,[7] characterized by contractures of finger joints with tight, waxy skin. There is a reported association with limited atlantoaxial movement and with difficult intubation.[8–10]

Autonomic neuropathy

Up to 50% of diabetic patients eventually develop autonomic neuropathy affecting both gastrointestinal and circulatory control. Impaired hemodynamic responses can be detected by standard tests, but these do not predict gastrointestinal problems such as gastroparesis.[11] Esophageal and gastric dysfunction may increase the risk of regurgitation at the induction of and recovery from anesthesia, and it should be noted that prokinetic drugs such as cisapride (no longer available in the UK) do not prevent this problem.[12–14] Severe bradycardia, hypotension, and cardiopulmonary arrest during anesthesia have been reported, and it has been shown that diabetic patients are at greater risk of undesirable cardiovascular events during surgery.[15–18]

It is interesting to note that 33% of (randomly selected) diabetic patients investigated by Williams and Morris[19] had impaired responses to hypercapnia and/or hypoxemia. These findings may reflect a manifestation of autonomic neuropathy, but a clear link has not been established. The possible relevance to anesthesia is self-evident.

Management of metabolic status before, during, and after scheduled surgery

Diabetic patients may present for surgery in stable therapeutic condition. Occasionally, however, patients with undiagnosed diabetes may present with acute surgical conditions.

It is generally accepted that, in the interests of general metabolic welfare, good wound healing, and resistance to infection, the objectives are (1) to maintain adequate plasma insulin levels in order to prevent catabolism with ketoacidosis and (2) to provide glucose intake sufficient to prevent hypoglycemia (~ 150 g per 24 h). However, there is little consensus as to how tightly the blood glucose should be controlled and even less as to how that might be achieved. As Alberti remarked (somewhat tartly in response to criticisms[20] of his own regimen), "The management of diabetes in patients undergoing surgery is a subject that has tended to generate heat rather than light, as occurs in so many other areas of clinical practice."[21] Alberti's recommendation that blood glucose should be controlled within the range 6.6–9.9 mmol L^{-1} (120–180 mg dL^{-1}) appears still to be widely accepted. However, in a recent review,[22] it has been argued that, since tight glycemic control is associated with better wound healing and a lower incidence of major complications, this should now be regarded as imperative and a goal which is attainable in most patients.

Type 1 diabetic patients should stop taking long-acting insulin preparations at least 24 h before surgery, converting to intermediate or soluble forms. Intermediate-acting insulin preparations may safely be continued until the evening before surgery.[21] On the morning of operation, the following methods may be considered for type 1 diabetic patients. All depend heavily for their safety on the regular estimation of blood glucose using bedside reflectance meters, with a formal program of staff training and quality assurance. Without such measures, ward measurements are likely to be both inaccurate and misleading.[23]

No insulin, no glucose

This method has the merit of simplicity, and is most unlikely to cause hypoglycemia. However, as the effects of the last preoperative dose of insulin decays, the inexorable process leading toward diabetic ketoacidosis begins. The preoperative blood glucose value may well be within the physiologic range (4.2–6.4 mmol L^{-1}), but intraoperative hyperglycemia is inevitable. Unless insulin and glucose are given very shortly after surgery, the stress response to surgery accelerates the catabolic process and the patient may rapidly become dehydrated and ketoacidotic. Nevertheless, this method is widely used for insulin-dependent patients who are to undergo brief, body surface procedures [such as dilation and curettage (D&C) or cystoscopy] which simply delay normal morning insulin and food intake by less than an hour.[24,25]

Partial morning dose of insulin (s.c.) with dextrose infusion

This traditional approach is based on custom rather than logic. The patient is not taking meals, and the dextrose solution provides caloric intake at a constant rate. Why, then, administer an evanescent hormone by intermittent subcutaneous (s.c.) injection – surely the least predictable method of parenteral administration? If hypoglycemia is to be avoided, each injection is certain to be preceded by a period of hyperglycemia. Walts *et al.* showed that, despite frequent blood glucose measurements, three commonly used techniques all failed to provide good glycemic control.[26]

Infusion of a glucose–insulin–potassium solution at a standard rate

In 1979, Alberti and Thomas proposed the use of a standard intravenous glucose–insulin–potassium (GIK) solution [500 mL of 10% glucose containing 10 U of soluble insulin with 1 g of KCl, to be administered at 100 mL h^{-1} (2 U h^{-1})].[27] They suggested that before surgery patients should be stabilized on a soluble insulin regimen, with the morning dose on the day of surgery omitted. The GIK infusion was to commence early on the morning of surgery, and the blood glucose monitored at 2–3 h and then before induction. If the blood glucose fell below 5 mmol L^{-1}, or increased to greater than 10 mmol L^{-1}, the bag of solution was to be replaced with one containing insulin 5 U or 15 U respectively. The blood glucose was to be checked 2- to 4-hourly, and the KCl content of the solution could be adjusted according to the serum K^+. The patient could revert to subcutaneous dosing when oral intake was resumed, with normal therapy resumed after 2–3 days.

The authors claimed that this technique was simple to use, effective in practice, and safe. Since the insulin and glucose were to be administered together, quite wide variations in administration rate would cause minimal changes in blood glucose. However, 5 years passed before they offered any supporting evidence, and when it came[28] it was unconvincing. The numbers in each group were tiny and the types of surgery undertaken varied widely. Their GIK infusion group (four patients) even contained a patient with pheochromocytoma, in whom major problems with glycemic control were to be anticipated (see below). Glycemic control was hardly better than in the "traditional" (i.e. reduced dose of soluble insulin by s.c. injection) group. Moreover, Bowen *et al.*[29] reported hypoglycemic incidents in 2 out of 27 patients undergoing a variety of scheduled procedures using the 1979 Alberti method, and suggested that no insulin be added to the bag when blood glucose is less than 5 mmol L^{-1}.

Despite Bowen *et al.*'s call for caution, Alberti's group increased the ratio of insulin to glucose in their GIK regimen and showed that it could achieve better glycemic control than a s.c. injection method, but that some failures did occur.[30]

The most recent version of the Alberti regimen[31] is set out in Table 48.1. Despite its obvious limitations, the method became popular, mainly because of simplicity of use and wide margin of safety.[20] Working in a hospital where the Alberti method has been standard practice for many years, these authors have found it easy and safe to use but frustrating in less stable patients, in whom frequent changes of solution may be required to maintain normoglycemia. If the standard solution is to be adhered to where possible, many patients will become moderately hyperglycemic by the end of surgery, and remain so in the early postoperative period. With patients undergoing major surgery who must rely on intravenous fluids for some days, care must be taken with fluid and electrolyte balance because 2.5 L of 10% glucose solution is infused per 24 h with an attendant risk of hyponatremia. The water load may be reduced by using 20% or even 50% glucose solution, but infusion into a central venous line then becomes essential. We remain concerned that the Alberti regimen continues to administer insulin to frankly hypoglycemic patients, and we suggest that the infusion be discontinued at blood glucose values below 5 mmol L^{-1}. Blood glucose measurements should then be repeated at 30-min intervals until 6.7 mmol L^{-1} is reached. Serum potassium should be checked 8-hourly and the potassium content of the solution adjusted as indicated. Particular care is required for patients with poor renal function.

Fixed-rate glucose infusion, with separate and adjustable infusion of insulin to maintain normoglycemia

Glucose must be administered at a rate sufficient to prevent ketosis, and

Table 48.1 *The Alberti GIK regimen for glycemic control during the perioperative period*[31]

Initial solution: 500 mL 10% glucose + 10 mmol KCl + 15 U insulin
Infuse at 100 mL h^{-1} (i.e. 3 U h^{-1})
Check blood glucose every 2 h

According to result:

Blood glucose mmol L^{-1}	Action
<6.5	Infuse solution containing 10 U insulin (2 U h^{-1})
>6.4 to <11.1	Infuse solution containing 15 U insulin (3 U h^{-1})
>11	Infuse solution containing 20 U insulin (4 U h^{-1})

Continue to adjust in 5-U steps as necessary

different groups have suggested rates ranging from 5 to 10 g h^{-1} (70-kg patient).[32,33]

Potassium supplementation is usually required, and the administration rate should be modified in the event of hypo- or hyperkalemia.

Watts *et al.*[34] found that insulin requirements varied very widely (0.5–5 U h^{-1}) during the perioperative period, and showed that a variable rate infusion could achieve normoglycemia in all patients. Based on the regimen proposed by Watts *et al.*, Hirsch *et al.*[35] set out a simple algorithm for insulin infusion which is easily followed by medical staff (Table 48.2).

Such regimens are capable of close control, but it must be accepted that separate administration of insulin and glucose increases the risk of insulin accidentally being given without glucose and causing severe hypoglycemia, or of infusion pumps being wrongly programmed. Alberti suggested that separate infusions of glucose and insulin were suitable for use in teaching hospitals, but that combined GIK infusions were more suitable for district general hospitals where, presumably, medical and nursing staff were more prone to error.[21] In truth, the choice of method is probably less important than the skill, organization, and coordination of the doctors and nurses involved.[36]

Closed loop controller: the artificial pancreas

Systems have been devised that can infuse glucose and insulin, as determined by an on-line glucose analyzer. Such systems are capable of very tight control to any stated blood glucose concentration. In most cases, such complexity is unnecessary and probably introduces more hazards than benefits. However, in cardiac surgery involving extracorporeal circulation, when insulin requirements may be very large, they may have a place.[37] They are, however, complex, expensive, demanding of technical supervision, and not yet a practicable proposition outside the research environment.

The type 2, noninsulin-dependent diabetic

These patients should stop taking long-acting hypoglycemic drugs some days before surgery, switching to shorter-acting drugs such as tolbutamide or glibenclamide.

In the case of patients undergoing minor surgery, one approach is to allow the patient to take an oral hypoglycemic on the morning of surgery, and then to infuse a 10% glucose solution to maintain normoglycemia until oral intake resumes.

However, it is common UK practice simply to omit both hypoglycemic drug and caloric intake on the morning of surgery.[25] If such patients are well controlled (i.e. fasting blood glucose < 11 mmol L^{-1}), we agree that they may safely be managed without further hypoglycemic medication until taking oral fluids and able to resume normal caloric intake (i.e. later the same day). It is, of course, essential that the blood glucose be checked at regular intervals, and active control instituted as necessary. If the fasting blood glucose level is greater than 11 mmol L^{-1}, active management with insulin and glucose is required if glycosuria (leading to osmotic dehydration), impaired wound healing, and impaired leukocyte function are to be prevented.[2] If the fasting blood glucose exceeds 14 mmol L^{-1}, we concur with Hirsch *et al.* that the risk of osmotic dehydration demands active management with glucose and insulin, however minor the surgery.[35]

All type 2 patients undergoing major surgery should be managed according to the standard diabetic regimen as for insulin-dependent diabetics.

Management of diabetic ketoacidosis prior to urgent or emergency surgery

Every anesthesiologist will encounter the type 1 diabetic patient, admitted as a surgical emergency, whose metabolic status has become highly deranged and may even be approaching ketoacidotic coma. Type 2 patients may also develop severe hyperglycemia leading to hyperosmolar coma. Treatment of both conditions is similar.

Except in the most pressing surgical circumstances (such as torrential and uncontrolled hemorrhage or the acutely compromised airway), such patients always require full stabilization before anesthesia and surgery can be contemplated. Many different regimens have been advocated, but all are based on insulin therapy with rehydration and electrolyte replacement. Dehydration and electrolyte loss may be severe, and large volumes of 0.9% saline solution may be required. Intravenous infusions of insulin are to be preferred because insulin has a plasma half-time of only a few minutes and absorption from subcutaneous depots (although much slower with half-time approximately 4 h) is highly variable in ketoacidotic patients.[38] Despite their widespread use for many years, large doses of insulin are not required, and the objective is to produce physiologic plasma insulin concentrations. For instance, Semple *et al.*[38] recommended a loading dose of insulin 8 U, followed by 8 U h^{-1}. Other authors have recommended insulin infusion rates as low as 2.4 U h^{-1}, showing that ketoacidotic patients stabilize within a few hours with a lower risk of hypoglycemia.[39] Glucose administration should recommence when the blood glucose level reaches 13 mmol L^{-1} in order to prevent a rapid overswing into hypoglycemia.

Table 48.2 *Insulin infusion algorithm for use prior to elective surgery (based on Hirsch* et al.[35] *with permission of the authors and* Anesthesiology*)*

Infuse glucose at 5 g h^{-1}, with potassium 2–4 mmol h^{-1}
Start insulin infusion at 0.5–1 U h^{-1}

Measure blood glucose hourly:

Blood glucose (mmol L^{-1})	Action
<4.5	Give 25 g glucose and stop insulin for 30 min; recheck blood sugar; restart insulin at 0.3–0.6 U h^{-1} when blood glucose > 6.7 mmol L^{-1}
4.5–6.6	Reduce insulin infusion by 0.3 U h^{-1}
6.7–10	No change
10.1–13.3	Increase insulin infusion by 0.3 U h^{-1}
>13.3	Increase insulin infusion by 0.5 U h^{-1}

Intravenous fluid requirements may exceed 10 L in the first 24 h, and potassium supplementation is required as potassium is driven back into the cells. Potassium should not, however, be given until the serum potassium falls below 5 mmol L^{-1}.[38] Metabolic acidosis is usually self-correcting, but the very severely acidotic patient (i.e. pH < 6.9) may require limited doses of sodium bicarbonate as a life-saving measure.[40]

As the blood glucose concentration declines, the acidosis resolves and the serum electrolytes normalize, and the contraindications to anesthesia and surgery diminish. In nonlife-threatening surgical situations, the ketoacidosis should be allowed to resolve fully and the patient stabilized on a GIK infusion before surgery is contemplated. In the case of the patient with pressing surgical problems, such as vascular or intra-abdominal emergencies, the surgeon and anesthesiologist must weigh the risks of delay against those of incomplete metabolic resolution compounded by the surgical stress response in deciding the optimum time for intervention.

Practical problems with insulin infusions

Anesthesiologists must be constantly aware of the danger presented by insulin administration without coadministration of glucose. When separate infusions are used, both insulin and glucose should be delivered by electronic pumps with operating alarm systems. Nurse- or anesthesiologist-monitored "drip set" infusions simply are not good enough. Where possible, the two channels should be common. Both pumps should take alternating current (a.c.) power from the same source (two-channel pumps are ideal), and the two delivery lines should join before reaching the patient.

Insulin is adsorbed onto glass or plastic surfaces, so that a very dilute solution may be even more dilute when it reaches the patient. The dangers associated with changing empty bags or syringes for fresh ones are obvious. Insulin adsorption can be prevented by adding human albumin (1 g per 100 mL) to the solution,[38] but this has raised concerns about blood-transmitted disease. In fact, since adsorption is both rapid and saturable, the problem may be minimized by priming the delivery system, waiting a few minutes, and then pumping out a volume equal to that of the delivery tubing. An alternative strategy is to place a high concentration of insulin in the syringe, so that the adsorbed fraction is much reduced and therefore less significant.

Organization of perioperative diabetic care

In the great majority of hospitals, the metabolic care of diabetic patients is managed by a diabetic team, using regimens devised in consultation with anesthesiologists and surgeons. Good coordination is mandatory because lack of communication between teams is responsible for the great majority of errors.

Anesthetic considerations

Anesthesiologists should consider the following issues, based on the authors' experience, when anesthetizing a diabetic patient:

- There is a greater than average risk that the patient will have coronary artery disease and renal impairment, and preoperative assessment should establish cardiovascular and renal status. Where patients have evidence of microalbuminuria, anesthesiologists may wish to avoid the use of potentially nephrotoxic drugs.[35]
- There is a strong case when assessing diabetic patients before major surgery for testing autonomic reflexes using R–R interval analysis and Valsalva and tilt tests.[18] Abnormal values indicating autonomic neuropathy will give warning of adverse hemodynamic events and impaired responses to physiologic stresses (such as blood loss and vascular occlusion) during surgery. Administration of spinal or extradural anesthesia in such patients may be especially hazardous.
- The medication record should be examined carefully to ensure that the diabetic regimen is, in fact, appropriate, and that the regular diabetic medication has been discontinued.
- The patient may be difficult to intubate. Patients with an abnormal "prayer sign" (inability to approximate the palmar surfaces of the fingers) may have "stiff joint" syndrome and should undergo detailed assessment of atlanto-occipital mobility.
- Diabetic autonomic neuropathy may also cause gastrointestinal problems such as disordered esophageal motility, gastroparesis, and hyperacidity, all of which may increase the risk of gastric reflux during anesthesia. This risk relates closely to that of difficult intubation.
- For a given glucose administration rate, insulin requirement may be expected to increase during surgery and may increase still further during the postoperative period.
- It is prudent to avoid the use of Hartmann's or other lactate-containing solutions because they may provoke hyperglycemia in both type 1 and 2 diabetic patients.[41] If they are to be used, then at the very least the glucose equivalence of the lactate should be regarded as part of the glucose intake.
- Because diabetic patients are less able to metabolize lipid emulsions,[42] caution should be exercised when considering the use of drugs in lipid emulsion form. Single doses of propofol are most unlikely to present any problem, but prolonged infusions for intensive care sedation may carry an increased risk of hyperlipidemia.[22]
- All diabetic patients must be monitored using regular blood glucose estimation. During anesthesia, estimation at 30-min intervals will give the anesthesiologist a clear indication of insulin and glucose requirements. Glucose concentrations in urine are retrospective and of significance only when glycosuria is present: they have no part to play in perioperative management. Since tight glycemic control is associated with better wound healing and a lower incidence of major complications, adherence to Alberti's permissible range of blood glucose concentrations (4.2–6.4 mmol L^{-1}) should be regarded as a clinical requirement.

DIABETES INSIPIDUS

Diabetes insipidus is a condition characterized by undersecretion or absent secretion of antidiuretic hormone (ADH, or arginine vasopressin) by the posterior part of the pituitary gland. It may be caused by trauma, by pituitary or hypothalamic tumors, or by inflammatory conditions such as sarcoidosis, or it may be familial. In addition to such "cranial" forms, secondary diabetes insipidus may be caused by a variety of conditions that increase renal resistance to vasopressin. It also occurs very occasionally in pregnancy, in which it is usually caused by excessive placental production of vasopressinase and by kidney disorders in which the renal tubule becomes resistant to the effects of ADH (so-called nephrogenic diabetes insipidus).[43,44]

When, in the healthy individual, blood osmolality increases, specialized receptors in the brain (osmoreceptors) detect the change and stimulate (1) thirst and (2) release of ADH from the posterior pituitary. ADH acts on the tubular system of the kidney to promote reabsorption of water from the renal tubule. Thus, the individual drinks more water and excretes more concentrated urine.

If the posterior pituitary fails to excrete ADH, there is profuse production of very dilute urine leading to increased blood osmolality and severe thirst. The patient responds by drinking large volumes of water. In such cases, it is not unusual for patients to drink more than 10 L of water per day, and to pass a similar volume of very dilute urine. If for any reason the patient is unable to drink freely (as would be the case when unconscious for example), the blood osmolality increases rapidly, leading to severe hypernatremia. When the serum sodium concentration exceeds 160–170 mmol L^{-1}, the hyperosmotic effect on brain cells may cause severe and irreversible cerebral damage.

Patients suffering from diabetes insipidus are treated with desmopressin (desamino-D-arginine vasopressin, or DDAVP), which is a long-acting analog of the natural hormone. This may be administered intravenously, intranasally in the form of snuff or atomizer, or orally.[45] The daily adult requirement ranges from 10 to 40 μg per day (intranasal spray) or 0.1–1.2 mg per day (oral tablets). Patients treated with regular and appropriate doses of desmopressin lead a perfectly normal life.

Overdose of desmopressin leads to reduced urine production. The resulting water retention causes reduced blood osmolality and hyponatremia. Mild degrees of water retention cause few symptoms, but severe excess causes cerebral edema with symptoms ranging from general lassitude to coma and convulsions. The neurologic picture is especially alarming when serum sodium declines rapidly because the adaptive mechanisms that occur with chronic hyponatremia do not operate.[46]

The anesthetic (i.e. perioperative) management of patients follows a common-sense approach:

- Patients continue to take their normal desmopressin dosage. If unable to take oral medication, an equivalent dose is administered intranasally or intravenously.
- Plasma concentrations of serum electrolytes, such as sodium and chloride, are measured preoperatively, so as to provide baseline normal values for that patient. In patients with cranial diabetes insipidus and intact thirst mechanisms, these would be expected to lie within the normal range.
- Accurate fluid balance charts are kept through the perioperative period to ensure that fluid intake continues to meet urine output.
- Serum electrolytes are monitored carefully. The serum sodium concentration provides vital information as the patient's kidney will not regulate urine output to compensate for under- or overhydration. Measurement of urinary osmolality shows how well the kidney is concentrating the urine, and may be very useful when the level of ADH activity is uncertain.
- Intravenous fluid therapy, when required, is regulated carefully so as to maintain accurate fluid balance and normal serum electrolyte concentrations.

If patients do become severely hyponatremic during the perioperative period, anesthesiologists should be aware of the dangers associated with rapid correction. Although this was at one time advocated on the grounds that cerebral exposure to hyponatremia must be minimized by prompt correction,[47] it is now recognized that rapid correction presents an even greater threat. Patients whose serum sodium concentration has been allowed to increase at a rate greater than 12 mmol per 24 h are likely to develop an osmotic demyelination syndrome, often described (not entirely accurately) as pontine myelinolysis.[48] This may develop over a period of several days (and often following an apparent improvement as the hyponatremia is corrected), presenting as fluctuation in the level of consciousness or even frank convulsions, and may be associated with both respiratory and cardiovascular disturbances. Patients then develop pseudobulbar palsy and a quadraparesis. In severe cases, patients may develop a "locked in" syndrome in which they remain fully conscious but are unable to move or communicate. Recovery is variable.

The osmotic demyelination syndrome can be prevented by slow correction of hyponatremia over several days, with close monitoring of serum electrolytes and urinary output.

THYROID DISEASE

The thyroid gland may be removed because it is overactive, enlarged and causing symptoms, cancerous, or because the patient has a genetic tendency to thyroid malignancy.

Thyrotoxicosis

Thyrotoxic patients may be managed medically or surgically. In the USA, radioactive iodine-131 is frequently used, but in the UK surgical treatment with partial or total thyroidectomy remains the most common approach.

It is essential that thyrotoxic patients are made euthyroid prior to surgery. Control is achieved with either carbimazole or propylthiouracil; both these thionamides inhibit the production of thyroid hormones. In the UK, a thionamide is usually accompanied by thyroxine in a "block and replace" regimen. In the days before surgery, inorganic iodine may be administered to reduce vascularity of the gland, although this practice is becoming less common. When used, it is important to schedule surgery within 3–8 days of commencement, after which vascularity may actually increase.

Retrosternal goiter

An enlarged thyroid gland can compress any of the structures surrounding it. Furthermore, if the gland grows downwards into the superior mediastinum, it can compress structures in the thoracic inlet. Airway symptoms are by far the most common; initially, the patient may complain of cough, hoarseness, or shortness of breath, frequently worse when lying down, and may progress to stridor.[49] The trachea may appear deviated or compressed on radiographs. Rarely, veins may be compressed, but the slow enlargement of most goiters allows collateral venous drainage to develop, thus preventing symptoms. The esophagus may be compressed, and such patients may complain of dysphagia. A more unusual problem is "downhill esophageal varices," caused by obstruction of the veins draining the upper third of the esophagus.[50] Nerves may also be affected. In particular, stretching the recurrent laryngeal nerve may cause vocal cord palsy, which usually responds to surgical removal of the gland.[51]

Thyroid malignancy

Follicular and papillary cancers arise from the follicular endothelium and medullary cancers from the parafollicular cells. The relatively rare medullary tumor releases calcitonin, and is often associated with hereditary conditions such as multiple endocrine neoplasia (MEN) type 2A, MEN type 2B, and familial non-MEN medullary thyroid cancer (FMTC).[52]

The lingual thyroid

The thyroid forms embryologically from the floor of the pharynx; occasionally, it may fail to migrate, leaving all or part of the gland at the junction of the anterior two-thirds with the posterior one-third of the tongue. This may cause airway obstruction and difficulties with airway maintenance during anesthesia. Preoperative treatment with thyroxine will shrink the gland and reduce the incidence of problems.[53]

Thyroid storm

Thyroid storm is a multisystem condition characterized by hyperpyrexia, tachycardia, dysrhythmias, heart failure, diarrhea, jaundice, agitation, psychosis, and coma. Between asymptomatic biochemical hyperthyroidism and thyroid storm lies a spectrum of severity, and whether or not the patient develops a crisis is dependent on many factors including age, intercurrent illness, and the rapidity of onset. It can be precipitated by many factors, including iodine ingestion (as in radiocontrast media), surgery, trauma, and parturition: "Storm is precipitated when the aggregate effect of these parameters surpasses the individual patient's ability to maintain adequate metabolic, thermoregulatory and cardiovascular compensatory mechanisms."[54] It should be noted that, just as thyrotoxicosis may present without gross physical signs, thyroid storm can present in an "apathetic" form with patients drifting into coma and death with very few signs to suggest the diagnosis.

Thyroid storm is associated with a high mortality rate and should be managed in an intensive care unit. Treatment is aimed at specific thyroid therapy and general supportive measures. Specific treatments include:

1 thionamide drugs, which inhibit conversion of T_4 to T_3 (the active form of thyroid hormone) within hours of starting treatment;
2 inorganic iodine, as either potassium iodide or ipodate (a radiocontrast medium), which inhibits thyroid hormone release;
3 steroids, which also inhibit T_3 synthesis;
4 plasmapheresis, which will remove circulating hormones from the blood (more than 99% of thyroid hormones are protein bound, so that simple plasma filtration is ineffective);
5 treatment of the precipitating cause.

General measures include temperature control and close attention to fluid balance. Anticoagulation may be indicated because pulmonary embolism has been reported. β-Adrenergic blocking agents (such as propranolol) may be used to control tachycardia and mental agitation. Despite the appearance of adrenergic system activation in thyroid storm, circulating catecholamines are reported to be normal and β-blockade may not be effective without other treatment.[55] Emergency thyroidectomy has been reported.[56]

Myxedema coma

Although patients may exist for many years with hypothyroidism, an intercurrent illness can precipitate multisystem failure and possibly death; this is decompensated hypothyroidism. Hypothermia, hyponatremia, bradycardia, low-voltage electrocardiogram (ECG), decreased myocardial contractility, hypoventilation, bone marrow depression, hypoglycemia, and increased transaminases are all found in myxedema coma. Management of these patients should take place in an intensive care unit; however, despite optimal treatment there is a high mortality rate. Treatment is specific and supportive.

Treatment of myxedema coma

Thyroid hormone may be replaced either as T_4 or T_3. Some 35–40% of T_4 is converted to T_3, the active form of the hormone, with the rest converted to an inactive form. Illness may inhibit conversion of T_4 to T_3 and so increase production of the inactive compound, as in the sick euthyroid syndrome. Controversy exists over whether replacement should be as T_3 or T_4, but whichever is used it must be given in small doses and with careful monitoring to avoid heart failure and myocardial infarction.

- Further heat loss should be prevented: active warming may precipitate hypotension because of the associated vasodilation and should be avoided.
- Fluids are the mainstay of cardiovascular management. These patients have reduced sensitivity to catecholamines owing to a downregulation of β-adrenergic receptors, so that inotropic drugs provoke dysrhythmias but may fail to produce any increase in cardiac output.
- Mechanical ventilation may be required because of hypoventilation.
- Treatment of the event which precipitated coma, which frequently is infection. It is of note that because of bone marrow suppression the white cell count may remain normal despite infection.
- Steroids are usually given because of the possibility of coexisting adrenal insufficiency.

If possible, surgery should be delayed in patients with hypothyroidism. However, in mild disease, there is no evidence to show that presurgical hormone treatment improves outcome.[57]

Pregnancy and thyroid disease

Untreated maternal hyperthyroidism or hypothyroidism is associated with high maternal and fetal mortality. For detailed information on this topic, readers are referred to specialized reviews.[58,59]

For further information on thyroid disease, readers are referred to Chapter 24 and recent reviews.[54,60,61]

Preoperative assessment of patients undergoing thyroid surgery

In addition to standard multisystem assessment, the patient should be examined for signs of hyper- or hypothyroidism and compression of neck or retrosternal structures. Careful assessment of intubation difficulty is essential.

Investigations should include full blood count (because the side-effects of thionamide drugs include agranulocytosis), thyroid function tests, chest radiography (for tracheal compression or deviation), ECG (for dysrhythmias or myocardial ischemia), and indirect laryngoscopy (to detect vocal cord lesions). Any patient with medullary thyroid cancer or multiple endocrine neoplasia should be screened for pheochromocytoma before proceeding to surgery.

Anesthesia for thyroid surgery

No particular anesthetic drugs have any advantage for thyroid surgery, and many techniques have been used. Intubation of the trachea may be *very* difficult, and this difficulty should be anticipated and appropriate equipment should be available. Failure to intubate a patient with a large goiter using the intubating laryngeal mask airway has been reported,[62] and anesthesiologists should be prepared to use a fiberoptic laryngoscope if required.

The authors prefer reinforced endotracheal tubes, which provide a guaranteed airway throughout and which do not kink. However, airway management using a laryngeal mask airway has been reported.[63] Standard monitoring is used. In addition, some authors have described recurrent laryngeal nerve monitoring, either bronchoscopically through a laryngeal mask airway[63] or with modified endotracheal tubes containing electrodes to detect impulses from laryngeal nerve stimulation. Commercial[64] and home-made[65] devices have been reported.

The patient's eyes should be protected; patients with Graves disease may have exophthalmia and so are at greater risk of corneal abrasion. Postoperative analgesia may include local anesthetic infiltration, nonsteroidal anti-inflammatory drugs, and opiates as required. The entire procedure can be carried out under local anesthesia.

Positioning is important to optimize surgical access; the neck is extended and the table placed in a 30° head-up tilt with the legs horizontal to prevent venous pooling. When assessing such patients before surgery, the authors ask them to tilt their head back as far as possible so that potential problems can be identified before anesthesia is induced. In the anesthetized patient, the neck should then be extended no further than the preanesthetic demonstration. It may be necessary to perform a sternal split to remove a substernal or mediastinal gland. Anesthesiologists should be aware that carotid sinus stimulation may lead to cardiovascular instability.

The major hazards of surgery are bleeding, damage to the recurrent laryngeal nerves, and inadvertent removal of the parathyroid glands leading to hypocalcemia.

Postoperative problems

In cases in which pressure on the trachea by the goiter has caused tracheomalacia, extubation may be followed by acute respiratory obstruction. Anesthesiologists must be aware of this problem, and careful assessment of the airway following extubation is essential.

Bleeding may cause a life-threatening emergency because a large hematoma in the neck can lead to airway obstruction of terrifyingly rapid onset. If a hematoma develops, the stitches or clips must be removed immediately, even on the ward if necessary, to allow evacuation of the clot.

Damage to the recurrent laryngeal nerves may lead not only to voice change but also to respiratory difficulties. Unilateral damage is frequently unnoticed because the opposite cord will compensate by moving across the midline, but bilateral damage may lead to airway obstruction. Complete transection of the nerve will result in the affected vocal cord coming to lie in the neutral position; if both nerves are divided, the opening between the cords may be insufficient for breathing. If the nerves are damaged but not actually divided, the adductors override the abductors and the cord becomes fixed in the midline; it follows that bilateral damage may lead to complete airway obstruction. Tracheostomy may be required until the nerves recover if they are only damaged, and permanently if they have been divided. Damaged recurrent laryngeal nerves commonly lead to litigation, and in one organization accounted for 4% of settlements in 1989.[63] Although the vocal cords can often be observed by direct laryngoscopy at the time of extubation, flexible laryngoscopy has been reported to be more successful, better tolerated, and associated with less cardiovascular stimulation.[66] Tracheomalacia may occur if the trachea has been compressed; this may cause a collapsing airway with complete closure during inspiration. This, too, may require reintubation followed by tracheostomy.

Hypocalcemia will occur if the parathyroid glands are removed or devascularized at the time the thyroid is removed. This is a relatively common complication (5.4% incidence during the postoperative period and 0.5% long term[67]).

Minimally invasive surgery has been reported and has been carried out both with[68] and without[69] gas insufflation. Day-case thyroid surgery has been successfully reported.[70]

For a more detailed account, readers are referred to a recent review.[71]

PARATHYROID DISEASE

Hyperparathyroidism

Hyperparathyroidism causes hypercalcemia, which in turn causes multisystem problems including polydipsia and polyuria, renal calculi, cardiac dysrhythmias, hypertension, left ventricular hypertrophy, hypovolemia, nausea, vomiting, constipation, peptic ulceration, pancreatitis, myopathy, bone disease, depression, and confusion.

Primary hyperparathyroidism (PHPT) occurs most commonly in women, and more than 90% of cases are due to a single adenoma. PHPT is also seen in patients with multiple endocrine neoplasia (MEN) syndromes.

For further information on parathyroid disease, readers are referred to Chapter 24, and to an authoritative review.[72]

Preoperative assessment

Mild hypercalcemia without cardiovascular involvement requires no special treatment during anesthesia. Severe hypercalcemia requires vigorous treatment prior to surgery; intravenous fluids will correct the hypovolemia and may rapidly reduce the calcium level. Loop diuretics will increase renal calcium excretion, but serum potassium and magnesium must be monitored and replaced appropriately. Hemodialysis is effective at removing calcium and may be necessary in patients with renal failure and hyperparathyroidism.

Elderly patients may be quite impaired by hypercalcemia and the outcome of treatment is good. Therefore, unless there are significant problems in other systems surgery should not be delayed.[73]

Renal failure in some patients will pose its own set of problems.

Anesthesia for parathyroid surgery

The problems are essentially similar to those presented by thyroid surgery. However, parathyroid adenomas do not grow large enough to cause pressure symptoms. Hypocalcemia may occur postoperatively as a result of preoperative treatment, or because affected bones may have increased affinity for calcium – so-called "hungry bones."

Hypoparathyroidism

This causes hypocalcemia and may be associated with multiple endocrine deficiency in which Addison's disease and pernicious anemia may be associated conditions.

Hypocalcemia causes tetany, and laryngeal spasm may also occur. Hyperventilation exacerbates hypocalcemia owing to the development of alkalosis.

Patients presenting for surgery who have hypoparathyroidism should receive calcium supplements intravenously to correct the hypocalcemia; otherwise, there are no particular problems with anesthesia or surgery.

Parathyroid disease in pregnancy

Hyperparathyroidism can lead to a high maternal and fetal morbidity rate.[74] Hypercalcemia may lead to neonatal tetany or stillbirth. The mother may suffer a hypercalcemic crisis after delivery, when the fetus, which has a high demand for calcium, no longer exerts a protective influence. Surgical treatment during pregnancy will prevent these complications.

Hypoparathyroidism also carries high fetal morbidity as a result of inadequate calcium supply. This is treated with calcium supplementation. Hyperventilation in labor will accentuate the hypocalcemia and regional analgesia is recommended.

ADRENAL DISORDERS

Adrenocortical insufficiency

Patients may present for surgery who (1) are taking corticosteroid drugs, either as replacement therapy or as treatment for specific conditions, (2) have recently been taking corticosteroids but are not currently doing so, or (3) have or are likely to develop corticosteroid deficiency. In all these cases, consideration must be given to steroid therapy during the perioperative period.

Patients who are currently taking corticosteroids

Although it has been traditional to increase steroid dosage during the perioperative period, there is no evidence to support such a strategy. As early as 1973, Kehlet and Binder[75] showed that patients on glucocorticoid therapy need only sufficient hydrocortisone to sustain physiologic plasma concentrations in order to avoid adrenocortical insufficiency. Kehlet[76] proposed a simple regimen for perioperative cover, involving a small (25 mg intravenously) dose of hydrocortisone at induction of anesthesia. In the case of minor, superficial surgery, this is sufficient until normal therapy is resumed. In the case of more major procedures, the initial dose is followed by a continuous infusion of hydrocortisone at 100 mg per 24 h, continued until the patient is able to resume normal steroid therapy. Subsequent studies by other groups have confirmed that no additional therapy is required.[77,78] A further reason for not escalating steroid dosage is the added risk of the patient developing steroid-related complications such as impaired wound healing, peptic ulceration, acute pancreatitis, bowel perforation, etc.

In their recent review, Nicholson and colleagues[79] point out that, in many cases, patients on steroid therapy depend on uninterrupted dosage; this is especially important for patients taking high doses for immunosuppression. They recommended that such patients should not take increased doses, but should be given the hydrocortisone equivalent of their current therapy throughout the perioperative period.

Patients on steroid therapy have no special anesthetic requirements, and a great variety of techniques may be used.

Patients who have recently discontinued corticosteroid therapy

These patients will include those who have a normal hypophyseal–pituitary–adrenal (HPA) axis and those who will have an impaired adrenal response to surgical stress. Following cessation of steroid therapy, normal adrenal responsiveness to ACTH usually returns within a few weeks, but in the absence of formal biochemical evidence should be assumed to be impaired for at least 2 months.[80] These patients should be managed using the same regimen as patients taking steroids.

The integrity of the HPA axis can be assessed by application of the short Synacthen test (SST), whereby a single 250-μg dose of Synacthen (a synthetic ACTH analog) is administered by intravenous (i.v.) injection and plasma cortisol is measured at 30 min.[81] Although there is no clear consensus as to the criteria for a normal result, and some false positives and false negatives do occur, it would appear that only very few patients achieving a plasma cortisol of 500 nmol L^{-1} will have an impaired stress response. Patients with normal SST values may safely be anesthetized without supplementary steroids. Nicholson and colleagues[79] proposed a simple set of criteria, based on those proposed by Kehlet,[76] for the guidance of clinicians (Table 48.3).

Patients who develop adrenocortical insufficiency

Any patient whose entire functioning adrenal cortex will be (or has been) surgically removed requires replacement steroid therapy. Hydrocortisone (25 mg) should be given as the last adrenal tissue is devascularized, followed by maintenance therapy at 100 mg day^{-1} until a regular oral regimen is established.

Critically ill patients, especially those developing multiple organ failure caused by sepsis, may develop acute adrenocortical insufficiency.[82,83] Since critically ill patients usually have elevated plasma cortisol concentrations, adrenal insufficiency may be associated with a wide range of values. The SST (see above) may be used to identify patients with decreased adrenocortical responsiveness. Because they require greater than normal plasma cortisol concentrations, treatment with hydrocortisone (400 mg day^{-1}) has been suggested.[84]

CUSHING SYNDROME

Cushing syndrome comprises the constellation of symptoms and signs that follow excessive adrenal corticosteroid secretion or administration. These include centripetal obesity, proximal muscle weakness, striae, poor wound healing, osteoporosis, hypertension, calcification of blood vessels, peptic ulceration, and diabetes mellitus. There also may be psychiatric changes ranging from depression to frank psychosis. The syndrome may be caused by adrenal tumors or by ACTH secreted by pituitary tumors or ectopic tumors such as oat cell carcinoma, bronchial carcinoid, medullary carcinoma of thyroid, carcinoma of pancreas, and pheochromocytoma.

Patients presenting for ablative surgery to pituitary or adrenals are likely to be treated with drugs such as metyrapone which not only suppress cortisol synthesis but also improve wound healing. In managing such patients, anesthesiologists should be aware that cortisol secretion may in fact be less than normal and that supplementation may be required.

Anesthetic management presents a variety of problems, many of which are related to comorbidity such as diabetes mellitus. The most important aspect is the management of plasma cortisol. Unless proved biochemically, it should not be assumed that patients do, in fact, have excessive plasma cortisol levels, so that it is the authors' practice to administer hydrocortisone supplements both during and after surgery. Those patients whose surgery leaves them with no functioning adrenal cortex should continue with standard replacement therapy, whereas those left with some adrenal tissue should continue on replacement therapy until it can be shown that they have a functional hypophyseal–adrenopituitary axis.

Cortisol-induced diabetes requires careful management during the perioperative period, as already discussed. An added complication is that, if surgery causes an abrupt reduction in serum cortisol, insulin sensitivity may show a similar increase, manifesting itself as a sharp reduction in insulin requirement.[85]

Some patients with long-standing Cushing syndrome present intubation difficulties, and all should be carefully assessed before induction of anesthesia. Patient positioning requires particular care because these patients have fragile bones, and thin skin, and are easily bruised.

Hyperaldosteronism (Conn syndrome)

Patients with Conn syndrome have an excess of aldosterone secreted by the adrenal cortex, caused either by hyperplasia or by an adenoma, leading to sodium (and water) retention, hypokalemia, and hypertension.[86] The last two may be severe and resistant to treatment. These patients usually present for adrenalectomy, and offer the anesthesiologist a number of problems.[87]

Despite preoperative potassium therapy the patient may have a persisting potassium deficit. This is because the intracellular deficit in a patient with chronic hypokalemia may exceed 500 mmol, so that replacement therapy may not achieve full correction. Anesthesiologists should be aware that chronic hypokalemia may present as generalized muscle weakness or cardiomyopathy.[88] Many of these patients also have abnormal glucose tolerance owing to impaired insulin secretion, which may require active management. Impaired renal function is common, and this may be due to the combined effects of hypertension and

Table 48.3 *Steroid treatment regimens (based on Nicholson* et al.,[79] *with permission of* Anaesthesia *and the authors)*

Patients currently taking steroids		
< 10 mg prednisone per day	Assume normal response	Continue current steroid medication. No additional steroid cover required
> 10 mg prednisone per day	Minor surgery	Usual steroid dosage until surgery; 25 mg hydrocortisone i.v. at induction
	Moderate surgery	Usual steroid dosage until surgery; 25 mg at induction + 100 mg day^{-1} for 24 h
	Major surgery	Usual steroid dosage until surgery; 25 mg at induction + 100 mg day^{-1} for 48–72 h
High-dose steroids, such as for immunosuppression		Continue current steroid dosage, if necessary in hydrocortisone equivalent
Patients who have discontinued steroid therapy		
< 3 months		Treat as if on steroids
> 3 months		No steroid cover required

chronic hypokalemia. If the patient remains hypokalemic at surgery, nondepolarizing muscle relaxants might be expected to have prolonged effects. The authors have never encountered this problem, but it is prudent to use a muscle relaxant with a short elimination half-time and low reliance on renal clearance, such as mivacurium or cisatracurium.

Anesthesiologists should be watchful for the patient whose potassium depletion has been corrected with excessive zeal and presents for surgery with hyperkalemia despite an underlying and intracellular deficit. The patient is likely to be taking antihypertensive drugs, probably in combination with spironolactone, and may have impaired baroceptor responses. Consequently, anesthetic agents and even modest blood loss are likely to cause hypotension, which may respond poorly to conventional measures. Anesthetic agents with negative inotropic effects, such as halothane, are best avoided, and intraoperative fluid replacement must be meticulous.

Occasionally, tumor handling will provoke an increase in blood pressure. However, this rarely requires active correction, and removal of the tumor is not usually followed by severe hypotension, as in patients with pheochromocytoma.

Even if one apparently normal gland is to remain, adrenalectomy may leave patients with at least temporarily impaired adrenocortical function. After the gland has been removed, it is prudent to commence low-dose replacement therapy, which can be discontinued postoperatively when a normal SST shows normal ACTH responsiveness. Removal of the tumor may be followed by hypoaldosteronism, so that sodium loss and potassium retention may be problems during the postoperative period. The hypertension persists, usually for many months.

PHEOCHROMOCYTOMA

Pheochromocytomas are catecholamine-secreting tumors derived from the primitive neural crest. They may occur in the adrenal medulla or at any site in the paraganglionic system from the base of the skull to the pelvis. Although most often benign, some 10% are malignant, showing both local invasion and metastases. They may be bilateral (10%). Some 13% are associated with the multiple endocrine neoplasia (MEN) syndrome type 2A (involving thyroid C cell, adrenal medulla, and parathyroid); in these cases, pheochromocytomas are more commonly bilateral and multiple. Uncommonly, pheochromocytomas also present in MEN type 2B (similar to type 2A, but including mucosal neurinoma and Marfan-like body habitus). In children, about 70% occur in boys, more commonly bilateral, extra-adrenal, and less commonly malignant. Pheochromocytoma may also present in association with von Recklinghausen's neurofibromatosis, von Hippel–Lindau syndrome, tuberous sclerosis, and Sturge–Weber syndrome. Familial cases of pheochromocytoma may present with no other endocrine abnormality.

Presentation

About 0.1% of hypertensive patients have pheochromocytoma, which may present in a variety of ways. Patients commonly present with headache, palpitations, pallor, flushing, sweating, nausea, and faintness. The hypertension may be continuous or episodic, and symptoms may be precipitated by actions such as bending and twisting. In bladder wall pheochromocytomas, a classic but unusual presentation takes the form of attacks precipitated by micturition. Typically, patients feel "drained" after each attack. Headache, palpitations, sweating, and hypertension are considered to be 90% predictive of pheochromocytoma.[89] In practice, such symptoms are often dismissed as psychologic or stress related, and the diagnosis may be missed until the patient presents with hypertension. Even worse, patients may suffer a whole series of major cardiovascular "events," only to suffer an unheralded intraoperative pheochromocytoma crisis. Excess catecholamines produce hyperglycemia, which may be mistaken for insulin-deficient diabetes mellitus.

Patients may present with acute medical emergencies such as heart failure, pulmonary edema, myocardial infarction, stroke, or abdominal pain with pseudo-obstruction or ischemic colitis. The onset of uterine contractions in labor may precipitate a pheochromocytoma crisis. Drugs such as β-adrenergic blockers, tricyclic antidepressants, monoamine oxidase inhibitors, metoclopramide, and naloxone may also precipitate a crisis. Anesthesia and surgery in unsuspected cases have a high reported mortality. In a postmortem series, 27% of patients with an undiagnosed pheochromocytoma died during or shortly after surgery.[90] Since the identification of the *RET* oncogene, some 25% of pheochromocytomas are detected by screening asyptomatic family members.[91]

Pheochromocytoma in pregnancy

Fortunately, this occurs rarely, but when pheochromocytoma does develop in pregnancy there is a high risk of maternal or fetal mortality or both.[92–95] Even vigorous fetal movements may be associated with hypertensive crises. Mortality rates decreased from 48% before 1969 to 17% between 1979 and 1987.[93]

For cases diagnosed during pregnancy, there is a clear choice between early intervention and conservative management until fetal viability permits elective cesarean section. Hamilton *et al.*[95] reported the use of α- and β-adrenergic blockade (prazosin and propranolol), followed by surgical removal of a pheochromocytoma at only 7 weeks' gestation, followed by an uneventful pregnancy with delivery at 37 weeks. Nitroglycerine was used to control hypertension during surgery in preference to sodium nitroprusside, on the grounds that the latter agent may reduce uterine blood flow. Since phenoxybenzamine may have teratogenic effects, it is best avoided in early pregnancy. Using the alternative approach, Takahashi *et al.*[96] describe a patient diagnosed at

29 weeks' gestation, for whom conservative treatment using labetolol continued until 35 weeks, at which time the fetus was successfully delivered and the tumor removed at the same operation. Patients may even commence labor with a large but unsuspected pheochromocytoma, as described by Strachan *et al.*,[97] in which case the circulation was successfully managed using i.v. phentolamine until delivery, followed by oral phenoxybenzamine until formal resection of the tumor 8 weeks later. In a patient subsequently proved to have a pheochromocytoma, Bullough *et al.*[98] successfully controlled blood pressure using a combination of magnesium and hydralazine.

Pheochromocytoma crisis

The clinical presentation may vary widely and be similar to that of malignant hyperpyrexia[99] or thyroid storm. The clinician faced with a patient with hypertension, which may alternate with hypotension, with developing heart failure, tachycardia, sweating, pulmonary edema, and acidosis with no other obvious cause should consider a diagnosis of pheochromocytoma. Another sign which may help to confirm the diagnosis is pupillary dilation due to high levels of catecholamines.[100] These tumors are rare but the cost of missing the diagnosis is high.

Emergency treatment will usually involve α-adrenergic blocking agents such as phentolamine, leading to longer-acting agents such as phenoxybenzamine or doxazosin. In the case of epinephrine (adrenaline)-secreting tumors, β-adrenergic blocking drugs such as propranolol may also be required. Magnesium infusions may be particularly useful, especially when the problem is compounded by cardiac failure.

Surgical aspects of pheochromocytoma

Until the mid-1920s, surgery for resection of pheochromocytoma was invariably fatal, but then Mayo[101] and Roux[102] performed successful operations. Although surgery remained hazardous for more than 50 years,[103] mortality rates are now very low.[104]

Conventionally, the tumor is approached with a midline, transverse, or flank incision, but laparoscopic approaches have also been described. Each technique presents its own problems for the anesthesiologist.

Formal laparotomy was the favored approach before accurate preoperative localization of the tumor was possible; this allowed the position of the tumor to be confirmed by palpation and observation of the blood pressure. Today, the position of the tumor is usually known accurately before surgery and a more focused approach is possible. Inflation of the abdomen with carbon dioxide for laparoscopy causes increased plasma norepinephrine (noradrenaline) concentrations in blood, even in healthy subjects.[105] In patients with pheochromocytoma, the increased intraperitoneal pressure may provoke the tumor, leading to marked increases in blood pressure. It is clear from case reports that careful patient preparation and very detailed hemodynamic monitoring is required if the anesthesiologist is to maintain good control.[106–108]

Laparoscopic surgery generally takes much longer than conventional surgery, but patients go home sooner. In an attempt to avoid the complications of bilateral adrenalectomy, partial excision has been carried out in patients with hereditary syndromes predisposing to pheochromocytoma, who are prone to bilateral disease.

Preparation for surgery and anesthesia

It should be remembered that use of radiocontrast media has been associated with pheochromocytoma crisis, so that patients must be fully protected before investigations such as arteriography are contemplated.

The mainstay of preoperative preparation has been α- and, if necessary, β-adrenergic blockade. The use of preoperative α-adrenergic blockade effectively reduces the wide blood pressure variations during anesthesia and also the occurrence of tachycardia and tachyarrhythmias.[109] Before the use of α-adrenergic blockade, surgical mortality and morbidity was high (40–60%). This declined to 0–6% with the use of adrenergic blockade. More recently, successful management of patients receiving no preoperative α-blockade has been reported.[104] However, Steinsapir *et al.*[110] reported two deaths in patients presenting unblocked for surgery, and these authors could not recommend such an approach.

Since the objective is to suppress all catecholamine-driven pressor activity, long-acting drugs are desirable. The choice lies between phenoxybenzamine, which has a noncompetitive mode of action, and competitive α_1-antagonists, such as prazosin and doxazosin.

Phenoxybenzamine is probably still the most commonly used preoperative treatment because once fully active it cannot be over-ridden by surges in plasma norepinephrine concentration. It does, however, have the disadvantage that if given in high dosage before surgery the patient may be refractory to norepinephrine during the early postoperative period. As yet, there have been no randomized trials to ascertain the correct dose or duration of blockade. Roizen *et al.*[111] proposed treatment for at least 10 days and until:

1 There are no marked symptoms.
2 Arterial pressure does not exceed 21.3/12 kPa (160/90 mmHg) on more than four measurements in 24 h.
3 Systolic blood pressure has decreased by at least 15% when moving from lying to standing position, but was more than 10.67/6 kPa (80/45 mmHg).
4 The ECG was free of changes in ST segment and T wave for 2 weeks.

The authors' choice is to monitor the patient with a 24-h blood pressure recording and to proceed when there are no blood pressure spikes exceeding 18.67/12 kPa (140/90 mmHg) and the heart rate is less than 100 beats per min.

The doses of phenoxybenzamine used have varied widely from a maximum of 60 to 320 mg day^{-1}.[112,113] Many patients with pheochromocytoma have a reduced circulating volume, and in some centers patients have been given preoperative blood transfusions in addition to α-adrenergic blockade in an attempt to correct this. In fact, it appears that with α-adrenergic blockade the circulating volume is restored to a normal or even supranormal value.[109] It is this increase which is thought to improve cardiovascular stability during surgery. There are many side-effects associated with the use of phenoxybenzamine, including postural hypotension, tachycardia (owing to blockade of presynaptic α_2-adrenoceptors), lethargy, blurred vision, nasal stuffiness, and dependent edema. These are minimized by low initial dosage, followed by increases as tolerated by the patient. It is advisable to counsel patients not to drive or undertake dangerous activities while receiving phenoxybenzamine. Treatment is continued until the day before surgery.

The selective α_1-antagonists prazosin and doxazosin have also been used in the management of pheochromocytoma. They do not block α_2-adrenergic receptors; thus, by allowing norepinephrine reuptake by nerve endings, the tachycardia seen with phenoxybenzamine does not occur.

However, not all clinicians have found prazosin to be as satisfactory as phenoxybenzamine.[112,114]

Citing a series of 18 successful cases since 1991, Prys-Roberts[115] has argued that doxazosin, a long-acting, competitive, and selective α_1-adrenergic blocking agent, is preferable to phenoxybenzamine when used in doses in the range 2–8 mg day^{-1}. He suggests that because doxazosin lacks α_2-blocking activity, many patients treated in this way do not require β-adrenergic blocking agents.

However, it is possible that the very high levels of catecholamines encountered during tumor handling may overcome the competitive inhibition of prazosin and doxazosin, whereas phenoxybenzamine-inhibited receptors are refractory to norepinephrine stimulation. We have continued to use phenoxybenzamine, believing that this agent has stood the test of time for very large numbers of patients and should be used until doxazosin can be shown to be superior in a large series.

Having established α-adrenergic blockade, β-adrenergic blockade may be necessary to control the tachycardia caused either by the α-adrenergic blockade or by the tumor itself. Traditional wisdom states that β-blockade must be introduced after α-blockade in order to prevent β-mediated vasoconstriction, and thus hypertension and pulmonary edema[116,117] Many patients with pheochromocytoma will have had their hypertension treated with β-adrenergic blocking drugs prior to diagnosis with apparently no ill effects, although some do report that they were "allergic" to this medication. Despite the theoretical problems, Russell *et al.*[112] and Mihm *et al.*[118] have successfully reported the use of "beta before alpha" blockade. Choice of drug is wide and, although propranolol is probably the most widely used, atenolol, metoprolol, and esmolol have all been used with success. Labetolol enjoyed a brief vogue as a combined α- and β-blocking agent, and we accept that it is appealing to use only one drug. However, the β-antagonist effects predominate, and it has been associated with the occurrence of pulmonary edema.[119] Today, it is little used.

Metyrosine acts as a false transmitter in the conversion of tyrosine to dopa, thus reducing the production of catecholamine by the tumor. The side-effects include somnolence, bizarre dreams, hallucinations, confusion, depression, psychosis, and crystalluria. It has been used with some success in combination with phenoxybenzamine and produced greater cardiovascular stability than α-blockade alone.[110]

Calcium channel blockers act by inhibiting calcium entry into the smooth muscle of the blood vessel, thus preventing vasoconstriction due to catecholamine action. Oral nifedipine followed by intravenous nicardipine has been successfully used by Colson *et al.*[120] for 19 patients.

There is no consistent advice on duration of blockade prior to surgery. It is probably more related to practical than technical considerations. Once the diagnosis of pheochromocytoma is seriously suspected, patients should receive α-adrenergic therapy to limit surges in arterial pressure and so prevent the occurrence of hypertensive encephalopathy, stroke, and heart failure.

Preanesthetic assessment

Management of these patients with difficulties requires cooperation between physician, surgeon, and anesthesiologist. Ideally, the anesthesiologist is involved in preoperative blockade and proceeds to surgery once he/she is sure that the patient is adequately prepared. This decision is not easily made by a physician who is not to face the intraoperative problems. Assessment includes ECG and echocardiography. These patients may develop a catecholamine cardiomyopathy, and it is important to identify this at an early stage.[121] Since β-adrenergic blockers may cause heart failure in patients with cardiomyopathy, dysrhythmias may need to be controlled with amiodarone.

Monitoring

Comprehensive monitoring is essential. This should include ECG, intra-arterial pressure, central venous pressure, arterial saturation, temperature, and urinary output. Pulmonary artery catheterization yields crucially important information in complex cases, especially those involving cardiomyopathy. The use of transesophageal echocardiography has been also been described.[122]

Anesthetic technique

Many different anesthetic techniques have been described in the literature, frequently reporting very small numbers of patients with no comparative groups. This suggests that the choice of drugs is less important than good technique and careful monitoring: "The anaesthetic objectives are to avoid provocation of catecholamine release by anaesthetic drugs or manoeuvres, to suppress the adrenergic response to surgical stimulation, and to minimise the haemodynamic responses to both tumour handling and devascularisation."[116] The authors use $0.5\,mg\,kg^{-1}$ temazepam for premedication, etomidate or propofol for induction of anesthesia, alfentanil to obtund the hypertensive response to intubation and surgical stimulation, vecuronium for neuromuscular blockade, and isoflurane for maintenance of anesthesia. All drugs are chosen as those least likely to release histamine or catecholamines. Drugs such as morphine, atracurium, pancuronium, succinylcholine (suxamethonium), and droperidol may prove to be safe in individual cases, but when safer and equally effective drugs are available it would seem logical to use these.

Fluid loading is the best protection against extreme hypotension after tumor removal and this should start at induction. Hypertension, especially during tumor handling, can be controlled by deepening anesthesia, infusion of sodium nitroprusside, phentolamine,[115] glyceryl trinitrate, or nicardipine. For many years, James[123–125] has promoted the use of magnesium sulfate on the grounds that it has many useful properties, including adrenergic agonist, vasodilator, and antiarrhythmic actions. Tachycardia or dysrhythmias can be treated with β-adrenergic blockers, such as propranolol or esmolol, or with lidocaine (lignocaine) or amiodarone. Following vascular isolation of the tumor, hypotension should be treated initially with intravenous fluids, while pressor agents such as norepinephrine or epinephrine should be used only if volume loading is ineffective or if peripheral vascular resistance is shown to be abnormally low. Anesthesiologists should be aware that fluid requirements may exceed greatly the measured blood loss during surgery. The authors have seen both low and high cardiac output in the early post-tumor excision phase, and choice and dosage of pressor agent can be guided by cardiac output measurement if a pulmonary artery catheter has been inserted.

Postoperative analgesia can be provided by either patient-controlled analgesia or a low thoracic epidural block. We favor the latter on the grounds of reduced somnolence, which may be caused by parenteral opioids.

The use of regional anesthesia alone or in combination with general anesthesia is rare in the literature, but it has been used successfully.[126,127] By blocking pain signals, it might be expected that regional techniques would lead to a decrease in catecholamine secretion; however, the major release is associated with tumor handling and is unaffected by the anesthetic effect. The vasodilation seen with sympathetic blockade is due to an effect on preganglionic sympathetic fibers, but circulating catecholamines act at blood vessel level and so overcome the blockade.

The patients may remain hemodynamically unstable for many hours, and therefore postoperative management should be in a high-dependency or intensive care facility.

Postoperative hypoglycemia

The excessive production of catecholamines by a pheochromocytoma results in inhibition of insulin release, while lipolysis and glycogenolysis further increase the blood glucose concentration. Many patients will be frankly diabetic before tumor removal. After removal of the catecholamine source, there is a rebound increase in insulin secretion with possibly continuing adrenergic blockade, which will prevent the normal stress response to hypoglycemia. Severe hypoglycemia is a major hazard during the first few postoperative hours, and may develop very rapidly.[128,129] Indeed, unless patients are monitored closely, the first indication may be loss of consciousness. Blood glucose measurements should be performed at least hourly for the first 12 h following surgery; the authors advocate 20-min intervals.

The patient with malignant pheochromocytoma

Patients with malignant pheochomocytoma with functioning secondary deposits may present for incidental surgery. Treatment for these patients is aimed at pharmacologic control of blood pressure and heart rate, and if necessary (or possible) tumor debulking to decrease tumor mass. High-dose metaiodoguanidine (MIBG) has been described, with the aim of inducing radioiodine tumor uptake and necrosis. Unfortunately, this approach has a low success rate (and is very expensive). Metyrosine may also be used for long-term tumor control,[110] but its side-effects may preclude this. Prazosin or doxazosin, which have fewer side-effects than phenoxybenzamine, may be used for the long-term treatment of hypertension. Management of these patients for anesthesia and surgery will be as for tumor excision.

The undiagnosed pheochromocytoma

Occasionally, patients undergoing surgery are found to have previously undiagnosed pheochromocytoma. This may occur when a tumor is found by the surgeon or dramatic changes in heart rate and/or blood pressure alert the anesthesiologist to consider pheochromocytoma as a cause. When the operation is far remote from the likely tumor site, as in a reported case involving craniotomy,[130] the anesthesiologist is faced with a difficult management problem that will require judicious use of drugs such as phentolamine or sodium nitroprusside to control the arterial pressure. Except where there is extreme tachycardia, the use of β-blockade in the acute situation is best avoided. Where surgery can reasonably be aborted, that is likely to be the wise option.

When the tumor is found to be surgically accessible, as in a laparotomy, the surgeon may decide to remove it. Although successful outcomes following such procedures have been reported,[131] we would urge caution. Since tumor handling in an unprepared patient is likely to cause very large increases in arterial pressure, followed by intractable hypotension after tumor excision, a safer option would be careful retreat followed by planned resection after confirmation of the diagnosis and proper pharmacologic preparation. Whatever the decided course of action, this must be made jointly by surgeon and anesthesiologist.

CARCINOID

Carcinoid is a tumor, usually of gut, arising from enterochromaffin cells, in the primitive neuroectoderm, that may metastasize (usually to the liver) and may synthesize a variety of chemical mediators. It may also derive from the primitive foregut, with primary tumors developing in lung or bronchus.

The appendix is the commonest site (36–46%), but only infrequently leads to metastases and carcinoid syndrome. Tumors in the ileum and jejunum (32%) metastasize frequently, as do those in the colon and rectum.[132]

Carcinoid tumors may release a number of chemical mediators, including 5-hydroxytryptamine (serotonin), kallikrein, bradykinins, calcitonin, prostaglandins, histamine, gastrin, and a variety of neuropeptides.[133] These include substance P, which is a powerful stimulator of gut activity and a far more potent vasodilator than bradykinin.[134] To make matters more complicated, the tumor may also contain monoamine oxidase, which deactivates serotonin before it can be released into the bloodstream. Such is the variation in mediator release among carcinoid patients that each must be considered as functionally unique.

When the tumor mass is large, especially in liver metastases, or when the tumor drains directly into the systemic venous system (as with lung primaries), as in some 25% of cases, patients may develop a characteristic syndrome of right-sided heart disease, bronchoconstriction, cyanosis, and circulatory disturbances associated with excessive release of serotonin.[135] Characteristically, patients suffer intermittent attacks of "flushing" over the upper body and face, which may be precipitated by foods, drugs (especially catecholamines), alcohol, excitement, anxiety, exercise, and environmental factors. During surgery, tumor handling is a potent cause. Diarrhea, which occurs in some 78% of patients, may be profuse and accompanied by abdominal pain, nausea, vomiting, and electrolyte disturbances.[136] Secondary cardiac involvement, such as pulmonary stenosis and tricuspid regurgitation, is characterized by superficial endocardial and valvular fibrosis.[137] Presumably, the left heart usually is unaffected because the concentration of mediators is greatly reduced by lung uptake.[138] Such patients usually have increased urinary output of the serotonin metabolite 5-hydroxyindoleacetic acid (5-HIAA) (normal range $< 37\,\mu$mol per 24 h).

Pharmacologic effects of serotonin and bradykinin

In anesthetized patients, serotonin causes hypertension and tachycardia. In the gastrointestinal tract, it causes increased motility leading to diarrhea. In the brain it is an important neurotransmitter, and the small quantities that cross the blood–brain barrier may cause somnolence with delayed recovery from anesthesia.[139] Serotonin also stimulates glycogenolysis to cause hyperglycemia.

Bradykinin is a potent vasodilator, and may be the main cause of hypotension associated with carcinoid flushing attacks. It also increases capillary permeability, leading to the peripheral edema that appears in many of these patients. It causes bronchoconstriction, which is a major feature of the flush attacks.

Pharmacologic control of patients with carcinoid syndrome

Antiserotonin drugs have been the mainstay of pharmacologic control (Table 48.4). These include methisergide, α-methyl-dopa, cyproheptadine (an antihistamine with antiserotoninergic actions), parachlorophenylalanine (a serotonin synthesis inhibitor), and chlorpromazine. These may be effective against diarrhea but not other manifestations. Ketanserin is an antagonist at 5-hydroxytryptamine type 2 receptors, and has been found useful in controlling unwanted hypertension.[140]

Kallikrein–bradykinin inhibitors have also been advocated. Aprotinin, which inhibits kallikrein synthesis, was reported to have been dramatically effective for one case,[139] but disappointing in others. It has, however, been used as part of an inhibitor cocktail for many cases. Anesthesiologists should be aware that this agent also inhibits both platelet aggregation and the intrinsic coagulation cascade, so that the antithrombotic effects of anticoagulant drugs may be enhanced.[141]

Antihistamines may also be useful for those cases in which the tumor releases significant quantities of histamine. Chlorpheniramine, cyproheptadine, and ranitidine may be effective.

In some patients, treatment with alpha- and beta-blocking agents has reduced the severity of flushing attacks, possibly because they are easily precipitated by epinephrine.[142] In others, it has been ineffective.

Somatostatin inhibits the physiologic release of growth hormone, thyrotropin, insulin, and glucagon. In the gut, it has a wide range of actions, reducing both endocrine and exocrine secretions, inhibiting motility, and reducing blood flow. This hormone, when injected, prevents the release of all active mediators from carcinoid tumors, and longer acting analogs such as octreotide (Sandostatin) have proved highly effective both in controlling the symptoms suffered by these patients and in reducing urinary 5-HIAA concentrations.[143] Somatostatin has a very short half-time in plasma (1–3 min), and so must be administered by continuous infusion.[144] Octreotide has a plasma half-time of 45 min

Table 48.4 *Drugs used in the management of carcinoid syndrome*

Target mediator	Inhibition of synthesis or release	Receptor inhibition	Antagonistic effect
Serotonin	Parachlorophenylalanine Phenoxybenzamine α-Methyl dopa Octreotide	Methysergide Cyproheptadine Chlorpromazine Ketanserin (S_2) Pizotifen Methotrimeprazine	Phentolamine Esmolol Propranolol
Kallikrein	Steroids ε-Aminocaproic acid Aprotinin Octreotide		
Histamine		Chlorpheniramine (H_1) Cyproheptadine (H_1) Ranitidine (H_2) Cimetidine (H_2)	

after i.v. injection, and is effective for at least 5 h after subcutaneous injection.[145] Doses of 200 μg to 1 mg daily may be required, with even greater doses when used to suppress carcinoid crisis.[146,147]

Surgical management of carcinoid tumors

Surgical management of the solitary primary tumor is simply to remove it, but disseminated tumors causing carcinoid syndrome present greater problems. Since the severity of symptoms is directly related to the mass of actively secreting tumor, surgical strategy is aimed toward reduction of the carcinoid biomass. Radical surgery to remove active tumor, at both primary and metastatic sites, can be highly effective.[148] In the case of very large metastatic tumors, devascularization or embolization procedures have been employed.[149,150] Aortic and/or mitral valve replacement may also benefit patients whose heart valves have been damaged by the disease.[137]

Anesthetic management of patients with carcinoid syndrome

Following the first reported fatality in 1952,[151] carcinoid syndrome presented anesthesiologists with severe difficulties because there were no drugs which could suppress all the circulatory and respiratory components of an intraoperative carcinoid crisis. Indeed, Mason and Steane,[152] in reviewing the literature up to 1976, noted that major hemodynamic changes occurred in 26 out of 40 reported cases, especially during tumor handling, and that bronchospasm and flushing were also significant problems despite the use of a variety of inhibitors. Two of these patients had died as a consequence of circulatory collapse, which even in the survivors had been refractory to conventional measures. At that time, the best anesthetic strategy was to pretreat patients with a cocktail of antiserotonin and antibradykinin drugs and to avoid the use of drugs likely to provoke carcinoid crisis.[150,152]

The introduction of octreotide has dramatically improved the situation, in terms of both preoperative preparation and intraoperative prevention of carcinoid crisis. In 1987, Marsh *et al.*[153] reported the successful use of octreotide in controlling a carcinoid crisis during anesthesia, and Roy *et al.*[146] reported its successful use in preventing intraoperative carcinoid crises by preoperative infusion. Although partially controlled by long-term parachlorophenylalanine therapy, the patient developed a preoperative crisis despite pretreatment with aprotinin and chlorpromazine, with ketanserin-resistant hypertension and severe bronchospasm. After 2 weeks of octreotide therapy, the patient subsequently underwent major surgery with no recurrence of serotoninergic manifestations. In the following year, Parris *et al.*[154] reported a second case in which circulatory and respiratory complications may have been prevented by octreotide pretreatment.

Preoperative preparation is important, and depends upon effective inhibition of tumor activity by octreotide therapy. Other drugs, such as aprotinin and cyproheptadine, may be used as required. Electrolyte abnormalities must be corrected and cardiac function optimized before operation is considered. As in pheochromocytoma, close teamwork between physician, surgeon, and anesthesiologist throughout the preparative period is essential. Similarly, the timing of surgery must be a team decision.

Since catecholamines are potent triggers of carcinoid crisis, there must be a high emphasis on careful, smooth anesthesia with avoidance of major hemodynamic changes. For premedication, benzodiazepines facilitate smooth and tranquil induction, and opioids are best avoided.[155] Octreotride (up to 500 μg) is administered with premedication to ensure minimal mediator release in the preinduction period. The preoperative administration of H_1 and H_2 antihistamines may also be useful, especially where the tumor is known to be histamine secreting.

As in the management of pheochromocytoma, it makes sense to avoid the use of anesthetic drugs that release trigger substances such as catecholamines or histamine. Thus, morphine, atracurium, and tubocurarine are contraindicated because of histamine-releasing potential when effective alternatives are readily available. Although succinylcholine has been used successfully in this context,[155] the initial fasciculations may provoke mediator release. It is best avoided unless intubation is expected to be unusually difficult.

Etomidate, which does not provoke histamine release, would appear to be the induction agent of choice, and in anxious patients may be preceded by i.v. midazolam. Since vecuronium is devoid of autonomic effects at clinical dosage and does not release histamine, it is the muscle relaxant of choice. Topical laryngeal spraying with lidocaine, combined with intravenous administration of fast-acting opioids such as remifentanil or alfentanil, prevent hypertensive responses to intubation. Hemodynamic responses to surgical stimuli can be prevented by continuous infusion of opioids such as fentanyl, alfentanil, or remifentanil, with the lack of persisting effects making the last particularly useful. Since cardiac reserve may be minimal, drugs and anesthetic agents with negative inotropic actions should be avoided or their doses kept to a minimum.

In most reported cases, anesthesia has been maintained using a balanced inhalational/opioid sequence. Successful use of a propofol infusion has also been reported.[147]

Management of hemodynamic disturbances during surgery

Small bolus doses (10–20 μg) of octreotide may be used (and repeated as required) when there is flushing or tumor-mediated hemodynamic disturbance. In the case of hypertensive events, ketanserin also may be useful. Tachycardia, if severe, may be treated using β-adrenergic blocking agents such as propranolol or esmolol. Hypotension requires vigorous fluid replacement therapy, guided by central venous or pulmonary artery wedge pressure. Recently, Cortinez[156] reported a patient whose severe hypotension during tumor resection became refractory to octreotide. Under such circumstances we would suggest the supplementary use of other inhibitors such as aprotinin. Vasopressors should not be used except in extreme circumstances because they may provoke further mediator release. However, Neustein and Cohen[137] have argued that, if hypotension is not caused by tumor mediators or by hypovolemia, epinephrine may be used very cautiously to increase the systemic vascular resistance.

Anesthesiologists should be aware that octreotide inhibits the secretion of many hormones, including both insulin and glucagon. High plasma concentrations of catecholamines and infusion of dextrose- or lactate-containing solutions may, therefore, lead to hyperglycemia. It is good practice to monitor blood glucose concentrations during surgery and during the early postoperative period, and if necessary to maintain normoglycemia by active management as described for diabetic patients.

Patient monitoring during anesthesia

Monitoring should, of course, include such standard measurements as ECG, pulse oximetry, capnography, and thermometry. Except where surgery is minor and blood loss is expected (by the anesthesiologist) to be minimal, monitoring should include direct arterial and central venous pressure measurement. In patients with poor cardiac function in whom central venous pressure may not provide useful information on volume requirements, use of a pulmonary artery flotation catheter should be considered. However, for patients with damaged heart valves, the benefits and risks must be considered carefully. If major hemodynamic or metabolic disturbances do occur, frequent arterial blood gas analyses are required.

Close observation should be continued into the postoperative period because several deaths have occurred during the recovery phase. It should be noted that, as with pheochromocytoma, conventional doses of opioids may cause marked somnolence and severe respiratory depression. Although conventional patient-controlled analgesia techniques may be used (avoiding morphine), regional analgesia has an obvious application and has been found to be both safe and effective.[155]

Although spinal or extradural anesthesia have been considered unwise owing to the risk of hypotension and the undesirability of administering vasopressor drugs,[152] Monteith and Roaseg[157] have shown that, with combined octreotide and inhibitor cover, extradural anesthesia can be used safely, at least for nontumor-involving surgery.

As with pheochromocytoma, anesthetic expertise with carcinoid syndrome comes with familiarity, and such patients should be managed by anesthesiologists with experience of this condition.

INSULINOMA

Insulin-secreting islet cell tumors may occur alone, or as part of the MEN type 1 syndrome. In the latter case, there is an association with parathyroid adenoma and carcinoid and pituitary tumors. Some 15% are malignant, and hepatic metastases may cause severe and intractable hypoglycemia.

From a physiologic point of view, these patients are hyperinsulinemic and may become dramatically so during tumor handling.

Insulin secretion may be suppressed using diazoxide, or with octreotide, as with carcinoid syndrome (see above). When octreotide is used, both insulin and glucagon secretion will be heavily suppressed, whereas catecholamine and cortisol secretion may be increased by surgical stimulation. At operation, a glucose infusion should be commenced as soon as "nil by mouth" begins, and careful cardiovascular monitoring is mandatory. Frequent estimations of blood glucose are essential throughout the perioperative period, and independent infusions of glucose and insulin are required to manage rapidly changing requirements.

Other hormone-secreting tumors of the gut, such as glucagonoma, gastrinoma, and somatostatinoma, may be encountered, and readers are referred to the comprehensive review by Holdcroft.[158]

REFERENCES

1. Reddi AS, Camerini-Davalos RA. Diabetic nephropathy: an update. *Arch Intern Med* 1990; **150:** 31–43.
2. McMurray JF. Wound healing with diabetes mellitus: better glucose control for better healing in diabetes. *Surg Clin North Am* 1984; **64:** 769–78.
3. Rayfield EJ, Ault MJ, Keusch GT, *et al.* Infection and diabetes: the case for glucose control. *Am J Med* 1982; **72:** 439–50.
4. Fowkes FGR, Lunn JN, Farrow SC, *et al.* Epidemiology in anaesthesia III: mortality risk in patients with coexisting physical disease. *Br J Anaesth* 1982; **54:** 819–25.
5. MacKenzie CR, Charlson ME. Assessment of perioperative risk in the patient with diabetes mellitus. *Surg Gynecol Obstet* 1988; **167:** 293–9.
6. Raucoules-Aim È, Roussel LJ, Rossi D, *et al.* Effects of severity of surgery on metabolic control and insulin requirements in insulin-dependent diabetic patients. *Br J Anaesth* 1995; **74:** 231–3.
7. Rosenbloom AL. Skeletal and joint manifestations of childhood diabetes. *Pediatr Clin North Am* 1984; **31:** 569–89.
8. Salzarulo HH, Taylor LA. Diabetic "stiff joint syndrome" as a cause of difficult endotracheal intubation. *Anesthesiology* 1986; **64:** 366–8.
9. Hogan K, Rusy D, Springman SR. Difficult intubation and diabetes mellitus. *Anesth Analg* 1988; **67:** 1162–5.
10. Reissell E, Orko R, Maunuksela EL, Lindgren L. Predictability of difficult laryngoscopy in patients with long-term diabetes mellitus. *Anaesthesia* 1990; **45:** 1024–7.
11. Lydon A, Murray C, Cooke T, *et al.* Evaluation of standard haemodynamic tests of autonomic function and HbA1c as predictors of delayed gastric emptying in patients with type 1 diabetes mellitus. *Eur J Anaesthesiol* 2000; **17:** 99–104.
12. Mulhall BP, O'Fearghail M. Diabetic gastroparesis. case report and review of the literature. *Anaesthesia* 1984; **39:** 468–9.
13. Schiller L. Gastrointestinal problems in diabetes. *Clin Diabetes* 1987; **5:** 128–42.
14. Reissel E, Orko R, Maunuksela EL, Lindgrern L. Increased volume of gastric contents in diabetic patients undergoing renal transplantation: lack of effect with cisapride. *Acta Anaesthesiol Scand* 1992; **36:** 736–40.
15. Triantafillou AN, Tsueda K, Berg J, Wieman TJ. Refractory bradycardia after reversal of muscle relaxant in a diabetic with vagal neuropathy. *Anesth Analg* 1986; **65:** 1237–41.
16. Page MM, Watkins PJ. Cardiorespiratory arrest and diabetic autonomic neuropathy. *Lancet* 1978; **1:** 14–16.
17. Ciccarelli LL, Ford CM, Tsueda K. Autonomic neuropathy in a diabetic patient with renal failure. *Anesthesiology* 1986; **64:** 283–7.
18. Burgos LG, Ebert TJ, Asiddao C, *et al.* Increased intraoperative cardiovascular morbidity in diabetics with autonomic neuropathy. *Anesthesiology* 1989; **70:** 591–7.
19. Williams JG, Morris AI. Respiratory responses of diabetics to hypoxia, hypercapnia and exercise. *Thorax* 1984; **39:** 529–34.
20. Hall GM, Desborough JP. Diabetes and anaesthesia – slow progress? *Anaesthesia* 1988; **43:** 531–2.
21. Alberti KGMM. Diabetes and surgery. *Anesthesiology* 1991; **74:** 209–11.
22. McAnulty GR, Robertshaw HJ, Hall GM. Anaesthetic management of patients with diabetes mellitus. *Br J Anaesth* 2000; **85:** 80–90.
23. Lawrence PA, Dowe MC, Perry EK, *et al.* Accuracy of nurses in performing capillary blood glucose monitoring. *Diabetes Care* 1989; **12:** 298–301.
24. Dunnett JM, Holman RR, Turner RC, Sear JW. Diabetes mellitus and anaesthesia. A survey of peri-operative management of the patient with diabetes mellitus. *Anaesthesia* 1988; **43:** 538–42.
25. Eldridge, Sear JW. Preoperative management of diabetic patients. Any changes for the better since 1985? *Anaesthesia* 1996; **51:** 45–51.
26. Walts LF, Miller J, Davidson MB, Brown J. Perioperative management of diabetes mellitus. *Anesthesiology* 1981; **55:** 104–9.

27. Alberti KGMM, Thomas DJB. The management of diabetes during surgery. *Br J Anaesth* 1979; **51:** 693–710.
28. Thomas DJB, Platt HS, Alberti KGMM. Insulin-dependent diabetes during the peri-operative period. An assessment of continuous glucose–insulin–potassium infusion, and traditional treatment. *Anaesthesia* 1984; **39:** 629–37.
29. Bowen DJ, Daykin AP, Nancekievill ML, Norman J. Insulin-dependent diabetic patients during surgery and labour. Use of continuous intravenous insulin–glucose–potassium infusions. *Anaesthesia* 1984; **39:** 407–11.
30. Christiansen CL, Schurizek BA, Malling B, *et al.* Insulin treatment of the insulin-dependent diabetic patient undergoing minor surgery. *Anaesthesia* 1988; **43:** 533–7.
31. Gill GV, Alberti K. The care of the diabetic patient during surgery. In: Alberti K, Zimmett P, DeFronzo RA, Keen H (eds). *International Textbook of Diabetes Mellitus*, 2nd edn. Chichester: John Wiley & Sons, 1997: 1243–53.
32. Pezzarossa A, Taddei F, Cimicchi MG, *et al.* Perioperative management of diabetic subjects: subcutaneous vs intravenous insulin administration during glucose-potassium infusion. *Diabetes Care* 1988; **11:** 52–8.
33. Husband DJ, Thai AC, Alberti KGMM. Management of diabetes during surgery with glucose-insulin-potassium infusion. *Diabetic Med* 1986; **3:** 69–74.
34. Watts NB, Gebhart SP, Clark RV, Phillips LS. Perioperative management of diabetes mellitus: steady-state glucose control with bedside algorithm for insulin adjustment. *Diabetes Care* 1987; **10:** 722–8.
35. Hirsch IB, McGill JB, Cryer PE, White PF. Perioperative management of surgical patients with diabetes mellitus. *Anesthesiology* 1991; **74:** 346–59.
36. Milaskiewicz RM, Hall GM. Diabetes and anaesthesia: the past decade. *Br J Anaesth* 1992; **68:** 198–206.
37. Elliott MJ, Gill GV, Home PD, *et al.* A comparison of two regimens for the management of diabetes during open heart surgery. *Anesthesiology* 1984; **60:** 364–68.
38. Semple PF, White C, Manderson WG. Continuous intravenous infusion of small doses of insulin in treatment of diabetic ketoacidosis. *Br Med J* 1974; **1:** 694–8.
39. Kidson W, Casey J, Kraegen E, Lazarus L. Treatment of severe diabetes mellitus by insulin infusion. *Br Med J* 1974; **1:** 691–4.
40. Marshall SM, Walker M, Alberti KGMM. Diabetic ketoacidosis and hyperglycaemic non-ketotic coma. In: Alberti KGMM, Zimmet P, DeFronzo RA, Keen H (eds). *International Textbook of Diabetes Mellitus,* 2nd edn. Chichester: John Wiley & Sons, 1997: 1215–29.
41. Thomas DJB, Alberti KGMM. Hyperglycaemic effects of Hartmann's solution during surgery in patients with maturity onset diabetes. *Br J Anaesth* 1978; **50:** 185–8.
42. Wicklmayr M, Rett K, Dietz G, Mehnert H. Comparison of metabolic clearance rates of MCT/LCT and LCT emulsions in diabetics. *J Parenteral Enteral Nutr* 1988; **12:** 68–71.
43. Durr JA, Hoggard JD, Hunt JM, Schrier RW. Diabetes insipidus in pregnancy associated with abnormally high circulating vasopressinase activity. *N Engl J Med* 1987; **316:** 1070–4.
44. Passanante AN. Diabetes insipidus and epidural analgesia for labor. *Anesth Analg* 1994; **80:** 837–8.
45. AAotBP. *Compendium of Datasheets*. London: Datapharm Publications, 2000: 432–3.
46. Grantham JML. The effect of hyponatraemia on the regulation of intracellular volume and solute composition. *Circ Res* 1984; **54:** 483–91.
47. Ayus JC, Olivero JJ, Frommer JP. Rapid correction of severe hyponatraemia with intravenous hypertonic saline solution. *Am J Med* 1982; **72:** 43–8.
48. Sterns RH, Riggs JE, Schochet SSJ. Osmotic demyelination syndrome following correction of hyponatraemia. *N Engl J Med* 1986; **314:** 1535–42.
49. Newman E, Shaha AR. Substernal goitre. *J Surg Oncol* 1995; **60:** 207–12.
50. Anders H-J. Compression syndromes caused by substernal goitres. *Postgrad Med J* 1998; **74:** 327–9.
51. Rowe-Jones JM, Rosswick RP, Leighton SE. Benign thyroid disease and vocal cord palsy. *Ann R Coll Surg Engl* 1993; **75:** 241–4.
52. Proye CAG, Nguyen HH. Current perspectives in the surgery of multiple endocrine neoplasias. *Aust NZ J Surg* 1999; **69:** 106–16.
53. Arancibia P, Veliz J, Barria M, Pineda G. Lingual thyroid: report of three cases. *Thyroid* 1998; **8:** 1055–7.
54. Burch HB, Wartofsky L. Life threatening thyrotoxicosis. *Endocrinol Metab Clin North Am* 1993; **22:** 263–77.
55. Anaissie E, Tohmè JF. Reserpine in propranolol resistant thyroid storm. *Arch Intern Med* 1985; **145:** 2248–9.
56. Hermann M, Richter B, Roka R, Freissmuth M. Thyroid surgery in untreated severe hyperthyroidism: perioperative kinetics of free thyroid hormones in the glandular venous effluent and peripheral blood. *Surgery* 1994; **115:** 240–5.
57. Bennett-Guerrero E, Kramer DC, Schwinn DA. Effect of chronic and acute thyroid hormone reduction on perioperative outcome. *Anesth Analg* 1997; **85:** 30–6.
58. Mestman JH. Hyperthyroidism in pregnancy. *Clin Obstet Gynaecol* 1997; **40:** 45–64.
59. Montoro MN. Management of hypothyroidism during pregnancy. *Clin Obstet Gynaecol* 1997; **40:** 65–80.
60. Nicoloff JT, LoPresti JS. Myxedema coma. *Endocrinol Metab Clin North Am* 1993; **22:** 279–90.
61. Edwards R. Thyroid and parathyroid disease. *Int Anesthesiol Clin* 1997; **35:** 63–83.
62. Wakeling HG, Ody A, Ball A. Large goitre causing difficult intubation and failure to intubate using the laryngeal mask airway: lessons for next time. *Br J Anaesth* 1998; **81:** 979–81.
63. Hobbiger HE, Allen JG, Greatorex RG, Denny NM. The laryngeal mask airway for thyroid and parathyroid surgery. *Anaesthesia* 1996; **51:** 972–4.
64. Barwell J, Lytle J, Page R, Wilkins D. The NIM-2 nerve integrity monitor in thyroid and parathyroid surgery. *Br J Surg* 1997; **84:** 854.
65. Mermelstein M, Nonweiler R, Rubinstein EH. Intraoperative identification of laryngeal nerves with laryngeal electromyography. *Laryngoscope* 1996; **106:** 752–6.
66. Lacoste L, Karayan J, Lehuedè MS, *et al.* A comparison of direct, indirect and fibreoptic laryngoscopy to evaluate vocal cord paralysis after thyroid surgery. *Thyroid* 1996; **6:** 17–21.
67. Pattou F, Combemale F, Fabre S, *et al.* Hypocalcaemia following thyroid surgery: Incidence and prediction of outcome. *World J Surg* 1998; **22:** 718–24.
68. Gagner M. Endoscopic subtotal parathyroidectomy in patients with primary hyperparathyroidism. *Br J Surg* 1996; **83:** 875.
69. Bellantone R, Lombardi CP, Raffaelli M, *et al.* Minimally invasive, totally gasless video-assisted thyroid lobectomy. *Am J Surg* 1999; **177:** 342–3.
70. Samson PS, Reyes FR, Saludares WN, *et al.* Outpatient thyroidectomy. *Am J Surg* 1997; **173:** 499–503.
71. Farling PA. Thyroid disease. *Br J Anaesth* 2000; **85:** 15–28.
72. Mihai R, Farndon JR. Parathyroid disease and calcium metabolism. *Br J Anaesth* 2000; **85:** 29–43.
73. Chen H, Parkerson S, Udelsman R. Parathyroidectomy in the elderly: do the benefits outweigh the risks? *World J Surg* 1998; **22:** 531–6.
74. Kort KC, Schiller HJ, Numann PJ. Hyperparathyroidism and pregnancy. *Am J Surg* 1999; **177:** 66–8.
75. Kehlet H, Binder C. Adrenocortical function and clinical course during and after surgery in unsupplemented glucocorticoid-treated patients. *Br J Anaesth* 1973; **45:** 1043–8.
76. Kehlet H. A rational approach to dosage and preparation of parenteral glucocorticoid substitution therapy during surgical procedures. A short review. *Acta Anaesthesiol Scand* 1975; **19:** 260–4.
77. Symreng T, Karlberg BE, Kågedal B, Schildt B. Physiological cortisol substitution of long-term steroid-treated patients undergoing major surgery. *Br J Anaesth* 1981; **53:** 949–54.
78. Friedman RJ, Schiff CF, Bromberg JS. Use of supplemental steroids in patients having orthopaedic operations. *J Bone Joint Surg* 1995; **77A:** 1801–6.
79. Nicholson G, Burrin JM, Hall GM. Peri-operative steroid supplementation. *Anaesthesia* 1998; **53:** 1091–104.
80. Plumpton FS, Besser GM, Cole PV. Corticosteroid treatment and surgery. 1. An investigation of the indications for steroid cover. *Anaesthesia* 1969; **24:** 3–11.
81. Wood JB, Frankland AW, James VHT, Landon J. A rapid test of adrenocortical function. *Lancet* 1965; **1:** 243–5.
82. Bouachour G, Tirot P, Gouello JP, *et al.* Adrenocortical function during septic shock. *Intensive Care Med* 1995; **21:** 57–62.
83. Duggan M, Browne I, Flynn C. Adrenal failure in the critically ill. *Br J Anaesth* 1998; **81:** 468–70.
84. Werbel SS, Ober KP. Acute adrenal insufficiency. *Endocrinol Metab Clin North Am* 1993; **22:** 303–28.
85. Mellor A, Harvey RD, Pobereskin LH, Sneyd JR. Cushing's disease treated by trans-sphenoidal selective adenomectomy in mid-pregnancy. *Br J Anaesth* 1998; **80:** 850–2.
86. Conn JW. Primary aldosteronism, a new clinical syndrome. *J Lab Clin Med* 1955; **45:** 3–17.
87. Winship SM, Winstanley JHR, Hunter JM. Anaesthesia for Conn's syndrome. *Anaesthesia* 1999; **54:** 564–74.
88. Funder JW. Aldosterone, salt and cardiac fibrosis. *Clin Exp Hypertension* 1997; **19:** 885–99.

89. Bravo EL, Gifford RW. Pheochromocytoma: diagnosis, localisation and management. *N Engl J Med* 1984; **311:** 1298–303.
90. Sutton MG, Sheps SG, Lie JT. Prevalence of clinically unsuspected phaeochromocytoma. Review of a 50 year autopsy series. *Mayo Clin Proc* 1981; **56:** 354–60.
91. Geoghegan JG, Emberton M, Bloom SR, Lynn JA. Changing trends in the management of phaeochromocytoma. *Br J Surg* 1998; **85:** 117–20.
92. Schenker JG, Granat M. Phaeochromocytoma and pregnancy – an updated appraisal. *Aust NZ J Obstet Gynaecol* 1982; **22:** 1–10.
93. Harper MA, Murnaghan GA, Kennedy L, *et al.* Phaeochromocytoma and pregnancy. Five cases and a review of the literature. *Br J Obstet Gynaecol* 1989; **96:** 594–606.
94. Pattison J, Harrop-Griffiths AW, Whitlock JE, Roberts JC. Caesarean section in a patient with haemoglobin SC disease and a phaeochromocytoma. *Anaesthesia* 1990; **45:** 958–9.
95. Hamilton A, Sirrs S, Schmidt N, Onrot J. Anaesthesia for phaeochromocytoma in pregnancy. *Can J Anaesth* 1997; **44:** 654–7.
96. Takahashi K, Sai Y, Nosaka S. Anaesthetic management for Caesarean section combined with removal of phaeochromocytoma. *Eur J Anaesthesiol* 1998; **15:** 364–6.
97. Strachan AN, Claydon P, Caunt JA. Phaeochromocytoma diagnosed during labour. *Br J Anaesth* 2000; **85:** 635–7.
98. Bullough AS, Karadia S, Watters M. Phaeochromocytoma: an unusual cause of hypertension in pregnancy. *Anaesthesia* 2001; **56:** 43–6.
99. Allen GC, Rosenberg H. Phaeochromocytoma presenting as acute malignant hyperthermia – a diagnostic challenge. *Can J Anaesth* 1990; **37:** 593–5.
100. Larson MD, Herman WC. Bilateral dilated nonreactive pupils during surgery in a patient with undiagnosed pheochromocytoma. *Anesthesiology* 1992; **77:** 200–2.
101. Mayo CH. Paroxysmal hypertension with tumour of retroperitoneal nerve. Report of a case. *JAMA* 1927; **89:** 1047–50.
102. von der Mühll R. *Contribution a l'etude des paragangliomes de la surrénal.* Lausanne: l'Universite de Lausanne, 1928.
103. Welbourn RB. Highlights from endocrine surgical history. *World J Surg* 1996; **20:** 603–12.
104. Ulchaker JA, Goldfarb DA, Bravo EL, Novick AC. Successful outcomes in pheochromocytoma surgery in the modern era. *J Urol* 1999; **161:** 764–7.
105. Myre K, Rostrup M, Buanes T, Stokland O. Plasma catecholamines and haemodynamic changes during pneumoperitoneum. *Acta Anaesthesiol Scand* 1998; **42:** 343–7.
106. Mann C, Millat B, Boccara G, *et al.* Tolerance of laparoscopy for resection of phaeochomocytoma. *Br J Anaesth* 1996; **77:** 795–7.
107. Jerwood C, Willis B. Tolerance of laparoscopy for resection of phaeochromocytoma. *Br J Anaesth* 1997; **78:** 775–6.
108. Joris JL, Hamoir EE, Hartstein GM, *et al.* Hemodynamic changes and catecholamine release during laparoscopic adrenalectomy for pheochromocytoma. *Anesth Analg* 1999; **88:** 16–21.
109. Stenström G, Kutti J. The blood volume in pheochromocytoma patients before and during treatment with phenoxybenzamine. *Acta Med Scand* 1985; **218:** 381–7.
110. Steinsapir J, Carr AA, Prisant LM, Bransome ED. Metyrosine and pheochromocytoma. *Arch Intern Med* 1997; **157:** 901–6.
111. Roizen MF, Horrigan RW, Koike M, *et al.* A prospective randomized trial of four anesthetic techniques for resection of pheochromocytoma. *Anesthesiology* 1982; **57:** A43.
112. Russell WJ, Metcalfe IR, Tonkin AL, Frewin DB. The preoperative management of phaeochromocytoma. *Anaesth Intensive Care* 1998; **26:** 196–200.
113. Stenström G, Haljamäe H, Tisell LE. Influence of pre-operative treatment with phenoxybenzamine on the incidence of adverse cardiovascular reactions during anaesthesia and surgery for phaeochromocytoma. *Acta Anaesthesiol Scand* 1985; **29:** 797–803.
114. Nicholson JP, Vaughn ED, Pickering TG, *et al.* Phaeochromocytoma and prazosin. *Ann Intern Med* 1983; **99:** 477–9.
115. Prys-Roberts C. Phaeochromocytoma – recent progress in its management. *Br J Anaesth* 2000; **85:** 44–57.
116. Hull CJ. Phaeochromocytoma – diagnosis, preoperative preparation and anaesthetic management. *Br J Anaesth* 1986; **58:** 1453–68.
117. Sloand EM, Taylor Thompson B. Propranolol-induced pulmonary edema and shock in a patient with pheochromocytoma. *Arch Intern Med* 1984; **144:** 173–4.
118. Mihm FG, Sandhu JS, Brown MD, Rosenthal MH. Short acting beta-adrenergic blockade as initial drug therapy in pheochromocytoma. *Crit Care Med* 1990; **18:** 673–4.
119. Navaratnarajah M, White DC. Labetolol and phaeochromocytoma. *Br J Anaesth* 1984; **56:** 1179.
120. Colson P, Ryckwaert F, Ribstein J, *et al.* Haemodynamic heterogeneity and treatment with the calcium channel blocker nicardipine during phaeochromocytoma surgery. *Acta Anaesthesiol Scand* 1998; **42:** 1114–19.
121. Gilsanz FJ, Luengo C, Conejero P, *et al.* Cardiomyopathy and phaeochromocytoma. *Anaesthesia* 1983; **38:** 888–91.
122. Ryan T, Timoney A, Cunningham AJ. Use of transoesophageal echocardiography to manage beta-adrenoceptor block and assess left ventricular function in a patient with phaeochromocytoma. *Br J Anaesth* 1993; **70:** 101–3.
123. James MFM. The use of magnesium sulfate in the anaesthetic management of pheochromocytoma. *Anesthesiology* 1985; **62:** 188–90.
124. James MFM. Use of magnesium sulphate in the anaesthetic management of phaeochromocytoma: a review of 17 anaesthetics. *Br J Anaesth* 1989; **62:** 616–23.
125. James MFM. Phaeochromocytoma – recent progress in its management. *Br J Anaesth* 2001; **86:** 594–5.
126. Cousins MJ, Rubin RB. The intraoperative management of phaeochromocytoma with total epidural sympathetic blockade. *Br J Anaesth* 1974; **46:** 78–81.
127. Liem TH, Moll JE, Booij LHDJ. Thoracic epidural analgesia in a patient with bilateral phaeochromocytoma undergoing coronary artery bypass grafting. *Anaesthesia* 1991; **46:** 654–8.
128. Levin H, Heifetz M. Phaeochromocytoma and severe protracted hypoglycaemia. *Can J Anaesth* 1990; **37:** 477–8.
129. Meeke RI, O'Keefe JD, Gaffney JD. Phaeochromocytoma removal and postoperative hypoglycaemia. *Anaesthesia* 1985; **40:** 1093–6.
130. Jones SE, Redfern N, Shaw IH, Baylis PH. Exaggerated cardiovascular response to anaesthesia – a case for investigation. *Anaesthesia* 1999; **54:** 882–4.
131. Greaves DJ, Barrow PM. Emergency resection of phaeochromocytoma presenting with hyperamylasaemia and pulmonary oedema after abdominal trauma. *Anaesthesia* 1989; **44:** 841–2.
132. Swensen SR, Snow E, Gaisford WD. Carcinoid tumours of the gastrointestinal tract. *Am J Surg* 1973; **126:** 818.
133. Rambaud JC, Hautefeuille M, Ruskone M, Jacquenod P. Diarrhoea due to circulating agents. *Clin Gastroenterol* 1986; **15:** 603–29.
134. Zinner MJ, Yeo CJ, Jaffe BM. The effects of carcinoid levels of serotonin and substance P on hemodynamics. *Ann Surg* 1984; **199:** 197–204.
135. Thorson A, Biörck G, Björkman G, Waldenström J. Malignant carcinoid of the small intestine with metastases to the liver, valvular disease of the right side of the heart, peripheral vasomotor symptoms, bronchoconstriction and an unusual type of cyanosis; clinical and pathologic syndrome. *Am Heart J* 1954; **47:** 795–817.
136. Creutzfeldt W, Stockman F. Carcinoids and carcinoid syndrome. *Am J Med* 1987; **82:** 4–16.
137. Neustein SM, Cohen E. Anesthesia for aortic and mitral valve replacement in a patient with carcinoid heart disease. *Anesthesiology* 1995; **82:** 1067–70.
138. Millward MJ, Blake MP, Byrne MJ, *et al.* Left heart involvement with cardiac shunt complicating carcinoid heart disease. *Aust NZ J Med* 1989; **19:** 716–17.
139. Déry R. Theoretical and clinical considerations in anaesthesia for secreting carcinoid tumours. *Can Anaesth Soc J* 1971; **18:** 245–63.
140. Houghton K, Carter JA. Peri-operative management of carcinoid syndrome using ketanserin. *Anaesthesia* 1986; **41:** 596–9.
141. Royston D. Aprotinin therapy. *Br J Anaesth* 1994; **73:** 734–7.
142. Ludwig GD, Cushard W, Bartuska D, *et al.* Effects of beta-adrenergic blockade in the carcinoid syndrome. *Arch Intern Med* 1968; **68:** 1188.
143. Kvols LK, Moertel CG, O'Connell MJ, *et al.* Treatment of the malignant carcinoid syndrome. Evaluation of a long-acting somatostatin analogue. *N Engl J Med* 1986; **315:** 663–6.
144. Sheppard M, Shapiro B, Pimstone B, *et al.* Metabolic clearance and plasma half-disappearance time of exogenous somatostatin in man. *J Clin Endocrinol Metab* 1979; **48:** 50–3.
145. Whitehouse I, Beglinger C, Ruttiman G, Gyr K. Inhibition of pentagastrin-stimulated acid secretion after subcutaneous injection of a new somatostatin analogue. *Gut* 1986; **27:** 141–6.
146. Roy RC, Carter RF, Wright PD. Somatostatin, anaesthesia and the carcinoid syndrome. *Anaesthesia* 1987; **42:** 627–32.
147. Pratila MG, Pratilas V. Propofol infusion in carcinoid syndrome [letter]. *Can J Anaesth* 1991; **38:** 943–4.
148. Stephen JL, Grahame-Smith DG. Treatment of the carcinoid syndrome by local removal of hepatic metastases. *Proc R Soc Med* 1972; **65:** 444.
149. Aune S, Schistad G. Carcinoid liver metastases treated with hepatic dearterialisation. *Am J Surg* 1972; **123:** 715.

150. Maton PN, Camilleri M, Griffin G, *et al.* Role of hepatic arterial embolization in the carcinoid syndrome. *Br Med J* 1983; **287:** 932–5.
151. Biörck G, Axen O, Thorson A. Unusual cyanosis in a boy with congenital pulmonary stenosis and tricuspid insufficiency. Fatal outcome after angiocardiography. *Am Heart J* 1952; **44:** 143.
152. Mason RA, Steane PA. Carcinoid syndrome: its relevance to the anaesthetist. *Anaesthesia* 1976; **31:** 228–42.
153. Marsh HM, Martin JK, Kvols LK, *et al.* Carcinoid crisis during anesthesia: successful treatment with a somatostatin analogue. *Anesthesiology* 1987; **66:** 89–91.
154. Parris WCV, Oates JA, Kambam J, *et al.* Pre-treatment with somatostatin in the anaesthetic management of a patient with carcinoid syndrome. *Can J Anaesth* 1988; **35:** 413–16.
155. Veall GRQ, Peacock JE, Bax NDS, Reilly CS. Review of the anaesthetic management of 21 patients undergoing laparotomy for carcinoid syndrome. *Br J Anaesth* 1994; **72:** 335–41.
156. Cortinez LI. Refractory hypotension during carcinoid resection surgery. *Anaesthesia* 2000; **55:** 505–6.
157. Monteith K, Roaseg OP. Epidural anaesthesia for transurethral resection of the prostate in a patient with carcinoid syndrome. *Can J Anaesth* 1990; **37:** 349–52.
158. Holdcroft A. Hormones and the gut. *Br J Anaesth* 2000; **85:** 58–68.

49

Anesthesia for dental and orofacial surgery

PENELOPE B HEWITT

General anesthesia for dental extractions has a long and interesting history. In 1844, a dentist, Horace Wells, saw a demonstration by Gardner Q Colton, a traveling chemist, of the effects of inhaling nitrous oxide. He noted that a young shop assistant under the influence of the gas knocked his shin and made it bleed but stated that he felt no pain. Wells then persuaded Colton to use nitrous oxide the next day for a dental extraction, with Wells as the patient, and it was a big success – "a new era in tooth pulling." This is vividly described, with extracts from contemporary reports and biographical details of those involved, in a chapter entitled "The crucial experiment, its eclipse and its revival" in Denis Smith's fascinating book on the history of nitrous oxide anesthesia.[1,2]

The first public and successful demonstration of ether anesthesia took place at the Massachusetts General Hospital on Friday 16 October 1846 when William Morton, a Boston dentist, used it for the painless removal of a tumor from a patient's neck. Then, when the news of the use of ether for anesthesia first arrived in London by means of a letter from Jacob Bigelow to Francis Boott, Boott arranged with James Robinson, a friend who was a dentist, to carry out their own experiments. The first use in the UK, following on from these experiments, was for the painless extraction of a wisdom tooth. In 1983, Ellis, of St Bartholomew's Hospital, procured the publication of a facsimile edition of James Robinson's 1847 *A Treatise on the Inhalation of the Vapour of Ether for the Prevention of Pain in Surgical Operations.* This gives a fascinating description of these innovative efforts.[3]

The dental profession in the UK took up this use of general anesthetic agents very rapidly. Even now that safe and effective local anesthetic techniques are readily available, a large proportion of the general public in the UK still seems to feel that any form of dental surgery is an indication for a "gas" or an "i.v." to "knock them out."

Interestingly, there was no specific chapter on anesthesia for dental surgery in the 1966 edition of this text (Wylie and Churchill-Davidson's *A Practice of Anaesthesia,* 2nd edition). However, in the chapter "The anaesthetic gases," the section on nitrous oxide had a detailed description of the technique for using nitrous oxide in dentistry.[4] This was an account of how a dental "gas" should be administered. The patient was settled comfortably, sitting in the dental chair, with the body tilted slightly backwards with the neck slightly extended and a mouthprop inserted. Induction was usually carried out with 100% nitrous oxide via a nasal mask, oxygen being added at the point of loss of consciousness or the onset of cyanosis. A slight increase in the pressure of the gases was found to be helpful at this stage. A small pack was inserted and placed at the back of the tongue to prevent blood and tooth fragments from being aspirated. The anesthesiologist supported the head and jaw during the extractions and sometimes introduced a mouth gag to allow the dental prop to be switched over to the other side. This was the generally accepted technique at that time. Consciousness normally returned within a few seconds to a minute and the patient was expected to walk from the dental chair within a few minutes. Occasionally, however, recovery was delayed. Bourne identified that this was not uncommon and that some patients suffered severe cerebral hypoxia resulting from being kept upright during an "undetected faint."[5]

RECENT REGULATIONS CONCERNING DENTAL ANESTHESIA AND SEDATION

The Poswillo Report, produced in the UK in 1990, saw the beginning of a major move to make general anesthesia in the community safer, particularly with regard to the level of experience of the anesthesiologist and the provision of proper equipment.[6]

In November 1998, the General Dental Council (GDC) issued revised guidance to dentists concerning general anesthesia.[7] This put the onus on both the referring dentist and the treating dentist to explain to the patient the alternatives to general anesthesia and the risks involved. It also laid down the criteria for ensuring that any general anesthetics would be administered by an individual on the General Medical Council Specialist Register as an anesthesiologist or by a properly supervised trainee or nonconsultant career grade doctor. This anesthesiologist must also have a trained assistant and adequate recovery facilities. The Royal College of Anaesthetists' publication of their *Position Paper on Standards and Guidelines for General Anaesthesia for Dentistry*, prepared by their Dental Anaesthesia Committee, enlarged upon this.[8] The implications of these reports for the relation between anesthesia and dentistry have been summarized in the Royal College of Anaesthetists' *Newsletter.*[9]

In 1999, the GDC amended the *Maintaining Standards: Guidance to Dentists on Professional and Personal Conduct* document with regard to the section on pain and anxiety control.[10] This states that conscious sedation can be an effective method of facilitating dental treatment and is normally used in conjunction with appropriate local anesthesia. Conscious sedation is defined as "A technique by which a drug or drugs produces a state of depression of the central nervous system enabling treatment to be carried out, but during which verbal contact with the patient is maintained throughout the period of sedation. The drugs and techniques used to provide conscious sedation should carry a margin of safety wide enough to render loss of consciousness unlikely." It also states that "The level of sedation must be such that the patient remains conscious, retains protective reflexes, and is able to understand and to respond to verbal commands."

The guidelines issued by the American Dental Society of Anesthesiology (ADSA; founded in 1954) differ from those applicable in the UK. In 1964, it established a Fellowship in General Anesthesia for those who had received 1 year or more, or the equivalent, of advanced training, or residency, in anesthesia and who had passed an oral examination. Oral surgeons with training of 3 years or more were eligible. Many states include Fellowship of the ADSA as a prerequisite for obtaining a permit to administer parenteral conscious sedation for dental procedures in the dental office. They also produce guidelines for teaching the comprehensive control of pain and anxiety in dentistry. In 1984, the ADSA began to support several 2-year "anesthesia residencies" for dentists, but only a few such courses materialized, and those tended to be lost to medical school graduates. Nevertheless, it is accepted that, in the USA, dental practitioners with appropriate training may use techniques of "deep sedation" involving combinations of analgesic and sedative drugs administered parenterally during which verbal contact is *not* maintained.[11] In the UK, this is not accepted as part of dental practice; when verbal contact is lost, this is regarded as *general anesthesia,* which is the realm of the specialist anesthesiologist.

GENERAL ANESTHESIA FOR EXODONTIA IN CHILDREN

The number of general anesthetics for dentistry has been found to be much higher in the UK than in other countries. General anesthesia was found in a survey to be unusual in other European countries, even for extractions in children under the age of 7 years.[12] In the UK, a visit to a dental practitioner because of toothache and the subsequent use of general anesthesia for a dental extraction is frequently a child's first experience of anesthesia. This practice makes it very important because it establishes the impression of anesthesia and anesthesiologists in the eyes of the public. It is essential that such encounters should be undertaken in a kind and thoughtful way, as well as with the same standards of care and safety as for any other use of anesthesia. Careful selection of "child-friendly" equipment, such as a reservoir bag with a picture of a teddy bear (see Fig. 49.1), transparent face masks with attractive scents, etc., can be used to make anesthetic interventions more acceptable.

It is also important that the dentistry to be undertaken is carefully planned. Nowadays, the "smash and grab" approach is not acceptable. If a general anesthetic is given for removal of severely decayed teeth, it is logical to review the remaining dentition so that future care may be planned. If a child is below the age at which they will be able to cooperate with dental fillings to other teeth, it may be better to provide a longer anesthetic in order to render the child "dentally fit" and avoid the need for a further anesthetic some months later. One study of 200 episodes (mean age of children, 5 years 4 months) showed that, out of 53 single-tooth extractions, 75% of the patients required subsequent treatment under a second general anesthetic for caries that had been charted at the first assessment but left untreated.[13]

Preoperative assessment and preparation must be carried out as for any other day-stay (ambulatory) anesthesia procedure and the patient must be weighed. The anesthesiologist should decide whether intravenous or inhalational induction of anesthesia would be preferable for each individual patient. This decision depends on the age of the patient, the likely ease or difficulty of venous puncture, the availability of EMLA (eutectic mixture of local anesthetics) cream or Ametop (amethocaine cream) application to reduce the pain, and the experience and attitude of the child and the parent(s).

Propofol with lidocaine (lignocaine) induction of anesthesia, for children over the age of 3 years, followed by maintenance with nitrous oxide, oxygen, and isoflurane with spontaneous ventilation is a simple and safe anesthetic. For children below 3 years of age, or those who are afraid of needles, sevoflurane induction is preferable. It has been shown that sevoflurane with nitrous oxide and oxygen provides satisfactory induction of anesthesia for children aged 1–12 years, but when used with oxygen alone there is a significantly higher incidence of excitement.[14] If sevoflurane is not available, halothane provides a smoother induction than isoflurane.[15] The induction with halothane is more rapid; when isoflurane is used, there is a higher incidence of coughing, breath holding, laryngospasm, and laryngospasm requiring treatment. *Maintenance* of anesthesia with halothane is not recommended for dental anesthesia because of the higher incidence of arrhythmias, and the greater proportion of these arrhythmias that are ventricular in origin.[16,17] In November 1999, The Committee on the Safety of Medicines in the UK advised that the use of halothane in pediatric dental anesthesia should be restricted to within hospitals only.[18,19] The incidence of arrhythmias in dental surgical patients who are anesthetized with halothane varies between 18% and 75%. One factor leading to these arrhythmias includes stimulation of the sympathoadrenal system via the fifth cranial nerve during dental extractions. The slowing of conduction in the atria, bundles of His, and ventricles in the presence of halothane may allow re-entrant activity to cause arrhythmias.

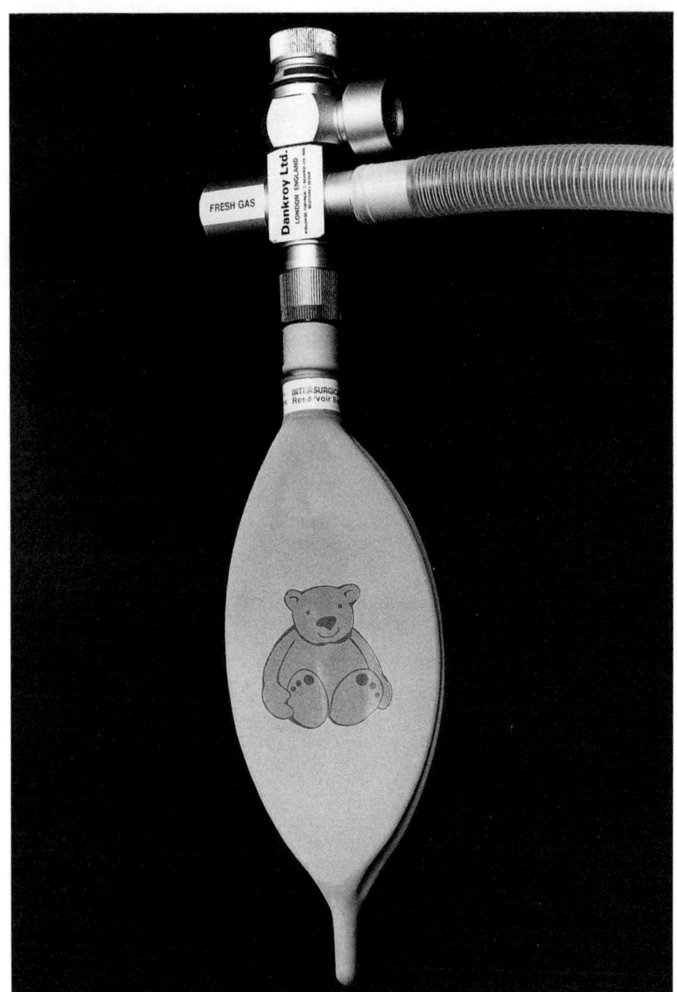

Figure 49.1 *Pediatric reservoir bag with "teddy bear" picture.*

When the procedure involves only simple extraction of anterior teeth, maintenance using a nasal mask is satisfactory, provided that the anesthesiologist and the dental surgeon are familiar with the technique. A safe system of propping the mouth open and using a pack as a screen across the mouth to stop any teeth or debris falling back into the pharynx, plus suction to prevent aspiration of blood into the larynx, must be used (Fig. 49.2). It has been suggested that anesthesia administered through a nasopharyngeal airway provides higher quality anesthesia and operating conditions than the traditional nasal mask.[20] Others, however, feel that the incidence of nasal bleeding (28%) that was reported was not acceptable.[21]

In the past, some practitioners anesthetized such patients for exodontia in the sitting position in a dental chair. Not only did this incur the danger of blood and secretions running down into the larynx but there was the additional risk of cerebral hypoxia consequent upon unrecognized fainting in this position.[5]

For multiple extractions of molar teeth, or any cases for which difficulty is anticipated either with the dentistry or maintenance of a clear airway, a reinforced laryngeal mask airway (LMA) should be used.[22,23] Figure 49.3 shows two sizes of reinforced laryngeal masks with, for comparison, one standard LMA. It can be seen that the reinforced tube leading to the reinforced LMAs is also longer and narrower than that of the same size of standard LMA. This enables the connection with the breathing system to be outside the field of the dental procedure and out of the way of the operator. A moistened pack should be carefully positioned above the LMA so that blood and dental debris do not enter the pharynx but distortion or displacement of the LMA must be avoided (see Figs 49.4 and 49.5).

An oral nonsteroidal anti-inflammatory analgesic drug (NSAID) may be administered preoperatively, or per rectum during the anesthetic (having previously explained this to parent/child and having obtained consent), to provide the initial postoperative analgesia. Acetaminophen (paracetamol) should be used if NSAIDs are contraindicated.

Trained members of staff are required to supervise safe recovery. Bleeding must have ceased and the child must be tested to be able to walk steadily, given adequate analgesia, and a clear fluid drink before being discharged home, supervised by a responsible adult and, preferably, not traveling by public transport. Details must be given to the parents about how to contact the hospital, dental unit, or general medical or dental practitioner for further advice, help, or treatment should the need arise.

Recommendations for provision of further analgesia must also be given to the parents. Acetaminophen (paracetamol) elixir (120 mg per 5 mL) is usually the best option; the dose is around 10–15 mg kg^{-1} body weight, which can be repeated every 4–6 h. Ibuprofen is also included in the dental formulary and may be useful when there is inadequate effect from acetaminophen, provided that the patient does not suffer from asthma, renal disease, a bleeding disorder, or any other potential contraindication to NSAIDs. A suspension containing 100 mg per 5 mL is available and the recommended dose for a 3- to 7-year-old child is 100 mg (5 mL) every 6–8 h and for an 8- to 12-year-old 200 mg (10 mL) every 6–8 h as required.

One study showed that 92% of children aged 5–15 years having tooth extraction under general anesthesia in general dental practice complained of symptoms associated with the surgery under general anesthesia.[24] Distress was noted in 20% of patients during induction and 33% during recovery. Continued crying was reported for 39% during the journey home and for 37% once home had been reached. Other symptoms included nausea, vomiting, sickness, and prolonged bleeding. Of the 80 patients in this study, six patients reported psychologic trauma 1 month after, three had nightmares, two had continuing bad memories, and one was depressed for several days.

ANESTHESIA FOR PATIENTS WITH SPECIAL NEEDS

There are many patients with mental, psychological, or physical problems for whom normal dental care under local anesthesia is not feasible.[25] They often have devoted carers who make enormous efforts to prevent dental caries developing, but procedures under general anesthesia may be required nevertheless. These are often carried out in day-stay units to minimize disruption to everyday care. Preoperative assessment requires expertise and common sense when deciding whether inpatient treatment is required and how the anesthetic care can best be managed.[26] Admission to hospital will be required for any general anesthetic when serious medical problems coexist.

Special needs patients require special care from experienced anesthesiologists.[27] Often, inhalational anesthesia is the only acceptable approach, even for large patients. Their regular carer may be the best person to help ensure maximum possible cooperation. An experienced dental team needs to decide a practical treatment plan that will fit into an acceptable timescale for day-stay care.[28]

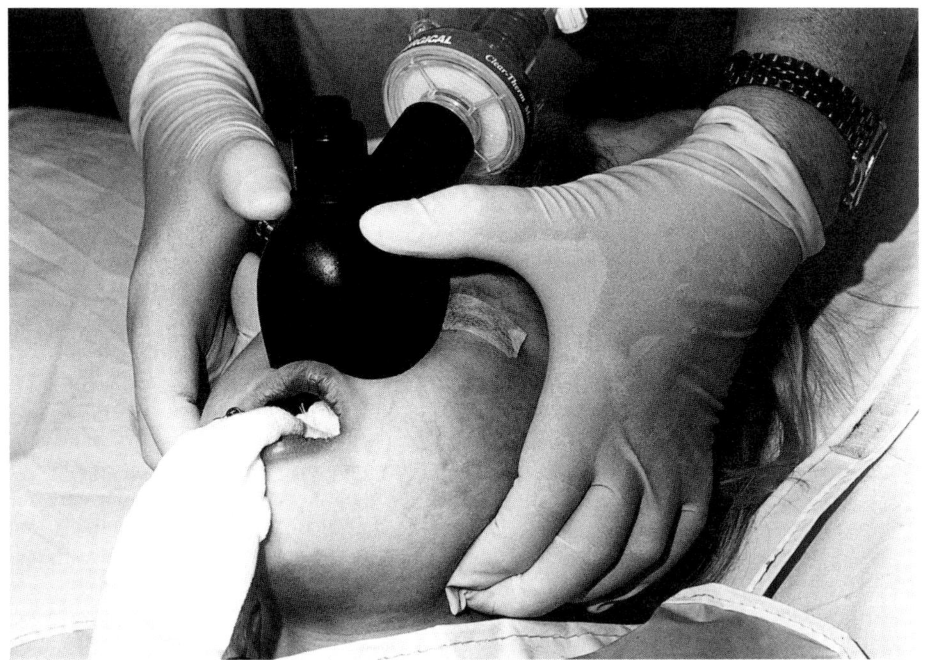

Figure 49.2 *Nasal mask in use, with mouth prop and pack.*

Figure 49.3 *Laryngeal mask airways (LMAs). Top, standard LMA; below, two sizes of reinforced LMA.*

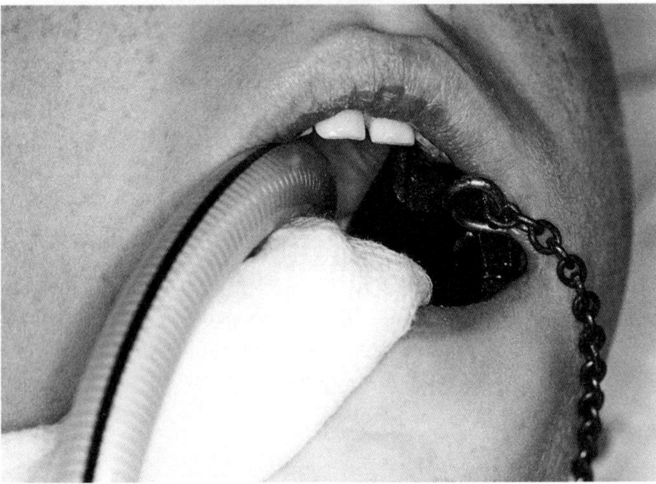

Figure 49.4 *LMA with mouth prop and pack positioned.*

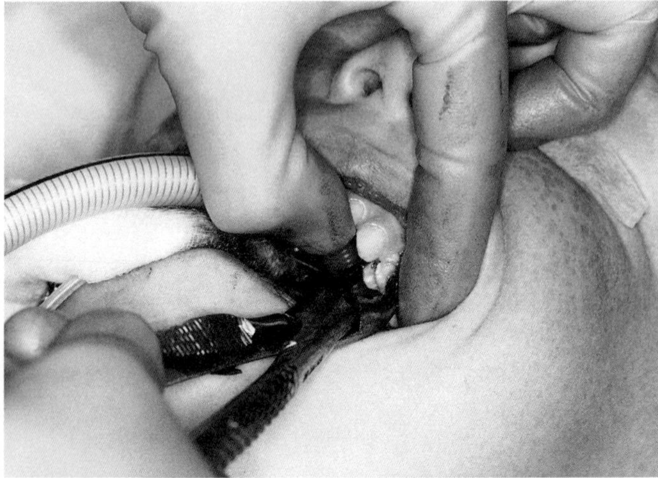

Figure 49.5 *Extraction of upper tooth, showing reinforced LMA and throat pack in position.*

DENTISTRY AND PATIENTS WITH CARDIAC DISEASE

Patients with congenital or acquired cardiac disease involving valvular lesions, or other causes of turbulent flow, are at risk of developing bacterial endocarditis. For many years, dental interventions, especially those involving extraction of teeth or procedures involving damage to the tissues with consequent bleeding, have been considered to be particularly to blame. A Working Party of the British Society for Antimicrobial Chemotherapy has drawn up recommendations for the use of antibiotic prophylaxis to cover dental procedures in patients with heart valve lesions, septal defects, patent ductus arteriosus, or prosthetic valves.[29–32] The recommendations are conveniently summarized in the *British National Formulary*.[33]

Dental procedures regarded as requiring antibiotic cover are extractions, scaling, and surgery involving gingival tissues. The antibiotic prophylaxis may be supplemented with 1% chlorhexidine gluconate gel or 0.2% chlorhexidine gluconate mouthwash used 5 min before the procedure.

For dental procedures under local or no anesthesia, patients who have not received more than a single dose of penicillin in the previous month, including those with a prosthetic valve (but not those who have had endocarditis), should be given 3 g oral amoxycillin 1 h before the procedure. A child less than 5 years old should be given one-quarter of the adult dose; a child aged 5–10 years should be given one-half the adult dose. Patients who are allergic to penicillin, or who have received more than a single dose of a penicillin in the previous month, should be given 600 mg oral clindamycin 1 h before the procedure; a child under 5 years old should be given one-quarter of the adult dose; a child aged 5–10 years should be given one-half of the adult dose. Patients who have had endocarditis should be given amoxycillin plus gentamicin, as for those under general anesthesia.

Patients with cardiac lesions with no special risk (including patients who have received no more than a single dose of a penicillin in the previous month) undergoing dental procedures under general anesthesia may be given 1 g intravenous (i.v.) amoxycillin at induction, then 500 mg oral amoxycillin 6 h later. A child under 5 years of age should be given one-quarter of the adult dose; a child aged 5–10 years should be given one-half the adult dose. Alternatively, 3 g amoxycillin can be given orally 4 h before induction, then a further 3-g oral dose as soon as possible after the procedure (a child less than 5 years old being given one-quarter of the adult dose; a child aged 5–10 years, one-half of the adult dose). Another alternative is 3 g oral amoxycillin plus 1 g oral probenecid 4 h before the procedure.

Patients at special risk (e.g. those with a prosthetic valve or who have had endocarditis) should be given 1 g i.v. amoxycillin plus 120 mg i.v. gentamicin at induction or 15 min before the procedure. Children younger than 5 years old should be given one-quarter of the adult dose of amoxycillin plus 2 mg kg^{-1} gentamicin; children aged 5–10 years should be given one-half the adult dose of amoxycillin with 2 mg kg^{-1} gentamicin. Patients who are allergic to penicillin, or who have received more than a single dose of penicillin in the past month, may be given 1 g i.v. vancomycin over at least 100 min then 120 mg i.v. gentamicin at induction or 15 min before the procedure (for a child under 10 years, use 20 mg kg^{-1} vancomycin plus 2 mg kg^{-1} gentamicin). Another option is to give 400 mg i.v. teicoplanin plus 120 mg gentamicin at induction or 15 min before the procedure; children under 14 years old should be given 6 mg kg^{-1} teicoplanin and 2 mg kg^{-1} gentamicin. The third option is clindamycin 300 mg over at least 10 min at induction or 15 min before the procedure then 150 mg oral or i.v. clindamycin 6 h later. For a child under 5 years of age, one-quarter of the adult dose should be given; for a child aged 5–10 years, one-half of the adult dose should be given.

However, much recent work suggests that many other less invasive procedures are likely to produce more bacteremia, especially when the presence of the organisms is summated over a period of time.[34] The literature reveals evidence that cumulative exposure over the course of 1 month to "physiologic" bacteremia from everyday events such as chewing and brushing teeth exceeded the "surgical" bacteremia from a dental extraction by a multiplication factor of 895! It has also been suggested that children are less likely than adults to develop bacterial endocarditis because prevalence is low in those younger than 20 years old. Perhaps the time has come to review the requirement for routine use of antibiotic cover for dental procedures in children. There will always be the risk of an anaphylactoid reaction, especially when the antibiotics are given intravenously. When antibiotics are given in association with general anesthesia, it is wise to give them either before the induction of anesthesia or after induction is complete, i.v. access and airway control having been secured, so that if a reaction does occur it can be identified and treated rapidly without other distractions.

ANESTHESIA FOR ORAL SURGERY

Removal of impacted third molars (wisdom teeth) is one of the most frequently performed operations in the UK National Health Service. In recent years, much attention has been given to deciding when this procedure is required and the level of priority that it should be given by healthcare purchasers and providers.[35] Many patients assume that these teeth will be removed under general anesthesia, but this is not essential. If the removal is unlikely to be difficult, and especially when only one side is affected, local anesthesia can be recommended. The dental surgeon can increase acceptance rates for nervous patients by providing conscious sedation to cover the procedure and provide some amnesia.

When general anesthesia is required, for difficult extractions or uncontrollably dental phobic patients, this can often be carried out as a day-stay procedure in accordance with normal guidelines. Preoperative medication with an NSAID and an antiemetic is helpful. When surgery may be difficult or prolonged, nasotracheal intubation is helpful and ensures a clear airway, protection against aspiration of blood or debris into the tracheobronchial tree, and controlled ventilation of the lungs. Preformed cuffed nasotracheal tubes (Fig. 49.6) are available for this purpose. A moistened throat pack is positioned in the oropharynx by the anesthesiologist after the trachea has been intubated.

If surgery is uncomplicated and there are no difficulties with the patient's airway, or medical problems, a reinforced LMA with a throat pack and spontaneous ventilation can be used.

Pain resulting from the extraction of impacted third molar teeth is a standard model for the investigation of analgesic efficiency. Consequently, there are numerous studies documenting their effects in these patients. Postoperative analgesia with NSAIDs alone has been shown to be effective after dental surgery, preoperative administration is more effective, and oral administration is effective.[36]

CONSCIOUS SEDATION FOR PROCEDURES UNDER LOCAL ANESTHESIA

Many patients have such serious phobias about intraoral procedures of any kind that they will not attend for treatment unless sedation or general anesthesia is available.

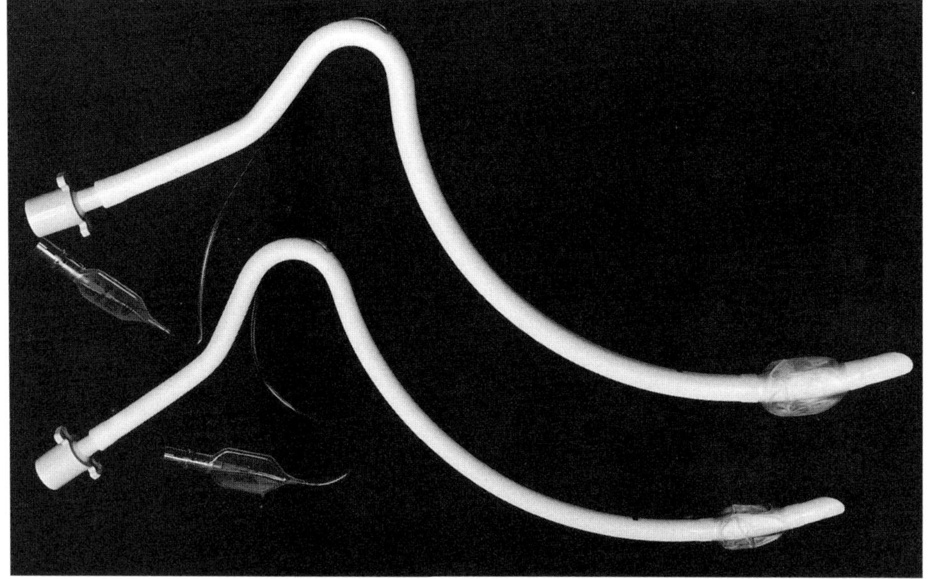

Figure 49.6 *Preformed, cuffed nasotracheal tubes.*

The recommended techniques involve either use of small, slowly administered incremental doses of a short-acting benzodiazepine (usually midazolam) or inhalation of a carefully controlled mixture of nitrous oxide with oxygen to provide inhalation sedation.[37] Inhalation sedation equipment, the most commonly used type being called a relative analgesia (RA) machine (Fig. 49.7), is specially designed so that the concentration of nitrous oxide in oxygen being administered can be carefully controlled and increased in a stepwise manner until the optimum effect is produced. It is not possible to reduce the administered oxygen concentration below 30% when this equipment is used. The patient can position the soft, but weighted, mask on his/her own nose to ensure that it is comfortable (Fig. 49.8). The effects are significantly enhanced by behavioral management techniques employed concomitantly by the dental practitioner.

Conscious sedation techniques are used to cover dental procedures being carried out under local anesthesia (LA).[38] It is the LA that provides the analgesia, therefore the problems of using systemic analgesic drugs can be avoided. Anesthesiologists may play a part in the training of dental practitioners who are learning to administer safe conscious sedation, e.g. the use of patient monitoring and the management of the effects of overdose. It is most important, however, that anesthesiologists do not confuse conscious sedation for dentistry with the levels of sedation used to ensure compliance with intermittent positive pressure ventilation of the lungs in an intensive care unit. Nor should they suggest use of the potentially hazardous combinations of opioids and benzodiazepines, which may be used for medical procedures, when LA is not feasible, as these are inappropriate in the dental setting in which LA is used to provide the analgesia![37]

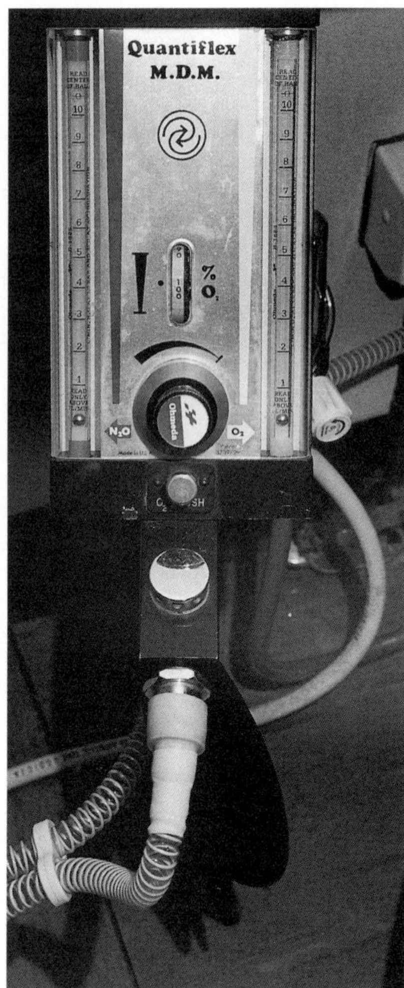

Figure 49.7 *Relative analgesia machine head for inhalation sedation.*

ANESTHESIA FOR MAXILLOFACIAL TRAUMA

This is often carried out as an emergency and for patients who may have multiple trauma, a full stomach, and bleeding into the upper air passages. These patients can provide a challenge for even the most experienced practitioners, and all appropriate precautions must be taken.[39–42] Airway control is the first priority.[43] Any patient who has sustained head trauma must be checked for possible neck injury. Great care must be taken to avoid movements that could endanger the integrity of the cervical spinal cord in such cases. Fiberoptic intubation may be the safest way to secure airway control without interfering with stabilization of an injured neck. It must also be remembered that even the greatest fiberoptic intubation expert cannot see the larynx through a pool of blood.

Postoperative airway care is equally important. It will often require high-dependency unit or intensive therapy unit care. If the jaws are wired together, wire cutters *must* always be kept at the bedside in case an emergency arises, e.g. vomiting, regurgitation, or bleeding into the pharynx, and the staff must be instructed and skilled in their use.

ANESTHESIA FOR ORTHOGNATHIC SURGERY

This surgery is carried out electively, may involve difficult intubation, and requires the same standards of postoperative care as outlined for patients following trauma when the jaws are wired together.

ANESTHESIA FOR MAJOR RESECTIONS (HEAD AND NECK CANCER SURGERY)

These can be very long and extensive procedures involving significant blood loss. Invasive cardiovascular monitoring techniques will often be required. Careful preoperative assessment is necessary when deciding on the method of airway control to be used.[44,45] If a large or friable cancerous lesion is near the laryngeal opening, a surgical tracheostomy may need to be established under local anesthesia prior to general anesthesia for resective surgery. Otherwise, cautious induction of anesthesia, maintaining spontaneous ventilation, is required until it can be ascertained that the larynx is visible on direct laryngoscopy. If this is not possible, awake fiberoptic intubation will be needed.[46] Postoperative intensive care for 48 h or more is often required before these patients can have tracheal extubation carried out safely.

CONCLUSIONS

In current practice we need to consider the circumstances in which general anesthesia is required for dentistry and the alternatives that are available. If a patient is apprehensive or has an absolute phobia about dental procedures being carried out with local anesthesia, how may they be managed? What is the safest and best way to administer general anesthetics to children or those with "special needs" who cannot cope with local anesthesia alone? When can oral surgery be carried out under local anesthesia, with or without sedation? What methods of airway control are safe and satisfactory while patients are undergoing exodontia or intraoral procedures? How should patients with maxillofacial trauma or those undergoing orthognathic procedures be managed? What are the special demands for those undergoing extensive resections for cancerous lesions?

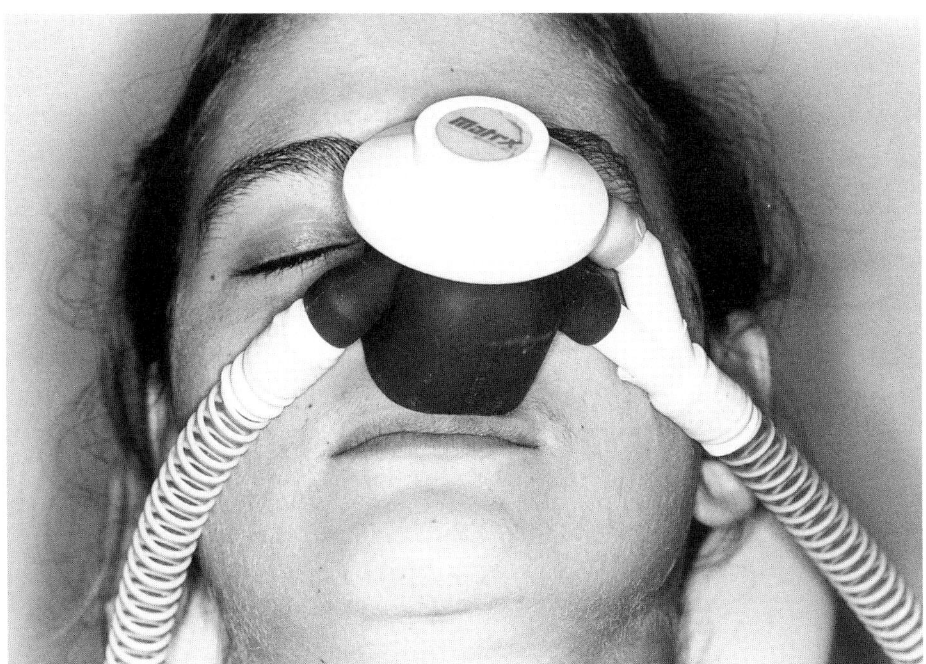

Figure 49.8 *Inhalation sedation mask in position.*

REFERENCES

1. Smith WDA. *Under the Influence: a History of Nitrous Oxide and Oxygen Anaesthesia*. London: Macmillan, 1982: 53–66.
2. Lee JA, Atkinson RS. *A Synopsis of Anaesthesia*, 7th edn. Bristol: John Wright, 1973: 6–7.
3. Ellis RH. *James Robinson on the Inhalation of the Vapour of Ether*. Eastbourne: Baillière Tindall, 1983.
4. Wylie WD, Churchill-Davidson CD. *A Practice of Anaesthesia*, 2nd edn. London: Lloyd-Luke, 1966: 245–51.
5. Bourne JG. Fainting and cerebral damage. A danger in patients kept upright during dental gas anaesthesia and after surgical operations. *Lancet* 1957; **2:** 499.
6. Poswillo D. *General Anaesthesia, Sedation and Resuscitation in Dentistry. Report of an Expert Working Party for the Standing Advisory Dental Committee*. London: Department of Health, 1990.
7. General Dental Council. *General Dental Council: Maintaining Standards: Guidance to Dentists on Professional and Personal Conduct. Amendment: General Anaesthesia and Resuscitation*. London: General Dental Council, 1998.
8. The Royal College of Anaesthetists. *Position Paper on Standards and Guidelines for General Anaesthesia for Dentistry*. London: The Royal College of Anaesthetists, 1999.
9. Wildsmith JAW. Anaesthesia and dentistry: a changing relationship. *Newsletter, The Royal College of Anaesthetists* 1999, **49:** 231–2.
10. General Dental Council. *General Dental Council: Maintaining Standards: Guidance to Dentists on Professional and Personal Conduct. Amendment: Pain and Anxiety Control*. General Dental Council, 1999.
11. Jacobsohn PH. Office anesthesia: past, present, and future considerations. In: Dembo JB, Trieger N (eds). *Inpatient and Outpatient Anesthesia and Sedation. Oral and Maxillofacial Surgery Clinics of North America*, 4 (4). Philadelphia: WB Saunders, 1992.
12. Davies MW, Nind D. Anaesthesia for exodontia in young children – a snapshot survey of European practice. *Anaesthesia* 1996; **51:** 713.
13. Harrison M, Nutting L. Repeat general anaesthesia for paediatric dentistry. *Br Dent J* 2000; **189:** 37–9.
14. Simmons M, Miller CD, Cummings CG, Todd JG. Outpatient paediatric dental anaesthesia: a comparison of halothane, enflurane and isoflurane. *Anaesthesia* 1989; **44:** 735–8.
15. Sarner JB, Levine M, Davis PJ, *et al*. Clinical characteristics of sevoflurane in children: a comparison with halothane. *Anesthesiology* 1995; **82:** 38–46.
16. Paris ST, Cafferkey M, Yate PM, *et al*. A comparison of sevoflurane and halothane for outpatient dental anaesthesia in children. *Br J Anaesth* 1997; **79:** 280–4.
17. Worthington LM, Flynn PJ, Strunin L. Death in the dental chair: an avoidable catastrophe? *Br J Anaesth* 1998; **80:** 131–2.
18. Committee on Safety of Medicines. Safety of halothane in dental anaesthesia in children – use to be restricted to hospitals only. CEM/CMO/99/19. London: Committee on Safety of Medicines, 1999.
19. Blayney MR, Malins AF, Cooper GM. Cardiac arrhythmias in children during outpatient general anaesthesia for dentistry: a prospective randomised trial. *Lancet* 1999; **354:** 1864–6.
20. Bagshaw ONT, Southee R, Ruiz K. A comparison of the nasal mask and the nasopharyngeal airway in paediatric chair dental anaesthesia. *Anaesthesia* 1997; **52:** 786–9.
21. Bass S, Maclachlan K. Paediatric chair dental anaesthesia. *Anaesthesia* 1997; **52:** 1230.
22. Bailie R, Barnett MB, Fraser JF. The Brain laryngeal mask: a comparative study with the nasal mask in paediatric dental outpatient anaesthesia. *Anaesthesia* 1991; **46:** 358–60.
23. Woodcock BJ, Michaloudis D, Young TM. Airway management in dental anaesthesia. *Eur J Anaesthiol* 1994; **11:** 397–401.
24. Bridgman CM, Ashby D, Holloway PJ. An investigation of the effects on children of tooth extraction under general anaesthesia in general dental practice. *Br Dent J* 1999; **186:** 245–8.
25. British Society of Dentistry for the Handicapped. *Guidelines for Standards of Dental Care for People with Disabilities*. London: British Society of Dentistry for the Handicapped, 1996.
26. Wilkinson PA. Anaesthesia for adult special needs patients undergoing dental treatment. *Proc Assoc Dent Anaesth* 1996; **14:** 31–4.
27. Haywood PT, Karalliedde LD, Erridge PL. General anaesthesia for disabled in the Department for Sedation and Special Needs Dentistry. *Proc Assoc Dent Anaesth* 1998; **16:** 13–19.
28. Erridge PL. An audit of standards for GA and sedation for dental care of patients with special needs. *Proc Assoc Dent Anaesth* 1996; **14:** 29–30.
29. British Society for Antimicrobial Chemotherapy Working Party Report. The antibiotic prophylaxis of infective endocarditis. *Lancet* 1982; **ii:** 1323–26 (see also: *Lancet* 1986, **1:** 1267. Lancet 1990, **355:** 88–9. Lancet 1992, **339:** 1292–93).
30. Endocarditis Working Party of the British Society for Antimicrobial Chemotherapy. Recommendations for endocarditis prophylaxis. *J Antimicrob Chemother* 1993; **31:** 437–8.
31. Prevention of Bacterial Endocarditis. Recommendations of the American Heart Association. *JAMA* 1997; **277:** 1794–801.
32. Littler WA, McGowan DA, Shanson DC. Changes to recommendations about amoxycillin prophylaxis for prevention of endocarditis. *Lancet* 1997, **350:** 1100.
33. British Medical Association & Royal Pharmaceutical Society of Great Britain. *British National Formulary*, 43. London: British Medical

Association & Royal Pharmaceutical Society of Great Britain, 2002: 257–8.
34. Roberts GJ. Dentists are innocent! "Everyday" bacteremia is the real culprit: a review and assessment of the evidence that dental surgical procedures are a principal cause of bacterial endocarditis in children. *Pediatr Cardiol* 1999; **20:** 317–25.
35. Jones CM, O'Brien K, Blinkhorn AS, Rood JP. Dentists' agreement on treatment of asymptomatic impacted third molar teeth: interview study. *Br Med J* 1997; **315:** 1204.
36. Guideline Working Group. *Guidelines for the Use of Non-steroidal Anti-inflammatory Drugs in the Perioperative Period*. London: The Royal College of Anaesthetists, 1998.
37. The Royal College of Surgeons of England. *Report of the Working Party on Guidelines for Sedation by Non-Anaesthetists. Commission on the Provision of Surgical Services, 1993*. London: The Royal College of Surgeons of England, 1993.
38. Meechan JG, Robb ND, Seymour RA. *Pain and Anxiety Control for the Conscious Dental Patient*. Oxford: Oxford University Press, 1998.
39. American Society of Anesthesiologists. Practice guidelines for management of the difficult airway: a report of the American Society of Anesthesiologists' task force on the management of the difficult airway. *Anesthesiology* 1993; **78:** 597–602.
40. Behringer EC, Anderson CT, Sanchez AF. Fibreoptics: evaluation of the difficult airway. In: Adams AP, Hewitt PB, Grande CM (eds). *Emergency Anaesthesia*, 2nd edn. London: Arnold, 1998: 89–112.
41. Williams JP, Krekorian TD. Neck trauma. In: Adams AP, Hewitt PB, Grande CM (eds). *Emergency Anaesthesia*, 2nd edn. London: Arnold, 1998: 186–96.
42. Shearer VE. Facio-maxillary, ear, nose and throat emergencies. In: Adams AP, Hewitt PB, Grande CM (eds). *Emergency Anaesthesia*, 2nd edn. London: Arnold, 1998: 197–215.
43. American College of Surgeons Committee on Trauma. *Advanced Trauma Life Support Course Manual*. Chicago: American College of Surgeons, 1989.
44. Ovassapian A. *Fiberoptic Airway Endoscopy and Critical Care*. New York: Raven Press, 1990: 135–48.
45. Dougherty TB, Nguyen DT. Anesthetic management of the patient scheduled for head and neck cancer surgery. *J Clin Anesthesiol* 1994; **6:** 74–82.
46. Supkis DE, Dougherty TB, Ngyuyen DT, Cagle CK. Anesthetic management of the patient undergoing head and neck cancer surgery. *Cancer Bull* 1995; **47:** 21–9.

FURTHER READING

Girdler NM, Hill CM. *Sedation in Dentistry*. Oxford: Wright, 1998.

Denbo JB, Trieger N. *Inpatient and Outpatient Anesthesia and Sedation. Oral and maxillofacial surgery clinics of North America*, 4 (4). Philadelphia: WB Saunders, 1992.

Meechan JG, Robb ND, Seymour RA. *Pain and Anxiety Control for the Conscious Dental Patient*. Oxford: Oxford University Press, 1998.

The Royal College of Surgeons of England Commission on the Provision of Surgical Services. *Guidelines for Sedation by Non-anaesthetists*. London: the Royal College of Surgeons of England, 1993.

50

Anesthesia for ENT procedures and laser surgery

DIRK G SNIJDELAAR AND D JOHN DOYLE

INTRODUCTION

Providing anesthesia for ear–nose–throat (ENT) procedures can be very challenging, in part because one deals with a wide variety of patients from young children with congenital deformities to the very elderly with significant comorbidity.

Preoperative evaluation

A thorough history is vital when assessing the anesthetic risk for the patient. Here, we mention only those points in the history that are of special concern to patients undergoing ENT surgery:

- Antibiotics, antihistamines, and aspirin are medications commonly used by ENT patients. Be aware that some cold medications and antihistamines contain aspirin, which may affect platelet function; this should be taken into account.
- Patients presenting for nasal surgery may have nasal obstruction, which can make ventilation by mask more difficult. Nasal polyps are more frequently found in patients with allergies and in those with cystic fibrosis.
- Chronic upper airway infections are very common in ENT patients. In particular, children presenting for myringotomy and tube insertion or tonsillectomy and adenoidectomy usually have some degree of chronic upper airway infection. In such cases, the presence of the chronic airway infection is not generally a strong reason to postpone the surgery because the infection can usually only be resolved by drainage of the middle ear fluid or removal of the tonsils and adenoids. Furthermore, no differences are found in perioperative morbidity in children with or without upper respiratory infection at the time of surgery (see Chapter 70).[1]
- Patients with cardiac valvular disease are at risk for endocarditis from recurrent streptococcal bacteremia from infected tonsils. These risks may dictate the need for tonsillectomy.
- Patients with an enlargement of the tongue or tonsils and/or adenoids are prone to the syndrome of obstructive sleep apnea (OSA).[2] This syndrome consists of periods of absent nasal and oral airflow during sleep despite continuing respiratory effort. This is at least partly due to backward tongue movement and pharyngeal wall collapse (glossoptosis) secondary to interference with the normal coordinated contraction of pharyngeal and hypopharyngeal muscles.[3] OSA is diagnosed by finding at least 30 episodes of apnea (of duration at least 10 s) in a 7-h study period. From an anesthetic viewpoint, OSA patients are particularly at risk for airway obstruction during the induction and recovery phases of anesthesia. Management options range from heightened clinical monitoring to the use of artificial airway devices (e.g. nasopharyngeal airway, Guedel airway), to carrying out induction, and to recovery in a sitting or semi-sitting or lateral position to minimize pharyngeal wall collapse.
- Most individuals with stridor need to undergo a direct laryngoscopic and bronchoscopic evaluation of the airway. Information must be gathered about the age of onset (in children), the likely cause, and the positions that make the stridor better or worse. The presence of wheezing, cyanoses, chest retraction, and nasal flaring should also be noted.
- In children with long-standing airway obstruction leading to hypoxemia and hypercarbia, cor pulmonale may develop. Electrocardiographic evidence of right ventricular hypertrophy and chest radiographs consistent with cardiomegaly may sometimes be found. Pulmonary artery hypertension leading to right ventricular dysfunction and cardiac dysrhythmias are possible outcomes.
- Patients presenting with hoarseness, stridor, and/or hemoptysis are usually booked for endoscopic evaluation or (as the diagnosis is established) for some form of head and neck surgery. The most common cause of these symptoms is cancer, caused by years of heavy drinking and/or smoking. Usually, these are elderly patients with significant comorbidity. Cardiovascular diseases, chronic obstructive pulmonary disease (COPD), malnutrition, anemia, and alcoholism can all be present.
- Zenker's diverticulum is an esophageal outpouching for which patients are sometimes referred to an ENT surgeon to seek a surgical repair. Because food and other material may settle in the diverticulum, there is a concern that any pouch material may find itself into the airway with the induction of anesthesia.[4] Some patients can manually empty the pouch themselves; others may benefit from suction catheter placement in the pouch prior to induction (easier said than done). One key thing to remember, however, is that the application of cricoid pressure (used during a rapid sequence induction) may actually dislodge any pouch contents into the oropharynx.

The airway

Of special importance in all ENT cases is the assessment of the airway. Before bringing the patient to the operating room (OR) one must establish whether problems can be expected in the management of the airway. Valuable information can be obtained from the chart. Notes about the presence of any airway disease (abscesses, tumor, infection), trauma to the airway, the presence of postsurgical or irradiation scarring, as well as information from previous anesthetic records will help in deciding whether a difficult airway can be expected. If indirect laryngoscopy is carried out before surgery, the surgeon can provide the anesthesiologist with extra information about the airway. Where available, computed tomography (CT) scans and magnetic resonance images (MRIs) of the airway may be reviewed together with the surgeon. The assessment of the airway is completed by a physical examination of the patient's airway (see Table 50.1).

If there is substantial doubt about the airway, one has to consider special techniques such as an awake fiberoptic intubation or performing a tracheotomy under local anesthesia before inducing anesthesia. For further discussion on the management of the patient with a difficult airway, the reader is referred to Chapter 28.

USE OF LARYNGEAL MASK AIRWAY FOR ENT SURGERY

The use of the laryngeal mask airway (LMA) has become more popular in ENT since the introduction of the flexible reinforced version. Compared with the standard LMA, the flexible reinforced LMA is more resistant to oropharyngeal instrumentation (e.g. mouth gag) and is less likely to be displaced during movement of the head. Furthermore, it can be connected to a breathing system at any angle.[5]

The main advantage of the use of the LMA is that it can be inserted blindly without the need to paralyze the patient. This makes it an important tool when securing the airway in the case of a difficult intubation, which is frequently encountered in ENT patients. After securing the airway with the LMA, a fiberoptic bronchoscope and a tube size 6 can be passed through the LMA when there is a need to intubate the trachea.[6]

In most ENT cases, coughing should be avoided because of the risk of (re)bleeding or displacement of grafts after ear surgery. Compared with an endotracheal tube, the LMA is better tolerated and can be left in place during the recovery period. In the case of an expected prolonged recovery (e.g. following some forms head and neck surgery), the trachea can be extubated and an LMA inserted to maintain a patent airway during the recovery period.[5] A Guedel airway may also be used for this purpose, but Dob *et al.*[7] have shown that the LMA provides easier airway maintenance, less coughing, and initially higher median S_pO_2 during recovery than the Guedel airway.

Table 50.1 *Physical examination of the airway*

General appearance of the patient: obesity, gross deformities
Listen and observe how the patient is breathing: stridor, wheezing, mouth breathing
Inspection of the chin and the mouth (frontally and in profile) Shape of the chin: micrognathia Mouth opening Loose teeth, caps, crowns, dentures, overbite Size of the tonsils Size and mobility of the tongue Obtain Mallampati score
Inspection of the nose Nasal obstruction, deviated septum, mucosal congestion
Inspection of the larynx and the neck (frontally and in profile) Presence of goiter Short neck Position of the trachea Mobility of the cervical spine Amount of extension at the atlanto-occipital joint Measure thyromental distance

Webster *et al.*[8] used the flexible reinforced LMA for intranasal surgery and compared its use with the use of an endotracheal tube. In their study, they found that the LMA provides a safe, protected airway with a smoother emergence from anesthesia than following tracheal intubation. No laryngospasm was noted after the removal of the LMA, whereas the incidence of laryngospasm in the group in which the endotracheal tube was removed while the patients were deeply anesthetized was 19%.

The use of the flexible reinforced LMA for tonsillectomy is more controversial. Although enthusiastic reports have been published by anesthesiologists,[5,9] the ENT surgeons seem to be less enthusiastic. Hern *et al.*[10] found that the use of an LMA for tonsillectomy resulted in an inferior surgical access and that the weight of tonsillar tissue excised is less. In addition, they found that the LMA has to be changed to an endotracheal tube during the procedure in 11.4% of the patients. Most problems with the use of the LMA for tonsillectomy (such as limited surgical access or obstruction of the airway) can be avoided by making sure that a proper size LMA is correctly positioned and (in case of obstruction) by using a smaller blade on the mouth gag.[5,11] This of course can only be achieved with the full cooperation of the surgeon.[12]

EAR SURGERY

Procedures such as stapedectomy, middle ear surgery (lasting less than 2 h), and premeatal surgery can be safely performed under local anesthesia with sedation in well-selected (cooperative) adult patients.[13] Local infiltration and topical instillation of local anesthetic – usually lidocaine (lignocaine) with epinephrine (adrenaline) – can provide blockade of the sensory innervation of the ear. Usually, the surgeon injects the local anesthetic, but both the surgeon and the anesthesiologist must keep track of the total amount of local anesthetic used in order to prevent toxic blood concentrations.

Sedation must be titrated to the patient's needs. If the patient is very anxious, a benzodiazepine premedication is often given. A small dose of intravenous (i.v.) fentanyl (0.5–1.0 $\mu g\ kg^{-1}$) or a small dose of i.v. propofol (0.3–0.5 $mg\ kg^{-1}$) can be given just before the injection of the local anesthetic. Repeated small doses of i.v. midazolam (0.02–0.03 $mg\ kg^{-1}$) or running a continuous propofol infusion (starting at 50 $\mu g\ kg^{-1}\ min^{-1}$) usually provides satisfactory sedation during the procedure. Giving supplemental oxygen is recommended, especially when propofol or midazolam is combined with opioids.[14]

General anesthesia is needed for ear surgery in children and for procedures such as tympanoplasty or mastoidectomy in adults. General anesthesia for ear surgery has its own set of considerations that need to be addressed.

Positioning

Patients are usually placed in a slightly reversed Trendelenburg position of 15–20°. This will lower the venous pressure and helps to provide the surgeon with a "dry" field. Sometimes, quite extreme degrees of rotation of the neck are needed to gain access to the surgical site. This can be dangerous in elderly patients with limited carotid blood flow secondary to stenosis of the carotid arteries; in these cases, turning the head may further decrease the blood flow. Also, in patients with Down syndrome[15] or with rheumatoid arthrosis[16] extreme rotation of the neck should be avoided because of the risk of C1–C2 subluxation.

Preservation of the facial nerve

Most types of major ear surgery require the identification of the facial nerve. Usually, the function of the facial nerve is monitored by using a nerve stimulator or by recording an electromyogram (EMG) from facial muscles, although other methods are available.[17] Facial nerve function is more easily monitored if deep muscle relaxation is avoided. This means that the use of muscle relaxant is best avoided, or that at least 30% of the muscle response (as measured by a twitch monitor) needs to be preserved. However, two studies[18,19] revealed that despite significant neuromuscular block, as measured by no response on stimulation of the ulnar nerve, facial nerve activity could still be detected on electrical stimulation; however, the anesthesiologist cannot depend on this.

Need for induced hypotension

In order to minimize bleeding (especially during microscopic surgery), it has long been advocated that one should induce deliberate hypotension (aiming at a mean blood pressure of around 6.67–7.33 kPa; 50–55 mmHg) by using drugs such as sodium nitroprusside, nitroglycerine, hydralazine, droperidol, trimetaphan, or beta-blockers. However, the use of controlled hypotension remains seriously controversial. For example, Tono *et al.*[20] showed that deliberate trimetaphan-induced hypotension has a potentially harmful effect on cochlear blood flow during otological surgery. Preckel *et al.*[21] found that, during middle ear surgery under isoflurane anesthesia, autoregulation of inner ear blood flow is lost during controlled hypotension.

In our experience, the best way to reduce bleeding during microscopic ear surgery is usually to combine the use of opioids with isoflurane in a nitrous oxide (N_2O)/oxygen (O_2) or air/O_2 mixture, titrated to maintain a systolic blood pressure of around 12 kPa (90 mmHg). Total intravenous anesthesia with propofol as the main agent can also be used. The advantages of using propofol for ear operations are its lower incidence of postoperative nausea and vomiting,[22] the reduction in blood pressure without a compensatory increase in heart rate,[23] the preservation of the autoregulation of inner ear blood flow during controlled hypotension,[21] and its excellent recovery profile.[22]

However, in the unparalyzed patient, significant amounts of propofol are often needed to prevent movement; this may add significantly to the cost of the anesthetic. Jellish *et al.*[24] showed that a propofol "sandwich technique" (propofol for induction and in the last 30 min of the surgery, isoflurane intraoperatively) is a useful and cost-effective technique. These anesthetic techniques, combined with a slight head-up position and topical application of epinephrine, usually provide the surgeon with good operating conditions.

When epinephrine is used, the maximum concentration should not exceed 1:100 000 or 10 μg mL^{-1}. Lower concentrations may also be acceptable since no differences where found in the degree of vasoconstriction with the use of concentrations as low as 1:400 000.[25,26] Keeping the concentration and total use of epinephrine as low as possible is important since it is known that the combined use of volatile agents (especially halothane) and epinephrine can induce cardiac arrhythmias.[27,28]

Nitrous oxide

Nitrous oxide is far more soluble than nitrogen, as evidenced by a blood–gas coefficient of 0.46 for nitrous oxide and 0.013 for nitrogen. This means that, during the use of nitrous oxide, the pressure in the middle ear and sinuses will rise because nitrous oxide will diffuse more rapidly into these nondistensible, air-filled cavities than nitrogen can be absorbed by the bloodstream. Normally, passive venting will occur through the Eustachian tube. However, in the case of malfunction of the Eustachian tube (e.g. as caused by previous surgery, inflammation, edema, enlarged adenoids), middle ear pressures can rise significantly during the use of nitrous oxide, possibly resulting in hearing loss or rupture of the tympanic membrane.[29,30] Also, after the discontinuation of nitrous oxide, the rapid reabsorption of the gas in the blood can lead to a negative middle ear pressure. This has been associated with serous otitis, stapes disarticulation, and temporary hearing loss. During tympanoplasty, nitrous oxide must be discontinued for 15–30 min (time depending on alveolar ventilation and fresh gas flow) before the application of the graft to avoid pressure-related dislodgment of the graft.

Myringotomy and tube insertion in children

Myringotomy and tube insertion for chronic serous otitis is one of the most common procedures performed in children. This procedure usually lasts only 5 min and can easily be carried out by using a potent volatile agent such as halothane (or sevoflurane[31,32]) with N_2O/O_2 by mask or alternatively with the use of a laryngeal mask.[33] No opioids are required as the pain can easily be managed by the intraoperative topical administration of lidocaine[34,35] and/or by using acetaminophen (paracetamol) or a nonsteroidal anti-inflammatory drug (NSAID).[31,36]

Postoperative nausea and vomiting

Ear surgery is known to have a high incidence of postoperative nausea and vomiting, therefore the use of a prophylactic potent antiemetic drug (metoclopramide, droperidol, dexamethasone, or one of the newer drugs such as ondansetron and granisetron[37–40]) should be part of the anesthetic protocol.

NASAL AND SINUS SURGERY

Nasal surgery procedures such as septoplasty, polyp removal, and reduction of fractured nasal bones can often be carried out safely by using local anesthetics combined with sedation.[41–44] For this purpose, different nerve blocks can be used; however, the most widely used method is still the topical application of cocaine.[45,46] Cocaine is a local anesthetic with vasoconstrictive properties. This agent provides analgesia, a "dry" surgical field, and shrinkage of the mucous membranes. As these properties are also of value during general anesthesia, the combined use is common practice.

Cocaine is known to have sympathomimetic side-effects and sensitizes organs to epinephrine by blocking reuptake at the synaptic level.[47] Different reports have been published describing major cardiovascular complications (e.g. ventricular fibrillation, myocardial infarction) after the use of topical cocaine, especially when combined with the use of topical epinephrine or with the use of halothane.[48–50] This has led Latorre and Klimek[51] to question whether cocaine still has a role in nasal surgery, since studies have shown that lidocaine with epinephrine and/or oxymetazoline are effective alternatives to cocaine.[52–54] If cocaine is still preferred, a 4% solution (without the addition of epinephrine!) with a maximum dose of 1.5 mg kg^{-1} or a total dose of 160 mg may be used.[55–57]

Potentially serious complications may arise if the patient moves during endoscopic sinus surgery; thus, general anesthesia is recommended. Adverse outcomes include entering the intracranial space, blindness, and damage to the internal carotid artery.[58] Paralyzing the patient is advised when the risk of complications from movement is high.

In patients who have had nasal surgery, blood present in the oropharynx at the time of extubation may lead to coughing and/or laryngospasm. Attempts at positive-pressure ventilation, should they be necessary, are complicated by concerns that tight application of a face mask over the patient's nose may damage the surgeon's handiwork. The following methods can help to make extubation uneventful. First, bleeding can be reduced by using topically applied vasoconstrictive drugs, a head-up position of 15–20°, and providing a mild degree of hypotension. Second, use of a throat pack intraoperatively (e.g. saline-soaked gauze) will reduce the amount of blood entering the glottis. Third, thorough suctioning of the oropharynx and nasopharynx prior to extubation will be of value (blood clots are often present in the vicinity of the soft palate). Finally, it may be safer to extubate the patient on his or her left side while wide awake.

In this context, special mention should be made of blood that may collect at the back of the soft palate during and after nasal surgery. Following extubation, clots from this site may fall into the glottis, leading to complete airway obstruction ("coroner's clot"). Thorough suctioning by both the nasal and oral routes will help to reduce the incidence of this problem.

TONSILLECTOMY AND ADENOIDECTOMY

Common indications for tonsillectomy include chronic or recurrent acute tonsillitis, peritonsillar abscess formation, and obstructive tonsillar hyperplasia. In children, and to a lesser extent in adults, adenoidal hyperplasia may lead to nasopharyngeal airway obstruction with its many potential consequences, and may necessitate surgical removal of the adenoids along with the tonsils.

Anesthetic management

Premedication may be used, but sedative premedication tends to be avoided in children with obstructive sleep apnea, intermittent obstruction, or very large tonsils. An antisialagogue such as glycopyrrolate or atropine is often included to reduce secretions. As blood in the pharynx may enter the trachea during the procedure, the supraglottic area is often packed with saline-soaked gauze. Blood loss is difficult to measure but can be quite significant. These patients should be well hydrated during and after surgery (e.g. 5 mL kg^{-1} h^{-1} for 3 h).[59] Propofol can be used for induction and maintenance of anesthesia in adults, whereas a volatile agent (halothane or sevoflurane) is commonly used in children. A short-acting muscle relaxant [succinylcholine (suxamethonium)] can be used for tracheal intubation.

Ideally, emergence from anesthesia should be peaceful and the patient should be awake and alert before being transferred to the recovery room. Also, the patient should be awake enough to be able to effectively clear oropharyngeal blood and secretions before removal of the endotracheal tube (or laryngeal mask airway). Spraying of local anesthetics on the surgical area has been shown to reduce the incidence of laryngospasm and postoperative stridor.[60]

Complications

The overall incidence of emesis after tonsillectomy can be as high as 70%,[61] from irritant blood in the stomach, interference of the gag reflex by inflammation and edema at the surgical site, and the administration of narcotic analgesics such as meperidine (pethidine). Prophylactic use of metoclopramide reduces the incidence of vomiting after tonsillectomy.[61]

The most serious complication of tonsillectomy is postoperative hemorrhage. Approximately 75% of postoperative tonsillar bleeding occurs within 6 h of surgery.[62] In adults, pharyngeal packs and cautery can be used in an effort to control the bleeding. In children, these methods are difficult to use because of restlessness and anxiety secondary to pain or fear at seeing blood. If all else fails, patients must return to the operating room for exploration and surgical hemostasis under anesthesia. Blood should be typed and cross-matched and, when possible, rehydration must be established before the induction of anesthesia. Large volumes of blood may be swallowed, so these patients must be considered to have a full stomach, and a rapid-sequence induction is recommended. A variety of laryngoscope blades and endotracheal tubes should be available at the time of induction. Furthermore, an additional person should be available to help in suctioning the blood.

Pain after adenoidectomy is usually minimal, but is often severe after tonsillectomy and seems to be related to the surgical technique used.[63] For children, liquid acetaminophen should be given[59] every 3–4 h at a dose of 10–15 mg kg^{-1}.

ENDOSCOPIC SURGERY

The typical patient presenting for an endoscopic procedure is an elderly patient with significant comorbidity and sometimes a compromised airway. This patient has to undergo a short procedure during which the surgical stimulation is highly variable and at times quite intense. Also, children may be booked for endoscopic procedures for evaluation of stridor. Common procedures include (micro-)laryngoscopy, esophagoscopy, and bronchoscopy. During endoscopic procedures, the airway has to be shared with the surgeon. For this reason, preoperative discussion with the surgeon about the method of providing oxygenation and ventilation during the procedure is critical.

Airway management

The vast majority of the vocal cord lesions are located in the anterior commissure area. Thus, in most (micro-)laryngoscopy cases using a tube with a small diameter will not interfere with the surgeon's visualization. For this purpose, special microlaryngeal tubes have been developed.[64] These tubes are as long as regular tubes but are stiffer and have a high-volume/low-pressure cuff. They come in different sizes up to an internal diameter of 6.0 mm. The advantages of using cuffed tubes are obvious: they provide protection of the airway against aspiration, they enable positive pressure ventilation and volatile agents to be used, and they enable monitoring of ventilation by spirometry and capnography. Disadvantages are limited surgical access to posterior lesions, less work space for the surgeon, and possible distortion of (pathologic) tissues during insertion of the tube.

An alternative to positive-pressure ventilation through a microlaryngeal tube is the use of jet ventilation. Two methods are available: manual and automated, high-frequency jet ventilation. The manual jet ventilator is connected to the laryngoscope through a side port. Inspiration is active and involves allowing oxygen from a high-pressure [70–350 kPa (525–2625 mmHg)] source to flow in for about 1.5 s. Expiration is passive and should last about 6 s. A hand is placed on the chest to allow for tactile monitoring of the motion of the chest wall. The jetted gas must have free egress, and jet ventilation can only be used when the vocal cords are visible through the laryngoscope. The chest has to rise and fall in parallel with the use of the jet ventilator to avoid air trapping and barotrauma. Manual jet ventilation has the disadvantage of inducing vibration of the vocal cords, and it may force blood or tumor tissue into the lungs.[65]

High-frequency ventilation uses a small catheter placed in the trachea. This catheter is connected to an automatic ventilator, which injects small quantities of oxygen (tidal volumes of 2–3 mL kg^{-1}) at rates of up to 400 breaths min^{-1}. This method provides good gas exchange and has proved to be a safe method.[66] Compared with the supraglottic ventilation of manual jet ventilation, high-frequency ventilation delivers the oxygen subglottically. The advantages of subglottic "jetting" are that blood and debris are not blown into the trachea, there is minimal movement of the vocal cords, and there is less concern over the alignment of the laryngoscope with the vocal cords.[67] However, the use of high-frequency jet ventilation is associated with a risk of barotrauma. Using pressure-sensing devices, which will shut off the ventilator if a preset airway pressure is reached, can reduce this risk.[68]

In the case of severe upper airway obstruction, jet ventilation using a percutaneous transtracheal catheter may be needed. This has proved to be an effective way of providing oxygenation in adults and large children.[69] In morbidly obese patients and in patients with poor pulmonary compliance, the use of any jet ventilation method is not recommended as it may lead to barotrauma. Furthermore, it has to be remembered that none of the jet ventilation methods provides protection of the airway against aspiration.

An apneic technique can be used for short endoscopic procedures such as a diagnostic laryngoscopy. With this method, the patient is ventilated by mask (or with an endotracheal tube) to an S_aO_2 of at least 98%. The mask or tube is then removed and the surgery is performed during a period of apnea. If the S_aO_2 begins to fall, ventilation is started again by mask or by reinsertion of the tube.

A final airway technique is to let the patient breath spontaneously during the procedure. This is a popular technique, especially for children, since it allows assessment of the dynamics of the trachea and/or bronchi, and also the movement of the vocal cords can be observed. This is important when determining the cause of stridor in young children.

The disadvantages of the apneic and spontaneous ventilation techniques are clear: there is no complete control or protection of the airway and ventilation can at times be suboptimal. During spontaneous ventilation, light planes of anesthesia may occur, resulting in laryngospasm.

Anesthetic technique

Short-acting anesthetics that allow for a smooth recovery with a quick return of airway reflexes are the drugs of choice for patients undergoing endoscopic procedures. Only very light premedication is recommended. A drying agent such as glycopyrrolate in a dose of 0.2–0.4 mg by intramusclar injection, 30–60 min before the start of the procedure, may be beneficial. A recommended anesthetic regimen is to induce the patient with propofol (2 mg kg^{-1}) and fentanyl (1–2 μg kg^{-1}) or alfentanil (10–20 μg kg^{-1}), followed by a continuous infusion of propofol. Muscle relaxation is usually necessary for the introduction of the endoscopic instruments and to provide the surgeon with an immobile surgical field. A succinylcholine drip or repeated injections of succinylcholine are commonly used for procedures lasting less than 30 min. Mivacurium or cisatracurium (by continuous infusion or intermittent administration) can be used for surgery that is expected to last longer than 30 min. Puura *et al.*[70] found that succinylcholine and mivacurium are economical to use during microsurgery of the larynx. Intermediate-acting muscle relaxants (rocuronium, vecuronium, atracurium) result in an unduly prolonged recovery time.

Small bolus doses of fentanyl or alfentanil can be given during periods of increased stimulation. Other methods used to blunt the sympathetic responses are the use of short-acting beta-blockers (especially esmolol) and the use of lidocaine, either for topicalization of the airway or intravenously (1–1.5 mg kg^{-1}).

Remifentanil is a potent, fast-acting, systemic μ-opioid with a rapid recovery profile (even after prolonged continuous infusion).[71] Based on this profile, it will likely become the opioid of choice for endoscopic procedures in the future. It has already been shown to effectively blunt the hemodynamic response of intubation.[72,73] To date, no large-scale studies have been published regarding its use in endoscopic procedures.

If spontaneous ventilation is needed or preferred during the endoscopic procedure, the patient is induced by mask with a volatile agent (usually halothane or sevoflurane) for children or with intravenous propofol for adults. Deeper planes of anesthesia are reached by letting the patients breathe a high concentration of a volatile agent by mask in 100% oxygen, combined with a low-dose, continuous, intravenous infusion of propofol.[74] After topical application of lidocaine (4%) to the airway, the endoscopic instruments can be introduced. Anesthesia is maintained by insufflation of the volatile agent in 100% oxygen via the sideport of the laryngoscope or bronchoscope.

Because of the highly variable surgical stimulation during endoscopic procedures, blood pressure may need to be monitored by means of an arterial line in patients with cardiovascular instability, even in procedures that are expected to last only several minutes.

LASER SURGERY

Laser (light amplification by stimulated emission of radiation) has become an important tool for the ENT surgeon performing microlaryngeal surgery or tracheobronchial surgery. Also, in ear[75] and nasal[76] surgery, the use of laser has become popular. Laser techniques enable the surgeon to concentrate high levels of energy on a small surface. This allows for very precise resection of tissue with the added advantage of almost immediately sealing blood vessels and lymphatics.

The most commonly used lasers are the carbon dioxide (CO_2), argon, Nd-YAG (neodymium yttrium–aluminum garnet), and KTP (potassium–titanylphosphate)/Nd-YAG laser types. The most important differences between these laser types are listed in Table 50.2. The energy from long-wavelength laser light, such as that from CO_2, is absorbed completely by water. This means that when the CO_2 laser hits tissue only the first few layers of cells will be vaporized, leaving the underlying layers intact. The argon laser and (KTP)/Nd-YAG are short-wavelength lasers. The energy from these types of lasers is less absorbed by water and penetrates tissue much deeper, producing more thermal coagulation than vaporization. Lasers are powerful tools, therefore special precautions have to be taken when using these devices.

Protecting the patient and operating room personnel

When a laser beam hits tissue, a plume of smoke and fine particulates is produced. Besides its unpleasant odor, the particulates have mutagenic and tetragenic potential. Although controversial, there are also concerns regarding the role of the smoke plume as a vector for transmission of viral infections.[77] Inhalation of the smoke is best avoided by using a smoke evacuator and wearing special "laser" masks.

A reflected or misdirected laser beam can also hit the patient's eyes or those of the operating room personnel. The CO_2 laser can cause corneal injury, whereas the retina is at risk when a Nd-YAG laser is used. The patient's eyes should be protected by first taping the lids shut and then applying wet sponges or eyepatches. Operating room personnel must wear appropriate goggles for the laser wavelength in use. Regular, clear eyeglasses can be sufficient when CO_2 is used because they are opaque to far-infrared light. Other lasers (with a shorter wavelength) require special goggles with color filters. To prevent eye damage to personnel entering the operating room, warning signs noting that a laser is in use should be placed on the outside of the door.

The intense heat produced by a focused laser beam can very easily ignite the surgical drapes. Covering the face of the patient (and the upper thorax) with wet towels can help to prevent a surgical drape fire.

Table 50.2 *Characteristics of commonly used lasers in ENT surgery*

Laser medium	Color	Wavelength (nm)	Output	Transmitted by fiberoptics?
CO_2	Far infrared	10 600	Continuous or intermittently pulsed	No
Nd-YAG	Near infrared	1064	Pulsed	Yes
KTP/Nd-YAG	Green	532	Pulsed	Yes
Argon	Green	515	Continuous or intermittently pulsed	Yes
	Blue	488		

Airway fires

A feared complication of laser-assisted airway surgery is the occurrence of an endotracheal tube fire. The incidence is estimated to be in the range 0.14–1.5%.[78] The occurrence of an airway fire can have devastating effects for the patient, and every precaution should be taken to prevent this.

Laser surgeons should also share the responsibility for fire prevention. They should set the laser power as low as possible (10–15 W) and use the noncontinuous mode. If possible, wet gauzes should be used to protect nontarget tissue in the surgical field and the cuff of the endotracheal tube.[79] Between repeated pulses of laser, sufficient time should be allowed to elapse to let the heat disperse.

Nitrous oxide and oxygen are known to support combustion. The inspiratory oxygen fraction ($F_{I}O_2$) should be kept as low as the patient's hemoglobin saturation allows (usually between 0.25 and 0.30). It is better to avoid the use of nitrous oxide and it is advised to use an air/O_2 mixture instead. Alternatively, a helium/O_2 mixture can be used because helium has a higher thermal conductivity and may delay ignition. This only seems to be true in the case of a fire ignited by a CO_2 laser and not by a KTP/Nd-YAG laser.[80]

All hydrocarbon-containing materials (such as plastics and rubber) can ignite when hit by a laser beam. Conflicting results have been published about the best construction material for the endotracheal tube to be used during laser surgery. Polyvinylchloride (PVC), silicone, and red rubber have all been recommended.[77] One may also wrap a mircolaryngeal tube with a metalized foil tape[81] or use specially designed "laser-resistant" tubes.

Wrapping a PVC tube with a special developed metallic foil wrap ("Laser Guard") protects the shaft of the tube (but not the cuff) from ignition during the use of CO_2, argon, and KTP/Nd-YAG laser.[82] The disadvantages of this metallic foil wrap are cost and the increased diameter of the tube. Although less effective and not Food and Drug Administration (FDA) approved, a less costly alternative is electric aluminum tape. Avoid wrinkles in the metallic foil wrap because the sharp edges can damage the airway mucosa.

A number of laser-resistant tubes are commercially marketed. These tubes are made from different materials (silicone, steel, aluminum) and provide protection against various types of laser energy. The "Laser Shield" (Xomed-Treace), "Laser-Trach" (Kendall-Sheridan), and "Fome-Cuff" (Bivona) provide protection against CO_2 laser only. The "Laser Flex" (Mallinckrodt) protects against CO_2 and KTP/Nd-YAG (not Nd-YAG!) lasers and has two separate cuffs. The Fome-Cuff has a foam-filled cuff that prevents collapse after puncture. The disadvantages of all of these specially designed tubes are their increased diameter, reduced flexibility, and greater cost than conventional endotracheal tubes.

Whichever type of tube is used it is recommended that the cuff is inflated with sterile saline to which methylene blue is added. In this way, a cuff rupture by a misdirected laser beam can be easily detected.[83] Also, ensure that the cuff is placed as far distally in the trachea as possible so that it is out of the "line of fire" of the laser.

An alternative method for providing oxygenation and ventilation is to use manual or high-frequency jet ventilation, as discussed above (Endoscopic procedures). The major advantage of jet ventilation is that it provides ventilation without a bulky, flammable tube in the surgical field. But, even with jet ventilation, airway fires can occur during the use of a laser.[84] Spontaneous ventilation can be used especially for airway laser surgery in children. The anesthetic technique for laser surgery is similar to that described for endoscopic procedures.

In the unfortunate circumstance that an airway fire does occur, first remove the tube as quickly as possible (Table 50.3). Ventilation should be stopped and the pharynx flushed with water. A source of water (e.g. 60-mL syringe filled with cold saline) should always be immediately available. As soon as the fire is extinguished, the patient must be ventilated by mask using 100% oxygen. In case of a difficult airway, it can be hazardous to remove the burning tube immediately. In such a situation, ventilation should be discontinued first, the tube and trachea flushed with water, a tube exchanger inserted through the lumen of the tube, the tube removed, and another endotracheal tube reinserted over the tube exchanger.

Direct laryngoscopic and rigid bronchoscopy can reveal any damage to the airway and allows for removal of any charred debris. In case of severe damage, a tracheotomy may be indicated. If there is only slight damage, the trachea must be reintubated with a conventional tube. One must not forget to also inspect the oropharynx and face for any burn-related injuries. Pulmonary damage from heat and/or smoke inhalation should be assessed by taking repeated arterial blood gas samples and repeated chest radiographs. Sometimes, prolonged intubation and ventilation is necessary. Late complications from airway fire include the formation of granulation tissue or stenosis in the larynx and/or trachea.

HEAD AND NECK SURGERY

Commonly performed procedures in patients with cancer of the head and neck include radical sinus surgery, parotidectomy, glossectomy, hemimandibulectomy, pharyngectomy, laryngectomy, and radical neck dissection. If immediate plastic reconstructive surgery is necessary (e.g. free flap), these procedures can sometimes last for up to 18 h. The following are the special considerations for anesthesia in head and neck surgery.

Table 50.3 *Airway fire protocol*

1. The following steps should be taken simultaneously:
   - Stop ventilation
   - Turn off oxygen and all the anesthetic gases
   - Deflate cuff and remove endotracheal tube
   - Flush pharynx with water to extinguish flames
2. Ventilate the patient by mask with 100% oxygen
3. Perform laryngoscopy and bronchoscopy to assess any airway damage and to remove debris
4. Reintubate the patient if airway damage is present

Positioning

Patients need to be placed on a well-padded table (e.g. "egg crate" mattress) to avoid pressure necrosis. A pillow placed under the knees will prevent overstretching of the legs. A slightly reversed Trendelenburg position will decrease the bleeding in the surgical field, although it has to be emphasized that this position will also increase the risk of venous air emboli.

Monitoring

Because of the length of the procedure, the possibility of substantial blood loss, and the usual presence of significant intercurrent disease, for major head and neck surgery most patients require arterial cannulation for blood pressure and blood gas monitoring. In most cases, a central venous catheter (antecubital or subclavian) is also inserted, although the routine insertion of a central venous line has been questioned.[85,86] A urinary catheter should be placed to measure the urine output. Priano *et al.*[87] found that perioperative urine output during radical neck dissection was not important for patients with normal renal function provided systemic hemodynamic responses were maintained.

Temperature can be monitored by using a rectal or axillary probe. During the microvascular part of the procedure, hypothermia (causing vasoconstriction) must be carefully avoided by using techniques such as a forced air warming blanket, warming all intravenous fluids, and warming and humidification of the anesthetic gases.

Intraoperative management

Usually, patients requiring extensive head and neck surgery need a tracheotomy. If the tracheostomy is established at the beginning of the procedure, an armored tube or laryngectomy tube is placed in the tracheostomy and sutured to the chest wall. At the end of the procedure, this is replaced with a definitive tracheostomy tube (e.g. Shiley).

During a parotidectomy or a neck dissection, the surgeon may request that muscle relaxants are not used so that nerves, such as the facial nerve or the spinal accessory nerves, may be identified.

Blood loss can be significant and should, therefore, be anticipated. In appropriate cases, hypervolemic or isovolemic hemodilution can be used to avoid using homologous blood.[88,89] During microvascular anastomosis of the blood vessels of the free flap, the hematocrit should ideally be maintained at a value of around 0.28–0.30 and the blood pressure maintained around baseline values.

Intraoperative and postoperative complications

In the first 2000 patients of the Australian Incident Monitoring Study,[90] 19 cases of air embolism were identified, 47% of which occurred during head and neck surgery. No embolism-related fatalities were reported. Rice and Gonzalez[91] observed easily visible bubbles in the jugular veins in 5 out of 12 consecutive patients undergoing supine radical neck surgery; in one case, a transient drop in blood pressure and in end-tidal CO_2 was noted. Although air embolism is a common occurrence during head and neck surgery, the morbidity and mortality seem to be quite low. Treatment is mainly supportive and includes discontinuation of nitrous oxide, flooding the surgical field with saline, Trendelenburg position and (if possible) left lateral position, and aspiration of air through a central venous catheter.

Manipulation of the carotid artery can cause a number of problems. Pressure on the carotid sinus can elicit a vagal reflex resulting in bradycardia and hypotension. Denervation of the carotid sinus and bodies has been associated with postoperative hypertension[92] and loss of hypoxic ventilatory response.[93] Patients with carotid atherosclerosis are at increased risk of stroke during neck surgery, and it has even been suggested that some patients need to have a prophylactic carotid endarterectomy.[94] Ablation of the right sympathetic stellate ganglion increases the QT interval of the electrocardiogram.[95] This is probably the reason for a prolonged QT interval after (radical) neck dissection. An acquired prolonged QT interval can lead to malignant arrhythmias,[96] although the incidence of this happening seems to be low.[97]

Following neck surgery, hematomas may form which can compress the trachea and lead to airway obstruction and suffocation. Specific management depends on the clinical circumstances, but a number of important considerations exist. First, immediate intubation may be necessary should respiratory embarrassment occur. Second, intubation may be difficult if hematoma formation distorts the airway anatomy, e.g. by causing deviation or compression of the trachea. Third, the use of muscle relaxants to facilitate intubation in this setting is especially hazardous; should intubation attempts fail in this setting, one cannot readily revert to spontaneous respiration. Finally, reopening the surgical incision with manual evacuation of the hematoma may help to reduce respiratory embarrassment and facilitate intubation.

TRACHEOTOMY: COMPLICATIONS AND CARE

A number of airway-related problems may arise in the immediate postoperative period after a tracheotomy has been performed. These include bleeding, subcutaneous emphysema, mediastinal emphysema, pneumothorax, airway obstruction, and hypoventilation. Late complications following tracheotomy include tracheal stenosis, tracheoesophageal fistula, tracheomalacia, and tracheal necrosis.

Bleeding, when it occurs after a tracheotomy, is usually minor, but even minor bleeding into the airway may lead to tracheal irritation and sometimes cause the patient to cough and buck vigorously. Major hemorrhage in the immediate postoperative period occasionally occurs as a result of bleeding from a large artery or vein (often the communicating branch of the superior thyroid artery). This situation requires immediate exploration of the surgical field. Major bleeding from the innominate artery may occur following erosion of this vessel by the distal end of the cannula in the presence of a mediastinal infection. One hint that the tracheostomy could be applying pressure to the innominate artery is the finding of pulsations in the tracheotomy cannula after initial insertion. If it is suspected that bleeding is from an innominate artery erosion, treatment includes inflating the tube cuff and pulling the tube assembly anteriorly to tamponade the bleeding. An oral tracheal tube should then be inserted for more definitive management of the airway, followed by repair in the operating room.

Subcutaneous and mediastinal emphysema leading to hypoventilation and hypoxemia may occur as a result of partial obstruction of the tracheostomy cannula when the wound has been closed too tightly. Under these conditions, air may be forced down fascial planes.

With long-term intubation, tracheomalacia, tracheal necrosis, and tracheal stenosis may occur, particularly when cuff pressures are chronically excessive. With tracheal necrosis or tracheomalacia, the airway may collapse with extubation or decannulation; surgical management (tracheoplasty) is often needed.

Changing fresh tracheostomy tubes

Changing a tracheostomy tube following a fresh tracheotomy is especially hazardous, but may be required because of a severe cuff leak or because of tube obstruction from the build-up of secretions. The main concern here is that the replaced tube may enter a false passage rather than enter the trachea. (This in itself is bad enough, but when the false passage is ventilated the resulting subcutaneous emphysema soon removes all possibility of easily re-establishing the airway.) This problem eventually diminishes as the tracheal stoma matures to form a well-defined and self-supporting orifice. However, this rigidity and tissue support is lacking in a fresh tracheostomy; with removal of the tube, the tissue just "collapses in" on itself to obscure the passage. Accordingly, the clinician should be familiar with certain precautions when dealing with a fresh tracheostomy tube. These precautions include:

1 For the first week or so, all tube changes should be carried out in the operating room by an experienced surgeon, with good lighting and with a full set of surgical instruments (cricoid hooks, etc.). An anesthesiologist should also be present in case intubation "from above" needs to be attempted as a last resort if the surgeons lose control of the airway.
2 Once the tracheostomy has begun to mature, it is no longer necessary to carry out tube changes in the operating room, but a full set of tracheotomy instruments (especially cricoid hooks) should still be available. Changing the tube over a tube changer may also be useful, but some find that this unnecessarily complicates matters.
3 Obviously, before any tube change, the patient should be preoxygenated with 100% oxygen.
4 The fiberoptic bronchoscope (FOB) may be potentially useful in confirming tracheal placement of a tracheostomy tube prior to attempting positive pressure ventilation that could lead to subcutaneous emphysema if the tube is in fact malpositioned.

EMERGENCIES

Laryngospasm

Laryngospasm is the protective reflex closure of the upper airway from spasm of the glottic musculature. This form of airway obstruction is especially common in children and is associated with light planes of anesthesia and the presence of foreign matter (e.g. blood or secretions) irritating the vocal cords. While laryngospasm can often be broken by deepening the depth of anesthesia with intravenous (i.v.) propofol or another i.v. agent, sometimes muscle relaxation (e.g. with succinylcholine 10–20 mg i.v.) is needed to allow the patient to be ventilated. Failure to deal with laryngospasm can result in significant periods during which the patient cannot be adequately ventilated and which result in hypoxemia and hypercarbia. Some patients who are able to generate very large negative inspiratory pressures in attempting to breathe against the obstruction may succumb to "negative-pressure pulmonary edema." A proactive approach for preventing/terminating laryngospasm and preventing hypoxemia and other complications is the mark of a seasoned anesthesiologist.

Acute epiglottitis

Epiglottitis is the most dreaded of airway infections, especially in children. Victims are usually children aged 2–6 years, often infected with *Haemophilus influenzae*. These children may appear to be systemically ill ("toxic"), perhaps with a fever and/or perhaps sitting up in a "tripod" position and drooling from difficulty with swallowing. Examining the child's airway may exacerbate the problem (by increasing airway edema), so tongue depressors and laryngoscopy are not options for the initial management. Anything that might cause the child to cry (e.g. needles) should, if possible, be avoided. Consequently (and for other reasons), the usual approach to management involves a careful inhalational induction with the child sitting in the anesthesiologist's lap and intubation of the child while he or she is breathing spontaneously under deep halothane or sevoflurane anesthesia. If at laryngoscopy the orifice through the glottis cannot be identified, one trick is to have someone compress the child's chest, thus generating a small bubble in the glottic opening that the anesthesiologist can aim for. In the past, patients were managed by emergency tracheostomy; however, contemporary management of children includes short-term nasal intubation and intravenous antibiotic therapy.[98,99]

Epiglottitis can also occur in adults (George Washington is said to have died from it), but the situation is less dreadful than in children because the adult airway is larger. Most anesthesiologists would use awake fiberoptic laryngoscopy when necessary to secure the airway in this situation. There is considerable disagreement concerning airway management in the adult; however, there seems to be a growing consensus that the majority of adults are adequately treated in an intensive care unit with inhaled mist, antibiotics, and corticosteroids and that tracheal intubation is necessary only if symptoms of respiratory distress develop.[100,101]

Retropharyngeal abscess

Retropharyngeal abscess[102] formation may occur from bacterial infection of the retropharyngeal space secondary to a tonsillar or dental infection. Untreated, the posterior pharyngeal wall may advance anteriorly into the oropharynx, resulting in a dyspnea and airway obstruction. Other clinical findings may include difficulty in swallowing, trismus, and a fluctuant posterior pharyngeal mass. An abscess cavity may be evident on lateral neck radiographs with anterior displacement of the esophagus and upper pharynx. Airway management may be complicated by trismus or airway obstruction. Because abscess rupture can lead to soiling of the trachea, contact with the posterior pharyngeal wall during laryngoscopy and intubation should be minimized. Incision and drainage is the mainstay of treatment. Tracheostomy is often, but not always, required.

Ludwig's angina

Ludwig's angina[103] is a multispace infection in the floor of the mouth. The infection starts with infected mandibular molars and spreads to sublingual, submental, buccal, and submandibular spaces. The tongue becomes elevated and displaced posteriorly, which may lead to loss of the airway, especially when the patient is placed in the supine position. An additional concern is the potential for abscess rupture into the hypopharynx (with possible lung soiling) either spontaneously or with attempts at laryngoscopy and intubation. Airway management options will depend on clinical severity, surgical preferences, and other factors (e.g. CT or MRI findings), but elective tracheostomy prior to incision and drainage remains the classic treatment modality (although many experts advocate fiberoptic intubation if at all possible).

Stridor

Stridor, or noisy inspiration from turbulent gas flow in the upper airway, is often seen in airway obstruction, and always commands attention. Wherever possible, attempts should be made to establish immediately the cause of the stridor (e.g. foreign body, vocal cord edema, tracheal compression by tumor, etc.). The first issue of clinical concern in stridor is whether or not intubation is immediately necessary. If intubation can be delayed for a period, a number of potential options may be considered, depending on the severity of the situation and other clinical details. These include:

- use of Heliox (70% helium, 30% oxygen);
- expectant management with full monitoring, oxygen by face mask, and positioning the head of the bed for optimum conditions (e.g. 45–90°);
- use of nebulized racemic epinephrine or cocaine (but not both together) in cases in which airway edema may be the cause of the stridor;
- use of dexamethasone (Decadron) 4–8 mg i.v. every 8–12 h in cases where airway edema may be the cause of the stridor.

Acknowledgment

Parts of this chapter have been modified from Doyle DJ, Arellano R. Medical conditions with airway implications. *Anesthesiol Clin North Am* 1995; **13:** 615–33.

REFERENCES

1. Tait AR, Knight PR. The effects of general anesthesia on upper respiratory tract infections in children. *Anesthesiology* 1987; **67:** 930–5.
2. Dodds C, Ryall DM. Tonsils, obesity and obstructive sleep apnoea. *Br J Hosp Med* 1992; **47:** 62–6.
3. Cadieux RJ, Kales A, Santen RJ, *et al.* Endoscopic findings in sleep apnea associated with acromegaly. *J Clin Endocrinol Metab* 1982; **55:** 18–22.
4. Meyer GW, Castell DO. Evaluation and management of diseases of the esophagus. *Am J Otolaryngol* 1981; **2:** 336–44.
5. Nair I, Bailey PM. Review of uses of the laryngeal mask in ENT anaesthesia. *Anaesthesia* 1995; **50:** 898–900.
6. Benumof JL. Use of the laryngeal mask airway to facilitate fiberscope-aided tracheal intubation. *Anesth Analg* 1992; **74:** 313–15.
7. Dob DP, Shannon CN, Bailey PM. Efficacy and safety of the laryngeal mask airway vs Guedel airway following tracheal extubation. *Can J Anaesth* 1999; **46:** 179–81.
8. Webster AC, Morley-Forster PK, Janzen V, *et al.* Anesthesia for intranasal surgery: a comparison between tracheal intubation and the flexible reinforced laryngeal mask airway. *Anesth Analg* 1999; **88:** 421–5.
9. Williams PJ, Bailey PM. Comparison of the reinforced laryngeal mask airway and tracheal intubation for adenotonsillectomy. *Br J Anaesth* 1993; **70:** 30–3.
10. Hern JD, Jayaraj SM, Sidhu VS, *et al.* The laryngeal mask airway in tonsillectomy: the surgeon's perspective. *Clin Otolaryngol Allied Sci* 1999; **24:** 122–5.
11. Gupta S, Kavan R. Mogera C. Matching appropriately sized reinforced laryngeal mask airways with Boyle–Davis gags for paediatric adenotonsillectomies. *Acta Anaesthesiol Scand* 1999; **43:** 789.
12. Howard-Griffin RM, Driver IK. Laryngeal mask airway in adeno-tonsillectomy in children. *Anaesthesia* 1996; **51:** 409.
13. Yung MW. Local anaesthesia in middle ear surgery: survey of patients and surgeons. *Clin Otolaryngol Allied Sci* 1996; **21:** 404–8.
14. Tucker MR, Ochs MW, White Jr RP. Arterial blood gas levels after midazolam or diazepam administered with or without fentanyl as an intravenous sedative for outpatient surgical procedures. *J Oral Maxillofac Surg* 1986; **44:** 688–92.
15. Harley EH, Collins MD. Neurologic sequelae secondary to atlantoaxial instability in Down syndrome. Implications in otolaryngologic surgery. *Arch Otolaryngol Head Neck Surg* 1994; **120:** 159–65.
16. Macarthur A, Kleiman S. Rheumatoid cervical joint disease – a challenge to the anaesthetist. *Can J Anaesth* 1993; **40:** 154–9.
17. Harper CM, Daube JR. Facial nerve electromyography and other cranial nerve monitoring. *J Clin Neurophysiol* 1998; **15:** 206–16.
18. Brauer M, Knuettgen D, Quester R. Doehn M. Electromyographic facial nerve monitoring during resection for acoustic neurinoma under moderate to profound levels of peripheral neuromuscular blockade. *Eur J Anaesthiol* 1996; **13:** 612–15.
19. Paloheimo M, Edmonds Jr HL, Wirtavuori K, Tammisto T. Assessment of anaesthetic adequacy with upper facial and abdominal wall EMG. *Eur J Anaesthiol* 1989; **6:** 111–19.
20. Tono T, Ueki Y, Nagata N, *et al.* Effects of trimetaphan-induced deliberate hypotension on human cochlear blood flow. *Acta Otolaryngol Suppl* 1998; **539:** 40–3.
21. Preckel MP, Ferber-Viart C, Leftheriotis G, *et al.* Autoregulation of human inner ear blood flow during middle ear surgery with propofol or isoflurane anesthesia during controlled hypotension. *Anesth Analg* 1998; **87:** 1002–8.
22. Jellish WS, Leonetti JP, Murdoch JR. Fowles S. Propofol-based anesthesia as compared with standard anesthetic techniques for middle ear surgery. *J Clin Anesth* 1995; **7:** 292–6.
23. Abdulatif M. Sodium nitroprusside induced hypotension: haemodynamic response and dose requirements during propofol or halothane anaesthesia. *Anaesth Intensive Care* 1994; **22:** 155–60.
24. Jellish WS, Leonetti JP, Fahey K, Fury P. Comparison of 3 different anesthetic techniques on 24-hour recovery after otologic surgical procedures. *Otolaryngol Head Neck Surg* 1999; **120:** 406–11.
25. O'Malley TP, Postma GN, Holtel M, Girod DA. Effect of local epinephrine on cutaneous bloodflow in the human neck. *Laryngoscope* 1995; **105:** 140–3.
26. Dunlevy TM, O'Malley TP, Postma GN. Optimal concentration of epinephrine for vasoconstriction in neck surgery. *Laryngoscope* 1996; **106:** 1412–14.
27. Johnston RR, Eger II EI, Wilson C. A comparative interaction of epinephrine with enflurane, isoflurane, and halothane in man. *Anesth Analg* 1976; **55:** 709–12.
28. Hayashi Y, Sumikawa K, Yamatodani A, *et al.* Myocardial epinephrine sensitization with subanesthetic concentrations of halothane in dogs. *Anesthesiology* 1991; **74:** 134–7.
29. Patterson ME, Bartlett PC. Hearing impairment caused by intratympanic pressure changes during general anesthesia. *Laryngoscope* 1976; **86:** 399–404.
30. Davis I, Moore JR, Lahiri SK. Nitrous oxide and the middle ear. *Anaesthesia* 1979; **34:** 147–51.
31. Davis PJ, Greenberg JA, Gendelman M, Fertal K. Recovery characteristics of sevoflurane and halothane in preschool-aged children undergoing bilateral myringotomy and pressure equalization tube insertion. *Anesth Analg* 1999; **88:** 34–8.
32. Bacher A, Burton AW, Uchida T, Zornow MH. Sevoflurane or halothane anesthesia: can we tell the difference? *Anesth Analg* 1997; **85:** 1203–6.
33. Watcha MF, Garner FT, White PF, Lusk R. Laryngeal mask airway vs face mask and Guedel airway during pediatric myringotomy. *Arch Otolaryngol Head Neck Surg* 1994; **120:** 877–80.
34. Derkay CS, Wadsworth JT, Darrow DH, *et al.* Tube placement: a prospective, randomized double-blind study. *Laryngoscope* 1998; **108:** 97–101.
35. Lawhorn CD, Bower CM, Brown Jr RE, *et al.* Topical lidocaine for post-operative analgesia following myringotomy and tube placement. *Int J Pediatr Otorhinolaryngol* 1996; **35:** 19–24.
36. Bean-Lijewski JD, Stinson JC. Acetaminophen or ketorolac for post myringotomy pain in children? A prospective, double-blinded comparison. *Paediatr Anaesth* 1997; **7:** 131–7.
37. Fujii Y, Saitoh Y, Tanaka H, Toyooka H. Combination of granisetron and droperidol in the prevention of nausea and vomiting after middle ear surgery. *J Clin Anesth* 1999; **11:** 108–12.
38. Fujii Y, Toyooka H, Tanaka H. Prophylactic anti-emetic therapy with granisetron, droperidol and metoclopramide in female patients undergoing middle ear surgery. *Anaesthesia* 1998; **53:** 1165–8.
39. Fujii Y, Toyooka H, Tanaka H. Prophylactic antiemetic therapy with a combination of granisetron and dexamethasone in patients undergoing middle ear surgery. *Br J Anaesth* 1998; **81:** 754–6.
40. Jellish WS, Leonetti JP, Fluder E, Thalji Z. Ondansetron versus droperidol or placebo to prevent nausea and vomiting after otologic surgery. *Otolaryngol Head Neck Surg* 1998; **118:** 785–9.
41. Srinivasan V, Arasaratnam RB, Jankelowitz GA. Day-case septal surgery under general anaesthesia and local anaesthesia with sedation. *J Laryngol Otol* 1995; **109:** 614–7.
42. Owen GO, Parker AJ, Watson DJ. Fractured-nose reduction under local anaesthesia. Is it acceptable to the patient? *Rhinology* 1992; **30:** 89–96.
43. Cook JA, McRae RD, Irving RM, Dowie LN. A randomized comparison of manipulation of the fractured nose under local and general anaesthesia. *Clin Otolaryngol Allied Sci* 1990; **15:** 343–6.
44. Waldron J, Mitchell DB, Ford G. Reduction of fractured nasal bones; local versus general anaesthesia. *Clin Otolaryngol Allied Sci* 1989; **14:** 357–9.
45. Rontal M, Rontal E, Anon JB. An anatomic approach to local anesthesia for surgery of the nose and paranasal sinuses. *Otolaryngol Clin North Am* 1997; **30:** 403–20.
46. Molliex S, Navez M, Baylot D, *et al.* Regional anaesthesia for outpatient nasal surgery. *Br J Anaesth* 1996; **76:** 151–3.
47. Smith RB. Cocaine and catecholamine interaction. A review. *Arch Otolaryngol* 1973; **98:** 139–41.
48. Ashchi M, Wiedemann HP, James KB. Cardiac complication from use of cocaine and phenylephrine in nasal septoplasty. *Arch Otolaryngol Head Neck Surg* 1995; **121:** 681–4.

49. Lormans P, Gaumann D, Schwieger I, Tassonyi E. Ventricular fibrillation following local application of cocaine and epinephrine for nasal surgery. *J Otorhinolaryngol Related Specialties* 1992; **54:** 160–2.
50. Chiu YC, Brecht K, DasGupta DS, Mhoon E. Myocardial infarction with topical cocaine anesthesia for nasal surgery. *Arch Otolaryngol Head Neck Surg* 1986; **112:** 988–90.
51. Latorre F, Klimek L. Does cocaine still have a role in nasal surgery? *Drug Safety* 1999; **20:** 9–13.
52. Tarver CP, Noorily AD, Sakai CS. A comparison of cocaine vs. lidocaine with oxymetazoline for use in nasal procedures. *Otolaryngol Head Neck Surg* 1993; **109:** 653–9.
53. Riegle EV, Gunter JB, Lusk RP, *et al.* Comparison of vasoconstrictors for functional endoscopic sinus surgery in children. *Laryngoscope* 1992; **102:** 820–3.
54. McClymont LG, Crowther JA. Local anaesthetic with vasoconstrictor combinations in septal surgery. *J Laryngol Otol* 1988; **102:** 793–5.
55. Liao BS, Hilsinger Jr RL, Rasgon BM, *et al.* A preliminary study of cocaine absorption from the nasal mucosa. *Laryngoscope* 1999; **109:** 98–102.
56. Greinwald Jr JH, Holtel MR. Absorption of topical cocaine in rhinologic procedures. *Laryngoscope* 1996; **106:** 1223–5.
57. Van Dyke C, Byck R. Cocaine. *Sci Am* 1982; **246:** 128–41.
58. Maniglia AJ. Fatal and major complications secondary to nasal and sinus surgery. *Laryngoscope* 1989; **99:** 276–83.
59. Riding KH. Otolaryngologic surgery. In: White PF (ed.). *Ambulatory Anesthesia & Surgery*. London: WB Saunders, 1997: 301–9.
60. Staffel JG, Weissler MC, Tyler EP, Drake AF. The prevention of postoperative stridor and laryngospasm with topical lidocaine. *Arch Otolaryngol Head Neck Surg* 1991; **117:** 1123–8.
61. Ferrari LR, Donlon JV. Metoclopramide reduces the incidence of vomiting after tonsillectomy in children. *Anesth Analg* 1992; **75:** 351–4.
62. Guida RA, Mattucci KF. Tonsillectomy and adenoidectomy: an inpatient or outpatient procedure? *Laryngoscope* 1990; **100:** 491–3.
63. Linden BE, Gross CW, Long TE, Lazar RH. Morbidity in pediatric tonsillectomy. *Laryngoscope* 1990; **100:** 120–4.
64. Pommerenke C, Lipp M, Collo J. The microlaryngeal tube – a new tube for direct laryngoscopy in the ENT field. *Anaesthesist* 1989; **38:** 144–6.
65. Crockett DM, Scamman FL, McCabe BF, *et al.* Venturi jet ventilation for microlaryngoscopy: technique, complications, pitfalls. *Laryngoscope* 1987; **97:** 1326–30.
66. Rouby JJ, Viars P. Clinical use of high frequency ventilation. *Acta Anaesthesiol Scand* 1989; **90** (Suppl.): 134–9.
67. Hunsaker DH. Anesthesia for microlaryngeal surgery: the case for subglottic jet ventilation. *Laryngoscope* 1994; **104:** 1–30.
68. Smith BE. Developments in the safe use of high frequency jet ventilation. *Br J Anaesth* 1990; **65:** 735–6.
69. Depierraz B, Ravussin P, Brossard E, Monnier P. Percutaneous transtracheal jet ventilation for paediatric endoscopic laser treatment of laryngeal and subglottic lesions. *Can J Anaesth* 1994; **41:** 1200–7.
70. Puura AI, Rorarius MG, Manninen P, *et al.* The costs of intense neuromuscular block for anesthesia during endolaryngeal procedures due to waiting time. *Anesth Analg* 1999; **88:** 1335–9.
71. Burkle H, Dunbar S, Van Aken H. Remifentanil: a novel, short-acting, mu-opioid. *Anesth Analg* 1996; **83:** 646–51.
72. Grant S, Noble S, Woods A, *et al.* Assessment of intubating conditions in adults after induction with propofol and varying doses of remifentanil. *Br J Anaesth* 1998; **81:** 540–3.
73. McAtamney D, O'Hare R, Hughes D, *et al.* Evaluation of remifentanil for control of haemodynamic response to tracheal intubation. *Anaesthesia* 1998; **53:** 1223–7.
74. Quintal MC, Cunningham MJ, Ferrari LR. Tubeless spontaneous respiration technique for pediatric microlaryngeal surgery. *Arch Otolaryngol Head Neck Surg* 1997; **123:** 209–14.
75. Wiet RJ, Kubek DC, Lemberg P, Byskosh AT. A meta-analysis review of revision stapes surgery with argon laser: effectiveness and safety. *Am J Otol* 1997; **18:** 166–71.
76. Kamami YV. Laser-assisted outpatient septoplasty results on 120 patients. *J Clin Laser Med Surg* 1997; **15:** 123–9.
77. Rampil IJ. Anesthetic considerations for laser surgery. *Anesth Analg* 1992; **74:** 424–35.
78. Hermens JM, Bennett MJ, Hirshman CA. Anesthesia for laser surgery. *Anesth Analg* 1983; **62:** 218–29.
79. Sosis MB. Saline soaked pledgets prevent carbon dioxide laser-induced endotracheal tube cuff ignition. *J Clin Anesth* 1995; **7:** 395–7.
80. AlHaddad S, Brenner J. Helium and lower oxygen concentration do not prolong tracheal tube ignition time during potassium titanyl phosphate laser use. *Anesthesiology* 1994; **80:** 936–8.
81. Sosis MB. Evaluation of five metallic tapes for protection of endotracheal tubes during CO_2 laser surgery. *Anesth Analg* 1989; **68:** 392–3.
82. Anonymous. Laser-resistant endotracheal tubes and wraps. *Health Devices* 1990; **19:** 112–39.
83. Sosis MB, Dillon FX. Saline-filled cuffs help prevent laser-induced polyvinylchloride endotracheal tube fires. *Anesth Analg* 1991; **72:** 187–9.
84. Wegrzynowicz ES, Jensen NF, Pearson KS, *et al.* Airway fire during jet ventilation for laser excision of vocal cord papillomata. *Anesthesiology* 1992; **76:** 468–9.
85. Jensen NF, Block RI. Vasopressin levels in major head and neck surgery. *Ear Nose Throat J* 1997; **76:** 87–4.
86. Jensen NF, Todd MM, Block RI, *et al.* The efficacy of routine central venous monitoring in major head and neck surgery: a retrospective review. *J Clin Anesth* 1995; **7:** 119–25.
87. Priano LL, Smith JD, Cohen JI, Everts EE. Intravenous fluid administration and urine output during radical neck surgery. *Head Neck* 1993; **15:** 208–15.
88. Van Hemelen G, Avery CM, Venn PJ, *et al.* Management of Jehovah's Witness patients undergoing major head and neck surgery. *Head Neck* 1999; **21:** 80–4.
89. Zahoor-ul-Haq-Mackay, Mehraj-ud-Din, Darzi MA, Chowdri NA. Experience with isovolemic hemodilution in extensive head and neck surgery. *Plast Reconstr Surg* 1995; **95:** 479–85.
90. Williamson JA, Webb RK, Russell WJ, Runciman WB. The Australian Incident Monitoring Study. Air embolism – an analysis of 2000 incident reports. *Anaesth Intensive Care* 1993; **21:** 638–41.
91. Rice JH, Gonzalez RM. Large visible gas bubbles in the internal jugular vein: a common occurrence during supine radical neck surgery? *J Clin Anesth* 1992; **4:** 21–4.
92. Celikkanat S, Akyol MU, Koc C, *et al.* Postoperative hypertension after radical neck dissection. *Otolaryngol Head Neck Surg* 1997; **117:** 91–2.
93. Moorthy SS, Sullivan TY, Fallon JH, *et al.* Loss of hypoxic ventilatory response following bilateral neck dissection. *Anesth Analg* 1993; **76:** 791–4.
94. Sprung J, Jones FD, Rosen JS, *et al.* Asymptomatic carotid stenosis and stroke during neck surgery. *Otolaryngol Head Neck Surg* 1996; **115:** 568–72.
95. Yanowitz F, Preston JB, Abildskov JA. Functional distribution of right and left stellate innervation to the ventricles. Production of neurogenic electrocardiographic changes by unilateral alteration of sympathetic tone. *Circ Res* 1966; **18:** 416–28.
96. Otteni JC, Pottecher T, Bronner G, *et al.* Prolongation of the Q-T interval and sudden cardiac arrest following right radical neck dissection. *Anesthesiology* 1983; **59:** 358–61.
97. Acquadro MA, Nghiem TX, Beach TP, *et al.* Acquired QT interval changes and neck dissections. *J Clin Anesth* 1995; **7:** 54–7.
98. Rhine EJ, Roberts D. Acute epiglottitis – revisited. *Paediatr Anaesth* 1995; **5:** 345–6.
99. Cressman WR, Myer 3rd CM. Diagnosis and management of croup and epiglottitis. *Pediatr Clin North Am* 1994; **41:** 265–76.
100. Crosby E, Reid D. Acute epiglottitis in the adult: is intubation mandatory? *Can J Anaesth* 1991; **38:** 914–18.
101. Rivron RP, Murray JA. Adult epiglottitis: is there a consensus on diagnosis and treatment? *Clin Otolaryngol Allied Sci* 1991; **16:** 338–44.
102. Gidley PW, Ghorayeb BY, Stiernberg CM. Contemporary management of deep neck space infections. *Otolaryngol Head Neck Surg* 1997; **116:** 16–22.
103. Fritsch DE, Klein DG. Ludwig's angina. *Heart Lung* 1992; **21:** 39–46.

51

Anesthesia for ophthalmic surgery

ANTHONY RUBIN

Ophthalmic surgery involves patients in all age groups and may be performed under local or general anesthesia. The neonate and infant present special problems, and may have associated congenital anomalies that influence anesthetic management. Most elderly patients have coincidental medical problems, especially cardiorespiratory disorders, arthritis, or diabetes mellitus, and may well be taking several drugs.[1–3] Although patients may be in a high-risk category, ophthalmic surgery is low risk with respect to general morbidity and mortality. Many procedures are suitable for day-case surgery, but the established criteria for the care of day-stay patients may need to be reviewed. This is because this type of surgery causes minimal blood loss and physiologic disturbance, a lack of fluid shifts, little impact on the stress response and frequently an absence of postoperative pain.

Ophthalmic surgery may be broadly divided into extraocular and intraocular procedures. The oculocardiac reflex is frequently seen during extraocular procedures, especially surgery for strabismus, but may occur during other types of eye surgery. Its mechanism must be understood, and it must be prevented, or recognized rapidly and treated. During intraocular surgery, vascular congestion must be avoided, and, as the globe is opened, intraocular pressure (IOP) needs to be controlled.

Detailed knowledge of the anatomy of the globe and orbit and its contents are essential for the safe practice of local anesthesia.

CHOICE OF ANESTHESIA

The trend over the last decade has been to increase the use of local anesthesia so that it is used in about 86% of cataract operations.[3] This has coincided with surgical and anesthetic advances. These include the more widespread use of small-incision phacoemulsification and folding lenses for cataract surgery, improvements in local anesthetic techniques, and increasing use of day-stay facilities. Regional anesthesia may be the technique of choice for the whole range of adult patients, not just for those who are deemed unfit to undergo general anesthesia. The patient must be able to lie still and to cooperate. Recovery time is shorter after regional anesthesia, the patient leaving promptly after the end of surgery, and there are savings with respect to space, equipment, and staffing. For longer operations, such as prolonged vitreoretinal surgery and surgery in young patients, such as surgery for strabismus, general anesthesia may be preferred. The choice is usually clear, but the views of the surgeon, anesthetist, and patient need to be considered.

Some authors have failed to demonstrate any difference in outcome between local or general anesthesia with respect to memory, cognitive function, oxygen saturation, or major morbidity or mortality.[4] Others have suggested that there may be less intraoperative oxygen desaturation, hemodynamic alteration, nausea and vomiting, and postoperative pain and stress response with local anesthesia.[5,6] After general anesthesia there is a greater rate of unplanned hospital admission and more males have urinary retention. Chest infection or thromboembolism is very rare after eye surgery owing to the immediate mobilization.

REGIONAL ANESTHESIA

The predominantly elderly patients tolerate local anesthesia very well, and the frequency of intercurrent disease[1,2] and multiple drug therapy makes the avoidance of general anesthesia more desirable. General anesthesia may be associated with an increase in the perioperative and immediate postoperative complications, and the possibility of straining or coughing during the awakening period is undesirable.

The local techniques are relatively simple, have a high success rate, and should result in excellent operating conditions with a wide margin of safety. Anesthesiologists are involved not only in a stand-by capacity to monitor, sedate, and occasionally resuscitate the patients, but actually to perform the blocks. With skilled administration of the blocks, the need for sedation is minimal and systemic complications may be anticipated and prevented rather than allowed to progress to crisis situations that then need urgent treatment. If emergencies do arise, the presence of an anesthesiologist allows for their rapid and appropriate treatment. Patients will usually expect to leave hospital within 30 min of the end of the operation, so postoperative monitoring is limited and iatrogenic complications are poorly tolerated.

Contraindications

Contraindications to local anesthesia for ophthalmic procedures include young age, an informed preference for general anesthesia, an anticipated lack of cooperation, severe involuntary movements, an inability to lie in the required position for surgery and relatively still, and the rare situations of allergy to local anesthetics or the presence of infection at the site of injection. Relative contraindications would be operations lasting more than an hour and a long myopic eye (above 26 mm) in which there might be an increased risk of globe perforation if sharp needle techniques are planned.[7,8] Anticoagulation within the therapeutic ratio for the condition for which the patient is being treated (international normalized ratio 1.5–3.5) is not considered a contraindication as the risk of stopping anticoagulants may exceed the risk of continuing their use.[9–11] However a less invasive technique such as topical or sub-Tenon's block may be preferred in anticoagulated patients.[12]

Preoperative assessment

For minor procedures under topical or simple infiltration anesthesia without sedation, little preparation is required. However, if a formal eye block or sedation is planned, detailed preoperative evaluation and preparation is desirable. The patient should be in optimal condition with special attention paid to the control of high blood pressure, heart failure, or diabetes mellitus. Protocols are required, and these should include the indications for investigations. Investigations that will not affect patient management should be discouraged.[13,14] Routine medical testing has not been shown to increase the safety of cataract surgery under local anesthesia.[15] As failure of these blocks is exceptionally rare if sufficient time is allowed, preoperative starvation is unnecessary.[16,17] However, in the event of failure of the block, the operation must be postponed rather than changing to a general anesthetic. Diabetics may therefore remain on their usual regimens. Their management is thereby simplified and early discharge made possible.

Full resuscitation equipment must be available, and an indwelling intravenous cannula should be inserted for the occasional administration of drugs for cardiovascular adjustment, respiratory stimulation, resuscitation, and mild sedation or to enable the lowering of intraocular pressure.

Sedation

Effective preoperative counseling and rapport increases patient confidence and reduces anxiety and the need for sedation. Fewer than 10% of patients should require sedation.[18] If sedation is required, the drugs must be selected carefully for safety and must never be used to cover inadequate local anesthetic blockade.[19] Very occasionally, drugs, for example midazolam 7 μg kg^{-1} and alfentanil 3 mg kg^{-1}, have been used to allay anxiety, to add analgesia, and to enhance, not diminish, cooperation. The patient must remain conscious and be able to respond to commands ("conscious sedation"). The use of an intravenous induction agent such as propofol in very low dosage has been described, and patient-controlled sedation is growing in popularity.[20] The intravenous route is preferred as this allows the agents to be titrated to the exact effect required. Drugs that work rapidly, wear off quickly, and do not accumulate are essential, as trained observers to watch over the outpatient once he or she has left the hospital will not be available.[21] Maintenance of verbal contact remains the most important guide to patient well-being, and an educated hand-holder is both reassuring to the patient and a route for information to be passed in both directions. If sedative drugs are used, an anesthesiologist should be in attendance.[11] The airway must remain clear, additional inspired oxygen should be provided, and respiration and gas exchange should be monitored. Monitoring with a pulse oximeter, an electrocardiograph (ECG), and noninvasive blood pressure recorder is also essential. Accumulation of carbon dioxide under the drapes has been described, and an open system of draping eliminates this possibility. In the oversedated patient, the risk of sudden uncontrolled movement is increased and occasionally leads to unnecessary complications of surgery. The anesthesiologist must ensure safe recovery from the effects of any sedation.

Anatomy

The orbit is a quadrilateral pyramid with the apex posteromedially and the base facing anteriorly. The lateral walls are at an angle of 45° to the medial wall, whereas the floors pass upwards at an angle of 5° (Fig. 51.1). The medial walls and roofs are vertical and horizontal respectively. The lateral orbital rim is 12–18 mm behind the cornea, allowing easy access from the inferolateral corner to the equator of the globe and the posterior part of the orbit. The apex, including the optic foramen, is in the same sagittal plane as the medial wall, and lies 42–54 mm from the inferior orbital rim. The orbit contains the globe, orbital fat, extraocular muscles, conjunctiva, nerves, and blood vessels. The volume of the orbit is about 30 mL, while that of the globe is about 6.5 mL. The globe, which lies closer to the roof of the orbit than the floor, is normally about 22–24 mm long but in myopic eyes may be longer than 30 mm. Longer eyes tend to have thinner sclerae and even swellings of the sclerae (staphylomata). They are therefore at greater risk of perforation by a needle.[7] The globe normally occupies the front half of the orbital cavity, and extends anteriorly beyond it. The clearance is greatest at the corners of the orbital cavity. The globe is separated from the other orbital structures by Tenon's fascia, which is covered by conjunctiva reflected on to the inner surface of the lids in the upper and lower fornices (Fig. 51.2). The orbital fat is divided into a central (intracone, retrobulbar) space and a peripheral (extracone, peribulbar) space by the muscle cone of the four recti muscles. However, the orbital fat is continuous through the cone, which is not well developed posteriorly. Thus, the cone does not act as a barrier to the spread of local anesthetic. As a result, solutions placed in the extracone space (peribulbar injection) enter the intracone space rapidly.[22]

All the nerves to the extraocular muscles and ciliary ganglion, as well as the branches of the ophthalmic division of the Vth nerve and the terminal branches of the VIIth nerve to the orbicularis oculi muscle, may be blocked by injections into the orbital fat. The optic, oculomotor (which supplies the superior, inferior and medial recti and the inferior oblique muscles), abducens (which supplies the lateral rectus muscle), and the nasociliary nerves (innervating the corneal and perilimbal conjunctiva) as well as the ciliary ganglion are all within the cone. The lacrimal, frontal, and infraorbital nerves (which supply the peripheral conjunctiva) and trochlear nerve (which supplies the superior oblique muscle) are outside the cone. The globe moves as a result of activity of the four recti muscles and the superior and inferior oblique muscles. The recti arise from the annulus of Zinn at the orbital apex and are

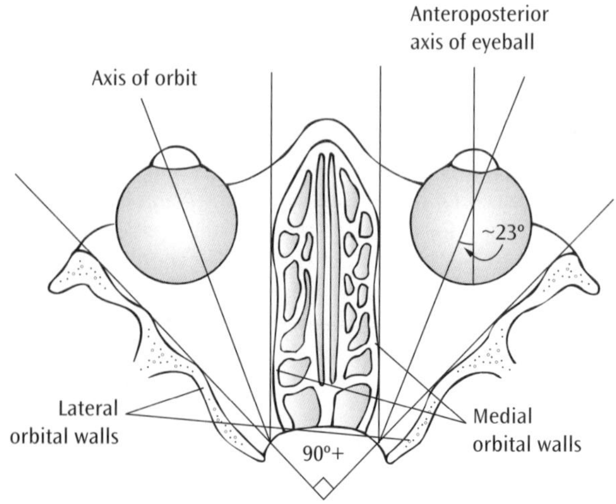

Figure 51.1 *Geometry of the orbits and eyes.*

Figure 51.2 *Schematic transverse section of the orbit. The dotted line represents the path and depth of penetration of a 30G sharp disposable needle traversing the medial check ligament and entering the medial compartment of the nasal side of the rectal muscle. (Modified and reprinted with permission from Winder* et al.[26]*)*

inserted into the globe just in front of the equator of the globe about 5–7 mm from the corneoscleral junction. The upper lid is controlled by the levator palpebrae superioris. The orbicularis oculi, which surrounds and squeezes the front of the eye, is supplied by the facial nerve. The least vascular parts of the orbital fat are the inferotemporal and nasal areas, and it is usual to make injections into one or both of these regions. The optic nerve, which in its intraorbital course is about 4 mm in diameter, enters the orbit through the optic foramen, passes anterolaterally for about 3 cm to enter the globe at its rear surface a little to the medial side of the center, and innervates the retina. The optic nerve is covered by a dural cuff, which contains a prolongation of the subarachnoid space right up to the sclera.

Techniques

Methods include:

1 topical;
2 subconjunctival injection;
3 sub-Tenon's block;
4 retrobulbar and facial nerve blocks;
5 combined retrobulbar/peribulbar block;
6 peribulbar block.

The aim should be complete anesthesia of the conjunctiva and globe, and a normal or soft eye. If complete akinesia of the globe, eyelids ,and orbicularis oculi muscle is required, akinetic methods such as retrobulbar, peribulbar, combinations, or sub-Tenon's blocks should be used. If akinesia is not required, topical methods or subconjunctival injections may suffice.

Topical

Many surgeons who use small-incision phacoemulsification for cataract surgery may not require akinesia, and the operation may be done using topical local anesthetic drops alone, usually amethocaine 1%, lidocaine (lignocaine) 4%, or bupivacaine 0.75%.[23,24] Satisfactory anesthesia results, although the iris is not anesthetized, but as there is no globe akinesia more patient cooperation is required, aided by the stabilizing effect of the two instruments within the eye. Anesthesia may be improved by the use of either intracameral (into the anterior chamber) preservative-free lidocaine[25,26] or local anesthetic-soaked sponges placed in the fornices,[27] or by the application to the eye of local anesthetic gel.[28] Very careful selection of patients and very skilled surgery are required if the technique is to be successful. The advantages are the avoidance of any needle-related complications, the lack of need for an eyepad postoperatively, and, as the local anesthetic wears off rapidly, more rapid recovery of sight. Oxybuprocaine (Benoxinate) 0.4% or proxymetacaine 0.5%, although having a shorter duration of action, are preferred to amethocaine prior to sub-Tenon's blocks or retrobulbar or peribulbar injections as they sting less.

Subconjunctival injection

Topical anesthesia combined with a small volume of local anesthetic (0.2–0.5 mL) injected under the conjunctiva close to the superior limbus will also produce good anesthesia but has no effect on the motor nerves to the globe or periorbital structures.[29] It is simple and very safe, but an isolated case of globe perforation has been described.[30]

Sub-Tenon's block

Sub-Tenon's block is a technique that has been reintroduced and is increasing rapidly in popularity as it involves the use of a blunt cannula rather than a sharp needle. Following administration of topical drops, a small incision is made in both the conjunctiva and Tenon's fascia with round-tipped scissors, usually in the inferonasal region about 5 mm from the limbus (Fig. 51.3). About 5 mL of local anesthetic with hyaluronidase is introduced via a blunt metal or plastic cannula passed around the eye to the posterior pole deep to the Tenon's fascia layer, which lies under the conjunctiva[31,32] (Fig. 51.4). There is evidence from B-scan ultrasonography that the solution tracks back to the retrobulbar space and acts there.[33] It is relatively painless, anesthesia is good, and akinesia follows the spread of the solution into the intracone space or along the muscle sheaths of the recti muscles.[34,35] The only common complications of sub-Tenon's block are chemosis and subconjunctival hemorrhage, but further experience and comparative trials are required to determine whether sub-Tenon's block avoids the risks associated with sharp needles, in particular retrobulbar hemorrhage and globe perforation. It may be particularly indicated for long eyes and in anticoagulated patients. Anesthesiologists as well as surgeons have adopted it in many centers.

Retrobulbar and facial nerve blocks

This combination was very popular in the past, but as the facial nerve endings may be blocked in the lids from within the orbit a separate facial nerve block is no longer required. The retrobulbar injection remains in wide use and is often performed on its own with higher volumes, or combined with a nasal peribulbar injection.[36,37]

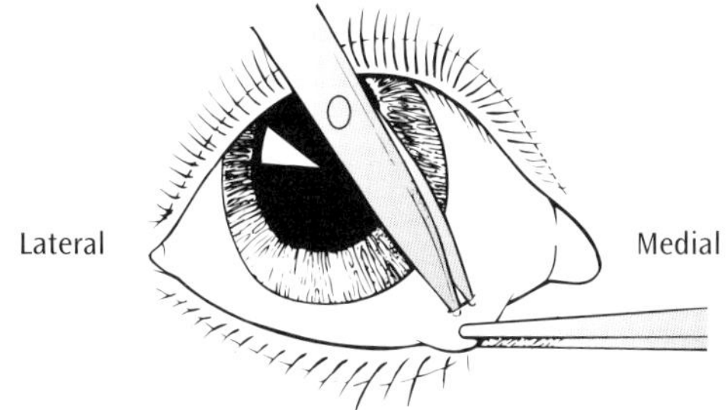

Figure 51.3 *Conjunctival incision in inferonasal quadrant.*

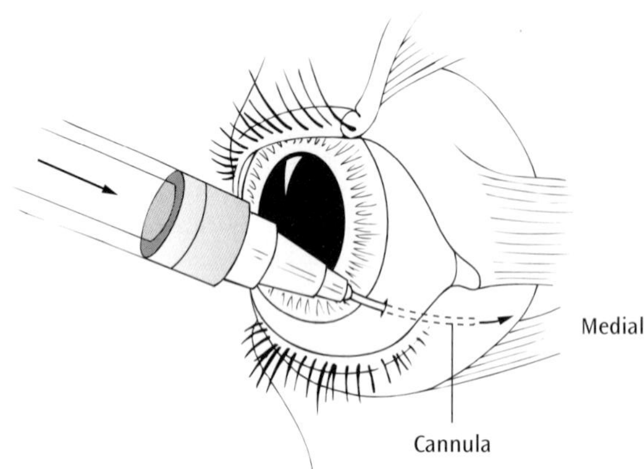

Figure 51.4 *Sub-Tenon's anesthesia.*

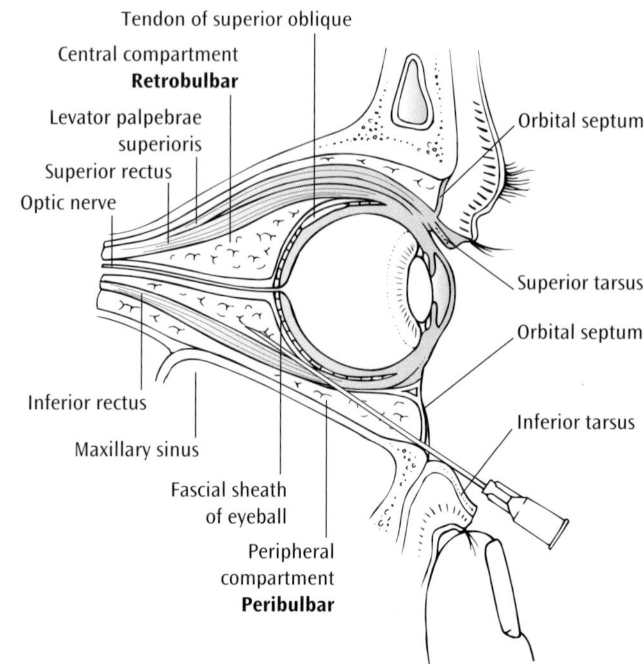

Figure 51.5 *Retrobulbar injection. (Reprinted with permission from Khoo* et al.[35]*)*

Combined retrobulbar/peribulbar block

For a retrobulbar block, the eye should look straight ahead in the primary gaze position, to prevent rotation of the optic nerve, vasculature, and posterior pole of the globe toward the inferotemporal needle.[38] The retrobulbar injection is made from the inferotemporal region of the orbit. It is convenient to go through the conjunctiva, which may be anesthetized with topical local anesthetic drops, and this route is therefore less painful than injection through the skin.[39] Occasionally, if the eye is very deepset, the orbital fissure is very narrow, or there is pronounced blepharospasm, access to the conjunctival fornix may be difficult. In such patients, it may be safer to go through the lower lid. Long needles, such as the 38 mm previously popular, must not be used as they have been shown to be able to reach the optic nerve in over 11% of the population.[40] Much shorter, sharper needles are now favored, and, although in theory there may be a greater chance of failing to recognize a globe perforation with a sharp needle, in practice this has not been demonstrated.[41,42]

Thus, a 25-gauge, 2.5-cm sharp needle is inserted with the bevel toward the globe, close to the lateral canthus, avoiding conjunctival vessels. The needle is then passed away from the globe, below it along the floor of the orbit, past the equator, and then upward and inward to the full depth of 2.5 cm. This will usually allow the needle tip to enter the cone just behind the rear of the globe (Fig. 51.5).

The tip of the needle should not cross the line of the lateral edge of the iris so that it cannot reach the optic nerve. After careful aspiration, 2–5 mL of solution may be injected, monitoring any proptosis and pressure rise, and stopping the injection if it rises excessively. A good sign of correct needle placement is the onset of ptosis during the injection. This may be used as an endpoint to limit the injection volume. Pressure should be applied once the needle has been removed to control any venous bleeding, to aid spread of the solution, and to lower IOP.[43] This volume should block all the relevant sensory nerves and the motor nerves to all structures, except perhaps the orbicularis oculi and the superior oblique, which are outside the muscle cone. When required, the orbicularis oculi is blocked by a nasal peribulbar injection,[44] in which the 25-gauge, 2.5-cm needle is inserted between the skin of the medial canthus and the caruncle and directed backward into the orbital fat parallel to the medial orbital wall for about 2 cm. The feel of going through the medial orbital septum (medial check ligament) is often detected (Figs 51.6 and 51.7). About 5 mL of solution is injected and will spread in the medial orbital fat to augment the effect of the retrobulbar block. It will also come forward above and below the medial orbital septum to fill the lids, where it blocks the terminal branches of that part of the VIIth nerve that supplies the orbicularis oculi.

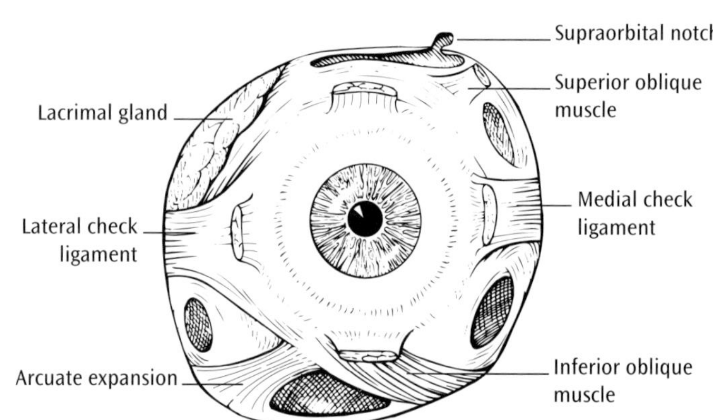

Figure 51.6 *Hemial orifices within the connective tissue diaphragm situated just anterior to the globe equator.*

Peribulbar block

Peribulbar block has been considered safer than retrobulbar block, as the needles are directed farther away from vital structures and are not necessarily inserted so deep.[45] However, there is little evidence to confirm its superiority compared with a shallow retrobulbar injection. The peribulbar block has in the past been performed with two injections through the skin, one inferotemporal and the other superonasal.[45] More recently, the technique has also been modified so that all the injections are made through the conjunctiva, which has been shown to cause less pain,[39] and the superonasal injection has been superseded by the nasal one described above.

The solution is deposited outside the cone rather than behind the globe and has a slower onset of effect (up to 25 min) (Fig. 51.8). A larger volume of local anesthetic (10–15 mL) is required to achieve complete akinesia, and supplementary injections are required more often (5–24% of patients).[46,47] There were fears that these larger volumes might cause

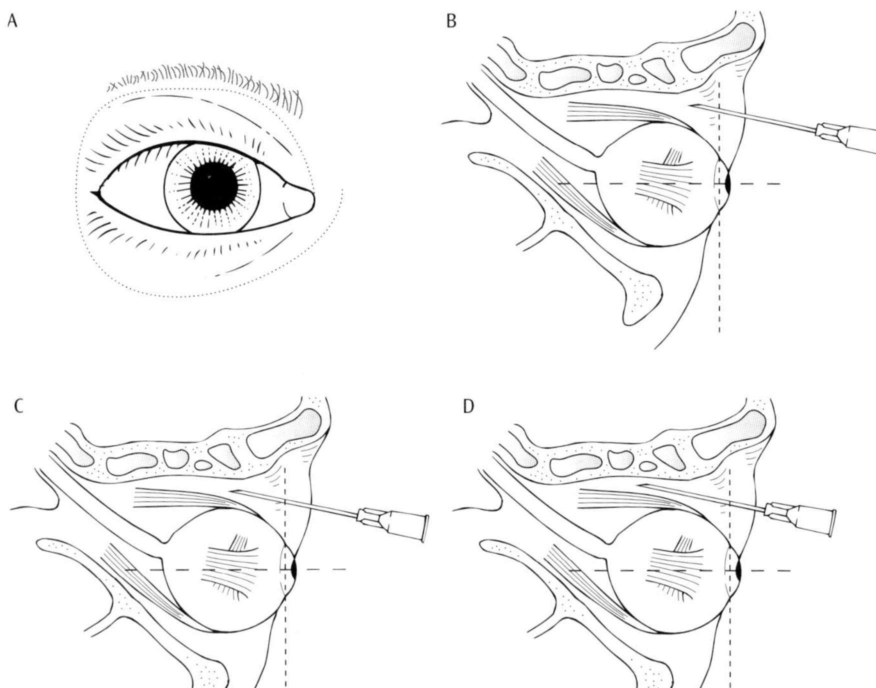

Figure 51.7 *Medial pericone block. B–D as seen from above. (Reprinted with permission from Gimbel Educational Services.)*

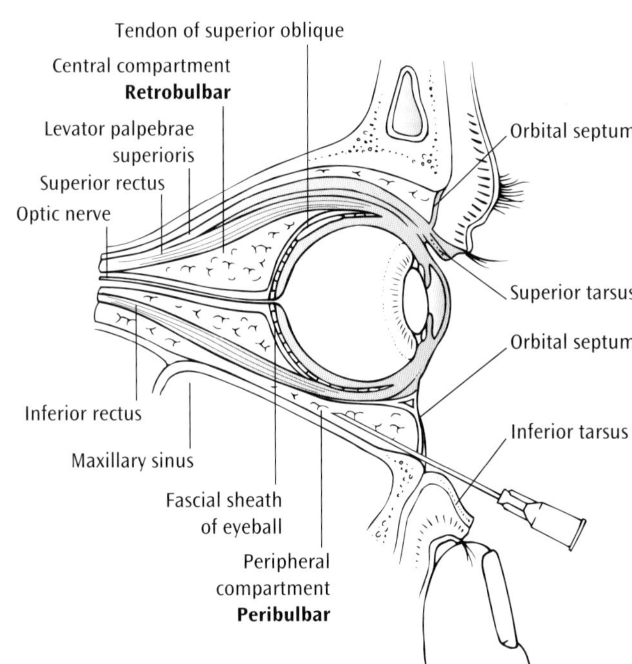

Figure 51.8 *Peribulbar injection. (Reprinted with permission Khoo* et al.[35]*)*

a sustained increase in IOP with risk to the retinal blood supply, but it has been shown that the pressure falls rapidly.[48] The local anesthetic acts after diffusion into the intracone space, which may begin within 2 min.[22] The inferotemporal injection is made in the conjunctival fornix close to the lateral canthus and about 2 mm from the sclera. A 25-gauge, 2.5-cm needle is inserted away from and then below the globe. No attempt is made to go up or in toward the muscle cone, and the needle need not go further than the equator of the globe. At least 5 mL of solution is usually injected while assessing orbital pressure; the injection should be stopped if orbital pressure rises excessively. Ninety percent of patients will also require a nasal injection to achieve complete akinesia. This is performed as has been described for the combined retrobulbar/peribulbar injection, inserting the needle medial to the caruncle and piercing the medial orbital septum before injecting 2–5 mL at a depth of about 2 cm. Indeed, 25% of patients will require even more injections in order to achieve adequate akinesia, and the choice of additional entry sites depends on the deficiencies of the block.[47] They may be inferotemporal or nasal through the conjunctiva, or superotemporal through the skin of the upper eyelid.

More recently, some have described using only a nasal injection with a 6–8 mL volume, but up to 50% of patients will require further injections.[49,50] Up to 30 min of gentle massage or a pressure device applied to the closed eye may be needed to allow for the absorption of the larger volumes of local anesthetic and a return to normal or low IOP. The applied pressure must be controlled to prevent postoperative ptosis or vascular impairment of the retina.

Pharmacology and choice of solution

The blocks may be preceded by administration of topical drops and a preliminary injection with a 1-cm, 30-gauge needle in the inferotemporal conjunctival fornix of 1–1.5 mL of a dilute solution of lidocaine (0.2%) in balanced salt solution. This solution does not sting on injection, and the definitive solution hurts less if it follows the preliminary injection, is warmed to body temperature, and is injected slowly. The ideal local anesthetic would be safe, painless to inject, and would have a rapid onset of dense sensory and motor block and a predictable duration of action. The onset time is, in part, a feature of the agent but also of the proximity at which it is placed to the target nerves. Thus, intraconal injections tend to work quicker and better than extraconal ones. The duration of effect also depends on the properties of the agent as well as on the mass used and whether additives such as epinephrine (adrenaline) or clonidine are used. High concentrations of local anesthetic seem to be required to ensure adequate penetration and intense motor block.

The traditional solution is an equal parts mixture of 2% lidocaine and 0.75% bupivacaine, giving rapid onset and long duration. Lidocaine 2%[51] and prilocaine 2%[52,53] are excellent agents if a duration of no longer than an hour is required. In the UK, higher concentrations of prilocaine are licensed only for dental use and appear to be contraindicated for eye blocks as they have been associated with optic nerve damage.[54] Epinephrine $5\,\mu g\,mL^{-1}$ and hyaluronidase $7.5\,i.u.\,mL^{-1}$ may be added freshly, and, although there is controversy over their effect, both may be beneficial in terms of spread, quality, and duration of block and reduction of pressure.[55–57] Clonidine $100\,\mu g$ has been added but also prolongs the motor block.[58] Both ropivacaine and levobupivacaine have been studied;[59–61] these are clinically as effective as racemic bupivacaine, and being S-enantiomers have the potential for reduced toxicity. However, the use of long-acting agents necessitates that the eye is padded until the anesthesia has worn off and is followed the next day by a high incidence of residual diplopia.

Adding bicarbonate to raise the pH of the local anesthetic causes a greater proportion of the drug to exist in the uncharged form. This results in more rapid onset, and may lessen the need for supplemental injections.[62,63]

Assessment of the block

The block should ensure anesthesia and akinesia, if required, must be assessed. Block of the levator palpebrae superioris is confirmed by the inability to open the eye, of the orbicularis oculi by the inability to squeeze the lids, and of the external ocular muscles by a failure to move the globe in any direction.

Care in the operating room

The patient must be made as comfortable as possible, often aided by careful attention to the position of the head and neck and a pillow under the knees to take the strain off the lumbar spine. Minimal monitoring should include oximetry and electrocardiography, and blood pressure measurements are desirable. Oxygen is usually administered under the drapes, which should be suspended off the patient's nose and mouth. If the patient is breathing only air, up to one-third will have oxygen saturations below 95%. Nasal cannulae with 2 L of oxygen may be preferred to piped oxygen under the drapes at 6–8 L min^{-1}.[64] The patient must be monitored by a trained member of staff, whose role is to provide reassurance and to explain some of the noises associated with modern cataract surgery. The patient must be encouraged to remain still and silent unless reporting a problem.

Complications

Systemic toxicity

Complications may be due to systemic toxicity of the local anesthetic or to the vasoconstrictor agents used and may follow an overdose or accidental intravenous injection. Allergic reactions to local anesthetic or hyaluronidase are seen very rarely. Severe systemic reactions may be associated with incidental problems of the cardiovascular system, including vasovagal and ischemic manifestations.

Subconjunctival edema (chemosis)

Chemosis often follows orbital injections or sub-Tenon's block but is of little significance. It usually disappears with gentle pressure and time.

Bruising (ecchymosis)

Ecchymosis is more likely if the injections are percutaneous but may also follow transconjunctival injections. Bruises do not interfere with surgery and do not pose any threat to the eye.

Hemorrhage

Orbital (retrobulbar) hemorrhage is a serious complication with an incidence of between 0.1% and 1.7%.[65] It is more likely to follow the use of longer needles as larger vessels are in the posterior orbit. It is identified by increasing proptosis, tight eyelids, periorbital and subconjunctival hemorrhage, and a dramatic increase in intraorbital pressure. The operation may have to be postponed, and urgent treatment may be required to prevent permanent loss of vision if the pressure causes occlusion of the central artery of the retina.[66]

Globe penetration or perforation

The needle may enter the globe (penetration) or pass right through it (perforation).[67] Myopic eyes which are longer and have a thinner sclera are at increased risk, as are those which have undergone previous retinal detachment surgery. The length of the globe is known following preparation for lens implantation. Detailed knowledge of the anatomy and an initial tangential approach with the bevel of the needle facing toward the globe help to reduce the incidence. Diagnosis may be suggested by pain, sudden loss of vision, hypotonia of the globe, a poor red reflex, or vitreous hemorrhage. It may follow both peribulbar and retrobulbar injections, but it should be a very rare event with an incidence not greater than about 1 in 15 000.[46]

Optic nerve complications

There is a small risk of direct damage to the optic nerve or injection or hemorrhage within the optic nerve sheath. Anatomical knowledge and the use of short 25-mm needles should make this complication most unlikely. Pressure on the optic nerve may also be a consequence of retrobulbar hemorrhage.[66] Some local anesthetic preparations, such as high concentrations of prilocaine, may be neurotoxic.[54]

Amaurosis (loss of vision)

The blocks may lead to temporary loss of vision. This is more frequent following a retrobulbar block, as more local anesthetic reaches the optic nerve, but may also occur following peribulbar blockade. The patient should be reassured that, on the one hand, retention of vision does not imply failure of block and that, on the other hand, loss of vision may occur but this will return as the block wears off.

Central spread of local anesthetic

Local anesthetic may be injected into the optic nerve sheath, which is a dural cuff communicating with the intracranial cavity. The globe must be looking straight ahead during insertion of the block so that the optic nerve remains in its normal position behind the globe and does not rotate toward the needle.[38] Symptoms include drowsiness, ipsilateral or contralateral loss of vision, convulsions, or respiratory or cardiovascular depression. Although symptoms occur most commonly soon after the injection, their onset may be delayed, so the patient must be carefully monitored to detect early signs and to institute prompt treatment as required.

External ocular muscle palsies

Ptosis may result from the surgery or from the local anesthetic injections or pressure applied to the globe. Muscle palsies may follow injection of high concentrations of local anesthetic directly into a muscle, the medial rectus and inferior oblique being the most common sites. These usually recover without treatment.

GENERAL ANESTHESIA

Intraocular pressure

IOP should be low or normal prior to surgical incision. High IOP or sudden rises must be avoided to minimize the risk of iris or lens prolapse, vitreous extrusion, or choroidal hemorrhage that might threaten vision. The normal IOP is between 8 and 16 mmHg (1 and 2 kPa),[68] although it is normally lower in infants and young children.[69] A value above 25 mmHg (3.3 kPa) is considered pathological. It may be measured by a corneal contact method with the Perkins applanation tonometer or by noncontact methods such as the pneumatic air puff technique. The applanation method depends on the force needed to flatten part of the surface of the eye, which is equal to the internal pressure. The pneumatic method uses a jet of air from a set distance at constant pressure to indent the cornea. The IOP is the balance between the extraocular muscle tone and the scleral rigidity, on the one hand, and the volume of the aqueous, vitreous, and choroidal vasculature on the other. It is also affected by the balance between aqueous humor production and drainage. It drains through the pupil and then it passes centrifugally toward the angle of the anterior chamber, and through the trabecular meshwork into the canal of Schlemm. From there it enters the episcleral veins, which drain into the jugular veins. Reduced drainage is the most common cause of raised IOP and glaucoma. Aqueous humor is produced at a rate of 2 μL min^{-1}, in an active process by the ciliary body involving carbonic anhydrase and cytochrome oxidase, and by simple filtration through the anterior surface of the iris. Its normal volume is only about 0.3 mL.

Carbonic anhydrase inhibitors such as acetazolamide act by decreasing aqueous production, whereas osmotic diuretics such as mannitol reduce vitreous volume. Thus, both lower IOP, but by different mechanisms. The IOP must not exceed the perfusion pressure in the optic nerve or choroidal vasculature, and special care must be taken if the patient has glaucoma, and starts with an elevated pressure.

Increased choroidal blood flow and IOP may push the posterior segment and capsule forward, and make the contents of the eye, such as the iris or vitreous, bulge out. A low pressure ensures that the posterior capsule of the lens, behind which is the vitreous face, remains concave and relaxed and is least likely to rupture. It also ensures maximum room behind the cornea for the safe removal of the lens material and its replacement with the prosthetic lens. A sudden increase in choroidal blood volume predisposes to choroidal hemorrhage.

IOP may be affected by physiologic factors, by drugs including anesthetic agents and muscle relaxants, and by the technique of anesthesia itself. External pressure on the eye by the anesthetic face masks, retractors, or increased extraocular muscle tone may cause a rise in IOP.

Effect of arterial pressure changes

A wide range of arterial blood pressure has little effect on the changes in IOP. The systolic blood pressure has to be well below 90 mmHg (12 kPa) before there is any related reduction in IOP. Sudden rises in arterial blood pressure may, however, produce a small and transient rise.

Effect of venous pressure changes

A rise in venous pressure, following an obstructed airway, coughing, sneezing, straining, breath-holding, vomiting, a Valsalva maneuver, or intermittent positive-pressure ventilation (IPPV) with positive end-expiratory pressure (PEEP), will cause a rise in IOP. Coughing may raise the intraocular pressure to 40 mmHg (5.3 kPa). Anything that prevents free venous return, such as something tight around the neck or the head-down position, will be transmitted to the vasculature of the eye and immediately raise the IOP.

Effect of changes in respiratory gases

The relation between arterial carbon dioxide tension (P_aCO_2) and IOP is linear.[70] As the P_aCO_2 rises, the choroidal blood flow and the IOP increase, and as it falls so the IOP falls. Thus, controlled ventilation of the lungs may be used to control IOP. Oxygen has little effect on IOP unless it is pathologically low, in which case the IOP may rise.

Effect of changes in posture

A head-up tilt of 15° enhances venous drainage, reduces choroidal blood flow, and lowers IOP to the same degree as hyperventilation to a P_aCO_2 of 3.5–4.0 kPa.

Effects of anesthetic and related drugs

Drugs used in anesthesia may affect IOP in different ways.[71] These may act on the central IOP control centers, or by relaxation of the external ocular muscle tone, or they may act via changes in cardiovascular or respiratory values. It is apparent that IOP is most likely to rise during induction and recovery.

Thus, it is obvious that there should be a smooth induction and maintenance of anesthesia. One should avoid airway manipulation such as insertion of laryngeal masks, laryngoscopy, and intubation until an adequate depth of anesthesia has been achieved. It is desirable to use a very slight head-up tilt, and ensure smooth extubation and recovery to keep the IOP low.

Local anesthetic injections may, because of the volume being injected into the relatively closed space around or behind the globe, cause a rise in IOP,[72] and retrobulbar hemorrhage may result in a dramatic and possibly dangerous rise.

Ocular preparations

Many drugs, used for their actions on the eye, may have systemic as well as local effects, and these need to be taken into account.[73] Drugs placed in the conjunctival sac are absorbed either directly or rapidly from the nasal mucosa after passing through the nasolacrimal duct, or from the stomach following swallowing. Mydriatics and cycloplegics, vasoconstrictors, miotics, drugs used to lower intraocular pressure, and antibiotics will be considered. Steroids and anti-inflammatory agents are also widely used for specific indications.

Mydriatics and cycloplegics

The pupil needs to be dilated before cataract and vitreoretinal surgery to provide a good view, to allow access for instruments, to aid the removal of the cataract and insertion of an intraocular lens, or to access the vitreous or retina. This is most frequently achieved by the administration of sympathomimetics and parasympatholytics, which are usually applied topically but very occasionally are injected under the conjunctiva. Phenylephrine, an α_1-receptor agonist, is used in a concentration of 2.5%, 5%, or 10%. A concentration of 2.5% may be preferred for children and for those adults who are hypertensive or have cardiac disease. Sympathomimetics should be avoided altogether in the presence of monoamine oxidase inhibitors. Systemic effects, which may follow absorption, include hypertension, headache, tachycardia, cardiac arrhythmias, fainting, and angina.[74] Clearly, the dose of these drugs should be limited, and it is preferable for these to be used with anticholinergic mydriatics such as cyclopentolate. Homatropine 1–5%, cyclopentolate 0.5–1%, and tropicamide 0.5–1% are rapid-onset, short-duration parasympatholytics. They rarely cause side-effects. Atropine is used when the pupil needs to be dilated for more prolonged periods of time, but repeated administration might lead to overdose and atropine poisoning. Hyoscine is an alternative to atropine but may cause confusion in the elderly. Parasympatholytics may cause a rise in IOP in patients with closed-angle glaucoma or in whom the anterior chamber is shallow.

Epinephrine 1 μg mL^{-1} is often added to the irrigating fluid during cataract surgery to maintain maximal pupillary dilation. No problems have been reported from this use. Mydricaine is a combination of atropine, epinephrine, and procaine and is occasionally injected under the conjunctiva to improve and maintain pupillary dilation. In addition to the local effect, it is absorbed very rapidly and has very potent side-effects, such as tachycardia, arrhythmias, and hypertension.

Miotics

Miotic drugs reduce the size of the pupil and change the trabecular meshwork to enhance aqueous drainage. Miotics act by a cholinergic or anticholinesterase mechanism. These drugs include pilocarpine 1–4%, carbachol 3%, neostigmine 2.5–5%, and ecothiopate applied topically, and miochol, which is injected directly into the anterior chamber. Bradycardia and hypotension are occasional side-effects.

Vasoconstrictors

Vasoconstrictors, such as cocaine or epinephrine, may be applied to the nasal mucosa to reduce bleeding during lacrimal surgery. They are rapidly absorbed and have a stimulating effect on the sympathetic nervous system. Caution is required when these drugs are used in hypertensive patients and in those being treated with tricyclic or monoamine oxidase inhibitor antidepressants. Local application of cocaine to the cornea causes vasoconstriction, which could lead to corneal opacity and make intraocular surgery very difficult but epinephrine is a suitable alternative.

Drugs used to lower intraocular pressure

Cholinergics, anticholinesterases, sympathomimetics, β-blockers, carbonic anhydrase inhibitors, and osmotic diuretics may all be given to lower IOP. Combinations of these drugs are used frequently. Cholinergic drugs, such as pilocarpine, constrict the ciliary muscle, and this helps to increase the drainage through the trabecular meshwork leading to the canal of Schlemm. The action of anticholinesterases such as ecothiopate and isoflurophate may persist for several weeks after the drug is stopped. These drugs may induce prolonged apnea by delaying hydrolysis of succinylcholine (suxamethonium) or mivacurium. This action persists for several weeks. Sympathomimetics, e.g. 0.5–2% epinephrine, increase aqueous outflow by an α-agonist action and decrease aqueous inflow through a β-agonist activity. They have local side-effects including stinging, rebound vasodilation, allergy, mydriasis, which can precipitate angle-closure glaucoma, and cystoid macular edema, and are less effective than cholinergics or β-blockers. β-Blockers reduce aqueous humor production, but some, such as timolol, carteolol, and levobunolol, being noncardioselective, may lead to bronchospasm, bradycardia, hypotension, or heart failure. Betaxolol, a more cardioselective β-blocker, may be preferred for patients at risk of bronchospasm. Many other types of drug, such as nitrates, calcium channel blockers, angiotensin-converting enzyme inhibitors, and α_2-agonists, are sometimes used to lower IOP.

Carbonic anhydrase inhibitors, such as acetazolamide, reduce aqueous production from the ciliary body but also, after an initial increase, decrease choroidal blood flow. Acetazolamide is given 6-hourly in an oral dose of 250–1000 mg or by slow intravenous injection in a dose of up to 500 mg. A diuresis may result and, if used for a prolonged period, hyponatremia, hypokalemia, and metabolic acidosis. An osmotic diuretic such as mannitol 20% has been given in a dose of up to 1–1.5 g kg^{-1} over 30–60 min. It acts by withdrawing fluid from the vitreous body; the effect persists for about 4–6 h, and an expansion of the intravascular volume may result, leading to circulatory overload and heart failure, an overdistended bladder, and, following the diuresis, dehydration. Mannitol is hypertonic, and toxic if it extravasates outside a vein and is rarely used. Sucrose 50%, 0.5–1 g kg^{-1} may be used as an alternative. It has a more rapid effect, usually within 5 min, and is less likely to produce a significant diuresis.

Gentle eye massage or the application of pressure-reducing devices such as the Honan balloon may also help to reduce IOP. These devices are generally used in conjunction with local anesthetic blocks.

Antibiotics

Antibiotics of the aminoglycoside group are known to prolong neuromuscular block, but this does not seem to be a problem with the small doses used locally in ophthalmology.

Techniques of general anesthesia

The aim should be a smooth induction and maintenance of anesthesia with stable and low IOP, avoidance or treatment of the oculocardiac reflex, a guaranteed airway, a motionless surgical field, and smooth emergence without coughing, straining, nausea, or vomiting. Early discharge is desirable and, in skilled hands, possible.[4,75] Obvious features are that the operations are in the head and neck region, are mostly microsurgical, and that complete immobility is normally required. Thus, airway control is mandatory, and laryngeal masks or endotracheal tubes must be positioned correctly and secured in such a way that they cannot become dislodged. All monitoring devices must be attached and the patient positioned on the table with special care to protect limbs, pressure points, and usually the other eye.

Cataract extraction and intraocular lens implantation is by far the most frequent operation, followed by surgery for glaucoma such as trabeculectomy. The following general points apply especially to these procedures, and the specific points of other operations will be discussed later.

Preoperative assessment

There is controversy in respect of the amount of preoperative evaluation and preparation that is required. Effective communication between the patient, nurse, ophthalmologist, and anesthesiologist and consultations with relevant practitioners as indicated should ensure that the patient is in optimal condition. A management plan should be established for anesthesia and the perioperative management of chronic medical problems. Nurse evaluation is becoming the most frequent method of assessment, and liaison with the anesthesiologist is essential so that acute illness is diagnosed and chronic medical problems, such as diabetes or hypertension, which are common, identified and controlled.[76]

Particular attention should also be paid to ischemic heart disease or cardiac failure, to any pre-existing arrhythmias, as well as to chronic obstructive airways disease and asthma. There is a known association between eye disease and other medical conditions, and care should be taken to look for metabolic and endocrine diseases and conditions affecting the neuromuscular system, such as dystrophia myotonica. Dislocation of the lens may occur in Marfan, Stickler, or Ehlers–Danlos syndromes. Many patients will be taking one or more drugs that might affect anesthesia, and relevant drugs should be continued during the operative period and any possible interactions anticipated. Patient age is no longer a factor as it has been shown that the complication rate correlates better with the number of associated diseases than with age.[77] Laboratory investigations and chest radiographs should be ordered when indicated. An ECG recording should be available for all patients older than 60 years. Any particular risks should be explained to the patient and real consent obtained.

Premedication

Premedication is rarely needed as many patients will be elderly and will be day-cases, but is indicated for some children and particularly for nervous adults. Benzodiazepines given intravenously lower IOP unless they result in significant respiratory depression, although oral administration has little effect on IOP. Anticholinergic drugs are unlikely to raise IOP,[78] even in patients with acute-angle glaucoma, but are rarely used except to prevent the oculocardiac reflex. Opioids, which increase the incidence of nausea and vomiting and respiratory depression, are rarely used for premedication. Both benzodiazepines and opioids may have excessive and prolonged actions in the elderly and, if used, should be titrated with care. Prophylactic antiemetics must be given to prevent any risk to the eye from postoperative vomiting.

Preparation

The preparation of the anesthetic equipment and the application of monitoring devices should in the UK follow the Royal College of Anaesthetists[79] and Association of Anaesthetists[80] guidelines. Monitoring is vital as the anesthesiologist does not have easy access to the airway and is usually positioned at the patient's side, and the surgery may take place in a darkened operating room.

Induction of anesthesia

All intravenous induction agents, except ketamine, which raises blood pressure, lower intraocular pressure, although etomidate and propofol seem to lower it more than thiopentone.[81–83] Propofol produces muscular relaxation and depression of airway reflexes and therefore seems to be the best agent prior to the insertion of a laryngeal mask airway. Recovery from propofol is rapid and is usually associated with a feeling of well-being. Total intravenous anesthesia may be used and, as long as the depth of anesthesia is adequate, is associated with a low IOP. Ketamine may be used for examination of the eye and for pressure measurement in children. However, the resulting increase in intraocular pressure, nystagmus, blepharospasm, and adventitious movements makes it unsuitable in other situations. The choice and dose of induction agent depend on age, physical status, and the perceived need for rapid recovery. An adequate depth of anesthesia is required as in light anesthesia the eye may look up, which may hinder surgery.

Muscle relaxants

IOP is raised rapidly by 6–12 mmHg (0.8–1.6 kPa) by succinylcholine, as a result of either increased tension in the tonic muscles, causing contracture of the extraocular muscles, or an increase in choroidal blood flow. The rise persists for up to 10 min.[84,85] Other adverse side-effects of succinylcholine include muscle pains. None of the suggested preventive measures, such as the use of priming doses, precurarization, or administration of benzodiazepines or lidocaine is consistently effective, and the drug should be avoided unless strongly indicated. All the non-depolarizing agents may be used as they either have no effect or in fact lower IOP. Atracurium, vecuronium, and mivacurium are all popular because of their short duration of action, controllability of the depth of neuromuscular block, rapid offset, and associated cardiovascular stability. Rocuronium has a more rapid onset than vecuronium but results in a small rise in blood pressure and heart rate. It may be indicated for the emergency penetrating eye injury.[86]

Airway control

An adequate depth of anesthesia and muscular relaxation is required before a laryngeal mask or endotracheal tube is passed. A small dose of opioid, for example 1 $\mu g\,kg^{-1}$ fentanyl or 10 $\mu g\,kg^{-1}$ alfentanil, or an α-agonist such as dexmedetomidine, may be used with propofol to obtund the pressor response to laryngoscopy and intubation in hypertensive patients and the consequent rise in IOP.[71,87,88] Spraying the vocal cords with lidocaine may attenuate but not abolish this pressor response to laryngoscopy and intubation.[89] A clear airway is mandatory, as even a minor obstruction will raise venous and intraocular pressure. The use of a laryngeal mask airway is no longer controversial, provided it is placed correctly. Many anesthesiologists consider these to be safe and avoid a difficult intubation. They cause less rise in intraocular and arterial pressure and heart rate during both insertion and removal, and the incidence of coughing or straining at the end is much lower than following the use of an endotracheal tube.[90–93] IPPV with low inflation pressures via the laryngeal mask is used by some anesthesiologists, but the risk of pulmonary aspiration of gastric contents is ever present. An endotracheal tube should be preferred to a laryngeal mask, especially if the patient is obese, has a history of regurgitation, or has low chest compliance, or if the laryngeal mask cannot be placed correctly or does not provide a reasonable air-tight seal. Difficult intubation is quite common in the elderly, and an accurate assessment of the airway and a plan to deal with failed intubation must be in place. The preferred endotracheal tube is a "south facing" preshaped "Rae," which allows the connection, filter, and gas sampling connector to be well away from the face, and does not require a catheter mount between it and the anesthetic circuit. All connections must be "locked" to prevent disconnection during surgery and the endotracheal tube or laryngeal mask, if used, should be firmly fixed with adhesive tape to prevent dislodgement.

Maintenance of anesthesia

Anesthesia may be maintained with inhalational agents, usually using low-flow methods,[94] or by continuous intravenous propofol. All of the currently available inhalational agents, with the possible exception of nitrous oxide, cause a fall in IOP, as does propofol.[83,95] Propofol may be given by infusion using a decremental scale or the target-controlled Diprifusor.[96] Some allow spontaneous ventilation with a laryngeal mask. Although, theoretically, the potential rise in carbon dioxide tension might raise the IOP, and higher concentrations of inhalational agents are more likely to lead to hypotension, this has not been found to occur in practice.[97] Others use controlled ventilation with normocarbia or even mild hypocarbia to a level of 30 mmHg (4 kPa) aided by the administration of muscle relaxants or a remifentanil infusion. Atracurium 0.5 $mg\,kg^{-1}$ and vecuronium 0.1 $mg\,kg^{-1}$ are the most widely used relaxants, and increments or a continuous infusion may follow the loading dose if the surgery is expected to be prolonged. A nerve stimulator with train-of-four enables the depth of neuromuscular block to be monitored accurately and ensures that increments are given to prevent any sudden offset. It also allows a more accurate assessment of the level of recovery from the relaxant drug. The most important factor remains smooth anesthesia without straining or coughing. Opioid analgesics are not often required as most of the operations are of short duration and not very stimulating and their use might increase the incidence of postoperative nausea and vomiting. However, analgesics may be required for extraocular or prolonged procedures.

Recovery

Normal doses of atropine or glycopyrronium and neostigmine may be used, and neuromuscular block must be completely reversed if it has not worn off spontaneously.

Extubation should be performed without excessive coughing, although the eye is usually safe as surgical incision and suturing techniques have improved. It is difficult in practice to prevent coughing unless the endotracheal tube is removed at a deep level of anesthesia, which adds to the risk by prolonging recovery. Some might wish to place a laryngeal mask behind the endotracheal tube as this will help to maintain the airway during the period after the tube has been removed at deeper levels of anesthesia and before the patient awakes. It has been shown that an etomidate–vecuronium–isoflurane combination is superior to propofol as it produces less hypotension and more rapid recovery.[75] The newer inhalational agents, such as desflurane and sevoflurane, have lower blood–gas solubility coefficients, and therefore ensure more rapid recovery, almost independent of duration of surgery.[98] This may be an advantage in reducing the time until the patient regains his or her protective reflexes. Adequate facilities for the observation and monitoring of patients must be provided until they are fit to leave the recovery room.[99] Oxygen should be given and particular care taken to detect respiratory depression, hypoxia, and failure of adequate reversal of neuromuscular blockade, arrhythmias, or hypotension.

Postoperative analgesia

Following intraocular surgery, most patients require only simple nonsteroidal analgesics such as paracetamol and diclofenac or ibuprofen, but more complex or extraocular surgery may result in pain requiring opioids or local anesthetic blockade. Attention should also be given to the prevention or treatment of postoperative nausea and vomiting.

Other ophthalmologic procedures

Pediatric ophthalmology

Pediatric eye disease is often associated with other congenital abnormalities that may affect anesthesia. The systemic effects of drugs given for ophthalmic purposes must be understood, and doses adjusted accordingly.[100]

Small babies may require examination under anesthetic, measurement of intraocular pressure or probing and syringing of the lacrimal ducts. They are frequently admitted as day-cases and, although the procedures may seem minor, for this age group the administration of the anesthetic demands that the full skills, facilities, and equipment are available. Ketamine may be preferred if intraocular pressure is to be measured as inhalation agents and hyperventilation are all likely to result in low readings. Ketamine may be given intramuscularly in a dose of 5–10 mg kg^{-1}, or more usually 1–2 mg kg^{-1} intravenously. Most pediatric surgery will require a laryngeal mask airway as it often takes longer than predicted, or endotracheal intubation as the lacrimal system communicates with the airway via the nasolacrimal duct. Babies may also present with congenital cataracts or glaucoma, which may be treated in any eye unit, and occasionally with ocular or orbital tumors, which are usually referred to specialized centers. The details of pediatric anesthesia are outside the scope of this chapter, but basic principles apply, the airway must be secured, and the oculocardiac reflex and postoperative nausea and vomiting are more often encountered than in adults. Ondansetron 0.1 mg kg^{-1} may be the antiemetic of choice.[101] Postoperative analgesia may usually be achieved without intramuscular injections by the use of paracetamol in high dose (up to 90 mg kg^{-1} 24 h^{-1}) and a nonsteroidal anti-inflammatory agent such as diclofenac or ibuprofen, all given by syrup or suppository.

Surgery for strabismus

Surgery for strabismus may be performed at all ages, but the majority of operations are carried out in children or young adults. Increasingly, babies are subjected to surgery as the chance of binocular vision increases if the squint is corrected early. Strabismus may occur in patients with cerebral palsy or a neuromuscular disease, and the rare possibility of masseter spasm or a malignant hyperthermia susceptibility should be considered. Squint surgery usually involves shortening of one muscle (resection) and lengthening of the opposite muscle (recession). An adjustable suture may be put in during the surgery but not adjusted until the patient can cooperate in the postoperative period. The adjustment may be possible with topical local anesthetic drops only, but this is often uncomfortable for the patient, and occasionally general anesthesia is required. There is a very high incidence of pain and nausea and vomiting after surgery for strabismus, and many advocate the routine use of antiemetics such as droperidol 0.075 mg kg^{-1}, metoclopramide 0.25 mg kg^{-1}, or ondansetron 0.1 mg kg^{-1} for these patients.[102] Surgery for squint requires airway control and protection against the oculocardiac reflex, which is most often precipitated by traction on the external ocular muscles.

Oculocardiac reflex

The oculocardiac reflex, first described by Aschner in 1908, is a sinus bradycardia, occasionally with bigeminy, ectopic beats, nodal rhythm, atrioventricular block, or asystole. It may follow pressure on the eye, traction on the extraocular muscles or other manipulation of the globe, or a rise in IOP. It is most commonly seen during surgery for strabismus but may also occur during surgery for retinal detachment or enucleation, or occasionally during the insertion of a superior rectus suture. The afferent loop is via the long and short ciliary nerves along trigeminal afferents, and the efferent loop is via the vagus nerves. It will be observed on the ECG or pulse counter or from the audible slowing of the pulse detected by the oximeter, and may be very dramatic, the rate being so slow that no cardiac complexes are seen on the ECG monitor. Although the reflex tends to fatigue rapidly and vagal escape occurs, it must be identified immediately and the stimulus removed. As it may occur in up to 90% of unpremedicated children having surgery for strabismus, a vagolytic such as atropine or glycopyrronium should be available, and many would advocate their prophylactic use.[103] Suitable doses would be atropine 0.02 mg kg^{-1} or glycopyrronium 0.01 mg kg^{-1}. Very occasionally, an associated oculorespiratory reflex may manifest as shallow breathing, bradypnea, or even respiratory arrest.[104]

Corneal grafting (keratoplasty)

These operations may take 2 h and were traditionally done under general anesthesia. Increasingly, they are undertaken with regional block anesthesia. Control of IOP is essential as the eye is open for some of the procedure.

Dacrocystorhinostomy

Dacrocystorhinostomy, in which the lacrimal sac is linked to the nasal mucosa, is a common procedure for opening the blocked nasolacrimal duct.[105] Bleeding is a problem, and the nasal mucosa may be prepared with a vasoconstrictor such as cocaine or epinephrine. Cocaine is very rapidly absorbed from the nasal mucosa and should not be used in a dose greater than 1.5 mg kg^{-1} as it has a stimulating effect on the sympathetic nervous system. Care must be taken with hypertensive patients and those taking tricyclic antidepressants and monoamine oxidase inhibitors. A topical dose of epinephrine should not exceed 0.5 mg.[106] Induced hypotension may be requested, and labetalol is commonly used. A throat pack should be used to protect the lower airway from aspiration of blood.

Recently, a minimally invasive endoscopically assisted and a laser procedure, both of which may be performed under topical and infiltration anesthesia alone, has been developed.[107,108]

Oculoplastic surgery

Oculoplastic operations on the lids are common and may be performed under local or general anesthesia. Most operations can be performed with infiltration local rather than nerve block anesthesia, and a safe dose of local anesthetic must not be exceeded. The local anesthetic is usually combined with epinephrine to reduce absorption and induce vasoconstriction. Sedation is often needed for younger patients, who are more likely to be anxious. If general anesthesia is required, it follows standard principles, bearing in mind that most of the procedures will be suitable for day-case surgery.

Orbital decompression and tumors

Orbital decompression operations may be required for the treatment of exophthalmos in patients with thyroid overactivity or for the removal of tumors. These operations may be associated with considerable blood loss and may require fluid replacement. The surgeon may request hypotensive anesthesia. The oculocardiac reflex may occur. Scanning may be required in the diagnostic phase and radiotherapy, which may be indicated for tumors and for children, will usually necessitate repeated general anesthesia. Special arrangements are required to allow the anesthesiologist to be outside the treatment area but able to observe the child and the monitors, and to return if necessary.

Vitreoretinal surgery

Vitreoretinal surgery is mostly performed under general anesthesia because of the duration of the surgery, but local anesthesia, which reduces the incidence of nausea and vomiting and postoperative pain, is increasingly used, alone or in combination with general anesthesia.[109–113] Factors to take into account are the longer duration of surgery, which is often repeated, the use of darkened operating room, and the possible administration of intraocular gas. Very insoluble gases such as sulfur hexafluoride may be injected to tamponade the retinal tear, and are retained for several days. The importance is that if nitrous oxide, which is 117 times more soluble than sulfur hexafluoride, is used, it will diffuse into the gas bubble, enlarging it up to three times.[114] This may compromise retinal blood flow. When the nitrous oxide is discontinued it will diffuse out of the bubble and there may be a sudden drop in IOP, and the tamponade effect of the bubble will cease. One solution is to avoid nitrous oxide altogether, by using total intravenous anesthesia with, for example, infusions of propofol and remifentanil and an air–oxygen mixture. Another is to discontinue the nitrous oxide at least 20 min before the gas is injected and to avoid the use of nitrous oxide within 5 days of a previous intravitreous air bubble or within 3–4 weeks of a sulfur hexafluoride injection. The patient may need to be kept in a particular position in the postoperative period to keep the bubble pressing on the detachment area.

Emergency ophthalmic surgery

Most injuries in the orbital region do not involve intraocular structures. Few require immediate surgery, and there is usually time for full assessment and preparation. Sometimes there are associated injuries, which require urgent intervention, and the eye injury should be considered in the choice of anesthetic technique and drugs. Local anesthesia may be considered, but if the pressure rises there is an increased potential for expulsion of intraocular contents.

Patients with injuries that penetrate the globe may require urgent surgery and are likely to have a "full stomach." Aspiration prophylaxis with antacids and an H_2-receptor antagonist should be used. The anesthesia technique employed has to achieve early airway protection from the risk of aspiration of gastric contents without causing a rise in IOP, vitreous loss, and further damage to the eye. A dilemma surrounds the need for succinylcholine, which is known to cause a rise in IOP but is considered to be an essential feature of the rapid sequence induction on account of its rapid onset, excellent intubating conditions, and short duration. There is little evidence that the transient rise in pressure [6–12 mmHg (0.8–1.6 kPa) for about 5 min] that follows succinylcholine is in fact detrimental to the eye, and laryngoscopy and intubation under light anesthesia will themselves raise the IOP more significantly. Attempts to reduce the harmful effects of succinylcholine include a priming dose of succinylcholine or pretreatment with diazepam or lidocaine, but these are not reliable. A review of 63 penetrating eye injuries failed to show any harmful effects when succinylcholine was used following pretreatment with a small dose of a nondepolarizing relaxant.[115] More recently, the combination of propofol and alfentanil prior to succinylcholine prevented a significant rise in IOP following intubation.[116] If succinylcholine is to be avoided, the patient must be intubated after administration of a nondepolarizing relaxant, such as vecuronium 0.2 mg kg^{-1}.[117] Rocuronium 1.0–1.5 mg kg^{-1} might be considered to be a better relaxant with a shorter onset time of about 1 min. The rise in IOP was less than with succinylcholine, and the intubating conditions at 1 min were the same.[118] However, the paralysis will last for about 1 h. Particular care must be taken if a difficult intubation is predicted or the patient also has other significant injuries, and a plan should be drawn up, carefully weighing up the advantages and disadvantages of the possible choices. Extubation should be carried out in the lateral position to reduce the risk of aspiration of gastric contents with the operated eye uppermost .

Anesthesia-related eye injuries

Iatrogenic eye injuries mostly relate to corneal injuries, of which 16% are permanent.[119] The anesthetized cornea must be protected by closing the eye and by padding it until sensation and motor function have returned. Damage to the eye may be associated with unexpected patient movement when instruments are in the eye. Serious sight-threatening injury may result with increased levels of patient financial compensation.

REFERENCES

1. Fisher SJ, Cunningham RD. The medical profile of cataract patients. *Clin Geriat Med* 1985; **1:** 339–44.
2. McKibbin M. The pre-operative assessment and investigation of ophthalmic patients. *Eye* 1996; **10:** 138–40.
3. Desai, P, Reidy, A, Minassian DC. Profile of patients presenting for cataract surgery in the UK: national data collection. *Br J Ophthalmol* 1999; **83:** 893–6.
4. Campbell DN, Lim M, Muir MK, *et al.* A prospective randomised study of local versus general anaesthesia for cataract surgery. *Anaesthesia* 1993; **48:** 422–8.
5. Barker JP, Robinson PN, Vafidis GC, *et al.* Local analgesia prevents the cortisol and glycaemic responses to cataract surgery. *Br J Anaesth* 1990; **64:** 442–5.
6. Barker JP, Vafidis GC, Robinson PN, *et al.* The metabolic and hormonal response to cataract surgery. A comparison between retrobulbar and peribulbar blockade. *Anaesthesia* 1993; **48:** 488–91.
7. Vohra SB, Good PA. Altered globe dimensions of axial myopia as risk factors for penetrating ocular injury during peribulbar anaesthesia. *Br J Anaesth* 2000; **85:** 242–5
8. Thind, GS, Rubin AP. Local anesthesia for surgery – no room for complacency. *Br J Anaesth* 2001; **86:** 473–6.

9. Kearon C, Hirsh J. Management of anticoagulation before and after elective surgery. *N Engl J Med* 1997; **336:** 1506–11.
10. Koopmans SA, van Rij G. Cataract surgery and anticoagulants. *Documenta Ophthalmol* 1996–7; **92:** 11–16.
11. The Royal College of Ophthalmologists and the Royal College of Anaesthetists. *Local Anaesthesia for Intraocular Surgery*. London, 2001.
12. Roberts CW, Woods SM, Turner LS. Cataract surgery in anticoagulated patients. *J Cataract Refractive Surg* 1991; **17:** 309–12.
13. Walters G, McKibbin M. The value of pre-operative investigations in local anaesthetic ophthalmic surgery. *Eye* 1997; **11:** 847–9.
14. Munro J, Booth A, Nicholl J. Routine pre-operative testing: a systematic review of the evidence. *Hlth Technol Assess* 1997; **1** (12).
15. Schein OD, Katz J, Bass EB, *et al.* The value of routine preoperative medical testing before cataract surgery. Study of Medical Testing for Cataract surgery. *N Engl J Med* 2000; **342:** 168–75.
16. Maltby J, Hamilton RC. Preoperative fasting guidelines for cataract surgery under regional anaesthesia. *Br J Anaesth* 1993; **71:** 167.
17. Steeds C, Mather SJ. Fasting regimes for regional ophthalmic anaesthesia: a survey of members of the British Ophthalmic Anaesthesia Society. *Anaesthesia* 2001; **56:** 638–42.
18. Eke T, Thompson JR. The National Survey of Local Anaesthesia for Ocular Surgery. 1. Survey methodology and current practice. *Eye* 1999; **13:** 189–95.
19. Wong DH, Merrick PM. Intravenous sedation prior to peribulbar anaesthesia for cataract surgery in elderly patients. *Can J Anesth* 1996; **43:** 1115–20.
20. Herrick IA, Gelb AW, Nichols B, Kirkby J. Patient-controlled propofol sedation for elderly patients: safety and patient attitude towards control. *Can J Anesth* 1996; **43:** 1014–18.
21. Fanning GL. Sedation techniques. *Ophthalmol Clin N Am* 1998; **11:** 73–85.
22. Ropo A, Nikki P, Ruusuvaara P, Kivisaari L. Comparison of retrobulbar and periocular injections of lignocaine by computerised tomography. *Br J Ophthalmol* 1991; **75:** 417–20.
23. Grabow HB. Topical anesthesia for cataract surgery. *Eur J Implant Refractive Surg* 1993; **5:** 200–1.
24. Fichman RA. Topical anesthesia. *Ophthalmol Clin N Am* 1998; **11:** 125–6.
25. Gills JP, Cherchio M, Raanan MG. Unpreserved lidocaine to control discomfort during cataract surgery using topical anesthesia. *J Cataract Refractive Surg* 1997; **23:** 545–50.
26. Koch PS. Anterior chamber irrigation with unpreserved lidocaine 1% for anesthesia during cataract surgery. *J Cataract Refractive Surg* 1997; **23:** 551–4.
27. Rosenthal KJ. Deep, topical, nerve block anesthesia. *J Cataract Refractive Surg* 1995; **21:** 499–503.
28. Assia EI, Pras E, Yehezkel M, *et al.* Topical anesthesia using lidocaine gel for cataract surgery. *J Cataract and Refractive Surg* 1999; **25:** 635–9.
29. Petersen WC, Yanoff M. Subconjunctival anesthesia: an alternative to retrobulbar and peribulbar techniques. *Ophthalmic Surg* 1991; **22:** 199–201.
30. Yanoff M, Redovan EG. Anterior eyewall perforation during subconjunctival cataract block. *Ophthalmic Surg* 1990; **21:** 362–3.
31. Stevens JD. A new local anaesthesia technique for cataract extraction by one quadrant sub-Tenon's infiltration. *Br J Ophthalmol* 1992; **76:** 670–4.
32. Bergman L, Berglin L, Algvere PV, *et al.* Limbal sub-Tenon's administration of retrobulbar anesthesia using a blunt irrigating cannula. *Ophthalmic Surg Lasers* 1996; **27:** 106–12.
33. Winder S, Walker SB, Atta HR. Ultrasonic localization of anesthetic fluid in sub-Tenon's, peribulbar, and retrobulbar techniques. *J Cataract Refractive Surg* 1999; **25:** 56–9.
34. Kapran Z, Uyar M, Eltutar K, Dincer N. One quadrant sub-Tenon's capsule anesthesia in anterior segment surgery. *Eur J Ophthalmol* 1996; **6:** 131–6.
35. Khoo BK, Lim TH, Yong V. Sub-Tenon's versus retrobulbar anesthesia for cataract surgery. *Ophthalmic Surg Lasers* 1996; **27:** 773–7.
36. Buttery R, Wise G. Conal anaesthesia: a new approach to retrobulbar anaesthesia. *Austral NZ J Ophthalmol* 1989; **17:** 63–9.
37. Meyer D, Hamilton RC, Loken RG, Gimbel HV. Effect of combined peribulbar and retrobulbar injection of large volumes of anesthetic agents on the intraocular pressure. *Can J Ophthalmol* 1992; **27:** 230–2.
38. Unsold R, Stanley JA, DeGroot J. The CT-topography of retrobulbar anesthesia. Anatomic–clinical correlation of complications and suggestion of a modified technique. *Albrecht von Graefes Archiv Klin Exp Ophthalmol* 1981; **217:** 125–36.
39. Sweeney EJ, Barber K, Prosser JA. A comparison of percutaneous and perconjunctival routes of administration of peri-ocular anaesthesia for day case cataract surgery. *Anaesthesia* 1993; **48:** 336–8.
40. Katsev DA, Drews RC, Rose BT. An anatomic study of retrobulbar needle path length. *Ophthalmology* 1989; **96:** 1221–4.
41. Callahan A. Ultrasharp disposable needles. *Am J Ophthalmol* 1966; **62:** 173.
42. Waller SG, Taboada J, O'Connor P. Retrobulbar anesthesia risk. Do sharp needles really perforate the eye more easily than blunt needles? *Ophthalmology* 1993; **100:** 506–10.
43. Bowman R, Liu C, Sarkies N. Intraocular pressure changes after peribulbar injections with and without ocular compression. *Br J Ophthalmol* 1996; **80:** 394–7.
44. Hustead, RF, Hamilton, RC, Loken, RG. Periocular local anesthesia: medial orbital as an alternative to superior nasal injection. *J Cataract Refractive Surg* 1994; **20:** 197–201.
45. Davis II DB, Mandel MR. Posterior peribulbar anesthesia: an alternative to retrobulbar anesthesia. *J Cataract Refractive Surg* 1986; **12:** 182–4.
46. Davis II DB, Mandel MR. Efficacy and complication rate of 16,224 consecutive peribulbar blocks. A prospective multicenter trial. *J Cataract Refractive Surg* 1994; **20:** 327–37.
47. Hamilton RC, Gimbel HV, Strunin L. Regional anesthesia for 12,000 cataract extraction and intraocular lens implantation procedures. *Can J Anesth* 1988; **35:** 615–23.
48. Joshi N, Reynolds A, Porter EJ, *et al.* An assessment of intraocular pressure during fractionated peribulbar block. *Eye* 1996; **10:** 565–8.
49. Brahma AK, Pemberton CJ, Ayeko M, Morgan LH. Single medial injection peribulbar anaesthesia using prilocaine. *Anaesthesia* 1994; **49:** 1003–5.
50. Ripart J, Lefrant J, Lalourcey L, *et al.* Medial canthus (caruncle) single injection periocular anesthesia. *Anesth Analg* 1996; **83:** 1234–8.
51. Oji E, Oji A. Bupivacaine and lignocaine for ophthalmic surgery. *Br J Ophthalmol* 1987; **71:** 66–8.
52. Coelho ET, Gomes EB, Martins HS, de Sousa B. Prilocaine: an old anesthetic agent and a new ophthalmic procedure. *Ophthalmic Surg* 1993; **24:** 612–16.
53. Henderson TR, Franks W. Peribulbar anaesthesia for cataract surgery: prilocaine versus lignocaine and bupivacaine. *Eye* 1996; **10:** 497–500.
54. Dorey SE, Gillespie IH, Barton F, MacSweeney E. Magnetic resonance image changes following optic nerve trauma from peribulbar anaesthesia. *Br J Ophthalmol* 1998; **82:** 586–748.
55. Nicoll JM, Treuren B, Acharya PA, *et al.* Retrobulbar anesthesia: the role of hyaluronidase. *Anesth Analg* 1986; **65:** 1324–8.
56. Abelson MB, Mandel E, Paradis A, George M. The effect of hyaluronidase on akinesia during cataract surgery. *Ophthalmic Surg* 1989; **20:** 325–6.
57. Bowman RJ, Newman DK, Richardson EC, *et al.* Is hyaluronidase helpful for peribulbar anaesthesia? *Eye* 1997; **11:** 385–8.
58. Gillart T, Bazin JE, Brandely C, *et al.* Effects of local clonidine for prolongation of akinesia after peribulbar block. *Anesthesiology* 1994; **81:** A941.
59. McLure HA, Rubin AP. Comparison of 0.75% levobupivacaine with 0.75% racemic bupivacaine for peribulbar anesthesia. *Anaesthesia* 1998; **53:** 1160–4.
60. Huha T, Ala-Kokko TI, Salomaki T, Alahuhta S. Clinical efficacy and pharmacokinetics of 1% ropivacaine and 0.75% bupivacaine in peribulbar anaesthesia for cataract surgery. *Anaesthesia* 1999; **54:** 137–41.
61. McLure HA, Rubin AP, Westcott M, Henderson H. A comparison of 1% ropivacaine with a mixture of 0.75% bupivacaine and 2% lignocaine for peribulbar anaesthesia. *Anaesthesia* 1999; **54:** 1178–82.
62. Zahl K, Jordan A, Sorensen B, Gotta AW. pH-adjusted lidocaine/bupivacaine mixture are superior for peribulbar anesthesia. *Anesthesiology* 1988; **69:** A368.
63. Zahl K, Jordan A, McCroarty J, Gotta AW. pH-adjusted bupivacaine and hyaluronidase for peribulbar block. *Anesthesiology* 1990; **72:** 230–2.
64. Risdall JE, Geraghty IF. Oxygenation of patients undergoing ophthalmic surgery under local anaesthesia. *Anaesthesia* 1997; **52:** 492–495.
65. Edge KR, Nicoll JM. Retrobulbar haemorrhage after 12,500 retrobulbar blocks. *Anesth Analg* 1993; **76:** 1019–22.
66. Kraushar MF. Seelenfreund MH. Freilich DB. Central retinal artery closure during orbital hemorrhage from retrobular injection. *Trans Am Acad Ophthalmol Otolaryngol* 1974; **78:** 65–70.
67. Duker JS, Belmont JB, Benson WE, *et al.* Inadvertent globe perforation during retrobulbar and peribulbar anesthesia. Patient characteristics, surgical management and visual outcome. *Ophthalmology* 1991; **98:** 519–26.
68. Martin XD. Normal intraocular pressure in man. *Ophthalmologica* 1992; **205:** 57–63.
69. Pensiero S, Da Pozzo S, Perrissutti P, *et al.* Normal intraocular pressure in children. *J Pediat Ophthalmol Strabismus* 1992; **29:** 79–84.

70. Samuel JR, Beaugie A. Effect of carbon dioxide on the intraocular pressure in man during general anaesthesia. *Br J Ophthalmol* 1974; **58:** 62–7.
71. Jantzen JP. Anaesthesia and intraocular pressure *Anaesthesist* 1988; **37:** 458–69.
72. Solomon R, Liu C, Sarkies N. IOP changes after peribulbar injection with or without compression. *Br J Ophthalmol* 1996; **80:** 394–7.
73. McGoldrick KE. Ocular drugs and anesthesia. *Int Anesthesiol Clin* 1990; **28:** 72–7.
74. Malhotra R, Banerjee G, Brampton W, Price NC. Comparison of the cardiovascular effects of 2.5% phenylephrine and 10% phenylephrine during ophthalmic surgery. *Eye* 1998; **12:** 973–5.
75. Moffatt A, Cullen PM. Comparison of two standard techniques of general anaesthesia for day-case cataract surgery. *Br J Anaesth* 1995; **74:** 145–8.
76. Milaskiewicz RM, Hall GM. Diabetes and anaesthesia: the past decade. *Br J Anaesth* 1992; **68:** 198–206.
77. Tiret L, Desmonts JM, Hatton F, Vourc'h G. Complications associated with anaesthesia – a prospective survey in France. *Can Anesth Soc J* 1986; **33:** 336–44.
78. Cozanitis DA, Dundee JW, Buchanan TAS, Archer DB. Atropine versus glycopyrrolate. A study of intraocular pressure and pupil size in man. *Anaesthesia* 1979; **34:** 236–8.
79. The Royal College of Anaesthetists. *Guidelines for the Provision of Anaesthetic Services.* London: The Royal College of Anaesthetists, 1999.
80. Association of Anaesthetists of Great Britain and Ireland. *Recommendations for Standards of Monitoring during Anaesthesia and Recovery.* London: Association of Anaesthetists of Great Britain and Ireland, 2000.
81. Mirakhur RK, Shepherd WF, Darrah WC. Propofol or thiopentone: effects on intraocular pressure associated with induction of anaesthesia and tracheal intubation (facilitated with suxamethonium). *Br J Anaesth* 1987; **59:** 431–6.
82. Mirakhur RK, Elliott P, Shepherd WF, Archer DB. Intraocular pressure changes during induction of anaesthesia and tracheal intubation. A comparison of thiopentone and propofol followed by vecuronium. *Anaesthesia* 1988; **43** (Suppl.): 54–7.
83. Guedes Y, Rakotoseheno JC, Leveque M, *et al.* Changes in intraocular pressure in the elderly during anaesthesia with propofol. *Anaesthesia* 1988; **43** (Suppl.): 58–60.
84. Cook JH. The effect of suxamethonium on intraocular pressure. *Anaesthesia* 1981; **36:** 359–65.
85. Lavery GG, McGalliard JN, Mirakhur RK, Shepherd WF. The effects of atracurium on intraocular pressure during steady state anaesthesia and rapid sequence induction: a comparison with succinylcholine. *Can Anesth Soc J* 1986; **33:** 437–42.
86. Robertson EN, Hull JM, Verbeek AM, Booij LH. A comparison of rocuronium and vecuronium: the pharmacodynamic, cardiovascular and intra-ocular effects. *Eur J Anaesthesiol* 1994; Suppl. 9: 116–21.
87. Jaakola ML, Ali-Melkkila T, Kanto J, *et al.* Dexmedetomidine reduces intraocular pressure, intubation responses and anaesthetic requirements in patients undergoing ophthalmic surgery. *Br J Anaesth* 1992; **68:** 570–5.
88. Mostafa SM, Lockhart A, Kumar D, Bayoumi M. Comparison of effects of fentanyl and alfentanil on intra-ocular pressure. A double-blind controlled trial. *Anaesthesia* 1986; **41:** 493–8.
89. Mostafa SM, Murthy BV, Barrett PJ, McHugh P. Comparison of the effects of topical lignocaine spray applied before or after induction of anaesthesia on the pressor response to direct laryngoscopy and intubation. *Eur J Anaesthesiol* 1999; **16:** 7–10.
90. Lamb K, James MF, Janicki PK. The laryngeal mask airway for intraocular surgery: effects on intraocular pressure and stress responses. *Br J Anaesth* 1992; **69:** 143–7.
91. Holden R, Morsman CD, Butler J, *et al.* Intra-ocular pressure changes using the laryngeal mask airway and tracheal tube. *Anaesthesia* 1991; **46:** 922–4.
92. Akhtar TM, McMurray P, Kerr WJ, Kenny GN. A comparison of laryngeal mask airway with tracheal tube for intra-ocular ophthalmic surgery. *Anaesthesia* 1992; **47:** 668–71.
93. Denny NM, Gadelrab R. Complications following general anaesthesia for cataract surgery: a comparison of the laryngeal mask airway with tracheal intubation. *J Roy Soc Med* 1993; **86:** 521–2.
94. Suttner S, Boldt J. Low-flow anaesthesia. Does it have potential pharmacoeconomic consequences? *Pharmacoeconomics* 2000; **17:** 585–90.
95. Holloway KB. Control of the eye during general anaesthesia for intraocular surgery. *Br J Anaesth* 1980; **52:** 671–9.
96. Sutcliffe NP, Hyde R, Martay K. Use of 'Diprifusor' in anaesthesia for ophthalmic surgery. *Anaesthesia* 1998; Suppl. 53: 49–52.
97. Myint Y, Singh AK, Peacock JE, Padfield A. Changes in intra-ocular pressure during general anaesthesia. A comparison of spontaneous breathing through a laryngeal mask with positive pressure ventilation through a tracheal tube. *Anaesthesia* 1995; **50:** 126–9.
98. Bailey JM. Context-sensitive half-times and other decrement times of inhaled anesthetics. *Anesth Analg* 1997; **85:** 681–6.
99. Yee DA, Rose DK, Cohen MM, Rogers KH. Recovery room events in eye patients: Should it influence your technique? *Can J Anesth* 1990; **37:** S80.
100. Palmer EA. How safe are ocular drugs in pediatrics? *Ophthalmology* 1986; **93:** 1038–40.
101. Davis PJ, McGowan Jr FX, Landsman I, *et al.* Effect of antiemetic therapy on recovery and hospital discharge time. A double-blind assessment of ondansetron, droperidol and placebo in pediatric patients undergoing ambulatory surgery. *Anesthesiology* 1995; **83:** 956–60.
102. Tramer M, Moore A, McQuay H. Prevention of vomiting after paediatric strabismus surgery: a systematic review using the numbers-to-treat method. *Br J Anaesth* 1995; **75:** 556–61.
103. Mirakhur RK, Jones CJ, Dundee JW, Archer DB. I.m. or i.v atropine or glycopyrrolate for the prevention of the oculocardiac reflex in children undergoing squint surgery. *Br J Anaesth* 1982; **54:** 1059–63.
104. Blanc VF, Jacob JL, Milot J, Cyrenne L. The oculorespiratory reflex revisited. *Can J Anesth* 1988; **35:** 468–72.
105. Tarbet KJ, Custger PL. External dacrocystorhinostomy. Surgical success, patient satisfaction, and economic cost. *Ophthalmology* 1995; **102:** 1065–70.
106. Nicholson KE, Rogers JE. Cocaine and adrenaline paste: a fatal combination? *Br Med J* 1995; **311:** 250–1.
107. Metson R, Woog JJ, Puliafito CA. Endoscopic laser dacrocystorhinostomy. *Laryngoscope* 1994; **104:** 269–74.
108. Szubin L, Papageorge A, Sacks E. Endonasal laser-assisted dacrocystorhinostomy. *Am J Rhinol* 1999; **13:** 371–4.
109. Benedetti S, Agostini A. Peribulbar anaesthesia in vitreoretinal surgery. *Retina* 1994; **14:** 277–80.
110. Brucker AJ, Saran BR, Maguire AM. Perilimbal anesthesia for pars plana vitrectomy. *Am J Ophthalmol* 1994; **117:** 599–602.
111. Gottfreothsdottir MS, Gislason I, Stefansson E, *et al.* Effects of retrobulbar bupivacaine on post-operative pain and nausea in retinal detachment surgery. *Acta Ophthalmol* 1993; **71:** 544–7.
112. Murat J, Chauvaud D. Evaluation of a simplified protocol of local regional anesthesia for the surgery of the posterior segment. *J Francais d'Ophthalmol* 1993; **16:** 254–8.
113. Simcock PR, Raymond GL, Lavin MJ, Whitley CJ. Combined peribulbar injection and blunt cannula infiltration for vitreoretinal surgery. *Ophthal Surg* 1994; **25:** 232–235.
114. Stinson TW III, Donlon JV Jr. Interaction of intraocular air and sulfur hexafluoride with nitrous oxide: a computer simulation. *Anesthesiology* 1982; **56:** 385–8.
115. Libonati MM, Leahy JJ, Ellison N. The use of succinylcholine in open eye surgery. *Anesthesiology* 1985; **62:** 637–40.
116. Zimmerman AA, Funk KJ, Tidwell JL. Propofol and alfentanil prevent the increase in intraocular pressure caused by succinylcholine and endotracheal intubation during a rapid sequence induction of anesthesia. *Anesth Analg* 1996; **83:** 814–17.
117. Abbott, MA, Samuel JR. The control of intra-ocular pressure during the induction of anaesthesia for emergency eye surgery. A high-dose vecuronium technique. *Anaesthesia* 1987; **42:** 1008–12.
118. Chiu CL, Jaias F, Wang CY. Effect of rocuronium compared with succinylcholine on intraocular pressure during rapid sequence induction of anaesthesia. *Br J Anaesth* 1999; **82:** 757–60.
119. Gild WM, Posner KL, Caplan RA, Cheney FW. Eye injuries associated with anesthesia: a closed claims analysis. *Anesthesiology* 1992; **76:** 204–8.

52

Anesthesia for patients with renal disease

JENNIFER M HUNTER

Anesthesia for patients with renal dysfunction has become commonplace since the advent of renal transplantation 40 years ago, but such patients may also require anesthesia for unrelated conditions and, therefore, present on any operating room list. Particularly if they have had renal dysfunction for several years, their medical history may be complex, and many systems may be affected. It is therefore important to take a full preoperative history and make an examination and to evaluate the drug therapy, which is often complex, that the patient is receiving. This chapter discusses the chronic dialysis techniques available to renal patients and the medical complications which these patients may suffer. The chapter will outline the preoperative preparation required and suggest the most appropriate anesthetic techniques to employ. It will deal mainly with the patient in end-stage renal failure undergoing supportive dialysis treatment, although the same basic principles are applicable to the patient with deteriorating renal function who has not yet reached this stage.

CHRONIC DIALYSIS TECHNIQUES

Patients in end-stage renal failure are either maintained on hemodialysis for periods of 4–6 h two or three times per week or use continuous ambulatory peritoneal dialysis (CAPD). Hemodialysis removes fluid and metabolic products from the plasma, replacing these with isotonic fluid and, if necessary, blood or plasma. The patient uses either an arteriovenous fistula in the arm or a prosthetic vein graft to connect up to the hemodialysis machine by an indwelling cannula. For short-term purposes, a two-channel central venous line may be inserted into a subclavian or jugular vein.

CAPD involves the insertion of a peritoneal dialysis catheter, which must be cared for daily using a strict aseptic technique. The patient slowly runs three or four 1-L bags of dextrose solution (1.36%) into the peritoneal cavity every 24 h, draining the fluid out before a new bag is commenced. The regular introduction of fluid into the peritoneal cavity irritates the omentum, increasing tissue vascularity. This produces a large area for the passive diffusion of the products of metabolism from the plasma into the peritoneal fluid. CAPD is easier for the patient than hemodialysis, allowing more freedom to travel, and is a much cheaper maintenance therapy. It has become a popular method of dialysis. Insulin can be added to the liter bags in diabetic patients, producing better control of blood sugar than intermittent injections. Excess fluid can be removed from the patient by the use of one high-osmolality dextrose (3.86%) bag every 24 h.

The main disadvantage of CAPD is the risk of peritonitis; adhesions form around the omentum, decreasing the efficacy of the technique. For this reason, a partial omentectomy is sometimes performed during surgical insertion of a CAPD catheter. If the infection cannot be cleared, resort must be made to hemodialysis. Because it is cheaper, CAPD has allowed more patients access to maintenance therapy. It is particularly useful in the elderly with cardiovascular disease, when hemodialysis may cause large swings in blood pressure and possibly induce attacks of angina.[1] CAPD has been shown to be as efficient as hemodialysis.[2]

MEDICAL PROBLEMS OF PATIENTS WITH RENAL DISEASE

Cardiovascular

Hypertension

Over 50% of adult patients with renal disease need treatment for hypertension, which is thought to be caused in part by excess renin production from the diseased kidney.[3] The increased blood pressure is often resistant to drug therapy and the patient may be taking two or more antihypertensives. Calcium antagonists, such as nifedipine and diltiazem, are frequently employed, as are β-blocking drugs, usually those with specific β_1-blocking properties such as atenolol or acebutalol. Angiotensin-converting enzyme (ACE) inhibitors such as captopril and enalapril have become increasingly popular in the management of patients with renal dysfunction, although, as these drugs are excreted in part through the kidney, the dose should be decreased. Vasodilators such as hydralazine may also be used, although this particular drug is better reserved for intravenous use in the acute state because of the high risk of side-effects when used chronically (e.g. symptoms similar to systemic lupus erythematosus). Hypertension is thought to be less marked in dialysis patients who have had bilateral nephrectomy, possibly because of the subsequent absence of renin production following removal of the kidneys.

The patient with renal dysfunction occasionally suffers from hypertension due to renal artery stenosis, especially if the patient has had a renal transplant. Hypertension from this cause is particularly difficult to treat with drug therapy; indeed, ACE inhibitors are recognized to precipitate a deterioration in renal function in these circumstances.[3] The possibility of renal artery stenosis being the cause of an intractable rise in blood pressure should be excluded using radiological techniques. It may be possible, if there is a stenosis, to perform an angioplasty. This is an invaluable radiologic technique as surgical intervention in such cases, although increasingly common, can be hazardous.[4] The difficulty in controlling the very high and labile blood pressure leads to a significant risk of a cerebrovascular accident during the perioperative period.

Peripheral vascular disease is also more common, and occurs at an earlier age, in patients with renal dysfunction.

Myocardial infarction

Myocardial infarction is 10 times more common in the renal transplant patient than in the general population of the same age and sex.[5] Episodes of angina are frequent, and intercurrent anemia is usually a contributory cause (see below). Myocardial arrhythmias may also follow and may be exacerbated by metabolic problems such as hyper- and hypokalemia and hypocalcemia.

Pulmonary edema

Pulmonary edema is a common problem in the patient with renal dysfunction for two reasons. First, the patient may simply be overloaded with fluid which he/she is unable to clear through the diseased kidney. The fluid therefore enters the interstitial tissues from the overloaded intravascular compartment; the process is potentiated by hypoproteinemia. Increased ventricular filling pressures lead to left heart failure and pulmonary edema.

Second, acute pulmonary edema may develop as a consequence of a myocardial infarction or myocardial ischemia, which are frequent incidents during the perioperative period in the renal patient.[5] More than half of renal failure patients presenting for transplantation are also in congestive (right) heart failure.[6]

Pericarditis

Pericarditis is not uncommon in patients with renal dysfunction and is sometimes accompanied by a pericardial effusion. Such problems are more common in the poorly controlled patient, who is overloaded with fluid, and can occur in the absence of infection. Such clinical signs must be taken seriously and anesthesia should, if possible, be delayed until the causal condition has been treated because of the risk of severe myocardial depression per- and postoperatively.

Biochemical

Potassium

Decreased excretion of this mainly intracellular electrolyte in the patient with compromised renal function frequently results in a chronic rise in total body potassium, which is largely resistant to drug therapy. Glucose and insulin or calcium resonium often induce only a transient improvement. The patient who presents for surgery with a high serum potassium should be dialyzed before anesthesia is induced. Surgical trauma, succinylcholine (suxamethonium), and hypercarbia all cause the serum potassium to rise, possibly at very fast rates, with the risk of cardiac arrhythmias and even ventricular fibrillation during surgery. High concentrations of potassium in some of the older preservation fluids used for transport of cadaveric kidneys (e.g. Collin's solution) could also induce hyperkalemia sufficient to cause cardiac arrest during renal transplantation.[7]

Higher plasma potassium levels are usually seen in patients on peritoneal rather than hemodialysis, probably because the technique is slightly less efficient.

Hypokalemia is unusual in the patient with renal dysfunction; it may be due to fluid overload in the anephric patient or to loop diuretics in the patient who still produces urine or has recently had a renal transplant. It must be remembered that nondepolarizing neuromuscular blocking drugs are potentiated by hypokalemia.

Sodium

Sodium is mainly an extracellular cation, in contrast with potassium. The serum level is therefore a more accurate estimate of the total body content. With proper dietary control of intake, and appropriate diuretic and dialysis therapy if necessary, the serum sodium can be managed easily. A rise in serum sodium is usually an indication of dehydration, rather than an excess of sodium ions; a fall is usually due to fluid retention, caused by excessive fluid intake and/or inadequate dialysis.

Calcium and phosphate

Patients with renal failure usually suffer from hypocalcemia and hyperphosphatemia, sometimes accompanied by the deposition of calcium in body tissues, in particular blood vessels. Heavily calcified arteries may be seen throughout the body on radiography and the coronary arteries may be involved. Affected vessels lose their power of autoregulation; patients with widespread vessel calcification are often intractably hypertensive and at high risk of myocardial infarction.

In contrast, the patient with a functioning renal transplant may develop hypercalcemia and hypophosphatemia in response to hypertrophy of the parathyroid glands and release of excess parathyroid hormone – *tertiary hyperparathyroidism*.[8] Hypercalcemia potentiates acetylcholine release from the presynaptic vesicles in the neuromuscular junction; thus, it potentiates neuromuscular transmission and decreases the potency of nondepolarizing neuromuscular blocking drugs, making adequate relaxation difficult to achieve when such patients present for surgery such as parathyroidectomy. Hypocalcemia, in contrast, by impairing acetylcholine release, might potentiate neuromuscular block.

Aluminum and magnesium

Although aluminum is not present in the body in large amounts, it can accumulate in those patients who are in chronic renal failure, especially if they are undergoing regular hemodialysis in an area with a high aluminum content in the tap water. This is more common in hard water, which contains a larger amount of aluminum salts. As patients with renal disease are also more prone to increased gastric acidity, they often consume large amounts of antacids. If these contain aluminum, for example aluminum trisilicate, then the plasma level may also rise. Aluminum may be deposited in the brain, causing confusion[9] and even epileptic fits. It decreases myocardial contractility and, in contrast with calcium, release of acetylcholine from the presynaptic membrane is reduced. Thus, neuromuscular block might be expected to be potentiated.

An excess of *magnesium* ions, also consumed in antacid therapy, may produce similar effects.

Acid–base changes

Renal impairment is associated with a failure to adequately excrete hydrogen ions. Accumulation results in a fall in intra- and extracellular pH, thus decreasing myocardial contractility and renal blood flow. The entry of hydrogen ions into the cell is accompanied by the movement of potassium ions out of the cells into the plasma, causing a further rise in serum potassium. Plasma bicarbonate levels fall – a useful indication of the severity of disease and of inadequate dialysis.

Glucose

The decreased excretion of glucose by the diseased kidney makes control of blood glucose difficult, especially in the insulin-dependent diabetic patient in renal failure or in the patient receiving drugs which increase blood glucose, e.g. corticosteroid therapy. Hyperglycemia increases the risk of infection in the postoperative patient. This is in part the reason why, before the advent of the immunosuppressant drug cyclosporine (cyclosporin A), when steroid therapy was commonplace, renal transplantation was less successful in the diabetic patient. A rise in blood sugar may be accompanied by a rise in serum potassium, making cardiac arrhythmias more likely.[10]

The diabetic patient in renal failure will probably have significant cardiac disease. These patients are at increased risk during anesthesia and need detailed preoperative assessment (see below). They may also have impairment of vision and, because of this, more effort is required to explain the details of anesthesia and surgery.

Albumin

Plasma albumin levels are often reduced in patients with renal disease. This may be due to hemodilution, to impaired synthesis if the patient is catabolic or malnourished, to an increased loss of protein through the diseased nephron, or to combinations of these factors. Alterations in plasma albumin may alter the degree of binding of many drugs. This is particularly relevant with drugs that are highly protein bound (98% or more), such as warfarin, diazepam, and phenytoin. Here, only 2% or less of the drug in the plasma is unbound, and thus free to have an effect. A small decrease in plasma albumin, and thus drug binding, can cause a significant increase in free drug available. An increase in unbound drug from 2% to 3% represents a 50% increase, and therefore markedly potentiates the drug effect. Most anesthetic agents are not predominantly bound to plasma albumin: neuromuscular blocking drugs are mainly bound to plasma globulins, although not to a significant degree.[11]

Hematologic

Anemia

Patients with renal disease are commonly anemic. The anemia is of the normochromic, normocytic type and is unresponsive to oral iron therapy. It is more severe in patients on hemodialysis than in those on peritoneal dialysis, possibly because of the increased trauma to the red blood cells that occurs with the former technique and the inevitable blood loss that occurs, to a small degree, every time a patient is subjected to hemodialysis. The anemia is thought to be due to decreased erythropoiesis resulting from decreased production of the hormone erythropoietin from the diseased kidney. Patients with polycystic renal disease, in which the kidneys are replaced by large cysts, may continue to produce the hormone and are less anemic.

Erythropoietin (EPO) is available commercially[12] and has become widely used for patients with chronic renal failure. This substance is genetically engineered and expensive to administer on a long-term basis. It rapidly raises the hemoglobin concentration, depleting iron stores if iron and folic acid are not administered simultaneously. The hemoglobin concentration will return to normal values over a period of 2–3 weeks, increasing the patient's sense of well-being, exercise tolerance, appetite, and libido. However, such rapid rises in hemoglobin concentration are not without problems: in 30–35% of patients, hypertension worsens, probably as a result of increased blood viscosity and peripheral resistance, and arteriovenous fistulae, used for hemodialysis, may thrombose. There is an increased risk of a cerebrovascular accident,[13] and 5% of patients develop epileptiform convulsions.[14] Liver function tests may become abnormal[15] and the serum potassium may rise,[16] probably as a result of improved appetite, although dialyzer clearance may be reduced by the increased hematocrit. An influenza-like illness may develop on starting therapy, although this does not seem to be due to antibody formation. The hemoglobin concentration should only be raised to about $10\,g\,dL^{-1}$ to optimize oxygen delivery to the tissues without excessively increasing blood viscosity.

It is difficult to determine a maintenance dose of erythropoietin once an optimal hemoglobin level has been achieved. Although erythropoietin was administered initially by the intravenous route, it is now used routinely by subcutaneous injection with a significant reduction in cost.[17]

Hemolysis

The red blood corpuscles of patients with renal disease have a shorter half-life than those of a healthy person who is not uremic; thus, if the cells of a patient with renal failure were to be given to a healthy patient, their half-life would increase. The increased hemolysis potentiates the normochromic anemia and depletes iron stores further.

Platelet dysfunction

Although the platelet count may be normal in the uremic patient, platelet dysfunction may occur (thrombasthenia), prolonging bleeding times and thus increasing the risk of hemorrhage during surgery, especially in the patient who has not been adequately dialyzed. The surgeon must be especially careful to control bleeding sites in the patient with renal failure.

Heparin

The use of this drug to control the bleeding time during hemodialysis may also potentiate blood loss if surgery is carried out soon afterwards. A heparin titer should be estimated before an antagonist is used, for there is always the risk of excessive coagulability if protamine is given in the absence of heparin.

Blood transfusion

It was once considered inappropriate to regularly transfuse the anemic patient with renal disease. The benefit of the (transient) rise in hemoglobin was thought to be outweighed by the risks of transmission of blood-borne infection, such as serum hepatitis, and of the presence of unwanted antigens on the surface of the transfused blood cells which could stimulate antibody production and subsequently lead to rejection of an allogeneic renal transplant. Preoperative transfusion is used more frequently now that there are improved techniques for screening donated blood, which reduces the risk of transmission of infection, and following studies that reported a better transplant survival in patients who had been regularly transfused with third-party blood in the months preceding transplantation.[18] In some transplant centers where live-related donor transplantation is carried out, there was a fashion for only using blood from the future donor for preoperative transfusion to reduce the risk of organ rejection, and third-party blood was avoided except in life-threatening circumstances. The kidney survival rates in those circumstances were impressive: over 90% at 1 year.[19] However, advances in immunosuppression have reduced the need for this interesting technique.

Tissue oxygenation

It is thought that there is a shift to the right of the oxygen dissociation curve in the anemic patient with renal disease, thereby increasing oxygen delivery to the tissues despite the low hemoglobin concentration. Increased delivery of oxygen may also be the result of an increase in cardiac output that may occur in the patient with renal failure. This is an additional reason for not attempting to raise the hemoglobin concentration to completely normal values with erythropoietin since this will increase cardiac workload.

PREOPERATIVE ASSESSMENT

In addition to a routine preoperative assessment, the following points need to be given particular attention in the patient with renal disease.

Hemoglobin concentration, platelet count, and white blood cell count

Hemoglobin concentration, platelet count, and *white blood cell count* must be measured. If the platelet count is less than 50 000 preoperatively, this should be investigated. It may be that more adequate dialysis is necessary, or that covert infection is present, which needs treating before surgery.

Blood cross-match

Patients with renal disease are frequently anemic, therefore it is often necessary to have blood cross-matched for surgery for which it would not normally be required in the case of a healthy patient. A hemoglobin level greater than $8\,g\,dL^{-1}$ may be considered normal in renal patients. As a result, such patients can lose up to 500 mL of blood during surgery before blood is given; for a lesser loss, crystalloids are appropriate. If the hemoglobin is in the range $5–8\,g\,dL^{-1}$, intraoperative blood loss should be replaced with blood. If the level is below $5\,g\,dL^{-1}$ preoperatively, then transfusion is required before surgery. This is usually carried out during hemodialysis if the patient is receiving such treatment to decrease the effect of the volume load, as fluid can be removed as necessary. Otherwise, care must be taken that the transfusion load does not precipitate left ventricular failure. A loop diuretic should accompany blood transfusion if the patient is still responsive to frusemide; in the patient on peritoneal dialysis, a high-dextrose (3.86%) bag may be needed to remove excess water.

Plasma sodium, potassium, bicarbonate, and urea

Plasma sodium, potassium, bicarbonate, and *urea* should always be checked on the *day* of surgery – the previous day's results are not good enough. Rapid changes can occur in these variables, making an immediate preoperative level essential. If the serum sodium is low ($<125\,mmol\,L^{-1}$) or the potassium level high ($>5.5\,mmol\,L^{-1}$), the patient needs further dialysis before surgery. If the plasma bicarbonate is reduced, drug or dialysis therapy is inadequate. Neuromuscular blocking drugs will have a prolonged effect in acidotic patients. The anesthetic agents will result in increased myocardial depression and a higher risk of postoperative complications. The acidosis should be treated prior to surgery.

Plasma albumin

Plasma albumin should be measured. A low value may be due to the dilutional effect of fluid overload or the presence of infection. Anesthesia induced in such circumstances carries an increased risk; drugs may have a prolonged action and pulmonary edema, especially at the end of anesthesia after a period of artificial ventilation, is more common.

Chest radiograph

A *chest radiograph* is mandatory before anesthesia in patients of all ages with severe renal dysfunction. It will give an indication of pulmonary congestion, especially in the upper lobes, well before frank pulmonary edema is present (Fig. 52.1A). Increased hilar markings may also be present before any clinical symptoms can be detected. Areas of pulmonary collapse may be present that may be asymptomatic, especially in the patient receiving immunosuppressive therapy.

Cardiac enlargement is common in patients with renal disease (Fig. 52.1B); it is usually associated with hypertension but is sometimes due to ischemic disease or to a pericardial effusion.

Electrocardiogram

An *electrocardiogram* (ECG) is necessary for these patients preoperatively. Cardiac enlargement, myocardial ischemia, evidence of previous myocardial infarction, and arrhythmias can be detected.

A

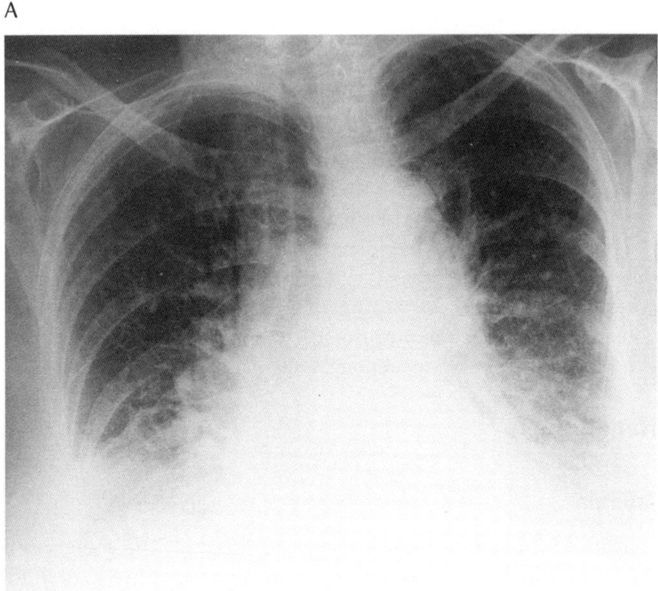

B

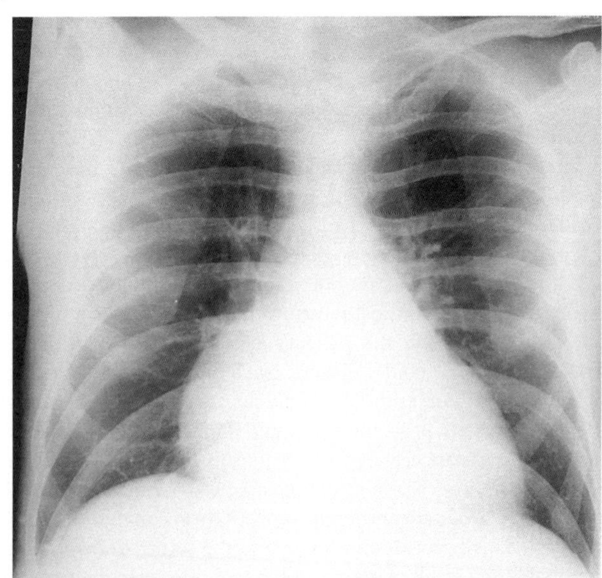

Figure 52.1 *(A) A preoperative chest radiograph of a woman with a failing renal transplant, presenting for insertion of a continuous ambulatory peritoneal dialysis (CAPD) cannula under general anesthesia. Note the increased pulmonary markings and bilateral pleural effusions, together with cardiac enlargement. (B) A preoperative chest radiograph of a man presenting for renal transplantation. Note the right and left ventricular enlargement.*

Drug therapy

This should be studied in detail. Most patients with significant renal disease are receiving oral iron, folic acid, sodium bicarbonate, and calcium and aluminum salts. They may be receiving diuretics (in which case, note the electrolyte status) and antihypertensive agents – if on beta-blocking drugs, particularly note the pulse rate. Be aware that more than two antihypertensive agents suggests that the problem is refractory and the blood pressure could be labile peroperatively and into the immediate postoperative period, especially if blood loss is significant.

Note whether the patient is receiving steroid therapy or other immunosuppressant drugs. Steroid cover will need to be increased preoperatively – it is useful to give the normal morning oral dose early on the day of surgery and then start 100 mg of hydrocortisone 6-hourly, intravenously or intramuscularly, at induction of anesthesia.

It should also be noted whether the patient is receiving the immunosuppressant *cyclosporine*[20] prior to surgery, or if it is planned to introduce this drug peroperatively by the intravenous route. Cyclosporine potentiates nondepolarizing neuromuscular blocking agents,[21] and therefore necessitates the use of neuromuscular monitoring peroperatively.

Cyclosporine, which is a more specific immunosuppressant than its predecessors azathioprine and the steroids, acts mainly on the T lymphocyte to suppress the immune response. It has improved graft survival significantly.[19,20] It is a fungal peptide which is metabolized in the liver by the cytochrome P450 enzyme system. It potentiates the action of other drugs metabolized by this enzyme system such as nifedipine, propofol, phenytoin, phenobarbital (phenobarbitone), and cimetidine. Unlike cortisone, it does not affect the control of blood sugar and has improved the success of transplantation in diabetic patients. But cyclosporine does have side-effects. It is nephrotoxic, and this can cause problems in achieving an appropriate maintenance dose and differentiating toxicity from acute rejection; it also causes gum hypertrophy, hirsutism, and, rarely, neurotoxicity.

Postoperative bacterial infections were common when steroids and azathioprine were used for immunosuppression after renal transplantation, but, with the advent of cyclosporine, atypical or viral infections are more frequently reported. Chest infections in renal transplant recipients taking cyclosporine, as a result of cytomegalovirus, *Mycoplasma pneumoniae, or Legionella pneumophila,* or influenzal pneumonia, may be sufficiently severe to require admission to an intensive therapy unit and artificial ventilation (Fig. 52.2).

Cyclosporine is a much more expensive maintenance immunosuppressant than steroids or azathioprine and, together with erythropoietin, has significantly increased the drug expenditure by renal transplant units. The original formulation (Sandimmun) has now been replaced by a microemulsion (Neoral).

Newer immunosuppressants

Tacrolimus has a mode of action similar to cyclosporine. It reduces steroid requirements, the need for antihypertensive drugs, and the serum cholesterol concentration. Early reports suggested that tacrolimus improved renal allograft survival compared with cyclosporine.[22] This has been disputed, although a meta-analysis did suggest that tacrolimus significantly reduced the incidence of acute rejection episodes compared with cyclosporine, but not graft survival.[23] An increased prevalence of diabetes mellitus occurred after transplantation if tacrolimus rather than cyclosporine was given for immunosuppression.

Long-term immunosuppression in transplant patients carries a higher risk of tumor formation than in the general population, with uncommon malignancies, such as lymphomas, presenting at an earlier age than would normally be expected (Fig. 52.3).

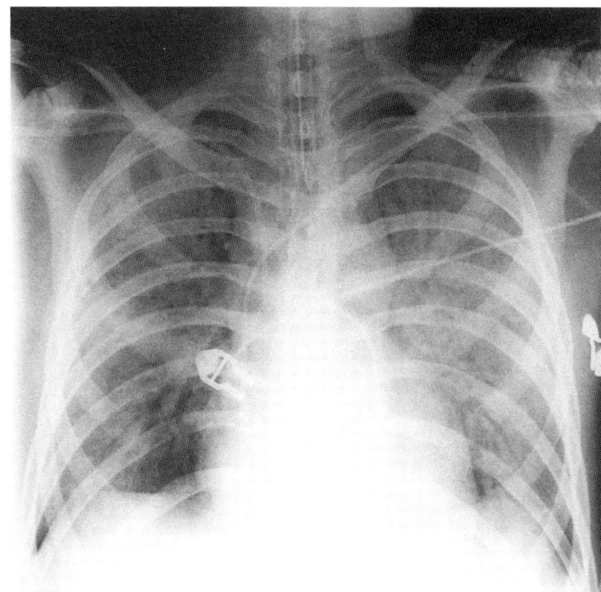

Figure 52.2 *A 17-year-old "transplant" patient receiving cyclosporine and prednisolone, who developed cytomegalovirus pneumonia in both lungs and required artificial ventilation. Air bronchograms, typical of adult respiratory distress syndrome, are visible in the left lung.*

Diabetes mellitus

Patients with insulin-dependent diabetes mellitus (IDDM) and significant renal impairment need careful perioperative supervision. If these patients are unable to respond to a fluid load with a diuresis, the Alberti regime is unsuitable as the patient would receive 100 mL h^{-1} of fluid. The additional potassium is also inappropriate. It is suggested that, for major surgery, the patient is established on a constant infusion of human insulin (1 unit mL^{-1}) via a separate pump, although possibly through the same intravenous cannula, from an infusion of dextrose given at a slow rate. The insulin infusion rate is adjusted as required. If 20% dextrose is tolerated without uncontrollable blood sugar levels, 40 mL h^{-1} should be given, but it may be necessary to use the same volume of only 10% or 5% dextrose during the stressful perioperative period to achieve good blood sugar control. The blood sugar should be measured at induction of anesthesia, then at least every hour, and again on recovery. It should be rechecked every 2–4 h in the postoperative period, and a sliding scale for intravenous or subcutaneous administration of insulin introduced.

If the patient is only undergoing very minor surgery, the morning dose of insulin may be omitted and a 5% dextrose infusion started at 40 mL h^{-1}, with the intention of giving the usual evening dose of insulin. If the patient has IDDM and is on CAPD, injecting insulin into the dialysis bags, then the insulin should be omitted from the overnight bag prior to surgery the next day. It will then be necessary to use the same per- and postoperative insulin regime as for the patient undergoing hemodialysis.

If the blood sugar level goes out of control in the patient with renal failure, then the serum potassium level may also change significantly. A rise in blood sugar will be accompanied by a rise in extracellular potassium; a fall in blood sugar by a fall in serum potassium.[10]

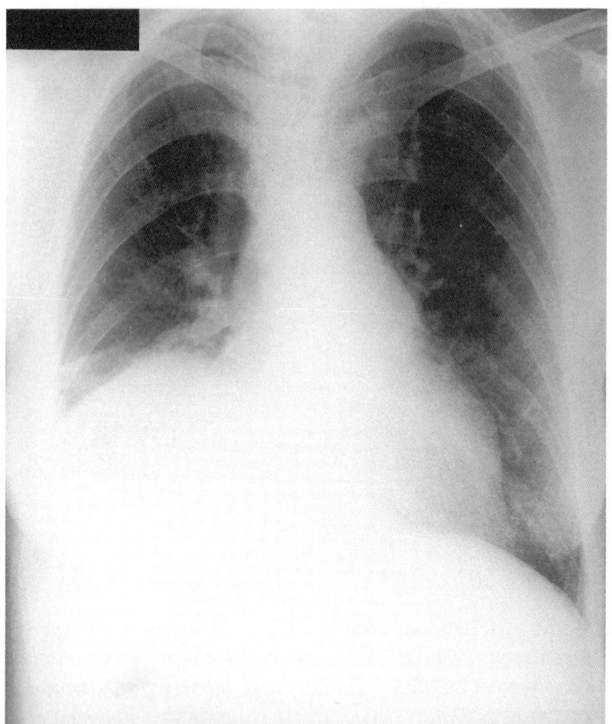

Figure 52.3 *Persistent right lower lobe collapse due to carcinomatosis in a 38-year-old renal transplant patient, with good renal function, who had been receiving steroid immunosuppression for 5 years. A vulval carcinoma with widespread metastases was present.*

Patient's weight

It is essential that this is recorded prior to surgery. These patients will know their "dry" weight and that, if it is raised, there is a need for further dialysis and fluid removal prior to surgery. Patients with chronic renal disease are often catabolic, especially if treatment is inadequate, and they have a reduced muscle mass. The dose of neuromuscular blocking drug required may therefore need to be reduced. All other anesthetic agents that are excreted through the kidney or which depress the myocardium should be used with caution (see below).

When was the patient last dialyzed?

This is a useful fact to note – if the patient only finished hemodialysis a few hours before surgery, he or she may be relatively hypovolemic, with the increased risk of hypotension on induction of anesthesia. If hemodialysis is due in the immediate future, the patient may be relatively overhydrated and dialysis may be preferable prior to surgery because of the increased risk of pulmonary edema in the perioperative period.

Previous general anesthetic

Details should be noted of any previous general anesthetic, in particular whether any problems of residual curarization occurred (see below). The previous anesthetic record should be obtained if possible.

Allergic reactions

Allergic reactions must also be detailed, although these are less common in the immunosuppressed, uremic patient than in the general population.

PERIOPERATIVE FLUID THERAPY

Perioperative fluid balance in the patient with renal disease must be guided by the degree of remaining renal function. It should not be forgotten that in all patients with renal disease it is still essential to replace insensible fluid loss. At least 40 mL h^{-1} of 5% dextrose is advisable if the patient is apyrexial. This should be increased by 5 mL h^{-1} for each degree (Celsius) increase in core temperature. Peroperative fluid loss should be replaced by normal saline solution. Two groups of patients can be identified.

The patient with a raised serum creatinine and continuing urine output

Patients with a raised serum creatinine and continuing urine output (usually less than 2 L day^{-1}) have a limited ability to concentrate urine. An adequate fluid volume must therefore be given postoperatively if an added solute load has been administered during surgery, frequently accompanied by a dose of a loop diuretic such as furosemide. It is essential to maintain a good urine output throughout the perioperative period. The use of 5% dextrose, at a rate of at least 80 mL h^{-1} postoperatively, will provide this water load without giving excess solute, in particular sodium ions, which will inhibit free water excretion. Potassium supplementation may be necessary.

It is preferable to pass a urinary catheter and to insert a central venous line in such patients prior to major surgery in order to facilitate management of perioperative fluid and electrolyte balance.

The anephric patient

These patients are maintained on dialysis and either pass no urine or empty their bladder only once every 2–3 days. They require that only insensible loss is replaced, together with any fluid loss suffered intra- or postoperatively. It is preferable to replace blood loss with blood or colloid, rather than with crystalloid solutions, to avoid the possibility of excess fluid load and pulmonary edema. A central venous catheter is essential if major surgery is being undertaken.

During renal transplantation it is important to maintain a good intravascular volume, allowing adequate perfusion of the transplanted kidney once the arterial clamps have been removed. A central venous pressure of at least +10 cmH_2O (1 kPa) from the anterior axillary line is recommended during intermittent positive pressure ventilation to increase left ventricular end-diastolic pressures and arterial blood flow. It is usual to administer an osmotic diuretic such as mannitol 0.5 g kg^{-1} intravenously before the transplanted kidney is perfused, or a loop diuretic such as furosemide, to promote urine output. A "low-dose" intravenous infusion of dopamine 2 μg kg^{-1} min^{-1} may also be used to increase renal blood flow.

SPECIFIC ANESTHETIC PROBLEMS IN RENAL PATIENTS

Gastric emptying

Uremia delays gastric emptying. The patient with renal disease, especially if not well managed preoperatively, should be considered to have a full stomach. The use of a rapid-sequence induction should be considered at the beginning of anesthesia, although the use of succinylcholine must be balanced against the rise in serum potassium which this drug will produce (see below).

Gastric acidity

Uremia produces an increase in gastric acidity. This, combined with the delayed gastric emptying, increases the risk and severity of aspiration pneumonia in these immunocompromised patients. Patients with renal dysfunction are often receiving regular antacid therapy. If H_2 antagonists are being administered, it must be remembered that these drugs are excreted in part through the kidney and have a greater intensity of effect and duration of action in renal failure. *Cimetidine* may cause confusion when given to these patients and is also contraindicated because it is a rare cause of bone marrow depression. This drug is an enzyme inhibitor, potentiating many other drugs metabolized by the cytochrome P450 system in the liver, including cyclosporine, beta-blocking agents, propofol, and antiepileptic drugs. *Ranitidine* is preferable, in reduced dosage. Antacids containing aluminum or magnesium should be avoided in patients with renal failure (see above).

Immunosuppression

Uremic patients with renal disease must be considered to be immunosuppressed even if they are not receiving immunosuppressive agents, such as steroids, azathioprine, or cyclosporine; this is part of the nature of their condition. The result is that these patients are more liable than the healthy patient to infection, possibly of an atypical variety, in the perioperative period. It is usual to administer a broad-spectrum antibiotic on induction of anesthesia, prior to major surgery. As Gram-positive cocci are a common commensal on the skin of patients with renal failure, it is important that an agent such as amoxycillin and clavulanic acid (Augmentin), which "covers" this group of bacteria, as well as Gram-negative organisms, is used.[24] Scrupulous attention to an aseptic technique is essential throughout surgery, and during the insertion of monitoring lines by the anesthesiologist.

Tuberculosis was more common in these patients than in the general population, especially if they were receiving steroid therapy. Although this can now be adequately treated, patient compliance is still necessary. This disease must be considered in all renal patients with a persistent chest infection, even if the chest radiograph findings are inconclusive. A suitable anesthetic technique, which allows adequate postoperative cleaning of all the equipment used, must be employed for the patient with tubercle in the sputum.

Serum hepatitis has long been a threat to patients undergoing hemodialysis and to attendant staff because of the repeated handling of blood-stained tubing. The regular screening of renal patients, at 6-monthly intervals, together with the use of disposable tubing on hemodialysis machines, has much reduced the risk of this potentially fatal disease.

Positive serology for *hepatitis C,* transmitted by blood transfusion before adequate screening procedures were available to detect it, is increasingly common in patients with chronic renal failure. No treatment is available and no suitable vaccination protects against it. Such patients should be treated as "high risk" during surgery.

Care of arteriovenous fistulae

The patient undergoing regular hemodialysis usually has an arteriovenous fistula established, if possible on the nondominant arm. This is the patient's "life line," which must be cared for diligently by the anesthesiologist. It should not be used for the injection of anesthetic drugs, which may cause venous irritation or thrombosis, nor for infusion of intravenous fluids. It is recommended that the fistula be well covered with gauze padding during surgery and that the arm is allowed to rest alongside the patient without being flexed, as this could also promote congestion and thrombosis. Significant falls in blood pressure may also decrease perfusion of the fistula and promote thrombosis.

Venous access

As patients with renal disease experience frequent blood sampling and may have had repeated vascular access surgery, venepuncture may be difficult. It is essential to have good venous access throughout anesthesia. The long-term use of central venous cannulae for hemodialysis in these patients is causing an increased incidence of stenosis in central vessels, such as the subclavian or internal jugular veins.

ANESTHESIA FOR PATIENTS WITH RENAL DISEASE

Premedication

As these patients have frequently undergone anesthesia, they may well be anxious prior to surgery and premedication is therefore indicated. As they know the perioperative routines, cooperation may be difficult, especially, for instance, if preoxygenation using a black face mask is indicated. As with all patients, a preoperative visit with full explanation of the planned procedure is more effective than any drug which may be administered to calm the patient and allay anxiety. It is recommended that all the patient's routine antihypertensive therapy and other important drugs be taken as usual on the day of surgery, even when the patient is being starved.

Sedatives

Sedatives are suitable premedication for these patients as they can be given orally, which is less unpleasant than by the parenteral routes. Benzodiazepines are particularly useful, often accompanied by night sedation, the evening before surgery. Antihistamine drugs are partially excreted by the kidney and their action will be potentiated by renal failure, sometimes causing excessive sedation.

Narcotic analgesics

Narcotic analgesics usually require the use of an intramuscular injection, which is more likely to produce a severe hematoma in these patients because of attendant clotting defects. These drugs are also more potent in the patient with renal failure (see below). They are not therefore the premedication of choice in this condition.

Vagal blockade

Vagal blockade is not appropriate in these hypertensive patients, even though they may be receiving a beta-blocking agent. It is preferable to have atropine or glycopyrrolate ready for intravenous use in the anesthetic room rather than administering such drugs prophylactically. Only when these drugs are indicated specifically, as for fiberoptic intubation to dry up secretions, should they be used. The resulting tachycardia promotes the pre-existing hypertension and may decrease coronary artery perfusion. In addition, the drying effect is unpleasant for the patient.

Steroid therapy

Steroid therapy may need to be increased to cover the stress response immediately prior to induction of anesthesia. It is again preferable to avoid an intramuscular injection and to give these drugs intravenously on arrival in the anesthetic room.

Induction of anesthesia

A rapid-sequence induction must be considered (see above), as should preoxygenation, if this can be accomplished without distressing the patient. Preoxygenation is particularly indicated if the patient is very anemic or has severe coronary artery disease.

Intravenous induction agents

Barbiturates are more potent in renal disease, in part because of the pre-existing myocardial problems.[25] Nevertheless, *thiopental (thiopentone)*, in reduced dosage and administered slowly, is the agent of choice. *Propofol* is likely to cause a greater fall in blood pressure than thiopental in all patients, but this decrease does not appear to be greater in patients with renal failure.[26] After a bolus dose, the plasma levels of propofol are similar in renal patients and healthy patients (Fig. 52.4), as are the pharmacokinetic parameters.[26] *Etomidate* may be considered if hypotension is a particular threat. This drug is not thought to have any significant immunosuppressive effect when used as a bolus dose and has less effect on the blood pressure than the barbiturates. It is more expensive than thiopental. *Ketamine* is not recommended in renal patients as its sympathomimetic properties may worsen the pre-existing hypertension and tachycardia.

Inhalational agents

An inhalational induction of anesthesia should be considered in the patient with renal failure with significant myocardial disease, possibly accompanied by an intravenous sedative or opioid analgesic. The more gradual onset of anesthesia allows more control of the blood pressure than an intravenous induction, although it has the disadvantage that the patient may not cooperate with the close application of a face mask. The use of a clear Perspex mask may help.

Cyclopropane, ether, and *trichloroethylene* are known to cause renal vasoconstriction, even in the denervated organ, and are contraindicated in these patients.[27,28] *Methoxyflurane*, which is metabolized significantly in the liver with the production of inorganic fluoride ions, has been reported to produce deposition of fluoride crystals in the kidney and is not therefore recommended.[29]

Although *halothane* potentiates the bradycardia produced by beta-blocking drugs, it will not alter renal perfusion unless the patient is hypotensive, hypovolemic, or hypercarbic, when renal blood flow will decrease further.[30] Halothane may also potentiate cardiac arrhythmias in the patient with myocardial ischemia and is a potent myocardial depressant. Despite this, it was used successfully as an adjuvant to artificial ventilation for many years in patients with renal disease.

Enflurane and isoflurane are less likely to cause myocardial depression than halothane. Both agents undergo some hepatic metabolism to produce fluoride ions, which are nephrotoxic, but this is significantly less with isoflurane than with enflurane.[31] There have been occasions when enflurane produced renal failure in patients with renal dysfunction,[32] and higher plasma inorganic fluoride levels have been reported in transplant patients receiving enflurane than in those receiving halothane anesthesia.[33] Isoflurane is the inhalational agent of choice in these patients, despite the risk of coronary artery steal in the presence of coronary artery disease.

Sevoflurane is particularly useful for inhalational induction for sick patients. Its rapid onset of effect and good tolerability allow a smooth induction of anesthesia.[34]

Sevoflurane is metabolized in the liver to compound A and inorganic fluoride. Both compounds are thought to be nephrotoxic – fluoride in plasma concentrations above 50 μmol L^{-1}. Such levels are reached in the plasma during prolonged sevoflurane anesthesia.[35] Although early studies suggest that sevoflurane is safe to use for patients with renal dysfunction,[36] more evidence is still required about its safety in this group of patients.

Desflurane is more irritant to the airways than sevoflurane. It is not therefore as suitable for inhalational induction of anesthesia even though it has a low blood gas-solubility coefficient. It undergoes much less metabolism than sevoflurane with minimal fluoride production, so should be appropriate as a maintenance agent during anesthesia for patients with chronic renal failure.

Neuroleptanalgesia

This technique has the benefits of providing cardiovascular stability and well-maintained renal blood flow.[37] *Fentanyl* only decreases renal blood flow in very high doses, of the order of 10–15 μg kg^{-1}.[37] The alpha-blocking activity of *droperidol* may be thought to be advantageous in maintaining renal blood flow; although in the doses usually used in clinical practice, this effect is probably not significant. Droperidol is excreted through the kidney and this long-acting drug may have a greater effect in patients with renal failure. Droperidol is no longer available in the UK.

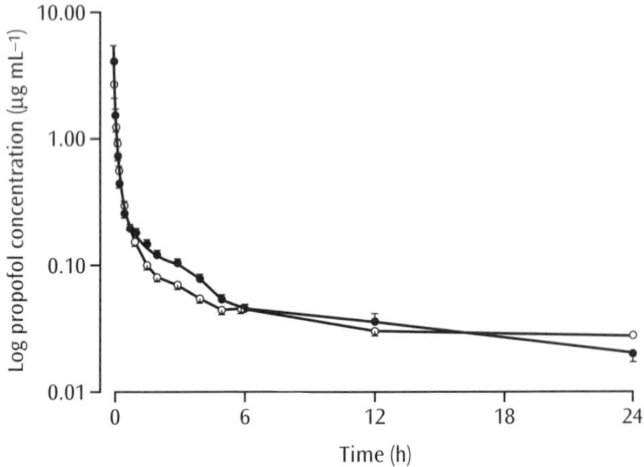

Figure 52.4 *The mean plasma propofol levels in a group of patients with renal failure (open circles) compared with healthy patients (filled circles). No significant difference is evident.[26] (Reprinted with kind permission of the editor of the* British Journal of Anaesthesia*).*

Narcotic analgesics

Although these drugs are primarily metabolized in the liver, the metabolites, some of which have potent analgesic properties, are excreted through the kidney and may cumulate in the presence of renal impairment, be it transient as in hypovolemia or permanent as in end-stage renal failure. *Morphine sulfate* is metabolized in the liver to morphine-3-glucuronide, morphine-3,6-glucuronide, and morphine-6-glucuronide. The pharmacokinetics of morphine itself are, therefore, little changed in the presence of renal impairment (Table 52.1), although the volume of distribution may be reduced possibly because of hypoproteinemia.[38] Morphine-6-glucuronide is a very potent analgesic and respiratory depressant and is thought to contribute significantly to the enhanced effect of morphine in the renal patient.[38] The dose of this drug should be reduced in these circumstances and care is required, particularly if repeated doses are used.

The main metabolites of *meperidine (pethidine)*, including normeperidine (norpethidine) and normeperidine acid, are also excreted through the kidney. Normeperidine possesses analgesic and respiratory depressant properties,[39] although not to as marked a degree as mor-

Table 52.1 *Morphine kinetics in renal transplant patients compared with healthy patients*[38]

	Renal	Healthy
Elimination half-life (min)	290	286
Clearance (mL min^{-1})	533	741
$V_{d(ss)}$ (L)	141	241**

**$P < 0.002$; $V_{d(ss)}$, volume of distribution at steady state.

phine-6-glucuronide. Meperidine is probably the analgesic of choice for these patients; morphine can be used if meperidine proves inadequate. Both drugs should be used in reduced dosage.

The clearance of *fentanyl* is little changed in renal failure;[40] as this drug has a shorter half-life than morphine or meperidine and its metabolites are inactive, it is the peroperative analgesic of choice. *Alfentanil* would appear to have a similar disposition in healthy patients and in those with renal failure,[41] but because of its short half-life it must be given by constant infusion for major surgery. *Buprenorphine*, which is also metabolized mainly in the liver, does not appear to cumulate in renal failure, although the inactive metabolites do.[42]

Remifentanil, which is metabolized in the plasma by nonspecific esterases, has unaltered pharmacokinetic and dynamic effects in patients with chronic renal failure compared with healthy controls.[43] However, its principal metabolite GB90291, which has 0.02% of the potency of remifentanil, has a much longer elimination half-life in anephric patients (26 h) than in a healthy group (1.5 h). Its steady-state plasma concentrations are predicted to be about 25 times higher in patients with renal failure. This metabolite may have a mild opioid effect in patients with renal failure.

Neuromuscular blocking agents

Succinylcholine

Although it has long been recognized that a single dose of succinylcholine will increase the serum potassium by about 0.5 mmol L^{-1} during halothane anesthesia,[44] this increase is thought not to be exaggerated by renal disease. The problem is that such patients may have a higher plasma potassium level before the succinylcholine is given and any rise may therefore be sufficient to cause cardiac arrhythmias and, rarely, cardiac arrest. The serum potassium must always be measured before succinylcholine is given to the patient with renal dysfunction, both in the operating room and in the intensive care unit. Succinylcholine remains the best muscle relaxant for a rapid-sequence intubation – it is the only such agent that allows endotracheal intubation within 1 min[45] and this is particularly relevant in the uremic patient with decreased gastric emptying.

Nondepolarizing muscle relaxants

The percentage excretion of these drugs through the kidney is shown in Table 52.2. With the older nondepolarizing agents that were excreted to a significant degree through the kidney, cumulation was a recognized problem, especially if repeated doses had been given or an increment was used to allow the surgeon to close the abdomen. These drugs are more potent in an acidotic state. If an inadequate reversal ensued after surgery, respiratory distress leading to carbon dioxide retention might cause respiratory acidosis in addition to the pre-existing metabolic acidosis, and thus apparently make worse any residual neuromuscular block. *Recurarization* has been reported in renal patients after the use of *tubocurarine*[46] and *pancuronium*.[47] As *gallamine*[48] is almost entirely excreted through the kidney, it is not surprising that reports of persistent curarization lasting for several days after the use of this drug in patients

Table 52.2 *The percentage excretion of various neuromuscular blocking drugs in the urine over 24 h*

	% Excretion
Succinylcholine (suxamethonium)	<10
Tubocurarine	66
Gallamine	>95
Pancuronium	60
Metocurine	52
Alcuronium	80
Atracurium	10
Vecuronium	20–30
Pipecuronium	64
Doxacurium	60
Mivacurium	<10
Rocuronium	33
Cisatracurium	15
Rapacuronium	?33

with renal failure also occurred. The use of gallamine in this condition is contraindicated. *Alcuronium*[49] and *metocurine* are also excreted through the kidney to a significant degree (Table 52.2).

With the advent of *atracurium* and *vecuronium*, the management of neuromuscular block in the patient with renal disease became more simple. Only 10% of a dose of atracurium is excreted by the kidney,[50] and although the relative contributions of Hofmann degradation and ester hydrolysis to the breakdown of atracurium in man are uncertain, it is thought that Hofmann degradation acts as a form of safety net in the absence of any organ function. Pharmacodynamic[51] and pharmacokinetic[52] studies have demonstrated no cumulation of atracurium in patients with renal failure, even if the drug is given by constant infusion for several days.[50]

Concern has been expressed that the metabolite of Hofmann degradation, *laudanosine*, which is known to produce cerebral irritation in animals and to be excreted in part through the kidney, may accumulate in the presence of renal dysfunction. Fahey and colleagues[53] did show a significant increase in plasma laudanosine levels in patients with renal failure given a bolus dose of atracurium compared with a control healthy group. The plasma laudanosine level was only of the order of 0.3 μg mL^{-1} in the renal group and that required to produce cerebral irritation in dogs is of the order of 14 μg mL^{-1}.[54] There is no risk of cumulation of laudanosine during general anesthesia. If atracurium is given by constant infusion for many days to patients who are critically ill with multiple organ failure in an intensive care unit, plasma levels of laudanosine will be higher, at up to 5 μg mL^{-1}.[50] No clinical reports have occurred of laudanosine causing convulsions in such circumstances, but it is not impossible to imagine that these may occur if large doses of atracurium are given to such patients for many days, perhaps in the presence of a low epileptic threshold, hypoxemia or metabolic disturbances.

Although vecuronium is excreted through the kidney to a greater extent than atracurium, excretion is still significantly less than with the older nondepolarizing drugs.[55] Cumulation is unlikely unless repeated doses are used. Potentiation of block may occur however if the patient is very acidotic. Several reports have occurred of persistent block when vecuronium is given repeatedly to patients in renal failure[56] or when it is given by constant infusion in the intensive therapy unit to patients with impaired renal function.[57] This may be due in part to cumulation of the active metabolite of vecuronium, 3-desacetylvecuronium, which is excreted through the kidney, has a long half-life, and has about 40% of the neuromuscular blocking potency of the parent drug.[58] It is preferable to give vecuronium in bolus doses to patients who are critically ill.

Pipecuronium, a steroidal muscle relaxant, and *doxacurium*, a benzylisoquinolinium derivative, although both free of cardiovascular effects, are excreted to a significant degree by the kidney (Table 52.2) and do not represent advances in the management of the patient in renal failure.[59,60]

Mivacurium is metabolized in the plasma by plasma cholinesterase, at 88% of the rate of succinylcholine. As cholinesterase levels may be reduced in patients with chronic renal disease, prolongation of block may be anticipated when these patients are given mivacurium. Phillips and Hunter[61] have demonstrated a direct relation in healthy patients and in patients with renal failure between the time to 5% recovery of the first twitch of the train of four (T1) after 0.15 mg kg^{-1} mivacurium and both plasma cholinesterase activity (Fig. 52.5) and the infusion dose of mivacurium required to keep the height of T1 at 5% (Fig. 52.6).

The pharmacokinetics of the three isomers of mivacurium in patients with renal dysfunction and end-stage renal disease have been described.[62] The two active isomers, *cis–trans* and *trans–trans* mivacurium, are unaffected by renal dysfunction, but the *cis–cis* isomer, which has only one-tenth of the neuromuscular potency of the two active isomers, does undergo renal excretion and has a reduced clearance in chronic renal failure. Plasma cholinesterase activity is the main determinant of the effect of mivacurium in patients with renal dysfunction.

Rocuronium, a steroidal nondepolarizing muscle relaxant with a rapid onset of action, has also been shown to have an increased duration of action in renal disease,[63] although other workers have not confirmed these findings. The pharmacokinetics of rocuronium are little changed in patients undergoing renal transplantation.[64] The volume of distribution is increased, and the elimination half-life prolonged but only slightly.

Cisatracurium is the 1R-*cis* 1′R-*cis* isomer of atracurium (which is a mixture of 10 stereo- and geometric isomers) and became available in 1997. It is more potent than atracurium (ED_{95} values 0.05 mg kg^{-1} and 0.23 mg kg^{-1} respectively). Cisatracurium has a longer onset of action (about 3 min) than atracurium, and a slightly longer duration of effect.[65] It is metabolized mainly by Hofmann degradation,[66] and only about 15% of a single dose is excreted in the urine in healthy patients.

As cisatracurium is more potent than atracurium, a smaller dose is given and less laudanosine is produced. After bolus doses of cisatracurium are given to patients in chronic renal failure, the mean peak laudanosine level is 30 ng mL^{-1}, which is 10 times less than after an equipotent dose of atracurium.[67] Laudanosine levels are also lower when cisatracurium, rather than atracurium, is given by continuous infusion to critically ill patients with renal dysfunction in the intensive care unit.[68] Peak plasma levels after cisatracurium (0.15 mg kg^{-1} h^{-1}) are 1.2 μg mL^{-1} compared with 4.3 μg mL^{-1} after atracurium 0.6 mg kg^{-1} h^{-1}. Cisatracurium is the neuromuscular blocking agent of choice for critically ill patients needing infusion of a relaxant for several days.

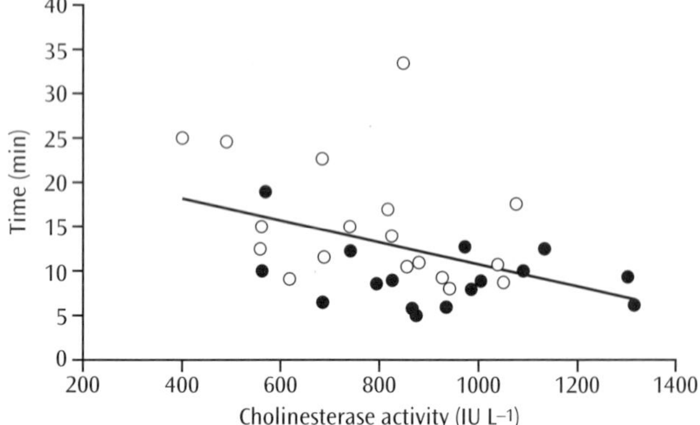

Figure 52.5 *The time to 5% recovery of the first twitch of the train of four (T1) is plotted against plasma cholinesterase activity in a group of patients with renal failure (open circles) and healthy patients (filled circles). There was a significant negative correlation between these variables* (r = –0.42; P < 0.02).[61]

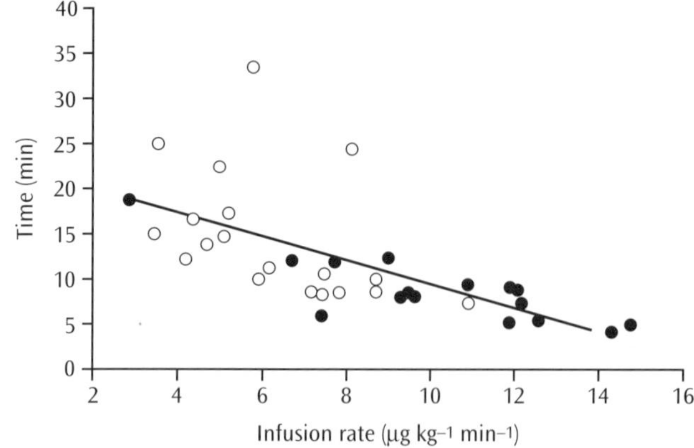

Figure 52.6 *The time to 5% recovery of T1 is plotted against the infusion rate of mivacurium required to maintain T1 at 5% in patients with renal failure (open circles) and healthy patients (filled circles)* (r = –0.447; P < 0.01).[61]

Cisatracurium stimulates less histamine release than atracurium, causing fewer adverse cardiovascular effects than the parent compound. It is therefore more suitable to use for patients with cardiovascular disease, including patients with renal failure.

Rapacuronium (Org 9487) was the latest aminosteroid neuromuscular blocking drug to be introduced. It is derived from vecuronium, but has a much more rapid onset of action that is similar to, if not faster than, an equipotent dose of rocuronium at 83 s.[69] It is more lipid soluble than other neuromuscular blocking drugs, and therefore has a larger volume of distribution. It is metabolized in the liver and excreted in the urine.[70] First reports suggest that the clearance of rapacuronium is reduced in patients with chronic renal failure.[71] Bronchospasm, hypotension, and tachycardia have been reported following the use of this drug, although it is not certain that these are due to histamine release. It has now been withdrawn from use in the USA.

It is essential to monitor neuromuscular block throughout surgery, whichever muscle relaxant is used during anesthesia for patients with renal dysfunction.

Reversal of residual neuromuscular blockade

Anticholinergic agents such as *atropine* and *glycopyrrolate* and anticholinesterases such as *neostigmine* and *edrophonium* are highly ionized, water-soluble substances; they are excreted to a significant extent through the kidney.[72,73] Their duration of action is therefore prolonged in patients with renal disease (Table 52.3).

The anticholinergics have shorter half-lives than the anticholinesterases; because the half-lives of both types of agent are approximately doubled in the presence of renal disease, the period of bradycardia produced by the anticholinesterases will be exaggerated. The bradycardia will be further potentiated in those patients receiving beta-blocking drugs.

Glycopyrrolate has less cardiac effect than atropine, therefore it is preferable to use it for the patient with cardiac problems and renal disease.

A suggested general anesthetic technique for the patient with renal disease presenting for major surgery is given in Table 52.4.

Table 52.3 *The effect of renal failure on the elimination half-life and clearance of neostigmine and edrophonium*[72,73]

	Neostigmine		Edrophonium	
	Elimination half-life (min)	Clearance ($mL\,kg^{-1}\,min^{-1}$)	Elimination half-life (min)	Clearance ($mL\,kg^{-1}\,min^{-1}$)
Healthy	77.8	16.7	110	9.6
Renal failure	181	7.8	304	3.9

Intraoperative monitoring

It is essential that electrocardiographic monitoring is commenced before induction of anesthesia and continued until the patient leaves the recovery room. Arterial oxygen saturation should also be monitored using a pulse oximeter throughout this period, together with heart rate and blood pressure. As these patients are anemic, higher inspired oxygen concentrations may be required, e.g. 40%, to provide adequate oxygen delivery to the tissues. End-tidal carbon dioxide concentration should be kept in the normal range to optimize renal blood flow.[30] Hypovolemia should also be corrected for the same reason. Accurate measurement of blood loss during surgery will aid the maintenance of correct fluid balance. For major surgery, central venous pressure monitoring is also essential. If the patient is expected to pass any urine during the procedure, a urinary catheter should be inserted and hourly measurements recorded throughout the perioperative period. Neuromuscular monitoring should be instigated after induction of anesthesia if a muscle relaxant is being used and continued until the patient is awake.

If major blood loss occurs, the patient's hemoglobin and serum potassium and sodium should be checked peroperatively and clotting studies carried out. The fall in hemoglobin may not be as great as anticipated because of pre-existing hemodilution. If the patient is an insulin-dependent diabetic, blood sugar should also be checked regularly (see above).

Postoperative monitoring in the recovery room

As patients with renal disease are usually anemic, oxygen therapy should be continued into the postoperative period for as long as is feasible, but at least for 24 h. It is now clear that periods of arterial desaturation are not infrequent during the first two postoperative nights;[74] as these patients are not only anemic, with decreased oxygen-carrying capacity, but also frequently have coronary artery disease, they must be at considerable risk of developing myocardial ischemia during this time. Electrocardiographic monitoring should be continued in the recovery room, combined with pulse oximetry.

Fluid balance should be charted at least every hour, taking into account the central venous pressure, urine output (if any), and fluid drainage. As many patients with end-stage renal failure live constantly on the brink of pulmonary edema, they rarely lie flat: they sleep propped up on several pillows. It is preferable to place them in their usual sitting position on recovery from anesthesia. If there is considerable risk of pulmonary edema, a chest radiograph is indicated.

The recovery room nurse should be informed of the site of an arteriovenous fistula to prevent the blood pressure inadvertently being taken on the same arm. Every attempt should be made to keep the patient warm as shivering, which is common for all patients postoperatively, frequently potentiates severe hypertension in the anephric patient during this unstable period.

Table 52.4 *A suggested general anesthetic technique for the adult patient with renal disease*

Premedication	Nitrazepam 5–10 mg orally the evening before surgery Diazepam 5–10 mg orally, 2–3 h preoperatively
Induction of anesthesia	Fentanyl 1.0 $\mu g\,kg^{-1}$ Thiopental 4–5 $mg\,kg^{-1}$ Atracurium 0.5 $mg\,kg^{-1}$ or cisatracurium 0.15 $mg\,kg^{-1}$ (or succinylcholine 1 $mg\,kg^{-1}$ if stomach full)
Maintenance of anesthesia	N_2O/40% O_2/isoflurane increments of fentanyl and atracurium/cisatracurium
Reversal of residual block	Glycopyrrolate 0.5 mg Neostigmine 2.5 mg

Succinylcholine (suxamethonium).

Local anesthesia for the patient with renal disease

Local analgesic drugs have a shorter duration of action in the acidic tissues of a patient with renal disease and therefore appear less efficacious, particularly when used for local infiltration.[75] The benefits of using local blocks in restricted areas such as the epidural space or spinal canal is questionable because of the increased risk of hemorrhage – there is undoubtedly a higher risk of a hematoma than in the healthy patient, with possibly permanent neurological consequences. In addition, these anxious patients often wish to be given a general anesthetic.

Vascular surgery is often required in the arm of patients with renal failure at a time, perhaps, when dialysis is proving inefficient because of difficulty with pre-existing vascular access. So, brachial plexus block may be useful for intraoperative management. The supraclavicular approach has the advantage of producing analgesia of the whole arm, which is particularly important if the surgeon works in the antecubital fossa or deltoid region. Infraclavicular blocks may fail to establish adequate analgesia in these areas. The disadvantage of the supraclavicular approach is the risk of puncturing the pleura, producing a pneumothorax in a high-risk patient.

Because of its longer duration of action, *bupivacaine* is more useful than lidocaine (lignocaine) if a brachial block is to be instigated; *lidocaine* may be insufficient to cover the length of what may become prolonged surgery. Bupivacaine does, however, have the disadvantage of a prolonged onset of action: 20 min or more may elapse before adequate block is established, especially if the drug is not injected close to the brachial plexus. Lidocaine may be mixed with the bupivacaine to reduce the delay with a potentiation of effect. It is recommended that for the supraclavicular approach 30 mL bupivacaine (0.25%), in three 10-mL aliquots, should be injected along the first rib as the three branches of the brachial plexus traverse it.

SUMMARY

The patient with chronic renal failure has a multiplicity of medical problems which all require careful assessment before anesthesia.

Cardiovascular pathology, anemia, biochemical disturbances, and diabetic therapy may need preoperative correction. Current drug therapy must be known in detail. Perioperative fluid balance needs close monitoring and adjustment.

Patients with chronic renal failure also have specific anesthetic problems, related to increased gastric acidity, delayed gastric emptying, immunosuppressive treatment, problems with vascular access, and care of arteriovenous fistulae.

Anesthesia should take account of the altered pharmacodynamics and pharmacokinetics of many anesthetic-related drugs in chronic renal failure patients. In particular, the altered effect of neuromuscular blocking drugs and opioid analgesics needs careful monitoring.

The indications for the use of local anesthetic drugs and their limitations in patients with chronic renal failure have been considered. The need for supplementary oxygen therapy postoperatively is emphasized.

REFERENCES

1. Williams AJ, Antao AJO. Referral of elderly patients with end-stage renal failure for renal replacement therapy. *Q J Med* 1989; **268:** 749–56.
2. Burton PR, Walls J. Selection – adjusted comparison of life expectancy of patients on continuous ambulatory peritoneal dialysis, haemodialysis and renal transplantation. *Lancet* 1987; **i:** 1115–19.
3. Legendre C, Saltiel C, Kreis H, Grunfeld J-P. Hypertension in kidney transplantation. *Klin Wochenschr* 1989; **67:** 919–22.
4. Weaver RA. Restoration of renal function by renal revascularisation. *West J Med* 1989; **151:** 189.
5. Gunnarsson R, Lofmark R, Norlander R, *et al.* Acute myocardial infarction in renal transplant recipients: incidence and prognosis. *Eur Heart J* 1984; **5:** 218–21.
6. Heino A, Orko R, Rosenberg PH. Anaesthesiological complications in renal transplantation: a retrospective study of 500 transplantations. *Acta Anaesthesiol Scand* 1986; **30:** 574–80.
7. Soulilou JP, Fillaudeau F, Keribin JP, Guenel J. Acute hyperkalaemia risks in recipients of kidney graft cooled with Collins solution. *Nephron* 1977; **19:** 301–4.
8. Horl WH, Riegel W, Wanner C, *et al.* Endocrine and metabolic abnormalities following kidney transplantation. *Klin Wochenschr* 1989; **67:** 907–18.
9. Smith I, Hyland K. Disturbance of cerebral function by aluminium in haemodialysis patients. *Lancet* 1989; **ii:** 501–2.
10. Goldfarb S, Cox M, Suiger I, Goldbert M. Acute hyperkalaemia induced by hyperglycaemia; hormonal mechanisms. *Ann Intern Med* 1976; **84:** 426–32.
11. Hunter JM. Resistance to non-depolarising muscle relaxants. *Br J Anaesth* 1991; **67:** 511–14.
12. Hambley H, Mufti GH. Erythropoietin: an old friend revisited. *Br Med J* 1990; **300:** 621–2.
13. Raine AEG. Hypertension, blood viscosity, and cardiovascular morbidity in renal failure: implications of erythropoietin therapy. *Lancet* 1988; **i:** 97–9.
14. Eschbach JW, Egrie JC, Downing MR, *et al.* Correction of the anemia of end-stage renal disease with recombinant human erythropoietin. *N Engl J Med* 1987; **316:** 73–8.
15. Bommer J, Alexiou C, Muller-Butil U, *et al.* Recombinant human erythropoietin therapy in haemodialysis patients – dose determination and clinical experience. *Nephrol Dial Transplant* 1987; **2:** 238–42.
16. Casati S, Passerini P, Campse MR, *et al.* Benefits and risks of protracted treatment with human recombinant erythropoietin in patients having haemodialysis. *Br Med J* 1987; **295:** 1017–20.
17. Stevens ME, Summerfield GP, Hall AA, *et al.* Cost benefits of low dose subcutaneous erythropoietin in patients with anaemia and end-stage renal disease. *Br Med J* 1992; **304:** 474–7.
18. Opelz G. The role of HLA matching and blood transfusions in the cyclosporine era. *Transplant Proc* 1989; **21:** 609–12.
19. Sells RA, Hillis A, Bone MJ, *et al.* Donor specific transfusion with and without cyclosporin A – a controlled clinical trial. *Transplant Proc* 1988; **10** (Suppl. 3): 270–3.
20. Calne RYC, White DJG, Thiru S, *et al.* Cyclosporin A in patients receiving renal allografts from cadaveric donors. *Lancet* 1978; **ii:** 1323–7.
21. Gramstadt L, Gjerlow A, Hysing ES, Rugstad HE. Interaction of cyclosporin and its solvent cremophor with atracurium and vecuronium. Studies in the cat. *Br J Anaesth* 1986; **58:** 1149–55.
22. Gjertson DW, Cecka JM, Terasaki PI. The relative effects of FK506 and cyclosporine on short- and long- term kidney graft survival. *Transplantation* 1995; **60:** 1384–8.
23. Knoll GA, Bell RC. Tacrolimus versus cyclosporin for immunosuppression in renal transplantation: meta-analysis of randomised trials. *Br Med J* 1999; **318:** 1104–7.
24. Evans CM, Purohit S, Colbert JW, *et al.* Amoxycillin – clavulanic (Augmentin) antibiotic prophylaxis against wound infections in renal failure patients. *J Antimicrob Ther* 1988; **22:** 363–9.
25. Dundee JW, Annis D. Barbiturate narcosis in uraemia. *Br J Anaesth* 1955; **27:** 114–23.
26. Kirvela M, Olkkola KT, Rosenberg PH, *et al.* Pharmacokinetics of propofol and haemodynamic changes during induction of anaesthesia in uraemic patients. *Br J Anaesth* 1992; **68:** 178–82.
27. Deutsch S, Pierce EC, Vandam LD. Cyclopropane effects on renal function in normal man. *Anesthesiology* 1967; **28:** 547–58.
28. Hamelburg W, Sprouse JH, Mahaffey JE, Richardson JE. Catechol amine levels during light and deep anesthesia. *Anesthesiology* 1960; **21:** 297–302.
29. Cousins MJ, Mazze RI, Kosek JC, *et al.* The etiology of methoxyflurane toxicity. *J Pharmacol Exp Ther* 1974; **190:** 530–41.
30. Hunter JM, Jones RS, Utting JE. Effect of acute hypocapnia on renal function in the dog artificially ventilated with nitrous oxide, oxygen and halothane. *Br J Anaesth* 1980; **52:** 197–8.
31. Chase RE, Holaday DA, Fiserova-Bergesova V, *et al.* The biotransformation of ethrane in man. *Anesthesiology* 1971; **35:** 262–7.
32. Eichhorn JH, Hedley-White J, Steinman TL, *et al.* Renal failure following enflurane anesthesia. *Anesthesiology* 1976; **45:** 557–60.
33. Wickstrom I. Enflurane anaesthesia in living renal transplantation. *Acta Anaesthesiol Scand* 1981; **25:** 263–9.
34. Thwaites A, Edmends S, Smith I. Inhalation induction with sevoflurane: a double-blind comparison with propofol. *Br J Anaesth* 1997; **78:** 356–61.
35. Higuchi H, Sumikura H, Sumita S, *et al.* Renal function in patients with high serum fluoride concentrations after prolonged sevoflurane anesthesia. *Anesthesiology* 1995; **85:** 449–58.
36. Conzen PF, Nuscheler M, Melotte A, *et al.* Renal function and serum fluoride concentrations in patients with stable renal insufficiency after anesthesia with sevoflurane or enflurane. *Anesth Analg* 1995; **81:** 569–75.
37. Hunter JM, Jones RS, Utting JE. Effects of acute hypocapnia on some aspects of renal function in anaesthetised dogs. *Br J Anaesth* 1979; **51:** 725–31.
38. Sear JW, Hand CW, Moore RA, McQuay HJ. Studies on morphine disposition: influence of renal failure on the kinetics of morphine and its metabolites. *Br J Anaesth* 1989; **62:** 28–32.
39. Armstrong PJ, Bersten A. Normeperidine toxicity. *Anesth Analg* 1986; **65:** 536–8.
40. Corall IM, Moore AR, Strunin L. Plasma concentrations of fentanyl in normal surgical patients and those with severe renal and hepatic disease. *Br J Anaesth* 1980; **52:** 101P.
41. Sear JW, Bower S, Potter D. Disposition of alfentanil in patients with chronic renal failure. *Br J Anaesth* 1986; **58:** 812P.
42. Hand CW, Sear JW, Uppington J, *et al.* Buprenorphine disposition in patients with renal impairment: single and continuous dosing with special reference to metabolites. *Br J Anaesth* 1990; **64:** 276–82.
43. Hoke JF, Shlugman D, Dershwitz M, *et al.* Pharmacokinetics and pharmacodynamics of remifentanil in persons with renal failure compared to healthy volunteers. *Anesthesiology* 1997; **87:** 533–41.
44. Paton WDM. The effects of muscle relaxants other than muscle relaxation. *Anesthesiology* 1959; **20:** 453–4.
45. Hunter JM, Jones RS, Utting JE. Use of atracurium during general surgery monitored by the train-of-four stimuli. *Br J Anaesth* 1982; **54:** 1243–51.
46. Riordan DD, Gilbertson AA. Prolonged curarisation in a patient with renal failure. *Br J Anaesth* 1971; **43:** 506–8.
47. Rouse JM, Galley RLA, Bevan DR. Prolonged curarisation following renal transplantation. *Anaesthesia* 1977; **32:** 247–51.
48. Jenkins IR. Three cases of apparent curarisation. *Br J Anaesth* 1961; **33:** 314–18.
49. Buzello W, Agoston S. Comparative clinical pharmacokinetics of tubocurarine, gallamine, alcuronium, pancuronium. *Anaesthetist* 1978; **27:** 313–18.
50. Shearer ES, O'Sullivan EP, Hunter JM. Clearance of atracurium and laudanosine in the urine and by continuous venovenous haemofiltration. *Br J Anaesth* 1991; **67:** 569–73.
51. Hunter JM, Jones RS, Utting JE. Use of atracurium in patients with no renal function. *Br J Anaesth* 1982; **54:** 1251–4.
52. Fahey MR, Fisher DM, Miller RD, *et al.* The pharmacokinetics and phar-

macodynamics of atracurium in patients with and without renal failure. *Anesthesiology* 1984; **61:** 699–702.
53. Fahey MR, Rupp SM, Canfell C, *et al.* Effects of renal failure on laudanosine excretion in man. *Br J Anaesth* 1985; **57:** 1049–51.
54. Hennis PJ, Fahey MR, Miller RD, *et al.* Pharmacology of laudanosine in dogs. *Anesthesiology* 1984; **61:** A305.
55. Lynam DP, Cronnelly R, Castagnoli KP, *et al.* The pharmacodynamics and pharmacokinetics of vecuronium in patients anesthetized with isoflurane with normal renal function or with renal failure. *Anesthesiology* 1988; **69:** 227–31.
56. Cody MW, Dormon FM. Recurarisation after vecuronium in a patient with renal failure. *Anaesthesia* 1987; **42:** 993–5.
57. Smith CL, Hunter JM, Jones RS. Vecuronium infusions in patients with renal failure in an ITU. *Anaesthesia* 1987; **42:** 387–93.
58. Segredo V, Matthay MA, Sharma ML, *et al.* Prolonged neuromuscular blockade after long term administration of vecuronium in two critically ill patients. *Anesthesiology* 1990; **72:** 566–70.
59. Caldwell JE, Claver Canfell P, Castagnoli KP, *et al.* The influence of renal failure on the pharmacokinetics and duration of action of pipecuronium bromide in patients anesthetized with halothane and nitrous oxide. *Anesthesiology* 1989; **70:** 7–12.
60. Cashman JN, Luke JJ, Jones RM. Neuromuscular block with doxacurium (BW A938U) in patients with normal or absent renal function. *Br J Anaesth* 1990; **64:** 184–92.
61. Phillips BJ, Hunter JM. The use of mivacurium chloride by constant infusion in the anephric patient. *Br J Anaesth* 1992; **68:** 492–8.
62. Head-Rapson AG, Devlin JC, Parker CJR, Hunter JM. Infusion pharmacokinetics and pharmacodynamics of the three isomers of mivacurium in health, in end-stage renal failure and in patients with impaired renal function. *Br J Anaesth* 1995; **75:** 31–6.
63. Cooper RA, Maddineni VR, Mirakhur RK, *et al.* Time course of neuromuscular effects and pharmacokinetics of rocuronium (Org 9426) during isoflurane anaesthesia in patients with and without renal failure. *Br J Anaesth* 1993; **71:** 222–6.
64. Szenohradszky J, Fisher DM, Segredo V, *et al.* Pharmacokinetics of rocuronium bromide (Org 9426) in patients with normal renal function or patients undergoing cadaver renal transplantation. *Anesthesiology* 1992; **77:** 899–904.
65. Boyd AH, Eastwood NB, Parker CJR, Hunter JM. The pharmacodynamics of the 1R *cis*-1′R *cis* isomer of atracurium (51W89) in health and chronic renal failure. *Br J Anaesth* 1995; **74:** 400–4.
66. Wastila WB, Maehr RB, Turner GL, *et al.* Comparative pharmacology of cisatracurium (51W89), atracurium and five isomers in cats. *Anesthesiology* 1996; **85:** 169–77.
67. Eastwood NB, Boyd AH, Parker CJR, Hunter JM. Pharmacokinetics of 1R *cis*–1′R *cis* atracurium besylate (51W89) and plasma laudanosine concentrations in health and chronic renal failure. *Br J Anaesth* 1995; **75:** 431–5.
68. Boyd AH, Eastwood NB, Parker CJR, Hunter JM. Comparison of the pharmacodynamics and pharmacokinetics of an infusion of cis-atracurium (51W89) or atracurium in critically ill patients undergoing mechanical ventilation in an intensive therapy unit. *Br J Anaesth* 1996; **76:** 382–8.
69. Wierda JM, van den Broek L, Proost JH, *et al.* Time course of action and endotracheal intubating conditions of ORG 9487, a new short-acting steroidal muscle relaxant: a comparison with succinylcholine. *Anesth Analg* 1993; **77:** 579–84.
70. Wierda JMKH, Beaufort AM, Kleef UW, *et al.* Preliminary investigation of the pharmacology of three short-acting nondepolarising neuromuscular blocking agents Org 9453, Org 9489 and Org 9487. *Can J Anaesth* 1994; **41:** 213–20.
71. Szenohradszky J, Caldwell JE, Wright PMC, *et al.* Influence of renal failure on the pharmacokinetics and neuromuscular effects of a single dose of rapacuronium bromide. *Anesthesiology* 1999; **90:** 24–35.
72. Morris R, Cronnelly R, Miller RD, *et al.* Pharmacokinetics of edrophonium and neostigmine when antagonising D-tubocurarine neuromuscular blockade in man. *Anesthesiology* 1981; **54:** 399–402.
73. Cronnelly R, Stanski DR, Miller RD, *et al.* Renal function and the pharmacokinetics of neostigmine in anaesthetised man. *Anesthesiology* 1979; **51:** 222–6.
74. Reeder MK, Goldman MD, Loh L, *et al.* Postoperative hypoxaemia after major abdominal vascular surgery. *Br J Anaesth* 1992; **68:** 23–6.
75. Orko R, Pitkanen M, Rosenberg PH. Subarachnoid anaesthesia with 0.75% bupivacaine in patients with chronic renal failure. *Br J Anaesth* 1986; **58:** 605–9.

FURTHER READING

Bastron RD, Deutsch S. *Anaesthesia and the Kidney*. New York: Grune and Stratton, 1976.

Bevan DR (ed.). *Renal Function in Anaesthesia and Surgery*. London: Academic Press, 1979.

Hunter JM. Recent advances in the management of renal disease: their relevance to the anaesthetist. *Curr Opin Anaesthesiol* 1990; **3:** 452–6.

Priebe H-J (ed.). *The Kidney in Anaesthesia*. International Anesthesiology Clinics. Boston: Little, Brown and Company, 1984.

Smith CE, Hunter JM. *Anaesthesia for Renal Transplantation: Relaxants and Volatiles*. International Anesthesiology Clinics. Boston: Little, Brown and Company, 1995: 69–92.

53

Anesthesia for surgery on the liver

MUZAFFAR FAROQUI

INTRODUCTION

The incidence of liver disease and mortality is increasing worldwide, probably because of an increase in alcohol consumption. Anesthesiologists may be called upon to care for patients for an unrelated condition or for a more specific procedure involving the liver itself. With improved survival following liver transplantation, even more patients are likely to present for surgery and anesthesia than in the past. A detailed assessment of these patients should focus on the following objectives:

1 type and extent of liver impairment;
2 extrahepatic effects of liver disease;
3 risk assessment for postoperative care.

ASSESSMENT OF LIVER FUNCTION

Jaundice

Jaundice can be easily missed in artificial light and is best seen in the sclera under natural light. As outlined in Chapter 17, a careful history of drug use, family history, blood transfusion, tattooing, alcohol intake, foreign travel or recent immigration, sexual orientation and contacts, and other occupational hazards is essential. Jaundice may be due to intrahepatic or extrahepatic obstruction to the flow of bile. Hepatocellular disease is diagnosed in one-quarter of the patients initially suspected of having biliary obstruction.[1] Intrahepatic obstruction may be caused by viral hepatitis or as a consequence of adverse drug reactions. The latter is discussed in detail in the section on postoperative jaundice.

A mildly jaundiced patient with simple biliary obstruction may not have many additional physical signs. In approximately 75% of patients with unexplained jaundice of 4 weeks' duration or longer the cause is an obstruction. Gallstones are usually accompanied by pain and pyrexia and may present as pancreatitis with or without jaundice. Weight loss could suggest a malignancy, whereas weight gain or abdominal distension should point to ascites. Abdominal pain or severe back pain with onset of diabetes should raise the suspicion of pancreatic malignancy. In obstructive jaundice, pruritus is a prominent symptom along with lethargy, nausea, and general malaise. Alteration in mental status and other neurological signs appear only with advanced hepatocellular damage.

Renal impairment is often noticed in jaundiced patients, possibly because of the release of endotoxins into the systemic circulation following long-standing biliary obstruction and infection.[2] With very high serum bilirubin levels ($>140\,\mu mol\,L^{-1}$), preoperative percutaneous drainage of the biliary tree under appropriate antibiotic cover has been recommended to prevent the occurrence of postoperative renal failure.[3] Preoperative oral bile salts have also been given to reduce the possibility of endotoxemia in obstructive jaundice and prevent associated renal failure.[4] Postoperative acute oliguric renal failure may be due to nephrotoxic bile salts and pigments, endotoxins, or inflammatory mediators.[5]

In addition to a raised bilirubin, alkaline phosphatase levels are also elevated. Simultaneous measurement of 5-nucleotidase helps to distinguish a rise in alkaline phosphatase associated with normal growth in adolescents from a pathological rise in liver disease.

The two enzymes rise in parallel in liver disease. Serum transaminase levels are moderately elevated except in the presence of cholangitis, when the rise is marked.

Noninvasive investigative techniques to find the cause of biliary obstruction include ultrasonic scanning, computed tomography, and magnetic resonance imaging.[6] Direct visualization of the bile and pancreatic ducts and the duodenal loop is possible with endoscopic examination, but areas proximal to the obstruction cannot be seen. Percutaneous introduction of dye into the intrahepatic biliary tree runs the risk of biliary peritonitis, sepsis, and hemorrhage.[7]

Cirrhosis

Cirrhosis is characterized by severe fibrosis and nodular regeneration of the hepatic parenchyma. Although there are many causes for cirrhosis, alcohol abuse is becoming the most prominent reason throughout the world. In particular, it is related to heavy consumption over a long period rather than occasional sprees.[8] Cirrhosis may also be caused by chronic active hepatitis of any type. Other less common causes for cirrhosis include hemochromatosis and primary biliary cirrhosis. Hemochromatosis is characterized by accumulation of iron within the hepatocytes,[9] a higher incidence of liver cancer,[10] and a high serum ferritin level, with a definitive diagnosis made by a liver biopsy.[11] Primary biliary cirrhosis predominantly affects women, with cholestasis progressing to fibrosis and frequently associated with osteoporosis, malabsorption, and autoimmune disease.[12] Patients with cirrhosis may be asymptomatic with almost normal liver function or they may present in a severely decompensated state with gross ascites, jaundice, and other signs and symptoms of liver failure. Clinical assessment should identify the degree of hepatocellular damage, the biochemical hepatic reserve, and the presence of portal hypertension. The severity of cirrhosis can be judged by clinical, biochemical, and histological investigations. The distortion of the normal hepatic cellular architecture leads to a mechanically obstructed blood flow, with portal venous pressure rising from an average of 0.9 kPa (7 mmHg) under normal conditions to 6.7 kPa (50 mmHg), and the creation of alternative collateral venous channels. Esophageal varices, prominent collateral veins radiating from the umbilicus, dilated rectal veins, and splenomegaly are associated with portal hypertension. The natural history of chronic liver disease is not necessarily one of unremitting and progressive deterioration, and it may be the stress of intercurrent surgery or other illness that renders it apparent.[13] When symptoms do occur, they tend to be vague, such as lethargy, malaise, dyspepsia, weight loss, and loss of libido. Physical signs can be completely absent or there may be such changes as white skin spots, paper-money skin, white nails, and palmar erythema. Occasionally, nonspecific signs such as finger clubbing and pigmentation may also be seen. A significant sign of cirrhosis is the presence of spider nevi on the face, upper body, and the arms. Spider nevi may also be transiently seen during pregnancy.

In cirrhosis due to alcohol abuse or hemochromatosis, the liver is often large, but in primary biliary cirrhosis and cryptogenic cirrhosis it is small and shrunken. Severe hepatocellular failure is characterized by jaundice, ascites, and encephalopathy. Lowered plasma oncotic pressure due to the failure of albumin synthesis and a rise in portal venous pressure leads to the formation of ascites. This relative depletion in intravascular volume triggers the renal tubules to retain sodium and water and thus encourages the formation of additional ascites. Ascites can develop acutely or may take months to become clinically obvious. The hepatorenal syndrome is commonly seen in patients with long-standing ascites and may be precipitated if brisk diuresis is achieved when treating patients with ascites.[14] Peritonitis as a result of spontaneous bacterial infection is seen in a small percentage of cirrhotic patients.

SYSTEMIC EFFECTS OF LIVER DISEASE

General condition

Not infrequently, ascites and generalized tissue edema mask a poor nutritional state. With advanced liver disease, there is considerable loss of muscle mass and power.

Cardiovascular system

Advanced cirrhosis is often associated with a hyperdynamic circulatory state, low peripheral vascular resistance, high cardiac output, and significant intrapulmonary and peripheral arteriovenous shunting. In alcoholic liver disease, left ventricular function may be impaired.[15] Clinical examination reveals the presence of tachycardia, flushed and warm extremities with a bounding pulse, capillary pulsation, and an ejection systolic murmur. A differential diagnosis of hypotension should include low peripheral vascular resistance, occult bleeding, and poor left ventricular function.

Respiratory system

Intrapulmonary shunts may be associated with hypoxemia, impaired hypoxic pulmonary vasoconstriction, and hyperventilation.[16] Nearly one-third of patients with decompensated cirrhosis have low $P_{a}O_2$ and are cyanosed. In advanced liver disease, impaired arterial oxygenation ranging from an increased alveolar–arterial gradient to severe hypoxemia is common. The severe form of impaired pulmonary function with chronic liver disease, absence of intrinsic cardiopulmonary disease, alveolar–arterial gradient of >2 kPa (15 mmHg), and evidence of intrapulmonary vascular dilation is referred to as the hepatopulmonary syndrome.[17,18] Absence of hypoxemia in the presence of end-stage liver disease and high shunt fraction may be due to an increased cardiac output leading to a decrease in arterio-mixed venous oxygen content difference and an increase in mixed venous oxygenation level.[19] Patients with ascites or significant hepatomegaly have basal atelectasis due to an increase in closing volume of the lungs. Chest infections are common and pleural effusions sometimes coexist with ascites.

Renal function

The effect of jaundice on renal function has already been commented on in Chapter 17. The link between preoperative jaundice and postoperative renal dysfunction is well known. In a series of 114 patients undergoing surgery on the liver, biliary tract, and the pancreas, 36 patients (17%) developed acute renal failure, compared with 1% of 78 patients who were not jaundiced preoperatively.[20] Deeply jaundiced elderly patients are more likely to develop postoperative oliguric renal failure than patients of similar age without jaundice.[21] In addition to jaundice, the preoperative serum creatinine level is a factor of major prognostic importance when identifying patients undergoing biliary tract surgery who are at risk of developing renal failure.[22]

Hepatorenal syndrome is a common complication in patients with progressive liver disease. It has been described as "a decrease in renal function which develops in a patient with serious liver disease in whom all other causes of renal dysfunction are excluded."[23] Severe renal vasoconstriction, intravascular volume depletion, peripheral vasodilation, and the presence of portal hypertension are possible contributory factors. Intravascular volume depletion or vigorous diuresis in a cirrhotic patient can precipitate hepatorenal syndrome. The chance of developing hepatorenal syndrome increases with progressive liver disease (Fig. 53.1),[24] and the longer the duration of the syndrome the higher the risk of dying (Fig. 53.2).[24] With established hepatorenal syndrome, the kidneys are more prone to damage, with volume depletion and nephrotoxic side-effects of drugs such as the nonsteroidal anti-inflammatory drugs (NSAIDs), aminoglycosides, and the contrast agents. The syndrome is characterized by progressive water retention, hyponatremia, azotemia, and oliguria due to a decrease in renal blood flow.[13]

Hemostatic function

Patients with liver disease may have prolonged bleeding time owing to the failure to produce clotting factors. Factors II, VII, IX, and X require vitamin K-dependent enzyme for their activity and therefore may respond to vitamin K administration. However, in the presence of parenchymal liver disease, this needs to be supplemented with fresh-frozen plasma. Slow administration of vitamin K is recommended as rapid intravenous injection has been reported to cause cardiovascular collapse.[25] Other factors involved in the hemorrhagic tendency include dilutional coagulopathy, an exaggerated fibrinolytic response, and metabolic problems such as hypothermia, acidosis, and hypocalcemia.[16] The enhanced fibrinolytic activity seen in cirrhosis may be due to an exaggerated response to vasoactive substances resulting from the delayed hepatic clearance of plasminogen, decreased synthesis of naturally occurring inhibitors, and activation of protein C.[16]

Neurological function

In alcoholic cirrhosis, cerebellar ataxia and peripheral neuropathy occur in the absence of encephalopathy. Hepatic encephalopathy may be pres-

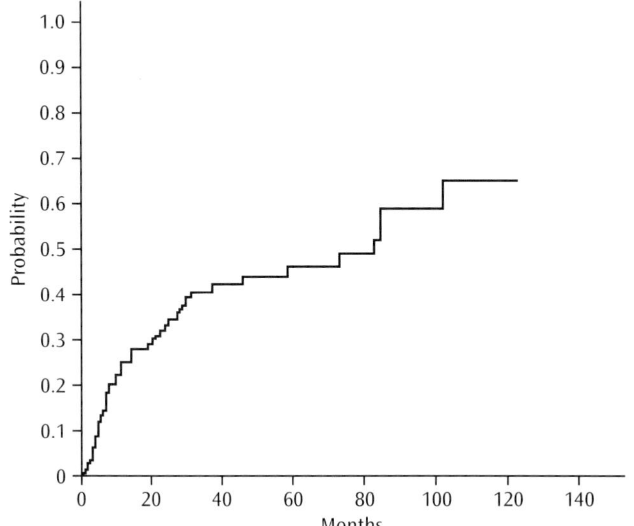

Figure 53.1 *Cumulative probability of developing hepatorenal syndrome from the onset of ascites in a series of 136 cirrhotic patients. (Reproduced from Ginès* et al.[24]*)*

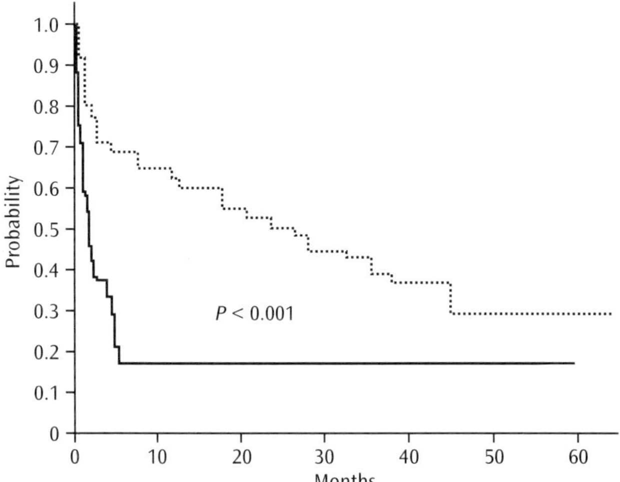

Figure 53.2 *Probability of survival in a series of 136 patients with cirrhosis and ascites, classified according to the presence (solid line;* n = 24*) or absence (dashed line;* n = 112*) of hepatorenal syndrome. (Reproduced from Ginès* et al.[24]*)*

ent in both severe acute and decompensated chronic liver disease with increasing portosystemic shunting. In its mild form, the symptoms are limited to personality changes, impaired intellect, and drowsiness, but in severe form dysarthria, incoordination, increased muscle tone with hyper-reflexia, a flapping tremor, and other signs of cerebral edema are noticeable. A detailed description is given later, in the section on acute liver failure.

Gastrointestinal system

In liver disease, gastrointestinal hemorrhage may be caused by the rupture of gastric and esophageal varices – the clinically important portosystemic shunts. Although common in alcoholic cirrhosis, these are not the only source;[26] endoscopy may be required to identify the source of bleeding. As in any other form of hypovolemia due to heavy blood loss, the initial management involves intravenous fluid therapy with appropriate fluids. In patients with persistent gastrointestinal (GI) bleeding in the presence of portal hypertension, other pharmacological or mechanical means may be required.

Vasopressin and octreotide are two of the agents used to lower portal venous pressure. Vasopressin causes arteriolar vasoconstriction of the splanchnic bed, but this action is not confined to gut vasculature alone as it causes coronary artery vasoconstriction and serious cardiovascular consequences including a fall in cardiac output. Octreotide, on the other hand, has fewer cardiovascular side-effects.[27]

For short-term control of variceal bleeding, as for example during transportation to specialized centers for definitive treatment, balloon tamponade with a Sengstaken–Blakemore tube is the mainstay of treatment. Injection of sclerosing agents directly into the varices controls the bleeding in the majority of patients, but with rebleeding this therapy becomes ineffective.[28] Increasingly, anesthesiologists are involved in the management of these patients for the creation of an intrahepatic portosystemic shunt. Using the transjugular approach, a communication is established using an expandable metallic stent between the hepatic and the portal veins within the hepatic parenchyma. Transjugular intrahepatic portosystemic shunt (TIPS) has proved to be an attractive alternative to the more invasive surgical procedure of portocaval shunt formation.[29]

Specific issues related to the gastrointestinal system in acute liver failure are covered later.

RISK ASSESSMENT

The principle of management of patients with well-compensated or decompensated liver disease is essentially the same, but for the latter there is a much reduced hepatic reserve. Child and Turcotte first described estimation of hepatic reserve and, by inference, operative risk and mortality.[30] Pugh and colleagues subsequently added the evaluation of prothrombin time to these clinical and laboratory indices.[31] Garrison and colleagues provided further clarification of these risk factors for patients with hepatic cirrhosis in 1984.[32] Tables 53.1, 53.2, and 53.3 give details of various risk-scoring systems. These systems may be helpful when making decisions about elective surgery.[33] The Child and Pugh classifications are easy to apply, and it has been suggested[13] that as a working rule only patients in Child's group A should be recommended for elective surgery; those in group B may be acceptable, but every effort should be made to correct abnormalities of nutrition, to raise the plasma albumin, and to correct anemia and clotting abnormalities. Patients in group C should be considered only for emergency surgery.

PERIOPERATIVE MANAGEMENT

Preoperative assessment

Essentially, the visit should be used to assess the severity of the patient's illness, the presence of complications associated with liver disease, and the likely impact of anesthesia and surgery. This will entail a detailed history from either the patient or the relatives, thorough physical examination of the patient, including the state of hydration, nutritional, and neurological status, and an assessment of the associated complications. In addition to liver function tests, clinical and laboratory investigations should include an assessment of cardiorespiratory, metabolic,and hematological impairment.

Table 53.1 *Clinical and laboratory classification of patients with cirrhosis in terms of hepatic functional reserve*

	Group A	Group B	Group C
Serum bilirubin (μmol L^{-1})	<40	40–50	>50
Serum albumin (g L^{-1})	>35	30–35	<30
Ascites	None	Easily controlled	Poorly controlled
Neurological disorder	None	Minimal	Advanced coma
Nutrition	Excellent	Good	Poor, wasting
Risk of operation	Good (5%)	Moderate (10%)	Poor (50%)

Child group A, 4–6 points; Child group B, 7–9 points; Child group C, 10–12 points.
Reproduced from Child and Turcotte.[30]

Table 53.2 *Grading of severity of liver disease*

Clinical and biochemical measurement	Points scored for increasing abnormalities		
	1	2	3
Encephalopathy (grade)	None	1 and 2	3 and 4
Bilirubin (μmol L^{-1})	<25	25–40> 40	
Albumin	35	28–35	<28
Prothrombin time (seconds prolonged)	1–4	4–6	>4

Reproduced from Pugh *et al.*[31]

Table 53.3 *Preoperative risk factors associated with increased postoperative mortality*

Serum albumin <3 g L^{-1}
Presence of infection
White blood cell count >10 000
Treatment with more than two antibiotics
Prothrombin time >1.5 s over control
Serum bilirubin >50 mmol L^{-1}
Presence of ascites
Malnutrition
Emergency surgery

Data from Browne[16] and Garrison *et al.*[32]

Short-acting oral benzodiazepines such as temazepam may be prescribed for anxiolysis in the absence of any neurological impairment. Patients suspected of having hepatic encephalopathy should not be given any long-acting central nervous system (CNS) depressants and opiates should be avoided.[34] As mentioned previously, vitamin K may need to be administered preoperatively. Optimal hydration in jaundiced patients or in those with hepatorenal syndrome requires careful intravenous fluid therapy and use of diuretics.

Anesthetic technique

Unlike the normal liver, the cirrhotic liver receives a greater proportion of its blood supply from the hepatic artery and the regeneration nodules are primarily supplied with arterial blood. It is therefore imperative to avoid hypotensive anesthetic techniques for these patients. Systemic hypoxemia and hypotension may result in severe hepatic necrosis and must be prevented at all costs. Owing to the presence of intrapulmonary shunts, a higher than normal concentration of oxygen should be administered.

Drug pharmacokinetics is altered in liver disease to a variable degree, especially in parenchymal disease. This mainly affects drugs with high extraction ratios, e.g. morphine, lidocaine (lignocaine). Most of the intravenous induction agents are metabolized by the liver, but the recovery from an induction dose depends on the redistribution of these drugs. Although the intrinsic clearance of thiopentone may be delayed, there is a concomitant reduction in its protein binding and therefore recovery is unaffected.[35] Patients with alcoholic liver disease may require a higher dose of thiopentone, possibly because of cross-tolerance between alcohol and barbiturates.[36] In well-compensated cirrhotic patients, recovery from propofol due to redistribution has been documented;[37] in addition, there is evidence of extrahepatic metabolism, as seen during the anhepatic phase of liver transplantation.[38] Although plasma pseudocholinesterase levels are reduced, they are seldom low enough to prolong the action of succinylcholine (suxamethonium).[39]

Atracurium is broken down by Hoffman degradation and its breakdown is independent of hepatic metabolism, therefore it is an ideal muscle relaxant in liver disease. However, patients with liver disease show increased resistance and a shorter duration of action with atracurium,[39] possibly because of increased binding to raised globulin levels. Vecuronium, which depends on the liver for elimination, has been shown to have a recovery time twice as long as normal even in mild disease.[40] However, in a dose less than 0.15 mg kg^{-1}, the kinetics and duration of action of vecuronium were unaffected in patients with cirrhosis.[41] The half-life of pancuronium was prolonged 1.6-fold in patients with extrahepatic cholestasis.[42]

The pharmacokinetic activity of fentanyl following a single dose in uncomplicated alcoholic cirrhosis is essentially normal,[43] but in end-stage liver disease the action becomes variable and cannot be predicted with accuracy.[44] Similarly, the elimination half-life of sufentanil following a single dose is unaltered.[45] Remifentanil is metabolized by nonspecific blood and tissue esterases and would therefore seem to be an ideal opiate for use in patients with liver disease. Various authors have investigated its use in patients with hepatic or renal disease.[46–48] Isoflurane is the inhalational agent of choice because hepatic oxygen supply is better preserved with this agent than with other volatile anesthetic agents.[49] Bito and Ikeda[50] reported minor elevations of bilirubin and transaminases with both isoflurane and sevoflurane anesthesia. Halothane was used in pediatric patients with cholestasis without any adverse hepatic consequences.[51]

Fluid balance requires meticulous attention, and invasive monitoring of intravascular fluid status is essential. Patients with ascites undergoing laparotomy lose a large amount of fluid rapidly with resultant hemodynamic instability. Concentrated albumin solutions should be infused to correct the protein loss associated with acute ascitic fluid drainage. If needed, fresh whole blood should be transfused in preference to stored blood to avoid hypocalcemia resulting from a reduced metabolism of the preservatives. Calcium chloride is given if the ionized calcium level falls. Fresh-frozen plasma in a dose of 12–15 mL kg^{-1} should be given to correct dilutional coagulopathy.

Temperature should be monitored throughout and appropriate

measures taken to prevent excessive heat loss. In surgical procedures involving exposure of thoracic or abdominal organs, heat loss is substantial. Measures include active patient warming, humidified inspired gases, and intravascular fluid warmers to prevent drastic falls in temperature.

In patients with history of excessive alcohol intake, other nonhepatic effects should be borne in mind. These include the presence of osteoporosis,[52,53] cardiomyopathy,[54] myocardial depression,[55] and altered immune status.[54]

Routine coagulation tests such as platelet count, prothrombin time, partial thromboplastin time, activated clotting time, and fibrin degradation products measure hypocoagulability and end with the formation of the first fibrin strand in plasma.[56,57] Furthermore, the physiological status of the patient (e.g. hypothermia, acidosis, hypocalcemia) is not taken into account. In addition, they do not measure the quality of the coagulation factors and there is a lag time of 30–60 min before the results become available.[58] Recently, the thromboelastogram (TEG) has re-emerged as a tool for use during surgery in patients with impaired hepatic function.[57–59] Whitten and Greilich[60] have recently reviewed the subject of thromboelastography. TEG has been advocated as a useful guide to transfusion therapy in cardiac surgery,[61,62] liver transplantation.[63–65] and intensive care.[66] The TEG measures the hemostatic process in whole blood from the start of clotting to the final stages of clot lysis, thereby monitoring both hypocoagulable states and fibrinolysis. The trace produced by the TEG allows a diagnosis to be made in respect of a lack of platelets, other clotting factors, or fibrinolysis (Fig. 53.3).[59]

In 1914, Goodpasture first described the presence of fibrinolysis in chronic liver disease.[67] To counter fibrinolytic activity, ε-aminocaproic acid[68] and antithrombin III have been shown to have some beneficial effect. In clinically stable cirrhosis, Schipper and Ten Cate confirmed the increased turnover of ^{125}I-labeled fibrinogen and its correction by antithrombin III.[69] Both thrombocytopenia and platelet dysfunction have been reported in liver disease,[70] and it is sometimes necessary to administer platelets if the count is below 70 000.

Postoperative management

The principle of management remains the same in the postoperative as in the intraoperative phase. Mild and reversible impairment of liver function is common in the postoperative period, possibly because of a reduction in hepatic blood flow with both regional and general anesthesia.[71,72] These changes are clinically insignificant, although in a small group of patients undergoing major surgery postoperative jaundice is present. The pathophysiology of this is discussed later, in the section on postoperative jaundice.

ANESTHESIA FOR LIVER TRANSPLANTATION AND LIVER SURGERY

Anesthesia for liver transplantation

Starzl *et al.*[73] carried out the first human liver transplant in Denver, Colorado, in 1963, and in 1967 Calne performed the first liver transplant in the UK at Addenbrooke's Hospital in Cambridge, UK.[74] Over the subsequent 17 years, the number of centers performing these procedures increased several-fold both in the USA as well as in Europe. The next major milestone, however, was the introduction of cyclosporine (cyclosporin A), an immunosuppressant, used experimentally in humans for renal graft survival in 1980. The liver graft survival increased dramatically from 35% to 78.6% at 1 year after the use of cyclosporine.[75,76] With further advances in immunosuppression, long-term survival and quality of life is markedly improved for transplanted patients.

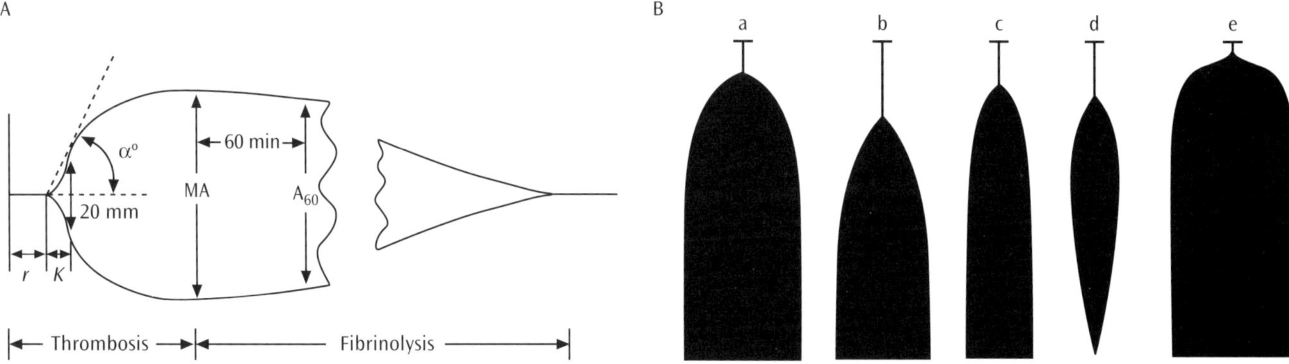

Figure 53.3 *Thromboelastography (TEG). (A) Quantification of TEG variables. Analysis of the thromboelastograph.* r = *reaction time (time from sample placement in the cuvette until TEG tracing amplitude reaches 2 mm) (normal range 6–8 min). This represents the rate of initial fibrin formation and is related functionally to plasma clotting factor and circulating inhibitor activity (intrinsic coagulation). Prolongation of the* r *time may be a result of coagulation factor deficiencies, anticoagulation (heparin), or severe hypofibrinogenemia. A small* r *value may be present in hypercoagulability syndromes.* K = *clot formation time (normal range 3–6 min), measured from time* r *to the point where the amplitude of the tracing reaches 20 mm. The coagulation time represents the time taken for a fixed degree of viscoelasticity to be achieved by the forming clot, as a result of fibrin build-up and cross-linking. It is effected by the activity of the intrinsic clotting factors, fibrinogen, and platelets. Alpha angle (α°) (normal range 50–60°) = angle formed by the slope of TEG tracing from the* r *to the* K *value. It denotes the speed at which the clot forms. Decreased values may occur with hypofibrinogenemia and thrombocytopenia. Maximum amplitude (MA) (normal range 50–60 mm) = greatest amplitude on the TEG trace and is a reflection of the absolute strength of the fibrin clot. It is a direct function of the maximum dynamic properties of fibrin and platelets. Platelet abnormalities, whether* qualitative *or quantitative, substantially disturb the MA.* A_{60} *(normal range = MA – 5 mm) = amplitude of the tracing 60 min after MA is achieved. It is a measure of clot lysis or retraction. The clot lysis index (CLI) (normal range > 85%) is derived as* $(A_{60}/MA) \times 100$ *(%). It measures the amplitude as a function of time and reflects loss of clot integrity as a result of lysis. (B) Specific hemostatic defects produce characteristic TEG traces. a, Normal trace. b, Hemophilia: marked prolongation of* r *and* K *times; decreased alpha angle. c, Thrombocytopenia: normal* r *and* rK *times; decreased MA (< 40 mm). d, Fibrinolysis: CLI < 85%. e, Hypercoagulability: short* r *time; increased MA; steep clot formation rate. (Reproduced from Mallet and Cox.*[59]*)*

In orthotopic liver transplantation, the donor liver is implanted in the normal anatomic position. However, in heterotopic liver transplantation the donor liver is placed within the abdominal cavity with the patient's native organ occupying the normal anatomic position.[77] It is difficult to accommodate an extra organ in the abdomen in a way that it receives arterial and portal blood and drains hepatic venous blood and bile. There is also the added danger of multiple anastomoses kinking or becoming otherwise compromised. Almost all the liver transplant procedures undertaken at present are orthotopic.

As described above, the liver is a complex organ involved with numerous synthetic and metabolic functions of the body. Whereas there is dialysis for renal replacement, the artificial heart for cardiac function, and various ventilatory modalities for the lungs, the complexities of hepatic function have, as yet, rendered this organ irreplaceable. Studies are ongoing to provide a short-term liver support system, although the results are not very encouraging. It is therefore imperative for survival that a liver diseased beyond its capacity to recover should be replaced with a healthy one.

Major indications for liver transplantation are shown in Table 53.4.

With advances in immunosuppression, anesthesia, and surgical management, liver transplantation has become increasingly successful, with contraindications limited to extrahepatic malignancy, active substance abuse, and active extrahepatic infection. However, published reports demonstrating successful transplants even in these groups continue to reduce the contraindications. Although extremes of age were a contraindication in the past, recent developments have shown encouraging graft survival in the old and the very young. Survival in recipients older than 50 years is similar at 5 years to that of younger adults.[78] Transplantation for alcoholic liver disease, viral hepatitis, and hepatic neoplasm remains controversial because of the high incidence of recurrence of the original disease.[79]

Surgical approach

Surgical access is gained via a wide, bilateral, subcostal incision with a xiphoid extension. The xiphoid process is removed to allow access to the suprahepatic abdominal vena cava and the main hepatic veins. The diseased organ is excised by dividing the hepatic artery, the portal vein, and the suprahepatic and the infrahepatic vena cava. The donor liver is then implanted in the same anatomic position, vascular anastomoses made, and the new organ reperfused. Duct-to-duct biliary anastomosis or Roux-en-Y choledochojejunostomy completes the procedure.

Limited availability of suitably sized pediatric livers has led to the development of techniques such as split grafts, in which a single donor organ may be split for multiple transplants. However, the incidence of complications is much higher with this technique. These include excessive bleeding,[80] tissue necrosis, and reduced survival rate in the recipients.[81] Sometimes, the left lobe of the liver is removed from a healthy living related donor and used as a graft. Potential donor morbidity and a lower survival rate in the recipients make this option less attractive. Gundlach and colleagues[82] have demonstrated 1-year survival following split liver and living related liver transplantation of 80.5% in adults and 84.3% in children. A higher incidence of hepatic artery thrombosis has also been reported in these procedures.[83]

The surgical procedure can be divided into three stages: (1) dissection phase to excise the diseased liver; (2) anhepatic phase, during which the donor liver is anastomosed; and (3) reperfusion phase. Even though the preoperative condition of the patient undergoing liver transplantation poses difficult problems common throughout these phases, some of the more specific ones pertaining to each of these are discussed in detail below.

Table 53.4 *Major indications for liver transplantation*

Adults
Primary biliary cirrhosis
Chronic active hepatitis
Primary hepatoma
Carcinoma of the hepatic ducts
Primary sclerosing cholangitis
End-stage cirrhosis
Metastatic carcinoid tumors

Children
Congenital biliary atresia
Familial intrahepatic cholestasis
Arteriohepatic dysplasia
Neonatal hepatitis
α_1-Antitrypsin deficiency
Wilson's disease
Tyrosinemia
Glycogen storage disease types I and IV

Anesthetic management

The clinical features and pathophysiology of liver disease have already been described in detail above and in the section on the physiology of liver. They are present in patients for liver transplantation to a variable degree. In particular, the involvement of other organ systems is important and is often seen as the presence of a hyperdynamic circulation with reduced peripheral vascular resistance, pulmonary hypertension, intrapulmonary shunts, and coagulation disorders including thrombocytopenia, renal impairment, portal hypertension, and its sequelae. Not infrequently, if there has been a recent deterioration, signs suggestive of acute liver failure such as hypoglycemia and a deteriorating level of consciousness may be present.

Cardiomyopathy can be associated with alcoholic liver disease or hemosiderosis, but it may be difficult to detect without an endomyocardial biopsy. Serum albumin level is often low, resulting in fewer binding sites for the drugs, an increase in the volume of distribution, and impaired drug metabolism and excretion (see above).

The basic principles of anesthetizing patients with liver disease have been described above. For a patient undergoing transplantation involving section and subsequent reanastomosis of major blood vessels, it is vital to establish adequate venous access for rapid transfusion. This can be achieved by insertion of at least two large-bore peripheral venous cannulae in the upper half of the body. Fluids administered through lower body cannulae are lost in the surgical field. Invasive hemodynamic monitoring should include systemic and pulmonary arterial catheters in addition to direct arterial pressure measurement. An arterial catheter should preferably be placed in the right brachial or right radial artery to obviate the distortion of the arterial waveform due to the mechanical compression of the left axillary artery by the return limb of a venovenous bypass circuit. Some centers also use a femoral artery catheter to monitor distal arterial pressure that may be compromised during transient abdominal aortic clamping during hepatic artery anastomosis. More sophisticated monitoring may be required in sicker patients. This includes transesophageal echocardiography, continuous cardiac output measurement,[84] mucosal pH measurement,[85] and the use of transcranial Doppler.[86]

Special attention should be paid to positioning the patient correctly with adequate padding because of the long surgical procedure. Injury to the brachial plexus can be minimized by arm abduction not exceeding 90°, with forearm supination and anterior flexion. Liver transplant patients have a higher incidence of brachial plexus neuropathy. The etiology, although multifactorial, includes cyclosporine toxicity and nerve compression from the axillary limb of the venovenous bypass circuit.[87]

Various anesthetic drugs have been used successfully for induction of anesthesia. However, an agent such as etomidate with minimal cardiovascular effects may be the most appropriate. "Rapid sequence" technique is recommended for patients with delayed gastric emptying as with gross ascites, active GI bleeding, or encephalopathy, and for those with a full stomach. As mentioned before, plasma pseudocholinesterase levels are reduced in liver disease but the resultant prolongation of succinylcholine effect is of no clinical significance. Altered pharmacokinetic responses to the nondepolarizing neuromuscular blockers in liver disease result in an increased initial dose requirement and a possible prolongation of effect. However, these effects are less pronounced with atracurium or cisatracurium. The rate of recovery from vecuronium[88] and rocuronium[89] has been used as an indicator of the function of the newly transplanted liver. Ventilation with added positive end-expiratory pressure of up to 5 cmH_2O (0.5 kPa) is used to prevent atelectasis and to reduce the risk of air embolism from the hepatic bed. Anesthesia is maintained with a mixture of oxygen-enriched air and isoflurane supplemented with opioids such as fentanyl, alfentanil, sufentanil, or remifentanil. Nitrous oxide should be avoided because of its potential for bowel distension and an increase in the size of an air embolus. Isoflurane is considered a safe inhalational agent for liver transplantation, as there is evidence that hepatic artery blood flow is substantially preserved, possibly by preservation of the autoregulation or as a result of profound vasodilation of the hepatic vasculature.[90,91]

Benzodiazepines should be used with caution in patients with cirrhosis, owing to an increased risk of excessive sedation resulting from reduced drug elimination and increased sensitivity.[92] They are relatively contraindicated in patients with incipient encephalopathy in whom γ-aminobutyric acid (GABA)-ergic neurotransmission may be increased by elevated levels of benzodiazepines.[93]

Body temperature is difficult to maintain with a large surface area of the body exposed for a long time. The use of efficient fluid warmers, heating blankets, heated humidifiers, and forced air warming devices is highly recommended. Large volumes of warmed blood and blood products may be required at high flow rates during the dissection phases of both liver transplantation and liver resection. Devices such as the Rapid Infusion System (RIS) (Hemonetics, Braintree, MA, USA) or Level I warming device (Level I Technologies, Rockland, MA, USA) meet these requirements. RIS incorporates a 3-L fluid reservoir, a 170-μm filter, a heat exchanger, a roller pump, a 40-μm filter, an infusion rate controller, and air detectors. When large blood loss is anticipated, a blood salvage system (Cell-Saver, Hemonetics) will help to reduce the demand on the blood bank for red cells. This can be connected directly to the reservoir of the RIS in a life-threatening emergency, and salvaged blood transfused directly into the patient.

Monitoring

The principles of monitoring a patient with liver disease have been described above. During liver transplantation, not only may hepatic blood flow be adversely affected by the surgical procedure but also hepatic surgery usually entails significant blood loss, large fluid shifts, cardiovascular instability, coagulation disorders, electrolyte and acid–base imbalance, and difficulty in maintaining body temperature. It is therefore essential that monitoring and therapy be based on knowledge of hepatic physiology and pathophysiology.

Cardiovascular monitoring needs to include multichannel electrocardiogram, invasive arterial blood pressure, and central venous and pulmonary artery pressure, with facilities for measuring cardiac output and other derived parameters. Ventilatory function should be monitored by pulse oximetry, end-tidal carbon dioxide analysis, and frequent blood gas analysis.

Immediate access to laboratory services is essential to monitor the rapid changes in electrolytes and coagulation profile. It is preferable to have a "minilaboratory" within the operating suite for a rapid "turnover" of results. Ionized calcium levels require close and frequent monitoring as citrate toxicity can occur rapidly with transfusion of large amounts of blood and blood products. Often, calcium may need to be administered as a constant infusion to maintain the ionized calcium level within the therapeutic range. Coagulation state should ideally be monitored by measuring prothrombin time, partial thromboplastin time, fibrinogen level, platelet count, and thrombin clotting time. A relatively rapid (30 min) and qualitative assessment of the state of coagulation can be obtained within the operating suite by using a thromboelastograph (TEG)[16,62] (see above). The TEG provides a graphic display of the clot formation and lysis. Calculated variables – reaction time, maximum amplitude, and clot formation and lysis rate – are displayed along with the normal ranges on a videomonitor. Diagnosis of altered coagulation and its effective treatment with blood components should be based on a balanced judgment of the results of standard tests and the TEG.

Neuromuscular monitoring with a nerve stimulator is recommended, especially if the muscle relaxants are administered by continuous infusion.

Blood sugar level should be monitored regularly. Hypoglycemia, although rarely seen, is an indication of severe liver failure.

Renal impairment (described above) may be intensified by physiological insults during the surgical procedure, by massive hemorrhage, by profound vasoconstriction, and by clamping of the major abdominal vessels such as the aorta and the inferior vena cava. Efforts should be made to preserve renal function by meticulous surgical technique, adequate and appropriate fluid administration, and maintenance of adequate cardiac output to ensure end-organ perfusion. Measures should include the use of furosemide, mannitol, and dopamine (DA) or dopexamine. Dopamine is commonly believed to possess renal preservatory effects in dosages of 2–3 $\mu g\,kg^{-1}\,min^{-1}$, although this effect has not been confirmed.[94–96] Dopexamine, on the other hand, has been shown to improve renal function, possibly because of the agonistic action at the renal vascular and tubular DA_1 receptors.[97]

Issues specific to the three phases

Dissection phase

This includes the dissection and isolation of the hepatic vasculature, the hilar structures, and the liver. Some centers use venovenous bypass to minimize the impact of hemodynamic instability associated with the various phases of liver transplantation. It is established by cannulation of the portal and the femoral veins. The draining blood passes through a centrifugal pump and is returned via the axillary vein (Fig. 53.4). The use of heparin or heparin-bonded tubing for the bypass circuit differs from center to center. The procedure marginally increases operating time and may contribute to heat loss.[98] Other complications include air and thromboembolism.[99] Blood loss, both insidious and obvious, can occur especially in patients with portal hypertension. Adhesions can be very extensive, tedious, and the cause of substantial blood loss. Large volumes of ascitic fluid may be lost, with resultant fluid shifts that need to be anticipated and corrected with appropriate fluids. Other factors that contribute to excessive hemorrhage include hemodilution, fibrinolysis,[100] deficiency of clotting agents, and the release of endogenous heparin-like substances.[101] In patients with clinically significant coagulopathy, abnormal TEG, and altered clotting results, attempts should be made to correct the defect as soon as possible. In addition drugs such as aprotinin, tranexamic acid, and conjugated estrogen have been recommended[102] to control hemorrhage. A meta-analysis of pharmacological strategies to decrease bleeding associated with cardiac surgery has demonstrated a reduction in the use of blood transfusion following the use of aprotinin.[103] Various investigators have investigated its role in liver transplantation.[104–107] A recent multicenter study has strongly recommended the use of aprotinin for adult patients undergoing liver transplantation.[108] Molenaar *et al.*[109] claim improved early graft survival

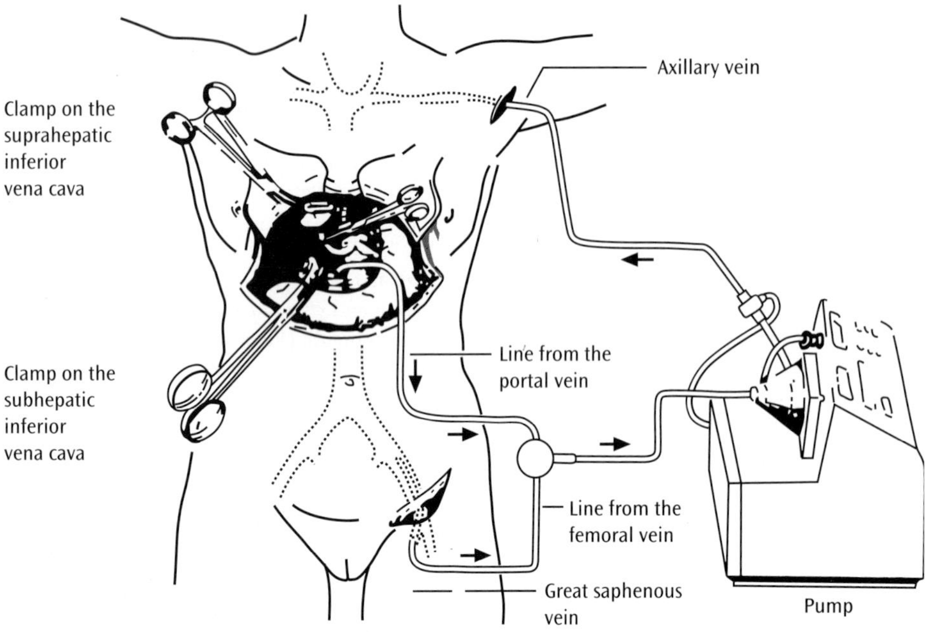

Figure 53.4 *Diagrammatic representation of venovenous bypass to reduce back-pressure on the gastrointestinal tract during inferior vena caval cross-clamping.*

in patients receiving aprotinin during orthotopic liver transplantation. In some centers, ε-aminocaproic acid is given by infusion from the start of the surgical procedure to prevent fibrinolysis. Surgical manipulation, especially around the major vessels, can lead to vascular compression, a reduction in venous return, and a fall in cardiac output. The patient is considered anhepatic once the hepatic blood vessels are ligated.

Anhepatic phase

Clamping the inferior vena cava leads to a substantial reduction in venous return in the absence of venovenous bypass, with a resultant fall in renal perfusion leading to oliguria. In patients with long-standing portal hypertension, this reduction is less marked because of a well-developed portosystemic collateral circulation. The decrease in cardiac output can be compensated by fluid loading with or without vasopressors. However, this exposes the patient to the additional risk of dilutional coagulopathy and, in the reperfusion phase, to the possibility of developing pulmonary edema.

The physiologic changes induced by venovenous bypass which runs throughout the anhepatic phase include a fall in body temperature, a decrease in both heart rate and arterial pressure, and an increase in central venous pressure.[98,110] A prolonged bypass period leads to an increase in hematocrit, colloid oncotic pressure, and serum osmolality. A severe and progressive metabolic acidosis suggests less than optimal perfusion of the lower half of the body.[111] Markers of renal perfusion are preserved with the use of bypass.[112,113]

Citrate toxicity, especially with rapid transfusion of blood and blood products such as fresh-frozen plasma, is pronounced owing to the absence of the normal metabolic activity of the liver. Judicious calcium administration is required to prevent hypocalcemia. Following caval anastomosis, portal bypass is discontinued to allow portal anastomosis to be completed. Venovenous bypass is then discontinued and the new graft reperfused. The anhepatic phase ends with "washing out" of the preservative solution prior to unclamping of vessels.

It is worthwhile considering the organ preservation and the mechanism of reperfusion injury before considering the reperfusion phase in detail.

Preservation

Donor organs were preserved in a solution with high potassium content until 1988. This preservative solution, Euro-Collins solution, allowed a maximum ischemia of 8 h for donor livers. In 1987, Jamieson *et al.*[114] reported that cold ischemia of canine and human homografts could be safely extended to at least 24 h with an infusate first described by Wahlberg *et al.*[115] in experiments on pancreas preservation. This University of Wisconsin preservation fluid (UW solution) has allowed liver transplantation to become a semielective procedure. Cofer *et al.*[116] have demonstrated improved enzyme function, decreased blood usage, and shorter hospital stays with UW solution. This improvement may be the result of the impermeants in the solution. Table 53.5 compares the constituents of the two solutions.

Reperfusion injury and syndrome

Meticulous care at the time of harvesting the donor liver, improved preservation during cold ischemia, and therapeutic measures aimed specifically at reducing reperfusion injury all help to improve graft function and survival. Free radical scavengers such as superoxide dismutase, catalase,[117] and mannitol have been used to reduce reperfusion injury. Greig *et al.*[118] have reported successful use of prostaglandin E_1 (PGE_1) in livers that appeared to be compromised at reperfusion. "Reperfusion syndrome" is the name given to cardiovascular instability following the release of vascular clamps. This is characterized by bradycardia, hypotension, dysrhythmias, and, ultimately, circulatory arrest. The hemodynamic instability can be seen in up to half the liver transplant procedures and is associated with a significant fall in systemic vascular resistance. Right ventricular dysfunction and a rise in pulmonary artery pressure have been reported.[119]

Reperfusion phase

Following reanastomosis of hepatic vessels, the "new" liver is cleared of residual preservation fluid, air, and other debris via the portal vein. Despite this "flushing," the release of the vascular clamp to establish portal venous continuity results in the release of blood rich in metabolic acids along with cold hyperkalemic preservative solution. We have observed "first flush" serum potassium levels as high as 35 mmol L^{-1} despite careful flushing of the donor liver prior to reperfusion. Using transesophageal echocardiography, Roberts *et al.*[120] have recorded a stream of air bubbles entering the heart. Other suggested mediators include endotoxins, nitric oxide, and prostaglandins. Although minor changes require no treatment, major instability demands vigorous resuscitative measures. Prophylactic atropine decreases the incidence

Table 53.5 *Composition of preservative solutions used to preserve donor livers*

	UW solution	Euro-Collins solution
Impermeants	Raffinose (30 mmol L^{-1}) Lactobionate (100 mmol L^{-1})	Glucose (194 mmol L^{-1})
Hydrogen ion buffers	KH_2PO_4 (25 mmol L^{-1})	KH_2PO_4 (15 mmol L^{-1}) K_2HPO_4 (42 mmol L^{-1}) $NaHCO_3$ (10 mmol L^{-1})
Colloids	Hydroxyethyl starch (5 g dL^{-1})	
Metabolites and others	$MgSO_4$ (5 mmol L^{-1}) Adenosine (5 mmol L^{-1}) Glutathione (3 mmol L^{-1}) Allopurinol (1 mmol L^{-1}) Insulin (1 u L^{-1}) Dexamethasone (8 mg L^{-1})	KCl (15 mmol L^{-1})
Osmolarity	320 mmol L^{-1}	335 mmol L^{-1}

Reproduced from Cofer *et al.*[116]

of bradycardia and sinus arrest. Calcium chloride is the drug of choice for management of acute hyperkalemia that can be clearly noticed with characteristic electrocardiogram (ECG) changes. In severe cases of reperfusion syndrome due to cardioactive mediators,[121] venous air embolism,[122] or pulmonary thromboembolism,[123-125] inotropic support may be needed to reverse myocardial depression.

Hepatic artery and biliary anastomosis complete the surgical procedure during this stage. Hemostasis and temperature maintenance become the primary concerns for the anesthesiologist. In some patients, reperfusion coagulopathy with fibrinolysis may occur. Transfusion of clotting factors such as fresh-frozen plasma, platelets, and cryoprecipitate may be required to correct the acute coagulation disorder. With the return of graft function, body temperature increases, acidosis is corrected, coagulation state returns to normal, serum potassium levels return to normal, and an increase in carbon dioxide is noticed.[126] Urine output improves even in patients with prior hepatorenal syndrome.[127] There is a gradual reduction in the need for inotropic support. Vigorous correction of intraoperative metabolic acidosis in the presence of a functioning graft can lead to postoperative metabolic alkalosis and difficulty in weaning from the ventilatory support. The optimal hematocrit to aim for without a risk of postoperative hepatic artery thrombosis is between 30% and 35%.

Postoperative management

Patients are electively ventilated in an intensive care unit during the immediate postoperative period. With a well-functioning graft and adequate analgesia, routine monitoring of vital signs and fluid balance is all that is required. Early tracheal extubation can be attempted in patients who are hemodynamically stable with good gas exchange and no evidence of coagulopathy. This "fast track" approach has resulted in major reductions in cost without any change in outcome.[128]

Routine biochemical measurements include blood sugar estimations, coagulation studies, and liver function tests. The patency of the hepatic artery is determined by Doppler ultrasonography. Early intervention in the event of hepatic artery thrombosis can salvage the graft and prevent the need for regrafting.[129] Graft malfunction due to injury or acute rejection is associated with a rise in liver enzymes [particularly aspartate aminotransferase (AST)], failure to correct the coagulation disorder, and a subsequent rise in serum bilirubin level. Patients are more prone to respiratory complications possibly because of pre-existing nutritional deficiencies, nosocomial infections,[130] intraoperative diaphragmatic injury, and the respiratory sequelae of massive transfusion. Other postoperative problems include continuing hemorrhage and the development of hypertension in about 50% of patients. The latter requires treatment with adrenergic blockers, angiotensin-converting enzyme (ACE) inhibitors, and diuretics.

Immunosuppression is started immediately upon arrival in the intensive care unit. Triple therapy with cyclosporine, azathioprine, and prednisolone is commonly used. Early rejection is treated with extra boluses of steroids or antibodies such as OKT3 or antilymphocytic globulin (ALG). Other immunosuppressants include macrolide antibiotics such as tacrolimus (FK506) and rapamycin. As in the case of cyclosporine, FK506 is highly nephrotoxic.

OTHER NONTRANSPLANT LIVER SURGERY

Apart from liver transplantation, an anesthesiologist may be called upon to provide anesthesia for procedures such as segmental resection of the liver or repair following hepatic trauma. In both, basic anesthetic considerations are similar to those outlined above for patients with liver disease and liver transplantation, but there are some significant differences.

Hepatic resection

Based on the distribution of the portal pedicles and the location of the hepatic veins, five segmental resections can be undertaken. These are right and left trisegmentectomy, right and left lobectomy, and left lateral segmentectomy. For smaller lesions, it is possible to undertake subsegmental or local wedge resections.

Intraoperative ultrasonography is used to define further the blood supply and to outline accurately the position of the intrahepatic lesions.[131]

The indications for hepatic resection are:

1 benign hepatic tumors;
2 metastatic lesion confined to resectable areas;
3 primary malignant tumors in resectable areas;
4 split liver grafts in living related transplants.

Hemorrhage, coagulation disorders, and metabolic changes are the primary problems encountered in these patients.

In patients with advanced tumors, two other approaches for liver resection have been described. These are *ex situ* and *in situ* hypothermic techniques. In the *ex situ* procedure, the patient is rendered anhepatic, as for liver transplantation, and the resection is completed on the bench. Despite venovenous bypass, significant metabolic and coagulation disorders are associated with this prolonged anhepatic phase.[132] In the *in situ* technique, the liver is isolated and perfused with hypothermic preservative solution, the hepatic artery is clamped, and rewarming is prevented by wrapping the liver in silver foil. Venovenous bypass is used to minimize the hemodynamic disturbances.

The major complications of hepatic resection are hepatic failure, hemorrhage, biliary leak and infection, with postoperative death largely attributable to hepatic failure.[133]

Hepatic trauma

Although the mortality from hepatic trauma has decreased considerably, from 66% during World War I to 9% during the Vietnam War,[134] uncontrolled hemorrhage continues to be the primary cause of death.[135] Ruptured liver is still the commonest missed diagnosis in multiple trauma.[136]

Clinical presentation depends upon the severity of hepatic trauma and on other associated injuries. Some patients may require detailed diagnostic work-up, including peritoneal lavage, computed tomography, and arteriography, whereas those with severe injury may present with profound hypotension and a distended abdomen requiring immediate surgical intervention. It is imperative that adequate resuscitation is undertaken as soon as possible. Facilities for rapid fluid administration with large-bore intravenous catheters in the upper half of the body must be obtained before surgery commences.

Oxygenation and control of the airway (especially in the unconscious patient) are of paramount importance. Anesthetic agents that cause minimal cardiovascular depression (e.g. etomidate or ketamine) combined with an opioid-relaxant technique are the drugs of choice.

Massive blood transfusion may be necessary to replace blood lost once the abdomen is opened. Transfusion alone may not be enough to maintain adequate perfusion of vital organs, and vasopressors may be required.

Other areas of concern during surgery include coagulation disorder, hypothermia, acidosis, and problems associated with any other injuries the patient may have. It is therefore essential that arterial blood gas analyses are carried out frequently and that electrolytes, glucose, ionized calcium, hematocrit, and clotting factor levels are measured on a regular basis.

Depending upon the extent of hepatic injury, the treatment options range from perihepatic packing to total hepatectomy and liver transplantation.

Postoperative complications include persistent coagulopathy, renal failure, local sepsis, systemic sepsis with or without adult respiratory distress syndrome, and features of multiple organ failure.

Anesthesia in patients after liver transplantation

With a well-functioning graft, the hepatic metabolic function returns to normal quickly, but changes in the volume of distribution may persist for a longer period. These patients are immunosuppressed and hence prone to infectious and malignant complications. In addition, interactions between immunosuppressants and anesthetic drugs, toxicity of the former, and special aspects of transfusion in transplanted patients should be borne in mind. Regional anesthesia and analgesia should be considered for patients with normal coagulation.

POSTOPERATIVE JAUNDICE

Minor and reversible changes are present postoperatively in up to 50% of patients. These changes can be detected with sensitive biochemical tests, but are of no clinical significance. Mild hepatic impairment is caused by a reduction in liver blood flow with both regional and general anesthesia,[72] and is usually not associated with any histological changes.[137] Following major surgery, mild jaundice is present in approximately 17% of patients and marked jaundice in 4%.[138] Twenty-five percent of patients develop jaundice in the postoperative period after cardiopulmonary bypass.[139] This condition is self-limiting, with no evidence of hepatocellular necrosis. Patients most at risk of developing postoperative complications are those with compromised preoperative liver function,[71,140] especially if subjected to hypotension, hypoxia, or sepsis.

Hayes and Bouchier[71] classified the causes of postoperative jaundice into patient and perioperative factors (Table 53.6). Their influence on bilirubin metabolism is illustrated in Fig. 53.5.

Hyperbilirubinemia without an elevated aminotransferase level is due to either an increased bilirubin production or a defect in its metabolism. The commonest defect in metabolism is seen in Gilbert's disease, which affects 3–7% of the population.[141] Other rare causes are Dubin–Johnson syndrome, Rotor syndrome, and Crigler–Najjar disease. Healthy adults produce 250–350 mg of bilirubin per day and can handle up to three times this load.[140] However, with excessive extravascular and/or intravascular hemodestruction, bilirubin loads may exceed this level. Extravascular erythrocyte breakdown from a 1-L hematoma can release approximately 5000 mg of bilirubin. Intravascular red cell destruction can occasionally result from hemolytic conditions such as glucose-6-phosphate dehydrogenase deficiency, cardiopulmonary bypass, artificial valves, and sickle cell disease, but is more commonly seen following large or multiple transfusions. Approximately 10% of 2-week-old stored blood will undergo hemolysis.[142] Following incompatible transfusion, hemolysis may be delayed and can occur any time from 2 to 21 days.[143] Delayed transfusion reactions occur following a second stimulus of transfused blood and may produce jaundice in the postoperative period several days after anesthesia.[140]

Cholestasis from both intra- and extrahepatic causes leads to hyperbilirubinemia with a mild-to-moderate rise in transaminase level. Extrahepatic obstruction following biliary surgery gives rise to an increase in bilirubin and alkaline phosphatase within 2–3 days of surgery; the aminotransferase rise follows later if obstruction persists.[140]

Table 53.6 *Causes of postoperative jaundice*

Patient factors
Congenital hemolytic disorders
Acquired hemolytic disorders
Pre-existing liver disease with or without portal hypertension
Coagulopathy
Gilbert syndrome
Sepsis
Perioperative factors
Anesthetic-induced reduction in liver blood flow
Bleeding
Hypotension
Blood transfusion
Biliary tree trauma
Viral hepatitis
Drugs
Halothane
Antibiotics
Nonsteroidal agents
Polypharmacy and drug interactions
Antihypertensives
Potential hemolytic agents

Reproduced from Hayes and Bouchier.[71]

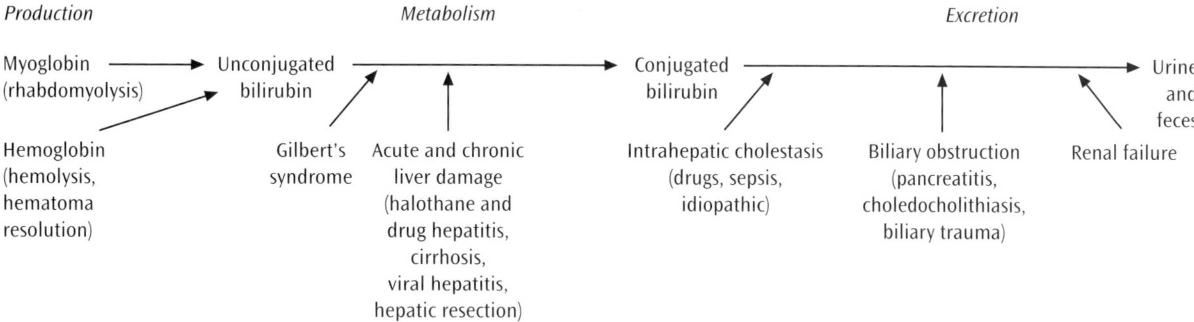

Figure 53.5 *Mechanisms of hyperbilirubinemia. (Reproduced from Hayes and Bouchier.[71])*

Postoperative cholecystitis and pancreatitis are rare causes of hepatic dysfunction. Postoperative cholecystitis has been reported to carry a mortality rate of 25%.[144] Cholecystitis is usually acalculous, may be complicated by gangrene of the gall bladder, and has a poor outcome.[145] High serum amylase levels confirm the diagnosis of pancreatitis.

Postoperative intrahepatic cholestasis follows lengthy and complicated surgical procedures involving multiple transfusions, episodes of hypotension, and hypoxia in the presence of sepsis. Conjugated bilirubin levels rise 2–7 days after surgery, with a moderate rise in alkaline phosphatase but without any increase in transaminase level, at least in the early stages. Liver biopsy shows dilated biliary canaliculi and bile casts with minimal hepatocellular damage and inflammation.[137,146] The symptoms usually resolve within 3 weeks. It is important to distinguish this condition from extrahepatic biliary obstruction.

Jaundice with an elevated serum transaminase level implies damage to hepatocytes. In its severe form it is associated with centrilobular hepatocellular necrosis and may lead to acute liver failure. Marked and sustained hypotension, hypoxemia, and sepsis are mainly responsible for hepatocyte damage. The severity of injury can often be correlated with the degree of hypoxemia and the duration of hypotension.[137,147] Vasopressors used to improve systemic blood pressure may accentuate the hepatic hypoperfusion.[148]

A similar though less acute and florid form of liver damage is encountered in patients with right-sided, congestive heart failure and in association with pneumonia.[149]

Viral hepatitis, usually hepatitis C, can be acquired during surgery. Before the introduction of effective screening of donated blood for hepatitis C, the incidence was quoted to be as high as 10% for those receiving transfusions.[150]

Drug-induced hepatocellular damage can be caused by a variety of agents. Up to 7% of adverse drug reactions are reported to be the result of drug-induced liver damage.[151] A list of potential hepatotoxic drugs and their mechanisms of hepatotoxicity is given in Table 53.7.[140] The presentation varies from asymptomatic to life threatening.

Adverse drug reactions can be divided into two groups: predictable and idiosyncratic.[152] Predictable drug reactions are dose dependent and appear above a certain level. The clinical picture is similar in all patients and can be reproduced in animal models and, hence, minimized by therapeutic rationale. On the other hand, idiosyncratic reactions are variable in presentation, are less predictable, and are not dose dependent. They may result from metabolic idiosyncracy or from activation of the immune system. Characteristics of predictable, idiosyncratic, and immune-mediated toxicity are given in Table 53.8.[152]

Hepatitis secondary to halothane use has been extensively reviewed.[140,141,152,153] Retrospective studies confirm an incidence of between 1 in 6000 and 1 in 20000; there is a higher incidence after repeated use, especially within a short time.[154–157] Prospective studies demonstrate two patterns of liver dysfunction: one is common, minor, and predictable; the other is rare, severe, and idiosyncratic and may be immune mediated.[158,159] Several studies have reported a rise in transaminase level in up to 25% of patients following anesthesia, but more so after halothane anesthesia.[160–163] Abnormal liver function tests may not be detectable until well into the second postoperative week.[162] An increase in glutathione-*S*-transferase is a sensitive and specific index of acute drug-induced hepatocellular dysfunction. Increased plasma concentrations have been reported after halothane but not after isoflurane anesthesia.[164,165] These studies also showed that halothane is associated with less liver damage when given under high (100%) oxygen tensions than at lower (30%) oxygen tensions. A mild subclinical form of liver dysfunction could be caused by the toxic products of halothane metabolism, possibly influenced by genetic and pre-existing enzyme factors[166] or by hepatic hypoxia in relation to oxygen demand.[153] The severe form can lead to fulminant hepatic failure. There have been only very rare reports of halothane hepatitis in children; there is no doubt, given the frequent use of halothane in pediatric anesthesia, that halothane hepatitis is much rarer in children than in adults.[153]

The presence of eosinophilia and autoantibodies have been proposed as diagnostic markers in hepatitis following halothane anesthesia.[167–171] The majority of patients with a clinical diagnosis of halothane hepatitis have serum antibodies that react with one or more specific liver microsomal proteins that have been covalently altered by the trifluroacetyl chloride metabolite of halothane. These serum antibodies are not found in patients with other types of liver failure,[171] but neither are they present in all patients for whom the clinical diagnosis of halothane hepatitis has been made.[170]

Hepatic dysfunction following enflurane anesthesia is rare, with a reported incidence of 1 in 800000;[153] and that following isoflurane is even more rare.[172,173]

The time of onset of jaundice in the postoperative period is given in Fig. 53.6, and a useful algorithm for its investigation in Fig. 53.7.

ACUTE LIVER FAILURE

Acute liver failure (ALF) is defined as severe hepatic dysfunction leading to encephalopathy or coagulopathy within 6 months of the first symptom. Rapid progression with encephalopathy developing within 8 weeks is referred to as fulminant hepatic failure (FHF).[174]

Worldwide, the commonest cause of ALF is viral hepatitis, although in some countries overdose of acetaminophen (paracetamol) taken with suicidal intent is the prime reason. Hepatotoxicity following therapeutic doses of acetaminophen has been reported in patients taking enzyme-

Table 53.7 *Drugs known to produce or suspected of producing liver damage and the resulting histological injury*

Drug	Injury pattern
Isoniazid, phenytoin, α-methyldopa	Viral hepatitis-like injury
Oxacillin, aspirin	Nonspecific hepatitis
Quinidine, allopurinol, phenylbutazone	Granulomatous hepatitis
α-Methyldopa, methotrexate, amiodarone, dantrolene	Chronic hepatitis
Chlorpromazine, erythromycin, estrogen	Cholestasis
Tetracycline, valproic acid, ethanol	Fatty liver changes
Oral contraceptives	Hepatic vein thrombosis
Anabolic steroids	Peliosis hepatitis

Reproduced from Frink and Brown.[140]

Table 53.8 *Classification of drug hepatotoxicity*

	Dose dependent	Onset	Response to challenge	Animal model	Immune features
Predictable	+	Rapid (days)	Rapid	+	–
Idiosyncratic metabolic	+/–	Variable (up to 1 year)	Delayed	+/–	–
Immune mediated	–	Variable (1 day to 12 weeks)	Rapid	–	+

Reproduced from Neuberger.[152]

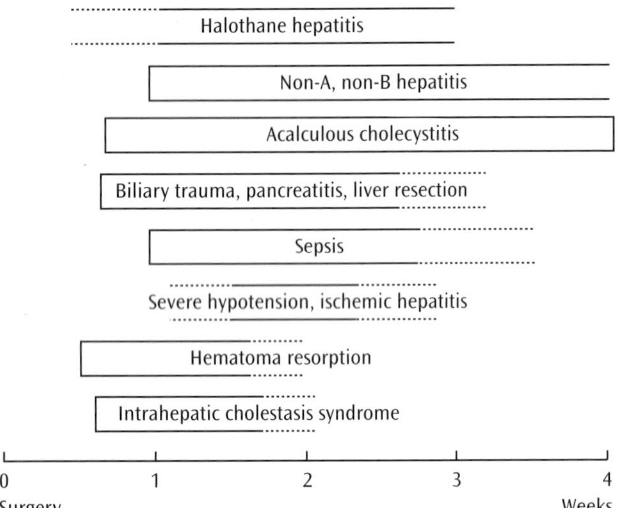

Figure 53.6 *Time-course of onset of postoperative jaundice. (Reproduced from Hayes and Bouchier.[71])*

inducing agents such as phenytoin or in patients who have a chronic use of alcohol.[175] ALF can also be part of generalized infection with cytomegalovirus, Coxsackievirus B, echovirus, Epstein–Barr virus, and herpes simplex virus. Rare causes of ALF include mushroom poisoning with *Amanita phalloides*, acute fatty liver of pregnancy, Wilson's disease, and Budd–Chiari syndrome.

Clinical features and management

The emphasis for the management of ALF is to minimize any damage to other organ systems that might lead to multiple organ failure, and to allow time for the regeneration and recovery of liver function or to procure a suitable graft for transplantation.

Encephalopathy and cerebral edema

Encephalopathy is graded, according to its severity, into four grades (Table 53.9).[176] Grades I and II, which do not progress, carry the best prognosis. Following ingestion of an overdose of acetaminophen, it takes 3–4 days for the signs of encephalopathy to appear. During the subsequent 24–48 h, there is rapid progression through the various stages. However, the onset is much more variable in patients with acute liver failure of viral origin. Cerebral edema, a major cause of death, is seen in 80% of patients with fulminant hepatic failure (FHF).[177] The signs and symptoms of raised intracranial pressure include systemic hypertension with episodes of bradycardia, hyperventilation, decerebrate posture, abnormal papillary reflexes, and impaired brainstem reflexes.

The precise pathogenic mechanisms responsible for encephalopathy in FHF are still not well understood, although various factors have been implicated. These include benzodiazepine agonists, increased aromatic amines, ammonia, phenols, mercaptans, and altered γ-aminobutyric acid levels. Basile *et al.*[93] demonstrated raised brain concentrations of 1,4-benzodiazepines in patients with FHF. Mullen *et al.*[178] have identified an endogenous benzodiazepine ligand with a molecular weight less than 10 000 in the cerebrospinal fluid of FHF patients. Flumazenil, a benzodiazepine antagonist, might therefore be considered to be of use for reversing the encephalopathy. However, it is recommended that, until a beneficial role for such agents is established, these should not be used in the presence of cerebral edema, as they are likely to aggravate the condition.[176]

Patients with grade III or IV encephalopathy should be intubated and ventilated and nursed in a head-up position with minimal stimuli. The main aim of the therapy is to maintain a cerebral perfusion pressure greater than 6.7 kPa (50 mmHg). Raised intracranial pressure can be controlled by hyperventilation in the acute stages, but sustained hyperventilation should be avoided as it may lower perfusion pressure. Bolus administration of mannitol 0.5 g kg^{-1} over 10 min is also effective in reducing intracranial pressure (ICP), and can be repeated in patients with normal renal function if the plasma osmolarity is below 320 mmol L^{-1}. In patients with renal impairment, ultrafiltration or intermittent hemofiltration may be required to remove two to three times the volume of mannitol infused. Sodium thiopentone in bolus doses of 185–500 mg followed by an infusion of 50–250 mg h^{-1} has been shown to be effective for patients with mannitol-resistant cerebral edema.[179] The use of sodium thiopentone does, however, make the interpretation of cerebral signs difficult and can preclude the diagnosis of brainstem death.

Coagulopathy

The liver produces most coagulation factors, apart from factor VIII. In acute liver failure, circulating levels of these factors are reduced, as is antithrombin III. The latter is an inhibitor of coagulation. In addition, an increase in the peripheral consumption of clotting factors leads to disseminated intravascular coagulation.[180] Thrombocytopenia with increased adhesiveness but impaired aggregation is also a feature of ALF.

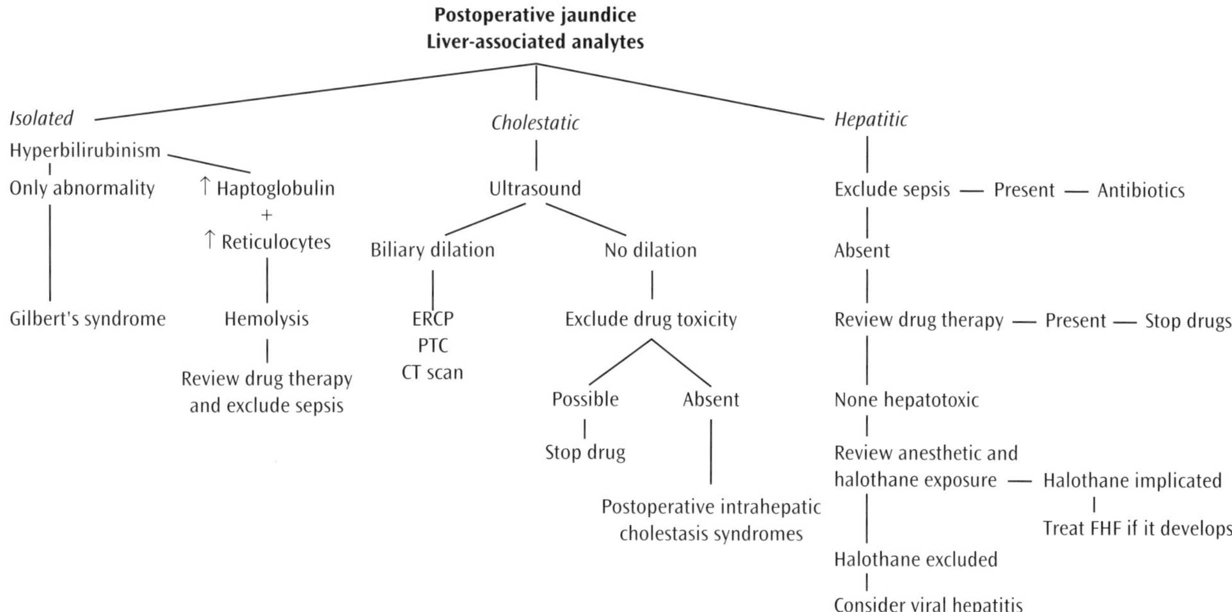

Figure 53.7 *Algorithm for investigation of postoperative jaundice. ERCP, endoscopic retrograde cholangiopancreatography; FHF, fulminant hepatic failure; PTC, percutaneous transhepatic cholangiogram. (Reproduced from Hayes and Bouchier.[71])*

Table 53.9 *Clinical features and grade of encephalopathy*

I	Mild or episodic drowsiness; impaired intellect, concentration, and psychomotor function, but rousable and coherent
II	Increased drowsiness with confusion and disorientation; rousable and conversable
III	Very drowsy, disoriented, responds to verbal commands, often agitated and aggressive
IV	Responds to painful stimuli at best, but may be unresponsive; may be complicated by evidence of cerebral edema

Reproduced from O'Grady and Williams.[176]

Prolongation of prothrombin time is commonly used as an indicator of liver damage, although a more sensitive marker might be a specific factor V assay. Factor V has the shortest half-life of all the clotting factors synthesized by the liver.

Fresh-frozen plasma and platelets can be transfused to correct the coagulopathy in the short term. The incidence of gastrointestinal bleeding can be significantly reduced with H_2-receptor antagonists or cytoprotective agents.

Hemodynamic effects

Patients in ALF have a raised cardiac output and a low systemic vascular resistance. Persistent hypotension, despite adequate volume replacement requiring inotropic support, is usually a poor prognostic indicator. Inotropes may, however, be needed to allow therapeutic measures such as hemodialysis or transplantation. Epinephrine (adrenaline), norepinephrine (noradrenaline), and vasopressin have all been used, but their use should be guided by derived hemodynamic parameters.

Cardiac dysrhythmias, although rare, are usually due to hypo- or hyperkalemia, hypoxia, acidosis, or mechanical irritation linked to the presence of central intravascular catheters.

Metabolic effects

Severe hypoglycemia sufficient to lead to brain damage is common in ALF. Infusion of 10–20% glucose may be needed to maintain normoglycemia. Metabolic acidosis is common with acetaminophen-induced ALF. Raised serum lactate levels result from poor tissue oxygen extraction[181] and, as in the case of severe metabolic acidosis, signify poor prognosis. Alkalosis of mixed origin is often associated with hypokalemia. Other metabolic changes that have been reported in patients with normal renal function include dilutional hyponatremia and hypophosphatemia.

Renal effects

The incidence of renal failure in patients with grade IV encephalopathy due to acetaminophen overdose has been reported to be around 75%, compared with 30% in other forms of ALF.[182] This difference may be due to a direct nephrotoxic effect of acetaminophen and often precedes encephalopathy. In patients with ALF arising from other causes, renal impairment develops when encephalopathy is advanced. Persistent oliguria despite adequate intravascular volume and low-dose dopamine infusion may require intermittent hemodialysis, especially in the presence of hyperkalemia and metabolic acidosis. The hemodynamic changes associated with hemodialysis may lead to surges in intracranial pressure with a consequent fall in cerebral perfusion.[183] Continuous hemodiafiltration is an effective alternative and causes minimal disturbance. Despite coagulopathy, low-dose heparin with epoprostanol infusion is necessary for hemodiafiltration.

Respiratory effects

Alkalosis due to hyperventilation is common in spontaneously breathing patients with ALF. Hypoxemia due to multifactorial etiology is also frequent in ALF. This includes aspiration of gastric contents (especially in patients with grade II or III encephalopathy), atelectasis, and intrapulmonary bleeding. Noncardiogenic pulmonary edema has also been recorded in patients with metabolic acidosis following acetaminophen overdose.

Sepsis

Rolando *et al.*[184] reported an 80% incidence of bacterial infection, the predominant organisms being *Staphylococcus aureus*, streptococci, and coliforms. Fungal infection, mainly due to *Candida* species, has also been reported.[185] This increased susceptibility in ALF is due to a compromised immune system with impaired neutrophil and Kupffer cell function and a deficiency in complement components and fibronectin. Surveillance with daily cultures and appropriate antibiotics for positive cultures is indicated, although the role of prophylactic broad-spectrum cover and selective decontamination of the digestive tract has not been established.

Other measures

Specific measures aimed at hepatocyte regeneration include charcoal hemoperfusion, therapy with insulin and glucagon, interferon, and prostaglandin E_1. Despite theoretical benefits, conclusive evidence has yet to be demonstrated. Measures such as plasmapheresis and exchange transfusion with transient improvement in encephalopathy have convinced some researchers about their efficacy. *N*-Acetylcysteine, a specific antidote for acetaminophen, has been shown to be effective when given within 8 h of an overdose.[186] *N*-Acetylcysteine may be a life-saving therapy as it restores the available stores of glutathione.[187] Evidence showing improved outcome exists to justify its use even when administered late.[188,189]

Orthotopic liver transplantation with survival rates of up to 80%[190–192] is a recommended therapeutic option.

The altered physiological state of ALF persists for some time into the post-transplant period; it is therefore essential to continue the preoperative therapy for some time after surgery.

VIRAL INFECTIONS AND THE LIVER

Viral hepatitis is a worldwide public health problem affecting hundreds of millions of people. Patients may present with acute infections or chronic sequelae such as chronic active hepatitis, cirrhosis, and primary liver cancer. Hepatocellular carcinoma is one of the 10 most common cancers in the world.

Viral hepatitis

Patients with viral hepatitis may be completely asymptomatic or complain of nonspecific symptoms such as anorexia, arthralgia, nausea and vomiting, lethargy, abdominal discomfort, and low-grade fever. Jaundice may be the presenting symptom in some patients.

Essentially, there are five main types of viral hepatitis. These are classed as hepatitis A, B, C, D, and E.

Hepatitis A

Hepatitis A is endemic throughout the world and is caused by a small RNA virus. It is spread by fecal–oral transmission and usually signifies poor sanitation and hygiene. People most at risk are staff and residents of mental institutions and day-care centers, sewerage workers, health-care workers, and military personnel. The incubation period is about 4 weeks, with maximal fecal viral shedding about 10 days after exposure and decreasing after the onset of jaundice. The patients are therefore infectious for several weeks after contracting the infection. Diagnosis is confirmed serologically by elevated levels of immunoglobulin (Ig) M antihepatitis A virus. This rise appears within a month of the infection and lasts 3–6 months. However, the rise in IgG antibody appears several months after the infection and persists indefinitely.

Uneventful recovery within weeks of the infection is the norm, with ALF reported in less than 0.5% of hospitalized cases.[176] Infections later in life have been associated with higher mortality.[193,194]

Hepatitis B

Hepatitis B virus (HBV) is a double-stranded DNA virus that causes the most common form of parenterally transmitted viral hepatitis. The acute disease has an incubation period of 1–6 months and clinical presentation ranges from an asymptomatic anicteric infection to ALF in about 4% of patients.[176] Diagnosis of hepatitis B is confirmed by the presence of hepatitis B surface antigen (HbsAg) and IgM antibody to hepatitis B core antigen. Persistent carriage of hepatitis B is defined as the presence of the hepatitis B surface antigen in the serum for more than 6 months. The presence of antibody to surface antigen that develops about 6 months after the infection is a sign of recovery and is thought to be protective against any future infection. Long-term viral replication may progress to cirrhosis and hepatocellular carcinoma. A serum marker of continuing replication, secreted by infected hepatocytes, is hepatitis B e antigen (HbeAg). Carriers of HBV who are also HbeAg positive have high concentrations of the virus in their blood and therefore are likely to be the source of occupational transmission.

Effective vaccination against HBV is recommended for those working in high-risk areas such as hospitals, residential institutions, and even for all newborns,[194] for their protection as well as to prevent the spread of the disease.

Hepatitis D

Hepatitis D virus (HDV) is a single-stranded RNA virus that requires hepatitis B virus for replication. Hepatitis B and D may be acquired simultaneously, resulting in a more severe form of hepatitis,[195] or hepatitis D may be a superadded infection in a patient already infected with hepatitis B. The latter can accelerate the course of chronic disease or render previously asymptomatic disease apparent.[194] Evidence of HDV infection was found in 43% of patients with HBV fulminant hepatic failure, compared with 19% of less severe cases.[196,197] IgM anti-HDV is present in both acute and chronic forms of the infection, with a high titer in chronic carriers indicting poor prognosis.[198] Patients with long-standing infection develop an IgG antibody.[199] Hepatitis D is very common among intravenous drug abusers.

Hepatitis C

Until recently, this used to be called non-A/non-B hepatitis. The virus responsible is a single-stranded RNA virus with an incubation period of between 1 and 4 months since transfusion. The largely presumptive diagnosis by exclusion has now been replaced by a sensitive serological test that can confirm the diagnosis in over 90% of chronic and more than 60% of acute cases. This has been made possible by the cloning of the viral genome.

Fulminant hepatic failure occurs in up to 5% of hepatitis C patients, with hepatitis C a predominant cause of late-onset hepatic failure.[176,200] Fifty percent of patients with hepatitis C infection progress to the chronic stage. Almost all cases of this infection are sporadic, except the water-borne variety occurring on the Indian subcontinent.[176]

Hepatitis E

Hepatitis E virus (HEV) is a single-stranded RNA virus that is thought to be the cause of enterically transmitted hepatitis C infection. HEV is an important cause of large epidemics in India, central and South-east Asia, the Middle East, parts of Africa, and the constituent countries of the former USSR.[194] The highest incidence is found in young adults, and mortality rates of 25% have been reported in the third trimester of pregnancy.

REFERENCES

1. O'Connor KW, Snodgrass PJ, Swonder JE, *et al.* A blinded prospective study comparing four current non-invasive approaches in the differential diagnosis of medical versus surgical jaundice. *Gastroenterology* 1983; **84:** 1498.
2. Bailey ME. Endotoxin, bile salts, and renal failure in obstructive jaundice. *Br J Surg* 1976; **63:** 774–8.
3. Pain JA, Cahill CJ, Bailey ME. Perioperative complications in obstructive jaundice. Therapeutic considerations. *Br J Surg* 1985; **72:** 942–7.
4. Cahill CJ. Prevention of postoperative renal failure in patients with obstructive jaundice – the role of bile salts. *Br J Surg* 1983; **70:** 590–5.
5. Kramer HJ. Impaired renal function in obstructive jaundice: roles of thomboxane and endothelin systems. *Nephron* 1997; **77:** 1.
6. Saini S. Imaging of the hepatobiliary tract. *N Engl J Med* 1997; **336:** 1889.
7. Zilly W, Liehr H, Hummer N. Chiba-needle percutaneous cholangiography – a method without risk to the patient? *Endoscopy* 1980; **12:** 12.
8. Morgan MY, Sherlock S. Sex-related differences among 100 with alcoholic disease. *Br Med J* 1977; **1:** 939.
9. Kent G, Popper H. Liver biopsy in diagnosis of hemochromatosis. *Am J Med* 1968; **44:** 837.
10. Niederau C, Fischer R, Sonnenberg A, *et al.* Survival and causes of death in cirrhotic and in noncirrhotic patients with primary haemochromatosis. *N Engl J Med* 1985; **313:** 1256.
11. Bacon BR. Diagnosis and management of haemochromatosis. *Gastroenterology* 1997; **113:** 995.
12. Kaplan MM. Primary biliary cirrhosis. *N Engl J Med* 1987; **316:** 512.
13. Strunin L. Preoperative assessment of hepatic function. *Bailliere's Clin Anaesthesiol* 1992; **6 (4):** 781–93.
14. Gabuzada GJ. Cirrhosis, ascites and edema. *Gastroenterology* 1970; **58:** 546.
15. Limas CJ, Guiha NH, Lekagul O, Cohn JN. Impaired left ventricular function in alcoholic cirrhosis with ascites. *Circulation* 1974; **49:** 755–60.
16. Browne DRG. Anaesthesia in impaired liver function. *Curr Anaesth Crit Care* 1990; **1:** 220–7.
17. Rodriguez-Roisin R, Agn A, Roca J. The hepatopulmonary syndrome: new name, old complexities. *Thorax* 1992; **47:** 897–902.
18. Rolla G, Brussino L, Bucca C. The hepatopulmonary syndrome. *Forum* 1998; **8:** 84–92.
19. Stenqvist O, Olausson M, Karlsen KL. Luxury lung perfusion in end-stage liver disease during liver transplantation. *Acta Anaesthesiol Scand* 1999; **43:** 447–51.
20. Allison MEM. The kidney and the liver. Pre- and post-operative factors. In: Blumgart LH (ed.). *Surgery of the Liver and the Biliary Tract.* London: Churchill Livingstone, 1988: 405–22.
21. Wait RB, Kahng KU. Renal failure complicating obstructive jaundice. *Am J Surg* 1989; **157:** 256.
22. Blamey SL, Fearon KCH, Gilmour WH, *et al.* Prediction of risk in biliary surgery. *Br J Surg* 1983; **70:** 535–8.
23. Boyer TD. Major sequelae of cirrhosis. In: Wyngaaden JB, Smith LH (eds). *Cecil, Textbook of Medicine*, 16th edn. Philadelphia, PA: WB Saunders, 1982: 804–8.
24. Gines P, Arroyo V, Rodes J. Treatment of ascites and renal failure in cirrhosis. *Bailliere's Clin Gastroenterol* 1989; **3:** 165–86.
25. Songy Jr KA, Layon AJ. Vitamin K-induced cardiovascular collapse. *J Clin Anesth* 1997; **9:** 514.
26. Novis BH, Duys P, Barbezat GO, *et al.* Fibre-optic endoscopy and the use of Sengstaken tube in acute gastrointestinal hemorrhage in patients with portal hypertension and varices. *Gut* 1976; **17:** 258.
27. Law AW, Gales MA. Octreotide or Vasopressin for bleeding esophageal varices. *Ann Pharmacother* 1997; **31:** 237.
28. Cello JP. Endoscopic management of esophageal variceal hemorrhage: injection, banding, glue, or a combination. *Semin Gastrointest Dis* 1997; **8:** 179.
29. Jalan R, Redhead DN, Hayes PC. Transjugular intrahepatic portosystemic stent shunt in the treatment of variceal hemorrhage. *Br J Surg* 1995; **82:** 1158.
30. Child III CG, Turcotte JG. Surgery and portal hypertension. In: Child III CG (ed.). *The Liver and Portal Hypertension.* Philadelphia, PA: WB Saunders, 1964: 50.
31. Pugh RNH, Murray-Lyon IM, Dawson JL. Transection of the oesophagus for bleeding oesophageal varices. *Br J Surg* 1973; **60:** 646–9.
32. Garrison RN, Cryer HM, Howard DA, Polk HC. Clarification of risk factors for abdominal operations in patients with hepatic cirrhosis. *Ann Surg* 1984; **199:** 648–55.
33. Alber I, Hartmann H, Bircher J, Creutzfeldt W. Superiority of Child–Pugh classification to quantitative liver function tests for assessing prognosis of liver cirrhosis. *Scand J Gastroenterol* 1989; **234:** 269–76.
34. Branch RA, Morgan MH, James J, *et al.* Intravenous administration of diazepam in patients with chronic liver disease. *Gut* 1976; **17:** 975.
35. Pandele G, Chaux F, Salvadori C, *et al.* Thiopental pharmacokinetics in patients with cirrhosis. *Anesthesiology* 1983; **59:** 123–6.
36. Loft S, Jenson V, Resaard S, Dyrberg V. Influence of moderate alcohol intake on thiopental anesthesia. *Acta Anaesth Scand* 1982; **26:** 22.
37. Servin F, Desmonts JM, Haberer JT, *et al.* Pharmacokinetics and protein binding of propofol in patients with cirrhosis. *Anesthesiology* 1988; **69:** 887.
38. Veroli P, O'Kelley B, Bertrand F, *et al.* Extrahepatic metabolism of propofol in man during the anhepatic phase of orthotopic liver transplantation. *Br J Anaesth* 1992; **68:** 183.
39. Gyasi HK, Naguib M. Atracurium and severe hepatic disease: a case report. *Can Anaesth Soc J* 1985; **32:** 161–4.
40. Hunter JP, Parker CJR, Bell CF, *et al.* The use of different doses of vecuronium in patients with liver dysfunction. *Br J Anaesth* 1982; **54:** 1267–9.
41. Arden JR, Lynman DP, Castagnoli KP, *et al.* Vecuronium in alcoholic liver disease: a pharmacokinetic and pharmacodynamic analysis. *Anesthesiology* 1988; **68:** 771.
42. Somogyi A, Shanks CA, Triggs EJ. Disposition kinetics of pancuronium bromide in patients with total biliary obstruction. *Br J Anaesth* 1977; **49:** 403.
43. Haberer JP, Schoeffler P, Couderc E, Duvaldestin P. Fentanyl pharmacokinetics in anaesthetised patients with cirrhosis. *Br J Anaesth* 1982; **54:** 1267–9.
44. Kang YG, Uram M, Shiu GK, *et al.* Pharmacokinetics of fentanyl in end stage liver disease. *Anesthesiology* 1984; **61:** 3A, A380.
45. Chauvin M, Ferrier C, Haberer JP, *et al.* Sufentanil pharmacokinetics in patients with cirrhosis. *Anesth Analg* 1989; **68:** 1.
46. Burkle H, Unbar S, Van Aken H. Remifentanil: a novel, short-acting, μ-opioid. *Anesth Analg* 1996; **83:** 646–51.
47. Tegeder I, Lotsch J, Geisslinger G. Pharmacokinetics of opioids in liver disease. *Clin Pharmacokinet* 1999; **37:** 17–40.
48. Dershwitz M, Hoke JF, Rosow CE, *et al.* Pharmacokinetics and pharmacodynamics of remifentanil in volunteer subjects with severe liver disease. *Anesthesiology* 1996; **84:** 812–20.
49. Gelman S, Fowler KC, Smith LR. Regional Liver circulation and function during isoflurane and halothane anesthesia. *Anesthesiology* 1984; **61:** 726–30.
50. Bito H, Ikeda K. Renal and hepatic function in surgical patients after low-flow sevoflurane or isoflurane anesthesia. *Anesth Analg* 1996; **82:** 173.
51. Wark H, Earl J, Cooper M, Overton J. Halothane in children with chronic liver disease. *Anesth Intensive Care* 1991; **19:** 9.
52. Bikle DD, Genant HK, Cann C, *et al.* Bone disease in alcohol abuse. *Ann Intern Med* 1985; **103:** 42.
53. Spencer H, Rubio N, Rubio E, *et al.* Chronic alcoholism. Frequently overlooked cause of osteoporosis in men. *Am J Med* 1986; **80:** 393.
54. O'Connor PG, Schottenfeld RS. Patients with alcohol problems. *N Engl J Med* 1998; **338:** 592.
55. Lang RM, Borow KM, Neumann A, *et al.* Adverse cardiac effects of acute alcohol ingestion in young adults. *Ann Intern Med* 1985; **102:** 742.
56. Howland WS, Schweizer O, Gould P. A comparison of intraoperative measurements of coagulation. *Anesth Analg* 1974; **53:** 657–63.
57. Zuckerman L, Cohen E, Vagher JP, *et al.* Comparison of thromboelastography with common coagulation tests. *Thromb Haemostasis* 1981; **46:** 752–6.
58. Kang YG. Monitoring and treatment of coagulation. In: Winter PM, Kang YG (eds). *Hepatic Transplantation. Anesthetic and Perioperative Management.* Westport, CT: Praeger Publishers, 1986: 151–73.
59. Mallett SV, Cox DJA. Thromboelastography. *Br J Anaesth* 1992; **69:** 621–30.
60. Whitten CW, Greilich PE. Thromboelastography: past, present, and future. *Anesthesiology* 2000; **92:** 1223–5.
61. Shore-Lesserson L, Manspeizer HE, DePerio M, *et al.* Thromboelastography-guided transfusion algorithm reduces transfusions in complex cardiac surgery. *Anesth Analg* 1999; **88:** 312–19.
62. Oshita K, Az-ma T, Osawa Y. Quantitative measurement of thromboelastography as a function of platelet count. *Anesth Analg* 1999; **89:** 296–9.
63. Kang YG, Martin DJ, Marquez J, *et al.* Intraoperative changes in blood coagulation and thromboelastographic monitoring in liver transplantation. *Anesth Analg* 1985; **64:** 888–96.
64. McNicol PL, Liu G, Harley ID, *et al.* Patterns of coagulopathy during

liver transplantation: experience with the first 75 cases using thromboelastography. *Anaesth Intensive Care* 1994; **22:** 659–65.
65. Hardings SA, Mallett SV, Peachey TD, *et al.* Use of heparinase modified thromboelastography in liver transplantation. *Br J Anaesth* 1997; **78:** 175–9.
66. Clayton DG, Miro AM, Kramer DJ, *et al.* Quantification of thromboelastographic changes after blood component transfusion in patients with liver disease in the intensive care unit. *Anesth Analg* 1995; **81:** 272–8.
67. Goodpasture EW. Fibrinolysis in chronic hepatic insufficiency. *Bull Johns Hopkins Hosp* 1914; **25:** 330–6.
68. Kang YG, Lewis JH, Navalgund A, *et al.* Epsilon-amino-caproic acid for treatment of fibrinolysis during liver transplantation. *Anesthesiology* 1987; **66:** 766–73.
69. Schipper HG, Ten Cate JW. Antithrombin III transfusion in patients with hepatic cirrhosis. *Br J Haematol* 1982; **52:** 25–33.
70. Thompson JN, Rotoli B. Endotoxins. The liver and haemostasis. In: Blumgart LH (ed.). *Surgery of the Liver and Biliary Tract.* London: Churchill Livingstone, 1988: 133–44.
71. Hayes PC, Bouchier IA. Postoperative jaundice. *Bailliere's Clin Gastroenterol* 1989; **3:** 485–505.
72. Becker SD, Lamont JT. Postoperative jaundice. *Semin Liver Dis* 1988; **8:** 183.
73. Starzl TE, Marchioro TL, Von Kaulla KN, *et al.* Homo-transplantation of the liver in humans. *Surg Gynecol Obstet* 1963; **117:** 659–76.
74. Calne RY, Williams R. Liver transplantation in man. 1. Observations on technique and organisation in five cases. *Br Med J* 1968; **4:** 535–40.
75. Starzl TE, Klintmalm GBG, Porter KA, *et al.* Liver transplantation with use of cyclosporin A and prednisolone. *N Engl J Med* 1981; **305:** 266–9.
76. Calne RY, Williams R, Lindop M, *et al.* Improved survival after orthotopic liver grafting. *Br Med J* 1981; **283:** 115–18.
77. Starzl TE, Marchioro TL, Porter KA. Progress in homo-transplantation of the liver. *Adv Surg (Chicago)* 1966; **2:** 295–370.
78. Starzl TE, Todo S, Gordon R, *et al.* Liver transplantation in older patients. *N Engl J Med* 1987; **316:** 484.
79. Van Thiel DH, Carr BI, Watsuki S, *et al.* Liver transplantation for alcoholic liver disease, viral hepatitis and hepatic neoplasms. *Transplant Proc* 1991; **23:** 1917–21.
80. Lichtor JL, Emond J, Chung MR, *et al.* Pediatric orthotopic liver transplantation: multifactorial predictions of blood loss. *Anesthesiology* 1988; **68:** 607.
81. Salt A, Barnes ND, Mowat AP, *et al.* Five year experience of liver transplantation in children. *Transplant Proc* 1990; **22:** 1514.
82. Gundlach M, Topp S, Broring D, Rogiers X. Split liver transplantation. *Ann Transplant* 2000; **5:** 38–42.
83. Bismuth H, Houssin D. Reduced-size orthotopic liver graft in hepatic transplantation in children. *Surgery* 1984; **95:** 367.
84. Greim CA, Roewer N, Thiel H, *et al.* Continuous cardiac output monitoring during adult liver transplant: thermal filament technique versus bolus thermodilation. *Anesth Analg* 1997; **85:** 483.
85. Welte M, Pichler B, Groh J, *et al.* Fulminant and late onset hepatic failure. *Br J Anaesth* 1996; **76:** 90.
86. Skak C, Rasmussen A, Kirkegaard P, *et al.* Cerebral oxygen saturation and blood flow during liver transplantation. *Anesth Analg* 1997; **84:** 730.
87. Whitten CW, Ramsay MAE, Paulsen AW, *et al.* Upper extremity neuropathy after orthotopic hepatic transplantation: a retrospective analysis. *Transplant Proc* 1988; **20:** 628–9.
88. Pittet JF, Denis M, Mentha G, *et al.* Vecuronium neuromuscular blockade reflects liver function during hepatic autotransplantation. *Anesthesiology* 1994; **81:** 168.
89. Marcel RJ, Ramsay MAE, Hein HA, *et al.* Duration of rocuronium-induced neuromuscular blockade during liver transplantation: A predictor of primary allograft function. *Anesth Analg* 1997; **84:** 870.
90. Gelman S, Fowler KC, Smith LR. Regional blood flow during isoflurane and halothane anesthesia. *Anesth Analg* 1984; **63:** 557–65.
91. Frink E, Morgan S, Coetzee A, *et al.* The effects of sevoflurane, halothane, enflurane and isoflurane on hepatic blood flow and oxygenation in chronically instrumented greyhound dogs. *Anesthesiology* 1992; **76:** 86–90.
92. Bakti G, Fisch HU, Karlaganis G, *et al.* Mechanics of the excessive sedative response of cirrhotics to benzodiazepines: model experiments with triazolam. *Hepatology* 1987; **7:** 629–38.
93. Basile AS, Hughes RD, Harrison PM, *et al.* Elevated brain concentrations of 1,4-benzodiazepines in fulminant hepatic failure. *N Engl J Med* 1991; **325:** 473–8.
94. Polson RJ, Park GR, Lindop MJ. The prevention of renal impairment in patients undergoing orthotopic liver grafting by infusion of low dose dopamine. *Anaesthesia* 1987; **42:** 15–19.
95. Arcas M, Pensado A, Gomez-Arnan J, *et al.* Renal failure in immediate post-operative phase after liver transplantation. In: *Proceedings of First Symposium of the International Society for Perioperative Care in Liver Transplantation*, 7th September, Pittsburgh, PA,1990.
96. Swygert TH, Roberts LC, Valek TR, *et al.* Effect of intra-operative low dose dopamine on renal function in liver transplant recipients. *Anesthesiology* 1991; **75:** 571–6.
97. Lokhandwala MF. Renal actions of dopexamine hydrochloride. *Clin Intensive Care* 1990; **1:** 163–74.
98. Paulsen AW, Whitten CW, Ramsay MAE, *et al.* Considerations for anesthetic management during veno-venous bypass in adult hepatic transplantation. *Anesth Analg* 1989; **68:** 489–96.
99. Khoury GF, Mann ME, Porot MJ, *et al.* Air embolism associated with veno-venous bypass during orthotopic liver transplantation. *Anesthesiology* 1987; **67:** 848.
100. Lewis JH, Bontempo FA, Awad SA, *et al.* Liver transplantation: Intraoperative changes in coagulation factors in 100 first transplants. *Hepatology* 1989; **9:** 710.
101. Kettner SC, Gonano C, Seebach F, *et al.* Endogenous heparin-like substances significantly impair coagulation in patients undergoing orthotopic liver transplantation. *Anesth Analg* 1998; **86:** 691.
102. Frenette L, Cox J, McArdle P, *et al.* Conjugated estrogen reduces transfusion and coagulation requirements in orthotopic liver transplantation. *Anesth Analg* 1998; **86:** 1183.
103. Levi M, Cromheecke ME, de Jonge E, *et al.* Pharmacological strategies to decrease excessive blood loss in cardiac surgery: a meta-analysis of clinically relevant endpoints. *Lancet* 1999; **354:** 1940–7.
104. Lentschener C, Benhamou D. Aprotinin during liver transplantation. *Br J Anaesth* 1996; **76:** 882.
105. Garcia-Huete L, Domenech P, Sabate A, *et al.* The prophylactic effect of aprotinin on intraoperative bleeding in liver transplantation: a randomised clinical study. *Hepatology* 1997; **26:** 1143–8.
106. Llamas P, Cabrera R, Gomez-Arnau J, Fernandez MN. Hemostasis and blood requirements in orthotopic liver transplantation with or without high dose aprotinin. *Haematologica* 1998; **83:** 338–46.
107. Porte RJ, Molenaar IQ. Aprotinin in liver transplantation. *Hepatology* 1998; **27:** 1169–71.
108. Porte RJ, Molenaar IQ, Begliomini B, *et al.* Aprotinin and transfusion requirements in orthotopic liver transplantation: a double-blind study. EMSALT Study Group. *Lancet* 2000; **15:** 1303–9.
109. Molenaar IQ, Veldman M, Begliomini B, *et al.* Improved early graft survival in patients receiving aprotinin during orthotopic liver transplantation. *Transplant Proc* 2001; **33:** 1345–6.
110. Khoury GF, Kaufman RD, Musich JA. Hypothermia related to the use of veno-venous bypass during liver transplantation in man. *Eur J Anaesthiol* 1990; **7:** 501–3.
111. Ramsay MAE, Swygert TH. Anaesthesia for hepatic trauma, hepatic resection and liver transplantation. *Bailliere's Clin Anaesthesiol* 1992; **6:** 863–94.
112. Brown M, Gunning T, Roberts C, *et al.* Biochemical markers of renal perfusion are preserved during liver transplantation with veno-venous bypass. *Transplant Proc* 1991; **23:** 1980–1.
113. Gunning TC, Brown MC, Swygert TH, *et al.* Peri-operative renal function in patients undergoing orthotopic liver transplantation. *Transplantation* 1991; **51:** 422–7.
114. Jamieson NV, Sundberg R, Lindell S, *et al.* Successful 24 to 30 hour preservation of the canine liver: a preliminary report. *Transplant Proc* 1988; **20:** 945–7.
115. Wahlberg JA, Love R, Landegaard L, *et al.* Seventy-two hour preservation of the canine pancreas. *Transplantation* 1987; **43:** 5–8.
116. Cofer JB, Klinkmalm GB, Howard TK, *et al.* A comparison of UW with Eurocollins preservation solution in liver transplantation. *Transplantation* 1990; **49:** 1088–93.
117. Adkinson D, Hollworth ME, Benoit JN, *et al.* Role of free radicals in ischaemic reperfusion injury to the liver. *Acta Physiol Scand* 1986; **548** (Suppl.): 101–7.
118. Greig PD, Woolf GM, Abecassis M, *et al.* Prostaglandin E for primary non-function following liver transplantation. *Transplant Proc* 1989; **21:** 3360–1.
119. Lichtor JL. Ventricular dysfunction does occur during liver transplantation. *Transplant Proc* 1991; **23:** 1924–6.
120. Roberts LC, Duke PK, Gottlich CM, *et al.* transesophageal echocardiography during orthotopic liver transplantation. *Anesthesiology* 1991; **75:** A388.

121. Bellamy MC, Salley HF, Webster NR. Changes in inflammatory mediators during liver transplantation. *Br J Anaesth* 1997; **79:** 338.
122. Prager MC, Gregory GA, Ascher NL, *et al.* Massive venous air embolism during orthotopic liver transplantation. *Anesthesiology* 1990; **72:** 198.
123. Ellis JE, Lichtor JL, Feinstein SB, *et al.* Right heart dysfunction, pulmonary embolism and paradoxical embolization during liver transplantation. *Anesth Analg* 1989; **68:** 777.
124. Navalgund AA, Kang Y, Sarner JB, *et al.* Massive pulmonary thromboembolism during liver transplantation. *Anesth Analg* 1988; **67:** 400.
125. Lustik SJ, Eichelberger JP, Chhibber A, *et al.* Torsade de pointes during orthotopic liver transplantation. *Anesth Analg* 1998; **87:** 300.
126. Paulsen AW, Brajtbord D, Klintmalm GB, *et al.* Intraoperative measurements related to subsequent hepatic graft failure. *Transplant Proc* 1989; **21:** 2337–8.
127. De Kock M, Laterre PF, Van Obbergh L. The effects of intraoperative intravenous clonidine on fluid requirements, hemodynamic variables and support during liver transplantation. *Anesth Analg* 1998; **86:** 468.
128. Mandell SM, Lockrem J, Kelly S. Immediate tracheal extubation after liver transplantation. *Anesth Analg* 1997; **84:** 249.
129. Klintmalm GB, Olson LM, Nery JR, *et al.* Treatment of hepatic artery thrombosis after liver transplantation with immediate vascular reconstruction: a report of three cases. *Transplant Proc* 1988; **20:** 610.
130. Park GR, Gomez-Arnan J, Lindop MJ, *et al.* Mortality during intensive care after liver transplantation. *Anaesthesia* 1989; **44:** 959–63.
131. Maknuchi M. Ultrasonically guided liver surgery. *Jpn J Ultrasonic Med* 1980; **7:** 45–9.
132. Grosse H, Pichlmayr R, Hansen B, *et al.* Specific anaesthetic problems in ex-situ resections of the liver. *Anaesthesia* 1990; **45:** 726–31.
133. Thompson HH, Thompkins RK, Longmire Jr WP. Major hepatic resections. A 25 year experience. *Ann Surg* 1983; **197:** 375–88.
134. Hardaway RM. Vietnam wound analysis. *J Trauma* 1978; **18:** 635.
135. Beal SI. Fatal hepatic haemorrhage: an unresolved problem in the management of complex liver injuries. *J Trauma* 1990; **30:** 163–9.
136. Royal College of Surgeons of England. *Report of the Working Party on the Management of Patients with Major Injuries.* London: RCSE, 1988.
137. LaMont JT, Isselbacher K. Postoperative jaundice. In: Wright R, Alberti KGMM, Karran S, Millward-Sadler GH (eds). *Liver and Biliary Disease*, 2nd edn. London: Bailliere Tindall/WB Saunders, 1984: 1367–77.
138. Evans C, Evans M, Pollock AV. The incidence and causes of postoperative jaundice. *Br J Anaesth* 1974; **46:** 520–5.
139. Chu C-M, Chang C-H, Liaw Y-F, Hsieh M-J. Jaundice after open heart surgery: a prospective study. *Thorax* 1984; **39:** 52–6.
140. Frink EJ, Brown BR. Postoperative hepatic dysfunction. *Bailliere's Clin Anaesthesiol* 1992; **6:** 931–52.
141. Owens D, Evans J. Population studies on Gilbert's syndrome. *J Med Genetics* 1975; **12:** 152–6.
142. Valeri CR. Viability and function of preserved red cells. *N Engl J Med* 1971; **284:** 81–6.
143. Solanki D, McCurdy PR. Delayed haemolytic transfusion reactions: an often-missed clinical entity. *JAMA* 1978; **239:** 729–31.
144. Howard RJ, Delaney JP. Postoperative cholecystitis. *Am J Dig Dis* 1972; **17:**213.
145. Johnson LB. The importance of early diagnosis of acute acalculous cholecystitis. *Surg Gynecol Obstet* 1987; **164:** 197–203.
146. LaMont JT, Isselbacher KJ. Postoperative jaundice. *N Engl J Med* 1973; **288:** 305–8.
147. Banks JG, Foulis AK, Ledingham IMcA, McSween RNM. Liver function in septic shock. *J Clin Pathol* 1982; **35:** 1249–52.
148. Richardson PDI, Withrington PG. Alpha- and beta-adrenoceptors in the hepatic portal vascular bed of the dog. *Br J Pharmacol* 1978; **62:** 376–7.
149. Dunn JD, Hayes P, Breenk S. The liver in congestive heart failure: a review. *Am J Med Sci* 1973; **265:** 174–89.
150. Aach RD, Szmuness W, Mosley JW, *et al.* Serum alanine amino-transferase of donors in relation to the risk on non-A, non-B hepatitis in recipients. The transfusion-transmitted viruses study. *N Engl J Med* 1981; **304:** 989–94.
151. Bass HM, Ockner RK. Drug-induced liver disease. In: Zakim D, Boyer TD (eds). *Hepatology – a Textbook of Liver Disease.* Philadelphia, PA: WB Saunders, 1990: 754–80.
152. Neuberger JM. Halothane and the implications of hepatitis. In: Kaufman L (ed.). *Anaesthetic Review*, 8. London: Churchill Livingstone, 1991: 179–94.
153. Ray DC, Drummond GB. Halothane hepatitis. *Br J Anaesth* 1991; **67:** 84–99.
154. Bottiger LE, Dalen E, Hallen B. Halothane-induced liver damage: an analysis of the material reported to the Swedish Adverse Drug Reaction Committee 1966–73. *Acta Anaesthesiol Scand* 1976; **20:** 40–6.
155. Inman WHW, Mushin WW. Jaundice after repeated exposure to halothane: an analysis of reports to Committee on Safety of Medicines. *Br Med J* 1974; **1:** 5–10.
156. Inman WHW, Mushin WW. Jaundice after repeated exposure to halothane: a further analysis of reports to Committee on safety of Medicines. *Br Med J* 1978; **2:** 1455–6.
157. Walton B, Simpson BR, Strunin L, *et al.* Unexplained hepatitis following halothane. *Br Med J* 1976; **1:** 1171–6.
158. Neuberger J, Williams R. Halothane anaesthesia and liver damage. *Br Med J* 1984; **289:** 1136–9.
159. Farrell GC. Mechanism of halothane induced liver injury. *J Gastroenterol Hepatol* 1988; **3:** 465–82.
160. Fee JPH, Black GW, Dundee JW, *et al.* A prospective study of liver enzyme and other changes following repeat administration of halothane and enflurane. *Br J Anaesth* 1979; **51:** 1133–41.
161. Trowell J, Peto R, Crampton-Smith A. Controlled trial of repeated halothane anaesthetics in patients with carcinoma of the cervix treated with radium. *Lancet* 1975; **1:** 821–4.
162. Wright R, Chisholm M, Lloyd B, *et al.* A controlled prospective study of the effect on liver function of multiple exposures to halothane. *Lancet* 1975; **1:** 817–20.
163. Stock JGL, Strunin L. Unexplained hepatitis following halothane. *Anesthesiology* 1985; **63:** 424–39.
164. Allan LG, Hussey AJ, Howie J, *et al.* Hepatic glutathione S-transferase release after halothane anaesthesia: open randomised comparison with isoflurane. *Lancet* 1987; **1:** 771–4.
165. Hussey AJ, Aldridge LM, Paul D, *et al.* Plasma glutathione S-transferase concentration as a measure of hepatocellular integrity following a single general anaesthetic with halothane, enflurane or isoflurane. *Br J Anaesth* 1988; **60:** 130–5.
166. Nomura F, Hatano H, Ohnishi K, *et al.* Effects of anticonvulsant agents on halothane-induced liver injury in human subjects and experimental animals. *Hepatology* 1986; **6:** 952–6.
167. Kenna JG, Neuberger J, Williams R. Identification by immunoblotting of three halothane-induced liver microsomal polypeptide antigens recognised by antibodies in sera from patients with halothane-associated hepatitis. *J Pharmacol Exp Ther* 1987; **242:** 733–40.
168. Satoh H, Gillette JR, Davies HW, *et al.* Immunochemical evidence of trifluroacetylated cytochrome P-450 in the liver of halothane-treated rats. *Mol Pharmacol* 1985; **28:** 468–74.
169. Satoh H, Martin BM, Schulick AH, *et al.* Human anti-endoplasmic reticulum antibodies in sera of patients with halothane-induced hepatitis are directed against a trifluroacetylated carboxylesterase. *Proc Natl Acad Sci USA, Medical Sciences* 1989; **86:** 322–6.
170. Bird GLA, Williams R. Detection of antibodies to a halothane metabolite hapten in sera from patients with halothane-associated hepatitis. *J Hepatol* 1989; **9:** 366–73.
171. Martin JL, Kenna JG, Martin BM, *et al.* Halothane hepatitis patients have serum antibodies that react with protein disulphide isomerase. *Hepatology* 1993; **18:** 858–63.
172. Stoelting RK, Blitt CD, Cohen PJ, Merin RG. Hepatic dysfunction after isoflurane anaesthesia. *Anesth Analg* 1987; **66:** 147–53.
173. Stoelting RK. Isoflurane and postoperative hepatic dysfunction. *Can J Anaesth* 1987; **34:** 223–6.
174. Trey C, Davidson C. *The Management of Fulminant Hepatic Failure.* New York: Grune & Stratton, 1970: 282–98.
175. Bray G, Mowat C, Muir D, *et al.* The effect of chronic alcohol intake on prognosis and outcome in paracetamol overdose. *Hum Exp Toxicol* 1991; **10:** 435–8.
176. O'Grady JG, Williams R. Management of acute hepatic failure. *Curr Anaesth Crit Care* 1990; **1:** 213–19.
177. O'Grady JG, Gimson AES, O'Brien CJ, *et al.* Controlled trials of charcoal haemoperfusion and prognostic factors in fulminant hepatic failure. *Gastroenterology* 1988; **94:** 1186–92.
178. Mullen KD, Martin JV, Mendelson WB, *et al.* Could an endogenous benzodiazepine ligand contribute to hepatic encephalopathy? *Lancet* 1988; **1:** 457–9.
179. Forbes A, Alexander GJM, O'Grady JG, *et al.* Thiopental infusion in the treatment of intracranial hypertension complicating fulminant hepatic failure. *Hepatology* 1989; **10:** 306–10.
180. O'Grady JG, Langley PG, Isola LM, *et al.* Coagulopathy of fulminant hepatic failure. *Semin Liver Dis* 1986; **6:** 159–63.
181. Bihari DJ, Gimson AES, Williams R. Cardiovascular, pulmonary and renal complications of fulminant hepatic failure. *Semin Liver Dis* 1986; **6:** 119–28.

182. O'Grady JG, Williams R. Management of acute liver failure. *Schweiz Med Wochenschr* 1986; **116:** 541–4.
183. Davenport A, Will E, Davidson A, *et al.* Changes in intracranial pressure during machine and continuous haemofiltration. *Crit Care Med* 1989; **12:** 439–44.
184. Rolando N, Harvey F, Braham J, *et al.* Prospective study of bacterial infections in acute liver failure: an analysis of fifty patients. *Hepatology* 1990; **11:** 49–53.
185. Rolando N, Harvey F, Braham J, *et al.* Fungal infections: a common unrecognised complication of acute liver failure. *Hepatology* 1991; **12:** 1–9.
186. Prescott L, Illingworth R, Critchley J, *et al.* Intravenous N-acetyl cysteine: the treatment of choice for paracetamol poisoning. *Br Med J* 1979; **2:** 1079–1100.
187. Acetylcysteine for acetaminophen overdose. *Med Lett* 1979; **21:** 98–100.
188. Harrison PM, Keays R, Bray GP, *et al.* Improved outcome of paracetamol induced fulminant hepatic failure by late administration of acetyl cysteine. *Lancet* 1990; **1:** 1572–3.
189. Keays R, Harrison PM, Wendon JA, *et al.* Intravenous acetyl cysteine and paracetamol induced fulminant hepatic failure: a prospective controlled trial. *Br Med J* 1991; **303:** 1026–9.
190. Vickers C, Neuberger J, Buckels J, *et al.* Transplantation of the liver in adults and children with fulminant hepatic failure. *J Hepatol* 1988; **7:** 143–50.
191. Emond JC, Aran PP, Whitington PF, *et al.* Liver transplantation in the management of fulminant hepatic failure. *Gastroenterology* 1989; **96:** 1583–8.
192. Schafer DF, Shaw BW. Fulminant hepatic failure and orthotopic liver transplantation. *Semin Liver Dis* 1989; **9:** 189–94.
193. Forbes A, Williams R. Increasing age – an important adverse prognostic factor in hepatitis A virus infection. *J R Coll Physicians (Lond)* 1988; **22:** 237–9.
194. Harrison TJ, Zuckerman AJ. Viral hepatitis. *Baillere's Clin Anaesthesiol* 1992; **6:** 759–817.
195. Rosina F, Saracco G, Rizzetto M. Risk of post transfusion infection with the hepatitis delta virus. A multicenter study. *N Engl J Med* 1985; **312:** 1488.
196. Smedile A, Farci P, Verme G, *et al.* Influence of delta infection on severity of hepatitis B. *Lancet* 1982; **2:** 945–7.
197. Govindarajan S, Chin KP, Redecker AG, Peters RL. Fulminant B viral hepatitis: role of delta agent. *Gastroenterology* 1984; **86:** 1417–20.
198. Farci P, Gerin JL, Aragona M, *et al.* Diagnostic and prognostic significance of the IgM antibody to the hepatitis delta virus. *JAMA* 1986; **255:** 1443.
199. Rizzetto M, Gocke DJ, Verme G, *et al.* Incidence and significance of antibodies to delta antigen in hepatitis B virus infection. *Lancet* 1979; **2:** 986.
200. Gimson AES, O'Grady J, Ede RJ, *et al.* Late-onset hepatic failure: clinical, serological and histological features. *Hepatology* 1986; **6:** 288–94.

54

Intra-abdominal laparoscopic surgery: anesthetic implications

ANTHONY J CUNNINGHAM AND NOREEN DOWD

HISTORICAL PERSPECTIVES

The modern age of laparoscopic surgery was ushered in with the incorporation of a miniature video camera attached to the eyepiece of a laparoscope, allowing multiple assistants to view the operative field from the same vantage point.[1] Gynecologic laparoscopic surgery has been routinely performed since the 1970s. In 1987, Phillipe Mouret described the first laparoscopic cholecystectomy in France; the first series was reported by Perissat *et al.*,[2] and the technique was introduced into the USA in 1988 by Reddick and Olsen.[3] Improved instrumentation allowed laparoscopic cholecystectomy to revolutionize upper abdominal surgery in the 1990s. Currently, laparoscopic gastroesophageal, hepatobiliary, colorectal, solid-organ renal/splenic procedures, and herniorrhaphy are routinely performed via minimal access techniques.

Laparoscopic surgical techniques have been rapidly accepted by surgeons worldwide, with published reports describing the benefits of less postoperative pain, reduced hospital stay, and an earlier return to work.[4] Until the late 1980s, morbidity and mortality were accepted as unavoidable aspects of the therapeutic process. The current realization that less invasive methods of treatment may reduce the risks of death and morbidity has given rise to the concept of "minimally invasive therapy" with the general aim to "minimise the trauma of the interventional process whilst still achieving a satisfactory therapeutic result."[5] A UK report commissioned by the Department of Health[6] to assess the implications of minimally invasive therapy did not favor the term "minimally invasive surgery," with its connotation of increased safety and minor procedure, preferring instead the term "minimal access surgery." The key feature of this technology-dependent surgery is that it produces significantly less trauma than does the conventional means of gaining access. The technology required is expensive, and its adoption has major implications for patient services, hospital design, operating room equipment, surgical specialty alignment, and training.[7]

Public perception that laparoscopic techniques were superior has led to the poorly controlled and audited introduction of laparoscopy-based surgical procedures. The percentage of cholecystectomies that are laparoscopic procedures climbed from 0% in 1987 to 80% in 1992.[8] A State of New York Department of Health memorandum reported 158 adverse incidents involving laparoscopic cholecystectomy between August 1990 and March 1992.[9] Seventy-two percent of these incidents required remedial open surgical repair of the injury/complication. As the demand grew for laparoscopy-based procedures, the demand for training also increased. Approximately 15 000 general surgeons were trained in new laparoscopic techniques in the USA between 1990 and 1992.[8] The Society of American Gastrointestinal Endoscopy Surgeons suggested guidelines for the credentialing, training, and determination of competence in laparoscopy techniques for their members.[10]

For more than a century, surgeons have upheld the legacy of William Halsted, who believed that each surgical advance should be based on thoughtful observation, laboratory experimentation, and carefully planned clinical trials. The evolution of laparoscopic cholecystectomy, however, represented a departure from traditional surgical development. The National Laparoscopic Surgery Registry was established in the USA in 1990 with the support of independent educational grants to help evaluate the acquisition of technical skills, the outcome analysis of new laparoscopic procedures, and cost–benefit assessments. The initial mission of the Registry was to collect, organize, and disseminate clinical data relevant to laparoscopic cholecystectomy, but this has been expanded to include all endocavity surgical procedures.[11]

The development and potential for advanced laparoscopic surgery, beyond laparoscopic cholecystectomy and diagnostic laparoscopy, was recently reviewed by Hunter.[12] Current limitations include a two-dimensional video image and the requirement for specialized surgical instrumentation. The laparoscopic port acts as a fulcrum that restricts the freedom of movement of the instruments.[1] The development of three-dimensional imaging and the expected introduction of flexible laparoscopes and robotics in the future will herald a new age in interventional surgery.[1,13] The implications for anesthesia will be far reaching. The physiologic effects of prolonged carbon dioxide (CO_2) insufflation into an endocavity combined with variations in positioning has a major impact on cardiopulmonary function, particularly in American Society for Anesthesiologists (ASA) grade III or IV patients.[14] Recent reports of "gasless laparoscopy" using an abdominal wall-lifting device may obviate the requirement for pneumoperitoneum.[15]

INTRA-ABDOMINAL LAPAROSCOPIC PROCEDURES

Cholecystectomy

Laparoscopic cholecystectomy (LC) involves changes in patient position from Trendelenburg to reverse Trendelenburg (rT), and intraperitoneal CO_2 insufflation (Fig. 54.1).

LC combines the benefit of completely removing the gall bladder with the advantages of shorter hospital stays, more rapid return to normal activities, less pain associated with the small, limited incisions, and

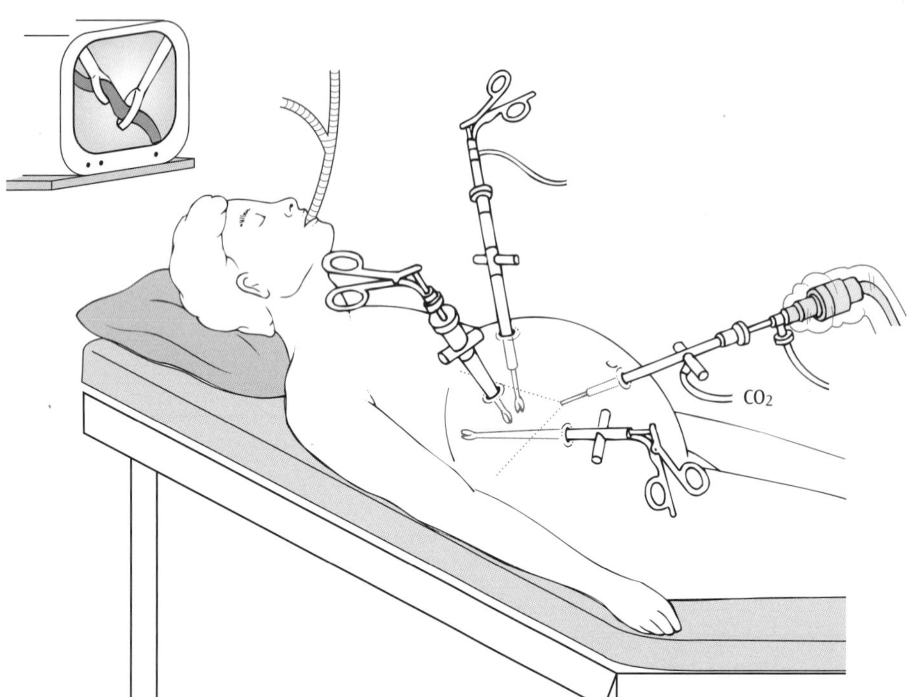

Figure 54.1 *Laparoscopic cholecystectomy: patient positioning and equipment.*

less postoperative ileus compared with the open laparotomy technique[16] (Table 54.1).

The Southern Surgeons Club,[17] in a prospective study of 1518 laparoscopic cholecystectomies performed by 59 surgeons in academic and private practice, defined a standard of care for the new procedure in 1991. Several other large series have also been reported from Europe[18] and North America.[19,20] Acute cholecystitis, obesity, and previous intra-abdominal surgery were initially considered to present difficult technical challenges. In late pregnancy, limited exposure was believed to compound the potential hazards of trocar insertion and the deleterious fetal effects of hypercarbia and pneumoperitoneum.

An impressive body of experience and literature has emerged confirming the safety and efficacy of laparoscopic cholecystectomy in the hands of experienced surgeons. Acute cholecystitis, despite concerns about technical difficulties with the associated edema, inflammation and necrosis, is no longer considered a contraindication to LC.[21] The conversion rate, however, is high, especially in patients >65 years with a history of biliary disease and an acute gangrenous gall bladder.[22] Although the incidence of symptomatic biliary disease in pregnancy is estimated at only 0.05%, the need for surgery in symptomatic patients is approximately 40%, and the risk of premature labor is inversely related to gestational age.[23] As with open cholecystectomy, conventional wisdom suggests delay until the postpartum period, if possible, when managing biliary colic in pregnancy. Recent case reports,[24] series,[25] studies,[26] and literature reviews[27] confirm that LC can be safely performed in all trimesters of pregnancy, with acceptable maternal and fetal morbidity. The available data suggest that the safety and efficacy of LC in pregnancy is increased by using the open Hasson technique for instrumentation, by limiting intra-abdominal pressure during the pneumoperitoneum, by using appropriate maternal and fetal monitoring, by ensuring adequate maternal oxygenation and normocapnia, by prevention of aortocaval compression by left tilt, and by the use of active antithromboembolism measures, including calf compression.

Table 54.1 *Potential benefits of laparoscopic cholecystectomy*

Comparison with traditional open cholecystectomy
Minimizes abdominal incision
Preserves diaphragmatic function
Potential benefits
Reduced adverse events
Pulmonary function preserved
Less postoperative ileus
Early ambulation
Economic benefits
Shorter hospital stay
Early return to work and normal activities

Careful audit of large series has highlighted problems unique to, or more commonly associated with, the laparoscopic approach in North American and Australian/New Zealand practice.[28,29] Pre-existing umbilical and ventral hernia defects are major risk factors for postoperative trocar site hernia formation. Critics of laparoscopic surgery cite the increased incidence of tumor recurrence at the trocar sites following LC in patients incidentally found to have carcinoma of the gall bladder. There is considerable controversy regarding the appropriateness of laparoscopy for the treatment of known malignant disease. However, recent data suggest that gall bladder cancer is an aggressive malignancy and that abdominal wall implantation is not increased with laparoscopic surgery but is more likely a manifestation of the aggressive nature of the tumor.[30] Bile duct injuries are more common after laparoscopy than after open cholecystectomy.[31] Furthermore, such injuries after laparoscopic cholecystectomy tend to be more extensive and higher in the duct system than those following open cholecystectomy, thus reducing the chance of a successful outcome from reconstruction. Roy *et al.*[32] undertook a case series review of 21 patients who sustained bile duct injuries during laparoscopic cholecystectomy in two tertiary care centers over a 2-year period. Misidentification of the common duct, resulting in accidental division or resection, and obstruction by hemoclips were the most common injuries. Pain, jaundice, and bile collections were the typical presenting features of injuries that became evident after laparoscopic cholecystectomy. Twenty of the 21 patients required Roux-en-Y hepaticojejunostomy for definitive treatment.

Laparoscopic surgery

- Acute cholecystitis, obesity, previous intra-abdominal surgery, and late pregnancy were initially contraindicated but are now considered safe in experienced hands.
- Laparoscopic cholecystectomy in known gall bladder malignancy is controversial.
- Endoscopic antireflux surgery (laparoscopic Nissen fundoplication) has been established. Patient selection is important to avoid unnecessary/inappropriate operations.
- Laparoscopic hernia repair and solid organ procedures are evolving.
- Diagnostic laparoscopy, particularly for acute appendicitis, is associated with a longer duration of surgery and shorter hospital stay. There are no differences in time to return to activity and work compared with open surgery.

Miscellaneous intra-abdominal procedures

The adoption of therapeutic endoscopy has triggered the single largest change in surgical practice for many decades. Proponents of the endoscopic approach claim that the minimally invasive aspect will decrease postoperative morbidity and allow patients to return to normal activity and work earlier than after a conventional open procedure.

Mellinger and Ponsky[33] highlighted the minimally invasive surgical literature in 1996. The list of procedures now commonly performed endoscopically has grown rapidly with gastric, antireflux, colonic, and renal surgery following appendectomy and inguinal hernia repair (Table 54.2).

Raiser and colleagues[34] reviewed the current status of minimally invasive antireflux surgery. They emphasized the importance of preoperative evaluation – endoscopy, biopsy, manometry, pH monitoring – in guiding patient selection for the most appropriate procedure and in avoiding unnecessary or inappropriate operative misadventures. A laparoscopic Nissen fundoplication may prove a cost-effective technique for patients with gastroesophageal reflux on long-term medical management, provided complication rates are comparable and surgical results are enduring. Interest in laparoscopic hernia repair continues, although conflicting reports have been published regarding its putative advantages over traditional surgical techniques. The laparoscopic surgical technique has evolved from external intraperitoneal only to transabdominal preperitoneal (TAPP) to totally extraperitoneal (TEP). Laparoscopic techniques involve the use of general anesthetic techniques, and the associated higher operative costs and complication rates may not offset the potential benefits of less postoperative pain.[35] Laparoscopic approaches to solid abdominal organs, especially the spleen, kidney, and adrenal gland, continue to be described. A comparative study of laparoscopic and open splenectomy reported by a group from the University of California at San Francisco noted equivalent blood loss, complication rates, transfusion requirements, and hospital costs.[36] Longer operative times, earlier return to regular diet, and shorter hospital stay were a feature of the laparoscopic group. Goletti and Buccianti[37] reported a mean operative time of 109 min and a median postoperative stay of 3 days in their series of 25 patients undergoing laparoscopic adrenalectomies.

Table 54.2 *Laparoscopic intra-abdominal surgical procedures*

Cholecystectomy
Vagotomy
Hiatus hernia repair
Diaphragmatic hernia repair
Appendectomy
Colectomy
Inguinal hernia repair
Nephrectomy
Adrenalectomy

Despite the significant advances in surgery over the past century, the diagnosis of acute appendicitis continues to present problems for clinicians. In 20% of patients with appendicitis, the diagnosis was missed initially, and the appendix was normal in 15–40% of those undergoing emergency surgery for suspected appendicitis.[38] In a prospective randomized study, the laparoscopic appendectomy technique was associated with longer duration of surgery, shorter hospital stay, and no differences in terms of time to return to activity and work compared with conventional open surgery.[39] Case reports, with associated literature reviews and editorial comments, highlighted concerns about trocar site recurrence following laparoscopic colectomy for colorectal cancer.[40,41] Preliminary experimental data confirmed a significantly increased incidence of diffuse carcinomatosis, even when performed for locally noninvasive tumors.[42]

PHYSIOLOGIC CHANGES AND COMPLICATIONS

Significant data have been accumulated about complications associated with laparoscopy.[43] The complications unique to laparoscopic cholecystectomy, reviewed by Strasberg and colleagues,[44] include bile duct injury and disruption of major blood vessels. Other problems relate to the cardiopulmonary effects of pneumoperitoneum, systemic CO_2 absorption, extraperitoneal gas insufflation, and venous gas embolism (Table 54.3).

Trocar insertion

Most laparoscopists consider that it is essential to establish a pneumoperitoneum during laparoscopy before a trocar and laparoscope can be introduced into the peritoneal cavity. In order to achieve a pneumoperitoneum, a Veress needle is introduced into the peritoneal cavity and CO_2 gas is insufflated. Injuries have been reported to occur as the Veress needle or trocar is introduced blindly through the abdominal wall prior to insertion of the laparoscope (Fig. 54.2). Such injuries have included bleeding from abdominal wall vessels, gastrointestinal tract perforations, hepatic and splenic tears, major vascular trauma, avulsion of adhesions, omental disruption, and herniation at the trocar insertion site.[45] Near the level of the umbilicus, both the medial vessels (superficial and inferior epigastric) and lateral vessels (superficial and deep circumflex iliac) are at risk of injury.[46] A "Hasson" minilaparotomy technique has been advocated for pneumoperitoneum creation to avoid injuries associated with blind Veress needle and trocar insertion.[47] In this open technique, the first or primary trocar is inserted through a minilaparotomy incision, and the potential complications of blind Veress needle and trocar insertion are avoided.

Gees and Holden[48] retrospectively reviewed 2201 laparoscopic procedures performed in a 3-year period in Columbus, Ohio, between 1992 and 1995. There were three major vascular injuries – the left common iliac vein, the right common iliac artery, and the left internal iliac artery – giving an incidence of 0.14%. Noga and colleagues[49] highlighted the role of the anesthesiologists in the early diagnosis of retroperitoneal hematoma – a potentially fatal complication of laparoscopic surgery.

Table 54.3 *Summary of potential cardiopulmonary changes during laparoscopic surgery*

Trendelenburg position	
Circulation	Heart rate
	Stroke volume
Respiration	Minute volume
	Work of breathing
	Lung volumes
	Gas exchange
Pneumoperitoneum	
Circulation	Venous return (cardiac filling pressures)
	Contractility (neural/humoral)
	Afterload
Respiration	Minute ventilation
	Airway pressure
	Lung volumes (FRC)
	Gas exchange (hypoxemia/hypercarbia)
Exogenous CO_2	
Circulation	Dysrhythmias
	Contractility
	Venous gas embolization
Respiration	Ventilation (dead space)
	CO_2 hemostasis
Reverse Trendelenburg	
Circulation	Venous return
	Afterload
Respiration	Lung volumes
	Work of breathing
	Minute ventilation
	Gas exchange

FRC, functional residual capacity.

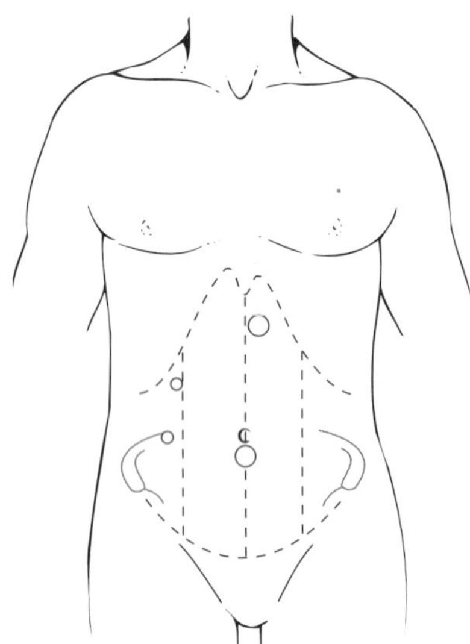

Figure 54.2 *Laparoscopic cholecystectomy: surgical incision sites.*

Patient position

During laparoscopic surgery, the patient is positioned to produce gravitational displacement of the abdominal viscera away from the surgical site. Gravity has profound effects on the cardiovascular and pulmonary systems. The head-down tilt of 10–20° commonly used both in gynecologic procedures and for the initial trocar insertion for laparoscopic cholecystectomy is accompanied by an increase in central blood volume[50] and a decrease in vital capacity and diaphragmatic excursion,[51] whereas the rT position favors improved pulmonary dynamics[52] but reduced venous return.[53,54] These changes associated with positioning may be influenced by the extent of the tilt,[55] the patient's age, intravascular volume status, associated cardiac disease,[56,57] anesthetic drugs administered, and ventilation techniques. The potential for inadvertent right mainstem bronchial intubation and hypoxemia associated with Trendelenburg positioning was highlighted by Wilcox and Vandam.[58] A subsequent case report confirmed this possibility.[59] The proposed mechanism is that the endotracheal tube, firmly secured at its proximal end to the mandible, does not always move along with the trachea as the diaphragm causes cephalad displacement of the lung and carina.[60] Prolonged laparoscopic surgery in the Trendelenburg position was recently complicated by brachial plexus injury.[61]

Creation of pneumoperitoneum

Creation of the pneumoperitoneum involves the intraperitoneal insufflation of CO_2 through a Veress needle while the patient is in a 15–20° Trendelenburg position. The potential difficulties that may be encountered during creation of pneumoperitoneum are outlined below.

Technical difficulties

Extraperitoneal insufflation of CO_2 is one of the most common complications of laparoscopy. The incidence of this complication has been reported to vary from 0.4% to 2%.[62] Such extraperitoneal insufflation may cause subcutaneous or retroperitoneal emphysema, prolonging surgery or causing its abandonment. Subcutaneous emphysema may occur if the tip of the Veress needle does not penetrate the peritoneal cavity prior to insufflation of gas. This may cause the insufflating gas to accumulate in the subcutaneous tissue or between the fascia and the peritoneum. Lew *et al.*[63] reported extensive subcutaneous emphysema, which involved the neck, chest, and abdomen and extended to the groin, attributed to subcutaneous insufflation of CO_2 from a poorly stabilized Veress needle.

Extraperitoneal insufflation has been associated with higher levels of CO_2 absorption than intraperitoneal insufflation and may be the cause of a sudden rise in $P_{ET}CO_2$ during the procedure.[64]

Pneumomediastinum and pneumothorax

Pneumothorax is a rare but potentially life-threatening complication of pneumoperitoneum. The history, pathogenesis, and management of such clinical situations were reviewed by Prystowsky and colleagues.[65] This complication occurs primarily on the right side. Insufflated gas may track around the aortic and esophageal hiatuses of the diaphragm into the mediastinum and then rupture into the pleural space. However, an anatomic basis for passage of gas into the thoracic cavity through a diaphragmatic defect is more likely. Commonly, these weak points or defects occur at the pleuroperitoneal hiatus or foramen of Bochdalek, the outer crus, or the esophageal hiatus. Pneumothoraces have been reported in association with subcutaneous emphysema and pneumomediastinum, whereas an isolated tension pneumothorax has been reported during laparoscopic cholecystectomy following trocar insertion and intraperitoneal CO_2 insufflation.[66] A congenital defect of the diaphragm (patent pleuroperitoneal canal) through which the insufflated gas passes into the thoracic cavity has been suggested as the underlying mechanism. Alternatively, a ruptured bleb or bulla could have produced the tension pneumothorax independent of the pneumoperitoneum.

Hasel *et al.*[67] reported three cases in which extravasation of CO_2 during laparoscopic cholecystectomy resulted in subcutaneous emphysema associated with pneumomediastinum, pneumoscrotum, pneumothorax, and ocular emphysema. It was assumed that intraperitoneal CO_2 traversed into the mediastinum via a defect in the diaphragm and into the scrotum along the spermatic cord through the inguinal canal. Excessively high intra-abdominal pressures during CO_2 insufflation may have contributed to these complications, which resolved uneventfully within 24 h.

Undetected pneumothorax/pneumomediastinum can be life threatening. The diagnosis should be considered in the presence of increased airway pressure, hemodynamic compromise, oxygen desaturation, or unexpected hypoxemia/hypercarbia. Subcutaneous emphysema of the neck, chest wall, and face should alert the anesthesiologist to the possibility of such associated complications. As soon as this possibility is suspected, a chest radiograph should be obtained to diagnose or rule out a pneumomediastinum or pneumothorax. If the hemodynamic status is unstable and if there is clinical evidence of a tension pneumothorax, chest tube decompression and abdominal deflation are indicated before obtaining a chest radiograph. Once the chest drain is in a satisfactory position, the abdomen can be insufflated and the procedure can be continued if the patient remains stable. If the pneumothorax is recognized near the end of the operation and the patient is stable, the surgery can be completed without therapeutic intervention. Once the abdomen is deflated, the CO_2 in the pleural cavity will be rapidly resorbed, obviating the necessity for a chest tube.

Cardiovascular effects

The extent of cardiovascular changes associated with creation of the pneumoperitoneum will depend on the interaction of factors, including positioning of the patient,[68] the intra-abdominal pressures obtained during insufflation,[69] and the neurohumoral effects of absorbed[70] CO_2 (Table 54.3). Preoperative cardiorespiratory status,[14] the intravascular volume,[71] and the anesthetic agents employed may also be significant.

The physiologic changes associated with laparoscopy and pneumoperitoneum in gynecologic surgery have been well described.[72,73] This patient population generally comprises healthy females undergoing short procedures in the Trendelenburg position. In comparison, abdominal laparoscopic surgery has been recommended for elderly and infirm patients who may not tolerate conventional surgery,[74,75] although the technique requires complicated positioning and increased operating time.[6]

The hemodynamic effects of CO_2 insufflation and rT positioning were comprehensively reviewed by Wahba and colleagues[76] in a meta-analysis of recent North American and UK literature. The dynamic physiologic changes that occur during laparoscopic abdominal surgery appear to have a phasic component. Joris *et al.*[77] used flow-directed pulmonary artery catheters to assess the effects of CO_2 insufflation to an intra-abdominal pressure of 1.87 kPa (14 mmHg) in healthy patients undergoing laparoscopic cholecystectomy. Cardiac index (CI) was reduced by 35–40% from baseline after induction of anesthesia and rT positioning, and further reduced to 50% of its preoperative value 5 min after the beginning of CO_2 insufflation. The CI gradually improved after 10 min of CO_2 insufflation. Other studies support this phasic change in hemodynamic function.[78,79] However, some investigators have documented an unchanged CI during insufflation of CO_2.[80,81]

The filling pressures of the heart, central venous pressure (CVP), and pulmonary artery occlusion pressure (PAOP) initially are reduced following induction of anesthesia and venous pooling in the rT position. Following CO_2 insufflation, the right- and left-sided filling pressures substantially increase.[14,77,82,83] The mechanical effects of insufflated CO_2 may explain some of these changes. Modern laparoscopic insufflators automatically terminate the gas flow when a preset intra-abdominal pressure (IAP) of 1.33–2 kPa (10–15 mmHg) is reached. The insufflated CO_2 compresses both the venous capacitance system and the arterial resistance vessels. The mechanical effect on the venous system will involve transiently increased venous return followed by a reduction.[84] However, it has been suggested that the increase in intra-abdominal pressure causes a proportionate increase in intrathoracic pressure and that this probably also contributes to the documented rise in CVP and PAOP.[85,86]

The compressive effects on the arterial vasculature result in a dramatic increase in calculated systemic vascular resistance (SVR), particularly during the initial phase of CO_2 insufflation. Mean arterial blood pressure (MABP) also rises substantially, reflecting the increased afterload with an associated deterioration in CI.[14,77,78] The magnitude of CI reduction is directly proportional to the insufflation pressure. Westerband *et al.*,[78] using impedance cardiography, reported a 30% reduction in CI and a 79% increase in SVR immediately after peritoneal insufflation to 2 kPa (15 mmHg). The safe upper limit of IAP insufflation was studied in an animal model investigating stepwise increases in IAP of 1.07 kPa (8 mmHg), 1.6 kPa (12 mmHg), and 2.13 kPa (16 mmHg). The threshold pressure that had minimal effects on hemodynamic function was found at an IAP of 1.6 kPa (12 mmHg). The authors recommend this pressure limit to avoid cardiovascular compromise during pneumoperitoneum.[69]

In a series of 13 otherwise healthy patients, Cunningham *et al.*[68] found that left ventricular function, as determined by transesophageal echocardiography, was preserved following CO_2 insufflation and patient position changes, despite variations in left ventricular loading conditions. However, CO_2 insufflation was associated with increases in left ventricular end-systolic wall stress, concomitant with increases in systemic arterial pressure. In addition, left ventricular end-diastolic volume decreased following rT positioning, indicating reduced venous return. Left ventricular ejection fraction was maintained throughout the study period in this investigation of otherwise healthy patients. However, it might reasonably be speculated that the aforementioned changes in left ventricular loading conditions might have had deleterious consequences in a patient population with significant cardiovascular disease.

Safran *et al.*[14] investigated ASA grade III/IV patients with severe heart disease. Cardiac output (CO) decreased and SVR and MABP increased following CO_2 insufflation. Significant reductions in mixed venous oxygen saturation ($S_{\bar{v}}O_2$) and oxygen delivery were noted in 50% of their patients. Feig and colleagues[87] documented significant increases in SVR, MABP, PAOP, and left ventricular stroke work index (LVSWI) occurring with insufflation pressures up to 2 kPa (15 mmHg) in 15 ASA grade III/IV patients. Persistent refractory acidemia and hypercarbia complicated four cases in the study. Two patients had significant cardiac arrhythmias requiring treatment during insufflation. Hypercarbia and respiratory acidosis may cause a decrease in myocardial contractility and a lowering of the arrhythmia threshold, particularly if the myocardium is already sensitized by the use of volatile anesthetic agents. Hypercarbia is reported to increase CO, MABP, heart rate, and plasma epinephrine (adrenaline) and norepinephrine (noradrenaline) levels.[88] Because the direct effects of hypercarbia include arteriolar dilation and myocardial depression, the overall change in cardiovascular function is thought to be mediated by the catecholamine release.

A number of case reports have described acute hypotension, hypoxemia, and cardiovascular collapse associated with laparoscopy.[89,90] Postulated causes included: (1) hypercarbia, which may induce dysrhythmias; (2) reflex increases in vagal tone due to excessive stretching of the peritoneum; (3) compression of the inferior vena cava, leading to decreased CO; (4) hemorrhage; and (5) venous gas embolism. The clinical conditions associated with venous CO_2 embolism during laparoscopy have also been described.[91,92] Venous CO_2 embolism in these cases was associated with profound hypotension, cyanosis, and asystole after creation of pneumoperitoneum. Beck and McQuillan[90] noted a sudden decrease in end-tidal CO_2 ($P_{ET}CO_2$) after 1 h of surgery in a fatal case of carbon dioxide embolism. The authors suggested that CO_2 could enter a tributary of the portal system during attempts at establishing the pneumoperitoneum. Rapid CO_2 exsufflation was reported to have precipitated acute hypotension, bradycardia, and hypoxemia.[93] Derouin and colleagues,[94] using TEE, observed CO_2 gas embolism in 11 out of 16 patients studied (five during peritoneal insufflation and six during gall bladder dissection). Cerebral arterial CO_2 embolism has been reported in a patient with an atrial septal defect.[95]

Renal and hepatic blood flow

Renal and hepatic blood flow may be influenced by intra-abdominal pressure, hypercarbia, and patient position. Head-up position and intraperitoneal pressure >1.6 kPa (12 mmHg) compromised hepatic and renal blood flow in an experimental animal study.[96] The level and duration of intra-abdominal pressures were responsible for elevations in serum bilirubin and hepatic transaminases during laparoscopic surgery.[97] Although no symptoms appeared in patients with normal hepatic function, patients with severe hepatic failure should probably not be subjected to prolonged laparoscopic procedures.

During pneumoperitoneum, the plasma concentrations of dopamine, vasopressin, epinephrine, norepinephrine, renin, and cortisol are noted to rise significantly.[98,99] The time-course of vasopressin and norepinephrine elevation is of particular importance. The plasma concentration–time-course profile parallels that of the change in CI, MABP, and SVR,[100,101] suggesting a possible cause–effect relation. It is probable that hypercarbia and pneumoperitoneum cause stimulation of the sympathetic nervous system and release of catecholamines.[101] The phasic restoration in CI may be as a result of the direct arteriolar vasodilatory effects of CO_2 and the effects of anesthetic agents on the SVR. Overall, the hemodynamic effects of pneumoperitoneum will generally be well tolerated by healthy individuals but will require careful evaluation in compromised patients.

Respiratory function

CO_2 homeostasis

Peritoneal gas insufflation is essential to facilitate exposure, visualization, and manipulation of intra-abdominal contents. Although nitrous oxide has been used for diagnostic gynecologic procedures, it is flammable when electrocautery is used. Helium has not been accepted because of its insolubility in blood and the possibility of embolic phenomena.[102] CO_2 has evolved as the insufflation gas of choice for laparoscopic surgery because of its efficacy and safety during electrocautery and laser surgery and its capability for pulmonary excretion.[81]

CO_2 insufflation into the peritoneal cavity increases arterial CO_2 tension, which is managed by increasing minute ventilation. The absorption of CO_2 from a closed cavity depends on its diffusibility and perfusion of the walls of that cavity and not on the rate of insufflation of the gas into the cavity.[103] Mullet *et al.*[104] hypothesized that the rate of CO_2 diffusion into the body depends on the duration and the site of CO_2 insufflation. They examined $P_{ET}CO_2$ tension and pulmonary CO_2 elimination during CO_2 insufflation under general anesthesia for gynecologic laparoscopy (intraperitoneal for 43 min), laparoscopic cholecystectomy (intraperitoneal for 125 min), and pelviscopy (extraperitoneal for 45 min). $P_{ET}CO_2$ and pulmonary CO_2 elimination increased in parallel from 8 to 10 min after the start of CO_2 insufflation. A plateau was reached 10 min later in patients having intraperitoneal insufflation, whereas $P_{ET}CO_2$ and pulmonary CO_2 elimination continued to increase slowly throughout CO_2 insufflation during pelviscopy.

Wittgen *et al.*[105] compared 20 healthy patients undergoing laparoscopic cholecystectomy with 10 ASA grade II/III patients. Compared with the healthy group, there were significant decreases in pH and increases in P_aCO_2 during pneumoperitoneum in the ASA grade III group, and this group also had significantly higher minute ventilation and peak inspiratory pressures than baseline values. Increasing minute ventilation in most cases will maintain P_aCO_2 within normal limits, but will inevitably lead to some increase in airway pressure. However, in ASA grade III or IV patients, P_aCO_2 may remain elevated despite adjusting minute ventilation to normalize $P_{ET}CO_2$.[87] Preoperative evaluation with pulmonary function tests demonstrating forced expiratory volumes less than 70% of predicted values and diffusion defects less than 80% of predicted values can identify patients at risk of developing hypercarbia and respiratory acidosis following pneumoperitoneum. Hall *et al.*[106] reported a case of acute profound hypercarbia occurring late in the procedure caused by CO_2 insufflation and first detected by capnography.

Intraoperative changes

Respiratory function changes occurring during laparoscopic cholecystectomy may differ from those reported during gynecologic laparoscopic procedures, probably because of the intra-abdominal nature of the surgery and the prolonged insufflation times required. Functional residual capacity (FRC) and lung compliance decrease with assumption of the supine position and cephalad shift of the diaphragm and with induction of general anesthesia.[107] However, the insufflation of intraperitoneal CO_2 may further exacerbate these changes. Lung and chest wall mechanical impedance increase with increasing intra-abdominal pressure.[108] The increase depends on body configuration and is greater when head down. These changes should be considered for patients in whom increases in impedance may be critical, such as obese patients and those with pulmonary disease.

Hypoxemia during laparoscopic abdominal surgery can have many causes, including a reduction in compliance, which may lead to diminished FRC relative to closing volume and $\dot{V}/\dot{Q}$ mismatch. Intraoperative hypoxemia is uncommon in healthy patients.[109,110] Joris *et al.*[77] found no significant increased intrapulmonary shunt despite reductions in CO and oxygen delivery in 20 healthy patients during laparoscopic cholecystectomy. We reported a case of intraoperative hypoxemia complicating laparoscopy in an obese patient with sickle hemoglobinopathy.[111] Hypoxemia may also be caused by regurgitation and aspiration of gastric contents. Duffy[112] reported gastric regurgitation in 2 out of 93 fasted patients undergoing laparoscopic gynecologic surgery. Similarly, during laparoscopic cholecystectomy, there are several factors that predispose to regurgitation, including the initial steep head-down tilt, insufflation of intraperitoneal gas, and mechanical pressure exerted on the abdomen by the surgical team. The hazards of intraoperative pneumothorax have already been described above.

Postoperative changes

There have been few prospective, randomized studies comparing laparoscopic and open cholecystectomy. Pulmonary dysfunction after open cholecystectomy is multifactorial and has been characterized as a restrictive pattern with a decrease in vital capacity and FRC. The common denominator is division of the abdominal musculature, which produces incisional pain, diaphragmatic dysfunction, and impairment of ventilatory mechanics. It has been suggested that laparoscopic surgery may reduce postoperative pulmonary complications by avoiding the restrictive pattern of breathing that usually follows upper abdominal surgery.

Schauer *et al.*[113] observed that, compared with patients undergoing open cholecystectomy, the laparoscopic procedure was associated with 30–38% less impairment of pulmonary function including FRC, forced expiratory volume in 1 s, maximum forced expiratory flow, and total lung capacity. Joris and colleagues[114] differentiated the influence of site of surgery, parietal trauma, intraoperative patient position, and pneumoperitoneum on pulmonary function and, by extension, clarified their roles in the pathophysiology of postoperative pulmonary dysfunction in females of normal body mass index and free of cardiopulmonary disease. Reductions in effort-dependent measures of pulmonary function – forced expiratory volume in 1 s (FEV_1), peak expiratory flow rate (PEFR), and vital capacity – were less than those usually associated with "open" cholecystectomy, and return to normal function was more rapid. While surgical trauma to the gall bladder is almost identical with open and laparoscopic techniques, the advantage of the latter may relate to the minimal trauma inflicted on the abdominal wall.[115] Postoperative residual pneumoperitoneum per se may not explain the diaphragmatic dysfunction observed after laparoscopic cholecystectomy. Visceral afferents originating in the gall bladder area or somatic afferents arising from the abdominal wall, which exert an inhibitory action on phrenic discharge, may be the cause of this diaphragmatic dysfunction. Erice and colleagues[116] concluded that the internal site of surgical intervention is the crucial variable determining diaphragmatic inhibition after they observed a decrease in maximum transdiaphragmatic pressure with laparoscopic cholecystectomy and not laparoscopic hernia repair.

Physiologic changes and complications

Patient position: head-down tilt of 10–20°

- ↓ Central blood volume, vital capacity, and diaphragmatic excursion.
- Inadvertent right mainstem bronchial intubation.
- Brachial plexus injury.

Creation of pneumoperitoneum

- Bile duct or major vessel injury.
- Subcutaneous/retroperitoneal emphysema.
- Pneumomediastinum/pneumothorax.

Cardiovascular effects

- No change or ↓ cardiac index, ↓CVP, ↓ PAOP after induction of anesthesia and rT.
- ↑ Venous return, ↑ intra-abdominal/intrathoracic pressure, ↑SVR, ↑ MABP with CO_2 insufflation.
- Left ventricular function preserved following CO_2 insufflation.
- ↑ Left ventricular end-systolic wall stress with increases in systemic arterial pressure.

Hypercarbia/CO_2 insufflation

- ↓Myocardial contractility.
- Dysrhythmias.
- Reflex increases in vagal tone with stretching of the peritoneum.
- Compression of the inferior vena cava, leading to decreased CO and venous gas embolism.

Renal and hepatic blood flow

- rT and intraperitoneal pressure > 1.6 kPa (12 mmHg) may ↓ hepatic and renal blood flow.

Respiratory function

- FRC and lung compliance ↓ with induction of general anesthesia and insufflation of CO_2.
- Lung and chest wall mechanical impedance ↑ with increasing intra-abdominal pressure.
- Potential regurgitation and aspiration of gastric contents.
- Postoperative diaphragmatic dysfunction (phrenic inhibition/residual pneumoperitoneum).

ANESTHETIC MANAGEMENT

A number of reviews have highlighted the anesthetic considerations for laparoscopic cholecystectomy, including anesthetic technique, intraoperative opioid and nitrous oxide administration, and appropriate monitoring.[117,118] The choice of anesthetic technique for upper abdominal laparoscopic surgery is mostly limited to general anesthesia because of patient discomfort associated with creation of the pneumoperitoneum and the extent of position changes associated with the procedure. Cuffed endotracheal tube placement will minimize the risk of acid aspiration if reflux occurs. Controlled ventilation is recommended because several factors may induce hypercarbia, including depression of ventilation by anesthetic agents, absorption of CO_2 from the peritoneal cavity, and mechanical impairment of ventilation by the pneumoperitoneum and the initial steep Trendelenburg position.

Following induction of anesthesia, a urinary catheter and nasogastric tube are placed. Bladder catheterization is undertaken to decompress the bladder and thus avoid trauma to intra-abdominal contents at the time of trocar insertion. Gastric decompression reduces the risk of visceral puncture, and may improve laparoscopic visualization and facilitate retraction of the right upper quadrants.[119] Data reported by Goodale and colleagues[84] suggest that the IAP increases with pneumoperitoneum lead to venous stasis. Measures to reduce stasis, such as pneumatic compressive stockings, may be indicated during these procedures. In general, local or regional anesthetic techniques have not been advocated for laparoscopic cholecystectomy or other upper abdominal laparoscopic procedures.

Anesthetic agents

Limited data are available concerning the impact of anesthetic management on postoperative outcome following laparoscopic cholecystectomy. Rose and colleagues[120] prospectively documented intraoperative critical observations and adverse outcomes in the recovery room for the first 101 patients undergoing laparoscopy at their institution. The authors compared the anesthetic management and outcome with patients undergoing open cholecystectomy. Intraoperative hypothermia (35 °C nasal/oral) and hypotension [systolic blood pressure < 10.67 kPa (80 mmHg)] were documented in 6.2% and 12.9% of patients undergoing laparoscopic cholecystectomy compared with 2.9% and 3.4%, respectively, for open cholecystectomy. Of those patients undergoing laparoscopic cholecystectomy, 31.4% had skin temperature recordings of 35 °C in the recovery room.

Most authors studying laparoscopic techniques have used balanced anesthetic techniques with oxygen, nitrous oxide, volatile anesthetic agents, relaxants, and opioids. Opioid or cholinergic agents have been reported to cause spasm of the sphincter of Oddi,[121] which can be antagonized by several drugs including naloxone,[122] glucagon,[123] and nalbuphine.[124] The advent of parenteral perioperative nonsteroidal anti-inflammatory drugs (NSAIDs) and the tendency for less postoperative pain associated with the laparoscopic approach may obviate perioperative narcotic administration.

Pain following laparoscopic surgery may result from tissue injury, nociceptor sensitization, and activation of central pathways. Michaloliakou and colleagues[125] used wound infiltration with local anesthesia and NSAIDs to attenuate peripheral pain and opioids for central pain modulation. This preoperative multimodal analgesic regime was associated with less postoperative pain, nausea, and vomiting and faster recovery/discharge.

Intraperitoneal (IP) administration of local anesthetics has been reported to reduce postoperative shoulder pain after minor gynecologic laparoscopic procedures. Experiences with IP local anesthetic administration after LC have ranged from significant reduction in postoperative pain during the first 48 h with 10 mL of 0.5% bupivacaine[126] to no effect in reducing postoperative pain, improving lung function or attenuating metabolic endocrine responses with 20 mL of 0.25% bupivacaine.[127] Joris and colleagues[128] investigated the time-course of parietal (abdominal wall), visceral, and shoulder pain following laparoscopic cholecystectomy. Visceral pain accounted for most of the discomfort after LC and was not attenuated by IP administration of 80 mL of 0.125% bupivacaine.

Postoperative nausea and vomiting are among the most common and distressing symptoms after laparoscopic surgery.[129] A highly potent and selective 5-hydroxytryptamine (5-HT_3) receptor antagonist, ondansetron, has proved to be an effective oral and intravenous (i.v.) prophylactic against postoperative emesis.[130]

Use of nitrous oxide

The use of nitrous oxide during laparoscopic surgery is controversial because of concerns regarding its ability to produce bowel distension during surgery and to increase postoperative nausea. The effects of nitrous oxide on bowel distension during surgery and bowel function after surgery was studied in 150 patients undergoing elective colonic surgery.[131] There was no difference between the air–oxygen group and the nitrous oxide–oxygen group in duration of anesthesia, distension of the bowel, and postoperative bowel function. The safety and efficacy of nitrous oxide specifically during laparoscopic cholecystectomy were investigated by Taylor *et al.*[132] There were no significant differences between the groups receiving air and nitrous oxide with respect to operating conditions or bowel distension. More importantly, there were no time-related changes in either variable during the course of surgery. Finally, the incidence of postoperative nausea and vomiting was similar in both treatment groups. However, a meta-analysis performed by Divatia and colleagues[133] noted that the omission of nitrous oxide reduced the risk of postoperative nausea and vomiting by 28%. In the subgroup analysis, the maximum effect of nitrous oxide omission was seen in female patients.

In summary, there is no conclusive evidence demonstrating a clinically significant effect of nitrous oxide on surgical conditions during laparoscopic cholecystectomy or on the incidence of postoperative emesis. With the caveats previously described, nitrous oxide therefore may still be a useful adjuvant during general anesthesia for this procedure.

Monitoring

Standard monitoring techniques are required for all patients undergoing laparoscopic surgery. $P_{ET}CO_2$ is most commonly used as a noninvasive substitute for P_aCO_2 in the evaluation of the adequacy of ventilation during laparoscopic cholecystectomy. Wahba and Mamazza[134] studied 28 otherwise healthy patients undergoing elective laparoscopic cholecystectomy to determine the increase in minute ventilation required to maintain the preinsufflation arterial CO_2 tension and whether $P_{ET}CO_2$ could safely be used as an index of P_aCO_2 and, therefore, the adequacy of ventilation during pneumoperitoneum. Increasing minute ventilation by 12–16% maintained the P_aCO_2 close to the preinsufflation levels. $P_{ET}CO_2$ was not a satisfactory noninvasive index of P_aCO_2 if it exceeded 5.47 kPa (41 mmHg) and if large volumes of CO_2 were insufflated. Otherwise, $P_{ET}CO_2$ proved to be a reasonable approximation of P_aCO_2 in these patients free from cardiopulmonary disease. In contrast, patients with preoperative cardiopulmonary disease demonstrated significant increases in P_aCO_2 not reflected by similar increases in $P_{ET}CO_2$ during insufflation.[135]

P_aCO_2 may be underestimated by $P_{ET}CO_2$ if there is a reduction in CO or an increase in $\dot{V}/\dot{Q}$ mismatch, and occasionally $P_{ET}CO_2$ may overestimate P_aCO_2.[135] In patients with significant cardiopulmonary disease, it would seem prudent to monitor P_aCO_2 levels at times during the procedure to avoid problems with hypercarbia and acidosis. Preoperative pulmonary function tests with low forced expiratory and vital capacity volumes and high ASA grouping can predict those patients at risk for developing hypercarbia and acidosis during laparoscopic cholecystectomy, but patient age and duration of surgery do not seem to be influencing factors.[136]

Invasive hemodynamic monitoring may be required in ASA grade III/IV patients in order to monitor the cardiovascular response to insufflation and institute therapy. Because the CO is inversely proportional to the insufflation pressure in the abdomen, gradual insufflation should be monitored by the anesthesiologist and a limit of 1.07–1.6 kPa (8–12 mmHg) set as maximal inflationary pressure. Limiting the rT tilt may attenuate the reduction in CO during pneumoperitoneum.[137] Refractory persistent hypercarbia, acidosis, and/or a reduction in S_vO_2 may necessitate exsufflation of the pneumoperitoneum or lowering of the insufflation pressure.[137] Finally, a decision to convert to an open procedure may be an important option in those patients with significant hemodynamic compromise.

SUMMARY

Minimally invasive therapy aims to minimize the trauma of any interventional process but still achieve a satisfactory therapeutic result. The development of "critical pathways," rapid mobilization, and early feeding have contributed towards the goal of shorter hospital stay. This concept has been extended to include LC and laparoscopic hernia repair.[138] Reports have been published confirming the safety of same-day discharge for the majority of LC patients.[139] The minimal access nature of the surgical insult and the lack of opioid administration may minimize postoperative hypoxemia and sleep disturbance.[140] However, we would caution against overenthusiastic ambulatory LC on the rational, but unproved, assumption that early discharge will lead to occasional delays in diagnosis and management of postoperative complications. A New South Wales group in Australia recently reported a 1.37% incidence of intensive care unit (ICU) admissions following 725 general surgical procedures.[141] Surgical complications were associated with delayed diagnosis and longer ICU admissions.

Endoscopic-assisted intra-abdominal procedures recently introduced include appendectomy, herniorrhaphy, adhesiolysis, antireflux and acid-reducing procedures, and intestinal resections. Case reports of bile duct injuries following laparoscopic cholecystectomy and unusual modes of colorectal, renal, and gall bladder carcinoma recurrence after laparoscopic-assisted surgery confirm the need for rigorous prospective study of these new procedures.

Intraoperative complications of laparoscopic surgery are mostly the result of traumatic injuries sustained during blind trocar insertion and physiologic changes associated with patient positioning and creation of the pneumoperitoneum. General anesthesia and controlled ventilation constitute the accepted anesthetic technique to reduce the increase in

P_aCO_2. Investigators have recently documented the cardiorespiratory compromise associated with upper abdominal laparoscopic surgery, and particular emphasis is placed on careful perioperative monitoring of ASA grade III/IV patients during insufflation. Setting limits on the inflationary pressure is advised in these patients. Anesthesiologists must maintain a high index of suspicion for complications such as gas embolism, extraperitoneal insufflation and surgical emphysema, pneumothorax, and pneumomediastinum.

Postoperative nausea and vomiting are among the most common and distressing symptoms after laparoscopic surgery. A highly potent and selective 5-HT_3 receptor antagonist, ondansetron, has proved to be an effective oral and i.v. prophylactic against postoperative emesis in preliminary studies. Opioids remain an important component of the anesthesia technique, although the introduction of newer potent NSAIDs may diminish their use. A preoperative multimodal analgesic regimen involving skin infiltration with local anesthesia, NSAIDs to attenuate peripheral pain, and opioids for central pain may reduce postoperative discomfort and expedite patient recovery/discharge. There is no conclusive evidence to demonstrate clinically significant adverse effects of nitrous oxide on surgical conditions during laparoscopic cholecystectomy or on the incidence of postoperative emesis. Laparoscopic cholecystectomy has proved to be a major advance in the treatment of patients with symptomatic gall bladder disease.

REFERENCES

1. Soper NJ, Brunt LM, Kerbl K. Laparoscopic general surgery (review article). *N Engl J Med* 1994; **330:** 409.
2. Perissat J, Collet D, Belliard R. Gallstones: laparoscopic treatment – cholecystectomy, cholecystotomy and lithotripsy – our own technique. *Surg Endosc* 1990; **4:** 1.
3. Reddick EJ, Olsen DO. Laparoscopy laser cholecystectomy, a comparison with mini lap cholecystectomy. *Surg Laparosc Endosc* 1990; **1:** 2.
4. Soper NJ, Barteau JA, Clayman RV, *et al.* Comparison of early postoperative results for laparoscopic versus standard open cholecystectomy. *Surg Gynecol Obstet* 1992; **174:** 114.
5. Wickham JEA. Minimally invasive surgery: future developments. *Br Med J* 1994; **308:** 193.
6. Working Group of Department of Health and the Scottish Department of Home Health. *Minimal Access Surgery: Implications for the NHS.* Edinburgh: HM Stationary Office, 1994.
7. Lawrence K. Minimal access surgery: harnessing the revolution. *Lancet* 1994; **1:** 308.
8. NIH Consensus Conference. Gallstones and laparoscopic cholecystectomy. *JAMA* 1993; **269:** 1018.
9. State of New York Department of Health. *Memorandum: Health Facilities Series H-18.* New York: State of New York Department of Health, 1992.
10. Society of American Gastrointestinal Endoscopic Surgeons (SAGES). Granting of privileges for laparoscopic general surgery. *Am J Surg* 1991; **161:** 324.
11. White JV. Registry of laparoscopic cholecystectomy and new and evolving laparoscopic techniques. *Am J Surg* 1993; **165:** 536.
12. Hunter JG. Advanced laparoscopic surgery. *Am J Surg* 1997; **173:** 14–18.
13. Satava RM. 3-D vision technology applied to advanced minimally invasive surgery systems. *Surg Endosc* 1993; **7:** 429.
14. Safran D, Sgambati S, Orlando III R. Laparoscopy in high risk cardiac patients. *Surg Gynecol Obstet* 1993; **176:** 548.
15. Smith RS, Fry WR, Tsoi EK, *et al.* Gasless laparoscopy and conventional instruments. *Arch Surg* 1993; **128:** 1102.
16. Grace PA, Quereshi A, Coleman J, *et al.* Reduced postoperative hospitalization after laparoscopic cholecystectomy. *Br J Surg* 1991; **78:** 160.
17. Southern Surgeons Club. A prospective analysis of 1518 laparoscopic cholecystectomies. *N Engl J Med* 1991; **324:** 1073.
18. Cuschieri A, Dubois F, Mouiel J, *et al.* The European experience with laparoscopic cholecystectomy. *Am J Surg* 1991; **161:** 385.
19. Litwin DEM, Girotti MJ, Poulin EC, *et al.* Laparoscopic cholecystectomy: trans-Canada experience with 2201 cases. *Can J Surg* 1992; **35:** 291.
20. Stoker ME, Vose JO, Meara P, Maini BJ. Laparoscopic cholecystectomy: a clinical and financial analysis of 280 operations. *Arch Surg* 1992; **127:** 589.
21. Lujan JA, Parrilla P, Robles R, *et al.* Laparoscopic cholecystectomy vs open cholecystectomy in the treatment of acute cholecystitis: a prospective study. *Arch Surg* 1998; **133:** 173–5.
22. Eldar S, Sabo E, Nash E, *et al.* Laparoscopic cholecystectomy for acute cholecystitis; prospective trial. *World J Surg* 1997; **21:** 540–5.
23. McKellar DP, Andersson CT, Bynton CJ. Cholecystectomy during pregnancy without fetal loss. *Surg Gynecol Obstet* 1992; **174:** 292–4.
24. Pucci RO, Seed RW. Case report of laparoscopic cholecystectomy in the third trimester of pregnancy. *Am J Obstet Gynecol* 1991; **165:** 401–2.
25. Amos JD, Schorr SJ, Norman PF, *et al.* Laparoscopic surgery during pregnancy. *Am J Surg* 1996; **171:** 435–7.
26. Curet MJ, Allen D, Josloff RK, *et al.* Laparoscopy during pregnancy. *Arch Surg* 1996; **131:** 546–551.
27. Halpern NB. Laparoscopic cholecystectomy in pregnancy: a review of published experiences and clinical considerations. *Semin Laparosc Surg* 1998; **5:** 129–34.
28. Lee VS, Chari RS, Cucchiaro G, Meyers WC. Complications of laparoscopic cholecystectomy. *Am J Surg* 1993; **165:** 527.
29. Deziel DJ, Millikan KW, Economou SG, *et al.* Complications of laparoscopic cholecystectomy: a national survey of 4,292 hospitals and an analysis of 77,604 cases. *Am J Surg* 1993; **165:** 9.
30. Ricardo AE, Feig BW, Ellis LM, *et al.* Gallbladder cancer and trocar site recurrences. *Am J Surg* 1997; **174:** 619–23.
31. Fletcher DR. Biliary injury at laparoscopic cholecystectomy: recognition and prevention. *Aust NZ J Surg* 1993; **63:** 673.
32. Roy AF, Passi RB, Lapointe RW, *et al.* Bile duct injury during laparoscopic cholecystectomy. *Can J Surg* 1993; **36:** 509.
33. Mellinger JD, Ponsky JL. Recent publications in laparoscopic surgery: an overview. *Endoscopy* 1996; **28:** 441–51.
34. Raiser F, Hinder RA, McBride PJ. The technique of laparoscopic Nissen fundoplication. *Chest Surg Clin North Am* 1995; **5:** 437–8.
35. Lawrence K, McWinnie D, Goodwin A. Randomized controlled trial of laparoscopic versus open repair of inguinal hernia. *Br Med J* 1995; **311:** 981–5.
36. Yee LF, Carvajal SH, de Lorimer AA. Laparoscopic splenectomy : the initial experience at the University of California. *Arch Surg* 1995; **130:** 874–7.
37. Goletti O, Buccianti P. Laparoscopic adrenalectomy. *J Laparoendosc Surg* 1995; **5:** 221–6.
38. Rao PM, Rhea TJ, Novelline RA, *et al.* Effect of computed tomography of the appendix on treatment of patients and use of hospital resources. *N Engl J Med* 1998; **338:** 141–6.
39. Martin LC, Puente I, Sosa JL. Open versus laparoscopic appendectomy: a prospective randomized comparison. *Ann Surg* 1995; **222:** 256–61.
40. Jacquet P, Averbach AM, Stephens AD, Sugerbaker PH. Cancer recurrence following laparoscopic colectomy. *Dis Colon Rectum* 1995; **38:** 1110–14.
41. Laparoscopic surgery for cure of colorectal cancer. *Surg Endosc* 1997; **11:** 797–9.
42. Le Moine MC, Navarro F, Burgel JS, *et al.* Experimental assessment of the risk of tumour recurrence after laparoscopic surgery. *Surgery* 1998; **123:** 427–31.
43. Nord HJ. Complications of laparoscopy. *Endoscopy* 1992; **24:** 693.
44. Strasberg SM, Sanabria JR, Clavien PA. Complications of laparoscopic cholecystectomy. *Can J Surg* 1992; **35:** 275.
45. Ponsky JL. Complications of laparoscopic cholecystectomy. *Am J Surg* 1991; **161:** 393.
46. Hurd WW, Pearl ML, DeLancey JO, *et al.* Laparoscopic injury of abdominal wall blood vessels: a report of three cases. *Obstet Gynecol* 1993; **82:** 673.
47. Hasson H. A modified instrument and method for laparoscopy. *Am J Obstet Gynecol* 1971; **70:** 886.
48. Gees J, Holden C. Major vascular injury as a complication of laparoscopic surgery: a review of three cases and review of the literature. *Am Surg* 1996; **62:** 377–9.
49. Noga J, Fredman B, Olsfanger D, Jedeikin R. Role of the anaesthetist in the early diagnosis of life-threatening complications during laparoscopic surgery. *Surg Laparosc Endosc* 1997; **7:** 63–5.
50. Miller AH. Surgical posture with symbols for its record on the anaesthetist's chart. *Anesthesiology* 1940; **1:** 241.
51. Schiller WR. The Trendelenburg position: surgical aspects. In: Martin JT (ed.). *Positioning in Anaesthesia and Surgery*, 2nd edn. Philadelphia, PA: W.B. Saunders, 1987: 117.
52. Don HF. The measurement of trapped gas in the lungs at functional residual capacity and the effects of posture. *Anesthesiology* 1971; **35:** 582.
53. Sonkodi S, Agabiti-Rosei E, Fraser R. Response of the renin–angiotensin–aldosterone system to upright tilting and to intravenous furosemide:

effect of prior metoprolol and propranolol. *Br J Clin Pharmacol* 1982; **13:** 341.
54. Williams GH, Cain JP, Dluly RG. Studies on the control of plasma aldosterone concentration in normal man: response to posture, acute and chronic volume depletion and sodium loading. *J Clin Invest* 1972; **51:** 1731.
55. Ward RJ, Danziger F, Bonica JJ. Cardiovascular effects of change of posture. *Aerospace Med* 1966; **37:** 257.
56. Kubal K, Komatsu T, Sanchala V. Trendelenburg position used during venous cannulation increases myocardial oxygen demands. *Anesth Analg* 1984; **63:** 239.
57. Pricolo VE, Burchard KW, Singh AK. Trendelenburg versus PASG application: Hemodynamic response in man. *J Trauma* 1986; **26:** 718.
58. Wilcox S, Vandam LD. Alas, poor Trendelenburg and his position! A critique of its uses and effectiveness. *Anesth Analg* 1988; **67:** 574.
59. Burton A, Steinbrook RA. Precipitous decrease in oxygen saturation during laparoscopic surgery. *Anesth Analg* 1993; **76:** 1177.
60. Brimacombe JR, Orland H. Endobronchial intubation during upper abdominal laparoscopic surgery in the reverse Trendelenburg position. *Anesth Analg* 1994; **78:** 607.
61. Gagnon J, Poulin EC. Beware of the Trendelenburg position during prolonged laparoscopic procedures. *Can J Surg* 1993; **36:** 505.
62. Kabukoba JJ, Skillern LH. Coping with extraperitoneal insufflation during laparoscopy: a new technique. *Obstet Gynecol* 1992; **80:** 144.
63. Lew JKL, Gin T, Oh TE. Anaesthetic problems during laparoscopic cholecystectomy. *Anaesth Intensive Care* 1992; **20:** 91.
64. Kendall AP, Bhatt S, Oh TE. Pulmonary consequences of carbon dioxide insufflation for laparoscopic cholecystectomies. *Anaesthesia* 1995; **50:** 286.
65. Prystowsky JB, Jerico BJ, Epstein HB. Spontaneous bilateral pneumothorax: complication of laparoscopic cholecystectomy. *Surgery* 1993; **114:** 988.
66. Seow LT, Khoo ST. Unilateral pneumothorax: an unexpected complication of laparoscopic cholecystectomy. *Can J Anaesth* 1993; **40:** 1000.
67. Hasel R, Arora SK, Hickey DR. Intraoperative complications of laparoscopic cholecystectomy. *Can J Anaesth* 1993; **40:** 459.
68. Cunningham AJ, Turner J, Rosenbaum S, Rafferty T. Transoesophageal echocardiographic assessment of haemodynamic function during laparoscopic cholecystectomy. *Br J Anaesth* 1993; **70:** 621.
69. Ishizaki Y, Bandai Y, Shimomura K, Abe H. Safe intraabdominal pressure of CO_2 pneumoperitoneum during laparoscopic surgery. *Surgery* 1993; **114:**549.
70. Rasmussen JP, Dauchot PJ, De Palma RG. Cardiac function and hypercarbia. *Arch Surg* 1978; **113:** 1196.
71. Ho HS, Saunders CJ, Corso FA, Wolfe BM. The effects of CO_2 pneumoperitoneum on haemodynamics in haemorrhaged animals. *Surgery* 1993; **114:** 381.
72. Alexander GD, Noe FE, Brown EM. Anaesthesia for pelvic laparoscopy. *Anesth Analg* 1969; **48:** 14.
73. Calverly RK, Jenkins LC. The anaesthetic management of pelvic laparoscopy. *Can Anaesth Soc J* 1973; **20:** 679.
74. Fried GM, Clas D, Meakins JL. Minimally invasive surgery in the elderly patient. *Surg Clin North Am* 1994; **74:** 375.
75. Carroll BJ, Chandra M, Phillips EH, Margulies DR. Laparoscopic cholecystectomy in critically ill cardiac patients. *Am Surg* 1993; **59:** 783.
76. Wahba RWM, Beique F, Kleiman SJ. Cardiopulmonary function and laparoscopic cholecystectomy. *Can J Anaesth*1995; **42:** 51.
77. Joris JL, Noirot DP, Legrand MJ, *et al.* Hemodynamic changes during laparoscopic cholecystectomy. *Anesth Analg* 1993; **76:** 1067.
78. Westerband A, Van De Water JM, Amzallag M. Cardiovascular changes during laparoscopic cholecystectomy. *Surg Gynecol Obstet* 1992; **175:** 535.
79. Reid CW, Martineau RJ, Hull KA, Miller DR. Haemodynamic consequences of abdominal insufflation with CO_2 laparoscopic cholecystectomy. *Can J Anaesth* 1992; **39:** A132.
80. Morris JJ, Perkins SR, Hein HAT, *et al.* Physiologic alterations during laparoscopic cholecystectomy in cardiac transplant patients. *Anesth Analg* 1995; **80:** S329.
81. Liu SY, Leighton T, Davis I. Prospective analysis of cardiopulmonary responses to laparoscopic cholecystectomy. *J Laparoendosc Surg* 1991; **1:** 241.
82. Iwase K, Takenaka H, Yagura A, *et al.* Hemodynamic changes during laparoscopic cholecystectomy in patients with heart disease. *Endoscopy* 1992; **24:** 771.
83. Fox LG, Hein Hat, Gawey BJ, *et al.* Physiological changes during laparoscopic cholecystectomy in ASA III & IV patients. *Anesthesiology* 1993; **79:** A55.
84. Goodale RL, Beebe DS, McNevin MP, *et al.* Hemodynamic, respiratory and metabolic effects of laparoscopic cholecystectomy. *Am J Surg* 1993; **166:** 533.
85. Smith I, Benzie RJ, Gordon NLM, *et al.* Cardiovascular effects of peritoneal insufflation of carbon dioxide for laparoscopy. *Br Med J* 1971; **3:** 410.
86. Joris J, Honore P, Lamy M. Changes in oxygen transport and ventilation during laparoscopic cholecystectomy. *Anesthesiology* 1992; **77:** A149.
87. Feig BW, Berger DH, Dougherty TB, *et al.* Pharmacological intervention can reestablish baseline hemodynamic parameters during laparoscopy. *Surgery* 1994; **116:** 733.
88. Rasmussen JP, Dauchot PJ, DePalma RG, *et al.* Cardiac function and hypercarbia. *Arch Surg* 1978; **113:** 1196.
89. Shifren JL, Adelstein L, Finkler NJ. Asystolic cardiac arrest: a rare complication of laparoscopy. *Obstet Gynecol* 1992; **79:** 840.
90. Beck DH, McQuillan PJ. Fatal carbon dioxide embolism and severe haemorrhage during laparoscopic salpingectomy. *Br J Anaesth* 1994; **72:** 243.
91. Clarke CC, Weeks DB, Gusdon JP. Venous carbon dioxide embolism during laparoscopy. *Anesth Analg* 1977; **56:** 650.
92. Root B, Levy MN, Pollack S, *et al.* Gas embolism death after laparoscopy delayed by trapping in the portal circulation. *Anesth Analg* 1978; **57:** 232.
93. Baraka A. Cardiovascular collapse after carbon dioxide exsufflation in a patient undergoing laparoscopic cholecystectomy. *Anesth Analg* 1994; **78:** 603.
94. Derouin M, Couture P, Boudreault D, *et al.* Detection of gas embolism by transoesophageal echocardiography during laparoscopic cholecystectomy. *Anesth Analg* 1996; **82:** 119–24.
95. Schindler E, Muller M, Kelm C. Cerebral carbon dioxide embolism during laparoscopic cholecystectomy. *Anesth Analg* 1995; **81:** 643–5.
96. Junghans T, Bohm B, Grundel K, *et al.* Does pneumoperitoneum with different gases, body positions, and intraperitoneal pressures influence renal and hepatic blood flow. *Surgery* 1997; **121:** 206–11.
97. Morino M, Giraudo G, Festa V. Alterations in hepatic function during laparoscopic surgery. *Surg Endosc* 1998; **12:** 968–972.
98. Aoki T, Tanii M, Takahashi K, *et al.* Cardiovascular changes and plasma catecholamine levels during laparoscopic surgery. *Anesth Analg* 1994; **78:** S8.
99. Felber AR, Blobner M, Goegler S. Plasma vasopressin in laparoscopic cholecystectomy. *Anesthesiology* 1993; **79:** A32.
100. Joris J, Lamy M. Neuroendocrine changes during pneumoperitoneum for laparoscopic cholecystectomy. *Br J Anaesth* 1993; **70:** A33.
101. Mealy K, Gallagher H, Barry M, *et al.* Physiological and metabolic responses to open and laparoscopic cholecystectomy. *Br J Surg* 1992; **79:** 1061.
102. Wolf Jr JS, Carrier S, Stoller S. Gas embolism: helium is more lethal than carbon dioxide. *J Laparendosc Surg* 1994; **4:**173.
103. Piiper J. Physiological equilibria of gas cavities in the body. In: Fenn WO, Rahn M (eds): *Handbook of Physiology. 3. Respiration*. Washington, DC: American Physiology Society, 1965: 1205.
104. Mullet CE, Viale JP, Sagard PE. Pulmonary CO_2 elimination during surgical procedures using intra- or extraperitoneal CO_2 insufflation. *Anesth Analg* 1993; **76:** 622.
105. Wittgen CM, Andrus CH, Fitzgerald SD. Analysis of the hemodynamic and ventilatory effects of laparoscopic cholecystectomy. *Arch Surg* 1991; **126:** 997.
106. Hall D, Goldstein A, Tynan E, Braunstein L. Profound hypercarbia late in the course of laparoscopic cholecystectomy: detection by continuous capnometry. *Anesthesiology* 1993; **79:** 173.
107. Wahba RWM. Perioperative functional residual capacity. *Can J Anaesth* 1991; **38:** 384.
108. Fahy B, Barnas G, Flowers J, *et al.* The effects of increased abdominal pressure on lung and chest wall mechanics during laparoscopic surgery. *Anesth Analg* 1995; **81:** 744–50.
109. Puri GD, Singh H. Ventilatory effects of laparoscopy under general anaesthesia. *Br J Anaesth* 1992; **68:** 211.
110. Brown DR, Fishburne JI, Roberson VO. Ventilatory and blood gas changes during laparoscopy with local anaesthesia. *Am J Obstet Gynecol* 1976; **124:** 741.
111. Cunningham AJ, Schlanger M. Intraoperative hypoxemia complicating laparoscopic cholecystectomy in a patient with sickle hemoglobinopathy. *Anesth Analg* 1992; **75:** 838.
112. Duffy BL. Regurgitation during pelvic laparoscopy. *Br J Anaesth* 1979; **51:** 1089.
113. Schauer PR, Luna J, Ghiatas AA, *et al.* Pulmonary function after laparoscopic cholecystectomy. *Surgery* 1993; **114:** 389.

114. Joris J, Kaba A, Lamy M. Postoperative spirometry after laparoscopy for lower abdominal or upper abdominal surgical procedures. *Br J Anaesth* 1997; **79:** 422–6.
115. McKeague H, Cunningham AJ. Postoperative respiratory dysfunction: is the site of surgery crucial? *Br J Anaesth* 1997; **79:** 415–16.
116. Erice F, Fox GS, Salib YM, *et al.* Diaphragmatic function before and after laparoscopic cholecystectomy. *Anesthesiology* 1993; **79:** 966.
117. Cunningham AJ, Brull SJ. Laparoscopic cholecystectomy: anaesthetic implications. *Anesth Analg* 1993; **76:** 1120.
118. Chui PT, Oh TE. Anaesthesia for laparoscopic general surgery. *Anaesth Intensive Care* 1993; **21:** 163.
119. Marco AP, YEO CJ, Rock P. Anaesthesia for a patient undergoing laparoscopic cholecystectomy. *Anesthesiology* 1990; **73:** 1268.
120. Rose DK, Cohen MM, Soutter DI. Laparoscopic cholecystectomy: the anaesthetist's point of view. *Can J Anaesth* 1992; **39:** 809.
121. Chesick KC, Black S, Hoye SJ. Spasm and operative cholangiography. *Arch Surg* 1975; **110:** 53.
122. McCammon RL, Viegas OJ, Stoelting RK. Naloxone reversal of choledochoduodenal sphincter spasm associated with narcotic administration. *Anesthesiology* 1978; **48:** 437.
123. Jones RM, Detmer M, Hill AB. Incidence of choledochoduodenal sphincter spasm during fentanyl-supplemented anaesthesia. *Anesth Analg* 1981; **60:** 638.
124. Humphrey HK, Fleming NW. Opioid induced spasm of the sphincter of Oddi apparently reversed by nalbuphine. *Anesth Analg* 1992; **74:** 308.
125. Michaloliakou C, Chung F, Sharma S. Preoperative multimodal analgesia facilitates recovery after ambulatory laparoscopic cholecystectomy. *Anesth Analg* 1996; **82:** 44–51.
126. Weber A, Munoz J, Garteiz D, *et al.* Use of subdiaphragmatic bupivacaine instillation to control postoperative pain after laparoscopic surgery. *Surg Laparosc Endosc* 1997; **7:** 6–8.
127. Rademaker BMP, Kalkman CJ, Odoom J, *et al.* Intraperitoneal local anaesthetics after laparoscopic cholecystectomy: effects on postoperative pain, metabolic responses and lung function. *Br J Anaesth* 1994; **72:** 263–6.
128. Joris J, Thiry E, Paris P, *et al.* Pain after laparoscopic cholecystectomy: characteristics and effect of intraperitoneal bupivacaine. *Anesth Analg* 1995; **81:** 379–84.
129. Malins AF, Field JM, Nesling PM, Cooper GM. Nausea and vomiting after gynaecological laparoscopy: comparison of premedication with oral ondansetron, metoclopramide and placebo. *Br J Anaesth* 1994; **72:** 231.
130. Raphael JH, Norton AC. Antiemetic efficacy of prophylactic ondansetron in laparoscopic surgery: randomised, double-blind comparison with metoclopramide. *Br J Anaesth* 1993; **71:** 845.
131. Krogh B, Jensen PJ, Henneberg SW, *et al.* Nitrous oxide does not influence operating conditions or postoperative course in colonic surgery. *Br J Anaesth* 1994; **72:** 55.
132. Taylor E, Feinstein R, White PF, Sopor N. Anaesthesia for laparoscopic cholecystectomy: is nitrous oxide contraindicated? *Anesthesiology* 1992; **76:** 541.
133. Divatia JV, Vaidya JS, Badwe RA, Hawaldar RW. Omission of nitrous oxide during anaesthesia reduces the incidence of postoperative nausea and vomiting. A meta-analysis. *Anesthesiology* 1996; **85:** 1055–62.
134. Wahba RWM, Mamazza J. Ventilatory requirements during laparoscopic cholecystectomy. *Can J Anaesth* 1993; **40:** 206.
135. Bhavani-Shanker K, Moseley H, Kumar AY, Delph Y. Capnometry and anaesthesia. *Can J Anaesth* 1991; **39:** 617.
136. Wittgen CM, Naunhein KS, Andrus CH, Kaminski DL. Preoperative pulmonary evaluation for laparoscopic cholecystectomy. *Arch Surg* 1993; **128:** 880.
137. Dhoste K, Karayan J, Lacoste L, *et al.* Haemodynamic changes during laparoscopic cholecystectomy in the elderly. *Br J Anaesth* 1993; **72:** A32.
138. Stevenson ARL. Ambulatory laparoscopic surgery: the patient's perspective in an inpatient world. *Aust NZ J Surg* 1998; **68:** 753–4.
139. Cuschieri A. Day-case (ambulatory) laparoscopic surgery. Let us sing from the same hymn sheet *Surg Endosc* 1997; **11:** 1142–4.
140. Rosenberg-Adamsen S, Skarbye M, Wildschiodtz G, *et al.* Sleep after laparoscopic cholecystectomy. *Br J Anaesth* 1996; **77:** 572–5.
141. Hayes C, Ambazidis S, Gani JS. Intensive care unit admissions following laparoscopic surgery: what lessons can be learned? *Aust NZ J Surg* 1996; **66:** 206–9.

55

Anesthesia for gynecologic, urologic, and laparoscopic procedures

TIMOTHY BLACK AND MIRJANA LOVRINCEVIC

INTRODUCTION

The anesthetic care of the gynecology and urology patient has come a long way. With the technologic revolution, even complicated procedures have become routine. Laparoscopy, laser surgery, and *in vitro* fertilization are commonplace. However, although, for the surgeon, the gynecologic operation is an ordinary event of usually simple dimension, for each patient a procedure is a unique experience.

The anesthesiologist must recognize and appreciate a strong emotional component when administering anesthesia to a patient undergoing urogenital surgery, because that influences the perioperative anesthetic plan. The patient must also be evaluated for coexisting medical problems, previous anesthetic complications, potential airway difficulties, and considerations relating to intraoperative positioning. This evaluation, coupled with the appreciation of the surgeon's needs, is used to formulate the anesthetic plan.

ANESTHESIA FOR GYNECOLOGIC SURGERY

Preoperative considerations

General considerations

Preoperative anxiety is essentially universal. It is usually the result of fear of the unknown or of what the patient imagines he or she will be forced to endure during the surgery and after. In the gynecologic patient, however, these issues are compounded by the nature of the organs involved. Patients often bear strong feelings of anger, guilt, embarrassment, or inadequacy. It is very important for the anesthesiologist to appreciate this issue, as the perioperative course might be significantly influenced. It has been shown that increased baseline anxiety is associated with autonomic dysfunction, cardiac arrhythmias, hypertension, decreased gastric motility, and increased intraoperative anesthetic requirements.[1] Preoperative visits are clearly helpful in alleviating anxiety and should be carried out whenever possible.[2,3] In addition to psychologic preparation, patients also benefit from premedication. Traditionally, goals for premedication are relief of apprehension, sedation, analgesia, amnesia, reduction of gastric fluid volume and acidity, prevention of nausea and vomiting, prevention of autonomic reflex responses, decreased minimum alveolar concentration (MAC), etc.[4,5] Premedication should fit the requirements of the individual patient in the same way as do anesthetic techniques.

Laboratory studies

It is essential that the laboratory investigation of a patient be limited to those diagnostic procedures that are appropriate to the findings elicited during the history and physical examination.[6] The decision to order electrolyte and creatinine analyses, coagulation studies, chemistry panels, an ECG, and chest radiographic films should be based on the evaluation of the patient.[7,8] Medical illnesses such as diabetes, hypertension, asthma, and hypothyroidism need to be optimally controlled before surgery. Specialty consultation is generally necessary for patients with pulmonary or cardiac disease[9,10] to be sure that the best preoperative condition is achieved and that the operative risk is acceptable.

Blood transfusion

A blood sample should be sent to the blood bank well in advance of the planned operative procedure so that the blood bank will have time to overcome any difficulty encountered in performing the intended crossmatch. For procedures in which blood loss is not anticipated, a type and screen is sufficient. Autologous blood use should be encouraged if the patient is in good general health.[11]

Prophylactic antibiotics

Prophylactic antibiotics are recommended for vaginal hysterectomy, and possibly are helpful for abdominal hysterectomy. They are not considered necessary for adnexal surgery when there is no evidence of previous pelvic infection. The drug of choice is generally cefazolin, 1 g before surgery. Patients with valvular heart disease, a history of endocarditis, a vascular graft, or implanted devices may require special antibiotic coverage.[12]

Positioning the patient

The lithotomy position is used frequently in gynecologic surgery.[13] The patient lies supine with each lower extremity flexed at the hip and knee, and both limbs are simultaneously elevated and separated so that the perineum becomes accessible to the surgeon. Hemodynamic changes can sometimes occur on elevation of legs into the stirrups, as this increases venous return to the heart. Similarly, problems with hypotension on lowering legs postoperatively are common. When the legs are to be lowered to the original supine position at the end of the procedure, they should first be brought together at the knees and ankles in the sagittal plane, and then lowered slowly together to the tabletop. This minimizes torsion stress on the lumbar spine that would occur if each leg were lowered independently. It also permits gradual accommodation to the increase in the circulatory capacitance, thereby avoiding sudden hypotension. If pressure on the nerve over fibula is not prevented by adequate padding or positioning, common peroneal nerve injury is possible.[14] It is manifested as an inability to dorsiflex the foot and loss of sensation over the dorsum of the foot. Hyperflexion of hip joint can cause femoral and lateral femoral cutaneous nerve palsy. Obturator and saphenous nerve injury are also complications of the lithotomy position.[15,16]

Frequently, some degree of head-down tilt is added to a lithotomy position.[17] Depending on the degree of head depression, the addition of tilt to the lithotomy position combines the worst features of both the lithotomy and the Trendelenburg postures. The weight of abdominal viscera on the diaphragm adds to whatever abdominal compression is produced by the flexed thighs of an obese patient or of one placed in an exaggerated lithotomy position. Consequently, the work of spontaneous ventilation is increased for an anesthetized patient. The ventilation–perfusion ratio deteriorates as a result of gravitational accumulation of blood in the poorly ventilated lung apices. During controlled ventilation, increased inspiratory pressures are needed to expand the lung.

Implications related to gynecologic malignancies

The type and extent of malignancy play a major role in determining the extent of preoperative preparation and intraoperative monitoring that the patient will require. The treatment history must be thoroughly evaluated. Most likely, these patients have had radiation therapy and chemotherapy and, perhaps, numerous surgical procedures. All of these factors impinge on the underlying physiologic status of the patient.

Bleeding and fluid shifts should be anticipated for any patient undergoing a definitive operation for cancer, whether it is for potential cure, debulking, or palliation. In that respect, the need for blood and blood products should be anticipated.

Chemotherapeutic agents used most commonly for the treatment of patients with gynecologic malignancies include *cis*-platinum, bleomycin, doxorubicin, and methotrexate.[18–20] *Cis*-platinum is used for the treatment of ovarian carcinoma. The primary dose-limiting toxicities are myelosuppression and renal toxicity. Preoperative evaluation as well as intraoperative management of these patients should focus on fluid and electrolyte balance as well as optimizing renal perfusion. Anesthetic agents that may be nephrotoxic should be avoided.

Bleomycin, used to treat cervical cancer and germ cell tumors of the ovary, is known to produce acute interstitial pneumonia and chronic fibrotic changes in the lung. In addition, it appears that bleomycin sensitizes lung to the toxic effect of oxygen and OH radicals, especially if F_IO_2 is kept >0.3. Baseline pulmonary function tests and arterial blood gas analysis are helpful in defining the patient's pulmonary status after bleomycin therapy. F_IO_2 needs to be maintained at the lowest level compatible with adequate oxygenation. Doxorubicin has been useful in treatment of endometrial and ovarian carcinomas. Its major side-effect is a dose-related cardiomyopathy, which might exist in an acute and chronic form. An acute form is characterized by relatively benign ECG changes that include ST–T changes and decreased voltage. The chronic form is characterized by progressive cardiac failure unresponsive to inotropic drugs that may be observed on serial echocardiogram (ECHO) studies.

Methotrexate is used in the treatment of ovarian cancer. The major toxic complications associated with this agent are gastrointestinal toxicity, impaired liver function manifested by elevated transaminases, and renal tubular injury characterized by a rising blood urea nitrogen (BUN) and serum creatinine with a decreasing urinary volume.

Preoperative laboratory studies should be individualized for each patient. Consultation with an oncologist might be needed in some cases.

ANATOMY AND INNERVATION

Nerves[21]

The pelvis is innervated by both the autonomic and somatic nervous systems. The autonomic nerves include both sympathetic (adrenergic) and parasympathetic (cholinergic) fibers and provide the primary innervation for genital, urinary, and gastrointestinal visceral structures and blood vessels.

Somatic innervation

The lumbosacral plexus and its branches provide motor and sensory somatic innervation to the lower abdominal wall, the pelvic and urogenital diaphragms, the perineum, and the hip and lower extremity. A visceral component, the pelvic splanchnic nerve, is also included (Table 55.1).

Autonomic innervation

Functionally, the innervation of the pelvic viscera may be divided into an afferent or sensory component and an efferent component: in reality, however, afferent and efferent fibers are closely associated in a complex network and cannot be separated anatomically.

Efferent innervation

The ovaries and part of the uterine tubes and broad ligament are innervated by the ovarian plexus.

The inferior hypogastric plexus is divided into three portions, representing distribution of innervation to the viscera: the vesical plexus, which innervates bladder and urethra; the hemorrhoidal plexus, which innervates rectum; and the uterovaginal plexus (Frankenhauser's ganglion), which provides innervation to uterus, vagina, clitoris, and vestibular bulbs.

Afferent innervation

Afferent fibers from the pelvic viscera and blood vessels traverse the same pathways to provide sensory input to the central nervous system. They are also involved in reflex arcs needed for bladder, bowel, and genital tract function. The afferent fibers reach the central nervous system to have their first synapse within posterior spinal nerve ganglia.

COMMON GYNECOLOGIC PROCEDURES[22,23]

From the anesthesiologist's point of view, gynecologic procedures can be divided into four major categories: transvaginal, perineal, intra-abdominal, and transabdominal (laparoscopic).[24] They are grouped according to the surgical site, position, and surgical technique and equipment used.

Transvaginal surgery

Dilation and curettage

This procedure is performed to diagnose and treat bleeding from uterine and cervical lesions, to complete an incomplete or missed spontaneous abortion, or to treat cervical stenosis. Either local, regional, or general anesthesia may be appropriate. If regional anesthesia is chosen, a T10

Table 55.1 *Somatic innervation of the abdomen and lower limb*

Nerve	Spinal segment	Innervation
Iliohypogastric	T12, L1	Sensory – skin near iliac crest, just above symphysis pubis
Ilioinguinal	L1	Sensory – upper medial thigh, mons pubis, labia majora
Lateral femoral cutaneous	L2, L3	Sensory – lateral thigh to level of knee
Femoral	L2, L3, L4	Sensory – anterior and medial thigh, medial leg and foot, hip, and knee joints Motor – iliacus, anterior thigh muscles
Genitofemoral	LI, L2	Sensory – anterior vulva (genital branch) middle/upper anterior thigh (femoral branch)
Obturator	L2, L3, L4	Sensory – medial thigh and leg, hip, and knee joints Motor – adductor muscles of thigh
Superior gluteal	L4, L5, S1	Motor – gluteal muscles
Inferior gluteal	L4, L5, S1, S2	Motor – gluteal muscles
Posterior femoral cutaneous	S2, S3	Sensor – vulva, perineum
Sciatic	L4, L5, S1, S2, S3	Sensory – much of leg, foot, lower extremity joints Motor – posterior thigh muscle, leg and foot muscles
Pudendal	S2, S3, S4	Sensory – perianal skin, vulva, and perineum, clitoris, urethra, vaginal vestibule Motor – external anal sphincter, perineal muscles, urogenital diaphragm

sensory level is appropriate for the provision of anesthesia for procedures in the uterus. Bupivacaine 0.75%, 10–15 mg in 7.5% dextrose, is used most commonly, while lidocaine, both 2% and 5%, has fallen our of favor in recent years as a result of numerous reports on transient neurologic symptoms that can occur in up to one-third of patients.[25–27] General anesthesia using O_2/N_2O plus a volatile anesthetic is frequently administered by face mask or laryngeal mask with the patient breathing spontaneously, provided that there are no contraindications such as a full stomach, obesity, severe anxiety, nausea, vomiting, or emergent surgery, in which case endotracheal intubation is required.

When bleeding may be expected, oxytocin is usually given i.v., not to exceed 20 U L^{-1}, and occasionally in cases of bleeding unresponsive to oxytocin. Ergonovine maleate is used i.m. or s.c. to promote uterine contraction and decrease the bleeding. An antibiotic such as doxycycline 100 mg i.v. is commonly used when infection is a likely result, as, for example, following an incomplete or missed abortion.

Laser therapy to vulva, vagina, and cervix

Laser therapy is indicated for preinvasive lesions of the vulva, vagina, or cervix. It destroys tissues by the selective application of light energy focused into a beam. The CO_2 laser has a sharply focused beam with a very narrow spot diameter and a high power density. This is perfect for cutting, and lateral tissue damage is minimized. The yttrium–aluminum–garnet (YAG) laser is able to penetrate tissue to a much greater depth than CO_2 laser energy. YAG energy scatters in tissue, so thermal damage is greater. Thus, this laser serves better as a coagulator of tissue and for debulking.

Most gynecologic laser procedures are done under local anesthesia and i.v. sedation, but general anesthesia and regional technique may also be used. If regional anesthesia is used, T10 sensory level is desirable.

Special attention should be given to protection against the eye injury, operating room fires, and aerosolization of viral particles during laser procedure. Goggles should be worn by the patient and all operating room personnel during laser use to prevent injury to eyes from the laser beam. If the patient is asleep, the eyes should be covered with saline-soaked gauze. It is always advisable to watch for improper handling of lasers as operating room fires can occur rapidly. Vaporization of condyloma may produce aerosolization of viral particles; thus, appropriate ventilation is suggested for smoke dispersal, and the use of a special laser surgical mask to trap virus-containing particles is recommended.

Perineal surgery

Radical vulvectomy

En bloc dissection of the inguinal–femoral region and the vulva is the current treatment for invasive vulval carcinoma. This surgery involves bilateral excision of lymphatic and areolar tissue in the inguinal and femoral regions, combined with removal of the entire vulva between the labia–crural folds, from the perineal body to the upper margin of mons pubis. If the large surgical wound is created, a skin graft may be necessary.

Patients with vulval carcinoma are typically elderly and have a high incidence of comorbidity. Careful preoperative assessment is needed in order to optimize the patient for the surgery. It is wise to have blood available for transfusion, as occasionally femoral vessels may be injured, requiring rapid blood replacement.

Both general and regional anesthesia can be used, alone or in combination. Although vulvectomy is not particularly painful for a prolonged period postoperatively, continuous epidural technique allows earlier ambulation with less sedation, especially for the elderly.

Operations for stress urinary incontinence

Stress incontinence is a symptom that describes involuntary loss of urine associated with sudden cough or strain. The incidence of genuine stress incontinence is less than 10% among women of childbearing age, but may approach 10–20% among postmenopausal patients.

There are currently two surgical approaches: suspension by the vaginal route and abdominal suspension procedures. The primary surgical treatment often involves a vaginal approach (Kelly urethral plication), especially when further vaginal surgery needs to be performed. Abdominal approaches (Marshall–Marchetti–Krantz, and Burch) are probably more successful in the long term.

Patients are usually past childbearing age, and need to be assessed for coexisting health problems. Both general and regional anesthesia can be used. A T10 sensory level is sufficient to provide anesthesia for procedures on the uterus and bladder, while a T4 level is recommended if the peritoneum is to be opened.

Care should be taken if the lithotomy position is being used to pad pressure points so as to prevent peroneal nerve injury (see Perioperative considerations).

Intra-abdominal operations

Hysterectomy

After cesarean section, hysterectomy is the most commonly performed operation in the USA. Common indications include dysfunctional uterine bleeding, adenomyosis, descent or prolapse of the uterus, uterine leiomyomas, and neoplastic diseases of the uterus or adjacent pelvic organs.

There are two surgical approaches: vaginal and abdominal. Often the approach is decided upon in the operating room, where a pelvic examination under anesthesia will determine the true uterine size and the presence of pelvic pathology.

General anesthesia is commonly used; however, regional anesthesia may be also appropriate for simple hysterectomies. A T4–6 sensory level is sufficient to provide anesthesia for procedures on the uterus.

Heavy blood loss may occur. Blood and evaporative losses are usually greater in patients undergoing abdominal, rather than vaginal, hysterectomy. For all these reasons it is wise to have blood products ready for transfusion. Autologous blood donation would be the best choice, but for many patients anemia may preclude this option.

Tubal ligation

In the USA, sterilization has become the most commonly used method of contraception among married couples. The procedure can be performed at any time but commonly follows cesarean section or vaginal delivery. The timing of tubal sterilization can influence the choice of anesthetic, the surgical approach, and the method of tubal occlusion.[28] Most tubal sterilizations performed after vaginal delivery are done by minilaparotomy; those not associated with birth are usually performed by laparoscopy or minilaparotomy.

Complications of general anesthesia are the leading cause of death attributed to sterilization in the USA. The risks inherent in general anesthesia are exacerbated by its use post partum and during laparoscopy. (A discussion about anesthetic considerations in the peripartum period is beyond the scope of this chapter.)

Sterilization by laparoscopy or minilaparotomy can be safely performed under local anesthesia and i.v. sedation. In this way, the patient avoids the risks associated with general anesthesia, spends less time sedated or anesthetized, and recovers more rapidly. Nausea and vomiting are less likely to occur, and the patient is awake to report symptoms that might indicate the occurrence of a complication.

ANESTHESIA FOR LAPAROSCOPIC SURGERY

Gynecologic surgery accounts for a large proportion of both in- and outpatient operating room procedures. Simple procedures such as dilation and curettage, evaluation under anesthesia, and hysteroscopy as well as more complicated procedures such as hysterectomy, laparoscopy, and major cancer surgery are also performed.

In recent years, the development of laparoscopy has resulted in far-reaching changes in surgical practice. Laparoscopic tubal surgery was first reported in 1962, but it was not until 1989 when reports of laparoscopic cholesystectomy appeared that the surgical subspecialties began to appreciate the value of laparoscopy and embrace its use.[29] Simultaneously, a major expansion in equipment technology and availability occurred. Today, laparoscopic evaluation and complicated surgical procedures are undertaken worldwide.

Operations that were once extremely painful, debilitating, and associated with large scars and prolonged recovery times now, as a result of laparoscopy, require only small incisions and brief hospital stays and are associated with shorter recovery times. These advantages lead to reduced healthcare costs, and patients return to useful employment and activity much sooner.

Today, as equipment and techniques improve, a greater number as well as more involved types of surgery are performed using laparoscopy. As a result of the frequency and complexity of much of this surgery, it is imperative that the anesthesiologist has a clear understanding of the procedure, the physiologic changes, and the potential complications.

Initiation of the operative procedure of laparoscopy

The first step is to establish a pneumoperitoneum. This is accomplished by making a small incision above or in the umbilicus and then inserting a Verres needle under manual control in the midline at a 30° downward angle toward the pelvis. This points the needle tip to a site below the bifurcation of the aorta, thereby minimizing the risk of arterial puncture. Decompression of the bladder with a catheter and the stomach with a gastric tube helps to avoid any puncture injury to these organs.

The correct placement of the needle tip in the peritoneal cavity is assured by several methods: the drop test, aspiration, and pressure measurement. After placement of the Verres needle in the peritoneal cavity, several drops of saline are placed in the hub of the needle and, if correctly placed, the needle will draw the saline into the cavity as a result of the subatmospheric intra-abdominal pressure. The needle is then aspirated to ensure that it is not intravascular and has not entered bowel. The Verres needle is then connected to the insufflator. A pressure reading of 0 to –5 mmHg reconfirms that the tip of the needle is in the peritoneal cavity. The insufflator's upper pressure limit is set to 15 mmHg. Carbon dioxide is instilled using a low rate of 1 L min^{-1} through the needle. The quadrants are percussed to ensure even distribution of the gas. Once an adequate pneumoperitoneum has been established (about 1.5 L) a higher flow rate is used (2–3 L min^{-1}) until the pressure limit of 15 mmHg has been reached.

The Verres needle is removed and a large (11 mm) cannula over a trocar is inserted through the umbilical incision. Modern trocars have retractable safety mechanisms so that, once through the abdominal wall, the sharp tip of the trocar is protected to prevent injury to intra-abdominal organs. Once in place, the trocar is removed, leaving the cannula in the intra-abdominal cavity. The automatic insufflator is attached and flow rates of 6–10 L min^{-1} are used to maintain a steady pneumoperitoneum (volume of 3–5 L). It is critical that the cannula delivering the pneumoperitoneum is sited intra-abdominally otherwise a rapid subcutaneous emphysema will occur.

An alternative to blind insertion of the needle is to perform a minilaparotomy with the trocar placed under direct vision, thereby avoiding many complications.[30]

Once the trocar is set, the laparoscope may be inserted and the abdominal contents inspected under direct vision. Other instruments and trocars may also be placed under direct vision.

Laparoscopic gynecologic surgery is very closely related to other intra-abdominal operations performed by other surgical subspecialties. With the growth in the cases involving laparoscopy there is also a growing need to be aware of the physiologic changes related to laparoscopic surgery. From this basic understanding, insight into the potential risks and complications encountered may be appreciated.

Insufflation

Laparoscopy of the upper and lower abdominal cavities makes use of gas insufflation to obtain improved views and access to surgical sites. Carbon dioxide became the standard because of its valuable properties. It is nonflammable, permitting safe electrocautery. It is also highly soluble in blood and tissue, thereby minimizing the dangers of gas embolization.[31] Automatic pressure limits are used on the insufflator to minimize the deleterious effects of raised intra-abdominal pressure. It is recommended that the pressures be set to no higher than 15 mmHg while maintaining appropriate gas volumes to obtain adequate views. Pressures greater than 5.3 kPa (40 mmHg) are known to cause circulatory and respiratory embarrassment.[32] The risk of CO_2 embolism and peritoneal and subcutaneous emphysema also increases when high pressures are used.[33]

Carbon dioxide homeostasis

Much interest has surrounded the homeostasis of carbon dioxide during laparoscopy. Serious derangements of respiratory parameters have been encountered during laparoscopy.

During controlled ventilation in the Trendelenburg position and with peritoneal insufflation giving an intra-abdominal pressure of 2 kPa (15 mmHg), there are significant increases in $P_{a}CO_2$, to 1.3 kPa (10 mmHg), and in $P_{A}CO_2$, to 0.5 kPa (4 mmHg), with a decrease in total lung compliance of 25%.[34]

Absorption of CO_2 occurs as indicated by an increase in end-tidal (ET) CO_2 under controlled ventilation. In the clinical state, the absorption of CO_2 appears to be modest and can be compensated for by a small increase in minute ventilation.

With the patient in the supine position, induction of general anesthesia and the increased intra-abdominal pressure during carbon dioxide insufflation lead to elevation of the diaphragm, thereby decreasing functional residual capacity (FRC) and lung compliance, while the resulting atelectasis leads to less effective minute ventilation, further increasing $P_{a}CO_2$.[35] This situation is made worse by the head-down (Trendelenburg) position and is somewhat attenuated by head-up tilt.[36] It should be noted that most respiratory parameters can be corrected and compensated by monitoring ET CO_2 and by increasing minute ventilation when controlled ventilation is used.

Although hypoxemia may also result from the alteration in respiratory mechanics, this is less common and is usually and easily compensated for by intraoperative increased $F_{I}O_2$. This problem may be more significant in older and debilitated patients.

Large, uncompensated increases in $P_{a}CO_2$ may occur during spontaneous ventilation. $P_{a}CO_2$ levels of 70 mmHg (9.3 kPa) have been documented under general anesthesia with spontaneous ventilation. Levels greater than 100 mmHg (13.3 kPa) have been documented when unlimited pressure insufflation was allowed.[37]

Abrupt and large increases in ET CO_2 suggest intravascular carbon dioxide embolism.

Venous CO_2 embolism

High solubility is an important advantage desirable of CO_2. In the event that small volumes of CO_2 are absorbed or gain intravascular access, these are unlikely to cause harm because they are absorbed and quickly excreted by the lungs. However, if larger bolus volumes pass unrecognized into the circulation, serious deleterious hemodynamic events may occur. Venous CO_2 embolism has been reported to occur intraoperatively and postoperatively and must be considered in the event of cardiovascular collapse.

An important etiologic factor in the development of venous CO_2 embolus is the use of high insufflating pressures (greater than 15 mmHg) In the presence of open venous channels following dissection or trauma and during the application of a constant-pressure pneumoperitoneum, CO_2 may easily gain intravascular access. This will, of course, occur instantaneously if the Verres needle penetrates a blood vessel.

Continuous monitoring of heart sounds, ET CO_2, and systolic blood pressure may provide early clues. Early signs of significant CO_2 embolism include falling systolic pressure, millwheel cardiac murmur, and cyanosis and desaturation evident on pulse oximetry. Initially with a small bolus, the ET CO_2 may increase abruptly. However, with a larger bolus causing a gas lock in the right heart or pulmonary artery outflow tract the ET CO_2 may fall. Carbon dioxide embolism with cardiovascular collapse is a true emergency and must be treated promptly. Immediate deflation of the pneumoperitoneum may prevent further progression.

Cardiovascular changes

Hemodynamic changes occur during laparoscopy and must be appreciated by the anesthesiologist. Peritoneal insufflation causes major hemodynamic alterations. These are characterized by a decrease in cardiac output (CO) in the presence of increases in total pulmonary resistance (TPR), peripheral vascular resistance (PVR), and arterial blood pressure. Early reports contained conflicting information about the alterations in cardiac output (CO). However, recent data clearly show that the initiation of peritoneal insufflation results in a decrease in CO of 25–30% regardless of patient tilt. This reduction in CO has been confirmed in echocardiography studies. This depression in CO remains throughout surgery regardless of surgical stimulation.[10]

The mechanism for the decreased CO is multifactorial. Increased intra-abdominal pressure with insufflation results in pooling of blood in the legs and reduces venous return to the inferior vena cava (IVC), which parallels the decrease in CO. Although right atrial pressure and pulmonary artery pressures increase during pneumoperitoneum, the consequent increase in intrathoracic pressure during the pneumoperitoneum decreases the transmural right atrial pressure, thereby decreasing venous return.[38]

Systemic vascular resistance (SVR) has been shown to increase during laparoscopic pneumoperitoneum. The increase in intra-abdominal pressure may contribute to compression of intra-abdominal arterioles and the aorta. However, this does not explain the entire increase in SVR. Humoral factors such as catecholamines, prostaglandins, renin–angiotensin, and vasopressin are responsible for a significant portion of this increase. The intra-abdominal organs appear to be very sensitive to increased intra-abdominal pressure, and a result is the release of these factors. The increase in mean aterial pressure (MAP) despite a drop in CO is explained by the rise in SVR.[39]

Anesthetic induction drugs depress the myocardium and may reduce cardiac index (CI) and MAP. Head-up tilt further decreases these parameters by reducing venous return, as evidenced by falls in pulmonary capillary wedge pressure (PCWP) and right atrial pressure (RAP). Consequently, CI and MAP may be further reduced.

When the myocardium is depressed, the increase in afterload becomes a significant factor. Great care and caution should be exercised when a patient with impaired cardiovascular function or hypovolemia is exposed to a pneumoperitoneum during laparoscopy.

A combination of transesophageal echocardiography (TEE) and invasive cardiovascular monitoring has been used to elucidate in detail the hemodynamic responses that occurred during laparoscopic colectomy in an elderly population with significant cardiopulmonary disease.[40]

Three distinct phases of hemodynamic change were demonstrated. Phase I, peritoneal insufflation after induction of anesthesia, resulted in significant increases in SVR and central venous pressure (CVP) and a decrease in CI. TEE confirmed these changes and revealed a decrease in ejection fraction (EF) of 16% and an increase in end-systolic area of 25%. Ventricular dysfunction occurred during an acute increase in afterload.

The second distinct phase of circulatory response to laparoscopy occurred when the Trendelenburg position was introduced. Increased preload (CVP) facilitated ventricular function to meet the demands of increased SVR, and EF and CI increased.

The third phase was seen at the end of the laparoscopy. This was a hyperdynamic state characterized by an increased heart rate and CI and a significant decrease in SVR. Echocardiographic analysis confirmed the higher EF. When the pneumoperitoneum was released, venous resistance was reduced, and the hormonal stimulation created by the pneumoperitoneum ceased, thereby allowing the SVR to fall.[40]

Following the pneumoperitoneum, steep head-up or head-down positions may be used to facilitate surgical view and access. The capacity of the elderly and patients with significant cardiovascular disease to tolerate these changes is of concern.

Arrhythmias

Cardiac arrhythmias may occur during laparoscopy with CO_2 and are thought to be related to respiratory acidosis, which leads to increased sympathetic outflow in the presence of halogenated anesthetic agents such as halothane, enflurane, isoflurane, and sevoflurane. Arrhythmias can be prevented in the presence of these agents by keeping the CO_2 in the normal range.[41]

Hypoxia also contributes to the occurrence of arrhythmias. Supplemental oxygen guided by careful monitoring of pulse oximeter values can avoid this problem.

Severe bradycardia and other arrhythmias may occur from vagal reflexes associated with stretching of the peritoneum during insufflation. These are uncommon but usually respond quickly to anticholinergics.[42]

The extension of laparoscopy to more complicated intra-abdominal procedures presents further concerns. Nowadays, more patients undergoing surgery are older than in the past and have coexisting medical conditions (hypertension, coronary artery disease, chronic obstructive pulmonary disease). These patients will present a challenge to the anesthesiologist of today and tomorrow as patients who are more compromised by disease undergo more complicated laparoscopic surgery.

Gastric reflux

High intra-abdominal pressure associated with a pneumoperitoneum may cause reflux of gastric contents. The use of general anesthesia combined with cuffed endotracheal tubes greatly reduces this risk. In addition, the use of a gastric tube to decompress the stomach further decreases the likelihood of reflux and aspiration.

The use of regional anesthesia with sedation or general anesthesia using a face mask or laryngeal mask airway increases the likelihood of reflux and the risk of aspiration of gastric contents. Treatment with H_2 blockers to increase gastric pH, and metoclopramide to help gastric emptying and increase lower esophageal tone, seems to be appropriate in these situations.

General considerations

A well-planned and well-executed general anesthetic with endotracheal intubation is by far the most common and safest approach and allows respiratory and cardiovascular stability to be maintained. The use of appropriate monitors is vital. The ET CO_2 monitor aids in the early diagnosis of underventilation and CO_2 embolization. The pulse oximeter guides the use of supplemental F_IO_2 and provides a warning of severe CO_2 emboli.

The use of nondepolarizing neuromuscular blockers can improve the operative procedure. Relaxation of the abdominal muscles will augment the pneumoperitoneum at lower insufflation pressures.[43] Likewise, with lower intra-abdominal pressures, the untoward side-effects and complications of raised intra-abdominal pressure may be reduced. The duration of laparoscopic procedures varies widely, and choosing an appropriate agent is important.

Most anesthetic plans today involve controlled ventilation, although there are reports of successful general anesthesia while the patient is breathing spontaneously.[44,45] It must be remembered that elevation of CO_2 may result from depression of the respiratory center by the general anesthetic drugs, depression of the respiratory mechanics by the pneumoperitoneum, and the use of the Trendelenburg position.

A report from the Centers for Disease Control has revealed that almost one-third of deaths associated with laparoscopic procedures are related to complications of general anesthesia without intubation.[46]

Regional anesthesia has been shown to be an effective and appropriate alternative to general anesthesia. It has been shown that respiratory parameters remain stable during epidural anesthesia.[47,48] However, the monitoring required during pneumoperitoneum and while in the Trendelenburg position can be stressful for patients.

Deep sedation of a patient under regional anesthesia may further reduce respiratory function and result in an inability to deal effectively with rising CO_2 levels. Similarly, failure to protect the airway can be catastrophic.

Laparoscopy under regional anesthesia is best suited for lower abdominal procedures. However, procedures in the upper abdomen have been managed effectively. Patients may have referred shoulder pain and difficulty in breathing when surgical sites are close to the diaphragm.

Laparoscopy under local anesthesia with i.v. sedation has been reported to be successful.[49] This technique is obviously limited to short, uncomplicated procedures.

ANESTHESIA FOR UROLOGIC PROCEDURES

The development of fiberoptic instrumentation and the introduction of flexible and rigid catheters for cystoscopy have made lower urinary tract evaluation and surgery easier to perform.

Cystourethroscopy may be performed in the outpatient setting using small-caliber flexible fiberoptic scopes under local anesthesia applied to the urethra, or it may involve regional and or general anesthesia using rigid scopes in the hospital setting. The level of anesthesia needed for urethroscopy involves S2–S4. Cystoscopy will require a higher level of anesthesia. Bladder innervation is T11 to L2 in the dome and S2–S4 for the lower tract. Parasympathetic innervation provides the motor supply to the bladder. Afferent parasympathetics fibers carry sensation of fullness and stretch. Pain, touch, and temperature sensation are carried in the sympathetic flow. Ureteroscopy can also be accomplished easily with these scopes, but the level of anesthesia required to attain adequate pain relief needs to be higher. Pain from the ureter and kidney is referred in the somatic distribution of the 10th thoracic through to the second lumbar segments: the low back, flank, ilioinguinal, and scrotal–labial areas. The prostate is also innervated from the lumbosacral area. The levels of regional anesthesia required for surgical procedures involving the different structures are:[50]

Ureter	T10
Bladder	T11
Prostate	T11–L2/S2–S4
Urethra	S2–S4

Transurethral prostatectomy (TURP)

TURP is a common procedure performed on elderly men with prostatic hypertrophy, either benign or neoplastic. The classic operation encompasses the use of a cystoscope with a cutting and coagulating wire loop to remove the prostatic tissue from its medial and lateral lobes. Irrigation is used throughout the procedure to distend the bladder, clear the operative field, and remove dissected tissue.

The prostate has large venous channels that are exposed during the procedure. Absorption of irrigant into these channels occurs and may lead to predictable complications depending on a number of factors. The amount of fluid absorbed is related to the hydrostatic pressure of the fluid (i.e. the height of the fluid above the venous channels) and the duration of the operation.[51] The longer the duration, the greater the opportunity to absorb fluid. Ten to thirty milliliters of irrigation fluid is absorbed per minute of surgery. Thus, the amount and type of fluid absorbed may produce complications.[52] As a result of this absorption, continuous shifts in fluids, electrolytes, and solutes occur.[53] The TURP syndrome is a direct complication of these processes.[54]

TURP syndrome

The TURP syndrome comprises cardiovascular and central nervous system alterations related to intravascular absorption of the irrigating solutions used.[55] Acutely altered states of consciousness and cardiovascular complications have been reported and listed below.[56]

Cardiovascular and central nervous system symptoms

The cardiovascular and CNS complications of the TURP syndrome are numerous:

- increased CVP apprehension/agitation;
- bradycardia;
- hypertension;
- cardiovascular collapse;
- ECG changes;
- angina;
- visual disturbances;
- disorientation;
- stupor;
- nausea;
- coma;
- seizures.

The CNS changes have been attributed to hyponatremia, hyperglycinemia, and hyperammonemia. Hyponatremia may occur with the use of any irrigating fluid. The last two occur only with glycine irrigation.

The TURP syndrome presents with altered states of consciousness and visual disturbances. The etiology is a metabolic encephalopathy. Mild symptoms to generalized seizures and coma may occur. Visual disturbances have been reported, but only when hyponatremia has occurred and glycine has been used as the irrigating fluid.[57] Diminished vision extending to blindness has been reported.[58] The onset may occur any time from 30 min after the start of surgery up to 6 h after surgery is completed. Vision usually returns to normal 2–12 h later.

The etiology of the TURP syndrome is related to intravascular absorption of the irrigating solution. Ideal irrigating fluids would be isotonic, nonhemolytic, nontoxic, and nonelectrolytic, would not be metabolized, would allow clear visibility, would not influence osmolality, would be rapidly excreted, and would be an osmotic diuretic.[59]

The irrigating fluid must be nonelectrolytic to ensure dispersal of the cautery loop current. Plain water is clear and allows excellent visibility but is hypotonic and can cause hemolysis when absorbed. Glycine, mannitol, sorbitol, and urea have all been added to irrigation fluids in an attempt to increase the osmolality to a value close to that of plasma. Ideally, irrigating solutions and their metabolites should be nontoxic. Mannitol is not metabolized but undergoes urinary elimination, causing osmotic diuresis. Sorbitol is metabolized to glucose and glycine and its metabolites may be more toxic than initially thought.[59]

During TURP, both intravascular and extravascular absorption occur. Factors influencing the absorption of fluid include:

- hydrostatic pressure of the irrigating fluid;
- number and size of the venous channels open;
- venous pressure in the prostate;
- duration of surgery;
- skill of the surgeon.

Intravascular absorption occurs when the pressure of the irrigating fluid exceeds the open venous sinusoid pressure.[60] Extravascular absorption occurs when perforation of the prostatic capsule occurs. The absorption affects serum homeostasis.

Hyponatremia results from intravascular absorption of large amounts of electrolyte-free solutions. Symptoms are related to the degree of hyponatremia and the speed with which this develops. Signs and symptoms related to low levels of serum sodium are shown in Table 55.2.

It should be noted that a decrease in serum sodium of 20–30 mequiv L^{-1} is roughly equivalent to absorption of 3–4 L of irrigating fluid.[55] The development of a severe TURP reaction requires a large amount of irrigation fluid to be absorbed relatively quickly. Extravascular sequestration and renal excretion diminish the effects of intravascular absorption. The signs and symptoms of metabolic encephalopathy associated with the TURP syndrome have been attributed to cerebral edema caused by hypotonicity and the toxicity of glycine breakdown products.

Glycine is commonly used in the irrigation fluid for TURP.[61,62] There is anecdotal evidence that incidence of CNS disturbance is higher with glycine than with other irrigants. Serum glycine concentrations have been reported to be increased 10-fold after TURP.[63] Glycine is an inhibitory neurotransmitter in the CNS and may act on receptors in the retina to cause blindness. CNS toxicity as a result of glycine absorption may occur in combination with hypotonicity, resulting in cerebral edema.

Glycine, being a simple amino acid, is metabolized to, among other things, ammonia. Raised levels of ammonia have been implicated in the pathogenesis of coma following TURP, independently of hyponatremia. Deterioration in cerebral function has been documented at ammonia concentrations exceeding 150 μmol L^{-1}.[64] Hyperammonemia causes an excess of inhibitory neurotransmitters and a deficit of excitatory transmitters, leading to coma.[65]

Treatment of the symptomatic patient after TURP will depend on the severity of the symptoms. Patients who exhibit nausea, vomiting, agitation, confusion, and/or visual disturbances should be monitored closely if there are no cardiovascular problems. Serum sodium should be monitored. A level of 120 mmol L^{-1} is the borderline between mild and severe reactions. Lasix should be given if there are signs of fluid overload. Most patients will diurese spontaneously and require no further treatment.[55] If visual disturbances are present, evaluation by an ophthalmologist would be prudent. However, there is no specific treatment for visual disturbances, and vision should return to normal over 24 h.[57]

Table 55.2 *Signs and symptoms of hyponatremia*

Serum sodium (mequiv L^{-1})	ECG changes	CNS changes
120	Widened QRS	Restlessness and confusion
115	Widened QRS/elevated ST segments	Nausea and/or semicoma
100	Ventricular tachycardia/ fibrillation	Seizures and coma or fibrillation possible

Severely symptomatic patients require acute and aggressive care. Other potentially treatable conditions must be considered and excluded. Immediate tests to evaluate metabolic coma must include blood glucose, complete electrolyte panel, BUN and creatinine, osmolality, glycine and ammonia, arterial blood gases, and an ECG. The presence of an acute hypotonic state, i.e. a serum sodium less than 120 mmol L^{-1}, in a severely symptomatic patient is life-threatening.[66] Therapy is directed toward increasing extracellular fluid tonicity, thereby shifting fluid from the intracellular to extracellular compartment and thus ameliorating cerebral edema. This may be accomplished with hypertonic saline when normal renal function is present or by dialysis when renal failure occurs.[67] There is no specific treatment for hyperammonemia or hyperglycinemia. Their concentrations should return to normal over 24 h. Neurological complications have been reported after rapid correction of hyponatremia. A rapid intracellular contraction could lead to a rapid decrease in intracellular volume and cerebral hemorrhage. Cerebral demyelination has also been reported after rapid correction in chronically hyponatremic patients.[68]

The CNS complications should be carefully monitored by the surgeon and the anesthesiologist. The resection time should be limited to 1 h if possible. The hydrostatic pressure of the irrigating fluid should not exceed 70 cmH_2O. The early detection of cerebral symptoms is facilitated by the use of a spinal anesthetic rather than general anesthetic. Hypotonic i.v. fluids should be avoided, especially when treating hypotension associated with a spinal anesthetic. This should be treated with vasopressors rather than large boluses of fluids. It is suggested that 0.9% saline is the ideal i.v. fluid for infusion during surgery.

Other complications of TURP

Perforation of the bladder may occur during TURP, and in most cases the perforation is extraperitoneal and is manifest by periumbilical, inguinal, and/or suprapubic pain. If the perforation extends to the intraperitoneal space, then acute abdominal symptoms may develop.

Bacteremia may develop perioperatively. The prostate harbors many bacteria, and these may escape into the bloodstream through the venous sinusoids. Bacteremia is usually treated easily. Septicemia may also occur and be manifest by fevers, chills, and tachycardia. In severe cases, septic shock with hypotension may develop.[20]

Abnormal bleeding may occur following TURP. This is thought to be due to systemic fibrinolysis caused by plasmin. The prostate releases plasminogen activator, which converts plasminogen to plasmin.[69]

Anesthesia for TURP

Spinal anesthesia is the technique of choice for TURP.[70] There is high patient acceptability and strong medical reasons for using this form of anesthesia. A moderate level, T10, is easily accomplished and provides excellent anesthesia for the patient and acceptable conditions for the surgeon. The signs and symptoms of the TURP syndrome or fluid overload can be watched for and ongoing progress observed.

General anesthesia can be used when contraindications to subarachnoid block are present. It is a safe and an acceptable alternative.[71] However, the clinical signs and symptoms of TURP syndrome will be masked. The results of blood chemistry, physical diagnosis, and ECG information must be relied upon intraoperatively and early postoperatively to assess the patient.

Lithotripsy

Extracorporeal shock wave lithotripsy (ESWL) is the treatment of choice for the disintegration of urinary stones in the ureter and kidney. The lithotripter comprises a spark plug as an energy source, an energy reflector and concentrator, and an ongoing method for viewing the stone by fluoroscopy and/or ultrasound. The energy produced by the spark plug is used to vaporize water and thereby create an external shock wave that can be focused in a water bath. The shock wave is passed from the water bath to the patient's body without loss of energy. When the wave encounters a stone (change in medium) it releases energy. Energy is also released at the point where the energy wave leaves the stone, thereby supplying double power to disintegrate the stone.[72,73]

The high-energy waves are focused on the ureter or the kidney. The lithotripter uses the R-wave of the ECG as the trigger for the shock wave. Cardiac arrhythmias related to the shock wave have been observed in 10–15% of patients undergoing ESWL. The wave is set on the R-wave to deliver the energy during the refractory period of the cardiac cycle. Arrhythmias may occur as a result of mechanical stimulation of the myocardium and the conduction system, leading to atrial and ventricular premature contraction, atrial fibrillation, supraventricular tachycardia, and ventricular tachycardia.[74,75]

The first lithotripters required the patient to be submerged in a water bath. Physiologic changes occur during lithotripsy when a patient is placed in a water bath. Cardiac preload is augmented, manifested by increase in CVP and PCWP associated with compression of the peripheral venous system. As a consequence, an increase in stroke volume of 30% and an increase in cardiac output of 30% occurs without a change in heart rate.[76]

Hydrostatic pressure on the chest decreases FRC by 30% and vital capacity by 20% and decreases tidal volume while the work of breathing increases. Ventilatory reserves are diminished and there is an increase potential for hypoxia.[77]

Newer lithotripters have eliminated the need for the water bath. They use a universal table to allow supporting procedures (e.g. fluoroscopy) to be performed simultaneously. The energy can be focused more precisely so that it is less painful. In spite of these developments, the procedure still requires analgesia and/or anesthesia.

There are several situations that require special consideration when planning lithotripsy. Women of childbearing age need to undergo a pregnancy test as pregnancy is an absolute contraindication to lithotripsy. Bleeding disorders and the use of anticoagulants are relative contraindications. Pacemakers in the chest are usually not a problem. Damage to abdominal pacemakers exposed to the energy shock wave has been reported.[78] Abdominal aortic aneurysms with calcium deposits as well as orthopedic prostheses are also relative contraindications and must be kept out of the path of the shock wave. Extreme obesity may prevent successful lithotripsy because of the obvious mechanical limitations. Lung tissue is especially susceptible to shock wave injury. Hemoptysis and pulmonary contusion with severe hypoxia in an adult have been reported.[79] It is suggested that Styrofoam padding be placed under a child to shield the lung bases from shock waves during ESWL.[80] The water temperature may also affect body temperature if not kept close to the physiologic range.[81,82]

The choice of anesthetic technique for ESWL has changed over the years. Initially, when a water bath was used, epidural anesthesia was the technique of choice,[83] although general anesthesia was also used successfully. With the advent of the modern lithotripters, i.v. sedation and/or general anesthesia is used. This seems to provide the easiest and most flexible regime.

Open surgical procedures in urology

Radical prostatectomy for the treatment of localized prostate cancer has become commonplace. Proponents of this procedure are influenced by the high likelihood of sparing the nerves and preventing impotence. The procedure requires the patient to be in an extreme position: supine in the Trendelenburg position with the kidney rest raised, with the back extended and the pubis lifted above the head. Fluid shifts leading to pooling in the dependent areas are common. Venous air embolism has also been reported.

The most common intraoperative complication is blood loss, which can be quite large. Many patients require transfusions. Presently, many operations are completed without the need for allogenic transfusions. Both hemodilution and predonation of blood have been found to be effective.

Nephrectomy and total cystectomy also can be associated with large amounts of blood loss. The need for special positioning for nephrectomy may be encountered.

REFERENCES

1. Maranets I, Kain ZN. Preoperative anxiety and intraoperative anesthetic requirements. *Anesth Analg* 1999; **89:** 1346–51.
2. Leigh JM, Walker J, Janaganathan P. Effect of preoperative anesthetic visit on anxiety. *Br Med J* 1997; **2:** 987–9.
3. Speir BR, Freeman MG. Psychological aspects of pelvic surgery. In: Rock JA, Thompson JD (eds). *Linde's Operative Gynecology*, 8th edn. Philadelphia: Lippincott–Raven Publishers, 1997: 33–44
4. Walsh J, Puig MM, Lovitz MA, Turndorf H. Premedication abolishes the increase in plasma beta-endorphin observed in the immediate preoperative period. *Anesthesiology* 1987; **66:** 402–5.
5. White PF. Pharmacologic and clinical aspects of preoperative medication. *Anesth Analg* 1986; **65:** 963–74.
6. Narr BJ, Warner ME, Schroeder DR, Warner MA. Outcomes of patients with no laboratory assessment before anesthesia and a surgical procedure. *Mayo Clinic Proc* 1997; **72:** 505–9.
7. Parker BM, Tetzlaff JE, Litaker DL, Maurer WG. Redefining the preoperative evaluation process and the role of the anesthesiologist. *J Clin Anesth* 2000; **12:** 350–6.
8. Smetana GW. Preoperative pulmonary evaluation. *N Engl J Med* 1999; **340:** 937–44.
9. Doyle RL. Assessing and modifying the risk of postoperative pulmonary complications. *Chest* 1999; **115:** 77S–81S.
10. Goldman L. Cardiac risk in noncardiac surgery: an update. *Anesth Analg* 1995; **80:** 810–20.
11. McFarland JG. Perioperative blood transfusions. *Chest* 1999; **115:** 113S–121S.
12. ASHP therapeutic guidelines on antimicrobial prophylaxis in surgery. *Am J Health Syst Pharm* 1999; **56:** 1839–88.
13. Martin J. Patient positioning. In: Barash PG, Cullen BF, Stoelting RK (eds). *Clinical Anesthesia*, 2nd edn. Philadelphia: Lippincott Co., 1992: 709–36.
14. Warner MA, Warner DO, Harper CM, *et al.* Lower extremity neuropathies associated with lithotomy positions. *Anesthesiology* 2000; **93:** 938–42.
15. Verdolin MH, Toth AS, Schroeder R. Bilateral lower extremity compartment syndromes following prolonged surgery in the low lithotomy position with serial compression stockings. *Anesthesiology* 2000; **92:** 1189–91.
16. Halliwill JR, Hewitt SA, Joyner MJ, Warner MA. Effect of various lithotomy positions on lower-extremity blood pressure. *Anesthesiology* 1998; **89:** 1373–6.
17. Fahy BG, Barnas GM, Nagle, SE, Flowers JL. Effects of Trendelenburg and reverse Trendelenburg postures on lung and chest wall mechanics. *J Clin Anesth* 1996; **8:** 236–44.
18. Selvin BL. Cancer chemotherapy: implications for the anesthesiologist. *Anesth Analg* 1981; **60:** 425–34.
19. Desiderio DP. Anesthetic–antineoplastic drug interactions. *Semin Anesth* 1993; **12:** 74–8.
20. Peppriell JE, Lema MJ. Preanesthetic considerations for the patient with cancer receiving cancer treatment. *Problems Anesth* 1993; **7:** 349–64.
21. Anderson JR, Genadry R. Anatomy and embryology. In: Berek JS, Adashi EY, Hillard PA (eds). *Novak's Gynecology*, 12th edn. Baltimore, MD: Williams & Wilkins, 1996: 84–90.
22. Edraki, B, Tens NN, Kapp DS. Gynecologic procedures. In: Jaffe RA, Samuels SI (eds). *Anesthesiologist's Manual of Surgical Procedures*, 2nd edn. Philadelphia: Lippincott, 1999: 537–98.
23. Dorsey JH. Application of laser gynecology. In: Rock JA, Thompson, JD. (eds). *Linde's Operative Gynecology*, 8th edn. Philadelphia, PA: Lippincott–Raven Publishers, 1997: 363–75.
24. Garfield JM, Muto MG, Bizzari-Schmid M. Anesthesia for gynecologic surgery. In: Rogers MC, Tinker JH, Covino BG, Longnecker DE (eds). *Principles and Practice of Anesthesiology*. Mosby: St Louis, MO, 1993: 2105–36.
25. Hampl KF, Schneider MC, Ummenhofer W, Drewe J. Transient neurologic symptoms after spinal anesthesia. *Anesth Analg* 1995; **81:** 1148–53.
26. Hampl KF, Heinzman-Wiedmer S, Luginbuehl I, *et al.* Transient neurologic symptoms after spinal anesthesia: a lower incidence with prilocaine and bupivacaine than with lidocaine. *Anesthesiology* 1998; **88:** 629–33.
27. Hampl KF, Schneider MC, Pargger H, *et al.* A similar incidence of transient neurologic symptoms after spinal anesthesia with 2% and 5% lidocaine. *Anesth Analg* 1996; **83:** 1051–4.
28. Bucklin BA, Smith CV. Postpartum tubal ligation: safety, timing, and other implications for anesthesia. *Anesth Analg* 1999; **89:** 1269–74.
29. Talamani MA, Gadaz TR. Laparoscopic approach to cholecystectomy. *Advanc Surg* 1991; **25:** 1–20.
30. Hasson H. A modified instrument and method for laparoscopy. *Am J Obstet Gynecol* 1971; **70:** 886.
31. Caverly RK, Jenkins LC. The anaesthetic management of pelvic laparoscopy. *Can Anesth Soc J* 1973; **20:** 679–86.
32. Kelman GR, Swapp GH, Smith I, *et al.* Cardiac output and arterial blood gas tension during laparoscopy. *Br J Anaesth* 1972; **44:** 1155–62.
33. Lew JKL, Gin T, Oh TE. Anesthetic problems during laparoscopic cholecystectomy. *Advanc Intensive Care* 1992; **20:** 91.
34. Versichelen L, Serreyn R, Rully G, Vandderkerckhave D. Physiologic changes during anesthesia administration for gynecologic laparoscopy. *J Reprod Med* 1984; **10:** 697–700.
35. Hodson C, McClelland RMA, Newton JR. Some effects of the peritoneal insufflation of carbon dioxide at laparoscopy. *Anaesthesia* 1970; **25:** 382–90.
36. Schiller WR. The Trendelenburg position: surgical aspects. In: Morton JT (ed.). *Positioning in Anesthesia and Surgery*, 2nd edn. Philadelphia, PA: WB Saunders, 1987: 117.
37. Lewis DG, Ryder W, Burn N, *et al.* Laparoscopy – an investigation during spontaneous ventilation under halothane. *Br J Anaesth* 1972; **44:** 685–91.
38. Joris JL, Noirot DP, Legrand MJ, *et al.* Hemodynamic changes during laparoscopic cholecystectomy. *Anesth Analg* 1993, **76:** 1067.
39. Joris J, Lamy M. Neuroendocrine changes during pneumoperitoneum for laparoscopic cholecystectomy. *Br J Anaesth* 1993; **70:** A33.
40. Harris HN, Ballytyne GH, Luther MA, Perrino AC. Alteration of cardiovascular performance during laparoscopic colectomy; a combined hemodynamic and echocardiographic analysis. *Anesth Analg* 1996; **83:** 482–7.
41. Harris MNE, Plateum OM, Crowther A. Cardiac arrhythmias during anesthesia for laparoscopy. *Br J Anaesth* 1984; **56:** 1213.
42. Carmichael DE. Laparoscopy – cardiac considerations. *Fertil Steril* 1971; **22:** 69.
43. Chassard D, Berrada K, Tournadre J, *et al.* The effects of neuromuscular block in peak airway pressure and abdominal elastance during pneumoperitoneum. *Anesth Analg* 1996; **82:** 525.
44. Swann DG, Spens H, Edwards SA, *et al.* Anesthesia for gynaecological laparoscopy – a comparison between the laryngeal mask airway and tracheal intubation. *Anaesthesia* 1993; **48:** 431.
45. Keneflick JP, Leader JR, Maltby JP, Taylor JP. Laparoscopy: blood gas values and minor sequelae associated with three techniques based on isoflurane. *Br J Anaesth* 1987; **59:** 189–94.
46. Peterson HB, DeStafano F, Rubin GL, *et al.* Deaths attributable to tubal sterilization in the United States, 1977–1981. *Am J Obstet Gynecol* 1983; **146:** 131.
47. Ciofolo MJ, Clergue F, Seebacher J, *et al.* Ventilatory effects of laparoscopy under epidural anesthesia. *Anesth Analg* 1990; **70:** 357–61.
48. Dohi S, Takeshum R, Hiroshi N. Ventilatory and circulatory responses to carbon dioxide and high sympathectomy induced by epidural blockade in awake humans. *Anesth Analg* 1986; **65:** 9–14.
49. Peterson HB, Hulka J, Spielman FJ, *et al.* Local versus general anesthesia for laparoscopic sterilization. *Obstet Gynecol* 1987; **70:** 903.
50. Taragho EA. Anatomy of the lower urinary tract. In: Walsh PC, Retik AB, Staurey TA, Vaughn ED (eds). *Campbell's Urology*, 7th edn. Philadelphia, PA: WB Saunders, 1998.
51. Marx GF, Orkin LR. Complications associated with transurethral surgery. *Anesthesiology* 1962; **23:** 802.
52. Emmet J, Gilbough JH, McLean P. Fluid absorption during transurethral resection: comparison of mortality and morbidity after irrigation with water and non-hemolytic solutions. *J Urol* 1969; **101:** 884.
53. Hahn RG. Relations between irrigation absorption rate and hyponatremia during transurethral resection of the prostate. *Acta Anaesthesiol Scand* 1988; **32:** 53–60.
54. Sunderrajan S, Bauer JH, Vopat RL, *et al.* Post transurethral prostatic resection hyponatremic syndrome: case report and review of the literature. *Am J Kidney Dis* 1984; **4:** 80.

55. Hatch PD. Surgical and anesthetic considerations in transurethral resection of the prostate. *Anaesth Intensive Care* 1987; **15:** 203.
56. Henderson DJ, Middleton RG. Coma from hyponatremia following transurethral resection of the prostate. *Urology* 1980; **15:** 267.
57. Kay MC, Kay J, Begun F, Yeung JE, Vision loss following transurethral resection of the prostate. *J Clin Neuro-ophthalmol* 1985; **5:** 273.
58. Creel DJ, Wang JM, Wong KC. Transient blindness associated with transurethral resection of the prostate. *Arch Ophthalmol* 1987; **105:** 1537.
59. Jenson V. The TURP syndrome. *Can J Anaesth* 1991; **38:** 90.
60. Desmond J. Complications of transurethral prostate surgery. *Can Anesth Soc J* 1970; **17:** 25.
61. Zucker JR, Bull AP. Independent plasma levels of sodium and glycine during transurethral resection of the prostate. *Can Anesth Soc J* 1984; **31:** 307.
62. Gecelter LG, Gascoigne H. Safety and efficacy of a 1.5 per cent glycine solution as an irrigation medium in prostatic surgery. *S Afr Med J* 1984; **65:** 693.
63. Hahn RG. Serum amino acid patterns and toxicity symptoms following the absorption of irrigant containing glycine in transurethral prostatic surgery. *Acta Anaesthesiol Scand* 1988; **32:** 493.
64. Hoekstra PT, Kahnoski R, McCamish MA, *et al.* Transurethral prostatic resection syndrome – a new perspective: encephalopathy with associated hyperammonemia. *J Urol* 1983; **130:** 704.
65. Roesch RP, Stoelting RK, Lingeman JE, *et al.* Ammonia toxicity resulting from glycine absorption during transurethral resection of the prostate. *Anesthesiology* 1983; **58:** 577.
66. Campbell H, Fincher M, Sklar A. Severe hyponatremia without severe hypo. osmolality following transurethral resection of the prostate in end-stage renal disease. *Am J Kidney Dis* 1988; **12:** 152.
67. Ayus JC, Oliverio JJ, Frommer JP. Rapid correction of hyponatremia with intravenous hypertonic saline solution. *Am J Med* 1982; **72:** 43.
68. Illowsky BP, Laureno R. Encephalopathy and myelinolysis after rapid correction of hyponatremia. *Brain* 1987; **110:** 855.
69. Hatch PD. Surgical and anesthetic considerations in transurethral resection of the prostate. *Anesth Intensive Care* 1987; **15:** 203.
70. Mebust WK, Holtgrieve HL, Cockett ATK, *et al.* Transurethral prostatectomy – immediate and post operative complications. *J Urol* 1989; **141:** 243.
71. Chung FF, Chung A, Meier RH, *et al.* Comparison of perioperative mental function after general anesthesia and spinal anesthesia with intravenous sedation. *Can J Anaesth* 1989; **36:** 382.
72. Rassweiler J, Henkel TO, Kohrmann KU, *et al.* Lithotripter technology: present and future. *J Endourol* 1992; **16:** 1,
73. Drach DW, Dretler S, Fair W, *et al.* Report of the United States cooperative study of extracorporeal shock wave lithotripsy. *J Urol* 1986; **135:** 1127.
74. Simon CA, LeHenzey NY, Baras E, *et al.* Cardiac arrhythmias during extracorporeal shock wave lithotripsy under general anesthesia. *Anesthesiology* 1986; **65 (3A):** A147.
75. Walts LF, Atlee JL. Supraventricular tachycardia associated with extracorporeal shock wave lithotripsy. *Anesthesiology* 1986; **65:** 521.
76. Behnia R, Shanks CA, Ovassapian A, *et al.* Hemodynamic responses associated with lithotripsy. *Anesth Analg* 1987; **66:** 354,
77. Bromage PR, Bonsu AK, El-Fagih SR, Husain I. Influence of Dornier HM3 system on respiration during ESWL. *Anesth Analg* 1989; **68:** 363.
78. Weber W, Back P, Wilddgans H, *et al.* Anesthetic considerations in patients with cardiac pacemakers undergoing extracorporeal shock wave lithotripsy. *Anesth Analg* 1988; **67:** S251.
79. Malhorta V, Rosen RJ, Slepian RL. Life threatening hypoxemia in an adult due to shock wave induced pulmonary contusion. *Anesthesiology* 1991; **75:** 529.
80. Tredrea CR, Pathak D, From RP, *et al.* Lung protection in children during extracorporeal shock wave lithotripsy. *Anesth Analg* 1987; **66:** S178.
81. Higgins TL, Miller EV, Roberts J. Accidental hyperthermia as a complication of extracorporeal shock wave lithotripsy under general anesthesia. *Anesth Analg* 1987; **66:** 389.
82. Malhorta V. Hyperthermia and hypothermia as complications of extracorporeal shock wave lithotripsy. *Anesthesiology* 198; 7**67:** 448.
83. Duvall JO, Griffith DP. Epidural anesthesia for extracorporeal shock wave lithotripsy. *Anesth Analg* 1985; **64:** 544.

56

Effects of anesthetic drugs on the mother and fetus

DAVID M DEWAN AND KENNETH E NELSON

The pregnant state alters the maternal response to anesthetic drugs and induces changes in maternal physiology which may influence anesthetic response and risk. The fetus may also be affected, either directly by drugs which cross the placenta or indirectly secondary to altered maternal hemodynamic changes. Thus, anesthetic management for nonobstetric surgery has two driving forces: maternal safety and fetal preservation. This chapter explores how maternal physiologic changes influence the maternal pharmacologic response to anesthesia, and the anesthetic effects on the fetus.

MATERNAL FACTORS

Respiratory system

Alveolar ventilation increases by 50–70% by term, whereas functional residual capacity (FRC) is reduced by approximately 20%. The increase in minute ventilation, along with the decrease in FRC, will speed the equilibration of the F_I to F_A ratio. Even though a mask induction is rarely if ever indicated during pregnancy, this effect can have clinical significance during general anesthesia. The more rapid equilibration of F_I to F_A can increase the likelihood of relative overdose during a period of overpressure.[1] Fetal asphyxia can accompany high concentrations of anesthetic vapors.[2] This accelerated induction of inhalation anesthesia is compounded by a 25–40% reduction in minimum alveolar concentration (MAC) during pregnancy.[3,4]

Cardiovascular system

Consistent with increased plasma volume, colloid oncotic pressure decreases as plasma protein concentration declines. Pedal edema may be a normal finding in late pregnancy. However, total protein stores may be higher, secondary to the large increase in blood volume, offering additional sites for drug binding. The alterations in protein binding appear to have little clinical significance for drug binding.

Importantly, anesthetic drugs or techniques which decrease systemic vascular resistance may unmask compensated cardiovascular alterations and threaten maternal cardiovascular stability and organ perfusion. The increased threat of supine hypotension among pregnant patients receiving spinal and epidural anesthesia-induced sympathectomy is well documented. For example, pharmacologic sympathectomy produces greater hypotension in pregnant than in nonpregnant patients,[5] demonstrating the purported exaggerated dependence on tone in the venous capacitance system.

Vasoactive treatment of decreased blood pressure in the parturient requires a different clinical approach from the nonpregnant patient because of the pregnant patient's changed responsiveness to vasoactive compounds. Sensitivity to exogenous vasopressors decreases during pregnancy, but responsiveness varies among vascular beds.[6] For example, ephedrine produces less vasoconstriction in the uterine vessels than other agents with α-agonist activity.[7] This response in the uterine bed differs from the effects of ephedrine on the femoral artery. This differential sensitivity offers fetal protection during indicated vasopressor treatment of hypotension. Other evidence suggests that low-dose neosynephrine, an agent with significant α-agonist activity, may safely be used to treat brief periods of maternal hypotension during regional anesthesia in term healthy patients. Baroreceptor reflex function increases during pregnancy, probably contributing to the decreased responsiveness to phenylephrine. Nevertheless, these findings are consistent with others indicating that the choice of vasopressor is relatively unimportant for the fetus, based on Doppler flow studies performed during cesarean sections.[8] According to these studies, hypotension has a far greater effect on flow than the choice of treatment agent. Very low-concentration epinephrine (adrenaline) infusions in pregnant patients may also not be harmful.[9]

Renal

Renal blood flow (RBF), renal plasma flow (RPF), and glomerular filtration rate (GFR) increase markedly during pregnancy. By 16 weeks' gestation, effective RPF increases by 75%.[10] Effective RPF may decline slightly in late pregnancy, and the decline is not related to patient position.[11] GFR remains elevated throughout pregnancy, resulting in an increased filtration fraction.

Importantly for the anesthesia provider, glycosuria can occur despite normal blood glucose levels.[12] Similarly, bicarbonate, creatinine, and blood urea levels decline during pregnancy. Blood urea nitrogen (BUN) levels may reach 8–9 mg mL^{-1}. Despite altered normal values, drug responses appear to be unchanged by altered renal function.

Hepatic

Other than a rise in alkaline phosphate activity secondary to placental production, liver enzymes remain normal. Plasma cholinesterase declines during pregnancy and slightly prolongs the duration of action of succinylcholine (suxamethonium) administered by weight. Mivacurium has also been used safely for cesarean section. Serum albumin concentrations fall. A greater plasma volume may be responsible in part for this fall. Despite reduced albumin concentrations, the response to anesthetic drugs is unchanged.

The effects of pregnancy on neuromuscular blocking drugs have recently been reviewed.[13] Atracurium has been used safely in pregnancy, and responses resemble those observed with nonpregnant patients. Vecuronium displays a more rapid onset and prolonged blockade, and its ED_{50} is decreased by 50% in pregnant rats. Altered hepatic blood flow may explain the rapid onset and prolongation of blockade provided by vecuronium and rocuronium. All may be used safely during pregnancy.

Response to anesthetic drugs

Pregnancy reduces the MAC significantly for the potent inhalation agents; MAC declines by approximately 25–40%. The 28% reduction in the MAC of isoflurane returns to near normal within 72 h post partum.[14] Elevated progesterone levels may contribute because both serum and cerebrospinal fluid (CSF) levels of progesterone increase during pregnancy, and intravenous progesterone can cause unconsciousness. Thiopental requirements also decline by 17–18%. This reduction in drug requirement appears at 7–13 weeks' gestation. Additionally, the volume of distribution and the elimination half-life of thiopental are prolonged. Propofol is not approved for use during pregnancy in the USA. However, propofol clearance may increase and its pharmacokinetics are not greatly altered by pregnancy.

There is a purported exaggerated response to local anesthetics during pregnancy. Subarachnoid requirements for spinal anesthesia decline by 33%, and epidural local anesthetic requirements decline by up to 30%. Factors proposed as explanation of the reduction are: (1) reduced CSF volume secondary to compression of the subarachnoid space by the enlarged epidural veins; (2) increased local anesthetic diffusion across membranes because of decreased serum bicarbonate and elevated CSF pH; (3) enhanced sensitivity of the nerves to local anesthetics related to elevated progesterone levels and anatomic changes.

Mechanical factors are disputed. Exaggerated lumbar lordosis during pregnancy, potentially promoting cephalad spread of spinal drugs, does not occur when patients are supine. However, a caudad shift of the apex of lumbar lordosis may promote cephalad spread. Other data contradict this: Abouleish[15] noted a 30% increase in spinal bupivacaine requirements for patients undergoing tubal ligation compared with patients undergoing cesarean section, and Datta *et al.*[16] also noted decreased lidocaine (lignocaine) requirements for cesarean sections and postpartum tubal ligation compared with nonpregnant patients. Simultaneously sampled CSF and serum progesterone levels were elevated, suggesting hormonal causes. However, more recently, Hirabyashi *et al.*[17] sampled CSF for progesterone in nonpregnant patients and in pregnant patients in the first, second, and third trimesters. Although spinal tetracaine demonstrated the greatest spread in the second and third trimesters of pregnancy, spread of anesthesia did *not* correlate with CSF progesterone levels, suggesting causes other than hormonal. Dietz and Jaffe[18] also demonstrated that pregnancy does not increase the susceptibility of spinal root axons to bupivacaine. Nevertheless, preterm pregnant patients require less spinal drug as gestation proceeds to term, and parturients with multiple gestation require lower doses of spinal drugs than singleton gestation, suggesting that pregnancy does decrease neuraxial drug requirements.

Data for epidurally administered local anesthetic are also conflicting. While Bromage[19] noted decreased requirements during pregnancy, Fragraeus *et al.*[20] identified that these changes existed in early pregnancy prior to uterine enlargement. Finally, Grundy and coworkers[21] noted no decreased drug requirements. Regardless, fractionation and titration of epidurally administered drugs render these conflicting data unimportant during epidural anesthesia.

In the past, concern has arisen over whether local anesthetic toxicity is enhanced by pregnancy. In 1985, bupivacaine was shown to cause complete respiratory arrest and cardiovascular collapse at a lower dose in pregnant than in nonpregnant ewes, despite similar doses required to cause CNS toxicity.[22] This evidence, combined with previous case reports of bupivacaine-related cardiovascular collapse in pregnant women, led clinicians to speculate that the pregnant state conferred an increased bupivacaine sensitivity. More recently, however, bupivacaine toxicity in pregnant ewes was reinvestigated in a blinded fashion using a larger number of animals (24 compared with 8) with the same 0.5 mg kg^{-1} min^{-1} intravenous infusion of bupivacaine.[23] No differences were noted between nonpregnant and pregnant animals in the doses or serum concentrations of bupivacaine required to elicit toxic manifestations. Additionally, mepivacaine, lidocaine, and ropivacaine do not exhibit enhanced toxicity in pregnant compared with nonpregnant animals. Therefore, the preponderance of evidence suggests that pregnancy itself does not enhance local anesthetic toxicity. Nevertheless, adequate testing for intravenous placement of epidural catheters and fractionation of local anesthetic doses define safe care.

PLACENTAL FACTORS

Placental anatomy and circulation

Understanding the function of the placenta is essential for the anesthesiologist caring for the pregnant woman. The placenta serves to connect the fetal with the maternal circulation, facilitating oxygen, nutrient, and waste transfer while simultaneously providing a "barrier" that prevents direct continuity between the fetal and maternal vascular systems. At term, the human placenta weighs approximately 500 g. It is disk shaped, 20 cm in diameter, and 2–3 cm thick. On the fetal side of the placenta, deoxygenated blood flows from the fetus to the placenta through two umbilical arteries and returns from the mother to the fetus through a single umbilical vein. Upon reaching the placenta, the umbilical arteries repeatedly branch out into the villous tree, progressively lose their smooth muscular walls, and become the capillary networks where exchange with the maternal circulation takes place. On the maternal side of the placenta, endometrial spiral arteries eject blood directly into the intervillous space to bathe the villous tree before returning passively to the maternal circulation through the endometrial veins.

Uterine blood flow determinants

Uterine blood flow (UBF) originates from both uterine and ovarian arteries, primarily from the former. Uterine blood flow increases throughout pregnancy from around 50–100 mL min^{-1} before pregnancy to over 500 mL min^{-1} in late pregnancy. Blood flow to the uterus can be described by:

Uterine blood flow = Uterine arterial pressure – Uterine venous pressure/uterine vascular resistance

Therefore, either an increased uterine vascular resistance or a decreased uterine perfusion pressure will decrease UBF. For example, compression of the maternal aorta and/or inferior vena cava by the gravid uterus can directly decrease UBF by increasing uterine venous pressure, or by decreasing arterial pressure. Indirectly, this aortocaval compression can decrease UBF by decreasing venous return to the heart, resulting in decreased maternal cardiac output and blood pressure.

Anesthetic factors decreasing uterine blood flow

The anesthetic effects on UBF can be measured experimentally by uterine and umbilical artery Doppler velocimetry in pregnant women, and clinically important effects can be identified with changes in fetal heart rate patterns.

Both regional anesthesia and general anesthesia can decrease UBF (Table 56.1), either directly or indirectly. Spinal and epidural anesthesia accompanied by hypotension indirectly reduce UBF by blockade of sympathetic efferent nerves responsible for maintaining vascular tone, reducing venous return, cardiac output, and blood pressure. The resulting placental hypoperfusion may lead to fetal hypoxia and lactic acidosis. However, multiple studies in both animals and humans have demonstrated that UBF does not decrease significantly as long as adequate maternal blood pressure is maintained with intravenous fluids and appropriate vasopressor drugs. Epidural anesthesia can directly reduce UBF by unintentional intravenous injection of local anesthetics, epinephrine, or other vasoconstricting drugs. The induction of general anesthesia can also result in a reduction in uterine blood flow either directly or indirectly. Barbiturates administered in sufficient dosage to cause systemic maternal hypotension will directly result in reduced uterine perfusion pressure. Laryngoscopy and intubation are associated with increased maternal blood pressure, which results from an acute rise in circulating catecholamines. The increased levels of catecholamines can indirectly reduce UBF by constricting uterine arteries. Similarly, inhalation anesthetics in high concentrations reduce maternal cardiac output, and when accompanied by hypotension can lead to fetal acidosis. Ketamine, unique among the general anesthetic induction agents, increases myometrial tone and could therefore potentially reduce UBF at high doses. However, 0.7 mg mL^{-1} ketamine in pregnant ewes increased myometrial tone without decreasing UBF.[24] The effect of ketamine on myometrial tone has been shown to decrease significantly in the third trimester.

Vasoconstrictors are commonly used to restore the blood pressure of obstetric patients during both general and regional anesthesia. The use of α_1-adrenergic agents such as phenylephrine and methoxamine will decrease UBF in spite of a normalized maternal mean arterial pressure (MAP). In contrast, ephedrine, a mixed α- and β-adrenergic agonist, will restore maternal MAP while increasing UBF. The effect of epinephrine on UBF has also been studied in animals and humans. Based on consistent findings of decreased UBF, epinephrine is not recommended as a routine treatment for hypotension in pregnancy. However, epinephrine remains popular as a test dose for excluding an intravenously placed epidural catheter, as the decreased UBF from a 5- to 20-μg bolus of epinephrine is a transient effect.

Oxytocin is a naturally occurring peptide that is commonly used to augment labor, and to induce rapid and forceful contraction of the uterus after delivery of the fetus and the placenta. Oxytocin can decrease uteroplacental blood flow by two mechanisms. First, bolus administration of large doses of oxytocin can cause vasodilation and hypotension, thereby indirectly reducing uterine blood flow. Second, oxytocin augments the duration and magnitude of uterine contractions, during which blood flow is reduced in proportion to the increased uterine venous pressure caused directly by the contraction itself.

Local anesthetics are frequently employed during labor and can potentially have very important effects on UBF. Severe fetal effects of local anesthetics injected for a paracervical block clearly illustrate the potential adverse effects of local anesthetics on UBF. Local anesthetics cause constriction of human uterine arteries *in vitro* and can alter systemic blood pressure when injected intravenously. Furthermore, intravenous local anesthetics will reduce UBF in pregnant ewes at arterial blood concentrations encountered in the clinical setting. The vasoconstricting property of some local anesthetics is felt to be responsible for adverse fetal effects caused by accidental intravenous injection of local anesthetic that was intended to remain in the epidural space. Fortunately, the amount of local anesthetic used for labor analgesia in a properly functioning lumbar epidural catheter should not be expected to lead to plasma levels sufficient to cause a significant decrease in UBF. Indeed, studies of Doppler velocimetry during bupivacaine epidural analgesia show no changes in uteroplacental blood flow.[25–28]

Placental exchange of drugs

Most anesthetic drugs cross the placenta by the process of passive diffusion, or passive transport, which depends on a concentration gradient, and requires no energy expenditure. Passive diffusion can occur directly through a lipid membrane or through protein channels in the membrane. The amount of any drug crossing the placenta by passive diffusion depends on the maternal to fetal plasma concentration gradient, and the duration of exposure to this gradient. Each drug possesses a different diffusion constant, which is determined by properties of the specific drugs such as molecular weight, degree of ionization, lipid solubility, and protein binding. Molecules that are 500 Da or less in size usually cross the placenta easily, and passive diffusion becomes proportionately slower for molecules that are larger in size. Since the placental barrier consists primarily of lipid membranes (syncytiotrophoblasts, stroma of the intervillous space, fetal capillary wall), the less ionized and more lipid-soluble drugs will cross more readily. Protein binding will limit the amount of free drug available for diffusion, and the more

Table 56.1 *Factors decreasing uterine blood flow*

Direct
Regional anesthesia – inadvertent i.v. injection of local anesthetic (high doses) or epinephrine
General anesthesia – hypotension on induction
Other – vasoconstrictors
Epinephrine
Phenylephrine
Methoxamine
Oxytocin – uterine hypertonus
Indirect
Regional anesthesia – hypotension from sympathectomy
General anesthesia – catecholamines from laryngoscopy and intubation
Other – drug-induced hypotension

i.v., intravenous; epinephrine (adrenaline).

protein bound a drug is in maternal plasma, the less should be expected to reach the fetal circulation.[29] Active transport of molecules differs from passive transport in that expenditure of cellular energy is required, and does not play a significant role in the transport of anesthetic agents across the placenta.

Methods of determining drug transfer

Although it is impractical to measure anesthetic drug transfer *in vivo*, several methods have been used in an attempt to better understand the characteristics of the placental transfer of anesthetic drugs used in pregnant women (Table 56.2). While animal models can be used to approximate the characteristics of anesthetic drug transfer in humans, the usefulness of such models is limited by interspecies differences in anatomy and physiology. Nevertheless, experimental animal work has led to a large part of our current understanding of placental transfer of anesthetic drugs.

Alternatively, human placentas can be used either in isolated anatomic sections or as isolated cotyledons which are perfused to simulate *in vivo* maternal and fetal circulations while measuring drug transfer across the "barrier." More sophisticated designs allow for up to 48 h of study by providing oxygen and nutrients to the placenta while removing carbon dioxide and waste products.

Finally, fetal to maternal (F/M) ratios of drugs can be compared at delivery by sampling both maternal arterial and umbilical venous blood (Table 56.3). Although this method has been used extensively and has provided valuable information, it is limited to providing a "snapshot" of conditions present at the time of delivery. This should be kept in mind during the subsequent discussions of F/M ratios of individual drugs.

Specific anesthetic agents will be discussed individually according to what is currently known about their placental transfer based on animal studies, *in vitro* placental perfusion, and F/M ratios. As a general rule, anesthetic drugs that are chosen for their quick onset and profound effects in the central nervous system will rapidly cross both the blood–brain barrier and the placental barrier.

Local anesthetics

The placental transfer of local anesthetics has been studied extensively. All commonly used local anesthetics have a molecular weight less than 300 Da, therefore their size alone does not impede placental transfer. Indeed, maternal intravenous injection of lidocaine appears in the fetal circulation of sheep within 1 min of injection;[30] in humans, bupivacaine can be detected in the fetal plasma, even after a bupivacaine spinal for cesarean section.[31] A more important determinant of transfer for local anesthetics is their degree of ionization. Most local anesthetics have a p*K* greater than physiologic pH. Nevertheless, the two values are sufficiently close that a significant proportion of the drug exists in both the ionized and unionized state, and at any given time transfer will depend upon the relative percentages, since only the unionized molecules pass freely. The relative inability of ionized local anesthetic to cross is illustrated by a phenomenon known as ion trapping. When the fetus is stressed by inadequate oxygen delivery, anaerobic metabolism results in the production of lactic acid, which will eventually lead to fetal acidosis. Unionized molecules of local anesthetic will pass easily from the maternal plasma, but once ionized in the fetal plasma they become "trapped," leading to accumulation in the fetus. Protein binding will also influence the amount of local anesthetic that can cross the placenta. Bupivacaine is up to 90% protein bound to maternal α_1-acid glycoprotein, and reported F/M ratios range from 0.3 to 0.6. In contrast, lidocaine, which is only about 20% bound to maternal plasma protein, exhibits an F/M ratio of 0.5–0.9.

Table 56.2 *Methods of determining placental drug transfer*

Human *in vivo* – only one study exists, using methohexital
Human placentas – whole or sectioned cotyledons
Human fetal-to-maternal ratios at birth
Animal studies – *in vivo*

Table 56.3 *Fetal-to-maternal (F/M) ratios of commonly used anesthetic drugs*

Drug	F/M ratio
Local anesthetics	
Bupivacaine	0.3–0.6
Lidocaine	0.5–0.9
Volatile inhalational agents	0.7
Intravenous induction agents	
Thiopental	0.96
Ketamine	1.26
Propofol	0.62–0.86
Etomidate	0.5
Diazepam	0.92
Midazolam	0.66
Opioids	
Fentanyl	0.6
Remifentanil	0.88
Morphine	0.9
Meperidine	0.61

Lidocaine (lignocaine); meperidine (pethidine).

Inhalational anesthetics

Inhalational anesthetics, including volatile agents and nitrous oxide, cross the placenta rapidly. Volatile inhalational anesthetics such as halothane and isoflurane measured in cord blood at cesarean section reveal F/M ratios of around 0.7, even with induction to delivery times of less than 12 min. Nitrous oxide also crosses rapidly, and exhibits F/M ratios similar to the volatile agents.

Intravenous induction agents

Thiopental is probably the most commonly used agent to induce general anesthesia for cesarean section in the USA. Its placental transfer has been studied extensively at cesarean section by comparing umbilical and maternal blood levels. High F/M ratios have been a consistent finding, with results as high as 0.96. Similarly, methohexital rapidly crosses the placenta, and maternal and fetal methohexital levels parallel each other.

Ketamine is a phencyclidine derivative that is often chosen to induce general anesthesia for obstetric patients when concern arises over hypovolemia. Ketamine can support blood pressure with its indirect sympathomimetic action. As in the case of thiopental, ketamine crosses quite rapidly and a peak F/M ratio of 1.26 occurs within 2 min of an intravenous bolus.

Propofol is a newer induction agent used in the UK but not yet approved for obstetric use in the USA, and has been used and studied less extensively than thiopental in the obstetric population. Just as maternal anesthesia is rapidly induced after intravenous bolus, propofol rapidly crosses the placenta. At cesarean section, F/M ratios have been reported in a range 0.62–0.86.

Etomidate was first described for the induction of anesthesia for cesarean section in 1978, and the researchers concluded that newborn clinical status was superior to that following thiopental induction.[32] In spite of this early enthusiasm, and an F/M ratio of 0.5 published in 1991,[33] further research and published clinical reports have been limited.

Benzodiazapines

Both *diazepam* and *midazolam* have been studied as induction agents for cesarean section. In two studies, 0.3 mg kg^{-1} diazepam was found to be similar to thiopental 3 mg kg^{-1} when comparing F/M ratios and Apgar scores. Ridd *et al.*[34] found F/M ratios of 1.73 and 0.92 for total and free plasma diazepam respectively. A dual-perfusion human placenta lobule study concurred that the transport fraction of diazepam is relatively high.[35] Conklin *et al.*[36] found that midazolam exhibited less placental transfer than diazepam in sheep. Similarly, F/M ratios for midazolam at cesarean section were 0.66, about 30% lower than thiopental. However, reports of slower induction times and significantly more neonatal depression than with thiopental make midazolam a less attractive choice for induction of general anesthesia for cesarean section.

Opioids

Fentanyl and *sufentanil* are now very commonly used for labor analgesia by both the epidural and intrathecal routes. Both drugs are very highly lipid soluble and are relatively small molecules, therefore they cross the placenta rapidly. Recent *in vivo* human placenta studies have shown that fentanyl exhibits more placental transfer than sufentanil, perhaps because of the placenta itself acting as a reservoir for sufentanil or because of greater maternal plasma protein binding. The site of injection is another important factor affecting the amount of placental transfer. Epidural administration can be expected to result in significantly less fetal exposure than an intravenous injection of the same dose.

Remifentanil is a newer opioid that is rapidly eliminated by esterase metabolism. Currently, only one study of remifentanil in obstetric patients exists, in which an F/M ratio of 0.88 has been reported.

Morphine is much less lipid soluble than both sufentanil and fentanyl, yet this opioid too crosses the placenta rapidly. Morphine is used spinally, epidurally, and even intravenously for labor analgesia. Hartvig *et al.*[37] demonstrated rapid fetal uptake of radiotracer-labeled morphine administered intravenously to monkeys. Even when given intrathecally, morphine can be measured in fetal blood.

Meperidine (pethidine) is very commonly used for labor analgesia via both the intravenous and intramuscular routes. Wilson *et al.*[38] reported an F/M ratio of 0.61 at delivery when meperidine was used for labor analgesia. However, the F/M ratio has been shown to vary from 0.35 to 1.5 depending on the time from dose to delivery, reaching a peak plateau value 1–5 h after maternal administration of meperidine.

Muscle relaxants, unlike induction drugs and narcotics, are unable to cross the placenta easily. These agents are large, highly polar drugs with a quaternary structure rendering them unlikely to pass through lipid membranes. Succinylcholine is most commonly used to facilitate tracheal intubation in pregnant women, and none can be detected in the umbilical venous blood of the neonate born to a mother who has been given less than 300 mg. Similarly, Dailey *et al.*[39] demonstrated low F/M ratios for nondepolarizing muscle relaxants, reporting an F/M ratio of 0.11 for vecuronium and 0.19 for pancuronium. A more recent study places the F/M ratio for vecuronium even lower, at 0.056.[40]

FETAL EFFECTS

Direct effects of anesthesia on the fetus

Some anesthetic agents can be shown to have some immediate effects on the fetus when administered to the pregnant mother. These effects are seen either at delivery or *in utero* with ultrasonic monitoring. Most of the fetal effects seen at delivery parallel those seen in the mother, such as the respiratory depressant effects of narcotics. Other effects can be seen by fetal heart rate monitoring, such as the loss of beat-to-beat variability and the sinusoidal pattern seen occasionally with narcotic administration, or even severe fetal bradycardia seen with spinal sufentanil. A single 50-μg dose of intravenous fentanyl can even be shown to have an adverse effect on the fetal biophysical profile. Induction agents used for cesarean section may cause fetal depression that will become evident upon delivery. Midazolam has been shown to cause more neonatal depression than propofol, and both cause more neonatal depression than thiopental.[41–43] Unless delivery of the fetus is imminent, as with cesarean section, the clinical relevance of these depressant effects of narcotics and induction agents is questionable. Although it has been suggested that volatile anesthetics will cause fetal depression that manifests in the neonate at cesarean section, this probably will occur only with prolonged incision-to-delivery times. In fact, Gambling *et al.*[44] found no difference in neonatal outcome up to 24 h between spinal block, sevoflurane, or isoflurane anesthesia. Fetal effects of nitrous oxide have been studied, and the potential for diffusion hypoxia at birth has been suggested but not proved. At doses approaching twice the MAC, however, significant *in utero* effects can be seen, with a decreased fetal cardiac output potentially causing fetal acidosis. Reports exist of maternally administered succinylcholine causing neonatal hypotonus, but this should only be expected either when unusually large doses are used or perhaps when a fetus has a pseudocholinesterase deficiency. The nondepolarizing muscle relaxants vecuronium, pancuronium, and rocuronium do not have clinically significant effects on the fetus or neonate under standard clinical circumstances.

Teratogenicity is defined as the propensity of a substance or etiologic factor to cause abnormalities of development, which manifest as structural or functional defects in the postnatal organism. Thalidomide also serves as an example of a drug that, despite being shown not to have teratogenic effects in animals, proved to be a potent teratogen in humans. Others, such as diethylstilbestrol, may have more subtle effects, requiring the offspring to reach reproductive age before manifestations are revealed. Both practical and ethical constraints prevent the teratogenicity of anesthetic agents being studied in humans. Therefore, current information comes from other sources, including animal studies, epidemiological studies in healthcare workers exposed to chronic subclinical levels of inhalational agents while pregnant, and outcome studies from women who have undergone anesthesia while pregnant.

Although no clear evidence exists to suggest that any of the currently used anesthetic induction agents, inhalational agents, narcotics, local anesthetics, or muscle relaxants are human teratogens, two specific examples deserve further discussion: nitrous oxide and benzodiazepines.

Nitrous oxide

The first evidence of nitrous oxide teratogenicity was published in 1967.[45] Subsequently, multiple studies on rodents confirmed the teratogenic potential of nitrous oxide. Various abnormalities have been produced, including skeletal and visceral malformations. Even when directly exposing rat embryos grown in culture to nitrous oxide, morphologic abnormalities are produced, demonstrating a direct effect on the embryonic tissue.[46] Furthermore, when xenon, a biologically inert gas with anesthetic properties similar to nitrous oxide, was compared with MAC-equivalent nitrous oxide exposure, anomalies occurred only in the rats anesthetized with nitrous oxide,[47] eliminating the likelihood that fetal abnormalities were a consequence of the maternal anesthetic state. Although the mechanism of nitrous oxide teratogenicity is not fully understood, it has been shown to inactivate methionine synthase via oxidation of vitamin B_{12}, which could lead to decreased DNA synthesis in the developing embryo. In spite of clear evidence for the teratogenicity of nitrous oxide in animals, no such evidence exists in women who have been exposed to nitrous oxide during surgery. It seems likely that the prolonged exposure to high concentrations of nitrous oxide required to cause abnormalities in animal embryos represents conditions which are not encountered under normal circumstances of clinical anesthesia. Even so, it is wise to carefully consider relative benefits and potential risks of using nitrous oxide in the pregnant woman during the period of embryogenesis.

Benzodiazepines

In 1975, both Saxen and Saxen[48] and Safra and Oakley[49] implicated an association between diazepam and oral clefts. Their studies were soon criticized for methodologic flaws, such as failure to control or to take into account other potentially important etiologic factors such as substance abuse, other drug use, medical conditions such as epilepsy and diabetes, and environmental exposure. Indeed, multiple subsequent studies have failed to verify the conclusions that they drew to explain the role of diazepam in the development of the oral cleft. Nevertheless, just as with nitrous oxide, it seems prudent to avoid the use of benzodiazepines early in pregnancy unless absolutely necessary or when alternatives are not available.

Chronic exposure in healthcare workers

The medical literature is replete with studies of chronic exposure of gestating animals to anesthetic and subanesthetic doses of inhalational agents, and the results are somewhat conflicting. Regardless of the conclusions of these animal studies, carried out mostly in rodents, their applicability to pregnant women working in an operating room or dentist's office is questionable. Occupational exposure to anesthetic gases has been cited in early epidemiologic studies as an important cause of both congenital anomalies and spontaneous abortion.[50–54] Upon careful critical analysis of these studies, however, it becomes clear that they suffer from flaws that make their conclusions dubious. For instance, the study reporting an increased incidence of miscarriage among dental workers drew conclusions based on questionnaires that are more likely to be returned by those women who have had reportable outcomes. Additionally, these studies failed to report or control for other factors known to increase the risks for reproductive problems, such as smoking, alcohol abuse, and other drug abuse. Then, in 1991, catecholamine levels were shown to be significantly elevated in pregnant healthcare workers when compared with nonworking pregnant controls, and it was suggested that this could be another factor contributing to an increased reproductive risk.[55] Subsequent epidemiologic studies failed to confirm the conclusions drawn by the reports published in the 1970s. In 1985, Ericson and Kallen[56] in Sweden and Hemminki *et al.*[57] in Finland found no statistically significant difference in miscarriage or malformations when comparing nurses exposed to anesthetic gases with a control group of nurses. Two years later, Spence[58] published a prospective survey that also found no differences in reproductive outcome when comparing female anesthesiologists with other female physicians. Yet the controversy continues. A recent meta-analysis performed using data from 19 previously published reports concluded that the overall risk for spontaneous abortion as much as doubles for women with a history of occupational exposure to waste gases.[59] Although the author suggests that modern gas scavenging has reduced or eliminated this risk, environmental levels of desflurane and sevoflurane in the recovery room and intensive care unit in 1998 were shown to exceed the legal limits for workplace concentrations prescribed by German maternity law.[60]

Nonobstetric surgery in pregnant women

Another source of data on the direct effects of anesthetic agents on the fetus are pregnant women who have undergone a surgical procedure during pregnancy. The surgery was in no case elective, and the indications range from liver transplantation to pheochromocytoma, with appendectomy and cholecystectomy being much more common. Cardiopulmonary bypass during pregnancy has also been described. Multiple studies have been published primarily in the form of retrospective reviews, and none has demonstrated an increased risk for anomalies.

A far greater concern for the anesthesiologist is the risk of *preterm labor*. An increased incidence of preterm labor has been a consistent finding in studies examining the risks of anesthesia in pregnant women. The risk of preterm labor increases when the surgery involves the abdomen or when surgery is performed in either the first or third trimester, and is as high as 21% after exploratory laparotomy.[61] Although one may hypothesize that the depressant effect of volatile agents on uterine muscle might make general anesthesia more "protective" against preterm labor than regional anesthesia, no evidence exists to suggest one technique is superior to the other. Consultation with an obstetrician and postoperative monitoring for preterm labor is strongly recommended, as tocolysis or emergent delivery may become necessary.

Indirect effects of anesthesia on the fetus

Although a great deal of attention has been given to teratogenicity and other direct effects of anesthetics on the fetus, the greatest risks posed by anesthesia are those that are indirect and are far more mundane. Fortunately, they are also for the most part preventable. The anesthesiologist caring for the pregnant patient must always be vigilant to assure adequate uteroplacental perfusion. The mechanisms have been described by which both regional anesthesia and general anesthesia can decrease blood pressure and therefore reduce UBF. If not rapidly treated, fetal distress and eventually asphyxia may result. During general anesthesia, hypoxemia can occur rapidly, especially upon induction and emergence. Fetal distress may be prevented by adequate preoxygenation prior to induction, and by using 100% oxygen upon emergence. The endotracheal tube should be removed only when the muscle relaxation has been reversed and the patient is known to be fully awake. Placement of the patient such that the uterus is displaced to the left can help alleviate the decreased UBF caused by aortocaval compression. Finally, both hypocarbia and hypercarbia can cause a decrease in UBF, and can be prevented by choosing appropriate minute ventilation. High peak airway pressures reached when giving inappropriately high tidal volumes can exacerbate the decrease in UBF caused by hypocarbia. The resulting high intrathoracic pressures can reduce preload to the heart, leading to systemic hypotension and decreased UBF.

REFERENCES

1. Moya F, Smith BE. Uptake distribution of placental transport of drugs and anesthetic. *Anesthesiology* 1965; **26:** 465–76.
2. Palahniuk RJ, Shnider SM. Maternal and fetal cardiovascular and acid–base changes during halothane and isoflurane anesthesia in the pregnant ewe. *Anesthesiology* 1974; **41:** 462–72.
3. Palahniuk RJ, Shnider SM, Eger II EI. Pregnancy decreases the requirement for inhaled anesthetic agents. *Anesthesiology* 1974; **41:** 82–3.
4. Gin T, Chan MTV. Decreased minimum alveolar concentration of isoflurane in pregnant humans. *Anesthesiology* 1994; **81:** 829–32.
5. Assali NS, Prystowsky H. Studies on autonomic blockade. I. Comparison between the effects of tetraethelamonium chloride (TEAC) and a high select of spinal anesthesia on blood pressure of normal and toxemic pregnancies. *J Clin Invest* 1950; **29:** 1354–66.
6. McLaughlin MK, Keve TM, Cooke R. Vascular catecholamine sensitivity during pregnancy in the ewe. *Am J Obstet Gynecol* 1989; **160:** 47–53.
7. Tong C, Eisenach JC. The vascular mechanism of ephedrine's beneficial effect on uterine perfusion during pregnancy. *Anesthesiology* 1992; **76:** 792–8.
8. Wright PM, Iftikhar M, Fitzpatrick KT, Moore J, Thompson W. Vasopressor therapy for hypotension during epidural anesthesia for cesarean section: effects on maternal and fetal flow velocity ratios. *Anesth Analg* 1992; **75:** 56–63.

9. Norris MC, Grieco W, Arkoosh VA. Does continuous intravenous infusion of low-concentration epinephrine impair uterine blood flow in pregnant ewes? *Reg Anesth* 1995; **20:** 206–11.
10. Dunlop W. Serial changes in renal haemodynamics during normal human pregnancy. *Br J Obstet Gynaecol* 1981; **88:** 1–9.
11. Ezimokhai M, Davison JM, Phillip PR, Dunlop W. Non-postural serial changes in renal function during the third trimester of normal human pregnancy. *Br J Obstet Gynaecol* 1981; **88:** 465–71.
12. Davison JM, Hytten FE. The effect of pregnancy on the renal handling of glucose. *Br J Obstet Gynaecol* 1975; **82:** 374–81.
13. Ward SJ, Rocke DA. Neuromuscular blocking drugs in pregnancy and the puerperium. *Int J Obstet Anesth* 1998; **7:** 251–60.
14. Chan MTE, Gin T. Postpartum changes in the minimum alveolar concentration of isoflurane. *Anesthesiology* 1995; **82:** 1360–3.
15. Abouleish E. Postpartum tubal ligation requires more bupivacaine for spinal anesthesia than does cesarean section. *Anesth Analg* 1986; **65:** 897–900.
16. Datta S, Hurley R, Naulty S, *et al.* Plasma and cerebral spinal fluid progesterone concentrations in pregnant and non-pregnancy women. *Anesth Analg* 1986; **65:** 950–4.
17. Hirabayashi Y, Shimizu R, Saitoh K, Fukuda H. Cerebral spinal fluid progesterone in pregnant women. *Br J Anaesth* 1995; **75:** 683–7.
18. Dietz FB, Jaffe RA. Pregnancy does not increase susceptibility to bupivacaine in spinal root axons. *Anesthesiology* 1997; **87:** 610–16.
19. Bromage PR. *Epidural Analgesia*. Philadelphia: W B Saunders, 1978: 525.
20. Fragraeus L, Urban BR, Bromage PR. Spread of epidural analgesia in early pregnancy. *Anesthesiology* 1983; **58:** 184–7.
21. Grundy EM, Zamora AM, Winnie AP. Comparison of spread of epidural anesthesia in pregnant and non-pregnant women. *Anesth Analg* 1978; **57:** 544–6.
22. Morishima HO, Pedersen H, Finster M, *et al.* Bupivacaine toxicity in pregnant and nonpregnant ewes. *Anesthesiology* 1985; **63:** 134–9.
23. Santos AC, Arthur GR, Wlody D, *et al.* Comparative systemic toxicity of ropivacaine and bupivacaine in nonpregnant and pregnant ewes. *Anesthesiology* 1995; **82:** 734–40.
24. Craft Jr JB, Coaldrake LA, Yonekura ML, *et al.* Ketamine, catecholamines, and uterine tone in pregnant ewes. *Am J Obstet Gynecol* 1983; **146:** 429–34.
25. Patton DE, Lee W, Miller J, Jones M. Maternal, uteroplacental, and fetoplacental hemodynamic and Doppler velocimetric changes during epidural anesthesia in normal labor. *Obstet Gynecol* 1991; **77:** 17–19.
26. Alahuhta S, Rasanen J, Jouppila R, *et al.* Uteroplacental and fetal haemodynamics during extradural anaesthesia for caesarean section. *Br J Anaesth* 1991; **66:** 319–24.
27. Huges AB, Devoe LD, Wakefield ML, Metheny WP. The effects of epidural anesthesia on the Doppler velocimetry of umbilical and uterine arteries in normal term labor. *Obstet Gynecol* 1990; **75:** 809–12.
28. Morrow RJ, Rolbin SH, Ritchie JW, Haley S. Epidural anaesthesia and blood flow velocity in mother and fetus. *Can J Anaesth* 1989; **36:** 519–22.
29. Wood M. Plasma binding and limitation of drug access to site of action. *Anesthesiology* 1991; **75:** 721–3.
30. Morishima HO, Heymann MA, Rudolph AM, *et al.* Transfer of lidocaine across the sheep placenta to the fetus. Hemodynamic and acid–base responses of the fetal lamb. *Am J Obstet Gynecol* 1975; **122:** 581–8.
31. Kuhnert BR, Zuspan KJ, Kuhnert PM, *et al.* Bupivacaine disposition in mother, fetus, and neonate after spinal anesthesia for cesarean section. *Anesth Analg* 1987; **66:** 407–12.
32. Houlton PJ, Downing JW, Buley RJ, Brock-Utne JG. Anaesthetic induction for caesarean section with etomidate compared with thiopentone. *S Afr Med J* 1978; **54:** 773–5.
33. Gregory MA, Davidson DG. Plasma etomidate levels in mother and fetus. *Anaesthesia* 1991; **46:** 716–18.
34. Ridd MJ, Brown KF, Nation RL, Collier CB. The disposition and placental transfer of diazepam in cesarean section. *Clin Pharmacol Ther* 1989; **45:** 506–12.
35. Guerre-Millo M, Rey E, Challier JC, *et al.* Transfer in vitro of three benzodiazepines across the human placenta. *Eur J Pharmacol* 1979; **15:** 171–3.
36. Conklin KA, Graham CW, Murad S, *et al.* Midazolam and diazepam: maternal and fetal effects in the pregnant ewe. *Obstet Gynecol* 1980; **56:** 471–4.
37. Hartvig P, Lindberg BS, Lilja A, *et al.* Positron emission tomography in studies on fetomaternal disposition of opioids. *Dev Pharmacol Ther* 1989; **12:** 74–80.
38. Wilson CM, McClean E, Moore J, Dundee JW. A double-blind comparison of intramuscular pethidine and nalbuphine in labour. *Anaesthesia* 1986; **41:** 1207–13.
39. Dailey PA, Fisher DM, Shnider SM, *et al.* Pharmacokinetics, placental transfer, and neonatal effects of vecuronium and pancuronium administered during cesarean section. *Anesthesiology* 1984; **60:** 569–74.
40. Iwama H, Kaneko T, Tobishima S, *et al.* Time dependency of the ratio of umbilical vein/maternal artery concentrations of vecuronium in caesarean section. *Acta Anaesthesiol Scand* 1999; **43:** 9–12.
41. Celleno D, Capogna G, Emanuelli M, *et al.* Which induction drug for cesarean section? A comparison of thiopental sodium, propofol, and midazolam. *J Clin Anesth* 1993; **4:** 284–8.
42. Bland BA, Lawes EG, Duncan PW, *et al.* Comparison of midazolam and thiopental for rapid sequence anesthetic induction for elective cesarean section. *Anesth Analg* 1987; **66:** 1165–8.
43. Celleno D, Capogna G, Tomassetti M, *et al.* Neurobehavioural effects of propofol on the neonate following elective caesarean section. *Br J Anaesth* 1989; **62:** 649–54.
44. Gambling DR, Sharma SK, White PF, *et al.* Use of sevoflurane during elective cesarean birth: a comparison with isoflurane and spinal anesthesia. *Anesth Analg* 1995; **81:** 90–5.
45. Fink BR, Shepard TH, Blandau RJ. Teratogenic activity of nitrous oxide. *Nature* 1967; **214:** 146–8.
46. Baden JM, Fujinaga M. Effects of nitrous oxide on day 9 rat embryos grown in culture. *Br J Anaesth* 1991; **66:** 500–3.
47. Lane GA, Nahrwold Ml, Tait AR, *et al.* Anesthetics as teratogens: nitrous oxide is teratogenic, xenon is not. *Science* 1980; **210:** 899–901.
48. Saxen I, Saxen L. Association between maternal intake of diazepam and oral clefts. *Lancet* 1975; **13:** 498.
49. Safra MJ, Oakley Jr GP. Association between cleft lip with or without cleft palate and prenatal exposure to diazepam. *Lancet* 1975; **13:** 478–80.
50. Cohen EN, Belville JW, Brown BW. Anesthesia, pregnancy, and miscarriage: a study of operating room nurses and anesthetists. *Anesthesiology* 1971; **35:** 343–7.
51. Knill-Jones RP, Moir DD, Rodrigues LV, Spence AA. Anaesthetic practice and pregnancy: controlled survey of women anaesthetists in the United Kingdom. *Lancet* 1972; **2:** 1326–8.
52. Cohen EN, Brown BW, Bruce DL, *et al.* Occupational disease among operating room personnel: a national study. *Anesthesiology* 1974; **41:** 321–40.
53. Cohen EN, Brown BW, Wu ML, *et al.* Occupational disease in dentistry and chronic exposure to trace anesthetic gases. *J Am Dent Assoc* 1980; **101:** 21–31.
54. Spence AA, Cohen EN, Brown BW. Occupational hazards for operating room-based physicians. *JAMA* 1977; **283:** 955–9.
55. Katz VL, Jenkins T, Haley L, Bowes Jr WA. Catecholamine levels in pregnant physicians and nurses: a pilot study of stress and pregnancy. *Obstet Gynecol* 1991; **77:** 338–42.
56. Ericson HA, Kallen AJ. Hospitalization for miscarriage and delivery outcome among Swedish nurses working in operating rooms 1973–1978. *Anesth Analg* 1985; **64:** 981–8.
57. Hemminki K, Kyronen P, Lindbohm ML. Spontaneous abortions and malformations in the offspring of nurses exposed to anaesthetic gases, cytostatic drugs, and other potential hazards in hospitals, based on registered information of outcome. *J Epidemiol Community Health* 1985; **39:** 141–7.
58. Spence AA. Environmental pollution by inhalation anaesthetics. *Br J Anaesth* 1987; **59:** 96–103.
59. Boivin JF. Risk of spontaneous abortion in women occupationally exposed to anaesthetic gases: a metaanalysis. *Occup Environ Med* 1997; **54:** 541–8.
60. Byhahn C, Westphal K, Strouhal U. Maternal protection law and exposure of personnel in the recover room and surgical intensive care unit by inhalation anesthetics. *Gesundheitswesen* 1998; **60:** 586–91.
61. Liang CC, Hsieh TT, Chang SD. Appendicitis during pregnancy. *Chang Keng I Hsueh* 1989; **12:** 208–14.

57

Obstetric anesthesia

RACHEL A FARRAGHER AND BHAVANI SHANKAR KODALI

Obstetric anesthesia has developed over the last 150 years, and has grown into a dominant specialty of its own. This parallels an important change in the philosophical thinking and attitude to the relief of pain in labor. The safety of obstetric anesthesia has increased, primarily as a result of the awareness of local anesthetic toxicity and the increased use of regional anesthesia. Maternal mortality directly related to anesthesia has dramatically decreased. This chapter outlines the safe conduct of analgesic and anesthetic techniques for parturients. Current opinion on the role of newer techniques, such as combined spinal–epidural analgesia and walking epidurals, is discussed. No techniques are immune to controversy. Thus, a section on current controversies in obstetric anesthesia has been included. The current thinking on the effect of regional anesthesia on both the progress and outcome of labor is detailed. As anesthesiologists working in general surgery may still encounter pregnant patients, we describe the principles of anesthesia for nonobstetric surgery during pregnancy. The anesthetic implications of pre-eclampsia are reviewed, and specific considerations for other high-risk obstetric patients are highlighted. Modern practice has resulted in a consistently diminishing incidence of maternal deaths that can be directly attributed to anesthesia.

HISTORY OF OBSTETRIC ANESTHESIA

Obstetric anesthesia has had a turbulent history since its first use in Scotland in 1847 when James Young Simpson administered diethyl ether to a woman during delivery.[1] Great opposition followed; this was a time when the concept of pain had theologic connotations and was not viewed as a biologic process. Despite controversy, physicians quickly incorporated anesthesia into clinical practice, largely as a result of patient demand. Queen Victoria received chloroform during childbirth in 1853.

In the early twentieth century, a technique of repeated morphine and scopolamine injections became popular. This twilight sleep often led to severe maternal and neonatal respiratory depression. In 1900, spinal cocaine was used for labor analgesia; 2 years later the first cesarean delivery under spinal anesthesia was performed in the USA. The subsequent frequent use of spinal anesthesia, often by inexperienced personnel and without monitoring, led to frequent complications and brought discredit on the technique. At the time, the mortality rate for cesarean deliveries performed under spinal anesthesia was reported to be 1 in 139. These negative experiences resulted in the abandonment of pain relief in obstetrics until the 1950s, a period often described as the dark age of obstetric anesthesia. During this time, natural childbirth and psychoprophylaxis became popular.[2]

Obstetric anesthetic research first emerged as a real endeavor more than 30 years ago.[3] Improvements in equipment design, advances in opioid and local anesthetic pharmacology, awareness of toxicity, and new techniques have brought us to the present time, and have made regional anesthesia the method of choice for labor analgesia. Of the 3 700 000 women estimated to give birth each year in the USA, 20–50% receive regional anesthesia during labor and delivery.[4]

PERIOPERATIVE CONSIDERATIONS BASED ON PHYSIOLOGIC CHANGES

There are five important physiologic changes that have direct bearing on the clinical anesthetic management of obstetric patients. These are (1) airway changes posing intubation difficulties; (2) metabolic and respiratory changes resulting in profound hypoxemia during apnea; (3) gastrointestinal changes predisposing the parturient to regurgitation and aspiration; (4) pressure effects of the gravid uterus on the aorta and inferior vena cava resulting in the supine hypotensive syndrome of pregnancy; and (5) mechanical, hormonal, and biochemical factors that can result in an increased spread of intrathecal and epidural drugs. These are discussed in greater detail in Chapter 21.

The incidence of failed endotracheal intubation is approximately 1:280 to 1:300 in obstetric patients.[5,6] This is considerably higher than in other surgical patients (1:2230).[6] The majority (41%) of maternal deaths attributed to anesthesia are a result of intubation difficulties and their consequences, such as failed ventilation and oxygenation, and/or pulmonary aspiration.[7,8] It is stated that most difficult intubations in obstetrics are unanticipated.[5,9] Furthermore, anesthesiologists must be aware that there are some obstetric patients whom they may never be able to intubate, irrespective of their experience. Failure to anticipate difficult to intubate patients before embarking on general anesthesia, and an inability to oxygenate a parturient with a difficult airway, contributes to significant anesthesia-related morbidity and mortality.[10,11] Pregnancy produces several changes that influence the airway. As the bony structures remain virtually unchanged, the problem resides with the soft tissues and their mobility, with perhaps secondary effects on the mobility of the bony structures.[12]

During pregnancy, capillary engorgement of the nasopharyngeal and laryngeal mucosa, disposition of fat, tongue enlargement, and increased venous pressure with subsequent tissue engorgement may not only reduce the dimensions of the pharyngeal space during intubation, but may also make elevation of the hyoid bone difficult during larngoscopy.[13] There is an increased incidence of class IV airways (37–56%)

among pregnant women at 38 weeks' gestation compared with nonpregnant women or women in early pregnancy.[14,15] Furthermore, the onset and progress of labor can induce edema of the oropharynx and change the airway classification from a Mallampati class I–II at the beginning to a class III–IV at the end of labor.[16,17] Pre-eclampsia further worsens the airway as a result of enhanced fluid accumulation in the larngopharynx.[18]

A careful airway evaluation must be performed in every parturient at risk for cesarean delivery, and should be repeated in those in whom labor is prolonged. In a study of 1500 parturients[19] requiring general anesthesia for cesarean delivery, only 16 out of 27 inadequate exposures occurred in class III or IV airways, with the remainder in class I and II. Thus, in addition to visualizing the oropharyngeal structures, other factors, such as obesity, neck mobility, short thyromental distance, protruding upper teeth, and excessive weight gain in pregnancy should be taken into account.[15,19] Adjuvant equipment should be readily available, in all anesthetizing locations, to manage an unanticipated difficult airway.

The enlarging gravid uterus can compress the inferior vena cava and abdominal aorta against the lumbar vertebrae. This results in reduced uteroplacental perfusion by three mechanisms: (1) decreased venous return reduces preload and cardiac output; (2) obstructed uterine venous drainage increases uterine venous pressure and decreases uterine perfusion pressure; and (3) compression of the aorta and common iliac arteries decreases perfusion pressure in the uterine arteries. It is, therefore, essential to maintain left uterine displacement in every parturient before and during cesarean delivery.[20]

Gastric stasis is a common phenomenon in pregnancy. It is due to the effects of progesterone, mechanical consequences of the growing uterus, and the pain, fear, and anxiety of labor. Pain and opioid administration during labor further decrease the rate of gastric emptying.[21] Gastric stasis predisposes parturients to gastroesophageal reflux and regurgitation, emesis, and pulmonary aspiration of gastric contents, particularly when airway reflexes are diminished. A gastric pH of 2.5, and gastric volume of greater than 0.4 $mL\,kg^{-1}$, or approximately 25 mL in the adult, poses an increased risk of aspiration pneumonitis. In one study, the presence of high gastric volume (>25 mL) and a low pH (<2.5) was observed in 2% of parturients who had oral antacid therapy, and 27% of parturients who had no antacid, or antacid within 4 h,[22] regardless of the time between the last meal and onset of labor. It is therefore prudent to take steps to reduce the volume and acidity of gastric contents in order to minimize the aspiration risk.

Oral antacids should be mandatory before the induction of anesthesia for all parturients. Thirty milliliters of 0.3 $mol\,L^{-1}$ sodium citrate, administered 1 h before induction of anesthesia for cesarean delivery, maintained gastric pH at >2.5 until the end of surgery[23,24]. Metoclopramide, a dopamine antagonist, increases lower esophageal sphincter (LES) tone, is a prokinetic, sensitizes gastric muscle to the effects of acetylcholine[25–27] and has central antiemetic effects. It can have significant effects on gastric volume as early as 15 min after administration.[28] Histamine (H_2) receptor antagonists, such as cimetidine and ranitidine, decrease basal gastric acid secretion and volume within 60–90 min, but have no effect on acid already secreted into the stomach. Oral cimetidine, 400 mg given 3–4 h preoperatively, followed by oral antacid 1–2 h before induction, has been shown to be more efficacious than either agent alone.[29] Anticholinergics, such as atropine 7 $\mu g\,kg^{-1}$ i.m. or glycopyrrolate 4 $\mu g\,kg^{-1}$, used in combination with oral antacid are six times more efficacious in reducing the number of parturients at risk of acid aspiration than oral antacid alone.[30] However, these agents decrease LES tone and increase the potential for gastroesophageal reflux.[31] It remains controversial as to at what gestational age and postpartum period intubation should be considered routine to protect the airway during general anesthesia. In practice, most anesthesiologists will secure the airway between 14 weeks of pregnancy and 48 h post partum, in the absence of other factors.

In the parturient, hemoglobin desaturation follows even brief periods of apnea, as a result of increased oxygen consumption and decreased pulmonary functional residual capacity. Apnea lasting 1 min has been found to reduce oxygen tension by 139 mmHg (18.5 kPa) in parturients, compared with 58 mmHg (7.7 kPa) in nonpregnant women.[32] This leads to two important clinical implications. Firstly, it is essential to begin mask ventilation early rather than persist with intubation attempts. Secondly, it is necessary to improve maternal oxygen reserve and neonatal outcome by adequate preoxygenation. Three minutes of preoxygenation, or four vital capacity breaths within 30 s of induction, satisfactorily increases maternal oxygenation. The latter technique is of particular value when fetal distress is present and rapid induction of anesthesia is necessary.[33]

Pregnancy is associated with increased central spread of local anesthetic, such that 30–50% less drug is required for a given level of spinal or epidural anesthesia. This may be due to mechanical, hormonal, and biochemical factors associated with pregnancy. Caval compression causes engorgement of the epidural venous plexus, reducing the compliance of the epidural space and decreasing spinal cerebrospinal fluid (CSF) volume.[34] Bearing-down during labor accentuates these effects. The exaggerated lumbar lordosis of pregnancy can further increase the spread of local anesthetic. Hormonal and biochemical factors contributing to a higher drug spread in pregnancy include progesterone, increased endorphin levels, lower CSF proteins, and decreased CSF buffering capacity.[25,35]

PREANESTHETIC ASSESSMENT OF THE PARTURIENT

The preanesthetic assessment of the parturient should be conducted in the same thorough fashion as for all patients. However, owing to the unpredictable nature of obstetrics, we are frequently confronted with acute cases, removing our ability to plan anesthetic care in advance. The antenatal visit is an ideal opportunity to identify any coexisting medical conditions, determine the influence of pregnancy on the patient, and to assess any potential anesthetic difficulties, allowing us to plan anesthetic options and care. This requires good communication with obstetricians and midwives. Most obstetric units have either a distinct preanesthetic assessment clinic or an arrangement to refer patients directly from the antenatal clinic to the obstetric anesthesia service for evaluation. The anesthesiologist must be familiar with the physiologic changes of pregnancy and their anesthetic implications.

Important factors to note in the history are indications for, and the urgency of, the procedure, fasting time, gestational age, fetal well-being, the presence of any pregnancy-related pathology (such as pre-eclampsia) and any contraindications to regional anesthetic techniques. Any sciatica or pregnancy-related backache should also be documented.

Specific considerations in the physical examination of a parturient should include anticipation of a difficult airway by means of a focused airway examination. Height and weight are measured to warn of potential technical difficulties with regional or general techniques. A neurologic examination prior to neuraxial blockade may be indicated by the history, and the lumbar region should be examined prior to regional techniques. A full blood count is considered routine, and additional investigations may be ordered as clinically indicated.

OBSTETRIC PAIN PATHWAYS

Labor pain has both visceral and somatic components. Pain during the first stage of labor is visceral in nature and results primarily from uterine contractions and dilation of the cervix. The lower uterine segment and the cervix have the same afferent supply as the body of the uterus.[36] Pain is transmitted by Aδ and C afferent nerve fibers, which travel with sympathetic nerves to the uterine and cervical plexuses; the pelvic (inferior hypogastric) plexus; and the middle and superior hypogastric and aortic plexuses. They then pass to the lumbar and lower thoracic sympathetic chain and terminate in the dorsal horn of the spinal cord at the T10 to L1 segments (see Fig. 57.1). As is typical of visceral pain, the pain of uterine contractions is referred to the dermatomes supplied by the same spinal cord segments that receive input from the uterus and cervix.[38] Parasympathetic innervation of the uterus does not appear to play a role in uterocervical pain mediation.

During the late first stage and throughout the second stage of labor, when the cervix is fully dilated, nociceptive stimulation continues from uterine body contractions and distension of the lower uterine segment. There is a progressive increase in somatic pain resulting from distension of the pelvic floor, vagina, and perineum by the descending fetus. Pain is transmitted primarily by the pudendal nerve, which is derived from the anterior primary divisions of sacral nerves S2, S3, and S4. Peripheral innervation of the perineum is provided by the ilioinguinal nerve and the genital branch of the genitofemoral nerve anteriorly and by the posterior femoral cutaneous nerve laterally. Like other somatic pain, the perineal pain is sharp and well localized.

During cesarean delivery, additional nociceptive pathways are involved in the transmission of pain. A horizontal Pfannenstiel incision is usual and involves the infraumbilical T11 to T12 dermatomes. During surgery, stretching of the skin may involve dermatomes 2–4 levels higher. Intraperitoneal manipulation and dissection involve poorly localized visceral pain pathways, therefore requiring a T4 level sensory block.

PAIN RELIEF DURING LABOR

Labor and delivery result in severe pain for many women. The McGill Pain Questionnaire ranks labor pain in the upper part of the pain scale between that of cancer pain and amputation of a digit.[39] Melzack *et al.*[40] also demonstrated that the severity of labor pain varies greatly, with nulliparous women experiencing greater pain. Studies suggest that severe labor pain is a predictor of dystocia,[41] and it is well known that an occiput-posterior position typically results in more pain. Furthermore, many women retrospectively devalue the intensity of their pain.[42]

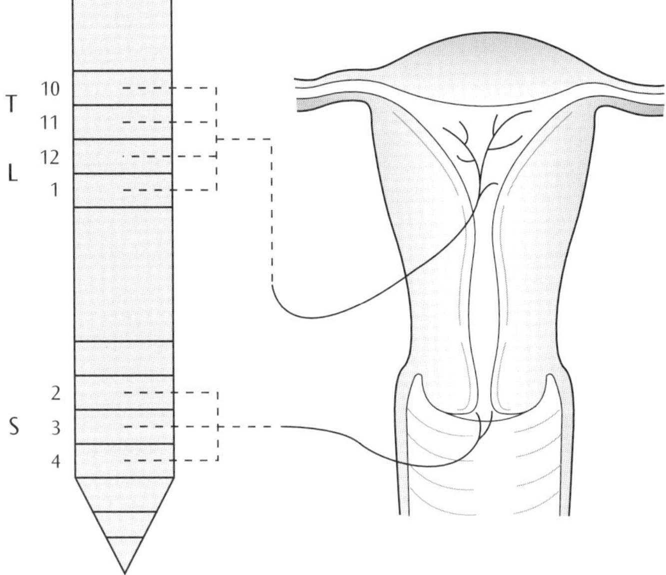

Figure 57.1 *Obstetric pain pathways. (From Datta[37] with permission.)*

Effects of labor pain

Painful contractions result in maternal hyperventilation, causing respiratory alkalosis, a leftward shift of the oxyhemoglobin dissociation curve, and increased maternal hemoglobin oxygen affinity. Hypocarbia also leads to hypoventilation between contractions, which may decrease maternal P_{aO_2}. There is a further increase in oxygen consumption during painful labor. These factors, in addition to hypocarbic uteroplacental vasoconstriction, are potential causes of fetal hypoxemia. Cardiac output increases by 10–25% and blood pressure by 5–20% with each contraction. Maternal plasma catecholamine concentrations are increased. Although most mothers and fetuses do not suffer harm as a result of these cyclic changes, effective analgesia likely provides an advantage for the high-risk parturient (those with pre-eclampsia or cardiac disease) and those with marginal uteroplacental circulation and function.

Antenatal education

In 1940, Eappen and Robbins[43] originated the concept of natural childbirth, teaching that relaxation techniques and the elimination of fear would prevent labor pain. Fernand Lamaze first introduced psychoprophylaxis. The Lamaze[44] method involves focusing on objects or breathing exercises to distract from pain, and allows for the use of conventional analgesic drugs. Although taught extensively, there is a lack of scientific validation of the efficacy of these methods. Patients have been found to be able to use coping techniques in the early first stage of labor, but less so as labor progresses. Prepared childbirth does not mean nonpharmacologic analgesia. Most modern instructors provide information about the elementary physiology of pregnancy and delivery, aim to reduce fear, teach relaxation and breathing exercises, and make a fair presentation of the advantages and disadvantages of various analgesic techniques. Patient expectation concerning labor influences the childbirth experience. Success should be defined as a positive childbirth experience, regardless of the mode of delivery, use of analgesia, or other arbitrary definitions. Well-informed patients are more likely to accept the interventions that may become necessary during labor.

Nonpharmacologic analgesic techniques

These techniques include the therapeutic use of heat and cold, hydrotherapy, vertical position, hypnosis, acupuncture, and transcutaneous electrical stimulation (TENS). Hot or cold compresses may be placed over the lower back or perineum to decrease pain perception. Proposed benefits of hydrotherapy include relaxation, reduced anxiety and pain, and increased efficiency of uterine contractions. Regarding the vertical position, one prospective randomized trial noted that walking neither shortened the first stage of labor nor reduced the need for oxytocin augmentation, use of analgesia, or operative delivery.[45] Ambulation may not produce shorter, less painful labor; rather, it may be that shorter, less painful labor allows continued ambulation. Hypnosis has been used for a long time for the relief of labor pain, but with a relatively small success rate. There has not been widespread use of acupuncture in obstetric patients, resulting in a lack of standardization of acupuncture points to be stimulated. Studies show conflicting results. TENS has been used for the relief of labor pain with varied success. Skin electrodes are placed over the T10–L1 spinal region bilaterally, and over the sacral area during the second stage of labor.

Ultimate success from the techniques described above depends greatly upon the motivation of the parturient, with the result that success varies and these modes have not been universally accepted. No nonpharmacologic technique consistently provides the quality of intrapartum pain relief that is provided by regional analgesia.

SYSTEMIC ANALGESIA IN LABOR

Inhalational analgesia

This technique involves the inhalation of subanesthetic concentrations of an agent while the mother remains awake with intact protective laryngeal reflexes. It can be used alone or in combination with other methods of analgesia. Entonox is a 50% mixture of nitrous oxide and oxygen and is delivered via a demand valve through a low-resistance breathing system. As it takes 45 s for the analgesic effect to be achieved, the parturient should start breathing Entonox at the start of a contraction, so that an adequate brain concentration can be achieved at the contraction peak. Deep, slow breathing and abstinence between contractions is encouraged. The parturient may breathe Entonox prior to expulsive efforts during the second stage. When properly applied, Entonox has been reported to provide significant pain relief in 50% of mothers.[46] At this concentration, nitrous oxide does not interfere with uterine activity.[47] Maternal cooperation is required as unscavenged nitrous oxide may cause environmental pollution. All apparatus must be checked regularly to avoid inhalation of 100% oxygen first, followed by nitrous oxide resulting from the gas mixture becoming separated, as may occur at low temperatures.

The efficacy of small concentrations of halothane, enflurane, isoflurane, and desflurane in labor, alone and in combination with nitrous oxide, has been demonstrated.[48–50] As the effects of inhalational agents and systemic opioids are additive, some practitioners express concern regarding potential loss of consciousness and aspiration. Entonox is the only method of inhalational analgesia in standard use; however, it is used much more commonly in Europe than in the USA.

Parenteral agents

There is free placental transfer of opioids, therefore their use in labor is a compromise between effective analgesia and unwanted side-effects. Morphine is associated with a higher incidence of neonatal respiratory depression than other opioids and is not a popular agent for obstetric patients. Opioids may result in a transient (30–60 min) loss of beat-to-beat variability of the fetal heart rate. Meperidine (pethidine) is the most commonly used opioid. It can be given in doses of 50–100 mg intramuscularly or 25–50 mg intravenously, every 2–4 h, with onset times of 45 and 5 min and maximum neonatal respiratory depression occurring at 3 h and 20 min respectively. Consequently, the best timing for birth would be within the first hour, or more than 4 h after maternal administration, depending on route of administration. Normeperidine (norpethidine) is an active metabolite that also crosses the placenta and is a potent respiratory depressant. A phenothiazine is often given with meperidine to diminish nausea and vomiting.

Fentanyl is a rapid-acting and short-lasting opioid with no active metabolites. Its peak effect occurs 3–5 min after intravenous use. Fentanyl 100 μg is equipotent to 10 mg morphine and 100 mg meperidine. Sufentanil, alfentanil, and remifentanil have been used in labor, but a dosing regimen has not been established for their systemic administration. Intravenous administration is superior to intramuscular injection as there is less variability in peak plasma concentrations and faster onset of analgesia.

Patient-controlled analgesia (PCA) is widely used in the management of postoperative pain and has been used for labor pain. Purported advantages of PCA include superior analgesia at lower doses, resulting in less maternal respiratory depression than with bolus administration, less placental transfer, less emesis, and higher patient satisfaction. Smaller, more frequent dosing should result in a more stable plasma concentration and a more consistent analgesic effect.[51] Owing to the fluctuating intensity of labor pain, small doses of opioids may not always be effective. Meperidine, fentanyl, and the mixed agonist/antagonist nalbuphine are the most frequently used opioids for PCA administration, with bolus doses of 10–15 mg, 10–25 μg, and 1–3 mg respectively.[52] Most studies have examined on-demand dosing only, without a continuous background infusion. PCA is an attractive alternative for labor analgesia in settings in which regional anesthesia is either unavailable or contraindicated.[53]

Butorphanol and nalbuphine are mixed agonist/antagonist opioids which are very popular, especially in the USA, for the relief of labor pain. These drugs do cause respiratory depression, but exhibit a ceiling effect with increasing doses. Butorphanol is associated with 75% incidence of transient sinusoidal fetal heart rate pattern.[54] For this reason, although benign, and because of maternal sedation, nalbuphine 10 mg i.v. has become the drug of choice at our institution.

Phenothiazines are often used in combination with opioids in obstetric patients for their anxiolytic and antiemetic properties. However, these agents can also cause a reduction in the beat-to-beat variability of the fetal heart rate. Promethazine 25–50 mg is the most commonly used and is a mild respiratory stimulant. Ketamine, a phencyclidine derivative, in doses of 10–20 mg intravenously produces good analgesia in 2–5 min without loss of consciousness. Doses up to 1 mg kg^{-1} do not cause fetal depression and have no effect on uterine tone. Although its short duration of action makes ketamine unsuitable for first-stage analgesia, it may be effective just prior to vaginal delivery or as an adjuvant to regional anesthesia. The potential for unpleasant psychomimetic effects must be borne in mind, but the incidence may be lower with lower doses.

EPIDURAL ANALGESIA IN LABOR

Neuraxial analgesia is the most effective and least depressant method of intrapartum pain relief in current practice.[55] Epidural analgesia offers great versatility in extent and duration of effect. Segmental lumbar analgesia can be tailored for the first stage and extended into the sacral segments for the second stage of labor.

Effects of epidural analgesia

By providing effective pain relief, epidural analgesia attenuates the adverse physiological responses to pain mentioned above. In addition, effective epidural analgesia reduces maternal catecholamine levels, increasing intervillous blood flow, and results in improved uteroplacental perfusion.[56] A greater effect is seen in patients with pre-eclampsia.[57] Local anesthetics, at clinically used concentrations, do not have a direct effect on uterine activity. Neonatal effects may occur, indirectly, from reduced uteroplacental perfusion due to hypotension. The duration and degree of maternal hypotension are important factors in fetal hypoxia and consequent neonatal neurobehavioral changes. The effects of epidural analgesia on the progress of labor are controversial and will be discussed later.

Indications

Epidural analgesia as a method of pain relief is most often requested by the patient; however, there are some women who will obtain particular benefit. Epidural analgesia blunts the hemodynamic effects of contractions and the associated pain response, which is desirable for patients with hypertensive disorders, asthma, diabetes, and cardiac and intracranial neurovascular disease. Epidural analgesia is specifically indicated when tracheal intubation is expected to be difficult or impossible, as the block can be extended should operative intervention become necessary. Obstetric indications include prolonged labor, oxytocin augmentation of labor, and any factors that place the parturient at high risk for cesarean section. Fetal indications include prematurity, breech presentation, and multiple gestation, as greater control of delivery is possible and the depressant effects of systemic opioids are avoided.

Contraindications

Contraindications to regional anesthesia in obstetric patients are similar to those in the general population. Absolute contraindications include infection over the site of placement, frank coagulopathy, hypovolemic shock, and patient refusal or inability to cooperate. There are several relative contraindications in the parturient. There relate to concerns about performing neuraxial blockade in bacteremic patients and subsequent development of meningitis and epidural abscess. Chorioamnionitis occurs in approximately 1% of pregnancies, and there are no good predictive factors for identifying the subgroup of febrile patients who are bacteremic.[58] It is our practice to administer regional anesthesia to these patients after appropriate antibiotic therapy is instituted. There is consensus that regional anesthesia is safe in parturients with recurrent genital herpes infection, in the absence of systemic symptoms. The risks and benefits of regional anesthesia must be determined on an individual basis.

Conduct of epidural analgesia

Epidural anesthesia in the parturient should be performed under the same standards as in the general surgical patient. Informed consent is obtained and intravenous access established. Resuscitation equipment should be immediately available. Blood pressure and heart rate (by electrocardiography or pulse oximetry) are monitored during initiation of block. Blood pressure should be recorded every 2 min after each dose and every 15 min thereafter. The fetal heart rate should be monitored, if possible, during epidural placement, and throughout the subsequent duration of epidural analgesia. During identification of the epidural space, the lateral position may have advantages in that orthostatic hypotension is less likely, continuous fetal heart rate monitoring is more often possible and it may be a more comfortable position for some, especially those in advanced labor. However, the skin-to-epidural space distance is greater in the lateral position. The sitting position may improve identification of the midline in obese patients, and one study has shown a reduced incidence of aortocaval compression in the sitting position compared with the left lateral position.[59] Maternal position does not appear to affect the incidence of complications of epidural placement.[60] Several studies have reported a lower incidence of inadequate block when using multiorifice catheters compared with single-endhole catheters.[61–63] After institution of the block, the parturient is nursed in the lateral position to avoid aortocaval compression, the effects of which may be exaggerated by sympathetic blockade.

Maintenance of epidural analgesia

A bilateral T10 sensory level of analgesia should be established at initiation of the epidural block. Thereafter, analgesia may be maintained by continuous infusion, intermittent bolus injection, or patient-controlled epidural analgesia (PCEA) of a dilute mixture of local anesthetic, combined with a narcotic. Several dosing regimens exist (Table 57.1).

Labor lasts several hours in most women. A continuous infusion of a dilute mixture offers the advantages of a stable level of analgesia, increased maternal hemodynamic stability, less risk of systemic local anesthetic toxicity, and a slower ascent of the level of anesthesia should intravascular or subarachnoid migration of the catheter occur. The use of dilute concentrations avoids loss of motor function. The intermittent technique needs reinforcement every 1–2 h; however, continuous techniques do not necessarily abolish the need for top-ups. Neonatal outcome is the same with both techniques. The superiority of either technique is controversial. Most studies suggest that the continuous technique results in the administration of a greater total dose of local anesthetic, but this does not result in greater maternal or umbilical venous drug concentrations at delivery.[73,74] One study has shown that the use of intermittent technique with a multiorifice catheter may provide better spread of drug and better labor analgesia. This is probably due to a fountain effect (drug exits through all pores during a bolus, whereas it exits only through the proximal pore during continuous infusion).[75] On the other hand, patient satisfaction is reportedly higher with continuous techniques.[74]

PCEA consists of intermittent demand dosing controlled by the patient, with or without a background continuous infusion. Bupivacaine

Table 57.1 *Commonly used continuous and patient-controlled infusion regimens*[64–72]

Technique	Drug	Concentration and dosage
Epidural continuous infusion	Bupivacaine	0.625–0.25% at 8–15 mL h^{-1}
Epidural continuous infusion	Ropivacaine	0.125–0.25% at 6–12 mL h^{-1}
Patient-controlled epidural analgesia (PCEA)	Bupivacaine	0.125%, 4 mL basal infusion, bolus dose 4 mL, lockout 20 min, maximum 16 mL h^{-1}
PCEA	Bupivacaine	0.125%, 0 mL basal infusion, bolus dose 3 mL, lockout 5–20 min, maximum 12 mL h^{-1}
PCEA	Bupivacaine + fentanyl 2 µg mL^{-1}	0.125%, 6 mL basal infusion, bolus dose 3 mL, lockout 10 min, maximum 24 mL h^{-1}
PCEA	Ropivacaine	0.125%, 6 mL basal infusion, bolus dose 4 mL, lockout interval 10 min, maximum 30 mL h^{-1}
Patient-controlled intravenous analgesia (PCA)	Fentanyl	10 µg h^{-1} continuous infusion + 10 µg bolus with 12 min lockout
PCA	Fentanyl	50 µg loading dose i.v., PCA bolus 20 µg, 3 min lockout
Continuous spinal analgesia	Bupivacaine	Initial dose (bupivacaine 0.25%, 1 mL + 25 µg fentanyl) followed by 1–2 mL h^{-1} (bupivacaine 0.125% + fentanyl 2 µg mL^{-1})
PCA	Fentanyl	25 µg fentanyl continuous infusion, PCA bolus 25 µg, 12 min lockout, 4-h maximum dose 600 µg
PCA	Nalbuphine	5 mg loading dose i.v., PCA bolus 1 mg, 6 min lockout, discontinue when cervix completely dilated

and ropivacaine have been used for this technique during labor.[64] PCEA results in a lower average hourly dose of local anesthetic than a continuous infusion.[65,66,76] However, there is a wide range of dose requirements among patients, and the ability to titrate dose to effect is an advantage of the PCEA technique. Increased patient satisfaction from a greater degree of autonomy is another potential benefit.

Whichever modality is used to maintain epidural analgesia, the patient must be assessed regularly. At our hospital, we personally assess our patients every 90 min and document maternal hemodynamics, fetal heart rate, sensory level, and degree of motor blockade.

Complications

Complications of epidural catheter insertion, epidural analgesia, and centrally administered opioids are the same in parturients as in the general population. Some are of particular relevance to obstetrics and will be discussed here. Hypotension and inadequate analgesia are the most common complications.

Hypotension

Uncorrected hypotension results in decreased uteroplacental perfusion, causing fetal hypoxemia and acidosis, and must be treated urgently. Prevention of hypotension includes intravenous prehydration and avoidance of aortocaval compression. Strategies aimed at the *in utero* resuscitation of the fetus include full lateral positioning the mother, supplemental oxygen, intravenous fluid bolus, and administration of ephedrine.

Inadequate analgesia

Inadequate epidural analgesia occurs in 1.5–5% of laboring patients, even in experienced hands. When the parturient complains of discomfort, the sensory level of analgesia to pinprick or alcohol should be assessed and the cervical dilation, stage of labor, uterine contraction, and fetal heart rate tracing noted. Factors to rule out include equipment problems (pump malfunction/disconnected tubing/empty reservoir bag) and a full bladder. The epidural catheter should be examined for migration by aspiration, test dose, and level at skin compared with that at time of insertion.

In cases of asymmetrical block, an additional bolus of local anesthetic may be given. Although there is no scientific evidence for a gravitational effect on epidural blockade, many anesthesiologists will administer this bolus dose with the inadequately blocked leg in the dependent position. If an inadequate block persists, the catheter may be partially withdrawn and reassessed or replaced (catheter deviated from midline or in anterior epidural space). Owing to the dilute infusions used, intravascular catheter migration is more likely to result in diminishing analgesia than systemic toxicity. A progressive increase in the sensory level of analgesia or significant motor blockade may indicate subarachnoid migration. In both situations, the catheter should be examined and replaced as necessary.

Patient discomfort may indicate progression to the second stage of labor. Sacral nerves are large-diameter, myelinated fibers that require a large volume of more concentrated local anesthetic solution for blockade. The patient may have high analgesic requirements. An occiput-posterior fetal head is associated with more severe pain, often felt in the back. An increased concentration and infusion rate may be used. Opioid boluses (50 μg fentanyl in saline) or PCEA may be considered. Severe, unrelenting pain despite an adequate sensory level and present between contractions may indicate placental abruption or uterine rupture (Crawford's sieve[77]).

Catheter type and depth of insertion may be important factors. Some studies suggest a higher rate of satisfactory block with multiorifice catheters. Shallow placement increases the chance of block failure due to movement out of the epidural space, and deep catheter insertion increases the chance of intravenous placement. One study observed an optimal insertion depth of 5 cm.[78] Catheters secured at the skin in the sitting position may be partially withdrawn on assuming the lateral position.[79]

Subdural injection of local anesthetic typically results in a high, but patchy block, cranial spread is more extensive, sacral analgesia may be absent, and there is less intense motor blockade.

It is advisable to use local anesthetics without narcotics when establishing the initial epidural blockade. Epidurally administered narcotics will produce analgesia without surgical anesthetic properties (masking effect); if operative delivery becomes necessary, the epidural may prove inadequate.

Accidental subarachnoid placement/injection

The incidence of dural puncture varies approximately between 0.2% and 2%. The subsequent incidence of postdural puncture headache (PDPH), resulting from a 16–18G needle puncture, may reach 76–87%, and 40% of affected patients may require an epidural blood patch.[80] Accidental subarachnoid injection of large volumes of local anesthetics results in rapid cardiorespiratory collapse, loss of consciousness, and ultimately brain death. If free flow of CSF occurs from the catheter, aspiration of at least 10 mL of CSF is recommended,[81] and lavage with preservative-free normal saline may help lower the amount and concentration of local anesthetic in the CSF. This may hasten the resolution of the total spinal block. If inadvertent dural puncture occurs during epidural needle placement, the catheter may be threaded and a continuous spinal technique employed, or the epidural may be resited at another interspace.

Accidental intravenous placement/injection

Reports of bupivacaine-induced cardiac arrest in 1979 stimulated the current interest in test procedures to detect i.v. placement. Vessel entry can occur on initial insertion of the epidural needle or catheter, or, again, due to migration of the catheter tip at any time during ongoing epidural therapy. The typical frequency appears to be in the range of 2% in the general population and between 7% and 8.5% in pregnant patients. The incidence of intravascular catheter placement can be reduced by injecting fluid through the epidural needle before catheter placement.[80] This emphasizes the need for vigilance when administering large drug doses through an indwelling epidural catheter for cesarean delivery. Accidental slow intravenous injection of local anesthetics results in subjective maternal symptoms of lightheadedness, apprehension, tinnitus, perioral paresthesia, and a metallic taste. Close attention to these prodromal symptoms will provide early warning of intravascular injection of local anesthetics and avoid their more dangerous toxic effects, such as seizures, ventricular dysrhythmias, and cardiac arrest.

Other complications

Major anesthesia-related neurologic complications are extremely rare, with a rate of 1:100 000.[82] Obstetric-related major complications, however, are more common, with a rate of 1:7000, and are associated with prolonged pushing, large babies, lithotomy position, and forceps delivery. The lumbosacral plexus and femoral and lateral femoral cutaneous nerves are the most frequently involved. Prospective studies have consistently shown that no causal relation exists between the use of epidural analgesia and the development of long-term postpartum backache.[83,84]

SPINAL ANALGESIA

In most cases, a single-shot subarachnoid injection of a local anesthetic is not suitable for the first stage of labor because of its finite duration, and multiple injections increase the risk of PDPH. Occasionally, it may be employed to provide analgesia in multiparous women presenting at an advanced stage of cervical dilation, when only one injection is anticipated. Continuous spinal analgesia can be provided via an intrathecal catheter. This technique has been used for patients in whom placement of an epidural catheter is problematic (morbid obesity, abnormal vertebral anatomy). Initial injection of 2.5 mg of bupivacaine with 25 μg of fentanyl is followed by infusion of the standard local anesthetic/opioid mixture, but at lower rates of 1–2 mL h^{-1}. The use of standard epidural kits for this technique increases the risk of PDPH, but such kits may be employed when an unintentional wet tap occurs. Intrathecal microcatheters were removed from the North American market in 1992 following several cases of permanent neurologic injury. These were probably due to maldistribution of hyperbaric lidocaine (lignocaine). Microcatheters continue to be used in Europe. All continuous spinal catheters must be labeled appropriately, and the sensory level and intensity of motor block must be monitored closely to avoid high spinal anesthesia.

COMBINED SPINAL–EPIDURAL ANALGESIA

The combined spinal–epidural (CSE) technique, whereby selected advantages of each technique are combined, has gained increasing popularity in recent years.[85] In this technique, a long spinal needle is placed through a properly sited epidural needle, CSF is obtained, medication is given intrathecally, and an epidural catheter is placed. This is the needle-through-needle technique. There are also several commercially available combined needle devices.

The advantages of a CSE technique are that it provides a rapid onset of profound analgesia[86] with sacral coverage, and includes the placement of an epidural catheter for use if the extent or duration of the spinal analgesia is inadequate. Maternal satisfaction is high.[87] The adjuvant use of neuraxial opioids allows for lower doses of local anesthetics to be used. This enhancement of analgesia comes without additive motor blockade or hypotension, except with meperidine, which, because of its unique local anesthetic-like properties, may result in motor block, hypotension, or loss of proprioception. It has been observed that subsequent epidural analgesia can be achieved with lower doses of local anesthetic than if prior intrathecal opioid had not been used. The presence of even a small-bore dural puncture may enhance the spread of subsequently administered epidural medications.[88] A CSE technique may also be adapted for cesarean delivery and is particularly useful if prolonged operative duration is anticipated.

Short-acting, lipid-soluble opioids such as fentanyl 10–25 μg or sufentanil 5–15 μg are given intrathecally, with a duration of analgesia of 90–120 min. During this period, the patient may ambulate with assistance. Because analgesic requirements are greater in advanced labor, the addition of a small dose of local anesthetic (2.5 mg of bupivacaine) to the intrathecal opioid provides rapid onset of more prolonged effective analgesia than opioid alone. Many patients receiving this combination are able to ambulate.

When should the epidural infusion be started? Some practitioners wait for the spinal block to resolve, but it is our practice to give 1 mL (2.5 mg) of bupivacaine with 25 μg of fentanyl intrathecally, followed by continuous epidural infusion of 0.125% bupivacaine with 2 μg mL^{-1} of fentanyl at 10 mL h^{-1}. This allows for a smooth transition between the spinal and epidural portions of analgesia. Addition of epinephrine (adrenaline) to the opioid/local anesthetic combination may provide prolonged analgesia.

The potential risks associated with the CSE technique include PDPH, subarachnoid catheter migration, opioid-related side-effects, fetal bradycardia, and potential problems posed by an untested catheter. Both the spinal and epidural component are associated with a risk of PDPH; however, several studies have demonstrated a lower incidence of wet tap with CSE than with routine epidural analgesia during labor. It is postulated that in cases of inconclusive loss of resistance with the epidural needle, the spinal needle can be used as a guide to assess the proximity of the dura from the tip of the advancing epidural needle. While subarachnoid migration of the epidural catheter is a theoretical risk, in practice this does not seem to be a common occurrence.[89] Intrathecal opioids are associated with dose-dependent side-effects such as nausea, vomiting, sedation, pruritus, and respiratory depression. These side-effects may be increased if the patient has already received systemic opioids, and the incidence is higher with morphine than fentanyl or sufentanil. It is strongly recommended that oxygen saturation be monitored with intrathecal opioid use.

No significant changes in neonatal Apgar scores[90] or neurobehavioral studies have been reported with clinically used doses of intrathecal or epidural opioids. There have been reports of fetal heart rate decelerations following CSE. The incidence of these changes is similar with standard epidural techniques, and may result from increased uterine tone due to abrupt decreases in maternal catecholamines, effects on uteroplacental blood flow, or rapid fetal descent. Finally, the use of CSE may cause some difficulty in the timely assessment of proper functioning of the epidural catheter. In situations in which a well-functioning epidural catheter is of high priority (such as an anticipated difficult airway), the CSE technique may not be ideal. However, recent evidence suggests that epidural catheters placed as part of a combined technique are at least as successful as, and possibly even more successful than, catheters placed for standard epidural techniques.[91–93]

AMBULATION AND NEURAXIAL LABOR ANALGESIA

The interest in ambulation derives, in part, from the hypothesis that the upright posture and ambulating may have beneficial effects on the progress of labor.[94] Ambulation does not improve labor outcome.[95] Uncomplicated and less painful labor permits ambulation, rather than vice versa. Although some parturients are capable of walking, some have no desire to do so once they receive adequate analgesia.[96] Initial concerns with ambulation were for maternal safety (hypotension, risk of injury) and fetal well-being. A typical walking CSE consists of intrathecal fentanyl 25 μg and/or 2.5 mg of bupivacaine followed by continuous epidural infusion of a dilute local anesthetic/opioid mixture, e.g. 0.0625–0.1% bupivacaine with fentanyl 2 μg mL^{-1}, which retains sensory and motor function adequate to ambulate.[96–98] Prior to allowing ambulation, the clinician should assess for orthostatic blood pressure changes, lack of motor block (e.g. a deep-knee bend), and retention of proprioceptive abilities (e.g. toe-pointing). The fetal heart rate may be monitored on an intermittent basis or via a telemetry unit. Patients should not walk unaccompanied.

ALTERNATIVE REGIONAL ANESTHETIC TECHNIQUES

Paracervical blocks inhibit nerve impulses from the uterine body and cervix by injecting local anesthetic submucosally, in the vagina, on either side of the cervix at the 3 o'clock and 9 o'clock positions. This technique provides pain relief only for the first stage of labor and is associated with an unacceptably high incidence (up to 33%) of fetal bradycardia. The close proximity of the injection site to the uterine artery is thought to result in uterine arterial vasoconstriction and high fetal blood levels of local anesthetic.

Lumbar sympathetic blocks are beneficial only for the first stage of labor, and are rarely used.

Pudendal nerve blocks are often combined with perineal infiltration of local anesthetic to provide perineal anesthesia during the second stage of labor. The pudendal nerves are blocked bilaterally while passing over the ischial spine. These blocks are performed by obstetricians, and are of value in situations in which epidural/spinal analgesia is unavailable or contraindicated.

Caudal anesthesia has been supplanted by epidural/spinal anesthesia.

ANESTHESIA FOR CESAREAN SECTION

The incidence of cesarean section has increased dramatically over the last 20 years. In 1980, cesarean sections accounted for 16.5% of all deliveries in the USA. This figure rose to 24.7% in 1988. The selection of an anesthetic technique for cesarean delivery depends on several surgical, anesthetic, and maternal factors. Surgical factors include the indication for, and therefore the degree of urgency of, delivery. Anesthetic considerations include anticipated ease of intubation, presence of a labor epidural catheter, contraindications to regional techniques, and potential for technical difficulties (obesity, spinal deformities). Maternal factors include consent and cooperation. When feasible, regional is preferred to general anesthesia because of its better safety profile. In a survey of anesthesia-related maternal deaths in the USA between 1979 and 1990,[99] the number of deaths involving general anesthesia was found to have remained stable, whereas the number of regional anesthesia-related deaths decreased after 1984. The case fatality ratio for general anesthesia was 2.3 times that for regional anesthesia before 1985, increasing to 16.7 times that after 1985. General anesthesia is still indicated for emergency cesarean delivery and when regional anesthesia has failed or is contraindicated. It is our practice to administer regional anesthesia for all elective and semiurgent procedures, reserving general anesthesia for the above situations. If difficulty with intubation is anticipated, a regional technique should be employed despite emergency. We encourage obstetricians and midwives to secure early anesthesia counseling in all high-risk obstetric patients (obesity, anticipated difficult airway). This facilitates discussion of anesthetic options with both the patient and obstetrician, and allows formulation of a suitable anesthetic care plan for labor and delivery. For example, we consider it prudent to institute epidural analgesia in early labor in patients in whom intubation is judged to be difficult, so that regional anesthesia can be used if emergent delivery is subsequently required. Regardless of the intended anesthetic technique, all patients undergoing cesarean delivery must receive gastric aspiration prophylaxis, as mentioned earlier.

Spinal anesthesia

The principal advantages of spinal anesthesia for cesarean delivery are its simplicity, speed, reliability, and minimal fetal exposure to depressant drugs. The parturient remains awake, and the hazards of aspiration are minimized. Furthermore, the neurobehavioral assessment of neonates born following spinal anesthesia is better than after general anesthesia with either thiopental or ketamine inductions.[100] Compared with epidural anesthesia, spinal anesthesia produces a denser sacral nerve root blockade, more motor block, and less shivering (5.5% vs. 42.2% respectively).[101]

Successful spinal anesthesia for cesarean delivery requires a T4 level block. This can be achieved with lidocaine 60–75 mg (duration of block 45–75 min) or bupivacaine 10–15 mg (duration of block 60–120 min) through a Whitacre/Sprotte (27 or 25/24 gauge) needle inserted into subarachnoid space at the L3–4 or L2–3 interspace. Both needles have a pencil-point tip, which reduces the incidence of PDPH. Fentanyl 10–20 μg may be added to the local anesthetic to enhance the quality of sensory blockade. Epinephrine (200 μg) can be added to prolong the duration of anesthesia.[102] An adequate bilateral level can be achieved with lumbar puncture performed in the right lateral position and immediate placement of the parturient in left semilateral position, using a wedge. This ensures adequate and symmetric local anesthetic distribution within the subarachnoid space.[25,103]

The disadvantages of spinal anesthesia include hypotension and intrapartum nausea and vomiting, possibility of PDPH, and limited duration of action (unless a continuous spinal technique is utilized). Maternal hypotension lasting more than 2 min should be avoided, as it may be associated with lower Apgar scores.[25,104] Recommended measures to decrease the incidence of hypotension include prehydration with 1000–1500 mL of lactated Ringer's solution, maintaining left uterine displacement during anesthesia, and prophylactic administration of 50 mg of ephedrine i.m. or 5–15 mg ephedrine i.v. boluses.[105–108] Ephedrine improves uterine circulation and fetal heart tracing when fetal hypoxia and hypercapnia follow hypotension from spinal anesthesia.[107] While phenylephrine and methoxamine impair uterine blood flow, these pressors can be safely used to maintain maternal blood pressure in the presence of ischemic heart disease or valvular stenosis.[109]

Nausea and vomiting can be extremely distressing for the mother. Datta *et al.*[110] showed that avoiding hypotension following induction of spinal anesthesia can result in 6.6- to 7-fold reduction in peripartum emetic symptoms. Presumably, hypotension results in relative brainstem hypoxia, triggering vomiting. Supplemental oxygen, despite hypotension, also decreases emetic symptoms.

Symptoms may also result from uterine or peritoneal traction during surgery. The level of anesthesia necessary for cesarean delivery results in vagal predominance in the upper gastrointestinal tract. Visceral pain from traction of abdominal visceral allows vagal afferents to trigger the vomiting center. This apparent autonomic imbalance, coupled with inadequate conduction blockade, may result in viscerally mediated emetic symptoms.

Thus, it is essential to provide dense sensory afferent blockade to modulate nociceptive afferents mediating visceral pain. This can be achieved with adequate local anesthetic dosage together with addition of intrathecal opioids that enhance the quality of the sensory blockade. Prophylactic antiemetics such as metoclopramide, droperidol, and scopolamine patches can be also used to reduce nausea and vomiting.[25]

A typical T4 block results in a loss of thoracic proprioception, and the patient may not appreciate her chest movement. The patient may become restless and complain of dyspnea. Reassurance will help to overcome this fear. Rarely, however, the patient may develop respiratory insufficiency with loss of protective airway reflexes, requiring rapid-sequence induction of general anesthesia and endotracheal intubation.

Epidural anesthesia

The advantages of epidural anesthesia for cesarean delivery over spinal anesthesia include a lower frequency, and severity, of maternal hypotension, avoidance of intentional dural puncture, and ability to extend the duration of block as desired. A combined spinal–epidural (CSE) can be used when the duration of surgery is uncertain. We do not use a CSE technique in parturients with an anticipated difficult airway because the epidural catheter remains untested until the spinal anesthesia has worn off. In these patients, we prefer to perform cesarean delivery under epidural analgesia.

Between 15 and 20 mL of 2-chloroprocaine (3%) with bicarbonate is a suitable local anesthetic agent for urgent cesarean delivery in parturients with a labor epidural catheter in place. As the placental transfer of chloroprocaine is minimal, it is not subjected to ion trapping at low pH and, therefore, is the preferred agent in the presence of fetal acidosis.[111] Two percent lidocaine with epinephrine (with or without bicarbonate) can be used for nonurgent and elective cesarean deliveries. Addition of 50 μg fentanyl to the local anesthetic enhances the quality of sensory analgesia. Bupivacaine provides excellent motor and sensory anesthesia for cesarean delivery. Because of its associated cardiotoxicity, 0.75% bupivacaine solution is no longer available for obstetric use. The 0.5% bupivacaine solution usually requires the addition of epinephrine or supplementation with 50 μg fentanyl to provide optimal conditions for cesarean delivery.[112] Bupivacaine and lidocaine have no adverse neonatal neurobehavioral effects when used over the short period required for cesarean delivery.[113,114]

The disadvantages of epidural compared with spinal anesthesia include slower onset of surgical anesthesia, greater likelihood of failure, greater incidence of shivering, accidental dural puncture, and accidental intravascular injection. There is a ninefold increase in shivering with epidural anesthesia compared with spinal anesthesia. This usually begins within 10 min of the onset of anesthesia.[115] Shivering increases oxygen consumption, carbon dioxide production, and cardiac work, which may contribute to an elevated maternal base deficit. Warm intravenous fluids and local anesthetic solutions, and the use of 50 μg fentanyl or sufentanil, can minimize postepidural shivering.[80]

General anesthesia

The use of general anesthesia for cesarean delivery has reduced dramatically over the past 20 years. A teaching hospital in the UK has reported a decrease in the general anesthesia cesarean section rate from 76% in 1982 to 7.7% in 1998.[116]

Two important factors should be considered when contemplating general anesthesia for cesarean delivery: (1) ability to intubate swiftly and (2) minimizing neonatal depression. Gastric aspiration prophylaxis is imperative in this setting, and the supine position with left uterine displacement should be employed before induction of anesthesia. It must be emphasized that great care must be exercised in positioning the parturient's head in a good sniffing position to facilitate intubation. Several folded bed sheets can be placed in a stepwise fashion from the back to the occiput to attain a good intubating position. In cases of anticipated difficult intubation, fiberoptic intubation or awake topicalization of the oropharynx and visualization of the larynx should be performed before induction of anesthesia.

After preoxygenation and denitrogenation, rapid-sequence induction of anesthesia is performed, typically with thiopental 5 mg kg^{-1} i.v., followed by succinylcholine 1.5 mg kg^{-1}. Cricoid pressure is maintained until endotracheal intubation is achieved and confirmed with bilateral air entry and CO_2 return on capnography. The short-handled Datta–Briwa laryngoscope[117] is particularly useful in preventing enlarged breasts from interfering with intubation.

Although the concentration of thiopental rises rapidly in the fetus [umbilical artery/umbilical vein ratio = 0.87 with induction-to-delivery (I–D) intervals of 8–22 min],[118] an awake baby is delivered. There are several reasons for this: (1) preferential uptake of thiopental by the fetal liver; (2) a higher relative water content of fetal brain; (3) rapid redistribution of thiopental in the mother, which rapidly reduces the maternal–fetal concentration gradient; (4) nonhomogeneity of blood flow in the intervillous spaces; and (5) progressive dilution by admixture with the various components of the fetal circulation.

Propofol is a suitable alternative to thiopental as an induction agent. It attenuates the pressor response to laryngoscopy and intubation more effectively than thiopental. Both agents result in similar Apgar and neonatal neurobehavior scores.[119] Ketamine 1 mg kg^{-1} is a good alternative for induction of general anesthesia, particularly in the presence of hypovolemia and hypotension. The indirect sympathomimetic properties of ketamine can help to support the circulation. However, if hypovolemia is severe, cardiac output and blood pressure can be reduced as a result of the direct myocardial depression produced by ketamine.[120]

We do not precurarize to prevent succinylcholine-induced fasciculations from raising intra-abdominal and intragastric pressure, because of a risk of partial paralysis from the small dose of nondepolarizing muscle relaxant. Furthermore, succinylcholine produces a more rapid and profound relaxation in the absence of precurarization in parturients. Parturients rarely fasciculate, and the incidence of muscle pains is lower than age-matched female controls. Anesthesia is maintained with isoflurane 0.5% in a 50% oxygen–nitrous oxide mixture. Inhalational agents are used to minimize the chances of maternal awareness. Muscle relaxation can be achieved with small doses of any nondepolarizing agent.

Maternal hyperventilation should be avoided as a maternal $P_{a}CO_2$ < 25 mmHg (3.3 kPa) may result in reduced uteroplacental perfusion and consequent fetal acidosis.[121] Hyperventilation and hypocarbia result in uterine artery vasoconstriction, reduced cardiac output secondary to increased intrathoracic pressure, and a leftward shift in the maternal oxyhemoglobin dissociation curve, impairing oxygen release from maternal blood to the fetus. Ventilation should be adjusted to a maternal $P_{a}CO_2$ of around 30 mmHg (4 kPa). Maternal $P_{a}CO_2$ end-tidal CO_2 difference is small [0.03 mmHg (0.004 kPa)], therefore end-tidal CO_2 is a good reflection of maternal $P_{a}CO_2$, and is an essential monitor.[122]

Narcotics are administered for analgesia, after delivery of the infant. At the conclusion of surgery, adequate neuromuscular recovery is confirmed with a peripheral nerve stimulator. The trachea is extubated with the patient awake, with intact pharyngeal reflexes, to safeguard against pulmonary aspiration.

Management of the unexpected difficult airway

As 50% of difficult intubations in obstetric practice occur unexpectedly, protocols dealing with the management of difficult airways should be in effect in every obstetric anesthesia location. In our institution, a code airway is called in the event of a difficult intubation. This summons, among others, a senior surgeon who can expeditiously perform a tracheotomy/tracheostomy, if required. The American Society of Anesthesiologists (ASA) and the ASA Task Force on Management of the Difficult Airway have developed guidelines to deal with unexpected airway difficulties.[123] Additional anesthetic assistance should be requested immediately. If intubation is initially unsuccessful, additional efforts are appropriate using different laryngoscopic blades and head positions, and, where possible, a further attempt by an experienced colleague, before considering the case to be difficult. If the trachea cannot be intubated, one should not persist with intubation, but begin mask ventilation *as parturients die from hypoxemia, not from failure to intubate*. If mask ventilation is unsuccessful, despite an oral airway, a laryngeal mask airway (LMA) or Combitube may be inserted to facilitate ventilation. We prefer an LMA as first choice because anesthesiologists have considerable experience with their use in routine practice. If ventilation cannot be accomplished despite LMA/Combitube (cannot intubate, cannot ventilate), transtracheal jet ventilation, cricothyrotomy, or tracheostomy has to be considered.

If ventilation is successful with a mask or an LMA (cannot intubate, can ventilate), the decision to continue anesthesia, or to wake the patient, is dependent on the indication for surgery.[124] If cesarean delivery is being performed for elective indications, there is no justification in jeopardizing the mother's life by continuing anesthesia without a tracheal tube. Alternatively, general anesthesia with mask/LMA can be continued when the mother's life is dependent on the completion of cesarean delivery (massive antepartum hemorrhage). In between these two extremes are indications for cesarean delivery that pose considerable dilemmas and require discussion between the obstetric and anesthetic services. For example, longstanding fetal distress showing good recovery between contractions does not warrant continuation of general anesthesia, and experience has shown that the vast majority of these fetuses can be delivered without detriment, under regional anesthesia, or after awake intubation.[124] However, severe fetal distress, not recovering between contractions, may lead to fetal death if general anesthesia is abandoned. General anesthesia may be continued in the presence of adequate ventilation and oxygenation. Fiberoptic intubation, through an LMA, can be considered under these circumstances. Additional anesthetic assistance and surgical help should continue until the termination of anesthesia has culminated in the safe recovery of the patient. Local infiltration and field block has been described, and is a potential last resort when spinal/epidural/general anesthetic techniques are not viable or have failed.[125,126]

Postoperative pain relief

Preservative-free morphine, 0.2 mg intrathecally or 3 mg epidurally, provides analgesia for 17–27 h following cesarean delivery. Postoperative life-threatening respiratory depression is a rare event when these doses are used. Occasionally, emesis and pruritis may be distressing postoperative side-effects, requiring treatment with the mixed opioid agonist–antagonists (nalbuphine) or the antagonist naloxone.[127]

Patient-controlled analgesia with meperidine or morphine has become a popular postoperative pain relief technique following general anesthesia. Meperidine has a rapid onset and causes less sedation, nausea, vomiting, and pruritus than morphine, but produces a lower neurobehavioral score on the third day of life.[120,121] This should not pose problems if meperidine is used for less than 24 h.

CONTROVERSIAL AREAS IN OBSTETRIC ANESTHESIA

Regional anesthesia in labor and pyrexia

The association between the use of regional anesthesia during labor and temperature elevation in the parturient has become extremely controversial in recent years. Several studies have noted an increase in maternal temperature associated with epidural analgesia.[128–130] The increase is mild, averaging 0.1 °C per hour, beginning several hours after the administration of epidural analgesia. In the above studies, there was no increase in the incidence of maternal or neonatal infection, suggesting noninfectious causes of elevated maternal temperature. Although women with other risk factors for fever – long labors, nulliparity, prolonged rupture of membranes – are more likely to request regional anesthesia, epidural analgesia was found to be an independent risk factor for developing fever in labor.[130] Increased length of labor raises the risk.

The mechanisms by which epidural analgesia produces maternal hyperthermia during labor remains unclear. There may be reduced dissipation of heat as a result of the inhibition of sweating with sympathectomy, and less heat loss from hyperventilation due to improved analgesia.[131] The high incidence of shivering among laboring women who receive epidural analgesia (up to 33%) may also result in thermogenesis.[132]

Another proposed mechanism for the increased maternal temperature is the possible presence of a subclinical infection. One study concluded that fever associated with epidural analgesia is due to unrecognized chorioamnionitis rather than the analgesia itself.[133]

What is the clinical significance of epidural-related intrapartum fever? Initial, often poorly constructed, studies showed an increased incidence of neonatal sepsis evaluations and antibiotic treatment in the setting of regional anesthesia. However, subsequent studies, have not found this.[134] A recent retrospective study, examining outcomes among noninfected infants, found that maternal pyrexia is associated with lower 1-min Apgar scores and neonatal hypotonia.[135] However, this study did not control for the risk factors for selecting epidural analgesia, which may confound the results. Furthermore, none of these outcomes reflects any lasting injury to the fetus. When pyrexia does occur, as in other clinical circumstances, efforts should be made to lower the temperature and identify and treat a presumed maternal infection. An association between epidural analgesia and intrapartum maternal temperature has been established, but epidural analgesia per se is not an indication for neonatal sepsis evaluation, and it has not changed our practice.

Progress of labor

The effect of epidural analgesia on the progress (duration) and outcome (mode of delivery) of labor has been a controversial issue for over a century and a half. James Young Simpson, who administered the first labor anesthetic, wrote in 1871 that "It will be necessary to ascertain anesthesia's precise effect, both upon the action of the uterus and on the assistant abdominal muscles; its influence, if any, upon the child; whether it has a tendency to hemorrhage or other complications."[1]

Clarification of this issue is difficult because of methodologic difficulties in study design when examining the relation between epidural analgesia and the progress of labor. Retrospective studies are severely limited because of selection bias: women who self-select epidural analgesia may be different from those who do not require analgesia. These women may be in greater pain, and this pain may be a sign of difficult labor and dystocia, and has been recognized as a risk for cesarean section.[136] Other factors associated with requests for an epidural include nulliparity, presentation at hospital in early labor, high fetal station, slow cervical dilation prior to analgesia, oxytocin administration, even prior to epidural placement, large fetuses, the presence of other obstetric and medical factors associated with operative delivery (poor fetal status, obesity), and great pain, especially in the latent phase.[137] Patients judged to be at high risk for operative vaginal or cesarean delivery may be encouraged to receive epidural analgesia, so that an epidural catheter is in place and tested for the anticipated surgery. In addition, obstetricians may be more likely to perform a forceps- or vacuum-assisted delivery in a patient with effective epidural analgesia.

Randomized trials have not completely clarified the issue of an association between epidural administration and the progress and outcome of labor. Placebo-controlled trials are practically impossible and probably unethical. Parenteral opioids are consistently inferior to epidural analgesia, and, as mode of delivery is a subjective obstetric decision, blinding is difficult. Crossover between epidural and opioid groups may be problematic. It is not known if patients who agree to be in a study in which analgesic method is randomly assigned are truly representative of all laboring patients or are a group for whom analgesia is not an important issue. Some studies have analyzed the data only for the protocol-compliant women (by the treatment they received instead of on an intent-to-treat basis). In essence, the patients selected their own group and the study becomes functionally a retrospective analysis. It must be recognized that factors unrelated to analgesia may also significantly affect the patient's course, including her obstetrician's practice pattern and obstetric complications. Thus, while an association may exist between epidural analgesia and the progress of labor, a causal relation cannot be claimed.

Is it ever too early?

In contrast to earlier uncontrolled studies, more recent randomized studies have found no difference between epidurals placed at 1 cm and parenteral opioids.[138] Two trials by Chestnut and coworkers[139,140] found no difference between early and late epidurals.

Any effect on cervical dilation?

Early retrospective studies found slower progress with epidurals, but with the bias noted above. A meta-analysis of 10 randomized trials found that the first stage of labor was prolonged by 42 min in patients receiving epidural analgesia compared with opioids.[144]

Effects on the second stage of labor

There may be an inhibition of the urge to push, but inhibition of ability to push is unlikely as maternal expulsive efforts are Valsalva maneuvers and are not impaired until high dense blocks are achieved. Epidurals could theoretically block the afferent limb of the Ferguson reflex (distension of the lower vagina causing oxytocin release). There may also be relaxation of the pelvic musculature. There is clear evidence that the pattern of fetal descent is altered in patients with epidural analgesia, and delaying maternal expulsive efforts for some time after full dilation does reduce the incidence of instrumental delivery.[142,143] Halpern *et al.*'s meta-analysis[141] found the second stage to be prolonged by 14 min in the epidural groups. Instrumental (forceps) delivery may be increased by up to twofold in the epidural groups. There is huge variation between institutions and obstetricians (0–80%), suggesting that obstetric practice is probably a dominant factor. Additionally, obstetricians may be more likely to perform a forceps- or vacuum-assisted delivery on a comfortable patient with relaxed pelvic musculature, perhaps for teaching purposes.[144]

Effect on the mode of delivery

This is the main issue of debate in recent years. In several trials in the 1990s women were randomly assigned to receive epidural analgesia or parenteral opioids. These studies[145,146] found higher rates of cesarean deliveries in the epidural groups. Several criticisms have been aimed at the first study. These include a lack of blinding, low crossover, and premature data analysis. When the data from the second study were analyzed on an intent-to-treat basis, no difference in the rate of operative delivery was observed.[147] Other studies found no difference in cesarean section rates in the epidural groups.[144,148,149] Meta-analysis confirmed these findings,[141] as did another study comparing combined spinal–epidurals with parenteral opioids.[150]

Catastrophe theory studies (also known as impact or sentinel event studies) have examined the operative delivery rates in institutions after the introduction of an on-demand epidural service. The assumption is that the patient population and obstetric practice styles are likely to change little compared with the sudden availability of epidural analgesia. One study reported no difference in cesarean delivery rate during a rise in epidural use from 10% to 57%.[151] Meta-analysis of seven such studies found no increase in cesarean rates with increased availability of epidural analgesia.[152] In summary, the findings of many well-conducted prospective, randomized trials in the last decade have confirmed the opinion of most anesthesiologists that epidural analgesia only minimally lengthens labor and does not increase the rate of cesarean section.

THE EPIDURAL TEST DOSE

Epidural catheter placement may be complicated by blood vessel or dural puncture. The purpose of the test dose is to give a dose of drug that allows recognition of intravenous or subarachnoid catheter placement but does not result in systemic toxicity or total spinal anesthesia. The ideal test dose should have high sensitivity and high specificity. The low doses of local anesthetics used in modern practice to initiate and maintain labor analgesia make the likelihood of systemic toxicity extremely low. However, untoward effects remain a significant risk with the larger doses required for anesthesia for cesarean delivery. The appropriate steps to ensure safe initiation of epidural anesthesia remain controversial.[153]

Currently suggested tests

Aspiration

Aspiration of the needle or catheter is the oldest recommendation, and may identify subarachnoid and intravascular placement. However, epidural veins are thin walled and collapse easily when subjected to negative pressure, and there are multiple reports of false negatives. Catheter type may be an important feature: higher false-negative rates have been reported with single-endhole catheters than with multiorifice catheters.[154] Some authors recommend observing for the passive flow of blood while holding the open catheter below the level of insertion.

Incremental injection

This is the mainstay of safe regional anesthesia practice. Theoretically, the patient should report subjective symptoms before blood local anesthetic concentration reaches the threshold for seizures.

Local anesthetic test injections

A 3-mL local anesthetic test dose is traditionally used to detect subarachnoid injection. Assessing for symptoms of central nervous system (CNS) irritability (tinnitus, perioral tingling, metallic taste, dizziness, changes in hearing, etc.) produced by subtoxic doses of local anesthetic has also been recommended as an indicator of unintentional i.v. injection. A larger amount of drug, e.g. the total milligram dose contained in 5 mL of drug (100 mg lidocaine, 25 mg bupivacaine), is probably required to produce these symptoms.

Epinephrine

The first well-studied epidural test dose of 3 mL of 1.5% lidocaine with 15 μg of epinephrine[155] (1:200 000) was designed as a convenient one-step test to simultaneously detect i.v. or intrathecal placements (addition of epinephrine negates the need for a 5 mL volume of local anesthetic, as above). Maternal heart rate response may be monitored by continuous ECG or pulse oximetry. There are several limitations to the use of epinephrine in parturients. Pregnancy alters a woman's sensitivity to chronotropes and vasopressors. The average parturient's heart rate increases by only 10 beats min^{-1} after 15 μg intravenously.[156] Cyclic changes in heart rate during labor may be confounding. Injecting the test dose between contractions, if possible, may limit this confusion.

Questions have arisen regarding the safety of epinephrine test doses. Epinephrine causes a significant rise in blood pressure that may be dangerous in women with hypertension (e.g. pre-eclampsia).[157] Fetal cardiac decelerations (as a result of uterine artery vasoconstriction and reduced blood flow) were reported in some women after i.v. epinephrine test doses, without adverse clinical outcome.[158] The epinephrine test dose has greater sensitivity than specificity, which may lead to unnecessary catheter replacements.[159]

Alternative test doses

Air (using precordial Doppler),[154] isoproterenol, ephedrine, and fentanyl have all been injected as epidural test doses.

No epidural test dose is perfect, and some authors have advocated only aspiration and incremental dosage,[160] but the administration of a test does focus the attention of the anesthesiologist on the early recognition of an intravascular or subarachnoid catheter. It is recommended that careful aspiration be performed and that a test dose be administered whenever a new catheter is placed and before administration of large doses of local anesthetic. Additionally, the patient should be monitored for objective and subjective signs of intravascular or intrathecal injection.

PRE-ECLAMPSIA AND OTHER CONDITIONS OF INTEREST

Pre-eclampsia is classically defined as a triad of hypertension, non-dependent edema, and proteinuria occurring after 20 weeks' gestation. Complications from pre-eclampsia and other hypertensive disorders of pregnancy are consistently listed among the most common causes of maternal death in virtually all developed countries. Pre-eclampsia occurs in 3–5% of pregnancies.[161] Mild disease is diagnosed by a sustained elevation of blood pressure to 140/90 mmHg (18.7/12 kPa), proteinuria in excess of 300 mg 24 h^{-1}, and the presence of edema. Pre-eclampsia is severe when any one of the following is present: blood pressure exceeding 160/110 mmHg (21.3/14.7 kPa), proteinuria of 5 g or more in 24 h, oliguria, cerebral or visual disturbances, pulmonary edema, epigastric or right quadrant pain, altered liver function, thrombocytopenia, fetal growth retardation and HELLP (*h*emolysis, *e*levated *l*iver enzymes and *l*ow *p*latelets) syndrome. Acute cocaine toxicity can mimic the signs and symptoms of pre-eclampsia. Labetalol and hydralazine remain the mainstays of antihypertensive management. Magnesium is used for seizure prophylaxis.

The etiology of pre-eclampsia is unknown, and several theories exist. There are three hallmarks of pre-eclampsia: vasoconstriction, reduced blood volume, and platelet aggregation. There is a relative reduction in the prostacyclin to thromboxane ratio, a deficiency in the production of nitric oxide, and an increase in endothelin-1. These factors lead to widespread vasoconstriction, increased systemic vascular resistance, and hypertension. The ensuing baroreceptor response causes increased sodium and water excretion by the kidney, with resultant hypovolemia and hemoconcentration. There are increased circulating levels of renin, angiotensin, aldosterone, and catecholamines. The pre-eclamptic patient is very sensitive to exogenously administered pressor agents (ephedrine etc.). There is reduced uteroplacental perfusion, decreased renal plasma flow, and oliguria. Proteinuria is secondary to altered glomerular permeability. The reduced plasma oncotic pressure leads to peripheral, pulmonary, cerebral, and laryngeal edema. Prostaglandin imbalance may cause platelet aggregation and activation of the clotting cascade. This is a multiorgan disease process.

The ultimate cure for pre-eclampsia is delivery of the placenta. In severe disease, this may entail delivery of a preterm infant, frequently by cesarean section. Furthermore, surgery is often performed emergently, e.g. for abruption. Epidural, spinal, and general anesthetic techniques have all been used successfully to manage severe pre-eclamptic patients. Epidural analgesia is the preferred method of pain relief in labor, and should be instituted early. It reduces the stress of labor, reduces maternal blood pressure, and can improve placental perfusion by reducing circulating catecholamines. It also provides an anesthetic route should cesarean section become necessary. The risks associated with neuraxial sympathetic blockade are hypotension and hemodynamic instability, which may have additional adverse effects on an already compromised renal blood flow and uteroplacental unit. Therefore, hypovolemia should be carefully corrected before induction of regional anesthesia, and pressor agents should be used judiciously.

Pre-eclampsia is associated with abnormal hemostasis, most commonly caused by thrombocytopenia and rarely because of disseminated intravascular coagulation. A lack of correlation between bleeding time and platelet count has been reported. However, there is a strong correlation between platelet count and the maximum amplitude (MA) of the thromboelastogram (TEG). The TEG measures overall coagulation, and MA is a reflection of platelet function. Studies have found that MA does not decrease until the platelet count falls to 70 000 mm^{-3}.[162,163] At what platelet count is it considered safe to administer regional anesthesia? This remains controversial. With due consideration of the risk–benefit ratio of regional anesthesia (and risk of hematoma) vs. general anesthesia (and risk of airway problems), a platelet count of 70 000 mm^{-3} is considered safe by most practitioners.

Formerly, spinal anesthesia was discouraged in severely pre-eclamptic patients because of the potential for precipitous changes in maternal hemodynamics. This rationale posed a problem when epidural anesthesia was not feasible in the time required before emergency cesarean section, leaving general anesthesia as the sole option. However, there is evidence in the recent literature to suggest that spinal anesthesia can be safely administered to patients with severe pre-eclampsia.[164,165]

There are several concerns regarding the use of general anesthesia in severely pre-eclamptic patients. There may be generalized airway edema, which can be severe enough to cause airway obstruction, and intubation difficulties. Small endotracheal tubes should be readily available. Repeated intubation attempts exacerbate edema and hypertension. It has been shown that pre-eclamptic patients, under general anesthesia, are at greater risk for airway difficulties.[8] In addition, cerebrovascular events cannot be monitored. It is important to attenuate the pressor response to laryngoscopy in order to avoid the potential risks of cerebral hemorrhage and pulmonary edema. Interactions with drug therapies must be borne in mind when administering general anesthesia, e.g. magnesium therapy potentiates the effects of muscle relaxants. The factors that dictate the need for invasive monitoring are complex and variable, and should be tailored according to the clinical status of the individual patient, regardless of the anticipated anesthetic technique.

Eclampsia is the occurrence of seizures in the setting of pre-eclampsia. It occurs in 0.05% of pregnancies. Management involves anticonvulsant therapy, adequate airway protection, and treatment of hypertension. Regional anesthesia is not contraindicated if coagulation is normal. General anesthesia is used for obtunded patients. The fact that 30% of patients may present with eclampsia or pre-eclampsia in the postpartum period must be remembered in the differential diagnosis of PDPH.

Other conditions of interest with specific anesthetic considerations are morbid obesity, gestational thrombocytopenia, idiopathic thrombocytopenia, scoliosis, and herpes simplex. These are considered in Table 57.2.

OBSTETRIC HEMORRHAGE

Obstetric hemorrhage remains a leading cause of maternal death. It is classified as antepartum (placenta previa, abruption) or postpartum (lacerations, uterine atony, retained products). Uncomplicated vaginal delivery is associated with an average blood loss of 500 mL and cesarean section with a loss of 800–1000 mL. The physiologic increase in blood volume and the hypercoaguable state, as well as the autotransfusion with labor contractions and postpartum involution of the uterus, have equipped the parturient to cope with the mandatory blood loss associated with delivery.

Management of hemorrhage is similar to other clinical situations, and early recognition of ongoing blood loss is essential. The increase in baseline heart rate and reduction in baseline blood pressure that occur during pregnancy may confound a diagnosis of hypovolemia. Uterine atony is the most frequent cause of postpartum hemorrhage, and management includes emptying the uterus and massage. Drug

Table 57.2 *Special anesthetic considerations*[166–171]

Morbid obesity	Preanesthetic evaluation during pregnancy
	Airway assessment
	Evaluation of associated cardiorespiratory abnormalities
	Early epidural placement and assurance of function
	Consider continuous spinal technique if epidural unsuccessful and airway anticipated to be difficult
	Several folded bed sheets can be placed in a stepwise fashion from the back to the occiput, to attain a good intubating position
	Large panus may cause hemodynamic instability after regional anesthesia
Gestational thrombocytopenia	Benign and no intervention is required
	No contraindication to regional anesthesia
Idiopathic thrombocytopenia	If platelet counts $<30–50\times10^9\,L^{-1}$ – treat with intravenous immunoglobulin and prednisolone to augment the platelet count
	A response is anticipated in about 24–48 h
	Platelet count $>70–75\times10^9\,L^{-1}$ – regional anesthesia is appropriate if good clinical hemostasis is observed
	Platelet count below $70\,000\times10^9\,L^{-1}$ – regional anesthesia can be considered; consider the risk–benefit ratio (risk of bleeding into spinal space less than risk of general anesthesia)
Scoliosis	Patients may have underlying neuromuscular abnormality
	Evaluation in the prenatal period for associated cardiorespiratory abnormalities, particularly if Cobb's angle $>30°$
	History of prior spinal fusion
	Technical difficulties for regional anesthesia are expected in the presence of scoliosis or prior spinal surgery and instrumentation
	Direct the epidural or spinal needle toward the convexity of scoliotic curve
	High incidence of inadequate, patchy, and unilateral block, and intravascular or intrathecal placement
Herpes simplex	No contraindication to spinal/epidural in patients with secondary herpes
	Safety of regional technique in patients with primary herpes infection remains unclear
	Epidural morphine may reactivate latent herpes simplex virus after cesarean delivery and thus the risks and benefits should be carefully weighed

treatments are not without side-effects; oxytocin is the first-line drug therapy and can cause hypotension and reflex tachycardia. Ergot alkaloids are administered intramuscularly and may cause hypertension and bradycardia. Prostaglandin $F_{2\alpha}$ is administered intramyometrially and may cause bronchospasm.

Internal iliac artery ligation, uterine artery embolization, and peripartum hysterectomy have been employed in situations of uncontrolled, life-threatening hemorrhage. Blood conservation methods, aimed at reducing transfusion of homologous blood, have been used in obstetrics. Antepartum autologous blood donation is not feasible because of the low number of parturients requiring transfusion and the difficulty in predicting those likely to require it. Acute normovolemic hemodilution has been used during cesarean section for abnormal placentation.[172] There have been concerns with the use of intraoperative blood salvage during cesarean section, regarding the potential for fetal or amniotic substances to cause amniotic fluid embolism or disseminated intravascular coagulation (DIC). Recent studies, however, have shown the safety of specific cell savers in this setting.[173]

There is no place for a regional anesthetic technique in the cardiovascularly unstable patient. However, the uterine relaxant effect of volatile agents must be borne in mind when general anesthesia is employed. In addition, intraoperative infusion of large volumes of fluid may increase airway edema, and may pose postextubation problems. The role of regional anesthesia in the setting of anticipated or potential hemorrhage, e.g. anterior placenta previa, is more controversial. A multi-institutional study concluded that epidural anesthesia was not contraindicated in this setting.[174]

NONOBSTETRIC SURGERY IN THE PREGNANT PATIENT

Up to 2% of pregnant women receive anesthesia for surgery each year. Cervical cerclage placement is probably the most common. Appendicitis occurs in 1:2000 people of child-bearing age. Laparoscopic procedures, e.g. cholecystectomy, have been performed successfully on pregnant patients (Table 57.3). Anesthetic considerations include maternal safety, fetal well-being, and continuation of pregnancy. Again, thorough knowledge of the physiologic changes of pregnancy is essential. Antacid prophylaxis and uterine displacement should be used when appropriate. Hypoxia, hypotension, hypercarbia, and hypovolemia should be avoided, as in any patient, regardless of the anesthetic technique employed.

With regard to fetal well-being, avoidance of teratogenic agents is paramount, and knowledge of the placental transfer of drugs is important. No anesthetic agent used in pregnancy, with the exception of cocaine, has been specifically linked to human teratogenicity. The drugs of most concern are nitrous oxide and the benzodiazepines. Animal studies have shown that nitrous oxide inhibits methionine synthetase, which can inhibit DNA synthesis in a developing fetus. This teratogenic effect can be prevented by the addition of fentanyl or halogenated agents to nitrous oxide,[179,180] suggesting that the adverse effects may be secondary to reduced uteroplacental blood flow. No adverse effects of nitrous oxide have been demonstrated in human pregnancy. Diazepam has been anecdotally associated with cleft lip abnormalities, but prospective analysis has failed to support this alleged teratogenic effect. A review article has been published recently relating to the use of

Table 57.3 *Anesthetic management of pregnant women for laparoscopy*[175–178]

Position	Left or right uterine displacement
Premedication	Oral sodium citrate, 30 mL; metoclopramide, 10 mg i.v.
Induction	Rapid-sequence induction (thiopental sodium and succinylcholine)
Ventilatory adjustments	To keep end-tidal $P\text{CO}_2$ between 32 and 34 mmHg
Positioning	Gradual changes to reverse Trendelenburg
Fetal heart rate monitoring	Around 16 weeks, pre- and immediate postoperative period
Insufflation technique	Open trochar method
Tocolysis	Terbutaline 0.25 mg subcutaneous, if needed
Hypotension	Increments of ephedrine, 5–10 mg
Postoperative period	Left/right uterine displacement, oxygen supplements, fetal heart rate monitoring

drugs in pregnancy.[181] The hemodynamic effects of drugs or techniques employed may result in an adverse intrauterine environment. Maternal blood pressure and normocarbia should be maintained to preserve uteroplacental blood flow.

Surgery during pregnancy has been associated with an increased incidence of premature labor and spontaneous abortion. The incidence is higher during lower abdominal and pelvic surgery. Tocodynamometry can be used intraoperatively, depending on the site of surgery, to monitor uterine contractions, and postoperatively to detect preterm labor, so that tocolytic therapy may be instituted. Prophylactic tocolysis is controversial. Doppler assessment of fetal heart tones is possible from 16 weeks on, and should be documented pre- and postoperatively. Continuous fetal heart rate monitoring intraoperatively prior to viability is controversial, but is warranted at viability and afterwards, if technically feasible. When used, the baseline rate should be monitored, as general anesthesia can abolish variability. Trained personnel should interpret the monitor.

Elective surgery should be postponed until delivery. Semielective surgery should be avoided during the period of organogenesis of the first trimester. In emergency cases, the anesthetic of choice depends on the site and extent of surgery. Where possible, regional anesthesia is advised.

CARDIOPULMONARY RESUSCITATION IN PREGNANCY

Although cardiopulmonary resuscitation (CPR) in pregnancy is rare, some differences unique to the pregnant patient do affect resuscitation efforts. In patients without cardiopulmonary risk factors, hemorrhage, hypovolemia, and cocaine intoxication are the most common causes. Intubation should be performed early, because of faster desaturation during apnea and a higher risk of aspiration. The high-output, low vascular tone state of pregnancy and aortocaval and iliac compression contribute to difficulties in perfusion with CPR. Basic life support guidelines for the pregnant woman clearly state the need for uterine displacement.[182] Bretylium and cardioplulmonary bypass should be considered in cases of suspected bupivacaine toxicity. At our hospital we have a policy of emergent cesarean section at 4 min into a cardiac arrest in a pregnant patient with a uterus larger than 20 weeks' size. The rationale is twofold. It is better for the mother as delivery of the fetus improves perfusion during CPR and may reduce neurologic injury. It is also better for the baby, as the earlier the delivery during cardiac arrest, the better the survival and the lower the brain damage.[183] Open chest massage may be considered after 15 min of closed-chest CPR, as most pregnant patients are healthy young women.

MATERNAL MORTALITY

In the UK, a Report on Confidential Enquiries into Maternal Deaths has been published for each triennium since 1952. In the last report, covering the years 1997–99, the baseline (direct and indirect) maternal mortality rate was 11.4 per 100 000 maternities.[184] The leading causes of death were thrombosis and thromboembolism, accounting for almost 33% of all direct maternal deaths, followed by hypertensive diseases of pregnancy, sepsis, deaths in early pregnancy (ectopic pregnancy), amniotic fluid embolism, and hemorrhage. Unlike other leading causes of direct deaths, the rate of maternal deaths from sepsis is slowly increasing (8.0 per million maternities, a rise from 6.8 per million maternities in the 1994–96 report). Deaths from amniotic fluid embolism have reduced by half compared with the earlier report (3.8 per million maternities compared with 7.7 per million). Deaths directly associated with hemorrhage also show a decrease (3.3 from 5.5 per million maternities); however, hemorrhage remains a dominant cause in developing countries.

Anesthesia was the third most common cause of maternal death in 1982. In the following years, deaths directly associated with anesthesia have fallen to 0.5 per million pregnancies in the 1994–96 report, the lowest figure in the preceding four triennia.[184] There was only one death directly due to an anesthetic. The reduction in the mortality has been attributed to a reduction in the use of general anesthesia and more exerienced supervision. There were three deaths attributed to anesthesia in the 1997–99 report, although still only accounting for 3% of direct maternal deaths.

One study in the USA has attempted to quantify and evaluate anesthesia-related pregnancy deaths by means of a national surveillance system and analysis of vital records.[99] The major finding was that the anesthesia-related maternal mortality rate declined from 4.6 per million live births in the period 1979–81 to 1.7 in 1988–90. The absolute number of deaths involving general anesthesia remained stable (with airway problems as the major factor), and, despite the increased utilization of regional anesthesia, there was a reduction in the absolute number of deaths (factors being local anesthetic toxicity and high spinal/epidural).

REFERENCES

1. Caton D. What a blessing she had chloroform. *The Medical and Social Response of the Pain of Childbirth from 1800 to the Present*. New Haven, CT: Yale University Press, 1999.
2. Gogarten W, Van Aken H. A century of regional analgesia in obstetrics. *Anesth Analg* 2000; **91:** 773–5.
3. Eisenach JC. Obstetric anesthesia: what have you done for us lately? *Anesthesiology* 1999; **91:** 907–8.

4. Hawkins JL, Gibbs CP, Orleans M, *et al.* Obstetric anesthesia work force survey, 1981 versus 1992. *Anesthesiology* 1997; **87:** 135–43.
5. Samsoon GL, Young JR. Difficult tracheal intubation: a retrospective study. *Anaesthesia* 1987; **42:** 487–90.
6. Lyons G: Failed intubation. Six years' experience in a teaching maternity unit. *Anaesthesia* 1985; **40:** 759–62.
7. Department of Health and Social Services. *Report on Confidential Enquiries into Maternal Death in England and Wales 1973–1975*. London: Department of Health and Social Services, 1976.
8. Department of Health and Social Services. *Report on Confidential Enquiries into Maternal Deaths in England and Wales 1982–1984*. London: Department of Health and Social Service, 1985.
9. Tunstall ME. Anaesthesia for obstetric operations. *Clin Obstet Gynaecol* 1980; **7:** 665–94.
10. Bannister F, Macbeth R. Direct laryngoscopy and tracheal intubation. *Lancet* 1944; **2:** 651–4.
11. Benumof JL. Management of the difficult adult airway with special emphasis on awake tracheal intubation. *Anesthesiology* 1991; **75:** 1087–110.
12. King TA, Adams AP. Failed tracheal intubation. *Br J Anaesth* 1990; **65:** 400–14.
13. Hytten F. Weight gain in pregnancy. In: Hytten F, Chamberlain G (eds). *Clinical Physiology in Obstetrics*. Oxford: Blackwell Scientific Publications, 1980: 193–233.
14. Pilkington S, Carli F, Dakin MJ, *et al.* Increase in Mallampati score during pregnancy. *Br J Anaesth* 1995; **74:** 638–42.
15. Bhavani-Shankar K, Krishna S, Moseley H. Airway changes in pregnancy (abstract). *Anesthesiology* 1997; **87:** A895.
16. Farcon EL, Kim MH, Marx GF. Changing Mallampati score during labour. *Can J Anesth* 1994; **41:** 50–1.
17. Bhavani-Shankar K, Bulich L, Kafiluddi R, *et al.* Does labor and delivery induce airway changes? (abstract). *Anesthesiology* 2000; **93:** A1072.
18. Brock-Utne JG, Downing JW, Seedat F. Laryngeal oedema associated with pre-eclamptic toxaemia. *Anaesthesia* 1977; **32:** 556–8.
19. Rocke DA, Murray WB, Rout CC, Gouws E. Relative risk analysis of factors associated with difficult intubation in obstetric anesthesia. *Anesthesiology* 1992; **77:** 67–73.
20. Milsom I, Forssman L, Biber B, *et al.* Maternal haemodynamic changes during caesarean section: a comparison of epidural and general anaesthesia. *Acta Anaesthesiol Scand* 1985; **29:** 161–7.
21. O'Sullivan GM, Sutton AJ, Thompson SA, *et al.* Noninvasive measurement of gastric emptying in obstetric patients. *Anesth Analg* 1987; **66:** 505–11.
22. Roberts RB, Shirley MA. Reducing the risk of acid aspiration during cesarean section. *Anesth Analg* 1974; **53:** 859–68.
23. Gibbs CP, Spohr L, Schmidt D. The effectiveness of sodium citrate as an antacid. *Anesthesiology* 1982; **57:** 44–6.
24. Dewan DM, Floyd HM, Thistlewood JM, *et al.* Sodium citrate pretreatment in elective cesarean section patients. *Anesth Analg* 1985; **64:** 34–7.
25. Lussos S, Datta S. Anesthesia for cesarean delivery. I. General considerations and spinal anesthesia. *Int J Obstet Anesth* 1993; **2:** 109–23.
26. Murphy DF, Nally B, Gardiner J, Unwin A. Effect of metoclopramide on gastric emptying before elective and emergency caesarean section. *Br J Anaesth* 1984; **56:** 1113–16.
27. Wyner J, Cohen SE. Gastric volume in early pregnancy: effect of metoclopramide. *Anesthesiology* 1982; **57:** 209–12.
28. Cohen SE, Jasson J, Talafre ML, *et al.* Does metoclopramide decrease the volume of gastric contents in patients undergoing cesarean section? *Anesthesiology* 1984; **61:** 604–7.
29. Okasha AS, Motaweh MM, Bali A. Cimetidine – antacid combination as premedication for elective caesarean section. *Can Anesth Soc J* 1983; **30:** 593–7.
30. Dewan DM, Wheeler AS, James FM, *et al.* Antacid anticholinergic regimens in patients undergoing elective caesarean section. *Can Anesth Soc J* 1982; **29:** 27–30.
31. Brock-Utne JG, Rubin J, McAravey R, *et al.* The effect of hyoscine and atropine on the lower oesophageal sphincter. *Anaesth Intensive Care* 1977; **5:** 223–5.
32. Archer Jr GW, Marx GF. Arterial oxygen tension during apnoea in parturient women. *Br J Anaesth* 1974; **46:** 358–60.
33. Norris MC, Dewan DM. Preoxygenation for cesarean section: a comparison of two techniques. *Anesthesiology* 1985; **62:** 827–9.
34. Marx GF. Regional analgesia in obstetrics. *Anaesthesist* 1972; **21:** 84–91.
35. Datta S, Hurley RJ, Naulty JS, *et al.* Plasma and cerebrospinal fluid progesterone concentrations in pregnant and nonpregnant women. *Anesth Analg* 1986; **65:** 950–4.
36. Bonica J. Peripheral mechanisms and of parturition pain. *Br J Anaesth* 1979; **51:** 3–9.
37. Datta S. *Obstetric Anesthesia Handbook*, 3rd edn. Philadelphia, PA: Hanley and Belfus, 2000.
38. McDonald J. Pain of childbirth. In: Loeser J (ed.). *Bonica's Management of Pain*, 3rd edn. Philadelphia, PA: Lippincott, Williams and Wilkins, 2001: 1388–414.
39. Melzack R, Taenzer P, Feldman P, Kinch RA. Labour is still painful after prepared childbirth training. *Can Med Assoc J* 1981; **125:** 357–63.
40. Melzack R, Kinch R, Dobkin P, *et al.* Severity of labour pain: influence of physical as well as psychologic variables. *Can Med Assoc J* 1984; **130:** 579–84.
41. Palmer S, Lobo A, Tinnell C. Pain and duration of latent phase labor predicts the duration of active phase labor (abstract). *Anesthesiology* 1996; **85:** A858.
42. Norvell KT, Gaston-Johansson F, Fridh G. Remembrance of labor pain: how valid are retrospective pain measurements? *Pain* 1987; **31:** 77–86.
43. Eappen S, Robbins D. Nonpharmacological means of pain relief for labor and delivery. *Int Anesthesiol Clin* 2002; **40**(4): 103–14.
44. Lamaze F. *Painless Childbirth*. Celestin LR trans. London: Burke, 1958.
45. Bloom SL, McIntire DD, Kelly MA, *et al.* Lack of effect of walking on labor and delivery. *N Engl J Med* 1998; **339:** 76–9.
46. Rosen M. Recent advances in pain relief in childbirth. I. Inhalation and systemic analgesia. *Br J Anaesth* 1971; **43:** 837–48.
47. Marx GF, Katsnelson T. The introduction of nitrous oxide analgesia into obstetrics. *Obstet Gynecol* 1992; **80:** 715–18.
48. Abboud TK, Shnider SM, Wright RG, *et al.* Enflurane analgesia in obstetrics. *Anesth Analg* 1981; **60:** 133–7.
49. Abboud TK, Gangolly J, Mosaad P, Crowell D. Isoflurane in obstetrics. *Anesth Analg* 1989; **68:** 388–91.
50. Swart F, Abboud T, Zhu J. Desflurane analgesia in obstetrics: maternal and neonatal effects (abstract). *Anesthesiology* 1991; **75:** A844.
51. McIntosh DG, Rayburn WF. Patient-controlled analgesia in obstetrics and gynecology. *Obstet Gynecol* 1991; **78:** 1129–35.
52. Podlas J, Breland BD. Patient-controlled analgesia with nalbuphine during labor. *Obstet Gynecol* 1987; **70:** 202–4.
53. Rosaeg OP, Kitts JB, Koren G, Byford LJ. Maternal and fetal effects of intravenous patient-controlled fentanyl analgesia during labour in a thrombocytopenic parturient. *Can J Anesth* 1992; **39:** 277–81.
54. Hatjis CG, Meis PJ. Sinusoidal fetal heart rate pattern associated with butorphanol administration. *Obstet Gynecol* 1986; **67:** 377–80.
55. Robinson JO, Rosen M, Evans JM, *et al.* Maternal opinion about analgesia for labour. A controlled trial between epidural block and intramuscular pethidine combined with inhalation. *Anaesthesia* 1980; **35:** 1173–81.
56. Hollmen AI, Jouppila R, Jouppila P, *et al.* Effect of extradural analgesia using bupivacaine and 2-chloroprocaine on intervillous blood flow during normal labour. *Br J Anaesth* 1982; **54:** 837–42.
57. Jouppila P, Jouppila R, Hollmen A, Koivula A. Lumbar epidural analgesia to improve intervillous blood flow during labor in severe preeclampsia. *Obstet Gynecol* 1982; **59:** 158–61.
58. Gibbs RS, Castillo MS, Rodgers PJ. Management of acute chorioamnionitis. *Am J Obstet Gynecol* 1980; **136:** 709–13.
59. Andrews PJ, Ackerman III WE, Juneja MM. Aortocaval compression in the sitting and lateral decubitus positions during extradural catheter placement in the parturient. *Can J Anesth* 1993; **40:** 320–4.
60. Stone PA, Kilpatrick AW, Thorburn J. Posture and epidural catheter insertion. The relationship between skill, experience and maternal posture on the outcome of epidural catheter insertion. *Anaesthesia* 1990; **45:** 920–3.
61. Dickson MA, Moores C, McClure JH. Comparison of single, end-holed and multi-orifice extradural catheters when used for continuous infusion of local anaesthetic during labour. *Br J Anaesth* 1997; **79:** 297–300.
62. Segal S, Eappen S, Datta S. Superiority of multi-orifice over single-orifice epidural catheters for labor analgesia and cesarean delivery. *J Clin Anesth* 1997; **9:** 109–12.
63. D'Angelo R, Foss ML, Livesay CH. A comparison of multiport and uniport epidural catheters in laboring patients. *Anesth Analg* 1997; **84:** 1276–9.
64. Owen MD, D'Angelo R, Gerancher JC, *et al.* 0.125% ropivacaine is similar

to 0.125% bupivacaine for labor analgesia using patient-controlled epidural infusion. *Anesth Analg* 1998; **86:** 527–31.
65. Gambling DR, Yu P, Cole C, *et al.* A comparative study of patient controlled epidural analgesia (PCEA) and continuous infusion epidural analgesia (CIEA) during labour. *Can J Anesth* 1988; **35:** 249–54.
66. Purdel J, Reid J, Thorburn J, Ashbury AJ. Continuous extradural analgesia: comparison of midwife top-ups, continuous infusions and patient controlled administration. *Br J Anaesth* 1992; **68:** 580–4.
67. Ferrante FM, Rosinia FA, Gordon C, Datta S. The role of continuous background infusions in patient-controlled epidural analgesia for labor and delivery. *Anesth Analg* 1994; **79:** 80–4.
68. Rayburn WF, Smith CV, Leuschen MP, *et al.* Comparison of patient-controlled and nurse-administered analgesia using intravenous fentanyl in labor. *Anesth Rev* 1991; **18:** 31–6.
69. Kleiman SJ, Wiesel S, Tessier MJ. Patient-controlled analgesia (PCA) using fentanyl in a parturient with a platelet function abnormality. *Can J Anesth* 1991; **38:** 489–91.
70. Douglas MJ. Alternatives to epidural analgesia during labor. *Can J Anesth* 1991; **38:** 421–4.
71. Rosaeg OP, Kitts JB, Koren G, Byford LJ. Maternal and fetal effects of intravenous patient-controlled fentanyl analgesia during labor in a thrombocytopenic parturient. *Can J Anesth* 1992; **39:** 277–81.
72. Podias J, Breland BD. Patient-controlled analgesia with nalbuphine during labor. *Obstet Gynecol* 1987; **70:** 202–4.
73. Li DF, Rees GA, Rosen M. Continuous extradural infusion of 0.0625% or 0.125% bupivacaine for pain relief in primigravid labour. *Br J Anaesth* 1985; **57:** 264–70.
74. Smedstad KG, Morison DH. A comparative study of continuous and intermittent epidural analgesia for labour and delivery. *Can J Anesth* 1988; **35:** 234–41.
75. Bhavani-Shankar K, Malov S, Hurley R, Datta S. Do rapidly administered intermittent epidural boluses provide better labor analgesia? (abstract). *Anesthesiology* 2000; **93:** A1071.
76. Curry PD, Pacsoo C, Heap DG. Patient-controlled epidural analgesia in obstetric anaesthetic practice. *Pain* 1994; **57:** 125–7.
77. Crawford JS. The epidural sieve and MBC (minimal blocking concentration): an hypothesis. *Anaesthesia* 1976; **31:** 1277–80.
78. Beilin Y, Bernstein HH, Zucker-Pinchoff B. The optimal distance that a multiorifice epidural catheter should be threaded into the epidural space. *Anesth Analg* 1995; **81:** 301–4.
79. Hamilton CL, Riley ET, Cohen SE. Changes in the position of epidural catheters associated with patient movement. *Anesthesiology* 1997; **86:** 778–84.
80. Lussos S, Datta S. Anesthesia for cesarean delivery. II. Epidural anesthesia, intrathecal and epidural opioids, venous air embolism. International *J Obstet Anesth* 1992; **1:** 208–21.
81. Covino BG, Marx GF, Finster M, Zsigmond EK. Prolonged sensory/motor deficits following inadvertent spinal anesthesia. *Anesth Analg* 1980; **59:** 399–400.
82. Scott DB, Hibbard BM. Serious non-fatal complications associated with extradural block in obstetric practice. *Br J Anaesth* 1990; **64:** 537–41.
83. Breen TW, Ransil BJ, Groves PA, Oriol NE. Factors associated with back pain after childbirth. *Anesthesiology* 1994; **81:** 29–34.
84. MacArthur AJ, Macarthur C, Weeks SK. Is epidural anesthesia in labor associated with chronic low back pain? A prospective cohort study. *Anesth Analg* 1997; **85:** 1066–70.
85. Rawal N, Van Zundert A, Holmstrom B, Crowhurst JA. Combined spinal–epidural technique. *Reg Anesth* 1997; **22:** 406–23.
86. Hepner DL, Gaiser RR, Cheek TG, Gutsche BB. Comparison of combined spinal–epidural and low dose epidural for labour analgesia. *Can J Anesth* 2000; **47:** 232–6.
87. Collis RE, Davies DW, Aveling W. Randomised comparison of combined spinal–epidural and standard epidural analgesia in labour. *Lancet* 1995; **345:** 1413–16.
88. Suzuki N, Koganemaru M, Onizuka S, Takasaki M. Dural puncture with a 26-gauge spinal needle affects spread of epidural anesthesia. *Anesth Analg* 1996; **82:** 1040–2.
89. Holmstrom B, Rawal N, Axelsson K, Nydahl PA. Risk of catheter migration during combined spinal epidural block: percutaneous epiduroscopy study. *Anesth Analg* 1995; **80:** 747–53.
90. Palmer CM, Maciulla JE, Cork RC, *et al.* The incidence of fetal heart rate changes after intrathecal fentanyl labor analgesia. *Anesth Analg* 1999; **88:** 577–81.
91. Norris M. Are combined spinal–epidural catheters reliable? *Int J Obstet Anesth* 2000; **9:** 3–6.
92. Eappen S, Blinn A, Segal S. Incidence of epidural catheter replacement in parturients: a retrospective chart review. *Obstet Anesth* 1998; **7:** 220–5.
93. Albright GA, Forster RM. The safety and efficacy of combined spinal and epidural analgesia/anesthesia (6,002 blocks) in a community hospital. *Reg Anesth Pain Med* 1999; **24:** 117–25.
94. Richardson MG. Regional anesthesia for obstetrics. *Anesthesiol Clin N Am* 2000; **18:** 383–406.
95. Nageotte MP, Larson D, Rumney PJ, *et al.* Epidural analgesia compared with combined spinal-epidural analgesia during labor in nulliparous women. *N Engl J Med* 1997; **337:** 1715–19.
96. Sia AT, Chong JL, Tay DH, *et al.* Intrathecal sufentanil as the sole agent in combined spinal–epidural analgesia for the ambulatory parturient. *Can J Anesth* 1998; **45:** 620–5.
97. Parry MG, Fernando R, Bawa GP, Poulton BB. Dorsal column function after epidural and spinal blockade: implications for the safety of walking following low-dose regional analgesia for labour. *Anaesthesia* 1998; **53:** 382–7.
98. Pickering AE, Parry MG, Ousta B, Fernando R. Effect of combined spinal-epidural ambulatory labor analgesia on balance. *Anesthesiology* 1999; **91:** 436–41.
99. Hawkins JL, Koonin LM, Palmer SK, Gibbs CP. Anesthesia-related deaths during obstetric delivery in the United States, 1979–1990. *Anesthesiology* 1997; **86:** 277–84.
100. Hodgkinson R, Bhatt M, Kim SS, *et al.* Neonatal neurobehavioral tests following cesarean section under general and spinal anesthesia. *Am J Obstet Gynecol* 1978; **132:** 670–4.
101. Helbo-Hansen S, Bang U, Garcia RS, *et al.* Subarachnoid versus epidural bupivacaine 0.5% for caesarean section. *Acta Anaesthesiol Scand* 1988; **32:** 473–6.
102. Abouleish EI. Epinephrine improves the quality of spinal hyperbaric bupivacaine for cesarean section. *Anesth Analg* 1987; **66:** 395–400.
103. Sprague DH. Effects of position and uterine displacement on spinal anesthesia for cesarean section. *Anesthesiology* 1976; **44:** 164–6.
104. Corke BC, Datta S, Ostheimer GW, *et al.* Spinal anaesthesia for Caesarean section. The influence of hypotension on neonatal outcome. *Anaesthesia* 1982; **37:** 658–62.
105. Wollman SB, Marx GF. Acute hydration for prevention of hypotension of spinal anesthesia in parturients. *Anesthesiology* 1968; **29:** 374–80.
106. Gutsche BB. Prophylactic ephedrine preceding spinal analgesia for cesarean section. *Anesthesiology* 1976; **45:** 462–5.
107. Hollmen AI, Jouppila R, Albright GA, *et al.* Intervillous blood flow during caesarean section with prophylactic ephedrine and epidural anaesthesia. *Acta Anaesthesiol Scand* 1984; **28:** 396–400.
108. Shnider SM, de Lorimier AA, Holl JW, *et al.* Vasopressors in obstetrics. I. Correction of fetal acidosis with ephedrine during spinal hypotension. *Am J Obstet Gynecol* 1968; **102:** 911–19.
109. Moran DH, Perillo M, LaPorta RF, *et al.* Phenylephrine in the prevention of hypotension following spinal anesthesia for cesarean delivery. *J Clin Anesth* 1991; **3:** 301–5.
110. Datta S, Alper MH, Ostheimer GW, Weiss JB. Method of ephedrine administration and nausea and hypotension during spinal anesthesia for cesarean section. *Anesthesiology* 1982; **56:** 68–70.
111. Brown Jr WU, Bell GC, Alper MH. Acidosis, local anesthetics, and the newborn. *Obstet Gynecol* 1976; **48:** 27–30.
112. Gaffud MP, Bansal P, Lawton C, *et al.* Surgical analgesia for cesarean delivery with epidural bupivacaine and fentanyl. *Anesthesiology* 1986; **65:** 331–4.
113. Kileff ME, James III FM, Dewan DM, Floyd HM. Neonatal neurobehavioral responses after epidural anesthesia for cesarean section using lidocaine and bupivacaine. *Anesth Analg* 1984; **63:** 413–17.
114. Datta S, Alper MH, Ostheimer GW, *et al.* Effects of maternal position on epidural anesthesia for cesarean section, acid-base status, and bupivacaine concentrations at delivery. *Anesthesiology* 1979; **50:** 205–9.
115. Chan VW, Morley-Forster PK, Vosu HA. Temperature changes and shivering after epidural anesthesia for cesarean section. *Reg Anesth* 1989; **14:** 48–52.
116. Johnson RV, Lyons GR, Wilson RC, Robinson AP. Training in obstetric general anaesthesia: a vanishing art? *Anaesthesia* 2000; **55:** 179–83.
117. Datta S, Briwa J. Modified laryngoscope for endotracheal intubation of obese patients. *Anesth Analg* 1981; **60:** 120–1.
118. Morgan DJ, Blackman GL, Paull JD, Wolf LJ. Pharmacokinetics and plasma binding of thiopental. II. Studies at cesarean section. *Anesthesiology* 1981; **54:** 474–80.
119. Lussos S, Datta S. Anesthesia for cesarean delivery. III. General anesthesia. *Int J Obstet Anesth* 1993; **2:** 109–23.
120. Horwitz LD. Effects of intravenous anesthetic agents on left ventricular function in dogs. *Am J Physiol* 1977; **232:** H44–8.

121. Levinson G, Shnider SM, DeLorimier AA, Steffenson JL. Effects of maternal hyperventilation on uterine blood flow and fetal oxygenation and acid–base status. *Anesthesiology* 1974; **40:** 340–7.
122. Shankar KB, Moseley H, Kumar Y, Vemula V. Arterial to end tidal carbon dioxide tension difference during caesarean section anaesthesia. *Anaesthesia* 1986; **41:** 698–702.
123. Practice guidelines for management of the difficult airway. A report by the American Society of Anesthesiologists' Task Force on Management of the Difficult Airway. *Anesthesiology* 1993; **78:** 597–602.
124. Harmer M. Difficult and failed intubations in obstetrics. International *J Obstet Anesth* 1997; **6:** 25–31.
125. Cooper MG, Feeney EM, Joseph M, McGuinness JJ. Local anaesthetic infiltration for caesarean section. *Anaesth Intensive Care* 1989; **17:** 198–201.
126. Ranney B, Stanage WF. Advantages of local anesthesia for cesarean section. *Obstet Gynecol* 1975; **45:** 163–7.
127. Abouleish E, Rawal N, Fallon K, Hernandez D. Combined intrathecal morphine and bupivacaine for cesarean section. *Anesth Analg* 1988; **67:** 370–4.
128. Fusi L, Steer PJ, Maresh MJ, Beard RW. Maternal pyrexia associated with the use of epidural analgesia in labour. *Lancet* 1989; **1:** 1250–2.
129. Camann WR, Hortvet LA, Hughes N, *et al.* Maternal temperature regulation during extradural analgesia for labour. *Br J Anaesth* 1991; **67:** 565–8.
130. Herbst A, Wolner-Hanssen P, Ingemarsson I. Maternal fever in term labour in relation to fetal tachycardia, cord artery acidaemia and neonatal infection. *Br J Obstet Gynaecol* 1997; **104:** 363–6.
131. Glosten B, Savage M, Rooke GA, Brengelmann GL. Epidural anesthesia and the thermoregulatory responses to hyperthermia–preliminary observations in volunteer subjects. *Acta Anaesthesiol Scand* 1998; **42:** 442–6.
132. Webb PJ, James III FM, Wheeler AS. Shivering during epidural analgesia in women in labor. *Anesthesiology* 1981; **55:** 706–7.
133. Dashe JS, Rogers BB, McIntire DD, Leveno KJ. Epidural analgesia and intrapartum fever: placental findings. *Obstet Gynecol* 1999; **93:** 341–4.
134. Camann W. Intrapartum epidural analgesia and neonatal sepsis evaluations: a casual or causal association? *Anesthesiology* 1999; **90:** 1250–2.
135. Lieberman E, Lang J, Richardson DK, *et al.* Intrapartum maternal fever and neonatal outcome. *Pediatrics* 2000; **105:** 8–13.
136. Hess PE, Pratt SD, Soni AK, *et al.* An association between severe labor pain and cesarean delivery. *Anesth Analg* 2000; **90:** 881–6.
137. Wuitchik M, Bakal D, Lipshitz J. The clinical significance of pain and cognitive activity in latent labor. *Obstet Gynecol* 1989; **73:** 35–42.
138. Philipsen T, Jensen NH. Epidural block or parenteral pethidine as analgesic in labour; a randomized study concerning progress in labour and instrumental deliveries. *Eur J Obstet Gynecol Reprod Biol* 1989; **30:** 27–33.
139. Chestnut DH, McGrath JM, Vincent Jr RD, *et al.* Does early administration of epidural analgesia affect obstetric outcome in nulliparous women who are in spontaneous labor? *Anesthesiology* 1994; **80:** 1201–8.
140. Chestnut DH, Vincent Jr RD, McGrath JM, *et al.* Does early administration of epidural analgesia affect obstetric outcome in nulliparous women who are receiving intravenous oxytocin? *Anesthesiology* 1994; **80:** 1193–200.
141. Halpern SH, Leighton BL, Ohlsson A, *et al.* Effect of epidural vs parenteral opioid analgesia on the progress of labor: a meta-analysis. *JAMA* 1998; **280:** 2105–10.
142. Goodfellow CF, Studd C. The reduction of forceps in primigravidae with epidural analgesia – a controlled trial. *Br J Clin Pract* 1979; **33:** 287–8.
143. Maresh M, Choong KH, Beard RW. Delayed pushing with lumbar epidural analgesia in labour. *Br J Obstet Gynaecol* 1983; **90:** 623–7.
144. Bofill JA, Vincent RD, Ross EL, *et al.* Nulliparous active labor, epidural analgesia, and cesarean delivery for dystocia. *Am J Obstet Gynecol* 1997; **177:** 1465–70.
145. Thorp JA, Hu DH, Albin RM, *et al.* The effect of intrapartum epidural analgesia on nulliparous labor: a randomized, controlled, prospective trial. *Am J Obstet Gynecol* 1993; **169:** 851–8.
146. Ramin SM, Gambling DR, Lucas MJ, *et al.* Randomized trial of epidural versus intravenous analgesia during labor. *Obstet Gynecol* 1995; **86:** 783–9.
147. Sharma S, Leveno K. Update: Epidural analgesia during labor does not increase cesarean births. *Curr Anesthesiol Rep* 2000; **2:** 18–24.
148. Sharma SK, Sidawi JE, Ramin SM, *et al.* Cesarean delivery: a randomized trial of epidural versus patient-controlled meperidine analgesia during labor. *Anesthesiology* 1997; **87:** 487–94.
149. Clark A, Carr D, Loyd G, Cook V, Spinnato J. The influence of epidural analgesia on cesarean delivery rates: a randomized, prospective clinical trial. *Am J Obstet Gynecol* 1998; **179:** 1527–33.
150. Gambling DR, Sharma SK, Ramin SM, *et al.* A randomized study of combined spinal–epidural analgesia versus intravenous meperidine during labor: impact on cesarean delivery rate. *Anesthesiology* 1998; **89:** 1336–44.
151. Impey L, MacQuillan K, Robson M. Epidural analgesia need not increase operative delivery rates. *Am J Obstet Gynecol* 2000; **182:** 358–63.
152. Segal S, Su M, Gilbert P. The effect of a rapid change in availability of epidural analgesia on the cesarean delivery rate: a meta-analysis. *Am J Obstet Gynecol* 2000; **183:** 974–8.
153. Mulroy MF, Norris MC, Liu SS. Safety steps for epidural injection of local anesthetics: review of the literature and recommendations. *Anesth Analg* 1997; **85:** 1346–56.
154. Leighton BL, Norris MC, DeSimone CA, *et al.* The air test as a clinically useful indicator of intravenously placed epidural catheters. *Anesthesiology* 1990; **73:** 610–13.
155. Moore DC, Batra MS. The components of an effective test dose prior to epidural block. *Anesthesiology* 1981; **55:** 693–6.
156. Colonna-Romano P, Lingaraju N, Godfrey SD, Braitman LE. Epidural test dose and intravascular injection in obstetrics: sensitivity, specificity, and lowest effective dose. *Anesth Analg* 1992; **75:** 372–6.
157. Hadzic A, Vloka J, Patel N, Birnbach D. Hypertensive crisis after a successful placement of an epidural anesthetic in a hypertensive parturient. *Reg Anesth* 1995; **20:** 156–8.
158. Leighton BL, Norris MC, Sosis M, *et al.* Limitations of epinephrine as a marker of intravascular injection in laboring women. *Anesthesiology* 1987; **66:** 688–91.
159. Norris MC, Ferrenbach D, Dalman H, *et al.* Does epinephrine improve the diagnostic accuracy of aspiration during labor epidural analgesia? *Anesth Analg* 1999; **88:** 1073–6.
160. Norris MC, Fogel ST, Dalman H, *et al.* Labor epidural analgesia without an intravascular "test dose". *Anesthesiology* 1998; **88:** 1495–501.
161. Roberts JM, Cooper DW. Pathogenesis and genetics of pre-eclampsia. *Lancet* 2001; **357:** 53–6.
162. Sharma SK, Philip J, Whitten CW, *et al.* Assessment of changes in coagulation in parturients with preeclampsia using thromboelastography. *Anesthesiology* 1999; **90:** 385–90.
163. Orlikowski CE, Rocke DA, Murray WB, *et al.* Thrombelastography changes in pre-eclampsia and eclampsia. *Br J Anaesth* 1996; **77:** 157–61.
164. Hood DD, Curry R. Spinal versus epidural anesthesia for cesarean section in severely preeclamptic patients: a retrospective survey. *Anesthesiology* 1999; **90:** 1276–82.
165. Wallace DH, Leveno KJ, Cunningham FG, *et al.* Randomized comparison of general and regional anesthesia for cesarean delivery in pregnancies complicated by severe preeclampsia. *Obstet Gynecol* 1995; **86:** 193–9.
166. Douglas MJ, Ballem PJ. Hematologic disorders. In: Gambling DR, Douglas MJ (eds). *Obstetric Anesthesia and Uncommon disorders.* Philadelphia, PA: WB Saunders, 1998: 307–31.
167. Crosby ET, Halpern SH. Obstetric epidural anaesthesia in patients with Harrington instrumentation. *Can J Anesth* 1989; **36:** 693.
168. Daley MD, Morningstar BA, Rolbin SH, *et al.* Epidural anesthesia for obstetrics and after spinal surgery. *Reg Anesth* 1990; **15:** 280.
169. Hubbert CH. Epidural anesthesia in patients with spinal fusion. *Anesth Analg* 1985; **64:** 843.
170. Bader AM, Camann WR, Datta S. Anesthesia for cesarean delivery in patients with herpes simplex virus type-2 infections. *Reg Anesth* 1990; **15:** 261–3.
171. Boyle RK. Herpes simplex labialis after epidural or parenteral morphine: a randomized prospective trial in an Australian obstetric population. *Anaesth Intensive Care* 1995; **23:** 433.
172. Grange CS, Douglas MJ, Adams TJ, Wadsworth LD. The use of acute hemodilution in parturients undergoing cesarean section. *Am J Obstet Gynecol* 1998; **178:** 156–60.
173. Bernstein HH, Rosenblatt MA, Gettes M, Lockwood C. The ability of the Haemonetics 4 Cell Saver System to remove tissue factor from blood contaminated with amniotic fluid. *Anesth Analg* 1997; **85:** 831–3.
174. Chestnut DH, Dewan DM, Redick LF, *et al.* Anesthetic management for obstetric hysterectomy: a multi-institutional study. *Anesthesiology* 1989; **70:** 607–10.
175. Steinbrook RA, Brooks DC, Datta S. Laparoscopic cholecystectomy during pregnancy. Review of anesthetic management, surgical considerations. *Surg Endosc* 1996; **10:** 511–15.
176. Bhavani-Shankar K, Steinbrook R. Anesthetic considerations for mini-

mally invasive surgery. In: Brooks D (ed.). *Current Review of Minimally Invasive Surgery*, 2nd edn. Philadelphia, PA: Current Medicine, 1998: 29–40.

177. Bhavani-Shankar K, Steinbrook RA, Brooks DC, Datta S. Arterial to end-tidal carbon dioxide pressure difference during laparoscopic surgery in pregnancy. *Anesthesiology* 2000; **93:** 370–3.
178. Shay DC, Bhavani-Shankar K, Datta S.: Laparoscopic surgery during pregnancy. *Anesthesiol Clin N Am* 2001; **19:** 57–67.
179. Mazze RI, Fujinaga M, Baden JM. Reproductive and teratogenic effects of nitrous oxide, fentanyl and their combination in Sprague–Dawley rats. *Br J Anaesth* 1987; **59:** 1291–7.
180. Mazze RI, Fujinaga M, Rice SA, *et al*. Reproductive and teratogenic effects of nitrous oxide, halothane, isoflurane, and enflurane in Sprague–Dawley rats. *Anesthesiology* 1986; **64:** 339–44.
181. Koren G, Pastuszak A, Ito S. Drugs in pregnancy. *N Engl J Med* 1998; **338:** 1128–37.
182. Guidelines 2000 for Cardiopulmonary Resuscitation and Emergency Cardiovascular Care. Part 8: advanced challenges in resuscitation: section 3: special challenges in ECC. The American Heart Association in collaboration with the International Liaison Committee on Resuscitation. *Circulation* 2000; **102:** 1229–52.
183. Katz VL, Dotters DJ, Droegemueller W. Perimortem cesarean delivery. *Obstet Gynecol* 1986; **68:** 571–6.
184. Department of Health and Social Services. *Why Mothers Die: Report on Confidential Enquiries into Maternal Deaths in the United Kingdom 1997–1999*. London: Department of Health and Social Services, 2001.

58

Neonatal anesthesia

JERROLD LERMAN

The neonate presents with some of the greatest challenges that anesthesiologists must face in clinical pediatric practice. Special anatomy, adaptive physiology, developmental pharmacology, and congenital as well as acquired pathology combine to produce a very complex set of conditions that the anesthesiologist must address. Medical and technological advances have pushed the gestational age at which preterm neonates are viable closer and closer to the 20-week date.[1–3] As a consequence, small size has added a serious technical challenge for anesthesiologists. In the past decade, our understanding of physiology and pharmacology as they relate to the neonate together with innovative technology have dramatically increased the margin of safety when anesthetizing neonates. Despite these innovations, perioperative morbidity and mortality in the neonate remain greater than in any other pediatric age group.[4,5] This chapter summarizes the salient considerations that the practicing clinician must master by merging the developmental changes in the neonate with scientific and technological innovations.

Before we begin, several terms merit definition. A neonate is defined as a baby whose postnatal age is 28 days or fewer, and an infant is one whose postnatal age is 12 months or fewer. A fullterm neonate is a baby whose gestational age at birth was 37 weeks or more, whereas a preterm neonate is one whose gestational age at birth was fewer than 37 weeks, i.e. 36 weeks' gestation or fewer.

ANATOMY AND PHYSIOLOGY

Central nervous system

Several anatomic features distinguish the central nervous system of the neonate from that of the adult, including a soft and pliable cranium, nonfused sutures, two open fontanels (the posterior fontanel closes by 6–9 months' postnatal age, whereas the anterior fontanel closes by approximately 18 months of age), a brain that is structurally complete but incompletely myelinated (until 2 years of age), a cerebral cortex that is poorly developed, a spinal cord that ends at L1 (compared with L4 in adults), and, in the case of the preterm neonate, fragile subependymal blood vessels. These features have important physiologic implications for the management of neonates under anesthesia.

The composition of the brain changes dramatically during early infancy.[6] In the neonate, the predominant constituent of the brain is water. Its proportion in the brain decreases steadily as cerebral myelin and protein concentrations increase throughout infancy and early childhood. This decreasing proportion of water in the brain is reflected in inverse changes in the partition coefficients of inhalational anesthetics.[7] The partition coefficients of inhalational anesthetics increase as the proportion of water in the brain decreases with increasing age.[7] The significance of the reduced solubility of anesthetics in the brain of neonates is twofold: (1) it contributes in part to the more rapid washin and washout of inhalational anesthetics from the brain of neonates compared with adults and (2) it may contribute to the altered requirements for inhaled anesthetics in this age group.

The blood–brain barrier in the neonate is immature at birth, thereby facilitating the passage of large, lipid-soluble compounds such as anesthetic drugs and free bilirubin into the brain. Although the blood–brain barrier comprises capillary endothelial walls without fenestrations, tight junctions, and an outer sheath of astrocyte foot processes, numerous compounds are transported from the blood to the brain via specialized transport mechanisms in the neonate. Maturation of the barrier occurs soon after birth.

One-third of the total cardiac output perfuses the brain in the neonate compared with one-seventh in the adult. However, cerebral blood flow (CBF) in the healthy neonate (30–40 mL per 100 g brain tissue per min) is less than it is in both adults (55 mL per 100 g per min) and children (65–100 mL per 100 g per min).[8] Cerebrovascular responsiveness to changes in carbon dioxide (CO_2) and oxygen (O_2) tensions are attenuated in the neonate. Although CBF is autoregulated over a wide range of arterial blood pressures in the healthy neonate, autoregulation is compromised in the asphyxiated preterm neonate.[9] In the latter, CBF is pressure passive, i.e. CBF varies directly with systemic mean arterial pressure. As CBF increases, intracranial pressure also increases, depending on the compliance of the brain. Autoregulation of CBF in the asphyxiated preterm neonate is restored at some time after the asphyxial insult, although when this occurs remains unclear.

Neural mechanisms responsible for the perception of noxious stimuli are present as early as week 6 of gestation.[10,11] Although these neural pathways have been known for some time to exist, the notion that they are developed and that neonates perceive and respond to noxious stimuli in a manner not unlike older children and adults was not widely appreciated until the 1980s. This has led to the development of guidelines and new interventions to prevent and manage pain in the neonate, including regional anesthesia and opioid administration as discussed below.

In addition to the development of a neural axis to stress and surgery, the neuroendocrine axis in the preterm neonate is also well developed. These neonates respond to ligation of the patent ductus arteriosus with increased epinephrine (adrenaline), glucose, and other mediators indicative of a neuroendocrine response.[12] Indeed, the addition of a single intravenous dose of fentanyl (10 µg kg^{-1}) to a light anesthetic was sufficient to significantly attenuate these responses to surgery. These data are consistent with our belief that neonates, both preterm and fullterm, require analgesia and anesthesia during and after surgery[12,13] and that inadequate levels of anesthesia can result in a marked stress response.[12,14,15]

Respiratory physiology

Embryologically, the lungs begin to develop by 4 weeks' gestation; lobar airways are formed by 5 weeks, segmental airways by 6 weeks, and subsegmental airways by 7 weeks. By 8 weeks, the epithelial cords, which will differentiate into the trachea and bronchi, have migrated caudally and ventrally into the mesenchyme accompanied by the budding pulmonary vasculature. By 16 weeks' gestation, the tracheobronchial tree has divided into 16 bronchial branches terminating in the terminal bronchiole or acinus. Failure to develop these 16 branches, whether because of a genetic defect or because of a space-occupying lesion (congenital diaphragmatic hernia), will result in pulmonary hypoplasia. Between 16 and 25 weeks' gestation, the lungs begin to adopt the characteristics of a potential gas exchange organ: pulmonary capillaries begin to interdigitate among the alveolar saccules and type II pneumocytes begin to form. Type II pneumocytes may actually be the nondifferentiated epithelial cells of the lungs, with type I cells deriving from these. As the lung grows, the type I cells become so thin they are no longer visible by light microscopy. In fact, in the mature adult lung, type I pneumocytes cover a 25-fold greater surface area of the lung than type II cells.

At 34–36 weeks' gestation, acini continue to proliferate into multiple branching saccules and true alveoli. The capillaries envelop the acini, the alveolar capillary membrane thins, and type II pneumocytes begin to secrete mature surfactant (phosphatidyl choline and phosphatidyl glycerol).

Dramatic changes occur within the lung with the first few breaths after delivery. Initial respiratory efforts generate extremely large negative intrapleural pressures (exceeding −9.33 kPa; −70 mmHg) in order to inflate the fluid-filled alveoli. As these powerful respiratory efforts continue, alveoli are recruited in increasing numbers with the assistance of the surface tension-lowering properties of endogenous surfactant. Most of the fluid within the alveoli is cleared rapidly through the upper airway, although any residual fluid is cleared slowly over the subsequent 24–72 h by transcapillary and translymphatic routes. Both inflation of the alveoli and clearance of alveolar fluid increase lung compliance during the first few days after delivery.

Control of respiration matures rapidly in the neonatal period. Exogenous CO_2 increases alveolar ventilation in the neonate, although the magnitude of the response is blunted in preterm infants.[16] The ventilatory response to CO_2 increases with both gestational age and postnatal age. The resting CO_2 tension in the neonate is less than it is in the adult; this leftward shift of the CO_2 ventilation response curve gradually develops into the adult response by 2 years of age. Unlike the response in the adult, hypoxemia (15% inspired O_2) in the preterm neonate attenuates the ventilatory response to CO_2.[17] This response dissipates by 2–3 months after birth.

The ventilatory response to hypoxemia in the neonate is more complex than the response to CO_2.[18] During the first 3 weeks after delivery, the ventilatory response to hypoxia depends on the temperature of the neonate: in the presence of normothermia, hypoxemia causes transient hyperventilation (via peripheral chemoreceptors) that is followed by a decrease in ventilation, whereas in the presence of hypothermia, hypoxemia decreases ventilation. Hyperventilation in response to hypoxia is poorly developed in the fullterm neonate and even less well developed in the preterm neonate. By the end of the first month after delivery, however, hypoxemia increases alveolar ventilation independent of the infant's temperature.

Two additional respiratory reflexes are present in the neonate: Head's paradoxical reflex and the Hering–Breuer reflex. The former describes the inspiratory response to partial inflation of the lung and the latter describes the initiation of passive exhalation that occurs after inflation of the lung. The respiratory pattern in some preterm neonates has been described as periodic, which is a breathing pattern that is punctuated by occasional episodes of apnea (5–15 s in duration). The incidence of these apneas is directly related to the degree of prematurity and, thus, immaturity of the respiratory control center. More than 70% of preterm infants display evidence of periodic breathing, with up to 50% experiencing prolonged apneic episodes. When the apneic episodes are prolonged (> 15 s), they may be accompanied by bradycardia and hemoglobin O_2 desaturation < 90%. Between apneic episodes, normal respiratory rates or tachypnea are present. These patterns may occur up to 52 weeks' postconceptual age. Although periodic breathing and apnea can occur in the fullterm neonate, they are rarely associated with perioperative complications. Effective management of apnea of prematurity includes phosphodiesterase inhibitors (such as oral theophylline). Perioperative therapy includes a single dose of 10 mg kg^{-1} parenteral caffeine base.[19]

The upper airway of the neonate differs in several respects from that of the adult.[20] The head is relatively large, the occiput is prominent, and the chin is retrognathic in the neonate. The size of the head and the prominence of the occiput naturally position the head in the "sniffing" position to facilitate tracheal intubation. The nasal passages are relatively narrow, predisposing them to obstruction in the presence of small amounts of secretions. The nasal passages, which account for more than 50% of the total resistance of the respiratory system, are of particular importance as the neonate is an obligate nasal breather. The tongue is relatively large and occupies much of the oropharynx. In contrast to the older child and adult, lymphoid tissue is scant in the upper airway in the neonate. Because the neck is short and the hyoid cartilage lies in close proximity to the thyroid cartilage, the larynx is situated more cephalad (at the C3–4 vertebral level) in the neonate than it is in the adult (at the C4–5 level). The epiglottis is long, floppy, and omega-shaped in the neonate in contrast to the short, broad, and flat epiglottis in the adult. It projects posteriorly at an angle of 45° to the base of the tongue compared with 15–25° in the adult. These anatomic features explain why the epiglottis must be lifted during laryngoscopy in the neonate.

The laryngeal inlet is recognized anatomically by the two pearly white vocal cords that lie immediately caudad to the epiglottis. The vocal cords are bow-shaped being cephalad anteriorly and rostral posteriorly in contrast with their flat orientation, perpendicular to the long axis of the trachea in the adult. The cricoid ring which is situated immediately below the vocal cords is the most critical anatomic feature of the airway in the neonate as (1) it is the only circumferentially solid cartilaginous structure within the airway, (2) it is funnel-shaped with the caudal aperture being the narrowest part of the airway in the neonate (3–5 mm in diameter) and (3) it is covered with loose pseudostratified columnar epithelium, which is susceptible to both inflammation and edema when it is irritated or traumatized.

The cricoid ring, the "Achilles heel" of the upper airway, is so named for being the most vulnerable structure within the upper airway in the neonate. When the epithelial lining of the ring is irritated or traumatized, such as in the presence of a viral infection of the upper respiratory tract or a tight-fitting tracheal tube, it becomes inflamed and edematous. As the epithelium swells, it encroaches on the lumen within the cricoid ring and may severely compromise airflow. Because the airflow in the upper airway is turbulent (Reynolds number > 2000) and the resistance to turbulent airflow is proportional to the fifth power of the radius, small amounts of swelling dramatically decrease the radius of the lumen, which in turn increases the resistance to airflow. For example, a twofold reduction in radius of the lumen increases the resistance to airflow by 32-fold. Thus, care must be taken to avoid trauma and irritation of the epithelial lining of the cricoid ring. The length of the trachea in the neonate is 4–5 cm and is supported by noncalcified, soft (compliant), cartilaginous tracheal rings. As in adults, the right bronchial angle is 32° to the axis of the trachea, whereas the left bronchial angle is 47° in the preterm and fullterm neonates.[21]

The ontogeny of the lower respiratory tract is relevant for anesthesiologists beginning about week 16 of gestation. By that time, the divisions of the airway are completed to the terminal bronchioles. Saccules, clusters of air sacs, begin to develop by 24 weeks' gestation, followed shortly thereafter with periacinar capillary proliferation. Alveoli begin to develop from these saccules at 32 weeks' gestation, increasing in number to approximately 20 million by term. The number of alveoli continues to increase after birth, reaching adult numbers, approximately 300 million, by 6 years of age. Two types of cells line the alveolar walls: type 1 and type 2 pneumocytes. Type 1 pneumocytes compose the structural lining of the alveoli. Type 2 pneumocytes first appear at 24 weeks' gestation and are responsible for the production of surfactant. Surfactant production begins in the second trimester, with increasing volumes of surfactant produced as the fetus approaches term.

Structurally, the lower airways and chest wall of the neonate suffer from several anatomic and structural disadvantages compared with those in the adult. The ribs are soft, noncalcified, and perpendicular to the vertebral column. They contrast with the ribs in the adult chest, which are calcified and bucket-handled. The increased compliance of the chest wall in the neonate decreases the efficiency of the respiratory effort. The intercostal muscles in the neonate are poorly developed, containing fewer type I high-oxidative fibers than children older than 2 years.[22] The elastin content of the pulmonary interstitium in the neonate is less than that in the adult, accounting in part for the greater closing capacity, greater lung compliance, and smaller intrapleural pressure (0 to −2 cmH_2O) in the neonate compared with the adult. This predisposes the neonate to intrapulmonary shunting of blood. Together, these differences place the fullterm neonate and the preterm neonate at risk for respiratory failure to an even greater extent.

The diaphragm is the primary muscle responsible for effective ventilation in the neonate. However, the diaphragm is also disadvantaged both anatomically and functionally. It has disproportionately fewer type I fast-oxidative muscle fibers than children aged 2 years. Thus, it is prone to fatigue.[22] The mechanical efficiency of the diaphragm is further compromised by the acute angle formed by the diaphragm and the abdominal wall. A protuberant abdomen pushes the diaphragm cephalad well beyond the optimal curvature for maximum contraction and increases the load against which the diaphragm must contract. These features act together to reduce the mechanical efficiency of the diaphragm and predispose it to fatigue and failure in the neonate.

The lung volumes in the neonate differ in several respects from the adult (Table 58.1). Although the number of alveoli increases during early childhood, the lung volumes in the neonatal period are small when adjusted for body weight and even smaller when adjusted for metabolic differences. The total alveolar surface area for gas exchange in the neonate is approximately 50-fold less than that in the adult: 2.8 m^2 compared with 150 m^2 in the adult even though the metabolic rate in the neonate is twice that in the adult (see below). Functional residual capacity (FRC) increases during the first 48 h after birth, reaching similar levels to those in the adult when normalized for weight. Despite the similarity in FRC between neonates and adults, closing volume exceeds the FRC and may explain, in part, the low arterial O_2 tensions observed in early infancy. Tidal volume in the neonate and adult are similar when normalized for body weight (Table 58.1). Dead space is also similar in the two age groups, being 30% of the tidal volume. The lung continues to mature throughout childhood and adolescence, reaching adult volumes by 18 years of age.

Table 58.1 *Normal pulmonary indices*

Index	Neonate	Adult
Oxygen consumption (mL kg^{-1} min^{-1})	6.4	3.5
Carbon dioxide production (mL kg^{-1} min^{-1})	6.0	3.0
Alveolar ventilation (mL kg^{-1} min^{-1})	130	60
Respiratory rate (breaths min^{-1})	35	15
Minute volume (mL kg^{-1} min^{-1})	200	90
Tidal volume (mL kg^{-1})	6	7
Vital capacity (mL kg^{-1})	35	70
Functional residual capacity (mL kg^{-1})	30	34
FRC/V_A ratio	0.23	0.57
Closing capacity (mL kg^{-1})	35	23
Total lung capacity (mL kg^{-1})	63	86

FRC, functional residual capacity; V_A, alveolar ventilation.

Spontaneous respiratory rate decreases as age increases: from peak values in the preterm (40–70 breaths min^{-1}) and fullterm neonate (35–40 breaths min^{-1}) to values in the adult (12–16 breaths min^{-1}). Alveolar ventilation also decreases as age increases from 100–150 mL kg^{-1} min^{-1} in neonates to 60 mL kg^{-1} min^{-1} in adults. This age-related decrease in ventilatory requirements reflects a parallel decrease in metabolic rate with age: O_2 consumption in the neonate, 7 mL kg^{-1} min^{-1}, is twice that in the adult, 3.5 mL kg^{-1} min^{-1}. Although respiratory rate in the awake neonate is rapid, alveolar ventilation is inefficient because of the reasons outlined above. Consequently, when the trachea is intubated and ventilation is controlled mechanically, normocapnia can be maintained in the neonate with healthy lungs, with tidal volumes of 10–15 mL kg^{-1} and low respiratory rates of 15–25 breaths min^{-1}. These data suggest that the major source of CO_2 production in the preterm neonate is the energy expended for spontaneous ventilation. For the neonate with poor respiratory gas exchange (as evidenced by hypercapnia or hypoxemia), respiratory rates in excess of the 15–25 breaths min^{-1} may be required.

Arterial blood gases change dramatically during the first 24 h after delivery. Arterial P_{O_2} increases from 4.66 kPa (35 mmHg) to 9.33 kPa (70 mmHg), P_{CO_2} decreases from 8.66 kPa (65 mmHg) to 5.06 kPa (38 mmHg), and pH increases from 7.20 to 7.36. These changes in blood gases reflect the changes in respiratory function in the early postnatal period.

Cardiovascular physiology

Embryologically, the four-chambered heart and great vessels are developed by 8 weeks' gestation. *In utero*, the right and left sides of the heart pump blood in parallel as follows: oxygenated blood returns from the placenta via the umbilical vein and follows one of two paths before entering the right atrium – approximately equal volumes of venous blood bypass the liver via the ductus venosus and pass through the liver. As the oxygenated blood flows from the inferior vena cava into the right atrium, one-third is preferentially shunted via the crista dividens through the foramen ovale to the left side of the heart and from there to the head, neck, and upper extremities. The remaining two-thirds of the oxygenated blood combines with all of the deoxygenated blood that returns via the superior vena cava, and enters the right ventricle and exits into the pulmonary artery. Ninety-three percent of the blood entering the pulmonary artery is then shunted through the ductus arteriosus into the descending aorta, whereas the remaining 7% enters the pulmonary artery.

During the transition to extrauterine life, the heart undergoes dramatic adaptive changes. Immediately after birth, however, these flow patterns change drastically as the right and left sides of the heart begin to pump blood in series rather than parallel. The change in the pattern of blood flow is facilitated by a precipitous decrease in the pulmonary vascular resistance that has been attributed, in part, to an increase in the alveolar O_2 tension as well as to a mechanical effect resulting from inflation of alveoli.

Pulmonary blood flow increases during this period from only 7% of the cardiac output *in utero* to 100% *ex utero*. As the pulmonary blood flow increases, the left atrial pressure increases until the pressure exceeds that in the right atrium. This pressure gradient across the atrial septum is sufficient to close the foramen ovale. Although functionally closed immediately after birth, the foramen ovale remains probe patent in approximately 50% of children less than 5 years of age. Moreover, high pressures within the right side of the heart (such as those that result from hypoxemia, a Valsalva maneuver, coughing, or crying) may prevent closure of the foramen ovale or reopen an already closed foramen, resulting in a right-to-left shunt.

The ductus arteriosus functionally closes within the first 24 h after birth. During this period, the closure of the ductus is reversible. Anatomic closure of the ductus, however, may not be complete for up to 4 weeks after birth in the fullterm neonate. At least five factors facilitate closure of the ductus arteriosus: O_2, norepinephrine (noradrenaline), epinephrine, acetylcholine, and bradykinin. Of these factors, O_2 is by far the most important determinant of the closure of the ductus. Several factors have been associated with relaxation of the smooth muscle of the ductus arteriosus, i.e. they delay or prevent closure of the ductus, including hypoxemia, acidosis, fluid overload, and prematurity. The sensitivity of ductal smooth muscle cells to oxidative phosphorylation in the presence of O_2 depends on the gestational age of the infant: the sensitivity of ductal smooth muscle to oxygen increases in parallel with gestational age.

If these factors are corrected and the ductus remains patent, the first-line therapy is indomethacin (prostaglandin synthetase inhibitor). If indomethacin fails, then surgical closure may be required. The sensitivity of the infant ductal smooth muscle to indomethacin is similar to the effect of O_2, i.e. the sensitivity increases with gestational age. In patients with congenital heart defects that are associated with critically low pulmonary blood flow, prostaglandin E_2 may be administered in order to prevent closure of the ductus until other shunts are in place to maintain pulmonary blood flow. Finally, the ductus venosus, an extracardiac shunt between the umbilical vein and the inferior vena cava, closes functionally within the first week after birth and anatomically within the first 2–3 months. A patent ductus venosus decreases the delivery of drugs to the liver and therefore may prolong their elimination half-life in the first few days after delivery.

The right and left ventricles are similar in size at birth. Within the first few days after birth, however, the thickness of the left ventricular wall increases dramatically in response to the increased workload, whereas the right ventricle wall thickness remains unchanged. By 3 months after birth, the mass of the left ventricle exceeds that of the right ventricle, approaching their relative proportions in adults. Ventricular muscle from fetal lambs is primarily cartilaginous in histology, with sparse contractile elements when compared with myocardium from adult sheep. This is reflected in decreased compliance and less active tension during stimulation of the ventricular myocardium.[23] Evidence has also been forthcoming to suggest that intracellular calcium flux and calcium sensitivity of the contractile proteins are decreased in the neonatal myocardium.[24,25] Together, these features limit myocardial contractility in the neonate.

Functionally, cardiac output depends on the product of heart rate and stroke volume. Stroke volume in turn depends on myocardial contractility, preload, and afterload. In preterm and fullterm neonates, heart rate is the primary determinant of cardiac output. Studies in fetal lambs demonstrated an important role for heart rate in the determination of cardiac output.[26] The low compliance of the ventricular myocardium in the neonate limits the role of preload in determining stroke volume. In response to hypoxemia, cardiac output increases via an increase in heart rate. In response to hypercapnia or lactic acidosis, stroke volume decreases. Afterload is determined by the resistance of the large arterial blood vessels and the tone of the peripheral vascular bed. Because sympathetic tone is poorly developed in the neonate, afterload is low in the neonate but increases in parallel with the increase in systemic blood pressure with aging. In summary, cardiac output in the neonate depends primarily on a rapid heart rate and to a lesser extent on an adequate preload and adequate myocardial contractility.

At birth, autonomic innervation of the heart (and peripheral arterial vasculature) is primarily parasympathetic with sparse innervation from the sympathetic nervous system. The balance of autonomic innervation matures as the child ages, with increasing innervation by the sympathetic nervous system in parallel with age.

Systolic arterial blood pressure and heart rate in infancy change dramatically with increasing age. In the fullterm neonate, systolic pressure is approximately 8.66 kPa (65 mmHg) by the first 24 h after delivery. It increases to 10 kPa (75 mmHg) in the first week after delivery, increases slowly to 12.66 kPa (95 mmHg) by 1 year of age and then reaches its apex of 15.33 kPa (115 mmHg) by 12 years of age. In the preterm neonate, 27–30 weeks gestational age (0.8–1.7 kg), the systolic pressure range is 6–7.33 kPa (45–55 mmHg). In contrast, heart rate increases during the perinatal period and then decreases with increasing age. At birth, the heart rate in the neonate is 120–175 beats min^{-1}, with the preterm having a more rapid heart rate. Heart rate increases to a maximum of 160 beats min^{-1} by the end of the neonatal period and then decreases steadily to 125 beats min^{-1} at 1–3 years and 80 beats min^{-1} by 8–12 years.

Circulating blood volume decreases with increasing age. Blood volume in the preterm neonate is greatest, 90–100 mL kg^{-1}, decreasing to 80 mL kg^{-1} in the fullterm neonate and then to 70 mL kg^{-1} by adulthood.

At birth, the concentration of hemoglobin (Hb) in blood is between 14 and 20 g dL^{-1} in the fullterm acyanotic neonate. The concentration of Hb decreases during infancy, reaching a nidus of 10 g dL^{-1} by 10–15 weeks in fullterm neonates and 8 g dL^{-1} by 4–8 weeks in preterm neonates. The decrease in Hb concentration in early infancy has been attributed, in part, to decreased erythropoiesis and a shortened lifespan of red cells. After reaching its nidus, Hb increases steadily throughout infancy reaching adult concentrations by the end of infancy.[27,28]

Not only does the concentration of Hb change throughout infancy but also the type of Hb changes. The concentration of HbF decreases from 95% at 30 weeks' gestation to 80% by 40 weeks, and then decreases steadily to 5% by 6 months after birth. The remainder of the Hb present in blood is predominantly HbA. Because 2,3-diphosphoglycerate binds poorly to the γ chains of HbF, HbF has a very high affinity for oxygen. This is reflected in the values of the P_{50} for the oxyhemoglobin dissociation curve during gestation and early infancy: 2–2.4 kPa (15–18 mmHg) in the preterm neonate, 2.58 kPa (19.4 mmHg) in the fullterm neonate, 4.13 kPa (31 mmHg) in the infant 8–12 months after delivery, and 3.69 kPa (27.7 mmHg) in the adult.[28] Although the low P_{50} in the fetus optimizes the uptake of oxygen from the placenta, it prevents its release at the tissue. Additional maneuvers that shift the oxyhemoglobin dissociation curve to the left (i.e. lower the P_{50}) include hyperventilation, hypothermia, and alkalosis. These may further limit the availability of oxygen and compromise tissue oxygenation. However, these disadvantages are offset, in part, by the increased hemoglobin concentration, expanded red cell volume, and greater cardiac output in the neonate, thereby assuring adequate oxygen delivery to tissues.

Fluid homeostasis and metabolic function

Total body water decreases with increasing gestational age, reaching 78% of body weight in the fullterm neonate (Fig. 58.1).[6] Total body water decreases steadily from birth, reaching 65% of body weight by 12 months of age, where it remains unchanged until adulthood. In contrast, the relative proportions of extra- and intracellular fluid change dramatically throughout gestation and the first few years after birth. Extracellular fluid decreases rapidly throughout gestation and during the first 12 months after birth, after which time the decrease is attenuated, reaching approximately 20% by 4 years of age. In contrast, intracellular fluid increases throughout gestation and during the first 2 months after birth. During the remainder of infancy, the proportion of intracellular fluid decreases until 12 months, after which time the proportion of intracellular fluid increases, reaching 50% by 4 years of age.

Renal function is immature at birth, particularly in the preterm neonate. Embryologically, a complete set of nephrons have formed in the fetal kidney by 36 weeks' gestation, although renal cortical development continues for several more months. At birth, renal function is characterized by a low glomerular filtration rate, low renal blood flow, and poor tubular function. Glomerular filtration rate (GFR) increases throughout gestational age, reaching 30% of the adult GFR in the term neonate.[29] Within the first week after birth, renal function dramatically improves: renal blood flow increases with a commensurate increase in GFR.

The fullterm neonate is limited in its ability to concentrate urine (maximum concentrating ability is 800 mosmol L^{-1}) to one-third that of the adult. The neonate is also limited in its ability to excrete a large water load, but this matures to adults levels by approximately 6 weeks of age.[30] These limitations in renal function may be explained by a low GFR and limited tubular secretion and by resorption of water, glucose, sodium, and bicarbonate. Although renal function matures rapidly in the first month of extrauterine life, tubular resorption does not reach adult levels until approximately 12 months of age.[31] Thus, the elimination half-lives of drugs that depend on the kidney for elimination may be prolonged in the neonate.

Hepatic function is also immature at birth. Carbohydrate reserves in the liver accumulate primarily during the third trimester of pregnancy and, consequently, are limited in the preterm neonate. Preterm neonates, particularly those stressed at birth, may require a 10% dextrose infusion in the early postnatal period to prevent hypoglycemia. Clinically significant hypoglycemia is defined as a blood glucose concentration $<30\,\mathrm{mg\,dL^{-1}}$ in the fullterm neonate and $<20\,\mathrm{mg\,dL^{-1}}$ in the preterm neonate during the first 3 days of extrauterine life. After the first 3 days, hypoglycemia is defined as a concentration $<40\,\mathrm{mg\,dL^{-1}}$. Treatment of acute hypoglycemia requires a bolus of $0.5\text{–}1.0\,\mathrm{g\,kg^{-1}}$ intravenous (i.v.) glucose followed by an infusion of $5\text{–}6\,\mathrm{mg\,kg^{-1}\,min^{-1}}$ as a maintenance infusion. Serial blood glucose concentrations should be monitored to prevent wide swings in the glucose concentration.

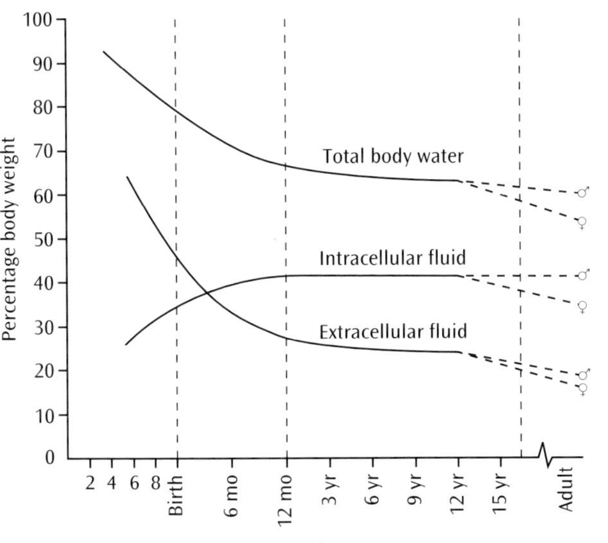

Figure 58.1 *Changes in total, extracellular, and intracellular body water throughout gestation and early infancy up to 16 years of age. (Reproduced with permission from Friis-Hansen.[6])*

Hepatic synthesis of the vitamin K-dependent clotting factors – II, VII, IX, and X – in the fullterm neonate is between 20% and 60% of adult values and less in the preterm neonate. As a result of the deficiency of these clotting factors, the prothrombin time is prolonged. Consequently, oral or parenteral vitamin K may be required at birth to augment the clotting cascade.

Hepatic metabolism of drugs in the neonatal period has been the subject of intense research during the past two decades. The following five points summarize our understanding of the biotransformation of drugs in the neonate:

1 The overall rates of drug biotransformation and elimination are slow in the neonate.
2 The overall rate of drug elimination from the neonate displays marked interindividual variability.
3 Enzyme systems responsible for drug biotransformation mature at different rates.
4 Drug biotransformation and elimination in the neonate depend on the pathophysiology present.
5 Alternative paths for biotransformation of drugs may be active in neonates.

The biotransformation of many drugs may be slower in the neonate than in the adult. Many enzyme systems in the liver are immature at birth.[32] The activity of phase 1 cytochrome P450-dependent mixed function oxidases is immature in the neonate, but matures to adult values by 6 months of age. However, these oxidases are not uniformly immature. Considerable variability exists in the efficiency of this group of enzymes, resulting in some drugs being transformed at rapid rates whereas others are transformed at slow rates. Furthermore, multiple isoforms of these enzymes may exist. These may result in dramatically different biotransformation rates for individual drugs with similar structures. Additionally, the activity of phase 2 reactions, which are primarily conjugative, matures at a variable rate: sulfation is mature by birth, whereas glucuronidation, acetylation, and glycination are quite immature at birth but mature by 1 year of age.[33,34]

The delivery of drugs to the liver may also be reduced in addition to the slow biotransformation of drugs in the neonate. Liver blood flow in the neonate is reduced in the presence of a patent ductus venosus and increased intra-abdominal pressure. Data from lambs indicate that the ductus venosus may remain patent for several days of extrauterine life.[35] Liver blood flow may also decrease further if intra-abdominal pressure increases after repair of a congenital lesion of the anterior abdominal wall.[36]

Several disease states may further compound the delayed elimination of drugs in the neonate. Congestive heart failure, hepatic disease, and renal insufficiency may delay the elimination of drugs. In the neonate, hypoxia and asphyxia further delay elimination of drugs, as evidenced by the accumulation of phenobarbital in perinatal asphyxia.

Based on these considerations, the elimination half-life of many drugs that depend on hepatic biotransformation may be significantly prolonged in the neonate. For preterm infants, the smaller the infant, the less mature the liver, then the less frequent repeat doses are required. Repeat doses or the dose for continuous infusion should be adjusted downward to preclude toxic concentrations of drugs. Sequential determinations of plasma concentrations of the drug or titration of end-organ effects may be useful to guide clinicians to the optimal dosing regimen.

Blood chemistry changes throughout gestation and postnatal life (Table 58.2). In the fullterm neonate, the serum concentration of sodium is similar to that in the adult. However, the normal serum concentration of potassium may be as great as 7.6 mequiv L^{-1}. Serum potassium concentration decreases after birth, reaching adult values during infancy. Hypocalcemia may occur in the first few days of life, particularly in the sick preterm neonate. Two mechanisms have been proposed to explain this hypocalcemia: poor transport of calcium across the placenta and inadequate levels of parathyroid hormone.[37] Hypocalcemia may be prevented by administering infusions of calcium when required.

Plasma protein concentrations also change with gestational and postnatal ages. Albumin concentration increases in parallel with age.[38] Similarly, α_1-acid glycoprotein concentrations increase with increasing age (Fig. 58.2).[39] With lower concentrations of α_1-acid glycoprotein in neonates than in adults, the free fraction and thus the volume of distribution of circulating opioids (fentanyl, alfentanil, and sufentanil)[40] and local anesthetics [lidocaine (lignocaine), bupivacaine] increase.

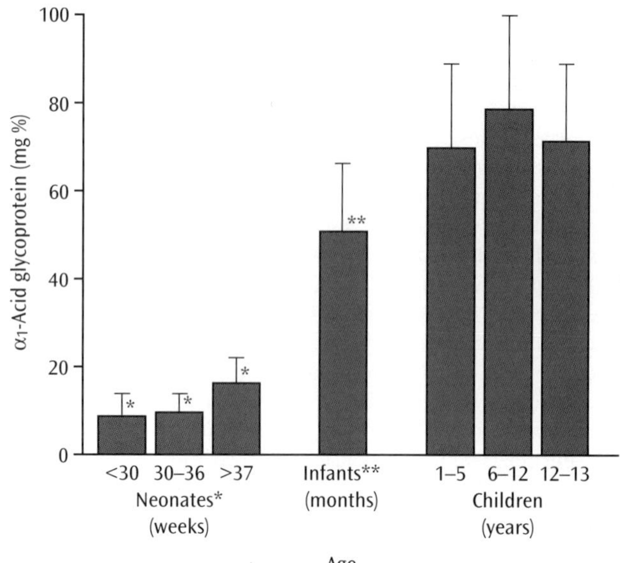

Figure 58.2 *Age and α_1-acid glycoprotein concentration. The concentration increased significantly with age (P < 0.001). (Adapted from data in Lerman* et al.[39]*)*

Metabolic and thermal homeostasis

The oxygen requirement by the neonate increases after birth from 5 mL kg^{-1} min^{-1} on day 1 to a zenith of 7–8 mL kg^{-1} min^{-1} by 1 week of age. This high oxygen consumption persists throughout infancy, but wanes during late childhood to adult levels of 3–4 mL kg^{-1} min^{-1}. The CO_2 production parallels these changes in oxygen consumption (Table 58.1). In the neonate, the respiratory quotient, V_{CO_2}/V_{O_2}, varies between 0.7 and 1.0 depending on internal and external influences.

Manifestations of the increased metabolic rate are reflected in the pulmonary and cardiac indices (Table 58.1). Alveolar ventilation and cardiac output are markedly increased compared with adults. For the most part, these increases are driven by increased respiratory and heart rates.

Basic energy requirements of the neonate are the likely cause of the increased metabolic rate deduced from oxygen consumption and CO_2 production. In the neonate, the basal energy requirement, 580 joules per day or 120 kcal kg^{-1} day^{-1}, is 3.5–5 times greater than that in adults, 146 joules per day or 35–50 kcal kg^{-1} day^{-1}. Glucose is the primary energy substrate for the brain and myocardium in the neonate. Endogenous stores of glucose in the form of glycogen are present in the liver of the neonate, but are limited in quantity. In the preterm neonate, hepatic glycogen stores may be even more marginal. Consequently, neonates, particularly critically ill neonates, have a limited reserve against hypoglycemia. Blood glucose levels less than 30–40 mg dL^{-1} in preterm and fullterm neonates must be maintained to preclude hypoglycemia. Similarly, calcium homeostasis is a fragile balance in the neonate. Critically ill preterm neonates and those neonates who require blood transfusions with citrated blood may be relatively hypocalcemic and require supplemental calcium.

Table 58.2 *Normal blood chemistry*

	Age	
	<1 month	**1–24 months**
Sodium (mmol L^{-1})	134–152	139–146
Potassium (mmol L^{-1})	5.0–7.7	3.0–6.0
Chloride (mmol L^{-1})	92–114	98–106
Calcium ion (mmol L^{-1})	2.2–2.5	2.2–2.5
Glucose (fasting) (mg dL^{-1})	40–90	60–100
Total protein (g dL^{-1})	5.9–8.5	6.1–7.9
Blood urea nitrogen (mg dL^{-1})	3–12	5–18
Osmolality (mosmol kg^{-1})	290–310	290–310

The axis responsible for the stress response in both the preterm and fullterm neonate is intact. Recent studies have shown that the stress response to birth results in a proinflammatory cytokine profile, as evidenced by increases in plasma interleukin 6 and tumor necrosis factor, not unlike the response in the adult.[14] In the presence of light anesthesia without opioid, significant derangements in the metabolic, catecholamine, and autonomic responses to surgery have been associated with serious sequelae that include circulatory instability, hyperglycemia, intraventricular hemorrhage, and acidosis.[12,15]

The neonate is limited in maintaining thermal neutrality. Thermal neutrality is the condition wherein the balance between heat loss and production maintains a prescribed temperature.[41] The range of thermal neutrality depends on the birth weight and postnatal age of the infant. For example, for a 3-kg neonate, thermal neutrality temperature decreases from 34 °C at birth to 32 °C by 10 days' postnatal age, whereas for a 1-kg neonate it decreases from 35.5 °C at birth to 33.5 °C at 10 days' postnatal age.[41] Heat loss is pronounced in the neonate, particularly in the preterm neonate, because (1) the surface area to body weight ratio is very large (body surface area to body mass ratio is 1400 cm kg^{-1} in very low birth weight infants compared with 250 cm kg^{-1} in adults), (2) skin is thin and subcutaneous tissue is scant, and (3) there is minimal motor function. Heat loss occurs through four mechanisms: radiation, convection, evaporation, and conduction losses. Of these mechanisms, radiation, convection, and evaporation heat losses account for approximately 75% of the total heat loss in the neonate.

If the temperature of the neonate decreases below that required for thermal neutrality, then oxygen and glucose consumption increase and acidemia may ensue. For example, oxygen consumption increases by 500% in response to a decrease in body temperature from 37 °C to 34 °C in the neonate. This may also precipitate right-to-left intracardiac shunting at the level of a patent ductus arteriosus or foramen ovale, which may further increase oxygen consumption and lead to hypoxemia and acidemia. To maintain thermal neutrality, the neonate tries to preserve and generate heat. The neonate can preserve heat by peripheral vasoconstriction similar to the adult. However, the neonate cannot shiver and, therefore, must rely on nonshivering thermogenesis.[42] This highly oxidative mechanism produces heat by burning brown fat (which composes 5% of the body weight) through a norepinephrine-dependent pathway. In the neonate, brown fat is located around the scapula, the back, and the kidneys.

In order to maintain thermal homeostasis and minimize the dependency on nonshivering thermogenesis, three pivotal measures should be instituted: the operating room should be warmed before the neonate arrives (≥27 °C), a forced air heater should be used once the neonate is draped, and a servo-controlled heater humidifier should be included in the breathing circuit (Fisher-Paykell, New Zealand) (temperature controlled in the range 37–40 °C). Other measures that may be used to supplement those listed above include covering the exposed head and extremities with a clear plastic sheet, focusing an overhead radiant heater onto the infant until he/she is covered with drapes, and using a heating blanket.

ANESTHESIA

In addition to a routine preanesthetic evaluation, the preoperative assessment of the neonate requires consideration of the gestational age at birth (extent of prematurity), the presence of congenital anomalies (cardiorespiratory defects), the assessment of the airway, severity of co-existent diseases (i.e. sepsis, chronic respiratory failure), and examination of laboratory indices.

Preoperative assessment

Fasting

Neonates who present for surgery within the first 24 h after birth have, for the most part, never been fed by mouth. In contrast, neonates who present for elective surgery up to the first 28 days after birth have been fed and must be fasted before surgery. In the latter instance, it is imperative that we review current guidelines.

The ontogeny of gastric acid secretion begins in the second trimester of pregnancy. Preterm neonates as young as 24 weeks' gestation secrete gastric acid to protect the gastric mucosa from bacteria and protein antigens.[43] At birth, gastric acid secretion is slow but increases throughout the first 24 h. As a consequence, gastric fluid pH at birth is high (pH 5.3), but decreases to approximately pH 4.0 by 8 h.[44] All neonates, including those born preterm, secrete sufficient quantities of acid during the first day after birth to decrease and maintain the gastric fluid at less than pH 4.0. In 22 preterm neonates who were investigated, gastric fluid pH was consistently less than 2.3 by 16 days after birth.[43]

The purpose of fasting before surgery is to decrease the risk of severe aspiration pneumonitis should regurgitation occur. Current evidence supports the notion that severe pneumonitis is possible if gastric fluid with a pH level <2.4 and a volume greater than 0.8 mL kg^{-1} is aspirated into the lungs.[45] Furthermore, other factors, including the presence of particulate matter, may exacerbate the lung injury.[46] Studies in children have demonstrated that fasting for more than 2 h after oral clear fluid ingestion does not decrease the risk of pneumonitis should aspiration occur.[47,48] This is likely attributable to the rapid passage of clear fluids out of the stomach. Consistent with these data, the American Society of Anesthesiologists (ASA) Task Force on Preoperative Fasting recommended a minimum interval of 2 h fasting after clear fluids.[49]

Fasting after breastfeeding is more complex than after clear fluids: not only is the emptying time after breastmilk delayed compared with clear fluids but also aspiration of breastmilk may be severely injurious to the lungs.[50] Cavell[51,52] demonstrated that the time to emptying for 50% of the ingested breastmilk in fullterm infants is about 20% longer than that in preterm infants (Fig. 58.3). Moreover, the emptying time for breastmilk is approximately fivefold longer than that for water. In surgical infants, Litman *et al.*[53] confirmed that fasting 2 h after breastfeeding was insufficient to empty the milk from the stomach. The consensus of the ASA Task Force on Preoperative Fasting was to recommend a 4-h fast after breastmilk.[49]

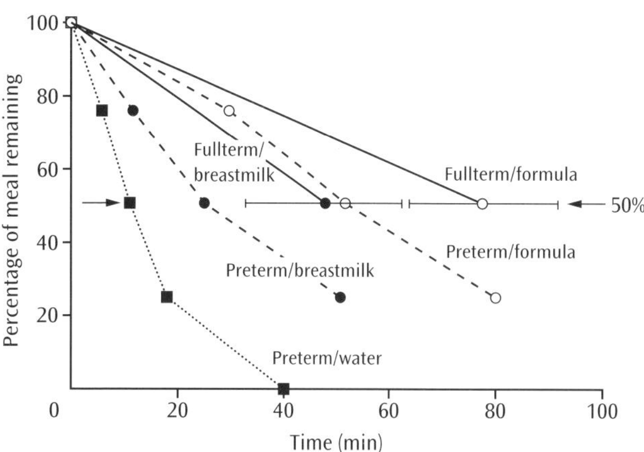

Figure 58.3 *Emptying times for clear fluids, breastmilk, and formula in preterm and fullterm neonates. (Adapted with permission from Cavell.[51,52])*

Unlike breastmilk, there is a wide variety of formula milk, each with a different composition. Published studies have established that the gastric emptying time of whey-based formulae is greater than that of casein-based formulae.[54] Cavell[51,52] demonstrated that the time to emptying for 50% of an ingested meal of formula was 20% longer than that for breastmilk. Moreover, data from the effects of the pulmonary aspiration of formula in rabbits' lungs suggested that formula may be at least as injurious to the lungs, if not more, as the pulmonary effects of breastmilk.[50] Consistent with these observations, the ASA Task Force recommended a 6-h fast after formula.[49]

Premedication

Most neonates do not require premedication before surgery. Atropine is no longer required as an antisialagogue premedicant in neonates. Premedication is usually indicated for those infants and children who experience separation anxiety. Separation anxiety is not a concern in the neonatal period, and therefore premedication is not required in this age group. Other drugs such as cardiac inotropes should be continued during the perioperative period.

Laboratory testing

The laboratory tests required before surgery in neonates depend on the severity of the intercurrent illness and pre-existing diseases. For neonates who are scheduled for elective minor surgery, such as inguinal hernia repair, laboratory tests may be restricted to a complete blood count and serum glucose concentration. For neonates with chronic illnesses or congenital defects, a complete blood count, electrolytes including glucose and albumin concentrations, clotting indices (prothrombin time, partial thromboplastin time, international normalized ratio) and platelet count should be investigated preoperatively. Renal function testing is not required in neonates who do not urinate in the first 24 h after birth as this is not an uncommon event. However, in the presence of other anomalies, congenital renal anomalies should be considered, particularly in the absence of urine output. Investigation of renal anomalies should include laboratory tests, serum potassium, blood urea nitrogen, and creatinine, as well as a renal ultrasound and intravenous pyelogram.

A precordial heart murmur, circulatory instability, or cyanosis point to a congenital heart defect. Approximately 30% of neonates who present with midline lesions, including tracheoesophageal fistula and omphalocele, will have a congenital heart defect ranging from a patent ductus arteriosus to hypoplastic left heart syndrome. A preoperative electrocardiogram and echocardiogram are required to establish a diagnosis.

AIRWAY

Management of the airway in the neonate depends on three considerations: patient, surgeon, and anesthesiologist. Although surgery is occasionally elective, the vast majority is emergent for neonates who are either already intubated or in whom intubation is required.

Examination of the airway usually reveals evidence of a difficult airway. Table 58.3 presents a synopsis of syndromes associated with airway difficulties; a complete listing can be found elsewhere.[56]

Depending on the surgical and patient requirements, the airway in the neonate can be maintained with a face mask, tracheal tube, or laryngeal mask airway (LMA) (Fig. 58.4). For preterm neonates who require general anesthesia, spontaneous ventilation is avoided because of their proclivity for periodic breathing and apnea during general anesthesia. Tracheal intubation is the optimal means to secure and maintain the airway in these neonates.

Management of the neonatal airway often presents one of the greatest problems for anesthesiologists. The size of face mask (0) and oral airway (0 and 00) for the neonate is often underestimated because of the disproportionate sizes of the head and body. An improperly sized oral airway could obstruct the upper airway: if too large, the airway could displace the epiglottis caudally into the larygneal inlet; if too small, the airway could displace the base of the tongue posteriorly, thereby obstructing the nasopharynx. In order to prevent obstruction of the airway by external compression, the anesthesiologist should confine all finger contact to the bony prominences of the face, although a significant proportion of neonates cannot breathe with their mouths closed. In order to adequately ventilate the lungs by mask, slight extension of the neck and subluxation of the temperomandibular joint from behind the pinna may be required.[57]

Table 58.3 *Disease states associated with a difficult airway*

Mask/spontaneous ventilation
Preterm infant
Crouzon syndrome
Apert syndrome
Choanal atresia
Micrognathia
Pierre Robin sequence
First arch syndrome
Treacher Collins syndrome
Goldenhar syndrome (either easy or extremely difficult)
Arthrogryposis
Macroglossia
Beckwith–Wiedemann syndrome
Congenital hypothyroidism
Down syndrome
Congenital lingual tumor/intraoral tumor
Cystic hygroma
Intraoral pathology
Congenital temperomandibular joint fusion/dysfunction
Laryngeal cyst, web
Laryngotracheal cleft
Microstomia

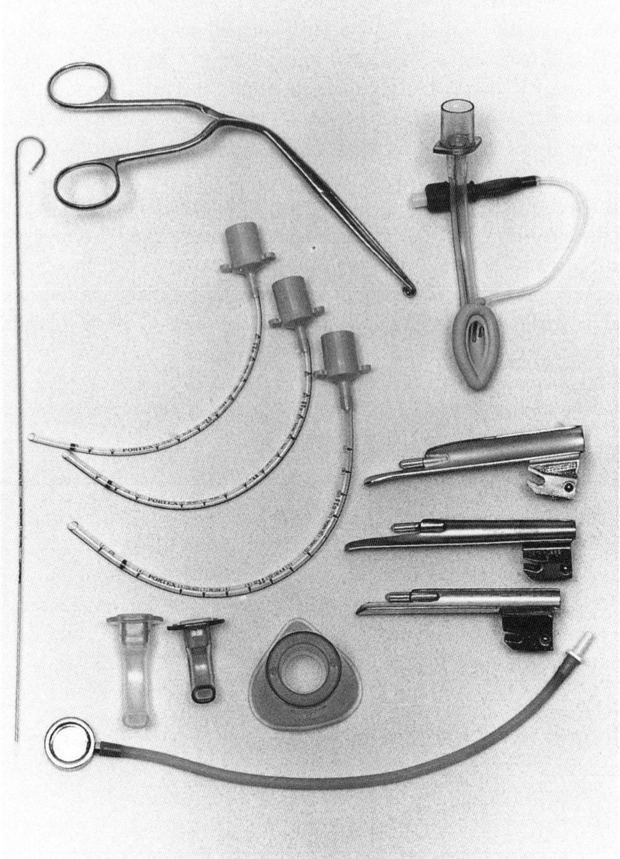

Figure 58.4 *Neonatal airway equipment. At the extreme left, is a 3-mm National Catheter tracheal tube stylet. Next to it, from top to bottom, are neonatal Magill forceps, tracheal tubes 2.5-, 3.0-, and 3.5-mm inner diameter, two oral airways, sizes 0 and 00, a size 0 Rusch clear plastic Rendell–Baker mask, and, at the bottom, a neonatal precordial stethoscope. On the right, viewing from top to bottom, is a size 1 laryngeal mask airway and three laryngoscope blades: Foregger 0, Wisconsin 0, and a modified Wisconsin 0. The modified Wisconsin 0 blade differs from the original blade in that the entire length of the inferior lip of the C-curve of the blade was removed to increase the view of the larynx in the very small infant's mouth. (Reproduced with permission from Lerman.[55])*

The laryngoscope blade should be introduced into the mouth at the right commissure, with the tongue completely displaced to the left of the blade. At no time during laryngoscopy should the tongue straddle the blade or appear on the right side of the blade. Once inside the mouth, the blade should be advanced with the tip aimed towards the midline. The novice anesthesiologist may find it easier to insert the blade into the esophagus and slowly pull it back, watching for the pearly white vocal cords to drop into view like the curtains at the end of a stage performance. The experienced anesthesiologist will insert the blade until he/she can lift the epiglottis with the tip of the blade while applying constant force along the axis of the laryngoscope handle via the elbow (not the wrist). For an awake or difficult intubation, a stylet that is molded into the shape of a hockey stick will help to direct the tube anteriorly towards the larynx. If the intubation is difficult (axes of the mouth and larynx cannot be aligned), the larynx may be displaced posteriorly by applying external pressure to the thyroid cartilage with the fifth digit of the hand that is performing laryngoscopy. For the extremely retrognathic mandible, a two-handed laryngoscopy may be employed in which the laryngoscope is manipulated with one hand while the second applies external pressure to the thyroid cartilage. Once the oral and laryngeal axes are aligned, a second person looks over the anesthesiologist's shoulder into the laryngeal inlet and inserts the tube.

Tracheal intubation in the neonate may be performed either awake or with general anesthesia.[56,58,59] In cases of planned elective surgery, the airway may be topicalized with local anesthetics and the neonate sedated/paralyzed.[58,60] Although many clinicians have shifted their practice from awake intubation to intubation under general anesthesia, the former offers several advantages: (1) spontaneous ventilation and a patent airway are maintained (if the intubation proves to be unexpectedly difficult, the anesthesiologist can pause and reassess the airway while the child continues to breathe) and (2) the airway is protected if the neonate regurgitates gastric contents.[58]

Critics of awake intubations have expressed concern over the oral trauma from multiple attempts at intubation – intracranial hemorrhage, uncontrolled hypoxemia and bradycardia, and unnecessary stress.[58] There is no evidence that intracranial complications have ever been associated with awake intubation in either the preterm or fullterm neonate. Anterior fontanel pressure, an estimate of intracranial pressure, measured during awake intubations was similar to the pressure reported when the neonate cried.[61]

Transient cardiorespiratory changes including hemoglobin desaturation and bradycardia during awake laryngoscopy have been reported, particularly when laryngoscopy and intubation are performed by inexperienced physicians. These effects can be attenuated by administering 0.02 mg kg^{-1} atropine i.v. preoperatively, by preoxygenating the lungs, and by using an oxyscope. Tracheal intubation performed under general anesthesia offers the advantages of intubating the trachea while the child is unresponsive and has obtunded reflexes, muted stress response, and the ability to control ventilation if necessary. For those not accustomed to managing the airway of the neonate, awake intubation is safe, reliable, and preferable, particularly in the absence of backup.

Neonates may be intubated by the oral or nasal route. For surgery in which the neonate can be extubated at the conclusion, an orotracheal tube may be used. For surgery in which the neonate must remain intubated postoperatively, a nasotracheal tube is preferred. The latter facilitates transport of the intubated neonate as well as nursing in the intensive care unit. It is helpful to warm the distal 2–3 cm of the nasal tube before inserting it to decrease the trauma of intubation. Small Magill forceps are usually required to direct the tube into the larynx.

Specialized equipment is required when managing the airway of a neonate. The Wisconsin straight blade (size 0 for preterm neonates and size 1 for fullterm neonates) is preferred for laryngoscopy and visualization of the larynx in neonates (Fig. 58.4). The fiberoptic Heine 0 blade is not ideally suited for use in preterm and fullterm neonates and infants as the tip of the blade is curved. For neonates with airways that may be difficult to intubate, fiberoptic flexible bronchoscopes (1.8–2.4 mm in diameter) with excellent optics are available. These bronchoscopes will accommodate tubes as small as 2.5 mm in diameter, but lack a suction port and are overly malleable. Two other techniques for establishing an airway in the neonate with a difficult airway include the LMA size 1 (see below) and digital intubation.[62]

Neonates who present with a potentially difficult airway (see Pharmacology) require the skills of a specialist anesthesiologist. When evaluating the airway, the difficult airway considerations always take precedence over the full stomach considerations. The airway may be secured while the neonate is either awake or anesthetized, the latter with an inhalational anesthetic. The choice of technique to secure the airway will depend on the airway anomaly (Fig. 58.5A and B): direct laryngoscopy, indirect visualization using a flexible fiberoptic bronchoscope, LMA to guide the tracheal tube, Trach-light, or rigid bronchoscopy may be used. A selection of uncut tubes of different sizes should be available as well as a stylet to mold the shape of the tube.

Tracheal tube size is selected on the basis of weight: for preterm neonates < 1500 g, a 2.5-mm inner diameter tube is used; for those > 1500 g, a 3.0-mm inner diameter tube; and for fullterm neonates, a 3.5-mm inner diameter tube. To anticipate a difficult airway, tubes that are 0.5-mm inner diameter smaller should also be available. The length of the tracheal tube in the fullterm neonate is 10–12 cm placed orally and 12–14 cm placed nasally.

Induction of anesthesia in neonates must be tailored to the clinical presentation. Most neonates who present with surgical emergencies are considered to be at risk for a full stomach and therefore require either an awake intubation or a rapid sequence induction to secure the airway. A rapid sequence induction includes: (1) preparation of intubating equipment and suction, (2) preoxygenation of the lungs, (3) rapid induction of anesthesia using one of sodium thiopentone, propofol, or ketamine (their pharmacology is discussed below), (4) application of cricoid pressure, (5) rapid onset of paralysis [either 2 mg kg^{-1} succinylcholine (suxamethonium) or 1 mg kg^{-1} rocuronium), and (6) intubation of the trachea without ventilating the lungs.

Atropine (0.02 mg kg^{-1}) should be given i.v. in conjunction with the induction agent and before succinylcholine. The use of a nondepolarizing relaxant such as rocuronium commits the anesthesiologist to controlled ventilation. Whether cricoid pressure should be part of the rapid sequence induction, particularly in the neonate, remains controversial. First, the use of cricoid pressure is not evidence based, i.e. studies have never established its effectiveness in preventing aspiration in patients with full stomachs. Second, the force required to occlude the esophagus in the neonate is unknown. Third, the application of cricoid pressure to the neck of the neonate may interfere with laryngoscopy and the speed at which the airway is secured. Instances of a difficult intubation have been reported with cricoid pressure in the neonate.[64] Although considered by many to be the quintessential maneuver in the rapid sequence induction, as described by Sellick,[65] this author submits that its role in a rapid sequence induction in neonates must be reconsidered only after an evidence-based approach evaluates its effectiveness.

Traditionally, the anesthetic technique for securing the airway in neonates with a tracheoesophageal fistula is an awake intubation followed by spontaneous ventilation until the chest is opened. More recently, both inhalational inductions with halothane or sevoflurane or intravenous inductions with controlled ventilation have become the fashion. Spontaneous ventilation is preferred for these neonates to avoid inadvertent gastric inflation with controlled ventilation. This author prefers an awake intubation and spontaneous ventilation with an inhalational anesthetic while gently assisting ventilation to assess the risk of gastric inflation. If spontaneous ventilation is maintained until the chest is opened, then even a large fistula between the trachea and the esophagus could be managed with assisted or controlled ventilation by asking the surgeon to apply a ligature to the fistula to prevent gastric inflation.

The introduction of the LMA offers an alternative to mask anesthesia in the neonate who is scheduled for minor surgery. The LMA size 1 can be used in neonates weighing up to 6.5 kg. The success rate for inserting the LMA in the neonate is less than in the adult, being 70% on the first attempt in the neonate compared with 95% in the adult.[66] Both direct fiberoptic bronchoscopy and magnetic resonance imaging have demonstrated that the epiglottis is not in its anatomic position in up to 75% of instances in infants and children, although this rarely results in an obstructed airway.[67] The high incidence of finding the epiglottis downfolded over the laryngeal inlet or within the bowl of the LMA is not surprising when one considers that the LMA was designed for the adult airway and simply scaled down in size to fit neonates, infants, and

A

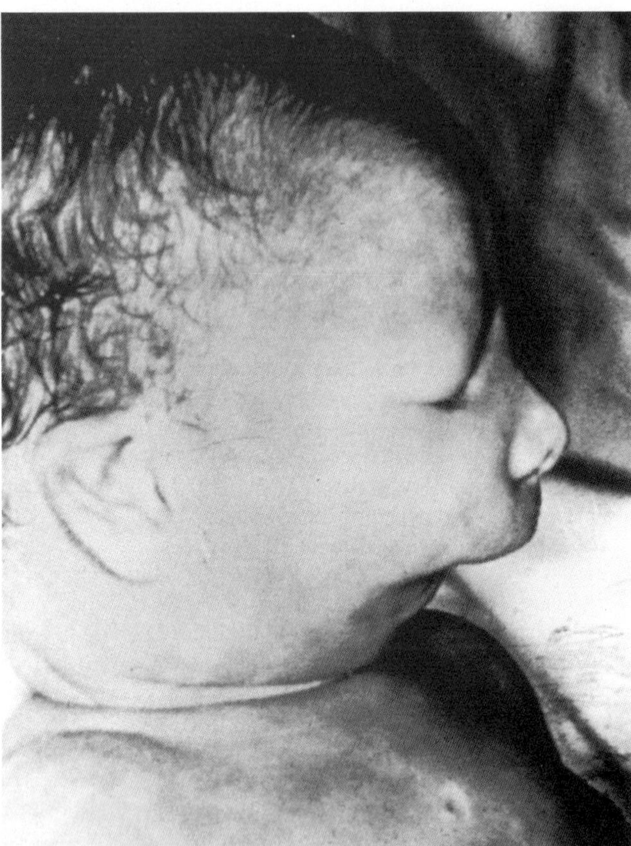

B

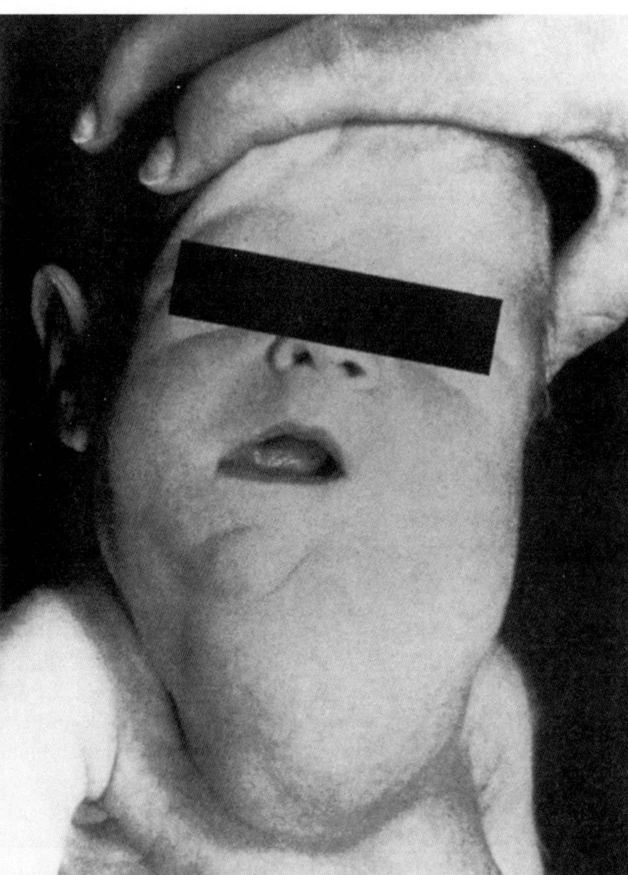

Figure 58.5 *(A) A fullterm neonate with bilateral first arch syndrome, a disease characterized by absence of the mandible and other structures derived from the first branchial arch. More common but less severe manifestations of this type of dysgenesis include Pierre Robin sequence and Treacher Collins syndrome. Awake intubation, inhalational induction, or tracheotomy are possible techniques that may be required to secure the airway in this neonate. (Reproduced with permission from Vener and Lerman.[63]) (B) A fullterm neonate with a large cystic hygroma. Although these masses appear extraoral, they may involve both the tongue and supraglottic structures. Usually, oral or nasal intubation is possible. Tracheotomy is usually impossible. (Reproduced with permission from Vener and Lerman.[63])*

children. Nonetheless, the role of the LMA in neonatal surgery will likely be limited because, in most instances, the airway must be secured to prevent aspiration and to facilitate positive pressure ventilation, neither of which can be assured with an LMA.

After tracheal intubation, ventilation may be controlled either manually or mechanically. Manual ventilation of neonatal lungs has been the tradition in many institutions because it allows a breath-by-breath estimation of changes in chest compliance.[68] Of course, the need for manual assessment of chest compliance to assure adequacy of ventilation predated modern noninvasive monitoring techniques (oximetry and capnography) and the widespread use of ventilators that are designed for use in neonates and infants. Moreover, manual ventilation limits the activities of the anesthesiologist, particularly during critical periods and may provide a false sense of security in detecting changes in compliance. Recent evidence from neonates indicates that the fresh gas flow and the experience of the anesthesiologist determine the success rate for detecting complete tube occlusions in which, under ideal conditions, 80% of the obstructions can be detected.[68]

Two ventilators are commonly used to ventilate the lungs of neonates: volume-limited/time-cycled and pressure-limited/time-cycled. Volume-limited/time-cycled ventilators deliver a fixed tidal volume that is based on the inspiratory time and inspiratory flow. These ventilators deliver a fixed tidal volume that is independent of the peak inspiratory pressures. Ventilators that are designed expressly for adults may be incapable of delivering the small tidal volumes that are required for neonates (25–45 mL). Some anesthesiologists have suggested that ventilators which deliver large tidal volumes can be adapted for use with neonates by interposing highly compliant tubing in the circuit to decrease the tidal volume delivered to the lungs. This author admonishes this practice because the inadvertent use of tubing that is far less compliant than recommended could result in overinflation and barotrauma of the lungs. In contrast to the volume-limited ventilators, a pressure-limited/time-cycled ventilator delivers a tidal volume that is limited by a peak pressure. As a result, the tidal volume varies directly with the compliance of the chest: as the compliance decreases, tidal volume also decreases, and vice versa. These ventilators should be used with caution during surgery when marked changes in chest compliance may occur as a result of the surgery. To account for changes in compliance when using a pressure-limited ventilator, the adequacy of alveolar ventilation can only be assured by using breath-by-breath capnography.

Pharmacology

With a greater understanding of the pharmacology of anesthetic drugs and their responses in neonates, clinicians have become much more adept at providing quality anesthetic care for these very small patients. This section summarizes the current state of knowledge of the pharmacology of anesthetic agents as they pertain to the neonate.

The uptake and distribution of inhalational anesthetics in neonates is more rapid than in adults for several reasons:

1 The ratio of alveolar ventilation to FRC ratio is 5:1 in neonates compared with 1.5:1 in adults. This difference is attributed to the two- to threefold greater metabolic rate in neonates compared with adults.[69]
2 A greater fraction of the cardiac output is distributed to the vessel-rich group, being 18% of the body weight in the neonate compared with only 6% in the adult.[69]
3 In the neonate, the lower protein and lipid concentrations in both blood[70,71] and tissues[7] (or conversely, the greater water content) reduce the solubilities of inhalational anesthetics in these tissues compared with those in adults (Fig. 58.6).

Together, these factors speed the rise of alveolar to inspired anesthetic partial pressures and facilitate a more rapid equilibration of anesthetic partial pressures in neonates compared with adults.[69,72] Hence, the washin and washout of these anesthetics will be rapid and will facilitate rapid control and adjustment of the desired concentration.

In 1969, Gregory *et al.*[73] first reported the relation between the MAC (minimum alveolar concentration), a measure of potency of inhalational agents, of halothane and age. They found that the MAC of halothane increased as age decreased from the elderly to neonates. The MAC of halothane reaches its zenith in the youngest age group, which comprises neonates and infants up to 6 months old. Based on these observations, one study cautioned against the use of halothane in neonates as it caused more hypotension than in older infants.[74] Two possible explanations were postulated to explain this effect of halothane in neonates: (1) the MAC values of halothane in neonates and older infants were not identical or (2) myocardial/vascular development was immature in the neonate. When the MAC of halothane was subsequently determined in neonates as a group distinct from older infants aged 1–6 months, the MAC in the former was 15–25% less than that in the latter.[75] Furthermore, when 1 MAC of inhalational anesthetics was administered, the incidence of hypotension and the decrease in heart rate in neonates were similar to those in infants.[76,77] The MAC (9.2 ± 0.02) values in fullterm neonates for the inhalational anesthetics in use today are: 0.87 ± 0.10% for halothane,[75] 1.60 ± 0.01% for isoflurane,[78] 9.0 ± % for desflurane,[76] and 3.3 ± 0.2% for sevoflurane.[77]

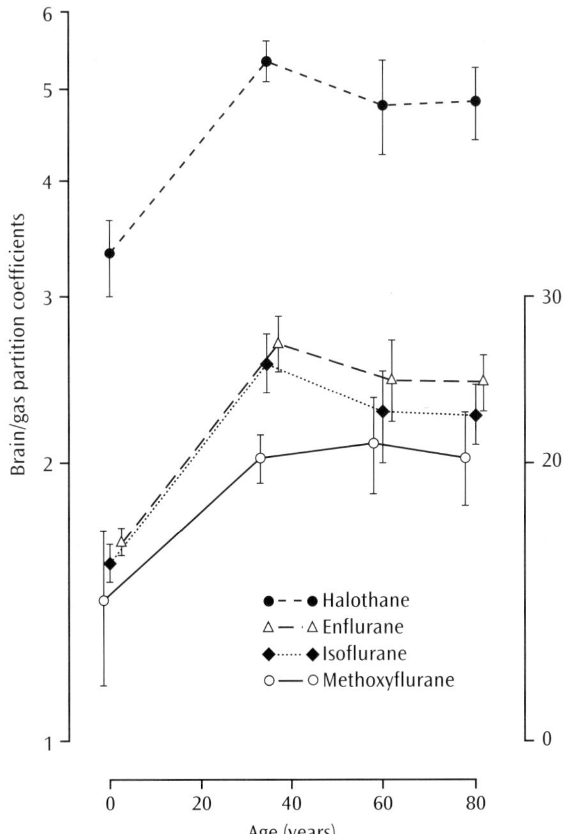

Figure 58.6 *Aging, between birth and adulthood, increases the solubility of inhalational anesthetics in human brain tissue. Brain–gas partition coefficients are plotted on a logarithmic scale. Data are means ± standard errors. (Reproduced with permission from Lerman* et al.[7]*)*

There is also evidence that the primary cause of the increased sensitivity of neonates to cardiodepression by inhalational anesthetics may be explained by immaturity of the cardiovascular system.[79,80] Using echocardiography, the cardiodepressant effects of halothane and isoflurane in concentrations up to 1.5 MAC in neonates were noted to be greater than in older infants.[81] The increased susceptibility of neonates to the depressant effects of inhalational anesthetics may be attributed, in part, to a decrease in myocardial contractile elements, decrease in calcium sensitivity of myocardial fibers,[80] and incomplete sympathetic innervation of the heart and vascular system. Evidence also indicates that both pressor and depressor baroresponses are depressed in the presence of isoflurane in the preterm and fullterm neonate.[79] These data suggest that, in the neonate, the magnitude of the cardiovascular depression by inhalational anesthetics at 1 MAC is similar to that reported in older infants, but that at concentrations in excess of 1 MAC it may be greater than in older infants.

In order to attenuate the cardiodepressant effects of inhalational anesthetics in neonates, heart rate should be maintained and preload should be optimized. Because neonates depend on a rapid heart rate to maintain cardiac output, cardiovascular depression, particularly in the presence of halothane, can be reversed or offset in part by intravenous atropine (0.02 mg kg^{-1}). To optimize preload, balanced salt solution or albumen, in a volume of 10–20 mL kg^{-1}, should be administered before anesthesia is induced. Neonates who have had cardiorespiratory dysfunction in the presurgical period often present to the operating room in a state of relative dehydration because of aggressively administered diuretic therapy or third-space fluid losses. After rehydration, but in the absence of atropine, systolic arterial pressure decreases by approximately 20–25% at 1 MAC halothane, desflurane, and sevoflurane compared with awake values, with either no changes or minimal decreases in heart rate.[75–77] Similar responses have been reported with 1 MAC of these anesthetics in infants 1–6 months of age.[76,77]

That the relations between the MAC values of isoflurane and desflurane and age were similar to that reported by Gregory *et al.*[73] for halothane is not surprising. What was unexpected was the lack of a relation between the MAC of sevoflurane and age in infants and children.[77] In the case of sevoflurane, MAC increases in a stepwise manner as age decreases: the MAC in neonates and infants aged 1–6 months is a constant 3.2%, and that in infants older than 6 months and in older children is 2.5%.[77] It remains unclear why the relation between the MAC of sevoflurane and age in childhood differs from that of the other inhalational anesthetics. Whether the conformational structure of sevoflurane, a methylisopropyl ether, or some other physicochemical characteristic is responsible for this unique relation between MAC of sevoflurane and age remains unclear.

The MAC of isoflurane decreases steadily in neonates as gestational age decreases to 24 weeks (Fig. 58.7).[13] Not only did this study characterize the relation between the MAC for isoflurane in preterm neonates and age, but it also confirmed the notion that neonates as young as 24 weeks' gestation respond to noxious stimuli in a predictable manner. Although several explanations have been posited to explain the age-dependent change in MAC in the perinatal period, including residual effects of

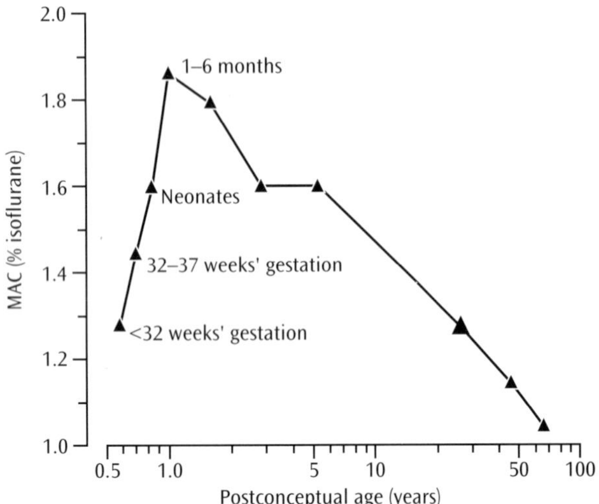

Figure 58.7 *The MAC of isoflurane and postconceptual age on a semilogarithmic scale. Postconceptual age was the sum of the mean postnatal age for each age group and 40 weeks. (Reproduced with permission from LeDez and Lerman.*[13]*)*

placentally transmitted female hormones, central nervous system substance P, and maturation of central nervous system, the cause still remains speculative.

Nitrous oxide is commonly used to supplement general anesthesia. However, nitrous oxide is infrequently used in neonates, particularly preterm neonates, who require emergency surgery and who are at risk of pulmonary or retinal complications from high oxygen tensions. The avoidance of nitrous oxide in neonates who have bowel obstruction or gas-filled closed spaces is well accepted.[82] However, its avoidance in neonates who are at risk of oxygen toxicity is less clear. It has been recommended that the $P_{a}O_2$ be limited to a maximum value of 10.66 kPa (80 mmHg), i.e. an $S_{a}O_2$ of 93%, to prevent the effects of oxygen toxicity. This value lies at the shoulder of the steep descending portion of the oxyhemoglobin dissociation curve. If nitrous oxide were used to maintain the arterial oxygen tension below this value, then any minor difficulty with the airway could lead to a rapid hemoglobin oxygen desaturation. This potential problem would be mitigated if nitrogen were used instead of nitrous oxide because the former is 34 times less soluble in blood than the latter. In these circumstances, nitrous oxide should be avoided and replaced with an air–oxygen mixture.

Several recent studies have focused on the pharmacology of intravenous anesthetic agents in the neonate. Sodium thiopentone is the oldest intravenous induction agent in clinical use. The dose requirement for thiopentone in infancy is similar to that for inhalational anesthetics, i.e. the ED_{50} (means ± standard errors of the mean) for thiopentone that ablates movement or coughing upon application of the face mask in the neonate (3.4 ± 0.2 mg kg^{-1}), is 60% less than that in the older infant aged 1–6 months (6.3 ± 0.7 mg kg^{-1}).[83] This difference may be explained in part by an increased free fraction of thiopentone in the neonate, the result of lower serum concentrations of proteins,[38,84] a more permeable blood–brain barrier,[85,86] and decreased anesthetic requirements because of an immature brain in the neonate compared with older infants. The effects of thiopentone on the cardiovascular system in the neonate are similar to those in the older infant aged 1–6 months.[83] Blood pressure and heart rate are maintained at the ED_{50} dose of thiopentone. In this author's experience, thiopentone does not depress cardiovascular function excessively in the neonate even at 1.5 times the ED_{50} provided it is administered after normovolemia has been established with or without intravenous atropine (0.02 mg kg^{-1}).

The dose requirements for propofol in neonates and older infants are similar to those reported for thiopentone. The dose of propofol that attenuates the lash reflex in the neonate is 3.5 mg kg^{-1}. Although propofol has not been approved for use in infants and children less than 3 years of age in North America, it remains the judgment of the consultant anesthesiologist whether or not to use propofol in this age group.

The use of ketamine in neonatal anesthesia has gradually ebbed over the past decade because of the increased use of propofol. Ketamine has a primary role as an induction agent in neonates, particularly in those with cyanotic heart defects or circulatory instability. Friesen and Henry[87] compared the circulatory responses of ketamine (2 mg kg^{-1}) with isoflurane (0.75%), halothane (0.50%), and fentanyl (20 μg kg^{-1}) for induction of anesthesia in healthy neonates. They found that all four anesthetics decreased systolic arterial pressure compared with control measurements, although the incidence of hypotension (> 25% decrease in arterial pressure) after ketamine was less than with the other three anesthetics. Ketamine has also been used intramuscularly (3–10 mg kg^{-1}) for minor surgery such as cleft lip suture removal. Its onset of action is 5–7 min and its duration is 20 min.

The hypnotics/sedatives diazepam and, more recently, midazolam, have been used to supplement opioid-based anesthesia and as sedative agents. Although dose–response curves for these drugs in neonates have not been established, this author uses a dose of 0.05–0.075 mg kg^{-1} for midazolam. Pharmacokinetic data for diazepam suggest that immature hepatic mixed function oxidases account for its prolonged elimination half-life (31 ± 2 h) in the neonate compared with that in the older child (18 ± 3 h).[88] Hence, supplementary doses of diazepam should be administered less frequently in the neonate than in the older child to prevent any cumulative effect. In preterm infants, the elimination half-life of diazepam is more than twice that in fullterm neonates.[88] Repeat doses of diazepam should be administered less frequently in fullterm neonates than in adults, and less frequently still in preterm neonates. The pharmacokinetics of midazolam in neonates have not been established.

In the past, opioids were used sparingly in neonates. However, with the appreciation of the ontogeny of pain pathways in the neonate[10,11] and our insight into the pharmacology of opioids in neonates, the use of opioids has increased in neonates. The use of morphine in the neonate has been limited by serious concerns for excessive respiratory depression.[89] The sensitivity of the neonate to morphine was attributed to several causes, including a greater permeability of the blood–brain barrier to morphine in the neonate than in the adult.[89,90] Morphine use has never been limited by cardiovascular effects: at a dose of 0.1 mg kg^{-1} there are no significant cardiovascular effects in the preterm neonate.[91]

The pharmacokinetics of morphine in neonates are characterized by a large interindividual variability – up to 10-fold.[90,92–94] This variability may be explained by age, hepatic enzyme maturation, liver blood flow, and type of surgery. However, even over brief intervals, marked interindividual variability in the pharmacokinetics of morphine has been reported.[95,96] Indeed, a meta-analysis of the literature concluded that the clearance of morphine increases with both gestational and postnatal age from 2.2 ± 0.7 mL kg^{-1} min^{-1} in preterm infants to 8.1 ± 3.2 mL kg^{-1} min^{-1} in term neonates to 24 ± 8.5 mL kg^{-1} min^{-1} in infants and children.[95,97] As clearance increases, the elimination half-life of morphine decreases with increasing age, such that the elimination half-life of morphine is 9.0 ± 3.4 h in preterm neonates, 6.5 ± 2.8 h in term neonates, and 2.0 ± 1.8 h in infants and children.[97,98] Evidence indicates that the preterm neonates is capable of metabolizing morphine, albeit at a slower rate than older infants.[97] Type of surgery also appears to affect the kinetics of morphine. Lynn *et al.*[99] demonstrated that neonates who underwent cardiopulmonary bypass showed 50% slower clearance of morphine than matched neonates not undergoing bypass. This may be attributed to differences in cardiac output or hepatic enzyme function. The infusion rate of morphine in neonates should account for the pharmacokinetic differences among age groups, although interindividual differences may also be profound. Based on a meta-analysis, guidelines have been proposed for the infusion of morphine in neonates: 2 μg kg^{-1} h^{-1} in preterm neonates, 7 μg kg^{-1} h^{-1} in term neonates, and 20 μg kg^{-1} h^{-1} in infants and children.[100]

The use of fentanyl in neonates undergoing surgery exceeds that of morphine. Pharmacokinetic and pharmacodynamic studies of fentanyl in neonates have characterized its actions as follows: (1) the pharmacokinetics of fentanyl in neonates are quite variable, (2) clearance is decreased, particularly within the first few days after birth and in those with increased intra-abdominal pressure, and (3) dose requirements of fentanyl in the neonate are less than those in the adult and appear to vary with the type of surgery.

The smaller dose requirement for fentanyl in neonates has been attributed to several factors, including a lower anesthetic requirement and increased free fraction (i.e. lower protein binding to both albumen and α_1-acid glycoprotein) of fentanyl in neonates than in older infants.[40] Preterm infants undergoing ligation of the patent ductus arteriosus require more fentanyl (30–50 μg kg^{-1}) than an older group of preterm and fullterm neonates (10–12.5 μg kg^{-1}) undergoing intra-abdominal surgery for approximately 90 min.[101,102] In more direct comparisons of specific surgical lesions, investigators noted that neonates with increased intra-abdominal pressure did not clear fentanyl as rapidly as neonates with normal intra-abdominal pressure.[103,104] Although limited by small sample sizes, studies of the dose requirements for fentanyl in the neonate with increased intra-abdominal pressure showed a reduced requirement for fentanyl compared with those with normal intra-abdominal pressure. This decreased requirement in neonates with increased intra-abdominal pressure was attributed, in part, to a prolonged elimination half-life of fentanyl due to decreased liver blood flow,[33] decreased cardiac output, and decreased clearance[33,104] compared with the adult.

In neonates with increased intra-abdominal pressure, 12.5 μg kg^{-1} fentanyl decreases heart rate and systolic arterial pressure by approximately 15%.[102] Similar doses of fentanyl also depress the baroresponse.[105] In most of these studies, fentanyl was administered slowly in incremental doses after intravenous volume loading with colloid or crystalloid. Atropine was used infrequently. Although a rapid heart rate remains an important determinant of an adequate cardiac output in neonates, the results of these studies indicate that a fentanyl/pancuronium anesthetic did not depress excessively the circulation in the euvolemic neonate.[101]

Alfentanil is a synthetic opioid similar in chemical structure to fentanyl, but differs in several characteristics: it is one-fourth as potent as fentanyl, is more highly protein bound (90%) to α_1-acid glycoprotein, and is less lipid soluble than fentanyl. These differences result in a smaller volume of distribution and therefore a prolonged elimination half-life compared with fentanyl. Alfentanil has a more rapid onset and shorter duration of action than fentanyl.[106] The pharmacokinetics of alfentanil (20 μg kg^{-1}) in preterm infants yielded a volume of distribution of 0.5 L kg^{-1}, an elimination half-life in excess of 5 h, and a clearance of 0.9 mL kg^{-1} min^{-1}.[107] The markedly prolonged elimination half-life in neonates compared with children and adults likely reflects a slower clearance in preterm infants. Hence, repeat doses of alfentanil are not required as frequently in preterm infants as in older children and adults. Alfentanil is metabolized rapidly in the liver by oxidative N,O dealkylation. The enzyme responsible for this metabolism may be immature in the preterm infant. If this is true, then low activity of this oxidative enzyme may explain in part the markedly prolonged clearance compared with adults. Like the pharmacokinetics of fentanyl in neonates, wide interindividual variability in the pharmacokinetics of alfentanil precludes simple dosing programs in neonates.[107] Alfentanil has been eclipsed by fentanyl in neonatal anesthesia.

Sufentanil is a fentanyl derivative that is 8–10 times more potent than fentanyl. The pharmacology of sufentanil is intermediate between fentanyl and alfentanil. Sufentanil undergoes extensive metabolism in the liver via O-demethylation and N-dealkylation. Pharmacokinetic studies in neonates and children have been limited to open heart surgery. Sufentanil has age-dependent kinetics: in neonates, a greater volume of distribution at steady state (V_{dss}) and delayed clearance lead to a prolonged elimination half-life compared with older infants and children.[108] Anand and Hickey[109] reported minimal metabolic and hemodynamic changes in neonates anesthetized with *very* high-dose (35–40 μg kg^{-1}) sufentanil for open heart surgery. Further evaluation is required in order to define the dose requirements and pharmacology of sufentanil in the neonate with normal cardiac anatomy.

Remifentanil is a new synthetic opioid that is rapidly inactivated by ubiquitous tissue esterases. With an elimination half-life of 5–7 min, remifentanil must be administered as a continuous infusion. Preliminary pharmacokinetic data for remifentanil in neonates are similar to those in adults: the elimination half-life in neonates is 4–6 min.[110] In adults, the elimination half-life is independent of the dose of remifentanil administered and the duration of the infusion. Infusion rates of remifentanil range from 0.025 to 1.0 μg kg^{-1} min^{-1} depending on the presence of adjunct agents such as inhalational anesthetics. At the conclusion of surgery, the rapid offset of analgesia after discontinuation of remifentanil necessitates either continuation of the infusion or the addition of another form of analgesia/opioid lest the neonate recover in extreme pain.

Succinylcholine is commonly used to facilitate tracheal intubation in the neonate. The ED_{95} in the neonate is twice that in the adult; thus, the intubating dose in the neonate is 1.5–2.0 mg kg^{-1} i.v. Succinylcholine is rapidly metabolized by plasma pseudocholinesterase. The speed of hydrolysis is rarely attenuated even in neonates with low plasma pseudocholinesterase activity, such as the critically ill preterm neonate or the neonate with hepatic dysfunction.[111] The contraindications to or complications from the use of succinylcholine in the neonate are the same as those in older children and adults.

Nondepolarizing muscle relaxants have been used for many years in pediatric patients, although their pharmacokinetics and pharmacodynamics in the neonatal period have been poorly understood. Fisher *et al.*[112] demonstrated that the dose requirement of *d*-tubocurarine in the neonate is similar to that in older children because of two off-setting factors: a greater sensitivity to neuromuscular blockade and a larger volume of distribution. Although the dose requirement of *d*-tubocurarine is similar in all age groups, repeat doses should be administered less frequently in the neonate to avoid accumulation. The newer intermediate-acting nondepolarizing muscle relaxants rocuronium, *cis*-atracurium, mivacurium, atracurium, and vecuronium have become very popular in clinical practice because their elimination half-lives are brief and the risk of accumulation is small.[113] However, there is marked variability in the sensitivity to and recovery from neuromuscular blocking agents in the neonatal and early infant period. Atracurium and vecuronium are two relaxants that have been the most studied in infancy. Data from clinical studies indicate that the dose requirements in neonates are markedly reduced compared with older children: the ED_{95} for vecuronium is 47 ± 11 μg kg^{-1} in neonates vs. 81 ± 12 μg kg^{-1} in children 3–12 years.[114]

There are no data for rocuronium, *cis*-atracurium, and mivacurium in neonates. When atracurium is administered on a surface area basis in neonates (which accounts for the differences in extracellular fluid volume and organ size), the doses are significantly reduced compared with those in adults.[115] Consequently, repeat doses of these relaxants should be administered less frequently in neonates than in older children. Since mivacurium depends on plasma pseudocholinesterase for termination of its activity, its elimination half-life may be prolonged in the preterm critically ill neonate whose plasma pseudocholinesterase activity may be reduced.

Both temperature and age also affect the duration of neuromuscular blockade in neonates: hypothermia and younger age independently prolong the duration of action of relaxants.[116,117] If repeat doses of these relaxants are required, then the neuromuscular blockade should be monitored using a supramaximal constant current nerve stimulator. Rapacuronium, the newest rapid-onset, short-acting nondepolarizing relaxant, was withdrawn from the US market in 2001 1 year after it was introduced because of reports of severe bronchospasm in infants, children, and adults as well as five deaths possibly related to the drug.[118]

Infusions of atracurium (400 μg kg^{-1} h^{-1}) and vecuronium (62 μg kg^{-1} h^{-1}) have been shown to be effective during balanced anesthesia in neonates.[119,120] Large variability in response to relaxants in neonates necessitates that these drugs be administered in small incremental doses or infusions and with continuous monitoring with a constant current nerve stimulator.[121] A complete listing of doses and infusion rates for these muscle relaxants may be found elsewhere.[121] The relaxant effect of all nondepolarizing muscle relaxants should be antagonized with an anticholinergic and an anticholinesterase at the termination of surgery, as described below.

Monitoring

Reliable and accurate monitoring of cardiorespiratory homeostasis in the neonate has been a challenge during anesthesia. Many of the recent advances in monitoring have required modification for use in the neonate.

Standard monitoring includes electrocardiogram, blood pressure, temperature, and precordial stethoscope. The electrocardiographic pads must maintain contact with the skin even in the presence of a warm humid environment. Furthermore, the area of the pads must be small in diameter and easy to apply to the extremities. The blood pressure cuff may be applied to either arm (unless the neonate is undergoing ligation of a patent ductus arteriosus or repair of coarctation of the aorta, in which case it must be applied to the right arm). Systolic pressure may be measured noninvasively either manually (with the assistance of a Doppler flow probe applied to the radial or brachial artery on the same extremity) or mechanically via a noninvasive blood pressure device. Because many of the mechanical devices are calibrated for the size of the patient, it is important to select the "neonate" mode for accurate measurements. Core temperature may be monitored in the nasopharynx, esophagus, rectum, or external auditory canal. Nasopharyngeal temperature is an accurate estimate of the central blood temperature. Esophageal temperature may not accurately reflect core temperature as it is affected directly by the temperature of the inspired gases. Rectal temperature usually reflects the core temperature but is slow to change. When the body temperature is measured in the external auditory canal (tympanic membrane), it accurately reflects the core temperature, but is not commonly used because of the risk of trauma to the tympanic membrane. Axillary temperature is rarely used in the neonate because of the difficulty in maintaining its position over the axillary artery. Our choices for the site for monitoring core temperature in neonates are nasopharynx and rectum.

The ability to measure the hemoglobin oxygen saturation (S_aO_2) continuously and noninvasively has been one of the greatest advances in pediatric anesthesia care of this century. S_aO_2 has proven to be an extremely sensitive early warning sign of impending hypoxia long before clinical signs are present.[122] The elegance of the oximeter lies in the simplicity of the principles upon which it was designed. These are detailed elsewhere.[123] The oximeter sensor may be attached to the neonate at any number of places, including the extremities (in the neonate, on the medial aspect of the hand or lateral aspect of the foot), ears, nose, and tongue.[123–125] The accuracy of this monitor is unaffected by the presence of fetal hemoglobin,[126] hyperbilirubinemia,[127,128] low oxygen saturation,[129] or anemia (hemoglobin > 15 g%).[130] However, the accuracy is affected by several factors, including met- and carboxyhemoglobinemia,[131] certain dyes and hues of nail polish,[132] extraneous infrared lights (radiant overhead heater), hypothermia, hypotension, and rapid acute arterial oxygen desaturation.[133] Consequently, S_aO_2 may not be accurate in cool neonates with poorly perfused extremities. In these instances, application of the oximeter to the ear or nose may yield accurate measurements. In addition, the oximeter sensor should be shielded from overhead radiant light. Movement artefact has precluded accurate measurements of S_aO_2 in neonates and older infants both before and after anesthesia as well as during induction of, and emergence from, anesthesia. However, new algorithms (Massimo) have virtually eliminated motion artifact, thus enabling accurate measurements in infants and children in spite of spontaneous movement.

Carbon dioxide partial pressure in blood can be estimated noninvasively by both transcutaneous and end-tidal techniques.[134,135] Although the advantages of transcutaneous monitoring systems are well known, transcutaneous monitors are not commonly used in the operating room because they require a calibration period, they respond slowly to changes in CO_2 partial pressure, and they do not provide breath-by-breath analysis of ventilation as do end-tidal gas analyzers.[135] The accuracy of end-tidal gas measurements depends on several factors,[135] including the type of capnometer, the location of the end-tidal gas sampling port within the circuit,[136] the type of circuit, and the presence of cardiorespiratory dysfunction.[137] Two types of capnometers are available: sidestream and mainstream capnometers. Sidestream capnometers continuously aspirate gas from the breathing circuit. For accurate readings, these analyzers must aspirate gas at a sufficient rate compared with the respiratory rate to sample the peaks and valleys of the CO_2 concentration.

Mainstream capnometers are placed within the circuit and analyze gas within the circuit as it passes through the sensor. These capnometers may provide accurate estimates of CO_2 tension but may be heavy relative to the weight of the circuit and add deadspace to the circuit. With a Mapleson D or F circuit, an aspirating capnometer will provide accurate end-tidal $P\text{CO}_2$ estimates in infants weighing < 12 kg provided that the gas is sampled from within the tracheal tube.[134,136] To sample end-tidal gas from within the tracheal tube, a 19G Vialon catheter may be inserted into the 3.0-mm-inner-diameter and 3.5-mm-inner-diameter tracheal tubes and a 21G catheter into 2.5-mm-inner-diameter tubes. These catheters are cut such that the tip of the catheter lies anywhere within the lumen of the tracheal tube.

Similar principles also apply for accurate end-tidal measurements of anesthetic gas concentrations. With circle circuits, gas may be sampled from anywhere within the lumen of the tracheal tube to minimize the dilutional effect of the fresh gas flow.

In the presence of right-to-left cardiac shunts, end-tidal CO_2 tensions do not correlate with arterial CO_2 tensions.[137] In contrast, with normal cardiac anatomy or left-to-right shunts, end-tidal CO_2 tension accurately reflects arterial tensions. End-tidal CO_2 tension does not accurately reflect the arterial tension in neonates with lung disease. Although end-tidal CO_2 tension may be used to follow trends, it should not be relied upon for accurate assessments of the adequacy of alveolar ventilation. In such cases, arterial blood gases should be analyzed to document the actual gas tensions.

Fluid and metabolic requirements

Fluid and metabolic requirements for the neonate reflect a high metabolic rate. Maintenance fluids such as D5/0.2%S should be administered at 4 mL kg^{-1} h^{-1} for the first 10 kg. In order to minimize the likelihood of fluid overload, maintenance fluids should be administered slowly, using an infusion pump. Supplemental glucose as a 10% solution (4–5 mg kg^{-1} min^{-1}) and calcium gluconate as a 10% solution

(2–3 mg kg^{-1} h^{-1}) may be required for preterm neonates and those fullterm neonates who are nutritionally deficient. Third-space losses (2–15 mL kg^{-1} h^{-1}) should be replaced with balanced salt solution, colloid (albumin or stored plasma), or a combination of the two. The latter may be particularly appropriate for the preterm neonate who is often hypoalbuminemic.

In some neonatal surgical lesions (such as gastroschisis and omphalocele), large volumes of third-space fluids must be replaced in order to maintain cardiovascular and renal homeostasis before and after surgery. The volume of third-space fluids required may be even greater than suggested above if the lesions are complicated by sepsis and coagulopathies. In the latter circumstances, fresh-frozen plasma and platelets may be required. Red cell transfusions are indicated for neonates during surgery when the hemoglobin concentration decreases to values less than 10 g dL^{-1}.

Overzealous fluid administration must be tempered with the risk of reopening the ductus arteriosus. The presence of a systolic murmur from a patent ductus arteriosus should be documented preoperatively. If large fluid shifts are expected during surgery (as in the case of a myelomeningocele repair with a large skin rotational flap) or a sacrococcygeal teratoma, then a central venous pressure monitor may be indicated.

Regional anesthesia

The role of regional anesthesia in the neonate both intraoperatively and postoperatively has attracted great interest in the past decade.[138] The most popular techniques performed by anesthesiologists are spinal and caudal blocks (see below). A complete discussion of other blocks, including ilioinguinal and iliohypogastric nerve blocks and penile blocks, can be found elsewhere.[139]

Spinal anesthesia has been used for repair of hernias, as well as ligation of ductus arteriosus and repair of tracheoesophageal fistulae.[140–142] Candidates for hernia repair under spinal anesthesia include preterm and ex-preterm infants with chronic lung disease for whom surgery is scheduled for less than 1 h in duration and the surgeons do not apply strong traction on the peritoneum during repair.

For ductus ligation and tracheoesophageal fistula repairs, the high spinal level required for analgesia necessitates instrumentation of the airway to preclude bradypnea or apnea.[142] The advantage of this technique is a decreased incidence of postanesthetic apnea in ex-preterm infants compared with a general anesthetic technique.[143] However, complications have been reported, particularly when the lower extremities are raised before the block has had time to fix, resulting in a high block.[144] In addition, inadequate anesthesia has occurred, resulting in the administration of a general anesthetic with the associated risks including postoperative apnea.[142] Unlike adults, neonates maintain a stable heart rate, blood pressure, and respiration during spinal anesthesia even without prehydration.[145] This has been attributed to a predominantly parasympathetic inhibition by the spinal block.

Because the spinal cord in the neonate may extend as far rostral as the T12–L3 level, spinal punctures should be performed at the L4–L5 level. This block may be administered with the neonate sitting or in the lateral decubitus position with the spine flexed maximally but the head extended to minimize the risk of airway obstruction. A 22G or 25G needle (with a stylette, i.e. Quincke needle) is inserted into the L4–L5 interspace under sterile conditions and the hyperbaric solution injected. The dose of tetracaine for lower abdominal surgery is 0.4–1.0 mg kg^{-1} (with an equal volume of 10% dextrose) or 3 mg kg^{-1} lidocaine. The dose of tetracaine for thoracic surgery (patent ductus arteriosus ligation) when a lumbar approach is used is even larger, varying inversely with weight. The average dose in one study[142] was 2.4 mg kg^{-1}. Despite this dose, 50% of the neonates required supplemental anesthesia. The large doses of local anesthetic required for spinal anesthesia in the preterm infant may be explained by the five- to sevenfold greater volume of cerebrospinal fluid per kg body weight compared with that in the adult. Tetracaine provides about 1 h of operating time, whereas lidocaine provides about one-half that duration. If the spinal anesthetic is supplemented with sedation, the probability of a postoperative apnea increases dramatically.[143]

Caudal analgesia is another neuroaxial regional technique that is used both intraoperatively and postoperatively.[146] These blocks are performed with the neonate in the decubitus position and under sterile conditions. A 24G Angiocath is inserted into the sacrococcygeal ligament of the neonate and 0.175–0.25% bupivacaine in a volume of 0.5–0.75 mL kg^{-1} is injected slowly. Other local anesthetics for caudal analgesia include lidocaine, 3% 2-chloroprocaine,[147,148] and 1 mg kg^{-1} 0.2% ropivacaine.[149] In the neonate, several cases of sudden onset of bradycardia or ventricular tachycardia have been reported after a single-dose administration of bupivacaine in the caudal space.[150] Although low serum concentrations of albumin and α_1-acid glycoprotein may increase the free fraction of bupivacaine,[39] these arrhythmias are likely attributable to the inadvertent intraosseous or intravascular injections.

Caudal blocks in neonates must be performed with great caution to avoid intravascular or interosseous injection of local anesthetic.[146] The thin tables of sacral bone in the neonate are easily punctured and bloody fluid may not be aspirable, thus making identification of the caudal space difficult to differentiate from the intraosseous space. Indwelling caudal catheters (Portex 19G) may be threaded through an 18G Intracath for continuous infusion of bupivacaine intra- and postoperatively. Berde[151] recommended that bupivacaine should not be infused in doses in excess of 0.2 mg kg^{-1} h^{-1} via the epidural route in neonates, although even this dose may result in an accumulation of bupivacaine in neonates after 48 h.[152] Bupivacaine undergoes hepatic degradation by aromatic hydroxylation, N-dealkylation, and amide hydrolysis. Immature enzyme systems in the neonate prolong the half-life of bupivacaine but reach adult levels of elimination by 3–6 months of age. This is due to the prolonged elimination half-life of bupivacaine in neonates. At this infusion rate, the plasma concentrations of bupivacaine remain within acceptable limits, although recent evidence indicates that, by 48 h, the plasma levels are still rising.

Supplemental medications have been used as adjuncts to caudal analgesia. Epinephrine has no clear effect on the duration of caudal block in infants and children. Clonidine (2 μg kg^{-1}) has prolonged the duration of block in children. However, reports have suggested that a single dose of clonidine in the caudal space might be associated with life-threatening postoperative apneas in term and preterm neonates.[153,154]

Emergence and pain management

At the termination of the anesthetic, extubation may be considered once the neonate has satisfied several criteria. The neonate should be normothermic, normocapneic or hypercapneic, the serum hemoglobin and electrolyte and glucose concentrations should be normal, and any residual neuromuscular blockade should be antagonized. Neuromuscular blockade should be antagonized in all neonates, preterm or fullterm, who received a nondepolarizing relaxant and whose trachea is to be extubated. Even with the use of modern short-acting neuromuscular blocking agents, recovery from paralysis in the neonate remains unpredictably variable, and any residual neuromuscular blockade may quickly lead to respiratory failure. Neostigmine (0.04–0.05 mg kg^{-1}) and atropine (0.02 mg kg^{-1}) should successfully antagonize the residual neuromuscular blockade within 10 min.

Emergence from inhalational anesthesia tends to follow three phases. In the first phase, the neonate begins to breathe, but respiration remains irregular and he/she coughs and strains on the tracheal tube. In the second phase, the neonate breathholds for a variable period, and it is at this time that the neonate is at greatest risk for hemoglobin oxygen desaturation. Finally, the neonate resumes regular respiration, begins to gag on the tracheal tube, flexes the hips, and contracts the rectus abdominis muscle.[155] When the neonate has achieved this final phase of recovery, extubation may be considered.

Postoperative management of the neonate depends on both the severity of the primary surgical condition and the associated medical problems. After minor surgery, the healthy fullterm neonate (less than 4 weeks of age) is monitored in the recovery room for 4 h with an apnea monitor, pulse oximeter, and electrocardiogram. Neonates may be transferred to a ward for overnight observation if the recovery stay is uneventful. At our institution, neonates are not discharged home on the day of surgery. Although postoperative apnea is rare in the fullterm neonate, several cases have recently been reported.[156–158] Postoperative apnea usually occurs within 6 h of discontinuation of anesthesia and does not lead to untoward outcomes. Because maturation of the respiratory control center is a continuous process with variability among individuals, it is not surprising that rare episodes of postoperative apnea do occur, even in the fullterm neonate.

In contrast, up to 20% of preterm neonates may develop postoperative apnea after general anesthesia.[159–162] The risk of postoperative apnea increases in the presence of anemia and decreases with increasing postconceptual age, i.e. the sum of gestational and postnatal age, in the preterm and ex-preterm infant. The pathogenesis of the postoperative apnea appears to be both central and obstructive in origin.[163] Infants with major organ dysfunction (congenital heart disease, severe respiratory distress, and major intracranial hemorrhage) are at greater risk of postoperative apnea. Caffeine ($10\,mg\,kg^{-1}$) during the anesthetic is recommended to those preterm infants at risk for a postoperative apnea.[19] A single dose of caffeine is sufficient for 18–24 h. When these neonates are extubated immediately after surgery, they are monitored in the recovery room for at least 4 h, and then admitted to a constant care suite and monitored with an apnea monitor for 24 h or at least 12 h after the last apneic episode. Following major surgery or for the critically ill neonate, these patients are transferred to the neonatal or pediatric intensive care and are weaned from the ventilator as rapidly as possible.

Perioperative pain management of the pediatric patient is a rapidly expanding area of interest (see Chapter 77). At the present time, however, our experience in pain management of the neonate is limited, except to say that neonates can mount both behavioral and neurohumoral responses to painful stimuli.[12,14,15] Intraoperative opioids and regional anesthesia may be administered to provide postoperative pain relief. Infiltration of local anesthetic solutions into the wound and in the wound edges is popular. Postoperative analgesic medications include acetaminophen (paracetamol) ($15–25\,mg\,kg^{-1}$ per rectum or per os) and codeine ($0.5–1.5\,mg\,kg^{-1}$ intramuscularly), although the latter is rarely given to infants weighing less than 4.5 kg. Morphine infusions are not commonly used because of the unpredictability of respiratory depression and side-effects (see above).

Recent research has increased our understanding of perinatal physiology and anesthesia for the neonate. Increased awareness of pharmacology in relation to the particular needs of the sensitive and rapidly developing neonate will continue to improve perioperative care.

REFERENCES

1. Piecuch RE, Leonard CH, Cooper BA, Sehring SA. Outcome of extremely low birth weight infants (500–999 grams) over a 12-year period. *Pediatrics* 1997; **100:** 633–9.
2. Yu VY. Developmental outcome of extremely preterm infants. *Am J Perinatol* 2000; **17:** 57–61.
3. Kinouchi K, Kitamura S. Improved viability of the low birth weight infant and the increasing needs for anaesthesia. *Paediatr Anaesth* 2001; **11:** 131–3.
4. Cohen MM, Cameron CB, Duncan PG. Pediatric anesthesia morbidity and mortality in the perioperative period. *Anesth Analg* 1990; **70:** 160–7.
5. Keenan RL, Boyan CP. Cardiac arrest due to anesthesia. An study of incidence and causes. *JAMA* 1985; **253:** 2372–7.
6. Friis-Hansen B. Changes in body water compartments during growth. *Acta Pediatr Scand* 1957; **110** (Suppl.): 49–54.
7. Lerman J, Schmitt-Bantel BI, Gregory GA, *et al*. Effect of age on the solubility of volatile anesthetics in human tissues. *Anesthesiology* 1986; **65:** 307–11.
8. Younkin DP, Reivich M, Jaggi J, *et al*. Noninvasive method of estimating human newborn regional cerebral blood flow. *J Cereb Blood Flow Metab* 1982; **2:** 415–20.
9. Lou H, Lassen NA, Friis-Hansen B. Impaired autoregulation of cerebral blood flow in the distressed newborn infant. *J Pediatr* 1979; **94:** 118–21.
10. Anand KJS, Hickey PR. Pain and its effects in the human neonate and fetus. *N Engl J Med* 1987; **317:** 1321–9.
11. Fitzgerald M. Development of pain pathways and mechanism. In: Anand KJS, McGrath PJ (eds). *Pain in Neonates*. Amsterdam: Elsevier, 1993: 19–37.
12. Anand KJS, Sippell WG, Aynsley-Green A. Randomised trial of fentanyl anaesthesia in preterm babies undergoing surgery: effects on the stress response. *Lancet* 1987; **i:** 243–8.
13. LeDez KM, Lerman J. The minimum alveolar concentration (MAC) of isoflurane in preterm neonates. *Anesthesiology* 1987; **67:** 301–7.
14. Protonotariou E, Malamitsi-Puchner A, Giannaki G, *et al*. Patterns of inflammatory cytokine serum concentrations during the perinatal period. *Early Hum Dev* 1999; **56:** 31–8.
15. Lago P, Benini F, Agosto C, Zacchello F. Randomised controlled trial of low dose fentanyl infusion in preterm infants with hyaline membrane disease. *Arch Dis Child Fetal Neonatal Ed* 1998; **79** (3): F194–7.
16. Frantz III ID, Adler SM, Thach BT, Taeusch Jr HW. Maturational effects on respiratory responses to carbon dioxide in premature infants. *J Appl Physiol* 1976; **41:** 634–8.
17. Rigatto H, de la Torre Verduzco R, Cates DB. Effect of O_2 on the ventilatory response to CO_2 in preterm infants. *J Appl Physiol* 1975; **39:** 896–9.
18. Brady JP, Ceruti E. Chemoreceptor reflexes in the new-born infant. Effects of varying degrees of hypoxia on heart rate and ventilation in a warm environment. *J Physiol (Lond)* 1966; **184:** 631–45.
19. Welborn LG, Hannallah RS, Fink R, *et al*. High-dose caffeine suppresses postoperative apnea in former preterm infants. *Anesthesiology* 1989; **71:** 347–9.
20. Eckenhoff JE. Some anatomic considerations of the infant larynx influencing endotracheal anesthesia. *Anesthesiology* 1951; **12:** 401–10.
21. Tsuneto S, Yamashita M, Miyamoto Y. Tracheo-bronchial angles in neonates. *Anesthesiology* 1987; **67:** 151.
22. Keens TG, Bryan AC, Levison H, *et al*. Developmental pattern of muscle fibers in human ventilatory muscles. *J Appl Physiol* 1978; **44:** 909–13.
23. Friedman WF. The intrinsic physiologic properties of the developing heart. *Prog Cardiovasc Dis* 1972; **15:** 87–111.
24. Hoerter J, Mazet F, Vassort G. Perinatal growth of the rabbit cardiac cell: possible implications for the mechanism of relaxation. *J Mol Cell Cardiol* 1981; **13:** 725–40.
25. Nakanishi T, Okuda K, Kamata K, *et al*. Development of myocardial contractile system in the fetal rabbit. *Pediatr Res* 1988; **22:** 201–7.
26. Rudolph AM, Heyman MA. Cardiac output in the fetal lamb: the effects of spontaneous and induced changes of heart rate on right and left ventricular output. *Am J Obstet Gynecol* 1976; **124:** 183–92.
27. O'Brien RT, Pearson HA. Physiologic anemia of the newborn infant. *J Pediatr* 1971; **79:** 132–8.
28. Delivoria-Papadopoulos M, Roncevic NP, Oski FA. Postnatal changes in oxygen transport of term, premature, and sick infants: the role of red cell 2,3-diphosphoglycerate and adult hemoglobin. *Pediatr Res* 1971; **5:** 235–45.
29. Guignard JP, Torrado A. Mazouni SM, Gautier E. Renal function in respiratory distress syndrome. *J Pediatr* 1976; **88:** 845–50.
30. Aperia A, Zetterstron R. Renal control of fluid homeostasis in the newborn infant. *Clin Perinatol* 1982; **9:** 523–34.
31. Spitzer A. Renal physiology and functional development. In: Edelman Jr CM (ed.) *Pediatric Kidney Disease*. Boston: Little Brown & Co., 1978: 25.
32. Zink J, Van Petten GR. Time course of closure of the ductus venosus in the newborn lamb. *Pediatr Res* 1980; **14:** 1–3.
33. Masey SA, Koehler RC, Buck JR, *et al*. Effect of abdominal distention on central and regional hemodynamics in neonatal lambs. *Pediatr Res* 1985; **19:** 1244–9.
34. Aranda JV, MacLeod SM, Renton KW, Eade NR. Hepatic microsomal drug oxidation and electron transport in newborn infants. *J Pediatr* 1974; **85:** 534–42.

35. Sereni F, Principi N. Developmental pharmacology. *Annu Rev Pharmacol* 1968; **8:** 453–66.
36. Levy G, Khanna NN, Soda DM, *et al*. Pharmacokinetics of acetaminophen in the human neonate: formation of acetaminophen glucuronide and sulfate in relation to plasma bilirubin concentration and D-glucaric acid excretion. *Pediatrics* 1975; **55:** 818–25.
37. Tsang RC, Light IJ, Sutherland JM, Kleinman LI. Possible pathogenetic factors in neonatal hypocalcemia of prematurity. *J Pediatr* 1973; **82:** 423–9.
38. Ehrnebo M, Agurell S, Jalling B, *et al*. Age differences in drug binding by plasma proteins: studies on human foetuses, neonates and adults. *Eur J Clin Pharmacol* 1971; **3:** 189–93.
39. Lerman J, Strong HA, LeDez KM, *et al*. Effects of age on the serum concentration of alpha-1 acid glycoprotein and the binding of lidocaine in pediatric patients. *Clin Pharm Ther* 1989; **46:** 219–25.
40. Meuldermans WEG, Hurkmans RMA, Heykants JJP. Plasma protein binding and distribution of fentanyl, sufentanil, alfentanil and lofentanil in blood. *Arch Int Pharmacodyn* 1982; **257:** 4–19.
41. Hey E, Katz G. The optimum thermal environment for naked babies. *Arch Dis Child* 1970; **45:** 328–34.
42. Perkins MN, Rothwell NJ, Stock MJ, *et al*. Activation of brown adipose tissue thermogenesis by the ventromedial hypothalamus. *Nature* 1981; **289:** 401–2.
43. Kelly EJ, Newell SJ, Brownlee KG, *et al*. Gastric secretion in preterm infants. *Early Hum Dev* 1993; **35:** 215–20.
44. Euler AR, Byrne WJ, Cousins LM, *et al*. Increased serum gastrin concentrations and gastric acid hyposecretion in the immediate newborn period. *Gastroenterology* 1977; **72:** 1271–3.
45. Raidoo DM, Rocke DA, Brock-utne JG, *et al*. Critical volume for pulmonary acid aspiration: reappraisal in a primate model. *Br J Anaesth* 1990; **65:** 248–50.
46. Knight PR, Rutter T, Tait AR, *et al*. Pathogenesis of gastric particulate lung injury: a comparison and interaction with acidic pneumonitis. *Anesth Analg* 1993; **77:** 754–60.
47. Crawford M, Lerman J, Christensen S, Farrow-Gillespie A. Effects of duration of fasting on gastric fluid pH and volume in healthy children. *Anesth Analg* 1990; **71:** 400–3.
48. Splinter WM, Stewart JA, Muir JG. Large volumes of apple juice preoperatively do not affect gastric pH and volume in children. *Can J Anaesth* 1990; **37:** 36–9.
49. American Society of Anesthesiologists Task Force on Preoperative Fasting. Practice guidelines for preoperative fasting and the use of pharmacologic agents to reduce the risk of pulmonary aspiration: application to healthy patients undergoing elective procedures. *Anesthesiology* 1999; **90:** 896–905.
50. O'Hare B, Lerman J, Endo J, Cutz E. Acute lung injury after instillation of human breast milk or infant formula into rabbits' lungs. *Anesthesiology* 1996; **84:** 1386–91.
51. Cavell B. Gastric emptying in infants fed human milk or infant formula. *Acta Paediatr Scand* 1981; **70:** 639–41.
52. Cavell B. Gastric emptying in preterm infants. *Acta Paediatr Scand* 1979; **68:** 725–30.
53. Litman RS, Wu CL, Quinlivan JK. Gastric volume and pH in infants fed clear liquids and breast milk prior to surgery. *Anesth Analg* 1994; **79:** 482–5.
54. Billeaud C, Guillet J, Sandler B. Gastric emptying in infants with or without gastro-oesophageal reflux according to the type of milk. *Eur J Clin Nutrition* 1990; **44:** 577–83.
55. Lerman J. Anesthesia for the preterm and fullterm neonate. In: Prys-Roberts C, Brown Burnell Jr R (eds). *International Practice of Anesthesia*, vol. 2. Oxford: Butterworth Heinemann, 1996: 2/103/9.
56. Steward DJ, Lerman J. *Manual of Pediatric Anesthesia,* 5th edn. New York: Churchill Livingstone, 2001: 85, 445–506.
57. Larson Jr CP. Laryngospasm – the best treatment. *Anesthesiology* 1998; **89:** 1293–4.
58. Duncan HP, Zurick HJ, Wolf AR. Should we reconsider awake neonatal intubation? A review of the evidence and treatment strategies. *Paediatr Anaesth* 2001; **11:** 135–45.
59. Whyte S, Birrell G, Wyllie J. Premedication before intubation in UK neonatal units. *Arch Dis Child Fetal Neonatal Ed* 2000; **82:** F38–41.
60. Barrington KJ, Byrne PJ. Premedication for neonatal intubation. *Am J Perinatol* 1998; **15** (4): 213–16.
61. Stow PJ, McLeod ME, Burrows FA, Creighton RE. Anterior fontanelle pressure responses to tracheal intubation in the awake and the anaesthetized infant. *Br J Anaesth* 1988; **60:** 167–70.
62. Hancock PJ, Peterson G. Finger intubation of the trachea in newborns. *Pediatrics* 1992; **89:** 325–7.
63. Vener DF, Lerman J. The pediatric airway and associated syndromes. In: Doyle DJ, Sandler AN (eds). *The Difficult Airway II. Anesthesiol Clin North Am* 1995; **13:** 610.
64. Georgescu A, Miller JN, Lecklitner ML. The sellick maneuver causing complete airway obstruction. *Anesth Analg* 1992; **74:** 457–9.
65. Sellick BA. Cricoid pressure to control regurgitation of stomach contents during induction of anaesthesia. *Lancet* 1961; **ii:** 404–6.
66. Dubreuil M, Laffon M, Plaud B, *et al*. Complications and fiberoptic assessment of size 1 laryngeal mask airway. *Anesth Analg* 1993; **76:** 527–9.
67. Goudsouzian NG, Denman W, Clevelant R, Shorten G. Radiologic localization of the laryngeal mask airway in children. *Anesthesiology* 1992; **77:** 1085–9.
68. Schily M, Koumoukelis H, Lerman J, Creighton RE. Can pediatric anesthesiologists detect an occluded tracheal tube in neonates? *Anesth Analg* 2001; in press.
69. Salanitre E, Rackow H. The pulmonary exchange of nitrous oxide and halothane in infants and children. *Anesthesiology* 1969; **30:** 388–94.
70. Lerman J, Gregory GA, Willis MM, Eger II EI. Age and the solubility of volatile anesthetics in blood. *Anesthesiology* 1984; **61:** 139–43.
71. Malviya S, Lerman J. Blood/gas solubilities of sevoflurane, isoflurane, halothane and serum constituent concentrations neonates and adults. *Anesthesiology* 1990; **72:** 793–6.
72. Steward DJ, Creighton RE. The uptake and excretion of nitrous oxide in the newborn. *Can Anaesth Soc J* 1978; **25:** 215–17.
73. Gregory GA, Eger II EI, Munson EW. The relationship between age and halothane requirement in man. *Anesthesiology* 1969; **30:** 488–91.
74. Diaz JH, Lockhart CH. Is halothane really safe in infancy? *Anesthesiology* 1979; **51:** A313.
75. Lerman J, Robinson S, Willis MM, Gregory GA. Anesthetic requirements for halothane in young children 0–1 month and 1–6 months of age. *Anesthesiology* 1983; **59:** 421–4.
76. Taylor RH, Lerman J. Minimum alveolar concentration of desflurane and hemodynamic responses in neonates, infants and children. *Anesthesiology* 1991; **75:** 975–9.
77. Lerman J, Sikich N, Kleinman S, Yentis S. Pharmacology of sevoflurane in infants and children. *Anesthesiology* 1994; **80:** 814–24.
78. Cameron CB, Robinson S, Gregory GA. The minimum anesthetic concentration of isoflurane in children. *Anesth Analg* 1984; **63:** 18–20.
79. Murat I, Lapeyre G, Saint-Maurice C. Isoflurane attenuates baroreflex control of heart rate in human neonates. *Anesthesiology* 1989; **70:** 395–400.
80. Murat I, Hoerter J, Ventura-Clapier R. Developmental changes in effects of halothane and isoflurane on contractile properties of rabbit cardiac skinned fibers. *Anesthesiology* 1990; **73:** 137–45.
81. Murray DJ, Forbes RB, Mahoney LT. Comparative hemodynamic depression of halothane versus isoflurane in neonates and infants: an echocardiographic study. *Anesth Analg* 1992; **74:** 329–37.
82. Eger II EI, Saidman LJ. Hazards of nitrous oxide anesthesia in bowel obstruction and pneumothorax. *Anesthesiology* 1965; **26:** 61–6.
83. Westrin P, Jonmarker C, Werner O. Thiopental requirements for induction of anesthesia in neonates and infants one to six months of age. *Anesthesiology* 1989; **71:** 344–6.
84. Kingston HGG, Kendrick A, Sommer KM, *et al*. Binding of thiopental in neonatal serum. *Anesthesiology* 1990; **72:** 428–31.
85. Kupferberg HJ, Way EL. Pharmacologic basis for the increased sensitivity of the newborn rat to morphine. *J Pharmacol Exp* 1963; **141:** 105–12.
86. Sanner JH, Woods LA. Comparative distribution of tritium labeled dihydromorphine between maternal and fetal rats. *J Pharmacol Exp* 1965; **148:** 176–84.
87. Friesen RH, Henry DB. Cardiovascular changes in preterm neonates receiving isoflurane, halothane, fentanyl, and ketamine. *Anesthesiology* 1986; **64:** 238–42.
88. Morselli PL, Principi N, Tognoni G, *et al*. Diazepam elimination in premature and full term infants and children. *J Perinatol Med* 1973; **1:** 133–41.
89. Way WL, Costley EC, Way EL. Respiratory sensitivity of the newborn infant to meperidine and morphine. *Clin Pharm Ther* 1965; **6:** 454–61.
90. Bhat R, Abu-Harb M, Chari G, Gulati A. Morphine metabolism in acutely ill preterm newborn infants. *J Pediatr* 1992; **120:** 795–9.
91. Rutter N, Evans N. Cardiovascular effects of an intravenous bolus of morphine in the ventilated preterm infant. *Arch Dis Child Fetal Neonatal Ed* 2000; **83** (2): F101–3.
92. Lynn AM, Slattery JT. Morphine pharmacokinetics in early infancy. *Anesthesiology* 1987; **66:** 136–9.
93. Choonara IA, McKay P, Hain R, Rane A. Morphine metabolism in children. *Br J Clin Pharmacol* 1989; **28:** 599–604.
94. Chay PCW, Duffy BJ, Walker JS. Pharmacokinetic-pharmacodynamic

relationships of morphine in neonates. *Clin Pharmacol Ther* 1992; **51:** 334–42.

95. Saarenmaa E, Neuvonen PJ, Rosenberg P, Fellman V. Morphine clearance and effects in newborn infants in relation to gestational age. *Clin Pharm Ther* 2000; **68** (2): 160–6.
96. Scott CS, Riggs KW, Ling EW, *et al.* Morphine pharmacokinetics and pain assessment in premature newborns. *J Pediatr* 1999; **135:** 423–9.
97. Kart T, Christrup LL, Rasmussen M. Recommended use of morphine in neonates, infants and children based on a literature review. Part 1. Pharmacokinetics. *Paediatr Anaesth* 1997; **7:** 5–11.
98. Pokela ML, Olkkola KT, Seppala T, Koivisto M. Age-related morphine kinetics in infants. *Dev Pharmacol Ther* 1993; **20:** 26–34.
99. Lynn A, Nespeca MK, Bratton SL, *et al.* Clearance of morphine in postoperative infants during intravenous infusion: the influence of age and surgery. *Anesth Analg* 1998; **86:** 958–63.
100. Kart T, Christrup LL, Rasmussen M. Recommended use of morphine in neonates, infants and children based on a literature review: Part 2-Clinical use. *Paediatr Anaesth* 1997; **7:** 93–101.
101. Robinson S, Gregory GA. Fentanyl-air-oxygen anesthesia for ligation of patent ductus arteriosis in preterm infants. *Anesth Analg* 1981; **60:** 331–4.
102. Yaster M. The dose response of fentanyl in neonatal anesthesia. *Anesthesiology* 1987; **66:** 443–5.
103. Koehntop DE, Rodman JH, Brundage DM, *et al.* Pharmacokinetics of fentanyl in neonates. *Anesth Analg* 1986; **65:** 227–32.
104. Gauntlett IS, Fisher DM, Hertzka RE, *et al.* Pharmacokinetics of fentanyl in neonatal humans and lambs: effects of age. *Anesthesiology* 1988; **69:** 683–7.
105. Murat I, Levron J-C, Berg A, Saint-Maurice C. Effects of fentanyl on baroreceptor reflex control of heart rate in newborn infants. *Anesthesiology* 1988; **68:** 717–22.
106. Bovill JG. Which potent opioid? Important criteria for selection. *Drugs* 1987; **33:** 520–30.
107. Marlow N, Weindling AM, Van Peer A, Heykants J. Alfentanil pharmacokinetics in preterm infants. *Arch Dis Child* 1990; **65:** 349–51.
108. Greeley WJ, de Bruijn NP. Changes in sufentanil pharmacokinetics within the neonatal period. *Anesth Analg* 1988; **67:** 86–90.
109. Anand KJS, Hickey PR. Halothane-morphine compared with high-dose sufentanil for anesthesia and postoperative analgesia in neonatal cardiac surgery. *N Engl J Med* 1992; **326:** 1–9.
110. Davis PJ, Ross AK, Henson LG, Muir KT. Remifentanil pharmacokinetics in neonates. *Anesthesiology* 1997; **87:** A1064.
111. Zsigmond EK, Downs JR. Plasma cholinesterase activity in newborns and infants. *Can Anaesth Soc J* 1971; **18:** 278–85.
112. Fisher DM, O'Keefe C, Stanski DR, *et al.* Pharmacokinetics and pharmacodynamics of D-tubocurarine in infants, children and adults. *Anesthesiology* 1982; **57:** 203–8.
113. Brandom BW, Stiller RL, Cook DR, *et al.* Pharmacokinetics of atracurium in anesthetized infants and children. *Br J Anaesth* 1986; **58:** 1210–13.
114. Meretoja OA, Wirtavuori K, Neuvonen PJ. Age-dependence of the dose–response curve of vecuronium in pediatric patients during balanced anesthesia. *Anesth Analg* 1988; **67:** 21–6.
115. Brandom BW, Woelfel SK, Cook DR, *et al.* Clinical pharmacology of atracurium in infants. *Anesth Analg* 1984; **63:** 309–12.
116. Nightingale DA. Use of atracurium in neonatal anaesthesia. *Br J Anaesth* 1986; **58:** 32S–36S.
117. Meakin G, Shaw EA, Baker RD, Morris P. Comparison of atracurium-induced neuromuscular blockade in neonates, infants and children. *Br J Anaesth* 1988; **60:** 171–5.
118. Meakin GH, Pronske EH, Lerman J, *et al.* Bronchospasm after rapacuronium in infants and children. *Anesthesiology* 2001; **94:** 926–7.
119. Kalli I, Meretoja OA. Infusion of atracurium in neonates, infants and children: a study of dose requirements. *Br J Anaesth* 1988; **60:** 651–4.
120. Meretoja OA. Vecuronium infusion requirements in pediatric patients during fentanyl-N_2O–O_2 anesthesia. *Anesth Analg* 1989; **68:** 20–4.
121. Cook DR, Davis PJ, Lerman J. Pharmacology of pediatric anesthesia. In: Motoyama EK, Davis PJ (eds). *Smith's Anesthesia for Infants and Children*, 6th edn. St Louis: Mosby 1996: 188–209.
122. Cote CJ, Goldstein EA, Cote MA, *et al.* A single-blind study of pulse oximetry in children. *Anesthesiology* 1988; **68:** 184–8.
123. Tremper KK, Barker SJ. Pulse oximetry. *Anesthesiology* 1989; **70:** 98–108.
124. Jobes DR, Nicolson SC. Monitoring of arterial hemoglobin oxygen saturation using a tongue sensor. *Anesth Analg* 1988; **67:** 186–8.
125. O'Leary RJ, Landon M, Benumof JL. Buccal pulse oximeter is more accurate than finger pulse oximeter in measuring oxygen saturation. *Anesth Analg* 1992; **75:** 495–8.
126. Durand M, Ramanathan R. Pulse oximetry for continuous oxygen monitoring in sick newborn infants. *J Pediatr* 1986; **109:** 1052–6.
127. Beall SN, Moorthy SS. Jaundice, oximetry, and spurious hemoglobin desaturation. *Anesth Analg* 1989; **68:** 806–8.
128. Veyckemans F, Baele P, Guillaume JE, *et al.* Hyperbilirubinemia does not interfere with hemoglobin saturation measured by pulse oximetry. *Anesthesiology* 1989; **70:** 118–22.
129. Deckardt R, Steward DJ. Noninvasive arterial hemoglobin oxygen saturation versus transcutaneous oxygen tension monitoring in the preterm infant. *Crit Care Med* 1984; **12:** 935–9.
130. Lee S, Tremper KK, Barker SJ. Effects of anemia on pulse oximetry and continuous mixed venous hemoglobin saturation monitoring in dogs. *Anesthesiology* 1991; **75:** 118–22.
131. Eisenkraft JB. Pulse oximeter desaturation due to methemoglobinemia. *Anesthesiology* 1988; **68:** 279–82.
132. Cote CJ, Goldstein A, Fuchsman WH, Hoaglin DC. The effect of nail polish on pulse oximetry. *Anesth Analg* 1988; **67:** 683–6.
133. Severinghaus JW, Naifeh KH, Koh SO. Errors in 14 pulse oximeters during profound hypoxia. *J Clin Monit* 1989; **5:** 72–81.
134. McEvedy BAB, McLeod ME, Mulera M, *et al.* End-tidal, transcutaneous, and arterial pCO_2 measurements in critically ill neonates: a comparative study. *Anesthesiology* 1988; **69:** 112–16.
135. Kirpalani H, Kechagias S, Lerman J. Technical and clinical aspects of capnography in neonates. *J Med Eng Technol* 1991; **15:** 154–61.
136. Badgwell JM, McLeaod ME, Lerman J, Creighton RE. End-tidal pCO_2 measurements sampled at the distal and proximal ends of the endotracheal tube in infants and children. *Anesth Analg* 1987; **66:** 959–64.
137. Burrows FA. Physiologic dead space, venous admixture, and the arterial to end-tidal carbon dioxide difference in infants and children undergoing cardiac surgery. *Anesthesiology* 1989; **79:** 219–25.
138. Bosenberg AT, Ivani G. Regional anaesthesia – children are different. *Pediatr Anaesth* 1998; **8:** 447–50.
139. Rice LJ. Regional anesthesia and analgesia. In: Motoyama EK, Davis PJ (eds). *Smith's Anesthesia for Infants and Children*, 6th edn. St Louis: Mosby 1996; 403–42.
140. Abajian JC, Mellish RWP, Browne AF, *et al.* Spinal anesthesia for surgery in the high-risk infants. *Anesth Analg* 1984; **63:** 359–62.
141. Gerber ACH, Baitella LC, Dangel PH. Spinal anaesthesia in former preterm infants. *Pediatr Anaesth* 1993; **3:** 153–6.
142. Williams RK, Abajian JC. High spinal anaesthesia for repair of patent ductus arteriosus in neonates. *Pediatr Anaesth* 1997; **7** (3): 205–9.
143. Welborn LG, Rice LJ, Hannallah RS, *et al.* Postoperative apnea in former preterm infants: prospective comparison of spinal and general anesthesia. *Anesthesiology* 1990; **72:** 838–42.
144. Wright TE, Orr RJ, Haberkern CM, Walbergh EJ. Complications during spinal anesthesia in infants: high spinal blockade. *Anesthesiology* 1990; **73:** 1290–2.
145. Oberlander TF, Berde CB, Lam KH, *et al.* Infants tolerate spinal anesthesia with minimal overall autonomic changes: analysis of heart rate variability in former premature infants undergoing hernia repair. *Anesth Analg* 1995; **80:** 20–7.
146. Bosenberg, AT. Epidural analgesia for major neonatal surgery. *Paediatr Anaesth* 1998; **8:** 479–83.
147. Henderson K, Sethna N, Berde CB. Continuous caudal anesthesia for inguinal hernia repair in former preterm infants. *J Clin Anesth* 1993; **5:** 129–33.
148. Tobias JD, Rasmussen GE, Holcomb III GW, *et al.* Continuous caudal anaesthesia with chloroprocaine as an adjunct to general anaesthesia in neonates. *Can J Anaesth* 1996; **53:** 69–72.
149. Wulf H, Peters C, Behnke H. The pharmacokinetics of caudal ropivacaine 0.2% in children. A study of infants aged less than 1 year and toddlers aged 1–5 years undergoing inguinal hernia repair. *Anaesthesia* 2000; **55:** 757–60.
150. Broadman LM. Complications of pediatric regional anesthesia. *Reg Anesth* 1996; **21** (6S): 64–70.
151. Berde CB. Convulsions associated with pediatric regional anesthesia. *Anesth Analg* 1992; **75:** 164–6.
152. Larsson BA, Lonnqvist PA, Olsson GL. Plasma concentrations of bupivacaine in neonates after continuous epidural infusion. *Anesth Analg* 1997; **84:** 501–5.
153. Breschan C, Krumpholz R, Likar R, *et al.* Can a dose of 2 μg/kg caudal clonidine cause respiratory depression in neonates? *Paediatr Anaesth* 1999; **9:** 81–3.
154. Bouchut JC, Dubois R, Godard J. Clonidine in preterm-infant caudal anesthesia may be responsible for postoperative apnea. *Reg Anesth Pain Med* 2001; **26:** 83–5.
155. Mason LJ, Betts EK. Leg lift and maximum inspiratory force, clinical signs

of neuromuscular blockade reversal in neonates. *Anesthesiology* 1975; **52:** 441–2.

156. Tetzlaff JE, Annand DW, Pudimat MA, Nicodemus HF. Postoperative apnea in a full-term infant. *Anesthesiology* 1988; **69:** 426–8.
157. Noseworthy J, Duran C, Khine HH. Postoperative apnea in a full-term infant. *Anesthesiology* 1989; **70:** 879–80.
158. Cote CJ, Kelly DH. Postoperative apnea in a full-term infant with a demonstrable respiratory pattern abnormality. *Anesthesiology* 1990; **72:** 559–61.
159. Steward DJ. Preterm infants are more prone to complications following minor surgery than are term infants. *Anesthesiology* 1982; **56:** 304–6.
160. Kurth CD, Spitzer AR, Broennle AM, Downes JJ. Postoperative apnea in preterm infants. *Anesthesiology* 1987; **66:** 483–8.
161. Malviya S, Swartz J, Lerman J. Are all preterm infants younger than 60 weeks postconceptual age at risk for postoperative apnea? *Anesthesiology* 1993; **78:** 1076–81.
162. Cote CJ, Zaslavsky A, Downes JJ, *et al.* Postoperative apnea in former preterm infants after inguinal herniorrhaphy. A combined analysis. *Anesthesiology* 1995; **82:** 809–22.
163. Kurth CD, LeBard SE. Association of postoperative apnea, airway obstruction, and hypoxemia in former premature infants. *Anesthesiology* 1991; **75:** 22–6.

59

Anesthesia for infants and children

GEORGE H MEAKIN AND LEILA G WELBORN

Pediatric anesthesia has evolved as a subspecialty because the needs of infants and young children are fundamentally different from those of adults. The provision of anesthesia for pediatric patients depends on a clear understanding of these needs and the psychological, anatomical, physiologic, and pharmacologic differences that underlie them. This chapter reviews the relevant differences between pediatric patients and adults, and outlines current methods of anesthesia for infants aged 1 month to 1 year and children aged 1–12 years. The special problems of neonatal anesthesia have been dealt with elsewhere.

FUNDAMENTAL DIFFERENCES

Psychological differences

Psychological development proceeds rapidly after birth. During the second month, the social smile appears, to be followed at 3 and 4 months by cooing and laughing respectively. By 6–8 months, infants recognize their mothers and become upset when separated from them. The second year is frequently a time of heightened frustration as the child submits to increasing social pressures to control bodily functions and behavior. Temper tantrums and breath-holding spells are common during this period and may reappear in times of stress in later preschool years. Emotional lability declines gradually throughout childhood, but this trend may reverse itself during adolescence, when the child must cope with the problems of sexual maturation and the desire for independence from parental influences.

Stress of hospitalization

Almost all children hospitalized for anesthesia and surgery experience stress. Most commonly, this is based on fear of separation from loved ones, exposure to the strange hospital environment, fear of painful procedures, fear of the operation itself, or fear of anesthesia. Fear of separation is the main focus of anxiety in preschool children, whereas older children may be equally worried about the prospect of painful procedures, surgery, or anesthesia.[1]

Many children are emotionally upset by their experiences in hospital and show behavioral changes when they return home. These changes include increased bed-wetting, nightmares, phobias, temper tantrums, hostility, and rebellion. The incidence of these problems is greatest in preschool children. The stress experienced by children in hospital and the subsequent behavioral changes can be reduced by appropriate psychological preparation, effective sedative premedication, and the supportive care of nursing staff and parents.[1,2]

Anatomical and physiologic differences

Size

The most striking difference between pediatric patients and adults is their size, and the variation in size with age. Size is usually measured by weighing patients, and therapies are prescribed as dose per kilogram. In some situations it may be impracticable to weigh the child and the weight must be estimated; the following formula provides average weights for children aged up to 12 years.

$$\text{Weight (kg)} = (\text{age} + 3) \times 5/2$$

Although it is convenient to express body size in terms of weight, many physiologic processes are related more closely to surface area.[3] As the surface area to weight ratio of the infant is approximately twice that of the adult (Fig. 59.1), metabolic rate, water, electrolyte, and ventilation requirements are proportionately greater when expressed on a weight basis. These differences decrease gradually throughout childhood.

Respiratory system

In infants and young children, the head is relatively large and the neck shorter than in the adult. These factors, together with the relatively large tongue, predispose to upper airway obstruction, and probably account for the greater use of tracheal intubation in these patients.

The infant glottis is situated opposite the C3–C4 intervertebral disk. By the age of 3 years it has descended to the C4–C5 interspace, where it remains until puberty, when it descends again to lie opposite the body of C5.[4] The epiglottis of the infant is longer and U-shaped posteriorly as opposed to the flat leaf-shape of the adult. Before puberty the narrowest part of the larynx is at the level of the cricoid ring.[5] While it is often stated that the larynx in infants occupies a more anterior position compared with that in adults, this difference is not striking.

Ventilation

Several anatomical differences make ventilation less efficient in the infant. The small diameter of the airways increases resistance to air flow, while the ribs are almost horizontal and contribute very little to breathing, which is almost entirely diaphragmatic. Also, the infant

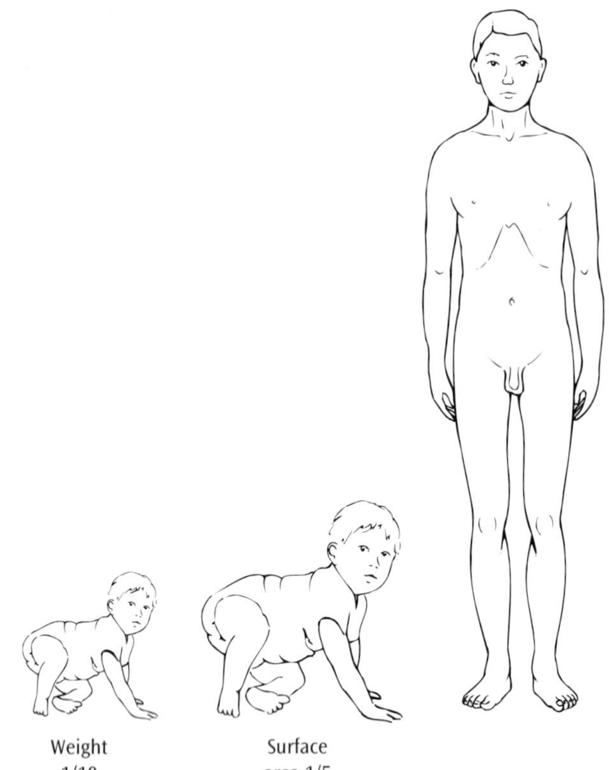

Figure 59.1 *Proportions of an infant aged 6 months relative to an adult, with respect to weight and surface area.*

diaphragm has fewer type I muscle fibers, rendering it susceptible to fatigue.[6]

Minimal oxygen consumption in the neonate is 7 mL kg^{-1} min^{-1}, or about twice the adult value.[7] This is reflected in an increase in the resting minute ventilation, which is about 200 mL kg^{-1} min^{-1} in the newborn compared with 100 mL kg^{-1} min^{-1} at puberty. As tidal volume remains constant at 7 mL kg^{-1} throughout life, the increased ventilation in younger patients is brought about by an increase in respiratory rate; this is an inefficient way of increasing ventilation because a proportion of the increase will be wasted ventilating respiratory dead space. Accordingly, the respiratory rate is approximately 30 breaths min^{-1} at birth, compared with 24 breaths min at 1 year and 12 breaths min in the adult.

In infants, the chest wall is more compliant than the lungs, with the result that the functional residual capacity (FRC) is reduced and small airways have an increased tendency to close at end-expiration.[8] In the awake state, there is evidence that infants use active mechanisms such as glottic closure (laryngeal braking) and premature cessation of expiration to maintain FRC above its true resting value. However, these mechanisms are not available during anesthesia, and airways closure may result in absorption atelectasis with ventilation–perfusion imbalance and hypoxemia. Inefficiency of ventilation and the tendency for atelectasis account for the greater use of controlled ventilation in infants, in whom the use of large tidal volumes (e.g. 10–12 mL kg^{-1}) and up to 5 cmH_2O end-expiratory pressure may be beneficial.

Control of respiration

The control of respiration involves biochemical and reflex mechanisms which are well developed in the healthy full-term infant: in these patients, the ventilatory response to increased concentrations of inspired CO_2 is proportionately similar to that in adults. In contrast, the response of the preterm infant to increased CO_2 is not well sustained, and the slope of the CO_2 response curve is decreased in infants displaying episodes of apnea. The incidence of apneic episodes in the ex-preterm infant is related to immaturity of the brain[9] and declines with increasing postconceptual (gestational + postnatal) age. Otherwise healthy ex-preterm infants with a gestational age of less than 44 weeks have been shown to be at increased risk of developing apnea following general anesthesia.[10–12] Accordingly, it has been recommended that all ex-preterm infants with gestational age less than 50 weeks undergoing general anesthesia, even those having minor surgery, should be monitored overnight for apnea.[12] Where there is significant coexisting disease it may be necessary to extend this policy to ex-preterm infants older than 50 weeks' gestational age.

Cardiovascular system

The mass of the heart doubles in the first 10 months of life while the body weight triples. Heart mass doubles again between the ages of 4–5 years and 12–13 years. At birth, the ratio of right to left ventricular wall thickness is about 0.4; relative hypertrophy of the left ventricle leads to the establishment of the adult ventricular ratio of 0.3 by age 2 years.[13]

The myocardium of the newborn contains less contractile tissue and more connective tissue than that of the adult. As the low compliance of the relaxed ventricles tends to limit the size of the stroke volume, the cardiac output of the newborn is to a large extent rate dependent. Reduced compliance and contractility of the ventricles also predisposes the infant heart to failure with increased volume load.

Cardiac output, heart rate, and blood pressure

The changes in resting cardiac output in infancy and childhood mirror those in pulmonary ventilation. Shortly after birth, resting cardiac output is about 200 mL kg^{-1} min^{-1}, declining gradually to 100 mL kg^{-1} min by adolescence.[14] As resting stroke volume remains fairly constant at about 1 mL kg^{-1}, the increased cardiac output in younger patients is achieved mainly by an increase in the heart rate; average values are 140 beats min^{-1}, at birth falling to 70 beats min^{-1} by puberty (Fig. 59.2).

Average systolic blood pressure at birth is 9.33 kPa (70 mmHg); it increases to 13.3 kPa (100 mmHg) by about 1 year, where it remains until 6–7 years. Thereafter, there is a gradual increase in systolic blood pressure to 16 kPa (120 mmHg) at puberty.

Autonomic control

Animal studies indicate that, although parasympathetic control of the cardiovascular system is well developed at birth, sympathetic control is immature. For example, it has been shown that the heart of the newborn rabbit is not fully innervated with sympathetic fibers, and the norepinephrine (noradrenaline) content of the cardiac sympathetic nerves is diminished.[15] Decreased sympathetic neural output may explain the normally reduced blood pressure in human infants and their increased susceptibility to reflex bradycardia and hypotension.

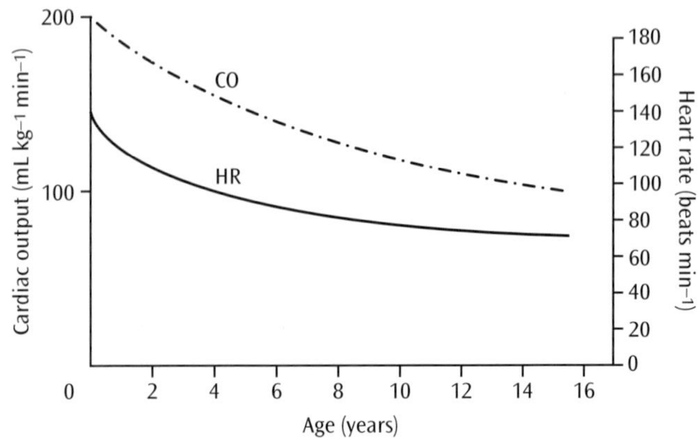

Figure 59.2 *Variation in cardiac output (CO) and heart rate (HR) with age.*

Furthermore, diminished baroreceptor activity in infants may reduce their ability to adapt to hypotension by an increase in heart rate.[16]

Causes of bradycardia

Potent causes of reflex bradycardia and hypotension in infants during anesthesia include laryngoscopy, tracheal intubation, tracheal suctioning, and traction on eye muscles and viscera. Bradycardia may also be caused by a variety of anesthetic drugs, including succinylcholine (suxamethonium), halothane, and neostigmine. These effects can be prevented or treated with intravenous atropine 20 $\mu g\,kg^{-1}$.

The blood

Average blood volume varies from 80 to 90 $mL\,kg^{-1}$ at birth depending on the amount of blood drained from the placenta before the cord is clamped. By 1 month of age the blood volume varies between 70 and 80 $mL\,kg^{-1}$, as in the adult.

Hemoglobin concentration

At birth the hemoglobin concentration ranges from 16 to 19 $g\,dL^{-1}$ and the red cell count is $3.74–6.54 \times 10^{12}\,L^{-1}$. These values are greater than the corresponding values in adults because the relatively hypoxic environment of the uterus stimulates the production of erythropoietin, which in turn triggers red cell production. After birth, there is a sharp fall in erythropoietin activity because of the greater availability of oxygen. As a result, the hemoglobin concentration and red cell count decline steadily to reach 9.5–11.0 $g\,dL^{-1}$ and $3.4 \times 10^{9}\,L^{-1}$, respectively, by 7–9 weeks, after which recovery begins. By 6 months, a mean hemoglobin of 12.5 $g\,dL^{-1}$ is achieved, which is maintained until 2 years of age. Thereafter, there is a gradual increase up to puberty.[17]

Oxygen delivery

At full term, 70–80% of hemoglobin in the circulating red cells is in the form of fetal hemoglobin (HbF), the remainder being adult hemoglobin (HbA). The changeover from HbF to HbA synthesis is probably genetically determined and occurs at around 32 weeks' gestational age, regardless of the time of birth. HbF has a higher affinity for oxygen, which is advantageous in the hypoxic intrauterine environment. However, after birth the persistence of HbF places the infant at a disadvantage because oxygen cannot be unloaded so easily in the tissues. In term infants, HbF is virtually all replaced by HbA by the age of 6 months and there is an increase in 2,3-diphosphoglycerate (2,3-DPG) levels; these changes shift the oxygen dissociation curve to the right. The net result is that, although hemoglobin concentration in the normal infant decreases in the first 3 months of life, oxygen delivery to the tissues increases progressively from birth to 8 months of age, when it achieves adult values.[17] These observations make the point that anemia should be judged by its effect rather than by any arbitrary concentration of hemoglobin. Increases in cardiac output or elevations in blood lactate are rarely seen in normal individuals until the hemoglobin concentration falls below 6 $g\,dL^{-1}$.[18]

The kidneys and fluid balance

Renal function is markedly diminished in the neonate because of low perfusion pressure and immature glomerular and tubular function. Nearly complete maturation of glomerular filtration and tubular function occurs by approximately 20 weeks after birth.[19] Complete maturation of renal function occurs by about 2 years of age. Thus, the ability to handle free water and solute loads may be impaired in the neonate, and the half-life of medications dependent on renal function for their excretion will be prolonged.[20]

Body fluids

At birth total body water constitutes 80% of body weight, but it falls dramatically to around 60% by the end of the first year (Fig. 59.3).[21] Most of this reduction is accounted for by a decrease in the extracellular fluid volume, which declines from 46% of the body weight at birth to 26% at age 1 year. There is a further gradual reduction in extracellular fluid volume throughout childhood, so that in the adult it constitutes about 16% of the body weight. The increased volume of extracellular fluid in infants compared with adults enables them to tolerate a somewhat greater degree of dehydration before developing clinical symptoms. It also provides a greater volume of distribution for highly ionized drugs such as muscle relaxants.

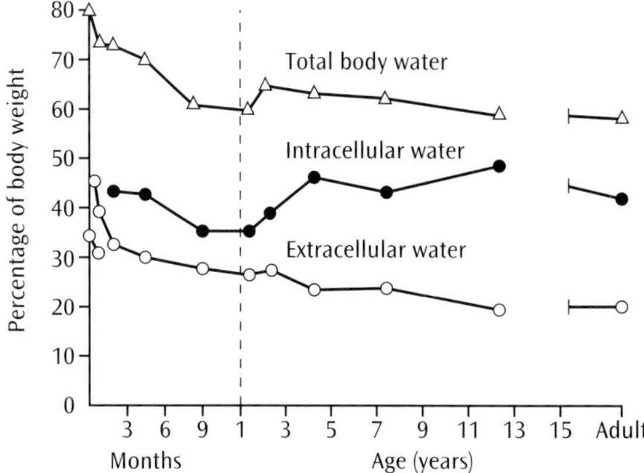

Figure 59.3 *Variation in body water compartments with age. (Reproduced with permission from Friss-Hansen.[21])*

Fluid and electrolyte requirements

Maintenance fluid and electrolyte requirements are related to metabolic rate. In general, 1000 mL of fluid is required for every 1000 calories expended. Requirements of sodium, potassium, and chloride are usually quoted as 30, 20, and 20 mmol per 1000 calories respectively, although quantities considerably in excess of these can be handled readily. Thus, normal maintenance requirements of both fluid and electrolytes will be satisfied by infusing a solution of one-fifth normal saline with 20 $mmol\,L^{-1}$ KCl at a rate equal to caloric expenditure. It is customary to make this solution isotonic by adding 4% dextrose. The dextrose provides only 16% of the total calorie requirement, but this is sufficient to prevent ketosis.

Holliday and Segar[22] related maintenance fluid and calorie requirements of hospitalized patients to body weight by a simple formula (Table 59.1). This formula is now the standard method of calculating hourly maintenance fluid requirements for infants and children. Because hourly infusion volumes are frequently small, it is useful to employ a volumetric intravenous infusion pump when administering intravenous fluids to infants and small children (Fig. 59.4).

Although it is infrequent, healthy children who have fasted for prolonged periods (longer than 15 h) can become hypoglycemic without showing symptoms. Contrary to accepted opinion, a "stress-induced" intraoperative increase in blood glucose does not occur in all patients. Some may show no change or even a further decrease in blood glucose postoperatively.[23] In such patients, infusion of dextrose 4% in one-fifth normal saline or dextrose 2.5% in lactated Ringer's solution at the rate recommended for maintenance will provide adequate glucose to prevent hypoglycemia.[24] If glucose is not included in the intraoperative infusion for patients who have fasted for an extensive

Table 59.1 *Maintenance fluid requirements*[22]

0–10 kg	4 $mL\,kg^{-1}\,h^{-1}$
10–20 kg	40 mL + 2 $mL\,kg^{-1}\,h^{-1}$ for each kg over 10
20–70 kg	60 mL + 1 $mL\,kg^{-1}\,h^{-1}$ for each kg over 20

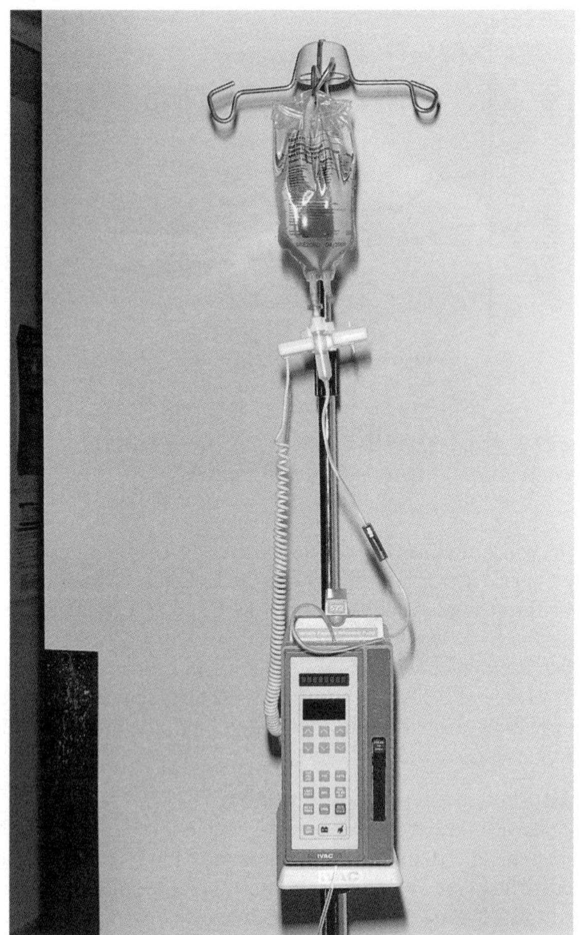

Figure 59.4 *A volumetric intravenous infusion pump (IVAC® Corporation).*

period, intraoperative monitoring of blood glucose levels (with portable devices such as a glucometer) is suggested.

Treatment of dehydration

Dehydration develops rapidly in infants and small children owing to the larger turnover of body fluid (Table 59.1). Depending upon the relative amounts of water and electrolyte (Na^+) lost it may be classified as iso-, hypo-, or hypernatremic.

In infants mild, moderate, and severe dehydration correspond to a loss of 5%, 10%, and 15% of body weight respectively (Table 59.2).[25] In older children and adults, these same degrees of dehydration correspond to a loss of 3%, 6%, and 9% of body weight. The total fluid deficit in liters equates with the weight loss in kilograms. Treatment consists of replacing the deficit with a solution of appropriate ionic composition.[26]

Moderate to severe dehydration, regardless of type, must be treated initially by rapid expansion of the extracellular fluid volume with normal saline. Normal saline 20–30 mL kg^{-1} is administered over the first hour or faster depending on the severity of circulatory compromise. If shock is present, 10–20 mL kg^{-1} salt-poor albumin may also be administered. Once the circulation has been restored and urine output established, one can proceed more slowly to treat the specific type of dehydration on the basis of serum electrolyte values.

The liver

The functional maturity of the liver is incomplete at birth. As the infant grows, the ability to metabolize medications increases rapidly in two ways: (1) hepatic blood flow increases, and more drug is delivered to the liver; and (2) the enzyme systems develop and are induced. In general, two types of reactions take place in the liver: phase I (nonsynthetic) reactions, such as oxidation, reduction, and hydrolysis; and phase II (synthetic) reactions, which involve conjugation with other molecules, notably glucuronide, glycine, and sulfate.[20] Oxidation and reduction are weak in the neonate but increase to adult levels within a few days; conjugation reactions take 1–3 months to develop. From the age of 3 months to 3 years, drug metabolism may actually be increased compared with that in adults, due either to increased microsomal enzyme activity or to the relatively large hepatic mass.

Thermoregulation

The ability of homeothermic animals to maintain a constant body temperature ensures that the enzyme systems responsible for bodily functions operate optimally over a wide range of environmental temperatures. Temperature control is achieved by reflex mechanisms integrated in the hypothalamus, which balance heat production and loss. In the older infant or child, a fall in body temperature is normally countered by an increase in metabolic rate, peripheral vasoconstriction, and shivering. Neonates and young infants have a reduced ability to shiver; in these patients, nonshivering thermogenesis (metabolism of brown fat) is the principal method of heat production.

During moderate to deep anesthesia, temperature control mechanisms are less effective or absent and body temperature tends to fall toward that of the environment. Under these circumstances, hypothermia is associated with a reduction in metabolic rate, oxygen consumption, respiratory rate, heart rate, cardiac output, and blood pressure. The potency of inhaled anesthetics is increased and the duration of action of muscle relaxants and opioids is prolonged. Postoperatively, metabolic activity is increased to restore body temperature. However, if the depressed respiratory and cardiovascular

Table 59.2 *Correlation of the intensity of clinical signs with the degree of dehydration. The correlation shown applies to isotonic dehydration in an infant. Modifications are required for hypertonic and hypotonic dehydration as well as for age*[25]

	Degree of dehydration		
	Mild	**Moderate**	**Severe**
Weight loss (fluid deficit)	5%	10%	15%
Skin turgor	↓	↓↓	↓↓↓
Mucous membranes	Dry	Very dry	Parched
Skin color	Pale	Gray	Mottled
Urine	Slight oliguria	Oliguria	Marked oliguria and azotemia
Pulse	±↑	↑	↑↑
Blood pressure	Normal	± Normal	Reduced

systems are unable to meet the greatly increased demands for oxygen at this time, hypoxemia and lactic acidosis will occur.

Prevention of heat loss

Infants are particularly at risk of accidental hypothermia during anesthesia owing to their small size, relatively large surface area, and increased ventilation requirements. These factors increase heat losses by conduction, convection, radiation, and evaporation. Heat loss from the body surface can be minimized by increasing the temperature of the operating room to 22–24 °C and keeping the infant covered as much as possible. Heat loss by evaporation of water in the respiratory tract can be reduced by warming and humidifying the anesthetic gases. Blood and other fluids for infusion should be warmed to 37 °C.

Warming devices Measures solely for the prevention of heat loss are rarely sufficient to maintain the body temperature of anesthetized infants above 36 °C. An overhead radiant warmer may be used after induction of anesthesia and before the surgical drapes have been applied. Intraoperatively, a warm water mattress may be used,[27] and additional heat may be supplied by circulating warm air under the surgical drapes.[28] Alternatively, a warm air mattress that performs both of these functions may be used (Fig. 59.5). The use of active warming devices usually allows the temperature of the operating room to be reduced to a more comfortable level for operating room personnel. In order to avoid thermal injury, radiant warmers should not be placed too close to the patient's skin and the working temperature of other warming devices should not exceed 39 °C.

PEDIATRIC ANESTHESIA PHARMACOLOGY

The response of the infant and child to medication is modified by many factors, including body composition, protein binding, body temperature, distribution of cardiac output, and maturation of the blood–brain barrier, liver, and kidneys.[29–32]

For the neonate, alterations in body composition have several clinical implications: (1) the greater volume of extracellular fluid provides a larger volume of distribution for highly ionized drugs and, therefore, a larger initial dose may be required to achieve the desired blood level (e.g. succinylcholine); (2) a decrease in amount of body fat results in an increase in the duration of action of nonionized drugs that depend on redistribution into fat for termination of their effects (e.g. thiopental); and (3) a reduced muscle mass results in an increase in the duration of action of drugs that redistribute into muscle (e.g. fentanyl). In addition, altered elimination may occur as a result of increased volume of distribution, immature hepatic and renal function, and reduced protein binding.

In general, the potency of many drugs is greater in neonates and infants and less in children when compared with adults. Similarly, most medications will have a prolonged elimination half-life in neonates and a shortened half-life in children aged over 2 years, which gradually lengthens toward adulthood. Thus, compared with adults, neonates and infants frequently require reduced drug doses while children require increased doses in relation to their body weight.

Inhaled anesthetics

Uptake and elimination of inhaled anesthetics is more rapid in pediatric patients than in adults. The principal reasons for this appear to be: (1) an increased level of ventilation in relation to FRC, resulting in an increase in the rate of washin to the lungs; (2) an increase in cardiac output in relation to body weight, which increases the rate of anesthetic equilibration in the tissues; and (3) reduced solubility of inhaled anesthetics in blood.[33,34] Thus, the ratio of alveolar to inspired halothane concentration at 20 min in infants aged 1–3 months is 0.83 compared with 0.59 in adults. The increased rate of equilibration in infants correlates with more rapid induction of anesthesia and earlier development of cardiovascular side-effects.[35]

Halothane

Although the use of halothane in Western countries has declined, it remains a standard agent for anesthesia in children. It has a sweet, nonpungent odor, allowing smooth induction and maintenance of anesthesia.[36] In addition, its relatively low blood–gas solubility coefficient (2.3) and high potency permit rapid onset and recovery (Table 59.3). Approximately 20% of absorbed halothane is metabolized in the liver, mainly by oxidation. This high degree of metabolism appears to be an important factor in the etiology of halothane hepatitis, which occurs in 1 in 10 000 to 1 in 30 000 adults exposed to the drug.[37] By contrast, halothane hepatitis is exceedingly rare in children; two

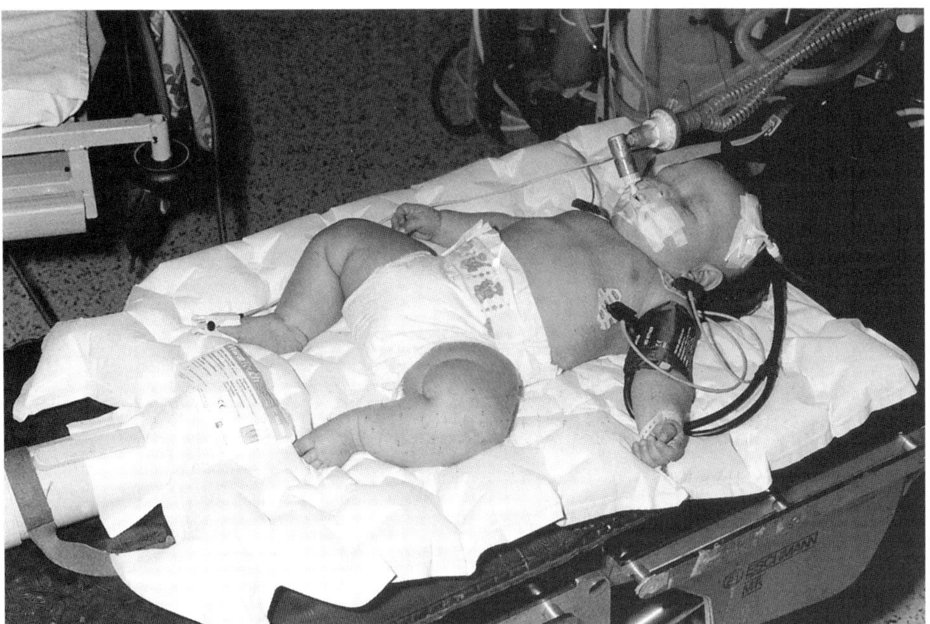

Figure 59.5 *A thermostatically controlled warm air mattress (Warm Touch® Mallinckrodt Medical).*

Table 59.3 *Properties of volatile anesthetic agents*

	Halothane	Isoflurane	Sevoflurane	Desflurane
Odor	Sweet, nonpungent	Markedly pungent, ethereal	Minimally pungent	Markedly pungent, ethereal
Blood–gas partition coefficient:				
Neonates	2.1	1.2	0.7	–
Adults	2.3	1.4	0.7	0.4
MAC (%)				
Neonates	0.9	1.6	3.3	9.2
Infants	1.2	1.9	2.5	9.9
Adults	0.8	1.2	2.0	6.0
Rate of metabolism (%)	20.0	0.2	2.0	0.02
Myocardial depression	++	+	?+	+
Peripheral vasodilation	+	++	?++	++
Respiratory depression	+	++	++	++

large retrospective studies from the UK and the USA revealed only three possible cases, none of which was fatal.[38,39]

The potency of halothane varies with age (Fig. 59.6). In neonates, the minimum alveolar concentration (MAC) of halothane is about 0.9%, but it increases rapidly to a maximum of 1.2% at 6 months and thereafter declines gradually to about 0.8% in the adult.[40,41] The lower MAC of halothane in neonates compared with infants may be related to immaturity of the central nervous system and attenuation of the pain response due to high levels of plasma peptides (β-endorphin and β-lipotropin).[40] The higher MAC in infants compared with older children and adults may be due to an increase in the brain water content.[42]

In a study of unpremedicated infants anesthetized with halothane, the incidence of significant hypotension (systolic blood pressure ≤70% control) was found to be increased in infants aged less than 16 weeks and even more so in neonates.[43] Transient bradycardia was also common, particularly in older infants. Indirect measurements of myocardial contractility suggest that the hypotension produced by halothane is primarily due to direct myocardial depression.[44] Neonates may be particularly susceptible to these effects owing to a reduction in the active tension of the myocardium, reduced compliance of the ventricles, and relative underdevelopment of the sympathetic innervation.[45] Bradycardia and hypotension due to halothane in infants can be prevented or treated by giving atropine 20 μg kg^{-1} i.v. or i.m.[46,47]

Isoflurane

Isoflurane is a halogenated methyl ether; it is one of a series of ether anesthetics developed in order to improve molecular stability and reduce metabolism compared with halothane. *In vivo* metabolism of isoflurane is about one-hundredth that of halothane (0.2%), and there have been no reports of hepatotoxicity in children.

Isoflurane has an irritant, ethereal odor that is associated with an increased incidence of airway problems such as coughing and laryngospasm during induction, maintenance, and recovery from anesthesia. Thus, despite its lower blood–gas solubility coefficient (1.4) compared with halothane, induction of anesthesia is significantly slower and recovery time is longer when the agent is used with spontaneous ventilation for relatively short surgical procedures.[36,48] However, when modified with halothane induction, isoflurane anesthesia was reported to have improved induction characteristics and more rapid recovery compared with halothane anesthesia alone, although the recovery characteristics were still somewhat less good with the halothane–isoflurane sequence than with halothane alone.[48]

The MAC of isoflurane varies with age in a similar way to that of halothane; thus, it is about 1.6% in neonates and 1.9% in infants aged 1–6 months, after which it declines gradually to approximately 1.2% in adults.[49] Further reductions in the MAC of isoflurane have been reported in premature infants. In infants born at 32 weeks' gestational age, the MAC of isoflurane is about 1.3%, whereas at 32–37 weeks it is 1.4%.[50] The suggested mechanisms for this variation are similar to those proposed for halothane.

In infants and children, equipotent concentrations of isoflurane and halothane produced similar reductions in blood pressure.[51,52] However, although heart rate was reduced by halothane, it was either unchanged or increased in infants anesthetized with isoflurane. Also, in contrast to halothane, the reduction in arterial blood pressure that occurs during isoflurane anesthesia appears to be largely the result of a decrease in peripheral resistance rather than myocardial depression. These studies suggest that, despite a similar reduction in blood pressure, isoflurane may be associated with greater cardiovascular reserve than halothane in infants and small children.[52]

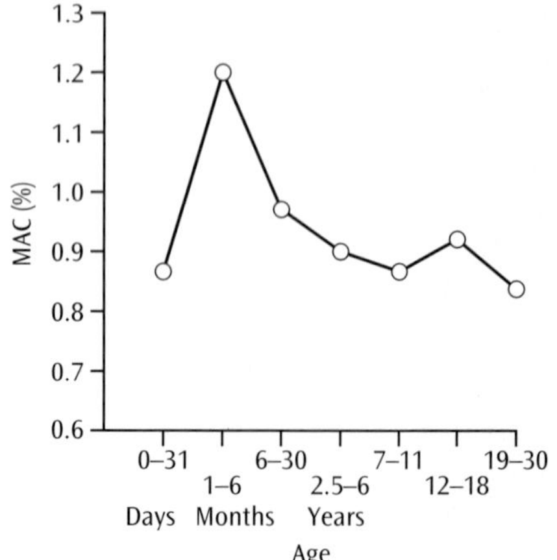

Figure 59.6 *Variation in MAC of halothane with age. (Data from Lerman* et al.[40] *and Gregory* et al.[41]*)*

Sevoflurane

Sevoflurane is one of two new ether anesthetics halogenated solely with fluorine (desflurane being the other). Fluorination reduces solubility in both fat and blood, thereby reducing anesthetic potency while increasing the rate of uptake and elimination.[53] Sevoflurane has a slightly pungent but not unpleasant odor, allowing smooth induction of anesthesia in infants and children.[54,55] As a result of its low blood solubility (Table 59.3), induction of anesthesia is more rapid with sevoflurane than with halothane, eyelash reflex being lost in 60–90 s.[55,56] Recovery is also more rapid after sevoflurane than halothane, although not as rapid as after desflurane.[55] Rapid emergence from sevoflurane anesthesia may be associated with increased agitation in children who have not received adequate analgesia.

As with other volatile anesthetics, the MAC of sevoflurane varies with age, being 3.3% in neonates, 2.5% in infants and children aged over 6 months, and 2.0% in adults. The cardiovascular responses to 1 MAC sevoflurane are similar to those reported for halothane and desflurane, the greatest reduction in systolic pressure occurring in newborns and infants.[55]

Areas of concern with sevoflurane are its relatively high rate of metabolism (2%) and instability with soda-lime. In pediatric studies, *in vivo* metabolism of sevoflurane after 60–90 min of anesthesia produced peak concentrations of fluoride ion ranging from less than one-third to two-thirds of the purported nephrotoxic level of 50 mmol L^{-1}.[54,55,57] Instability with soda-lime results in the formation of compound A, another nephrotoxic substance.[58] Although levels of compound A, sufficient to cause nephrotoxicity in rats (50 ppm), have been found in circle systems during low-flow (0.5–1.0 L min^{-1}) anesthesia with sevoflurane, these are generally much lower and there have been no reported cases of nephrotoxicity in humans.[59,60] In view of the potential for compound A-induced nephrotoxicity, the Food and Drug Administration of the USA initially prohibited the use of sevoflurane in rebreathing systems with fresh gas flow rates less than 2 L min^{-1}.[58] However, this ruling was subsequently relaxed and the package insert for the USA currently states that sevoflurane should not be used in a fresh gas flow < 1.0 L min^{-1} and should not be applied at this flow rate for more that 2 MAC hours. Several other countries (including the UK) have no such restrictions.

Desflurane

Desflurane is produced by replacing the single chorine atom of isoflurane with fluorine.[53] Like isoflurane, it has a markedly pungent ethereal odor, making it unsuitable for inhalation induction of anesthesia in children owing to a high incidence of airway complications.[61,62] However, by virtue of its lower solubility in blood (Table 59.3), recovery from anesthesia maintained with desflurane is faster than that maintained with halothane[63] or sevoflurane.[55]

The MAC of desflurane varies with age in a manner similar to that of halothane and isoflurane, being 9.2% in neonates, 9.9% in infants aged 6–12 months, and thereafter declining gradually to 6.0% in adults.[64] In the same study, the hemodynamic responses to 1 MAC desflurane in neonates and infants were found to be similar to those reported for halothane. Metabolism of absorbed desflurane is difficult to measure (approximately 0.02%) and the drug is stable with soda-lime.[53] As it provides stable conditions of anesthesia with rapid recovery, desflurane may be a useful agent for maintenance of anesthesia in infants and children. Its high cost may be mitigated by the use of low flow rates in a circle system.

Nitrous oxide

Nitrous oxide is sweet-smelling, nonirritant, nonflammable anesthetic gas. Its low potency (MAC 105%) precludes is use as a sole anesthetic, but it is a useful adjunct to potent volatile anesthetic agents during induction and maintenance of anesthesia. A low blood–gas partition coefficient of 0.47 results in rapid uptake and elimination, and there is little, if any, biotransformation.

At equipotent anesthetic concentrations, nitrous oxide is approximately half as potent as halothane in depressing the cat myocardium.[65] Occasionally, premature and sick neonates may not tolerate the cardiovascular effects of nitrous oxide, in which case air may be substituted as a carrier gas for oxygen. The main contraindications to nitrous oxide are the presence of air pockets within the body (e.g. bowel obstruction, diaphragmatic hernia, lobar emphysema, Eustachian tube obstruction) and the need for a high inspired oxygen tension.

Intravenous anesthetics

Thiopental is a short-acting barbiturate which, when given intravenously, produces smooth induction of anesthesia in one arm-brain circulation time. There are no significant differences in distribution kinetics[66] or apparent recovery times between children and adults. The dose of thiopental varies with age (Fig. 59.7).[67,68] In neonates, the ED_{50} sleep dose is only 3.5 mg kg^{-1}, but it increases rapidly to around 7 mg kg^{-1} in infants aged 1–6 months, thereafter declining gradually throughout infancy and childhood. Thus, it appears that neonates require 4–5 mg kg^{-1}, infants 7–8 mg kg^{-1}, and children 5–6 mg kg^{-1} 2.5% thiopental for fast, reliable induction of anesthesia. The reduced requirements in neonates compared with older infants can be explained by a decrease in plasma protein binding.[69] The increased requirements in infants and children compared with adults (usual adult dose 4 mg kg^{-1}) may be due to their increased cardiac output, as this would be expected to reduce the first-pass concentration of thiopental arriving at the brain. Induction doses of thiopental may be reduced by up to 50% by sedative premedication.[70]

The most important side-effects of thiopental are respiratory and cardiovascular depression. Apnea lasting a few seconds and followed by a period of respiratory depression is common after an induction dose. Induction of anesthesia with thiopental is accompanied by a 15–23% reduction in arterial blood pressure in healthy infants and children, which is secondary to depression of myocardial contractility.[71] Thiopental should be avoided in children who are dehydrated, have lost a significant amount of blood, or are in heart failure, as clinically significant hypotension may be produced. Other side-effects seen with an induction dose of thiopental include hiccups, coughing, and laryngospasm. Extravasation of thiopental can cause tissue injury – probably secondary to its alkalinity.

Methohexital is a short-acting barbiturate administered intravenously at a concentration of 1% and a dose of 1–2 mg kg^{-1}. Muscular twitching and hiccups may occur due to central nervous system excitation. Methohexital has a shorter elimination half-life than thiopental and this is reflected in shorter recovery times in children undergoing brief surgical procedures.[72] Cardiovascular and respiratory effects of methohexital are similar to those of thiopental.

Propofol is an alkylphenol formulated as a 1% solution in a white soyabean oil, egg phosphatide, and glycerol emulsion. It is a rapid-acting hypnotic agent with no analgesic properties. Propofol is highly lipophilic and protein bound. It is rapidly distributed and redistributed throughout the body compartments. The dose requirement for propofol is higher in unpremedicated children than in adults because the volume of the central compartment is 50% larger and the clearance

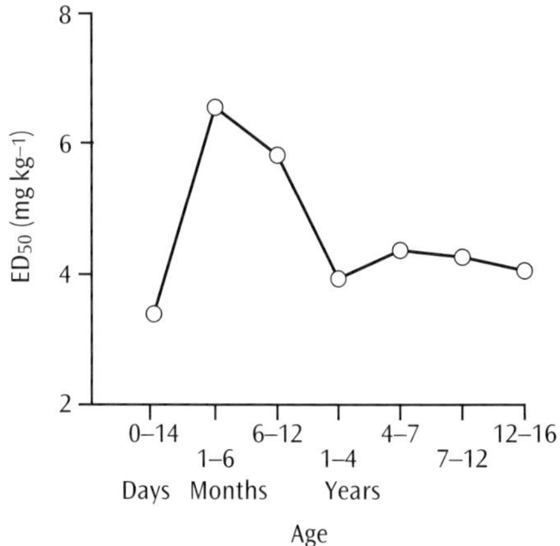

Figure 59.7 *Variation in the ED_{50} sleep dose of thiopental with age. (After Westrin* et al.[67] *and Jonmarker* et al.[68] *with permission.)*

is 25% higher in children.[73] The induction dose ranges from 2.5 to 4 mg kg^{-1}.[73–76] Pain may occur on injection[77] but can be minimized by using a large vein, administering the solution more slowly, or injecting lidocaine (lignocaine) before the propofol.[78] The minimum effective dose of lidocaine for this purpose in children is 0.2 mg kg^{-1} followed by 3 mg kg^{-1} propofol.[77,79,80] Propofol produces rapid, smooth induction with a low incidence of serious adverse effects.[81–84] Recovery time after propofol is shorter than that after thiopental[79,85] and similar to that after methohexital.[72] Propofol induction can produce respiratory depression, apnea, and breath-holding[74,77] Cardiovascular effects include decreases in blood pressure and heart rate.[86] Involuntary movements may be seen with propofol induction in children. They are usually caused by an inadequate induction dose and early stimulation.[84] Because of its prompt wake-up characteristics and antiemetic effects, propofol has displaced short-acting barbiturates as the induction agent of choice for outpatients in many centers.[87,88] The versatility of propofol, which also can serve as a maintenance anesthetic agent by continuous infusion (100–300 μg kg^{-1} min^{-1}), increases its utility in outpatient surgery. Strict aseptic technique is recommended in handling propofol because sepsis has been reported after contamination of the intralipid preparation.[89]

Opioids

Morphine

Morphine remains the most commonly used opioid for the management of severe pain in children and the standard with which other potent analgesics should be compared. It is the only naturally occurring opioid in clinical use and the only member of this group that is poorly lipid soluble (octanol–water coefficient 1.4). Although only a small proportion of a given morphine dose passes the blood–brain barrier in older infants and children, there is evidence that morphine passes this barrier more easily in neonates.[90] Morphine is metabolized mainly by conjugation with glucuronide in the liver. Deficiency of the microsomal enzymes responsible for glucuronide conjugation may be responsible for a prolongation of clinical effect in infants aged less than 6 months.[91]

For control of postoperative pain, morphine is usually administered by continuous intravenous infusion or patient-controlled analgesia (PCA). In view of its long half-life, a loading dose must first be administered, and this is usually done during the surgical procedure. In general, an infusion regimen comprising a loading dose of 100 μg kg^{-1} followed by a maintenance dose of 25 μg kg^{-1} h^{-1} provides excellent intraoperative and postoperative analgesia for children and infants aged over 6 months [92] Infants age less than 6 months require reduced doses of morphine, possibly as a result of increased brain uptake and/or reduced plasma clearance.[90,91] In neonates undergoing relatively brief (45 min) procedures, a single dose of 25 μg kg^{-1} usually provides adequate intraoperative and postoperative analgesia. After more prolonged and more complex surgery, postoperative analgesia may be supplemented with a continuous infusion of morphine 5–10 μg kg^{-1} h^{-1}. It is recommended that all infants aged less than 6 months receiving morphine infusions should be nursed in a high-dependency area and monitored with continuous pulse oximetry.[93,94]

Fentanyl

Fentanyl is a synthetic, lipid-soluble opioid agonist that is 50–100 times more potent than morphine. Because of its lipid solubility, a single dose of fentanyl has a more rapid onset and shorter duration of action than morphine. When fentanyl is administered in multiple doses or as an infusion, progressive saturation of peripheral tissue sites will lead to prolonged duration of action.[95] In the study by Singleton *et al.*,[96] the volume of distribution of fentanyl was similar, but the plasma clearance and elimination half-life were greater in infants than in adults. As fentanyl is metabolized by the liver, the higher clearance rate in infants may be attributed to a higher hepatic blood flow. Infants older than 3 months have been shown to be no more sensitive than adults to the respiratory depressive effects of fentanyl.[97] In these patients, and in older children, fentanyl is usually administered in a dose of 1–2 μg kg^{-1} at the start of anesthesia followed by further bolus doses as clinically indicated, or by a continuous infusion of 1 μg kg^{-1} h^{-1}. Much higher doses may be used when controlled ventilation is planned postoperatively (e.g. in cardiac surgery patients). Fentanyl administration may be associated with chest wall rigidity severe enough to limit adequate ventilation. In infants it may cause bradycardia but does not depress cardiovascular function.[98]

Alfentanil

Alfentanil is a rapid-acting opioid with short duration of analgesic action. The brief duration of action of alfentanil is the result of its redistribution to inactive tissue sites and hepatic metabolism. Unlike fentanyl, continuous infusion or repeated doses of alfentanil does not result in cumulative effects.[99] However, alfentanil is dependent on hepatic function for clearance. Bolus doses of alfentanil can cause bradycardia and chest wall rigidity in all age groups. The initial dose of alfentanil is 25 μg kg^{-1} followed by an average infusion rate of 0.5 μg kg^{-1} min^{-1}.

Remifentanil

Remifentanil is a new ultrashort-acting, synthetic opioid. Its methyl ester linkage makes the drug susceptible to metabolism by nonspecific blood and tissue esterases.[100] Pharmacokinetic studies in adults demonstrate that the drug has a small volume of distribution, a rapid distribution phase, and a terminal elimination half-life of 3–10 min. Preliminary pharmacokinetic reports in children 2–12 years of age suggest a pharmacokinetic profile similar to that of adults. The initial dose of remifentanil is 1 μg kg^{-1} followed by an average infusion rate of 0.25 μg kg^{-1} min^{-1}.

Neuromuscular blocking drugs

The use of neuromuscular blocking drugs has significant advantages in pediatric anesthesia, but responses may differ markedly from those in adults. In general, neonates and infants appear to be clinically sensitive to nondepolarizing neuromuscular blocking drugs and resistant to depolarizing drugs.[101]

The infant's sensitivity to nondepolarizing drugs may be explained by immaturity of the neuromuscular system, notably a reduction in the availability of acetylcholine in motor nerves.[102,103] However, the clinical significance of this sensitivity may not be great owing to the larger volume of distribution of neuromuscular blocking drugs in infants (reflecting the larger extracellular fluid volume). The increased requirement of succinylcholine by pediatric patients is probably the result of an increase in its volume of distribution. As a general rule, the elimination of nondepolarizing relaxants that are metabolized in the plasma (e.g. succinylcholine, atracurium, mivacurium) does not vary greatly with age, but the elimination of drugs that depend upon hepatorenal function (e.g. the aminosteroidal relaxants vecuronium and rocuronium) appears to be delayed in the first 12 months of life.[104]

Succinylcholine

Succinylcholine is the only depolarizing muscle relaxant in clinical use. Structurally, it resembles two molecules of acetylcholine joined back to back by an ester linkage. A unique combination of rapid onset and short duration of action make it especially useful for rapid sequence and emergency intubations.

Dose–response studies suggest that infants should receive 3 mg kg^{-1} and children 2 mg kg^{-1} succinylcholine for intubation.[105] These doses produce 95% neuromuscular block in about 35 s followed by 90% recovery in approximately 10 min.[106] As elimination of succinylcholine depends on hydrolysis by plasma cholinesterase, a deficiency in this enzyme may result in prolonged block.

The unique mode of action of succinylcholine (sustained depolarization) and its activity at muscarinic acetylcholine receptors are responsible for a large number of side-effects, including histamine release, muscle fasciculation, muscle rigidity, postoperative muscle pain, raised intraocular and intracranial pressure, and cardiac dysrhythmias. Less common but more serious side-effects include anaphylactoid reactions, hyperkalemia (especially in patients with muscle disease, denervation injury, burns, etc.) and malignant hyperthermia (in susceptible patients). Bradycardia, due to the action of succinylcholine on the sinoatrial node, is especially common in infants, in whom it is most reliably attenuated by prior administration of atropine 20–30 µg kg^{-1} i.v.[107] In view of its poor side-effect profile, the use of succinylcholine should probably be reserved for emergency intubation or when it is necessary to secure the airway immediately.[108]

Atracurium

Atracurium is a bisquaternary benzylquinolinium diester with an intermediate duration of clinical action. In contrast to some other nondepolarizing drugs, the plasma clearance of atracurium has been found to be greater in infants than in older children (9.1 vs. 5.1 mL kg^{-1} min^{-1}).[109] This feature probably relates to the fact that the major route of elimination of atracurium is chemical biodegradation in the plasma (Hofmann reaction).[110] As with other relaxants, the volume of distribution was increased in infants compared with older children (0.18 vs. 0.14 L kg^{-1}), but the net result of these changes was a reduction in elimination half-time (13.6 vs. 19.1 min).

When compared during nitrous oxide narcotic anesthesia, the ED_{95} of atracurium was found to be significantly less in neonates and infants than in children (119 and 163 vs. 195 mg kg^{-1}).[111] Following a standard dose of atracurium 0.5 mg kg^{-1}, 95% depression of twitch occurred more rapidly in neonates than in children (0.9 vs. 1.4 min), whereas recovery to 10% of the control twitch height occurred more rapidly in neonates compared with the other two groups (22.7 vs. 29.7 and 28.6 min). Prompt recovery in all age groups is the main advantage of atracurium when used in pediatric anesthesia.

The adverse effects associated with atracurium relate mainly to histamine release.[112] This commonly results in a macular rash or erythema along the course of the vein of injection, which may subsequently spread peripherally. Occasionally, the rash may be accompanied by more serious histamine-mediated effects such as hypotension, tachycardia, or bronchospasm. The cardiovascular changes are dose related and usually occur at doses greater than $2 \times ED_{95}$.

Mivacurium

Mivacurium is structurally similar to atracurium but has a shorter duration of action owing to its metabolism by plasma cholinesterase. When compared during halothane anesthesia, there is no significant difference in the ED_{95} or clinical duration of action of mivacurium between infants and children.[113–116] As with atracurium, the absence of prolonged activity of mivacurium in infants compared with children may be due to an increase in plasma clearance that parallels the expected increase in volume of distribution. Following doses of 0.15–0.2 mg kg^{-1} in infants and children, onset of complete block occurs in 1.4–1.9 min, while 25% recovery of twitch occurs in 8.5–9.4 min.[113,116] Thus, mivacurium is an alternative to succinylcholine when profound neuromuscular block of short duration is required but rapid onset of action is unnecessary. Mivacurium, like atracurium, has significant histamine-releasing properties which may be evident at therapeutic doses;[114] accordingly, the standard dose of 0.2 mg kg^{-1} should not be exceeded. The duration of action of mivacurium may be prolonged in infants with plasma cholinesterase deficiency.[116]

Vecuronium

Vecuronium is a monoquaternary aminosteroidal relaxant that is largely eliminated via the liver. In a pharmacokinetic study undertaken in infants, children, and adults, the plasma clearance of vecuronium did not to vary with age but the volume of distribution was greater in the infants than in the other two groups.[117] As a result, the mean residence time (a parameter similar to half-time of elimination) was also increased in infants compared with the older age groups (66 vs. 34 and 52 min).

When measured during nitrous oxide–oxygen–narcotic anesthesia, the ED_{95} of vecuronium was significantly lower in neonates and infants than in older children (48 and 47 vs. 81 µg kg^{-1}).[118] In a subsequent study, a standard intubating dose of 100 µg kg^{-1} maintained over 90% neuromuscular blockade for almost an hour in infants compared with only 18 min in children.[119] Therefore, it would appear that vecuronium is a *long-acting* muscle relaxant in infants, in agreement with the increased residence time observed in this age group. Vecuronium-induced neuromuscular block is characterized by a lack of histamine release and marked cardiovascular stability in all age groups.

Rocuronium

Rocuronium (*r*apid-*on*set *curonium*) is a desacetoxy analog of vecuronium with a rapid (1–2 min) onset of action, probably related to its reduced potency.[120] As with vecuronium, the ED_{95} of rocuronium is significantly lower in infants than in children (248 vs. 396 µg kg^{-1}),[121] whereas the duration of clinical effect following a standard intubating dose of 0.6 mg kg^{-1} is longer (42 vs. 27 min).[122,123] However, unlike vecuronium, rocuronium retains the characteristics of an intermediate duration relaxant in infants (clinical duration < 50 min). A dose of 0.6 mg kg^{-1} produces 90% depression of EMG twitch in 37 s in infants and 48 s in children without significant changes in blood pressure or heart rate. Rocuronium may therefore be an alternative to succinylcholine when rapid tracheal intubation is desired.

Antagonism of muscle relaxants

Any residual nondepolarizing neuromuscular blockade at the conclusion of anesthesia should be antagonized by an anticholinesterase, the usual drugs being neostigmine or edrophonium. Pharmacologic reversal of profound neuromuscular blockade is usually unsatisfactory and should not be attempted.[124] In the presence of 10% recovery of twitch height, 35 µg kg^{-1} neostigmine or 0.7 mg kg^{-1} edrophonium will provide maximal antagonism in all age groups (Fig. 59.8).[125] For convenience, and to provide a margin of safety, somewhat larger doses of 50 µg kg^{-1} neostigmine or 1 mg kg^{-1} edrophonium are usually given. Atropine 20 µg kg^{-1} or glycopyrrolate 10 µg kg^{-1} should be administered before, or with, the anticholinesterase to prevent muscarinic effects.

PREOPERATIVE PREPARATION

Psychological preparation

Psychological preparation is an important aspect of preoperative care, especially for younger children. Vetter[126] has shown that children aged 2–6 years are over five times more likely to have significant preoperative anxiety than are older children. Parental anxieties concerning the surgical procedure may be profound and can also be transmitted to the child.[127] Special pamphlets, books, videos, animated events – such as puppet show – and a guided tour of the facility before the day of surgery have been found to reduce the anxiety, misunderstanding, and mistrust of both children and parents.

On admission to hospital, every effort must be made to help the child to adjust to the new environment. Decorations should be appropriate and a selection of toys should be available in every ward. In addition, the child should be encouraged to bring a favorite toy or treasure from home. The child's nickname, as used at home, should be entered in the nursing notes and used by his carers.

The preoperative visit of the anesthesiologist affords an important opportunity to provide reassurance to both child and parents. The child will be reassured by an anesthesiologist who has a sympathetic manner, explains the proposed procedure simply, and avoids words that may cause alarm. Parents will be reassured by an anesthesiologist who shows a genuine interest in the child's well-being. In hospitals with appropriate facilities, separation anxiety may be avoided by inviting a parent to accompany the child at induction of anesthesia.

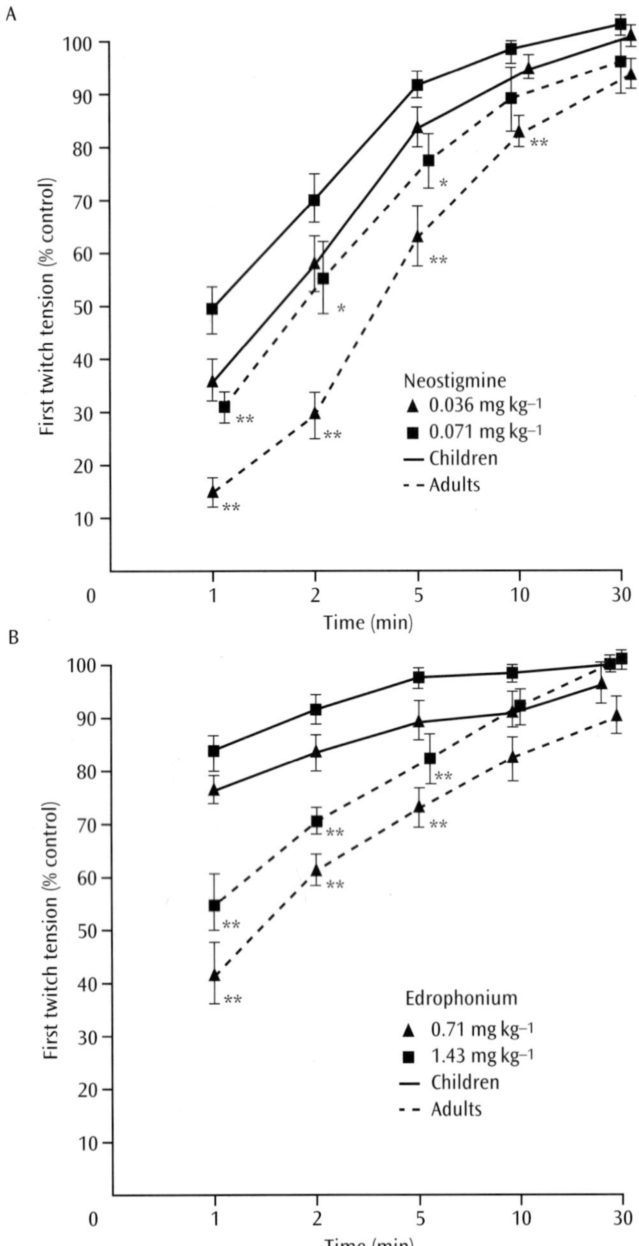

Figure 59.8 *Recovery of first-twitch tension as a percentage of control in pediatric patients and adults after one of two doses of neostigmine (A) or edrophonium (B). Significant differences between pediatric and adult subjects after same dose of antagonist:* *$P<0.05$; **$P<0.01$.[128]

Anesthetic assessment

History

A full medical history should be taken, paying particular attention to previous illnesses and operations, current medications, allergy, and any unusual syndrome with anesthetic implications. Parents of infants should be asked whether the child was born at term and whether he or she breathed immediately after birth. Infants born prematurely, especially those with a history of apneic periods, are more likely to develop apnea following anesthesia and should not be accepted for day-case procedures until they are at least 50 weeks' gestational age.[12]

In the case of older children it is important to note whether the weight given on the child's notes is appropriate for his or her age. This will give and indication of growth and may influence the selection of anesthetic equipment (e.g. size of tracheal tube). The average weights of children aged 1–12 years may be calculated using the formula given on p. 965.

Several studies have shown that children with a history of upper respiratory tract infection (URTI) within 4 weeks of operation, or who have symptoms of URTI preoperatively, are at increased risk of respiratory complications such as laryngospasm, bronchospasm, atelectasis, and hypoxemia during or after anesthesia.[128] In view of the seriousness of these complications, it is usual to postpone elective surgery for 4–6 weeks. However, bearing in mind that some small children have 5–10 URTIs per year, this may not always be practical. Moreover, many of the children with recurrent symptoms will be suffering from allergy. In these cases, it is appropriate to discuss situation with the parents and the surgeon to obtain a balanced view of the risks and benefits of proceeding with the surgery. Where a decision is made to proceed, it may be wise to control the airway using an endotracheal tube to minimize the risk of coughing or laryngospasm during anesthesia. Postoperatively, the patient will require supplemental oxygen and careful monitoring, which should include pulse oximetry.

Examination

The head and neck should be examined to detect loose deciduous teeth and signs of potentially difficult tracheal intubation. Signs of potentially difficult intubation include limited mouth opening, micrognathia, a large tongue, or noisy breathing. The presence of high temperature (38 °C), cough, malaise, and audible chest signs suggests lower respiratory tract infection. Elective anesthesia should be postponed for a least 4–6 weeks to allow hyperactive airways to return to normal.[129]

Investigations

Routine preoperative investigations should not be required in healthy children undergoing relatively minor surgery.[130] Groups of patients at risk of significant anemia will require a hemoglobin estimation. These include infants, patients with chronic disease, children with signs and symptoms suggesting anemia and children at risk of a hemoglobinopathy. Children at risk of hemoglobinopahy should also undergo a Sickledex test, which, if positive, should be followed by hemoglobin electrophoresis to determine the type of hemoglobin present. Hemoglobin estimation and cross-matching will be required prior to major surgery if significant blood loss is anticipated. Other investigations, such as chest radiography, ECG, serum urea and electrolytes, coagulation tests, etc., should be ordered only when clinically indicated. Children with complex medical problems may need referral to an appropriate specialist for investigation or treatment.

Assessment of risk

Based on the medical history, examination, and investigations, a formal assessment of the risk of anesthesia should be made and entered into the patient's notes. This is most easily accomplished using the American Society of Anesthesiologists (ASA) classification. In addition, it may be advisable to note any special precautions that are considered necessary for the safe conduct of anesthesia.

Preoperative fasting

Preoperative fasting is required to minimize residual gastric volume at induction of anesthesia and reduce the risk of pulmonary aspiration of gastric contents.[131] The duration of fast required depends on the nature of the last intake. In adults, solid food leaves the stomach in a linear fashion with time and 10–30% may be left after 6 h.[132] Liquid contents leave the stomach in an exponential pattern. The half-time for water is about 12 min, which implies that 95% of ingested water will leave the stomach in 1 h. In babies, breast milk leaves the stomach more rapidly than formula milk. The half-time for breast milk is about 25 min, whereas that for formula is 51 min.[133,134]

Recent evidence suggests that the free intake of clear fluids (defined as those through which it is possible to read newsprint) up to 2 h preoperatively does not affect the pH or volume of gastric contents at induction of anesthesia in children[135–139] or adults.[140,141] Although there have been relatively few studies in infants, these suggest that infants may be allowed clear fluids up to 2 h and breast milk 4 h preoperatively.[142,143] There is also evidence that infants aged less than 3 months may safely be given infant formula (cow's milk) up to 4 h preoperatively.[142] By contrast, there is little evidence to support a reduction in the traditional 6 h fasting time for cow's milk or solid food in older infants and children.[144] Table 59.4 reflects current practices in many hospitals regarding fasting times for pediatric patients.[145]

Premedication

Premedicant drugs are often used to reduce the stress of anesthesia and surgery and the attendant risk of postoperative behavioral disturbances. A wide variety of drugs and routes of administration have been described, reflecting both the preferences of individual anesthesiologists and the specific needs of the child.[146–155] Sedative premedication is rarely indicated for infants aged less than 6 months, as they appear relatively undisturbed when separated from their mothers. This group may also have increased sensitivity to the respiratory and cardiac depressant effects of sedative drugs. Because most children fear needles, the intramuscular route should be avoided whenever possible. In a recent postal survey of US anesthesiologists, about 80% of respondents reported that they premedicated their pediatric patients using the oral route; 8% used the intranasal route, 6% the intramuscular route, and 3% the rectal route. More than 80% of respondents routinely used midazolam as a premedicant; the remainder used mainly ketamine (4%) and transmucosal fentanyl (3%).[156]

Midazolam can be administered by a variety of routes. Because of the decrease in bioavailability of the drug, doses must be significantly higher when using the oral and rectal routes than with other routes. Oral doses of 0.5–0.75 mg kg^{-1},[146–148,153,157] nasal doses of 0.2–0.3 mg kg^{-1},[150,151,158] and rectal doses of 0.4–0.5 mg kg^{-1}[159,160] have been found to sedate children adequately. Oral midazolam is the most popular premedication for pediatric patients despite its bitter taste. This can be masked somewhat by mixing it with a small amount of fruit juice. It takes approximately 20 min to be effective.

Ketamine 2 mg kg^{-1} by intramuscular injection is occasionally useful for the very apprehensive or combative child who will not take an oral premedicant and refuses to cooperate at induction of anesthesia. This dose provides adequate sedation for mask acceptance in approximately 3 min and is not associated with excessive salivation or emergence delirium.[161] Ketamine can also be administered orally in a dose of 6 mg kg^{-1},[149] or nasally when the dose is 3 mg kg^{-1}.[150]

Oral transmucosal fentanyl citrate (OTFC) is prepared by dissolving fentanyl in a sucrose solution that is molded into a lozenge. A stick is then attached, making it resemble a lollipop (Oralet®). It is available in a range of doses. Onset of action is 20–30 min with a 30-min duration of action in a dose of 15–20 μg kg^{-1}.[152,154,162] Fentanyl is most effective when it is absorbed through the oral mucosa; swallowing the drug decreases its effect because first-pass metabolism through the liver is high. Respiratory rate decreases in 10 min and requires constant observation and monitoring. The disadvantages of OTFC are a high incidence of pruritus and vomiting and occasional desaturation. Because of these side-effects, OTFC should only be administered in a monitored clinical setting. The principal advantages of OTFC are that it decreases intraoperative and postoperative analgesic requirements and does not delay discharge from the hospital.

Sufentanil administered nasally in a dose of 1.5–3 μg kg^{-1} has been successful in sedating children within 10 min.[163,164] The disadvantages include a burning sensation in the nose and decreases in chest wall compliance and oxygen saturation. Advantages include a reduced need for intraoperative and postoperative analgesics and fewer delays in discharge from the hospital.

Methohexital may be administered rectally in a sedating dose of 20–30 mg kg^{-1} (10% solution). It also serves as an induction medication. The onset of action is 7–10 min.[165] One advantage of sedation is decreased separation anxiety. Disadvantages include defecation after rectal administration, airway obstruction, and hypoventilation, which requires close observation.

PRACTICAL MANAGEMENT OF ANESTHESIA

Induction of anesthesia

The choice of agent and technique must be based on the needs of the individual patient. Avoidance of needles is considered a major advantage of inhalational induction in younger children, while older children and adolescents often prefer an intravenous induction.

Table 59.4 *Preoperative fasting times for different types of liquids and solids*[145]

	Minimum fasting period (h)			
	Clear fluids	**Breast milk**	**Formula or cow's milk**	**Solids**
Infants and children aged over 3 months	2	4	6	6
Infants aged less than 3 months	2	4	4	6

Inhalation induction

Sevoflurane is now the drug of choice for inhalation induction in many centers because of its minimal pungency and relatively low blood solubility, which allows rapid induction of anesthesia. Scented face masks (e.g. Sweet Dreams®, King Systems Corporation) are more acceptable to children than standard face masks and help to hide the smell of sevoflurane. A combination of nitrous oxide (70%) in oxygen (30%) is given initially to allow the patient to become obtunded. At this stage, 8% sevoflurane can usually be introduced without any reaction from the patient and unconsciousness will be produced after 4–6 breaths. In addition to increasing the speed of induction, the use of 8% sevoflurane may result in less excitation than an incremental technique.[166]

Halothane is still the drug of choice for inhalation induction in some centers, although its smell may be more difficult to mask than that of sevoflurane. In view of the profound cardiovascular effects of halothane, especially in infants, an incremental technique is usually employed. Following the administration of 70% nitrous oxide in oxygen, halothane concentration is increased in 0.5% increments every three to five breaths. Consciousness is usually lost after 1–2 min. This incremental technique may occasionally be associated with an exaggerated excitement phase.

Intravenous induction

Speed is a major advantage of intravenous induction. The induction agent is usually injected in a dorsal hand vein via a small-gauge cannula or butterfly needle (22–25 s.w.g.). It is important to be successful on the first attempt so that the child's confidence in the anesthesiologist is not damaged. Local anesthetic preparations such as prilocaine–lidocaine cream (EMLA®) or amethocaine gel (Ametop gel®) are effective in reducing the pain of venipuncture, thereby facilitating intravenous induction.[167,168]

Airway maintenance and tracheal intubation

Correct head positioning is the first step to successful tracheal intubation. Unlike adults, infants and children should be intubated with the head in a neutral position, the occiput resting directly on the trolley or operating table. Raising the head on a low pillow (as for adults) does not improve the view of the larynx because there are fewer intervertebral joints above the larynx that can be flexed.[4] The most effective maneuver is the application of external pressure at the level of the cricoid cartilage to push the larynx into view. In the first instance this pressure should be applied by the anesthesiologist, using the right hand. Pressure applied blindly by an assistant often displaces the small larynx laterally, obscuring the view. Having achieved the best view, the anesthesiologist should ask the assistant to press in the same place and then adjust the assistant's hand, if necessary, before attempting intubation.

Laryngoscope blades

In infants, a flat laryngoscope blade, such as the infant Magill, which passes posterior to the epiglottis, may be more suitable than a curved one, as it flattens out the curvature of the epiglottis and can be used to lift it forward to expose the larynx. In children aged over 1 year, laryngoscopy can usually be accomplished using a medium-sized curved blade, such as the Mackintosh blade, with the tip placed in the vallecula. The laryngoscope should be inserted gently into the mouth, taking care to avoid trapping the lips between the teeth and the laryngoscope blade. It is equally important not to lever the laryngoscope blade against the upper teeth to avoid dislodging or breaking them.

Tube size

As the narrowest part of the larynx before puberty is the cricoid ring,[5] cuffed tracheal tubes are not usually required for infants and children. The use of an excessively large tube may result in postintubation croup;[169] however, the view that an appropriately sized tubes should allow a leak when 20–25 cmH_2O pressure is applied has recently been challenged.[170] Whatever the outcome of this debate, it is clear that an appropriately sized tracheal tube should pass easily through the cricoid ring and not leak excessively in the working range. The following formula may be used as a guide to tracheal tube sizes in children aged 2 years and over:

$$\text{Tube size (mm ID)} = [\text{age (years)}/4] + 4.5$$

When using the above formula any quarter sizes should be rounded down. Tube sizes used for infants and children aged less than 2 years must be memorized. It is useful to recall that a neonate weighing 3 kg will usually require a size 3-mm tube, whereas premature and low-birthweight babies may require a size 2.5-mm tube. The remaining sizes up to 2 years may then be interpolated.

Tube length

Tracheal tubes should be cut to a length that allows the tip of the tube to reach the mid-tracheal point while 2–3 cm protrudes from the mouth for fixation. The following formula may be used to estimate orotracheal tube length in children aged over 2 years:

$$\text{Orotracheal tube length (cm)} = [\text{age (years)}/2] + 13$$

Orotracheal tube lengths for patients aged less than 2 years must be memorized. Here it is useful to recall that the appropriate length for neonate is usually 10 cm, while that for a 1-year-old is 12 cm; other tube lengths can then be interpolated. Some disposable tubes have depth markings 2 cm from the patient end to indicate adequate insertion of tube into the trachea. Correct positioning of the tracheal tube should be checked by capnography and auscultation of the lung fields.

Laryngeal mask airway (LMA)

The LMA (Intavent®) is a soft, mask-shaped bowl positioned in the pharynx above the opening of the larynx. It is inserted into anesthetized patients without the need for muscle relaxant, direct visualization, or laryngeal instrumentation. Selecting the appropriate-sized LMA for a pediatric patient may require some experience; Table 59.5 gives guidelines based on the manufacturer's recommendations. Before insertion, the cuff of the LMA should be completely deflated so that its tip forms a thin wedge that can pass between the epiglottis and the posterior pharyngeal wall. The rear surface of the LMA should be lubricated to facilitate its easy passage along the palate. With the patient in the "sniffing position," the LMA is firmly pressed against the roof of the mouth and advanced down behind the tongue and into the pharynx. Following full insertion, the cuff is inflated to stabilize the mask, which is then taped in place, similar to an endotracheal tube.

Maintenance of anesthesia

The goals for maintenance of anesthesia include provision of adequate anesthesia and operating conditions for the surgeon, maintaining physiologic homeostasis, and providing appropriate fluid administration to maintain adequate circulating blood volume. The types of anesthetic techniques that can be used have increased with the availability of more rapid-onset and shorter-acting anesthetic, analgesic, and muscle

Table 59.5 *Laryngeal mask sizes for children*

Patient weight	Mask size	Maximum inflation volume (mL)
10–20 kg	2	10
20–30 kg	2.5	15
30–50 kg	3	20
50 kg and over	4	30

relaxant drugs. The use of local or regional blocks can reduce anesthetic and analgesic requirements and provide for a rapid pain-free emergence from anesthesia.

In general, infants are poor candidates for anesthesia with spontaneous ventilation because of poor pulmonary mechanics and increased susceptibility to the cardiovascular depressant effects of volatile anesthetic agents. These patients are likely to benefit from a combination of tracheal intubation and balanced anesthesia with full doses of muscle relaxants, controlled ventilation, minimum concentrations of volatile anesthetics, and reduced doses of opioids. Older children undergoing surgery of more than 45 min duration will also benefit from balanced anesthesia. However, children undergoing surgery lasting less than 30–40 min may be allowed to breath spontaneously a mixture of 66% nitrous oxide in oxygen and a volatile anesthetic agent, supplemented, where appropriate, with an opioid analgesic, local infiltration, or a regional block.

Anesthetic breathing systems

Anesthetic breathing systems may be classified broadly into those that do not contain a chemical means of absorbing carbon dioxide and those which are equipped with such units.[171] In the past, concerns about resistance to breathing and apparatus dead space with the use of absorber systems led pediatric anesthesiologists to use mainly nonabsorber breathing systems;[173,174] however, attitudes are changing and there is a renewed interest in the use of the circle absorber system in pediatric practice. This change may be attributed to several factors: (1) increased concerns about economy and environmental pollution; (2) improvements in the design of anesthetic machines and ventilators; (3) the increasing availability and use of multigas analyzers; and (4) the desire to use standard anesthetic breathing equipment for patients of all ages. The breathing systems of greatest importance to pediatric anesthetists are the T-piece system and the circle system.

T-piece system

The original Ayre's T-piece system consisted of a light metal T-tube with a main lumen of 1 cm diameter, and a smaller side tube at right angles to the main lumen through which the anesthetic gas mixture was introduced: a length of rubber tubing attached to the open end of the T-piece acted as a reservoir for anesthetic gases.[174] In 1950, Jackson Rees[175] modified the system by attaching an open tailed bag to the reservoir tube, in order to facilitate controlled ventilation (Fig. 59.9). The advantages of the T-piece include its simplicity, convenience, and compact size. The small size results in a low compression volume, which is an advantage when hand ventilating patients with small tidal volumes and low lung compliance. Accordingly, the T-piece remains popular for induction of anesthesia and for anesthesia of short duration when low-flow techniques are not appropriate.

In common with other nonabsorber breathing systems, the T-piece systems rely on an adequate fresh gas flow to eliminate CO_2. During spontaneous ventilation, a fresh gas flow greater than twice the minute volume is required to eliminate rebreathing completely.[176,177] However, favorable changes in the respiratory waveform during anesthesia, and the fact that small amounts of rebreathed gas may be accommodated in the dead space at end inspiration, mean that significant physiologic changes are unlikely to occur provided the fresh gas flow is greater than 1.5 times the minute volume.[177,178] As minute volume is usually depressed to two-thirds of normal during inhalation anesthesia, it appears that a flow equal to the normal minute volume, being 1.5 times the patient's actual minute volume, should be sufficient to prevent significant rebreathing. In practice, the use of a fresh gas flow 25% greater than the normal minute volume flow [$\dot{V}_F = \sqrt{wt}$ (kg) L min^{-1}] simplifies calculations and provides a margin of safety.[179]

Carbon dioxide rebreathing is of less consequence during controlled ventilation as respiration will not be stimulated and the administrator can control $P_{A}CO_2$ by increasing ventilation. Under these conditions, efficiency is best defined in terms of the fraction of the fresh gas flow that takes part in gas exchange.[180] During controlled ventilation with the ratio of minute volume to fresh gas flow greater than 1.5, fractional utilization of fresh gas with a T-piece system is 0.72[181] and a fresh gas flow approximately equal to the normal minute volume [$\dot{V}_F = 0.8 \times \sqrt{wt}$ (kg) L min^{-1}] is sufficient to maintain normocapnia.[182]

Circle system

The circle system is the only absorber breathing system in common use. In general, it consists of afferent and efferent breathing tubes, a reservoir bag, and a spill valve; carbon dioxide removal is effected by a chemical absorber unit and one-way flow around the system is achieved using two unidirectional valves. The major advantages of the circle system include

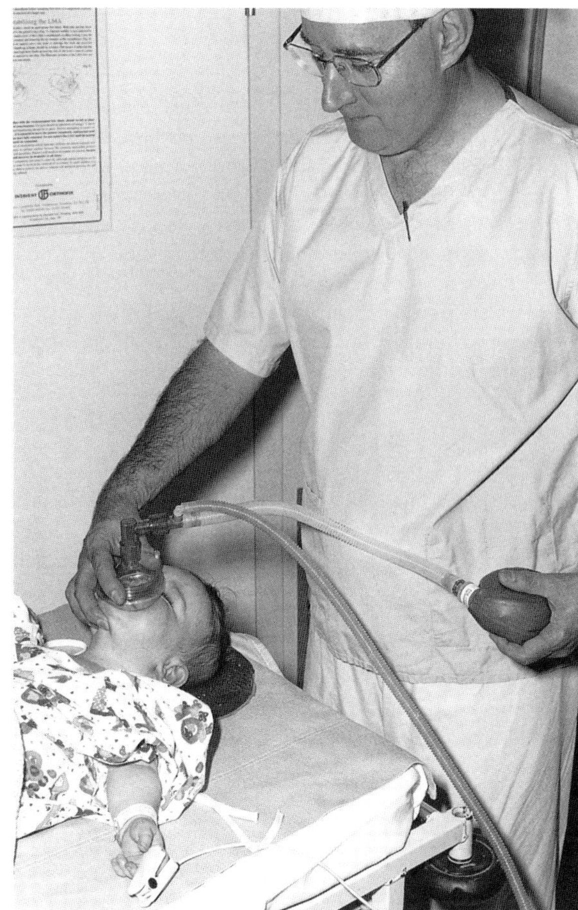

Figure 59.9 *Manual ventilation of an infant using the Jackson Rees T-piece.*

economical use of anesthetic gases, conservation of heat and moisture, and reduced atmospheric pollution,[183] although it seems likely that these advantages will be achieved only when the fresh gas flow is reduced to 1.0 L min^{-1} or less.[184]

A recent review provided little support for the opinion that circle systems impose an excessively high resistance to breathing in infants and children, although it appears that the mechanical dead space imposed by some Y-piece connectors can be excessive.[185] Physiologic factors such as muscle fatigue, inefficient ventilation, and a tendency to lung collapse may have been responsible for some of the respiratory problems observed previously in pediatric patients breathing spontaneously from these systems. It appears that, providing ventilation is controlled in neonates, and either controlled or assisted in infants, a standard adult circle system fitted with low-dead-space connectors, small-bore tubing, and a reduced-capacity reservoir bag is suitable for maintenance of anesthesia for patients of all ages (Fig. 59.10).[185]

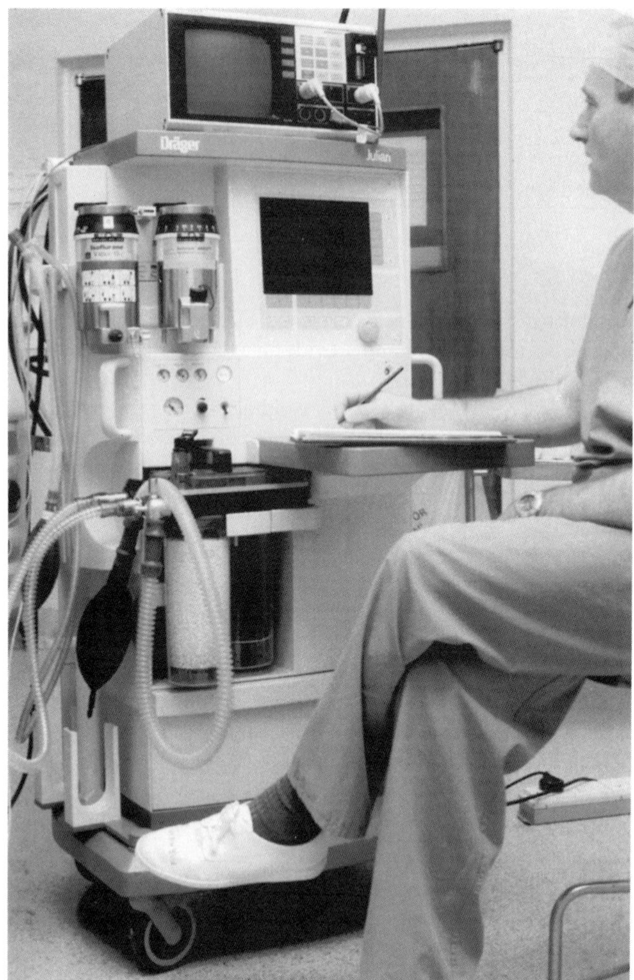

Figure 59.10 *A modern anesthetic workstation incorporating a circle absorber system (Drager Julian®). The standard 22-mm breathing tubes have been replaced by 15-mm lightweight tubes to reduce bulk. The use of a 1-L reservoir bag in place of the standard 2-L bag enables better visual assessment of spontaneous respiration possible in children aged over 1 year.*

Monitoring

Direct observation of the patient is the most important method of monitoring. Monitoring the color, chest movements, breath sounds, and arterial pulse provides information about the patient's oxygenation, ventilation, and circulation. Limb movement, lacrimation, or sweating may indicate that anesthesia is too light.

Routine instrumental monitoring should include a precordial or esophageal stethoscope to monitor continuously heart and breath sounds, a blood pressure cuff of suitable width, pulse oximeter, electrocardiogram, temperature, end-tidal CO_2, and a peripheral nerve stimulator if muscle relaxants are administered.

Intraoperative fluid therapy

An intravenous infusion should be established for all but minor procedures. With the recent reduction in fasting times, patients scheduled for elective surgery should not present for anesthesia with a significant fluid deficit, and in many cases maintenance fluid requirements only need be given. During major surgery, a balanced salt solution, such as Ringer's lactate, should be given to replace extracellular fluid translocated into the surgical site (third space loss). The magnitude of the third space loss will depend upon the degree of trauma associated with the surgery. Estimates vary from 1 to 10 mL kg^{-1} h^{-1}, being highest for intra-abdominal procedures. Translocation is greatly reduced after 2–3 h.[186]

Blood loss

Assessment of blood loss is essential. For relatively minor procedures, blood loss can usually be estimated by visual inspection of the suction bottle and surgical swabs; for more major surgery, swab weighing or colorimetry may be required. In general, blood loss less than 10% of the blood volume (estimated at 80 mL kg^{-1}) either requires no replacement or can be replaced by crystalloid solution. Losses between 10% and 20% can be replaced by colloids or blood, but losses over 20% must be replaced by blood. The adequacy of blood replacement should be assessed with regard to the patient's blood pressure, pulse, and the central venous pressure.

Regional analgesia

Regional anesthesia, used intraoperatively as a supplement to general anesthesia, decreases the dosage of general anesthetic required for surgery, resulting in rapid, pain-free recovery and early ambulation and discharge. The blocks and techniques chosen should have minimal side-effects and not interfere with motor function.

Caudal block with 0.25% bupivacaine, in a dose of 0.75–1 mL kg^{-1} for inguinal hernia repair or orchidopexy and 0.5 mL kg^{-1} for circumcision and hypospadias repair, has been effective. For volumes over 20 mL the bupivacaine is diluted to 0.19%. Analgesia lasts 4–6 h.[187] Higher bupivacaine concentrations (0.3% and 0.375%) offer no advantage over a 0.25% concentration. A 0.125% bupivacaine solution was reported to produce the same quality and duration of postoperative analgesia as a 0.25% concentration, and the lower concentration resulted in less motor blockade.[188]

Ilioinguinal and iliohypogastric nerve block achieved by infiltrating 0.25% bupivacaine medial to the anterior superior iliac spine has been used successfully for pediatric patients undergoing inguinal hernia repair or orchidopexy.[189] Others reported that caudal analgesia and ilioinguinal nerve blocks are safe and effective in controlling postoperative pain in children.[190]

Penile nerve block infiltration of epinephrine (adrenaline)-free 0.25% bupivacaine (1–3 mL) or epinephrine-free 1% lidocaine (1 mL) in newborns around the nerves at the base of the penis provides excellent postoperative analgesia.[191]

Emergence from anesthesia

When a balanced anesthetic technique has been used, the volatile anesthetic should be discontinued just before the conclusion of surgery, and any residual neuromuscular blockade reversed with an anticholinesterase. Subsequently, the patient should be ventilated with 100% oxygen, the oropharynx should be suctioned, and the patient should be extubated when fully awake, as indicated by spontaneous eye opening or grimacing. Following anesthesia with spontaneous ventilation, extubation may be performed with the child deeply anesthetized or fully awake. It is not advisable to extubate children during light anesthesia as laryngeal spasm may result; therefore, if extubation is to be performed "deep," it is probably safer to continue the volatile anesthetic until after the child has been extubated. The tube is removed after oropharyngeal suctioning, an oropharyngeal airway is inserted, and the child is given 100% oxygen to breathe.

If, despite the precautions outlined above, laryngeal spasm occurs following extubation, it can usually be overcome by administering oxygen by continuous positive pressure via a firmly applied face mask. Laryngeal spasm that fails to respond to this treatment should be managed by giving succinylcholine 2 mg kg^{-1} i.v or 4 mg kg^{-1} i.m. followed by oxygenation and reintubation.

POSTOPERATIVE CARE

Once the anesthesiologist is satisfied that adequate spontaneous ventilation is present following cessation of anesthesia, the child should be turned into the lateral position and transported, breathing oxygen, to the postanesthesia recovery room.

Recovery room protocol

On arrival in the recovery room, details of the operative procedure and any special instructions should be given to the nurse assuming care of the child. Recovery room care includes attention to the airway, provision of oxygen therapy, monitoring of pulse, respiration, and blood pressure, and the completion of a postanesthetic recovery chart. Recovery nurses should be trained to detect early changes in respiration or circulation and be able to initiate treatment while the anesthesiologist is summoned. The use of a recovery scoring system provides a means of determining the duration of stay in the recovery room, although this will also depend on the general condition of the patient.[192] When the child is awake, one or more parents may be invited to join them in the recovery room prior to their eventual return to the surgical ward.

Problems during recovery

Hypoxemia

The introduction of the pulse oximeter has shown that transient hypoxemia is common in apparently healthy infants and children during recovery from anesthesia.[193] As a result of this, it is recommended that oxygen be administered routinely to all pediatric patients until they are awake and able to maintain an oxygen saturation greater than 95% in air. In order to reduce the risk of retinopathy in newborn and premature infants with a gestational age less than 44 weeks, the inspired oxygen concentration should be adjusted to maintain an oxygen saturation between 90% and 95% [$P_{aO_2} \geq 9.33$ kPa (70 mmHg)].

Postoperative apnea

Postoperative apnea (>20 s) is a particular problem in newborn and preterm infants with a gestational age less than 44 weeks.[10–12] In the interests of safety, it is advisable to monitor all ex-premature surgical infants of gestational age less that 50 weeks overnight for postoperative apnea.[12] The majority of apneic episodes in infants following anesthesia respond readily to manual stimulation or brief manual ventilation with oxygen. Mechanical ventilation is required occasionally to treat repeated prolonged apnea.

Nausea and vomiting

Postoperative nausea or vomiting is a relatively frequent and unpleasant complication of anesthesia in infants and children and a major cause of delayed discharge from the postanesthesia recovery room or unscheduled admission for day-surgery patients.[194] The incidence of postoperative vomiting in children has been reported to be 10–35% in children.[195,196] The incidence seems to be much higher in patients after certain types of surgery, such as strabismus, adenotonsillectomy, and orchidopexy surgery.[195,197]

Antiemetics may be given before, during, and after surgery for the prevention of postoperative nausea and vomiting. Metoclopromide 0.15–0.25 mg kg^{-1} is efficacious in preventing vomiting in children after strabismus surgery or tonsillectomy.[198,199] Ondansetron (a 5-HT_3-receptor antagonist), in a dose of 0.05–0.1 mg kg^{-1}, is effective in reducing the incidence and severity of vomiting in children after tonsillectomy and is free of extrapyramidal side-effects.[200,201] Total intravenous anesthesia with propofol is associated with rapid recovery and a reduced incidence of postoperative emesis in children undergoing strabismus surgery.[202]

Postintubation croup

The incidence of postintubation croup has declined dramatically since the introduction of disposable, sterile, implant-tested endotracheal tubes. The most common cause is the use of a tube that is too large for the trachea, and signs of obstruction are usually obvious within 1 h of extubation.[169] Initial treatment consists of inhalation of cold mist and oxygen. If moderate symptoms persist, inhalation of nebulized epinephrine, 0.5 mL of a 2.25% racemic epinephrine diluted to 3 mL with normal saline, or 5 mL of 1/1000 epinephrine, may give transient relief.[203,204] Very few patients will require reintubation, but all require observation in hospital for 12–24 h.

Postoperative pain relief

The use of wound infiltration, regional blocks, and morphine to supplement anesthesia, as previously described, will usually provide analgesia for several hours postoperatively. Subsequent analgesic requirements will depend upon the extent of the surgery. Following minor surgical procedures, oral acetaminophen (paracetamol) 15 mg kg^{-1} 6 h^{-1} (maximum 1000 mg), codeine phosphate 0.5 mg kg^{-1} 6 h^{-1} (maximum 30 mg) and ibuprofen 5 mg kg^{-1} 6 h^{-1} (maximum 400 mg) may be given either alone or in combination. After more major surgery continuous infusion of a potent opioid analgesic such as morphine may be required .

Postoperative fluids

When drinking is delayed or impossible postoperatively because of the surgical condition, normal maintenance fluid and electrolytes should be given as described earlier. In addition, extracellular fluid (ECF) loss due to nasogastric aspiration or fistulous drainage should be replaced with a balanced salt solution. Blood loss should be monitored and replaced if necessary. Potassium replacement should not be necessary for the first 24 h.

REFERENCES

1. Visintainer MA, Wolfer JA. Psychological preparation for surgical pediatric patients: the effect on children's and parent's stress responses and adjustment. *Pediatrics* 1975; **56:** 187–202.
2. Eckenhoff J. Relationship of anaesthesia to postoperative personality changes in children. *Am J Dis Child* 1953; **86:** 587–91.
3. Harris JS. Special pediatric problems in fluid and electrolyte therapy in surgery. *Ann NY Acad Sci* 1957; **66:** 966–75.
4. Westhorpe RN. The position of the larynx in children and its relationship to the ease of intubation. *Anesth Intens Care* 1987; **15:** 384–8.
5. Eckenhoff JE. Some anatomic considerations of the infant larynx influencing endotracheal anesthesia. *Anesthesiology* 1951; **12:** 401–10.
6. Keens TG, Bryan AC, Levinson H, Ianuzzo CD. Developmental patterns of muscle fibre types in human ventilatory muscles. *J Appl Physiol* 1978; **44:** 909–13.
7. Scopes JW. Metabolic rate and temperature control in the human baby. *Br Med Bull* 1966; **22:** 88–91.
8. Mansell A, Bryan C, Levinson H. Airway closure in children. *J Appl Physiol* 1972; **33:** 711–14.
9. Henderson-Smart DJ, Pettigrew AG, Campbell DJ. Clinical apnea and brainstem neural function in preterm infants. *N Engl J Med* 1983; **308:** 353–7.
10. Welborn LG, Ramirez N, Oh TH, *et al.* Postanesthetic apnea and periodic breathing in infants. *Anesthesiology* 1986; **65:** 658–61.
11. Welborn LG. Post-operative apnoea in the former preterm infant: a review. *Paediatr Anaesth* 1992; **2:** 37–44.
12. Malviya S, Swartz J, Lerman J. Are all preterm infants younger than 60 weeks postconceptual age at risk for postanesthetic apnea? *Anesthesiology* 1993; **78:** 1076–81.
13. Lentner C (ed.). *Giegy Scientific Tables:* Vol. 5 *Heart and Circulation*. Basle: Ciba-Geigy Corporation, 1990: 65–9.
14. Rudolph AM. *Congenital Diseases of the Heart.* Chicago: Year Book Medical Publishers, 1974: 28.
15. Friedman WF, Pool PE, Jacobowitz D, *et al.* Sympathetic innervation of the developing rabbit heart. *Circ Res* 1968; **23:** 25–32.
16. Gregory GA. The baroresponses of preterm infants during halothane anaesthesia. *Can Anesth Soc J* 1982; **29:** 105–7.
17. Letski EA. Anaemia in the neonate. In: Hann IM, Gibson BES, Letsky EA (eds). *Fetal and Neonatal Haematology*. London: Baillière Tindall, 1991: 51–86.
18. Oski FA. Designation of anaemia on a functional basis. *J Pediatr* 1973; **83:** 353–4.
19. Spitzer A. The role of the kidney in sodium homeostasis during maturation. *Kidney Int* 1982; **21:** 539–45.
20. Morselli PL. Clinical pharmacokinetics in neonates. In: Gibaldi M, Prescott L (eds). *Handbook of Clinical Pharmacokinetics*. New York: Adis Health Science Press, 1983: 79–97.
21. Friis-Hansen B. Body water compartments in children: changes during growth and related changes in body composition. *Pediatrics* 1961; **28:** 169–81.
22. Holliday MA, Segar WE. The maintenance need for water in parenteral fluid therapy. *Pediatrics* 1957; **19:** 823–32.
23. Welborn LG, McGill WA, Hannallah RS. Perioperative blood glucose concentrations in pediatric outpatients. *Anesthesiology* 1986; **65:** 543–7.
24. Welborn LG, Hannallah RS, McGill WA. Glucose concentrations for routine intravenous infusion in pediatric outpatient surgery. *Anesthesiology* 1987; **67:** 427–30.
25. Dell RB. Pathophysiology of dehydration; normal acid base regulation. In: Winters RW (ed.). *The Body Fluids in Pediatrics.* Boston: Little, Brown, 1973: 142.
26. Ellis D, Avner ED. Fluid and electrolyte disorders in pediatric patients. In: Puschett JB (ed.). *Disorders of Fluid and Electrolyte Balance.* New York: Churchill Livingstone, 1985: 217.
27. Goudsouzian NG, Morris RH, Ryan JF. The effects of a warming blanket on the maintenance of body temperatures in anesthetized infants and children. *Anesthesiology* 1973; **39:** 351.
28. Nightingale P, Meakin G. A new method for maintaining body temperature in children. *Anesthesiology* 1986; **65:** 447–8.
29. Besunder JB, Reed MD, Blumer JL. Principles of drug biodisposition in the neonate: a critical evaluation of the pharmacokinetic–pharmacodynamic interface (Part I). *Clin Pharmacokinet* 1988; **14:** 189–216.
30. Morselli PL, Franco-Morselli R, Bossi L. Clinical pharmacokinetics in newborns and infants. In: Gibaldi M, Prescott L (eds). *Handbook of Clinical Pharmacokinetics.* New York: Adis Health Science Press 1983, Section II, 98–141.
31. Ehrnebo M, Agurell S, Jalling B, Boreus LO. Age differences in drug binding by plasma proteins: studies on human foetuses, neonates and adults. *Eur J Clin Pharmacol* 1971; **3:** 189–93.
32. Wood M. Plasma drug binding: implications for anesthesiologists. *Anesth Analg* 1986; **65:** 786–804.
33. Salanitre E, Racknow H. The pulmonary exchange of nitrous oxide and halothane in infants and children. *Anesthesiology* 1969; **30:** 388–94.
34. Lerman J. Pharmacology of inhalational anaesthetics in infants and children. *Paediatr Anaesth* 1992; **2:** 191–203.
35. Brandom BW, Brandom RB, Cook DR. Uptake and distribution of halothane in infants: In vivo measurements and computer simulations. *Anesth Analg* 1983; **62:** 404–10.
36. Fisher DM, Robinson S, Brett CM, *et al.* Comparison of enflurane, halothane, and isoflurane for diagnostic and therapeutic procedures in children with malignancies. *Anesthesiology* 1985; **63:** 647–50.
37. Hubbard AK, Gandolfi AJ, Brown BR. Immunological basis of anesthetic-induced hepatotoxicity. *Anesthesiology* 1988; **69:** 814–7.
38. Wark HJ. Postoperative jaundice in children – the influence of halothane. *Anaesthesia* 1983; **38:** 237–42.
39. Warner LO, Beach TP, Garvin JP, Warner EJ. Halothane and children: the first quarter century. *Anesth Analg* 1984; **63:** 838–40.
40. Lerman J, Robinson S, Willis MM, Gregory GA. Anesthetic requirements for halothane in young children 0–1 month and 1–6 months of age. *Anesthesiology* 1983; **59:** 421–4.
41. Gregory GA, Eger EI II, Munson ES. The relationship between age and halothane requirement in man. *Anesthesiology* 1969; **30:** 488–91.
42. Cook DR, Brandom BW, Shiu G, Wolfson BW. The inspired median effective dose, brain concentration at anesthesia, and cardiovascular index for halothane in young rats. *Anesth Analg* 1981; **60:** 182–5.
43. Diaz JH, Lockhart CH. Is halothane really safe in infancy? *Anesthesiology* 1979; **57:** S313.
44. Tibballs J, Malbezin S. Cardiovascular changes during deep halothane anaesthesia in infants and children. *Anaesth Intens Care* 1988; **16:** 285–91.
45. Friedman WF. The intrinsic physiologic properties of the developing heart. *Progr Cardiovasc Dis* 1972; **15:** 87–111.
46. Friesen RH, Lichtor JL. Cardiovascular depression during halothane anesthesia in infants: a study of three induction techniques. *Anesth Analg* 1982; **61:** 42–5.
47. Friesen RH, Henry DB. Cardiovascular changes in preterm neonates receiving isoflurane, halothane, fentanyl and ketamine. *Anesthesiology* 1986; **64:** 238–42.
48. Pandit UA, Steude GM, Leach AB. Induction and recovery characteristics of isoflurane and halothane anaesthesia for short outpatient operations in children. *Anaesthesia* 1984; **40:** 1226–30.
49. Cameron CB, Robinson S, Gregory GA. The minimum anesthetic concentration of isoflurane in children. *Anesth Analg* 1984; **63:** 418–20.
50. Le Dez KM, Lerman J. The minimum alveolar concentration (MAC) of isoflurane in preterm neonates. *Anesthesiology* 1987; **67:** 301–7.
51. Wolf WJ, Neal MB, Peterson MD. The hemodynamic and cardiovascular effects of isoflurane and halothane anesthesia in children. *Anesthesiology* 1986; **64:** 328–33.
52. Murray D, Vandewalker G, Matherne GP, Mahoney LT. Pulsed doppler and two-dimensional echocardiography: Comparison of halothane and isoflurane on cardiac function in infants and small children. *Anesthesiology* 1987; **67:** 211–17.
53. Eger EI II. New inhalational agents – desflurane and sevoflurane. *Can J Anesth* 1993; **40:** R3-R5.
54. Muto R, Miyasaka K, Takata M, *et al.* Initial experience of complete switchover to sevoflurane in 1550 children. *Paediatr Anaesth* 1993; **3:** 229–33.
55. Lerman J, Sikich N, Kleinman S, Yentis S. The pharmacology of sevoflurane in infants and children. *Anesthesiology* 1994; **80:** 814–24.
56. Davis PJ, Lerman J, Welborn L, *et al.* Emergence and recovery from sevoflurane in pediatric ambulatory patients: a multicentre study. *Anesthesiology* 1993; **79:** A1165.
57. Cousins MJ, Mazze RI. Methoxyflurane nephrotoxicity: a study of dose–response in man. *J Am Med Assoc* 1973; **225:** 1611–6.
58. Mazze RI, Jamison RL. Low-flow (1 l/min) sevoflurane: is it safe? *Anesthesiology* 1997; **86:** 1225–7.
59. Frink Jr EJ, Malan TP, Morgan SE, *et al.* Quantification of the degradation products of sevoflurane in two CO_2 absorbents during low-flow anesthesia in surgical patients. *Anesthesiology* 1992; **77:** 1064–9.
60. Kharasch ED, Thorning D, Garton K, *et al.* Role of renal cysteine conjugate β-lyase in the mechanism of compound A nephrotoxicity in rats. *Anesthesiology* 1997; **86:** 160–71.
61. Taylor RH, Lerman J. Induction, maintenance and recovery characteristics of desflurane in infants and children. *Can J Anesth* 1992; **39:** 6–13.

62. Zwass MS, Fisher DM, Welbourn LG, *et al.* Induction and maintenance characteristics of anesthesia with desflurane and nitrous oxide in infants and children. *Anesthesiology* 1992; **76:** 373–8.
63. Davis PJ, Cohen IT, McGowan FX, Latta K. Recovery characteristics of desflurane *versus* halothane for maintenance of anaesthesia in pediatric ambulatory patients. *Anesthesiology* 1994; **80:** 298–302.
64. Taylor RH, Lerman J. Minimum alveolar concentration (MAC) of desflurane and hemodynamic responses in neonates, infants and children. *Anesthesiology* 1991; **75:** 975–9.
65. Price HL. Myocardial depression by nitrous oxide and its reversal by calcium. *Anesthesiology* 1976; **44:** 211–5.
66. Sorbo S, Hudson RJ, Loomis JC. The pharmacokinetics of thiopental in pediatric surgical patients. *Anesthesiology* 1984; **61:** 666–70.
67. Westrin P, Jonmarker C, Werner O. Thiopental requirements for induction of anesthesia in neonates and in infants 1–6 months of age. *Anesthesiology* 1989; **71:** 344–6.
68. Jonmarker C, Westrin P, Larsson S, Werner O. Thiopentone requirements for induction of anesthesia in children. *Anesthesiology*, 1987; **67:** 104–7.
69. Kingston HG, Kendrick A, Sommer KM, *et al.* Binding of thiopental in neonatal serum. *Anesthesiology* 1990; **72:** 428–31.
70. Duncan BBA, Zaimi F, Newman GB, *et al.* Effect of premedication on the induction dose of thiopentone in children. *Anaesthesia* 1984; **39:** 426–8.
71. Tiballs J, Malbezin S. Cardiovascular responses to induction of anaesthesia with thiopentone and suxamethonium in infants and children. *Anaesth Intens Care* 1988; **16:** 278–84.
72. Sharples A, Shaw EA, Meakin G. Recovery times following induction of anaesthesia with propofol, methohexitone, enflurane or thiopentone in children. *Paediatr Anaesth* 1994; **4:** 101–4.
73. Marsh B, White M, Morton N, Kenny GNC. Pharmacokinetic model-driven infusion of propofol in children. *Br J Anaesth* 1991; **67:** 41–8.
74. Hannallah RS, Baker SB, Casey W, *et al.* Propofol: effective dose and induction characteristics in unpremedicated children. *Anesthesiology* 1991; **74:** 217–19.
75. Patel DK, Keeling PA, Newman GB, Radford P. Induction dose of propofol in children. *Anaesthesia* 1988; **43:** 949–52.
76. Westrin P. The induction dose of propofol in infants 1–6 months of age and in children 10–16 years of age. *Anesthesiology* 1991; **74:** 455–8.
77. Morton NS, Wee M, Christie G, *et al.* Propofol for induction of anaesthesia in children. A comparison with thiopentone and halothane inhalational induction. *Anaesthesia* 1988; **43:** 350–5.
78. Morton NS. Abolition of injection pain due to propofol in children. *Anaesthesia* 1990; **45:** 70.
79. Mirakhur RK. Induction characteristics of propofol in children: comparison with thiopentone. *Anaesthesia* 1988; **43:** 593–8.
80. Cameron E, Johnston G, Crofts S, Morton NS. The minimum effective dose of lignocaine to prevent injection pain due to propofol in children. *Anaesthesia* 1992; **47:** 604–6.
81. Purcell-Jones G, Yates A, Baker JR, James IG. Comparison of the induction characteristics of thiopentone and propofol in children. *Br J Anaesth* 1987; **59:** 1431–6.
82. Servin F, Desmonts JM, Haberer JP, *et al.* Pharmacokinetics and protein binding of propofol in patients with cirrhosis. *Anesthesiology* 1988; **69:** 887–91.
83. Valtonen M, Iisalo E, Kanto J, Tikkanen J. Comparison between propofol and thiopentone for induction of anaesthesia in children. *Anaesthesia* 1988; **43:** 696–9.
84. Borgeat A, Popovic V, Meier D, Schwander D. Comparison of propofol and thiopental/halothane for short-duration ENT surgical procedures in children. *Anesth Analg* 1990; **71:** 511–15.
85. Puttick N, Rosen M. Propofol induction and maintenance with nitrous oxide in paediatric outpatient dental anaesthesia. A comparison with thiopentone-nitrous oxide-halothane. *Anaesthesia* 1988; **43:** 646–9.
86. Short SM, Aun CST. Haemodynamic effects of propofol in children. *Anaesthesia* 1991; **46:** 783–5.
87. Borgeat A, Wilder-Smith OH, Saiah M, Rifat K. Subhypnotic doses of propofol possess direct antiemetic properties. *Anesth Analg* 1992; **74:** 539–41.
88. Martin TM, Nicolson SC, Bargas MS. Propofol anesthesia reduces emesis and airway obstruction in pediatric outpatients. *Anesth Analg* 1993; **76:** 144–8.
89. Bennett SN, McNeil MM, Bland LA, *et al.* Postoperative infection traced to contamination of an intravenous anesthetic, propofol. *N Engl J Med* 1995; **333:** 147–54.
90. Kupferberg HJ, Way EL. Pharmacologic basis for the increased sensitivity of the newborn rat to morphine. *J Pharmacol Exp Ther* 1963: **141:** 105–12.
91. Lynn AM, Slattery JT. Morphine pharmacokinetics in early infancy. *Anesthesiology* 1987; **66:** 136–9.
92. Lynn AM, Opheim KE, Tyler DC. Morphine infusion after pediatric cardiac surgery. *Crit Care Med* 1984; **12:** 863–6.
93. Pounder DR, Steward DJ. Postoperative analgesia: opioid infusions in infants and children. *Can J Anesth* 1992; **39:** 969–74.
94. Catley DM, Thornton C, Jordan C, *et al.* Pronounced, episodic oxygen desaturation in the postoperative period: its association with ventilatory pattern and analgesic regimen. *Anesthesiology* 1985; **63:** 20–8.
95. Murphy MR, Olson WA, Hug CC. Pharmacokinetics of ^{3}H-fentanyl in the dog anesthetized with enflurane. *Anesthesiology* 1979; **50:** 13–19.
96. Singleton MA, Rosen JI, Fisher DM. Plasma concentrations of fentanyl in infants, children and adults. *Can J Anesth* 1987; **34:** 152–5.
97. Hertzka RE, Gauntlett IS, Fisher DM, Spellman MJ. Fentanyl-induced ventilatory depression: effects of age. *Anesthesiology* 1989; **70:** 213–18.
98. Hickey PR, Hansen DD, Wessel DL, *et al.* Pulmonary and systemic responses to fentanyl in infants. *Anesth Analg* 1985; **64:** 483–6.
99. Marlow N, Weindling AM, Van Peer A, Heykants J. Alfentanil pharmacokinetics in preterm infants. *Arch Dis Child* 1990; **65:** 349–51.
100. Feldman PL, James MK, Brackeen MF, *et al.* Design, synthesis, and pharmacological evaluation of ultrashort-to long-acting opioid analgesics. *J Med Chem* 1991; **34:** 2202–8.
101. Stead AL. The response of the newborn infant to muscle relaxants. *Br J Anaesth* 1955; **27:** 124–30.
102. Wareham AC, Morton RH, Meakin GH. Low quantal content of the endplate potential reduces safety factor for neuromuscular transmission in the diaphragm of the newborn rat. *Br J Anaesth* 1994; **72:** 205–9.
103. Meakin G, Morton RH, Wareham AC. Age-dependent variation in response to tubocurarine in the isolated rat diaphragm. *Br J Anaesth* 1992; **68:** 161–3.
104. Meakin G. *Neuromuscular Blocking Drugs in Paediatric Anaesthesia.* Interface Series: Organon Teknika, 1998.
105. Meakin G, McKiernan EP, Morris P, Baker RD. Dose–response curves for suxamethonium in neonates, infants and children. *Br J Anaesth* 1989; **62:** 655–8.
106. Meakin G, Walker RWM, Dearlove OR. Myotonic and neuromuscular blocking effects of increased doses of suxamethonium in infants and children. *Br J Anaesth* 1990; **65:** 816–18.
107. Goudsouzian NG. Turbe del ritmo cadiaco durante intubazione tracheale nei bambini. *Acta Anaesthesiol Ital* 1981; **32:** 293–9.
108. Hopkins PM. Use of suxamethonium in children. *Br J Anaesth* 1995; **75:** 675–7.
109. Brandom BW, Stiller RL, Cook DR, *et al.* Pharmacokinetics of atracurium in anaesthetized infants and children. *Br J Anaesth* 1986; **58:** 1210–3.
110. Stenlake JB, Waigh RD, Urwin J, *et al.* Atracurium: conception and inception. *Br J Anaesth* 1983; **55:** 3S–10S.
111. Meakin G, Shaw EA, Baker RD, Morris P. Comparison of atracurium-induced neuromuscular blockade in neonates, infants and children. *Br J Anaesth* 1988; **60:** 171–5.
112. Bevan DR, Bevan JC, Donati F. *Muscle Relaxants in Clinical Anaesthesia.* Chicago: Year Book Medical Publishers, 1988: 148–151.
113. Goudsouzian NG, Alifimoff JK, Eberly C, *et al.* Neuromuscular and cardiovascular effects of mivacurium in children. *Anesthesiology* 1989; **70:** 237–42.
114. Woelfel SK, Brandom BW, McGowan FX, Cook DR. Clinical pharmacology of mivacurium in pediatric patients less than two years old during nitrous oxide–halothane anesthesia. *Anesth Analg* 1993; **77:** 713–20.
115. Sarner JB, Brandom DW, Woelfel SK, *et al.* Clinical pharmacology of mivacurium chloride (BW B1090U) in children during nitrous oxide–halothane and nitrous oxide-narcotic anesthesia. *Anesth Analg* 1989; **68:** 116–21.
116. Goudsouzian NG, Denman W, Schwartz A, *et al.* Pharmacodynamic and hemodynamic effects of mivacurium in infants anesthetized with halothane and nitrous oxide. *Anesthesiology* 1993; **79:** 919–25.
117. Fisher DM, Castagnoli BA, Miller RD. Vecuronium kinetics and dynamics in anaesthetized infants and children. *Clin Pharmacol Ther* 1985; **37:** 402–6.
118. Meretoja OA, Wirtavuori K, Neuvonen PJ. Age-dependence of the dose–response curve of vecuronium in pediatric patients during balanced anaesthesia. *Anesth Analg* 1988; **67:** 21–6.
119. Meretoja OA. Is vecuronium a long-acting neuromuscular blocking agent in neonates and infants? *Br J Anaesth* 1989; **62:** 184–7.
120. Bowman WC, Rodger IW, Houston J, *et al.* Structure–action relationships among some desacetoxy analogues of pancuronium and vecuronium in the anesthetized cat. *Anesthesiology* 1988; **69:** 57–62.
121. Taivainen T, Meretoja OA, Erkola O, *et al.* Rocuronium in infants, children and adults. *Anesthesiology* 1994; **81:** A1074.

122. Woelfel SK, Brandom BW, Cook DR, Sarner JB. Effects of bolus administration of ORG-9426 in children during nitrous oxide-halothane anesthesia. *Anesthesiology* 1992; **76:** 939–42.
123. Woelfel SK, Brandom BW, McGowan FX, *et al.* Neuromuscular effects of 600 mg.kg-1 of rocuronium in infants during nitrous oxide-halothane anaesthesia. *Paediatr Anaesth* 1994; **4:** 173–7.
124. Gwinnutt CL, Walker RMW, Meakin G. Antagonism of intense atracurium-induced neuromuscular blockade in children. *Br J Anaesth* 1991; **67:** 13–16.
125. Meakin G, Sweet PT, Bevan JC, Bevan DR. Neostigmine and edrophonium as antagonists of pancuronium in infants and children. *Anesthesiology* 1983; **59:** 316–21.
126. Vetter TR. The epidemiology and selective identification of children at risk for preoperative anxiety reactions. *Anesth Analg* 1993; **77:** 96–9.
127. Bevan JC, Johnston C, Haig MJ, *et al.* Preoperative parental anxiety predicts behavioural and emotional responses to induction of anaesthesia in children. *Can J Anesth* **1990:** 37; 177–82.
128. Cohen MM, Cameron CB. Should you cancel the operation when a child has an upper respiratory tract infection? *Anesth Analg* 1991; **72:** 282–8.
129. Empey DW, Laitinen LA, Jacobs L, *et al.* Mechanisms of bronchial hyperreactivity in normal subjects after upper respiratory tract infection. *Am Rev Respir Dis* 1976; **113:** 131–9.
130. Steward DJ. Screening tests before surgery in children. *Can J Anesth* 1991; **38:** 693–5.
131. Mendelson CL. The aspiration of stomach contents into the lungs during obstetric anesthesia. *Am J Obstet Gynecol* 1946; **53:** 191–205.
132. Heading RC. Gastric motility and emptying. In: Sircus W, Smith AN (eds). *Scientific Foundations of Gastroenterology.* London: Heinemann, 1980**:** 287–96.
133. Cavell B. Gastric emptying in preterm infants. *Acta Paediatr Scand* 1979; **68:** 527–31.
134. Cavell B. Gastric emptying in infants fed human milk or infant formula. *Acta Paediatr Scand* 1981; **70:** 639–41.
135. Sandhar BK, Goresky GV, Maltby JR, Shaffer EA. Effect of oral liquids and ranitidine on gastric fluid volume and pH in children undergoing outpatient surgery. *Anesthesiology* 1989; **71:** 327–30.
136. Splinter WM, Steward DA, Muir JG. The effect of preoperative apple juice on gastric contents, thirst, and hunger in children. *Can J Anesth* 1989; **36:** 55–8.
137. Schreiner MS, Triebwasser A, Keon TP. Ingestion of liquids compared with preoperative fasting in pediatric outpatients. *Anesthesiology* 1990; **72:** 593–7.
138. Splinter WM, Schaefer JD. Unlimited clear fluid ingestion two hours before surgery does not affect volume or pH of stomach contents. *Anaesth Intens Care* 1990; **18:** 522–6.
139. Nicolson SC, Dorsey AT, Schreiner MS. Shortened preanesthetic fasting interval in pediatric cardiac surgical patients. *Anesth Analg* 1992; **74:** 694–7.
140. Phillips S, Hutchinson S, Davidson T. Preoperative drinking does not affect gastric contents. *Br J Anaesth* 1993; **70:** 6–9.
141. Soreide E, Holst-Larsen H, Reite K, *et al.* Effects of giving water 20–450 mL with oral diazepam premedication 1–2 h before operation. *Br J Anaesth* 1993; **71:** 503–6.
142. Van der Walt JH, Floate JA, Murrell D, *et al.* A study of preoperative fasting in infants aged less than three months. *Anaesth Intens Care* 1990; **18:** 527–31.
143. Litman RS, Wu CL, Quinlivan JK. Gastric volume and pH in infants fed clear fluids and breast milk prior to surgery. *Anesth Analg* 1994; **79:** 482–5.
144. Meakin G, Dingwall AE, Addison GM. Effects of fasting and oral premedication on the pH and volume of gastric aspirate in children. *Br J Anaesth* 1987; **59:** 678–82.
145. Meakin GH, Murat I. Immediate preoperative preparation. In: Hatch DJ, Sumner E (eds). *Paediatric Anaesthesia.* London: Edward Arnold, 1999: 71–95.
146. McMillan CO, Spahr-Schopfer IA, Sikich N, *et al.* Premedication of children with oral midazolam. *Can J Anesth* 1992; **39:** 545–50.
147. Van der Walt JH, Jacob R, Murrell D, Bentley M. The perioperative effects of oral premedication in children. *Anaesth Intens Care* 1990; **18:** 5–10.
148. Parnis SJ, Foate JA, Van der Walt JH, *et al.* Oral midazolam is an effective premedication for children having day-stay anaesthesia. *Anaesth Intensive Care* 1992; **20:** 9–14.
149. Gutstein HB, Johnson KL, Heard MB, Gregory GA. Oral ketamine preanesthetic medication in children. *Anesthesiology* 1992; **76:** 28–33.
150. Davis PJ, Tome JA, McGowan Jr FX, *et al.* Preanesthetic medication with intranasal midazolam for very brief pediatric surgical procedures: effect on recovery and hospital discharge times. *Anesthesiology* 1995; **82:** 2–5.
151. Karl HW, Keifer AT, Rosenberger JL, *et al.* Comparison of the safety and efficacy of intranasal midazolam or sufentanil for preinduction of anesthesia in pediatric patients. *Anesthesiology* 1992; **76:** 209–15.
152. Feld LH, Champeau MW, Van Steenis CA, Scott JC. Preanesthetic medication in children: a comparison of oral transmucosal fentanyl citrate versus placebo. *Anesthesiology* 1989; **71:** 374–7.
153. Feld LH, Negus JB, White PF. Oral midazolam preanesthetic medication in pediatric outpatients. *Anesthesiology* 1990; **73:** 831–4.
154. Friesen RH, Lockhart CH. Oral transmucosal fentanyl citrate for pre-anesthetic medication of pediatric day surgery patients with and without droperidol as a prophylactic antiemetic. *Anesthesiology* 1992; **76:** 46–51.
155. Lin SM, Liu K, Tsai SK, Lee TY. Rectal ketamine versus intranasal ketamine as premedicant in children. *Ma Tsui Hsueh Tsa Chi Anaesthesiol Sinica* 1990; **28:** 177–83.
156. Kain ZN, Mayes LC, Bell C, *et al.* Premedication in the United States: a status report. *Anesth Analg* 1997; **84:** 427–32.
157. Kanto J. Benzodiazepines as oral premedicants. *Br J Anaesth* 1981; **53:** 1179–88.
158. Wilton NCT, Leigh J, Rosen DR, Pandit UA. Preanesthetic sedation of preschool children using intranasal midazolam. *Anesthesiology* 1988; **69:** 972–5.
159. Saint-Maurice C, Mesistelman C, Rey E, *et al.* The pharmacokinetics of rectal midazolam for premedication in children. *Anesthesiology* 1986; **65:** 536–8.
160. De Jong PC, Verburg MP. Comparison of rectal to intramuscular administration of midazolam and atropine for premedication of children. *Acta Anaesthesiol Scand* 1988; **32:** 485–9.
161. Hannallah RS, Patel R. Low-dose intramuscular ketamine for anesthesia pre-induction in young children undergoing brief outpatient procedures. *Anesthesiology* 1989; **70:** 598–600.
162. Nelson PS, Streisand JB, Mulder SM, *et al.* Comparison of oral transmucosal fentanyl citrate and an oral solution of meperidine, diazepam, and atropine for premedication in children. *Anesthesiology* 1989; **70:** 616–21.
163. Helmers JH, Noorduin H, Van Peer A, *et al.* Comparison of intravenous and intranasal sufentanil absorption and sedation. *Can J Anesth* 1989; **36:** 494–7.
164. Henderson JM, Brodsky DA, Fisher DM, *et al.* Preinduction of anesthesia in pediatric patients with nasally administered sufentanil. *Anesthesiology* 1988; **68:** 671–5.
165. Kestin IG, McIlvaine WB, Lockhart CH, et al. Rectal methohexital for induction of anesthesia in children with and without rectal aspiration after sleep: A pharmacokinetic and pharmacodynamic study. Anesth Analg 1988; **67:** 1102–4.
166. Sigston PE, Jenkins AMC, Jackson EA, *et al.* Rapid inhalation induction in children: 8% sevoflurane compared with 5% halothane. *Br J Anaesth* 1997; **78:** 362–5.
167. Gajraj NM, Pennant JH, Watcha MF. Eutectic mixture of local anaesthetics (EMLA®) cream. *Anesth Analg* 1994; **78:** 574–83.
168. Lawson RA, Smart NG, Morton NS. Evaluation of an amethocaine gel preparation for percutaneous analgesia before venous cannulation in children. *Br J Anaesth* 1995; **75:** 282–5.
169. Koka BV, Jeon IS, Andre JM, *et al.* Postintubation croup in children. *Anesth Analg* 1977; **56:** 501–5.
170. Khalil SN, Mankarious R, Campos C, *et al.* Absence or presence of a leak around tracheal tube may not affect postoperative croup in children. *Paediatr Anaesth* 1998; **8:** 393–6.
171. Conway CM. Anaesthetic breathing systems. *Br J Anaesth* 1985; **57:** 649–57.
172. Stephen CR, Slater HM. Agents and techniques employed in pediatric anesthesia. *Anesth Analg* 1950; **29:** 254–62.
173. Adriani J, Griggs T. Rebreathing in pediatric anesthesia: recommendations and descriptions of improvements in apparatus. *Anesthesiology* 1953; **14:** 337–47.
174. Ayre P. The T-piece technique. *Br J Anaesth* 1956; **28:** 520–3.
175. Jackson Rees G. Anaesthesia in the newborn. *Br Med J* 1950; **2:** 1419–22.
176. Mapleson WW. The elimination of rebreathing in various semi-closed anaesthetic systems. *Br J Anaesth* 1954; **26:** 323–32.
177. Meakin G, Coates AL. Evaluation of rebreathing with the Bain circuit during anaesthesia with spontaneous ventilation. *Br J Anaesth* 1983; **55:** 487–96.
178. Willis BA, Pender JW, Mapleson WW. Breathing in a T-piece: volunteer and theoretical studies of the Jackson-Rees modification of Ayre's T-piece during spontaneous respiration. *Br J Anaesth* 1975; **47:** 1239–46.
179. Meakin G. Fresh gas requirement of the T-piece systems. *Br J Anaesth* 1986; **58:** 935.

180. Conway CM. Alveolar gas relationships during the use of semi-closed rebreathing anaesthetic systems. *Br J Anaesth* 1976; **48:** 865–9.
181. Rose DK, Froese AB. The regulation of $PaCO_2$ during controlled ventilation of children with a T-piece. *Can Anesth Soc J* 1979; **26:** 104–13.
182. Meakin G, Jennings AD, Beatty PCW, Healy TEJ. Fresh gas requirements of an enclosed afferent reservoir breathing system during controlled ventilation of children. *Br J Anaesth* 1992; **68:** 43–7.
183. Waters RM. Clinical scope and utility of carbon dioxide filtration in inhalation anesthesia. *Anesth Analg* 1924; **3:** 20–2.
184. Baum JA, Aitkenhead AR. Low-flow anaesthesia. *Anaesthesia* 1995; **50** (Suppl.): 37–44.
185. Meakin GH. Low-flow anaesthesia in infants and children. *Br J Anaesth* 1999; **83:** 50–7.
186. Bennet EJ. Fluid balance in the newborn. *Anesthesiology* 1975; **43:** 210–24.
187. Eyers RL, Bishop W, Oppenheim RC, Brown TCK. Plasma bupivacaine concentrations in children during caudal epidural analgesia. *Anaesth Intens Care* 1983; **20:** 11–14.
188. Wolf AR, Valley RD, Fear DW, *et al*. Bupivacaine for caudal analgesia in infants and children: the optimal effective concentration. *Anesthesiology* 1988; **69:** 102–6.
189. Shandling B, Steward DJ. Regional analgesia for postoperative pain in pediatric outpatient surgery. *J Pediatr Surg* 1980; **15:** 477–80.
190. Hannallah RS, Broadman LM, Belman A, *et al*. Comparison of caudal and ilioinguinal/iliohypogastric nerve blocks for control of post-orchiopexy pain in pediatric ambulatory surgery. *Anesthesiology* 1987; **66:** 832–4.
191. Soliman MG, Tremblay NA. Nerve block of the penis for postoperative pain relief in children. *Anesth Analg* 1978; **57:** 495–8.
192. Steward DJ. Outpatient pediatric anesthesia. *Anesthesiology* 1975; **43:** 268–76.
193. Motoyama EK, Glazener CH. Hypoxaemia after general anaesthesia in children. *Anesth Analg* 1986; **65:** 267–72.
194. Patel RI, Hannallah RS. Anesthetic complications following pediatric ambulatory surgery: a 3-year study. *Anesthesiology* 1988; **69:** 1009–12.
195. Steward DJ. Experiences with an outpatient anesthesia service for children. *Anesth Analg* 1973; **52:** 877–80.
196. Rita L, Goodarzi M, Seleny F. Effect of low dose droperidol on postoperative vomiting in children. *Can Anesth Soc J* 1981; **28:** 259–62.
197. Guida RA, Matucci KF. Tonsillectomy and adenoidectomy: an inpatient or outpatient procedure? *Laryngoscope* 1990; **100:** 491–3.
198. Broadman LM, Ceruzzi W, Patane PS, *et al*. Metoclopramide reduces the incidence of vomiting following strabismus *Surg* in children. *Anesthesiology* 1990; **72:** 245–8.
199. Ferrari LR, Donlon JV. Metoclopramide reduces the incidence of vomiting after tonsillectomy in children. *Anesth Analg* 1992; **75:** 351–4.
200. Litman RS, Wu LL, Catanzaro FA. Ondensetron decreases emesis after tonsillectomy in children. *Anesth Analg* 1994; **78:** 478–81.
201. Watcha MF, Bras PJ, Cieslak GD. Pennant JH. The dose–response relationship of ondansetron in preventing postoperative emesis in pediatric patients undergoing ambulatory surgery. *Anesthesiology* 1995; **82:** 47–52.
202. Watcha MF, Simeon RM, White PF, Stevens JL. Effect of propofol on the incidence of postoperative vomiting after strabismus surgery in pediatric outpatients. *Anesthesiology* 1991; **75:** 204–9.
203. Jordan WS, Graves CL, Elwyn RA. New therapy for post-intubation laryngeal edema and tracheitis in children. *J Am Med Assoc* 1970; **212:** 585–8.
204. Remington S, Meakin G. Nebulised adrenaline 1:1000 in the treatment of croup. *Anaesthesia* 1986; **41:** 272–5.

60

Anesthesia for the elderly

STANLEY MURAVCHICK

INTRODUCTION

Advances in nutrition, public health, education, and social services during the twentieth century produced extraordinary increases in human longevity. In all industrialized societies, increased life expectancy and reduced mortality from chronic age-related disease continue to enlarge that fraction of the surgical patient population considered elderly. Although they represent only 10–15% of all Americans, individuals 65 years of age or older undergo almost one-third of the 25 million surgical procedures performed annually in the USA. Overall, older Americans also consume about one-third of all health expenditures and fully one-half of the $140 billion annual US federal healthcare budget. The surgical demographics are very similar in Europe and in Japan. Therefore, these apparently beneficial changes have further amplified the fiscal impact of the increasing *per capita* healthcare costs that already represented a formidable burden for modern societies. Consequently, unless intentionally limited to pediatrics or obstetrics, every anesthesiologist in contemporary practice eventually becomes a subspecialist in geriatric medicine with a special responsibility for delivering cost-effective healthcare to older adults. The sections that follow define the current concepts of aging that are relevant to anesthetic practice and discuss the distinction between aging and age-related disease, perioperative assessment of the elderly patient, and practical aspects of anesthetic management and outcome in geriatric surgical patients.

GERONTOLOGY

Gerontology is the broadest term applied to studies of aging.[1] Biogerontologists usually limit their scope to the physiologic and biochemical, rather than the socioeconomic, aspects of aging. Although many gerontologists study human aging exclusively, others have extended their interests down to a cellular or subcellular level, and therefore this discipline may encompass the study of nonhuman organisms. In contrast, "geriatrics," a term with origins early in the last century,[2] is more specific because it describes the medical subspecialty that focuses upon care of the elderly patient. Geriatricians are physicians who specialize in the care of the elderly patient. However, there is no consensus regarding the starting point of the human geriatric era. Physiologic markers that may have some clinical value for establishing or confirming "biologic age" or for predicting an individual's proximity to death include physical stature, changes in sleep pattern, reduced heart rate variability, loss of visual acuity, or increases in summed sensory deficits, reduction of nerve electrical impulse conduction velocity, changes in immune function, or alteration of β-adrenoceptor responsiveness. However, it remains unclear whether the geriatric era has a discrete beginning, or whether any one physiologic marker can identify a patient as having become "elderly." Therefore, birthdate or other simple chronologic descriptors for agedness remain the most widely accepted criteria, both for identifying elderly patients and for selecting patients for studies of aging. For clarity and consistency within this chapter, therefore, the terms "elderly" and "geriatric" will be used synonymously to describe human subjects who, by arbitrary convention, have entered the seventh decade. Some specialists in this area further distinguish those in the ninth decade of their lives and beyond as "aged."

Any experienced clinician and all geriatricians are well aware that the elderly patient does not belong to a surgical subpopulation that is medically or physically homogeneous. People are never more alike than they are at birth, nor more different or unique than when they enter the geriatric era. As they age, adult patients exhibit an increasingly complex array of unique physical responses to environmental and socioeconomic conditions and to concurrent disease states. Survival to adulthood and beyond permits the full expression of genetic differences between individuals that might not be expressed within shorter lifespan intervals (Fig. 60.1). Therefore, precise assessment and appropriate management of the elderly surgical patient represents a great challenge to all medical healthcare providers. Perhaps more than for any other medical specialty, increased interpatient variability is a hallmark of geriatric medicine.

Studies of human aging are further complicated by difficulties in discriminating clearly between aging itself, the consequences of age-related disease, and the cohort-specific effects that make data from cross-sectional studies ambiguous. Cross-sectional studies measure physiologic parameters simultaneously in young and in elderly subjects, so changes owing to undiagnosed age-related disease may be erroneously attributed to age itself. Similarly, this experimental design cannot be controlled for cohort-specific factors such as nutritional and environmental history, genetic background, or prior exposure to infectious agents. Many of the "classic" cross-sectional studies of aging in the gerontologic literature must be reconsidered because data from cross-sectional studies rarely permit unambiguous conclusions regarding the effect of age itself on any one measured physiologic parameter.

Some biogerontologists feel that processes of aging can be unequivocally identified only when a longitudinal study is used to supplement carefully performed cross-sectional studies. For some measurements, such as glomerular filtration, data from longitudinal studies validated the results of earlier cross-sectional investigations.[3] However, longitudinal studies of human aging require an arbitrary chronologic "starting point" for the geriatric era that may change significantly during the

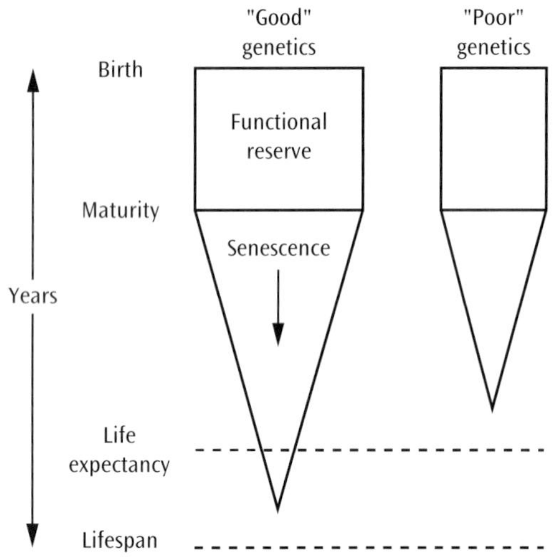

Figure 60.1 *Lifespan describes maximum attainable age. Conceptually, the duration of senescence in a benign environment, and therefore lifespan itself, increases in proportion to the degree of functional reserve as determined by a favorable genetic profile. Observed life expectancy for a population of individuals is a measure of typical or average longevity and includes those with a "poor" genetic profile as well as those individuals who die of external, nongenetic causes.*

duration of the study itself because of increases in life expectancy.[4] These studies also have intrinsic sources of error.[5] In addition, the validity and utility of the data they generate are subject to the evolution or revision of physiologic concepts and measurement techniques over the long time period required to study human aging. Consequently, some of the statements and conclusions presented here represent substantial revision of the "conventional wisdom" taught only a few years ago.

CONCEPTS OF AGING

Lifespan is an idealized, species-specific biologic parameter that quantifies maximum attainable age under optimal environmental conditions. Historical anecdote suggests that human lifespan has remained constant at 110–115 years for at least the past 20 centuries.[6] In contrast, life expectancy is an empirical estimate of typical longevity under prevailing or predicted circumstances. Advances in medical science and health care have improved life expectancy dramatically in industrialized societies and increased their relative "agedness" but do not appear to have altered human lifespan. In fact, the mechanisms that control the aging process and determine lifespan remain unknown. Perhaps because gerontology is a relatively new discipline, theories of aging have been presented from various individual perspectives, many without any logical relation or interconnection. In general, however, theories of aging fall into two major categories. One group can be described as stochastic because it is essentially time and probability dependent. In contrast, the nonstochastic group includes theories proposing that there are "biologic clocks" or "life pacemakers" for each species.[7] A nonstochastic theory usually involves a neuroendocrine or immune mechanism because the pacemaker tissue or organ must itself have widespread interaction with all other organ systems to effect processes of aging throughout the organism.

The "error–catastrophe" theory of aging is a stochastic concept that postulates that random errors of protein synthesis due to faulty nucleic acid transcription or translation accumulate and eventually compromise cellular function and produce the physical signs of aging. However, there is little evidence that the individual cells of older subjects contain more defective protein than do young cells. This theory also fails to explain the dramatically different patterns of aging that are seen in various animal species that share a common ecosystem and are exposed to similar catabolic environmental forces such as ionizing radiation. Similarly, a "genetic wear and tear" theory of aging proposes that recurrent damage to nuclear deoxyribonucleic acid (nDNA) eventually exhausts intrinsic intracellular capacity for nuclear chromosomal repair, leading to a critical loss of cellular and tissue elements. Although there is a general correlation between species longevity and nDNA repair capacity, there is no firm evidence that the ability to recover from random nDNA damage is, in fact, progressively or universally compromised in older human subjects.[8]

However, investigations of oxidative phosphorylation in aging mitochondria suggest that progressive increases in the incidence of defects within mitochondrial DNA (mDNA) may lead to a decline in bioenergetic capacity[9] and a progressive reduction in the efficiency with which free radical species that form within the mitochondria during aerobic metabolism are scavenged from the cytosol of aging cells. Free radicals and other reactive oxygen metabolites damage the unsaturated fatty acid and nucleic acid components of cells and cross-link protein molecules, eventually compromising cellular microarchitecture.[10] Superoxide dismutase (SOD), the most important endogenous enzymatic scavenger of free radical species, is present in higher concentrations within human cells than in the cells of species with a shorter lifespan. A relatively recent proposal[11] suggests that, in fact, cellular aging is due to mDNA damage and diffuse bioenergetic failure in the mitochondria of metabolically active tissues (Fig. 60.2). A mechanism consisting of progressive failure of a genetically determined capacity to clear random damage to mDNA by free radicals is compatible with both stochastic and nonstochastic theories[12] and falls within the larger concept[13] that aging reflects a lifetime of oxidative stress. Perhaps this explains observations that ingestion of antioxidants may increase longevity, at least under experimental conditions.

ORGAN FUNCTION AND RESERVE

Processes of aging are usually distinguishable from age-related disease by the fact that they are universally present in all members of an elderly population and, in longitudinal studies of aging subjects, become progressively more apparent with increasing chronologic age. Aging is a universal and progressive physiologic phenomenon characterized by degenerative changes in both the structure and the function of organs and tissues. It produces many physical manifestations by reducing connective tissue flexibility and elasticity or by leading to the degeneration of highly structured molecular arrangements within specialized tissues such as the lens of the eye. At the tissue level, cross-linking, glycosylation, or similar dysfunctional interactions occur in the elastic elements of cardiovascular and pulmonary structures as well as in the basement membrane proteins of the kidney.[14]

At one time, the functional consequences of aging at an organ level were represented graphically as linear declines. The decrement from maximum function was shown as beginning in young adulthood and continuing inexorably downward thereafter. However, more current concepts describe a complex, nonlinear process that is first apparent following the peak of somatic maturation, in the fourth decade of human life. Subsequent decrements of function in most organs are relatively subtle during the middle adult years, but then become progressively more dramatic during the traditional years of geriatric senescence.[15] At every age, the competence of integrated organ system function varies considerably from one patient to the next, even in the absence of disease. Elderly patients who maintain greater than average functional capacities are said to be "physiologically young." When function declines at an

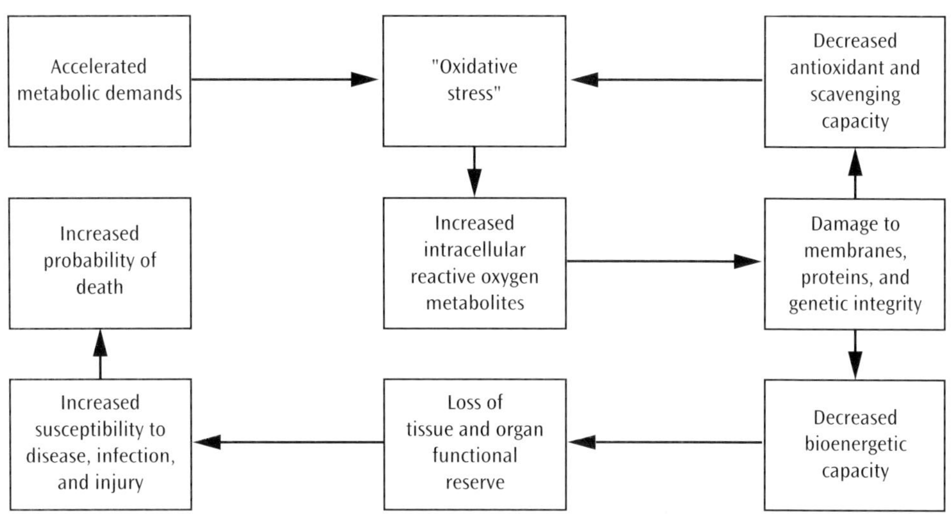

Figure 60.2 *In older adults, declining antioxidant and free radical scavenging functions increase the reactive oxygen metabolites that damage mitochondrial machinery, compromising bioenergetic capacity at a cellular level and increasing the likelihood of death. This cycle of injury and bioenergetic failure may be an expression of "oxidative stress."*

earlier age, or at a more rapid rate, elderly patients can be considered "physiologically old" (Fig. 60.3).

In healthy geriatric patients, however, maximum organ system functional capacity at all ages is greater than the basal level of activity, at rest. The difference between maximum capacity and basal levels of function is organ system functional reserve (Fig. 60.4), a "safety margin" available to meet the additional demands for cardiac output, carbon dioxide excretion, or protein synthesis imposed upon the patient by trauma or disease or by surgery, healing, and convalescence. Cardiopulmonary functional reserve, for example, can be quantified and assessed clinically using various exercise or maximal stress tests. However, there is, at present, no comparable approach to assessment of renal, hepatic, immune, or nervous system functional reserve. It is by this mechanism that the functional reserve of these organ systems is reduced in elderly patients and susceptibility of elderly patients to stress- and disease-induced organ system decompensation occurs.

Just as in young adult surgical patients, routine preoperative testing protocols are of low yield and expensive. Even when the results fall outside the normal range they rarely alter the plan for perioperative management. Therefore, preoperative testing of elderly surgical patients should not consist of "screening" tests determined by patient age alone but instead should be directed by physical status, disease, and the specific surgical procedure (Fig. 60.5). Preoperative laboratory data are of greatest value when used to quantify or define disorders and impairment already suggested or identified by medical and surgical history and by physical examination.[16] Although any type of preoperative testing may be appropriate to further characterize an identified disorder or to manage a patient having a specific surgical procedure, only the electrocardiogram appears to be sufficiently cost-effective, specific, and sensitive in a general geriatric surgical patient population to warrant routine preoperative application.[17]

Elderly patients account for 30% of all drug prescriptions, approximately twice the rate expected from their representation in the general population, and they consume 40% of all over-the counter medications.[18] One-half of all adults aged 75 years or older takes at least two different types of medication for the purpose of treating an age-related disease. Although it is appropriate to maintain elderly patients perioperatively on all medications needed to effectively control the symptoms of their disorders, especially cardiovascular, neurologic, and metabolic disease, some drug interactions may complicate perioperative management or make the pharmacokinetics of drugs used perioperatively less predictable.[19] Drug interactions are a form of iatrogenic disease. The high prevalence of disease in an elderly surgical patient population exposes

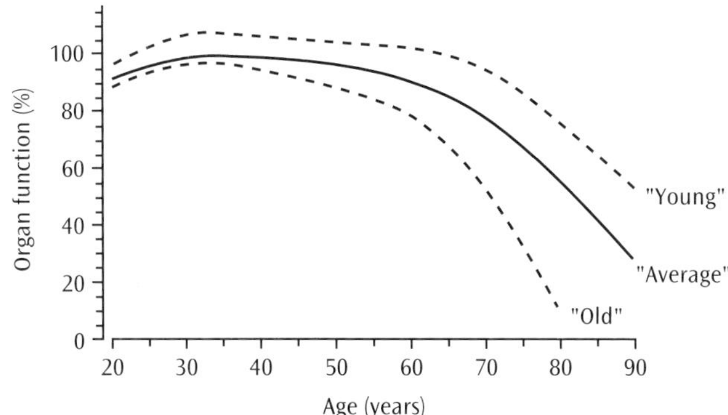

Figure 60.3 *Variability in the rate at which maximal organ system function declines with increasing age explains the presentation of patients as physiologically "young" or "old."*

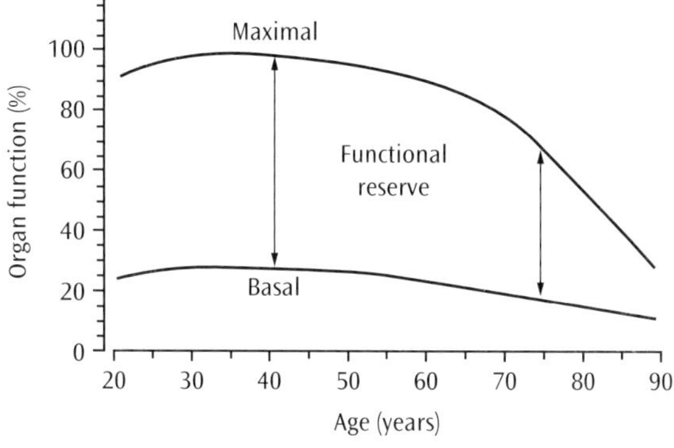

Figure 60.4 *Organ system "functional reserve" is the difference between basal and maximal organ system function. Functional reserve declines markedly within increasing age. Maximal function, modeled here after maximal aerobic capacity in trained athletes, is far more variable than basal function, but aging inevitably reduces functional reserve even in individuals who are physiologically "young." The configuration of the curve for basal function is adapted from longitudinal measurements of total basal metabolic rate.*

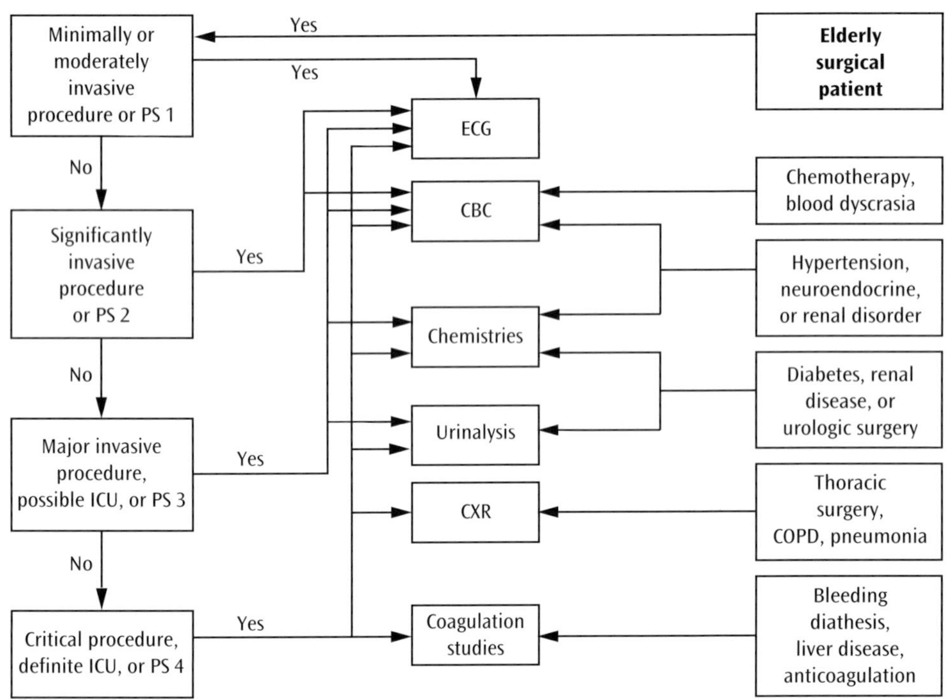

Figure 60.5 *Preoperative testing for elderly surgical patients should be clinically directed as indicated by both the physical status of the patient (PS), the site and invasiveness of the surgical procedure, and the likelihood of a need for intensive care unit (ICU) disposition. Electrocardiogram (ECG) alone may suffice for active, healthy elderly patients having minimally invasive procedures, but additional studies such as complete blood count (CBC) and chest radiograph (CXR) may be added as needed or as suggested by medical or surgical history or by clinical judgment. This schematic is shown for conceptual purposes and should not be considered as definitive for all elderly patients. COPD, chronic obstructive pulmonary disease.*

them not only to the stigmata of the disorders themselves, but also to the risks of polypharmacy from the drugs used for medical therapy (Fig. 60.6). Adverse drug interactions are due to the additive, synergistic, or antagonistic actions of multiple drugs sharing common sites of action, or to unexpected changes in the duration of drug effects. They occur far more often than in young patients, primarily because polypharmacy is common in older adults and because reduced hepatic and renal functional reserve prolongs both the desired and the unwanted effects of medications taken by older adults.

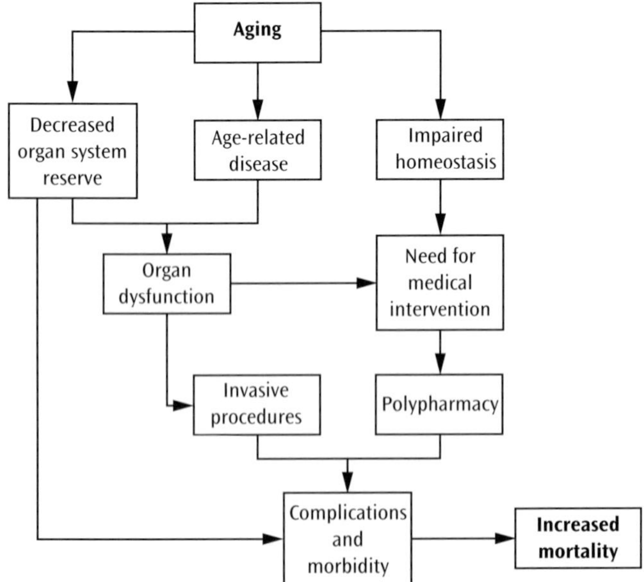

Figure 60.6 *Increased morbidity and a greater likelihood of perioperative mortality in elderly surgical patients reflects the interaction of the effects of aging on organ system functional reserve and the consequences of both age-related disease and its therapy. Polypharmacy and the need for invasive medical intervention further amplify the likelihood of adverse outcome and perioperative death.*

CARDIOPULMONARY SYSTEMS

The classic data suggesting that aging produces an irreversible depression of cardiac output are contradicted by more recent studies of fit and active elderly subjects in whom demand for cardiopulmonary function is maintained through daily exercise. In young and elderly alike, therefore, integrated cardiopulmonary function responds appropriately to physical activity and to variations in metabolic demand.[20] The modest decrease in resting cardiac index observed in healthy elderly subjects is not evidence of inexorable degenerative change. Rather, it represents an appropriate response to the reduced metabolic requirements associated with age-related atrophy of skeletal muscle and the loss of lean tissue mass.[21] In effect, aging simply produces a progressively smaller aerobic machine. Under conditions of submaximal demand, rates of myocardial shortening and ventricular pressure generation – two indices of myocardial contractility – appear to remain uncompromised by increasing age, at least until the eighth decade.

Although many aged individuals compete successfully in a variety of strenuous athletic events, aging does impose significant limitations upon maximal heart rate, maximal cardiac output, and maximal aerobic capacity that can be achieved during strenuous physical exercise. It reduces the cardiac end-organ response to β-adrenoceptor stimulation. In the elderly patient, increases in cardiac output are accomplished largely by increased left ventricular diastolic volume and augmented ventricular preload (Fig. 60.7) with little enhancement of ejection fraction.[22] Mechanical compensatory mechanisms predominate over changes in heart rate mediated by adrenoceptor activation or baroreflex activity.[23] However, a stiffer, less compliant ventricular and atrial myocardium also impairs ventricular filling.[24] Diastolic dysfunction is a common cause of significant cardiac failure in older adults who have no evidence of systolic compromise,[25] especially if the atrial kick of sinus rhythm is lost.[26] Thus, relatively small decreases in venous return such as those produced by positive pressure ventilation, surgical hemorrhage,

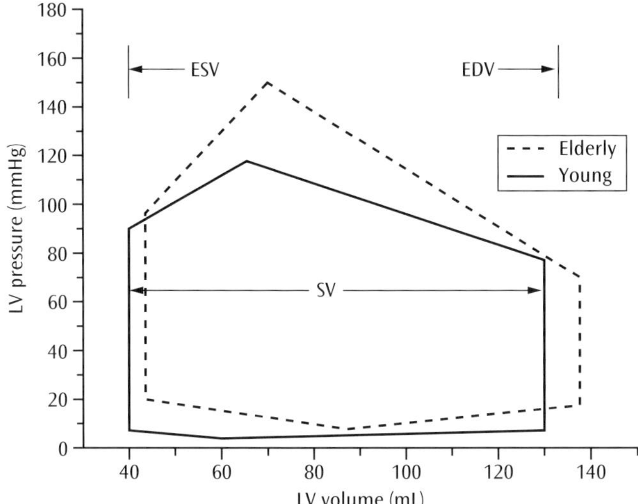

Figure 60.7 *Left ventricular pressure–volume loops for basal cardiac output in active, nonsedentary young (solid line) and older adults (broken line) demonstrate that age-related increases in chamber size (increased end-systolic and end-diastolic volumes; ESV and EDV respectively) and myocardial stiffness increase intraluminal pressures during diastole and delay the passive phase of ventricular filling in older subjects, with little change in stroke volume (SV). Consequently, aging alters ventricular hemodynamics by greatly increasing dependence upon atrial contraction for the maintenance of normal stroke volume.*

or venodilator drugs may significantly compromise stroke volume. With limited reflex-mediated ability to increase heart rate, hypotension can be frequent and severe both intraoperatively and postoperatively in older surgical patients. Conversely, rates of intravenous fluid administration that would be modest for young adults may, in the geriatric patient, produce increases in atrial and pulmonary artery pressure sufficiently large to disrupt the balance of forces that control lung water, precipitating congestive heart failure and pulmonary edema.

Virtually all longitudinal studies confirm the universal nature of progressive, gender-independent arterial hypertension, a phenomenon due to fibrotic replacement of elastic tissues within the walls of arteries. The ability of the aorta and large arteries to store hydraulic energy is compromised, increasing the vascular impedance to cardiac ejection, raising cardiac workload, and ultimately producing symmetrical left ventricular hypertrophy. For any given stroke volume, loss of compliance increases arterial pulse pressure, particularly the systolic pressure component. Large stroke volumes and stiff arteries produce the familiar "overshoot" characteristic of radial artery waveform tracings in older adults as well as the large discrepancies between blood pressure values obtained by invasive as opposed to occlusive cuff techniques for determining blood pressure.

Age-related loss of tissue elasticity is ubiquitous, involving the lung as well as the cardiovascular system. Loss of lung elastic recoil is a primary anatomic mechanism by which aging exerts deleterious effects on pulmonary gas exchange. With increasing age, lung elasticity declines,[27] probably from elastin degeneration and cross-linking. As a result, elderly individuals may experience emphysema-like increases in lung compliance. However, because calcification and stiffening of the thorax also reduces chest wall compliance, total pulmonary compliance is essentially unchanged,[28] and there is only a small increase in functional residual capacity (FRC).

Aging does significantly compromise ventilatory mechanics, however. Costochondral calcification makes the thorax more rigid and increases the work of breathing. Maximal breathing capacity is significantly reduced. Vital capacity is progressively compromised because residual volume increases at the expense of inspiratory and expiratory reserve volumes (Fig. 60.8). In elderly subjects, there may be small airway closure at a lung volume close to FRC if the patency of small airways is compromised.[29] Age-related breakdown of alveolar septae reduces total alveolar surface area, limiting gas exchange and progressively increasing both anatomic and alveolar dead space. These changes in the physical properties of the lungs are nonuniform. Therefore, ventilation/perfusion mismatching with increased shunting and dead space may occur, the effect of which may be accentuated by anesthetic-induced impairment of hypoxic pulmonary vasoconstriction.

The moment-to-moment control of ventilation and the response to changes in pH and respiratory gases appear to be unchanged in healthy and alert elderly subjects.[30] However, the cardiovascular and the ventilatory stimulation normally mediated by reflex mechanisms in response to imposed hypoxia or hypercarbia are delayed in onset, and of considerably smaller magnitude, in geriatric patients. Elderly subjects also experience a higher incidence of transient apnea and episodic respiration when given narcotics,[31] for reasons that are not completely understood. They may also be more sensitive to the respiratory depression produced by non-narcotic drugs such as the benzodiazepines.

Narcotic-induced rigidity of the chest wall occurs more frequently in older than in younger adults.[32] Protective laryngeal reflexes require a greater threshold stimulus magnitude,[33] increasing the risk of aspiration pulmonary injury in older patients, especially if the level of consciousness is depressed. Consequently, geriatric surgical patients are clearly at greater risk of unrecognized respiratory failure in the typical postoperative setting of residual anesthetics and pain therapy.[34] Supplemental inspired oxygen, enhanced monitoring, and continued observation of the adequacy of oxygenation and ventilation are essential in this surgical subpopulation.

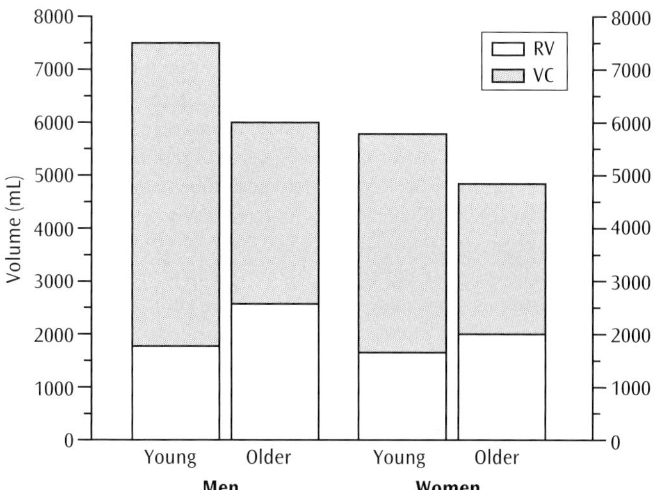

Figure 60.8 *Aging increases residual volume (RV, open bars) and compromises vital capacity (VC, shaded bars) in both men and women. These changes in VC and the decline in stature associated with aging are responsible for the "typical" age-related loss of total lung capacity (TLC, the sum of RV and VC) shown here. Although some data suggest that, unlike total vital capacity, specific vital capacity (mL cm^{-1} of height) is relatively independent of age itself, most predictive spirometric formulae assume that specific vital capacity is also progressively reduced with increasing age.*

HEPATORENAL FUNCTION

Aging produces a marked reduction in liver size. As much as 40–50% of hepatic tissue mass may involute by the age of 80, with liver blood flow proportionally reduced. There is progressive redistribution of perfusion away from the splanchnic vascular bed.[35] Loss of well-perfused hepatic tissue appears to play the major role in age-related declines in rates of drug clearance for those anesthetics and adjuvants that require hepatic biotransformation, especially those that utilize a "first-pass" mechanism.[36] The duration of the clinical effect of these intravenous agents may be further prolonged if their primary or secondary metabolites subsequently undergo renal elimination.

However, there is little qualitative change in hepatocellular function with advancing age. In normal individuals, microsomal and nonmicrosomal enzyme activity appears to be well preserved, and both microsomal and nonmicrosomal enzymatic activities, expressed per gram of hepatic tissue, are virtually the same in biopsy specimens taken from elderly as from young adults,[37] although hepatic synthesis of plasma cholinesterase is deficient in many elderly men.[38] Older women are better able to maintain their enzymatic function at levels near those seen in young adults, and are more likely than men to exhibit the smoking-induced enzyme induction that can produce enhanced rates of drug biotransformation. Although adequate to meet the requirements for normal coagulation, hepatic capacity for protein synthesis is nevertheless significantly reduced by the eighth decade of life.[39]

Normal plasma concentrations of transaminase and other hepatocyte-derived enzymes are similar to those of young adults, but the sulfobromophthalein (bromsulphalein; BSP) retention test is prolonged with increasing age, approaching the upper limit of normal in the seventh decade of life in individuals.[40] Hepatic biotransformation and protein synthesis, adequate to meet modest increases in metabolic demand, may easily be overwhelmed by the metabolic response to trauma, disease, or surgical intervention, especially if associated with arterial hypotension, low cardiac output, hypothermia, or direct hepatic injury.[41] Overt hepatic dysfunction and failure appear in about 4% of elderly surgical patients, but more subtle degrees of hepatic compromise and limited hepatic functional reserve produce many postoperative complications and may require supportive therapy and intensive care.[42]

Aging alters renal function. About 20% of renal tissue mass is lost by the eighth decade, and more than one-third of glomeruli and their associated nephron tubular structures disappear. Therefore, glomerulotubular balance is relatively well maintained; however, in 10–20% of the remaining glomeruli, sclerosis impairs effective filtration by producing dysfunctional continuity between afferent and efferent glomerular arterioles.[43] Tubular diverticuli are also common and permeability to water may be increased, compromising urinary concentrating ability. Total renal plasma flow eventually falls to about one-half of that of young adults, and there is a virtually linear decline in glomerular filtration rate (GFR) of 6–8% per decade of life during adulthood. Active tubular secretion and reabsorption of drugs and other solutes also is reduced, and the elimination half-time ($t_{1/2b}$) of virtually every anesthetic drug and metabolite normally cleared by renal mechanisms is prolonged in elderly patients, especially in those with pre-existing renal dysfunction.

Much of this age-related renal compromise is undetected by routine laboratory "screening" tests because loss of skeletal muscle mass, especially in men, significantly reduces creatinine load. Therefore, serum creatinine concentrations are the same as those of young adults. Yet even in the absence of defined or suspected renal disease, older patients have marked impairment of the ability to concentrate urine and conserve free water. Excretion of a free water load is also markedly delayed. Diminished thirst, poor diet, and the use of diuretic agents to decrease age-related hypertension also make intravascular and intracellular dehydration a more common finding of the preoperative examination of elderly patients. Thus, under normal circumstances, while there is sufficient residual renal function to avoid gross azotemia or uremia, the renal functional reserve needed to withstand imposed water and electrolyte imbalance in elderly patients is minimal.[44] Geriatric surgical patients do not appear to require a unique fluid replacement protocol, but their limited renal functional reserve requires meticulous calculation and monitoring of fluid and electrolyte balance. Acute renal failure is responsible for at least one-fifth of the perioperative mortality in elderly surgical patients.[45] Reduced renal tissue vascularity increases the risk of renal ischemia if cardiac output is depressed, especially for geriatric patients taking nonsteroidal anti-inflammatory agents. These and other cyclo-oxygenase enzyme inhibitors reduce the normal renal vasodilator activity of endogenous prostacyclin.

BODY COMPOSITION, BLOOD, AND IMMUNE FUNCTION

Age-related changes in body composition are universal, progressive, and essentially irreversible. From young adulthood through late middle age, men typically gain about 12 kg of adipose tissue but lose about 8 kg of skeletal muscle mass. Eventually, accelerating loss of muscle and atrophy of central organs combined with loss of subcutaneous fat produce a significant fall in total body weight in aged men (Fig. 60.9). In women, atrophy of lean tissue mass and bone resorption as a result of osteoporosis are essentially offset by increasing body fat. These changes in body composition reduce the basal metabolic requirements for aging patients by 10–15% compared with their young adult counterparts. The reduction in rate of body heat production and simultaneous age-related impairment of the thermosensitivity and efficiency of autonomic thermoregulation also increase the risk of inadvertent hypothermia: intraoperative decreases in core body temperature average almost 1 °C h^{-1}, about twice that observed in young adults under similar circumstances. In addition, the time needed for spontaneous rewarming postoperatively appears to increase in direct proportion to the patient's age.[46,47]

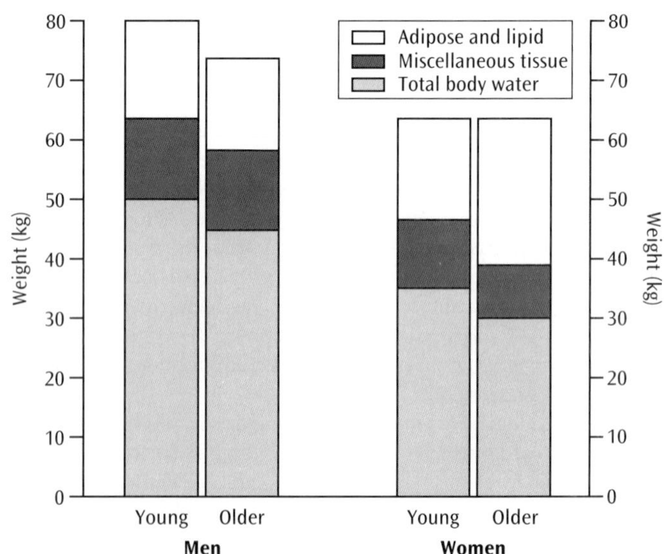

Figure 60.9 *Age-related changes in body composition are now known to be gender specific. In women, increases in body lipid actually offset osteoporosis and the loss of lean tissue mass and intracellular water, with little change in total body weight. In men, more accelerated loss of skeletal muscle mass without compensatory increase in fat produces a modest drop in total body weight by the eighth decade or later.*

Although muscle loss may be minimized by vigorous exercise and increase in body fat tempered by diet, these changes reflect the unavoidable consequences of reduced testosterone, thyroid hormone, and other endogenous modulators of tissue metabolism as much as they reflect individual lifestyle and the environment. Loss of skeletal muscle mass is also associated with progressive impairment of the ability to handle an intravenous glucose challenge, in large part because this tissue and the liver normally provide storage for carbohydrates. However, age-related glucose intolerance may be due to progressive impairment of insulin function or subtle antagonism of its effect on these target tissues. Both the timing and the magnitude of insulin release itself appear to remain normal.[48] In any case, intravenous fluid replacement using glucose-containing solutions should be limited to environments that permit frequent measurement of blood sugar levels. In older subjects of either gender, virtually all age-related changes in body water are limited to intracellular compartments. Plasma volume, red cell mass, and extracellular fluid volumes are well maintained in nonhypertensive elderly individuals who maintain adequate levels of daily physical activity.[49]

Age-related changes in body composition have a significant impact on the pharmacokinetic processes of drug elimination that occur during anesthesia. Changes in body composition influence anesthetic pharmacokinetic behavior because they increase the fraction of body mass that acts as a reservoir for lipid-soluble drug molecules. If the distribution volume of a narcotic or lipid-soluble agent is significantly enlarged, the time required for its subsequent elimination is increased even if clearance from plasma remains unchanged. If, in addition, the elimination clearance of a drug from plasma is impaired because of age-related loss of hepatic mass or reduced renal perfusion, the elimination half-life will be increased more than would be expected solely from reduced hepatic and renal drug clearance (see Chapter 2).[50] Only molecules with particularly high solubility in specialized lipid compartments such as brain and spinal cord or those with very high receptor affinities demonstrate unchanged steady-state distribution volumes when administered to elderly patients.

Despite the common observation of ecchymotic lesions on the skin of the extremities of many elderly individuals as a result of age-related increases in the fragility of cutaneous blood vessels, aging actually enhances platelet-mediated hemostasis.[51] Although stress and other factors that impair fibrinolysis may play an important etiologic role,[52,53] there are also small "prethrombotic"[54] increases in several intrinsic clotting factors that may help to explain the increased risk of pulmonary thromboembolism in the elderly surgical subpopulation.[55] In general, however, although bone marrow, spleen, and other hematopoietic reserve tissues are reduced, the effect of aging is rarely sufficient to alter either day-to-day hemostasis or the acute hematologic responses to incidental injury or mild stress. Erythropoietin levels are generally normal, but may be easily depressed by infection.[56] Standard hematologic screening tests such as hemoglobin concentration, hematocrit, and white cell count and differential are also well within the relatively wide range of "normal" values for young adults, and hemoglobin concentrations of 13.5–16.0 g dL^{-1} are considered normal.[57] Anemia, defined as a hemoglobin value less than 12 g dL^{-1}, is not a condition of aging, but is a symptom of age-related disease that is more common in older adults than in the general adult population.

In fit elderly subjects, even in the absence of disease, the older adult exhibits some general characteristics of decreased immune responsiveness (see Chapter 23).[58] The quantitative age-related change in thymic mass and the progressive alteration of thymic cellular composition both play a central role in senescence of the adaptive immune system, primarily T-lymphocyte-mediated responses.[59–61] However, aging appears to have little effect upon phagocytic activity. Older adults are particularly predisposed to streptococcal pneumonia, meningitis, and septicemia. Infection or sepsis, notoriously occult in geriatric surgical patients, is second only to cardiac failure as a cause of morbidity and mortality.

CENTRAL NERVOUS SYSTEM

Clearly, age-related changes in nervous system function have direct and important implications in the anesthetic plan for an elderly patient. Aging appears to compromise nervous system functional reserve and to alter the response to anesthetic agents and perioperative stress far more than it alters day-to-day function. Aging is associated with selective attrition of cerebral and cerebellar cortical neurons[62] and with progressive neuronal loss within certain areas of the thalamus, locus ceruleus, and basal ganglia. In normal elderly subjects, there is also a generalized reduction in neuron density.[63] Brain mass typically declines 30% by the age of 80 years, with atrophy most evident in the gray matter. The fraction of intracranial volume occupied by brain tissue falls from 92% to 82% over the same time period, with the most rapid reduction in brain mass and the greatest rate of compensatory increase in cerebrospinal fluid occurring after the sixth decade. Remaining neurons are less densely layered and have markedly simplified synaptic interconnections.[64] Aging is associated with depletion of catecholamines, serotonin, acetylcholine, and other brain neurotransmitters because of attrition of neurotransmitter-synthesizing tissues and a generally reduced rate of biochemical synthesis.[65] Transmitter destruction by endogenous synaptic catabolic enzymes, in contrast, appears to occur at an accelerated rate.

Aging produces generalized deafferentation as a result of progressive increases in the activation thresholds needed for the special sense organs responsible for vision, hearing, touch, joint position sense, smell, and peripheral pain and temperature (Fig. 60.10). Nevertheless, global integrated nervous system functions such as intelligence, personality, and memory are similar to those of young adults, although there may be moderate compromise of the "fluid" intelligence required for most tests of cognitive function or rapid retrieval of stored information.[66]

The intrinsic mechanisms by which the brain closely couples neuronal activity, metabolism, and blood flow remain grossly intact,[67] at least in the absence of disease, as does cerebrovascular responsiveness to carbon dioxide.[68] The blood–brain barrier also is functionally intact. Therefore, in healthy elderly individuals, reduced cerebral blood flow is an appropriate response to decreased cerebral metabolic demands,[69] and not, as was once believed, a manifestation of inevitable, senile "hardening of the arteries." Specific brain and spinal cord blood flow and oxygen consumption (both expressed per 100 g of brain tissue) exhibit a slight,

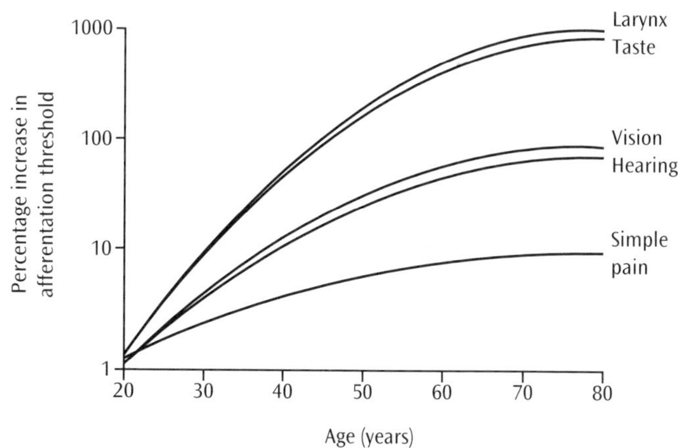

Figure 60.10 *Age-related processes of central and peripheral deafferentation produce logarithmic increases in the thresholds for virtually all sensory modalities.*

parallel decline, especially in women, and glucose utilization falls at a slightly faster rate. Overall, global or hemispheric brain blood flow reaches its maximum value in the fourth decade of life and thereafter is reduced 20–40% by the age of 80 years.[70]

Many elderly patients with impaired cognition of uncertain etiology may have hypothalamic–pituitary–adrenal axis dysregulation and elevated basal cortisol levels. In a self-enhancing cycle, aging within the central nervous system leads to selective hippocampal cell loss. Neuronal attrition in the hippocampus produces symptoms of impaired cognition as well as activation of the hypothalamic–pituitary–adrenal axis owing to removal of the hippocampal regulatory action of these responses. The resulting increase in plasma cortisol further accelerates hippocampal cell loss and perpetuates the stress–injury cycle. In fact, the change in cortisol levels over time may predict cognitive deficits in a healthy elderly population.[71] High levels of stress-related glucocorticoids produced in response to tissue injury, pain, or the psychosocial consequences of disability may actually produce or accelerate cognitive decline in aged adults in whom nervous system tissue and neurotransmitter reserve is most severely reduced.[72]

However, the most common nervous system disorders seen in a geriatric population – parkinsonism and Alzheimer's dementia – reflect specific neurotransmitter deficits. Their prevalence may be amplified by the normal processes of neurotransmitter depletion that occur with advancing years even in normal subjects. Cerebrovascular disease seems to be the most common etiology for the remainder of age-related nervous disorders: typically, 6% of the geriatric surgical population present at time of surgery with a history of cerebral vascular accident. Stroke or other neurologic ischemic phenomena account for 3% of perioperative mortality in these patients. The reduced central nervous system functional reserve of elderly patients amplifies the effects of even low residual tissue levels of anesthetic agents. Therefore, although metabolic abnormalities must be excluded, prolonged depression of consciousness, disorientation, autonomic instability, hyper-reflexia, or other manifestations of acute postoperative nervous system dysfunction in elderly patients are usually produced by the residual effects of the anesthetic drug.

PERIPHERAL AND AUTONOMIC NERVOUS SYSTEM

Older subjects experience loss of peripheral, motor, sensory, and autonomic nerve fibers and diffuse axonal "drop out," with subsequent reduction in both afferent and efferent nerve conduction velocities and some reduction in the rate of signal processing within the brainstem and spinal cord. Aging also produces a deterioration in electrical conduction along efferent motor pathways. Peripheral motor nerve conduction velocity falls[73] by approximately $0.15\,m\,s^{-1}\,year^{-1}$, and impairment of corticospinal transmission increases the time needed between intention and onset of voluntary motor activity. There is a loss of many afferent conduction pathways in the peripheral nervous system and spinal cord, and a reduced velocity and amplitude of evoked electrical potentials in those remaining.[74] Generalized and progressive deafferentation may be further accelerated by degenerative changes at specialized sense organs. For example, there is an almost exponential fall in the density of pain-sensing Meissner's corpuscles in the skin of elderly individuals.

Peripherally, impaired proximodistal protoplasmic transport of amino acids and neuropeptides within nerve axons produces disseminated neurogenic atrophy, a proliferation of muscle endplates, and upregulation of peripheral nicotinic cholinergic receptors. Thickening of the postjunctional membrane and its spread beyond the usual endplate areas because of age-related deficiency of cyclic guanosine monophosphate (GMP) also result in the generation of atypical extrajunctional cholinergic receptors.[75] This increase in number and variety of cholinergic receptors at the endplate and surrounding areas offsets the age-related decline in the number and the density of motor neuron/endplate units. Therefore, despite loss of skeletal muscle mass, dose requirements for competitive neuromuscular blocking drugs are not reduced, and, in fact, are frequently slightly increased. Neurogenic skeletal muscle atrophy also impairs dynamic strength, control, and ability to maintain steadiness of the skeletal muscles in the extremities, although isometric muscle strength appears to be well maintained.[76]

Viewed from a neuroendocrine perspective, aging can also be thought of as a progressive hyperadrenergic state. Plasma concentrations of epinephrine (adrenaline) and norepinephrine (noradrenaline) are elevated two- to fourfold, both at rest and in response to exercise-induced physical stress in elderly subjects.[77] Nevertheless, neurons in sympathoadrenal pathways, as in the rest of the peripheral nervous system, are subject to cellular attrition, and adrenal tissue mass and cortisol secretion decline at least 15% by the age of 80.[78] In elderly patients, high levels of catecholamines are rarely apparent clinically because aging also produces a marked depression of autonomic end-organ responsiveness. There is significant impairment of the ability of β-agonists to enhance the velocity and force of cardiovascular contraction[79] and general impairment of maximal chronotropic responses to isoproterenol.[80] This endogenous β-adrenergic blockade of aging may reflect simple attrition of adrenoreceptors, reduced affinity for agonist molecules, or a compromise in adenylate cyclase activation because of decreased cell membrane fluidity.[81] The demonstration of a decreased affinity of the aging β-adrenoreceptor for both agonist and antagonist molecules, however, suggests that qualitative, not quantitative, changes are predominant.

The more complex, integrated autonomic reflex responses that maintain cardiovascular and metabolic homeostasis so closely in young adults are also progressively impaired in elderly individuals. Baroreflex responsiveness, the vasoconstrictor response to cold stress, and beat-to-beat heart rate responses following postural change in elderly subjects grow progressively less rapid in onset, smaller in magnitude, and less effective in stabilizing blood pressure under a variety of circumstances.[82] The autonomic nervous system in the elderly patient is, in effect, "under-damped" and less effectively self-regulated, permitting wider variation from homeostatic set-points and delayed restabilization during stress. Therefore, anesthetic agents that disrupt end-organ function or reduce plasma catecholamines, or techniques such as spinal or epidural anesthesia that produce a rapid pharmacologic sympathectomy, are more likely to cause arterial hypotension in elderly than in young patients.[83,84] If exaggerated endogenous autonomic activity compensates for significant end-organ disease as, for example, in elderly patients with congestive heart failure, then any anesthetic-related "disintegration" of autonomic homeostasis can have abrupt, hemodynamically catastrophic consequences.

ANESTHESIA REQUIREMENTS

The age-related changes within the nervous system described above are measurable and consistent, but their net effect on consciousness and on generalized, pain-related neurologic function in healthy elderly subjects is complex and hard to predict. Anesthetic requirement under equilibrium conditions are determined by pharmacodynamics and can be quantified and compared using the concept of median effective dose (ED_{50}). Beginning in young adulthood, MAC (minimum alveolar concentration), the ED_{50} equivalent for inhalational anesthesia, declines linearly with increasing age (Fig. 60.11). Typically, an 80-year-old patient requires only two-thirds to three-quarters of the anesthetic concentration needed to produce similar effects in a young adult. This reduction in the pharmacodynamic requirement for general anesthetics is independent of the inhalational agent selected and has been observed for the newest[85] as well as for the older inhalational agents.[86,87] Therefore,

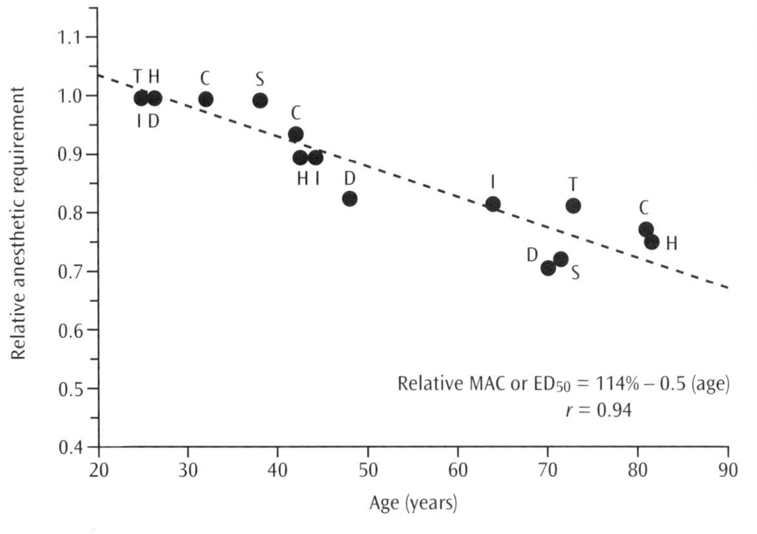

Figure 60.11 *Despite many differences in chemical structure and clinical pharmacology, relative anesthetic requirement (MAC or ED_{50}) declines both for inhalational (C, D, H, I, S) and for intravenous (T) anesthetics. The consistency of this age-related decline in unsedated human subjects suggests that it is due to a common fundamental neurophysiologic expression of aging.*

the decrease in MAC with aging probably reflects fundamental neurophysiologic changes within the brain, perhaps reduced neuron density or altered concentrations of brain neurotransmitters. Anesthetic requirement may, in fact, be a quantifiable measure of the functional reserve of the central nervous system.[88]

Some of the reported age-related changes in requirement for intravenous anesthetics may simply be the result of higher than expected initial plasma concentrations of these drugs during the early phases of their redistribution from plasma to body tissues.[89] Thus, the reduced bolus dose requirements for intravenous agents such as thiopental[90] may be explained, in least in part, by age-related early or "alpha-phase" pharmacokinetic changes rather than by pharmacodynamic factors.[91] However, other studies of the relation between drug effect and plasma concentration for benzodiazepines and for the effects of near steady-state infusions of narcotics and propofol also support the concept that aging alters the pharmacodynamic responses of elderly individuals. The reduction in anesthetic requirement is similar to that observed for inhalational agents.[92]

The classic two- and three-compartment models used for pharmacokinetic analysis of intravenous anesthetics have also been less predictive of actual clinical responses of older subjects than had been hoped,[93] leading to extensive re-evaluation of assumptions that age simply alters the size of the "lipophilic" and "hydrophilic" drug disposition volumes.[94] Classic pharmacokinetic parameters such as elimination clearance may have less to do with the termination of clinical drug effects than was once assumed. Drugs such as fentanyl,[95] thiopental,[96] and propofol[97] behave as short-acting anesthetics in both younger and older adults because their clinical effects are dissipated initially not by elimination but by redistribution to other sites within the body. Modification of traditional pharmacokinetic compartment models with emphasis upon altered rates of transfer between compartments, rather than the size or the number of the compartments themselves, may be needed for inhalational[98] as well as for intravenous agents to provide more accurate predictions of drug dispositions in elderly subjects (see Chapter 2). The mechanism of altered rates of intercompartmental transfer is presently unknown.

The elderly patient has long been known to have decreased segmental dose requirements for local anesthetics during epidural analgesia.[99] This may reflect arteriosclerotic changes in the anatomy of the epidural space, but higher sensory levels also occur in spinal anesthesia when a fixed drug dose and volume protocol is followed. This suggests age-related impairment of the clearance of drug from the intrathecal or the epidural space.[100–102] In any case, the role of amplification, modulation, and selectivity of afferent input within the spinal cord, thalamus, and perhaps at other locations within the aging nervous system has yet to be studied adequately to permit broad generalizations regarding aging and susceptibility to pain.[103] Clinical evidence actually suggests that elderly patients, especially women,[104] have elevated thresholds for discrete and superficial discomfort,[105] but are more vulnerable and sensitive to severe or visceral pain if it is associated with protracted illness or the prospect of debilitation.

The dosages of classic competitive drugs such as curare, pancuronium, vecuronium, or atracurium needed to produce initial nondepolarizing neuromuscular blockade have been shown to be either virtually unchanged or increased only slightly in the elderly patient.[106] These pharmacodynamic requirements reflect the quality and quantity of cholinoceptor dynamics at the neuromuscular junction, not skeletal muscle mass itself. Cholinoceptor upregulation appears to offset declining prejunctional acetylcholine mobilization. The duration of neuromuscular blockade, however, is significantly prolonged for those drugs that are dependent upon organ-based elimination because clearance declines dramatically with increasing age.[107] The exceptions to this pattern are atracurium and cisatracurium – drugs that undergo spontaneous organ-independent hydrolysis in plasma at rates indistinguishable from those in young adults.[108] The dynamics and the efficacy of antagonism or "reversal" of nondepolarizing neuromuscular blockade by neostigmine are also essentially unchanged.[109] For any given level of pre-existing neuromuscular blockade, the choice of reversal agent, and not patient age, determines the speed and the completeness of recovery of neuromuscular transmission.

DECISION-MAKING, RECOVERY, AND OUTCOME

With increasing numbers of elderly surgical patients has come better understanding and awareness of the need for review of the basic principles of patient autonomy and self-determination in medical decision-making, including the right to refuse treatment or resuscitation. There is no basis for a general assumption that the elderly patient is less competent to make these often difficult decisions than is his young adult counterpart, but advanced directives can do much to eliminate ambiguity with regard to establishing a patient's wishes and, thereby, determine the course of acute hospitalization and subsequent healthcare options. Physicians and other healthcare providers are not only wise to consider these issues carefully but also are ethically bound to individualize their actions based on each patient's expressed or implied requests, but must of course not break the law.

Overall, perioperative morbidity and mortality begins to increase progressively during the years that follow young adulthood and somatic maturity. Eventually, the likelihood of adverse outcome becomes three- to fourfold that of young adult surgical patients.[110] The factors that make mortality more common in older patients than in young adults are complex and inter-related. Much of this increase is due to the high prevalence of disease seen in every elderly patient cohort.[111,112] In fact, site of surgery and the severity of pre-existing disease as assessed by physical status remain far more powerful predictors of surgical complications than does age itself (Figs 60.12 and 60.13).[113,114]

Therefore, there is probably no patient who should be considered "too old" for surgery. However, clinical experience with increasing numbers of octogenarian,[115–117] nonagenarian, and even older[118,119] geriatric patients needing surgery has made it apparent that, at this end of the geriatric spectrum, the continuing erosion of organ system functional reserve by processes of aging may be associated with a doubling of perioperative risk for a wide variety of surgical procedures. Preoperative malnutrition or hypoalbuminemia, or the development of a negative protein balance perioperatively, may also have predictive value with regard to surgical mortality for elderly patients. The metabolic response of elderly patients to tissue injury is sluggish. Ability to ambulate promptly after surgery and overall aerobic capacity are fundamental determinants of uncomplicated surgical recovery, but these cannot be achieved in older adults simply by giving injections of growth hormone or increasing parenteral protein replacement.[120]

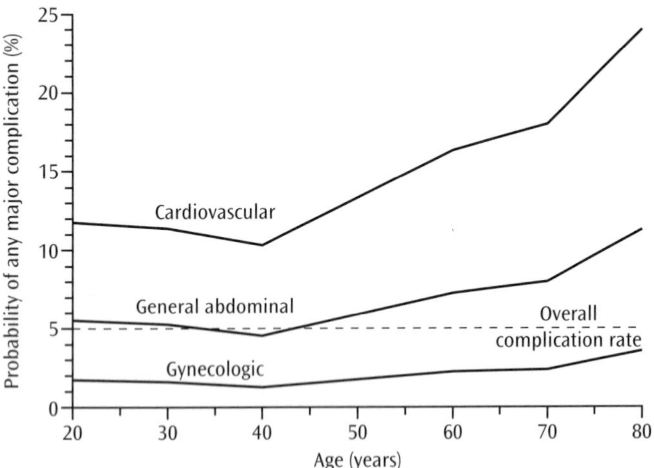

Figure 60.12 *Even more for the elderly surgical patient than for his younger counterpart, the site of surgery is a primary determinant of the probability of major perioperative morbidity. Prospective study of almost 14 000 patients undergoing elective surgery suggests that complications from gynecologic procedures occur less frequently than the average for all surgeries (broken line) well into the geriatric era, but cardiovascular and upper abdominal surgery produce a progressively greater probability of major complications in older adults.*

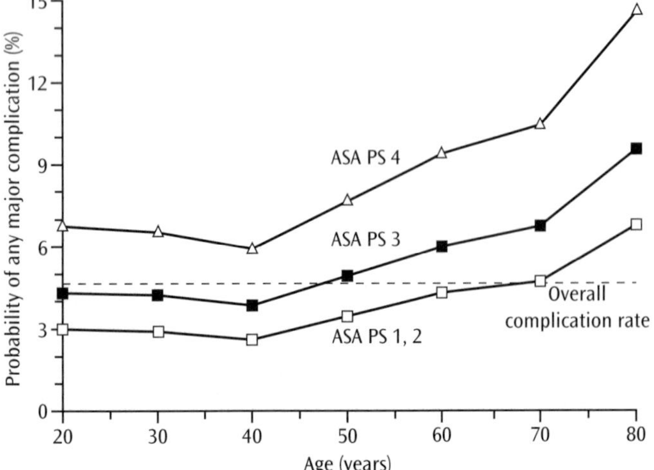

Figure 60.13 *The probability of a severe cardiovascular or pulmonary adverse outcome, estimated prospectively from a large series of surgical patients, is more dependent upon physical status (PS) than upon age.*

All anesthetic techniques are appropriate and in widespread use for geriatric surgical patients. None appears to have general advantages for the elderly surgical patient with regard to survival.[121] Some approaches such as regional anesthesia for hip surgery are associated with specific benefits such as reduction of thromboembolism.[122–125] However, even for outpatient surgery, when rapid ambulation and prompt recovery is essential, careful and appropriate general anesthesia is a safe and widely practiced anesthetic option. The use of newer intravenous agents such as remifentanil[126,127] and cisatracurium[128] minimize dependence upon organ system functional reserve for drug elimination, and inhalation agents such as sevoflurane provide very rapid recovery of consciousness even in the aged adult. Numerous retrospective and prospective clinical studies have arrived at the same conclusion: there are no significant differences in perioperative survival or major morbidity that are attributable directly to the choice of anesthetic agents or to the anesthetic technique selected.

Local anesthesia or regional techniques performed without intravenous sedation may significantly improve postoperative mental function immediately after surgery,[129,130] although nerve palsies, residual paresthesiae, and other neuropraxias associated with regional anesthesia are more common in older than in young adults.[131,132] There appear to be no significant differences in the incidences of many common minor neurologic sequelae of general anesthesia such as nausea and vomiting, myalgia, or dizziness, although a greater fraction of elderly patients demonstrate prolonged postoperative confusion following anesthesia than do their younger counterparts.[133] Even when anesthetic management is appropriate and surgical convalescence uncomplicated, the return of cognitive function to preoperative levels after a prolonged general anesthetic may require 5–10 days.

It is of greater concern that recently published findings show that psychometrically defined postoperative cognitive dysfunction is a measurable adverse outcome 3 months after otherwise uncomplicated surgery in 10–15% of patients 60 years of age or older who have had major procedures and a hospital stay of 4 or more days.[134] This suggests that, at least in older adults with reduced central nervous system functional reserve, either the process of general anesthesia or the drugs used to produce narcosis may have sufficient short-term effects upon the metabolic and neurotransmitter functions of neuronal tissue to produce neurologic injury. However, perioperative environmental factors such as chronic medication and drug interaction,[135] disorientation due to sensory deprivation,[136] or the disruption of normal routine needed to maintain "implicit" memory may also explain the high incidence of postoperative cognitive impairment in older surgical patients. There is also extensive neuroendocrine and sympathoadrenal stress produced by major surgery and tissue injury.

Therefore, surgical procedures in the elderly require a disproportionately large share of societal and institutional healthcare resources. Routine postoperative hospitalization and intensive care, especially after major trauma, are frequently protracted and may be complicated by infection, poor wound healing, and, in critically ill elderly patients, by multiple organ system failure. Aged skin and bones are fragile, joints are stiff, and the range of motion is limited, so the physical management of even fit elderly patients requires special attention, and extended rehabilitation may be required to permit discharge from hospital. Bleeding diatheses, hypercoagulable states,[137] and bacterial infection[138] are more likely in older than in younger adults if stress responses are sustained during a difficult recovery.

An anesthetic plan that includes suppression of neuroendocrine stress with an α_2-adrenergic agonist such as dexmedetomidine or clonidine[139] or a postoperative epidural for sympathectomy[140] and analgesia[141] may be of value. This agent may accelerate rewarming,[142] promote healing,[143] reduce cardiovascular and pulmonary demands, and eliminate the long periods of stress due to inadequate analgesia because of unrealistic fears of narcotic side-effects.

REFERENCES

1. Schneider EL, Rowe JW (eds). *Handbook of the Biology of Aging*, 3rd edn. San Diego: Academic Press, 1990: 439.
2. Nascher IL. *Geriatrics. NY Med J* 1909; **90:** 358–9.
3. Rowe JW, Andres R, Tobin JD, *et al*. The effect of age on creatinine clearance in men: a cross-sectional and longitudinal study. *J Gerontol* 1976; **31:** 155–63.
4. Louis TA, Robins J, Dockery DW, *et al*. Explaining discrepancies between longitudinal and cross-sectional models. *J Chron Dis* 1986; **39:** 831–9.
5. Xu X, Laird N, Dockery DW, *et al*. Age, period, and cohort effects on pulmonary function in a 24-year longitudinal study. *Am J Epidemiol* 1995; **141:** 554–66.
6. Schneider EL, Reed Jr JD. Life extension. *N Engl J Med* 1985; **312:** 1159–68.
7. Hayflick L. The biology of human aging. *Am J Med Sci* 1973; **265:** 433–45.
8. Schneider EL. Aging processes. In: Abrams WB, Beers MH, Berkow R (eds). *The Merck Manual of Geriatrics*, 2nd edn. Whitehouse Station, NJ: Merck and Co., 1995: 419–24.
9. Linnane AW, Marzuki S, Ozawa T, Tanaka M. Mitochondrial DNA mutations as an important contributor to ageing and degenerative diseases. *Lancet* 1989; **1:** 642–5.
10. Yu BP (ed.). *Free Radicals in Aging*. Boca Raton, FL: CRC Press, 1993: 303.
11. Ozawa T. Genetic and functional changes in mitochondria associated with aging. *Physiol Rev* 1997; **77:** 425–64.
12. Jazwinski SM. Longevity, genes, and aging. *Science* 1996; **273:** 54–9.
13. Sohal RS, Weindruch R. Oxidative stress, caloric restriction, and aging. *Science* 1996; **273:** 59–63.
14. Bailey AJ, Robins SP, Balian G. Biological significance of the crosslinks of collagen. *Nature (Lond)* 1974; **251:** 105–9.
15. Muravchick S. *Geroanesthesia: Perioperative Management of the Elderly Patient*. Chicago: Mosby-Year Book Medical Publishers, 1997: 306.
16. Prause G, Ratzenhofer-Komenda B, Smolle-Juettner F, *et al*. Operations on patients deemed "unfit for operation and anaesthesia:" what are the consequences? *Acta Anaesth Scand* 1998; **42:** 316–22.
17. Golub R, Cantu R, Sorrento JJ, Stein DH. Efficacy of preadmission testing in ambulatory surgical patients. *Am J Surg* 1992; **163:** 565–71.
18. Schechter BM, Erwin WG, Gerbino PP. The role of the pharmacist. In: Abrams WB, Berkow R (eds). *The Merck Manual of Geriatrics*. Rahway, NJ: Merck Sharp & Dohme, 1990: 193–9.
19. Larson EB, Kukull WA, Buchner D, Reifler BV. Adverse drug reactions associated with global cognitive impairment in elderly persons. *Ann Intern Med* 1987; **107:** 169–73.
20. Rodeheffer RJ, Gerstenblith G, Becker LC, *et al*. Exercise cardiac output is maintained with advancing age in healthy human subjects: cardiac dilatation and increased stroke volume compensate for diminished heart rate. *Circulation* 1984; **69:** 203–13.
21. Tzankoff SP, Norris AH. Effect of muscle mass decrease on age-related BMR changes. *J Appl Physiol* 1977; **43:** 1001–6.
22. Aronow WS, Stein PD, Sabbah HN, Koenigsberg M. Resting left ventricular ejection fraction in elderly patients without evidence of heart disease. *Am J Cardiol* 1989; **63:** 368–9.
23. Duke PC, Wade JG, Hickey RF, Larson CP. The effects of age on baroreceptor reflex function in man. *Can Anesth Soc J* 1976; **23:** 111–24.
24. Folkow B, Svanborg A. Physiology of cardiovascular aging. *Physiol Rev* 1993; **73:** 725–64.
25. Bryg RJ, Williams GA, Labovitz AJ. Effect of aging on left ventricular diastolic filling in normal subjects. *Am J Cardiol* 1987; **59:** 971–74.
26. Wei JY. Age and the cardiovascular system. *N Engl J Med* 1992; **327:** 1735–9.
27. Cohn JE, Donoso HD. Mechanical properties of lung in normal men over 60 years old. *J Clin Invest* 1963; **42:** 1406–10.
28. Mittman C, Edelman NH, Norris AH, Shock NW. Relationship between chest wall and pulmonary compliance and age. *J Appl Physiol* 1965; **20:** 1211–16.
29. Wahba WM. Influence of aging on lung function – clinical significance of changes from age twenty. *Anesth Analg* 1983; **62:** 764–76.
30. Peterson DD, Pack AI, Silage DA, Fishman AP. Effects of aging on ventilatory and occlusion pressure responses to hypoxia and hypercapnia. *Am Rev Resp Dis* 1981; **124:** 387–91.
31. Kaiko RF, Wallenstein SL, Rogers AG. Narcotics in the elderly. *Med Clin North Am* 1982; **66:** 1079–89.
32. Bailey PL, Wilbrink J, Zwanikken P, *et al*. Anesthetic induction with fentanyl. *Anesth Analg* 1985; **64:** 48–53.
33. Pontoppidan H, Beecher HK. Progressive loss of protective reflexes in the airway with the advance of age. *JAMA* 1960; **174:** 2209–13.
34. Kitamura H, Sawa T, Ikezono E. Postoperative hypoxemia: the contribution of age to the maldistribution of ventilation. *Anesthesiology* 1972; **36:** 244–52.
35. Geokas MC, Haverback BJ. The aging gastrointestinal tract. *Am J Surg* 1969; **117:** 881–92.
36. Wilkinson GR, Shand DG. A physiological approach to hepatic drug clearance. *Clin Pharmacol Ther* 1975; **18:** 377–90.
37. Woodhouse KW, Mutch E, Williams FM, *et al*. The effect of age on pathways of drug metabolism in human liver. *Age Aging* 1984; **13:** 328–34.
38. Shanor SP, Van Hees GR, Baart N, *et al*. The influence of age and sex on human plasma and red cell cholinesterase. *Am J Med Sci* 1961; **242:** 357–61.
39. Kampmann JP, Sinding J, Moller-Jorgensen I. Effect of age on liver function. *Geriatrics* 1975; **30:** 91–5.
40. Thompson EN, Williams R. Effect of age on liver function with particular reference to bromsulphalein excretion. *Gut* 1965; **6:** 266–9.
41. Young VR, Steffee WP, Pencharz PB, *et al*. Total human body protein synthesis in relation to protein requirements at various ages. *Nature* 1975; **253:** 192–4.
42. Carli F, Emery PW, Freemantle CAJ. Effect of perioperative normothermia on postoperative protein metabolism in elderly patients undergoing hip arthroplasty. *Br J Anaesth* 1989; **63:** 276–82.
43. McLachlan MSF. The ageing kidney. *Lancet* 1978; **2:** 143–6.
44. Rowe JW, Shock NW, DeFronzo R. The influence of age on the renal response to water deprivation in man. *Nephron* 1976; **17:** 270–8.
45. Kumar R, Hill CM, McGeown MG. Acute renal failure in the elderly. *Lancet* 1973; **1:** 90–1.
46. Morrison RC. Hypothermia in the elderly. *Int Anesthesiol Clin* 1988; **26:** 124–33.
47. Frank SM, Beattie C, Christopherson R, *et al*. Epidural versus general anesthesia, ambient operating room temperature, and patient age as predictors of inadvertent hypothermia. *Anesthesiology* 1992; **77:** 252–7.
48. Davidson MB. The effect of aging on carbohydrate metabolism: a review of the English literature and a practical approach to the diagnosis of diabetes in the elderly. *Metabolism* 1979; **28:** 688–705.
49. Fulop Jr T, Worum I, Csongor J, *et al*. Body composition in elderly people. *Gerontology* 1985; **31:** 6–14.
50. Richey DP, Bender AD. Pharmacokinetic consequences of aging. *Annu Rev Pharmacol Toxicol* 1977; **17:** 49–65.
51. Yokoyama M, Kusui A, Sakamoto S, Fukuzaki H. Age-associated increments in human platelet alpha-adrenoceptor capacity; possible mechanism for platelet hyperactivity to epinephrine in aging man. *Thromb Res* 1984; **34:** 287–95.
52. Dormandy JA, Edelman JB. High blood viscosity: an aetiological factor in venous thrombosis. *Br J Surg* 1973; **60:** 187–90.
53. Britton B, Hawkey C, Wood W, Peele M. Stress – a significant factor in venous thrombosis? *Br J Surg* 1974; **61:** 814–20.
54. Currie MS, Rao MK, Blazer DG, Cohen HJ. Age and functional correlations of markers of coagulation and inflammation in the elderly: functional implications of elevated crosslinked fibrin degradation products. *J Am Geriatr Soc* 1994; **42:** 738–42.
55. Kakkar VV. Diagnosis, prevention, and treatment of venous thromboembolism. *Int Anesthesiol Clin* 1985; **23:** 157–72.
56. Joosten E, Van Hove L, Lesaffre E, *et al*. Serum erythropoietin levels in elderly inpatients with anemia of chronic disorders and iron deficiency anemia. *J Am Geriatr Soc* 1993; **41:** 1301–4.

57. Zauber NP, Zauber AG. Hematologic data of healthy very old people. *JAMA* 1987; **257:** 2181–4.
58. Miller RA. The aging immune system: primer and prospectus. *Science* 1996; **273:** 70–4.
59. Hirokawa K, Makinodan T. Thymic involution: effect on T-cell differentiation. *J Immunol* 1975; **114:** 1659–64.
60. Sparrow D, Silbert JE, Rowe JW. The influence of age on peripheral lymphocyte count in men: a cross-sectional and longitudinal study. *J Gerontol* 1980; **35:** 163–6.
61. Stoy PJ, Roitman-Johnson B, Walsh G, *et al.* Aging and serum immunoglobin E levels, immediate skin tests, and RAST. *J Allergy Clin Immunol* 1981; **68:** 421–6.
62. Devaney KO, Johnson HA. Neuron loss in the aging visual cortex of man. *J Gerontol* 1980; **35:** 836–41.
63. Katzman R, Terry RD. Normal aging of the central nervous system. In: Katzman R, Terry RD (eds). *The Neurology of Aging.* Philadelphia: FA Davis, 1983: 15–50.
64. Feldman ML. Aging changes in the morphology of cortical dendrites. In: Terry RD, Gershon S (eds). *Neurobiology of Aging.* New York: Raven Press, 1976: 211–27.
65. McGeer EG, McGeer PL. Age changes in the human for some enzymes associated with metabolism of catecholamines, GABA, and acetylcholine. *Adv Behav Biol* 1975; **16:** 287–305.
66. Macht ML, Buschke H. Speed of recall in aging. *J Gerontol* 1984; **39:** 439–43.
67. Lassen NA, Ingvar DH, Skinhoj E. Brain function and blood flow. *Sci Am* 1978; **239:** 62–71.
68. Yamamoto M, Meyer JS, Sakai F, Yamaguchi F. Aging and cerebral vasodilator response to hypercarbia. *Arch Neurol* 1980; **37:** 489–96.
69. Creasey H, Rapoport SI. The aging human brain. *Ann Neurol* 1985; **17:** 2–10.
70. Kety SS. Human cerebral blood flow and oxygen consumption as related to aging. *J Chron Dis* 1956; **3:** 478–86.
71. Meaney MJ, O'Donnell D, Rowe W, *et al.* Individual differences in hypothalamic-pituitary-adrenal activity in later life and hippocampal aging. *Exp Gerontol* 1995; **30:** 229–51.
72. O'Brien JT. The "glucocorticoid cascade" hypothesis in man: prolonged stress may cause permanent brain damage. *Br J Psychiatry* 1997; **170:** 199–201.
73. Dorfman LJ, Bosley TM. Age-related changes in peripheral and central nerve conduction in man. *Neurology* 1979; **29:** 38–44.
74. Beck EC, Dustman RE, Schenkenberg T. Life span changes in the electrical activity of the human brain as reflected in the cerebral evoked response. *Adv Behav Biol* 1975; **16:** 175–92.
75. Betz H, Changeux JP. Regulation of muscle acetylcholine receptor synthesis in vitro by cyclic nucleotide derivatives. *Nature* 1979; **278:** 5706.
76. Larsson L. Morphological and functional characteristics of the ageing skeletal muscle in man. *Acta Physiol Scand* 1978; **457** (Suppl.): 1–36.
77. Ziegler MG, Lake CR, Kopin IJ. Plasma noradrenaline increases with age. *Nature* 1976; **261:** 333–4.
78. Kaack B, Ordy JM, Trapp B. Changes in limbic, neuroendocrine and autonomic systems, adaptation, and homeostasis during aging. *Adv Behav Biol* 1975; **16:** 209–31.
79. Guarnieri T, Filburn CR, Zitnik G, Lakatta EG. Contractile and biochemical correlates of beta-adrenergic stimulation of the aged heart. *Am J Physiol* 1980; **239:** H501–8.
80. Vestal RE, Wood AJJ, Shand DG. Reduced adrenoceptor sensitivity in the elderly. *Clin Pharmacol Ther* 1979; **26:** 181–6.
81. Dax EM. Receptors and associated membrane events in aging. *Rev Biol Res Aging* 1985; **2:** 315–36.
82. Collins KJ, Exton-Smith AN, James MH. Functional changes in autonomic nervous responses with aging. *Age Aging* 1980; **9:** 17–24.
83. Coe AJ, Revanas B. Is crystalloid preloading useful in spinal anaesthesia in the elderly? *Anaesthesia* 1990; **45:** 241–3.
84. Carpenter RL, Caplan RA, Brown DL, *et al.* Incidence and risk factors for side effects of spinal anesthesia. *Anesthesiology* 1992; **76:** 906–16.
85. Nakajima R, Nakajima Y, Ikeda K. Minimum alveolar concentration of sevoflurane in elderly patients. *Br J Anaesth* 1993; **70:** 273–5.
86. Gregory GA, Eger II EI, Munson ES. The relationship between age and halothane requirement in man. *Anesthesiology* 1969; **30:** 488–91.
87. Rampil IJ, Lockhart SH, Zwass MS, *et al.* Clinical characteristics of desflurane in surgical patients: minimum alveolar concentrations. *Anesthesiology* 1991; **74:** 429–33.
88. Muravchick S. Immediate and long-term nervous system effects of anesthesia in elderly patients. *Clin Anesthesiol* 1986; **4:** 1035–45.
89. Avram MJ, Krejcie TC, Henthorn TK. The relationship of age to the pharmacokinetics of early drug distribution: the concurrent disposition of thiopental and indocyanine green. *Anesthesiology* 1990; **72:** 403–11.
90. Muravchick S. Effect of age and premedication on thiopental sleep dose. *Anesthesiology* 1984; **61:** 333–6.
91. Arden JR, Holley FO, Stanski DR. Increased sensitivity to etomidate in the elderly: initial distribution versus altered brain response. *Anesthesiology* 1986; **65:** 19–27.
92. Scott JC, Stanski DR. Decreased fentanyl and alfentanil dose requirements with increasing age. A simultaneous pharmacokinetic and pharmacodynamic evaluation. *J Pharmacol Exp Ther* 1987; **240:** 159–65.
93. Hull CJ. How far can we go with compartmental models? *Anesthesiology* 1990; **72:** 399–402.
94. Homer TD, Stanski DR. The effect of increasing age on thiopental disposition and anesthetic requirement. *Anesthesiology* 1985; **62:** 714–24.
95. Singleton MA, Rosen JI, Fisher DM. Pharmacokinetics of fentanyl in the elderly. *Br J Anaesth* 1988; **60:** 619–22.
96. Stanski DR, Maitre PO. Population pharmacokinetics and pharmacodynamics of thiopental: the effect of age revisited. *Anesthesiology* 1990; **72:** 412–22.
97. Kirkpatrick T, Cockshott ID, Douglas EJ, Nimmo WS. Pharmacokinetics of propofol (Diprivan) in elderly patients. *Br J Anaesth* 1988; **60:** 146–50.
98. Strum DP, Eger II EI, Unadkat JD, *et al.* Age affects the pharmacokinetics of inhaled anesthetics in humans. *Anesth Analg* 1991; **73:** 310–18.
99. Bromage PR. Ageing and epidural dose requirements. Segmental spread and predictability of epidural analgesia in youth and extreme age. *Br J Anaesth* 1969; **41:** 1016–22.
100. Sharrock NE. Epidural dose responses in patients 20 to 80 years old. *Anesthesiology* 1978; **49:** 425–8.
101. Veering BT, Burm AGL, Vletter AA, *et al.* The effect of age on systemic absorption and systemic disposition of bupivacaine after subarachnoid administration. *Anesthesiology* 1991; **74:** 250–7.
102. Cameron AE, Arnold RW, Ghoris MW, Jamieson V. Spinal analgesia using bupivacaine 0.5% plain: variation in the extent of block with patient age. *Anaesthesia* 1981; **36:** 318–22.
103. Harkins SW, Chapman CR. Detection and decision factors in pain perception in young and elderly men. *Pain* 1976; **2:** 253–8.
104. Hapidou EG, DeCatanzaro D. Responsiveness to laboratory pain in women as a function of age and childbirth pain experience. *Pain* 1992; **48:** 177–81.
105. Procacci P, Bozza G, Buzzelli G, Della Corte M. The cutaneous pricking pain threshold in old age. *Gerontol Clin* 1970; **12:** 213–18.
106. Shanks CA. Pharmacokinetics of the nondepolarizing neuromuscular relaxants applied to calculation of bolus and infusion dosage regimens. *Anesthesiology* 1986; **64:** 72–86.
107. McLoed K, Hull CJ, Watson MJ. Effects of ageing on the pharmacokinetics of pancuronium. *Br J Anaesth* 1979; **51:** 435–8.
108. Sarooshian SS, Stafford MA, Eastwood NB, *et al.* Pharmacokinetics and pharmacodynamics of cisatracurium in young and elderly adult patients. *Anesthesiology* 1996; **84:** 1083–91.
109. Muravchick S. Age does not change the dynamics of atracurium reversal. *Anesthesiology* 1990; **73** (Suppl.): A384.
110. Filzwieser G, List WF. Morbidity and mortality in elective geriatric surgery. In: Lunn JN, Mushin WW (eds). *Mortality Associated with Anaesthesia.* London: Nuffield Provincial Hospital Trusts, 1982: 75–82.
111. Pedersen T, Eliasen K, Henriksen E. A prospective study of mortality associated with anaesthesia and surgery: risk indicators of mortality in hospital. *Acta Anaesthesiol Scand* 1990; **34:** 176–82.
112. Lewin I, Lerner AG, Green SH, *et al.* Physical class and physiologic status in the prediction of operative mortality in the aged sick. *Ann Surg* 1971; **174:** 217–31.
113. Marx GF, Mateo CV, Orkin LR. Computer analysis of postanesthetic deaths. *Anesthesiology* 1973; **39:** 54–8.
114. Forrest JB, Rehder K, Cahalan MK, Goldsmith CH. Multicenter study of general anesthesia. III. Predictors of severe perioperative adverse outcomes. *Anesthesiology* 1992; **76:** 3–15.
115. Salomon NW, Page US, Bigelow JC, *et al.* Coronary artery bypass grafting in elderly patients; comparative results in a consecutive series of 469 patients older than 75 years. *J Thorac Cardiovasc Surg* 1991; **101:** 209–17.
116. Plecha FR, Bertin VJ, Plecha EJ, *et al.* The early results of vascular surgery in patients 75 years of age and older: an analysis of 3259 cases. *J Vasc Surg* 1985; **2:** 769–74.
117. Elayda MA, Hall RJ, Reul RM, *et al.* Aortic valve replacement in patients 80 years of age and older; operative risks and long-term results. *Circulation* 1993; **88** (Part II): 11–6.
118. Cohen JR, Johnson H, Eaton S, *et al.* Surgical procedures in patients during the tenth decade of life. *Surgery* 1988; **104:** 646–51.
119. Whittle J, Steinberg EP, Anderson GF, *et al.* Mortality after elective total hip arthroplasty in elderly Americans; age, gender, and indication for surgery predict survival. *Clin Orthop Rel Res* 1993; **295:** 119–26.

120. Clevenger FW, Rodriguez DJ, Demarest GB, *et al*. Protein and energy tolerance by stressed geriatric patients. *J Surg Res* 1992; **52:** 135–9.
121. Sutcliffe AJ, Parker M. Mortality after spinal and general anaesthesia for surgical fixation of hip fractures. *Anaesthesia* 1994; **49:** 237–40.
122. Wickstrom I, Holmberg I, Stefansson T. Survival of female geriatric patients after hip fracture surgery: a comparison of 5 anaesthetic methods. *Acta Anaesthesiol Scand* 1982; **26:** 607–14.
123. Valentin N, Lomholt B, Jensen JS, *et al*. Spinal or general anaesthesia for surgery of the fractured hip? *Br J Anaesth* 1986; **58:** 284–91.
124. Davis FM, Woolner DF, Frampton C, *et al*. Prospective, multi-centre trial of mortality following general or spinal anaesthesia for hip fracture surgery in the elderly. *Br J Anaesth* 1987; **59:** 1080–8.
125. Hole A, Terjesen T, Breivik H. Epidural versus general anaesthesia for total hip arthroplasty in elderly patients. *Acta Anaesthesiol Scand* 1980; **24:** 279–87.
126. Westmoreland CL, Hoke JF, Sebel PS, *et al*. Pharmacokinetics of remifentanil (GI87084B) and its major metabolite (GI90291) in patients undergoing elective inpatient surgery. *Anesthesiology* 1993; **79:** 893–903.
127. Minto CF, Schnider TW, Egan TD, *et al*. Influence of age and gender on the pharmacokinetics and pharmacodynamics of remifentanil. *Anesthesiology* 1997; **86:**10–23.
128. Wright PMC, Ornstein E. Pharmacokinetics, pharmacodynamics and safety of cisatracurium in elderly patients. *Curr Opin Anaesth* 1996; **9** (Suppl 1.): S30–S33.
129. Chung F, Meier R, Lautenschlager E, *et al*. General or spinal anesthesia: which is better in the elderly? *Anesthesiology* 1987; **67:** 422–7.
130. Chung FF, Chung A, Meier RH, *et al*. Comparison of perioperative mental function after general anaesthesia and spinal anaesthesia with intravenous sedation. *Can J Anaesth* 1989; **36:** 382–7.
131. Hampl KF, Heinzmann-Wiedmer S, Luginbuehl I, *et al*. Transient neurologic symptoms after spinal anesthesia. *Anesthesiology* 1998; **88:** 629–33.
132. Martinez-Bourio R, Arzuaza M, Quintana JM, *et al*. Incidence of transient neurologic symptoms after hyperbaric subarachnoid anesthesia with 5% lidocaine and 5% prilocaine. *Anesthesiology* 1998; **88:** 624–8.
133. Tzabar Y, Asbury AJ, Millar K. Cognitive failures after general anaesthesia for day-case surgery. *Br J Anaesth* 1996; **76:** 194–7.
134. Moller JT, ISOPCD Investigators. Long-term postoperative cognitive dysfunction in the elderly: ISPOCD1 study. *Lancet* 1998; **351:** 857–61.
135. Jolles J, Verhey FR, Riedel WJ, Houx PJ. Cognitive impairment in elderly people; predisposing factors and implications for experimental drug studies. *Drugs Aging* 1995; **7:** 459–79.
136. O'Keefe ST, Ni Conchubhair A. Postoperative delirium in the elderly. *Br J Anaesth* 1994; **73:** 673–87.
137. Yardumian A, Machin SJ. Hypercoagulable states. *Int Anesthesiol Clin* 1985; **23:** 141–55.
138. Harbrecht PJ, Garrison RN, Fry DE. Role of infection in increased mortality associated with age in laparotomy. *Am Surg* 1983; **49:** 173–8.
139. Ghignone M, Noe C, Calvillo O, Quintin L. Anesthesia for ophthalmic surgery in the elderly: the effects of clonidine on intraocular pressure, perioperative hemodynamics, and anesthetic requirement. *Anesthesiology* 1988; **68:** 707–16.
140. Stefansson T, Wickstrom I, Haljame H. Effect of neurolept and epidural analgesia on cardiovascular function and metabolism in the geriatric patient. *Acta Anaesthesiol Scand* 1982; **26:** 386–92.
141. Ready LB, Loper KA, Nessly M, Wild L. Postoperative epidural morphine is safe on surgical wards. *Anesthesiology* 1991; **75:** 452–6.
142. Carli F, Gabrielczyk M, Clark MM, Aber VR. An investigation of factors affecting postoperative rewarming of adult patients. *Anaesthesia* 1986; **41:** 363–9.
143. Kiecolt-Glaser JK, Marucha PT, Malarkey WB, *et al*. Slowing of wound healing by psychological stress. *Lancet* 1995; **346:** 1194–6.

61

Anesthesia for organ transplantation

LEONARD L FIRESTONE AND SUSAN FIRESTONE

Transplantation is now a routine part of clinical practice. Bone, tendon, cartilage, and fascia were used early on to provide a relatively inert framework for healthy native cells. Cornea, blood vessels, heart valves, and certain endocrine tissues appear to be, to some extent, immunologically isolated and therefore can successfully be transplanted. Bone marrow is used to replace the hematopoietic system. More recently, transplantation of parenchymous, vascularized organs, including the kidneys, liver, heart, and lungs, has finally achieved the status of preferred therapeutic option for end-stage visceral disease. Anesthesiologists involved in transplantation provide care for organ donors, prospective recipients, or transplant patients who require further surgery. To do so competently, specialized knowledge is required in a diversity of disciplines such as transplantation immunology, organ preservation, biomedical ethics, and the physiology of brain death.

ANESTHESIA CARE OF ORGAN DONORS

In the USA, most organs for transplantation are derived from brain-dead donors through voluntary programs established by state and federal law. Some states have also enacted "required request" legislation, obliging hospital personnel to ask the family of a brain-dead patient to grant permission for organ donation. In the USA, organs are distributed through a nationwide organ and transplantation network developed, under federal contract, by the United Network for Organ Sharing (UNOS). UNOS is also responsible for collecting data, reporting statistics, and educating the public about organ donation and transplantation.[1]

Brain death is usually a consequence of catastrophic neurologic injury after blunt head trauma (most often from motor vehicle accidents), penetrating head injury (from gunshot wounds), or intracranial hemorrhage (cerebrovascular accidents). In general, suitable donors will not have sustained prolonged periods of circulatory compromise or septicemia. Donors are screened for infectious processes that would disqualify organ donation, including serologic evidence of hepatitis B or human immunodeficiency virus infection, as well as active toxoplasmosis, herpes, or tuberculosis. In contrast, most transplant centers will use organs obtained from donors with prior cytomegalovirus (CMV) infection for recipients with previous CMV exposure.

Autoimmune disease, in general, has not been a criterion for disqualification of donors, despite a report that idiopathic thrombocytopenic purpura can be transmitted by liver transplantation.[2] Cardiac donors are usually younger than 50 years of age and without pre-existing myocardial or coronary artery disease, although older donor hearts have been successfully transplanted. Myocardial contractility must be adequate as judged by echocardiography, and there should be no history of use of intracardiac injections or high doses of inotropes. Hepatic function tests are useful to screen potential liver donors who may have abused drugs or alcohol. Urinalysis and cultures, blood urea nitrogen, and creatinine levels are standard tests for potential kidney donors. However, given that there are currently > 75 000 people waiting for an organ,[3] and some 6000 will die while waiting this year, more compromised donor organs may make their way into patient care.

Viscera for transplantation are also obtained from living donors. Almost all viscera derived from living donors are kidneys, although partial liver and lung resections have been performed to create reduced size allografts for relatively few recipients. Living donors must be closely related to recipients if there is to be any benefit; human leukocyte antigen (HLA) identity between donor and recipient results in significantly greater graft survival than even a partially matched organ.[4]

Diagnosis of brain death

Heart transplantation in the late 1960s drove the need for a uniform definition of brain death. Before that time, retrieval of kidneys, which are tolerant of a short period of warm ischemia, was performed after cessation of the donor's heartbeat. Several legislative efforts were initiated to address the issue, until a special panel of medical consultants (President's Commission for the Study of Ethical Problems in Medicine and Biomedical and Behavior Research) issued a report that defined brain death as "irreversible cessation of all function of the entire brain, including the cortex and brainstem, determined in accordance with accepted medical standards."[5] The concept of brain death is now widely recognized in Western societies, although the medical standards of its determination have been the subject of much debate.

Cerebral cortical function is deemed absent when no spontaneous movement or response to noxious external stimuli can be elicited by an experienced physician (Table 61.1). However, studies supporting these physical findings are often obtained in accordance with local "medical standards," which may include electroencephalography or cortical blood flow determinations. An electrically silent (flat) electroencephalogram is consistent with the diagnosis of brain death, although residual activity may still be found after cessation of cerebral blood flow.[6] Four-vessel cerebral angiography is the gold standard to establish brain death,[7] but less invasive methods, such as transcranial Doppler and xenon-enhanced computed tomography, are widespread substitutes.

Brainstem infarction is indicated by loss of reflexes mediated by bulbar cranial nerve and respiratory nuclei. These include the direct

Table 61.1 *Criteria for the diagnosis of brain death*

Loss of cerebral cortical function
No spontaneous movement
Unresponsive to external stimuli

Loss of brainstem function
Absent respiratory reflex (apnea test)
Absent cranial nerve reflexes
Pupillary light reflex
Corneal reflex
Oculocephalic reflex
Oculovestibular reflex
Atropine resistance

Supporting studies
Electroencephalography
Cerebral flow studies
Angiography
Transcranial Doppler examination
Xenon computed tomography scan

pupillary light reflex (absent when bright light fails to constrict the homolateral pupil); the oculocephalic reflex (absent when ocular position is fixed during rotation of the head – "doll's eyes"); the corneal reflex (absent when lightly touching the cornea fails to elicit a blink); and the oculovestibular reflex (absent when irrigation of the external auditory canal with ice water fails to produce nystagmus – "cold caloric test"). Respiratory reflexes are assessed by the apnea test. In most protocols, after a period of mechanical ventilation on 100% oxygen, the ventilator is disconnected (although oxygen is still supplied) and respiratory effort is judged by serial determinations of P_aCO_2. By this means, an accurate assessment of respiratory brainstem function can be obtained during 10 min of observation if the patient remains otherwise physiologically stable.

Irreversibility is essential to the diagnosis of brain death and is established by the lack of improvement in the neurologic examination for 12–24 h. Factors that may confound this diagnosis include generalized seizures, centrally active drug effects, hypothermia, and cardiovascular or metabolic instability, because all may reversibly depress brain function. Therefore, it is also important that the cause of brain death is known and sufficient to account for this diagnosis. In young children, the potential for recovery from neurologic insults may be less predictable than in adults, so it is recommended that an experienced pediatric neurologist be consulted to evaluate these young brain-injured patients.

Physiologic derangements with brain death

Brain death is frequently accompanied by marked physiologic instability, and treatment is often necessary to maintain the viability of donor organs (Table 61.2). Hypotension, hypoxemia, or arrhythmias may be part of the pathogenesis of brain death, or else a consequence of brainstem infarction. Hypotension results from the loss of descending vasomotor control and is exacerbated by hemorrhage, massive diuresis from diabetes insipidus or radiographic dyes, or dehydration therapy for cerebral edema.

Treatment consists of restoration of intravascular volume with colloid and crystalloid solutions, and, if necessary, vasopressin administration (Pitressin 0.5–15 U h^{-1}) or vasoactive drug infusion. Because phenylephrine may diminish splanchnic perfusion and thereby jeopardize abdominal donor organs, dopamine (2–5 mg kg^{-1} min^{-1}) is recommended for blood pressure support in this setting. Hypoxemia may follow from overzealous fluid administration during resuscitation attempts, atelectasis, aspiration, pneumothorax, pulmonary contusion, or pneumonia. The F_IO_2, minute volume of ventilation, and positive end-expiratory pressure (PEEP) are usually adjusted to maintain systemic arterial saturation in excess of 95%.

Table 61.2 *Common physiologic derangements after brain death*

Condition	Cause
Hypotension	Hypovolemia (diabetes insipidus, hemorrhage)
Hypoxemia	Neurogenic shock Neurogenic pulmonary edema Pulmonary contusion Pneumonia Gastric aspiration Fluid overload
Hypothermia	Hypothalamic infarction Exposure dysrhythmia (especially bradycardia) Intracranial injury or herniation Hypothermia Hypoxia Electrolyte abnormality Myocardial contusion, ischemia

Atrial and ventricular arrhythmias, as well as varying degrees of conduction blockade, have been noted after brain death.[8] Etiologies include intracranial hypertension, vagal nucleus infarction, myocardial ischemia or contusion,[9] hypothermia, and abnormal pH or serum electrolytes. Bradycardia is resistant to atropine but responds to direct-acting chronotropic agents (e.g. dopamine, isoproterenol).

Numerous endocrine responses have been associated with brain death, including diabetes insipidus. This diagnosis is confirmed when polyuria is accompanied by relative hyposmolarity of the urine (300 mosmol L^{-1}) despite serum hyperosmolarity (310 mosmol L^{-1}) and hypernatremia (serum sodium 150 mequiv L^{-1}). Treatment consists of replacement of free water losses while restoring normal serum electrolyte and osmolarity values, and infusion of aqueous vasopressin [Pitressin, 0.5–15 U h^{-1} intravenously (i.v.)]. Infrequently, catecholamine and cortisol levels are markedly elevated, and thyroid hormone (T_3) or insulin activity reduced after brain death. However, there is no consistent pattern; therefore, replacement therapies are not routinely used.

Donor operation

Anesthesia care for multiple organ retrieval should continue the focus on maintenance of donor organ perfusion and oxygenation begun in the intensive care unit. Although cortical and brainstem function is absent, both visceral and somatic reflexes that can lead to physiologic responses during the procedure may be present. For example, reflex pressor responses may accompany surgical stimuli and can jeopardize the renal microvasculature. Vasodilator infusion is sufficient treatment because general anesthetics are unnecessary under these circumstances. Reflex neuromuscular activity mediated by spinal somatic reflexes is suppressed with relaxants.

After surgical preparation in the supine position, a midline incision is made from the suprasternal notch to the pubic symphysis, followed by sternotomy. Once exposed, the liver is freed of its ligamentous attachments to the diaphragm. To minimize warm ischemic time and surgical trauma to the harvested viscera, the typical donor operation involves regional cooling and preservation of organs *in situ*, followed by *en bloc* removal. Thus, after the abdominal aorta is encircled with a ligature above the celiac artery, either the splenic or inferior mesenteric vein is cannulated and the liver is flushed through the portal system with cold preservative solution.

The donor is then systemically heparinized and the abdominal aorta is cannulated, cross-clamped, and perfused with cold preservative. This cools the donor's kidneys and liver, and, once the ureters are dissected and divided, *en bloc* graft nephrectomy can be accomplished by transecting the aorta and inferior vena cava (IVC) above and below the renal pedicles. The hepatic artery and common bile duct are then divided and the donor liver can now be removed. Donor cardiectomy begins once *in situ* preservation of the abdominal viscera is begun; further details about the cardiac donor procedure are found in the section on Heart transplantation. After all donor organs are removed, ventilatory and circulatory support is discontinued and the anesthesiologist's involvement ends. Death is always certified before the donor procedure and is not considered to have occurred in the operating room.

ORGAN PRESERVATION

Organ transplantation depends on the temporary separation of a donor organ from a blood supply and protection from ischemia while *ex vivo*. Organ-sharing networks are based on distant procurement, which may extend the period of ischemia to the biologically tolerable limit. The protection strategy combines hypothermia to decrease metabolism with preservative solutions of specific electrolyte composition to maintain cellular integrity. These solutions may also contain chemical additives that are cryoprotective and prevent cellular swelling, vasospasm, and build-up of toxic metabolites and provide a source of energy.

Preservation strategies are based on the control of the adverse cellular events that follow ischemia and reperfusion. Preventing these chain reactions is the rationale for using free radical scavengers (e.g. mannitol and superoxide dismutase) and synthesis blockers (allopurinol) as additives to preservative solutions.

Preservation solutions

Collins *et al.*[10] first developed a series of isotonic flushing solutions for renal preservation. Their compositions usually resembled that of intracellular fluid (i.e. low sodium and high potassium), which was shown to diminish renal cortical respiration. Other additives included heparin, phenoxybenzamine, and procaine, all meant to prevent agonal vasospasm and thrombosis in cadaver kidneys. Today, among the most widely used kidney flushing solutions in the USA and Europe is a modified Collins solution, termed Euro-Collins (Table 61.3). Euro-Collins solution is modestly hyperosmotic, does not contain additives, and supports kidney viability *ex vivo* for more than 48 h.[13]

The high metabolic rate of the liver makes it relatively vulnerable to ischemia, and its large bulk prevents rapid, uniform cooling during procurement. As a consequence, the most common cause of postoperative hepatic graft dysfunction is ischemic injury. UW (University of Wisconsin) solution[11] was shown to extend hypothermic preservation of donor livers for at least 24 h *ex vivo*, and possibly longer. The key additives in UW solution (see Table 61.3) include lactobionate and raffinose, which are used as impermeants to suppress hypothermia-induced cellular swelling.

Protection of the heart is based on cellular metabolic arrest and uniform cooling, both of which prevent the generation of cytotoxic free radicals.[14] Techniques that provide myocardial protection, particularly cardioplegia, were developed in parallel with heart transplantation and greatly facilitated distal procurement.[12] Compared with other preservative regimens, cardioplegia solutions (see Table 61.3) were shown to reduce the need for inotropic support after implantation[12] and are now generally used for *ex vivo* myocardial preservation. Under laboratory conditions, cardioplegia is able to preserve cardiac function for up to 24 h. However, in humans, the practical limit of ischemic time is 4–6 h.[12]

Table 61.3 *Organ preservation solutions*

Solution	Amount per liter
Euro-Collins solution[a]	
Potassium	115 mequiv
Sodium	10 mequiv
Chloride	15 mequiv
Bicarbonate	10 mequiv
Dihydrogen phosphate	15 mequiv
Monohydrogen phosphate	85 mequiv
Measured osmolality	375 mosmol
pH (4 °C)	7.25
University of Wisconsin (UW) or Beezer's solution[b]	
K^+ lactobionate	100 mmol
KH_2PO_4	25 mmol
Adenosine	5 mmol
$MgSO_4$	5 mmol
Glutathione	3 mmol
Raffinose	30 mmol
Allopurinol	1 mmol
Tosulin	100 units
Penicillin	40 units
Dexamethasone	8 mg
Hydroxyethyl starch	50 g
Osmolality	320–330 mosmol
pH (4 °C)	7.4
Crystalloid cardioplegia[c]	
Potassium	30 mequiv
Sodium	25 mequiv
Chloride	30 mequiv
Bicarbonate	25 mequiv
Dextrose	50 g
Mannitol	12.5 g
Osmolality	440 mosmol
pH (4 °C)	8.1–8.4

a. "Modified" Euro-Collins contains 5 mL L^{-1} of 50% glucose and 1 g L^{-1} of magnesium sulfate. Adapted with permission from Collins *et al.*[10]
b. Adapted with permission from Belzer and Southard JH.[11]
c. Adapted with permission from Hardesty *et al.*[12]

TRANSPLANTATION IMMUNOLOGY

Tissue derived from a (nontwin) donor of the same species for transplantation is termed an *allograft*. When an immunocompetent recipient is confronted with foreign antigens present on the cell surfaces of an allograft, an immune response occurs. All elements of a recipient's immune system contribute to the response provoked by transplanted tissue; these include humoral factors (immunoglobulins secreted by B lymphocytes as well as complement proteins) and cellular elements (T cells, other leukocytes, and macrophages). For a more complete review, see Chapter 23. T lymphocytes play a primary role in the immune response by initial antigen recognition and ultimate allograft destruction. On the basis of their specific reactivity to certain monoclonal antibodies or their cell-surface antigens, T lymphocytes can be subdivided into at least four subpopulations:[15] cytotoxic T cells, helper T cells, delayed hypersensitivity T cells, and suppressor T cells. All are important participants in the reaction to foreign tissue.

The cell-surface glycoproteins that establish the immunologic identity of donor tissues are termed the *major histocompatibility complex* (MHC) antigens. Class I MHC antigens, also called HLA-A, -B, and -C, are found on all nucleated cells. These are the classic transplantation antigens as well as the primary targets for cytotoxic cells. Class II MHC antigens, also termed HLA-DR, -DO, and -DP, are located on activated

T cells, B cells, dendritic cells, and macrophages, and are the primary targets for helper T cells. There is an enormous diversity of alleles at the chromosomal loci encoding for the HLA antigens, and this accounts for the varying degrees of HLA matching observed. Finally, the major blood group antigens (ABO) are particularly potent transplantation antigens, such that organs transplanted into patients with known preformed isohemagglutinins against the donor blood type can be expected to provoke the most rapid form of rejection (hyperacute rejection) because of thrombosis in the microvasculature (Fig. 61.1).

Mechanisms of allograft rejection

Unless suppressed, the immune response to transplanted tissue begins with the recognition of the donor antigens as foreign or "nonself," proceeds with proliferation of immunocompetent cells, and culminates in an effector phase. Briefly, recognition involves a binding reaction between an immunogenic histocompatibility antigen present on the surface of the allogeneic (donor) cell and a receptor on the surface of a helper or cytotoxic T cell. After T cells are bound, accessory macrophages secrete "monokines," notably interleukin 1 (IL-1), to further

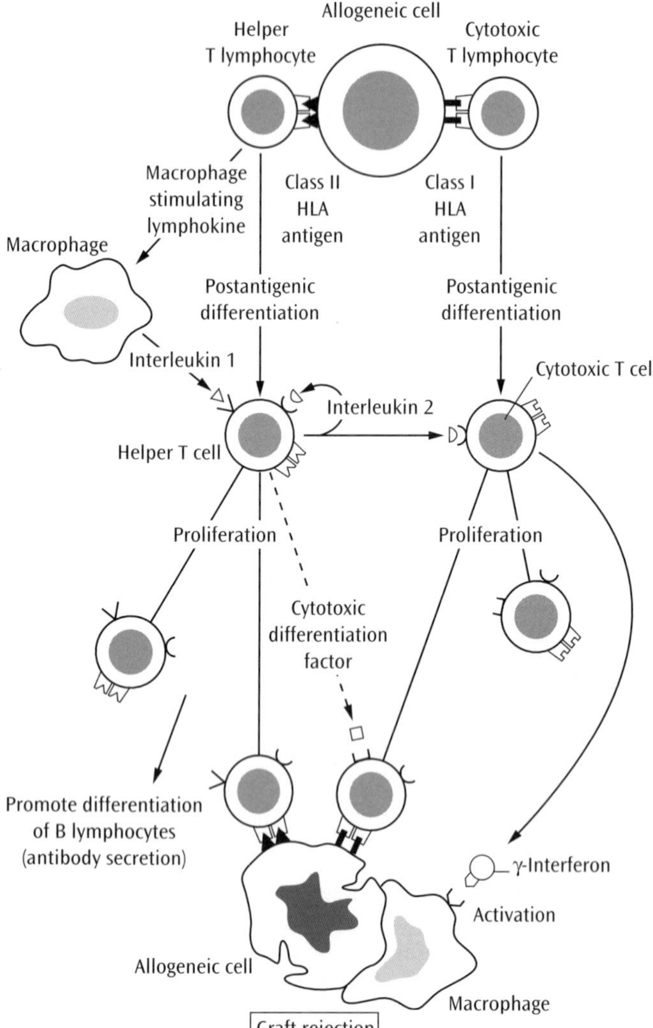

Figure 61.1 *Immune response to allogeneic tissue. The cellular and humoral events that make up the immune cascade are illustrated, starting with recognition of an allogeneic (foreign) cell by T lymphocytes at the top of the figure. See text for details. HLA, human leukocyte antigen. (Reprinted with permission from Strom.[16])*

enhance T-cell activation. IL-2 and other lymphokines are secreted by helper T cells, promoting lymphocyte proliferation and differentiation. Differentiated lymphocytes, in turn, secrete effector molecules, including γ-interferon, which activate and enlist macrophages and leukocytes to cooperate in the process of graft rejection.

Clinical immunology of organ transplantation

Hyperacute rejection of renal allografts, characterized by microvascular thrombosis rapidly followed by graft necrosis, occurs in the presence of major blood group (ABO) incompatibilities. However, like blood transfusion, kidneys from type O donors can be transplanted into compatible, nonidentical (A, B, or AB) recipients. In some centers, ABO-incompatible, living-related donor kidney transplants are performed with good results, but only under special immunosuppression protocols that include splenectomy, plasmapheresis, donor-specific platelet transfusion, and cyclosporine (cyclosporin) administration. The importance of HLA histocompatibility matching in kidney transplantation is controversial; HLA-incompatible, living-related donor transplantation yields excellent results, but survival rates of HLA-matched cadaver allografts are superior. The presence of preformed cytotoxic antibodies to the donor's T lymphocytes (antilymphocyte antibodies) increases the risk of hyperacute rejection and usually precludes kidney transplantation.[13] One other immunologic parameter that may affect renal allograft survival is the panel-reactive antibody (PRA). In this test, cross-match testing is carried out between the patient's serum and donor cells to detect the presence of preformed antibodies. It has been reported that patients with lymphocytotoxic antibodies that react against more than 50% of the random test panel have a greater rate of rejection.[17]

Donor-specific ABO isoagglutinins may induce hyperacute reactions of cardiac allografts;[18] thus, ABO matching is considered to be essential. The role of HLA matching in heart transplantation is more controversial. Some studies indicate that HLA mismatching does not correlate with the number of cardiac rejection episodes or survival,[19] whereas others find that HLA mismatching is clinically important.[17] However, until the tolerable donor heart ischemic time is extended beyond the present 4–6 h, full, prospective histocompatibility matching and PRA screening will remain impractical and limit their application.

In contrast to the heart and kidneys, hyperacute rejection has not been reported to occur in liver allografts,[20] supporting the assertion that the liver is resistant to such antibody-mediated injury.[21] Consequently, liver transplantation is often performed despite major ABO incompatibility, although the risk of subsequent rejection is elevated.[22] When ABO matching is carried out, short-term survival is better with ABO-identical than with ABO-compatible, nonidentical allografts, and the longer term trend is similar.[23] There does not seem to be any relation between either HLA matching or T-cell cross-match and allograft survival.

In summary, the distribution of renal allografts depends mostly on immunologic factors such as ABO match, HLA histocompatibility, T-cell cross-match, and PRA profile. In contrast, except for ABO matching, the distribution of donor livers and hearts depends more on factors such as size compatibility and medical urgency than on immunologic criteria.

Mechanisms of immunosuppression

In clinical practice, the immune response must be controlled to avoid allograft rejection. Immunosuppressant drugs have been developed for this purpose, but their use is accompanied by significant morbidity. Because of side-effects and toxicities (as discussed in Evaluation of patients with a prior organ transplant), immunosuppression is warranted only for grafts essential for life. For example, a thyroid allograft would be inappropriate because it is easily substituted by medication.

Ideally, immunosuppressants should inhibit only that lymphocyte subset directed against donor-specific alloantigens, but the drugs in current use are immunologically nonspecific. Antirejection regimens usually combine low doses of several agents to provide superior immunosuppression and to minimize side-effects.

Glucocorticoids

Glucocorticoids (Table 61.4) are potent anti-inflammatory agents and have been a mainstay in almost all immunosuppressive regimens. These agents decrease macrophage production of IL-1, a critical factor in helper T-cell development.[24] In addition, T-cell secretion of IL-2 is also diminished, preventing clonal expansion of helper and cytotoxic T cells.[25]

Azathioprine is an imidazole derivative of 6-mercaptopurine, an analog of the purine hypoxanthine. Thioinosinic acid, a metabolite of azathioprine, competes with inosinic acid for conversion to xanthylic acid, an essential substrate for *de novo* purine synthesis required for production of both DNA and RNA. As a result, protein synthesis and both T- and B-lymphocyte proliferation are inhibited.[26]

Cyclosporine, tacrolimus, mycophenolate, and rapamycin

Cyclosporine is a lipophilic undecapeptide antibiotic isolated from a soil fungus that virtually revolutionized viscera transplantation by making it feasible routinely to achieve results comparable to those obtained in transplants between identical twins. Its major target is the T cell, which is inhibited from elaborating key lymphokines such as IL-2.[27] Cyclosporine also prevents activation of helper T cells by foreign antigens and inhibits the production of IL-1 by macrophages.

Tacrolimus (FK 506) and rapamycin are newer macrolide antibiotic immunosuppressants. Both are highly potent and may have somewhat more immunospecificity and less toxicity than cyclosporine. These agents diminish activation and proliferation of T cells as well as lymphokine production, but do so through distinct intracellular signaling pathways.

Mycophenolate mofetil is hydrolyzed to mycophenolic acid, which inhibits the enzyme inosine monophosphate dehydrogenase. In turn, this disrupts guanosine nucleotide synthesis in T and B lymphocytes, reducing their ability to proliferate during an immune response.[28]

Table 61.4 *Mechanisms of immunosuppressant action*

Agent	Main effect(s)
Glucocorticoids	Decrease IL-1 production from macrophages (reducing effectiveness of T-helper cells) Decrease IL-2 production from T cells (reducing clonal expansion of T-helper and cytotoxic cells)
Azathioprine	Inhibits DNA and RNA synthesis (reducing lymphocyte proliferation)
Cyclosporine	Prevents T-helper cell activation by antigen Inhibits elaboration of T-cell-derived factors, particularly IL-2
Tacrolimus (FK 506)	Inhibits T-cell production of IL-2 Inhibits production of IL-2 receptors on T cells Prevents B-cell activation
Antilymphocyte globulin	Diminishes populations of both T and B lymphocytes
OKT3	Inactivates T cells and prevents reactivation

IL, interleukin.

Whether its immunospecificity and toxicity profiles are better than those of the aforementioned compounds remains to be seen from accumulating clinical experience.

Antilymphocyte globulin and OKT3

Antilymphocyte globulin (ALG) is a polyclonal antibody produced by immunizing animals with human lymphoid cells and isolating the immunoglobulin G (IgG) fraction from resulting antisera. ALG seems rapidly to diminish the availability of activated T lymphocytes, interrupting the chain of events leading to rejection. ALG may also have a sustained effect on T-cell proliferation, perhaps by promoting formation of nonspecific suppressor T cells.[29] Similarly, the OKT series of murine monoclonal antibodies directed against T-cell-surface antigens are added to some immunosuppression regimens to treat rejection. OKT3 is specifically directed against the T3 (CD3) complex on the surface of mature T lymphocytes. The T3 complex is located adjacent to the T-cell receptor involved in recognition of foreign antigens; binding of OKT3 blocks the recognition of MHC antigens and, consequently, the immune response cascade. Administration of OKT3 also results in removal of opsonized T cells by the reticuloendothelial system.

GENERAL PREANESTHETIC EVALUATION OF TRANSPLANT CANDIDATES

The general indication for organ transplantation is failure of medical or other surgical management to enhance the quality of life for patients with end-stage organ disease or significantly to improve their chances for long-term survival. Because major organ transplantation procedures are now associated with reasonably low perioperative mortality rates, this option is considered in virtually all such cases.

The major contraindications to organ transplantation are: incurable malignancy; the presence of another debilitating or uncontrolled systemic disease; active, poorly controlled infection; and physical or social factors that would either impede recovery or lead to recurrent disease (Table 61.5). Rather than being considered absolute, these criteria are under continuous evaluation in light of new information. For example, diabetes mellitus was formerly considered to contraindicate organ transplantation, but many diabetic patients have now undergone renal transplantation and 1-year allograft survival is the same as for non-diabetic patients. Patients with diabetic nephropathy now constitute the largest segment of adults who undergo renal transplantation. Similarly, many elderly patients have undergone heart transplantation with results that are similar to those for younger subpopulations.

Candidates for organ transplantation often manifest physical findings or laboratory abnormalities indicative of secondary organ involvement (e.g. hepatomegaly consequent to right ventricular failure). It is important to verify that such findings do not represent a coexistent primary disease process (which might disqualify potential recipients) and to bear in mind that compromised organs may be especially vulnerable to acute insults. Because recipients will be immunosuppressed, occult infection (e.g. tuberculosis) should assiduously be ruled out. For the same reason, it is standard to order CMV-negative blood for transfusion

Table 61.5 *General contraindications to viscera transplantation*

Incurable malignancy
Other major systemic illness
Old ("physiologic") age
Active systemic or incurable infection
Significant obesity
Current alcohol, drug, or tobacco abuse
Evidence of emotional instability or lack of supportive social milieu

unless recipients are seropositive. On occasion, technical feasibility may become the overwhelming source of concern (e.g. with atypical vascular anatomy or body habitus, or multiple previous surgeries).

Because of the shortage of suitable donor organs, patients may remain on a waiting list for many months while their conditions continue to deteriorate. Interval changes, as well as corresponding alterations in their medical regimens, should be ascertained. The urgency of surgery may, by necessity, influence the acceptability of an available donor organ.

With organs for which the safe ischemic time is less than 24 h, transplantation procedures are usually performed under emergency circumstances. The patient to receive the organ may have eaten recently and arrives in the operating room without the benefit of premedication. The remaining management considerations are specific to the particular type of transplantation procedure, as discussed in the following sections.

KIDNEY TRANSPLANTATION

Approximately 10 000 renal transplantations are performed each year in the USA. This comprises 5–10% of patients with end-stage renal disease who are otherwise dependent on dialysis. Dialysis is clearly effective in prolonging life, but considerable morbidity and mortality are associated with its use. For example, in 1988, the 1-year mortality rate after renal transplantation was 5%; in some studies, the yearly mortality rate of patients on chronic dialysis is at least twice as high.[30]

Renal transplantation is a highly successful procedure. According to data from the national organ procurement and transplantation network UNOS, cadaveric renal allografts have a 1-year survival rate of 81%, whereas the same statistic for living-related donor organs is 91%.[31] Studies from large centers indicate that longer term graft survival is also similarly favorable, as are other measures of outcome. In adults with end-stage renal disease, kidney transplantation improves the quality of life[32] while remaining cost-effective.[33] For these reasons, renal transplantation has become the treatment of choice for end-stage renal disease, with its growth limited only by the supply of available donor organs.

Pathophysiology of end-stage renal disease

End-stage renal disease can result from numerous causes (Table 61.6), all of which ultimately lead to the uremic syndrome. In uremia, patients are unable to regulate the volume and composition of their body fluids, resulting in fluid overload, acidemia, and imbalance of electrolytes such as potassium, phosphorus, magnesium, and calcium. In addition, there is usually evidence of secondary dysfunction in other organ systems (Table 61.7). Even patients maintained by dialysis may have peripheral neuropathy, pericardial or pleural effusions, renal osteodystrophy, and gastrointestinal (GI) as well as immunologic dysfunction.

Specific indications and contraindications

A large proportion of adults with end-stage renal disease are candidates for kidney transplantation. Aside from the general contraindications to viscera transplantation (see Table 61.5), relative contraindications specific to renal transplantation are disease processes likely to recur in the transplanted kidney. Hemolytic uremic syndrome, membranoproliferative glomerulonephritis, and metabolic derangements that produce toxic deposits in the kidney (e.g. gout, oxalosis, cytinosis) fall into this group. In practice, however, patients with such disorders may derive years of benefit from transplantation, and thus at many centers are still considered eligible. Similarly, diabetic nephropathy can also recur in allografts, but diabetes mellitus is no longer considered a contraindication to renal transplantation.

Table 61.6 *Etiology of end-stage renal disease in renal transplant recipients[a]*

Etiology	Total cases (%)
Diabetic glomerulonephropathy	43.6
Other glomerulonephritides	23.2
Polycystic kidney disease	5.8
Chronic pyelonephritis	5.4
Obstructive uropathy	3.4
Alport syndrome	2.1
Lupus nephritis	1.6
Miscellaneous, including unknown	14.9

a. Data derived from 2591 cases at the University of Minnesota performed between 1963 and 1990. (Adapted with permission from Belani and Palaliniuk.[34])

Table 61.7 *Common pathophysiologic consequences of end-stage renal disease*

Organ system	Consequence
Nervous system	Peripheral neuropathy Lethargy–coma
Hematologic	Anemia Diminished erythrocyte survival Platelet dysfunction Shift in P_{50} of oxyhemoglobin dissociation curve
Cardiovascular	Congestive heart failure Pericarditis Hypertension Dysrhythmias (abnormal electrolytes) Capillary fragility
Pulmonary	Pleural effusions Pulmonary edema
Musculoskeletal	Generalized muscle weakness Renal osteodystrophy Metastatic calcification Gout, pseudogout
Gastrointestinal	Nausea, vomiting Ileus Peptic and colonic ulceration
Endocrine	Pancreatitis Glucose intolerance
Integument	Pruritus Hyperpigmentation
Immunologic	Impaired cellular immunity

Adapted with permission from Belani and Palaliniuk.[34]

Preanesthetic considerations

Because the tolerable ischemic time for kidneys is at least 48 h,[13] cadaver allografts may be transplanted semielectively. With living-related donation, renal transplantation is an elective procedure. In either case, sufficient time is available for ABO matching, cross-matching of the recipient's serum with donor lymphocytes, and, at some institutions, HLA tissue typing. Likewise, dialysis may precede transplantation to correct serious electrolyte and volume derangements. After dialysis, it is important to ascertain the net volume status of patients; the final hematocrit, electrolyte, and bicarbonate levels; and whether there is any residual heparin effect. The serum potassium should be normal, and the serum calcium supplemented if $<7\,mg\,dL^{-1}$ to prevent tetanus. Most uremic patients, even those on dialysis, have hemoglobin levels in the $6–8\,g\,dL^{-1}$ range. However, in chronically anemic patients, compensatory changes promote tissue oxygen unloading and, on this basis alone, preoperative transfusion is not mandatory. But transfusion may enhance allograft survival; thus, it has become a standard part of the preoperative regimen at some centers. On occasion, pleural or pericardial effusions may require treatment if there is functional impairment; in patients on chronic steroids, preoperative administration of full replacement doses of glucocorticoids should be considered.

Because many adult recipients are diabetic, the possibility of coexistent ischemic heart disease is usually evaluated by exercise stress testing and, if indicated, coronary angiography. Diffuse coronary disease has not been considered a contraindication to renal transplantation, provided that ventricular function is not seriously diminished and the patient is willing to assume the added risk. In such patients, appropriate invasive monitoring (arterial and pulmonary artery catheters) is warranted; in all others, a central venous pressure catheter is sufficient to monitor intravascular volume for optimal renal perfusion. Finally, transplanted kidneys, particularly those derived from cadaver donors, may not be functional immediately, so it is vital to protect existing arteriovenous fistulas or other routes for postoperative hemodialysis or peritoneal dialysis.

Donor procedure and related considerations

The procedure used for harvesting abdominal viscera from cadaver donors is reviewed in the section on Anesthesia care of organ donors. If the cadaver is brain dead but the circulation is intact, harvesting may proceed at leisure through the transperitoneal route. If the circulation fails, however, the kidneys must be rapidly removed and flushed with preservative solution to minimize warm ischemic time.

Living donors are the source of 20% of the kidneys transplanted in the USA and 60% of those in Europe. Because results with unrelated living donors are no better than those achieved with cadaver donors, living donors are virtually always close relatives. Most are healthy adults because any significant systemic disease increases the risk of general anesthesia and surgery, giving rise to ethical conflicts. For similar reasons, donors who are 45 (male) or 50 years (female) of age usually undergo noninvasive studies to detect occult coronary ischemia. The use of living-related donors has gained widespread acceptance because the overall incidence of serious perioperative morbidity in this population is small (2%), and deaths are extremely rare.[35] Furthermore, long-term follow-up studies indicate that donors have no greater risk of renal failure or hypertension.[36]

Before surgery, donors undergo renal arteriography and intravenous (i.v.) pyelography and are screened for ABO blood group compatibility and CMV titer. Then, 2–4 weeks before the procedure, several units of blood are donated for autologous transfusion. During the night preceding harvesting, donors are hydrated with crystalloid solutions to promote an active diuresis, and, at the time of nephrectomy, a minimum urine output of $1\,mL\,min^{-1}$ is achieved by means of mannitol and furosemide. The timing of the donor and recipient procedures is coordinated so that the kidney's ischemic interval is minimized. Heparin is administered systemically before removal of the organ from the donor, which is then flushed free of blood with a cold crystalloid solution and transplanted immediately.

Anesthesia induction for recipients

Diabetic patients can have delayed gastric emptying, therefore rapid induction may be warranted. Provided the serum potassium is normal after recent dialysis, there is no contraindication to the use of succinylcholine (suxamethonium). Drugs that are highly protein bound (e.g. thiopental) should be administered in reduced dosages. Further discussion of the kinetics and dynamics of drugs in renal failure patients is found elsewhere in this textbook.

Central venous catheters are useful for the reasons discussed earlier, but are usually inserted after induction. Many renal transplant recipients are moderately hypertensive and maintained on combinations of appropriate medications. Most have recently been dialyzed and are volume depleted. Thus, the possibility of synergistic interactions between strongly vasodilating anesthetics (e.g. isoflurane), antihypertensives (e.g. hydralazine, diltiazem, captopril), and hypovolemia should be considered.

Anesthesia and surgical procedures

Although regional anesthetic techniques have been advocated by some, the use of general anesthesia is more common. With general anesthesia, there is superior control of ventilation, which becomes particularly important when surgical retraction is close to the diaphragm. In addition, the duration of renal transplant procedures in most centers makes regional techniques impractical. Enflurane and sevoflurane are seldom chosen because their biotransformation results in inorganic halides that are nephrotoxic. Nitrous oxide is often omitted to avoid distension of the bowel, particularly in children, so either opioids and benzodiazepines are used in combination or a potent inhaled agent is used alone.

Atracurium and vecuronium are the preferred muscle relaxants because they are least dependent on renal metabolism, although laudanosine, a metabolite of atracurium, may accumulate in patients with end-stage renal disease.[37] Laudanosine increases the minimum alveolar concentration of halothane in laboratory animals, but does not seem to cause an analogous clinical effect in humans. The response to vecuronium may be variable in renal failure, and, because it is not clear precisely when renal metabolic function is restored after transplantation, neuromuscular monitoring is highly recommended.

In adults, the kidney is implanted retroperitoneally in the upper pelvis using a paramedian lower abdominal approach; in children weighing $<20\,kg$, abdominal implantation is the rule. Revascularization of the allograft in adults involves anastomoses of the renal vessels to an iliac vein and artery. This necessitates clamping the common iliac vessels, resulting in lower extremity ischemia, usually for less than 60 min. After the anastomoses are complete, the circulation is restored to the allograft and lower extremities. To promote renal perfusion, a high-normal blood pressure is achieved by reducing the depth of anesthesia, bolus administration of crystalloid, or temporary dopamine infusion. When the vascular clamps are released, renal preservative solution and the venous drainage from the legs are also released into the circulation. These effluents are relatively rich in potassium and acid metabolites, but in adults have little systemic effect. The final stage of the procedure involves ureteral implantation for urinary drainage.

Postoperative management

Varying periods of oliguria or anuria due to acute tubular necrosis are associated with cadaveric renal transplantation in approximately one-third of cases; thus, fluids must be administered judiciously to reduce the risk of postoperative pulmonary edema. In contrast, the ischemic time for organs derived from living-related donors is minimal and urine flow is usually immediate. Emergence is often accompanied by both pain and hypertension, which are particularly hazardous in diabetic patients with coexistent ischemic heart disease. In such cases, preparations should be made to administer potent analgesics (e.g. by epidural catheter) and antihypertensives in the recovery room, if myocardial ischemia is to be avoided. Other early postoperative complications include atelectasis, bleeding and thrombosis of vascular anastomoses, urinary obstruction or leak, and, rarely, gastric aspiration. Hyperacute rejection may also occur and lead to anuria; definitive diagnosis requires a renal biopsy. This complication has become rare because both ABO matching and cross-matching of the recipient's serum to donor lymphocytes are routinely performed.

Immunosuppression with "triple therapy" (cyclosporine, azathioprine, prednisone) is usually begun before transplantation of living-related donor organs or after transplantation of cadaveric kidneys. Long-term complications of renal transplantation related to immunosuppression are discussed in the section Evaluation of patients with a prior organ transplant.

LIVER TRANSPLANTATION

Medical treatment for chronic end-stage liver disease is supportive but does little to prolong or improve the quality of life, particularly after serious complications (e.g. GI bleeding, coma, uremia) develop. In acute hepatic failure, the salvage rate with medical treatment is between 5% and 20%.[38] In contrast, in the cyclosporine era, the overall 1-year survival rate of orthotopic liver recipients is 76%, with an allograft survival rate of 69%.[31] Longer term survival is also comparatively high (Fig. 61.2). Moreover, the quality of life for a high proportion of transplantation survivors is markedly improved.

The yearly rate of liver transplantations in the USA has reached approximately 2500, although it has been argued that more than twice that number are needed. The overwhelming majority of these procedures are orthotopic, involving native hepatectomy and implantation of the donor organ in anatomic position in the right upper quadrant. Heterotopic (also called auxiliary) transplantation, where the donor liver is implanted adjacent to the native liver, which is left *in situ*, has been used on rare occasion for reversible hepatic failure and in patients too frail for the orthotopic procedure.

Pathophysiology of end-stage liver disease

The liver has numerous synthetic and metabolic functions; thus, end-stage liver disease has ramifications that extend to virtually every other organ system (Table 61.8). In disease processes that destroy the normal hepatic architecture, portal hypertension results and extensive venous collaterals develop in the abdominal wall, mesentery, retroperitoneum, and GI tract. Aside from the significant morbidity associated with hemorrhage from esophageal varices, the extensive network of arteriovenous communications results in low systemic vascular resistance and high cardiac output. Intrapulmonary shunting is also seen frequently in patients with end-stage liver disease,[40] leading to hypoxemia that is exacerbated by pleural effusions and bibasilar atelectasis from abdominal distension. Renal function may be impaired secondary to hepatorenal syndrome or prerenal azotemia. Ascites develops as a result of venous hypertension, decreased albumin synthesis, and sodium and water retention from a relative excess of aldosterone and antidiuretic hormone. Treatment often consists of diuretics, which in turn may cause electrolyte and acid–base derangements and intravascular volume depletion. Blood coagulation is abnormal because synthesis of the hepatically derived clotting factors (I, fibrinogen; II, prothrombin; V; VII; IX; X) and clearance of fibrinolyric factors are compromised. Hypersplenism may also secondarily diminish the platelet count markedly. Eventually, even the central nervous system is affected, resulting in a progressive toxic encephalopathy and cerebral edema, which presage death.

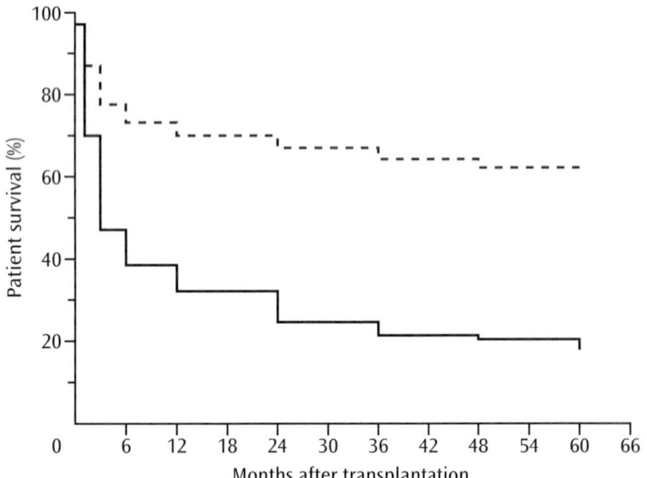

Figure 61.2 *Survival of liver transplant recipients treated before and after the availability of cyclosporine. Data are derived from 170 "before" (solid line) and 125 "after" (dashed line) recipients. Survival is calculated using the life-table method. (Reprinted with permission from Starzl* et al.[39]*)*

Specific indications and contraindications

The decision to transplant is difficult to base on objective liver function test results because these values vary considerably according to the specific pathologic process. Instead, the degrees of medical, social, and psychological impairment are considered in combination, then

Table 61.8 *Common pathophysiologic consequences of end-stage liver disease*

Organ system	Consequence
Central nervous	Encephalopathy (mild confusion → coma) Brain edema (fulminant hepatitis)
Cardiovascular	Hyperdynamic circulation Reduced systemic resistance Increased plasma volume Pericardial effusion
Pulmonary	Pleural effusion Interstitial edema (hypoalbuminemia) Atelectasis Ventilation–perfusion mismatch and shunting
Gastrointestinal	Esophageal varices Ascites Portal hypertension Delayed gastric emptying
Hematologic	Reduced clotting factor levels Anemia Thrombocytopenia (hypersplenism) Reduced clearance of fibrinolytic substances and tissue plasminogen activators
Endocrine	Glucose intolerance Diminished glycogen stores
Renal	Oliguria (hepatorenal syndrome, prerenal azotemia) Hyponatremia (diuretics, increased antidiuretic hormone activity) Hypokalemia (poor nutrition, diuretics, intestinal losses)

balanced against the mortality associated with conservative management. Ideally, liver transplantation is undertaken before the degree of organ failure becomes severe and the patient incapacitated, to reduce perioperative morbidity.

There is little debate that liver transplantation is indicated for nonmalignant end-stage liver disease that will not recur in the hepatic graft. Most often, this procedure is used to treat benign parenchymal diseases, including postnecrotic cirrhosis and any of the causes of acute liver failure or cholestatic processes (e.g. primary biliary cirrhosis or biliary atresia in children; Table 61.9). In all, more than 60 disease entities have now been successfully treated by liver transplantation. Transplanting in the presence of a disease when recurrence is a possibility is somewhat more controversial, considering the limited supply of donor organs. Alcoholic cirrhosis was once considered an absolute contraindication to transplantation, but multidisciplinary care and careful selection have led to results with Laennec's cirrhosis that are similar to those with other liver diseases. Similarly, transplantation for cirrhosis from hepatitis B virus infection has proved to be beneficial for many patients despite the inability to prevent infection in the donor liver. Advanced age was also once a contraindication, but recipients older than 50 years have been shown to have a 5-year survival rate after transplantation, which is similar to that of younger adults.[41]

Treatment of hepatic cancers by transplantation is being studied at several centers and is the subject of considerable debate. Patients with primary liver and bile duct cancers, as well as hepatic metastases from GI and endocrine tumors, have undergone liver transplantation with varying durations of remission.[42,43] But recurrence of tumor is the rule, so transplantation is usually reserved for selected cases with isolated tumors and deteriorating liver function. If hepatic function remains preserved in the presence of a liver tumor, major hepatic resection is the recommended alternative.

Other possible contraindications relate to specific surgical obstacles, including thromboses of major abdominal veins and scarring from multiple abdominal procedures. However, the successful use of vein grafts and accumulation of practical experience with the transplantation procedure have rendered even these contraindications obsolete.

Table 61.9 *Preoperative pathologic diagnoses in liver transplant recipients*[a]

Disease	Number of cases
Parenchymal	
Postnecrotic cirrhosis	348
Alcoholic cirrhosis	76
Acute liver failure	54
Budd–Chiari syndrome	18
Congenital hepatic fibrosis	9
Cystic fibrosis	6
Neonatal hepatitis	8
Hepatic trauma	3
Cholestatic	
Biliary atresia	217
Primary biliary cirrhosis	186
Sclerosing cholangitis	100
Secondary biliary cirrhosis	25
Familial cholestasis	16
Inborn errors of metabolism	114
Tumors	
Benign	10
Primary malignant	60
Metastatic	8

a. Data derived from 400 pediatric and 858 adult recipients of liver transplants at the University of Pittsburgh, 1981–8. (Adapted with permission from Starzl *et al.*[39])

Preanesthetic considerations

Candidates for liver transplantation present a broad clinical spectrum, ranging from chronic fatigue with mild jaundice to coma with multiorgan failure. Hepatic encephalopathy may be reversible; thus, the timing of liver transplantation can be critical to outcome. Emergency transplantation for fulminant hepatic failure can have a salvage rate of 55–75%[44] provided that symptoms have not progressed to grade 4 encephalopathy. Without transplantation, most causes of fulminant hepatic failure are associated with much poorer prognoses.

Certain uncommon diseases treated by liver transplantation have additional implications for anesthesiologists. For example, after transplantation for Budd–Chiari syndrome, which typically is associated with extensive hepatic venous thrombosis, patients may require anticoagulation. In children with an even rarer disorder, Crigler–Najjar syndrome (bilirubin uridine diphosphate-glucuronyl transferase deficiency), drugs that interfere with bilirubin binding to albumin (e.g. barbiturates) should be avoided.

Many of the physiologic derangements associated with end-stage liver disease are not correctable until after transplantation. Therefore, the major emphasis in the preanesthetic evaluation should be on identifying the most important areas of physiologic compromise and treating only those that threaten the safe induction of anesthesia. For example, pleural effusions may be responsible for profound hypoxemia, and, despite clotting abnormalities, preoperative thoracentesis may be a necessity. However, defects in coagulation are usually not corrected at this point unless there is active hemorrhage. If blood product administration is essential, but limited by oliguric hypervolemia, hemofiltration has been used in parallel to the venovenous bypass circuit.

Preparation of fluid-warming units, gas circuit humidifiers, warming blankets, and nonconductive wraps for the head and extremities is essential before induction; otherwise, hypothermia will rapidly result from transfusion, convective and evaporative losses from exposure of abdominal organs, diminished hepatic energy production, and implantation of a cold donor organ of large thermal mass. A thromboelastograph is also assessed at many centers as a relatively rapid means to elucidate a need for specific blood product replacement under conditions of massive transfusion.

Finally, as a result of the primary disease process or subsequent multiple transfusions, recipient serologies may be positive for hepatitis A, B, or C. The healthcare team should be aware of the potential for infectious contamination and take appropriate precautions (see Chapter 70).

Anesthesia induction

Liver transplantation involves transection and reanastomosis of several major venous structures (portal vein and IVC), and the ability to transfuse rapidly is vital to successful outcome. At least two large-bore peripheral venous cannulae should be inserted, one of which is 8.5 French units to facilitate the use of a rapid transfusion device. Because major shifts in intravascular volume are common and reperfusion of the donor liver has been associated with hypotension, invasive monitoring with arterial and pulmonary artery catheters is standard. Both radial and femoral artery catheters are often placed because distal arterial flow may be compromised by aortic clamps during hepatic artery anastomoses. The balance of the monitoring array is similar to that used for any critically ill patient undergoing a major general surgical procedure.

Patients with end-stage liver disease have numerous reasons for delayed gastric emptying, such as ascites or active upper GI bleeding.

Therefore, aspiration precautions are mandatory and induction of general anesthesia should proceed by either a rapid sequence technique or, in patients with hemodynamic instability or significant hypovolemia, awake intubation.

Anesthesia and surgical procedures

Anesthesia is maintained by agents that preserve splanchnic flow (e.g. opioids or isoflurane) combined with muscle relaxants, except in cases of fulminant hepatic failure in which the possibility of intracranial hypertension contraindicates potent inhaled agents. Nitrous oxide is not contraindicated but is usually avoided because of its ability to distend the bowel and increase the size of gas bubbles entrained in the circulation. Pharmacokinetic alterations associated with end-stage liver disease are complex and have been reviewed.[45] The net effect of these factors for nondepolarizing muscle relaxants is to increase the loading dose requirements and prolong the durations of action. In contrast, fentanyl kinetics are not markedly changed.[46] Although well-preserved liver allografts can rapidly begin to metabolize drugs,[47] many of the pharmacokinetic changes (e.g. diminished serum albumin, enlarged volumes of distribution) persist beyond the transplantation procedure.

The orthotopic procedure involves replacing the diseased native liver with a cadaveric organ in the most anatomic position possible. It consists of three stages: the preanhepatic, anhepatic, and neohepatic stages (Table 61.10).

The preanhepatic stage involves dissection of the structures of the porta hepatis and mobilization of the native liver. Cardiovascular instability is common during this phase because of hypovolemia from acute third-space losses (ascites) and hemorrhage from venous collaterals in the body wall and mesentery. Citrate-induced hypocalcemia, hyperkalemia from rapid transfusion and hemolysis, embarrassment of venous return from retraction, or precipitous drops in intra-abdominal pressure and consequent venous pooling also contribute to hemodynamic instability. During sudden volume shifts, previously asymptomatic pericardial effusions may reduce cardiac output, so they are often drained under direct vision. Hemorrhage may be exacerbated by clotting factor deficiencies or hemodilution, and by fibrinolysis. These defects should be treated as specifically as is feasible using either conventional studies (prothrombin time, partial thromboplastin time, bleeding time, fibrinogen, fibrin split product levels, and platelet count) or thromboelastography. Rapid infusion systems designed to deliver prewarmed fluids or blood products at a rate of up to $1.5\,L\,min^{-1}$ are used routinely (Fig. 61.3). Line pressure monitors, filters, air detectors, and fluid-level sensors are built into the device to minimize trauma to the blood and to prevent transfusion of air. Blood salvaging ("autotransfusion") systems, which collect and wash extravasated blood, are also used, provided that there is no active infection or malignancy.

Metabolic acidosis may accompany hypotension and persist in the absence of hepatic metabolic function. Sodium bicarbonate is used for treatment, although if acidosis is severe, THAM [tromethamine (tris(hydroxymethyl)aminomethane)] is an alternative that avoids hyperosmolar hypernatremia.[47] Oliguria is also common in this phase, and once prerenal causes are ruled out, aggressive treatment with osmotic or potent loop diuretics, as well as renal-dose dopamine ($2.5\,mg\,kg^{-1}\,min^{-1}$), is begun.

The anhepatic stage begins when the native diseased liver is removed after transection of its blood supply (hepatic artery and portal vein), as well as occlusion of the suprahepatic and infrahepatic portions of the IVC. If large esophageal varices seem at high risk for rupturing during IVC clamping, a Sengstaken–Blakemore tube may be placed temporarily. To avoid drastic decreases in venous return and cardiac output, as well as venous congestion in the lower body, bowel, and kidneys, many centers use a venovenous bypass system. The venovenous circuit drains blood from the portal and femoral veins and routes it extracorporeally to the axillary vein. A centrifugal pump propels blood through the circuit at a flow rate 20–50% of usual total systemic flow. The circuit makes use of heparin-bonded tubing, which at the flow rates typically used obviates the need for systemic heparinization. Although venous bypass may help to preserve renal function, it may not improve overall morbidity and mortality[49] and can lead to venous air embolism and thrombosis. The use of venous bypass can also prolong the procedure and contribute to heat loss. Moreover, support of cardiac output with positive inotropes may still be required.

Removal of the native liver and implantation of the allograft usually require vigorous retraction near the diaphragm, decreasing respiratory compliance, and causing atelectasis and hypoventilation. Adding PEEP and raising inspiratory pressures may help to minimize these effects. Because of the lack of liver metabolic function during the anhepatic phase, citrate intoxication from rapid transfusion is a more likely possibility, and calcium must be infused to maintain the ionized calcium level above $1.0\,mmol\,L^{-1}$. Calcium chloride is often chosen, but even in the absence of hepatic function, calcium gluconate has effectively treated ionized hypocalcemia. Progressive hyperkalemia may be treated with an insulin infusion, despite the absence of liver, but metabolic acids, including lactate, remain largely uncleared during the anhepatic period.

The neohepatic or postreperfusion stage begins with reanastomoses of the major vascular structures. Before removal of all clamps, the allograft is flushed of air, debris, and preservative solution with blood released from the portal vein. Despite this, subsequent final unclamping can cause release of a large load of potassium and metabolic acids into the circulation. Dysrhythmias, hypotension, and cardiac arrest may ensue, and the anesthesiologist should be prepared to treat the underlying metabolic causes specifically. Inotropic support may be needed to treat hypotension stemming from myocardial depression

Table 61.10 *Overview of the orthotopic liver transplantation procedure*

Phase	Surgical procedures	Physiologic changes
Preanhepatic	Dissection of porta hepatis Release of hepatic attachments	Third-space losses (as hepatis cites) Hemorrhage (venous collaterals)
Anhepatic	Clamp hepatic aorta, portal vein Venovenous bypass (adults) Clamp IVC Retraction on diaphragm	Obstruction of venous return Oliguria (venous congestion) Atelectasis, decreased compliance
Neohepatic	Anastomosis of IVC Flush hepatic allograft Anastomosis of portal vein, hepatic artery Biliary drainage procedure	Hemorrhage (coagulopathy) Citrate intoxication Hyperkalemia Hypothermia Metabolic acidosis

IVC, inferior vena cava.

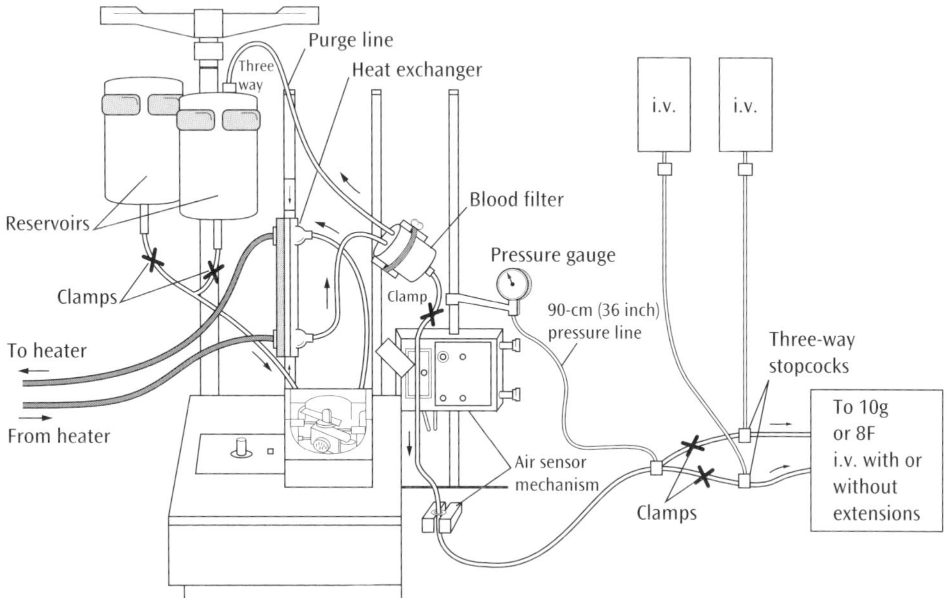

Figure 61.3 *Rapid infusion system used during liver transplantation at the University of Pittsburgh. (Reprinted with permission from Kang* et al.[48]*)*

by putative vasoactive mediators, or right-heart failure from venous air embolism. Appearance of significant end-tidal nitrogen from venous air embolism by mass spectroscopy is useful to differentiate between these alternatives. Pulmonary thromboembolism has also been reported to be a cause of cardiovascular collapse during reperfusion.[50,51]

Once the allograft begins to function, hemodynamic and metabolic stability is gradually restored. The need for inotropic support usually diminishes, and urine output improves even in patients with prior hepatorenal syndrome.[52] Clotting parameters can usually be normalized with specific replacement therapy, and fibrinolysis controlled with, ε-aminocaproate (Amicar). The procedure ends with some form of biliary reconstruction, either direct bile duct anastomosis or a Roux-en-Y choledochojejunostomy (Fig. 61.4).

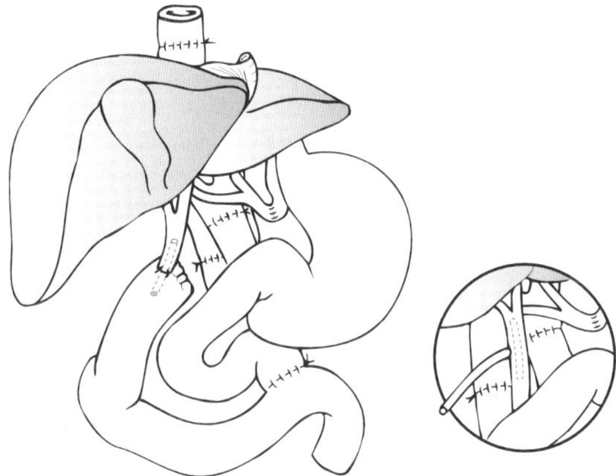

Figure 61.4 *Biliary reconstruction after orthotopic liver transplantation. Biliary drainage can be accomplished via a Roux-en-Y (choledochojejunostomy) or "duct-to-duct" anastomosis (inset). (Reprinted with permission from Starzl* et al.[39]*)*

Postoperative management

In a well-functioning allograft, metabolic acids, including lactate, continue to be metabolized and systemic alkalosis may result. Meticulous postoperative pulmonary toilet is vital and may be complicated by injury to the diaphragm, nosocomial pneumonia, adult respiratory distress syndrome from massive transfusion, and weakness from nutritional deficiencies. Primary nonfunction of the allograft is now a rare complication of liver transplantation, perhaps because of the widespread use of UW solution for preservation. Recovery from primary nonfunction has occurred, but most often retransplantation has been necessary.

The full immunosuppression regimen of cyclosporine or tacrolimus, azathioprine, and prednisone is begun in the early postoperative period, yet rejection episodes are still common and may be treated with the monoclonal antibody OKT3. Other complications include biliary or vascular anastomotic leaks, abdominal abscesses, and thrombosis of the hepatic artery or portal vein. As in other patients on long-term immunosuppression with cyclosporine, recipients are also at risk for development of lymphoproliferative malignancies and opportunistic infections (see Evaluation of patients with a prior organ transplant). Cases of transplantation for hepatitis B or neoplasms may also be complicated by recurrence of the original disease.[53]

HEART TRANSPLANTATION

It is estimated that as many as 14 000 patients per year in the USA alone could benefit from heart transplantation.[49] However, after rapid growth in the mid-1980s, the number of heart transplantations per year has now reached a plateau of approximately 3000 cases worldwide because of the limited availability of donor organs. The orthotopic procedure has accounted for the overwhelming majority of cases.

Growth in heart transplantation has been encouraged by dramatic increases in survival. Before the introduction of cyclosporine, the 1-year survival rate was approximately 40%. In the 1990s, cyclosporine, coupled with intensive immunologic surveillance by endomyocardial biopsy and aggressive antirejection treatment with lymphocyte-specific monoclonal antibodies, has boosted overall survival rates of orthotopic transplant recipients worldwide to >80% at 1 year and >70% at 5 years.[54] Individual centers have reported survival rates to be as high as 90% at 4 years.[55] Other outcome variables, such as quality of life, are favorable as well.

Pathophysiology of end-stage heart disease

End-stage heart disease may result from either congenital or acquired diseases of the heart or vascular system. The leading causes include ischemic and valvular disease and primary cardiomyopathy. Depending on the cause, a varying period of physiologic adaptation precedes the onset of decompensation, which is usually manifested by congestive heart failure. Once this symptom is present, the overall 5-year survival rate is less than 50%, although patients with rapidly progressive symptoms seem even less likely to survive.[56] Dysrhythmias and laboratory evidence of pump failure (e.g. low ejection fraction) are also associated with a relatively poorer prognosis.

As the left ventricle fails, the main compensatory mechanism is an increase in left ventricular end-diastolic volume, which enhances resting myocardial fiber length and promotes more effective fiber shortening. Such changes restore stroke volume, at the cost of increasing left atrial pressure and producing pulmonary venous congestion. Other compensations include elevation in catecholamines and increased renin production, resulting in salt and water retention.

Progression of the underlying pathophysiologic process eventually reduces ejection fraction and results in severe congestive heart failure refractory to conventional drug therapy. At this point, some patients may still be ambulatory, but have little functional reserve; others are not ambulatory because of dyspnea or dependence on i.v. inotropes, mechanical circulatory support, or mechanical ventilation. Protracted periods of low cardiac output compromise other vital organ functions (e.g. passive congestion of the liver and prerenal azotemia) and may culminate in inadequate perfusion to the heart itself, initiating a final, irreversible, downward spiral. Patients may enter a transplant program during any of these stages, or even after mechanical circulatory support with an intra-aortic balloon or ventricular assistance device becomes necessary. Interestingly, survival rates remain relatively high in patients requiring mechanical circulatory support as a bridge to transplantation, even in those receiving a temporary artificial heart.[54]

Specific indications and contraindications

The indication for heart transplantation is fulfilled when New York Heart Association class IV status (severely compromised) and prognosis (guarded despite therapy) persist despite maximal medical therapy. The typical candidate is a 40- to 60-year-old man with a pretransplantation diagnosis of ischemic cardiomyopathy and left ventricular ejection fraction of < 20%. The other common diagnoses are idiopathic cardiomyopathy and viral cardiomyopathy; end-stage congenital heart disease accounts for the remainder. In the latter group, the congenital defect is often associated with a cardiomyopathy secondary to long-standing cyanosis or myocardial hypertrophy, making further palliation impossible.

The list of contraindications has undergone considerable evolution in the last decade and will probably continue to do so. For example, the upper age limit was formerly 50 years. However, substantial numbers of older patients have now undergone this procedure without disproportionate morbidity, and, as a consequence, "physiologic" rather than chronologic age is now emphasized when deciding on candidacy. Diabetes mellitus has also been an absolute contraindication; however, it now seems that even insulin-dependent diabetic patients can be successfully immunosuppressed without the aid of steroids, and short-term results seem favorable. A history of cancer was once an absolute contraindication as well, but strict exclusion on this basis became obsolete as true long-term cures for certain malignancies (e.g. Hodgkin's lymphoma) were demonstrated. The presence of certain systemic diseases may also contraindicate heart transplantation; for example, the cardiomyopathy accompanying sarcoidosis could respond to medical therapy, and amyloidosis might recur in the donor organ.

Severe, irreversible pulmonary hypertension remains one of the few absolute contraindications to orthotopic heart transplantation because the right ventricle of a normal donor heart is unable acutely to cope with a markedly elevated, fixed, pulmonary vascular resistance and rapidly decompensates. The precise level of pulmonary hypertension deemed unacceptable is still a matter of debate: the traditional values are 6–8 Wood units [0.8–1.1 kPa (6–8 mmHg) ($L\,min^{-1}$), or in metric resistance units, 480–640 $dyne\,s\,cm^{-5}$], or a transpulmonary gradient (mean pulmonary artery pressure–mean pulmonary capillary wedge pressure) of 1.3–2 kPa (10–15 mmHg). If irreversible pulmonary hypertension is present, heterotopic heart transplantation is one option, although, more recently, as long as suitable organs are available, heart–lung transplantation is preferred.

Preanesthetic considerations

Given the candidacy criteria, the recipient's other vital organs are usually not seriously impaired. However, low cardiac output may lead to chronic passive liver congestion and oliguria, and there may be corresponding physical signs and abnormal laboratory values (Table 61.11).

Candidates for heart transplantation are usually maintained on oral or i.v. inotropes (e.g. digoxin, amrinone), vasodilators (captopril, amrinone), and diuretics, and, when appropriate, antidysrhythmics. Patients with large, dilated hearts and low cardiac output are prone to form intracardiac thrombi and, therefore, are anticoagulated with warfarin. In such cases, fresh-frozen plasma is required following cardiopulmonary bypass, and appropriate arrangements should be made before induction. Blood products should be CMV free for patients without antibody evidence of prior exposure, considering the likelihood and morbidity of CMV viremia in immunosuppressed recipients. Bacterial pneumonia is relatively common early after heart transplantation, so preparation of the anesthesia machine with a fresh, sterile breathing circuit and bacterial filter seems prudent. It has not been found necessary to sterilize tracheal intubation equipment, although, at most institutions, factory-sterilized disposable endotracheal tubes are standard.

Some transplantation candidates have previously undergone coronary bypass or other thoracic or mediastinal procedures. If so, they are likely to require more than the usual time for insertion of vascular catheters and cannulation for cardiopulmonary bypass. To avoid unnecessary prolongation of donor organ ischemic times, the surgical and anesthesia teams must factor in these potential sources of delay.

Donor procedure and related considerations

Cardiac harvesting is best carried out simultaneously with the harvesting of abdominal viscera. This approach, which involves local perfusion with preservative solutions after cross-clamping the abdominal and thoracic aortae, avoids inadvertent cardiac arrest before cardiectomy and damage to the allograft. Donor cardiectomy begins with pericardiotomy, after which the epicardial coronary arteries are grossly palpated for plaques. The aorta and both venae cavae are dissected, and, after systemic heparinization, the superior vena cava is ligated and the IVC and a pulmonary vein are transected. The heart is then exsanguinated, and cardioplegia is administered through the aortic root. After cardiac arrest, the aorta is cross-clamped, the heart is topically cooled, and the remaining pulmonary veins are individually transected. Finally, the great arteries are divided, and the heart is rinsed and examined for a

Table 61.11 *Pathophysiologic consequences of dilated cardiomyopathy*

Organ system	Consequence
Pulmonary	Pulmonary venous congestion Interstitial edema
Renal	Prerenal azotemia Oliguria
Hepatic	Chronic passive congestion Hepatomegaly Ascites
Central nervous	Confusion (low cardiac output)
Endocrine	Elevated serum catecholamine Elevated renin levels

patent foramen ovale or valvular lesions and then placed in a sterile plastic bag containing cold saline, which, in turn, is placed inside an insulated cooler. In laboratory studies, hearts have been preserved for as long as 24 h with excellent subsequent graft function. Currently, however, the generally accepted limit on human donor heart ischemic time (measured from the time the cross-clamp is applied to the time of cross-clamp removal after implantation) is 4–6 h.[57] In view of this limited duration, the only immunologic matching performed prospectively is ABO compatibility.

Cardiac trauma, cardiac arrest, hypoxemia, and excessive requirement for exogenous catecholamines may render a potential donor's heart unacceptable for transplantation. However, as long as there is echocardiographic evidence of good contractility, such criteria do not necessarily mandate exclusion. In most transplantation centers, there is no absolute age limit for eligibility as a heart donor, but in donors older than 40 years careful physical examination at the time of harvest is essential to avoid transplanting organs with significant coronary lesions.

Anesthesia induction

Candidates are often on the transplant list for extended periods and build up considerable apprehension. Despite this, preoperative sedation must be used judiciously because residual cardiac performance depends on elevated endogenous catecholamines. The monitoring regimen used by most heart transplantation centers includes intra-arterial and pulmonary artery pressure monitoring. Although avoidance of sepsis is important, conventional aseptic techniques for catheter insertions have proved to be sufficient.[58] Pulmonary artery catheterization is routinely performed through the right internal jugular vein and does not seem to jeopardize access for future endomyocardial biopsies. Correct pulmonary artery catheter positioning is often more difficult in this population owing to severe orthopnea (necessitating a semisitting position), cardiac dilation (promoting intraventricular coiling), tricuspid regurgitation, atrial fibrillation or other arrhythmias, or congenital vascular anomaly. Once the catheter is placed, a long, sterile sheath is always used because this catheter is pulled back to "central venous pressure position" before caval cannulation.

Whether already in the hospital or newly admitted through the emergency department, most of these patients have recently eaten and, thus, require rapid inductions. There have been numerous descriptions of anesthetic techniques,[59–61] all based on agents compatible with the pathophysiology of end-stage heart disease. In one study of induction regimens, a combination of 0.3 mg kg^{-1} etomidate, 10 µg kg^{-1} fentanyl, and 1.5 mg kg^{-1} i.v. succinylcholine was shown rapidly to produce adequate intubating conditions without significant cardiovascular depression.[62] Anesthesia can then be maintained using a regimen compatible with extremely poor ventricular function [e.g. O_2/35–75 µg kg^{-1} i.v. fentanyl (total) + 0.3 mg i.v. scopolamine].

After induction, tracheal intubation is accomplished without specially sterilized laryngoscopy equipment, and broad-spectrum prophylactic antibiotics and the immunosuppressant azathioprine are infused. Patients with end-stage heart disease are often exquisitely sensitive to changes in preload or afterload; thus, hypotension may stem from relatively small degrees of hypovolemia or alterations in systemic vascular resistance. Because one or both ventricles are usually extremely noncompliant, filling pressures may not accurately reflect intracavitary volumes, so transesophageal echocardiography can be especially helpful in maintaining cardiovascular stability.

Surgery and cardiopulmonary bypass

In the prepump phase of the orthotopic procedure, manipulation of the heart is minimized to avoid dislodging any intracardiac thrombi. After individual cannulation of the venae cavae as well as the aorta, cardiopulmonary bypass is initiated and the patient is cooled as for conventional cardiac procedures (26–30 °C). During cooling, the diseased heart is excised, leaving an atrial cuff containing the caval and pulmonary venous orifices and long remnants of the aorta and pulmonary artery. The donor heart's back wall (atrium) is trimmed appropriately, then anastomosed with the recipient's atrial remnant. Special care must be taken to keep the anterior wall of the donor heart cold even during posterior wall anastomosis because warming may contribute to poor right ventricular function later. The heart is then filled with cold saline to displace most of the air, the aorta is anastomosed, and after de-airing once again, the cross-clamp is removed (ending the ischemic time). Often, electromechanical activity resumes spontaneously and, finally, the pulmonary artery anastomosis is completed (Fig. 61.5). A more recently introduced variation, the complete atrioventricular heart transplantation operation, involves bicaval anastomoses with preservation of the entire donor atria. The principal advantage seems to be a lower prevalence of tricuspid regurgitation.

For the heterotopic procedure (Fig. 61.6), after sternotomy, a right pleuropericardial flap is created. When cardiopulmonary bypass is initiated, the native heart undergoes cardioplegic arrest for myocardial protection, and the donor heart is placed in the right thorax anterior to the compressed lung. The donor and recipient superior venae cavae and right atria are incised and sutured together, and the donor's aorta is sutured end to side to the recipient's ascending aorta. The donor's pulmonary artery is then connected to the recipient's main pulmonary artery by means of a Dacron graft.

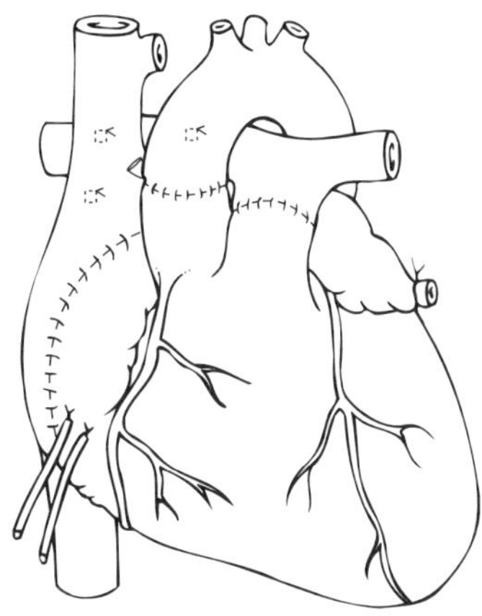

Figure 61.5 *Sites of anastomoses after the mid-atrial excision orthotopic cardiac transplantation procedure. (Reprinted with permission from Reitz* et al.[63]*)*

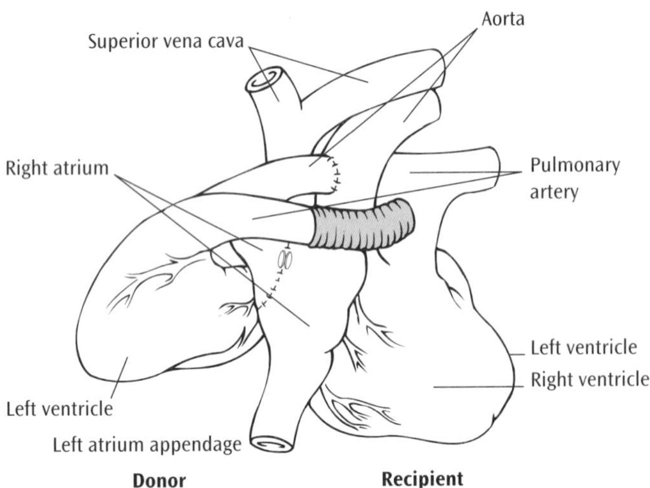

Figure 61.6 *Heterotopic transplantation of a donor heart. (Reprinted with permission from Cooper and Lanza.[64])*

Because many patients with end-stage heart disease are maintained on diuretics, mannitol or furosemide may be necessary to maintain a urine flow. In some cases, these patients may have markedly expanded blood volumes and benefit from hemoconcentration on bypass. At many centers, just before release of the aortic cross-clamp, to reduce the possibility of hyperacute immune response, 500–1000 mg i.v. methylprednisolone is administered. Immediately after release of the aortic cross-clamp, slow junctional rhythms or arteriovenous nodal dysfunction is relatively common. An infusion of either isoproterenol or another catecholamine with positive chronotropic effects is often begun temporarily to support heart rate. Most of these dysrhythmias resolve, but a small percentage do persist after surgery, even in the absence of rejection. Ultimately, approximately 5% of recipients require implantation of a permanent pacemaker, although the balance of survivors do not seem particularly prone to other serious dysrhythmias.

Immediately before weaning from cardiopulmonary bypass, the posterior anastomosis is rechecked because leaks in this area are difficult to repair later. After final de-airing, the superior vena caval cannula is removed, the pulmonary artery catheter advanced and repositioned, and the serum ionized calcium restored to normal. If heart rate is less than 60–70 beats per min, epicardial electrodes are placed and pacing is begun.

Cardiac performance is often mildly compromised immediately after heart transplantation, and many transplantation centers routinely use inotropic infusions to wean patients from cardiopulmonary bypass. Although there have been reports of exaggerated effects, in practice, responses to catecholamine infusions seem qualitatively similar to those in other cardiac surgical patients.[65] Further discussion of the physiology and pharmacology of cardiac denervation can be found in the section on Evaluation of the patient with a prior organ transplant.

Markedly elevated pulmonary vascular resistance is a contraindication to orthotopic transplantation, but transient pulmonary vasospasm can occur during weaning, even in patients with previously normal pulmonary artery pressures, producing life-threatening right-heart failure. Prostaglandin E_1 (PGE_1), at infusion rates between 0.025 and 0.2 mg kg^{-1} min^{-1}, has been shown effectively to unload the right heart,[66] although simultaneous norepinephrine (noradrenaline) or phenylephrine infusion may be required to support systemic vascular resistance. Elevated pulmonary vascular resistance often falls within hours of the procedure,[67] allowing PGE_1 infusions to be discontinued; however, as a last resort, mechanical right ventricular assistance has been used for varying periods with success.[68]

Postoperative management

The short-term management goals in the intensive care unit include cardiovascular support and prevention of rejection and infection. Most patients receive triple immunosuppression (cyclosporine–azathioprine–prednisone) and, at some centers, OKT3. The sources of fever or pulmonary infiltrates are sought aggressively. Early in the postoperative period, bacterial pneumonias with typical nosocomial organisms are encountered. Later, opportunistic infection with CMV, *Pneumocystis*, or *Legionella* may occur, and transbronchoscopic brushing may be necessary to establish the etiology. There may be bradydysrhythmias or atrioventricular block in this period, with temporary pacing required. Persistently low cardiac output may result from rejection or from reperfusion injury, and endomyocardial biopsy may be the only means to establish the diagnosis.

Excessive mediastinal bleeding and coagulopathy may be encountered in patients who have previously undergone a cardiac surgical procedure and are treated in the conventional fashion. If hemodynamic stability is maintained, evidence of mild organ compromise present before transplantation will gradually disappear. If, however, the transplanted heart functions poorly, organs with preoperative impairment may rapidly decompensate.

HEART–LUNG TRANSPLANTATION

Heart–lung transplantation is the procedure of choice for patients with end-stage lung disease complicated by irreversible right ventricular failure or end-stage congenital heart disease with secondary pulmonary vascular involvement (Eisenmenger syndrome). Specific pathologic diagnoses in recipients have included primary pulmonary hypertension, emphysema, multiple pulmonary emboli, cystic fibrosis, and granulomatous and fibrotic diseases of the lung. Suitable donor blocs are in extremely short supply because both the lungs and heart must fulfill the criteria for acceptability (see Other viscera transplantation procedures). Such blocs consist of the entire heart and lungs, including a tracheal segment long enough to facilitate anastomosis. Distal procurement is made feasible by flushing the harvested bloc with modified Euro-Collins or UW solution, to which PGE_1 or other pulmonary vasodilator may be added.

Considerations for monitoring and induction of anesthesia are in general similar to those for heart transplantation, but air trapping during ventilation and pulmonary hypertension are additional factors that may lead to hemodynamic instability. Difficulty with the airway during induction can result in hypercarbia or hypoxia and further elevate pulmonary vascular resistance.

Patients with congenital heart disease may have bidirectional intracardiac shunts, which can become predominantly right-to-left and lead to profound hypoxemia. Such shunts may also lead to paradoxical air emboli, so bubbles in i.v. tubing should be scrupulously avoided. Chronically cyanotic patients are often severely polycythemic (hematocrit >60%) and manifest clotting derangements. Under these circumstances, phlebotomy and hemodilution may be beneficial. In all recipients, large endotracheal tubes are preferred to facilitate therapeutic bronchoscopies.

In the prebypass phase, surgical dissections may be complicated by extensive pleural adhesions; however, once on bypass, *en bloc* implantation is relatively straightforward and accomplished by sequential tracheal (or bibronchial), right atrial, and aortic anastomoses. The phrenic, vagus, and recurrent laryngeal nerves may be damaged by both dissection and topical cooling, and must be protected. The tracheal anastomosis usually involves some technique to prevent dehiscence, such as a "telescope" anastomosis or wrapping the suture line with vascularized omentum. Re-expansion of transplanted lungs may require bronchoscopy to relieve mechanical obstruction by secretions; occasionally, bronchodilators are useful to treat bronchospasm. Because of the extensive mediastinal and pleural dissection, the early postbypass period may be complicated by hemorrhage leading to coagulopathy. Pulmonary compliance and gas exchange may deteriorate during this time because of pulmonary hemorrhage or inadequate preservation, and the use of PEEP is often required.

After surgery, rejection episodes are relatively common and are characterized by infiltrates, fever, and deteriorating gas exchange. Pulmonary allografts may be rejected without significant abnormalities in endomyocardial specimens,[69] so low cardiac output is not necessarily a symptom of rejection. Recipients are also highly susceptible to bacterial pneumonia, which presents with the same clinical picture as rejection; bronchoalveolar lavage or transbronchial biopsy may be necessary for definitive diagnosis. A dreaded problem soon after heart–lung transplantation is dehiscence of the tracheal or bronchial suture lines, which can lead to fatal mediastinitis. Later, bronchiolitis obliterans develops in a significant proportion of survivors. The etiology is unknown, but this condition is associated with a progressive decline in exercise tolerance. Bronchiolitis obliterans and the physiology of transplanted lungs are discussed further in the section on Other viscera transplantation procedures.

In the future, heart–lung transplantation will probably have even fewer indications, as experience with isolated lung transplantation accumulates. The latter operation will then be used in patients with end-stage lung disease before right ventricular failure becomes irreversible and necessitates the combined heart–lung procedure.

LUNG TRANSPLANTATION

End-stage lung disease from destruction of the pulmonary parenchyma or vasculature is a leading cause of disability and death among adults. Several lung transplantation operations have been developed to treat end-stage lung disease, each having certain conceptual and practical advantages. These include the heart–lung, *en bloc* double-lung, single-lung, and bilateral sequential single-lung procedures. In the setting of chronically elevated pulmonary vascular resistance with right ventricular failure, heart–lung transplantation is usually chosen. However, when cardiac performance is preserved, isolated lung transplantation has been shown to be of benefit to carefully selected patients with end-stage lung disease[70] (Table 61.12).

End-stage pulmonary parenchymal diseases are restrictive, obstructive, or infectious. Briefly, restrictive lung diseases are characterized by interstitial fibrosis with a loss of lung elasticity and compliance. Most fibrotic diseases are idiopathic, but they may also be caused by an inhalation injury or immune/inflammatory processes. Interstitial lung disease may affect the blood vessels as well, so pulmonary hypertension is often found. Functionally, diseases in this category are associated with diminished lung volumes and diffusion capacity, but preserved air flow rates. Respiratory muscle strength is usually excellent because the work of breathing is chronically elevated.

The most common cause of end-stage obstructive lung disease is smoking-induced emphysema, but other causes include asthma and several comparatively rare congenital disorders. Among these, α_1-antitrypsin deficiency is associated with severe bullous emphysema in the fourth or fifth decade of life. With obstructive diseases, airway resistance is elevated, expiratory flow rates are diminished, air trapping may be prominent, and ventilation–perfusion mismatching severe.

Table 61.12 *Pathologic diagnoses in lung transplant recipients*[a]

Diagnosis	Number
Chronic obstructive pulmonary disease	20
α_1-Antitrypsin deficiency	19
Cystic fibrosis	8
Pulmonary hypertension	8
Pulmonary fibrosis	7
Bronchiectasis	2
Eosinophilic granuloma	1
Lymphangiomyomatosis	1

a. Data derived from 66 consecutive patients who underwent lung transplantation at Barnes Hospital, St Louis, between July 1988 and January 1991. (Adapted with permission from Trulock *et al.*[71])

The common infectious etiologies of end-stage lung disease include cystic fibrosis and bronchiectasis. Cystic fibrosis, which occurs in 1 out of every 2000 live births in the USA, produces mucus plugging of peripheral airways, chronic bronchitis, and bronchiectasis. Smoking and environmental exposures may also lead to bronchiectasis.

End-stage pulmonary vascular disease may be a consequence of primary pulmonary hypertension, which is a relatively rare disease of unknown etiology characterized by marked elevation of pulmonary vascular resistance from hyperplasia of the muscular pulmonary arteries and fibrosis of smaller arterioles. Congenital heart disease with Eisenmenger syndrome and diffuse arteriovenous malformations are other causes of destruction of the pulmonary arterial bed.

The general indications for transplantation with any of the end-stage lung diseases are progressive exercise intolerance, increasing oxygen requirements, and carbon dioxide retention. Other factors favoring the transplantation option are recurrent need for phlebotomy and increasing physical and social debilitation. The timing of surgery depends on the rate of functional deterioration and ability of the right ventricle to tolerate the progression of pulmonary hypertension. Considering the limited supply of donor organs, specific contraindications to lung transplantation include severe debilitation, neuromuscular disease, or mechanical ventilator dependence (because respiratory muscle strength is crucial to recovery); severe chest deformity or pleural disease (complicating surgical procedures and postoperative ventilation); advanced right ventricular failure; or glucocorticoid dependence (because healing of airway anastomoses is impeded by steroids).

The choice of lung transplantation procedure is based largely on the consequences of leaving the native lung *in situ*. For example, single-lung transplantation is not an option if infection or severe bullous emphysema is present in the contralateral lung. Infection would cross-contaminate the healthy transplanted lung, and severe bullous disease in the native lung could lead to gross ventilation–perfusion mismatching and shifting of the mediastinum. Instead, double-lung transplantation would be chosen for such cases. Similarly, double-lung transplantation may also lead to better functional outcomes in the treatment of end-stage pulmonary hypertension.[70,72] The other major factor influencing the choice of procedure is the relative rate of perioperative complications. For example, single-lung transplantation is feasible without cardiopulmonary bypass and is seldom complicated by bleeding diatheses. In contrast, *en bloc* double-lung transplantation mandates cardiopulmonary bypass with full systemic heparinization and extensive mediastinal dissection – both risk factors for development of postoperative coagulation defects. Another advantage of single-lung transplantation is that it makes use of bronchial anastomoses, which heal with significantly fewer complications than the tracheal repairs typical of the *en bloc* double-lung procedure. Bilateral sequential lung transplantation, an alternative to *en bloc* double-lung transplantation, combines advantages by using bibronchial anastomoses and avoiding cardiopulmonary bypass.

Donor lungs

Donor lungs may be jeopardized by massive fluid resuscitation, aspiration, contusion, and exposure to nonphysiologic oxygen tensions because most organ donors are trauma victims. Ideally, the donor's history should indicate early tracheal intubation with no evidence of aspiration, minimal fluid administration in the course of resuscitation, and absence of chest tubes, pleural diseases, or tracheostomy at any time. Suitable donors should have a minimal alveolar–arterial O_2 gradient [i.e. a P_aO_2 of > 53.3 kPa (400 mmHg) while breathing 100% O_2, or 13.3 kPa (100 mmHg) on 40% O_2/5 cmH_2O PEEP], as well as a clear chest radiograph and sputum examination within 2 h of harvesting.[73] If bronchoscopy fails to demonstrate any pathologic process, i.v. glucocorticoids and antibiotics are administered and the lungs harvested. Because both the heart and lungs may be harvested from the same donor, a method has been developed for cardiectomy without jeopardizing the use of the lungs. First, the heart is removed, but a cuff of left atrium is left attached to the donor lungs. The trachea is then stapled and divided at its midpoint, and the lungs removed *en bloc* and immersed in cold preservative solution. In some centers, before removal, the donor is treated with a pulmonary vasodilator (e.g. PGE_1) to improve the distribution of a large volume of either a blood-based or intracellular-type cold crystalloid preservative solution, infused through the pulmonary artery. Finally, the lungs may be inflated before immersion in preservative solution and stored for transportation.

Preanesthetic considerations

Preanesthetic considerations for lung recipients have been described previously.[74–77] Briefly, size matching is achieved by comparing the vertical and transverse radiologic chest dimensions of the donor and recipient. Organs are also matched on the basis of ABO compatibility, but because the need for histocompatibility is still unknown and the tolerable ischemic time for the lung is relatively short (approximately 4 h), HLA matching is carried out only in retrospect. Preoperative pulmonary function and right-heart catheterization studies, ventilation–perfusion scans, and arterial blood gas values are helpful to predict the difficulties likely to be encountered during and after induction. For example, diminished expiratory flow rates and air trapping may exacerbate hypoxemia and hypercapnia and lead to hemodynamic instability during mask ventilation and after tracheal intubation. Elevated pulmonary artery pressures may indicate a likelihood that cardiopulmonary bypass will be necessary because right ventricular failure can suddenly result when one-lung ventilation or ligation of a pulmonary artery is begun. Even in the absence of pulmonary hypertension, many centers recommend "pump standby" for these cases because gas exchange is so precarious. Clearly, both systemic and pulmonary arterial pressure monitoring are vital during lung transplantation procedures, although profound dyspnea may make internal jugular cannulation difficult before induction. Pulmonary artery catheters should be inserted through a sterile sleeve to allow withdrawal during the anastomosis and subsequent repositioning. Finally, candidates may have recently undergone weaning from glucocorticoids, but "stress doses" are avoided in the perioperative period to protect from systemic sepsis or suture line dehiscence.

Single-lung transplantation

The single-lung transplantation procedure involves pneumonectomy and implantation of a new lung, sometimes preceded by mobilization of the omentum with its vascular pedicle for bronchial wrapping. If the native lungs are equally impaired and no pleural scarring is present, the left lung is often chosen for transplantation for technical reasons: the native right pulmonary veins are less accessible than those on the left, the recipient's left bronchus is longer, and the left hemithorax can more easily accommodate a somewhat oversized donor lung. Most surgeons prefer that the lung to be removed is collapsed during dissection; both bronchial blockers and double-lumen endobronchial tubes have been used for this purpose. Because the right upper lobe bronchial orifice is relatively close to the origin of the mainstem bronchus, left-sided endobronchial double-lumen tubes have been recommended for both right and left single-lung transplants as well as for the bilateral sequential operation.

For the induction of anesthesia by the rapid-sequence technique, drugs that do not release histamine or depress the myocardium are usually preferred (e.g. etomidate, vecuronium). Nitrous oxide is avoided in patients with bullae or elevated pulmonary vascular resistance and when 100% oxygen is needed to maintain acceptable arterial saturation. Both high-dose opioids and potent inhaled agents, supplemented with long-acting relaxants, have been used successfully for the maintenance of anesthesia.

With the onset of one-lung ventilation, acute deterioration in gas exchange or hemodynamics is the rule. Strategies for improving oxygenation under these circumstances include the use of PEEP in the dependent lung, continuous positive airway pressure or high-frequency ventilation in the nondependent lung, or ligation of the (nondependent) pulmonary artery. If pulmonary artery pressures rise sharply at this point, right ventricular failure may ensue. Vasodilators or inotropes may diminish right-heart strain; if not, one-lung ventilation should be abandoned. Similarly, if hemodynamics or systemic arterial saturations deteriorate when the pulmonary artery is clamped in anticipation of pneumonectomy, cardiopulmonary bypass may be necessary.

Immediately before implantation, the donor lung is trimmed to match the size of the recipient bronchus, branch pulmonary artery, and atrial cuff containing the orifices of the pulmonary veins. While attempting to keep the allograft cold, the atrial, pulmonary artery, and bronchial anastomoses are completed in sequence. The circulation is then restored to the donor lung, ending the ischemic interval; however, until ventilation to the allograft is restarted, systemic arterial saturation suffers. Flexible bronchoscopy is prudent at this stage to visualize the anastomosis directly or reinflate the allograft by removing secretions or blood from the airway. Once the anastomosis is secure, a pedicle of omentum with its blood supply intact may be brought into the chest and wrapped around the bronchial anastomosis. Finally, after the chest is closed, the supine position can be restored and the endobronchial tube exchanged for a standard endotracheal type (except if "split" ventilation is planned).

Double-lung transplantation

Double-lung transplantation is most often used in patients with primary pulmonary hypertension or cystic fibrosis. The *en bloc* operation is performed in the supine position, and because both lungs are replaced at once, cardiopulmonary bypass is mandatory. Cardioplegic arrest is used to accomplish anastomosis of the left atrial cuff containing all four pulmonary venous orifices. The airway is typically interrupted at the level of the trachea, so a standard endotracheal tube is suitable. Because systemic arterial supply to the trachea is permanently interrupted, an omental wrap may be added. The extensive retrocardiac dissection required often leads to cardiac denervation and postoperative bleeding that is difficult to control.[78]

Bilateral sequential single-lung transplantation was introduced to treat the same spectrum of patients as the *en bloc* procedure, but obviates the need for cardiopulmonary bypass and tracheal anastomosis. Access to the hilar structures is gained in the supine position through a rather extensive incision that includes a transverse sternotomy ("clamshell" incision; Fig. 61.7). Another relative disadvantage is that serial implantation results in a longer ischemic time for the second allograft.

Postoperative management

Postoperative management of patients after isolated lung transplantation involves intensive respiratory support and differentiating between lung infection and rejection using transbronchial biopsies obtained by flexible bronchoscopy.[80] Early respiratory insufficiency may be due to pulmonary venous (anastomotic) obstruction or possible reperfusion injury, which is characterized by large alveolar–arterial oxygen gradients, poor pulmonary compliance, and parenchymal infiltrates despite low cardiac filling pressures. Mechanical ventilation with PEEP is essential, but in consideration of new airway anastomoses, inflation pressures are kept to a minimum. $F_{I}O_2$ values are also maintained at the lowest levels compatible with acceptable oxygen saturation. After single-lung transplantation for an obstructive disease, the endobronchial tube may be left in place for several days, and special respiratory support in the form of split (individual lung) ventilation used to avoid overinflation of the native lung, gross ventilation–perfusion mismatching, and shifting of the mediastinum.

The lung is unique among transplanted viscera because it is exposed to the external environment. Lymphatic disruption, poor mucociliary function, and the presence of suture lines across the airway are other factors increasing the susceptibility of transplanted lungs to infection. In the first postoperative month, bacteria are the most frequent cause of pneumonia; nosocomial Gram-negative organisms constitute the bulk of isolates.[81] After this period, CMV pneumonitis becomes more common, particularly if lungs from a CMV-seropositive donor are used in a seronegative recipient.[73] There is a high rate of acute rejection episodes after lung transplantation, which on clinical grounds alone are often difficult to distinguish from infection. This distinction is vital, however, because steroid boluses used to treat rejection may worsen pneumonia or promote systemic sepsis. Bronchoalveolar lavage fluid or sputum specimens obtained by fiberoptic bronchoscopy may be helpful in diagnosing an infectious etiology; transbronchial or, occasionally, open lung biopsy is needed to establish the diagnosis of rejection. Hemorrhage is a complication that most frequently occurs after *en bloc* double-lung transplantation, particularly in patients with pleural disease or Eisenmenger syndrome with extensive mediastinal vascular collaterals. The recurrent laryngeal, phrenic, and vagal nerves are jeopardized during lung transplantation, and injury complicates the process of weaning from mechanical ventilation. Primary healing occurs with most bronchial anastomoses; rarely, bronchial fistulae lead to stenoses that can be successfully treated by silicone stents and dilation. In contrast, tracheal anastomotic leaks often lead to fatal mediastinitis.

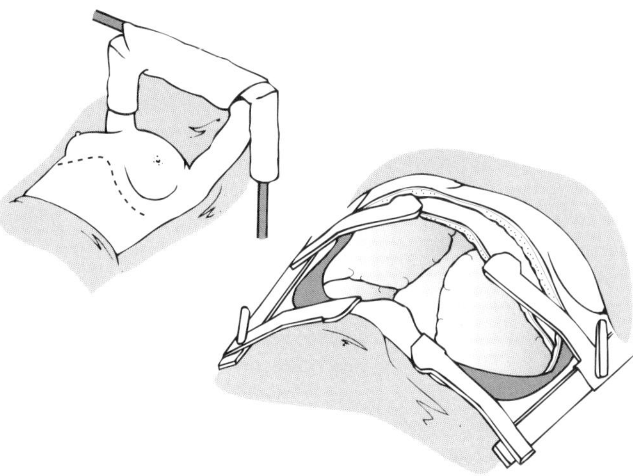

Figure 61.7 *Positioning and surgical approach for bilateral sequential lung transplantation. The incision consists of bilateral anterior thoracotomies with a transverse sternotomy. After insertion of vascular catheters, the patient's arms are wrapped and suspended from the ether screen. (Reprinted with permission from Cooper and Patterson.[80])*

Long-term complications include lung infections with opportunistic organisms, such as *Pneumocystis carinii* and *Candida albicans*. Bronchiolitis obliterans, a pathologic condition characterized by luminal destruction of small respiratory bronchioles, has been noted after heart–lung transplantation,[82] but so far seems less common after single-lung transplantation. Outcome results of lung transplantation series from specialized centers are promising. The Washington University Lung Transplantation Group[71] has reported on a series of 69 procedures and found the actuarial survival at 1 year to be 90% after single-lung transplantation and 82% after the bilateral sequential operation. Pulmonary function tests, pulmonary arterial pressure and resistance, arterial blood gases, and exercise capacities all improved significantly after operation. In an earlier analogous series from Toronto, there were no ventilatory limitations or significant desaturation during exercise testing noted in lung transplantation survivors .

OTHER VISCERA TRANSPLANTATION PROCEDURES

There is considerable interest in transplantation of the pancreas and small intestine, particularly in view of the sizable patient populations that stand to benefit. These are relatively fragile viscera, and optimal preservation regimens and implantation procedures have yet to be defined.

Pancreas transplantation

There are as many as 20 000 new cases of type 1 (juvenile onset, insulin dependent) diabetes mellitus in the USA each year.[83] This disease destroys the insulin-producing pancreatic β cells by an inflammatory process. The microangiopathy that results from diabetes is among the leading causes of blindness and renal failure.

Pancreatic transplantation by surgical means was first attempted in the mid-1960s, and by 1989 the annual rate of such cases reported to the International Pancreas Transplantation Registry was 554.[84] At specialized centers, the operative mortality rate was low (≤1%), the 1-year survival rate was at least 90%, and normoglycemia and insulin independence was achieved in 50–70% of cases at 1 year.[85] In many of these cases, patients received both kidney and pancreas allografts, which seemed to prevent the recurrence of diabetic nephropathy in the transplanted kidney,[86] as well as some of the other microvascular complications.

Pancreatic transplantation is usually reserved for diabetic patients with the most severe and rapidly progressive complications in view of the considerable side-effects of immunosuppression. Preoperative screening consists of thorough evaluation of the organ systems most affected by diabetes; metabolic studies, including a glucose tolerance test; and urine and serum C-peptide levels ("connecting" peptide is cleaved from proinsulin before secretion into the circulation); glycosylated hemoglobin levels (an index of glycemic control during preceding months); and insulin and islet cell antibodies. Ultrasonography of the gallbladder is conducted to rule out cholelithiasis. In addition to tight preoperative plasma glucose control, mechanical and antibiotic bowel preparation is usually undertaken.

Most pancreatic transplantations are accomplished using the bladder drainage technique. This involves extraperitoneal pancreatic placement and exocrine drainage by duodenocystostomy. After surgery, patients seldom require intensive care, although assiduous control of plasma glucose using an insulin infusion is recommended. Once oral feeding is resumed, insulin is unnecessary unless allograft function is lost. A major advantage of the bladder drainage technique is the ability to monitor allograft exocrine function, which deteriorates during episodes of rejection. Urinary pH may fall, reflecting a decrease in pancreatic bicarbonate secretion, and urinary amylase may diminish. Other postoperative complications include graft thrombosis and intra-abdominal infection.

Pancreatic islet transplantation, in which only the required cell type is introduced, has undergone numerous clinical trials.[87] In this procedure, which does not require surgical intervention, just the islets are isolated by cell separation techniques then infused into the portal vein. In some cases, islet cells may become fully functional over several weeks and restore insulin independence;[87] in others, insulin requirement has been reduced but not eliminated.

Multiviscera transplantation

Simultaneous replacement of multiple digestive organs, known as the *cluster operation*, has been introduced to treat two diseases: short gut syndrome and locally confined GI tumors. With short gut syndrome from any cause, parenteral feeding may lead to liver failure, and *en bloc* transplantation of the liver combined with the pancreas, stomach, duodenum, and jejunum (Fig. 61.8) has met with some success. In children, multiviscera transplantation is performed primarily for short gut syndrome resulting from necrotizing enterocolitis or midgut volvulus.

Tumors such as hepatomas and cholangiocarcinomas, as well as carcinomas of the proximal GI tract or pancreas, have also been treated by cluster operation after upper abdominal exenteration. Without surgery, the prognosis for these cancers is uniformly dismal, and even partial resections combined with chemotherapy or radiation offer little improvement in overall survival. In contrast, although experience is still limited, multiviscera transplantation is associated with 1-year survival rates of 70% (with sarcomas or GI-derived neuroendocrine tumors) or 44% (primary liver cancers).[89]

Anesthetic management of cluster surgery has been reviewed in detail.[90] Briefly, the types and doses of previous chemotherapy should be ascertained during the preoperative visit because some agents have long-lasting toxic effects on the heart or kidneys. Hormone-secreting tumors, producing carcinoid crisis, can be suppressed with octreotide acetate, a somatostatin analog; with ketanserin, a serotonin antagonist; or by arterial embolization. During surgery, the management issues are similar to those for liver transplantation alone, namely massive transfusion, coagulopathies, hypothermia, electrolyte abnormalities, and the use of venovenous bypass for systemic venous return. Postoperative complications include a high incidence of rejection, particularly of the small bowel, sepsis from loss of the intestinal barrier, and graft-versus-host disease. The likelihood of graft-versus-host disease is proportional to the length of intestine transplanted, presumably reflecting the quantity of lymphoid tissue contained in the wall of this organ.

TRANSPLANTATION IN CHILDREN

The clinical manifestations of end-stage organ disease in children are in general similar to those in adults; however, the pathologic processes leading to organ failure often differ. For example, the etiology of end-stage renal disease noted in the pediatric population (Table 61.13) differs markedly from that for the general population (see Table 61.6). During childhood, developmental anomalies and genetic defects, anatomic or functional (i.e. inborn errors of metabolism), may lead to end-stage organ disease. Congenital anomalies may be confined to a single organ system (e.g. reflux nephropathy) or be part of a constellation of abnormalities. For example, in Alagille syndrome, end-stage liver disease is accompanied by congenital heart disease, hypercholesterolemia, and renal dysfunction. Clearly, awareness of such syndromes is necessary to anticipate coexistent pathologic processes in other organ systems.

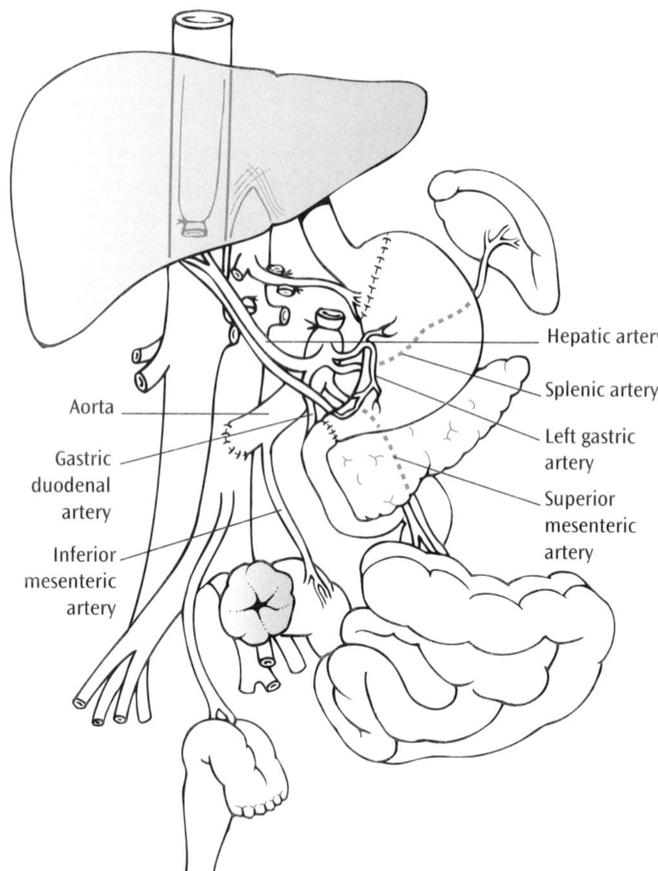

Figure 61.8 *Schematic representation of the recipient procedure for multiviscera transplantation. (Reprinted with permission from Starzl* et al.[88]*)*

Ethical considerations

The ethics of transplantation are also somewhat different in the pediatric age group. The legally adopted criteria for brain death are not universally accepted as applicable in the immediate neonatal period, so organ donation from this population is controversial. Size considerations place additional constraints on the organ-matching process in children, exacerbating the shortages. To remedy this, procedures for living-related donation have been developed for kidney transplantation, and, more recently, liver and lung transplantation. Although living-related renal transplantation has gained acceptance because of its particular benefits for children, the liver and lung procedures are more controversial owing to higher morbidity and mortality in the donors. Other ethical dilemmas, such as whether transplantation can provide truly long-term survival and whether transplanted organs grow and develop normally in children, remain unresolved. In addition, long-term immunosuppression with cyclosporine increases the risk for development of a lymphoproliferative malignancy, perhaps related to Epstein–Barr virus infection or reactivation. Although the overall incidence is reasonably low, the shift to earlier presentation of aggressive malignancies raises new concerns.

Table 61.13 *Pathologic diagnoses in pediatric renal transplant recipients at the University of Minnesota*[a]

Diagnosis	Total cases (%)
Obstructive	16.8
Renal uropathy hypoplasia	15.3
Glomerulonephritis	15.3
Congenital nephrotic syndrome	8.5
Steroid-resistant nephrotic syndrome	7.2
Medullary cystic disease	4.5
Pyelonephritis	4.1
Hemolytic uremic syndrome	4.0
Alport syndrome	2.6
Oxalosis	2.3
Miscellaneous, including unknown	19.4

a. Data derived from a total of 531 cases performed between 1963 and 1990. (Adapted with permission from Belani and Palaliniuk.[34])

Renal transplantation

Although pharmacologic agents combined with dialysis can be used to treat end-stage renal disease in children, medical management has an overall high morbidity rate and adversely affects growth and development.[91] Children treated medically during their maximum growth years show a marked decrease in eventual height and weight,[92] as well as cognitive development,[93] compared with control subjects. Early transplantation seems to reduce the severity of these problems,[94,95] justifying the current recommendation "expectantly" to transplant children with progressive renal insufficiency, sometimes even before dialysis is required.

The most common diseases leading to renal transplantation in children are related to congenital anomalies and acquired nephropathies. A group of miscellaneous diseases account for the remainder (Table 61.13). Living-related renal transplantation is most often carried out in children and confers significant advantages: both short- and long-term mortality rates are improved, and graft survival is superior, perhaps because the risk of minor antigenic mismatch is reduced. Organ survival in children receiving a living-related donor kidney approaches 100% at 1 year and 70% at 10 years.[96] Because perioperative mortality and renal rejection are greater in infants, current practice is to avoid transplantation until later in childhood.

In contrast to adults, pediatric renal transplantation relies on intra-abdominal placement of the organ. This allows adult-sized kidneys to be transplanted into very small children and increases the size of the donor pool. During surgery, however, placement of the allograft can acutely cause hypothermia and sequester relatively large proportions of the child's blood volume. As a consequence, hypotension can occur. To prevent this, fluid boluses and vasoactive infusions are used to maintain systemic blood pressure in the high-normal range. As in adults, living-related donor kidneys usually function at once, whereas cadaver kidneys may take hours to resume urine production. Fluid management must take this into account. In either case, adult kidneys initially produce adult-sized volumes of urine, so maintenance fluids must be adjusted accordingly.

Liver transplantation

Approximately 20% of the orthotopic liver transplantations performed worldwide are in children, and most recipients are younger than 5 years of age.[97] Biliary atresia is by far the most common cause of liver failure in this population (Table 61.14). This is followed by inborn errors of metabolism, which include disorders such as α_1-antitrypsin deficiency, glycogen storage diseases, Wilson's disease, and tyrosinemia. The last three conditions primarily involve biochemical defects in hepatocytes and are, therefore, considered cured by liver transplantation.

Several aspects of the orthotopic liver transplantation procedure are unique to children. For example, patients with biliary atresia have usually undergone prior decompression with a Kasai (choledochojejunostomy) procedure, and this may complicate abdominal dissection during the preanhepatic phase of liver transplantation as well as later biliary reconstruction. Venovenous bypass is not feasible in patients weighing < 20 kg, so the lower body venous congestion that accompanies portal vein and IVC occlusion often leads to oliguria and intestinal complications in this group. An oversized allograft may sequester a substantial proportion of the blood volume, increase the risk of excessive potassium release after reperfusion, and lead to severe hypothermia. In children whose temperature falls below 34 °C, lavage of the peritoneal cavity with warm saline is effective in raising core temperature.

The limited availability of suitably sized organs for small patients has prompted the development of techniques for transplanting part of a liver. Figure 61.9 illustrates the technique that is used to create a reduced-size ("split") liver and enable one donor liver to be used for multiple patients. There is a significantly higher complication rate with this method, including greater blood loss, risk of organ necrosis, and diminished patient survival, so it is usually reserved for patients who are rapidly deteriorating. Living-related (partial) liver donation has also been promoted by the contention that up to one-half of pediatric liver transplantation candidates die while awaiting a suitable organ. However, in view of the potential for donor morbidity and the relatively reduced survival of recipients of reduced size livers, few centers offer this option.

The overall 1-year survival rate in children after orthotopic liver transplantation is 70–75%, but results for younger (< 3 years) and smaller (< 12 kg) patients are not as good (45–50% 1-year survival rate).[97,100] This discrepancy probably stems from two factors: the greater incidence of hepatic artery thrombosis in small children, which in turn is related to arterial size, and the use of reduced size livers.

Heart transplantation

Cardiac transplantation for congenital heart disease is the major indication for this procedure in children younger than 5 years of age. In older children, dilated cardiomyopathy remains most common. However, mortality rates for the young remain higher than for older children and adults (25% vs. 10% 30-day mortality respectively),[101] which results in lower overall survival. Cardiac-related complications are responsible for most early deaths, stemming from the presence of complex vascular anatomy, previous cardiac surgery, and elevation of pulmonary vascular resistance. The last factor is a well-recognized contraindication to heart transplantation in adults, but it is often difficult to accurately quantify

Table 61.14 *Pathologic diagnoses in pediatric orthotopic liver transplant recipients*[a]

	Total cases (%)
Biliary atresia	44
α_1-Antitrypsin deficiency	20
Other inborn errors of metabolism	10
Other obstructive disease (e.g. Alagille and Byler syndromes)	12
Miscellaneous	14

a. Data derived from 50 pediatric orthotopic liver transplant recipients at Children's Hospital of Pittsburgh between 1981 and 1983. (Adapted with permission from Borland *et al.*[98])

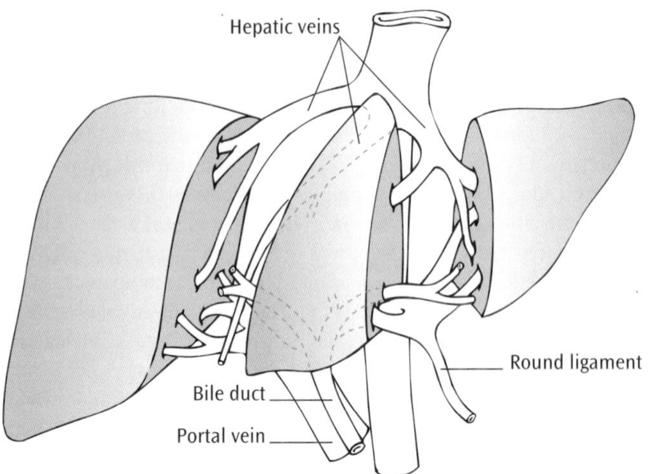

Figure 61.9 *A schematic for* ex vivo *dissection of an adult liver to create reduced size liver allografts with vascular supplies and biliary orifices. Donor iliac arteries or veins are used as needed to extend the vessels. (Adapted and reprinted with permission from Broelsch* et al.[99]*)*

in infants. If pulmonary vascular resistance is fixed at a high level, the normal allograft's right ventricle cannot acutely adjust to the increased afterload, and refractory right-heart failure ensues. Long-term survival may also be limited by an accelerated form of coronary atherosclerosis, as is seen in adults.

Generally accepted indications for heart transplantation in newborns include aortic atresia and hypoplastic left-heart syndrome. If reconstruction of the aortic arch is required, profound hypothermia and circulatory arrest are usually necessary. Positional or size discrepancies of the great vessels and abnormal arrangements of systemic or pulmonary venous return can complicate these procedures, and have so far limited overall survival rates for neonates to 66% at 1 year.[102]

A scientifically provocative aspect of transplantation unique to neonates is that the immature immune system seems relatively tolerant of foreign antigens.[103] By several criteria, the neonatal immune response to allograft tissue is attenuated, although the response to infective organisms and active immunization is comparatively intact. The mechanisms responsible are unclear, but may involve neonatal suppressor cells or maternal cells that enter the circulation during gestation.

Other viscera transplantation procedures

Rarely, heart–lung transplantation is indicated before early adulthood for cystic fibrosis, Eisenmenger syndrome, or primary pulmonary hypertension. Isolated lung transplantation may offer the only chance of survival to children with severe developmental anomalies of the lung, including cystadenomatous malformations and congenital diaphragmatic hernia with pulmonary hypoplasia or, in older children, cystic fibrosis. The scarcity of suitable donor organs has led to instances of living-related lung donation, but the merits of this approach have yet to be fully evaluated.

Multiviscera transplantation, which combines liver and small bowel transplantation, has been tried in children with short gut syndrome (as a result of necrotizing enterocolitis or midgut volvulus) further complicated by hepatic failure after long-term hyperalimentation. So far, intra-abdominal infection and repeated episodes of bowel rejection have limited survival, and thus the approach is still considered experimental.

EVALUATION OF PATIENTS WITH A PRIOR ORGAN TRANSPLANT

Transplant recipients may return for a staged repair (e.g. bile duct reconstruction after liver transplantation) or for entirely unrelated surgery. They may also present with a surgical illness superimposed on organ rejection, in which the usual signs and symptoms are masked. Immunosuppression increases the risk of opportunistic infection, so many recipients are maintained on a fixed dose combination of trimethoprim–sulfamethoxazole, which is effective in preventing such illnesses.[104] Postoperative bacterial infections are also more common in this group, so an attempt should be made to minimize exposure to nosocomial sources, such as urinary and intravascular catheters, and mechanical ventilators. Immunosuppressants also have numerous other adverse effects that can influence perioperative management.

Immunosuppressant side-effects and toxicities

Although immunosuppressants are usually administered in combination to diminish the risk of dose-related toxicity from any single agent, significant morbidity is still associated with their use (Table 61.15).

Glucocorticoids

Glucocorticoids produce glucose intolerance, cushingoid habitus, fragility of the integument, aseptic necrosis, and exacerbation of peptic ulcer disease. Yet, attempts to eliminate them from immunosuppression regimens usually have not met with success, with the possible exception of neonatal heart transplant recipients. Chronic glucocorticoid use is also associated with adrenal suppression. Although some authors advocate administration of preoperative stress doses of glucocorticoids, this has been shown to be unnecessary in at least one large series of surgical patients following renal transplantation.[105]

Table 61.15 *Immunosuppressant side-effects and toxicities*

Agent	Side-effect/toxicity
Glucocorticoids	Adrenal suppression Glucose intolerance Cushingoid appearance Integument fragility Aseptic necrosis Peptic ulceration
Azathioprine	Anemia Thrombocytopenia Leukopenia Pancreatitis Hepatitis Decreased nondepolarizing relaxant requirement
Cyclosporine	Glomerulosclerosis (elevation of blood urea tacrolimus nitrogen, creatinine) Hypertension Hepatotoxicity Neurotoxicity Enhanced renal sensitivity to insults
Antilymphocyte globulin	Leukopenia Thrombocytopenia Systemic symptoms
OKT3	Systemic symptoms Increased susceptibility to cytomegalovirus infections

Azathioprine

Azathioprine is a myelosuppressant, producing anemia, thrombocytopenia, and occasionally marrow aplasia. It has also been associated with hepatitis, alopecia, and GI upset and, through an allergic mechanism, pancreatitis. Azathioprine has been reported to increase the requirement for nondepolarizing relaxants to a modest degree, probably by presynaptic inhibition of phosphodiesterase in the motor nerve terminal.[106]

Cyclosporine and tacrolimus

Cyclosporine is both acutely and chronically nephrotoxic, producing interstitial renal fibrosis and tubular atrophy. Chronic toxicity is common, leading to elevations in blood urea nitrogen and creatinine levels, as well as systolic and diastolic hypertension. Management with conventional antihypertensives is usually successful, but the kidneys of such patients may be more vulnerable to acute insults, such as radiographic dye- or hypotension-induced nephropathy. Cyclosporine may be hepatotoxic, producing hyperuricemia, gingival hypertrophy, or seizures and neurotoxicity at high serum levels. The toxicity profile of tacrolimus seems to be qualitatively similar.

Antilymphocyte globulin and OKT3

Antilymphocyte globulin is a polyclonal antibody, and as such is "contaminated" with antibodies other than those directed against lymphocytes. This antilymphocyte globulin may give rise to marked leukopenia and thrombocytopenia, and systemic symptoms such as fever, chills, pruritus, GI upset, and even frank serum sickness. The first dose of OKT3 is frequently followed by systemic symptoms such as fever, dyspnea, and nausea, unless patients are pretreated with hydrocortisone, acetaminophen (paracetamol), and diphenhydramine. Subsequent reactions are less pronounced. OKT3 has also been associated with episodes of pulmonary edema, aseptic meningitis, and an unusually high incidence of CMV infection.

Early after transplantation, bacterial infections related to wound infection, urinary catheters, and pneumonia are most common (e.g. with *Staphylococcus aureus*, *Escherichia coli*, and *Streptococcus pneumoniae* respectively). After 1 month, immunosuppressed patients become vulnerable to opportunistic infections (*P. carinii* pneumonia, herpes zoster infections, and CMV viremia).[107] These episodes need not be fatal and can be overcome if diagnosis is rapid and treatment specific. The most common viral infection is CMV, which can occur as a primary infection from contaminated blood or allograft tissue in seronegative recipients, or as reactivated infection in seropositive patients.

Immunosuppressed patients are also more likely to have one of several histologically distinct types of lymphoproliferative malignancy. For example, the incidence of B-cell lymphoma in patients with renal allografts is approximately 350-fold higher than that seen in the normal age-matched population, and the same is probably true for cardiac recipients. Some studies have documented a causal role for Epstein–Barr virus,[108] and it is speculated that cyclosporine may diminish the cytotoxic response of suppressor T cells to autologous Epstein–Barr virus-infected B cells. Unfortunately, the mortality rate associated with these malignancies is relatively high; in one series, the 5-year mortality rate was 37%.[109]

Other preanesthetic considerations

Transplant recipients depend on immunosuppressants to avoid rejection, and these regimens must be restarted soon after surgery. If oral intake is expected to be delayed, appropriate parenteral formulations should be used. Certain drugs used in the perioperative period may inhibit the cytochrome P450 system and interfere with metabolism of cyclosporine (e.g. cimetidine), whereas others may induce the P450 enzymes and decrease cyclosporine levels (e.g. phenobarbital and phenytoin). Cyclosporine also increases the hypnotic duration of pentobarbital in laboratory animals,[110] but it does not increase the requirement for inhaled agents.[111] Such effects may be pharmacokinetic in origin. Cyclosporine has also been reported to prolong the action of pancuronium,[112] but controlled data are lacking.

The transplant population is also particularly prone to bacterial pneumonia and CMV viremia, so early extubation of the trachea is an important goal after any surgical procedure, and the use of CMV-negative blood is mandatory. In addition, intravascular catheterization is used only when specifically indicated, although standard aseptic cannulation techniques seem sufficient.

Anesthesia after kidney transplantation

Although renal transplantation is usually highly successful, some recipients still require dialysis. Thus, it is important to ascertain the degree of residual renal impairment and treat such patients accordingly. If the allograft is functional, renal excretion of drugs may be expected to be similar to that through native kidneys.

Many of these patients are diabetic and return to the operating room for ophthalmologic or peripheral vascular procedures. Perioperative complications leading to loss of the renal allograft are uncommon,[105,113] but sepsis is a major cause of morbidity. Management of blood glucose may be complicated by steroid immunosuppressants and fever; in such cases, insulin infusions are often necessary.

Because kidney recipients are maintained on cyclosporine, other agents with nephrotoxic potential (e.g. enflurane) are usually avoided. Cyclosporine may render allografts particularly sensitive to insults, so maintaining a brisk urine flow during anesthesia is recommended. During long procedures, this may justify the use of central venous pressure and urinary catheters.

Anesthesia after liver transplantation

In a well-functioning liver allograft, common biochemical pathways for drug metabolism are unimpaired. Provided that the metabolic and synthetic functions of the transplanted liver are also intact, the anesthetic care of these patients differs little from that of any other visceral transplant recipient. Within the first 2 months after liver transplantation, the most common surgical procedures are exploratory laparotomy for biliary leak or abscess drainage, or open liver biopsy. Regional anesthesia is avoided unless the coagulation profile has returned to normal. The likelihood of ileus or elevated intra-abdominal pressure indicates the use of rapid-sequence induction. Later, patients may require biliary reconstruction procedures.

Anesthesia after heart transplantation

Heart transplant recipients return to the operating room for non-cardiac surgery with some regularity. Such procedures do not always immediately follow the transplantation, but, instead, occur months or even years later. Overall, 25–30% of these patients will require a general surgical procedure within 2 years of transplantation.[114,115] Infectious causes for surgery (e.g. drainage of abscesses) can clearly be attributed to immunocompromise, but a relatively high incidence of cholecystitis is unexplained. In addition to these common general surgical problems, orthopedic procedures are frequently required secondary to joint complications arising from chronic steroid use. Despite numerous case reports of cardiac recipients undergoing noncardiac surgery, there are no prospective data addressing the risks of anesthesia in this physiologically unique population.

During orthotopic heart transplantation, the aorta and the main pulmonary artery are transected (see Fig. 61.6). As a result, the cardiac plexus is divided, resulting in autonomic afferent and efferent denervation. Myocardial tissue obtained from hearts transplanted for as long as 12 years fails to reveal evidence of abundant reinnervation.[116] Some of the nerve cells present in such specimens probably represent postganglionic parasympathetics because significant amounts of acetylcholine do remain.[116] Although early canine studies indicated that implanted hearts underwent efferent reinnervation and thus regained autonomic control,[117] in humans, with rare exception, studies of transplanted heart rate responses to exercise and respiratory stimuli[116,118–120] indicate that autonomic efferent denervation is permanent. Afferent reinnervation may occur in some cases, as suggested by clinical and biochemical criteria.[121]

In the absence of rejection or significant pulmonary hypertension, long-term follow-up studies after heart transplantation have demonstrated that, despite denervation, the resting stroke volume and indices of myocardial contractility are often normal[122] or only subtly reduced.[123] However, with demands for increased cardiac output (e.g. during exercise), the response of the denervated heart is demonstrably different (Fig. 61.10). In the normally innervated heart, immediate increases in cardiac output are mediated by elevation in heart rate with little change in stroke volume. In contrast, the denervated heart responds to such demands by increases in stroke volume rather than in heart rate. Cardiac recipients are thus preload dependent and must have adequate central volume to meet the demands of stress or anesthetic techniques that redistribute vascular volume to the periphery.

The denervated heart eventually can manifest increases in heart rate, albeit with some delay (Fig. 61.11). In cardiac transplant recipients, the maximal achievable pulse rate during exercise develops more slowly than in control subjects, and the return of heart rate to baseline is slower. The delay in achieving a maximal heart rate corresponds to the time required for secretion and circulation of adrenal catecholamines, and the slow return is probably related to the absence of vagal input.

As a consequence of the mid-atrial orthotopic surgical technique, the transplant recipient retains remnants of the native atria, and the electrocardiogram may contain both donor and native P-waves. Because the sinus node is normally under the continual influence of autonomic (vagal) nerves, the rate of the transplanted atria usually exceeds that of the native atria.[126] With parasympathetic activation (e.g. by visceral traction including laryngoscopy or drug effects), the native atrial rate may diminish, but the transplanted heart rate remains unchanged because vagal input is absent. In contrast, sympathetic stimulation (whether from hypoxemia, hypercapnia, hypotension, or pain) can still increase the donor heart's sinus rate, although, importantly, such responses are delayed. In contrast to effects on the sinoatrial node, denervation usually does not alter the arteriovenous conduction time or affect ventricular conduction.[127]

By 3 years, approximately 30% of survivors have multivessel coronary stenoses[128] (Fig. 61.12). These lesions are diffuse, concentric narrowings of the coronary lumen, and are thought to arise from areas of immune-mediated endothelial damage. In some cases, lesions are amenable to angioplasty or surgical bypass, but, often, myocardial ischemia and infarction limit the useful life of the allograft. Although the ability of these patients to perceive angina pectoris has been documented,[121] afferent innervation seems to be lacking in most, rendering episodes of myocardial ischemia silent. Thus, diagnostic electrocardiographic monitoring is essential throughout the perioperative period, and paroxysmal dyspnea, which may be the only indication of ischemia, should be regarded as an ominous symptom.

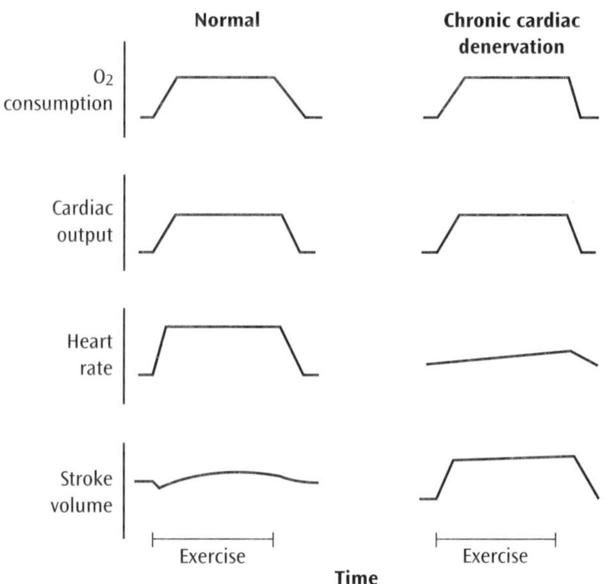

Figure 61.10 *Schematic representation of the cardiac physiologic responses to moderate supine exercise in humans. Responses of normal subjects are represented on the left; those following cardiac denervation are on the right. (Reprinted with permission from Kent and Cooper T.[124])*

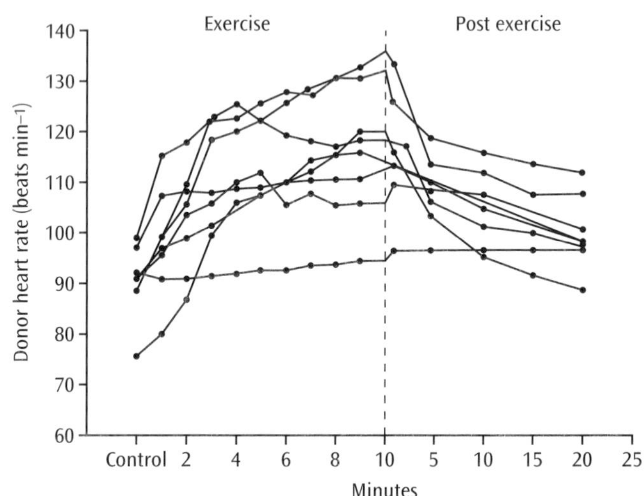

Figure 61.11 *Donor heart rates during supine bicycle exercise by eight patients 1 year after heart transplantation. The rates of achieving a maximal pulse are slower than in patients with innervated hearts. "Control" refers to measurements made at the start of exercise. The postexercise scale is compressed. (Reprinted with permission from Stinson* et al.*[125])*

Clearly, drugs that act indirectly on the heart fail to produce their typical effects after denervation; for example, administration of atropine or pancuronium does not elevate heart rate (Table 61.16), although neostigmine can cause bradycardia in this population.[131] In contrast, agents that act directly on myocardium or cardiac conduction tissues manifest their usual effects; for example, isoproterenol increases contractility and heart rate, whereas propranolol has the opposite effects.

Digoxin, which has mixed direct–indirect actions,[131] acts only directly after transplantation. An i.v. bolus of digoxin fails to alter either

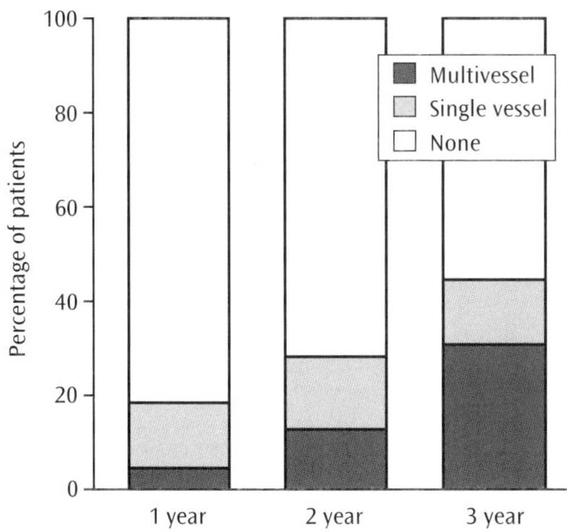

Figure 61.12 *Life-table analysis showing the risk, in humans, for development of coronary artery disease over the first 3 years after cardiac transplantation. (Reprinted with permission of the authors and the American Heart Association. From Uretsky* et al.[129]*)*

the functional or effective refractory periods of the atrioventricular node,[131] whereas it significantly increases the refractory period in normal patients. This suggests that the acute, chronotropic effects of digoxin are vagotonic and depend on intact autonomic innervation. When treated chronically with digoxin, cardiac transplant recipients demonstrate an inotropic response from a direct effect independent of autonomic innervation.

Norepinephrine is another cardioactive drug with somewhat atypical effects in this population. Infusions at conventional doses may be accompanied by more pronounced chronotropic effects than usual, through a direct β-adrenergic receptor-mediated effect on the sinus node that is normally masked by vagal reflexes. Cardiac transplant recipients with previous longstanding heart failure may also have a persistently blunted response to α-adrenergic agonists.[132] This probably results from adjustment of the peripheral vasculature or the baroreceptors to chronically elevated catecholamine levels. Finally, there is electrophysiologic evidence of moderate supersensitivity to adenosine after transplantation.[133]

Cardiac rejection may be superimposed on the surgical illness and may be the cause of low cardiac output and dysrhythmias. Rejection can, thus, impair responses to the stress of surgery and anesthesia. Endomyocardial biopsy may be necessary for definitive diagnosis of rejection, and aggressive immunotherapy with high-dose steroids or antilymphocyte globulin started in the perioperative period.

Table 61.16 *Altered responses to common cardiovascular drugs after cardiac denervation*

Drug	Response
Atropine	No vagolytic effect
Pancuronium	No vagolytic effect
Edrophonium	No vagotonic effect
Ephedrine	Less cardiostimulatory effect
Nifedipine	No depression of nodal conduction
Digoxin	No acute vagotonic effect
Norepinephrine	Enhanced β-stimulatory effect
Phenylephrine	Diminished vasoconstrictive effects with longstanding heart failure

Norepinephrine (noradrenaline).

FUTURE TRENDS

Since its inception, viscera transplantation has been limited by a shortage of suitable donor organs. For patients with end-stage renal disease, this has meant longer periods on dialysis with greater costs and morbidity, but for prospective heart and liver recipients there is a 10–40% mortality rate while awaiting transplantation. One remedy lies in further improvements in organ preservation because prolonging tolerable organ ischemic time increases the potential donor pool. The size of this pool will also increase as the criteria for donor acceptability expand (e.g. to include older donors, donors with certain systemic diseases, and terminally ill and fetal donors). Other approaches to deal with the limited supply of organs include cellular transplantation, in which healthy allograft cells derived from one organ may be infused into multiple recipients, and xenotransplantation from genetically "humanized" animals.

Optimizing the use of the available donor organs will also be important. For example, early application of isolated lung transplantation could make the heart–lung procedure obsolete and allow each heart–lung bloc to serve several patients. Accelerated atherosclerosis is a major factor limiting the useful lifespan of donor hearts; development of an effective therapy would represent a major breakthrough.

For the foreseeable future, immunosuppressant drugs will continue to be necessary to prevent the response to foreign tissue antigens. Development of agents with greater immunoselectivity and reduced toxicity is of the highest priority. Noninvasive methods to diagnose organ rejection would also substantially improve the quality of life for transplantation survivors. Longer term approaches to the problem of rejection currently under investigation include induction of tolerance to foreign antigens by promoting cell migration and "chimerism;" definition of the most critical elements for histocompatibility; and development of better "rescue" drugs once rejection has begun.

REFERENCES

1. United Network for Organ Sharing (UNOS): UNOS receives federal contract to develop OPTN. *UNOS Update* 1986; **2:** 1.
2. Friend PJ, McCarthy U, Fib RS, *et al.* Transmission of idiopathic (autoimmune) thrombocytopenic purpura by liver. *Ann Thorac Surg* 1986; **41:** 520.
3. United Network for Organ Sharing (UNOS) website: http://www.unos.org, 2001.
4. Simmons RL, Canafax DM, Fryd DS, *et al.* New immunosuppressive drug combinations for mismatched and cadaveric renal transplantation. *Transplant Proc* 1986; **18** (Suppl. 1): 76.
5. Guidelines for the Determination of Death. Report of the medical consultants on the diagnosis of death to the President's Commission for the Study of Ethical Problems in Medicine and Biomedical and Behavioral Research. *JAMA* 1981; **246:** 2184.
6. Grigg MM, Kelly MA, Celesia GG, *et al.* Electroencephalographic activity after brain death. *Arch Neurol* 1987; **44:** 948.
7. Lynn J. Diagnosis of brain death. *JAMA* 1983; **250:** 612.
8. Logigian EL, Ropper AH. Terminal electrocardiographic changes in brain-dead patients. *Neurology* 1985; **35:** 915.
9. Vaghadia H. Atropine resistance in brain dead organ donors. *Anesthesiology* 1986; **65:** 711.
10. Collins GM, Bravo-Shuarman M, Teraskai P. Kidney preservation for transplantation: initial perfusion and 30 hours ice storage. *Lancet* 1969; **2:** 1219.
11. Belzer FO, Southard JH. Principles of solid organ preservation by cold storage. *Transplantation* 1988; **45:** 673.
12. Hardesty RL, Griffith BP, Deep GM, *et al.* Improved cardiac function using cardioplegia during procurement and transplantation. *Transplant Proc* 1983; **15:** 1253.
13. Baron P, Heil J, Condie R, *et al.* 96-Hour renal preservation with silica gel precipitated plasma cold storage versus pulsatile perfusion. *Transplant Proc* 1990; **22:** 464.
14. Downey JM. Free radicals and their involvement during long-term myocardial ischemia and reperfusion. *Annu Rev Physiol* 1990; **52:** 487.

15. Reinherz EL, Sclossman SF. The differentiation and function of human T-lymphocytes. *Cell* 1980; **19:** 821.
16. Strom TB. Immunosuppressive agents in renal transplantation. *Kidney Int* 1984; **26:** 353.
17. Opelz G. Effect of HLA matching, blood transfusions, and presensitization in cyclosporine-treated kidney transplant recipients. *Transplant Proc* 1985; **17:** 2179.
18. Weil R, Clarke DR, Iwaki Y, *et al.* Hyperacute rejection of a transplanted human heart. *Transplantation* 1981; **32:** 71.
19. Stinson EB, Payne R, Griepp RB, *et al.* Correlation of histocompatibility matching with graft rejection and survival after cardiac transplantation in man. *Lancet* 1971; **2:** 459.
20. Starzl TE, Tzakis A, Makowka U, *et al.* The definition of ABO factors in transplantation: Relation to other humoral antibody states. *Transplant Proc* 1987; **19:** 4492.
21. Gordon RD, Iwatsuki S, Esquivel CO, *et al.* Liver transplantation across ABO blood groups. *Surgery* 1986; **100:** 342.
22. DeThetris AJ, Jaffe R, Tzakis A, *et al.* Antibody-mediated rejection of human orthotopic liver allografts: a study of liver transplantation across ABO blood group barriers. *Am J Pathol* 1988; **132:** 489.
23. Gordon RD, Fung JJ, Markus B, *et al.* The antibody crossmatch in liver transplantation. *Surgery* 1986; **100:** 705.
24. Snyder DS, Unanue ER. Corticosteroids inhibit immune macrophage's Ia expression and interleukin-1 production. *J Immunol* 1982; **129:** 1803.
25. Dupont E, Wybran J, Toussant C. Glucocorticosteroids and organ transplantation. *Transplantation* 1984; **37:** 331.
26. Keown PA, Stiller CR. Kidney transplantation. *Surg Clin North Am* 1986; **66:** 517.
27. Kahane BD. Cyclosporine. *N Engl J Med* 1989; **321:** 1725.
28. Sollinger HW. Update on preclinical and clinical experience with mycophenolate mofetil. *Transplant Proc* 1996; **28:** 24.
29. Maki T, Simpson M, Monaco MP. Development of suppressor T cells by antilymphocyte serum treatment in mice. Transplantation 1982; **34:** 376.
30. Hull AR, Parker TF. Proceedings from the Morbidity, Mortality and Prescription of Dialysis Symposium, Dallas, Texas, Sept. 15–17, 1989. *Am J Kidney Dis* 1990; **15:** 375.
31. United Network for Organ Sharing. *United Network for Organ Sharing Newsletter* January 21, 1991.
32. Evans RW, Manninen DL, Garrison LP, *et al.* The quality of life of patients with end-stage renal disease. *N Engl J Med* 1985; **312:** 553.
33. Eggers PW. Effect of transplantation on the Medicare end-stage renal disease program. *N Engl J Med* 1988; **318:** 223.
34. Belani KG, Palaliniuk RJ. Kidney transplantation. In: Firestone LL (ed.). *Anesthesia and Organ Transplantation*. Boston: Little, Brown, 1991: 17.
35. Bay WH, Herbert LA. The living donor in kidney transplantation. *Ann Intern Med* 1987; **106:** 719.
36. Spital A, Spital M, Spital R. The living kidney donor: alive and well. *Arch Intern Med* 1986; **146:** 1993.
37. Fahey MR, Rupp SM, Canfell C, *et al.* Effect of renal failure on laudanosine excretion in man. *Br J Anaesth* 1985; **57:** 1049.
38. Bernuau J, Rueff B, Benhamon JP. Fulminant and subfulminant liver failure: definition and causes. *Semin Liver Dis* 1986; **6:** 97.
39. Starzl TE, Demetris AJ, van Thiel DH. Liver transplantation. *N Engl J Med* 1989; **321:** 1014, 1092.
40. Krowka MJ, Cortese DA. Pulmonary aspects of chronic liver disease and liver transplantation. *Mayo Clin Proc* 1985; **60:** 407.
41. Starzl TE, Todo S, Gordon R, *et al.* Liver transplantation in older patients. *N Engl J Med* 1987; **316:** 484.
42. Starzl TE, Todo S, Tzakis A, *et al.* Abdominal organ cluster transplantation for the treatment of upper abdominal malignancies. *Ann Surg* 1989; **210:** 374.
43. Makowka L, Tzakis AG, Massaferro V, *et al.* Transplantation of the liver for metastatic endocrine tumors of the intestine and pancreas. *Surg Gynecol Obstet* 1989; **168:** 107.
44. Bismuth H, Samuel D, Gugenheim J, *et al.* Emergency liver transplantation for fulminant hepatitis. *Ann Intern Med* 1987; **107:** 337.
45. Howrie DL, Burckart GJ. Drug disposition in organ transplantation. In: Cook DR, Davis PJ (eds). *Anesthetic Principles for Organ Transplantation*. New York: Raven Press, 1994: 55.
46. Haberer JP, Schoeffler P, Coudere E, *et al.* Fentanyl pharmacokinetics in anaesthetized patients with cirrhosis. *Br J Anaesth* 1982; **54:** 1267.
47. Rosenberg PH, Oikkonen MP, Orko RH, *et al.* A transplanted liver rapidly begins to metabolize enflurane in humans. *Anesth Analg* 1984; **63:** 1131.
48. Kang YG, Martin DJ, Marquez J, *et al.* Intraoperative changes in blood coagulation and thromboelastographic monitoring in liver transplantation. *Anesth Analg* 1985; **64:** 888.
49. Wall WJ, Grant DR, Duff JH, *et al.* Blood transfusion requirement and renal function in patients undergoing liver transplantation without venous bypass. *Transplant Proc* 1987; **19** (Suppl. 3): 17.
50. Ellis JE, Lichtor JL, Feinstein SB, *et al.* Right heart dysfunction, pulmonary embolism and paradoxical embolization during liver transplantation. *Anesth Analg* 1989; **68:** 777.
51. Navalgund AA, Kang Y, Sarner JB, *et al.* Massive pulmonary thromboembolism during liver transplantation. *Anesth Analg* 1988; **67:** 400.
52. Iwatsuki S, Popovtzer MM, Corman JL, *et al.* Recovery from "hepatorenal syndrome" after orthotopic liver transplantation. *N Engl J Med* 1973; **289:** 1155.
53. Starzl TE, Demetris AJ. Candidacy, original disease, and outcome. In: Starzl TE, Demetris AJ (eds). *Liver Transplantation*. Chicago: Yearbook Publishers, 1990: 119.
54. Griffith BP, Hardesty RI, Kormos RI, *et al.* Temporary use of the Jarvik-7 total artificial heart before transplantation. *N Engl J Med* 1987; **316:** 130.
55. Paulsen AW, Whitten CW, Ramsay MAE, *et al.* Considerations for anesthetic management during veno-venous bypass in adult hepatic transplantation. *Anesth Analg* 1989; **68:** 489.
56. Massie BM, Conway M. Survival of patients with congestive heart failure: past, present, future prospects. *Circulation* 1987; **75:** 11.
57. Watson DC, Reitz BA, Baumgartner WA, *et al.* Distant heart procurement for transplantation. *Surgery* 1979; **86:** 56.
58. Walsh TR, Syttendorf J, Dummer S, *et al.* The value of protective isolation procedure in cardiac allograft recipients. *Ann Thorac Surg* 1989; **47:** 539.
59. Keats AS, Strong JM, Girigis KZ, *et al.* Observations during anesthesia for cardiac homotransplantation in ten patients. *Anesthesiology* 1969; **30:** 192.
60. Fernando NA, Keenan RI, Boyan CP. Anesthetic experience with cardiac transplantation. *J Thorac Cardiovasc Surg* 1978; **75:** 531.
61. Demas K, Wyner J, Mihm FG, *et al.* Anaesthesia for heart transplantation. *Br J Anaesth* 1986; **58:** 1357.
62. Waterman PM, Bjerke R. Rapid-sequence induction technique in patients with severe ventricular dysfunction. *J Cardiothorac Anesth* 1988; **2:** 602.
63. Reitz BA, Fowles RE, Ream AK. Cardiac transplantation. In: Ream AT, Fogdall RP (eds). *Acute Cardiovascular Management*. Philadelphia: JB Lippincott, 1982: 549.
64. Cooper DKC, Lanza LP. *Heart Transplantation: The Present Status of Orthotopic and Heterotopic Heart Transplantation*. Lancaster: MTP Press, 1984.
65. Cannon DS, Rider AK, Stinson EB, *et al.* Electrophysiological studies in the denervated transplanted human heart. II. Response to norepinephrine, isoproterenol, and propranolol. *Am J Cardiol* 1975; **36:** 859.
66. Armitage JM, Hardesty RI, Griffith BP. Prostaglandin E1: an effective treatment of right heart failure after orthotopic heart transplantation. *J Heart Transplant* 1987; **6:** 348.
67. Bliatia SJS, Kirshenbaum M, Shemin RJ, *et al.* Time course of resolution of pulmonary hypertension and right ventricular remodeling after orthotopic cardiac transplantation. *Circulation* 1987; **76:** 819.
68. Fonger JD, Borkon AM, Baumgartner WA, *et al.* Acute right heart failure following heart transplantation: improvement with PGE1 and right ventricular assist. *J Heart Transplant* 1986; **5:** 317.
69. Griffith BP, Hardesty RI, Trento A, *et al.* Asynchronous rejection of heart and lungs following cardiopulmonary transplantation. *Ann Surg* 1985; **40:** 488.
70. Arcasoy SM, Kotloff RM. Lung transplantation. *N Engl J Med* 1999; **340:** 1081.
71. Trulock EP, Cooper JD, Kaiser LR, *et al.* The Washington University–Barnes Hospital experience with lung transplantation. *JAMA* 1991; **266:** 1943.
72. Miyoshi S, Trulock EP, Schaefers HJ, *et al.* Cardiopulmonary exercise testing after single and double lung transplantation. *Chest* 1990; **97:** 1130.
73. Griffith BP, Zenati M. The pulmonary donor. *Clin Chest Med* 1990; **11:** 217.
74. Conacher ID. Isolated lung transplantation: a review of problems and guide to anesthesia. *Br J Anaesth* 1988; **61:** 468.
75. Conacher ID, McNally B, Choudhry AK, *et al.* Anaesthesia for isolated lung transplantation. *Br J Anaesth* 1988; **60:** 588.
76. Gayes JM, Giron L, Nissen MD, *et al.* Anesthetic considerations for patients undergoing double-lung transplantation. *J Cardiothorac Anesth* 1990; **4:** 486.
77. Thomas BJ, Siegel UC. Anesthetic and postoperative management of single-lung transplantation. *J Cardiothorac Vasc Anesth* 1991; **5:** 266.

78. Schaefers H-J, Waxman MB, Patterson GA, *et al*. Cardiac innervation after double lung transplantation. *J Thorac Cardiovasc Surg* 1990; **99:** 22.
79. Cooper JD, Patterson GA. Isolated lung transplantation. In: Kapoor AS, Laks H, Schroeder JS *et al.* (eds). *Cardiomyopathies and Heart–Lung Transplantation*. New York: McGraw-Hill, 1991: 429.
80. Bierman MI, Stein KU, Stuart RS, *et al*. Critical care management of lung transplant recipients. *J Intensive Care Med* 1991; **6:** 135.
81. Dauber JH, Paradis IL, Dummer JS. Infectious complications in pulmonary allograft recipients. *Clin Chest Med* 1990; **11:** 291.
82. Burke CM, Theodore J, Dawkins ED, *et al*. Post-transplant obliterative bronchiolitis and other late lung sequelae in human heart–lung transplantation. *Chest* 1984; **86:** 824.
83. National Diabetes Data Group. Diabetes in America. NIH publication no. 85-1467. Washington, DC: US Department of Health and Human Services, August 1985.
84. Sutherland DER, Gilliugham K, Moudry-Munns KC. Registry report on clinical pancreas transplantation. *Transplant Proc* 1991; **23:** 55.
85. Sutherland DER, Dunn DL, Goetz FC, *et al*. A 10-year experience with 290 pancreas transplants at a single institution. *Ann Surg* 1989; **210:** 274.
86. Bilous RW, Mayer SM, Sutherland DER, *et al*. The effects of pancreas transplantation on the glomerular structure of renal allografts in patients with insulin-dependent diabetes. *N Engl J Med* 1989; **321:** 80.
87. Tzakis AG, Ricordi C, Alejandro R, *et al*. Pancreatic islet transplantation after upper abdominal exenteration and liver replacement. *Lancet* 1990; **336:** 402.
88. Starzl TE, Rowe MI, Todo S, *et al*. Transplantation of multiple abdominal viscera. *JAMA* 1989; **261:** 1449.
89. Tzakis AG, Todo S, Madariaga J, *et al*. Upper abdominal exenteration in transplantation for extensive malignancies of the upper abdomen: an update. *Transplantation* 1991; **51:** 727.
90. DeWolf A. Multiviscera and pancreas transplantation. In: Firestone LU (ed.). *Anesthesia and Organ Transplantation*. Boston: Little, Brown, 1991: 111.
91. Turcotte JG, Campbell DA, Dafoe DC, *et al*. Pediatric renal transplantation. In: Cerelli GJ (ed.). *Organ Transplantation and Replacement*. Philadelphia: JB Lippincott, 1988: 349.
92. Warady B, Kriley M, Farrell S, *et al*. Growth and development of infants with end-stage renal disease receiving long-term peritoneal dialysis. *J Pediatr* 1988; **112:** 714.
93. McGraw ME, Haka-Ikse K. Neurologic developmental sequelae of chronic renal failure in infancy. *J Pediatr* 1985; **106:** 579.
94. Ingelfinger J, Grupe W, Harmon W, *et al*. Growth acceleration following renal transplantation in children less than 7 years of age. *Pediatrics* 1981; **68:** 255.
95. Fennell K, Rasbury W, Fennell E, *et al*. Effects of kidney transplantation on cognitive performance in a pediatric population. *Pediatrics* 1984; **74:** 273.
96. Van Meurs IP, Terasaki PI, Cecka JM, *et al*. A report from the UNOS scientific renal transplant registry. *Transplant Proc* 1991; **23:** 53.
97. Gordon RD, Bismuth H. Liver transplant registry report. *Transplant Proc* 1991; **23:** 58.
98. Borland LM, Roule M, Cook DR. Anesthesia for pediatric orthotopic liver transplantation. *Anesth Analg* 1985; **64:** 117.
99. Broelsch CE, Edmond JC, Whitington PF, *et al*. Application of reduced-size liver transplants as split grafts, auxiliary orthotopic grafts, and living related segmental transplants. *Ann Surg* 1990; **212:** 368.
100. Salt A, Barnes AP, Mowat R, *et al*. Five years' experience of liver transplantation in children. *Transplant Proc* 1991; **22:** 1514.
101. Iriett JM, Kay MP. The registry of the International Society for Heart Transplantation: seventh official report, 1990. *J Heart Transplant* 1990; **9:** 323.
102. Starnes V, Oyer P, Bernstein D, *et al*. Heart and heart–lung transplantation in the first year of life. *J Heart Lung Transplant* 1991; **10:** 162.
103. Bailey U, Kahan B, Nehlsen-Cannarella S. The neonatal immune system: window of opportunity? *J Heart Lung Transplant* 1991; **10:** 828.
104. Gryzan S, Paradis IL, Zeevi A, *et al*. Unexpectedly high incidence of *Pneumocystis carinji* infection after lung-heart transplantation: implications for lung defense and allograft survival. *Am Rev Respir Dis* 1988; **137:** 1268.
105. Leapman SB, Vidne BA, Butt KM, *et al*. Elective and emergency surgery in renal transplant patients. *Ann Surg* 1976; **183:** 262.
106. Dretchen KU, Morgenroth VH, Standaert FG, *et al*. Azathioprine: effects on neuromuscular transmission. *Anesthesiology* 1986; **45:** 604.
107. Dummer JS. Infectious complications of transplantation. In: Thompson ME (ed.). *Cardiac Transplantation*. Philadelphia: FA Davis, 1990: 163.
108. Hanto DW, Simmons RI, Najarian JS. Epstein–Barr virus-induced lymphoproliferative diseases in renal allograft recipients. *J Heart Transplant* 1984; **3:** 121.
109. Nalesnik MA, Locker J, Jaffe R, *et al*. Clonal characteristics of posttransplant lymphoproliferative disorders. *Transplant Proc* 1988; **20:** 280.
110. Cirella VN, Pantuck CB, Lee YJ, *et al*. Effects of cyclosporine on anesthetic action. *Anesth Analg* 1987; **66:** 703.
111. Firestone LU, Martin T, Liu P, *et al*. The effect of cyclosporine on the potencies of general anesthetics. *Anesth Analg* 1990; **70:** 8105.
112. Crosby E, Robblee JA. Cyclosporine–pancuronium interaction in a patient with a renal allograft. *Can J Anaesth* 1988; **35:** 300.
113. Bakkaloglu M, Hamilton DNH, MacPherson SG, *et al*. Morbidity and mortality in renal transplant patients after incidental surgery. *Br J Surg* 1978; **65:** 228.
114. Steed DL, Brown B, Reilly JI, *et al*. General surgical complications in heart and heart–lung transplantation. *Surgery* 1985; **98:** 739.
115. Colon R, Frazier OH, Kahan BD, *et al*. Complications in cardiac transplant patients requiring general surgery. *Surgery* 1988; **103:** 32.
116. Kaye MP. Denervation and reinnervation of the heart. In: Randall WC (ed.). *Nervous Control of Cardiovascular Function*. New York: Oxford University Press, 1984: 278.
117. Dong E, Hurley EJ, Lower RR, *et al*. Performance of the heart two years after autotransplantation. *Surgery* 1964; **56:** 270.
118. Pope SE, Stinson EB, Daughters GT, *et al*. Exercise response of the denervated heart in long-term cardiac transplant recipients. *Am J Cardiol* 1980; **46:** 213.
119. Mason JW, Harrison DC. Electrophysiology and electropharmacology of the transplanted human heart. In: Narula OS (ed.). *Cardiac Arrhythmias: Electrophysiology, Diagnosis and Management*. Baltimore, MD: Williams & Wilkins, 1979: 66.
120. Kavanagh T, Yacoub MH, Mertens DJ, *et al*. Cardiorespiratory responses to exercise training after orthotopic cardiac transplantation. *Circulation* 1988; **77:** 162.
121. Stark RP, McGinn AL, Wilson RE. Chest pain in cardiac-transplant recipients. *N Engl J Med* 1991; **324:** 1791.
122. Stinson EB, Griepp RB, Clark DA, *et al*. Cardiac transplantation in man. VIII. Survival and function. *J Thorac Cardiovasc Surg* 1970; **60:** 303.
123. Verani MS, George SE, Leon CA, *et al*. Systolic and diastolic ventricular performance at rest and during exercise in heart transplant recipients. *J Heart Transplant* 1988; **7:** 145.
124. Kent K, Cooper T. The denervated heart: a model for studying autonomic control of the heart. *N Engl J Med* 1974; **291:** 1017.
125. Stinson EB, Griepp RB, Schroeder JS, *et al*. Hemodynamic observations one and two years after cardiac transplantation in man. *Circulation* 1972; **45:** 1183.
126. Cannom DS, Graham AF, Harrison DC. Electrophysiologic studies in the denervated transplanted human heart: response to atrial pacing and atropine. *Circ Res* 1973; **32:** 268.
127. Firestone LU. Autonomic influence on cardiac performance: lessons from the transplanted (denervated) heart. *Int Anesthesiol Clin* 1988; **27:** 283.
128. Uretsky BF. Physiology of the transplanted heart. In: Thompson ME (ed.). *Cardiac Transplantation*. Philadelphia: FA Davis, 1990: 21.
129. Uretsky BF, Murali B, Reddy PS, *et al*. Development of coronary artery disease in cardiac transplant patients receiving immunosuppressive therapy with cyclosporine and prednisone. *Circulation* 1987; **76:** 827.
130. Beebe DS, Shumway SJ, Maddock R. Sinus arrest after intravenous neostigmine in two heart transplant recipients. *Anesth Analg* 1994; **78:** 779.
131. Goodman DJ, Rossen RM, Cannom DS, *et al*. Effect of digoxin on A-V conduction: studies in patients with and without autonomic innervation. *Circulation* 1975; **51:** 251.
132. Borow EM, Neumann A, Arensman FW, *et al*. Cardiac and peripheral vascular responses to adrenoreceptor stimulation and blockade after cardiac transplantation. *J Am Coll Cardiol* 1989; **14:** 1229.
133. Ellenbogen KA, Thames MD, DiMarco JP, *et al*. Electrophysiological effects of adenosine in the transplanted human heart. *Circulation* 1990; **81:** 821.

62

Anesthesia for the outpatient

JAMES B MAYFIELD AND CARL E ROSOW

Over the last 15 years, there has been an explosive growth in the trend to provide cost-effective care in the practice of medicine. The worldwide increase in anesthesia for ambulatory surgery is an increasingly important part of that trend. Currently, over 70% of all elective surgery in the USA and the UK is performed on an outpatient basis, and this is likely to increase in response to economic pressures in the healthcare market. European countries are experiencing a steady increase in ambulatory procedures, although recent unfavorable economic conditions have slowed the pace of adoption. Despite vastly different social systems and economic forces affecting healthcare delivery, same-day surgery is gaining acceptance in countries such as Brazil (over 15%) and China (2–3%).

AMBULATORY SURGERY: FACILITIES AND ADVANTAGES

In the earliest days of anesthesia, both nitrous oxide and ether were used for ambulatory (outpatient) dental extractions. Pediatric ambulatory anesthesia was first reported by Nicoll[1] in 1909, and in 1916 Ralph Waters opened the first outpatient clinic in Sioux City, Iowa. This free-standing clinic was so successful that in 1918 he was able to move into a prime city center location.[2] In 1962, at the University of California at Los Angeles, a formal ambulatory surgical program began, followed by similar programs at George Washington University in 1966 and Providence, Rhode Island, in 1968. In 1969, the first successful free-standing surgical center was opened in Phoenix, Arizona, by Wallace Reed and John Ford. By 1985, 7.3 million operations in the USA (34% of total elective procedures) were performed on an ambulatory basis. In 1990, this figure had climbed to over 11 million, and in 1994 over 16 million ambulatory operations accounted for 61.3% of all elective procedures performed in the USA.

It was not until the economic constraints of the 1970s and 1980s led to a large increase in ambulatory surgery that the subspecialty of ambulatory anesthesia finally emerged. In 1984, the Society of Ambulatory Anesthesia (SAMBA) was formed in the USA. Currently, a significant portion of residency training in anesthesiology consists of procedures done on an ambulatory basis. Many residency training programs also offer extra fellowship training in the techniques of ambulatory anesthesia. In 1995, the International Association for Ambulatory Surgery (IAAS) held its organizational meeting in Brussels, Belgium, for the purpose of facilitating worldwide development in ambulatory surgical practices. The American Society of Anesthesiologists (ASA) has recently amended its guidelines for ambulatory anesthesia and surgery (see Appendix 62.1).

Facilities

Ambulatory surgery units may be either attached to a hospital (integrated unit), free standing, or office based. Some integrated units have a separate ward for pre- and postoperative care but use the main operating rooms. This may reduce initial capital costs but the outpatients may be canceled at short notice to make way for emergency procedures. Integrated units may avoid this by having either a separate block of operating rooms or a separate building in the hospital grounds. Specialized procedures need not be performed in the main ambulatory facility, e.g. vascular access surgery may be performed in renal units. Some free-standing units have facilities for overnight observation following procedures such as laparoscopic cholecystectomy or knee ligament reconstruction, following which a period of time close to trained medical assistance is available.

The facility design and layout is an integral part of the overall efficiency of any surgical unit. A preoperative evaluation center and holding area that is close to the operating suite, but completely separate from recovery areas, is preferable. To allow patient traffic to flow smoothly, both the postanesthesia recovery unit (phase 1 PACU) and postrecovery lounge (PRL or phase 2 PACU) should be in very close proximity to the operating suites. The phase 2 PACU should ideally be located close to the patient changing areas, which should have separate entrances to avoid impeding the flow of preoperative and postoperative patients. A separate pediatric area with appropriate decor and toys can make the entire operative experience more pleasant for children, parents, and other adult patients.

Primarily driven by financial concerns, office-based ambulatory surgery has seen a dramatic increase over the past 5 years. Common office-based procedures include cosmetic and reconstructive plastic surgery, oral surgery, and some gynecological procedures. The convenience, low overhead costs, and relative autonomy from hospitals continue to attract more procedures into the office. However, even for minor surgical procedures, the anesthesia required should be held to the same strict standards of care that apply to hospital-based and free-standing surgical centers. Backup emergency care must usually be arranged with nearby hospitals. With the growth of minimally invasive surgery likely to continue, office-based ambulatory anesthesia will expand at a rate depending on regional needs and economical considerations.[3,4]

Advantages of ambulatory surgery

Ambulatory surgery offers a wide variety of advantages to all parties involved: patients, surgeons, insurance companies, and surgery facilities. Patients and their relatives experience less disruption to their personal lives and a more rapid return to daily activities. Patients are able to recover at home in familiar surroundings, thus providing an additional psychosocial benefit. There is a reduced risk of nosocomial complications such as wound infections, deep venous thrombosis, pulmonary embolism, ileus, and pneumonia.[5–8]

The cost of surgery on an ambulatory basis has been estimated to be 25–75% less than a similar inpatient procedure, in part because of less preoperative testing, a reduced need for ancillary services, a reduced demand for postoperative medications, and a more efficient use of equipment and operating rooms. However, a study completed in 1984 showed that 30% of women undergoing laparoscopic surgery would have preferred to stay overnight.[9] With the recent improvements in both surgical and anesthetic techniques, patient acceptance of and satisfaction with ambulatory surgery have increased. In a recent prospective study only 2.5% of patients ($n = 2730$) were dissatisfied with their ambulatory surgical experience.[10] The most common reason for dissatisfaction was personal preference for inpatient care. Only 1.1% were dissatisfied with anesthesia specifically. Of those dissatisfied with anesthesia, most problems were due to intraoperative adverse outcomes, inadequate anesthesia, and lack of communication.

PATIENT SELECTION FOR AMBULATORY SURGERY

Patient selection criteria

Successful ambulatory surgery requires careful selection of patients, operative procedures, and available facilities. Proper planning will minimize cancellations and unexpected admissions and allow for easy access to inpatient services when necessary. There continues to be controversy over which patients are appropriate for ambulatory surgery. Selection criteria should include the overall medical health of the patient (ASA physical status criteria), age, social factors, the surgical procedure, and the limitations of the healthcare providers and surgical facility.

General medical health

In the past, only young healthy patients were considered appropriate for ambulatory surgery. However, experience involving outpatients with chronic medical problems has led to the acceptance in the USA of ASA physical status III and IV patients. In a 1984 prospective study of 18 000 patients, Natof[11] found those with pre-existing disease to have the same complication rate as healthy patients. This surprising finding was attributed to good patient selection following a thorough preoperative screening and close communication between the surgeon, anesthesiologist, and the primary care physician. In 1987, the Federated Ambulatory Surgery Association (FASA) concluded from a survey of over 87 000 patients that there was no significant relation between cause and effect for pre-existing disease and the incidence of perioperative complications in the ambulatory patient.[12] A study done at the Mayo Clinic with nearly 40 000 patients concluded that major morbidity occurred less often in the ambulatory surgical population than in the age- and gender-matched population not having surgery. The study also found no obvious relation between ASA physical status and major morbidity or mortality after ambulatory surgery.[13]

Influence of age

Extremes of age should no longer be considered a deterrent to ambulatory surgery. Few studies have shown any increase in morbidity with increasing age. By avoiding admission for these older patients the postoperative confusion that occurs in up to half of elderly inpatients may be reduced. However, special attention must be paid to discharge planning because recovery of fine motor function and cognitive skills following general anesthesia or sedation is slower in the elderly.

Children are usually well suited for ambulatory surgery, and those treated on a same-day basis have less psychological disturbance than those admitted on the day before and discharged on the day after surgery.[14] These children also require less additional attention in the first week after discharge home and have fewer sleep disturbances.[15] The very young and preterm infants are a special case. There is an increased risk of postoperative apnea for up to 12 h after general anesthesia. Although this was initially reported in premature infants under 10 weeks postnatal age, increased risk appears to persist up to 46–55 weeks postconceptual age.[16,17] There remains some controversy over the appropriate guidelines for premature infants having ambulatory surgery. When in doubt, inpatient care is recommended for any ex-premature infant younger than 60 weeks postconceptual age. Children with bronchopulmonary dysplasia should be considered at risk as long as their symptoms persist.

Surgical procedures

Ideally, surgical procedures for the ambulatory patient should be completed in a reasonable amount of time and they should not require blood transfusion or create excessive fluid shifts. Anticipated postsurgical management and pain control should be simple enough to be handled by patients in their own homes. The number and type of surgical procedures performed on an ambulatory basis continues to increase. In the past, procedures expected to last longer than 60–90 min were not scheduled because it was assumed that a long anesthetic would mandate a prolonged recovery. However, oral, plastic, general, gynecological, and orthopedic surgery procedures lasting 2–4 h are now being routinely performed successfully in many ambulatory facilities in the USA. Meridy,[18] in a retrospective analysis, found no correlation between duration of anesthesia and the recovery time. With current fast-acting anesthesia drugs and new monitors, patients are consistently able to recover faster with fewer side-effects than just 5 years ago.

Social factors

Patients should live within a reasonable distance of the surgery unit and have a responsible person available to care for them during the first postoperative night. Although no recommendations currently exist that are applicable to all situations, medical staff should have guidelines for what is considered reasonable and safe in their own environment. In today's technological environment, it may be reasonable to assume that patients have access to a telephone should a problem arise. Socioeconomic conditions and education level within a patient population can vary tremendously and hospital or surgery center staff should make certain that patient instructions are actually understood. Instructions should be free from language barriers. In addition to translation services for patients who cannot provide their own, instructions written in the surrounding community's predominant languages should be available.

PREOPERATIVE EVALUATION

Historically, surgery in the ambulatory setting was meant to be more convenient for patients and surgeons, and much more efficient in terms of overall cost and total resources consumed. One way, in particular, that efficiency can be maintained is through the appropriate use of preoperative assessment and laboratory evaluation.

Medical evaluation

Cancellations from inadequate preparation can be reduced by having medically complicated patients seen by an anesthesiologist prior to the day of surgery. Those patients contacted by telephone during business or evening hours also have a lower cancellation rate and are less likely to need admission. However, it is not always possible or practical to have all patients regardless of medical condition seen prior to surgery. Many institutions find alternative ways to achieve the same goals. Surgeons can be asked to screen their patients at the initial office visit prior to scheduling surgery. Patients who are deemed physical status ASA I or II, who do not require laboratory testing, and are not overly anxious about the anesthesia, can be seen by the anesthesiologist on the day of surgery. To save time, patients may be asked to complete a questionnaire on general health, past surgical procedures, drug and allergy history, and family history. This process may be automated using a computer. These computer-based programs may facilitate the health screening process, and provide recommendations regarding appropriate laboratory tests. This approach has been shown to reduce the number of tests ordered and result in considerable cost savings. In the near future, interactive screening processes will almost certainly become available over the Internet.

Medical laboratory test selection

Preoperative testing should be based on the patient's age, history, and examination. Indiscriminate laboratory testing produces a large number of false-positive or random abnormal results, most of which are ignored by the anesthesiologist. On the other hand, physicians may pursue or treat borderline or false-positive abnormalities that can lead to patient harm with no benefit. One such study showed that 1 in every 2000 preoperative tests led to patient harm because of the ensuing workup, whereas only 1 in 10000 tests led to patient benefit.[19] Similarly, over 99% of electrocardiograms (ECGs) and chest radiographs currently requested have no influence on patient management.[20]

Healthy (ASA I) male patients under the age of 40, undergoing ambulatory surgery, usually do not require routine laboratory testing. A hemoglobin or hematocrit is appropriate for females of child-bearing age, and possibly for children under the age of 5 years. ECGs are generally obtained for men over 40 and women over 50 years. Routine chest radiographs are probably only needed for patients over 70 years. Otherwise, testing should be based on a patient's history and physical examination and the proposed surgical procedure. Please refer to Chapter 26 for suggested guidelines that can be used along with a careful history and physical examination when ordering preoperative laboratory tests. An accurate history and good clinical judgment will provide for the most appropriate preoperative testing.

PREOPERATIVE CONSIDERATIONS AND MEDICATIONS

Considerations for preoperative fasting

There are several documented drawbacks to preoperative fasting:

1 About 50% of ambulatory patients complain of hunger or thirst following an overnight fast. This may increase preoperative anxiety.
2 One in seven young women who fasted overnight prior to elective surgery in the afternoon had a serum glucose concentration less than 2.5 mmol L^{-1}.
3 Children tend to go to bed earlier, producing a longer overnight fast. Of children who fast overnight, one in five fast for 16 h or more, and up to 9% may be hypoglycemic.

Optimal guidelines for preoperative oral intake are still being debated. Since prolonged fasting does not guarantee an empty stomach at the time of induction, several investigators have questioned the value of the usual overnight fast, or even a 4–5 h fast prior to elective surgery.[21] In adults, 150 mL of coffee or orange juice ingested 2–3 h before induction of general anesthesia has no significant effect on residual gastric volume or pH. Also, the length of fasting has no significant effect: gastric fluid volume and pH are similar when intervals of less than 3 h, 3–4.9 h, 5–8 h, and "nothing by mouth after midnight" are compared.

There are data to suggest that intake of oral fluids may dilute gastric secretions and actually stimulate gastric emptying. In children, preoperative administration of apple juice (3 mL kg^{-1}) has decreased gastric volume, thirst, and hunger. Furthermore, administration of ranitidine (2 mg kg^{-1}) with orange juice (5 mL kg^{-1}) 2–3 h preoperatively resulted in a decrease in both volume and acidity of gastric contents.[22] Therefore, the arbitrary restriction of fluids after midnight prior to elective surgery appears to be unwarranted. Only those patients suspected, or known, to be at risk for delayed gastric emptying (those with diabetes, hiatal hernia, gastroesophageal reflux, and gastric outlet obstruction) should be considered for a prolonged fast that may otherwise cause stress and discomfort without any clear benefit. If a patient is scheduled for afternoon surgery it is reasonable to allow them to ingest clear fluids (black coffee, clear tea, water, fruit juice without pulp, or carbonated beverages) on the morning of surgery.

Recent practice guidelines have been published by the ASA task force on preoperative fasting (Table 62.1).[23] These recommend a fasting period for clear liquids of 2 h for all patients. The task force also recommends a fast from breast milk of 4 or more hours, and from infant formula of 4–6 h for neonates and infants. For solids and nonhuman milk the guidelines recommend a fast of 6 or more hours prior to elective procedures requiring general anesthesia, regional anesthesia, or monitored anesthesia care. However, in a busy ambulatory surgical practice, care must be taken to allow time for unforeseen scheduling conflicts, or normal surgical start-time variations.

Prevention of aspiration

The incidence of pulmonary aspiration in ambulatory surgical patients is very low (1 in 35000).[24] However, several studies have found that 40–60% of ambulatory patients would be defined as "high risk" for aspiration pneumonitis by the traditional criteria (gastric volume more than 25 mL with pH less than 2.5) despite an overnight fast. Although ambulatory patients were initially reported to have significantly higher residual gastric volumes than inpatients, this has not been confirmed in more recent studies. These concerns have led to the evaluation of a variety of premedication regimens to reduce the risk of aspiration pneumonitis. It has been suggested that all patients receiving general anesthesia by mask should be protected against the acid component of pulmonary aspiration injury with an H_2-antagonist. However, very few of the ambulatory centers in the USA routinely use prophylactic antacid or antisecretory medication. In elective gynecological patients neither anxiety nor benzodiazepine premedication has a clinically important impact on gastric content.[25]

The ASA task force on preoperative fasting has recommended no routine use of gastrointestinal stimulants, gastric acid secretion blockers, antacids, antiemetics, anticholinergics, or combinations of these medications for patients who have no apparent increased risk for pulmonary aspiration. However, for patients who are at high risk, several different medications are effective.

The H_2-receptor antagonists cimetidine and ranitidine are both effective in decreasing the number of patients "at risk" for pulmonary aspiration. Ranitidine may be preferable because of its longer period of protection. Ranitidine may be given orally or parenterally, with peak

Table 62.1 *Preoperative fasting guidelines*

	Clear liquids	Breast milk and infant formula	Solids
Neonates	2 h	>4 h	>6 h
Infants and children	2 h	4–6 h	>6 h
Adults	2 h	–	>6 h

effects occurring within 2 h. Oral ranitidine given with coffee or orange juice 2–3 h prior to induction of anesthesia produces lower residual gastric volumes, higher pH values, and less thirst than fasting alone.[26]

Metoclopramide has been shown to reduce gastric volume in outpatients without altering the pH. Use of metoclopramide in combination with an H_2-antagonist drug has been advocated to decrease postoperative emesis and further reduce the risk of aspiration pneumonitis. However, studies have failed to demonstrate a significant advantage of this combination over an H_2- receptor antagonist alone.[26,27] Metoclopramide may offer an additional protective effect as a result of its ability to increase lower esophageal sphincter tone and thus may have a role in diabetic and pregnant outpatients.

Sodium citrate, a nonparticulate oral antacid, is less effective in raising pH than the H_2-antagonists and can increase gastric volume.[28] However, sodium citrate may be useful in combination with metoclopramide when little time is available prior to the surgery.[29]

Premedication for adults

There is considerable debate about the use of premedication for adult outpatients. Premedication is not used routinely in many ambulatory surgery facilities because anesthesiologists believe that the use of centrally acting depressants will significantly prolong recovery. The indications for preoperative medications are similar to those for inpatients and include anxiolysis, sedation (especially for pediatric patients), analgesia, amnesia, vagolysis, and prophylaxis against postoperative emesis and aspiration pneumonitis. Anxiety is related to previous anesthetic experience and the type of operation. Oral surgery patients may be particularly anxious and often desire anxiolytic premedication. Healthy patients' anxiety may not be reduced by meeting the anesthesiologist prior to the day of surgery or outside the operating room immediately prior to the procedures.

The judicious use of premedication for ambulatory patients can be beneficial, and in most prospective studies premedication does not prolong recovery to street fitness,[30] although coordination and reaction times may be impaired for 5–12 h.[30,31] Some studies have even found a decrease in recovery times with analgesic or antiemetic premedication.[32,33] Premedication with sedative or analgesic drugs does not appear to increase the percentage of outpatients at risk of aspiration pneumonitis.[34]

The rapid onset of action and water solubility of midazolam offer a number of advantages for ambulatory surgery. This agent may be given intramuscularly 30–60 min before surgery or, preferably, intravenously in the induction room. Midazolam (1–2 mg) given intravenously prior to induction of general anesthesia reduces anxiety and increases amnesia without prolonging the recovery room stay.[35] However, when compared with placebo, it is associated with impaired postoperative psychomotor skills. Although larger doses are required because of first-pass metabolism, midazolam given orally has been reported to be highly effective for adults, as well as for children.

Temazepam is an effective oral premedication for ambulatory surgery. Temazepam (20 mg) produces a similar degree of anxiolysis and sedation as midazolam (7.5–10 mg) and does not affect recovery compared with placebo.[36] However, temazepam produces less perioperative amnesia than does midazolam. Furthermore, although postoperative sedation is similar, patients given temazepam are more sleepy and retire to bed earlier following surgery.[37] Lorazepam provides good amnesia and may have antiemetic effects but is generally considered too long acting for outpatient anesthesia. While oral triazolam can produce effective sedation and amnesia, it may be less effective than diazepam or midazolam for reducing anxiety and may lead to more residual sedation at the time of discharge.

Opioid analgesics for premedication

The routine use of opioid analgesics for premedication has been criticized unless the patient is experiencing acute or chronic pain. Use of traditional opioid premedicant combinations [e.g. papaveretum–hyoscine, meperidine (pethidine)–atropine] may increase the incidence of postoperative nausea and vomiting. The agonist–antagonist nalbuphine produces good sedation and smooth induction but has similar postoperative side-effects. The use of small doses of the potent opioid analgesics (e.g. fentanyl at 0.5–1 $\mu g\,kg^{-1}$, sufentanil at 0.1–0.2 $\mu g\,kg^{-1}$) prior to induction of general anesthesia reduces the intravenous anesthetic requirement and may actually reduce recovery times. Sufentanil (0.15 $\mu g\,kg^{-1}$) reduces preoperative anxiety and provides more satisfactory induction, maintenance, and recovery from anesthesia than morphine, meperidine, or fentanyl.[38] However, the use of these potent rapid-acting opioids still increases the incidence of postoperative nausea and vomiting.[39–41]

Premedication for children

Oral midazolam (0.05–0.075 $mg\,kg^{-1}$) provides good sedation and reduces children's levels of anxiety at induction of anesthesia without increasing the time to discharge or overnight stay. Intranasal and rectal midazolam are also highly effective routes of administration, if the child will tolerate them. Oral transmucosal fentanyl citrate (OTFC) reliably induces preoperative sedation and facilitates inhalation induction of anesthesia. It is also useful for painful procedures done with sedation alone. However, it may produce a significant decrease in respiratory rate and peripheral blood oxygen saturation and an increase in postoperative nausea and vomiting. Pruritus may also be a significant problem. Chloral hydrate (40 $mg\,kg^{-1}$ p.o.) is reported to increase the number of children who are calm or asleep at induction of anesthesia compared with midazolam (0.05 $mg\,kg^{-1}$ p.o.), alprazolam (0.005 $mg\,kg^{-1}$ p.o.), or placebo. Postoperative behavior and the incidence of vomiting are similar in all cases.[42] Ketamine (2 $mg\,kg^{-1}$) given intramuscularly to uncooperative children permits inhalation induction with halothane after 2–3 min. Although early recovery time is unaffected, home discharge was delayed by an average of 13 min in one study.[43]

The expansion of ambulatory surgery has made it difficult to provide an unhurried preoperative visit to the hospital. Children and their parents may visit when the facilities are otherwise unused. This may take the form of a "Saturday club" and include a puppet show. Other anesthesiologists have made videotapes showing the operating rooms and explaining the risks of anesthesia. Children's fears during the induction period may be minimized by play-oriented preoperative teaching. It is helpful to allow parents to comfort their child during induction to relieve the child's anxiety and produce a smoother induction of anesthesia. If it is planned to have a parent present at induction, it is important to educate the parent about normal operating room procedure and what to expect from his or her child.

ANESTHETIC MANAGEMENT AND TECHNIQUES

The ideal anesthetic for ambulatory surgery should produce a rapid and smooth onset of action, intraoperative amnesia and analgesia, good surgical conditions, and a short recovery period free from side-effects. Although many ambulatory procedures are performed under general anesthesia, peripheral nerve blocks and regional techniques can be used for a variety of urological, gynecological, and orthopedic procedures. Sedative–analgesic drugs can be valuable supplements to local anesthetic techniques during monitored anesthesia care. The practice of ambulatory anesthesia often requires a combination of these techniques.

Monitoring

Outpatients require the same basic equipment as inpatients for delivery of anesthetic drugs, and to ensure appropriate surgical conditions and intraoperative safety. Standard intraoperative monitoring equipment includes an electrocardiograph, a noninvasive blood pressure measurement device, a pulse oximeter, and a capnograph. Temperature monitoring is important for patients undergoing general anesthesia with known triggers for malignant hyperthermia. The use of electroencephalogram (EEG)-based consciousnesss monitors to titrate the sedative and hypnotic effects of anesthetic agents reduces drug consumption, allows for faster emergence, reduces time required for recovery, and increases the number of patients eligible to bypass the postanesthesia care unit.

Intravenous fluids

Children undergoing procedures lasting less than 15 min and which do not require the administration of intravenous drugs or fluids (i.e. myringotomy and eye examination under anesthesia) may not require intravenous access. Hypoglycemia does not occur in healthy children or adults who have fasted for less than 15 h.[44] However, during longer cases, or if a patient has had a prolonged fast (over 15 h), an intravenous line should be started and may be used for maintenance of fluid and administration of perioperative medications. The benefit of fluid administration during brief ambulatory procedures is unproved. However, Cook *et al.*[45] found that both sodium lactate and glucose solutions produced significant improvement in variables that reflected hydration.

Management of the airway

Anesthesia for ambulatory surgery requires a variety of airway management techniques because of the wide variety of surgical procedures. Alternatives to endotracheal intubation are preferred for most ambulatory procedures, since sore throat is a common cause of minor morbidity in this setting. Sore throats are more common if the patient is allowed to breathe spontaneously after intubation, but the incidence is not influenced by deep or light extubation.[46,47] Airway maintenance using a face mask or laryngeal mask airway (LMA) may reduce the incidence of postoperative sore throat.

Endotracheal intubation is a safe and time-honored approach to management of the airway. Although there are risks with the procedure, i.e. dental and soft-tissue injury, in the hands of an experienced clinician major trauma is rare. Although few ambulatory procedures require a secure airway, patients undergoing laparoscopy are intubated because gas insufflation and the Trendelenburg position are believed to increase the risk of regurgitation and hypoventilation. However, in some units these patients are not intubated. These centers report that spontaneous ventilation via a face mask in the Trendelenburg position does not result in significant hypercapnia or acidosis in nonobese patients, nor is it associated with reflux of gastric contents except in patients with hiccups.[21] By avoiding laryngoscopy and intubation, the amount of anesthetic drugs administered is decreased and there is a faster recovery with fewer minor side-effects.

The LMA offers several advantages for ambulatory procedures. Insertion does not require use of muscle relaxation, or use of a laryngoscope. Insertion may be easier than with endotracheal intubation. Indeed, the LMA plays a significant role in the ASA difficult airway management algorithm. The LMA offers a hands-free approach to airway management, allowing the anesthesiologist to complete other tasks. There is a decrease in hemodynamic changes during both induction and emergence, and a reduced work of breathing compared with the use of the endotracheal tube. It is also suitable for use in children of all ages. Reported complications from the LMA and their incidence include dysphagia (38%), sore throat (16%), and hoarseness (6%).[48] The LMA does not offer the same airway protection as an endotracheal tube so it is usually inappropriate for patients with symptomatic gastroesophageal reflux or gastric outlet obstruction and in patients who are significantly obese or pregnant.

The cuffed oropharyngeal airway (COPA) is a relatively new device that is as easy to insert as the LMA. However, it has been demonstrated that the LMA offers significant advantages over the COPA in most aspects of airway management. The COPA occasionally requires additional chin support to relieve airway obstruction and is more prone to become dislodged than the LMA. The COPA was, however, associated with a lower incidence of sore throat, suggesting that it may cause less pharyngeal trauma.[49,50]

Management of the airway in any facility in which anesthesia is performed should include the immediate availability of emergency airway equipment. Various types of laryngoscope blades, LMAs, oral airways, and a jet ventilator are recommended. In addition, a fiberoptic bronchoscope that can be used for difficult intubation should be readily available.

Monitored anesthesia care

In 1966, Shane described an "intravenous amnesia" technique involving the use of small incremental doses of barbiturates, opioids, anticholinergics, and neuroleptics.[51] Intravenous sedative and analgesic drugs are often used in conjunction with local anesthesia, especially by oral and plastic surgeons, to reduce the discomfort of local anesthesia injections and recall of intraoperative events. Most oral surgery outpatients prefer local anesthesia with sedation to local anesthesia alone, and patient satisfaction is directly related to the level of intraoperative sedation. Appropriate end-points for "sedation" and "sedation/analgesia" were recently approved by the ASA (see Appendix 62.2). Although the ASA guidelines use the term "conscious sedation," it is often an inappropriate descriptor and should probably be abandoned.[52]

Effective sedation techniques for analgesia can also be applied as alternatives to general anesthesia in the ambulatory setting. However, because of the risk of ventilatory depression, respiratory monitoring and supplemental oxygen are usually required. Clinically significant hemoglobin desaturation may occur in up to 40% of patients who do not receive supplemental oxygen during sedation techniques, although it has also been observed in patients who receive local anesthesia alone. These risks must be taken into consideration when assessing the safety of doing a procedure under local anesthesia with sedation. Achieving an optimal balance between patient comfort and safety requires careful titration of sedative and analgesic drugs, appropriate monitoring of the cardiovascular, respiratory, and central nervous systems, and, most importantly, good communication between the anesthesiologist, patient, and surgeon.

Drugs used in monitored anesthesia care

Benzodiazepines

Benzodiazepines are the drugs most widely used to produce sedation and amnesia during monitored anesthesia care (MAC). Diazepam has active metabolites and a very long elimination half-life (24–48 h), which is increased in elderly patients. When used during MAC, midazolam may offer some advantages over other benzodiazepines. This agent has a slower onset of action, but usual doses produce more effective amnesia than diazepam. Although the difference between diazepam and midazolam is minimal after a single dose, multiple doses will reveal the benefits of the shorter half-life of midazolam. Recovery from similar levels of intraoperative sedation is more rapid following midazolam than diazepam. Oral midazolam has been used for conscious sedation in ambulatory patients undergoing minor procedures and is associated with greater patient and physician acceptance than intravenous diazepam. Other agents have distinct disadvantages when used for MAC. Sublingual lormetazepam is as effective as parenteral benzodiazepines for conscious sedation, but has been found to be less acceptable to patients.[53] Lorazepam has a slow onset of action that precludes careful titration and a prolonged duration of amnesia could delay discharge.

Flumazenil is a specific benzodiazepine antagonist that may be used to reverse the residual sedative and amnesic effects of benzodiazepines after inadvertent overdose. This antagonist will not reverse the effects of opioids in a benzodiazepine–opioid mixture. Flumazenil also may not completely reverse the depression of hypoxic drive produced by midazolam.[54] The short half-life of this drug (1–2 h) may allow recurrence of sedation after discharge.[54,55]

Opioid analgesics

During MAC, the addition of an opioid analgesic to a benzodiazepine significantly improves patient comfort during local anesthesia and greatly increases the sedative effect. For example, midazolam and fentanyl may be combined by first sedating the patient with midazolam (1–3 mg) intravenously followed by small aliquots of fentanyl (25–50 μg) given as needed. Benzodiazepine–opioid combinations cause synergistic depression of ventilatory drive. Benzodiazepines reduce the hypoxic drive and opioid analgesics reduce both hypercapnic and hypoxic drive, and the combination can produce life-threatening apnea if not managed carefully. Agonist–antagonist opioids, such as nalbuphine and butorphanol, produce effective sedation when given alone, and they are less likely to produce severe ventilatory depression than fentanyl. Unfortunately, dysphoria can also occur when they are combined with midazolam, and the incidence of nausea, vomiting, and hypoxia is higher than with midazolam alone. When more profound sedation is required, a nalbuphine and methohexital or propofol combination can also be highly effective. Carefully titrated, an alfentanil or remifentanil infusion by itself can produce substantial analgesia with somewhat less sedation and ventilatory depression than the benzodiazepine–opioid combinations. Techniques such as these can rapidly progress to general anesthesia and may produce significant impairment of airway reflexes. These should only be used by individuals with proper training in airway management and the use of rapid-acting anesthetic drugs.

Ketamine

Ketamine has been used for sedation during MAC, but it may cause marked cardiovascular stimulation. Unpleasant psychomimetic emergence reactions may occur, but these may be reduced if the patient is first sedated with a benzodiazepine. Midazolam is occasionally combined with low-dose ketamine (0.25–0.5 mg kg^{-1}). One study suggested that midazolam is preferable to diazepam in this combination as it provides more profound intraoperative sedation, anxiolysis, and amnesia, and higher overall patient acceptance.[56] Amnesia with midazolam and ketamine combination may persist into the postoperative period.

Propofol

Propofol infusions during MAC are highly effective in producing rapid, smooth, and controllable sedation. Propofol sedation has become a very popular technique for MAC in many centers for ambulatory surgery. It is easily titratable and produces antiemetic and mood-elevating effects. With very low infusion rates (25–50 μg kg^{-1} min^{-1}), sedation can be achieved without the addition of benzodiazepines or opioid medications, thereby facilitating a more rapid recovery. The overall quality of intraoperative sedation is similar to a midazolam infusion, but the use of propofol results in a much quicker recovery of cognitive function.[57] The propofol infusion should be given into a large vein (e.g. the antecubital or cephalic vein) to minimize pain on injection. Propofol used alone in sedative–hypnotic doses does not usually cause respiratory depression, although the hypoxic ventilatory drive is depressed. Care must be taken to avoid oversedation and the creation of a general anesthetic.

Regional anesthesia techniques

Regional anesthesia offers many advantages to the ambulatory patient. The side-effects of general anesthesia and tracheal intubation are avoided, the risks of aspiration pneumonitis are minimized, post-anesthesic nursing care and patient recovery times may be reduced, and analgesia may be provided well into, and sometimes beyond, the early postoperative period.[58,59] In most instances, the use of a peripheral nerve block may allow patients to be safely discharged much earlier than if they underwent general anesthesia. Prolonged analgesia from a peripheral nerve block may be a great advantage for patient comfort. However, when a patient is ready for discharge and the arm or leg is still numb, great care must be taken to instruct the patient in the proper care of the extremity while normal sensation is still lacking. Patients need to be reassured that sensation will return and given oral pain medication to take when pain begins. Although some studies suggest that there may be fewer postoperative complications in patients receiving regional anesthesia, there is continued debate over whether it is truly safer than general anesthesia.

In children, a regional block performed immediately after induction of general anesthesia can reduce the anesthetic requirement, provide postoperative analgesia, and allow more rapid recovery. Caudal epidural anesthesia is an effective technique for children undergoing lower abdominal, perineal, and lower extremity procedures. Combined ilioinguinal and iliohypogastric nerve block or caudal epidural block reduce pain following herniotomy or herniorrhaphy. Postcircumcision pain may be reduced by a dorsal block of the penis, a subcutaneous ring block, or topical local anesthetic ointment.

Spinal anesthesia (subarachnoid block)

Spinal anesthesia is useful for lower extremity, urological, some gynecological, and hernia procedures. However, many clinicians do not promote the use of spinal anesthesia for ambulatory patients because of the fear of postdural puncture headache (PDPH) and local anesthesia-induced transient radicular irritation (TRI). The perceived lack of a good alternative to lidocaine (lignocaine) for short-duration spinal anesthesia, without the risk of TRI (as high as 16–20%), has been the subject of recent controversy. Typically the pain from TRI begins within 24 h of spinal anesthesia, and lasts for approximately 2 days. TRI is amenable to rest and oral analgesics. Hyperbaric lidocaine, both 5% and 2%, has the highest incidence of TRI.[60] Bupivicaine and mepivicaine do not seem to be associated with TRI, and both are currently acceptable for spinal anesthesia for ambulatory patients.

The risk of PDPH in ambulatory patients appears to be of foremost concern among clinicians and patients. Ambulatory patients receiving spinal anesthesia may be at increased risk for PDPH compared with inpatients. In general, the use of smaller gauge (27 G), noncutting needles can reduce the incidence of PDPH, and these are preferable for ambulatory patients. If PDPH does occur, the initial measures of hydration, caffeine, oral analgesics, and bedrest are still the first line of treatment. For patients failing to respond to conservative therapy, an epidural blood patch is highly effective and has been administered on an ambulatory basis.

Common adjuvants to local anesthetics include epinephrine (adrenaline) and opioids. Epinephrine (0.2 mg) prolongs lidocaine and bupivicaine spinal anesthesia by approximately 30 min but may delay time to voiding by 50–80 min.[61] Fentanyl (20–25 μg) and sufentanil (10 μg) prolong both lidocaine and bupivicaine spinals by approximately 30 and 60 min respectively, without any effect on motor blockade or bladder function.[61]

Epidural anesthesia

Epidural anesthesia has been advocated in lower abdominal and lower extremity procedures such as abdominoplasty and knee ligament reconstruction. An epidural performed with a short-duration local anesthetic in combination with wound infiltration with a prolonged-action agent (0.5% bupivicaine) can provide rapid recovery from the epidural and significant postoperative pain relief, allowing for more rapid discharge. Continuous lumbar epidural anesthesia with lidocaine has been used successfully for ambulatory knee arthroscopy and lithotripsy. Continuous thoracic epidural anesthesia has been used for ambulatory oncological and reconstructive breast surgery. In addition to the continuous-infusion epidural, a single-shot technique using 2% lidocaine, with or without epinephrine, is also useful for a wide range of procedures. Caudal epidural anesthesia can be employed in anorectal surgery and some gynecological procedures. In our experience, these epidural techniques, when used by experienced practitioners, usually take no longer to perform, result in fewer hemodynamic changes, have a lower incidence of PDPH or urinary retention, and may provide for a faster recovery when compared with spinal anesthesia.

Brachial plexus blockade

Ambulatory procedures on the upper extremity, including the shoulder, can be performed under brachial plexus blockade using the interscalene, infraclavicular, or axillary approaches. In recent evaluations of brachial plexus anesthesia, all three of these approaches have been shown to be reliable and safe. The infraclavicular and axillary approaches are preferred for surgery on the elbow, forearm, and hand, while the interscalene block is more commonly used for shoulder surgery.

In one series surgical anesthesia was achieved in 97% of patients receiving an interscalene block ($n = 266$) and 93% receiving an axillary block ($n = 242$). The incidence of postoperative complications was low, with only one patient in each group experiencing neuropraxia beyond 4 weeks.[62] The coracoid technique for infraclavicular brachial plexus block has been shown to be very effective, while avoiding the neurovascular structures in the neck, and minimizing the risk of pneumothorax. In skilled hands, however, the method of brachial plexus blockade probably makes no clinically significant difference.

Intravenous regional anesthesia

For ambulatory procedures on a single extremity, the intravenous regional block (Bier's block) is a simple and very reliable technique. Although there may, theoretically, be complications from local anesthesia toxicity, this block is generally considered safe when performed by clinicians familiar with the technique and the appropriate doses. In a survey of North American anesthesiologists, the most commonly used medication was 0.5% lidocaine (40–50 mL in the average adult arm), using a double tourniquet with cuff pressures of 33.3 kPa (250 mmHg) or 13.3 kPa (100 mmHg) above the systolic blood pressure.[63] Other medications used in addition to lidocaine included ketorolac and clonidine, both of which have been reported to improve the quality of anesthesia. Intravenous regional anesthesia of the leg requires a larger volume of solution and higher cuff pressures. For these reasons it is not frequently used.

Miscellaneous nerve blocks

The "3-in-1" block (femoral, obturator, and lateral femoral cutaneous nerves) provides adequate anesthesia for ambulatory knee arthoscopy and gives excellent postoperative analgesia. Popliteal sciatic nerve block may be used for procedures in the lower leg and foot. In one study, this block was sufficient to provide surgical anesthesia in 92% of patients; supplemental anesthesia was required in 5%, and general anesthesia was required in 3% of cases. Overall satisfaction with the perioperative analgesia was evaluated in 466 patients: 95% were completely satisfied, 4% expressed moderate reservations, and 1% expressed major reservations.[64] Nerve blocks at the ankle, wrist, or digits can provide excellent anesthesia and are easy to perform. In a busy ambulatory unit regional blocks can be performed in the preoperative holding area in advance of the actual surgery, thereby maintaining efficiency.

Local anesthesia infiltration

Infiltration of the operative site with solutions of local anesthetic is simple, safe, and provides satisfactory conditions for many outpatient operations including vasectomy, orchidopexy, hydrocele, and spermatocele surgery. Transurethral resection of the prostate has been performed under local anesthesia. Inguinal herniorrhaphy under field block has excellent patient acceptance and few postoperative complications. Ambulatory knee arthroscopy and breast biopsies are frequently performed under local anesthesia. The use of a retrobulbar block instead of general anesthesia for ophthalmological surgery has many advantages including a marked reduction in postoperative emesis. Although only relatively superficial operations can be performed with local infiltration or field block, wound infiltration with local anesthesia will decrease incisional pain in the recovery room. The use of topical local anesthetic creams and aerosols can provide effective postoperative analgesia.

General anesthesia techniques

The delivery of safe and effective general anesthesia with minimal side-effects and a rapid recovery is essential in a busy ambulatory surgery unit. General anesthesia remains the most widely used technique for ambulatory patients because of its popularity with patients, surgeons, and anesthesiologists. There are many components of the anesthetic plan that can be tailored for the ambulatory patient to provide for a safe, efficient, and pleasant operative experience.

Intravenous induction

Induction of general anesthesia is usually accomplished with a rapid-acting intravenous anesthetic agent. These agents are safe, although they are associated with a variety of minor side-effects that take on added significance in the ambulatory environment. Thiopental is usually associated with a rapid induction of anesthesia without significant side-effects. However, psychomotor recovery is sometimes delayed and prolonged subjective feelings of tiredness and drowsiness are drawbacks to its use in ambulatory patients. Methohexital is associated with slightly shorter awakening and recovery times than thiopental and its pharmacokinetic profile makes administration by continuous infusion possible. However, recovery of fine motor skills may not be complete until 6–8 h after induction. Methohexital may also cause pain on injection, involuntary muscle movements, and hiccupping. The use of a small dose of a rapid-acting opioid analgesic (i.e. sufentanil or remifentanil) can minimize these side-effects without prolonging recovery.

Etomidate may be used for induction and maintenance of general anesthesia during short ambulatory procedures. The rate of recovery is more predictable than with thiopental and compares favorably with methohexital. Disadvantages of etomidate include pain on injection, a high incidence of postoperative nausea and vomiting, myoclonic movements, and transient suppression of adrenal steroidogenesis. The tendency to cause postoperative nausea and vomiting make this drug much less useful for the ambulatory patient.

Although a very uncommon practice, midazolam alone can be used as an intravenous induction agent. The dose required for hypnosis can vary remarkably between patients. The onset of action is slower in ambulatory patients and recovery is prolonged compared with the barbiturates. Recovery following midazolam is significantly slower and associated with a lower level of psychomotor function than following propofol.[65] Flumazenil given at the end of surgery can speed recovery following midazolam induction, but it may not permit earlier discharge since the duration of reversal is less than 60 min.

Induction of anesthesia with propofol is associated with a greater decrease in blood pressure and heart rate than with either thiopental or methohexital, but this disadvantage is offset by a more rapid and dramatically improved quality of recovery with fewer postoperative side-effects. Propofol has many qualities that make it suitable for ambulatory anesthesia. It may be used in the elderly patient but the dose should be reduced.[66] Pain on injection can be significant, but this may be reduced by the addition of lidocaine, the use of a large vein, or by cooling the propofol to 4 °C. The direct antiemetic effect of propofol may also offer a significant advantage. The improved recovery profile of propofol may be negated somewhat if anesthesia is maintained with the moderately soluble volatile agents (i.e. halothane, enflurane, and isoflurane), leading some to question whether its advantages justify the increased expense. However, propofol shows significant advantages over thiopental in both recovery profile and diminished side-effects, regardless of the maintenance agent.

Inhalational induction

In adult patients in whom intravenous access may be very challenging an excellent alternative to intravenous induction is the use of inhaled anesthetics. There can also be economic advantages in the use of inhalational induction, which saves the cost of an intravenous agent. The combination of an intravenous agent for induction and an inhalational agent for maintenance of brief procedures is associated with a slightly prolonged recovery compared with the use of an inhalational agent alone. Some have advocated the routine use of this technique in adults, but it seems likely that most patients will prefer an intravenous induction. An inhalation induction should not normally be used for patients with symptomatic gastroesophageal reflux.

In children, an inhalational induction is a useful alternative to the standard intravenous induction techniques. Unfortunately, inhalational inductions are frequently more time-consuming, and many children object to the face mask and the pungent smell of the inhaled agents. In cooperative children these problems can be reduced by the use of the single-breath induction technique.[67] Halothane and sevoflurane are popular choices for inhalational induction, because they lack pungency and are relatively nonirritating. Sevoflurane is associated with shorter induction times and fewer cardiorespiratory problems than halothane, enflurane, or isoflurane. Desflurane is too irritating to be used in this manner. In children this agent is also associated with a higher incidence of coughing and larygospasm on induction.

In toddlers, young children, and some mentally retarded children, methohexital (20–30 mg kg^{-1}) can be administered rectally prior to entering the operating room. However, the recovery time may be prolonged after this premedication. Small doses of ketamine (2–4 mg kg^{-1} intramuscularly) can also produce a rapid onset of anesthesia without cardiorespiratory depression and with relatively little effect on recovery time. This technique is useful for induction of an uncooperative child, however home readiness will be delayed when larger doses (e.g. 6–10 mg kg^{-1} intramuscularly) are combined with a volatile anesthetic.[68] In addition, recurrent dreams or flashbacks have been reported several weeks after ketamine administration in children who did not receive benzodiazepine premedication.

Volatile anesthetic agents have traditionally been considered to be superior to intravenous agents for maintenance of anesthesia during outpatient surgery, although there seems little basis for such a generalization. With almost all modern anesthetic agents, the time to awakening after brief anesthesia does not differ by more than a few minutes. The advantages of the newer agents such as propofol, sevoflurane, and desflurane seem to be in the more rapid attainment of late recovery milestones, i.e. ambulation. Studies have suggested that the higher costs of these drugs may be offset by the benefits of "fast tracking" or bypassing the phase 1 PACU and rapid discharge from the hospital. Dexter and Tinker[69] concluded that PACU economics are determined by the number of patients admitted to the unit rather than choice of anesthetic drugs. Significant savings can be achieved by timing patient arrival or by fast tracking to reduce the peak requirement of PACU nurses. It should be noted that any real cost savings requires a commitment from anesthesia, surgery, and nursing to utilize the extra time or reduce some other expenditure.

Nitrous oxide

The use of a volatile agent in combination with nitrous oxide (60–70%) in oxygen remains the most popular technique for maintenance of general anesthesia. The extremely low blood gas partition coefficient of nitrous oxide and the diminished requirement for more soluble agents contribute to the rapid recovery from anesthesia. Some investigators have found an association between nitrous oxide and postoperative nausea and vomiting,[70,71] but other studies have challenged these findings.[72] Certainly, the combination of nitrous oxide and an opioid analgesic as part of a balanced anesthetic technique increases these side-effects.[73]

Isoflurane

Isoflurane has a higher solubility than desflurane and sevoflurane, but this difference is probably minimal for brief procedures. Its cost is currently a distinct advantage over the newer agents. The induction of anesthesia with isoflurane is associated with an increased incidence of coughing and laryngospasm compared with halothane or enflurane and is judged to be much less pleasant than induction with sevoflurane.[74]

Desflurane

Desflurane has a blood–gas partition coefficient (0.42) very similar to that of nitrous oxide and it has a very rapid washin and washout. The time required for the end-tidal concentration to decrease by 50% is 2.5 min for desflurane compared with 9.5 min for isoflurane. Induction of anesthesia with desflurane is rapid but associated with a high incidence of airway irritation, especially in children. Compared with isoflurane, desflurane is associated with more rapid initial awakening and less impairment of cognitive function. Psychomotor recovery following desflurane for induction and maintenance of anesthesia is better than that following propofol for induction and maintenance. However, desflurane is associated with a higher incidence of nausea than propofol. Given its favorable early recovery profile, desflurane would appear to be a useful alternative to other volatile anesthetics in ambulatory patients, although its respiratory irritant properties make it unlikely to find much use an induction agent. The unique advantage of desflurane for outpatients is primarily related to its extremely fast washout, allowing patients the opportunity for faster discharge.

Sevoflurane

Sevoflurane has low blood–gas solubility, which provides for rapid induction and recovery times. The nonirritating odor of sevoflurane makes a gaseous induction much easier for most patients to tolerate. As stated previously, inhalational induction with sevoflurane and nitrous oxide in oxygen is not associated with coughing or laryngospasm. In children undergoing outpatient procedures, induction with sevoflurane in oxygen produces more rapid emergence and a significantly shorter postoperative recovery time than halothane. In adults, induction with sevoflurane and nitrous oxide is more rapid than with enflurane and nitrous oxide but early recovery times are similar. Emergence times following propofol or sevoflurane induction and sevoflurane maintenance are similar and more rapid than a propofol–isoflurane–nitrous oxide technique. However, late recovery times are similar. Serum fluoride levels following sevoflurane anesthesia correlate with exposure in MAC-hours, although there does not appear to be any evidence of abnormal renal function following clinical use.[75] The advantages of sevoflurane in ambulatory surgery are a smooth and rapid inhalational induction and less airway irritation in patients with reactive airways.

Opioid analgesics

Opioid analgesics play a very significant role in any surgical practice, and an ambulatory surgical practice is no exception. All opioids have common action and side-effect profiles; however, there is a wide range of duration – from the ultrashort-acting remifentanil to extremely long-acting preparations of morphine. Opioids are used as premedicants, coinduction agents, intravenous analgesics, and postoperative analgesics. When given prior to or during general anesthesia, opioids can reduce the requirement for sedative or hypnotic drugs and thereby improve recovery times and psychomotor function.[76] All opioids are accompanied by fairly predictable side-effects, including drowsiness, nausea and vomiting, and respiratory depression. Using smaller doses of the more potent and faster acting opioids, and with judicious use of antiemetic medications, opioids play an integral part in ambulatory perioperative care practice.

Although morphine and meperidine still have a place in ambulatory anesthesia, they have generally been replaced by the more potent, faster onset, and shorter-acting opioid analgesics such as fentanyl, sufentanil, alfentanil, and remifentanil. Fentanyl is the only one of these commonly used for premedication, and all are used to attenuate the cardiovascular responses to laryngoscopy and tracheal intubation and to supplement an inhaled anesthetic agent during maintenance of general anesthesia. Smaller doses of these agents are also given either by bolus or as a continuous infusion during procedures requiring only MAC or the performance of regional or local anesthetic blocks.

The extremely rapid onset and short duration of action of alfentanil make it particularly useful for ambulatory anesthesia. Many studies have shown a more rapid emergence and recovery of psychomotor function after alfentanil compared with fentanyl. The small volume of distribution and short terminal half-life of alfentanil make it particularly suitable for administration by continuous infusion. The addition of alfentanil improves anesthetic conditions after both propofol and thiopental–enflurane anesthesia. Alfentanil may be combined with methohexital or propofol to produce total intravenous anesthesia.

It is now realized that sufentanil may actually have a shorter duration than alfentanil when given by infusion. Use of a sufentanil infusion for maintenance of ambulatory general anesthesia with nitrous oxide has been associated with less nausea and reduced postoperative pain than fentanyl.

Fentanyl is commonly used as an adjuvant for ambulatory anesthesia. When used as a premedication, it has been shown to decrease the total dose of propofol on induction of general anesthesia. However, there was no improvement in recovery time or in the subjective assessment of quality of anesthesia. During short gynecological procedures, the addition of fentanyl (50 μg) does not affect recovery from a propofol–nitrous oxide technique. This dose does not seem to increase postoperative nausea and vomiting or decrease the requirement for postoperative analgesics.[77]

Remifentanil is an esterase-metabolized μ-opioid agonist with an effective biologic half-life of 3–5 min regardless of the total dose or duration of infusion.[78,79] A potent opioid with no accumulation even after prolonged infusion, remifentanil has become very useful in providing profound analgesia, even for short cases, without affecting recovery. However, there is no evidence that the use of remifentanil leads to earlier recovery or discharge. Its short duration is a definite disadvantage if significant postoperative pain is anticipated and additional postoperative analgesics will usually be required.[80]

The choice of opioid is usually based on the desired duration of effect. If a strong analgesic effect is desired for an extremely brief period of time, this may best be achieved by bolus administration of a fentanyl derivative. Alfentanil or remifentanil would have a slight advantage in this circumstance. However, fentanyl would be a better choice if analgesia needs to be maintained into the postoperative period. If a strong analgesic effect is to be maintained by repeated bolus injections or a continuous infusion, remifentanil, sufentanil, or alfentanil would be the best choices. Finally, if the patient needs moderate analgesia for 2 h or more, an injection of meperidine or morphine is a reasonable alternative to multiple boluses of fentanyl or sufentanil.[81,82] Increasingly painful procedures, such as laparoscopic cholecystectomy and anterior cruciate ligament repair, are being done on an ambulatory basis, and these patients may need significant postoperative analgesia. The use of older long-acting opioids may be most appropriate for these cases.

Nonopioid analgesic medications

The desire to reduce the side-effects of opioid analgesics for the ambulatory patient has led to the use of alternative analgesic adjuvants, i.e. nonsteroidal anti-inflammatory drugs (NSAIDs), α_2-agonists, and local anesthetics. A balanced approach to postoperative pain management is extremely important in the ambulatory setting. The combination of local anesthesia infiltration at the surgical site and a nonopioid adjuvant can have a significant influence on unexpected admission rate, postoperative nausea and vomiting, and the overall recovery process. For example, infiltration of the mesosalpinx with bupivicaine 0.5% decreases the analgesic requirement after laparoscopic tubal ligation, and, likewise, intra-articular bupivicaine 0.5% reduces the opioid requirements and facilitates earlier mobilization following arthroscopy.[83,84] Both ketorolac (60 mg) and naproxen (550 mg p.o.) reduced postoperative pain, emetic side-effects, and recovery times following laparoscopy and tubal ligation.[85]

Neuromuscular blocking agents

The judicious use of appropriate muscle relaxants can decrease the total anesthetic requirement and thereby shorten recovery times.[86] However, care should be taken when choosing agents for use with ambulatory patients. Prior to the introduction of intermediate-acting nondepolarizing muscle relaxants, a succinylcholine (suxamethonium) bolus and infusion were frequently used during ambulatory anesthesia. Administration of succinylcholine may be associated with muscle pain lasting up to 4 days after the procedure.[87] However, factors other than the succinylcholine may also contribute to these myalgias.[88] Although the use of nondepolarizing agents has been shown to reduce the incidence of myalgias in several studies, this is not a universal finding.[89]

Given the many choices of drugs for muscle relaxation for ambulatory patients, the longer-lasting agents may not be an appropriate option. For example, for patients receiving both pancuronium and a volatile anesthetic, the time to full reversal of neuromuscular function was significantly increased compared with rocuronium, vecuronium, and atracurium.[90]

Rocuronium is a fast-onset, intermediate-acting nondepolarizing muscle relaxant which provides an acceptable alternative to succinylcholine for tracheal intubation. However, its duration of action is similar to that of vecuronium, so the need for reversal agents is increased following short procedures.[91,92] Liver disease increases the duration of action significantly and prolonged duration has been reported in the elderly.

Mivacurium is extensively metabolized by plasma cholinesterase and therefore offers rapid spontaneous recovery without the need for reversal drugs. The onset of action (3.5 min) is slower than with succinylcholine or rocuronium, and this agent may stimulate histamine release following rapid bolus injection.[93] Duration of action, normally about 25 min, may be increased in individuals with reduced plasma cholinesterase activity.[94]

Cisatracurium, the *R*-cis configuration of atracurium, is an intermediate-duration nondepolarizing agent that undergoes primarily Hoffman elimination. It therefore has no clinically significant degradation from either the kidney or the liver. Cisatracurium has an onset time of 3–5 min after an ED_{95} dose, a clinical duration of about 45 min, and a greater than 70% recovery at 65 min. It has little tendency to accumulate after repeated doses. Patients undergoing more prolonged ambulatory procedures may benefit from the predictable recovery and may not require reversal agents.

Vecuronium, an analog of pancuronium, has an intermediate duration of action, and a near absence of cardiovascular effects. With its predictable recovery profile, it has been used for patients undergoing ambulatory procedures requiring moderate-duration relaxation and who would benefit from very stable cardiovascular conditions.[95] Vecuronium is taken up by the liver and excreted in bile, which accounts for the reported prolonged elimination in patients with liver disease. In common with the other intermediate-acting agents, vecuronium may not require reversal after longer ambulatory procedures.

Total intravenous anesthesia

Please refer to Chapter 39 for full details of total intravenous anesthetic (TIVA) techniques. Such methods are now quite popular for short ambulatory cases. The introduction of propofol and remifentanil has allowed for an extremely fast recovery when compared with some of the conventional inhalation techniques. TIVA results in a more rapid recovery than after enflurane–N_2O or isoflurane–N_2O inhalation techniques. However, with the introduction of sevoflurane and desflurane, two highly insoluble inhalation anesthetics, the differences in recovery profile are significantly minimized.[96]

At present, propofol and alfentanil are the most widely used agents in ambulatory TIVA regimens. However, with increasing duration of surgical procedures, the accumulation of alfentanil may increase the risk of prolonged recovery. Remifentanil, unlike other opioids, is rapidly metabolized by hydrolysis of its ester linkage so that its total clearance is unaffected by the duration of infusion.[78] It is therefore uniquely suited to provide a rapid and predictable emergence and is becoming an increasingly popular choice for ambulatory TIVA. Remifentanil may be given in higher doses than other opioids without prolonged recovery. This allows the anesthesiologist to achieve greater suppression of the responses to surgical stimuli, although it may predispose to hypotension and bradycardia.

Current infusion pump technology for TIVA is such that past problems of pump failure have been minimized. In addition to newer infusion pumps, CNS monitoring technology has added the ability to titrate accurately the TIVA hypnotic agent. A reduction in the time needed for recovery may then result.

POSTANESTHETIC CARE MANAGEMENT

In the ambulatory unit it is important to consider, along with the initial anesthetic plan, a plan for optimal recovery, with the shortest duration and with minimum postoperative side-effects. Anesthesiologists in the ambulatory unit must have their patient's recovery in mind during the entire perioperative period. Of course, some problems will inevitably be related to the surgery itself, and postoperative morbidity can be significantly reduced by minimizing the physiologic responses to surgical trauma.

Even after a brief general anesthetic, patients can have significant postoperative problems, therefore experienced recovery room staff play an important role during the recovery process. For example, episodes of oxygen desaturation may occur following brief general anesthetics, despite the use of supplemental oxygen. However, these episodes may be reduced significantly when experienced staff, trained in airway management, are present.

Patients continue to experience postoperative symptoms after ambulatory surgery irrespective of the anesthetic technique used. Tracheal intubation results in a higher incidence of airway-related complaints and greater morbidity. Side-effects after general anesthesia may be reduced by simple maneuvers, for example the use of airway heating and passive heat and moisture exchangers to decrease postoperative shivering after longer ambulatory procedures. The use of intraoperative local anesthetics to reduce postoperative pain, and prophylactic antiemetics for those with a high risk of postoperative nausea and vomiting, may also reduce the incidence of postoperative problems.

Prevention of nausea and vomiting

Postoperative nausea and vomiting (PONV) remains a common problem after general anesthesia and can delay discharge or result in unexpected hospital admission. The incidence continues to be in the 20–30% range despite some of the newer medications.[97] PONV is unpleasant for both patients and staff, and occasionally can be dangerous. At the very least, it can disrupt the smooth progression of patients through the ambulatory care unit. When one also considers the added costs of the antiemetic drugs, PONV can add a significant cost to the entire perioperative process. Factors that increase the incidence of PONV include certain types of surgery (e.g. laparoscopy, orchidopexy, and strabismus surgery), the use of assisted ventilation with a face mask (especially by junior anesthesiologists), the use of certain anesthetic and analgesic medications (e.g. fentanyl, etomidate, isoflurane, and nitrous oxide), and postoperative hypotension.[98] The patient's body habitus, medical condition, sex, and age will also influence the incidence of PONV. Many different pharmacologic and nonpharmacologic regimens for the treatment of PONV have been evaluated, including acupuncture and acupressure.

Recent studies have suggested that the risks of PONV can be predicted using validated mathematical models. In one study, 2722 adult patients were studied prospectively and found to have four predictors of PONV: female gender, history of PONV or motion sickness, nonsmoking, and the use of postoperative opioids.[99] In a separate study, 17 638 consecutive adult ambulatory surgical patients were studied prospectively over a 3-year period. Age, sex, smoking status, previous incidence of PONV, type of anesthesia, duration of anesthesia, and type of surgery were all independent predictors of PONV (Table 62.2). A 10-year increase in age decreased the likelihood of PONV by 13%. The risk for men was one-third of that for women. A 30-min increase in the duration of anesthesia increased the likelihood of PONV by 59%. General anesthesia increased the likelihood of PONV 11 times compared with other types of anesthesia. Compared with patients having urologic or neurosurgical procedures, patients having plastic or orthopedic shoulder surgery had a sixfold increase in the risk for PONV.[100] It is little surprise that studies disagree on the influence of any one factor (e.g. anesthetic agent) when so many others need to be controlled. Knowing the predictors of PONV and identifying patients at high risk may allow effective and cost-efficient antiemetic administration and prophylaxis for patients having ambulatory surgery.

Antiemetic drugs

Causes of PONV are multifactorial and can result from stimulation of dopamine, serotonin, muscarinic, cholinergic, histamine, and opioid receptors. Most older antiemetic drugs (droperidol, prochlorperazine) are dopamine antagonists and may cause sedation, dysphoria, or extrapyramidal side-effects. However, some of the newer serotonin antagonists produce few side-effects. Routine prophylaxis of PONV is a subject of some debate, but it should be considered for patients at high risk for PONV. Prophylaxis may be indicated for patients with two or more of the predictors for PONV (Table 62.3).[101] There are also indications that a multiple modality approach is successful, with a 92% success rate (no PONV) for the combination of droperidol and ondansetron.[102]

Droperidol has arguably been our cheapest and most effective antiemetic, but the recent restrictions introduced by the US Food and Drug Administration (FDA) have made it difficult to use the drug in typical ambulatory surgery. Droperidol, like many other drugs, inhibits the cardiac potassium channel, Ikr, and causes dose-related prolongation of the QTc interval. Such an effect can increase the risk for a dangerous or fatal dysrhythmia such as torsades de pointes. In 2001, a series of adverse event reports from Europe described dysrhythmias and cardiovascular toxicity following droperidol treatment, primarily when high doses (10–50 mg) were administered for therapy of acute psychosis. The FDA inserted a "black-box" warning in the drug labeling stating that droperidol should be used only when other therapies had failed. Even more important from an ambulatory surgical perspective, the agency mandated a pretreatment ECG to document a normal QTc interval and 2–3 h of continuous ECG monitoring after the last dose. This last requirement makes it very difficult to use droperidol efficiently in a rapid-turnover ambulatory surgical practice.

The regulations seem illogical to many clinicians: droperidol has been in use for 40 years without reports of dysrhythmias. The doses normally used for PONV do not affect the QTc interval and are much lower than the doses formerly used routinely in anesthesia. The adverse event reports prompting this action included only a handful at relevant doses, and in our opinion the information was insufficient to ascribe specific toxicity to droperidol. At present, droperidol is still an approved drug, and clinicians may elect to use it for patients for whom the benefits seem sufficient. Typical adult doses for prophylaxis or treatment are 7.5–15 $\mu g\,kg^{-1}$. Pediatric doses of 5–15 $\mu g\,kg^{-1}$ are effective in decreasing nausea and vomiting following orthopedic or dental surgery, but larger doses (50–75 $\mu g\,kg^{-1}$) may be necessary following strabismus surgery. Restrictions have not been placed on droperidol in most countries, and it is conceivable that some of the US restrictions and requirements may be dropped or modified in the future. For this reason we have retained droperidol as a treatment option in Table 62.3, even though its use will be very likely to be limited in some places. Droperidol is no longer available in the UK.

Although Handley found metoclopramide (0.25 $mg\,kg^{-1}$) to be as effective as droperidol (0.075 $mg\,kg^{-1}$) in children following strabismus surgery,[101] other studies have failed to confirm metoclopramide's antiemetic action.[102] The differences in response may relate in part to varying dosages, routes, and timing of the administration. Metoclopramide may be most effective when given at the end of anesthesia upon arrival in the recovery room, or in combination with other antiemetics.

Antihistamine (H_1-receptor antagonist) and anticholinergic medications have also been used for PONV. Although the antihistamine medications have not been well studied for ambulatory patients, the older ones all have significant sedative effects that can be problematic. The most common antihistamines used for inpatient PONV include promethazine, hydroxyzine, and diphenhydramine. Transdermal scopolamine has been approved for treatment of motion sickness and reduces the incidence of PONV in ambulatory gynecological surgery. However, the use of scopolamine is limited by a troublesome side-effect profile that includes sedation, delirium, visual changes, and xerostoma. A single dose of dexamethasone (4–8 mg i.v.) is effective for PONV prophylaxis (but not treatment), particularly when it is combined with other antiemetics.[104]

Selective serotonin-3 (5-HT_3) receptor antagonists decrease the

Table 62.2 *Patients at high risk of postoperative nausea and vomiting (PONV)*

- Age < 50 years
- Female
- History of PONV or motion sickness
- Nonsmoking
- Certain types of surgery (ear, nose, and, throat; plastic; gynecological)
- Requirement for perioperative narcotics
- Duration of general anesthesia > 90 min

Complied from Apfel[101] and Sinclair.[102]

Table 62.3 *Recommendations for postoperative nausea and vomiting (PONV) prophylaxis*

	PONV high-risk procedure (e.g. laparoscopy)	PONV low-risk procedure (e.g. knee arthroscopy)
Low-risk patient	Droperidol 0.6–1.25 mg on induction	No prophylaxis recommended
High-risk patient	Droperidol 0.6–1.25 mg on induction and ondansetron 4 mg before wakeup	Droperidol 0.6–1.25 mg on induction

From Sun,[110] McKenzie and Lim,[104] and Massachusetts General Hospital Department of Anesthesia and Critical Care staff manual.

emetic symptoms associated with cancer chemotherapy and radiotherapy and prevent and treat PONV without many troublesome side-effects. Ondansetron (4 mg intravenously), granisetron (20 μg kg^{-1}), and dolasetron (12.5 mg intravenously) are effective in the prevention and treatment of PONV without producing significant side-effects.[105] Tropisetron, a long-acting 5-HT_3 antagonist available outside the USA, is effective in the prevention of PONV after gynecological surgery.[106]

There is no evidence that a single antiemetic – at any dose – can achieve more than 60–70% prevention of nausea and vomiting. The multicenter investigational trials of ondansetron and dolasetron found very shallow dose–response curves for both PONV prophylaxis and treatment. This means, for example, that the effect of 1 mg ondansetron was not much less than that of 8 mg.[107] Administering more than 4 mg is not likely to result in a greater therapeutic benefit. As stated previously, complete response rates as high as 92% can be achieved by combining 5-HT_3 antagonists with droperidol. Of course, the older drugs are significantly cheaper, and the substitution of a drug such as ondansetron or dolasetron for droperidol has major cost implications for hospitals.

A large trial comparing low-dose droperidol with ondansetron for PONV prophylaxis found no major difference in efficacy or side-effects.[108] It is possible that the 5-HT_3 antagonists may have an advantage in the treatment of established PONV. This often requires higher antiemetic doses, and older drugs such as droperidol, prochlorperazine, and phenergan can produce significant sedation and prolong PACU stay. These agents may still be good choices when symptoms are persistent, since protracted nausea and vomiting can also delay discharge.

There has been some debate about the optimal timing of prophylactic antiemetics. One study suggests that giving ondansetron at the end of surgery is the most effective.[109] However, there is by no means complete agreement on this issue. All of the approved agents have a relatively long duration of action (12 h or greater), so it seems most logical to give them sufficiently early to ensure that a pharmacologic effect is present before emergence from anesthesia.

Fast tracking ambulatory recovery

With the increased use of the newer, short-acting anesthetic agents, including desflurane, sevoflurane, remifentanil, ketorolac, and propofol, some patients meet PACU discharge criteria before arriving in the PACU. When patients are awake and oriented in the operating room and are able to sit up with stable vital signs, minimal pain or bleeding, and no nausea, they may be eligible to go directly to the phase 2 PACU (postrecovery lounge). Bypassing the phase 1 PACU is often called fast tracking. Fast tracking facilitates earlier discharge times, with continued patient safety and satisfaction.

Fast tracking patients also has potential economic advantages for a busy ambulatory surgical facility. The phase 2 PACU does not require the presence of an expensive monitor for each patient and the nursing staff can be maintained with a lower ratio of registered nurses to nursing aides. The overall time for the recovery process can be significantly shortened. Patients appreciate being able to leave the surgical facility sooner and continue their recovery in the comfort of their own homes.

Not every patient can or should be fast tracked. Some patients require a period of observation to check for surgical complications, and some may not feel ready to sit in a chair. The process of fast tracking a patient may be slightly different for different surgical facilities. At our institutions the fast-tracked patient has one set of vital signs taken when he or she arrives in the phase 2 PACU. A brief evaluation is made to see if postsurgical and anesthesia side-effects remain minimal. The patient is then encouraged to sit in a lounge-type chair and offered something simple to eat and drink. Length of stay in the phase 2 PACU is patient specific. If the patient experiences any change during this recovery period, i.e. increased pain or bleeding, nausea or vomiting, he or she should be returned to the phase 1PACU for continued monitoring and treatment.

Table 62.4 *Standard Aldrete scoring system*

Activity	Score
Ability to move	
Four extremities	2
Two extremities	1
No extremities	0
Respiration	
Able to breathe deeply and cough freely	2
Dyspnea, shallow, or limited breathing	1
Apneic	0
Circulation	
Preoperative blood pressure (BP), kPa (mmHg):	
BP±20 mmHg of preanesthesia level	2
BP±20 to 50 mmHg of preanesthesia level	1
BP±50 mmHg of preanesthesia level	0
Consciousness	
Fully awake	2
Arousable on calling	1
Not responding	0
Color	
Normal	2
Pale, dusky, or blotchy	1
Cyanotic	0

A total score of 10 indicates that the patient is in optimal condition for discharge

From Aldrete JA, Kroulik D. A postanesthesia recovery score. *Anesth Analg* 1970; **49:** 924–34.

Discharge criteria

The accurate assessment of recovery of cognitive and psychomotor function is important in determining the appropriate time for discharge after ambulatory surgery. The recovery room nurse, the surgeon, and the anesthesiologist, as well as the patient (and the responsible escort), all play important roles in determining when a "home-ready" state has been achieved. There are several sets of standardized discharge criteria [e.g. Aldrete, the postanesthesia discharge scoring system (PADS)]. These recovery "scores" are useful in that they allow documentation of objective measurements of clinical recovery (Table 62.4). Most ambulatory units have developed variations of these for use in their own circumstances. A wide variety of psychomotor tests have also been used to assess recovery following general anesthesia or sedation (e.g. Trieger test, digit symbol substitution test). Most of these tests are too complex and time-consuming to use in a busy clinical setting but can provide information to help develop practical discharge criteria. Simple tests of memory and sensorimotor coordination appear to be the most useful indices of recovery.

Additional criteria must be applied to patients who undergo neuraxial regional anesthesia. Prior to discharge patients should ideally have recovered motor and sensory function. Once the sensory deficits have resolved, residual sympathetic blockade and orthostatic hypotension are rarely a problem on ambulation. It has been suggested that patients may be safely discharged when they have two successive orthostatic mean arterial pressure decreases of 10% or less after a spinal anesthetic.

However, several studies have reported recovery of sympathetic activity before complete regression of the subarachnoid block.[110] Prior to ambulation, patients should ideally have intact perianal sensation (S4–S5), the ability to plantar flex the foot, and normal proprioception in the big toe.

While the use of a checklist is appropriate to determine when patients may be discharged from the day-surgery unit, the criteria should be regularly reviewed. For example, it is no longer considered necessary for every patient to drink prior to discharge: children forced to drink before discharge have a higher incidence of vomiting and a longer stay in the recovery unit.[111] Urination as a criterion for discharge is controversial. However, it is customary to require patients to void after urologic procedures and spinal anesthesia.

Prior to discharge, pain should be controlled with oral medication. Pain medication should also be an integral part of recovery at home. In one study, only 38% of patients were able to return to their usual activities on the day after surgery. The most important factors determining the delay in return to normal activity were a feeling of general malaise (57%) and the degree of surgical pain experienced (38%).[112]

Patients should be given written instructions on discharge, including details of whom to contact if they experience any problems. Patients who have had general anesthesia or sedation cannot be relied upon to remember verbal instructions. In many day-surgery units in the USA, patients are routinely contacted the following day by telephone to allow assessment of the postdischarge recovery.

SUMMARY

The basic principles of ambulatory surgery were originally applied to healthy children and adults undergoing "minor operations." There is increasing evidence that arbitrary limits placed on the type of surgery, age of patients, duration of operation, preoperative fasting period, and selection of perioperative medication may be unwarranted. However, many controversies remain unresolved. Over the past decade, an increasing number of "high-risk" patients have presented for outpatient surgery, making proper patient selection and evaluation increasingly important. More information is required about the optimal anesthetic techniques for managing outpatients with significant pre-existing diseases or those at the extremes of age.

It is obvious that there is still much to learn about anesthesia for ambulatory surgery. In many situations, recovery times are still too long and the incidence of common side-effects remains too high. A major limiting factor in outpatient surgery at present is inadequate postoperative pain management. The rational use of available combinations of anesthetic drugs and equipment will provide for a rapid and smooth induction, excellent intraoperative conditions, and a rapid recovery with minimal side-effects. The incidence of anesthetic-related side-effects (e.g. drowsiness, headache, nausea, sore throat, myalgia, and dizziness) may be reduced depending on the premedication, the anesthetic technique, and the skill of the anesthesiologist. With the availability of more rapid and shorter-acting anesthetic, analgesic, and muscle relaxant drugs, as well as improved techniques for administering these drugs (e.g. the laryngeal mask airway and simplified infusion pumps), the care that we provide to our expanding outpatient population should continue to improve in the future.

Acknowledgment

Portions of this chapter were adapted from Chapter 68 by Christopher D Newson, Michael H Nathanson, and Paul F White in the previous (sixth) edition of this book.

APPENDIX 62.1 GUIDELINES FOR AMBULATORY ANESTHESIA AND SURGERY, APPROVED BY THE AMERICAN SOCIETY OF ANESTHESIOLOGISTS (ASA) HOUSE OF DELEGATES ON 11 OCTOBER 1973 AND LAST AMENDED ON 21 OCTOBER 1998

The American Society of Anesthesiologists (ASA) endorses and supports the concept of Ambulatory Anesthesia and Surgery. ASA encourages the anesthesiologist to play a leadership role as the perioperative physician in all hospitals, ambulatory surgical facilities, and office-based settings.

These guidelines apply to all care involving anesthesiology personnel administering ambulatory anesthesia in all settings. These are minimal guidelines, which may be exceeded at any time based on the judgment of the involved anesthesia personnel. These guidelines encourage high quality patient care, but observing them cannot guarantee any specific patient outcome. These guidelines are subject to periodic revision, as warranted by the evolution of technology and practice.

I ASA Standards, Guidelines, and Policies should be adhered to in all settings except where they are not applicable to outpatient care.

II A licensed physician should be in attendance in the facility or, in the case of overnight care, immediately available by telephone at all times during patient treatment and recovery and until the patients are medically discharged.

III The facility must be established, constructed, equipped, and operated in accordance with applicable local, state, and federal laws and regulations. At a minimum, all settings should have a reliable source of oxygen, suction, resuscitation equipment, and emergency drugs. (Specific reference is made to the *ASA Guidelines for Nonoperating Room Anesthetizing Locations.*)

IV Staff should be adequate to meet patient and facility needs for all procedures performed in the setting and should consist of:
- A Professional staff:
  - 1 Physicians and other practitioners who hold a valid license or certificate are duly qualified
  - 2 Nurses who are duly licensed and qualified
- B Administrative staff
- C Housekeeping and maintenance staff

V Physicians providing medical care in the facility should assume responsibility for credentials review, delineation of privileges, quality assurance, and peer review.

VI Qualified personnel and equipment should be on hand to manage emergencies. There should be established policies and procedures to respond to emergencies and unanticipated patient transfer to an acute care facility.

VII Minimal patient care should include:
- A Preoperative instructions and preparation
- B An appropriate preanesthesia evaluation and examination by an anesthesiologist prior to anesthesia and surgery. In the event that nonphysician personnel are utilized in the process, the anesthesiologist must verify the information and repeat and record essential key elements of the evaluation.
- C Preoperative studies and consultations as medically indicated
- D An anesthesia plan developed by an anesthesiologist and discussed with and accepted by the patient
- E Administration of anesthesia by anesthesiologists, other qualified physicians, or nonphysician anesthesia personnel medically directed by an anesthesiologist
- F Discharge of the patient is a physician responsibility
- G Patients who receive other than unsupplemented local anesthesia must be discharged with a responsible adult

H Written postoperative and follow-up care instructions
I Accurate, confidential, and current medical records

From the ASA website: www.asahq.org/Standards/04.html.

APPENDIX 62.2 DEFINITION OF GENERAL ANESTHESIA AND LEVELS OF SEDATION/ANALGESIA,[a] APPROVED BY THE AMERICAN SOCIETY OF ANESTHESIOLOGISTS (ASA) HOUSE OF DELEGATES ON 13 OCTOBER 1999

Sedation (anxiolysis) is a drug-induced state during which patients respond normally to verbal commands. Although cognitive function and coordination may be impaired, ventilatory and cardiovascular functions are unaffected.

Moderate sedation/analgesia ("Conscious Sedation") is a drug-induced depression of consciousness during which patients respond purposefully[b] to verbal commands, either alone or accompanied by light tactile stimulation. No interventions are required to maintain a patent airway and spontaneous ventilation is adequate. Cardiovascular function is usually maintained.

Deep sedation/analgesia is a drug-induced depression of consciousness during which patients cannot be easily aroused but respond purposefully[b] following repeated or painful stimulation. The ability to independently maintain ventilatory function may be impaired. Patients may require assistance in maintaining a patent airway and spontaneous ventilation may be inadequate. Cardiovascular function is usually maintained.

General anesthesia is a drug-induced loss of consciousness during which patients are not arousable, even by painful stimulation. The ability to independently maintain ventilatory function is often impaired. Patients often require assistance in maintaining a patent airway, and positive-pressure ventilation may be required because of depressed spontaneous ventilation or drug-induced depression of neuromuscular function. Cardiovascular function may be impaired. Because sedation is a continuum, it is not always possible to predict how an individual patient will respond. Hence, practitioners intending to produce a given level of sedation should be able to rescue patients whose level of sedation becomes deeper than initially intended. Individuals administering moderate sedation/analgesia ("Conscious Sedation") should be able to rescue patients who enter a state of deep sedation/analgesia, while those administering deep sedation/analgesia should be able to rescue patients who enter a state of general anesthesia.

a. Monitored anesthesia care does not describe the continuum of depth of sedation, rather it describes "a specific anesthesia service in which an anesthesiologist has been requested to participate in the care of a patient undergoing a diagnostic or therapeutic procedure."
b. Reflex withdrawal from a painful stimulus is *not* considered a purposeful response.

From the ASA website: www.asahq.org/Standards/04.html.

REFERENCES

1. Nicoll JH. The surgery of infancy. *Br Med J* 1909; **2:** 753–4.
2. Waters RM. The downtown anesthesia clinic. *Am J Surg* 1919; **33:** 71–3.
3. Committee on Quality Assurance in Office-Based Surgery. *Medical Society of the State of New York Survey on Office-Based Surgery and Invasive Procedures.* New York: New York State Public Health Council, October 1998.
4. Moss E. Revelations: New Jersey office regulations adopted. *American Society of Anesthesiologists Newsletter* 1998; **62** (8): 17–19, 22.
5. Zoutman D, Pearce P, McKenzie M, Taylor G. Surgical wound infections occurring in day surgery patients. *Am J Infect Control* 1990; **18:** 277–82.
6. Manian FA, Meyer L. Comprehensive surveillance of surgical wound infections in outpatient and inpatient surgery. *Infect Control Hospital Epidemiol* 1990; **11:** 515–20.
7. Oesch A. Indications for and results of ambulatory varices therapy. *Therapeutische Umschau* 1991; **48:** 692–6.
8. Federated Ambulatory Surgery Association. *Special Study 1.* Alexandria, VA: Federated Ambulatory Surgery Association, 1986.
9. Kurer FL., Walsh DB. Gynecological laparoscopy: clinical experiences of two anesthetic techniques. *Br J Anaesth* 1984; **56:** 1207–10.
10. Tong D, Chung F. Predictive Factors in global and anesthesia satisfaction in ambulatory surgical patients. *Anesthesiology* 1997; **87:** 856–64.
11. Natof HE. Pre-existing medical problems. Ambulatory surgery. *Illinois Med J* 1984; **166:** 101–4.
12. Federated Ambulatory Anesthesia Association. *Special Study 1.* Alexandria, VA: Federated Ambulatory Anesthesia Association, 1987.
13. Warner MA. Major morbidity and mortality within one month of ambulatory surgery and anesthesia. *JAMA* 1993; **270:** 1437–41.
14. Campbell IR, Scaife JM, Johnstone JM. Psychological effects of day case surgery compared with inpatient surgery. *Arch Dis Child* 1988; **63:** 415–17.
15. Astfalk W, Warth H, Leriche C. Day case surgery in childhood from the parents' point of view. *Eur J Pediatr Surg* 1991; **1:** 323–7.
16. Liu LMP, Cote CJ, Goudsouzian NG, *et al.* Life-threatening apnea in infants recovering from anesthesia. *Anesthesiology* 1983; **59:** 506–10.
17. Kurth CD, Spitzer AR, Broemile AM, Downes JJ. Postoperative apnea in preterm infants. *Anesthesiology* 1987; **66:** 483–8.
18. Meridy HW. Criteria for selection of ambulatory surgical patients and guidelines for anesthetic management: a retrospective study of 1553 cases. *Anesth Analg* 1982; **61:** 921–6.
19. Apfelbaum J. How frequently do asymptomatic patients benefit from the pursuit of abnormalities in their preoperative test results? *Anesthesiology* 1990; **73:** A1254.
20. Wyatt WJ, Reed DN Jr, Apelgren KN. Pitfalls in the role of standardized preadmission laboratory screening for ambulatory surgery. *Am Surg* 1989; **55:** 343–6.
21. Roberts Q, Goodman NW. Gastro-oesophageal reflux during elective laparoscopy. *Anaesthesia* 1990; **45:** 1009–11.
22. Sandhar B, Goresky GV, Maltby JR, Shaffer EA. Effect of oral liquids and ranitidine on gastric fluid volume and pH in children undergoing outpatient surgery. *Anesthesiology* 1989; **71:** 327–30.
23. Report by the American Society of Anesthesiologists Task Force on Preoperative Fasting. Practice guidelines for preoperative fasting and the use of pharmacologic agents to reduce the risk of pulmonary aspiration: application to healthy patients undergoing elective procedures. *Anesthesiology* 1999; **90:** 896–905.
24. Olsson GL, Hallen B, Hambraeus-jonzon K. Aspiration during anaesthesia: a computer-aided study of 185 358 anaesthetics. *Acta Anaesthesiol Scand* 1986; **30:** 84–92.
25. Haavik PE, Soreide E, Hofstad B, Steen PA. Does preoperative anxiety influence gastric fluid volume and acidity? *Anesth Analg* 1992; **75:** 914.
26. Maltby A, Reid CRG, Hutchinson A. Gastric fluid volume and pH in elective inpatients. Part II: Coffee or orange juice with ranitidine. *Can J Anaesth* 1988; **35:** 16–19.
27. Pandit SK, Kothary SP, Pandit UA, Mirakhur RK. Premedication with cimetidine and metoclouprumide. Effect on the risk factors of acid aspiration. *Anaesthesia* 1986; **41:** 486–92.
28. Foulkes E, Jenkins LC. A comparative evaluation of cimetidine and sodium citrate to decrease gastric acidity: effectiveness at the time of induction of anaesthesia. *Can Anaesth Soc J* 1981; **28:** 29–32.
29. Manchikanti L, Grow JB, Colliver JA, *et al.* Bicitra R (sodium citrate) and metoclopramide in outpatient anesthesia for prophylaxis against aspiration pneumonitis. *Anesthesiology* 1985; **63:** 378–84.
30. Jakobsen H, Hertz JB, Johansen JR, *et al.* Premedication before day surgery. A double-blind comparison of diazepam and placebo. *Br J Anaesth* 1985; **57:**300–5.
31. Korttila K, Linnoila M. Psychomotor skills related to driving after intramuscular administration of diazepam and meperidine. *Anesthesiology* 1975; **42:** 685–91.
32. White PF, Chang T. Effect of narcotic premedication on the intravenous anesthetic requirement. *Anesthesiology* 1984; **61:** A389.
33. Doze VA, Shafer A, White PR. Nausea and vomiting after outpatient anesthesia – effectiveness of droperidol alone and in combination with metoclopramide. *Anesth Analg* 1987; **66:** S41.
34. Manchikanti L, Canella MG, Hohlbein Q, Colliver JA. Assessment of effect

of various modes of premedication on acid aspiration risk factors in outpatient surgery. *Anesth Analg* 1987; **66:** 81–4.
35. Taylor E, Ghouri AF, White PF. Midazolam in combination with propofol for sedation during local anesthesia. *J Clin Anesth* 1992; **4:** 213–16.
36. Turner GA, Paech M. A comparison of oral midazolam solution with temazepam as a day case premedicant. *Anaesth Intensive Care* 1991; **19:** 365–8.
37. Short TG, Galletly DC. Double-blind comparison of midazolam and temazepam as oral premedicants for outpatient anaesthesia. *Anaesth Intensive Care* 1989; **17:** 1514.
38. Pandit SK, Kothary SP. Intravenous narcotics for premedication in outpatient anaesthesia. *Acta Anaesthesiol Scand* 1989; **33:** 353–8.
39. Horrigan RW, Moyers JR, Johnson BR, *et al.* Etomidate vs. thiopental with and without fentanyl – a comparative study of awakening in man. *Anesthesiology* 1980; **52:** 362–4.
40. Craig J, Cooper GK Sear JW. Recovery from daycase anaesthesia. Comparison between methohexitone, althesin and etomidate. *Br J Anaesth* 1982; **54:** 447–51.
41. White PF, Sung M-L, Doze VA. Use of sufentanil in outpatient anesthesia – determining an optimal preinduction dose. *Anesthesiology* 1985; **63:** A202.
42. Anderson B, Exarchos K, Brown TC. Oral premedication in children: a comparison of chloral hydrate, diazepam, alprazolam, midazolam and placebo for day surgery. *Anaesth Intensive Care* 1990; **18:** 185–93.
43. Hannallah RS, Patel RI. Low-dose intramuscular ketamine for anesthesia pre-induction in young children undergoing brief outpatient procedures. *Anesthesiology* 1989; **70:** 598–600.
44. Stafford M, Jeon A, Pascucci R. Pre and post-induction blood glucose concentrations in healthy fasting children. *Anesthesiology* 1985; **63:** A350.
45. Cook R, Anderson S, Riseborough M, Bloog CE. Intravenous fluid load and recovery. A double-blind comparison in gynaecological patients who had day-care laparoscopy. *Anaesthesia* 1990; **45:** 826–30.
46. Fassoulaki A, Sarantopoulos C. Minor complications of general anesthesia in a series of 1220 patients: the influence of mode of ventilation. *Acta Anaesthesiol Belg* 1991; **42:** 157–63.
47. Patel RL Hannallah RS, Norden J, *et al.* Emergence airway complications in children: a comparison of tracheal extubation in awake and deeply anesthetized patients. *Anesth Analg* 1991; **73:** 266–70.
48. Rieger A, Brunne B, Striebel HW. Intracuff pressures do not predict laryngopharyngeal discomfort after use of the laryngeal mask airway. *Anesthesiology* 1997; **87:** 63–67.
49. Greenberg RS, Brimacombe J, Berry A, *et al.* A randomized controlled trial comparing the cuffed oropharnygeal airway and the laryngeal mask airway in spontaneously breathing anesthetized adults. *Anesthesiology* 1988; **88:** 970–77.
50. Brimacombe JR, Brimacombe J. A comparison of the laryngeal mask airway and cuffed oropharyngeal airway in anesthetized adult patients. *Anesth Analg* 1998; **87:** 147–52.
51. Shane SM. Intravenous amnesia for total dentistry in one sitting. *J Oral Surg* 1966; **241:** 27–32.
52. Cote CJ. Conscious sedation: time for this oxymoron to go away! *J Pediatr* 2001; **139:** 15–17.
53. O'Boyle CA, Barry H, Fox E, *et al.* Controlled comparison of a new sublingual lormetazepam formulation and i.v. diazepam in outpatient minor oral surgery. *Br J Anaesth* 1988; **60:** 419–25.
54. Gross JB, Blouin RT, Zandsberg S, Conard PF. Effect of flumazenil on ventilatory drive during sedation with midazolam and alfentanil. *Anesthesiology* 1996; **85:**713–20.
55. Ghouri AF, Ramirez Ruiz MA, White PF. Effect of flumazenil on recovery after midazolam and propofol sedation. *Anesthesiology* 1994; **81:** 333–9.
56. Scarborough DA, Bisaccia E, Swensen RD. Anesthesia for outpatient dermatologic cosmetic surgery: midazolam-low dosage ketamine anesthesia. *J Dermatol Surg Oncol* 1989; **15:** 658–63.
57. White PF, Negus JB. Sedative infusions during local and regional anesthesia: a comparison of midazolam and propofol. *J Clin Anesth* 1991; **3:** 32–9.
58. Bridenbaugh LD. Regional anaesthesia for outpatient surgery – a summary of 12 years experience. *Can Anaesth Soc J* 1983; **30:** 548–52.
59. Philip BK, Covino BG. Local and regional anesthesia. In: Wetchler BV (ed.). *Anesthesia for Ambulatory Surgery*, 2nd edn. Philadelphia: JB Lippincott, 1985: 309–65.
60. Pollock JE. Prospective study on the incidence of transient radicular irritation in patients undergoing spinal anesthesia. *Anesthesiology* 1996; **84:** 1361–7.
61. Vaghadia H. Spinal anesthesia for outpatients: controversies and new techniques. *Can J Anaesth* 1998; **45:** R64–R70.
62. Lanz E. The extent of blockade following various techniques of brachial plexus block. *Anesth Analg* 1983; **62:** 55–8.
63. Henderson CL. A North American survey of intravenous regional anesthesia. *Anesth Analg* 1977; **85:** 858–63.
64. Singelyn FJ. Popliteal sciatic nerve block aided by a nerve stimulator: A reliable technique for foot and ankle surgery. *Reg Anesth* 1991; **16:** 178–281.
65. Norton AC, Dundas CR. Induction agents for day-case anaesthesia. A double-blind comparison of propofol and midazolam antagonized by flumazenil. *Anaesthesia* 1990; **45:** 198–203.
66. Dundee JW, McCollum JSC, Robinson FP, Halliday N. Elderly patients are unduly sensitive to propofol. *Anesth Analg* 1986; **65:** S43.
67. Wilton NCT, Thomas VL. Single breath induction of anaesthesia using a vital capacity breath of halothane, nitrous oxide and oxygen. *Anaesthesia* 1986; **41:** 472–6.
68. Meyers EF, Charles R. Prolonged adverse reactions to ketamine in children. *Anesthesiology* 1978; **49:** 39–40.
69. Dexter F, Tinker JH. Analysis of strategies to decrease postanesthesia care unit costs. *Anesthesiology* 1995; **82:** 94–101.
70. Melnick BM, Johnson LS. Effects of eliminating nitrous oxide in outpatient anesthesia. *Anesthesiology* 1987; **67:** 982–4.
71. Muir JJ, Warner MA, Offord KP, *et al.* Role of nitrous oxide and other factors in producing postoperative nausea and vomiting. A randomized and blinded prospective study. *Anesthesiology* 1986; **66:** 513–18.
72. Korttila K, Hovorka J, Erkola 0. Nitrous oxide does not increase the incidence of nausea and vomiting after isoflurane anesthesia. *Anesth Analg* 1987; **66:** 761–5.
73. Alexander GD, Skupski JN, Brown EM. The role of nitrous oxide in postoperative nausea and vomiting. *Anesth Analg* 1984; **63:** 175.
74. Muzi M. Induction of anesthesia and tracheal intubation with sevoflurane in adults. *Anesthesiology* 1996; **85:** 536–43.
75. Smith L, Ding Y, White PF. Comparison of induction, maintenance, and recovery characteristics of sevoflurane–N_20 and propofol–sevoflurane–N_20 with propofol–isoflurane–N_20 anesthesia. *Anesth Analg* 1992; **74:** 253–9.
76. Cooper GM, O'Conner M, Mark J, Harvey J. Effect of alfentanil and fentanyl on recovery from brief anaesthesia. *Br J Anaesth* 1983; **55:** S179–S182.
77. Cade L, Ross AW. Is fentanyl effective for postoperative analgesia in day-surgery? *Anaesth Intensive Care* 1992; **20:** 38–40.
78. Burkle H, Dunbar S, van Aken H, *et al.* Remifentanil: A novel, short acting μ-opioid. *Anesth Analg* 1996; **83:** 646–51.
79. Dershwitz M, Randel GL, Rosow CE, *et al.* Initial clinical experience with remifentanil, a new opioid metabolized by esterases. *Anesth Analg* 1995; **81:** 619–23.
80. Philip BK, Scuderi PE, Chung F, *et al.* Remifentanil compared with alfentanil for ambulatory surgery using total intravenous anesthesia. The Remifentanil/Alfentanil Outpatient TIVA Group. *Anesth Analg* 1997; **84:** 515–21
81. Vuyk J, Mertens MJ, Olofsen E, *et al.* Propofol anesthesia and rational opioid selection: determination of optimal EC_{50}–EC_{95} propofol–opioid concentrations that assure adequate anesthesia and a rapid return of consciousness. *Anesthesiology* 1997; **87:** 1549–62.
82. White PF, Shafer A. Clinical pharmacology and uses of injectable anesthestic and analgesic drugs. In: Wetchler BV (ed.). *Problems in Anesthesia.* Philadelphia: JB Lippincott, 1988: 37–54.
83. Alexander CD, Wetchler BV, Thompson RE. Bupivacaine infiltration of the mesosalpinx in ambulatory surgical laparoscopic tubal sterilization. *Can J Anaesth* 1987; **34:** 362–5.
84. Smith I, Van Hemelrijck J, White PF, Shively R. Effects of local anesthesia on recovery after outpatient arthroscopy. *Anesth Analg* 1991; **73:** 536–9.
85. Comfort VK, Code WE, Rooney W, Yip RW. Naproxen premedication reduces postoperative tubal ligation pain. *Can J Anaesth* 1992; **39:** 349–52.
86. Herbert M, Healy TEJ, Bourke JB, *et al.* Profile of recovery after general anaesthesia. *Br Med J* 1983; **286:** 1539–42.
87. Brindle GF, Soliman MG. Anaesthetic complications in surgical outpatients. *Can Anaesth Soc J* 1975; **22:** 613–19.
88. Zahl K, Apfelbaum JL. Muscle pain occurs after outpatient laparoscopy despite the substitution of vecuronium for succinylcholine. *Anesthesiology* 1989; **70:** 408–11.
89. Trepanier CA, Brousseau C, Lacerte L. Myalgia in outpatient surgery: comparison of atracurium and succinylcholine. *Can J Anaesth* 1988; **35:** 255–8.
90. Baurain MJ, Hoton J. Is recovery of neuromuscular transmission com-

plete after the use of neostigmine to antagonize block produced by rocuronium, vecuronium, atracurium and pancuronium? *Br J Anaesth* 1996; **77:** 496–9.

91. Tang J. Comparison of rocuronium and mivacurium to succinylcholine during outpatient laparoscopic surgery. *Anesth Analg* 1996; **82:** 994–8.
92. Mayer M, Doenicke A, Hofmann A, Peter K. Onset and recovery of rocuronium (ORG 9426) and vecuronium under enflurane anaesthesia. *Br J Anaesth* 1992; **69:** 511–12.
93. Basta SJ. Clinical pharmacology of mivacurium chloride: a review. *J Clin Anesth* 1992; **4:** 153–63.
94. Petersem RS, Bailey PL, Kalameghan R, Ashwood ER. Prolonged neuromuscular blockade after mivacurium. *Anesth Analg* 1993; **76:** 194–6.
95. Booth MG, Marsh B, Bryden FM, *et al.* A comparison of the pharmacodynamics of rocuronium and vecuronium during halothane anaesthesia. *Anaesthesia* 1992; **47:** 832–4.
96. Fredman B. Sevoflurane for outpatient anesthesia: a comparison with propofol. *Anesth Analg* 1995; **81:** 823–8.
97. Watcha MF, White PF. Postoperative nausea and vomiting. Its etiology, treatment and prevention. *Anesthesiology* 1992; **77:** 162–84.
98. White PF, Shafer A. Nausea and vomiting: causes and prophylaxis. *Semin Anesth* 1987; **6:** 300–8.
99. Apfel C. A simplified risk score for predicting postoperative nausea and vomiting. *Anesthesiology* 1999; **91:** 693–700.
100. Sinclair, D. Can postoperative nausea and vomiting be predicted? *Anesthesiology* 1999; **91:** 109–18.
101. Handley, AJ. Metoclopramide in the prevention of postoperative nausea and vomiting. Br J Clin Pract 1967; **21:** 460–2.
102. McKenzie R, Lim TN. Droperidol/ondansetron combination controls nausea and vomiting after tubal ligation. *Anesth Analg* 1996; **83:** 1218–22.
103. Cohen SE, Woods WA, Wyner J. Antiemetic efficacy of droperidol and metoclopramide. *Anesthesiology* 1984; **60:** 67–9.
104. McKenzie R, Tantisira B, Karambelkar DJ, *et al.* Comparison of ondansetron with ondansetron plus dexamethasone in the prevention of postoperative nausea and vomiting. *Anesth Analg* 1994; **79:** 961–4
105. Graczyk S. Intravenous dolasetron for the prevention of postoperative nausea and vomiting after outpatient laparoscopic gynecologic surgery. *Anesth Analg* 1997; **84:** 325–30.
106. Zomers PJW, Lanagerberg CJM, de Bruijin KM. Tropisetron for postoperative nausea and vomiting after gynaecological surgery. *Br J Anaesth* 1993; **71:** 677–80.
107. Pearman MH. Single dose intravenous ondansetron in the prevention of postoperative nausea and vomiting. *Anaesthesia* 1994; **49** (Suppl): 11–15.
108. Fortney JT, Gan TJ, Graczyk S, *et al.* A comparison of the efficacy, safety, and patient satisfaction of ondansetron versus droperidol as antiemetics for elective outpatient surgical procedures. S3A-409 and S3A-410 Study Groups. *Anesth Analg* 1998; **86:** 731–8.
109. Sun R. The effect of timing of ondansetron administration in outpatients undergoing otolaryngologic surgery. *Anesth Analg* 1997; **84:** 331–6.
110. Wetchler BV. Problem solving in the post anesthesia care unit. In: Wetchler BV (ed.). *Anesthesia for Ambulatory Surgery*, 2nd edn. Philadelphia: JB Lipincott, 1985: 375–436.
111. Schreiner, MS. Should children drink before discharge from day-surgery? *Anesthesiology* 1992; **76:** 528–33.
112. Philip, BK. Ambulatory anesthesia. *Semin Surg Oncol* 1990; **6:** 177–83.

63

Anesthesia for offsite procedures

M KEITH BRESLAND, MARK L THOMAS, AND W LAWRENCE ROY

INTRODUCTION

The introduction of modern drugs and portable monitoring systems has prompted anesthesiologists to leave the sheltered operating room (OR) workplace and provide care in remote offsite locations. Physicians and patients who in the past may not have had access to anesthetic care are now aware of the option. The recognition of the need for improved pain management has sponsored the move of anesthetic care beyond the OR. These out-of-OR expeditions are often complicated by the unexpected, and are clearly now the domain of the anesthesiologist. Infants and children are most often the patients who benefit from these out-of-OR initiatives. Indeed, much of the information contained in this chapter will pertain to the pediatric sedation/anesthesia experiences of the authors.

The early days of the sedation service at The Hospital for Sick Children, Toronto, Canada, consisted of the occasional consultation regarding appropriate sedation medication for the problematic patient.

What has evolved is the peripatetic (a person who walks from place to place) anesthesiologist[1] – an appropriate term applied to anesthesiologists providing care in offsite locations. Any department of anesthesia contemplating involvement in such a program should first consider the essential criteria for offsite anesthesia:[1]

- *Applicability*. Is it appropriate to actually provide the service?
- *Ability*. Does an anesthesiologist necessarily have to be present?
- *Affordability*. What is the cost and is it justifiable?
- *Availability*. Can your department actually provide the resources?
- *Affability*. Is it the desire of the cardiac catheterization laboratory or the magnetic resonance imaging (MRI) suite that an anesthesiologist provides the care?
- *Accountability*. Will the department oversee quality assurance and measurement of outcomes?
- *Altruism*. Are you providing a service because you get paid or are you getting paid because you provide a service?

PATIENT SELECTION

Patients are generally American Society of Anesthesiologists (ASA) grade I or II and do not require intubation. The offsite locations are generally adjacent to the hospital wards and clinics and are some distance from the postanesthesia care unit. If the anesthesia/sedation is to be provided in an offsite location, the recovery of patients will very likely occur there as well. Thus, patients should be uncomplicated, the duration of procedures brief, and the patients awake and not requiring significant postoperative analgesia. Patients with significant cardiac, respiratory, or neurological disease or those with a potential for significant bleeding or with unstable cervical spine should be managed in a formal OR. The need for postsedation/postanesthesia recovery should be assessed in advance of treatment. If the patient requires the skills and facilities of a postanesthesia care unit, safety suggests that patients should not be sedated at a remote site for subsequent transfer to an area adjacent to the main OR.

DEFINITIONS

An anesthesiologist must provide care when deep sedation and/or general anesthesia are required. When conscious sedation is required, the need for qualified personnel, sophisticated monitoring, and extended recovery are perhaps reduced, thus the cost, time, and organization are also diminished. Frequently, the term conscious sedation is applied when, in fact, deep sedation/general anesthesia is actually being provided.[2]

Conscious sedation

Conscious sedation is a medically controlled state of depressed consciousness that:

1 allows protective reflexes to be maintained;
2 retains the patient's ability to maintain a patent airway independently and continuously;
3 permits an appropriate response by the patient to physical stimulation or verbal command, e.g. "Open your eyes."[3]

Who should provide and supervise conscious sedation?

The American Academy of Pediatrics' (AAP) Committee on Drugs[3] states that an individual must be competent to use, and be capable of managing complications associated with, such techniques. A responsible physician should be available for both preoperative assessment and postsedation management. Expertise in airway management is essential. Personnel must be able to identify signs of early and late airway complications. Abilities should include the maintenance of an airway during spontaneous ventilation and intermittent positive pressure ventilation with a mask and a self-inflating resuscitation bag. Previous exposure to methods required to secure the airway is mandatory.

Some centers have chosen to write their own guidelines rather than adopt those of the AAP.[3] Some of these new protocols may set out lenient guidelines with regard to fasting, monitoring, and appropriate personnel. The confusing term conscious sedation may create some of the misunderstanding. A patient who sustains a painful stimulus will purposefully withdraw and indeed utter some displeasure. A comatose patient may be able to withdraw from painful stimulation. Unskilled and unqualified personnel unaware of the planes of sedation and anesthesia may well be monitoring anesthetized patients. Any center constructing guidelines should include the following warning:

> Those physicians utilizing these drugs alone or in combination should be familiar with these agents and aware of their potential respiratory complications.

Deep sedation

Deep sedation is a medically controlled state of depressed consciousness or unconsciousness from which a patient may not be aroused. It may be accompanied by a partial or complete loss of protective reflexes, and includes the inability to maintain a patent airway independently and respond purposefully to physical stimulation or verbal command.[3]

Who should provide and supervise deep sedation?

The term "conscious sedation" continues to be applied to far deeper levels of sedation. Coté[4] has eloquently summarized the issue when referring to conscious sedation. He writes, "This phrase is an oxymoron that should be removed from the medical literature. When caring for children, particularly when they have to remain quiet for any length of time, one must induce pharmacologic coma; – let us be honest and call deep sedation exactly what it is and take proper care of these deeply sedated patients."

Our medical colleagues have unrealistic expectations: because an anesthesiologist is present, the "conscious sedation" should be dramatic, i.e. the patients will be motionless. Moreover, anesthesiologists may be uncomfortable with patients who are reacting to pain and will administer additional medication, so that the patient lies still and unconscious. The need for an anesthesiologist in this setting is obvious.

The sedation guidelines (internal document) produced by the Harvard Medical School's Department of Anesthesia note that "the minimum number of personnel shall be two – the operator and the monitor (an assistant trained to monitor appropriate physiologic parameters and to assist in any supportive or resuscitation measures required). Such personnel will be available to the patient from the time of administration of sedative medication until the recovery is judged adequate, or the care of the patient is transferred to personnel performing recovery care."

Postanesthesia recovery nurses with pediatric education and experience are required. Often, patients sedated or anesthetized in offsite locations do not recover in a postanesthesia care unit. Nurses providing such care should be comfortable managing the pediatric airway and skilled in basic resuscitation techniques. Postsedation discharge criteria are given in Table 63.1.

General anesthesia

If one moves not very far along a continuum, general anesthesia is by definition very close to that of deep sedation:[3] "a medically controlled state of unconsciousness accompanied by a loss of protective reflexes including the inability to maintain a patent airway independently and respond purposefully to physical stimulation or verbal command."

Table 63.1 *Postsedation discharge criteria*[a]

Cardiovascular function and airway patency are satisfactory and stable
Patient is easily aroused and protective reflexes are intact
Patient can talk (if age appropriate)
Patient can sit up unaided (if age appropriate)
Very young or handicapped children – the presedation level of responsiveness should be achieved
The state of hydration is adequate

a. Guidelines for monitoring and mangement of pediatric patients during and after sedation for diagnostic and therapeutic procedures. *Pediatrics* 1992; **89:** 1110–15.

Who should provide and supervise general anesthesia?

Your plastic surgeon or your dentist?[5] A cynical question – the correct answer is an anesthesiologist!

FACILITY

Early in the development of satellite anesthesia at The Hospital for Sick Children, Toronto, departmental members traveled to various wards with a cart containing all the needed drugs and equipment required to provide conscious and deep sedation.

However, as demands increased, anesthesia staff grew weary of the need to travel from site to site. The need for nitrous oxide in these procedures became apparent, and thus the need for adequate room ventilation in these locations also became evident. Offsite anesthesia procedure suites were, therefore, developed adjacent to the sites of care. Each of these locations was built to OR specifications, according to the *Guidelines to the Practice of Anaesthesia* produced by the Canadian Anaesthetists' Society.[6]

MAGNETIC RESONANCE IMAGING

The provision of anesthesia and sedation in the MRI suite raises a series of challenges. In order to obtain high-quality images, patients need to remain immobile within the confined space of the magnetic core for at least 20 min. Large numbers of patients (Table 63.2) are unable to do this without adjuvant sedation or general anesthesia.

Once selected as in need of such help, the ensuing requirement for adequate monitoring and management according to strict guidelines[3] is obligatory. Equipment used for both the provision and monitoring of anesthesia must be nonferromagnetic and must function normally within the strong magnetic field.

Magnetic resonance imaging basic physics

Magnetic resonance imaging relies on the application of a powerful (0.05–2.0 tesla) magnetic field that results in the nuclei of the tissue being examined to align either parallel or antiparallel to that field.[7] The application of a second, superimposed oscillating magnetic field results

Table 63.2 *Categories of patient requiring anesthesia or sedation for magnetic resonance imaging*

Patient category	Requirement
Pediatric	Sedation or anesthesia
Developmental delay or psychiatric	Education, sedation, or anesthesia
Intensive care	Intubation and intermittent positive pressure ventilation
Raised intracranial pressure	Beware carbon dioxide retention with sedation

in minute oscillations of the aligned nuclei, thus inducing a small current specific to the type of nucleus under examination. By grading the strength of the applied signal throughout thin slices of tissue, an overall picture can be built of the entire tissue.

Clearly, ferromagnetic objects exposed to such strong fields will experience considerable pull proportional to their mass. Even weakly ferromagnetic objects such as metallic make-up or tattoos can distort the image or be heated by the field to the point of causing burns. There are also concerns that such fields can alter cell physiology such as altering bone fracture healing and erythrocyte morphology,[8] although the clinical significance of these is yet to be determined. A field above 30 gauss may also erase magnetic strip data such as that stored on computer disks and credit cards. During scanning, the noise level may reach 95 decibel and earplugs should be worn, even by anesthetized patients, to avoid cochlea damage. There are groups of patients in whom MRI is contraindicated because of the potential hazard of implanted ferromagnetic devices or objects. These are summarized in Table 63.3.

Monitoring equipment for magnetic resonance imaging

In complying with minimum monitoring standards,[9] a balance must be struck between loss of image quality due to electromagnetic interference from monitoring equipment and degradation of the monitor signal quality as a result of the powerful magnetic field. There are several monitoring systems that are nonferromagnetic and therefore compatible with use in the MRI.[10]

Electrocardiogram

Blood flowing through the aorta will produce a voltage that is maximal at 90° to the direction of flow according to Faraday's law. When superimposed upon the native electrocardiogram (ECG) signal, this can cause artifactual peaking of the T-wave. Strategies have been proposed by several authors to combat this problem.[11,12] These include placing the electrodes in the center of the field, keeping the wires together to avoid loops forming and, when using chest leads, favoring V5 and V6 as these are the furthest from the induced aortic voltage and most aligned to the QRS axis. ECG leads leaving the scanner can act as antennae, causing difficulty with quality of both monitor and scan signals. Telemetric ECG has been used[13] in an attempt to circumvent this problem and is now available commercially. A liquid crystal display should be used to avoid distortion of a cathode ray trace by the magnet. Cardiac motion artifacts can be widely eliminated by timing the scan to the ECG (ECG gating).

Pulse oximetry

Accurate monitoring is notoriously difficult since the signal is grossly distorted by the generated radiofrequencies of the scanner. However, the oximetry signal can be filtered to improve its quality. The signal in the Nellcor N-200 is preamplified prior to filtering, resulting in less loss of signal amplitude within the filter. Furthermore, this monitor can be ECG gated to improve pulse recognition.

Capnography

Inline sampling is not possible because the motor within the sampler tends to overheat and because the sampler would grossly distort the image. Side-stream sampling should be used but necessitates a long sampling set to keep the monitor beyond the 30-tesla line.

Blood pressure

Indirect measurement is possible by using nylon connectors rather than the standard ferromagnetic connectors. An extended length of tubing to the base unit will also be required. However, some damping of the signal will inevitably result from this length of tubing. Invasive monitoring is possible, but in order to minimize damping the transducer must be kept as close to the patient as the field will allow. The transducer will thus be within the 30-tesla line, even in the most concentrated of fields, and therefore has to be radiofrequency filtered to limit interference. MRI equipment compatibility is summarized in Table 63.4.

A study examining scan quality in awake volunteers with or without standard monitoring found that ASA minimum standards can be achieved without appreciable image degradation.[9]

Anesthetic equipment for magnetic resonance imaging

Beyond the 50-gauss line, anesthetic and monitoring equipment should work normally. The distance from the scanner at which this line can be drawn depends upon both the strength of the magnet and the presence of shielding. However, even with an unshielded scanner, monitoring equipment should work normally outside the scanning room. The argument for not using such a remote system is that a disconnection, distension of long ventilator tubing, and distortion of signals from long monitoring lines are all more likely. Within the 50-gauss line, nonferromagnetic equipment should be used, and there are several brands of all type of equipment available (Table 63.5). Patients can be transported on aluminum or high-grade stainless-steel trolleys to and from the scanner, although care must be taken not to cross the 50-gauss line with ferromagnetic oxygen cylinders.

Interventional magnetic resonance imaging

Increasingly, procedures are now being carried out during the MRI, including laparotomies and craniotomies with intermittent imaging to allow accurate tumor resection. The scanners are horseshoe shaped in design, with one side open to allow access to the patient. The same principles in anesthetic management apply for these operations as for scans alone, although the scan times can be significantly longer. Titanium instruments are used and patient access is extremely limited. The challenge of maintaining normothermia is even greater not only

Table 63.3 *Implanted devices or objects representing a contraindication to magnetic resonance imaging*

Implanted devices	Comments	Reference
Cardiac pacemaker	Reed switch malfunction reported	63
Metal eye splinter/shrapnel	Blindness has been reported	64
Vascular clips, intrauterine contraceptive devices, penile implant	Devices vary in compatibility	For a list of compatible equipment, see reference 65
Interventional radiology device (coil/stent)		
Orthopedic device (prosthetic joint, wire plate)		

Table 63.4 *Monitoring equipment requirements for magnetic resonance imaging (MRI)*

Monitor	Ideal requirements for MRI monitors
ECG	Liquid crystal screen, high-impedance graphite electrodes and leads, avoid loops of wire, optical links available
Blood pressure	Oscillotonometer with nonferrous gauge (long tubing may affect accuracy); ferrous-poor monitors available
Respiratory gas	Outside unit with long sampling line; qualitative analysis within scanner possible
Temperature	Skin temperature-sensing strips; burns have been reported with probes
Pulse oximeter	Nonferromagnetic model

ECG, electrocardiogram.

Table 63.5 *Magnetic resonance imaging-compatible anesthetic equipment*

Anesthetic equipment	Comments
Laryngoscope	Standard batteries are highly magnetic; plastic scopes with paper- or aluminum-covered lithium cells are available
Stylet	Copper model available
Endotracheal tube	Spring within valve cuff may distort image; nonmagnetic version is available. Avoid reinforced tubes and metal connectors
Laryngeal mask airway	Spring within valve cuff may distort image; a nonmagnetic version is available
Ventilator	Available
Anesthetic machine	Several nonmagnetic machines are available; note that aluminum cylinders are required
Infusion pumps	Infusion pumps have been used at the 30-gauss line, but extension sets are recommended to minimize the field effect on motor function; the need for long extension lines may exclude patients requiring high-dose inotropes
Self-inflating bags	Valveless with no magnetic parts
Suction	Wall-mounted with 10-m tubing
Defibrillators	Cathode ray tube and batteries will malfunction within the 30-gauss line; resuscitation should preferably be carried out outside the magnetic field

because of the difficulties in measuring temperature accurately but also because of the logistics of warming fluids.

Sedation/anesthesia for magnetic resonance imaging

Criteria for selection for general anesthesia versus sedation are outlined at the beginning of this chapter, but several sedation protocols are in use with varying failure rates. Of particular interest is a Wisconsin study in which introduction of a dedicated sedation program improved scan success and reduced scan time in a pediatric population. Thiopental (4 mg kg^{-1}) was the most frequently employed agent (54% of patients) followed by chloral hydrate (40–80 mg kg^{-1} in 27% of patients), whereas midazolam (0.3–0.5 mg kg^{-1}) was used in only 15% of children.[14] Extreme caution must be exercised in the application of all sedation protocols as success is more a function of careful case selection and appropriate staffing than it is the adoption of a particular pharmacological cocktail.

Several units use high-dose chloral hydrate (50–100 mg kg^{-1}),[15] although major respiratory complications have been reported in Leigh's encephalopathy.[16] Chloral hydrate seems less effective for children aged 4 years or less, whereas other agents may be more appropriate.[17]

Supplementary intravenous (i.v.) diazepam (Diazemuls) may be given under the direction of a skilled pediatric resuscitator up to a maximum of 0.1 mg kg^{-1} for those sedated with chloral hydrate, temazepam, or droperidol.

For each of these patient groups, the scan requirement is immobility. In order to achieve this safely, the anesthesiologist must be assured that the airway and breathing are adequately maintained. Sedation requirements inevitably and correctly err on the side of caution in this regard, with a resultant failure rate requiring progression to general anesthesia. Several sedation protocols have been advocated, but with each of them emphasis should be placed on the presence of the attending staff and monitoring levels of safe sedation within the scanning environment.

If the indication for scanning under general anesthesia is for suspected raised intracranial pressure or if general anesthesia is indicated for a patient with a potentially full stomach, then intubation with positive pressure ventilation is required. Maintenance with a volatile-based anesthetic and with a propofol infusion have both been employed. However, with the latter, dose requirement can be unpredictable,[18] and infusion pumps may malfunction near the field. The use of laryngeal masks in the setting of MRI is gaining in popularity, with the caveat that continued security of the airway must be ensured. The effect of increasing the length of the expiratory limb of the Ayre's T-piece has been studied.[19] Ventilation of lung models with a 10-m breathing system results in only minimal decreases in tidal volume as a result of circuit compliance, and thus remote (outside the scanner) ventilation can be used.

Contrast enhancement

Scan quality can be significantly enhanced by the use of gadolinium. This agent is renally cleared with an elimination half-life of 90 min. There is only one case report of death due to anaphylaxis in a 67-year-old woman,[20] making this an extremely safe agent especially when compared with other contrast media.

Recurring issues and magnetic resonance imaging

1 Consent. Occasionally, consent is not secured by the radiologist as no intervention is contemplated. Preanesthetic assessment must include confirmation of verbal and/or written consent for sedation/anesthesia.
2 Need for deep sedation/anesthesia. Anesthesia is occasionally requested without the benefit of prior assessment as many of these patients travel from distant locations. Often, a child may cooperate fully with the addition of parental presence and/or conscious sedation.
3 Requests for anesthesia assistance following failed conscious sedation is a common occurrence. In the past, these patients have not fasted, thus the option of elective deep sedation/anesthesia was unavailable. As many diagnostic imaging departments now adhere to published sedation guidelines, this group of patients (failed

conscious sedation) are at least fasting when assistance is requested. The dilemma is whether one should defer until another date, recommend additional sedation, or provide anesthetic support.

COMPUTED TOMOGRAPHY SCANNING

The computed tomography (CT) scan itself is painless, but immobility is essential for good image definition. Children, patients with movement disorders or impaired mentation, or those who are acutely ill and require invasive monitoring may all require an anesthesiologist to provide sedation/anesthesia in the CT scan room.

Modern CT scan rooms have been designed and built with anesthetic requirements taken into account. These include piped in anesthetic gas outlets and suction units available for use with an anesthetic machine and ventilator. An anesthetic supply cart, fully equipped with drugs, airway adjuncts, laryngoscopes, syringes, etc. should be positioned within easy reach together with a full monitoring stack placed where it can be viewed through the window from outside the scan room. Some modern scanners have closed circuit television imaging of the patient as they lie within the tube, allowing constant observation of continuing chest wall movement.

Patient monitoring

The basic monitoring standards[6] apply to the CT suite, as they do to any "remote" area within the hospital where heavy sedation/anesthesia is being administered. As mentioned previously, it may be difficult at times to view the patient directly, especially if the anesthesiologist removes him/herself from the scan room for their own protection. It is imperative that the monitoring equipment is easily viewed, is working correctly with alarm functions appropriately set, and that these alarms are acted upon promptly. The anesthesiologist must ensure that the patient is positioned safely, with pressure points padded, and that no part of the patient is at risk as the scan table moves in and out of the scanner. Similarly, the breathing circuit, i.v. tubing, and monitoring equipment should all be checked to ensure adequate freedom over the full range of table movement.

Anesthetic considerations

There is now a broad range of indications for use of CT imaging, and anesthesiologists may have to adapt their techniques depending on whether the patient is elective or an emergency trauma victim with ongoing blood loss or raised intracranial pressure. These latter patients must be treated as if they have full stomachs, and therefore sedation is not an option. These patients should be scanned fully awake or be intubated following a rapid sequence induction – *remember to stabilize the cervical spine prior to laryngoscopy and intubation.* Intubation and ventilation is the preferred choice in any unstable head-injured patient since the airway is controlled, allowing manipulation of P_{O_2} and P_{CO_2} to minimize secondary brain injury.

The majority of patients undergoing CT imaging will be outpatients requiring preanesthetic evaluation on the day of the procedure. A full medical history and examination should be secured, with particular attention to the individual's pathology and any implications for the anesthetic technique. For example, a head CT implies the possibility of a mass lesion and, therefore, potential for raised intracranial pressure. Respiratory depression and resultant increased cerebral blood flow may contraindicate the use of a sedative technique in this situation.

CT scans of the thorax or abdomen are often performed to assess the extent of a tumor mass. Careful assessment will highlight the patient's physiological reserve, nutritional status, and any compromise of cardiovascular or respiratory function. It is important to assess whether the tumor mass is compressing an airway or a major vessel. With abdominal CT scans, recommendations include tissue opacification with both oral and intravenous contrast medium.[21] The oral contrast would normally be given within 1 h of the planned procedure, thus leaving the anesthesiologist with the dilemma of managing a patient for a CT scan who technically has not fasted.

Historically, radiologists have been the physicians most commonly involved in the sedation of children in the radiology department[22] and often rely on a single regime with a clinical history of safety. There is very little evidence in the literature of complications arising from these "full stomach" sedations; however, as more anesthesiologists become responsible for the care of the patients in CT, a more interventional approach to managing the airway will undoubtedly follow, for better or worse!

Anesthetic/sedative drug regimens

Propofol has now gained widespread acceptance as a useful sedative/anesthetic agent in the radiology suite.[23] Merola *et al.*[24] reported a zero complication rate in a series of 324 patients who received propofol for sedation during radiological imaging. However, they do not recommend its use for children under 1 year of age.

Chloral hydrate is another popular sedative used frequently for nonpainful imaging. It is given orally in a dose of 50 mg kg^{-1}. Vade *et al.*[25] report 100% success for sedation of children having CT examinations with chloral hydrate alone or supplemented with hydroxyzine. Mild hypoxia (S_{pO_2} 90–95%) is reported in 9% of the children under 1 year, whereas moderate to severe hypoxia occurred in 0.5% of children studied. They concluded that chloral hydrate sedation provides effective and safe sedation for children if the AAP guidelines for patient selection, monitoring, and management are followed.[3]

Pereira *et al.*[26] compared chloral hydrate, intramuscular pentobarbital, and intravenous pentobarbital, concluding that i.v. pentobarbital provided faster and superior quality sedation for CT scan. The incidence of desaturation is increased in patients receiving i.v. pentobarbital and chloral hydrate; however, only i.v. pentobarbital is associated with severe and prolonged desaturation.

A 1990 survey[22] found that in the USA only 2% of sedated examinations were carried out in the presence of an anesthesiologist, whereas 55% of cases were in the presence of a radiologist and 27% of cases were supervised by a nurse. Clearly, anesthesiologists cannot attend all sedated cases, but whoever assumes responsibility must ensure appropriate patient selection, correct patient evaluation and drug choice, and be able to safely monitor and resuscitate cases should the need arise.

Hematology and oncology procedures

Childhood cancer is uncommon, with an incidence in the USA of 1 in 333 for those under 20 years of age compared with a figure of 1 in 3 for adults.[27] Nevertheless, between the ages of 1 and 14 years, malignant disease is the second most common cause of death after accidents. Acute lymphoblastic leukemia is the commonest childhood malignancy, being 23.3% of the total.[27] The initial diagnosis requires a bone marrow aspiration to differentiate between acute lymphoblastic (80%) and acute myeloblastic leukemia. This initial investigation necessitates the first in a series of sedations/general anesthetics for the child that, during the course of their treatment, will involve several lumbar punctures and possible repeat aspirations of the bone marrow.

Historically, these procedures were performed in treatment rooms, often without the presence of an anesthesiologist, and commonly involved the use of ketamine as the main sedative agent. Following the introduction of propofol, ketamine use is in decline. The presence of personnel with anesthetic skills is essential for all of these procedures. Bone marrow aspiration in particular is extremely painful, and the use of the newer short-acting opiates such as remifentanil in combination with propofol is an area of expanding interest. A eutectic mixture of local anesthetic (EMLA) cream is also used to good effect when applied at least 1 h prior to lumbar puncture to allow a reduction in the anesthetic/sedative requirement.

The services of an anesthesiologist in the setting of hematology/oncology are almost exclusively confined to the pediatric population. The use of remote anesthetizing locations obviates the need for repeat visits to the OR and may also reduce the cost of treatment. Parent and patient preference for less threatening locations has also sponsored development of these offsite treatment areas. The procedure site at The Hospital for Sick Children, Toronto, has been situated adjacent to the outpatient clinic, inpatient hospital ward, and the recovery/observation unit. This location has increased efficiency and parent/patient satisfaction. The department of anesthesia now provides sedation/anesthesia for 2000 procedures per year at this location.

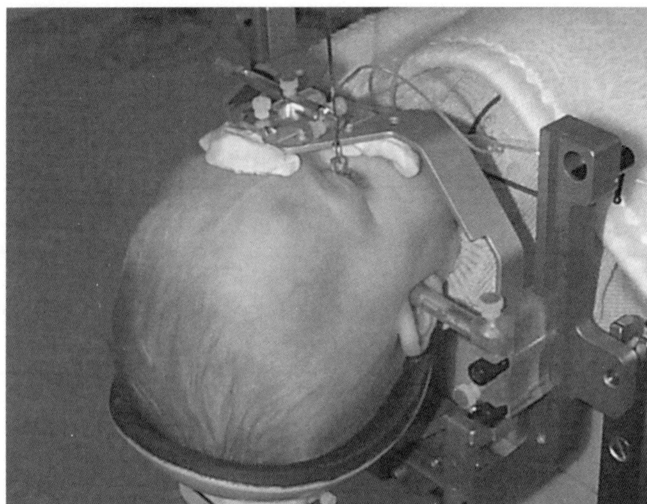

Figure 63.1 *Stereotactic radiation. A 9-month-old infant undergoing stereotactic radiation for retinoblastoma. The patient was anesthetized with intravenous propofol and room air. All monitors were in place. Three video cameras displayed monitor images outside the radiation suite.*

Radiotherapy

Daily therapy during a 2- to 3-week course of treatment for radiosensitive tumors requires complete immobility for the duration of the dose. The first treatment involves fitting a bracket or cast to allow similar positioning during subsequent treatments. Deep sedation with midazolam or propofol[23] is often adequate since these procedures are not painful and daily use of the laryngeal mask for repeat anesthetics has also been used without complications.[28] If prone positioning is required, or if there is raised intracranial pressure, then intubation and positive pressure ventilation may be required. The use of ketamine in this latter group may be contraindicated because of the possibility of raised intracranial pressure. Considerations for stereotactic surgery are shown in Table 63.6. See also Fig. 63.1.

Interventional radiology

An increasing number of ever more complex procedures are being carried out by interventional radiologists.[29] These range from the embolization of an arteriovenous malformation (AVM) in asymptomatic patients to the control of subarachnoid bleeding in a critically ill patient. A range of neuropathologies is amenable to interventional treatment.[30] These can be divided into AVMs of the brain, dura, and spine; arteriovenous fistulae; aneurysms; and tumors. Interventional radiologists are also involved in the placement of long-term percutaneous intravenous catheters, in gastrostomies, and in extracranial angiography and embolization.

For arteriovenous malformations, embolic material is placed transvascularly, usually via the femoral artery. This technique can also be used to reduce the vascularity of tumors prior to surgical excision. The latter usually employs fine polyvinyl particles mixed with contrast. For AVMs, detachable platinum coils are often introduced.[31] Although sclerosants and polymerizing substances (glue) are preferred by some clinicians, ischemia, thromboembolism, and hemorrhage have all been reported. Preoperative assessment should concentrate on commonly associated pathologies, especially hypertension in association with subarachnoid hemorrhage. Preoperative investigation should include clotting studies as heparin is often used perioperatively to prevent embolization distal to the treated lesion.

Table 63.6 *Considerations for stereotactic radiosurgery*

Removal of head frame in urgent situations requires wrench and previous experience
Vomiting may occur following radiation to the fourth ventricle
Linear accelerator moves as the table rotates – potential for disruption of anesthetic and/or monitoring equipment
Head frame may interfere with airway access

Local anesthetic with sedation has been used, but requires an extremely cooperative patient capable of lying relatively still, possibly for several hours. Furthermore, prolonged procedures and oversedation can occur, and thus general anesthesia has several advantages. Mild hyperventilation to a $P_{a}CO_2$ of 4–4.5 kPa has been shown to improve angiographic images;[32] however, this must be weighed against the inverse steal phenomenon that may occur to the noncarbon dioxide-responsive circulation of an AVM. As catheters pass the carotid sinus, arrhythmias may occur, in particular bradycardia. Further cardiovascular instability can occur upon embolization of the lesion, although this is most often temporary. The femoral catheter is removed at the end of the procedure and direct arterial pressure applied for at least 10 min to avoid hemorrhage. Avoidance of coughing on extubation is clearly desirable, although this must be balanced against being assured that consciousness has been regained prior to extubation. The major interventional complication is hemorrhage, which if slight can be treated with protamine and antihypertensives. Note that the administration of protamine[33,34] is not without complication. Severe fatal reactions following administration have been reported.

Endoscopy suite

Traditionally, endoscopists have administered sedation to the majority of their patients, usually in the form of a combination of benzodiazepines and narcotics. However, a subgroup of patients (mainly pediatric) is perceived to be at higher risk, and the anesthesiologist is involved increasingly. Note that bronchoscopy is rarely undertaken in an offsite location.

Gastrointestinal endoscopy

The initial step, as always, should be a careful evaluation of the patient preprocedure. Many of these patients are being investigated for achalasia, esophageal stricture, or severe erosive esophagitis secondary to reflux, all of which would dictate the need for airway protection during sedation. The adequacy of standard fasting regimens has recently been questioned[35] in terms of achieving the "desirable" values: gastric volume of 0.4 mL kg^{-1} or less with a gastric pH level of 2.5 or more. The authors noted fewer than half of fasted pediatric patients actually achieve these values, consequently gastric aspiration is of high concern. The insertion of a gastroscope is stimulating, often causing patients to retch or hiccup. Appropriate airway equipment (endotracheal tubes, laryngoscope, and wall suction) should be readily available.

A benzodiazepine is generally used when sedation is required for gastroscopy, although propofol appears to have a more suitable pharmacokinetic profile. Carlsson *et al.*[36] found that adult patients receiving propofol (0.6 mg kg^{-1} bolus, followed by repeat doses of 50%) tolerated endoscopy better, reached a deeper maximum level of sedation, and recovered more rapidly than those receiving 0.06 mg kg^{-1} i.v. midazolam. They concluded that although propofol facilitated gastroscopy to a greater extent it was a more demanding agent to administer. High- and low-dose topical anesthesia have also been assessed [topical pharyngeal lidocaine (lignocaine) 30 mg or 100 mg] for use in gastroscopy in otherwise unsedated adult patients;[37] although the high-dose lidocaine reduced patient discomfort, a large proportion of the subjects (37%) stated that they would request sedation for a subsequent procedure.

Upper endoscopy has been available to the pediatric population for some years, and the anesthetic for it has been evolving over that time.[38] The most common indications seen at our institution for children requiring upper endoscopy studies are abdominal pain, vomiting, dysphagia, caustic ingestion, and foreign body. Colonoscopy is generally indicated for the investigation of malabsorption, diarrhea, and inflammatory bowel disease. Patients with the gastrointestinal (GI) disorders shown in Table 63.7 are not appropriate for offsite care as they are at increased risk of aspiration of gastric contents.

Conscious sedation for children under 12 years of age for upper GI endoscopy is often inadequate, thus deep sedation or general anesthesia is more appropriate for these younger patients. Propofol has taken its place as a cornerstone anesthetic agent for ambulatory anesthesia. Propofol administration for GI endoscopy in small children is often at dosages that lead to deep sedation and/or anesthesia. It is rapid in onset, short acting, and has a good recovery profile. It may be used with a bolus technique or as an infusion. An added plus to this drug is its apparent antiemetic properties. At The Hospital for Sick Children, Toronto, propofol has become the standard, either as a solitary agent or in combination with midazolam. Patients are rarely intubated in the offsite endoscopy suite. Indeed, if intubation is required, the procedure is reassigned to the main OR suite. A review of 136 patients concluded that colonoscopy performed under general anesthesia in children is a very safe procedure, is preferred by the patient, and is felt to be superior to sedation.[39]

Topical application of local anesthetics to the pharyngeal structures must be considered, especially for those patients in whom a minimum of anesthetic agents are required. These agents improve tolerance and make examination easier.[40] Administration of glycopyrrolate reduces secretions, which are copious during upper endoscopy. Our experience with pediatric patients for gastroscopy has allowed us to develop a method of deep sedation/anesthesia for these occasions. Generally, these ASA I/II patients, who do not have significant esophageal disease, are administered a bolus of propofol (2–3 mg kg^{-1}) followed by a propofol infusion at a rate of 100–150 μg kg^{-1} min^{-1}. Monitoring in these patients is essential. All standard monitors (ECG, blood pressure, pulse oximetry) should be applied to all patients.

Table 63.7 *Contraindications for gastrointestinal endoscopy in offsite anesthesia locations*

Achalasia
Esophageal stricture or narrowing
Severe erosive esophagitis
Intestinal pseudo-obstruction
Scleroderma with esophageal involvement
Oropharyngeal discoordination

Colonoscopy may be perceived as less challenging than gastroscopy to the anesthesiologist because there is neither shared airway nor pathologies of the upper GI tract. However, the procedure is not without risks to the patient. In a recent study,[41] arterial oxygen desaturation occurred in 45% of adult patients, with ECG evidence of myocardial ischemia demonstrated in 11%. In the pediatric population, the anesthetic technique for colonoscopy at our institution consists of propofol/fentanyl/oxygen. The profound sedation/anesthesia and rapid rate of recovery have provided for high patient and parent satisfaction. Our anesthetic technique has evolved from a conscious sedation protocol utilizing intravenous diazepam and meperidine (pethidine). The use of propofol improved the adequacy of sedation, reduced the incidence of respiratory depression requiring intervention, and reduced the mean length of stay after the procedure.

Recovery

Recovery area monitoring is vital. In a study of 475 adult patients who received sedation for an endoscopic procedure, the incidence of oxygen desaturation was 24% in the recovery phase, with the majority occurring within the first 10 min.[42] To maximize patient safety, a coordinated effort is required by the anesthesiologist, the endoscopist, and the unit nursing staff. Patients with multisystem disease and those considered high risk because of underlying pathophysiological conditions should be recovered in a designated postanesthesia care unit (PACU) facility. Therefore, such patients are managed in the main OR rather than the offsite endoscopy suite. These patients are then transferred directly to the adjacent postanesthesia care unit.

Burn dressing changes

The burned patient will probably undergo multiple procedures in the months and years following his or her injury, the majority of which will be relatively minor debridements and dressing changes. The equipment and nursing expertise available in the burn unit makes it the ideal place to perform these procedures efficiently and with minimal distress to the patient.

Procedural pain is commonly undertreated, with up to 84% of adult patients reporting extremely intense pain levels during procedures.[43] Similar undertreatment of pain occurs in the pediatric setting,[44] children being much more likely to receive little or no analgesic during procedures. Opioid administration is the mainstay of procedure-related pain management in all age groups. It should be borne in mind that opioid pharmacokinetics are altered in the burned patient both immediately and for weeks to months after the injury. Osgood and Szyfelbein[44] document that the volume of distribution and elimination half-life of morphine appear to be significantly reduced in burned children compared with controls.

In our institution, with a pediatric only population, patients are usually managed with combinations of nitrous oxide/oxygen, propofol, and narcotic with or without midazolam. For the child without i.v. access, oral transmucosal fentanyl citrate (OTFC) has become popular and has proven to be safe and effective in providing sedation and analgesia for painful procedures.[45] The nausea and vomiting associated with OTFC during other applications has not been a problem for patients undergoing burn dressing changes. Ketamine is widely used as an anesthetic and analgesic for burned patients.[46] It has an intense analgesic effect, producing a "dissociative" anesthetic state in which ventilation and airway reflexes are largely preserved, although it is associated with increased pharyngeal and tracheobronchial secretions. (Prophylactic administration of an antisialagogue is recommended.)

Anesthetic issues for dressing change

The extent of the burn will affect the length of the procedure and the positioning of monitoring on the patient. If the burn involves the neck or face, then airway management may be a problem (specialized equipment should be available, e.g. laryngeal mask airway, fiberoptic scope). These patients are not managed in an offsite location. When patients require lengthy debridement, additional nursing personnel are essential to reduce anesthesia and treatment time. Because these units do not enjoy the same staff allocations as an OR, there may often be prolonged treatment intervals. All measures must be undertaken to reduce treatment time. Fasting for burned patients with high caloric requirements has been waived for patients receiving continuous gastrojejunal tube feeds. The feeds are continued until just before induction of sedation/anesthesia. There has been no increased morbidity, and recent investigations suggest that there may not be an increased risk of aspiration.[47] For burned patient considerations, see Table 63.8.

EMERGENCY DEPARTMENT

Today's anesthesiologist can expect to be called to the modern emergency department with increasing frequency not only to assist in the management of trauma but also as an expert in sedation/anesthesia. Minor surgical and procedural undertakings are performed on a semielective basis within the sometimes chaotic setting of the emergency department. Provision of sedation in such a setting is complicated by the absence of fasted patients, the need for sedative agents that confer almost no postprocedural sedation, and the inconsistent presence of an expert in sedation and airway management. If called upon to sedate a patient in these surroundings, it is important that the anesthesiologist satisfies him/herself that adequate provision has been made in terms of equipment, monitoring, personnel, and trained assistance as specified in the sedation guidelines produced by the AAP in the USA[3] or by the Royal College of Anaesthetists in the UK.

Emergency department anesthetic regimens

Different sedative regimens have been evaluated for use during simple painful procedures, such as laceration suturing. Midazolam in a dose of 0.5 mg kg^{-1} given orally is effective in 76% of children,[48] with an onset time of 15 min compared with 10 min when administered nasally.[49] This route is associated with increased difficulty of administration. Hart *et al.*[50] highlight the need for a high level of monitoring for patients receiving conscious sedation. They compared i.v. fentanyl with i.v. fentanyl–midazolam and intramuscular (i.m.) meperidine–promethazine–chlorpromazine (MPC) used for painful emergency department procedures. They concluded that all three regimens produce adequate sedation and analgesia, but also a relatively high incidence of subclinical respiratory depression (20% of patients receiving fentanyl, 23% of patients receiving fentanyl–midazolam, and 11% of patients receiving MPC) as detected by $ET_{CO_2} \geq 6.7$ kPa (50 mmHg). Also, MPC administration resulted in a significantly delayed discharge from the emergency department.

Table 63.8 *Considerations for burned patients*

Organ system failures
Smoke inhalational injury associated with carbon monoxide and/or cyanide poisoning
Hypermetabolic state develops which is proportional to the area of burn
Anemia secondary to the burn itself, blood sampling, and the procedures performed
Erythrocyte half-life is shortened
Platelets may initially decrease but return to normal within 7 days
Clotting factors generally decrease
Renal failure varies from 0.5% to 38%, being more common with larger area burns
Immune function is impaired
Increased incidence of gastric mucosal ulceration
Pharmacokinetic and pharmacodynamic properties of drugs are altered
Hypoalbuminemia leads to reduced protein binding of drugs

Chudnofsky[51] demonstrated the safety and efficacy of using flumazenil for the reversal of midazolam-induced sedation in emergency department patients given a combination of fentanyl and midazolam to facilitate the performance of short, painful procedures. Intramuscular ketamine in a dose of 4 mg kg^{-1} has been found to produce acceptable sedation in 98% of patients undergoing brief emergency department procedures.[52] Transient airway complications occurred in 1.4%, but were quickly identified and treated without intubation or sequelae. Moderate to severe recovery agitation has been noted in 1.6% of patients, with a median time to discharge of 110 min. Similar results have been achieved with intravenous ketamine in a dose of 1.5 mg kg^{-1} with no serious complications noted,[53] but vomiting, ataxia, and agitation have been described in a few cases.

Chloral hydrate, with its wide margin of safety, appears to be particularly well suited to emergency department requirements.[54] It is administered in a dose of 25–50 mg kg^{-1} orally, with the time to sedation being 20–60 min and to recovery being 20–60 min. Chloral hydrate sedation is appropriate for wound repair, foreign body removal, and abscess drainage in the emergency department.

Propofol has gained acceptance as a useful drug in the emergency department. Swanson *et al.*[55] have described the use of continuous propofol infusion after an initial dose of fentanyl (2 μg kg^{-1}) for a range of procedures. The only side-effects noted were pain on injection, one episode of hypotension, and two episodes of apnea (both < 30 s). The patients reported 97% satisfaction with the sedation produced, and the authors concluded that propofol, given its rapidity of onset and elimination, may become a useful agent for i.v. sedation in the emergency department.

Another useful and effective technique for the cooperative patient is the use of self-administered nitrous oxide in 50% oxygen. Self-administration prevents oversedation, and the effect is rapidly lost once inhalation stops. Pain relief is reasonable and side-effects are few (nausea, vomiting, disinhibition), but the technique does require diligent attention by the patient to maintain a tight face mask seal and to provide enough inspiratory effort to trigger the valve of the nitrous oxide/oxygen apparatus.

Closed forearm fracture manipulation in the emergency department

This often requires some form of anesthesia or sedation. A combination of sedation and i.v. regional anesthesia may be the most desirable approach to forearm fracture in children[56] since the diminished need for sedation combined with the profound analgesia of an intravenous block requires that the patient only be observed for a brief period following the fracture reduction. An alternative to i.v. sedation and/or i.v. regional anesthesia is the hematoma block, which has been shown to be both safe and effective in selected patients.[57,58] Some have also suggested the use of self-administered 50% nitrous oxide and 50% oxygen for the provision

Table 63.9 *Recommended conscious sedation drug dosages for children*

Drug	Dosage
Chloral hydrate	50–100 mg kg^{-1} p.o. or p.r.; maximum dose 2 g
Diazemuls	0.1 mg kg^{-1} i.v.
Diazepam	0.2 mg kg^{-1} p.o.
Midazolam	0.05 mg kg^{-1} i.v.; dose may be repeated once p.r.n.; maximum dose 0.15 mg kg^{-1} i.v.
Midazolam	0.5–0.75 mg kg^{-1} p.o. for children < 20 kg; 0.3–0.5 mg kg^{-1} p.o. for children > 20 kg
Morphine	0.05–0.1 mg kg^{-1} i.v.; this dose may be repeated once after 15 min
Morphine	0.3 mg kg^{-1} p.o.
Flumazenil	10 μg kg^{-1} i.v. over 15 s; wait 1–3 min; if necessary, dose may be repeated up to four times at 1- to 3-min intervals to a total dose of 50 μg kg^{-1}. If resedation occurs, doses may be repeated every 20 min, or the effective dose may be given hourly as infusion
Narcan	The administration of narcan (0.01–0.10 mg kg^{-1} i.v.) should be reserved for emergency use, i.e. severe obtundation and respiratory depression; following the administration of narcan, patients must be cared for in a constant care setting and discharged only when they are fully awake and a minimum time of 3 h has elapsed
Pentobarbital	4.0–5.0 mg kg^{-1} i.v. to a maximum of 100 mg; 6.0 mg kg^{-1} i.m. for children < 15 kg; 5.0 mg kg^{-1} i.m. for children ≥ 15 kg

Physicians utilizing these drugs alone or in combination should be familiar with these agents and aware of their potential respiratory complications.
p.o., per os; p.r., per rectum; i.v., intravenous; p.r.n., *pro re nata*; i.m., intramuscularly.

of pain relief during manipulation of closed forearm fractures. Pain relief is useful, and the incidence of complications is low with easy administration.[59] The provision of monitoring and moment-to-moment observation are essential measures when utilizing this technique.[60]

Our institution has assembled a patient strategy of utilizing midazolam/morphine and nitrous oxide/oxygen for the management of fractured forearms. To date there have been few complications and useful pain relief. The combination of oral midazolam 0.50 mg kg^{-1} and nitrous oxide/oxygen has been studied.[61] No airway complications have been encountered; however, some children have been deeply sedated or reached early levels of general anesthesia. Most of these patients are not fasted, thus caution and preparation are essential. The goal for these cases must be that of conscious sedation. Physicians, parents, and patients should be advised that these patients will not be asleep nor will they be completely pain free. Recovery is also an issue for these patients.

SUMMARY

Departments of anesthesia can provide monitored anesthetic care (deep sedation) such that the patient sleeps through the procedure and is awake and alert within minutes of its completion. Many patients have been subjected to uncomfortable and painful procedures with minimal preparation, with little sedation and lots of "OK anesthesia," i.e. "OK, OK you'll be fine" or "We will be done in just a minute." One articulate pediatric subspecialist has written[5] "I would like to see the problem [sedation of children] turned over to experts in the field. We can then concentrate on the procedure itself – I contend that this is safer for the patient."

The recommended conscious sedation drug dosages are shown in Table 63.9.

REFERENCES

1. Proctor L. The peripatetic anesthesiologist. *Curr Opin Anesthesiol* 1998; **11:** 283–4.
2. Maxwell LG, Yaster M. The myth of conscious sedation. *Arch Pediatr Adolesc Med* 1996; **150:** 665–7.
3. Anonymous. American Academy of Pediatrics Committee on Drugs: guidelines for monitoring and management of pediatric patients during and after sedation for diagnostic and therapeutic procedures. *Pediatrics* 1992; **89** (6 Pt 1): 1110–15.
4. Coté CJ. Monitoring guidelines: do they make a difference? *Am J Roentgenol* 1995; **165:** 910–12.
5. Hassall E. Should pediatric gastroenterologists be i.v. drug users? *J Pediatr Gastroenterol Nutr* 1993; **16:** 370–2.
6. CAS. CAS guidelines to the practice of anesthesia. *Can J Anaesth* 1998; **45** (10): 6–7.
7. Menon DK, Peden CJ, Hall AS, *et al.* Magnetic resonance for the anaesthetist. Part I. Physical principles, applications, safety aspects. *Anaesthesia* 1992; **47:** 240–55.
8. Tobias MSD. Magnetic resonance imaging. In: Rogers M (ed.). *Current Practice in Anesthesiology*, 2nd edn. St Louis, MO: Mosby, 1990: 169.
9. Jorgensen NH, Messick Jr JM, Gray J, *et al.* ASA monitoring standards and magnetic resonance imaging. *Anesth Analg* 1994; **79:** 1141–7.
10. Peden CJ, Menon DK, Hall AS, *et al.* Magnetic resonance for the anaesthetist. Part II. Anaesthesia and monitoring in MR units. *Anaesthesia* 1992; **47:** 508–17.
11. Wendt RED, Rokey R, Vick GWD, Johnston DL. Electrocardiographic gating and monitoring in NMR imaging. *Magn Reson Imaging* 1988; **6:** 89–95.
12. Dimick P, Helvig E, Heimbach D, *et al.* Anesthesia-assisted procedures in a burn intensive care unit procedure room: benefits and complications. *J Burn Care Rehabil* 1993; **14:** 446–9.
13. Roth JL, Nugent M, Gray JE, *et al.* Patient monitoring during magnetic resonance imaging. *Anesthesiology* 1985; **62:** 80–3.
14. Hollman GEM. Results of a pediatric sedation program on head MRI scan success rates and procedure duration times. *Clin Pediatr* 1995; **June:** 300–5.
15. Menon DGA. Anaesthesia and sedation for diagnostic procedures. *Curr Opin Anesthesiol* 1994; **7:** 495–9.
16. Greenberg SB, Faerber EN. Respiratory insufficiency following chloral hydrate sedation in two children with Leigh disease (subacute necrotizing encephalomyelopathy). *Pediatr Radiol* 1990; **20:** 287–8.
17. Greenberg SB, Faerber EN, Aspinall CL, Adams RC. High-dose chloral hydrate sedation for children undergoing MR imaging: safety and efficacy in relation to age. *Am J Roentgenol* 1993; **161:** 639–41.
18. MacIntyre PA, Sury MR. Is propofol infusion better than inhalational anaesthesia for paediatric MRI? *Anaesthesia* 1996; **51:** 517.
19. Jackson E, Tan S, Yarwood G, Sury MR. Increasing the length of the expiratory limb of the Ayre's T-piece: implications for remote mechanical ventilation in infants and young children. *Br J Anaesth* 1994; **73:** 154–6.
20. Jordan RM, Mintz RD. Fatal reaction to gadopentetate dimeglumine. *Am J Roentgenol* 1995; **164:** 743–4.
21. Kaufman RA. Technical aspects of abdominal CT in infants and children. *Am J Roentgenol* 1989; **153:** 549–54.
22. Keeter S, Benator RM, Weinberg SM, Hartenberg MA. Sedation in pediatric CT: national survey of current practice. *Radiology* 1990; **175:** 745–52.
23. Martin LD, Pasternak LR, Pudimat MA. Total intravenous anesthesia with propofol in pediatric patients outside the operating room. *Anesth Analg* 1992; **74:** 609–12.
24. Merola C, Albarracin C, Lebowitz P, *et al.* An audit of adverse events in children sedated with chloral hydrate or propofol during imaging studies. *Paediatr Anaesth* 1995; **5:** 375–8.
25. Vade A, Sukhani R, Dolenga M, Habisohn-Schuck C. Chloral hydrate sedation of children undergoing CT and MR imaging: safety as judged by American Academy of Pediatrics guidelines. *Am J Roentgenol* 1995; **165:** 905–9.
26. Pereira JK, Burrows PE, Richards HM, *et al.* Comparison of sedation regimens for pediatric outpatient CT. *Pediatr Radiol* 1993; **23:** 341–4.

27. Osborn I. Pediatric malignancies and anesthesia. *Anesthesiol Clin North Am* 1998; **16:** 667–88.
28. Waite K, Filshie J. The use of a laryngeal mask airway for CT radiotherapy planning and daily radiotherapy. *Anaesthesia* 1990; **45:** 894.
29. Porche V. Anesthetic considerations in radiologic procedures performed outside the operating room. *Cancer Bull* 1995; **47**.
30. Canter M. Therapeutic embolization of neurovascular lesions. *Anesthesiol Clin North Am* 1993; **91** (11): 157–95.
31. Parry TIP, Molyneux A. Anaesthesia for interventional radiology. *Curr Anaesth Critical Care* 1997; **8:** 275–8.
32. Dallas SH, Moxon CP. Controlled ventilation for cerebral angiography. *Br J Anaesth* 1969; **41:** 597–602.
33. Sharath MD, Metzger WJ, Richerson HB, *et al.* Protamine-induced fatal anaphylaxis. Prevalence of antiprotamine immunoglobulin E antibody. *J Thorac Cardiovasc Surg* 1985; **90:** 86–90.
34. Levy JH. Hemostatic agents and their safety. *J Cardiothorac Vasc Anesth* 1999; **13** (4 Suppl. 1): 6–11; discussion 36–7.
35. Ingebo KR, Rayhorn NJ, Hecht RM, *et al.* Sedation in children: adequacy of two-hour fasting. *J Pediatr* 1997; **131** (1 Part 1): 155–8.
36. Carlsson U, Grattidge P. Sedation for upper gastrointestinal endoscopy: a comparative study of propofol and midazolam. *Endoscopy* 1995; **27:** 240–3.
37. Mulcahy HE, Greaves RR, Ballinger A, *et al.* A double-blind randomized trial of low-dose versus high-dose topical anaesthesia in unsedated upper gastrointestinal endoscopy. *Aliment Pharmacol Ther* 1996; **10:** 975–9.
38. Balsells F, Wyllie R, Kay M, Steffen R. Use of conscious sedation for lower and upper gastrointestinal endoscopic examinations in children, adolescents, and young adults: a twelve-year review. *Gastrointest Endosc* 1997; **45:** 375–80.
39. Dillon M, Brown S, Casey W, *et al.* Colonoscopy under general anesthesia in children. *Pediatrics* 1998; **102** (2 Part 1): 381–3.
40. Campo R, Brullet E, Montserrat A, *et al.* Topical pharyngeal anesthesia improves tolerance of upper gastrointestinal endoscopy: a randomized double-blind study. *Endoscopy* 1995; **27:** 659–64.
41. Holm C, Christensen M, Rasmussen V, *et al.* Hypoxaemia and myocardial ischaemia during colonoscopy. *Scand J Gastroenterol* 1998; **33:** 769–72.
42. Poser G, Ladik S. Oxygen saturation post-gastroscopy and post-colonoscopy. *Gastroenterol Nurs* 1995; **18** (4): 128–32.
43. Perry S, Heidrich G. Management of pain during debridement: a survey of U.S. burn units. *Pain* 1982; **13:** 267–80.
44. Osgood PF, Szyfelbein SK. Management of burn pain in children. *Pediatr Clin North Am* 1989; **36:** 1001–13.
45. Lind GH, Marcus MA, Mears SL, *et al.* Oral transmucosal fentanyl citrate for analgesia and sedation in the emergency department. *Ann Emerg Med* 1991; **20:** 1117–20.
46. Reich DL, Silvay G. Ketamine: an update on the first twenty-five years of clinical experience. *Can J Anaesth* 1989; **36:** 186–97.
47. Fischer CJM, Gottschlich M. Perioperative enteral nutrition in pediatric burn patients. *Anesthesiology* 1995; **83:** A1164.
48. Davies FC, Waters M. Oral midazolam for conscious sedation of children during minor procedures. *J Accid Emerg Med* 1998; **15** (4): 244–8.
49. Connors K, Terndrup TE. Nasal versus oral midazolam for sedation of anxious children undergoing laceration repair. *Ann Emerg Med* 1994; **24:** 1074–9.
50. Hart LS, Berns SD, Houck CS, Boenning DA. The value of end-tidal CO_2 monitoring when comparing three methods of conscious sedation for children undergoing painful procedures in the emergency department. *Pediatr Emerg Care* 1997; **13** (3): 189–93.
51. Chudnofsky CR. Safety and efficacy of flumazenil in reversing conscious sedation in the emergency department. Emergency Medicine Conscious Sedation Study Group. *Acad Emerg Med* 1997; **4:** 944–50.
52. Green SM, Johnson NE. Ketamine sedation for pediatric procedures. Part 2. Review and implications. *Ann Emerg Med* 1990; **19:** 1033–46.
53. Dachs RJ, Innes GM. Intravenous ketamine sedation of pediatric patients in the emergency department. *Ann Emerg Med* 1997; **29:** 146–50.
54. Binder LS, Leake LA. Chloral hydrate for emergent pediatric procedural sedation: a new look at an old drug. *Am J Emerg Med* 1991; **9:** 530–4.
55. Swanson ER, Seaberg DC, Mathias S. The use of propofol for sedation in the emergency department. *Acad Emerg Med* 1996; **3:** 234–8.
56. Olney BW, Lugg PC, Turner PL, *et al.* Outpatient treatment of upper extremity injuries in childhood using intravenous regional anaesthesia. *J Pediatr Orthop* 1988; **8:** 576–9.
57. Furia JP, Alioto RJ, Marquardt JD. The efficacy and safety of the hematoma block for fracture reduction in closed, isolated fractures. *Orthopedics* 1997; **20:** 423–6.
58. Kendall JM, Allen PE, McCabe SE. A tide of change in the management of an old fracture? *J Accid Emerg Med* 1995; **12:** 187–8.
59. Gregory PR, Sullivan JA. Nitrous oxide compared with intravenous regional anesthesia in pediatric forearm fracture manipulation. *J Pediatr Orthop* 1996; **16:** 187–91.
60. Selbst SM, Henretig FM. The treatment of pain in the emergency department. *Pediatr Clin North Am* 1989; **36:** 965–78.
61. Litman RS, Berkowitz RJ, Ward DS. Levels of consciousness and ventilatory parameters in young children during sedation with oral midazolam and nitrous oxide. *Arch Pediatr Adolesc Med* 1996; **150:** 671–5.
62. Cote CJ. Sedation for the pediatric patient. A review. *Pediatr Clin North Am* 1994; **41:** 31–58.
63. Hayes DL, Holmes Jr DR, Gray JE. Effect of 1.5 tesla nuclear magnetic resonance imaging scanner on implanted permanent pacemakers. *J Am Coll Cardiol* 1987; **10:** 782–6.
64. Kelly WM, Paglen PG, Pearson JA, *et al.* Ferromagnetism of intraocular foreign body causes unilateral blindness after MR study. *Am J Neuroradiol* 1986; **7:** 243–5.
65. Shellock FG, Morisoli S, Kanal E. MR procedures and biomedical implants, materials, and devices: 1993 update. *Radiology* 1993; **189:** 587–99.

PART IV

Perioperative and Intensive Care

Critical Care Management

Pain Management (Section Editor – Mark Lema)

64

Metabolism and the metabolic response to trauma

IAIN T CAMPBELL AND RODERICK A LITTLE

This chapter describes the normal relations between the body's supply of and demand for protein and energy and the homeostatic adjustments that take place when these relations are disturbed by trauma and/or sepsis, together with the principles of the methods used to measure these changes. Details of the provision of metabolic (nutritional) support for such an episode are given in Chapter 65.

ENERGY

Energy is defined as the ability to do work. The unit of energy is the joule (J), defined as the work done when a force of 1 newton (N) moves through a distance of 1 m. In the living organism, energy is derived from the oxidation of foodstuffs, principally carbohydrate, fat, and protein. The summary equations for these processes are given in Table 64.1. Oxygen is consumed, carbon dioxide and water are produced, and energy is released in discrete packages, via a number of intermediary steps, mostly in the form of adenosine triphosphate (ATP).[1]

Energy in the equations in Fig. 64.1 is given as units of heat – kilocalories (kcal); the kilocalorie is defined as 1000 calories, the amount of heat required to heat up 1 g of water by 1 °C. Heat is a form of energy; the relation between the (kilo-) joule and the (kilo-) calorie is given by the mechanical equivalent of heat:

1 kcal = 4.18 kJ

The kilocalorie has been the traditional unit in energy metabolism; in the early metabolic studies, heat production was technically the easiest parameter to measure. With the institution of the SI system of units 40 years ago, the kilocalorie was supposed to be replaced by the kilojoule, but there has been some user resistance and both units remained, although the kilocalorie is now used less and less.

The energy production represented in Table 64.1 applies to molar quantities of the various nutrients. Energy values provided per gram of nutrient oxidized are given in Table 64.2. The values vary slightly with the precise nature of the carbohydrate, fat, or protein being oxidized, so these figures should be considered as average values. Starch, for example, provides 4.1 kcal g^{-1} and glucose 3.75 kcal g^{-1}. Carbohydrates and fat are oxidized completely to carbon dioxide and water, and they provide the same amount of energy when oxidized (burnt) outside the body as when metabolized. Protein, on the other hand, is incompletely oxidized by the body, and energy (and nitrogen)-containing products of protein metabolism are excreted in the urine, principally as urea, but also as creatinine, uric acid, and some as ammonia, the last particularly during starvation (see below). The amount of protein oxidized over a given period can be assessed from urinary nitrogen excretion (see below).

WHOLE-BODY ENERGY AND SUBSTRATE METABOLISM

The equations in Fig. 64.1 represent the fundamental processes whereby energy is released: oxygen is consumed and energy and carbon dioxide are produced. Energy expenditure can thus be measured by measuring the energy (heat) released, although this is cumbersome, as it requires the subject to be confined in an insulated room for periods in excess of 24 h; the technique is known as direct calorimetry. It is now more usual to measure oxygen consumption ($\dot{V}O_2$) and carbon dioxide production ($\dot{V}CO_2$) and make assumptions about the energy release that consumption of a given amount of oxygen denotes; this approach is known as indirect calorimetry. The precise methodology for measuring gas

Table 64.1 *Oxidation of carbohydrate, fat, and protein*

$$1\ \text{glucose} + 6O_2 \xrightarrow[5.03\ \text{kcal L}^{-1}\ O_2]{RQ = 1.0} 6CO_2 + 6H_2O + 673\ \text{kcal (2.81 MJ)}$$

$$1\ \text{palmitate} + 23O_2 \xrightarrow[4.68\ \text{kcal L}^{-1}\ O_2]{RQ = 0.7} 16CO_2 + 16H_2O + 2398\ \text{kcal (10.0 MJ)}$$

$$1\ \text{amino acid} + 5.1O_2 \xrightarrow[418\ \text{kcal L}^{-1}\ O_2]{RQ = 0.8} 4.1CO_2 + 0.7\text{urea} + 2.8H_2O + 475\ \text{kcal (1.98 MJ)}$$

Gas volumes are at STPD.
RQ = (CO_2 produced/O_2 consumed).

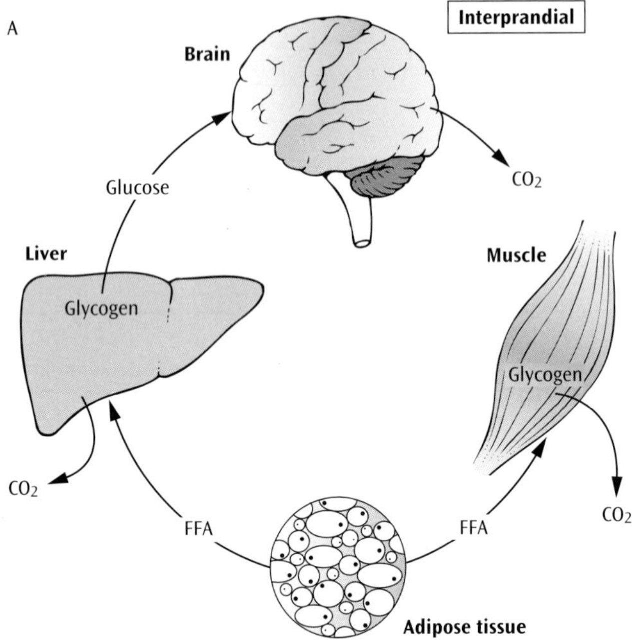

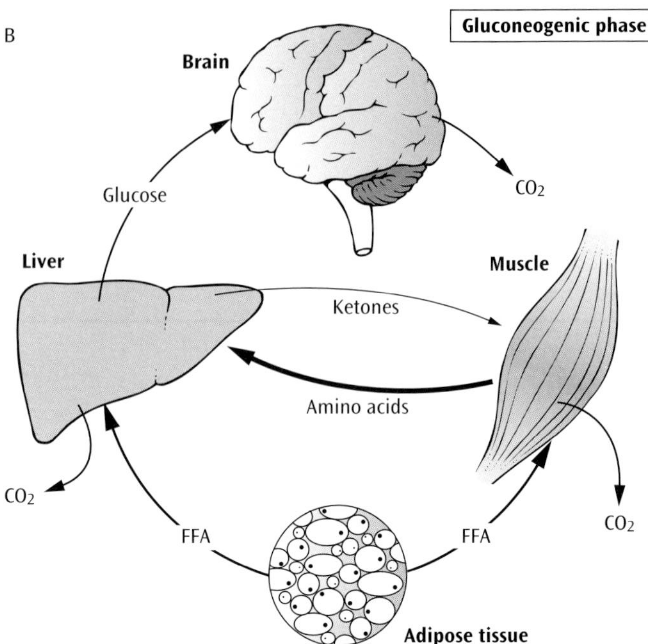

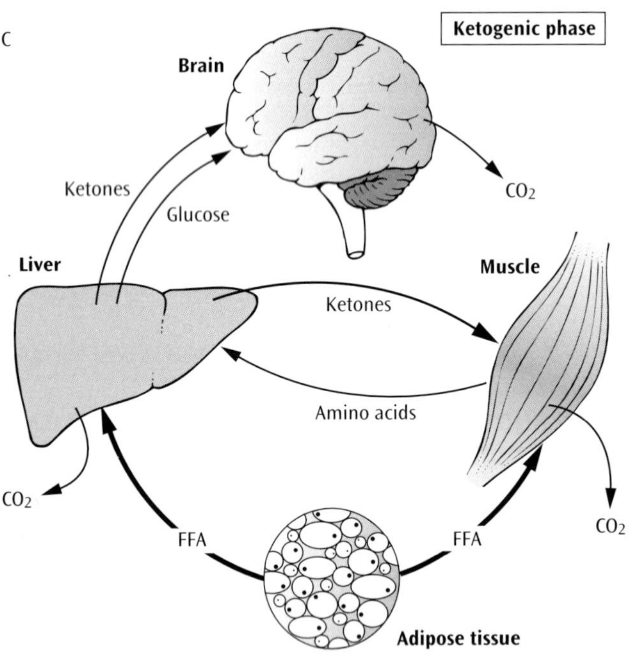

Figure 64.1 *Changes in substrate oxidation in the metabolic adaptation to starvation. (A) Interprandial glycogen stores, present in liver and muscle, maintain blood glucose (liver) and provide glucose for the brain and energy substrate for muscle. (B) Gluconeogenic phase. At 24–48 h to 7–14 days, glycogen stores are exhausted. Nervous tissue requires glucose as provided mainly by gluconeogenesis from amino acids derived from protein (muscle) breakdown. The liver starts to make ketones. (C) Ketogenic phase. Nervous tissue partially adapted to ketone oxidation. Peripheral tissues obtain energy requirements from oxidation of fatty acids (FFA).*

Table 64.2 *Energy values of the various foodstuffs*

1 g of carbohydrate	4 kcal	16.7 kJ
1 g of protein	4 kcal	16.7 kJ
1 g of fat	9 kcal	37.6 kJ

exchange is beyond the scope of the present discussion, but it involves the measurement of inspired and mixed expired gas concentrations and inspired and expired volumes. Less carbon dioxide is normally produced than oxygen is consumed (Fig. 64.1) so the expired volume is normally less than the inspired volume.

Consumption of 1 L of oxygen denotes the expenditure of 4.6–5.0 kcal (19.2–20.9 kJ) of energy, 4.6 kcal (19.2 kJ) when only fat is metabolized and 5.0 kcal (20.9 kJ) with carbohydrate metabolism. When glucose is oxidized, the ratio of carbon dioxide produced to oxygen consumed is 1 (Fig. 64.1); with fat, the figure is 0.7. This ratio is known as the respiratory quotient (RQ) and its normal range is 0.7–1. The precise value is a linear function of the percentage energy expenditure derived from fat and carbohydrate oxidation respectively.

The urinary excretion of 1 g of nitrogen reveals the oxidation of 6.25 g of protein (Fig. 64.1).[2] Energy expenditure and quantities of carbohydrate, fat and protein oxidized over a given period can thus be calculated from measurements of oxygen consumption, carbon dioxide production, and urinary nitrogen excretion made over that period. In clinical practice, urinary nitrogen is rarely measured because of technical difficulties. A value can be derived from urinary urea and an assumption can be made that 80% of the urinary nitrogen is present as urea; the true value is very variable, from 60% to 100%, but for clinical purposes this is probably acceptable. When calculating energy expenditure only, protein metabolism can be ignored.

RQ is a biochemical concept at the tissue level and cannot actually be measured. What is measured is gas exchange ($\dot{V}O_2$, $\dot{V}CO_2$) at the mouth. This is more correctly termed the respiratory exchange ratio (RER) and is affected by factors other than substrate metabolism, particularly anything that might alter respiratory patterns. Hyperventilation will produce an apparent increase in carbon dioxide production, albeit transient. Likewise, hypoventilation resulting from administration of, for example, an opiate will produce carbon dioxide retention and an apparent transient fall in carbon dioxide production relative to oxygen consumption and a transient decrease in respiratory exchange ratio. Other factors that may affect RER in clinical practice are disturbances in acid–base metabolism, in which a metabolic acidosis increases and alkalosis decreases RER, and body temperature. Carbon dioxide is more soluble than oxygen; a decrease in body temperature depresses RER and a rise elevates it. Any sort of instrumentation around the face used to measure $\dot{V}O_2$ and $\dot{V}CO_2$, such as face masks, nose clips, and mouth pieces, may disturb breathing patterns, most commonly inducing hyperventilation. If any conclusions are to be drawn about substrate metabolism from measurements of gas exchange, the measurements have to be made for a minimum of 30 min.

ENERGY EXPENDITURE IN MAN

Energy is expended in fulfilling basal requirements (maintenance of cell membrane potentials, work of breathing, beating of the heart, etc.), muscle contraction (activity, shivering) and the energy associated with the digestion and assimilation of food, known as dietary-induced thermogenesis. In adult man any increase in expenditure due to cold exposure in defense of body temperature is due to increases in muscle tone and ultimately shivering. The thermoneutral ambient temperature for naked man starts at about 27–28 °C. Below this temperature, heat production increases by the mechanisms just discussed, i.e. shivering or an increase in muscle tone. In practice, the thermoneutral temperature is modified also by clothing and/or bed coverings. The mechanisms of heat production in adult man are in contrast with those of the neonate and the hibernating rodent (see below). Body temperature affects metabolism and in the healthy individual metabolic rate rises by 13% for every 1 °C increase in body temperature.

The largest single component of 24-h energy expenditure is "basal" expenditure and, in a bedbound inactive individual, may account for 95–100% of it. In a heavy laborer or professional athlete, it may account for only 50%. "Basal" energy expenditure classically is measured in the absence of any stimuli that raise expenditure, i.e. with the subject at rest, after an overnight fast, and in a thermoneutral environment. Basal metabolic rate can also be calculated from any one of a number of standard formulae. They vary slightly, but all of these include measures of body size (height and weight), age (metabolic rate decreases with age), and gender. For a given body size, women have a lower metabolic rate than men because of their greater amount of fat, which is less metabolically active than lean tissue and is also a better insulator.

Nonshivering thermogenesis

In the hibernating rodent, and in the newborn human, energy expenditure can be increased by sympathetic activation of brown adipose tissue – so-called nonshivering thermogenesis. The mechanism is associated with changes in mitochondrial function and ATP synthesis. Increased conductance of protons occurs through the inner mitochondrial membrane and, instead of the energy associated with this movement going to form ATP, energy is released as heat – oxidative phosphorylation is described as uncoupled. The adipose tissue is brown because of the high concentration of (uncoupled) mitochondria and, in the rat, is found in a large depot between the scapulae. In the human, it is found above the kidneys, around the great vessels at the base of the heart and around the vertebral vessels. Nonshivering thermogenesis is a method of thermoregulation in rodents and the very young but does not occur in man beyond the age of 6 months.

BODY COMPOSITION

Energy intake in the form of food (ingested or infused intravenously) in excess of requirements results in an increase in body mass. In the healthy individual this is manifest principally as an increase in body fat or adipose tissue. If energy intake is less than expenditure, because either expenditure is increased and/or intake is decreased, body mass is lost. The relative changes in adipose and lean tissue depend on the circumstances in which disturbances in intake and expenditure have occurred, and are due to factors as yet poorly defined. In health, these include voluntary dieting, perhaps accompanied by varying degrees of exercise. In sepsis, trauma, and many forms of malignant disease, appetite is depressed and a diminution in voluntary intake occurs as well as a decrease in voluntary activity, and often the presence of an acute-phase response leads to a breakdown of lean tissue and an increase in gluconeogenesis (see later).

The human body is made up principally of fat, protein, and minerals such as the calcium salts in bone, but is commonly thought of as a two-compartment model, variously called fat mass and fat-free mass or adipose tissue and lean body mass. The two sets of terms are not synonymous. They do approximate to each other, but lean body mass contains structural fat such as in the nervous systems and cell membranes. The lean tissue element represents the body's metabolically more active tissue, and fat or adipose tissue represents an energy store. Such a model has obvious limitations; it implies a uniform and static structure with metabolic activity confined to the lean tissue element, which is obviously not true. Despite this, there is a need to differentiate degrees of leanness and fatness between individuals as well as changes in body mass and lean tissue mass within individuals. This type of two-compartment model, in the absence of a more satisfactory and practical alternative, is the one most widely used.

Little more than 50 human bodies have been analyzed and the details published. These include those dissected in the nineteenth century.[3,4] Muscle contributes on average about 50% of the lean body mass and bone about 21%. The skin constitutes about 8% and the remainder – internal organs, etc. – about 21%.

MEASUREMENT OF BODY COMPOSITION

All techniques for measuring body composition *in vivo* are of necessity indirect and make assumptions about the distribution of certain elements within the body, or the density of the two compartments referred to above. Most assume a normal state of hydration. Body weight is the usual index of body mass but takes no account of the relative proportions of fat and lean tissue. Body weight normally varies by 0.5 kg from day to day, but changes of up to 1 kg due to variation in body water are regarded as normal.[5] In disease states, these figures are larger; patients retain up to about 3 L of fluid after major surgery. Patients in intensive care in multiple organ failure often retain about 10 L. Figures of up to 35 L have been described.

An index of body mass which takes height into account is the body mass index (BMI). This is given by:

$$\text{BMI} = \text{wt (kg)}/[\text{height (m)}]^2$$

The normal range is 18–25. Above 25, the individual is said to be "overweight," and over 30 to be obese; at figures of 10–12, survival is starting to be threatened.

Densitometry and skinfold thickness

Percentage body fat can be calculated from body density. The relation is described by the equation

$$\text{Percent fat} = (a/\text{body density} - b) \times 100$$

This relation was originally derived empirically but can be derived from first principles. The constants a and b depend on the density of lean tissue and fat, which in turn depends on the temperature at which the measurements are made. At 37 °C the density of fat-free mass is normally assumed to be 1.1 kg L^{-1} and fat to be 0.9 kg L^{-1}. With these assumptions, the values of a and b are 4.95 and 4.5 respectively.

Prediction equations have been derived empirically relating skinfold thickness measurements to body density. Body density is derived from underwater weighing allowing for, or measuring, residual gas in the lungs and gastrointestinal tract. The equations most widely used are those of Durnin and Womersley.[6] The skinfold sites most commonly measured are: (1) over the biceps, (2) the triceps muscles, (3) just below the inferior angle of the scapula, and (4) just above the iliac crest in the midline.

In routine clinical practice, mid-upper arm circumference is a useful index of lean body mass, and triceps skinfold alone of body fat. From these two measurements, two other indices of lean body mass – arm muscle area and arm muscle circumference – can be derived.[7]

Other measures of body composition

Lean body mass can also be derived from total body water using isotope dilution with tritiated or deuterated water and the assumptions are made that (1) all of the total body water is contained in the lean body mass and (2) total body water constitutes 73% of lean body mass.[8] A noninvasive variation of body water measurement is total body impedance or resistance, which consists of measuring the resistance to an alternating current (impedance) run between electrodes placed on the hands and the feet. A number of relatively inexpensive microprocessor-run instruments are now available which will produce an estimate of body fat from impedance. Although impedance is a fairly precise measurement, the figure produced for body fat does rather depend on the make of the instrument. The algorithms used are commercially sensitive.

Total body potassium is an indicator of lean tissue mass, although like body water it is subject to changes with illness. It can be measured in a total body counter; naturally occurring ^{40}K emits gamma rays that can be detected. The most accurate and reliable method of measuring total body protein is by measuring total body nitrogen using neutron activation analysis and assuming that 1 g of nitrogen represents 6.25 g of protein. The technique consists of making the body radioactive by firing neutrons at it and measuring the gamma radiation emitted, which is specific for the various elements in the body. Although probably the most reliable, particularly in the acutely ill individual, it is not generally available, is cumbersome, and involves quite large doses of radiation. It has, however, given some of the best data on changes in body composition in critical illness.

Dual-energy X-ray absorptiometry (DXA), normally used for assessing bone density, can also be used to assess body composition (i.e. fat and lean tissue masses). It is extremely precise (reproducible) and the radiation dose is very low, but again the answers one gets depend on the machine. Again the algorithms used are commercially sensitive.

STARVATION

Trauma and sepsis are often accompanied by varying degrees of undernutrition. Starvation is defined as a lack of exogenous energy substrate and may be relative or absolute. Following injury, appetite is depressed and spontaneous intake is often inadequate to meet protein and energy requirements. The normal metabolic responses to starvation or semistarvation are modified by trauma and sepsis in ways that will be described but, in order to understand these modifications, a knowledge of the response to simple starvation is desirable.[9]

Energy and protein requirements are normally derived from the dietary intake; 10–20% of energy comes from oxidation of protein, with fat and carbohydrate providing the remaining 80–90% in roughly equal proportions. Food consumed in excess of immediate requirements is stored – carbohydrate as glycogen in the liver and muscle, fat as adipose tissue. Amino acids consumed in excess of requirements for protein synthesis are deaminated and the amino group metabolized, principally to urea. The carbohydrate residues from amino acid deamination are used as energy, or go to form new glucose via hepatic or renal gluconeogenesis, or are synthesized into fat.

Most tissues derive their energy requirements from a mixture of carbohydrate, fat, and proteins as discussed above, but some, such as nervous tissue, red cells, and hemopoietic tissue, as well as wound tissue, are obligatory consumers of glucose. During starvation, adaptive processes are all directed toward the conservation of energy and protein. Glycogen stores are small and are exhausted in 24–48 h (Fig. 64.1B). Only liver glycogen contributes to the maintenance of blood glucose, the glycogen in muscle being used only by the muscle itself. However, glycolysis in some circumstances, such as severe exercise or "shock," results in the formation of lactate, which diffuses into the bloodstream and may be converted to glucose by the liver.

When glycogen stores are exhausted, glucose requirements are met by the synthesis of glucose from amino acids, glycerol, and lactate – the process of gluconeogenesis (Fig. 64.1B), and urinary nitrogen excretion increases accordingly. Most of the body's tissues, particularly muscle, including cardiac muscle, derive their energy from fat oxidation, and as the glycogen stores run out there is an increase in lipolysis, fatty acids, and glycerol being released from adipose tissue stores. The initial stimulus to this is a decline in insulin and a reciprocal rise in glucagon that occurs when blood glucose falls. The liver starts to synthesize ketones – acetoacetate and β-hydroxybutyrate – from fatty acids, and these ketones are metabolized by peripheral tissues and the central nervous system, which, in the fully adapted state, derives about 50% of its energy requirements from ketones (Fig. 64.1C). Initially, however, the nervous system can only obtain its energy requirements from glucose oxidation; as the glycogen stores run out glucose is obtained via gluconeogenesis mainly from amino acids. Body protein (principally muscle) is broken down, urinary nitrogen increases, and lean tissue is lost, resulting in an inevitable loss in function. As keto-adaptation takes place, the amount of protein broken down and contributing to gluconeogenesis diminishes. Urinary nitrogen excretion, which rises slightly during the first week of starvation from 8–10 g day^{-1} to 10–12 g day^{-1}, now diminishes to 2–5 g day^{-1}. Protein breakdown diminishes with the increasing use of ketones, from around 75 g day^{-1} during the first few days to 20 g day^{-1} by week 3. Total glucose consumption by the brain decreases from 140 to 40 g day^{-1}. As starvation progresses, the proportion of the nitrogen excreted as urea diminishes and that excreted as ammonia rises. Glutamine is involved in the ammonia synthesis, and this enhances the ability of the kidney to cope with the excretion of the various fixed acids that accompany tissue breakdown. These changes in substrate metabolism are summarized in Fig. 64.1A–C.

Fat and protein stores in an individual of normal build last about 60–70 days, although there are cases on record of very obese individuals

Table 64.3 *Phases of the metabolic response to trauma*

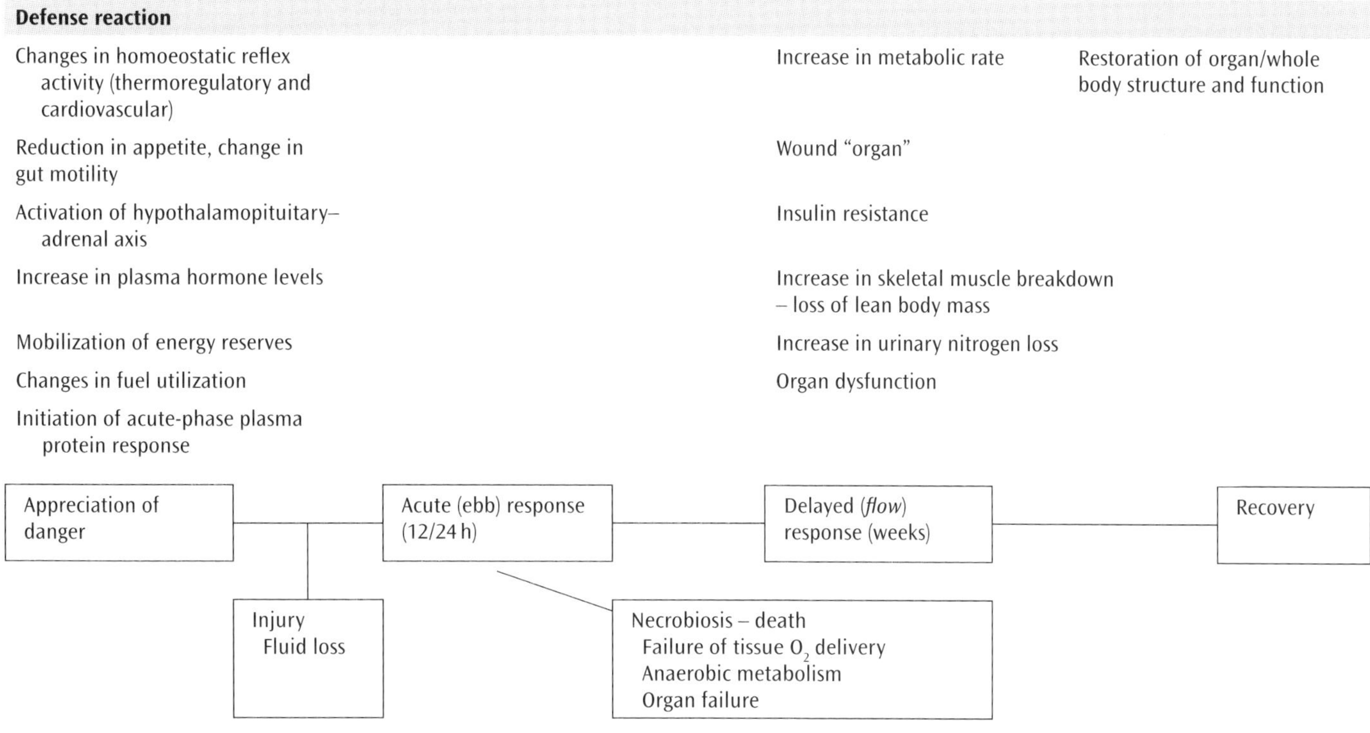

Defense reaction		
Changes in homoeostatic reflex activity (thermoregulatory and cardiovascular)	Increase in metabolic rate	Restoration of organ/whole body structure and function
Reduction in appetite, change in gut motility	Wound "organ"	
Activation of hypothalamopituitary–adrenal axis	Insulin resistance	
Increase in plasma hormone levels	Increase in skeletal muscle breakdown – loss of lean body mass	
Mobilization of energy reserves	Increase in urinary nitrogen loss	
Changes in fuel utilization	Organ dysfunction	
Initiation of acute-phase plasma protein response		

surviving without food for over a year. Fat in the form of adipose tissue represents the energy store. Protein, however, as well as being a "store" of gluconeogenic precursors, constitutes the structure and function of the body, so any diminution in protein mass represents a diminution in function.

Energy is conserved by a decrease in energy expenditure brought about by a decrease in resting metabolism and by a decrease in spontaneous activity. Over time, there is an absolute decrease in resting metabolic rate of about 40%, but also a loss of body weight; when the decrease in energy expenditure is corrected for the loss in weight the decrement in energy expenditure is nearer 20%. The fall in resting metabolism is due to a decrease in mass of some of the metabolically more active tissues in the body such as the liver and the gastrointestinal tract, particularly the gastrointestinal mucosa, which tends to become atrophic; this can cause problems when a normal intake is resumed. There is a loss of skeletal and heart muscle mass and a decrease in heart rate. With starvation, sympathetic nervous activity diminishes and circulating levels of epinephrine (adrenaline) and norepinephrine (noradrenaline) decrease.

The hormonal responses to fasting are well characterized. Low insulin levels caused by the decrease in blood glucose result in an increase in glucagon, which provokes hepatic glycogenolysis, the initiation of gluconeogenesis, and the breakdown of body protein. Glucagon increases over the first 24–48 h then decreases and by day 10 has reverted to prefasting values. Growth hormone, in the absence of energy intake, is a catabolic and lipolytic hormone and is seen to rise in the first 24–48 h, then decreases over the ensuing 10–20 days. Catecholamines and sympathetic activity diminish. Triiodothyronine levels decrease, and this probably contributes in part to the fall in energy expenditure.

METABOLIC RESPONSES TO TRAUMA AND SEPSIS[10]

Classically the metabolic response to injury has been classified into two phases, the "ebb" phase and the "flow" phase (Table 64.3). In the former, a period immediately following injury, metabolic activity is reduced, body temperature may be depressed, and spontaneous activity is diminished. There is an increase in substrate availability but a decreased ability to utilize it, and insulin secretion is inhibited. The "flow" phase is a period of increased metabolic activity, of regeneration and repair and an increase in body temperature. Appetite is depressed and the body derives its energy requirements, at least in part, from endogenous stores of fat and protein, but there is an ongoing need for glucose by tissues such as the central nervous system and wound tissue. The process of gluconeogenesis meets this ongoing requirement. The liver, and to an extent the kidney, synthesize glucose out of a number of gluconeogenic precursors, such as lactate and glycerol, but most significant are the amino acids released from the peripheral breakdown of lean tissue. Body protein is broken down and there is an increase in excretion of the nitrogen-containing products of protein metabolism, principally urea. Any use of endogenous protein as a metabolic fuel results in a loss of structure and a diminution in function. As the organism recovers it enters the "anabolic" phase, food intake increases, lean tissue is laid down, and activity and function return toward normal, initially with a reduced body mass.

Study of the response to trauma has the advantage that there is a clearly defined starting point and the factors responsible for its initiation can be investigated. Metabolic responses to sepsis are broadly similar to those seen in trauma, but it is often difficult to decide exactly when a patient becomes septic. If the traumatic or septic insult is overwhelming or blood loss is massive, and treatment not instituted, or homeostatic mechanisms are unable to cope because of, for example, a preceding period of illness or malnutrition, organ systems fail and the organism dies by a process that has been called necrobiosis.[11]

The ebb phase

A common misconception is that the "ebb" phase immediately after injury represents the period before resuscitation and thus implies that the metabolic responses at this time are secondary to circulatory hypovolemia and a failure of oxygen delivery. This is not so; a failure of oxygen transport is the hallmark of necrobiosis, whereas the ebb phase is a complex neuroendocrine response[12,13] characterized by a mobilization of energy reserves and changes in the central control of a number of homeostatic reflexes. The ebb phase can be transient or persist for 24 h or more. It includes the pattern of physiologic and metabolic changes associated with the preparation for "fight-or-flight" (the defense or alerting reaction) on which are superimposed the responses to fluid loss from the circulation and/or tissue damage and pain associated with injury.

Thermoregulation

In the experimental animal, major changes in thermoregulation occur after injury. Rosenthal and his colleagues[14] did the first systematic studies in the 1940s. They noted that following hemorrhage mice (treated with saline) were unable to maintain body temperature when transferred from an ambient temperature of 26–29 °C to 18 °C. The fall in body temperature could be prevented or reversed by either the administration of 100% oxygen or the intravenous injection of whole blood.[14] The conclusion was that the effect of hemorrhage on body temperature was secondary to changes in oxygen delivery. However, a very different picture was seen following tissue injury when the fall in body temperature (and oxygen consumption) on transfer to the lower ambient temperature could not be corrected by increasing tissue oxygen delivery.[15] These studies suggested that tissue injury, in some way which could not be related to a change in oxygen delivery, impaired heat production on cold exposure.

A more complete description of these changes in body temperature and heat production during the ebb phase showed, in the rat, an inhibition of thermoregulatory heat production resulting from an activation of noradrenergic neurons in the hindbrain, from which axons descend in the ventral noradrenergic bundle to liberate norepinephrine in the region of the dorsomedial nucleus of the hypothalamus. The changes can be initiated by nociceptive stimuli triggered by the application of tourniquets to the hindlimb and they are exacerbated by fluid loss from the circulation. However, thermoregulatory heat production can be stimulated in such injured animals if the ambient temperature is lowered sufficiently.[15]

The inhibition of thermoregulatory heat production by limb ischemia in the rat involves both skeletal muscle and brown adipose tissue. Lower temperatures have to be applied to the skin or the hypothalamus to induce shivering in skeletal muscle, and the ambient temperature at which heat transfer from interscapular brown adipose tissue commences is reduced for injured animals. The thermogenic activity of brown adipose tissue is also decreased shortly after scalding injury in the rat.[16] However, after both types of injury, brown adipose tissue thermogenesis could be activated by the injection of exogenous norepinephrine, strongly supporting the suggestion that the reduction in heat production in the "ebb" phase of the response to injury in experimental animals is due to a change in central control rather than a change in peripheral effector mechanisms. These inhibitory effects of injury affect the mechanisms of heat loss as well as of heat production.

The evidence for a similar pattern of "ebb" phase in man is not nearly so convincing. Core and whole body temperatures, the latter calculated from the core and mean skin values, are reduced acutely after accidental injury and the reduction is directly related to the severity of the injury.[17] It was also noted following accidental injury that patients did not shiver when their body temperatures fell below the normal threshold for the onset of shivering. It is difficult to be sure that the changes in man are central in origin because in the most severely injured plasma lactate concentrations are elevated and impairment of oxygen transport cannot be excluded. There is, however, some evidence for a change in thermoregulatory control at this time in that in man the normal relation between core temperature and the selection of an ambient temperature that maximizes thermal comfort is lost and all subjects select a high temperature irrespective of body temperature.[18]

There is no convincing evidence for a reduction in metabolic rate in man shortly after accidental trauma, although values as low as 55% of predicted basal have been measured after severe injuries.[19] Oxygen consumption calculated from the data provided by Cournand and his colleagues[20] suggested that heat production is maintained in critically injured patients, even before resuscitation, at higher than normal values.[21] Oxygen consumption calculated from a modification of the Fick equation showed that it was above normal in 10 and reduced in only 2 out of 16 patients vigorously resuscitated shortly after severe multiple injuries,[21] a trend that was supported by direct measurements of oxygen consumption in a group of critically ill patients in the emergency room.[22] There is also no evidence for a reduction in metabolic rate immediately following surgery (data reviewed by Barton *et al.*[23]). In fact there is often a rise in metabolic rate at this time, which cannot be simply explained as a response to intraoperative cooling.[24]

After burn injury, children rapidly develop a pyrexia and not a fall in body temperature as would be expected from both experimental work[25] and clinical studies with adults described above. The increase in body temperature and heat content is maximal within the first 12 h following injury and is due to an upward resetting of metabolic control rather than the use of occlusive dressings and a high ambient temperature.[26,27] In such children, body temperature was positively related to plasma levels of interleukin 6 (IL-6). Interleukin 1 (IL-1) was not detectable in plasma at this time but was found, together with IL-6, in high concentrations in blister fluid.[28] Thus it is possible that IL-6 produced by macrophages and endothelial cells activated by burning injury may have a role in the mediation of the acute hypermetabolic response to such injuries in children, perhaps involving the central release of prostaglandins, which, in turn, influence hypothalamic thermoregulatory control. This suggestion is supported by the reduction in core temperature elicited in burned children by acetaminophen (paracetamol), a cyclo-oxygenase inhibitor.[29] IL-6 has also been detected in the plasma of adult burned patients.[30]

In summary, there does seem to be good experimental evidence for a reduction in body temperature and heat production during the ebb-phase response to injury which is not due to failure of oxygen transport but a change in central metabolic control. However, the clinical evidence for such a response is not nearly so convincing, and what data there are suggest that metabolic rate at this time is increased, not decreased. This apparent discrepancy may be explained by differences between species in the relative importance of heat loss and heat production for thermal homeostasis. As discussed above, injury inhibits the efferent pathways for both heat loss and heat production and so, although an animal such as the rat, which depends mainly on heat production, might be expected to show an inhibition of heat production after injury, an animal such as man, in whom heat loss predominates, might be expected to show an inhibition of heat loss. Indeed, there is some evidence that heat loss is inhibited acutely following burn injury in children[31] and lower limb fractures in adult man.[18]

Hormonal changes

The hypothalamic–pituitary–adrenal axis is perhaps the most thoroughly investigated response to injury. Nociceptive stimuli increase via a complex series of neuronal interactions involving 5-HT, GABA, and the opioids and the release of corticotrophin-releasing factor (CRF) by the parvocellular nuclei of the posterior hypothalamus. CRF is secreted into the capillary plexus of the hypophyseal portal system and is then carried to the adenohypophysis, where it stimulates adrenocorticotrophic hormone (ACTH) secretion. CRF is the main stimulus for ACTH production, but vasopression released concomitantly from the neurohypophysis following activation of the magnocellular (supraoptic) nuclei of the hypothalamus[32] is also involved.[33] ACTH stimulates the secretion of cortisol from the adrenal cortex, although the relation between plasma ACTH and cortisol concentration, acutely after injury, is complex.[34] Plasma cortisol, both free and bound, concentrations are higher after injuries of moderate severity than after minor trauma, but more severe injuries are associated with lower concentrations. This cannot be attributed to low ACTH levels; after severe injury plasma ACTH concentrations are raised to around the concentration needed for maximal stimulation of the adrenal cortex and reduced perfusion of the adrenal cortex may be important.

Growth hormone, the endorphins, and prolactin, secreted by the anterior pituitary, are released acutely after injury, and once again the relations with severity are complex.[34] The plasma concentrations of thyrotrophic hormone (TSH) appear to be normal immediately after injury, and although triiodothyronine (T_3) may start to fall at this time changes in the control of thyroid hormone concentrations are a feature of the flow phase. The release of vasopression from the posterior pituitary is increased in the ebb phase and its plasma concentration is directly related to the severity of the injury.[35]

The other major component of the neuroendocrine response to injury is a consequence of the increased activity of the sympathetic nervous system. As mentioned above, many of the afferent inputs associated with the appreciation of danger, fluid loss from the circulation, and tissue damage are integrated within the hypothalamus which, in turn, modifies the activity of the preganglionic sympathetic neurons in the anteromediolateral columns of the spinal cord. Increased activity of the sympathetic nervous system leads to the release of norepinephrine from postganglionic nerve fibers and epinephrine from adrenal medullary cells, which are analogous to postganglionic neurons. Acutely after injury there are rapid increases in the plasma concentrations of norepinephrine, epinephrine, and dopamine which are directly related to the severity of the injury.[36,37] The increases are sufficient to influence the secretion of other hormones and, as will be discussed below, the mobilization of energy substrates. Plasma insulin concentrations are often low acutely after severe injuries despite a marked hyperglycemia, and this is a result of a suppression of insulin secretion by adrenaline acting on α-adrenergic receptors.[38] In contrast, the secretion of glucagon is stimulated by raised catecholamine concentrations, this time by a β-adrenergic receptor mechanism,[39] and, as expected, glucagon levels after injury are raised.[12]

An increase in central adrenergic activity may be involved in the increase in plasma prolactin levels after surgery.[40] The role that prolactin plays in the response to injury is unclear, although it may be involved in increasing glucocorticoid secretion[41] and it has also been shown to be immunostimulatory.[42]

Metabolic changes

The increased activity of the sympathetic nervous system acutely after injury leads to mobilization of energy substrates, stimulating glycogenolysis and lipolysis. The main stimulus for breakdown of glycogen in both skeletal muscle and liver is epinephrine (adrenaline), although glucagon and vasopressin may also have a role in the liver. This glycogenolysis leads to hyperglycemia either directly due to liberation of glucose or indirectly, via the Cori cycle in the liver, from lactate released from the skeletal muscle. The hyperglycemia, which is directly related to the severity of injury,[43] is potentiated after severe injuries by the reduction in glucose utilization in skeletal muscle following the inhibition of insulin secretion by raised epinephrine levels and by the development of intracellular insulin resistance. The mechanism of this early insulin resistance is still unclear although both glucocorticoids and cytokines may be involved.

The changes in carbohydrate metabolism in the "ebb" phase can be interpreted as defensive. In addition to providing fuel for fight or flight, the hyperglycemia may also play a role in the compensation of post-traumatic fluid loss, both through the mobilization of water associated with glycogen and through its osmotic effects. The decrease in glucose clearance associated with insulin resistance can also be considered protective in that it prevents the wasteful use of the mobilized glucose, which is an essential fuel for the brain and the wound, at a time when a supply of nutrients may be limited.

Plasma concentration of nonesterified fatty acids (NEFAs) and glycerol are also raised after injury, reflecting the mobilization of triacylglycerol stores in adipose tissue. The relation with severity, however, is also complex; for example, NEFA concentrations are lower after severe than after moderate injuries. This may be related to either metabolic (e.g. stimulation of re-esterification within adipose tissue by the raised lactate levels associated with severe injury) or circulatory (e.g. poorer perfusion of fat depots) factors.

Although the major changes in protein metabolism following injury are associated with the flow phase (see below), the acute-phase plasma protein response[44] is initiated during the ebb phase. A number of plasma proteins increase in concentration [e.g. C-reactive protein (CRP) and fibrinogen], although there is always a lag of approximately 6 h before changes are seen. The cytokine IL-6 released from activated macrophages etc. after injury may be responsible for inducing the hepatic synthesis of such acute-phase proteins.[45] After surgery, the rise in IL-6 precedes that of CRP and a weak but significant relation has been demonstrated between their serum levels.[46] Such a delay or lag is not seen for the proteins that show an acute-phase decrease in concentration after injury. The rapid fall for example in albumin concentration cannot be attributed to a reduction in its rate of synthesis but is due to changes in its distribution between intra- and extravascular compartments secondary to an increase in microvascular permeability.[44,47] There is also a reduction in plasma amino acid concentration after, for example, major surgery, and a marked negative correlation has been found between the plasma concentrations of IL-6 and glutamine.[48]

The flow phase (Fig. 64.2)

Increases in metabolic rate and core temperature are characteristic features of the "flow" phase. The increase in metabolic rate is said to be directly related to the severity of injury.[49] The largest increases have been reported after major burns (>40% total body surface area) treated by exposure,[50] although the introduction of early excision and grafting of such wounds has reduced the hypermetabolism. The increases in oxygen consumption in the critically ill are associated with improved survival.[51] Any increase in metabolic rate has to be met by an increase in tissue oxygen delivery secondary to an increase in minute ventilation, cardiac output, and tissue blood flow. If a patient is unable to achieve these increases unaided then assistance with, for example, mechanical ventilation and the administration of inotropes is indicated. An increase in the extraction of the delivered oxygen by the tissue is also important, although it has been calculated that if the oxygen saturation of mixed venous blood falls below 30% then reoxygenation in the lungs may not be completed and this leads to a progressive arterial hypoxemia.[52] This problem would be exacerbated if pulmonary gas exchange were impaired – a common problem in the critically ill.

When metabolic rates are measured in patients who would be expected to show a marked flow-phase response (e.g. 1 week after a major head injury or with sepsis complicating intra-abdominal surgery), they are often close to predicted basal levels. This apparent discrepancy is related to problems with energy expenditure prediction in patients who would have been bedridden for a period and/or have lost weight (especially lean body mass) because of their catabolic state and inadequate nutritional support. Thus, a hypermetabolic state is superimposed on conditions that tend to lower energy expenditure.

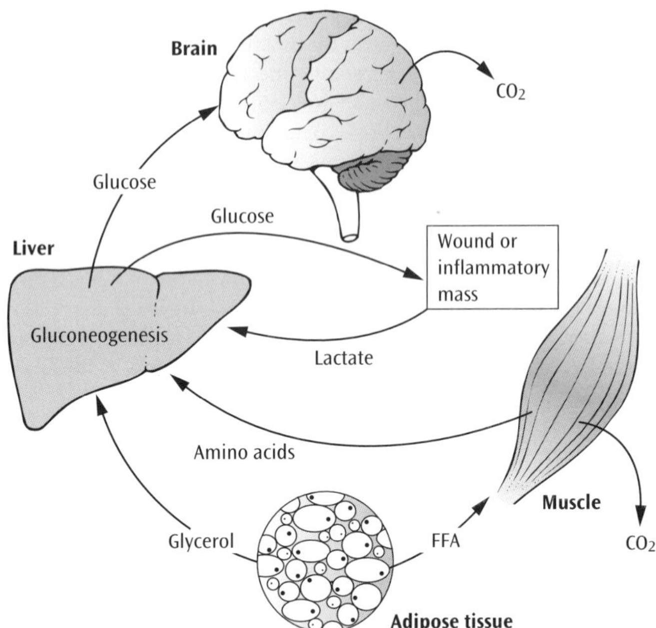

Figure 64.2 *Metabolism in severe trauma and serious sepsis. Peripheral tissues obtain energy requirements from FFA oxidation. The wound and inflammatory tissue obtains energy via glycolysis, with the resulting lactate being recirculated to the liver for gluconeogenesis. Glucose needed by the brain is synthesized from lactate, amino acid is released by protein, and glycerol is released by adipose tissue.*

The pathogenesis of the hypermetabolism is unclear although a number of factors have been proposed, and it is quite possible that they may all contribute, although their relative roles may depend on the underlying clinical condition. An upward central resetting of metabolic control is strongly suggested by the studies of Wilmore and colleagues.[53] They have found that an increase in energy expenditure occurred in burned patients even at ambient temperatures within the thermoneutral range. This was not secondary to an increased afferent cold input stimulating metabolism; in fact, the burned patient at this time is warm both peripherally and centrally. It seems most likely that the burn wound triggers a cytokine/prostanoid "cascade" that elicits an increase in sympathetic nervous system activity. Plasma catecholamine concentrations are raised during the "flow" phase following burns, and combined α- and β-adrenergic blockade reduces the hypermetabolic response to such injuries.[53] It should be noted, however, that although plasma catecholamine levels are raised during the hypermetabolic phase of the response to burning injury, and also to a lesser extent following severe head injuries, they are close to normal at a similar time after major nonhead injuries.[10]

It has been suggested that one mechanism by which catecholamines may stimulate energy expenditure is by an increase in substrate cycling. This is a process in which, although there is no change in the amount of either substrate or its metabolic products, ATP is used and energy expenditure has to be increased for its resynthesis. Two such cycles, glycolysis–gluconeogenesis and triglyceride–fatty acid, have been shown to be increased during the period 9–48 days following severe 60–95% burns. The increase in the triglyceride–fatty acid cycle is due to β-adrenergic stimulation.[54] The contribution that such "cycling" makes to total energy expenditure is difficult to assess, but an estimate has been made of at least 15%.[54]

An increase in sympathetic activity will also stimulate brown adipose tissue thermogenesis in the small mammal and its activity is increased concomitantly with an increase in whole-body oxygen consumption following a scald injury in the rat. Its role in energy balance in adult man is controversial. There is little evidence for its importance under normal conditions. However, it has been reported to become important in a number of situations in which circulating catecholamines are increased for some time,[55] for example during chronic cold exposure or after the development of a pheochromocytoma, but the situation after severe injury or sepsis is unknown.

As alluded to previously, the severely injured are frequently not fed for a number of days following their accident. This may, perhaps surprisingly, contribute to the increase in heat production during the flow phase as a period of starvation enhances the thermogenic response to glucose.[56]

A feature of the flow phase is increased catabolism of lean tissue, and there has been considerable debate about the contribution this makes to the increase in heat production.[57] Early predictions that the hypermetabolism could be fully explained by the thermic effect of protein metabolism[58] have not been substantiated. It now seems that the contribution of protein oxidation to total heat (energy) production is no more than 20–30%, even in patients with multiple injuries or in those receiving burns of up to 60% of body surface area.[59] The situation may be different after head injuries, when values of up to 34% have been calculated,[60–62] although some of these data have to be interpreted with caution as a number of the patients were treated with dexamethasone, which augments the catabolic response to head injury.[63]

The evaporation of water from the surface of a burned wound or an area of granulation tissue will increase energy expenditure. For example, the energy cost of the latent heat of evaporation of a transcutaneous water loss of 3 L day^{-1}, which is not unusual after severe burns,[64] will increase energy expenditure by over 1500 kcal day^{-1}. The impact of this evaporative water loss on energy balance can be reduced by the application of impermeable dressings or by raising ambient temperature to reduce dry heat losses. However, although such maneuvers may ameliorate the hypermetabolism associated with a burn injury, they do not abolish it. Indeed, Wilmore has agreed that the evaporative water loss is not the cause of the hypermetabolism, but instead acts as a convenient route for the dissipation of the excess calories generated by an upward setting of metabolic control.[49] It has also been suggested that the increased oxygen consumption associated with enhanced reactive oxygen generated by macrophages contributes to the hypermetabolism.[65]

The hypermetabolism does not seem to affect the body uniformly; thus, as discussed below, following a burn the wound itself may be the main site of an increased metabolic rate.[66] As part of the systemic inflammatory response associated with major trauma, however, it has been demonstrated that the splanchnic region appears to be the main site of the hypermetabolic response.[67]

The wound may be the most important influence on heat production in the "flow" phase, and it has been suggested that the wound (e.g. burn, fracture site, abscess, etc.) should be considered as an extra organ "grafted" onto the body by injury/infection.[66] It is a heterogeneous tissue consisting of polymorphonuclear leukocytes, monocytes, fibroblasts, and endothelial and epithelial cells, all of which are metabolically very active. The wound has a large blood supply, which is not under neural control, and indeed much of the increase in cardiac output during the "flow" phase may be directed to the wound.[66] One feature of the wound very relevant to a discussion of metabolic rate is the ability of monocytes and endothelial cells to produce cytokines.[68]

The burn wound involving a limb has been studied extensively and shown to be a consumer of large amounts of glucose and to a lesser extent of oxygen.[69] The glucose is converted to lactate in the presence of oxygen (i.e. aerobic glycolysis) but, as less ATP is generated by glycolysis than by oxidative phosphorylation in order to meet the energy demands of the wound, a large amount of glucose has to be taken up and converted to lactate. The lactate produced is carried to the liver, where it is reconverted to glucose. This is an energy-consuming process, which is reflected in an increase in hepatic oxygen consumption.[70] Thus, the wound becomes a user of glucose at a time when other tissues, such as skeletal muscle, reduce their uptake of glucose secondary to insulin resistance[71] (Fig. 64.2). Thus, it can be seen that the wound may increase whole-body heat production in two ways. First, there is the increase in the peripheral glucose–lactate cycle and, second, the wound acts as a focus for triggering the cytokine–prostanoid "cascade," which, as discussed above, may lead to a central upward resetting of metabolic control.

Metabolic changes

Whole-body protein turnover is increased after injury, with the balance between synthesis and breakdown being modified by the severity of injury and the influence of nutritional intake on synthesis.[72] Thus, increasing severities of injury cause increasing rates of both synthesis and breakdown, whereas undernutrition reduces synthesis. However, after the most severe injuries the increase in breakdown predominates and cannot be counteracted by even the most aggressive nutritional support.[73]

The most obvious site for the net increase in protein breakdown is skeletal muscle, although it is likely that, just as in starvation, muscle in the diaphragm, the wall of the gut, and the heart is also affected. The breakdown of myofibrillar protein is reflected by an increase in urinary excretion of 3-methylhistidine, which is directly related to the amount of damaged muscle rather than to the injury severity score (ISS).[74] However, the use of 3-methylhistidine as a specific marker of skeletal muscle breakdown is complicated by its liberation from other organs such as the gut.[75] The increase in urinary creatinine after injury is, however, directly related to ISS, although much of the creatinine comes from muscle distant to the site of injury, emphasizing the general nature of the catabolic flow phase.[76]

The increase in proteolysis provides amino acids as precursors for hepatic gluconeogenesis. Although the plasma levels of a number of amino acids, such as alanine, fall at this time, their hepatic extraction is increased because of increases in hepatic blood flow.[23] The increase in hepatic gluconeogenesis at a time when plasma concentrations of glucose and insulin are increased is one of the facets of insulin resistance discussed in more detail below. One amino acid of particular interest is glutamine, the intracellular concentration of which falls from its normally high levels after injury/sepsis.[77,78] Glutamine released from muscle is an important fuel for the lymphocytes and macrophages activated by injury. Also, it has recently been implicated in the maintenance of the gut mucosa,[79] the integrity of which is compromised after injury and which may have a role in enhancing insulin-mediated glucose metabolism.[80]

Hyperglycemia and inappropriately high plasma insulin concentrations are features of the flow phase, although an exception to this pattern may be seen after very severe injuries, such as burns, when the prolonged rise in plasma catecholamine concentration maintains adrenergic suppression of insulin secretion. There is also an exaggerated pancreatic insulin response to glucose, which may be related to the increased plasma concentration of arginine, an insulin secretagogue.[81] The concomitant elevations in plasma glucose and plasma insulin concentration are the hallmarks of insulin resistance, which involve both liver and muscle. Also, hepatic glucose production is not inhibited as expected by hyperglycemia and hyperinsulinemia during the flow phase. There is an increase in glucose turnover at this time, although because of the prevailing insulin resistance the peripheral utilization of glucose is less than expected from the raised glucose and insulin concentrations (see review by Barton *et al.*[23]).

This impairment in glucose disposal has been demonstrated using glucose/insulin clamp techniques after thermal and nonthermal injuries, and also in septic surgical patients.[82–85] As expected, part of insulin resistance is found in uninjured skeletal muscle,[71] suggesting changes in both the receptor binding of insulin and in the intracellular pathways.[86] Recent work using glucose clamp methodology has produced evidence that the insulin resistance seen in septic patients with multiple organ failure is due to impairment of the ability to store glucose. The ability to use it as a metabolic fuel appears to be relatively normal.[87] This finding has since been confirmed by others in surgical patients with abdominal sepsis, but using slightly different techniques.[88]

An important role has been suggested for the counterregulatory hormones (cortisol, epinephrine, glucagon, and growth hormone) in the pathogenesis of insulin resistance. The plasma concentrations of all these hormones are elevated at some time during the response to injury.[12] Infusion of glucagon, epinephrine, and cortisol over a 3-day period mimics some of the features of the flow phase – peripheral insulin resistance and increases in metabolic rate and urinary nitrogen excretion.[89,90] These responses were enhanced if the volunteers were also injected intramuscularly with the inflammatory agent etiocholanolone, which induces IL-1 production.[91] However, the plasma concentrations of the counterregulatory hormones needed to elicit this pattern of response are closer to those found in the acute "ebb" phase rather than in the "flow" phase, when the endogenous levels of these hormone are falling to or close to normal, except after the most severe injuries. The suggestion is that other humoral factors may have a role and the cytokines are likely candidates.[92] They are able to reproduce, by central and peripheral mechanisms, many of the acute- and flow-phase responses to injury, such as changes in the plasma concentrations of stress hormones,[93] acute-phase protein synthesis,[45] central resetting of metabolic activity,[94] stimulation of pituitary–adrenal cortex axis,[95] and changes in glucose homeostasis.[96,97] A role for IL-1 acting via prostaglandin E_2 in the stimulation of muscle proteolysis has also been proposed,[98] although this has not been supported by more recent studies using recombinant IL-1.[99] Although it is perhaps an oversimplification to assume that any single cytokine is predominant, they may, by acting collectively in a coordinated way, both locally (e.g. IL-1) and systemically (e.g. IL-6 and TNF), be very important. Once glucose has been taken up during the "flow" phase, it seems that in those receiving low-dose glucose infusions or those receiving enteral carbohydrate its rate of oxidation is increased.[82,100] The "insulin resistance" commonly observed appears to be due to impairment of the ability to store glucose, as described earlier.

Leptin, a peptide secreted by adipose tissue, has also been implicated in the metabolic disturbances associated with the flow phase. It increases resting energy expenditure, mediates satiety and correlates negatively with insulin sensitivity.[101,102] However, although animal studies have shown that endotoxin increases circulating leptin concentrations,[103] the evidence that it has a role in trauma or septic patients is not convincing.[104,105]

Early in the flow phase, fatty acids are released, often in excess of their rate of oxidation, and it has been suggested that the hepatic re-esterification of the excess may contribute to fatty infiltration of the liver.[106] As the flow phase progresses, plasma NEFA concentrations fall as the sympathetic drive to lipolysis wanes, although after major injuries, such as severe burns, they may remain high.[82,107] Fatty acid oxidation is, however, greater than expected from the plasma NEFA concentration.[82,108] Turnover, which is normally directly proportional to concentration, is also disproportionately increased,[109] although there is no clear relation between NEFA turnover and oxidation. The turnover of endogenous and of infused triacyglycerol is also enhanced in the hypermetabolic state.[109–111] Injury causes similar changes in the relation between the turnover and the plasma concentration of glycerol. Thus, in patients with burns, glycerol turnover is increased in relation to its concentration and also to the turnover of NEFA, implying increased re-esterification within adipose tissue.[54]

In the fasted uninjured subject, fat oxidation is suppressed by insulin released by the intravenous administration of large amounts of glucose. However, in hypermetabolic patients this suppression is incomplete and fat oxidation continues.[23] The reason for this continuing preferential oxidation of fat is not known, but it is an important factor to be considered when planning nutritional support for the injured/septic patient.

PROVISION OF NUTRITIONAL SUPPORT IN TRAUMA, SEPSIS, AND MULTIPLE ORGAN FAILURE

It is self-evident that unless nutritional support is provided, the injured body will derive its energy and protein requirements entirely from its endogenous reserves of fat and (structural) protein. Energy requirement (expenditure) can be assessed either by measuring it or by estimating "basal" requirements from weight, age, height, and sex, using one of a number of standard formulae and adding correction factors for injury, sepsis, and burns (discussed earlier). Expenditure can be measured using indirect calorimetry. Formerly a research tool, there are now instruments available that enable this technique to be used in routine clinical practice.[112,113] A major potential problem, however, is in extrapolating from a brief period of measurement to a "true" 24-h expenditure. Most hospital patients are relatively inactive so, if several discrete measurements are made over a period, it is a reasonable assumption in this population that measured expenditure will reflect true 24-h expenditure.

Problems arise also in measuring energy expenditure in patients requiring high inspired oxygen concentrations. In measuring oxygen consumption, inspired and mixed expired gas concentrations are measured, as discussed earlier. Inspired and expired volumes (V_I and V_E) can also be measured, but it is more usual to measure only one and calculate the other from the inspired and expired nitrogen concentration (N_I and N_E respectively), i.e. the non-O_2 non-CO_2 gas concentrations. Thus, $V_E = V_I \times N_I/N_E$. This assumes a steady state and that net "nitrogen" exchange is zero. As the inspired oxygen concentration (F_IO_2) increases, it is obvious that the amount of "nitrogen" in the system decreases, and in practice with most commercial instruments the system ceases to function at an F_IO_2 of about 0.7,[114] above which it is more accurate to measure inspired and expired volumes separately.[115]

The conventional recommendations for nutritional support have in the past been to cover basal requirements, and added an factor for stress requirements, plus 25% for "anabolism and weight gain."[116] Relative requirements for protein (nitrogen) and energy can be calculated on the basis of 1 g N per 200 kcal nonprotein energy for the unstressed patient, 1 g N per 150 kcal for the uncomplicated surgical patient, and a figure of 1 g N per 100 kcal for the septic patient or the patient in multiple organ failure. These recommendations have, on the whole, been based on first principles, and very little work has been done to determine what contribution nutritional support makes to the maintenance, or gain, of lean or even fat tissue. Septic or injured patients will oxidize glucose in response to its administration – intravenously or enterally. The maximum rate of oxidation of exogenous glucose in severe burn injury has been shown to be $5\,\mathrm{mg\,kg^{-1}\,min^{-1}}$.[117] Exogenous protein (amino acids) stimulate protein turnover and oxidation. Protein given at rates much in excess of $1.5\,\mathrm{g\ day^{-1}}$ increase net protein catabolism. With the accompanying stimulation of metabolic rate, body temperature, and urea production, this must be considered undesirable.[118]

In the septic or traumatized patient, rates of gluconeogenesis are about twice those seen in normal controls.[119] Provision of energy substrate suppresses gluconeogenesis completely in the normal individual, but in the septic patient it decreases by only 50%. So, theoretically, the most one could expect in providing nutritional support for the severely stressed patient would be to decrease gluconeogenesis and the rate of lean tissue breakdown but not to stop it completely.[119] Septic patients fed around $42\,\mathrm{kcal\,kg^{-1}}$ lean body mass per day over 2 weeks with amino acids equivalent to $20\,\mathrm{g\,N\ day^{-1}}$ showed a decrease in total body protein stores of 12.5%. Body composition measurements were made by *in vivo* neutron activation analysis. Energy expenditure was not measured but body fat increased.[73] Another study[120] showed that lean tissue as denoted by mid-upper arm circumference wasted away at rates that were independent of the level of energy intake relative to expenditure.

Surprisingly, it is only recently that any effort has been made to examine systematically changes in body composition after elective major surgery. After uncomplicated major surgery, Hill[121] showed that without any artificial nutritional support 3 kg of weight was lost over 2 weeks, then regained over 3 months, with many patients going on to overshoot their pre-illness weight by 2–3 kg owing to accumulation of fat. The 3-kg weight loss was composed of 1.4 kg of fat, 0.6 kg of protein, and 1 kg of water. Many patients felt unduly fatigued postoperatively. Most had recovered by 1 month and those with severe preoperative weight loss were generally better by 3 months, although events other than pure protein loss appear to be involved.[122]

Measurements of energy expenditure in patients who have suffered trauma, elective surgery, or burns show an elevation in metabolic rate proportional to the severity of the pathologic insult. In the patient suffering multiple organ failure, this does not appear to be the case. Patients, on average, have a measured energy expenditure generally about 120–130% of predicted basal, but with a very wide spread of individual values that are not related to normal clinical scores or other markers of severity of illness.[123–125] The only way to assess energy expenditure in these patients is to measure it either using indirect calorimetry, as discussed earlier, or by calculating $\dot{V}O_2$ using cardiac output measurements and measurements of mixed venous and arterial oxygen content – the so-called reverse Fick technique. Not surprisingly, energy expenditure in many instances is related to the degree of disturbance/sedation/paralysis/spontaneous activity,[125] but no studies as yet have examined the relation between the level of sedation/muscular activity and measured 24-h energy expenditure.

Gluconeogenesis persists in the septic state and also in the patients with multiple organ failure despite apparently adequate levels of nutrient intake. The largest source of endogenous amino acids is obviously muscle, and the amino acids released in the greatest quantities from muscle are alanine and glutamine. Glutamine is a primary fuel for the gut and for the immune system and macrophages and is the most abundant intramuscular free amino acid, accounting for 60% of the free amino acid pool. The size of the pool diminishes under conditions of trauma and sepsis. Protein breakdown within the muscle releases the branched-chain amino acids. Their amino groups transfer to pyruvate to form alanine and α-ketoglutarate to form glutamine. Alanine is a major gluconeogenic precursor, and glutamine, in addition to being a metabolic fuel for the gut and the immune system, also releases ammonia in the kidney, where it has a major role in acid–base regulation and the excretion of hydrogen ions.

Over the last 10–15 years, much evidence has accumulated from animal work that a variety of stimuli – shock, sepsis, burn injury, etc. – affect the integrity of the gastrointestinal tract such that endotoxins, and bacteria leak into the portal and systemic circulations and start a generalized inflammatory reaction. The phenomenon is more severe in the presence of malnutrition. The assumption has been made that this occurs also in man, but apart from a degree of bacteremia, found to correlate with the severity of shock (hypotension), there has been no direct evidence to support this supposition. The nutrition of the gastrointestinal mucosa, however, is obtained from the lumen of the bowel, and with the realization that providing parenteral nutritional support deprived the gut of nutrition, and made worse any potential for translocation of bowel contents, there has been a move to provide artificial nutritional support enterally whenever possible. Apart from being cheaper and more "physiologic," it was thought it might damp down the severity of any accompanying inflammatory response. Again, there has been no direct evidence to support this, but a number of studies have shown a lower incidence of septic complications with early enteral feeding after surgery for abdominal trauma compared with parenteral nutritional support, but no difference in mortality.[126–128] The same has been shown also for enteral nutritional support following elective abdominal surgery[129,130] but the feeding does have to be started early. Whether or not this beneficial effect is due directly to an effect on intestinal translocation is not known.

There has also been much interest in recent years in so-called "immunologically enhanced" feeds, supplementing them with glutamine, arginine, nucleotides and *n*-3 fatty acids. Arginine and the nucleotides enhance immune function, n-3 fatty acids alter the structure of cell membranes and affect ecosanoid generation, and glutamine has the beneficial effects on the gastrointestinal mucosa and on lymphocytes referred to earlier. A number of studies have shown beneficial effects of immunomodulatory diets on critically ill patients after major trauma and major surgery in terms of reductions in septic complications, length of intensive care unit stay, and on various parameters of immune function,[131,132] although two recent studies failed to show any benefit.[133,134]

In a more heterogeneous ICU population, use of an immunologically enhanced feed has shown reductions in the number of ventilator days and length of hospital stay,[135] while the use of glutamine alone has shown similar results.[136] Supplementation of intravenous feeding with glutamine has produced a reduction in mortality in patients 6 months after ICU discharge.[137]

It is clear that as a result of the metabolic changes described above the traditional supply of apparently adequate protein and energy alone has not been enough to preserve lean body mass in critically ill patients. In fact, as yet there is little evidence that in the very severely ill it even attenuates the rate of loss. It is becoming apparent that the injured and septic individual has specialized nutritional requirements, as indicated by the results with the specialized feeds (glutamine, nucleotides, *n*-3 fatty acids, etc.) referred to above, possibly along with the need for some pharmacologic means of modifying metabolism. The subject has been reviewed recently,[138,139] and the relative merits of various substances discussed, as well as the potential for muscle stimulation, growth hormone, and the so-called anabolic steroids. Growth hormone has repeatedly been shown to have beneficial effects on nitrogen balance in elective surgical patients, particularly when given hypocaloric feeds, but not when used as an adjuvant to full parenteral nutrition. Several trials of growth hormone used to induce "anabolism" in severely ill patients on intensive care were abandoned because of excess mortality in the trial groups. Growth hormone stimulates protein synthesis, and it has been shown that, whereas elective surgical patients have depressed rates of whole-body protein synthesis, patients in mutiple organ failure in the ICU have elevated rates of both synthesis and degradation.[140] Such agents may have a role in the recovery phase of critical illness, and possibly in malnourished individuals with less severe injury, but probably not in those at the more severe end of the illness severity spectrum.

Recent work[141] has demonstrated that the aggressive use of insulin in a heterogeneous group of intensive care patients to maintain blood glucose levels between 80 and 110 mg 100 mL^{-1} (4.4–6.1 mmol L^{-1}) was associated with a dramatic increase in mortality. The authors attributed this to the avoidance of the deleterious effects of hyperglycemia on neutrophil and macrophage function and the overcoming of a relative resistance of peripheral tissues to insulin.[141] Martinez and Allison,[142] however, have pointed out that insulin has a wide range of physiologic effects, including the promotion of glycogen and protein synthesis. It also restores cell membrane function. In critical illness there is a decrease in cell membrane potential; potassium is lost from the cell and sodium enters – the so-called "sick-cell syndrome."[143] Zierler[144] pointed out nearly 40 years ago that glucose, insulin, and potassium would restore cell membrane potentials toward normal by promoting the translocation of K^+ into the cells and the extrusion of Na^+. Thus, a generalized restoration of cell membrane function could be another explanation for this improvement in outcome.

REFERENCES

1. Flatt JP. Energetics of intermediary metabolism. In: *Assessment of Energy Metabolism in Health and Disease*. Columbus, OH: Ross Laboratories, 1980: 77–87.
2. Lee HA, Hartley TF. A method of determining daily nitrogen requirements. *Postgrad Med J* 1975; **51:** 441–5.
3. Clarys JP, Martin AD. The concept of adipose tissue-free mass. In: Norgan NG (ed.). *Human Body Composition and Fat Distribution*. Wageningen: Euro Nut, 1985: 49–63.
4. Knight GS, Beddoe AH, Streat SJ, Hill GL. Body composition of two human cadavers by neutron activation and chemical analysis. *Am J Physiol* 1986; **250:** E179–85.
5. Adam JM, Best TW, Edholm OG. Weight changes in young men. *J Physiol* 1961; **156:** 38P.
6. Durnin JVGA, Womersley J. Body fat assessed from total body density and its estimation from skinfold thickness: measurements on 481 men and women aged 16 to 72 years. *Br J Nutr* 1974; **32:** 77–97.
7. Fidanza F (ed.). *Nutritional Status Assessment: A Manual for Population Studies*. London: Chapman & Hall, 1991.
8. Shizgal HM. Body composition and nutritional support. *Surg Clin North Am* 1981; **61:** 729–41.
9. Cahill GF. Starvation in man. *N Engl J Med* 1970; **282:** 668–75.
10. Frayn KN. Hormonal control of metabolism in trauma and sepsis. *Clin Endocrinol* 1986; **24:** 577–99.
11. Stoner HB. Metabolism after trauma and in sepsis. *Circ Shock* 1986; **19:** 75–87.
12. Barton RN. The neuroendocrinology of physical injury. *Baillière's Clin Endocrinol Metab* 1987; **1:** 355–74.
13. Gann DS, Amaral JF. Endocrine and metabolic responses to injury. In: Schwartz SI, Shires GT, Spence FT (eds). *Principles of Surgery*. New York: McGraw-Hill, 1988: 1–68.
14. Tabor H, Rosenthal SM. Body temperature and oxygen consumption in traumatic shock and haemorrhage in mice. *Am J Physiol* 1947; **149:** 459–64.
15. Stoner HB. Studies on the mechanism of shock: the impairment of thermoregulation by trauma. *Br J Experiment Pathol* 1969; **50:** 125–38.
16. Rothwell NJ, Little RA, Rose JG. Brown adipose tissue activity and oxygen consumption after scald injury in the rat. *Circ Shock* 1991; **33:** 33–6.
17. Little RA, Stoner HB. Body temperature after accidental injury. *Br J Surg* 1981; **68:** 221–4.
18. Little RA, Stoner HB, Randall P, Carlson G. An effect of injury on thermoregulation in man. *Q J Exp Physiol* 1986; **71:** 295–306.
19. Little RA, Stoner HB, Frayn KN. Substrate oxidation shortly after accidental injury in man. *Clin Sci* 1981; **61:** 789–91.
20. Cournand A, Riley RA, Bradley SE, *et al*. Studies of the circulation in clinical shock. *Surgery* 1943; **13:** 964–95.
21. Edwards JD, Redmond AD, Nightingale P, Wilkins G. Oxygen consumption following trauma – a reappraisal in severely injured patients requiring mechanical ventilation. *Br J Surg* 1988; **75;** 690–2.
22. Skootsky SA, Abraham E. Continuous oxygen consumption measurement during initial emergency department resuscitation of critically ill patients. *Crit Care Med* 1988; **16:** 706–9.
23. Barton RN, Frayn KN, Little RA. Trauma, burns and surgery. In: Cohen RD, Lewis N, Alberti KGMM, Denman AM (eds). *The Metabolic and Molecular Basis of Acquired Disease*, Vol. I. London: Baillière Tindall, 1990: 684–717.
24. Carli F, Aber VR. Thermogenesis after major elective surgical procedures. *Br J Surg* 1987; **74:** 1041–5.
25. Little RA. The impairment of thermoregulation by trauma during the first days of life of the rabbit. *Biol Neonate* 1974; **24:** 363–74.
26. Childs C. Fever in burned children. *Burns* 1998; **1114:** 1–6.
27. Childs C, Stoner HB, Little RA, Davenport PJ. A comparison of some thermoregulatory responses in healthy children and in children with burn injury. *Clin Sci* 1989; **77:** 425–9.
28. Childs C, Ratcliffe RJ, Holt I, *et al*. The relationship between interleukin-1, interleukin-6 and pyrexia in burned children. In: Dinarello CA, Kluger M, Powanda M, Oppenheim J (eds). *Physiological and Pathological Effects of Cytokines – Progress in Leukocyte Biology*. New York: Alan R Liss, 1990; 295–300.
29. Childs C, Little RA. Acetaminophen (paracetamol) in the management of burned children with fever. *Burns* 1988; **14:** 343–8.
30. Guo Y, Dickerson C, Chrest FJ, *et al*. Increased levels of circulating interleukin-6 in burn patients. *Clin Immunol Immunopathol* 1990: **54:** 361–71.
31. Childs C, Stoner HB, Little RA. Cutaneous heat loss shortly after burn injury in children. *Clin Sci* 1992; **83:** 117–26.

32. Gann DS, Lilly MP. The endocrine response to injury. *Prog Crit Care Med* 1984; **1:** 15–47.
33. Buckingham JC. Hypothalamic-pituitary responses to trauma. *Br Med Bull* 1985; **41:** 203–11.
34. Barton RN, Stoner HB, Watson SM. Relationships among plasma cortisol, adrenocorticotrophin and severity of injury in recently injured patients. *J Trauma* 1987; **27:** 384–92.
35. Anderson ID, Forsling ML, Little RA, Pyman JA. Acute injury is a potent stimulus for vasopressin release. *J Physiol* 1989; **416:** 28P.
36. Davies CL, Newman RJ, Molyneux SG, Grahame-Smith DG. The relationship between plasma catecholamines and severity of injury in man. *J Trauma* 1984; **24:** 99–105.
37. Frayn KN, Little RA, Maycock PF, Stoner HB. The relationships of plasma catecholamines to acute metabolic and hormonal responses to injury in man. *Circ Shock* 1985; **16:** 229.
38. Frayn KN, Maycock PF, Little RA, *et al.* Factors affecting the plasma insulin concentration shortly after accidental injury in man. *Arch Emerg Med* 1987; **4:** 91–9.
39. Porte D, Robertson RP. Control of insulin secretion by catecholamines, stress and the sympathetic nervous system. *Fed Proc* 1973; **32:** 1792–6.
40. Noel GL, Suh HK, Stone J, Frantz AG. Human prolactin release during surgery and other conditions of stress. *J Endocrinol Metab* 1972; **35:** 1–10.
41. Drago F, Amir S, Continellao G, *et al.* In: *Prolactin, Basic and Clinical Correlates*. Macleod RM, Thorner MO, Scapagnini U (eds). Italy: Libviana Press, 1985: 609–614.
42. Reichlin S. Neuroendocrine-immune reaction. *N Engl J Med* 1992; **329:** 1246–1253.
43. Stoner HB, Frayn KN, Barton RN, *et al.* The relationships between plasma substrates and hormones and the severity of injury in 277 recently injured patients. *Clin Sci* 1979; **56:** 563–73.
44. Fleck A. Nutrition, protein metabolism and fluid balance. In: Kox W, Gamble J (eds). *Baillière's Clinical Anaesthesiology – Fluid Resuscitation 2.* London: Baillière Tindall, 1989: 625–48.
45. Gauldie J, Richards C, Harnish G, *et al.* Interferon beta 2/B-cell stimulatory factor type 2 shares identity with monocyte-derived hepatocyte-stimulating factor and regulates the major acute plasma protein response in liver cells. *Proc Natl Acad Sci USA* 1987; **84:** 7251–5.
46. Cruickshank AM, Fraser WD, Burns HJG, *et al.* Response of serum interleukin-6 in patients undergoing elective surgery of varying severity. *Clin Sci* 1990; **79:** 161–5.
47. Fleck A, Colley CM, Myers MA. Liver export proteins and trauma. *Br Med Bull* 1985; **41:** 265–73.
48. Parry Billings M, Newsholme EA, Baigrie R, *et al.* Effects of major and minor surgery on plasma glutamine and cytokine concentrations. *Proc Nutr Soc* 1992; **51:** 107A.
49. Wilmore DW. *The Metabolic Management of the Critically Ill.* New York: Plenum Press, 1977.
50. Matsuda T, Clarke N, Hariyani GD, *et al.* The effect of burn wound size on resting energy expenditure. *J Trauma* 1987; **27:** 115–118.
51. Shoemaker WC. Hemodynamic and oxygen transport patterns in septic shock: physiologic mechanisms and therapeutic implications. In: Sibbald WJ, Sprung CL (eds). *Perspectives on Sepsis and Septic Shock.* Fullerton, CA: Society of Critical Care Medicine, 1986: 203–34.
52. Dantzker DR. The influence of mixed venous P02 on arterial oxygenation. In: Vincent JL (ed.). *Uptake in Intensive Care and Emergency Medicine* – update 1990. Berlin: Springer-Verlag, 1990: 131–7.
53. Wilmore DW, Long JM, Mason AD, *et al.* Catecholamines: mediator of the hypermetabolic response to thermal injury. *Ann Surg* 1974; **180:** 653–68.
54. Wolfe RR, Herndon DN, Jahoor F, *et al.* Effect of severe burn injury on substrate cycling by glucose and fatty acids. *N Engl J Med* 1987; **317:** 403–8.
55. Lean MFJ, James WPT. Brown adipose tissue in man. In: Trayhurn P, Nicholls DG, (eds). *Brown Adipose Tissue.* London: Edward Arnold, 1986; 339–65.
56. Mansell PI, Fellows IW, MacDonald IA. Enhanced thermogenic response to epinephrine after 48-h starvation in humans. *Am J Physiol* 1990; **258** (Regulatory, Integrative and Comparative Physiology 27): R87–93.
57. Little RA. Heat production after injury. *Br Med Bull* 1985; **41:** 226–31.
58. Cuthbertson DP. Alterations in metabolism following injury. Part 1. *Injury* 1980; **11:** 174–89.
59. Duke JH, Jorgensen SB, Broell JR, *et al.* Contribution of protein to caloric expenditure following injury. *Surgery* 1970; **68:** 168–74.
60. Clifton GI, Robertson CS, Grossman RG, *et al.* The metabolic response to severe head injury. *J Neurosurg* 1984: **60:** 686–96.
61. Dickerson RN, Guenter PA, Gennarelli TA, *et al.* Increased contribution of protein oxidation to energy expenditure in head-injured patients. *J Am Coll Nutr* 1990; **9:** 96–8.
62. Hadfield JM, Little RA. Substrate oxidation and the contribution of protein oxidation to energy expenditure after severe head injury. *Injury* 1992; **23:** 183–6.
63. Greenblatt SH, Long CL, Blakemore WS, *et al.* Catabolic effect of dexamethasone in patients with major head injuries. *J Parenter Enteral Nutr* 1989; **1:** 372–6.
64. Davies JWL. *Physiological Responses to Burning Injury*. London: Academic Press, 1982.
65. Vlessis AA, Goldman RK, Trunkey DD. New concepts in the pathophysiology of oxygen metabolism during sepsis. *Br J Surg* 1995; **82:** 870–876.
66. Wilmore DW. The wound as an organ. In: Little RA, Frayn KN (eds). *The Scientific Basis for the Care of the Critically Ill.* Manchester: Manchester University Press, 1986: 45–59.
67. Takala J. Regional contribution to hypermetabolism following trauma. In: Little RA and Wernerman J (eds). *Energy Metabolism in Trauma. Baillière's Clinical Endocrinology and Metabolism.* London: Baillière Tindall, 1997; 617–628.
68. Fong U, Moldawer LL, Shires GT, Lowry SF. The biologic characteristics of cytokines and their implications in surgical injury. *Surg Gynecol Obstet* 1990; **170:** 363–78.
69. Wilmore DW, Goodwin CW, Aulick LH, *et al.* Influence of the burn wound on local and systemic responses to injury. *Ann Surg* 1977; **186:** 444–58.
70. Wilmore DW, Goodwin CW, Aulick LH, *et al.* Effect of injury and infection on visceral metabolism and circulation. *Ann Surg* 1980; **192:** 491–502.
71. Henderson AA, Frayn KN, Galasko CSB, Little RA. Dose–response relationships for the effects of insulin on glucose and fat metabolism in injured patients and control subjects. *Clin Sci* 1991; **80:** 25–32.
72. Clague MB, Keir MJ, Wright PD, Johnston IDA. The effects of nutrition and trauma on whole-body protein metabolism in man. *Clin Sci* 1983; **65:** 165–75.
73. Streat SJ, Beddoe AH, Hill GL. Aggressive nutritional support does not prevent protein loss despite fat gain in septic intensive care patients. *J Trauma* 1987; **27:** 262–6.
74. Threlfall CJ, Stoner HB, Galasko CSB. Patterns in the excretion of muscle markers after trauma and orthopedic surgery. *J Trauma* 1981; **21:** 140–7.
75. Rennie MJ, Millward DJ. 3-Methylhistidine excretion and the urinary 3-methylhistidine/creatinine ratio are poor indicators of skeletal muscle protein breakdown. *Clin Sci* 1983; **65:** 217–25.
76. Threlfall CJ, Maxwell AR, Stoner HB. Post-traumatic creatinuria. *J Trauma* 1984; **24:** 516–23.
77. Vinnars E, Bergstrom J, Furst P. Influence of the postoperative state on the intracellular free amino acids in human muscle tissue. *Ann Surg* 1975; **182:** 665–71.
78. Milewski PJ, Threlfall CJ, Heath DF, *et al.* Intracellular free amino acids in undernourished patients with or without sepsis. *Clin Sci* 1982; **62:** 83–91.
79. O'Dwyer ST, Smith RJ, Hwang TL, Wilmore DW. Maintenance of small bowel mucosa with glutamine enriched parenteral nutrition. *J Parenter Enteral Nutr* 1989; **13:** 579–85.
80. Borel MJ, Williams PE, Jabbour K, *et al.* Parenteral glutamine infusion alters insulin-mediated glucose metabolism. *J Parenter Enteral Nutr* 1998; **22:** 280–285.
81. Fajans SS, Floyd JC, Knopf RF, Conn JW. Effect of amino acids and proteins on insulin secretion in man. *Recent Prog Horm Res* 1967; **23:** 617–62.
82. Frayn KN, Little RA, Stoner HB, Galasko CSB. Metabolic control in non-septic patients with musculoskeletal injuries. *Injury* 1984; **16:** 73–9.
83. Black PR, Brooks DC, Bessey PQ, *et al.* Mechanisms of insulin resistance following injury. *Ann Surg* 1982; **196:** 420–35.
84. Brookes DC, Bessey PQ, Black PR, *et al.* Post-traumatic insulin resistance in uninjured forearm tissue. *J Surg Res* 1984; **37:** 100–7.
85. White RH, Frayn KN, Galasko CSB, Little RA. Hormonal and metabolic responses to glucose infusion in sepsis studied by the hyperglycemic glucose clamp technique. *J Parenter Enteral Nutr* 1987; **11:** 345–53.
86. Kahn CR. Insulin resistance, insulin sensitivity, and insulin unresponsiveness: a necessary distinction. *Metabolism* 1978; **27** (Suppl. 2): 1893.
87. Green CJ. Campbell IT, O'Sullivan E, *et al.* Septic patients in multiple organ failure can oxidize infused glucose, but non-oxidative disposal (storage) is impaired. *Clin Sci* 1995; **89:** 601–9.
88. Saeed M, Carlson GL, Little RA, Irving MH. Selective impairment of glucose storage in human sepsis. *Br J Surg* 1999; **86:** 813–21.
89. Bessey PQ, Watters JM, Aoki TT, Wilmore DW. Combined hormonal infusion simulates the metabolic response to injury. *Ann Surg* 1984; **200:** 264–80.
90. Gelfand RA, Matthews DE, Bier DM, Sherwin RS. Role of counterregula-

tory hormones in the catabolic response to stress. *J Clin Invest* 1984; **74:** 2238–48.

91. Watters JM, Bessey PQ, Dinarello CA, *et al.* Induction of interleukin-1 in humans and its metabolic effects. *Surgery* 1985; **98:** 298–306.
92. Chang HR, Bistrian B. The role of cytokines in the catabolic consequences of infection and injury. *J Parenter Enteral Nutr* 1998; **22:** 156–166.
93. Van der Poll T, Romijn JA, Endert R, *et al.* Tumor necrosis factor mimics the metabolic response to acute infection in healthy humans. *Am J Physiol* 1991; **261:** E457–65.
94. Dinarello C. Interleukin-1. *Rev Infect Dis* 1984; **6:** 51–6.
95. Roh MS, Drazenovich KA, Barbose JJ, *et al.* Direct stimulation of the adrenal cortex by interleukin-1. *Surgery* 1987; **102:** 140–6.
96. Del Rey A, Besedovsky H. Interleukin-1 affects glucose homeostasis. *Am J Physiol* 1987: **253:** 794–8.
97. Tredget EE, Yong Ming UY, Zhong S, *et al.* Role of interleukin-1 and tumor necrosis factor on energy metabolism in rabbits. *Am J Physiol* 1988; **255:** E760–8.
98. Clowes GHA, George BC, Villee CA, Saravis CA. Muscle proteolysis induced by a circulating peptide in patients with sepsis or trauma. *N Engl J Med* 1983; **308:** 545–52.
99. Moldawer LL, Svaninger G, Gelin J, Lundholm KG. Interleukin-1 and tumor necrosis factor do not regulate protein balance in skeletal muscle. *Am J Physiol* 1987; **253:** C766–73.
100. Long CL, Spencer JL, Kinney JM, Geiger JW. Carbohydrate metabolism in man: effect of elective operations and major injury. *J Appl Physiol* 1971; **31:** 110–116.
101. Campfield IA, Smith FJ, Guisez Y, *et al.* Recombinant mouse *ob* protein P: evidence for a peripheral signal linking adiposity and neural central networks. *Science* 1995; 26.
102. Kennedy A, Getys TW, Watson P, *et al.* The metabolic significance of leptin in humans. *J Endocrinol Metab* 1997; **82:** 1293–9.
103. Grunfeld C, Zhao C, Fuller J, *et al.* Endotoxin and cytokines induce expression of leptin and *ob* gene product in hamsters. *J Clin Invest* 1996; **97:** 2152–7.
104. Jeevanandam M, Begay CK, Petersen SR. Plasma leptin levels in trauma patients: effect of adjuvant recombinant human growth hormone in intravenously fed mutiple trauma patients. *J Parenter Enteral Nutr* 1998; **22:** 340–6.
105. Carlson GL, Saeed M, Little RA, Irving MH. Serum Leptin concentrations and their relation to metabolic abnormalities in human sepsis. *Am J Physiol* 1999; **276:** E658–62.
106. Wolfe RR. Substrate metabolism in anaesthesia and critical care. In: *Topics in Anaesthesia and Critical Care. Metabolism and Artificial Nutrition in the Critically Ill.* Guarnieri G and Iscara F (eds). Berlin: Springer, 1999: 3–10.
107. Batstone GF, Alberti KGMM, Hinks L, *et al.* Metabolic studies in subjects following thermal injury. Intermediary metabolites, hormones and tissue oxygenation. *Burns* 1976; **2:** 207–25.
108. Birkhahn RH, Long CL, Fitkin DL, *et al.* A comparison of the effects of skeletal trauma and surgery on the ketosis of starvation in man. *J Trauma* 1981; **21:** 513–518.
109. Nordenstrom J, Carpentier YA, Askanazi J, *et al.* Free fatty acid mobilisation and oxidation during total parenteral nutrition in trauma and infection. *Ann Surg* 1983; **198:** 725–35.
110. Wilmore DW, Moylan JA, Helmkamp GM, Pruitt BA. Clinical evaluation of 10 per cent intravenous fat emulsion for parenteral nutrition in thermally injured patients. *Ann Surg* 1973; **178:** 503–13.
111. Wolfe RR, Shaw JHF, Durkot MJ. Effects of sepsis on VLDL kinetics: responses in basal state and during glucose infusion. *Am J Physiol* 1985; **248:** E732–40.
112. Regan CJ, Snowdon SL, Campbell IT. Laboratory evaluation and use of the Engstrom Metabolic Computer in the Clinical setting. *Crit Care Med* 1990; **18:** 871–7.
113. Takala J, Keinanen O, Vaisanen P, Kari A. Measurement of gas exchange in intensive care: laboratory and clinical validation of a new device. *Crit Care Med* 1989; **17:** 1041–7.
114. Ultman JS, Bursztein S. Analysis of error in the determination of respiratory gas exchange at varying FIO_2. *J Appl Physiol* (Respiratory, Environmental, Exercise Physiology) 1981; **50:** 210–216.
115. Svensson KL, Sonander HG, Stenqvist O. Validation of a system for measurement of metabolic gas exchange during anaesthesia with controlled ventilation in an oxygen consuming lung model. *Br J Anaesth* 1990; **64;** 311–319.
116. Blundell JE, Campbell I, Catalano P, *et al.* Report of the IDECG Working Group on the modulating effect of stressors on the upper and lower limits of lipid and carbohydrate intake. *Eur J Clin Nutr* 1999; **53** (Suppl. 1): S127–181.
117. MacBurney M, Wilmore DW. Rational decision-making in nutritional care. *Surg Clin North Am* 1981; **61:** 571–82.
118. Blundell JE, Campbell IT, Catalano P, *et al.* Report of the IDECG working group on the modulating effect of stressors on the upper and lower limits of lipid and carbohydrate intake. *Eur J Clin Nutr* 1999; **53** (Suppl. 1): S179–181.
119. Shaw JHF, Sklein S, Wolfe RR. Assessment of alanine, urea and glucose interrelationships in normal subjects and in patients with sepsis with stable isotope tracers. *Surgery* 1985; **97:** 557–62.
120. Green CJ, Campbell IT, McClelland P, *et al.* Energy and nitrogen balance and changes in midupper-arm circumference with multiple organ failure. *Nutrition* 1995; **11:** 739–46.
121. Hill GL. *Disorders of Nutrition and Metabolism in Clinical Surgery.* Edinburgh: Churchill Livingstone, 1992: 19–32.
122. Editorial. Postoperative fatigue. *Lancet* 1979; **1:** 84–5.
123. Dickerson RN, Vehe KL, Mullen JL, Feurer ID. Resting energy expenditure in patients with pancreatitis. *Crit Care Med* 1991; **19:** 484–90.
124. Weissman C, Kemper M, Hyman AI. Variation in the resting metabolic rate of mechanically ventilated critically ill patients. *Anesth Analg* 1989; **68:** 457–61.
125. Weissman C, Kemper M, Elwyn DH, *et al.* The energy expenditure of the mechanically ventilated critically ill patient. An analysis. *Chest* 1986; **89:** 254–9.
126. Kudsk KA, Croce MA, Fabian TC, *et al.* Enteral versus parenteral feeding: effects on septic morbidity after blunt and penetrating abdominal trauma. *Ann Surg* 1992; **215:** 503–511.
127. Moore FA, Moore EE, Jones TN, *et al.* TEN versus TPN following major abdominal trauma – reduced septic morbidity. *J Trauma* 1989; **29:** 916–922.
128. Moore FA, Feliciano DV, Andrassy RJ, *et al.* Early enteral feeding compared with parenteral reduces septic postoperative complications. The results of a meta-analysis. *Ann Surg* 1992; **216:** 172–183.
129. Beier-Holgerson R, Boesby S. Influence of postoperative enteral nutrition on postsurgical infections. *Gut* 1996; **39:** 833–837.
130. Carr CS, Ling KDE, Boulos P, Singer M. Randomised trial of safety and efficacy of immediate postoperative enteral feeding in patients undergoing gastrointestinal resection. *Br Med J* 1996; **312:** 869–873
131. Kudsk KA, Minard G, Croce MA, *et al.* A randomized trial of isonitrogenous enteral diets after severe trauma- and immune-enhancing diet reduced septic complications. *Ann Surg* 1996; **224:** 531–540.
132. Kenler AS, Swails WS, Driscoll DF, *et al.* Early enteral feeding in postsurgical cancer patients: fish oils, structured lipid-based polymeric formula versus a standard polymeric formula. *Surgery* 1996; **223:** 316–333.
133. Mendez C, Jurkovich GJ, Garcia I, *et al.* Effects of an immune enhancing diet in critically injured patients. *J Trauma* 1997; **42:** 933–940.
134. Saffle JR, Wiebke G, Jennings K, *et al.* Randomized trial of immune enhancing enteral nutrition in burn patients. *J Trauma* 1997; **42:** 793–800.
135. Atkinson S, Sieffert E, Bihari D. A prospective, randomized, double-blind, controlled clinical trial of enteral immunonutrition in the critically ill. *Crit Care Med* 1998; **26:** 1164–1172.
136. Houdijk AP, Rijnsburger ER, Jansen J, *et al.* Randomised trial of glutamine-enriched enteral nutrition on infectious morbidity in patients with multiple trauma. *Lancet* 1998; **352:** 772–776.
137. Jones J, Palmer TEA, Griffiths RD. Randomised clinical outcome study of critically ill patients given glutamine supplemented enteral nutrition. *Nutrition* 1999; **15:** 108-
138. Griffiths RD, Hinds CJ, Little RA. Manipulating the metabolic response to injury. *Br Med Bull* 1999; 181–195.
139. Rennie M. Anabolic agents for the critically ill. *Br J Intensive Care* 1999; **9:** 177.
140. Arnold J, Campbell IT, Samuels TA, *et al.* Increased whole body protein breakdown predominates over increased whole body protein synthesis in multiple organ failure. *Clin Sci* 1993; **84:** 655–661.
141. Van den Berghe G, Wouters P, Weekers F, *et al.* Intensive insulin therapy in critically ill patients. *N Engl J Med* 2001; **354:** 1359–67.
142. Martinez A, Allison SP. Insulin revisited. *Clin Nutr* 2003; **22**: 7–15.
143. Flear CTG. Electrolyte and body water changes after trauma. *J Clin Pathol* 1970; **23** (Suppl. 4): 16–21.
144. Zierler KL. Possible mechanisms of insulin action on membrane potential and ion fluxes. *Am J Med* 1970; **40**: 735–9.

65

Nutritional support

SIMON P ALLISON

The anesthesiologist may be faced with providing nutritional support in two situations: first, in the perioperative period, for patients who come to surgery in a malnourished state or who become malnourished as a result of postoperative complications; second, in the intensive care unit. Although the average length of stay of patients in intensive care units is only a few days, there are a few whose illness is so severe that they require prolonged ventilatory support and are consequently unable to eat for long periods.

MALNUTRITION

Form and function

Obese patients are often required by the surgeon to lose weight in order to facilitate surgery. The loss of 10% of the body weight with a properly supervised reducing diet may have a beneficial effect in such patients and may even improve surgical outcome. On the other hand, the initially slim or mesomorphic patient who is unable to eat properly because of disease is in an entirely different category. Total starvation for 3 weeks results in 15% weight loss.[1] Starvation for 9 weeks causes 38% weight loss and a 30% mortality from malnutrition alone.[2,3] Periods of total or partial starvation for 2–3 weeks are not uncommon in hospital practice and may be superimposed upon weight loss before admission. The accelerated catabolism associated with acute illness or injury may further exacerbate tissue loss. Just as important, however, weight loss beyond 8% causes functional deterioration in ways that impair recovery from disease and multiply its complications.[4] The classic Minnesota study by Keys and his colleagues in the 1940s[5] showed that young men who underwent a 24-week period of voluntary partial starvation lost 24% of their body weight and suffered profound physical and psychologic changes that had not returned to normal after a 16-week period of refeeding. They became depressed and irritable, and suffered muscle weakness with a severe reduction in their fitness score. Muscle wasting and weakness from starvation affects particularly the fast-twitch fibers and hence the respiratory muscles, including the diaphragm, impairing respiratory function and the ability to cough and clear secretions.[6–17] Malnutrition also reduces respiratory drive.[15] In contrast, nutritional support has facilitated weaning from ventilators[18] as well as improving muscle strength[6,10,19] and allowing more rapid recovery from orthopedic injuries.[20] Increased susceptibility to infection has always been a prominent feature of famines, highlighted in the studies carried out by the Jewish physicians in the Warsaw ghetto[21] and by more recent studies showing impaired immune function and increased infection rates with undernutrition.[22–24] The Warsaw studies described reduced cardiovascular and gastrointestinal function, with lowered blood pressure, decreased cardiac output, and achlorhydria, among other features. Acute illness and malnutrition may impair not only the digestive functions of the gut but also the barrier it imposes to infection.[25–28] With severe weight loss and a body mass index (BMI) below 18, pancreatic enzyme production declines, which, when combined with bowel dysfunction, may result in maldigestion and malabsorption.[29] Gastrointestinal functions may be protected by nutritional support, particularly when given by the enteral route,[30] although parenteral feeding supplemented by glutamine may also protect gut function.[31–34] Cardiovascular reflexes have been studied following injury and shown to be impaired,[35] thereby inhibiting compensatory responses to blood loss. More than 48 h starvation may also impair the vasoconstrictor response to cold, reducing heat conservation.[36] Loss of body mass is associated with reduced thermogenic response to cold, whereas feeding and recovery in weight restore these thermoregulatory responses to normal.[37,38] Malnutrition also contributes to increased surgical risk and slower recovery from surgery.[10,24,39–43] Wound healing is also impaired but, as Windsor *et al.*[41] showed, this relates even more to poor food intake and a metabolic state of starvation than to absolute reductions in body composition, emphasizing the role of the wound as an organ with its own particular metabolic requirements.

As weight loss proceeds, the various compartments of the body change at different rates.[10] Keys and colleagues[5] showed that, by 24 weeks of partial starvation, fat mass was reduced by over 60% and fat-free mass by 16%. Because of accelerated protein catabolism, the loss of lean body mass in the injured and acutely ill may be proportionately greater than this. The Minnesota study[5] also showed that the absolute extracellular fluid volume remains unchanged, or is only moderately reduced, although as body mass shrinks it increases as a proportion of body weight. Both prolonged starvation and the response to injury confer an inability to excrete an excess salt and water load,[5,21,44–48] and put both depleted and sick patients at risk of salt and water overload unless their intake is carefully controlled. The kidneys of such patients are incapable of compensating for the errors of the doctor prescribing intravenous fluids.

As well as starvation and the response to injury, immobility also contributes to muscle wasting. Studies have shown how, in healthy normal subjects, immobilization in bed can produce negative nitrogen balance and muscle wasting.[49] Conversely, mobilization and exercise enhance protein synthesis and restore wasted muscles. This consideration applies particularly to patients who spend prolonged periods paralyzed on ventilators in the intensive care unit. Muscle anabolism in such patients cannot be achieved by feeding alone, and the sooner the patient can be weaned from the ventilator and mobilized, the sooner will muscle mass be restored. Anoxia also inhibits protein synthesis, thereby contributing to loss of lean mass.[50]

Malnutrition also has other important consequences. A number of studies have shown that 40% of patients have some degree of malnutrition on admission, and in half of these it is severe.[51] This goes largely unrecognized because of failure of doctors and nurses to understand the importance of nutrition.[52] The nutritional state of patients also tends to deteriorate while in hospital through lack of adequate nutritional care.[51] Catering in many hospitals is ill-adapted to the needs of the sick, resulting in food wastage rates in excess of 40% and food intakes of less than 80% of requirements.[53–55] A recent review[56] has shown a direct relation between the degree of undernutrition and the length of hospital stay, as well as a reduced length of stay with early and adequate intervention. The delayed recovery from illness associated with inadequately treated malnutrition has therefore economic as well as clinical consequences. The nutrition-related problems faced by the surgical or critically ill patient are summarized in Table 65.1 with their causes, consequences, and treatment.

BENEFITS OF TREATMENT

It is one thing to show that starvation and weight loss are associated with measurable changes in structure and function. It is another to show that nutritional support not only reverses these changes but also results in significantly improved clinical outcome, at reasonable cost in resources and without excessive complications. Feeding during illness may produce improvements in nitrogen balance, anthropometric measurements, and weight (chiefly due to fluid gain) without producing any measurable improvement in outcome. In the severely malnourished, however, improvements in function due to feeding may be more clinically significant and occur before any increase in body mass.[10,18] Reviews and meta-analyses published between 1984 and 1987[57–59] concluded that there was no evidence of benefit from nutritional support in patients with mild-to-moderate nutritional depletion and that the evidence for benefit in severely malnourished patients was suggestive but required confirmation. Many trials were criticized for their design, methodology, patient selection, and inadequate numbers. Since then, a large number of trials have shown improved outcome with nutritional support in appropriate patients. A more recent meta-analysis of perioperative feeding[60] concluded that the routine use of postoperative parenteral nutrition in those without antecedent malnutrition conferred no benefit, and may even be harmful. In those with prior malnutrition, however, perioperative feeding appeared to confer benefit.[3,61,62] Results of trials may be critically dependent on patient selection, timing, route, and content of feeds. The outcome measures used are also important. Lower mortality is desirable, but may not be achievable or ascertainable in a condition with an already low mortality. Useful outcome measures are infectious and other complications, antibiotic use, functional improvement, rate of recovery, length of stay, and costs. Tucker[56] carried out an audit in 20 hospitals throughout the USA and showed not only a close correlation between poor nutritional status and longer hospital stay, but also a direct relation between early nutritional intervention and shorter hospital stay.

Nutritional care of the surgical patient

Nutritional care of the surgical patient can be considered in four phases.

Preoperative

With recent weight loss of more than 10%, combined with physiologic dysfunction, there is evidence that a period of preoperative nutritional support, continued into the postoperative period, has a beneficial effect on outcome.[60] Much will depend on the urgency to undertake surgery and the patient's circumstances. If carried out at home rather than in hospital, preoperative nutritional support is more economically feasible.

Perioperative

The policy of fasting patients overnight before surgery, which brings patients to surgery in a metabolically starved state, has been shown to increase postoperative insulin resistance and catabolic response.[63] Conversely, a glucose drink administered 2 h preoperatively not only clears the stomach rapidly but results in diminished postoperative insulin resistance, improved nitrogen balance, and shorter hospital stay.[64] It is clearly desirable, therefore, to maintain the surgical patient in a hormonally and metabolically fed state at the time of operation.

Postoperative

The routine use of nasogastric tubes for gastric decompression and drainage, combined with "nil-by-mouth" regimens and intravenous fluids, has been shown, at least in small and distal bowel surgery, to be largely unnecessary and even harmful.[63,65–67] Comparing conventional treatment with one employing oral intake from the first day, no nasogastric suction and no intravenous fluids, Wara and Hessov[67] showed that, with the latter protocol, gastrointestinal function returned earlier, with no greater incidence of vomiting or complications. More recently, he and colleagues have used oral intake from the first day combined with low thoracic epidural analgesia (avoiding opiate-induced ileus) and aggressive mobilization, and have shown better preservation of muscle mass and strength with more rapid convalescence and earlier discharge.[68,69] The current consensus is to provide postoperative nutritional support by whatever means possible for patients who were significantly malnourished preoperatively and to all patients whose oral intake remains minimal for more than 7–10 days postoperatively. Artificial nutritional support should be continued until daily oral intake exceeds 60% of nutritional requirements.

A number of apparently conflicting trials have addressed the routine use of postoperative nutritional support for patients undergoing abdominal surgery, using the oral, enteral, and parenteral routes, with both standard and modified feeding formulae.[66] In studies from Rana *et al.*[70] and Keele *et al.*,[71] unselected patients were given oral supplements from the sixth postoperative day, resulting in a reduction in postoperative infections and other complications, improved muscle strength, and shorter hospital stay. The average preoperative weight loss in these patients was 7%. In contrast, MacFie and colleagues[72] found no benefit from the routine use of both pre- and postoperative oral supplements in a population of patients whose average BMI was 23 and mid-arm muscle circumference was 25 cm. One possible explanation of these differing results is that the patient populations were nutritionally different from the beginning. Another is the variation in the proportion of supplement actually ingested over that prescribed, so that, in some cases, treatment had an insignificant impact on total nutritional intake. There is a theoretical reason why orally ingested food might be superior to tube feeding, which bypasses the cephalic and oral responses, as saliva has potent antibacterial properties that could be important in relation to infectious complications.[66]

One of the earliest trials to show the benefit of enteral feeding was carried out in elderly women after surgery for fractured neck of the femur.[20] Patients were divided by anthropometric means into normal,

Table 65.1 *Nutritional and metabolic problems of the perioperative and critical care patient*

Problem	Cause	Effect	Treatment
Anorexia/appetite change	Mental and physical disease Pain Changes in taste and smell, e.g. with aging Drugs, e.g. antibiotics	Weight loss Specific deficiencies	Targeted menu Treat depression Regional analgesia if possible Change/stop drugs Oral supplements Artificial nutrition
Fasting/starvation	Investigative procedures Surgery Poor catering practice Anorexia	Weight loss Specific deficiencies Changes in hormonal, metabolic, and tissue function	Avoid where possible Review catering and feeding policy Glucose 2 h preoperatively
Catabolism	Injury/trauma Surgery Inflammation Infection Fever Starvation	Accelerated loss tissue, particularly lean mass Specific deficiencies, e.g. in burns	Minimize catabolic stimuli, e.g. pain, fever Feeding and correction of specific deficiencies (Immunonutrition) (Anabolic hormones)
Weight loss	Anorexia Fasting/starvation Catabolism	Loss of cell mass Loss of organ function Immobility Depression/apathy More complications Longer hospital stay	Nutritional support Mobilization Treat underlying disease
Immobility	Disease Treatment	Loss of lean mass Thromboembolism	Control pain Physiotherapy Early mobilization
Gastrointestinal dysfunction	Disease Maldigestion Surgery Drugs, e.g. opiates, antibiotics Microflora	Malabsorption Gastrointestinal failure Malnutrition Fluid and electrolyte deficits	Nutritional support
Fluid, electrolyte, and protein losses from wounds, burns, fistulae, abscesses, drains, aspiration	Trauma Infection Surgery	Fluid, electrolyte, mineral, and nutritional deficits	Replace/maintain fluid and electrolytes Nutritional support Octreotide (fistulae)
Sodium and water overload	Residual from resuscitation Mismanagement	Respiratory and wound complications Gastrointestinal dysfunction Edema	Diuretics Albumin (if plasma volume deficit) Spironolactone

thin (1–2 SD below the reference range) and very thin (>2 SD below the reference range). The thin and very thin groups were randomized to receive ward diet or ward diet plus 1000 kcal in the form of supplementary overnight nasogastric tube feed. Rehabilitation to mobility was 10 days in the normal group, not significantly affected by feeding in the thin group, but reduced from 23 to 16 days in the very thin group. These results have been confirmed in a smaller study using oral supplements.[73] Studies following abdominal surgery have been conflicting. Beier-Holgersen[74] placed nasojejunal tubes at the time of laparotomy and began feeding a diet giving 1000–1500 kcal from the first postoperative day, with a reduction in infectious complications. In contrast, Heslin *et al.*[75] showed no benefit, but intake in their patients was only 400 kcal per day. Sharpe *et al.*[76] showed clear benefit of early postoperative nasojejunal feeding following liver transplantation with a reduction in rejection rates from 44% to 7% and of hospital stay from 31 to 22 days. Kudsk[77] also found striking benefit from this modality in patients following major abdominal trauma. The effect of treatment in reducing infections and antibiotic usage was further enhanced when an "immune-enhancing" formula was used. There is clear evidence, therefore, of benefit from enteral feeding in certain groups of patients. Further studies of enteral feeding are needed to define its use postoperatively, although this is well established in the patient, with a functional GI tract, unable to take normal food for longer than 7–10 days. In upper gastrointestinal surgery, the placement of a feeding jejunostomy during the surgery allows ready access to the gut in high-risk patients. It has been suggested that the enteral route is superior to the parenteral route by preventing mucosal atrophy, diminishing bacterial translocation, enhancing the function of the gut-associated lymphatic tissue, and being cheaper and with fewer complications.[66] Although this may be so in some patients, a recent review[78] suggests that the clinical evidence to support this contention is sparse. It is reasonable, however, when nutritional support is indicated, to use the enteral route when feasible, having recourse to parenteral nutrition when it is not. Again, parenteral nutrition benefits the undernourished patient with gastrointestinal dysfunction, but its routine use in the surgical patient may produce no benefit or a worse outcome in the absence of malnutrition. Two important studies again highlight the fact that the effect of continuing nutritional support, using oral supplements, into the postdischarge period is critically dependent on case selection. Jensen and Hessov[79] showed weight gain but no functional or clinical benefit from this practice in an unselected group of patients undergoing surgery. In contrast, Beattie *et al.*[80] showed clear benefit, in terms of recovery, in patients who were selected because they were significantly malnourished.

Critical care

As far as the patient requiring critical care is concerned, there is no evidence of benefit from the routine feeding of patients who spend brief periods in the intensive care unit.[81] Following major trauma or burns, however, significant benefit has been demonstrated from early nutritional support with mineral and micronutrient supplements,[82] and enteral feeds, particularly using so-called immune-enhancing diets.[77,83] Again, in this group of patients, prolonged gastrointestinal dysfunction remains an indication for parenteral nutrition in which the use of additional special substrates such as glutamine[84] may add further benefit. The beneficial effects of feeding may be negated by excess administration of energy (see below).

In all techniques of artificial nutrition, benefit is critically dependent on the expertise with which they are conducted. Inexpert technique results in higher complication rates and consequently less benefit.[3,85–88]

Summary

From a consideration of the evidence outlined, it is suggested that the broad indications and guidelines for nutritional support are as follows:

1 Continuing recent weight loss of 10% or more. Preoperative treatment should be given where appropriate (at home if possible) and continued into the postoperative period.
2 Continuing inadequate oral intake for more than 7–10 days postoperatively.
3 The presence of disease whose known natural history predicts accelerated catabolism and poor intake for 7 days or more. In a patient with burns, or severe pancreatitis, or following major trauma, for example, no time should be wasted in starting nutritional support once the initial resuscitation phase is over, even in the absence of prior malnutrition.
4 Moderate malnutrition is more significant in the presence of catabolic disease. The presence of both constitutes an indication for early nutritional support.
5 Patients undergoing major surgery should receive glucose, orally if possible, intravenously if not, 2 h preoperatively, and oral intake should be resumed without delay postoperatively. The unnecessary use of drip and suck regimens should be avoided, and when these prove necessary they should be discontinued as soon as possible.
6 Oral supplements should be used when possible. When swallowing or anorexia is problematic, enteral feeding should be given into the stomach or small bowel, using immune-enhancing formulae in major trauma or severe critical illness. Parenteral feeding should be used when gastrointestinal dysfunction precludes the enteral route.

MEASUREMENT

Nutritional screening and assessment

The simple practical techniques for screening and assessment that may be carried out in any hospital are discussed here. For the more sophisticated measurements used for research purposes, the reader is referred to appropriate texts. A protocol for rapid initial screening on admission by nurses should be used in all hospitals to detect patients at risk.[55,87,88] This may consist of minimal data derived from simple questions such as "have you lost weight recently – if so, how much?," and "has your appetite or food intake changed recently?."[52] Several scoring systems have also been devised with more or less similar criteria.[89] The recently published Danish guidelines[90] embody a combined score for severity of malnutrition and disease severity linked to a protocol for action and referral to a dietitian or the nutrition team. In Table 65.2, I have adapted the Danish Protocol to aid clinical decision making in respect of nutritional support. This includes recording of height, weight, and BMI where possible, and/or arm anthropometry. A more detailed nutritional assessment of those deemed at risk should then be carried out by a dietitian or clinician. Weekly monitoring and review of nutritional status should be carried out on all patients in hospital for 7 days or more. The parameters of weight, hemoglobin, plasma proteins, and skin immune response have been variously combined in the form of so-called nutritional indices, which have been shown to correlate with postoperative complications.[91] Such derived values should more properly be designated as surgical "risk indices," as they reflect the severity of the disease (reflected by serum albumin or hemoglobin levels) as well as malnutrition, without separating the two components as in the Danish system. On the other hand, the presence of disease or the prospect of major surgery, radiotherapy or chemotherapy enhances the clinical significance of even moderate malnutrition.

Weight

The serial measurement and recording of weight is of the greatest value.[3,10,39,90,91] If this can be related to the patient's remembered or previously recorded weight, the percentage weight loss can be estimated. Involuntary weight loss of 5–10% in the previous 3 months indicates moderate, and more than 10% severe, malnutrition. Weight can also be related to skeletal length using measurement of height or demi-span[92] (measured from the suprasternal notch to the web between the third and fourth fingers with the arm outstretched). Dividing weight in kilograms by height squared in meters, a BMI can be derived, with a normal range of 18.5–25. Alternatively, the patient's weight and height can be related to tables from relevant normal populations of the same age and sex. The wide variation in normal values makes them valuable for epidemiologic purposes, but not always for the assessment of the individual. Weight is also affected in the short term by the state of hydration. In the postoperative period, fluid retention and edema may conceal true tissue weight loss unless such factors are allowed for.[93] During treatment, long-term weight gain in the absence of edema may reflect true tissue gain, whereas day-to-day changes in weight may be the best measures of fluid balance. Knowing the weight has additional value not only for calculating the dose of drugs, but also for estimating the patient's metabolic rate and nutritional and fluid requirements.

Voluntary oral intake

The simple estimation of voluntary postoperative oral intake has been validated by Hessov[94] and has shown to be a useful clinical tool.[41,95,96] Meguid *et al.*[96] have described the "inadequate oral nutrient intake period" (IONIP), and shown that, in the postoperative period, those who fail to achieve an oral intake greater than 60% of their estimated requirements by the tenth day postoperatively tend to do badly and should be considered for artificial nutritional support. The help of an experienced dietitian is invaluable in this respect in providing appropriate, palatable, and nutritionally dense food[97–99] supplemented by snacks[100] and/or oral supplements.[101,102]

Table 65.2 *Nutrition risk score*

Score	Degree of malnutrition		Disease severity
0	Normal	Weight loss < 5% in 3 months Normal function Previous week food intake > 80% requirements BMI 20–26	No disease
1	Mild	Weight loss 5% in 3 months Normal function Previous week food intake 60–80% requirements	Chronic medical – cirrhosis, renal failure, COPD, diabetes, cancer Surgical – hip fracture, cholecystectomy, laparoscopy, amputation Minor postoperative complications
2	Moderate	Weight loss 5–10% in 3 months Function normal or moderately impaired Previous week food intake 25–60% requirements BMI 18–20% and/or MAC/TSF 5–15th centile	Medical – severe pneumonia, long-stay geriatric, stroke, malignant hematology Surgical – major abdominal, thoracic, or vascular surgery Chemotherapy, radiotherapy
3	Severe	Weight loss > 10% in 3 months Function markedly impaired Previous week food intake 25% requirements BMI < 18 and/or MAC/TSF < 5th centile and/or multiple micronutrient/mineral deficiencies	Major trauma and burns. Head injury Major postoperative complications Sepsis with temperature > 38 °C Critical care (APACHE score > 10) Severe pancreatitis Bone marrow/liver/heart/lung transplant

Protocol: Combine nutrition score 0–3 with disease severity score 0–3. If combined score is 3 or more, take necessary action or refer to dietitian or nutrition team as appropriate and start nutritional treatment, oral (normal food or oral supplements), enteral, or parenteral, or a combination of these as appropriate, giving sufficient to meet nutritional goals. If score 3, reassess weekly. If malnutrition score 2 but major surgery, radiotherapy, or chemotherapy impending, consider proactive nutritional support.
Adapted from Danish Guidelines 1999.

Anthropometry and body composition

The simple measurement with a tape of mid-arm circumference (MAC), half-way between the acromion and the olecranon, combined with the measurement of triceps skinfold thickness (TSF), gives an estimate of body composition and the relative amounts of fat and muscle.[10,103–106] Values can be compared with centile tables for the relevant age group and sex. The measurement of TSF, in particular, requires some skill, and there can be a 20% interobserver variation in unskilled hands.[105] MAC is a fairly robust measurement, however, and can be useful in clinical practice. Both may be affected by the patient's state of hydration. A bedside estimate of body composition may be obtained by the bioimpedance method, although the errors that occur in unstable or very sick patients can affect its accuracy.[106] In clinical practice, it probably adds little to the measurements already described.

Functional parameters

Preservation of function is the main goal of nutritional support and determinant of outcome. Some assessment of the changes in body function consequent upon change in composition is therefore an essential part of nutritional assessment and of monitoring the response to nutritional support.[3,10,18,20,107,108] As weight loss and even a BMI in the 18–20 range are not incompatible with health in some cases, it is important to obtain some estimate of how far such changes have affected function. Hill[10,107] and Jeejeebhoy[19] have shown that skeletal and respiratory muscle strength decline as protein–energy malnutrition worsens, and respond positively and rapidly to nutritional support. Klidjian *et al.*[108] showed also that muscle strength measured by hand dynamometry is one of the best predictors of surgical complications, and is improved by good nutrition. Some measures of immunologic competence may also be useful. In normal clinical practice, the lymphocyte count is easy to measure, but skin tests to antigens, although being of research interest, probably add little to the other parameters. In the nutritional assessment of the surgical patient, therefore, some attempt should be made to record not only changes in body composition, but also their functional correlates of muscle strength, respiratory function, and immune competence.

Biochemical and hematologic measurements

The concentration of the serum albumin and of the shorter half-life protein thyroid-binding prealbumin (TBPA) have been cited as nutritional parameters, despite the fact that with starvation alone they remain unchanged. Their concentration falls postoperatively or in the presence of acute illness or inflammation due to changes in distribution rather than metabolism.[3,20,109] Excessive crystalloid administration also dilutes serum albumin, which returns toward normal with diuresis of the extracellular fluid overload.[93] Recovery to normal levels may, however, be delayed by malnutrition and assisted by nutritional support.[20] Similarly, a fall in hemoglobin levels may reflect a deficiency of hematinics, e.g. B_{12}, folate, and iron, or more usually severity of disease or blood loss. Such measurements are therefore more useful in monitoring the response to treatment than in deciding whether nutritional support is needed in the first place.

The measurement of vitamin, mineral, and trace elements is particularly helpful in certain patients, e.g. those with severe gastrointestinal disease, and guide treatment of deficiencies in these important nutrients. Similarly, hematologic values are an important part of the full assessment of the surgical patient.

The concentration of creatinine in serum and its 24-h excretion in the urine correlate with lean mass. The serum concentration may rise above the normal range in weight-lifters or body-builders, but may fall below the normal range in patients who have lost lean mass through illness and/or starvation. The blood urea concentration also falls with declining protein turnover. The 24-h urinary creatinine excretion as a ratio of the expected value for a normal adult of the same sex and height has been termed the creatinine–height index and is a useful measure of change in muscle mass.

Summary

Measurements of weight and its change, anthropometrics, and oral intake, combined with simple functional assessment, form the basic parameters upon which the decision to give nutritional support is based, although the severity of accompanying disease should also be considered in a combined scoring system, as even moderate malnutrition may indicate the need for nutritional support in the presence of continuing catabolic illness. A suggested clinical definition of malnutrition and disease severity is summarized in Table 65.2, with a scoring system to guide decision making. Malnutrition may be defined as "a state of energy, protein or other specific nutrient deficiency that produces a measurable change in body function, is associated with a worse outcome from illness and is specifically reversible by nutritional treatment." This definition covers protein–energy malnutrition as well as single or multiple deficiency of micronutrients but excludes conditions of "suboptimal nutrition" where no prior malnutrition exists in a traditional sense but the patient benefits from additional substrate to meet the extra metabolic demands of illness, e.g. glucose perioperatively or immune-enhancing diets in critical illness.

A simple admission screening protocol to detect patients at nutritional risk should be carried out by nursing staff, followed by more detailed nutritional assessment by a clinician or dietitian. Changes in hematologic and biochemical measurements are useful adjuncts, especially to detect micronutrient, mineral, or electrolyte disorders. Their regular measurement also forms a vital part of the monitoring of the response to treatment. All these parameters must be interpreted in the light of a knowledge of the natural history of the underlying disease and its pathophysiologic effects.

TREATMENT

Treatment goals

In the past, hyperalimentation regimens containing large amounts of glucose were used in an attempt to bludgeon the catabolic response to injury into reverse and to try and achieve positive energy and nitrogen balance. These regimens proved counterproductive for several reasons. First, it was found that, although nutritional support can help to reduce net nitrogen balance and tissue loss, it cannot switch off the catabolic response to injury until the underlying disease resolves. Second, the administration of glucose at a rate greater than 6 mg kg^{-1} min^{-1} results not only in hyperglycemia, which may increase infection risk, but also in increased oxygen consumption and carbon dioxide production, thereby worsening the problems of respiratory failure.[110–112] Third, although lean mass continued to dissolve through catabolism and immobility, fat mass increased and a fatty liver developed, with abnormal liver function tests and jaundice from cholestasis. Accordingly, a more conservative approach was adopted for critical care patients, in whom energy intake was matched to energy consumption, or even, in the acute phase of illness, set at a hypocaloric level. Indeed, several positive trials of nutritional support for postoperative and critical care patients have used an initial regimen whose total energy content was modest, i.e. 18–20 kcal kg^{-1}.[74,77] As described above, one of the responses to trauma is the inability to excrete an excess salt and water load[44,45] Nutritional support is inseparable from the administration of water, electrolytes, and minerals. Careful attention should therefore be paid to the proper balance of these nutrients, as excess or lack can affect clinical outcome adversely. As the patient enters the anabolic or convalescent phase of illness and starts to be mobile, the capacity to diurese salt and water returns.[45] The patient is also able to take larger amounts of energy and protein and to use them for the resynthesis of lost tissue. The treatment goals, therefore, in the early phase of illness are, first, to maintain cellular and tissue function, second, to minimize the additional catabolic effects of starvation, third, to maintain the patient in a metabolically fed state, as fasting has been shown to have deleterious effects on the patient undergoing surgery and, last, to avoid the toxic effects of nutrient or fluid and electrolyte excess. In the anabolic or convalescent phase, mobilization should be combined with increasing food intake, particularly by the oral route, to achieve early restoration of lost tissue and normal function. The achievement of these goals depends on the timing, content, and route of administration of feeds and the skill and attention with which nutritional support is conducted.

Content of feeds

Energy

With modern management of surgical and critical care patients, it is rare to find measured energy expenditures much in excess of 1.3× basal or resting metabolic rate[10,113,114] estimated by Harris and Benedict or Schofield (see Table 65.3).[115,116] In catabolic patients with prolonged illness, it is desirable to measure energy expenditure by indirect calorimetry as, under these circumstances, the error in its estimation using the above equations may be larger than in the normal individual.[113] However, such measurements are demanding in technical time and skill if they are to be performed accurately and in general clinical practice good management can be achieved by estimation rather than measurement. As described above, beneficial effects have been obtained following surgery and major trauma using short periods of relatively hypocaloric feeding. In the acute phase of illness, even after severe burns, many experienced clinicians give an energy intake (including protein and nonprotein energy sources) of 1.3–1.5 times the estimated resting expenditure, and for short periods in the early stage of feeding as little as 1.0× estimated expenditure. In most patients, this equates to an intake of 25–35 kcal total energy per kilogram per day. Diet-induced thermogenesis means that the patient fed by whatever route has an energy expenditure approximately 10% higher than that of the fasted individual. Also, for every 1 °C rise in temperature, there is a 13% increase in metabolic rate. In the past, these considerations have been combined with fudge factors for severity of illness, but the errors inherent in these approximations have led most clinicians in recent years to adopt the simpler approach described above. In the postoperative surgical patient, any increase in metabolic rate due to illness is more than offset by a 20–30% reduction in total energy expenditure due to immobility. During the anabolic or convalescent phase of illness, when the patient is starting to be mobile, energy intakes can be increased to meet the demands of tissue synthesis and of activity.

It is usual practice to provide between 30% and 50% of nonprotein

Table 65.3 *Calculation of energy expenditure using Schofield equations[81] (weight in kg; BMR in kcal per 24 h[a])*

Age (years)	Male	Female
15–18	BMR = 17.6 × weight + 656	BMR = 13.3 × weight + 690
18–30	BMR = 15.0 × weight + 690	BMR = 14.8 × weight + 485
30–60	BMR = 11.4 × weight + 870	BMR = 8.1 × weight + 842
> 60	BMR = 11.7 × weight + 585	BMR = 9.0 × weight + 656

a. Multiply kilocalories by 4.184 to obtain kilojoule equivalents.

energy from fat to reduce the toxic effects of carbohydrate excess. Suggested maximum administration rates of the various substrates used for parenteral nutrition are summarized in Table 65.4. Rates of administration above these either produce no additional benefit or are associated with toxic effects. Although these considerations apply primarily to parenteral nutrition, the rate of administration of feed by the oral or enteral route is usually constrained by gastrointestinal tolerance.

In the past, most lipid emulsions for parenteral use have contained long-chain triglycerides (LCTs), excess administration of which may lead to hypertriglyceridemia and other undesirable consequences, particularly in the case of children. Medium-chain fatty acids, being independent of the carnitine shuttle for entry into mitochondria, can be cleared more rapidly and provide a useful source of energy. Similarly, although ω-6 fatty acids may enhance the inflammatory response, the ω-3 fatty acids found in fish oils may diminish it and have some clinical advantages. Structured lipid emulsions, in which LCT/MCT and ω-3 fatty acids are linked to the same glycerol molecule, may prove superior in critical care patients, although unequivocal evidence for this is not yet available.

Although MCT-containing enteral feeds may have limited application, the use of triglycerides with monounsaturated fatty acid, e.g. oleic, may allow the carbohydrate content of enteral feeds to be reduced for diabetics and result in lower plasma lipids and improved diabetic control.[116] ω-3 fatty acids have been used as a component of immune-enhancing diets used following major trauma and during critical care.

Nitrogen/protein

As described above, nitrogen balance is influenced by severity of catabolic illness and the degree of mobility. It is also influenced by both energy and nitrogen intake, as well as the quality of administered protein or the spectrum and proportion of amino acids used in various feeds. If energy requirements are satisfied, then in health a minimum protein intake of 0.7 g per kg per day has been recommended by the World Health Organization. This is insufficient for most patients, however, who require 1–1.5 g of protein per kg per day, or 0.15–0.25 g of nitrogen per kg per day (1 g of nitrogen is equivalent to 6.25 g of protein). In the acute phase of catabolic illness, even when energy requirements are fully satisfied, nitrogen intakes above 0.25 g per kg per day seldom produce any increase in nitrogen balance, but merely an increase in urea synthesis and output (see Table 65.4). On the other hand, during convalescence, higher nitrogen intakes may be tolerated and, when combined with adequate energy intakes and physical activity, will result in useful resynthesis of lean mass.

The relation between energy and nitrogen intake has been described in terms of the nonprotein energy–nitrogen ratio of feeds. In normal subjects, a ratio as high as 300:1 may maintain nitrogen balance, whereas in a critically ill patient one of between 100:1 and 150:1 may be more appropriate. This illustrates the fact that protein requirements during illness increase by a proportionally greater amount than those of energy.[110]

Table 65.4 *Suggested maximum substrate administration rates in catabolic patients*

Substrate	$mg\,kg^{-1}\,min^{-1}$	$g\,kg^{-1}\,day^{-1}$	$g\,day^{-1}$	60-kg man ($kcal\,day^{-1}$)
Glucose	5	7.8	468	1800
Fat	1.3	1.5	100	900
Protein/AAs		1.5	90	400
Nitrogen		0.25	15	
Max. total				3100

From Allison.[55]

In considering the quality of protein, egg protein is used as a reference value for first-class protein, and the adequacy of amino acid spectrum and content should be judged against this. Certain amino acids are difficult to provide in parenteral solutions, unless as dipeptides, as they are relatively unstable, e.g. glutamine, or insoluble, e.g. cysteine. These considerations are particularly important in growing children, in whom, for example, an adequate supply of sulfhydryl-containing amino acids is important.

Minerals and micronutrients

Space does not allow full treatment of this subject, and readers are referred to appropriate texts. Large losses of gastrointestinal fluids may result in sodium, potassium, magnesium, selenium, and zinc deficiencies. Zinc, copper, and selenium losses are excessive following major burns, and supplements of these have proved beneficial.[82] Most enteral feeds have an adequate spectrum of vitamins and trace elements, but some are deficient in these. Proprietary supplements are available for parenteral use (see Table 65.5). In some conditions, however, additional amounts of individual nutrients may be needed, e.g. because of increased folate requirements and relatively low levels of this vitamin in some preparations. It is our practice to administer 15 mg of folate intramuscularly once per week by patients receiving parenteral nutrition.

Methodology

Having made the clinical decision to provide nutritional support, how should it be given and what should be the composition of the feed? Before answering such questions, it is first necessary to consider how nutritional support should be organized, as the sporadic and occasional use of the more technically demanding forms of artificial nutrition can be fraught with complications when conducted by the inexpert. Any anesthesiologist wishing to take an interest in this field should be associated with a hospital nutrition team, whose members should include doctors, nurses, dietitians, and pharmacists. With parenteral nutrition, for example, it has been shown that the formation of a nutrition team working to agreed standards and protocols results in a reduction in catheter sepsis rates from 28% to under 3%, of mechanical problems from 24% to 6%, and of metabolic problems from 30% to 12%.[3,84,85]

Table 65.5 *A typical standard parenteral feed for maintenance feeding to give 2400 kcal and 14 g of nitrogen in 2.5 L*

1000 mL of amino acid solution to give 14 g of nitrogen and 400 calories;
500 mL of 20% lipid emulsion to give 1000 kcal and 7.5 mmol phosphate;
1000 mL of 26% glucose/electrolyte/mineral solution, to give:

Energy	100 kcal
Na^+	120 mmol
K^+	80 mmol
Mg^{2+}	7.5 mmol
Phosphate	10 mmol
Calcium	7.5 mmol
Chloride	240 mmol
Fluoride	0.05 mmol
Iodide	0.001 mmol
Zinc	0.12 mmol
Copper	0.02 mmol
Manganese	0.005 mmol
Molybdenum	0.002 mmol
Selenium	0.0005 mm

Additional fat- and water-soluble vitamins
Multiply kilocalories by 4.184 to obtain kilojoule equivalents

Costs per day and per patient are also reduced.[3] A standard recording system should be used to allow regular audit of the equipment and feed used, and of complications and costs. By careful attention to such detail, septic complications may be reduced to zero and satisfactory cost-effectiveness and cost benefit demonstrated.[3]

In deciding upon the route of administration of feed, the rules are simple. If the gut works, try to use it. If the patient can swallow, try oral supplements or, failing this, some form of enteral tube feeding. Parenteral nutrition is the treatment of prolonged gastrointestinal dysfunction, in the same sense that dialysis is the treatment of renal failure.

Normal food

As described above, our own and other studies of both medical and surgical patients have shown that 35–40% of food supplied is left and wasted, resulting in intakes of energy, protein, and other nutrients less than 70% of that required to maintain balance.[53–55] Fortified meals and targeted menus have resulted in improved intake and less wastage.[55,97–100] Catering practices, therefore, need to be reviewed and menus made more appropriate to the needs of the sick. It should be remembered that hospital food is part of the treatment and not just a hotel service.[55]

Oral supplements

These should not be made a substitute for inadequate provision of palatable food for patients able to eat. On the other hand, they have proved their benefit, particularly in the postoperative patient, for whom the traditional postoperative drip and suck regimens have been challenged as described above. A more aggressive and effective approach by nurses and dietitians toward oral feeding may be the most cost-effective way of providing nutritional support for most surgical patients, although this method is clearly impractical for those in the intensive care unit.

Enteral tube feeding

Many elderly patients, in particular, are slow to recover their appetite postoperatively, even though bowel function has returned. Although many will respond to oral supplements, a few benefit from a period of fine-bore nasogastric tube feeding. Patients with swallowing difficulties may be managed similarly, although, if tube feeding needs to be continued for longer than 1–2 weeks, a feeding gastrostomy or jejunostomy should be considered.[118–123] With obstructive lesions of the upper gastrointestinal tract, causing severe weight loss, there may be a case for a period of preoperaive tube feeding. The insertion of a jejunostomy or gastrostomy allows feeding to be carried out at home, which is particularly important for patients with inoperable obstructive lesions.

The technique of using nasogastric or nasoenteral fine-bore tubes is well known but a few points are worth emphasizing.[124] It is important to select a good-quality tube, preferably of polyurethane, with side holes and a flexible guide wire that is removed easily. The internal diameter of the tube need not be greater than 2–3 mm for adequate feeding. After insertion of the tube, a radiograph to ascertain its position is necessary only for those with impaired consciousness or gag reflex. Auscultation for bubbles in the epigastrium when air and water are syringed down the tube is usually sufficient in the conscious patient. Reversal of the Luer fittings with male fitting on the tube and the female fitting on the giving set prevents accidental connection of the feeding line with an intravenous catheter. We favor continuous pumped feeding, although this may be carried out intermittently both for convenience and to allow the gastric pH to fall to bactericidal levels.[125]

Overnight nasogastric tube feeding is a valuable technique for some patients, allowing freedom to exercise and take oral feed during the day. We have found that this method may result in a disinhibition of appetite in anorectic patients, accelerating the return to a full oral diet.[126] This is quite contrary to the inhibition that might be expected, and its mechanism is uncertain, although gastrointestinal hormones may have some part to play, as intravenous feeding has the opposite effect. A sterile feed should be used and the giving sets and reservoirs changed daily, particularly for patients during intensive care, because enteral feeding has been incriminated in cross-infections and even in fatalities.[127–129]

Gastrostomy and jejunostomy[123]

Gastrostomies and jejunostomies may be inserted during surgery. Many a patient undergoing upper gastrointestinal surgery could have been saved from having to undergo intravenous feeding by the prophylactic insertion of one of these tubes at operation. With prolonged gastric outlet obstruction, for example, it is invaluable to have a jejunostomy in place to help with postoperative management. The Delaney type of fine-bore jejunostomy is to be preferred, inserted via a wide-bore needle and tunneled in the bowel wall, with the entry site sewn to the anterior abdominal wall. Such tubes can be used for long periods of time and are effective and unobtrusive. Infection is the major complication, but this is uncommon in skilled hands and usually responds to antibiotics.

Gastrostomies may also be inserted by the percutaneous endoscopic gastrostomy technique described by Ganderer and colleagues.[118,119] A gastroscope is passed and a second operator observes the gastroscope light in the epigastrium, directing the local anesthetic to this area, which is then punctured with a large cannula until the endoscopist observes the point of the cannula within the stomach. A nylon thread is passed through this, grasped by the endoscopy forceps and brought up through the mouth. To the thread is attached a narrow-bore gastrostomy tube with a flange. The second operator then pulls the nylon thread back through the epigastric cannula until the gastrostomy tube appears on the outside and the flange fits snugly against the gastric mucosa. An external flange is then put in place to anchor the tube and a hub is attached for connection with the giving set. The internal part of the gastrostomy tube may be short and end in the stomach itself. Some tubes have a long tail, however, which can then be threaded by the endoscopist through the pylorus and round into the jejunum, overcoming problems of gastric outlet obstruction and hopefully diminishing the amount of reflux. Instead of the "pull" technique described above, "push" techniques under radiologic control are also available.

Content of feed

For most enteral tube feeding, a standard defined formula whole-protein feed is all that is required. Such feeds contain a balanced proportion of protein, carbohydrate, and fat, with adequate supplies of vitamins, minerals, and trace elements. Where constipation is a problem, fiber-containing feeds may be advantageous, and, in some cases, diarrhea is improved by the addition of fiber. We have not used an elemental diet (amino acids rather than whole protein) for many years, although there are some patients, particularly those with a jejunostomy, for whom a peptide feed appears to be tolerated better. There is some evidence that high-fat, low-carbohydrate feeds give a lower respiratory quotient (RQ), make less demand for gas exchange, and are therefore advantageous when patients are being weaned off ventilators. Others maintain that a reduction in caloric intake is just as effective. As with parenteral nutrition, it is customary to supply half the nonprotein energy as fat and half as carbohydrate. The use of disease-specific feeds and of special substrates has created a whole new discipline of pharmacologic nutrition. The indications for these are beginning to be defined, with clinical benefit having been demonstrated in several studies of critically ill patients. The main benefits appear to be improved gut function and enhancement of immune tissue activity with protection against infection.

Complications[124–133]

Whichever technique is used, the slow continuous or intermittent administration by pump diminishes many of the complications of reflux, nausea, and diarrhea associated with the bolus method. If diarrhea still occurs, it is often in association with broad-spectrum antibiotics, which should be stopped if possible. Otherwise the addition of loperamide or codeine phosphate syrup is effective. In cases both of constipation and of diarrhea, the use of a fiber-containing feed may also be helpful. In the intensive care unit, there has been a shift in emphasis from parenteral to enteral feeding on the grounds of cost-effectiveness and the reported complications of the former method, although the evidence for these has been challenged.[76] In many cases, combined enteral and parenteral feeding allows inadequate total nutrient intake with the benefits of some enteral nutrient.

Enteral feeding has been advocated to maintain bowel function and the integrity of the mucosal barrier against infection,[66] but it is not without its problems, apart from those which have already been mentioned. The most potentially serious problem is that of aspiration pneumonia. Aspiration has been variously reported as occurring in 4–74% of patients.[131–133] The different rates reported are due to the differences in the sensitivity of the methods employed, and the type of patients studied. Ibanez *et al.*,[131] using a highly sensitive isotope method that picks up even minor degrees of aspiration, studied the difference in aspiration rate between the supine and the semirecumbent (30–45°) position. Without a nasogastric tube, 50% of supine patients had some aspiration. This was reduced to 12% by semirecumbency. With a 5.5-mm-diameter nasogastric tube in place, the aspiration rate in the supine position rose to 81%, compared with 35% in the semirecumbent position. It is not clear whether rates of aspiration would have been reduced by narrower bore tubes, used in many units. Another important study, by Strong *et al.*,[132] using physical signs and chest radiograph, showed an aspiration rate of 30–40% of patients, and also that there was no improvement when nasoduodenal rather than nasogastric tubes were used. Another study, by Mullan and colleagues,[133] again using physical signs supported by chest radiograph, found only a 4.4% aspiration rate and remarked that not only was the condition uncommon but it was also usually benign in its effect. Our own practice is to use a wide-bore tube initially and to infuse 30 mL per hour, aspirating 4-hourly to ensure that gastric emptying is taking place. Once this is established, the tube is replaced by a fine-bore tube and the feed administered at gradually increasing rates. Much is made of the osmolality of feeds, and it has been suggested that a dilute feed should be used initially. It is, however, moles delivered per unit time rather than per unit volume that is important, and a slowly delivered feed is swiftly diluted by the large volume of gastrointestinal juice. Contaminated feeds have been reported as a cause of significant infection in enterally fed patients.[128,129] It is important, therefore, particularly for intensive care patients, to use sterile feeds straight from the container and to change the reservoir and giving set each day. Metabolic complications are unusual, provided that an appropriate feed is given and fluid balance is maintained. Hyperosmolar states have been reported, due to inadequate water intake, excess nitrogen administration, or excess carbohydrate in glucose-intolerant patients.

Parenteral feeding

When Wretlind introduced his amino acid solution, Aminosol, and his fat emulsion, Intralipid, in the 1950s, he designed the feeds to be isotonic and to be given via a peripheral vein. Because fat emulsions were unavailable in the USA, concentrated glucose was the only energy source available for intravenous feeding. It was the contribution of Dudrick *et al.*[134] to introduce Aubaniac's method of central venous catheterization to parenteral feeding, and this is the standard method now adopted throughout the world, although, with improved technique, there has been a swing back to peripheral vein feeding in some centers.[135]

This method, of course, requires that the patient has adequate and accessible peripheral veins. New techniques, using fine pediatric Silastic cannulae, nitrate patches to dilate the vein, and heparin with hydrocortisone to prevent thrombophlebitis, have allowed the use of the same catheter site for many days whereas, previously, the cannula had to be re-sited every 24–48 h. It is not yet clear whether, with the new cannulae, the use of hydrocortisone and heparin is strictly necessary. Central venous catheterization via the jugular, or via the subclavian, is a technique that is too well known to warrant repeating here. For details of the technique, the reader is referred to appropriate texts.[136] Some points, however, need emphasis. A low level of mechanical complications at the time of insertion depends very much on the skill and experience of the operator. It has been the custom in our nutrition team to confine the insertion of lines to two or three doctors with particular experience of the technique. With the use of a strict aseptic technique and protocols, central venous catheters may be safely inserted on the ward. It is not where it is done that matters, but who does it and how it is done.

The development of new plastic materials has greatly improved the complication rate of central lines. The modern polyurethane catheters and the infusion of less hypertonic materials have reduced trauma and thrombosis in the large veins. For long-term feeding (i.e. more than 3 months), we use the slightly wider-bore cuffed Hickman or Broviac lines. The lines are always tunneled, not to prevent infection but to anchor them firmly and prevent displacement. The addition of a small extension tubing allows the changing of giving sets to take place well away from the insertion site. If possible, lines should be dedicated to feeding and not used for other purposes, although this is an ideal that is sometimes difficult to achieve in unstable patients in the intensive care unit. Trials have shown that the use of triple-lumen lines does not really reduce the infection rate when they are used for multiple purposes.[137] Such devices may be convenient, but it must recognized that they are likely to become infected and withdrawn within 7–14 days. The alternative is to have one line dedicated to feeding and a second line on the opposite side for other purposes. Apart from the skill and meticulous care of the operator who inserts the line, the success of intravenous feeding depends crucially upon the subsequent nursing management. No one, not even medical staff, should be allowed to touch the line apart from the nurses who have been specially trained in the protocols required. By adopting this policy, in our own and in other centers, a catheter sepsis rate of zero in the nutrition ward has been achieved, whereas in the intensive care unit it is running at about 5%.[3] Careful audit over the years has allowed us to modify our protocols so that, with prolonged postoperative feeding, the catheter entry sites are cleaned and dressed and the giving set is changed only once per week, without any increase in complications and with a considerable reduction in costs.[3] In the intensive care unit, especially if lines are used for more than one purpose, changes of giving set and site dressing may need to be more frequent. New techniques in the pharmacy have also contributed to improved efficiency.

Following the pioneering work of Solassol and Joyeux in France,[138] it has become possible to mix glucose, amino acids, fat emulsions, and micronutrients in a single large plastic bag and for the resulting mixture to be stable over several days. This is not only much more convenient than the multiple bottle technique used previously but also greatly reduces both the demands on nursing time and the opportunities for introducing infection. This "big bag" all-in-one technique is now accepted generally as the method of choice.

Content of feed

In contrast with enteral feeding, amino acid rather than protein solutions are much more effective. Some of the earlier hydrolysates contained peptides, and recent work has shown that these are not only effective but, as described above, also allow the delivery of important but relatively insoluble or unstable amino acids such as cystine and glutamine.[139] Although the amino acids should be included in the calculation of total energy intake, most of this is supplied in the form of glucose solutions and fat emulsions in roughly equicaloric proportions. This allows the avoidance of carbohydrate overload with the consequences described above, and recognizes the fact that, in sepsis, fat may be oxidized preferentially.[140,141] Both the response to injury and diabetes are associated with glucose intolerance, which may necessitate either reducing the rate of carbohydrate administration or the use of insulin, guided by the algorithm described by Woolfson.[142] The majority of stable patients can be fed with a standard feed, an example of which is shown in Table 65.5. Requirements for micronutrients and minerals are better understood,[143] and excellent preparations are available commercially. The provision of nutrients or the amounts of water and electrolytes and minerals may have to be varied according to clinical circumstances, as described above.

Complications[144]

The subject of preventing catheter infections has already been addressed. If the patient develops a fever and catheter sepsis is suspected, it is important to take blood cultures through the line as well as peripherally. The line is then heparin locked and systemic antibiotic therapy with vancomycin and netilmicin is commenced, pending catheter culture results. If *Staphylococcus epidermidis* (the usual contaminant) is identified, the line can be sterilized using antibiotic. If *Staphylococcus aureus* or fungi are identified, the line should always be removed. Fibrinous obstructions of the line can usually be cleared with a urokinase lock, but, if in doubt, remove the catheter and replace it. Venous thrombosis is now uncommon in short-term feeding.

Lack of stimulation of the gall bladder results in the formation of sludge and gall stones, which may present problems with prolonged intravenous feeding. This can be prevented by the intermittent use of cholecystokinin or by the infusion of fatty food into the duodenum. Excess carbohydrate or total calorie loads may also be associated with abnormalities of liver function tests, fatty liver, and cholestasis. Amino acids, a balance of fat and carbohydrate, and the avoidance of overfeeding are protective. Intra-abdominal sepsis is frequently associated with abnormal liver function tests. The finding of such abnormalities does not constitute a reason for stopping the feeding, but should stimulate a review of the feeding prescription. With appropriate prescription of feeds and adequate monitoring, other metabolic complications are infrequent. In stable patients, regular weighing, fluid balance charts, and once- or twice-weekly hematology and biochemical screening are usually sufficient, although more frequent measurements may be required in the intensive care unit.

NUTRITIONAL PHARMACOLOGY

This extremely important subject can only be summarized briefly here, and the reader is urged to keep abreast of the rapidly growing literature in the field.[145–147] First, it may be described as the use of techniques that modify the metabolic response to injury and therefore reduce the nutritional requirements of patients below those described in the past. Examples of this are the use of epidural analgesia per- and postoperatively,[144] as well as nursing in a warm environment, control of infection, proper fluid replacement, and improved techniques of anesthesia and surgery. Second, and more commonly, this term refers to physiologic substrates or hormones with nutritional support in amounts in excess of normal physiologic requirements in order to produce a specific effect in one or more organs.

Special substrates

Special substrates may be administered singly by the oral, enteral, or parenteral route, or combined in so-called immune-enhancing diets.[77,145] One of the problems in interpreting the results of studies using a combination of substrates is to determine which of them has been responsible for beneficial or other effects. The beneficial effects or otherwise of each substrate may also vary according to the phase of illness. At the peak of acute inflammation, substrates which act as precursors for inflammatory cytokines or for nitric oxide could theoretically produce harmful effects, despite their immunomodulatory properties, although at a later stage of the illness their immune-enhancing properties may be beneficial. We may begin to see more sophisticated combinations of these substrates to be used at different phases of the natural history of disease. Following trauma and surgery, intracellular and extracellular levels of glutamine fall, making it conditionally essential because of its importance in the metabolism of intestinal mucosa and immune cells. Similarly, L-arginine acts as a precursor for nitric oxide. These two amino acids can stimulate a variety of host defenses, modulate tumor cell metabolism, increase wound healing, and reduce nitrogen losses after trauma.[146] The ketoanalog of glutamine, α-ketoglutarate, has been combined with ornithine (convertible to arginine) to raise glutamine levels, improve nitrogen balance, and support resistance to infection. Its use in burned patients not only improves nutritional parameters, but also improves healing.[148] Improved growth in undernourished children has also been demonstrated.[149] Glutamine in parenteral nutrition has shown benefit in critical care[84] and also following bone marrow transplantation and burns.[150] Nucleotides have theoretical benefits but there is no evidence for their clinical efficacy. ω-3 fatty acids prevalent in fish oils may have beneficial anti-inflammatory effects, whereas ω-6 fatty acids may be proinflammatory. The properties and uses of these in patients have been extensively reviewed elsewhere.[145] ω-3 fatty acids on their own have been used successfully to reduce inflammation and in combination as part of immune-enhancing diets. They are also being introduced into lipid emulsions for parenteral use. The role of micronutrients and antioxidants in this context has been reviewed recently and is, as yet, uncertain.[151] Creatine and β-adrenergic agents have anabolic properties in muscle but their role in patients is untested.

Hormones[147]

Somatostatin preparations, e.g. octreotide, are of value in blocking the hormonal stimulus to upper gastrointestinal secretions and reducing the volumes of gastric aspirate or output from small bowel or pancreatic fistulae, thereby reducing the requirement for fluid replacement.

Growth hormone, insulin, and other growth factors have been used for their anabolic effects on protein metabolism. Although the use of growth hormone in some critically ill adult patients has been associated with increased mortality, protein economy and wound healing have been improved without adverse effects in adults and children with burns.[147] The use of insulin to reduce protein catabolism was described many years ago[152,153] and reinvestigated more recently by Sakurai *et al.*,[154] who showed, in catabolic patients, a specific effect to stimulate amino acid uptake by muscle cells, increasing their intracellular content and enhancing protein synthesis. Insulin was also shown to cause salt and water diuresis in fluid overloaded burned patients[155] as well as in those with diuretic-resistant heart failure.[156] High-dose insulin to maintain normoglycemia has recently been shown to improve outcome in critical illness.[157,158]

ETHICAL AND LEGAL ASPECTS[159–161]

Clinical decision making and actions in nutritional support as well as other fields are increasingly being influenced by ethical considerations of beneficence, nonmaleficence, and autonomy and justice, as well as the law. Important recent cases in the courts have involved withholding or withdrawing fluid or nutritional support. The three publications referred to review most important aspects of the subject and are recommended reading.

INTEGRATED NUTRITIONAL SUPPORT[162–165]

As this chapter has emphasized, nutrition is only part of a protocol of integrated care, since each intervention affects nutrition, and nutrition in turn affects function in several organ systems, and, hence, the need for or response to other treatment, e.g. antibiotics. Salt and water excess, for example, not only increase respiratory and other complications,[162] but impair return of gastrointestinal function and the ability to eat postoperatively.[163] Opiates cause similar problems.

A good example of the integrated approach is the evidence-based Enhanced Recovery after Surgery (ERAS) program developed for colorectal surgery by Scandinavian surgeons.[164] This includes preoperative assessment, an oral glucose load[165] within 4 h preoperatively, epidural analgesia,[69] and both oral intake and early mobilization within 24 h of surgery. Nasogastric tubes are avoided unless absolutely necessary and intravenous fluids are kept to a minimum.

Examples

A few examples may help to illustrate some of the practical points discussed in this chapter.

Example 1

A 55-year-old obese woman, weighing 80 kg, was admitted to hospital complaining of a week's history of increasing muscle weakness. A diagnosis of Guillain–Barré syndrome was made and, because of increasing difficulty in breathing due to muscle weakness, the patient was transferred to the intensive care unit for artificial ventilation, which, from our knowledge of the disease, we expected to last for several weeks. Swallowing would therefore be difficult, although the gastrointestinal tract would continue to function. The patient was initially overweight but, although this might be some protection against starvation, it would not prevent the catabolic effects of the disease upon her lean body mass. Muscle wasting would also be exacerbated by the neuropathy and by immobilization.

From the equations in Table 65.1, her basal metabolic rate was calculated to be 6200 kJ (1490 kcal) per day. In view of the fact that she had a modest degree of catabolism and was immobile, her energy requirements for maintenance should lie between 1 and 1.3 times the estimated basal metabolic rate (BMR), i.e. approximately 1600 kcal per day.

A nasogastric tube was passed, and first 30 mL and then 60 mL of water were infused; 4-hourly aspiration produced only 50 mL in 4 h, and adequate gastric emptying was therefore presumed. The tube was then replaced by a fine-bore feeding tube and an enteral feed containing 4.2 kJ (1 kcal) per milliliter was administered, initially at a rate of 30 mL per hour, increasing until 1600 mL per day was achieved. The patient was nursed in a semirecumbent position to minimize reflux, and the feed given for 8-h periods with a gap of up to 4 h in between.

Example 2

A young man was admitted with acute asthma of such severity as to require ventilation. It seemed likely from previous experience that this would be necessary for only 24–48 h before his bronchospasm responded to medical treatment. It was likely, therefore, that he would be back on a normal oral intake within a few days, and no nutritional support needed to be considered.

Example 3

A woman of 23 years with a 2-year history of ulcerative colitis developed a severe exacerbation, during which she lost 15% of her body weight and failed to respond to medical treatment. Abdominal distension and discomfort was observed, with continuing blood-stained diarrhea. It was considered that she was in danger of perforation, and, rather than giving preoperative nutritional support, she was taken to the operating room for emergency colectomy, with the intention of giving intravenous feeding postoperatively. However, on the second postoperative day she began to take fluids by mouth and appeared well and apyrexial. It was therefore decided to monitor her oral intake over the next few days and to ensure that it reached adequate level, not only for maintenance but also to restore lost body tissue. Full restoration of lean body mass and full restoration of physical fitness were likely to take between 2 and 3 months.

Example 4

A man of 28 years, weighing 65 kg and previously fit, suffered 40% full-thickness burns and inhaled toxic fumes, resulting in respiratory failure shortly after admission. Ventilatory support was necessary for a period of 3 weeks before recovery, and for the first week an ileus was present. In view of his catabolic state and the likelihood that he would be unable to take food by mouth for more than 10 days, no time was wasted following the shock phase in starting nutritional support intravenously. From the formulae in Table 65.1, his basal metabolic rate was calculated as 7000 kJ (1665 kcal) per day. Although he was immobilized on a ventilator, he had major burns with pulmonary complications. Although, ideally, the metabolic rate of such patients should be measured for accurate balance, a practical approach was taken, assuming his requirements to be 1.5 times the estimated BMR, i.e. 10 000 kJ (2400 kcal) per day. The nitrogen intake would need to be at the upper end of the range, i.e. 0.25–0.3 g per kg per day. The upper figure was chosen to give 19.5 g of nitrogen, or 120 g of protein a day. Because he had an ileus, intravenous feeding was necessary, and a central line was passed. Using the prescription in Table 65.5 as a basis, 4180 kJ (1000 kcal) could be found from 500 mL of 20% fat emulsion, the nitrogen intake from 1.5 L of the amino acid solution gave 21 g of nitrogen and an additional 2110 kJ (504 kcal), whereas the 1 L of 26% glucose would make up the total to 10 500 kJ (2504 kcal), which was near enough to the estimated target.

Despite an apparently adequate intake being maintained for the 3 weeks in the intensive care unit, the patient was returned to the burns unit suffering from muscle wasting and weakness. This was mistakenly assumed to be metabolic in origin, whereas it was almost certainly mechanical and had resulted from being paralyzed on a ventilator for 3 weeks. An attempt was made to reverse this by a high-nitrogen nasogastric feed – apparently given with insufficient water, for the patient developed a rising blood urea and a hyperosmolar syndrome. This resolved rapidly when the nitrogen intake was reduced and the water intake was increased. Adequate oral intake was resumed soon after this, and the patient made an uninterrupted recovery.

Example 5

A 70-year-old woman of normal weight (45 kg) had lost 12 kg in weight following a laparotomy, complicated by intra-abdominal sepsis and prolonged inability to eat. For convenience, she was given the standard intravenous feed shown in Table 65.5 but, in the middle of the night, she developed shortness of breath, which was mistakenly diagnosed as pulmonary embolus. The diagnosis became clear when the appropriate calculation showed that this patient was receiving 290 kJ kg^{-1} (69 kcal kg^{-1}), more than twice her estimated requirement. Apart from the effect of this caloric load, which increased her metabolic rate, she was receiving glucose 5.2 kg min^{-1}. The combined effect of these was to increase the demands for gas exchange, so that with her weakened respiratory muscles the sensation of shortness of breath became intolerable. The moral of this story is that the calculation should be made at the beginning.

Example 6

A 60-year-old woman of normal weight (50 kg) developed bowel symptoms, losing 3 kg in weight. A sigmoid carcinoma was resected but anastomotic breakdown led to postoperative intra-abdominal sepsis and colonic fistula. Three weeks postoperatively she had received no food by mouth and only dextrose and salt solutions intravenously. Her weight had fallen to 46 kg, but she was noted to be extremely edematous with a serum albumin of 18 g L^{-1}. From this picture and clinical evidence, it was concluded that she had a reduced plasma volume but with an expanded interstitial fluid volume. It was also estimated that, with the edema, her true weight was near 40 kg, giving a total weight loss of 20%. Accordingly, salt-free albumin and frusemide (furosemide) were given intravenously, a central venous catheter was inserted, and a low-salt feed was begun. Her BMR was calculated using an estimated real weight of 40 kg to be 4250 kJ (1016 kcal) per day. She was bedbound, which probably canceled out the metabolic effect of her raised temperature of 38 °C. Because the aim at this stage was not only to improve function but to gain tissue, it was decided to give a total energy intake of just over 1.5 times her resting BMR using parenteral nutrition consisting of 2 L of salt-free solution containing 12 g of nitrogen, 4180 kJ (1000 kcal) from fat emulsion, and 2500 kJ (600 kcal) from glucose. During the first 10 days, there was a steady fall in weight and rise in serum albumin as the excess salt and water load was excreted and fluid was redistributed. Subsequently, after the sepsis had been treated and the patient mobilized, the feed was continued and resulted in a continuous and steady real tissue weight gain of 1 kg per week. After 4 weeks, the fistula had resolved and the patient was able to take sufficient by mouth, thereby allowing the central venous catheter to be withdrawn.

SUMMARY AND CONCLUSIONS

Starvation and weight loss are associated with increased morbidity and mortality from disease. Trials of efficacy show benefits from perioperative nutritional support in patients with antecedent weight loss. In major surgery and critical illness, benefits have been shown, particularly from early enteral nutrition in the postoperative or postinjury phase. There is increasing evidence for the use of a special substrates, and even anabolic hormones as an adjunct to nutritional therapy following major trauma and burns. A practical approach to nutritional assessment is described using changes in weight, simple anthropometric measures, and voluntary food intake, combined with functional assessment. With such measurements and a knowledge of the natural history of the disease, a rational decision can be made on when to start nutritional support, which is then carried out in the simplest and most effective way possible. With adequate training, protocols, and care, enteral and parenteral feeding can be carried out in the perioperative period or in the intensive care unit effectively and without undue complications or excessive cost. When things go wrong, it is not usually because of failure to understand the complexities, but because the simple rules have not been observed.

REFERENCES

1. Benedict FG. *A Study of Prolonged Fasting*. Publication No. 203. Washington, DC: Carnegie Inst., 1915.
2. Love G. Weight loss during hunger strike, 1992 (personal communication).
3. Allison SP. The uses and limitations of nutritional support. *Clin Nutr* 1992; **11:** 319–30.
4. Kinney JM. The influence of calorie and nitrogen balance on weight loss. *Brit J Clin Prac* 1988; **42** (Suppl. 63): 114–20.
5. Keys A, Brozek J, Henschel A. *The Biology of Human Starvation*. Minneapolis, MN: University of Minnesota Press, 1988.
6. Russell DM, Pendergast PJ, Darby PL, *et al.* A comparison between muscle function and body composition in anorexia nervosa: the effect of refeeding. *Am J Clin Nutr* 1983; **38:** 229–37.
7. Russell DM, Walker PM, Leiter LA, *et al.* Metabolic and structural changes in muscle during hypocaloric dieting. *Am J Clin Nutr* 1984; **39:** 503–13.
8. Pichard C, Jeejeebhoy KN. Muscle dysfunction in malnourished patients. *Quart J Med* 1988; **260:** 1021–45.
9. Church JM, Choong SY, Hill GL. Abnormalities of muscle metabolism and histology in malnourished patients awaiting surgery: effect of a course of intravenous nutrition. *Br J Surg* 1984; **71:** 563–9.
10. Hill GL. *Disorders of Nutrition and Metabolism in Clinical Surgery*. Edinburgh: Churchill Livingstone, 1992.
11. Arora NS, Rochester DF. Effect of body weight and muscularity on human diaphragm muscle mass, thickness and area. *J Appl Physiol* 1982; **52:** 64–70.
12. Kelsen SG, Ference M, Kapoor S. Effects of prolonged undernutrition on structure and function of the diaphragm. *J Appl Physiol* 1985; **58:** 1354–9.
13. Lewis MI, Sieck GC, Fournier M, Belman MJ. Effect of nutritional deprivation on diaphragm contractility and muscle fibre size. *J Appl Physiol* 1986; **60:** 596–603.
14. Lewis MI, Sieck GC. Effect of acute nutritional deprivation on diaphragm structure and function. *J Appl Physiol* 1990; **68:** 1938–44.
15. Doekel Jr RC, Zwillich CW, Scroggin CH. Clinical semi-starvation: depression of hypoxic ventilatory response. *N Engl J Med* 1976; **295:** 358–61.
16. Kelly SM, Rosa A, Field S, *et al.* Inspiratory muscle strength and body composition in patients receiving total parenteral nutrition therapy. *Am Rev Respir Dis* 1984; **130:** 33–7.
17. Murciano D, Armengauk MH, Rigand D, *et al.* Effect of renutrition on respiratory and diaphragmatic function in patients with severe mental anorexia. *Annu Rev Respir Dis* 1990; **141:** A 547.
18. Bassili HR, Deitel M. Effect of nutritional support on weaning patients off mechanical ventilation. *J Parenteral Enteral Nutr* 1981; **5:** 161–3.
19. Jeejeebhoy KN. Bulk or bounce – the object of nutritional support. *J Parent Gut Nutr* 1988; **12:** 539–49.
20. Bastow MD, Rawlings J, Allison SP. Benefits of supplementary tube feeding after fractured neck of femur: a randomised controlled trial. *Br Med J* 1983; **287:** 1589–92.
21. Winick M (ed.) *Hunger Disease: Studies by the Jewish Physicians in the Warsaw Ghetto*. New York: Wiley, 1979.
22. Shizgal HM. Nutrition and immune function. *Surg Ann* 1981; **12:** 15–29.
23. Chandra RK. Immunity and infection. In: Kinney JM, Jeejeebhoy KN, Hill GL, Owen OE (eds). *Nutrition and Metabolism in Patient Care*. Philadelphia: WB Saunders, 1988: 598–604.
24. Windsor JA, Hill GL. Risk factors for postoperative pneumonia: the importance of protein depletion. *Ann Surg* 1988; **208:** 209–14.
25. Deitch EA, Winterton J, Li M, Berg R. The gut as a portal of entry for bacteremia: role of protein malnutrition. *Ann Surg* 1987; **205:** 681–90.
26. Berg RD. Translocation of indigenous bacteria from the intestinal tract. In: Hentges DJ (ed.). *Human Intestinal Microflora in Health and Disease*. New York: Academic Press, 1983.
27. Fiddian-Green RG. Studies in splanchnic ischaemia and multiple organ failure. In: Maston A, Bulkley G, Fiddian-Green RG, Haglund U (eds). *Splanchnic Ischaemia and Multiple Organ Failure*. London: Edward Arnold, 1989: 339–48.
28. Alexander JW. Nutrition and translocation. *JPEN* 1990; **14** (Suppl): S170–4.
29. Winter TA, Lemmer E, O'Keefe SJD, Ogden JM. The effect of severe undernutrition, and subsequent refeeding on digestive function in human patients. *Eur J Gastroenterol Hepatol* 2000; **12:** 191–6.
30. Levine GM, Deren JJ, Steiger E, Zinno R. Role of oral intake in maintenance of gut mass and disaccharidase activity. *Gastroenterology* 1974; **67:** 975–82.
31. Burke DJ, Alverdy JC, Aoys E, Moss GS. Glutamine supplemented TPN improves gut immune function. *Arch Surg* 1989; **124:** 1396–9.

32. Souba WW, Henskowitz K, Sallourn RM, *et al*. Gut glutamine metabolism. *JPEN* 1990; **14** (Suppl.): S45–50.
33. Alverdy JC, Aoys E, Moss GS. TPN promotes bacterial translocation from the gut. *Surgery* 1988; **104:** 185–90.
34. Moore F, Feliciano D, Andrassy R, *et al*. Enteral feeding reduces postoperative septic complications. *JPEN* 1991; **15** (Suppl.): S22.
35. Little RA and Stoner HB. Effect of injury on the reflex control of pulse rate in man. *Circulatory Shock* 1983; **10:** 161–71.
36. Macdonald IA, Bennett T and Sainsbury R. The effect of a 48-hour fast on the thermoregulatory responses to graded cooling in man. *Clin Sci* 1984; **67:** 445–52.
37. Fellows IW, Macdonald IA, Bennett T, Allison SP. The effect of undernutrition on thermoregulation in the elderly. *Clin Sci* 1985; **69:** 215–22.
38. Mansell PI, Fellows IW, Macdonald IA, Allison SP. Restoration of normal thermoregulation following weight gain in undernourished patients. *Quart J Med* 1990; **76:** 817–29.
39. Studley HO. Percentage of weight loss, a basic indication of surgical risk in patients with chronic peptic ulcers. *J Amer Med Ass* 1936; **106:** 458–60.
40. Windsor JA, Hill GL. Weight loss with physiologic impairment – a basic indication of surgical risk. *Ann Surg* 1988; **207:** 290–6.
41. Windsor JA, Knight GS, Hill GL. Wound healing response in surgical patients: recent food intake is more important than nutritional status. *Br J Surg* 1988; **75:** 135–7.
42. Christiansen T, Kehlet H. Postoperative fatigue and changes in nutritional status. *Br J Surg* 1984; **71:** 473.
43. Schroeder DS, Hill GL. Postoperative fatigue; a prospective physiological study of patients undergoing major abdominal surgery. *Aust NZ J Surg* 1991; **61:** 774–9.
44. Wilkinson AW, Billing BH, Nagy C, *et al*. Excretion of chloride and sodium after surgical operations. *Lancet* 1948; **1:** 640.
45. Moore FD. *Metabolic care of the surgical patient*. Philadelphia, PA: Saunders, 1959.
46. Starker PM, Lasala PA, Askanazi J, *et al*. The influence of preoperative total parenteral nutrition upon morbidity and mortality. *Surg, Gynaecol Obstet* 1986; **162:** 569–74.
47. Clark RG. Postoperative water and sodium metabolism. In: Little RA, Frayn KN (eds). *The Scientific Basis for the Care of the Critically Ill*. Manchester: Manchester University Press, 1986.
48. Sitges-Serra A, Arcas G, Guirao X, Garcia-Domingo M, Gil MH. Extracellular fluid expansion during parenteral refeeding. *Clin Nutr* 1992; **11:** 63–9.
49. Schønheyder F, Heilskov NSC, Olesen K. Isotopic studies on mechanism of negative nitrogen balance produced by immobilization. *Scand J Clin Lab Invest* 1954; **6:** 178–88.
50. Leverve X. Metabolic and nutritional consequences of chronic hypoxia. *Clin Nutr* 1998; **17:** 241–251.
51. McWhirter JP. Pennington CR. Incidence and recognition of malnutrition in hospital. *BMJ* 1994; **308:** 945–8.
52. Lennard-Jones JE, Arrowsmith H, Davison C, *et al*. Screening by nurses and junior doctors to detect malnutrition when patients are first assessed in hospital. *Clin Nutr* 1995; **14:** 336–40.
53. Stephen AD, Beigg CL, Elliot ET, *et al*. Food provision, wastage and intake in elderly hospital patients. *Proc Nutr Soc* 1997; **56:** 220A.
54. Stephen AD, Beigg CL, Elliot ET, *et al*. Food provision, wastage and intake in medial, surgical and elderly hospitalized patients. *Clin Nutr* 1997: **16** (Suppl. 2): 4.
55. Allison SP (ed.) *BAPEN Report. Hospital Food as Treatment*. Maidenhead: British Association for Parenteral and Enteral Nutrition, 1999.
56. Tucker H. Cost containment through nutrition intervention. *Nutrition Reviews* 1996; **54:** 111–21.
57. Koretz RL. Is perioperative support of demonstrated value? Negative. In: Gitnick G (ed.). *Controversies in Gastroenterology*. Edinburgh: Churchill Livingstone, 1984: 253.
58. Koretz RL. Nutritional support: how much for how much? *Gut* 1986; **27:** SI, 85–95.
59. Detzky AS, Baker JP, O'Rourke K, Goel V. Perioperative parenteral nutrition; a meta analysis. *Ann Inter Med* 1987; **107:** 195–203.
60. Satyanarayana R, Klein S. Clinical efficacy of perioperative nutrition support. *Current Opinion in Clinical Nutrition and Metabolic Care* 1998; **1:** 51–8.
61. Veterans Affairs Total Parenteral Nutrition Study Group. Perioperative total parenteral nutrition in surgical patients. *N Engl J Med* 1991; **325:** 525–32.
62. Von Meyenfeldt MF, Meijerink WJHJ, Rouflart MMJ, *et al*. Perioperative nutritional support: a randomised clinical trial. *Clin Nutr* 1992; **11:** 180–6.
63. Hessov I, Ljungqvist O. Perioperative oral nutrition. *Curr Opin Clin Nutr Metab Care* 1998; **1:** 29–33.
64. Ljungqvist O, Nygren J, Thorell A. Modulation of post-operative insulin resistance by pre-operative carbohydrate loading. *Proc Nutr Soc* 2002; **61** (3): 329–36.
65. Bengmark S. Progress in perioperative enteral tube feeding. *Clin Nutr* 1998; **17:** 1–8.
66. Silk DBA, Green CJ. Perioperative nutrition: parenteral versus enteral. *Curr Opin Clin Nutr Metab Care* 1998; **1:** 21–7.
67. Wara P, Hessov I. Nutritional intake after colorectal surgery: a comparison of a traditional and a new postoperative regimen. *Clin Nutr* 1985; **4:** 225–8.
68. Henriksen MG, Hansen HV, Hessov I. Early oral nutrition after elective colorectal surgery. Influence of balanced analgesia and enforced mobilisation. *Nutrition* 1999; 2002; **18**: 263–7.
69. Kehlet H. Modification of responses to surgery and anaesthesia by neural blockade. In: Cousins MJ, Bridenhagh PO (eds). *Clinical Anaesthesia and Management of Pain*. Philadelphia: JB Lippincott, 1987.
70. Rana SK, Bray J, Menzies Gow N, *et al*. Short term benefits of postoperative oral dietary supplements in surgical patients. *Clin Nutr* 1992; **11:** 337–44.
71. Keele AM, Bray MJ, Emery PW, *et al*. Two phase randomised controlled clinical trial of postoperative oral dietary supplements in surgical patients. *Gut* 1997; **40:** 393–99.
72. MacFie J, Palmer D. oral dietary spplements before and after surgery. *Nutrition* 2001; **17** (2): 186.
73. Delmi M, Rapin C-H, Bengoa JM, *et al*. Dietary supplementation in elderly patients with fractured neck of femur. *Lancet* 1990; **335:** 1, 1013–16.
74. Beier-Holgersen R, Boesby S. Influence of postoperative enteral nutrition on postsurgical infections. *Gut* 1996; **39:** 833–35.
75. Heslin MJ, Latkany L, Leung D, *et al*. A prospective randomized trial of early enteral feeding after resection of upper GI malignancy. American Surgical Association Abstract, 1997, 117th Meeting, April 17–19th, Quebec City, Canada.
76. Sharpe MD, Pikul J, Lowdnes R, *et al*. Early enteral feeding (EEF) reduces incidence of early rejection following liver transplantation (Abstract). Joint Congress of Liver Transplantation, London, 1995.
77. Kudsk KA, Minard G, Groce MA, *et al*. A randomized trial of isonitrogenous enteral diets after severe trauma. An immune-enhancing diet reduces septic complications. *Ann Surg* 1996; **224:** 531–43.
78. Lipman TO. Grains or veins. Is enteral nutrition really better than parenteral nutrition? A look at the evidence. *JPEN* 1998; **22:** 167–182.
79. Jensen MB, Hessov I. Randomization to nutritional intervention at home did not improve postoperative function, fatigue or well being. *Br J Surg* 1997; **84:** 113–118.
80. Beattie AH, Prach AT, Baxter JP, Pennington CR. The change in nutritional status after surgery: the influence of oral supplements. *Clin Nutr* 1999; **18** (Suppl. 1): 19.
81. Heyland DK, Macdonald S, Keefe L, Drover JW. Total parenteral nutrition in the critically ill patient; a meta-analysis. *JAMA* 1998; **280:** 2013–19.
82. Berger MM, Spertini F, Shenkin A, *et al*. Clinical, immune and metabolic effects of trace element supplements in burns: a double-bind placebo-controlled trial. *Clin Nutr* 1996; **15:** 94–96.
83. Zaboga GP. Immune enhancing enteral diets: where's the beef. *Crit Care Med* 1996; **26:** 1143–6.
84. Griffiths RD, Jones C, Allan Palmer TE. Six month outcome of critically ill patients given glutamine supplemented parenteral nutrition. *Nutrition* 1997; **13:** 295–302.
85. Elia M. Artificial nutritional support in clinical practice. *J Roy Coll Phys Lond* 1993; **27:** 8–15.
86. Lennard-Jones JE (ed.). King's Fund Report. *A Positive Approach to Nutrition as Treatment*. London: King's Fund Centre, 1992.
87. Sizer T (ed.) *BAPEN Report. Standards and Guidelines for Nutritional Support of Patients in Hospitals*. Maidenhead: British Association for Parenteral and Enteral Nutrition, 1996.
88. ASPEN. Standards for nutrition support: hospitalised patients. *Nutr Clin Pract* 1995; **10:** 208–218.
89. Strattan RJ, Green CJ, Elia M. *Disease Related Malnutrition – An Evidence-based Approach to Treatment*. Oxford: CAB International, 2003.
90. Danish Association for Parenteral and Enteral Nutrition. In: Pedersen AN, Ovesen LM (eds). *Recommendations for Food in Public Institutions in Denmark*. Copenhagen: Danish Ministry of Food and Agriculture, 1999.
91. Clark RG, Karatzas T. Preoperative nutritional status. *Br J Clin Pract* 1988; **42** (Suppl. 63): 2–7.
92. Lehmann AB, Bassey EJ, Morgan K, Dalloso HM. Normal values for

weight, skeletal size and body mass indices in 890 men and women aged over 65 years. *Clin Nutr* 1991; **10:** 18–22.

93. Lobo DN, Bjarnason K, Field J, *et al.* Changes in weight, fluid balance and serum albumin in patients referred for nutritional support. *Clin Nutr* 1999; **18:** 197–201.
94. Hessov I. Detecting deficient energy and protein intake in hospital patients: a simple recording method. *BMJ* 1988; **1:** 1667–8.
95. Hackett AF, Yeung CK, Hill GL. Eating patterns in patients recovering from major surgery: a study in voluntary food intake and energy balance. *Br J Surg* 1979; **66:** 415–18.
96. Meguid MM, Campos ACL, Meguid V, *et al.* IONIP, a criterion of surgical outcome and patient selection for perioperative nutritional support. *Br J Clin Pract* 1988; **63** (Suppl.): 8–14.
97. Stephen AD, Beigg CL, Elliot ET, *et al.* A recipe for improving the nutritional intake in elderly hospital patients. *Proc Nutr Soc* 1998; 57(**3**): 89A.
98. Ödlund-Olin A, Österberg P, Hadell K, *et al.* Energy-enriched hospital food to improve energy intake in elderly patients. *JPEN* 1996; **20:** 93–7.
99. Kondrup J, Bak L, Stenbaek Hansen B, *et al.* Outcomes from nutritional support using hospital food. *Nutrition* 1998; **14:** 319–21.
100. Gall MJ, Grimble GK, Reeve NJ, Thomas SJ. Effect of providing fortified meals and between-meal snacks on energy and protein intake of hospital patients. *Clin Nutr* 1998; **17:** 259–264.
101. Larsson J, Unosson M, Ek A-C, *et al.* Effect of dietary supplement on nutritional status and clinical outcome in 501 geriatric patients – a randomised study. *Clin Nutr* 1990; **9:** 179–84.
102. Potter JM, Roberts MA, Reilly JJ, McColl JH. An evaluation of protein energy supplementation in medically ill admissions to a geriatric unit. *Proc Nutr Soc* 1998; **57:** 88A.
103. Durnin JVGA, Womersley J. Body fat assessed from body density and its estimation from skinfold thickness: measurements on 481 men and women aged from 16–72 years. *Br J Nutr* 1974; **32:** 77–9.
104. Collins JP, McCarthy ID, Hill GL. Assessment of protein nutrition in surgical patients – the value of anthropometrics. *Am J Clin Nutr* 1979; **32:** 1527–30.
105. Bastow MD. Anthropometrics revisited. *Proc Nutr Soc* 1982; **41:** 381.
106. Elia M. Body composition analysis: an evaluation of two component models, multicomponent models and bedside techniques. *Clin Nutr* 1992; **11:** 114–27.
107. Hill GL. Body composition research: implications for the practice of clinical nutrition. *JPEN* 1992; **16:** 197–218.
108. Klidjian AM, Foster KJ, Kammerling RM, *et al.* Relation of anthropometric and dynamometric variables to serious postoperative complications. *Br Med J* 1980; **281:** 899–901.
109. Fleck A. Plasma proteins as nutritional indicators in the perioperative period. *Br J Clin Pract* 1988; **42** (Suppl. 63): 20–4.
110. Burke JF, Wolfe RR, Mullaney CJ, *et al.* Glucose requirements following burn injury. *Ann Surg* 1979; **190:** 274–85.
111. Bursztein S, Elwyn DH, Askanazi J, Kinney JM. *Energy Metabolism, Indirect Calorimetry and Nutrition.* Baltimore, MD: Williams and Wilkins, 1993.
112. Askanazi J, Carpentier YA, Elwyn DH, *et al.* Influence of total parenteral nutrition on fuel utilisation in injury and sepsis. *Ann Surg* 1980; **191:** 40–6.
113. Shaw-Delanty SN, Elwyn DH, Askanazi J, *et al.* Resting metabolic expenditure in injured septic and malnourished adult patients on intravenous diets. *Clin Nutr* 1990; **9:** 305–12.
114. Goran MI, Peters EJ, Herndon DN, Wolfe RR. Total energy expenditure in burned children using the doubly labelled water technique. *Am J Physiol* 1990; **259** (4 Part 1): E576–85.
115. Harris JA, Benedict FG. *A Biometric Study of Basal Metabolism in Man.* Publication No. 279. Washington, DC: Carnegie Institute of Washington, 1919.
116. Schofield WN. Predicting basal metabolic rate, new standards and review of previous work. *Hum Nutr Clin Nutr* 1985; **39C** (Suppl. 1.5): 41.
117. Wright J. TPN and EN in diabetes. *Curr Opin Clin Nutr Metab* 2000; **3:** 5–10.
118. Gauderer MWL, Ponsky JL, Izant RJ. Gastrostomy without laparotomy: a percutaneous endoscopic technique. *J Paediatr Surg* 1980; **15:** 872–5.
119. Ponsky JL, Gauderer MWL. Percutaneous endoscopic gastrostomy: a non-operative technique for feeding gastrostomy. *Gastrointest Endosc* 1981; **27:** 9–11.
120. Park RHR, Allison MC, Lang J, *et al.* Randomised comparison of percutaneous endoscopic gastrostomy and nasogastric tube feeding in patients with persisting neurological dysphagia. *Br Med J* 1992; **304:** 1406–9.
121. Wicks C, Gimson A, Vlavianos P, *et al.* Assessment of the percutaneous endoscopic gastrostomy feeding tube as part of an integrated approach to enteral feeding. *Gut* 1992; **33:** 613–16.
122. Hull MA, Rawlings J, Murray FE, *et al.* An audit of outcome of long-term enteral nutrition using percutaneous endoscopic gastrostomy. *Lancet* 1993; **340:** 869–72.
123. Rombeau JL. Feeding by tube enterostomy. In: *Atlas of Nutritional Support Techniques.* Rombeau JL, Caldwell MD, Forlaw L, Guenter PA (eds). Boston and Toronto: Little Brown, 1989: 107–82.
124. Silk DBA. Towards the optimisation of enteral nutrition. *Clin Nutr* 1987; **6:** 61–74.
125. Jacobs S, Chang RWS, Lee B, *et al.* Continuous enteral feeding: a major cause of pneumonia among ventilated intensive care patients. *JPEN* 1990; **14:** 353–6.
126. Bastow MD, Rawlings J, Allison SP. Overnight nasogastric tube feeding. *Clin Nutr* 1985; **4:** 7–11.
127. Bastow MD. Complications of enteral nutrition. *Gut* 1986; **27(S1):** 51–5.
128. Bastow MD, Greaves P, Allison SP. Microbial contamination of enteral feeds. *Hum Nutr Appl Nutr* 1982; **36A:** 213–17.
129. Casewell MW. Nasogastric feeds as a source of Klebsiella infection for intensive care patients. *Res Clin Forums* 1979; **1:** 101–5.
130. Maynard ND, Bikari DJ. Postoperative feeding. *BMJ* 1991; **303:** 1007–8.
131. Ibanez J, Penafiel A, Raurich JM, *et al.* Gastro-oesophageal reflux in intubated patients receiving enteral nutrition: effect of supine and semi-recumbent positions. *JPEN* 1992; **16:** 419–28.
132. Strong RM, Condon SC, Solinger MR, *et al.* Equal aspiration rates from post-pylorus and intragastric placed small-bore nasoenteric feeding tubes: a randomised prospective study. *JPEN* 1992; **16:** 59–63.
133. Mullan H, Roubenoff RA, Roubenoff R. Risk of pulmonary aspiration among patients receiving enteral nutrition support. *JPEN* 1992; **16:** 160–4.
134. Dudrick SJ, Wilmore DW, Vars HM, *et al.* Long term total parenteral nutrition with growth, development and positive nitrogen balance. *Surgery* 1968; **64:** 134–4.
135. Macfie J, Nordenstrom J. Full circle in parenteral nutrition. *Clin Nutr* 1992; **11:** 237–9.
136. Caldwell MD, Pomp A. In: Rombeau JL, Caldwell MD, Forlaw L, Guenter PA (eds). *Atlas of Nutritional Support Techniques.* Boston: Little Brown, 1989, 193–299.
137. Clark-Christoff N, Watters VA, Sparks W, *et al.* Use of triple-lumen subclavian catheters for administration of total parenteral nutrition. *JPEN* 1992; **16:** 403–7.
138. Solassol C, Joyeux H. In: Fischer JE (ed.). *Total Parenteral Nutrition.* Boston: Little Brown, 1976.
139. Stehle P, Zander J, Mertes N, *et al.* Effect of parenteral glutamine peptide supplements on muscle glutamine loss and nitrogen balance after major surgery. *Lancet* 1989: 231–33.
140. Greenberg GR, Marliss EB, Anderson GH, *et al.* Protein sparing therapy in postoperative patients. *N Engl J Med* 1986; **294:** 1411–16.
141. Nordenstrom J, Askanazi J, Elwyn DH, *et al.* Nitrogen balance during total parenteral nutrition. *Ann Surg* 1983; **197:** 27–33.
142. Woolfson AMJ. An improved method for blood glucose control during nutritional support. *JPEN* 1981; **5:** 436–40.
143. Shenkin A, Fell GS. Micronutrients. In: Woolfson AMJ (ed.). *Biochemistry in Hospital Nutrition.* Edinburgh: Churchill Livingstone, 1986: 83–122.
144. Pennington CR. Parenteral nutrition: the management of complications. *Clin Nutr* 1991; **10:** 133–7.
145. Immunonutrition Symposium. *Nutrition* 1998; **14:** 563–647.
146. Heys SD, Walker LG, Smith I, Eremin O. Enteral nutritional supplementation with key nutrients in patients with critical illness and cancer. A meta-analysis of randomized controlled clinical trials. *Ann Surg* 1999; **229:** 467–477.
147. Proceedings of ASPEN's 23rd Clinical Congress Research Workshop. Anabolic hormones in nutrition support. *JPEN* 1999; **23** (Suppl.).
148. Donati L, Ziegler F, Pongelli G, Signorini MS. Nutritional and clinical efficacy of ornithine α-ketoglutarate in severe burns. *Clin Nutr* 1999; **18:** 307–11.
149. Moukarzel A, Goulet O, Cynober L, Ricour C. Positive effects of ornithine alpha-ketoglutarate in paediatric patients on parenteral nutrition and failure to thrive. *Clin Nutr* 1993; **12:** 59–60.
150. Ziegler TR. L-glutamine enriched parenteral nutrition in catabolic patients. *Clin Nutr* 1993; **12:** 65–6.
151. Shenkin A. Micronutrients in adult nutritional support: requirements and benefits. *Curr Opin Clin Nutr Metab Care* 1998; **1:** 15–19.
152. Hinton P, Allison SP, Littlejohn S, Lloyd J. Insulin and glucose to reduce catabolic response to injury in burned patients. *Lancet* 1971; **1:** 767.
153. Woolfson AMJ, Heatley RV, Allison SP. Insulin to inhibit protein catabolism after injury. *N Engl J Med* 1979; **300:** 14.
154. Sakurai Y, Aarsland A, Herndon DN, *et al.* Stimulation of muscle protein

synthesis by long term insulin infusion in severely burned patients. *Ann Surg* 1995; **222:** 283–297.

155. Hinton P, Allison SP, Littlejohn S, Lloyd J. Electrolyte changes after burn injury and the effect of treatment. *Lancet* 1973; **1:** 218.
156. Allison SP, Morley CJ, burns-Cox CJ. Insulin, glucose and potassium in the treatment of congestive heart failure. *Br Med J* 1972; **3** (828): 675–8.
157. Van den Berghe G, Wouters P, Weeks F, *et al*. Intensive insulin therapy in critically ill patients. *N Engl J Med* 2001; **345** (19): 1359–670.
158. Martinez-Riquelme AE, Allison SP. Insulin revisited. *Clin Nutr* 2003; **22:** 7–15.
159. Lennard-Jones JE. *BAPEN Report. Ethical and Legal Aspects of Clinical Hydration and Nutritional Support*. Maidenhead: British Association for Parenteral and Enteral Nutrition, 1999.
160. Herrmann VM. Nutrition support: ethical or expedient, and who will choose? *JPEN* 1999; **23:** 195–202.
161. MacFie J. Ethical and legal considerations in the provision of nutritional support to the perioperative patient. *Curr Opin Clin Nutr Metab Care* 2000; **3:** 23–9.

66

Ventilator management

PHILIP D LUMB AND LEON D WRIGHT

PRINCIPLES OF MECHANICAL VENTILATION

Periodic inflation of the lungs can maintain life in the absence of spontaneous ventilation. Elisha breathed life into the lungs of the Shunamite woman's son [2Kings IV: 34], and mouth-to-nose resuscitation of the newborn has long been standard practice in animal husbandry. In the 1500s, using the pig and the pregnant canine, Andreas Vesalius[1] demonstrated that it was possible to maintain cardiopulmonary function in an open chest preparation. In order to prevent lung collapse, he cannulated the trachea with the nozzle of a pair of bellows and rhythmically inflated the lungs under positive pressure. He also vividly showed the development of ventricular fibrillation when the lungs were left uninflated, describing cardiac function as "undulating, creeping and distorted."

In 1788, Charles Kite,[2] a surgeon from Gravesend, UK, described bellows resuscitation that involved endotracheal or laryngeal intubation with a metal tube. He used this apparatus to ventilate the drowned, or the apparently drowned, who were rescued from the River Thames. He believed that his method was superior to other commonly employed resuscitation techniques not only because it provided demonstrably improved ventilation, but also because the stomach was less likely to become distended with air. This apparatus appears to have been of vital benefit in artificial ventilation, because mouth-to-mouth resuscitation was the usual method of treating the "apparently dead." When mouth-to-mouth resuscitation was being used, he recommended prophylactic pressure on the cricoid cartilage ("upper-most ring of the trachea") to avoid air being blown down the esophagus.

In the 1880s, enhanced surgical expectation, stimulated by greatly improved outcome from abdominal surgical procedures, prompted attempts to invade the thoracic cavity. Rudolph Matas[3] summarized the technical problems involved as follows: "while great progress has been accomplished in a better appreciation and control of septic conditions and better results have been obtained from this reason alone, the dangers from pneumothorax remain practically an unchanged factor in the mortality." He continued to opine that "until the risk of seriously interfering with respiratory function by inducing acute collapse of the lung is clearly eliminated, or is reduced to a safe minimum, the analogy between the pleura and the peritoneum will never exist."[3] His suggestion was to use the laboratory technique of artificial ventilation as a method of maintaining the patient's respiration during intrathoracic procedures. Toward the end of the nineteenth century, artificial ventilation had become established laboratory practice, often facilitated with the use of curare, as it seemed to give so much more satisfactory "anesthesia" than chloroform, which stopped the canine heart, or ether, which could cause a dog to vomit for days. The development of the modern anesthetic machine, and the introduction of cuffed endotracheal tubes by Magill after World War I, led to endotracheal intubation and, initially, manual ventilation becoming the standard method of overcoming the "pneumothorax problem."

In the 1920s, Dr Cecil K Drinker, Professor of Physiology at the Harvard School of Public Health, became involved in the resuscitation of accident victims in the Boston electrical generator and gas-producing plant.[4] With his advice, his brother Philip Drinker[5,6] developed a tank respirator, which was first successfully used in 1929 on a child with bulbar poliomyelitis. This was the beginning of long-term respiratory care, and the apparatus became known as the "iron lung" or negative-pressure ventilator. Negative-pressure ventilation remained the predominant type of ventilation until the mid-1950s. The patient was placed inside a metal cylinder with the head exposed, and an airtight collar around the neck sealed the body from atmospheric pressure. When a vacuum was applied to the chamber, the resultant negative pressure caused passive airflow through the open larynx into the lungs. Exhalation was passive and resulted when the vacuum was released and chamber pressure returned to atmospheric. A modification of the technique, the cuirass ventilator, applied negative external pressure to the rib cage only in order to induce inspiratory flow.[7] It was hoped that the cuirass would be more easily applied and permit nursing care and other access to the patient. Initially these ventilators used a hard shell, hence the name, which was later replaced with a flexible shell to improve patient comfort. In general, negative-pressure ventilators are bulky and poorly tolerated, and have not been proven to be effective for patients with end-stage chronic obstructive pulmonary disease (COPD),[8-10] although newer modifications of the cuirass device are useful for some chronic, home ventilation applications. Modern application of negative-pressure ventilation may include support for those patients with tracheomalacia or for whom placement of cuffed endotracheal tubes is contraindicated.

EARLY VENTILATORS IN ANESTHESIA

The stimulus of open thoracic surgery, with its requirement for positive-pressure ventilation to maintain lung expansion, stimulated the clinical use of muscle relaxants. The tedium and inefficiency of hand ventilation during long operations led to the development of the mechanical anesthetic ventilator in the 1930s and 1940s.[4] Initially these were pressure limited, but soon "bag-in-bottle," volume-cycled varieties emerged on both sides of the Atlantic. European anesthesiologists began to use and appreciate controlled ventilation; their American counterparts were wedded to "assisted respiration" in a nonparalyzed patient. The concept that the educated hand of a trained anesthesiologist squeezing the bag just as the patient inspired was superior to controlled mechanical ventilation was strongly believed and taught by some to be a better method of maintaining pulmonary function, especially when muscle relaxants were not used. The abolition of spontaneous breathing necessitating mechanical ventilation was feared, despite the documented acidosis that frequently occurred in these patients. This practice was not surprising considering that some anesthesiologists believed that *d*-tubocurarine was a diaphragm-sparing muscle relaxant and that patients would tolerate assisted spontaneous, diaphragmatic ventilation, despite peripheral neuromuscular blockade. Another and more appropriately based fear was the explosive danger inherent in using cyclopropane and ether in the presence of electrically driven mechanical devices. This situation was overcome with the development of nonelectric, nonspark-producing, pneumatically powered ventilators for use in the operating room. Mechanical ventilators timed by fluidic logic boards became ubiquitous in operating rooms in which flammable anesthetic agents were used. Positive-pressure ventilation was the most logical method for providing controlled ventilation for surgery because of the problems associated with negative-pressure ventilation, most specifically related to equipment characteristics and resultant lack of surgical access.

THE COPENHAGEN POLIO EPIDEMIC (1952)

The poliomyelitis epidemic of 1952 created a medical crisis in Scandinavia. In Copenhagen, at the height of the epidemic, 50–60 new cases requiring mechanical ventilatory support were diagnosed every day.[11] There were an inadequate number of negative-pressure ventilators ("iron lungs") available to cope with the emergency requirement for such a large number of patients. A multidisciplinary team was established under the leadership of Bjorn Ibsen, an anesthesiologist familiar with ventilating paralyzed surgical patients with positive-pressure techniques, to respond to the problem. With Lassen (an epidemiologist) and Astrup, who provided the laboratory back-up, the first multidisciplinary intensive care unit was established specifically to provide acute ventilatory support. Their work and success established the basis for care of the patient with respiratory failure needing mechanical ventilatory support.[12] Ibsen, Lassen, and Astrup defined the multidisciplinary team; an anesthesiologist, an epidemiologist, and an ear, nose, and throat surgeon working with help from an excellent and capable STAT laboratory. Later, radiologists and physiotherapists were incorporated into the Copenhagen team. Today, the modern multidisciplinary intensive care unit (ICU) team is composed of critical care nurses, subspecialty trained physicians from several core disciplines, pharmacists, epidemiologists, respiratory therapists, consultant and primary care physicians, and a myriad of other individuals. Their collaboration is responsible for creating the requisite environment necessary to insure a positive outcome for patients with complex diseases.

It was during similar epidemics that recurred in 1953 and even more virulently in 1954 that positive-pressure ventilation, which had recently been introduced,[13] became the method of choice to support patients with respiratory failure. Tank ventilators were abandoned because there were not enough of them, they were cumbersome, and they limited access to the patient, thereby prohibiting necessary nursing and medical care and increasing patient morbidity and mortality. The improved clinical results obtained with positive-pressure ventilation were a great tribute to Bjorn Ibsen and his team. They not only reduced the mortality of bulbar poliomyelitis from 80% to 25% but also established the practice for the critical care management of the acutely ill patient in use today. The experience of the Copenhagen team quickly led to the adoption of positive-pressure ventilation through a cuffed endotracheal or tracheotomy tube as the standard means for managing the patient with respiratory failure throughout Europe and the British Commonwealth. The USA did not follow the same path and continued using tank ventilators until about 1960.

Positive-pressure ventilators operate by providing a cyclic, greater than atmospheric pressure to the upper airway, usually through a cuffed endotracheal or tracheotomy tube. The positive (superatmospheric) pressure gradient created between the upper airway and lungs pushes gas through the airways. Conventional positive-pressure ventilation is identified with respiratory rates up to 60 breaths per minute. Rates higher than 60 breaths per minute are designated as high-frequency positive-pressure ventilation (HFPPV).

The first positive-pressure ventilators were designed to inflate the lungs until a preset pressure was reached; this was termed pressure-cycled ventilation. For any given pressure, the generated tidal volume and peak inspiratory flow varied with the impedance of the respiratory system. The earliest ventilators delivered preset tidal volumes at a selected rate. Pressure and volume were generated irrespective of patient effort, and muscle relaxants were commonly employed to minimize patient–ventilator disharmony. Clinical practice supported the use of large tidal volume ventilation with intermittent "sighs" (a supernormal tidal volume of 15–25 $mL\,kg^{-1}$); the nonparalyzed patient better tolerated this ventilatory strategy, probably because lung J-receptors were appropriately stimulated. An early modification to controlled mechanical ventilators incorporated negative-pressure sensors in the inspiratory limb, which enabled the patient's inspiratory effort to trigger the predetermined positive-pressure gas flow. This design was intended to provide synchronized mechanical assistance coincident with the patient's spontaneous respiratory efforts. In a lung with normal or constant compliance, the change in volume as a result of a change in pressure is predictable, and a preset inflation pressure generates the same lung volume over successive breaths. However, an increase in impedance changes the relation between pressure and volume and may produce a fall in minute ventilation with resultant CO_2 retention and possible hypoxemia. Pressure-controlled ventilation is, therefore, limited by changes in the mechanical properties of the lungs.[14–18] When lung compliance decreases, constant pressure generates a lower tidal volume. Conditions that decrease tidal volume are poorly compliant lungs or chest wall, reduced inspiratory effort, or increased airway resistance. Volume-cycled ventilation delivers a constant alveolar volume despite changes in the mechanical properties of the lungs (compliance). The lung is inflated with a constant flow rate, which produces a linear increase in lung volumes.[19–21] However, the lung volume increase is often obtained at the expense of requiring high peak inflation pressures. Pressure-limited ventilation is believed to minimize mechanical ventilator induced barotrauma, the development of pneumothorax, pneumomediastinum, subcutaneous emphysema, pneumatocele or any collection of extra-alveolar air. For a number of years, discussion focused on safety issues with respect to pressure-limited vs. volume-cycled ventilation. It was felt that the higher peak inflation pressures generated by volume-cycled devices caused pulmonary barotrauma. Recent opinion favors the theory that barotrauma is more likely caused by alveolar overdistension (excessive stretch), repetitive alveolar opening and closing, or excessive stress at the margin between aerated and atelectatic regions, rather than by overpressure as reflected in the peak inflation pressure. This is borne out by earlier experiments in which animals were ventilated at high peak pressures while chest wall expansion, and thus alveolar distension, was controlled by placing restrictive casts around the chest wall.[22–24] The resulting high pressures were not associated with a significant increase in barotrauma, supporting overdistension as the likely inciting event. Also, Macklin and Macklin[25] described the probable mechanism of mechanical ventilation-induced pneumothorax as overdistension resulting in rupture of alveolar walls adjacent to pulmonary vessels. Gas enters the peribronchial sheath and proceeds to proximal dissection into the mediastinum. Mediastinal gas can then rupture through the pleura, causing pneumothorax. This mechanism appeals logically because high inflation pressures have not been reproduced in the alveoli, and alveolar anatomy favors overdistension with resultant gas extravasation along neurovascular bundles as the proximate cause of barotrauma.

During volume-cycled ventilation, pressure in the proximal airway initially increases abruptly. This is followed by a gradual incremental and continuous pressure rise throughout the remainder of lung inflation. The relation between pressure and flow is a product of alveolar elastance. Pressure in individual alveoli demonstrates only a gradual increase throughout inflation. The initial abrupt increase in pressure (peak airway pressure) is the result of flow resistance in the proximal airways and gas delivery system including the ventilator tubing and endotracheal or tracheotomy tube. An increase in airway resistance increases the initial rise in airway pressures, and higher inflation pressures are required to deliver the desired inflation volume. Changes in the mechanical properties of lungs that result in increased inflation pressures are atelectasis, edema, or bronchoconstriction. Alveoli are not exposed to these higher pressures if lung compliance is normal. If lung compliance (distensibility) decreases, the alveoli will be exposed to the higher pressures, and both alveolar and proximal airway pressures will be increased. The increase in alveolar pressure in noncompliant lungs can lead to pressure-induced lung injury. In order to match more closely the inflation pattern to compliance changes, most ventilators permit several inspiratory flow patterns ranging from sine wave, increasing or decreasing ramp, and square wave patterns, all with constant gas flow throughout the inspiratory cycle. Few data exist that support use of defined flow patterns in specific disease states, and recently ventilator usage algorithms have been developed in an attempt to create rational plans for managing complex patients.

Positive-pressure ventilation has an influence on right and left ventricular preload and afterload.[26] Transmural pressure, the pressure across the vessel wall, is determined by the difference in alveolar pressure and pulmonary capillary hydrostatic pressure. Transmural pressure determines the preload and afterload of the ventricles. In normal lung tissue, an increase in intrathoracic pressure will not affect transmural pressure because the increase in alveolar pressure is completely transmitted into the pulmonary capillaries. When lung compliance decreases, external alveolar pressure increase and subsequent increases in pulmonary capillary hydrostatic pressure result in an increase in the transmural pressure, i.e. the pressure measured across the vessel wall. This results in an increase in extravascular lung water or interstitial pulmonary edema. Pathologic conditions associated with this type of lung injury are pulmonary edema and pneumonia.

Positive intrathoracic pressure decreases preload as a result of increased pressure on the outer surface of the heart, compression of pulmonary vessels, and reduced right heart filling. The dilated right ventricle pushes against the interventricular septum, reducing the size of the left ventricle, a phenomenon known as ventricular interdependence. The ventricular compression that results during positive-pressure ventilation impedes diastolic filling, and cardiac output will decrease when positive-pressure ventilation impedes venous return and biventricular volumes during diastole.

The same compression that impedes right ventricular diastolic filling will facilitate left ventricular emptying during systole. The afterload, or impedance to ventricular emptying, is a function of systolic transmural pressure, and increasing the transmural pressure produces a greater pressure gradient, thereby facilitating ejection. The increase in the pressure gradient will overcome impedance or afterload, if ventricular filling is not decreased by positive-pressure ventilation. Thus, there is an increased cardiac output only if preload is maintained or increased. In summary, right ventricular preload is reduced and afterload is increased during positive-pressure ventilation, the former because increased intracardiac pressure impedes diastolic filling. Concomitantly, by expanding alveoli to a greater volume than normally encountered, mechanical ventilation effectively stretches the pulmonary capillary bed, thereby decreasing its cross-sectional area and increasing its resistance proportionately. This results in increased resistance to right ventricular ejection. Conversely, the afterload to the left ventricle is decreased because the increased transmural pressure is relatively greater than that (seen by the ventricle) in the abdomen. This effectively reduces the impedance to left ventricular ejection. These findings support volume augmentation during initiation of mechanical ventilation, especially following administration of negative inotropes and vasodilators (e.g. anesthetic agents).

Initially, large lung volumes were employed in an attempt not only to prevent alveolar collapse,[27] but also to increase comfort in the conscious mechanically ventilated patient. Prior to the advent of mechanical ventilators that permitted spontaneous ventilation, patients required heavy sedation in order to tolerate controlled mechanical ventilation. Ventilation with large tidal volumes and sighs were tolerated better and permitted patient management with less sedation. Theoretically, this may be explained by excitation of the lung stretch or J-receptors. These receptors are understimulated at lower tidal volumes, causing a sensation of air hunger despite adequate minute ventilation. Over a period of time, large tidal volume ventilation became the standard of care. Routine tidal volumes were set at 10–15 $mL\,kg^{-1}$ during volume-cycled ventilation. Additions of sigh breaths increased the volume further (15–30 $mL\,kg^{-1}$, 6–12 times per hour). Recently, recommendations have been established for "lung-protective ventilation," which uses a lower tidal volume in an attempt to minimize pulmonary barotrauma secondary to excessive alveolar distension, repetitive alveoli opening and closing, or excessive stress at the margin between aerated and atelectatic regions. Table 66.1 compares the two techniques.

Either of these techniques is appropriate for individuals with normal lungs requiring mechanical ventilation during elective surgery. However, the traditional large tidal volume delivery of 10–15 $mL\,kg^{-1}$ (normal adult lung volumes are 5–7 $mL\,kg^{-1}$) can result in hyperinflation of noncollapsed lung segments in patients with acute lung injury or acute respiratory distress syndrome (ARDS). These patients have a smaller aerated volume than those patients with uninjured lungs (termed baby lungs); additional lung volume is recruited utilizing advanced ventilatory techniques including use of the prone position, inhaled nitric oxide, partial liquid ventilation, and inverse ratio ventilation (see below).[28] Inflation volumes are distributed preferentially to regions of normal lung with surfactant activity and, therefore, tend to overinflate the areas of nondiseased lung. The pathologic result is stress tears in the alveolar walls and adjacent pulmonary capillaries resulting from hyperinflation of normal lung tissue.[29,30] The secondary damage to pulmonary capillaries can result in a leaky capillary type of pulmonary edema. Thus, alveolar damage leads to pulmonary interstitial emphysema, pneumomediastinum, or pneumothorax. Alveolar damage can result from excessive pressure or excessive volumes (Bray).

Peak airway pressures should be minimized to reduce the risk of alveolar overdistension, because high airway pressures have been associated with barotrauma. There is a growing consensus that the main determinant of alveolar overdistension is the end-inspiratory lung volume.[31] Lung-protective ventilation reduces lung volumes to 6–8 $mL\,kg^{-1}$ ideal body weight, eliminates the sigh, and uses positive end-expiratory pressure (PEEP) to prevent lung collapse. The goal is to keep plateau pressures below 3.5 kPa (35 cmH_2O). Lower inflation volume can result in CO_2 retention and is termed "permissive hypercapnia." It is not known whether or not sighs are needed to prevent atelectasis during mechanical ventilation with conventional tidal volumes and PEEP. Periodic stretching is thought to stimulate surfactant production and release, thereby preventing atelectasis.[32]

Ventilation parameters	Traditional	Lung protective
Inflation volumes	10–15 mL kg^{-1}	5–8 mL kg^{-1}
Mechanical sighs	Rate 6–12 h^{-1}; 15–30 mL kg^{-1}	None
End inspiration	Peak pressure < 50 mmHg	Plateau pressure < 35 mmHg (Hoppin)
Positive end-expiratory	When needed $F_{I}O_2$ <0.60	5–15 cmH$_2$O
ABG	pH 7.36–7.44	pH 7.20–7.44 hypercapnia

ABG, arterial blood gas. 1 kPa = 7.5 mmHg; 1 kPa = 10 cmH$_2$O.

Table 66.1 *Comparison of "traditional" and "lung-protective" ventilatory techniques*

MONITORS OF PULMONARY MECHANICS

During spontaneous breathing, pulmonary function tests are used to measure the mechanical properties of the lungs. During positive-pressure ventilation proximal airway pressures are used to monitor the mechanical properties of the lungs.[33,34] Peak airway pressure, measured at the inlet to the upper airway, is a function of inflation volume, flow rate, resistance of the mechanical and biologic systems involved, and elastance (the elastic recoil of the lung and chest wall). At constant inflation volume and flow rate (volume ventilation), peak airway pressure becomes a function of resistance and elastance:

$$P_{(\text{peak})} = P_{(\text{res})} + P_{(\text{el})}$$

Plateau pressure or static airway pressure is an elastance function of the lungs and chest wall. No airflow is present during the period of plateau pressure measurement, therefore the derived pressure is not a flow resistance function. When the airway is occluded at end-inspiration, flow falls to zero and the airway pressure drops from peak pressure to elastance pressure (end inflation, or static or, plateau pressure). $P_{(\text{el})}$ represents the static elastic recoil pressure of the respiratory system at end-inflation volume. The difference between peak airway pressure and plateau pressure represents resistance to gas flow and distribution through the lungs. Recovery from acute lung injury may be inferred when peak and plateau pressures begin to approximate one another. Zero end-expiratory pressure (ZEEP) is reached in the absence of pulmonary hyperinflation when alveolar pressure approximates to atmospheric. The elastic recoil of the respiratory system drives passive expiration ($P_{(\text{el})}$). In the presence of either intrinsic lung disease or extrinsic, ventilator circuit applications, ZEEP is not attained and residual alveolar positive pressure may further compromise circulatory function.

PATTERNS OF ASSISTED VENTILATION

Since the development of positive-pressure ventilation during the recurrent poliomyelitis epidemics in the early 1950s, there have been numerous methods of assisted ventilation.[14,35,36] A review of the commonly used methods follows, with indications and contraindications for each application.

Controlled ventilation (CV)

The first and least sophisticated method of positive-pressure ventilation involves intermittent, time-cycled, volume-limited lung inflation. The ventilator delivers a preselected tidal volume at a specified rate (breaths per minute) and inspiratory flow rate and pattern (L min^{-1}), thereby controlling the ratio between inspiration and expiration. The patient neither initiates a breath nor influences operator-selected ventilator settings; this is defined as controlled ventilation (time-cycled initiation of a positive-pressure deflection unresponsive to a patient-initiated negative-pressure deflection). This type of ventilation is used during general anesthesia. The patient is paralyzed to eliminate unsynchronized respiratory effort, to eliminate diaphragmatic movement, to decrease abdominal and thoracic muscular tone, and to decrease peak airway pressure necessary for full lung inflation. Muscle relaxants paralyze proximal airway musculature, thereby decreasing resistance to gas flow and generated peak airway pressure.

Assist control ventilation (ACV)

A pattern of volume-cycled lung inflation during which the patient can initiate a breath (usually triggered by a negative-pressure deflection in the circuit) at which the ventilator delivers the preset volume (positive-pressure deflection) is termed assist control ventilation (ACV). The negative pressure produced by the patient's inspiratory effort opens a pressure-activated valve, enabling the ventilator to deliver the preset machine breath. The ventilator is sensitized to respond to the patient's respiratory effort, measured as a negative pressure in the ventilator circuit. If a negative-pressure deflection is not sensed, the ventilator defaults to a timed ventilatory cycle, ensuring adequate minute ventilation. In the A/C mode, the ventilator assists patient-initiated inspiratory efforts by delivering a preset tidal volume and, in the absence of patient effort, defaults to a volume-cycled, rate-controlled ventilator. Usually the mechanically delivered tidal volumes exceed normal spontaneous breaths, therefore more time is required to empty the lungs following mechanical breaths.[36] The I/E ratio, inspiratory time to expiratory time, is maintained between 1:2 and 1:4. A ratio below 1:2 may not allow the lung to empty completely. Decreasing the inspiratory time will decrease time for lung inflation and may increase peak inflation pressure unnecessarily.

Indications for ACV may include patients with respiratory muscle weakness and a history of left ventricular dysfunction. This mode of ventilation has largely been replaced by more sophisticated techniques developed over the past few years, because of the danger of uncontrolled hyperventilation and auto cycling.

The undesirable effects of ACV are hyperventilation and respiratory alkalosis, which results from the patient's inability to control minute alveolar ventilation (each sensed negative inspiratory effort stimulates delivery of the ventilator tidal volume), an increased work of breathing, and hyperinflation due to inadequate emptying time. Auto-PEEP (or intrinsic PEEP) accompanies alveolar hyperinflation and is a direct result of incomplete emptying of alveolar units. Auto-PEEP increases the inspiratory work required to generate a sensed negative inspiratory pressure. A negative pressure is required to open the pressure-activated valve that initiates the machine breath. The increased work of breathing, as a result of auto-PEEP, is due to the increased effort required to initiate a machine breath.

The contraction of the diaphragm is initiated by the brainstem respiratory neurons that fire in periodic bursts throughout life.[37] During patient-initiated spontaneous respiratory effort, the diaphragm triggers the ventilator and the contraction continues for the duration of the burst activity. With ACV, the diaphragm contracts with each breath, so that the energy expended for breathing is considerable[38] and may approximate to 25% of the patient's metabolic expenditure in some disease states. This is compared with the normal work of breathing of between 3% and 5% of the basal metabolic rate.

Intermittent mandatory ventilation (IMV)

Using this method, periodic volume-cycled breaths at a preset rate are delivered; however, the patient is able to breathe spontaneously between delivered volumes. It is interesting to note that early Engstrom ventilators permitted spontaneous breathing because a "fail-safe" mechanism permitted room air entrainment into the ventilator circuit if pipeline oxygen or air pressure decreased. This provision permitted spontaneous ventilation as well as providing a room air gas source for mechanical ventilation. Its efficacy was not recognized at the time, and the method was formally developed and introduced in 1971 for neonates to address the problem of rapid breathing and associated hyperventilation seen with ACV. The patient was permitted to remain tachypneic without mandatory mechanically assisted tidal volumes per breath. The patient is connected to an oxygen source through two parallel pathways. The circuits consist of a volume-cycled ventilator in parallel with a specially constructed reservoir that supports the high gas delivery flow requirements during spontaneous breathing. The patient-generated negative pressure opens a one-way valve and an effort-dependent tidal volume is extracted from the reservoir circuit. The delivered gas is at the same F_IO_2, humidity, and extrinsic positive end-expiratory pressure as that delivered during the mechanical breaths.

In the absence of spontaneous effort, the ventilator delivers a preset, volume-limited breath to the patient and closes the one-way valve to the reservoir bag. Each spontaneous breath does not trigger a machine breath, therefore the risks of hyperinflation and respiratory alkalosis are reduced.

Some patients may not tolerate IMV well because ventilator inhalation is time-cycled and can occur during spontaneous exhalation. In order to correct this problem, simple IMV was improved by synchronizing ventilator inhalation with a patient-initiated negative pressure inspiratory effort. This prevented spontaneous exhalation occurring during positive-pressure inflation and subsequent breath "stacking," thus reducing the danger of mechanical breaths causing excessively high peak inflation pressures. In both SIMV and IMV modes, a machine breath is delivered in the absence of patient effort. However, with SIMV, if the machine breath coincided with the patient's spontaneous effort, then the spontaneous breath triggers a machine breath.

The machine breath delivered with the SIMV mode is similar to that in the IMV and assist control modes. The machine delivers a timed breath in the absence of patient effort – ventilator-sensed negative-pressure trigger, IMV – or delivers a breath as result of a patient trigger when the timed breath coincides with patient effort, similar to ACV. The significant difference is that each patient breath does not trigger a machine breath. Indications for SIMV include management of patients with evidence of hyperinflation and overventilation; it is commonly used following elective surgical procedures in an attempt to permit normal inspiratory effort and patient comfort.

The disadvantage of SIMV is increased work of breathing imposed by the compression inefficiencies of the ventilator circuitry, which cause gas delivery delays in the pressure-sensing valve systems, and a tendency to decrease cardiac output. The increased work of breathing is a result of spontaneous breathing through a high-resistance circuit (tracheal tube and ventilator tubing) and can lead to respiratory fatigue (Sassoon). Increased work of breathing leads to muscle fatigue and promotes ventilator dependency. This is exacerbated by application of PEEP or development of auto-PEEP because of the relatively greater patient inspiratory effort required to generate adequate negative pressure to activate the supplemental gas flow circuit. The increased work of breathing with the SIMV mode can result in increased CO_2 production. It is important to recognize that normalized blood gases in this setting may conceal, inappropriately, a situation in which the patient's work of breathing is increased significantly. A pressurized gas source that assists spontaneous respiratory effort and overcomes the increased work of breathing caused by mechanical valves and tubing associated with mechanical ventilation, called "pressure support," has been added to limit the increased work of breathing.

In patients with left ventricular dysfunction and adequate blood volume, the positive-pressure effects of mechanical ventilation outweigh its negative effects on cardiac output. When filling pressure is adequate, positive-pressure ventilation will decrease left ventricular afterload, resulting in an increased cardiac output.[39,40] In most cases and when initiated and maintained correctly, SIMV increases rather than decreases cardiac output.

Pressure-controlled ventilation (PCV)

The risk of ventilator-induced lung injury has renewed interest in PCV, because peak airway pressures are maintained lower than in volume-cycled patterns. Therefore, there is theoretically less risk of developing ventilator-induced barotrauma. Major advantages relate to the inspiratory flow pattern; inspiratory flow decreases exponentially during lung inflation to keep the airway pressures at the operator preset value.[41,42] Decreasing inspiratory flow pattern reduces peak airway pressures and improves gas exchange.

In the PCV mode, it is possible to set and maintain inverse I/E ratio ventilatory patterns. Inverse I/E ratios are used for patients with poor compliance in order to improve oxygenation. The prolonged inflation time can help prevent alveolar collapse. Prolonged inflation times decrease required gas flow delivery rates, thereby reducing peak inspiratory pressure. The prolonged inflation decreases time available for lung emptying and can lead to developing auto-PEEP (or intrinsic PEEP) and may cause significant reduction in cardiac output. Inverse ratio pressure-controlled ventilation is independent of patient effort and participation; it is one of the indications for muscle relaxant use in ICU ventilation. This mode is best suited for patients with compromised lung mechanics unresponsive to conventional lung recruitment methods and requires the patient to be sedated and paralyzed.

Pressure support ventilation (PSV)

Pressure support augmented breathing allows the patient to determine/control the inflation volume and respiratory cycle duration. This mode is used to augment spontaneous breathing, not as a mode to provide full ventilatory support. Spontaneous (negative pressure) inspiratory effort results in delivery of a preset, continuous peak airway pressure below the levels required for full mechanical ventilatory support. The usual level of pressure support ranges from 0.5 to 2 kPa (5 to 20 cmH_2O); pressures of 1.5 kPa (15 cm H_2O) or less are most commonly applied. The ventilator is adjusted as needed to keep the inflation pressure constant, usually by increasing inspiratory flow rate. When the patient's inspiratory flow rate falls below 25% of the ventilator-supported peak inspiratory flow rate, the augmented breath is terminated. PSV circuitry recognizes and synchronizes with the patient's inspiratory effort, thereby permitting the patient to dictate the duration and total volume of lung inflation.

As noted above, PSV helps overcome the resistance of breathing through ventilator circuits. Resistance increases the work of breathing with a ventilator. During a ventilator wean, pressure support will decrease the work of breathing and may facilitate a more rapid wean with reduced ventilator-related fatigue. PSV can also be used as a non-invasive mode of mechanical ventilation.[42] In this case, PSV is delivered through a specialized face mask or nasal mask using pressures of 2 kPa [20 cmH_2O (BiPap)].

High-frequency ventilation (HFV)

HFV is the delivery of small tidal volumes (equal to or less than the anatomic dead space) at high rates. Four methods of HFV have been developed: high-frequency positive-pressure ventilation (HFPPV); high-frequency jet ventilation (HFJV); high-frequency oscillation (HFO); and high-frequency chest wall compression (HFCWC) (see Table 66.2).

HFV was developed to reduce the risk of barotrauma and cardiovascular compromise and to improve pulmonary gas exchange. Mean airway pressure and peak airway pressures are reduced. CO_2 elimination is maintained with tidal volumes as low as 50–75 mL; however, oxygenation is not always improved. In some applications, HFV is used with conventional modes to promote bronchopulmonary toilet and to preserve oxygenation at lower inspired oxygen concentrations than possible with either technique alone.

Indications include laryngeal and tracheal surgery, emergency airway management, bronchopleural fistula, and infant and adult respiratory distress syndrome.

Disadvantages include high gas utilization; difficulty in monitoring tidal volume, $F_{I}O_2$, $P_{ET}CO_2$, and airway pressures; insufficient alarms; aspiration; poor humidification; no scavenging of gas; and possible barotrauma.

Positive end-expiratory pressure

When the inhaled lung volume is completely exhaled, the expiratory airflow ceases at the end of expiration, i.e. termed the end-expiratory point or end expiration. When alveolar pressure at end-expiration is equivalent to atmospheric pressure, it is termed the zero point. When the alveolar pressure at end-expiration is above the zero point, it is referred to as positive end-expiratory pressure (PEEP). If a pressure-limiting device is added to the expiratory limb of the ventilator, i.e. *extrinsic*, to stop exhalation at a preselected pressure, then the resultant positive pressure above the zero point is designated PEEP. PEEP displaces the entire pressure waveform in an upward direction and increases mean intrathoracic pressure. When using peak airway pressures and plateau pressures to measure lung mechanics, the effect of PEEP on proximal airway pressures is important to consider. The amount of PEEP must be subtracted from the peak end-inspiratory pressure to determine the intrinsic lung characteristics responsible for the measured pulmonary static compliance.

PEEP prevents alveoli from collapsing and may reopen collapsed lung segments. PEEP improves gas exchange by decreasing intrapulmonary shunting and, when appropriately applied, increases pulmonary compliance. The improved gas exchange increases arterial $P_{a}O_2$ and permits a therapeutic decrease in $F_{I}O_2$. (Nitrogen does not diffuse across the alveolar–capillary membrane, thereby helping to maintain alveolar integrity. By reducing $F_{I}O_2$, the normal alveolar nitrogen concentration is restored and alveolar stability improved.) One of the major uses of PEEP is to decrease the toxic effects of oxygen.

The effect of PEEP on cardiac output will determine whether increased arterial oxygenation ($S_{a}O_2$) is associated with an increase in systemic oxygenation. An increase in arterial oxygenation should never be used as the endpoint of PEEP application. If the application of PEEP does not reduce cardiac output, an increase in arterial oxygen saturation will be associated with an increase in systemic oxygen transport. However, if PEEP reduces cardiac output, then an increased arterial $P_{a}O_2$ will not correlate with an increase in systemic oxygenation, and may be associated with a net decrease in oxygen transport and availability. The point at which PEEP application best improves systemic oxygenation without a decrease in cardiac output was initially characterized by Fairley as *best PEEP*.

The effects of PEEP on oxygenation and cardiac output cannot be evaluated immediately. Usually, assessment of incremental changes in PEEP level is made 15 min after a new level is reached. In order to evaluate systemic oxygen transport, determinations of cardiac output and arterial oxygen saturation are necessary. Oxygen transport is calculated as the product of cardiac output (CO or Q) × arterial oxygen content ($C_{a}O_2$), where $C_{a}O_2 = [\text{Hemoglobin}] \times 1.39 \times S_{a}O_2 + 0.0031 \times P_{a}O_2$. From this relation, it is understandable that, although a significant increase in oxygen saturation may occur with the application of PEEP, a concomitant decrease in cardiac output may negate any overall benefit and compromise systemic oxygen delivery.

Additionally, evaluation of mixed venous oxygen saturation may help in the management of critically ill patients in whom minor changes in PEEP may prove beneficial. The mixed venous oxygen saturation represents the circulatory oxygen reserve following systemic tissue oxygen extraction. A decrease in mixed venous oxygen saturation often parallels a fall in cardiac output and may provide early information to augment clinical management strategies.

Application of PEEP is indicated in numerous clinical situations. Despite early concerns about the association of PEEP with pulmonary barotrauma, it is now recognized that recruitment/de-recruitment sequences are potentially more likely to cause lung damage than maintenance of a reasonable functional residual capacity (FRC) at the end of expiration. It is in this context that PEEP is best evaluated. Lung recruitment continues during inspiration and may not be complete until end inspiration. Proponents of large tidal volume ventilation argued that the beneficial effects of lung recruitment outweighed the potential for pulmonary damage. To a certain extent the argument has merit, but if the pressure–volume curves of the healthy and diseased lung are compared, a rational accommodation between the two positions can be reached.

In healthy lung, the inspiratory curve is linear until near total lung capacity; during expiration, lung volume does not markedly decrease with the initial change in pressure, causing hysteresis (Fig. 66.1). This is contrasted with the situation in ARDS (Fig. 66.2). Note that volume change during initial inflation is minimal because of atelectasis, and much of the pressure effect is in reopening collapsed alveoli. A point in the curve at which lung expansion becomes linear is defined as P_{flex} and indicates early lung recruitment. On the expiratory curve, similar changes are noted from the normal lung, and a point is reached at which lung volume decreases markedly, the point of maximum curvature (PMC_{ex}).

Kacmarek[43] has suggested that PEEP may be applied using the values of P_{flex} and PMC_{ex} to determine the minimum level of PEEP required to maintain alveolar volume (P_{flex}) and the target PEEP necessary to achieve maximum recruitment (PMC_{ex}). Pressure–volume loops are analyzed easily on modern ventilators and, in most cases, the difference between the two values is relatively small. Very high PEEP levels are unnecessary if careful attention is paid to minimize alveolar de-recruitment at end-inspiration.

Table 66.2 *Comparison of high-frequency ventilatory support modes*

	HFPPV	HFJV	HFO	HFCWC
Frequency	1–2 Hz	2–6 Hz	2–15 Hz	2–15 Hz
Cycles per min	60–110	110–400	400–2400	400–2400
Tidal volume	3–5 mL kg^{-1}	2–5 mL kg^{-1}	–	–

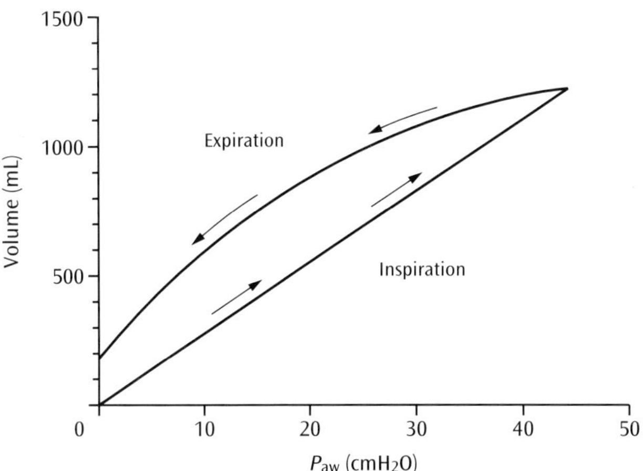

Figure 66.1 *Pressure–volume curve of the total respiratory system in the healthy lung. The inspiratory curve is linear until near total lung capacity; during expiration, lung volume does not markedly decrease with the initial change in pressure, causing hysteresis.*

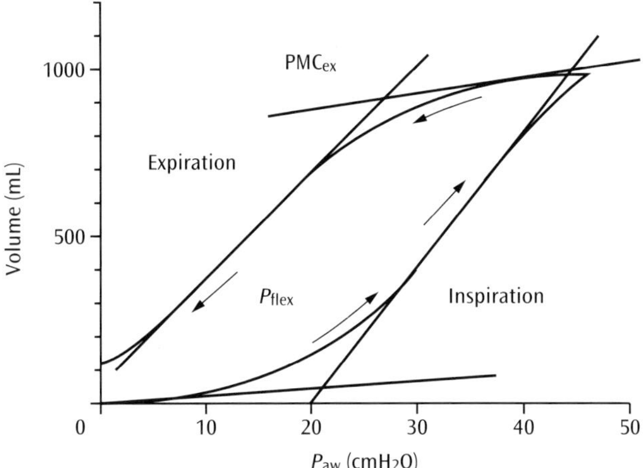

Figure 66.2 *Pressure–volume curve of the total respiratory system in ARDS. In early inspiration, little volume is delivered in spite of pressure increases because of lung collapse.* P_{flex} *is that part of the curve where the slope increases, identifying early lung recruitment. During expiration, the point where lung volume markedly decreases is defined as the point of maximum curvature* (PMC_{ex}).

Kacmarek[43] has suggested a useful ventilatory strategy as follows:

Management of PEEP:

- P_{flex} (minimum PEEP needed): 1–1.5 kPa (10–15 cmH_2O);
- PMC_{ex} (maximum PEEP required): 1.5–2 kPa (15–20 cmH_2O);
- target PEEP: ~1.5 kPa (15 cmH_2O) in early ARDS;
- recruitment maneuver: 3.5–4 kPa (35–40 cmH_2O CPAP for 30–40 s);
- inadequate PEEP: Po_2 decreases over 1–2 h after recruitment maneuver;
- F_{IO_2}: decrease before PEEP (F_{IO_2} 0.5 before PEEP decreased).

Indications for PEEP:

1 Decrease toxicity associated with high F_{IO_2} levels; most effective in patients with stiff lungs and/or diffuse disease.
2 Low-volume ventilation (5–8 mL kg^{-1}). Note: PEEP is applied to minimize alveolar collapse and should be above the inflection point in pressure-cycled ventilation that is associated with the point of distal airway closure.
3 Obstructive lung disease.[44]

PEEP is recommended with low tidal volumes to prevent lung injury with repetitive opening and closing of the lungs.[45] Controversial applications of PEEP include trying to reduce lung edema and mediastinal bleeding.

The use of PEEP to replace the effect of the larynx in intubated patients led to the concept of physiologic PEEP. All individuals approximate atmospheric pressure at end-expiration, and the concept of "physiologic PEEP" is suspect. However, in the postoperative patient, translaryngeal intubation is associated with airway collapse and atelectasis, perhaps because the patient is unable to cough and apply expiratory retard in an attempt to maintain functional residual capacity. In this setting, PEEP application may improve the patient's postoperative comfort and aid in weaning from mechanical ventilatory assistance. The patient will often delineate his/her optimal ventilator settings, and the practitioner should be responsive to this subjective commentary.

Continuous positive airway pressure (CPAP)

Spontaneous breathing during which positive airway pressure is maintained throughout the respiratory cycle is called continuous positive airway pressure (CPAP). Theoretically, the patient should not have to generate a negative airway pressure to receive gas flow for spontaneous inspiration. However, owing to the inefficiency of ventilator circuits, CPAP may also increase the work of breathing. Despite theoretic disadvantages, the net result is elimination of a significant component of the extra work of breathing involved in generating negative pressure associated with conventional ventilation.

In the presence of spontaneous or intrinsic PEEP, patient generation of a large negative airway pressure is required for inhalation, thereby increasing the work of breathing. Intrinsic PEEP is intra-alveolar pressure measured above the zero point not associated with an extrinsic pressure device. Patients with significant lung disease, obstruction, or bronchospasm are at risk of developing significant levels of intrinsic or auto-PEEP because of delayed alveolar emptying. Cardiac output may be depressed significantly in this setting, and the risk of ventilator-associated pulmonary barotrauma increases.

CPAP can also be applied in the nonintubated patient utilizing a specialized face mask or nasal mask. The nasal method is popular for the treatment of obstructive sleep apnea. Therapeutic effect is obtained when the CPAP splints open the upper airways during negative-pressure breathing. Nasal CPAP (nCPAP) can also be used to ameliorate blood gas abnormalities and dyspnea associated with acute exacerbation of COPD. Recently, Kindgen-Mills *et al.*[46] described successful support of spontaneously breathing patients with oxygen saturation deficit managed successfully with nCPAP. In a series of 20 extubated patients exhibiting hypoxemia following thoracic or thoracoabdominal operations, 18 were successfully managed with 0.8–1 kPa (8–10 cmH_2O) nCPAP, avoiding reintubation.[46] It is suggested that this therapeutic strategy may avoid complications of prolonged intubation in specific cases. Combined with mechanical support (BiPap; see below), noninvasive methods of respiratory support are gaining popularity in the postoperative intensive care setting.

Airway pressure release ventilation (APRV)

APRV is a new mode of ventilation, in which CPAP is released temporarily to permit passive exhalation. The goal is to facilitate exhalation and appropriate alveolar emptying and cycling based on the lung's compliance elastic properties. In conventional ventilation, end-expiration is associated with the lowest pressure measured in the ventilator circuit. In APRV, end-expiration is associated with a superatmospheric pressure that, when acutely withdrawn (released), initiates exhalation through the lung's intrinsic geometry and elastance. Reapplication of the end-expiratory pressure causes inhalation. Therefore, APRV periodically augments exhalation by reducing levels of CPAP. It is reported to reduce barotrauma and minimizes the adverse hemodynamic effects of positive-pressure ventilation. APRV employs higher pressures than conventional CPAP and can be used as an alternative ventilatory mode for patients with acute respiratory failure.[47]

A specific form of APRV, BiPAP, used in conjunction with nasal CPAP, may be used in some cases of respiratory insufficiency associated with sleep apnea. This technique has shown recent promise in maintaining ventilatory function in patients with impending respiratory failure, often following thoracic surgery. Unlike IPPB (see below), BiPAP provides appropriate support and may permit patient management without intubation.

Intermittent positive-pressure breathing (IPPB)

IPPB is a noninvasive method of assisting ventilatory effort previously popular in postoperative settings. Based on the intraoperative observation that extrinsic positive-pressure lung expansion reduced atelectasis in the open thorax, devices were developed to provide positive-pressure lung inflation with patient-generated inspiratory effort. Although extrinsic positive pressure expands alveoli in the open chest, transpulmonary pressure gradients are altered in the normal physiologic state. When alveoli are returned to ZEEP following positive-pressure expansion in the closed chest condition, alveolar recruitment is not maintained. This technique has now been replaced with bedside incentive spirometry. This recruitment strategy forces maximum alveolar expansion by maintaining peak inspiratory lung volume through voluntary patient effort. Maintenance of alveolar volume in this manner helps prevent and/or reverse postoperative atelectasis and improves pulmonary function.

The majority of patients who require mechanical ventilation have ventilatory failure, an inability to exchange air, oxygenate the blood, or expire CO_2. Possible causes include sedation from medication, general anesthesia, drug overdose, and chest wall deformity or airway disease. These patients usually require intubation if the CO_2 is greater than 6.7 kPa (50 mmHg) and pH less than 7.30. A smaller number of patients require ventilation due to hypoxemia, defined as a P_aO_2 less than 6.7 kPa (50 mmHg) on 100%. These patients are often able to maintain ventilation but cannot maintain oxygenation. Causes include pneumonia, aspiration, ARDS, and pulmonary emboli. The ventilator setting is chosen to optimize oxygenation and acid–base status. Tidal volumes of 6 mg kg^{-1} are associated with decreased ICU stays and lower infection rates. An arterial blood gas is drawn 30 min after either the patient has been placed on mechanical ventilation or the ventilator settings have been changed to determine oxygenation and ventilation. Important parameters to follow are peak airway pressure and static airway pressures. High peak airway pressures occur with bronchospasm, inappropriate ventilator settings, or pneumothorax. Static airway pressure is measured during the last second of expiration by adding an inspiratory pause prior to initiation of the next breath. Static airway pressures reflect underlying properties of the lung. Static airway pressures are increased in the following disease processes that stiffen the lungs: ARDS, pulmonary edema, pneumonia, increase in tidal volume, or fibrosis. Static airway pressure decreases with emphysema due to loss of lung parenchyma. (Note: the most common complication of mechanical ventilation is barotrauma.)

Anesthesiology's primary mode of mechanical ventilation in the

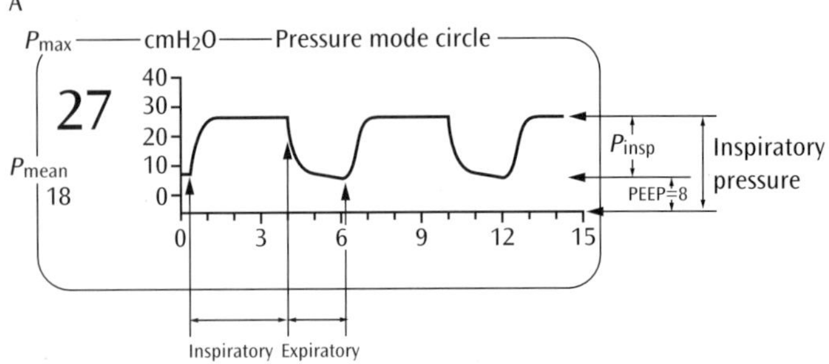

B

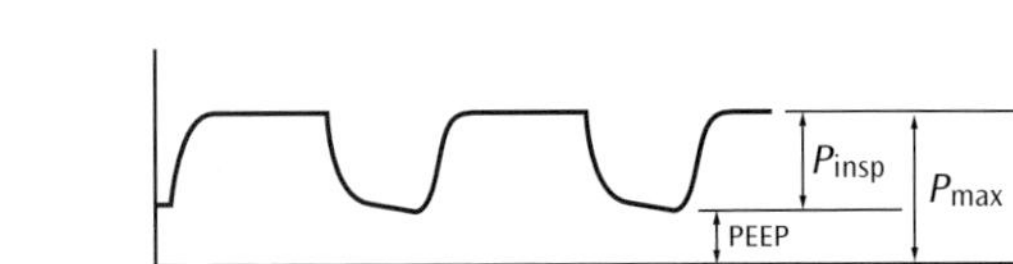

Figure 66.3 *(A and B) Pressure mode waveforms are depicted and should be compared and contrasted with the volume mode displays reproduced in Fig. 66.4A and B. Inspiratory and expiratory times are depicted, and the different pressure applications should be noted. In the paralyzed patient with normal lungs, either mode is acceptable. However, surgical positioning requirements and intra-abdominal or thoracic retraction and/or surgery requires use of higher than normal pressures to insure adequate tidal volume excursion. Unlike ICU ventilators, anesthesia machines are less likely to function adequately in the presence of significantly reduced pulmonary compliance. Although newer models are available with increased pressure-generating capacity, nonetheless it is occasionally necessary to use the patient's ICU ventilator in the operating room to insure adequate ventilation and maintenance of PEEP. Anesthetic strategies must be accommodated for this purpose. (Reproduced with permission from Datex-Ohmeda.)*

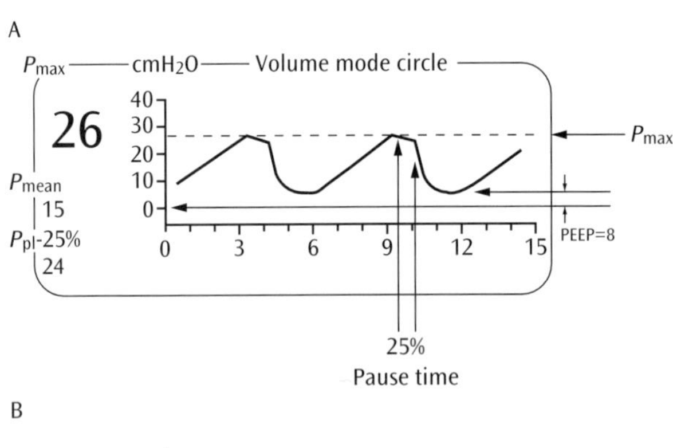

B

Pinsp

Pmax

PEEP

Figure 66.4 *Refer to legend for Fig. 66.3. (Reproduced with permission from Datex-Ohmeda.)*

operating room is volume controlled, with operator-defined peak pressure limitation in the paralyzed patient. For the majority of patients, this is appropriate and maintains pulmonary expansion in the face of specific surgical requirements, especially in upper abdominal and thoracic surgery. The waveform differences in gas delivery are depicted in Figs 66.3 and 66.4. Note that not only is the inspiratory pressure rate of rise more rapid in the pressure control mode, but also the mean intrathoracic pressure is higher. In the ICU, this is beneficial for preserving alveolar volume, but in the paralyzed patient, this waveform selection could adversely affect cardiac output secondary to negative impact on right atrial filling. When supine, the paralyzed diaphragm's downward deflection in response to positive pressure is influenced by the passive weight of abdominal content pressing upward. This leads to enhanced ventilation in the anterior or superior segments, whereas perfusion is preferentially directed inferiorly. This creates a situation in which accentuated ventilation–perfusion mismatch may develop during the course of long operations (Fig. 66.5).

WEANING THE PATIENT FROM THE VENTILATOR

Is the patient awake and responsive? It is important to establish that the patient has the ability to follow commands and cooperate with verbal instructions to perform a vital capacity maneuver and cough, and that the patient has an intact gag reflex. The patient must have a normal minute ventilation (6–8 L min^{-1}), normal work of breathing, PEEP 0.5 kPa (5 cmH_2O), and acceptable gas exchange.

Many of the bedside parameters in current use have a poor predictive value (see Table 66.3). Minute ventilation incorrectly predicted the weaning outcome in 40–50% of patients. The best predictors for successful weaning are the maximum inspiratory pressure generated by the patient and the ratio of respiratory frequency to tidal volume. The strength of the diaphragm and other inspiratory muscle can be evaluated by having the patient exhale to residual volume and inhale as forcefully as possible against a closed valve. In one study, 40% of the patients with a value less negative than 2 kPa (20 cmH_2O) did not wean from the ventilator. Rapid and shallow breathing is common in patients who fail to wean from the ventilator. An index of rapid and shallow breathing is the ratio of respiratory rate to tidal volume (RR/V_T). The ratio is normally less than 50 breaths min^{-1} L^{-1} and often exceeds 105 in the patient who fails to wean successfully. This test has a predictive value of 95% for failure to wean. A value of below 105 had a predictive value of 80% for successful weaning.

Anesthesiologists usually wean and extubate patients in the operating room following short-term interventions. Importantly, patients who have been intubated for extended periods and with poor nutritional reserves present a significant challenge for the critical care staff. However, in all cases, the following simple suggestions may prevent extubation complications.

1 The patient should be normothermic. This prevents unexpected respiratory acidosis should the compromised patient shiver following extubation and be unable to generate the additional ventilatory capacity necessary to maintain normal acid–base status.
2 The patient should demonstrate the ability to follow simple commands. Specifically, the patient should open his/her mouth and protrude the tongue on command. Patients capable of this maneuver are unlikely to obstruct on extubation. This is especially important in edentulous patients with unsupported pharyngeal soft tissues. Occasionally, such patients develop airway obstruction that may be alleviated by padding the buccal mucosa and restoring normal intra-oral anatomy.
3 Patients with suspected airway edema should be able to breathe around an occluded endotracheal tube with the cuff deflated. If this is not possible, consider continued significant laryngeal or tracheal edema that may become problematic if the translaryngeal tube is removed prematurely. This technique may help determine when to extubate nasally intubated patients with "wired" jaws.
4 On peak inspiration, the patient should be asked to hold his/her breath. Although many patients will be unable to perform this maneuver, it is indicative of adequate pain relief and muscle strength for extubation. In those patients with upper abdominal or thoracic wounds, pain management is an important adjunct to successful weaning from mechanical ventilatory assistance.

There are three general approaches to withdrawing ventilator support. Two involve initiating periods of spontaneous breathing interspersed with periods of ventilatory support. The other method involves a gradual reduction in the fraction of total support provided by the ventilator (IMV wean). The two methods of intermittent spontaneous breathing trials are known as T-piece trials with either pressure support and/or full resumption of mechanical support. The method of gradual reduction in rate is accomplished by reducing the mandatory number of breaths in an IMV circuit.

The T-piece is an on–off method of supplying supplemental

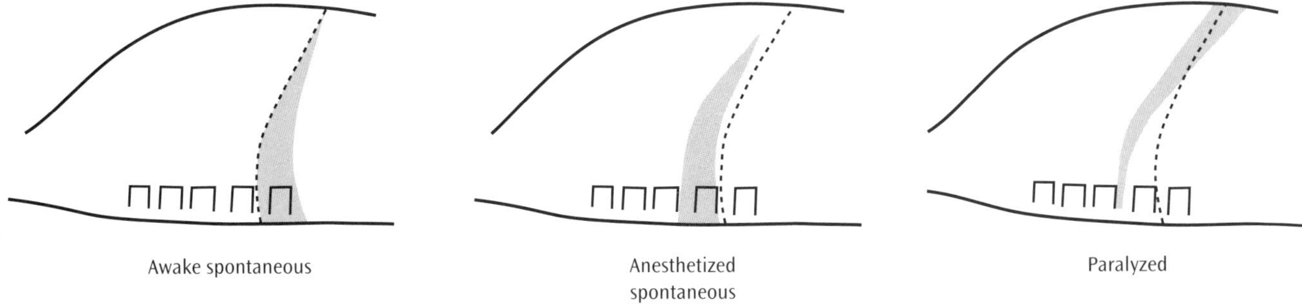

Figure 66.5 *These three examples show the benefits of spontaneous ventilation over mechanical ventilation in a paralyzed patient. In an awake, supine patient, active diaphragmatic contraction causes more volume increase in the posterior basal segments of the lung. Under anesthesia, the distribution of ventilation does not change, but an erosion of total pulmonary volume is seen. This occurs at the expense of the expiratory reserve volume, although ventilation–perfusion ratios are not altered initially. In paralyzed humans, greater changes are seen as ventilation–perfusion ratios throughout the lung are altered. The reasons for these changes are as follows: (1) Approximately a 2.5 kPa (25 cmH_2O) gradient exists between the anterior abdominal wall and the back owing to the weight of the abdominal contents pressing against the posterior diaphragmatic surface. (2) Diaphragmatic displacement is governed by the law of Laplace, which provides that pressure = tension/radius. Therefore, in the anterior diaphragmatic segments with a larger radius of curvature, diaphragmatic tension is less and displacement per unit pressure greater. Thus, anterior segments move more freely and lead to the large change in volume distribution seen in the diagram. (3) Positive-pressure breathing reduces venous return to the right heart and may reduce cardiac output, further reducing perfusion in anterior lung segments. (From Froese AB, Bryan AC. Effects of anesthesia and paralysis in diaphragmatic mechanics in man.* Anesthesiology *1974;* **47:** *242.)*

Table 66.3 *Bedside weaning parameters*

Parameters	Bedside weaning parameter: Normal adult range	Threshold for weaning
$P_{a}O_2/F_{I}O_2$	>400	200
Tidal volume	5–7 mL kg^{-1}	5 mL kg^{-1}
Respiratory rate	14–18 min^{-1}	40 min^{-1}
Vital capacity	65–75 mL kg^{-1}	10 mL kg^{-1}
Minute ventilation	5–7 L min^{-1}	10 L min^{-1}
Maximum inspiratory	>−90 cmH$_2$O (F) >−120 cmH$_2$O (M)	−25 cmH$_2$O
Frequency–volume ratio	<50 min^{-1} L^{-1}	100 min^{-1} L^{-1}

1 kPa = 10 cmH$_2$O.

oxygen to the mechanically unassisted endotracheal tube. Patients are disconnected from the ventilator for variable but gradually increasing time intervals. Between trials, full resumption of mechanical support is advocated to avoid patient fatigue. This method theoretically improves respiratory muscle conditioning. The interval off the ventilator is increased until the patient is extubated. This occurs in most cases when the patient tolerates spontaneous breathing for 24 h. If patients fail they are returned to full mechanical ventilatory support until they can tolerate another trial. The gas is delivered to the T-piece at a high flow rate for two reasons: first, this prevents the patient from inhaling room air from the exhalation side of the apparatus and, second, it carries the exhaled gases away to prevent rebreathing. The drawback with system is the increased work of breathing created by spontaneous breathing through an endotracheal tube and, furthermore, the translaryngeal tube prevents the patient from maintaining the lungs at maximal inspiration.

A pressure support wean or CPAP overcomes this problem by adding positive pressure to the system in order to eliminate work of breathing and provide pulmonary support at end-expiration. The goal is to provide enough pressure to overcome resistance of the ventilator circuit without augmenting the patient's spontaneous inflation volumes, called minimum pressure support. Minimum pressure support is equal to the peak inspiratory flow rate during spontaneous breathing and the resistance to inspiratory flow during mechanical ventilation. The same time interval used to wean a patient with a T-piece is used for a pressure wean.

IMV provides a predetermined number of breaths each minute and allows the patient to breathe spontaneously. Thus, the patient is gradually weaned from the ventilator by decreasing the rate of the ventilator to zero. However, the end result of IMV weaning is a T-piece trial. Therefore, most use the T-piece wean, which has a better rate of successful weans than the IMV wean.

SUMMARY

This discussion has focused on those aspects of mechanical ventilatory support most directly involving the anesthetist. Critical care techniques and technologies such as extracorporeal membrane oxygenation (ECMO) and permissive hypercapnia have been omitted from the discussion not because of lack of importance, but rather from lack of routine application.

The relation between pulmonary ventilation and perfusion is important and is of necessity altered with the initiation of mechanical ventilation. The normal cyclical changes in negative pressure are changed to positive with concomitant decrease in right ventricular preload and increased afterload. This is further compounded in the operating room by the use of anesthetic agents acting as both negative inotropes and vasodilators, further compromising cardiac function. Finally, the insult is also exacerbated with the use of neuromuscular blocking agents that further alter ventilation–perfusion inequality and compromise hemoglobin oxygen loading in the alveolar capillaries.

Anesthesiologists manage these complex interactions with judicious fluid therapy, careful ventilatory management, and, whenever possible, restoration of spontaneous breathing. Careful attention to the pathophysiology of pulmonary function and dysfunction will improve the ability to manage clinical situations in which positive-pressure mechanical ventilatory support is required to support a failing physiology.

The necessity to initiate mechanical ventilation may be precipitated by pathologic, therapeutic, or pharmacologic requirements. The selection of a particular technique depends upon the primary diagnosis and anticipated duration of support. Mechanical support of the lung through ventilation must not be confused with respiration, the exchange of oxygen and carbon dioxide at the cellular level. All routinely used mechanical ventilatory techniques provide a controllable, humidified oxygen source under positive pressure administered cyclically. The volume delivered per breath is controlled either by pressure or volume limits.

Until recently in adult critical care, volume-cycled ventilators were preferred to pressure-cycled devices because they could be relied upon to deliver preset tidal volumes for those patients with reduced pulmonary compliance. However, in the last few years low tidal volume ventilation has become the standard of care for long-term ventilatory management. This change has been occasioned by the recognition that the proximate cause of pulmonary barotrauma resulting in pneumothorax is overdistension of alveoli with subsequent rupture and dissection of gas along bronchoalveolar segments.

Pressure-controlled or regulated ventilation is, therefore, increasingly utilized as a primary support mode. In this technique, tidal volume is curtailed by operator set limits for tidal volume (approximately 8 mL kg^{-1} – see above) or at a peak inflation pressure consistent with the patient's underlying ventilatory history and pathology. Lower tidal volumes and/or decreased inflation pressures have necessitated greater tolerance in defining acceptable $P_{a}CO_2$ and pH levels in the critically ill or patients requiring long-term ventilatory support. Chronic weaning programs attempt to match cardiopulmonary physiologic capacity with intellectual tolerance; the physician must recognize that "normal" arterial blood gases are defined in patient context, and not as idealized values to be attained prior to separation form mechanical support.

The anesthesiologist is charged with the responsibility of supporting ventilation in two often widely disparate environments. The majority of anesthetic ventilation is of short duration and precipitated by the intraoperative use of anesthetic agents including narcotics, inhalation vapors, and muscle relaxants. Their duration is often only marginally greater than that of the surgery itself, and in most elective cases not involving the lung parenchyma extubation is anticipated within a few hours following completion of surgery. Mechanical ventilation in this setting is relatively simple, and it is more important to guard against therapeutic misadventure than to be concerned about difficult weaning problems. Synchronized IMV is an appropriate technique, and because of anticipated short-term requirement tidal volumes in the 10–12 mL kg^{-1} range are acceptable. Pressure support and PEEP are added as indicated, usually to improve patient comfort and expedite weaning. Larger tidal volumes and addition of PEEP may be indicated in these patients in order to insure that the lungs are maintained above FRC and do not undergo repetitive cycles of closing and reopening because of inadequate support. This concept was demonstrated by Amato *et al.*[48] when they described two levels of PEEP: the maximum PEEP required to maintain FRC vs. the minimum PEEP needed to prevent alveolar collapse at end-expiration. Obviously, the ideal setting for individual patients must rest between these two values, but the concept remains important for the patient recovering from uncomplicated surgery. Also, it is important to understand that normal lung subjected to PEEP will distend preferentially to collapsed lung units. Therefore, before applying PEEP, it is important to attempt alveolar recruitment. No specific recommendations exist, but suggestions have included maintaining a high CPAP level [3–4 kPa (30–40 cmH_2O) for up to 30 s in the absence of hemodynamic compromise]. Despite this recommendation, seldom is a lung-recruiting maneuver employed prior to increasing PEEP levels.

In diseased lungs, greater attention must be paid to minimizing pressure and/or volume damage to the already compromised lung. Therefore, comparatively smaller tidal volumes to minimize peak inflation pressure have become the standard of management in this setting, although it remains important to minimize de-recruitment/collapse/re-recruitment cycles for the same reasons detailed above.

An appropriate ventilatory strategy is always to prepare the patient for rapid weaning and extubation. Adequate levels of analgesia, sedation, and occasionally paralysis are important adjuncts to this process and beyond the scope of this chapter. It must be recognized, however, that the patient's pharmacologic requirements may impact negatively on the ability to pursue a vigorous weaning strategy. In appropriate circumstances, use of regional anesthetic techniques to manage postoperative or post-trauma pain may expedite resumption of effective spontaneous ventilation and expedite weaning. In order to separate a patient from ventilatory assistance, a number of requirements must be met. For the routine postoperative patient, normothermia, hemodynamic stability with stable coagulation status, adequate analgesia, absence of residual neuromuscular blockade, and return of cognitive function are important and relatively easy to assess prior to extubation. Similar parameters in chronically ventilated patients with underlying pulmonary pathology, either chronic or as a result of acute respiratory dysfunction, are more difficult to assess. In these cases, careful attention to the amount of respiratory support that is required to maintain oxygenation and ventilatory function is important. Nutritional status and metabolic requirements are important; normally, the metabolic cost of breathing represents 3–5% of total caloric expenditure. In the patient suffering from ARDS, the metabolic cost of pulmonary function may exceed 25% of caloric expenditure. Therefore, the patient's recovery from any acute and/or stabilization of chronic disease states must be assessed carefully and extubation delayed until controllable factors are optimized. Home ventilatory support techniques and equipment are becoming increasingly sophisticated and appropriate for minimally supervised use and offer either temporary or permanent solutions for patients being weaned from ICU machines and transferred out of the ICU and hospital. They are used primarily in situations in which the patient is suffering from ventilatory dysfunction and is able to manage unsupported for short periods of time.

Mechanical techniques for the support of the ventilatory function of the failing lung are undergoing continuous appraisal and change. Although this chapter has introduced the various support modes and techniques available, it does not purport to be the *sine qua non* of clinical integration. It is important to realize that the failing lung requires continuous clinical assessment and, subsequently, changes in ventilatory strategy are likely to be necessary. The astute clinician will try to follow clinical ventilatory guidelines and track performance throughout the course of a patient's illness. Any deviation from a well-established protocol should be documented and justified. In this manner, an individual patient's progress can be judged in the greater context of disease-specific anticipated outcome; appropriate intervention for deviations from expected progress are more likely to be made in this setting.

REFERENCES

1. Vesalius A. *De Humani corporis. Libri septem*. Basel: Oporinus, 1543: 658.
2. Kite J. *An Essay on Recovery of the Apparently Dead*. London: Dilly, 1877.
3. Matas R. On the management of acute traumatic pneumothorax. *Am J Med* 1902; **3:** 97–103.
4. Mushin WW, Rendell-Baker L, Thompson WP, *et al. Automatic Ventilation of the Lungs*, 3rd edn. Oxford: Blackwell Scientific Publications, 1980: 191–222.
5. Drinker P, Khann CF. The use of a new apparatus for the prolonged administration of artificial respiration. I. A fatal case of poliomyelitis. *JAMA* 1929; **92:** 1658–60.
6. Drinker P, Shaw L. An apparatus for the prolonged administration of artificial respiration: a design for children and adults. *J Clin Invest* 1929; **7:** 229–47.
7. Holtacker TR, Loosbrock LM, Gracey DR. The use of the chest cuirass in respiratory failure of neurologic origin. *Respir Care* 1989; **27:** 271.
8. Levy RD, Cosio MG, Gibbons L, *et al.* Induction of sleep apnoea with negative pressure ventilation in patients with chronic obstructive lung disease. *Thorax* 1992; **47:** 612.
9. Shapiro SH, Ernst P, Gray-Donald K, *et al.* Effect of negative pressure ventilation in severe chronic obstructive pulmonary disease. *Lancet* 1992; **340:** 1425.
10. Hill NS. Clinical application of body ventilation. *Chest* 1986; **90:** 897.
11. Lassen HCA. A preliminary report on 1952 Polio epidemic. *Lancet* 1953; **1:** 37–41.
12. Ibsen B. The anaesthetist viewpoint in the treatment of respiratory complications in poliomyelitis during the epidemic in Copenhagen. *Proc R Soc Med* 1954; **47:** 72–4.
13. Engstrom CG. Treatment of respiratory paralysis by the Engstrom University Respirator. *Br Med J* 1954; **2:** 666–9.
14. Slutsky AS. American College of Chest Physicians' Consensus Conference on Mechanical Ventilation. *Chest* 1993; **104:** 1833–59.
15. Tobin MJ. Mechanical ventilation. *N Engl J Med* 1994; **330:** 1056–61.
16. Marini JJ. Pressure-targeted, lung protection ventilation support in the acute lung injury. *Chest* 1994; **105** (Suppl.): 109S–115S.
17. Gammon RB, Strickland Jr JH, Kennedy Jr KI, Young Jr KR. Mechanical ventilation: a review for internist. *Am J Med* 1995; **99:** 553–62.
18. Shapiro BA, Peruzzi WT. Changing practices in ventilation management: a review of the literature and suggested clinical correlation. *Surgery* 1995; **117:** 121–33.
19. Bates JH, Rossi A, Milic-Emili J. Analysis of the behavior of the respiratory system with constant inspiratory flow. *J Appl Physiol* 1985; **58:** 1840.
20. Hubmayr RD, Gay PC, Tayyab M. Respiratory system mechanics in ventilated patients: techniques and indications. *Mayo Clin Proc* 1987; **62:** 358.
21. Sassoon CSH Mechanical ventilation design and function. The trigger variable. *Respir Care* 1992; **37:** 1056.
22. Polak B, Adams H. Traumatic air embolism in submarine escape training. *US Naval Med Bull* 1932; **30:** 165–77.
23. Caldwell EJ, Powell RD, Mullooly JP. Interstitial emphysema: a study of physiology factors involved in experimental induction of lesion. *Am Rev Respir Dis* 1970; **102:** 516–25.
24. Dreyfuss D, Soler P, Basset G, Saumon G. High inflation pressure pulmonary edema: respective effects of high airway pressure, high tidal volume, and positive end-expiratory pressure. *Am Rev Respir Dis* 1988; **137:** 1159–64.
25. Macklin MT, Macklin CC. Malignant interstitial emphysema of the lungs and mediastinum as in important occult complication in many respiratory disease and other conditions: an interpretation of the clinical literature in the light of laboratory experiment. *Medicine* 1944; **23:** 281–358.
26. Pinsky MR. Cardiovascular effects of ventilation support and withdrawal. *Anesth Analg* 1994; **79:** 567–76.

27. Bendixen HH, Egbert LD, Hedley-White J, *et al. Respiratory Care*. St Louis, MO: Mosby, 1965: 137–53.
28. Gattinoni L, Pesenti A. ARDS: the nonhomogeneous lung facts and hypothesis. *Intensive Crit Care Dig* 1987; **61:** 1.
29. Costello ML, Mathieu-Costello OA, West JB. Stress failure of alveolar epithelial cells studied by scanning electron microscopy. *Am Rev Respir Dis* 1992; **145:** 1446–1455.
30. Costello ML, Mathieu-Costello OA, West JB. Are pulmonary capillaries susceptible to mechanical stress? *Chest* 1994; **105** (Suppl.): 102S–107S.
31. ACCP. Consensus Conference on Mechanical Ventilation. *Chest* 1993; **104:** 1833.
32. Davis K, Branson RD, Campbell RS, *et al*. The addition of sighs during pressure support ventilation: is there a benefit? *Chest* 1993; **104:** 867.
33. Tobin MJ. Respiratory monitoring. *JAMA* 1990; **264:** 244–51
34. Marini JJ. Lung mechanics determinations at the bedside: instrumentation and clinical application. *Respir Care* 1990; **35:** 669–96.
35. Sassoon CSH, Mahutte K, Light RW. Ventilation modes: old and new. *Crit Care Clin* 1990; **6:** 605–634.
36. Rasanen J. Mechanical ventilatory support: time for appraisal. *Int Crit Digest* 1991; **10:** 3–5
37. Fernandez R, Blanch L, Antigas A. Respiratory center activity during mechanical ventilation. *Crit Care Clin* 1990; **6:** 635–61.
38. Marini JJ. Strategies to minimize breathing effort during mechanical ventilation. *Crit Care Clin* 1990; **6:** 661–73.
39. Pinsky, MR. Cardiovascular effects of ventilation support and withdrawal. *Anesth Analg* 1994; **79:** 567–76.
40. Mathru M, Rao TL, El-Etr AA, Pifarre R. Hemodynamic response to changes in ventilation patterns in patients with normal and poor left ventricular reserve. *Crit Care Med* 1982; **10:** 423–6.
41. Shelledy DC, Rau JL, Thomas-Goodfellow L. A comparison of the effect of assist-control, SIMV, and SIMV with pressure-support on ventilation, oxygen consumption, and ventilatory equivalent. *Heart Lung* 1995; **24:** 67–75.
42. Rappaport SH, Shinper R, Yoshihara G, *et al*. Randomized, prospective trial of pressure-limited versus volume controlled ventilation in severe respiratory failure. *Crit Care Med* 1994; **22:** 22–32.
43. Brochard L, Mancebo J, Wysocki M, *et al*. Noninvasive ventilation for acute exacerbation of chronic obstructive pulmonary disease. *N Engl J Med* 1995; **338:** 817–22.
44. Edward P, Ingenito KR, Jeffrey M. PEEP in ARDS. In: Kacmarek RM (ed.). *Mechanical Ventilatory Support*. Drazen: Harrisons on Line, modified June 21, 1999.
45. Pinsky MR. Through the past darkly: ventilatory management of patients with chronic obstructive pulmonary disease. *Crit Care Med* 1994; **22:** 1714–17.
46. Marini JJ. Pressure-targeted, lung-protective ventilation support in acute lung injury. *Chest* 1994; **105** (Suppl.): 109S–115S.
47. Kindgen-Mills D, Buhl R, Gabriel A, *et al*. Nasal continuous positive airways pressure – a method to avoid intubation in postoperative high-risk patients with severe nonhypercapnic oxygenation failure. *Chest* 2000; **117:** 1106–11.
48. Cane R, Peruzzi WT, Shapiro BA. Airway pressure release ventilation in acute respiratory failure. *Chest* 1991; **100:** 460–3.

67

Critical care

CARLOS KUREK AND PETER NIGHTINGALE

OVERVIEW

Intensive care has been defined as "a service for patients with potentially recoverable diseases, who can benefit from more detailed observation and treatment than is generally available in general wards and departments."[1] Critical care has successfully evolved to become a medical and nursing specialty in itself, as a result of the progressive achievement in treating life-threatening conditions. Today, sophisticated equipment and technology allow the critical care team to prolong survival and promote recovery among patients suffering from life-threatening, critical illnesses.

The multidisciplinary team

Patients admitted to the intensive care unit (ICU) are suffering from increasingly complex problems; in addition, the ability to treat them has improved. As a result, many more specialties are becoming actively involved in the process of intensive care. As well as physicians and nurses, the multidisciplinary team may include members from the disciplines of respiratory therapy, nutritional support, clinical pharmacy, pastoral care, ethics, radiology, and infectious diseases, to name just a few. Today, no single physician can provide the complex care that patients with rapidly changing conditions need, and thus a multidisciplinary approach has become necessary. In the USA, the healthcare accreditation body, the Joint Committee on Accreditation of Healthcare Organizations (JCAHO), requires hospitalized patients to receive interdisciplinary care.[2] The Society of Critical Care Medicine's recommendations for intensive care unit design for delivery of level I critical care services include considerations for a team approach to care.[3]

The complex interactions between the team members have led to different models of delivery of care, depending on the needs of individual institutions and the availability of services. One such model is the "closed unit," in which an ICU team is responsible for admission, discharge, and overall management of patients. The admitting physician provides input and is always contactable, but the responsibility for medical care remains with the ICU team. Usually, in a closed unit, all members of the multidisciplinary team conduct the patient rounds, providing an opportunity for input from the different specialists. At the other extreme, the "open unit" model is the one in which the admitting physician remains in charge of the management of the patient, consulting with the ICU specialist and other services as necessary. Although a matter of controversy, the team approach to care has proven to be cost-beneficial and to improve outcome in mechanically ventilated patients.[4] Moreover, the presence of a fully trained intensivist in charge of the care improves outcome.[5–7]

Does this patient need an ICU bed?

Hospital resources are not infinite, nor are ICU beds. As a limited resource, the allocation of beds must be rational and well justified. That, however, is easier said than done. In the USA, patients have in the past been admitted freely to the ICU, among other reasons for financial incentives and fear of litigation. The question of appropriateness of admission has become critical in the last few years, since the shift to a prospective payment system has placed great financial pressure on the ICU. Traditionally a profit center, the ICU has become a cost center for the hospital, forcing the clinician to scrutinize the admissions more carefully. In some cases the need for critical care services is obvious, i.e. a patient in septic shock. However, often the case is not clear-cut. To quote Kirton and Civetta:[8] "Life was simpler when we believed we could characterize patients as too well, too sick, and just right for intensive care." In general, ICU patients should need either frequent or continuous monitoring, intensive nursing care or close physician observation. Broadly stated, in deciding whether a patient requires a "unit bed" the following two questions should be answered: What kind of need does the patient have that will not be met in a regular ward? How will the provision of that care affect the outcome of the patient? Answering the first question is much easier than answering the second, particularly in the case of terminally ill patients, for whom critical care may be considered "futile," or elective low-risk postoperative admissions. Many intensive care units have a set of admission and discharge criteria that provide a framework for the decision-making process of bed allocation. Those criteria should be evidence based, fit the particular need of the population served, and have the approval of the physicians involved in the care of the patients. The criteria should always allow for flexibility because, despite attempts to base decisions on hard scientific evidence, the practice of medicine is still an art, and the goal of therapy should be individually tailored. The American College of Critical Care Medicine and the Society of Critical Care Medicine have published guidelines for admission, discharge, and triage of adult patients in the ICU.[9] Moreover, changes and advances in the medical or surgical management of some conditions may have an impact on the need for intensive care. Patients undergoing carotid endarterectomy have been routinely admitted to the ICUs in the USA. However, admission criteria have changed significantly in the last few years, based on published evidence that conclusively demonstrates the safety of discharge to the regular ward after a period of observation in the recovery room.[10–12]

Ethical considerations and withdrawal of support

The support of vital organ functions is the basis of modern critical care. Life-sustaining therapy is always provided in the initial belief that the patient will recover and the support provided will be withdrawn. The provision of invasive and potentially harmful therapeutic interventions such as mechanical ventilation, renal replacement therapy, inotropic support, etc. is consistent with two principles that guide the practice of medicine: preserving life and alleviating suffering. However, frequently it comes to pass that the physician believes that if the patient survives his or her quality of life will be unacceptably poor, and thus a conflict between those two principles develops.[13] At this point the question arises as to whether interventions should be either withheld or withdrawn, with death being the inevitable outcome. What is the appropriate course of action? The problem is compounded by the disparity of opinion among different providers faced with the problem.

In a study performed in Canada, nurses, attending staff, and ICU nurses were presented with 12 clinical scenarios and asked for their personal opinion as to whether support should be withdrawn. In only one scenario did more than 30% of the respondents choose the same therapeutic action.[14]

In the USA, the principle of autonomy carries a great deal of weight. This principle establishes the right of the patient to consent to or refuse any therapy. Based on this principle, withholding or withdrawal of support must be discussed with the patient. In fact, often the patient, but more frequently the family, initiates the request to withdraw support. Unfortunately, in many cases, the patient is unable to make an informed decision, and the physician and the family are left to deal with the difficult problem.[15–17] In order to avoid this emotionally charged situation, two solutions can be put into practice. Advance directives (also called living wills) establish the patient's wishes in a broad way to guide the caregivers; alternatively, the patient may appoint in advance a healthcare proxy, a person designated to make decisions on his or her behalf. Given the success in prolonging life in the modern ICU, it is not surprising that withdrawal of support precedes death more and more frequently in ICUs.[18] The Society of Critical Care Medicine has published a consensus statement addressing the problem of futility in critical care.[19]

SCORING SYSTEMS

Although clinicians integrate statistical information and personal experience when establishing a prognosis for an individual patient, that prediction is subjective by nature. When applied to a population of patients with certain conditions in a particular unit, a more objective evaluation is needed. That is the role of scoring systems in the ICU. They are designed to enable a complex medical condition to be expressed numerically by weighing certain variables, which are summed to give an overall score. Their use in ICUs is becoming commonplace.

The majority of the systems developed serve the purpose of outcome prediction. The scoring systems serve four major purposes: research, administrative purposes, evaluation of ICU performance, and assessment of individual patient prognosis (Table 67.1).[20]

Many scoring systems are specific for certain clinical conditions and enable prediction of outcome for individual patients. The vast majority that are described below are nonspecific, which expands their scope of use beyond the prediction of outcome to benchmarking in the individual ICU.

Therapeutic Intervention Scoring System (TISS)

This is the most common scoring system used for resource allocation.[21,22] It is not designed to predict outcome, as it quantifies nursing, medical, and technologic support activity. TISS consists of 76 procedures assigned a score from 1 to 4, and it is used as a nonspecific system for assessing ICU activity and expenditure. It assigns points to therapeutic interventions, not to specific physiologic abnormalities, and reflects nursing and medical intensity of care.

Acute Physiology and Chronic Health Evaluation (APACHE)

The original APACHE score was described in 1981. A refined version, which has found wide acceptance, is the APACHE II scoring system.[23] It consists of two parts: the Acute Physiology Score (APS), comprising a sum of 12 physiologic variables, and the Chronic Health Evaluation.

The score is computed after 24 h of ICU care, using the worst values for each of the recorded variables. APACHE II is the most commonly used system worldwide (Fig. 67.1). Although originally validated only in the USA, it has been tested in different settings for validation,[24,25] and applied to a variety of patient populations[26] with mixed results.[27] The Intensive Care Society undertook a prospective validation of the APACHE II system in 35 hospitals in the UK and Ireland.[28,29] Early reports stressed the variability of the case mix in the units studied, and this was important when comparing crude hospital mortality. The overall *goodness of fit* of the American APACHE II equation was good when applied to the British and Irish data but did not apply uniformly to specific groups of patients. Thus, the use of the American equation could advantage or disadvantage individual units in comparison with others, depending on their case mix. Although the APACHE II system has been accepted worldwide as a general indicator of severity of illness for patients admitted to the ICU, it is recognized to have inherent problems.[30] These often reflect the lack of rules and definitions in data collection, such as lead time bias (therapy before admission) and assessment of the Glasgow Coma Scale (GCS). The diagnostic groups are limited in scope, and variations in classification can have major effects on the calculated risk of death.

APACHE III[31]

The APACHE scoring system has been further refined and extended to overcome many of its shortcomings, and has been tested in large databases.[32–34] The number of variables has been increased, statistical modeling has been used to derive and weight the variables of interest, functional physiologic reserve is better delineated, and resuscitation before admission is accounted for. APACHE III is used in a dynamic fashion with daily scoring and the use of TISS. The system is considerably more complex than its predecessor, but the improvement in correct classification is only modest when applied to populations of patients other than those in the original US setting.[35] Unfortunately, the coefficients for the diagnostic categories are not in the public domain and the expense of purchasing the system from the authors has limited its widespread acceptance.

Simplified Acute Physiology Score (SAPS and SAPS II)

The original SAPS score[36] (a modification of the APACHE score) was later modified and weighted by statistical modeling. Centers in the USA, Canada, and Europe took part in the data collection.[37] Recent research tends to show the need for customization to improve the performance of the system.[38,39]

Table 67.1 *Potential uses of severity of illness scoring systems (from Gregoire and Russell[20] with permission)*

Uses of scoring systems in randomized, controlled trials (RCTs) and clinical research
To compare different RCTs and clinical studies
To determine sample size
To do stratified randomization (a priori subgroups identification, stratification for severity of illness)
To assess success of randomization
To assess treatment effects in subgroups (*post hoc* subgroup identification)
To compare study patients to patients in clinicians' practices

Uses of scoring systems for administrative purposes
To describe resource utilization in the ICU
To describe acuity of illness
To relate resource utilization to acuity of care
To guide reimbursement and budget of an ICU

Uses of scoring systems to assess ICU performance
Quality assurance
To assess performance of an ICU in general or for a specific disease category
To assess performance of an ICU overtime
To compare individual intensivists' performance
To assess the performance of a therapeutic intervention
Comparison of ICU performance in different categories of hospitals, countries, etc.
Performance for different ICU administrative characteristics (open/closed unit, communication, ICU director task, etc.)
Effectiveness

Uses of scoring systems to assess individual patient prognosis and to guide care
Triage of patients
Decisions regarding intensity of care
Decisions to withhold and withdraw care

The Mortality Probability Model II (MPM II)

This is a predicting tool based on two sets of variables: the MPM 0 and MPM 24.[40] The model was developed based on data from 19 124 admissions to ICUs in 12 countries. The MPM 0 consists of 15 variables and is applied to patients on admission. The MPM 24 adds eight more variables measured 24 h after admission, and is applied to patients who remain in the ICU after 24 h. Both the MPM 0 and MPM 24 demonstrated a good degree of discrimination in the original description.

MECHANICAL VENTILATION IN THE ICU

Indications for mechanical ventilation

The indication for positive-pressure ventilation (Table 67.2) is very straightforward in some situations, such as an episode of apnea in a patient with head injury. However, more often, the situation is less clear cut. Among the most common reasons to institute ventilatory support is hypoxia refractory to high-flow supplemental oxygen, or hypoxemia with fatigue and hypoventilation with a rising $P\text{CO}_2$. Although clinical judgment is required to make the decision to intubate, reasonable criteria include a $P\text{O}_2$ of 50 mmHg or less in a patient breathing a mixture with at least 50% oxygen and/or a $P\text{CO}_2$ of greater than 50 mmHg. Patients with neuromuscular disorders who cannot cough and clear secretions and comatose or severely obtunded patients may be intubated and placed on a ventilator in order to protect the airway. The GCS is frequently used to make a decision in such patients. A GCS score of 7 or less is an indication for intubation.

Available modes of mechanical ventilation

The techniques available for respiratory support have increased as a result of advances in technology, improved understanding of the pathophysiology of acute respiratory failure, and a realization of the possible benefits of various modes of ventilation. Unfortunately, many of the new modes have been introduced merely on the basis of technical ability rather than as a result of a defined clinical need or demonstrable advantage to the patient. Two major modalities of ventilatory support are available today: noninvasive, in which a device is applied to the patient's face, and invasive, which involves intubation of the airway. Whether the initial mode of ventilation uses a mask or an endotracheal tube, the clinician at the bedside should be vigilant and flexible. The initial settings may need to be modified, remembering that the goal is to reverse the abnormalities that motivated the need for ventilatory support, avoid complications, and achieve maximum patient comfort.

Noninvasive ventilatory support

The use of noninvasive positive-pressure ventilatory support (NIPPV) allows intubation to be avoided in patients with a variety of conditions.[41,42] The technique involves applying a tight-fitting mask to the nose, or, if the patient cannot tolerate this, a face mask. Different levels of positive pressure are applied, allowing for different levels of pressure support in inspiration/expiration.

Among patients with chronic obstructive pulmonary disease, the use of the technique has had a major impact, decreasing the need for endotracheal intubation and shortening the length of ICU stay.[43,44] However, NIPPV has many limitations, including the patient–device interaction. The mask fit maybe deficient, and the presence of leaks accounts for

Physiologic variable	High abnormal range				Low abnormal range				
	+4	+3	+2	+1	0	+1	+2	+3	+4
Temperature–rectal (°C)	≥ 41°	39–40.9°		38.5–38.9°	36–38.4°	34–35.9°	32–33.9°	30–31.9°	≤ 29.9°
Mean arterial pressure–mmHg	≥ 160	130–159	110–129		70–109		50–69		≤ 49
Heart rate (ventricular response)	≥ 180	140–179	110–139		70–109		55–69	40–54	≤ 39
Respiratory rate (nonventilated or ventilated)	≥ 50	35–49		25–34	12–24	10–11	6–9		≤ 5
Oxygenation: A_2DO_2 or P_aO_2 (mmHg) a. F_{IO_2}>0.5 record A–$_aDO_2$	≥ 500	350–499	200–349		< 200				
b. F_{IO_2}<0.5 record only P_aO_2					PO_2 > 70	PO_2 61–70		PO_2 55–60	PO_2 < 55
Arterial pH	≥ 7.7	7.6–7.69		7.5–7.59	7.33–7.49		7.25–7.32	7.15–7.24	< 7.15
Serum sodium (mmol L^{-1})	≥ 180	160–179	155–159	150–154	130–149		120–129	111–119	≤ 110
Serum potassium (mmol L^{-1})	≥ 7	6–6.9		5.5–5.59	3.5–5.4	3–3.4	2.5–2.9		< 2.5
Serum creatinine (mg per 100 mL) (double point score for acute renal failure)	≥ 3.5	2–3.4	1.5–1.9		0.6–1.4		< 0.6		
Hematocrit (%)	≥ 60		50–59.9	46–49.9	30–45.9		20–29.9		< 20
Total WBC (10^3 per mm^3)	≥ 40		20–39.9	15–19.9	3–14.9		1–2.9		< 1
Glasgow coma score (GCS): score = 15 minus actual GCS									
A Total **acute** physiology score (APS): sum of the 12 individual variable points									
Serum HCO_3 (venous mmol L^{-1}) (not preferred, use if no ABGs)	≥ 52	41–51.9		32–40.9	22–31.9		18–21.9	15–17.9	nn < 15

B Age points:
Assign points to age as follows:

Age (years)	Points
≤44	0
45–54	2
55–64	3
65–74	5
≥ 75	6

C Chronic health points

It the patient has a history of severe organ system insufficiency or is immunocompromised assign points as follows:
A. For nonoperative or emergency postoperative patient–5 points
OR
B. For elective postoperative patient–2 points

Definitions

Organ insufficiency or immunocompromised state must have been evident prior to hospital admission and conform to the following criteria:
Liver: biopsy-proven cirrhosis and documented portal hypertension; episodes of past upper GI bleeding attributed to portal hypertension; or prior episodes of hepatic failure/encephalopathy coma.
Cardiovascular—New York Association class IV: severe limitation of exercise tolerance; symptoms are present at rest.
Respiratory: chronic restrictive, obstructive, or vascular disease resulting in severe exercise restriction, i.e. unable to climb stairs or perform household duties; or documented chronic hypoxia, hypercapnia, secondary polycythemia, severe pulmonary hypertension (> 40 mmHg), or respirator dependency.
Renal: receiving chronic dialysis.
Immunocompromised: the patient has received therapy that suppresses resistance to infection, e.g. immunosuppression, chemotherapy, radiation, long-term or recent high-dose steroids, or has a disease that is sufficiently advanced to suppress resistance to infection, e.g. leukemia, lymphoma, AIDS.

APACHE II SCORE

Sum of A + B + C

A APS points ____
B Age points ____
C Chronic health points ____
Total APACHE II ____

Figure 67.1 *APACHE II worksheet.*

Table 67.2 *Some indications for intubation and mechanical ventilation in acute respiratory failure*

Clinical	Biochemical
Impending apnea	P_{aO_2} < 50 mmHg on high F_{IO_2}
Paradoxical respiration	Pulse oximeter < 90% on F_{IO_2} > 50%
Obvious fatigue	Rising P_{CO_2}
Persistent tachypnea	High P_{CO_2} in metabolic acidosis
Variable respiratory rate	
Absent protective reflexes	
Threat of airway obstruction	

many failed attempts to use the technique. Patient cooperation and the very limited ability to use sedation are other limitations.

Invasive positive-pressure ventilation

Invasive positive-pressure ventilation is usually divided into the so-called "conventional modes" available in any modern ventilator and "unconventional modes," which have more specific indications and require more sophisticated hardware. See Chapter 66 for more details.

Is this patient ready to be weaned from the ventilator?

Mechanical ventilation is instituted as part of the delivery of anesthesia, and sometimes is prolonged into the ICU stay. When mechanical ventilation is used in this fashion, its discontinuation is not a major problem and can be done as soon as the patient is awake (provided no other relevant factors are at play).

However, in patients who undergo a prolonged period of mechanical ventilation, weaning from ventilatory support can pose a real challenge. Two major problems arise in that regard. The first problem is to decide *when* the patient is ready. The second one is *how* to wean.

Deciding when to wean remains an empirical task in most settings, and it is up to the clinician to decide when the patient is "ready to be tested." There is great variability among physicians in terms of their perception that the patient will tolerate a weaning trial. The lack of a standardized approach leads to delays in withdrawing mechanical support, potentially adding morbidity and increasing costs. The institution of a readiness protocol, in which patients are initiated on a weaning trial as soon as they meet predetermined criteria, has been found to be effective. One such protocol, published by Horst *et al.*,[45] allows the respiratory therapist to place the patient on a weaning trial when the patient meets pre-established criteria. Such an approach has led to a significant decrease in ventilator hours and length of stay, and significant financial savings.

What criteria should be used to determine when to initiate a trial of weaning? Extensive research has been conducted in the area, and several predictive indices of successful discontinuation of support have been proposed. Yang and Tobin[46] prospectively studied several predictive indices for weaning. The authors found that the most accurate index was the so-called rapid shallow breathing index. The index divides the respiratory frequency over the tidal volume using a calibrated spirometer attached to the endotracheal tube, while the patient breaths room air spontaneously for a minute. If the result of the 1-min trial was more than 100 breaths min^{-1}/tidal volume in liters the patients had a 95% likelihood of failing a weaning trial. Conversely, if the results were less that 100 breaths min^{-1}/tidal volume in liters patients had an 80% likelihood of success. Other indices that are frequently used in clinical practice were found to have significant less positive and negative predictive value (Table 67.3).

The second problem is how to wean a patient from the ventilator. There are as many recipes as there are physicians, and none of them has conclusively been proven to be better than others. Weaning using decreasing levels of pressure support or decreasing levels of synchronized intermittent mandatory ventilation (SIMV) is acceptable. Interestingly, the "tried and true" daily trial of spontaneous breathing is even more successful than other, more complicated, schemes.[47]

In short, individual units should develop a set of criteria to decide *when* to test the patient. Every patient who meets criteria should be tested to evaluate readiness to wean (such as a daily evaluation using the rapid shallow breathing index or other predicting tool). If the patient successfully completes the test, undergo a weaning trial, through a standardized protocol, such as the one presented in Fig. 67.2.

Patients who fail and are found to be difficult to wean should be approached by a multidisciplinary team.[4]

SEDATION AND NEUROMUSCULAR BLOCKING AGENTS IN THE ICU

Sedation in the ICU

Patients admitted to an ICU are usually confined to a bed 24h per day, attached to an array of monitors and a variety of invasive lines and draining devices. Their movement is limited, and alarms go off frequently. Physicians and nurses can walk into the room throughout the day and night, and communication, particularly in intubated patients, is fragmented at best. Not surprisingly, patients are anxious, confused, and scared. Thus, sedation is necessary for all but a few patients admitted to the unit. The ideal sedation plan should include anxiolysis, amnesia, and also analgesia, as many patients will have postoperative pain, pain resulting from procedures performed in the unit, or an underlying painful condition (i.e. cancer).

The degree of sedation/analgesia should be tailored to each patient individually. Choosing an appropriate sedative/analgesic schedule requires an understanding of the patient's underlying condition. Patients may be agitated or confused by reasons other than just being in the ICU, and those conditions may carry significant morbidity in themselves. The temptation to label the patient as having "ICU psychosis" should be avoided, as it implies that the ICU stay is responsible for the patient's state, that the condition can be ignored, and that sedation to the point of pharmacologic coma is the only answer.

The list of conditions that cause confusion is very extensive, but medications prescribed in the ICU are a frequent culprit, among them agents with anticholinergic properties, such as antiparkinsonian and antihistamine drugs. Cimetidine and other medications that inhibit the cytochrome P450 enzyme system and steroids have also been frequently implicated. The same drugs used for sedation, analgesia, and anxiolysis (barbiturates, opiates, and benzodiazepines) can cause confusion as well. Many conditions that complicate the postoperative course can cause clouding of consciousness (delirium), especially in the elderly patient. Pulmonary embolism, pneumonia, sepsis, and myocardial infarction frequently present as confusion. Electrolyte imbalance, acid–base disorders, and hepatic and renal failure can also cause confusion and anxiety as the initial clinical sign.

Once the underlying cause is addressed, or if the indication for sedation is very clear-cut (i.e. an awake patient fully oriented on ventilatory support), a therapeutic plan is in order. Attempts should always be made to enhance communication, frustrating as the experience may be for the physician and the patient. Involvement of close family members may, in itself, have a therapeutic effect. When pharmacologic interventions are considered, the minimum dose that provides the therapeutic effect must be used. "Heavy" sedation to the point of complete detachment from the environment used to be the preferred technique, particularly in ventilated patients.[48] That strategy, however, puts the patient at risk for oversedation or prolonged sedation, and the minimum dose that will provide comfort and still allow the patient to respond to command is recommended. Multiple studies have addressed the differences between different schedules and compared therapeutic options.[49,50] Traditionally, a combination of a benzodiazepine and narcotic analgesic has been used. Lorazepam and midazolam are the most commonly used benzodiazepines, while fentanyl and morphine are among the most commonly employed narcotics. Propofol is also a very useful agent for sedation in the ICU. However, reports of hypertriglyceridemia may limit its use for long-term infusion. The use of this agent has recently been reviewed.[51]

Table 67.3 *Accuracy of the indexes used to predict weaning outcome (from Yang and Tobin[46] with permission)*

Index	Sensitivity	Specificity	Positive predictive value	Negative predictive value
Minute ventilation	0.78	0.18	0.55	0.38
Respiratory frequency	0.92	0.36	0.65	0.77
Tidal volume	0.97	0.54	0.73	0.94
Tidal volume/patient's weight	0.94	0.39	0.67	0.85
Maximal inspiratory pressure	1.00	0.11	0.59	1.00
Dynamic compliance	0.72	0.50	0.65	0.58
Static compliance	0.75	0.36	0.60	0.53
P_{aO_2}/P_{AO_2} ratio	0.81	0.29	0.59	0.53
Frequency/tidal volume ratio	0.97	0.64	0.78	0.95
CROP index	0.81	0.57	0.71	0.70

CROP index, compliance rate oxygenation pressure index.

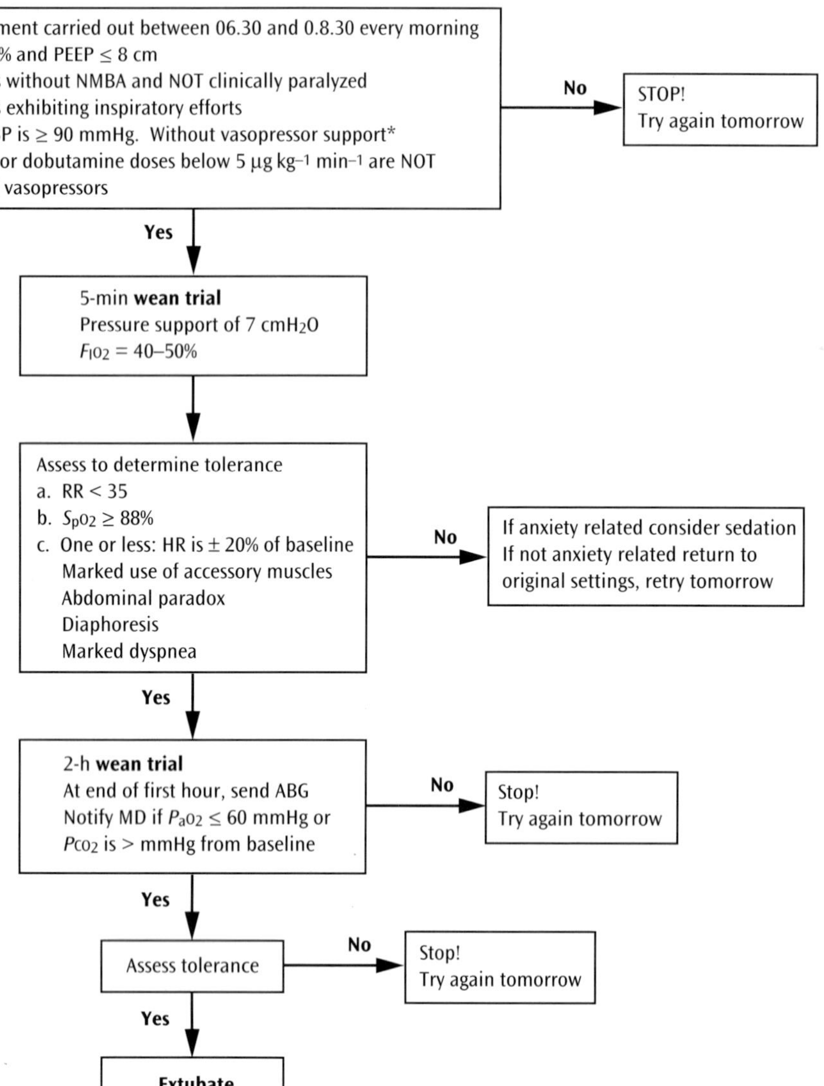

Figure 67.2 *Example of a simplified weaning protocol.*

The choice of agent has more to do with the prevailing conditions in the particular ICU than with the characteristics of the agents themselves. For example, the population served (predominance of short-term postoperative cardiac patients vs. long-term trauma patients) and the economic considerations (different cost schemes in different regions or countries) may sway the selection toward one drug or another. A loading dose followed by an intravenous infusion is the optimum method of delivery. Infusion of the drugs is titrated to effect, to avoid oversedation.[52] Interruptions of the infusion at scheduled daily intervals are suggested, in order to prevent accumulation of the infused drugs and prolonged effect. One of the most common methods of assessment of the level of sedation is the Ramsay scale (Table 67.4).[53] Although this assessment does not provide information on the quality of the sedation, it is simple to use.

Neuromuscular blocking agents in the ICU

The use of muscle relaxants in the ICU was once very common. The purported advantages include lower oxygen consumption, control of intracranial pressure, supplementation of some forms of ventilator strategies (permissive hypercapnia, inverse inspiratory–expiratory ratio), and facilitation of bedside procedures. However, in the early 1990s, several reports of prolonged paralysis in the ICU appeared in the literature.[54,55] The reports linked paralysis with the administration of steroid nucleus blocking agents, but reports implicating nonsteroidal neuromuscular blocking agents soon followed.[56] Two forms of prolonged paralysis have been described. In the first, the cause appears to be the inability to excrete active metabolites. In the other, a poorly understood interaction with the receptor at the neuromuscular junction is the likely basis for the complication. The correct application of neuromuscular blocking agents requires the use of a nerve stimulator and monitoring of the degree of paralysis by means of any of the accepted monitoring strategies used in anesthesia. In the USA, the use of nerve stimulators was in the past infrequent. A survey conducted in 1991 found that neuromuscular blockade[57] was routinely monitored in only 4% of ICUs. We believe that the use of neuromuscular blocking agents in the ICU should be restricted to very few and specific situations. Furthermore, the use of these drugs should be preceded by an educational effort and training in the use of nerve stimulators, to avoid the occurrence of harmful neuromuscular weakness.

Table 67.4 *ICU sedation score (from Ramsay* et al.[53] *with permission)*

Patient awake	
1	Patient anxious and agitated or restless, or both
2	Patient cooperative, orientated and tranquil
3	Patient responds to command only
Patient asleep	
4	Brisk response
5	Sluggish response
6	No response

Asleep level is dependent on the patient's response to a light glabellar tap or loud auditory stimulus.

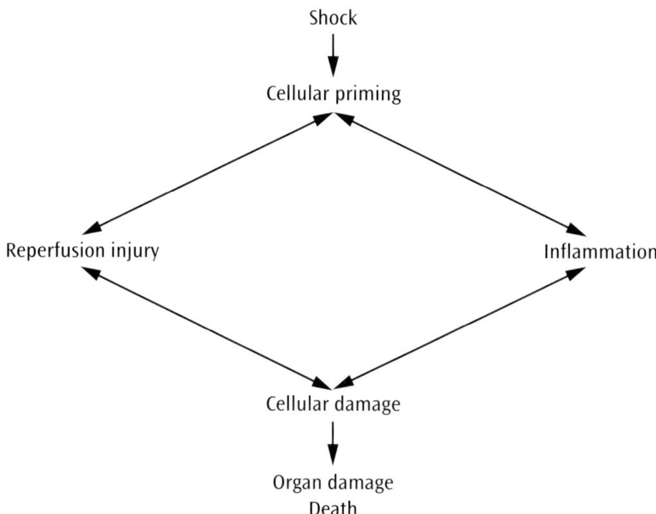

Figure 67.3 *A new paradigm for traumatic shock (from Waxman[61] with permission).*

SPECIAL INTENSIVE CARE-REQUIRING SYNDROMES

Systemic inflammatory response syndrome (SIRS)

This term was originally coined by Bone *et al.*[58] in an attempt to describe and characterize the observed systemic response to infection. The original aim was to improve the ability to make an earlier bedside detection of sepsis, to facilitate early medical intervention, and to allow standardization of research protocols. At the time, the term SIRS was defined as more than one of the following: (1) a body temperature greater than 38 °C or less than 36 °C; (2) a heart rate greater than 90 beats min^{-1}; (3) tachypnea, manifested by a respiratory rate greater than 20 breaths min^{-1}, or hyperventilation, as indicated by a P_aCO_2 of less than 32 mmHg; and (4) an alteration in the white blood cell count to more than 12 000 mm^{-3} or a less than 4000 mm^{-3}, or the presence of more than 10% immature forms ("bands"). The criteria are very broad, and the authors themselves recognized the limitations. Many other conditions may meet more than one of the above criteria and still not represent a systemic inflammatory response.

What is the underlying process that leads to SIRS? Originally, the clinical features of the syndrome were attributed to sepsis. However, it is clear today that, although sepsis and the byproducts of invading micro-organisms can trigger the syndrome, multiple pathologic states can lead to this condition. Burns, trauma, and shock of multiple etiologies can also trigger SIRS. At the cellular level, the initiating event is believed to be an alteration in cellular function as a consequence of transient oxygen deprivation (dysoxia).[59] In this setting, intracellular acidosis along with several alterations in cell function ensue (Fig. 67.3).[60] These include increased intracellular sodium and water and a decrease in the transmembrane potential. Although cells can survive a severe hypoxic insult for extended periods of time, the adaptive changes the insult initiates (termed "hypoxic priming"[61]) may lead to injury following reinstitution of more physiologic conditions (ischemia–reperfusion).

This state occurs upon restoring oxygen delivery to the cells. It is believed that during the dysoxic period ATP is not replenished, and an increase in precursors of reactive oxygen species occurs. Cells are then "primed" by ischemia and have the potential to produce increased numbers of oxygen free radicals during reoxygenation. The free radicals injure the cells directly, by causing damage to cell and organelle membranes, denaturation of proteins, and disruption of chromosomes. They also lead to activation of inflammation by multiple mechanisms. Oxidant injury appears to rapidly activate polymorphonuclear leukocytes (PMNs).[62] It also activates macrophages to release cytokines, including tumor necrosis factor (TNFα), interleukin 1β, interleukin 8, and platelet-activating factor (PAF). These cytokines amplify the inflammatory response by further activation of PMNs. The biochemical events surrounding the inflammatory response can be outlined, although significant uncertainty remains. TNFα, IL-1β, and IL-8 are proinflammatory cytokines, whereas IL-10 modulates or downregulates the acute inflammatory response but may enhance a chronic monocytic inflammatory response. IL-6 is also responsible for many of the acute-phase responses associated with stress. After the initial insult, TNFα, IL-1β, and IL-8 promote neutrophil adhesion and release of proteolytic enzymes, oxygen radicals, and arachidonate mediators. They also promote the release of other cytokines that act to perpetuate the inflammatory process, as well as those that retard the inflammatory response. Secondary inflammatory mediators (cytokines, prostaglandins, leukotrienes, and proteases) are released[63] secondary to neutrophil recruitment and activation.

The neuroendocrine stress response also plays an active role. Several hormones and neuropeptides have a significant role during the inflammatory challenge.[64] Although some areas are controversial, this mechanism would be the underlying mechanism responsible for the clinical expression of the SIRS, which can precede multiple organ system failure (MOSF).

Much research has been conducted into the role of the gastrointestinal (GI) tract as the initiator of the SIRS process. It has been hypothesized that poor GI tract perfusion leads to increased intestinal wall permeability, with bacterial translocation and gut-derived endotoxemia further promoting the metabolic derangement seen in MOSF. Experimental studies in animals support the concept that in the face of a severe insult the gut becomes very sensitive to ischemia–reperfusion injury. Such injury impairs the mechanical barrier of the intestinal mucosa, leading to translocation of bacteria and endotoxin, a process that would result in the release of inflammatory mediators and SIRS. Although there is an extensive body of experimental and clinical evidence to support a role of the gut in SIRS,[65] its function as the mechanism for maintaining the pathogenic process associated with SIRS and MOSF has been questioned, and therapies such as selective decontamination of the GI tract have failed to improve survival.[66]

Unfortunately, there is no clinical test that can accurately predict or signal the start of the dysoxic state and its consequences. Measurement of blood lactate levels is controversial, and the presence of elevated lactate levels would imply a much later stage of the dysoxic state. Furthermore, normal blood lactate levels do not ensure the presence of adequate tissue oxygenation. Measurements of regional blood flow are available, such as the gastric tonometer, which indicates the adequacy of aerobic metabolism at the level of the mucosal lining of the stomach.

This technique has been found to be useful as a marker of inadequate regional flow during resuscitation.[67]

Further, there is doubt as to whether the problem is always the inadequate *utilization* of oxygen. Certainly, in low-flow states such as hypovolemic shock, the dysoxic state is the consequence of poor perfusion. Clinically, hypotension, tachycardia, and oliguria are late markers of established poor cardiac output. However, in certain pathologic states, such as sepsis, regional maldistribution of blood flow more than low flow itself is the cause of the dysoxia.[68,69] Animal studies also suggest that an impairment in the utilization of oxygen may be involved in the genesis of the dysoxic state.[70] This process is now being studied, and the management of patients at risk for impaired oxygen utilization is very important. Avoidance of dysoxia by ensuring adequate oxygen delivery and aggressive correction of low or maldistributed flow states is paramount: "resuscitation delayed is resuscitation denied."

How should patients undergoing a catastrophic insult that leads to poor perfusion be treated? Since the classic work of Shoemaker *et al.*[71] it has been hypothesized that patients develop an "oxygen debt", which can be calculated clinically.[72] Shoemaker *et al.* argue that traditional endpoints of resuscitation (normalization of heart rate and blood pressure) are achieved in both survivors and nonsurvivors of critical illness and, therefore, lack reliability as outcome predictors. It is also observed that survivors achieve supranormal values of oxygen delivery (DO_2) and consumption (VO_2). In 1988, Shoemaker *et al.*[73] proposed that supranormal values of oxygen delivery should be achieved in order to improve the outcome after shock states. This group published the results of a randomized study of 58 patients and demonstrated that mortality and morbidity could indeed be reduced if the cardiac output and oxygen delivery values were used to target additional therapy. Since this controversial report, multiple studies have been published addressing the question of supranormal oxygen delivery in shock states of different etiologies, with mixed results. Depending on the population studied, the methodology to achieve the supranormal oxygen delivery values, and the endpoint of therapy selected, the studies reported an improvement in outcome,[74,75] no effect,[76] or an increase in mortality.[77,78] The identification of patients who may benefit from this kind of goal-oriented resuscitation remains elusive.

Although multiple therapeutic goals have been published, identification of poor oxygen delivery appears to be a critical first step. It can be achieved by any means available in the setting in which the clinician is working, such as measurement of cardiac output and index, gastric tonometry, mixed venous oxygen saturation, oxygen extraction ratio, etc. If a decision is made to increase oxygen delivery to supranormal values once optimal fluid resuscitation has been performed, the therapeutic hemodynamic endpoints should be individualized. While an oxygen delivery of 600 $mL\,min^{-1}\,m^{-2}$ has been advocated,[74,75] this may be too much for elderly patients and, in trying to achieve increased oxygen delivery, other complications, such as myocardial ischemia and infarction, may ensue. On the other hand, that endpoint may be too conservative for young, healthy trauma patients. An excellent review on the subject has been published.[79]

Multiple organ system failure (MOSF)

The term defines a clinical condition characterized by multiple dysfunction of organs or systems to the point of needing sophisticated measures of support available in the ICU. MOSF usually develops in the ICU, and it is simply the consequence of treatment of individual organ failure. The ability to support pulmonary gas exchange, renal function, and hemodynamic homeostasis, as well as advances in enteral and parenteral nutrition, frequently leads to a prolonged course with a significant risk for sequential failure of other systems. The syndrome may also be immediately preceded by SIRS, after an initial injury (the so-called one-hit model) in which the inflammatory cascade described previously continues unabated during the ICU stay. Today, MOSF is one of the leading causes of prolonged stay and mortality in the ICU.

MOSF may also be precipitated by an event during the ICU stay, such as an infection, intra-abdominal catastrophe needing surgery, etc. (two-hit model). The sequence or timing of organ failure does not follow any clearly identified pattern. The available treatment of MOSF is supportive, and consists of therapies aimed at individual organs, replacing or supporting those that have failed, i.e. renal replacement therapy, mechanical ventilation, inotropic support of the heart, combined with prevention of possible complications such as malnutrition, line sepsis, and ventilator-associated pneumonia. However, as the knowledge of the pathophysiologic process increases, new therapies aimed at underlying mechanisms have emerged.

As much of the injury in reperfusion is caused by oxygen free radicals, attempts at increasing the antioxidant capacity of the patient have been tested. There is a solid body of evidence in animals that supports the supplementation of antioxidants in different models of ischemia–reperfusion.[80] Among the therapies tested in animal studies are the administration of xanthine oxidase inactivators, including sodium tungsten,[81] allopurinol,[82] and folate.[83] Aprotinin, a serine protease inhibitor, is used clinically to decrease blood loss in heart surgery, and has also shown promise as an agent to decrease oxidant stress by increasing antioxidant defenses.[84] In humans, protocols aimed at ameliorating ischemia–reperfusion and the incidence of SIRS have been tested. One such protocol, directed at trauma patients in the University of Miami, includes intravenous lidocaine (lignocaine), folate, vitamin C, selenium, mannitol, glutamine, acetylcysteine and vitamins A and E, among other agents.[85,86]

Another potential line of therapy involves the modulation of the cytokine cascade. This approach to therapy has been tested clinically in patients with sepsis, given the predisposition of septic patients to suffer from SIRS-MOSF. Multiple anti-cytokine therapies have been tested. These include anti-TNF receptor antibodies,[87,88] anti-TNF antibodies,[89,90] IL-1 receptor antagonists,[91,92] and PAF receptor antagonist.[93] Overall, the attempt to neutralize the cytokine bioactivity in MOSF demonstrates only a small, nonsignificant trend toward improved survival. In view of the documented role of cytokines in the process, and some evidence from animal studies of the effectiveness of anti-cytokine therapy,[94] the lack of success in this area so far possibly indicates that the redundancy of the system makes the attack on a single molecule insufficient to obtain a clinically important result. Treatment of SIRS-MOSF at this point therefore consists of good ICU care, support of the individual organs, and prevention of complications.

Acute respiratory distress syndrome (ARDS)

Acute respiratory distress syndrome (ARDS) is very common in the ICU setting. This syndrome was first described more than 30 years ago.[95] Since then, extensive research has been conducted investigating the epidemiology, pathophysiology, and management of the condition. One recurrent problem, however, has been the lack of a standard definition of the syndrome. In 1992, a European–American Consensus Committee on ARDS was formed to focus on issues of definition, mechanisms, risk factors, etc. The report[96] acquired great significance because a definition of the syndrome was established, as well as a definition of the term "acute lung injury" (ALI) (Table 67.5).

Many conditions can lead to the development of ARDS. Sepsis, aspiration of gastric contents, trauma, multiple transfusions, pneumonia, and smoke inhalation as well as other pulmonary insults have been implicated in its genesis. Irrespective of the cause, the triggering event often does not involve the lungs primarily. For example, ARDS is in many cases the pulmonary manifestation of SIRS in its progression

Table 67.5 *Recommended criteria for acute lung injury (ALI) and acute respiratory distress syndrome (ARDS) (from Bernard* et al.[96] *with permission)*

	Timing	Oxygenation	Chest radiograph	Pulmonary artery wedge pressure
ALI criteria	Acute onset	$P_ao_2/F_io_2 \leq 300$ mmHg (regardless of PEEP level)	Bilateral infiltrates seen in frontal chest radiograph	≤ 18 mmHg when measured or no evidence of left atrial hypertension
ARDS criteria	Acute onset	$P_ao_2/F_io_2 \leq 200$ mmHg (regardless of PEEP level)	Bilateral Infiltrates seen in frontal chest radiograph	≤ 18 mmHg when measured or no evidence of left atrial hypertension

to MOSF. Although the pathologic picture has been referred to as diffuse alveolar damage,[97] it has become clear that the damage is far from uniform.[98] Areas of normal lung architecture are mixed with areas with airspace disease. This finding has significant therapeutic implications.

From the pathologic point of view, two well-defined stages have been identified. In the early stage, all patients exhibit increased permeability of the alveolar–capillary membrane with accumulation of protein-rich fluid in the alveolar space.[99,100] This edema fluid also contains white and red blood cells. Hyaline membranes are often formed. This phase is followed by a fibroproliferative stage over the next 7–14 days, when repair is initiated but pulmonary fibrosis, capillary obliteration, and pulmonary hypertension can also develop.

Clinically, hypoxemia is the hallmark of the syndrome. Areas of very low ventilation–perfusion ratio due to the alveolar edema cause the severe intrapulmonary shunt. Patients are tachypneic, with a rapidly worsening picture, characterized radiologically by bilateral infiltrates in the chest radiograph. Patients almost always require mechanical ventilatory support. Management of this condition includes general supportive care, nutrition, avoidance of line sepsis, etc. Most patients undergo mechanical ventilation for a prolonged period of time. Several pharmacologic agents directed against the perceived underlying pathogenic mechanism have also been tested in the treatment.

Mechanical ventilation is a potential source of iatrogenic damage. However, significant progress has been made in this area, and the prognosis of the patient is much more dependent on comorbidities or the potential development of extrapulmonary complications, rather than the ARDS itself. Since areas of significant damage are not available for gas exchange, the area of effective ventilation is limited. The use of the classic settings of a ventilator (e.g. 10–15 mL kg^{-1} tidal volume) results in overdistension of the units that are spared. Consequently, those alveoli are exposed to trauma caused by the therapeutic maneuver designed to treat the pulmonary syndrome.

Originally thought to be a pressure-related injury, ventilator-induced lung injury may be more related to the distension itself (volotrauma) than to the pressure applied. Hernandez *et al.*[101] tested the hypothesis by subjecting young rabbits to mechanical ventilation at high pressures. Rabbits were divided into three groups: closed chest, open (excised lungs) chest, and closed chest with a full body plaster cast. The results revealed a significant increase in the capillary filtration coefficient in the open lung and virtually no change in the rabbits covered with a cast, suggesting that distension, and not pressure, is the pathogenic mechanism of the ventilator-induced injury.

In humans, Roupie *et al.*[102] demonstrated, using pressure–volume curves, that plateau pressures were above the upper inflexion point (the point at which an increase in pressure does not result in an increase in volume, indicating near-maximal stretching) in 80% of patients with ARDS when ventilated with tidal volumes of 10 mL kg^{-1}. These findings suggest that this tidal volume is excessive. Given the strength of these data, the so-called lung protective strategy has been advocated. The principle is based on the use of low tidal volumes and limited airway pressure to avoid overdistension and high end-expiratory pressure (PEEP) to maximize the recruitment and patency of alveolar units. The use of high PEEP also may prevent the damage caused by the repetitive opening and closing of the alveoli. The results of such a strategy have been mixed, with some reports showing higher rates of weaning[103,104] and shorter periods of mechanical ventilation. The inevitable consequence of the above-mentioned strategy is a rise in $P\text{CO}_2$. However, no attempts are made to increase ventilation (permissive hypercapnia; Table 67.6), leading to respiratory acidosis. The consequences of hypercapnia have been reviewed.[105,106]

The only formal contraindication to the institution of a ventilation strategy that involves permissive hypercapnia is the presence of increased intracranial pressure, given the powerful vasodilatory activity of CO_2 in the cerebral vessels. Additionally, patients need to be sedated to blunt the ventilatory response to hypercapnia. Another supportive measure to improve oxygenation is to place the patient in the prone position with the aim of improving ventilation in dependent areas of the lung, which have been shown to consolidate in severe ARDS.[107–109]

Several pharmacologic strategies based on the pathophysiology of the syndrome have emerged. Among them, the replacement of surfactant[110] and nitric oxide (NO) therapy[111] has been proposed to treat ARDS and ALI. As surfactant is lost early in the inflammatory process, leading to alveolar collapse, replacement by insufflation into the lungs has been advocated. Surfactant therapy is well established for newborns with respiratory distress syndrome (RDS). Trials in adults have shown improved survival when protein-rich, bovine surfactant was used.[112] However, a larger trial using synthetic surfactant failed to demonstrate improvement.[113] More research in the area of protein-rich surfactant is needed before a clinical recommendation can be issued.

NO is synthesized in a variety of cells and acts as an intracellular or extracellular messenger. By its action on cyclic guanosine 3,5′-monophosphate (cGMP), NO causes smooth muscle relaxation and when produced by endothelial vascular cells leads to vasodilation. The vasodilatory effects have been used in ARDS, to improve oxygenation and decrease shunt.[111] When delivered by inhalation, it reaches the better ventilated lung units, where it spreads to the smooth muscle of the pulmonary vessels as well. The resultant vasodilation preferentially increases perfusion to the well-ventilated areas, decreasing the shunt and improving oxygenation.[114] It will also cause a decrease in pulmonary vascular resistance.[115]

Outcome studies, however, produced controversial results. In a cohort study of septic patients with ARDS, responders to NO exhibited an improved survival that did not reach statistical significance (67% vs. 40%).[116] In a multicenter, double-blinded, placebo-controlled study, Dellinger *et al.*[117] enrolled 177 patients to receive different doses of

Table 67.6 *Application of permissive hypercapnia for acute lung injury (modified from Dries*[105] *with permission)*

Ventilator parameters	Other measures
Inspired oxygen fraction < 0.6	Sedation
Rate < 30 breaths min^{-1}	Reduce CO_2 production
Tidal volume 4–7 mL kg^{-1}	Consider base administration
Peak airway pressure < 35 cmH$_2$O	
Plateau airway pressure < 30 cmH$_2$O	
PEEP 7–15 cmH$_2$O	
Minimal I/E ratio 1:1	

NO and placebo. There were improvements in intermediate outcome parameters (i.e. days off mechanical ventilation) in one group of patients, but no improvement in survival.

Liquid ventilation

This term applies to a modality of ventilation that includes the use of a perfluorocarbon (PFC), an inert substance with very low surface tension and high respiratory gas solubility. The strategy involves the use of PFC to fill up the lungs (total liquid ventilation or TLV) or the use of PFC to fill up a volume equal to the functional residual capacity, and apply conventional gas ventilation.[118] The strategy is called perfluorocarbon-associated gas exchange (PAGE). This therapy has demonstrated improvement in gas exchange in lung injury models and in humans. It is hypothesized that the ability of PFC to recruit atelectatic areas and improve lung compliance may be the basis of its therapeutic action.[119] Furthermore, PFC may also have anti-inflammatory actions in the lung. Initial experience with the use of partial liquid ventilation has been reported in humans, with improvement in gas exchange and compliance.[120]

As the understanding of the cytokine cascade has become better understood[121,122] many trials of anticytokine therapy have been conducted for sepsis (see above), with disappointing results. The effect of anti-cytokine therapy has not been specifically studied in ARDS.

The presence of highly reactive oxygen species is kept under control by different antioxidant mechanisms in the normal lung. However, those may be overwhelmed in ARDS. Attempts to increase the natural antioxidant defenses (catalase, superoxide dismutase, etc.) result in a decrease in the duration of ALI.[123] Finally, the delivery of oxygen to patients with ARDS is common, to avoid hypoxemia. However, in the inflammatory milieu of the injured lung, the administration of oxygen can increase the local inflammatory process.[124,125] Oxygen should be administered to patients with ARDS as necessary to prevent hypoxemia, and only in the minimal dose possible, which has to be determined individually. As a guideline, the F_{IO_2} should be set to keep the hemoglobin oxygen saturation above 90%.

Ventilator-associated pneumonia (VAP)

Patients who receive mechanical ventilation make up a significant percentage of any ICU population. Ventilator-associated pneumonia (VAP) (see also Chapter 70) is a frequent complication of ventilatory support, and one accompanied with significant mortality. In fact, VAP is such a common event that the clinician should consider not *if* pneumonia may occur, but *when* it will occur."[126] The incidence of VAP has been estimated from 9% to 21% in patients with respiratory failure of different origins, and is more frequent in patients with ARDS.[127,128] Frequent as it may be, however, VAP is a very difficult diagnosis to make, and both overdiagnosis and underdiagnosis are frequent. VAP is defined as bacterial pneumonia developing in patients with acute respiratory failure who have been receiving mechanical ventilation for at least 48 h.[129] Classical clinical criteria for the diagnosis of pneumonia in patients receiving mechanical ventilation, as compiled by Meduri,[130] include radiographic appearance of a new or progressive pulmonary density, fever, leukocytosis, purulent tracheobronchial secretions, and tracheal aspirate Gram stain showing more than 25 leukocytes and fewer than 10 squamous epithelial cells per low-power field, with recovery of a potential pathogen.

The problem in applying clinical criteria such as the ones mentioned above to patients receiving mechanical ventilation is that many other conditions can cause a similar clinical picture. Colonization of the upper airway with Gram-negative bacteria is common after even a short period of mechanical ventilation.[131] The presence of the endotracheal tube impairs mucociliary and mechanical clearance from the lower airways, which quickly become covered by a biofilm that is colonized.[132] Changes in plain radiographs and computed tomography consistent with pneumonia are also seen in atelectasis, pulmonary hemorrhage, pulmonary edema, ARDS, and other pulmonary syndromes. Purulent secretions are common in tracheal aspirates but may originate in the upper respiratory tract, and the area of the trachea above the endotracheal tube cuff serves a "catch basin" for oral or nasopharyngeal secretions. Finally, fever and leukocytosis may be absent in VAP patients. In short, when strict diagnostic criteria are used, less than half of the patients who meet the clinical criteria are found to have VAP.[133,134]

Other diagnostic tools have been developed to overcome the lack of specificity of the clinical diagnosis. Among them, the protected specimen brush (PSB) and bronchoalveolar lavage (BAL) are the most important. The protected specimen brush consists of a fiberoptic bronchoscope with a double-catheter system and an occluding plug (designed to bypass the upper airway and avoid contamination) and is used to obtain a specimen from the area suspected to be infected. Quantitative culture is used to differentiate between colonization and infection, the cut-off point being 10^3 colony-forming units (CFU) mL^{-1}. The accuracy of the technique has been confirmed by evaluating postmortem histologic and microbiologic lung features in the same lung area.[135] The reported sensitivity of PSB ranges from 88% to 100% and specificity from 60% to 100%.[136–138] Quantitative BAL involves the use of a fiberoptic bronchoscope, which is wedged in a distal airway. Sequential instillation and aspiration of a physiologic solution follows. BAL samples a large area of the lung (approximately 10^6 alveoli) and recovers 5–10 times the number of organisms obtained by PSB. A CFU count of 10^4 mL^{-1} is diagnostic.[139] The reported sensitivity ranges from 76% to 100% and specificity from 82% to 100%.[140–142] The use of nondirected nonbronchoscopic techniques has been advocated, mostly based on expense, convenience, and potential morbidity of the bronchoscopic techniques. The correlation between nonbronchoscopic, protected aspirates of the airway and the above-mentioned techniques is good.[143]

What, then, is the best diagnostic approach? The issue is very relevant, as timely identification and treatment of VAP may improve survival.[128] However, BAL fluid might have a role in excluding pneumonia in the ventilated patient. The method developed by Meduri *et al.*,[144] using a systematic diagnostic protocol, maybe the most rational approach at the present time to an elusive diagnosis that carries a significant morbidity and cost.

REFERENCES

1. King's Fund. Intensive care in the United Kingdom. *Anesthesia* 1989; **44:** 428–31.
2. Joint Committee on Accreditation of Healthcare Organizations. *Comprehensive Accreditation Manual for Hospitals: The Official Handbook* 1998. Standard TX 1.2.
3. Task Force on Guidelines, Society of Critical Care Medicine: Guidelines for categorization of services for the critically ill patient. *Crit Care Med* 1991; **19:** 279–85.
4. Cohen IL, Bari N, Strosberg MA, *et al.* Reduction of duration and cost of mechanical ventilation in an intensive care unit by the use of a ventilator management team. *Crit Care Med* 1991; **19:** 1278–84.
5. Hanson CW, Deutshman CS, Anderson HL, *et al.* Effects of an organized critical care service on outcomes and resource utilization: a cohort study. *Crit Care Med* 1999; **27:** 270–4.
6. Brown JJ, Sullivan G. Effect on ICU mortality of a full-time critical care specialist. *Chest* 1989; **96:** 127–9.
7. Reynolds HN, Haupt MT, Thill-Baharozian, *et al.* Impact of critical care physician staffing on patients with septic shock in a university hospital medical intensive care unit. *JAMA* 1988; **260:** 3446.
8. Kirton OC, Civetta JM. Setting objectives: perspectives for care. In: Civetta JM, Taylor RW, Kirby RR (eds). *Critical Care*, 3rd edn. Philadelphia, PA: Lippincott-Raven, 1997: 23.
9. Task force of the American College of Critical Care Medicine and the

Society of Critical Care medicine. Guidelines for intensive care unit admission, discharge and triage. *Crit Care Med* 1999, **27:** 633–8.

10. Rigdon EE, Monajjem N, Rhodes RS. Criteria for selective utilization of the intensive care unit following carotid endarterectomy. *Ann Vasc Surg* 1997; **11:** 20–7.
11. Morasch MD, Hirko MK, Hirasa T, *et al.* Intensive care unit after carotid endarterectomy: a prospective evaluation. *J Am Coll Surg* 1996; **183:** 387–92.
12. Melissano G, Castellano R, Mazzitelli, *et al.* Safe and cost effective approach to carotid surgery. *Eur J Vasc Surg* 1997; **14:** 164–9.
13. Young EWD. Life and death in the ICU: ethical considerations. In: Civetta JM, Taylor RW, Kirby RR. (eds) *Critical Care*, 3rd edn. Philadelphia, PA: Lippincott-Raven, 1997: 64.
14. Cook DJ, Guyatt GH, Jaeschke R, *et al.* Determinants in Canadian health care workers of the decisions to withdraw life support in the critically ill. *JAMA* 1995; **273:** 703–8.
15. Council on Ethical and Judicial Affairs, American Medical Association. Decisions near the end of life. *JAMA* 1992; **267:** 2229–33.
16. American Thoracic Society. Withholding and withdrawing life sustaining therapy. *Am Rev Respir Dis* 1991; **144:** 726–31.
17. Brody H, Campbell ML, Faber-Langendoen K, *et al.* Withdrawing intensive life-sustaining treatment – recommendations for compassionate clinical management. *N Engl J Med* 1997; **336:** 652–7.
18. Prendergast TJ, Luce JM. Increasing incidence of withholding and withdrawal of life support from the critically ill. *Am J Respir Crit Care Med* 1997; **155:** 15–20.
19. Consensus statement of the Society of Critical Care Medicine's Ethics Committee regarding futile and other possibly inadvisable treatments. *Crit Care Med* 1997; **25:** 887–91.
20. Gregoire G, Russell JA. Assessment of severity of illness. In: Hall JB, Schmidt GA, Wood LDH (eds). *Principles of Critical Care*, 2nd edn. New York, NY: McGraw Hill, 1998: 57.
21. Cullen DJ, Civetta JM, Briggs BA, *et al.* Therapeutic Intervention Scoring System. A method for quantitative comparison of patient care. *Crit Care Med* 1974; **2:** 57–62.
22. Keene AR, Cullen DJ. Therapeutic Intervention Scoring System. Update 1983. *Crit Care Med* 1983; **11:** 1–3.
23. Knaus WA, Draper EA, Wagner DP, *et al.* APACHE II: a severity of disease classification system. *Crit Care Med* 1985; **13:** 818–829.
24. Jacobs S, Change RW, Lee B, Lee B. Audit of intensive care: a 30 month experience using the Apache II severity of disease classification system. *Int Care Med* 1988; **14:** 567–574.
25. Kruse JA, Thill-Baharozian MC, Carlson RW. Comparison of clinical assessment with APACHE II for predicting mortality risk in patients admitted to a medical intensive care unit. *JAMA* 1988; **260:** 1739–42.
26. Dobkin JE, Cutler RE. Use of APACHE II classification to evaluate outcome of patients receiving hemodialysis in an intensive care unit. *Western J Med* 1988; **149:** 547–50.
27. Fedullo AJ, Swinburne AJ, Wahl GW, *et al.* APACHE II score and mortality in respiratory failure due to cardiogenic pulmonary edema. *Crit Care Med* 1988; **16:** 1218–21.
28. Rowan KM, Kerr JH, Major E, *et al.* Intensive Care Society's APACHE II study in Britain and Ireland. I. Variations in case mix of adult admissions to general intensive care units and impact on outcome. *Br Med J* 1993; **307:** 972–7.
29. Rowan KM, Kerr JH, Major E, *et al.* Intensive Care Society's APACHE II study in Britain and Ireland-II: Outcome comparisons of intensive care units after adjustment for case mix by the American method. *Br Med J* 1993; **307:** 977–81.
30. Godhill David R, Sumner A. Outcome of intensive care patients in a group of British intensive care units. *Crit Care Med* 1998; **26:** 1337–45.
31. Knaus WA, Wagner DP, Draper EA, *et al.* The APACHE III prognostic system. Risk prediction of hospital mortality for critically ill hospitalized adults. *Chest* 1991; **100:** 1619–36.
32. Pappachan JV, Millar B, Bennett ED, *et al.* Comparison of outcome from intensive care admission after adjustment for case mix by the APACHE III prognostic system. *Chest* 1999; **115:** 802–10.
33. Zimmerman JE, Wagner DP, Draper EA, *et al.* Evaluation of acute physiology and chronic health evaluation III predictions of hospital mortality in an independent database. *Crit Care Med* 1998; **26:** 1317–26.
34. Bastos PG, Sun X, Wagner DP, *et al.* Application of the APACHE III prognostic system in Brazilian intensive care units: a prospective multicenter study. *Int Care Med* 1996; **22:** 564–70.
35. Beck DH, Taylor BL, Millar B, Smith GB. Prediction of outcome from intensive care: a prospective cohort study comparing Acute Physiology and Chronic Health Evaluation II and III prognostic systems in a United Kingdom intensive care unit. *Crit Care Med* 1997; **25:** 9–15.
36. Le Gall JR, Loirat P, Alperovitch A, *et al.* A simplified acute physiology score for ICU patients. *Crit Care Med* 1984; **12:** 975–7.
37. Le Gall JR, Leweshow S, Saulnier F. A new Simplified Acute Physiology Score SAPS II based on a European/North American Multicenter Study. *JAMA* 1993; **270:** 2957–63.
38. Moreno R, Morais P. Outcome prediction in intensive care: results of a prospective, multicenter, Portuguese study. *Int Care Med* 1997; **23:** 177–86.
39. Apolone G, Bertolini G, D'Amico R, *et al.* The performance of SAPS II in a cohort of patients admitted to 99 Italian ICUs: results from GiViTI. Gruppo Italiano per la Valutazione degli interventi in Terapia Intensiva. *Int Care Med* 1996; **22:** 1368–78.
40. Lemeshow SD, Teres D, Klar J, *et al.* Mortality Probability Models (MPM II) based on an International cohort of Intensive Care Unit Patients. *JAMA* 1993; **270:** 2478–86.
41. Stewart TE, Meade, MO, Cook, DJ, *et al.* Evaluation of a ventilation strategy to prevent barotrauma in patients at high risk for acute respiratory distress syndrome. *N Engl J Med* 1998; **338:** 355–61.
42. Conti G, Marino P, Cogliati A, *et al.* Noninvasive ventilation for the treatment of acute respiratory failure in patients with hematologic malignancies: a pilot study. *Int Care Med* 1988; **24:** 1283–8.
43. Varon J, Walsh GL, Fromm Jr RE. Feasibility of noninvasive mechanical ventilation in the treatment of acute respiratory failure in postoperative cancer patients. *J Crit Care* 1998; **13:** 55–7.
44. Hilbert G, Gruson D, Gbikpi-Benissan G, Cardinaud JP. Sequential use of noninvasive pressure support ventilation for acute exacerbations of COPD. *Int Care Med* 1997; **23:** 955–61.
45. Horst H, Mathilda MD, Mouro D, *et al.* Decrease in ventilation time with a standardized weaning process. *Arch Surg* 1998; **133:** 483–8.
46. Yang KL, Tobin MJ. A prospective study of indexes predicting the outcome of trials of weaning from mechanical ventilation. *N Engl J Med* 1991; **324:** 1445–50.
47. Esteban A, Frutos F, Tobin MJ, *et al.* A comparison of four methods of weaning patients from mechanical ventilation. *N Engl J Med* 1995; **332:** 345–50.
48. Merriman HM. The techniques used to sedate ventilated patients. *Int Care Med* 1981; **7:** 217–24.
49. Cernaianu AC, DelRossi AJ, Flum DR, *et al.* Lorazepam and midazolam in the intensive care unit: a randomized, prospective, multicenter study of hemodynamics, oxygen transport, efficacy, and cost. *Crit Care Med* 1996; **24:** 222–8.
50. Chamorro C, de Latorre FJ. Montero A, *et al.* Comparative study of propofol versus midazolam in the sedation of critically ill patients: results of a prospective, randomized, multicenter trial. *Crit Care Med* 1996; **24:** 932–9.
51. Miller LJ, Wiles-Pfeifler R. Propofol for the long-term sedation of a critically ill patient. *Am J Crit Care* 1998; **7:** 73–6.
52. Shafer A. Complications of sedation with midazolam in the intensive care unit and a comparison with other sedative regimens. *Crit Care Med* 1998; **26:** 947–56.
53. Ramsay MA, Savege TM, Simpson BR, *et al.* Controlled sedation with alphaxalone/alphadolone. *Br Med J* 1974; **2:** 256.
54. Kupfer Y, Namba T, Kaldawi E, *et al.* Prolonged paralysis after long term infusion of vecuronium. *Ann Intern Med* 1992; **117:** 484–6.
55. Segredo V, Caldwell JE, Miller R. Persistent paralysis in critically ill patients after long term administration of vecuronium. *N Engl J Med* 1992; **327:** 524–8.
56. Watling S, Dasta J. Prolonged paralysis in intensive care unit patients after the use of neuromuscular blocking agents: a review of the literature. *Crit Care Med* 1994; **22:** 884–93.
57. Hansen-Flaschen JH, Brazinsky S, Basile C, *et al.* Use of sedating drugs and neuromuscular blocking agents in patients requiring mechanical ventilation for respiratory failure: a national survey. *JAMA* 1991; **266:** 2870–5.
58. Bone RC, Balk RA, Cerra FB, *et al.* ACCP/SCCM Consensus Conference. Definitions of sepsis and organ failure and guidelines for the use of innovative therapies in sepsis. *Chest* 1992; **101:** 1644–55.
59. Connett R, Honig C, Gayeski T, *et al.* Defining hypoxia: a systems view of VO_2, glycolysis, energetics, and intracellular PO_2. *J Appl Physiol* 1990; **68:** 833–42.
60. Gores G, Nieminen A, Wray B, *et al.* Intracellular pH during "chemical hypoxia" in cultured rat hepatocytes. *J Clin Invest* 1989; **83:** 386–96.
61. Waxman K. Shock: ischemia, reperfusion and Inflammation. *New Horiz* 1996; **4:** 153–60.
62. Seekamp A, Mulligan MS, Till GO, *et al.* Requirements for neutrophil products and L-arginine in ischemia–reperfusion injury. *Am J Pathol* 1993; **142:** 1217–26.

63. Wheeler AP, Bernard GR. Treating patients with severe sepsis. *N Engl J Med* 1999; **340:** 207–14.
64. Chrousos GP. The hypothalamic–pituitary–adrenal axis and immune mediated inflammation. *N Engl J Med* 1995; **332:** 1351–62.
65. Deitch EA, Rutan R, Waymack JP. Trauma, shock and gut translocation. *New Horiz* 1996; **4:** 289–99.
66. Van Saene HKF, Stoutenbeek CC, Stroller JK. Selective decontamination of the digestive tract in the intensive care unit: current status and future prospects. *Crit Care Med* 1992; **20:** 691–703.
67. Chang MC, Cheatham ML, Nelson LD, *et al.* Gastric tonometry supplements information provided by systemic indicators of oxygen transport. *J Trauma* 1994; **37:** 488–94.
68. Winslow C, Dorinsky PM. Regional blood flow distribution in endotoxin treated dogs: modification by ibuprofen. *J Crit Care* 1994; **9:** 159–68.
69. Fink MP, Cohn SM, Lee P, *et al.* Effect of Lipopolysaccharide on intestinal intramucosal hydrogen ion concentration in pigs: evidence of gut ischemia in a normodynamic model of septic shock. *Crit Care Med* 1989; **17:** 641–6.
70. Unno N, Wang H, Menconi MJ, *et al.* Inhibition of inducible nitric oxide synthase ameliorates endotoxin-induced gut mucosal barrier dysfunction in rats. *Gastroenterology* 1997; **113:** 1246–57.
71. Shoemaker WC, Montgomery ES, Kaplan E, *et al.* Physiologic patterns in surviving and non surviving shock patients. *Arch Surg* 1973; **106:** 630–6.
72. Shoemaker WC, Appel PL, Kram HB. Role of oxygen debt in the development of organ failure, sepsis and death in high risk surgical patients. *Chest* 1992; **102:** 208–15.
73. Shoemaker WC, Appel PL, Kram HB, *et al.* Prospective trial of supranormal values of survivors as therapeutic goals in high-risk surgical patients. *Chest* 1988; **94:** 1176–86.
74. Boyd O, Grounds RM, Bennett ED. A randomized clinical trial of the effect of deliberate perioperative increase of oxygen delivery on mortality in high risk surgical patients. *JAMA* 1993: **270:** 2699–707.
75. Yu M, Burchell S, Hasaniya N, *et al.* Relationship of mortality to increasing oxygen delivery in patients > 50 years of age: a prospective, randomized trial. *Crit Care Med* 1998; **26:** 1011–19.
76. Gattinoni L, Brazzi L, Pelosi P, *et al.* A trial of goal-oriented hemodynamic therapy in critically ill patients. *N Engl J Med* 1995; **333:** 1025–32.
77. Hayes MA, Yau EHS, Timmins AC, *et al.* Response of critically ill patients to treatment aimed at achieving supranormal oxygen delivery and consumption: relationship to outcome. *Chest* 1993; **103:** 886–95.
78. Hayes MA, Timmins AC, Yau EHS, *et al.* Elevation of systemic oxygen delivery in the treatment of critically ill patients. *N Engl J Med* 1994; **330:** 1717–22.
79. Yu M. Oxygen transport optimization. *New Horiz* 1999; **7:** 46–53.
80. Sies H. Strategies of antioxidant defense. *Eur J Biochem* 1993; **215:** 213–19.
81. Nielsen VG, Tan S, Baird MS, *et al.* Gastric intramucosal pH and multiple organ injury: impact of ischemia–reperfusion and xanthine oxidase. *Crit Care Med* 1996; **24:** 1339–44.
82. Deitch EA, Specian RD, Grisham MB, *et al.* Zymosan-induced bacterial-translocation: a study of mechanisms. *Crit Care Med* 1992; **20:** 782–8.
83. Manning A, Bernier M, Crome R, *et al.* Reperfusion-induced arrhythmias: a study of the role of xanthine oxidase-derived free radicals in the rat heart. *J Mol Cell Cardiol* 1988; **20:** 35–45.
84. Nader-Djalal N, Davidson BA, Kurek CJ, *et al.* Aprotinin restores superoxide dismutase activity in acute inflammatory lung injury. *Anesthesiology* 1998; **89(3A):** A1380.
85. Hudson-Civetta J, Civetta J, Kirton OC, *et al.* Mitigating increased severity of illness in trauma patients (Abstract). *Crit Care Med* 1998; **26** (Suppl.): A94.
86. Kirton OC, Civetta J, Hudson-Civetta J. Gastric intramucosal pH driven resuscitation and antioxidants. Normalized pHi is associated with high survival (Abstract). *Crit Care Med* 1998; **26** (Suppl.): A142.
87. Abraham E, Glauser MP, Butler T, *et al.* P55 tumor necrosis factor receptor fusion protein in the treatment of patients with severe sepsis and septic shock. Ro 45–2081 Study Group. *JAMA* 1997; **227:** 1531–8.
88. Fisher CU, Agosti JM, Opal SM, *et al.* Treatment of septic shock with the tumor necrosis factor receptor: Fc fusion protein. *N Engl J Med* 1997; **334:** 1697–702.
89. Cohen J, Carlet J. INTERSEPT: an international, multicenter, placebo-controlled trial of monoclonal antibody to human tumor necrosis factor-alpha in patients with sepsis. International Sepsis Study Group. *Crit Care Med* 1996; **24:** 1431–40.
90. Abraham E, Anzueto A, Gutierrez G, *et al.* Double blind randomized controlled trial of monoclonal antibody to human tumor necrosis factor in treatment of septic shock. *Lancet* 1998; **351:** 929–33.
91. Fisher CJ, Dhainaut JF, Opal SM, *et al*: Recombinant human interleukin 1 receptor antagonist in the treatment of patients with sepsis syndrome. Phase III rhIL 1ra Sepsis syndrome study Group. *JAMA* 1994; **271:** 1836–43.
92. Opal SM, Fisher CJ, Dhainaut FJ. Confirmatory Interleukin 1 receptor antagonist in severe sepsis: a phase III, randomized, double-blind, placebo controlled, multicenter trial. *Crit Care Med* 1997; **25:** 1115–24.
93. Dhainaut JF, Tenaillon A, Hemmer M, and the BN 52021 Sepsis Investigator Group. Confirmatory platelet activating factor receptor antagonist trial in patients with severe gram negative bacterial sepsis: a phase III, randomized, double-blind, placebo-controlled, multicenter trial. *Crit Care Med* 1998; **26:** 1963–71.
94. Folkesson HG, Matthay MA, Hebert CA, *et al.* Acid aspiration induced lung injury in rabbits is mediated by interleukin 8 dependent mechanisms. *J Clin Invest* 1995; **96:** 107–16.
95. Ashbaugh DG, Bigelow DB, Petty TI, *et al.* Acute respiratory distress in adults. *Lancet* 1967; **2:** 319–23.
96. Bernard GR, Artigas A, Brigham KL, and the consensus committee. The American–European Consensus Conference on ARDS. Definitions, Mechanisms, Relevant Outcomes, and Clinical Trial Coordination. *Am J Respir Crit Care Med* 1994; **149:** 818–24.
97. Rinaldo JE, Rogers RM. Adult respiratory distress syndrome: changing concepts of lung injury and repair. *N Engl J Med* 1982; **306:** 900–9.
98. Gattinoni L, Bombino M, Pelosi P, *et al.* Lung structure and function in different stages of severe adult respiratory distress syndrome. *JAMA* 1994; **271:** 1772–6.
99. Brigham KL, Meyrick B. Endotoxin and lung injury. *Am Rev Respir Dis* 1986: **133:** 913–27.
100. Matthay MA, Wiener-Kronish JP. Intact epithelial barrier function is critical for the resolution of alveolar edema in humans. *Am Rev Resp Dis* 1990; **142:** 1250–7.
101. Hernandez LA, Peevy KJ, Moise AA, *et al.* Chest wall restriction limits high airway pressure-induced lung injury in young rabbits. *J Appl Phys* 1989; **66:** 2364–8.
102. Roupie E, Dambrosio M, Servillo G, *et al.* Titration of tidal volume and induced hypercapnia in acute respiratory distress syndrome. *Am J Resp Crit Care Med* 1995; **152:** 121–8.
103. Amato MBP, Barbas CSV, Medeiros DM, *et al.* Beneficial effects of the "open lung approach" with low distending pressures in acute respiratory distress syndrome: a prospective randomized study on mechanical ventilation. *Am J Respir Crit Care Med* 1995; **152:** 1835–46.
104. Amato, MBP, Barbas CSV, Medeiros D, *et al.* Effect of a protective-ventilation strategy on mortality in the acute respiratory distress syndrome. *N Engl J Med* 1998; **338:** 347–54.
105. Dries DJ. Permissive hypercapnia. *J Trauma* 1995; **39:** 984–9.
106. Feihl F, Perret C. Permissive hypercapnia. How permissive should we be? *Am J Resp Crit Care Med* 1994; **150:** 1722–37.
107. Gattinoni L, Pelosi P, Vitale G, *et al.* Body position changes redistribute lung computed tomographic density in patients with acute respiratory failure. *Anesthesiology* 1991; **74:** 15–23.
108. Stocker R, Neff T, Stein S, *et al.* Prone positioning and low-volume pressure limited ventilation improve survival in patients with severe ARDS. *Chest* 1997; **111:** 1008–17.
109. Jolliet P, Bulpa P, Chevrolet JC. Effects of the prone position on gas exchange and hemodynamics in severe acute respiratory distress syndrome. *Crit Care Med* 1998; **26:** 1977–1985.
110. Lewis JF, Jobe AH. Surfactant and the adult respiratory distress syndrome. *Am Rev Resp Dis* 1993; **147:** 218–33.
111. Roissant R, Falke K, Lopez F, *et al.* Inhaled nitric oxide for the adult respiratory distress syndrome. *N Engl J Med* 1993; **328:** 399–405.
112. Gregory TJ, Longmore WJ, Moxley MA, *et al.* Bovine surfactant therapy for patients with acute respiratory distress syndrome. *Am J Respir Crit Care Med* 1997; **155:** 1309–15.
113. Anzueto A, Baughman RP, Guntupalli KK, *et al.* Aerosolized surfactant in adults with sepsis-induced acute respiratory distress syndrome. Exosurf Acute Respiratory Distress Syndrome Study Group. *N Engl J Med* 1996; **334:** 1417–21.
114. Gerlach H, Roissaint R, Pappert D, *et al.* Time course and dose response on nitric oxide inhalation for systemic oxygenation and pulmonary hypertension in patients with adult respiratory distress syndrome. *Eur J Clin Invest* 1993; **23:** 499–502.
115. Puybasset L, Rouby JJ, Mourgeon E, *et al.* Factors influencing cardiopulmonary effects of inhaled nitric oxide in acute respiratory failure. *Am J Respir Crit Care Med* 1995; **152:** 318–28.
116. Krafft P, Fridrich P, Fitzgerald RD, *et al.* Effectiveness of nitric oxide inhalation in septic ARDS. *Chest* 1996; **109:** 486–93.
117. Dellinger RP, Zimmerman JL, Taylor RW, *et al.* Effects of inhaled nitric

oxide in patients with acute respiratory distress syndrome: results of a randomized phase II trial. Inhaled Nitric Oxide in ARDS Study Group. *Crit Care Med* 1998; **26:** 15–23.

118. Fuhrman BP, Paczan PR, Defrancisis M. Perfluorocarbon associated gas exchange. *Crit Care Med* 1991; **19:** 712–22.
119. Tooley R, Hirschl RB, Parent A, *et al.* Total liquid ventilation with perfluorocarbons increases pulmonary end-expiratory volume and compliance in the setting of lung atelectasis. *Crit Care Med* 1996; **24:** 268–73.
120. Hirschl RB, Pranikoff T, Wise C, *et al.* Initial experience with partial liquid ventilation in adult patients with the acute respiratory distress syndrome. *JAMA* 1996; **275:** 383–9.
121. Donnelly TJ, Meade P, Jagels M, *et al.* Cytokine, complement and endotoxin profiles associated with the development of the adult respiratory distress syndrome after severe injury. *Crit Care Med* 1994; **22:** 768–76.
122. Kiehl MG, Ostermann H, Thomas M, *et al.* Inflammatory mediators in bronchoalveolar lavage fluid and plasma in leukocytopenic patients with septic shock-induced acute respiratory distress syndrome. *Crit Care Med* 1998; **26:** 1194–9.
123. Bernard GR, Wheeler AP, Arons MM, *et al.* A trial of antioxidants N-acetylcysteine and procysteine in ARDS. *Chest* 1997; **112:** 164–72.
124. Nader-Djalal N, Knight PR, Davidson BA, *et al.* Hyperoxia exacerbates micro-vascular lung injury following acid aspiration. *Chest* 1997; **112:** 1607–14.
125. Knight PR, Kurek C, Davidson BA, *et al.* Acid aspiration increases sensitivity to increased ambient oxygen concentrations. *Am J Physiol Lung Cell Mol Physiol* 2000; **278:** L1240–7.
126. Garrard CS, A'Court CD. The diagnosis of pneumonia in the critically ill. *Chest* 1995; **108:** 17S–25S.
127. Craven DE, Steger KA, Barat LM, *et al.* Nosocomial pneumonia: epidemiology and infection control. *Int Care Med* 1992; **18:** 510–17.
128. Torres A, Aznar R, Gatell JM, *et al.* Incidence, risk and prognostic factors of nosocomial pneumonia in mechanically ventilated patients. *Am Rev Respir Dis* 1990; **142:** 523–8.
129. Pingleton SK, Fagon JY, Leeper KV. Patient selection for clinical investigation of ventilator associated pneumonia: Criteria for evaluating diagnostic techniques. *Chest* 1992; **102:** 553–8.
130. Meduri UG. Diagnosis and differential diagnosis of ventilator associated pneumonia. *Clin Chest Med* 1995; **16:** 61–93.
131. Johanson Jr WG, Pierce AK, Sanford JP, *et al.* Nosocomial respiratory infections with gram negative bacilli. The significance of colonization of the respiratory tract. *Ann Int Med* 1972; **7:** 701–6.
132. Inglis TJ, Millar MR, Jones G, *et al.* Tracheal tube biofilm as a source of bacterial colonization of the lungs. *J Clin Microbiol* 1989; **7:** 2014–18.
133. Meduri GU, Mauldin GL, Wunderkind RG, *et al.* Causes of fever and pulmonary densities in patients with clinical manifestations of ventilator associated pneumonia. *Chest* 1994; **106:** 221–35.
134. Fagon JY, Chastre J, Hance AJ, *et al.* Evaluation of clinical judgment in the identification and treatment of nosocomial pneumonia in ventilated patients. *Chest* 1993; **103:** 547–53.
135. Chastre J, Fagon JY, Bornet M, *et al.* Evaluation of bronchoscopic techniques for the diagnosis of nosocomial pneumonia. *Am Rev Respir Dis* 1995; **152:** 231–40.
136. Baughman RP, Thorpe JE, Staneck J, *et al.* Use of the protected specimen brush in patients with endotracheal or tracheostomy tubes. *Chest* 1987; **91:** 233–5.
137. Chastre J, Fagon JY, Soler P, *et al.* Diagnosis of nosocomial bacterial pneumonia in intubated patients undergoing ventilation: Comparison of the usefulness of the bronchoalveolar lavage and the protected specimen brush. *Am J Med* 1988; **85:** 499–506.
138. Chastre J, Vian F, Brun P, *et al.* Prospective evaluation of the protected specimen brush for the diagnosis of pulmonary infection in ventilated patients. *Am Rev Respir Dis* 1984; **130:** 924–9.
139. Meduri GU, Chastre J. The standardization of bronchoscopic techniques for VAP. *Chest* 1992; **102:** 557–64.
140. Guerra LF, Baughman RP. Use of bronchoalveolar lavage to diagnose pneumonia in mechanically ventilated patients. *Crit Care Med* 1990; **18:** 169–73.
141. Violan JS, De Castro FR, Luna JC. Comparative efficacy of bronchoalveolar lavage and telescoping plugged catheter in the diagnosis of pneumonia in mechanically ventilated patients. *Chest* 1993; **103:** 386–90.
142. Chastre J, Fagon JY, Bornet M, *et al.* Comparison of the usefulness of bronchoalveolar lavage and the protected specimen brush for diagnosing nosocomial bacterial pneumonia. *Am Rev Respir Dis* 1992; **145:** A542.
143. Rumbak MJ, Bass RL. Tracheal aspirate correlates with protected specimen brush in long term ventilated patients who have clinical pneumonia. *Chest* 1994: **106:** 531–4.
144. Meduri GU, Mauldin GL, Wunderkind RG, *et al.* Causes of fever and pulmonary densities in patients with clinical manifestations of ventilator associated pneumonia. *Chest* 1994; **106:** 221–35.

68

Thermal injury: anesthesia, analgesia, and intensive care

KEITH C JUDKINS AND W DAVID LORD

INTRODUCTION

A lot has changed during the last decade or two in the clinical management of the burned patient. There has been much research into wound healing, and improved treatment possibilities have been developed, including better techniques of skin substitution and grafting. Length of stay in hospital is much shorter, infections are fewer, and outcomes are more satisfactory when measured in terms of functional recovery. Efforts are now being focused on injury prevention, improved psychologic well-being for the recovered burn victim, more confident return to work or school, and reintegration into society.[1]

One of the most important achievements of the recent past has been better understanding of the relation between burn surgery and high-quality intensive care, a symbiosis that enhances the potential for survival of the massively burned patient or of the burn complicated by inhalation injury, previous comorbidity or associated trauma, and reduces length of stay for many patients.[2] Aggressive resuscitation and early surgical intervention have resulted in survival of patients with the severest of injuries. Continuing treatment with early physiotherapy and techniques of contracture control, such as compression by pressure garments, have resulted in better cosmetic and functional repair. Morbidity and mortality from thermal injury is however increased by the presence of pre-existing respiratory, metabolic, or endocrine disease or additional trauma such as fractures.

Children

Children, in contrast, free from degenerative disease, are capable of an extraordinary degree of repair. Successful management depends on strong overall direction, and the active involvement of many medical and paramedical disciplines is required. It is now impossible to consider intensive care in severe burn injury separately from the provision of anesthesia and analgesia in support of surgery to the burn wound. The role of the anesthesiologist as a member of the burn care team in the management of a survivable burn is therefore pivotal. The concept of the anesthesiologist as a "perioperative care consultant" is nowhere better illustrated than in the care of the burned patient, encompassing the activities listed in Table 68.1.

In this chapter, paragraphs of particular relevance to care of children are subheaded. Exhortations to tailor treatment to the specific needs of children are, however, to be found throughout the text.

DEMOGRAPHICS AND CAUSATION

It is estimated that each year in the UK there are approximately 14 000 thermal injuries that necessitate hospital admission. This probably represents only a fraction of the burns that occur in the community, most of which are trivial. A similar "tip-of-the-iceberg" picture is obtained in the USA, where the hospitalization rate is about one million, and indeed in most other countries. Less than 15% of patients needing hospital treatment are burned sufficiently severely to need referral to a burn center, and, of these, up to 10% may require intensive care during some part of their stay; 45% or so are children, most of whom are under 3 years old. The commonest causes of thermal injury are listed in Table 68.2.

Scalds

Scalds are common in children and in the elderly. Over 85% of small children admitted have suffered scalds, usually from common household sources of hot liquid, such as cups of tea or coffee, kettles, and saucepans.

Flame burns

Flame burns are less common than scalds, usually arising from house fires, and are frequently major, sometimes life-threatening, and almost always accompanied by smoke inhalation. Electrical faults, unextinguished cigarettes, cookers, domestic open fires, and naked flames such as candles have all been identified as causes of house fires, but one of the commonest is children playing with matches. In the UK, legal and industry standards (British Standards Institute, BSI) for children's clothing material and the reduction in open fires in homes has dramatically reduced the incidence of flame injury. However, the current trend for wearing T-shirts and unconventional night attire has resulted in a recent increase in flame burns, because these garments are not covered by the legislation.

Adolescents, especially boys, experiment with fire, fireworks, and flammable liquids resulting in sometimes extensive deep injury. In adults, thermal injury sometimes has an industrial cause, but it occurs more frequently in association with frailty or neglect due to age, psychiatric illness, or substance abuse. More exotic causes include barbecues or the inappropriate use of petrol to aid ignition of a bonfire. Self-immolation with petrol or other accelerants is fortunately less common but usually severe.

Table 68.1 *Aspects of burn care in which the anesthesiologist's contribution is significant*

At the district/community hospital	• Initial assessment and resuscitation of burned patients at the local hospital • Transportation of moderate and major burns to appropriate burn care services • Anesthesia and analgesia for minor burns in the district hospital context and in plastic surgery units, including provision of training • Recognition of danger symptoms in minor burns
In the specialized burn center	• Full assessment and resuscitation of patients with major and complex burns and recognition of complications • Intensive care for adult and pediatric major burns, particularly treatment of respiratory tract injury (upper airway obstruction and smoke inhalation), including training • Anesthesia for modern burn surgery, including children, and including training • Provision of pain relief in burn treatment facilities for acute and background pain, for pain after surgery, and for dressings changes and procedures, including training

Table 68.2 *Causes of thermal injury*

Scalds
Flame burns
Explosions
Contact burns
Chemical burns
Electrical injury
Ionizing radiation
Nonaccidental injury

Electrical burns

Electrical burns vary from small but very deep burns to the hand or mouth caused when a small child investigates the mains electricity to massive injury from high-tension electricity caused, for instance, when a teenager goes train-surfing. Low-tension injuries are rarely dangerous but may cause disability or disfigurement that must be minimized by appropriate surgical treatment. In contrast, high-tension injuries cause extensive deep tissue injury, which may be belied by a moderate area of skin burn. Deep tissue damage is caused by a combination of microvascular coagulation and high heat intensity in tissues of greater electrical resistance, typically bone, so that adjacent deep muscle dies. Major nerve trunks may be damaged, leading to varying degrees of paralysis. Other serious complications include a high risk of renal failure caused by massive release of tissue hemochromagens, compartment syndrome due to swelling of affected muscle groups, and spinal shock if the spinal cord is affected.

High-tension electrical burns are always serious until proved otherwise, and invasive monitoring is almost always needed. Emergency fasciotomy can save limbs; rigorous fluid resuscitation guided by invasive monitoring will often save lives. Urgent surgery is needed to debride all damaged deep tissues. This may have to be repeated daily until no more die-back of ischemic tissue is identified.

Flash burns

Flash burns, caused by explosion accidents or electrical arcing (no direct contact), are the result of high temperatures at short duration. They are usually more superficial than flame injuries, but may be associated with other injury such as blast damage to the lung.

Chemical burns

Chemical burns differ from other causes only in their initial management, which must include immediate and thorough first aid. These are fortunately rare, but the anesthesiologist may be called to the emergency department to assist in initial management; a brief outline of specific care is given in Table 68.3. Hydrofluoric acid burns present particular problems because of the high penetration of the fluoride ion, which chelates calcium, causing severe pain and risk of cardiac arrest if sufficient is absorbed to reach the heart.[3]

Table 68.3 *Specific treatment notes for chemical burns*

General
Always protect yourself – wear rubber gloves and other protection as appropriate
Except as indicated below, first aid includes copious irrigation with running water
Antidotes (sodium bicarbonate for acids and weak vinegar for alkalis) must be used with caution as some reactions are exothermic; a phosphate buffer solution is safer but water is most readily available
Avoid secondary injury by making sure that all care personnel are protected from contact with the chemical on the patient – wear gloves
Phosphorus
First aid using water does not stop burning while the phosphorus is in the wound
Pick out phosphorus with forceps (helped by using 1% copper sulfate solution, which turns the phosphorus particles black)
Beware: the above may cause systemic copper toxicity if used on a large area
Phenol
Irrigation with copious running water will help remove the phenol
Water/saline soaks are contraindicated as they enhance phenol absorption through skin
Polyethylene glycol soaks may assist removal of phenol from skin
Do not treat ingestion by drinking water: enhances absorption. Activated charcoal
Hydrofluoric acid
Immediate irrigation with cold water
Removal of finger- or toenails if the acid has penetrated beneath
Calcium gluconate gel rubbed in continuously until pain is relieved
Intra-arterial calcium gluconate 10% if injury is distal (relieves pain, may preserve part)
10% calcium gluconate under the wound is advocated (not proved effective)
Serum calcium levels may become dangerously low; must be measured frequently
Once hydrofluoric acid has penetrated the superficial layers of the skin, the only way to remove it may be immediate excision of the wound

Radiation burns

Radiation burns are very rare, usually small, and usually caused by excessive deep X-ray therapy. They heal slowly and graft take is often poor. Cover using a flap (local, or microvascular free tissue transfer) may be necessary, with skin graft to the flap donor site.

Contact burns

Contact burns occur at both ends of the age spectrum: the newly ambulant child who reaches up and places a hand on a cooker ring or the elderly person with diminished sensation who collapses at home against a domestic radiator and is unable to get up again quickly, becoming slowly cooked in the part of the body in contact with the radiator.

Nonaccidental injury (NAI)

NAI is most often seen in children, although a frail or demented adult may occasionally be admitted whose injury has been caused by the actions of a long-term family carer who has reached the end of her tether – the great majority of such carers are women. In some minority populations, an "accidental" injury is sometimes accompanied by an inconsistent history that raises a suspicion of assault by a relative (usually the husband) or of self-immolation, both as an expression of marriage difficulties. It is rare for these suspicions to be corroborated by hard evidence, which is a pity because the opportunity for support and counseling is lost. Care must never be compromised in the light of suspected or actual assault, especially if the alleged perpetrator is also injured.

NAI in children

This can rouse strong emotions in staff. Objectivity is important, and is one of the strengths of good legislation such as the UK Children's Act 1989, which prioritizes proper support for the child before apportionment of blame. The provisions of the Act may be triggered by any member of staff and are pursued through a clearly defined process, separate from but parallel to the clinical care of the child. The perpetrator may be a single mother at the end of her tether, or a jealous or vindictive boyfriend. Exasperation and ignorance feature more often than open cruelty. Typical NAI includes holding the child in an over-hot bath [which causes a typical pattern of damage, including buttock sparing, "sock pattern" injury to the feet (Fig. 68.1), and lack of splash injury]; cigarette burns to various body parts, typically hands, face, and genitals; holding the child's hand or face to a cooker ring or iron. Clues to the nonaccidental nature of the wound can be found in its appearance, the implausibility of the history, inconsistencies in the history from one family member to another, or abnormal emotions in the child to one or all family members. The wound alone cannot prove NAI; other pieces of evidence must be taken into account. The family is already known to social services more often than not. Sibling rivalry may occasionally be an important factor (the patient in Fig. 68.1 is in fact such a case).

Pediatricians normally lead the process of child protection investigation, but the anesthesiologist can sometimes provide valuable information from observing the interactions of a parent with the child during intensive care or at the time of surgery.

A word about emotions

Anesthesiologists are not immune from feelings of anger or other strong emotional reactions, including revulsion, when faced with major burn injuries, especially if nonaccidental. These can arise at any time, catching even experienced staff unawares. The irregularity with which major burns present can also induce stress. Death after weeks or sometimes months of hard and difficult work is a personal loss, for one has come to know the patient and the family. It is important that such reactions are acknowledged and dealt with outside the clinical situation, with professional help if necessary, if the affected person is to maintain his or her effectiveness within the team. Much support can be obtained within the team, and is usually given and received almost without being noticed for what it is. Recognizing those rare occasions when professional help is needed is difficult, but necessary if long-term damage to health is to be avoided. On the other hand, the rewards in seeing horribly burned victims recover both personality and function more than make up for the more negative moments.

CLASSIFICATION AND PROGNOSIS IN THERMAL INJURY

It is customary to classify thermal injury by depth and by percent of the total body surface area (% total body surface area, TBSA) burned. Prognosis is related to the area burned, the proportion of burn that is full thickness, the age of the patient, and the presence of inhalation injury.[4] Although comorbidity and other injuries influence prognosis, they are difficult to separate from these four factors. Various attempts have been made to measure prognosis, the most thorough of which for some time was that of Bull.[5] Much has changed since this work:

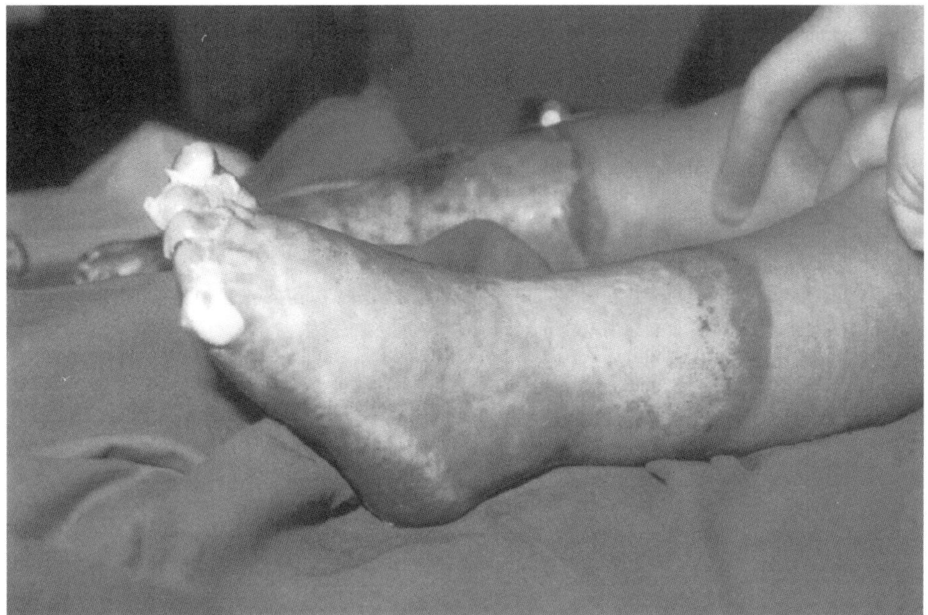

Figure 68.1 *"Sock pattern" distribution of deep scald following nonaccidental injury.*

intensive care has advanced, surgical approaches are more aggressive and effective. Their mortality probability chart, still frequently referred to, must be interpreted with caution therefore: a burn center achieving a comparative mortality of 1.0 vs. Bull should look to its laurels, especially in respect of uncomplicated moderate to major burns in fit, younger patients, especially children.

The age of the patient as a prognostic factor probably links to physiologic age just as it does in general intensive care, although few studies make the distinction between that and chronologic age. There is, however, good evidence that comorbidity at any age makes the prognosis worse.[4] In massive burns with smoke inhalation, ability to restore core temperature after cooling at initial assessment[6] or during surgery or dressings changes[7,8] is linked to prognosis in otherwise similar injuries, which may indicate a failure to mount an adequate metabolic response to the burn. There are, however, no foolproof indicators of prognosis, and the initial care philosophy should be that all burn-injured patients are capable of surviving. Decisions about lethality of injury and in favor of comfort care should be made carefully over time, guided usually by considerations not directly related to the severity of the burn.[9]

Death during resuscitation is now a very rare event. Most deaths are associated with late septic complications and with respiratory injury, and the greatest reduction in mortality in recent years has occurred in patients under 40 years with massive burns since the advent of aggressive early surgery to remove the burn wound.[4] This is heavily dependent on being able to close the wound, and in major burns availability of donor sites is limited, making immediate autograft impossible. Cadaver skin (fresh, cryopreserved, or glycerol preserved) is therefore used, or artificial skin substitutes. These are usually expensive, although cheaper alternatives can be developed in some circumstances.[10] Cultured epithelial autografts may help to achieve final wound healing, especially following massive burns when donor sites are scarce, but are also expensive and are beyond the scope of this chapter.

Classification of the severity of smoke inhalation injury is fraught with error because of the heterogeneous nature of the injury, although there have been attempts.[11] Prognosis is poorer in patients with a burn that is complicated by inhalation injury. This has been specifically investigated by Shirani *et al.*,[12] who report a low mortality in isolated smoke inhalation injury, rising to 40% when there is also a significant cutaneous burn. If pneumonia supervenes, the mortality rises to 80%. Other studies indicate less reduction in mortality by early surgery when inhalation injury is present than when the burn is uncomplicated.[13] The main mode of death remains, as ever, septic complications leading to multisystem organ failure.[4,14] The patient with inhalation injury has a much larger total injury, a second focus for sepsis in the injured lung, and invasive treatment and monitoring with sedation. All these increase exposure to nosocomial infection risk and diminish immunocompetence. It is not surprising therefore that smoke inhalation mortality has proved less accessible than the cutaneous wound to improved treatment. Excision and immediate cover of the wound can be very demanding in a major burn but are not technically difficult and can be undertaken at an early stage; in contrast, "excision and grafting" (heterotransplant) of the injured lung is reserved for extreme cases of lung failure only.

PATHOPHYSIOLOGY

The burn wound

The physiologic changes that follow burn injury were extensively studied over many years, culminating in a thorough review by Davies.[15] Among other things, it was determined that patients with thermal injury require about 0.5 mmol kg^{-1} per %TBSA burn of sodium in the first 24 h after injury. As has been understood for many years,[16] capillary leak occurs, which allows proteins to enter the extracellular compartment. With capillary integrity impaired, plasma proteins no longer exert their colloid osmotic effect. Further leak of fluid into edematous areas is therefore promoted until capillary integrity returns to normal. The most osmotically active substance in this circumstance is the most plentiful particle in solution, sodium.

A burn is a coagulative or colliquative lesion of the surface layers of the body, which varies in the area injured and the depth of the wound. The tissues affected are "cooked," their protein denatured, and their cellular structure disrupted. Altered proteins, membrane lipoprotein complexes (LPCs), and other chemicals are liberated into the surrounding tissue. The body recognizes these as foreign and mounts an inflammatory response in defense. The process, summarized in Fig. 68.2, is the subject of much research at the present time. Many factors are involved, including thromboxanes, leukotrienes, and the interleukins. The free radicals, superoxide anion (O_2^{-}), hydrogen peroxide (H_2O_2), and hydroxyl ion (OH^-), are also implicated. "Clumping" of white cells reduces blood flow to damaged but potentially viable areas under the burn (the "zone of stasis"), a process exacerbated by thromboxane A_2 (a smooth muscle constrictor). An interaction between the capillary endothelium and the leukocyte is probably the prime mover in the process, causing white cells to marginate in the capillary and extrude into the interstitium. There is potential in the first 24 h therefore for "wound conversion," or deepening of the burn. The complement cascade is activated in major injuries, probably the main stimulus for the systemic metabolic response. Some authors have suggested there is a specific "burn toxin" (probably a ligand of skin lipoprotein complexes) that triggers the inflammatory response and the subsequent immunosuppression and hypercatabolism.[17,18]

The leaky vascular endothelium caused by these influences is readily permeable to all intravascular substances with the exception of red blood cells. The control of the microcirculation is modified by release of local and circulating mediators such as histamine, bradykinin, and vasodilator prostaglandins. The net effect is an increase in extracellular fluid and pressure, resulting in reduced oxygen transport to damaged cells. Hypotension will exacerbate ischemia caused by locally mediated capillary shunting or vasoconstriction. The vessels under the burn are equally permeable to crystalloids and colloids, therefore the timescale of edema formation depends on cardiac output rather than the type of resuscitation fluid.

The eschar of deep circumferential burns is inelastic so will not swell outward as edema develops. Edema, in these circumstances, will cause venous and then arterial compression, producing acute ischemia and possibly limb loss, relieved only when the inelastic full-thickness burn is incised down to deep fascia by escharotomy.

It is logical to postulate that the magnitude of the response, whatever its causes, is proportional to the area of the interface between burn and living tissue, and this view is supported by the relation between burn size and mortality at any given age.[4,5] Burn depth is best expressed in descriptive terms, because the old descriptions of "degrees" of injury suffer from variance in interpretation in different countries. The injury may be described as "superficial," which affects the epidermis mainly, "partial thickness," which describes a dermal injury and can be shallow or deep, or "full thickness," in which all layers of the skin are involved. These are depicted in Fig. 68.3. Complex full-thickness injuries are those in which subcutaneous tissues such as muscle are involved. Depth of injury is of only minor importance in guiding immediate fluid resuscitation but is crucial for prognosis and in deciding surgical management.

If the burn is large, sufficient mediators are produced to give a significant "dose" to unburned organs and tissues. Capillary leak is therefore stimulated at these locations, leading to formation of nonburn edema. A decrease in cell transmembrane potential resulting in an

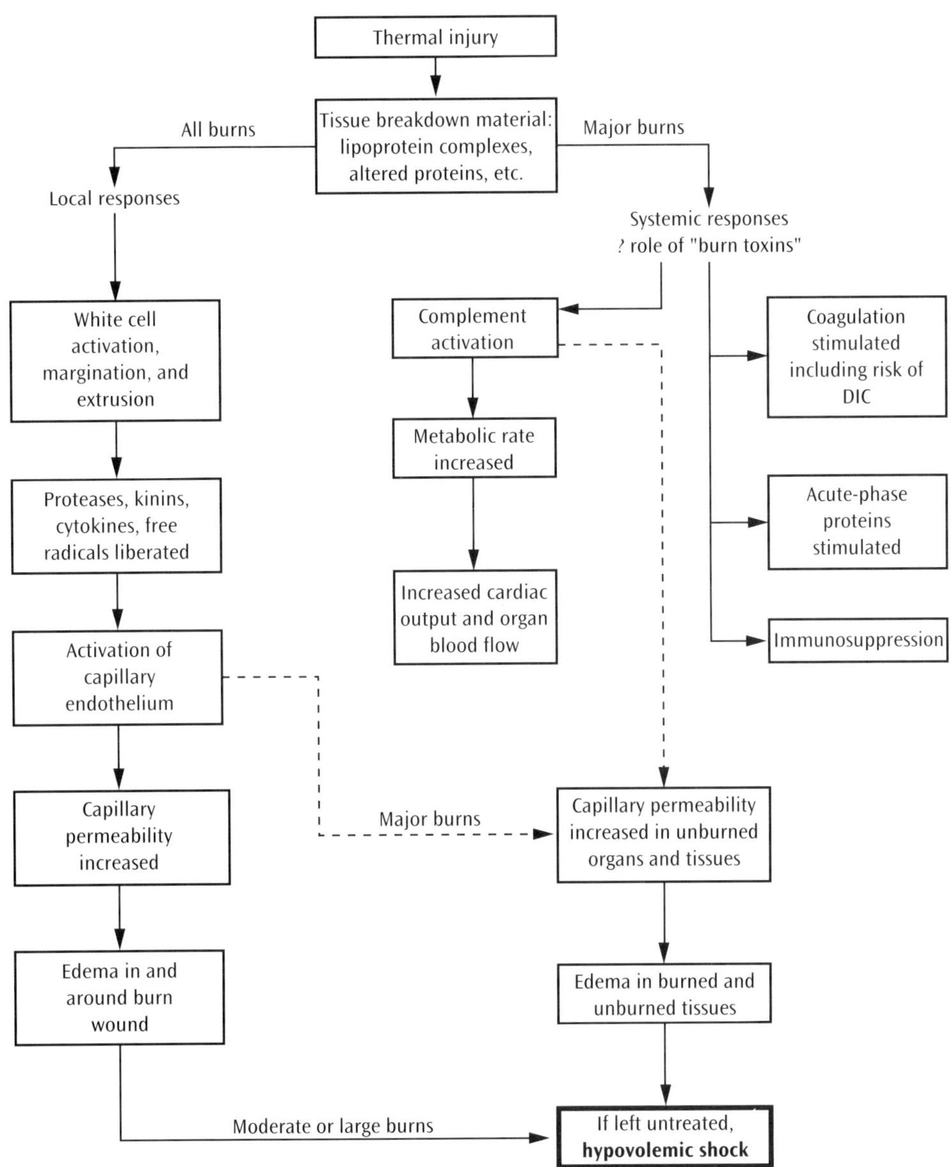

Figure 68.2 *The pathophysiologic response following thermal injury. DIC, disseminated intravascular coagulation.*

intracellular shift of sodium and water has also been suggested, making multiorgan failure increasingly likely the larger the burn. Crystalloid resuscitation leads to increased nonburn edema even in minor burns because there are no molecules big enough to confine the fluid to the vascular compartment. The exact significance of this for outcome has not been studied, although there are suggestions emerging that massive burns are at risk of compartment syndrome in unburned limbs, from this cause.[19] The rationale for fluid therapy is discussed in more detail below.

The respiratory tract

The pathophysiologic process in inhalation injury is broadly the same as that in the burned skin.[20] Because the structure and functions of the organ are different, the clinical effects are also very different (Fig. 68.4). In the upper airway, swelling is greater than in the skin because the submucosal areolar tissue is loose. Airway obstruction is likely, particularly when the pharynx, or larynx, is involved. In children, the clinical effect is proportionately more serious because the child's airways are much narrower than those of the adult.

Children

Cricoid edema can be demonstrated in most children with moderate and major burns even if the airway is not directly injured. This necessitates a reduction in tracheal tube size for age in the region of 0.5–1 mm, for both anesthesia and intensive care. The combination of burn and nonburn edema can be particularly dangerous around the head and neck, where massive and progressive edema will cause swelling of the face, tongue, and supraglottic structures. The edema reaches its peak at 24–36 h and subsides over 2 or 3 days.

The noxious fire environment

The consequences of smoke inhalation are mediated by the various components of smoke, some of which are listed in Table 68.4. Organic radicals are released irrespective of the combustible material. Some are intensely irritant, such as the aldehyde acrolein, whereas others have widespread activity on smooth muscle and the cardiovascular system. Some of these radicals are undoubtedly direct cellular toxins. Inorganic compounds, such as sulfur dioxide, nitrogen dioxide, chloride and phosphate radicals, become hydrated in the lung to form their corresponding

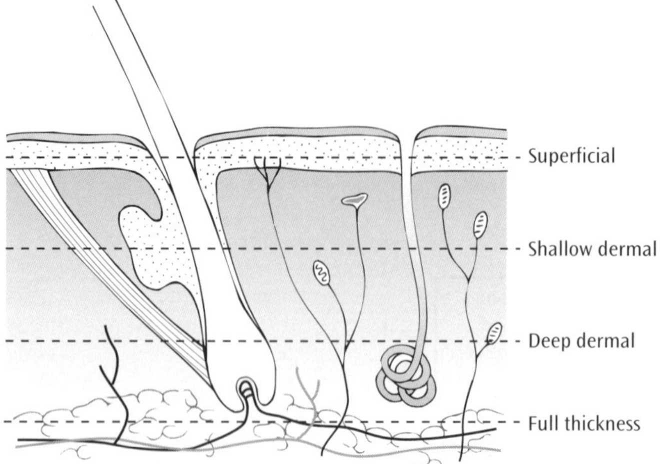

Figure 68.3 *Section through skin showing depths of thermal injury. (Reproduced and adapted by kind permission of Smith & Nephew Medical Limited.)*

Table 68.4 *Some constituents of smoke*[139]

Low oxygen	Aldehydes	Hydrogen chloride
High carbon dioxide	Acrolein	Hydrogen sulfide
Carbon monoxide	Acrylonitriles	Phosgene
Hydrogen cyanide	Isocyanates	Ammonia
Carbon particles	Formaldehyde	

acids. These organic and inorganic substances are adsorbed on to the surface of soot to be steadily released once inside the bronchial tree.[21] The soot becomes seared on to the mucosa, causing continuing damage. In the absence of ciliary activity, soot does not appear on endobronchial suction until bronchorrhea commences some 24 h after the insult.

The presentation and pathology of smoke inhalation have been extensively reviewed.[22–27] Inhalation of smoke causes a chemical burn to the lower airways and to the type 1 pneumocytes of the lung.[28] Edema of the bronchial mucosa, protein exudation, alveolar destruction, and necrotizing bronchitis follow. Bronchospasm, both true due to inflammatory mediators, particularly thromboxane A_2, and false due to mucosal edema, is common. Soot blocks small airways, leading to focal areas of collapse and hyperinflation in the lung. Mucosal secretions are rich in polymorphonuclear cells (PMNs) and the exudate is in consequence fibrinous. Mingled with debris, soot, and sometimes blood

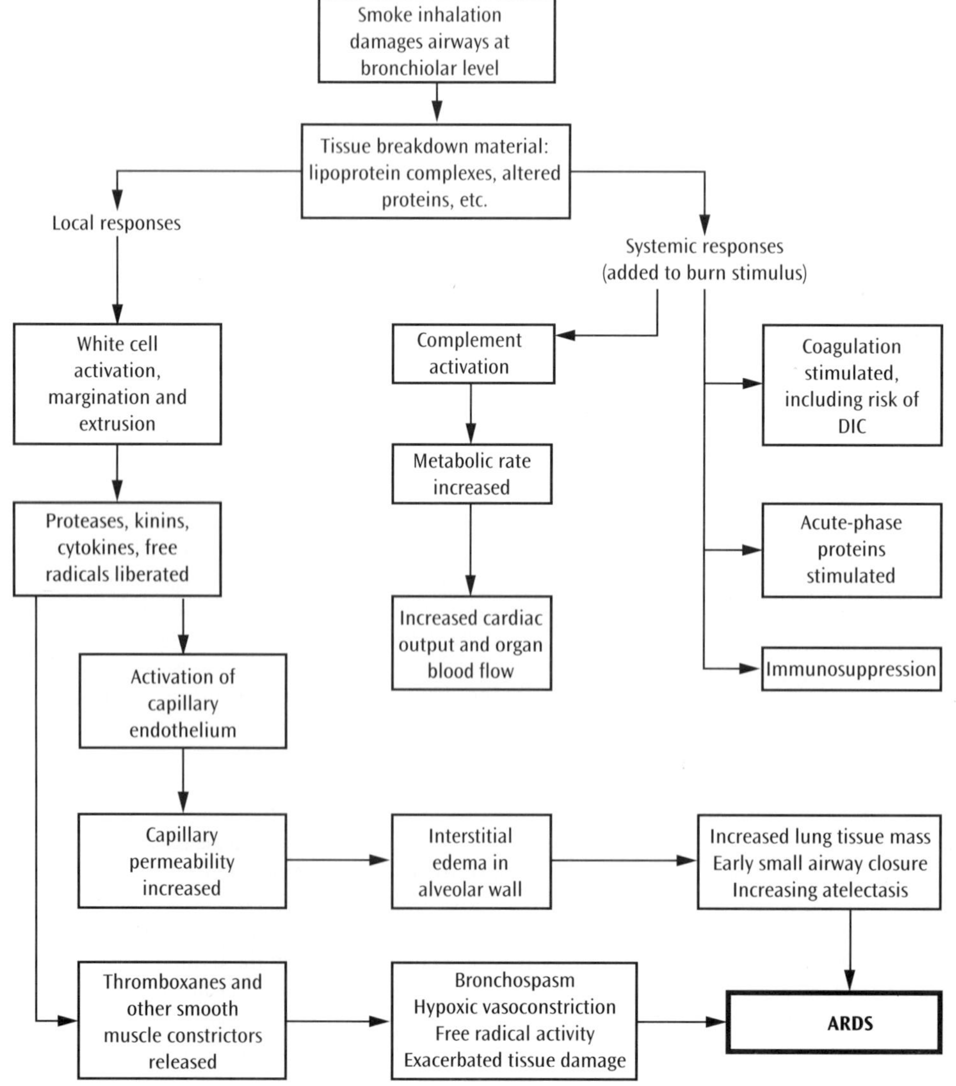

Figure 68.4 *Respiratory pathophysiology following smoke inhalation. DIC, disseminated intravascular coagulation; ARDS, acute respiratory distress syndrome.*

clots, the exudate forms into "casts," which can lead to obstruction of segmental bronchi and, occasionally, sudden catastrophic tracheal tube blockage (Fig. 68.5).

As well as injury to type 1 pneumocytes, smoke inhalation triggers an inflammatory cascade that sets up the sequence outlined in Fig. 68.4. Free radicals formed in inadequately oxygenated alveoli exacerbate the damage. Attempts have been made to modify these responses with anti-inflammatory drugs and the iron chelator desferrioxamine,[29] but with little demonstrable success to date. The injured lung is susceptible to secondary infection, and contributes significantly to the total "dose" of inflammatory mediators circulating in the body.[30] In addition, the smoke-injured patient has suffered an acute hypoxic episode, massive hypercarbia, carbon monoxide and cyanide poisoning, as well as an acute lung injury. It is not surprising that inhalation injury remains a major contributor to mortality in thermal injury.

Should the patient survive, long-term consequences can include increased bronchoreactivity and impaired lung function, with bronchiolitis obliterans and a lifetime of bronchiectasis a likely occurrence for children.[31–33]

RESUSCITATION

There is no good reason why the emergency assessment of the burned patient should differ from that afforded any other victim of trauma. It is only by thorough history taking, examination, and investigation that all factors requiring treatment will be identified with confidence. In thermal injury, these include:

- the cutaneous burn;
- heat damage to the upper airway;
- smoke inhalation injury;
- concurrent illnesses that may have contributed to the cause;
- other injuries, including alcohol or drug intoxication;[34]
- nonaccidental injuries.

A full ABC primary survey followed by systematic review must be undertaken. *It is essential* to keep the patient warm during this external examination because burned patients lose heat rapidly by evaporation from the burn wounds. The environment should verge on being uncomfortably hot for clinical staff if heat loss is to be minimized.

Airway

As indicated earlier, heat injury to the mouth, pharynx, or larynx can lead to airway obstruction. Upper airway injury is most often associated with facial, particularly circumoral, burns, although absence of these does not rule out the possibility in any patient extricated from a house fire. Singed nasal hairs may be visible. Upper airway injury can occur in isolation, but is often associated with smoke inhalation. If lips, tongue, and face are swollen, these will not only produce obstruction but will also increase the risk of aspiration of secretions, by restricting swallowing. Later in the healing process, sloughs of epiglottic mucosa may threaten to obstruct the airway. Figure 68.6 shows the view on laryngoscopy (post intubation) in a typical, though not particularly severe, upper airway burn.

Signs of potential airway obstruction include hoarseness of voice at an early stage, followed by stridor and respiratory distress. If there is a significant cutaneous burn requiring intravenous resuscitation, there will be more swelling and the need for intubation will be greater,[35] especially if resuscitation is crystalloid based. Intubation, if needed, should be undertaken early because swelling will impede access for laryngoscopy if the face is burned, and will stiffen the neck tissues; a grade 1 intubation can degenerate quite quickly to a grade 3 or 4. On the other hand, intubation itself is not without risk so should not be undertaken solely because there are facial burns. The need for intubation may be urgent but it is not an emergency unless stridor is present. There is always time for inspection of the larynx under gaseous general anesthesia, e.g. halothane or sevoflurane in oxygen. The anesthesiologist should take time to ensure the patient is at a deep level, which will be maintained for longer using halothane than using sevoflurane. Emergency tracheotomy may be impossible if the neck is badly burned, or at best it will be much more difficult, again emphasizing the need to assess and intubate calmly and with more than one game plan in mind.

An anesthesiologist should ensure that intubation is carried out in an unhurried manner, with all tools for difficult airway access to hand – including fiberoptic laryngoscopy, but only if the operator is skilled in the technique. Awake inspection and intubation may be possible if the patient is cooperative, otherwise anesthesia should be induced by spontaneous inhalation of a volatile anesthetic in oxygen, and the larynx should be inspected. If there is no visible sign of injury, the patient may be allowed to wake up. However, if there is any doubt at all about the condition of the pharynx or larynx, the patient should be intubated under deep anesthesia using a high-volume, low-pressure cuffed tracheal tube. These points are summarized in Fig. 68.7. The nasal route is better tolerated, but the oral route is acceptable. If intubated nasally, application of a topical antimicrobial cream as a lubricant (e.g. mupirocin, Bactroban®) reduces the chance of carrying nasal commensals into the trachea. The tube should then be fixed firmly so that risk of accidental extubation is minimized.[36] Accidental extubation at a time when facial swelling is maximum is highly dangerous, especially in children. Once the patient

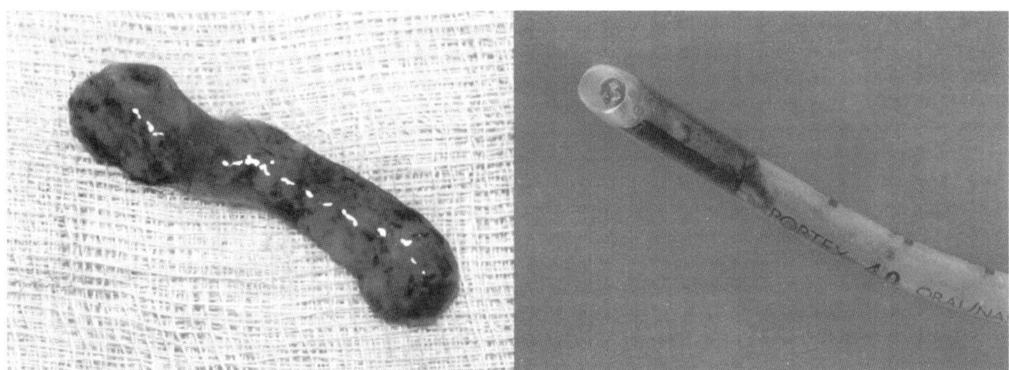

Figure 68.5 *Casts: the left-hand picture shows a cast removed at bronchoscopy; the right-hand picture shows a child's tube blocked by a cast.*

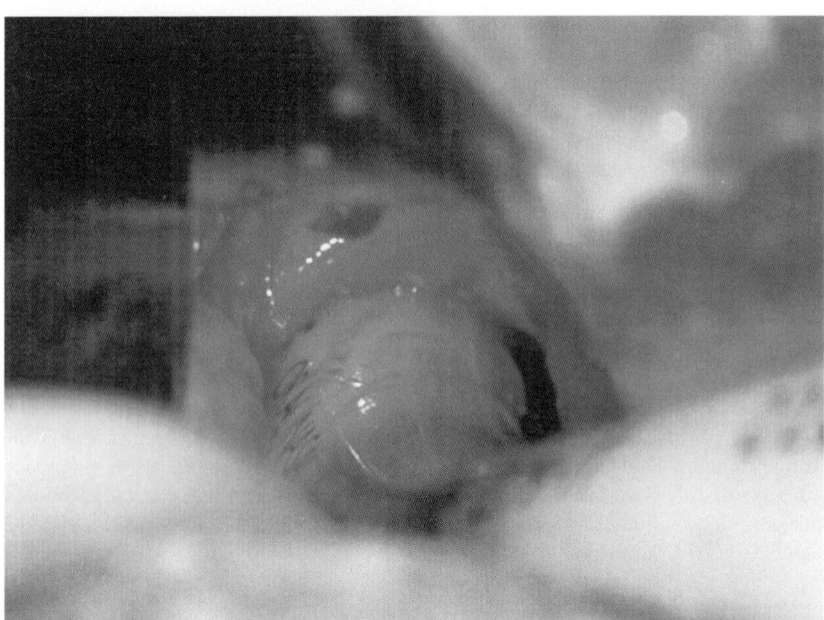

Figure 68.6 *The view of a burned upper airway on laryngoscopy. Note the swollen and, in places, necrotic epiglottis.*

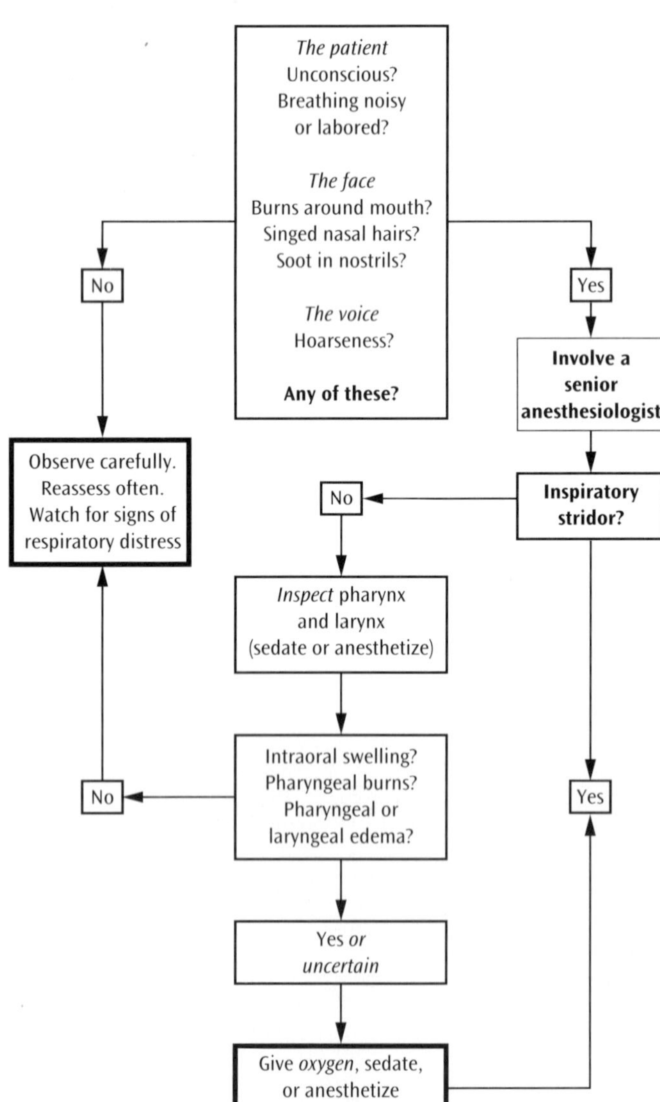

Figure 68.7 *Sequence for intubation of the patient who may have upper airway burns.*

is settled and oxygenation is good, a nasogastric tube should be passed and the stomach emptied.

Security of the tube must be achieved in a manner that allows adequate mouth toilet, does not cause chafing of the burn wound or accumulation of infected debris, and prevents accidental extubation. Sticky tape comes loose very quickly, ribbon ties become encrusted or contaminated, and external ties do not always prevent outward migration of the tube as the face swells. Fixing a nasal tube by external ties is notoriously difficult. In children, good fixation can be achieved using a wire support and a forehead bandage which may be included in dressings. In adults, one author (KCJ) employs variants of the technique described[37] by using a nasogastric tube looped around the back of the soft palate (Fig. 68.8).

Rapid-sequence induction is strongly discouraged for intubation in these circumstances. The stomach may be full, but regurgitation is minimized if spontaneous breathing is maintained and a slight head-up tilt is established before induction. Intubation is carried out under deep anesthesia. If a relaxant is given, the risk of regurgitation rises immediately and substantially. Succinylcholine (suxamethonium) is probably not contraindicated in the first 24 h (see Pharmacology section, below), but its use is usually inappropriate. If a relaxant is given at any stage, the ability to ventilate using a mask and airway or a laryngeal mask must be established first, to avoid a "can't intubate – can't ventilate" catastrophe. Transtracheal jet ventilation or an emergency tracheotomy may not be available as options if the neck is burned, but should be prepared for in case the situation becomes desperate. If there is no significant lung injury, spontaneous respiration should be encouraged as soon as possible, as high ventilatory pressures will tend to increase neck and face swelling by increased venous pressure. Nursing the patient with the upper body elevated a little will help resolution of cervicofacial edema by facilitating venous return.

Children

There is a high incidence of croup-type symptoms in the preschool child who presents with thermal injury. This may be related to a higher incidence of upper respiratory tract infection (URTI) in the child with a scald injury – the URTI probably makes the child fractious, precipitating injury. In addition, a consistent manifestation of nonburn edema in children is a deposition of edema at the cricoid ring. Injury to the head or pretracheal neck will exacerbate this edema. Complete airway

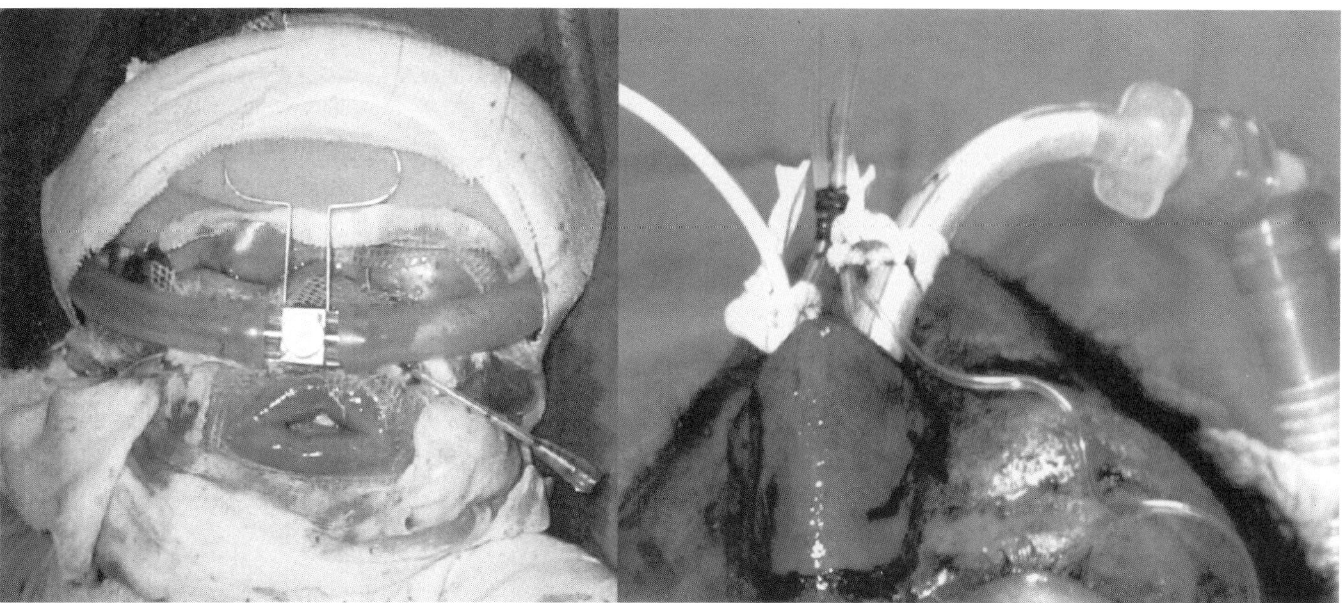

Figure 68.8 *Fixation of the tube when the face is burned: child (left) and adult (right). See text.*

obstruction is possible in children with simple scalds in whom ingestion or inhalation of hot liquid has not occurred.[35]

Tracheal tubes for children commonly need to be reduced in diameter by at least 0.5 mm for routine burns anesthesia. This same reduction in size should be made for prolonged intubation to preserve mucosal perfusion at the edematous cricoid ring in an attempt to reduce the incidence of postextubation stridor.[38] The nasal tube should be cut to allow extra intratracheal length, thus allowing for facial swelling. A recently evaluated technique advocates that the tube is passed through the cords to the same distance in centimeters that the diameter is in millimeters, i.e. 5 cm for a 5.0-mm-internal-diameter tube.[39] A further 0.5–1 cm should be added to the nasotracheal tube length to allow for increase in edema.

Breathing

Unless smoke inhalation is very severe, symptoms and signs may be slight in the first few hours.

Diagnosis

Diagnosis of smoke inhalation is made initially from the history, which will include elements such as rescue from smoke, or fire in an enclosed space. On examination, there may be soot in the mouth and nose. Bronchospasm may be present, and a harsh, dry cough is likely. Petechial hemorrhages on the anterior chest (if unburned) indicate violent coughing at the scene, and are not uncommon in children affected by smoke. Other signs such as bronchorrhea and carbonaceous sputum are related to the pathologic development of the injury so are not often seen immediately. Chest radiograph is often completely normal initially but becomes a significant indicator as the condition develops.[11]

Diagnosis is confirmed by blood gases, co-oximetry and bronchoscopy (Fig. 68.9). Blood gases may initially be normal. Early changes in alveolar–arterial oxygen difference on serial blood gases indicate the onset of interstitial parenchymal edema as the inflammatory response develops. A carbon monoxide level taken within 1 h after injury is strongly indicative of smoke inhalation if it exceeds 10%. Bronchoscopy not only confirms the diagnosis of inhalation but also gives a good indication of severity from the degree of soot soiling, reddening or pallor, edema of the mucosa, and areas of mucosal separation and bleeding.

Progression

The patient has suffered an acute hypoxic and hypercarbic episode in an atmosphere containing irritants, corrosives, and poisons (Table 68.4). Progression to acute respiratory distress (ARDS) is likely. It has been shown that early application of positive pressure support improves outcome.[40,41] In the absence of a large (> 10% TBSA) cutaneous burn, an expectant approach can be adopted, although even in these minor injuries continuous positive airway pressure (CPAP) by mask or tracheal tube is beneficial. In moderate and major injuries, full ventilation is usually required and must be accompanied by positive end-expiratory pressure (PEEP); 1 kPa (10 cmH_2O) is a good starting point.

The P_aO_2/F_IO_2 (*P*/*F*) ratio in predicting injury severity and therefore possible outcome was examined by Brown *et al.*[11] In a review of 120 patients with inhalation injury, those with *P*/*F* ratios greater than or equal to 300 after resuscitation were found to be more likely to survive than those with ratios less than 300. The *P*/*F* ratio had no value when obtained before resuscitation.

Carbon monoxide and cyanide

Carbon monoxide (CO) levels must be measured as soon after injury as possible, to achieve the best estimate of the exposure dose. Extrapolation from the measured blood level to give an estimate of the level at time of injury can be performed using a standard nomogram. Cyanide (CN) is derived from modern synthetics such as plastics and furniture foam. CN estimation is unavailable in most emergency departments. In a high proportion of patients rescued from house fires, cyanide inhalation can be assumed, especially if the carbon monoxide level is high.[42]

The clinical significance of CO and CN exposure is less easy to judge; both are frequently overrated but neither should be dismissed lightly. There is no doubt that chronic exposure to low levels of CO can lead to significant neurologic damage, nor that hyperbaric oxygen is of proved benefit in this circumstance. In smoke inhalation, however, high doses of CO have been inhaled for remarkably short periods of time. The presence of carbon dioxide (CO_2) in smoke (levels of 12–20% have

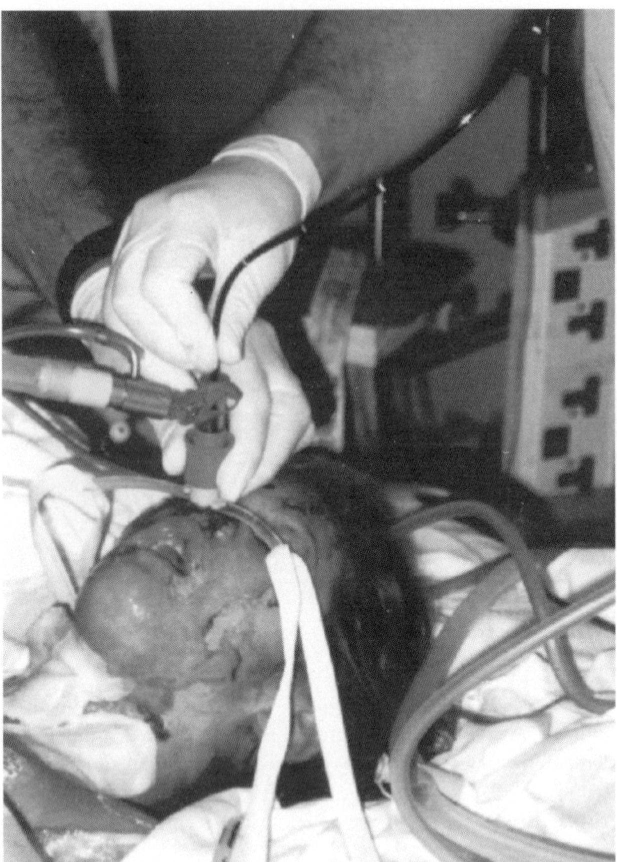

Figure 68.9 *Bronchoscopy in a child with smoke inhalation injury – used for diagnosis and to assist secretion removal by lavage.*

been recorded) ensures CO_2 narcosis within a minute or two, so that the time window for escape from smoke is short and is further reduced by the incapacitation of violent coughing and hypoxia. Therefore, although blood levels are often very high, the *dose* of CO inhaled is probably quite small and is largely contained in the vascular compartment. Inhalation of high-dose oxygen is mandatory to displace this CO from the hemoglobin quickly, and is usually instituted at the scene by the fire brigade. High blood CO levels are a further indication for elective positive-pressure ventilation, and 100% oxygen should be given until blood CO levels are negligible and acid–base status is normal. However, hyperbaric oxygen, which is considered in more detail later in this chapter, is not usually indicated in most burn victims with smoke inhalation.

Circulation

A brief history

Up to and including World War II, most patients with burns affecting more than 20% body surface area were at mortal risk from acute renal failure. Fluid infusion was used but was ill defined until the early 1950s, when several groups of workers devised formulae that would guide resuscitation. This led to the Parkland (or Baxter) formula in the USA, and the Mount Vernon (or Muir and Barclay) formula in the UK, among others. Neither formula was subjected to randomized controlled study or published as an original paper in a peer-review journal, but both have stood the test of time. These formulae were based on animal work in primates and subprimates, and validation was based on clinical experience in thousands of patients over many years. The "controls" were historical: burns patients who used to die before fluid resuscitation was used no longer died. It became clear that burn-associated renal failure and consequent death were avoidable unless systemic sepsis and multiorgan failure intervened. Successful treatment of the latter would await development of modern intensive care 20 years or so later.

The nature of burn shock

The formation of edema leads to loss of fluid from the intravascular compartment.[43] A 5% burn loses approximately 200 mL of fluid into the wound in the first 4 h, and the body is quite capable of making up this deficit from normal physiologic reserves. On the other hand, a 15% burn will lose 500 mL or more in the first 4 h and a similar amount each subsequent 4 h. If untreated, this will eventually lead to significant shock. A 30% burn injury will manifest clinical shock within the first 4 h, having lost between 1000 mL and 1200 mL of fluid in that time. However, because the extent of injury and the extent of the inflammatory response is proportional to the area of burn, it is possible to anticipate these losses and minimize the damage they might cause. So, burn shock resuscitation consists not so much in treatment as in prevention – "catch up and keep up."

This is in sharp contrast with hemorrhagic shock, which has to be managed retrospectively, using invasive monitoring. Burn shock has a physiologic cause (the inflammatory response), a predictable evolution (exponential recovery over 24–48 h), and a slower onset than hemorrhagic shock. Burn shock can be anticipated by assessing the burn size, treated prospectively by formula-guided fluid infusion, and the treatment audited by clinical monitoring in most cases; 90% or more of burn-injured patients can be so managed if meticulous care is taken. To some degree, especially following major injuries, there is maintenance of the inflammatory response by the presence of large amounts of burn tissue so that recovery is never complete until the wound has been adequately treated by excision and wound cover.

In most patients with smoke inhalation and in patients following massive burns, cardiac output becomes unpredictable, as is so in any patient with the systemic inflammatory response syndrome (SIRS). Cardiac index is low in the early hours after injury, and this is greater than would be expected from fluid loss alone. Cardiac poisons such as CO and CN, intracellular fluid shifts, circulating inflammatory, mediators (tumor necrosis factor, TNF, has been specifically implicated),[44] and possibly burn toxin reduce cardiac contractility. If cardiac function is already impaired by previous disease, the effect of injury on cardiac function becomes even less predictable.[45] Inflammatory and metabolic changes, however, lead to an early increase in oxygen demand, which, with increased circulating catecholamines, drives cardiac output upwards by 24 h onward. These conflicting influences result in the cardiac output not always matching demand. Some studies suggest that following major burns, invasive monitoring and goal-directed resuscitation can improve outcome.[46]

Practicalities of fluid resuscitation

Venous access

Good peripheral venous access is essential, and should be achieved quickly before estimating burn surface area. In major burns, two cannulae, or a 14G peripheral cannula plus good central venous access, must be established.

Children

The ease of venipuncture varies with the size of the child and the area of injury. At initial resuscitation, peripheral vasoconstriction through pain, fear, cold, and hypovolemia can make vascular access extremely difficult. The choice is, in order, the dorsum of hand, the long saphenous vein in the foot, the external jugular, or any visible vein. This will obviously depend on the area injured, the skill of the practitioner, and the level of sedation of the child. Where percutaneous venous access is impossible and surgical cut-down is delayed, the intraosseous route can be used to infuse fluid under pressure in children up to 8 years.[47]

Reuscitation formulae

The formulae most commonly used for anticipating fluid requirements following thermal injury are given in Table 68.5. All fluid regimens allow for decreasing losses with time from the injury. The fluid used is governed by a wealth of historical data but little well-controlled evidence. The choice of fluid is not thought to be critical, provided it contains an adequate amount of sodium.[15] Whichever formula is chosen, it is used only for initiating resuscitation. Thereafter, it is important not to be a slave to figures but to treat the patient according to response. However, by anticipating fluid loss and treating prospectively in this way, a degree of fine tuning only is required to keep the patient physiologically stable.

The burn surface area on which the calculation is based is assessed using the Wallace Rule of 9s or, more accurately, a chart (Fig. 68.10) on which the burn area can be mapped. The latter enables the observer to draw the area of burn, estimate the amount of burn in each part of the drawing, and add up the total of body surface area burned. It also takes into account the differences in body surface area between adults and children.

Fluid infusion

Intravenous fluid resuscitation is required for all burns greater than 15% TBSA in adults over 12 years and less than 60 years. Fluid handling differs for children compared with adults, and evaporative losses are greater because of a larger body surface to weight ratio. In infants, renal function is less mature. The elderly are often chronically "dry" before the accident happens, whether from diuretic therapy, inadequate intake, deteriorating renal function, or other causes. For these reasons, intravenous fluid is needed for burns greater than 10% TBSA in children under 12 years and in the elderly. Full-thickness burns greater than 5% should be observed very carefully, in case toxins or hemochromagens released from damaged deep tissues compromise renal function. Intravenous fluids should be given to any burned patient unable to tolerate oral fluids.

In the light of the pathophysiologic process described above, fluid therapy should be sufficient to support circulating volume to maintain flow to vital organs. Because of the capillary leak, resuscitation initially makes edema worse,[48] regardless of the type of fluid used. The effect of over-resuscitation on organ function has not been investigated, but logic suggests that it would be detrimental. There is some anecdotal evidence that large volumes of crystalloid can cause compartment syndrome in unburned limbs due to nonburn edema, and this has some support from animal work.[19] The message would seem to be that too much fluid is as bad as too little, though there is scant evidence as to what constitutes "too much."

The kidneys and their supporting hormonal systems respond sensitively to changes in circulating volume, more so than any other organ except, arguably, the gut. Release of hormones that conserve sodium and water occurs early after burn injury, even if resuscitation is started promptly.[49] The body cannot therefore respond to an excess water load, so it is important that water given is sufficient only to balance the sodium administered and to support metabolic needs. Very hypotonic solutions are therefore inappropriate. Ringer's lactate (Hartmann's or LR) solution is slightly hypotonic and therefore delivers enough metabolic water for daily needs as well as achieving resuscitation. Children have higher metabolic water needs than adults due to greater evaporative losses, so they always need extra metabolic water at 1500 mL per m^2 body surface per day. Plasma protein solutions are isotonic for sodium, so extra metabolic water should be considered, at normal maintenance rates. Whichever solutions are used, sufficient solution must be given to maintain vital organ function but no more, because excess will merely exacerbate edema.

Colloid

Although there is an immense accumulated experience on the use of colloids for burned patients, most of it suggests that natural colloids can be used safely in uncomplicated burns; there is little good evidence to justify their use over crystalloid and a scant evidence base to guide their use in critical care management of thermal injury.

The Muir and Barclay resuscitation formula (M&B) was devised from historical data on several thousand patients using freeze-dried plasma as the main resuscitation fluid.[50] When this became unavailable, substitution with human plasma protein fraction and, later, 4.5% human albumin solution (HAS) was made. It is clear from the early literature that less fluid was needed to resuscitate burned patients when plasma was used in comparison with Ringer's lactate (LR) solution.[15] Subsequent studies showed that 25–30% more fluid was needed to achieve the same result using these solutions,[51] so they clearly behave differently, probably because of smaller average molecular size. Because LR is slightly hypotonic and provides its own metabolic water component, the Parkland formula is a single-infusion model, whereas M&B requires an additional infusion of dextrose or dextrose–saline. In the early stages, the behavior of HAS probably differs little from that of LR. However, patients treated solely with crystalloid end the resuscitation period with much lower serum albumin levels. The significance of this for outcome is not clear.

So how should colloids be used in burned patients? In moderate burns, where the response to injury is mostly local, there is no difference in outcome between crystalloid and colloid resuscitation. Crystalloid is cheaper, so it makes sense to use this method for all patients with

Table 68.5 *Commonly used burns resuscitation formulae*

Formula title	First 24 h	Second 24 h (traditional)
Parkland (Baxter) *Fluid*: Lactated Ringer's solution	3–4 mL per kg per %TBSA, half in first 8 h, half in second 16 h, from time of injury	2 mL per kg per %TBSA plus 0.5 mL per kg per %TBSA of 5% albumin
... in practice:	0.25 mL per kg per %TBSA, for each hour after injury, for first 8 h post burn	Adjusted according to clinical response
Mount Vernon (Muir and Barclay) *Fluid*: Plasma (HAS requirement ~25% more)	0.5 mL per kg per %TBSA during each *period* after injury (periods: 4, 4, 4, 6, and 12 h)	Plasma at 0.5 mL per kg per %TBSA over 12 h, maintenance fluid thereafter
	Basal metabolic water at standard rates, as dextrose 5%	

Both formulae are derived from retrospective analysis of successful fluid resuscitation in large numbers of patients. Neither formula should be followed slavishly. They identify a starting point; the rate should be adjusted over time according to clinical and other monitoring.

Chart for estimating severity of burn wound

To use this chart:

[shaded box] Draw, then shade in, all burned areas (ignore simple erythema)

1. **Draw the burned area as accurately as possible**. *Do not worry about distinguishing between deep and shallow burns at this stage* – we will do that at the burn center.
REMEMBER: the drawing is 2D, the body is 3D; take this into account when drawing the burn.
2. Work out total burn in *each chart area*, using the percentages on the figure or in the table.
3. *Add up the percentage of total body surface area burned (%TBSA).*

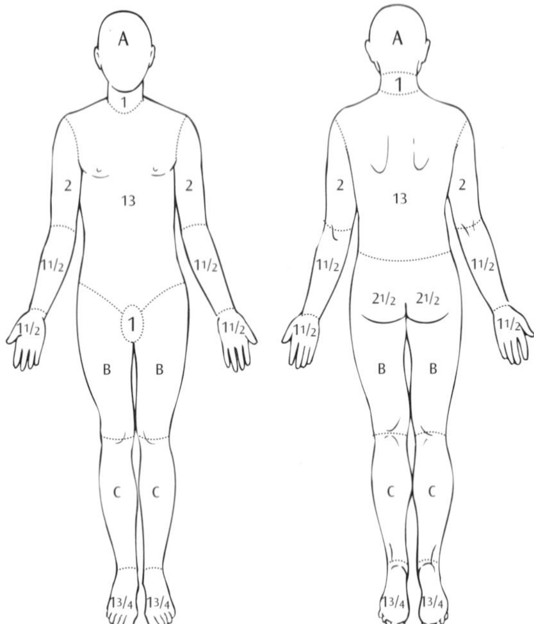

Region	Front	Back
Head		
Neck		
Trunk		
Right upper arm		
Right lower arm		
Right hand		
Left upper arm		
Left lower arm		
Left hand		
Buttocks		
Perineum		
Right thigh		
Right lower leg		
Right foot		
Left thigh		
Left lower leg		
Left foot		
Subtotals		
Total		

Relative percentage of body surface area affected by growth

Area	Age 0	1	5	10	15	Adult
A=1/2 of head	9 1/2	8 1/2	6 1/2	5 1/2	4 1/2	3 1/2
B=1/2 of one thigh	2 3/4	3 1/4	4	4 1/2	4 1/2	4 3/4
C=1/2 of one leg	2 1/2	2 1/2	2 3/4	1 1/4	3 1/4	3 1/2

Figure 68.10 *Emergency room chart for estimating area of body surface burned.*

moderate injuries. By empirical tradition, colloid (as plasma historically, nowadays albumin or hydroxyethyl starch) is given in the second 24 h when the Parkland formula is used (Table 68.5). Crystalloid will leak into normal tissue as well as burned tissue, so significant nonburn edema can be expected,[52] which usually resolves quickly.

Paradoxically, for major burns, the differences between crystalloid and colloid resuscitation diminish because of the massive capillary leak triggered in all tissues by circulating inflammatory mediators. Fluid shifts are massive, however, resulting in considerable weight gain.[52] All fluids given distribute evenly across the extracellular compartment. In the first 8 h, therefore, the Parkland formula offers a reliable method of resuscitation at modest cost. If a colloid is necessary in the early phase, it should probably be one with a large molecule, such as the hydroxyethyl starches. However, the tendency of some starches to remain in the tissues for many years suggests that they should be used sparingly. After 24 h, the Parkland formula advocates the addition of plasma to the regimen, as discussed earlier. There is no clear evidence that M&B resuscitation using HAS is detrimental in most burned patients, and its abandonment by some is based more on grounds of cost than perception of harm.

Children

In children, nonburn edema may risk airway narrowing at the cricoid ring, and this risk is clearly greater if crystalloid is used. Therefore, in the UK it is felt strongly that the M&B formula using HAS remains the method of choice for children.

Other solutions

Other solutions for resuscitation offer no benefit in most circumstances over LR or HAS, and may be detrimental. Strongly hypertonic saline solutions (e.g. 640 mmol sodium per liter) have been used to minimize volumes infused in major burns and demonstrated initial promise, but have been shown more recently to have no advantage over LR,[53] and in animals to carry a higher risk of renal failure.[54] Slightly hypertonic saline (210 mmol L^{-1}, made by adding 100 mL of 8.4% sodium bicarbonate per liter of LR) seems to lack this drawback and may confer added benefit by alkalinizing the urine and thus minimizing deposition of hemoglobin and myoglobin released from burned tissues in the renal tubules. Gelatine solutions have a smaller molecular size than HAS so will behave little differently from LR in the first 24 h, at increased cost. Use of colloids for burns requiring intensive care is discussed below (see Intensive care).

Clinical monitoring

Most burned patients are well managed by clinical monitoring. Patients with massive burns, smoke inhalation, other injuries, or chronic illnesses almost always need more complex monitoring (see Intensive care section). Urine flow gives a good indication of renal function, an hourly output of 0.75 ± 0.2 mL per hour being adequate. The urine produced will be concentrated because injury triggers release of excess antidiuretic hormone, natriuretic peptide, and other regulators that conserve water.[55]

The osmolality of the urine should be measured: adequate resuscitation volumes will have an osmolality between 500 and 900 mosmol L^{-1}. Low volume and high osmolality indicate inadequate resuscitation; low volume and low osmolality indicate impaired renal tubule function, which should initially suggest a serious fluid deficit but may indicate poor cardiac output from other causes. If there is a poor response to a fluid challenge, invasive monitoring [central venous pressure (CVP) or pulmonary artery catheter (PAC), depending on severity] may unmask the problem and allow confident treatment before acute tubular necrosis occurs. Changes in urine osmolality occur 4 h or more before a rise in serum creatinine and can be checked hourly by the nurses in the burns unit, almost eliminating the risk of renal failure in early burn care.

Other monitoring includes measurement of blood pressure and heart rate, and frequent assessment of capillary refill. Measurement of peripheral temperature is prone to substantial errors but, nevertheless, the trend in core–peripheral temperature difference is a useful indicator of the adequacy of capillary filling when considered alongside other parameters. Packed cell volume will rise if resuscitation is inadequate, but is unreliable as a main indicator because the preinjury level is unknown, hemoconcentration is inevitable in the early hours, and red cell destruction following major deep burns reduces the base level in a nonmeasurable manner. Plasma electrolytes and full blood count should be measured at frequent intervals, at least 6-hourly. No single measurement is sufficient on its own to determine the adequacy of resuscitation. Staff must make frequent assessments of progress and adjust volumes infused accordingly. Dramatic changes in fluid flow rates are unnecessary unless incipient renal failure is suspected.

The secondary survey

By this time, the condition of most burned patients will be well diagnosed. The burn presents one further hazard: constriction of major vessels in the limbs or restriction of thoracic respiratory excursion as edema develops. Escharotomies may be required to preserve perfusion to a distal limb or to relieve thoracic restriction. These must be done by someone well trained in the technique, and can usually be left until arrival in the burns unit unless transfer is delayed significantly.

A full history should be obtained from any relatives or ambulance staff present, which, combined with a thorough secondary survey, will reveal any contributory problems such as pre-existing disease or nonburn injuries.[56] Illnesses which may have contributed to the injury include epilepsy, diabetes (hypo- or hyperglycemia), and cardiovascular disease including heart, blood pressure, strokes, and transient ischemic attacks. Psychiatric illness may precipitate suicide by self-immolation or, more commonly, may contribute to a lower than average awareness of risk. Alcohol or drug abuse is a common accompaniment to thermal injury, especially if violence has been a component in the etiology, and these may adversely affect prognosis.[57]

All ages are susceptible to associated injuries, which are surprisingly quite rare but must on no account be ignored because their treatment may be much more urgent than that of the burn wound. Explosions cause shrapnel and blast damage, the latter to the eardrums and particularly to the lungs. Explosions occur in house fires as flammable materials vaporize in the extreme heat generated. Falling debris may cause direct trauma, including head injury. The patient who has jumped to escape, or been thrown by a blast (Fig. 68.11), may have sustained a skeletal injury. Any history of loss of consciousness at the scene is important, although its cause is more likely to be a combination of hypoxia, carbon dioxide narcosis, and CO intoxication than head injury.

Children

Fortunately, children are largely unaffected by comorbidity, but children with congenital illness, diabetes, epilepsy, or learning difficulties are more vulnerable than their peers. Social deprivation plays a part in a high proportion of pediatric burns. Children are vulnerable as toddlers when all kinds of dangers become unexpectedly reachable, and as teenagers (especially boys) when the urge to experiment with fire is often not tempered by common sense.

TRIAGE AND TRANSFER

The burn unit

Thermal injuries vary from tiny to massive, and fortunately the majority are trivial – although not so for the patient if disabled or disfigured

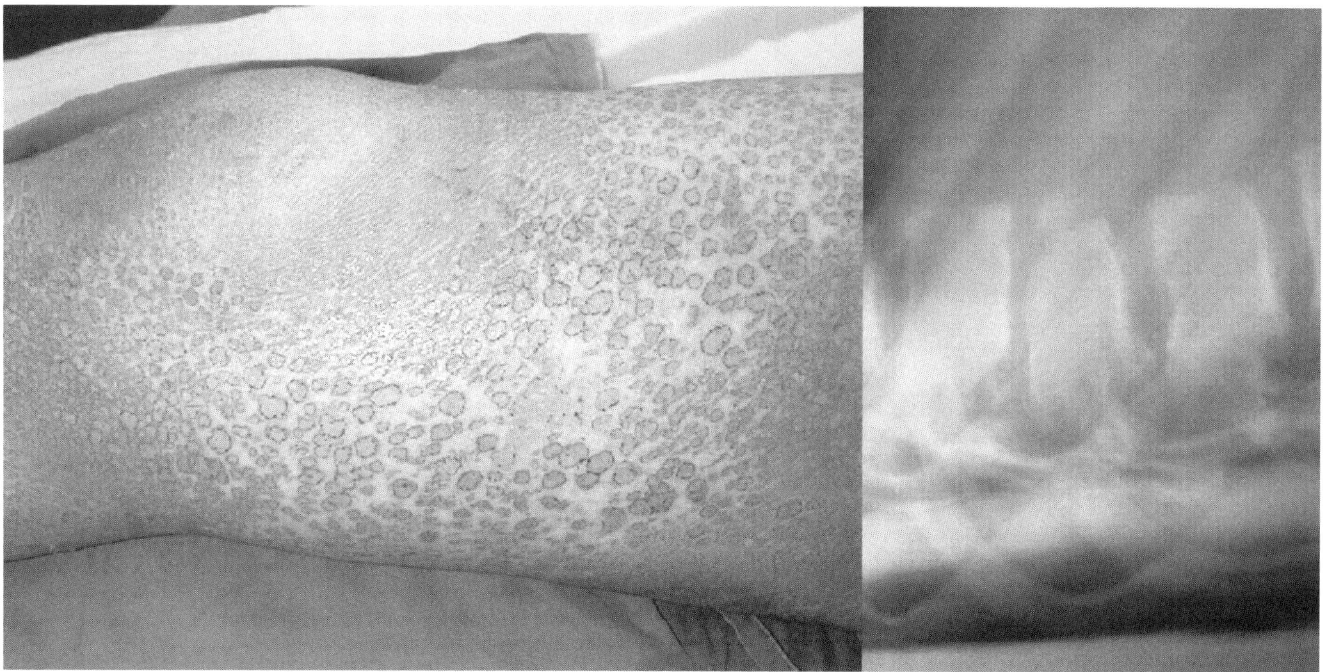

Figure 68.11 *Superficial flash burn (left) in a patient with associated spinal injury (right)*

for life. Those in this group who require hospital treatment can often be managed as outpatients with dressings. A proportion of these will need grafting or flap repair, for which they should ideally be referred to a plastic surgeon. Burns that do not heal within 10 days qualify for such referral, to ensure optimal surgery for best possible functional outcome.

Burn units were developed in the 1950s to provide particular support and concentrate specialist expertise in the management of critical or complex injuries. Definitions are generally loose, resulting in some anomalies. For instance, by accepted criteria, a "critical" burn is one that is surgically critical, needing expert attention and, in some cases, fluid resuscitation. Only a small proportion of these patients are "critically ill" in the sense that an intensive care clinician would define the term. Equally unhelpful is the tendency to refer to all burns as either "minor" (small burns that may need surgical help) or "major" (any burn big enough to need fluid resuscitation).

A more informative classification for the anesthesiologist in these days of intensive and high-dependency care is given in Table 68.6. This separates patients fairly crudely into four injury severity groups according to age, %TBSA, comorbidity, and associated injury. The basis for this is theoretical, but broadly accords with the experience of one author's (KCJ) own burn center: patients in groups 1 and 2 always survive and do well if treated appropriately; mortality is significant in group 3 but the majority of patients should survive if good surgical management and (when necessary) intensive care are delivered concurrently; and burned patients in group 4 have a very high but not 100% mortality.

Burned patients always need good burn care: in addition, some need good intensive care and children need good pediatric care.[58] Lack of the first two can have fatal consequences; lack of the third is undesirable but rarely dangerous. Burn care facilities must have a good intensive care facility near enough to permit well-timed wound surgery alongside first-class intensive care, without the need to move the patient long distances down corridors. A dedicated burn ICU is an attractive concept but may not maintain sufficient throughput to justify its existence, unless it serves a very large catchment population.

Children

Ideally, children should have access to a pediatric intensive care unit (PICU) but, if unavailable, the pediatric expertise can be imported according to locally agreed protocol. It is unacceptable to transfer a burned child away from a burn ICU facility to a PICU if the necessary burn surgery expertise is not available on the same site as the PICU.

Criteria for referral

The usual UK criteria for referral to a burn unit accord very closely with those devised by the American Burn Association. These include factors listed in Table 68.7. A key requirement of any burn unit is to have access to a wide range of support disciplines: medicine, including elderly care; general and trauma surgery; microbiology and full laboratory facilities; radiology and imaging; dietetics; physiotherapy; occupational therapy; psychology; anesthesia; pain relief and intensive care; and – for children – pediatrics, pediatric anesthesia, and (for a very few cases) pediatric intensive care. Multidisciplinary ward rounds and care including contribution by anesthesiologists should be the norm.

Transportation

Once assessed and stabilized according to accepted trauma care standards, patients fulfilling burns unit admission criteria will need to be transferred. In some parts of the world, burn centers operate retrieval programs. How is transfer to be achieved? Are there advantages in helicopter transfer over longer distances – such as 40 miles?[59] Most transfers take place by road ambulance, with the sending hospital providing a transfer team. Moderate injuries needing just fluid resuscitation can often be accompanied by a competent nurse, who should take care to monitor vital signs en route and ensure the infusion is kept running. Patients with major burns should also be accompanied by a doctor, who should be an anesthesiologist if the patient is intubated.

It is to be hoped that clearer standards for the transfer of burned patients will be devised, to include:

Table 68.6 *Classification of burn injury into four categories according to complexity of physiologic response*

Injury severity group	Burn	Other factors
Minor	Burn 15% TBSA in adults Burn 10% TBSA in age 12 years or >65 years	Intravenous fluid resuscitation rarely needed Expert surgery may be required, e.g. hands Rare potential for lethal complications, e.g. toxic shock syndrome Anesthetic challenge if face burned
Moderate	Burn > minor, <30% TBSA	All minor burns in: Children <1 Adults >55 Comorbidity 1× in a minor burn
Major	Burn >30%, <50% TBSA	Moderate burns in: Children <1 Adults >55 Comorbidity 2× in a minor burn Smoke inhalation, any burn <30% Associated injury, any burn <30%
Complex major	Burn >50% TBSA	Major burns in: Children <1 Adults >55 Comorbidity 3× or more in a minor burn Smoke inhalation, any burn >30% Associated injury, any burn >30%

Smoke inhalation turns any burn into a major injury. Patients with burns greater than 5% TBSA, or with hand or face burns, frequently require high-dependency levels of nursing care for four-fifths of their stay because of dressings, operative care, comorbidity factors, and extremes of age. (Source: Pinderfields Burn Center data.)

Table 68.7 *Typical criteria for referral to a burn center*

ALL extensive burns, *including* scalds, assessed as:
> 10% of TBSA[a] in patients younger than 12 years or older than 60 years
> 15% of TBSA in patients aged 12–60 years
Full-thickness burns > 5% of TBSA, all ages
Inhalation injury, suspected or actual, associated with any burn
Major electrical burns, especially lightning and high-tension injuries
Any burn of any size about which the referring hospital is unhappy, e.g.
Burn patients with associated trauma or pre-existing illness
Deep circumferential burns of an extremity or the chest
Burns of the face, hands, feet, or perineum, or across joints
Chemical burns, fat burns, industrial injuries
Any burn of any size, which the referring hospital does not have the expertise to treat, including ability to refer to a plastic surgeon.
Other causes of extensive skin loss, e.g. toxic epidermal necrolysis.

a. TBSA= total body surface area.

- ambulance requirements, including equipment, for transferring those who have suffered major burns;
- staff numbers and appropriate experience;
- protocols for treatment prior to and during transfer;
- any special considerations for helicopter transfer.[60]

In the meantime, standards for transfer of critically ill burns can mirror those well reviewed by Wallace and Ridley.[61]

Children

The few children with massive injuries may in future be transferred to a specialist pediatric burn center allied to a PICU in a major hospital, as in the USA. If so, there may be only a handful of transfers required in the UK and helicopter transfer will become the norm.

INTENSIVE CARE

All patients receiving fluid resuscitation must be cared for in a high-dependency environment, so that response to treatment can be monitored hourly and adjusted frequently as needed. Children with any significant thermal injury should be managed in a high-dependency environment. A high level of monitoring is required to detect deterioration in condition as early as possible, including airway edema and toxic shock syndrome. Patients needing more than simple fluid resuscitation, i.e. respiratory or cardiovascular support, or whose fluid resuscitation cannot be monitored by clinical means (see below), must be treated in an intensive care environment.

Fluid resuscitation in massive injury

Most fluid resuscitation in burns can be delivered according to formula, adjusted according to clinical response, and guided by noninvasive monitoring. Complex or mixed injuries, however, are less predictable (see The nature of burn shock, above). Pulmonary artery catheter insertion and monitoring should be considered early in the management of any burn greater than 50% TBSA and in smoke inhalation associated with a significant cutaneous burn, especially if resuscitation fluid requirements exceed prediction by more than 30%, blood pressure is not maintained despite apparently adequate vascular filling, or there are other indicators that cardiac function may be impaired.[62,63] In these circumstances, inotropic support guided by oxygen delivery parameters may be the best line of treatment.[46]

Because the genesis of burn shock is relatively slow, physiologic responses maintain filling pressures until fluid losses are significant. Central venous pressure monitoring may therefore be deceptively unhelpful unless interpreted with great care. Infusing fluids, especially crystalloids, to maintain an arbitrary filling pressure in the presence of a massive capillary leak may cause excess fluid to be administered and unnecessarily exacerbate nonburn edema. It is dangerous to institute central venous access in a small child via the internal jugular, subclavian, or femoral vein without general anesthesia.

The Cochrane Collaboration has suggested that there is a possible risk to critically ill patients in using colloids,[64] particularly albumin.[65] Most burned patients receiving LR or HAS are not critically ill and fluid infusion is intended to prevent them becoming so, therefore it is unlikely that these studies are relevant to the initial management of the burned patient. There is some weak evidence[66] that, in patients in whom the lung is damaged, albumin will become trapped in the lung interstitium when a capillary leak reverts. It is therefore wise to use all colloids with caution and for well-identified and monitored clinical reasons in patients with massive or complex injuries, particularly those with smoke inhalation.

Inhalation injury

Patients with smoke inhalation have an extra focus of capillary leak, so fluid losses are greater. It used to be argued that the smoke-injured patient should be managed "dry" to minimize exacerbation of interstitial pulmonary edema. There is no doubt that patients with a cutaneous burn and smoke inhalation suffer a greater degree of ARDS than those with smoke inhalation alone, but this is due to the greater inflammatory response experienced by the lung. Evidence exists that inadequate fluid resuscitation makes the lung injury worse.[67] In practice, whether crystalloids or colloids are used, fluid requirements in burns with smoke inhalation are up to 25% greater than when smoke injury is absent, and may be predictive of severity.[68]

The case for hyperbaric oxygen (HBO) therapy following smoke inhalation is not supported by evidence drawn from robust literature.[69] Hyperbaric facilities are not readily available and transfer to the nearest chamber will delay institution of definitive burn care. Many HBO chambers do not safely allow critically ill patients to be monitored during treatment. Therefore, care may be sacrificed to a treatment of questionable value. HBO is therefore impractical for most patients suffering smoke inhalation, although high-dose oxygen (100%) is always indicated because it shortens the half-life of CO to less than 40 min compared with 240 min in room air. There are possible exceptions: (1) long exposure to low levels of smoke where something may have been smoldering for some time; (2) any patient exhibiting signs of neurologic deficit; and (3) anyone rescued from a domestic explosion that may be the culmination of a long-standing gas leak. In these circumstances, the HBO chamber should be brought to the patient in the burn center if at all possible.

Likewise, specific treatment of cyanide poisoning is not indicated unless there are signs of persistent tissue poisoning as the total *dose* inhaled is likely to be low. The half-life of cyanide is short and treatment should be given at the scene of the fire when this is practical. A single dose of sodium thiosulfate is the safest treatment, or (if available, as in France but not in the UK) cyanocobalamin.[70] Sodium nitrite may induce profound vasodilation, exacerbating hypovolemia, and should therefore be used cautiously.[70]

Intensive care management aims to address the cardinal elements of smoke inhalation injury, by:

- bronchoalveolar lavage to remove as much smoke-damaged material and mucus as possible;[24]
- the use of nebulized heparin and acetylcysteine to encourage mucolysis and free radical scavenging;[71,72]

- positive airway pressure to keep small airways open;[41]
- vigorous treatment of bronchospasm;[24]
- rigorous attention to sterile technique – pneumonia doubles the mortality;
- minimal safe sedation – if possible, coughing should not be abolished.

Positive-pressure support of breathing is essential, and should cover the whole respiratory cycle.[41] In patients with mild smoke inhalation, spontaneous breathing can be supported by CPAP.[40] Following more severe injuries, full ventilation is usually needed and as high a level of PEEP as can be tolerated should be applied (see Pathophysiology section above). Some authors have applied high-frequency ventilation techniques with significant success.[26,73] The common factor with all treatment modalities seems to be maintenance of a high mean airway pressure while avoiding high peak pressures that risk barotrauma. Active humidification of inspired gases is essential, to assist in mobilizing tenacious and often copious secretions.

Nasal intubation or tracheotomy permits lighter levels of sedation than oral intubation. To minimize the risk of bacterial contamination of the tube during its passage through the nose, it can be lubricated using mupirocin cream.[74] Bronchoalveolar lavage using normal saline and suction should be undertaken every hour for 12 h or until secretions are clear of soot.

The rationale for using heparin derives from studies in animals.[75,76] It was first studied by intravenous administration, but its use by nebulizer is effective not only in improving pulmonary microcirculation but also in minimizing cast formation.[71] Nebulized heparin 5000 units in 5 mL of saline every 4 h is alternated with nebulized *N*-acetylcysteine 3–5 mL of 20% every 4 h. Blood coagulation should be monitored during therapy with nebulized heparin, although abnormalities may equally be caused by the SIRS response to the burn. Doses should be calculated pro rata by weight in children. *N*-acetylcysteine is usefully followed *immediately* by 2.5–5 mg of nebulized salbutamol, to treat smoke-induced bronchospasm prospectively and because acetylcysteine often itself stimulates bronchospasm.

Antibiotics should be administered with great caution because of the risk of inducing resistance. Narrow-spectrum drugs active against common respiratory commensals should be used initially – flucloxacillin or erythromycin – and more powerful agents substituted when indicated. All antimicrobial therapy should be given as advised by the microbiologist, who has knowledge of the flora commonly found in that community, hospital and unit, and of the normal pattern of colonization in burned patients.

The lungs should be auscultated daily as a minimum, and a chest radiograph ordered as indicated and at least every other day. Blood gas estimation is required 4- to 6-hourly; sputum cultures every 24 h. Regular, vigorous chest physiotherapy should be delivered as indicated by secretions but at least 6-hourly. Suction and other airway handling techniques should be meticulously sterile to reduce the risk of nosocomial pneumonia. Some authors have suggested that selective digestive decontamination reduces mortality in smoke inhalation,[77] but the evidence is not robust.

Children

The following are indications for ventilatory support, in children especially but not exclusively, in addition to direct respiratory injury:

- significant injury to the head and neck;
- major burns, to allow nursing and analgesia;
- respiratory failure due to increased metabolism, infection, or physical compromise affecting chest compliance;
- following major excision to allow equilibration of fluid distribution;
- incipient septicemia with pulmonary shunting;
- cerebral irritation secondary to inappropriate fluid deposition.

Recent work suggests that, if the particulate elements in smoke are removed, the sequence of events which leads to progressive pulmonary deterioration does not occur.[21] At Manchester, in 1993, when one author (WDL) routinely commenced diagnostic bronchoscopy, an attempt was made to remove and neutralize the soot, by lavage and suction at bronchoscopy. Aliquots of isotonic sodium bicarbonate are added at hourly intervals thereafter, until no more soot is returned on physiotherapy and suction at between 48 and 72 h (Figs 68.9 and Fig. 68.12). After that, the bicarbonate is exchanged for similar volumes of normal saline to facilitate slough removal. An infant will receive 5 mL and a larger child up to 10 mL, combined with vigorous physiotherapy. No deleterious effects of this continuing lavage have been identified. The expected deterioration of pulmonary function and radiograph appearance does not appear to occur. Referring casualty units are advised to commence sodium bicarbonate instillation as soon as possible and before transfer to the burns unit. Should inhalation be found not to have occurred on bronchoscopy, bicarbonate is stopped. Although verifiable evidence of benefit cannot as yet be shown, there have been no fatalities from pulmonary causes in 15 child victims of house fires treated in this way.

Toxic shock syndrome in children

This relatively rare condition is important because it is a cause of mortality following superficial cutaneous burns often of a quite small area. It is more commonly associated with menstruation and tampon use, but

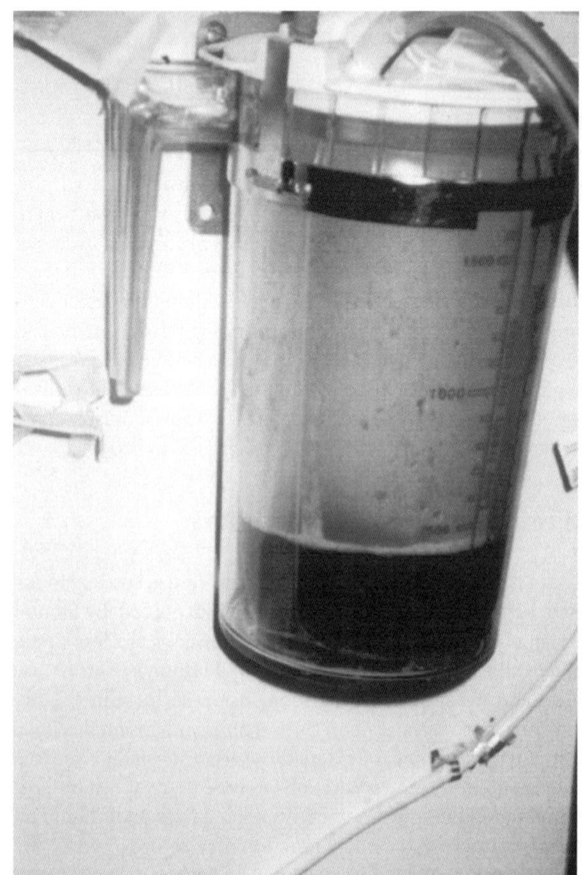

Figure 68.12 *The results of bronchial lavage: returned bicarbonate with adsorbed toxins and blood.*

it should be considered when any child suffers a deterioration in general condition out of proportion to the cutaneous injury.[78,79] Diagnosis depends on fulfilling five out of the six criteria given in Table 68.8.

A striking feature is desquamation of palms and soles during the recovery phase. An initially superficial burn will often be found to have increased in depth. Diagnosis may be difficult initially because of high primary temperature but cerebral and gastrointestinal signs present earlier than cardiovascular signs. The illness is secondary to colonization of a superficial perfused burn with *Staphylococcus aureus* of phage type 59/29 in patients who have no natural immunity. Blood cultures for the organism are negative, the condition being produced by absorption of toxin. Successful treatment depends on recognition before cardiovascular deterioration is established. β-Lactamase-resistant antibiotics should be prescribed but may alter the course of the illness only when given early. Prophylaxis with antistaphylococcal ointment or parenteral antistaphylococcal antibiotics has been used in some centers.

Intensive monitoring of cardiovascular parameters and support of the circulation initially with fresh-frozen plasma has been found to be effective early therapy. In the presence of adequate colloid infusion, inotropic support may be required depending on cardiovascular variables. Unfortunately, in severe cases, tachyphylaxis to these catecholamines may be found with fulminating metabolic acidosis.

METABOLIC CHANGES

The metabolic response to burn injury[80,81] is triggered by the effect of inflammatory mediators on the complement cascade and includes increased secretion of catecholamines, glucagon, and glucocorticoids. These lead to an increase in metabolic rate accompanied by pyrexia, particularly in children (38–39 °C is common), and suppression of immune responses. Cardiac output rises two- to fivefold, following the initial fall alluded to above (see The nature of burn shock, above). The metabolic impact of a 10% burn is roughly equivalent to a single fracture or a mild fever, whereas a 35% burn mirrors multiple trauma or severe sepsis. Burns greater than 35% TBSA are unique in the severity of their metabolic impact, being accompanied by a resting metabolic rate of up to twice normal. Lean body mass is used as a substrate for energy, leading to a high rate of catabolism for which adequate supplementation of nutrition is essential.

Table 68.8 *Toxic shock syndrome in burned children; diagnosis depends on fulfilling five out of the six criteria given*

1 Temperature of 38.9 °C or above
2 Erythematous macular rash (occasionally petechial)
3 Systolic blood pressure less than 12 kPa (90 mmHg) or less than 5th percentile for ages in children
4 Involvement of three or more organ systems, i.e.
Gastrointestinal: vomiting and/or watery diarrhea at onset of illness
Mucous membranes: vaginal, oropharyngeal, or conjunctival hyperemia
Muscular: severe myalgia and or CPK level twice normal
Renal: blood urea or creatinine level twice normal and/or urinary sediment with sterile pyuria (more than five white blood cells per high-powered field)
Hepatic: total bilirubin, SGOT or SGPT at least twice the upper limit of normal
Hematology: thrombocytopenia of less than 100 000 mm^{-3}
CNS: disorientation or alterations in consciousness without focal findings in the absence of hypotension and hyperpyrexia
Cardiopulmonary: hypoxia, ARDS, or myocardial depression (cardiac index less than 3.3 $L\,min^{-1}\,m^{-2}$)
5 Metabolic: serum calcium less than 7.0 $mg\,dL^{-1}$, serum phosphate less than 2.5 $mg\,dL^{-1}$, and total serum protein less than 5 $mg\,dL^{-1}$
6 Reasonable evidence of absence of systemic infection

Release of inflammatory mediators in large amounts into the circulation inevitably poses the potential for organ failure,[82] which can be in single organs or in more than one – multisystem organ failure (MSOF). These effects are not specific to burns, and are usually afforded the title systemic inflammatory response syndrome (SIRS). SIRS can be triggered by the burn, smoke inhalation injury, any associated injuries, or systemic sepsis, as well as major surgery such as is necessary to remove the burn wound.

Specific organ systems

The gut

Blood flow to the gut may be impaired during the shock phase following major burns. Measurement of intragastric pH by tonometry ought therefore to be a useful tool when assessing the adequacy of early resuscitation but, in practice, it has not found favor, largely because of the practical difficulties in interpreting results.

Curling's ulcer used to be an uncommon but potentially lethal complication of burns, but its incidence has declined since the routine use of antiulcer prophylaxis and, more recently, early enteral feeding.

There is good evidence that early nutrition[83] – started within 12 h of injury, usually by the enteral route – furnishes the following benefits:

- It maintains the integrity of the gut mucosa.[84]
- It reduces the intensity of the metabolic response.[84]
- It reduces the infection risk posed by bacterial translocation across the gut wall.[85,86]
- It reduces the complications associated with enteral feeding, especially diarrhea.[87]
- In practice, early enteral feeding almost eliminates the need for parenteral nutrition, which does not afford the same intestinal mucosa protection, does not reduce the metabolic response,[84] and carries a higher associated mortality.[88]

Feeding can usually be achieved using a fine-bore nasogastric tube, but some patients, especially those with complications such as smoke inhalation, benefit from the use of a jejunal tube introduced endoscopically. Those with major burns may benefit from the addition of extra specific nutrients including the semiessential amino acids arginine and glutamine, and ω-3 polyunsaturated fatty acids. There is some evidence that these further enhance the protection of intestinal mucosal integrity.[84]

The kidney and liver

In both these organs, blood flow is increased following moderate or major burns. The effects of specific mediators such as hemochromagens in the kidney have been described earlier (see Pathophysiology section). Fluid shifts in the early hours after injury can impair function of both organs, particularly the kidney; hepatic transaminases may be transiently elevated. Inflammatory mediators impose a risk of failure on all organs, the kidney being most sensitive, whereas the liver rarely signals failure except in end-stage multisystem organ failure. Alterations in plasma protein production are precipitated by changes in metabolism and the reactions to injury of the immune system: albumin production is decreased in favor of acute-phase proteins such as α_1-acid glycoprotein.[89]

It is tempting to replenish albumin in the face of a low serum level. Although lower measured levels are associated with a poorer outcome, there is good evidence that giving exogenous albumin does not improve this situation,[90] in children at least, and indeed the Cochrane study of 1998[65] suggests the reverse. Although albumin should therefore not be given to treat a low serum level per se, it may be considered of value for patients demonstrating detrimental effects of low albumin. It is arguable that administration in these circumstances should be guided by measurement of colloid osmotic pressure but, in practice, most clinicians are reluctant to allow the serum albumin to fall below $10\,g\,L^{-1}$ ($1\,g\,dL^{-1}$). There is little hard research information to guide the clinician in this context, hence the largely empirical approach to albumin use in most centers.

The brain

It is surprising that survivors of smoke inhalation only rarely exhibit significant neurologic damage, given the acute hypoxia at the scene and the cellular hypoxia consequent on asphyxia through laryngospasm and bronchospasm, and the tissue effects of carboxyhemoglobin and possibly cyanide. A varying degree of cerebral hypoxia is always associated with smoke inhalation and may contribute to the high mortality. It could be hypothesized that specific injury to the thermoregulatory center accounts for the observed inability of a few patients to generate heat in response to hypothermia, but this is not supported by evidence.

Children

The child particularly may suffer some loss of higher functions, and when most severely affected may become decorticate. Changes in cerebral perfusion, as a result of low cardiac output and high venous pressures secondary to high intrathoracic pressures required for ventilation, exacerbate the injury in both adults and children. If the inhalation is complicated by cutaneous injury, erratic and inaccurate fluid resuscitation will cause excessive cerebral edema. In these situations, some authors suggest the use of intracranial pressure monitoring as this allows optimal control of both resuscitation and cerebral perfusion pressure.[91]

The hematologic system and coagulation

The white cell count usually falls initially, due probably to depletion as part of the initial response to injury. After a few days, the white cell count may remain suppressed but is more commonly increased as part of the inflammatory response to injury. Red cells are destroyed in vessels beneath and adjacent to burned tissue. Their formation is subsequently suppressed, and red cell fragility increased. For platelets, the pattern is of an initial thrombocytopenia, which can be very severe, followed by a thrombocytosis developing during the second week.

A cyclical pattern of change is usually seen in coagulation following a burn.[92] In minor and moderate burns, these changes are rarely significant unless systemic infection occurs, when disseminated intravascular coagulation (DIC) is possible. SIRS following major burn injury or smoke inhalation may also trigger DIC. Initially the level of measurable coagulation factors falls, an effect probably caused by dilution during resuscitation. Later, thrombogenicity is increased.

The immune system and sepsis

Major thermal injury damages the body's largest immune organ – the skin. Further, the injury has significant deleterious effects on systemic immunocompetence. It is not surprising that infection and its complications remain the most significant factor in the events leading to the death of burned patients.[4]

Given the potential for SIRS described above, and the need to treat infection promptly in immunocompromised burn patients, it is important to distinguish SIRS due to the burn from sepsis. Unfortunately, the signs of SIRS and systemic sepsis are almost indistinguishable. The keyword in this context is therefore "vigilance," constantly being on the lookout for change – in gut function, renal function, mental state, wound appearance or culture, pattern of pyrexia (up, down, swinging), blood gases, especially arterial oxygen and pH, coagulation status, or any other variable: if it has changed, infection should be high on the list of possible reasons.

Wound cultures should be taken at each dressings change, which informs the nature of wound colonization, so suggesting best immediate antimicrobial treatment if infection is suspected. Invaded orifices, especially lung and bladder, should also be cultured regularly. Blood cultures should be taken when any change raises the possibility of infection as the cause.

ANESTHESIA FOR BURN PROCEDURES

Pharmacology

The behavior of all drugs used in anesthesia is affected by changes in cardiac output, plasma proteins, and volume of distribution that occur following a burn. These changes are nonspecific, occurring in response to any major trauma, but their magnitude is greater following major burns than in any other injury, mirroring the general metabolic changes described above. Changes in organ function influence the metabolism and excretion of drugs, and alterations in receptor structure or function can be demonstrated. All this means that both the pharmacokinetics and the pharmacodynamics of drugs used for anesthesia or intensive care are potentially affected in burned patients.

Neuromuscular blocking agents

Abnormalities in the response to depolarizing and nondepolarizing relaxants in thermally injured patients, including, and perhaps especially, children, have been recognized for many years.[93] Upregulation of the skeletal muscle acetylcholine receptors occurs, which is clinically demonstrable from the third day post injury and lasts for up to 3 years following the injury. This increase in receptors is thought to be responsible for the sensitivity to succinylcholine with concomitant excessive potassium release and for the development of resistance to nondepolarizing relaxants, and has been succinctly reviewed by Martyn *et al.*[94] (Fig. 68.13).

Muscle relaxation is commonly required to facilitate the control of ventilation in intensive care and during anesthesia for surgical excision. From approximately 3 days post burn, it is thought that extreme sensitivity to the effects of succinylcholine occurs,[95] with the risk of a massive hyperkalemic response. This reaction precludes the use of succinylcholine for a prolonged period following injury.

In the first week following injury, changes in cardiac output, plasma proteins, and distribution volume may increase requirements for all nondepolarizing relaxants. Following this acute period, progressive resistance is experienced with all relaxants proportionate to the size of cutaneous burn. Before the advent of vecuronium and atracurium, dimethyl tubocurarine in a dose of $1\,mg\,kg^{-1}$ was the relaxant of choice because of its low intrinsic anticholinergic activity. The absence of anticholinergic activity and completeness of reversal have established atracurium and vecuronium as the currently most frequently used agents. Atracurium will be required in a dose of $0.3\,mg\,kg^{-1}$ in the first week, rising to twice this dose in burns of 20–60% TBSA. Burns greater than 70% TBSA may require $3\,mg\,kg^{-1}$.[96] The time-course of effect of atracurium is similar to that in nonburned patients, as are the plasma clearance and half-life. The maximum twitch depression is smaller, not being abolished in many cases although intubating conditions are unaffected with recovery to 50% of twitch height in a significantly shorter period.[97] Similar resistance has been demonstrated to vecuronium.[98]

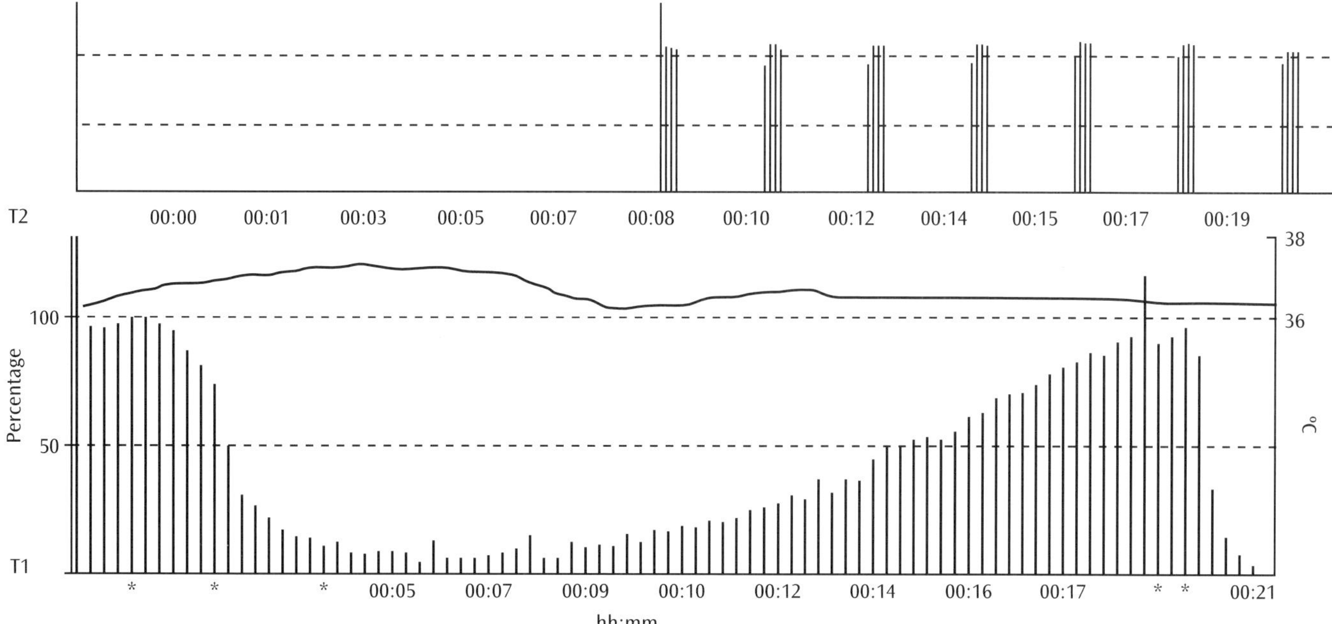

Figure 68.13 *A myo-accelograph following a normal dose of nondepolarizing relaxant, in this case rocuronium, showing incomplete twitch suppression and shortened duration of action.*

Rocuronium is a derivative of vecuronium with an onset of action similar to that of succinylcholine. It has an intermediate duration of action and demonstrates cardiovascular stability.[99,100] Its use in infants and children has been evaluated, and it has been used in intensive care as a continuous infusion.[101] Its use in children with burns is soon to be reported. The rapid onset of action may be of value when the airway must be gained rapidly and the potential for less tachyphylaxis and duration of action makes it a suitable choice in intensive care.

Other drugs

The action, metabolism, and clearance of any drug are a function of the route of administration, its degree of ionization, the proportion bound to protein, the volume of distribution, its affinity for its receptor, the number and sensitivity of receptors, the means by which it is degraded or conjugated, and the route of excretion. All of these may be affected following major injury, especially burns. Space does not allow an exhaustive account here. There are still many unknowns, and this topic is an important area for research.

The muscle relaxants are a good example of drugs the behavior of which is influenced by changes in receptor pharmacology following a burn. The actions of other drugs are influenced following burns by the various physiologic responses to injury. Shifts in fluid distribution may alter the pattern of distribution of some drugs, especially in the early days after injury. Changes in hepatic enzyme function caused by the metabolic response and increased hepatic blood flow can influence the degradation or conjugation of some drugs (e.g. diazepam, opiates). Drugs which are highly protein bound will become more or less bioavailable for a given dose, depending on whether they bind mainly to albumin (e.g. diazepam, vancomycin[102]) or to α_1-acid glycoprotein (e.g. alfentanil[103]). Drugs excreted via the kidney will usually be eliminated more rapidly (e.g. cimetidine), unless renal function is impaired. In any given instance, several of these factors can combine.

For example, most anesthesiologists find in practice that the dose of opiate drugs required for burned patients is greater than in other instances, yet published evidence does not fully support this view.[104] Many factors are in play, including the complex pharmacology of opiate receptors and the wide variation in plasma levels needed to produce equivalence of analgesia, and more research is undoubtedly needed to answer this conundrum. In the case of antibiotics, higher than normal doses of aminoglycosides are needed to achieve therapeutic levels, so that a priming dose 50% greater than normal is recommended for major burns, as well as regular monitoring. Other antibiotics exhibit variable penetration into burn tissue, so that doses at the top of the therapeutic range are recommended. Three-times-a-day dosage of the histamine antagonist cimetidine is needed to achieve adequate elevation of gastric pH, but normal dosing of ranitidine suffices.[105]

By far the best approach to drug administration in anesthesia or intensive care for burned patients therefore is to titrate dose against carefully monitored effects, but a knowledge of the known physiology and pharmacology is important. Whenever possible, effective dosage should be monitored by measurement of effect (e.g. muscle relaxants), plasma level estimation (e.g. gentamicin), and where necessary by monitoring function of the organs of elimination (liver or kidney). At the end of the day "the proper dose of any drug is enough" (J H Drysdale) but not too much.

TIMING AND METHOD OF SURGERY

Conservative treatment that allows eschar separation followed by serial skin grafting is now a thing of the past except perhaps for the sick elderly with small area burns.[13] Even in small burns, active surgical management minimizes infection, reduces hospital stay, and improves the final cosmetic or functional result. The timing of surgery is a matter of judgment to be made by an experienced burn surgeon and anesthesiologist in careful discussion. When the patient is uncomplicated, the decision is guided by the nature and extent of the wound. For mostly superficial burns, practice varies between early excision and grafting, and expectant treatment. The benefits of the former in terms of shorter lengths of stay are offset by more extensive excisions and imposition of a second wound, i.e. the donor site. The expectant approach allows shallow wounds to heal for 10 days, then grafts the remainder before 2 weeks. The result is a slightly longer hospital stay, a similar cosmetic result, and a smaller operation and donor site. Delay of necessary surgery beyond 2 weeks produces a much worse cosmetic result.

Extensive mixed or full-thickness wounds will not heal spontaneously in a reasonable timescale and remain substantial nidi for infection. The goal is to excise all but very superficial components within 1 week after injury. Burns of less than 15% TBSA are excised in one procedure. In more extensive burns, the surgical policy varies between burn centers, but it is now common to excise up to 30% TBSA in one sitting, commencing at day 2 and repeating frequently until the whole wound is excised.[106] A few centers excise massive burns in one long procedure, starting within the first 24 h; there is as yet no clear evidence that this significantly reduces mortality compared with serial excision. It is certainly more readily achieved in children than in adults. However timed, there is now no doubt that early wound excision saves lives.[13] It has been shown to:

- reduce the inflammatory stimulus;
- reduce metabolic demand;
- minimize infection risks, and;
- reduce length of stay;
  - but it is very demanding on all staff... *and*:
  - temporary wound cover is needed (freeze-dried or glycerolized cadaver skin, or artificial materials (Biobrane™, Dermagraft™, Integra™ for instance).

Intensive care is therefore an indication for early surgery, not an impediment to it, but the patient must be in a stable condition.

The method of excision is usually one of two: tangential shave excision or full-thickness diathermy-assisted excision (Fig. 68.14). The first traditionally is usually more bloody as it relies on the occurrence of profuse capillary bleeding as a sign that healthy tissue has been reached. Blood loss can be reduced by infiltrating epinephrine (adrenaline) under the eschar, but this makes determination of the depth of excision less certain, as it requires an experienced surgical eye. Diathermy excision of fascia sheds much less blood and is generally less traumatic overall. It is still therefore the method of choice during massive excisions for extensive full-thickness burns in which the priority is to save life. When followed by serial skin grafting, it invariably gives a cosmetically poor result, although artificial dermis substitutes such as Integra™ can markedly improve cosmetic and functional outcome – but at substantial cost.

These factors are important for the anesthesiologist when deciding the mode and likely duration of anesthesia, also the anticipated blood requirement. It is important to be aware that excision of vascular or intricate sites, such as the face or hands, is likely to take longer and require more blood.

Preoperative assessment and preparation

The patient is often at one extreme or other of age, i.e. an infant, a child, or an elderly person. Adults are often those with chronic illness, epilepsy, or occasionally other injuries, and may be chronic abusers of alcohol or drugs. It is important therefore to properly assess the patient, as with any patient presenting for surgery. It is also essential to be told the proposed extent of surgery contemplated, although this may be adjusted in the operating room according to findings and the patient's initial response to surgery. Third, it is necessary to assess the extent of the burn, its metabolic effect, and the presence of sepsis.

The aim is to take the patient to the operating room, stabilized if necessary in intensive care, to remove the source of metabolic stress by surgical excision and return the patient with the least physiologic disturbance. Given the maximum 7-day window of opportunity for early surgical management without excessive blood loss or before invasive sepsis, a good reason is required for postponement. Contraindications for surgery are :

- inadequate resuscitation;
- abnormal electrolytes;
- respiratory or metabolic acidosis;
- abnormal clotting studies;
- incipient septicemia;
- unexplained rapid temperature change;
- changed consciousness level;
- instability in respiratory or cardiovascular parameters.

Therefore, it is important to get on top of these problems during early resuscitation. Further, a wound culture of β-hemolytic streptococ-

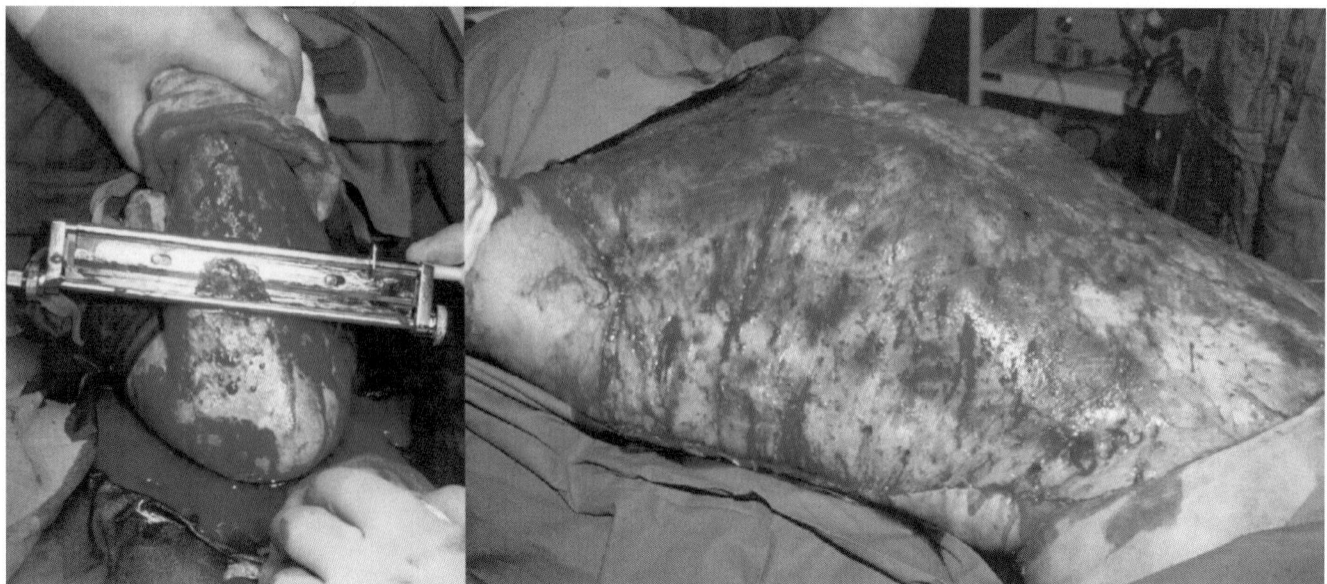

Figure 68.14 *Excising the burn wound. Tangential shave excision (left). Note the amount of blood loss. Diathermy excision to fascia of a full-depth wound (right).*

cus or *Staphylococcus aureus* will usually delay surgery because they are both known to lyse grafted skin. Any condition that would benefit from a further 24-h active treatment will also suggest delay. Preoperative anemia will be, in part, dilutional in the early days, but levels below 8 g dL^{-1} should be corrected before surgery. There is a high incidence of upper respiratory tract infections among the toddler age group, which may be an etiological factor in the accidental scald. Surgery should not be postponed because of upper respiratory tract or chest infections provided any necessary antibiotics have been started. Pyrexia of up to 39 °C and fleeting or maculopapular rashes are frequently seen in the thermally injured child, and even in adults a mild pyrexia is common in the absence of infection.

Premedication

The use or otherwise of premedication in adults is a matter of personal preference for the anesthesiologist; there are no hard rules.[107] A calm, reassuring visit is often sufficient for adults. If need be, a sedative premedication, an antiemetic, and/or a measure to reduce gastric acidity (e.g. ranitidine) can be prescribed in patients at appropriate risk. Full explanations must be given, however, of the procedure envisioned, the probability that this will be one of a series of procedures, and of the strong possibility of pain postoperatively. Reassurance must be offered that pain will be treated vigorously and promptly, and it is good for the anesthesiologist's credibility when explaining this if past experience is of high-quality pain relief. A high standard of meticulous anesthesia and analgesia brings quick rewards; merely adequate standards have a habit of coming back to haunt. All the anesthesiologists providing anesthesia to a burns unit will find that it is in their mutual interests to adopt common protocols for anesthesia and pain relief.

Children

In contrast with adults, preoperative sedation is desirable for children to reduce the stress of fasting, transport to the operating room, and induction of anesthesia. Sedation, amnesia, and sufficient drying of secretions will be provided by a premedicant dose of trimeprazine supported, if necessary, by a further dose of intravenous morphine at induction. Atropine is not required to dry secretions or for its vagolytic effect. The routine administration of atropine to pyrexial and tachycardic children may be deleterious and will confuse the response to changing intravascular volume and temperature control. EMLA™ [a eutectic mixture of lidocaine (lignocaine) and prilocaine] or amethocaine (Ametop™) cream applied to a suitable area of skin will reduce pain if venipuncture is contemplated.

Parental presence is encouraged whenever possible during induction. We have found the presence of a parent very supportive, provided there is adequate time for preparation. A greater proportion of parents become upset once the child has lost consciousness as compared with nonburns surgery. We would therefore suggest the presence of a second parent or other supporter during induction. Active involvement of parents throughout the management of the child with burns is regarded as essential and contributes to reduction of morbidity and mortality.[108] In some units, play specialists have been included in the induction process, because their skills of distraction through targeted play can assist in maintaining calm. They should serve as a supplement to, but never a substitute for, parents unless the parent is unable or unwilling to accompany the child.

On occasion a child will exhibit extreme distress at the prospect of induction of anesthesia. This is most common for a child around adolescence and associated with a degree of poor graft survival and extended hospitalization. Such a child will react noisily and aggressively at any movement or therapy. Following discussion with the child, confidence may be improved by the administration of a light general anesthetic in the bed before transport to theatre fully monitored by the anesthesiologist. Nasal or oral ketamine has been used in particularly fractious children but may cause prolonged sedation and/or unpleasant emergence side-effects.

Fasting

Nutrition is a core objective for burns therapy. Oral, nasogastric, or nasojejunal feeding is instituted early. Accepted guidelines for preoperative fasting[109] can apply but prolonged starvation must be avoided, and nutrition restarted as soon as possible after surgery. More than 2 h of preoperative starving markedly impairs that day's nutrition intake.[110]

Controversy exists as to whether tube feeding needs to be stopped several hours before surgery, and there is evidence that it can be continued safely until 1 h beforehand.[110] A feeding tube will affect the integrity of the lower esophageal sphincter, making regurgitation more likely but, if absorption of the steady trickle flow of feed has been good with zero aspirates, there should be nothing in the stomach to regurgitate. It is becoming increasingly common, therefore, for tube feeds to be continued almost up to the start of anesthesia. In some centers, including that of one author (KCJ), enteral feeds are continued for those with major burns requiring intensive care throughout the operation without reported detriment so far. Caution must be exercised for those patients lying prone during the procedure and the lack of a tracheal cuff requires that feeding should always be stopped in the case of children, to prevent airway soiling, which occurs even when there is minor regurgitation.

Prophylaxis

Antithrombotic prophylaxis should be considered, balancing the hypercoagulable state of the major burn with the risk of DIC, and the potential for deep vein thrombosis in any hypoambulant patient against the risk of hematoma formation under grafts or skin substitutes.

Antibiotic prophylaxis is necessary for any patient who has remaining unexcised burn greater than 2 days old and who is not already receiving antibiotics, to minimize the potential for bacteremia during wound excision. A single dose only should be given, on induction of anesthesia. The choice of antibiotic should be guided by wound cultures and known bacterial flora in the unit; if these are not available, a broad-spectrum antibiotic active against common Gram-positive organisms and *Pseudomonas aeruginosa* should be chosen.

The anesthetic

The anesthesiologist's priorities are to maintain cardiovascular stability, conserve body heat, and provide analgesia and if necessary sedation which lasts into the postoperative period and beyond. A large number of agents, parenteral and volatile, with a wide margin of safety and which do not depress myocardial function, are available, making for safe possibilities in young and old alike. The options for anesthesia are therefore governed largely by ability to access the airway and the requirements of the anticipated surgery. For inhalational induction in children or needle-phobic adults, sevoflurane has improved on the qualities of halothane.[111] Intravenous induction may be achieved with pentothal or propofol. Anesthesia is then supported by an appropriate narcotic, of which the ephemeral agents alfentanil or remifentanil have proved very effective and may obviate the need for muscle relaxation.

A recurrent question exists over the role of succinylcholine. Prior to the upgrading of the neuromuscular junction, demonstrable from day 3 following injury, succinylcholine produces no deleterious rise in serum potassium and could be used. Rocuronium in appropriate dose would appear to offer an advantage should neuromuscular blockade be required (see under Airway above).

Intravenous induction agents

Pentothal or propofol[112] provides rapid induction of anesthesia for both adults and children. The dose of each may have to be increased secondary to a hyperdynamic circulation and increased volume of redistribution, and this situation may persist after the acute period.[113,114] For brief procedures, propofol may facilitate earlier positioning of a laryngeal mask. The low incidence of nausea and vomiting and the rapid and complete recovery provide an indication for use of propofol when regular dressings are required.

Ketamine continues to have a role in premedication for children via the oral, rectal, and nasal routes, and for induction in some centers.[107] It may be used exclusively for dressings. Propofol is superior in many respects,[115] especially for adults (see Analgesia section).

Intubation

The size and type of tracheal tube is determined by standard principles, bearing in mind that a reinforced tube may be needed if the head is to be turned or the patient's position is altered during the procedure. Circumstances may dictate a smaller tube than otherwise estimated. Intubation may be more difficult than usual if the neck or face has been burned; a difficult intubation kit and strategy should be a normal part of a burn room's armamentarium. Fiberoptic intubation is a valuable technique for these circumstances, but only in experienced hands, remembering that stiffness or distortion of face, neck, or oropharyngeal tissues may impede even this technique when the patient is asleep. Good psychologic preparation must precede awake fiberoptic intubation. The problems potentially encountered when intubating a major burn are legion.

The key is: anticipate the worst situation, ensure expert assistance, think ahead, oxygenate well, and stay calm throughout. Then, after intubation, achieve firm fixation of the tube. This may require some imagination if the face is burned (see Fig. 68.8). Direct thermal injury to the face and neck will result in difficulty in securing the airway because of facial maceration or dressings preventing adequate seal of a mask, to deep burns causing restriction to mouth opening or, if over the submental region, difficulty in displacing the tongue forward for intubation. The favored method of intubation in these circumstances in children is under direct vision using a fiberoptic bronchoscope but there are several other techniques described.[116]

The laryngeal mask airway (LMA) in burns

This device must rank as the most effective and useful device for control of the airway since the introduction of endotracheal intubation. After initial caution, it has been adopted by the anesthetic community for use in a variety of situations including pediatric practice.[117] It allows treatment of facial injury while maintaining the airway,[118] avoiding repetitive laryngeal instrumentation. The mask is tolerated at light levels of anesthesia and is suitable for sedation or anesthesia using propofol as the sole agent. Although it protects the larynx from aspiration of substances in the mouth, it does not prevent aspiration of stomach contents, and should not be used for more major surgery when complete control of the airway is necessary and when there is a danger of displacement with the frequent changes of position during the surgery. Capnography is essential to confirm correct placement.

A very major advantage is the ability to maintain the difficult airway while deepening the anesthetic or as an aid to intubation with or without the fiberoptic bronchoscope.[116] When there is difficulty in securing the airway, spontaneous ventilation should be maintained. The mask can be used with care, however, with intermittent positive-pressure ventilation, should laryngeal paralysis be required.[119] Peak airway pressures should be maintained as low as possible to avoid inflation of the stomach. The airway can be left *in situ* until the return of consciousness, allowing the administration of oxygen without a face mask or nasal catheter that might disturb grafts.

Control of the intravascular compartment

The main intraoperative concerns are control of intravascular volume, preservation of oxygen-carrying capacity, and maintenance of coagulation. The amount of blood loss will depend on several factors, including extent and method of excision, timing of surgery, and the part of the body involved. Judicious use of tourniquets, infiltration of epinephrine, and choice of dressing for the donor site, all help to reduce blood loss.

Burn vascularity rises toward the end of the first week, leading to excessive loss thereafter. After 3 weeks, some healing has occurred and, when slough is removed, granulation tissue is found to cover the deep dermal injury. Burns of intricate areas such as hands and feet lose a considerable amount of blood unless part of the excision is performed under tourniquet. Neck and face injuries rarely have to be shaved but bleeding cannot be controlled by pressure dressings. Temporary bandaging and application of calcium alginate (Kaltostat™) reduce ooze from donor sites.

Blood loss can be reduced by infiltration of epinephrine or by the application of epinephrine-soaked swabs; solutions at 1:100 000 or as dilute as 1:500 000 are effective. Up to $10\,\mu g\,kg^{-1}$ has been used with halothane for children without cardiac arrhythmia.[120] Vasopressin has been used similarly.[121] The risk of cardiac arrhythmias is less if a volatile agent other than halothane is used. Surgeons have become much more discriminating when shaving a burn of mixed depth, resulting in much less blood loss than in the days of early tangential burn excision when a child with a 10% burn could expect to lose one-third to one-half of a blood volume.[122]

Attitudes to transfusion have changed, as have estimates of red cell mass necessary for healing. The possibility of transmitting infection and inducing antibody formation with stored blood products has resulted in a re-evaluation of transfusion therapy in recent years. The need to maintain a hemoglobin concentration of $10\,g\,dL^{-1}$ or a hematocrit of 30% has been disputed. Some centers have allowed the hemoglobin to fall as low as $6.5\,g\,dL^{-1}$ before transfusion without adverse effects.[123] Burns of intricate areas such as the hands and feet lose a considerable amount of blood unless part or all of the excision is performed with the use of a tourniquet; the surgeon must be experienced in determining by color alone the distinction between burned and healthy tissue in the absence of capillary bleeding. Transfusion policy should take into account further postoperative ooze and the failure of erythropoiesis until healing is established. If blood loss is continuing, a healthy margin should be allowed and the hemoglobin should be maintained above $10\,g\,dL^{-1}$. A higher red cell mass will be appropriate for patients compromised by the catabolic state or pyrexia with concomitant demands on oxygen delivery.

Assessment of the blood loss associated with early tangential excision has been made at approximately 2% of blood volume for each percentage burn shaved[124] and formulas have been developed to assess the transfusion requirements to cover losses from the burn and the donor areas.[125] Adequate supplies of blood and blood products should be available in the hospital. Modern cross-matching techniques provide fully compatible products in 30 min. Provided there is an adequate specimen for further cross-match, a conservative estimate of blood requirements can be made, which should be in the order of one unit for every 10% of cutaneous burn. Packed red blood cells in optimal additive solution (SAGM) have the advantages of high cell survival and 2,3-diphosphoglyceride levels in addition to being more readily available.

However, intraoperative estimation of blood loss is notoriously difficult. Washing of swabs and colorimetric estimation is too slow. Individual swab weighing provides reasonable accuracy if swabs are not presoaked, but they frequently are. The most accurate method is clinical observation of hemodynamic parameters, especially heart rate, combined with serial hematocrit or hemoglobin estimations. These can be performed on a drop of blood in the operating room, using a microcentrifuge or optical hemoglobin meter. CVP measurement is valuable during major excisions but is not without hazard, especially for children. Access for CVP measurement via the neck or subclavian approach will be impossible until burns in these areas have been excised. The only available access is often the groin.

Prevention of pathologic bleeding

In the absence of inherited disease or anticoagulant therapy, most burned patients do not exhibit coagulopathy. The systemic inflammatory response syndrome triggered by major burns is capable of inducing disseminated intravascular coagulation, and lesser degrees of coagulopathy do occur in susceptible patients. In major burns, platelet counts commonly fall during the first week or so but, by 10 days, a thrombocytosis is frequently seen. Similarly, early reduction in clotting factors may be followed by laboratory evidence of hypercoagulability. It is therefore important to measure coagulation regularly and, when normal, to cover operative procedures with active prophylaxis against thromboembolism.

If whole blood is used for replacement, factor deficiency, particularly factors V and VIII, is unlikely to occur unless three blood volumes or more have been replaced. As packed red cells contain minimal factors, pathologic bleeding will occur much earlier. Empirical replacement of these by giving fresh-frozen plasma, when 30% of each blood volume has been lost, will minimize problems. Should massive blood loss be expected, alternate fresh-frozen plasma and packed cells can be given from the outset, maintaining oxygen-carrying capacity and coagulability. It is also important, however, to measure coagulation and platelets periodically during major excisions if one or more blood volumes are lost.

Conduct of anesthesia

The aim of the anesthesiologist is to provide optimal conditions for surgery with minimal physiologic disturbance. The maintenance of a full hyperdynamic circulation avoiding peripheral vasoconstriction is essential as this facilitates accurate discrimination between superficial and deep dermal injury and thus avoids excessively deep excision. This state will only exist in the presence of adequate fluid replacement and good anesthesia. Suppression of the response to surgical stimulus, temperature maintenance and avoidance of hypocarbia are essential.

Venous access should usually be secured before any anesthetic intervention. Adequate peripheral veins may be difficult to find. Primary sites for induction in order of ease of access are dorsum of hand, ventral wrist, dorsum of foot, antecubital fossa, and, finally, in the baby, the scalp. A larger vein will be required for volume replacement: in order, the long saphenous, the antecubital fossa, the external jugular, and then the central sites, internal jugular, subclavian, and, finally, femoral. A cut-down should be performed following failure to gain adequate percutaneous venous access capable of sustaining rapid infusion rates.

Inhalational induction is indicated when there is actual or potential airway obstruction. Preoxygenation and partial denitrogenation is advisable. Children can sometimes display an educated preference for inhalational induction, or this may be the safest and most efficient method for the restless or fractious child. Halothane, because of its potency and low incidence of laryngeal irritation, has previously been the agent of choice. Sevoflurane in oxygen is likely to replace halothane in pediatric practice for induction, although concern has been expressed about adequacy of depth for laryngoscopic and bronchoscopic procedures.[111] Subsequent laryngeal mask insertion will then free the anesthesiologist to undertake cannulation prior to intubation in the uncommon cases when this is impossible before induction.

Monitoring should be commenced prior to induction. In the case of a child, as much monitoring as is possible should be in use but without causing distress. Minimum monitoring would include pulse oximetry, ECG and noninvasive blood pressure, with an end-tidal carbon dioxide analyzer available to confirm intubation. A urinary catheter will often already be *in situ*. Unless there is a specific indication for inhalational induction, intravenous induction is the most rapid and convenient method and, in the absence of hypovolemia, it provides rapid and safe induction.

If the patient is not already intubated, tracheal intubation may be performed orally, using a cuffed tube in adults or the child after puberty. Careful choice of uncuffed tube size for smaller children is needed to avoid trauma to the cricoid mucosa, as noted previously. Adequate fixation must be assured; for the child, a mouth pack will provide further security. A note should be made of any edema, erythema, sloughs, or soot in the supraglottic or glottic area seen during laryngoscopy.

The maintenance of anesthesia thereafter is a matter of preference by the anesthesiologist, taking the patient's condition into account as well as the needs of surgery. Monitoring should be established in harmony with the extent of excision required and the condition and needs of the patient, but may be tricky to achieve. Access for invasive monitoring may be difficult, and placement of pulse oximeter and ECG electrodes often requires ingenuity and imagination.[126] Noninvasive blood pressure, ECG, pulse oximeter, and end-tidal carbon dioxide monitoring are an essential minimum.

Supplements

Because of the requirements for adequate anesthesia, no single agent fulfills all requirements intraoperatively. Volatile agents are potent and convenient but their vasodilator effects are terminated with the end of the anesthetic to be replaced by vasoconstriction. Their characteristics are discussed in detail elsewhere in this book (see Chapter 33). The agent of choice for anesthesia for burn surgery is one which affords the least cardiovascular disturbance. Halothane has been used for repeated anesthesia in the management of burns in children without adverse effects. However, it produces peripheral vasodilation and depresses cardiac output and, in the presence of the slightest hypovolemia, peripheral perfusion will be seriously compromised. Sevoflurane has a low blood–gas partition coefficient, and it provides more rapid induction with greater patient acceptability associated with a similar or lower incidence of laryngeal irritability,[127] and a lower incidence of cardiovascular side-effects.[128] Sevoflurane is replacing halothane for burn pediatric practice, although concern has been expressed about the adequacy of anesthetic depth for laryngoscopic and bronchoscopic procedures.[111] Sevoflurane produces less myocardial sensitization to epinephrine, which is now routinely used in soaks and by infiltration to suppress blood loss.

Isoflurane and enflurane, used for adults, are associated with reduced oxygen requirements, cardiac index, mean arterial pressure, and pulmonary artery pressure without a change in systemic and pulmonary vascular resistance.[129] Isoflurane protects cardiac output and peripheral blood flow in children.[130] Its ability to produce laryngeal irritation renders it unacceptable as an agent for inhalational induction in the emergency situation when the airway must be secured in the shortest possible time. Therefore, either agent can be used as a supplement during surgery for burns, provided that laryngospasm is unlikely at emergence.

Narcotics suppress the hemodynamic response to surgical stimulus, and reduce the requirements for volatile agents and neuromuscular blocking agents. Fentanyl administered in a dose of 10 μg kg^{-1} before the onset of surgery ensures suppression of tachycardia during the harvesting of donor skin. Adequate spontaneous respiration will occur after 1 h with no evidence of postoperative respiratory depression. Patients are monitored both routinely and closely in a high-dependency environment. If postoperative ventilation is to be continued, an infrequent need, repeated boluses of fentanyl should be administered to prevent a tachycardia.

When a high inspired oxygen is required, unconsciousness should be assured with a combination of volatile agent and narcotic or narcotic and propofol infusion to maintain suppression of the hemodynamic response. Initial studies would appear to indicate that the dose requirements of propofol for induction and maintenance of adequate anesthesia are greater than those for nonburned adults and children, but especially for children.[114] Both alfentanil and remifentanil have been used in the maintenance of anesthesia for burn surgery.[112] Remifentanil has a reduced incidence of postoperative narcosis[131] but, because of its ephemeral action, it should be replaced with a longer-acting narcotic prior to emergence from anesthesia.

Heat conservation

The greatest care must be taken to avoid the patient cooling below the preoperative temperature as metabolic activity with concomitant calorie loss and increased oxygen consumption will be necessary during the postoperative period.[132] The patient should be covered with drapes, gamgee or foil, and protected from draughts. Radiant heaters provide heat during the insertion of intravascular lines or debridement prior to surgery.

Depending on the size of the burn and the degree of preoperative pyrexia, the ambient operating room temperature must be maintained between 29 °C and 34 °C. Local warming should be provided by a warming blanket maintained at no greater than 1 °C above skin temperature. Further heat and moisture can be conserved by using a condenser humidifier for short procedures, or a hot water humidifier for more prolonged procedures. All fluids should be warmed prior to infusion. When working at these high temperatures, the surgical and nursing team should be sent for frequent breaks to maintain concentration.

Postoperative care

Postoperatively, the patient should ideally be returned to a room with a thermoneutral ambient temperature of between 30 °C and 34 °C to minimize metabolic drive, but the use of a hot-air blanket produces this environment for the patient without undue discomfort for staff. Close observation is required to watch for blood loss by monitoring vital signs for at least 24 h, and by checking dressings for blood seeping through. Good analgesia is mandatory (see below), and nausea must also be anticipated and treated vigorously. A poor postoperative experience will increase anxiety for the subsequent procedures that the patient will undoubtedly require, especially a child, making future management very difficult. Fears are easier to prevent than to cure.

Anesthesia and analgesia for change of dressings

The requirement for general anesthesia for the changing of dressings or wound toilet has reduced in recent years. Techniques of analgesia using sedatives, narcotics, or inhalational or intravenous agents prove adequate in most situations. Ketamine has in the past been widely recommended for dressing changes and, used carefully in subanesthetic doses (1 mg kg^{-1}), is still of value. The duration of sedation and a number of disturbing psychologic sequelae, however, can make it unacceptable in practice.

Premixed nitrous oxide 50%/oxygen 50% (Entonox) by continuous flow in the young child or demand flow in older children and adults, supplemented if necessary by narcotics with or without sedatives, provides adequate conditions accepted by patient and nursing staff in the majority of cases. Children familiar with this technique will more readily accept gaseous induction of anesthesia.

General anesthesia is reserved for major burns, for the very young child, or for intricate dressings, e.g. to the hand, which take a considerable time. In this situation, anesthesia may be required on several occa-

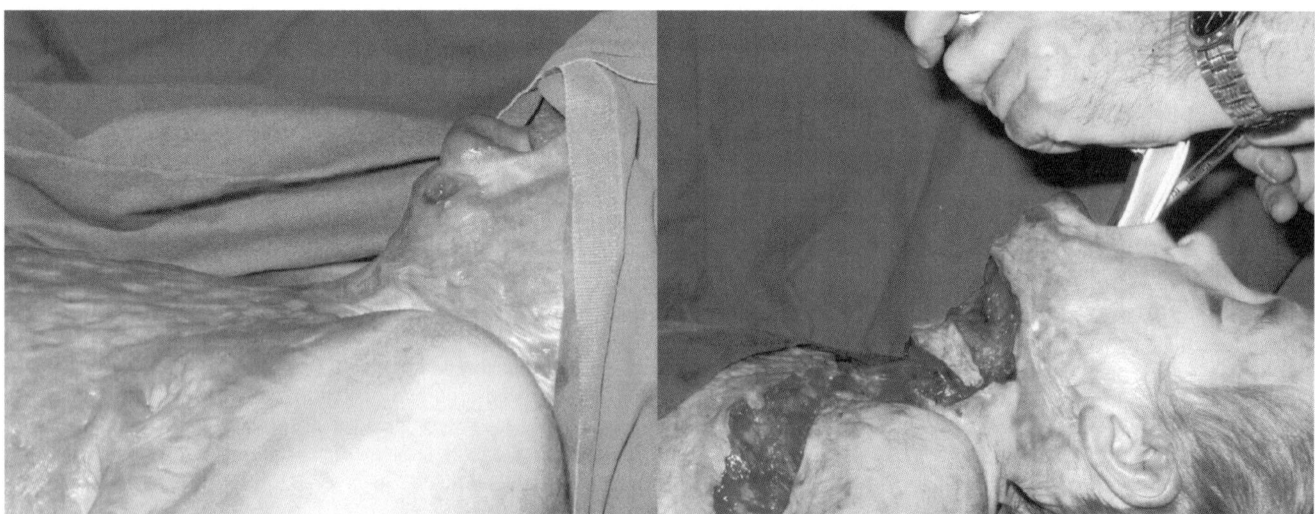

Figure 68.15 *Surgical release of a moderately severe neck contracture prior to inserting a full-thickness graft: before (left) and after (right) Note the extra neck extension achieved, allowing a grade 1 intubation.*[140]

sions separated by 2–3 days. Excessive sedation following anesthesia is neither necessary nor desirable as oral nutrition will be compromised.

A small number of patients who are healing in part by granulation may require sequential soaking and dressing in the bath. These patients exhibit a great deal of physical and mental debility. The anesthesiologist can play a vital supportive role ensuring adequate analgesia and stress relief. Techniques such as continuous propofol sedation have proved not only satisfactory but beneficial in this respect,[115] maintaining patient morale and ensuring comfort which may contribute positively to healing. Adequate analgesia sessions must be planned into the job descriptions of anesthesiologists having a major interest in anesthesia for burns, to support the day-to-day care of patients undergoing procedures outside the operating room. In children, the play specialist has a vital role to play in providing confidence, support, and play distraction for the child undergoing painful procedures and may be of great assistance to the anesthesiologist in this respect.

Anesthesia for reconstructive procedures

Following survival from a major burn, or from any burn involving the limbs, face, or genitalia, the patient may present for reconstructive surgery requiring many procedures over many years. The challenges that face the anesthesiologist are interesting and are offset by the chance to see progress in recovery over time, an opportunity rarely seen by the anesthesiologist working with other disciplines.

The anesthesia required is usually remarkably straightforward unless the face, neck, or airway is compromised in any way. The severely contracted neck is a particular problem, which may be best managed using a mask or laryngeal mask until the contracture has been surgically released before intubation (Fig. 68.15).

Additionally, these patients may be suffering or recovering from a raft of psychologic disorders, including post-traumatic stress disorder or depression. Needle phobia is common in children and may not be at all obviated by use of local analgesia creams, because the child anticipates hurt – he or she has been there before! Veins may be difficult to locate in burned limbs, commonly making gaseous induction prior to intravenous cannulation a necessary compromise to minimize distress.

PAIN RELIEF

Analgesia and sedation in general burn care

The provision of adequate analgesia and, when necessary, sedation, is of paramount importance from admission, following surgery and to facilitate dressings changes. The variability of injury and patient response, both pharmacologically and emotionally, necessitate close monitoring and adjustments and modification of technique, which include pharmacologic and nonpharmacologic methods.[133,134] The pain experience for the burned patient is outlined in Fig. 68.16, together with some of the treatments used.

On admission, the patient, especially if a child, is not only in pain but is also frightened. The most adequate management is administration of narcotic analgesia, with emotional support from relatives or friends, staff and parents of acutely distressed children.

Morphine sulfate should be given intravenously initially in a dose of up to $0.2\,mg\,kg^{-1}$. Intramuscular administration should be avoided as it will be associated with variable initial absorption and effect to be followed by a cumulative effect on return of perfusion of the muscles. Repeated intramuscular injection will risk fear of needles, especially but by no means exclusively by children. Should the first dose prove insufficient, a further incremental dose will be required within 10 min, when the initial dose has had sufficient time to take effect. Once adequate sedation and analgesia have been attained in the acute phase, further analgesia can be maintained by intravenous bolus injection, continuous background infusion at $0.05\,mg\,kg^{-1}\,h^{-1}$, or patient-controlled analgesia. This latter device can be used to give a background infusion with nurse-administered bolus administration to children, which provides further analgesia instantly, as the nurse deems it necessary.

A similar regimen may be used in the postoperative period. Increments of intravenous morphine as above may be given by experienced and accredited recovery nurses immediately on waking, to control pain before maintenance analgesia is started. Provided the patient is sufficiently conscious and, if a child, of an age to comprehend the principles of patient-controlled analgesia (PCA), there would appear to be no reason to deny the benefits that it provides. Children as young as 4 years have successfully used this technique, which has been shown to have a high index of safety.[135] Current techniques of control of acute pain in children have been recently reviewed.[136] The practical problems of using PCA for patients with burned hands can be overcome by alternative trigger devices produced by some companies, but more usually by using a continuous infusion. The latter must be well monitored for respiratory depression if overdose is to be anticipated and avoided.

Local analgesic techniques have increased in popularity in both adult and pediatric burns practice. Infiltration of donor sites and topical application of bupivacaine have been used. Theoretical considerations of limitation by toxicity seem not to be a problem in practice. Regional blockade is helpful in limited burns, brachial plexus blockade for the arm, and leg blocks for the lower leg and foot or for thigh donor sites. A single caudal epidural injection of 0.25% bupivacaine $1\,mL\,kg^{-1}$ for the child produces excellent analgesia below the umbilicus and gives a degree of sensory suppression facilitating sleep. Continuous extradural infusions are only rarely used because of the possibility of infection.

Acetaminophen (paracetamol) has been administered in response to rises in temperature. Studies have shown that acetaminophen administered orally or rectally is ineffective in reducing the pyrexia associated with burn injury in the child.[137] Acetaminophen, ibroprofen, and diclofenac, however, may be used successfully as an adjuvant to analgesia in the healing phase of burns. Concerns over renal function, platelet function, and duration of administration limit their use in the elderly or in patients with known impairment of renal function.

Intensive care

It is difficult to assess the requirements for analgesia and sedation in the patient requiring prolonged ventilation. Our current practice is to administer an analgesic and a sedative in combination, and any of those used in general intensive care is suitable accompanied by appropriate monitoring including level of sedation by one of the accepted techniques such as the Newcastle sedation score. High doses of opiates may apparently be needed; anecdotal evidence is available that tachyphylaxis can be attenuated by coadministration of $1–1.5\,mg\,kg^{-1}\,h^{-1}$ of ketamine.[138] Further opiate or sedative by bolus or adjustment of infusions, as appropriate, is given on the assessment of hemodynamic response to physiotherapy and endotracheal suction or motor response on breakthrough of neuromuscular blockade.

Children

In addition to analgesia, the uncomfortable and fractious child may require background sedation. This can be provided by trimeprazine, $2–3\,mg\,kg^{-1}$ three times daily, if required. This drug is effective in reducing the itching experienced in the recovery phase. Benzodiazepines are very variable in their effects, so should trimeprazine prove inadequate chloral hydrate may be more suitable. The aim is not to render the child unconscious but to provide a comfortable, calm child who will respond to and benefit from the presence of parents, who are also in a tense and emotional state.

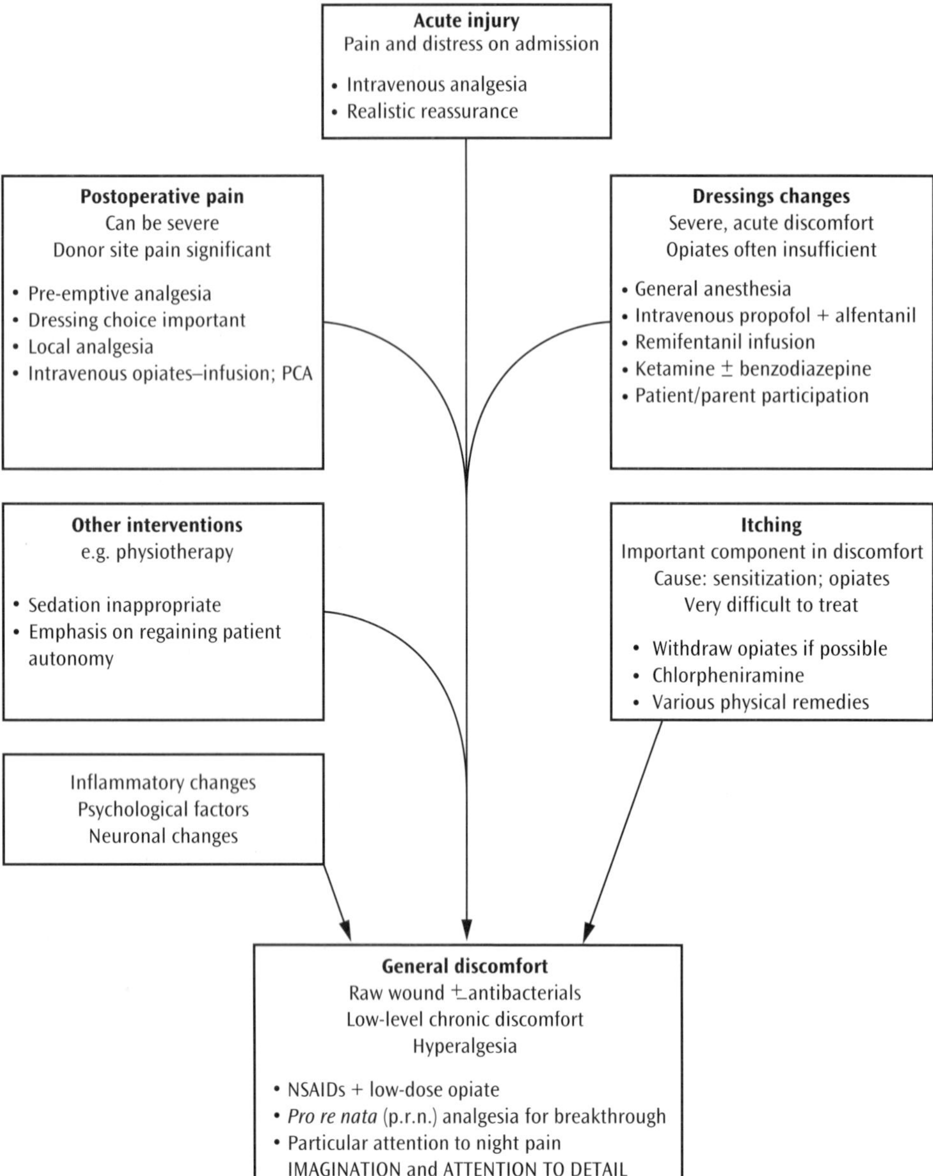

Figure 68.16 *Schematic representation of the pain experience in burns and possible focused treatment strategies in nonventilated patients. See text for fuller description.*

Background pain

It is beyond the scope of this chapter to address in detail the management of background pain for the burned patient over long periods. This is reviewed elsewhere.[134] Suffice to emphasize that it is in no-one's interests, least of all the patient's, and including the anesthesiologist's, for the patient to suffer unnecessary pain on the ward between the frequent interventions of modern burn care. There should be protocols for pain treatment that include guidance on drugs, doses, methods of administration in children and adults, monitoring pain, tailoring of dose to pain experience, and the place and value of nonpharmacologic methods. Drugs used include opiates (oral or parenteral), nonsteroidal anti-inflammatory drugs (NSAIDs), and mild analgesics such as acetaminophen. Combination analgesics are often more effective than single agents. High doses are not often needed because pain levels are not often high, but regular administration with an additional breakthrough prescription may manage the experience better than as required medication only. Because treatment may be required over long periods, potential side-effects (e.g. renal impairment using NSAIDs) must be known, diligently anticipated, and prevented or treated. Nausea in particular must be vigorously managed as it will impair vital nutrition intake. Lastly, pruritus is a very distressing and sometimes disabling symptom of the healing burn for which there are few effective remedies, but withdrawal of opiate medication can sometimes help if pain levels allow.

REFERENCES

1. Judkins K, Pike H. Prevention and rehabilitation: the community faces of burn care. *Burns* 1998; **24:** 594–8.
2. Munster AM, Smith-Meek M, Sharkey P. The effect of early surgical intervention on mortality and cost-effectiveness in burn care, 1978–91. *Burns* 1994; **20:** 61–4.
3. Matsuno K. The treatment of hydrofluoric acid burns. *Occup Med (Oxf)* 1996; **46:** 313–17.
4. Ryan CM, Schoenfeld DA, Thorpe WP. Objective estimates of the probability of death from burn injuries. *N Engl J Med* 1998; **338:** 362–6; editorial 387–8.
5. Bull JP. Revised analysis of mortality due to burns. *Lancet* 1971; **ii:** 1133–4.
6. Platt AJ, Aslam S, Judkins K, Phipps AR, Smith GL. Temperature profiles during resuscitation predict survival following burns complicated by smoke inhalation injury. *Burns* 1997; **23:** 250–5.
7. Shiozaki T, Kishikawa M, Hiraide A, *et al.* Recovery from postoperative

hypothermia predicts survival in extensively burned patients. *Am J Surg* 1993; **165:** 326–30; discussion 331.
8. Shiozaki T, Hiraide A, Shimazu T, *et al.* Differences in body temperature changes during dressing change in surviving and non-surviving burned patients. *Br J Surg* 1995; **82:** 784–6.
9. Platt AJ, Phipps AR, Judkins K. Is there still a place for comfort care in severe burns? *Burns* 1998; **24:** 754–6.
10. Keswani MH, Patil AR. The boiled potato peel as a burn wound dressing: a preliminary report. *Burns Incl Therm Inj* 1985; **11:** 220–4.
11. Brown DL, Archer SB, Greenhalgh DG, *et al.* Inhalation injury severity scoring system: a quantitative method. *J Burn Care Rehabil* 1996; **17:** 552–7.
12. Shirani KZ, Pruitt Jr BA, Mason Jr AD. The influence of inhalation injury and pneumonia on burn mortality. *Ann Surg* 1987; **205:** 82–7.
13. Herndon DN, Barrow RE, Rutan RL, *et al.* A comparison of conservative versus early excision. Therapies in severely burned patients. *Ann Surg* 1989; **209:** 547–52; discussion 552–3.
14. Peck MD, Heimbach DM. Does early excision of burn wounds change the pattern of mortality? *J Burn Care Rehabil* 1989; **10:** 7–10.
15. Davies JWL. *Physiological Responses to Burning Injury*, 1st edn. London: Academic Press, 1982.
16. Sørensen B, Sejrsen P. Saline solutions in the treatment of burn shock. *Acta Chir Scand* 1965; **129:** 239–42.
17. Sparkes BG, Gyorkos JW, Gorczynski RM, Brock AJ. Comparison of endotoxins and cutaneous burn toxin as immunosuppressants. *Burns* 1990; **16:** 123–7.
18. Sparkes BG. Mechanisms of immune failure in burn injury. *Vaccine* 1993; **11:** 504–10.
19. Deb S, Martin B, Sun L, Ruff P, *et al.* Resuscitation with lactated Ringer's solution in rats with hemorrhagic shock induces immediate apoptosis. *J Trauma* 1999; **46:** 582–8; discussion 588–9.
20. Lentz CW, Peterson HD. Smoke inhalation is a multilevel insult to the pulmonary system. *Curr Opin Pulm Med* 1997; **3:** 221–6.
21. Lalonde C, Demling R, Brain J, Blanchard J. Smoke inhalation injury in sheep is caused by the particle phase, not the gas phase. *J Appl Physiol* 1994; **77:** 15–22.
22. Herndon DN, Barrow RE, Linares HA, *et al.* Inhalation injury in burned patients: effects and treatment. *Burns Incl Therm Inj* 1988; **14:** 349–56.
23. Desai MH, Rutan RL, Herndon DN. Managing smoke inhalation injuries. *Postgrad Med* 1989; **86:** 69–70, 73–6.
24. Demling RH. Smoke inhalation injury. *New Horiz* 1993; **1:** 422–34.
25. Ruddy RM. Smoke inhalation injury. *Pediatr Clin North Am* 1994; **41:** 317–36.
26. Fitzpatrick JC, Cioffi Jr WG. Ventilatory support following burns and smoke-inhalation injury. *Respir Care Clin North Am* 1997; **3:** 21–49.
27. Lee-Chiong Jr TL. Smoke inhalation injury. *Postgrad Med* 1999; **105:** 55–62.
28. Burns TR, Greenberg SD, Cartwright J, Jachimczyk JA. Smoke inhalation: an ultrastructural study of reaction to injury in the human alveolar wall. *Environ Res* 1986; **41:** 447–57.
29. Demling R, LaLonde C, Ikegami K. Fluid resuscitation with deferoxamine hetastarch complex attenuates the lung and systemic response to smoke inhalation. *Surgery* 1996; **119:** 340–8.
30. Demling R, Lalonde C, Youn YK, Picard L. Effect of graded increases in smoke inhalation injury on the early systemic response to a body burn. *Crit Care Med* 1995; **23:** 171–8.
31. Fogarty PW, George PJ, Solomon M, Spiro SG, Armstrong RF. Long term effects of smoke inhalation in survivors of the King's Cross underground station fire. *Thorax* 1991; **46:** 914–18.
32. Desai MH, Mlcak RP, Robinson E, *et al.* Does inhalation injury limit exercise endurance in children convalescing from thermal injury? *J Burn Care Rehabil* 1993; **14:** 12–16.
33. Mlcak R, Cortiella J, Desai M, Herndon D. Lung compliance, airway resistance, and work of breathing in children after inhalation injury. *J Burn Care Rehabil* 1997; **18:** 531–4.
34. Swenson JR, Dimsdale JE, Rockwell E, *et al.* Drug and alcohol abuse in patients with acute burn injuries. *Psychosomatics* 1991; **3:** 287–93.
35. Zak AL, Harrington DT, Barillo DJ, *et al.* Acute respiratory failure that complicates the resuscitation of pediatric patients with scald injuries. *J Burn Care Rehabil* 1999; **20:** 391–9.
36. Achauer BM, Mueller G, Vanderkam VM. Prevention of accidental extubation in burn patients. *Ann Plast Surg* 1997; **38:** 280–2.
37. Chay S, Board PN, Lawler PG. A safe, simple and effective technique for securing nasojejunal tubes in the intensive care unit [letter]. *Anaesthesia* 1999; **54:** 715–16.
38. Kemper KJ, Benson MS, Bishop MJ. Predictors of postextubation stridor in pediatric trauma patients. *Crit Care Med* 1991; **1**): 352–5.
39. Freeman JA, Fredricks BJ, Best CJ. Evaluation of a new method for determining tracheal tube length in children. *Anaesthesia* 1995; **50:** 1050–2.
40. Davies LK, Poulton TJ, Modell JH. Continuous positive airway pressure is beneficial in treatment of smoke inhalation. *Crit Care Med* 1983; **11:** 726–9.
41. Cox Jr CS, Zwischenberger JB, Traber DL, *et al.* Immediate positive pressure ventilation with positive end-expiratory pressure (PEEP) improves survival in ovine smoke inhalation injury. *J Trauma* 1992; **33:** 821–7.
42. Baud FJ, Barriot P, Toffis V, *et al.* Elevated blood cyanide concentrations in victims of smoke inhalation. *N Engl J Med* 1991; **325:** 1761–6.
43. Shirani KZ, Vaughan GM, Mason Jr AD, Pruitt Jr BA. Update on current therapeutic approaches in burns. *Shock* 1996; **5:** 4–16.
44. Horton JW, Baxter CR, White DJ. Differences in cardiac responses to resuscitation from burn shock. *Surg Gynecol Obstet* 1989; **168:** 201–13.
45. Giroir BP, Horton JW, White DJ, *et al.* Inhibition of tumor necrosis factor prevents myocardial dysfunction during burn shock. *Am J Physiol* 1994; **267:** H118–24.
46. Barton RG, Saffle JR, Morris SE, *et al.* Resuscitation of thermally injured patients with oxygen transport criteria as goals of therapy. *J Burn Care Rehabil* 1997; **18:** 1–9.
47. Goldstein B, Doody D, Briggs S. Emergency intraosseous infusion in severely burned children. *Pediatr Emerg Care* 1990; **6:**195.
48. Clark Jr WR, Nieman GF, Goyette D, Gryzboski D. Effects of crystalloid on lung fluid balance after smoke inhalation. *Ann Surg* 1988; **208:** 56–64.
49. Crum RL, Dominic W, Hansbrough JF, *et al.* Cardiovascular and neurohumoral responses following burn injury. *Arch Surg* 1990; **125:** 1065–9.
50. Traber DL, Pollard V. Pathophysiology of inhalation injury. In: Herndon DN (ed.). *Total Burn Care*, 2nd edn. London: WB Saunders Company, 2002: 175–83.
51. Murison MS, Laitung JK, Pigott RW. Effectiveness of burns resuscitation using two different formulae. *Burns* 1991; **17:** 484–9.
52. Du GB, Slater H, Goldfarb IW. Influences of different resuscitation regimens on acute early weight gain in extensively burned patients. *Burns* 1991; **17:** 147–50.
53. Gunn ML, Hansbrough JF, Davis JW, *et al.* Prospective, randomized trial of hypertonic sodium lactate versus lactated Ringer's solution for burn shock resuscitation. *J Trauma* 1989; **29:** 1261–7.
54. Huang PP, Stucky FS, Dimick AR, *et al.* Hypertonic sodium resuscitation is associated with renal failure and death. *Ann Surg* 1995; **221:** 543–54; discussion 554–7.
55. Aikawa N, Wakabayashi G, Ueda M, Shinozawa Y. Regulation of renal function in thermal injury. *J Trauma* 1990; **30:** S174–8.
56. Dougherty W, Waxman K. The complexities of managing severe burns with associated trauma. *Surg Clin North Am* 1996; **76:** 923–58.
57. Grobmyer SR, Maniscalco SP, Purdue GF, Hunt JL. Alcohol, drug intoxication, or both at the time of burn injury as a predictor of complications and mortality in hospitalized patients with burns. *J Burn Care Rehabil* 1996; **17:** 532–9.
58. Nguyen TT, Gilpin DA, Meyer NA, Herndon DN. Current treatment of severely burned patients. *Ann Surg* 1996; **223:** 14–25.
59. Kee SS, Ramage CM, Mendel P, Bristow AS. Interhospital transfers by helicopter: the first 50 patients of the Careflight project. *J Roy Soc Med* 1992; **85:** 29–31.
60. Bristow AS, Toff NJ. Medical helicopter systems – recommended minimum standards for patient management. *J Roy Soc Med* 1991; **84:** 242–4.
61. Wallace PGM, Ridley SA. ABC of Intensive care: transport of critically ill patients. *Br Med M* 1999; 319(368–71).
62. Dries DJ, Waxman K. Adequate resuscitation of burn patients may not be measured by urine output and vital signs. *Crit Care Med* 1991; **19:** 327–9.
63. Reynolds EM, Ryan DP, Sheridan RL, Doody DP. Left ventricular failure complicating severe pediatric burn injuries. *J Pediatr Surg* 1995; **30:** 264–9; discussion 269–70.
64. Schierhout G, Roberts I. Fluid resuscitation with colloid or crystalloid solutions in critically ill patients: a systematic review of randomised trials. *Br Med J* 1998; **316:** 961–4.
65. Anon. Human albumin administration in critically ill patients: systematic review of randomised controlled trials. Cochrane Injuries Group Albumin Reviewers. *Br Med J* 1998; **317:** 235–40.
66. Goodwin CW, Dorethy J, Lam V, Pruitt BA. Randomized trial of the efficacy of crystalloid and colloid resuscitation on hemodynamic response and lung water following thermal injury. *Ann Surg* 1983; **197:** 520–29; discussion 529–31.
67. Herndon DN, Traber DL, Traber LD. The effect of resuscitation on inhalation injury. *Surgery* 1986; **100:** 248–51.
68. Lalonde C, Picard L, Youn YK, Demling RH. Increased early postburn

fluid requirements and oxygen demands are predictive of the degree of airways injury by smoke inhalation. *J Trauma* 1995; **38:** 175–84.

69. Brannen AL, Still J, Haynes M, *et al.* A randomized prospective trial of hyperbaric oxygen in a referral burn center population. *Am Surg* 1997; **63:** 205–8.
70. Hall AH, Kulig KW, Rumack BH. Suspected cyanide poisoning in smoke inhalation: complications of sodium nitrite therapy. *J Toxicol Clin Exp* 1989; **9:** 3–9.
71. Fitzpatrick JC, Cioffi Jr WG. Diagnosis and treatment of inhalation injury. In: Herndon DN (ed.). *Total Burn Care*, 1st edn. London: WB Saunders Company, 1996: 184–92.
72. Suter PM, Domenighetti G, Schaller MD, *et al.* N-acetylcysteine enhances recovery from acute lung injury in man. A randomized, double-blind, placebo-controlled clinical study. *Chest* 1994; **105:** 190–4.
73. Cioffi Jr WG, Rue LWD, Graves TA, *et al.* Prophylactic use of high-frequency percussive ventilation in patients with inhalation injury. *Ann Surg* 1991; **213:** 575–80; discussion 580–2.
74. Mackie DP, van Hertum WA, Schumburg TH, *et al.* Reduction in *Staphylococcus aureus* wound colonization using nasal mupirocin and selective decontamination of the digestive tract in extensive burns. *Burns* 1994; **20:** S17–18.
75. Brown M, Desai M, Traber LD, *et al.* Dimethylsulfoxide with heparin in the treatment of smoke inhalation injury. *J Burn Care Rehabil* 1988; **9:** 22–5.
76. Cox Jr CS, Zwischenberger JB, Traber DL, *et al.* Heparin improves oxygenation and minimizes barotrauma after severe smoke inhalation in an ovine model. *Surg Gynecol Obstet* 1993; **176:** 339–49.
77. Mackie DP, van Hertum WA, Schumburg T, *et al.* Prevention of infection in burns: preliminary experience with selective decontamination of the digestive tract in patients with extensive injuries. *J Trauma* 1992; **32:** 570–5.
78. Davis TC, Griffin NK. The consequences of toxic shock syndrome in an 18-month-old boy with 20% scalds. *J Roy Soc Med* 1996; **89(2):** 115–116.
79. Judkins K. Toxic shock syndrome and burns [letter; comment]. *J R Soc Med 1996*; **89:** 538–9.
80. Wallace BH, Caldwell Jr FT, Cone JB. The interrelationships between wound management, thermal stress, energy metabolism, and temperature profiles of patients with burns. *J Burn Care Rehabil* 1994; **15:** 499–508.
81. Khorram-Sefat R, Behrendt W, Heiden A, Hettich R. Long-term measurements of energy expenditure in severe burn injury. *World J Surg* 1999; **23:** 115–22.
82. Huang YS, Li A, Yang ZC. A prospective clinical study on the pathogenesis of multiple organ failure in severely burned patients. *Burns* 1992; **18:** 30–4.
83. McDonald WS, Sharp Jr CW, Deitch EA. Immediate enteral feeding in burn patients is safe and effective. *Ann Surg* 1991; **213:** 177–83.
84. Alexander JW, Gottschlich MM. Nutritional immunomodulation in burn patients. Crit Care Med 1990; **18** (Suppl. 2): S149–53.
85. Gianotti L, Nelson JL, Alexander JW, *et al.* Post injury hypermetabolic response and magnitude of translocation: prevention by early enteral nutrition. *Nutrition* 1994; **10:** 225–31.
86. Baron P, Traber LD, Traber DL, *et al.* Gut failure and translocation following burn and sepsis. *J Surg Res* 1994; **57:** 197–204.
87. Chiarelli A, Enzi G, Casadei A, *et al.* Very early nutrition supplementation in burned patients. *Am J Clin Nutr* 1990; **51:** 1035–9.
88. Herndon DN, Barrow RE, Stein M, *et al.* Increased mortality with intravenous supplemental feeding in severely burned patients. *J Burn Care Rehabil* 1989; **10:** 309–13.
89. Hiyama DT, von Allmen D, Rosenblum L, *et al.* Synthesis of albumin and acute-phase proteins in perfused liver after burn injury in rats. *J Burn Care Rehabil* 1991; **12:** 1–6.
90. Greenhalgh DG, Housinger TA, Kagan RJ, *et al.* Maintenance of serum albumin levels in pediatric burn patients: a prospective, randomized trial. *J Trauma* 1995; **39:** 67–73; discussion 73–4.
91. Kay S, Samba Siva Rao G, Lord D. Intracranial pressure monitoring in the burnt and asphyxiated child. *Burns* 1986; **12:** 212–13.
92. Lawrence C, Atac B. Hematologic changes in massive burn injury. *Crit Care Med* 1992; **20:** 1284–8.
93. Bush GH. The use of muscle relaxants in burnt children. *Anaesthesia* 1964; **19:** 231–8.
94. Martyn JA, White DA, Gronert GA, *et al.* Up-and-down regulation of skeletal muscle acetylcholine receptors. Effects on neuromuscular blockers [see comments]. *Anesthesiology* 1992; **76:** 822–43.
95. Brown TC, Bell B. Electromyographic responses to small doses of suxamethonium in children after burns. *Br J Anaesth* 1987; **59:** 1017–21.
96. Mills AK, Martyn JA. Evaluation of atracurium neuromuscular blockade in paediatric patients with burn injury. *Br J Anaesth* 1988; **60:** 450–5.
97. Marathe PH, Dwersteg JF, Pavlin EG, *et al.* Effect of thermal injury on the pharmacokinetics and pharmacodynamics of atracurium in humans. *Anesthesiology* 1989; **70:** 752–5.
98. Mills AK, Martyn JA. Neuromuscular blockade with vecuronium in paediatric patients with burn injury. *Br J Clin Pharmacol* 1989; **28:** 155–9.
99. Motsch J, Leuwer M, Bottiger BW, *et al.* Dose-response, time-course of action and recovery of rocuronium bromide in children during halothane anaesthesia. *Eur J Anaesthesiol* (Suppl) 1995; **11:** 73–8.
100. Meretoja OA, Taivainen T, Erkola O, *et al.* Dose-response and time-course of effect of rocuronium bromide in paediatric patients. *Eur J Anaesthesiol* (Suppl) 1995; **11:** 19–22.
101. Tobias JD. Continuous infusion of rocuronium in a paediatric intensive care unit. *Can J Anaesth* 1996; **43**: 353–7.
102. Zokufa HZ, Solem LD, Rodvold KA, *et al.* The influence of serum albumin and alpha 1-acid glycoprotein on vancomycin protein binding in patients with burn injuries. *J Burn Care Rehabil* 1989; **10:** 425–8.
103. Macfie AG, Magides AD, Reilly CS. Disposition of alfentanil in burns patients. *Br J Anaesth* 1992; **69:** 447–50.
104. Furman WR, Munster AM, Cone EJ. Morphine pharmacokinetics during anesthesia and surgery in patients with burns. *J Burn Care Rehabil* 1990; **11:** 391–4.
105. Martyn JA, Bishop AL, Oliveri MF. Pharmacokinetics and pharmacodynamics of ranitidine after burn injury. *Clin Pharmacol Ther* 1992; **51:** 408–14.
106. Caldwell Jr FT, Wallace BH, Cone JB. Sequential excision and grafting of the burn injuries of 1507 patients treated between 1967 and 1986: end results and the determinants of death. *J Burn Care Rehabil* 1996; **17:** 137–46.
107. Coté CJ. Preoperative preparation and premedication. *Br J Anaesth* 1999; **83:** 16–28.
108. Benians RC. The influence of parental visiting on survival and recovery of extensively burned children. *Burns Incl Therm Injury* 1988; **14:** 31–4.
109. Phillips S, Daborn AK, Hatch DJ. Preoperative fasting for paediatric anaesthesia. *Br J Anaesth* 1994; **73:** 529–36.
110. Pearson KS, From RP, Symreng T, Kealey GP. Continuous enteral feeding and short fasting periods enhance perioperative nutrition in patients with burns. *J Burn Care Rehabil* 1992; **13:** 477–81.
111. Hatch DJ. New inhalation agents in paediatric anaesthesia. *Br J Anaesth* 1999; **83:** 42–9.
112. Aun CST. New intravenous agents. *Br J Anaesth* 1999; **83(1):** 29–41.
113. Coté CJ, Petkau AJ. Thiopental requirements may be increased in children reanesthetized at least one year after recovery from extensive thermal injury. *Anesth Analg* 1985; **64:** 1156–60.
114. Murat I, Billard V, Vernois J, *et al.* Pharmacokinetics of propofol after a single dose in children aged 1–3 years with minor burns. Comparison of three data analysis approaches. *Anesthesiology* 1996; **84:** 526–32.
115. Mills DC, Lord WD. Propofol for repeated burns dressings in a child. *Burns* 1992; **18:** 58–9.
116. Frei FJ, Ummenhofer W. Difficult intubation in paediatrics. *Paediatr Anaesth* 1996; **6:** 251–63.
117. Haynes SR, Morton NS. The laryngeal mask airway: a review of its use in paediatric anaesthesia. *Paediatr Anaesth* 1993; **3:** 65.
118. Russell R, Judkins KC. The laryngeal mask airway and facial burns [letter]. *Anaesthesia* 1990; **45:** 894.
119. Frei FJ, Wengen DF, Rutishauser M, Ummenhofer W. The airway endoscopy mask: useful device for fibreoptic evaluation and intubation of the paediatric airway. *Paediatr Anaesth* 1995; **5:** 319–24.
120. Karl HW, Swedlow DB, Lee KW, Downes JJ. Epinephrine-halothane interactions in children. *Anesthesiology* 1983; **58:** 142–5.
121. Achauer BM, Hernandez J, Parker A. Burn excision with intraoperative vasopressin. *J Burn Care Rehabil* 1989; **10:** 375–8.
122. Mann R, Heimbach DM, Engrav LH, Foy H. Changes in transfusion practices in burn patients. *J Trauma* 1994; **37:** 220–2.
123. Sittig KM, Deitch EA. Blood transfusions: for the thermally injured or for the doctor? *J Trauma* 1994; **36:** 369–72.
124. Housinger TA, Lang D, Warden GD. A prospective study of blood loss with excisional therapy in pediatric burn patients. *J Trauma* 1993; **34:** 262–3.
125. Brown RA, Grobbelaar AO, Barker S, Rode H. A formula to calculate blood cross-match requirements for early burn surgery in children. *Burns* 1995; **21:** 371–3.
126. Cote CJ, Daniels AL, Connolly M, *et al.* Tongue oximetry in children with extensive thermal injury: comparison with peripheral oximetry. *Can J Anaesth* 1992; **39:** 454–7.

127. Eger EI. New inhalational agents desflurane and sevoflurane. *Can Anaesth* 1993; **40:** 3–5.
128. Piat V, Dubois MC, Johanet S, Murat I. Induction and recovery characteristics and hemodynamic responses to sevoflurane and halothane in children. *Anesth Analg* 1994; **79:** 840–4.
129. Gregoretti S, Gelman S, Dimick A, Bradley Jr EL. Hemodynamic changes and oxygen consumption in burned patients during enflurane or isoflurane anesthesia. *Anesth Analg* 1989; **69:** 431–6.
130. Wolf WJ, Neal MB, Peterson MD. The hemodynamic and cardiovascular effects of isoflurane and halothane anesthesia in children. *Anesthesiology* 1986; **64:** 328–33.
131. Davis PJ, Lerman J, Suresh S, *et al.* A randomized multicenter study of remifentanil compared with alfentanil, isoflurane, or propofol in anesthetized pediatric patients undergoing elective strabismus surgery. *Anesth Analg* 1997; **84:** 982–9.
132. Demling RH, Lalonde C. Oxygen consumption is increased in the post-anesthesia period after burn excision. *J Burn Care Rehabil* 1989; **10:** 381–7.
133. Osgood PF, Szyfelbein SK. Management of burn pain in children. *Ped Clin North Am* 1989; **36:** 1001–13.
134. Judkins K. Pain management in the burned patient. *Pain Rev* 1998; **5:** 133–46.
135. Gaukroger PB, Chapman MJ, Davey RB. Pain control in paediatric burns – the use of patient-controlled analgesia. *Burns* 1991; **17:** 396–9.
136. Morton NS. Prevention and control of pain in children. *Br J Anaesth* 1999; **83:** 118–29.
137. Childs C, Little RA. Paracetamol (acetaminophen) in the management of burned children with fever. *Burns* 1989; **14:** 343–8.
138. Cederholm I, Bengtsson M, Bjorkman S, *et al.* Long term high dose morphine, ketamine and midazolam infusion in a child with burns. *Br J Clin Pharmacol* 1990; **30:** 901–5.
139. Prien T, Traber DL. Toxic smoke compounds and inhalation injury: a review. *Burns Incl Therm Inj* 1988; **14:** 451–60.
140. Kreulen M, Mackie DP, Kreis RW, Groenevelt F. Surgical release for intubation purposes in postburn contractures of the neck. *Burns* 1996; **22:** 310–12.

FURTHER READING

Herndon DN (ed.). *Total Burn Care,* 2nd edn. Philadelphia, PA: WB Saunders Co., 2002.

Settle JAD (ed.). *Principles and Practice of Burn Management.* London: Churchill Livingstone, 1996.

69

Head injury

TOBIAS CLAUSEN AND ROSS BULLOCK

INTRODUCTION

The brain is the organ on whose integrity the life and, perhaps more importantly, the unique personality of every individual is dependent. A variety of traumatic events ranging from car accidents to falls may endanger integrity and function of the brain temporarily or permanently in a fraction of a second and therefore alter drastically the course of life for the affected individual.

We cannot influence the initial damage after it has happened but we can try (and it is our responsibility) to treat conditions that promote further damage and might thus be able to help to preserve or restore the personality of an individual. This chapter outlines the role of the anesthesiologist in this complex process. Although we try to base all information, explanations, and recommendations in this chapter on established current medical knowledge, we intend to offer ideas rather than to present dogmas. Medical knowledge, especially in the area of brain trauma research, is in constant change; today's truth may be obsolete tomorrow. Therefore, we would like to encourage the reader to view the topic from different perspectives, to think of it as a "building under continuous construction" and to apply his/her own ideas.

Although the term "head injury" is widely used among clinicians and medical researchers, there seems to be no agreed definition. Generally, head injury is considered to be the result of a mechanical force acting on the head, which may potentially cause functional or structural damage to the brain. A head injury with an intact dura mater is called *closed head injury*, whereas an *open head injury* denotes direct or indirect connection between the brain and the extracorporeal environment.

The anesthesiologist is frequently the first physician to see the head-injured patient as he or she is often part of the ambulance team (at least in many European countries). He/she is often responsible for the handling of the patient in the emergency room, and is required to take care of the anesthesia in the operating room. Furthermore, the anesthesiologist is often responsible for the management of the patient in the intensive care unit (ICU). Hence, the importance of an extensive knowledge of the pathophysiology and treatment of severe head injury for anesthesiologists cannot be understated. This is underlined by the fact that the improvement in the outcome of severely head-injured patients over the last two decades has resulted especially from improvements in early resuscitation, as well as improved intensive care, both of which require active participation on the part of the anesthesiologist.

PATHOPHYSIOLOGY OF SEVERE HEAD INJURY

The term head injury does not describe a single entity. In reality, we have to deal with a multitude of clinical pictures caused by different pathologic events. The pathogenic mechanisms involved are numerous and often poorly understood. No two "head injuries" are the same. This chapter is designed to characterize the common pathophysiologic mechanisms as well as their pathologic correlates.

Although this section focuses on damage to the brain, we have to take into account that other parts of the head may also sustain damage, requiring the special attention of the anesthesiologist. Epipharyngeal bleeding and damage may lead to severe pulmonary aspiration, especially in unconscious patients. Possible injuries of the cervical spinal column put the patient at high risk of a spinal cord injury and constitute a major risk of endotracheal intubation. It is important to keep in mind that the brain can be severely damaged without any skull fractures or visible superficial wounds.[1]

There are several classifications of head injuries. Two of these are of major clinical importance. The first focuses upon the severity of the head injury, according to the Glasgow coma scale (GCS), with significant implications for treatment (see Preclinical management). The other distinguishes between primary and secondary injury according to the time-course of events.

Primary and secondary injury

Primary brain damage is defined as the damage to neurons (especially axonal damage), astrocytes, and cerebral blood vessels resulting from brief applications of shearing forces, with consequent tissue deformation, at the time of injury.

Secondary brain damage may be defined as delayed damage to cerebral tissue as a result of harmful ionic shifts, hypoxia, ischemia, cerebral edema, elevated intracranial pressure (ICP), infection, seizures, and other less clearly understood mechanisms.

Both primary and secondary brain damage can be either diffuse or focal depending on its spatial pattern.

Primary brain damage is believed to be irreversible and, therefore, not amenable to therapy. Prevention strategies, for vehicles, driver safety, and the environment, are thus very important. Secondary brain damage, however, develops after the primary event and follows events such as hypotension or intracranial hypertension. These result in cerebral ischemia, and, following respiratory dysfunction, in hypoxemia, or by other less fully understood mechanisms involving biochemical cascades. Treatment is designed mainly for the prevention of events triggering secondary brain damage, or "blockade" of cellular pathways that can lead to delayed neuronal death (e.g. apotosis).

Biomechanical aspects of head injury

Head injury is caused by mechanical forces acting on the head. In effect, two situations are possible: either the head injury results from the impact of a moving object on the stationary head (e.g. a club) or the moving head strikes a stationary object (e.g. the ground or a car windshield). From a physical point of view, it is less important whether the head or the "object" is moving. More essential are the relative velocities of these two and the force and duration of the impact. In either case, an acceleration or deceleration of the brain will be the consequence. This results in brief, transient shearing forces on the intracranial tissue (neuronal, glial, vascular, connecting tissue), potentially causing axonal injury, or diffuse or focal bleeding. Axonal damage may be independent of vascular damage and is typically associated with axonal swelling ("retraction balls"), a sign of disturbed axonal transport due to a collapse of the intracytoplasmic microtubular system.[2] The recognition that axonal injury develops sequentially, over hours and days, and not immediately,[3] is of considerable clinical importance, as it suggests that therapeutic intervention may in some cases alleviate the extent of damage (Fig. 69.1).

As shearing forces are directly caused by acceleration or deceleration, damage to intracranial tissue is possible even without any impact.[4] This is seen especially following high-speed aircraft crashes. An impact of an object on the head (or vice versa), however, may additionally produce local deformation of the skull, with the possibility of bone fracture and the potential for local brain tissue damage by bone fragments or rupture of adjacent blood vessels. Furthermore, the skull can be transiently deformed at the site of impact without fracture and return subsequently to its normal shape by elastic recoil. Considerable damage to the underlying cerebral tissue may result.[5,6] This mechanism strips the dura from the overlying skull, to cause epidural hematomas. Skull fractures do not necessarily occur at the location of impact. Basal skull fractures can often be detected in patients when the actual blow occurred somewhere over the calvarium. These patients often suffer hemorrhage from one of the external auditory canals.

Significant brain surface damage may occur on the side opposite to the impact. This kind of injury has been defined as "contrecoup". Several mechanisms have been suggested to explain the development of such contrecoup injuries. Courville postulated that short-duration negative pressures, attributable to cavitation effects resulting from relative brain motion within the skull, cause this phenomenon,[7] whereas Shatsky and coworkers proposed that the irregular bone anatomy of the anterior fossa, as well as the relative movements of the brain against these structures, might play a role in the etiology of contrecoup injuries.[6]

Importantly, the site of the impact has considerable influence on the outcome of head-injured patients. Patients affected by a frontal impact often suffer significantly less brain damage than patients involved in lateral collisions of similar force.[8]

Main pathologic manifestations

Impact of the head injury on cellular function

Although current knowledge of events at the cellular level is still rather limited, encouraging progress has been made during recent years. At the moment of injury, shearing forces of different magnitude and duration act on the intracranial tissues, that is, among others, neuronal and glial cells, and blood vessels. Neurons (as well as astrocytes) are highly specialized cells. Their cell membrane surface is not only large, because of the multitude of dendritic processes, but it also contains a large number of transmembrane proteins – most of these form ion channels (voltage gated and agonist gated). The functionality of these ion channels – as of virtually all functional proteins – depends vitally on their three-dimensional conformation.

Recent studies suggest strongly that transient mechanical deformation of at least some ion channel types might cause a leakage of Na^+ and Ca^{2+} ions into the cell and K^+ ions out of the cell.[9–11] This process can last for several hours[11] and may have various consequences.

The loss of resting membrane potential and the subsequent depolarization following Na^+ influx can cause the massive release of excitatory neurotransmitters immediately after injury. (Other possible explanations for the neurotransmitter increase include leakage from

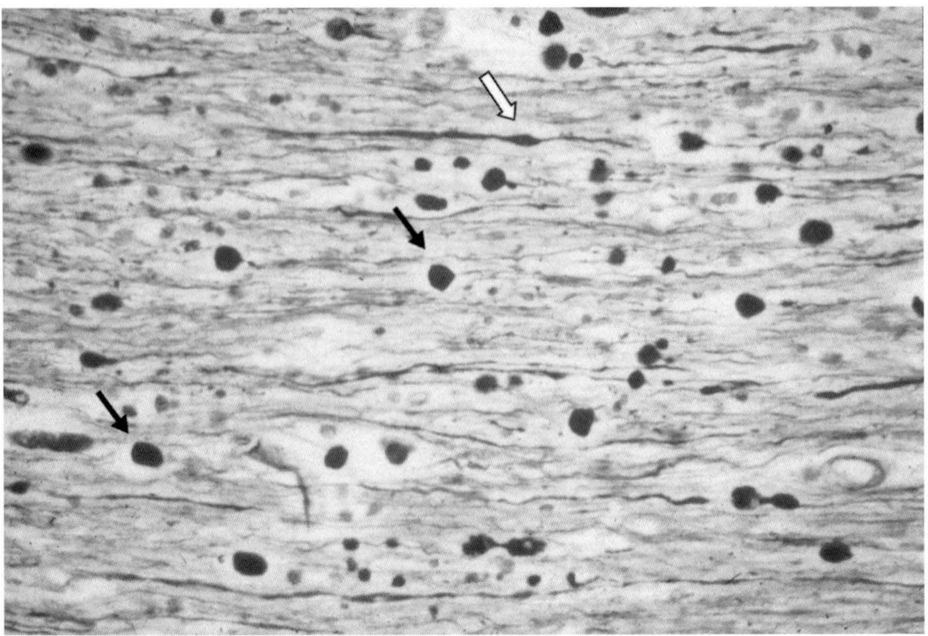

Figure 69.1 *Diffuse axonal injury (Marchi silver staining). Note the number of "retraction balls" (black arrows). The hollow arrow indicates the early formation of axonal swelling.*

damaged cells or diffusion from other sites of injury.[12,13]) The excitatory neurotransmitters so released, especially glutamate and aspartate, in turn may cause depolarization of adjacent neurons, resulting in further Na^+ and Ca^{2+} entry into the cell and K^+ efflux into the extracellular fluid.

Additional intracellular Ca^{2+} may be released from the endoplasmic reticulum, due to partial damage to the cytoskeleton by the shearing forces. The rapid increase in cytosolic Ca^{2+} concentration is also capable of interfering with mitochondrial function, thus disturbing oxidative metabolism and leading to energy failure. An alternative way to produce ATP is by anaerobic glycolysis. Unfortunately, this pathway is far less effective than its aerobic counterpart and results in a massive accumulation of lactate and a consecutive decrease in brain pH. If the neuron is unable to produce enough ATP to maintain basal metabolism, cell death results.

Furthermore, extremely high intracellular Ca^{2+} concentrations may alter the activity of several enzymes. This is particularly harmful if free radical quenchers, such as superoxide dismutase, are inactivated, causing cellular damage by free radicals. Free radicals are highly reactive molecules, owing to an unpaired electron on the outer shell. These oxidants are normal byproducts of oxidative metabolism, and fulfill various physiologic functions. However, in high concentrations these reactive species may react with almost all cellular structures, e.g. membrane proteins, enzymes, ribosomal proteins or RNA, nuclear DNA, and therefore cause considerable cellular dysfunction. To protect the cell from these potentially deleterious effects, highly reactive species are usually compartmented in small vesicles, such as peroxisomes, or confined in mitochondria. Additionally, intracellular enzyme systems, e.g. superoxide dismutase and xanthine oxidase, are capable of degrading free radicals, to keep their cytosolic levels under control. Trauma can disrupt peroxisomes and increase their generation, especially during postischemic reperfusion. Raised intracellular calcium concentrations inactivate protective enzyme systems at least in part. An increase in intracellular calcium also activates pathways, leading to delayed neuronal cell death, or "apoptosis" after head trauma.

The considerable ion shift between intra- and extracellular spaces causes an imbalance in ionic homeostasis. In order to restore ionic homeostasis, astrocytes take up K^+ ions along with water to preserve osmolality. The potassium buffering by the astrocytes therefore serves as a compensation mechanism but may result in rapid astrocyte swelling, the major cause of cytotoxic edema, and raised ICP (see below). As a consequence of the swelling of astrocytes, the lumina of cerebral capillaries may be compressed, especially by the astrocyte end feet processes and, therefore, substrate supply and disposal of waste products in the affected brain area might be additionally compromised.

Astrocytes not only serve as a buffer for potassium, they also take up neurotransmitters' extracellular space.[14] Both processes, as well as re-establishment of neuronal resting membrane potential by ATP-dependent membrane Na^+/K^+ exchangers, are extremely energy consuming. At the same time, the substrate supply, especially for oxygen and glucose, may be impaired because of a disturbed microcirculation. The subsequent increase in anaerobic glycolysis further depletes extracellular glucose.

There is now evidence that astrocytes may actually "feed" neurons in situations of an increased energy demand as long as there is sufficient oxygen for the neurons to utilize lactate.[14] Recently, several researchers have suggested that astrocytes metabolize glucose to lactate via anaerobic glycolysis, using the resulting ATP to maintain ion homeostasis, whereas the lactate produced seems to serve as the preferred oxidative energy substrate for the neurons during neuroexcitation caused by high extracellular glutamate levels.[14] Elevated extracellular brain lactate levels can be seen in patients after severe head injury, even in the presence of sufficient oxygen. Whether the extracellular acidosis caused by the increase in extracellular lactate concentration is deleterious remains to be established. However, likely impaired cellular functions might occur at lower pH levels (Fig. 69.2).[15,16]

Why exactly are these cellular processes important to the anesthesiologist? Previously, it was assumed that the main damage to the patient's cerebral tissues occurs at the time of impact and therefore is not amenable to therapy. In fact, between 30% and 40% of the patients who will

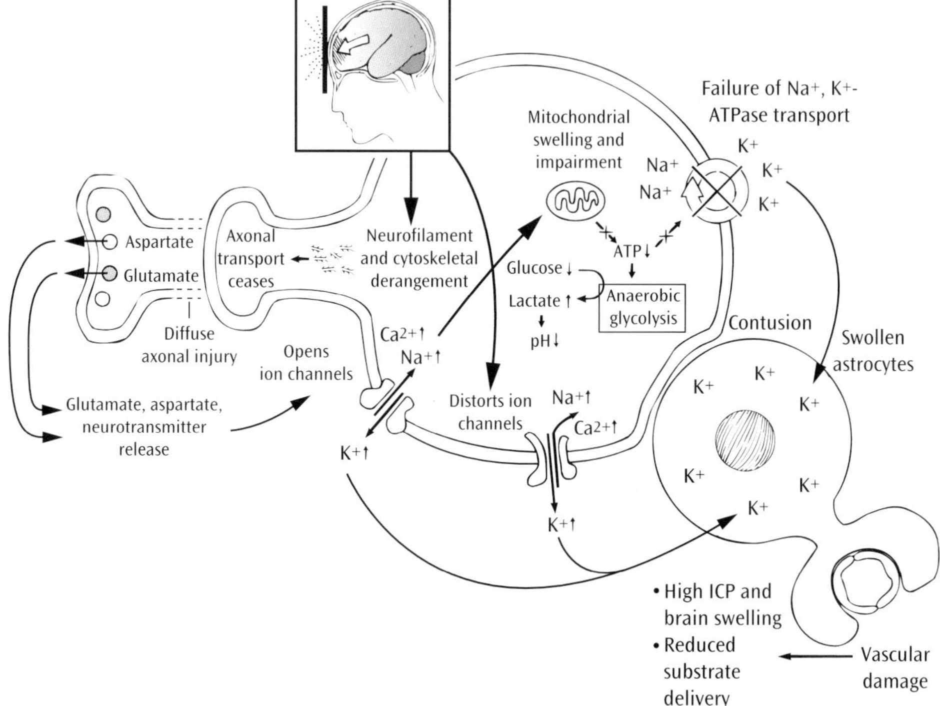

Figure 69.2 *Impact of traumatic brain injury (TBI) on cellular function.*

die after severe head injury experience a lucid interval following trauma. This observation suggests that the primary insult promotes a secondary brain damage that might be decreased with interventions.

In order to achieve this, it is essential to understand the underlying mechanisms of cellular pathologic physiology described above. Many aspects of this complex process, following severe head injury, are unknown to us. For instance, we do not really know what causes apoptosis, or which part of the cascades leading to secondary brain damage may be amenable to therapy, among many others. Even although we may not be able to completely prevent secondary brain damage, we may be able to reduce its incidence with better understanding of its origins.

Brain swelling

Post-traumatic enlargement of the brain mass may be caused either by brain edema or by vascular engorgement, but the former is probably far more important. Both processes are multifactorial and appear to contribute to the development of brain swelling during the time-course after injury (Fig. 69.3).

Brain edema

An increased extra- or intracellular water content is termed brain edema. Brain edema may be caused by different pathophysiologic mechanisms and is thus classified into different types. However, the various causes of edema are not usually found in isolation following head injury, but in combination depending on the nature of the head injury. For example, cerebral edema is especially marked as focal edema around contusions.

Cytotoxic edema

In cytotoxic edema, the intracellular water content is markedly increased. Energy depletion with consecutive failure of the Na^+,K^+-ATPase, as well as stimulation of the neurons due to massive glutamate release after head injury, as discussed above, are believed to be causal. These changes result in an influx of Na^+ and Ca^{2+} into neurons and an efflux of K^+ out of neurons into the extracellular fluid. In order to preserve ionic homeostasis, astrocytes take up K^+ ions from the extracellular fluid. To maintain osmolality, water is also shifted into the astrocytes, leading to astrocyte swelling.

Magnetic resonance imaging (MRI) and brain water measurement techniques demonstrate that transient cytotoxic edema is extremely common, probably universal, following severe head injury.[17]

Vasogenic edema

Severe head injury often causes brief, transient impairment of the blood–brain barrier function. Thus, water, ions, and high-molecular-weight substances (plasma proteins) flow into the extracellular space. This probably persists for an hour or so following diffuse injury, but is much more prolonged around a hematoma or a contusion, where it may persist for many days.[18] The accumulation of proteins increases the oncotic pressure in the extracellular space, potentially causing further water influx even after the blood–brain barrier has been repaired.

As the hydrostatic pressure gradient is a major driving force between the vessel and extracellular space (see hydrostatic edema), patients with disturbed blood–brain barrier function are at risk of developing or aggravating vasogenic edema during periods of excessive high blood pressure.[19]

Osmotic edema

A decreased blood osmotic pressure (as well as an increased osmotic pressure in the cerebral extracellular space) leads to an inflow of free water into the extracellular space, even through an intact blood–brain barrier. Iatrogenic reduction of the serum osmolality by excessive infusion of hypotonic or glucose water solutions is a leading cause in producing osmotic brain edema. Inadequate secretion of antidiuretic hormone (ADH) is another possible, but rare, cause.

Hydrostatic edema

Not only the gradient in the osmotic pressure, but also the gradient in the hydrostatic pressure, acts as a driving force for fluid shifts between the intravascular and the cerebral extracellular space. If either the hydrostatic pressure within the brain tissue is decreased, e.g. after decompressive surgery, or the intravascular hydrostatic pressure is increased, free water may diffuse into the brain tissue. The most important reasons for a significantly elevated hydrostatic pressure in the cerebral capillaries after severe head injury are impaired autoregulation mechanisms and surges of high blood pressure.

Interstitial edema

Disturbances in the drainage of cerebrospinal fluid (CSF) may result in a periventricular water accumulation. Although traumatic intraventricular hematomas may impair CSF drainage, interstitial edema is not frequently seen acutely after head injury, except when posterior fossa masses are present. Occlusion of CSF drainage may occur via the Pacchionian granulations days after head injury, due to subarachnoid

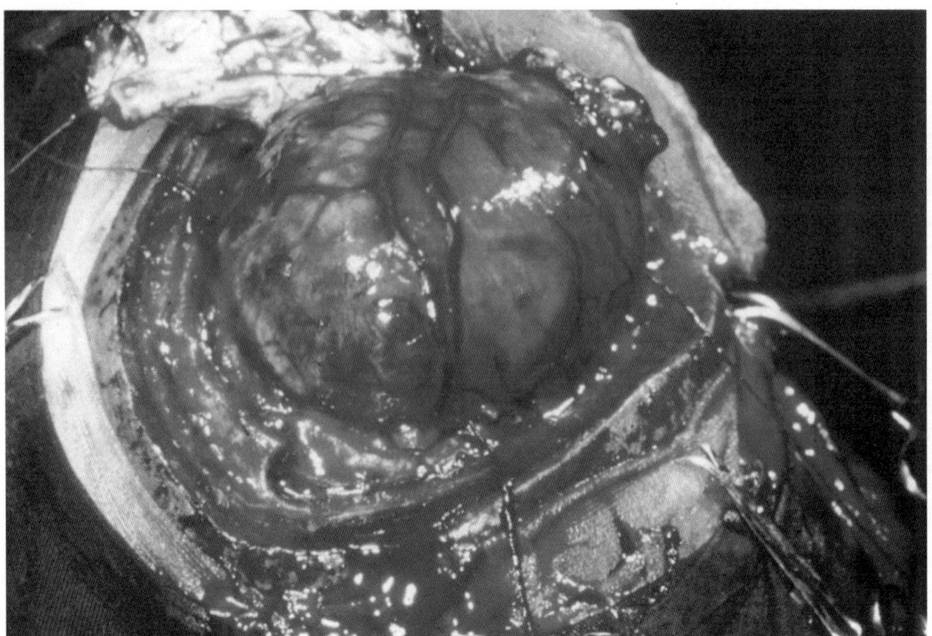

Figure 69.3 *Massive intraoperative brain swelling.*

hemorrhage. This may result in a "communicating" hydrocephalus and edema.

Although any of these edema types may occur in the head-injured patient, there is strong evidence that the major component of early brain edema is cytotoxic rather than vasogenic. However, the significance of vasogenic edema increases after the second day after injury, especially around contusions. Therefore, some treatment strategies for brain edema might be more advantageous than others at different times after head injury.

Vascular engorgement

Cerebrovascular dilation, probably due to vasomotor paralysis, or postischemic reperfusion, manifests chiefly as venous congestion and usually develops 24 h after the insult. During the first 24 h, ischemia is common and is believed to be an important factor in the pathophysiology of raised ICP,[20] superimposed upon prior cytotoxic swelling.

The pathophysiologic role of vasodilation in the development of raised ICP has misled intensivists into hyperventilation therapy. Although hyperventilation can increase ischemia, excessive (as opposed to moderate) hyperventilation is still, unfortunately, widely used to treat increased ICP.

Ischemic brain damage

Ischemic-type brain damage is seen in 85–90% of severely head-injured patients who die,[21] especially in those who have demonstrated a raised ICP and/or arrive at hospital hypotensive, hypoxic, or both.[22–24] There is a very high mortality in severely head-injured patients with both hypoxia and hypotension (Fig. 69.4).

Traumatic intracranial hematomas

Different types of hematomas can be found following head injury. Epidural hematomas (EDH) are due to rupture of meningeal arteries or venous sinuses between the skull bone and the dura mater, when the dura mater separates from the bone, as it deforms and at impact. As epidural hematomas may grow relatively slowly, patients may deteriorate gradually after a lucid interval. Small and moderate-sized epidural hematomas can increase their volume up to 150% within the first 2 weeks after injury, underlining the importance of diagnostic head CT scans in all patients following a head injury, and "concussion" of greater than a few minutes.

The rupture of subdural bridge veins, as well as large brain tissue contusions or lacerations, may lead to acute subdural hematoma. In rare cases, subdural hematomas follow the rupture of small superficial cortical arteries. Acute subdural hematoma and cerebral contusion with adjoining intracerebral hematoma is termed a "burst lobe phenomenon" and most frequently involves the frontal or the temporal lobes. Patients with "burst lobes" often deteriorate 72–96 h after injury because of massive swelling of the injured brain tissue. Mortality rates after acute subdural hematoma are reported to be between 30% and 90%. This poor outcome is associated with ischemic brain tissue damage beneath the subdural hematoma.[21] It has been postulated that this ischemic damage is mainly due to an increased ICP impairing the cerebral perfusion. Early removal of the acute subdural hematoma can dramatically reverse global ischemia and reduce the mortality. Furthermore, brain stem dysfunction after acute traumatic subdural hematoma is reversed by early surgical evacuation of the hematoma. However, mechanical compression of the underlying brain tissue alone does not fully explain the extent of ischemic tissue damage and the consecutive brain edema as hemispheric swelling may occur even beneath a thin subdural hematomas. Another possible mechanism contributing to the massive brain swelling beneath subdural hematomas may be an "excitotoxic" edema due to massive neurotransmitter release.

Even though subarachnoid hemorrhage is the most common form of post-traumatic hemorrhage, it is typically of minor clinical significance. However, this injury, when severe, may cause vasospasm and delayed ischemia. Cortical contusion may cause subarachnoid hemorrhages and may become an important factor in the pathogenesis of ischemia. Generally, subarachnoid hemorrhage increases the risk of cerebral vasospasm, which must be taken into consideration. These patients might benefit from nimodipine treatment.[25,26]

Bleeding within the cerebral tissue caused by head injury is termed intracerebral hemorrhage. This usually denotes lesions of 2 cm or larger in size rather than more diffuse vascular injury or contusions. The origin of traumatic intracerebral hematomas is most likely to result from rupture of smaller vessels within the brain tissue at the time of injury. Traumatic intracerebral hematomas can also develop later and, therefore, may not appear on the initial CT scan. These delayed traumatic

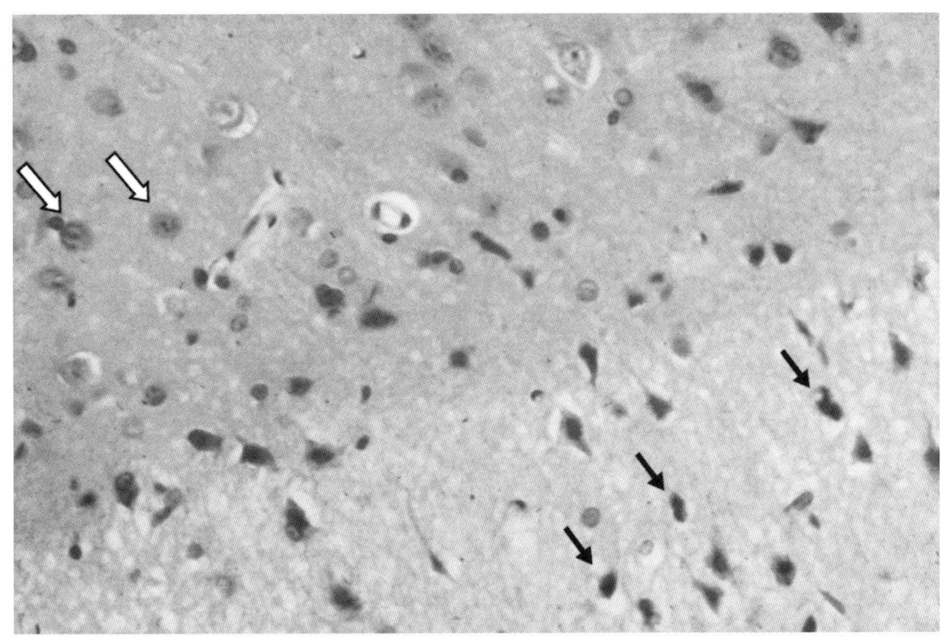

Figure 69.4 *Ischemic brain damage (hematoxylin and eosin staining). Note the dying/dead shrunken neurons (black arrows) in contrast with normal neurons (hollow arrows).*

intracerebral hematomas are especially common when a coagulopathy is present, such as warfarin therapy or disseminated intravascular coagulation (DIC).

Multiple small intracerebral bleeding sites may also coalesce to form larger hematomas. As in the case of all major space-occupying lesions, intracerebral hematomas may increase ICP, thereby compromising local or global cerebral blood flow (CBF), causing mechanical damage to the brain tissue, resulting finally in herniation.

A common finding in the CT scan of head-injured patients is hematomas within the ventricles. These traumatic intraventricular hemorrhages (IVH) may be due to the rupture of small vessels in the periventricular walls, the choroid plexus, the septum pellucidum, the corpus callosum, or extensions of intracerebral hematomas. Blood clots in the third or fourth ventricle may occlude the flow of cerebrospinal fluid, thereby contributing to a rise in ICP and secondary ischemic injury. Massive bleeding into the ventricles may also act as a space-occupying lesion. Prognosis is especially poor following this type of lesion. However, intraventricular thrombolytics have been successfully used in these patients.

Numerous small petechial hemorrhages spread throughout large parts of the brain, especially in the white matter, often visible only under the microscope, represent diffuse vascular injury. This is associated with a very poor outcome. The pathophysiologic mechanisms of diffuse vascular injury are believed to involve diapedesis of blood cells as well as alterations of the endothelial cell membranes.[27] The majority of these patients succumb rapidly and do not usually reach a medical center alive.

Shearing forces within the brain stem at the time of injury may lead to brain stem lesions. These "bleeds" are often combined with widespread diffuse axonal injury. Although most of those lesions are small and difficult to detect, early detection using imaging often determines the outcome of these patients. Isolated brain stem lesions are rare, and more usually occur in combination with damage to other regions of the brain.

In addition to the primary injury, secondary brain stem lesions often develop as a complication of raised ICP and herniation. Increased intracranial supratentorial pressure results in compression of the brain stem at the tentorial hiatus, and vascular damage results from avulsion of the basilar artery perforator vessels, from the brainstem itself, as it descends, along the clivus (Duret hemorrhages); death results, secondary to paralysis of the respiratory and vasomotor centers (Fig. 69.5).

Factors responsible for ischemic brain damage – ICP, cerebral perfusion pressure, cerebral blood volume, and cerebral blood flow

The relations among ICP, cerebral perfusion pressure (CPP), cerebral blood volume (CBV), and CBF are discussed in Chapter 44. We would like to briefly review this crucial subject, especially elaborating on aspects of importance for head-injured patients.

The human brain is enclosed in the rigid cranial shell. Any increase in one of the intracranial compartments will lead to an increase in ICP if not compensated by a volume decrease of another component. The most common reasons for increases in ICP after head injury are the development of brain edema and/or an intracranial space-occupying lesion. Vasodilation, either compensatory or due to vasoparalysis, is a less significant factor. Usually several factors contribute to the ICP rise at the same time.

Unlike other tissues, the brain is unable to store significant amounts of either oxygen or glucose, and, therefore, depends crucially on an adequate CBF. The CBF, in turn, is a function of the CPP (mean arterial blood pressure minus ICP), cerebrovascular resistance, and the rheologic properties of the blood. A drastically elevated ICP causes a

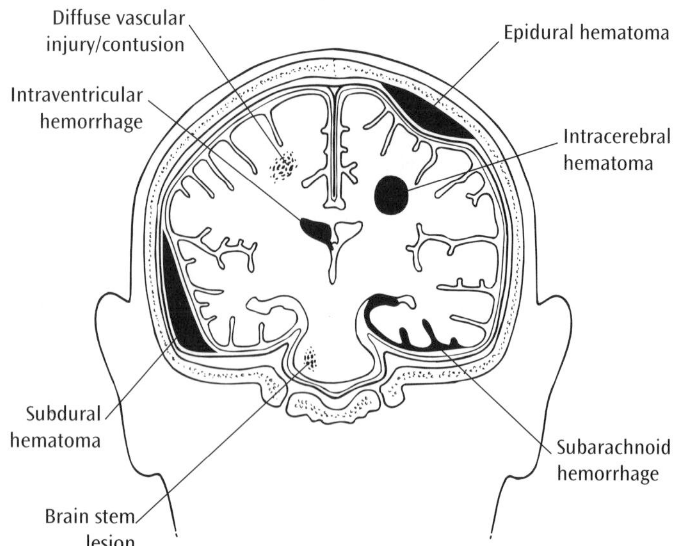

Figure 69.5 *Traumatic intracranial hematomas/contusions.*

decrease in the CPP unless the mean arterial blood pressure (MAP) increases appropriately. A decrease in the MAP will reduce the CPP. Although the normal brain is able to maintain an almost constant blood flow over a wide perfusion pressure range (between approximately 50 and 150 mmHg/6.7 and 20.0 kPa in healthy individuals), autoregulation may be impaired after head injury, making these head-injured patients even more likely to develop cerebral ischemia. If the CPP falls below a certain threshold, CBF decreases the supply of oxygen and glucose as well as the disposal of waste products, endangering brain tissue integrity and global or brain function.

The normal uninjured brain tolerates cortical blood flow reduction down to 20 mL $100g^{-1}$ min^{-1} without a major dysfunction. At blood flow values below 20 mL $100g^{-1}$ min^{-1}, consciousness is lost rapidly. If CBF is reduced to less than 18 mL $100g^{-1}$ min^{-1}, neurons switch to the less efficient anaerobic metabolism, and failure of ATP-dependent ion exchangers and subsequent loss of ionic homeostasis occurs. CBF values of less than 18 mL $100g^{-1}$ min^{-1} are not unusual after traumatic brain injury, and occur in approximately one-third of severely head-injured patients early after injury.[28] Furthermore, regional blood flow reductions to about 18 mL $100g^{-1}$ min^{-1} are frequently seen around contusions and intracerebral hematomas.[28] When flow declines to below 10 mL $100g^{-1}$ min^{-1}, loss of membrane integrity follows, with a massive influx of Ca^{2+} ions, resulting in cell death.

Interestingly, neurons seem to be more vulnerable to ischemic episodes than astrocytes. Although both cell types undergo ischemic necrosis during extreme ischemia (< 10 mL $100g^{-1}$ min^{-1} for more than 60 min), selective neuronal loss, by apoptosis or necrosis, may occur during less pronounced ischemia (15–18 mL $100g^{-1}$ min^{-1} for 30 min). The effect of progressively decreased CBF on neuronal function and brain tissue integrity depends on the duration of the blood flow reduction itself, and its intensity. Brief episodes (< 2 h) of insufficient CBF may be tolerated without irreversible deficit if blood flow is restored subsequently.

These data stress the importance of maintaining an adequate CPP. However, although a CPP of about 60–70 mmHg (7.9–9.3 kPa) is adequate,[29] there is some disagreement in this respect.[30] The "optimal" CPP may vary from patient to patient, and may possibly fluctuate in the same patient over time. According to the hemodynamic phases after head injury, the maintenance of a CPP of 60 mmHg (7.9 kPa) or more seems to be appropriate at least during the first 24 h. Optimal control of cerebral perfusion might become available through the development of bedside CBF monitoring systems.

A large elevation in ICP causes brain compression against rigid intracranial structures, such as the foramen magnum, the tentorium, or the falx. This can lead to significant mechanical damage to parts of the brain, with brain death as the final consequence. The compression of the brain stem against the foramen magnum results in impairment of vital vegetative centers, such as the vasomotor and the respiratory centers. Such events occur rapidly with posterior fossa hematomas. Therefore, an important goal in the treatment of head-injured patients is to try to avoid large increases in ICP, as is often seen after traumatic brain injury.

PREHOSPITAL MANAGEMENT

The management of the severely head-injured patient begins at the accident site. Although conditions there are usually not optimal, several important goals of early treatment have to be accomplished. Aspects of the management of these multitrauma patients are extensively described in Chapter 42. We will discuss the aspects associated with brain trauma here.

At the site, if the patient has to be transferred to a safe place immediately, the principles of transport of patients with possible vertebral column injuries must be employed. Whenever there is doubt, the patient's head should be fixed with a rigid collar and a spinal support board should be applied until vertebral injuries have been radiologically excluded.

At the same time, the vital functions of the patient must be evaluated and resuscitation should be initiated if necessary. The importance of adequate oxygenation is recognized, especially in head-injured patients, and, therefore, all unconscious patients should be intubated as early as possible, and ventilated with 100% oxygen until arrival in a medical center. Unfortunately, a relatively high percentage of head trauma patients are inadequately ventilated and, therefore, still suffer from hypoxemia during the crucial first hour after injury. Intubation, with pharmacologic sedation, analgesia, and muscular paralysis, to secure an airway and ventilate the patient is therefore indicated. Furthermore, intubation reduces the risk of aspiration. Hyperventilation should be avoided during the first hour after injury to avoid a reduction in impaired CBF, which is present in a high proportion of patients. Hypoventilation must also be avoided because hypercarbia might increase the ICP.

The maintenance of an adequate arterial blood pressure (MAP >90 mmHg/12.0 kPa) is equally important, as is airway care. In order to infuse fluid and/or for application of vasopressors, at least one or more large-bore intravenous lines must be placed. Colloids, as well as isotonic crystalloid solutions, are suitable choices. Hypotonic or glucose-containing solutions should be avoided. Fluid should be rapidly administered to bring the central venous pressure to about 10 cmH_2O (1 kPa) ; 3–5 L may be needed over the first 12–24 h.

While resuscitating the patient, a brief assessment of basic neurologic functions should be performed to assess a possible brain injury. The GCS is by far the most common classification used, owing to its practicability and its ability to predict the outcome of head-injured patients. Basically, the GCS takes the patient's reaction (eye opening, verbal response, motor response – spontaneously or to external stimuli) after trauma into consideration (Table 69.1).

Although the GCS is of considerable practical value as a means to evaluate the severity of head injuries, it does not indicate the underlying pathologic mechanisms. Even patients with initially high scores may deteriorate later and therefore need to be monitored closely at least during the first 24 h. Additionally, the neurologic assessment should also include the pupillary reactions (light response, size, and symmetry).

Adequate analgesia, or analgesia and sedation, must be provided although these drugs might influence neurologic examination. The first assessment of brain function and the GCS should be completed, if possible, before administration of these drugs. Appropriate analgesia is also essential for comatose patients. So as not to limit the clinician's ability to neurologically examine the patient, pharmacologic intervention should be limited as far as possible. Short-acting opioids, such as alfentanil, and sedatives, such as midazolam or propofol, should be titrated carefully. A short-acting opioid, etomidate, and succinylcholine (suxamethonium) appear to be optimal for intubation. Importantly, the drug-induced changes in neurologic function disappear only minutes after discontinuation of a remifentanil infusion.

Table 69.1 *Glasgow coma scale (GCS)*

Eye opening
4 = spontaneously
3 = to speech
2 = to pain
1 = none
Verbal response
5 = oriented
4 = confused
3 = inappropriate
2 = incomprehensible words
1 = none
Motor response
6 = obeys commands
5 = localized to pain
4 = withdraws to pain/normal flexion
3 = abnormal flexion to pain
2 = extension to pain
1 = none

Each response is evaluated separately then the scores are added to give a total score (= GCS).

The neurologic assessment should be repeated during the transfer to a medical center and thereafter. At this early stage, this may be the only way to detect deterioration. The minimum monitoring during the transfer to a medical center comprises ECG, noninvasive blood pressure, pulse oximetry and, if possible, end-tidal P_{CO_2} measurement.

A very important aspect in the primary "handling" of potentially severely head-injured patients is the choice of the appropriate medical center, which must have the neurosurgical facilities to comprehensively monitor and treat patients with severe head injury. Simply "unloading" the patient at the nearest available hospital with an emergency center might considerably delay adequate treatment and, furthermore, expose the patient to the risk of another interhospital journey (Table 69.2).

ACUTE CLINICAL MANAGEMENT IN THE EMERGENCY ROOM SETTING

The primary goals after the arrival of a potentially head-injured patient at an emergency medical center are stabilization of all vital systems, establishment of comprehensive monitoring of vital functions, precise diagnosis and initiation of treatment based on the diagnosis, in order to prevent secondary damage (Table 69.3).

After stabilization of cardiovascular and respiratory functions, diagnostic evaluation must be initiated without delay. Computed tomography (CT) of the head, including the first two cervical vertebrae, and a conventional radiograph of the cervical spinal column in two planes, and a chest radiograph are mandatory. According to the result of the CT scan, head injury patients may be divided into six subgroups (Marshall groups, Table 69.4).

The results of the initial examination determine the further management of the patient. Immediate neurosurgical intervention is indicated when large epidural, subdural, and intracerebral hematomas are present,

Table 69.2 *Goals of preclinical management*

Goals of preclinical management
Stabilization of vital functions
Evaluation of consciousness and injury pattern
Stabilization of the vertebral column
Adequate pain treatment
Gathering of useful information about the injury mechanism
Transport of the patient to an adequate medical center, close monitoring of vital and neurologic functions

Table 69.3 *Goals of clinical management*

Goals of clinical management
Stabilization of vital functions
Comprehensive monitoring of vital functions
Precise diagnosis
Acute surgical treatment of major mass lesions and hematomas
Adequate pain treatment
Transfer to a specialized ICU

in order to prevent secondary damage caused by increased ICP and impaired CBF. Massive brain swelling, especially in young patients, may also benefit from early craniotomy, with duroplasty. Depressed skull fractures or open-skull fractures with dural tears require early surgery, although this may be delayed for 4–6 h unless bleeding heavily or accompanied by a hematoma. In all cases of open head injury, antibiotic therapy should be started without delay (e.g. 2 g ceftriaxone every 8–12 h i.v.). Even without the need for immediate neurosurgical intervention after admission of the head-injured patient, the establishment of an ICP sensor or ventriculostomy should be considered as soon as possible.

In general, major extracranial injuries, which present 40–50% of the time, such as major retroperitoneal, intra-abdominal or intrathoracic bleeding, should be operated upon *before* craniotomy, unless a large hematoma is present intracranially. If necessary, both procedures may also be performed simultaneously. However, life-threatening extracranial injuries should be treated first if simultaneous surgery is not feasible.

Necessary monitoring in the emergency room includes invasive blood pressure monitoring, ECG, and end-tidal CO_2 partial pressure. An arterial line as well as a central-venous catheter should be placed in the emergency room, as these provide crucial information about the cardiovascular and blood gas status and, therefore, help to stabilize the patient. Serum electrolytes, glucose, hemoglobin, hematocrit, creatinine, urea, plasma osmolality, as well as the coagulation status and arterial blood gases, should be determined soon after admission of the patient. Blood should be cross-matched. After determination of the arterial blood gas status, the inspired oxygen fraction (F_iO_2) should be decreased according to the arterial oxygen partial pressure (P_aO_2).

Every severely head-injured patient should be transferred to a specialized ICU either after surgery or immediately from the emergency room if early surgery is not indicated.

ANESTHESIA

The main objectives of anesthesia in head-injured patients are to prevent secondary brain damage by optimizing cerebral perfusion and oxygenation and to achieve optimal surgical conditions for the neurosurgeon, primarily by preventing brain swelling and vascular engorgement.

Practical anesthesia

Induction

Every severely head-injured patient should already be intubated by the time he or she is brought into the operating room. If for some reason this is not the case, the patient needs to be intubated without further delay. The possibility of a cervical column instability, as well as an increased aspiration risk, has to be taken into consideration. As fiberoptic intubation is usually not an option in comatose patients, the neck should be secured with the help of an assistant by gentle in-line traction during the intubation process. To minimize the risk of aspiration, a rapid-sequence induction should be performed. After a "precurarization dose" of a nondepolarizing muscle relaxant (e.g. 0.01 $mg\,kg^{-1}$ vecuronium) and breathing of 100% oxygen for 4 min, an induction dose of etomidate (0.3 $mg\,kg^{-1}$) or thiopental (3–5 $mg\,kg^{-1}$) is administered, followed by succinylcholine (1.5 $mg\,kg^{-1}$). Next, the cricoid cartilage is pressed slightly toward the esophagus by an assistant. After 60 s, the trachea is intubated. Immediately after inflating the cuff and confirmation of the correct tube location, the pressure on the cricoid cartilage can be released.

Several forms of a "modified" rapid-sequence induction are possible. Rocuronium (0.6–1.0 $mg\,kg^{-1}$) may be used as an alternative to succinylcholine; priming with vecuronium is not then necessary. Good intubation conditions are usually achieved 60–90 s after administration of rocuronium. In order to prevent ICP increases during intubation, either minor doses of an opioid (e.g. 1–4 $\mu g\,kg^{-1}$ of fentanyl) or lidocaine (1.5 $mg\,kg^{-1}$) may be administered intravenously.

Table 69.4 *Traumatic Coma Data Bank: CT classification (Marshall score)*

1	Diffuse injury I	No visible intracranial pathology seen on CT scan
2	Diffuse injury II	– cisterns are present – midline shift: 0–5 mm – no high/mixed density lesion >25 cc – may include bone fragments or foreign bodies
3	Diffuse injury III (swelling)	– cisterns are compressed or absent – midline shift: 0–5 mm – no high/mixed density lesion >25 cc – may include bone fragments or foreign bodies
4	Diffuse injury IV (shift)	– midline shift: >5 mm – no high/mixed density lesion >25 cc
5	Evacuated mass lesion	Any lesion surgically evacuated.
6	Nonevacuated mass lesion	High/mixed density lesion >25 cc that is not surgically evacuated

Maintenance

Although so far there is no anesthesiologic regime that has proved superior over the others in regards to the maintenance of anesthesia in head-injured patients, the regime outlined below seems reasonable in the light of current knowledge. As propofol (3–10 mg kg^{-1} h^{-1}) does not cause vasodilation, it may have some advantages over volatile anesthetics as a way to maintain sedation. However, apart from theoretical considerations, no practical disadvantages of either isoflurane or its newer relative, sevoflurane, in moderate doses combined with opioids, have been detected so far. Any combination with nitrous oxide should be avoided because of the influence of this drug on CBV, ICP, and CBF. In patients with cardiovascular concerns, benzodiazepines may be preferred because of a negligible effect on cardiac inotropy.

Sufficient analgesia should be provided by opioids (fentanyl, sufentanil, remifentanil), which may be administered continuously or intermittently (Table 69.5).

Muscle relaxation can be achieved by intermittent or continuous administration of nondepolarizing relaxants (Table 69.6). Adequate relaxation prevents coughing and therefore sudden increase in ICP, as well as sudden and potentially deleterious movement of the patient. However, relaxation must always be accompanied by appropriate sedation and analgesia.

Standard monitoring

Standard monitoring of head-injured patients during neurosurgery includes invasive ("zeroed" at the level of the mastoids) and noninvasive arterial blood pressure, central venous pressure, ECG, pulse oximetry, body temperature, fluid balance (input–urinary output), end-tidal CO_2, and neuromuscular monitoring. Hemoglobin, hematocrit, serum glucose, serum electrolytes, coagulation status, serum osmolarity, and arterial blood gases should be determined intermittently (e.g. every 2 h). When the cranium is open, ICP monitoring is not usually needed, as pressure will equilibrate to atmospheric, unless there is massive brain swelling. However, for nonintracranial surgery in the severely head-injured patient, ICP monitoring should always be established as soon as possible, often in the operating room, during the noncranial procedure, unless a coagulopathy is present.

Optional monitoring

Optional monitoring depends on the special situation of the patient as well as of the resources of the medical center. The jugular venous oxygen saturation (S_jO_2) provides information about the balance between oxygen supply and oxygen demand. It can be determined either intermittently or continuously with a special sensor probe. An S_jO_2 of less than 55% is considered pathologic. It can be caused by a decreased oxygen supply (decreased CBF due to hyperventilation or insufficient CPP; hypoxemia or anemia) or, rarely, by an increased oxygen demand (seizures, hyperthermia). The causes should be treated accordingly. An increase of the S_jO_2 over 75% may be caused by a major shunt area, e.g. large infarctions. Unfortunately, the method is prone to erroneous readings, therefore S_jO_2 values should be confirmed and interpreted cautiously. If patients are in a sitting position, an ultrasound Doppler probe should be positioned either intraesophageally or precardially in order to detect possible air embolism early (Table 69.7).

Table 69.5 *Dosage of opioids during neurosurgery after traumatic brain injury*

Fentanyl	Intermittently: 0.5–2.5 μg kg^{-1} Continuously: 2–10 μg kg^{-1} h^{-1}
Sufentanil	Intermittently: 0.1–0.5 μg kg^{-1} Continuously: 0.3–1.0 μg kg^{-1} h^{-1}
Remifentanil	Continuously: 0.1–0.5 μg kg^{-1} min^{-1} (very variable, depending on propofol dosage and surgical stimulation)

Table 69.6 *Dosage of muscle relaxants during neurosurgery after traumatic brain injury*

Atracurium	Intermittently: 100–200 μg kg^{-1} Continuously: 6–8 μg kg^{-1} min^{-1}
Mivacurium	Intermittently: 100–150 μg kg^{-1} Continuously: 4–8 μg kg^{-1} min^{-1}
Rocuronium	Intermittently: 75–150 μg kg^{-1} Continuously: 8–11 μg kg^{-1} min^{-1}
Vecuronium	Intermittently: 30–50 μg kg^{-1} Continuously: 1–2 μg kg^{-1} min^{-1}

Controlled ventilation

A positive end-expiratory pressure (PEEP) of 5 cmH_2O (0.5 kPa) usually does not impair the cerebrovenous outflow and helps to avoid pulmonary atelectasis, thereby improving arterial oxygenation. F_IO_2 should be adjusted to achieve an arterial PO_2 of > 100 mmHg (13.3 kPa). Tidal volume and ventilation should be set to achieve an arterial PCO_2 of about 35 mmHg (4.7 kPa) in order to prevent vascular engorgement and to improve surgical conditions. If the anesthesia is maintained with a volatile anesthetic, mild hyperventilation (arterial PCO_2 30–35 mmHg/4.0–4.7 kPa) is useful for the prevention of anesthesia-induced vasodilation. If the jugular venous oxygen saturation falls below 55% and other causes such as hyperthermia, anemia, hypoxemia or an insufficient CPP have been excluded, ventilation settings should be adapted to aim at a slightly higher P_aCO_2. Hypercarbia, however, must be avoided at all costs.

Intraoperative cardiovascular management

One of the main goals of the anesthesiologic management of head-injured patients is the maintenance of an adequate CBF. Direct continuous CBF measurements during neurosurgery are not routinely feasible; therefore, the anesthesiologist has to use CPP and S_jO_2 as a guide. The optimal CPP is between 70 and 80 mmHg (9.3 and 10.7 kPa), but varies between individuals. Either systemic arterial hypotension or increased ICP may cause decreases in the CPP. If hypotension is caused by a fluid deficit, intravascular volume must be replaced. Depending on hematocrit (≥30%), either erythrocytes, fresh-frozen plasma, plasma expanders (ideally human albumin), or isotonic electrolyte solutions should be infused cautiously. Hyperinfusion may theoretically promote the formation of brain edema, although the risks of

Table 69.7 *Monitoring of severely head-injured patients in the operating room*

Standard monitoring
Arterial blood pressure (invasive and noninvasive)
Central venous pressure
Intracranial pressure
Cerebral perfusion pressure (MAP–ICP)
Heart rate and rhythm (ECG)
Core body temperature
Fluid balance (Foley catheter)
End-tidal CO_2
Repeated blood gas analysis
Laboratory analysis: hemoglobin, hematocrit, serum electrolytes, glucose, coagulation status
Optional monitoring
Electrophysiologic examination
Jugular venous oxygen saturation

hypovolemia are greater. Glucose-containing solutions should only be administered in cases of hypoglycemia. Hypotonic solutions should be avoided at all costs. The total fluid balance should be slightly positive. If hypotension is due to either impaired cardiac contractility or insufficient systemic vascular resistance, vasopressors such as epinephrine (adrenaline) (0.05–0.1 $\mu g\,kg^{-1}\,min^{-1}$), norepinephrine (noradrenaline) (0.05–0.2 $\mu g\,kg^{-1}\,min^{-1}$), dopamine (3–9 $\mu g\,kg^{-1}\,min^{-1}$), or dobutamine (3–9 $\mu g\,kg^{-1}\,min^{-1}$) should be used accordingly, either alone or in an appropriate combination. Bolus administration of vasopressors should be avoided to prevent potentially deleterious ICP peaks.

Hypertension must be treated cautiously as it may be a compensatory response resulting in an adequate CBF, in the presence of high ICP (Cushing's reflex). Antihypertensive drugs with only minor direct effects on cerebral vessels, such as urapidil or labetalol, should be preferred.

Management of increased ICP

Increased ICP is usually due to edema, vascular engorgement, or intracranial hematomas. Craniotomy results in adequate pressure relief. Any hematomas, and sometimes swollen damaged brain tissue, e.g. a burst lobe, may be removed surgically. If the increase in ICP is caused by vascular engorgement, mild hyperventilation (P_aCO_2 30–35 mmHg/4.0–4.7 kPa) is useful, but should not be prolonged for more than 30 min. Edema can be reduced by the use of mannitol (0.25–0.5 $g\,kg^{-1}$) infused over 10 to 20 min. Mannitol should not be administered if the serum osmolarity is higher than 320 $mosmol\,kg^{-1}$.

If the brain bulk protrudes after craniotomy, even although the CPP is adequate and stable, mild hyperventilation is being applied, and mannitol has been given, the administration of thiopental (0.25–0.5 $mg\,kg^{-1}$) may be considered, and a CT scan, or intraoperative ultrasound, may be useful for the exclusion of an intraoperative hematoma at another intracranial site.

Postoperative management

Patients who have been conscious prior to the neurosurgery (e.g. hematoma removal) may be awoken and extubated postoperatively after an adequate and cautious weaning period with effective spontaneous ventilation and if an adequate airway has been ensured.

However, most head injury patients do not fulfill these criteria. Early emergence from sedation and extubation is contraindicated if the patient was unconscious or suffering from impaired consciousness prior to surgery, if a significant brain edema is present, or if there are other major injuries that will need to be surgically treated. Hypothermic patients must be *slowly*(!) rewarmed to normothermia before ceasing anesthesia and weaning from the respirator. Clonidine (75 μg slowly, i.v.) may help to avoid stress and shivering during the rewarming period, which may lead to a rise in ICP. All severely head-injured patients must be transferred to a specialized ICU postoperatively.

Special pharmacology

There is no "gold standard" for the anesthesiologic management of patients with traumatic brain injury. Nevertheless, it is essential for the anesthesiologist who deals with head-injured patients to have a comprehensive knowledge of the pharmacologic properties of anesthetics, especially with regard to their impact on brain function.

Volatile anesthetics

Volatile anesthetics (haloflurane, isoflurane, enflurane) increase ICP at normocapnia. This can be prevented almost completely by hypocapnia.

All volatile anesthetics increase CBF. Traumatic brain injury may interfere with regional cerebrovascular autoregulation. The vasodilating effects of volatile anesthetics may lead to redistribution of the blood flow toward less impaired brain regions. However, whether this postulated "steal effect" is of any clinical significance is debatable.

The quantitatively different effects of halothane, enflurane, and isoflurane on CBF and cerebral metabolism[31–40] led to the conclusion that isoflurane would be the "best" volatile anesthetic because it seemed to have the least influence on CBF. However, more recent studies indicate that the influence of halothane, enflurane, and isoflurane on CBF may vary between different regions of the brain. The overall effect on global CBF seems to be the same for all three substances (mild vasodilation) but blood distribution within the brain is altered in a different manner.

As cerebral metabolic activity decreases during anesthesia with halothane, enflurane, or isoflurane, and while CBF increases simultaneously, volatile anesthetics appear to "uncouple" CBF from cerebral metabolism. However, rather than "uncouple" metabolism and blood flow, volatile anesthetics seem to increase the slope of the curve to a greater angle.[41] That is, with increasing concentrations of a volatile anesthetic, the same metabolic activity will be associated with higher CBF values. In other words, for a given concentration (MAC) of a volatile anesthetic, the relation between blood flow and metabolism remains linear, but the "sensitivity" of the CBF for alterations in metabolism has changed. This has been shown in several studies.[41] Much higher concentrations (>2 MAC for halothane) might cause real "uncoupling" between metabolism and CBF.[42]

Whether the more recently developed volatile anesthetics desflurane and sevoflurane are in fact superior to isoflurane for neuroanesthesia has still to be proved. In clinical practice, they seem to have some advantages such as faster onset time and easier controllability, owing to their physical properties (lower blood–gas solubility). Unlike the other volatile anesthetics, sevoflurane might be able to decrease CBF slightly,[43–46] an advantage during neurosurgery.

Nitrous oxide

The use of nitrous oxide during neurosurgery is still practiced; however, nitrous oxide increases both CBF and ICP considerably, as well as CBV, without decreasing cerebral metabolic activity significantly. Nitrous oxide might even increase the $CMRO_2$.[47] Unlike other volatile anesthetics, this CBF rise cannot be prevented by mild hyperventilation.[48] Both effects are undesirable during neurosurgery in head-injured patients. Therefore, the use of this agent cannot be recommended after head injury or following a subarachnoid hemorrhage.

Intravenous sedative and hypnotic anesthetics

Barbiturates

Barbiturates are probably the most extensively examined anesthetic agents with respect to their effect on cerebral metabolism and CBF. Thiopental, the typical example, decreases CBF by a reduction in cerebral metabolic activity and $CMRO_2$. The CBF reduction seems to be coupled to the reduction in $CMRO_2$, and neither appears to be in a linear relation to the thiopental dose. A relatively high grade of metabolic suppression – as much as 40% – can be accomplished with reasonably small thiopental blood concentration. Further increases in the thiopental dose could result in increasing side-effects (especially reduced blood pressure, tracheobronchial mucociliary clearance, and leukocyte function) without a further significant reduction of the cerebral metabolism. Even in very high doses, barbiturates do not seem to interfere with cerebrovascular autoregulation or CO_2 reactivity. Although the various barbiturates in clinical use vary in their pharmacokinetic behavior, their pharmacodynamics appears to be consistent.

Etomidate

Etomidate reduces ICP, cerebral metabolism, and CBF, but, unlike barbiturates and propofol, CBF decreases faster than metabolic activity, indicating that etomidate might cause vasoconstriction additionally by an as yet unknown mechanism. In predisposed patients, etomidate might cause seizures even in small doses.

Propofol

With an action similar to that described for barbiturates, propofol reduces cerebral metabolic activity (down to 40% of normal values) and CBF. Propofol is known to decrease arterial blood pressure when administered too quickly, or in high concentrations, and hypotension is a major risk for head trauma patients. However, if the drug is given in appropriate doses, and if fast bolus injections are avoided, propofol provides several advantages for neurosurgical patients compared with other hypnotics. For instance, a thorough neurologic examination is possible relatively soon after discontinuation of a propofol infusion, an essential in management of head-injured patients.

Benzodiazepines

Benzodiazepines such as diazepam or midazolam decrease cerebral metabolic rate, and blood flow moderately.

Midazolam is useful for the long-term sedation of head-injured patients; however, it hinders a clinical neurologic evaluation more than propofol. Since reversal of benzodiazepines (e.g. with flumazenil) may increase CBF and therefore ICP, this procedure should be applied with special caution in head-injured patients (e.g. when coma may be due either to benzodiazepines or to head injury).

Analgesic drugs

Opioid

Most clinically used opioids (remifentanil, sufentanil, alfentanil, fentanyl, morphine) decrease cerebral metabolism, as well as CBF, dose dependently. However, these effects are significant only in relatively high doses of these opioids. The frequency of the EEG pattern is reduced simultaneously but does not reach the isoelectric level. Despite the effect of opioids on cerebral metabolism and blood flow, it has been reported that these substances might actually increase ICP, even when the arterial $P\text{CO}_2$ is controlled.[49]

Remifentanil, a recently introduced synthetic ultrashort-acting opioid, might have advantages over other opioids as a result of its very good controllability. In the final analysis, however, more clinical experience is necessary with this drug in severely head-injured patients.

Ketamine

Ketamine markedly increases CBF and ICP. These effects are even more pronounced in spontaneously breathing patients, without control of arterial $P\text{CO}_2$. Ketamine has been considered especially dangerous for head-injured patients because of these properties. More recent results regarding the effect of ketamine on CBF and ICP are consistent;[50] however, this drug's use in patients with severe head injury is still a concern, as even brief ICP increases may cause secondary ischemia.

Muscle relaxants

Depolarizing relaxants (succinylcholine)

Even although this fast-onset muscle relaxant is well known to increase ICP in humans, this effect can be prevented by "precurarization" with nondepolarizing relaxants, such as vecuronium or pancuronium. Therefore, succinylcholine use may have an important role.

The first contact between the anesthesiologist and the severely head-injured (and often polytraumatized) patient usually occurs under emergency conditions. Under these circumstances, a fast and swift intubation is absolutely necessary: first, because of the high risk of aspiration and, second, in order to secure the airway rapidly and to establish adequate ventilation. The consequences of prolonged hypoxia and hypercarbia on the injured brain are far more detrimental than the short, transient rise in ICP which may be caused by succinylcholine. More recently developed fast-acting nondepolarizing drugs such as rocuronium might be useful, but this remains to be established.

Nondepolarizing muscular relaxants

To our knowledge, nondepolarizing muscular relaxants do not significantly influence ICP, CBF, or CBV in typical doses.

INTENSIVE CARE

In general, the management of severely head-injured patients in the ICU should follow the same strategy as used for other critically ill patients. However, certain aspects of traumatic brain injury need to be specifically addressed. These include special monitoring requirements, as well as causes of deterioration that develop after traumatic brain injury. As elevated ICP is the most frequent and serious problem in severely head-injured patients, its treatment will be discussed in more detail.

Monitoring

The main goal when monitoring the severely head-injured patient is the early detection of states that potentially endanger a favorable outcome, such as high ICP, hypotension, hypoxemia, ischemia, hyperglycemia, and hyperthermia. As some of these conditions are unlikely to be detected with standard monitoring, further techniques may be necessary to adequately manage severely head-injured patients.

Unlike other organs, the number of routinely measurable parameters of cerebral physiology remains limited, despite the advances in neuroanesthesia during the last two decades. Unfortunately, there are no brain equivalents to the Swan–Ganz catheter and the echocardiograph!

Except in specialized centers with more sophisticated cerebral monitoring techniques, the neurointensivist depends on ICP measurement, CPP calculation, jugular venous blood saturation, CT scans, and repeated neurologic observations to evaluate the condition of the injured brain. In addition, the standard monitoring parameters for critically ill patients such as invasive arterial blood pressure, central venous pressure, ECG, pulse oximetry, core body temperature, end-tidal CO_2 pressure, urinary output, and calculation of the fluid balance are mandatory. Electrophysiologic techniques, such as EEG and evoked potentials, may also be helpful to assess damage especially to the brain stem.

ICP monitoring

ICP can be monitored via ventriculostomy catheters, and intraparenchymal or subdural sensors. Subdural sensors usually underestimate the real ICP value. Electronic intraparenchymal sensors generally accord well with ventricular ICP. The relation between MAP, ICP, CPP, and CBF, as well as the importance of maintaining an adequate CBF, have been discussed previously.

CBF monitoring

Although we can accurately measure CBF intermittently by means of xenon CT/CBF, there is clinically no well-validated continuous CBF monitor for use at the bedside. Recently, however, three methods have become available for continuous "semiquantitative" estimation of changes in CBF:

1 Continuous transcranial Doppler velocity measurement. This relies upon an elastic head holder that can immobilize a TCB probe, such that repeated velocity measurements can be made noninvasively in the middle cerebral artery. However, this is only a crude index of true CBF.
2 Thermal diffusion CBF – the "Carter" Flowtronics probe. This is a flat catheter (about 6 mm × 35 mm × 1 mm), which is laid upon the cortex, at craniotomy, and provides semiquantitative, continuous local CBF data, for the cortex under the probe.
3 Continuous laser Doppler flow probes. These may be only 1–2 mm in diameter, allowing use via a "bolt". The data obtained are dependent on local conditions, at the site of placement.

The measurement of jugular venous oxygen saturation, either intermittently or via the "Oximetrix®" sensor, may be helpful for the estimation of the balance between cerebral oxygen supply and demand. Either an impaired oxygen supply or an increased oxygen demand may cause a decrease in the jugular venous oxygen saturation. As oxygen supply and CO_2 removal are functions of CBF, measurement of jugular venous oxygen saturation as well as jugular venous oxygen and CO_2 partial pressure may be helpful to assess global CBF. A jugular venous oxygen saturation below 55% is considered pathologic and may indicate impaired cerebral perfusion, a decreased arterial oxygen content (anemia, hypoxemia), or, in rare cases, an increased cerebral oxygen consumption (seizures, hyperthermia). An unusually high jugular venous oxygen (>75%) saturation may reflect functional shunting, as occurs when large parts of the brain do not consume oxygen any more, such as in infarction and brain death. However, this monitoring technique only provides global information about the oxygen supply–demand balance; it is unable to detect disturbances in minor tissue areas that may be important despite their smaller size. Furthermore, the current sensor technique for continuous measurement of oxygen saturation in the jugular bulb is troubled by a high rate of poor-quality data and requires repeated recalibrations (Table 69.8).[51]

More sophisticated and relatively expensive monitoring techniques include xenon CT/CBF measurements, high-resolution imaging of brain metabolism via positron emission tomography, and direct monitoring of oxygen, CO_2 partial pressure, pH, and temperature continuously by means of special tissue sensors. Measurement of biochemical parameters, such as glucose, lactate, pyruvate, and glutamate, in the cerebral extracellular fluid via microdialysis is also a promising tool for the future management of severely head-injured patients but, currently, this is being evaluated at research centers.

Treatment strategies for high ICP

ICP values of 8–10 mmHg (1–1.3 kPa) are considered normal, but levels below 15 mmHg are acceptable after thermal brain injury (TBI). Therapy should aim to achieve an ICP of less than 20 mmHg (2.7 kPa), unless the CPP is not considerably lower than 70 mmHg (9.3 kPa). Occasional slightly higher ICP values are acceptable as long as the CPP is over 70 mmHg (9.3 kPa) and there is no indication of herniation.

Conventional therapies

These are usually applied in a stepwise manner (see Fig. 69.6).

Step 1: sedation

Adequate sedation is an important part of ICP control, especially in agitated patients. Although different sedative regimes are possible, as discussed earlier, propofol may be preferred because of the rapid emergence after discontinuation of the drug. If propofol is used in moderate doses (2–5 $mg\,kg^{-1}\,h^{-1}$) and bolus doses are avoided, and the patient is normovolemic, the risk of inducing hypotension is minimized. Continuous application of an opioid is usually required to achieve satisfactory analgesia in traumatized patients. Pain must be avoided as this triggers stress reactions, abnormal motor responses, and high ICP.

Table 69.8 *Monitoring of severely head-injured patients in the ICU*

Standard monitoring
Clinical examination
Arterial blood pressure
Central venous pressure
Intracranial pressure
Cerebral perfusion pressure (MAP–ICP)
Heart rate and rhythm (ECG)
Core body temperature
Fluid balance (Foley catheter)
End-tidal CO_2
Repeated blood gas analysis
Laboratory analysis: hemoglobin, hematocrit, serum electrolytes, glucose, creatinine, urea, plasma osmolality, plasma proteins, coagulation status
Optional monitoring
Electrophysiologic examination
Jugular venous oxygen saturation
Intermittent CBF measurements via xenon/CBF computed tomography
Cerebral microdialysis
Cerebral tissue O_2, CO_2, pH and temperature monitoring (Neurotrend® sensor)

Step 2: moderate head-up posture

Changes in the CBV may alter ICP. A decrease in CBV may result in a decrease in ICP. This goal can be reached by facilitating the outflow of venous blood from the head. This is possible, as approximately 90% of the cerebral blood is located in the postcapillary cerebrovenous system. A simple way to achieve this is by avoiding venous congestion (i.e. avoiding extreme lateral rotation of the head or full extension of the neck) and maintaining a modest head-up position for the patient; an angle of 30° above horizontal appears to be optimal. Higher angles seem to reduce mean cerebral arterial blood pressure more than ICP, thereby possibly impairing CPP.

Step 3: ventricular drainage

The installation of a ventriculostomy catheter has almost become a standard in the management of severely head-injured patients. It not only provides the means for accurate measurement of the ICP, but it is also useful for the treatment of elevated ICP, by CSF drainage. The intermittent ventricular drainage of CSF may help to decrease high ICP via spatial compensation. However, fast drainage of larger volumes of CSF risks a shift of brain components. The rapid drainage of CSF, especially via a lumbar catheter, may lead to brain stem compression in patients with space-occupying lesions and is, therefore, strictly contraindicated for these patients.

Step 4: osmotherapy

Especially when elevated ICP is caused by cerebral edema, increasing blood osmolality and, thus, shifting water from brain tissue into the blood is helpful. The optimal drug for this purpose should neither be able to cross the blood–brain barrier nor be metabolized or influence metabolism. The polyalcohol mannitol fulfills these conditions to a high degree, but not perfectly. To decrease ICP, 0.25–0.5 $g\,kg^{-1}$ mannitol (20–25% solution) is administered intravenously. Immediately after administration, ICP may increase slightly due to vasodilation. ICP decrease usually starts 10–20 min after administration, reaches its maximum after 30–90 min, and lasts up to 6 h.

Before repeatedly administering mannitol, serum osmolality should be analyzed and renal function checked; mannitol should not be given if the serum osmolality is higher than 320 $mosmol\,kg^{-1}$ or if renal failure is present.

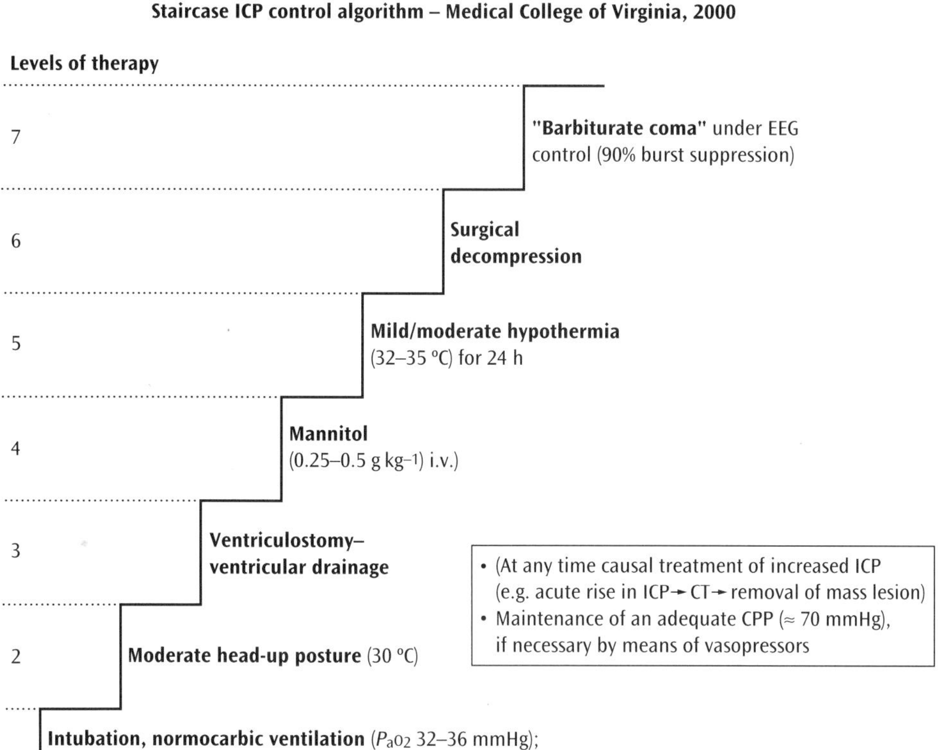

Figure 69.6 *Treatment of increased ICP (staircase algorithm).*

One drawback to the use of mannitol is that the blood–brain barrier is frequently disturbed after traumatic brain injury. As a consequence, mannitol may diffuse into the cerebral tissue, accumulate there, and increase local tissue osmolality. This can promote further edema development, and contribute to the "rebound phenomenon," leading to an ICP increase 6–12 h after mannitol administration, as well as to the loss of the therapeutic effect of mannitol after 3–4 days. Therefore, the use of mannitol in severely head-injured patients should be restricted to the treatment of acutely increased ICP; the drug should be administered in the least possible amount and not be given "prophylactically" on a regular basis in order to prevent brain edema.

Recently, hypertonic saline solutions (e.g. 5% NaCl) have become fashionable for the acute management of traumatized patients with severe head injury. They may also be useful as a "rescue therapy" for high ICP, unresponsive to mannitol.

Step 5: hypothermia

Lowering body temperature decreases cerebral metabolism and, as a consequence, CBF and ICP are also reduced. The reduction in energy needs of the brain may help to overcome an impaired supply of oxygen especially in the early phase after severe head injury. An improvement in behavioral outcome and tissue integrity was achieved by hypothermia in an animal TBI model.[52] Furthermore, hypothermia attenuates the release of excitatory amino acids after brain trauma and seems to provide a high degree of protection against secondary injury. An increase in brain tissue oxygen tension and a trend toward improved outcome was seen in patients.[53]

However, hypothermia has been associated with a variety of severe complications, such as arrhythmia, coagulopathies, and increased infections. These complications are less severe and less frequent when a core body temperature of 32–34 °C is maintained (moderate/mild hypothermia) and if the hypothermia does not persist for more than 24–48 h.

Despite some encouraging results, many questions regarding the therapeutic value of hypothermia for head-injured patients remain unanswered. A multicenter phase 3 trial of prophylactic hypothermia has been halted, with no evidence of benefit apparent at the time of writing this chapter. Therefore, we have applied hypothermia only as part of our "staircase model" for the treatment of otherwise therapy-resistant high ICP (see Fig. 69.6).

Hypothermia can be achieved either via active cooling (gel packs, air convection systems) or via pharmacologic downregulation of core body temperature [e.g. acetaminophen (paracetamol)], or both. Employment of hypothermia requires close cardiovascular and temperature monitoring as well as sedation of noncomatose patients, and neuromuscular paralysis, to prevent shivering.

To minimize complications, only mild-to-moderate hypothermia (32–34 °C) should be applied and maintained for no longer than 24–48 h. Normal core body temperature should be re-established very slowly, at least over 12 h. The patient needs especially close attention during the rewarming as complications such as rises in ICP occur most frequently in this phase.

On the other hand, there are much clearer indications that *hyper*thermia exerts deleterious effects on the recovery after traumatic brain injury.[54] Thus, elevated core body temperatures above normal should be treated aggressively in order to avoid further brain damage.

Step 6: surgical decompression

The early evacuation of all major space-occupying lesions, such as epidural or subdural hematomas, amenable to surgical intervention is the treatment of first choice in the therapy of elevated ICP.

However, in cases of otherwise uncontrollable ICP increases, without operable mass lesions, e.g. due to edema, a surgical decompression with temporary removal of a large area of skull bone and an extensive duroplasty has yielded favorable results.[55] Clearly, decompression must be performed *before* irreversible secondary global ischemic damage has occurred, due to high ICP, and reduced CPP. Criteria for the procedure, in our institution, thus include:

1 at least one functioning pupil;
2 EEG, or evoked potential, evidence of cerebral function (in the presence of neuromuscular paralysis);
3 viable brain stem appearances on CT (absent hemorrhage, normal density, or CBF, by xenon CT);
4 age under 65 years.

Step 7: barbiturates

As discussed above, barbiturates decrease the cerebral metabolic rate and decrease CBF in regions with intact metabolism–flow coupling. The CBF decrease is due to vasoconstriction, with reduction in the CBV, and also results in a reduction in ICP. Barbiturates should be administered with extreme care, under EEG control, and titrated to 90% suppression of EEG activity. A "zero line" EEG should be avoided.

Although barbiturates have proved useful for the control of ICP in several studies, they have failed to demonstrate improved outcome after severe head injury.[56] This may be due to the relatively high rate of side-effects, especially hypotension. A small and not very well-defined subset of patients with otherwise intractable ICP elevation benefits from barbiturate therapy. Barbiturates have other significant side-effects, especially for the immune, cardiovascular, and respiratory systems.

Therefore, we start ICP treatment with barbiturates only if all other methods have failed, and closely monitor cardiovascular function, via a Swan–Ganz catheter, and respiratory function. Blood pressure support with catecholamines is almost always necessary to maintain an adequate CPP.

In general it is important, if possible, to understand the pathophysiologic mechanisms underlying a rise in ICP before starting any therapy. Deleterious effects may result otherwise; for example, if the elevated ICP is due to an intracranial hematoma, mannitol may actually expand the hematoma volume by decreasing the volume of the unaffected brain tissue, allowing more bleeding. Thus, frequent CT scans have become a mainstay of management of high ICP.

The role of hyperventilation

Although controversial, hyperventilation is still very popular for the treatment of elevated ICP, despite strong evidence against its use. Hyperventilation-induced decreases in arterial carbon dioxide tension (P_aCO_2) cause vasoconstriction and therefore reduce CBV. Even a relatively small decrease in CBV may result in a significant reduction in ICP. The question, however, is whether hyperventilation reduces CBF even more than CBV. Several studies have shown a detrimental effect of hyperventilation after human severe head injury. Even moderate hyperventilation ($P_aCO_2 \approx 30$ mmHg/4.0 kPa), although decreasing ICP and increasing CPP significantly, has been demonstrated to reduce brain tissue oxygen tension. Chronic hyperventilation as part of ICP management also did not show any significant advantages compared with normoventilation, in severely head-injured patients.[57] Hyperventilation might be especially harmful during the first 24 h after trauma.

Therefore, at present hyperventilation is not recommended as a standard in the treatment of increased ICP. Maintaining an arterial PCO_2 of between 32 and 36 mmHg (4.3 and 4.8 kPa) seems to be a safe and reasonable guideline.

The role of steroids in ICP management after TBI

Although steroids may play a role in the treatment of edema-related rises in brain tumor patients, they have failed repeatedly to show any beneficial effects in the treatment of head-injured patients. As steroids are associated with various side-effects, among them hyperglycemia, and predispose to enhanced infection, which may be especially harmful in head-injured patients, their use in the treatment of TBI must be considered obsolete.

Lund therapy

The basis of the "Lund therapy" for the treatment of severely head-injured patients is the assumption that the elevated ICP is mainly due to vasogenic and hydrostatic edema under the conditions of an impaired cerebrovascular autoregulation and a disturbed blood–brain barrier. The inaugurators of this therapy concept argue that any increase in the intracapillary hydrostatic pressure must lead to a shift of water and plasma proteins into the cerebral tissue, thereby causing vasogenic extracellular edema or leading to a deterioration in the existing edema. The "Lund protocol" aims to reduce extravascular fluid passing across the impaired blood–brain barrier. Basic therapeutic principles of this concept are:

1 Evacuation of space-occupying lesions.
2 Reduction in the CBV by dihydroergotamine cerebrovenous vasoconstriction.
3 Reduction in the capillary hydrostatic pressure, by reduction of the cardiac output (through metoprolol), arterial dilation (via clonidine), and precapillary vasoconstriction (using low-dose thiopental). Therefore, it is suggested that a relatively low CPP (50–70 mmHg/6.7–9.3 kPa) should be maintained until cerebrovascular autoregulation and blood–brain barrier integrity have recovered.
4 Normalization of the oncotic pressure by means of human serum albumin.

The therapy concept considers ICP values of between 20 and 25 mmHg (2.7 and 3.3 kPa) to be acceptable.

Unfortunately, this approach is based upon assumptions about the pathophysiology of the edema. Cytotoxic edema is of considerably greater importance than vasogenic edema and, moreover, all the available evidence suggests that, except in the proximity to contused regions, the blood–brain barrier is only very briefly and transiently open, before the patient comes under medical care. Furthermore, this therapy is far more likely to induce secondary ischemia, due to low CPP, and ensuing hypoperfusion. Supporting evidence is necessary before this therapy concept can be recommended for general use.

Hyperglycemia

Hyperglycemia leads to a poorer outcome in head-injured patients, and following a stroke, and therefore should be avoided. Hypoglycemia, on the other hand, may also endanger substrate supply to the brain and must also be avoided.

Neurogenic pulmonary edema

Approximately 20% of all severely head-injured patients develop pulmonary edema without a primarily cardiovascular cause or (known) aspiration. This phenomenon, which has also been observed in patients with a subarachnoid hemorrhage, stroke, seizures, and meningitis, is termed neurogenic pulmonary edema (NPE) and is probably the most frequent and severe extracranial complication in brain trauma patients with a GCS of 8 or less. The risk is higher for patients with large unevacuated mass lesions or a pronounced midline shift, implying a brainstem causation. NPE has been found in 32% of head injury patients who died at the scene, and in 50% of those patients who died within 96 h after injury. Patients with NPE are approximately three times more likely to die or to survive in a vegetative state.

The NPE usually develops within the first 12 h after injury. Its main clinical signs are poor arterial oxygenation, frothy edema fluid coming from the endotracheal tube, and diffuse alveolar, interstitial infiltration on the chest radiograph and low filling pressures measured by right heart catheters. Several mechanisms, such as adrenergic discharge and endothelial dysfunction as well as neurogenic depletion of surfactant, have been suggested to be the cause of NPE. None of these explanations is satisfactory.

Neurogenic pulmonary edema is best treated in the way in which adult respiratory distress syndrome (ARDS) is treated, with fluid restriction, diuretics, and PEEP ventilation. It is of utmost importance to achieve adequate oxygenation in order to prevent secondary brain damage. The placement of a Swan–Ganz catheter can help to distinguish neuronal pulmonary edema from other causes of edema, and can be used to direct fluid and catecholamine therapy, if necessary, and to exclude cardiogenic causes, such as pericardial tamponade and myocardial infarction.

SUMMARY

The treatment of the severely head-injured patient begins at the accident site. Goals of the *preclinical management* are stabilization of vital functions, evaluation of consciousness and injury pattern, stabilization of the vertebral column, sufficient pain treatment, and transport of the patient to an adequate medical center. *Early clinical management* comprises further stabilization and comprehensive monitoring of vital functions, a precise diagnosis (via special examinations, such as CT) as well as adequate pain treatment. Major space-occupying lesions must be surgically evacuated as early as possible in order to prevent secondary damage. All severely head-injured patients need to be transferred to a specialized ICU.

Post-traumatic *brain swelling* may be caused either by brain edema or, to a lesser degree, by vascular engorgement. Both processes are multifactorial and appear to contribute to the development of brain swelling during the time-course following injury. *Brain edema* is thus classified into different types: the two most important are the cytotoxic edema and the vasogenic edema. Depending on the type of injury, a combination of different edema types can be found after head injury.

The main objectives of *anesthesia* in head-injured patients are to prevent secondary brain damage by optimizing cerebral perfusion and oxygenation and to achieve optimal surgical conditions for the neurosurgeon. Of special importance is the maintenance of an adequate CPP (70–80 mmHg/9.3–10.7 kPa) throughout the surgery.

The *intensive care management* of severely head-injured patients should routinely follow the same rationales as for other critically ill patients. Important goals in the management of patients in the ICU are the prevention, early detection, and efficient treatment of states that potentially endanger a favorable outcome after head injury. These include raised ICP, hypotension, hypoxemia, ischemia, hyperglycemia, and hyperthermia.

Increased ICP above 15–20 mmHg (2–2.7 kPa) should be treated according to a staircase algorithm (see Fig. 69.6). However, it is important to understand that the pathophysiologic mechanisms underlying a rise in ICP arise before therapy is started. It is necessary to avoid the deleterious effects of the therapy (Fig. 69.7).

In several centers dedicated to management of severe head injury, mortality rates have consistently fallen over recent years despite our failure to successfully introduce a specific drug therapy for traumatic brain injury. This improvement in outcome is especially the result of improvements in the early resuscitation, as well as improved intensive care. With intense application of techniques such as those described above, reductions in mortality should be achievable whenever dedicated neuroanesthesiologists and other neuroclinical care providers are given adequate resources to treat their TBI patients.

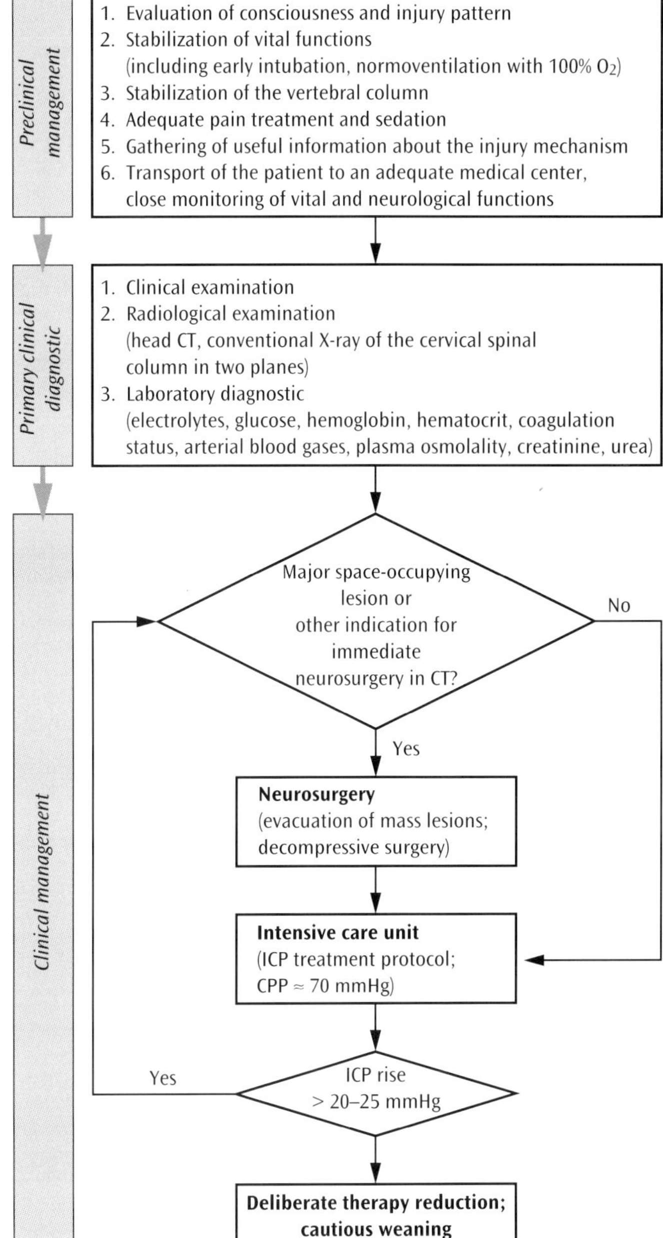

Figure 69.7 *General algorithm for the management of severely head-injured patients.*

REFERENCES

1. Gennarelli AT. Analysis of head injury severity by AIS-80. 24th Annual Conference, Morton Grove, IL: American Association for Automotive Medicine, 1980: 147–155.
2. Pettus EH, Christman CW, Giebel ML, Povlishock JT. Traumatically induced altered membrane permeability: its relationship to traumatically induced reactive axonal change. *J Neurotrauma* 1994; **11**: 507–22.
3. Povlishock JT. Traumatically induced axonal injury: pathogenesis and pathobiological implications. *Brain Pathol* 1992; **2**: 1–12.
4. Ommaya AK, Schatsky SA, Awae DC, *et al*. The role of whiplash in cerebral contusion. 10th Stapp Car Crash Conference, Society of Automotive Engineers, New York, 1966: 314–24.
5. Gurdjian ES. Recent advances in the study of the mechanism of impact injury of the head: a summary. *Clin Neurosurg* 1972; **19**: 1–42.
6. Shatsky SAAWAE, DE, *et al*. Traumatic dislocations of the primate head and chest: correlation of biomechanical, radiological and pathological

data. 18th Stapp Car Crash Conference, Society of Automotive Engineers, Warrendale, PA, 1974: 351–81.

7. Courville CB. Coup-contrecoup mechanism of cranio-cerebral injuries. *Arch Surgery* 1942; **45**: 19–43.
8. Simpson DA, Ryan GA, Paix BR, *et al.* Brain injuries in car occupants: a correlation of impact data with neuropathological findings. International Research Council on the Biomechanics of Impacts, Bron, France, 1991: 89–100.
9. Sachs F. Mechanical transduction by membrane ion channels: a mini review. *Mol Cell Biochem* 1991; **104** (1–2): 57–60.
10. Bowman CL, Ding JP, Sachs F, Sokabe M. Mechanotransducing ion channels in astrocytes. *Brain Res* 1992; **584** (1–2): 272–86.
11. Tavalin SJ, Ellis EF, Satin LS. Mechanical perturbation of cultured cortical neurons reveals a stretch-induced delayed depolarization. *J Neurophysiol* 1995; **74:** 2767–73.
12. Bullock R, Zauner A, Woodward JJ, *et al.* Factors affecting excitatory amino acid release following severe human head injury. *J Neurosurg* 1998; **89:** 507–18.
13. Di XH, Watson, JC, Bullock, MR. Excitotoxic damage in neurotrauma: fact or fiction. *Restorative Neurol Neurosci* 1996; **9:** 231–41.
14. Pellerin L, Magistretti PJ. Glutamate uptake into astrocytes stimulates aerobic glycolysis: a mechanism coupling neuronal activity to glucose utilization. *Proc Natl Acad Sci USA* 1994; **91:** 10625–9.
15. King LR, McLaurin RL, Knowles Jr HC. Acid–base balance and arterial and CSF lactate levels following human head injury. *J Neurosurg* 1974; **40:** 617–25.
16. Siesjo BK. Pathophysiology and treatment of focal cerebral ischemia. Part II: Mechanisms of damage and treatment. *J Neurosurg* 1992; **77:** 337–54.
17. Barzo P, Marmarou A, Fatouros P, *et al.* Magnetic resonance imaging-monitored acute blood–brain barrier changes in experimental traumatic brain injury. *J Neurosurg* 1996; **85:** 1113–21.
18. Kushi H, Katayama Y, Shibuya T, *et al.* Gadolinium DTPA-enhanced magnetic resonance imaging of cerebral contusions. *Acta Neurochir Suppl* 1994; **60:** 472–4.
19. Klatzo I. Pathophysiological aspects of brain edema. *Acta Neuropathol* 1987; **72:** 236–9.
20. Rosner M. Cyclic CSF pressure waves causally related to systemic arterial blood pressure. In: Avezaat CJJ, van Einhove M, Maas AIR, Tans JTJ (eds). *Intracranial Pressure VIII*. Berlin: Springer-Verlag, 1993.
21. Graham DI, Adams JH, Doyle D. Ischaemic brain damage in fatal non-missile head injuries. *J Neurol Sci* 1978; **39** (2–3): 213–34.
22. Chesnut RM, Marshall LF, Klauber MR, *et al.* The role of secondary brain injury in determining outcome from severe head injury. *J Trauma* 1993; **34** (2): 216–22.
23. Chesnut RM, Marshall SB, Piek J, *et al.* Early and late systemic hypotension as a frequent and fundamental source of cerebral ischemia following severe brain injury in the Traumatic Coma Data Bank. *Acta Neurochir Suppl* 1993; **59:** 121–5.
24. Gentleman D. Causes and effects of systemic complications among severely head injured patients transferred to a neurosurgical unit. *Int Surg* 1992; **77:** 297–302.
25. Harders A, Kakarieka A, Braakman R. Traumatic subarachnoid hemorrhage and its treatment with nimodipine. German tSAH Study Group. *J Neurosurg* 1996; **85** (1): 82–9.
26. A multicenter trial of the efficacy of nimodipine on outcome after severe head injury. The European Study Group on Nimodipine in Severe Head Injury. *J Neurosurg* 1994; **80:** 797–804.
27. Maxwell WL, Irvine A, Adams JH, *et al.* Response of cerebral microvasculature to brain injury. *J Pathol* 1988; **155:** 327–35.
28. Schroder ML, Muizelaar JP, Bullock MR, *et al.* Focal ischemia due to traumatic contusions documented by stable xenon-CT and ultrastructural studies. *J Neurosurg* 1995; **82:** 966–71.
29. Rosner MJ. Introduction to cerebral perfusion pressure management. *Neurosurg Clin N Am* 1995; **6:** 761–73.
30. Asgeirsson B, Grande PO, Nordstrom CH. A new therapy of post-trauma brain oedema based on haemodynamic principles for brain volume regulation. *Intensive Care Med* 1994; **20:** 260–7.
31. Boarini DJ, Kassell NF, Coester HC, *et al.* Comparison of systemic and cerebrovascular effects of isoflurane and halothane. *Neurosurgery* 1984; **15:** 400–9.
32. Eintrei C, Leszniewski W, Carlsson C. Local application of ^{133}Xenon for measurement of regional cerebral blood flow (rCBF) during halothane, enflurane, and isoflurane anesthesia in humans. *Anesthesiology* 1985; **63:** 391–4.
33. Hansen TD, Warner DS, Todd MM, *et al.* Distribution of cerebral blood flow during halothane versus isoflurane anesthesia in rats. *Anesthesiology* 1988; **69:** 332–7.
34. Madsen JB, Cold GE, Eriksen HO, *et al.* CBF and CMRO2 during craniotomy for small supratentorial cerebral tumours in enflurane anaesthesia. A dose-response study. *Acta Anaesthesiol Scand* 1986; **30:** 633–6.
35. Madsen JB, Cold GE, Hansen ES, Bardrum B. The effect of isoflurane on cerebral blood flow and metabolism in humans during craniotomy for small supratentorial cerebral tumors. *Anesthesiology* 1987; **66:** 332–6.
36. Madsen JB, Cold GE, Hansen ES, *et al.* Cerebral blood flow and metabolism during isoflurane-induced hypotension in patients subjected to surgery for cerebral aneurysms. *Br J Anaesth* 1987; **59:** 1204–7.
37. Michenfelder JD, Sundt TM, Fode N, Sharbrough FW. Isoflurane when compared to enflurane and halothane decreases the frequency of cerebral ischemia during carotid endarterectomy. *Anesthesiology* 1987; **67:** 336–40.
38. Scheller MS, Todd MM, Drummond JC. Isoflurane, halothane, and regional cerebral blood flow at various levels of PaCO2 in rabbits. *Anesthesiology* 1986; **64:** 598–604.
39. Todd MM, Drummond JC. A comparison of the cerebrovascular and metabolic effects of halothane and isoflurane in the cat. *Anesthesiology* 1984; **60:** 276–82.
40. Young WL, Prohovnik I, Correll JW, *et al.* Cerebral blood flow and metabolism in patients undergoing anesthesia for carotid endarterectomy. A comparison of isoflurane, halothane, and fentanyl. *Anesth Analg* 1989; **68:** 712–17.
41. Maekawa T, Tommasino C, Shapiro HM, *et al.* Local cerebral blood flow and glucose utilization during isoflurane anesthesia in the rat. *Anesthesiology* 1986; **65:** 144–51.
42. Kuramoto T, Oshita S, Takeshita H, Ishikawa T. Modification of the relationship between cerebral metabolism, blood flow, and electroencephalogram by stimulation during anesthesia in the dog. *Anesthesiology* 1979; **51** (3): 211–17.
43. Conzen PF, Vollmar B, Habazettl H, *et al.* Systemic and regional hemodynamics of isoflurane and sevoflurane in rats. *Anesth Analg* 1992; **74** (1): 79–88.
44. Kitaguchi K, Ohsumi H, Kuro M, *et al.* Effects of sevoflurane on cerebral circulation and metabolism in patients with ischemic cerebrovascular disease. *Anesthesiology* 1993; **79:** 704–9.
45. Manohar M. Regional brain blood flow and cerebral cortical O2 consumption during sevoflurane anesthesia in healthy isocapnic swine. *J Cardiovasc Pharmacol* 1986; **8:** 1268–75.
46. Scheller MS, Nakakimura K, Fleischer JE, Zornow MH. Cerebral effects of sevoflurane in the dog: comparison with isoflurane and enflurane. *Br J Anaesth* 1990; **65:** 388–92.
47. Sakabe T, Kuramoto T, Inoue S, Takeshita H. Cerebral effects of nitrous oxide in the dog. *Anesthesiology* 1978; **48** (3): 195–200.
48. Todd MM. The effects of $P_a\text{co}_2$ on the cerebrovascular response to nitrous oxide in the halothane-anesthetized rabbit. *Anesth Analg* 1987; **66:** 1090–5.
49. Sperry RJ, Bailey PL, Reichman MV, *et al.* Fentanyl and sufentanil increase intracranial pressure in head trauma patients. *Anesthesiology* 1992; **77:** 416–20.
50. Cavazzuti M, Porro CA, Biral GP, *et al.* Ketamine effects on local cerebral blood flow and metabolism in the rat. *J Cereb Blood Flow Metab* 1987; **7:** 806–11.
51. Kiening KL, Unterberg AW, Bardt TF, *et al.* Monitoring of cerebral oxygenation in patients with severe head injuries: brain tissue PO2 versus jugular vein oxygen saturation. *J Neurosurg* 1996; **85:** 751–7.
52. Clifton GL, Jiang JY, Lyeth BG, *et al.* Marked protection by moderate hypothermia after experimental traumatic brain injury. *J Cereb Blood Flow Metab* 1991; **11** (1): 114–21.
53. Marion DW, Obrist WD, Carlier PM, *et al.* The use of moderate therapeutic hypothermia for patients with severe head injuries: a preliminary report [see comments]. *J Neurosurg* 1993; **79:** 354–62.
54. Dietrich WD, Alonso O, Halley M, Busto R. Delayed posttraumatic brain hyperthermia worsens outcome after fluid percussion brain injury: a light and electron microscopic study in rats. *Neurosurgery* 1996; **38:** 533–41; discussion 541.
55. Polin RS, Shaffrey ME, Bogaev CA, *et al.* Decompressive bifrontal craniectomy in the treatment of severe refractory posttraumatic cerebral edema. *Neurosurgery* 1997; **41** (1): 84–92; discussion 92–4.
56. Ward JD, Becker DP, Miller JD, *et al.* Failure of prophylactic barbiturate coma in the treatment of severe head injury. *J Neurosurg* 1985; **62:** 383–8.
57. Muizelaar JP, Marmarou A, Ward JD, *et al.* Adverse effects of prolonged hyperventilation in patients with severe head injury: a randomized clinical trial. *J Neurosurg* 1991; **75:** 731–9.

70

Transmission of infection

ALAN R TAIT AND PAUL R KNIGHT

A major clinical challenge facing anesthesiologists today is to develop ongoing strategies to improve the quality of patient care, satisfaction, and medical outcome. In the past, infection control was considered low priority among anesthesiologists. However, with the expanding role of the anesthesiologist as the "total perioperative physician," the increasing number of invasive procedures performed by anesthesiologists, and with the increase in the prevalence of emerging diseases, stringent attention to infection control practices has now become of paramount importance.

Successful control of infection in the perioperative period requires not only application of infection control practices, but also a thorough understanding of the relation between the host and the pathogen. This understanding is important as many perioperative anesthetic practices and procedures can impact upon the incidence of postoperative infectious complications by altering mechanisms that control the equilibrium of this relation. For these reasons, the anesthesiologist must adhere to the principles of infection control and have a basic understanding of how anesthesia and surgery can affect the entry, infectivity, antigenicity, and pathogenicity of an invading microorganism.

Of growing concern, too, is the transmission of blood-borne and airborne pathogens from an infected patient to the anesthesiologist. Anesthesiologists are now exposed to an increasing number of patients who are at risk for, or who are infected with, human immunodeficiency virus (HIV), hepatitis B and C, and tuberculosis. This has heightened the awareness of the anesthesiologist to the possibility of occupational transmission and has led to the institution of national and international standards to reduce the potential for infection in the work place.

This chapter examines the subject of infectious disease as it applies to anesthetic practice in the perioperative period. We will discuss the epidemiology of infectious disease as it relates to the perioperative environment, and briefly review the mechanisms of the immune system responsible for host defenses and examine how these systems may be altered by anesthesia and surgery. In addition, we will describe a number of the most important nosocomial infections, discuss the technical aspects of infection control, and review the standards for prevention of occupational transmission of blood-borne and airborne pathogens.

EPIDEMIOLOGY

Approximately 70% of all acute illness can be attributed to infectious agents.[1] Nosocomial infections are estimated to occur in approximately 5% of patients in the USA, increasing the average length of hospital stay by 4 days and causing an estimated 60 000 deaths per year.[2] Nosocomial infections are primarily bacterial and are particularly prevalent in patients with decreased immune function. Viral infections are estimated to cause only 5% of nosocomial infections, but can cause significant morbidity in the immunocompromised patient. These infections typically reflect the seasonal patterns of viral disease in the community.

Transmission of hospital-acquired infections typically occurs by direct inoculation via one of the following routes:

1 the respiratory tract, following contact with an infected individual, placement of endotracheal tubes, inhalation of airborne pathogens, contamination of respiratory therapy and/or anesthesia equipment, or aspiration of oropharyngeal, or gastric contents;
2 the urinary tract, from indwelling catheter placement and/or surgery;
3 the skin and mucous membranes, from direct contact with infectious lesions or material, or as a result of surgery, trauma, or burns;
4 the skin and mucous membranes, from direct contact with infectious lesions or material, or as a result of surgery, trauma, or burns;
5 via the placement of grafts and prostheses.

Control of nosocomial infections should be directed at interrupting the infectious cycle. Use of barrier precautions, attention to aseptic technique, and strict compliance with other infection control practices, such as handwashing and sterilization/disinfection of equipment, are important in denying a portal of entry for microorganisms. Recognition of the interactions between anesthesia, immunology, and infection may be critical in optimizing patient management and subsequent outcome.

There is also a responsibility for anesthesiologists to protect themselves from occupational acquisition of disease. Following the advent of the acquired immunodeficiency syndrome (AIDS) epidemic, the increasing incidences of hepatitis C virus (HCV), and the omnipresent hepatitis B virus (HBV), the "Bloodborne Pathogen Standard" was established to protect the healthcare worker (HCW) from occupational exposure to blood-borne pathogens. At the core of the standard was the concept of universal precautions, which is now accepted as the primary means of protecting the HCW from occupational exposure to blood and bodily fluids. More recently, with the resurgence of tuberculosis throughout the world, the concept of universal precautions was expanded to include exposure to airborne pathogens. The term "standard precautions" is now used to reflect this change.

Typically, occupational transmission of disease from the patient to HCW occurs via the following routes:

1 parenteral exposure to infected blood, blood products, or blood-containing bodily fluids via a contaminated needlestick or other penetrating injury;

2 mucocutaneous exposure to infected blood, blood products, or bodily fluids, e.g. blood splash to the conjunctiva;
3 the respiratory system from exposure to airborne pathogens, e.g. tuberculosis;
4 direct contact from touching or from large-droplet spread.

To reduce the risk of bidirectional transmission of disease, the patient's underlying disease and/or immune status must be known. Thus, anesthesiologists must learn to adopt a high index of suspicion for patients who present for surgery with evidence of infection of unknown etiology or risk factors for disease. Furthermore, anesthesiologists must be familiar with standard precautions and be motivated to comply with them.

The interrelation of factors that predispose the patient to infection is outlined in Fig. 70.1.

PATHOGENESIS OF INFECTION

Resistance to infection

Although a cause–effect relation between anesthesia practice and the development of nosocomial infection is difficult to quantify, there are many aspects of practice that may predispose the patient to infection. Violation of the patient's natural protective barriers, poor infection control practices, and the use of anesthetic agents and drugs which may compromise the patient's immune system can all contribute to the development of a nosocomial infection. The purpose of this section is to review the ways in which anesthesia practice may contribute to the development of infection in the hospitalized patient and, as such, should not be considered a formal review of the immune system.

The first line of host defense is to deny a portal of entry for the microorganism. The initial integumentary barriers include the skin, conjunctiva, mucous membranes, and endothelial linings of the gastrointestinal and genitourinary tracts. The skin provides both a mechanical barrier to infection by virtue of its low water content, mild acidity, and constant desquamation and a chemical barrier owing to the secretion of long-chain fatty acids and the presence of resident nonpathogenic microbial flora. The mucous membranes possess special defenses in that many of their secretions, e.g. tears and cervical mucus, contain bacteriostatic agents such as lysozyme. Violation of these barriers by surgery, trauma, burns, or placement of intravascular catheters permits access of infectious agents into the body.

The endothelial linings of the genitourinary and gastrointestine secrete mucus that contains various proteins that are inhibitory to microbial growth. Bacteriocidal enzymes such as lysozyme, and specific secretory immunoglobulins that directly destroy or inhibit invading microbial agents. Damage to the endothelial linings of the gastrointestinal and urinary tracts as a result of disease, e.g. renal calculi, or abrasions by urinary catheters, can facilitate the entry of pathogenic agents.

Barrier protection of the upper airway involves the nasal hair and the labyrinthine effect of the nasal anatomy. The mucociliary clearing system protects the lower respiratory tree by ciliary propulsion of unwanted particles cephalad; 90% of deposited material is cleared within 1 hour via this process. However, volatile anesthetics and analgesics depress this ciliary activity and the cough reflex.[4] Mucus and saliva containing

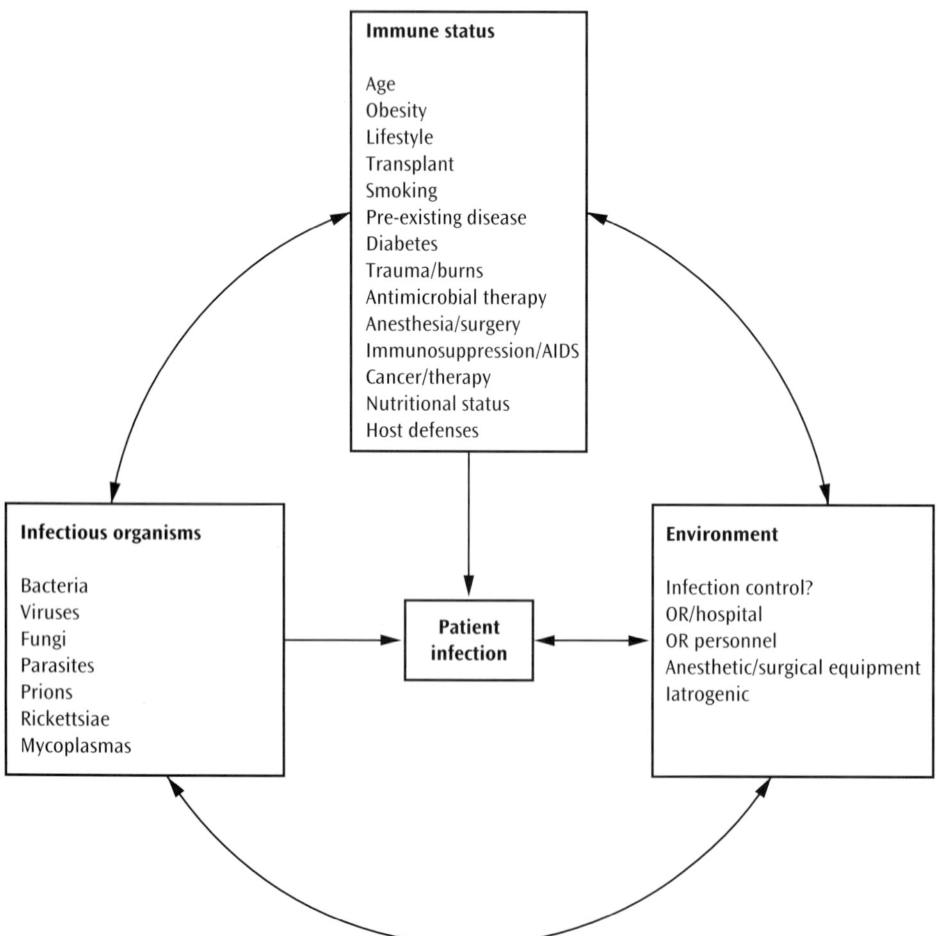

Figure 70.1 *Schematic representation of the interrelation of factors that predispose the patient to infection in the operating room (OR). Note that infection may be bidirectional between patient and personnel.*

IgA antibodies, lysozyme, and lactoferrin are important in preventing attachment of microorganisms and as bacteriostatic agents.

The respiratory tract is of special concern to the anesthesiologist owing to the possibility of mechanical trauma associated with airway instrumentation. Placement of airway devices and the use of non-humidified air may interfere with the normal ciliary clearing system. Furthermore, obtunded reflexes during anesthesia may allow for the regurgitation of acidic and/or particulate gastric contents that may damage the respiratory epithelium and ciliary blanket.

Once microorganisms gain a portal of entry, they are subjected to a number of nonadaptive (innate) and adaptive host responses. Three major factors determine their success in establishing an infection. The first is the microorganism's ability to enter the patient and survive (infectivity) and the second is the ability of the host to mount an immune/inflammatory response (antigenicity or immunogenicity). These two factors determine the microorganisms' invasiveness and how well they will spread systemically or to contiguous regions. The third factor is the microorganism's virulence or ability to produce pathology (pathogenicity). The microorganism's invasiveness and/or virulence depends on where it successfully enters the body, the inoculum size, the host's immune status, and the environment at the point of inoculation.

Having penetrated the host's integumentary barriers, invading microorganisms are subjected to innate nonspecific defense mechanisms. These are mobilized in response to chemoattractants such as cytokines that are produced by microbial activity at the site(s) of inoculation. These chemoattractants are produced by injured tissues and macrophages in response to microbes, microbial products, or products of tissue injury and can stimulate the recruitment of other phagocytes (macrophages, neutrophils, and eosinophils) as well as natural killer (NK) cells. Complement via the alternative pathway may also be activated in a nonadaptive sense and result in direct bacterial killing and activation of phagocytosis by leukocytes using a combination of low pH, digestive enzymes, and the production of highly reactive oxygen-free radicals. The acute inflammatory (acute phase) response, which is initiated by this sequence of events, promotes further recruitment of inflammatory cells, augments humoral activity, and enhances tissue damage.

The final adaptive line of defense is acquired and includes both humoral and cellular components. The humoral arm of the adaptive response involves the production and release of immunoglobulins (IgG, IgA, IgE, IgM, IgD) by plasma cells following differentiation from a subset of B lymphocytes.

Immunoglobulins may directly damage or inhibit the ability of the microorganism to be invasive or pathogenic by binding to key proteins on the microorganism's surface and/or by neutralizing substances released by the microorganism, which are responsible for the agents virulence (i.e. endotoxin). Antibodies also enhance the antimicrobial activity of nonadaptive responses such as complement activation and phagocytosis.

The cellular response to infection is mediated by a subset of specific lymphocytes that are directly cytotoxic to foreign cells. Like the B cell, the cytotoxic T lymphocytes require interaction with macrophages to recognize specific antigens on foreign cells.

Effects of anesthesia and surgery on the resistance to infection

It is well known that anesthesia and surgical stress alter the response of a number components of the immune system. However, although these changes have been well documented, their ability to alter clinical outcome (negatively or positively) is more difficult to assess.

Alterations to both the adaptive and nonadaptive host defenses occur following anesthesia and surgery.[3,4] Surgically induced changes correlate with the extent of trauma. For example, tissue injury, ischemia caused by tourniquets and hemostatic occlusion of vessels, and maldistribution of blood flow due to hypovolemia and/or vasoactive mediators can all activate proinflammatory responses and neurohumoral reflexes, including catecholamines, corticosteroids, and prostanoids. Increases in systemic corticosteroid levels promote IL-10 (interleukin 10) responses while inhibiting production of IL-1β, IL-2, tumor necrosis factor (TNF-α), IL-6, IL-8, and interferon (IFNγ).[5] Increases in the stress response by surgery may, however, be tempered by the effects of anesthesia. For example, anesthetics may directly alter immune/inflammatory responses and attenuate the stress response by decreasing cortisol, catecholamine, and cytokine levels.[6,7] Differentiation of direct vs. indirect effects of anesthetic agents indicates that general anesthetics directly inhibit cellular immune responses, even when surgical "stress" is controlled by neural blockade.

The balance of cytokine responses is clearly altered by anesthesia and surgery. Trauma-induced increases in TNF-α and IL-1β levels can stimulate generation of transforming growth factor (TGF-β) and IL-6, leading to elaboration of prostaglandin E_2 (PGE_2). PGE_2 suppresses macrophage growth antigen presentation, and increased catecholamine levels alter the sensitivity of macrophages to PGE_2. Macrophage phagocytosis, antigen presentation, expression of class II major histocompatibility complex, and membrane-bound IL-1β activity are all decreased by surgery.[8] Enhanced IL-10 production is also promoted by trauma-induced IL-6, TGF-β, and TNF-α. Evidence of increased T2 phenotypic cytokine activity is present following surgery. For example, inhibition of IFNγ-mediated activation of lymphocyte cytotoxicity occurs in both patients and mice exposed to anesthesia with or without surgery.[9,10] Additionally, decreased hypersensitivity reactions, NK cell activity, and mixed lymphocyte responses have been reported.

Anesthesia and surgery may also decrease the total number of T lymphocytes in the peripheral blood and alter the ratio of T helper cells. B lymphocytes are not decreased to the same extent, and antibody responses appear to be better maintained than the cellular responses.[8] Experimentally in mice, and in patients following anesthesia and surgery, a soluble mediator(s) has been detected, which decreases the cytotoxicity of lymphocytes and monocytes. Mediator inhibition of NK cell cytolytic responses is associated with increased lung metastases in mice.[11] Recent reports suggest that this soluble mediator may be IL-4 or IL-10.[12,13] Thus, there is much evidence to support the hypothesis that anesthesia and surgery promote T2 phenotypic responses.[12] Experimentally, enhancing T2 phenotypic responses following pulmonary bacterial challenge leads to decreased clearance and increased mortality.[14]

Blood transfusions are an important aspect of anesthesia practice; however, transfusions have been shown to decrease cytotoxic lymphocyte production, tumor necrosis factor levels, and NK activity.[15] Furthermore, blood transfusions have been associated with an increased risk for tumor recurrence and infection.[16]

NOSOCOMIAL INFECTIONS

Nosocomial respiratory tract infections

Pneumonia, second only to urinary tract infections, is the leading cause of hospital-acquired infection, accounting for 10–20% of all nosocomial infections and up to 50% of infection-associated mortality.[17] In one study, 75% of patients with bacterial pneumonia became infected following surgery.[18] A number of risk factors have important implications for anesthesia practice. A principal concern is the association of pneumonia with the placement of an endotracheal tube and mechanically assisted ventilation. The incidence of respiratory tract infections in patients requiring an endotracheal tube can be as high as 17–20%.[19] Additionally, the risk of acquiring ventilator-associated pneumonia (VAP) increases by as much as 1% per day. Seeding of oropharyngeal organisms into the trachea may occur during passage of the tube. Bacteria may also aggregate on the surface of the endotracheal tube forming a biofilm or glycocalyx that may actually protect the bacteria from host defenses.[18] These aggregates, however, may also become dislodged and embolize distally, setting up a focus of infection. The endotracheal tube may also facilitate infection by acting as a conduit that bypasses the mucociliary "blanket." Pooling of secretions around the cuff of the endotracheal may also provide a haven for colonizing bacteria. Endotracheal tube-induced mechanical abrasion and irritation of the respiratory mucosa, impairment of normal laryngeal function leading to an increased risk of aspiration of upper respiratory tract secretions, and bacterial flora and/or gastric contents may also be important in the pathogenesis of postoperative pneumonia.

Although ventilators alone are not considered an important source of bacterial spread, breathing circuits can become heavily contaminated with microorganisms from the patient's oropharynx and trachea. Single-use disposable circuits or disinfection of components of the breathing system after each use are, however, equally effective in preventing cross-infection between patients. Use of bacterial and/or viral filters has been advocated to prevent contamination;[20,21] however, their ability to prevent transmission of nosocomial infections requires further evaluation.[22,23]

Recent studies have identified a number of additional risk factors for the development of nosocomial pneumonia. These include persons greater than 70 years of age, altered mental status (particularly closed-head injuries with placement of intracranial pressure monitors), thoracoabdominal procedures, underlying chronic lung disease, history of large-volume aspiration, trauma, perioperative use of antibiotics, and obesity. Other factors include 24-h ventilator circuit changes, contaminated anesthesia or respiratory therapy equipment, stress ulcer prophylaxis with cimetidine, presence of a tracheostomy[24] or nasogastric tube, and recent bronchoscopy.[18]

Approximately 60% of nosocomial infections are caused by aerobic Gram-negative bacteria, in particular the Enterobacteriaceae and *Pseudomonas* spp. (see Table 70.1). *Staphylococcus aureus* (10–20% of infections) and *Streptococcus pneumoniae* (3–8%) are also important. The prognosis associated with infection with Gram-negative bacteria, particularly *Pseudomonas,* is considerably worse than that associated with infection with Gram-positive bacteria, which, in turn, is worse than that associated with viral pneumonia.[25] Interestingly, although rare, *Legionella* spp. in some hospitals may cause over 30% of lower respiratory infections. Older and immunocompromised patients have a high mortality rate from legionnaires' disease.[18]

Nosocomial viral infections represent approximately 20% of all pneumonia cases[21] and may be an important source of morbidity and mortality in immunocompromised patients. Most of these are caused by influenza virus, respiratory syncytial virus (RSV), and parainfluenza virus. Nosocomial fungal pulmonary infections represent approximately 4% of nosocomial pneumonias. *Aspergillus* sp., in particular, has been shown to cause severe illness in patients undergoing bone marrow transplants and chemotherapy. Less common agents responsible for less than 1% each of nosocomial pneumonias include *Cryptococcus, Mycoplasma pneumoniae, Moraxella catarrhalis, Hemophilus influenzae, Pneumocystis pneumoniae*, and cytomegalovirus (CMV).

Although many nosocomial pneumonias are polymicrobial, an infectious agent cannot be identified as the etiologic source in up to 40% of hospital-acquired pneumonias. Guidelines have now been formulated because of the difficulty in diagnosing nosocomial pneumonias. These include techniques such as bronchoalveolar lavage and quantitative culture of protected-specimen brushing.

Although the pathogenesis of nosocomial pneumonia results primarily from aspiration of bacteria colonized from the oropharynx, nosocomial pneumonia may also develop as a result of inhalation of aerosols containing infective nuclei, bacteremia, and aspiration or translocation of gastrointestinal bacterial flora. Colonization of the upper airway with Gram-negative bacilli is dependent on several factors which include: (1) the length of time spent in the hospital; (2) the use of antibiotics; (3) underlying pulmonary disease; (4) the presence of azotemia; and (5) endotracheal intubation and/or nasogastric suctioning. Bacterial factors that promote the colonization of Gram-negative bacilli include the presence of pili, epithelial cell receptors, fibronectin on the mucosal surface, and the protease content in the oral cavity.[26] Use of antacids and histamine-2 blockers that raise gastric pH may result in an overgrowth of Gram-negative rods in the stomach. Recently, however, sucralfate, a cytoprotective drug that protects the gastric mucosa without raising pH, has been shown to be effective in lowering the risk of pneumonia.[27]

Postoperative wound infections

Between 500 000 and 920 000 surgical wound infections occur annually in the USA.[28] Postoperative surgical infections result primarily from direct inoculation of pathogenic microorganisms from the patient's skin flora, from infected host tissue, and from contaminated surgical equipment or personnel. Airborne contamination and hematogenous–lymphatic seeding may also result in infection. The pathogenesis of these infections involves several factors, including nutritional status, extremes of age, obesity, underlying disease, presence of diabetes, steroid therapy, and level of host immunity. Wound-related factors include the degree of tissue trauma and presence of foreign material, whereas microbial factors include the concentration and virulence of the microbes and antibiotic use.[28]

Surgical or accidental trauma and iatrogenic injury (e.g. pressure) result in edema, which limits blood flow and diminishes the efficacy of the acute nonadaptive immune response. Established bacteria can release compounds that inhibit neutrophil and macrophage functions such as phagocytosis. Local trauma to the skin predisposes the injured dermis to a cellulitis and subsequent deep bacterial tissue invasion. Subcutaneous infections, abscesses, myositis, and hematogenous spread may result from this process.

Surgical procedures are classified as clean, clean contaminated, or contaminated. The most common microorganisms associated with surgical wounds are *S. aureus,* enterococci, and coagulase-negative staphylococci. The distribution of microbial pathogens, however, is clearly dependent on the source of contamination (e.g. GI, respiratory).

Prevention of surgical- and/or pressure-related infections should focus on the use of good clean technique and limiting the amount of local pressure when positioning the patient. Pressure-induced breakdown of the skin in susceptible parts of the body is prevented by proper body placement and padding of bony prominences and other areas of focused pressure. Although appropriate antibiotic prophylaxis has been shown to be efficacious, the issue of routine prophylaxis remains contentious, given the increasing demands to reduce hospital costs. Since the late 1800s, the surgical face mask has become a standard element of good infection control practice. However, despite the fact that face masks have been shown to reduce the dissemination of airborne bacteria from the nose and mouth, their ability to reduce surgical wound infections has been questioned.[29,30] In one study, the rate of postoperative wound infections was 4.7% for operations performed with unmasked personnel (surgical and anesthesia) and 3.5% when face masks were used.[29] Ironically, the importance of the surgical face mask today may be less to do with protecting the patient from infection than

Table 70.1 *Causes of nosocomial pneumonia*

Agent	Incidence	Source of contamination	Associated findings
Common etiologic agents			
Gram-positive bacteria			
Staphylococcus aureus	14.6%	Upper respiratory tract flora	Seen in elderly and debilitated patients or in patients after a viral infection
Streptococcus pneumoniae	< 3%	Upper respiratory tract flora	Most common cause of community-acquired pneumonias; also seen in patients with chronic obstructive pulmonary disease and following influenza virus infections
Gram-negative bacteria			
Pseudomonas aeruginosa	17.2%	Colonization of respiratory tract from environmental sources	Primarily a nosocomial pneumonia seen in patients with cystic fibrosis, burn patients, patients on long-term antibiotics, steroids, immunosuppressive drugs. and patients with long-term hospital stays
Klebsiella spp.	7.4%	Colonization of respiratory tract from environmental sources	Primarily a nosocomial pneumonia associated with altered states of consciousness, aspiration pneumonitis, patients on antibiotics, steroids, or antimetabolites
Enterobacteriaceae spp.	10.4%	Colonization of upper respiratory tract from gastrointestinal tract flora with aspiration into the lower respiratory tract	As above
Escherichia coli	6.4%	As above	As above
Serratia marcescens	4.5%	Environmental sources	As above
Proteus spp.	4.2%	Environmental sources	As above
Hemophilus influenzae	6.4%	Airborne, environmental sources	Most common in patients with chronic lung disease. Vaccine now available
Respiratory syncytial virus (RSV)	Hospital endemic; may account for up to 40% of infant nosocomial pneumonias in isolated settings	Exposure of infectious droplets from an infected person	Can be a major source of morbidity and mortality in hospitalized children in isolated locations
Legionella pneumophila	Hospital endemics may account for 4–30% of nosocomial pneumonias in isolated settings	Contamination of potable water. Air-conditioning units	Associated with an underlying illness, older males who smoke, or patients on immunosuppressive drugs – tends to occur in isolated outbreaks
Less common etiological agents			
Moraxella catarrhalis *Mycoplasma pneumoniae* *Aspergillus* Influenza A Cytomegalovirus *Pneumocystis carinii*	< 1% each		
Fungi	4%		
Unknown etiology	~40%		

in protecting the healthcare worker from inadvertent contact with blood or secretions from a patient infected with hepatitis or HIV.

Percutaneous intravascular infections

In the USA, more than 25 000 patients per year develop device-related bacteremias.[31] Local cellulitis, abscess formation, septic thrombophlebitis, and endocarditis may also occur.

Access of bacteria following intravascular line placement may follow contamination of the device insertion site by endogenous bacterial flora on the skin, contamination of the infusate, contamination at hub junctions, contamination of air inlet and in-line filters, and contamination of accessory devices such as transducers, manometers, i.v. piggybacks, and stopcocks.

Factors that predispose to intravascular infections include: (1) suppressed immune states (extremes of age, chemotherapy, severe illness, blood dyscrasias); (2) changes in normal skin function (burns, psoriasis, alteration of normal microbial flora); (3) hygiene of medical personnel (handwashing); (4) spread from other infected loci; (5) catheter risk factors: composition (plastic/Teflon > steel, stiff > flexible, thrombogenicity), size (large bore > small bore), and use (balloon-tipped > percutaneous, multilumen > single lumen); and (6) placement site (central > peripheral, femoral > subclavian), duration of placement (72 h or more > less than 72 h), type (cutdown > percutaneous, emergent > elective), and the skill of person inserting the catheter. Virtually all perfusates are capable of supporting bacterial growth, particularly lipid-based solutions and parenteral nutrition solutions. Recently, a number of cases of bacterial contamination of propofol have been described.[32]

Bacterial colonization of the skin at the device insertion site is the greatest associated risk factor for local infection. In total, 50–66% of device-related infections are due to *Staphylococcus* spp. *Pseudomonas* and *Corynebacterium* spp. may also produce local infection from colonization of the skin, *Klebsiella*, *Enterobacter*, *Serratia*, and *Citrobacter* spp. from contaminated infusate, and *Streptococcus*, *Staphylococcus*, and less commonly *Escherichia* spp. from other infected loci. *Candida* infections often result from contaminated parenteral nutrition solutions. Bacteria trapped by in-line filters may also serve as sources of sepsis by releasing endotoxins[33] that can initiate the proinflammatory cytokine cascade (e.g. TNF, IL-1, IL-6).

Clinical diagnosis of catheter-associated infections requires a high index of suspicion for fever of unknown origin, a positive blood culture for *Staphylococcus*, *Candida* or unusual microorganisms, and bacteremia or septicemia unresponsive to antimicrobial therapy. A presumptive diagnosis may be made based on the presence of bacteremia or sepsis in a patient with an indwelling intravascular line and no other source of infection, cellulitis or phlebitis at the catheter site, > 15 microbial colonies from the cultured catheter tip, resolution of fever following removal of the catheter, clustered infections by infusate-related microorganisms, or evidence of distal septic thrombi.

Bacteremia and septicemia

Bacteremia is defined as the presence of bacteria in the blood as confirmed by culture. In general, bacteremia is a transient phenomenon, but takes on greater significance for patients with endocarditis and intravascular infections. Septicemia is generally considered a more serious symptomatic state.

Besides percutaneous intravascular catheters, bacteremias may also occur when mucosal surfaces such as those lining the oropharyngeal cavity and the large intestine are traumatized or instrumented. Bacteremia may also occur following seeding from the urogenital tract or gastrointestinal and respiratory systems, or from pre-existing infections in these areas. Furthermore, translocation of normal gut flora such as *Escherichia coli* into the bloodstream may occur in patients following long-term parenteral nutrition.

Bacteremias have also been described following transfusion of contaminated blood products, drug infusates such as propofol, and parenteral nutrition solutions and have been associated with mortality rates as high as 35%.[34] *Pseudomonas* is the most important etiologic agent, accounting for as many as 28% of such infections.[34] *Yersinia enterocolytica* may proliferate in packed red blood cells stored at 4 °C and produce significant sepsis in the recipient.[35] Other bacteria associated with transfusion-related infections include *Escherichia coli*, *Serratia marcescens*, and *Staphylococcus* spp.

In terms of anesthetic practice, airway-related bacteremias are increased in the patient who is difficult to intubate, requires a double-lumen endotracheal tube, or undergoes rigid bronchoscopy. In addition, nasal placement of an endotracheal tube in patients with sinusitis may serve to seed the lower respiratory tract. The anesthesiologist can reduce the risk of bacteremia by scrupulous attention to aseptic technique, including handwashing and use of sterile gloves, skin preparation, catheter insertion and fixation, and appropriate care when infusing fluids and injecting drugs into the circuit during intravascular catheter placement.

A diagnosis of Gram-negative bacteremia and septicemia carries with it very high mortality. Care must be taken during laryngoscopy to minimize any trauma to the patient's oropharyngeal mucosa and to ensure proper handling and cleaning of the laryngoscope blades following use in patients who are the most likely to have Gram-negative bacterial colonization of the oropharynx, .

Although *E. coli* septicemias are common, other agents such as *Klebsiella*, *Enterobacter*, *Serratia* and *Pseudomonas* spp. are also important. *Pseudomonas* septicemia has the highest mortality rate of all the Gram-negatives and is often seen in the immunosuppressed patient or burn victim. Other than *S. aureus*, Gram-positive bacteremias do not carry as high a mortality. *Staphylococcus* and group A β-hemolytic *Streptococcus* are the most common Gram-positive pathogens to be isolated from blood cultures and generally result from the placement of intravascular catheters.

Candida, the fungal agent most frequently isolated from blood cultures, is found primarily in immunocompromised patients. *Candida* fungemias generally occur iatrogenically from placement of intravascular devices and pressure-monitoring devices.[36]

Endocarditis

Infective endocarditis (IE) is an infection involving the endocardial surface of the heart, particularly the heart valves. Infections of arterio-arterial and arteriovenous shunts and coarctation of the aorta may also be included in this diagnosis. Although difficult to assess, the incidence of IE ranges between 0.16 and 5.4 cases per 1000 admissions.[37]

The prodrome to the development of IE is an alteration in the endocardial surfaces and valves. Surface changes resulting from blood turbulence, metabolic changes, or trauma provide a nidus for fibrin and platelet deposition, and result in the formation of a nonbacterial thrombotic endocarditis (NBTE). Risk factors for NBTE include cardiac and Swan–Ganz catheters, rheumatic heart disease, malignancy, and uremia. Bacterial colonization of NBTE encourages further deposition of fibrin and platelets and the formation of vegetations that may affect valve function and/or be released as emboli. Colonization of pre-existing NBTE typically follows a transient bacteremia. This may occur following trauma to heavily colonized mucosal surfaces (e.g. dental extractions, periodontal surgery, tonsillectomy, and urethral dilation). Classically, the organisms associated with IE are the streptococci, staphylococci, and enterococci, although some Gram-negative bacteria and *Candida* have been isolated.

Patients with congenital or valvular heart disease, patients with pacemaker wires, and those with intravascular shunts are at increased risk for developing IE. Intravenous drug abusers, especially cocaine users, are at significant risk for IE involving the tricuspid valve. Nosocomial endocarditis is associated with the placement of pacemakers, dialysis shunts, and intravenous catheters and may represent up to 28% of all cases of IE. Patients who have an increased risk for contracting IE should be given prophylactic antibiotics immediately before surgery.[38] Recommended therapy is based on the type of procedure and the most likely associated organism. For most procedures, oral amoxicillin (2 g, 1 h before procedure) or parenteral ampicillin (2 g, i.m. or i.v. 30 min prior to procedure) provide adequate coverage. Other regimens may include clindamycin, cephalexin, vancomycin, gentamicin, and azithromycin.

Nosocomial urinary tract infections

Approximately 80% of urinary tract infections result following placement of an urethral catheter and a further 5–10% as a result of manipulation of the genitourinary tract. Unlike nosocomial pneumonias, which are often polymicrobial, approximately 95% of urinary tract infections are due to a single bacterial species. The most commonly isolated organism is *E. coli* followed by *Pseudomonas, Klebsiella, Proteus, Staphylococcus*, and *Enterobacter* spp.

Use of a closed system to collect urine dramatically decreases the incidence of bacteriuria; however, even with a closed system, bacteriuria will occur in almost all patients by 30 days. The duration of catheterization poses the greatest risk of bacteriuria. It has been estimated that for every day that a urinary catheter is in place the risk of infection increases by 3–10%.[39] The majority of urinary tract infections are caused by the patient's own endogenous intestinal flora, which migrates across the perineum and colonizes the periurethral area and enters the bladder during insertion of the catheter or by migration along the catheter lumen. The urethral catheter acts as a haven for colonizing bacteria, which are retained in a biofilm on the catheter surface. Furthermore, colonization of the catheter by urease-producing organisms may result in crystallization and blockage of the lumen.

Additional risk factors for the development of nosocomial urinary tract infections include female gender, diabetes, lack of antibiotic prophylaxis, contaminated equipment, poor catheter care and attention to hygienic practice, colonization of the drainage bag, and abnormal serum creatinine levels. Although most bacteriurias are asymptomatic, approximately 30% of patients will exhibit symptoms. Bacteremias account for approximately 15% of all nosocomial bloodstream infections. Mortality from urinary tract-originated bacteremias is less than 15% and is almost always confined to immunocompromised patients. Although antibiotics have been shown to decrease the incidence of urinary tract infections, their use prophylactically to postpone bacteriuria is not usually indicated because of concerns regarding bacterial resistance, cost, and side-effects.

THE INFECTED PATIENT

Pre-existing respiratory tract infections

Patients who present for surgery while harboring a respiratory tract infection may be at increased risk of intraoperative and postoperative complications. The increased secretions and airway reactivity that often accompany these infections can increase the risk of airway complications intraoperatively and arterial oxygen desaturation postoperatively. Furthermore, the potential for the development of postoperative pneumonia in patients presenting with an upper respiratory tract infection (URI) is of major concern.

Although the majority of these infections are viral, there are several bacterial infections that are important, including otitis media, gum and other maxillofacial abscesses, acute or chronic sinusitis, and bacterial pharyngitis. These may result in increased airway reactivity and serve to seed the lower respiratory tract by either aspiration or inoculation during placement of airway devices, inhibition of the normal bronchial toilet, or positive-pressure ventilation.

When evaluating the patient with pharyngitis, it is important to differentiate between viral and bacterial etiologies. The majority of cases of bacterial pharyngitis are due to group A β-hemolytic streptococci (e.g. *Streptococcus pyogenes*). Approximately 0.5% of all URIs are complicated by sinusitis. Sinusitis may develop into severe craniofacial or brain abscesses. Purulent discharge from the sinuses may also be aspirated into the lower respiratory tract. The most common etiologic agents of sinusitis are *Streptococcus pneumoniae, Hemophilus influenzae*, and *Moraxella catarrhalis*.

Otitis media is one of the most common diseases of childhood. Over 66% of children have had one or more episodes of otitis media by the age of 3 years. The majority of infections are due to *S. pneumoniae* and *H. influenzae* and are generally easily treated with antibiotics. Other infections of the oral cavity and neck may also be important as they may cause airway obstruction and/or may contain pus. Examples of these types of infections include Ludwig's angina, parotitis, and cervical adenitis.

Viral nasopharyngitis (the common cold) accounts for approximately 95% of all URIs. In the USA, adults average 2–4 colds per year and children 6–8 colds.[40] Approximately 40% of cases of the common cold are caused by rhinoviruses, of which there are 100 immunotypes. However, nasopharyngitis can also be caused by several other virus types including coronavirus, parainfluenza virus, adenovirus, influenza virus, and RSV.

Other important respiratory tract infections include acute laryngitis, bronchitis, bronchiolitis, acute pneumonia, laryngotracheobronchitis (croup), and epiglottitis. Croup accounts for approximately 10–15% of lower respiratory tract disease in children.[41] It causes inflammation of the subglottic region and is characterized by dyspnea and stridor on inspiration. The primary causative agent of croup is parainfluenza virus.

Bronchiolitis is another important infection particularly in children less than 2 years of age. Up to 75% of cases of bronchiolitis are caused by RSV. Care should be taken to avoid anesthetizing children with RSV because of the increased reactivity of the airways.

Laryngitis causes hyperemia and edema of the larynx and may be of viral or bacterial origin. Further mechanical irritation may make the edema worse.

Epiglottitis is a rapidly progressive cellulitis of the epiglottis caused by *H. influenzae* and is a true anesthetic emergency. When epiglottitis is suspected, a definitive diagnosis should be confirmed only in a location in which endotracheal intubation and emergency tracheostomy can be performed by skilled personnel. A cherry red epiglottis is pathognomonic in establishing the diagnosis. Bacterial tracheitis may mimic epiglottitis, but usually occurs in older children. Fortunately, the recent widespread use of the *H. influenzae* type b polysaccharide vaccine (Hib) has resulted in a dramatic reduction in the incidence of this disease.[42]

Approximately 58–89% of patients presenting with acute community-acquired pneumonia have at least one underlying disease, and up to 36% will have some form of immunosuppression.[43] This is important to recognize when evaluating the patient preoperatively.

When a patient presents for surgery with a lower respiratory tract infection or a severe URI, elective surgery should be canceled if at all possible. As studies suggest that altered airway reactivity can continue for 4–6 weeks following a respiratory tract infection, it would seem prudent to forgo elective anesthesia and surgery for at least 4 weeks after cessation of symptoms.

Human immunodeficiency virus (HIV)

As of December 1997, 641 086 cases of AIDS had been reported to the Centers for Disease Control (CDC). Furthermore, present estimates indicate that 2 million individuals in the USA and 23 million worldwide may be infected with HIV.[44]

HIV, the causative agent of AIDS, is an RNA virus in the lentivirus subfamily of retroviruses. To date, two major forms of HIV have been identified, HIV 1 and 2. The primary targets for HIV are the $CD4^+$ T lymphocytes, although monocytes and macrophages may also support viral replication. The initial or window phase of the infection follows exposure, during which the patient is infectious but may not have seroconverted. Within 1 week of the initial exposure, the individual may experience an acute flu-like illness characterized by fever, lymphadenopathy, rash, and fatigue. During this period, there may be an initial rapid depletion of the $CD4^+$ T cells and, often, accompanying viremia. Typically, seroconversion occurs within 2–6 weeks of exposure, but may not occur for 6 months or longer. Therefore, individuals with risk factors for HIV infection should not donate blood. Following the initial phase there is a latent period that may last for up to 10 years or more. However, this period ends when the CD4+ T cells levels again begin to decline. Monitoring of these levels is important in gauging the immune status of the patient. Indeed, a CD4+ T-cell count of less than 200 mm^{-3} (normal = 1 000 mm^{-3}) is now part of the case definition of AIDS even in the absence of symptoms. This late or symptomatic stage is characterized by numerous recurrent opportunistic infections, lymphadenopathy, weight loss, and, in some cases, neurologic manifestations such as dementia and peripheral neuropathy.

Since the formal discovery of AIDS in 1981, a number of risk factors have been established for the disease. Reports issued by the CDC suggest that approximately 48% of cases occur via male homosexual–bisexual contact; 26% are due to intravenous drug abuse; 4% and 39% of cases among men and women, respectively, arise from heterosexual contact; and 1% of cases are due to receipt of contaminated blood or blood products. Approximately 8% of cases are of undetermined etiology. Occupational transmission of HIV accounts for approximately 0.1% of AIDS cases. Approximately 91% of pediatric (< 13 years) AIDS cases result from perinatal infection.

As of December 1997, the CDC had received reports of 54 HCWs in the USA with documented occupational transmission of HIV and 132 with possible transmission. Of those with documented transmission, 46 (85%) had a percutaneous exposure, five (9.3%) had mucocutaneous exposures, and two (3.7%) had both types of exposure. One individual had an unknown route of exposure, and 49 out of the 54 HCWs were exposed to blood from an HIV-infected patient. The total number of individuals with occupationally acquired HIV, however, is probably higher, as many cases are not reported.[45] Risk factors that are believed to influence occupational transmission of HIV include: (1) factors related to the exposure, e.g. route, depth of inoculation, type of contamination (blood, bodily fluid), and concentration of virus; (2) patient (donor) factors, e.g. stage of HIV illness, presence of viremia, use of antiviral chemotherapy; and (3) HCW (recipient) factors, e.g. lack of skin integrity, inadequate first aid following exposure, immune status, and concurrent viral infection. Although there are no definitive reports, an apparent case of occupational transmission of HIV to an anesthesiologist has been reported[46] following an accidental needlestick during placement of a central venous catheter. The estimated risks of acquiring HIV from a needlestick or mucocutaneous exposure are 0.31% and 0.09% respectively. Based on data from a recent study, approximately 1138 anesthesiologists may have received an accidental needlestick from an HIV-infected patient.[47] Assuming an infection rate of one seroconversion per 200 needlesticks, at least five anesthesiologists may have become infected by this means.

Hepatitis viruses

Hepatitis B virus (HBV)

Among unvaccinated individuals, hepatitis B virus (HBV) poses the greatest risk to the HCW. It is estimated that 140 000–320 000 infections occur each year in the USA, resulting in 8400–19 000 hospitalizations and 140–320 deaths per year. Among HCWs, an estimated 8700 HBV infections occur annually in the USA and, of these, approximately 400–440 require hospitalization and 200 die from acute or chronic HBV infection.[48] In total, 5–10% of persons infected with HBV become chronic carriers.

Occupational transmission of HBV can occur following exposure to minute amounts of blood so that rates of transmission via needlestick injury are high, estimated at between 10% and 35%. Among anesthesiologists, the rates of HBV seroconversion following exposure have been estimated at between 12.7% and 48.6%.[48] A vaccine for HBV is available and has proved efficacious. Among healthy adults, seroconversion rates following vaccination are between 89% and 100%.[49] Since 1985, use of the vaccine and modification of high-risk behavior has resulted in a 55% decrease in the incidence of the disease. The present thrust to vaccinate children and adolescents should further decrease the risk of disease. In instances when the vaccine is unavailable or contraindicated, immune globulin is the treatment of choice.

Hepatitis C virus (HCV)

Hepatitis C virus, also known as parenteral non-A, non-B hepatitis, now presents a serious threat to the HCW. It is estimated that 150 000–180 000 HCV infections occur each year in the USA, of which 2% are reported among HCWs exposed to blood.[50] The fact that approximately 85% of those infected will become chronic carriers is of particular concern. HCV is most efficiently transmitted by repeated or large percutaneous exposures to blood. A major cause of post-transfusion hepatitis, HCV is now also a major source of infection among intravenous drug users. However, a number of studies have identified occupational transmission of HCV. In one study,[50] 23 out of 1677 (1.4%) hospital employees in a community hospital were seropositive for HCV. The incidence among physicians was 2.4%, with accidental needlestick injuries cited as the principal mode of occupational transmission. The risk of seroconversion following percutaneous exposure to HCV infected blood is estimated to be approximately 3.5% and appears to increase with the size of the needle (hollow bore) and the amount of the inoculum. However, in one study, the risk of transmission following a contaminated needlestick injury was as high as 10%.[51]

Transmission of HCV has also been demonstrated via a blood splash to the conjunctiva,[52] and a series of patient-to-patient transmissions in Australia implicated contamination of an anesthetic breathing circuit.[53] To date, there is no vaccine available for protection against the hepatitis C virus, and postexposure prophylaxis with immune globulin does not appear to prevent seroconversion. Postexposure protocols should include education regarding further transmission of the disease and 6-month follow-up testing for anti-HCV activity.

Hepatitis A virus (HAV)

An estimated 125 000–200 000 HAV infections occur annually in the USA. In Europe and the USA, prevalence in young adults varies between 30% and 70% but is less than 10% in small children. HAV produces an acute disease with a mortality rate below 0.5%. Transmission is primarily via the fecal–oral route. A vaccine is available which is highly effective although pre- and postexposure prophylaxis with immune globulin can also be used.

Hepatitis D virus (delta agent, HDV)

HDV is a defective single-stranded RNA virus that requires simultaneous infection with HBV to replicate. Frequently, this occurs when a chronic carrier of HBV is exposed to the delta agent.[54] Persons with HDV–HBV co-infection tend to have a more severe infection with a higher risk of fulminant hepatitis (2–20%) and a greater chance of developing chronic liver disease and cirrhosis (70%-80%) than patients with HBV alone. For the HCW, percutaneous exposures offer the greatest risk; therefore, attention to standard precautions and care in handling sharp devices is imperative. Co-infection of HBV–HDV can be prevented by vaccination for HBV; however, superinfection of HDV in a person with chronic HBV cannot be prevented.

Hepatitis E virus (HEV)

HEV is the major etiologic agent in enterically transmitted non-A, non-B hepatitis throughout the world. Transmission of HEV is by the fecal–oral route and, although person-to-person transmission appears to be uncommon, nosocomial transmission has occurred.

Hepatitis G virus (HGV)

Hepatitis G virus accounts for 0.3% of acute viral hepatitis. An estimated 900–2000 infections occur annually in the USA, of which 90–100% develop into chronic infections. High-risk groups include transfusion recipients and intravenous drug users. Although HGV has not been cited as an occupational pathogen, its blood-borne route of transmission may present a risk for accidental needlestick injuries.

Tuberculosis

Tuberculosis remains one of the leading causes of morbidity and mortality throughout the world. According to the World Health Organization, approximately 30 million people will have died from tuberculosis in the period from 1990 to 1999.[55] From the early 1950s to 1984, the incidence of tuberculosis in the USA decreased to approximately 5.3% per year. However, in the period between 1985 and 1992 the overall incidence unexpectedly increased by nearly 20%. Much of this increase was attributed to the burgeoning HIV epidemic and the concomitant appearance of multidrug-resistant *Mycobacterium tuberculosis* (MDR-TB).

The increased pattern of disease and the mode of airborne spread via droplet nuclei posed an immediate challenge to the HCW. In 1991, the CDC reported a cluster of seven hospital outbreaks of MDR-TB, resulting in a case fatality of 72–89%.[56,57] In another report, 31% of susceptible HCWs seroconverted following exposure to a patient with active tuberculosis. Although there are no reported cases of occupational transmission of tuberculosis to an anesthesiologist, anesthesiologists, by virtue of their participation in procedures that may induce coughing, such as bronchoscopy and endotracheal intubation, are undoubtedly at risk. Vaccination with bacille Calmette Guérin (BCG) is available and, despite its unpredictable efficacy, it is still used in many parts of the world.

Herpesviruses

Herpes simplex virus (HSV)

Herpes simplex viruses (HSV) are among the most ubiquitous infectious agents in man. Two distinct serotypes of this DNA virus exist. HSV-1 is extremely common in childhood and is transmitted primarily via the oral route. Once infected, the virus remains dormant throughout life, residing in the sensory ganglia that innervate the primary site of infection. Activation of the infection may occur following a number of stimuli, including stress and immunosuppression. Active lesions generally occur around the mouth, lips, and skin above the waist. Anesthesiologists may be particularly vulnerable to herpetic whitlow following unprotected contact with open lesions from an infected patient.[58] Thus, anesthesiologists should wear gloves when in contact with the oral mucosa of infected patients and maintain good handwashing practices. Furthermore, primary HSV-1 has been reported following mouth-to-mouth resuscitation. HSV-2 is most often transmitted venereally or following vaginal delivery of the newborn.

HSV may be associated with significant morbidity and mortality in patients who are immunocompromised. Transplant patients in particular frequently excrete HSV-1 in throat washings and, therefore, pose a risk to the anesthesiologist during manipulation of the patient's airway.[59] Severe infections among transplant patients are thought to be due to iatrogenic suppression of cell-mediated immunity.

Patients may also be at risk of acquiring HSV from an infected anesthesiologist. Infected personnel should be appropriately protected or should avoid treating patients during exacerbations. Fortunately, the virus is particularly susceptible to changes in environment and universal precautions are generally sufficient to prevent transmission.

Oral acyclovir has proven efficacious in reducing the frequency and severity of the infection. Vidarabine has also been shown to helpful in patients with herpes encephalitis and neonatal herpes infections.

Varicella-zoster virus (VZV)

Varicella-zoster virus (VZV) is a highly contagious member of the herpesvirus family. VZV causes two distinct clinical diseases. Varicella (chickenpox) is a highly contagious primary infection occurring mostly in childhood. A more localized form of the disease known as herpes zoster (shingles) forms the second spectrum of the disease and occurs mostly in the elderly.

Direct contact and airborne and droplet spread are the primary mechanisms of transmission. Typically, most nosocomial outbreaks are limited to children and immunocompromised patients. VZV in patients with compromised immune systems carries significant morbidity and mortality. In one study, one-third of children with lymphoproliferative malignancies developed progressive VZV disease with multiorgan involvement.[60] The mortality in this population of patients is approximately 15–18%.[60] When managing the patient with shingles or varicella, the anesthesiologist should wear a mask in addition to gloves and, if nonimmune, should avoid contact with the patient altogether.

Recently, a live varicella vaccine has been approved although long-term issues of safety and efficacy have yet to be determined.[61] For HCWs, the American Medical Association (AMA) has recommended vaccination of susceptible HCWs at risk of occupational acquisition of the disease.[62]

Cytomegalovirus (CMV)

In total, 60–80% of individuals over the age of 30 years possess the CMV antibody. Occupational transmission of CMV appears to be limited;[63] however, anesthesiologists who are pregnant should avoid contact with infected patients. Infection appears to occur following direct, intimate contact with the excretor or with contaminated secretions including urine, saliva, respiratory secretions, tears, feces, breast milk, semen, and cervical secretions. The risk of transfusion related CMV is 2.5% per unit of blood given. Infants infected with CMV and immunocompromised patients undergoing chemotherapy or organ transplantation are the principal reservoirs in hospitals. CMV infections can be particularly serious among immunocompromised patients and may predispose these patients to fatal opportunistic infections. Prevention of occupational transmission should focus on good hygienic precautions.

Epstein–Barr virus (EBV)

Epstein–Barr virus is most commonly associated with infectious mononucleosis, but has also been implicated with Burkitt's lymphoma and chronic fatigue syndrome. Although outbreaks of EBV have been described in the hospital setting,[64] the risk of occupational transmission is limited. Transmission occurs via intimate oral contact, and less frequently via blood transfusion, solid organ transplantation, and bone marrow donations. Prevention should be aimed at attention to hygienic practices, standard precautions, and handwashing.

Human herpesvirus 6 and 7 (HH-6 and HH-7)

Recently, two other herpesviruses, human herpesviruses 6 and 7 (HH-6, HH-7), have been identified. HH-6 is the etiologic agent in roseola infantum, which may present as a risk for nosocomial infection in pediatric wards.[65] HH-7 has recently been identified in saliva but, as yet, has not been associated with nosocomial disease.

PROTECTION OF THE HEALTHCARE WORKER

Prevention of occupational transmission of infection in anesthesiology practice

Blood-borne pathogens

In response to the increasing concern regarding occupational exposure of HCWs to blood-borne pathogens, the CDC issued a series of guidelines aimed at reducing transmission of these diseases.[66] Subsequently, the Occupational Health and Safety Administration (OSHA) issued "The Bloodborne Pathogen Standard."[67] This mandated that all employers should implement an exposure plan to protect the HCW and ensure accurate documentation of exposures and follow-up protocols.

The OSHA standard incorporates the concept of universal precautions, which assumes that all patients are infected and that barrier techniques be used to avoid contact with the patient's blood and body fluids. However, in 1996, the concept of universal precautions was expanded to include other routes of infection, e.g. airborne. This new definition was termed "standard" precautions and applies to any exposure to blood and blood products, semen, vaginal fluids, cerebrospinal fluid, synovial, pleural, pericardial, peritoneal and amniotic fluids, saliva in dental procedures, and any bodily fluid visibly contaminated with blood. Furthermore, nonintact skin, mucous membranes, unfixed tissue or organs from living or dead persons, and HIV-containing laboratory specimens should be considered as part of these "standard" precautions.[68] The risks of exposure to occupational pathogens are detailed in Table 70.2.

The standard precaution policy requires the use of barrier precautions such as gloves, face-shields, eye protection, and gowns to prevent skin and mucous membrane exposure to blood and bodily fluids. However, the choice of barrier precautions should be commensurate with the level of anticipated risk of exposure. For example, 98% of anesthesiologists' exposures to blood could have been prevented by the use of gloves.[69] Typical exposures for the anesthesiologist might include percutaneous placement of indwelling catheters, tracheal intubation and suctioning, bronchoscopy, and endoscopy.

According to the CDC, 80% of all occupational exposures to blood-borne pathogens occur following a contaminated needlestick. Risk factors associated with exposure via this route include the volume and number of infectious particles in the inoculum, and the depth of the injection.[70] The use of hollow-bore (particularly large gauge) needles poses a greater risk than use of solid suture needles.

In one survey, 36.7% of anesthesiologists reported having received at least one contaminated needlestick injury within the previous 12 months.[45] Additionally, in a recent multicenter study by Greene *et al.*[71], 74% resulted from injury from a hollow-bore needle and 74% were preventable. The authors projected that in 30 years, 17 and 155 anesthesiologists in the USA would contract HIV and HCV, respectively, following a contaminated percutaneous injury.

The Bloodborne Pathogen Standard recommends that needles should never be bent, broken, or recapped, and should be placed in puncture-proof containers after use. However, one survey indicated that 69.8% of anesthesiologists recapped needles on a frequent basis. Recently, a number of manufacturers have developed disposable syringe and needle systems that avoid the need to recap. Also, several needleless systems for the administration of drugs have been developed. Other methods of occupational transmission include dissemination of papillomavirus in the smoke from laser surgery and the aerosolization of infected blood and tissue during invasive orthopedic procedures.

In a survey of emergency nurses, universal precautions were followed only 16.5% of the time.[72] Indeed, the CDC suggests that 40% of all occupational exposures to HIV could have been avoided if universal guidelines had been employed. Reasons for noncompliance suggest that HCWs are too busy, do not always anticipate blood contact, or consider the patient low risk,[73] or that barrier supplies are not always readily available.[74]

Airborne pathogens (tuberculosis)

The CDC has developed guidelines for prevention of airborne transmission,[75] which focus on: (1) early diagnosis by ensuring access and availability of diagnostic tests; (2) source controls or prevention of transmission at the source, i.e. the patient, e.g. use of personal respirators and patient isolation; (3) engineering controls including negative

Table 70.2 *Occupational risk of important pathogens*

Organism	Source	Transmission	Prevention	Approximate risk
Human immunodeficiency virus (HIV)	Infected blood, blood products or bodily fluids	Needlesticks, contact with mucous membranes, open cuts or sores	Avoid needlesticks, standard precautions	0.3% needlestick 0.09% mucocutaneous
Hepatitis B virus (HBV)	See HIV	See HIV	Avoid needlesticks, standard precautions, immunization	10–35%
Hepatitis C virus (HCV)	See HIV	See HIV. Contaminated anesthesia equipment?	Avoid needlesticks, standard precautions No vaccine available	3.5%
Herpes simplex virus (HSV)	Infected fluid from open lesions	Contact with mucous membranes, open cuts or sores	Gloves, handwashing	Minimal, herpetic whitlow important
Varicella-zoster virus (VSV)	Respiratory secretions/droplets	Respiratory tract, direct contact	Masks, gloves, handwashing, immunization	Minimal
Cytomegalovirus (CMV)	Secretions, blood	Direct contact, associated with transfusions and transplants	Masks, gloves. Avoid contact if pregnant	Minimal
Tuberculosis	Infectious droplet nuclei	Airborne	HEPA respirator, negative-pressure environment BCG	Low

pressure patient environments, ultraviolet light sources, high-efficiency particulate air filters (HEPAs), and personal respirators; (4) sterilization and disinfection of equipment; (5) screening that includes regular (at least annual) tuberculin (Mantoux) testing; and (6) chemoprophylaxis and BCG vaccination when appropriate.

Surgery for patients with tuberculosis should be delayed until the patient is no longer infectious. Patients are considered no longer infectious if they have received antituberculosis medications and have had three consecutive negative sputum smears taken on different days. In case of urgency, surgery should be performed in operating rooms with negative pressure ventilation and as few personnel as possible. Anesthesiologists should wear HEPA respirators (individually fitted) that meet the N95 standard issued by the National Institute for Occupational Safety and Health. To prevent contamination of the anesthesia machine, a HEPA filter should be placed between the Y-connector and the mask or other airway device. Bacterial filters placed on the expiratory port of the ventilator may also prevent spread of the tubercle bacilli into the atmosphere.

Postoperative care of the tuberculous patient should occur, where possible, in a recovery room with negative pressure ventilation. If this is not feasible, the patient should remain in the operating room until safe transfer to a suitable isolation room is possible.

Prophylaxis following occupational exposure to blood-borne pathogens

Following an accidental needlestick or other sharps injury, the HCW should immediately seek first aid. Having cleaned the wound, the exposure must be reported to the employee health service for counseling and a recommendation for postexposure prophylaxis (PEP). The rationale for PEP is based on a perceived window of opportunity following exposure that offers a chance to prevent, or at least, attenuate the ensuing viremia. In one study, PEP with zidovudine (ZDV, 1 g day^{-1} for 3–4 weeks) was administered to 31 HCWs infected following percutaneous exposure and resulted in a decrease in the odds of HIV seroconversion of 79%.[76] Although ZDV remains the first-order drug for most HIV-PEP, combinations of ZDV with other nucleosides such as lamivudine (3TC; Epivar) and the new protease inhibitors such as indinavir (IDV) have been shown to be highly effective. International consensus now recommends treatment for 4 weeks with ZDV in combination with 3TC.[77] International guidelines recommend the addition of protease inhibitors for all significant exposures; however, the USA recommends their use only for high-risk exposures or when resistance to ZDV is suspected.[76]

In general, PEP should only be recommended for HCWs following exposures associated with a high likelihood of HIV transmission. HCWs with lower risk exposures should be offered PEP after ascertaining the risk/benefit of treatment. PEP for HCWs with negligible risk is not justified at this time. PEP should be instituted, if possible, within 1–2 h following exposure and continued for a minimum of 4 weeks. HIV antibody tests should be performed at baseline, 6 weeks, 3 months, and 6 months, and HCWs should be monitored for side-effects if on PEP. It may also be prudent for exposed workers to be tested for HBV and HCV at 6 weeks post exposure.

Postexposure prophylaxis for HBV is recommended for accidental percutaneous or permucosal exposures. Unvaccinated HCWs should receive HB immunoglobulin (0.06 mL kg^{-1}, i.m.) followed immediately by HBV vaccine at 0, 1, and 6 months.

Immunization of healthcare workers

The Advisory Committee on Immunization Practices (ACIP) and the Hospital Infection Control Practices Advisory Committee (HIPAC) have formulated a number of recommendations for the vaccination and protection of HCWs.[78] Diseases for which immunization is strongly recommended include HBV, influenza, measles, mumps, rubella, and varicella. BCG vaccination may also be warranted in areas where tuberculosis is endemic. Other vaccinations that may be indicated include HAV vaccine, meningococcal polysaccharide vaccine, typhoid vaccine, and vaccinia (smallpox) vaccine. Other vaccine-preventable diseases include tetanus, diphtheria, and pneumococcal diseases.

Anesthetic considerations for the infected patient

General dogma indicates that anesthesia is contraindicated for patients who present for surgery with an acute infection. Nowhere is this more evident than for the patient who presents with a URI. In one study, children with URIs were found to be two to seven times more likely to experience perioperative respiratory-related adverse effects than asymptomatic children, and 11 times more at risk if the patients had their tracheas intubated.[79] Our own findings, however, indicate no increase in perioperative complications for children with acute uncomplicated URIs undergoing minor surgery.[80]

Changes in airway reactivity, particularly in the recovery phase of the URI, and increased secretions may predispose the patient to intraoperative laryngospasm, bronchospasm, apnea, stridor, and blockage of the endotracheal tube. Postoperatively, patients may experience oxygen desaturation, atelectasis, postintubation croup, and pneumonia. Younger age and presence of an endotracheal tube appear to place the patient at increased risk. A recent study, however, suggests that placement of a laryngeal mask airway (LMA) results in less bronchospasm and fewer respiratory events than an endotracheal tube.[81] Based on our research, we believe that otherwise healthy patients presenting with acute uncomplicated URIs in which the secretions are clear and the patient is afebrile may be considered candidates for surgery. Similarly, patients with allergic or vasomotor rhinitis or patients with chronic rhinitis appear to be at no greater risk of perioperative complications. Patients who present with a bacterial infection, sinusitis, severe nasopharyngitis, fever greater than 38 °C, productive cough or flu- or croup-like symptoms should have their surgery delayed for a minimum of 4 weeks. Recommendations for the management of these patients include regional techniques, use of a mask or LMA instead of an endotracheal tube, hydration, humidified gases, and antisialagogues.

Anesthesia for the patient with AIDS poses a challenge to the anesthesiologist as these patients frequently present with multiorgan disease. In addition to the numerous opportunistic infections, many AIDS patients have decreased pulmonary function due to *Pneumocystis carinii* infection or tuberculosis. Neurologic function may also be affected, leading to dementia, seizures, and peripheral neuropathies. These findings may be important in decisions to use regional techniques. AIDS patients who present with wasting syndrome due to persistent diarrhea may be hypovolemic and have electrolyte imbalances. An increased risk of Addison's disease has also been noted in these patients. Furthermore, autopsy studies of AIDS patients describe multiple cardiac lesions including, pericardial effusion, fibrinous pericarditis, right ventricular hypertrophy, and evidence of Kaposi's sarcoma in the pericardium and myocardium.[82]

THE IMMUNOCOMPROMISED PATIENT

Pneumonia accounts for up to 40% of deaths in children and adults with cancer.[83] Furthermore, 35% of renal transplant recipients develop pneumonia in the first year following transplantation,[84] and approximately 64% of acute leukemia patients die from bacteremias originating in the lungs. Approximately 50% of bone marrow recipients and 25% of liver transplant patients will develop pneumonia. *P. aeruginosa*, *E. coli* and *Klebsiella pneumoniae* are the principal etiologic agents identified in immunocompromised patients with pneumonia.

Immunocompromise may also occur following iatrogenic disruption of the patient's integumentary barriers or suppression of the immune system by administration of immunosupressive drugs and/or radiation. Granulocytopenia and defects in phagocytosis occur in patients with acute leukemia, aplastic anemia, and bone marrow transplantation, and those on myelosuppressive therapy. These patients are prone to infections of the lung, oropharynx, perianum, and skin by Gram-negative bacilli, Gram-positive cocci, and *Candida* and *Aspergillus*. Pneumonia with *H. influenzae* or *Streptococcus* is prevalent in patients with humoral dysfunction associated with agammaglobulinemia, multiple myeloma, and chronic lymphocytic leukemia. Cellular immune dysfunction occurs with lymphoma, transplantation, AIDS, and cytotoxic drug administration, such as azathioprine, cyclosporine, and corticosteroids. These patients are prone to infections such as *Listeria monocytogenes* and *M. tuberculosis*, and numerous dimorphic fungal and herpesvirus infections. Opportunistic infections in this group of patients also include *Pneumocystis* pneumonia, HSV, VZV, CMV, tuberculosis, oral candidiasis, EBV, and CNS toxoplasmosis. Patients with severe combined immunodeficiency syndrome (SCID) have an absence of both humoral and cell-mediated immunity associated with marked lymphopenia, thymic abnormalities, and a lack of immunoglobulin. Patients who have tumors that obstruct natural passages and those with brain tumors that result in a loss of gag reflex may also be at increased risk of pulmonary infection. Finally, patients who are elderly, obese, or diabetic, or who smoke or have poor nutritional status are also at risk for infection.

Animal studies suggest that pulmonary metastases are increased following general anesthesia.[85] It has also been shown that in the immediate postoperative period lymphocyte cytotoxicity is diminished. This may have serious consequences for the immune-suppressed patient. Pretreatment of immunocompromised surgical patients with immune adjuvant may reverse these changes and decrease infections.[9] Blood transfusions may also contribute to a decrease in immune competency.[86] The immunosuppressive effect increases with the number of transfusions (see Chapter 23).

Throughout this chapter, emphasis has been placed on the importance of compliance with standard precautions, handwashing, and other infection control practices. Nowhere is this more important than in caring for the immunocompromised patient. HSV, for example, is troublesome to the healthy individual, but may be life-threatening in someone with poor immune function. In a survey of hygienic practices among anesthesiologists, 92% and 16% of respondents administered anesthesia while harboring a respiratory or HSV infection respectively.[87]

Aggressive antibiotic therapy in the immunocompromised host may alter the normal bacterial flora and increase the risk of nosocomial infections. Immunocompromised patients may also be malnourished, hypovolemic, and have electrolyte imbalances. Adjustments to anesthetic drug doses and hydration may be required in these patients. Patients who have been unable to eat may require early institution of enteral feeding following surgery, to avoid translocation of gut flora into the bloodstream.

PREVENTION OF PATIENT INFECTIONS

Infection control in anesthesia practice

Disinfection/sterilization of equipment

Anesthesia equipment may become contaminated as a result of direct contact with patients' blood and/or bodily fluids, contact with contaminated personnel, splashes from surgical procedures, airborne contamination, and poor infection control techniques in general. Although most anesthesia equipment today comes as sterile, disposable, single-use units designed for convenience and as a means to reduce cross-contamination and transmission of infection, there is still debate regarding the efficacy of using disposable vs. reusable items.[88]

In 1972, Spaulding[89] proposed that medical equipment should be categorized as critical, semicritical, and noncritical, based on the level of potential exposure and risk of infection. Items designated as critical include all those that are normally sterile, for example intravascular catheters, syringes, and needles, which make contact with areas of the body. These items must be sterile at the time of use. Semicritical items include those that come in contact with mucous membranes but do not ordinarily penetrate body surfaces. These include laryngoscope blades, oral and nasal airways, masks, temperature probes, and breathing circuits. Semicritical items should be subject to high-level disinfection.

Pulse oximeter probes, stethoscopes, blood warmers, ECG electrodes, blood pressure cuffs, the exterior of the anesthesia machine, and other types of equipment that do not normally come into contact with the patient or only touch unbroken skin satisfy Spaulding's noncritical classification. These should be cleaned with a detergent or disinfectant (low-level disinfection) at the end of the day or when obviously contaminated.

In general, routine sterilization or disinfection of the insides of the anesthesia machine is not required; however, valves and soda-lime canisters should be cleaned and disinfected with each change of absorbent. In one study, 25% and 44%, respectively, of circle systems and ventilators were contaminated. The working surfaces of anesthesia records should also be disinfected after each patient use. In one study, 51% of anesthesia records for coronary and vascular procedures were soiled and 36% tested positive for blood contamination.[90]

Sterilization implies the killing of all microorganisms, whereas disinfection, depending on the level (high, intermediate, or low), destroys vegetative organisms but not necessarily all bacterial and fungal spores or viruses. Sterilization usually involves the application of heat and pressure or gases to kill microorganisms. Steam sterilization employing saturated steam under pressure is recommended for a wide range of articles, including metal, cloth, glass and some thermoresistant plastics. Once used extensively, ethylene oxide (EtO) gas has been declared a health hazard by OSHA and a number of new techniques have been introduced to replace its use. These include radiosterilization, vapor-phase hydrogen peroxide (VPHP), VPHP/gas plasma discharge, low-temperature steam/formaldehyde, chlorine dioxide gas, and paracetic acid.[91]

High-level disinfectants include glutaraldehyde preparations, chlorine dioxide, hydrogen peroxide, and paracetic acid. Intermediate-level disinfectants include phenolic compounds, iodophors, and chlorine compounds. Low-level disinfectants include quaternary ammonium compounds and some phenolics and iodophors.

HBV can survive at 25 °C and drying for 1 week, but is killed by steam sterilization at 121 °C and 793 kPa for 20 min.[2] HBV is inactivated by 2% glutaraldehyde, 70% isopropyl alcohol, and 500 p.p.m. free chlorine from sodium hypochlorite. HIV is fairly labile and susceptible to many commonly used disinfectants (e.g. household bleach).[92]

Preventing infection during insertion of intravascular catheters

Placement of percutaneous catheters may serve as a route to introduce infection. Handwashing is central to infection control and standard precautions. During experimental rhinovirus infections, transmission of the virus occurs in 73% of cases via the hands and only 8% via sneezing and coughing.[93] Handwashing by anesthesiologists must be maintained before and after each patient contact, contact with blood or bodily fluids, and after glove use. In one study, 58% of anesthesiologists reported washing their hands after each patient contact, and 85% reported using aseptic technique for catheter placement.[87]

Preparation of the skin using a broad-spectrum antiseptic prior to catheter placement is important to prevent introduction of skin microflora into the wound. Examples of these include 1% iodine and 70% alcohol, chorhexidine, or iodophors. As discussed, the choice, site, and use of the catheter may be important in reducing the potential for infection. Catheters should be firmly secured and covered with a sterile dressing. Arterial catheters should not be exchanged over guidewires.

Administration sets and monitoring systems should be sterile and manipulated as little as possible. Transducer domes should not be reused and should be replaced together with continuous-flow devices every 48–72 h. Adequate pressure should be maintained by nonglucose-containing flush systems to prevent retrograde flow of blood. Stopcocks and injection ports should be kept free of blood and kept covered with a sterile cap when not in use.[94]

Preventing drug and medication contamination

Single-use ampules should be drawn up as close as possible to the time of use as bacteria can proliferate in solutions open to the atmosphere. Bacterial and fungal infections have been reported following contamination of propofol. Additionally, nosocomial outbreaks of bacterial and viral infections may occur following contamination of multidose vials.[95,96] Drugs should not have exceeded their expiration date, and aseptic technique should be used, including cleaning the rubber septum with alcohol and using a sterile needle and syringe to reduce the risk of infection. All drugs drawn up into a syringe should be administered as soon as possible or discarded within 24 h. Syringes, needles, infusion sets, and solutions should never be used on multiple patients. In one report, six patients contracted acute HBV infections from a reused syringe that had been in contact with a contaminated stopcock from a hepatitis B carrier.[97] Other studies describe patient-to-patient transmission of HIV and HBV from reused syringes.[98,99] Despite this, almost 20% of anesthesiologists report reusing syringes on a frequent basis.[85]

Preoperative blood screening

Approximately 10–20% of the 12 million units of blood collected and transfused annually in the USA are associated with adverse reactions.[100] Today, fewer than 5% will develop post-transfusion hepatitis and, of these, 90% will be HCV positive.[101] At the onset of the AIDS epidemic, transfusion-related HIV infections accounted for approximately 2% of all cases, however with the advent of improved donor screening, volunteer rather than paid donors, and the use of autologous blood donation, the risk of transmission of HIV from transfused blood and blood products is now estimated to be between 6.5×10^{-6} and 2.8×10^{-4} per unit.[102]

Preoperative chemoprophylaxis

It is important that anesthesiologists are aware of how to optimize the patient's prophylactic antibiotic management. Chemoprophylaxis prior to surgery is used in situations in which there is a high likelihood of exposure to pathogenic organisms. These include gastrointestinal or genitourinary surgery and surgery in patients with valvular heart disease, who are at risk for bacterial endocarditis. In general, a single dose of an antimicrobial agent given 30 min or less before skin incision provides adequate coverage. Unless there is obvious contamination, postoperative doses are generally unnecessary. Table 70.3 describes recommended prophylaxis regimens for the most common pathogens encountered by the surgical patient.

Antiviral prophylaxis may be important for patients who are immunocompromised. The most common antiviral agent used today is acyclovir. This deoxyguanosine analog has been shown to be most effective against HSV and VZV infections. Other important antiviral agents include amantadine (influenza), ganciclovir (CMV), zidovudine (HIV), and interferon-α2b (chronic HBV, HCV).

Table 70.3 *Preoperative chemoprophylaxis*

Type of surgery	Likely pathogens	Recommended drugs	Adult dosage
Cardiac	*S. epidermidis, S. aureus, Corynebacterium*, enteric Gram-negative bacteria	Cefazolin *or* cefuroxine *or* vancomycin	1–2 g, i.v. 1–2 g, i.v. 1 g, i.v.
Gastrointestinal	Enteric Gram-negative bacilli, enterococci, anaerobes	Cefoxitin *or* cefotetan *or* cefazolin	1–2 g, i.v. 1–2 g, i.v. 1–2 g, i.v.
Vascular	*S. aureus, S. epidermidis*, streptococci, enteric Gram-negatives, *Clostridia*	Cefazolin *or* vancomycin	1–2 g, i.v. 1 g, i.v.
Orthopedics	*S. aureus, S. epidermidis*	Cefazolin *or* vancomycin	1–2 g, i.v. 1 g, i.v.
Neurosurgery	*S. aureus, S. epidermidis*	Cefazolin *or* vancomycin	1–2 g, i.v. 1 g, i.v.
Obstetrics/ gynecology	Enteric Gram-negatives, anaerobes, enterococci, group B streptococci	Cefazolin *or* cefotetan *or* cefoxitin	1–2 g, i.v. 1–2 g, i.v. 1 g, i.v.
ENT	Anaerobes, enteric Gram-negatives, *S. aureus*	Clindamycin and gentamicin	600–900 mg, i.v. 1.5 mg kg^{-1}, i.v.
Ophthalmology	*S. epidermidis, S. aureus*, streptococci, enteric Gram-negatives, *Pseudomonas*	Gentamicin, ofloxacin, tobramycin, ciprofloxacin *or* neomycin–gramicidin–polymyxin B	Multiple topical drops over 2–24 h

Adapted from *The Medical Letter*, 1999; **41** (1060): 75–80.

EPIDEMIOLOGIC INVESTIGATION OF AN INFECTIOUS OUTBREAK FOLLOWING SURGERY

Clusters of cases involving infection among surgical patients or operating room personnel should be evaluated to determine if an outbreak or epidemic exists. The primary objectives of the investigation are to determine a diagnosis, and a common source, and to identify ways to prevent further transmission of the pathogen.

Consider an example in which four surgical patients develop fever (>39.4°C) and surgical wound infection within 12–72h of surgery. As this cluster of infections would be considered unusual, it is necessary to determine the etiologic agent responsible and whether a common source was apparent. A typical outbreak investigation would include the following steps:

1. Based on the patients' presenting symptoms and the timing of the onset of symptoms, make a differential diagnosis. The most common etiologic agents implicated in surgical wound infections include (in order): *S. aureus*, enterococci, coagulase-positive staphylococci, *E. coli*, and *P. aeruginosa.*
2. Examine the characteristics of the outbreak in terms of:
   - a person: age, sex, type of surgical procedure;
   - b place: did exposure occur in a common place, e.g. operating room?
   - c time: time of suspected exposure (surgery), onset of symptoms – an epidemic curve should be constructed to determine the possibility of a common agent.
3. Culture patients to determine etiologic agent and phage type.

Results from the initial findings of our hypothetical outbreak determined that all patients had undergone surgery in the same operating room on the same day. *S. aureus* was isolated from all patients and all had the same phage type, suggesting a common exposure.

Given this information, the next steps would be to:

4. Conduct a preliminary analysis to determine if a common source of infection exists and the potential vehicles/vectors, i.e. person-to-person, iatrogenic. Seek a common denominator and any unusual or secondary cases.
5. Formulate a causal hypothesis based on the available information, e.g. the etiologic agent, the source of infection, periods of exposure.
6. Test the hypothesis. Are there significant differences in attack rates between those exposed and those who were not? Was the source common to all patients? Examine the environment of exposure, e.g. anesthesia equipment, personnel.

In our hypothetical scenario, the one common factor was that all infected patients had received a propofol infusion that had been used for all patients by the same anesthesiologist. Given this information, culture of both the anesthesiologist and the used propofol ampule (if available) should be conducted to determine if *S. aureus* contamination had occurred and whether it was the same phage type as that isolated from the patient. Culture of unopened ampules of propofol from the same batch should also be performed to determine if the contamination was intrinsic (from manufacturer) or extrinsic (from contamination after opening). If there was no evidence of intrinsic contamination, did the contamination occur through poor infection control practices by the anesthesiologist?

7. Conclusions from the investigation: base conclusions on all the pertinent evidence and not on a single circumstance. Identify populations at risk and plan strategies for future prevention and control. This scenario is based on a true outbreak and emphasizes the importance of single-use administration of anesthetic drugs and the need for careful attention to aseptic technique.

In general, successful investigations of a disease outbreak involve good detective work utilizing an initial differential diagnosis and a final diagnosis from accurate clinical and laboratory information. Epidemic curves should be generated to identify cases in terms of times of onset and exposure. Attack rates, i.e. the number of persons exposed to the suspected etiologic agent who become infected, should be calculated to correlate exposure with outcome. In the case of a geographic or specific distribution of cases, spot maps should be generated to track them.

Successful verification involves demonstration that (a) there is a significant difference in the attack rates between individuals exposed to the suspected etiologic agent and those not exposed and (b) either there is a common source to all infected cases or that no other mode of transmission could account for the person and place distribution of the cases. Failure to confirm a diagnosis usually results from poor test execution or from an incorrect initial hypothesis. Under these circumstances, the hypothesis should be restated and tested again.

CONCLUSION

Over the last decade or more, the practice of anesthesiology has expanded to encompass the entire perioperative experience. Today, anesthesiologists are not simply limited to care of the patient during the intraoperative and immediate postoperative periods but have expanded their roles to include anesthesiologist-managed preanesthetic clinics and intensive care units. Furthermore, anesthesiologists, like practitioners of any other specialty, are faced with a consumer-driven need for cost-effective, high-quality healthcare and patient satisfaction.

Anesthesiologists are also now presented with an increasing number of patients who are at risk for, or who are infected with, a number of infectious diseases and/or who are immunosuppressed. Practices and procedures performed by anesthesiologists may result in either direct transmission of infection to the patient or an increased susceptibility of the patient to nosocomial infection. Successful perioperative control of infection requires not only application of sound infection control practices for the protection of the patient, but also strict compliance with occupational standards for the anesthesiologist's own protection. For these reasons, the anesthesiologist should not only be able to apply the principles of infection control, but also have a basic familiarity with how an infection becomes established, what factors influence this process, and how this infection produces pathogenicity. An understanding of these processes can facilitate the development of strategies to care for patients presenting with acute infections, or for those who are at an increased risk for developing an infectious illness postoperatively. The days of the empirically derived clinical doctrine and the technician approach to the infected patient will not serve if we are to make any impact on improving outcome and the overall quality of care in the perioperative setting.

REFERENCES

1. Hall, CB. Nosocomial viral respiratory infections: perennial weeds on pediatric wards. *Am J Med* 1981; **70:** 670–6.
2. Leu H, Kaiser DL, Mori M, *et al.* Hospital-acquired pneumonia: attributable mortality and morbidity. *Am J Epidemiol* 1989; **129:**1258–67.
3. Ayala A, Ertel W, Chaudry IH. Trauma-induced suppression of antigen presentation and expression of major histocompatibility class II antigen complex in leukocytes (editorial). *Shock* 1996; **5:** 79–90.
4. Sheeran P, Hall GM. Cytokines in anaesthesia. *Br J Anaesth* 1997; **78:** 201–19.
5. Wan S, Le Clerc JL, Vincent JL. Inflammatory response to cardiopulmonary bypass: mechanisms involved and possible therapeutic strategies. *Chest* 1997; **112:** 676–92.
6. Pirttikangas CO, Salo M, Peltola O. Propofol infusion anaesthesia and the immune response in elderly patients undergoing ophthalmic surgery. *Anaesthesia* 1996; **51:** 318–23.

7. Le Cras AE, Galley HF, Webster NR. Spinal but not general anesthesia increases the ratio of T helper 1 to T helper 2 cell subsets in patients undergoing transurethral resection of the prostate. *Anesth Analg* 1998; **87:** 1421–5.
8. Oladimeji M, Grimshaw AD, Baum M, *et al*. Effect of surgery on monocyte function. *Br J Surg* 1982; **69:** 145–6.
9. Markovic SN, Knight PR, Murasko DM. Inhibition of interferon stimulation of natural killer cell activity in mice anesthetized with halothane or isoflurane. *Anesthesiology* 1993; **78:** 700–6.
10. Kutza J, Gratz I, Afshar M, Murasko DM. The effects of general anesthesia and surgery on basal and interferon stimulated natural killer cell activity of humans. *Anesth Analg* 1997; **85:** 918–23.
11. Markovic SN. Murasko DM. Role of natural killer and T cells in interferon induced inhibition of spontaneous metastases of the B16F10L murine melanoma. *Cancer Research*. 1991; **51:** 1124–8, 1991.
12. Decker D, Schondorf M, Bidlingmaier F, *et al*. Surgical stress induces a shift in the type-1/type-2 T-helper cell balance, suggesting down-regulation of cell-mediated and up-regulation of antibody-mediated immunity commensurate to the trauma. *Surgery* 1996; **119:** 316–25.
13. Chaudry IH, Wichmann MW, Ayala A. Immunological alterations following hemorrhagic shock: considerations for resuscitation with blood substitutes. In: Rudolf AS, Rabinovici R, Fenerstein GZ (eds). *Red Blood Cell Substitutes*. New York: Marcel Dekker, 1998: 166–72.
14. Standiford TJ, Huffnagle GB. Cytokines in host defense against pneumonia. *J Invest Med* 1997; **45:** 335–45.
15. Waymack JP, Miskell P, Gonce S. Alterations in host defense associated with inhalation anesthesia and blood transfusion. *Anesth Analg* 1989; **69:** 163–8.
16. Chung M, Steinmetz OK, Gordon PH. Perioperative blood transfusion and outcome after resection for colorectal carcinoma. *Br J Surg* 1993; **80:** 427–32.
17. Torres A, Aznar R, Gatell JM, *et al*. Incidence of risk and prognosis of nosocomial pneumonia in mechanically ventilated patients. *Am Rev Respir Dis* 1990; **142:** 523–8.
18. Centers for Disease Control. Guidelines for prevention of nosocomial pneumonia. *Morbidity and Mortality Weekly Report* 1997; **46** (RR-1): 1–79.
19. Garibaldi RA, Britt MR, Coleman ML, *et al*. Risk factors for postoperative pneumonia. *Am J Med* 1981; **70:** 677–80.
20. American Association of Nurse Anesthetists. Infection control procedures for anesthesia equipment. In: *Infection Control Guide*, 2nd edn. Park Ridge, IL: American Association of Nurse Anesthetists, 1993: 12–28.
21. Centers for Disease Control. Draft guidelines for preventing the transmission of tuberculosis in health-care facilities. *Federal Register* 1993; **58:** 52810–54.
22. Berry AJ, Nolte FS. An alternative strategy for infection control of anesthesia breathing circuits: a laboratory assessment of the Pall HME filter. *Anesth Analg* 1991; **72:** 651–5.
23. Hogarth I. Anesthetic machine and breathing system contamination and the efficiency of bacterial/viral filters. *Anaesth Intensive Care* 1996; **24:** 154–63.
24. Craven DE, Kunches LM, Kilinsky V, *et al*. Risk factors for pneumonia and fatality in patients receiving continuous mechanical ventilation. *Am Rev Respir Dis* 1986; **133:** 792–6.
25. Pennington JE. Nosocomial respiratory infection. In: *Principles and Practice of Infectious Disease*, 3rd edn. New York: Churchill Livingstone, 1990: 2199–205.
26. Abraham SN, Beachey EH, Simpson WA. Adherence of *Streptococcus pyogenes*, *Escherichia coli*, and *Pseudomonas aeruginosa* to fibronectin-coated and uncoated epithelial cells. *Infect Immun* 1983; **41:** 1261–8.
27. Eddleston JM, Vohra A, Scott P, *et al*. A comparison of the frequency of stress ulceration and secondary pneumonia in sucralfate- or ranitidine-treated intensive care unit patients. *Crit Care Med* 1991; **19:** 1491–6.
28. Kernodle DS, Kaiser AB. Postoperative infections and antimicrobial prophylaxis. In: Mandell GL, Bennett JE, Dolin R (eds). *Principles and Practice of Infectious Diseases,* 4th edn. New York: Churchill Livingstone, 1995: 2742–56.
29. Tunevall TG. Postoperative wound infections and surgical face masks: a controlled study. *World J Surg* 1991; **15:** 383–8.
30. Mitchell NJ, Hunt S. Surgical face masks in modern operating Ors – a costly and unnecessary ritual? *J Hosp Infect* 1991; **18:** 239–42.
31. Henderson DK. Bacteremia due to percutaneous intravascular devices. In: Mandell GL, Bennett JE, Dolin R (eds). *Principles and Practice of Infectious Diseases,* 4th edn. New York: Churchill Livingstone, 1995: 2587–99.
32. Centers for Disease Control. Postsurgical infections associated with an extrinsically contaminated intravenous anesthetic agent: California, Illinois, Maine, and Michigan. *Morbidity Mortality Weekly Rep* 1990; **39:** 426.
33. Rusmin S, DeLuca P. Effect of antibiotics and osmotic change on the release of endotoxin by bacteria retained on intravenous in-line filters. *Am J Hosp Pharm* 1975; **32:** 378–80.
34. Morduchowicz G, Pitlik SD, Huminer D, *et al*. Transfusion reactions due to bacterial contamination of blood and blood products. *Rev Infect Dis* 1991; **13:** 307–14.
35. Centers for Disease Control and Prevention. Update: *Yersinia enterocolytica* bacteremia and endotoxin shock associated with red blood cell transfusions-United States, 1991. *Morbidity Mortality Weekly Rep* 1991; **40:** 176–8.
36. Nielsen H, Stenderup J, Bruun B. Fungemia in a university hospital 1984–1988. Clinical and mycological characteristics. *Scand J Infect Dis* 1991; **23:** 275–82.
37. Harris SL. Definitions and demographic characteristics. In: Kaye D (ed.). *Infective Endocarditis*. New York: Raven Press, 1992: 1.
38. Prevention of bacterial endocarditis. *Medical Letter* 1984; **26:** 3–4.
39. Garibaldi RA, Mooney BR, Epstein BJ, Britt MR. An evaluation of daily bacteriologic monitoring to identify preventable episodes of catheter-associated urinary tract infection. *Infect Control* 1982; **3:** 466–70.
40. Gwaltney JM, Henley JO, Simon G, Jordan WS. Rhinovirus infections in an industrial population: I, The occurrence of illness. *N Engl J Med* 1966; **275:** 1261–80.
41. Breese Hall C. Acute Laryngotracheobronchitis (Croup). In: Mandell GL, Bennett JE, Dolin R (eds). *Principles and Practice of Infectious Diseases*, 4th edn. New York: Churchill Livingstone, 1995: 573–9.
42. Adams WG, Deaver KA, Cochi SL, *et al*. Decline of childhood Haemophilus influenzae type b (Hib) disease in the Hib vaccine era. *JAMA* 1993; **269:** 221–6.
43. Fang GD, Fine M, Orloff G, *et al*. New and emerging etiologies for community-acquired pneumonia with implication for therapy: a prospective multicenter study of 359 cases. *Medicine* 1990; **69:** 307–16.
44. Centers for Disease Control. World AIDS day: December 1, 1997. *Morbidity Mortality Weekly Rep* 1997; **46:** 1085.
45. Tait AR. Prevention of HIV and HBV transmission among anesthesiologists: a survey of anesthesiology practice. *Anesthesiology* 1994; **79:** 623–8.
46. Busby J. Through the valley of many shadows: HIV infected physicians. *Texas Med* 1991; **87:** 36–46.
47. Rosenberg AD, Bernstein DB, Bernstein RL, *et al*. Accidental needlesticks: do anesthesiologists practice proper infection control precautions? *Am J Anaesthesiol* 1995; **22:** 125–32.
48. Berry AJ, Greene ES. The risk of needlestick injuries and needlestick-transmitted diseases in the practice of anesthesiology. *Anesthesiology* 1992; **77:** 1007–21.
49. Havlichek Jr D, RosenmanK, Simms M, Guss P. Age-related hepatitis B seroconversion rates in health care workers. *Am J Infect Control* 1997; **25:** 418–20.
50. Polish LB, Tong MJ, Co RL, *et al*. Risk factors for hepatitis C virus infection among health care personnel in a community hospital. *Am J Infect Control* 1993; **21:** 196–200.
51. Mitsui T, Iwano K, Masuko K, *et al*. Hepatitis C virus infection in medical personnel after needlestick accident. *Hepatology* 1992; **16:** 1109–14.
52. Ippolito G, Puro V, Petrosillo N, *et al*. Simultaneous infection with HIV and Hepatitis C virus following occupational conjunctival blood exposure (letter). *JAMA* 1998; **280:** 28.
53. Chant K, Kociuba K, Munro R, *et al*. Investigation of possible patient-to-patient transmission of hepatitis C in a hospital. *New South Wales Public Health Bull* 1994; **5:** 47–52.
54. Rizzetto M. The delta agent. *Hepatology* 1983; **3:** 729–37.
55. Raviglione MC, Snider DE, Kochi A. Global epidemiology of tuberculosis. Morbidity and mortality of a worldwide epidemic. *JAMA* 1995; **273:** 220–6.
56. Pearson ML, Jereb JA, Frieden TR, *et al*. Nosocomial transmission of multidrug-resistant *Mycobacterium tuberculosis*: a risk to patients and health care workers. *Ann Intern Med* 1992; **117:** 191–6.
57. Griffith DE, Hardeman JL, Zhang Y, *et al*. Tuberculosis outbreak among healthcare workers in a community hospital. *Am J Respir Crit Care Med* 1995; **152:** 208–11.
58. Orkin FK. Herpetic whitlow: occupational hazard to the anesthesiologist. *Anesthesiology* 1970; **33:** 671–3.
59. Johnson JR, Egaas S, Gleaves CA, *et al*. Hepatitis due to herpes simplex virus in marrow-transplant recipients. *Clin Infect Dis* 1992; **14:** 38–45.
60. Feldman S, Hughes WT, Daniel CB. Varicella in children with cancer: seventy-seven cases. *Pediatrics* 1975; **56:** 388–97.

61. Weibel RE, Neff BJ, Kuter BJ, *et al.* Live-attenuated varicella virus vaccine. Efficacy trials in healthy children. *N Engl J Med* 1984; **310:** 1409–15.
62. Lyznicki JM, Bezman RJ, Genel M. Report on the Council of Scientific Affairs, American Medical Association: Immunization of health-care workers with varicella vaccine. *Infect Control Hosp Epidemiol* 1998; **19:** 348–53.
63. Dworsky ME, Welch K, Cassady G, Stagno S. Occupational risk for primary cytomegalovirus infection among pediatric caseworkers. *N Engl J Med* 1983; **309:** 950–3.
64. Ginsburg C, Henle G, Henle W. An outbreak of infectious mononucleosis among the personnel in an outpatient clinic. *Am J Epidemiol* 1976; **104:** 571–5.
65. Yamanishi K, Okuno T, Shiraki K, *et al.* Identification of human herpesvirus 6 as a causal agent for *Exanthem subitum*. *Lancet* 1988; **1:** 1065–7.
66. Centers for Disease Control. Guidelines for the prevention of Human immunodeficiency virus and hepatitis B virus to health-care and public safety workers. *Morbidity Mortality Weekly Rep* 1989; **38:** (S6).
67. Occupational Safety and Health Administration. Occupational Exposure to Bloodborne Pathogens. OSHA 3127, 1996 (revised).
68. Centers for Disease Control and Prevention. Guidelines for isolation precautions in hospitals. *Infect Control Hosp Epidemiol* 1996; **17:** 53–80.
69. Kristensen M, Sloth E, Jensen TK. Relationship between anesthetic procedure and contact of anesthesia personnel with patient body fluids. *Anesthesiology* 1990; **73:** 619–24.
70. Berry AJ. Injury prevention in anesthesiology. *Surg Clinics North Am* 1995; **75:** 1123–32.
71. Greene ES, Berry AJ, Jagger J, *et al.* Multicenter study of contaminated percutaneous injuries in anesthesia personnel. *Anesthesiology* 1998; **89:** 1362–72.
72. McCray E, Martone WJ. Preventing HIV exposure among patients and staff. *AIDS Patient Care* 1987: **Sept.:** 32–34.
73. Tait AR, Voepel-Lewis T, Tuttle DB, Malviya S. Compliance with standard precautions for the prevention of occupational transmission of blood- and airborne pathogens: a survey of post-anesthesia nursing practice. *J Continuing Educ Nurs* 2000; **31:** 38–44.
74. Gruber M, Beavers FE, Johnson B, *et al.* The relationship between knowledge about acquired immunodeficiency syndrome and the implementation of universal precautions by registered nurses. *Clin Nurse Specialist* 1989; **3:** 182–5.
75. Centers for Disease Control. Guidelines for preventing the transmission of *Mycobacterium tuberculosis* in health care facilities. *Morbidity Mortality Weekly Rep* 1994; **43:** RR-13.
76. Centers for Disease Control. Case-control study of HIV seroconversion in health-care workers after percutaneous exposures to HIV-infected blood: France, United Kingdom, and United States, January 1988–August 1994. *Morbidity Mortality Weekly Rep* 1995; **44:** 929–33.
77. Centers for Disease Control. Notice to readers update: provisional public health service recommendations for chemoprophylaxis after occupational exposure to HIV. *Morbidity Mortality Weekly Rep* 1996; **45:** 468–72.
78. Centers for Disease Control. Immunization of health-care workers: Recommendations of the ACIP and the HICPAC. *Morbidity Mortality Weekly Rep* 1997; **46** (RR-18): 1–42.
79. Cohen MM, Cameron CB. Should you cancel the operation when a child has an upper respiratory tract infection? *Anesth Analg* 1991; **72:** 282–8.
80. Tait AR, Knight PR. The effects of general anesthesia on upper respiratory tract infections in children. *Anesthesiology* 1987; **67:** 930–5.
81. Tait AR, Pandit UA, Voepel-Lewis T, *et al.* Use of the laryngeal mask airway in children with upper respiratory tract infections: a comparison with endotracheal intubation. *Anesth Analg* 1998; **86:** 706–11.
82. Lewis W. AIDS: Cardiac findings from 115 autopsies. *Prog Cardiovasc Dis* 1989; **32:** 207–15.
83. Hughes WT. Fatal infections in childhood leukemia. *Am J Dis Child* 1971; **122:** 283–7.
84. Murphy JF, McDonald FD, Dawson M, *et al.* Factors affecting the frequency of infection in renal transplant recipients. *Arch Intern Med* 1976; **136:** 670–7.
85. Lundy J, Lovett EJ, Conran P. Pulmonary metastases, a potential biologic consequence of anesthetic-induced immunosuppression by thiopental. *Surgery* 1977; **82:** 254–6.
86. Waymack JP, Fernandes G, Cappelli PJ, *et al.* Alterations in host defense associated with anesthesia and blood transfusion: II. Effect on response to endotoxin. *Arch Surg* 1991; **126:** 59–62.
87. Tait AR, Tuttle DB. Preventing perioperative transmission of infection: a survey of anesthesiology practice. *Anesth Analg* 1995; **80:** 764–9.
88. du Moulin GC, Hedley-Whyte J. Bacterial interactions between anesthesiologists, their patients, and equipment. *Anesthesiology* 1982; **57:** 37–41.
89. Spaulding EH. Chemical disinfection and antisepsis in the hospital. *J Hosp Res* 1972; **9:** 5–31
90. Merritt WT, Zuckerberg AL. Contamination of the anesthetic record. *Anesthesiology* 1992; **77:** A1102.
91. Rutala WA. APIC guideline for selection and use of disinfectants. *Am J Infect Control* 1990; **18:** 99–117.
92. Favero MS, Boyland EA. Microbiologic considerations: disinfection and sterilization strategies and the potential for airborne transmission of bloodborne pathogens. *Surgical Clin North Am* 1995; **75:** 1071–89.
93. Gwaltney JM, Moskalski PB, Hendley JO. Hand-to-hand transmission of rhinovirus colds. *Ann Intern Med* 1978; **88;** 463–7.
94. Dryden GE, Brickler J. Stopcock contamination. *Anesth Analgesia* 1979; **58:** 141–2.
95. Alter MJ, Ahtone J, Maynard JE. Hepatitis B virus transmission associated with a multiple-dose vial in hemodialysis unit. *Ann Intern Med* 1983; **99:** 330–3.
96. Bawden JC, Jacobsen JA, Jackson JC, *et al.* Sterility and use patterns of multiple-dose vials. *Am J Hosp Pharmacol* 1982; **39:** 294–7.
97. Froggatt JW, Dwyer DM, Stephens MA. Hospital outbreak of hepatitis B in patients undergoing electroconvulsive therapy. Interscience Conference on Antimicrobial Agents and Chemotherapy, 1991: 347; 157.
98. Trepanier CA, Lessard MR, Brochu JG, Denault PH. Risk of cross-infection related to the multiple use of disposable syringes. *Can J Anesth* 1990; **37:** 156–9.
99. Chant K, Lowe D, Rubin G, *et al.* Patient-to-patient transmission of HIV in private consulting surgical consulting rooms. *Lancet* 1993; **342:** 1548.
100. Walker RH. Special report: Transfusion risks. *Am J Clin Pathol* 1987; **88:** 374–8.
101. Alter MJ, Hadler SC, Judson FN, *et al.* Risk factors for acute non-A, non-B hepatitis in the United States and association with hepatitis C virus infection. *JAMA* 1990; **264:** 2231–5.
102. Nelson KE, Donahue JG, Munoz A, *et al.* Transmission of retroviruses from seronegative donors by transfusion during cardiac surgery. A multicenter study of HIV-1 and HTLV-I/II infections. *Ann Intern Med* 1992; **117:** 554–9.

71

Hyperbaric physiology and medicine

JAMES D MARTIN, STEPHEN R THOM, AND RODERIC G ECKENHOFF

The number of people being exposed to hyperbaric environments has increased. This is a result of an increase in the use of hyperbaric oxygen therapy, an increase in the popularity of underwater diving, and the continued necessity for pressurized (Caisson) construction techniques. An understanding of human tolerance of hyperbaric environments and an appreciation of the unique aspects of medical care under pressurized conditions is therefore important. The anesthesiologist's expertise in gas physics and physiology, oxygen delivery, and acute care monitoring makes it both natural and necessary that the anesthesiologist has a basic understanding of the physiologic and practical considerations of man's exposure to hyperbaria. Indeed, anesthesiologists have been intimately involved in the operation and management of hyperbaric medicine centers throughout the world.

This chapter is directed at the anesthesiologist with no background in hyperbaric medicine. The first section covers the physiology of exposure to hyperbaric environments; the second discusses the indications, rationale, and risks of hyperbaric oxygen therapy, including the practicalities of patient care in a hyperbaric chamber.

PHYSIOLOGIC IMPLICATIONS OF HYPERBARIC EXPOSURE

Exposure to hyperbaric conditions necessarily involves three phases – compression, stable pressure, and decompression – and the physiologic implications follow this organization reasonably well. This section will divide the important physiologic effects into those occurring as a result of compression and habitation at increased pressure, and those occurring as a result of decompression.

Compression and stable pressure phase

The physical alterations present in hyperbaric conditions include: (1) an increase in hydrostatic pressure; (2) an increase in the partial pressure of the surrounding and inspired gases; and (3) an increase in gas density. Although this division is useful for the purposes of discussion, it is important to note that these physical alterations are not entirely distinct, and the physiologic consequences represent a summation of their influences. For example, the neurological consequences of exposure to very high pressure represent the effects of both increased partial pressures of the inspired gases and increased hydrostatic pressure itself.

Increased hydrostatic pressure

Hydrostatic or hydraulic pressure is mechanical pressure by itself, to be distinguished from gas partial pressure (see below). The effect of hydrostatic pressure depends on magnitude and the site affected. Table 71.1 lists the units commonly used for expression of pressure.

One of the more common problems experienced by those undergoing hyperbaric exposure, and which is primarily due to hydrostatic pressure, is *barotrauma*.[1] This is a consequence of the omnidirectional conduction of pressure in liquids that contain gas spaces (such as the body). If this gas space communicates freely with the external pressurized environment, molecules of gas or liquid can be admitted to equalize the pressure gradient. However, if this communication does

Table 71.1 *Pressure units and conversions*

1 atm = 1.013247 bar
1 atm = 101.3247 kPa
1 atm = 14.6959 p.s.i.
1 atm = 760.00 torr[a]
1 atm = 33.08 f.s.w.
1 atm = 10.13 m.s.w.
1 bar = 100.000 kPa
1 bar = 100 000 Pa[a]
1 bar = 14.50377 p.s.i.
1 bar = 750.064 torr
1 bar = 32.646 f.s.w.[b]
1 bar = 10.00 m.s.w.
1 f.s.w. = 3.063 kPa
1 f.s.w. = 22.98 torr
1 m.s.w. = 10.000 kPa[c]
1 m.s.w. = 1.450 p.s.i.
1 m.s.w. = 75.01 torr
1 p.s.i. = 6894.76 Pa[a]
1 p.s.i. = 51.7151 torr
1 p.s.i. = 2.251 f.s.w.
1 MPa = 10.000 bar
1 torr = 133.322 Pa[a]

a. Signifies a primary definition from which the other equalities were derived.
b. Primary definition for f.s.w.; assumes a density for seawater of 1.02489 g mL^{-1} at 4 °C (the value often used for depth gauge calibration).
c. Primary definition for m.s.w.; assumes a density for seawater of 1.01972 g mL^{-1} at 4 °C.

Reprinted with permission from *Undersea Biomedical Research*.

not exist, the unequalized pressure gradient will attempt to compress the gas space, the significance of which depends on the anatomy. For example, because intestinal walls are highly deformable, compression of any contained gas has minimal consequences. On the other hand, because gas spaces in the head or chest have limits on compression (or expansion; see below), important consequences exist. A pressure gradient across the bony sinus walls can be transmitted only through the blood or lymphatics. Therefore a painful, blood-filled sinus is the frequent result of pressurization without osteal patency. A similar injury may occur in the middle ear but, because only the thin tympanic membrane separates pressurized and nonpressurized space, rupture may occur when eustachian (pharyngotympanic) tube dysfunction does not allow pressure equalization from the nasopharynx. Patients with marginal eustachian tube function may develop serous otitis media with repeated exposure to pressure.[2] Though not recommended for underwater activity, systemic or topical decongestants may be useful in the maintenance of eustachian tube and osteal patency in a controlled hyperbaric environment. Myringotomy is occasionally required in circumstances in which "dry" pressure exposure is necessary.

Compression barotrauma of the chest is infrequent, owing to the absolute requirement for airway patency and to the compressible nature of the chest and lung. In the absence of ventilatory activity (during a breath-hold dive, for example), the limits of chest wall compression require a cephalad movement of the diaphragm and translocation of blood into the chest in an attempt to equalize the transthoracic pressure gradient. However, as the duration of such gradients is usually limited to only a few minutes, the physiologic consequences are small. Pulmonary barotrauma is most dangerous during decompression, and will be discussed later.

A more subtle form of compression, barotrauma is commonly referred to as *compression arthralgia.* As one is compressed to greater than 6 atmospheres absolute (ATA – the sum of the atmospheric and hydrostatic pressure in $kg\,cm^{-2}$), increased joint crepitance and arthralgias may occur. The mechanism for this effect is obscure, but the rapidity of its development implies that a compressible space (gas?) normally exists in or around the joint, the collapse of which can sufficiently distort the joint anatomy to produce pain and crepitance.

The final effect of hydrostatic pressure to be discussed here is the neurologic consequence of exposure to very high pressure. Both animals and humans experience a generalized excitation of the central nervous system (CNS) on exposure to pressures greater than about 10 ATA. A constellation of symptoms including tremors, visual disturbances, tinnitus, and seizures has been referred to as the high-pressure nervous syndrome (HPNS) and has represented a significant impediment to human tolerance of high-pressure environments.[3] The mechanism of this pressure-induced disorder is thought to be the result of specific pressure-sensitive proteins or receptor complexes in the CNS. HPNS can, in part, be controlled or masked by CNS-depressing agents, and the anesthetic "inert" gases (see below). HPNS may be closely related to, or possibly the mechanism of, pressure reversal of anesthesia,[4] a functional competition between excitatory and depressant sites in the CNS. HPNS (and pressure reversal of anesthesia) is rarely encountered in clinical practice, as it is a feature of pressure exposures in excess of those normally experienced by patients undergoing hyperbaric oxygen therapy (<6 ATA), by underwater divers (<7 ATA), or by pressurized construction workers (<3 ATA).

Increased partial pressure of inspired gases

Henry's law predicts that exposure to increased atmospheric pressure will increase the concentration (tension) of gas dissolved in the liquid phase. Because the biologic activity of any gas is related to its tension in the blood or tissues, exposure to increased pressure should have significant physiologic effects. The gases to be considered in this section are oxygen, carbon dioxide, the inert gases, and contaminant gases.

Oxygen

The scientific basis for breathing oxygen under hyperbaric conditions has evolved considerably since the inception of Henshaw's "Domicilium" in 1662.[5] This British clergyman could not have foreseen the intricate effects of hyperbaric oxygen therapy on the biochemical reactions in various organs, which are only now being elucidated. The fundamental physical event leading to these effects is the increased concentration of dissolved oxygen in the blood and tissues (see the section on Hyperbaric oxygen therapy below). At 2.8 ATA, the plasma contains a dissolved volume of oxygen equal to the mean O_2 extraction rate of the body. This results in fully saturated hemoglobin in the venous circulation. Tissue oxygen tension is not elevated as much, however, because of diffusion barriers, oxygen utilization, oxygen-induced vasoconstriction, and the poor solubility of oxygen in plasma. Table 71.2 lists *in vivo* oxygen tension measurements in a variety of tissues with increasing inspired oxygen partial pressure, demonstrating the modest increase in oxygen tension, especially in diseased tissues. Even though oxygen is poorly soluble in plasma, sufficient quantities can be dissolved at 3 ATA to meet metabolic needs in the complete absence of hemoglobin.

As with any other drug, oxygen has a therapeutic dose range. While this range varies with clinical indication, hyperbaric oxygen exposures are toxic to various organ systems. This toxicity is based on duration, inspired oxygen pressure, and individual susceptibility.[7] Pulmonary effects of oxygen are generally encountered at a lower $P\text{O}_2$ value, while central nervous system toxicity limits exposures above 3.0 ATA.

Pulmonary toxicity

The lung is continuously exposed to the highest $P\text{O}_2$ of any organ, and is the first to demonstrate toxicity with normobaric (1 ATA) exposures. Normobaric oxygen inhalation for as little as 6–8 h decreases tracheal mucous velocity, and nonspecific respiratory symptoms begin in as little as 12 h in normal humans.[8–10] Pulmonary function changes, nausea, vomiting, anorexia, and occasionally orthostasis are prominent symptoms with exposures of greater than 24 h. Survival time of normal primates in 100% oxygen is in excess of a week, with death the result of pulmonary edema and, ironically, hypoxia. The development and rate of progression of pulmonary oxygen toxicity are directly related to the inspired oxygen partial pressure ($P_I\text{O}_2$), such that substantial signs and symptoms are apparent in normal human subjects after 3–5 h of exposure to 2.0 ATA oxygen.[11] Considerable individual differences in oxygen sensitivity exist.

The maximum nontoxic ($P_I\text{O}_2$) has not been established, but prolonged exposures to 0.5 ATA produce few symptoms in normal subjects, and even allow recovery from acute lung injury in animals and humans.[12] Between 0.21 and 0.50 ATA, physiologic, biochemical, and anatomical changes occur, but are considered to be adaptive rather than pathological. Absorption atelectasis is not an important contributor to pulmonary oxygen toxicity, demonstrated by the usual progression of toxicity in humans breathing air at 5.0 ATA.[13] Therefore, prolonged hyperbaric exposure at pressures greater than approximately 3 ATA should have an $F_I\text{O}_2$ below that of air, so that a $P_I\text{O}_2$ of less than 0.5 ATA is produced.

The treatment of pulmonary oxygen toxicity relies on decreasing the $P_I\text{O}_2$ and providing supportive measures. There are currently no specific pharmacologic approaches to treatment. Dramatic improvements in oxygen tolerance have been produced with prior exposure to sublethal hyperoxia in some species;[14] paradoxically, hypoxic pre-exposure can also result in increased resistance to the toxic effects of oxygen.[15] Human oxygen tolerance has been shown to be significantly increased by brief

Table 71.2 *Tissue oxygen tension, in kPa (and mmHg), with increasing inspired oxygen pressure*

		Rat tibia		Human		
ATA O_2	Rat brain	Normal	Osteomyelitis	Muscle	Subcutaneous tissue	Myonecrosis phlegmon
0.2	4.5 (34)	6.0 (45)	2.8 (21)	3.9 (29)	4.9 (37)	6.7 (50)
1.0	12.0 (90)	–	–	7.9 (59)	7.1 (53)	14.7 (110)
2.0	32.5 (244)	42.8 (321)	13.9 (104)	29.5 (221)	29.5 (221)	33.3 (250)
3.0	60.3 (452)	–	–	–	–	44.0 (330)

ATA, atmospheres absolute. Reproduced, with permission, from Thom.[6]

interruptions of oxygen inhalation with an approximately normoxic gas,[16] a technique commonly employed in hyperbaric oxygen therapy. In animals, adaptation has been associated with increased cellular antioxidant enzyme levels, proliferation of alveolar type II cells, and increased alveolar surfactant levels.[17–19]

Central nervous system

Central nervous system oxygen toxicity is not usually observed with inhaled oxygen partial pressures of less than 2.0 ATA.[20] It may occur before pulmonary toxicity at pressures above 3.0 ATA, and, like pulmonary toxicity, there is wide variation in individual sensitivity. Oxygen toxicity of the CNS is characterized by convulsions, which may be preceded by visual symptoms or muscular twitching. Exercise and hypercapnia accelerate the onset of symptoms, probably due to cerebrovasodilation and increased delivery of oxygen to the brain. CNS oxygen toxicity is rapidly reversible with decreases in the $P_{I}O_2$ and permanent or residual sequelae have not been reported.

In addition to toxicity, increased oxygen partial pressures may have subtle physiologic effects. Oxygen inhalation at 1 ATA or above causes a small and immediate respiratory depression in normal subjects, presumably due to loss of tonic chemoreceptor activity.[21] However, this is soon followed by an increase in ventilation, due to an increase in tissue carbon dioxide tensions.[22] The increased tissue CO_2 tension is a result of decreased elimination of carbon dioxide; the increased concentration of oxyhemoglobin in the venous blood during oxygen inhalation implies a decreased concentration of deoxyhemoblobin, an important component of venous CO_2 buffering. Oxygen inhalation may also cause absorption atelectasis in lung regions with poor ventilation because of the absence of nitrogen.

The cardiovascular effects of oxygen inhalation are usually of little consequence. Heart rate and cardiac output are slightly reduced with little change in blood pressure, presumably because of oxygen-induced vasoconstriction. Pulmonary artery pressures are decreased somewhat by the removal of that component of pulmonary artery tone maintained by regional alveolar hypoxia.

A final and more practical result of increased oxygen concentration and partial pressure relates to fire risk, and is discussed in more detail later, in the section Risks of hyperbaric oxygen therapy.

Carbon dioxide

At constant atmospheric CO_2 fractional concentration, the $P_{I}CO_2$ and related physiologic effects increase with elevated pressure. For example, a normally well-tolerated atmosphere containing a CO_2 concentration of about 1% (~1.1 kPa or ~8 mmHg), if compressed and inhaled at 5 ATA, would produce approximately the same physiologic effect as breathing 5% CO_2 at 1 ATA. However, this does not mean that expired CO_2 is more dangerous at 5 ATA than at 1 ATA; end-tidal CO_2 concentration would be about 1% at 5 ATA, because the *partial pressure* of about 5.3 kPa (40 mmHg) is maintained.

Increased CO_2 partial pressures (over about 7.3 kPa or 55 mmHg) produce subjective hyperpnea and dyspnea as well as headache due to increased cerebral blood flow. Higher partial pressures can produce CNS depression, and are often accompanied by significant acidosis. Inhalation of atmospheres with increased $P_{I}CO_2$ may have opposing direct and indirect effects on the cardiovascular system. Activation of the sympathetic nervous system with increases in blood catecholamine concentration occurs at moderate $P_{I}CO_2$, while opposing direct depressant effects on tissues, such as cardiac and vascular muscle, may occur simultaneously. The cerebral circulation, which does not have functionally important sympathetic innervation, undergoes dilation with increased $P_{I}CO_2$. This cerebral vasodilation may explain the increased incidence of CNS oxygen toxicity in high CO_2 atmospheres and during exercise, a matter of importance during hyperbaric oxygen therapy. In general, however, the threshold for convulsions from other causes is elevated by increased $P_{I}CO_2$. CO_2 concentration is usually monitored in chamber atmospheres, and most hyperbaric chambers are well ventilated because of the important physiologic effects of breathing increased $P_{I}CO_2$.

Nitrogen, helium, and other inert gases

Most of the "inert" gases produce CNS depression at high partial pressure. For example, nitrogen is essentially anesthetic at pressures greater than about 30 ATA, and other gases have an anesthetic potency which approximately follows their solubility in lipid (Table 71.3).

Although these anesthetic partial pressures are produced by hyperbaric exposures of much greater magnitude than those used for hyperbaric oxygen therapy or for underwater diving, more subtle CNS effects may be observed at lower pressures. Nitrogen narcosis is a well-known malady among scuba divers breathing air at depths greater than about 100 feet of sea water (f.s.w.) (4 ATA), equivalent to 30.6 meters of sea water (m.s.w.) (306.2 kPa), resulting in euphoria and an impairment of judgment.[3] To minimize these CNS effects at high pressure, other inert gases have been substituted for nitrogen. Helium, in part because of its very low solubility, has such a low anesthetic potency that the pressures required to produce CNS depression exceed those required to produce HPNS in animals; depression has not been observed. Low concentrations of nitrogen (5%) have been added to the helium/oxygen atmospheres used for very high-pressure exposures to control or mask the CNS excitation of HPNS. Such "trimixes" have been used successfully for manned pressure exposures of about 70 ATA.[3] The use of hydrogen as a diluent gas for exposure to high pressure has received recent attention because of an intermediate narcotic potency between nitrogen and helium and a lower density than nitrogen. Unfortunately, it is dangerous because mixtures containing more than about 5% oxygen are explosive.

A final and important implication of an increased partial pressure of the inert gases is that the blood and tissue content of dissolved gas is also increased. The magnitude of the increase depends upon the pressure and duration of exposure and on the solubility of the inert gas. The kinetics and route of elimination of this additional inert gas are of fundamental importance to tolerance of decompression (see under Decompression sickness later).

Table 71.3 *Narcotic potency of gases*

Gas	Molecular wt	Lipid solubility[a]	Estimated MAC[b]
He	4	0.017	>180
Ne	20	0.022	>150
H_2	2	0.036	81
N_2	28	0.076	44
Ar	40	0.140	0.19
Kr	84	0.430	6.2
Xe	131	1.700	0.8

a. Ostwald coefficient at 37° C.
b. Minimum alveolar concentration for lack of movement with noxious stimulation. For Ne and He, this has not been observed, and the values given are estimates based on lipid solubility. For H_2, N_2, Ar, and Kr, the values were determined in animals;[3] Xe MAC was determined in humans.[23]

Contaminants

Carbon monoxide and various hydrocarbons sometimes contaminate compressed gas mixtures, and their toxicity will be magnified when compressed and inhaled. Rigorous standards for scrubbing and filtering compressed gases destined for human inhalation have greatly reduced the probability of significant intoxication. Compressor air intakes need to be well away from sources of contaminants, such as motor and fume hood exhausts; to reduce hydrocarbons, compressor lubrication is often accomplished with water or soaps.

Increased gas density

An increase in pressure leads to an increase in inspired gas density. The physiologic considerations of increased gas density simplify to two: respiration and thermal regulation. More practical sequelae, such as speech distortion, may also occur but are not discussed further here.

The respiratory effects of increased gas density are primarily flow related. Gas flow in the proximal airways (and of course in any external gas circuits such as tracheal tubes) is largely turbulent, and turbulent gas flow is inversely related to gas density. The relation between gas flow and density is exponential:

$$Y = BX^{-0.45}$$

where Y is the flow rate at density X ($g\,L^{-1}$), B is the flow rate at 1 ATA (1 ATA density: $1.1\,g\,L^{-1}$) and the exponent is an experimentally derived value for humans over a wide range of inhaled gas densities.[14,24] As an example, peak flow rates are decreased by about 50% at 5 ATA as compared with 1 ATA, reducing maximal ventilatory rates, and thereby the maximal sustainable workload. Because of helium's low density, its substitution for nitrogen in high-pressure atmospheres allows a preservation of peak flow rates. This application is similar to the rationale for using helium/oxygen mixtures at 1 ATA in the therapy of a large airway obstruction. It is important to note, however, that the viscosity of helium is somewhat greater than that of nitrogen, and therefore flow under viscosity-dependent conditions (laminar flow in small distal airways) might be compromised. For example, helium inhalation may actually decrease gas flow in patients with severe bronchoconstriction.

Gas exchange in distal airways and alveoli occurs primarily by diffusion, and an increase in gas density may have important effects on diffusion. This would manifest as an increase in the alveolar–arterial gradient for oxygen, due primarily to an imprecise calculation of P_{AO_2} and increased heterogeneity (layering) in the respiratory regions of the airways. Human studies have been unable to demonstrate this effect, although it is likely to exist at very high gas density.

Heat capacity and conductivity of a gas are proportional to the density. Thus, pressurized environments will cause an increase in heat loss from patients. The use of helium in such environments exacerbates this situation because of its uniquely high thermal conductivity. However, a common misconception is that the high thermal conductivity of helium increases *respiratory* heat loss in addition to that lost from the skin. Because respiratory gas is generally heated to body temperature, regardless of composition, the heat *capacity*, and not *conductivity*, is the relevant index. The heat capacity of helium is less than that of air (taking density into account), so inhalation of helium/oxygen mixtures may actually reduce the respiratory component of overall heat loss as compared with nitrogen/oxygen.

Decompression

Returning from pressure to 1 ATA (or from 1 ATA to altitude) can result in at least two problems: barotrauma and decompression sickness (DCS). While the former is more common, similarity in manifestations may be confused in their more serious forms.

Barotrauma

In order to achieve equalization of gas spaces at pressure (see above), an increased number of gas molecules (increased density – gas molecules per unit volume) must occupy the gas space in order to counter increasing ambient pressures. The "gas space" encompasses physiologic (lungs, sinuses, eustachian tubes, etc.) as well as artificial (masks, hoods, helmets) chambers. These gas molecules must then leave on decompression, or the space will be at increased pressure relative to the environment. Gas egress normally occurs more easily than entry, but occasionally the sinus ostia, eustachian tube, or bronchiole becomes obstructed and gas becomes trapped. The increased pressure resulting from expanding trapped gas is predicted by Boyle's law (P is pressure and V is volume):

$$P_1V_1 = P_2V_2$$

Thus:

$$V_1 = (P_2/P_1)V_2$$

produces effects that depend upon the anatomy of the region. Elevated pressure in a sinus causes pain, mucosal ischemia, and occasionally hyperasthesia in areas supplied by nerves traversing the spaces. In a space bounded by more flexible walls, such as the alveolus, elevated pressure may cause distension and possibly rupture. The resultant pulmonary barotrauma may then cause pneumothorax, or the gas may dissect through tissue planes to cause pneumomediastinum, subcutaneous emphysema, or gas embolism.[1,25] The last is most dangerous because the gas may enter a pulmonary vein and become directly arterialized. Depending on gas volume, position, and hemodynamics, the emboli may become widely distributed; of most concern is gas that enters the cerebral or coronary circulations (see below under Hyperbaric oxygen therapy). Such gas emboli may cause ischemia directly, as well as trigger a variety of mediator and humoral effects through bubble–blood and bubble–endothelium interactions.

Cerebral gas embolism is usually characterized by a sudden onset of unconsciousness or hemiplegic symptoms during or rapidly following a decompression. Immediate hyperbaric oxygen therapy (HBOT) is usually curative, but delay may reduce the chance of success. It is difficult to identify a predisposition to pulmonary barotrauma, but any condition that can produce "air-trapping" in the lung, such as the presence of blebs, bullae, or very poorly ventilated regions, should be considered to increase the risk of pulmonary barotrauma during decompression. Inadequate training and panic may also predispose to pulmonary barotrauma because of breath holding during decompression.

Decompression sickness

As predicted by Henry's law (where X represents the inspired gas, P is ambient pressure, and t is time):

$$\%X = [P(X)/P(t)] \times 100$$

increasing ambient pressure results in increasing gas dissolution in both the blood and the peripheral tissues. As a result, hyperbaric exposure leads to an increased tissue content of inert gas (typically nitrogen). Brief (1–2 h) exposures usually allow sufficient time for only the well-perfused (termed "fast tissues") compartments to equilibrate with the new partial pressure of inert gas, while exposures of greater than about 6–12 h are required for all of the tissues to equilibrate (saturate). Of course, the rate of saturation of tissues with an inert gas depends on both the pressure and the time of exposure. This is represented by the Hempleman exposure index (Q):

$$Q = P(\sqrt{t})$$

where P represents the ambient pressure and t is the exposure time. Complete saturation of all tissues may take much longer, but it is not certain whether gas in these very slowly equilibrating compartments contributes to the pathophysiology of DCS.

On decompression, the inert gas gradient is reversed and the tissues eliminate gas. This normally occurs via release as dissolved gas in the same manner as uptake, but it is possible that the reduction in ambient pressure is large and rapid enough to produce tissue or blood inert gas tensions that exceed their solubility at that pressure and temperature. Thus, the *rate of separation* of inert gas from peripheral tissue may result in the formation of a bubble (an insoluble gas phase), either stationary "autochthonous" in tissue or mobile in lymph or blood. Initially, mobile bubbles are probably small (~100 μm), but they grow and aggregate in areas of sluggish blood flow. There is now general agreement that both the stationary and the mobile gas bubbles are the primary etiology of the DCS syndromes,[26] but the mechanisms linking bubbles and symptoms are poorly appreciated.

The manifestations of the syndrome known as DCS are sufficiently undesirable as to leave no doubt that its prevention is far more desirable than its cure. Therefore, prior to a discussion of the pathogenesis, symptomatology, and treatment of this illness, a brief review of its prevention is appropriate. During the last century, considerable effort has gone into the development of decompression routines that limit the degree of tissue supersaturation to some arbitrary point that correlates with a low incidence of symptoms. This is generally accomplished by controlling the rate of decompression so that a given inert gas tension (maximum or "M" value) is never exceeded in some mathematically defined compartment – often the 360 min half-time tissue. This concept allows the construction of decompression schedules or tables that specify the maximum allowable time at any pressure for which normal decompression rates can be used (no-decompression limits), and which also specify how decompression must be modified when this time limit is exceeded. The success of such routines is shown by the low incidence of DCS in sport diving – estimated at about 1 in 10 000 exposures.[27] A more tightly regulated (but possibly more stressed) diving community, the military, is estimated to have a higher overall incidence of about 1 in 100, though under-reporting in the sport diving and commercial diving communities likely represents a significant problem. Nevertheless, military scientists are establishing new decompression schedules and tables that are based on a statistical treatment of accumulated world experience and that are flexible depending on the acceptable degree of risk.[28] Clearly, the decompression tables that have been developed have greatly minimized the incidence of injury from decompression events, but the reader should realize that these are merely mathematical models – the mechanism by which bubble cavitation leads to tissue injury remains to be fully demonstrated.

Aside from the use of controlled decompression rates to prevent DCS, enhanced removal of inert gas from tissues may also be accomplished by the use of elevated inspired concentrations of oxygen. An example of this is the denitrogenation procedures used by astronauts prior to hypobaric exposures (analogous to decompression of those exposed to hyperbaric exposures). In this case, the gradient for inert gas elimination is optimized without a change in ambient pressure and, thus, inert gas is eliminated while still in the dissolved form. This concept is also routinely used in hyperbaric exposures. For example, chamber attendants who have been exposed to pressure (breathing air) for prolonged periods may breathe oxygen for an hour prior to decompression to reduce the tissue content of dissolved inert gas. Oxygen decompression procedures are also used in underwater diving but usually limited to highly regulated situations, such as in military or industrial operations.

The introduction of Doppler ultrasound techniques to monitor the mobile gas phase (bubbles) has led to the discovery that many, and perhaps most, decompressions are accompanied by easily detected venous bubbles in humans.[29,30] Arterial bubbles have been detected as well, although rarely. Because most of these bubbles are unaccompanied by symptoms, the term "silent bubbles" has been applied – although it has not been established whether subclinical gas phase formation is actually benign. The dose–response relation for decompression magnitude and bubble formation has been described for humans, and it is remarkable how small an inert gas gradient is necessary.[30] The decompression ED_{50} for detection of bubbles is equivalent to only about 12 f.s.w. Importantly, bubbles have been detected by ultrasound in about 10% of people decompressing from exposures at which supersaturation does not exist. This may have important implications for the mechanism of bubble formation, suggesting that at least some of the bubbles produced during decompression arise from pre-existing gas spaces, perhaps micronuclei stabilized in hydrophobic crevices.[31] Regardless, it is important to recognize that the initial etiology of DCS, the gas bubble, is present in most decompressions, and that the appearance of symptoms probably depends on the rate and volume of evolved gas, and also on location. Finally, it should be emphasized that, despite the apparent invariant physical forces responsible for bubble formation, there is pronounced individual variation in the ability to form the gas phase after a decompression. The source of this differential tendency is poorly understood, but clearly moves the mechanism of bubble formation out of the realm of simple physical models that incorporate only exposure parameters.

The pathophysiologic link between bubble cavitation and symptoms is not clear, but is likely to be multifactorial. Gas may expand *in situ*, causing tissue distortion, dysfunction, and pain, or may become lodged in the vasculature, causing ischemia. Such obstruction may be venous, as in the case of low-flow systems such as spinal venous plexus, or may be arterial through the (uncommon) passage of gas emboli through the pulmonary circulation or through right-to-left shunts. Aside from a direct mechanical disruption of blood flow, the gas bubbles may cause a variety of indirect effects on the vasculature and tissue through interactions at the blood–bubble interface (complement and/or coagulation activation, for example) or between the bubble and endothelium. The sequestration of leukocytes in the CNS (suggesting a leukocyte–endothelial cell interaction) has recently been demonstrated in an animal model after a provocative decompression profile.[32] The importance of these indirect factors is suggested by the positive correlation between DCS symptoms and the predetermined reactivity of the complement system in animals.[33] Thus, another layer of physiologic heterogeneity with respect to *reaction to a gas phase* is superimposed on the heterogeneity of *gas phase formation*, resulting in such large variation in response to a decompression that the response appears to be essentially random. The apparent randomness of decompression outcome is the motivation for the current statistical approach to designing decompression procedures. This practice is, however, changing rapidly as we begin to uncover the molecular and biochemical cascades leading to tissue injury after bubble formation and cavitation.

HYPERBARIC OXYGEN THERAPY

The past 15 years have marked a dramatic refinement and clarification of the appropriate indications for HBOT. Prior to the final decade of last century, the use of HBOT had been somewhat limited because of the expense of constructing and maintaining the complex facility, the lack of recognized training pathways for personnel, and incomplete acceptance by the general medical community. Enhanced design of larger "multiplace" hyperbaric chambers (accommodating 2–14 patients/staff breathing 100% oxygen by mask or endotracheal tube) has maximized the utilization of available space and allowed the affordable addition of this invaluable clinical tool to university and larger tertiary care centers. Efficient monoplace hyperbaric chambers (sized for a single patient in a supine position with a 100% oxygen internal environment) are increasingly filling a critical need in regional and community hospitals.

At the time of writing, plans to formalize the education of hyperbaric physicians had culminated in the first board examination in hyperbaric medicine in 1999. Expanding fellowship positions for anesthesia/critical care, emergency, and surgically trained physicians leading to this certification have solidified the safe, rational use of HBOT. The thorough education of competent hyperbaric physicians, coupled with expanding clinical and animal studies, has led to an increased acceptance and utilization of HBOT by the general medical community. Though theory and animal studies are used as the rationale for prescribing hyperbaric oxygen in some of its current indications, many of the clinical scenarios for which HBOT is the standard of care are now well supported by appropriate studies, and the list is growing. This section provides a brief summary of the indications and rationale, and a description of equipment, procedures, risks, and some practical considerations of care in a pressurized environment. Detailed protocols are available in the Further reading section of this chapter.

Indications

Elegant animal studies have recently provided insight into the biochemical pathways through which HBOT exerts its effect. Though far from complete, our understanding of the widely varied applications of HBOT is growing rapidly. Pertinent clinical studies have further tailored hyperbaric therapy protocols to particular insults. In a basic sense, this therapeutic modality exerts the mechanical effect of hyperbaria and the physiologic effect of hyperoxia.[34] Though the principal goal of HBOT is to increase tissue oxygen tension, it can produce a myriad of effects, including reduction of air and gas embolism, increased leukocyte killing ability, augmented red cell flexibility, inhibition of selected anaerobic toxins, and reduction of tissue edema. HBOT has the added effects of preservation of intracellular adenosine triphosphate (ATP), increased fibroblast growth and collagen formation, tissue capillary angiogenesis, and termination of lipid peroxidation.[35]

One extremely valuable method of organizing the indications for HBOT is to consider conditions of regional or global hypoxia (Table 71.4). Another group of indications takes advantage of the fact that specific microorganisms are oxygen intolerant. Lastly, the increase in hydrostatic pressure inherent in HBOT provides an important part of the rationale for its use in gas lesion diseases. Perhaps the most inclusive means of discussing the application of HBOT is to consider acute or emergent vs. chronic conditions.

Emergent indications

Carbon monoxide/cyanide

HBOT has proved indispensable in the treatment of global hypoxic insults such as carbon monoxide (CO) and cyanide (CN) intoxications. Carbon monoxide poisoning is the leading cause of deaths due to poisoning in the USA, though reports of its morbidity and mortality have varied greatly.[36] CO, a colorless, tasteless, and odorless product of incomplete hydrocarbon combustion, is an extremely common poison. It interferes with oxygen delivery and utilization because of its high affinity for hemoglobin, the leftward shift of the oxyhemoblobin dissociation curve, and the interaction with specific cellular proteins (e.g. cytochrome oxidase), especially under hypoxic conditions. The result is tissue hypoxia, manifest usually as neurologic depression and occasionally hemodynamic instability. In fact, acute mortality from CO poisoning appears to be secondary to ventricular dysrhythmias related to the hypoxic stress of elevated carboxyhemoglobin (COHb). The concurrent release of hydrogen cyanide gas during industrial and house fires compounds the hypoxic insult by direct cellular mechanisms.[37]

Survivors of acute carbon monoxide intoxication are at risk for the development of delayed neurologic sequelae (DNS), which includes quantifiable cognitive deficits, short-term memory difficulties, dementia, variation in personality, parkinsonism, paralysis, chorea, cortical blindness, peripheral neuropathy, incontinence, and psychosis.[38,39] Manifestations of DNS (occurring 2–40 days post exposure) are not adequately attributed to hypoxia alone.[40] Animal studies have suggested that oxidative stress resulting from free radical generation may significantly contribute to the development of delayed neurologic injury.[41] The formation of COHb in the body leads to hypoxia as well as myocardial impairment.[42,43] The decrement in cardiac output and resultant hypotension during acute CO exposure may augment the recently described sequestration of leukocytes (secondary to β_2-integrin-mediated adherence to CNS endothelial cells) and subsequent endothelial damage.[44] Severely decreased cardiac output (hypotension with decreased tissue perfusion) has led to cerebral hypoperfusion in several animal models as manifested by transient loss of consciousness.[42,45] It has been suggested that a greater degree of DNS has been associated with those CO exposures resulting in unconsciousness.[7,46]

Treatment of victims of carbon monoxide poisoning with HBOT is based upon the increased concentration of dissolved oxygen molecules to a level that sufficiently meets the cerebral oxygen requirement in the absence of hemoglobin. Elevated oxygen concentrations in blood achieved with this therapy compete with CO molecules for hemoglobin (and other protein) binding sites, speed the elimination of CO, and

Table 71.4 *Indications for hyperbaric oxygen after CO poisoning*

Generally accepted criteria	Criteria for consideration
Syncope	COHb level over 20% to 25%
Severe neurologic symptoms on presentation: coma, seizures, focal neurologic findings, GCS < 15	Pregnancy, especially if symptomatic or with a COHb level over 15–20%
Persistent neurologic findings after several hours of oxygen therapy (i.e. mental confusion, visual disturbance, ataxia)	Abnormal neuropsychiatric examination
Myocardial ischemia by history or ECG	
Cardiac dysrhythmias (ventricular, life-threatening)	

ECG, electrocardiogram; GCS, Glasgow coma scale.

appear to inhibit progression of vascular injury via leukocyte interactions. Though HBOT is now accepted as the definitive treatment for CO poisonings,[47] controversy remains regarding the severity of exposure warranting treatment in a hyperbaric environment. It is important to bear in mind that the level of carboxyhemoglobin in the blood (%COHb) does not correlate with the degree of CO intoxication,[48] nor does it assist in assessing short- or long-term prognosis.[49–51] Most authors agree that the decision to employ HBOT rests with clinical symptoms (both immediate and on arrival at the emergency department) as well as the duration of both the exposure and the presentation to medical attention (Table 71.4). A similar rationale exists for the use of hyperbaric oxygen in cyanide poisoning but, because pure cyanide exposure is rare and effectively treated by conventional antidote therapy, HBOT should be reserved for refractory cases, or cases of mixed CO/CN intoxication, not uncommon following smoke inhalation.

Carbon monoxide elimination is based on the fraction of inspired oxygen (F_IO_2), individual metabolism, duration of exposure, and minute ventilation. The half-life of COHb (with the patient breathing room air) is between 4 and 6 h. If the patient is receiving normobaric 100% oxygen, the half-life of COHb drops to 40–90 min. Breathing oxygen under hyperbaric conditions (generally 2.8 ATA) reduces the COHb half-life to 15–30 min.[52] The immediate concerns of concomitant injuries such as burns and airway compromise secondary to altered Glasgow coma scale (GCS), smoke inhalation, and/or trauma should be addressed as soon as possible after a CO exposure. Hyperbaric oxygen treatment (if selected) should be initiated as soon as possible after stabilizing the patient in the emergency room. Most studies conclude that HBOT is most effective in the prevention of DNS, as well as acute neurologic deficits, when administered within 6 h of the exposure. It should be noted that, though some authors suspect that hyperbaric oxygen may adversely influence fetal physiology (transient closure of the ductus arteriosus, for example), the demonstrated benefits (for both mother and fetus) are considered to outweigh the theoretical risk. A high risk of spontaneous abortion and fetal limb malformations, cranial deformities, and cognitive deficits has been associated with maternal CO poisoning.[53–55] As there are currently no standard guidelines for the treatment of pregnant patients with HBOT, the physician should consider the previously stated elevated incidence of birth defects as well as the fact that maternal COHb level does not accurately represent fetal hemoglobin or tissue intoxication.[56] The reader is referred to Table 71.4 for an approach to the treatment of CO toxicity in pregnant women.

Acute anemia

Severe, acute anemia is another emergent indication for the use of HBOT, but only in a limited respect.[57] At 2.5–3.0 ATA inspired oxygen, sufficient arterial oxygen content is dissolved in plasma to meet metabolic needs, making hyperbaric oxygen useful in life support until red cells become available for transfusion, or until adequate red cell mass is generated endogenously. This therapy might be employed for the occasional patient who holds religious beliefs against the transfusion of blood products and who develops a life-threatening anemia, or the patient in whom cross-matching difficulties exist. However, because the toxicity of oxygen (see below) depends on its partial pressure and not content, this indication for hyperbaric oxygen is limited to only several hours of continuous therapy, or to patients for whom intermittent treatment is sufficient to bolster a marginal oxygen delivery.

Myonecrosis

Clostridial myonecrosis (gas gangrene) is the product of clostridrial invasion in the hypoxic environment of a necrotic wound. Gas gangrene caused by *Clostridium perfringens* is a fulminant infection that requires emergency measures to combat the profound shock and mortality that occurs without appropriate treatment. Anaerobic infections often develop in poorly oxygenated, ischemic areas as a result of an inadequate host response. Thus, there is a substantial overlap between infections amenable to HBOT and the group of indications classified as "regional hypoxia."

Clostridial myonecrosis is a rapidly progressive, life-threatening infection, in large part because of the series of exotoxins (largely the α toxin) produced by the microorganism. These exotoxins propagate tissue necrosis, destroy red blood cells, and impede local host defenses. The elevated oxygen tensions possible through HBOT lead to both the inhibition of toxin production by these bacteria and the inactivation of circulating toxin.[58] Another mechanism by which HBOT appears to resolve clostridial infections is by augmentation of leukocyte oxidative killing mechanisms, which operate only when the oxygen tension is above 4 kPa (30 mmHg).[59]

Prior to 1960, optimal management of gas gangrene included surgical debridement and antibiotic therapy. A wide variety of mortality rates from this infection were reported during that time (ranging from 30% to 70%). Boerema and Brummelkamp[60] reported a 95% survival rate after the addition of HBOT (seven 2-h exposures at 3 ATA over a 3-day interval) to conventional therapy. Subsequent incorporation of HBOT into the management of this infection has yielded a dramatic improvement in mortality. Rapid diagnosis is essential, and HBOT should be used early and frequently in the treatment regimen and in combination with parenteral antibiotics and surgery.

Necrotizing fasciitis and Fournier's gangrene

HBOT has also been advocated for use in the treatment of necrotizing soft tissue infections such as necrotizing fasciitis.[61] Though typically more slowly progressive than clostridial infections, the bacteria that cause necrotizing fasciitis and Fournier's gangrene also produce gas in tissue and are highly invasive and extremely aggressive. They also carry high reported mortality rates from 33% to 67% in the absence of HBOT.[61–63] Necrotizing soft-tissue infections are commonly caused by mixed flora, and are treated adequately in many cases with antibiotics and surgical debridement. These infections are rare, difficult to classify, and subject to the variety of underlying medical conditions that result in tissue hypoxia in a compromised host.[64] As such, difficulties with randomization into treatment populations, as well as ethical concerns in the face of high mortality, have prevented controlled clinical trials.

A markedly decreased mortality rate from necrotizing soft-tissue infections has been reported with the use of HBOT as an adjunct to conventional therapy (12–25%).[64–66] In extensive or more rapidly progressive cases, typified by Fournier's gangrene,[65] hyperbaric oxygen may produce a sufficient increase in local oxygen tension to allow a host response, but, as in the case of gas gangrene, is still to be considered an adjunct to conventional measures.

Crush injuries

Other examples of regional hypoxic insults for which hyperbaric oxygen has been successfully employed are crush injuries and following traumatic vascular compromises of the extremities. These injuries result in severe tissue edema and ischemia in areas not relieved by arterial revascularization. With the rationale that, in addition to improved oxygenation, the high arterial oxygen tension has the added benefit of causing a modest vasoconstriction (without compromising oxygen delivery), HBOT may reduce the post-traumatic edema and the possibility of compartment syndrome.

Thermal burns

Similarly, a reduction in edema, increased capillary angiogenesis and rate of epithelialization, augmented resistance to infection, and prevention of conversion from partial to full thickness injury has led many physicians to employ HBOT for patients with thermal burns. Various animal models have illustrated the benefits of hyperbaric oxygen in the treatment of experimentally induced burns.[67–69] A prospective randomized double-blinded clinical trial of burn patients with an involvement of 10–50% body surface area (BSA) revealed a 35% reduction in fluid requirements (in the first 24 h of hospitalization) as well as decreased average healing times (20 days vs. 44 days) in patients receiving hyperbaric oxygen treatment.[70–72] A decrease in the cost of hospitalization (hospital days, surgical procedures, and burn care) has been reported for this application of HBOT.[73,74]

Gas lesion disease

There are two principal types of gas lesion disease for which hyperbaric oxygen is a primary mode of therapy. The first, *decompression sickness*, has been discussed extensively above, and will be combined here with the second, *gas embolism*, because of the similarity of treatment rationale, despite the different initiation and pathophysiology.

Gas embolism is an acquired condition, whereby gas is admitted to the vasculature and circulation. This may occur as a result of pulmonary barotrauma or a wide variety of iatrogenic or traumatic causes: surgery, catheters, trauma, abortions, and orogenital sex.[75] The effects of gas embolism are related to the gas volume, the rate of administration, and its ultimate location. For example, small volumes of air admitted through an intravenous line (< 50 mL) will most likely be trapped efficiently by the pulmonary circulation, and cause little or no effect. On the other hand, much smaller volumes of gas admitted to the arterial side can cause catastrophic effects if distributed to the coronary or cerebral circulations. Venous emboli may be arterialized either through functional right-to-left shunts or in the presence of pulmonary hypertension, which may be precipitated by the venous embolism itself. Vascular obstruction and ischemia are the primary results of gas embolization, but humoral influences arising from interactions at the blood–bubble interface or at the endothelial surface may play an important vasoactive role.

DCS is a unique form of gas (micro) embolization due to *endogenous* production of gas bubbles.[27] Though occasionally reported in aviators who experience a sudden ("explosive") decrease in cabin pressure, DCS typically plagues both military and recreational divers. As the density of water far exceeds that of air, ambient pressure in water changes much more dramatically with relatively minor changes in depth. In fact, most of the disorders faced by the more than 4 million trained divers in the USA relate directly to these augmented alterations in ambient pressure[76] (see earlier discussion).

As previously mentioned, bubble cavitation in the vasculature may lead to tissue distension, mechanical obstruction, and activation of complement and inflammatory mediators, as well as leukocyte sequestration in end organs.[77,78] The manifestations of DCS are highly variable, and have been categorized classically using observed symptoms. Type 1 DCS has been considered a milder form of the disease involving joint and muscular pain, as well as vague, nonspecific complaints such as unusual fatigue. A more severe insult involving neurologic deficits (parasthesiae, ataxia, paraplegia, and seizure) has been labeled type 2 DCS. Several types of DCS have been categorized based on the anatomic region primarily affected. For example, inner ear involvement, which may result in tinnitus, hearing loss, and vertigo, has been termed "the staggers." A particularly fulminant and life-threatening pulmonary form of DCS characterized by dyspnea, substernal pain, and pulmonary edema has been referred to as "the chokes." A wide variety of other symptoms may occur, the result of arterial embolization of bubbles to heart, brain, or other vital organs. In addition, a chronic form of DCS has been described and is more common with repetitive or prolonged low-pressure (2–3 ATA) exposures, such as those experienced by pressurized Caisson workers. This form presents as an aseptic osteonecrosis, usually of the long bones (humerus, femur), years after the pressure exposures. The patient's history may contain repeated diagnoses of DCS. The mechanism is not completely clear, but probably involves bubble formation in the marrow cavity, elevating medullary pressure and causing ischemia.[79] It is important to realize that these represent *clinical* classifications only – even very mild hyperbaric exposures can result in the formation of bubbles. In practical terms, almost every type experienced by divers forms an insoluble gas phase (bubble), though the amount (*grade*) of bubbles is usually not sufficiently significant to result in overt symptoms. In this light, DCS can be viewed as a continuum of asymptomatic to severely symptomatic involvement.

Because the therapy of DCS is specific and unique, and because the symptoms are often nonspecific, accurate and rapid diagnosis is desirable, but difficult. Of most importance is a recent history of hyperbaric exposure. DCS symptoms do not start during the compression or stable pressure phase of an exposure – they begin during the decompression (usually late) or soon afterwards. Occasionally, symptoms may not be apparent to the patient for as much as 24 h after surfacing, but the majority of cases are noted within 12 h after decompression. Although the parameters of the hyperbaric exposure represent important historical information by which the chance of having DCS and its expected severity can be gauged, they cannot establish a diagnosis. Likewise, the presence of Doppler-detected gas phase cannot establish the diagnosis, because of the high incidence of false positives. The diagnosis of DCS rests primarily on the history of symptom onset during or shortly after a decompression.

The rationale for HBOT is founded in the two principal components of the treatment: pressure and hyperoxia. Hydrostatic pressure will cause a decrease in volume of the emboli, and the hyperoxia may improve oxygen delivery to tissue downstream of the obstructing emboli. The hyperoxia also maximizes the gradient for elimination of the gas (generally nitrogen) in the emboli. There is also recent evidence that HBOT may impede leukocyte sequestration and resultant oxygen radical species generation by inhibiting the leukocyte–β_2-integrin interaction with the vascular endothelium.[33] Or course, for hyperbaric therapy to be effective, rapid institution is essential – most treatment failures are probably due to the late use of hyperbaric therapy.

Nevertheless, though rapidity of administration remains an important determinant of a successful outcome, symptom resolution coincident with HBOT as long as a week after the pressure exposure has been reported.[80] This raises a dilemma in the postsurgical patient with suspected gas embolism in that the lack of emergence from anesthesia may be multifactorial; gas embolism may be relegated to a late diagnosis of exclusion.

For understandable ethical reasons, randomized clinical trials of hyperbaric oxygen for this indication (either gas embolism or DCS) have not been conducted. Nevertheless, the rapidity of symptom resolution coincident with the application of pressure, combined with numerous animal studies of both DCS and gas embolism, is compelling evidence for the continued use of hyperbaric oxygen in the gas lesion diseases.

Chronic indications

Irradiated tissue

Hyperbaric oxygen has been shown to be of benefit in more chronic examples of regional hypoxia, such as *osteoradionecrosis*, particularly of the head and neck. In addition to its therapeutic effects, radiation therapy can damage surrounding healthy tissue, leaving these areas without appropriately functioning osteoblasts or fibroblasts.[81] Osteoradionecrosis occurs as a result of the radiation-induced obliterative endarteritis, and has been estimated to occur in up to 10% of patients receiving radiation therapy for carcinoma.[82] It is characterized by aseptic necrosis, loss of tissue integrity, large hypoxic and hypocellular areas, and, occasionally, pathological fractures. Resultant friability and breakdown of this tissue increases the risk of infection (both cellulitis and osteomyelitis).

Prior to the use of HBOT for this indication, the remission rate for patients suffering from osteoradionecrosis was very poor. A protocol developed by Marx[83] suggested that patients with loss of tissue integrity following radiation therapy be subjected to an initial course of HBOT, followed by surgical debridement of the affected area and a postoperative course of hyperbaric oxygen.

Treatment of this disease with hyperbaric oxygen has been shown to promote repair and neovascularization of necrotic bone and to significantly improve covering of exposed bone and the efficacy of any subsequent surgery.[84] The mechanism for enhanced angiogenesis is not yet clear but is likely to involve improved macrophage and fibroblast function.[85] HBOT has also been successful in the treatment of other radiation-associated injury such as radiation cystitis and proctitis.[86]

Osteomyelitis

As alluded to in the above paragraph, osteomyelitis (particularly that which has not responded to conventional therapy) has been successfully treated with hyperbaric oxygen.[87] The rationale for treatment is similar to that of the infections discussed under "Emergent indications" in that oxygen tension in the area of infection is increased, leukocyte and osteoclast function improved, and bacterial susceptibility to antibiotics improved. Several animal studies have demonstrated the efficacy of HBOT in increasing osseous repair and augmenting osteoclast activity, but no randomized human trials have been conducted to date.[88,89] In general, oxygen is not directly bacteriostatic to most microorganisms associated with osteomyelitis at less than 10 ATA, although anaerobes are occasionally involved. A classification system based on anatomical location and host factors has been developed[90] and is useful when determining which types of osteomyelitis hyperbaric oxygen may benefit.

Compromised graft/flap

Although not indicated for the routine surgical graft or flap, HBOT has been shown to improve the survival of those which are clearly compromised after surgery. Numerous well-controlled animal and human studies have demonstrated improved graft/flap survival with intermittent hyperbaric oxygen for 1–3 days.[91,92]

Miscellaneous infections

Hyperbaric oxygen has also been used to treat life-threatening fungal infections, such as rhinocerebral mucormycosis, based on a similar rationale as that for the other infections previously discussed. Although the published reports of this application are few, the results have been encouraging in a disease with high mortality.

Hyperbaric chambers

Hyperbaric oxygen is administered in a hyperbaric chamber, of which there are two basic types – monoplace (Fig. 71.1) and multiplace (Fig. 71.2). The modern monoplace chamber is transparent acrylic, can accommodate a single patient and is usually pressurized with oxygen: the patient does not require a mask. The primary advantages of the monoplace chamber are cost and space requirements. The multiplace chamber is usually steel (some are aluminum), can accommodate more than two people, and is pressurized with air while the patient breathes oxygen from a tight-fitting mask or circuit. The multiplace chamber is suitable for critically ill patients requiring ventilation, monitoring, and constant attendance. However, even the monoplace chamber can be equipped with a full range of monitoring and critical care capability. The pressure and duration of HBOT depends on the indication, and ranges from 2 to 6 ATA for 2–6 h. Serious DCS or gas embolism may require prolonged, continuous "saturation" protocols when symptoms worsen during the decompression phase of conventional regimens. The $P_{\mathrm{I}}\mathrm{O}_2$ in most hyperbaric oxygen protocols rarely exceeds 2.8 ATA. Emergency indications for HBOT, such as CO poisoning or DCS, generally require only two or three separate chamber treatments, whereas problem wounds often require 40 or more daily sessions in the hyperbaric chamber. Detailed treatment protocols may be found in the entries listed in the Further reading section.

Practical aspects of care in a chamber

Monitoring of patients undergoing hyperbaric therapy is usually accomplished by maintaining the electrical components outside the chamber (for fire safety) and passing the electrode or transducer cables through electrically insulated passthroughs in the chamber wall. Necessary electrical equipment in the chamber should never be connected to or disconnected from line voltage during pressurization, to prevent sparks. Such equipment may also be purged continuously with low flows of nitrogen or helium to surround the electrical components with a low oxygen atmosphere. Cathode ray tube (CRT) monitors may not tolerate the additional pressure, although they may be placed outside a chamber viewport for viewing by inside personnel. The small battery-operated, liquid crystal display monitors appear to tolerate hyperbaric conditions well and have a minimal fire risk and are now being used inside chambers.

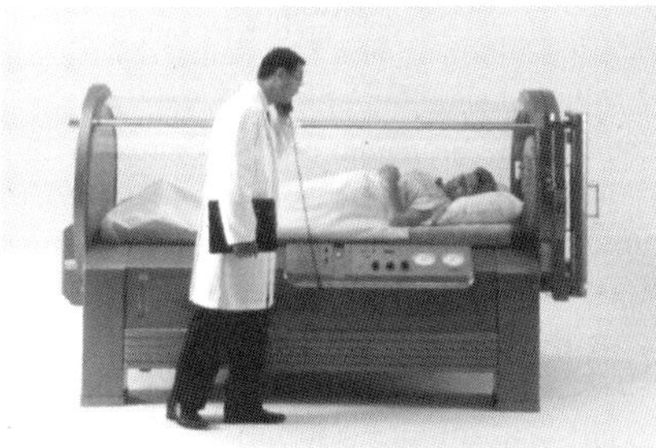

Figure 71.1 *A monoplace chamber. Photograph courtesy of Sechrist Industries Inc.*

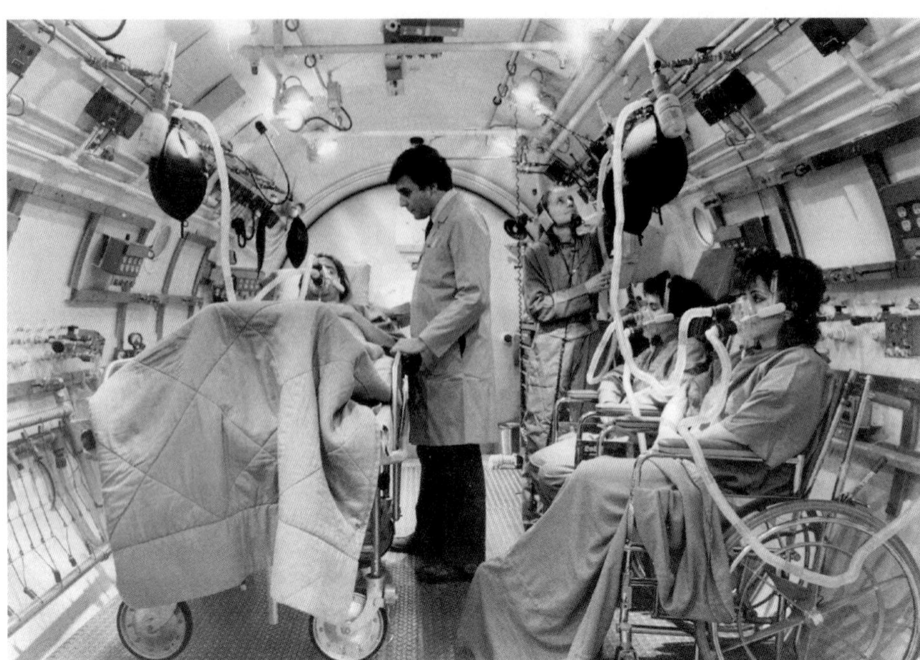

Figure 71.2 *A multiplace chamber at the University of Pennsylvania Institute for Environmental Medicine.*

Electrical defibrillation in a hyperbaric chamber is controversial, because of the possibility or poor skin contact, arcing, and risk of fire. In addition, because of the largely metal environment, attendants are at risk of shock. Many hyperbaric centers require that the chamber be decompressed prior to the use of a defibrillator. This causes some unique decompression problems for the attendants if the therapy has been prolonged. However, the latency of bubble formation and onset of DCS symptoms is sufficient to allow a brief (5–10 min) excursion to 1 ATA for defibrillation, with a subsequent return to pressure.[93]

The use of intravenous infusions and invasive monitoring in monoplace chambers is difficult, but appropriate equipment and experience are accumulating. This is much simplified in the multiplace chamber, in which normal equipment may be used with minor modification. For example, flexible bags are preferred over glass bottles for intravenous transfusion so that a pressure gradient between the chamber atmosphere and the fluid reservoir does not occur. If bottles must be used (a nitroglycerin infusion, for example), the attendant must ensure that the gas space above the liquid is in constant communication with the chamber atmosphere. Battery-driven syringe pumps are probably the best alternative for intravenous drug infusion in the hyperbaric chamber. Gas-filled pressure bags for arterial catheters must be checked during and after compression (refilled) and vented during decompression. Other closed, gas-filled devices that must be carefully monitored are the tracheal tube cuff and face mask seal, both of which may be filled with an incompressible medium such as water or saline instead of air so that over- or underexpansion does not occur and result in injury or leakage. An exception is the gas-filled balloon on flow-directed pulmonary artery catheters; this balloon is best left deflated with the filling port open to the atmosphere during hyperbaric therapy.

Positive-pressure ventilation may be performed with self-inflating bags, although volume-cycled ventilators are preferred.[94] A means of monitoring expired minute volume is required, as changes may occur with the alterations in ambient pressure. Peak ventilatory pressures should also be monitored, because the increased gas density at pressure may require large increases in the ventilatory pressure to achieve reasonable flow rates and minute volumes. Expired gas from all such patient breathing circuits should be collected and exhausted directly to the outside of the chamber to maintain a chamber oxygen concentration of less than about 23% (multiplace chamber).

Blood sampling at pressure is conducted as at sea level, and the sample slowly decompressed to 1 ATA in an airlock. Blood gas analysis is optimally conducted with the analyzer in the chamber and calibrated at pressure. When in-chamber equipment is not available, the sample can be analyzed after decompression. However, even small bubbles in the sample may lead to large errors in the $P_{a}O_2$. The $P_{a}CO_2$ in such samples is normally well preserved, because of the normal tension and large buffering and solubility of this gas.

Although the effects of intravenous sedatives/hypnotics, analgesics, and muscle relaxants are probably more predictable and their use more intuitive than with inhalational agents in these unusual environments, it is useful to understand how the delivery of an anesthetic vapor at pressure may differ from that at sea level. The vapor pressure of a liquid is independent of barometric pressure, so the saturated vapor pressure of isoflurane, for example, is about 34.7 kPa (260 mmHg) at room temperature, whether at 3000 m (10 000 feet) altitude or at 2.8 ATA in a hyperbaric chamber. Therefore, depending on the density and viscosity dependence of the proportioning valve in the agent-specific vaporizers, approximately the equivalent *partial pressure* of the anesthetic gas as that indicated on the calibrated dial for sea level will be delivered at increased pressure.[95,96] A similar situation exists for vaporizers of the copper kettle variety: normal anesthetic effects will be obtained by using standard flow ratios to the vaporizer. The delivered gas *concentration* (volume percent) will depend directly on atmospheric pressure but, as the pharmacologically relevant parameter is the partial pressure, the change in concentration is unimportant. While calculations predict that a slight deviation from indicated partial pressures may exist, it is important to remember that individual variation in response to the volatile anesthetic agents is substantially larger than the variation in vaporizer output in altered pressure environments, making their use possible with normal vigilance. Rotameter flowmeters, because of their density dependence, will overestimate gas flows slightly during hyperbaric therapy. Nitrous oxide is rarely used in chambers because the primary indication for HBOT is the delivery of 100% oxygen. In general, the indications for general anesthesia in a hyperbaric chamber are few and injectable agents are preferred. The pressure range used for clinical HBOT has not been associated with any demonstrable change in the pharmacokinetic or pharmacodynamic properties of the drugs likely to be used in such settings.

Risks of hyperbaric oxygen therapy

Barotrauma

Aural barotrauma is the most common risk or complication of hyperbaric therapy, and is almost always due to the compression phase. It can be minimized by the use of topical or systemic vasoconstrictors or, in specific cases, by myringotomy. Pulmonary barotrauma during hyperbaric therapy is rare but should be suspected when any significant chest or hemodynamic symptoms occur during or shortly after the decompression; if suspected, decompression should be stopped and pneumothorax treated with a chest tube. If evidence of gas embolism exists, the appropriate hyperbaric oxygen protocol should be initiated. Pre-existing pneumothorax should be treated with chest tube drainage prior to starting hyperbaric therapy to prevent the development of tension pneumothorax during decompression due to continued air leak.

Decompression sickness

DCS is unlikely to occur to the patient who breathes 100% oxygen during most of the therapy; little nitrogen (or other inert gas) uptake occurs. The chamber attendants, on the other hand, generally breathe air during the therapy, so substantial nitrogen uptake occurs and they are at risk of DCS. However, because HBOT protocols have been designed to limit nitrogen uptake by the attendants, this risk is small. If an attendant becomes unavoidably involved in a prolonged therapy, the decompression rate can be decreased to meet the decompression obligation, or oxygen inhalation can be used prior to and during decompression.

Oxygen toxicity

CNS oxygen toxicity is possible with the exposures normally used for HBOT. Generally, an inspired oxygen pressure of less than 3 ATA is used, and the incidence of CNS symptoms in resting patients is reported to be less than 1 in 10 000 patient therapies.[18] The risk may be higher with exertion or in hypercapnic patients, as discussed above. The primary manifestation of CNS oxygen toxicity is seizure activity, which may be preceded by muscular twitching or visual symptoms (narrowing of visual fields). Termination of oxygen inhalation and protection from injury are usually sufficient therapy. Because of the possibility of airway obstruction and breath holding during seizure activity, concurrent decompression may increase the risk of pulmonary barotrauma and gas embolism; changes in chamber pressure should await cessation of seizures. In susceptible patients, anticonvulsant therapy may reduce the probability of oxygen-induced convulsions during HBOT.

Pulmonary symptoms of oxygen toxicity are more predictable than those of the CNS, and are more slowly progressive. Significant symptoms in healthy subjects may develop in 8–10 h of continuous oxygen inhalation at 2 ATA,[8] but this is shortened to 3–4 h at 3 ATA. Intermittent air breathing during HBOT has been shown to substantially extend pulmonary oxygen tolerance, and it is now standard practice to include 5–15 min air "breaks" at regular intervals during oxygen breathing. Oxygen inhalation limits have been established so that the risk of toxicity in prolonged or unusual hyperbaric therapy protocols can be estimated, and modified if necessary. Pulmonary symptoms attributable to oxygen toxicity are readily reversible when the P_{IO_2} is decreased below 0.5 ATA,[13] and long-term sequelae have not been reported. Similarly, pulmonary sequelae of chronic daily therapy have not been detected.[97]

Visual function

Progressive myopia has been observed in some patients during prolonged daily therapy, presumably due to effects of either oxygen or pressure on lens shape or refractive index. It is usually reversed within days to weeks after completion of therapy.[98] A baseline ophthalmological examination is generally obtained prior to the initiation of an extended course of therapy. Cataract development has been associated with unusually prolonged of therapy, such as 150–200 daily exposures to 2.0–2.5 ATA, and does not reverse after cessation of therapy. Finally, the neonatal retina is sensitive to oxygen; prolonged exposure to even 1 ATA may induce retrolental fibroplasia.[99]

Other risks and side-effects

Claustrophobia may be a significant problem for isolated patients, especially in monoplace chambers, and they may require sedation for successful therapy. Sedation must be used cautiously in the spontaneously breathing patient receiving HBOT, however, because hypoventilation and hypercapnia may lower the threshold for oxygen-induced seizures.

The increased concentration and partial pressure of oxygen increases the risk of *fire*. In monoplace chambers, which are compressed with oxygen, scrupulous attention to elimination of sources of ignition is required. Because the multiplace chamber is compressed with air, and as the rate of combustion is related primarily to *fractional concentration* (volume percent) and not *partial pressure* of oxygen, the risk is less. In any case, limitation of flammable items and sources of ignition is necessary. Although most chambers have automatic fire-control systems, these should not be relied upon to stop a fire in an oxygen-enriched atmosphere.

REFERENCES

1. Wolf HK, Moon RE, Mitchell PR, Burger PC. Barotrauma and air embolism in hyperbaric oxygen therapy. *Am J Forensic Med Pathol* 1990; **11:** 149–53.
2. Fernau JL, Hirsch BE, Derkay C, *et al.* Hyperbaric oxygen therapy: effect on middle ear and eustachian tube function. *Laryngoscope* 1992; **102:** 48–52.
3. Bennett PB. Inert gas narcosis and the high pressure nervous syndrome in man. In: Bennett PB, Elliott DH (eds). *The Physiology and Medicine of Diving*, 3rd edn. San Pedro: Best, 1982: 239–96.
4. Wann KT, MacDonald AG. Actions and interactions of high pressure and general anesthetics. *Prog Neurobiol* 1988; **30:** 271–307.
5. Henshaw In: Simpson, A. (ed). *Compressed Air as a Therapeutic Agent in the Treatment of Consumption, Asthma, Chronic Bronchitis and Other Diseases.* Edinburgh: Sutherland and Knox, 1857.
6. Thom SR. Hyperbaric oxygen therapy. *J Intens Care Med* 1989; **4:** 58–74
7. Clark JM. Oxygen toxicity. In: Bennett PB, Elliott DH (eds). *The Physiology and Medicine of Diving*, 3rd edn. San Pedro: Best, 1982**:** 200–38.
8. Clark JM. Pulmonary limits of oxygen tolerance in man. *Exp Lung Res* 1988; **14:** 897–910.
9. Deneke SM, Fanburg BL. Normobaric oxygen toxicity of the lung. *N Engl J Med* 1980; **303:** 76–86.
10. Sackner MA, Landa J, Hirsch J, Zapata A. Pulmonary effects of oxygen breathing. *Ann Intern Med* 1975; **82:** 40–3.
11. Clark JM, Lambertsen CJ. Rate of development of pulmonary oxygen toxicity in man during oxygen breathing at 2.0 ATA. *J Appl Physiol* 1971; **30:** 739–52.
12. Cheney FW, Huang TW, Gronka R. The effects of 50% oxygen on the resolution of pulmonary injury. *Am Rev Respir Dis* 1980; **122:** 373–9.
13. Eckenhoff RG, Dougherty JH, Messier A, *et al.* Progression of and recovery from pulmonary oxygen toxicity in humans exposed to 5 ATA air. *Aviat Space Environ Med* 1987; **58:** 658–67.
14. Kravetz G, Fisher AB, Forman HJ. The oxygen-adapted rat model: tolerance to oxygen at 1.5 and 2 ATA. *Aviat Space Environ Med* 1980; **51:** 775–7.
15. Frank L. Protection from oxygen toxicity by pre-exposure to hypoxia: lung antioxidant enzyme role. *J Appl Physiol* 1982; **53:** 475–82
16. Hendricks PL, Hall DA, Hunter WL, Haley PJ. Extension of pulmonary oxygen tolerance in men at 2 ATA by intermittent oxygen exposure. *J Appl Physiol* 1977; **42:** 593–9.

17. Crapo JD, Barry BE, Foscue HA, Shelburne J. Structural and biochemical changes in rat lungs occurring during exposures to lethal and adaptive doses of oxygen. *Am Rev Respir Dis* 1980; **122:** 123–43.
18. Coursin DB, Cihla HP, Will JA, McCreary JL. Adaptation to chronic hyperoxia. Biochemical effects and the response to subsequent lethal hyperoxia. *Am Rev Respir Dis* 1987; **135:** 1002–6.
19. Holm BA, Matalon S, Finkelstein JN, Notter RH. Type II pneumocyte changes during hyperoxic lung injury and recovery. *J Appl Physiol* 1988; **65:** 2672–8.
20. Davis JC. Hyperbaric medicine: patient selection, treatment procedures, and side effects. In: Daves JC, Hunt TK (eds). *Problem Wounds: The Role of Oxygen.* New York: Elsevier, 1988: 225–35.
21. Roberton WG, Hargreaves JJ, Herlocher JE, Welch BE. Physiologic response to increased oxygen partial pressure. II. Respiratory studies. *Aerospace Med* 1964; **35:** 618–22.
22. Lambertsen CJ. Chemical control of respiration at rest. In: Mountcastle VB (ed.). *Medical Physiology*, 14th edn, vol 2. St Louis: CV Mosby, 1980: 1774.
23. Cullen SC, Eger EI, Cullen BF. Observations on the anaesthetic effect of the combination of xenon and halothane. *Anesthesiology* 1969; **31:** 305–9.
24. Wood LDH, Bryan AC. Effect of increased ambient pressure on flow volume curve of the lung. *J Appl Physiol* 1969; **27:** 4–8.
25. Dutka AJ. Air or gas embolism. In: Camporesi EM, Barker AC (eds). *Hyperbaric Oxygen Therapy: A Critical Review.* Bethesda, MD: Undersea and Hyperbaric Medical Society, 1991: 1–10.
26. Hallenbeck JM, Anderson JC. Pathogenesis of the decompression disorders. In: Bennett PB, Elliott DH (eds). *The Physiology and Medicine of Diving.* London: Baillière Tindall, 1982: 435–60.
27. Gilliam BC. Evaluation of decompression sickness incidence in multi-day repetitive diving for 77 680 sport dives. In: Lang MA, Vann RD (eds). *Proceedings of the American Society of Underwater Sciences. Repetitive Diving Workshop*, Costa Mesa, CA: American Academy of Underwater Sciences, 1992: 219–26.
28. Kelleher PC, Thalmann ED, Survanshi SS, Weathersby PK. Verification trial of a probabilistic decompression model. *Undersea Biomed Res* 1992; **19:** A123.
29. Spencer MP. Decompression limits for compressed air determined by ultrasonically detected blood bubbles. *J Appl Physiol* 1976; **40:** 229–35.
30. Eckenhoff RG, Olstad CE, Carrod GE. Human dose–response relationship for decompression and endogenous bubble formation. *J Appl Physiol* 1990; **69:** 914–18.
31. Tikuisis P. Modeling the observations of *in vivo* bubble formation with hydrophobic crevices. *Undersea Biomed Res* 1986; **13:** 165–80.
32. Martin JD, Beck G, Treat JR, Thom SR. Leukocyte sequestration as a consequence of decompression stress. *Undersea Hyperbaric Med* 1999; **26** (Suppl.): 58.
33. Ward CA, McCullough D, Fraser WD. Relation between complement activation and susceptibility to decompression sickness. *J Appl Physiol* 1987; **62:** 1160–6.
34. Grim PS, Gottlieb LJ, Boddie A, Batson E. Hyperbaric oxygen therapy. *J Am Med Assoc* 1990; **263:** 2216–20.
35. Kindwall EP. Uses of hyperbaric oxygen therapy in the 1990s. *Cleveland Clin J Med* 1992; **59:** 517–528.
36. Hardy KR, Thom SR. Pathophysiology and treatment of carbon monoxide poisoning. *Clin Toxicol* 1994; **32:** 613–29.
37. Ernst A, Zirbak J. Carbon monoxide poisoning. *N Engl J Med* 1998; **22:** 1603–8.
38. Tomaszewski CA, Thom SR. Use of hyperbaric oxygen in toxicology. *Emerg Med Clin N Am* 1994; **12:** 437–59.
39. Choi SH. Delayed neurological sequelae in carbon monoxide intoxication. *Arch Neurol* 1983; **40:** 433–5.
40. Thom SR. Carbon monoxide-mediated brain lipid peroxidation in the rat. *J Appl Physiol* 1990; **68:** 997–1003.
41. Meilin S, Rogatsky GG, Thom SR, *et. al.* Effects of carbon monoxide on may be mediated by nitric oxide. *J Appl Physiol* 1996; **81:** 1078–83.
42. Cramlet SH, Erickson HH, Gorman HA. Ventricular function following carbon monoxide exposure. *J Appl Physiol* 1975; **39:** 482–6.
43. Halebian B, Robinson N, Barie P, *et al.* Whole body oxygen utilization during acute carbon monoxide poisoning and isocapneic nitrogen hypoxia. *J Trauma* 1986; **26:** 110–17.
44. Thom SR. Xanthine dehydrogenase conversion to oxidase and lipid peroxidation in brain after carbon monoxide poisoning. *J Appl Physiol* 1992; **73:** 1587–7.
45. Ginsberg MD, Myers RE, McDonaugh BF. Experimental carbon monoxide encephalopathy in the primate. II. Clinical aspects, neuropathology and physiologic correlation. *Arch Neurol* 1974; **30:** 209–16.
46. Smith JS, Broudm S. Morbidity from acute carbon monoxide poisoning at three year follow-up. *Br Med J* 1973; **1:** 318–21.
47. Hampson NB (ed.). *Hyperbaric Oxygen Therapy: 1999 Committee Report.* Kensington, MD: Undersea and Hyperbaric Medical Society, 1999.
48. Myers RM, Snyder SK, Lindberg S, *et al.* Valuae of hyperbaric oxygen in suspected carbon monoxide poisoning. *J Am Med Assoc* 1981; **246:** 2478–80.
49. Raphael JC, Elkharrat D, Jars-Guincestre, MC, *et al.* Trial of normobaric and hyperbaric oxygen for acute carbon monoxide intoxication. *Lancet* 1989; **2:** 414–19.
50. Mathieu D, Nolf M, Purocher A, *et al.* Acute carbon monoxide poisoning: risk of late sequelae and treatment by hyperbaric oxygen. *Clin Toxicol* 1985; **23:** 315–24.
51. Sokal JA, Kralkowska E. The relationship between exposure duration, carboxy-hemoglobin, blood glucose, pyruvate and lactate and the severity of intoxication in 39 cases of acute carbon monoxide poisoning in man. *Arch Toxicol* 1985; **3:** 196–9.
52. Pace N, Strajman E, Walker EL. Acceleration of carbon monoxide elimination in man by high pressure oxygen. *Science* 1950; **111:** 652–4.
53. Thom SR. Smoke inhalation. *Emerg Med Clin N Am* 1989; **7:** 371–87.
54. Caravati EM, Adams CJ, Joyce SM, *et al.* Fetal toxicity associated with maternal carbon monoxide poisoning. *Ann Emerg Med* 1988; **17:** 714–17.
55. Longo LD. The biologic effects of carbon monoxide on pregnant woman, fetus and newborn infant. *Am J Obstet Gynecol* 1977; **1:** 69–103.
56. Longo LD, Hill EP. Carbon monoxide uptake and elimination in fetal and maternal sheep. *Am J Physiology* 1977; **232:** H324–H330.
57. Hart GB, Lennon PA, Strauss MB. Hyperbaric oxygen in exceptional acute blood loss anemia. *J Hyperbaric Med* 1987; **2:** 205–10
58. Van Unnik AM. Inhibition of toxin production in *Clostridium perfringens in vitro* by hyperbaric oxygen. *Antonie van Leeuwenhoek* 1965; **31:** 181–6.
59. Mandell G. Bacteriocidal activity of bacteriocidal activity of aerobic and anaerobic polymorphonuclear neutrophils. *Infect Immun* 1974; **9:** 337–41.
60. Boerema I, Brummelkamp WH. Treatment of anaerobic infections by the introduction of pure oxygen under a pressure of 3 atmospheres. *Nederl Tijdschr V Geneesk* 1960; **104:** 2548.
61. Bakker DJ. Pure and mixed aerobic and anaerobic soft tissue infections. *Hyperbaric Oxygen Rev* 1985; **6:** 65–9.
62. Gozal D, Ziser A, Shupak A, *et al.* Necrotizing fasciitis. *Arch Surg* 1985; **121:** 233–5.
63. Zanetti CL. Necrotizing soft tissue infection and adjunctive hyperbaric oxygen. *Chest* 1988; **92:** 670–1.
64. Weiss RD, Van Meter KW. The applications of hyperbaric oxygen therapy in emergecy medicine. *Am J Emerg Med* 1992; **10:** 558–68.
65. Riegels-Nielsen P, Hesselfeldt-Nielsen J, Ganz-Jensen E, *et. al.* Fournier's gangrene: five patients treated with hyperbaric oxygen. *J Urol* 1984; **132:** 918–920.
66. Ziger A, Girsh Z, Gozal D, *et al.* Hyperbaric oxygen therapy for Fournier's gangrene. *Crit Care Med* 1985; **13:** 773–4.
67. Ketchum SA, Zubrin JR, Thomas AN, Hall AD. Effect of hyperbaric oxygen on small first, second and third degree burns. *Surg Forum* 1967; **18:** 65–7.
68. Ketchum SA, Thomas AN, Hall AD. Angiographic studies of the effect of hyperbaric oxygen on burn wound revascularization. In: Wadan J, Iwa T (eds). *Proceedings of the Fourth International Congress on Hyperbaric Medicine.* Tokyo: Igaku Shoin, 1970; 383–94.
69. Korn HN, Wheeler ES, Miller JA. Effect of hyperbaric oxygen on second-degree burn wound healing. *Arch Surg* 1977; **112:** 732–7.
70. Hart GB, O'Reilly RR, Broussard ND, *et. al.* Treatment of burns with hyperbaric oxygen. *Surg Gynecol Obstet* 1974; **139:** 693–6.
71. Nin AC, Yang C, Lee HC, *et. al.* Burns treated with adjunctive hyperbaric oxygen therapy: A comparative study in humans. *J Hyperbaric Med* 1987; **2:** 75–85.
72. Clark JM. Hyperbaric oxygen therapy. In: Crystal RG, West JB (eds). *The Lung.* Philadelphia: Lippincott-Raven Publishers, 1977: 2667–76.
73. Waisbren BA, Schultz D, Collentine G, Banaszak E. Hyperbaric oxygen in severe burns. *Burns* 1987; **8:** 176–9.
74. Cianci P, Lueders H, Lee H, *et al.* Adjunctive hyperbaric oxygen reduces the need for surgery in 0–80% burns. *J Hyperbaric Med* 1988; **3:** 87–101.
75. Pierce EC. Cerebral gas embolism with special reference to iatrogenic accidents. *Hyperbaric Oxygen Rev* 1980; **1:** 161–84.

76. Braun F, Krishel S. Environmental emergencies. *Emerg Med Clin N Am* 1997; **15:** 451–60.
77. Kizer KW, Neuman TS. Meeting the challenge of scuba diving emergencies: recognition, resuscitation, and recompression. *Emerg Med Rep* 1991; **12:** 151–60.
78. Leitch DR, Green RD. Pulmonary barotrauma in divers and the treatment of cerebral arterial gas embolism. *Aviat Space Environ Med* 1986; **57:** 931–938.
79. Lehner CE. Dive profiles and adaptation: pressure profiles target specific tissues for decompression injury. In: Lang MA, Vann RD (eds). *Proceedings of the American Academy of Underwater Sciences. Repetitive Diving Workshop.* Costa Mesa, CA: American Academy of Underwater Sciences, 1992: 203–17.
80. Myers RAM, Bray P. Delayed treatment of serious decompression sickness. *Ann Emerg Med* 1985; **14:** 254–7.
81. Marx RE. Osteoradionecrosis: a new concept of its pathophysiology. *J Oral Maxillofac Surg* 1983; **41:** 283–88.
82. Epstein JB, Wong FW, Stevenson-Moore P. Osteoradionecrosis: clinical experience and proposal for classification. *J Oral Maxillofac Surg* 1987; **45:** 104–10.
83. Marx RE. A new concept in the treatment of osteoradionecrosis. *J Oral Maxillofac Surg* 1988; **41:** 351–7.
84. Marx RE, Johnson RP. Problem wounds in oral and maxillofacial surgery: the role of hyperbaric oxygen. In: Davis JC, Hunt T (eds). *Problem Wounds: The Role of Oxygen.* New York: Elsevier, 1988: 65–123.
85. Knighton DR, Hunt TK, Scheuestuhl H, *et. al.* Oxygen tension regulates the expression of angiogenesis factor of macrophages. *Science* 1983; **221:** 1283–5.
86. Weiss JP, Boland FP, Mori H, *et. al.* Treatment of radiation-induced cystitis with hyperbaric oxygen. *J Urol* 1985; **134:** 352–54.
87. Strauss MB. Refracotry osteomeylitis. *J Hyperbaric Med* 1987; **2:** 147–59.
88. Triplett RG, Branham GB, Gillmore JD, Lorber M. Experimental mandibular osteomyelitis: therapeutic trials with hyperbaric oxygen. *J Oral Maxillofac Surg* 1982; **40:** 640–46.
89. Niinkoski J, Penttinen R, Kulonen E. Effect of hyperbaric oxygen on fracture healing in the rat: a biochemical study. *Calcif Tissue Res* 1970; **4** (Suppl.): 115–16.
90. Cierny G, Mader JT, Pennick JJ. A clinical staging system for adult osteomyelitis. *Contemp Orthoped* 1985; **10:** 17–37.
91. Bowersox JC, Strauss MB, Hart GB. Clinical experience with hyperbaric oxygen therapy in the salvage of ischemic skin flaps and grafts. *J Hyperbaric Med* 1986; **1:** 141–9.
92. Perrins DJ. The effect of hyperbaric oxygen on ischemic skin flaps. In: Grabb WC, Myers MB (eds). *Skin Flaps.* Boston: Little, Brown, 1975: 53–63.
93. Eckenhoff RG, Parker JW. Latency in the onset of decompression sickness on direct ascent from air saturation. *J Appl Physiol* 1984; **56:** 1070–5.
94. Moon RE, Bergquist LV, Conklin B, Miller JN. Monaghan 225 ventilator use under hyperbaric conditions. *Chest* 1986; **89:** 846.
95. Satterfield JM, Russell GB, Graybeal JM, Richard RB. Anesthetic vaporizer performance under hyperbaric conditions. *Undersea Biomed Res* 1989; **16:** A43.
96. Severinghaus J. Committee report. Hyperbaric oxygenation: anesthesia and drug effects. *Anesthesiology* 1965; **26:** 812–24.
97. Rusca F, Garetto G, Ambrosio F, *et al.* HBO therapy and pulmonary function tests. *Undersea Biomed Res* 1991; **18:** A196.
98. Lyne AJ. Ocular effects of hyperbaric oxygen. *Trans Ophthalmol Soc N Z* 1978; **98:** 66–8.
99. Patz A. Effect of oxygen on immature retinal vessels. *Invest Ophthalmol* 1965; **4:** 988–99.

72

Management and complications of commonly ingested and inhaled poisons

JOHN A HENRY

GENERAL PRINCIPLES

The anesthesiologist usually becomes involved in the management of the acutely poisoned patient in three sets of circumstances: first, when called on to assist in the assessment or management of a sick or unconscious patient in the emergency department; second, following cardiopulmonary arrest due to poisoning; and, third, in the management of poisoned patients who have been referred to the intensive therapy unit.

Poisons information or control centers are a useful resource found in many cities in most countries. They are available for emergency consultations regarding diagnosis and therapy. They form a practical information source for the doctor who does not possess the necessary knowledge or who is perplexed by a confusing or complicated case.

POISONS AND THE OXYGEN PATHWAY

Most of the poisonings that the anesthesiologist sees involve the oxygen pathway, which covers the delivery of oxygen from the inspired air to cellular respiration. A severe reduction in the oxygen content of the inspired air will cause acute hypoxemia, producing collapse and coma. Interference with the mechanics of respiration by poisons may result in hypoxemia and hypercapnia. Disturbance of oxygen transfer may produce hypoxemia. Even if the oxygen content of the air is not diminished, and respiration is functioning adequately, disturbances to either process may prevent oxygen reaching its intracellular site of action. Further down the pathway, the oxygen-carrying capacity of the blood may be reduced by the presence of carboxyhemoglobin or methemoglobin or, more rarely, by acute hemolysis. Cardiac output may be reduced by a number of poisons that cause cardiac arrhythmias, or depress the contractility of the heart, or cause extreme vasodilation. The final step by which poisons may interfere with the oxygen pathway is by blockage of the cytochrome enzyme chain by toxins such as cyanide and hydrogen sulfide. The ultimate outcome of interference with the pathway is cellular hypoxia, which may lead to cell death. These effects and the main poisons involved are outlined in Table 72.1.

Immediate assessment

The doctor should avoid the danger of being so concerned about the reversal of the poisoning as to overlook the immediate care of the patient. It is essential to check at once whether the patient's respiration and cardiac output are adequate. A rapid inspection will indicate whether the patient's life is in immediate danger. Respiratory depression is a feature of poisoning by sedative, hypnotic, and narcotic drugs as well as by many chemical toxins. Blood gas estimation and measurement of the minute and tidal volumes are important in the management of the comatose, collapsed, or convulsing patient, as controlled ventilation may be needed at any stage. Pupil size and reaction are also an important part of the diagnostic assessment. It should be noted that there are many causes of widely dilated or fixed pupils in poisoned patients (see Table 72.2), which could lead to difficulty in diagnosis. The severely poisoned patient must be managed as any other critically ill patient, and cardiopulmonary stabilization is the immediate objective. Once the patient's immediate condition is stable, attention can be paid to assessing the type and severity of poisoning, so as to draw up a management plan.

Diagnosis of poisoning

It is important to obtain a history from the patient before deterioration occurs or consciousness is lost. Relatives or the ambulance crew may also be able to help, by describing the patient's behavior or the circumstances in which he/she was found, and by providing evidence such as tablets, syringes, or a suicide note. It is essential to search the patient's clothing for clues and to look for evidence of other metabolic, endocrine, and neurologic diseases (such as uremia, myxedema, diabetes, and epilepsy).

The clinical features of poisoning may be specific for the toxin but are often nonspecific. Clinical examination may reveal a picture characteristic of poisoning by a certain type of agent. The main ones are summarized in Table 72.3. Evidence may be provided by the smell of the patient's breath. Solvents, cyanide, hydrogen sulfide, carbamates, acetone, and many other agents produce characteristic odors that may help in diagnosis. The smell of alcohol is unreliable as it is mainly due to congeners and may be present at clinically insignificant levels or virtually absent at severely toxic levels. A breath alcohol meter may be helpful for diagnosis. If there is any doubt as to whether the apparently intoxicated patient has a significant head injury, the policy should be to anesthetize and control the patient's ventilation so that a computed tomography (CT) or magnetic resonance imaging (MRI) brain scan can be carried out.

Further clues to poisoning include the evidence of self-injection: injection marks, "tracks," and abscesses may be found during the initial assessment. Inspection of the mouth and throat may show traces of tablet residues or signs of corrosion.

Table 72.1 *Some major causes of blockade of the oxygen pathway due to poisoning, with mechanisms and typical values*

Cause	Mechanism	Effect
Asphyxiant gases (e.g. butane, methane, carbon dioxide, nitrogen)	Hypoxic gas mixture	Reduced inspired oxygen fraction (F_IO_2) (normal 0.21)
Respiratory depression (e.g. opioids, barbiturates, other sedatives, and hypnotics) Respiratory muscle disorders: paralysis (e.g. organophosphates, botulinum toxin) or spasm (e.g. strychnine, phencyclidine)	Failure of ventilation (type II respiratory failure)	Reduced alveolar oxygen tension (P_AO_2) (normal 13.3 kPa)
Aspiration pneumonitis Adult respiratory distress syndrome (e.g. paraquat)	Failure of oxygen transfer (type I respiratory failure)	Reduced arterial oxygen tension (P_aO_2) (normal 10–13.3 kPa)
Carboxyhemoglobin (carbon monoxide) Methemoglobin (e.g. nitrites) Hemolysis (e.g. arsine, stibine)	Loss of functioning hemoglobin	Reduced arterial oxygen content (C_aO_2) (normal 18–21 mL dL^{-1})
Myocardial depressants (e.g. beta-blockers, tricyclic antidepressants, dextropropoxyphene)	Reduced cardiac output	Reduced tissue oxygen delivery ($\dot{Q}O_2$) (normal 12–16 mL kg^{-1} per min)
Chemical asphyxiants (cyanide, hydrogen sulfide)	Block of cytochrome enzyme chain	Reduced tissue oxygen consumption ($\dot{V}O_2$) causing failure of oxidative metabolism (normal 3–4 mL kg^{-1} min^{-1})
Any or several of the above		Cell death

Table 72.2 *Effects of poisons on pupil size*

Widely dilated or fixed dilated pupils
- Cerebral hypoxia due to cardiorespiratory insufficiency or arrest
- Hypoxic cerebral damage
- Cerebral hypoxia due to cellular poisons, cyanide, hydrogen sulfide
- Severe hypothermia
- Poisons causing blindness: quinine, methanol
- Amphetamines, cocaine, monoamine oxidase inhibitors
- Anticholinergic agents

Small or pinpoint pupils
- Opioids
- Organophosphates
- Chloral hydrate
- Sodium valproate

Laboratory diagnosis

In many cases, it will be unnecessary to carry out any specialized laboratory investigations in order to confirm or quantify the poison involved. The history and the clinical state of the patient may be sufficient, or the patient may be recovering when seen. In some cases, however, a definitive diagnosis of poisoning may need to be made by laboratory analysis of specimens taken from the patient or of material found on or beside the patient (see Table 72.3). The usual samples required are blood (which should be separated and saved as plasma except when whole blood is required, as for example in carbon monoxide, mercury, and lead poisoning), gastric aspirate, and urine. However, in all cases, patient samples should be obtained on admission and saved in case subsequent analyses are needed. When there is adequate clinical evidence that a certain agent or group of agents is involved, and the knowledge acquired from chemical analysis is not going to alter the management of the patient, urgent analysis is not required. In cases where prolonged cardiopulmonary resuscitation is continuing, urgent toxicologic analysis may confirm the substance involved and help in making a decision on how long to persevere with efforts at resuscitation. The usual indications for urgent analyses are for those cases in whom the management of the patient will be affected by the result, e.g. in the use of active procedures to remove the poison or in the use of specific antidotes. Poisoning occurs through a wide range of mechanisms, many of which can be arrested or reversed by treatment with antidotes. Those most likely to be needed are listed in Table 72.4.

In every comatose patient suspected of self-poisoning by drugs, it is common practice to obtain laboratory measurements of plasma salicylate and acetaminophen (paracetamol), as these may have been taken together with another agent and may be overlooked. However, in very rare cases, massive overdose of acetaminophen alone may be the cause of the coma.

Emergency department management

The anesthesiologist may be called to the emergency department for assessment of ventilatory status or to carry out intubation for protection of the airway while gastric lavage is carried out in the unconscious patient. Ventilatory status should be assessed, as in Chapter 14, and the decision made as to whether the patient requires intubation and/or mechanical ventilation. The main problem to bear in mind is that the poisoned patient's condition may suddenly deteriorate at any time, with complications such as vomiting, convulsions, or cardiac/respiratory deterioration. Frequent close monitoring is required above all for the poisoned patient.

Elimination procedures

Gastrointestinal decontamination

Emetics are of little use in preventing absorption of ingested poisons. Although an emetic such as syrup of ipecacuanha induces vomiting very effectively, there is little evidence for its effectiveness in removing significant amounts of ingested poison, and its use has been largely discarded. Although gastric lavage may be shown very occasionally to remove large amounts of an ingested drug or poison, there is little documentation for its effectiveness. However, gastric lavage is the only means of emptying the stomach in the unconscious patient, in which case the airway will need to be protected. Oral activated charcoal is widely used either alone or in combination with emesis or gastric lavage in order to reduce drug absorption. There is considerable evidence for its effectiveness, especially when given shortly after ingestion. It is accepted that the dose of charcoal should be at least 10 times that of the dose of poison ingested; otherwise the dose is based on the amount likely to be tolerated: $1\,g\,kg^{-1}$ body weight in an infant or child and $25–50\,g\,kg^{-1}$ body weight for an adult. This applies to a single dose given shortly after ingestion. However, there is evidence that repeated doses of activated charcoal may be effective in removing poisons that have delayed absorption from the gastrointestinal tract (modified release preparations and salicylates) and those with a small volume of distribution, particularly theophylline, phenobarbital, salicylates, and carbamazepine. At the same time, there has been no convincing demonstration that repeated doses of activated charcoal shorten the time spent in the intensive therapy unit. The other gastrointestinal decontamination method that should be borne in mind is whole-gut lavage, in which the bowel is irrigated via a nasogastric tube with an isotonic solution, such as that used for preparing the intestine for radiologic procedures. This effectively clears the gut of ingested toxins that are potentially toxic yet are not easily removed by other means. These include the overdose of sustained-release preparations, heavy metal salts, iron or lithium ingestions, and swallowed packets of illicit drugs. The procedure is well tolerated and adverse effects are unlikely.[1]

Removal from the bloodstream

Hemodialysis is effective in removing many drugs and poisons from the bloodstream. The most important indications are salicylate poisoning, when hemodialysis additionally helps to correct metabolic disturbances, ethylene glycol, methanol, phenobarbital, lithium, and theophylline. When possible, hemodialysis should be used in preference to peritoneal dialysis or continuous arteriovenous hemoperfusion, which, though effective at supporting renal function, are less effective in removing toxins. Charcoal or resin hemoperfusion is effective in removing a wide range of drugs and poisons but is rarely indicated; its most important use is in severe theophylline overdose.

Cardiopulmonary resuscitation

The most urgent measure for the patient who is apneic or pulseless is to re-establish ventilation and circulation by cardiopulmonary resuscitation. Once this has been performed effectively, the opportunity may be taken to tackle the cause of the problem. In some cases, antidotes are available, which can be effective in reversing the effects of the poisoning during the course of cardiopulmonary resuscitation. Examples include naloxone, atropine, cyanide antidotes, and digoxin-specific Fab antibody fragments (FAB) (see Table 72.4). Other poisons are capable of producing cardiac arrest, intractable arrhythmias, or pulseless electrical activity (PEA), which cannot be reversed by resuscitative measures or inotropic agents. In these cases, it may be worth persisting with active cardiopulmonary resuscitation for several hours until spontaneous cardiac output recovers, while the drug or poison is metabolized by the body. There have been several case reports of the successful use of prolonged external chest compression in tricyclic antidepressant poisoning, when the patient had severe hypotension or asystole.[2] It has also been used successfully in poisoning by beta-blockers, quinine, chloroquine, and digoxin, local anesthetic toxicity, and also in hypothermia, which may complicate many types of poisoning. Prolonged resuscitative efforts are therefore indicated in many types of poisoning that are refractory to other treatments, to allow time for drug redistribution, metabolism, and clearance. Extracorporeal circulation may be used when circumstances permit.[3]

Management of hypotension and pulseless electrical activity (PEA)

Agents with a potent negative inotropic effect are sometimes taken as a means of self-poisoning. The usual clinical picture is one of profound hypotension, and the depression of myocardial function may be such that cardiac output is insufficient to maintain adequate cerebral perfusion. Many of these cases develop electromechanical dissociation (see Chapter 71), and a variety of agents may be responsible. Treatment for these patients should be aggressive, as PEA due to poisoning has a better prognosis than when due to other causes, and successful reversal is a common occurrence after acute poisoning. Cardiogenic pulmonary edema may occur but is rarely severe, presumably because both left and right ventricles are equally depressed. Coma, hypoxemia, and metabolic acidosis may persist despite adequate ventilation with a high inspired oxygen content. Convulsions may occur. Correction of hypovolemia and inotropic support are required, with mechanical support of the circulation by external chest compression, for cases in which cardiac output is judged to be inadequate and unresponsive to inotropic support. Extracorporeal membrane oxygenation may also be used to provide support in extreme cases.

In some cases of poisoning with cardiodepressant drugs, specific treatments are helpful. This is particularly true of poisoning with β-adrenergic antagonists, which respond rapidly to glucagon or isoprenaline. Propoxyphene poisoning can cause severe cardiac depression unresponsive to naloxone; the patient may present with severe hypotension, seizures, and electrocardiographic abnormalities. Inotropic support is often required, and dopamine appears to be effective.[4] Many other drugs and poisons (see Table 72.5) can cause severe myocardial depression, although the response to inotropic agents is less well documented.

Hypovolemia and relative hypovolemia respond to volume repletion, whereas negatively inotropic agents can be managed with positively inotropic drugs, specific antidotes, and, where necessary, external chest compressions.

Hypothermia

Hypothermia presenting with hypotension, hypotonia, fixed dilated pupils, and a metabolic acidosis must be included in the differential diagnosis of poisoning, and profound hypothermia can be indistinguishable from death.[5,6] Hypothermia also commonly accompanies poisoning by narcotics, tricyclic antidepressants, and sedative and hypnotic drugs, especially if ethanol has also been ingested. The rectal temperature should be taken with a low-reading thermometer. Temperatures as low as 20–22 °C are compatible with complete recovery by poisoned patients, and the prognosis is generally better than in hypothermia secondary to an underlying medical condition.

An important clinical feature of severe hypothermia is that the pupils are often fixed and dilated even when drugs that constrict the pupils, such as opioids, are responsible. Therefore, this finding does not necessarily indicate hypoxic cerebral damage and should not deter from attempts at resuscitation. Hyperkalemia is associated with low probability of survival.[7] The management of hypothermia is controversial, but relatively rapid rewarming should be the rule. Prolonged external chest compression has been used successfully when serious cardiac arrhythmias or asystole have occurred during hypothermia.

Hyperthermia

The traditional method of treating hyperthermia is to attempt to accelerate heat loss by tepid sponging and fanning. Cooling using extracorporeal circulation and peritoneal dialysis have also been used, and this is appropriate for many causes of hyperthermia, including severe anticholinergic poisoning. In many toxic hyperthermic states, the mechanisms involved are complex. Hyperthemia due to monoamine oxidase inhibitor poisoning is dealt with later in this chapter. Several

Table 72.3 *Analyses that may be required in the management of the poisoned patient*

Toxin or measurement	Indications for measurement	Interpretation
Amphetamines (including MDA and MDMA)	Abuse	Near patient or laboratory tests can confirm exposure
Carbamazepine	1. Overdose	Severe toxicity over 25 mg L^{-1}
	2. Therapeutic monitoring	Therapeutic range 1.5–9 mg L^{-1}
Carboxyhemoglobin	1. Carbon monoxide inhalation	May confirm exposure and indicate severity (normal1%)
	2. Smoke-exposed fire victims	Carboxyhemoglobin over 12% indicates potential for pulmonary damage
	3. Methylene chloride exposure	Carbon monoxide is a metabolite of methylene chloride (dichloromethane)
Chloroquine	Accidental or deliberate overdose	May confirm ingestion and indicate potential toxicity
Cholinesterase (RBC)	1. Acute poisoning with organophosphates	RBC cholinesterase 20% of normal indicates significant exposure (usually by ingestion)
	2. Chronic exposure to organophosphates	RBC cholinesterase 50% of normal helps to confirm exposure but is poor guide to severity
Digoxin	1. Digoxin or digitoxin overdose	High levels shortly after ingestion indicate the need to obtain Fab antibody The result from a sample taken over 6 h after ingestion may be used to calculate the dose of Fab required
	2. Detecting digitalis immunoactivity in cardiac glycoside plant ingestion	May be used to confirm ingestion but is not a guide to severity
	3. Detecting digitalis toxicity in therapeutic use	To confirm toxicity or undertreatment. Hypokalemia may cause signs of toxicity with digoxin levels in the therapeutic range
Drug abuse screen	1. Suspected acute toxicity	May confirm diagnosis
	2. Medicolegal indications	May be used to confirm abstinence (sample collection must be supervised)
	3. Employment screening	May exclude from certain types of employment
Ethanol	1. Severe intoxication	Very high concentrations (over 4 g L^{-1}) in a severely obtunded patient may be an indication for hemodialysis
	2. Intoxication (actual or possible) in head-injured patients	Low concentrations (under 1.5 g L^{-1}) help to exclude ethanol as a cause of behavioral disturbance or altered consciousness level
	3. Monitoring of treatment of methanol or ethylene glycol intoxication	Blood ethanol should be maintained between 1 and 2 g L^{-1} to inhibit alcohol dehydrogenase
Ethylene glycol	Suspected toxicity	High levels (over 500 mg L^{-1}) are an indication for ethanol or fomepizole administration and possibly active elimination (hemodialysis)
Iron	Overdose	Serum iron over 55 μmol L^{-1} is potentially toxic. Desferrioxamine challenge test may be indicated
Lead	1. Clinical suspicion of poisoning	May confirm toxicity and indicate need for antidote therapy. Toxic concentration over 3.4 μmol L^{-1}
	2. Monitoring industrial exposure	Normal values up to 1.0 μmol L^{-1}. Over 1.4 μmol L^{-1}, monitoring required. Over 3.4 μmol L^{-1}, toxic, unfit for work
Lithium	1. Acute overdose	Plasma levels may confirm ingestion and indicate possible toxicity, but clinical manifestations are main guide to toxicity and the need for hemodialysis (patient may be asymptomatic with plasma lithium over 5 mmol L^{-1}, depending on time since ingestion)
	2. Therapeutic monitoring	Therapeutic range 0.7–1.2 mmol L^{-1}. Toxicity in therapeutic use can occur at over 1.5–2 mmol L^{-1} [often due to interactions with diuretic or nonsteroidal anti-inflammatory drug (NSAID) therapy]. Over 4 mmol L^{-1} severely toxic
Methanol	Suspected toxicity	High levels (over 200 mg L^{-1}) are an indication for ethanol or fomepizole administration and possibly active elimination (hemodialysis) or folinic acid therapy
Opioids	1. Overdose	Near patient or laboratory tests confirm exposure
	2. Abuse	Near patient or laboratory tests confirm exposure
	3. Toxicity in renal failure patients	Requires measurement of morphine 6-glucuronide

Osmolality (plasma)	Suspected methanol or ethylene glycol ingestion	Depending on time since ingestion, normal osmolality (preferably osmolar gap) can exclude potentially toxic ingestion. The osmolar gap can indicate severity. As a rapid guide, plasma osmolality of over 350 mosmol L^{-1} (methanol) or 370 mosmol L^{-1} (ethylene glycol) indicates the need to commence ethanol or fomepizole regimen and measure implicated substance(s)
Acetaminophen	1. Acetaminophen overdose	High concentrations are an indication for antidote administration according to nomogram
	2. Comatose patient with suspected drug overdose	To exclude co-ingestion of acetaminophen
Paraquat	Suspected ingestion (or other route of exposure)	Plasma paraquat levels can confirm ingestion and severity of exposure. Positive urine dithionite test confirms exposure Dithionite test may be carried out on plasma – if positive, confirms massive ingestion
Phenobarbitone	1. Overdose	Severe toxicity over 50 mg L^{-1}
	2. Abuse	Levels may be in the range 30–60 mg L^{-1} with minimal impairment
	3. Therapeutic monitoring	Normal range 5–30 mg L^{-1}
Phenytoin	1. Overdose	Severe toxicity over 50 mg L^{-1}. Over 95 mg L^{-1} potentially fatal
	2. Following overdose to decide when therapy should be resumed	Normal range 7–20 mg L^{-1}, 50% of patients show side-effects at over 30 mg L^{-1}
	3. Therapeutic monitoring	
Quinine	1. Overdose	Toxic levels > 10 mg L^{-1}
	2. Monitoring of malaria therapy	Toxic levels > 15 mg L^{-1}
Salicylate	1. Salicylate overdose	Provides an indication of severity and action to be taken. May indicate need for hemodialysis (over 700 mg L^{-1})
	2. Comatose patient with suspected drug overdose	To exclude co-ingestion of salicylate
	3. Therapeutic monitoring in rheumatology	Upper normal range 250 mg L^{-1}. Toxic levels > 500 mg L^{-1}
Solvents (volatile substances)	1. Suspected poisoning in an unconscious patient	May provide diagnosis
	2. Behavioral disturbance or suspected abuse	May confirm exposure
	3. Industrial exposure	Tests can confirm excessive exposure
Theophylline	1. Acute overdose	High concentrations (over 80 mg L^{-1}) in a severely symptomatic patient (convulsions, cardiac arrhythmias) may be an indication for hemoperfusion
	2. Therapeutic monitoring	Severe toxicity may occur at 30 mg L^{-1} during regular therapy
Toxicology screen	1. Suspected acute poisoning in an unconscious patient	May provide diagnosis
	2. Behavioral disturbance due to suspected abuse or poisoning	May provide diagnosis
	3. Confirmation of brainstem death when drug administration is known or suspected	Presence of potentially toxic concentrations of drugs prevents diagnosis of brainstem death
Tricyclic antidepressants	1. Overdose	Drug plus metabolite over 1 mg L^{-1} indicates potentially serious toxicity
	2. Therapeutic monitoring	Drug plus metabolite between 50 and 300 $\mu g L^{-1}$ is the usual therapeutic range. Some patients are fast metabolizers and have low levels despite high doses

Table 72.4 *Commonly used antidotes in poisoning*

Poison	Antidote	Mechanism of action	Dosage regimen
Anticholinergic agents	Physostigmine	Cholinesterase inhibitor	2 mg i.v. over 5 min, continue with an infusion of 4–6 mg hourly (adult dose)
Anticoagulants (warfarin type)	Vitamin K (phytomenadione)	Competitive antagonist at site of prothrombin manufacture in liver	2–5 mg i.v. adult, 0.4 mg kg^{-1} child
Benzodiazepines	Flumazenil	Competitive antagonist at benzodiazepine receptors	Initially 0.2 mg i.v. over 30 s. Further doses of 0.5 mg can be given over 30 s at 60-s intervals to a total dose of 3 mg
Beta-blockers	Glucagon	Stimulates myocardial adenylate cyclase	5 mg i.v. over 1 min followed by an infusion of 1–10 mg h^{-1}
	Isoprenaline	Competitive antagonist at β-receptors	10–50 mg min^{-1} i.v.
Carbon monoxide	Oxygen (normobaric or hyperbaric)	Competitive displacement of carbon monoxide from hemoglobin and cytochrome molecules	Administer as high an inspired oxygen as possible until carboxyhemoglobin concentration falls below 5%. Consider hyperbaric oxygen in severe cases
Cyanide	Dicobalt edetate	Chelates cyanide ions	300 mg i.v. over 3 min
	Sodium nitrite	Forms methemoglobin, which combines with cyanide	10 mL of 30% solution i.v. over 10 min
	Sodium thiosulfate	Substrate for enzymatic detoxification of cyanide	50 mL of 25% solution i.v. over 10 min
	Hydroxocobalamin	Combines with cyanide to form cyanocobalamin	4 g i.v.
	Oxygen (normobaric or hyperbaric)	Competitive substrate binding	Administer a high inspired oxygen until clinical recovery occurs
Digoxin and digitoxin	Fab antibody fragments	Antidote forms an inert complex with poison	Dose should match the estimated dose of ingested digoxin
Ethylene glycol	Ethanol Fomepizole	High affinity for alcohol dehydrogenase, slow toxic metabolite production	Ethanol dose given should be sufficient to maintain plasma ethanol level at 1–2 g L^{-1} or fomepizole, two 30-min infusions daily, initial dose 15 mg kg^{-1}
Heavy metals: leads, mercury, arsenic	DMSA (2,3-dimercaptosuccinic acid)	Chelating agent	30 mg kg^{-1} 8-hourly for 5 days then 20 mg kg^{-1} 12-hourly for 14 days
(Note: the last three chelating agents are now seldom used. DMSA and DMPS are first choice)	DMPS (sodium 2,3-dimercaptopropane-sulfonate)	Chelating agent	Chronic: 100 mg three times per day
	Sodium calcium edetate	Chelating agent	Acute: 250 mg every 4 h for 24 h then 250 mg every 6 h for the next 24 h
	Dimercaprol	Chelating agent	Up to 40 mg kg^{-1} twice daily by i.v. infusion repeated every 48 h until lead falls below toxic level
	Pencillamine	Chelating agent	Mercury: 2.5–3 mg kg^{-1} deep i.m. injection 4-hourly for 2 days, two to four times on third day, one to two times daily for up to 10 days Lead: 0.5–1.5 g per day orally for 1–2 months or until lead level falls below toxic level
Hydrofluoric acid	Calcium gluconate	Forms an inert complex (calcium fluoride)	For burns: calcium gluconate (10%) 0.25–0.5 mmol kg^{-1}, up to 25 mmol kg^{-1}
Iron salts	Desferrioxamine	Chelating agent	In severe iron poisoning (plasma iron > 90 mmol L^{-1}) up to 15 mg kg^{-1} per hour reduced to keep the total i.v. dose under 80 mg kg^{-1} in each 24 h
Methanol	Ethanol Fomepizole	High affinity for alcohol dehydrogenase, slow toxic metabolite production	As for ethylene glycol (above)

Methemoglobin	Methylene blue	Cofactor for reduction of methemoglobin by NADPH	0.2 mL kg^{-1} of 1% solution (i.e. 2 mg kg^{-1}) slowly i.v. over 5 min, repeated as necessary to a maximum of 6 mg kg^{-1}
	Ascorbic acid	Reducing agent	1 g per 24 h i.v. or orally
Opioid analgesics (including heroin)	Naloxone	Competitive antagonist at opioid receptors	0.8–1.2 mg i.v. (children 0.2 mg). Repeat if respiratory depression (assessed by respiratory rate and minute volume) is not reversed within 1–2 min. Continue with an infusion of half the amount required to produce a response over 30 min
Organophosphates	Atropine	Competitive antagonist at acetylcholine receptors	2 mg i.v. (i.m. or s.c. in less severely poisoned patients) followed by 2-mg doses at 5- to 10-min intervals until clinical features of full atropinization become apparent (dry mouth is the most reliable sign)
	Pralidoxime	Cholinesterase reactivator	1 g i.v. (in 100 mL saline over 30 min) repeated every 4 h for 24 h in severe cases
Acetaminophen	Acetylcysteine	Replenishes hepatic glutathione stores	300 mg kg^{-1} i.v. over 16 h in three reducing doses
	Methionine	Replenishes hepatic glutathione stores	2.5 g orally every 4 h for 12 h (total 10 g)
Thallium	Berlin blue	Chelating agent	250 mg kg^{-1} per day orally in divided doses. Ideally given until thallium level is 10 mg L^{-1} in blood and urine

Table 72.5 *Factors contributing to hypotension and pulseless electrical activity (PEA) in poisoning*

Causes	Agents
Relative hypovolemia	
Vasodilation	Central nervous depressants Vasodilators Nitrates
Anaphylaxis	Calcium antagonists Drug hypersensitivity Bee stings
Hypovolemia	
Vomiting	Many agents
Hematemesis	Theophylline, iron
Sweating	Salicylates, MAOIs, amphetamine
Hyperventilation	Salicylates
Metabolic disorders	
Metabolic acidosis Hypoxemia Hypothermia	Many causes
Negative inotropic agents	
Cardiac drugs	Quinidine Disopyramide Flecainide β-Adrenergic antagonists
Antirheumatic/antimalarial	Chloroquine Quinine Halofantrine
Anesthetics and analgesics	Propoxyphene Local anesthetic agents
Psychoactive agents	Tricyclic antidepressants Phenothiazines
Volatile substances	Toluene, petroleum vapor, etc.
Others	Digoxin Carbon monoxide Cyanide Terminally due to many causes

MAOI, monoamine oxidase inhibitor.

other conditions deserve mention. Malignant hyperthermia, with hyperpyrexia, muscle rigidity, and metabolic acidosis, can be triggered in susceptible people by a number of agents including halothane and succinylcholine (suxamethonium). In neuroleptic malignant syndrome, hyperthermia, muscle rigidity, and mental disturbances occur in patients taking neuroleptic drugs, usually phenothiazines or butyrophenones. This syndrome has a mortality of 20–30%[8] but treatment with dantrolene may be effective.[9]

In each of these conditions, there appears to be a sudden loss of control of intracellular ionized calcium, which leads to the formation of short and rigid actinomyosin. The reaction can become self-sustaining, because heat reduces the calcium requirement for excitation–contraction coupling. The excess calcium may also be absorbed by mitochondria, where it can uncouple oxidative phosphorylation, leading to further heat production. The appropriate pharmacologic approach is to decrease muscle contraction and heat production by giving dantrolene, $1\,mg\,kg^{-1}$ repeated at 5- to 10-min intervals, to a maximum of $10\,mg\,kg^{-1}$. External cooling should be avoided if it is likely to lead to cutaneous vasoconstriction, which could be counterproductive for the patient with massive overproduction of heat.

Severe metabolic disturbances

Many poisons produce metabolic disturbances that can cause a deterioration in the patient's condition and which require immediate attention. An arterial blood gas estimation is therefore urgently indicated in every severely poisoned or deeply comatose patient. The most common abnormality is an anion gap metabolic acidosis, which may be caused by a number of poisons. In addition to specific treatments, sodium bicarbonate should be given to correct the acidosis. Hypokalemia may result from a shift in potassium into the cells in chloroquine and theophylline poisoning. Hyperkalemia indicates a poor prognosis for injured patients.

Severe hyperkalemia may also occur in digoxin poisoning, and the management of this complication is described later in this chapter. Hypocalcemia is common in severe ethylene glycol poisoning associated with metabolic production of oxalic acid. Other metabolic and electrolyte disturbances should be dealt with as indicated.

Methemoglobinemia

Many drugs and chemicals can cause mild to moderate methemoglobinemia, which is usually well tolerated. However, the more important causes of life-threatening methemoglobinemia include aniline, sodium or potassium nitrite, and sodium and potassium chlorate. Inhalation of nitrites (e.g. butyl nitrite) for abuse is unlikely to cause symptomatic methemoglobinemia, but ingestion could cause severe methemoglobinemia.[10,11]

It should be noted that methemoglobinemia may be iatrogenic, e.g. sodium nitrite given for cyanide poisoning. In most cases, the proportion of methemoglobin does not rise to 30% and is not life-threatening. In severe acute methemoglobinemia, the patient becomes comatose and flaccid, may have cardiac arrhythmias and convulsions, and may progress to cardiorespiratory arrest. Methemoglobinemia should be suspected if the skin has a grayish or blue cyanosed appearance: the blood may have a dark or chocolate-brown color. This color change occurs with methemoglobin concentrations of 15–20%, but clinical symptoms only appear at levels over 20–30%, whereas consciousness is not likely to be lost at under 50%. Death is common at methemoglobin concentrations of over 70%. In addition to supportive measures, which should include 100% oxygen, methemoglobinemia can be reversed by the administration of methylene blue. It should be given only in symptomatic cases, or to those with over 40% methemoglobinemia. When the cause is due to chlorate poisoning, methylene blue is unlikely to reverse the methemoglobinemia, although ascorbic acid (1 g per 24 h) can be given. In severe cases, exchange transfusion can be used, and hyperbaric oxygen, if available, may allow sufficient oxygen to be transported in the plasma to maintain life.

POISONING DUE TO SPECIFIC AGENTS

Sedative and hypnotic agents

Many drugs and poisons have sedative or hypnotic effects, so that central nervous depression may occur in proportion to the severity of exposure. Symptoms may progress through drowsiness, hallucinations, nystagmus, coma, flaccidity, hypotension, and respiratory depression. There may be further problems due to other properties of the poison, and convulsions, cardiac arrhythmias, and cardiac depression may occur with some agents, notably tricyclic antidepressants. Close observation and aggressive supportive care are the key features of management. Patients with no response to painful stimuli are at greatest risk of a fatal outcome, and obviously require airway protection and careful monitoring of respiratory function in case mechanical ventilation should be required. In contrast with the slowed respiratory rate associated with opioid drugs, respiratory depression due to sedative and hypnotic agents manifests itself not as a slowing of respiratory rate but as a reduction in tidal volume. A reduced minute volume and deteriorating blood gas values are an urgent indication for mechanical ventilation.

Sedative and hypnotic aspects

Benzodiazepines

The benzodiazepines are widely thought to be nonfatal in overdose, but deaths do occur, mainly due to respiratory depression, aspiration of vomit, or hypothermia. In most cases, the coma amounts to a deep sleep with an adequate gag reflex, preserved tendon reflexes, and response to painful stimuli. Concomitant toxicity from acetaminophen and salicylate should be excluded. Patients rarely need management in the intensive therapy unit, but coma may be deep, especially if the drug has been co-ingested with ethanol, opioids, barbiturates, or tricyclic antidepressants. The question may arise as to whether flumazenil should be given in treatment or as a diagnostic test. Reversal of symptoms may help to narrow the differential diagnosis and confirm benzodiazepine ingestion. Although widely used for reversing benzodiazepine anesthesia, one should be aware that reversal of benzodiazepine toxicity may provoke convulsions due to benzodiazepine withdrawal or a co-ingested tricyclic antidepressant.[12] In general, it should not be given routinely, but only in carefully considered circumstances. A clinical response should be evident within 5–15 min and largely complete by 30 min; large doses (in excess of 5 mg) may sometimes need to be given. Flumazenil is ineffective for ethanol poisoning.

Chloral preparations

Although regarded as relatively mild hypnotic drugs, chloral hydrate and chloral betaine are rapidly reduced to trichloroethanol, which has an elimination half-life of 8–10 h, and overdoses of 3 g or more may cause coma (often with meiosis), respiratory depression, convulsions, hypotension, and cardiac arrhythmias, including multifocal ventricular tachycardia and ventricular fibrillation. Repeated doses of oral activated charcoal may be effective in enhancing elimination of trichloroethanol, and charcoal hemoperfusion should be considered in severe cases.

Gas and smoke inhalation

The history provided by witnesses may indicate that the victim has been exposed to toxic gases, fumes, smoke, or vapor. When this is suspected, 100% oxygen should be administered while blood is assayed for carbon monoxide and other possible toxic agents, as well as arterial gas estimation, hematology, and blood chemistry.

It is important to establish the causative agent as soon as possible, as treatments differ. Poisoning by carbon monoxide and cyanide should be treated as described elsewhere in this chapter.

Exposure to asphyxiant gases demands full resuscitation and measures designed to prevent the sequelae of hypoxia. Simple asphyxiants act by reducing the proportion of oxygen in the inspired air (Table 72.1). Many gases, such as hydrogen, helium, methane, propane, petroleum vapor, carbon dioxide, and nitrogen may be responsible. The duration and severity of hypoxia play a critical part in determining the symptoms and outcome. An atmosphere of less than 6–8% oxygen will rapidly produce coma and cardiorespiratory collapse due to cerebral hypoxia. With gases heavier than air, there may be several victims, as each tries to rescue the others without using breathing apparatus.

Exposure to other gases should be treated on their merits. Water-soluble irritant gases (such as CS or CN gas or ammonia) produce severe watering of the eyes and upper respiratory tract irritation and coughing, but resuscitation is not usually required and symptomatic measures are sufficient. Pepper sprays produce similar symptoms. On the other hand, water-insoluble gases such as acrolein or phosgene tend to reach the lungs and may cause bronchoconstriction and pulmonary edema, often after a latent interval, so that the patient should be observed for at least 24 h. Carboxyhemoglobin levels and a careful clinical assessment are important in deciding the severity of smoke exposure. Cyanide toxicity may occur in fire victims[13] and an elevated plasma lactate concentration may indicate toxicity in patients without severe burns.

Gases such as arsine and stilbine can cause minimal symptoms on inhalation but may produce severe hemolysis and hemoglobinuria, sometimes presenting as renal failure 24 h or more after exposure. Accidental or intentional inhalation of volatile substances, especially chlorinated hydrocarbons, may result in deep coma, hyporeflexia, and cardiac arrhythmias, which may progress to ventricular fibrillation. Treatment is symptomatic; a β-blocking drug such as esmolol or atenolol may help to control arrhythmias.

Carbon monoxide

Carbon monoxide exposure produces cerebral hypoxia secondary to its reversible combination with hemoglobin to form carboxyhemoglobin. Symptoms are often poorly related to the blood carboxyhemoglobin content, which depends on the duration of exposure, time since exposure, and the treatment given. Throbbing headache, vomiting without diarrhea, lethargy, and hyperventilation are typical in the early stages and may progress to convulsions, coma, hypoventilation, bradycardia, and cardiovascular collapse. When there is a history suggestive of exposure to carbon monoxide, the diagnosis usually presents little difficulty but, in many cases, the diagnosis may not be apparent and the possibility of carbon monoxide poisoning should be borne in mind, especially when several people are affected with headache, vomiting, and collapse. In the elderly, carbon monoxide toxicity may also present as a cerebrovascular accident or myocardial infarction. The source of exposure is usually inhalation of products of combustion. In domestic incidents, there may be a faulty appliance or a blocked flue. Motor exhaust gas inhalation is the cause of many suicidal deaths. The prognosis is grave in severe poisoning. Because of the high affinity of carbon monoxide for hemoglobin, a few breaths at high concentrations can be fatal; 1% carbon monoxide in air can kill within a few minutes. There are no reports of recovery by patients who have required cardiopulmonary resuscitation following a cardiac or respiratory arrest.

Treatment consists of removal from the source of exposure and administration of 100% oxygen immediately, after taking an anticoagulated whole blood sample for carboxyhemoglobin estimation. The pregnant patient or any patient who has had symptoms suggestive of severe poisoning (including any degree of neurologic impairment) should be treated with hyperbaric oxygen if it is available. Hyperbaric oxygen is effective in reducing long-term mental impairment following carbon monoxide poisoning and is therefore indicated. A further advantage is that, in addition to shortening the half-life of carboxyhemoglobin, hyperbaric oxygen may prevent late neurologic sequelae.[15]

Cholinesterase inhibitors

Organophosphates inhibit cholinesterase, causing features of cholinergic toxicity. In peacetime, the most serious poisoning is by ingestion of an organophosphate insecticide, which often represents attempted suicide. Cutaneous absorption and inhalation of sprays rarely cause serious toxicity. "Nerve gases" such as sarin and tabun can cause severe toxicity after minimal exposure. Early symptoms are vague but the characteristic effects soon become apparent. Mild to moderate poisoning may cause headache, blurred vision, meiosis, excessive salivation, lacrimation, sweating, bradycardia, wheezing, and lethargy. The patient should be kept under observation for at least 24 h. Severe poisoning may additionally cause coma, hypotension, convulsions, and respiratory muscle paralysis.

Atropine should be given in large doses: 2–4 mg intravenously (children 0.05 mg kg^{-1}) every 10 min until atropinization is achieved and it can be seen that secretions are inhibited or pupils have become dilated. Atropine therapy should be continued for a minimum of 48 h, and the patient should be observed for at least 72 h, as relapse may occur due to delayed intestinal absorption.

Although the pulse rate is characteristically slowed in this type of poisoning, it may become rapid due to sympathetic compensation, so that the pulse rate is less useful as a guide than the other signs of atropinization. Pralidoxime (a specific cholinesterase reactivator) 1 g (children 20–40 mg kg^{-1}) in 100 mL saline over 30 min intravenously should ideally be started within 4 h of exposure. Following this, enzyme inactivation becomes less reversible, and pralidoxime is unlikely to have any effect after 24–36 h. The dose should be reduced if there is renal impairment. Pralidoxime is ineffective in poisoning by carbamate-type cholinesterase inhibitors (e.g. neostigmine or pesticides such as carbaryl).

Treatment should obviously be given without waiting for laboratory confirmation of the diagnosis, but the results may indicate the severity of the poisoning and the likely duration of treatment. Plasma or red cell cholinesterase can be measured; the latter is a more reliable indicator. A reduction to 50% of normal is diagnostic of organophosphate exposure but not of toxicity, and less than 10% usually indicates severe poisoning. It has been shown that patients may relapse after apparent recovery. One reason for relapse is that treatment has not been given for long enough. The other main reason is because of muscle cell necrosis. This is termed the "intermediate syndrome."[16] There may be widespread muscle weakness, and the muscles of respiration are often affected, leading to respiratory failure, which requires mechanical ventilation. Recovery eventually occurs, but it may be up to 2 weeks before the patient can be weaned off the ventilator.

Iron

Accidental ingestion of iron tablets is relatively common in young children, but serious toxicity and death are rare. Iron is highly corrosive and in overdose destroys the mucosal barrier to iron absorption. This can lead to metabolic, cardiovascular, and hepatic complications if the amount of free iron in the plasma exceeds its iron-binding capacity. The clinical course of iron poisoning can be divided into four clinically and pathologically distinct phases. The first phase, which occurs shortly after ingestion and usually resolves within 6–8 h, consists of gastrointestinal symptoms, mainly acute vomiting and diarrhea, and sometimes hematemesis. This may be severe enough to lead to drowsiness, lethargy, and shock with metabolic acidosis. This phase usually resolves spontaneously but may require supportive treatment.

The second phase is a "silent interval" of apparent recovery, which may be followed by the third phase at around 24–48 h after ingestion. Metabolic acidosis, shock, coma, convulsions, hypoglycemia, hepatic necrosis, cardiac failure, and acute tubular necrosis characterize this phase. Finally, several weeks after apparent recovery there may be stricture formation or pyloric stenosis resulting from corrosive injury (the fourth phase).

Treatment is aimed at preventing or reducing iron absorption, chelating absorbed iron with desferrioxamine, correcting metabolic disturbances, and providing supportive care. A radiograph of the abdomen should be taken as soon as possible, and this may reveal the extent of ingestion, as undissolved iron salts are radiopaque. Activated charcoal does not adsorb iron, but orally administered desferrioxamine (5–10 g) may help to reduce toxicity. The serum iron concentration should be measured at around 4 h post ingestion in order to assess the severity of poisoning and decide on the need for chelation therapy. A serum iron of 55–90 μmol L^{-1} is considered potentially toxic, between 90 and 180 μmol L^{-1} may be associated with severe toxicity, and over 180 μmol L^{-1} is potentially fatal. A useful diagnostic test is to carry out a desferrioxamine challenge test, which consists of giving desferrioxamine intramuscularly in a single dose of 50 mg kg^{-1}. The urine should be observed: if it develops a red or port-wine color, this indicates that there is an excess of free iron in the body, and that desferrioxamine treatment should be started. The usual dose is 15 mg kg^{-1} h^{-1} to a maximum of 80 mg in 24 h. Treatment can be discontinued when the urine color returns to normal. Desferrioxamine is not contraindicated after iron overdose in pregnant patients.

Cyanide

Cyanide poisoning can be rapidly fatal. It may be inhaled as hydrogen cyanide, or enter the body by ingestion or cutaneous absorption of cyanide salts, or intestinal hydrolysis of cyanogenic glycosides. Severe toxicity may develop within seconds of inhalation but may be delayed if salts are taken on a full stomach or following ingestion of cyanogenic glycosides or salts such as gold cyanide.

Cyanide acts as a chemical asphyxiant, combining with cytochromes and rapidly blocking cellular oxygen utilization so that cerebral function and circulation are soon impaired, with the development of a metabolic acidosis. Venous blood tends to have a high oxygen saturation, because of reduced cellular oxygen uptake, and one clinical sign of cyanide poisoning is that there may be little color difference between retinal veins and arteries on ophthalmoscopy. Early signs include hyperventilation and tachycardia, but coma, cyanosis, and convulsions may soon follow. A high inspired oxygen (or hyperbaric oxygen if available) is an effective treatment, although its mode of action is unclear; it may be a case of simple competition for binding sites. When the diagnosis is certain, dicobalt edetate (300 mg in 20 mL) can be given intravenously over 3 min, repeated if necessary, and is a highly effective antidote. However, if the patient is not poisoned, use of this antidote can produce severe anaphylactoid reactions with laryngeal edema and convulsions. The safest course of action is to give the antidote only if the patient's level of consciousness is deteriorating. Another group of antidotes (nitrites such as sodium nitrite) act by producing methemoglobin, each molecule of which can bind four cyanide ions in the bloodstream. Intravenous sodium thiosulfate (25 mL of a 50% solution intravenously) is nontoxic and acts by providing a substrate for the enzyme rhodanese to neutralize cyanide, producing sodium thiocyanate. Its disadvantage is that it is too slow acting for use in acute poisoning as it acts by facilitating the natural detoxification mechanism, but it is a safe adjunct to any of the other cyanide antidotes. Hydroxocobalamin is a recent, useful addition to the range of cyanide antidotes. It acts by combining in a 1:1 ratio with cyanide ions to inactivate them, forming cyanocobalamin, which is excreted in the urine. It is nontoxic and can therefore be given if the diagnosis is uncertain: it can also be administered outside hospital. The main disadvantage is the large dose required (4 g given intravenously).[17]

Subacute or chronic cyanide toxicity can also occur during prolonged nitroprusside therapy. The main clinical feature is a metabolic acidosis – if none is present then cyanide toxicity can be ruled out. In this case, a relatively rapid improvement should occur after the intravenous administration of sodium thiosulfate. Other cyanide antidotes are not indicated in this case.

Methanol

Patients poisoned with methanol, although initially asymptomatic for up to 60 h following ingestion, may present with profound coma, fixed, dilated pupils with retinal hemorrhages or papilledema, and profound metabolic acidosis. If the patient has reached this stage of toxicity, it is very probable that severe cerebral damage has already occurred, and recovery is unlikely. No patient who has required cardiopulmonary resuscitation has recovered.

In all cases of symptomatic methanol poisoning, assessment and urgent treatment are needed. The important measures are to correct the metabolic acidosis with sodium bicarbonate and to protect the body from further enzymatic transformation of methanol to formic acid, which is the agent mainly responsible for its metabolic, cerebral, and ocular toxicity. The usual treatment is to give ethanol by mouth or, if necessary, by intravenous infusion. Ethanol has a greater affinity for alcohol dehydrogenase than methanol and hence inhibits its metabolism to formaldehyde, which is converted by aldehyde dehydrogenase to formic acid. Fomepizole (4-methyl pyrazole) is a recently introduced alternative to ethanol.[18] A single 30-min intravenous infusion inhibits alcohol dehydrogenase for 12 h, so that the drug needs only to be given twice daily, and it also avoids the need for repeated ethanol estimations; the main drawback is its cost.

Hemodialysis can, if necessary, be used to remove methanol from the circulation. Furosemide may be given to enhance formic acid excretion. Another approach is to speed metabolism of formic acid via the dihydrofolate reductase pathway by administration of folinic acid.

If the patient has taken a single dose of methylated spirits or surgical spirit, the main toxicity will be that of ethanol and the small amount of methanol present will not cause a problem as its metabolism will be slowed due to the ethanol present. On the other hand, prolonged or repeated consumption of alcoholic drinks containing even a small proportion of methanol can lead to serious poisoning by the accumulation of methanol. Epidemics of fatal methanol have resulted from the use of illicit liquor containing excessive amounts of methanol.

Ethylene glycol

Ethylene glycol is a common constituent of automobile antifreeze. When ingested, it tends initially to cause signs of alcoholic intoxication followed later by tachycardia, pulmonary edema, convulsions, and acute renal failure. Metabolic acidosis, leukocytosis, hypocalcemia, and oxalic acid crystalluria are characteristic. Oxalate crystal deposition in the central nervous system may cause meningism. The main principles of treatment are to correct the acidosis, delay the metabolism of ethylene glycol to toxic metabolites by administering ethyl alcohol or fomepizole[19] (with a similar regime to the treatment of methanol poisoning above), and hasten elimination by using hemodialysis when blood levels of ethylene glycol are sufficiently high. Hemodialysis may also be required to support renal function.

Chloroquine

In overdose, this drug, which is used both as an antimalarial and an antirheumatic, can produce hypokalemia (often $<2\,\mathrm{mmol\,L^{-1}}$), coma, and cardiovascular collapse. Although many drugs in overdose produce deep coma before cardiac toxicity occurs, chloroquine overdose may produce collapse from profound hypotension or cardiac arrhythmias with minimal or no depression of consciousness beforehand. Later, severe hyperkalemia may ensue, particularly if potassium salts have been given to correct the hypokalemia. It was found by chance in Africa that patients who had taken an overdose of diazepam plus chloroquine fared better than those who had taken chloroquine alone and, although its mode of action is unclear, diazepam therapy is part of the treatment regimen. Resuscitation should be aggressive and the use of norepinephrine (noradrenaline) and diazepam may be life saving.[20] Active removal methods such as hemoperfusion and hemodialysis are ineffective.

Cardioactive drugs

Cardiac glycosides

Acute poisoning with cardiac glycosides such as digoxin, digitoxin, or plants such as foxglove, *Thevetia peruviana* ("yellow oleander"), or oleander (*Nerium oleander*) can produce cardiac arrhythmias, and hyperkalemia, each of which can be fatal. If the patient presents within 4 h of ingestion, gastric lavage should be performed and activated charcoal left in the stomach to adsorb the cardiac glycoside and thus reduce intestinal absorption. For digoxin overdose, plasma digoxin levels should be measured urgently, bearing in mind that the concentration peaks within 1–2 h, and that potentially toxic levels cannot be readily interpreted until 6 h after ingestion, when tissue distribution is complete. Even in plant poisonings, a measured digoxin concentration by immunoassay, although of no help in quantifying the toxin, may be used to confirm ingestion. However, as soon as there is a real suspicion of a large overdose from the history, clinical features of toxicity (arrhythmias, heart block, or a raised or increasing plasma potassium), or digoxin assay results, arrangements should be made to obtain digoxin-specific Fab antibodies urgently in case life-threatening toxicity should develop. These Fab fragments of sheep antidigoxin immunoglobulin molecules bind with high affinity to digoxin and other cardiac glycosides, thus removing the poison from receptor sites in the tissues. Apart from measuring digoxin levels, the most decisive investigations are the electrocardiogram, digoxin assay, and plasma potassium; a plasma potassium concentration of over $5\,\mathrm{mmol\,L^{-1}}$ is a strong indicator of potential toxicity.

β-Adrenoreceptor antagonists, lidocaine (lignocaine), amiodarone, or phenytoin may be useful in treating cardiac arrhythmias, and insulin plus glucose can be used as a short-term measure for hyperkalemia. A pacing wire should be inserted if second- or third-degree heart block develops. Direct current countershock should be used for ventricular fibrillation. If these measures fail to restore an adequate cardiac output, the circulation can be supported with external chest compression pending the arrival of Fab antibodies, which should reverse the clinical features of cardiac glycoside poisoning within 20–30 min.[21] The dose (in milligrams) of antibody can be calculated from the amount of digoxin ingested [dose (mg)$\times$60] or the plasma digoxin concentration [concentration ($\mathrm{g\,L^{-1}}$ or $\mathrm{ng\,mL^{-1}}$)$\times$0.34$\times$weight of patient in kilograms]. If the dose required cannot be calculated and treatment indicated, a speculative dose of 300 mg (five ampules) can be given, and further doses of 200 mg can be added depending on the response. Overdosage with the antibody is at worst likely to cause hypokalemia if treatment for hyperkalemia has already been given, or might precipitate fast atrial fibrillation or cardiac failure if the patient was taking digoxin for control of these disorders. Allergic reactions do not appear to be a problem. Once Fab antibodies have been given, plasma digoxin assay results are likely to be unreliable.[22]

Beta-blocking drugs

In overdose, β-adrenergic antagonists can cause hypotension, bradycardia, cyanosis, coma, and convulsions.[23] Deaths can occur with propranolol, oxprenolol, sotalol, and acebutolol but are extremely rare with other β-adrenergic blocking drugs. In severe cases, hypotension may be marked and PEA may occur. Electrical conduction disturbances (first-degree atrioventricular block and widened QRS lead prolongation complexes) are common. Sotalol can also cause ventricular arrhythmias, including torsades des pointes, which should respond to overdrive pacing or infusion of isoproterenol (isoprenaline).

After correction of hypovolemia, the most appropriate treatment is to give either an intravenous bolus of glucagon (5 mg), followed by an infusion of 1–5 mg h^{-1}, or an intravenous infusion of isoproterenol of 10–100 μg min^{-1}. The response should be assessed by the improvement in blood pressure, rather than by change in the pulse rate, and the isoproterenol infusion rate should be increased until the blood pressure improves. When asystole or PEA occur, external chest compression should be used. Once the patient comes under medical care, full recovery is usually the rule, provided hypoxic cerebral damage has not already occurred.

Calcium antagonists

Overdose of calcium channel blockers can cause severe cardiac depression, which may be fatal. Management with intravenous fluids, glucagon, calcium gluconate, dopamine, dobutamine, and norepinephrine has been tried, but results are frequently disappointing. Recently, hyperinsulinemia and euglycemia have been proposed, and seem to produce a marked improvement, although the mechanism of action of this regime is not clear. The regime is 0.5 units $insulin^{-1}$ kg body weight h^{-1}, 10% dextrose 100 mL h^{-1}.[24]

Theophylline

Theophylline is usually prescribed in sustained-release formulations, so that symptoms of overdose may develop gradually over 6–12 h. Vomiting, hematemesis, hyperventilation, tachycardia, cardiac arrhythmias, convulsions, and coma may occur. Hypokalemia and hyperglycemia are the most common biochemical findings. Plasma theophylline levels do not correlate well with symptoms, and so are a poor guide to the severity of toxicity in acute overdose. Patients with levels of 150 mg L^{-1} may have minimal symptoms, whereas severe poisoning may be associated with levels of 60 mg L^{-1}. Accumulation from chronic overdosage may cause toxicity with theophylline levels of 30–60 mg L^{-1}.

When the patient presents early, severe toxicity should be prevented by giving oral activated charcoal and carrying out whole bowel lavage, using metoclopramide or ondansetron in sufficient doses to inhibit vomiting. If the patient has already developed severe toxicity, the same measures should be used, plus full supportive care. In the nonasthmatic patient, intravenous propranolol (5–10 mg i.v. over 1 h) will reverse the metabolic and cardiovascular changes but, in the asthmatic patient, potassium replacement is more appropriate, as propranolol might precipitate bronchospasm. Another alternative is to give an infusion of esmolol, as this β–blocking drug has a very short half-life and can be stopped at the first hint of bronchospasm. Hemofiltration or charcoal hemoperfusion or may be indicated in cases with intractable vomiting or severe metabolic or cardiovascular toxicity.[25]

Antidepressants and lithium

Tricyclic antidepressants

Acute overdose with tricyclic antidepressants is a common cause of admissions following poisoning to intensive therapy units. Ironically, in most cases they have been prescribed to treat depressed and potentially suicidal patients.

The mechanisms of toxicity are complex and are due to at least three main pharmacologic effects. These are: (1) a "quinidine-like" or "membrane-stabilizing" effect due to sodium channel blockade; (2) an anticholinergic effect; and (3) a variety of other neurotransmitter effects, including blockade of norepinephrine uptake at adrenergic synapses, producing initial stimulation followed by α-adrenergic blockade. The most important of these toxic mechanisms is the quinidine-like effect that slows sodium flux into cells and is the mechanism underlying cardiac toxicity.

Clinical features

There may be initial agitation and hallucinations, giving way to deepening coma. The neurologic state may be confusing. The patient may be flaccid, but sometimes the tendon reflexes are brisk, with an extensor plantar response and dysconjugate gaze.

Pupils are often mid-size rather than widely dilated. Convulsions are common and respiratory depression may occur. The most serious and potentially fatal complications are cardiac arrhythmias (most commonly atrioventricular block, ventricular tachycardia, and ventricular fibrillation, which may be followed by asystole) and profound hypotension, which may amount to PEA. These can be further aggravated by hypoxemia (Fig. 72.1). A sinus tachycardia and a widened QRS complex are common. The electrocardiogram (ECG) frequently shows a right bundle branch block pattern, and a QRS duration of over 100 ms[26] is regarded as the best indicator of risk of cardiac toxicity. The electrocardiographic changes are so typical that a right bundle branch block pattern in a patient presenting with unconsciousness should raise the

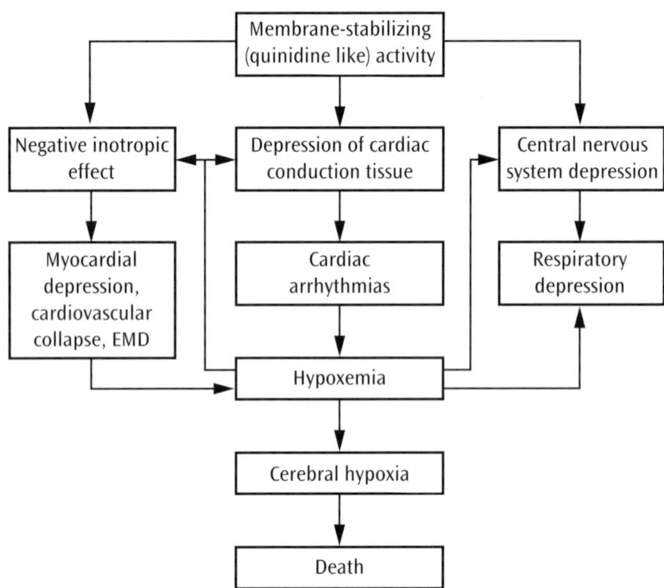

Figure 72.1 *Mechanisms by which membrane-stabilizing activity of drugs and poisons may lead to fatal toxicity in man.*

suspicion of a tricyclic antidepressant overdose. Plasma levels of tricyclic drugs do not correlate well with the severity of toxicity, although there is little danger of severe poisoning if concentrations of drug and metabolite combined are less than 100 mg L^{-1}.

Management

Cardiopulmonary status must be assessed urgently and resuscitation commenced if necessary. The most important message about this type of poisoning is that it is potentially reversible, provided hypoxic cerebral damage has not occurred. Full recovery can be hoped for even after prolonged external chest compression, which may be necessary when profound hypotension or cardiac arrhythmias are unresponsive to treatment. Supportive care will be required for the comatose patient, and ventilatory support may be needed for respiratory depression.

As the anticholinergic effects of these drugs cause delayed gastric emptying, it is worth performing gastric lavage up to 12 h after ingestion in a seriously poisoned patient. Activated charcoal should then be given via the lavage tube, because as little as 10 g can absorb a potentially fatal amount of antidepressant. Further doses should also be given, as although they have a large volume of distribution and are unlikely to be removed by back-diffusion through the gut ("gastrointestinal dialysis"), there is considerable biliary excretion and reabsorption of tricyclic antidepressants, which can be interrupted by administration of repeated doses of activated charcoal.[27]

In the management of cardiac arrhythmias and hypotension, alkalinization to an arterial pH of approximately 7.5 is effective and should constitute first-line therapy. A sodium bicarbonate infusion (0.5–2.0 mmol kg^{-1} given rapidly and repeated when necessary) may help to correct hypotension and control cardiac arrhythmias or convulsions. Its mechanism of action is controversial but may involve decreased free drug concentration due to pH-related change in protein binding or may be due to a direct cardiac effect. Hypotension not corrected by volume challenge may respond to sodium bicarbonate. An α-antagonist such as norepinephrine may also be of value; mixed α- and β-agents such as dopamine may increase the hypotension. In PEA and intractable hypotension, physical support of the heart with external chest compression may be required. Cardiac arrhythmias may respond to phenytoin, atenolol, or lignocaine, but negative inotropic drugs such as diopyramide, quinidine, and procainamide that prolong cardiac intervals are contraindicated. Direct current shock will be required for ventricular tachycardia or fibrillation, and cardiac pacing may be necessary for bradyarrhythmias causing hypotension. Patients without signs of cardiac toxicity after 6 h of observation do not require extended cardiac monitoring. Monitoring may be discontinued when the patient has regained consciousness and has had a normal ECG for 24 h. Metabolic disturbances (principally metabolic acidosis or hypokalemia) should be corrected. Metabolic acidosis following convulsions or hypoperfusion may enhance cardiac toxicity. Once adequate oxygenation is assured, convulsions should be treated with diazepam in the first instance and phenytoin if they persist. As the anticholinergic effects of tricyclic antidepressants do not cause serious toxicity, the use of physostigmine is no longer recommended. Administration of physostigmine in tricyclic poisoning has produced asystole in human beings.[28]

Monoamine oxidase inhibitors

Several drugs and foods are prohibited for patients taking monoamine oxidase inhibitors to prevent the well-known "cheese" reaction, which consists of a sudden and severe rise in blood pressure due to the release of norepinephrine.[29] The hypertensive crisis may be accompanied by headache, vomiting, and neurologic signs, and is best managed by prompt antihypertensive therapy, ideally by α-adrenergic blockade with a drug such as phentolamine. Overdose of monoamine oxidase inhibitors does not usually produce a hypertensive crisis unless the patient deliberately provokes a reaction. Following an overdose, symptoms usually build up over 12–24 h, with muscle twitching progressing to widespread muscle spasm, trismus, and opisthotonus. The blood pressure may vary between hypotension and moderate hypertension. There is usually a sinus tachycardia, the skin is hot to the touch, and sweating is profuse. The pupils are fixed and dilated. The core temperature may rise steeply, leading to death from hyperthermia. The muscle spasms may lead to rhabdomyolysis, which can cause renal failure. Disseminated intravascular coagulation is a known complication.

Management

Rapid intravenous infusion of fluid usually restores the blood pressure and reduces the pulse rate. The continued muscle contraction causes excessive heat production, and the body temperature may rise to a point at which hyperthermia is fatal, unless muscle relaxants are given. Sedation with diazepam is of little use. If the rectal temperature rises above 39 °C, the patient should be electively paralyzed with a muscle relaxant such as alcuronium or pancuronium and mechanically ventilated for 12–24 h to correct hyperthermia and prevent rhabdomyolysis. The temperature usually falls rapidly, without the need for any further measures, because the body's thermoregulatory mechanism is usually able to reduce body temperature once the overproduction of heat has been controlled. External cooling is of little help as heat generation due to profound muscle contraction exceeds heat loss. Hypotension is usually due to hypovolemia, but a low dose of dopamine can be tried if fluid replacement fails to restore blood pressure.

Selective serotonin reuptake inhibitors

This group of drugs has now largely superseded older antidepressants as first-line therapy. Overdose may cause a mild serotonin syndrome, whereas interactions with monoamine oxidase inhibitors or MDMA ("ecstasy") can cause a very marked serotonin syndrome.[30] Although the syndrome may be mild and transient, the patient may develop trismus, opistotonus, and hyperthermia, with the risk of disseminated intravascular coagulation. Severe cases will need to be managed by paralysis and ventilation, and dantrolene should be considered.

Lithium

Lithium salts are widely used to treat bipolar or manic–depressive disorders. This metal is eliminated by kidneys, and therefore reduced renal function can lead to accumulation. The therapeutic range is narrow (plasma concentrations between 1.0 and 1.4 mmol L^{-1}; blood should not be collected into a lithium heparin tube), and toxicity in therapeutic use can be caused by changes in fluid or electrolyte balance (particularly due to reduction in fluid intake or increased fluid loss from diarrhea or vomiting). Diuretic therapy or nonsteroidal anti-inflammatory drugs (NSAIDs) may also reduce lithium excretion and provoke toxicity. Symptoms of toxicity include confusion, agitation, drowsiness, tremor, hyperreflexia, hypertonia, ataxia, vomiting, convulsions, and, rarely, electrocardiographic changes, diabetes insipidus, and acute renal failure. In acute poisoning, plasma lithium levels of over 5 mmol L^{-1} may be associated with minimal symptoms, and the elimination half-life is relatively rapid.[31] The development of marked neurologic symptoms such as tremor is an indication for active elimination following an acute overdose. Deaths from lithium poisoning are not common, but neurologic impairment may be permanent.

Management

Gastric lavage may be appropriate to remove any lithium remaining in the stomach, but whole bowel lavage is probably more effective. Lithium is not adsorbed by activated charcoal. Lithium is excreted by the kidneys, and a good urine output should be ensured. Urinary alkalinization does not increase excretion of lithium.

Hemodialysis should be considered for a symptomatic patient with a high plasma lithium concentration following an acute overdose. Although well removed by hemodialysis, lithium has a large volume of distribution, a "rebound" rise in plasma concentrations may occur, and repeated dialysis may be necessary. Peritoneal dialysis is not recommended.

Original antipsychotic agents

The original antipsychotic agents were mainly phenothiazines and butyrophenones. The main problems that occur with these drugs are: dystonic reactions, cardiac arrhythmias, neuroleptic malignant syndrome, and toxicity from overdose.

Acute dystonia may occur following a single dose of a phenothiazine and often consists of spasm of the tongue and jaw muscles, torticollis, and sometimes oculogyric crisis. It is commoner in young female patients. The patient is usually conscious but frightened. Reassurance is essential, and a small intravenous dose of diazepam may help. Procyclidine 5–10 mg intravenously usually causes resolution of the dystonic reaction.

Cardiac arrhythmias and sudden death can occur when high doses of antipsychotic drugs are used. It is most commonly recognized with chlorpromazine, but may occur with any of this group of drugs. It probably occurs because of ventricular fibrillation, but may also occur due to severe hypotension. The ECG in these patients may show a long Q-T interval, and torsades des pointes may occur. Increasing the heart rate by atrial overdrive pacing or infusion of isoprenaline will decrease the risk of potentially fatal arrhythmias.

The neuroleptic malignant syndrome consists of relatively acute onset of a change in mental state, with confusion, muscle rigidity, hyperthermia, sweating, lactic acidosis, and rhabdomyolysis, occurring within hours or months of commencing therapy with a phenothiazine or butyrophenone drug. The syndrome may present acutely, and in some cases it may run a prolonged course with a differential diagnosis of febrile conditions. The mortality is often quoted as 20%. The drug treatment of choice is intravenous dantrolene.

An acute overdose of one of the older antipsychotic agents may cause coma, convulsions, respiratory depression, and hypotension. There may be hypothermia or hyperthermia. The ECG commonly shows a prolonged Q-T interval and arrhythmias may occur. Symptoms may only become severe 12–24 h after ingestion. Management is mainly supportive. Intravenous sodium bicarbonate, as for tricyclic antidepressant poisoning, is often effective. Atrial overdrive pacing may correct torsades des pointes unresponsive to antiarrhythmic agents.

Newer antipsychotic agents

The newer or atypical antipsychotic agents (risperidone, clozapine, quetiapine, olanzapine, ziprasidone, and sertindole) have now largely replaced the traditional agents as first-line drugs for the treatment of schizophrenia. Most patients who take an overdose of atypical antipsychotic drugs will remain asymptomatic or develop only mild to moderate toxicity. Death is very unusual. Toxic effects begin within 1–2 h after ingestion and peak by 4–6 h. Toxicity is variably characterized by depression of the central nervous and respiratory systems, meiosis or mydriasis, hypertension or orthostatic hypotension, sinus tachycardia, agitation, delirium, anticholinergic effects, and, rarely, seizures and arrhythmias. Management is supportive.[32]

Anticonvulsants

Anticonvulsant overdose is most commonly encountered in epileptics. In this case, serial measurements of plasma concentrations of the drug should be made, so that dosage can be restarted, in order to prevent seizures, when the plasma concentration has fallen into the therapeutic range.

Phenytoin

This drug has dose-dependent elimination kinetics, and phenytoin toxicity can occur after regular therapy with inappropriately high doses, or from acute overdose. Clinical features include cerebellar ataxia, confusion, and vomiting. Deep coma and respiratory depression are rare. Excessively rapid intravenous administration can cause cardiac arrest due to the propylene glycol vehicle; this does not occur with fosphenytoin. Gastric lavage, repeated doses of activated charcoal, and supportive care are the best means of treatment. Forced diuresis, hemodialysis, and hemoperfusion are not necessary.

Phenobarbital

Phenobarbital overdose causes prolonged deep coma, and its elimination half-life in overdose may be from 50 to over 100 h. Pupil size changes from time to time. There may be respiratory depression, vasodilation, and hypotension. Cardiac output is proportional to depth of coma. Ileus due to "intestinal narcosis" may cause further absorption of drug deepening of coma as signs of recovery become apparent. Treatment with repeated doses of activated charcoal may shorten the elimination half-life of phenobarbital. Alkaline diuresis with dopamine has been used but, if poisoning is very severe, hemodialysis or hemoperfusion is the most effective way of removing the drug and shortening the duration of toxicity.

Sodium valproate

Overdose of this drug causes gastrointestinal symptoms, ataxia, irritability, drowsiness, and coma. Pupils are constricted. A dose greater than 25 g (adult), or plasma concentrations exceeding 1000 mg L^{-1}, may result in convulsions and cerebral edema. Management is supportive.[33]

Carbamazepine

In overdose, there may be delay in the onset of symptoms due to the cholinergic effect of the drug, enterohepatic circulation, bezoar formation, or accumulation of an epoxide metabolite. As late relapse may occur, close monitoring is necessary. Symptoms include drowsiness, ataxia, coma, and myoclonus. The stomach should be emptied, and repeated doses of activated charcoal may increase elimination. Although many of the symptoms of carbamazepine overdose are similar to those of the tricyclic antidepressants, this drug has a small volume of distribution (1 kg L^{-1}), and charcoal hemoperfusion may be effective. Plasma levels of the drug should be obtained urgently, and repeated 4- to 6-hourly in case of delayed or prolonged absorption. Toxic effects may be noted at 12 mg L^{-1}, but patients with plasma concentrations of under 60 mg L^{-1} can be managed symptomatically. The epoxide metabolite should be measured in severe cases if possible.

Analgesic drugs

The opioid drugs are considered below, under Drug abuse. Apart from these, the most important cause of serious poisoning from analgesics occurs with acetaminophen and the aspirin group of drugs. In general, the other nonsteroidal drugs have much lower toxicity. Ibuprofen has remarkably low toxicity in overdose. Mefenamic acid is unusual in that overdose may result in convulsions that are usually brief.

Acetaminophen (paracetamol)

Deaths are rare in comparison with its extremely wide use. The anesthesiologist should be aware that, although safe in therapeutic use, acetaminophen overdose may lead to severe hepatoxicity and nephrotoxicity. Diagnosis of risk depends on the accepted nomogram for plasma acetaminophen level against the time since ingestion. However, acetaminophen plasma concentrations may be misleading in patients with cytochrome enzyme induction by agents such as phenytoin, carbamazepine, rifampicin, and phenobarbital. This is the main reason for the introduction of a second line on the nomogram, so that high-risk patients are given treatment at lower plasma levels.

Late-presenting or untreated acetaminophen poisoning may result in hepatic or renal failure, and liver transplantation may be the final resource when supportive care fails.[34]

Drug and substance abuse

Opioid analgesics

Misuse of any drug can cause a variety of serious medical complications but toxicity from the opioids is a common problem. They are readily available as analgesics, cough medicines, and antidiarrheal agents and are widely misused, mainly as heroin (diamorphine). Heroin abuse is common in the UK and results in over 900 deaths per year. Many of these are due to respiratory failure or aspiration of vomit after the first use of the drug, but experienced users may die from loss of tolerance after a period of abstinence. The dose required may fall by 10- to 100-fold over as short a period of abstinence as 2 weeks or less, so that a single dose which previously produced euphoria could prove fatal within minutes.

The classic signs of opioid toxicity consist of depressed consciousness (which may amount to profound coma), small or pinpoint pupils [meperidine (pethidine) is an exception to this, and the atropine in Lomotil, a combination of diphenoxylate and atropine, may also cause dilated pupils], and respiratory depression. The respiratory depression is characteristic, and consists of a slowing of respiration with terminal apnea. The initial management consists of immediate attention to the airway and ensuring adequate ventilation. Once the patient is not in immediate danger of death, naloxone should be given; a dose of 0.8–2.0 mg intravenously will usually produce a change in respiratory rate, pupil size, and state of consciousness within 1 min. A partial response may be related to the size of the overdose, in which case further intravenous bolus doses of naloxone to a maximum of 4–6 mg should be given. Failure to respond may be due to the presence of other central nervous depressant agents, hypothermia, or hypoxic cerebral damage. Pethidine, buprenorphine, and propoxyphene may require large doses of naloxone. The fact that the patient may be an opioid addict is no contraindication to the use of naloxone; opioid withdrawal is not fatal, whereas opioid toxicity can easily kill. The presence of other sedative or hypnotic drugs, hypothermia, hypoxic cerebral damage, or other causes of coma may mask the response to naloxone. Diamorphine has a short elimination half-life of about 2 h, so prolonged treatment may not be needed. Some other drugs, such as buprenorphine, dihydrocodeine, methadone, and dextropropoxyphene, have considerably longer elimination half-lives, so that a longer recovery period should be anticipated.

Once the diagnosis of opioid toxicity has been confirmed by administration of naloxone, the choice can be made between continuing reversal with an infusion of naloxone sufficient to maintain adequate spontaneous breathing and controlled ventilation pending recovery as the drug is metabolized. As a rough guide, twice the amount of naloxone required to produce the initial response should be given over the first half-hour, and subsequent doses should be titrated against the patient's condition. The patient who regains consciousness may insist on leaving but should be restrained because the duration of action of naloxone (20–30 min) is shorter than the half-life of most opioid drugs, and the patient may relapse. Complications of heroin overdose include a chemical pneumonitis due to aspiration of vomit, noncardiogenic pulmonary edema, and nontraumatic rhabdomyolysis. Infective complications of intravenous drug abuse include lung abscesses, septicemia, right-sided endocarditis, hepatitis B and C infection, and HIV infection.

Cocaine

Cocaine toxicity produces widespread vasospasm and marked hypertension, and the commonest hospital presentation is chest pain, which usually resolves without intervention. Patients may also present with confusion, convulsions, myocardial infarction, acute heart failure, or cerebral hemorrhage. There is no specific antidote, but diazepam in adequate doses usually diminishes most features of toxicity. Control of blood pressure with intravenous nitrates is essential. Aspirin should be given to the patient complaining of chest pain. Other management is supportive. Cocaine is known to lead to premature atheroma[35] and cocaine abuse should be suspected in any young patient with myocardial infarction. Over one-third of patients with dissecting aortic aneurysms in a USA series had used cocaine.[36]

Amphetamine sulfate and methamphetamine

The amphetamines are frequently abused for their stimulant effect. Amphetamine sulfate may be injected, inhaled, or taken orally. Methamphetamine ("ice") usually comes in the form of crystals, which are smoked, and is about 20 times as potent as amphetamine sulfate, but has similar effects. The main complications of amphetamine toxicity include tachycardia and hypertension, convulsions, hyperthermia, rhabdomyolysis, and renal failure. Myocardial infarction and cerebral hemorrhage have been reported. There is no specific pharmacologic antidote, and management is mainly supportive. Sedation and anticonvulsants will be needed for the patient who is agitated or convulsing. Acid urine markedly shortens the elimination half-life of amphetamine by increasing its renal excretion. However, if there is suspicion of rhabdomyolysis, for example after repeated seizures, myoglobinuria, or if the plasma creatine phosphokinase (CPK) is raised, then alkalinization of the urine is more appropriate in order to prevent myoglobinuric renal failure.

Hallucinogenic amphetamines: MDMA ("ecstasy"), MDA, and MDEA

MDMA (3,4-methylenedioxymethamphetamine), also known as "ecstasy," "XTC," or "E," is an amphetamine derivative with different properties to those of amphetamine. MDMA is metabolized to 3,4-methylenedioxyamphetamine (MDA, "Adam"), which is also an abused drug. There are several related drugs, including 3,4-methylenedioxyethamphetamine (MDEA, "Eve"). MDMA was first patented in 1914 and was briefly used as a mood-modifying agent, but was banned in the USA in 1985. In the usual dose (up to 150 mg orally), it has few adverse effects in the majority of people, but sudden death from ventricular fibrillation has been reported.[37] Some users develop trismus and muscle pain and stiffness. When the drug is used as a "dance drug" it can lead to prolonged dancing without adequate fluid replacement. Collapse and convulsions may occur and hyperthermia may lead to disseminated intravascular coagulation and myoglobinuric renal failure. Initial investigation should include measurement of fibrin degradation products, plasma CPK, and urine myoglobin. Initial management consists of urgently restoring fluid volume to facilitate thermoregulation, together with the use of dantrolene if the body temperature is over 39 °C or if there is established heatstroke.[38]

Hyponatremia is a further complication of MDMA ingestion when large amounts of fluid are also ingested, but without exertion to induce sweating. The clinical pattern consists of initial vomiting and disturbed behavior, followed by drowsiness, agitation, and convulsions. Drowsiness, a mute state, and disorientation may persist for up to 3 days. The neurologic dysfunction is caused by hemodilution, with a rapid fall of serum sodium, leading to intracellular movement of water and subsequently to cerebral and possibly pulmonary edema. It has been shown that secretion of antidiuretic hormone is markedly increased following administration of 40 mg MDMA in healthy volunteers.[39]

It thus appears that this inappropriate production of antidiuretic hormone is not an idiosyncratic effect of MDMA but is a predictable pharmacologic effect. Most patients seem to make a steady recovery without neurologic sequelae once they reach medical care. Fluid restriction is indicated and any administration of fluids should be avoided if there is any suspicion of hyponatremia, but the use of intravenous mannitol, loop diuretics, or hypertonic saline may be considered.

LSD (lysergic acid diethylamide)

LSD is a synthetic hallucinogen that may occasionally bring the patient to the intensive therapy unit because of hypertension or cardiac arrhythmias, or because of accidents or suicide attempts. If the patient is hallucinating or violent, chlorpromazine may be effective, but large doses may lower blood pressure, depressing cardiac function.

Gamma-hydroxybutyrate

This substance, known as "GHB," "GBH," "liquid X," and "liquid E," has been used as a body-building substance, anesthetic agent, and sedative. More recently, it has become a drug of abuse, as it produces an alcohol-like euphoric intoxication. Overdose may lead to confusion, dizziness, drowsiness, vomiting, and coma. Muscle tremors and spasms may occur and patients are often hypothermic. As GHB has a short half-life (20–30 min), the patient may recover within minutes from a deep unresponsive coma. A fatal outcome is highly unlikely and management is supportive. It has been shown that physostigmine may reverse GHB toxicity, but it is not an established antidote.[40] Regular users develop tolerance, taking the drug every 1–3 h around the clock, and may experience a marked discontinuation syndrome within 3 h of the last dose. Treatment is by sedation.[41]

Volatile substance abuse

Volatile substance abuse (solvent abuse, "glue sniffing") causes about 150 deaths per year in the UK. The main substances abused are toluene, a constituent of impact adhesives, and butane in lighter fuels. The main causes of death are either a direct effect on the heart, causing ventricular fibrillation, hypotension, respiratory depression, or aspiration of vomit. Inhalation of butane may cause hypoxia due to an asphyxiant effect.[42] The very low temperature may cause collapse due to a vagal effect. Management consists essentially of resuscitation, ensuring an airway, and providing oxygen; the effects are usually short-lived. As these agents sensitize the myocardium to norepinephrine, cardiac arrhythmias may respond to intravenous administration of a beta-blocker such as esmolol or atenolol.

Drug couriers

Drug couriers ("body packers") smuggle drugs by bodily concealment. This can be by swallowing condoms, plastic bags, or vials of drug (usually heroin, cocaine, or amphetamine), or by rectal or vaginal concealment. Leakage may result in severe toxicity, and the patient may be moribund when seen. There is usually a history of a recent plane journey. Abdominal radiograph may be revealing.[43] Heroin toxicity can be treated with large doses of naloxone. Cocaine toxicity has no specific antidote, but most complications can be prevented or diminished in severity by the administration of large doses of diazepam. Sodium nitroprusside is probably the most useful agent in a patient with a hypertensive crisis or neurologic complications. Removal by whole bowel lavage is appropriate if packages have not ruptured. Surgical removal may be the only way to prevent worsening toxicity when rupture of a drug package has led to severe symptoms.[44]

REFERENCES

1. Tenenbein M. Position statement: whole bowel irrigation. American Academy of Clinical Toxicology; European Association of Poisons Centres and Clinical Toxicologists. *J Toxicol Clin Toxicol* 1997; **35:** 753–62.
2. Orr DA, Bramble MG. Tricyclic antidepressant poisoning and prolonged external cardiac massage during asystole. *BMJ* 1981; **283:** 1107–8.
3. Auzinger GM, Scheinkestel CD. Successful extracorporeal life support in a case of severe flecainide intoxication. *Crit Care Med* 2001 **29:** 887–90.
4. Krantz T, Thisted B, Strom J, *et al.* Severe, acute propoxyphene overdose treated with dopamine. *Clin Toxicol* 1985; **23:** 347–52.
5. Nozaki R, Ishibashi K, Adachi N, *et al.* Accidental profound hypothermia. *N Engl J Med* 1986; **315:** 1680.
6. Gilbert M, Busund R, Skagseth A, *et al.* Resuscitation from accidental hypothermia of 13.7 °C with circulatory arrest. *Lancet* 2000; **355:** 375–6.
7. Schaller M, Fischer M, Perret M. Hypokalemia. *JAMA* 1990; **264:** 1462–5.
8. Guze B, Baxter LR. Current concepts; neuroleptic malignant syndrome. *N Engl J Med* 1985; **313:** 163–6.
9. Ward A, Chaffman MO, Sorkin EM. Dantrolene. A review of its pharmacodynamic and pharmacokinetic properties and therapeutic use in malignant hyperthermia, the neuroleptic malignant syndrome and an update of its use in muscle spasticity. *Drugs* 1986; **32:** 130–68.
10. Wright RO, Lewander WJ, Woolf AD. Methemoglobinemia: etiology, pharmacology, and clinical management. *Ann Emerg Med* 1999; **34:** 646–56.
11. Stambach T, Haire K, Soni N, Booth J. Saturday night blue: a case of near fatal poisoning from the abuse of amyl nitrite. *J Accid Emerg Med* 1997; **14:** 339–40.
12. Votey SR, Bosse GM, Bayer MJ, Hoffman JR. Flumazenil: a new benzodiazepine antagonist. *Ann Emerg Med* 1991; **20:** 181–8.
13. Baud F, Barriot P, Tottis V, *et al.* Elevated blood cyanide concentrations in victims of smoke inhalation. *N Engl J Med* 1991; **325:** 1761–6.
14. Weaver LK, Hopkins RO, Chan KJ, *et al.* Hyperbaric oxygen for acute carbon monoxide poisoning. *N Engl J Med* 2002; **347:** 1057–67.
15. Thom SR, Taber RL, Mendiguren II, et al. Delayed neuropsychologic sequelae after carbon monoxide poisoning: prevention by treatment with hyperbaric oxygen. Ann Emerg Med 1995; **25:** 474–80.
16. Senanayake N, Karalliedde L. Neurotoxic effects of organophosphorus insecticides. An intermediate syndrome. *N Engl J Med* 1987; **316:** 761–3.
17. Borron SW, Baud FJ. Acute cyanide poisoning: clinical spectrum, diagnosis, and treatment. *Arm Hig Rada Toksikol* 1996; **47**(3): 307–22.
18. Brent J, McMartin K, Phillips S, *et al.* Fomepizole for the treatment of methanol poisoning. *N Engl J Med* 2001; **344:** 424–9.
19. Brent J, McMartin KE, Phillips S *et al.* 4-Methylpyrazole (fomepizole) for the treatment of ethylene glycol poisoning. *N Engl J Med* 1999: **340:** 832.
20. Riou B, Barriot P, Rimailho A, Baud FJ. Treatment of severe chloroquine poisoning. *N Engl J Med* 1988; **318:** 1–6.
21. Smith TW, Butler Jr VP, Haber E, *et al.* Treatment of life-threatening digitalis intoxication with digoxin-specific Fab antibody fragments. Experience in 26 cases. *N Engl J Med* 1982; **307:** 1357–62.

22. Gibb I, Adams PC, Parnham AJ, Jennings K. Plasma digoxin: assay anomalies in Fab-treated patients. *Br J Clin Pharmacol* 1983; **16:** 445–7.
23. Weinstein RS. Recognition and management of poisoning with beta adrenergic blocking agents. *Ann Emerg Med* 1984; **13:** 1123–31.
24. Boyer EW, Shannon M. Treatment of calcium-channel-blocker intoxication with insulin infusion. *N Engl J Med* 2001; **344:** 1721–2.
25. Henderson JH, McKenzie CA, Hilton PJ, Leach RM. Continuous venovenous haemofiltration for the treatment of theophylline toxicity. *Thorax* 2001; **56:** 242–3.
26. Boehnert MT, Lovejoy FN. Value of the QRS duration versus the serum drug level in predicting seizures and ventricular arrhythmias after an acute overdose of tricyclic antidepressants. *N Engl J Med* 1985; **313:** 474–9.
27. Swartz CM, Sherman AJ. The treatment of tricyclic antidepressant overdose with repeated charcoal. *J Clin Psychopharmacol* 1984; **4:** 336–40.
28. Pentel P, Peterson CD. Asystole complicating physostigmine treatment of tricyclic antidepressant overdose. *Ann Emerg Med* 1980; **9:** 588–90.
29. Lippmann SB, Nash K. Monoamine oxidase inhibitor update: potential adverse food and drug reactions. *Drug Safety* 1990; **5:** 195–204.
30. Sporer KA. The serotonin syndrome. Implicated drugs, pathophysiology and management. *Drug Safety* 1995; **13:** 94–104.
31. Dyson EH, Simpson D, Prescott LF, Proudfoot AT. Self-poisoning and therapeutic intoxication with lithium. *Hum Toxicol* 1987; **6:** 325–9.
32. Burns MJ. The pharmacology and toxicology of atypical antipsychotic agents. *Clin Toxicol* 2001; **39:** 1–14.
33. Dupuis RE, Lichtman SN, Pollack GM. Acute valproic acid overdose: clinical course and pharmacokinetic disposition of valproic acid and metabolites. *Drug Safety* 1990; **5:** 65–71.
34. Bernal W, Wendon J, Rela M, *et al*. Use and outcome of liver transplantation in acetaminophen-induced acute liver failure. *Hepatology* 1998; **27:** 1050–5.
35. Karch SB, Green GS, Young S. Myocardial hypertrophy and coronary artery disease in male cocaine users. *J Forensic Sci* 1995; **40:** 591–5.
36. Hsue PY, Salinas CL, Bolger AF, *et al*. Acute aortic dissection related to crack cocaine. *Circulation* 2002; **105:** 1592–5.
37. Dowling GP, McDonough ET, Bost RO. 'Eve' and 'Ecstasy': a report of five deaths associated with the use of MDEA and MDMA. *JAMA* 1987; **257:** 1615–17.
38. Henry JA, Jeffreys, Dawling S. Toxicity and deaths from 3,4-methylenedioxymethamphetamine ('ecstasy'). *Lancet* 1992; **1:** 384–7.
39. Henry JA, Fallon JK, Kicman AT, *et al*. Low dose MDMA ("ecstasy") induces vasopressin secretion. *Lancet* 1998; **351:** 1784.
40. Caldicott DG, Kuhn M. Gamma-hydroxybutyrate overdose and physostigmine: teaching new tricks to an old drug? *Ann Emerg Med* 2001; **37:** 99–102.
41. Sivilotti, MLA, Burns MJ, Aaron CK, *et al*. Pentobarbital for severe gamma butyrolactone withdrawal. *Ann Emerg Med* 2001; **38:** 660–6.
42. Flanagan RJ, Ruprah M, Meredith TJ, Ramsey JD. An introduction to the clinical toxicology of volatile substances. *Drug Safety* 1990; **5:** 359–83.
43. Lancashire MJ, Legg PK, Lowe M. Surgical aspects of international drug smuggling. *BMJ* 1988; **296:** 1035–7.
44. Bulstrode N, Banks F, Shrotria S. The outcome of drug smuggling by 'body packers': the British experience. *Ann R Coll Surg Engl* 2002; **84:** 35–8.

73

Management of cardiac and respiratory arrest

CHARLES W OTTO

The earliest developments in modern cardiopulmonary resuscitation (CPR) came as the result of attempts to treat cardiac arrest occurring in the operating room. The operating room still remains the location where CPR has the highest rate of success. Cardiac arrest occurs approximately seven times for every 10 000 anesthetics.[1] The cause for the arrest is anesthesia related approximately 4.5 times for every 10 000 anesthetics, but mortality from these arrests is only 0.4 per 10 000 anesthetics. Thus, resuscitation is successful approximately 90% of the time in anesthesia-related cardiac arrests.

Application of CPR to the arrest victim has spread from the operating room to the rest of the hospital and to the community at large. Over the past 40 years, CPR has become widely practiced, facilitated by the efforts of the American Heart Association, European Resuscitation Council, International Red Cross, and many other organizations around the world. Guidelines for the practice of CPR, encompassing the latest scientific evidence and expert opinions, are published periodically.[2] These organizations also develop courses at different levels of complexity for teaching CPR to lay people, and to medical and paramedical personnel. The two levels of CPR care are referred to as basic life support (BLS) for ventilation and chest compressions without additional equipment, and advanced cardiac life support (ACLS) for using all modalities available for resuscitation.

As an expert in resuscitation, the anesthesiologist is expected to be able to teach and lead these teams of CPR practitioners. To do so requires a thorough knowledge of the pathophysiology, pharmacology, and techniques of CPR. The purpose of this chapter is to discuss the scientific background upon which current CPR practice is based, not merely to review the protocols from BLS and ACLS courses. It will focus exclusively on circumstances when cardiac and respiratory arrest victims are different from victims of other cardiovascular crises.

OVERVIEW

In the USA, cardiovascular disease accounts for 50% of the annual mortality in adults or approximately 1 million yearly deaths, with one-half due to coronary artery disease.[2] The majority of deaths from coronary disease are sudden deaths, with approximately two-thirds occurring outside the hospital. The severity of the underlying cardiac disease is the major determining factor in the success or failure of resuscitation of these victims. Of the factors under control of the rescuers, poor outcomes are associated with (1) long arrest times before CPR is begun; (2) prolonged ventricular fibrillation without definitive therapy; and (3) inadequate coronary and cerebral perfusion during CPR.

Brain adenosine triphosphate (ATP) is depleted after 4–6 min if there is no blood flow, although it returns to nearly normal within 6 min of starting CPR. Studies in animals suggest that good neurologic outcome may be possible from 10- to 15-min periods of normothermic cardiac arrest if good circulation is promptly restored. In clinical practice, survival is dependent on the rapid institution of resuscitation attempts, especially in out-of-hospital arrest. Outcome is improved when CPR is begun by bystanders. Optimum survival from ventricular fibrillation is obtained only if basic CPR is started within 4 min and defibrillation applied within 8 min.[3] The longer a heart fibrillates, the more difficult is defibrillation. Early defibrillation is so important that it should take precedence over all other resuscitative efforts if the diagnosis of ventricular fibrillation can be made and defibrillation equipment is available.[4]

In cities with an effective rapid response emergency medical system for out-of-hospital cardiac arrests, initial resuscitation rates of 40% and survival to hospital discharge of 10–15% may be possible.[4] A better outcome might be expected for in-hospital arrests because of rapid response times and expert personnel. However, overall rates for initial resuscitation and survival to discharge from in-hospital arrest are approximately 40% and 10% respectively.[5]

Concurrent illnesses of hospitalized patients reduce the likelihood of survival and the arrest victim is more likely to be elderly, a factor that may reduce survival. Outside the operating suite, the best initial resuscitation rates are found in the intensive care unit (ICU), whereas the best survival rates are for patients arresting in the emergency department. The cause of arrest associated with the best outcome and the most common cause of out-of-hospital arrest is ventricular fibrillation secondary to myocardial ischemia. This initiating event is less common in hospitalized patients. When applying CPR, attention to the details of effective resuscitation is important. However, it should always be remembered that CPR is only symptomatic therapy. Thus, so much attention should not be paid to the mechanics of CPR that search for a treatable cause of the arrest is forgotten.

BASIC LIFE SUPPORT

Basic life support consists of those elements of resuscitation that can be performed without additional equipment: airway management, ventilation, and chest compressions. Common practice is to approach a victim with the ABC (airway–breathing–circulation) sequence, although the CAB sequence has been used in some countries with similar results. The full sequence for initiating CPR in an apparent arrest victim is given in Table 73.1. However, if complete resuscitation equipment and expertise in its use is available, the overall priorities of resuscitation may dictate altering this sequence (Table 73.2).

AIRWAY MANAGEMENT

The goal of airway management during cardiorespiratory arrest is the same as during general anesthesia: provide a clear path for respiratory gas exchange while minimizing gastric insufflation and the risk of pulmonary aspiration. Airway maintenance in an unconscious patient is a basic part of anesthetic practice and all the techniques learned for use during anesthesia are applicable to the cardiac arrest victim. Just as in the operating room, the most commonly used technique for opening the airway is the "head tilt/chin lift" method. If this is ineffective, the "jaw thrust" maneuver is frequently helpful. Oropharyngeal and nasopharyngeal airways are useful for helping maintain an open airway in patients who are not intubated. Care must be used to ensure that they are correctly inserted and that they do not worsen airway obstruction. Insertion in the semiconscious can induce vomiting or laryngospasm.

Through the years, it has become obvious that effective airway management during CPR is a major problem, even for medical professionals. Many individuals cannot manage effectively a self-inflating resuscitation bag and mask. Larger tidal volumes at lower pressures are delivered by mouth-to-mouth or mouth-to-mask ventilation.[6] The bag and mask apparatus is more effective if two individuals manage the airway: one to hold the mask and maintain the airway and one to squeeze the bag.[7] In the hands of adequately trained personnel, the laryngeal mask airway (LMA) and esophageal tracheal combitube (ETC) provide superior ventilation to the bag and mask apparatus and are recommended alternatives. Of course, none of these allows the degree of airway control obtained with an endotracheal tube. Endotracheal intubation should be carried out in all resuscitations lasting more than a few minutes if a skilled laryngoscopist is available. However, it should not be performed until adequate ventilation by other means (preferably with supplemental oxygen) and circulation by chest compressions have been established (Table 73.2).

Table 73.1 *Sequence of basic life support*

1 Determine unresponsiveness
2 Activate emergency medical services or code team
3 Position victim supine on firm surface
4 Open airway
5 Determine absence of breathing
6 Perform ventilation: two breaths
7 Determine absence of pulse or signs of circulation
8 Initiate chest compression
9 Alternate 15 compressions with two breaths

Table 73.2 *Procedural priorities during CPR[a]*

1 Diagnose ventricular fibrillation and defibrillate
2 Open airway
3 Begin ventilation
4 Begin chest compressions
5 Administer supplemental oxygen
6 Obtain intravenous access
7 Administer epinephrine or vasopressin
8 Assess adequacy of CPR efforts
9 Intubate trachea
10 Additional drug therapy

a. Most important to least important interventions assuming that all necessary equipment and expertise are available.

Foreign body airway obstruction

In 1998 in the USA, the National Safety Council reported that foreign body airway obstruction accounted for approximately 1.2 deaths per 100 000 of the population, compared with 1.7 for drowning, 16.5 for motor vehicle crashes, and 198 for coronary heart disease.[2] However, few subjects in CPR have caused more controversy than the management of this emergency. Total airway occlusion by a foreign body must be considered in any victim who suddenly stops breathing, and who becomes cyanotic and unconscious. It occurs most commonly during eating and usually is due to food, especially meat, impacting in the laryngeal inlet, at the epiglottis, or in the vallecula. Factors contributing to choking include poorly chewed pieces of food, poor dentition or dentures, and elevated blood alcohol levels. Sudden death in restaurants from this cause is frequently mistaken for a myocardial infarction, leading to the label "cafe coronary."

Total airway obstruction is characterized by the inability to speak, cough, or breathe. There is complete lack of air movement despite respiratory efforts. Cyanosis and loss of consciousness occur quickly and cardiac arrest will follow within minutes. Partial airway obstruction is characterized by rasping or wheezing respirations accompanied by coughing. The voice may be weak or speaking may be impossible. If air exchange appears good and coughing is forceful, no intervention in the patient's attempts to clear the airway should be made. If the obstruction cannot be cleared, definitive care with extraction under controlled circumstances in a medical facility may be necessary. If the cough weakens or cyanosis intervenes, the patient should be treated as if there were complete obstruction.

Recommended treatments for airway obstruction have ranged from back blows to subdiaphragmatic abdominal thrusts (Heimlich maneuver) to sternal thrusts to finger sweeps to grasping with instruments. No one technique is always successful and each may be successful when another has failed.[8] Mothers and friends have been pounding on the backs of choking victims for centuries. In 1974, Heimlich proposed abdominal thrusts as a better method of relieving airway obstruction.[9] A subsequent report suggested that the sternal thrusts of cardiac compression were at least as effective as abdominal thrusts.[10] Experimental studies show that a normal cough produces better air movement and higher airway pressures than any artificial maneuver. Abdominal and sternal thrusts produce only modest elevations in airway pressure but can induce a high volume and flow of exhaled air that may move the obstructing object into the pharynx. Back blows produce little air flow or volume, but result instantaneously in very high airway pressures, considered helpful in dislodging an impacted obstruction. There continues to be no convincing evidence that any single technique is superior to the others.

The European Resuscitation Council recommends five back blows as the initial maneuver followed by abdominal thrusts, if necessary. However, because of confusion in teaching multiple techniques (especially to the lay public), the American Heart Association has chosen to emphasize the abdominal thrust maneuver (with chest thrusts as an alternative for pregnant and massively obese victims) for adults and children.[2] This recommendation is made on the basis that the abdominal thrust is at least as effective as other techniques and teaching one method simplifies education. For infants less than 1 year old, the American Heart Association recommends five back blows with the infant in the head-down position followed by five chest thrusts, if necessary.

Abdominal thrusts in the awake victim are applied in the sitting or standing position. The rescuer reaches around the victim from behind, placing the fist of one hand in the epigastrium between the xiphoid and umbilicus. The fist is grasped with the other hand and a quick upward thrust is given in the epigastrium. In the unconscious, thrusts are applied by kneeling astride the victim, placing the heel of one hand in the epigastrium and the other on top of the first. The thrust should be in the midline and care should be taken that the xiphoid is not pushed into the abdominal contents.

With the massively obese or women in advanced pregnancy, sternal thrusts may be safer and more effective than abdominal thrusts. In the erect victim, the chest is encircled from behind as in the abdominal maneuver, but the fist is placed in the midsternum. In the supine victim, thrusts are applied from the side with the hands in the same position as for external cardiac compressions.

If back blows are used, they should be applied directly over the thoracic spine between the scapulae. They must be delivered with force. The head-down position may help move the obstructing object into the pharynx with this maneuver.

Whatever technique is used, each individual maneuver must be delivered as if it will relieve the obstruction. If the first attempt is unsuccessful, repeated attempts should be made because hypoxia-induced muscular relaxation may allow success eventually. Complications of the thrust maneuvers include lacerations of the liver and spleen, fractured ribs, gastric rupture, and regurgitation.

In the unconscious victim, if these maneuvers are unsuccessful, dislodging the obstruction manually should be tried. The tongue and jaw are grasped between the thumb and fingers and pulled forward. A finger of the other hand is inserted along the cheek and attempts are made to dislodge the object laterally. Care must be taken not to push the object deeper into the larynx. Direct visualization of the object can also be successful. In the absence of a laryngoscope and forceps, ordinary instruments (such as a tablespoon and ice tongs) may be used. However, blind grasping with instruments is rarely successful and may cause damage to tonsils or other tissue. Finally, if the object cannot be dislodged, a cricothyroidotomy may be life saving.

VENTILATION

The standard approach to the unresponsive victim is to follow opening the airway with ventilation (Tables 73.1 and 73.2). If the airway remains patent, chest compressions cause substantial air exchange. Early studies in anesthetized humans suggested that the airway would not remain open in the unconscious,[11,12] leading to the teaching that airway control and artificial ventilation must accompany chest compressions. However, data from the Belgian CPCR Registry have demonstrated that 14-day survival and neurologic outcome are the same if bystanders initiate full BLS or only do chest compressions. Both lead to substantially better survival than if the bystanders only do mouth-to-mouth ventilation or attempt no CPR.[13,14] Studies in the more controlled setting of the animal laboratory also raise questions about the importance of ventilation during BLS. In a swine model of up to 5 min of untreated fibrillatory cardiac arrest, comparison of 10 min of standard BLS with chest compressions without airway control or ventilation demonstrated that all successfully resuscitated animals in both groups survived for 24 h and were neurologically normal.[15–18] A separate study using an asphyxial cardiac arrest model found a markedly improved 24-h outcome when ventilation was added to chest compressions during BLS.[19] These observations suggest that when arrest is witnessed, and likely to be of cardiac (rather than respiratory) cause, and intubation is available within a short time, closed-chest compressions alone may be as efficacious as compressions and mouth-to-mouth ventilation. If these preliminary studies are confirmed, BLS teaching could be considerably simplified, potentially resulting in improved rates of bystander CPR.

Currently, if the unconscious victim is not making respiratory efforts after an open airway is established, rescue breathing to assist ventilation is recommended. Mouth-to-mouth or mouth-to-nose ventilation is the most expeditious and effective method immediately available. Although inspired gas with this method will contain approximately 4% carbon dioxide and only 17% oxygen (composition of exhaled air), it is sufficient to maintain viability. Published surveys have documented that professional and lay rescuers are reluctant to provide mouth-to-mouth ventilation for unknown victims of cardiac arrest, primarily related to a fear of infectious disease.[20–22] That risk is actually very small. Only 15 reports of CPR-related infections were published between 1960 and 1998 and no reports of HIV, HBV, hepatitis C, or cytomegalovirus were found.[23] Mouth-to-face shield and mouth-to-mask (especially with a one-way valve) breathing are effective alternatives that may reduce the fear of infection. If the mask is fitted with a nipple adaptor, a flow of oxygen can also supplement inspired oxygen concentration. The self-inflating resuscitation bag with mask also can be used with or without supplemental oxygen. If a rescuer is unable or unwilling to perform mouth-to-mouth ventilation for an adult victim of apparent cardiac arrest, chest compression-only CPR should be provided rather than performing no attempt at rescue.

Physiology of ventilation during CPR

In the absence of an endotracheal tube, the relative distribution of gas between the lungs and stomach during mouth-to-mouth or bag–valve–mask ventilation will be determined by the impedance to flow into each compartment. In the respiratory compartment, the lung–thorax compliance will be the major factor. Impedance to flow into the stomach will be determined primarily by esophageal opening pressure. Although there are no specific data during human CPR, it is likely that the opening pressure of the esophagus is no higher than it is under anesthesia (approximately 20 cmH_2O). In experimental animals, esophageal pressure decreases from 28 to 4 mmHg (3.7 to 0.5 kPa) during 15 min of cardiac arrest without CPR, whereas the lung–thorax compliance decreases by 30% over the same time.[24]

Insufflation of air into the stomach during resuscitation leads to gastric distension, impeding ventilation, and increasing the danger of regurgitation and gastric rupture. If gastric insufflation is to be avoided, inspiratory airway pressures must be kept low. A major cause of increased airway pressures and gastric insufflation is partial airway obstruction by the tongue and pharyngeal tissues. Meticulous attention to maintaining an open airway is necessary during rescue breathing. To cause an obvious rise in the chest of most adults, a tidal volume of 10 $mL\,kg^{-1}$ (600–900 mL) will be needed. Even with an open airway, a relatively long inspiratory time is necessary to administer this volume at low pressure. Thus, rescue breaths should be given over 2.0 s during a pause in chest compressions. If supplemental oxygen is available, such as with a bag-mask apparatus, tidal volumes can be lowered to 6–7 $mL\,kg^{-1}$ (400–600 mL), further reducing the risk of gastric distension. A useful aid to minimizing gastric insufflation is the use of cricoid pressure (Sellick maneuver). Pressure applied over the anterior arch of the cricoid cartilage can prevent air from entering the stomach at airway pressures up to 100 cmH_2O (10 kPa).

Technique of rescue breathing

Using the head tilt/chin lift method of maintaining an open airway, mouth-to-mouth ventilation is administered by using the hand on the forehead to pinch the nose. The rescuer takes a breath, seals the victim's mouth with his or her mouth, and exhales, watching for the chest to rise. When both hands are being used with the jaw thrust, the cheek can be used to seal the nose. For mouth-to-nose ventilation, the rescuer's lips surround the nose and the lips are held closed. For exhalation, the rescuer removes his or her mouth from the victim, listening for escaping air and taking a breath. When initiating resuscitation, two to five breaths should be given and breathing should be continued at a rate of 10–12 breaths per minute. During chest compressions, a pause for two breaths (2 s per breath) should be made after each 15 compressions whether there are one or two rescuers. Exhalation can occur during the next compressions.

The best way to ensure adequate ventilation without gastric distension is endotracheal intubation. It is indicated during any prolonged resuscitation. However, other aspects of the resuscitation that might lead to a restoration of spontaneous circulation should not be delayed for intubation (Table 73.2). Once an endotracheal tube is in place, ventilation can proceed without concern for gastric distension or synchronizing ventilation with chest compressions. Blood flow during CPR slows rapidly when chest compressions are stopped and recovers slowly when they are restarted. Consequently, following intubation, no pause should be made for ventilation: ventilation should be approximately 12 breaths per minute without regard for the compression cycle.

CIRCULATION

Physiology of circulation during closed-chest compressions

Two theories have been proposed to explain the mechanism by which closed-chest compressions cause blood to flow through the circulatory system.[25,26] They are not mutually exclusive, and which theory is more feasible in humans continues to be actively investigated.

Cardiac pump mechanism

With the original description of closed-chest cardiac massage in 1960, Kouwenhoven *et al.*[25] suggested that the heart was compressed between the sternum and spine, resulting in increased intraventricular pressure, closing of the atrioventricular valves, and ejection of blood into the lungs and aorta. During the relaxation phase, negative intrathoracic pressure caused by expansion of the thoracic cage facilitates blood return and aortic pressure results in aortic valve closure and coronary perfusion. This has come to be known as the cardiac pump theory of blood flow during CPR. Support for this theory comes from echocardiography studies that show reduction in ventricular size and mitral valve closure with chest compression during the early stages of CPR. In addition, CPR techniques that incorporate direct sternal compressions, compared with techniques that raise intrathoracic pressure without sternal compressions, result in better tissue blood flow and survival in animals.[27,28]

Thoracic pump mechanism

A few early investigators questioned the cardiac pump mechanism, and many practitioners have questioned the ability of rescuers to depress the sternum enough to compress the heart in very large victims. In 1976, Criley *et al.*[29] reported a patient undergoing cardiac catheterization who simultaneously developed ventricular fibrillation and an episode of cough-hiccups. With every cough-hiccup, a significant arterial pressure was noted and the patient never lost consciousness even though CPR was not performed. This description of "cough CPR" led to further investigations[30] and codification of the thoracic pump theory of blood flow during CPR.[26] According to this theory, all intrathoracic structures are compressed equally by the increase in intrathoracic pressure resulting from sternal compression. Backward flow through the venous system is prevented by valves in the subclavian and internal jugular veins and by dynamic compression of the veins at the thoracic outlet. Thicker, less compressible vessel walls prevent collapse on the arterial side. The heart acts as a passive conduit with the atrioventricular valves remaining open during chest compression.

A number of studies and observations support the thoracic pump theory.[31] Angiography during a cough has shown blood flowing through the left heart into the aorta without cardiac compression. Maneuvers that raise intrathoracic pressure (such as simultaneous ventilation and chest compression or abdominal binding) increase arterial pressure and carotid blood flow compared with standard CPR. Artificial circulation adequate to maintain viability can be accomplished with simultaneous ventilation and inflation of vests surrounding the chest and abdomen in experimental animals.

It seems clear that fluctuations in intrathoracic pressure play a significant role in blood flow during CPR. It is also likely that the cardiac pump mechanism contributes under some circumstances. Which mechanism predominates probably varies from patient to patient and may vary even during the resuscitation of the same patient.

Distribution of blood flow during CPR

Whatever the actual mechanism of blood flow, cardiac output is severely reduced during closed-chest compressions, ranging from 10% to 33% of prearrest values in experimental animals. Total blood flow also tends to decrease with time during CPR, although changes in technique and the use of epinephrine (noradrenaline) may help sustain cardiac output. Nearly all of the cardiac output is directed to organs above the diaphragm. Brain blood flow is 50–90% of normal and myocardial blood flow 20–50% of normal, whereas lower extremity and abdominal visceral flow is reduced to less than 5% of normal. All flows tend to decrease with time but the relative distribution of flow does not change. Epinephrine improves flow to the brain and heart, whereas flow to organs below the diaphragm is unchanged or further reduced.

Physiology of gas transport during CPR

During CPR, measurement of blood gases reveals an arterial respiratory alkalosis and a venous respiratory acidosis because the arterial $P\text{CO}_2$ is reduced and the venous $P\text{CO}_2$ is elevated. The cause of these changes is the reduced cardiac output. During the low-flow state of CPR, excretion of CO_2 (milliliters of CO_2 min^{-1} in exhaled gas) is decreased from prearrest levels approximately to the same extent as cardiac output is reduced. This reduced CO_2 excretion is due primarily to shunting of blood flow away from the lower half of the body. The exhaled CO_2 reflects only the metabolism of the part of the body that is being perfused. In the nonperfused areas, CO_2 accumulates during CPR. When normal circulation is restored, the accumulated CO_2 is washed out and a temporary increase in CO_2 excretion is seen.

Although CO_2 excretion is reduced during CPR, the mixed venous partial pressure of CO_2 ($P_{\bar{v}}\text{CO}_2$) is usually increased.[32] Two factors account for this elevation. Buffering acid causes a reduction in serum bicarbonate, so that the same blood CO_2 content results in a higher $P_{\bar{v}}\text{CO}_2$. In addition, the mixed venous CO_2 content is elevated. When flow to a tissue is reduced, all the CO_2 produced fails to be removed and CO_2 accumulates, raising the tissue partial pressure of CO_2. This allows more CO_2 to be carried in each aliquot of blood and mixed venous CO_2 content increases. If flow remains constant, a new equilibrium is established at which all CO_2 produced in the tissue is removed but at a higher venous CO_2 content and partial pressure. In contrast with the venous blood, arterial CO_2 content and partial pressure ($P_a\text{CO}_2$) are usually reduced during CPR. This reduction accounts for most of the observed increase in arterial–venous CO_2 content difference. Thus, despite the marked reduction in cardiac output, maintaining ventilation results in very efficient CO_2 removal.

Decreased pulmonary blood flow during CPR causes lack of perfusion to many nondependent alveoli. The alveolar gas of these lung units has no CO_2. Consequently, mixed alveolar CO_2 (i.e. end-tidal CO_2) will be very low and correlate poorly with arterial CO_2. However, end-tidal CO_2 does correlate well with cardiac output during CPR. As flow increases, more alveoli become perfused, there is less alveolar dead space, and end-tidal CO_2 measurements rise.

Technique of closed-chest compression

Cardiac arrest must be assumed in the absence of signs of circulation in an unconscious patient. After opening the airway and providing two ventilations, look for signs of circulation, such as breathing, coughing, movement, or a pulse in the major arteries (carotid, femoral, axillary), before starting chest compressions. If weak circulation exists in a patient with a primary respiratory arrest, pulses may return after adequate ventilation and compressions may not be necessary.

Standard chest compression technique consists of the rhythmic application of pressure over the lower half of the sternum. For compressions to be effective in providing blood flow to the brain and heart, the patient must be on a firm surface with the head level with the heart. The rescuer should stand or kneel at the side of the patient so that the hips are on a level with the victim's chest. The heel of one hand is placed on the lower sternum and the other hand placed on top of the first. Care must be taken that the xiphoid is not pressed into the abdomen, as this can lacerate the liver. Pressure on the ribs or costal cartilages rather than the sternum increases the risk of rib fracture. The elbows should be locked in position with the arms straight and the shoulders over the hands. Using the weight of the entire upper body, the compression is delivered straight down with enough force to depress the sternum 3.5–5 cm. Following maximal compression, pressure is released completely from the chest, but the hands stay in contact with the chest wall, maintaining proper hand position for the next thrust.

Chest compressions should be performed at a rate of 100 per minute. These are most effective if the compression and relaxation phases of the cycle are equal in length. This 50% compression time is easier to achieve at faster compression rates. With one or two rescuers providing CPR, it is recommended that 15 compressions be followed by a pause for two ventilations (2 s each) followed by 15 more compressions. When the airway is controlled by an endotracheal tube, breaths at a rate of 12 per minute should be interposed between chest compressions without a pause for ventilation.

Alternative techniques of circulatory support

Better understanding of circulatory physiology during CPR, especially involving the thoracic pump mechanism, has generated several proposed alternatives to standard CPR techniques. Most are intended to provide better hemodynamics and, thus, to improve survival or to extend the duration during which CPR can successfully support viability. Unfortunately, none has proven reliably superior to standard techniques and no improvement in survival from cardiac arrest has been consistently demonstrated.[33]

Closed-chest techniques

According to the thoracic pump theory, maneuvers that increase intrathoracic pressure during chest compression should improve blood flow and pressure.[30] Several methods for raising intrathoracic pressure during CPR have been studied, including simultaneous ventilation and compression, abdominal binding with compression, and the pneumatic antishock garment. Early results indicated improved aortic pressures and carotid blood flows with these techniques.[30] The increase in pressure was expected to improve myocardial and cerebral perfusion. Unfortunately, the elevation in right atrial, intraventricular, and intracranial pressure is equal to or greater than the rise in aortic pressure. The net result is no improvement or diminution of myocardial and cerebral perfusion pressures and blood flows. Studies of these techniques have failed to demonstrate consistently improved resuscitation success or survival in animals[27,28] or humans.[34]

Another alternative technique, commonly called high-impulse CPR, is based more on the cardiac pump mechanism.[35] Using relatively short compressions with moderately high force results in cardiac output being directly related to the rate of compressions. The optimal cardiac output and coronary blood flows are obtained with a compression rate of 120 per minute in this experimental model. This technique is quite similar to the standard technique, and many of the results from studies of high-impulse CPR have been incorporated into the currently recommended chest compression technique. Emphasis now is placed on ensuring adequate sternal depression. Recommended compression rates have been increased to 100 per minute. The faster rate and focus on sternal depression result in shorter compressions with relatively high force.

Other techniques continue to be actively investigated. The pneumatic CPR vest relies entirely on the thoracic pump mechanism of blood flow.[31] With this technique, thoracic and abdominal vests containing pneumatic bladders are inflated simultaneously with positive-pressure ventilation. Experimental animal studies have shown excellent hemodynamics and the ability to maintain viability for prolonged periods. A small clinical study found better aortic and coronary perfusion pressure with the vest but survival was not improved.[36] Large-scale randomized trials are now being conducted.

The technique of interposed abdominal compression CPR (IAC-CPR) uses an additional rescuer to apply manual abdominal compressions during the relaxation phase of chest compressions.[37] Abdominal pressure is released when chest compression begins. Although animal studies suggested better hemodynamics with this technique, there was no improvement in survival.[27] A large randomized trial of IAC-CPR in out-of-hospital human arrest found no improvement in survival compared with standard CPR.[38] Two smaller studies have reported improved survival from in-hospital cardiac arrest with this technique.[39] The safety of IAC-CPR has been established. Further studies will be needed to establish out-of-hospital efficacy.

The latest proposed alternative technique to receive extensive investigation is called active compression–decompression CPR (ACD-CPR).[40] With this technique, CPR is performed with a suction device applied to the chest over the sternum, allowing active decompression. Animal and human studies have often shown improvement in resuscitation hemodynamics. One in-hospital preliminary study found improved immediate resuscitation with the device but no difference in survival.[41] Two early out-of-hospital trials found no difference in immediate resuscitation or survival.[42,43] One recent randomized trial in France found improved outcome in out-of-hospital arrest with the technique.[44] However, a large study in Canada involving in-hospital and out-of-hospital arrests found no difference in immediate resuscitation or survival.[45] Two new devices are undergoing preliminary investigations. The impedance threshold valve lowers intrathoracic pressure, enhancing venous return during CPR.[46] Phased chest and abdominal compression CPR is a combination of ACD- and IAC-CPR.[47]

Invasive techniques

Much of the effort spent improving current CPR techniques and investigating new techniques was prompted by the hope that better blood flows would extend the time during which CPR can support viability. Unfortunately, the results have been disappointing. Despite the occasional success of prolonged resuscitation efforts, it appears that closed-chest compressions can sustain most patients only for 15–30 min. If successful restoration of spontaneous circulation has not occurred in that time, the results are dismal. In contrast with the closed-chest techniques, two invasive maneuvers have been shown to be able to maintain cardiac and cerebral viability during long periods of cardiac arrest. In animal models, open-chest cardiac massage and cardiopulmonary bypass (through the femoral artery and vein using a membrane oxygenator) can provide better hemodynamics and myocardial and cerebral perfusion than closed-chest techniques. Prompt restoration of blood flow and perfusion pressure with cardiopulmonary bypass can provide resuscitation with minimal neurologic deficit after 20 min of fibrillatory cardiac arrest in canines. However, to be effective, these techniques must be instituted relatively early (probably within 20 to 30 min).[48] If open-chest massage is begun after 30 min of ineffective closed-chest compressions, there is no better survival even though hemodynamics are improved.[49] The need to apply these maneuvers early in an arrest obviously limits the application. In-hospital arrests are circumstances in which the necessary expertise may be available to apply these techniques. However, there is an appropriate reluctance to apply such invasive maneuvers until it is clear that closed-chest techniques are ineffective. Unfortunately, at that point it may be too late for invasive methods to be successful as well. Before invasive procedures can play a greater role in modern CPR, a method must be developed to predict, early in the resuscitation, which patients will respond and which will not respond to closed-chest compressions.

Assessing the adequacy of circulation during CPR

There is an obvious need to assess whether ongoing CPR is generating adequate myocardial and cerebral blood flow for viable resuscitation. The traditional method is to palpate the carotid or femoral pulse during chest compressions. However, a palpable pulse primarily reflects systolic blood pressure. Mean blood pressure correlates better with cardiac output, and diastolic pressure is the major determinant of coronary perfusion. Nevertheless, palpation of the pulse remains the only assessment tool available during basic life support.

Successful resuscitation in experimental models is associated with myocardial blood flows of 15–30 mL min^{-1} 100 g^{-1}.[50] Obtaining such flows relies on closed-chest compressions generating adequate cardiac output and coronary perfusion pressure. During CPR, coronary perfusion occurs primarily during the relaxation phase (diastole) of chest compression. The critical myocardial blood flow is associated with aortic "diastolic" pressure exceeding 40 mmHg (5.3 kPa) and myocardial perfusion pressure (aortic diastolic minus right atrial diastolic pressure) exceeding 25 mmHg (3.3 kPa) in animal models.[50–53] One report has confirmed similar findings in humans, noting that all patients with successful return of spontaneous circulation have coronary perfusion pressures higher than 15 mmHg (2.0 kPa).[54] When invasive pressure monitoring is available during CPR, it should be used to guide resuscitation efforts. If pressures are below these levels, adjustments should be made to improve chest compressions and/or additional epinephrine or vasopressin should be administered. However, obtaining pressures above the critical levels does not ensure success. Damage to the myocardium from underlying disease may preclude survival no matter how effective the CPR efforts. Regardless, vascular pressures below these levels are associated with poor results even in patients who may be salvageable.

Although invasive pressure monitoring may be the ideal, exhaled end-tidal CO_2 is an excellent noninvasive guide to the effectiveness of standard CPR. Carbon dioxide excretion during CPR with an endotracheal tube in place is dependent primarily on flow rather than ventilation. As alveolar dead space is large during low-flow conditions, end-tidal CO_2 is very low [frequently < 10 mmHg (1.3 kPa)]. If cardiac output increases, more alveoli are perfused and end-tidal CO_2 rises [usually to > 20 mmHg (2.6 kPa) during successful CPR]. When spontaneous circulation resumes, the earliest sign is a sudden increase in end-tidal CO_2 to greater than 40 mmHg (5.3 kPa). Within a wide range of cardiac outputs, end-tidal CO_2 during CPR correlates with coronary perfusion pressure, cardiac output, initial resuscitation, and survival.[55–57] Two studies have shown that end-tidal CO_2 measured during human CPR can predict outcome.[57,58] No patient with an end-tidal $CO_2 < 10$ mmHg (1.3 kPa) could be successfully resuscitated. In the absence of invasive pressure monitoring, end-tidal CO_2 monitoring can be used to judge the effectiveness of chest compressions.[59] Attempts should be made to maximize the value by alterations in technique or drug therapy. Sodium bicarbonate administration results in the liberation of CO_2 in the venous blood and a temporary rise in end-tidal CO_2. Therefore, end-tidal CO_2 monitoring will not be useful for judging the effectiveness of chest compressions for 3–5 min following bicarbonate administration.

ADVANCED CARDIAC LIFE SUPPORT

Advanced cardiac life support encompasses all those cognitive and technical skills that are necessary to restore spontaneous circulatory function when simple support does not result in resuscitation. In addition to BLS skills, it includes use of adjunctive equipment and techniques for assisting ventilation and circulation, electrocardiographic (ECG) monitoring with arrhythmia recognition and defibrillation, establishment of intravenous access, and drug therapy. A number of aspects of ACLS have been discussed in the preceding sections, especially regarding adjuncts for airway management, ventilation, and alternative methods of chest compression.

DEFIBRILLATION

Duration and electrical pattern of fibrillation

Ventricular fibrillation is the most common ECG rhythm in adult cardiac arrest. The longer fibrillation continues, the more difficult it is to defibrillate and the less likely is successful resuscitation. The fibrillating heart has high oxygen consumption, increasing myocardial ischemia and decreasing the time to irreversible cell damage. The only effective treatment for this dysrhythmia is electrical defibrillation, and the sooner it is applied, the higher the rate of successful resuscitation.[4,60] Thus, conversion of ventricular fibrillation to a rhythm capable of restoring spontaneous circulation should be the first priority of any resuscitation attempt (Table 73.2).

The amplitude and frequency (coarseness) of the fibrillatory waves on the ECG may reflect the severity and duration of the myocardial insult and, thus, have prognostic significance.[61] Low-voltage and low-frequency fibrillation is associated with poor outcome. Increasing myocardial ischemia results in less vigorous fibrillation, reduced amplitude and frequency of electrical activity, and more difficult defibrillation. Catecholamines with β-adrenergic activity, such as epinephrine, increase the amplitude of the electrical activity but have no influence on the ability to defibrillate.[60,62] Consequently, defibrillation should not be postponed for any other therapy but should be carried out as soon as the rhythm is diagnosed and the equipment is available. The importance of early defibrillation has been demonstrated in numerous studies.[3,4] The application has been made much easier by the development of automatic external defibrillators (AEDs) that recognize ventricular fibrillation, charge automatically, and give a defibrillatory shock. The AEDs allow minimally trained individuals to incorporate defibrillation into BLS skills, including public access defibrillation.[4]

Defibrillators: energy, current, and impedance

The defibrillator is a variable transformer that stores a direct current in a capacitor until discharged through the electrodes. The waveform of most clinically used defibrillators is a monophasic, damped sinusoid (MDS), although some are designed to deliver trapezoidal or near-square waves. Implantable defibrillators use multipulse, multipathway defibrillation, but such techniques have had conflicting results in transthoracic defibrillation. Recently, biphasic, truncated, exponential (BTE) waveforms have been introduced for transthoracic defibrillation. This is the waveform used in AEDs and it allows successful defibrillation at lower energies than MDS waveforms.[63]

Defibrillation is accomplished by the electrical current passing through a critical mass of myocardium, causing simultaneous depolarization of the myofibrils. However, the output of most defibrillators is indicated in energy units (joules or watt-seconds). The relations among energy, current and impedance (resistance) are given by the following equations (standard units are indicated):

$$\text{Energy (joules)} = \text{power (watts)} \times \text{duration (s)} \quad (73.1)$$

$$\text{Power (watts)} = \text{potential (volts)} \times \text{current (amperes)} \quad (73.2)$$

$$\text{Current (amperes)} = \text{potential (volts)}/\text{resistance (ohms)} \quad (73.3)$$

$$\text{Current}^2\text{ (amperes)} = \text{energy (joules)}/[\text{resistance (ohms)} \times \text{duration (s)}] \quad (73.4)$$

From these equations it can be determined that as the impedance between the paddle electrodes increases, the delivered energy will be reduced. For consistency, the energy level indicated on most commercially available defibrillators is the output when discharged into a 50-ohm load. Even at a constant delivered energy, equation 73.4 indicates that delivered current will be reduced as impedance increases. At high impedance and relatively low energy levels, current could be too low for defibrillation. Optimum success of defibrillation is obtained by keeping impedance as low as possible.

Transthoracic impedance during human defibrillation has been measured at between 15 and 143 ohms.[64] Many of the important factors in minimizing transthoracic impedance are under the control of the rescuers. Resistance decreases with electrode size, so large paddles (>8 cm in diameter) should be used. The greatest impedance is between the metal electrode and skin. This can be reduced slightly by the use of saline-soaked gauze pads or ECG electrode cream. However, the lowest resistance is obtained with the specially designed defibrillation gels or pastes. Self-adhesive defibrillation/monitor pads also work well when carefully applied. Firm paddle pressure of at least 11 kg reduces resistance by improving electrode–skin contact and by expelling air from the lung. Transthoracic impedance is reduced by successive shocks. This factor may partially explain why additional shocks of the same energy may succeed when previous shocks did not, although its clinical importance has been questioned.[64]

The average transthoracic impedance in human defibrillation is 70–80 ohms. If relatively high-energy shocks (>300 J) are used with reasonable attention to proper technique, resistance is probably of little clinical significance. For lower-energy shocks, great care should be taken to minimize resistance. Recently, defibrillators have been developed which measure transthoracic impedance before the shock by passing a low-level current through the chest during the charge cycle. Although not widely available, this technology may allow current-based defibrillation by adjusting the delivered energy for the measured resistance.[65]

Energy requirements and adverse effects

The incidence and severity of myocardial damage from defibrillation in humans is not clear. Repeated high-level shocks in animals result in dysrhythmias, ECG changes and myocardial necrosis. Whether such injuries occur in humans is unknown, although slight elevations in creatine kinase MB fractions have been reported after cardioversions with high energies. It would seem prudent to keep energy levels as low as possible during defibrillation attempts.

There is a general relation between body size and energy requirements for defibrillation. Children need lower energies than adults, perhaps as low as $0.5\,\text{J kg}^{-1}$, although the recommended pediatric dose is $2\,\text{J kg}^{-1}$.[66] However, over the size range of adults, body size does not seem to be a clinically important variable. Multiple studies have now demonstrated that using relatively low-level initial shocks in adults is as successful as beginning with higher energy.[67] Therefore, it is currently recommended that the initial shock be given at 200 J followed by a second shock at 200–300 J if the first is unsuccessful. If both fail to defibrillate the patient, additional shocks should be given at 360 J.

PHARMACOLOGIC THERAPY

The discussion in this section will be confined to the use of drugs during CPR attempts to restore spontaneous circulation. Management of shock, dysrhythmias, and metabolic disturbances when there is effective mechanical function of the heart will be discussed in other chapters. During cardiac arrest, drug therapy is secondary to other interventions (Table 73.2). Chest compressions, airway management, ventilation, and defibrillation, if appropriate, should take precedence over medications. Establishing intravenous access and giving drugs should come after other interventions are established. The reason for making drugs a secondary intervention is that they contribute little to resuscitation attempts in many circumstances. Effective chest compressions, ventilation, and defibrillation are most important. Of the drugs used during CPR, only epinephrine and other vasopressors are usually acknowledged as being useful in helping to restore spontaneous circulation.

Routes of administration

The preferred route of administration of all drugs during CPR is intravenous and the doses listed in Table 73.3 are for intravenous use. The most rapid and highest drug levels occur with administration into a central vein. Therefore, when a central venous catheter is available during a cardiac arrest, it should be used for drug therapy. However, intravenous administration is also effective and is preferred for starting an infusion during resuscitation because placement of a central line usually necessitates stopping CPR. In children, the intraosseous route is also effective. Sites in the upper extremity and neck are necessary because of the paucity of blood flow below the diaphragm during CPR. Drugs administered in the lower extremity may be extremely delayed or may not reach the sites of action. Even in the upper extremity, drugs may require 1–2 min to reach the central circulation. Onset of action may be speeded if a drug bolus is followed by a 20- to 30-mL bolus of intravenous fluid.

Epinephrine, vasopressin, lidocaine (lignocaine), and atropine do not injure the lungs and can be absorbed from the tracheal mucosa. Therefore, if intravenous access cannot be established, the endotracheal route provides an alternative for these drugs following intubation. Sodium bicarbonate should not be given by this route. The time to effect and drug levels achieved after endotracheal administration are

Drug	Adult	Infant and child
Epinephrine (adrenaline)	1 mg	0.01 mg kg^{-1}
(If dose fails, may consider)	3–7 mg	0.1 mg kg^{-1}
Vasopressin	40 units	Not recommended
Amiodarone	300 mg	5 mg kg^{-1}
Lidocaine (lignocaine)	1.5 mg kg^{-1}	1 mg kg^{-1}
Atropine	1 mg	0.02 mg kg^{-1}
Sodium bicarbonate	1 mequiv kg^{-1}	1 mequiv kg^{-1}

Table 73.3 *Advanced cardiac life support drug doses*

very inconsistent during CPR. Studies have demonstrated that volumes of 5–10 mL need to be delivered to have reasonable uptake. It is likely that higher doses of the drugs need to be used via this route; currently, 2–2.5 times the intravenous dose is recommended. Studies conflict on whether deep injection is better than simple instillation in the tube.

Catecholamines and vasopressors

Mechanism of action

The only drugs generally accepted as being useful during CPR are the vasopressors.[68] Epinephrine has been used in resuscitation since the 1890s and has been the vasopressor of choice in modern CPR since the studies of Redding and Pearson in the 1960s.[69,70] The efficacy of epinephrine lies entirely in its α-adrenergic properties.[53] Peripheral vasoconstriction leads to an increase in aortic diastolic pressure, causing an increase in coronary perfusion pressure and myocardial blood flow. It is tempting to invoke the β-adrenergic properties of cardiac stimulation to explain the success of epinephrine. However, animal studies demonstrate that all strong vasopressors (α-adrenergic agonists and nonadrenergic vasoconstrictors) are equally successful in aiding resuscitation regardless of the β-adrenergic potency. β-Adrenergic agonists without α-activity are no better than placebo. α-Adrenergic blockade precludes resuscitation, whereas β-adrenergic blockade has no effect on the ability to restore spontaneous circulation. Although it is generally believed that the ability of epinephrine to increase the amplitude of ventricular fibrillation (a β-adrenergic effect) makes defibrillation easier, animal studies demonstrate that epinephrine does not improve the success of or decrease the energy necessary for defibrillation.[60,62] Furthermore, retrospective clinical studies have shown no effect of epinephrine on defibrillation success.[61] Because other drugs have not definitively been shown to be superior, epinephrine remains the vasopressor of choice in CPR. It should be administered whenever resuscitation has not occurred after adequate chest compressions and ventilation have been started and defibrillation attempted, if appropriate. Any other agent with strong vasopressor properties [phenylephrine, norepinephrine (noradrenaline), methoxamine, dopamine, vasopressin] is an acceptable alternative if epinephrine is unavailable.

When added to chest compressions, epinephrine helps develop the critical coronary perfusion pressure necessary to provide enough myocardial blood flow for restoration of spontaneous circulation. If invasive monitoring is present during CPR, adequacy of myocardial blood flow can be judged by the vascular pressures. If arterial diastolic pressure is less than 40 mmHg or coronary perfusion pressure is less than 20 mmHg, better chest compression technique and/or more vasoconstriction is needed. In the absence of such monitoring, the dose of epinephrine must be chosen empirically. The standard dose used for many years has been 1.0 mg intravenously or approximately 0.01–0.02 mg kg^{-1}.

In the 1980s, dose–response studies in swine suggested that doses of 0.1–0.2 mg kg^{-1} were necessary to improve hemodynamics to levels compatible with successful resuscitation,[71] leading to speculation that higher doses of epinephrine in human CPR might improve myocardial and cerebral perfusion and improve the success of resuscitation. There are several case reports and a series of children (with historical controls) that demonstrated return of spontaneous circulation when large doses (0.1–0.2 mg kg^{-1}) of epinephrine were given to patients in whom resuscitation with standard doses had failed.[72,73] Subsequently, in a swine cardiac arrest model, two randomized, blinded studies of standard and high-dose epinephrine found no difference in 24-h survival or neurologic status.[74,75] Clinically, initial or escalating high-dose epinephrine has occasionally improved return of spontaneous circulation (ROSC) and early survival. However, eight adult prospective randomized clinical studies involving over 9000 cardiac arrest patients have found no improvement in survival to hospital discharge or neurologic outcome, even in subgroups, when initial high-dose epinephrine is compared with standard doses.[76–83]

Additionally, the β-adrenergic effects of epinephrine are potentially deleterious during cardiac arrest. In the fibrillating heart, epinephrine increases oxygen consumption and decreases the endocardial–epicardial blood flow ratio, an effect not seen with methoxamine.[84] Myocardial lactate production in the fibrillating heart is unchanged after epinephrine administration during CPR, suggesting that the increased coronary blood flow does not improve the oxygen supply–demand ratio. Large doses of epinephrine increased death in swine early after resuscitation due to tachyarrhythmias and hypertension, an effect partially offset by metoprolol treatment.[74] Despite these theoretical considerations, survival and neurologic outcome studies have shown no difference when epinephrine is compared with a pure α-agonist (methoxamine or phenylephrine) during CPR in animals or humans,[85,86] and there was no evidence of worse outcome with high-dose epinephrine in the studies comparing standard and high doses in humans.[76–83]

High doses of epinephrine apparently are not needed as initial therapy for most cardiac arrests and the excessive adrenergic stimulation could be deleterious under some circumstances. The successful case reports of high-dose epinephrine were in patients with prolonged CPR and the high doses were given as "rescue" therapy when standard doses had failed. This may be the appropriate place for higher doses of epinephrine in CPR practice. Certainly, there is an extremely large individual variation in response to catecholamines administered during CPR. Current recommendations are to give 1 mg intravenously every 3–5 min in the adult. If this dose seems ineffective, higher doses (3–8 mg) should be considered.

Vasopressin

The newest addition to the pharmacologic armamentarium in CPR is arginine vasopressin. It is administered as an alternative to epinephrine in a dose of 40 units i.v. Vasopressin is a naturally occurring hormone (antidiuretic hormone) that, when administered in high doses, is a potent nonadrenergic vasoconstrictor, acting by stimulation of smooth muscle V_1-receptors. It is usually not recommended for conscious patients with coronary artery disease, because the increased peripheral vascular resistance may provoke angina. The half-life in the intact circulation is 10–20 min, and longer than epinephrine during CPR.

Animal studies have demonstrated that vasopressin is as effective or more effective than epinephrine in maintaining vital organ blood flow during CPR.[87-89] Repeated doses during prolonged CPR in swine were associated with significantly improved rates of neurologically intact survival compared with epinephrine and placebo.[90] Postresuscitation myocardial depression and splanchnic blood flow reduction are more marked with vasopressin than epinephrine, but they are transient and can be treated with low doses of dopamine.[91] Preliminary clinical studies indicate that vasopressin is as effective as epinephrine, but have not definitively shown it to be superior. A small randomized, blinded study comparing vasopressin and standard-dose epinephrine in 40 patients with out-of-hospital ventricular fibrillation found improved 24-h survival with vasopressin but no difference in ROSC or survival to hospital discharge.[92] A larger, clinical trial of 200 inpatients found no difference between the drugs in survival for 1 h or to hospital discharge (I Stiell, personal communication). In this study, response times were short, indicating that CPR outcome achieved with both vasopressin and epinephrine in short-term cardiac arrest may be similar. The hemodynamic effects of vasopressin, compared with epinephrine, are especially impressive during long cardiac arrests. Thus, vasopressin may find most use in CPR during prolonged resuscitation.

Amiodarone, lidocaine (lignocaine), and bretylium

After epinephrine, the most effective drugs during CPR are those used to suppress ectopic ventricular rhythms. Amiodarone, lidocaine, and bretylium are used during cardiac arrest to aid defibrillation when ventricular fibrillation is refractory to electrical countershock therapy or when fibrillation recurs following successful conversion. However, no antiarrhythmic agent has been shown superior to electrical defibrillation or more effective than placebo in the treatment of ventricular fibrillation. Consequently, defibrillation should not be withheld or delayed for drug therapy but should be applied at the earliest possible time when treating ventricular fibrillation.

Amiodarone is a pharmacologically complex drug with sodium, potassium, calcium, α- and β-adrenergic blocking properties that is useful for treatment of atrial and ventricular dysrhythmias. Amiodarone can cause hypotension and bradycardia when infused too rapidly, but less so than bretylium. This can usually be prevented by slowing the rate of drug infusion, or treated with fluids, vasopressors, chronotropic agents, or temporary pacing. There have been two randomized placebo-controlled clinical trials demonstrating improved admission alive to hospital with amiodarone treatment, although there was no difference in survival to discharge.[93,94] This is more evidence of efficacy than exists for lidocaine or bretylium, suggesting that amiodarone should now be first-line treatment for shock-resistant fibrillation. In cardiac arrest, amiodarone is initially administered as a 300-mg rapid infusion. Supplemental infusion of 150 mg can be repeated as necessary for recurrent or resistant dysrhythmias to a maximum daily dose of 2 g.

Lidocaine is primarily an antiectopic agent with few hemodynamic effects. It tends to reverse the reduction in ventricular fibrillation threshold caused by ischemia or infarction. It depresses automaticity by reducing the slope of phase 4 depolarization and reducing the heterogeneity of ventricular refractoriness. Lidocaine is an alternative to amiodarone when ventricular tachycardia or ventricular fibrillation has not responded to or has recurred following epinephrine and defibrillation. However, it has no proved short- or long-term efficacy in cardiac arrest. It has fewer immediate side-effects and is cheaper than amiodarone. To rapidly achieve and maintain therapeutic blood levels during CPR, relatively large doses are necessary. An initial bolus of 1.5 mg kg^{-1} should be given and additional boluses of 0.5–1.5 mg kg^{-1} can be given every 5–10 min during CPR, up to a total dose of 3 mg kg^{-1}. Only bolus dosing should be used during CPR, but an infusion of 2–4 mg min^{-1} can be started after successful resuscitation.

Bretylium has been called a primary antifibrillatory drug because it reduces the chances for re-entry to occur between ischemic and normal areas of myocardium. Similar to lidocaine, it reverses the reduction in fibrillation threshold caused by ischemia. Unlike lidocaine, bretylium has significant hemodynamic effects when administered intravenously. It causes the release of norepinephrine from adrenergic nerve endings. With a normal circulation, this results in tachycardia, hypertension, and increased contractility. After approximately 20 min, blockade of the uptake and release of norepinephrine from the nerve terminal begins, an effect that peaks 45–60 min after drug administration. This blockade can lead to profound hypotension. Although bretylium has some theoretical advantages over lidocaine for use during cardiac arrest, direct comparison of the drugs in clinical trials has found no differences in resuscitation success or survival.[95,96] The initial dose is 5 mg kg^{-1} by intravenous bolus. The dose can be increased to 10 mg kg^{-1} and repeated at 5-min intervals for a total dose of 30–35 mg kg^{-1}. Because of the side-effects, the availability of other agents, and the limited supply of the drug, bretylium has been removed from the most recent ACLS treatment algorithms.

Atropine

Atropine sulfate enhances sinus node automaticity and atrioventricular conduction by its vagolytic effects. Its primary use during cardiac arrest is when the ECG shows a pattern of asystole or slow idioventricular rhythm. Animal and human studies provide little evidence that atropine actually improves outcome from asystolic or bradysytolic arrest.[97,98] The predominant cause of asystole and pulseless electrical activity (PEA) is severe myocardial ischemia. Excessive parasympathetic tone probably contributes little to these rhythms during cardiac arrest in adults. Even in children, the significance of autonomic tone during arrest is doubtful. The most effective treatment for asystole or PEA is improvement in coronary perfusion and myocardial oxygenation with chest compressions, ventilation, and epinephrine. However, cardiac arrest with these rhythms has a very poor prognosis. As atropine has few adverse effects, it can be tried in arrest refractory to epinephrine and oxygenation. The recommended dose is 1.0 mg intravenously, repeated every 3–5 min up to a total of 0.04 mg kg^{-1}. Full vagolytic doses may be associated with fixed mydriasis following successful resuscitation confounding neurologic examination. Occasionally, a sinus tachycardia following resuscitation may be due to use of atropine during CPR.

Sodium bicarbonate

Although sodium bicarbonate was used commonly during CPR in the past, there is little evidence to support its efficacy. Current practice restricts its use primarily to arrests associated with hyperkalemia, severe pre-existing metabolic acidosis, and tricyclic antidepressant or phenobarbital overdose. It may be considered for use in protracted resuscitation attempts after other modalities have been instituted. The use of sodium bicarbonate during resuscitation has been based on the theoretical considerations that acidosis lowers fibrillation threshold and respiratory acidosis impairs the physiologic response to catecholamines. One early animal study found improved success of resuscitation from ventricular fibrillation when bicarbonate therapy was added to epinephrine.[70] Most subsequent studies have been unable to demonstrate improvement in success of defibrillation or resuscitation with the use of bicarbonate.[99-102] The observation that metabolic acidosis develops very slowly during CPR may explain the absence of effect of buffer therapy. Acidosis does not become severe for 15–20 min of cardiac arrest.[32,103,104]

Current recommendations for restricting sodium bicarbonate during CPR are based on the documented complications from excessive use. Metabolic alkalosis, hypernatremia, and hyperosmolarity are well documented after administration of bicarbonate during resuscitation.[104,105]

These abnormalities are associated with low resuscitation rates and poor survival. However, if sodium bicarbonate is given judiciously according to standard recommendations, no significant metabolic abnormalities should occur.[106] When bicarbonate is used during CPR, the usual dose is 1 mequiv kg^{-1} initially, with additional doses of 0.5 mequiv kg^{-1} every 10 min. However, dosing of sodium bicarbonate should be guided by blood gas determination, whenever possible.

Studies describing the physiology of CO_2 transport during CPR have focused interest on the effects of administering bicarbonate during resuscitation.[32,103] As discussed in the above section on physiology of gas transport during CPR, tissue acidosis during CPR is caused primarily by the low blood flow and accumulation of CO_2 in the tissues. Intravenous sodium bicarbonate combines with hydrogen ions to produce carbonic acid, which dissociates into CO_2 and water. The $P\text{CO}_2$ in blood is temporarily elevated until the excess CO_2 is eliminated through the lungs. Carbon dioxide readily diffuses across cell membranes and the blood–brain barrier, whereas bicarbonate diffuses much more slowly. Thus, it is possible that sodium bicarbonate administration could result in a paradoxical worsening of intracellular and cerebral acidosis by further raising intracellular and cerebral CO_2 without a balancing increase in bicarbonate. Direct evidence for this effect has not been found. One older study demonstrated an elevation in cerebrospinal fluid $P\text{CO}_2$ and reduction in pH when very large doses of bicarbonate were given.[107] A more recent study found no changes in spinal fluid acid–base status with clinically relevant doses.[108] Similarly, measurement of myocardial intracellular pH during bicarbonate administration did not detect a worsening acidosis.[109] Therefore, paradoxical acidosis from sodium bicarbonate remains a concern primarily on theoretical grounds.

Calcium salts

With normal cardiovascular physiology, calcium increases myocardial contractility and enhances ventricular automaticity. Consequently, it has been advocated for years as a treatment for asystole and PEA. An early report of success in four children following open-heart surgery[110] was bolstered by the animal studies of Redding and Pearson,[69] demonstrating moderate success with calcium chloride in asphyxial arrest. However, Redding's studies actually showed vasopressors to be more successful than calcium. More recent animal studies have not found calcium to improve resuscitation or electromechanical coupling. In 1981, Dembo questioned the efficacy of calcium in cardiac arrest and reported dangerously high serum calcium levels (up to 18.2 mg dL^{-1}) during CPR.[111] Subsequently, several retrospective studies and prospective clinical trials examined the efficacy of calcium during out-of-hospital human cardiac arrest.[112,113] Results showed that calcium was no better than placebo in promoting resuscitation and survival from asystole or PEA. Consequently, calcium may be helpful during cardiac resuscitation only if hyperkalemia, hypocalcemia, or calcium channel blocker toxicity is present. There are no other indications for its use during CPR. If calcium is administered, the chloride salt (2–4 mg kg^{-1}) is recommended because it produces higher and more consistent levels of ionized calcium than other salts.

DO NOT RESUSCITATE ORDERS

Over the past two decades, CPR has become the standard of medical care when an individual is found apparently dead. During the same time period, terminally ill patients have become increasing concerned about inappropriate application of life-sustaining procedures, including CPR. Consequently, do not attempt resuscitation (DNR) orders and other limitations of medical treatment have become more common. They are generally accepted, even welcomed, by healthcare workers. However, the operating room is the one area of the hospital where DNR orders continue to cause ethical conflicts between medical personnel and patients.[114,115]

The patient's right to limit medical treatment, including refusing CPR, is firmly established in modern medical practice based on the ethical principle of respect for patient autonomy. A terminally ill patient can reject heroic measures such as resuscitation and still choose palliative therapy. If a surgical intervention will ameliorate symptoms or cure a different problem and will improve the patient's quality of life, there is no reason why this treatment should be withheld. However, the same patient reasonably may desire to maintain the DNR status during surgery to avoid heroic measures that only prolong death. An operative intervention may increase the risk of cardiac arrest. Thus, this is the time that the DNR order provides the greatest protection against unwanted intervention. The patient may not want the burden of surviving resuscitation in worse condition than previously. In fact, he or she may view the possibility of death under anesthesia as especially peaceful.

Despite these rather strong arguments for treating a DNR status in the operating room the same way it is treated elsewhere in the hospital, most operating room personnel are, at least, a little uneasy caring for these patients. Many assume or require that DNR orders be suspended during the perioperative period. There are multiple reasons for the reluctance to accept DNR status during surgery and anesthesia. Many interventions commonly used in the operating room (mechanical ventilation, vasopressors, antiarrhythmics, blood products) may be considered forms of resuscitation in other situations. The only modalities that may not be considered routine are cardiac massage and defibrillation. Therefore, the specific interventions included in a DNR status must be clarified with specific allowance made for methods necessary to perform anesthesia and surgery. Many, but not all, cardiac arrests in the operating room are related to a surgical or anesthetic complication. In addition, resuscitation under these circumstances is highly successful.[1] Based on the ethical principle of nonmaleficence (*primum non nocere* – first, do no harm), surgeons and anesthesiologists have a tremendous sense of responsibility for what happens to patients in the operating room. Because this is an interventional procedure, the physicians are highly diligent in monitoring and managing changes in the patient's status. Honoring a DNR under these circumstances is frequently viewed as failure to treat a reversible process and, therefore, tantamount to killing. This can be an ethically sound view if the cause of arrest is readily identifiable, easily reversible, and treatment is likely to allow the patient to fulfill the objectives of coming to surgery.[114]

There are ethically sound arguments on both sides of the issue of whether DNR orders should be upheld in the operating room. For the individual patient, conflicts can usually be resolved by communication among the patient and caregivers. A mutual decision usually can be reached to suspend or severely limit a DNR order in the perioperative period if the patient understands (1) the special circumstances of perioperative arrest; (2) that interventions are brief and usually successful; and (3) that the physicians supports both the patient's goals in coming to surgery and the patient's values in desiring not to prolong death.

POSTRESUSCITATION CARE

The major factors contributing to mortality following successful resuscitation are progression of the primary disease and cerebral damage suffered as a result of the arrest. Active management following resuscitation appears to mitigate postischemic brain damage and improve neurologic outcome without increasing the number of patients surviving in a vegetative state.[116] When flow is restored following a period of global brain ischemia, three stages of cerebral reperfusion are seen in the ensuing

12 h. These are multifocal areas of the brain with no-reflow immediately following resuscitation. Global hyperemia occurs within 1 h followed quickly by prolonged global hypoperfusion.

Postresuscitation support is focused on providing stable oxygenation and hemodynamics in order to minimize any further cerebral insult. A comatose patient should be maintained on mechanical ventilation for several hours to ensure adequate oxygenation and ventilation. Restlessness, coughing, or seizure activity should be aggressively treated with appropriate medications including neuromuscular blockers, if necessary. Arterial Po_2 should be maintained above 100 mmHg (13.3 kPa) and moderate hypocapnia [P_aco_2 25–35 mmHg (3.3–4.7 kPa)] may be helpful. Blood volume should be maintained at normal levels and moderate hemodilution to a hematocrit of 30–35% may be helpful. A brief 5-min period of hypertension to mean arterial pressure of 120–140 mmHg (16–18.7 kPa) may help overcome the initial cerebral no-reflow. This frequently occurs secondary to the effects of epinephrine given during CPR. However, both prolonged hypertension [>110 mmHg (14.7 kPa)] and hypotension are associated with a worsened outcome. Hyperglycemia during cerebral ischemia is known to result in increased neurologic damage. Thus, it seems prudent to control glucose in the 100–300 mg dL^{-1} range.

In contrast with general supportive care, specific pharmacologic therapy directed at brain preservation has not been shown to have further benefit. Some animal trials of barbiturates were promising, but a large multicenter trial of thiopental found no improvement in neurologic status when this drug was given following cardiac arrest.[115] Similar results have been found with calcium channel blockers with no apparent improvement in human trials. Currently, there is no evidence that any specific pharmacologic agent will improve neurologic outcome following resuscitation from cardiac arrest.

As opposed to pharmacologic intervention, recent studies have demonstrated that therapeutic hypthermia in comatose survivors of cardiac arrest will improve survival and neurologic outcome.[117,118] It is now recommended that unconcious adult patients with spontaneous circulation after out-of-hospital cardiac arrest should be cooled to 32–34 °C for 12–24 h when the initial rhythm was ventricular fibrillation (VF). For any other rhythm, cardiac arrest in hospital, or pediatric patients such cooling may also be beneficial but specific evidence of efficacy does not currently exist.

REFERENCES

1. Olsson GI, Hallen B. Cardiac arrest during anaesthesia. A computer-aided study of 250 543 anaesthetics. *Acta Anaesthesiol Scand* 1988; **32:** 653–64.
2. Emergency Cardiac Care Committee and Subcommittees, American Heart Association. Guidelines 2000 for cardiopulmonary resuscitation and emergency cardiovascular care. International consensus on science. *Circulation* 2000; **102** (Suppl. I): I-1–I-370
3. Eisenberg MS, Bergner L, Hallstrom A. Cardiac resuscitation in the community. Importance of rapid provision and implications for program planning. *JAMA* 1979; **241:** 1905–7.
4. Weaver WD, Hill D, Fahrenbruch CE, *et al.* Use of the automatic external defibrillator in the management of out-of-hospital cardiac arrest. *N Engl J Med* 1988; **319:** 661–6.
5. Taffet BE, Teasdale TA, Luchi RJ. In-hospital cardiopulmonary resuscitation. *JAMA* 1988; **260:** 2069–72.
6. Harrison RR, Maull KI, Keenan RL, *et al.* Mouth-to-mask ventilation: a superior method of rescue breathing. *Ann Emerg Med* 1982; **11:** 74–6.
7. Hess D, Baran C. Ventilatory volumes using mouth-to-mouth, mouth-to-mask, and bag valve mask techniques. *Am J Emerg Med* 1985; **3:** 292–6.
8. Redding JS. The choking controversy: critique of evidence on the Heimlich maneuver. *Crit Care Med* 1979; **7:** 475–9.
9. Heimlich HJ. Pop goes the cafe coronary. *Emergency Med* 1974; **6:** 154–5.
10. Guildner CW, Williams D, Subtich T. Airway obstructed by foreign material: the Heimlich maneuver. *J Am Coll Emerg Physicians* 1976; **5:** 675–7.
11. Safar P, Escarraga LA, Elam JO. A comparison of the mouth-to-mouth and mouth-to-airway methods of artificial respiration with the chest-pressure arm-lift methods. *N Engl J Med* 1958; **258:** 671–7.
12. Safar P. Failure of manual respiration. *J Appl Physiol* 1959; **14:** 84–8.
13. Bossaert L, Van Hoeyweghen R. The Cerebral Resuscitation Study Group. Bystander cardiopulmonary resuscitation (CPR) in out-of-hospital cardiac arrest. *Resuscitation* 1989; **17** (Suppl.): S55–S69.
14. Van Hoeyweghen RJ, Bossaert LL, Mullie A, *et al.* Quality and efficiency of bystander CPR. *Resuscitation* 1993; **26:** 47–52.
15. Berg RA, Kern KB, Sanders AB, *et al.* Bystander cardiopulmonary resuscitation: Is ventilation necessary? *Circulation* 1993; **88:** 1907–15.
16. Berg RA, Wilcoxson D, Hilwig RW, *et al.* The need for ventilatory support during bystander cardiopulmonary resuscitation. *Ann Emerg Med* 1995; **26:** 342–50.
17. Berg RA, Kern KB, Hilwig RW, *et al.* Assisted ventilation does not improve outcome in a porcine model of single-rescuer bystander cardiopulmonary resuscitation. *Circulation* 1997; **95:** 1635–41.
18. Berg RA, Kern KB, Hilwig RW, *et al.* Assisted ventilation during 'bystander' CPR in a swine acute myocardial infarction model does not improve outcome. *Circulation* 1997; **96:** 4364–71.
19. Berg RA, Hilwig RW, Kern KB, *et al.* Simulated mouth-to-mouth ventilation and chest compressions ('bystander' CPR) improves outcome in a swine model of prehospital pediatric asphyxial cardiac arrest. *Crit Care Med* 1999; **27:** 1893–9.
20. Ornato JP, Hallagan LF, McMahan SB, *et al.* Attitudes of BCLS instructors about mouth-to-mouth resuscitation during the AIDS epidemic. *Ann Emerg Med* 1990; **19:** 151–6.
21. Brenner BE, Kauffman J. Reluctance of internists and medical nurses to perform mouth-to-mouth resuscitation. *Arch Intern Med* 1993; **153:** 1763–9.
22. Locke CJ, Berg RA, Sanders AB, *et al.* Bystander cardiopulmonary resuscitation: concerns about mouth-to-mouth contact. *Arch Intern Med* 1995; **155:** 938–43.
23. Mejicano GC, Maki DG. Infections acquired during cardiopulmonary resuscitation: estimating the risk and defining strategies for prevention. *Ann Intern Med* 1998; **129:** 813–18.
24. Melker RJ. Recommendation for ventilation during cardiopulmonary resuscitation: Time for change? *Crit Care Med* 1985; **13:** 882–3.
25. Kouwenhoven WB, Jude JR, Knickerbocker GG. Closed-chest cardiac massage. *JAMA* 1960; **173:** 1064–7.
26. Babbs CF. New versus old theories of blood flow during CPR. *Crit Care Med* 1980; **8:** 191–5.
27. Kern KB, Carter AB, Showen RL, *et al.* Twenty-four-hour survival in a canine model of cardiac arrest comparing three methods of manual cardiopulmonary resuscitation. *J Am Coll Cardiol* 1986; **7:** 859–67.
28. Kern KB, Carter AB, Showen RL, *et al.* Comparison of mechanical techniques of cardiopulmonary resuscitation: survival and neurologic outcome in dogs. *Am J Emerg Med* 1987; **5:** 190–5.
29. Criley JM, Blaufuss AH, Kissel GL. Cough-induced cardiac compression. Self-administered form of cardiopulmonary resuscitation. *JAMA* 1976; **236;** 1246–50.
30. Rudikoff MJ, Maughan WL, Effrom M, *et al.* Mechanisms of blood flow during cardiopulmonary resuscitation. *Circulation* 1980; **61:** 345–52.
31. Criley JM, Niemann JT, Rosborough JP, Hausknecht M. Modifications of cardiopulmonary resuscitation based on the cough. *Circulation* 1986; **74** (Suppl. IV): IV-42–IV-50.
32. Weil MH, Rackow EC, Trevino R, *et al.* Difference in acid–base state between venous and arterial blood during cardiopulmonary resuscitation. *N Engl J Med* 1986; **315:** 153–6.
33. Ewy GA. Alternative approaches to external chest compression. *Circulation* 1986; **74** (Suppl. IV): IV-98 - IV-101
34. Kirscher JP, Fine EG, Weisfeld ML, *et al.* Comparison of prehospital conventional and simultaneous compression-ventilation cardiopulmonary resuscitation. *Crit Care Med* 1989; **17:** 1263–9.
35. Maier GW, Newton JR, Wolfe JA, *et al.* The influence of manual chest compression rate of hemodynamic support during cardiac massage: high-impulse cardiopulmonary resuscitation. *Circulation* 1986; **74** (Suppl. IV): IV-51–IV-59.
36. Halperin HR, Tsitlik JE, Belfand M, *et al*: A preliminary study of cardiopulmonary resuscitation by circumferential compression of the chest with use of a pneumatic vest. *N Engl J Med* 1993; **329:** 762–6.
37. Babbs CF, Tacker WA. Cardiopulmonary resuscitation with interposed abdominal compression. *Circulation* 1986; **74** (Suppl. IV): IV-37–IV-41.
38. Mateer JF, Stueven HA, Thompson BM, *et al.* Pre-hospital IAC-CPR versus

standard CPR: paramedic resuscitation of cardiac arrests. *Am J Emerg Med* 1985; **3:** 143–6.

39. Sack JB, Kesselbrenner MB, Bregman D. Survival from in-hospital cardiac arrest with interposed abdominal counterpulsation during cardiopulmonary resuscitation. *JAMA* 1992; **267:** 379–85.
40. Cohen TJ, Tucker KJ, Lurie KG, *et al.* Active compression-decompression: a new method of cardiopulmonary resuscitation. *JAMA* 1992; **267:** 2916–23.
41. Cohen TJ, Goldner BG, Maccaro PC, *et al*: A comparison of active compression-decompression CPR for cardiac arrests occurring in the hospital. *N Engl J Med* 1993; **329:** 1918–21.
42. Lurie, KG, Shulta, JJ, Callaham, ML, *et al*: Evaluation of active compression-decompression CPR in victims of out-of-hospital cardiac arrest. *JAMA* 1994; **271:** 1405–11.
43. Schwab TM, Callaham ML, Madsen CD, *et al.* A randomized clinical trial of active compression-decompression CPR vs. standard CPR in out-of-hospital cardiac arrest in two cities. *JAMA* 1995; **273:** 1261–8.
44. Plaisance P, Lurie KG, Vicaut E, *et al.* A comparison of standard cardiopulmonary resuscitation and active compression-decompression resuscitation for out-of-hospital cardiac arrest. *N Engl J Med* 1999; **341:** 569–75.
45. Stiell IG, Herbert PC, Wells GA, *et al.* The Ontario trial of active compression-decompression cardiopulmonary resuscitation for in-hospital and prehospital cardiac arrest. *JAMA* 1996; **275:** 1417–23.
46. Lurie KG, Mulligan KA, McKnite S, *et al.* Optimizing standard cardiopulmonary resuscitation with an inspiratory impedance threshold valve. *Chest* 1998; **113:** 1084–90.
47. Tang W, Weil MH, Schock RB, *et al.* Phased chest and abdominal compression-decompression: a new option for cardiopulmonary resuscitation. *Circulation* 1997; **95:** 1335–40.
48. Sanders AB, Kern KB, Atlas M, *et al.* Importance of the duration of inadequate coronary perfusion pressure on resuscitation from cardiac arrest. *J Am Coll Cardiol* 1985; **6:** 113–18.
49. Kern KB, Sanders AB, Badylak SF, *et al.* Long term survival with open-chest cardiac massage after ineffective closed-chest compression in a canine preparation. *Circulation* 1987; **75:** 498–503.
50. Ralston SH, Voorhees WD, Babbs CF. Intrapulmonary epinephrine during prolonged CPR: improved regional blood flow and resuscitation in dogs. *Ann Emerg Med* 1984; **13:** 79–86.
51. Redding JS. Abdominal compression in cardiopulmonary resuscitation. *Anesth Analg* 1971; **50:** 668–75.
52. Sanders AB, Ewy GA, Taft TV. Prognostic and therapeutic importance of the aortic diastolic pressure in resuscitation from cardiac arrest. *Crit Care Med* 1984; **12:** 871–3.
53. Otto CW, Yakaitis RW. The role of epinephrine in CPR. A reappraisal. *Ann Emerg Med* 1984; **13:** 840–3.
54. Paradis NA, Martin GB, Rivers EP, *et al.* Coronary perfusion pressure and the return of spontaneous circulation in human cardiopulmonary resuscitation. *JAMA* 1990; **263:** 1106–13.
55. Sanders AB, Atlas M, Ewy GA, *et al.* Expired PCO_2 as an index of coronary perfusion pressure. *Am J Emerg Med* 1985; **3:** 147–9.
56. Sanders AB, Ewy GA, Bragg S, *et al.* Expired PCO_2 as a prognostic indicator of successful resuscitation from cardiac arrest. *Ann Emerg Med* 1985; **14:** 948–52.
57. Sanders AB, Kern KB, Otto CW, *et al.* End-tidal carbon dioxide monitoring during cardiopulmonary resuscitation. A prognostic indicator for survival. *JAMA* 1989; **262:** 1347–51.
58 Levine RL, Wayne MA, Miller CC: End-tidal carbon dioxide and outcome of out-of-hospital cardiac arrest. *N Engl J Med* 1997; **337:** 301–4.
59. Kern KB, Sanders AB, Raife J, *et al.* A study of chest compression rates during cardiopulmonary resuscitation in humans. The importance of rate-directed compressions. *Arch Intern Med* 1992; **152:** 145–9.
60. Yakaitis RW, Ewy GA, Otto CW, *et al.* Influence of time and therapy on ventricular defibrillation in dogs. *Crit Care Med* 1980; **8:** 157–63.
61. Weaver SC, Cobb LA, Dennis D, *et al.* Amplitude of ventricular fibrillation waveform and outcome after cardiac arrest. *Ann Intern Med* 1985; **102:** 53–5.
62. Otto CW, Yakaitis RW, Ewy GA. Effects of epinephrine on defibrillation in ischemic ventricular fibrillation. *Am J Emerg Med* 1985; **3:** 285–91.
63. Bardy GH, Marchlinski FE, Sharma AD, *et al.* Multicenter comparison of truncated biphasic shocks and standard damped sine wave monophasic shocks for transthoracic ventricular defibrillation. *Circulation* 1996; **94:** 2507–14.
64. Kerber RE, Grayzel J, Hoyt R, *et al.* Transthoracic resistance in human defibrillation. Influence of body weight, chest size, serial shocks, paddle size and paddle contact pressure. *Circulation* 1981; **63:** 676–82.
65. Lerman BB, DeMarco JP, Haines DE. Current-based versus energy-based ventricular defibrillation: a prospective study. *J Am Coll Cardiol* 1988; **12:** 1259–64.
66. Gutgesell HP, Tacker WA, Geddes La, *et al.* Energy dose for defibrillation in children. *Pediatrics* 1976; **58:** 898–901.
67. Weaver WD, Cobb LA, Copass MK, Hallstrom AP. Ventricular defibrillation-a comparative trial using 175-J and 320-J shocks. *N Engl J Med* 1982; **307:** 1101–6.
68. Otto CW. Cardiovascular pharmacology. II. The use of catecholamines, pressor agents, digitalis, and corticosteroids in CPR and emergency cardiac care. *Circulation* 1986; **74** (Suppl. IV): IV-80–IV-85.
69. Redding JS, Pearson JW. Evaluation of drugs for cardiac resuscitation. *Anesthesiology* 1963; **24:** 203–7.
70. Redding JS, Pearson JW. Resuscitation from ventricular fibrillation (drug therapy). *JAMA* 1968; **203:** 255–560.
71. Brown CG, Werman HA, Davis EA. The effects of graded doses of epinephrine on regional myocardial blood flow during cardiopulmonary resuscitation in swine. *Circulation* 1987; **75:** 491–7.
72. Koscove EM, Paradis NA. Successful resuscitation from cardiac arrest using high-dose epinephrine therapy: report of two cases. *JAMA* 1988; **259:** 3031–4.
73. Goetting MG, Paradis HA. High-dose epinephrine improves outcome from pediatric cardiac arrest. *Ann Emerg Med* 1991; **20:** 22–6.
74. Berg RA, Otto CW, Kern KB, *et al.* High dose epinephrine results in greater early mortality following resuscitation from prolonged cardiac arrest in pigs: a prospective randomized study. *Crit Care Med* 1994; **22:** 282–90.
75. Berg RA, Otto CW, Kern KB, *et al.* A randomized, blinded trial of high-dose epinephrine versus standard-dose epinephrine in a swine model of pediatric asphyxial cardiac arrest. *Crit Care Med* 1996; **24:** 1695–1700.
76. Linder KH, Ahnefeld FW, Prengel AW. Comparison of standard and high-dose adrenaline in the resuscitation of asystole and electromechanical dissociation. *Acta Anaesthesiol Scand* 1991; **35:** 253–6.
77. Stiell IB, Hebert PC, Weitzman BN, *et al.* High-dose epinephrine in adult cardiac arrest. *N Engl J Med* 1992; **327:** 1045–50.
78. Brown CG, Martin DP, Pepe PE, *et al.* A comparison of standard-dose and high-dose epinephrine in cardiac arrest outside the hospital. *N Engl J Med* 1992; **327:** 1051–55.
79. Callaham M, Madsen CD, Barton CW, *et al.* A randomized clinical trial of high-dose epinephrine and norepinephrine vs. standard-dose epinephrine in prehospital cardiac arrest. *JAMA* 1992; **268:** 2667–72.
80. Lipman J, Wilson W, Kobilski S, *et al.* High-dose adrenaline in adult in-hospital asystolic cardiopulmonary resuscitation: a double-blind randomized trial. *Anaesth Intensive Care* 1993; **21:** 192–196
81. Choux C, Gueugniaud PY, Barbieux A, *et al.* Standard doses versus repeated high doses of epinephrine in cardiac arrest outside the hospital. *Resuscitation* 1995; **29:** 3–9.
82. Sherman BW, Munger MA, Foulke GE, *et al.* High-dose versus standard-dose epinephrine treatment of cardiac arrest after failure of standard therapy. *Pharmacotherapy* 1997; **17:** 242–7.
83. Gueugniaud PY, Mols P, Goldstein P, *et al.* A comparison of repeated high doses and repeated standard doses of epinephrine for cardiac arrest outside the hospital. *N Engl J Med* 1998; **339:** 1595–1601.
84. Livesay JJ, Follette DM, Fey KH, *et al.* Optimizing myocardial supply/demand balance with alpha-adrenergic drugs during cardiopulmonary resuscitation. *J Thorac Cardiovasc Surg* 1978; **76:** 244–51.
85. Brillman JC, Sander AB, Otto CW, *et al.* A comparison of epinephrine and phenylephrine for resuscitation and neurologic outcome of cardiac arrest in dogs. *Ann Emerg Med* 1987; **16:** 11–17.
86. Silvast T, Saarnivaara L, Kinnunen A, *et al.* Comparison of adrenaline and phenylephrine in out-of-hospital CPR: a double-blind study. *Acta Anaesthesiol Scand* 1985; **29:** 610–13.
87. Lindner KH, Brinkmann A, Pfenninger EG, *et al.* Effect of vasopressin on hemodynamic variables, organ blood flow, and acid–base status in a pig model of cardiopulmonary resuscitation. *Anesth Analg* 1993; **77:** 427–33.
88. Lindner KH, Prengel AW, Pfenninger EG, *et al.* Vasopressin improves vital organ blood flow during closed-chest cardiopulmonary resuscitation in pigs. *Circulation* 1995; **91:** 215–21.
89. Wenzel V, Lindner KH, Krismer AC, *et al.* Repeated administration of vasopressin, but not epinephrine, maintains coronary perfusion pressure after early and late administration during cardiopulmonary resuscitation in pigs. *Circulation* 1999; **99:** 1379–85.
90. Wenzel V, Lindner KH, Krismer AC, *et al.* Survival with full neurologic recovery and no cerebral pathology after prolonged resuscitation in pigs. *J Am Coll Cardiol* 2000; **35:** 527–31.
91. Prengel AW, Lindner KH, Keller A, Lurie KG. Cardiovascular function during the postresuscitation phase after cardiac arrest in pigs: a com-

parison of epinephrine versus vasopressin. *Crit Care Med* 1996; **24:** 2014–19.

92. Lindner KH, Dirks B, Strohmenger HU, *et al.* Randomized comparison of epinephrine and vasopressin in patients with out-of hospital ventricular fibrillation. *Lancet* 1997; **349:** 535–37.
93. Kudenchuk PJ, Cobb LA, Copass MK, *et al.* Amiodarone for resuscitation after out of hospital cardiac arrest due to ventricular fibrillation. *N Engl J Med* 1999; **341:** 871–6.
94. Dorian P, Cass D, Schwarz B, *et al.* Amiodarone as compared with lidocaine for shock-resistant ventricular fibrillation. *N Engl J Med* 2002; **346:** 884.
95. Haynes RE, Chinn TL, Copass MK, Cobb LA. Comparison of bretylium tosylate and lidocaine in management of out of hospital ventricular fibrillation: a randomized clinical trial. *Am J Cardiol* 1981; **48:** 353–6.
96. Olson DW, Thompson BM, Darin JC, Milbrath MH. A randomized comparison study of bretylium tosylate and lidocaine in resuscitation of patients from out-of-hospital ventricular fibrillation in a paramedic system. *Ann Emerg Med* 1984; **13:** 807–10.
97. Coon GA, Clinton JE, Ruiz E. Use of atropine for brady-asystolic prehospital cardiac arrest. *Ann Emerg Med* 1981; **10:** 462–7.
98. Stueven HA, Tonsfeldt DJ, Thompson BM, *et al.* Atropine in asystole: human studies. *Ann Emerg Med* 1984; **13:** 815–17.
99. Minuck M, Sharma GP. Comparison of THAM and sodium bicarbonate in resuscitation of the heart after ventricular fibrillation in dogs. *Anesth Analg* 1977; **56:** 38–45.
100. Guerci AD, Chandra N, Johnson E, *et al.* Failure of sodium bicarbonate to improve resuscitation from ventricular fibrillation in dogs. *Circulation* 1986; **74** (Suppl. IV): IV-75–IV-79.
101. Federiuk CS, Sanders AB, Kern KB, *et al.* The effect of bicarbonate on resuscitation from cardiac arrest. *Ann Emerg Med* 1991; **20:** 1173–7.
102. Vukmir RB, Bircher NG, Radovsky A, Safar, P. Sodium bicarbonate may improve outcome in dogs with brief or prolonged cardiac arrest. *Crit Care Med* 1995; **23:** 515–19.
103. Weil MH, Grundler W, Yamaguchi M, *et al.* Arterial blood gases fail to reflect acid–base status during cardiopulmonary resuscitation. a preliminary report. *Crit Care Med* 1985; **13:** 884–5.
104. Bishop RL, Weisfeldt ML. Sodium bicarbonate administration during cardiac arrest. Effect on arterial pH, Pco_2, and osmolality. *JAMA* 1976; **235:** 506–9.
105. Mattar JA, Weil MH, Shubin H, *et al.* Cardiac arrest in the critically ill. II. Hyperosmolal states following cardiac arrest. *Am J Med* 1974; **56:** 162–8.
106. White BC, Tintinalli JE. Effects of sodium bicarbonate administration during cardiopulmonary resuscitation. *JACEP* 1977; **6:** 187–190.
107. Berenyi KG, Wolk M, Killip T. Cerebrospinal fluid acidosis complicating therapy of experimental cardiopulmonary resuscitation. *Circulation* 1975; **52:** 319–324.
108. Sanders AB, Otto CW, Kern KB, *et al.* Acid–base balance in a canine model of cardiac arrest. *Ann Emerg Med* 1988; **17:** 667–71.
109. Kette F, Weil MH, von Planta M, *et al.* Buffer agents do not reverse intramyocardial acidosis during cardiac resuscitation. *Circulation* 1990; **81:** 1660–6.
110. Kay JH, Blalock A. The use of calcium chloride in the treatment of cardiac arrest in patients. *Surg Gynecol Obstet* 1951; **93:** 97–102.
111. Dembo DH. Calcium in advanced life support. *Crit Care Med* 1981; **9:** 358–9.
112. Stueven HA, Thompson BM, Aprahamian C, *et al.* Calcium chloride: reassessment of use in asystole. *Ann Emerg Med* 1984; **13:** 820–2.
113. Stueven HA, Thompson BM, Aprahamian C, *et al.* The effectiveness of calcium chloride in refractory electromechanical dissociation. *Ann Emerg Med* 1985; **14:** 626–9.
114. Cohen CB, Cohen PJ. Do-not-resuscitate orders in the operating room. *N Engl J Med* 1991; **325:** 1879–82.
115. Walker RM. DNR in the OR. Resuscitation as an operative risk. *JAMA* 1991; **266:** 2407–12.
116. Abramson NS, Safar P, Detre KM, *et al.* Randomized clinical study of cardiopulmonary-cerebral resuscitation: thiopental loading in comatose cardiac arrest survivors. *N Engl J Med* 1986; **314:** 397–403.
117. Bernard SA, Gray TW, Buist MD, *et al.* Treatment of comatose survivors of out-of-hospital cardiac arrest with induced hypothermia. *N Engl J Med* 2002; **346:** 557–63.
118. The Hypothermia after Cardiac Arrest Study Group. Mild therapeutic hypothermia to improve neurologic outcome after cardiac arrest. *N Engl J Med* 2002; **346:** 549–56

74

Acute postoperative pain

DAVID JAMES AND DOUGLAS JUSTINS

INCIDENCE

Pain is a common human experience, a symptom frequently encountered in clinical practice that is usually associated with actual or impending tissue damage.[1] Pain is a consistent and predominant complaint of most individuals following most surgical interventions. "Failure to relieve pain is morally and ethically unacceptable."[2] Adequate pain relief could be considered a basic human right.

The true enormity of the problem can only be surmised, as epidemiological data are lacking. Clinical surveys dating back to the 1950s suggest that there is an on-going silent pandemic of poorly managed acute postoperative pain, with up to 75% of patients describing their pain as moderate to severe in these circumstances.[3] This scourge similarly affects the UK,[4] where:[5]

> … a visit to most postoperative wards will show the time-honoured ritual of inadequate postoperative pain management. Patients expect ineffective postoperative pain relief, and their carers ensure that they are not disappointed.

These disadvantaged patients are often unable to breathe adequately, cough effectively, move enough even to tend to their own daily needs or participate in their own rehabilitation, and experience feelings of helplessness, fear, anxiety, low mood, and loss of control.[6] The causes of this failure are multiple, systemic, and complex; the low-priority status afforded to postoperative pain transcends all strata of healthcare systems, ultimately reflecting poor understanding of the subject. Healthcarers prefer to ignore the problem, abdicate responsibility, or rely on outdated and often misguided beliefs, myths, traditions, dogma, anecdote, and prejudice. These past failures have prompted various professional and governmental bodies to address this issue.[7] It is our belief that healthcarers have, first and foremost, a moral and ethical obligation to help all patients manage their pain adequately, which may lead to better "outcomes" for both the patient and the healthcare system.

Acute postoperative pain does not discriminate on the basis of gender or age: children appear to fare little better than adults,[8,9] and the extent of the problem in other clinical arenas, e.g. trauma, medicine, and general practice, can only be imagined.

DEFINITION

Pain is not a straightforward sensory "perception" (biological process); pain is an "experience," as the physiological sensation is inseparable from the associated emotional distress. Thus, pain is always a neuropsychological phenomenon that has an unpleasant intrusive nature; is associated with threat of or actual tissue damage; and disrupts normal physiological and psychological homeostasis, manifesting clinically as organ dysfunction and altered human behavior. Pain is best defined as "an unpleasant sensory and emotional experience associated with actual or potential tissue damage, or described in terms of such damage."[10] This definition emphasizes that the experience of pain has two inseparable elements processed in parallel by the nervous system, i.e. sensory (nociception) and affective (emotional), and that pain can be experienced without discernible physical cause, i.e. injury or disease. Pain is always a subjective experience; individuals learn the application of the word through experiences related to injury in early life. "Pain behaviors" describe how an individual in pain interacts with his or her immediate environment. Typically, this might involve a range of actions such as talking about pain, moaning, grimacing, limping, taking analgesics, going to the doctor, collecting compensation, etc. Pain must not be confused with suffering; the latter is a state of emotional distress associated with events that threaten the biological and/or psychosocial integrity of the individual. Suffering often accompanies severe pain but can occur in its absence.[11]

ETIOLOGY

The long-held notion that pain encountered clinically is "perceived" in direct proportion to the stimulus intensity is outdated. This is based on an anatomical model of pain, in which noxious impulses are conducted along fixed neural pathways (so-called "hard-wired") from source to consciousness. We now accept that no such linear relation exists, which is reflected by our poor ability to predict the severity and course of the acute postoperative pain experienced by individual patients. The nature of the surgery,[12] and to a lesser extent the surgical technique,[13] do offer us some predictive ability to this end.[14–16] However, the great variability of individuals' complaint of pain, pain behaviors, and response to pain management strategies, even in identical clinical circumstances, reflects the multidimensional nature of the pain experience, with variable contributions made by physiological, psychological, social/environmental, and pharmacological factors (Table 74.1 and Fig. 74.1). The contribution made by age to the complaint of pain is unclear, but the postoperative opioid requirements of adult patients appears to decrease with age.[17]

Table 74.1 *Factors affecting variability of clinical pain complaint, behaviors, and response to management*

Biological factors
The flow of nociceptive impulses is dynamic or modifiable by:
- Sensitization of peripheral and central nociceptors in response to prolonged or excessive noxious stimuli, so "amplifying" the response characteristics of the system to subsequent noxious stimuli
- Modulation or "dampening" of nociceptors at various points along their passage to consciousness
- Eliciting local and general motor and autonomic reflexes

Psychological factors
- Affective: the intrinsic emotional response to a noxious stimulus is influenced by pre-existing affective dysfunction and personality traits
- Cognitive: understanding the nature, cause, purpose, and consequences of the pain, together with learned influences (coping style, previous pain experiences and culture)

Social/environmental factors
The gain derived from an individual's interactions with family, work, community, and healthcarers, together with the immediate context (battlefield or lonely cold bed)

Pharmacological factors
Pharmacokinetic and pharmacodynamic variability

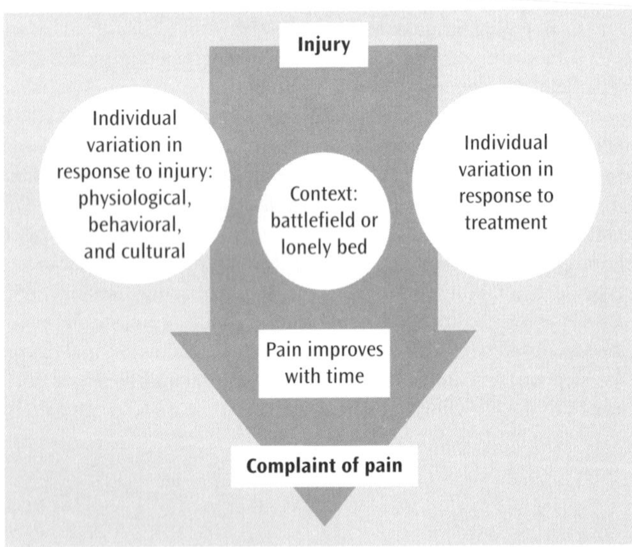

Figure 74.1 *Factors influencing the pain reported by patients. (From McQuay* et al.[85] *with permission.)*

CLASSIFICATIONS

We make no attempt to outline the detailed pathophysiology of pain and nociception in the following sections. We describe only some integrated aspects of nociception; reference to standard texts is recommended.[18–20]

Physiological and clinical pain

Physiological pain

Minimal tissue injury (a brief noxious stimulus) such as a pinprick *activates* high-threshold nociceptors (Aδ- and C-fibers), which convey this information to the first relay in the spinal cord. Second-order neurons then project rostrally, principally via the spinothalamic and spinoreticular tracts. The magnitude of the nerve impulses may be modulated at points along its pathway. This is simple neural processing and has little to do with the pain experienced clinically; it is probably an alerting mechanism. There is good correlation between nociceptor discharges and the pain experienced.

Clinical pain

Greater tissue injury (more severe or prolonged noxious stimulus) *activates* the same high-threshold nociceptors while the local tissue inflammatory response *sensitizes* these same nociceptors, increasing their sensitivity to stimulation (peripheral sensitization). The increasing nociceptive "traffic" entering the spinal cord increases the sensitivity of the central components of the nociceptors (central sensitization).[21,22] Clinical pain is conveniently classified as nociceptive or neuropathic.

Nociceptive pain

Nociceptive pain represents normal neural processing (nociceptor activation and sensitization) in response to tissue injury and associated inflammatory response, e.g. surgical trauma. Clinically, this process is manifested as primary and secondary hyperalgesia and allodynia. There is poor correlation between nociceptor discharges and pain perception.[23] Hyperalgesia and allodynia may have a protective function, limiting stimulation of the injured area and thereby assisting the healing process.[24] They also demonstrate that nociception is a dynamic process, the intensity of which depends on the "past history" of the injury site and not just the magnitude of the current stimulus. Furthermore, the allodynia associated with secondary hyperalgesia demonstrates that pain can be produced in normal subjects by the activation of low-threshold mechanoreceptors, albeit in the context of a previous injury in this instance.

Neuropathic pain

Neuropathic pain represents an abnormal pain state with dysfunctional neural processing secondary to peripheral and/or central neural damage. This damage may be a direct physical insult that damages the structure of the nociceptors, e.g. cutting a nerve, or caused by alterations in the structure and function of the nociceptors secondary to a prolonged and intense barrage of neural activity. The pain can be spontaneous, triggered by innocuous stimuli, or an exaggerated response to minor noxious stimuli. There is no correlation between injury and pain perceived and pain may differ significantly in character between patients. Psychological, socioenvironmental and possibly genetic elements may then operate to maintain the painful state.

Somatic and visceral pain

Features typical of somatic and visceral pain are outlined in Table 74.2. Visceral nociceptors travel to the spinal cord by way of the sympathetic chain with considerable overlap from various organs as the fibers converge, explaining many diagnostic errors that occur in relation to visceral pain. There is also convergence of visceral and somatic nociceptors at the spinal cord level, explaining why visceral pain is often referred to cutaneous areas and initiates viscerosomatic and somaticovisceral reflexes. Peripheral and central sensitization may be a feature common to both somatic and visceral structures.

Acute and chronic

Acute pain is pain of recent onset and probable limited duration; it usually has an identifiable temporal and causal relation with injury or disease. This is distinct to chronic pain, which is pain that persists for longer periods of time, often beyond the time it takes for an injury to

Table 74.2 *Characteristics of somatic and visceral pain*

Somatic pain
- Arises from skin and deep somatic structures (muscles, bones, etc.)
- Well localized
- Sharp
- Often constant (sometimes periodic)

Visceral pain
- Cannot be evoked from all viscera
- Poorly localized
- Dull and vague
- May be colicky, cramping, squeezing
- Referred often to somatic areas

heal, frequently there may not be any clearly identifiable cause.[1] Pain that recurs often as part of a disease process e.g. rheumatoid arthritis is usually classified as chronic pain.

PHYSIOLOGICAL AND PSYCHOLOGICAL EFFECTS OF ACUTE INJURY

From a young age everybody learns to associate pain with injury; individuals' normal response to injury is, initially, to remove themselves from harm's way and then to protect the injured area while healing occurs. This "injury response" manifests clinically as altered organ functions and behaviors and may benefit the individual's short-term survival,[25] but if prolonged may slow or even prevent recovery.[26] Surgery causes tissue injury; generally, the more radical surgery, the greater the tissue injury.[27] Biological systems are largely unable to distinguish the cause of the tissue injury, eliciting broadly similar physiological and psychological responses.[28] Surgery is "controlled" tissue injury which, nevertheless, results in alteration in organ functions and behaviors. Although safe and effective postoperative pain relief is principally provided for humanitarian reasons, it may be possible to reduce organ dysfunctions and improve postoperative patient outcome by reducing the physiological and psychological responses to tissue injury (Table 74.3).[29]

Physiological effects

Cardiovascular

Severe acute pain increases heart rate, blood pressure, systemic and coronary vascular resistances, and cardiac output, mediated by the sympathetic nervous system. Cardiac work and myocardial oxygen consumption increase, while myocardial oxygen delivery decreases. The imbalance of myocardial oxygen supply and demand may result in myocardial ischemia, infarction, and failure, a situation made worse by coexistent hypoxemia, coronary artery disease, and anxiety. These adverse effects may be reduced by epidural blockade of the cardiac sympathetic fibers (T1 to T5) with local anesthetic.[30–33] Clinical evidence that epidural blockade reduces the risk of adverse cardiac outcomes in "high-risk" surgical patients is controversial,[34,35] although myocardial ischemia has been noted on cessation of epidural analgesia in this group of patients.[36] Thoracic epidural blockade has, however, been shown to improve the myocardial oxygen supply, reducing myocardial ischemia, in both animal models[37,38] and clinically,[39] and has been associated with improved indices of myocardial function in patients with unstable angina.[40–44] It is unknown if epidural blockade is able to influence the incidence of adverse cardiovascular outcome in the longer term, e.g. by beta-adrenoreceptor blockade with atenolol.[45]

Table 74.3 *Biological responses to tissue injury*

Hyperalgesia and allodynia
Catabolism
Sympathetic stimulation
Hypercoagulability
Immunosuppression
Organ systems dysfunction
Psychological dysfunction

Respiratory

The pain associated with chest and abdominal surgery can cause significant postoperative respiratory dysfunction. Involuntary spinal reflexes cause increased skeletal muscle tone around the injury site. The effects of this "muscle splinting" are made worse by voluntary reductions in thoracic and abdominal respiratory muscle excursions, which, coupled with diaphragmatic dysfunction, cause reductions in lung volumes (tidal volumes, vital capacity, functional residual capacity) with regional lung collapse (atelectasis) and reduced alveolar ventilation, culminating in hypoxemia and hypercapnia. Likewise, the patient's ability to cough is reduced, secretions are retained, and chest infection may ensue.[46] The increasing respiratory rate, in an attempt to maintain normal gas exchange, significantly increases metabolic rate with consequent increased requirement for oxygen and metabolic substrates; hyoxemia is made worse and respiratory muscle fatigue supervenes. The vicious circle accelerates the patient toward respiratory failure. Poorly managed severe acute pain following peripheral surgery that renders the patient immobile is also associated with significant respiratory dysfunction and infective complications (hypostatic pneumonia), initially affecting the lung bases.[47] A recent meta-analysis of randomized controlled trials found that, compared with conventional analgesic delivery, epidural opioid analgesia produced clinically significant beneficial effects on arterial oxygen saturation and on the incidence of atelectasis.[48] Epidural blockade with local anesthetics has the potential to improve pulmonary function, but at present confirmatory data are insufficient to draw this conclusion.

Thromboembolic

Epidural blockade may reduce the incidence of both vascular graft occlusion after peripheral arterial surgery[35,49] and deep venous thrombosis and pulmonary embolism following hip surgery.[50] These effects may be related to improved arterial and venous lower limb blood flow,[51] changes in blood coagulability, fibrinolysis, and earlier postoperative patient mobilization. The systemic absorption of local anesthetic agents used for neural blockade may itself have an antithrombotic effect.[52]

Gastrointestinal and genitourinary

Sympathetic activity associated with severe pain may increase intestinal secretions and smooth muscle sphincter tone and decrease gastrointestinal motility (gastric stasis and paralytic ileus). Opioids may contribute significantly to gastric stasis,[53] while epidural blockade may significantly reduce gut transit time,[54] notably when using local anesthetic agents but not epidural opioid.[55–60] Ileus is a major problem postoperatively and may delay surgical recovery and hospital discharge. Early enteral feeding has been shown to reduce the surgical stress response, reduce postoperative septic complications, and improve wound healing.[60] Maximum benefit is likely to be gained if epidural blockade with local anesthetic is continued for several days postoperatively and opioid dose minimized by using a multimodal analgesic regimen. Interestingly, intravenous lidocaine (lignocaine) appears to speed the return of bowel function after radical prostatectomy, as well as reducing pain and shortening hospital stay.[53] Sympathetic activity increases bladder sphincter tone and possibly urinary retention; unfortunately, opioids have the same effect. We could find no evidence that pain is associated with reductions in renal and hepatic blood flow.

Neuroendocrine and metabolic

Along with sympathetic nervous system stimulation,[61] tissue injury leads to a metabolic response due to the increased secretion of catabolic hormones and decreased secretion or action of anabolic hormones and cytokines (Table 74.4). A transient hypometabolic phase ("ebb phase") occurs initially, characterized by reduced metabolic rate. This is followed by a hypermetabolic phase ("flow phase") characterized by elevated metabolic rate (with consequent increases in oxygen consumption and cardiac output) and catabolism. The latter causes a negative nitrogen balance due to loss of muscle protein.[62,63] The "flow phase" may last from days to weeks depending on not just the magnitude of the surgery, but the occurrence of complications such as infection, blood loss, tissue hypoxia and acidosis, hypothermia, pre-existing protein–calorie deficits, and anxiety.

It has been suggested that epidural block with local anesthetic agents is the most effective way of reducing the metabolic response to surgery and postoperative morbidity and mortality, and increasing speed of recovery.[59,64–68]). The reduced metabolic response, using this technique, is more pronounced following lower abdomen and lower limb procedures than following upper abdominal and thoracic procedures, possibly because of our inability to completely block afferent neural impulses in the latter case. To gain the maximum effect, in this context, the epidural block probably needs it to be maintained for at least 48–72 h postoperatively.[25,59,65] Neuraxial opioids used alone appear to be less efficient in reducing the metabolic response.[59] Conventional systemic analgesia, with the exception of high-dose opioids, has little or no modifying influence on the metabolic response to surgery.

Immunological

Surgical injury is known to be associated with immune dysfunction and expression of acute-phase proteins. Neural blockade appears to exert a slight influence on immunocompetence, although the mechanisms involved are unclear. Immune system dysfunction may increase the occurrence of infective complications and tumor recurrence.[69]

Table 74.4 *The endocrine and metabolic response to tissue injury*

Endocrine

- Catabolic due to rises in adrenal corticotrophic hormone (ACTH), cortisol, antidiuretic hormone (ADH), growth hormone, catecholamines, renin, angiotensin II, aldosterone, glucagon, interleukin 1 (IL-1)
- Anabolic due to decreases in insulin, testosterone

Metabolic

- Carbohydrate (hyperglycemia, glucose intolerance, insulin resistance) due to:
  - Increases in hepatic glycogenolysis (catecholamines and glucagon) and gluconeogenesis (cortisol, glucagon, growth hormone catecholamines, free fatty acids)
  - Decreases in insulin secretion/effect
- Protein (muscle protein catabolism and synthesis of acute-phase proteins) due to increased cortisol, catecholamines, glucagon, IL-1
- Fat (increased lipolysis and oxidation) due to increased catecholamines, cortisol, glucagon, growth hormone

Water and electrolyte balance

Retention of sodium and water, excretion of potassium, increased transcellular fluid due to increases in catecholamines, aldosterone, ADH, cortisol, angiotensin II

Persistent postoperative pain

Neuropathic pain as a cause of acute postoperative pain is frequently overlooked and often untreated.[70,71] This pain may persist long after apparent tissue healing and present as an array of clinical syndromes[72] which broadly divide into neuralgias, complex regional pain syndromes, and deafferentation syndromes. It may be possible to reduce the incidence of the persistent pains that are associated with the deliberate transection of large nerves that occurs when limbs are amputated.[73] More commonly, surgical incisions are invariably associated with damage to smaller peripheral nerves, the damage ranging from neuropraxia to complete nerve transection. The pathophysiological basis for developing persistent pain in these circumstances is covered in standard texts. Many and varied types of surgical interventions have been associated with persistent pain that can be long-lasting, severe, and debilitating for the sufferer, difficult to manage, and consume considerable healthcare resources. Notorious procedures include lateral thoracotomy,[74] cholecystectomy, nephrectomy, radical mastectomy, varicose vein stripping, inguinal herniorrhaphy, episiotomy, upper limb and facial procedures. Predisposing patient factors may include genetics, middle and old age, and pre-existing pain.[73,75]

Psychological responses[76,77]

Adverse psychological effects may not be in sharp focus in the postoperative period but are nonetheless harmful and may have physiological consequences. Acute severe pain causes changes in several ways.

Behavior

Typical behavioral responses include self-absorption and concern, withdrawal from interpersonal contact, increased sensitivity to all external stimuli, grimacing, posturing, reduced activity, moaning, and seeking help and attention. Extremes of behavior can occur in response to social/environmental factors, often for some "gain" from family, work, community, and healthcare systems.

Affect

Initially, feelings of fear (exacerbated by uncertainty, inappropriate beliefs, and expectations) and anxiety predominate, followed by feelings of helplessness, loss of control, and depression if the pain remains unrelieved. Anger and resentment may supervene if it is believed that pain relief is being withheld. These effects are exacerbated by the sleep deprivation that accompanies unrelieved severe acute pain. This state may also unmask premorbid tendencies for anxiety, hostility, depression, or preoccupation with health and occasionally provoke an acute psychotic reaction.

CLINICAL ASSESSMENT OF ACUTE PAIN

We know pain to be a uniquely personal symptom with no reliable objective signs, so we have to accept individuals' "self-report" of the severity of the pain they are experiencing. While pain may cause observable nonverbal behavioral changes,[78] we should strenuously resist the temptation of using these signs to estimate the severity of individual's pain, as clinical staff tend to overestimate low and underestimate high levels of the pain indicated by patients.[79] The terms "pain threshold" and "pain tolerance" should also not be confused; the former is used in laboratory experiments and is the level at which 50% of stimuli are recognized as painful and is defined in terms of the stimulus, not the pain, which limits its clinical application. The latter is the greatest level of pain a subject is prepared to tolerate; it is the subjective experience of the individual and is a better clinical tool. Accepting the self-reported pain score allows reliable *within-patient* comparisons but not *between-patient* comparisons of both pain severity and any response to pain management interventions. A variety of "self-reporting" pain severity scoring systems are used for adults (Table 74.5); they correlate well and are generally reliable.[80] These methods are easily adapted to estimate other aspects of pain management, e.g. pain relief score or expectations and experiences. It is important that patients understand the method used, what is being assessed, and why, and that the same method continues to be used to ensure reliability and avoid confusion.

Postoperative acute pain severity should be "scored" and recorded both at rest and on movement at regular intervals (Table 74.6). The frequency of assessments should depend on clinical circumstances (Table 74.7), increasing in frequency when pain is poorly managed or management is escalating. Pain severity scores cannot be viewed in isolation: they must be considered and recorded along with a sedation score (Table 74.8) and the traditional ward observations of temperature, pulse rate, blood pressure, and respiratory rate. These six observations constitute a minimum data set that should be recorded contemporaneously on a single bedside chart. Recording acute postoperative pain is, itself, the most likely way to improve the safety and effectiveness of acute pain management in individual patients.[15,81,82] This approach has to be adopted when sophisticated and invasive techniques are employed, such as epidural infusions and intravenous patient-controlled analgesia (PCA) techniques, where the risks of adverse effects are highest.[83] It needs to be emphasized that patients should have realistic expectations of what pain relief they can expect; it not generally possible, or indeed desirable, to "remove" pain entirely. The aim of pain management is to help patients tolerate their pain, i.e. to remove the associated suffering. Unexpected increases in pain severity postoperatively may herald the onset of complication, e.g. peritonitis, compartment syndromes, or neuropathic pain, so a detailed clinical assessment should be undertaken in all patients with escalating pain severity to identify the cause and direct subsequent management.

The above methods of pain assessment have to be adapted for patients with special needs, e.g. children and hearing-impaired and cognitively impaired patients. Pain severity scales for children are available,[84] while scales need to be modified for patients whose educational or cultural background differs from that of their carer or who do not have English as their first language.

MANAGEMENT OF ACUTE POSTOPERATIVE PAIN

The goal of postoperative pain management is to reduce an individual patient's pain to a tolerable level with minimal or no associated suffering or distress. Postoperative pain management relies heavily on pharmacological interventions, but acute postoperative pain management should also utilize the beneficial effects of physical and psychological interventions to provide a "package" of care."[85] Care has to exercised when using "alternative" or "complementary" interventions given the paucity of available evidence on safety and effectiveness, but any "relaxation" technique (e.g. aromatherapy, reflexology) that a patient has confidence in should be encouraged. The rational approach to the management of acute postoperative pain, like all medical interventions, is to use the highest quality evidence available.[85] We have attempted to use only the highest levels of evidence available, where such evidence is available. The relative strengths of different types of primary study used to make decisions about clinical interventions have be classified in rank order[86] and subsequently modified[87] (Table 74.9). A number of evidence-based resources on pain topics have recently been published,[87,88] and a

Table 74.5 *Simple pain scoring systems*

Categorical rating scales (CRS)
Frequently used to assess postoperative pain because it is a widely applicable verbal method that can employ different descriptors of pain, e.g. no pain, mild pain, moderate pain, severe pain

Visual analog scale (VAS)
Employs a 10-cm drawn line with the left anchor point descriptor labeled "no pain" and the right-sided equivalent labeled "worst possible pain" (Fig. 74.2). It requires patients to mark their current pain severity on the continuum. The VAS score is the measured distance from the "no pain" point to the pain estimate

Verbal numerical rating scale (VNRS)
Asks patients to estimate their pain severity as a number, "0" being no pain and "10" being the worst possible pain

Table 74.6 *Simple method of scoring acute pain*

Believe the patient about the severity of the pain he or she is experiencing

Avoid interpreting the severity of a patient's pain unless he or she is unable to give a subjective report. In this case, an estimate of the pain severity can be made by observing the patient at rest and when moving or moved

Sleep is a desirable event. It is not necessary to wake a patient to assess pain score provided that staff are "satisfied" with the patient's continuing condition, If doubt exists, gently disturb the patient and assess the response

Score the pain by asking the patient to estimate the pain at rest and during deep breathing or on performing a standard movement as either:
0 = none
1 = mild
2 = moderate
3 = severe
Record this score

Table 74.7 *Minimum assessment intervals*

5-min intervals following:
- Bolus injections of i.v. opioids or epidural local anesthetics with or without opioid
- Increasing rates of i.v. or epidural infusions

2-h intervals for the first 24–48 h postoperatively
4-h intervals as absolute minimum thereafter

Table 74.8 *Simple method of scoring sedation*

0 = none (patient alert)
1 = mild (patient may be sleepy but easy to rouse)
2 = moderate (frequently drowsy but still fully rousable)
3 = severe (difficult to rouse)
S = sleeping normally
Sedation is an earlier sign of opioid-induced respiratory depression

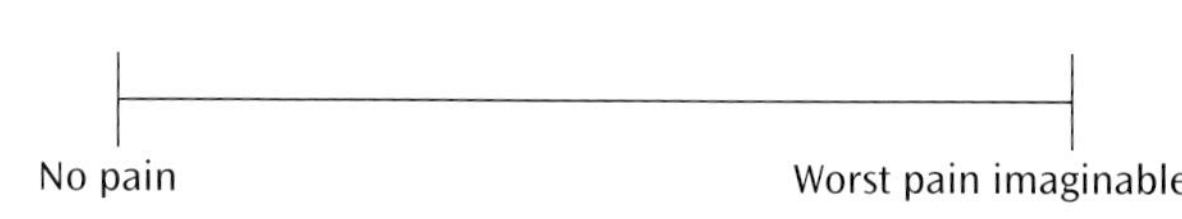

Figure 74.2 *Visual analog scale.*

Table 74.9 *Types and strengths of evidence*

Type	Strength
I	Strong evidence from at least one systematic review of multiple well-designed randomized controlled trials
II	Strong evidence from at least one properly designed randomized controlled trial of appropriate size
III	Evidence from well-designed trials without randomization, single-group pre–post, time series, or matched case–control studies
IV	Evidence from well-designed nonexperimental studies from more than one research center or research group
V	Opinions of respected authorities, based on clinical evidence, descriptive studies, or reports of expert committees

continually updated database of pain reviews is available through the Internet at http://www.jr2.ox.ac.uk/Bandolier/painres/MApain.html.

Traditionally, postoperative pain has been managed with intramuscular injection of opioids administered in fixed doses on patient request. This method is still prevalent[89] despite the well-known inadequacy of this approach.[90] Just as the "complaint of pain" varies between patients in similar circumstances and within patients in different circumstances, the same is true of their response to pain management interventions. Adequate acute postoperative pain management in individual patients is rarely difficult; this should be a generic skill possessed by all doctors, and should be "simple, clinically appropriate and evidence based."[85] However, the real challenge is to adequately manage this pain of populations of patients, so that all patients undergoing surgical interventions can benefit.

PHARMACOLOGICAL STRATEGIES TO MANAGE ACUTE PAIN

We make no attempt to outline the detailed pharmacology of individual drugs in the following sections; reference to standard pharmacology texts is recommended.[19,91]

Systemic analgesia

Opioids

These are the most commonly used drugs for the management of acute postoperative pain. It is undoubtedly still true that most patients receive inadequate doses because of an underestimation of the pain, overestimation of the duration of action of opioids, and the fear about the risk for abuse,[92] which simply reflects a lack of education and training. Opioid is the preferred term and refers to any substance, natural or synthetic, that acts as an agonist at opioid receptors.[91] Opioid receptors appear to be located supraspinally, spinally, and in peripheral tissues. Morphine is the prototype opioid agonist with which the potency of all others are compared.

Prescribing opioids

Ideally, opioid administration should start with an appropriate prescription (agent, dose, frequency, and route of administration) individualized for each patient. The patient's response (pain relief and adverse effects) should then be repeatedly monitored and the prescription altered accordingly to maximize analgesia and minimize side-effects – titration of drug against clinical effect.[87] Individual opioid requirements in the postoperative period vary considerably (up to 10-fold), and in adults age has been shown to be a better predictor than weight of opioid requirements in the first 24 h after surgery,[17] according to the formula: average first 24-h maintenance PCA morphine requirements in patients after major surgery aged between 20 and 70 years of age = 100 – age in years. This relation can be used as a guide to prescribing opioids by either parenteral or enteral routes.

The effectiveness of single-dose morphine, 10 mg, used for moderate to severe postoperative pain has been shown to be similar to each of the following: oral acetaminophen (paracetamol) 1000 mg, oral acetaminophen 1000 mg and codeine 60 mg, ibuprofen 400 mg and diclofenac 50 mg.[87] Initially, this may appear to reflect poorly on morphine, but its efficacy can be improved by titrating the drug to analgesic effect. Meperidine (pethidine) is a drug that should be used with caution in high doses or over prolonged periods of time, as its metabolite norpethidine can accumulate and has central nervous system effects.

Routes of administration

General considerations The route chosen to administer opioids should be:

1 Appropriate.[85] Access to parenteral and enteral routes will vary throughout the postoperative period. Oral therapy is simple and noninvasive but has limited application in the early postoperative phase, when patients may be fasting or unable to absorb oral medications as a result of gastric stasis, ileus, or vomiting. Absorption from intramuscular and subcutaneous injections will be reduced if peripheral perfusion is poor (i.e. in hypovolemia and hypothermia), leading to inadequate analgesia. In addition, there may be formation of depot of analgesic that may be absorbed at a later time when perfusion improves.
2 Safe. The safety of the route chosen is assessed by the balance of risk factors:
   a the patient's acute physiological status and comorbidities;
   b concurrent medications;
   c availability of specialized equipment;
   d availability of trained staff.
3 Effective, which is achieved by individualizing the dose and dosing intervals and applies to the administration of opioids by any route. Lack of flexibility in dose schedules has often meant that intermittent and "p.r.n." (as needed) methods of pain relief have been ineffective when given by any route. Intermittent administration is associated with marked variations in plasma concentration. As a result, patients may swing between pain with subtherapeutic concentrations and side-effects following a bolus dose, with little time spent within the therapeutic range (Fig. 74.3). Frequent assessment of the patient's pain severity and response to treatment rather than strict adherence to a dose regimen is required to ensure adequate analgesia.

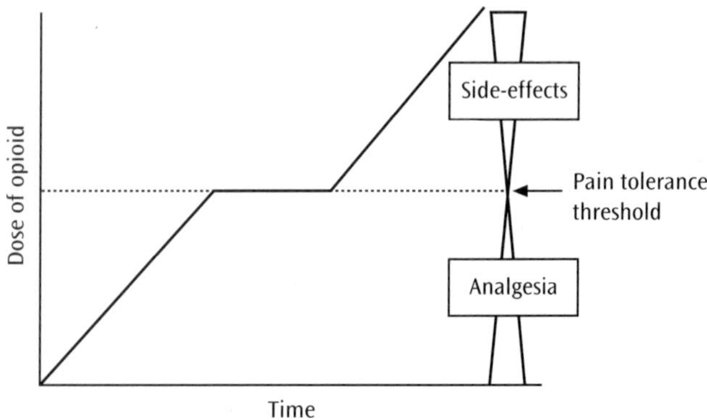

Figure 74.3 *Titration of opioids to effect. (Adapted from McQuay and Moore.[87])*

Oral route (p.o.) The oral route is a very effective way to administer opioids and is generally used when the patient is able to tolerate fluids freely. Weaker opioids such as codeine and dihydrocodeine are often used for pain of moderate severity, and there is an increasing trend to use oral morphine preparation for severe pain, which may be converted to long-acting preparations when this pain is ongoing but with a fairly stable morphine requirement. Many patients fall into "analgesic gaps" after surgery. The first gap occurs when parenteral administration is replaced by enteral administration, as the latter is often inadequate. The other gap is between good hospital-based analgesia (parenteral opioids and regional techniques) and community-based analgesia (simple oral analgesia at home).[93] Oral controlled-release opioids given in low dosage with a short-acting opioid prescribed as rescue medication may be used to bridge these gaps. The safety of this regimen depends on the resumption of gastrointestinal function before the oral opioid is given.[94]

Intramuscular (i.m.) route Intramuscular injections have been the traditional mainstay of postoperative pain management. Dose intervals should be long enough to ensure that a dose has had its maximum effect before another dose is given, but short enough to ensure that the patient receives further analgesia if required. The effectiveness of this route may be improved by prescribing the opioid according to the patient's age and titrating according to response "2-hourly" as required.[95]

Subcutaneous (s.c.) route Opioids may be administered by this route as intermittent injection or continuous infusion. A small cannula can be placed subcutaneously to avoid frequent skin punctures and risk of needlestick injuries, and can remain in place for several days.[95] There appears to be little difference between the s.c. and i.m. routes for morphine administration intermittently when comparing its absorption,[96] side-effect profiles, and degree of analgesia, although patients express a strong preference for the s.c. route.[97] Continuous infusions provide stable plasma levels and avoid bolus effects (i.e. toxicity at peak concentration and/or pain breakthrough at the trough concentration). This route is widely used in the treatment of severe cancer pain and may have applications in some postoperative patients, particularly if intravenous access is unavailable. Morphine, hydromorphone, and diamorphine are suitable for subcutaneous infusion as all cause little local tissue irritation. As dose requirements increase, it may be necessary to use more concentrated solutions to keep the infusion rate to a minimum.

Intravenous (i.v.) route To ensure safe and effective analgesia, intermittent i.v. opioid injections should be administered at lower doses but more frequently than i.m./s.c. opioids, with close monitoring of the effects. The advantage of this technique is that smaller and more frequent i.v. doses allow easy titration of dose to response as the effects are more rapid, predictable, and readily observable. This approach is most suitable in the following situations:

1 On postoperative care units (POCUs) to obtain initial and rapid pain relief (rescue analgesia) and in high-dependency units (HDUs) or intensive care units (ICUs). It should not be routinely be used on general wards because of the risk of rapidly developing life-threatening side-effects.
2 To provide analgesia for patients who are hypovolemic or hypotensive, in whom there is potentially poor uptake of drug from muscle or subcutaneous tissue.
3 To provide relief for episodes of "incident pain" (e.g. dressing changes, physiotherapy).

At our institution we recommend using i.v. bolus injection of morphine, 1–2.5mg every 5 min as required, to gain rapid control of severe acute pain until pain relief is achieved. The total dose needed for this "titration" is a guide to the subsequent dose requirements. Patients must be closely observed and continuously monitored during the titration.

Continuous intravenous infusions (i.v.i.) of opioids are used to avoid the "peaks and troughs" in blood concentrations associated with intermittent administration. Safe and effective administration of i.v.i.s requires reliable infusion devices and frequent assessment and monitoring of patients by trained staff, with appropriate adjustment of infusion rates and administration of bolus doses. It is a technique that should be reserved for HDU or ICU environments. To reach 95% of the final steady-state concentration for drugs given by infusion requires five half-lives (up to 20 h for morphine). Increasing the infusion rate alone in response to inadequate analgesia will result in considerable delays in achieving analgesia and the potential danger of further rising opioid concentrations once analgesia has been attained. If analgesia is inadequate, an increase in blood opioid concentration is best achieved by administrating a small bolus dose before increasing the infusion rate. The response to any change in dose must be carefully and frequently assessed as opioid administration continues with infusions regardless of the conscious state of the patient.

Patient-controlled analgesia (PCA) Patient control is fundamental to achieving satisfactory pain relief. "Patient-controlled analgesia" refers to the use of a sophisticated infusion device activated by the patient to self-administer small doses of intravenous opioids.

This technique has advantages as it overcomes the wide variation in patients' analgesic requirements and allows patients to balance their own comfort with any side-effects of opioids. PCA provides better patient satisfaction and improved respiratory function than conventional routes for administration of opioids.[98] Used in "PCA mode only," with no background infusion, the possibility of sedated patients receiving further opioids is minimized. In adults, background infusions increase the amount of opioid delivered and increase the risk of side-effects without significantly improving analgesia.[99] However, for patients with opioid tolerance undergoing surgery, adding a background infusion to the PCA is a reasonable choice – the infusion rate should be derived from the patient's current daily opioid requirement.[95] Adequate preoperative patient instruction is essential if PCA is to be successful; the suitability of this technique for the individual patient can be gleaned at this time (i.e. understanding and motor skills). PCA is usually used to administer medication by the i.v. route (i.v.-PCA) but may be used to deliver opioids subcutaneously (s.c.-PCA) or epidurally (PCEA). Commonly prescribed initial values for i.v.-PCA are listed in Table 74.10.[95]

The safety, appropriateness, and effectiveness of the PCA technique is improved by:

1 supervision by an acute pain service;[100]
2 training of the staff using the equipment;[101]
3 adequate maintenance of equipment;
4 appropriate preprinted guidelines that aim to standardize prescribing, clinical management, documentation, and patient monitoring, although some flexibility in prescribing is required in order to meet individual patients' needs for analgesia.[102]

Novel routes

Sublingual The potential for more rapid onset following sublingual rather than oral administration would benefit patients with intermittent, breakthrough, or incident pain. However, the lack of available formulations and the inability to deliver high doses limits the role of sublingual administration for constant severe pain.

Transmucosal Oral transmucosal fentanyl citrate (OTFC; fentanyl incorporated into a palatable, flavored solid matrix) has been evaluated as a preanesthetic medication in children and found to be effective. The average onset of pain relief is within 9.5 min, but, in addition to transmucosal absorption, gastric absorption (which is slower) also

Table 74.10 *Commonly prescribed initial values for i.v.-PCA*

Variable	Value
Loading dose	0 mg (i.e. zero)
Bolus dose	Morphine 1 mg Diamorphine 0.5 mg Fentanyl 20 μg
Concentration	Variable (ideally standardized)
Dose durations	Usually "stat"
Lock-out period	5 min
Background infusion	0 mg h^{-1} (although there are exceptions, e.g. opioid-tolerant patients)
Four-hour limit	30 mg of morphine or equivalent per 4 h

contributes to plasma levels. Side-effects of nausea and vomiting and preoperative reductions in oxygen saturation limit the clinical usefulness of this preparation. It is not currently available in the UK.

Transdermal Transdermal therapeutic systems (TTS) allow continuous parenteral administration of drug without needles or infusion devices. Lipid-soluble drugs are suitable (e.g. fentanyl). Transdermal fentanyl patches are available with different delivery rates ranging between 25 and 100 μg h^{-1}. Current patches have a slow onset and offset of action, and absorption continues for up to 72 h while the patch is in place, all of which limit the usefulness of these preparations in routine postoperative pain management. Caution should be taken with disposal as significant amounts of residual drug remain in the patch.

Rectal The rectal route may be used when the oral route is not available, e.g. due to nausea or vomiting, It should clearly be avoided for patients with painful perianal lesions or diarrhea. Doses similar to oral doses should be commenced, and then titrated according to response.

Intranasal Intranasal PCA opioid metered inhalers with a lockout period are being evaluated, and nasal spray formulations of fentanyl are in the offing.

Adverse effects of opioids

The principal adverse effects of opioids are listed in Table 74.11. Most side-effects of opioids are dose dependent. The management options available are:

1 Reduce the dose provided satisfactory analgesia can be maintained.
2 Administer symptomatic treatment, e.g. antiemetics for vomiting.
3 Change to another opioid, but generally equianalgesic doses of different opioids have similar adverse effect profiles, apart from a higher incidence of pruritus that has been noted with morphine.[103]

Table 74.11 *Side-effects of opioids*

Sedation
Pruritus
Nausea and vomiting
Slowing of gastrointestinal function
Urinary retention
Respiratory depression
CNS effects
Euphoria
Hallucinations
Miosis
Muscle rigidity
Metabolite toxicity
Allergy
Tolerance

Respiratory depression and hypoxemia The fear of respiratory depression and hypoxia dominates the use of opioids in ward environments, often leading to inadequate prescription of opioids. Respiratory depression can generally be avoided with careful titration of the opioid to its analgesic effect and individualization of the dose required. Clinically, pain tends to antagonize opioid-induced respiratory depression, and in human volunteers pain has been shown to stimulate respiration and attenuate morphine-induced respiratory depression.[104]

The risk of respiratory depression is increased by:

1 absolute overdose of opioid;
2 concurrent use of other hypnotic drugs, e.g. benzodiazepines;
3 pre-existing comorbidities, e.g. respiratory (including sleep apnea syndromes), renal and hepatic dysfunction, hypovolemia, raised intracranial pressure.

Respiratory depression associated with opioids is a late and unreliable sign; sedation is a better indicator of opioid overdose.[105] During "normal sleep" a patient should be rousable!

Postoperative episodic hypoxemia without respiratory depression has been noted in patients receiving opioids, not necessarily in excessive doses. It may be due to intermittent upper airway obstruction not dissimilar to that seen in sleep apnea syndromes. The falls in pulse oximetry readings can be profound.[106] Unfortunately, pulse oximetry is an unreliable indicator of respiratory depression, especially when supplemental oxygen is employed.[107,108] Conversely, hypoxemic episodes may also occur when pain itself restricts adequate ventilation coupled with the residual effects of anesthesia and surgery.[109] As significant background and/or intermittent hypoxemia may occur for a number of days postoperatively, notably during sleep,[110] supplemental oxygen is recommended for at least the first 48–72 h following major surgery and in elderly or high-risk patients.[111] This may be of vital importance to high-risk patients because of the link between postoperative hypoxemia and myocardial infarction.[112]

Metabolite toxicity Meperidine (pethidine) is N-demethylated to an active metabolite, normeperidine, which in turn is hydrolyzed to normeperidinic acid. Accumulation of normeperidine is associated with excitatory effects ranging from nervousness to tremors, twitches, multifocal myoclonus, and seizures. Meperidine should probably not be used for more than 72 h for the management of postoperative pain because of the risk of normeperidine accumulation. However, the evidence for this risk is not strongly documented.[113] Normeperidine toxicity has also been reported in patients receiving patient-controlled meperidine.[114] Renal dysfunction increases the half-life of norpethidine (15–30 h) and so increases the risk of normeperidine accumulation. Naloxone does not reverse, and may aggravate, normeperidine toxicity.

Morphine is metabolized in the liver to morphine 3-glucuronide (M3G) and morphine 6-glucuronide (M6G). M6G has similar affinity for μ receptors as morphine but has 10 times the potency.[115] With renal dysfunction, accumulation of M6G may contribute to analgesia and prolonged sedation. M3G has no affinity for the μ receptor, may antagonize the action of morphine at supraspinal sites, and has been postulated to cause myoclonic jerks and hyperalgesia in patients receiving very high doses of morphine.[116–118] Chronic morphine administration, impaired renal function, and age greater than 70 years have all been associated with higher ratios of morphine metabolites to morphine.[119,120]

Cardiovascular effects Opioids have variable cardiovascular effects depending on the agent employed and the dose and route of administration. Generally, the effects of opioids on blood pressure will depend on:

1 intravascular volume status;
2 degree of sympathetic nervous system activation.

Opioids may reduce a previously raised sympathetic tone and result in decreased blood pressure, if intravascular volume is depleted. Morphine may result in vasodilation; meperidine is associated with an increased heart rate.

Nausea and vomiting Postoperative nausea and vomiting (PONV) is both common and distressing for many patients. While it is a well-recognized adverse effect of opioids, PONV has a multifactorial etiology as listed in Table 74.12.[120,121] Antiemetic drugs act via a number of different mechanisms:

1 At the vomiting center:
   a centrally acting anticholinergic agents atropine and scopolamine;
   b antihistamines cyclizine and promethazine.
2 At the chemoreceptor trigger zone:
   a the neuroleptic drugs haloperidol, droperidol, and prochlorperazine block the dopamine-2 (D_2) receptor;
   b metoclopramide acts peripherally to enhance gastric emptying, and centrally at D_2 receptors to reduce vomiting;
   c ondansetron and granisetron act on specific 5-hydroxytryptamine-3 (5-HT_3) receptors and have been shown to be very effective for control of postoperative and cytotoxic drug-induced nausea and vomiting.[120–124]

A number of general measures may be employed in the management of PONV, including:

1 adequate hydration;
2 maintenance of adequate blood pressure;
3 avoiding excessive movement in the immediate postoperative phase;
4 reducing the patient's anxiety.

Allergy True allergy to opioids is very uncommon. The term is often misused in relation to opioids when patients describe another dose-related adverse effect.

Tolerance Tolerance can be defined as the phenomenon in which an organism becomes less susceptible to the effect of a drug as a result of its prior administration. Declining opioid responsiveness observed with chronic use has a number of causes, including tolerance; the other factors are listed in Table 74.13. Surgical review is needed if opioid requirements increase rapidly postoperatively as any increase in pain may be due to surgical complications, e.g. development of an intra-abdominal catastrophe, lower limb ischemia, and compartment syndrome, and not assumed to be due to tolerance, especially at an early stage. Once any threat to life or limb has been excluded, a decrease in analgesic effect of the opioid should be managed by increasing its dose, which only becomes a problem if limiting side-effects occur before analgesic doses are achieved.

Table 74.12 *Etiology of PONV*

Type of surgery performed
Gastrointestinal disorders (inflammation, gastric stasis, or bowel obstruction)
Chemical factors (drugs or metabolic disorders)
Raised intracranial pressure
Vestibular imbalance
Psychological factors

Table 74.13 *Causes of declining opioid responsiveness*

Tolerance
Increased activity in nociceptive pathways from disease progression
Evolution of neuropathic pain
Psychological processes
Changes in pharmacokinetic factors
Plasticity of opioid mechanisms

Addiction There is no evidence that the use of opioids in opioid-naive patients suffering acute severe pain increases their likelihood of developing opioid addiction and drug-seeking behavior. The incidence has been assessed to be 0.03%.[125–127]

Acetaminophen and nonsteroidal anti-inflammatory drugs (NSAIDs)

Acetaminophen (paracetamol)

Acetaminophen is effective for mild to moderate pain, and as an adjunct to opioids in more severe pain.[87,128] While it has analgesic and antipyretic effects, it is not generally considered to be anti-inflammatory. Its mechanism of action is unclear, but it may act by inhibiting the cyclo-oxygenase enzyme in the central nervous system, sparing the peripheral equivalent.[129]

Single doses of more than 100 mg kg^{-1} may result in severe liver damage, hypoglycemia, and acute tubular necrosis, and the contraindications to its use are restricted to patients with liver dysfunction, but at what level of dysfunction it should be avoided is unclear. Acetaminophen has few side-effects and can be used when NSAIDs are contraindicated. An intravenous preparation in the form of the precursor proacetaminophen (proparacetamol) (2 g of the precursor is converted to 1 g of acetaminophen) is commercially available but not licensed for clinical use in the UK. It may be more effective than oral acetaminophen[130] and has opioid-sparing effect.[131]

NSAIDs

The initial use of NSAIDs for managing acute postoperative pain was based on a desire to improve analgesia without incurring the adverse effects associated with using opioids, while recognizing the potential adverse effects of the drugs themselves.[132,133] The efficacy of a number of NSAIDs in managing postoperative pain has been confirmed: indomethacin,[134] tenoxicam,[135,136] ketorolac,[137–141] diclofenac,[87,140,142] and ibuprofen.[87] The relative effectiveness of different routes of administration is unclear,[87] but the oral route is preferable when available.[85] Topical NSAIDs may be useful in some situations.[87] They are useful for managing pain following minor surgery,[143] but when used alone they are not sufficient to manage severe pain,[144,145] whether given pre-emptively or not.[146,147] However, their efficacy as components of "multimodal analgesia" is established.[59,148,149]

The Royal College of Anaesthetists has published guidelines for the use of NSAIDs in the perioperative period based on a comprehensive structured review of the published evidence.[150] Among its conclusions are the following "grade A" conclusions, i.e. those "based on the strongest evidence available, including at least one randomized trial as part of the body of literature of overall good quality."

1 NSAIDs are not sufficiently effective as the sole agent after major surgery in most patients.
2 NSAIDs are often effective after minor or moderate surgery.
3 NSAIDs often decrease opioid requirement. A significant reduction in opioid side-effects has been noted in a few studies only.
4 The quality of opioid-based analgesia is often enhanced by NSAIDs.
5 NSAIDs increase bleeding time, and some studies have shown increased blood loss.

The guidelines point out that many clinically important drug interactions are associated with the use of NSAIDs, thus:

1 pharmacokinetic interactions with warfarin, lithium, oral hypoglycemics, phenytoin, methotrexate, digoxin, aminoglycosides, cyclosporin, tacrolimus, and probenicid;
2 pharmacodynamic interactions with antihypertensive drugs, anticardiac failure therapy, and anticoagulants.

Adverse effects of NSAIDs

NSAIDs have been administered to several million patients worldwide without complication,[151] but it is a class of drugs with a fearsome reputation for adverse effects. These adverse effects are potentially so serious that the contraindications to their use and correct dosage must be respected,[152] and patients with known risk factors for NSAID-related adverse effects should not be given these drugs in the perioperative period. The adverse effects may be commoner in the elderly. The route of administration chosen does not affect the occurrence of these adverse effects.

Gastrointestinal effects[153] The potential for NSAIDs to cause gastric ulceration is well known; what is less appreciated is that these data generally relate to chronic use of these agents. The risk of gastropathy with the short term use of these drugs is unknown. Clearly, it would be ill-advised to prescribe these agents to patients with previous histories of gastric ulceration and bleeding, but where a clinical benefit is perceived by including NSAIDs, some form of gastric protection would be advisable, e.g. misoprostinol.

Asthma[154] The association of NSAIDs and asthma is confusing and is not now generally regarded as a major concern. A small group of patients who suffer from aspirin sensitivity and nasal polyps may develop severe brochospasm in association with NSAIDs.

Renal effects NSAIDs given at the time of surgery have demonstrable effects on renal prostaglandins.[155] Case reports have attributed the development of unexplained acute renal failure to the use of ketorolac.[156] Other risk factors for this outcome include concomitant use of nephrotoxic antibiotics,[157] raised intra-abdominal pressure (such as occurs at laparoscopy), hypovolemia, and an age greater than 65 years. Ketorolac given for less than 5 days may not increase the rate of acute renal failure, but the risk increases with longer duration of therapy.[151]

Platelet function effects NSAIDs potentially have the ability to increase clinical bleeding by their ability to inhibit platelet function;[158] generally their antiplatelet effects are of no clinical consequence despite elevation of skin bleeding times.[159,160] The antiplatelet effect of aspirin is reported not to increase the risk of performing central neuraxial blocks, including epidurals.[161–163]

Newer NSAIDs

Traditional NSAIDs exert their effects by inhibiting all forms of the cyclo-oxygenase enzyme. Recently an inducible form of the enzyme, cyclo-oxygenase-2 (Cox-2) has been described.[164] It appears that Cox-2 is induced by a number of factors, including surgical and other tissue trauma, endotoxin, IL-1, and hypoxia.[165] In contrast, Cox-1 is constitutively expressed and is thought to be responsible for normal physiological prostaglandin production in many tissues (e.g. cytoprotection of the gastric mucosa and aspects of renal tubular function). A new class of NSAIDs has been developed that selectively inhibit the Cox-2 enzyme (inducible form) while sparing the constitutive form of the enzyme (Cox-l).[166,167] Meloxicam, a new commercially available Cox-2 NSAID, has been shown to be as effective an analgesic as diclofenac in patients with osteoarthritis of the knee,[168] and the incidence of gastrointestinal symptoms is halved in patients receiving meloxicam compared with diclofenac.[169] A meta-analysis involving 1100 patient–years of treatment with meloxicam showed improved gastrointestinal safety but similar renal and liver toxicity compared with conventional NSAIDs.[170] Nimesulide is another selective Cox-2 inhibitor with equivalent analgesic activity to conventional NSAIDs but with reduced gastrointestinal side-effects.[171,172] The safety and effectiveness of these agents in the management of acute postoperative pain is yet to be established.

Adjuvant agents in the management of pain

Adjuvant agents are commonly used in the management of numerous pain syndromes, including neuropathic pain. Type I evidence supporting their effectiveness exists.[87] The major classes of drugs used include:

1 tricyclic antidepressants, e.g. amitriptyline. doxepin, nortriptyline and dothiepin;[173]
2 traditional anticonvulsants, e.g. phenytoin, carbamazepine, sodium valproate;
3 "new" anticonvulsants, e.g. lamotrigine, vigabatrin, gabapentin;
4 "membrane stabilizers," e.g. lidocaine (lignocaine), mexilitine, flecainide);
5 corticosteroids;
6 central nervous system stimulants, e.g. dexamphetamine;
7 anxiolytics;
8 α_2-adrenergic agonists (clonidine);
9 *N*-methyl-D-aspartate (NMDA) antagonists, e.g. ketamine, dextromethorphan.

Locoregional anesthesia

Locoregional nerve blockade (the word blockade implies the use of local anesthetic agents) has wide applicability in the management of acute postoperative pain. The techniques employed are varied, ranging from simple wound infiltration to continuous neural blockade using indwelling catheters. A single bolus injection of local anesthetic around a peripheral nerve truck can give many hours of analgesia, but may also only serve to delay the onset of pain. Greater benefit is obtained by the use of continuous catheter techniques that allow analgesia to be maintained for prolonged periods using either repeated bolus injection or continuous infusion of a solution containing local anesthetic.

Peripheral blockade

Interpleural analgesia[174]

Interpleural analgesia has been successfully used for the management of unilateral pain following thoracic and upper abdominal surgery. It has been shown to improve postoperative respiratory function when compared with systemic opioids, although chest drains or intrapleural fluid collections can reduce its effectiveness.[175] Optimal pain relief may require supplementation with other analgesics by other routes.

Plexus and individual nerve blocks

The commonest techniques employed to assist postoperative pain management include brachial plexus blocks and femoral nerve blocks. Effective pain relief in both cases can be achieved by either bolus injection or continuous infusion of a local anesthetic solution within the investing facial sheaths. Femoral nerve blocks are useful for management of pain and muscle spasm following knee surgery.

Wound infiltration

Wound infiltration seems to be maximally effective when used in small adult wounds and in pediatric surgery, but infiltrating large adult wounds with local anesthetic is of less certain benefit. However, a subset of these trials did show benefit when large doses or volumes of local anesthetic were infiltrated into deeper wound structures (fascia, peritoneum, or muscle) rather than just subcutaneously.[176]

Neuraxial blockade

Epidural and intrathecal analgesic techniques have the potential to improve postoperative analgesia and modify physiological changes associated with surgery. Strong evidence indicates that postoperative epidural analgesia significantly reduces the incidence of pulmonary morbidity.[48] When combined with active postoperative rehabilitation programmes,[69] epidural analgesia may improve overall patient outcome. However, these techniques have rare but important risks associated with the technique itself and the drugs used. Thus, a risk–benefit assessment must be made for each individual patient, and the availability of appropriately safe postoperative care (adequate facilities and trained staff) must be considered before choosing these techniques for acute postoperative pain management.

Epidural and intrathecal anesthetics should be administered and managed by an anesthesiologist or trained members of an acute pain service. Selection of an appropriate route of administration (intrathecal vs. epidural) and site of catheter insertion (lumbar vs. thoracic epidural) should be based on individual patient factors, the intraoperative surgical requirements, and the planned postoperative analgesic regimen. If local anesthetics and a lipid-soluble opioid are to be administered postoperatively, an epidural catheter should be placed as close as possible to the level of the dermatomes affected by the surgical incision.[177] Epidural analgesia is most usually administered by continuous infusion, but PCEA appears to be safe and effective even in the general ward environment.[178]

Large audits of epidural analgesia show the safety of the technique to be equivalent to traditional analgesic methods when coordinated by an acute pain service with appropriate patient monitoring.[179–183] Epidural and intrathecal analgesic techniques can be safely managed on general wards if a number of measures are routinely adopted:

1 Patients are regularly reviewed by an anesthesiologist or trained members of an acute pain services.
2 An anesthesiologist is always available for consultation or management of complications.
3 Nursing staff have received specific training and education about the management of these methods and potential adverse effects.
4 Appropriate standardized prescribing, management, documentation, and monitoring guidelines are established.

Routine monitoring should be performed and documented at a frequency determined by clinical circumstances, and should consist of:

1 standard minimum data set of ward observations, including pain score, sedation score, respiratory rate, pulse rate, and blood pressure;
2 some assessment of motor and sensory block;
3 checking catheter skin puncture site for signs of inflammation/infection, leakage, and catheter dislodgement.

Agents used for neuraxial analgesia

Local anesthetic

Local anesthetics administered into the region of the neuraxis reversibly block nerve impulse conduction in nociceptive afferent and sympathetic efferent pathways, producing segmental analgesia and sympathetic block. The systemic absorption of these drugs also potentially reduces the physiological responses to surgery.

Opioids

Opioids administered into the region of the neuraxis produces selective segmental analgesia by blocking opioid receptors in the dorsal horn.[18,184] The analgesic actions and duration of effect of neuraxial opioids parallels the cerebrospinal fluid (CSF) concentrations rather than plasma concentrations of the drugs. Lower doses of opioids are required when given via the neuraxial route than via the systemic route, so side-effects may be reduced. However, plasma concentrations of the opioid may be significant and contribute to early analgesia, particularly following epidural administration of lipophilic agents such as fentanyl. Epidural opioids have been shown to be more effective when used in combination with local anesthetic to produce a synergistic analgesic action and reduce the required dose and side-effects associated with either the local anesthetic or opioid alone.[59] Some studies have been unable to show any advantage with opioids administered alone around the neuraxis compared with systemic administration. Episodic postoperative hypoxemia has been observed following both routes, and the stress response to surgery is only partially attenuated by opioids alone.[185]

Opioid uptake after epidural injection may follow at least four routes:

1 diffusion through the dural membrane of the spinal root cuff into the CSF and to the dorsal horn of the spinal cord and thence to the brain via cephalad migration in CSF;
2 possible direct transfer from the epidural space to the spinal cord via spinal radicular arteries;[186]
3 vascular uptake into the bloodstream and into the systemic circulation;
4 diffusion into surrounding lipophilic tissues that lack opioid receptors.

The physicochemical properties of different opioids result in differences in distribution, duration of effect, and side-effect profile when these agents are administered around the neuraxis. The hydrophilic agents, e.g. morphine, have a longer residence time in the CSF and are associated with cephalad migration. This has the advantage of prolonging the duration of analgesia following a single dose (12–24 h); in addition, the epidural catheter tip does not need to be close to the source of nociceptive impulses (e.g. lumbar epidural injection may provide analgesia for thoracic level pain). Because of its long residence in neural tissue, morphine has the potential for delayed respiratory depression 12–24 h after the last dose. Lipophilic agents, such as fentanyl, exhibit less migration and more segmental analgesia. The duration of action is also shorter and administration by an infusion with attention to the spinal level of the epidural catheter tip is required. The lipophilic opioid sufentanil has a segmental spread in the CSF and has been used safely on the ward when guidelines were followed.[187–189]

Nonopioid spinal analgesics

There is obviously much interest in developing new "magic bullets" targeted at spinal nonopioid receptors involved with the modulation of nociception. Clonidine, while not a new drug, appears to have synergistic analgesic action when coadministered spinally with opioids, but with side-effects including hypotension, bradycardia, and sedation. Midazolam, a GABA-A receptor agonist, has been shown to have analgesic properties. Neostigmine produces analgesia when administered spinally, but dose–response data and side-effect profiles are not fully elucidated. The spinal analgesic action, side-effects, and toxicology of NSAIDs, amitriptyline and other novel chemical compounds are currently under investigation.

Adverse effects of neuraxial techniques

The myriad of potential adverse effects associated with neuraxial analgesia at first seem somewhat daunting. They broadly divide into catheter related and drug related. It would be fair to say that serious sequelae, such as permanent neurological damage or mortality solely attributable to the epidural, are very rare, but must be borne in mind before embarking on the procedure. Most of the potential adverse effects can be avoided if patients are closely monitored by their carers, who in turn have a clear understanding about all aspects of epidural management.

Catheter-related adverse effects

1 Dural puncture: the rate of inadvertent dural puncture during epidural insertion is 0.6–1.3%. The likelihood of developing a posdural puncture headache varies between 16% and 86% as multiple factors are involved (e.g. needle size, patient age).
2 Serious neurological injury occurs very rarely in association with lumbar epidural analgesia. This is also true for insertion at the thoracic level,[190] which is similar to the incidence of occurrence following general anesthesia.[191]
3 Epidural hematoma: this is a confused and complicated subject; thankfully, clinically significant epidural hematomata occur rarely in association with epidural analgesia. The risk is increased by impaired hemostasis at the time of epidural catheter insertion or removal. The risk may also be increased by the concurrent use of prophylactic low-dose heparin or low-molecular-weight heparin.[192] To minimize the risk of this outcome, guidelines specify:
   a the use of minimal effective doses of anticoagulant given at appropriate intervals;
   b insertion and removal of epidural catheters separated by at least an entire half life of the anticoagulant used, timed from the last dose of anticoagulant given.[193–195]
4 Epidural abscess or meningitis are rare complications but require early detection and urgent surgical intervention to minimize the risk of permanent neurological sequelae.

Drug-related adverse effects

Local anesthetic effects consist of:

1 cardiovascular and central nervous system toxicity due to absolute local anesthetic overdose or intravascular injection;
2 urinary retention;
3 total spinal analgesia if excessive local anesthetic doses are administered intrathecally rather than epidurally;
4 variable hemodynamic effects of sympathetic blockade, postural hypotension;
5 motor block using higher concentrations of local anesthetic, which impairs mobilization, and which in combination with sensory block may contribute to the development of pressure areas.

Opioid-related adverse effects include the following:

1 Respiratory depression can occur with all spinally administered opioids, if given in excessive doses. The risk of delayed respiratory depression is greatest with morphine as its hydrophilic structure results in long transit time in the CSF with cephalad migration to the brainstem and prolonged residence in neural tissue.
2 Pruritus, nausea, and urinary retention are most frequent with morphine and less likely following fentanyl, but the incidence varies in different studies.

Outcomes following epidural anesthesia and analgesia

Currently, definitive evidence demonstrating clearly the ability of epidural analgesia to improve the postoperative outcome of any group of patients is unavailable. This is due to inherent problems associated with studying such a subject, namely recruiting sufficient numbers of patients and ensuring adequate standardization of patient groups from the point of view of surgical type, site of epidural catheter insertion, and type and duration of analgesic agent administered. Existing evidence suggests that the perioperative epidural technique using local anesthetic agents may offer the best possibility of reducing adverse postoperative outcomes, most notably in high-risk patients undergoing major surgery.[185] It is unrealistic to suppose that addressing an isolated factor, such as pain, associated with surgical outcome is likely to succeed. Recovery should not be a passive process but an active process of rehabilitation. Postoperative management should be considered as a "package," including superb analgesia using neuraxial blockade with local anesthetic as part of a "multimodal" approach, early instigation of enteral nutrition, early mobilization, close supervision of fluid balance, and close attention to cardiorespiratory function.[6]

Multimodal analgesia[196–198]

Sometimes referred to as "balanced analgesia," multimodal analgesia is an approach to pain management that uses a combination of drugs with different modes of action, possibly administered by different routes, to achieve improved pain relief with a reduction in the incidence and severity of side-effects. A large variety of individual analgesic drug combinations have been used in this way. Generally, where no contraindication exists, one drug is selected from each of the major classes of drugs with analgesic actions and administered systemically or locoregionally as appropriate.[102] A typical prescription for postoperative pain relief would incorporate regular acetaminophen (orally or rectally) plus regular NSAID (orally or rectally) as "baseline analgesia," with either systemic opioid or a locoregional infusion of a solution containing local anesthetic and opioid.

The nonopioid analgesics contribute significantly to multimodal analgesia by their opioid-sparing effect, so reducing the side-effects associated with these drugs,[59,148,199,200] and by their ability to provide pain relief on movement by virtue of including local anesthetic agents, so allowing earlier mobilization.[69,102] However, the benefit of multimodal analgesia to overall patient outcome (reduction in morbidity and mortality) has only been hinted at by existing observations.[201–203] Clearly, postoperative recovery comprises a complex system of interrelated variables, of which pain is only one, so it would be naive to anticipate that good pain management alone could improve overall patient outcome.[69] However, multimodal analgesia after major surgery may reduce costs.[200]

Pre-emptive analgesia

In essence, pre-emptive analgesia is a theoretical construct whereby the severity of pain that an individual experiences is reduced if some intervention can be applied before this noxious stimulus. It is an attempt to prevent or reduce the peripheral and central sensitization of nociceptors.[21,204] The potential advantages of this idea are significant: reduced opioid requirements, earlier return to normal activities, and fewer adverse outcomes. Initial data from animal studies were convincing, but clinical evidence in humans after surgery has either been equivocal or has failed to support the concept.[205–210] However, a recent human volunteers study did demonstrate a pre-emptive effect .[211] Again, it is probably naive to suppose that an isolated preoperative intervention would prevent the processes of sensitization occurring, as nociception continues for some time after surgery because of the inflammatory response at the site of tissue injury. If pre-emptive therapy is to be successful, it must include a strategy for modulating the prolonged nociceptive activity well into the postoperative period.[21]

NONPHARMACOLOGICAL STRATEGIES TO MANAGE ACUTE PAIN

An array of psychological and physical therapies have been used in the management of acute postoperative pain, though the evidence supporting their effectiveness is mainly at the level of opinion.

Psychological therapies

Psychological therapies include a range of therapies based on cognitive–behavioral techniques. They have been used very successfully in preparing patients for painful procedures including surgery and for helping to manage postoperative pain and distress. The principal techniques used are relaxation training, procedural information, cognitive coping methods, and behavioral instructions.[212]

Physical therapies

Physical therapies are greatly underutilized and poorly researched, while potentially they have many advantages.

Physiotherapy

The importance of the ward physiotherapists for postoperative patient care cannot be overemphasized. Ward staff themselves can undertake simple physiotherapy maneuvers that can have a material effect on the postoperative course of the patients under their care.

- Breathing exercises can significantly improve pain management and physiological parameters.
- Simple wound support during coughing, straining, and mobilization can provide a sense of control, so reducing fear and anxiety.

These interventions are inexpensive, easy to learn, and teach and hardly time-consuming to perform. This instruction should start preoperatively, and supportive and reassuring reminders should continue postoperatively.

Hot and cold applications may seem rather "old-fashioned," but may modify a patient's experience of pain by reducing muscle spasm and decreasing congestion in an injured area. Cold applications are used initially to decrease tissue injury response; later, heat is used to facilitate perfusion of injured tissue.

Massage and exercise are used to stretch and regain muscle and tendon length, while immobilization of fracture sites has profound pain-relieving effect in the short term.

TENS

A recent systematic review of studies of TENS in postoperative pain relief found no benefit compared with placebo.[213]

Acupuncture

A number of randomized, controlled studies have suggested that acupuncture results in a reduction in both pain and analgesic drug consumption following dental and abdominal surgery.[214,215]

SOME DIFFICULT PAINS AND SOME DIFFICULT PATIENTS

Management of pain associated with pediatric surgery

The acute postoperative pain management in children has been reported to need improvement.[8] Many children generally receive inadequate amounts of opioids, notably after painful surgical procedures.[216,217] Once again the problem revolves around the same myths and fears that have thwarted adult patients, with a few extra for good measure, including: "children experience less pain than adults;" "neonates don't experience or remember pain;" "children cannot localize or describe their pain;" and "pain is character building for children." As for adults, there is no evidence that the use of opioids for treatment of severe pain in children leads to opioid dependence or addiction. There is overwhelming evidence that all of the neurophysiological components required to experience pain are present by mid-gestation in the human fetus, and that these components are active by the time viable preterm birth occurs.[218]

There can be no doubt that good postoperative management of acute pain in children is challenging not because the individual's unique experience of pain is different from that in adults, but because the expression (verbal and behavior) and assessment of pain in children is more complex than in adults, being dependent on age, developmental level, previous pain experiences, medical, psychological, social and cultural factors, and pharmacological variability factors (notably in neonates). Pain management has to take these factors into consideration and utilize both pharmacological and nonpharmacological strategies as in adults. Good analgesia should be attained in the recovery room before discharge to the ward or home in the case of day-case surgery. As in adult practice, postoperative analgesia using the oral route is preferable.

Clinical assessment of pain in children

Any assessment should always include a careful history and examination. The pain rating scale chosen should be appropriate for the age and development of the child. Scales variously take account of physiological variables, behavioral observation, and self-reporting to rate children's pain. Self-reporting of pain appears to be reliable in children over 4 years of age[219,220] and numerous pain rating scales have been devised for neonates (e.g. CRIES[221]), and younger children (e.g. modified visual analog scales such as the poker chip tool[222] and Wong–Baker faces[223]). Valuable information can be gleaned by observing nonverbal behavioral cues, remembering that a quiet, withdrawn child may be in severe pain, which, over time, may suggest an increase in pain intensity. Physiological signs, such as tachycardia, may play a key role in very young children but need to be interpreted in the clinical context. Pain ratings provided by parents or regular carers are valid and reliable,[224] and the ability to console children may help to distinguish pain from other causes of distress such as parental separation, an unfamiliar environment, and hunger and thirst with fasting.

Pharmacological strategies

The choice of drug therapy for managing postoperative pain is influenced by the child's age, type of surgery, presence of comorbidities, and postoperative care environment. Generally:

1. Pain following minor surgery can usually be managed with oral acetaminophen and NSAIDs. If acetaminophen is used as the sole analgesic, higher doses are required.[225] For day-case patients, parents need to be given sufficient information to manage residual pain.
2. For major surgery, parenteral opioids remain the mainstay of postoperative pain management. Local anesthetic blocks initiated pre- and intraoperatively are being increasingly used for pain management following major surgery.

Systemic analgesia

Nonopioid analgesia

Acetaminophen (paracetamol) Acetaminophen is a safe and effective analgesic agent in children and infants (including for short courses at recommended doses in neonates)[226] administered orally or rectally. For acute postoperative pain it can be used as part of a "multimodal" approach. It has a good safety record and appears to be safe up to 100 mg kg^{-1} day^{-1} in children and up to 60 mg kg^{-1} day^{-1} in neonates.

NSAIDs Diclofenac (0.5–1 mg kg^{-1} 8-hourly orally) or ibuprofen (4–10 mg kg^{-1} 6- to 8-hourly orally) are frequently used in children. The contraindications to their use are the same as for adult patients. Aspirin should be used with caution because of the risk of precipitating Reye's syndrome. Few data are available on the parenteral use of NSAIDs in children.

Opioid analgesia

Opioid administration in children requires routine repeated monitoring, including a pain score and sedation score in addition to the traditional routine ward observation: heart rate, respiratory rate (and effort), blood pressure, and temperature.[227] As in adults, a decrease in respiratory rate may be a late sign of opioid-induced respiratory depression. Pulse oximetry is a valuable adjunct to clinical observation. Respiratory depression may be greater with pethidine than with morphine at equianalgesic doses.[228] We feel that, as in adults, morphine is the drug of first choice, with fentanyl as an alternative when morphine is absolutely or relatively contraindicated. The neurotoxicity of meperidine's metabolite normeperidine should, in our opinion, eliminate its use in children and adults. Side-effects should be managed with similar agents to those used for adults, remembering that young children may have difficulty expressing subjective symptoms, such as pruritus, nausea, and constipation.

In the past, minimal amounts of opioids were administered to infants intraoperatively because of concerns about respiratory and hemodynamic side-effects. The pharmacokinetics of opioids are widely variable among preterm and full-term neonates and infants, with increased elimination half-life[229–231] as the cytochrome P450 enzyme system in the liver does not reach maturity until several months after birth. Young infants (notably premature neonates and those with neurologic abnormalities or pulmonary disease) are susceptible to apnea and respiratory depression, which may be exacerbated by opioids, so the initial and infusion dose for infants up to 6 months of age should be reduced.[232] Infants who are treated with opioid analgesia should be cared for and monitored by experienced staff in an appropriate environment, operating within clear clinical guidelines and with access to immediate respiratory support facilities and resuscitation equipment. The long-term effects of opioids on pain pathway development are unknown.[233]

Oral route Codeine is commonly used for mild to moderate pain and step-down analgesia (converting from parenteral to enteral routes of administration) at a dose of 0.5–1.0 mg kg^{-1} 4- to 6-hourly. Codeine has good oral bioavailability and is converted to morphine; about 10% of adults lack the converting enzyme. Constipation is a frequent complaint with regular dosing and should be treated prophylactically. Ideally, codeine should be used in conjunction with nonopioid analgesics such as acetaminophen and NSAIDs ("multimodal analgesia"). Morphine sulfate may be used in the management of continuing acute pain states, e.g. burns. Slow-release morphine preparations may be used in these situations when the daily morphine dose is stable, using the normal preparation for breakthrough pain.

Intramuscular route Parenteral administration may be needed in the postoperative period, but intermittent i.m. injections provide poor analgesia and are painful and frightening for children. This route may be of use for a single dose of opioid if the pain is severe and no other route of administration is available.

Subcutaneous route Morphine has similar absorption characteristics if given by the s.c. or i.m. routes. Morphine administered via an indwelling s.c. cannula (inserted while the child is anesthetized)[234] offers advantages for postoperative pain management in children as it seems to satisfy nurses, patients and parents alike and is flexible as it may be used for intermittent injections[234] and continuous infusion.[235] This route requires adequate peripheral perfusion and is not recommended in a shocked or hypothermic child.

Intravenous route Opioids can be administered by this route as:

1 intermittent boluses in recovery, high-dependency, or intensive care environments with morphine in a dose of 0.03–0.05 mg kg^{-1}, until the child is comfortable;
2 continuous infusion of morphine (0.01–0.04 mg kg^{-1} h^{-1}) for children over 6 months of age,[236–238] which avoids the plasma morphine variations associated with intermittent administration.

Patient-controlled analgesia (PCA) Intravenous PCA provides safe and effective analgesia for children as young as 5 years of age[239] and is possibly more effective than intermittent i.m. injections in the older child.[240] It can be used as it is in adults, e.g. an intravenous bolus dose of morphine 0.01–0.02 mg kg^{-1} with a 5-min lock-out period. Postoperative analgesia may be improved, without increasing the side-effects, by including a small background infusion (e.g. morphine 5 μg kg^{-1} h^{-1}).[241] As with adults, the safety and effectiveness of the technique are likely to be maximized if clear and repeated instruction in its use is provided, the patient alone activates the PCA machine, and regular assessment of pain and its side-effects is undertaken. PCA may be unsuitable for children less than 5 years old, older children with developmental delay, those with altered levels of consciousness, and those unable to understand the idea of PCA, and care should be exercised in children who have renal failure (using a lower bolus dose, close monitoring, and no background infusion). Side-effects are managed in a similar way as in adults.

Locoregional analgesia

Locoregional techniques are increasingly used in children and infants (including neonates) for anesthesia and postoperative analgesia. The anatomical differences of children must be borne in mind when performing locoregional techniques, with close adherence to mass of local anesthetic agent used if toxicity is to be avoided. The volume of local anesthetic solution required to achieve a satisfactory locoregional block in children is relatively larger (on a body weight basis) than in adults. This is due to anatomical differences (notably around the neuraxis), and technical problems associated with accurate needle placement in anesthetized infants and children. Despite the need for large volumes, the concentration of local anesthetic agents required is usually lower as individual nerves are smaller, internodal distance is shorter, and there is less myelin in the very young. In clinical practice, it is usual to calculate the maximum dose that can be used and then derive the final concentration from the volume required to achieve a block, taking into account any supplemental analgesia (such as local infiltration) that may be required. Generally, there are no special requirements for the postoperative care of patients receiving routine locoregional "single-shot" analgesia, although parents need to be made aware of the likely duration of blockade and any precautions that may be required. However, caudal blocks may prevent discharge after day-case surgery due to the problem of leg weakness and inability to void urine.

Peripheral nerve blocks

Wound infiltration with local anesthetic agents may be used as an adjunct to postoperative analgesia after many surgical procedures in children and adults, and as the sole analgesic technique for many minor day-case procedures. Bupivacaine 0.25% is frequently used for this purpose, there being no evidence that higher concentrations achieve better or prolonged analgesia. Ropivacaine may become the agent of choice by virtue of its lower potential for cardiotoxicity and lesser motor blockade. Ilioinguinal and iliohypogastric block provides good postoperative analgesia after groin surgery,[242] while "single-shot" or continuous infusion analgesia is possible for femoral nerve, interpleural, brachial plexus, and lumbar plexus block. EMLA® cream can do much to reduce the pain and fear of injections for painful procedures such as lumbar puncture, combined if necessary with sedation. It should be applied generously under an occlusive dressing at least an hour before the procedure. EMLA should be used with care in the newborn infant, and application restricted to one site per day as there is potential for methemoglobinemia secondary to prilocaine absorption. Its use in the first week of life in premature neonates of less than 32 weeks' gestation is not recommended.[243]

Neuraxial analgesia

Epidural analgesia Continuous epidural infusions are safe and effective for postoperative analgesia in children after thoracic, abdominal, urological, and orthopedic procedures, provided there is close monitoring by experienced staff in an appropriate environment operating with clear clinical guidelines. The hemodynamic and respiratory effects appear minimal compared with adults.[244] There is currently limited information on the pharmacokinetics of such infusions, but maximum local anesthetic doses must be adhered to,[245,246] e.g. bupivacaine 0.125% with fentanyl 1–2 $\mu g\,mL^{-1}$ at 0.4 $mL\,kg^{-1}\,h^{-1}$ in infants and children and bupivacaine 0.1% with fentanyl 1 $\mu g\,mL^{-1}$ in newborn infants at 0.25 $ml\,kg^{-1}\,h^{-1}$. Infants under 1 year of age should receive continuous cardiorespiratory monitoring, and regular observation should include pain score, sedation score, extent of motor blockade and cardiorespiratory parameters, as well as checking the infusion rate. All infusions should be delivered with an appropriate volumetric pump, and ideally solutions for epidural infusion should be prepared within a central sterile suite under the supervision of a pharmacist. An anesthesiologist should be available on site to deal with any problems, in particular inadequate analgesia due to block regression. The overall management should remain under the care of the anesthesiologist initiating the block, with appropriate on-call anesthetic cover after hours, preferably within the context of an acute pain service.

Caudal analgesia This is a simple and versatile way of administering drugs into the epidural space for both intra- and postoperative analgesia. Prolonged sacral analgesia in inpatients can be achieved by supplementation with caudal morphine 20–30 $\mu g\,kg^{-1}$, provided that appropriate facilities are available for respiratory monitoring. The analgesic blockade can be extended by placement of a caudal epidural catheter and the use of an infusion, as for lumbar epidural analgesia. The maximum dose of bupivacaine used in "single-shot" techniques such as caudal blocks,[247] i.e. 3 $mg\,kg^{-1}$ results in acceptable blood levels, but should be reduced to a maximum of 2.5 $mg\,kg^{-1}$ in the neonate. The addition of epinephrine (adrenaline) to bupivacaine does not appear to reduce absorption (as it does for lidocaine) and therefore does not permit a larger dose to be used; however, epinephrine has been shown to significantly prolong caudal blockade in infants and younger children.[248] Recent experience supports the safety of caudal clonidine (1–2 $\mu g\,kg^{-1}$) as an adjunct,[249,250] while the effects of clonidine and other agents on the duration of caudal block are being evaluated.[251] The advantages of other agents, e.g. ketamine, provide a mild caudal analgesia that is sometimes inadequate in this situation unless large doses are used.

Psychological strategies

Children's fear and anxiety of impending surgical procedures may be reduced by psychological preparation.[252–255] It would also seem sensible to familiarize the children with environments, equipment, and procedures preoperatively and maintain the child in contact with parents or carers up to the induction of anesthesia, which may decrease postoperative pain.[256–258] Premedication should be given by the least painful route, when possible along with the use of EMLA patches.

Pediatric pain service

The same principles apply in pediatrics as in adults when establishing a pediatric acute pain service.[84]

Acute neuropathic pain

Neuropathic pain can be defined as pain associated with injury, disease, or surgical section of the peripheral or central nervous system. It is underdiagnosed in all acute pain contexts and has a variety of clinical presentations. The management of acute neuropathic pain[175,259] is problematic. As with nociceptive pain, complete relief of pain is unlikely to occur, the realistic goal being to remove the associated suffering or reduce the pain experienced to an acceptable level for that patient. This type of pain may be only partially relieved by opioids (opioid-resistant pain). The pharmacological agents chosen to help manage acute neuropathic pain are extrapolated from those used to treat chronic neuropathic pain. These drugs are the anticonvulsants, e.g. carbamazepine and the tricyclic antidepressants. Corticosteroids are effective for short-term relief of neuropathic pain with particular application for pain associated with spinal cord compression, usually in combination with radiotherapy.[260]

Amputees[261]

Amputation of limbs and removal of viscera are sometimes associated with painful sequelae, which are commonly described as phantom pains. Other painful and nonpainful neurological phenomena are also associated with amputated limbs, e.g. stump pains.

As many as 60–80% of amputees may complain of phantom limb pain shortly after limb removal, with about 10% suffering persistent, severe, often incapacitating, pain. The syndrome is not influenced by age, gender, or pathology requiring amputation. It is less common in young children and congenital amputees. There are conflicting reports associating the preamputation pain with phantom pain. The onset of the pain is often within week of amputation and is believed to gradually diminish with time (years). The pain is usually intermittent, often occurring at least daily; only a few patients are in constant pain. The duration of attacks is usually measured in seconds, minutes, or hours; rarely days. The character of the pain is variously described most often as shooting, pricking, or boring as well as stabbing, squeezing, throbbing, and burning. The pain is usually located distally in the amputated limb. The experience of pain can be modulated by attention–distraction, anxiety, autonomic events, and environmental conditions. Rarely, the occurrence of the pain has been reported following spinal anesthesia in previously pain-free patients.

Almost all amputees experience stump pain immediately after amputation. In between 5% and 21% of patients, pain may persist despite apparent healing of the stump. The pain is variously described as pressing, throbbing, burning, squeezing, stabbing, or like electric shocks localized to the stump's posterior aspect close to the scar. These pains are easily precipitated by stimulating the stump, e.g. pressing on tender neuromata. Spontaneous stump movements which are painful are reported. There may be an association between stump and phantom pain.

The underlying mechanisms are not fully defined, but clearly amputation is the severest form of nerve injury and involves a combination of peripheral, spinal, and supraspinal mechanisms, which is reflected in the fact that persisting phantom limb pain is difficult to manage, causes significant distress to the sufferer, and consumes significant amounts of healthcare resources. A discussion of the management of chronic phantom pain is beyond our remit, but it may be the case that perioperative management of amputees employing neuraxial (notably epidural)

Table 74.14 *Terms used for opioid-tolerant patients*

Addiction is a psychological state that translates into drug-seeking behaviors and is marked by compulsion, loss of control over use, and ongoing use despite physical or social harm
Physical dependence refers to the development of withdrawal phenomena after cessation or antagonism of a drug
"*Pseudoaddiction*" is a term that has been coined to describe patients who exhibit drug-seeking behavior, resembling addiction, in response to unrelieved pain

and peripheral neural blockade may help to reduce the incidence of phantom limb and stump pains; however, unfortunately, the evidence is conflicting. Whether preamputation patients benefit (in terms of a lower incidence of developing phantom and stump pains) from neuraxial analgesia that spans the perioperative period is, on current evidence, debatable. There can be no doubt that patients presenting for amputations that have rest pain of ischemic origin, which is often opioid insensitive, should for humanitarian reasons be offered continuous epidural analgesia for the perioperative period.

Management of acute pain in opioid-tolerant patients[95]

Generally, two groups of patients are opioid tolerant:

1 patients who use/abuse opioids for their psychological effects;
2 patients receiving long-term opioids treatment for chronic or cancer pain.

Confusing the terminology defined in Table 74.14 can lead to catastrophic breakdowns of patient–healthcarer relationships to the detriment of all concerned. The term "pseudoaddiction" characterizes those patients who demand opioids and invariably enter into conflict with their healthcarers simply because their prescribed pain relief is inadequate, a not infrequent situation among cancer patients.[262]

Both these groups of patients frequently exhibit opioid tolerance, i.e. a decrease in the sensitivity to opioids so that progressively larger doses are needed to obtain the same effect. Tolerance to the respiratory-depressant effects of opioids also develops. This "physical dependence" on opioids will be manifested as a withdrawal (or abstinence) syndrome if the drug is acutely ceased or antagonized. The clinical features of an opioid withdrawal syndrome include yawning, sweating, lacrimation, rhinorrhea, anxiety, pupillary dilation, piloerection, and chills ("cold turkey"), tachycardia, hypertension, nausea and vomiting, cramping abdominal pains, and diarrhea. Development of opioid withdrawal syndrome postoperatively can potentially affect patient outcome seriously. This is not the time for healthcarers to indulge in moral indignation or exert personal prejudices and deprive these patients of their continuing "baseline" opioid requirements and additional opioids to relieve the acute postoperative pain. This is also not the time to embark on an "opioid addiction rehabilitation program."

The clinical management of these patients in the context of acute postoperative pain is often difficult and challenging. Generally, the management plan should:

1 Identify the group to which the patient belongs and the extent of the problem.
2 Accept that any pain scoring system is not likely to be reliable. Opioid abusers in particular often have very unrealistic expectations of what constitutes pain relief and report high pain scores while heavily sedated.
3 Design a management plan (and all staff should adhere to it) with ward staff and the patient as soon as possible; these patients should be identified preoperatively. The patient should be assured that the staff aim to give good pain relief but that patient safety is paramount! Meperidine should be avoided at ever-higher doses as it may precipitate normeperidine toxicity. There is a high prevalence of coexisting substance abuse, e.g. of alcohol and benzodiazepines.
4 Calculate the baseline opioid requirements of cancer and chronic pain sufferers from all oral opioids used.
5 Transfer back to oral opioid as soon as practical, using a long-acting opioid. Opioid abusers can recommence their preoperative methadone dosage with oral morphine for residual acute pain.
6 Set expected goals of dosage, route of administration, and time frame with the patient.
7 The goal for opioid abusers should be discharge on methadone into the care of a drug and alcohol service. Unfortunately, not all opioid abusers will want to enter a methadone program.

Intravenous PCA with opioids is now regarded as useful for both groups of patients. Baseline opioid requirements can be provided by a background infusion (to prevent withdrawal) and additional opioid required to manage the acute postoperative pain can be provided by an increased bolus requirement with the usual lockout period. The baseline and acute pain requirements can be provided by the oral route once it is re-established. Patients given high doses of opioids for any reason for as little as 7–10 days may exhibit a withdrawal syndrome on acute cessation of the drug. In the context of acute postoperative pain, as the acute pain subsides a natural opioid "weaning" process occurs as less opioid is required day by day. The clinical features of withdrawal can be prevented by dose reductions of 10–25% daily depending on the chronicity of the use.

Day-case surgery

The numbers of patients receiving day-case surgery has risen steadily in the last 20 years. Undoubtedly, this rise has yielded economic savings, but is also offers advantages to the patient. The quality of day-case surgery and anesthesia is judged not just by immediate hospital recovery but by recovery in the community. Good recovery requires a swift return to "street fitness" and ongoing freedom from pain, nausea, vomiting, and other complications. Good pain management after day-case surgery is challenging and has not always been satisfactory. Surveys have found that about 30% of patients suffer moderate to severe pain in the first 24 h after day-case surgery.[263,264] Other studies have shown that pain is a common reason for delayed discharge and unplanned hospital admission after day-case surgery[265,266] as well as a common reason for patients to consult their general practitioner.[267] Analgesic techniques used in day-case surgery should ideally be safe (especially when administered at home), effective, devoid of side-effects, and cost-effective. No single technique exists that will satisfy these requirements, and in practice analgesia is best achieved by a combination of drugs and techniques (multimodal analgesia).

ACUTE PAIN SERVICES

Currently there are three ways to deal with the problem of globally poor acute postoperative pain management: pin our hopes to magic pharmacological bullets; ignore the problem; or maximize the efficiency of our existing resources by developing multidisciplinary acute pain services (APS)[2] capable of delivering safe and effective postoperative pain management for all patients. As health consumer expectations and healthcare costs are rising,[268] the first two solutions are not viable.

If we intend to provide good-quality acute postoperative pain management for *all* our patients, we have to reappraise this component of healthcare – we have to fundamentally change the traditional system for the provision of analgesia in this circumstance.[82] The inadequacies of this "traditional system" have already been outlined; it was also noted that these inadequacies reflects a number of shortcomings in this system, not least of which is the large numbers of patients requiring pain relief. Reliance on the "high-tech" pain interventions[105] will benefit only a small number of patients and, unsupervised, may increase the rates of critical incidents and adverse outcomes.

Adopting the increasingly popular "multidisciplinary team" is an ideal model for an acute pain service.[2,269] Unfortunately, generally less than half of hospitals have developed any kind of service,[270–274] despite numerous recommendations encouraging this strategy.[2,105,275–280] Where acute pain services have been established, the "quality" of postoperative pain management is judged to have improved. It has been stated that any hospital undertaking major surgery should have an acute pain team that is able to identify individual patients' pain needs throughout the perioperative period. This approach offers a real possibility of being able to deal with the large numbers of patients involved yet being able to "individualize" their pain management.

We have adopted this idea at our institution, which annually undertakes over 30 000 inpatient surgical procedures, and have developed a multidisciplinary acute pain service that is nurse led and anesthesiologist supervised. Our operational policy is to empower the ward staff to work with their patients to provide individual pain management. This is achieved by providing:

1 The knowledge required, in the form of an educational and training program for all healthcarers, as a service's principal role.[15,82]
2 The tools, in the form of clinical guidelines covering:
   a prescribing analgesic medications;
   b pain assessment and documentation
   c ongoing pain management including discharge;
   d management of complications.
3 The back-up support:
   a a 24-h consultation service for pain-associated problems outside the parameters set by the clinical guidelines;
   b routine review of patients receiving "high-tech" pain interventions, i.e. locoregional drug infusions and i.v.-PCA;
   c administration, documentation, and consultation with other healthcare providers.
4 The feedback to improve, in the form of regular and systematic quality reviews of:
   a audit of patients expectations and experiences of their postoperative pain management;
   b audit of achievement of educational and training objectives;
   c database of clinical referrals;
   d database of critical incidents;
   e database of capital equipment.
5 The research and development to modify and adapt to patients' needs.

REFERENCES

1. Ready LB, Edwards WT (eds). *Management of Acute Pain: A Practical Guide.* Taskforce on Acute Pain. Seattle, WA: IASP Publications, 1992.
2. Royal College of Surgeons of England/College of Anaesthetists. *Commission on the Provision of Surgical Services: Report of the Working Party on Pain after Surgery.* London: Royal College of Surgeons of England/College of Anaesthetists, 1990.
3. EuroPain Task Force. *European Minimum Standards for the Management of Postoperative Pain.* UK: Pegasus Health International, 1998.
4. Bruster S, Jarman B, Bosanquet N, *et al.* National survey of hospital patients. *Br Med J* 1994; **309:** 1542–6.
5. Hamer M. Postoperative pain relief – time to take our heads out of the sand? *Anaesthesia* 1991; **46:** 167–8.
6. Breivik H. Benefits, risks and economics of post-operative pain management programmes. In: Breivik H (ed.). *Baillière's Clinical Anaesthesiology. Post-operative Pain Management* 1995; **9:** 403–22.
7. Wulf H, Neugebauer E. Guidelines for postoperative pain therapy. *Curr Opin Anaesthesiol* 1997; **10:** 380–5.
8. Mather L, Mackie J. The incidence of postoperative pain in children. *Pain* 1983; **15:** 271.
9. Beyer JE, DeGood DE, Ashley LC, Russell GA. Patterns of postoperative analgesic use with adults and children following cardiac surgery. *Pain* 1983; **17:** 71.
10. International Association for the Study of pain. Pain terms: a list with definitions and notes on usage. *Pain* 1979; **6:** 249–52.
11. Chapman CR, Gavrin J. Suffering: the contributions to persistent pain. *Lancet* 1999; **353:** 2233–7.
12. Parkhouse J. The incidence of postoperative pain. *Br J Anaesth* 1961; **33:** 345.
13. Freiha F, Zeineh S. Dorsal approach to upper urinary tract. *Urology* 1983; **21:** 15–16.
14. Rawal N. Postoperative pain and its management. In Raj PP (ed.). *Practical Management of Pain*, 2nd edn. Malvern, PA: Mosby–Year Book, 1992: 367.
15. Gould TH, Crosby DL, Harmer M, *et al.* Policy for controlling pain after surgery: effect of sequential changes in management. *Br Med J* 1992; **305:** 1187–93.
16. Rawal N. *Management of Acute and Chronic Pain.* London: BMJ Books, 1997.
17. Macintyre PE, Jarvis DA. Age is the best predictor of postoperative morphine requirements. *Pain* 1995; **64:** 357–64.
18. Cousins MJ, Bridenbaugh PO (eds). *Neural Blockade in Clinical Anesthesia and Management of Pain*, 3rd edn. Philadelphia, PA: Lippincott-Raven, 1998.
19. Wall PD, Melzack R (eds). *Textbook of Pain*, 4th edn. London: Churchill Livingstone, 1999.
20. Ekblom A, Rydh-Rinder M. Pain mechanisms: anatomy and physiology. In: Rawal N (ed.). *Management of Acute and Chronic Pain.* London: BMJ Books 1997: 1–22.
21. Woolf CJ, Chong MS. Preemptive analgesia – treating postoperative pain by preventing the establishment of central sensitisation. *Anesth Analg* 1993; **77:** 362–79.
22. Woolf CJ. Recent advances in the in the pathophysiology of acute pain. *Br J Anaesth* 1989; **63:** 139–46.
23. Dickenson AH. Central acute pain mechanisms. *Ann Med* 1995; **27:** 223–7.
24. Woolf CJ. Somatic pain – pathogenesis and prevention. *Br J Anaesth* 1995; **75:** 169–76.
25. Kehlet H. Modification of responses to surgery by neural blockade: clinical implications. In: Cousins MJ, Bridenbaugh PO (eds). *Neural Blockade in Clinical Anesthesia and Management of Pain*, 2nd edn. Philadelphia, PA: JB Lippincott, 1988: 145–88.
26. Van den Berghe G. Acute and prolonged critical illness as different neuroendocrine paradigms. *J Clin Endocrinol Metab* 1998; **83:** 1827–34.
27. Chernow B. Hormonal responses to a graded surgical stress. *Arch Intern Med 1987*; **147:** 1273–8.
28. Cousins MJ. Acute pain and the injury response. *Reg Anesth* 1989;**16:** 162–76.
29. Kehlet H. Postoperative pain relief: what is the issue? *Br J Anaesth* 1994; **72:** 365.
30. Sjogren S, Wright B. Cardiovascular changes during epidural blockade. *Acta Anaesthesiol Scand* 1972; **46** (Suppl.): 5.
31. Hoar PF, Hickey RF. Systemic hypertension following myocardial revascularisation: a method of treatment using epidural anesthesia. *J Cardiovasc Surg* 1976; **71:** 859.
32. Kumar B, Hibbert GR. Control of hypertension during aortic surgery using lumbar extradural blockade. *Br J Anaesth* 1984; **56:** 797.
33. Meissner A, Rolf N, Van Aken H. Thoracic epidural anaesthesia and the patient with heart disease: benefits, risks and controversies. *Anesth Analg* 1997; **85:** 517–28.
34. Yeager MP, Glass DD, Neff RK, Brinck-Johnsen T. Epidural anesthesia and analgesia in high-risk surgical patients. *Anesthesiology* 1987; **66:** 729–36.
35. Tuman KJ, McCarthy RJ, March RJ, *et al.* Effects of epidural anesthesia and analgesia on coagulation and outcome after major vascular surgery. *Anesth Analg* 1991; **73:** 696–704.
36. Garnett RL, MacIntyre A, Lindsay P, *et al.* Perioperative ischemia in aortic

surgery: combined epidural/general anesthesia and epidural analgesia vs general and IV analgesia. *Can J Anesth* 1996; **43:** 769–78.
37. Vik-Mo H, Ottesen S, Renck H. Cardiac effects of thoracic epidural analgesia before and during acute coronary artery occlusion in open chest dogs. *Scand J Clin Lab Invest* 1978; **38:** 737–46.
38. Klassen GA, Bramwell RS, Bromage PR, Zborowska-Sluis DT. Effect of acute sympathectomy by epidural anesthesia on the canine coronary circulation. *Anesthesiology* 1980; **52:** 8–15.
39. Reiz S, Ostman M. Coronary hemodynamic effects of general anesthesia and surgery. *Reg Anesth* 1982; **7:** S8–18.
40. Blomberg S, Curelaru J, Emmanuelsson H, *et al.* Thoracic epidural anaesthesia in patients with unstable angina pectoris. *Eur Heart J* 1989; **10:** 437.
41. Blomberg S, Emmanuelsson H, Richstein SE, *et al.* Thoracic epidural anaesthesia and central haemodynamics in patients with unstable anginal pectoris. *Anesth Analg* 1989; **69:** 558–62.
42. Koch M, Blomberg S, Emmanuelsson H, *et al.* Thoracic epidural anaesthesia improves global and regional left ventricular function during stress induced myocardial ischaemia in patients with coronary heart disease. *Anesth Analg* 1990; **71:** 625.
43. Olausson K, Magnusdottir H, Lurje L, *et al.* Anti-ischaemic and anti-anginal effects of thoracic epidural anesthesia versus those of conventional medical therapy in the treatment of severe refractory unstable angina. *Circulation* 1997; **96:** 2178–82.
44. Blomberg S, Emmanuelsson H, Kvist H, *et al.* Effects of thoracic epidural anesthesia on coronary arteries and arterioles in patients with coronary artery disease. *Anesthesiology* 1990; **73:** 840–7.
45. Mangano D, Layug EL, Wallace A, Tateo I. Effect of atenolol on mortality and cardiovascular morbidity after non-cardiac surgery. Multicenter Study of Perioperative Ischemia Research Group. *N Engl J Med* 1996; **335:** 1713–20.
46. Craig DB. Postoperative recovery of pulmonary function. *Anesth Analg* 1981; **60:** 46.
47. Modig J. Respiration and circulation after total hip replacement surgery: a comparison between parenteral analgesics and continuous lumbar epidural block. *Acta Anaesthesiol Scand* 1976; **20:** 225–36.
48. Ballantyne JC, Carr DB, deFerranti S, *et al.* The comparative effects of postoperative analgesic therapies on pulmonary outcome: cumulative meta-analyses of randomised controlled trials. *Anesth Analg* 1998; **86:** 598–612.
49. Christopherson R, Beattie C, Frank SM, *et al.* The Perioperative Ischemia Randomised Anesthesia Trial Study Group: perioperative morbidity in patients randomised to epidural or general anesthesia for lower-extremity vascular surgery. *Anesthesiology* 1993; **79:** 422–34.
50. Modig J, Borg T, Karlstrom G, *et al.* Thromboembolism after hip replacement: role of epidural and general anesthesia. *Anesth Analg* 1983; **62:** 174–80.
51. Modig J, Malmberg P, Karlstrom G. Effects of epidural versus general anaesthesia on calf blood flow. *Acta Anaesthesiol Scand* 1980; **24:** 305.
52. Gourdine SB, Fisher HA, Kaufman Jr RP, *et al.* Intravenous lidocaine speeds the return of bowel function, decreases postoperative pain, and shortens hospital stay in patients undergoing radical retropubic prostatectomy. *Anesth Analg* 1998; **86:** 235–9.
53. Nimmo WS. Effects of anaesthesia on gastric motility and emptying. *Br J Anaesth* 1984; **56:** 29–37.
54. Ahn H, Bronge A, Johanson D, *et al.* Effect of continuous epidural analgesia on gastro-intestinal motility. *Br J Surg* 1988; **75:** 1176–8.
55. Scheinin B, Asantila R, Orko R. The effect of bupivacaine and morphine on pain and bowel function after colonic surgery. *Acta Anaesthesiol Scand* 1987; **31:** 161–4.
56. Thoren T, Sundberg A, Wattwil M, *et al.* Effects of epidural bupivacaine and epidural morphine on bowel function and pain after hysterectomy. *Acta Anaesthesiol Scand* 1989; **33:** 181–95.
57. Wattwil M, thoen T, Hennerdal S, Garvill JE. Epidural analgesia with bupivacaine reduces postoperative paralytic ileus after hysterectomy. *Anesth Analg* 1989; **68:** 353–8.
58. Thorn SE, Wattwil M, Naslund I. Post-operative epidural morphine, but not epidural bupivacaine, delays gastric emptying on the first day after cholecystectomy. *Reg Anesth* 1992; **17:** 91–4.
59. Wiebalck A, Brodner G, Wan Aken H. The effect of adding sufentanil to bupivacaine for postoperative patient-controlled epidural analgesia. *Anesth Analg* 1997; **85:** 124–9.
60. Liu S, Carpenter RL, Mackey DC, *et al.* Effects of peri-operative analgesic technique on rate of recovery after colon surgery. *Anesthesiology* 1995; **83:** 757–75.
61. Riles TS, Fisher FS, Schaefer S, *et al.* Plasma catecholamines concentrations during abdominal aortic aneurysm surgery: the link to perioperative myocardial ischaemia. *Ann Vasc Surg* 1993; **7:** 213–19.
62. Weissman C. The metabolic response to stress: an overview and update. *Anesthesiology* 1990; **73:** 308–27.
63. Wilmore DW. Alterations in protein, carbohydrate, and fat metabolism in injured and septic patients. *J Am Coll Nutr* 1983; **2:** 3.
64. Kehlet H. Effect of pain relief on the surgical stress response. *Reg Anesth* 1996; **21:** 37–9.
65. Kehlet H. Modification of responses to surgery by neural blockade: clinical implications. In: Cousins MJ, Bridenbaugh PO (eds). *Neural Blockade in Clinical Aesthesia and Management of Pain*, 3rd edn. Philadelphia, PA: Lippincott-Raven, 1998: 129–75.
66. Bromage PR. 50 years on the wrong side of the reflex arc. *Reg Anesth* 1996; **21:** 1–4.
67. Brandt MR, Fernades A, Mordhorst R, Kehlet H. Epidural analgesia improves postoperative nitrogen balance. *Br Med J* 1978; **1:** 1106–8.
68. Jorgensen L, Raasmussen LS, Nielsen PT, *et al.* Antithrombotic efficacy of continuous extradural analgesia after knee replacement. *Br J Anaesth* 1991; **68:** 8–12.
69. Kehlet H. Acute pain control and accelerated postoperative surgical recovery. *Surg Clin N Am* 1999; **79:** 431–43.
70. Hayes C, Molloy AR. Neuropathic pain in the perioperative period. *Int Anesthesiol Clin* 1997; **35(2):** 67–81.
71. White CL, Le Fort SM, Amsel R, Jeans ME. Predictors of the development of chronic pain. *Res Nurse Hlth* **1997: 20:** 309–18.
72. Mersky H. Classification of chronic pain. Descriptions of chronic pain syndromes and definition of pain terms. *Pain* 1986; **3:** S1–225.
73. Back S, Noreng MF, Tjellden NU. Phantom limb pain in amputees during the first 12 months following amputation, after preoperative lumbar epidural blockade. *Pain* 1988; **33:** 287–301.
74. Katz J, jackson M, Kavanagh BP, *et al.* Acute pain after thoracic surgery predicts long-term post-thoracotomy pain. *Clin J Pain* 1996; **12:** 50–5.
75. Cousins MJ, Reeve TS, Glynn CJ, *et al.* Neurolytic lumbar sympathetic blockade: duration of denervation and relief of rest pain. *Anesth Intensive Care* 1979; **7:** 121–35.
76. Peck C. Psychological factors in acute pain management. In: Cousins MJ, Phillips GD (eds). *Acute Pain Management*. Edinburgh: Churchill Livingstone, 1986: 251–74.
77. Chapman CR, Turner JA. Psychological control of acute pain in medical settings. *J Pain Symptom Manage* 1985; **1:** 9–20.
78. Cesaro P, Ollat H. Pain and its treatments. *Eur Neurol* 1997; **38** (N3): 209–15.
79. Sjostrom B, Haljjamae H, Dahlgren LO, Lindstrom B. Assessment of postoperative pain: impact of clinical experience and professional role. *Acta Anaesthesiol Scand* 1997; **41:** 339–44.
80. Murphy DF, Donald A, Power C, *et al.* Measurements of pain: a comparison of the visual analogue with a non visual scale. *Clin J Pain* 1988; **3:** 197–9.
81. Hamer M, Davies KA. The effect of education, assessment and a standardised prescription on postoperative pain management. *Anaesthesia* 1998; **53:** 424–30.
82. Rawal N, Berggren L. Organisation of acute pain services: a low cost model. *Pain* 1994; **57:** 117–23.
83. Bates DW, Cullen DJ, Laird N, *et al.* Incidence of adverse drug events and potential adverse drug events. *JAMA* 1995; **274:** 29–34.
84. Lloyd-Thomas AR, Howard R. A pain service for children. *Paediatr Anaesth* 1994; **4:** 3–15.
85. McQuay H, Justins D, Moore A. Treating acute pain in hospital. *Br Med J* 1997; **314**: 1535.
86. Guyatt GH, Sackett DL, Sinclair JC, *et al.* Users' guide to the medical literature. IX. A method of grading health care recommendations. *JAMA* 1995; **274:** 1800–4.
87. McQuay HJ, Moore RA. *An Evidence-Based Resource for Pain Relief*. New York, NY: Oxford University Press.
88. *Acute Pain Management: Scientific Evidence*. Canberra: NHMRC, 1999.
89. Nierhaus A, Am Esch JC. Postoperative pain management. *Pain Rev* 1997;**4:** 149–57.
90. Lavies N, Hart L, Rounsefell B, Runciman W. Identification of patient, medical and nursing staff attitudes to postoperative opioid analgesia: stage 1 of a longitudinal study of postoperative analgesia. *Pain* 1992; **48:** 313–19.
91. Stoelting RK. *Pharmacology and Physiology in Anesthetic Practice,* 2nd edn. Philadelphia, PA: JB Lippincott, 1991.
92. Marks RM, Sachar EJ. Undertreatment of medical inpatients with narcotic analgesics. *Ann Intern Med* 1973; **78:** 173–81.
93. *Provision of Pain Services*. London: Association of Anaesthetists of Great Britain and Ireland and The Pain Society, 1997.

94. Pinnock CA, Derbyshire DR, Achola KG, Smith G. Absorption of controlled release morphine sulphate in the immediate postoperative period. *Br J Anaesth* 1986; **58:** 868–71.
95. Macintyre P, Ready LB. *Acute Pain Management: a Practical Guide*. London: WB Saunders, 1996.
96. Semple TJ, Upton Rn, Macintyre PE. Morphine blood concentrations in elderly postoperative patients following administration via an indwelling subcutaneous cannula. *Anaesthesia* 1996; **52:** 318–23.
97. Cooper IM. Morphine for postoperative analgesia; a comparison of intramuscular and subcutaneous routes of administration. *Anaesth Intensive Care* 1996; **24:** 574–8.
98. McArdle CS. Continuous and patient controlled analgesic infusions. In: Doyle E (ed.). *1986 International Symposium on Pain Control*. London: RSM International Congress and Symposium Series No. **123:** 17–22.
99. Owen H, Plummer J. Patient-controlled analgesia: current concepts in acute pain management. *CNS Drugs* 1997; **8:** 203–18.
100. Stacey BR, Rudt TE, Nelhaus D. Management of patient-controlled analgesia: a comparison of primary surgeons and a dedicated pain service. *Anesth Analg* 1997; **85:** 130–4.
101. Kreitzer JM, Kirschenbaum LD, EisenKraft JB. Safety of PCA devices. *Anesthesiology* 1989; **70:** 881.
102. Breivik H, Hogstrom H, Niemi B, *et al.* Safe and effective post-operative pain relief: introduction and continuous quality-improvement of comprehensive pain management programmes. In: Breivik H (ed.). *Baillière's Clinical Anaesthesiology Post-operative Pain Management* 1995; **94:** 23–60.
103. Woodhouse A, Hobbes AFT, Mather LE, *et al.* A comparison of morphine, pethidine and fentanyl in the postsurgical patient-controlled environment. *Pain* 1996; **64:** 115–21.
104. Borgbjerg FM, Nielsen K, Franks J. Experimental pain stimulates respiration and attenuates morphine-induced respiratory depression. *Pain* 1996; **64:** 123–8.
105. Ready LB, Oden R, Chadwick HS, *et al.* Development of an anesthesiology-based postoperative pain service. *Anesthesiology* 1988; **68:** 100–6.
106. Jones JG, Sapsford DJ, Wheatley RG. Postoperative hypoxaemia: mechanisms and time course. *Anaesthesia* 1990; **45:** 566–73.
107. Bulow HH, Linnemann M, Berg H, *et al.* Respiratory changes during treatment of postoperative pain with high-dose transdermal fentanyl. *Acta Anaesthesiol Scand* 1995; **39:** 835–9.
108. Cately DM, Thornton C, Jordan C, *et al.* Pronounced episodic oxygen desaturation in the postoperative period: its association with ventilatory pattern and analgesic regimen. *Anesthesiology* 1985; **63:** 20–8.
109. Miller L, Gertel M, Fox GS, *et al.* Comparison of the effect of narcotic and epidural analgesia on postoperative respiratory function. *Am J Surg* 1976; **131:** 291.
110. Beydon L, Hassapopoulos J, Quera MA, *et al.* Risk factors for oxygen desaturation during sleep after abdominal surgery. *Br J Anaesth* 1992; **69:** 137–42.
111. Reeder MK, Goldman MD, Loh L, *et al.* Postoperative hypoxaemia after major abdominal vascular surgery. *Br J Anaesth* 1992; **68:** 23–26.
112. Mangano DT, Browner WS, Hollenberg M, *et al.* Long-term cardiac prognosis following non-cardiac surgery. The study of Postoperative Ischaemia Group. *JAMA* 1992; **268:** 233–9.
113. Kaiko RF, Roley KM, Grabinski PY, *et al.* Central nervous system excitatory effects of meperidine in cancer patients. *Ann Neurol* 1983; **13:** 180–5.
114. Stone PA, Macintyre PE, Jarvis DA, *et al.* Norpethidine toxicity and patient controlled analgesia. *Br J Anaesth* 1993; **71:** 738–40.
115. Abbott FV, Palmour RM. Morphine-6-glucoronide: analgesic effects and receptor binding profile in rats. *Life Sci* 1988; **43:** 1685–95.
116. Bartlett SE, Dodd PR, Smith MT. Pharmacology of morphine and morphine-3-glucoronide at opioid, excitatory amino acid, GABA and glycine binding sites. *Pharmacol Toxicol* 1994; **31:** 410–22.
117. Bartlett SE, Cramond M, Smith MT. The excitatory effects of morphine-3-glucoronide are attenuated by LY274614, a competitive NMDA receptor antagonist, and by midazolam, an antagonist at the benzodiazepine site on the GABA receptor complex. *Life Sci* 1994; **54:** 687–94.
118. Davies G, Kinswood C, Street M. Pharmacokinetics of opioids in renal dysfunction. *Clin Pharmacol* 1996; **31:** 410–22.
119. Osborne R, Joel R, Grebenik K, *et al.* The pharmacokinetics of morphine and morphine glucuronides in kidney failure. *Clin Pharmacol Ther* 1993; **54:** 158–67.
120. Andrews PLR. Physiology of nausea and vomiting. *Br J Anaesth* 1992; **69:** 2–20.
121. Watcha MF, White PF. Postoperative nausea and vomiting: its etiology, treatment and prevention. *Anesthesiology* 1992; **77:** 162–84.
122. Leeser J, Lip H. Prevention of postoperative nausea and vomiting using ondansetron, a new selective 5-HT3 receptor antagonist. *Anesth Analg* 1991; **72:** 751–5.
123. Watcha MF, Smith I. Cost-effectiveness analysis of anti-emetic therapy for ambulatory surgery. *J Clin Anesth* 1994; **6:** 370–7.
124. Paxton LD, McKay AC, Mirakrhur RK. Prevention of nausea and vomiting after day case gynaecological laparoscopy. *Anaesthesia* 1995; **50:** 403–6.
125. Chapman CR, Hill HF. Prolonged morphine self-administration and addiction liability. *Cancer* 1989; **63:** 1636–44.
126. Foley KM. Controversies in cancer pain: medical perspective. *Cancer* 1989; **63** (Suppl.): 2257–65.
127. Porter J, Jick H. Addiction rare in patients treated with opioids. *N Engl J Med* 1980;**302:** 123.
128. Schug SA, Sidebottom DA, McGuinnety M. Acetaminophen as an adjunct to morphine by patient-controlled analgesia in the management of acute postoperative pain. *Anesth Analg* 1998; **87:** 368–72.
129. Bannwarth B, Demotesmainard F, Schaeverbeke T, *et al.* Central analgesic effects of aspirin-like drugs. *Fundament Clin Pharmacol* 1995; **9:** 1–7.
130. Jarde O, Boccard E. parenteral versus oral route increases paracetamol efficacy. *Clin Drug Invest* 1997; **14:** 474–81.
131. Peduto VA, Ballabio M, Stefanini S. Efficacy of proparacetamol in the treatment of postoperative pain – morphine sparing effect in orthopedic surgery. *Acta Anaesthesiol Scand* 1998;**42:** 293–8.
132. Kweekel-De Vries WJ, Spierkijk J, *et al.* A new soluble acetylsalicylic acid derivative in the treatment of postoperative pain. *Br J Anaesth* 1974; **46:** 133–5.
133. Reasbeck PG, Rice ML, Reasbeck JC. Double blind controlled trial of indomethacin as an adjuvant to narcotic analgesia after major abdominal surgery. *Lancet* 1982; **ii:** 115–18.
134. Turner GA, Gorringe J. Indomethacin as adjunct analgesia following open cholecystectomy. *Anaesth Intensive Care* 1994; **22:** 25–9.
135. Elkahim M, Nafie M. Intravenous temoxicam for analgesia during caesarean section. *Br J Anaesth* 1995; **74:** 643–6.
136. Vandermeulen EP, Van Aken H, Vermylen J. Intravenous administration of temoxicam 40mg for postoperative analgesia; a double blind, placebo controlled multicentre study. *Eur J Anaesth* 1997; **14:** 250–7.
137. Gilils JC, Brogden RN. Ketorolac: a reappraisal of its pharmacodynamic and pharmacokinetic properties and therapeutic use in pain management. *Drugs* 1997; **53:** 139–88.
138. Power I, Noble DW, Douglas E, *et al.* Comparison of intramuscular ketorolac, trometerol and morphine sulphate for pain relief after cholecystectomy. *Br J Anaesth* 1990; **65:** 448–55.
139. Brown CR, Mazzulla JP, Mok MS, *et al.* Comparison of repeat doses of intramuscular ketorolac tromethamine and morphine sulphate for analgesia after major surgery. *Pharmacotherapy* 1990; **10:** 455–505.
140. Kostamovaara PA, Hendolin H, Kokki H, Nuutinen LS. Ketorolac, diclofenac and ketoprofen are equally efficacious for pain relief after total hip replacement surgery. *Br J Anaesth* 1998; **81:** 369–72.
141. Etches RC, Warriner CB, Badner N, *et al.* Continuous intravenous administration of ketorolac reduces pain and morphine consumption after total hip or knee arthroplasty. *Anesth Analg* 1995; **81:** 1175–80.
142. Gillberg LE, Harsten AS, Stahl LB. Preoperative diclofenac sodium reduces post-laparoscopy pain. *Can J Anesth* 1993; **40:** 406–8.
143. Jakobsson J, Rane K, Davidson S. Intramuscular NSAIDs reduce postoperative pain after minor outpatient anaesthesia. *Eur J Anaesthesiol* 1996; **13:** 67–71.
144. Power I, Chambers WA, Greer IA, *et al.* Platelet function after intramuscular diclofenac. *Anaesthesia* 1990; **45:** 916–19.
145. Cepeda SM, Vargas L, Ortegon G, *et al.* Comparative analgesic efficacy of patient controlled analgesia with ketorolac versus morphine after elective intra abdominal operations. *Anesth Analg* 1995; **80:** 1150–3.
146. Espinet A, Henderson DJ, Faccenda KA. Does pre-incisional thoracic extradural block combined with diclofenac reduce postoperative pain after abdominal hysterectomy? *Br J Anaesth* 1996; **76:** 209–13.
147. Buggy J, Wall C, Carton EG. Pre-operative or postoperative diclofenac for laparoscopic tubal ligation. *Br J Anaesth* 1994; **73:** 767–70.
148. Power I, Bowler GM, Pugh GC. Ketorolac as a component of balanced analgesia after thoracotomy. *Br J Anaesth* 1994; **72:** 224–6.
149. Pavy TJG, Gambling DR, Merrick PM, *et al.* Rectal indomethacin potentiates spinal morphine after caesarean section. *Anaesth Intensive Care* 1995; **23:** 555–9.
150. Royal College of Anaesthetists. *Guidelines for the Use of Non-steroidal Anti-inflammatory Drugs in the Perioperative Period*. London: Royal College of Anaesthetists, 1998.
151. Merry A, Power I. Perioperative NSAIDs: towards greater safety. *Pain Rev* 1995; **2:** 268–91.
152. Strom BL, Berlin JA, Kinman JL, *et al.* Parenteral ketorolac and risk of

gastrointestinal and operative site bleeding: a postmarketing survey. *JAMA* 1996; **69:** 451–6.
153. Power I. Aspirin-induced asthma. *Br J Anaesth* 1993; **71:** 619–21.
154. Power I, Cumming AD, Pugh GC, *et al.* Effect of diclofenac on renal function and prostacyclin generation after surgery. *Br J Anaesth* 1992; **69:** 224–6.
155. Smith K, Halliwell RMT, Lawrence S, *et al.* Acute renal failure associated with intramuscular ketorolac. *Anaesth Intensive Care* 1993; **21:** 700–3.
156. Jaquenod M, Ronnhedh C, Cousins MJ, *et al.* Factors influencing ketorolac-induced perioperative renal dysfunction. *Anesth Analg* 1998; **86:** 1090–7.
157. Feldman HI, Kinman JL, Berlin JA, *et al.* Parenteral ketorolac; the risk for acute renal failure. *Ann Intern Med* 1997; **126:** 193–9.
158. James DN, Fernandes JR, Calder I, Smith M. Low-dose aspirin and intracranial surgery. A survey of the opinions of consultant neuroanaesthetists in the UK. *Anaesthesia* 1997; **52:** 169–72.
159. Power I, Chambers WA, Greer IA, *et al.* Platelet function after intramuscular diclofenac. *Anaesthesia* 1990; **45:** 916–19.
160. Rodgers RP, Levin J. Bleeding time: a guide to its diagnostic and clinical utility. *Arch Pathol Lab Med* 1990; **114:** 1187–8.
161. Anonymous. Clasp – a randomised trial of low-dose aspirin for the prevention and treatment of pre-eclampsia among 9,364 pregnant women. *Lancet* 1994; **343:** 619–29.
162. Horlocker TT, Wedel DJ, Schroder DR, *et al.* Pre-operative anti-platelet therapy does not increase the risk of spinal haematoma associated with regional anaesthesia. *Anesth Analg* 1995; **80:** 303–9.
163. Smith MS, Muir H, Hall RI. Peri-operative management of drug therapy – clinical considerations. *Drugs* 1996; **51:** 238–59.
164. Vane JR, Bakhle YS, Botting RM. Cyclooxygenases 1 and 2. *Annu Rev Pharmacol Toxicol* 1998; **38:** 97–120.
165. Fosslien E. Adverse effects of non-steroidal anti-inflammatory drugs on the gastro-intestinal system. *Ann Clin Lab Sci* 1998; **28:** 67–81.
166. Laneuville O, Breuer DK, Dewitt DL, *et al.* Differential inhibition of human endoperoxide H synthases -1 and -2 by non-steroidal anti-inflammatory drugs. *J Pharmacol Exp Ther* 1994; **271:** 927–34.
167. Hawkey CJ. Future treatments for arthritis: new NSAIDs, NONSAIDs, or no ASAIDs? *Gastroenterology* 1995; **109:** 614–16.
168. Lund B, Distel M, Bluhmki E. A double blind, randomised, placebo-controlled study of efficacy and tolerance of meloxicam treatment in patients with osteo-arthritis of the knee. *Scand J Rheumatol* 1998; **27:** 32–7.
169. The HSG, Lund B, distel MR, *et al.* A double blind, randomised trial to compare meloxicam 15mg with diclofenac 100mg in the treatment of osteo-arthritis of the knee. *Osteoarthritis Cartilage* 1997; **5:** 283–8.
170. Furst DE. Meloxicam – selective cox-2 inhibition in clinical practice. *Semin Arthritis Rheum* 1997; **26:** 21–7.
171. Rabasseda X. Nimesulide – a selective cyclooxygenase 2 inhibitor antiinflammatory drug. *Drugs Today* 1996; **2:** 1–23.
172. Famaey JP. In vitro and in vivo pharmacological evidence of selective cyclooxygenase-2 inhibition by nimesulide – an overview. *Inflamm Res* 1997; **46:** 437–46.
173. McQuay H, Tramer M, Nye BA. A systematic review of antidepressants in neuropathic pain. *Pain* 1996; **68:** 217–27.
174. Murphy DF. Interpleural analgesia. *Br J Anaesth* 1993; **71:** 426–34.
175. Frenette L, Boudreault D, Guay J. Interpleural analgesia improves pulmonary function after cholecystectomy. *Can J Anaesth* 1991; **38:** 71–4.
176. Dahl JB, Moinche S, Kehlet H. Wound infiltration with local anaesthetic for postoperative pain relief. *Acta Anaesthesiol Scand* 1994; **38:** 7–14.
177. Breivik H, Niemi H, Haugtomt H, Hogstrom H. Optimal epidural analgesia: importance of drug combinations and correct segmental site of injection. In: Breivik H (ed.). *Baillière's Clinical Anaesthesiology, Postoperative Pain Management.* 1995; 9493–512.
178. Liu SS, Allen HW, Olsson GL. Patient-controlled epidural analgesia with bupivacaine and fentanyl on hospital wards: prospective experience with 1,030 surgical patients. *Anesthesiology* 1998; **88:** 688–95.
179. Ready LB, Loper KA, Nessly M. Postoperative epidural morphine is safe on surgical wards. *Anesthesiology* 1991; **75:** 452–6.
180. Schug SA, Torrie JJ. Safety assessment of postoperative pain management by an acute pain service. *Pain* 1993; **55:** 387–91.
181. Scott DA, Beilby DS, McClymont C. Postoperative analgesia using epidural infusions of fentanyl and bupivacaine: a prospective analysis of 1,014 patients. *Anesthesiology* 1995; **83:** 727–37.
182. Tanaka K, Watanabe R, Harada T. Extensive application of epidural anesthesia and analgesia in a university hospital; incidence of complications related to technique. *Reg Anesth* 1993; **18:** 34–38.
183. Breivik H. Prolonged postoperative epidural analgesia: how to make it work safely and effectively. *Acta Anaesthesiol Scand* 1996; **109** (Suppl.): 173–4.
184. Cousins MJ, Mather LE. Intrathecal and epidural administration of opioids. *Anesthesiology* 1984; **61:** 276–310.
185. Liu S, Carpenter RL, Neal JM. Epidural anesthesia and analgesia: their role in perioperative outcome. Anesthesiology 1995; **82:** 1474–506.
186. Bernards CM. Flux of morphine, fentanyl, and alfentanil through rabbit arteries in vivo: evidence supporting a vascular route for redistribution of opioids between the epidural space and the spinal cord. *Anesthesiology* 1993; **78:** 1126–31.
187. Hansdottir V, Woestenborghs R, Norberg G. The cerebrospinal fluid and plasma pharmacokinetics of sufentanil after thoracic or lumbar epidural administration. *Anesth Analg* 1995; **80:** 724–9.
188. Hansdottir V, Bake B, Norberg G. The analgesic efficacy and adverse effects of continuous epidural sufentanil and bupivicaine infusion after thoracotomy. *Anesth Analg* 1996; **83:** 394–400.
189. Hansdottir V, Woestenborghs R, Norberg G. The pharmacokinetics of continuous epidural sufentanil and bupivicaine infusion after thoracotomy. *Anesth Analg* 1996; **83:** 401–6.
190. Giebler SJ. Incidence of neurological complications related to thoracic epidural catheterisation. *Anesthesiology* 1997; **86:** 55–63.
191. Kroll DA, Caplan RA, Posner K, *et al.* Nerve injury associated with anesthesia. *Anesthesiology* 1990; **73:** 202–7.
192. US Food and Drug Administration. *FDA Public Health Advisory Committee Report.* December 1997.
193. Tryba M, Wedel DJ. Central neuraxial block and low-molecular-weight heparin (enoxaparin): lessons learned from two different dosage regimens in two different continents. *Acta Anaesthesiol Scand* 1997; **41:** 100–4.
194. Horlocker TT, Wedel DJ. Spinal and epidural blockade and perioperative low molecular weight heparin: smooth sailing on the Titanic. *Anesth Analg* 1998; **86:** 115–36.
195. Vandermeulen EP, Van Aken H, Vermylen J. Anticoagulants and spinal–epidural anesthesia. *Anesth Analg* 1994; **79:** 1165–77.
196. Kehlet H, Dahl JB. Postoperative pain. *World J Surg* 1993; **17:** 215–19.
197. Kehlet H, Dahl JB. The value of "multimodal" or "balanced" analgesia in postoperative pain treatment. *Anesth Analg* 1993; **77:** 1048–56.
198. Brodner G, Pogtatzki E, Van Aken H, *et al.* A multimodal approach to control postoperative pathophysiology and rehabilitation in patients undergoing abdominothoracic esophagectomy. *Anesth Analg* 1998; **96:** 228–34.
199. Schulze S, Roikjaer O, Hasselstrom L, *et al.* Epidural bupivicaine and morphine plus systemic indomethacin eliminates pain but not the systemic response and convalescence after cholecystectomy. *Surgery* 1988; **103:** 321–7.
200. Dahl JB, Rosenberg J, Dirkes WE, *et al.* Prevention of postoperative pain by balanced analgesia. *Br J Anaesth* 1990; **64:** 518–20.
201. Moiniche S, Hjortso NC, Hansen BL, *et al.* The effect of balanced analgesia on early convalescence after major orthopaedic surgery. *Acta Anaesthesiol Scand* 1994; **38:** 328–35.
202. Moniniche S, Dahl JB, Rosenberg J, *et al.* Colonic resection with early discharge after combined subarachnoid–epidural analgesia, preoperative glucocorticoids and early postoperative mobilisation and feeding in a pulmonary high-risk patient. *Reg Anesth* 1994; **19:** 352–6.
203. Bardram L, Funch-Jensen P, Jensen P, *et al.* Recovery after laparoscopic colonic surgery with epidural analgesia and early oral nutrition and mobilisation. *Lancet* 1995; **345:** 763–4.
204. McQuay H. Pre-emptive analgesia. *Br J Anaesth* 1992; **69:** 1–3.
205. Tverskoy M, Cozacov C, Ayache M, *et al.* Postoperative pain after inguinal herniorrhaphy with different types of anesthesia. *Anesth Analg* 1990; **70:** 29–35.
206. Rice ASC. The relative effects of analgesic therapy administered before, during or after surgical injury. *Semin Neurosci* 1995; **7:** 245–51.
207. Dahl JB, Hansen BL, Hirortso NC, *et al.* Influence of the timing of the effect of continuous extradural analgesia with bupivicaine and morphine after major abdominal surgery. *Br J Anaesth* 1992; **69:** 4–8.
208. Dierking GW, Dahl JB, Kanstrup J, *et al.* Effect of pre- vs postoperative inguinal field block on postoperative pain after herniorrhaphy. *Br J Anaesth* 1992; **68:** 344–8.
209. Dahl JB, Daugaard JJ, Ramussen B, *et al.* Immediate and prolonged effects of pre- versus postoperative epidural analgesia with bupivicaine and morphine on pain at rest and during mobilisation after total knee arthroplasty. *Acta Anaesthesiol Scand* 1994; **38:** 557–61.
210. Aguilar JL. Absence of an early pre-emptive effect after thoracic extradural bupivicaine in thoracic surgery. *Br J Anaesth* 1996; **76:** 72–6.
211. Pedersen JL, Crawford ME, Dahl JB, *et al.* Effect of preemptive nerve

block on inflammation and hyperalgesia after human thermal injury. *Anesthesiology* 1996; **84:** 1020–6.

212. Johnston M, Vogele C. Benefits of psychological preparation for surgery: a meta-analysis. *Ann Behav Med* 1993; **15:** 245–56.
213. Carroll D, Tramer M, McQuay H, *et al.* Randomisation is important in studies with pain outcomes: systematic review of transcutaneous electrical nerve stimulation in acute postoperative pain. *Br J Anaesth* 1996; **77:** 798–803.
214. Christensen PA, Noreg P, Andersen PE, *et al.* Electroacupuncture and postoperative pain. *Br J Anaesth* 1989; **62:** 258–62.
215. Sung YF, Kutner MH, Cerine FC, *et al.* Comparison of the effects of acupuncture and codeine on postoperative dental pain. *Anesth Analg* 1977; **56:** 473–8.
216. Foster RL, Hester NO. Administration of analgesics for children's pain. *Pain* (Suppl. **5**): S27.
217. Schechter NL, Allen DA, Hanson K, *et al.* Status of pediatric pain control: a comparison of hospital analgesic usage in children and adults. *Pediatrics* 1986; **77:** 11–15.
218. Fitzgerald M. Developmental neurobiology of pain. In: Wall PD, Melzack R (eds). *Textbook of Pain*, 4th edn. London: Churchill Livingstone, 1999: 235–51.
219. Maunuksela EL, Olkkola KT, Korpela R. Measurement of pain in children with self-reporting and behaviour assessment. *Clin Pharmacol Ther* 1987; **42:** 137–41.
220. Finley GA, McGrath PJ. *Measurements of Pain in Infants and Children. Progress in Pain Research and Management*, Vol. 10, Seattle, WA: IASP, 1998.
221. Krechel SW, Bildner J. CRIES: a new neonatal postoperative pain measurement score. Initial testing of validity and reliability. *Paediatr Anaesth* 1995; **5:** 53–61.
222. Hester NO, Foster RL. Measurement of pain in children: generalisability and validity of the Pain Ladder and Poker Chip Tool. In: Tyler DC, Krane EJ (eds). *Advances in Pain Research and Therapy: Pediatric Pain,* Vol. 15. New York, NY: Raven Press, 1990: 79–84.
223. Whaley L, Wong D. *Nursing Care of Infants and Children*, 4th edn. St Louis, MO: Mosby-Yearbook, 1991.
224. Wilson GA, Doyle E. Validation of three paediatric pain scores for use by parents. *Anaesthesia* 1996; **51:** 1005–7.
225. Anderson BJ, Woolard GA, Holford NHG. Pharmacokinetics of rectal paracetamol after major surgery in children. *Paediatr Anaesth* 1996; **24:** 669–73.
226. Berde CB. Pediatric postoperative pain management. *Pediatr Clin N Am* 1989**; 36:** 921–40.
227. Morton NS. Development of a monitoring protocol for the safe use of opioids in children. *Paediatr Anaesth* 1993; **3:** 179–84.
228. Hamunen K. Ventilatory effects of morphine, pethidine and methadone in children. *Br J Anaesth* 1993; **70:** 414–18.
229. Lynn AM, Slattery JT. Morphine pharmacokinetics in early infancy. *Anesthesiology* 1987; **66:** 136–9.
230. Choonara I, Ekbom Y, Lindstrom B, *et al.* Morphine sulphate in children. *Br J Clin Pharmacol* 1990; **30:** 897–900.
231. Barrett DA, Elias-Jones AC, Rutter N, *et al.* Morphine pharmacokinetics after diamorphine infusion in prem ature neonates. *Br J Clin Pharmacol* 1991; **32:** 31–7.
232. McRorie TI, Lynn AM, Nespeca MK, *et al.* The maturation of morphine clearance and metabolism. *Am J Dis Childh* 1992; **146:** 972–6.
233. Aynsley-Green A. Pain and stress in infancy and childhood – where to now? *Paediatr Anaesth* 1996; **6:** 167–72.
234. Lamacraft G, Cooper MG, Cabaletto BP. Subcutaneous cannulae for morphine boluses in children: assessment of a technique. *J Pain Symptom Manage* 1997; **13:** 43–9.
235. McNicol LR. Postoperative pain in children using continuous subcutaneous morphine. *Br J Anaesth* 1993; **71:** 396–9.
236. Bray RJ. Postoperative analgesia provided by morphine infusion in children. *Anaesthesia* 1983; **38:** 1075–8.
237. Hendrickson M, Myre L, Johnson DG, *et al.* Postoperative analgesia in children: a prospective study of intermittent intramuscular injections versus continuous intravenous infusion of morphine. *J Pediatr Surg* 1990; **25:** 185–91.
238. Lynn AM, Opein KE, Tyler DC. Morphine infusion after pediatric cardiac surgery. *Crit Care Med* 1984;**12:** 863–6.
239. Caukroger PB, Chapman MJ, Davey RB. Pain control in paediatric burns – the use of patient-controlled analgesia. *Burns* 1991;**17:** 396–9.
240. Berde CB, Lehn BM, Yee JD, *et al.* Patient-controlled analgesia in children and adolescents: a randomised, prospective comparison with intramuscular administration of morphine for postoperative analgesia. *J Pediatr* 1991;**118:** 460–6.
241. Doyle E, Harper I, Morton NS. Patient-controlled analgesia with low-dose background infusions after lower abdominal surgery in children. *Br J Anaesth* 1993; **71:** 818–22.
242. Trotter C, Martin P, Youngson G, *et al.* A comparison between ilioinguinal–iliohypogastric nerve block performed by the anaesthetist or surgeon for postoperative analgesia following groin surgery in children. *Paediatr Anaesth* 1995; 5: 363–7.
243. Gourrier E, Karoubi P, El Hanache A, *et al.* Use of EMLA cream in a department of neonatology. *Pain* 1996; **68:** 431–4.
244. Murat I, Delleur MM, Esteve C, *et al.* Continuous extradural anaesthesia in children – clinical and haemodynamic implications. *Br J Anaesth* 1987**; 69:** 1441.
245. Berde CB. Convulsions associated with pediatric anesthesia [editorial]. *Anesth Analg* 1992; **75:** 164–6.
246. Eyres Rl. Local anesthetic agents in infancy. *Paediatr Anaesth* 1995; **22:** 213–18.
247. Eyres RL, Bishop W, Oppenheimer R, *et al.* Plasma bupivacaine concentration in children during caudal anaesthesia. *Anaesth Intensive Care* 1983; **11:** 20–2.
248. Warner MA, Kunkel SE, Offord SO, *et al.* The effects of age, epinephrine and operative site on duration of caudal analgesia in pediatric patients. *Anesth Analg* 1987; **66:** 995–8.
249. Jamali S, Monin S, Begon C, *et al.* Clonidine in pediatric caudal anesthesia. *Anesth Analg* 1994; **78:** 663–6.
250. Constant I, Gall O, Gouyet L, *et al.* Addition of clonidine or fentanyl to local anaesthetics prolongs the duration of surgical analgesia after single shot caudal clock in children. *Br J Anaesth* 1998; **80:** 294–298.
251. Cook B, Grubb DJ, Aldridge LA, *et al.* Comparison of the effects of adrenaline, clonidine and ketamine on the duration of caudal analgesia produced by bupivacaine in children. *Br J Anaesth* 1995; **75:** 698–701.
252. Ferguson BF. Preparing young children for hospitalisation: a comparison of two methods. *Pediatrics* 1979; **64:** 656–64.
253. McGrath MM. Group preparation of pediatric surgical patients. *Image* 1979; **11:** 52–62.
254. Visintalner M, Wolfer J. Psychological preparation for pediatric surgical patients: the effects on children's and parents' stress responses and adjustment. *Pediatrics* 1975; **56:** 187–202.
255. Woffer J, Visintainer M. Prehospital psychological preparation for tonsillectomy patients: effects on children's and parents' adjustments. *Pediatrics* 1979; **64:** 646–655.
256. Hannallah RS, Rosales JK. Experience with parents' presence during anaesthesia induction in children. *Can Anesth Soc J* 1983; **30:** 286–9.
257. Johnston CC, Stevens B, Craig KD, *et al.* Parental presence during anesthesia induction. *Assoc Operating Room Nurses J* 1988;**47:** 187–194
258. Schofield N, White J. Interrelations between children, parents, premedication and anaesthetists in paediatric day stay surgery. *Br Med J* 1989; **299:** 1371–5.
259. McQuay H, Carrol D, Jadad AR, *et al.* Anticonvulsants drugs for the management of pain: a systematic review. *Br Med J* 1995; **311:** 1047–52.
260. Boogerd W, van der Sande JJ. Diagnosis of spinal cord compression in malignant disease. *Cancer Treat Rev* 1993; **19:** 129–150.
261. Jensen TS, Nikolajsen L. Phantom pain and other phenomena after amputation. In: Wall PD, Melzack R (eds). *Textbook of Pain*, 4th edn. London: Churchill Livingstone, 1999: 799–814.
262. Weissman DE, Haddox JD. Opioid pseudoaddiction: an iatrogenic syndrome. *Pain* 1989; 363–6.
263. The Audit Commission of England and Wales. *A Short Cut to Better Services: Day Surgery in England & Wales*. London: HSMO, 1990.
264. Hawkshaw D. A day surgery patient follow-up. *Br J Nurs* 1994; **3:** 348–50.
265. Fancourt-Smith PF, Hornstein J, Jenkins LC. Hospital admissions from the hospital day care centre of Vancouver General Hospital 1977–1987. *Can J Anesth* 1990; **37:** 699–704.
266. Gold BS, Kitz DS, Lecky H, *et al.* Unanticipated admission to the hospital following ambulatory surgery. *JAMA* 1989; **262:** 3008–10.
267. Fraser RA, Hotz SB, Hurtig JB, *et al.* The prevalence and impact of pain after day-care tubal ligation surgery. *Pain* 1989; **39:** 189–201.
268. Breivik H. Cost-effectiveness of postoperative pain management. *European Society of Anaesthesiologists Refresher Course Lectures*, Vol. 1, 183–8.
269. *The Anaesthesia Team*. London: Association of Anaesthetists of Great Britain and Ireland, 1998.
270. *Professional Roles in Anaesthetics: A Scoping Study*. London: NHS Executive, 1996.
271. *Anaesthesia Under Examination*. Report of the National Audit Commission. Oxford: National Publications, 1997.
272. Rawal N, Allvin R. Acute pain services in Europe: a 17-nation survey of

105 hospitals – the EuroPain Acute Pain Working Party. *Eur J Anaesthesiol* 1998; **15:** 354–63 (also reported as Rawal N. *Reg Anesth* 1995; **20:** S85).
273. Semple P, Jackson IJB. Postoperative pain control. A survey of current practice. *Anaesthesia* 1991; **46:** 1074–6.
274. Zimmerman DL Stewart J. Postoperative pain management and acute pain service activity in Canada. *Can J Anesth* 1993; **40:** 568–75.
275. US Department of Health and Human Services. *Acute Pain Management. Clinical Practice Guidelines.* AHCPR Publications No. 92-0032, 1992.
276. International Association for the Study of Pain (IASP). Management of acute pain. In: Ready LB, Edwards WT (eds). *A Practical Guide Task Force.* Seattle, WA: IASP Publications, 1992.
277. Faculty of Anaesthetists and Royal Australasian College of Surgeons. *Statement on Acute Pain Management.* Faculty of Anaesthetists and Royal Australasian College of Surgeons, 1991.
278. Ready LB, Ashburn M, Caplan RA, *et al.* Practice Guidelines for Acute Pain Management in the Perioperative Setting – a report of the American Society of Anesthesiologists Task Force on Pain Management, Acute Pain section. *Anesthesiology* 1995; **82:** 1071–81.
279. Wheatley RG, Madej TH, Jackson IJB, *et al.* The first years experience of an acute pain service. *Br J Anaesth* 1991; **67:** 353–9..
280. Cartwright PD, *et al.* Introducing an acute pain service. *Anaesthesia* 1991; **46:** 188–91.

75

Chronic pain management

MICHEL Y DUBOIS, CHRISTOPHER GHARIBO, AND ALLEN H LEBOVITS

INTRODUCTION

Chronic pain is one of the most common complaints that brings patients to a physician's office. Despite remarkable progress in the last 20 years in understanding pain mechanisms, and the advent of new therapies for chronic pain, this condition is still poorly treated. The main reason for undertreatment is largely that chronic pain is a highly complex phenomenon, a symptom of a multitude of medical conditions, each of which needs to be recognized and specifically treated. Pain has been defined by the International Association for the Study of Pain (IASP) as "an unpleasant sensory and emotional experience associated with actual or potential tissue damage or described in terms of such damage." Pain is a subjective sensation (medical diagnoses rely on the patients' reports), but one also must find objective signs of the pain complaints. Pain becomes "chronic" when the complaint persists beyond a reasonable time for an injury to heal, usually 3–6 months; it can be provoked by a chronic pathologic process that causes a continuous complaint, or the pain may recur at intervals, for months or years. Contrary to acute pain, chronic pain never has a protective biologic function, but it has an adverse effect that usually imposes severe physical, emotional, and environmental stresses on the individual.

Pain is a major public health problem. In the USA, 50 million Americans are partially or totally disabled by pain. Approximately 45% of all Americans have persistent pain at some point in their lives. Headaches and low back pain are the most common forms of chronic intractable pain. Headaches alone account for 150 million lost workdays; 22% of work-related injuries in the USA involve back pain, which is the second leading cause of work loss.[1]

Among several medical specialties involved in the management of chronic pain, anesthesiologists have taken the lead in evaluation and treatment. Over the last half-century, enormous effort has gone into organizing the practice of pain medicine. The knowledge base required in anesthesiology training has increased significantly during the last few years. Similarly, pain medicine has become a major subspecialty of anesthesiology. At the same time, chronic pain management has created daunting challenges for modern anesthesiologists, not only in the understanding of the mechanisms of pain but also in its evaluation and treatment, with associated psychological, social, and economic issues. The anesthesiologist pain specialist has seen his or her role widen into a new type of practice closer to conventional primary care. Although bringing his or her own expertise, the physician usually needs to interact closely with other specialists, as part of an integrated team, in order to coordinate the patient's treatment.

This chapter will summarize the basic knowledge necessary to understand the mechanisms of chronic pain and will provide a foundation for the evaluation and treatment of this condition.

PATHOPHYSIOLOGY OF CHRONIC PAIN

Classically, pain is separated into two major classes:

1 normal or nociceptive pain, which includes acute, subacute, and inflammatory pain;
2 abnormal or pathophysiologic pain, principally neuropathic, deafferentation, and central pain.

Nociceptive pain results from noxious stimuli and inflammation in otherwise intact tissues. Pathophysiologic pain, as observed in chronic pain, is associated with injury to neural tissue and reflects abnormal functioning of the pain system. Injury to neural elements may sometimes result in the loss of ability to perceive pain and under certain conditions may cause pain, allodynia (pain evoked by normally nonpainful stimuli), or hyperalgesia (exaggerated pain from a normally painful stimulus). It is essential to understand the basic mechanisms of nociception before dealing with the more complex mechanisms responsible for chronic pain states. If a noxious stimulation persists, irreversible alterations in nociceptor sensitivity may occur and lead to spontaneous firing of neural fibers and major changes in the reaction of the central nervous system (CNS) to sensory input.

The four processes that make up nociception are:[2]

1 transduction, when noxious stimuli are transformed into electrical impulses at the sensory endings of the nerve;
2 transmission of the impulse via the sensory nervous system;
3 modulation, which is the modification of the nociceptive transmission by a number of neural inferences;
4 perception, which is the subjective sensory and emotional experience of pain that occurs at the cortical level.

Nociceptors are the receptors that respond to intense, potentially tissue-damaging stimuli that exist throughout the body.[3] They can be found in the skin in the form of: (1) high-threshold mechanoreceptors, which are primarily responsive to intense mechanical stimuli (strong pressure) but may also respond to high temperatures after sensitization – their signal is conveyed through myelinated A-delta fibers; and (2) polymodal receptors, whose signal is conveyed by unmyelinated C-fibers and which respond to a variety of chemical, mechanical, and thermal stimuli. Nociceptors are also found in other structures such as muscles, tendons, joints, tooth pulp, and cornea, where they respond to a variety of stimuli (stretch, chemical, thermal changes, or electrical). In visceral organs, there is little evidence that specialized pain receptors exist. Inflammation, ischemia, stretching, dilation, or spasm of hollow viscera may produce severe pain through visceral afferent fibers, which accompanies sympathetic efferent axons, activating dorsal horn neurons. This usually creates a poorly localized pain, with referred pain due to viscerosomatic integration (i.e. back pain in chronic pancreatitis or left arm pain in angina).

If inflammation or repeated tissue injury occurs, nociceptors may become sensitized. This phenomenon is mediated by several endogenous chemical substances, such as bradykinin, histamine, and 5-hydroxytryptamine (serotonin). Local release of prostaglandins potentiates the action of bradykinin and acts as a sensitizer to the nociceptors. Prostaglandins originate from a cascade of reactions, starting with phospholipids from cell membranes which form arachidonic acid via phospholipase A_2; arachidonic acid is itself transformed into cyclic endoperoxides through cyclo-oxygenase (COX) action, and then into prostaglandin I_2 and prostaglandin E_2 and $F_{2\alpha}$.[4]

The termination of the primary afferent fibers in the spinal dorsal horn represents the next essential step of pain processing. Nociceptive afferent fibers terminate in the dorsal horn on the same side of the body as the dorsal root ganglion, where the primary sensory neural cell bodies are located. The unmyelinated C-fibers terminate primarily in the Rexed laminae 1, whereas the thinly myelinated A-delta fibers end in lamina 1 and 3–5. Two types of second-order nociceptive spinal projection neurons have been identified in the spinal cord: (1) the wide dynamic range (WDR) neurons and (2) the nociceptive-specific (NS) neurons. WDR cells are situated in deeper laminae (V) of the dorsal horn than NS neurons and receive input not only from nociceptive afferent fibers but also from low-threshold A-beta fibers. They may therefore be activated by both noxious and non-noxious stimuli. WDR neurons receive convergent input from skin, muscle, and viscera, which may account for "referred pain". NS neurons respond only to noxious stimuli and are found in the superficial lamina of the dorsal horn. They have neurophysiologic properties very distinct from WDR neurons. Neural impulses from both WDR and NS second-order neurons cross the midline near the level of the cell bodies and form a bundle of ascending fibers in the contra- and anterolateral spinal region (spinothalamic tract) reaching the brainstem and diencephalon.

Noxious inputs are *modulated* at the spinal level. The publication of the "gate control" theory by Melzack and Wall suggested that input of normally non-nociceptive fibers, such as A-beta low-threshold fibers, inhibited the response of WDR neurons to nociception. In fact, several neural transmitters were later identified in the spinal cord as being released by intrinsic spinal neurons. Neural transmitters play a major role in the modulation of nociceptive input. In addition to the locally produced modulation in the dorsal horn, descending systems exist, originating in various brainstem locations, which modulate both peripheral input and output of the neural cells. In chronic pain, the transmission modalities of the nociceptive system are changed and create what is called *"neuronal plasticity"*.[5] Following a noxious stimulus of sufficient intensity and duration, the pain signaling of neurons for a given stimulus may be increased. When a sustained partial depolarization of the dorsal horn renders the cell membrane increasingly susceptible to afferent input by repetitive stimulation of the small unmyelinated afferent fibers, a *"windup phenomenon"* is observed.

At the same time that there is an increase in discharge evoked by a given stimulus, there is also an expansion of the receptive field size and an increase in spontaneous discharge rate. The overall phenomenon is known as *"central sensitization"*.[6] Excitatory amino acids (EAAs), such as glutamate and aspartate, are the principal nociceptive neural transmitters. Receptors to these EEAs are located in the dorsal horn and include *N*-methyl D-aspartate (NMDA) receptors. These NMDA receptors, existing largely on WDR neurons, are enabled by repetitive release of glutamate or substance P and are responsible for the windup phenomenon. The prolonged increase in sensitivity of the spinal cord is initiated mostly by the NMDA receptors and is mediated by several intracellular mechanisms. They include increased intracellular calcium, production of nitric oxide, production of prostaglandins, and early immediate gene transcription. Prolonged excitation and release of EEAs can lead to neuronal damage and may produce irreversible CNS dysfunction.

The dorsal horn normal function has both excitatory modulators and inhibitory modulators. Among excitatory modulators are tachykinins, such as substance P, which enables the NMDA receptor, and dynorphin, an endogenous opioid, which, in certain concentrations, is antianalgesic. Inhibitory modulators include glycine and gamma amino butyric acid (GABA), which play a major role in descending inhibition; enkephalins, which are endogenous opioids released near the primary afferent nerve terminal in the dorsal horn and have both a presynaptic and postsynaptic mode of action; serotonin (5-HT) and norepinephrine (NE) (noradrenaline), important neurotransmitters in descending inhibitory pathways (NE provides spinal analgesia mediated by α-adrenergic receptors); and adenosine receptors, which also modulate dorsal horn nociceptive transmission (Fig. 75.1).

The somatosensory *ascending pathways* are primarily represented in the spinothalamic tract. This is still considered to be the most important pain projection pathway to the brain with neurons that respond to noxious stimulation. The cell origins of the spinothalamic tract are located in laminae 1 and 5. The pathway has a lateral portion, which mainly involves discriminative functions such as location, intensity and duration of the painful stimulus, and a medial portion, which entails the autonomic and unpleasant emotional aspects of pain. These tracts project in different parts of the thalamus (medial and posterior nuclei), which in turn project to specific cortical regions.[7]

Evidence for a *descending pathway*, which represents the supraspinal control of nociception, has been known for years. Several experiments using either electrical stimulation of periaqueductal gray (PAG) in the midbrain or microinjection of morphine in the same area have produced widespread analgesia in animals and humans. Descending endogenous pain-inhibitory pathways have also been identified. They involve connections from the PAG area to the nucleus raphe magnus and the reticular formation. Adrenergic and serotonergic nerve fibers have been identified descending from these two locations down to the spinal dorsal horn cells. Other neural transmitters, such as GABA or acetylcholine, are also likely to be involved in the descending inhibition. It is interesting to know that these descending pain control mechanisms are affected by environmental factors such as physical stress, anxiety, emotional distress, or depression, all of which can reduce or increase the pain threshold.[8]

Two separate pain syndromes require further explanation:

1 *Neuropathic pain.*[9] This is created by a spontaneous discharge from injured peripheral nerves and has been demonstrated experimentally in induced neuromas. This activity is generated at the site of injury and at the dorsal root ganglion (DRG), and is enhanced by sympathetic stimulation or NE. It has been shown that, in this condition, A fibers lose their myelin and C-fibers lose their Schwann cell sheath. This allows the spread of the electrical impulse between axons and the spread of abnormal neural activity proximally and distally. It may also involve new neurons, such as sympathetic afferents and mechanoreceptor afferents, which are not usually directly involved in nociception. When a peripheral nerve activity has been lost, there may be increased sensitivity in the dorsal horn and/or in the spinothalamic tract and/or in thalamic cells.

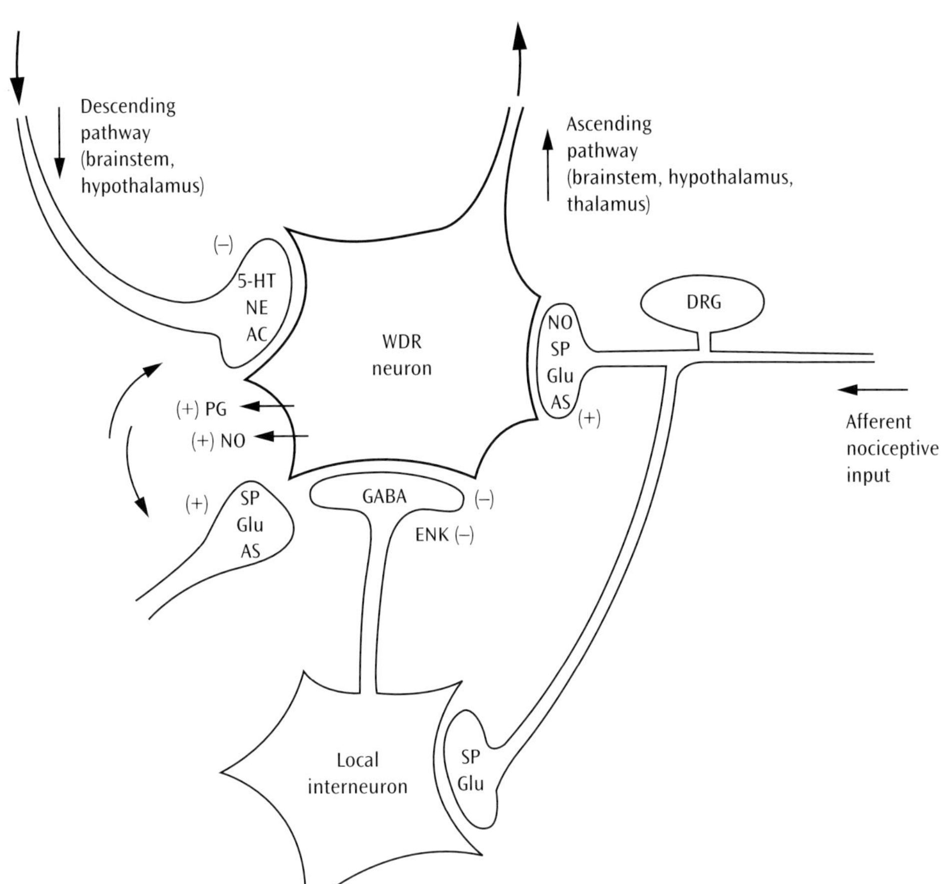

Figure 75.1 *Simplified representation of dorsal horn functional organization, with examples of neurochemical modulators. Mediators to nociception can be (1) excitatory, such as neurokinin A (NK), substance P (SP), excitatory amino acids (EAA), aspartate (AS) and glutamate (Glu) (both SP and EAA activate NMDA receptors), nitric oxide (NO), and prostaglandins (PG); or (2) inhibitory, such as GABA, glycine, enkephalins (ENK), norepinephrine (NE), serotonin (5-HT), and acetylcholine (AC). DRG, dorsal root ganglion.*

2 *Sympathetically maintained pain.* The sympathetic nervous system affects pain perception. There is evidence for sympathetically mediated sensitization of mechanoreceptors, and it is postulated that, when combined with the sensitization of the WDR neurons in the dorsal horn, it may be responsible for the mechanical allodynia associated with sympathetic dystrophy. Because of damage associated with neuropathic pain (see above), "cross-talk" may occur between sympathetic afferents and nociceptor axons.[10]

In summary, spinal neurons that signal pain are dynamic, and their output is modulated by segmental and descending control mechanisms. The sensation of pain involves a complex interaction of excitatory and inhibitory neural transmitter mechanisms. Although the anterolateral spinothalamic system is the primary pain-signaling channel, there is a medial, lemniscal, high-speed system in the dorsal column, usually transmitting nonpainful sensory signals, the role of which may also result in disturbances leading to chronic pain.

EVALUATION OF THE CHRONIC PAIN PATIENT

Medical evaluation

The evaluation of the chronic pain patient is an essential step in determining the pathophysiology responsible for the chronic pain state. After evaluation, the physician may label the patient's pain as "organic" if a specific pathology explaining the pain complaint is found or "psychogenic" (or functional) when the exact physical origin of the pain is not found. It is essential that from the outset the physician recognizes that the pain as described by the patient is *real* because "pain is whatever the experiencing person says it is occurring whenever he/she says it does."[11]

The pain practitioner who is accustomed to treating patients with chronic pain will quickly recognize the importance of psychosocial factors contributing to the patient's complaint, especially if the pain has persisted for a long period. An early evaluation by a pain psychologist is usually necessary to assess the importance of these factors; this may also lead to referral to a psychiatrist for associated psychopathology such as anxiety and depression often encountered in chronic pain patients. A psychological consultation should not be the last resort, after the physician has been unable to identify an organic cause for the pain, as this will only serve to aggravate the sense of hopelessness the patient may have of his or her condition. Psychosocial factors must be identified early in the workup as they can complicate the evaluation and the management of the patient's pain and may lead to endless and costly workups, which will likely prove negative and frustrating for both the professional evaluator and the patient. Medical evaluation must start with a detailed *questionnaire* to elicit the characteristics of the pain, i.e. its location, onset, quality, radiation, response to previous treatments, etc. Its intensity can be quantified using different available pain scales. The questionnaire should also establish a thorough history of the patient's past, not only medical but also personal, professional, social, economic, psychological, and emotional. The questionnaire is usually completed by the patient prior to or during the first visit. The physician should also request and closely examine previous medical records concerning past pain diagnoses and treatments. *Physical examination* must also be complete and systematic. Most often, depending on the type of pain complaint, it will consist of a standard review of systems, with particular emphasis on neurologic and musculoskeletal examinations. By looking in detail at sensory and motor systems, deep tendon reflexes, gait analysis, and range of motion, by palpation of tender zones or trigger points, the physician seeks to correlate the pain complaint with abnormal findings.

Imaging techniques [i.e. plain radiograph, computed tomography (CT) scan, magnetic resonance imaging (MRI)] may be helpful, especially if their findings explain the pain complaints and correlate with the results of the physical examination. In many cases, however, this relation is not found, and this can add to the frustrations of the examining physician. Some tests, such as MRI, may not only fail to provide any useful information but, because of the test's exquisite sensitivity, lead to false assumptions (e.g. the image of a bulging disk in the spine at a level that corresponds to the location of the pain complaint, but which can hardly explain the severity of the pain). This technique, therefore, should not constitute part of the routine screening but should be requested only as the result of significant clues from the physical examination and the history of the pain complaint. Electromyography (EMG) performed at least 2 weeks after the onset of a radiculopathy may be a valuable diagnostic adjuvant.

It is always important to remember that most patients with chronic pain experience an increasing degree of frustration related to the inability of the healthcare system to identify and treat their illness. As a rule, they will manifest anger, anxiety, and depression, which require careful psychological assessment and sometimes a psychiatric evaluation. Before initiating a treatment plan and interventions, such as surgery or nerve blocks or long-term pharmacotherapy, it is important to evaluate the psychological profile of the chronic pain patient.

Psychological evaluation

The objectives of the psychological evaluation of the patient with chronic pain are to:

1. determine the degree of psychological adaptation to chronic pain, which includes mood state, coping skills, effect on family, and, particularly, level of physical functioning;
2. evaluate the patient's premorbid psychological state and personality factors and its effect on onset and etiology of pain;
3. establish the role of psychological factors in the etiology, maintenance, and exacerbation of pain;
4. formulate a DSM-IV diagnosis;
5. predict outcome of invasive procedures such as surgical implantation of spinal cord stimulators or continuous infusion pumps;
6. determine which psychological and medical interventions would be most appropriate for which patients;
7. identify environmental reinforcers of chronic pain and illness behaviors such as family, litigation status, and disability insurance status;
8. evaluate the likelihood of the development of chronic pain-related disability.

The standard pain center evaluation protocol utilizes a pain questionnaire, a structured clinical interview, pain assessment measures that include pain intensity rating scales and the McGill Pain Questionnaire,[12] and a psychological evaluation of the patient. The pain questionnaire should be designed to yield objective clinical outcome measures, and include information such as demographic characteristics, pain descriptors, what makes the pain better or worse, interference with sleep, and circumstances causing the onset of pain. Also included typically is a review of prior interventions and their efficacy, current and past medication use, litigation and compensation status, job status and enjoyment, and interference of pain on various aspects of life.

The clinical interview is ideally suited to review the patient's pain complaints, onset of pain and relation to trauma, prior medical and psychiatric history, prior alcohol and drug usage, current marital and family environment, current functional level, utilization of coping skills, disability status, motivational level to return to work, secondary gain issues, and ability to sleep. The clinical interview also affords the opportunity to evaluate the patient's beliefs and cognitions about their pain.

Measures of psychological status include two assessments of mood state. The Beck Depression Inventory[13] is one of the most widely used tests with chronic pain patients because it is a relatively quick measure of depression, a mood state closely linked with chronic pain. The Spielberger State-Trait Anxiety Inventory (STAI)[14] is the most widely used measure of anxiety, a construct that is not used as extensively as depression is with chronic pain patients but, nevertheless, a very important one with pain patients. The Minnesota Multiphasic Personality Inventory (MMPI, MMPI-2),[15] one of the most widely used and researched tests of all time, is used quite extensively with chronic pain patients. The MMPI is a 566-question true–false test that evaluates the presence of psychopathology through three validity scales (the degree to which respondents may be trying to distort their true persona) and 10 clinical scales: hypochondriasis, depression, hysteria, psychopathic deviance (history of antisocial behavior and nonconformance), paranoia, psychasthenia (obsessive–compulsive tendencies as well as anxiety), schizophrenia, hypomania, masculinity–femininity, and social introversion. Other commonly used measures include the Symptom Checklist 90-Revised (SCL-90R),[16] a commonly used assessment of psychological symptom patterns, which evaluates nine "symptom dimensions": somatization, obsessive–compulsive, interpersonal sensitivity, depression, anxiety, hostility, phobic anxiety, paranoid ideation, and psychoticism. The Coping Strategies Questionnaire[17] is designed to evaluate how pain patients cope with their pain.

As pain management has become more technologically sophisticated and aggressive in its approach, one of the more common uses of the psychological evaluation has been to determine the appropriateness of a potential candidate, based on a set of predetermined psychosocial characteristics. Nelson *et al.*,[18] conducting a meta-analysis of the literature on this topic, concluded that patients should be excluded from implantable spinal cord stimulators if they have active psychosis, suicidality, untreated major depression, somatization disorder, alcohol or drug dependency, compensation/litigation, disincentive to recovery, lack of social supports, or cognitive deficits. Additional considerations for exclusion include unusual pain ratings, personality disorders, physical incongruence, a high elevation on the depression scale of the MMPI, or elevations on four or more MMPI scales.

Patients appreciate being listened to, rather than being dismissed as having imaginary pain. The experienced clinician needs to take his or her pain questionnaire, clinical interview, and psychological assessment measures, and apply them together with sound clinical judgment in formulating a diagnosis and treatment plan that is individually geared to that patient.

COMMON CHRONIC PAIN SYNDROMES

Low back pain

Back pain affects 60–80% of the adult population in the USA and is experienced by virtually everybody at some point in their lives.[19] Up to 90% of the episodes of acute low back pain resolve spontaneously, regardless of therapy.[20] The chronic low back pain that affects the remaining 10% of adults represents one of the greatest challenges to conventional medicine.

Sources of back pain

The differential diagnosis of low back pain is vast (Table 75.1). The majority of low back pain is caused by mechanical processes that develop with years of poor posture and age-related degenerative changes. The spinal structures that can be major contributors to low back pain are intervertebral disks, zygapophysial joints, posterior longitudinal ligament, nerve roots, dura, and ligamentum flavum.[21] The spine and its attached elements degenerate simultaneously, resulting in pain that may originate from multiple sources. The most common examples include

Table 75.1 *Causes of low back pain*

Muscle sprain/strain
Herniated nucleus pulposus
Degenerative disk disease
Annular fissure/tear
Zygapophysial joint arthropathy
Spinal central canal or foraminal stenosis
Osteoarthritis of the hip
Spondylolisthesis
Ankylosing spondylitis
Epidural abscess hematoma
Diskitis
Osteomyelitis
Primary or metastatic cancer
Referred: abdominal aortic aneurysm, pancreatitis, renal colic, etc.

muscle sprains and strains, osteoarthritis of the lumbosacral spine, and other anatomical abnormalities such as herniated nucleus pulposus, degenerative disk disease, and spinal stenosis. The typical low back pain patient often suffers from more than one musculoskeletal diagnosis and presents with multiple pain generators. Extraspinal lumbosacral radiculopathy is extremely rare, occurring in 1 out of 1000 patients.[22] Therefore, it is important to not miss the less frequent but more serious etiologies such as cancer, abdominal aortic aneurysm, fractures, or epidural infection.

Treatment and role of spinal injections in the low back pain patient

In 1994, the Agency for Health Care Policy and Research (AHCPR) in the USA published guidelines acknowledging that over 90% of low back pain episodes improve spontaneously within 4 weeks of onset, regardless of treatment. The Agency recommended against diagnostic tests, including imaging studies, for low back pain within the first 4–6 weeks.[23]

Although bed rest is widely recommended in the medical literature for the treatment of low back pain, it has been shown to impede recovery.[24,25] Prolonged inactivity and deconditioning propagate the conditions underlying the low back pain, making recovery more difficult. Currently, maintenance of the patient's activity and work status, participation in a physical rehabilitation program, and pharmacologic pain management have become the cornerstones of treating low back pain patients. A patient with low back pain that has persisted beyond a 4-week period should be referred to a multidisciplinary pain center in order to provide the patient with sufficient pain control, allow physical therapy, and allow reversal of the physical deconditioning that insidiously develops.

The general consensus is that diagnostic and therapeutic spinal injections are incorporated in the following groups of patients:

1 patients who have not improved after 4 weeks of conservative therapy utilizing modalities such as oral medications and physical therapy;
2 patients whose symptoms are significant enough to necessitate more definitive pain control;
3 patients who cannot tolerate or have contraindications to oral medications;
4 Patients who, due to excessive pain, are unable to engage in effective physical rehabilitation.

Lumbosacral radiculopathy

Lumbar spine lesions that result in inflammation or entrapment of the lumbar nerve root(s) can cause back and leg pain. Such lesions include herniated nucleus pulposus, internal disk disruptions such as annular tears, foraminal stenosis, and failed back surgery syndrome. The clinical presentation needs to be distinguished from that of predominantly low back pain with referred leg pain. A referred leg pain presentation will be associated with a greater degree of low back pain that somatically radiates to the posterior aspect of the thigh to the level of the knee. A radicular leg pain presentation will exhibit greater leg than back pain, with radiation down the leg in a radicular distribution with signs of nerve root tension and motor, sensory, and reflex nerve dysfunction. Herniated disks create dural inflammation.[26] The release of intradiskal phospholipase A_2 into the epidural space initiates a chemical cascade that results in production of prostaglandins and other inflammatory mediators in the epidural space. The result is an intense inflammatory reaction of the dura, intervertebral disk, posterior longitudinal ligament, and the nerve roots, causing hypersensitization of nociceptive nerve endings.[27] The majority of disk herniations are posterolateral and occur at L4–5 and L5–S1 levels, therefore affecting the nerve roots on one side of the spine.[28] The end result is low back and radicular leg pain that is due to inflammation or compression of the posterior division of the spinal nerve root.

Lumbar zygapophysial joint syndrome

Lumbar zygapophysial joint syndrome is due to degenerative changes of the posterior column resulting in low back, buttock, and referred leg pain with or without radiculopathy. If there is joint hypertrophy, particularly of the superior articular process, the resulting foraminal stenosis may also produce lumbar radiculopathy. As demonstrated by Bogduk and others, the capsule and synovium of the lumbar zygapophysial joints are richly innervated with nociceptive nerve endings.[29,30] Pain sensation is transmitted via medial branches that have their origin in the posterior ramus of the spinal nerve root.[31] Multiple studies have demonstrated that low back pain can be produced by injection of a physiologic irritant such as hypertonic saline into the zygapophysial joints.[32,33] This back pain has been shown to be relieved by subsequent injection of local anesthetics.[34] In the absence of a herniated disk and spinal instability, lumbar zygapophysial joints along with the intervertebral disk are believed to be responsible for a large percentage of undiagnosed back pain conditions.[35] Generally, patients complain of axial pain that radiates to the buttocks and the hamstring muscles. Pain is commonly aggravated by prolonged sitting, standing, and hyperextension and rotation of the lumbar spine. Physical examination reveals reproduction of the patient's pain with direct palpation of the suspected joints as well as during movements that produce loading of the zygapophysial joints, such as simultaneous lumbar hyperextension and lateral bending. Unless there is concomitant nerve root or spinal cord irritation, the neurologic examination is normal.

Spinal stenosis

Spinal stenosis is a general term for congenital and acquired stenotic disorders of the spine where narrowing of the bony frame surrounding the neural structures takes place. The stenosis can affect the central spinal canal and/or the lateral intervertebral foramen.[36] The narrowing of the central canal and the intervertebral foramens can be caused by disorders such as short pedicle syndrome, spondylolisthesis, osteoarthritis of the spine, zygapophysial joint hypertrophy, ligamentum flavum hypertrophy, and degenerative disk disease. Sometimes the process is iatrogenic such as following lumbar fusion or laminectomy, when the fibrous scarring can cause compression of the dural, neural, and vascular structures. Spinal stenosis is commonly multifactorial and affects several vertebral levels. The constricting effect exerted on the nerves is also exerted on the surrounding veins, causing venous congestion and venous hypertension. The resultant backpressure compromises the perfusion pressure and can result in neural ischemia. Regardless of the etiology, spinal stenosis may not clinically manifest for years and may surface together with symptoms of a disk herniation.

Failed back surgery/postlaminectomy syndrome

Patients with this syndrome form one of the most difficult to treat groups of chronic pain patients seen in pain clinics. The pain experienced in this syndrome exhibits strong nociceptive and neuropathic characteristics. The pain may be sharp and shooting, whereas at other times it may be burning and dysesthetic. The back and leg pain may be constant, or only with certain positions or during activity. The symptomatology is variable. Patients may have diskogenic pain, lumbar zygapophysial joint syndrome, spinal stenosis, accelerated degenerative disk disease, ligamentum flavum hypertrophy, arachnoiditis, and neurogenic pain alone or in combination. The pathophysiology is iatrogenic and due to development of fibrous scarring following fusion or laminectomy, which can cause inflammation and/or compression of the dural, neural, and vascular structures. Intraoperative and/or postoperative nerve damage, spinal instability, and recurrence of disk herniation are also possible etiologies. The physical examination findings depend on the underlying pathophysiology. Often, the spinal range of motion is markedly diminished. Neurologic deficits may be localized to the level and side of spinal surgery or to the surrounding vicinity.

Myofascial pain syndrome

Myofascial pain syndrome[37] is a soft-tissue disorder that creates pain to tender areas within muscle groups. Symptoms can suggest other musculoskeletal conditions such as muscle strains or sprains, and fibromyalgia. Diagnosis is made on the determination of clinical trigger points on examination. Trigger points are painful regions in a taut band of muscle that produce referenced pain with application of pressure. The painful area usually feels like a "rope". These trigger points are usually created by events such as trauma or prolonged tension from poor posture. Local prolonged ischemia may trigger the formation of subsequent fibrosis. Therapeutic modalities include passive stretching of the affected muscle group with cold spray, compression massage, and trigger point injection, which usually use a dry needle, or injection of 0.5% lidocaine (lignocaine) at the location of the trigger point. Botulinum toxin injections have also been successfully used. Once the local spasm has been treated, physical therapy is an essential part of the treatment of myofascial pain syndrome.

Headaches

Headache is one of the most frequent complaints presented to physicians. It is estimated that in the USA 45 million people suffer with chronic recurrent headaches severe enough to cause impairment or require medical treatment. Headaches can be secondary or primary. Secondary headaches are related to underlying disease processes such as infection, trauma, hemorrhage, tumor, and systemic disease. Primary headaches are defined as having no identifiable etiology, structural or disease related; they include migraine, cluster, and tension-type headaches.[38] *Migraine* is "classic" when preceded by visual symptoms such as spots, tunnel vision, or numbness or paresthesia in one side of the body. The "aura" – not always present – is followed by an intense crescendo, usually unilateral and retro-ocular, of pounding, pulsating, or throbbing head pain. Photophobia, nausea, or vomiting may accompany migraine, which is usually resolved without lasting complication. Approximately two out of three migraines occur in women. The precise cause of migraine is unknown. It is a neurovascular headache. Its mechanism is associated with the cranial perivascular inflammation mediated through the trigeminal nerve with alteration in cerebral blood perfusion. Neurochemical transmitter release is usually hypothesized. Simple analgesics may sometimes abort a migraine attack but usually other medications are necessary, such as cerebral vasoconstrictors, serotonin antagonists, nonsteroidal anti-inflammatory drugs (NSAIDs), and, in rare cases, narcotics. Prevention therapy after a thorough evaluation is the best treatment.

Tension-type headaches are the most common headaches. These headaches can be episodic, usually occurring on both sides of the head with pressing, squeezing, sensitivity to light or sound, and a mild-to-moderate intensity. A headache may last from several hours to several days and there is no evidence of underlying disease process. Tension headaches are usually associated with disorders of the pericranial muscles or with spinal nerve dysfunction, such as cervical radiculopathy. Peripheral nociceptors, which are inside the neck muscles or ligaments, are being activated. Treatment is usually a combination of simple analgesics and nonpharmacologic intervention, such as stress management, muscle relaxation, and biofeedback.

Cluster headache is a rare excruciating headache. It is usually a severe unilateral orbital or temporal pain, which lasts from a few minutes to 2–3 h. Attacks frequency varies but the headaches usually occur in cycles separated by pain-free periods; they are most prevalent in young men. Cluster headache pathophysiology is unknown. The treatment consists of withdrawal of trigger agents when identified, and abortive medications similar to the ones used in migraine headaches. Again, preventive treatment, once a thorough evaluation has been carried out, is best for this condition.

These most common headaches do not present any evidence of underlying disease process or structural pathology. They must, however, be differentiated from headaches associated with head trauma, vascular disease, or intracranial pathology, and from all systemic or regional diseases that may affect the head and upper neck.

Complex regional pain syndromes I and II

Complex regional pain syndrome (CRPS) is a form of neuropathic pain that commonly involves the upper or lower extremities; however, it can also involve the head, back, shoulders, and viscera. The old denominations "reflex sympathetic dystrophy" and "causalgia" have been renamed by IASP as "CRPS type I" and "CRPS type II" respectively. The symptoms and signs of CRPS type I and II overlap and clinical presentation is similar. CRPS type II is distinguished from CRPS type I as the former diagnosis can only be made when there is an identifiable nerve lesion in addition to a spectrum of sensory, motor, autonomic, and trophic changes:

- *Sensory disturbances.* Persistent pain following injury, which is present long after the injury has apparently healed, is one of the hallmark signs of CRPS. The reported pain is disproportionate in duration, severity, and distribution to what would be expected from the original injurious event. The pain is spontaneous, constant, diffuse, burning, and deep. It can be exacerbated by gentle touch, cold, heat, passive and active motion, damp weather, and emotion. Sensory findings can include allodynia, dysesthesia, and hyperalgesia.
- *Motor disturbances.* The assessment of muscle strength may not be possible due to the patient discomfort encountered in examining the affected area. The patient's reluctance to engage the area in active movement ultimately leads to muscle atrophy and weakness. Tremors of the affected area may also be present.
- *Autonomic disturbances.* Generalized swelling, hyperhidrosis, color changes, and temperature differences between the affected side and the normal side are commonly evident in the early stages of the

disease. The affected limb may be episodically warmer or colder than the contralateral limb, with associated changes in skin color.[39] This is due to abnormal vasomotor and sudomotor regulation of the affected limb by the autonomic nervous system.

- *Trophic changes*. These begin to occur almost immediately and become prominent in the later stages of the disease. They are partly the result of the patient's effort to protect the affected limb from any movement or contact at all costs. For example, the patient's reluctance to physically engage the painful area leads to atrophic changes on the joints and tendons in addition to muscle atrophy, leading to range of motion limiting contractures. Thinning of the skin, hair loss or overgrowth, and hypertrophic nails are later developments of the disease.

As soon as the diagnosis of CRPS has been considered, the patient should be evaluated by a multidisciplinary pain treatment facility that has experience in treating this syndrome. Timely intervention is of the essence. There is a critical window of opportunity during the early stages of the disease that must be best utilized. The therapeutic elements include rehabilitative, pharmacologic, psychological, and procedural approaches. Some patients progress to requiring inpatient stays for concomitant pain management and physical rehabilitation. Spinal cord stimulation and intrathecal drug therapy are last resorts for this difficult to treat syndrome.

Postherpetic neuralgia

Postherpetic neuralgia (PHN) results in pain of intractable nature that develops as a sequela of *acute herpes zoster (AHZ)* infection (shingles). Pain from AHZ resolves usually within 3–4 weeks, and whenever the pain of AHZ lasts longer than 4–6 weeks PHN should be suspected. In AHZ, the large myelinated fibers are preferentially destroyed over the smaller, unmyelinated fibers in the dorsal root ganglion and the dorsal horn. Therefore, as the disease progresses, the proportion of nonmyelinated fibers over the myelinated fibers progressively increases.[40,41] It has been postulated that pain processing by small fibers, which is normally impeded by large myelinated fibers, is compromised in PHN. Consequently, damaged small fibers spontaneously fire without modulatory effects from the larger inhibitory myelinated fibers, resulting in the intractable pain state of PHN. The incidence of PHN dramatically increases with each passing decade over 50 years of age, and it is generally considered to be a pain condition of the elderly and the immunosuppressed populations. Published reports have mentioned incidences as high as 30–40% of patients over the age of 60 years.[42,43] Octagenarians and patients with depressed cell-mediated immunity are susceptible to the spread of the virus to the adjacent dermatomes as well as spread to the visceral and other areas within the CNS where further complications can occur.

When the rash and persistent pain of AHZ extends beyond a 4- to 6-week period, the diagnosis of PHN is strongly considered. Patients will typically report unilateral pain in a dermatomal distribution. Thoracic dermatomal involvement is most common (50%), followed by facial and cervical locations. Physical examination will reveal areas of hyperpigmentation and scarring in the areas of the prior vesicular eruptions. Allodynia, dysesthesias, and hyperesthesias are commonly present.

Ultimately, the patient will exhibit pain-induced disruption of social activities, mood, depressed affect, and poor sleep. PHN is one of the most difficult conditions encountered by physicians. The serial failure of various therapies and the ongoing agonizing pain and suffering will cause many patients to consider suicide as an option. Therefore, in addition to pharmacologic, physical, and interventional modalities of management, the psychological and psychiatric needs of the patient need to be addressed concomitantly.

Orofacial pain

Orofacial pain can be encountered in a variety of medical conditions.[44] As with other chronic pain syndromes, it is important to avoid the pitfall of symptom management in the absence of diagnoses. Trigeminal neuralgia is an orofacial pain syndrome of neuropathic origin, which is defined as a sudden, usually unilateral, stabbing, recurrent pain, felt in the distribution of one or more branches on the fifth cranial nerve. In most cases, no cause is found, although in a small proportion of patients, trigeminal nerve root compression, usually by a vascular structure, can be found and released neurosurgically. Paroxysmal pain attacks may be extremely severe and, if left untreated, may lead the patient to severe depression and even suicide. Between episodes, sensation is essentially normal. Trigeminal neuralgia is usually treated by anticonvulsant medications such as gabapentin or carbamazepine. In severe refractory cases, radiofrequency lesioning of the trigeminal ganglion will result in symptom relief. Trigeminal neuralgia may also be the result of trauma, surgery, or peripheral lesions. Herpes zoster can affect the ganglion or one of the divisions of the trigeminal nerve. In addition to medical treatment, treatment of postherpetic neuralgia can be helped by local anesthetic nerve injection and techniques of neurolytic blockade.

Peripheral mandibular disorders can create facial pain and are related to, or referred to, the temporomandibular joint. Pain is usually aggravated by movements of the mandible. On palpation, muscles around the joint and the joint itself are usually tender, if not painful. Treatment is usually the treatment of the myofascial component, with stress-relieving techniques and medications. Many other causes of facial pain exist, including what is labeled "atypical facial pain", neuroma, facial trauma, glossopharyngeal neuralgia, and superolaryngeal neuralgia. Because facial pain may be due to a variety of causes and its diagnosis may be difficult, the treatment should be a multidisciplinary effort, coordinating the efforts of several specialists including a dental consultant, psychologist, anesthesiologist, and neurologist.

THERAPEUTIC MODALITIES

Diagnostic nerve blocks and spinal injections

The performance of a thorough history, physical examination and utilization of data provided by radiographs, MRI, and EMG may still leave the physician unable to identify with reasonable certainty the structures responsible for pain production. Pain-generating structures of the lumbosacral spine commonly produce clinically overlapping presentations. For example, the clinical picture of lumbar zygapophysial joint syndrome can mimic lumbosacral radiculopathy and, frequently, it is difficult to distinguish between low back and leg pain caused by hip abnormalities from that produced by lumbosacral pathology. These diagnostic uncertainties, associated with MRI findings that may be misleading, can be aided by diagnostic nerve and spinal injections such as paravertebral nerve root block, medial branch block, and diskography.[45,46]

Therapeutic nerve blocks and spinal injections

The therapeutic effects of spinal injections are a combination of the primary physiologic changes that result from the procedure and the secondary results arising from the enhanced pain control that allow other treatments (Table 75.2).[47] A wide spectrum of direct effects may provide therapeutic benefit. For example, most investigators believe that the predominant benefit of epidural steroids is their anti-inflammatory effect, although their neurolytic effect on unmyelinated C-fibers has also been demonstrated.[48,49] Local anesthetic injections may break the cycle of pain–spasm–ischemia, and high-volume injections may result in lysis of peridural adhesions and irrigation of inflammatory mediators. Pain relief after therapeutic spinal injections, although usually temporary, provides an opportunity for the patient to regain physical function and reverse the debilitating effects of chronic pain.

Examples of techniques used

Stellate ganglion nerve block

The cell bodies originating in the anterolateral horn of the spinal cord from T1 to L2 provide the spinal contribution to the sympathetic chain. Sympathetic fibers destined for the head and neck originate from T1 and T2 segments, whereas the sympathetic contribution to the upper extremity originates from T2–T8. The stellate ganglion is formed by the union of inferior cervical ganglion and the first thoracic ganglion. Although its location is variable, the stellate ganglion commonly lies anterior to C7 and T1 vertebrae. Direct contributions from the T2–T3 gray rami to the brachial plexus, which bypass the stellate ganglion, explain the potential failure of an apparently successful stellate ganglion block. The result would be failure to cause complete upper extremity sympathectomy and inadequate relief of the sympathetically maintained pain. Common indications for stellate ganglion block include CRPs type I and II, postherpetic neuralgia of the face and upper extremity, Raynaud's disease, occlusive vascular disease of the upper extremity, and vascular headaches.

Technique

The patient is placed supine on the table with a pillow under the shoulder blades to provide for slight extension of the neck. A peripheral venous line is placed. The head is maintained midline and the neck is allowed to relax. The area is prepared antiseptically. Vital monitoring and baseline temperature readings in the upper extremities are obtained. The cricoid cartilage, which corresponds to the level of the C6 vertebral body, is palpated. Lateral palpation from the cricoid cartilage should allow the palpation of the Chassaignac's tubercle (transverse process of C6) and the carotid artery. The carotid artery is retracted laterally and a 22-G 3″ needle is advanced perpendicularly until it makes contact with the Chassaignac's tubercle at C6. Once the bone is contacted, the needle tip is lifted 2–3 mm off the periosteum. A gentle aspiration is performed to test for the presence of blood or cerebrospinal fluid and, if negative, 5–10 mL of local anesthetic is injected to provide sympathectomy to the upper extremity and face. Less than 1 mL of local anesthetic injected in to the vertebral artery can result in seizures. Injection of a full complement of local anesthetic intrathecally will result in a total spinal block.

Table 75.2 *Proposed advantages of spinal injections*

Anti-inflammatory effect at the injection site
Neurolytic effect on the unmyelinated C-fibers
Lysis of peridural adhesions
Interruption of the cycle of pain–spasm–ischemia
Washout of mediators of inflammation
Radiofrequency thermocoagulation
Appropriate drug is delivered to the appropriate area
Immediate compatibility with other therapeutic modalities such as physical and psychosocial rehabilitation
Decreased oral analgesic use
Pain relief is provided without CNS depression
Relatively short outpatient procedures
Well tolerated by the vast majority of patients
Low risk when performed by experienced physicians

The skin temperature of the affected area is monitored for evidence of a sympathetic block. Sympathectomy to the face is evaluated by the presence of a Horner's syndrome (miosis, ptosis, and enophthalmos), injection of the conjunctiva, and nasal congestion. Sympathectomy to the upper extremity is evaluated by observing for the presence of venodilation and a temperature rise of greater than 2 °C on the ipsilateral upper extremity. Neurologic examination should not reveal radicular deficits if the injection is to be used for diagnostic purposes.

Lumbar sympathetic nerve block

The spinal contribution to the sympathetic chain ends at L2, but the sympathetic chain continues to the coccyx, ending with the ganglion impar. The lumbar sympathetic chain is located in the anterolateral portion of the vertebral bodies bilaterally. The sympathetic contribution to the lower extremity arises from the cell bodies originating in the anterolateral horn of the spinal cord from T10 to L2. The segment of the sympathetic chain that carries the sympathetic fibers to the lower extremities resides alongside L2, L3, and L4 vertebral bodies bilaterally. In the lumbar region, the psoas muscle separates the sympathetic chain from the somatic nerves.

The lumbar sympathetic block is used for diagnosis and treatment of sympathetically maintained pain conditions such as CRP types I and II, postherpetic neuralgia, and vascular diseases. A local anesthetic block under fluoroscopy should always precede a neurolytic injection into the same area. The use of fluoroscopy and contrast medium is a must to ensure a proper lumbar sympathetic block and minimize the chance of an injection into an undesired compartment.

Technique

The patient is placed in a prone position and a peripheral venous line is started. Vital signs monitoring, including temperature readings from both lower extremities, is carried out. Fluoroscopic images are obtained to identify the desired vertebral body and align the vertebral endplates. A 22-G 6″ needle is advanced toward the anterolateral portion of the vertebral body at its midpoint (Fig. 75.2); 5–15 mL of local anesthetics can be used. Sympathectomy is evaluated post injection by observing a temperature rise of greater than 2 °C on the ipsilateral leg. Neurologic examination should not reveal radicular deficits if the injection is to be used for diagnostic purposes.

Lumbar interlaminar epidural steroid injections

Interlaminar epidural steroids can provide up to 3 months of pain relief in up to 60–90% of patients.[50,51] Often, this period of response is adequate for these patients to engage in and complete their physical rehabilitation. There is evidence that the success rate and duration of analgesic effect is highly dependent on the selection criteria used as well as the successful integration of the procedure with a rehabilitation program. Saal and Saal[51] successfully treated 52 patients, with obvious indication for lumbar disk surgery, with integrated and progressive physical therapy and selective epidural nerve blocks. Fifty of these patients had *good* to *excellent* outcomes in terms of pain reduction and activity level; 48 were able to return to work. The lack of confirmation that the medication is actually delivered to the affected spinal level, side, and nerve root can compromise the efficacy of this technique. Therefore, utilization of fluoroscopy is fast becoming the standard of care in the performance of lumbar epidural steroid injections. Epidural steroids are best indicated in patients with low back pain with radicular symptoms and signs who have not improved after 4 weeks of a conservative therapy program. It has an excellent safety record, although complications such as vasovagal reactions, epidural abscesses, hematomas, postdural puncture headaches, and nerve damage may occur.

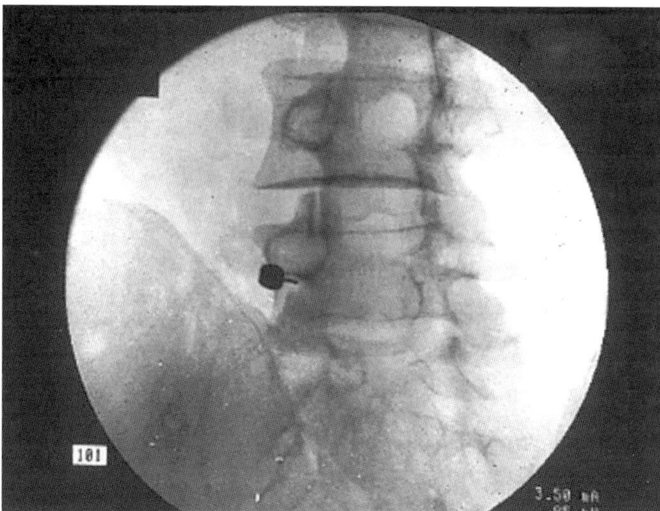

Figure 75.2 *Anteroposterior view of a lumbar sympathetic block. Needle tip at anterolateral aspect of L2, after 2 mL of contrast has been injected.*

Fluoroscopic interlaminar epidural steroid injection: technique

If fluoroscopy is being used, the patient lies prone with a pillow under the abdomen to maximize the interlaminar opening. Fluoroscopic imaging is obtained to identify the desired spinal level . The superior border of the lower lamina at its midpoint is the target point. The skin and tissue overlying the target point are anesthetized and an epidural needle is advanced toward the epidural space. Loss of resistance to air or the hanging drop technique can be utilized. If myelographic contrast is injected it commonly spreads ipsilaterally due to the presence of a dorsal midsagittal band (Fig. 75.3); 6–10 mL of local anesthetic and steroids is injected. The patient is asked to maintain a pain diary and is re-evaluated at 1 week. If only partial relief is obtained, a second injection can be scheduled.

Lumbar transforaminal epidural steroid injection

The transforaminal approach utilizes fluoroscopy to guide a needle into the intervertebral foramen on one side. The solution is injected directly onto the dural sleeve and then spreads transforaminally into the lumbar epidural space, potentially covering a greater area of nerve root inflammation than can be achieved by the interlaminar approach. A transforaminal nerve root injection has the potential to anesthetize the nerve roots and the dorsal root ganglion above and below the injected level, dura, posterior longitudinal ligament, and the innervation of the intervertebral disk. Therefore, relief of axial and/or radicular pain often occurs.

Fluoroscopic transforaminal epidural steroid injection: technique

The patient is placed prone on the table with a pillow under the abdomen to maximize the opening of the intervertebral foramen. Fluoroscopic images are obtained to align the vertebral endplates and identify the desired nerve root level and side. Oblique live fluoroscopy is obtained until the pedicle is positioned over the lower superior articular process.

The target point is the 6 o'clock position of the pedicle. The skin and tissue overlying this target are anesthetized and a 22-G needle is advanced toward the pedicle under intermittent fluoroscopic guidance. A lateral view is obtained to ensure that the needle tip rests below the midpoint of the pedicle (Fig. 75.4). The needle tip should rest within the "safe triangle" made up of the nerve root medially, the bony pedicle superiorly, and the lateral border of the foramen laterally (Fig. 75.5). The radiographic contrast should spread through the foramen to the central epidural space (Fig. 75.6). A 3-mL injectate comprising local anesthetic and steroids is injected per level. No more than 120 mg of triamcinolone should be injected during a session. The patient is asked to maintain a pain diary and is re-evaluated at 1 week. If only partial relief is obtained, a second injection can be scheduled.

Intra-articular zygapophysial joint injections

Intra-articular zygapophysial joint injections provide several months of pain relief at best. Their major role is to provide the patient with a period of pain control to allow effective physical rehabilitation.[52] There is no good evidence that intra-articular zygapophysial joint injections aid in the diagnosis of lumbar zygapophysial joint syndrome or help prognosticate the success of lumbar medial branch radiofrequency rhizotomy. These requirements are better met by lumbar medial branch blocks. Also, the zygapophysial joint space may be obliterated in the presence of extensive arthritis. The incidence of inability to enter the zygapophysial joint during attempted injections can be as high as 38%.[53] Under any circumstances, injection into a zygapophysial joint with absorbed synovium is without benefit.

Technique

The patient lies prone, with a pillow under the abdomen to maximize the intra-articular opening. An anteroposterior fluoroscopic view is obtained to identify the desired spinal level and side. Oblique fluoroscopy is obtained until the intra-articular opening of the target zygapophysial joint is maximized. A common target point is the midpoint of the zygapophysial joint. The skin and tissue overlying the target point are anesthetized and a 22-G needle is advanced into the capsular joint under radiographic guidance. The lumbar zygapophysial joints have a limited volume of 1.5 mL; a minimal (0.2 mL) amount of myelographic contrast material should be injected (Fig. 75.7). The 1.5 mL of a local anesthetic and steroid mixture is injected. The patient is evaluated post injection for degree of pain relief by engaging in activities that are known to produce the low back pain, such as lumbar hyperextension or rotation. A neurologic examination helps to ascertain the degree of extra-articular spread of the injection. The patient is asked to maintain a pain diary and is re-evaluated at 1 week.

Lumbar medial branch blocks and radiofrequency rhizotomy

Lumbar medial branch nerve blocks have been proposed as a tool to diagnose lumbar zygapophysial joint syndrome and prognosticate the success of radiofrequency denervation of the zygapophysial joints. The nerve supply to the implicated zygapophysial joints is blocked with local anesthetic and an assessment is made as to whether this has produced an improvement in the patient's pain condition.

Lumbar medial branch block: technique

The patient lies prone on the fluoroscopy table and an anteroposterior view is obtained to identify the desired spinal levels and side. The target point is the most medial and superior part of the transverse process, at its junction with the superior articular process. The skin overlying the target point is anesthetized and a 22-G needle is incrementally advanced under intermittent radiographic guidance until the superomedial aspect of the transverse process is contacted (Fig. 75.8). A lateral view of the spine is obtained to ensure that the needle has not been advanced excessively anteriorly to pass over the intervertebral foramen. Lumbar medial branch nerve blocks do not have a provocative component. The injection of limited local anesthetic volumes is imperative to minimize the spread of the anesthetic to the adjacent spinal nerve roots and

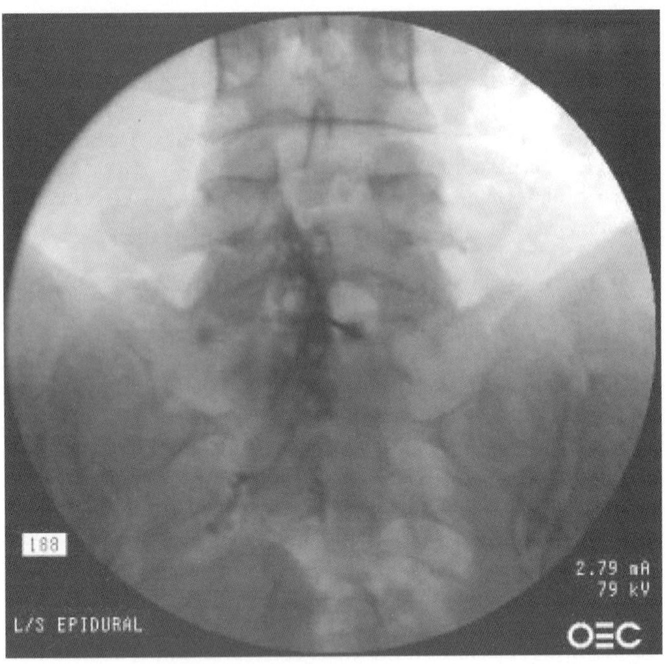

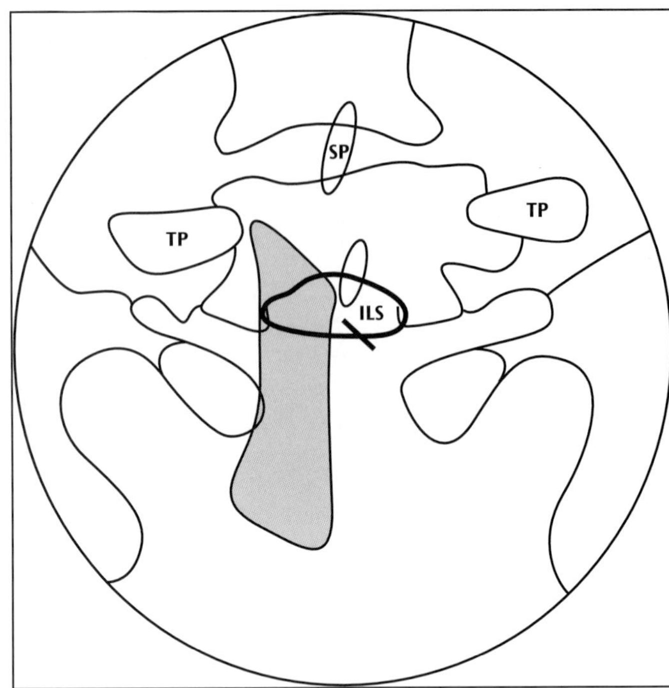

Figure 75.3 *An anteroposterior fluoroscopic view of an L5–S1 interlaminar epidural steroid injection. The needle tip is several millimeters to the left and the injection of 3 mL of myelographic contrast produces solely a left-sided epidurogram. A nonfluoroscopic technique would not ensure medication delivery to the correct level and side. ILS, interlaminar space; TP, transverse process; SP, spinous process.*

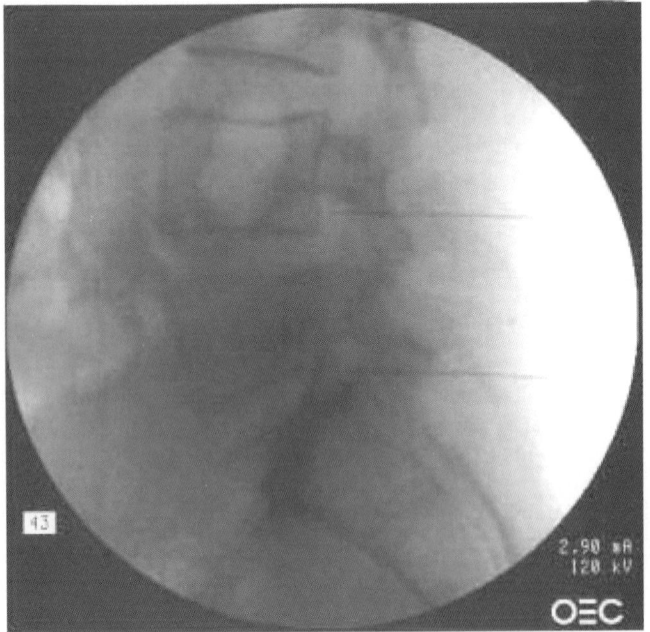

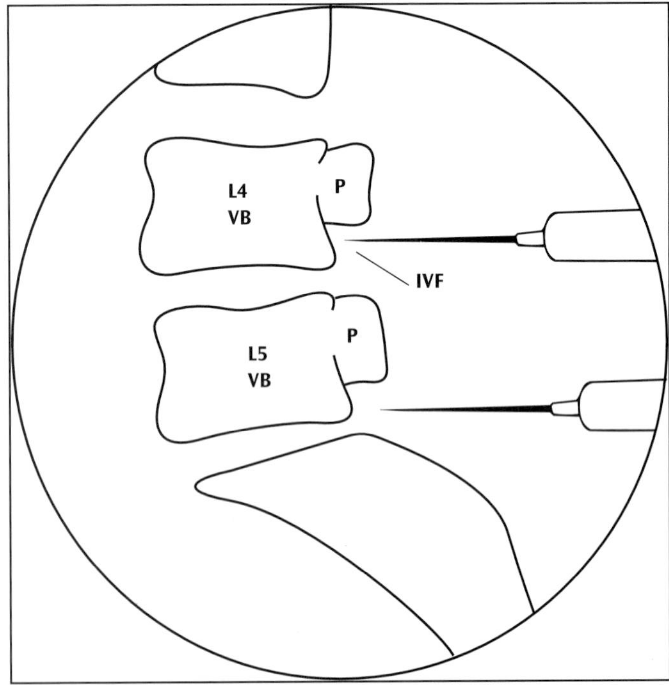

Figure 75.4 *A lateral view of a left L4 and L5 transforaminal epidural injection. The upper needle at the L4 intervertebral foramen is positioned properly. The needle at the L5 intervertebral foramen is positioned too caudad. See Fig. 75.5. VB, vertebral body; IVF, intervertebral foramen; P, pedicle.*

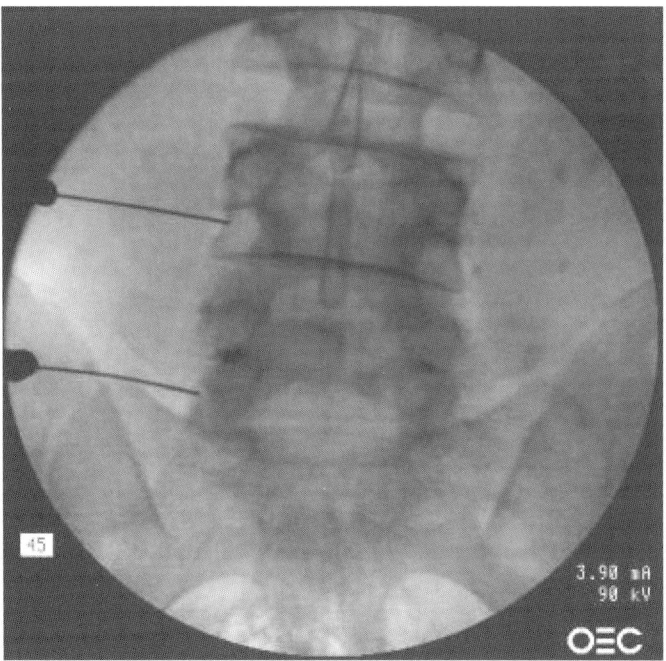

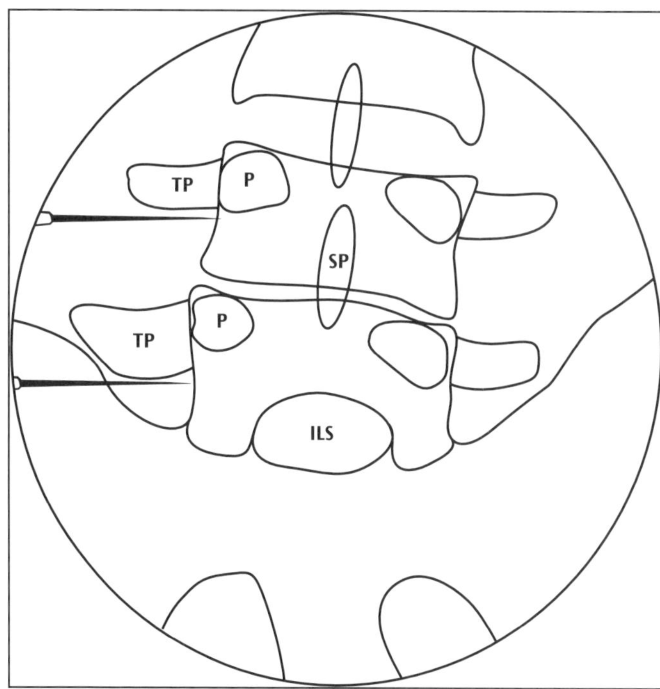

Figure 75.5 *An anteroposterior fluoroscopic view of the left L4 and L5 transforaminal epidural injection shown in Fig. 75.4. The needle tip is several millimeters into the intervertebral foramen at both levels. The L4 needle is positioned within the safe triangle; however, the L5 needle is deflected caudad by the transverse process. SP, spinous process; TP, transverse process; P, pedicle; ILS, interlaminar space.*

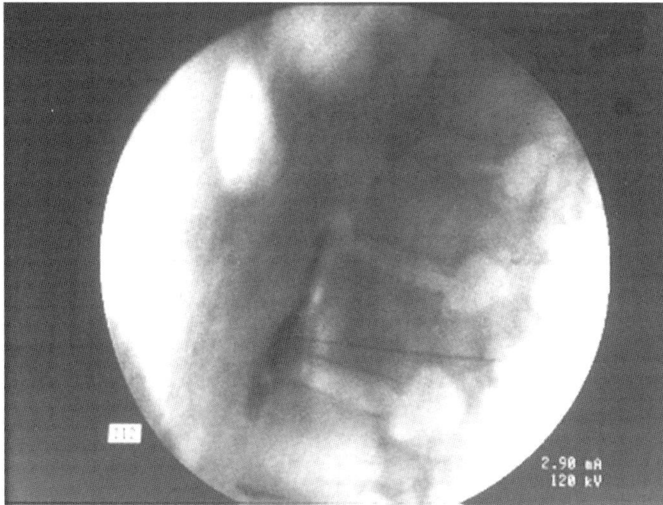

Figure 75.6 *An oblique view of a transforaminally placed needle at the right S1 foramen after a 0.5-mL myelographic contrast injection has produced a confirming neurogram.*

therefore minimize the incidence of false positives. 0.4 mL of 0.5% bupivacaine can be injected at each level to provide for adequate neural blockade of long enough duration to assess the patient's response. The patient is evaluated neurologically and for degree of pain relief post injection by performing the motions that are known to produce their pain. Numbness or weakness of a lower extremity indicates spread to spinal nerve roots and invalidates the findings. The patient is asked to maintain a pain diary for the day of the injection and is re-evaluated at 1 week. Pain improvement of greater than 50% during active and passive motion for the expected duration of the local anesthetic, without leg numbness or weakness, is an indication to proceed with radiofrequency rhizotomy of the zygapophysial joint.

Central nervous system electrical stimulation

Techniques stimulating the nervous system are among the treatments used to control chronic pain. A common technique is transcutaneous electrical nerve stimulation (TENS), which appears to activate peripheral A-beta fibers, which themselves modulate A-delta and C nociceptive fibers at the level of the spinal dorsal horn and produce central inhibitory effects. TENS units are advocated mostly for the relief of pain secondary to neuropathic conditions such as postherpetic neuralgia, neuritis, radiculopathy, or peripheral nerve injuries. It is also indicated for all types of musculoskeletal pain.[54] Its long-term efficacy has been questioned. TENS is widely used because of low risks of serious side-effects.

Epidural spinal cord stimulation (or dorsal column stimulation) is used for highly selected patients with intractable pain, for whom all more conservative treatments have failed.[55] Patients most likely to respond to such treatment are patients with failed back surgery syndrome, sometimes complicated by arachnoiditis, monoradiculopathy, and reflex sympathetic dystrophy of extremities. Patients who may benefit from this technique are selected according to a standard protocol that includes factors such as pain etiology, response to previous treatments, and psychological profile. When selected, they undergo a temporary stimulation trial: one or two electrodes are introduced in the epidural space above the area of pain and connected to an external stimulator. If this temporary trial produces significant and sustained pain relief (stimulation should produce paresthesias over the painful area), the patient is then a candidate for an implantable system. Several kinds of electrodes are available; some require a surgical implantation, whereas others can be inserted percutaneously. In the permanent system, the

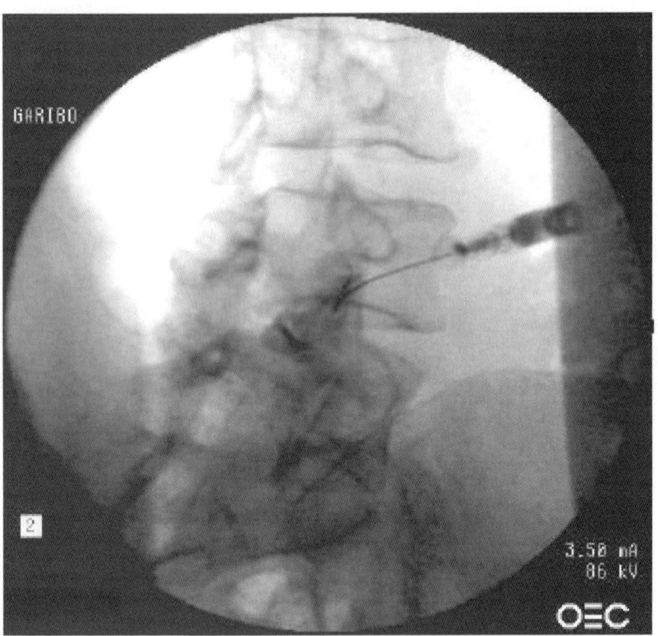

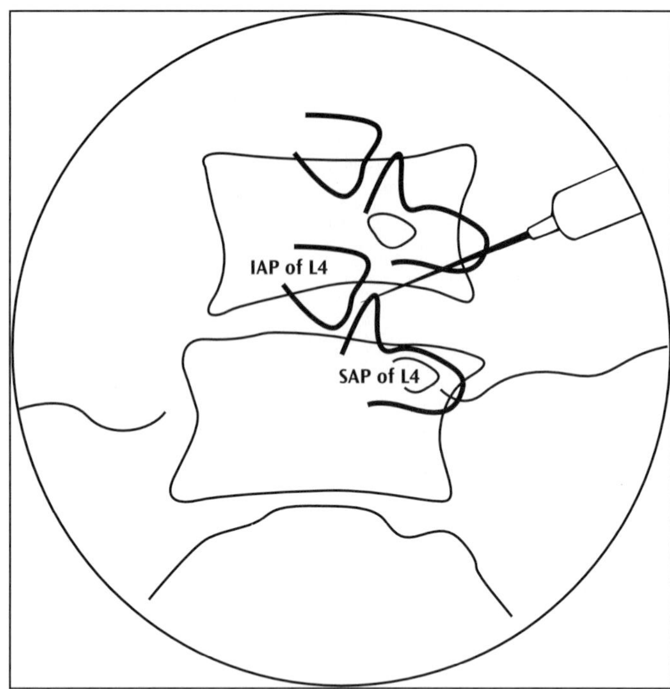

Figure 75.7 *An oblique fluoroscopic view of an L4-L5 intra-articular zygapophysial joint injection. The needle hub has been pulled to one side to allow visualization of the joint space. Injection of 0.2 mL of myelographic contrast produces a confirming arthrogram. IAP, interior articular process; SAP, superior articular process.*

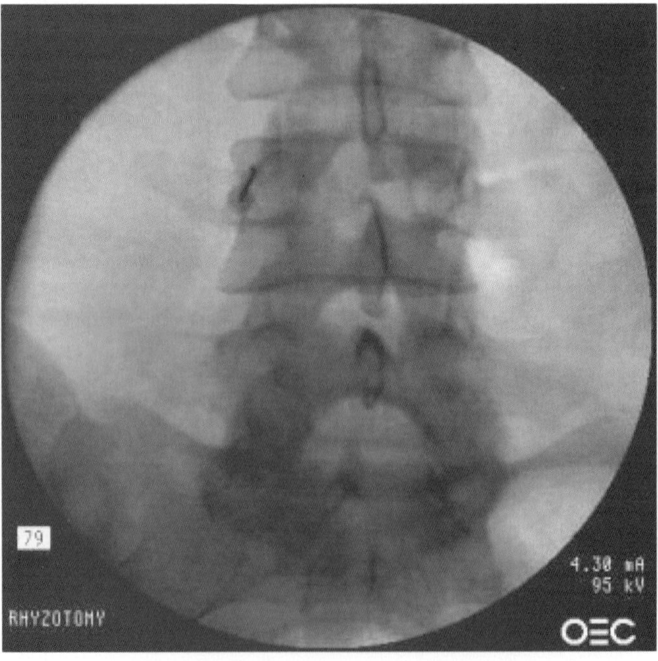

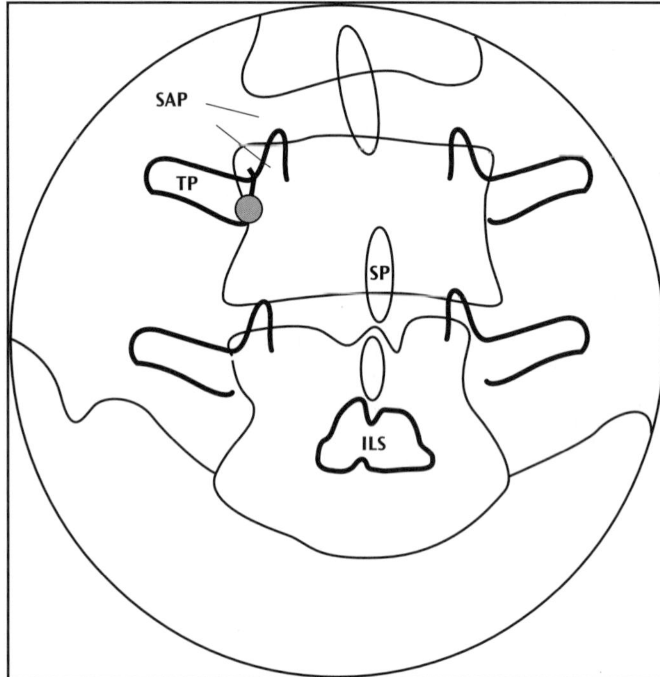

Figure 75.8 *A slightly oblique view of a needle placed over the L3 medial branch lying at the junction of the L4 superior articular and transverse process. SP, spinous process; TP, transverse process; ILS, interlaminar space; SAP, superior articular process.*

electrodes are attached to an internal receiver or generator. Patients can activate or deactivate the device at will, which provides pain relief whenever it is required. Results have shown that over a 20-year period, this technique, when applied in well-selected patients, is not only as good but probably better than major reconstructive surgery. Indications of new areas of application for this treatment currently being tested are peripheral vascular disease and refractory angina pectoris. Spinal cord stimulation is an effective nondestructive technique for the control of intractable pain in a few carefully selected patients, as part of a multidisciplinary approach.

Implanted spinal drug delivery systems

For the last 20 years, neuraxial drug therapy has increased in popularity. Spinally administered morphine was used first to provide intense analgesia without excessive systemic side-effects.[56] Today, opioid and nonopioid neuraxial therapy is used successfully to treat chronic intractable pain as well as spasticity. Available technology allows this treatment to be continued for years if necessary. Although it has been shown to be highly effective in cancer pain, the long-term administration of intraspinal opioid for chronic nonmalignant pain is still controversial. Patient selection criteria are an object of debate. The use of this technique in chronic nonmalignant pain may be life long, and patient selection for such a technique should be cautious. Inclusion criteria should take into consideration the fact that the pain may or may not be responsive to opioid treatment. Psychopathology, a history of addiction, and secondary gain issues are classic exclusion criteria. Although the major risks usually associated with systemically administered opioids, such as respiratory and behavioral effects (addiction), are usually not present with intrathecal chronic opioid delivery, the technique presents a significant number of side-effects, especially the development of tolerance, which make the technique difficult to use and may limit its usefulness. More interesting is the recent introduction of nonopioid substances for chronic intrathecal use. Increasingly, the α-$_2$-adrenergic agonist clonidine is being used, especially in cases of chronic neuropathic pain. Baclofen has also been used very successfully for pain-associated spasticity, particularly from spinal cord injury. Many other drugs have been, and are being, used intrathecally. It must be noted, however, that most of these drugs or combinations of these drugs have not been tested for prolonged intrathecal administration. In the USA, most of these drugs are used according to Food and Drug Administration (FDA) label recommendations. The system uses an intrathecal catheter connected to a pump, which is implanted subcutaneously, usually on one side of the abdomen. There are two types of pumps, one with fixed-rate drug delivery, which does not allow easy alteration in dosing, and the other fully programmable, communicating with a laptop computer through telemetry. Although these drugs and experience with them are now limited, this treatment may present a unique window of opportunity for patients with chronic intractable pain, as experience accumulates and new compounds are developed.

Use of the above-described implantable devices should be limited to highly selected patients, but also should be restricted to pain centers that are fully prepared to screen for appropriate patients, provide a safe implantation technique, and follow implanted patients closely for the duration of the entire treatment. Such a service requires special training, dedicated personnel, and adequate facilities.

MEDICATIONS USED FOR CHRONIC PAIN MANAGEMENT

Analgesics are among the most widely prescribed medications. Analgesics come from a variety of pharmacologic families, and can be very efficient in treating pain, but a detailed knowledge of their pharmacodynamics and pharmacokinetics is required in order to avoid side-effects and complications. Many variables are involved in the efficacy of these drugs, especially if they are administered for a prolonged duration, such as often occurs in chronic pain management. It is essential to realize the difference between the use of medication in acute pain and chronic pain. In acute pain, when there is usually an obvious tissue injury, medications are used during the acute phase until the pain is cured. Chronic pain is rarely cured, but usually only alleviated by different means, including medications. This pain relief, which may be only partial, is aimed at facilitating functional recovery of the patient, not at trying to get rid of the pain completely. As a rule, analgesics are one component of a multimodality treatment, in conjunction with others, which may address – in addition to the physical pain (e.g. nerve blocks) – other nonphysical pain, using emotional, cognitive, and rehabilitative techniques. Each chronic pain patient must have a long-term treatment plan in which medications, whenever they are used, are "helpers," and patients who receive the prescribed medications must be closely followed up. Most chronic pain patients, when medications are indicated, receive nonopioid analgesics, sometimes complemented with adjuvants. In some highly selected cases, opioid analgesics may also be used.

Nonopioid analgesic

Acetaminophen (paracetamol) is an analgesic antipyretic equipotent to aspirin. It is the first line of treatment for mild to moderate pain. Acute overdose or prolonged administration may create hepatotoxicity.

Nonsteroidal anti-inflammatory drugs are commonly used medications in the management of chronic pain. NSAIDs constitute a wide group of compounds of differing chemical structure.[57] They all have similar pharmacologic and clinical effects and side-effects. They inhibit cyclo-oxygenase, an enzyme that catalyzes the conversion of arachidonic acid to several types of prostaglandins. Prostaglandins play an important role in the central sensitization encountered during chronic pain (see above text). Therefore, they can be particularly useful in chronic pain states with inflammatory mechanism, windup phenomenon, central pain, and bone pain. Recently, new NSAIDs ("*COX-2 inhibitors*") have appeared which have a more selective action on COX-2 isozymes. It was found that COX-1 –a subgroup of COX– is necessary in order to protect the patient from significant side-effects from NSAIDs. These side-effects may occur in different degrees with most COX nonspecific NSAIDs: *gastropathy*, a known side-effect, may be responsible for major complications. Prostaglandins participate in the protection of the gastric mucosa and their inhibition may create a whole array of digestive symptoms. Also, oral NSAIDs may create direct irritation of the gastric mucosa. NSAIDs may also impair *hemostasis*. NSAIDs inhibit platelet COX irreversibly, such as with aspirin, or temporarily, with most other NSAIDs. Therefore, bleeding time may be increased. All NSAIDs compete with other anticoagulants, and patients receiving both must be carefully monitored. Another adverse effect of NSAIDs, also related to impaired prostaglandin synthesis, is *nephrotoxicity*. The blockade of prostaglandin synthesis in the kidney may result in an acute decline in renal blood flow, particularly obvious in people with pre-existing renal dysfunction, such as in heart failure, cirrhosis, or hypovolemia. NSAIDs can also lead to fluid retention and impaired response to diuretics. Finally, a variety of other adverse reactions, although rare, may also be seen, including hepatic, dermatologic, cognitive, and allergic. Examples of widely used NSAIDs are given in Table 75.3.

Tramadol hydrochloride is a short-acting analgesic, which has a partially opioid-mediated mechanism, binding modestly to the μ-receptor. It inhibits the uptake of norepinephrine and serotonin and, as such, has a unique place among analgesics. It has been shown to be efficient for controlling moderate pain and is usually considered as a weak opioid, without the abuse potential or the physical dependence

Table 75.3 *Nonsteroidal anti-inflammatory drugs (NSAIDs)*

Drugs	Maximum suggested p.o. daily dose (mg)	Frequency of administration
Acetaminophen (paracetamol)	650	q 4 h
Aspirin	650	q 4 h
Diclofenac	75	t.d.
Diflunisal	500	t.d.
Etodolac	400	t.d.
Ibuprofen	800	q.d.
Indomethacin	50	q.d.
Ketoprophen	75	q.d.
Ketorolac[a]	10	q.d.
Choline magnesium trisalicylate	1500	t.d.
Nabumetone	1000	t.d.
Naproxen	500	t.d.
Piroxicam	40	q.d.
Sulindac	200	b.d.
Selective COX-2 inhibitors		b.d.
Celecoxib	400	q.d.
Rofecoxib	50	

a. The i.v./i.m. dose is 30 mg q 6 h.

usually associated with opioids. The most common adverse effects are dizziness, nausea, and constipation.

Opioid analgesics

Although opioids are now widely accepted for the treatment of cancer pain, there is still a significant resistance within the medical community to the long-term use of opioids for chronic nonmalignant pain. The reasons usually put forward are: the possibility of developing addiction, likelihood of tolerance with a resulting loss of the drug's efficacy, dosage escalation that may lead to cognitive side-effects and decrease in overall function, and the fear of action against physicians by regulatory agencies. Increased experience has shown that a highly selected group of patients with chronic nonmalignant pain may benefit from the long-term administration of opioids. Classically, the population less likely to respond to opioids is patients with neuropathic pain, pre-existing cognitive impairment, psychological comorbidity, or a history of drug abuse. In addition to the development of physical dependence, opioids have a number of side-effects, including cognitive impairment, sedation, nausea, constipation, insomnia, and sexual dysfunction. The preceding factors are not absolute contraindications to the use of opioids, but necessitate a thorough knowledge of the pharmacology of these drugs and a close follow-up of treated patients. When initiating an opioid treatment in a chronic nonmalignant pain patient, it may be useful for the physician and the patient to agree, usually in writing, a clear description of the responsibilities of each, in order to reduce the probability of iatrogenic complications.

The advent of long-acting opioids has facilitated the use of opioids for chronic pain because the potential for abuse of these drugs is small (fewer psychotropic effects). Generally, long-term opioid prescriptions are reserved for use when other conservative treatment options have failed.[58] It is essential that only one physician be in charge of the treatment, providing the required information to the patient and establishing the behavioral rules and responsibilities of the patient. The degree of pain relief, functional improvement, and side-effects must be assessed on a regular basis. Oral administration is usually the first line of treatment in most patients, but many alternative routes of administration are available, including rectal, transdermal, sublingual, transmucosal, systemic (s.c. and i.v.), and spinal. Agonist opioids are usually used, whether naturally occurring opioids, such as morphine and codeine, semisynthetic opioids, such as hydromorphone or oxycodone, or synthetic opioids, such as methadone, propoxyphen, or fentanyl. Because of their plateau effect, their limited potency, and their side-effects, partial agonist and agonist–antagonist opioids are rarely used in the management of chronic pain. A list of commonly used opioids, with equivalent doses and length of action, is given in Table 75.4.

Adjuvants

Medications which are not primarily indicated in the control of pain have been found to be helpful as "adjuvants" in the management of chronic pain. Knowledge of the drugs is important because they may be used efficiently in treating neuropathic pain, a condition that is known to be difficult to treat with common analgesics or opioids.[59]

Antidepressants, particularly tricyclic antidepressants, have been used in chronic pain management in the last 20 years. Tricyclic antidepressants produce analgesia (especially in neuropathic pain) at doses of one-half to one-third of that required for antidepressant activity. They act by blocking the reuptake of serotonin, dopamine, and epinephrine. They also commonly produce sedation and may be used as sleeping aids in chronically sleep-deprived pain patients. They are typically started at a low dose, well under the antidepressant dosage. Anticholinergic side-effects are commonly encountered, such as constipation or dry mouth. The most commonly used drugs are amitriptyline, doxepin, imipramine, and nortriptyline.

Anticonvulsants are also useful in the management of chronic nonmalignant pain, again especially that of neuropathic origin. Anticonvulsants are a heterogeneous group of drugs, which depress abnormal neuronal discharges and raise the threshold for nerve activation. These compounds are membrane stabilizers on all neuronal membranes, altering sodium, calcium, and potassium fluxes, which are associated with action potentials. Phenytoin and carbamazepine have been used for many years to treat trigeminal neuralgia, which is characterized by sudden brutal attacks of sharp, lancinating pain. They are also used in other neuropathic pain conditions, such as postherpetic neuralgia, phantom limb pain, or diabetic neuropathy. Newer drugs, such as lamotrigin or gabapentin, are now commonly used for the above conditions. All these drugs are usually used at full anticonvulsant

Table 75.4 *Examples of opioids, with equivalent doses between routes of administration, and between drugs, i.e. all estimated doses are equivalent to 10 mg i.v. morphine*

Generic name	Route of administration	Equivalent dose	Range duration of action (h)
Morphine	p.o.	30 mg	3–4
	i.v.	10 mg	3–4
	Epidural	1 mg	6–24
Hydromorphone	p.o.	7.5 mg	3–4
	i.v.	1.5 mg	3–4
	Epidural	0.2 mg	10–16
Meperidine (pethidine)	p.o.	300 mg	3–6
	i.v.	75 mg	3–4
	Epidural	20 mg	4–8
Fentanyl	Transmucosal	100 μg	3–4
	Transdermal	a	72
	i.v.	100 μg	2–4
	Epidural	20 μg	6–10
Methadone	p.o.	20 mg	6–8
	i.v.	10 mg	6–8
Oxycodone	p.o.	30 mg	3–6
Levorphanol	p.o.	4 mg	4–8
	i.v.	2 mg	4–8
Codeine	p.o.	200 mg	4–5
Hydrocodone	p.o.	30 mg	3–4

a 25 μg h^{-1} corresponds approximately to a 26-h dose of 45–135 mg p.o. morphine and 15–40 mg i.v. morphine.

dosage. They can all cause cognitive impairment and sedation, which necessitates careful titration, starting with one-third to one-quarter of the full therapeutic dose.

Chronic administration of carbamazepine has been associated with pancytopenia and requires regular hematologic monitoring.

Anxiolytics, sedatives, and *hypnotics* are among of the most widely prescribed medications, and it is not unusual to find chronic pain patients taking any or all of them. These drugs are usually found useful for short-term indications but there is little benefit to using them in the long-term management of chronic pain. Among them, the benzodiazepines are most often used, especially as anxiolytics and to treat insomnia and muscle spasm. The risk of dependence and withdrawal symptoms is a significant barrier in their routine usage. Skeletal *muscle relaxants*, which act by depressing polysynaptic reflexes in the CNS, are sometimes used for muscle spasm. Baclofen (GABA-B receptor agonist), tizanidine, cyclobenzaprine, and carisoprodol are examples of such compounds. They all carry the risk of sedation and decreased function.

PSYCHOLOGICAL MODALITIES

The psychological intervention with the patient who has chronic pain is an integral part of the multidisciplinary approach to pain management. The most commonly utilized approach today is the cognitive–behavioral modality. The general goal of cognitive–behavioral treatment strategies is to reconceptualize patients' beliefs about their pain from an uncontrollable medical symptom to a belief that pain can be under their control.[60] The initial step is educating the patient about the relation between mind and body. The level and extent of this step depends on the patient's defensiveness and his/her level of knowledge and attitudes about mind–body approaches. The mainstay of this approach, however, is relaxation training, which helps patients by distracting them from their pain, reducing autonomic reactivity, and enhancing a sense of self-control. Relaxation training can be accomplished through several techniques: (1) guided imagery, (2) progressive muscular relaxation, (3) biofeedback, and (4) hypnosis.

1 Guided imagery has the patient focus on a multisensory imaginary scene. Typically, the image is elicited from the patient, and the psychologist guides the patient through the image, substituting sensations such as warmth or numbness for pain. Diaphragmatic breathing is an important part of the relaxation experience, distracting the patient even further.
2 In progressive muscular relaxation, patients are taught to alternately tense and relax individual muscle groups throughout the body.[61] Patients learn to recognize and differentiate feelings of tension and relaxation.
3 Biofeedback is a particularly effective modality for teaching chronic pain patients relaxation as well as self-regulation of physiologic processes. In a comparison of EMG biofeedback with cognitive–behavioral therapy and with conservative medical intervention, 57 patients with chronic back pain as well as 21 patients with temporomandibular disorders were evaluated.[62] At 24 months, only the biofeedback group maintained significant reductions in pain severity, interference, affective distress, and use of the healthcare system.
4 Hypnosis is another particularly effective therapeutic technique with pain patients. It not only teaches patients relaxation but also enables patients to experience an analgesic reinterpretation of their pain, experiencing numbness, for example, instead of pain. In a famous study by Spiegel and Bloom,[63] women with metastatic breast carcinoma pain undergoing weekly group therapy with self-hypnosis had significantly lower pain ratings over 1 year than a control group.

In addition to education and relaxation training, an essential part of the cognitive–behavioral approach is cognitive restructuring. With this technique, patients are taught to identify maladaptive negative thoughts that pervade their thinking and to replace them with more adaptive positive thoughts. The maladaptive thoughts often take the form of statements about oneself or illness that are negative, overgeneralizing, or catastrophizing. Psychotherapy also plays an essential role in the psychological intervention with pain patients. Group therapy is a frequently practiced method, as is supportive therapy, psychoanalytic psychotherapy, and family therapy.

COMPLEMENTARY MEDICINE AND PAIN MANAGEMENT

In two seminal studies by Eisenberg *et al.*,[64,65] the increasing use of complementary medicine techniques are well documented, with pain being identified as the most common problem for which these methods are used. More patient consultations take place with providers of complementary medicine than with conventional primary care physicians. Approximately one-third of Americans uses complementary modalities for various illnesses associated with pain. The most frequently used complementary modalities are chiropractic treatment, therapeutic massage, relaxation techniques, and acupuncture.

People with back, neck, and shoulder pain are the most common users. Those with headaches, stress, and anxiety disorders, as well as chronic musculoskeletal and rheumatologic disorders, are also frequent users.[65]

Most patients use complementary therapies as adjuncts to conventional therapies. If patients are not completely satisfied with conventional medical treatment, they seek out alternative practitioners as a way to supplement their conventional treatment.[66] This is particularly true of patients with chronic pain, as effective pain management continues to be unsatisfactory in many cases.

Although several research studies have demonstrated the effectiveness of acupuncture, chiropractic, and mind–body techniques with chronic pain patients, the evidence is equivocal. A review of the literature on treatments for low back pain by the US Agency for Health Care Policy and Research found that chiropractic was effective for the treatment of acute low back pain but the data were insufficient to judge its efficacy for chronic low back pain. A National Institutes of Health (NIH) technology assessment conference on the efficacy of mind–body approaches for the treatment of chronic pain and insomnia found "strong" to "moderate" evidence to support the use of relaxation techniques, hypnosis, cognitive–behavioral therapy, and biofeedback (particularly with headaches) in reducing chronic pain.[67] Davies *et al.*[68] concluded that pain clinics applying the full range of therapies offered the best symptomatic relief to patients with chronic pain.

Pain specialists need to be aware of the different alternative methods, and be open minded in their referral of these approaches. However, it should be realized that although conventional medicine has safeguards from governmental agencies, particularly in the USA, complementary medicine lacks any guidelines.

PAIN CLINIC ISSUES

Multidisciplinary approach to pain management

The multidisciplinary evaluation and treatment approach is widely practiced today and is considered to be the standard of care in pain management.[70] The evaluation and treatment of chronic pain patients has evolved from unidimensional to multidimensional models, and the utility of these approaches has increased exponentially. Since the formation of the first multidisciplinary pain center in 1961 by John Bonica at the University of Washington, over 350 such centers have been instituted in the USA, as listed by the American Pain Society.[70] A multidisciplinary pain center is a facility in which comprehensive treatment is provided by a team of healthcare professionals including physicians, physical therapists, occupational therapists, nurses, and psychologists.[71]

Turk and Stieg[72] prefer the term "interdisciplinary," which implies team interactions and communication and is different from the mere serial involvement of different specialists. Indeed, effective sharing of information among team members is essential. A major advantage of the team approach is that a broad base of knowledge and expertise is available, which can facilitate a team analysis of the etiology of the pain and the appropriate treatment approach.

Although the treatment of a patient with chronic pain mandates a comprehensive evaluation of the medical as well as psychological contributors to the causes of the pain, many patients are still evaluated and treated with a unimodal, strictly medical approach. This, unfortunately, often leads to iatrogenic effects, such as failed surgical interventions, and the restriction of activity. Additionally, failure to evaluate chronic pain patients for maladaptive behaviors, for example drug-seeking behaviors or addictive personality traits, can lead to pharmacologic disasters with attendant side-effects and exacerbation of pain. Another example of psychological issues that can be overlooked without a comprehensive psychological evaluation are patterns of somatization. These can lead to repeated medical interventions by all too willing pain specialists, and further contribute to medical and psychological morbidity. Therefore, in the USA, the Commission on Accreditation of Rehabilitation Facilities (CARF) accredits chronic pain programs that are interdisciplinary in both their evaluation and treatment of patients, and require, as part of the core pain team, a psychologist or psychiatrist.

Despite CARF criteria and the widely accepted standard of care, many third-party payers in the USA still refuse to cover multidisciplinary treatment, based on doubts regarding the efficacy and cost-effectiveness of treatment as well as an out-of-date notion of a physical–mental dichotomy.[73] Multidisciplinary pain center treatments do, however, result in greater clinical effectiveness and cost saving than the alternatives.[73] A recent report estimated outpatient multidisciplinary pain center treatment costs per patient as $8100[74], considerably less than the $15 000 estimate for back surgery[75] and the present cost estimate of $26 000 for conventional, nonsurgical medical treatment of chronic pain for the year prior to treatment at a multidisciplinary pain center.[73] Despite generally treating patients with highly complex problems who have often been previously refractory to treatment and iatrogenically injured, there have been numerous outcome studies demonstrating the efficacy of multidisciplinary treatment centers in: (1) reducing pain intensity – a meta-analysis of 65 studies ($n = 3089$) reports an average pain reduction of 20% following treatment at a multidisciplinary center; (2) management of opioid medications – at 1 year follow-up patients treated at a multidisciplinary pain center had reduced their opioid use from 69% to 22% compared with patients not treated (81% to 75%);[76] (3) return to a more optimal functional level – patients treated at a multidisciplinary pain center averaged a 65% increase in physical activity compared with 35% in patients treated in a standard manner;[77] and (4) healthcare utilization – one study reports a 36% reduction in pain-related clinic visits in the first year following treatment at a multidisciplinary pain center.[78] In total, there appear to be more data supporting the efficacy and cost-effectiveness of multidisciplinary treatment than for surgical procedures or conventional medical treatment for chronic pain.[73]

Treating the addicted pain patient

Among the most difficult chronic pain patients is the one who presents with a current or past history of addiction to illicit substances, alcohol, or prescription drugs. These patients can often wreak havoc in a pain clinic, severely testing the physician–patient boundaries, and eliciting strong emotional reactions in healthcare providers. The increasingly accepted management of chronic nonmalignant pain with opioid therapy underscores the importance of understanding the nature of opioid addiction.[79]

A recent survey of pain knowledge and attitudes of nearly 700 healthcare providers in three hospitals found a correct response rate of only 56%, with the addiction knowledge-related items responded to least correctly;[80] 72% of providers agreed incorrectly with the item "25% of patients receiving narcotics around the clock become addicted," when, in fact, the prevalence rate of opioid addiction in patients with chronic pain is much lower than the prevalence of substance use disorders in the population at large. The unwarranted fear of addiction is a misunderstood concept in pain management that can lead to the undertreatment of pain, a problem that has been well documented in AIDS and cancer patients.[81–84]

It is important to understand four often misunderstood concepts: (1) tolerance is the need for increasing doses to maintain effects; (2) physical dependence is an abstinence syndrome (withdrawal) following abrupt dose reduction; (3) although tolerance and physical dependence are normal pharmacologic phenomena, addiction is an abnormal psychological and behavioral syndrome characterized by loss of control over drug use, compulsive drug use, continued use despite harm to the user, and aberrant behavior such as theft, sale, hoarding of drugs, acquisition from several sources, and concurrent abuse of alcohol or other drugs; (4) addiction needs to be distinguished from pseudoaddiction, which refers to the distress and aberrant drug-related behaviors that can occur in the context of undertreated cancer pain.[85] The aberrant behaviors in pseudoaddiction disappear when an effective analgesic intervention is administered.

Treatment considerations for the addicted patient with chronic pain include the utilization of a multidisciplinary team approach with the inclusion of a provider with expertise in addiction medicine. A careful evaluation of the substance use history of the patient as well as documentation and direct communication with all providers of the patient who might write prescriptions is essential. Patients must be carefully monitored for the development of aberrant drug-related behaviors, with frequent visits (which also enable the prescription of small quantities of drugs), regular urine toxicology screens, and inquiries of significant others regarding the patient's drug use. A prerequisite for treatment is the use of a written contract that explicitly delineates the provider's expectations of the patient and the consequences of aberrant drug use. Contract stringency, such as how to deal with "lost" prescriptions or early refills, should be based on the level of concern regarding aberrant behaviors. Although management of the addicted patient with pain is very complex, it needs to be undertaken in a sensitive and nonjudgmental manner, with full knowledge and expertise of all of the issues.

Ethics in pain management

The formation of ethics committees by the American Pain Society and the American Academy of Pain Medicine reflects the growing concern about and significance of ethical issues in pain management. As the specialty of pain management has grown and developed, ethical challenges have emerged owing to factors such as managed care, increasingly invasive interventions, and state regulations. There are also characteristics of chronic pain patients that can lead to ethical dilemmas:

1 The inherent difficulty of "curing" chronic pain can lead practitioners, as well as patients, to be overly aggressive in their approaches, which can lead to significant side-effects or iatrogenic injuries, such as failed back surgery syndrome.
2 Pre-existing psychopathology may lead to a patient reacting to pain or to a failure in its relief. Iatrogenic injury may significantly affect treatment because the pain may not be taken seriously or may be treated too aggressively.
3 End-of-life issues and palliative care, which have received much publicity, pose enormously challenging ethical dilemmas for the pain practitioner. Pain, one of the most common reasons for assisted suicide or euthanasia, places the pain practitioner at the forefront of these issues.
4 The relation between the patient and physician in the chronic pain arena can be quite difficult because of the complexity of pain and prior failed attempts at relief, which can lead to anger on the part of the patient and frustration on the part of the provider. Emotional reactions can lead to a suspension of objective decision making.
5 Most interventions implemented today by pain centers have not been demonstrated in a scientifically rigorous manner to be efficacious. The use of unproved methods in pain management, as well as the growing popularity and acceptance by the medical community of complementary techniques that are used most often for pain,[65] places the pain provider in the moral dilemma of using or referring patients for unproved techniques.
6 The vulnerable, often desperate, nature of many pain patients makes them very susceptible to trying anything that all-too-willing practitioners might do. The issue can also be phrased as "when is aggressive intervention compassionate understanding and effort and when is it taking advantage of a vulnerable patient?"
7 The preceding issue becomes more pronounced when considering the increasing economic pressures on pain clinics. The advent of managed care in the USA, with its rejections of and lengthy delays in getting authorization, as well as its limitations on reimbursement, has changed the practice of pain management. This has increased the incentives to do more invasive and profitable interventions.
8 Many chronic pain patients are in litigation as a result of the onset of their pain, which may have been a motor vehicle accident, or an accident at work. Litigation is a very powerful secondary gain issue, which may consciously or subconsciously reinforce pain, illness behavior, and healthcare utilization. It often works against the goals of treatment; the ethical dilemma becomes whether or how to treat the patient in the face of such a powerful reinforcer of pain.
9 The worker's compensation system in the USA presents the treatment provider with many ethical conflicts, such as whether to treat a patient for whom authorization has been delayed or denied, return to work delays and difficulties, and the subjective medical judgments of medical physicians paid by the compensation system.

The International Association for the Study of Pain has published ethical guidelines for pain management.[86] The clinical care section focuses on the professional power and responsibility of the provider, which needs to be used in a supportive rather than abusive manner, and that the needs of patients take precedence over the needs of clinicians. The guidelines also recognize the existence of "vulnerable" groups such as those who cannot communicate verbally (infants, the elderly, those in an intensive care unit), cancer patients (the need to understand opioid pain control and the differences between addiction, dependence, tolerance, and pseudoaddiction), dying patients, and economically disadvantaged patients. The guidelines also acknowledge the moral responsibility for appropriate pain care and the need for an interdisciplinary approach.

Bioethical principles commonly encountered in pain management include beneficence (i.e. the obligation to do good), nonmaleficence (i.e. the obligation not to harm), respect for patient autonomy (i.e. the right of patients to make their own decisions), and justice (i.e. the right of all patients to equal services).[87] Specific ethical dilemmas in pain management include the undertreatment of pain because of:

1 The fear of addiction or lack of knowledge on the part of the health-care provider[80] and the patient.
2 Insurance denial of treatment and reimbursement conflicts such as different reimbursement rates for different patients and for different procedures. Do providers spend more time with more profitable patients and do more profitable interventions? This is not in the best interest of all patients and calls into question the bioethical principle of justice.
3 Special populations such as substance abusers, children, and the elderly tend to be undertreated due to biases and lack of knowledge of appropriate assessment and treatment methods with these populations.

In addition to the undertreatment of pain, additional ethical dilemmas that pain providers face include: (1) the lack of therapeutic standards of care to help guide the practitioner in choosing which therapy to initiate, which can be exacerbated even more when the patient demands a specific therapy; (2) management of pain at the end of life, with the very complex issues of advanced directives, living wills, and do-not-resuscitate orders; (3) the use of placebos in the clinical care of patients; (4) the growing use of largely unproved complementary techniques in pain management.

Proposed solutions for ethical dilemmas in pain management are unfortunately much briefer than the challenges themselves. Ethics strategies are largely preventive in nature and include discussing with colleagues all major decisions regarding ethical conflicts before any action is taken. Other subjects for discussion include currently accepted pain practice modalities, and complex end-of-life care issues. Additional ethics solutions include reviewing the informed consent process and improving communication with patients (which can improve compliance and avoid malpractice litigation), and third-party payers (which can reduce denials and delays in authorization and reimbursement). Finally, many institutions have formed ethics committees; it is always better to consult with one when faced with an ethical conflict than to be called before the committee after the fact.

Acknowledgment

Author Christopher Gharibo, MD, would like to thank Gisela Aydin for her review of the manuscript and valuable comments, many of which are incorporated herein.

REFERENCES

1. Waddell G. The epidemiology of low back pain. In: *The Back Pain Revolution.* London: Churchill Livingstone, 1998: 69–84.
2. Fields H. *Pain.* New York: McGraw-Hill, 1987.
3. Bonica JJ. Anatomic and physical basis of nociceptive and pain. In: *The Management of Pain.* Philadelphia: Lea and Febiger, 1990: 28–94.
4. Raja SN, Meyer RA, Ringkaup M, Campbell JN. Peripheral neural in changing of nociception. In: *The Textbook of Pain*, 4th edn. London: Churchill Livingstone, 1999: 11–57.
5. Doubell TP, Marion RJ, Woolf, CJ. The dorsal hour: late dependent sensory processing, plasticity and the generation of pain. In: *The Textbook of Pain.* London: Churchill Livingstone, 165–81.
6. Yaksh TL. Central pharmacology of nociceptive transmission. In: *The Textbook of Pain*, 4th edn. London: Churchill Livingstone, 1999: 253–308.
7. Raj PP. Pain mechanisms. In: *Pain Medicine, A Comprehensive Review.* St Louis, MO: Mosby-Year Book Publishers, 1996: 12–23.
8. Fields HL, Bashbaum AJ. Central nervous system mechanisms of pain modulation. *Textbook of Pain.* London: Churchill Livingstone, 1999: 309–29.
9. Woolf CJ, Marion RJ. Neurophatic pain. Etiology, symptoms, mechanisms and management. *Lancet* 1999; **353:** 1959–64.
10. Scadding JW. Complex regional pain syndrome. In: *The Textbook of Pain.* London: Churchill Livingstone, 1999: 835–49.
11. McCaffrey, M. Nursing practice theories related to cognition, bodily pain and man-environment interactions. *University of California at Los Angeles Students' Store*, 1968.
12. Melzack R. The McGill Pain Questionnaire: major properties and scoring methods. *Pain* 1975; **1:** 277–99.
13. Beck AT, Rush AJ, Sha BF, Emery G. *Cognitive Therapy of Depression.* New York: Guilford, 1979.
14. Spielberger CD. *Manual for the State-Trait Anxiety Inventory.* Palo Alto, CA: Consulting Psychologists Press, 1983.
15. Butcher NB, Dahlstrom WG, Graham JR, *et al. MMPI-2, Manual for Administration and Scoring.* Minneapolis, MN: University of Minnesota Press, 1989.
16. Derogatis LR. *The SCL-90R: Administration Scoring and Procedures Manual I.* Baltimore, MD: Clinical Psychometrics Research, 1977.
17. Rosenstiel AK, Keefe FJ. The use of coping strategies in chronic low back pain patients: relationship to patient characteristics and current adjustment. *Pain* 1983; **17:** 33–44.
18. Nelson DV, Kennington M, Novy DM. Psychological selection criteria for implantable spinal cord stimulators. *Pain Forum* 1996; **5:** 93–103.
19. Frymoyer JW, Cats-Baril WL. An overview of the incidences and costs of low back pain. *Orthop Clin North Am* 1991; **22:** 263–71.
20. Quebec Task Force on Spinal Disorders.: Scientific approach to the assessment and management of activity-related spinal disorders. *Spine* 1987; 12S16.
21. Derby RD, Bogduk N, *et al.* Precision percutaneous blocking procedures for localizing spinal pain. *Pain Digest* 1993; **3:** 89–100.
22. Kleiner JB, Donaldson III WF, Curd JG, *et al.* Extraspinal causes of lumbosacral radiculopathy. *J Bone Joint Surg* 1991; **73:** 817.
23. Bigos S, Bowyer O, Braen G, *et al.* Acute low back problems in adults. In: *Clinical Practice Guidelines No. 14. AHCPR Publication No. 95–0642.* Rockville, MD: Agency for Health Care Policy and Research, Public Health Service, US Department of Health and Human Services, December 1994.
24. Deyo RA, Diehl AK, Rosenthal M. How many days of bed rest for acute low back pain? A randomized clinical trial. *N Engl J Med* 1986; **315:** 1064–70.
25. Malmivaara A, Hakkinen U, Aro T, *et al.* The treatment of acute low back pain – bed rest, exercises or ordinary activity? *N Engl J Med* 1995; **332:** 351–5.
26. Rydevik B, Brown MD, Lundborg G. Pathoanatomy and pathophysiology of nerve root compression. *Spine* 1984; **9:** 7.
27. McMarron RF, Wimpee MW, Hudkins PG, *et al.* The inflammatory effect of nucleus pulposus. A possible element in the pathogenesis of low back pain. *Spine* 1987; **12:** 760–4.
28. Deyo RA, Loeser JD, Bigos SJ. Herniated lumbar intervertebral disk. *Ann Intern Med* 1990; **112:** 598.
29. Bogduk N, Twomey LT (eds). The facet joints (Chapter 3) In: *Clinical Anatomy of the Lumbar Spine*, 2nd edn. Australia, Churchill Livingstone, 1995: 27–34.
30. Giles LG, Harvey AR. Immunohistochemical demonstration of nociceptors in the capsule and synovial faults of lumbar zygapophysial joints. *Br J Rheumatol* 1987; **26:** 362–4.
31. Bogduk N. The innervation of the lumbar spine. *Spine* 1983; **8:** 286.
32. Hirsch C, Ingelmark B, Muller M. The anatomical basis for low back pain. *Acta Orthop Scand* 1963; **33:** 1.
33. Mooney V, Robertson J. The facet syndrome. *Clin Orthop* 1976; **115:** 149–56.
34. McCall IW, Park WM, O'Brien JP. Induced pain referral from posterior lumbar elements in normal subjects. *Spine* 1979; **4:** 441–6.
35. Badgley CE. The articular facets in relation to low back pain and sciatic radiation. *J Bone Joint Surg* 1941; **23:** 481–96.
36. Onel D, Sari H, Donmez C. Lumbar spinal stenosis: clinical/radiologic therapeutic evaluation in 145 patients. *Spine* 1993; **18:** 291–8.
37. Long SP, Kephart W. Myofascial Pain Syndrome. In: Ashburn MA, Rice LR (eds). *The Management of Pain.* London: Churchill Livingstone, 1999: 299–321.
38. Bana DS, Headaches. In: Aronoff GM (ed.). *Evaluation and Treatment of Chronic Pain.* Baltimore: MD: Williams & Wilkins, 1999: 147–76.
39. Blumberg H. A new clinical approach for diagnosing reflex sympathetic dystrophy. *Pain Research and Clinical Management*, vol. 4. Proceedings of the 6th World Congress on Pain, Amsterdam: Elsevier, 1991: 399–403.
40. Noordenbos W. Problems pertaining to the transmission of nerve impulses which give rise to pain. *Pain* 1959; **1:** 4–10, 68–80.
41. Watson CPN, Deck HJ, Morshead C, *et al.* Post herpetic neuralgia: further post post mortem studies of cases with and without pain. *Pain* 1991; **44:** 105–17.

42. Ragozzino MW, Melton III LJ, Kurland LT, *et al*. Population based study of herpes zoster and its sequelae. *Medicine* 1982; **61:** 310–16.
43. Boon R. Efficacy and safety of famcicclovir in the treatment of herpes zoster. *Presented at the Second International Conference on the Varicella Zoster Virus*. Paris, 1995.
44. Haddox JD, Biondi DM. Facial Pain. In: Abram SE, Haddox, JD (eds). *The Pain Clinic Manual*, 2nd edn. Philadelphia: Lippincott Williams & Wilkins, 2000: 201–12.
45. Jensen MC, Brant-Zawadzki MN, Obuchowski N, *et al*. Magnetic resonance imaging of the lumbar spine in people without back pain. *N Engl J Med* 1994; **331:** 69–73.
46. Boden SD, Davis DO, Dina TS, *et al*. Abnormal magnetic-resonance scans of the lumbar spine in asymptomatic subjects. *J Bone Joint Surg* 1990; **72** (A): 403.
47. Gharibo C. Spinal injections in diagnosis and treatment of low back pain. *Prog Anesthesiol* 1999: **12** (24): 423–40.
48. Devor M, Govrin-Lippman R, Raber P. Corticosteroids suppress ectopic neural discharge originating in experimental neuromas. *Pain* 1985; **22:** 127–37.
49. Johansson A, Hao J, Sjolund B. Local corticosteroid application blocks transmission in normal nociceptive C-fibres. *Acta Anaesthesiol Scand* 1990; **34:** 335–8.
50. Weinstein SM, Herring SA, Derby R. Corticosteroid application blocks transmission in normal nociceptive C-fibers. *Acta Anasthesiol Scand* 1990; **34:** 335–8.
51. Saal JA, Saal JS. Nonoperative treatment of herniated lumbar intervertebral disc with radiculopathy. An outcome study. *Spine* 1989; **14** (4): 431–7.
52. Merry A, Schug SA, Rogers A. Epidural steroid injections for sciatica and back pain: A meta-analysis of controlled clinical trials. *Reg Anesth* 1996; **21** (2S): 64.
53. Lynch MC, Taylor JF. Facet joint injection for low back pain. *J Bone Joint Surg* 1986; **68** (B): 138.
54. Hansson PH, Lundeberg T. TENS, vibration and acupuncture as pain-relieving measures. *Textbook of Pain*. London: Churchill Livingstone, 1999: 1341–51.
55. Bedder MD. Spinal cord stimulation and intractable pain: patient selection. In: Weldman S, Williams A (eds). *Interventional Pain Management*. Philadelphia: WB Saunders, 1996: 412–18.
56. Carr DB, Cousins MJ. Spinal route of analgesia: neural blockade. In: Cousins MJ, Bridenbaugh, PO (eds). *Clinical Anesthesia and Management of Pain*, 3rd edn. Philadelphia: Lippincott-Raven, 1998.
57. Brune K, Zeilhofer HU. Antipyrectic (non-narcotic) analgesics. In: *Textbook of Pain*. London: Churchill Livingstone, 1999: 1139–53.
58. Portenoy RK. Opioid therapy for chronic non-malignant pain: current status in progress. In: Fields HL, Liebeskind, JC (eds). *Pain Research and Management*, vol. 1. Seattle: IASP Press, 1994.
59. Haddox JD. Coanalgesic agents. In: Raj PP (ed.). *Pain Medicine: A Comprehensive Review*. St Louis, MO: Mosby Year Book, 1996: 142–53.
60. Bradley LA. Cognitive-behavioral therapy for chronic pain. In: Gatchel RJ, Turk DC (eds). *Psychological Approaches to Pain Management*. New York: Guilford Press, 1996: 131–47.
61. Lebovits AH, Bassman LE. Psychological aspects of chronic pain management. In: Lefkowitz M, Lebovits AH, Wlody D, Rubin S (eds). *A Practical Approach to Pain Management*. Boston, MA: Little Brown, 1996: 124–8.
62. Flor H, Birbaumer N. Comparison of the efficacy of EMG biofeedback, cognitive-behavior therapy and conservative medical interventions on the treatment of chronic musculoskeletal pain. *J Consult Clin Psychol* 1993; **61:** 653–8.
63. Spiegel D, Bloom J. Group therapy and hypnosis reduce metastatic breast carcinoma pain. *Psychosomatic Med* 1983; **45:** 333–9.
64. Eisenberg DM, Kessler RC, Foster C, *et al*. Unconventional medicine in the United States: prevalence, costs, and patterns of use. *N Engl J Med* 1993; **328:** 246–52.
65. Eisenberg DM, Davis RB, Ether SL, *et al*. Trends in alternative medicine use in the US, 1990–1997 *JAMA* 1998; **280:** 1569.
66. Berman BM, Swyers JP. Applying alternative medical approaches to managing chronic pain syndromes: if not now, when? *APS Bulletin* 1998; **March/April:** 4–6.
67. NIH Technology Assessment Panel on Integration of Behavioral and Relaxation Approaches into the Treatment of Chronic Pain and Insomnia. Integration of behavioral and relaxation approaches into the treatment of chronic pain and insomnia. *JAMA* 1996; **276:** 313–18.
68. Davies HTO, Crombie IK, Brown JH, Martin C. Diminishing returns or appropriate strategy?: an analysis of short-term outcomes after pain clinic treatment. *Pain* 1997; **70:** 203–8.
69. Lebovits AH. Chronic pain: the multidisciplinary approach. *Int Anesthesiol Clin* 1991; **29:** 1–7.
70. American Pain Society. *1996 Pain Facilities Directory*. Glenview, IL: American Pain Society, 1996.
71. Turk DC, Stacey BR. Multidisciplinary pain centers in the treatment of chronic pain. In: Fromeyer JW, Ducker TB, Hadler NM, Ksotuik JP, Weinstein JN, Whitecloud III, TS (eds). *The Adult Spine: Principles and Practice*, 2nd edn. New York: Raven 1997: 253–74.
72. Turk DC, Stieg RL. Chronic pain: the necessity of interdisciplinary communication. *Clin J Pain* 1987; **3:** 163–7.
73. Okifuji A, Turk DC, Kalauokalani D. Clinical outcome and economic evaluation of multidisciplinary pain centers. In: Block AR, Kremer EF, Fernandez E (eds). *Handbook of Pain Syndromes-Biopsychosocial Perspectives*. New Jersey, PA: Lawrence Erlbaum Associates, 1999: 77–97.
74. Marketdata Enterprises. *Chronic Pain Management Programs: A Market Analysis*. Valley Stream, New York: Marketdata Enterprises, 1995.
75. Fromeyer JW, Durett CL. The economics of spinal disorders. In: Fromeyer JW, Ducker TB, Hadler NM, Ksotuik JP, Weinstein JN, Whitecloud III, TS (eds). *The Adult Spine: Principles and Practice*, 2nd edn. New York: Raven, 1997: 143–50.
76. Tollison CD. Comprehensive treatment approach for lower back workers' compensation injuries. *J Occup Rehabil* 1991; **1:** 281–7.
77. Flor H, Fydrich T, Turk DC. Efficacy of multidisciplinary pain treatment centers: a meta-analytic review. *Pain* 1992; **49:** 221–30.
78. Caudill M, Schnabble R, Zuttermeister P, *et al*. Decreased clinic use by chronic pain patients: response to behavioral medicine intervention. *Clin J Pain* 1991; **7:** 305–10.
79. Portenoy RK. Opioid therapy for chronic nonmalignant pain: a review of the critical issues. *J Pain Symptom Manage* 1996; **11:** 203–17.
80. Lebovits AH, Florence I, Bathina R, *et al*. Pain knowledge and attitudes of health care providers: practice characteristic differences. *Clin J Pain* 1997; **13:** 237–43.
81. Lebovits AH, Lefkowitz M, McCarthy D, *et al*. The prevalence and management of pain in patients with AIDS: a review of 134 cases. *Clin J Pain* 1989; **5:** 245–8.
82. Lebovits AH, Smith G, Maignan M, Lefkowitz M. Pain in hospitalized patients with AIDS: Analgesic and psychotropic medications. *Clin J Pain* 1994; **10:** 156–61.
83. Breitbart W, Rosenfeld BD, Passik SD, *et al*. The undertreatment of pain in ambulatory AIDS patients. *Pain* 1996; **65:** 239.
84. Cleeland C, Gonin R, Hatfield A, *et al*. Pain and its treatment in outpatients with metastatic cancer. *N Engl J Med* 1994; **330:** 592.
85. Weissman DE, Haddox JD. Opioid pseudoaddiction-an iatrogenic syndrome. *Pain* 1989; **36:** 363.
86. Fields HL. Ethical standards in pain management and research. In: Fields HL (ed.). *Core Curriculum for Professional Education in Pain*. Seattle, WA: IASP Press, 1995; 117–23.
87. Beauchamp TL, Childress JF. *Principles of Biomedical Ethics*, 4th edn. Oxford: Oxford University Press, 1994.

76

Cancer pain

OSCAR A de LEON-CASASOLA AND MARK J LEMA

INTRODUCTION

Advances in cancer treatment continue to lengthen survival among cancer patients. As patients' lives are prolonged, the need for effective pain control to improve the quality of life has gained increased importance. The chief complaint of patients with advanced cancer is often pain. The incidence of pain varies depending upon the type of neoplasm, stage, and extent of spread. Although various investigators have tried to define the prevalence of pain in cancer patients, the lack of objective diagnostic tests for pain has led to figures ranging from 20–50% of all patients in early stages to 55–95% in the later stages.[1] Thus, pain is a common symptom of cancer patients and, next to incurability, it is the most feared complication. With the current therapeutic modalities available to the clinician about 80–90% of cancer pain can be controlled.[2] However, recent studies show that the majority of cancer pain, especially in women, members of ethnic minorities, and the elderly, is undertreated by cancer specialists.[3,4] Major barriers to effective cancer pain control include (1) inadequate assessment by practitioners, (2) under-reporting of pain by patients and families, (3) practitioners' lack of knowledge regarding current treatment, (4) lack of accountability for effectively treating pain, (5) fear of over-regulation by government officials, and (6) inadequate reimbursement for pain treatment or excessive administrative demands by healthcare providers.

Inadequate assessment of pain by physicians and nurses was demonstrated by Ho[5] to be one of the most important causes of treatment failure. Widespread misconceptions and knowledge deficits have also been shown to cause this poor assessment by healthcare providers. Many patients or families are reluctant to report pain because they are (1) afraid the tumor has spread, (2) wish to save opioids for when pain worsens, (3) are concerned about addiction, and (4) do not want to distract oncologists from curing the cancer.

In an attempt to rectify the problems, guidelines for the treatment of cancer pain have been developed by the World Health Organization, the American Society of Anesthesia, and the Agency for Health Care Policy and Research.[6,7]

PATHOPHYSIOLOGY OF CANCER PAIN

Causes of cancer pain

There are essentially four different causes of pain in cancer patients: acute cancer-related pain, chronic cancer-related pain, chronic nonmalignant pain in opioid-tolerant patients, and end-of-life pain.

Several classic studies have assessed the types of cancer pain seen in pain clinics.[8–10] Approximately 60–80% of all patients have tumor-related pain. Between 20% and 30% have treatment-related pain, and 10–15% have pain unrelated to the cancer. Twycross and Fairfield[9] found that about 80% of cancer patients coming to their clinic had two or more anatomically distinct pain sites, and one-third had four or more pain sites.

Classification of cancer pain

Cancer pain is classified according to pain duration and pain quality. Pain duration denotes the degree of chronicity. The three temporal conditions are acute pain, chronic pain, and incidental pain (joint pain, arthralgias) which occurs on movement. A pathophysiologic component is also described: somatic (nociceptive) pain, visceral pain, neuropathic pain, central pain, and sympathetic pain.

Somatic pain

Somatic pain results from the activation of nociceptors in peripheral or deep tissues. C- and Aδ-fibers transmit pain sensation from the periphery to the dorsal horn and eventually cephalad through the spinothalamic tract to various parts of the midbrain and neocortex. The quality of this pain is described as a well localized, aching or gnawing. Bone pain, muscle pain, and postoperative pain are common causes of this condition.

Visceral pain

When visceral structures are stretched, compressed, invaded, or distended, a poorly localized noxious pain is reported. Patients often describe the pain as deep, squeezing, crampy, and colic in nature. Referred pain, also known as a viscerosomatic reflex, such as shoulder complaints occurring when the diaphragm is invaded by hepatic tumor, and nausea and vomiting are common associated conditions. Pancreatic and colon carcinomas often produce this condition.

Neuropathic pain

Direct injury to neural tissue from tumor infiltration erosion or from cancer therapies such as vinca alkaloids, platinol compounds, radiation, or surgery can result in a noxious, intractable sensation. Associated sensory, motor, and autonomic deficits can accompany the symptoms of burning, squeezing, and paroxysmal sharp pain. Examples of this pain include brachial and lumbar plexopathies and post-thoracotomy pain syndrome. A high incidence of patient suffering is associated with neuropathic pain.

Central pain

Conditions that affect the central nervous system, usually involving second- or third-order neurons, can produce a central pain condition typified by abnormal sensibility to both pain and temperature (hyperalgesia). Examples include neoplastic lesions along the spinothalamic tract, thalamic or cerebral cortex projections, postherpetic neuralgia, and phantom limb syndrome.

Sympathetic pain

Although not commonly seen in cancer patients with pain, this condition can occur after pathologic fractures, thrombosis due to hypercoaguable states, and lymphedema of extremities. This condition is typified by constant burning, allodynic pain (pain in response to normally stimuli), with associated sudomotor (sweat gland neural activity) and vasomotor changes, edema, and coldness of the affected area.

Cancer pain syndromes

While clinicians classify pain according to its onset, duration, and nature, cancer pain is often experienced as several different types, with combined somatic and neuropathic being the most frequent.[11] During the course of the disease, the character of pain will change as the result of tumor progression or regression after treatment. These changes may occur rapidly and serve to illustrate the dynamic nature of cancer pain.

Acute pain

Pain is often the presenting symptom of a patient with cancer. If it occurs early in the disease, patients may endure high levels of pain in the expectation that adequate anticancer therapy will relieve their symptoms. If it occurs late in the course, pain often signifies disease recurrence, which is associated with anxiety, apprehension, and suffering. Acute pain may result from direct tumor involvement such as bony metastasis or visceral distension.

Pain also is associated with diagnostic procedures such as blood sampling, lumbar puncture, bone marrow biopsy, angiography, and endoscopy. Many patients undergo surgery for tissue diagnosis or for removal of the tumor; such procedures can involve extensive dissection, resulting in profound acute pain. Postoperative pain can persist after surgery for tumor recurrence and may be complicated in patients tolerant to opioids. The different types of acute cancer pain syndromes are described by Cherny and Portenoy.[12]

Anticancer therapy is frequently associated with painful sequelae such as skin burns, mucositis, pharyngitis, esophagitis, cystitis, or proctitis after radiation therapy. Similarly, with drug chemotherapy, some patients experience mucositis, myalgias, gastrointestinal distension, or local irritation from tissue extravasation of the agent. Acute pain caused by the treatment occasionally progresses to chronic pain. Usually, acute pain is self-limiting and is most effectively treated with opioid analgesics and nonsteroidal anti-inflammatory drugs (NSAIDs).

Chronic pain related to cancer

If the acute cancer pain does not subside with initial therapy, patients experience pain of a more constant nature, the characteristics of which vary with the cause and the involved sites. An accurate diagnosis is essential to providing appropriate treatment. Chronic cancer pain syndromes are described by Cherny and Portenoy.[12]

Chronic pain related to cancer can be considered according to the following categories.

Tumor-induced pain

The nature and severity of pain caused by tumor growth depends on the structures that are involved. It may occur at the site of the primary tumor or site of metastasis, or be referred to a distant site (e.g. pain from a spinal tumor).

Somatic pain from invasion of bone is the most common cause of cancer pain.[9,13] It is usually constant, with a gradual increase in intensity. The most common sites of metastasis are the spine, base of the skull, pelvis, and long bones, with multiple sites often existing. Metastases to vertebral bodies cause a dull and aching pain that, if located in the lumbar area, is exacerbated by lying or sitting and is often relieved by standing. Associated radicular pain or other neurologic signs such as weakness or numbness often accompany the pain. In the sacral area, bowel and bladder dysfunction often occur. It is essential to make an accurate and early diagnosis to minimize permanent neurologic deficit. Magnetic resonance imaging studies are more accurate than either computed tomography, bone scans, or radiographs for demonstrating bone metastases that produce neurologic dysfunction.

Tumor invasion of abdominal and pelvic organs manifests as visceral pain that is diffuse, poorly localized, and referred to dermatomes supplied by the corresponding spinal cord segments (e.g. midline thoracic back pain in pancreas cancer). Tumors often grow into a hollow viscus, causing obstruction, or may directly affect viscera such as colon, liver, pancreas, spleen, and kidney, resulting in organ dysfunction. Pain therefore arises as a result of distension and stretching of the mucosa or organ capsule or by direct tumor infiltration. Pain occurs frequently in pancreatic cancer, but largely depends on the location of the tumor in that organ. In one series,[14] 72% of patients with tumors in the head of the pancreas had pain, compared with 87% of patients with tumors in the body or tail. However, pain in the latter group is more likely to occur late in the disease.

Tumor compression or infiltration of peripheral nerves frequently causes a constant burning with hyperpathic, hypoesthetic, or dyesthetic pain in the area of sensory loss.[15] This syndrome, when associated with tumor infiltration of the brachial plexus, is called the Pancoast syndrome. Pain often arises initially in the shoulder and posterior arm in the distribution of C8 to T1 dermatomes. As it becomes progressively more severe, the pain extends to the medial part of the arm and hand. An associated Horner syndrome indicates the involvement of the sympathetic chain (stellate ganglion) in the paravertebral space.[16] The features of causalgia with associated vasomotor changes develop occasionally.

Lumbosacral (L5–S1) plexus involvement in patients with urinary, colonic, or gynecologic malignancies produces pain in the anterior thigh or groin if the upper lumbar (L1–3) plexus is involved or pain from the posterior part of the leg to the heel if the lower lumbosacral plexus is involved.[15] Perianal sensory loss associated with dull, aching, midline pelvic pain indicates sacral plexus involvement.

Chemotherapy-induced pain

Several of the commonly used chemotherapy agents occasionally result in the development of chronic pain problems. The vinca alkaloids, platinols, and taxol in therapeutic doses can cause peripheral neuropathy.[17] The features include pain and tenderness in muscles and joints. Aseptic necrosis of bone, usually in the femoral or humeral head, is also a side-effect of chronic steroid use. Pain usually precedes radiologic changes.

Mucositis occurs as a sequela to chemotherapy such as cyclophosphamide and after radiation therapy. The severity of this oral pain may make swallowing extremely difficult. The patient requires parenteral fluid support, analgesics, and prepared liquids such as BMX solution, which contains benadryl, maalox, and viscous xylocaine.

Radiation therapy-induced pain

Ionizing radiation, often used as a therapeutic modality for pain, can also be the primary therapeutic intervention for certain tumor types or an adjuvant to surgery or chemotherapy. However, pain problems, which may be short term or delayed, may arise after irradiation. Occasionally, they manifest as chronic and intractable pain syndromes. Determinants of toxicity include the total dose (in Gray units) delivered, whether fractionization was used, prior irradiation and chemotherapy, concurrent infection, and the underlying tissue vascularization.[18]

The early problems results from painful mucosal thinning or ulceration and include oral mucositis, esophagitis, and perineal pain. Injury to the small intestine causes cramping and abdominal distension. Fistulae may also develop.[19] Myelopathy resulting from damage to the spinal cord may be transient, with the onset delayed up to 4 months after irradiation and perhaps regressing in 2–36 weeks. If progressive, the myelopathy begins 5–13 months after irradiation. Pain, an early symptom in 15% of patients,[13] may be localized to the area of damage, referred with associated muscle weakness and painful dysesthesias,[16] or rarely progress to complete transverse myelopathy.

Fibrosis of a neural plexus poses a difficult diagnostic problem, because it can mimic the presentation of a recurrent tumor. The most commonly involved nerves are those of the limbs and brachial plexus. In these regions, pain can occur as early as 6 months after therapy or be delayed for up to 20 years. A previous history of radiation treatment with local skin changes, lymphedema of the limb, or evidence of radiation necrosis of bone without documented tumor recurrence aids in the diagnosis. Although rare, painful tumors can develop at the site of irradiation as late as 20 years after therapy. These are peripheral nerve tumors that produce burning, aching pain in the distribution of the involved nerve. When these tumors are surgically extirpated, a painful phantom syndrome usually develops.

Postsurgical pain syndromes

Pain after thoracotomy

After thoracotomy, pain develops in the distribution of the intercostal nerves in a small number of patients as a result of partial or complete injury by retractors, sutures, wires, or transection.[20] Pain most often develops 1–2 months after the surgery and is described as constant in the area of sensory loss, with occasional lancinating pain. This condition may be accompanied by dysesthesia at the scar and hyperesthesia in the surrounding area. Movement usually exacerbates the pain, often resulting in a frozen shoulder because of decreased joint motion. Other sequelae include disuse atrophy of the arm or, rarely, reflex sympathetic dystrophy.

Pain after mastectomy

Patients who have undergone radical mastectomy may develop pain in the posterior part of the arm, axilla, and anterior chest wall as a result of damage to the intercostobrachial nerve.[20] Pain typically develops 1–2 months after the operation and is tight, constricting, and burning in nature. Patients tend to keep the arm in a flexed position close to the chest wall, because movement exacerbates the pain, and a frozen shoulder may develop from reduced joint motion. Reports of phantom breast pain occasionally appear in the literature.[21]

Pain after radical neck dissection

Pain can arise as a result of radical neck dissection. This pain is characterized as being constant, with dysesthesia and shock-like sensation resulting from the interruption of the cervical plexus nerves and peripheral nerves serving those areas.[22]

Phantom limb pain

Phantom limb pain occurs in a significant number of patients after amputation in limbs and usually manifests as a burning and cramping sensation in the area of the original limb. It can easily be differentiated from stump pain, which occurs at the site of the amputation, and can be elicited by palpation or percussion of the stump area.[23]

Pain unrelated to cancer

Approximately 3% of the pain syndromes that occur in cancer patients have no relation to the underlying cancer or cancer treatment.[13] Most commonly, pain is caused by degenerative disk disease, arthritis, fibromyalgia, or migraine and has often predated the diagnosis of cancer. In these patients, pain does not necessarily signify recurrent disease or metastases. However, a chronic illness behavior has already developed in many of these patients, and they require careful assessment and early psychologic intervention.

CANCER PAIN AND OPIOID-TOLERANT PATIENTS

Opioid-tolerant pain patients are a challenging group for treatment. They may have used opioids illicitly in the past but are no longer using them. Many are reluctant to take opioids for their cancer pain, fearing an addiction potential. These patients require support and an understanding of the necessity to treat the pain. The liberal use of adjuvant therapies allowing for decreased opioid doses can also be beneficial.

Some patients remain actively involved in illicit drug use, making it difficult to evaluate and to treat them. The diagnosis of cancer and pain may lead them to increase their drug use in an attempt to manage their anxiety and depression. Their complaints are often misinterpreted as a request for more drugs, and they are best managed where pain, rehabilitation, and psychotherapy specialists can provide appropriate and adequate therapy. These patients may sell part of their prescriptions and seek additional pills.

Actions that are suggestive of addiction or drug diversion include overt selling of prescription drugs, prescription forgery, drug stealing, concurrent alcohol abuse, repeated dose escalations despite multiple warnings, multiple sources for obtaining prescriptions, deterioration at work/home with social withdrawal, resistance to change therapy, and repeated calls after hours for emergency prescription refills.[24]

Cancer pain that develops in patients who have been taking opioids for other medical conditions requires higher doses of opioids.[25] In these cases, the use of adjuvants and early intervention with block techniques or the use of more potent opioid receptor agonists may avoid dose escalation without good pain control.[26] Patients who use over 50 mg of oral morphine for more than 3 months require three times more drug for a three times longer duration than opioid-naive patients after surgery.[25]

ASSESSMENT OF CANCER PAIN

Assessment of cancer pain begins with a thorough understanding of the complex nature of pain. The International Association for the Study of Pain in 1979 defined pain as "an unpleasant sensory and emotional experience associated with actual or potential tissue damage or described in terms of such damage." This definition stresses the importance of the emotional and suffering aspects of pain. Derogatis *et al.*[27] found that the incidence of cancer-related pain was 39% in those who had a psychiatric diagnosis and 19% in those without mental impairment. In studies by Bond,[28,29] cancer patients were noted to have increased levels of hypochondriasis and neuroticism. This group was able to show restoration to a normal personality with the relief of pain. It has also been noted that uncontrolled pain is a major factor in the suicide of patients with cancer.[30,31]

Woodforde and Fielding[32] found that patients who were emotionally disturbed did not respond as well to therapy and died sooner than their counterparts who were not in pain and who were emotionally stable. Additionally, Wells and Bjorksten[33] showed that patients with depressive symptoms or a depressive disorder are more likely to be disabled and have pain. These studies demonstrate that the relief of pain goes beyond reducing the nociceptive component of pain and has a bearing on patient outcome. All too often, psychologic variables are proposed to explain continued pain or lack of response to therapy, when medical factors have not been adequately addressed.[34]

Clinical assessment

Treatment failure can often be directly attributed to an inadequate assessment by the physician of the patient with cancer pain. Initial treatment should be based on pain etiology and type of pain. A detailed analysis of each patient's pain condition should form the basis of rational therapy.[35]

Prior to beginning treatment, the clinician should perform a detailed history and physical examination. In a combined retrospective and prospective study, 20% of the 276 patients seen by the pain service received primary antineoplastic therapy based on the pain evaluation, and another 6% received antibiotics.[36] These investigators determined that a comprehensive pain evaluation represents an important opportunity to define the underlying pathology and thereby clarify prognosis or alter treatment strategy.

Based on the findings of the examination, diagnostic studies should be ordered; a preliminary diagnosis, treatment goals, and a treatment plan are then established. Following the initial evaluation, on subsequent visits, the patient's status should be reassessed, as tumor growth is a dynamic and evolving process.

History and physical examination

To determine what further testing a patient may require, the location, quality, and duration of the patient's pain should be elicited. A complete review of the past medical history and what, if any, therapeutic measures have been previously tried to relieve the pain may provide valuable information when developing a treatment plan. In addition to pain, most patients with cancer pain have numerous other symptoms.[37,38] They often suffer from insomnia, depression, fatigue, anxiety, anger, anorexia, and also the side-effects of therapeutic interventions such as nausea and vomiting, dysphasia, headache, pruritus, constipation, and light-headedness. It is essential to take into account all these symptoms when developing a therapeutic plan, as these impact on the quality of life and most are amenable to therapy.

Physical examination should include a complete neurologic examination. Neurologic deficits from direct tumor invasion or compression are common and are frequently painful. The examination should also be directed toward determining if any therapeutic blocks will benefit the patient in an adjunctive manner.

Pain intensity

One of the most difficult aspects of pain control is the accurate assessment of pain intensity.[39] Although intensity is difficult to gauge, it is important because it provides a basis for developing a treatment plan and evaluating the effectiveness of therapeutic interventions. Also, if a patient's pain level increases during treatment, it may indicate disease progression, which needs to be diagnosed, with consideration of further antitumor therapy. Some of the best methods available to us are verbal or visual analog pain scales and the McGill Pain Questionnaire. The Memorial Pain Assessment Card is easy to use and can distinguish pain intensity from both pain relief and global suffering.[40]

Even though two patients may estimate their pain scores to be equally high, the cause may be quite disparate (bruised knee vs. compound fracture). It is important to acknowledge that both are subjectively experiencing severe pain while their causes are treated quite differently (NSAIDs vs. opioids).

Diagnostic testing

The patient's prior test results should be reviewed, preferably using procedures such as computed tomography (CT), magnetic resonance imaging (MRI), bone scan, scopings, and staging procedures to assess the location and extent of the tumor. Additional testing may be necessary depending on the findings of the history, physical examination, and previous tests. In one study, over two-thirds of patients underwent diagnostic tests at the request of the pain service.[36] The most commonly ordered tests were plain radiographs, CT scans of the body, myelography, and MRI or CT of the head. Diagnostic testing may also be painful at times (e.g. lumbar puncture, electromyography, and scopings). These tests should be ordered only if the results are likely to alter therapy. Positioning and transport of patients in pain is poorly tolerated, and attempts should be made to minimize any incidental pain by premedicating patients in advance of moving them.

Treatment strategies

Following a thorough review of the patient's medical condition, a preliminary treatment plan should be established. Treatment plans often vary depending on prognosis, extent of disease, physical condition, age, and survivability. In patients undergoing active cancer therapy, immediate relief of pain is the most important aspect of the plan. It is also critically important to assess functional status and quality of life issues. Pain relief sufficient to allow the patient to tolerate diagnostic and therapeutic interventions should also be provided. For patients with far advanced disease, the treatment plan should be formulated and based on the wishes of the patient and family. Ensuring that the patient is comfortable is not only an important aspect of management, but also the primary "therapy" at this point. Provisions for supportive care, including nursing and psychological services, should be made available to the patient and family as part of a comprehensive treatment plan. The involvement of hospice in the patient's care must also be considered.

Goals

After establishing a treatment plan as part of the initial evaluation, the patient's expectations in terms of pain control should be discussed. Often, patients have unrealistic goals and may not fully understand the extent of the disease or prognosis. This situation may result from failure by the primary care physician to communicate with the patient or from the patient's denial of the medical condition. The help of the primary care physician should be obtained if one of the above conditions exists.

Cancer is a disease that not only impacts the individual but also affects the patient's friends and family. Attempts should be made to allay their fears while stressing that all attempts will be made to ensure that their loved ones do not suffer. Moreover, therapies provided to patients in the home environment by family members should not be regarded as "free" care. The average cost to families in lost wages and direct expenses amounts to approximately $2500.00 annually (USA). Over-the-counter medications can be more expensive than prescription co-payment options, so it is advisable to ask patients about the type of prescription payment insurance or coverage patients carry.

TREATMENT OPTIONS

In most cases, pain initially can be adequately relieved by the administration of either pharmacologic or invasive therapies and by adopting a multidisciplinary approach to supportive care.

Oral and parenteral analgesia

Pharmacotherapy is the most widely used method of pain control. The three categories of analgesic medications that are commonly available are NSAIDs, opioid analgesics, and adjuvant agents. The analgesic ladder was originally developed by the Cancer Relief Program of the World Health Organization[41] and has become a widely accepted method of drug selection. The initial approach for patients with mild to moderate pain is to use an NSAID, with addition of an adjuvant agent if indicated. If this does not provide adequate relief, if the pain increases or is severe on presentation, an opioid should be instituted, with or without an NSAID or adjuvant drug.

Nonsteroidal anti-inflammatory drugs

The peripheral effects of an NSAID inhibit the enzyme cyclo-oxygenase, decreasing tissue levels of a number of eicosanoids, which are the inflammatory mediators that are capable of sensitizing peripheral nociceptors in the skin.[42] NSAIDs have an anti-inflammatory action and inhibit bone tumor growth by inhibiting prostaglandin E_2 release. These agents may also have a centrally mediated analgesic effect.[43]

Acetaminophen's analgesic action is by inhibition of nitric oxide synthetase; it works at both central and spinal sites[44] and is similar in efficacy to aspirin. Acetaminophar is often classified as an NSAID but has no peripheral anti-inflammatory action.

The NSAIDs demonstrate a therapeutic ceiling dose, above which further dose increments provide little increase in analgesia. However, toxicity increases with larger doses, and includes nausea, gastritis, and platelet dysfunction. NSAIDs should therefore be used with caution in patients with peptic ulcer disease or a bleeding tendency.

Recently, cyclo-oxygenase 2 (COX-2-specific inhibitors have become available for patients in whom regular NSAIDs are contraindicated because of gastritis, ulceration, or platelet dysfunction. Celecoxib and rofecoxib provide satisfactory analgesia when compared with traditional NSAIDs such as ibuprofen.[45,46]

The efficacy of NSAIDs in cancer pain can usually be evaluated after 1 week, when doses may be increased if a response has occurred. However, if there is no initial response, sometimes the use of a different NSAID chemical formulation is efficacious. There may also be an advantage in using a nonacetylated salicylate if nausea develops. These drugs appear to cause less gastrointestinal irritation and interference with platelet function.

Opioid analgesics

Opioid analgesics are the mainstay of therapy for cancer pain. The objective when using these drugs is to control pain while minimizing distressing side-effects. The success of this therapy depends on the expertise of the prescriber, who must have a knowledge of the nuances of pharmacologic features among various opioids and experience in their use to make an appropriate selection for each patient.

Agonist–antagonist agents are not effective in the treatment of cancer pain because of their ceiling effect of analgesia, potential to precipitate withdrawal, and associated psychotropic side-effects with increasing dosage. The pure opioid agonists should be used exclusively, and prescribed for patients with moderate pain on the second step of the analgesic ladder. These drugs include codeine, oxycodone, and hydrocodone, and they are usually available in combination with acetaminophen, aspirin, or ibuprofen. Because of their nonopioid analgesic component, escalation of dosage is restricted to about 4–5 g of NSAID daily for aspirin or acetaminophen compounds to prevent renal or hepatic dysfunction. Ibuprofen-containing compounds are generally restricted to 3200 mg daily.

The availability of oxycodone alone, which is about the same potency as morphine when given orally, also makes it a third-step opioid. It is possible to titrate the dosage of oxycodone without restriction to treat more intense pain.

Patients who do not respond to second-step opioids are switched to opioids on the third step of the ladder, most often morphine, hydromorphone, oxycodone, or fentanyl. Morphine has been used extensively worldwide, and has been endorsed by the World Health Organization.[41] It is also available in several formulations, lending itself to administration by different routes. Sustained-release medication which can be administered orally two or three times daily is available. Oxycodone and hydromorphone are also available in sustained-release formulations. Fentanyl is available in a transdermal delivery system and as a lozenge in doses of 200–1600 μg for transmucosal absorption. Because of the individual variations in response, or in patients in whom one agent has been used for months, it is worthwhile trying a different opioid, if inadequate analgesia occurs with morphine.

Meperidine is a frequently used opioid for acute pain but is generally not employed for cancer pain. With long-term use, the accumulation of normeperidine occurs. This toxic metabolic is associated with myoclonus, tremulousness, hallucinations, and seizures.[47]

When the physician selects a route for administration, factors such as gastrointestinal upset or obstruction, outpatient versus inpatient setting, as well as patient compliance should be considered. Oral administration is preferred and is the most economical route. Some medications may be given rectally when doses by both routes are considered equivalent. Transdermal and transmucosal administration of fentanyl effectively bypasses the oral route. Other potential routes of administration include subcutaneous, especially in a home or hospice setting, and intravenous, which is used frequently in hospitalized patients with severe pain who require rapid dose titration.

A widely accepted principle for the effective management of cancer pain with opioids is dosage administration at fixed intervals on an around-the-clock basis. This approach provides sustained analgesia and avoids the peak and trough effects of medication when the drug given as needed, i.e. after pain returns. Additional opioids should also be available for breakthrough pain at all times during the course of treatment when sustained-release agents are used. Doses must be titrated to the patient's need, thereby avoiding side-effects from overdosing or persistent pain from inadequate analgesia.

Adjuvant therapy

Adjuvant medications are used in conjunction with oral or parenteral analgesics. They may have inherent analgesic action, potentiate the effect of the opioid analgesics, or improve mood, sleep, nausea, anxiety, and somnolence.

The tricyclic antidepressants are known to have analgesic action, treat depression, improve sleep, and benefit patients with neuropathic pain, especially those with dysesthesias. The tertiary amines (e.g. amitriptyline, doxepin) are often a first line of therapy owing to a greater analgesic effect. If these agents cause excessive sedation, a secondary amine (e.g. desipramine, nortriptyline) can be used. Anticonvulsant drugs (e.g. neurontin, carbamazepine, clonazepam, phenytoin) and the antispasmodic baclofen are helpful for patients with lancinating pain. Mexiletine, with action similar to the local anesthetic lidocaine, is now used for neuropathic pain secondary to cancer following previous success in the treatment of diabetic neuropathy.[48]

Corticosteroids may be useful adjuvants and improve analgesia, mood, and appetite in the short term.[49] These compounds are especially beneficial for patients with bone pain and for those with pain due to nerve trunk or spinal cord compression. Other medications that occasionally benefit patients are the benzodiazepines (anxiolytics) for patients in whom pain is accompanied by anxiety, haloperidol for the management of confusion, and phenothiazine for nausea and anxiety.

Transdermal delivery

The transdermal therapeutic system with a fentanyl patch has simplified the concept of continuous parenteral administration of opioid by using a noninvasive method. This system has proved to be beneficial for the treatment of cancer pain, with high patient preference.[50,51] Fentanyl is the only available opioid that can be administered by this method because of its high lipid solubility. The transdermal therapeutic system with fentanyl contains a drug reservoir and rate-controlling membrane that allows fentanyl to diffuse slowly into the dermal layer, where it accumulates.

After initial application of the patch, serum levels gradually increase to peak concentration in 12–24 h, and effective analgesia occurs as early as 6 h.[52] The patches are marketed in 25, 50, 75, and 100 $\mu g h^{-1}$ dosages and are applied for 72 h. Because these dosages are additive, a patient requiring 150 $\mu g h^{-1}$ transdermal fentanyl may have two 75 $\mu g h^{-1}$ patches or one 50 $\mu g h^{-1}$ and one 100 $\mu g h^{-1}$ patch applied. Some patients may experience only 48–60 h of analgesia before requiring a new patch. Titration of dosage is slower than by conventional oral or parenteral routes, and breakthrough medication must be available. However, this system provides a convenient method of continuous opioid delivery, and bypasses the gastrointestinal tract. Transdermal delivery is particularly advantageous for patients with head and neck tumors or esophageal cancer, or for those with gastrointestinal involvement by tumor, vomiting, or obstruction.

Patient-controlled analgesia

Patient-controlled analgesia allows patients to treat their own pain by self-parenteral administration of prescribed doses of opioids using a small, sophisticated, programmable, computerized pump. This technique has been widely used in the management of postoperative pain and has been developed in response to the undertreatment of pain in hospitalized patients.[53] Intravenous or subcutaneous routes are used in the hospital or the home setting. The pump can be programmed to deliver a continuous infusion, in addition to which the patient can administer bolus injections at a preset dose and time interval. There appears to be no difference in the effects on respiratory function compared with other therapies.[26]

This mode of delivery is useful when the oral route is unavailable, when the total dose required is excessive, when the beneficial effects of increased patient control are desirable, or when there is a need for immediate relief of breakthrough pain.[54]

Rapid relief and ease of dose titration for patients with severe exacerbations of cancer pain can be used in the home setting. However, with the increasing use of fentanyl patches, many patients are now able to achieve good pain control without patient-controlled analgesia, a more expensive technique in the home setting.

Neurosurgical procedures

With the development of the multidisciplinary approach to pain management and with an increasing range of available pharmacologic agents, fewer patients require surgical intervention. The aim of this therapeutic modality is to interrupt the nociceptive pathways in the peripheral nerves or at certain sites in the neuraxis.

The most commonly performed surgical procedure for cancer pain relief is anterolateral cordotomy, which targets the spinothalamic tract. This procedure can be performed by an open technique, which is associated with significant morbidity. The complications include hemiparesis, urinary retention, and sexual impotence. Percutaneous cordotomy has largely replaced the open method and is usually performed during local anesthesia by advancing a thermal coagulation probe under fluoroscopic guidance. It is not effective for the relief of neuropathic pain because of a central mechanism and has only limited use for the alleviation of visceral pain. Immediate and complete pain relief is achieved in 60–80% of patients,[55] but this decreases to 40–50% at 6–12 months. Many patients in whom pain recurs also have paresthesias or develop dysesthesias.

Another neurosurgical technique occasionally employed is implantation of an Ommaya reservoir connected to an intracerebroventricular catheter for relief of centrally mediated pain.[56] Rarely, rhizotomy, dorsal root entry zone (DREZ) lesioning, commissurotomy, and dorsal root ganglionectomy are used to interrupt pain neural pathways.[57]

Intraspinal therapies

Intraspinal administration of opioids is frequently used for the treatment of pain, especially pain not controlled with oral medications. Opioids can be delivered by the spinal or epidural routes, and the advantages include profound analgesia, often at a much lower opioid dose without the motor, sensory, or sympathetic block associated with intraspinal local anesthetic admnistration.[58]

However, combinations of low-dose opioids given epidurally with a local anesthetic act synergistically to produce effective analgesia while decreasing the side-effects. Opioids can be delivered by intermittent bolus injection or by continuous infusion. Morphine is the most commonly used opioid, although hydromorphone has also been successfully used.

Three systems employed for chronic intraspinal opioid administration include percutaneous tunneled epidural catheters, tunneled epidural or spinal catheters connected to subcutaneously implanted injection ports, and implanted spinal infusion pump systems. Implantable pumps, although more convenient and less likely to cause infection, are more costly if life expectancy is only 3–6 months.[59]

Tolerance to chronic intraspinal administration of opioids can occur and is managed by increasing doses, changing to another opioid, or substituting local anesthetic for a short period. Other side-effects include pruritus, urinary retention, somnolence, myoclonus, catheter infection, and, rarely, respiratory depression.

Clonidine can be used via the epidural or the spinal routes and provides an additive analgesic effect. It is also useful when there is a neuropathic component to the pain.[60] Small amounts of local anesthetic can act synergistically, reducing opioid dosages four- to 10-fold while still sparing motor or sensory blockade.[61,62]

Regional blocks

Patients suffering from cancer pain localized to a certain body area which manifests as peripheral neuralgia or visceral pain are excellent candidates for regional block with neurolytic agents. These techniques are also appropriate for patients who are extremely ill or debilitated.

Commonly used neurolytic substances are 3–12% phenol or 25–100% alcohol. These agents are thought to act by causing Wallerian degeneration of the nerve fiber by means of protein denaturation and destruction of the myelin sheath.[63]

When peripheral neurolysis is indicated in the management of malignant pain, neural interruption is implemented proximal to the source of irritation. The sensory receptive fields of peripheral nerves overlap and therefore blocks of neighboring segments are advisable, especially in the case of intercostal nerves. A diagnostic block with a local anesthetic is considered essential by many in order to evaluate the therapeutic effect and the impact of the resulting motor deficit following neurolyses. Accurate needle placement can avoid damage to adjacent structures and may be achieved easily with nerve stimulation devices or CT guidance. This is especially true for cranial and cervical nerve blocks. Transient postinjection neuritis may occur, and subsequent regeneration of peripheral nerves may be accomplished by neuritis or neuroma formation.

The autonomic nervous system is largely responsible for visceral nociception. A diagnostic block of a sympathetic or parasympathetic nerve plexus establishes the relative contribution of autonomic and visceral pain. It may also determine whether repeated blocks with a local anesthetic or a neurolytic agent will be beneficial. Ultralong-acting non-neurolytic local anesthetics are currently being examined and offer an exciting new approach to this technique.

Stellate ganglion block

The stellate (cervicothoracic) ganglion lies anterior to the lateral process of the C7 vertebra. Sympathetic nerve conduction to the ipsilateral head and upper extremity is interrupted by a block of this ganglion. Because of the proximity to other vital structures, many clinicians are reluctant to perform neurolytic blocks in this area. However, serial blocks with local anesthetic or neurolytic agents in dilute concentrations (3–6% phenol) after a diagnostic local anesthetic block have been employed.[64] Potential complications include intravascular injection of the vertebral artery, phrenic and superior laryngeal nerve block, and, rarely, intrathecal injection.[33]

Interpleural phenol blocks

The role of interpleural analgesia (IPA) in both acute and chronic pain management is still undergoing clinical scrutiny. Original work with this technique showed that IPA could provide analgesia for patients with subcostal incisions and fractured ribs.[65,66]

The technique for insertion of an interpleural catheter is relatively easy and an epidural tray can be utilized. Local anesthetics (0.5% bupivacaine or 2% lidocaine) have been traditionally utilized via intermittent bolus or a continuous infusion. Recently, interpleural phenol[67] has been described as an alternative for the treatment of visceral pain associated with esophageal cancer. In addition, unpublished findings suggest that this is an effective technique for the treatment of visceral pain associated with cancer of liver, biliary tree, stomach, and pancreas. Currently a multicenter study is under way to determine the efficacy of this block for the treatment of pain associated with the above-mentioned malignancies (H Silva, R Plancarte, and OA de Leon-Casasola, unpublished results).

Drugs and dosing

For neurolytic blocks, the utilization of increasing concentrations of phenol is recommended. As patients with cancer of the esophagus or the chest wall frequently suffer pleural effusions, several injections through a catheter may be indicated. Initially, 10 mL of 6% phenol is recommended, and progressive increase up to 10% according to the results is encouraged because the pleural effusion acts as a diluting agent. However, further experience with patients with pleural effusions suggest that administration of 5–10 mL of 6% phenol will achieve adequate results (H Silva, R Plancarte, and OA de Leon-Casasola, unpublished results).

For analgesia associated with cancer, a continuous infusion of 0.25–0.375% bupivacaine (8–10 ml h^{-1}), or intermittent bolus doses of 0.5% bupivacaine (10–15 mL every 8 h) also provide adequate analgesia. However, if the high concentration of bupivacaine is chosen, the risk of toxicity is greater. Thus, the use of 0.375–0.5% ropivacaine for a continuous infusion, and 0.5% ropivacaine, 10–15 ml every 8 h, would be a better choice in these patients. The investigation ultralong-acting agents may also gain a role in this therapeutic strategy in the future.

Complications

The use of IPA has been associated with the following complications:

1 pneumothorax (incidence of 2%[5]);
2 phrenic nerve palsy (avoid bilateral blocks) with respiratory failure;
3 systemic effects from drug absorption;
4 lung injury when a rigid catheter is utilized.[68]

Efficacy

There is no outcome information to determine the efficacy of this block in the treatment of visceral pain.

Celiac plexus block

The celiac plexus is situated retroperitoneally in the upper abdomen. It is at the level of the T12 and L1 vertebrae, anterior to the crura of the diaphragm. It surrounds the abdominal aorta and the celiac and superior mesenteric arteries.

The plexus is composed of a network of nerve fibers from both the sympathetic and parasympathetic systems. It contains two large ganglia that receive sympathetic fibers from the three splanchnic nerves (greater, lesser, and least). The plexus also receives parasympathetic fibers from the vagus nerve. The autonomic supply to the liver, pancreas, gallbladder, stomach, spleen, kidneys, intestines, and adrenal glands, as well as to the blood vessels, arises in the celiac plexus.

Indications

The indications for celiac plexus block are:

1 pain of acute or chronic pancreatitis;[69]
2 visceral pain from cancer in the upper abdomen.[70]

Drug and dosing

For neurolytic blocks, 50–100% alcohol, 20 mL per side, is utilized. Injected by itself, alcohol can produce severe pain. Thus, it is recommended that initially 5–10 mL of 0.25% bupivacaine should be injected 5 min prior to the injection of alcohol or that 100% alcohol is diluted by 50% with local anesthetic (0.25% bupivacaine). Phenol in a 10% final concentration may also be used and has the advantage of being painless on injection. Both agents appear to have the same efficacy.

Complications

Complications associated with celiac plexus blocks appear to be related to the technique used, retrocrural, transcrural,[71,72] or transaortic.[73] In a prospective, randomized study of 61 patients with cancer of the pancreas, Ischia *et al.*[73] compared the efficacy and the incidence of complications associated with three different approaches to celiac plexus neurolysis. Orthostatic hypotension was found to be more frequent in patients who underwent a retrocrural (50%) or splanchnic nerve block technique (52%) than in those who were treated with an anterocrural approach (10%). In contrast, transient diarrhea was more frequent in patients treated with an anterocrural approach (65%) than in those undergoing a splanchnic nerve block technique (5%), or by the retrocrural approach (25%). The incidence of dysesthesia, interscapular back pain, reactive pleurisy, hiccupping, or hematuria was not statistically different among the three groups.

The incidence of complications from neurolytic celiac plexus blocks was recently determined by Davis[74] in 2730 patients undergoing blocks between 1986 and 1990. The overall incidence of major complications, such as paraplegia or bladder and bowel dysfunction, was 1 in 683 procedures. However, the report did not relate which approach or approaches were utilized for the performance of the blocks.

Important aspects in the diagnosis and management of specific complications include:

1 Malposition of the needle should always be ruled out by radiologic imaging before the injection of a neurolytic agent, as the needle's tip may be intravascular, in the peritoneal cavity, or in a viscus. Imaging techniques currently used include biplanar fluoroscopy, CT or ultrasound. However, no study has evaluated the superiority of one technique over the others. Wong and Brown[75] have suggested that the use of radiologic imaging does not alter the quality of the block or the incidence of complications based on a retrospective study of 136 patients with pancreatic cancer pain treated with a celiac plexus block with or without radiologic control of the position of the needle's tip. However, the number of patients in whom radiologic imaging was performed was not stated. Assuming that radiologic imaging was used in half of the patients, the upper 95% confidence limit for complications is 5%.[76]
2 Orthostatic hypotension may occur in 1–3% of patients after the block for up to 5 days. Treatment includes bedrest, avoidance of sudden changes in position, and fluid replacement. Once compensatory vascular reflexes are fully activated, this side-effect disappears. Wrapping of the lower extremities from the toe to the upper thighs with elastic bandages has been used with success for patients who develop orthostatic hypotension and need to ambulate during the first week after the block.
3 Backache may result from (a) local trauma during the needle placement, resulting in a retroperitoneal hematoma, (b) alcohol irritation of the retroperitoneal structures, or (c) injury to the lumbar plexus. In patients with backache hematocrit should be measured at least twice with a 1-h interval. If there is a decrease in the hematocrit, radiologic imaging is indicated to rule out a retroperitoneal hematoma. A urine analysis positive for red blood cells suggests renal injury.
4 Retroperitoneal hemorrhage is rare, but has also been reported. Thus, in patients who present with orthostatic hypotension, one must rule out hemorrhage before assuming that it is a physiologic response to the block. Patients who present with backache and orthostatic hypotension after a celiac plexus block should be admitted to the hospital for serial hematocrit monitoring. If a low or a decreasing hematocrit is demonstrated, patients should undergo radiologic evaluation to rule out injury to the kidneys, the aorta, or other vascular structures. A surgical consultation should be obtained as soon as is feasible.
5 Diarrhea may occur due to the autonomic block of the bowel. Treatment includes hydration and antidiarrheal agents. Oral loperamide is a good choice, although any anticholinergic may be used. Matson *et al.*[77] have reported near-fatal dehydration from diarrhea after this block. Thus, in debilitated patients, diarrhea must be treated aggressively.
6 Abdominal aortic dissection has also been reported.[78,79] The mechanism of aortic injury is direct damage with the needle during the performance of the block. As expected, the anterocrural approach is more frequently associated with this complication. Thus, if there is evidence of atherosclerotic disease of the abdominal aorta, it would seem appropriate to avoid this technique.
7 Paraplegia and transient motor paralysis has occurred after celiac plexus block.[80–85] Current thinking is that these neurologic complications may occur as a result of spasm of the lumbar segmental arteries that perfuse the spinal cord.[86] In fact, canine lumbar arteries undergo contraction when exposed to low concentrations of alcohol.[87] Thus, if there is evidence of significant atherosclerotic disease of the aorta, suggesting the possibility of circulatory compromise in spinal cord, alcohol may not be the best choice. However, paraplegia after the use of phenol has been reported,[88] suggesting that other factors, such as direct vascular or neurologic injury, or retrograde spread to the spinal cord, may also come into play. The possibility of such serious complications makes the use of radiologic imaging during the performance of the block essential.

Efficacy

Two randomized controlled trials[70,89] and one prospective study[90] have evaluated the efficacy of celiac plexus neurolysis for pain due to cancer of the upper abdomen. One of the studies evaluated the efficacy of three different approaches to celiac plexus neurolysis for pancreatic cancer in a prospective, randomized fashion.[70] In this study, 48% (29/61) of patients experienced complete pain relief after the neurolytic block. The remainder (32 or 52%) required further therapy for residual visceral pain as a result of technical failure in 15 patients (20%) or neuropathic/somatic pains in 17 patients (28%). The other study[89] compared the procedure with oral pharmacologic therapy in 20 patients. The author concluded that celiac plexus neurolysis resulted in a reduction in visual analog pain scores equal to that achieved by therapy with a NSAID–opioid combination. However, opioid consumption was significantly lower in the group of patients who underwent neurolysis than in the group receiving oral pharmacologic therapy during the 7 weeks of the study. Moreover, the incidence of side-effects was greater in the group of patients receiving oral pharmacologic therapy than in those in the block group.

In another prospective, nonrandomized study,[90] 41 patients treated according to the World Health Organization (WHO) guidelines for cancer pain relief were compared with 21 patients treated with a neurolytic celiac plexus block. The authors concluded that this technique was effective in the management of pancreatic cancer pain.

As one of the two studies that used a randomized controlled design compared different approaches to the celiac plexus and had no control group,[71] and the other compared the procedure with an analgesic drug,[89] it was not possible to estimate the success rate of this technique. In contrast, the results of a meta-analysis that evaluated the results of 21 retrospective studies in 1145 patients concluded that adequate to excellent pain relief could be achieved in 89% of patients during the first 2 weeks after the block.[91] Partial to complete pain relief continued in approximately 90% of the patients who were alive at 3 months and in 70–90% of patients from the 3-month follow-up to the time of death. Moreover, the efficacy was similar for patients with pancreatic cancer and in those with other intra-abdominal malignancies of the upper abdomen. However, these results were based on retrospective evaluations that may not have yielded reliable information, or may be subjected to publication bias. In addition, statistical techniques used for the analysis had to account for the heterogeneity resulting from the patient selection criteria, technical differences in the performance of the blocks, choice of neurolytic agents and doses, diversity in the tools for the evaluation of pain, goals of therapy, etc. Thus, the meta-analysis must be interpreted with caution as the results could be overly enthusiastic.

New perspectives

As previously discussed, oral pharmacologic therapy with oral opioids, NSAIDs, and coadjuvants is frequently used for the treatment of cancer pain. However, there is evidence to suggest that chronic use of high doses of opioids may have a negative effect on immunity.[92] Thus, analgesic techniques that reduce opioid consumption can have positive effects on patient outcomes. Lillimoe *et al.*[93] found in a prospective, randomized trial that patients with nonresectable cancer of the pancreas who received a splanchnic neurolysis survived longer than patients who did not. These findings may be the result of lower opioid use in the group of patients randomized to neurolysis resulting in (a) better preserved immune function and (b) a reduced incidence of side-effects such as nausea and vomiting, which allows patients to gain better nutrition. This hypothesis is currently being tested in a prospective, randomized trial.

Superior hypogastric plexus block

Cancer patients with tumor extension into the pelvis may experience severe pain unresponsive to oral or parenteral opioids. Moreover, some patients may complain of excessive sedation or other side-effects that limit the acceptability and usefulness of oral opioid therapy. Thus, a more invasive approach may be needed to control pain and improve their quality of life.

Both pelvic pain associated with cancer and chronic nonmalignant conditions may be alleviated by blocking the superior hypogastric plexus.[94–96] Analgesia to the organs in the pelvis is possible because the afferent fibers innervating these structures travel in the sympathetic nerves, trunks, ganglia, and rami. Thus, a sympathectomy for visceral pain is analogous to a peripheral neurectomy or dorsal rhizotomy for somatic pain. A recent study has suggested that, even in advanced stages, visceral pain is an important component of the cancer pain syndrome experienced by patients with cancer of the pelvis.[96] Thus, percutaneous neurolytic blocks of the superior hypogastric plexus should offer relief to patients with advanced pelvic cancer.

The superior hypogastric plexus is situated in the retroperitoneum, bilaterally extending from the lower third of the fifth lumbar vertebral body to the upper third of the first sacral vertebral body. The technique for the blockade has been described elsewhere.[94–97]

Complications

A combined experience of more than 200 cases from the Mexican Institute of Cancer, Roswell Park Cancer Institute, and MD Anderson Cancer Center has failed to detect neurologic complications associated with this block.[96]

Efficacy

The effectiveness of the block was originally demonstrated by documenting a significant decrease in pain scores via a visual analog pain scale (VAPS).[94] In this study, it was shown that the block was effective in reducing VAPS scores in 70% of patients with pelvic pain associated with cancer.[94] The great majority of the patients enrolled had a diagnosis of cervical cancer. In a subsequent study, 69% of the patients experienced a decrease in VAPS scores. Moreover, a mean daily opioid morphine use was reduced by 67% (from 736 ± 633 to 251 ± 191 mg day^{-1}) in the success group and by 45% in the failure group (from 1443 ± 703 to 800 ± 345 mg day^{-1}).[95]

In a more recent multicentric study, 159 patients with pelvic pain associated with cancer were evaluated. Overall, 115 patients (72%) achieved satisfactory pain relief after one or two neurolytic procedures. Mean opioid use decreased by 40% from 58 ± 43 to 35 ± 18 equianalgesic mg day^{-1} morphine 3 weeks after treatment in all studied patients. This decrease in opioid consumption was significant for both the success group (from 56 ± 32 to 32 ± 16 mg day^{-1}) and the failure group (from 65 ± 28 to 48 ± 21 mg day^{-1}).[96] Success was defined in these two studies as the ability to reduce opioid consumption by at least 50% in the 3 weeks following the block and a decrease in the pain scores below 4/10 on the VAPS.[95,96]

In a recent case report,[97] the efficacy of the superior hypogastric plexus block in a patient with severe chronic nonmalignant penile pain after transurethral resection of the prostate was reported. Although the patient did not receive a neurolytic agent, a diagnostic block performed with 0.25% bupivacaine and 20 mg of methylprednisolone acetate was effective in relieving the pain for more than 6 months. The usefulness of this block for chronic benign pain conditions has not been assessed.

Ganglion impar block

The ganglion impar is a solitary retroperitoneal structure located at the level of the sacrococcygeal junction. This ganglion marks the end of the two sympathetic chains.

Visceral pain in the perineal area associated with malignancies may be treated effectively by neurolysis of the ganglion impar (Walther's).[98] Patients who will benefit from this blockade will frequently present with vague and poorly localized pain that is burning in character and frequently accompanied by sensations of burning and urgency. However, the clinical value of this block is not clear as the published experience is limited.

Complications

No complications have been reported with this block.

PRACTICAL MANAGEMENT CONSIDERATIONS

Some practical applications regarding the treatment of cancer pain patients may assist those starting cancer pain programs.[99] The physicians should determine if the prescribed therapy is compatible with the patient's home, social, and economic environments:

1. Is the patient capable of self-care?
2. Does the family support this daily care?
3. Is there a home care agency nearby that knows of this therapy and is willing to participate?
4. Are the local physicians agreeable to overseeing the primary physician's therapy?
5. Is there a 24-h hotline for pain patients having problems with the prescribed therapy?
6. Are the drugs, physical therapy, radiation therapy, or occupational therapy readily available in the patient's home town?
7. New techniques should not be introduced for out-of-town patients.
8. New complaints of pain must be treated seriously, assuming a recurrence of disease.
9. The cost of therapy must be considered:
   - a Has a trial or oral or parenteral therapy been considered before invasive catheters or pumps?
   - b Were inexpensive NSAIDS used before expensive NSAIDs?
   - c Therapies requiring many return trips to the operating room should be avoided.
   - d Inclusion and exclusion criteria should be applied for the use of implantable pumps.
10. Has a thorough biopsychosocial assessment been performed to address the suffering component of pain?

CONCLUSION

The management of patients with cancer pain can be a challenging task, even for physicians trained in cancer pain management. The use of a systematic approach for the assessment of such pain can simplify management. Without a thorough assessment, the possibility of misdiagnosis and undertreatment exists. Appropriate and frequently timed assessments form the basis for the development of an effective pain treatment plan. An understanding of the various etiologies of cancer and the different types of pain that they can produce is essential for the provision of appropriate therapeutic intervention. Finally, a multidisciplinary approach addressing pain, anger, anxiety, depression, and associated symptoms is essential in providing for the best quality of life during this life-threatening experience.

REFERENCES

1. Bonica JJ. Cancer pain. In: Bonica JJ (ed.). *The Management of Pain*, 2nd edn. Philadelphia, PA: Lea & Febiger, 1990: 401.
2. Stjernsward J, Eeoh N. The scope of the cancer pain problem. In: Foley KM, Bonica JJ, Ventafridda V (eds). *Advances in Pain Research and Therapy*, vol. 16. Second International Congress on Cancer Pain. Philadelphia, PA: Lippincott-Raven, 1990: 9.
3. Cleeland CS, Sonin R., Hatfield AK, *et al.* Pain and its treatment in outpatients with metastatic cancer. *N Engl J Med* 1994; **330:** 592–6.
4. Bernabi R, Gambassi G, Lapan K, *et al.* for the SAGE Study Group. Management of pain in elderly patients with cancer. *JAMA* 1998; **279:** 1877–82.
5. Ho RCS. Pain in the cancer patient. *Cancer J Clin* 1994; **44:** 259.
6. World Health Organization. *Cancer Pain Relief.* Geneva: WHO, 1986.
7. US Department of Health and Human Services. *Clinical Practice Guideline No. 9: Management of Cancer Pain*. Washington, DC: US Department of Health and Human Services, 1994.
8. Coyle N, Adelhardt J, Foley KM, *et al.* Character of terminal illness in the advanced cancer patient: pain and other symptoms during the last four weeks of life. *J Pain Symptom Manage* 1990; **5:** 83–93.
9. Twycross RG, Fairfield S. Pain in far-advanced cancer. *Pain* 1982; **14:** 303–10.
10. Kanner RM, Foley KM. Patterns of narcotic drug use in a cancer pain clinic. *Ann NY Acad Sci* 1981; **362:** 161–72.
11. Zech DFJ, Grand S, Lynch J, *et al.* Validation of World Health Organization Guidelines for cancer pain relief: a 10-year prospective study. *Pain* 1995 **63:** 65–6.
12. Cherny NI, Portenoy RK. The management of cancer pain. *CA Cancer J Clin* 1994: **44:** 262–303.
13. Foley KM. Pain syndromes in patients with cancer. In: Swerdlow M, Ventafridda V (eds). *Cancer Pain*. Boston, MA: MPT Press, 1987: 45–54.
14. Buncher CR. Epidemiology of pancreatic cancer. In: Moossa AR (ed.). *Tumors of the Pancreas*. Baltimore, MD: Williams & Wilkins, 1980: 415–27.
15. Bonica JJ, Benedetti C. Management of cancer pain. In: Moossa AR, Robson MC, Schimpff SC (eds). *Comprehensive Textbook of Oncology*. Baltimore, MD: Williams & Wilkins, 1986: 443–77.
16. Bonica JJ, Ventafridda V., Twycross RG. Cancer pain. In: Bonica JJ (ed.). The *Management of Pain*, 2nd edn, vol. 1. Philadelphia, PA: Lea & Febiger, 1990: 400–60.
17. Payne R. Post chemotherapy and post radiation pain syndromes. In: Foley KM (ed.). *Management of Cancer Pain. Syllabus of the Postgraduate Course of Memorial Sloan-Kettering Cancer Center*. New York, NY: Memorial Sloan-Kettering Cancer Center, 1985: 58–64.
18. Chapman CR. Pain related to cancer treatment. *J Pain Symptom Manage* 1988: **3:** 188–93.
19. Palmer JJ. Radiation myelopathy. *Brain* 1972; **95:** 109–22.
20. Kanner R. Postsurgical pain syndromes. In: Foley KM (ed.). *Management of Cancer Pain. Syllabus of the Postgraduate Course of Memorial Sloan-Kettering Cancer Center*. New York, NY: Memorial Sloan-Kettering Cancer Center, 1985: 65–72.
21. Weinstein S, Vetter RJ, Serson EA. Phantoms following breast amputation. *Neuropsychologia* 1970; **3:** 185–97.
22. Sist T, Lema MJ. Head and neck cancer pain. *Curr Rev Pain* 1997, **1:** 1–6.
23. Kao J, Wesolowski JA, Lema MJ. Phantom pain – current insights into its neuropathophysiology and therapy. *Pain Digest* 1997; **7:** 333–45.
24. Portenoy RK. Opioid therapy for non-malignant pain. In: Fields HL, Liebeskind JC (eds). *Pharmacological Approaches to the Treatment of Chronic Pain: New Concepts and Critical Issues. Progress in Pain Research and Management*, vol. 1. Seattle, WA: IASP Press, 1994: 267.
25. De Leon-Casasola OA, Myers DP, Donaparthi S, *et al.* A comparison of postoperative epidural analgesia between patients with chronic cancer taking high doses of oral opioids versus opioid-naïve patients. *Anesth Analg* 1993; **76:** 302–7.
26. Lema MJ. Cancer pain management: an overview of current therapeutic regimens. *Semin Anesth* 1993; **12:** 109–17.
27. Derogatis LR, Marrow GR, Fetting J. The prevalence of psychiatric disorders among cancer patients. *JAMA* 1983; **249:** 751.
28. Bond MR, Pearson IB. Psychological aspects of pain in women with advanced cancer of the cervix. *J Psychom Res* 1969; **13:** 13.
29. Bond MR. The relationship of pain to the Eysenck Personality Inventory, Cornell Medical Index and Whitely Index of Hypochondriasis. *Br J Psychiatry* 1971; **119:** 671.
30. Cleeland CS. The impact of pain on the patient with cancer. *Cancer* 1984; **58** (Suppl.): 2635.
31. Bolund C. Suicide and cancer. II. Medical and care factors in suicide by cancer patients in Sweden, 1973–1976. *J Psychosoc Oncol* 1985; **3:** 17.
32. Woodforde JM, Fielding JR. Pain and cancer. In: Weisenberg M (ed.). *Pain, Clinical and Experimental Perspectives*. St. Louis, MO: Mosby, 1975: 326.
33. Wells DG, Bjorksten AR. Monoamine oxidase inhibitors revisited. *Can J Anesth* 1989; **36:** 67.
34. Breibart W. Psychiatric management of cancer pain. *Cancer* 1989; **63:** 2336.
35. Banning A, Sjogren P, Henriksen H. Pain causes in 20 patients referred to a multidisciplinary cancer pain clinic. *Pain* 1991; **45:** 45.
36. Gonzales GR, Elliot KH, Portenoy RK, Foley KM. The impact of a comprehensive evaluation in the management of cancer pain. *Pain* 1991; **47:** 141.
37. Reuben DB, Mor V, Hiris J. Clinical symptoms and length of survival in patients with terminal cancer. *Arch Intern Med* 1998; **148:** 1586.
38. Coyle N, Adelhardt J, Foley KM, Portenoy RK. Character of terminal illness in the advanced cancer patient: pain and other symptoms during last four weeks of life. *J Pain Symptom Manage* 1990; **5:** 83.
39. Maguire P. The psychological and social sequelae of mastectomy. In: Howell JG (ed.). *Modern Perspectives in the Psychiatric Aspects of Surgery*. New York, NY: Brunner/Mazel, 1976: 390.
40. Fishman B, Pasternak S, Wallenstein SL, *et al.* The memorial pain assessment card: a valid instrument for the evaluation of cancer pain. *Cancer* 1987; **60:** 1151.
41. World Health Organization. *Cancer Pain Relief.* Geneva: World Health Organization, 1986: 18–19.
42. Vane JR. Inhibition of prostaglandin synthesis as a mechanism of action for aspirin-like drugs. *Nature New Biol* 1971; **231:** 232–5.
43. Willer JC, De Broucker T, Bussel B, *et al.* Central analgesic effect of ketoprofen in humans: electrophysiological evidence for a supraspinal mechanism in a double-blind and cross-over study. *Pain* 1989; **38:** 1–7.
44. Piletta P, Porchet HC, Dayer P. Central analgesic effect of acetaminophen but not of aspirin. *Clin Pharmacol Ther* 1991; **49:** 350–4.
45. Stichenoth DO, Wagner B, *et al.* Effects of meloxicam and indomethacin on cyclo oxygenase pathways in healthy volunteers. *J Invest Med* 1997; **45:** 44–9.
46. Wolfe, MM, Lichtenstein DR, Singh G. Gastrointestinal toxicity of nonsteroidal antiinflammatory drugs. *N Engl J Med* 1999; **340:** 1888–99.
47. Kaiko RF, Foley KM, Graninski PY, *et al.* Central nervous system excitatory effects of meperidine in cancer patients. *Ann Neurol* 1983; **13:** 180–5.
48. Dejgard A, Petersen P, Kastrup J. Mexiletine for treatment of chronic painful diabetic neuropathyl. *Lancet* 1988; **1:** 9–11.
49. Bruera E, Roca E, Cedaro L, *et al.* Action of oral methylprednisolone in terminal cancer patients: a prospective randomized double-blind study. *Cancer Treat Rep* 1985; **69:** 751–4.
50. Miser A W, Narang PK, Dothage JA, *et al.* Transdermal fentanyl for pain control in patients with cancer. *Pain* 1989; **37:** 15–21.
51. Maves TJ, Barcellos WA. Management of cancer pain with transdermal fentanyl: phase IV trial. University of Iowa. *J Pain Symptom Manage* 1992; **7** (Suppl. 3): 558–62.
52. Plezia PM, Kramer TH, Linford J, *et al.* Transdermal fentanyl: pharmacokinetics and preliminary clinical evaluation. *Pharmacotherapy* 1989; **9:** 2–9.
53. Burns JW, Hodsman NB, McLintock TT, *et al.* The influence of patient characteristics on the requirements for postoperative analgesia. A reassessment using patient-controlled analgesia. *Anesthesia* 1989; **44:** 2–6.
54. Ferrell BR, Nash CC, Warfield CC. The role of patient-controlled analgesia in the management of cancer pain. *J Pain Symptom Manage* 1992; **7:** 149–54.
55. Lahuerta J, Lipton SA, Wells JCD. Percutaneous cervical cordotomy: results and complications in a recent series of 100 patients. *Ann R Coll Surg Engl* 1985; **67:** 41–4.
56. Ballantyne JC, Carr DB, Berkey CS, *et al.* Comparative efficacy of epidural, subarachnoid, and intracerebroventricular opioids in patients with pain due to cancer. *Reg Anesth* 1996, **21:** 542–56.
57. Lema MJ. Invasive procedures for cancer pain. *Pain Clinical Updates* 1998; **6:** 1–4.
58. Plummer JL, Cherry DA, Cousins MJ, *et al.* Long-term spinal administration of morphine in cancer and non-cancer pain: a retrospective study. *Pain* 1991; **44:** 215–20.
59. Bedder MD, Burchiel K, Larson A. Cost analysis of two implantable narcotic delivery systems. *J Pain Symptom Manage* 1991; **6:** 368–73.
60. Eisenach JC, DuPen S, DuBois M, *et al.* and the Epidural Clonidine Study

Group: Epidural clonidine analgesia for intractable cancer pain. *Pain* 1995; **61:** 391–9.

61. Maves TJ, Gebhart GF. Antinociceptive synergy between intrathecal morphine and lidocaine during visceral and somatic nociception in the rat. *Anesthesiology* 1992; **77:** 1186–200.
62. Penning JP, Yaksh TL. Interaction of intrathecal morphine with bupivacaine and lidocaine in the rat. *Anesthesiology* 1992; **77:** 1186–200.
63. Myers RR, Katz J. Neuropathology of neurolytic and semidestructive agents. In: Cousins MJ, Bridenbaugh PO (eds). *Neural Blockade in Clinical Anesthesia and Management of Pain*, 2nd edn. Philadelphia: JB Lippincott, 1988: 1031–51.
64. Lofstrom JB, Cousins MJ. Sympathetic neural blockade of upper and lower extremity. In: Cousins MJ, Bridenbaugh PO (eds). Neural Blockade in Clinical Anesthesia and Management of Pain, 2nd edn. Philadelphia, PA: JB Lippincott, 1988: 461–500.
65. Reiestad FL, Stromskag KE. Interpleural catheter in the management of postoperative pain. A preliminary report. *Reg Anesth* 1986; **11:** 89.
66. Rocco A, Reiestand F, Gudman J, *et al.* Intrapleural administration of local anesthetics for pain relief in patients with multiple rib fractures. Preliminary report. *Reg Anesth* 1987; **12:** 10–14.
67. Lema MJ, Myers DP, de Leon-Casasola OA. Interpleural phenol therapy for the treatment of chronic esophageal cancer pain. *Reg Anesth* 1992; **17:** 166–70.
68. Stromskag KE, Reiestad F, Holmquist EVO, *et al.* Intrapleural administration of 0.25%, 0.375%, and 0.5% bupivacaine with epinephrine after cholecystectomy. *Anesth Analg* 1988; **67:** 430–44.
69. Rykowski JJ, Hilgier M. Continuous celiac plexus block in acute pancreatitis. *Reg Anesth* 1995; **20:** 528–32.
70. Ischia S, Ischia A, Polati E, Finco G. Three posterior percutaneous celiac plexus block techniques: a prospective randomized study in 61 patients with pancreatic cancer pain. *Anesthesiology* 1992; **76:** 534–40.
71. Singer RC. An improved technique for alcohol neurolysis of the celiac plexus block. *Anesthesiology* 1982; **56 :**137–41.
72. Hilgier M, Rykowski JJ. One needle transcrural celiac plexus block: single shot, or continuous technique, or both. *Reg Anesth* 1994; **19:** 277–83.
73. Ischia S, Luzzani A, Ischia A, Faggion S. A new approach to the neurolytic block for coeliac plexus: the transaortic technique. *Pain* 1983; **16:** 333–41.
74. Davis DD. Incidence of major complications of neurolytic coeliac plexus block. *J Roy Soc Med* 1993; **86:** 264–6.
75. Wong GY, Brown DL. Celiac plexus block for cancer pain. *Techniques Reg Anesth Pain Manage* 1997; **1:** 18–26.
76. Hanley JA, Lippman-Hand A. If nothing goes wrong, is everything all right. *JAMA* 1983; **249:** 1743–5.
77. Matson JA, Ghia JN, Levy JH. A case report of a potentially fatal complications associated with Ischia's transaortic method of celiac plexus block. *Reg Anesth* 1985; **10:** 193–6.
78. Sett SS, Taylor DC. Aortic pseudoaneurysm secondary to celiac plexus block. *Ann Vasc Surg* 1991; **5:** 88–91.
79. Kaplan R, Schiff-Keren B, Alt E. Aortic dissection as a complication of celiac plexus block. *Anesthesiology* 1995; **83:** 632–5.
80. Galizia EJ, Lahiri SK. Paraplegia following coeliac plexus block with phenol. *Br J Anaesth* 1974; **46:** 539–40.
81. Lo JN, Buckley JJ. Spinal cord ischemia a complication of celiac plexus block. *Reg Anesth* 1982; **7:** 66–8.
82. Cherry DA, Lamberty J. Paraplegia following coeliac plexus block. *Anaesth Intensive Care* 1984; **12:** 59–72.
83. Woodham MJ, Hanna MH. Paraplegia after coeliac plexus block. *Anaesthesia* 1989; **44:** 487–9.
84. Van Dongen RTM, Crul BJP. Paraplegia following coeliac plexus block. *Anaesthesia* 1991; **46:**862–863.
85. Jabbal SS, Hunton J. Reversible paraplegia following coeliac plexus block. Anaesthesia 1992; **47:** 857–8.
86. Wong GY, Brown DL. Transient paraplegia following alcohol celiac plexus block. *Reg Anesth* 1995; **20:** 352–5.
87. Brown DL, Rorie DK. Altered reactivity of isolated segmental lumbar arteries of dogs following exposure to ethanol and phenol. *Pain* 1994; **56:** 139–43.
88. Galizia EJ, Lahiri SK. Paraplegia following coeliac plexus block with phenol. *Br J Anaesth* 1974; **46:** 539–40.
89. Mercadante S. Celiac plexus block versus analgesics in pancreatic cancer pain. *Pain* 1993; **52:** 187–92.
90. Ventafridda GV, Caraceni AT, Sbanotto AM, *et al.* Pain treatment in cancer of the pancreas. *Eur J Surg Oncol* 1990; **16:** 1–6.
91. Eisenberg E, Carr DB, Chalmers TC. Neurolytic celiac plexus block for the treatment of cancer pain: a meta-analysis. *Anesth Analg* 1995; **80:** 290–5.
92. Yeager MP. Morphine inhibits spontaneous and cytokine-enhanced natural killer cell cytotoxicity in volunteers. *Anesthesiology* 1995; **83:** 500–8.
93. Lillimoe KD, Cameron JL, Kaufman HS, *et al.* Chemical splachnicectomy in patients with unresectable pancreatic cancer. *Ann Surg* 1993; **217:** 447–57.
94. Plancarte R, Amescua C, Patt RB, Aldrete JA. Superior hypogastric plexus block for pelvic cancer pain. *Anesthesiology* 1990; **73:** 236–9.
95. de Leon-Casasola OA, Kent E, Lema MJ. Neurolytic superior hypogastric plexus block for chronic pelvic pain associated with cancer. *Pain* 1993; **54:** 145–51.
96. Plancarte R, de Leon-Casasola OA, El-Helealy M, *et al.* Neurolytic superior hypogastric plexus block for chronic pelvic pain associated with cancer. *Reg Anesth* 1997; **22:** 562–8.
97. Rosenberg SK, Tewari R, Boswell MV, *et al.* Superior hypogastric plexus block successfully treats severe penile pain after transurethral resection of the prostate. *Reg Anesth Pain Med* 1998; **23:** 618–20.
98. Plancarte R, Amescua C, Patt RB. Presacral blockade of the ganglion of Walther (ganglion impar). *Anesthesiology* 1990; **73:** A751.
99. Lema MJ. A compassionate approach to pain management in the terminally ill patient. *Hosp Med* 1998; **34:** 11–21.

77

Treatment of pain in children

BRENDA GOLIANU AND ELLIOT J KRANE

The history of pain management in children is rather unfortunately described as underdiagnosis, misinterpretation, and undertreatment. Several reasons contribute to this needless suffering. First, the very survival of the child is frequently in question, relegating pain treatment to a subsidiary, often ignored, role. Second, there is inadequate pharmacologic information and experience regarding analgesics use in children. Third, scant information is available for assessing a child in pain, and the assessment of pain in the newborn or preverbal child is quite difficult. The adequate assessment of pain must precede an intervention in order to provide effective medication for children.

Evidence suggests that children not only experience pain but feel it more acutely than adults. There are also serious physiologic sequelae to undertreated pain that affect morbidity and mortality, including excess pulmonary complications, delayed wound healing, and delayed recovery.[1]

Pediatric pain management is challenging, and one of the frontiers of modern anesthesiology. This chapter will outline the fundamentals of diagnosis and managing pain in children.

PAIN ASSESSMENT

In order to manage pain successfully, it is imperative to measure it effectively, as the "fifth vital sign." Without periodic nursing assessment of pain, just as with other vital signs, the efficacy of therapy cannot be determined.

Pain assessment may be divided into three components: self-reporting for verbal children, behavioral assessment for both preverbal and verbal children, and assessment of physiologic parameters.

Self-reporting

For verbal children, the faces scale (Fig. 77.1)[2] or visual analog scale are best introduced preoperatively, and the child is told that postoperatively he or she will be asked to rate pain using this tool. This type of assessment has been shown to have good intrapatient reliability and to correlate well with pharmacologic interventions in the predicted direction.

Behavioral assessment

Behavioral cues include crying, grimacing, or fussiness. Children may, on the other hand, express the presence of pain by being uncharacteristically still in order to avoid its exacerbation, or by withdrawing or regressing behaviorally. Often, parents can be very helpful in identifying small deviations from the child's baseline behavior that may represent pain. It is important to realize, however, that many other environmental factors may contribute to a child's discomfort. Restriction of mobility, because of attachment to intravenous catheters or monitors or the presence casts, cold, a dirty diaper, a strange hospital environment, the absence of loved ones, hunger, and exhaustion can all contribute to an unhappy child.

An experienced nurse or parent can usually address this differential diagnosis and take the appropriate comforting steps. One method frequently used is to very gently tap the infant over an area distant from the surgical site. The gently, rhythmic pressure will often distract and calm a child. The hand is then gradually moved directly over the surgical dressing. If the now calmed child suddenly expresses discomfort by his or her behavior then the cause is likely to be pain related.

Assessment of physiologic parameters

Observational pain scales that rely upon observation of infant behavior include the CRIES score (Table 77.1),[3] the Pain Assessment Tool (PAT),[4] and, most recently, the FLACC (Table 77.2).[5]

When assessing pain in newborns, it is important to remember that the procedure is significantly different from assessment of pain in adults. The classic description of pain as "an emotional and sensory experience" depends upon individuals' ability to describe their experience. Thus, individuals who are unable to describe or rate their pain, such as neonates, infants, or adults who are verbally or cognitively impaired, can be severely undertreated. Anand and Craig[6] describe pain as "an inherent quality of life that appears early in ontogeny to serve as a signaling system for tissue damage." With this definition, behavioral and physiologic responses are considered valid pain indicators. Pain must be observed and assessed by others in these individuals; thus, the assessment is also dependent on the knowledge and personal experience of the observer.

A number of neonatal pain assessment scales have been created which incorporate physiologic and behavioral indicators for measurement of pain. The most popular of these is the Premature Infant Pain Profile, illustrated in Table 77.3.[7] Other commonly used scales include the Neonatal Infant Pain Scale (NIPS).[8] These scales aim at measuring pain experienced by the patient. Specific scales have also been designed for the measurement of withdrawal and abstinence in the neonate. This may be due to the maternal use of opioids or iatrogenically incurred during treatment for sedation as part of the course of intensive care unit

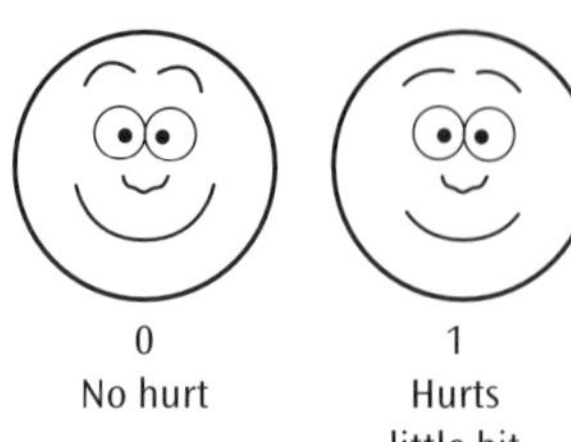
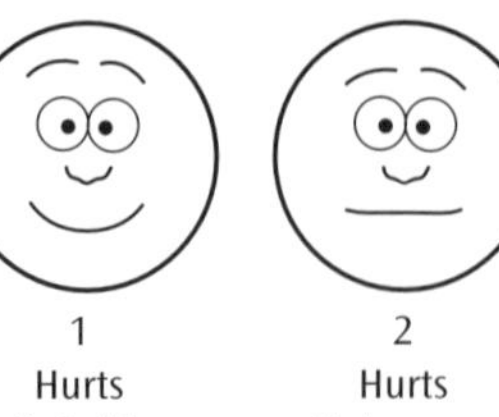

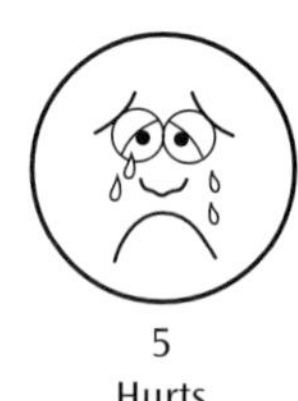

Figure 77.1 *FACES pain scale. (From Wong DL, Hockenberry-Eaton M, Wilson D,* et al. *Wong's Essentials of Pediatric Nursing, 6th edn. St Louis: Mosby, 2001: 1301. Copyrighted by Mosby, Inc. Reprinted by permission.)*

Table 77.1 *CRIES neonatal postoperative pain measurement score*

	0	**1**	**2**
(a) Summary			
Crying	No	High-pitched	Inconsolable
Requires O_2 for saturation >95%	No	<30%	>30%
Increased vital signs	Heart rate (HR) and blood pressure (BP) the same as or less than preoperative values	HR or BP increased by up to 20% of preoperative value	HR or BP increased by more than 20% of preoperative value
Expression	None	Grimace	Grimace/grunt
Sleepless	No	Wakes at frequent intervals	Constantly awake
(b) Coding tips for using CRIES			
Crying	The characteristic cry of pain is *high-pitched* If no cry or cry that is not high-pitched, score 0 If cry is high-pitched but baby is easily consoled, score 1 If cry is high-pitched and baby is inconsolable, score 2		
Requires O_2 for saturation >95%	Look for *changes* in oxygenation. Babies experiencing pain manifest decreases in oxygenation as measure by Tco_2 or oxygen saturation If no oxygen is required, score 0 If >30% O_2 is required, score 1 If 30% O_2 is required, score 2 (Consider other causes of changes in oxygenation such as atelectasis, pneumothorax, oversedation)		
Increased vital signs	Note: Take blood pressure last as this may waken the child, causing difficulty with other assessments. Use baseline preoperative parameters from a nonstressed period. Multiply baseline HR by 0.2 and then add this to baseline HR to determine the HR, which is 20% over baseline Do likewise for BP. Use mean BP If HR and BP are both unchanged or less than baseline, score 0 If HR or BP is increased but increase is 20% of baseline, score 1 If either one is increased >20% over baseline, score 2		
Expression	The facial expression most often associated with pain is a grimace. This may be characterized by brow lowering, eyes squeezed shut, deepening of the nasolabial furrow, open lips and mouth If no grimace is present, score 0 If grimace alone is present, score 1 If grimace and noncry vocalization grunt are present, score 2		
Sleepless	This parameter is scored based on the infant's state during the hour preceding this recorded score If the child has been continuously asleep, score 0 If he or she has awakened at frequent intervals, score 1 If he or she has been awake constantly, score 2		

Neonatal pain assessment tool developed at the University of Missouri-Columbia. Copyright S Krechel, MD, and J Bildner, RNC, CNS.

(ICU) care. Finnegan *et al.*[9] first described a scale of abstinence. This has subsequently revised by Franck and Vilardi[10] for the use of weaning in the ICU setting.

THE PHYSIOLOGY OF PAIN IN THE INFANT AND CHILD, AND ITS CONSEQUENCES

As stated, pain is defined as "an unpleasant sensory and emotional experience associated with actual or potential tissue damage or described in terms of such damage."[11] Between the initiation of tissue damage and the perception of pain that follows there occurs a complex series of physiologic events, collectively termed *nociception*. Nociception can be divided into four processes:

- transduction;
- transmission;
- modulation;
- perception.[12]

Table 77.2 *FLACC scale*

Categories	Score 0	1	2
Face	No particular expression or smile	Occasional grimace or frown, withdrawn, uninterested	Frequent to constant quivering chin, clenched jaw
Legs	Normal position or relaxed	Uneasy, restless, tense	Kicking, or legs drawn up
Activity	Lying quietly, normal position, moves easily	Squirming, shifting back and forth, tense	Arched, rigid, or jerking
Cry	No cry (awake or asleep)	Moans or whimpers; occasional complaint	Crying steadily, screams or sobs, frequent complaints
Consolability	Content, relaxed	Reassured by occasional touching, hugging, or being talked to, distractable	Difficult to console or comfort

Each of the five categories is scored from 0 to 2, which results in a total score between 0 and 10.

Table 77.3 *Premature Infant Pain Profile*[7]

Process	Indicator	0	1	2	3	Score
Chart	Gestational age	36 weeks and more	32 weeks to 35 weeks, 6 days	28 weeks to 31 weeks, 6 days	28 weeks and less	
Observe infant for 15 s	Behavioral state	Active/awake Eyes open, facial movement	Quiet/awake Eyes open, no facial movement	Active/sleep Eyes closed, facial movement	Quiet/sleep Eyes closed, no facial movement	
Observe baseline Heart rate ___ Oxygen saturation ___						
Observe Infant for 30 s	Heart rate maximum ___	0–4 beats min^{-1} increase	5–14 beats min^{-1} increase	15–24 beats min^{-1} increase	25 beats min^{-1} or more increase	
	Oxygen saturation minimum ___	0–2.4% decrease	2.4–4.9% decrease	5.0–7.4% decrease	7.5% or more decrease	
	Brow bulge	None 0.9% of time	Minimum 10–39% of time	Moderate 49–69% of time	Maximum 70% of time or more	
	Eye squeeze	None 0.9% of time	Minimum 10–39% of time	Moderate 49–69% of time	Maximum 70% of time or more	
	Nasolabial furrow	None	Minimum 10–39% of time	Moderate 49–69% of time	Maximum 70% of time or more	
					Total score	

Scoring method for the PIPP
Familiarize yourself with each indicator and how it is to be scored by looking at the measure.
Score gestational age (from the chart) before you begin.
Score behavioral state by observing the infant for 15 s immediately before the event.
Record baseline heart rate and oxygen saturation.
Observe the infant for 30 s immediately following the event. You will have to look back and forth from the monitor to the baby's face. Score physiologic and facial changes seen during that time and record immediately following the observation period.
Calculate the final score.

Transduction refers to the process in which noxious stimuli are translated into electrical signals at the sensory nerve endings and transmitted to the spinal cord. The nerves involved, called primary afferent nociceptors, are of two types: Aδ and C. Aδ-fibers are myelinated, rapidly conducting fibers (10–40 m s^{-1}), ending in specialized nerve endings (high-threshold mechanoreceptors). Aδ-fibers are primarily responsible for sensations of well-localized, sharp, stabbing pain, otherwise known as "first pain." Aδ-fibers have a high threshold for firing in response to mechanothermal stimuli, but once activated they dramatically increase their firing rate as the stimulus intensity increases.

C-polymodal fibers are unmyelinated fibers ending in free nerve endings. They respond to noxious mechanical, thermal, and chemical stimuli at a much slower rate (< 2 m s^{-1}),[13] giving rise to pain characterized as dull, aching, burning, and poorly localized. This pain is known as "second pain" because it is usually perceived slightly after the first pain sensation. Substances that mediate and intensify the stimulation of these nerve endings include bradykinin, prostaglandins, leukotrienes, substance P, acetylcholine, histamine, hydrogen ions, and potassium.

Sensitization is the process by which activation of neural impulses occurs at a lower than normal threshold of activation. Both Aδ and C-polymodal nociceptors are capable of sensitization. C-polymodal nociceptors may also widen their receptive fields, and are capable of prolonged discharge relative to the stimulus duration.

In addition to the above-mentioned mediators, the sympathetic system may itself be sensitized and may activate primary afferent neurons (Fig. 77.2). This may involve norepinephrine (noradrenaline) and other substances acting at α_2-adrenoreceptors on the afferent neurons. This phenomenon is certainly present in the early stages of the complex regional pain syndromes (CRPS I and II) but may also play a role in acute tissue trauma in the absence of nerve injury.[14]

Transmission (Fig. 77.3) refers to propagation of the impulse through

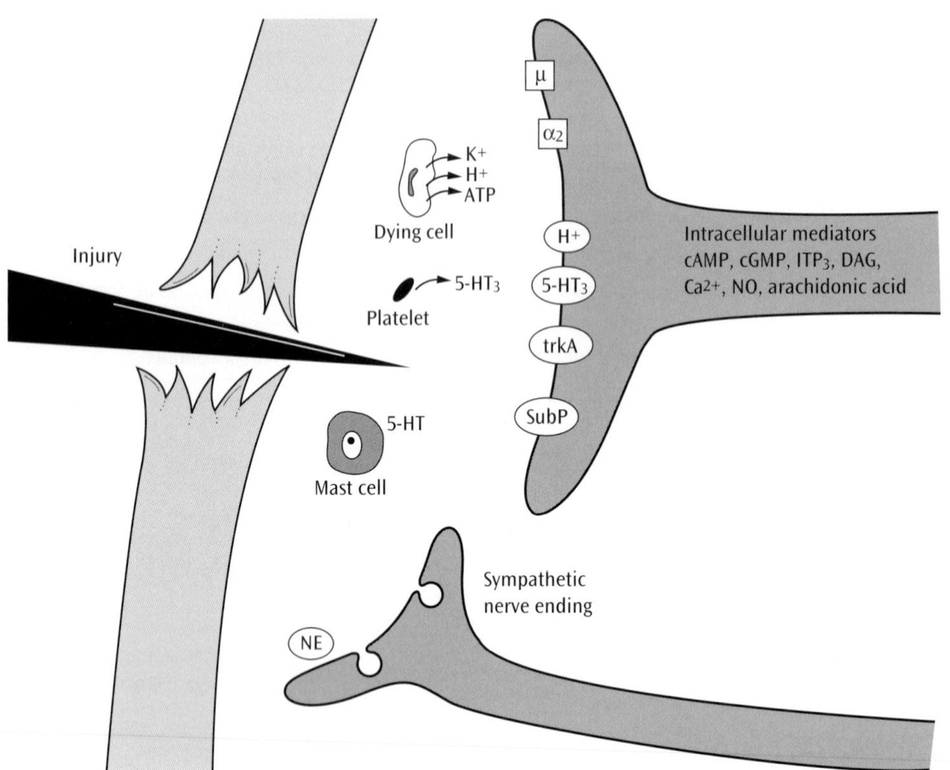

Figure 77.2 *Pain transduction in the periphery. Both the peripheral and autonomic nervous systems are integrally involved in the transmission of nociception, and many chemical mediators have been identified that trigger nociceptive impulses, including potassium and hydrogen ions, ATP, serotonin (5-HT), substance P, and norepinephrine (NE).*

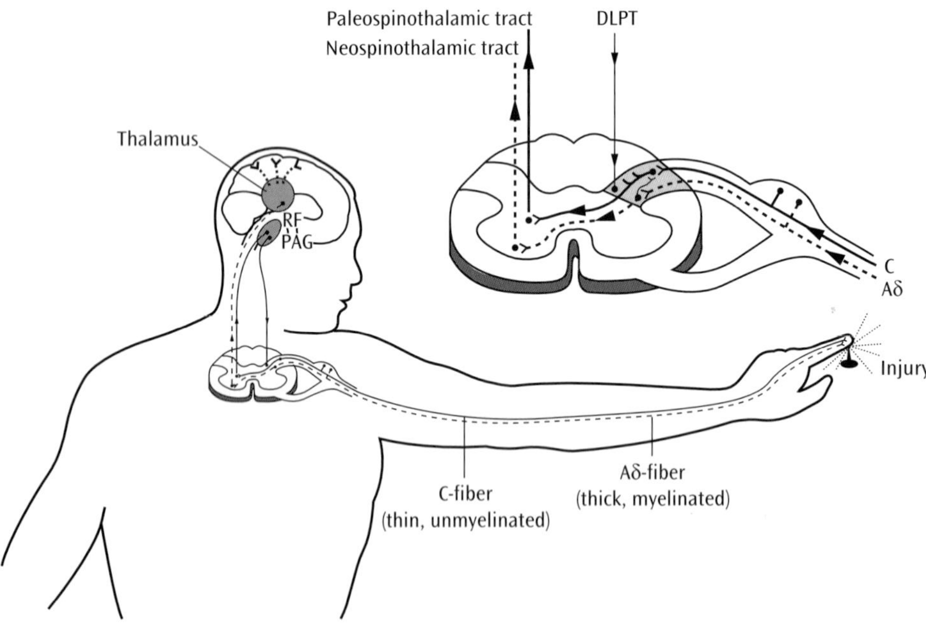

Figure 77.3 *Pain transmission. Primary nociceptive afferents synapse in the dorsal horn of the spinal cord with wide dynamic range (WDR) neurons. Descending inhibition of nociception modulates the excitability of the WDR neuron by the primary afferent.*

the sensory nervous system via primary afferent fibers, which synapse in the dorsal horn of the spinal cord, and second-order neurons in the lamina of the dorsal horn, ascending neurons projecting to brainstem, thalamus, and thalamocortical projections.

Modulation denotes the alteration of nociceptive information by endogenous mechanisms. This modulation may result in either attenuation or amplification of the initial signal. Perhaps the most important of these sites is the dorsal horn of the spinal cord. Modulation occurs between interneurons, as well as via pathways of descending inhibition originating in the thalamus and brainstem. Neurons within these pathways release inhibitory neurotransmitters, including norepinephrine, serotonin, γ-aminobutyric acid (GABA), glycine, and enkephalin, which block the release of substance P, glutamate and other excitatory neurotransmitters (Fig. 77.3).

Perception reflects the impact of the nociceptive information upon the existing psychological framework. Perception is the emotional and physical experience of pain. That experience then changes the framework itself, and thereby affects subsequent painful experiences.

All of the anatomical, physiological, and biochemical prerequisites for the perception of pain are present in the neonate.[15] In fact, the neonatal nervous system may be less effective at blocking painful stimuli because it has larger receptor fields, higher concentrations of

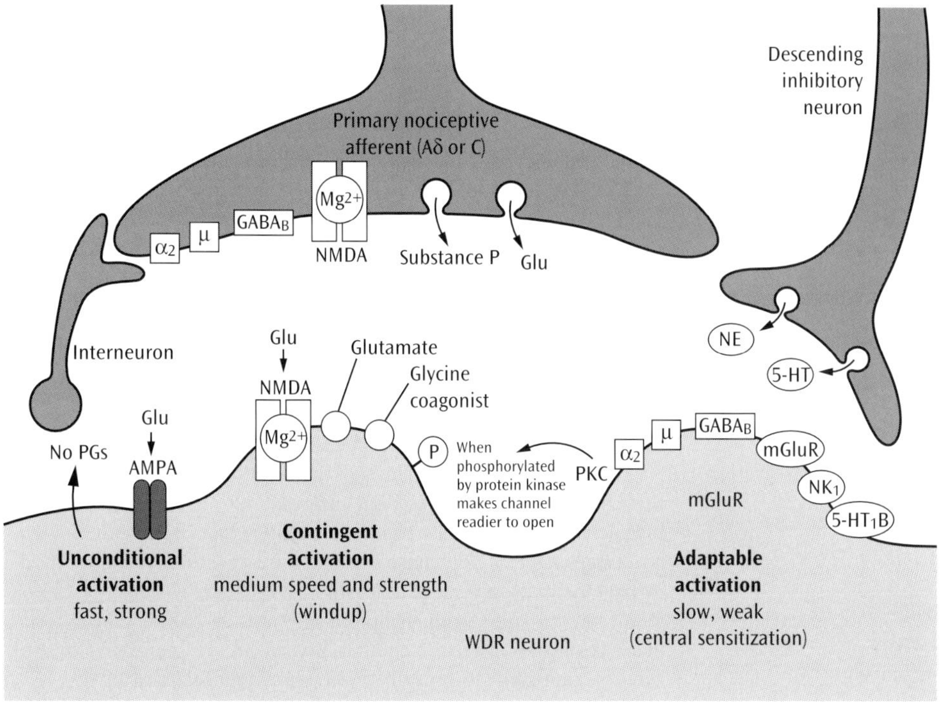

Figure 77.4 *Dorsal horn physiology. Input from the primary nociceptive neuron is processed in the dorsal horn by descending inhibition, interneurons, and WDR neuron activity. Opioids act at the primary neuron terminal but also affect mGluRs and may thereby affect central sensitization. Please note that there are also α_2-receptors on both primary afferents as well as interneurons and WDR neurons.*

(and more diffuse) receptor sites for substance P, and less developed descending inhibitory pathways than the adult nervous system.[16,17] In addition, because it is in a state of active development, the neonatal and infant nervous system has a high level of "plasticity."[18]

Painful experiences during this period may influence the final architecture of the adult brain in subtle and presently undefined ways.[19] These changes may be avoided with appropriate treatment. In a study comparing pain response at the time of fourth- and sixth-month vaccination of circumcised and uncircumcised infants, Taddio *et al.*[20] found that circumcised children had significantly higher pain scores than uncircumcised infants. Among the circumcised group, children who had received EMLA for vaccination showed an attenuated response to subsequent vaccination.

The practice of using regional nerve blocks and analgesics to provide "pre-emptive analgesia" has gained increased popularity. By "treating" pain before it has occurred, hypersensitization of the central nervous system (CNS) may be reduced, leading to a reduction in long-term pain perception.[21,22] If the central nervous system, does not "see" the nociceptive input, it will not undergo the phenomenon of centrally mediated hyperexcitability known as "central sensitization." Central sensitization may contribute to acute pain as well as the creation of chronic neuropathic pain states.

Although central sensitization involves modulation of the primary afferent terminal as well as interneurons in the dorsal horn, the most important elements are found at the level of the wide dynamic range (WDR) neurons, which are concentrated in lamina V of the dorsal horn. Nerve transmission in the dorsal horn begins with afferent stimuli causing release of aspartate, glutamate, substance P, and other neurotransmitters from the primary afferent. Glutamate then activates the AMP-A receptor, which results in a rapid and complete depolarization. These changes then elicit membrane depolarization in the WDR neuron. Then *N*-methyl-D-aspartate (NMDA) receptors, also found in WDR neurons, are activated more slowly (within seconds) and allow facilitated conduction and summation of action potentials. This initial activation of the NMDA receptor is referred to as "windup." Windup is an early and important component of central sensitization. With continued nociceptive input, the process then continues with the activation of other receptors, together referred to as the metabotropic glutamate receptors (mGluRs). These receptors require minutes to hours to become activated and begin a chain of translational events mediated by second-messenger systems (Fig. 77.4).

One of the key events is the phosphorylation of the NMDA receptor itself via protein kinase C. This phosphorylation then further increases the activity of the NMDA receptor and propagates the cycle of central sensitization. These events, however, can be intensely modulated by opioids, α_2-agonists, NMDA antagonists, norepinephrine, and gabaminergic, serotonergic, and other agents. The clinical applications of these findings are still being developed, but the effects will likely be far-reaching.

In one study, patients who received dextromethorphan, an NMDA antagonist, required fewer analgesics following hysterectomy than patients who did not receive it.[23] McQuay *et al.*[24] showed that, in patients undergoing surgery, opioid premedication with regional anesthesia resulted in increased time to postoperative analgesic request, as well as reduced overall need for analgesics. Patients who had received 72 h of epidural blockade prior to lower limb amputation had both less pain postoperatively and less phantom limb pain at 1-year follow-up.[25] Studies have also shown that regional anesthesia can modify the hemodynamic and endocrine response of infants to major surgical stimuli.[26,27]

PHYSIOLOGIC CONSEQUENCES OF PAIN

Noxious stimuli lead to activation of the physiologic stress response and to significant adverse changes in multiple organ systems including the cardiovascular, respiratory, metabolic, renal, hemostasis, and immune systems (Table 77.4).[28] These changes are found to be more pronounced in neonates, and higher plasma concentrations are required to produce clinical signs of analgesia compared with older age groups.[29,30] Appropriate analgesia ameliorates some of these responses to stress, and has been shown to lead to decreased complications perioperatively.[31–33]

How should we use our understanding of nociception in the management of acute pain in children? The most effective pain management is a poly- or multimodal strategy that prevents or diminishes all

Table 77.4 *Physiologic consequences of noxious stimuli*

Metabolic	Hypermetabolism Hyperglycemia Protein catabolism Lipolysis
Cardiovascular	Increased blood pressure Increased heart rate Increased cardiac output
Respiratory	Increased oxygen consumption Decreased tidal volume Decreased FRC *V*/*Q* mismatch Decreased cough Diaphragmatic splinting
Other physiologic responses	Decreased gut motility Gastric acid secretion Sodium and free water retention SIADH Hypercoagulability Increased fibrinolysis Altered immune function Cytokine production

the elements of nociception. This approach includes inhibition of the peripheral inflammatory response to tissue injury (nonsteroidal anti-inflammatory drug administration), neural blockade of transmission of pain impulses (regional anesthesia), prevention of "central sensitization" (administration of regional anesthetics and NMDA antagonists prior to tissue injury), enhancement of descending inhibitory pathways (neuraxial administration of opioids and/or α-adrenergic agonists), and prevention and management of anxiety (preoperative teaching and postoperative anxiolysis).

PHARMACOLOGIC TREATMENT OF PAIN

Therapeutic interventions in the management of acute pain are divided into nonpharmacologic and pharmacologic techniques.

Pharmacologic interventions include nonopioid medications such as acetaminophen (paracetamol) and nonsteroidal anti-inflammatory drugs (NSAIDs); opioids [morphine, meperidine (pethidine), etc.]; local anesthetics; and unconventional analgesics. A discussion of each of these will follow.

Nonopioids

Acetaminophen

Acetaminophen was first introduced in 1893. It is an antipyretic with weak analgesic properties. It uniquely blocks prostaglandin synthesis centrally and not peripherally. This accounts for its antipyretic as well as its analgesic properties, and explains why acetaminophen does not interfere with platelet aggregation or adhesiveness. The antipyretic effect is believed to be exerted via the hypothalamus, yet the analgesic effect may be spinally mediated, involving NMDA receptors and substance P.[34] Because acetaminophen is a weak analgesic, it has a "ceiling" effect, that is if pain is not controlled by standard acetaminophen dosing adding more drug will not produce more analgesia. Consequently, it is best used in the treatment of mild to moderate pain or as a component of multimodal therapy in patients with more severe pain.

In children, the loading dose required to produce a therapeutic blood level is 20 $mg\,kg^{-1}$ orally or 40 $mg\,kg^{-1}$ rectally.[35] Maintenance doses of 10–15 $mg\,kg^{-1}$ orally and 15–20 $mg\,kg^{-1}$ rectally can be continued as long as the drug is needed. The daily maximum is 90 $mg\,kg^{-1}\,day^{-1}$ regardless of the route used.[36] Neonates are at higher risk for toxicity due to immaturity of the hepatic cytochrome P450 metabolism system. Toxicity is seen at dosages of 300 $mg\,kg^{-1}\,day^{-1}$ and consists of hepatocellular necrosis secondary to binding by highly reactive electrophilic arylating metabolites. Hepatic and/or renal disease, malnutrition, and dehydration increase the risk of toxicity. Medications that induce the P450 system may also increase the risk of toxicity.

Nonsteroidal anti-inflammatory agents (NSAIDs)

Nonsteroidal anti-inflammatory agents inhibit peripheral cyclo-oxygenase and decrease prostaglandin production. In addition, NSAIDs may act centrally. The NSAIDs are more potent analgesics than acetaminophen and are excellent analgesics for mild to moderate pain. Like acetaminophen, they exhibit a "ceiling effect." They can, however, be quite useful as adjuvants to opioid treatment in the multimodal management of severe pain (Table 77.5), thereby reducing opioid requirements and diminish opioid-related side-effects. The NSAIDs that are approved for use in children in the USA are ibuprofen (Motrin®, Advil®), naproxen (Naprosyn®), and tolmentin (Tolectin®).

Other nonapproved NSAIDs frequently used in children are diclofenac (Voltaren®) and ketorolac (Toradol®). Ketorolac is the only commonly prescribed parenteral NSAID in North America. It is prescribed in doses of 0.5 $mg\,kg^{-1}$ and is given intravenously every 6 h (maximum dose 30 mg). Because it is a nonspecific cyclo-oxygenase inhibitor, it affects platelet binding, may cause gastric ulcers, may increase postoperative bleeding, and is occasionally of concern in cases where bone fusion is needed. Regardless of NSAID used or method of administration, the onset of pain relief following administration of these drugs is 20–30 min.

Opioids

Opioids produce their analgesic activity by mimicking the actions of endogenous opioid peptides at specific receptors in the CNS. Endogenous opioids all contain the amino acid sequence Tyr-Gly-Gly-phenyl. They include metenkephalin, β-endorphin, and dynorphin.

There are three main types of opioid receptors, each with its own subtypes:

1 mu (μ_1 and μ_2);
2 delta (δ_1 and δ_2);
3 kappa (κ_{1-4}).

These receptors are G-protein coupled and show considerable homology to one another.[37] Agonist binding to the μ- and δ-receptors depresses cyclic AMP formation. All three receptors induce membrane hyperpolarization through the activation of a K^+ channel and concurrent inhibition of a voltage-sensitive Ca^{2+} channel, which depresses terminal release of neurotransmitter from the cell, creating a powerful receptor mediated inhibition.[38]

Most commonly used opioids – morphine and codeine, for example – bind to the μ-receptor. Activation at the μ_1 receptor is responsible for supraspinal analgesia, whereas μ_2 activation leads to the undesired effects of respiratory depression, cardiovascular depression, and decreased gastrointestinal motility.[39] β-endorphin is the most potent of the endogenous opioids, binding at both μ_1 and μ_2 receptors. It is generated from the cleavage of pro-opiomelanocortin and released in a 1:1 ratio with adrenocorticotrophic hormone (ACTH). It binds to the hypothalamus, periaqueductal gray, and locus ceruleus.

Table 77.5 *Mixed oral opioid–nonopioid regimens*

Medication	Ingredients	Usual dosage
Hydrocodone and acetaminophen elixir (Lortab®)	Hydrocodone 7.5 mg and acetaminophen 500 mg per 15 mL	Hydrocodone 0.15 mg kg^{-1} per dose orally every 4–6 h
Hydrocodone and acetaminophen (Vicodin®, Lorcet®)	Hydrocodone 5 mg and acetaminophen 500 mg per tablet	As above
Acetaminophen and codeine elixir (Tylenol® with codeine elixir)	Acetaminophen 120 mg and codeine 12 mg per 5 mL	Codeine 1 mg kg^{-1} per dose orally every 4–6 h
Acetaminophen and codeine tablet (Tylenol® #2, #3, #4)	Acetaminophen 300 mg and codeine 15, 30, 60 mg per tablet	As above

The enkephalins are the primary endogenous ligands of the δ-receptor, and are primarily responsible for spinal analgesia. Enkephalins are found not only in areas known to be involved with nociception, but also in the gastrointestinal (GI) tract, the sympathetic nervous system, and the adrenal medulla. Dynorphin is the prototypic ligand for the kappa receptor. Activation of the κ-receptor results in segmental spinal analgesia and sedation. Most of mixed agonist antagonist opioids (e.g. butorphanol, nalbuphine) used in common practice bind to the κ-receptor.

Physiologic effects of opioids

At equipotent doses, all μ-agonist opioids (e.g. morphine, fentanyl, meperidine, codeine) produce similar physiologic effects and side-effects. They do, however, have different duration of action following equipotent dosing, and this fact to be taken into consideration when changing drug regimens. In addition, there can be incomplete cross-tolerance such that a patient who is not receiving much benefit from a morphine infusion may derive significant benefit from an equipotent fentanyl or hydromorphone infusion.

Respiratory

All opioids, not just codeine, are potent antitussives. Opioids depress minute ventilation by depressing the brain's response to carbon dioxide. Primarily they reduce respiratory rate, but at higher doses they also depress tidal volume. In terminally ill patients this effect is used to treat "air hunger." In acute pain management and in opioid abuse it is responsible for the most feared opioid-induced side-effects, namely respiratory depression, apnea, and death. When prescribed and administered for pain, respiratory depression is extremely rare and occurs most commonly when opioids are used concurrently with sedatives.[40] Indeed, the fear of inducing respiratory depression should never be used as an excuse not to treat pain. Rather, opioids should be incorporated into a rational plan of care for the patient.

Cardiovascular

Opioids have few hemodynamic side-effects. They do not affect the contractile state of the heart; nor do they alter cardiac output. With the exception of meperidine, which produces tachycardia, all opioids can cause dose-dependent, asymptomatic bradycardia. Morphine is a vaso- and venodilator. It affects preload and afterload by relaxing vascular smooth muscle and by releasing histamine from mast cells. This may produce mild hypotension, particularly in hypovolemic patients. Histamine release is seen to a lesser extent with codeine and meperidine and not at all with hydromorphone, fentanyl, or sufentanil. The hypotensive effects of the opioids can be minimized by slow infusion and maintaining an adequate intravascular volume.

Gastrointestinal

Opioids universally decrease gastrointestinal motility by decreasing peristalsis in the small intestine and large intestine and by increasing tone in the pyloric sphincter, ileocecal valve, and anal sphincter. Indeed, opioids were first used for the treatment of diarrhea (dysentery). Thus, opioid use is always associated with constipation and necessitates the use of stool softeners or stimulants whenever they are prescribed for more than a day or two. Unlike other opioid-induced side-effects, the body does not accommodate to these effects over time.

In addition, all μ-agonist opioids, *including meperidine*, can cause spasm of the sphincter of Oddi. This can be a problem in patients with pancreatitis, cholelithiasis, or sickle cell disease. Opioids are also associated with nausea and vomiting, caused by binding to the chemoreceptor trigger zone in the brainstem. This troublesome side-effect can be treated with metoclopramide (a dopamine antagonist), ondansetron (a 5-HT_3 antagonist), diphenhydramine (an antihistamine), nalbuphine (a mixed agonist–antagonist), or by a low-dose naloxone infusion, typically 0.5–1 μg kg^{-1} h^{-1}.

Genitourinary

Opioids cause increased tone of the detrusor muscle of the bladder, leading to urinary retention, which may require bladder catheterization. This side-effect may be seen regardless of route of opioid administration, but is seemingly more common after neuraxial administration.

Tolerance

Continued exposure to an opioid often results in the need for higher doses to achieve the same clinical effect. This phenomenon is known as *tolerance* and usually begins within 7–21 days after beginning opioid therapy. Shorter-acting, more lipophilic agents such as fentanyl may lead to tolerance faster than longer-acting, hydrophilic agents such as morphine. On the other hand, animal experimental evidence suggests that tolerance develops less with opioids with high receptor affinity, such as sufentanil. There is some degree of cross-tolerance between opioids, although it is incomplete. Patients who are becoming tolerant to morphine, for example, may benefit from a change to a drug with increased binding affinity such as hydromorphone.

Physical dependence

Sudden cessation of opioid medication after continued therapy may lead to the development of *abstinence* syndrome, or *withdrawal*. These symptoms can develop after as little as 5–7 days of therapy. Symptoms occur within 24 h of discontinuation and peak at 72 h. Symptoms include tachycardia, lacrimation, yawning, sneezing, coryza, nausea, vomiting, hypertension, restlessness, and insomnia. Tolerance and withdrawal appear to be linked. A child who develops tolerance can be expected to withdraw if opioids are suddenly stopped. However, this does not mean that the child is "addicted" to opioids. We do not consider a child who is physically dependent upon corticosteroids, insulin, or β-agonists "addicted." Why should we with opioids?

Addiction

Addiction is defined by the World Health Organization (WHO) as "a … *psychologic* and sometimes also physical state, resulting from the interactions between a living organism and a drug, characterized by behavioral and other responses that always include a compulsion to take the drug on a continuous or periodic basis in order to experience its psychic effects, and sometimes to avoid the discomfort of its absence. Tolerance may or may not be present." The DSM IV guidelines specify criteria for "substance dependence," defining psychological dependence or addiction as: taking a substance in larger amount than originally intended, spending a great deal of time in obtaining the substance, giving up important social, occupational or recreational activities in order to use the substance, and continuing to use the substance in spite of worsening of physical or psychological problems.[41]

In other words, addiction is a psychiatric disease associated with excessive self-medication against medical advice and compulsive and often criminal acquisition of drug. In the case of children legitimately treated with opioids for pain, addiction is extraordinarily rare[42] and concerns regarding addiction should never influence the analgesic care of children.

Mixed agonist–antagonists

An agonist has maximal physiologic effect at the binding site, e.g. morphine. An antagonist occupies and blocks the site but has no physiologic action, e.g. naloxone. A partial agonist occupies the site but has submaximal physiologic activity even at high doses, e.g. buprenorphone. A mixed agonist–antagonist has agonist effects at some receptors and antagonist effects at others, e.g. nalbuphine. Mixed agonist–antagonists opioids produce analgesia primarily at the κ-receptor. They have a ceiling effect and produce limited respiratory depression. In patients who are physically dependent on opioids, these drugs can induce withdrawal symptoms. In our experience, agonist–antagonists have their greatest utility for the treatment of opioid-induced side-effects, including nausea and vomiting, sedation, and pruritus. Agonist–antagonists generally reverse these effects without reversing analgesia.

Opioid (μ) agonists

Opioids are more the same than they are different. In selecting an opioid for clinical use, pharmacokinetic considerations include:

- route of administration;
- clearance;
- volume of distribution;
- unbound drug fraction;
- water/fat partition coefficient;
- pK_a;
- degree of ionization; and
- the bioavailability of oral dosing.

Many tables have been designed to provide guidelines for equianalgesic dosing (Table 77.6). These tables are based on single doses and do not reflect the use of drug over time. For example, 10 mg of morphine is frequently said to be equivalent to 100 μg of fentanyl, and 10 mg of methadone. However, fentanyl will reach peak effect within 5–10 min and will be redistributed by the body shortly thereafter, thereby terminating its analgesic effect. The duration of action of methadone is 8–16 h. While equianalgesic tables are useful in drug dose selection, other pharmacokinetic variables must be taken into account too.

Morphine

Morphine is the gold standard against which all other opioids are compared. It is the most widely used opioid for the management of acute pain in children and adults. It is hydrophilic and does not cross the blood–brain barrier well. It also has poor oral bioavailability (20–30%), which necessitates a larger oral dose when converting from parenteral to enteral routes of drug administration. In spite of these limitations, it is probably the most widely studied opioid in children.[43] In addition to oral, i.v., i.m., and s.c. routes, morphine can be administered in nebulized, epidural, and intrathecal formulations.

Morphine is metabolized in the liver by microsomal mixed-function oxygenases that require the P450 system. Two metabolites are morphine 6-glucuronide (which is active and more potent than morphine) and morphine 3-glucuronide (which is inactive but competes competitively with morphine at binding sites). These metabolites are renally excreted; thus, morphine (and opioids which are metabolized into morphine, such as codeine and methadone) must be used with caution in patients with renal failure because the active metabolite will accumulate in the blood. Morphine induces histamine release, and must be used carefully in patients with asthma or atopy. It also leads to vasodilation, and therefore may produce hypotension in hypovolemic patients. Side-effects of morphine (and all other opioids at equipotent doses) include decreased mental alertness, respiratory depression, hypotension, bradycardia, nausea, vomiting, pruritus, urinary retention, and, at high doses, myoclonus and seizures. The immature P450 system and decreased renal clearance of the neonate result in a prolonged metabolic half-life. In addition, the immature blood–brain barrier may result in higher morphine concentration in the brain of neonates.[44] Seizures have been reported in newborns at dosages considered "standard" for other age groups, 0.1 mg kg^{-1}.[45]

Fentanyl

Fentanyl is highly lipid soluble, equilibrates rapidly at the effector site, and has no active metabolites. There is increased clearance of fentanyl in children 3–12 months of age compared with adults, but a prolonged elimination half-life. Fentanyl can be administered i.v., i.m., s.c., transmucosally (Fentanyl Oralet®, Actiq®), and transdermally (Duragesic®) (see below). It is most commonly used for short painful procedures, but it can also be used for postsurgical and burn pain relief. Fentanyl is administered either in frequent boluses or (more often) as a continuous intravenous infusion. Tolerance and dependence develop rapidly when fentanyl is administered by continuous infusion. This is a very common problem in newborn infants who are treated for respiratory failure in the neonatal intensive care unit (NICU).

Meperidine

Meperidine (Demerol®) has one-tenth the analgesic potency of morphine. At equipotent doses, it has the same side-effect profile as

Table 77.6 *Intravenous equianalgesic ratios (based on single dosing)*

Drug	Relative potency	Intravenous loading dose
Meperidine (pethidine)	0.1	0.5–1 mg kg^{-1}
Morphine	1	0.05–0.1 mg kg^{-1}
Methadone	1	0.05–0.1 mg kg^{-1}
Hydromorphone	5	0.01–0.02 mg kg^{-1}
Fentanyl	50–100	0.5–1 μg kg^{-1}
Sufentanil	500–1000	0.025–0.05 μg kg^{-1}

morphine. It offers no advantages over morphine in terms of spasm of the sphincter of Oddi, bowel motility, or respiratory depression. The primary metabolite of meperidine, via *N*-demethylation, is normeperidine (norpethidine). This compound has one-half the analgesic activity of meperidine, is renally cleared, and can cause hallucinations, agitation, and seizures. Finally, meperidine interacts catastrophically in patients taking monoamine oxidase (MAO) inhibitors for depression. In these patients, meperidine may cause the neurolept malignant syndrome, a life-threatening condition manifested by hyperpyrexia, acidosis, shock, and death. Because of its drug interactions and toxic metabolite, we rarely prescribe meperidine for acute (or chronic) pain.

Hydromorphone

Hydromorphone is 3–6 times more potent that morphine, and 2–7 times more lipid soluble. It has no active metabolites, making it useful for use in patients with renal failure. The half-life of elimination is 3–4 h. It is anecdotally associated with fewer side-effects (e.g. nausea, vomiting, and pruritus) than morphine. Like morphine, it is very versatile and can be administered i.v., s.c., p.o., p.r., or in the epidural and intrathecal spaces.

Methadone

Although primarily thought of as a drug to treat and maintain opioid-addicted or -dependent patients, methadone can be a very useful agent in the treatment of acute and chronic pain. Because it has a half-life of 19 h, methadone can be used as an alternative to continuous opioid infusions. When used for acute pain, an intravenous loading dose of 0.1–0.2 $mg\,kg^{-1}$ is given followed by titration of 0.05 $mg\,kg^{-1}$ until satisfactory analgesia is achieved. Supplemental doses of 0.05–0.1 mg may be given every 8–12 h.[46] Oral or i.v. methadone is also useful in weaning patients who have developed opioid dependence.

Codeine, oxycodone, and hydrocodone

Codeine, oxycodone (the opioid in Tylox® and Percocet®) and hydrocodone (the opioid in Vicodin® and Lortab®) are opioids that are frequently used to treat pain in children and adults, particularly for less severe pain or when patients are being converted from parenteral opioids to enteral ones. Codeine, oxycodone, and hydrocodone are most commonly administered in the oral form, usually in combination with acetaminophen (Tylox®, Percocet®, Vicodin®, Lortab®, Codeine #1,2,3, and 4) or aspirin. Codeine can cause severe nausea. Many patients claim they are "allergic" to it because of this common side-effect. There are far fewer nausea and vomiting problems with oxycodone and hydrocodone. Indeed, because of this, oxycodone and hydrocodone are now our preferred oral opioids.

Codeine, hydrocodone, and oxycodone have a bioavailability of approximately 60% following oral ingestion. The analgesic effects occur as early as 20 min following ingestion and reach a maximum at 60–120 min. The plasma half-life of elimination is 2.5–4 h. Codeine undergoes nearly complete metabolism in the liver prior to its final excretion in urine. Approximately 10% of codeine is metabolized into morphine, and it is this 10% that is responsible for all of codeine's analgesic effect. Interestingly, approximately 10% of the US population cannot metabolize codeine into morphine, and in these patients codeine will have no analgesic effects.

Codeine is prescribed typically in a dose of 0.5–1 $mg\,kg^{-1}$. Elixirs, which are available in virtually every pharmacy, contain 120 mg of acetaminophen and 12 mg of codeine per teaspoon (5 mL). Codeine and acetaminophen are also available as compounded tablets, e.g. Tylenol® #1, 2, 3, or 4. Although it is an effective analgesic when administered parenterally, intramuscular codeine has no advantage over morphine or meperidine. Intravenous administration of codeine is associated with serious complications including apnea and severe hypotension, probably secondary to histamine release. Therefore, we do not recommend the intravenous administration of this drug in children.

Hydrocodone is prescribed in a dose of 0.05–0.15 $mg\,kg^{-1}$. The elixir is available as 2.5 mg per 5 mL combined with acetaminophen 167 mg per 5 mL. It is available as a tablet in doses between 2.5 and 10 mg, combined with 500–650 mg of acetaminophen. Oxycodone is prescribed in a dose of 0.05–0.1 $mg\,kg^{-1}$. The elixir, as 1 $mg\,mL^{-1}$, is not available in most pharmacies. In tablet form, oxycodone is commonly available as Tylox® (500 mg acetaminophen and 5.0 mg oxycodone) and as Percocet® (325 mg acetaminophen and 5 mg oxycodone). *In all combination preparations, beware of inadvertently administering a hepatotoxic acetaminophen dose when increasing doses for uncontrolled pain.* Acetaminophen toxicity may result from a single toxic dose, from repeated ingestion of large doses of acetaminophen (e.g. in adults, 7.5–10 g daily for 1–2 days, children 60–420 $mg\,kg^{-1}\,day^{-1}$ for 1–42 days), or from chronic ingestion.

Oxycodone and morphine are also available without acetaminophen in a sustained-release formulation for use in chronic, not acute, pain. As in the case of all time-released tablets, sustained-release oxycodone or morphine must be swallowed whole. Thus, these preparations cannot be administered to patients who cannot swallow tablets or who are fed through a gastric tube. Also note that in patients with rapid GI transit, sustained-release preparations may not be predictably absorbed (liquid methadone may be an alternative).

Neonatal considerations in the administration of opioids

Opioids can cause increased respiratory depression (including apnea) and seizures in the neonate, even when administered in doses that are safe to use in older children. The blood-brain barrier is immature at birth and is more permeable to morphine. The P450 microsomal enzyme system is immature at birth but matures quickly after birth regardless of gestational age. In addition, neonates have an increased unbound fraction of morphine (80% vs. 20%), which increases CNS sensitivity to the drug. Finally, there is decreased clearance of morphine. For all of these reasons, neonates less than 2 months of age who are receiving opioids should initially be placed in a monitored setting until the pharmacodynamic response to opioids has been judged to be safe.

Continuous intravenous opioid infusions

Patients with moderate or severe acute pain who cannot take oral medications, and who are not candidates for either patient-controlled analgesia (PCA) or spinal or epidural analgesia, should receive either continuous intravenous opioids via an infusion or around the clock bolus administration, not p.r.n. (*pro re nata*, or to give as needed). The anticipated level of pain drives the selected dose and method of intravenous opioid administration.

The first step in prescribing a continuous opioid infusion is to estimate the degree of pain and discomfort the patient is likely to experience, and to use that estimation to determine the amount of opioid that will be required. For the purpose of simplicity, the following discussion will be limited to continuous morphine infusions, but other opioids can be easily substituted by using equianalgesic ratios to determine the dose.

It is often necessary when treating patients with continuous infusions of opioids to establish a therapeutic blood level using bolus (loading) doses first. Reliance on the infusion alone to establish a therapeutic blood level will take five half-lives or, in the case of morphine, 10–24 h. Therefore, the first step in initiating a morphine infusion is to administer a loading dose of morphine as needed to establish patient comfort – generally 0.05–0.15 mg kg^{-1}. The second step is to initiate a continuous infusion of morphine. Generally speaking, the effective dose will be between 10 and 30 μg kg^{-1} h^{-1} depending on the severity of the painful stimulus. Doses less than 20 μg kg^{-1} h^{-1} are rarely associated with respiratory depression, while doses over 20 μg kg^{-1} h^{-1} may result in CO_2 retention unless mitigated by pain.

Dosing for the chronically ill, opioid-tolerant child requiring a new intervention

An important exception needs to be made regarding the child with chronic illness, often cancer, who may be on chronic opioid therapy and require a painful intervention. Following surgical intervention, a child will often require an approximately threefold increase in opiate dosing. If sedation is performed, the child will likewise have significantly increased medication requirements, often exceeding the parameters for standard sedation services. These patients are best referred for anesthesia consultation prior to their procedure. Where possible, the administration of a regional technique may significantly reduce the opioid requirement. However, care should be taken to ensure that patients are not suddenly taken off all opioid medication. Rather they may be provided with a moderate dose of PCA in order to be able to deliver additional doses as necessary.

Patient-controlled analgesia, parent-controlled analgesia, and nurse-controlled analgesia

The rationale for PCA is the following: the most common analgesic order, "p.r.n." leads to episodes or cycles of pain followed by "rescue" dosing of an analgesic. The episodes of pain that occur between analgesic administration lead to increased anxiety. The relatively large doses of opioids used to "rescue" the child are typically followed by periods of excessive sedation. PCA uses frequent administration of "mini" doses of analgesics initiated by the patients themselves, thereby eliminating the peaks and valleys of analgesia and pain. Overall, improved satisfaction results from patient control over medicine. Typically, PCA use is associated with less total analgesic use than conventional p.r.n. dosing. Therefore, there are less severe and fewer side-effects. PCA eliminates the need for nurses to "record" and administer analgesic medications with each patient demand. Children as young as 6 or 7 years of age can use PCA effectively. A rule of thumb is "if a child can play video games, he or she can master the use of PCA." Family members and nurses are generally not permitted to activate the PCA device (i.e. "*parent*-controlled analgesia"). In special circumstances, however, and with adequate parental education, this can be appropriate.

Relative contraindications to PCA use include the inability to use the PCA button effectively, for either physical or cognitive reasons, patient desire not to assume responsibility over analgesic administration, or a history of substance abuse. Nurses instructed in the use of PCA devices may be permitted to activate the PCA as they would otherwise be responsible for p.r.n. dosing ("*nurse*-controlled analgesia").

Unconventional analgesics

Injury or degeneration of nerves in the periphery or the pain pathway in the CNS causes neuropathic pain. Because of the loss of normal nerve conduction pathways and inhibitors of descending modulators of nociception, conventional analgesic medications are most often only partially effective, or are wholly ineffective in alleviating associated pain.

The creation of abnormal CNS nociceptive pathways devoid of CNS opioid receptors in neuropathic pain states, and the spontaneous activity of injured and regenerating neurons, requires a therapeutic approach to pain that differs radically from the management of more conventional nociceptive pain. Experience has shown that the use of membrane-stabilizing drugs, tricyclic antidepressants, and anticonvulsants, rather than NSAIDs, opioids, and other conventional analgesics, is quite effective in children.

Membrane stabilizers

Intravenous lidocaine

Lidocaine (lignocaine) has been shown to be beneficial in the treatment of neuropathic pain states by acting at sodium channels in reducing ectopic impulse firing. Intravenous lidocaine has also been shown to be a predictor of the efficacy of mexiletine in the treatment of neuropathic pain.[47]

Much of the pediatric pharmacokinetic information on intravenous lidocaine comes from empiric treatment of seizures. A review article by Walker and Slovis[48] on the use of lidocaine for the treatment of status epilepticus showed that, to establish and maintain therapeutic serum levels, an average intravenous bolus of 1.5–2.2 mg kg^{-1} with a maintenance infusion was required for adults, and 3.5 mg kg^{-1} h^{-1} to a maximum of 300 mg h^{-1} for children. Because neonates have a volume of distribution 2.5 times that of adults, a maintenance infusion for neonates of 4–6 mg kg^{-1} h^{-1} is required. Cardiovascular and CNS toxicity (seizures) occur with doses greater than 6 mg kg^{-1}.

Lidocaine infusions can be used to treat a variety of neuropathic pain states, including postoperative nerve injury pain, cancer pain that has neuropathic qualities, and pain due to CRPS. It also has utility in the management of non-neuropathic pain that is difficult to treat by conventional means, such as the pain of mucositis.[49,50]

Reports about the use of lidocaine for treatment of neuropathic pain states in children are few. Wallace and others used intravenous lidocaine to control pain after anti-GD2 antibody therapy in children with neuroblastoma.[51] Yet, lidocaine is useful for treatment of pediatric neuropathic conditions. In the treatment of neuropathic pain, we usually utilize a bolus dose of 1 mg kg^{-1} and maintenance infusion beginning at 1 mg kg^{-1} h^{-1}. Subsequent changes are guided by serum levels, obtained every 8 h. Serum lidocaine levels should be monitored, and the lidocaine infusion adjusted to achieve levels between 2–5 μg mL^{-1}. Patients with hepatic or renal insufficiency will, of course, need lower doses (typically halving the dosage of bolus or infusion) to prevent toxicity.

Anticonvulsants

Gabapentin

Gabapentin is an interesting compound that was originally synthesized as a GABAergic drug to treat spasticity. It was found to be more effective as a potent anticonvulsant. Animal studies show that gabapentin is effective for treating partial seizures and generalized tonic–clonic seizures. At this time, the mechanism of action of this agent is unclear. Gabapentin may enhance extracellular GABA levels by reversing GABA transport in a unique way, by enhanced reversal of GABA transport, and by increasing the activity of glutamic acid decarboxylase, a synthetic enzyme necessary for the production of GABA. The compound does not reduce voltage-sensitive sodium channels or affect NMDA receptors. On a biochemical level, gabapentin may inhibit a branched-chain amino acid transferase, ultimately resulting in a decreased level of glutamate, an excitatory amino acid that may be important in nerve transmission. Increased activity of glutamate dehydrogenase and glutamic acid decarboxylase has also been noted, further decreasing levels of glutamate.

Finally, gabapentin has been found to act at the α_2-dependent delta subunit of L-type Ca^{2+} channels, primarily in the hippocampus.[51]

Regarding the treatment of pain in the pediatric population, reports are few, limited mostly to case reports and small series.[52] Since the initiation of gabapentin use, however, its clinical utility has far outpaced the published data. In part this may be due to the relative paucity of agents useful in treating neuropathic pain, and the significant side-effects of these traditional agents. In many clinics, gabapentin is frequently used as a first- or second-line agent for the treatment of neuropathic pain, initially at 10 mg kg^{-1} daily and gradually escalating over several weeks to a maximum of 50 mg kg^{-1} daily.

Side-effects of gabapentin are generally minimal when a gradual increase in dosage is adopted. However, a clear dose–side-effect relation does not always exist. Commonly seen side-effects include sedation, fatigue, dizziness, headache, and ataxia. Some reports describe hyperactivity, irritability, and agitation in children with seizures being treated with gabapentin. In the authors' clinical experiences with the use of gabapentin for children, only one case of aggravation of aggressive behavior in a child with a previous history of such behavior has been documented.

The most important clinical characteristics of gabapentin are its relatively few side-effects or dose-limiting factors. (In fact, no ED_{50} has been defined for gabapentin.) The compound is not metabolized and does not induce hepatic enzymes. Elimination is by renal clearance, and dosages should therefore be adjusted proportionally to creatinine clearance in consultation with a nephrologist. Children tolerate doses of 15–30 mg kg^{-1} day^{-1} on a t.i.d. schedule. The dose may be titrated up to 70 mg kg^{-1} day^{-1} as side-effects permit.[53]

Sodium valproate

Valproic acid is an antiepileptic drug that has been used to treat neuropathic pain states and associated mood disturbances. The drug also seems to be effective for management of migraine headaches, but because of significant side-effects is not usually a first-line agent.

The mechanism of action of sodium valproate is unclear. The drug has a wide spectrum of anticonvulsant applications, therefore multiple mechanisms of action are proposed. Loscher[54] describes at least three mechanisms. Sodium valproate increases GABA synthesis and release, which may partially explain efficacy in treating central pain. Valproate also attenuates neuronal excitation induced by NMDA-type glutamate receptors. NMDA receptors have some correlation with centralization of neuropathic pain states or the "wind-up" phenomenon. Moreover, valproate has direct effects on excitable membranes and acts as a membrane stabilizer, similar to intravenous lidocaine and mexiletine.

Valproate is available in an oral tablet, syrup, and rectal suppository. Dosing starts at 10–15 mg kg^{-1} day^{-1} to a maximum of 30–60 mg kg^{-1} day^{-1}. The drug has a half-life in children of 6–18 h with a peak effect in 4 h after administration. Plasma concentration does not correlate with toxicity, seizure control, or analgesia. Valproate is protein bound (80–95%) and metabolized by glucuronidation and other oxidative pathways.

Adverse effects can be significant. Typical toxic effects within the first several months include anorexia, nausea/vomiting, sedation, and weight gain or loss. Valproate may cause hepatotoxicity and hepatic dysfunction in 5–30% of patients. Other less common adverse effects include hyperammonemia, pancreatitis, and platelet dysfunction. For these reasons, sodium valproate is not a first-line agent. Liver function tests should be performed prior to initiation of sodium valproate treatment and then every month for the next 6 months. Symptoms such as malaise, lethargy, gastrointestinal symptoms, and easy bruising may indicate liver dysfunction and lead to immediate laboratory evaluation and discontinuation of the drug.[55]

Carbamazepine

Carbamazepine is an earlier antiepileptic used to treat neuropathic pain via sodium channel blockade. Carbamazepine can be administered in oral (100–200 mg) and suspension formulations (100 mg per 5 mL). Recommended dosing schedules for children > 6 years start at 10 mg kg^{-1} day^{-1} in two divided doses to a usual maintenance dose of 15–30 mg kg^{-1} day^{-1} in 2–4 divided doses per day. Blood levels (therapeutic 4–12 μg mL^{-1}) can be obtained but do not necessarily correlate with analgesia for neuropathic pain.

Metabolism and adverse effects are significant with carbamazepine. Carbamazepine is hepatically metabolized, limiting its usefulness patients with hepatic insufficiency. Moreover, adverse effects are common, including hematologic (aplastic anemia, agranulocytosis), cardiovascular (congestive heart failure, syncope, arrhythmias), CNS (sedation, dizziness, fatigue, slurred speech, ataxia) and even hepatitis.[56] A complete cell count should be obtained prior to initiating this antiepileptic and should be repeated every 3–6 months. Although a classic neuropathic pain treatment, carbamazepine is no longer a first-line drug, particularly for a child or adult who may have hematologic alterations or hepatic dysfunction.

Antidepressants

Tricyclic antidepressants (TCAs)

Most antidepressants take 4–6 weeks to reach full antidepressant effect, but their onset in treating pain conditions is usually much shorter. TCAs have multiple mechanisms of action, including membrane stabilization, activation of descending inhibitory pain pathways, and a local anesthetic effect at the peripheral nerves, as well as having affective input in the limbic system.

The pharmacology of tricyclic antidepressants is well defined. All tricyclic antidepressants have equal analgesic efficacy at therapeutic dosages. The mechanism of action of tricyclic antidepressants is via serotonin and norepinephrine reuptake inhibition. Each TCA has varying degrees of action on CNS serotonin and norepinephrine levels, depending on whether the drug is a secondary or tertiary compound.

A special concern in TCA therapy is cardiovascular sudden death. As early as 1990 in *The Medical Letter*, and as recently as 1997, reports of the sudden death of children have raised concerns of life-threatening arrhythmias.[57,58] The review by Wilens *et al.* suggests that sudden deaths in TCA-treated children may be idiosyncratic. Desipramine and imipramine, in particular, seem to produce greater changes in baseline ECG, specifically increased QRS duration.

While the use of TCAs should be approached with caution, these drugs can be a very effective adjuvant in the treatment of neuropathic pain. Our practice is to obtain a baseline ECG prior to initiating TCA therapy, and to repeat an ECG after reaching a dose of 1 mg kg^{-1} per day.

Typical side-effects of TCAs are dose related and include antihistaminic (H_1 and H_2) effects such as sedation and increased gastric pH, antimuscarinic effects such as dry mouth and impaired visual accommodation, weight gain, urinary retention, constipation, α-adrenergic blockade resulting in orthostatic hypotension, and a quinidine-like effect promoting QRS widening (especially seen with amitriptyline).

Selective serotonin uptake inhibitors (SSRIs)

Although SSRIs are extremely useful for the management of situational or organic depression, in the chronic pain patient, whether child or adult, they have no primary use as analgesics at this time.

Spinal α-adrenergic agonists

Clonidine

Recent studies using clonidine in central and peripheral blockade show that it is coanalgesic when used with either local anesthetics or opioids in epidural, intrathecal, or peripheral blocks. Clonidine is thought to have applications in the treatment of chronic pain, particularly neuropathic pain. Finally, intrathecal administration of clonidine has been shown to reduce intractable muscle spasms in patients with spinal cord injuries.

α_2-Receptors are located on primary afferent terminals (both peripheral and spinal endings) in the superficial laminae of the dorsal horn of the spinal cord, and within several brainstem nuclei. The analgesic effect of clonidine may be at all three sites, with each site's relative contribution to its analgesic effect being unclear. Most studies support a direct and primary spinal analgesic action of clonidine. The relative potency of epidural clonidine to intravenous clonidine is 2:1. Clonidine has a lipophilicity similar to fentanyl. The duration of analgesia of epidural clonidine is 3–5 h, whereas intrathecal administration of clonidine results in a peak effect within 30–60 min and has a duration of up to 6 h.

Clonidine increases the release of acetylcholine at the dorsal horn. This enhances sensory and motor block of C and A-δ fibers by local anesthetics by increasing potassium conductance.

Adverse effects of clonidine include:

- Dose-dependent decrease in blood pressure. Action at the nucleus tractus solitarius and locus ceruleus decreases peripheral sympathetic tone. Further action at the lateral reticular nucleus causes hypotension and an antiarrhythmogenic action. Neuraxial administration inhibits sympathetic preganglionic neurons in the spinal cord, and heart rate may decrease secondary to a depression in atrioventricular nodal conduction.
- Sedation. This side-effect is localized to the activity in the locus ceruleus. The sedation is dose dependent between 50 and 900 μg regardless of route of administration. Clonidine has a rapid onset of sedation within 20 min. In adults, an infusion of epidural clonidine of 30 μg h^{-1} does not produce more sedation than epidural placebo or epidural morphine.
- Endocrine depression. Clonidine reduces but does not suppress neurohormonal secretion.

Clonidine alone does not induce respiratory depression or potentiate respiratory depression from opioids.

With regards to the pediatric literature, most studies have been performed using clonidine in combination with a bupivacaine epidural analgesia in the acute pain setting. Motsch *et al.*[59] studied a group of 40 children undergoing minor surgical procedures. He found that combined caudal analgesia with bupivacaine and clonidine (5 μg kg^{-1}) was superior to local anesthetic alone, as determined by both duration and intensity of analgesia. However, children had decreased blood pressure and sedation for the first three postoperative hours. This observed effect is consistent with the known duration of epidural clonidine in adults. Other authors have studied caudal analgesia using bupivacaine and clonidine, 1–2 μg kg^{-1}, with bupivacaine. This dose of clonidine was seen to decrease mean arterial pressure but not to cause bradycardia or respiratory depression.[13,60,61]

Techniques of intrathecal or spinal infusions of clonidine are beyond the scope of this review. The experience in adult cancer patients with intractable pain suggests an initial dose of 30–150 μg followed by a continuous infusion of 8–400 μg day^{-1}. Extrapolation from experience in adults suggests an initial dose of epidural clonidine of 1–2 μg kg^{-1} should also be appropriate either in the subarachnoid or epidural spaces, followed by an infusion of 0.02–0.05 μg kg^{-1} h^{-1}, titrating as needed to a maximum of 0.2 μg kg^{-1} h^{-1} while observing for undesired hemodynamic effects or sedation.

NONPHARMACOLOGIC TREATMENT OF PAIN

Nonpharmacologic techniques include distraction techniques (hypnosis, guided imagery), psychotherapy, physical and occupational therapy, transcutaneous electrical nerve stimulation (TENS), acupuncture, and massage. These tools frequently reduce both pain and anxiety, may reduce the need for opioid or other analgesics, and may thereby reduce drug-induced side-effects such as nausea and vomiting.

Unfortunately, the time and staff required to make these interventions work are often unavailable or are underutilized because of a lack of training, time, and a desire by the medical and nursing staffs to implement them. Additionally, these techniques are frequently viewed by third-party insurance carriers as "alternative" to mainstream medicine, and are reimbursed poorly if at all by insurance companies in spite of demonstrated efficacy.[62–69] Nevertheless, they should be considered in the care of more complicated patients, and especially in the care of chronic pain patients who require frequent interventions.

It is important to provide a realistic expectation of the possibilities of pain management, explaining that there may well be residual pain or discomfort in spite of the best efforts of the medical staff to combat pain, but that in the setting of acute traumatic or surgical pain continued recovery would be expected over the next few days. The reinforcement of reasonable expectations, the avoidance of maladaptive behaviors in the child and family, the elimination of secondary gain phenomena, and the development of improved coping and distraction skills are generally accomplished by an experienced psychotherapist.

Acupuncture

Acupuncture is becoming increasingly recognized in the treatment of a variety of chronic pain syndromes. The practice of acupuncture is based on placing specialized small needles in the skin in specific locations for the purpose of unblocking stuck energy or *chi*. In China it has been practiced for more than 2500 years. It also has a more than 100-year history in both Europe and the USA. Recently, however, it has come into the spotlight as an alternative treatment for many chronic pain conditions.

The mechanism of action of acupuncture remains unclear, although there is increasing evidence that CNS effects are involved. In an elegant study by Cho *et al.*,[62] a vision-related acupoint located on the lateral aspect of the foot was shown to result in activation of occipital lobes as visualized by functional magnetic resonance imaging (fMRI). Pomeranz and Nguyen[63] and He[64] showed that acupuncture analgesia is blocked by naloxone, implicating endogenous opioid effects.

There are also peripheral phenomena at work. Reichmanis *et al.*[65] systematically demonstrated that electrical resistance at acupuncture loci was significantly lower than in the surrounding tissue. In spite of these significant advances, however, the question remains to be elucidated. "Doctor, how is it that a needle in my foot cures my headache?"

In 1997, the National Institutes of Health (NIH) issued a consensus statement endorsing its use in the clinical setting and encouraging further basic and clinical research.[66] Promising results using acupuncture were found in diverse conditions such as postoperative nausea and vomiting, postoperative dental pain, tennis elbow, stroke rehabilitation, fibromyalgia, low back pain, menstrual cramps, and headache. In the pediatric population, nonmedical interventions are frequently considered earlier in the treatment paradigm as both parents and physicians are still reluctant to introduce medications for chronic use for the management of pain arising from benign conditions.

Although clinically it has become a frequently used modality, few studies exist regarding its use in children. One interesting study done by Schwarz *et al.*[67] looked at the stress response in premature infants undergoing ophthalmologic examination for retinopathy of prematurity. It was found that patients undergoing acupuncture had significantly reduced stress response, as measured by salivary cortisol levels. Another report describes the successful treatment of cyclic vomiting in a young child.[68] In the treatment of chronic pain conditions, acupuncture is generally well tolerated by children.[69] In fact, acupuncture may be more effective in children than adults, requiring fewer needles and achieving faster response (YC Lin, personal communication). Complications of acupuncture include bleeding, infection, pneumothorax, and vasovagal response. Acupuncture should only be performed by practitioners trained in the technique, using sterile and disposable needles.

REGIONAL BLOCKADE FOR TREATMENT OF PAIN

Epidural, intrathecal, and major nerve blocks

The practice of nerve blocks and regional anesthesia forms an integral part of pediatric pain management. The advantages are several.

1 It enables administration of putative pre-emptive analgesia.
2 Nerve blocks decrease or obviate the need for i.v. medications that can cause excessive sedation.
3 Nerve blocks can allow a lighter plane of general anesthesia.
4 Nerve blocks are both diagnostic and therapeutic interventions for chronic pain.

In theory, any nerve or neuraxial block that can be performed in adults can also be performed in children, provided the size and developmental anatomical and physiologic considerations are taken into account.

Central neuraxial blockade

Central neuraxial blockade has been in use in children since at least the early 1900s.[70] In most of the twentieth century, it was considered safer than the general anesthesia available at that time. As better techniques of general anesthesia became available, and with the advent of epidural anesthesia, spinal anesthesia became less frequent.

Today regional anesthetics have a place in the management of in a wide variety of surgical procedures, both because of its intraoperative benefits but more so for the superb postoperative pain relief that ensues.

General principles

All blocks may be performed in children with the appropriate indication. To ensure successful epidural blocks in pediatric patients, the anesthesiologist should be familiar with basic anatomical, physiologic, pharmacologic, and psychological differences between pediatric and adult patients.

The salient differences between children and adults that need to be remembered are as follows:

- Anatomical differences. The anatomical targets of the block are smaller and closer to nearby neurovascular structures. Caudally, the spinal cord and dural sac extend two or three interspaces lower in the infant than in the child or adult.
- Physiologic differences. Ostensibly because children and infants have little resting sympathetic tone, neuraxial blocks rarely produce hypotension in children less than 10 years. Crystalloid volume loading should therefore not be performed.
- Pharmacologic differences. Because children have a larger extracellular water space relative to body mass, and therefore the steady-state volume of distribution is higher, the maximum permissible dose of amide local anesthetics is somewhat higher, but clearance is longer. In addition, the duration of effect of local anesthetics, regardless of their site of injection, is somewhat shorter than in adults. For this reason, as much as 3 mg kg^{-1} bupivacaine, or 10 mg kg^{-1} lidocaine, may be injected without the production of systemic toxicity.[71–73]
- In newborns, in whom α_1-acid glycoprotein levels in the blood are reduced in comparison with older infants and adults, the maximum amide local anesthetic dose should be reduced by about 50% to compensate for decreased serum protein binding.[74]
- Of all the differences between children and adults, the most profound one is that blocks usually require a general anesthetic or deep sedation in children, and thus arises the controversy regarding the safety of performing blocks in anesthetized subjects who cannot express the presence of a paresthesia or report symptoms of accidental intravascular injection.[75,76]

Test doses are as important in children as adults, but when blocks are performed in the presence of general anesthesia their reliability may well be decreased. For example, during halothane administration, the injection of lidocaine and epinephrine (adrenaline) intravenously may increase blood pressure and reduce heart rate, rather than produce the expected tachycardia following a test dose, and prior administration of 0.01 mg kg^{-1} atropine increases the reliability of test doses.[77] Sevoflurane shows a similar response, but it is less pronounced. Using the criterion of systemic blood pressure greater than or equal to 2 kPa (15 mmHg) for a positive response, sevoflurane anesthesia showed 95% sensitivity compared with 71% for halothane. Interestingly, T-wave changes (25% increase or decrease) showed a 100% sensitivity with sevoflurane.[78,79] In spite of incomplete reliability, the test dose does offer a possible additional margin of safety. We recommend its use.

The same general indications and contraindications exist for regional anesthesia in the pediatric population as in the adult.

Contraindications

Absolute contraindications to neuraxial blocks include a lack of informed consent, the presence of an uncorrected coagulopathy, hemodynamic instability, infection at the proposed block site, and for neuraxial blocks, increased intracranial pressure (ICP). Relative contraindications include progressive neurologic disease and systemic septicemia.

Caudal epidural block

Indications

Indications for caudal epidural block include surgery or injuries below the diaphragm, especially infraumbilical, perineal pain syndromes, and complex regional pain syndromes (CRPS) involving the distal lower extremity.

Contraindications

Contraindications to caudal epidural block include sacral deformities and perianal surgery.

Equipment

The technique requires:

1 for a single-shot technique, a 20–22G Angiocath;
2 a 20G epidural catheter;
3 an 8G Angiocath;
4 sterile towels.

Note that using a nonstyleted catheter may introduce a plug of dermal tissue into the epidural space, resulting in a subsequent epidermoid tumor years or decades later.[80] For this reason, precautions should be taken to avoid this, such as preincising the skin with a larger-bore needle before inserting the needle to be used to enter the caudal space.[81]

Technique

With the patient in the decubitus or semiprone position, and with

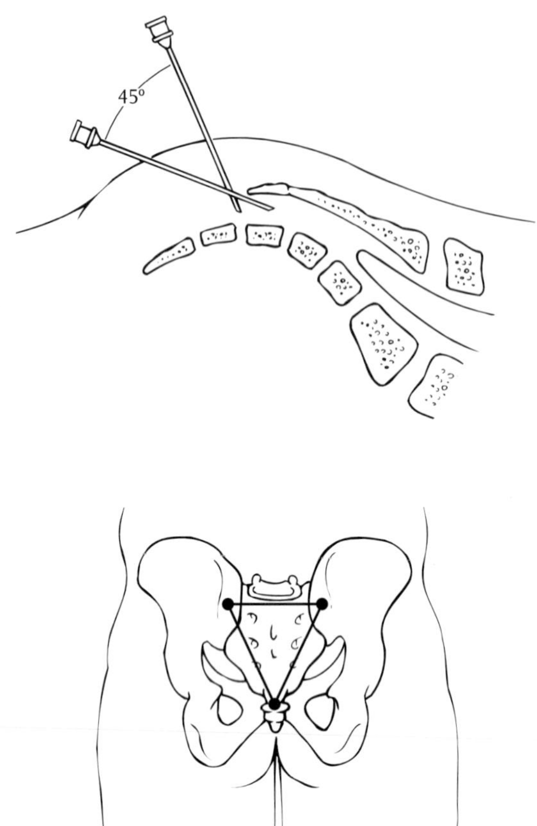

Figure 77.5 *Sacral anatomy. The most reliable indicator of the location of the sacral hiatus in children is an equilateral triangle connecting the posterior superior iliac spines to the hiatus (lower panel). Correct needle entry for a caudal block is initially about 66° to the skin until the sacral ligament is pierced, following which the needle may be advanced at a shallower angle.*

the knees drawn toward the chest, palpate the posterior superior iliac spines and visualize an equilateral triangle with the posterior superior iliac spine (PSIS) as the upper two vertices (Fig. 77.5). The lower apex of the triangle identifies the sacral ligament between the sacral cornua. The most common mistake is to insert the needle too far caudally. The needle should be inserted at 45° to the skin in a sagittal plane in the midline. A distinctive "give" or "pop" will be felt as the needle passes the sacral ligament and enters the caudal space. The needle should be advanced only 1–2 mm further and then the catheter passed or the drug injected after an appropriate test dose is administered. The dosage is 0.1mL kg^{-1} of 1.5% lidocaine with 1:200 000 epinephrine up to 3 mL (adult dose).

Drug selection/dose

The optimum drug combination is 0.25% bupivacaine and 1.5% lidocaine. The recommended dose depends on the level of the block. For block at the T10 dermatomal level, the recommended dose is 0.5 mL kg^{-1}, and for the T6 dermatomal level 1–1.2 mL kg^{-1}. The maximum dose is 3.5 mg kg^{-1} bupivacaine and 10 mg kg^{-1} lidocaine.

If injection is being performed through a catheter, follow the guidelines for lumbar or thoracic epidural block.

Lumbar or thoracic epidural block

Indications

Lumbar or thoracic epidural block is indicated for any surgery below the clavicles.

Contraindications

Contraindications include spinal deformity and bacteremia.

Equipment

The procedure requires an 18G 5-cm Tuohy needle and a 20G epidural catheter.

Technique

The patient is placed in a lateral decubitus position with knees to the chest. A Tuohy needle with glass syringe containing 3 mL of normal saline is inserted in the desired interspace. The epidural space is encountered at 1.2–2.5 m, depending on the age of the child, and may be accurately predicted by the formula:

$$\text{Epidural space depth (mm)} = 18 + 1.5 \times \text{age (years)}$$

The epidural catheter may be tunneled subcutaneously laterally to the flank or abdominal wall to permit it to remain securely *in situ* for several days, to an extended period of time (Fig. 77.6).

Drug selection/dose

The drug combination of choice is 0.25% bupivacaine plus 1.5% lidocaine at a dose of 0.5 mL kg^{-1}. For lumbar block a bolus of 0.5 mL kg^{-1} is followed by infusion of 0.25 mL $kg^{-1} h^{-1}$. For thoracic block a bolus of 0.25 mL kg^{-1} is followed by an infusion of 0.15 mL $kg^{-1} h^{-1}$.

Subarachnoid (spinal) block

Indications

Generally, this technique is performed only in children who were premature babies undergoing herniorrhaphy, circumcision, etc. in whom general anesthesia and/or sedatives may cause significant pulmonary sequelae yet muscle relaxation is needed (Fig. 77.7). There is also a role for subarachnoid injection for the diagnosis and management of pain syndromes or the administration of intraoperative analgesics to augment general anesthesia, particularly morphine and clonidine.

Contraindications

Contraindications include spinal deformity and bacteremia.

Equipment

The procedure requires a spinal tray and a 3-cm, 26G needle for infants, a 5-cm needle for children, and a 7-cm needle for adolescents.

Drug selection/dose

The agent of choice is tetracaine with epinephrine, 1 mg kg^{-1} for children up to 5 kg, 0.75 mg kg^{-1} for children up to 10 kg, and 0.5 mg kg^{-1} for children over 10 kg.

Upper extremity blocks

Many children have injuries or pain syndromes, or require surgery of the upper extremity for fractures, repair of congenital deformities, finger reimplantation, burn treatment, etc. Blocks of the upper extremity provide excellent analgesia, protect delicate repairs from patient movement, and, in the case of vascular injuries or repairs, reduce arterial spasm.

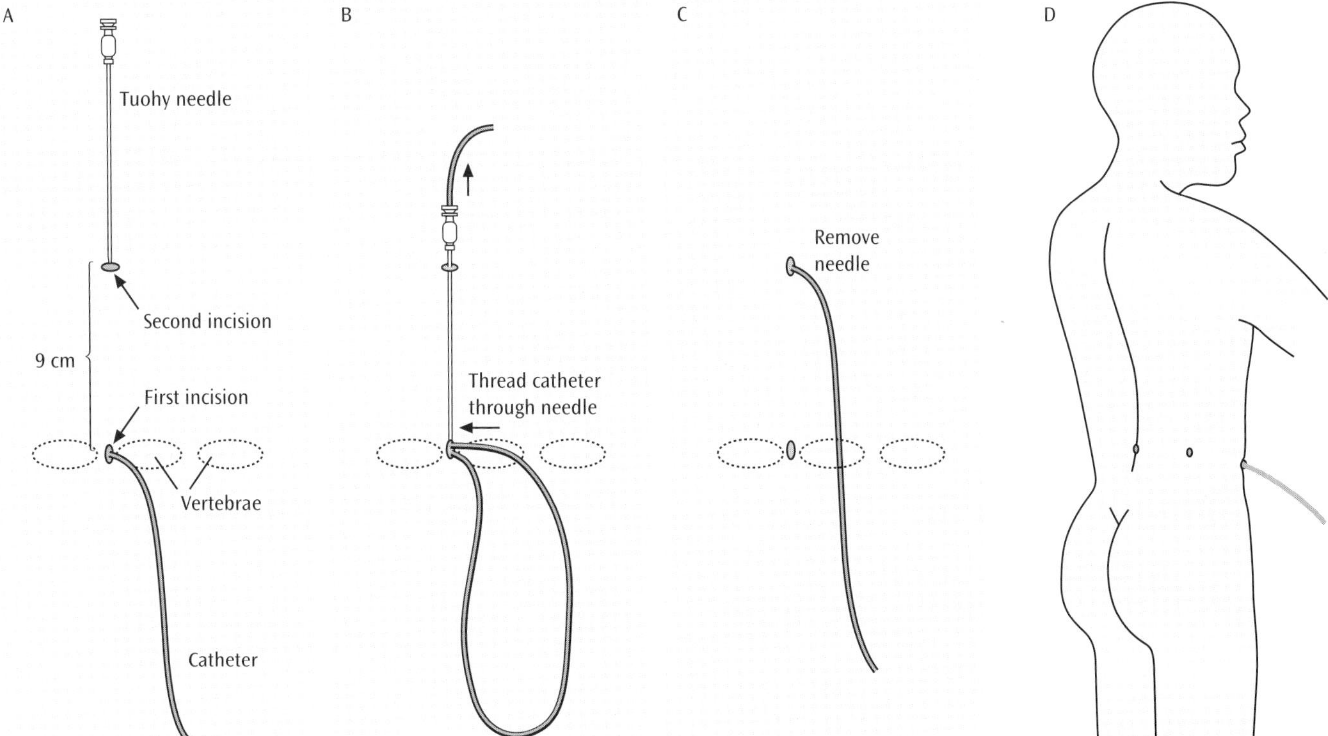

Figure 77.6 *Tunneling an epidural catheter. A, demonstrates the catheter placed into the epidural space, and a second puncture made with the Tuohy needle 9 cm lateral to the insertion site. B, demonstrates the Tuohy needle inserted from the second puncture site subcutaneously to the original insertion site, with the catheter threaded into the needle in order to bring it out of the second puncture (C). In this fashion, one to three further subcutaneous tunnels are made and the catheter ultimately exits the body over the abdominal wall (D). (From Aram* et al.[82]*)*

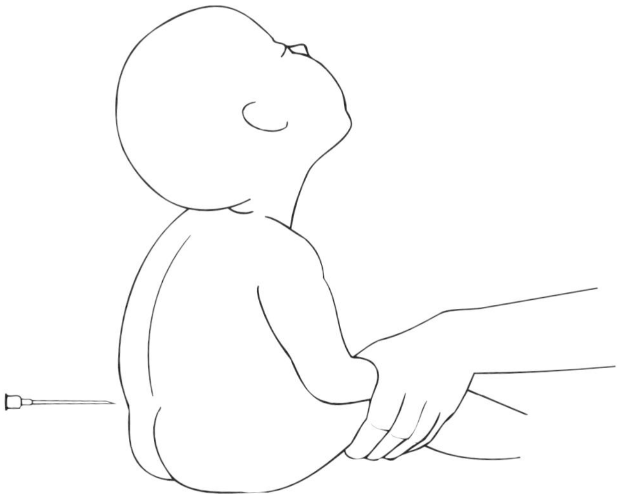

Figure 77.7 *Positioning for subarachnoid block. When subarachnoid blocks are performed on awake infants, adequate curvature of the lumbar spine can be obtained without neck flexure, which often results in inadvertent airway obstruction.*

Axillary block (C5–T1)

Indications

Indications for axillary block are as described above.

Contraindications

Generally, injuries or surgery that carry a significant risk of neurovascular injury and neuropraxia should not be managed with nerve blocks in order to facilitate a complete peripheral nerve examination by the clinician. In this way, a nerve injury may be detected in a timely manner for repair. Typical examples of this in pediatrics are supracondylar and condylar fractures of the elbow, which are often associated with ulnar nerve injuries.

Equipment

A nerve stimulator capable of delivering currents of 1 mA may be used. Butterfly needles (23G and 25G) are suitable block needles, or a 4-cm (1.5-inch) 25G spinal needle or insulated beaded block needle may be used.

Technique

Two techniques work best in our experience. Without a nerve stimulator, the axillary artery is compressed against the humerus with the nondominant hand; the needle is inserted through a skin wheal over the axillary artery, directing the needle tip just inferiorly to the axillary pulse (inferior trunk leads to ulnar nerve). When the sheath is entered, as detected by a slight "give" of the needle, half of the total intended dose is injected. The needle is then withdrawn to just under the skin and is redirected just superior to the pulse, and the remainder of the dose is injected (superior trunk leads to median/musculocutaneous nerves).

In the second technique, the nerve bundles are identified by a nerve stimulator, and one half of the dose is injected at each nerve. When the output of the stimulator is ~0.5–0.7 mA the needle tip is near enough to anesthetize the target reliably. If, during either technique, the artery is accidentally punctured, the needle is deliberately directed through the artery while continuously aspirating. When blood can no longer be withdrawn, half the dose is injected behind the artery to anesthetize the posterior trunk, the radial nerve.

During surgical procedures, to ablate all tourniquet pain, it is necessary also to anesthetize the intercostobrachial nerve, which runs subcutaneously in the axilla. Drug is injected subcutaneously, 2–5 cm caudal to the previous needle entry site over the axillary pulse.

Drug selection/dose

For a long-duration blockade, the drug of choice is 0.5% bupivacaine with epinephrine, 0.5 mL kg^{-1}. For a block of fast onset and medium duration, 2% lidocaine plus crystalline tetracaine, 5 mg per 10 mL of lidocaine, with epinephrine, 0.5 mL kg^{-1}, is preferred. For short-duration block, 2% lidocaine without epinephrine, 0.5 mL kg^{-1}, is recommended.

Interscalene approach (C4–T1, especially C4–C7 roots)

Indications

Indications include surgery or pain syndromes of the shoulder.

Contraindications

See Axillary block.

Equipment

See Axillary block. A nerve stimulator should be used.

Technique

The child's head is turned slightly to the opposite side, with the neck in slight extension. Landmarks are identified: the cricoid cartilage, the lateral border of the sternocleidomastoid muscle, the groove between the scalene muscles just posterior to the sternocleidomastoid border. A needle is inserted over the interscalene groove at the level of the cricoid, keeping the needle perpendicular to the skin in all planes. When hand contraction is seen with 0.5–0.6 mA of stimulating current, and negative aspiration is confirmed , a test dose is injected, followed by the remainder of the dose. Injection at too shallow a depth will produce Horner's syndrome and phrenic nerve anesthesia. Insertion in too cephalad direction can result in the needle entering an intervertebral foramen and produce high spinal blockade.

Drug selection/dose

See Axillary block.

Supraclavicular approach

This technique is not used in children because of the relatively high rise of the cupola of the lung and the greater subsequent risk of pneumothorax.

Infraclavicular approach

Indications

Indications include surgery of the forearm and hand.

Contraindications

See Axillary block.

Equipment

See Axillary block. A nerve stimulator should be used.

Technique

The head should be positioned midline with the arms down at the side. This block is especially helpful when abduction of the arm is difficult because of pain, as from a fracture. Landmarks include the coracoid process, clavicle, and anterior axillary line. The coracoid process is identified, and the site marked medially and inferiorly 2 cm. The needle should be inferior to the clavicle and just medial to the anterior axillary line. A groove is palpated here. Insert the needle to a depth of approximately 2 cm toward the axilla, while aspirating continuously. Needle insertion in the medial direction carries the risk of a pneumothorax.

Lower extremity blocks (L2–L4)

The major advantages of selective lower extremity blocks over lumbar or caudal epidural blocks are their increased duration of effect (10–12 h vs. 2–4 h) and the fact that patients will still be able to weight bear on one leg after the block, which facilitates their transfer in and out of bed, in and out of the family car, etc. Thus, these blocks may be safely performed on outpatients, whereas neuraxial blocks should probably not be performed on outpatients too large for the parents to easily carry in arms in and out of the car, home, etc. Furthermore, many children over 5 or 6 years of age are quite distressed by the numbness and paralysis following neuraxial blocks in spite of one's best efforts to prepare them for this sensation.

Femoral nerve block (L2–L4)

Indications

Indications for block of the anterior branch of the femoral nerve include surgery or pain of the anterior lateral thigh, femur fractures, quadriceps muscle biopsy, etc. The posterior branch gives rise to the saphenous nerve and block is indicated for surgery of or injury to the medial part of lower leg and the medial aspect of ankle. Note that the medial aspect of the knee is innervated by the obturator nerve, not the femoral nerve.

Contraindications

Contraindications to femoral nerve block include local adenopathy, local infection, sepsis, etc.

Equipment

A nerve stimulator capable of delivering currents of 1 mA may be used. Butterfly needles (23G or 25G)are suitable block needles, or a 6.5-cm (2.5-inch), 25G spinal needle or (insulated) beaded block needle with an extension attached may be used.

Technique

The femoral arterial pulse is identified below the inguinal ligament, and the needle is inserted just lateral to the pulse. It is surprising how superficial the nerve is. If a nerve stimulator is used, the needle is positioned to obtain quadriceps contractures at ~0.5–0.6 mA. Otherwise, the needle should be close enough to the artery to pulsate when disconnected from a syringe. Seventy-five percent of the dose is injected at the approximate depth of the arterial pulse and while moving the needle from that point to the subcutaneous tissues. One-fourth of the dose is reserved for a subcutaneous fan injection from a point 1 cm medial and inferior to the anterior superior iliac spine in order to anesthetize the lateral femoral cutaneous nerve.

Drug selection/dose

For long-duration block, 0.5% bupivacaine with or without epinephrine, 0.5 mL kg^{-1}, is recommended. For block of fast onset and medium duration, 2% lidocaine plus crystalline tetracaine, 5 mg per 10 mL of lidocaine, with or without epinephrine, 0.5 mL kg^{-1}, is preferred.

Fascia iliaca block (L2–L4)[83]

Indications

See Femoral nerve block. This block anesthetizes the obturator nerve, lateral femoral cutaneous nerve, and femoral nerve with one injection.

Contraindications

Contraindications to fascia iliac block include local adenopathy and local skin infection.

Equipment

The procedure requires a 6.5-cm (2.5-inch), 25G spinal needle or block needle.

Technique

The inguinal ligament is trisected in its length from the pubis to the anterior superior iliac spine, and the needle is inserted 0.5–1 cm below the juncture of the middle and lateral thirds of the ligament, directing the needle at 90° to the skin. A fascial plane will be punctured and a loss of resistance to injection will occur as the needle crosses the fascia latta. The needle is then further advanced until a second loss of resistance is felt as the fascia iliaca is pierced: then, while exerting pressure just caudal to the needle site, the dose is injected. The needle is withdrawn, and the groin "massaged" to encourage further proximal spread of local anesthetic.

Drug selection/dose

For long-duration block, 0.375% bupivacaine plus epinephrine, 0.7 mL kg^{-1}, is recommended. For block of fast onset and medium duration, lidocaine 2% plus crystalline tetracaine, 5 mg per 10 m, plus epinephrine, 0.7 mL kg^{-1}, is preferred. If combined with a sciatic block, the total bupivacaine dose should not exceed 3.2 mg kg^{-1}.

Popliteal block (continuation of sciatic nerve L4–S3)

Indications

Indications for popliteal block include surgery or pain in the lateral side of lower leg, tibia/fibula, lateral aspect of ankle, and the entire foot.

Contraindications

Contraindications include local skin infection.

Equipment

The procedure requires a 6.5-cm (2.5-inch), 25G spinal needle or (insulated) beaded block needle. A nerve stimulator may be used.

Technique

With the patient in the decubitus or prone position, and the knee straight, the bifurcation of the biceps femoris muscle is identified. This forms the apex of the popliteal fossa. The arterial pulse may be identified in slender patients. If so, the popliteal nerve lies lateral to the artery, in a slight depression. The local anesthetic may be blindly injected lateral to the pulse, or a nerve stimulator may be used to identify the nerve more accurately. Because there are no septations or sheaths in the space, the block will be effective either way.

Drug selection/dose

For a prolonged-duration block, 0.5% bupivacaine, with or without epinephrine, 0.5 mL kg^{-1}, is recommended. For block of fast onset and medium duration, 2% lidocaine plus crystalline tetracaine, 5 mg per 10 mL of lidocaine, with or without epinephrine, 0.5 mL kg^{-1}, is preferred. If combined with a sciatic block, the total bupivacaine dose should not exceed 3.2 mg kg^{-1} by using 0.375% bupivacaine for each block.

Sciatic nerve block (L4–S3)

Indications

Indications for sciatic nerve block include surgery of the lateral side of the lower leg, tibia/fibula, lateral aspect of ankle, and entire foot. In addition to the territory covered by the popliteal fossa block, a conventional sciatic nerve block anesthetizes the posterior aspect of the thigh.

Contraindications

Contraindications include local skin infection.

Equipment

The procedure requires an 8.5-cm (3.5-inch), 25G spinal needle or insulated block. A nerve stimulator may be used.

Technique

The patient is placed in the lateral decubitus position with the operative extremity on top, leg slightly flexed at hip and knee. A line is drawn from the PSIS to the greater trochanter of the femur; the hip is flexed so that the axis of the femur aligns with this line. From the midpoint of this line a second perpendicular line, 3 cm in length, is drawn caudally. The block needle is inserted at the end of the second line perpendicular to the skin until it contacts bone (ischial spine), and is "walked" off the bone toward the PSIS. The needle tip is positioned to achieve maximum contraction of a distal leg muscle while stimulating with 0.5–0.6 mA. The anticipated depth of the sciatic nerve may be predicted from the following formula in children of average size:[84]

$$\text{Depth (mm)} = \text{weight (kg)} + 5/\text{age (years)}$$

Drug selection/dose

For long-duration block, 0.5% bupivacaine, with or without epinephrine, 0.5 mL kg^{-1}, is recommended. For block of fast onset and medium duration, 2% lidocaine plus crystalline tetracaine, 5 mg per 10 mL of lidocaine, with or without epinephrine, 0.5 ml kg^{-1}, is preferred.

Management of epidural infusions

For effective pain management in hospitalized children with indwelling epidural catheters, preprinted order forms are very helpful to ensure a comprehensive and consistent approach to monitoring, assessment, adjustment of infusions, and treatment of side-effects (Table 77.7). Accessibility of a treating pain physician is essential, as are regular educational programs for the nursing staff.

In the case of the pediatric population, we believe that arterial oxygen hemoglobin saturation monitoring should be routinely used for at least the first 24 h of epidural treatment. Naloxone should be available at or near the bedside if hydrophilic epidural opioids such as morphine sulfate are administered.

Typically, a combination of a dilute local anesthetic and an analgesic is used for continuous or intermittent bolus administration in the epidural space. The continuous infusion technique, while requiring an electronic infusion device, eliminates the "peaks and valleys" of analgesia associated with intermittent techniques, and reduces the demand on nursing personnel.

The maximum safe infusion dose of local anesthetics has not been definitively established in children. Generally, the prevailing practice has been guided by the implicit dose ceilings derived from several case reports of local anesthetic toxicity in children.[85–87] Table 77.8 outlines appropriate starting and maximum doses for drugs commonly used in epidural infusions in children.

Once the epidural infusion is determined to be functioning as predicted, infusions are managed according to protocol. The functioning of the epidural infusion can be gauged by ease of placement, the results of test dosing, reduction in anesthetic requirement during surgery, patient comfort at end of surgery, determination of sensory level if the patient is cooperative, gentle stimulation of the surgical incision without the production of pain, examination of the catheter entry site, absence of back pain with injection, minimal or no leakage of fluid at the catheter site, and the response to epidural bolus doses of anesthetic or analgesic.

The recurrence of pain after the initiation of the infusion may be treated by a second bolus dose of anesthetic equal to the amount

Table 77.7 *Elements of standard epidural orders*

Essential elements	Example of order
Patient data	Epidural orders: patient weight = 28 kg
Drug selection	☑ Bupivacaine 0.1% + clonidine 0.5 μg mL^{-1} ☐ Bupivacaine 0.1% + hydromorphone 5 μg ml^{-1}
Drug dose	Infuse continuously at 0.3 mL^{-1} kg^{-1} h^{-1} (8.4 mL h^{-1})
Vital signs specific to epidural analgesia	Routine measurement of vital signs, plus assign sedation scale every 4 h Continuous pulse oximetry for 24 h
p.r.n. medications	☑ Breakthrough pain: bolus 0.3 mL kg^{-1} of epidural infusion fluid via epidural catheter (8 mL) and increase infusion by 1 mL h^{-1} ☑ Nausea and vomiting: ondansetron 0.1 mg kg^{-1} (3 mg) i.v. every 8 h ☑ Pruritus: diphenhydramine 7 mg i.v. every 8 h
Emergency medications	In the event of inability to arouse or oxygen saturation $<$92%, administer naloxone 0.01 mg kg^{-1} (0.28 mg) i.v. and notify the Pain Management Service immediately
Contact information	Pain Management Service contacts: Resident: Dr Jekyll, beeper 12345 Attending: Dr Hyde, beeper 56789 Nurse Ratchett, beeper 54321

i.v., intravenously; p.r.n., as required.

Table 77.8 *Epidural drug infusion doses*

Drug	Starting dose	Approximate maximum dose
Lidocaine	0.25%, 0.5 mg kg^{-1} h^{-1}	2 mg kg^{-1} h^{-1}
Bupivacaine	0.1%, 0.2 mg kg^{-1} h^{-1}	0.5 mg kg^{-1} h^{-1}
Levo-bupivacaine	0.1%, 0.2 mg kg^{-1} h^{-1}	0.5 mg kg^{-1} h^{-1}
Ropivacaine	0.1%, 0.2 mg kg^{-1} h^{-1}	0.5 mg kg^{-1} h^{-1}
Morphine	3 μg kg^{-1} h^{-1}	7.5 μg kg^{-1} h^{-1}
Fentanyl	0.25 μg kg^{-1} h^{-1}	0.67 μg kg^{-1} h^{-1}
Hydromorphone	0.5 μg kg^{-1} h^{-1}	1.25 μg kg^{-1} h^{-1}
Clonidine	0.1 μg kg^{-1} h^{-1}	0.8 μg kg^{-1} h^{-1}

previously infused per hour, followed by an increase in the infusion of 20–25%.

Patient-controlled epidural infusions are appropriate for children, using the same subject selection guidelines that would guide the selection of patients for intravenous patient-controlled analgesia.

Side-effects are not uncommon in children with the administration of epidural opioids.[88] Nausea and vomiting are the most common, and are treated with metaclopromide (0.1 mg kg^{-1}) or ondansetron (0.1 mg kg^{-1}). In children without bladder drainage, monitoring for bladder distension is necessary; urinary retention is treated with catheterization as necessary. Pruritus, another common side-effect of spinal or epidural opioids, may be treated with nalbuphine 0.05 mg kg^{-1} per dose, diphenhydramine 0.5 mg kg^{-1}, or a low-dose naloxone infusion (0.1 μg kg^{-1} h^{-1}).

A number of adjuvant medications are helpful in managing residual pain and discomfort while an epidural infusion is being administered:

- Acetaminophen 10–15mg kg^{-1} every 6 h orally or rectally.
- Ketorolac, 0.5 mg kg^{-1} i.v.
- Low-dose benzodiazepines are helpful for the management of situational anxiety in children. Low-dose benzodiazepines are additionally very useful to reduce muscle spasms in children with spasticity, and to eliminate hypnogogic myoclonus secondary to administration of opioids. Suitable alternatives for these indications are midazolam (10 μg kg^{-1} h^{-1} continuous intravenous infusion), diazepam (0.05 mg kg^{-1} orally every 6 h), or lorazepam (0.05 mg kg^{-1} intravenously every 8 h).

Transcutaneous electrical nerve stimulation, guided imagery, acupuncture, and psychological counseling may be considered but frequently prove unsuccessful in the setting of severe acute pain.

MANAGEMENT OF CHRONIC PAIN

Complex regional pain syndromes (CRPS) are a related group of disorders of neuropathic pain. They include CRPS-1 and CRPS-2. CRPS-1, formerly known as reflex sympathetic dystrophy, is a syndrome that usually develops after an initiating noxious or traumatic event but is not limited to the distribution of a single peripheral nerve and is apparently disproportionate to the inciting event. It is associated at some point with evidence of edema, changes in skin blood flow, abnormal sudomotor activity in the region of the pain, allodynia, and hyperalgesia. The site is usually the distal aspect of an affected extremity or with a distal to proximal gradient."[89]

CRPS-2 is a similar syndrome that follows injury to a major nerve root, unlike CRPS-1, in which no obvious nerve injury exists. These syndromes are described in other chapters of this book. We will focus on the pediatric presentations and treatments.

Few reports describe CRPS in children. In the largest case series, there was a marked predominance of girls over boys (6–8:1), and the majority of cases involved the lower extremity (61 out of 70).[90]

Symptoms of CRPS in children are similar to the presentations in adults in that they involve four major symptom types: (1) sensory abnormalities, (2) vascular changes, (3) trophic changes, and (4) motor and functional abnormalities. These changes may wax and wane but are usually progressive in the absence of treatment. As is typical of adults, the severity of symptoms is usually out of proportion to the magnitude of the inciting event, which may be quite innocuous indeed. In children, the inciting insult is usually a sports or repetitive stress injury.

The sensory abnormalities always involve pain, typically neuropathic pain, but may also involve muscle twitching, uncomfortable numbness (anesthesia dolorosa), or other unusual sensations. At times patients report that these sensations are more disturbing than the pain itself, and cases of self-mutilation have been described, in an attempt by the patient to attenuate these unpleasant and unnatural sensations. Neuropathic pain includes allodynia (pain in response to an otherwise innocuous stimulus), hyperesthesia (a mildly painful stimulus perceived as very painful), hypoesthesia (sensation that is less than it should be), and hyperpathia (increasing pain with a steadily repeating, otherwise nonpainful stimulus – e.g. repeated stroking of the skin with a swab).

Vascular changes include abnormal temperature of the extremity, either hot or, more typically, cold, in comparison with the contralateral extremity. The extremity may also exhibit increased or decreased sudomotor activity (sweating). Significant edema may be present. Trophic changes include changes in hair, increased nail growth, and skin changes. Muscle atrophy may also be seen in more advanced stages.

Motor and functional abnormalities include loss of strength in the extremity, largely related to disuse, restricted range of motion, and loss of fine motor movements.

The focal point of management of CRPS is aggressive and frequent physical therapy, designed to remobilize the affected extremity, restore flexibility and strength, and to desensitize the skin. However, this is frequently difficult to accomplish in more advanced cases, especially in children, and in these cases pharmacologic management becomes necessary.

Because of the usually unrelenting course of CRPS, the untoward side-effects of opioids, and the refractory nature of the pain to opioid therapy, unconventional analgesics are first deployed. The mainstay of treatment has become tricyclic antidepressants, gabapentin, and mexiletine, either singly or in combination. Cases refractory to oral pharmacologic therapy become candidates for more invasive techniques designed to impart a sympathetic block.

Chemical sympathectomy of an extremity may be achieved by one of three techniques:

1 Intravenous regional anesthesia. In this technique, bretyllium 2 mg kg^{-1}, ketorolac 1 mg kg^{-1}, and 0.5% lidocaine, 2.5–5 mg kg^{-1}, are injected into a distal vein of the affected extremity using a Bier block technique. The tourniquet is allowed to remain inflated for 30–60 min, and is then deflated. Pain relief is diagnostic of CRPS if the technique is applied without local anesthetic, and pain relief usually lasts well beyond the expected pharmacologic duration of action of any of the injected agents.
2 Epidural blockade. For CRPS of the lower extremities, placement of an epidural catheter and infusion of dilute local anesthetic will result in a distal sympathetic block and alleviation of pain. However, some patients may also experience a sensory or motor block limiting their mobility and ability to participate in physical therapy. This technique is generally not utilized for CRPS of the upper extremity, in which a cervical epidural catheter would be required.
3 Regional sympathectomy. Either a single-shot sympathectomy or a catheter technique may be used to treat unilateral CRPS of the upper extremity (stellate ganglion block) or lower extremity (lumbar sympathetic block).The advantage of this technique is long-lived analgesia and restoration of circulation, and the absence of sensory or motor block. However, for bilateral disease, bilateral blocks are generally considered to be unwise. The technique for performing these blocks is considered elsewhere in this textbook.

HEADACHE

Headache is one the most frequent presenting complaints to the pediatric pain clinic. Types of headache encountered in children include migraine headaches with or without aura, tension headaches, cluster headaches, and headaches caused by organic disease, an important subset. These include tumors (bearing in mind that brain tumors are the most common solid malignancy of childhood), ear and sinus infections, CNS infections such as meningitis, obstructive sleep apnea, and underlying neurologic dysfunction.

Of the various causes of nonmalignant headaches in children, migraine is both the most common and the most frequently underdiagnosed etiology. Overall, migraine prevalence among children between 5 and 15 years of age is between 2.7% and 10%,[91,92] and has been increasing over the past 20 years.[93] Until age 11–12 the frequency in males is approximately equal to that in females. After puberty, the prevalence assumes the 3 to 1 female to male ratio that is seen in adults.

There are multiple triggers in children that lead to acute migraines. These include dietary factors, strong visual and auditory stimuli (such as video or computer games), motion sickness, and sleep disturbances. There is also a strong genetic predisposition to migraine, making it up to four times more likely in cases in which there is a positive family history.[94] There is a slightly increased risk of epilepsy in children with migraine.[95]

Diagnosis should be based on a thorough history and physical examination to assess neurologic involvement and rule out organic disease. Headache triggers should be evaluated as well as social stressors and family history. Indicators for further diagnostic investigations include increasing frequency of headaches, headaches associated with vomiting, headaches that wake one up from sleep or early-morning headaches, lack of family history, neurologic findings, increasing headache with coughing, sneezing, and straining, and change of personality or habits. Because of the frequency of CNS malignancies in children, some form of radiologic imaging is usually performed before the diagnosis of migraine is entertained.[96]

Childhood migraines are usually associated with photophobia and phonophobia and may be associated with premonitory aura, but true visual auras are rare. Lack of sleep, stress, and hormonal changes in adolescence can be major triggers. In children, bilateral pain is common, and acute migraine is often associated with coincident severe abdominal pain and vomiting, known as abdominal migraine.[97,98]

Migraine management in children involves a multidisciplinary approach including biofeedback, relaxation therapy, and medical management. A headache diary is mandatory to identify triggers and monitor progress. In a study comparing nonpharmacologic treatment with medical interventions, it was found that nonpharmacologic treatment was more effective, and that the effects could still be observed at the 10-year follow-up.[99,100]

Initial pharmacologic abortive treatments include acetaminophen (paracetamol), ibuprofen, naproxen, Midrin®, dihydroergotamine, nasal lidocaine, CNS serotonin agonists (sumatriptan, naratriptan, etc.), and occasionally opioids when other therapies fail. Midrin® is an over-the-counter mixture of three compounds: acetaminophen 325 mg, isometheptane mucate 65 mg (a mild vasoconstrictor), and dichloral phenazone (a mild sedative). It can be used in children as young as 7 years of age. Addition of a small dose of caffeine, such as is found in a caffeinated carbonated beverage (about 40 mg of caffeine), can be effective in enhancing the effects of any of the above-mentioned abortive agents. Second-line abortives include butalbital compounds

(Fiorinal® and Fioricet®) and acetylsalicylic acid. Fiorinal® contains butalbital 50 mg, aspirin 325 mg, and caffeine 40 mg. Doses start at half a tablet for 7- to 8-year-olds, which may be repeated in 1–2 h to a maximum dose of one tablet per day. At age 9–10 the dosage is increased to one tablet per day and the maximum is increased to two tablets per day. Side-effects include nervousness, fatigue, lightheadedness, nausea, dizziness, and euphoria.

Third-line abortive agents include dihydroergotamine (DHE) nasal spray, DHE intravenous infusions, and parenteral corticosteroids. Dihydroergotamine has been used since 1945. It is generally considered a very safe medication and can be effective for migraine headaches refractory to all other treatments, so-called "status migraine," and is used as follows:

- premedication with metoclopramide 15 min prior to start of infusion to prevent nausea and vomiting;
- DHE i.v., 3 mg in 1000 mL of normal saline, at 42 mL h^{-1};
- metoclopramide 10 mg i.v. in 50 mL of normal saline over 30 min every 8 h p.r.n. nausea for six doses;
- diphenoxylate with atropine (Lomotil), one or two t.i.d. p.r.n. diarrhea;
- if excessive anxiety, jitteriness (akathisia), or dystonic reactions occur, benztropine (Cogentin) 1 mg i.v.;
- if significant nausea occurs at any time, reduce DHE infusion rate to 21–30 mL h^{-1}.

The infusion may be continued for up to 7 days, at which time transition to oral DHE should take place.

Antiemetics frequently need to be incorporated into the above regimens. Frequently used agents include Tigan® (trimethobenzamide), Phenergan® (promethazine), and Zofran® (ondansetron). The last is manufactured as a sublingual tablet in 4- and 8-mg strength, and is very well tolerated by children with refractory nausea and vomiting.

Prophylactic migraine therapy is warranted in children having more than one attack per month, and of such severity that the child's daily activities are significantly affected. Prophylactic medications include cyproheptadine (Periactin®), propranolol (Inderal®), amitriptyline (Elavil®), nortriptyline (Pamelor®), and trazodone (Desyrel®).

Although poorly understood, there is an intimate connection between serotonin receptor physiology and migraine headaches, nausea and vomiting syndromes, and recurrent abdominal pain. 5-HT receptors are prevalent in the CNS as well as the GI tract. As many as seven subreceptors have been identified. 5-HT_3 antagonists are used to prevent emesis, especially following chemotherapy and postoperative situations. 5-HT_4 agonists show prokinetic properties and are useful in management of gastroparesis and functional dyspepsia. The 5-HT_{1D} receptor agonist sumatriptan is used for migraine headache and in cyclic vomiting syndrome. These are active areas of research.[101]

Acupuncture can be an effective prophylactic modality for migraine headaches.[102] In the authors' experience, it is effective for children, provided they are able to tolerate the procedure. Practicing acupuncture in children requires that a bond of trust be established between practitioner and patient. Ample time must be allowed for preparation of the child and family. The child will often reflect adult perceptions. Treatments should be performed once or twice a week. The number of needles can gradually be increased from one or two to five or six as necessary. Effects are usually seen within 1–2 months after therapy is begun; however, responses that are more dramatic are sometimes seen. Acupuncture should be combined with other therapies in a multidisciplinary approach. It is often possible to decrease or eliminate other medications as treatment progresses. Once a plateau is reached, the treatments are reduced to once a month, or as necessary to maintain the therapeutic effects. In general, children respond faster and more profoundly than do adults to acupuncture therapy.

MANAGEMENT OF SPECIFIC PEDIATRIC PAIN STATES

Sickle cell disease pain

Patients with sickle cell disease frequently suffer from both acute vaso-occlusive crises as well as chronic pain. Frequent episodes of pain often render them tolerant to narcotics. Superimposed surgical pain may lead to very high narcotic requirements, leading to increased side-effects, including nausea, itching, and the possibility of respiratory depression. High anxiety may further complicate the scenario. In addition, sickle cell patients may have end-organ disease, including renal insufficiency or decreased hepatic clearance, rendering them more susceptible to accumulation of toxic metabolites, at times leading to respiratory depression and even death.[103] In the acute perioperative period, patients are at additional risk of vaso-occlusive crisis.

The optimal overall management strategy for acute sickle cell crisis is early intervention utilizing a multidisciplinary approach. Maximization of nonmedical resources available will help to minimize anxiety surrounding frequent hospitalizations. A patient care plan outlining the plan of treatment clarifies expectations for both the provider and the patient and eases the transition should a physician not immediately familiar with the patient be providing the care. The mainstay of therapy for sickle cell crises has conventionally been opioid therapy. However, nonsteroidal agents such as ketorolac can have a significant opioid-sparing effect.

The use of epidural anesthesia can be very effective for treatment of refractory pain in the chest, abdomen, hips, or lower extremities. This technique minimizes the need for oral or i.v. opioids, and enhances respiratory function and oxygenation.[104]

Neuropathic pain

Neuropathic pain encompasses a variety of pain types, including nerve injury states, complex regional pain syndromes, and phantom limb pain. It generally represents a state of injury, damage, or activation of the mechanisms of pain transmission without necessarily having significant tissue injury. This conditions results in hyperactivity or altered activity of the nervous system and can be associated with a particular type of debilitating and chronic pain. Neuropathic pain involves activation of the nociceptive pathways without necessarily involving the peripheral nociceptors. The result is a state of abnormal sensory potential. The continued pain experienced then further serves as a stimulus, creating increasingly abnormal synaptic connections in the central nervous system. These synapses may not be responsive to the normal descending inhibition pathways that modulate the normal perception of pain, and are usually refractory to treatment using opioids and nonsteroidal agents.

The pain of neuropathic states has one or more of the following qualities:

1. It may be burning, stabbing, or shooting.
2. There may be allodynia – pain experienced with simple touch of the affected area.
3. There may be hyperesthesia – increased touch sensation (i.e. light touch is experienced as heavy).
4. There may be hypoesthesia – decreased sensation to normal touch.
5. There may be hyperpathia – repetitive touch leads to progressively increased pain.

CRPS-1 and -2 fall in the category of neuropathic pain. In additions to the qualities mentioned above, there are associated autonomic changes:

- increased or decreased blood flow to the extremities;
- trophic changes of the skin and nails;
- increased or decreased hair growth;
- increased or decreased sweating.

Medications that allay neuropathic pain include tricyclic antidepressants, membrane-stabilizing agents such as lidocaine, mexiletine and anticonvulsants such as carbamazepine, sodium valproate, and, more recently, gabapentin. These are discussed in detail in the section on pharmacology above.

Much work remains to be done about understanding the synergy that is often found clinically in the utilization of medications for neuropathic pain. For example, gabapentin has recently been shown to be synergistic with morphine sulfate in healthy volunteers. Its good safety profile suggests a possible use in perioperative pain management. Combining low doses of several types of medications such as a tricyclic antidepressant, gabapentin, and a nonsteroidal anti-inflammatory agent, one is often able to achieve a superior result and decreased side-effect profile. Little is known about the mechanisms of this synergy. Gabapentin is well established in the treatment of pediatric neuropathic pain, and can be effectively combined with other agents such as tricyclic antidepressants, opioids, and nonsteroidal agents without adverse effects.

Cancer pain

Cancer pain is a complex phenomenon and an active area of investigation. Assessing cancer pain is made more difficult because of the difficulty in assessing the child's developmental level. In addition to age, chronic illness often results in considerable regression in developmental milestones.

Pain is one of the most feared consequences of cancer. Most commonly, this pain is due to bony or soft-tissue involvement of the tumor, mucositis, or neuropathy. Patients frequently require multiple procedures, including surgery, lumbar punctures, bone marrow aspirates, percutaneous access procedures, and others. One must treat both the pain and the anxiety associated with these procedures. This process requires adequate preparation and explanation, in addition to

Table 77.9 *Withdrawal scale for the newborn. (Courtesy of Children's Hospital Oakland, Oakland, CA)*

Analgesia/sedation orders (drug/dose/frequency)			
Date			
Drug			
Administration time			
Dose or frequency ↑ or ↓			
Choose one			
Crying/agitated 25–50% of interval	2		
Crying/agitated > 50% of interval	3		
Choose one			
Sleeps 25% of interval	3		
Sleeps 26–75% of interval	2		
Sleeps > 75% of interval	1		
Choose one			
Hyperactive Moro	2		
Markedly hyperactive Moro	3		
Choose one			
Mild tremors, disturbed	1		
Moderate/severe tremors, disturbed	2		
Other indicators			
Increased muscle tone	2		
Temperature 37.2–38.4 °C	1		
Temperature > 38.4 °C	2		
Respiratory rate > 60 (extubated)	2		
Suction > twice/interval (intubated)	2		
Sweating	1		
Frequent yawning (>3–4/interval)	1		
Sneezing (> 3–4/interval)	1		
Nasal stuffiness	1		
Emesis	2		
Projectile vomiting	3		
Loose stools	2		
Watery stools	3		
Total score			
Adjusted score			
Initials of person scoring			

Directions: Score each guideline every 2–4 h. A score greater than 8–12 may indicate withdrawal.

instruction in nonmedical techniques such as deep breathing, guided imagery, distraction, and play therapy. Pain must be assessed at each level of treatment utilizing an age-appropriate method.

In the pharmacologic management of cancer pain, the World Health Organization (WHO) ladder of pharmacologic intervention should be used.[105] For mild to moderate pain, a nonopioid, such as an NSAID or acetaminophen, is appropriate. For moderate to severe pain, transition to a weak opioid such as codeine, hydrocodone, or oxycodone together with a NSAID or acetaminophen is appropriate. For lumbar punctures and central venous port access procedures, EMLA cream applied 1 h before provides effective analgesia.[106] For severe pain, strong opioids are needed. The standard opioid for comparison is morphine, because of its excellent safety profile and extensive experience in its utilization. Other potent opioids, as described previously, include hydromorphone, oxycodone, fentanyl, and methadone. At times, change from one opioid to another, even at equianalgesic doses, can provide improved analgesia and improved side-effect profile. This phenomenon may be due to different populations of subreceptors present.[107]

The method of administration must be varied as necessary, utilizing enteral or intravenous routes if appropriate. A small number of patients require massive infusions of intravenous opioids to control their pain. At all stages of treatment, use of adjuvant medications is appropriate to improve analgesia or minimize side-effects. To counteract sedation associated with large doses of opioids, psychostimulants such as dextroamphetamine or methylphenidate may be useful.[108]

For patients in whom these methods fail, epidural or intrathecal administration may be possible, depending on the location of the pain.[109,110]

Prior to insertion of an epidural or intrathecal catheter, the location of metastatic lesions must be clarified with appropriate imaging such as computed tomography (CT) or magnetic resonance imaging (MRI), coagulation parameters must be verified and normalized as much as possible, and platelet count must be optimized. An epidural or intrathecal catheter is inserted on a trial basis, and tunneled under the skin. This helps to reduce the chance of accidental dislodgement, and may help to reduce chances of infection, extending the lifetime of the catheter.

Infusions usually incorporate a combination of agents to maximize pain relief through synergy while minimizing side-effect profile. In the case of epidural infusions, a mixture of local anesthetic, opioid, and clonidine can be used. In the case of intrathecal infusions, opioid and clonidine can be used at any time during the treatment process. However, local anesthetic must be reserved during the terminal phase of disease process due to potential neurotoxicity of long-term infusions. Other regional blocks such as brachial plexus, celiac plexus, and hypogastric plexus blocks may also be useful in the management of cancer pain, depending on the location of the tumor and nature of the pain.[111]

Pain in newborn infants

Newborn infants are exposed to a variety of noxious stimuli and painful procedures. A study by Barker and Rutter[112] reported that, among 54 infants consecutively admitted to the NICU, more than 3000 procedures were carried out.

Evidence shows that painful stimuli may have long-lasting consequences on the developing nervous system of the premature infant.[113] A number of nonpharmacologic interventions have been shown to be effective at promoting stability in physiologic indicators, growth, and behavioral state in the preterm infant. These processes include the use of sucrose, swaddling, and rocking.[114–116]

Many pharmacologic interventions have, of course, also been shown to be helpful. These include the use of analgesics such as acetaminophen, opioids such as morphine and fentanyl, and sedatives such as midazolam and chloral hydrate. Useful local anesthetics include EMLA cream for venipuncture, lumbar punctures, and heel sticks. Regional techniques such as dorsal penile nerve blocks for circumcision and epidural catheters for major abdominal and thoracic surgical procedures are becoming increasingly utilized in clinical practice.[117,118] In addition, the anesthesiologist may be called upon as a consultant in the treatment of neonatal pain and in the assessment of withdrawal and weaning of sedative and analgesic infusions.

Clinical signs of opioid withdrawal primarily involve the CNS, the GI system, and the autonomic system (Table 77.9). Neurologic symptoms include high-pitched crying, irritability, hyperactive reflexes, tremors, exaggerated Moro reflex, seizures, and intraventricular hemorrhage. GI symptoms are poor feeding, vomiting, uncoordinated sucking, and diarrhea. Autonomic signs include fever, mottling, sweating, and nasal stuffiness.[119]

Other conditions can mimic opioid withdrawal and should be evaluated. These include benzodiazepine withdrawal, hypoxia, hypercarbia, and metabolic abnormalities such as hypocalcemia, hypoglycemia, and hypomagnesemia.

Management includes nonpharmacologic interventions such as gentle handling and minimizing stimulation as well as pharmacologic measures. Infusions should be approximately 10% per day, with close evaluation. Alternatively, the patient can be transitioned to methadone, starting at approximately 30% of hourly morphine sulfate equivalent, and given b.id. by bolus infusion over 30 min to minimize hemodynamic effects. The oral route, if tolerated, is preferable to intravenous administration. Clonidine can also be used orally at 3–4 μg kg^{-1} to minimize withdrawal symptoms.[120] Additional p.r.n. doses of morphine sulfate for breakthrough pain or withdrawal symptoms should be allowed.

CONCLUSION

Pain management is an integral part of the management of complex diseases, as well as of end-of-life care. In the pediatric population, anesthesiologists have taken a lead in the management of pain for both invasive procedures and perioperative care as well as end-of-life issues.

REFERENCES

1. Anand KJS. Relationships between stress responses and clinical outcome in newborns, infants and children. *Crit Care Med* 1993; **21:** S358–9.
2. Wong DL, Hockenberry-Eaton M, Wilson D, et *al. Wong's Essentials of Pediatric Nursing*, 6th edn. St. Louis, MO: Mosby–Yearbook, 2001: 1301.
3. Krechel SW, Bildner J. CRIES: a new neonatal post-operative pain measurement score. Initial testing of validity and reliability. *Pediatr Anesth* 1995; **5:** 53–61.
4. Hodgkinson K, Bear M, Thorn J, *et al.* Measuring pain in neonates: evaluating an instrument and developing a common language. *Austral J Advanc Nurs* 1994; **12:** 17–22.
5. Merkel SI, Voepel-Lewis T, Shayevits JR, *et al.* The FLACC: A Behavioral Scale for Scoring Postoperative Pain in Young Children. *Pediatr Nurs* 1997; **23:** 293–7.
6. Anand KJS, Craig KD. New perspectives on the definition of pain. *Pain* 1996; **67:** 3–6.
7. Stevens B, Johnston CC, Petryshen P, *et al.* Premature Infant Pain Profile. Development and initial validation. *Clin J Pain* 1996; **12:** 13–22.
8. Lawrence J, Alcock D, McGrath P, *et al.* The development of a tool to assess neonatal pain. *Neonatal Network* 1997; **12:** 59–66.
9. Finnegan LP, Connaughton Jr JF, Kron RE, *et al.* Neonatal abstinence syndrome: assessment and management. *Addictive Dis* 1975; **2:** 141–58.
10. Franck L, Vilardi J. Assessment and management of opioid withdrawal in ill neonates. *Neonatal Network* 1995; **14:** 39–48.
11. Mersky H. Classification of chronic pain: description of chronic pain syndromes and definition of pain terms. *Pain* 1986; **3:** S1.
12. Fields HL. *Pain*. New York, NY: McGraw-Hill, 1987: 1–78.

13. Jamali S, Monin S, Begon C, *et al.* Clonidine in pediatric caudal anesthesia. *Anesth Analg* 1994; **78:** 663–6.
14. Janig W, Levine JD, Michaelis M. Interactions of sympathetic and primary afferent neurons following nerve injury and tissue trauma. *Progr Brain Res* 1996; **113:** 161–84.
15. Anand KJS, Menon G, Narsinghari U, *et al.* System analgesic therapy. In: Anand KJS, Stevens BJ, McGrath PJ (eds). *Pain in Neonates,* 2nd edn. *Pain Research and Clinical Management*, Vol. 10. Amsterdam: Elsevier Science, 2000: 159–88.
16. Fitzgerald M, McIntosh N. Pain and analgesia in the newborn. *Arch Dis Child* 1989; **64:** 441–3.
17. Majcher TA, Means LJ. Pain management in children. *Semin Pediatr Surg* 1992; **1:** 52–64.
18. Plotsky PM, Bradley CC, Anand KJS. Behavioral and neuroendocrine consequences of neonatal stress. In: Anand KJS, Stevens BJ, McGrath PJ (eds.) *Pain in Neonates,* 2nd edn. *Pain Research and Clinical Management*, Vol. 10. Amsterdam: Elsevier Science, 2000: 77–99.
19. Anand KJS, Carr DB. The neuroanatomy, neurophysiology, and neurochemistry of pain, stress, and analgesia in newborns and children. *Pediatr Clin N Am* 1989; **36:** 795–822.
20. Taddio A, Katz J, Ilersich AL, *et al.* Effect of neonatal circumcision on pain response during subsequent vaccination. *Lancet* 1997; **349:** 599–603.
21. Woolf CJ. Somatic pain–pathogenesis and prevention. *Br J Anaesthesiol* 1995; **75:** 169–76.
22. Kissin I. Preemptive analgesia: terminology and clinical relevance. *Anesth Analg* 1994; **79:** 809–10.
23. Henderson DJ, Withington BS, Wilson JA, *et al.* Perioperative dextromethorphan reduces postoperative pain after hysterectomy. *Anesth Analg* 1999; **89:** 399–402.
24. McQuay HJ, Carroll D, Moore RA. Postoperative orthopedic pain – the effect of opioid premedication and local anaesthetic blocks. *Pain* 1988; **33:** 291–5.
25. Bach S, Noreng MF, Tjellden NU. Phantom limb pain in amputees during the first 12 months following limb amputation after preoperative lumbar epidural blockade. *Pain* 1988; **33:** 297–301.
26. Murat I, Walker J, Esteve C, *et al.* Effects of lumbar epidural anaesthesia on plasma cortisol levels in children. *Can J Anesthesiol* 1988; **35:** 20–4.
27. Wolf AR, Doyle E, Thomas E. Modifying infant stress responses to major surgery: spinal vs. extradural vs. opioid analgesia. *Paediatr Anaesth* 1998; **8:** 305–11.
28. Anand KJS. Relationships between stress responses and clinical outcome in newborns, infants and children. *Crit Care Med* 1993; **21:** S358–9.
29. Yaster M. The dose response of fentanyl in neonatal anesthesia. *Anesthesiology* 1987; **66:** 433–5.
30. Chay PCW, Duffy BJ, Walker JS. Pharmacokinetic-pharmacodynamic relationships of morphine in neonates. *Clin Pharmacol Ther* 1992; **51:** 334–42.
31. Brandt MR, Fernandes A, Mordhorst R, *et al.* Epidural analgesia improves nitrogen balance. *Br Med J* 1978; 1106–8.
32. Williamson PS, Williamson ML. Physiological stress reduction by a local anesthetic during newborn circumcision. *Pediatrics* 1983; **71:** 36–40.
33. Anand KJS, Hickey PR. Halothane-morphine compared with high-dose sufentanil for anaesthesia and postoperative analgesia in neonatal cardiac surgery. *N Engl J Med* 1992; **326:** 1–9.
34. Bjorkman R, Hallman KM, Hedner J, *et al.* Acetaminophen blocks spinal hyperalgesia induced by NMDA and substance P. *Pain* 1994; **57:** 259–64.
35. Lin YC, Sussman HH, Benitz WE. Plasma concentrations after rectal administration of acetaminophen in preterm neonates. *Paediatr Anaesth* 1997; **7:** 457–9.
36. Shann F. Paracetamol: when, why and how much? *J Pediatr Child Hlth* 1993; **29:** 84–5.
37. Uhl GR, Childers S, Pasternak G. An opiate-receptor gene family reunion. *Trends Neurosci* 1994; **17:** 89–93.
38. Yaksh TL. Pharmacologic and mechanisms of opioid analgesic activity. *Acta Anaesthesiol Scand* 1997; **41:** 94–111.
39. Ferrante FM. Principles of opioid pharmacotherapy: practical implications of basic mechanisms. *J Pain Symptom Manage* 1996; **11:** 265–73.
40. Yaster M, Nichols DG, Deshpande JK, *et al.* Midazolam–fentanyl intravenous sedation in children: case report of respiratory arrest. *Pediatrics* 1990; **86:** 463–7.
41. American Psychiatric Association. *Diagnostic and Statistical Manual of Mental Disorders,* 4th edn. Washington, DC: American Psychiatric Association, 1998: 178–179.
42. Porter J, Jick J. Addiction is rare in patients treated with narcotics [letter]. *N Engl J Med* 1980; **302:** 123.
43. Payne R. Factors influencing quality of life in cancer patients: the role of transdermal fentanyl in the management of pain. *Semin Oncol* 1998; **3:** 47–53.
44. Way WL, Costley EL, Way EL. Respiratory sensitivity of the newborn infant to meperidine and morphine. *Clin Pharmacol Ther* 1965; **6:** 454–61.
45. Reeh PW, Kocher L, Jung S. Does neurogenic inflammation alter the sensitivity of unmyelinated nociceptors in the rat? *Brain Res* 1986; **384:** 42–50.
46. Berde CB. Pediatric Postoperative Pain Management. *Pediatr Clin N Am* 1989; **36:** 921–40.
47. Galer BS, Harle BS, Rowbotham MC. Response to intravenous lidocaine infusion predicts subsequent response to oral mexiletine: a prospective study. *J Pain Symptom Manage* 1996; **12:** 161–7.
48. Walker L, Slovis C. Lidocaine in the treatment of status epilepticus. *Acad Emerg Med* 1997; **4:** 918–22.
49. Lin YC, Sentivany-Collin S. The analgesic response to intravenous lidocaine in the treatment of mucositis pain. *Anesthesiology* 2000; **93:** A1258.
50. Wallace MS, Lee J, Sorkin L, *et al.* Intravenous lidocaine: effects on controlling pain after anti-GD2 antibody therapy in children with neuroblastoma – a report of a series. *Anesth Analg* 1997; **85:** 794–6.
51. McLean M. Gabapentin. Epilepsia 1995; **36:** S73–S86.
52. Wheeler DS, Vaux KK, Tam DA. Use of gabapentin in the treatment of childhood reflex sympathetic dystrophy. *Pediatr Neurol* 2000; **22:** 220–1.
53. Bourgeois B. Antiepileptic drugs in pediatric practice. *Epilepsia* 1995; **36:** S34–45.
54. Loscher W. Valproate: a reappraisal of its pharmacodynamic properties and mechanism of action. *Progressive Neurobiol* 1999; **58:** 31–59.
55. Committee on Drugs. Valproic acid: benefits and risks. *Pediatrics* 1982; **70:** 316–19.
56. Kong K. Carbamazepine-induced hepatitis in a patient with cervical myelopathy. *Arch Phys Med Rehabil* 1996; **77:** 305–6.
57. Wilens T, Biederman J, Baldessarini RJ, *et al.* Cardiovascular effects of therapeutic doses of tricyclic antidepressants in children and adolescents. *J Am Acad Child Adolesc Psychiatry* 1996; **35:** 1491–501.
58. Varley C, McClellan J. Case study: two additional sudden deaths with tricyclic antidepressants. *J Am Acad Child Adolesc Psychiatry* 1997; **36:** 390–4.
59. Motsch J, Bottiger B, Bach A, *et al.* Caudal clonidine and bupivacaine for combined epidural and general anaesthesia in children. *Acta Anaesthesiol Scand* 1997; **41:** 877–83.
60. Ivani G, Bergendahl H, Lampugnani E, *et al.* Plasma levels of clonidine following epidural bolus injection in children. *Acta Anaesthesiol Scand* 1998; **42:** 306–11.
61. Klimscha W, Chiari A, Michalek-Saubere A, *et al.* The efficacy and safety of a clonidine/bupivacaine combination in caudal blockade for pediatric hernia repair. *Anesth Analg* 1998; **86:** 54–61.
62. Cho ZH, Chung SC, Jones JP, *et al.* New findings of the correlation between acupoints and corresponding brain cortices using functional MRI. *Proc Natl Acad Sci USA* 1998; **95:** 2670–3.
63. Pomeranz B, Nguyen P. Naloxone blocks acupuncture analgesia and causes hyperalgesia: endorphin is implicated. *Life Sci* 1979; **191:** 1757–62.
64. He L. Involvement of endogenous opioid peptides in acupuncture analgesia. *Pain* 1987; **31:** 99–121.
65. Reichmanis M, Marino A, Becker R. Electrical correlates of acupuncture. *IEEE Trans Biomed Eng* 1975; **22:** 533–5.
66. *NIH Consensus Statement*, Vol. 15, No. 5, 3–5 November 1997. Bethesda, MD: NIH.
67. Schwarz L, Bauchner H, Blocker R, *et al.* Salivary cortisol as an indicator of stress in premature infants: The effect of electrical stimulation of acupuncture meridians in blunting this response. *Med Acupuncture* 1999; **10:** 27–30.
68. Lin YC. Acupuncture may treat cyclic vomiting syndrome. *Anesthesiol News* May 2000; 24.
69. Kemper KJ, Sarah R, Silver-Highfield E, *et al.* On pins and needles? Pediatric pain patients' experience with acupuncture. *Pediatrics* 2000; **105:** 941–7.
70. Gray HS. Study of spinal anaesthesia in infants and children. *Lancet* 1909; **25:** 913–17.
71. Ecoffey C, Desparmet J, Maury M, *et al.* Bupivacaine in children: pharmacokinetics following caudal anesthesia. *Anesthesiology* 1985; **63:** 447–8.
72. Epstein RH, Larijani GE, Wolfson PJ, *et al.* Plasma bupivacaine concentrations following ilioinguinal–iliohypogastric nerve blockade in children. *Anesthesiology* 1988; **69:** 773–6.
73. Murat I, Montay G, Delleur MM, *et al.* Bupivacaine pharmacokinetics

during epidural anaesthesia in children. *Eur J Anaesthesiol* 1988; **5:** 113–20.
74. Mazoit JX, Denson DD, Samii K. Pharmacokinetics of bupivacaine following caudal anesthesia in infants. *Anesthesiology* 1988; **68:** 387–91.
75. Bromage PR, Benumof JL. Paraplegia following intracord injection during attempted epidural anesthesia under general anesthesia. *Reg Anesth Pain Med* 1998; **23:** 104–7.
76. Krane EJ, Dalens BJ, Murat I, *et al.* The safety of epidurals placed during general anesthesia. *Reg Anesth Pain Med* 1998; **23:** 433–8.
77. Desparmet J, Mateo J, Ecoffey C, *et al.* Efficacy of an epidural test dose in children anesthetized with halothane. *Anesthesiology* 1990; **72:** 249–51.
78. Tanaka M, Nishikawa T. The efficacy of a simulated intravascular test dose in sevoflurane-anesthetized children: a dose–response study. *Anesth Analg* 1999; **89:** 632–7.
79. Kozak-Langenecker SA, Marhofer P, Jonas K. Cardiovascular criteria for epidural text dosing in sevoflurane and halothane-anesthetized children. *Anesth Analg* 2000; **90:** 579–83.
80. Goldschneider KR, Brandom BW. The incidence of tissue coring during the performance of caudal injection in children. *Reg Anesth Pain Med* 1999; **24:** 553–6.
81. Krane EJ. Spinal epidermoid tumors: will a forgotten complication rise again? *Reg Anesth Pain Med* 1999; **24:** 494–6.
82. Aram L, Krane EJ, Kozloski LJ, *et al.* Tunneled epidural catheters for prolonged analgesia in pediatric patients. *Anesth Analg* 2001; **92:** 1432 8.
83. Dalens B, Vanneuville G, Tanguy A. Comparison of the fascia iliaca compartment block with the 3-in-1 block in children. *Anesth Analg* 1989; **69:** 705–13.
84. Dalens B, Tanguy A, Vanneuville G. Sciatic nerve blocks in children: comparison of the posterior, anterior, and lateral approaches in 180 pediatric patients. *Anesth Analg* 1990; **70:** 131–7.
85. McCloskey JJ, Haun SE, Deshpande JK. Bupivacaine toxicity secondary to continuous caudal epidural infusion in children. *Anesth Analg* 1992; **75:** 287–90.
86. Mevorach DL, Perkins FM, Isaacson SA. Bupivacaine toxicity secondary to continuous caudal epidural infusion in children. *Anesth Analg* 1993; **77:** 1305–6.
87. Berde, C B. Toxicity of local anesthetics in infants and children. *J Pediatr* 1993; **122:** S14–20.
88. Krane, E J, Tyler D C, Jacobson LE. The dose response of caudal morphine in children. *Anesthesiology* 1989; **71:** 48–52.
89. Merskey H, Bogduk N. *Classification of chronic pain*. Seattle, WA: IASP Press, 1994.
90. Wilder RT, Berde CB, Wolohan M, *et al.* Reflex sympathetic dystrophy in children. Clinical characteristics and follow-up of seventy patients. *J Bone Joint Surg* 1992; **74:** 910–19.
91. Metsahonkala L, Sillanpaa M. Migraine in children: an evaluation of IHS criteria. *Cephalgia* 1994; **14:** 285–90.
92. Abu-Arafeh I, Russell G. Prevalence of headache and migraine in school children. *Br Med J* 1994; **309:** 765–9.
93. Metsahonkala L, Sillanpaa M, Tuominen J. Outcome of early school age migraine. *Cephalgia* 1997; **17:** 662–5.
94. Russell MB, Olesen J. Increased familial risk and evidence of genetic factor in migraine. *Br Med J* 1995; **311:** 541–4.
95. Singh R, Macdonell R A, Scheffer IE, *et al.* Epilepsy and paroxysmal movement disorders in families: evidence for shared mechanisms. *Epileptic Disorders* 1999; **1:** 93–9.
96. Edgeworth J, Bullock P, Bailey A, *et al.* Why are brain tumors still being missed? *Arch Dis Child* 1996; **74:** 148–51.
97. Welch, K M. Scientific basis of migraine: speculation on the relationship to cyclic vomiting. *Dig Dis Sci* 1999; **44:** 26S–30S.
98. Symon, D N. Is cyclical vomiting an abdominal form of migraine in children? *Dig Dis Sci* 1999; **44:** 23S–5S.
99. Sartory G, Muller B, Metsch J, *et al.* A comparison of psychological and pharmacological treatment of pediatric migraine. *Behav Res Ther* 1998; **36:** 1155–70.
100. Dooley J, Bagnell A. A prognosis and treatment of headaches in children: a ten-year follow-up. *Can J Neurol Sci* 1995; **22:** 47–9.
101. Hasler WL. Serotonin receptor physiology. *Dig Dis Sci* 1999; **44:** 108S-13S.
102. Vincent CA. A controlled trial of the treatment of migraine by acupuncture. *Clin J Pain* 1989; **5:** 305–12.
103. Gerber N, Apseloff G. Death from a morphine infusion during a sickle cell crisis. *J Pediatr* 1993; **123:** 322–5.
104. Yaster M, Tobin JR, Billett C, *et al.* Epidural analgesia in the management of severe vaso-occlusive sickle cell crisis. *Pediatrics* 1994; **93:** 310–15.
105. World Health Organization. *Cancer Pain Relief and Palliative Care.* Geneva: World Health Organization, 1990.
106. Miser AW, Goh TS, Dose AM, *et al.* Trial of a topically administered local anesthetic MLA cream for pain relief during central venous port accesses in children with cancer. *J Pain Symptom Manage* 1994; **9:** 259–64.
107. Pasternak GW. The molecular biology of mu opioid analgesia. In: Devor M, Rowbotham MC, Wiesenfeld-Hallin Z (eds). *Progress in Pain Research and Management.* Seattle, WA: IASP Press, 1999: 147–62.
108. Yee JD, Berde CB. Dextroamphetamine or methylphenidate as adjuvants to opioid analgesia for adolescents with cancer. *J Pain Symptom Manage* 1994; **9:** 122–5.
109. Collins JJ, Grier HE, Kinney HC, *et al.* Control of severe pain in children with terminal malignancy. *J Pediatr* 1995; **126:** 653–7.
110. Collins JJ, Grier HE, Sethna NF, *et al.* Regional anesthesia for pain associated with terminal pediatric malignancy. *Pain* 1996; **65:** 63–9.
111. Cooper MG, Keneally JP, Kinchington D, *et al.* Continuous brachial plexus neural blockade in a child with intractable cancer pain. *J Pain Symptom Manage* 1994; **9:** 277–81.
112. Barker DP, Rutter N. Exposure to invasive procedures in neonatal intensive care unit admissions. *Arch Dis Child* 1995; **72:** 47–8.
113. Grunau RE. Long-term consequences of pain in human neonates. In: Anand KJS, Stevens BJ, McGrath PJ (eds). *Pain in Neonates,* 2nd edn. *Pain Research and Clinical Management*, Vol. 10. Amsterdam: Elsevier Science, 2000: 55–76.
114. Stevens B, Johnston C, Franck L, *et al.* The efficacy of developmentally sensitive behavioral interventions and sucrose for relieving procedural pain in very low birth weight neonates. *Nurs Res* 1999; **48:** 35–43.
115. Fearon I, Kisilevsky B, Hains SMJ, *et al.* Swaddling after heel lance. Age specific effects on behavioral recovery in preterm infants. *J Dev Behav Pediatr* 1997; **18:** 222–32.
116. Korner A, Thoman EB. The relative efficacy of contact and vestibular-proprioceptive stimulation on soothing neonates. *Child Dev* 1972; **2:** 443–53.
117. Lander J, Brady-Fryer B, Metcalfe JB, *et al.* Comparison of ring block, dorsal penile nerve block, and topical anesthesia for neonatal circumcision. *JAMA* 1997; **278:** 2157–62.
118. Sethna NF, Koh JL. Regional anesthesia and analgesia. In: Anand KJS, Stevens BJ, McGrath PJ (eds). *Pain in Neonates*, 2nd edn. New York, NY: Elsevier Science, 2000: 189–201.
119. Santhanam S, Anand KJS. Opioid tolerance in neonates: mechanisms, diagnosis, assessment and management. *Semin Perinatol* 1998; **22:** 425–33.
120. Hoder EL, Leckman JF, Ehrenkranz R, *et al.* Clonidine in neonatal narcotic-abstinence syndrome. *N Engl J Med* 1981; **305:** 1284.

PART V

Anesthesia and Society – Section editor: Peter Cohen

78

Medicolegal aspects of anesthesia: an American perspective

DONALD A KROLL

The practice of medicine has many interfaces with the law. These occur because the State is responsible for the protection of its citizens and regulates the behavior of citizens with respect to society. The degree to which the State regulates a person or group reflects the balance among the values of the people, the perceived need for regulation, and the relative consequences of the acts of a person or group. Health care is highly valued by the people; there is, therefore, a perception of great need to regulate the behavior of physicians and hospitals because the consequences of a physician's actions are serious for the patient. It should not be surprising, therefore, that the State monitors a physician from the moment of matriculation to a medical school to the moment practice ceases. Such monitoring takes the form of licensing, practice regulation by business and professional codes, required reports, National Practitioner Database maintenance, and determining the conditions for reimbursement of services to State-sponsored patients.

The State also makes provisions under its civil codes, which enable its citizens to resolve disputes about the extent and quality of services rendered. If the question concerns a civil wrongdoing, tort law applies. Negligence is one type of tort, and malpractice is one type of negligence. Increasingly complex forms of healthcare delivery are leading to increased activity in the application of contract law to the practice of medicine. This, in turn, increases the interest of the State in protecting the rights of its citizens with respect to the business of medicine, and an increased application of antitrust laws to medical practice.

New technologies continually emerge and are applied to the practice of medicine. The application of a new technology may create new interfaces between medicine and jurisprudence. In some cases, the interface may broadly overlap with ethics and economics, such as occurs with transplantation surgery and fetal interventions, whereas in others there is an overlap with business law, such as the use of computerized databases in healthcare delivery. The introduction of a new technology may change the standards of anesthetic practice, as has been the case with pulse oximetry.

The practice of anesthesia is neither insulated from, nor immunized against, the dynamic evolution of medical jurisprudence. Anesthesiologists have been in the forefront of change in some areas, but only indirectly involved in others. A detailed discussion of all aspects of the interface of law and medicine is beyond the scope of this chapter, but there are some recurring issues of interest to anesthesiologists, and some dynamically evolving issues of major importance to the practice of anesthesia. This chapter provides an overview of the medicolegal aspects of anesthesia practice from an American perspective. It is of some importance to discuss the American legal and healthcare delivery systems for readers who may not be familiar with them. The subsequent sections will deal first with nonmalpractice issues, and then with malpractice in anesthesia.

THE AMERICAN LEGAL SYSTEM

The issues presented in this chapter will be bewildering to the non-American reader unless there is at least a cursory description of the American legal system. Medical practice in the USA is governed not only by laws and statutes, but also by a variety of rules and regulations that have the force of law. Executive orders and administrative regulations are not laws in the sense of being enacted by a legislative body, but have the same compliance requirements as laws because the agency promulgating them was empowered to do so by a legislative body or the United States Constitution. The Constitution's Tenth Amendment established broad latitude for the individual states to self-govern. This is why the specific laws governing the conduct of a physician vary from state to state. The derivation of laws will be addressed superficially in the appropriate sections and the reader is referred elsewhere for a detailed discussion of the sections of the Constitution pertinent to medicine.[1] The day-to-day practice of anesthesia is influenced far more heavily by rules and regulations derived from these sources than by malpractice law.

In addition to the statutory law discussed above, the American legal system also provides a body of case law, which represents the legal principles derived from judicial decisions. Most American case law is derived from English common law principles. Common law refers to those unwritten laws grounded in custom and sanctioned by usage. Under this system, people have certain rights and obligations in their interactions with other people. When a person believes that someone has violated his or her rights, they may sue under the civil law system. Civil liability implies a wrongful act against a person's rights, whereas criminal liability implies a wrongful act against society. The term "person" refers to a legally recognized entity, which may be a corporation or group. In practice, the two areas of civil liability of importance to physicians are contract law and tort law.

Under the American system of jurisprudence, malpractice is a civil wrongdoing (tort), specifically the tort of negligence. Although other legal theories have been applied to medical malpractice, the tort of negligence is the basis for virtually all malpractice claims. Under negligence theories, the conduct of the defendant is measured against arbitrary standards of reasonableness and prudence, which, in the case of physician conduct, are determined by other physicians (expert witnesses). The rationale for the requirement of expert testimony is that the scope of medical knowledge is beyond the scope of knowledge of lay jurors, and hence requires interpretation.

In order to be successful in a malpractice action, the patient-plaintiff must prove each of the four elements of negligence:

1 *Duty* – the patient-plaintiff must prove that the anesthesiologist owed him or her a particular duty or obligation.
2 *Breach of duty* – the patient-plaintiff must show that the anesthesiologist failed to fulfill his or her obligation.
3 *Causation* – the patient-plaintiff must demonstrate that a reasonable close causal relation exists between the anesthesiologist's acts and the resultant injury.
4 *Damages* – the plaintiff must show that actual damage resulted because of the acts of the anesthesiologist.

Proof of each of these elements is essential if the plaintiff is to prevail. Proof in civil law differs from proof in criminal law: in a civil procedure one need only prove that something is more likely to be true than not (a 51% probability is sufficient to establish "preponderance of evidence"), whereas criminal law requires that certainty be "beyond a reasonable doubt." Each of these elements will be discussed in greater detail in the sections to follow. The American Society of Anesthesiologists (ASA) has also published a concise monograph on the topic of malpractice liability.[2]

THE AMERICAN HEALTHCARE DELIVERY SYSTEM

The delivery of anesthetic care occurs in public and private hospitals and in freestanding surgery centers and offices. Anesthesiologists may be reimbursed on a fee-for-service (FFS) basis or be paid a salary. Recent trends toward *managed care*, a new system of reimbursement, have embroiled anesthesiologists in legal battles to retain their hospital privileges and prevent replacement by new groups. It is therefore important to understand the development of managed care medicine.

Managed care medicine

There is only one true reason for the push toward managed care systems – cost containment. It has been said that the death knell for FFS medicine was sounded when the automobile industry discovered that it was spending more for health care than for for steel. In 1960, health care consumed 5.2% of the gross national product (GNP). By 1980, it was 9.1% of the GNP, and in 1986 had increased to 10.9% of GNP. We are currently in the teens. Expressed in another way, the average per capita cost of a worker's medical bills has increased from $142 in 1960 to $1054 in 1980, $1724 in 1985, and $3217 in 1990. It was projected to be over $15 000 by the turn of the century. Clearly, both the federal government and the private sector are strongly motivated to curb what they view as runaway healthcare costs. Even although physician reimbursement accounts for only 20% of all costs, physicians are viewed as the decision makers in the process, and hence the controllers of costs. Thus, the central thrust of the cost containers has been directed at modifying physician behaviors through utilization review mechanisms (audit) and changing the economic driving forces for physicians by capitated payment schemes.

As anesthesiologists do not control the decision to operate but are needed once a decision has been made by the surgeon, they have no effective bargaining power in the process. This is why there was a major move by the Health Care Finance Administration (HCFA) in the mid-1980s to consider the "hospital-based" physicians as part of hospital services and subject to a Diagnosis-Related Group (DRG) payment system, a form of capitated payment. This was coupled to an attempt to make the assignment of Medicare cases mandatory (see below).

The two extremes of healthcare reimbursement are represented by fully *retrospective* FFS, on the one hand, and fully *prospective* capitated payment on the other. These are functional descriptors of the process, and there are business forms that have developed to follow these functions. The sole-proprietor private practitioner exemplifies FFS, whereas the staff Health Maintenance Organization (HMO) characterizes capitated payment. As third-party payers began attempting to extend the perceived cost advantages of the HMO toward the FFS sector, several new organizational forms appeared that could fulfill this function. These organizations – preferred provider organizations (PPOs), independent practice associations (IPAs), and networks, along with the traditional HMO – constitute what has become known as "managed care" systems. The functional distinction is that FFS provides healthcare services but not financing, whereas managed care systems provide both services and financing. The distinction between an HMO and other managed care systems is that an HMO requires that only plan member physicians may be used, whereas other forms such as a PPO provide incentives to use plan member physicians and hospitals in the form of lower cost to the patient. It is anticipated that, within a very few years, organizations that provide financing without services (the classical indemnity health insurance plans) will cease to exist. These changes in healthcare insurance have fundamentally altered the *business* of medicine by changing the physician's customer from the patient to the payer.

In managed care medicine, the potential patient selects an insurance plan offered by an employer or may purchase one privately. Federal law requires (within certain limits) that both public and private employers with 25 or more employees offer their employees the option of HMO membership. In 1990, 37% of all employers offered a PPO option. This federal requirement is undoubtedly responsible for large part of the rapid growth of HMO enrollment in the late 1980s, the majority of which is accounted for by IPA HMOs rather than group HMOs.

The selection of a plan by the patient is driven by cost unless there is a significant quality issue. The incentive to patients is that, by giving up autonomy of provider selection, their costs are less. The greater the loss of autonomy, the greater the personal savings. Many patients view PPOs or other managed care schemes as the best balance between provider selection and cost. This is why managed care plans advertise that they have the greatest number of highly skilled physicians and quality hospitals in their plan; they are trying to appeal to their customers (patients and businesses) by emphasizing that the loss of selection autonomy is minimal or of no importance.

Once enrolled in a managed care plan, a patient may receive a particular anesthesiologist's services only if the anesthesiologist is a member of the plan, or if the patient is willing to pay a substantial surcharge out of his or her own pocket. From a practical perspective, the only way a hospital or physician group may influence the patient is at the initial plan selection stage, or by providing a service unavailable elsewhere.

Although the healthcare reimbursement industry has been able to adapt by creating new business forms, physicians have been slow to respond. Perhaps this is a greater problem for anesthesiologists because they tend to work alone and are unaccustomed to collaborative efforts. The result is that disorganized individuals have little strength against a well-organized PPO. The PPO may control a large share of the local market, whereas the individual physician controls only a tiny fraction of the care delivery. The formation of IPAs is, in a sense, the physician's answer to the power of large PPOs. By joining together, physicians hope to control a greater share of the delivery and gain negotiating power.

NONMALPRACTICE MEDICOLEGAL ISSUES

Contracts

A contract is a legally enforceable agreement between two or more persons in which there is an exchange of promises to either do or not do something. The term "persons" may mean individuals or groups of individuals or corporate entities. Although there are many types of contracts that may be important to anesthesiologists, contract issues are generally becoming major factors in the relation between the anesthesiologist and the hospital.

The ASA regards the practice of anesthesia as the practice of medicine, and specifically excludes the idea that it may be considered as an institutional service. The ASA has taken the position that anesthesiologists, in common with other physicians, must be free to enter whatever contractual relations they wish but, as a general principle, the ability of an anesthesiologist to practice in a hospital in which other clinical departments have "open" staffs should not be arbitrarily restrained by requirements to join a group or enter into a financial arrangement with the hospital. Hospital administrators would prefer to consider the practice of anesthesia as a hospital service and contract with anesthesiologists for the provision of this service. Anesthesiologists who are unwilling to enter into contracts with hospitals may face the loss of their privileges, although this has been difficult because of "due process" protection. The Fifth and Fourteenth Amendments to the Constitution mandate that individuals may not be directly or indirectly deprived of their rights by either state or federal government without due process of law. Because hospitals receive a great deal of federal funding, and are considered to participate in interstate commerce, medical staff privileges could not be revoked without due process.

Mandatory assignment

The federal government is a large provider of health insurance through Medicare and Medicaid plans. The effect of reimbursement decisions by a federal or state provider carries all the weight of any other administrative decree and is effectively a law. The penalties for practices incompatible with or not participating in these administrative regulations are severe because the governmental agency may link the availability of funds for hospitals to the agreement to provide services at the rate specified. Initially, only hospital costs were included in these plans, but there have been attempts at the federal and state level to link acceptance of Medicare assignments to the retention of licensure. The net effect of these approaches will be the prospective determination of physician fees by a governmental agency and the requirement that physicians accept what is offered. It seems fairly obvious that the fee offered will be substantially less than what the physician would otherwise charge. These attempts have been thwarted so far because the Constitution allows only a state to regulate business activities within the state. Thus, granting and regulating medical licensure is a state and not a federal function. In a sense, linking licensure to the acceptance of federally funded patients at predetermined fees is a generalized form of what individual hospitals have attempted by means of "economic credentialling."

Economic credentialling

In any business system there are external factors to be considered that may serve to thwart even the best of plans. In anesthetic practices, the most dangerous of these external influences is the threat of economic credentialling. This term refers to attempts by hospitals or medical staffs to withdraw the privileges of anesthesiologists who refuse to accept large discounts in their reimbursement. In some cases, entire groups of anesthesiologists have been replaced. The hospital administration, of course, attempts to disguise this maneuver using inadequate performance by the existing group as an excuse and, in some cases, has been able to present good evidence to establish the truth of this claim.

In recent years, there have been several legal cases that have clearly established the liability of hospitals for the negligence of physicians who have been granted practice privileges in the hospital. Hospitals are expected to maintain quality control and establish peer review mechanisms to monitor the quality of care given by physicians. Hospital administrators have reasoned that, if the hospital is to be held responsible for the acts of physicians, it should have control over the actions of the physicians with authority to discipline when appropriate. Most of the cases in which a hospital has replaced an anesthesia group have been successful because the hospital was able to demonstrate a quality assurance basis for the maneuver.

Membership in an IPA or PPO may actually make the process of group displacement for economic reasons easier. The contractual arrangements with IPAs and PPOs depend on the physicians being members of an economic bargaining organization separate and distinct from the medical staff. There is, therefore, no longer any requirement for due process. The due process protection clauses, almost always required in hospital by-laws as a precondition for the receipt by the hospital of state and federal funds, may not apply to anesthesiologists as members of the PPO or IPA. Once involved in this type of arrangement, there is no protection for the anesthesiologist against forced fee reductions in subsequent contracts; similarly, there is no protection of medical staff privileges. This means that a physician may be effectively barred from practice without medical staff privileges ever being revoked. Anesthesiologists might be perfectly free to practice in the hospital, except for the fact that no patients are referred to them because their membership in the economic unit has been terminated. A more direct approach is to include a clause in the contract stipulating that removal from the contracting unit automatically results in revocation of medical staff privileges.

Antitrust laws

Antitrust laws are becoming more important due to developments in exclusive service contracts, managed care medicine, and the Health Care Quality Improvement Act. The possibility of antitrust liability is of more than theoretical importance to the anesthesiologist: damages awarded in antitrust cases may be triple the amount of the actual damages, and malpractice insurance does not cover this type of liability.

The foundation of antitrust law is the Sherman Antitrust Act of 1890, although several other statutes such as the Federal Trade Commission Act and the Clayton Act are significant for the practice of medicine. Section 1 of the Sherman Act considers any contract, combination, agreement, or understanding that unreasonably restrains trade in interstate commerce to be unlawful. Section 2 deals with monopolies. As virtually any contract or agreement between individuals or businesses is designed to "restrain trade" in some fashion, there has never been a literal interpretation of the Sherman Act, and it is precisely the requirement for interpretation that has caused the most confusion. Thus, antitrust liability is difficult to assess in advance and often appears capricious in the final determination because of the overwhelming importance of the specific facts of each case.

The "learned professions" were exempted from Sherman Act provisions initially because the interpretation of the words "commerce or trade" did not include the provision of professional services. Ironically, we owe the application of antitrust law to *medicine* to a landmark case involving minimum fee setting in the *legal* profession, an abuse that eliminated the learned professions' exemption in general. It is obvious that medicine is involved in interstate commerce; one need only consider the patient's domicile, location of hospital suppliers and insurance carriers, or the involvement of hospitals themselves. This leaves two major areas of interpretation; what constitutes a concerted activity and when does restraint become unreasonable.

Concerted activities

A single individual cannot act in restraint of trade because such activity can exist only with two or more legal entities that interact by means of a contract, combination, or conspiracy. There have been many interpretations based upon individual cases, but membership in a professional association has been held to be sufficient to satisfy the requirements for liability. Although professional associations are entitled to exclude members for reasons of competence or ethics, forbidding association with a particular group may be viewed as a boycott, especially when applied to economic competitors. This has been the basis of antitrust cases involving disputes between anesthetic groups and nurse anesthesiologists (a section 2 violation), and the 1979 challenge to the ASA's Relative Value Scale (a section 1 violation). There is little doubt that membership in an economic unit such as a PPO or IPA would satisfy the concerted activities requirement, and there is ample precedent that organized group practices likewise qualify.

Unreasonable restraint

Not all restraint of trade is "unreasonable." There are two tests that may be applied. The per se rule applies when the activity is so likely to restrict competition that all one must prove is that the activity existed. There is no need to prove that any actual restraint occurred, although mitigating gains in efficiency may be considered. Price fixing and market allocations are considered per se violations, but group boycotts and tying arrangements are now generally considered under the "rule of reason."

Under *rule of reason* analyses, the court will weigh the anticompetitive effect against the potentially legitimate purpose of the restraint. Application of the *rule of reason* analysis to medical practice has been restricted to cases where the discriminatory behavior was based upon the so-called "patient care defense."[3] As the application of this type of analysis to section 1 cases involving the healthcare industry increases, so does the importance of determining proof of market power, because actual harm to competition must be shown. It is difficult to demonstrate harm caused by the actions of a single group unless the group has clear market power.

Exclusive contracts

There have been several antitrust cases involving exclusive service contracts with hospitals. In a maneuver that may be related to economic credentialling (see above), the hospital first disallows practice by anesthesiologists who are not members of the group with whom it has a contract. The excluded anesthesiologist then alleges that the group has established an illegal monopoly by tying the provision of anesthesia care within the hospital to membership in the group. The hospital responds that quality patient care may be assured only by establishing an exclusive contract.

It must be proved that the hospital requires patients who use its operating rooms to purchase anesthesia services solely from the group in order to establish a tying arrangement. No tying arrangement exists unless it limits the number of anesthesiologists to members of the group.

Whether or not the hospital has market power is also important. If it can be shown that the hospital has sufficient market power to force patients to select only from their group, then the per se rule against tying arrangements might apply. It would not be a sufficient defense that the restraint was adopted to improve patient care (a *rule of reason* approach).

Economic bargaining units

PPOs may be formed by brokers, purchasers, or providers. Broker-type PPOs are not likely to have antitrust problems as long as they avoid appearing to become the agent of either the purchaser or providers. Purchaser PPOs may encounter price fixing or group boycott antitrust problems if more than one purchaser is involved in control of the PPO. Even a single purchaser PPO might encounter exclusive dealing, territorial restraint, or tying arrangement problems, particularly if it has market power.

A provider-sponsored PPO is most at risk for antitrust problems if it is viewed as a horizontal arrangement among competing providers. If it is viewed as a joint venture, it becomes a single legal entity and no concerted activity can be shown.

IPAs and other novel types of economic bargaining units will be analyzed under the same principles as a provider PPO. The IPA must be viewed as a bona fide joint venture that offers some new capabilities. The restraints in question must be reasonably related to the function of the joint venture, and the overall market power of the joint venture must not be so large as to be excessively anticompetitive.

Antitrust immunity

As membership in a professional association may be sufficient evidence of concerted activity, and professional associations are increasingly involved in lobbying activities, it is significant that lobbying efforts are protected from antitrust litigation. The *Noerr–Pennington Doctrine*[3] exempts individuals or groups seeking to influence government action or legislation even if their sole purpose is anticompetitive. Efforts to influence private associations are not exempt.

The second area of immunity is peer review activity under the *State Action Doctrine.*[4] Under the State Action Doctrine, hospitals have a common law duty to exercise care in selecting a qualified medical staff. States regulate and supervise the process and, therefore, the hospital will be immune as long as it actively supervises the policies, and the policies are clearly articulated and expressed. The Health Care Quality Improvement Act of 1986 (HCQIA) was a direct result of an antitrust action involving hospital peer review activities, and attempts to define the conditions under which peer review is exempt. The Act contains provisions that serve to broaden the applicability of the State Action Doctrine to include all medical peer review, but also to specify standards of fairness for peer review.

The HCQIA also, in an attempt to protect the public from incompetent physicians, established the *National Practitioner Data Bank for Adverse Information on Physicians and Other Health Care Practitioners.*

The National Practitioner Data Bank (NPDB)

Although the NPDB was established as part of HCQIA in 1986, full promulgation into law did not occur until 1989, and implementation was delayed even longer. In its final form, the Act also included requirements of the Medicare/Medicaid Patient and Program Protection Act of 1987.

The NPDB was established by the HCQIA as a nation-wide information system, although licensure of physicians is a proper function of the states because moving from one state to another was a recognized method of avoiding loss of medical livelihood in the face of pending legal action against a practitioner. The NPDB was designed to provide state licensing boards and hospitals with an improved means of detecting adverse information about physicians.[5]

Mandatory data entry became effective on 1 September 1990; its long-term effects remain to be determined. Although it clearly may be able to provide appropriate information to credentialling and licensing bodies, its ultimate utility depends on accurate reporting. For example, a physician may resign from a hospital prior to adverse action having been taken and thus avoid being reported to the NPDB. On the other hand, the name of a blameless physician who settles a malpractice case to avoid protracted litigation will be made available to the NPDB. Efforts to modify some of the provisions of the HCQIA continue, and it is therefore likely that the details of mandatory reporting criteria will change.

Malpractice issues

The germination of a lawsuit

All patients may be considered as potentially litigious. There are several factors that will determine whether or not a patient will become a plaintiff, and several others that will determine whether the lawsuit will be successful. The idea that there is a subset of patients who are more likely to sue than others is probably inaccurate. The so-called "professional plaintiff" is very rare.

Perhaps the most direct evidence of a litigious patient is a patient who is currently involved in a malpractice lawsuit, or has been a plaintiff in a prior malpractice case. However, unless a physician asks the question directly, or the patient volunteers the information, there is no way to determine the legal history of a patient.

A second category of patients who may be likely to sue are those who have had an adverse outcome from previous care, or who have had improper or questionable care. This might include delayed or improper diagnosis, delayed treatment, improper therapy, or an adverse reaction to treatment. Such patients may not yet have initiated a lawsuit but, depending upon the degree of injury or damages, they may be considered as highly likely to sue. Even though the current physicians may not have been directly involved in the initial injury, *all* physicians whose names appear in the chart may be sued.

There are other clues that may indicate that a particular patient is more likely to sue. Any patient who appears hostile to a physician or the hospital may be considering a lawsuit. Patients who take copious notes or tape record an interview are suspect, as are those who exhibit "physician-shopping" behavior or have numerous admissions to different hospitals for the same complaint. Unusually demanding patients and those who insist upon inappropriately dictating treatment choices may be impossible to satisfy, and therefore likely to sue.

The overriding factor that determines whether or not patients sue a physician is their satisfaction with the care provided. No patient comes to a physician with the intent of instituting a lawsuit; they come with the expectation of receiving good medical care for their problems. Only unhappy patients sue their physicians. The satisfaction of the patient is influenced by many factors, and there are physician, patient, media, attorney, and economic causes of the increasingly litigious patient population. Depersonalization of health care, unrealistic patient expectations induced by lay medical literature and the media, and the perception of a pro-plaintiff legal system all contribute to the problem.

On the other hand, the degree of injury and anticipated award are probably the major factors in the likelihood of a lawsuit. The greater the claim for damages, the greater the probability of a lawsuit. Stated simply, if no harm has come to the patient, the probability of a successful lawsuit is small. Barring the occurrence of the million-dollar anesthetic disaster, the anesthesiologist may be able to directly influence the probability of a lawsuit. It has been estimated that only one out of eight negligent acts results in a lawsuit. The prevention of a lawsuit in the face of an adverse outcome is a function of risk management.

Risk management strategies[5]

Improve the physician–patient relationship

Communication with the patient is essential. This requires both talking and listening, with a willingness to listen being the more important. It is important to give patients the opportunity to ask questions and to make sure that their consent to proceed is as fully informed as possible. It is also important to be truthful in assessing risks and benefits in order to avoid offering guarantees of safety or efficacy or warranties of treatment.

Anesthesiologists are more likely to be sued than primary care physicians for several reasons. Perhaps the most significant is that the patient is (hopefully) unaware of us for most of the time we are caring for them. Any physician–patient relationship is, of necessity, quickly established and even more quickly forgotten. Except for pediatric surgery, there is very little, if any, involvement with the patient's family. As a result, the anesthesiologist is not always recognized as a dedicated and skilled physician. It is much easier to blame the anesthesiologist for a less than perfect outcome than to blame the surgeon or internist who may have spent hours at the patient's bedside and offered comfort and consolation to a worried or bereaved family. Although the obvious solution would be to extend our involvement with the patient and the patient's family, it is impractical in most cases to make daily visits to every patient during their hospitalization, or to increase the duration of preoperative visits sufficiently to include a discussion of every conceivable eventuality, every remotely possible complication, and every alternative method or technique.

However, anesthesiologists aware of these problems may certainly be sensitive to the needs of patients who seem unusually anxious, ill, or prone to a specific complication. Spouses and family members may be informed separately of risks when patients clearly request not to be informed. This is more of a "public relations" technique than a legal safeguard, but it is effective in that it establishes good rapport with the family, and may have substantial medicolegal "prophylactic" value. It must be remembered that, from a legal point of view, in informing a spouse or family member, the anesthesiologist is not relieved from the burden of informing the patient unless the spouse or family member is the patient's legal guardian.

Even if the anesthesiologist does not personally conduct a full physical examination or take a complete history, the patient should be told that his or her condition is known about from other sources, and the medical record should include this information in the preoperative note. Active follow-up is essential and fully explanations should be offered. The anesthesiologist who gives the impression of being unconcerned or uninterested when a complication that may be related to anesthesia occurs may suffer a lawsuit.

It is also important for the physician to project a professional image to patients. Appearance and demeanor at the bedside are major contributors toward establishing this image. If patients and their families have the initial impression that the physician is sloppy, flippant, careless, or poorly informed, they are not likely to be very forgiving of a less than perfect outcome. Likewise, it is important to guard against careless conversation in the hospital corridors and operating rooms.

If it becomes apparent, after the preoperative interview with the patient, that a reasonable physician–patient relationship cannot be established, the anesthesiologist should consider very carefully whether or not to provide the anesthetic care. The option of refusing may not be available in an emergency. Nevertheless, there will be situations in which it would be unwise to become involved. One example is the patient who insists upon dictating the type of anesthetic, despite the anesthesiologist's best judgment. A similar situation occurs when the patient's religious beliefs prohibit the use of blood products. Anesthesiologists who cannot, in conscience, agree with these wishes should not make promises that they have no intention of keeping; rather, if at all possible, they should refer the patient to a physician willing to grant the patient's request. There are obviously other situations that could arise. The important point is that anesthesiologists avoid situations in which their ability to provide the best possible care is compromised.

Another valid reason for an anesthesiologist refusing to provide care for a patient is lack of necessary skill, experience, equipment, or facilities to deliver adequate care.

Adhere to a "standard of care"

One of the tests of negligence is whether or not the anesthesiologist adhered to the standard of care in treating the patient. The standard is most often determined retrospectively by review of the records. It may therefore not be feasible in all cases to know what the "standard" is. In practical terms, this requires that one keeps current in knowledge and provides medical care consistent with this knowledge. This does not mean that the anesthesiologist must be continually on the cutting edge of medical research, but it does require that one be aware of, and conform to, accepted guidelines for the provision of anesthesia care. The ASA has published guidelines for the practice of anesthesia, and the anesthesiologist may be judged in accordance with these guidelines, departmental standards, or published hospital procedures.

In terms of medical and anesthetic management, adhering to the standard of care requires that the choice of agents and techniques is appropriate, and that the anesthesiologist is competent in the use of these agents and techniques. It is necessary to know the contraindications for the use of drugs and anesthetic agents. An anesthesiologist who uses a barbiturate to induce anesthesia in patients with acute porphyria or who gives succinylcholine (suxamethonium) to a burned patient or to a quadriplegic, or who uses halothane in the presence of elevated hepatic enzymes following the previous use of the agent is likely to be sued successfully. If, on the other hand, one is prudent in the choice of agents, the likelihood of a successful legal action will be decreased.

The appropriately chosen agents and techniques must be used appropriately. As a general rule, an anesthetic record showing that vital signs were maintained within a reasonable range for the patient is evidence of the appropriate conduct of anesthesia.

Keep good records

The importance of good record keeping cannot be overemphasized. It is of little benefit in legal terms to have delivered good anesthetic care if it is impossible to identify each component of an anesthetic procedure and when it was performed. The record may have to be defended years after the case was completed, long after the specifics of the case have been forgotten. A general rule is that "*if it wasn't written, it wasn't done.*" When an incident occurs during the conduct of anesthesia, or at any time during the care of the patient, the facts should be documented in the medical record. Avoid using terms such as "inadvertently" that convey a message of guilt or negligence. Do not make written comments that admit wrongdoing, or are accusatory of others. Simply record the pertinent facts about the incident as accurately and completely as possible, including observations such as skin color, color of blood in the field, auscultatory findings, or other information not typically charted on the anesthetic record. If the problem occurred during the course of a regional or conduction technique, indicate the areas of anesthesia or spinal level of somatic block. It is often helpful to include differential diagnosis of the problem in a note on the chart, the laboratory tests or observations performed to make a diagnosis, and the treatments initiated. A frequent complaint is that there is no time to write notes while responding to an emergency situation. The solution is to write a "perioperative" note as soon as possible, making reference to the approximate times of the events. Such records, written at the time of occurrence, are invaluable in distinguishing between a bad result or known complication and actual negligence. Although it should be obvious to every physician that records should *never* be altered after the fact, instances of record alteration continue to occur. These suspicious records can never be used in defense, and may result in the success of a defendable legal case or even criminal prosecution for fraud. If an error is made in record keeping, a line should be drawn through the error, leaving it legible, and the correction initialed, with the time and date noted.

Respond appropriately when an incident occurs

In addition to documenting the facts, there are other options that may help prevent legal action. The most important is to ensure that, once an adverse occurrence has occurred, optimal medical care is provided. Consultation should be obtained when appropriate to ensure that all diagnostic and therapeutic steps have been taken and that the continued care of the patient is provided by the most suitable specialists. An important, and frequently overlooked, maneuver is to seek the opinion of another anesthesiologist in a timely fashion. When one is asked to help another anesthesiologist in an emergency, and it is believed that the patient may suffer harm because of the incident, then you should be willing to make a note on the record verifying the events.

Many hospitals have begun to use a system of risk management whereby specially trained personnel are available to intervene when a question of liability arises. These individuals are described by various titles such as "patient–staff relations," "patient advocates," "ombudsmen," or "risk management coordinators." They may be under the administrative supervision of the hospital attorney or hospital administration. Such personnel should be notified immediately of any incidents that occur. They will help to collect information about the incident, offer support for the patient and the patient's family, and act as liaison between the family and the medical staff involved. They may be invaluable in decreasing the likelihood of a lawsuit, or the damages eventually awarded.

The malpractice insurance carrier should be notified of any events that may lead to a lawsuit. Many companies require such notification as part of the insurance contract. It is most unlikely that one would be adversely affected by giving notice of an incident to an insurance carrier.

The anesthesiologist should continue to maintain professional contact with the patient during hospitalization after any incident that might be related to anesthesia. The anesthesiologist's role is that of a consultant to the primary care physicians. Failure to do so might be construed as abandoning the patient, and certainly will serve to demonstrate lack of interest in and disregard for the patient's welfare. If the incident is clearly unrelated to the anesthetic care, this should be made clear in the medical record, along with the reasons supporting this view, and the fact that the services of the anesthesiologist as a consultant are no longer required but will be available should the need arise.

Recognize malpractice "prodromes"

Anesthesiologists may first become suspicious about a pending lawsuit when they receive letters from former patients or requests for medical records from attorneys. Until a *complaint* has been served, no lawsuit has been actually filed, and the events are potentially reversible. If an anesthesiologist has any suspicion, the first step will be to notify the insurance carrier, sending copies of all relevant correspondence. The insurer may then be able to advise on how to proceed. Most of the "angry letter" complaints from former patients are meritless claims, or claims for very low damages; claims with merit and potentially high-dollar awards will in all probability be in the hands of a plaintiff's attorney. An example of a low-cost claim is the request for payment of dental bills accrued a year after an uneventful anesthetic. This type of nuisance claim is unlikely to result in a lawsuit, but the anesthesiologist may feel compelled to offer a settlement to avoid further interaction with the former patient. If it is decided to offer a settlement privately, this should be done only after consultation with an attorney who can ensure that the appropriate releases from further liability are obtained. In addition, the insurance carrier must be advised of your decision; failure to notify the company may result in voiding insurance coverage for this event. If, after consultation with the insurer, it is decided to ignore the claim, a polite letter explaining that no offer can be made in settlement for a meritless claim should be sent. The response should not be hostile or inflammatory. The goals are to explain why there is no liability for the claim and to reduce the chance of a lawsuit being filed. It is important not to appear unsympathetic or callous toward the patient, but direct correspondence with the patient should be kept to a minimum. It is generally best to work through the insurer or attorney.

A request by a plaintiff's attorney for records may be a cause for anxiety, but should not be construed as meaning that a lawsuit will be filed. The insurance carrier should be notified, as it may wish to review the medical records and be provided with the medical facts of the case. Other than following the instructions of your insurer, there is little else to do at this point. It is likely that nothing more will be heard about the case unless there is a genuine question of malpractice. In any event, it is pointless to become overly anxious. It is necessary for the patient to sign an authorization for the release of medical records. Records must be not changed, nor should the records be added to by writing a covering letter. As anesthesiologists, with the exception of those who operate pain clinics, usually keep no detailed records apart from those that are included as part of the patient's medical record, it is unlikely that there will be much to send in response to such a request. In general, requests for medical records do not include business records and billing statements are not required.

Avoid vicarious liability

Instructions to ward nurses, circulating nurses, or others may expose the anesthesiologist to vicarious liability. Such situations occasionally arise in positioning the patient, attaching electrocautery grounding pads, or in the use of various warming devices, when nerve damage or burns may occur. The anesthesiologist may be considered to be supervising and liable for the actions of anyone acting upon his/her instructions.

The anesthesiologist should not agree to supervise anyone who is incompetent. This may seem obvious but the reality of the situation is that well-entrenched personnel may be very hard to remove because of institutional policies or politics. If it is believed that someone who must be supervised is incompetent, supervision must be very close, such as by double-checking preoperative findings, specifying all agents and techniques to be used, and being present in the operating room during the entire case. Such extreme "supervision" may preclude involvement in other cases, but this must be weighed against the possibility of preventing injury to a patient with its attendant professional and emotional costs. The department and/or hospital administration should be consulted in order that incompetence can be documented. No-one, except in a teaching hospital, should be supervised who is not fully trained and certified. Anesthetic "technicians" or "aides" are not qualified to provide direct patient care and should never be expected to function in that capacity. The ASA specifies that the only personnel who may provide direct patient care under supervision are residents, student nurse anesthesiologists, and certified registered nurse anesthesiologists.

Do not agree to supervise more simultaneous cases than you can safely handle. There are differences of opinion regarding how many cases may be supervised by a single anesthesiologist; however, if you are supervising so many cases that you are unavailable during an emergency, or have not been supervising closely enough to prevent an adverse result, successful malpractice litigation may result. It may not matter that the result might have been the same even if the anesthesiologist had been present for the entire case. Issues of inadequate supervision and patient abandonment are hard to defend.

Notification of a lawsuit

An anesthesiologist may receive a notice of intent to sue within a specified period of time, or may receive a summons and complaint that outlines the alleged wrongdoing. In either case, the first action is to notify the malpractice insurance carrier. There is a finite period of time for a response to the summons, and the assistance of an attorney will be required. Failure to respond within the specified time will result in a directed decision for the plaintiff, and the malpractice carrier will not be responsible for payment if it has not been notified. Upon notification, the insurer will appoint an attorney to represent the physician.

The anesthesiologist should refrain from discussing the case with anyone other than the attorney, as certain statements may be discoverable (see Discovery, below) and used by the plaintiff during the trial. Attorney–client discussions are protected as privileged communications.

Access to the patient's medical records for the purpose of reviewing the anesthetic or notes is permissible, but the temptation to add notes or improve upon the record by way of an additional explanation must be avoided. The plaintiff's attorney has already obtained a copy of the medical record, and any alterations after notification of a lawsuit will be introduced at trial as evidence of negligence.

It is uncommon to obtain legal representation other than that provided by the insurer, but there are some circumstances for which it may be prudent. The physician may require private counsel when there is a conflict between the interests of the insurer and the physician. Such a situation may arise when the potential damages exceed the policy limits, thus exposing the physician's personal assets to risk. Another such conflict might arise if the physician's privileges or licensure are at risk as issues separate from the lawsuit. Finally, the physician may not have confidence in the attorney provided by the carrier, and may ask for a substitute. The relationship between the physician and the attorney will probably extend over 1–2 years, or even longer in complicated cases, during the process of discovery, so it is important that the relationship is sound.

Discovery

After the complaint is answered, both sides begin the process known as "discovery." The purpose of discovery is to ascertain the "facts" of the case in preparation for trial or settlement. It is important to consider briefly what constitutes a fact in a malpractice trial. When two opposing sides arrive at radically different views of the events and their significance, there must be two sets of "facts." One set of facts will eventually be "proved" to be true, and the other will be rejected. It is the responsibility of the jury to decide which facts to believe. Juries are, for this reason, called "triers of fact." Judges may also act as triers of fact before a case goes to trial. In a civil case, a "fact" is "proved" whenever it is determined that its truth is *more likely than not*. Both sides attempt to determine their strengths and weaknesses during discovery. A strength is a fact that is favorable and a weakness is a fact that is unfavorable.

The medical record is the primary source of the facts. Observations and descriptions written at the time of the event are the most credible sources of information. A trier of fact will believe what is written before believing what is said. It is assumed that the record was contemporaneous, and, therefore, the notes were completed before any adverse outcome was known. Because there is no logical reason to have lied, the records are generally trusted.

A second source of facts is the testimony of those who witnessed the event. The anesthesiologist may testify that something that was not recorded was done or seen. This is not as believable as the medical record because it relies upon specific recall of events that may have happened in the remote past. Opposing attorneys will often follow up this type of recollection with a series of questions about the case that preceded or followed the case in question in order to establish that the anesthesiologist's memory is incomplete. It is also true that such recollections tend to be self-serving and are not trusted by triers of fact.

A third source of facts is the usual practice pattern of the anesthesiologist. The anesthesiologist did not record something, has no independent recall of the specific case, but asserts that he or she must have done something because that is part of a routine. This obviously does not have great credibility. The maxim that "if it isn't written, it wasn't done" is difficult to overcome.

A fourth source of facts is expert witness testimony. Experts are necessary because the subject of medicine is held to be beyond the knowledge or understanding of lay jurors, and therefore requires interpretation. Experts will review the entire medical record, not just the anesthesia record, and may also review the depositions of the physicians involved. An excellent perioperative note that includes details of the event may certainly mitigate against a poor or incomplete anesthetic record, but does not substitute for a good anesthetic record. It has been the author's experience that the order of credibility is:

1 the anesthesia record and notes;
2 the expert's interpretation;
3 specific recall;
4 usual and customary practice.

Although a deposition or statement by the defendant anesthesiologist will provide evidence from recall and usual practices that are less credible than the record or the expert's testimony, the deposition is of critical importance in establishing the strength of the defense. In a system in which a "fact" is "true" once it is believed, the credibility of the physician is of major importance.

Deposition testimony

The defendant anesthesiologist's testimony is taken on behalf of the plaintiff, and is conducted by the plaintiff's attorney. The defense already knows what the physician will say. The plaintiff's attorney will attempt to uncover facts favorable to the plaintiff to ascertain the defense position on the issues in question. Typically, all the defendants in the case will be represented by counsel at the deposition and, in cases in which the anesthesiologist may wish to "criticize" the hospital or the surgeon, may have substantial interest in protecting their clients from adverse testimony.

The deposition is usually arranged to take place at a mutually agreeable time and place. The time of the deposition should be set such that the defendant is well rested and there should be sufficient time allowed so that there is no need to rush. In general, it is better to have the deposition at the office of the defense attorney than at the physician's office. An observant plaintiff's attorney may learn from the diplomas on the wall, the books on the shelf, or the neatness of the office, matters that he or she would otherwise not be entitled to know.

Prior to the deposition, the defense attorney should meet the anesthesiologist to explain the conduct of the procedure, what to bring, and what to wear.

Depositions usually begin with introductory comments by the plaintiff's attorney regarding the conduct of the deposition. These are general statements about the need to speak slowly and clearly, understanding the questions, and waiting until the question is fully asked before answering. There will then be a series of questions about the credentials of the anesthesiologist. It helps to have a current curriculum vitae and to be familiar with the dates of training, license, and certifications.

One of the purposes of the deposition is to give the plaintiff's attorney an opportunity to assess the defendant as a witness; therefore, dress and demeanor are important. Conservative, professional attire creates a better impression than casual or flamboyant dress. A serious but relaxed and calm demeanor gives the impression of competence. Questions may be asked, or postures adopted, by the plaintiff's lawyer designed to intimidate or elicit anger. Showing anger or hostility will give the impression that the physician has poor self-control. The plaintiff's attorney may welcome the opportunity to demonstrate that the witness is pompous or arrogant, has inadequate knowledge, or is evasive and unresponsive.

It is wise to pause for a moment before answering a question to allow for any interposed objections to be stated. Answers should be brief, and to the point. Do not embellish or expand upon the question asked. If a "yes"' or "no" is sufficient, stop there. Do not anticipate the questions. If a question is vague or ambiguous, ask to have it rephrased. If a question is not understood, always ask for clarification.

Expert witnesses

The courts have recognized that certain topics are beyond the knowledge and experience of most jurors. They demand that witnesses be called so that the jury can benefit from the expertise and opinions of uninvolved parties for the interpretation of the facts. Witnesses who are allowed to give opinions are called expert witnesses. All other witnesses are restricted in testimony to what was actually observed or done.

An expert witness must first be qualified by the court. The qualifications of experts are established by their training and experience. All that is required in most jurisdictions is that the medical expert is a licensed physician who professes familiarity with the standard of practice of anesthesiologists. Occasionally, a physician who is not a practicing anesthesiologist will be called to testify in a case involving anesthesia. The rules vary from state to state and by discipline. For example, in California only an emergency medicine physician may testify against another emergency medicine physician. No other specialty receives this statutory protection. Academic appointments, published papers, memberships in societies, and prestigious positions, although useful in establishing the power of the expert to influence a jury, are not necessary to be qualified by a court as an expert.

THE ELEMENTS OF NEGLIGENCE

Duty

In simple terms, establishing duty means that the anesthesiologist had an obligation to the patient. This obligation is proved by the existence of a physician–patient relationship. Once the anesthesiologist has agreed to provide care for the patient, then the physician–patient relationship exists. Therefore, duty is usually not a major issue in malpractice. The exception occurs when the anesthesiologist acts as a *good Samaritan* or rescuing physician in the event of an emergency situation. In most states, *good Samaritans* have statutory immunity from malpractice lawsuits.

Anesthesiologists accept all the general duties owed by any physician to any patient, and a specific duty to adhere to the standards of practice of anesthesia. General duties include an appropriate examination of the patient, obtaining consultations when necessary, obtaining informed consent, keeping good records, and providing appropriate follow-up care. As the trend toward outpatient and same-day surgery has grown, so have the medicolegal problems of anesthesiologists in fulfilling these general duties. It may be difficult to prove that an anesthesiologist who first saw a patient on a stretcher outside the operating room conducted an appropriate evaluation. The establishment of preoperative screening clinics is one solution to the problem, but has the drawback that the liability for injuries that occur increases because of an improper evaluation by the anesthesiologist who actually conducted the evaluation. The anesthesiologist providing intraoperative care must rely on the evaluation of another anesthesiologist. If no anesthesiologist has evaluated the patient, the situation is more tenuous because an internist or surgeon may not be aware of the information required for the conduct of an anesthetic.

Another problem arises from the general duty to provide appropriate follow-up care. An anesthesiologist ordering a chest radiograph as part of a preoperative evaluation may be responsible, either personally or, more likely, through consultation, for following up any abnormalities detected. This has nothing to do with being an anesthesiologist – it arises from being the ordering physician.

Patients have the right to self-determination regarding their bodies and what is done to them (see Chapter 80). In order for them to make such decisions, the law imposes upon physicians a duty to inform the patient of material risks associated with the planned procedures. In order to be successful in a malpractice action based upon the duty to obtain informed consent, the patient/plaintiff must prove three things:

1 The physician failed to disclose material risks and dangers *inherently* and *potentially* involved in the procedure.
2 The unrevealed risks actually materialized and were the proximate cause of the injuries sustained.
3 A reasonable person would have decided against the treatment had the dangers been disclosed.

Three distinct tests are applied to determine the informed consent requirements: the reasonable physician standard, the reasonable patient standard, and the subjective patient standard. Most states have adopted the reasonable patient standard; under this test, a risk is considered to be material when a reasonable person in the circumstances of the patient would be likely to attach significance to the risk(s) when deciding whether or not to forgo the treatment. The duty to disclose risks is based not upon the physician's practice (or upon expert witness testimony), but rather upon the patient's need for full disclosure of serious risks and the feasible alternatives in order to make an intelligent and informed choice.

Certain inherent risks apply to all patients without regard to their individual condition, whereas other dangers depend to a great extent upon the individual patient. For example, the risk of dental damage is inherently present whenever tracheal intubation is performed. The risks of a myocardial infarction or stroke are potentially present with a greater degree of probability in patients with vascular disease.

A special circumstance is imposed when there are nonmedical risks associated with a procedure. The two issues with the highest public awareness in this regard are HIV and drug testing. In both situations, the common theme is that the test results may affect the patient's ability to work, obtain insurance, or be free from discriminatory practices. Additional standards for informed consent and confidentiality are imposed because of these special risks. Given the evolving nature of the law in these areas, it would be advisable to obtain the patient's consent for drug or HIV testing if the test is to be performed electively prior to surgery. On the other hand, if the tests are indicated for the proper diagnosis and treatment of an adverse reaction, then the burden of obtaining special informed consent is reduced. Nevertheless, if the patient is able to give consent, then it is always a good idea to obtain it.

The standard of care

The specific duty owed by an anesthesiologist is to adhere to the standards of practice for the administration of anesthetic care. Practice standards change over time, but there is no longer a locality rule for specialists. In almost all cases, adherence to the standard of care is established by expert witness testimony. Because it is impossible to delineate specific standards for all aspects of medical practice and all eventualities, the test that is applied is whether or not the conduct of the anesthesiologist was reasonable and prudent. The conduct of the anesthesiologist need be neither state of the art nor the best possible care, and it is not necessary that it even be what the majority of anesthesiologists would do. It only has to be reasonable and prudent behavior under the specific circumstances. It is not sufficient, however, that the anesthesiologist acted to the limits of his or her potential, acted in good faith, or did what was considered normal in their hospital or the hospital down the street. On the other hand, to be considered a standard something must be universally applicable. Although an anesthesiologist or a department or a hospital may elect to hold themselves to a higher level of conduct or expertise than elsewhere, they cannot unilaterally hold anyone else to that standard. If an expert witness fails to understand that "standard of care" implies the lowest level of acceptable practice, no matter how well intentioned or altruistic he or she may be, they may do great injustice to the defense of the case.

The standard of care may also be determined by written policies of a department, a hospital, an accrediting organization, or a professional society. It is imperative that written policies be unambiguous, enforceable, and agreed to by all who practice under them. If an injury occurs because of failure to comply with a written standard, the occurrence of a breach of duty is obvious.

Breach of duty

If an anesthesiologist either does something that should not have been done or fails to do something that should have been done, there is a breach of duty, and the anesthesiologist's conduct will have fallen below an acceptable standard of practice. The breach of duty is the specific act that was unreasonable or imprudent under the circumstances.

The fact that an injury occurred is not sufficient evidence that a breach of duty has occurred, as this would imply a warranty or guarantee of a successful outcome. An honest mistake in diagnosis or treatment or an error in judgement "will not form the basis of liability in the absence of additional affirmative evidence that the physician's conduct deviated from an acceptable standard of care."[6]

It is also not sufficient to show that an alternative treatment was available, or for the expert to assert that he or she would have done things differently. As long as the act of omission or commission was within an acceptable standard of care by even a respectable minority of anesthesiologists, then no breach will have occurred.

Causation

The breach of the standard of care must be tied to the injury. The link between the breach and the injury is known as the proximate cause of the injury. Proximate cause is not identical with the medical cause of the injury. It is the event that sets in motion a chain of events that leads to the injury. There may be a series of events rather than a direct relation between the breach and the injury. The law, therefore allows for one out of two tests of this link. The method used varies from state to state.

The first test is the "but for" test. If the injury would not have occurred *but for* the acts of the anesthesiologist, then, provided that application of the test is just and fair, proximate cause is established. Under this doctrine, if there were other factors that might have led to the same injury, then the test is false, and no proximate cause is established.

The second test is the "substantial factor" test. Under this doctrine the act need not be the only possible cause of the injury, it must only be shown to have been a *substantial factor* in causing the injury. This test is less favorable to the physician defendant because recovery of damages is not prevented by the presence of other possible causes as is the case with the "but for" test.

Damages

The term "damages" as generally used applies to the injuries sustained by the patient, and is usually understood to refer to the translation of the injuries into an economic figure. It is obvious that, although the legal system cannot restore injured patients to their previous state of health, it can compensate them with money. The amount of money awarded is the damages, and should have a close relation to the degree of injury sustained and the results of such injury.

There are two types of compensatory damages: general damages and special damages. *General damages* occur as a result of the injury but may be intangible. Pain and suffering, humiliation, anxiety, and derivative claims such as loss of consortium are examples of general damages. *Special damages* have a measurable value and are imposed to compensate for such things as actual medical expenses, future expenses, loss of wages and earning capacity, and rehabilitation costs.

Much attention has been directed toward tort reforms that place a limit on the award of general damages. Although largely applauded by physicians and decried by attorneys, such measures have relatively little effect on damages because the majority of damages are special damages, and the cap may not apply when wrongful death has occurred.

In cases of gross misconduct, the law also allows for exemplary or punitive damages. These damages are awarded in excess of the compensatory damages, as a punishment, or in order to make an example of the case as a warning to other anesthesiologists. Malpractice insurance typically does not cover punitive or exemplary damages.

Damages are decided by a jury after the amounts allowed have been described by the judge. There has been a trend toward increased awards in medical malpractice cases, even after adjusting for inflation, and there has been an increased variability in awards for similar cases. This has been attributed in part to the reduction in jury size in some states from 12 to six members.[7] Similar cases tried before juries with 12 members will result in more consistent decisions than if the case were tried by six-member juries.

An additional factor has been the publicity that a multimillion dollar award gains for the plaintiff's attorney. What is often not appreciated is that these sums may represent the total estimated award over the lifetime of the patient – i.e. a structured settlement. The actual cost of purchasing the annuity is far less.

Closing a case: dismissal, settlement, or trial verdict

Once a lawsuit has been filed with the courts, some form of court document is required to terminate the physician defendant's liability. Approximately 1 in 10 lawsuits is carried through to a jury trial. The reason for this low percentage is that, if negligence actually occurred, this will usually become obvious during the discovery phase. If the physician was negligent, the insurer would much rather settle the case for a reasonable amount than risk a high jury award.

The plaintiff might refuse to settle, hoping for a very high jury award. If there was no negligence, a small settlement might be offered because the cost of defense is higher than the settlement, or the physician/anesthesiologist may be released with the promise not to attempt recovery of attorneys' fees. It is very unprofitable for the plaintiff's attorney to pursue lawsuits that they have little chance of winning; in a contingency fee system, the attorney must bear all the costs.

If the plaintiff fails to establish sufficient facts in the case, the defense may file a motion with the court for *summary judgment* by the judge in favor of the defendant physician/anesthesiologist. From the physician's point of view, a summary judgment is superior to a settlement as it vindicates him/her of the charges. Because a summary judgment eliminates the possibility of a trial by jury on the issues of the case, judges are reluctant to grant these motions unless there is clear and irrefutable evidence that the case against the defendant has no merit. In order to block such a motion, the plaintiff must find one physician/anesthesiologist willing to state that negligence had occurred.

The practical wisdom that "settlements should be made whenever it is cheaper to settle" may no longer be true as there is no minimum payment threshold for reporting in the National Practitioner Database. Physicians are more reluctant to approve settlements when they know that a mandatory report will follow. The fact that insurers must report all payments made on behalf of a physician to the National Practitioner Database may result in a decline in token settlements.

The physician is "released" from liability if a settlement is made, as the patient abandons the claim of malpractice. The patient executes a release document and is barred from making any further claims against the physician.

Even if a case proceeds to a trial, settlement offers may be made up to the time a verdict is reached. As a general rule, cases go to trial only when both sides think they have a good chance of winning. A victory does not necessarily require a favorable verdict; it may only mean a lower monetary cost than would have been required to settle. If the case is complicated or emotionally charged, jury selection may be crucial to the outcome, and the attorneys may wait until after the jury is selected before they estimate their chances of winning. Most cases that go all the way through the process to the point of a jury verdict are decided in favor of the physician defendant. This is not really surprising as the burden of proof rests with the plaintiff.

The adversarial legal system in malpractice: personalization of the process

The American judicial system is based upon the belief that "justice" is best served by having each side represented by lawyers whose sole responsibility is to their client. Thus, there are no ethical or moral restraints placed upon an attorney with respect to the opposing side; in fact, failure to do everything legally possible to discredit the opposing side would be considered unethical. This competition between opposing counsel, each side presenting its own version of the facts and the law, is supposed to enable the judge or jury to determine the truth and arrive at a just verdict. Physicians who fail to understand the adversarial system are vulnerable to personalization of the process. The legal system, therefore, reinforces any pre-existent self-doubts, guilt feelings, or simple remorse about the bad outcome.

Bargaining in the malpractice process is an integral part of the discovery phase leading to a determination of whether to settle or go to trial. The critical issue for the attorneys and insurance companies is limitation of the damages. It is simple economics and good business to minimize losses. At this point, physician defendants are actually not major players in the game. They have relatively little control over the events, even although convinced that their concept of professional self worth is being bargained away in the process. Physician defendants who believe they are innocent of any wrongdoing are particularly likely to want public vindication and exoneration. Such personalization of process may interfere with the expeditious settlement of the case and, in the extreme case, refusal to cooperate with the insurer may result in cancellation of coverage.

On the other hand, anesthesiologist defendants who realize that they made an error will find the process of discovery agonizing – every plaintiff's expert will make the same accusations over and over again. Defendants will be told repeatedly, on the record and in great detail, exactly how and when they made the mistake. This is part of the adversarial system, but it may cause or exacerbate depression in almost any defendant.

It is not surprising, given the high stakes involved, that depression may occur at virtually any point in the process. Only the most callous and uncaring physician could fail to be saddened by the death or serious injury of a patient. When the charge is made that the physician's negligence directly caused the outcome, it becomes difficult to continue in the belief that the tragedy was unavoidable, or unforeseeable, or occurred despite the best that medicine had to offer.

Anesthesiologists are at least as likely as other physicians to experience job-related stress. They may be at an increased risk relative to other medical specialties because of the solo practice nature of anesthesia and, sometimes, their perceived isolation from mainstream medicine. Anesthetic-related injuries are probably more likely to be disabling or lethal than injuries that occur during care by other specialties, and the emotional trauma, guilt, and self-doubts will be therefore be more severe. The adversarial system of malpractice litigation, by its very nature, causes substantial additional stress. Anesthesiologists involved in malpractice lawsuits should become familiar with the system, learn what to expect, and avoid taking the proceedings personally.[8]

Asset protection

A malpractice lawsuit may expose a physician's personal assets to risk. The most common means of protecting personal assets is the purchase of malpractice insurance.

There are three basic types of malpractice insurance: occurrence, claims made, and umbrella. An *occurrence* policy requires only that the insurance be in effect at the time of the incident. This makes it difficult for insurers to estimate the degree of risk to which they are exposed to at any given point in time. Most policies today are based upon *claims made*. A *claims made* policy differs from an *occurrence policy* – it must be in effect not only at the time of the occurrence, but also when a claim is made. This has resulted in the need for "nose" and "tail" coverage, and mandates a clear definition of what constitutes a claim. Tail coverage is commonly provided when a physician leaves practice or changes carriers. It typically extends coverage with the company beyond the statute of limitations for filing a lawsuit. Nose coverage is less common, but is offered by some companies to provide retroactive coverage when the physician purchases a new policy. Some companies allow notification of an incident to count as a claim. Physicians changing to another company may flood the insurer with reports of all incidents that might even remotely turn into a lawsuit in an attempt to avoid purchasing tail coverage. Some companies require notification of intent to sue, or the filing of a lawsuit, before a claim could be made.

Umbrella coverage is used to insure against the possibility of exceeding the limits of coverage provided by the primary policy. This type of insurance is of value if the anesthesiologist practices in a high-risk specialty and is concerned with potential liability for extraordinarily high damages. In most such cases, there are multiple defendants who share in the damages and structured settlements. For practical purposes, policies providing 1 million dollars in coverage for a single claim and 3 million dollars in any year are adequate.

The malpractice insurance industry is complex,[9] and there are many factors to consider when purchasing a policy. As the primary purpose of insurance is the protection of personal assets, it is important that the physician has confidence in the company. The least expensive policy does not always provide adequate peace of mind and financial security. Although a detailed discussion of all variables cannot be provided in this chapter, some general guidelines may be useful.

The financial security of the company is of prime importance. The failure of some liability carriers has exposed physicians to substantial personal risk. As a general rule, newer companies with an unproven "track record" are less secure than those with more years of experience. New companies may not be able to select good-risk physicians, may not have acquired large capital reserves, or may not be well enough known to qualify for the lowest rates for reinsurance. These added uncertainties may be covered by making the policies assessable. Should the company suffer excessive losses, subscribing physicians may be assessed a surcharge. The need to assess a surcharge depends upon the reserves and net worth of the company. A rule of thumb for the structure of reinsurance relative to policy limits is that the retained risk on any one policy should not exceed 10% of the surplus (net worth). A company's assets should be evaluated for adequacy, liquidity, and the risk of its investments. If the total net retained annual premium income exceeds four times its surplus, a company may be too heavily leveraged. In other words, the company may be relying upon new premium dollars to pay for losses incurred. Such arrangements are inherently unstable, as in any other pyramid scheme.

Once the financial security of an insurer is established, the physician should consider the quality of the services offered. This may be evaluated by references from insured physicians as well as by marketing brochures. An ongoing risk management and educational program is desirable. Requiring higher standards of practice or advanced monitoring may indicate that the company has high underwriting standards. The company should retain high-quality legal counsel, and be able to provide the names of the firms. Finally, the company should be responsive and accessible to the anesthesiologist.

There are many methods other than insurance that may be used to shelter personal assets from risk.[10] As a general rule, any asset owned by the physician may be seized to satisfy a debt owed by the physician. The most obvious way to protect an asset is to transfer its ownership to another party. The *Uniform Fraudulent Conveyance Act* effectively precludes any transfer of assets that occurs in the face of a debt or lawsuit. In practical terms, this requires preplanning and will make it very hard to avoid payment of any pending obligations. Assets may be transferred to entities such as trusts, partnerships, or corporations, or to individuals such as family members. It is important to keep in mind that transferring ownership of an asset may also result in loss of control over that asset. In the case of a mortgaged asset such as your home or other property, ownership transfer may be deemed a sale and require repayment of any loans in full to the lender.

There are many types of trusts that are distinguished by legal differences enabling them to act in different ways in response to events, but all trusts require that the assets are owned by the trust rather than by individuals. Therefore, any income from the asset goes into the trust, and the beneficiaries of the trust may have legally enforceable rights of ownership.

Normally, partners are liable for the acts of other partners as long as they are carried out within the scope of the partnership business. In contrast, members of a corporation are usually not personally responsible for the debts of the corporation. Unfortunately, unless the rules of maintaining a corporation are strictly adhered to, the court may treat the corporation as a partnership and "pierce the corporate veil" to reach the personal assets of the shareholders.

Transfers to individuals such as a spouse or children will result in loss of control of the asset by the physician/anesthesiologist. In the event of a divorce or other family difficulty, the physician will probably lose the asset altogether.

The major asset of many physicians/anesthesiologists is their home. There are special provisions for protecting the home in some states, but there is great variability in the means by which this may be accomplished. The options available will vary from state to state.

There are ways for physicians to protect their assets, but there are advantages and disadvantages for each method, and state laws that will determine which methods are available. Competent individual legal advice is imperative.

SUMMARY

This chapter has outlined the American system of medical jurisprudence in broad terms as it relates to the practice of anesthesia. It is not intended to be, and should not be used as, a substitute for competent legal counsel. The intent has been to provide the reader with sufficient descriptive information to enable physicians/anesthesiologists to understand the important medicolegal issues that regulate or influence their practice. There are several textbooks devoted to medical jurisprudence, which go into far greater detail with respect to the specialty of anesthesia[11–13] or the laws of specific states.[6,14–15] They also provide reference material for the many specific legal subjects such as vicarious liability, product liability, and the doctrine of *res ipsa loquitur* (the facts speak for themselves) that concern anesthesiologists under special circumstances, in addition to discussions of the many ethical dilemmas facing anesthesiologists.

Finally, it is important to recognize that, as multifaceted as the interfaces of law and medicine may be, the legal system addresses only a portion of a larger problem. If anesthesiologists always and undeniably did the right things under all circumstances, then there would never be any question of whether or not their care was reasonable and prudent. There are differences of opinion regarding the appropriateness of care that may be resolved on many levels with different intended outcomes. Peer review, quality assurance, risk management, and utilization review look at different aspects of the larger question of whether or not the correct things were done. A malpractice lawsuit is not a substitute for these activities and properly addresses only the issue of whether or not a plaintiff is entitled to receive a monetary award damages done. Thus, it is inherently backward looking and contingent upon the details of the specific case. The true value in understanding medicolegal principles lies in the recognition that the central issue is quality of care, and in the prospective application of these principles to influence decisions. The anesthesiologist should ask him-/herself the question "Can I adequately explain what I am about to do to a jury of lay people?" This is one way of answering the broader question "Is this the right thing to do for this patient under these circumstances?"

REFERENCES

1. Peters JD, Fineberg K, Kroll DA. *The Law of Medical Practice in Michigan*. Ann Arbor, MI: Health Administration Press, 1981: 21–5.
2. Kroll, DA. *Professional Liability and the Anesthesiologist*. Park Ridge, IL: American Society of Anesthesiologists, 1987.
3. Gilmore DA. The antitrust implications of boycotts by health care professionals: professional standards, professional ethics and the First Amendment. *Am J Law Med* 1988; **14** (2,3): 221–48.
4. McDowell TN, Rainer JM. The State Action Doctrine and the Local Government Antitrust Act: the restructured public hospital model. *Am J Law Med* 1988; **14** (2,3): 171–219.
5. Kroll DA. What to do when sued for malpractice. Part I. Prodromes of a lawsuit. *Am Soc Anesthesiol Newsletter* 1986; **50** (1): 7.
6. LeBlang TR, Basanta WE, Peters JD, *et al*. *The Law of Medical Practice in Illinois*. Rochester, NY: Lawyers Cooperative Publishing, 1986: 573.
7. Saks MJ. In search of the 'lawsuit crisis'. *Law Med Healthcare* 1986; **14** (2): 77–9.
8. Kroll, DA. The trauma of malpractice suits. *Semin Anesth* 1989: **8** (4): 347–52.
9. MacKenzie, RA. Professional liability insurance. In: Dornette WHL (ed.). *Legal Issues in Anesthesia Practice*. Philadelphia, PA: FA Davis, 1991: Chapter 29.
10. Kroll DA. Litigation and anesthesia: why does it happen and what to do if involved. In: *40th Annual Refresher Course Lectures and Clinical Update Program 115*. Park Ridge, IL: American Society of Anesthesiologists, 1989.
11. Peters JD, Fineberg K, Kroll DA, Collins V. *Anesthesiology and the Law*. Ann Arbor, MI: Health Administration Press, 1983.
12. Dornette, WHL. *Legal Issues in Anesthesia Practice*. Philadelphia, PA: FA Davis, 1991.
13. Peters JD, Fineberg K, Kroll DA. *The Law of Medical Practice in Michigan*. Ann Arbor, MI: Health Administration Press, 1981.
14. Post BL, Peters BM, Stahl SP, *et al*. *The Law of Medical Practice in Pennsylvania and New Jersey*. Rochester, NY: Lawyers Cooperative Publishing, 1984.
15. Woodside III FC, Lawson NA, Lyden DR, *et al*. *The Law of Medical Practice in Ohio*. Rochester, NY: Lawyers Cooperative Publishing, 1989.

79

The anesthesiologist's duty of care: a British perspective

CHRISTOPHER J HULL AND LORD BRENNAN

In the UK, an anesthesiologist owes a duty of care toward his or her patient. This is a legal concept, having nothing to do with clinical care. Indeed, chartered accountants have exactly the same duty of care toward their clients, who indeed may include anesthesiologists. Having accepted that duty, the professional person is obliged to fulfill it, while (in private practice) the client is equally bound to meet any reasonable charges. The duty encompasses the anesthesiologist's obligation to attend a patient, to warn of likely hazards, and, if it is in the patient's best interests, to apply such technical procedures as are appropriate. The standard of care to be provided is defined by a legal yardstick: the so-called Bolam test. This was established in *Bolam* v. *Friern HMC* in 1957, and has since become the fundamental and guiding principle on the standard of care in medical negligence.[1] Readers should note that following the publication of new civil procedure rules in 1999, plaintiffs are now referred to as claimants, and that for clarity this term will be used throughout.

THE BOLAM TEST – *BOLAM* v. *FRIERN HMC*

As well as being fundamental to the anesthesiologist's duty of care, this case is of particular interest because it involves anesthesia. In 1954 a mentally ill patient was "advised" by a consultant psychiatrist that electroconvulsive therapy (ECT) was necessary. A standard consent form was completed, but this did not make mention of any risk of injury. Since ECT in 1954 was often conducted without the benefit of neuromuscular blockade (or, for that matter, anesthesia of any kind), that omission might seem odd by today's standards. The patient underwent repeated ECT without benefit of anesthesia or relaxant drugs, and the only precaution against injury was jaw support and a male nurse standing on each side, presumably to prevent him being thrown off the couch by the force of his convulsions. During the second treatment the patient sustained a fracture, and he subsequently sued the hospital claiming compensation for his injury. He claimed that muscle relaxants should have been used, but that if they were not he should have been manually restrained to minimize injury and warned beforehand that injury was a possible consequence. All these claims were denied. At trial it was stated that the risk of fracture and other injury was well known, and that anesthetics with muscle relaxation were widely used as a protective measure (no suggestion, of course, that such techniques helped to mitigate the terror of repeated, unmodified ECT). However, contrary evidence was heard to the effect that the risk of fracture was, in fact, quite small, and that the method used had been standard practice at that hospital. Furthermore, it was claimed that the risks associated with anesthesia were just as great as (albeit different from) those of injury in the unmodified method. Only under special circumstances, therefore, was anesthesia used, and Mr Bolam was not such a case. Similarly, it was stated that manual control of patients undergoing unmodified ECT was by no means a universal practice, and that warning patients of possible injury would be likely to dissuade them from undergoing treatment!

Faced with two seemingly irreconcilable views, Mr Justice McNair held that there were at least two quite distinct schools of thought, all perfectly respectable and applied by practitioners of equal standing. He could find no reason to prefer one such school of thought over the others, and on that basis enunciated the celebrated principle in his directions to the jury:

> The test is the standard of the ordinary skilled man exercising and professing to have that special skill ... A doctor is not negligent if he is acting in accordance with a practice accepted as proper by a responsible body of medical men skilled in that particular art, merely because there is a body of opinion that takes a contrary view.

Not surprisingly, the jury found for the defendant. By today's standards that might seem to be a perverse decision, as the risks of anesthesia for ECT must be uncommonly small compared with those of physical injury. However, the case must be seen in the context of 1954 practice, whereby the anesthetic might well have been administered by a doctor with little or no anesthetic training.

In *Sidaway* v. *Bethlem Royal Hospital Governors* (1985)[2] Lord Scarman restated the test:

> A doctor is not negligent if he acts in accordance with the practice accepted at the time as proper by a responsible body of medical opinion, even though other doctors adopt a different practice.

The test is applied to diagnosis,[3] to advice,[2] and to treatment.[4] Liability is determined by the practice and medical thinking at the time of the alleged negligence rather than at the date of trial.[5]

Of course, the original concept leaves great scope for interpretation in individual cases, especially in deciding the precise meaning of *proper* and *responsible*. In *Gold* v. *Haringey Health Authority* (1987),[6] the *Bolam* principle was expressed in uncompromising terms, i.e. that the *practice regarded as proper by a responsible body of medical men* would be accepted uncritically, regardless of context or clinical wisdom. So long as the body of opinion was regarded as responsible, the court would not inquire further as to the reasoning behind that opinion.

Thus, an anesthesiologist who, in the early 1970s, maintained anesthesia during the predelivery phase of cesarean section using only 50%

nitrous oxide in oxygen, but subsequently faced a claim that the patient had suffered pain and awareness as a consequence of his or her negligence, had a clear defense in showing that a very substantial number of consultant anesthesiologists would have done likewise. It would not be necessary to demonstrate the *wisdom* of so doing, but simply that the practice was considered reasonable by that body of anesthesiologists.

There must, of course, be limits to doctors defending ludicrous clinical decisions on the sole ground that others could be found who would have done the same, and *Gold* was not slavishly followed. Indeed, the pendulum swung decisively toward critical analysis of expert opinions in the recent case of *Bolitho* v. *City and Hackney HA*.[7] Henceforth it is *Bolitho* rather than *Gold* that should be followed. Such is the importance of this case to anesthesiologists that it must be discussed in some detail.

THE BOLITHO CASE

In 1984 2-year-old Patrick Bolitho was admitted to hospital suffering from croup, having undergone surgery for patent ductus arteriosus only 1 month earlier. He was discharged after 4 days in a pediatric ward but then, on the following day, was readmitted in some respiratory distress. The following lunchtime Patrick became very wheezy and very pale. The ward sister directly asked Dr X, the pediatric senior registrar, to see him urgently. Patrick was then seen to be walking about the ward with normal color. About 1 h later, with Dr X not having attended, Patrick became distressed once again. Dr X, who by now had started an afternoon clinic, said that she would ask Dr Y, a pediatric senior house officer (SHO), to attend Patrick. Dr Y also failed to attend. Once again, Patrick recovered rapidly and was seen to be playing quite happily. Thirty minutes later Patrick suffered a respiratory and then cardiac arrest which, despite resuscitation, resulted in severe cerebral damage and later his death. It was claimed that he should have been intubated after the first episode and certainly after the second, and that had this been done he would not have suffered the third and disastrous event. The defense argued that this would have required anesthesia and would have been neither desirable nor necessary. Dr X said that she would not have intubated Patrick even if she had attended him. The trial judge was faced with pediatric experts having diametrically opposed views on the intubation issue. One would have intubated Patrick, while the other would not. He ruled for the defense, holding that it had not been shown that any competent doctor would have intubated Patrick after the first or second episodes, so that the pediatricians' failure to attend did not bear on the outcome.

The claimant appealed on the grounds that risk–benefit analysis, had it ever been considered by Dr X, would have been strongly in favor of intubation. It was also argued that a defense expert, Dr Z, had not been reliable or representative of a body of professional opinion. The appeal judges ruled that it was for the claimant to show that Dr X would have intubated had she attended, and to show that failure to do so was negligent. It was left to one dissenting appeal judge to point out that Patrick suffered a cardiac arrest for want of medical attention, and that what Dr X *would* have done was not the key issue. It was what *should* have been done had any competent doctor attended. In rejecting the appeal, the court appeared to be saying that Dr X was not negligent because, had she attended, she would not have intubated Patrick and so would not have prevented the subsequent disaster. No-one, it seems, was to blame.

The House of Lords concurred with regard to the trial judge's reasoning. However, there was a secondary argument concerning the pediatric expert, Dr Z, and this provoked the Lords to review the very basis of the Bolam defence before rejecting the appeal. Lord Browne-Wilkinson pointed out that:

> ... there are cases where, despite a body of professional opinion sanctioning the defendant's conduct, the defendant can properly be held liable for negligence. In my judgement that is because, in some cases, it cannot be demonstrated to the judge's satisfaction that the body of opinion relied upon is reasonable or responsible. ... if in a rare case it can be demonstrated that the professional opinion is not capable of withstanding logical analysis, the judge is entitled to hold that the body of opinion is not reasonable or responsible.

The *Bolitho* judgment does not, as has been suggested, diminish the importance of *Bolam* as a yardstick for medical negligence cases. Indeed, it re-emphasizes the views expressed by Lord Scarman in *Sidaway*, and clarifies what he meant by *"a responsible body of opinion."*

The *Bolitho* case is of very direct interest to anesthesiologists, as this was an all too familiar clinical scenario in which the one clinician able to resolve a problem was not even aware that it existed. It appears to the authors that Patrick suffered brief periods of respiratory obstruction caused by sticky secretions but was normal between events. A pediatric senior registrar (or SHO) would not have had the skills to intubate a wide-awake and highly mobile 2-year-old, and without anesthetic training would have been grossly negligent to try (as would have been the pediatric expert witnesses). Her only proper course of action, having assessed Patrick's condition, was to seek the urgent services of a duty anesthesiologist. Because she failed to do either, Patrick was attended only by nursing staff, who were unable to rescue him when he suffered a respiratory arrest. In the authors' view Patrick did not require intubation after the first or second episodes (as per Dr Z), but after the first (and certainly the second) episode he should have been moved to a place of safety (i.e. an intensive care unit), where, in the event of any sudden obstruction, his airway could be cleared and if necessary intubated by an anesthesiologist or intensivist with the required training and skill so to do. Seen in those terms, the result is at variance with good clinical practice. Moreover, the trial judge's finding (upheld on appeal) that the dangers of intubation justified a "wait and see" approach (thus providing a Bolam defence) without hearing any anesthetic evidence does seem surprising.

In *Marriot* v. *West Midlands RHA*,[8] the Court of Appeal upheld the trial judge's conclusion that the defense expert evidence was not what reasonable prudence required.

A CONTRACT TO TREAT?

In private medical practice, the duty of care is based upon the contract (real or implied) between a professional person and his or her client. The patient–doctor relationship commences when the anesthesiologist accepts any kind of clinical responsibility for the patient concerned. Of course, much depends upon the nature of the professional relationship between surgeon and anesthesiologist. If they work together on a regular basis, such that by common consent Dr X anesthetizes Mr Y's patients on a Wednesday afternoon, a list of names from Mr Y's secretary a few days earlier may be sufficient to establish his professional responsibility toward those patients. In the case of a more casual relationship, whereby Mr Y (or his secretary) telephones Dr X with a request to attend and anesthetize Mrs Z, Dr Z has no obligations whatever until and unless agreeing to do so. Even then, his responsibility is to attend and assess the patient and to offer professional advice. At that stage he has made no commitment to anesthetize the patient but simply to do that which is in the patient's best interests. If, for instance, the patient requires further preoperative investigation before safe anesthesia can be contemplated (as might apply in the case of a young woman presenting for varicose vein surgery who has clinical signs of anemia but no hemoglobin estimation), his duty toward that patient is clearly set: he must explain the need for additional tests to both patient and surgeon and ensure that the former has a clear understanding of the risks involved.

If an anesthesiologist in private practice is sufficiently unwise as to give an express guarantee as to outcome, that becomes part of the contract. Thus, if the anesthesiologist expressly guarantees that the patient will not suffer pain and awareness during surgery, but in the event that patient does so suffer, it matters not whether he or she was negligent as clearly there was breach of contract and the patient must be compensated accordingly.

A DUTY TO PROVIDE

In hospital practice, the situation is more complicated, because the ultimate duty of care is borne by the clinical provider, be it health authority or NHS trust. The provider has a clear duty to ensure that its employed doctors are adequate in both quantity and quality. In addition, it is more than likely that the provider also makes express warranty as to the adequacy of clinical care in its contract with the budget-holding purchasers.

In appointing anesthesiologists at any grade, the employer must fulfill his duty of care (and perhaps contractual obligations too) by ensuring that the process is conducted properly in terms of the statutory instrument (i.e. the Whitley terms and conditions of service). Posts must be advertised and appointments advisory committees must be properly constituted if it is to be shown subsequently that all reasonable steps had been taken to ensure an appointee's suitability for the post.

In the case of short-term or locum posts, many hospitals have taken a far more relaxed view of their obligations. It has become commonplace for locum consultant posts to be offered to doctors who do not even hold the FRCA (or equivalent), let alone a certificate of accreditation or completion of specialist training. It has not been unknown for locum anesthesiologists to be hired, even at consultant level, without seeking formal references and without any formal check of their medical qualifications or postgraduate diplomas. Such doctors then have been assigned clinical duties without any assessment of their clinical skills, and disasters have followed. The clinical director who instigates or even sanctions such a process in the interests of maintaining some kind of clinical service may be highly vulnerable in law. His or her employer is likely to find that any economies made by such appointments are likely to prove very expensive, in both financial and human terms.

Anesthesiologists themselves have a duty toward their patients, but there is no contract, real or implied. Thus, if a patient is scheduled to undergo panproctocolectomy on a scheduled operating list and is anesthetized by a senior house officer with 6 months' anesthetic experience, a mishap occurring as result of that doctor's inexperience might well be regarded as evidence of negligence on the part of the employer (i.e. the health authority or NHS trust).

Generally, however, individual clinicians must expect to answer for their own clinical decisions and actions. It is particularly important to note that they are likely to be judged by the standards of the posts in which they are employed. Thus, the actions of an SHO are judged by the standard of technical proficiency (and appreciation of his or her own limitations) and a duty to consult seniors where appropriate that would be expected of an average SHO, and those of a consultant by the standard to be expected of a consultant. This point should be well understood by anesthesiologists with limited formal training who are appointed to locum consultant posts, and also by their employers. Although such a doctor may have but 2 years' training and a Diploma in Anesthetics (DA), in the event of error or mishap he or she will be judged as a consultant. The likely cost of a major settlement should deter all but the most foolhardy clinical directors from making such appointments.

Equally, the law will probably require that a trainee be judged by the same standard as would more experienced anesthesiologists. This is on the basis that there should be an effective system of training and supervision so that the trainee can and should call on the help of an experienced colleague when required. Thus, trainees should be adequately supervised and they must be made aware of their duty to seek advice where appropriate.

A DUTY TO ATTEND AND ASSESS

It is quite obvious that an anesthesiologist cannot make an informed judgment as to an individual patient's fitness for anesthesia or to the type of anesthetic procedure to be employed without careful preoperative assessment.

The assessment should establish the medical history, with particular emphasis on previous anesthetic procedures. Records of such procedures may give valuable indications of special risks such as difficult intubation, adverse drug reactions, etc. Patients who have not previously been anesthetized should be asked about their family history, which may reveal potential problems such as succinylcholine (suxamethonium) apnea, sickle cell disease, or malignant hyperpyrexia.

Physical examination should identify any abnormalities of physique that might influence the choice of technique, together with particular risk factors such as cardiovascular or respiratory disease. No matter what anesthetic technique is planned, the assessment should always include a formal consideration of dentition and probable intubation difficulties. This should be self evident, because the need to intubate may develop both suddenly and unexpectedly. Under such circumstances the discovery of a mouth full of loose and rotten teeth together with severe limitation of mandibular movement may transform an emergency into a disaster.

The assessment should include discovery of all essential documentation, including the results of essential preoperative tests. In the event that such results are not available, it should be remembered that a measured but unreported preoperative serum potassium concentration of 7.5 mmol L^{-1} would be difficult to explain in the event of cardiac arrest occurring during the induction of anesthesia.

A DUTY TO EXPLAIN

Having established all the relevant facts, the anesthesiologist now has a clear duty to give the patient an explanation of what he or she intends to do, and to explain the nature of likely hazards. This cannot be accomplished satisfactorily at the doors of the operating room, and requires that the anesthesiologist who is to administer the anesthetic visits the patient some time before surgery. Obviously, there are limits to such a policy, as in the case of emergency surgery, when the opportunities for preoperative discussion and explanation may be very limited. In day-case surgery, too, the very short period between admission and surgery may preclude an effective preoperative visit. Under such circumstances the value of a preadmission anesthetic clinic is self-evident.

Anesthesiologists who intend to use spinal anesthesia alone must tell patients that they are to remain awake during surgery; but must they also inform patients of possible severe headache or even of major neurologic complications? Here the lines are less clearly drawn, but the strength of duty is clearly related to the probability of these complications occurring.

This principle was clearly established in the celebrated case of *Sidaway v. Bethlem Royal Hospital Governors*,[2] wherein a patient suffered major neurologic sequelae (of which she had not been warned) following a neurosurgical procedure. In the House of Lords, Lord Bridge observed:

> ... the Judge might in certain circumstances come to the conclusion that disclosure of a particular risk was so obviously

> necessary to an informed choice on the part of the patient that no reasonably prudent medical man would fail to make it.

He went on to explain that a procedure known to carry a 10% risk of some serious complication would be so regarded. In the same case in the Court of Appeal, Lord Donaldson went even further:

> ... a judge would be entitled to reject a unanimous medical view if he were satisfied that it was manifestly wrong and that the doctors must have been misdirecting themselves as to their duty in law.

He expressed a view that the key definition in the *Bolam* test should be reworded as:

> The duty is fulfilled if the doctor acts in accordance with a practice rightly accepted as proper by a body of skilled and experienced medical men.

His words paved the way for *Bolitho*, which 12 years later made clear that the views of a body of professional practitioners must be expected to withstand critical analysis.

As, in reasonably skilled hands, using modern needles and drugs, severe headache occurs in much less than 1% of patients, the duty to inform would not seem to be strong. In the case of major neurologic sequelae, it must be even weaker. However, by common consent the great majority of anesthesiologists would respond positively to any patient making a direct request for information. Thus, if asked for the exact risk of major sequelae, they would tell the patient, to the best of their knowledge, the odds of such an event occurring.

The same obligation rests on the anesthesiologist in the case of an anesthetic procedure that results in some adverse outcome. There is a clear duty to inform the patient, so far as possible, as to the cause of the accident. Indeed, a civil wrong may be committed in failing so to do.

However, it should be noted that the rigid Bolam interpretation set by *Gold* v. *Haringey HA*[6] was reinforced by the Court of Appeal in *Blythe* v. *Bloomsbury HA*,[9] in which it was held that a patient's direct request for information regarding possible risks of drug treatment could, quite properly, be disregarded if it was the contemporary practice of a responsible body of doctors so to do. Clearly, in this respect anesthesiologists working in the UK might appear to have far greater discretion than do their colleagues in the USA, who have almost none. In English law what should be said to the patient ultimately depends upon the characteristics of the particular patient and a reasonable medical judgment of the extent of the information that should be given to that patient.

A DUTY TO ENSURE THAT THE PATIENT CONSENTS TO TREATMENT

Having established that a patient has been properly informed of the planned surgical and anesthetic procedures, it is essential that consent be obtained. Normally, this involves the patient signing a witnessed declaration that a proper explanation has been given and that he or she consents to the surgical procedure set out above. In the case of a child aged less than 16, the parent or guardian signs the form. However, minors may be considered competent to give their own consent if they have sufficient understanding and intelligence to make that decision.[10]

Most hospital consent forms are somewhat vague with regard to anesthesia, and often refer to "local or general anesthesia." From a legal point of view, the essential step is to establish that the patient, while of sound mind, does consent to the procedure. Thus, verbal consent may be perfectly satisfactory so long as there are witnesses who may be relied upon to establish the fact at some later date. However, it should be borne in mind that in the event of a legal claim 3 or more years after the event, finding those witnesses and establishing direct recollection of the consent procedure may be a formidable undertaking. Clearly, a retrievable document is to be preferred. But, it is *not* satisfactory to rely upon a signature obtained from an elderly and heavily sedated patient sitting on a trolley in the operating room reception area *sans* teeth or spectacles when it is discovered that consent has not been obtained! Under such circumstances a patient would be in no fit state to give informed consent, and there would be no certainty that anyone had explained anything.

Occasionally, a patient refuses consent for a procedure that is judged to be necessary or even life saving. Because such patients may, at some later date, give an entirely different account of events, it is essential that such refusal be documented and witnessed with just as much care as consent itself. A documented refusal should be preserved in the case records.

CONSENT FOR RESEARCH PROCEDURES

Where research procedures are to be part of or associated with the conduct of anesthesia, special considerations apply. It is essential that the patient has a full understanding:

1 of what is experimental and what is not;
2 as to whether any part of the planned procedure is subject to randomization and, if so, what are the randomized alternatives;
3 that refusal to participate will not detract from the adequacy of his or her anesthetic care;
4 that consent for research may be withdrawn at any time.

Quite properly, most ethics committees insist on the use of patient information sheets written in lay English, with consent forms that are quite separate from those used for the surgical procedure itself. It is good practice for a research protocol to be explained and consented by one of the research team rather than the anesthesiologist who is to administer the anesthetic itself.

A DUTY TO PROVIDE SAFE ANESTHESIA

All doctors who describe themselves as anesthesiologists or are employed as such, should be capable of delivering safe, effective anesthesia. In order to do so they must:

1 Use anesthetic equipment that is fully functional, properly maintained, and, above all, safe. Today, it might be difficult to justify the use of an anesthetic machine capable of delivering oxygen-free gas mixtures or having a carbon dioxide rotameter calibrated up to 2 L min^{-1}.
2 Use monitoring equipment that warns of unsafe gas mixtures, inadequate blood oxygen saturation, inappropriate pulmonary ventilation, cardiac arrhythmias, and abnormalities in heart rate, blood pressure, or temperature.
3 Check that all equipment is fully functional, with particular attention paid to any items which have just returned from service or repair.
4 Be able to demonstrate adequate training for the post they hold. In the case of trainees this is self-evident, but even in the case of highly experienced clinicians continuing education is essential if skills are to be maintained and developed through the course of a professional lifetime.
5 Be physically capable of delivering a high-quality service to patients. It is inappropriate that any patient should unknowingly trust their lives to the care of a doctor who is exhausted, sick, demented, or under the influence of alcohol or other inebriants.
6 Use techniques that lie within the limits of currently accepted practice. Thus, anesthesiologists who rely upon 50% nitrous oxide

to ensure their patient's insensibility might find themselves called upon to justify that decision in defence of an awareness claim.

7 Keep an adequate written record of the anesthetic procedure and of physiologic monitoring data. Any hard-copy printouts from monitoring devices should be labeled with the patient's name and date, then attached to the anesthetic record. A vexatious claim may easily be discounted by reference to a good-quality clinical record with a wealth of detail to demonstrate the anesthesiologist's diligence. Conversely, poor note-taking may be taken by a judge as indicative of an unexplained carelessness, consistent with the claimant's explanation of events.[11] This is particularly important in the case of patients complaining that they have been aware and in pain during surgery under "general anesthesia." Such a claim may be impossible to defend unless the anesthesiologist can produce a contemporaneous record showing what agents he used and in what concentrations or doses they were administered. Indeed, this difficulty prompted the Medical Protection Society to voice the following warning in its 1987 Annual report:

> If members (whenever possible) ensure that they adhere to accepted techniques, and keep full anesthetic notes (including details of preoperative assessment, gas flows, delivery volumes, physiological parameters, circuit used, and the concentration of volatile agents selected, together with timing and usage), then and only then, may it be possible to defend a claim that awareness was due to negligence on the part of the anesthetist.

8 Ensure that their responsibilities are limited to caring for a single patient at any one time. Any anesthesiologist who by intent managed two anesthetized patients simultaneously would have no possible defence if misfortune were to befall either of them.

9 Ensure that the patient enjoys their undivided attention at all times. At its most basic level this requires that they be present throughout the procedure. In the event of any hazardous incident occurring in their absence, they might have to prove that their actions were at all times in the patient's best interest. As the patient's safety during the maintenance phase of anesthesia may well depend on anesthetic vigilance, they should not permit any distractions. Clearly, this depends upon individual circumstances, but it might well preclude inappropriate banter with or between other members of the operating room team, conversation with visitors, or teaching activities unrelated to the immediate welfare of the patient concerned. The practice of playing music in the operating room may be a dangerous distraction.

10 Ensure that if an inexperienced trainee is to administer the anesthetic there is close supervision such that the patient enjoys exactly the same standard of care as would have been provided by a consultant anesthesiologist. Inadequate supervision forms a major element of many negligence claims and, although not part of the direct chain of causation, may influence a judge strongly in favor of the claimant.

11 Ensure that they maintain proper care of their patients until they may be handed safely over to the care of a nurse. This will depend upon local circumstances, since patients may be passed to the care of a fully trained recovery nurse at a far earlier stage than to a student nurse with no recovery training whatever.

12 Wherever possible follow accepted clinical practice. However, it should be noted that where an anesthesiologist does not follow the accepted method of treatment (if indeed one exists) that is not necessarily evidence of negligence. In the Scots case of *Hunter* v. *Hanley*[12] the Court said:

> Even substantial deviation from normal practice may be warranted by the particular circumstances. To establish liability by a doctor when deviation from normal practice is alleged, three facts require to be established. First of all it must be proved that there is a usual and normal practice, secondly it must be proved that the defendant has not adopted that practice, and thirdly (and this is of crucial importance) it must be established that the course the doctor adopted is one which no professional man of ordinary skill would have taken if he had been acting with ordinary care.

13 When using new techniques, ensure that patients give informed consent to any new treatment which exposes them to risks of which they should be aware. Patients should not be subjected to unacceptable risk. A new technique must be justified as to its reasonable use in any particular case. If it results in damage to the patient that ought not to have occurred with the exercise of reasonable care, the doctor will be liable in negligence, as occurred in *Landau* v. *Werner*[13] and *Naylor* v. *Preston Health Authority*.[14]

A DUTY TO TELL WHEN THINGS GO WRONG

Just as anesthesiologists have a clear duty to warn their patients of likely dangers and complications associated with the planned course of action, they also have a duty to inform patients when those complications have occurred. Failure to do so, especially when some error has been made, may itself provide grounds for legal action.[13,14] Many patients discover that an error has been made only when they experience the result of that error. An obvious example is the patient who discovers that he has one fewer dental crown than on admission but cannot get any kind of explanation as to what has happened to it. When such events occur it is always better to tell the patient immediately, before he or she has time to become angry. In the great majority of cases patients become claimants only because no-one will tell them what happened. In the case of intraoperative awareness, the need for absolute honesty is paramount. Any denial or evasion on the part of the anesthesiologist is likely to intensify the mental trauma suffered by the patient, and may indeed contribute to the onset of a post-traumatic stress disorder.

FAILURE TO FULFILL THE DUTY OF CARE

If a patient suffers some accidental damage in the course of an anesthetic procedure, he or she may claim that this occurred as a direct consequence of negligence on the part of the anesthesiologist. Legal action may be brought against the anesthesiologist and/or the employer in pursuit of compensation for the damage.

Because (1) the introduction of NHS indemnity makes it no longer necessary to establish the liability of every doctor involved and (2) individual doctors may be difficult to identify and subsequently locate, it has become commonplace for health authorities and trusts to be named as defendants, with the negligence alleged as committed by their servants or agents. Such civil actions can succeed only if a number of strictly defined criteria can be met:

1 The patient suffered damage in the course of clinical management.
2 The anesthesiologist had a duty of care with respect to that patient.
3 The anesthesiologist failed, in one or more respects, to fulfill his or her duty of care.
4 The failing(s) caused the damage.

The onus of proof lies with the claimant, who must demonstrate *on the balance of probability* that the above conditions have been met. Such actions, if they cannot be settled by negotiation, are heard by a judge sitting alone. Damages are assessed as financial compensation for pain and suffering, and for both past and future financial loss. Their intention, in as much as money can compensate for suffering, is to restore the claimant to the position he or she would have been in had the tort not occurred. There is no provision for punitive or exemplary damages in English or Scottish law, so that the award must be seen as compensation, not punishment. Such cases often depend upon a judgment as to what standard of clinical care was to be expected of the anesthesiologist concerned, and to this end the judge hears expert witnesses from both claimant and defense. There is an implicit assumption in our adversarial system that the truth will emerge as somewhere between the opposing views.

RES IPSA LOQUITUR

Occasionally, an event occurs which is so far outside the natural expectation of events that the claimant may claim that it could have happened only as a result of negligence. Thus, if it is agreed that an anesthetized and intubated patient suffered an undetected accidental disconnection causing severe hypoxic cerebral damage, it is difficult to imagine any explanation that would not involve negligence. The claimant then may invoke the legal doctrine of *res ipsa loquitur*, meaning, quite literally, *the thing speaks for itself.* Under such circumstances the onus of proof may pass to the defendant, who then must demonstrate, on the balance of probabilities, that the accident did *not* occur as a result of his or her negligence. This may be achieved by demonstrating at least one plausible and non-negligent cause of the damage and by showing that there was no error in technique or clinical judgment.

This principle applied in *Saunders* v. *Leeds Western HA*,[15] in which a previously healthy 4-year-old child suffered a cardiac arrest in the course of an uncomplicated anesthetic. Mr Justice Mann held for the claimant on the grounds that healthy children do not, in the ordinary course of events, suffer such catastrophes without premonitory signs being evident from properly conducted physiologic monitoring, and that the defendants had not adequately discharged their burden of proof to show a non-negligent explanation. He held that, under those circumstances, the claimant did not need to demonstrate the specific cause of the cardiac arrest.

In a more recent case (*Ratcliffe* v. *Plymouth & Torbay HA, Exeter & N Devon HA*[16]), an adult male patient developed serious right-sided neurologic signs from the waist downward after an uncomplicated combined general and spinal anesthetic for surgery to his ankle. Several years later, spinal cord lesions at T9 and at T11–12 were demonstrated by magnetic resonance imaging (MRI), and it was claimed that the anesthesiologist must have injected the bupivacaine solution into the spinal cord at T12–L1, thus causing severe neurologic damage. The anesthesiologist produced clinical records to show that he *had* injected at the correct spinal interspace (L3–4), and pointed out that the claimant's neurologic condition could have been caused by nonsystemic vasculitis, a rare disease that could have been triggered by the operation. The trial judge rejected a claimant submission that *res ipsa loquitur* applied in this case, on the grounds that no prima facie case of negligence had been established. The Court of Appeal discussed previous applications of *res ipsa loquitur* in some detail, and agreed that it did not apply in cases such as this in which there was no direct inference of negligence from the facts. The Court of Appeal noted that the trial judge had believed the anesthesiologist but rejected the hypothetical chain of causation offered by the claimant, and ruled that he had been right to do so. Clearly, the courts will not regard *res ipsa loquitur* as a simple claimant strategy aimed at passing the onus of proof to the defendant simply upon the existence of a bad outcome.

THE CHAIN OF CAUSATION

Often it is assumed that, if an anesthesiologist is in some respect negligent *and* the patient sustains damage of some kind, then that patient has grounds for making a claim. This is true only when it can be shown that the negligence actually *caused* or *materially contributed to* the damage. Thus, a patient who suffers pain and awareness during cesarean section because her anesthesiologist had relied upon an empty isoflurane vaporizer has an excellent prospect of success. However, if instead of pain and awareness during surgery the patient claims that she suffered postoperative jaundice as a result of his incorrect choice of anesthetic agent, his undoubted negligence with regard to the vaporizer has no causative link with the supposed damage and her claim must fail.

Even if there is a feasible chain of causation, the claimant remains in severe difficulties unless he or she can show that on the balance of probabilities it was what actually happened. Thus, if there are alternative explanations, albeit less likely, which have not properly been excluded, causation has not been established. This principle is well illustrated by the case of *Wilsher* v. *Essex HA*, wherein a premature baby was accidentally exposed to high oxygen concentrations and subsequently developed retinal fibrosis.[17] As cause and effect appeared obvious at trial, judgment was given in favor of the claimant with £116 000 damages. At appeal the judgment was affirmed. However, in the House of Lords it was argued that there were five other pathological conditions which could, possibly, have resulted in similar retinal damage and had not been excluded.[18] Thus, despite the apparent etiologic link between the hyperoxia and the damage, it was held that causation had not been established and the appeal was allowed. It was for the claimant to prove the *specific* causative link between the negligence and the injury.

CRIMINAL CHARGES

A tort is a civil wrong in which the state has no direct interest. Libel, slander, defamation, breach of contract, and professional negligence are all torts. In certain circumstances, however, an anesthesiologist's actions may go beyond that limit. If, for instance, some procedure is performed in direct contravention to the patient's wishes, and then results in physical harm, he or she may be accused of assault and battery.

If it appears that a patient's death was caused by an anesthesiologist's criminal neglect or reckless behavior, a charge of manslaughter may be brought. An obvious scenario would be that in which a patient suffered hypoxic cardiac arrest following accidental circuit disconnection while the anesthesiologist took an unauthorized coffee break. At an even more sinister level, if it can be proved that an anesthesiologist actually intended to cause a patient's death (however noble the motivation, as may occur in the case of a terminally ill patient in uncontrolled agony) he or she may find themselves accused of murder. Fortunately, such events are rare and likely never to trouble the typical anesthesiologist.

REFERENCES

1. *Bolam* v. *Friern Hospital Management Committee* [1957] 2 All England Law Reports 118; [1957] 1 Weekly Law Reports 582.
2. *Sidaway* v. *Bethlem Royal Hospital Governors and others* [1985] 1 All England Law reports 643. House of Lords.
3. *Whitehouse* v. *Jordan* [1981] 1 Weekly Law Reports 246.
4. *Maynard* v. *West Midlands Region Health Authority* [1984] 1 Weekly Law Reports 634.
5. *Roe* v. *Ministry of Health* [1954] 2 Queens Bench 66.

6. *Gold* v. *Haringey Health Authority* [1987] 2 All England Law Reports 888.
7. *Bolitho* v. *City and Hackney Health Authority* [1997] Lloyd's Law Reports Medical [1998] 1 26. House of Lords.
8. *Marriot* v. *West Midlands RHA* [1999] Lloyd's Law Reports Medical 23.
9. *Blythe* v. *Bloomsbury Health Authority.* [1987] The Times 5 February. Court of Appeal.
10. *Gillick* v. *West Norfolk & Wisbech Area Health Authority and the DHSS* [1985] 3 All England Law Reports 402. House of Lords.
11. *Skelton* v. *Lewisham and North Southwark Health Authority* [1997] QBD Lloyds Law Reports Medical 8 324.
12. *Hunter* v. *Hanley [1955] Sessions (Scottish) Cases 200.*
13. *Landau* v. *Werner.* [1961] 105 Solicitors Journal 1008.
14. *Naylor* v. *Preston Health Authority.* [1987] 2 All England Law Reports 643.
15. *Saunders* v. *Leeds Western Health Authority and another* (1984). [1993] 4 Medical Law Reports.
16. *Ratcliffe* v. *Plymouth & Torbay Health Authority, Exeter & North Devon Health Authority.* [1998] Court of Appeal. Lloyds Law Reports Medical 162.
17. *Wilsher* v. *Essex Area Health Authority* [1986] 3 All England Law Reports 801.
18. *Wilsher* v. *Essex Area Health Authority* [1988] 1 All England Law Reports 871. House of Lords.

80

Informed consent: an American legal and ethical perspective

PETER J COHEN

> What is man, that thou art mindful of him?...
> For thou hast made him a little lower than the angels, and hast crowned him with glory and honour.
> Thou madest him to have dominion over the works of thy hands; and thou hast put all things under his feet...
>
> Psalm 8: 4–6 (King James Version)

> We the People of the United States, in Order to...secure the Blessings of Liberty to ourselves and our Posterity, do ordain and establish this Constitution for the United States of America.
>
> Constitution of the United States, Ratified 1788

> Every human being of adult years and sound mind has a right to determine what shall be done with his own body; and a surgeon who performs an operation without his patient's consent, commits an assault, for which he is liable in damages.
>
> Judge Benjamin Cardozo, *Schloendorff* v. *The Society of the New York Hospital* 211 NY 125, 129 (1914)

These ringing statements, their origins separated by centuries, set forth the philosophical basis for an Anglo-American consensus: competent patients must be *informed* and must *consent* before any physician may "lay hands" upon them. The concept of informed consent is, indeed, a paradigm truly reflecting the way in which we look upon ourselves, and the laws of the UK and the USA, derived from similar traditions, are a reflection of our deep belief epitomizing humans as rational beings responsible ultimately for the care of their bodies.

This chapter is neither a legal text nor law review article; rather, it is intended to provide the reader with a rationale for the requirement for and application of informed consent in today's medical practice. I will frequently quote a court's holding (decision), as its words often speak eloquently to the concepts that this chapter hopes to develop.

Common law has long recognized the civil wrong or injury (tort) of *battery* – the offensive touching of another's person. An affirmative defense to alleged battery is consent; if this is to prevail, the consenting person must have known the consequences of and reasons for the actions agreed to.

THE SCOPE OF DISCLOSURE

The term "informed consent" first appeared in a US judicial opinion in 1957.[1] The plaintiff, having developed lower extremity paraplegia after aortography under general anesthesia, claimed lack of prior knowledge that such a devastating complication could result from the procedure. In a one-paragraph discussion, buried in a decision of over 13 pages, the court was clear and unmistakable in announcing what the law requires of a physician:

> [The defendant admitted] that the details of the procedure and the possible dangers therefrom were not explained...[It is] the duty of a physician to disclose to the patient all the facts which mutually affect his (*sic*) rights and interests and of the surgical risk, hazard and danger, if any. A physician violates his duty to his patient and subjects himself to liability if he withholds any facts which are necessary to form the basis of an intelligent consent by the patient to the proposed treatment. Likewise the physician may not minimize the known dangers of a procedure or operation in order to induce his patient's consent...[The physician must render] full disclosure of facts necessary to an *informed consent* (author's italics).

Three years later, a state Supreme Court found that a patient may have a cause of action if a known risk was not disclosed *even if the treatment met medical standards of care*.[2] The holding is important for two reasons: (1) it proposed a "professional practice standard"; and (2) it made clear that (in the USA) it is the jury that decides whether sufficient and accurate information had been given to the patient when the question is one of fact rather than of law:

> [The patient's decision must be based on] such disclosure as a reasonable medical practitioner would make under the same or similar circumstances...[A] physician violates his duty to his patient and subjects himself to liability for malpractice, where no immediate emergency exists...if he makes no disclosure of significant facts within his knowledge which are necessary to form the basis of an intelligent consent by the patient to the proposed form of treatment.
>
> Whether or not a physician has advised his patient of the inherent risks and hazards of a proposed form of treatment is a question of fact concerning which lay witnesses are competent to testify...It is only when the facts concerning the actual disclosures made to the patient are ascertained, or ascertainable by the trier of fact [jury], that the expert testimony of medical witnesses is required to establish whether such disclosures are in accordance with those which a reasonable medical practitioner would make under the same or similar circumstances.

Should it be medical custom that sets the standards for what must be disclosed to the patient? Or should the knowledge provided by the physician be judged on the basis of whether it was appropriate for a "reasonable patient?" Just 2 years after promulgation of the *reasonable physician* standard, the United States Supreme Court declined to review (and thus affirmed) a decision of the Court of Appeals for the District of Columbia.[3] This decision is a beautiful articulation of the rationale supporting a policy that physicians disclose all material information to the extent that would satisfy the hypothetical *reasonable patient*. After all, *doctors* are *teachers* with a professional obligation to educate their patients. In the end, it is the patient who should determine what information is needed, not the custom of the medical profession:

> The record we review tells a depressing tale. A youth troubled only by back pain submitted to an operation without being informed of the risk of paralysis incidental thereto [which did, indeed, occur with paralysis of] the lower half of his body...Despite extensive medical care, he has never been what he was before.
>
> [The physician testified that] paralysis can be anticipated "somewhere in the nature of 1 percent"...a risk he termed "a very slight possibility." He felt that communication of that risk to the patient is not good medical practice because it might deter patients from undergoing needed surgery and might produce adverse psychological reactions which could preclude the success of the operation.
>
> True consent to what happens to one's self is the informed exercise of a choice, and that entails an opportunity to evaluate knowledgeably the options available and the risks attendant upon each. The average patient has little or no understanding of the medical arts, and ordinarily has only his physician to whom he can look for enlightenment with which to reach an intelligent decision. From these almost axiomatic considerations springs the need, and in turn the requirement, of a reasonable divulgence by physician to patient to make such a decision possible.
>
> There are, in our view, formidable obstacles to acceptance of the notion that the physician's obligation to disclose is either germinated or limited by medical practice...[We cannot] ignore the fact that to bind the disclosure obligation to medical usage is to arrogate the decision on revelation to the physician alone. Respect for the patient's right of self-determination on particular therapy demands a standard set by law for physicians rather than one which physicians may or may not impose upon themselves.
>
> In our view, the patient's right of self-decision shapes the boundaries of the duty to reveal. That right can be effectively exercised only if the patient possesses enough information to enable an intelligent choice. The scope of the physician's communications to the patient, then, must be measured by the patient's need, and that need is the information material to the decision.

The right to receive information about the risks and benefits of *not* undergoing treatment is as germane as the obligations already discussed. Thus, in 1980 a California court held that patients must be appraised of the hazards of not undergoing treatment:[4]

> This court must decide whether a physician's failure to inform a patient of the material risks of not consenting to a recommended pap smear, so that the patient might make an informed choice, may have breached the physician's duty of due care to his patient, who died from cancer of the cervix.
>
> [T]he need for disclosure is not lessened because patients reject a recommended procedure. Such a decision does not alter what has been termed the "fiducial qualities" of the physician–patient relationship since patients who reject a procedure are as unskilled in the medical sciences as those who consent.

THE RIGHT TO REFUSE

Everything said to this point assumes that a patient possesses an appropriate *decision-making capacity*. However, how should physicians act when a patient's decision appears totally "irrational?" It may be tempting to term any such patient *incompetent*; however, this is a judicial decision and not within the purview of the medical profession. In contrast, physicians are always obliged to assess their patients' *decision-making capacity*, whether or not their two viewpoints coincide. Waisel and Truog have nicely distinguished decision-making ability and competence:[5]

> The ability to participate in care decisions is called decision-making capacity. This is distinct from the legal concept of competency, which only a judge has the authority to determine. Decision-making capacity, on the other hand, can and should be assessed by anesthesiologists and other clinicians. Evidence that a person can make a decision includes the ability to understand the current situation, to use relevant information, and to communicate a preference supported by reasons. Decision-making capacity may vary relative to age, situation, mental status, and level of risk in the decision.

Physicians who are seriously concerned with a patient's embarking on a hazardous course in refusing recommended therapy may seek a judicial remedy. However, consistent with the above discussion, American courts are loath to contravene a patient's judgment unless there is clear evidence of incompetence. And failure to follow a physician's recommendations, even to the point of death, does not constitute incompetence per se.

Consider a paradigm case involving a 77-year-old widow with gangrene in the right lower leg. Although her physicians all recommended amputation, she refused to consent. Her daughter petitioned for appointment as temporary guardian with authority to consent to the procedure. Once again, the court was clear in formulating the rights of competent patients to decide what happens to their bodies, as they are capable of appreciating the nature and consequences of their actions. This patient was such an individual with:

> ... the right under the law to refuse to submit either to medical treatment or a surgical operation [and] therefore her leg may not be amputated unless she consents to that course of action.
>
> [S]he has exhibited a high degree of awareness and acuity when responding to questions concerning the proposed operation. She has made it clear that she does not wish to have the operation even though that decision will in all likelihood lead shortly to her death.
>
> The law protects her right to make her own decision to accept or reject treatment, whether that decision is wise or unwise... Even though we may consider [her] beliefs unwise, foolish or ridiculous, in the absence of an overriding danger to society we may not permit interference therewith...[Her] decision may be regarded by most as unfortunate, but on the record in this case it is not the uninformed decision of a person incapable of appreciating the nature and consequences of her act [and] we are all of the opinion that the operation may not be forced on her against her will.[6]

Although other clinicians may face a variety of manifestations of the right to refuse therapy, the question of an adult Jehovah's Witness is the one with which anesthesiologists are most familiar. Whereas there will always be wide disagreement among thoughtful physicians, the following articulate judicial opinion is worth considering. Judge Burger based his opinion on a decision rendered by the United States Supreme Court over three decades previously, in which Justice Brandeis had stated:[7]

> The makers of our Constitution undertook to secure conditions favorable to the pursuit of happiness. They recognized the significance of man's spiritual nature, of his feelings and of his intellect. They knew that only a part of the pain, pleasure and satisfactions of life are to be found in material things. They sought to protect Americans in their beliefs, their thoughts, their emotions and their sensations. They conferred, as against the Government, the right to be left alone – the most comprehensive of rights and the right most valued by civilized man.

Burger enlarged upon Brandeis' philosophy, formulating an approach consistent with what has already been said, and which many will find appealing today:[8]

> Nothing in this utterance suggests that Justice Brandeis thought an individual possessed these rights only as to sensible beliefs, valid thoughts, reasonable emotions, or well-founded sensations. I suggest he intended to include a great many foolish, unreasonable and even absurd ideas which do not conform, such as refusing medical treatment even at great risk.

The right of competent patients to refuse transfusion for themselves does not necessarily extend to their right to dictate therapy of their children. Over a half a century ago, the United States Supreme Court clearly articulated this concept:[9]

> Parents may be free to become martyrs themselves. But it does not follow they are free, in identical circumstances, to make martyrs of their children before they have reached the age of full and legal discretion when they can make that choice for themselves.

PERSONAL AUTONOMY IS NOT A UNIVERSAL BELIEF

The right to refuse is not confined to therapy alone; patients may decline the opportunity to receive pertinent information and waive their right to consent. In some societies, the cultural norm is for the individual to defer to the family or community when matters of great import are at stake. For members of some cultures, being informed of the possibility of death is considered to be equivalent to dying itself.[10]

> In traditional Navajo culture, it is held that thought and language have the power to shape reality and to control events. Discussing the potential complications of diabetes with a newly diagnosed Navajo patient may, in the view of the traditional patient, result in the occurrence of such complications...In the Navajo view of the world, language is not a mirror of reality, reality is a mirror of language.

Sensitivity to the ways in which different groups address these significant ethical questions does not mean denying the importance of informed consent in the Anglo-American ethos. Rather, it acknowledges the right of autonomous humans to consent *not* to receive certain information and *not* to make their own decisions but, instead, to defer these matters to others.[11]

> Allowing patients to choose a family-centered decision-making style does not mean abandoning our commitment to individual autonomy or its legal expression in the doctrine of informed consent. Rather, it means broadening our view of autonomy so that respect for persons includes respect for the cultural values they bring with them to the decision-making process.

Practicing anesthesiologists ought not be surprised when confronted with cultures grounded in viewpoints not subscribing to the dominance of personal autonomy. Those who worry that deferring to another cultural norm may set the stage for a successful suit, may find solace in the following legal analysis, an approach which may be equally well applied to a devout Jehovah's Witness who has refused transfusion:

> Would US tort law compel physicians to press information on patients despite their culturally based desire not to be informed? Since the boundaries of the duty to reveal are shaped by the patient's right of self-determination, it follows logically that the patient can decide whether to receive full information or whether disclosure should be made to the family. Courts have expressly determined that physicians should not be liable for failure to disclose resulting from the patient's specific request not to be informed...[Thus, the law rationally permits] a standard of disclosure guided by the patient's desire not to receive information. Whether that choice is wise – whether having the information is beneficial or burdensome – depends on the patient's own values.[12]

THE PHYSICIAN'S DUTY NOT TO INFORM

Are there instances in which a sympathetic physician may find it necessary *not* to inform a patient? The term *therapeutic privilege* refers to the rare instance in which just this situation arises. Interestingly enough, this concept was well elaborated in what this chapter has termed "a beautiful articulation of the rationale" for informed consent. The court's scholarly decision discussed two exceptions to the requirement for informed consent:[13]

> The first comes into play when the patient is unconscious or otherwise incapable of consenting, and harm from a failure to treat is imminent and outweighs any harm threatened by the proposed treatment...
>
> The second exception obtains when risk-disclosure poses such a threat of detriment to the patient as to become unfeasible or contraindicated from a medical point of view... The physician's privilege to withhold information for therapeutic reasons must be carefully circumscribed, however, for otherwise it might devour the disclosure rule itself. The privilege does not accept the paternalistic notion that the physician may remain silent simply because divulgence might prompt the patient to forgo therapy the physician feels the patient really needs. That attitude presumes instability or perversity for even the normal patient, and runs counter to the foundation principle that the patient should and ordinarily can make the choice for himself. Nor does the privilege contemplate operation save where the patient's reaction to risk information, as reasonably foreseen by the physician, is menacing. And even in a situation of that kind, disclosure to a close relative with a view to securing consent to the proposed treatment may be the only alternative open to the physician.

INFORMED CONSENT AND CLINICAL INVESTIGATION

When a patient or volunteer is given the opportunity to participate in a research protocol, the considerations already discussed obviously continue to apply. However, there are additional factors to contemplate. Remember that clinical studies may be "nontherapeutic," i.e. of no clinical benefit to the individual subject. In addition, even if the investigation may have a therapeutic effect, the patient may be randomly assigned to a placebo arm. These factors must be made explicit to the proposed subject.

As a direct result of a history of significant ethical abuses (e.g. the Tuskegee Study), the United States Congress promulgated several statutes. These set forth certain requirements that must be followed in all federally funded research, as well as any study that will develop data to be submitted to the Food and Drug Administration (FDA). The National Research Act of 1974 created the National Commission for the Protection of Human Subjects of Biomedical and Behavioral Research. This requires the Department of Health, Education and Welfare to publish regulations for the protection of human subjects, including requirements for informed consent and review of research by institutional review boards (IRBs). In its important publication, the *Belmont Report*, the Commission promulgated its views of the ethical basis of human research.[14]

The *Common Rule* makes explicit the requirement that all research supported, conducted, or regulated by federal agencies must be reviewed by an IRB.[15] IRBs are responsible for ensuring that the consent of all research subjects is informed and voluntary, that risks to the participants are minimized related to the significance of the investigators' goals, and that the participants' rights and welfare are protected. An IRB's membership must include individuals representing the public (e.g. attorneys, clergy, ethicists, or private citizens) as well as those possessing knowledge allowing them to evaluate risks and benefits of projects under consideration. It is essential that the IRB functions independently of its associated institution.

When contemplated research protocols involve *vulnerable populations* (e.g. prisoners,[16] children,[17] individuals who are decisionally impaired, a fetus or embryo, members of minority groups), the IRB has a responsibility for considerably increased scrutiny of risks, benefits, and potential coercion, the guidelines of which are spelled out in federal regulations.

At the present time, these federal mandates do not apply to privately funded human clinical research as long as the data will not be submitted to the FDA. Whether this will be changed and ethical protection extended to all research subjects is a matter of current debate.

SUMMARY

The requirement for informed consent, a heritage that mandates a respect for human autonomy, is derived from centuries of Anglo-American Common Law. This concept acknowledges that all competent individuals have the right to make decisions concerning what is done to their bodies, and that they can be furnished with information adequate to allow them to make a considered judgment. Despite the simplicity of this philosophy, it is frequently associated with major misconceptions, termed *myths* by Meisel and Kuczewski.[18] These myths include the beliefs that (1) a signed consent form is informed consent; (2) informed consent is a medical *Miranda Warning*; (3) patients need full disclosure about treatment only if they consent; and (4) patients must be told everything about treatment. However, in truth:

1 Consent forms are used as a matter of routine in both treatment and research settings because many hospital administrators, physicians, and their attorneys see these forms as providing protection against liability, despite the fact that they actually provide little protection.
2 Just as police [in the USA] are required to tell criminal suspects that "you have a right to remain silent, you have a right to a lawyer...," some physicians believe that informed consent been obtained if they warn patients of the risks of treatment. Certainly, patients should be told about the risks of treatment. Admittedly, it is difficult to know what risks must be disclosed, but the approach to informed consent that we advocate makes this less important. Rather than focusing on risks, the focus needs to be on therapeutic options; knowledge of one's options alone, however, is not meaningful unless one also knows the range of consequences of choosing each option.
3 In fact, physicians are obligated to obtain not only informed consent but also informed refusal. This is not as silly as it might at first appear, when one recalls that the most important part of informed consent is information about options and their consequences and a refusal of treatment is a choice to do nothing, which has predictable consequences too.
4 Actually, the law requires only that patients be given a *reasonable* amount of information... .[Depending on the jurisdiction,] patients must be given the information that a reasonable physician would disclose [or provided with] that amount and kind of information that a reasonable *patient* would find material to making a decision about treatment.

For medical professionals, the opportunity to interact with their patients and discuss risks, benefits, and therapeutic options offers both a challenge and fulfillment. If approached with skill, reason, and compassion, this responsibility can only serve to instill trust, perhaps the most important feeling that can be shared between the physician and the patient.

REFERENCES

1. *Salgo* v. *Leland Stanford, Jr. University Board of Trustees*, 317 P.2d 170, 181 (1957).
2. *Natanson* v. *Kline*, 354 P.2d 670, 671–3 (Kan) (1960).
3. *Canterbury* v. *Spence*, 464 F.2d 772, 776, 778, 780, 783–4, 786 (DC Cir), *cert.* denied, 409 US 1064 (1972).
4. *Truman* v. *Thomas*, 611 P.2d 902, 903, 906 (1980).
5. Waisel DV, Truog RD. Informed consent. *Anesthesiology* 1997; **87:** 968–78.
6. *Lane* v. *Candura*, 376 N.E. 2d 1232, 1233, 1235, 1236 (1978).
7. *Olmstead* v. *United States*, 277 U.S. 438, 478 (1928), (dissenting opinion).
8. Application of the President & Directors of Georgetown College, Inc., 331 F.2d 1010, 1017 (1964) (dissenting opinion).
9. *Prince* v. *Massachusetts*, 321 US 158, 170 (1944).
10. Cerrese, JA, Rhodes LA. Western bioethics on the Navajo reservation: benefit or harm? *JAMA* 1995; **274:** 826–9.
11. Blackhall LJ, Murphy ST, Frank G, *et al.* Ethnicity and attitudes toward patient autonomy. *JAMA* 1995; **274:** 820–5.
12. Gostin LO. Informed consent, cultural sensitivity, and respect for persons. *JAMA* 1995: **274:** 844–5.
13. *Canterbury* v. *Spence*, 464 F.2d 772, 788–9 (DC Cir), *cert.* denied, 409 U.S. 1064 (1972).
14. National Commission for Protection of Human Subjects of Biomedical and Behavioral Research. The Belmont Report: Ethical Principles and Guidelines for the Protection of Human Subjects in Research. OPRR Reports. Bethesda, MD: National Institutes of Health, 1979.
15. 56 Federal Register, 18 June 1999; 45 Code of Federal Regulations (CFR) 46.
16. 56 Federal Register, 18 June 1999; 45 Code of Federal Regulations (CFR) 46, Subpart C.
17. 56 Federal Register, 18 June 1999; 45 Code of Federal Regulations (CFR) 46, Subpart D.
18. Meisel A, Kuczewski M. Legal and ethical myths about informed consent. *Arch Intern Med* 1996; **156:** 2521–6.

81

Consent to medical treatment: the legal influences affecting the British perspective

THOMAS E J HEALY

In this chapter I shall trace the evolution of our present understanding of the law applied to consent. I shall do this by examining some important legal cases drawn from the courts in the English-speaking democracies. The central element in all of these is the complaint "I was not told that this might happen." The English-speaking democracies employ a similar legal approach, i.e. common law or the law of precedent, when deciding between the opposing sides in a dispute. The decisions taken in the different countries, although not binding in the other countries, are accorded persuasive authority and may be used in support of argument in the courts.

The duty of care owed by one person to another, when the relationship between the two individuals exposes one of them to danger, expects that the other must take reasonable care to protect the one placed in danger. In this we see the foundations of the "neighbor" principle and an expression of "the duty of care." Lord Atkin[1] held that the duty of care applies to:

> ... persons who are so closely and directly affected by my act that I ought reasonably to have them in contemplation as being so affected while I am directing my mind to the acts or omissions which are called into question.

and

> You must take reasonable care to avoid acts or omissions which you can reasonably foresee would be likely to injure your neighbour.

More recently, Lord Oliver[2] held:

> the three requirements of proximity, justice and reasonableness, and degree of foreseeability might be regarded as facets of the same thing.

Namely, were the consequences of a defendant's, e.g. an anesthesiologist's, action, i.e. loss and injury to the claimant (plaintiff), reasonably foreseeable, was there a relationship of proximity between the defendant and the claimant and would it be "just and reasonable" for a duty to be imposed on the defendant for the advantage of the claimant? While it was the view of the courts that duty itself should not be defined, except in relation to the circumstances of each case, anesthesiologists can take no consolation from this apparent lack of clarity. The courts have no difficulty in recognizing that it is just and reasonable to conclude that an anesthesiologist has a duty of care (see Chapter 79) to his or her patient, that the relationship is one of proximity, and that damage due to a breach in the duty, i.e. negligence, is foreseeable.

The duty of care (see Chapter 79) extends to all the medical interactions between a doctor and a patient and therefore includes ensuring that the patient has given consent to the treatment.

The standard of care in the UK was established in a landmark English case[3] in which the "Bolam" principle was recognized:

> (A doctor) is not guilty of negligence if he acted in accordance with a practice accepted as proper by a responsible body of medical men skilled in that particular art.

The right of patients to give or to withhold consent to treatment is an expression of their human freedom and must be respected by doctors. It is a component of their duty of care even if the reasons for the patient withholding consent are irrational.

In an earlier and more paternalistic society, patients were less questioning, less educated, and more submissive to those in authority, such as members of the medical profession, and it was accepted that the doctor knew best. Today, an autonomous patient's right to make decisions, even those with which the doctor disagrees, is fully respected in the English-speaking countries, and in many others. Indeed, it is a *legal requirement* that a patient's wishes be accepted by his or her doctors. Should a physician sincerely believe that these wishes do not accord with the accepted standards of medical practice, but be unable to convince the patient of this, the physician is obliged to withdraw from the case after finding a suitable substitute.

The need for a doctor to obtain consent from a patient is a new concept that was not mentioned in the Hippocratic Oath.[4] The Oath even prohibited disclosure of information to the patient,[5] but the Nuremberg Code highlights the need to obtain consent.[6]

Bristow J in *Chatterton* v. *Gerson*[7] examined the claim by a woman that treatment for pain in a postoperative scar in the groin had caused numbness in her right leg. The claimant alleged that she had not been warned about this possibility. Bristow J held that:

> Once the patient is informed in broad terms of the nature of the procedure which is intended and gives consent, the consent is real. The cause of the action on which to base a claim for failure to go into risks and implications is negligence not trespass ... but he ought to warn of what may happen by misfortune however well the operation is done.

Lord Scarman,[8] an English Law Lord, speaking in court, held that:

> A doctor who operates without the consent of his patients is, save in cases of emergency or mental disability, guilty of the civil wrong of trespass to the person; he is also guilty of the criminal offence of assault.

The General Medical Council in the UK recently considered the case of a consultant cardiologist who was accused of treating a child without the permission of the child's parents. Sir Herbert Duthie,[9] chairman of the committee, said:

> Consent to treatment is an essential part of the contract of trust between patients and doctors. Doctors must do their best to explain to patients the treatments which are proposed and to obtain their patients' consent. Where, subsequently, further procedures are considered necessary, the doctor must seek additional consent.

The common law principles expressed in the laws of the UK are also reflected in and reflect the laws of the USA, Canada, Australia, and New Zealand. The legal decisions taken in these English-speaking nations have generated and expressed a common legal view and are therefore used in this chapter to explain a shared interpretation and understanding of the meaning and application of consent. The principles are those which express a general behavior with which "the man in the street" would immediately agree. The principles are not new.

Judge Cardoso expressed these clearly in a landmark legal case in the USA[10] in 1914:

> Every human being of adult years and sound mind has a right to determine what shall be done with his own body; and a surgeon who performs an operation without the patient's consent commits an assault.

Consent, to have legal meaning, must be based on appropriate information. The patient must understand the reasons why a particular treatment is offered, the chances of success, the risks involved both with and without treatment, and, when available, the alternative treatments. The right of a patient to be informed about all the risks of the surgical treatment resulted in the development of the "doctrine of informed consent" in some jurisdictions in the USA. It was accepted also by the Supreme Court of Canada,[11] in a case in which a patient claimed that the surgeon had failed to inform him about the risk of surgery to the carotid artery. The decision of the Ontario Court of Appeal was that the doctor had been negligent because he had failed to disclose a risk inherent in the treatment.

How does a physician decide what, and how much, information it is appropriate to convey to achieve informed consent? Considerable diversity of opinion is obvious when we consider several judicial decisions. Whether the answer is couched in terms of the physician's perspective or that of patients in general, or depends on the specific individual patient, is subject to debate.

Canadian jurisprudence is typified by the comments of Laskin CJ in *Reibl* v. *Hughes*,[11] quoted by Lord Bridge in the landmark English case *Sidaway* v. *Bethlem Royal Hospital* 1985,[8] who held that the principle of informed consent would not be served by allowing the physician complete discretion in what information to share with the patient:

> To allow expert medical evidence to determine what risks are material and hence should be disclosed and, correlatively, what risks are not material is to hand over to the medical profession the entire question of the scope of the duty of disclosure, including whether there has been a breach of that duty.

In contrast is the English position, set out in *Sidaway* v. *Governors of Royal Bethlem Hospital*[8] and confirmed in an appeal to the House of Lords: the information that was deemed appropriate depended more on what the doctor felt the patient needed to know.

The claimant in *Sidaway*[8] had been warned by the surgeon that there was the possibility of damage to a nerve root and was informed about the consequences if this occurred. However, the surgeon failed to mention that there was also a 1% chance of damaging the spinal cord, which would be within 3 mm of the operation site, with the obvious possibility that there might be very serious consequences. The claimant was unable to sustain a claim against the surgeon based on negligent performance of the operation. She contended that the surgeon had been in breach of a duty owed to warn her of all possible risks of the operation and as a result of this omission she had not been able to give "informed consent." The trial judge, using the test of "action in accordance with accepted medical practice," dismissed the claim.

The Court of Appeal upheld the decision, holding that the doctrine of informed consent based on full disclosure of all the facts to the patient was not the appropriate test under English law. A majority of the House of Lords,[8] Lord Scarman dissenting, held that the question of a doctor's duty of care and his or her omission to warn a patient of the inherent risks of proposed treatment should be determined by applying the Bolam test of duty.[3] In spite of the decision, it seems that Lord Scarman saw more clearly the future direction in legal thought related to consent.

Lord Bridge argued in detail, drawing examples from many common law legal cases, not all from UK jurisdictions. He noted that in the judgment in the Canadian case (Reibl v. Hughes)[11] Robinson J held that the decisions cannot be left to be determined by the doctors:

> Respect for the patient's right of self determination on particular therapy demands a standard set by law for physicians rather than one which physicians may or may not impose on themselves.

However, in the case in which he was making his judgment (*Sidaway*), Lord Bridge accepted that he could not properly reject the conclusion to which unchallenged medical evidence led in the application of the Bolam test.

Lord Templeman set forth a point of view that allowed the physician (rather than the patient) to decide what information was material:

> An obligation to give a patient all the information available to the doctor would often be inconsistent with the doctor's contractual obligation to have regard to the patient's best interests. Some information might confuse, other information might alarm the patient ... the doctor must decide in the light of his training and experience and in the light of his knowledge of the patient what should be said and how it should be said ... where the patient's life and health are at stake, the patient must make the final decision.

Nonetheless, he acknowledged that the physician was also obliged to consider the patient's point of view:

> At the end of the day, the doctor, bearing in mind the best interests of the patient and bearing in mind the patient's right of information, which will enable the patient to make a balanced judgement, must decide what information should be given to the patient and in what terms that information should be couched.

Lord Keith did not add to Lord Bridge's finding.

Lord Diplock considered that:

> The merit of the Bolam test is that the criterion of the duty of care owed by a doctor to his patient is whether he acted in accordance with a practice accepted as proper by a body of responsible and skilled medical opinion.

Lord Scarman, who dissented from the majority opinion, adopted the transatlantic view that:

> In my judgement the merit of the propositions enunciated in Canterbury and Spence[12] is that, without excluding medical evi-

> dence, they set a standard and formulated a test of the doctor's duty, the effect of which is that the court determines the scope of the duty and decides whether the doctor has acted in breach of his duty … If the doctor fails to warn where the risk is such that in the court's view a prudent person in the patient's situation would have regarded it as significant, the doctor is liable.
>
> My Lords I think the Canterbury propositions reflect a legal truth which too much judicial reliance on medical judgement tends to obscure. In a medical negligence case where the issue is as to the advice and information given to the patient as to the treatment proposed, the available options, and the risk, the court is concerned primarily with the patient's right. The doctor's duty arises from his patient's right.

In *Salgo* v. *Leland Jr. University Board of Trustees*,[13] a patient who suffered paralysis following translumbar aortography sued the medical staff for negligently performing the investigation because they had not warned him about the risks. The court decided that the doctors had a duty to reveal:

> … any facts which are necessary to form the basis of an intelligent consent by the patient to the proposed treatment.

This American decision concerning informed consent draws close to the English and Scottish view that consent must protect the autonomy of the patient by disclosing the risks involved and the information necessary to consent. Lord Scarman, in *Sidaway* v. *Bethlem Royal Hospital Board of Governors*,[8] dissenting from the House of Lords decision, introduced the concept that the yardstick was not necessarily medical opinion but what a reasonable patient would want to know about the material risks.

This view has influenced Australian legal opinion because, in addition to taking account of clinical practice, it leaves it open for the court to decide on the "reasonable patient" issue. Justice Wilcox, in *E* v. *Australian Red Cross Society*,[14] held:

> The views of King in F v R[15] and Lord Scarman's dissenting view in the Sidaway case is to be preferred to rigid reliance on common (medical) practice. Whilst evidence of the practice usually adopted by persons in the position of the defendant (doctor/dentist) will generally be of great assistance and often decisive, the way must be left open to a plaintiff/complainant (patient) to persuade the court that the practice does not ensure an adequate standard of care.

It appears that the delicate compromise established in this case between clinical practice and the significant risk that a reasonable patient would want to know about is ahead of practice in the UK and draws close to *Canterbury* v. *Spence*,[12] an earlier court decision in the USA.

The view held in some American States was well expressed in *Canterbury* v. *Spence*[12] and concerns the need to disclose all material risks to which the patient might attach importance. In this case the patient, who was 19 years old, was recommended to have a laminectomy. The patient's mother was told that the operation was no more serious than any other operation and the patient did not ask about the operation or the risks. However, the patient suffered severe neurologic sequelae. She developed incontinence and difficulty in walking and complained that she should have been warned. The judge held:

> It is the right of the patient, not the doctor, to determine the direction in which his interests lie. The patient must be given the information to chart his course, to understand the therapeutic alternatives and their dangers.

The Canterbury court[12] enunciated four principles:

1 The root premise is the concept that every human being of adult years and of sound mind has a right to determine what shall be done with his body.
2 The consent is the informed exercise of a choice, and that entails an opportunity to evaluate knowledgeably the options available and the risks attendant on each.
3 The doctor must, therefore, disclose all "material risks;" what risks are "material" is determined by the "prudent patient" test, which was formulated by the court. "[a] risk is … material when a reasonable person, in what the physician knows or should know to be the patient's position, would be likely to attach significance to the risk or cluster of risks in deciding whether or not to forgo the proposed therapy."
4 The doctor, however, has what the court called a "therapeutic privilege."

It appears that the decision taken in *E* v. *Australian Red Cross Society*[14] prepared the way for a further understanding of the common law in Australia. The claimant in *Rogers* v. *Whittaker*,[16] heard in a court in New South Wales, underwent surgery to improve the sight in her right eye, which had been damaged by a penetrating eye injury when she was 9 years old. She expressed worry about any adverse consequences and, in particular, although she did not ask any questions about the possibility of damage to her good eye, she specifically asked the surgeon to protect it! After surgery she developed sympathetic ophthalmia in her good left eye and lost her sight in that eye. The operation failed to improve the sight in her blind right eye with the result that she was now blind in both eyes. There was no doubt that if she had known about the danger of sympathetic ophthalmia she would not have had the surgery.

Mrs Whittaker considered that the surgeon was negligent because he had not told her about the danger to her good eye. The surgeon believed that the risk was 1/14 000 and did not consider it necessary to tell his patient about sympathetic ophthalmia because the risk was so small. Mrs Whittaker contended that, had she known about the possibility, she would not have undergone the operation. During the legal argument that followed the surgeon claimed that his actions were in accordance with the "Bolam" principle[3] established in English law.

The patient, on the other hand, argued that the Bolam principle should not apply because this principle allowed the doctors and not the courts to decide whether there had been a failure in "the duty of care." The Australian court wisely decided that, in spite of the opinion of a responsible body of doctors, a trial judge must be free to decide whether or not disclosure of a risk is so necessary that no prudent doctor would fail to explain this to his or her patient.

We can see here the relation between duty of care and consent. This woman's prime concern was the protection of the sight in her good eye. In giving her consent she needed to be sure that no damage to her good eye might result. The possibility of damage to her good eye was the most important of her anxieties; it was central to her state of mind and therefore was relevant to the doctor's duty of care.

In a recent case in Wales, in which a patient underwent a revision decompression of his spine and a meningomyelocele repair, the surgeon failed to tell the claimant about the other treatment options and about the risks involved. His Honour Judge Graham Jones entered judgment for the claimant because, in his view, if the claimant had been given the information he would not have agreed to the surgery.[17]

Sometimes disclosure of information may pose a serious threat of psychologic detriment, i.e. damage, to the patient. In this case, the doctor may claim therapeutic privilege and withhold information. This concept, enunciated in the American court, was used in an English court *Re L (refusal of treatment)*[18] in the case of a patient whose sheltered lifestyle made it likely that she would not understand the seriousness of her situation.

In an interesting Canadian case, *Stoffberg* v. *Elliott*,[19] consent was not obtained as a result of an oversight, leading to an action of assault (not negligence). The judge directed the jury that consent to such surgical and medical treatment as the doctors might think necessary is not implied simply from the fact of going into hospital. On the other hand, consent may be implied for a physical examination, such as auscultation of the chest, by the act of undressing.

When oral consent is given by the patient the doctor must record: "This is what I said and this is what the patient (name) said."

When a written consent is obtained, the form must not be altered after it has been signed by the patient. The consent must be obtained before sedation, before the procedure and without coercion by the doctor. In the case of parental consent for children to receive treatment in England, the Children Act of 1989 confirms parental responsibility:

> ... all rights, duties, powers, responsibilities and authority which by law a parent has in relation to the child and his property ...

There are, however, limits to parental power.

The powers of a parent, to consent or not, exist for the good of the child, as seen through the eyes of the law. We see here both an ethical issue and a legal issue.

The judge Lord Eldon,[20] in the famous English case *Wellesley* v. *Duke of Beaufort* (1827), expressed the law using the best interests of the child approach, and in doing so expressed the "duty of care" to a child, which can never be expected to change:

> ... not to risk damage to children.

The law is designed to protect the best interests of the child, and the unchanging approach has been clearly restated in the American Supreme Court.[21] Particular notice may be taken of the religious views of the parent or surrogate when these affect the decision taken by the parent, surrogate or the person acting as a proxy for a child. These decisions may be respected unless, as in the case of a refused blood transfusion by a Jehovah's witness, they endanger the life of the child.

> Parents may become martyrs themselves but they are not free to make martyrs of their children.

A child may be considered competent to make decisions affecting his or her own care but, although a child's wishes may be properly held, they may nonetheless be ignored, as in *Re E*,[22] in which a 15-year-old boy, a Jehovah's witness, refused to have a blood transfusion. The judge accepted that his wish was honest and that he understood the consequences but ordered that the boy be given a blood transfusion:

> I respect this boy's faith but I cannot ignore the possibility that in later years he may suffer some diminution in his conviction.

It is important to consider those patients who by virtue of mental disease are unable to give a real consent. In *Re C (refusal of medical treatment)*,[23] Dr Eastman, a forensic psychiatrist, took the view that the ultimate conclusion should be reached by weighing in the scales the preservation of life against the autonomy of the patient. If the patient's capacity to decide is unimpaired autonomy weighs heavier, but the further capacity is reduced the lighter autonomy weighs.

Mental capacity was considered in a Law Commission consultation paper,[24] in which it was concluded that:

> ... a mentally disordered person should be considered unable to take the medical treatment decision ... if ... unable to understand an explanation in broad terms and simple language of the basic information for taking it, including information about the reasonably foreseeable consequences of taking or failing to take it, or is unable to retain the information for long enough to take an effective decision.

Of course, the reverse is also true, i.e. if a patient can understand the explanation, recognizes the consequences of the decision, and can retain the information long enough to make the decision, then, even if the patient is detained under the Mental Health Act 1983 autonomy demands that he or she has the right to take the treatment decision (enforcement of sections of the Mental Health Act 1983 other than sections 57 and 58 does not need consent, but section 63 overarches both when immediately necessary to save life).

In *Re C (refusal of medical treatment)*,[23] the claimant, years after admission to Broadmoor (a secure hospital prison in the UK) for a knife attack, developed gangrene and did not want an amputation. He had a small chance of survival without an amputation but preferred to risk dying now with two legs than have a few extra years with one cut off. The court complied with his wishes, respecting his right to self-determination and considered that, although he was a chronic paranoid schizophrenic, he had the capacity to make the treatment decision. However, the court would not have considered him to have capacity to decide for or against treatment for the mental condition that resulted in his admission to the hospital prison.

Clinical research presents a quite different problem, but the application of the principles of duty of care remain: there must be no coercion; there must be permission from the local ethics research committee; the implications, such as lack of predictability, must be discussed with the patient; research must never be against the interests of the patient; and, in the case of children and incompetent adults, it is wise to consult the Mental Incapacity Research Committee, the research councils, the professional bodies, and defense organizations.

It is also wise to obtain the patient's permission to publish the results obtained. There is evidence that some patients are distressed that information about them has been disclosed without their consent.[25,26]

The Human Rights Act 1998[27] came into force in the UK in 2000 and incorporates into the law of the UK the rights and freedoms expressed in the European Convention of Human Rights. It is likely that the Act will affect the day-to-day practice of medicine. Articles 2 and 3 confer absolute rights. The particular Articles likely to affect health care are:

- Article 2 concerns the right to life. An important issue is how the application of Article 2 will affect doctors' judgment as to whether or not to prolong the life of a dying or unconscious patient at all costs, or to withdraw hydration and nourishment from those in persistent vegetative state. How does it affect the rights of an unborn fetus? Will the English laws that allow abortions in the third trimester in cases of handicap be immune from the Act?[28] It is also feasible that Article 2 might be invoked in the case that death or injury to a patient could have been avoided by the presence of appropriate resources or a more senior doctor.[29]
- Article 3, the prohibition of inhuman and degrading treatment, has many possible ramifications that may affect research, particularly treatments that might be considered experimental. It may be possible to demonstrate the absence of consent if the patient is not told that the treatment is experimental. This Article may also influence the present discussions and decisions relating to euthanasia.
- Article 5, the right to liberty and security of the person, is qualified by exceptions that affect those of unsound mind.
- Article 8 concerns the right to privacy and family life. It is in Article 8 that we can identify the requirement that hospitals must provide patients with essential information about proposed treatments. Article 8 establishes the legal principle underlying a doctor's professional obligation to provide information essential for the patient's informed consent to the proposed treatment.

The rights afforded by the Human Rights Act 1998, apart from those conferred by Article 2 and 3, are not absolute, although the UK parliament will be able, if it chooses, to pass legislation restricting individual freedoms. The Act may nonetheless be expected to increase the opportunities for patients to obtain information.

As the interaction between common law decisions unfolds in the English-speaking jurisdictions and further interacts in the case of the UK with the European Human Rights Act 1998, it seems increasingly likely that "informed consent"' is likely to change from the view taken previously in the jurisdictions in the UK, i.e. "what the doctor decides you should know" to the interpretation more common in the USA, where patients are told "everything."[30]

In an excellent review[31] Andrew Smith has drawn attention to the relation between information, the use and choice of words, and the emotional effect of information and choice as follows:

> Doctors sometimes need to be reminded that words do not simply convey facts; they evoke feelings too. Although patient information is designed to provide information, the emotional effects that some words have on some people cannot be ignored. Second, information allows choice. We know that many more patients want to be informed about their treatment than want to make choices about their treatment,[32] but choice is impossible without information. Third, information is required to support the process of granting and obtaining consent.[33]

Conclusion

Consent may be summarized under three headings:

1 capacity, i.e. the ability to understand and remember the information given by the doctor;
2 information, i.e. to have confidence in the information and to understand the reasons for the proposed treatment;
3 voluntariness, i.e. consent must be given freely without coercion or fraud.

Consent must not be considered to be a single event. It is an agreement between the doctor and the patient. It is the result of an ethical and a legal process and defines the patient's state of mind. However, consent freely given may be equally freely withdrawn. The doctor must remember that to obtain consent for treatment is a component of the duty of care and is an ethical and legal responsibility.

In an excellent review[31] Andrew Smith has drawn attention to the relation between information, the use and choice of words, the emotional effect of information and choice as follows:

> Doctors sometimes need to be reminded that words do not simply convey facts; they evoke feeling too. Although patient information is delivered to provide information, the emotional effect that some words have on some people cannot be ignored. Second, information allows choice. We know that many more patients want to be informed about their treatment than want to make choices about that treatment,[32] but choice is impossible without information. Third, information is required to support the process of granting and obtaining consent.[33]

REFERENCES

1. *Donoghue* v. *Stevenson* [1932] AC 562.
2. *Caparo Industries plc* v. *Dickman* [1990] ALL ER 568 (HL).
3. *Bolam* v. *Friern Hospital Management Committee* [1957] 1 WLR 582.
4. Edelstein L. The Hippocratic Oath: text, translation and interpretation. In: Temkin Q, Tempkin CL (eds). *Ancient Medicine Selected Papers of Ludwig Edelstein*. Baltimore, MD: Johns Hopkins University Press, 1967: 3–64.
5. Veatch RM. *Abandoning Informed Consent*. Hastings Centre Report, March–April 1995.
6. *Encyclopedia of Bioethics*, s.v. "Nuremberg Code, 1946" quoted in the Hastings Centre Report (see reference 5).
7. *Chatterton* v. *Gerson* [1981] 1 ALL ER 25.
8. *Sidaway* v. *Board of Governors of the Bethlem Royal Hospital* [1985] 1 ALL ER 643.
9. Consultant suspended for not getting consent for cardiac procedure. *Br Med J* 1998; **316:** 955.
10. *Schloendorff* v. *The Society of the New York Hospital* 211 NY 125, 129, (1914).
11. *Reibl* v. *Hughes* 1980; 114 DLR(3d) 1 Can SC.
12. *Canterbury* v. *Spence*, 464 F.2d 772 (DC, 1972).
13. *Salgo* v. *Leland Stanford Jr, University Board of Trustees*, 317, P 2d 170 (Cal, 1957).
14. *E* v. *Australian Red Cross Society* 1991; ATPR 41085.
15. *F* v. *R* 1983; 33 SASR 198.
16. *Rogers* v. *Whittaker* (HCAus) [1993] 4 Med LR 79.
17. *Chinchen* v. *University Hospital Wales*, 8 November 2001. Reported in *Medical Litigation* 2001; December, p. 5.
18. *Re L (Refusal of Treatment)* Family Division. Quoted in *Medical Law Monitor* 1998; **5(10)**.
19. *Stoffberg* v. *Elliott* [1923] CPD 148, 46 Digest(Repl) 417,600.
20. *Wellesley* v. *Duke of Beaufort* [(1828) 2 B/I NS 124, 4ER 1078].
21. *Prince* v. *Massachusetts*, 321 US 158, 170 (1944).
22. *Re E (a minor)* 1990; 9 BMLR 1.
23. *Re C (refusal of medical treatment)* [1994] 22BML 13.
24. Law Commission No. 129 (1993) *Mentally Incapacitated Adults and Decision Making Medical Treatment*. London: HMSO.
25. Smith R. Informed consent: edging forwards (and backwards) *Br Med J* 1998; **316:** 949–51.
26. Snider D. Patient consent for publication and the health of the public. *JAMA* 1997; **278:** 624–6.
27. *Human Rights Act* 1998. London: Stationery Office, 1998.
28. Milne C. The Human Rights Act 1998. *J MDU* 1999; **15:** 18.
29. Human Rights. *The Personal and Medical Injuries Law Letter* 2000; July.
30. Why the human rights act matters to doctors. Definitions of informed consent and negligence may be challenged and lack of resources will not excuse poor care. *Br Med J* 2000; **321:** 780–1.
31. Smith AF. Patient information, risk and choice (editorial). *Anaesthesia* 2003; **58:** 409–11.
32. Coulter A. *The Autonomous Patient: Ending Paternalism in Medical Care*. London: The Nuffield Trust, 2002.
33. Department of Health. *Good Practice in Consent Implementation Guide: Consent to Examination or Treatment*. London: The Stationery Offfice, 2001.

FURTHER READING

Seeking Patient's Consent: The Ethical Considerations. London: General Medical Council.

Information and Consent for Anaesthesia. London: Association of Anaesthetists of Great Britain and Ireland.

The MDU's Guide to Consent to Treatment. London: MDU Services Ltd.

The Law Commission (Law Comm. no. 231) *Mental Incapacity*. Item 9 of the fourth programme of law reform: mentally incapacitated adults 1995. London: HMSO.

82

Stress and the anesthesiologist

MAIRE P SHELLY AND CHARLES E GRANGER

INTRODUCTION

We are all stressed; indeed, we need stress to develop both as individuals and as a species. We tend to think of stress as negative, producing psychological and physiologic ill health. Stress, however, also has a positive side, enabling us to respond effectively in new situations and to learn from them. Anesthesia and intensive care are regarded as stressful areas. In this chapter, we will review the current knowledge on the effects of stress on ourselves and on people with whom we work. We will also suggest ways of minimizing the harmful effects of stress.

WHAT IS STRESS?

There are many definitions of stress. At its simplest level, stress is a response to a new stimulus. The response, however, will vary with each individual and depends on previous experience and individual perceptions.

This is because we learn from each experience and interpret new experiences in terms of old ones. Stress is currently thought to be a dynamic system of stimulus and response that takes into account the individual's perception of the stimulus and that person's ability to respond effectively. Stress, therefore, may be positive and allow personal development and learning, but an individual unable to respond effectively to a stimulus will experience negative effects, or strain.

The response of the body to psychological stress is the same as its response to physiologic stress. Individuals taking their first parachute jump demonstrate a classic fight-or-flight response[1] with increased heart rate, respiratory rate, and plasma concentrations of epinephrine (adrenaline) and norepinephrine (noradrenaline). Psychological and physiologic stress also produce changes in the white cell count.[2,3] Immediately after a first parachute jump, the white cell count increases, but it then decreases to significantly below baseline values 1 h later. In conjunction with this change, the number and activity of natural killer cells increase as the stress response is at its height and then decrease to below baseline level.

Although a single stimulus is a stress, we usually reserve the term for a repeated or persisting stimulus that challenges us to adapt in some way. The stimulus represents a real or perceived danger and continues to trigger a fight-or-flight response after the first exposure. We adapt to the persisting stimulus by developing a resistance to it, so that the stimulus produces the same fight-or-flight response but we stop noticing it. If the stimulus persists further, however, then we become exhausted. This stage of exhaustion, or burnout, occurs when the fight-or-flight response to the stimulus becomes exaggerated or abnormal, so that we can no longer ignore it. The response is fundamentally fear or anger or a mixture of the two, but the manner of its expression will vary with the individual. Frequently observed responses are listed in Table 82.1.

So, we can summarize stress as being a response to a stimulus, but there are factors within each individual that mediate our response to that stimulus and will determine the outcome. Different people will find different stimuli stressful, and we all require different levels of stimulation in our lives. Stress is maximal when there is change, even an apparently pleasant one.[4] Maintaining sufficient stimulation to avoid boredom, without overstimulation to the stage of exhaustion, is the balance we need.

What we usually mean by the term "stress" is a pattern of strain produced by excessive urgency or pressure. This explains its negative connotation. Stress occurs when an individual perceives that there is an imbalance between the demands on them and their ability to meet these demands. Excessive stress – or insufficient stress – causes physical harm and may lead to psychological problems.[5] The harm may be the result not just of the stress itself but also the method of dealing with it. Although a fight-or-flight response is appropriate in the face of a physical threat, it may not be of use, or may even be harmful, if the threat is psychological or intellectual.

Table 82.1 *Responses to excessive stress*

Behavioral responses to excessive stress
Increased irritability or aggression
Anxiety or depression
Self-destructive or dangerous behavior
Obsessive or compulsive behavior, e.g. excessive working
Increased smoking
Increased alcohol intake
Increased drug usage
Physical responses to excessive stress
Altered heart rate or rhythm
Hypertension
Weight loss or gain
Sleep disturbance
Personal responses to excessive stress
Intellectual impairment
Poor concentration
Lack of judgment
Lack of creativity

STRESS IN PATIENTS

Patients about to undergo anesthesia and surgery are almost inevitably anxious. There are several reasons for this, but the underlying fears are most commonly fear of the unknown and fear of not being in control. These fears reflect the stress of the circumstances – the patient is in a new situation and does not know whether or not he or she can deal with it. Measures to reduce stress, therefore, should be aimed at reducing anxiety by making the experience less "new" and by giving the patient as much control as possible.

Fear of the unknown

Fear of the unknown can be reduced by giving the patient information and making the experience less unknown. For patients, a lack of information about anesthesia is common and may be a source of anxiety.[6] Giving the patient information about what to expect often reduces anxiety and stress around the time of surgery.[7] For instance, patients visited preoperatively by an operating room nurse had significantly less anxiety than a control group who had not been visited.[8]

However, it is not simply offering information that is important: patients' anxiety is reduced not simply by the information itself but by their satisfaction with the information.[9] This works both ways because patients given information about their treatment are also more satisfied with the treatment itself.[10] Satisfaction with information can be increased in several ways. Generally, patients are more satisfied with information delivered personally rather than indirectly, such as via a telephone call, although this is still better than no information.[11] The desire of any individual for information will depend on many different factors. For instance, different ethnic groups want both different amounts of information and different information. Any information given should be delivered in a way that respects cultural and religious differences. In general, women tend to want more information than men, divorcees more than single or married people, and individuals with a relative who has undergone surgery previously require more information than those without.[12]

Giving information may treat the cause of preoperative anxiety, but there are other ways of dealing with the anxiety itself, the most obvious being giving an anxiolytic drug preoperatively. Administration of the benzodiazepine midazolam, for instance, reduces both subjective anxiety levels[13] and the endocrine response to anxiety.[14] Relaxation techniques such as guided imagery are also effective, significantly reducing both preoperative and postoperative anxiety and analgesic requirements, and increasing satisfaction.[15]

Fear of lack of control

Fear of lack of control can be reduced by encouraging patients to participate in decisions about their management. Listening to their fears and understanding them is crucial to this. It may help patients to know that these fears are not uncommon and not as irrational as they may seem. Although reassurance may do little to reduce fear, it may still be useful, particularly if the patient is seen afterwards and the successful outcome re-emphasized.

An effective way of giving patients control of their pain and analgesia is to use a patient-controlled analgesia (PCA) machine. As well as providing effective analgesia, a PCA machine can reduce the levels of a patient's postoperative anxiety and stress.[16] Other drugs can be delivered in a similar way. A study of patient-controlled anxiolysis using a PCA machine to deliver midazolam or a placebo demonstrated that midazolam significantly reduced patient anxiety.[17] Simple measures also work: playing music and allowing the patient to choose the music played can reduce perioperative anxiety.[18,19]

Intensive care

Patients on the intensive care unit (ICU) are physiologically stressed by their illness. This is an appropriate response to their illness; indeed, we augment this response by infusing catecholamines. Etomidate was used for sedation in an attempt to reduce the level of physiologic stress experienced by critically ill patients. This regimen led to an increase in mortality from 25% to 69%.[20] The significant increase was the result of a direct suppression of adrenocortical function by etomidate. The immunosuppressant effect of this reduced the patients' ability to respond to the stress of their critical illness.

Critically ill patients cannot communicate effectively during their illness, so we can only establish their level of psychological stress retrospectively by talking with those who have survived similar situations. Several studies[21,22] have investigated patients' memories of intensive care. Among the memories there may be a high incidence of anxiety, depression, passivity, boredom, and fatigue – all stress-related symptoms. This information has been used to justify sedation, but perhaps these patients require support and sensitivity to their stress rather than sedation.

Boredom is an interesting stress-related symptom. Too much stimulation will lead to stress,[23] but too little stimulation is also stressful. Both sensory deprivation and sensory overload can cause the kind of psychological problems seen after discharge from the ICU.

The outcome of psychological stress in critically ill patients is difficult to assess. Some survivors of intensive care develop a post-traumatic stress disorder that requires treatment. Post-traumatic stress disorders can be minimized by allowing individuals to express their anxieties at the time. This is difficult in critically ill patients because of tracheal intubation and other bars to communication. There are few intensive care follow-up clinics, so patients are rarely followed up by the intensive care team after discharge. Studies from the intensive care follow-up clinics that do exist indicate high levels of anxiety and depression in their former patients.[24]

STRESS IN RELATIVES

The relatives of a patient in hospital are usually stressed also. Relatives often feel that they have no control over the circumstances; therefore, they may be even more stressed than the patients themselves. One study investigated stress levels in the relatives of patients undergoing routine, elective surgery, mostly as day cases.[25] Although this type of surgery is regarded as routine and straightforward by staff, the study demonstrated considerable anxiety and stress levels, particularly in older relatives and those with a lower educational level. The anxiety levels detected in relatives of patients undergoing routine elective surgery were higher than in relatives of patients undergoing coronary artery bypass surgery[26,27] and in mothers of hospitalized children.[28]

The parents of children about to undergo anesthesia and surgery are under stress: in one study, 47% had anxiety scores that indicated an anxiety-related illness.[29] The approach to reducing parental anxiety is similar to that for reducing anxiety in patients. Information plays a vital role, and allowing the parents and the child to watch a video of the procedure before induction of anesthesia reduces anxiety.[30]

On the ICU, the relatives of patients are, perhaps, the group most obviously and most negatively stressed. We understand this stress because relatives are faced with a new situation in a strange environment. The level of stress experienced by a patient's relatives is high – up to 75% have a Hospital Anxiety and Depression score that indicates the possibility of an anxiety-related illness. The level of stress is also related to the initial severity of the patient's illness.[31] Some stress is, therefore, based on fact and may be modified by accurate information. Support is vital for the relatives of critically ill patients.[31,32] The ICU staff can give effective support, but the effectiveness of support given by friends and other relatives will depend on their own response to the patient's illness.

During the course of a patient's critical illness, the stress levels of their family will change. Relatives have the highest stress score on the patient's admission to the ICU, and this score tends to reduce and then plateau as time goes on.[33] This is the stage of resistance as relatives become familiar with the ICU and its routines; the stimulus remains but becomes unnoticed. As patients recover, so the relatives' stress levels usually increase again. The stress score for relatives when the patient is recovering are significantly higher than for those when the patient's condition was unchanged or deteriorating. The reasons for this are unclear. We may, however, be discharging patients to less well-staffed wards where they are aware of and need their family's support, at a time when their families are least able to offer that support.[34] There is anecdotal evidence that the relationships patients have with their families undergo significant changes after an episode of intensive care. However, there is no information on the psychological sequelae of these changes.

STRESS IN STAFF

In contrast with the paucity of information on stress in patients and their relatives, data on staff stress, particularly nursing staff, are more widely available. Occupational stress in different groups within a hospital has been measured[35,36] using the occupational stress indicator.[37] Sources of stress for nursing staff included their working relationships, their career and level of achievement, and the structure of the organization, whereas doctors and managers tended to be less stressed by these factors. Both doctors and nurses were stressed with conflicts between home and work. The intensity of stress was reflected in the number of times coping strategies were used. The outcome of this stress at work was mostly in the areas of achievement and a perception of being valued. Managers and doctors had relatively high scores, indicating that they have achieved their aims and feel valued. Nurses and therapists had significantly lower scores than doctors and managers, indicating that they lack a sense of achievement and do not feel valued. Technicians had the lowest scores of all for achievement and a sense of being valued. This may reflect their lack of direct patient contact.[36]

ANESTHESIA

A career in medicine tends to attract conscientious individuals,[38] and many doctors have a type A personality[39] that renders them susceptible to stress. Anesthesiologists may suffer particularly from occupational stress.[40] Both male and female anesthesiologists have significantly higher rates of early retirement and death in post than other groups of doctors.[41,42] Trainees, especially female trainees, have high stress scores,[43] and both trainee and consultant anesthesiologists have one of the highest suicide rates among doctors, who themselves have one of the highest suicide rates in society.[42,44,45]

A survey of anesthesiologists indicated that 30% of anesthesiologists felt stressed a lot of the time, and 5% all the time. Although 33% were severely stressed, 7% described themselves as more than severely stressed.[5] The stressful elements for these anesthesiologists included:

- lack of control at work, 42%;
- administrative responsibilities, 42%;
- work/home conflict, 35%;
- strained professional relationships, 25%;
- work overload, 24%;
- money, 14%;
- teaching responsibilities, 6%;
- difficult work, 6%;
- peer review, 4%;
- potential litigation, 3%.

For anesthesiologists, there are particular risk factors for stress at work. Their work pattern is largely unpredictable and dependent on others. This may produce a permanently high level of anxiety. In addition, there is a risk that demands will be made on them which will force them to go beyond their real or perceived limits. The knowledge that any mistake may contribute to a patient's death is an ever-present anxiety.

The sources of stress will vary with the individual, but common traits appear. Stress is commonly caused by environmental, interpersonal, and personal factors (see Table 82.2), although there is significant overlap.[5]

INTENSIVE CARE UNIT STAFF

Intensive care units are often perceived as stressful places to work in, but this view is usually held by those working in other areas rather than ICU staff themselves. In fact, ICU nurses are more positive about their work than non-ICU nurses.[35] They feel that their work is more significant and more complex, and affords more opportunities than non-ICU nursing, but there is no difference in the amount of pressure they experience. Intensive care nurses feel that they have more autonomy and that their work is less task oriented and more patient oriented. Intensive care nurses also have more job satisfaction and, as an objective measure of this, they have a lower rate of absenteeism.

In general, individuals find a working environment with the right amount of stimulation for them; the problem is often controlling that stimulation so that it does not increase to stressful levels. The clinical aspects of health care are almost absent from lists of major stresses reported by nurses and doctors; organizational and interpersonal factors are consistently cited as the most stressful aspects of working in the health service.[36]

An investigation into occupational stress in staff on a single ICU[46] illustrates this point. Most clinical aspects of intensive care were not perceived as stressful, confirming that staff select for themselves an environment where they get what they need. Many work stressors constitute a satisfying challenge rather than a cause of distress; indeed,

Table 82.2 *Examples of sources of stress*

Environmental
Lack of control of work patterns
Unpredictable work pattern
Emergency work
Continuing medical education/examinations
High professional standards
Irregular working hours
Sleep deprivation
Interpersonal
Difficult relationships with colleagues
Time pressures
Marital problems
Bereavement
Illness
Unemployment
Personal
Impending litigation
Complaints
Time

unemployment and retirement are frequently associated with increased rates of stress-related problems.

In this study,[46] several factors influenced stress levels:

- The more senior the individual, the more stressed he or she was likely to be. A reason for this may be that more senior staff take on roles for which they do not feel adequately trained. Training increases competency and reduces stress. A lack of training adds to the stress of a job by increasing uncertainty and a sense of responsibility.
- Individuals with partners or children were less likely to be stressed. This is a finding reproduced in other studies. A possible reason is that people who have different roles may be satisfied in one role and that decreases the pressure on them to succeed in another role.
- Nurses appeared to have difficulty knowing where they fit in and how to get on in their career. Doctors have a greater sense of where they are in their career and what their role is. Nursing staff suffered from more stress than the medical staff, and this was reflected in a lower level of job satisfaction.

Compared with other groups, ICU staff suffer more stress from their perception of their career development and from organizational bureaucracy, they cope with stress in more emotional than logical ways, and they are less satisfied with the quality of their work relationships.[46]

Doctors and nurses are stressed by different factors. Many studies also suggest a lower level of stress in medical staff. Although this may be true, other evidence suggests the opposite.[5] One reason why such studies do not reflect stress in doctors may be their low response rate. Stress generates problems such that nonresponders may not reflect (or represent) responders. They may not have completed the questionnaire because of being busy or lack of time – signs of stress and exhaustion rather than a lack of stress. This low response rate may reflect a denial of stress rather than its absence.

Another possible reason for doctors failing to report stress is that more doctors than nurses have type A behavior patterns. Individuals with these patterns characteristically have a need to be in control and may have a high level of anxiety. They also obtain greater job satisfaction and perceive less pressure at work than those without type A characteristics. As they have an apparently protective effect on the individual's perception of stress, doctors usually report less occupational stress, and have less sick leave than nurses. Unfortunately, this protective effect is more apparent than real in the long term. Type A individuals characteristically suppress symptoms of fatigue and may sacrifice their own and their families' social needs to their pursuit of a successful career; a study of burnout in intensivists indicated this pattern.[47] Whereas the respondents had high scores for personal achievement, scores for emotional exhaustion were also high, indicating that burnout was common. Although finding some stress fulfilling, type A individuals may be exactly those people who have the least effective coping mechanisms for dealing with stress over a period of time. As a result, they are at risk of physical and psychological morbidity.[48]

OUTCOME OF STRESS

Although stress may have a positive outcome, with the individual learning from the experience, we often associate stress with a negative outcome. This occurs when the stressful stimulus, or stimuli, is repeated and the individual's usual coping strategies are either overcome or cannot be employed effectively. When the usual coping mechanisms are unavailable, negative mechanisms, such as excessive drug or alcohol intake or denial, may develop.[49]

The results of occupational stress in ICU staff have been studied. Reported personal responses include fatigue, increased irritability, increased smoking, and increased alcohol intake.[50,51] There is also a significant inverse correlation between stress levels and job satisfaction, and a strong association between individuals' perceived level of occupational stress and the amount of sick leave that they require.

In a survey of stress among doctors generally, the British Medical Association found significant consequences of stress;[52] 70% of respondents claimed that stress had adversely affected their work, with 37% saying it had impaired their judgment. Personal life had also been affected (see Table 82.3).

Addiction and substance abuse is a particular concern among anesthesiologists because of the availability of drugs.[53] In a survey of 247 training programs in anesthesia in the USA, 74% of programs had at least one suspected incident of drug dependence.[54] There were 334 identified cases of drug dependence in anesthesiologists, of whom 30 (9%) died of drug overdose. The physical consequences of stress are more difficult to quantify, but a Finnish study correlated a demanding work environment with a predisposition to an over-reactive blood pressure and a 10–40% greater thickening of the carotid arteries over 4 years.[55]

STRESS MANAGEMENT

Some causes of stress can be removed, or the individual removed from them. More often, the individual's reaction to the stressor is addressed. Stress may be reduced by modifying or controlling the response to stress or giving the individual new resources so that a greater range of responses is available to them.

Although reducing the stress of a particular circumstance is important, it is also vital to learn to manage stress better in the future. Identifying the nature, causes, and effects of stress will help individuals to recognize stress at an earlier stage and to manage it more effectively.

Modifying the response to stress

A starting point for modifying individuals' response to stress is to help them toward a realization that they are stressed and that they can change their response to the situation that produced this. Developing self-esteem is often an important part of the process. It is also important that individuals have a realistic concept of their area of influence. Some things they can change and some things they cannot, and the only person they can change is themselves.

The "macho" culture within medicine is responsible for the illusion that all doctors should be able to do everything. This culture also makes it more difficult for doctors to ask for and receive help. Doctors are fallible and human, like everybody else. Reviewing the pressures to perform to perfection at all times and to avoid failure at all costs may be helpful.

Developing coping strategies

The way we deal with stress is the result of a complex interaction of factors, including our own personality and coping skills, our experience of previous stressors and current levels of fatigue, distraction, or frustration, our social and occupational support, and, not least, the nature of the stressor itself. People feel stressed when their own coping strategies

Table 82.3 *Effects of stress*

Difficulty sleeping	70%
Loss of libido	40%
Physical illness	35%
Increased alcohol intake	35%
Contemplated suicide	21%
Drug misuse	4%

are inadequate. Developing existing strategies and creating new ones is an essential part of stress management.

Communication skills

Communicating effectively with others is a vital stress management skill. Many stressful circumstances arise because of avoidable misunderstandings.

Other useful communication skills are:

- assertiveness;
- negotiation;
- saying "no;"
- dealing with aggression;
- conflict resolution;
- dealing with anxiety and fear.

Time management

Circumstances frequently become stressful because of a perceived lack of time. Time management techniques may contribute to reduce the effect of this cause. The most important aspect of time management is to identify goals by maintaining vision and by setting priorities.

Relationships

Although the relationships established at work are important, the achievement of personal relationships is essential for stress management. Talking through a situation with somebody removed from it can put the situation into perspective. In addition, successful personal relationships make the need for successful work relationships less acute.

Hobbies

Preserving personal time is vital as this allows a balance in life to be maintained and stress reduced. An enjoyable hobby provides an area of personal control as well as acting as a diversion. Physical activity and relaxation may also encourage physical health. Achieving a balance between work, exercise, relaxation, and personal development will replace stress with well-being.

CONCLUSION

Stress is not uncommon and therefore it is essential to manage stress effectively. The hospital environment is stressful and the people, staff, and patients in a hospital will inevitably be stressed. Effective clinical management often includes managing a crisis or emergency. Staff may be familiar with the emergency plan, but patients and their relatives will not. Dealing with stressed people is stressful in itself.

It is important to accept that others are stressed and to be tolerant of this. At the same time, it is important to support rather than rescue the stressed individual. This maintains perspective. Ultimately, only the individual themselves can solve their problems – others can offer help and support but not long-term solutions. A stressed individual may come to depend on a rescuer; this does not manage their stress and but does increase the stress for the rescuer.

Perhaps most important is the need to acknowledge our own stress. If we are unaware of our own stressors, we cannot help or support others effectively and this may affect our clinical management. As we become more aware of our own stress patterns, so we learn to manage them more effectively and to help our colleagues by showing them how to manage stress.

REFERENCES

1. Schedlowski M, Jacobs R, Alker J, *et al.* Psychophysiological, neuroendocrine and cellular immune reactions under psychological stress. *Neuropsychobiology* 1993; **28:** 87–90.
2. Schedlowski M, Jacobs R, Stratmann G, *et al.* Changes of natural killer cells during acute psychological stress. *J Clin Immunol* 1993; **13:** 119–25.
3. Pederson BK, Tvede N, Hansen FR, *et al.* Modulation of natural killer cell activity in peripheral blood by physical exercise. *Scand J Immunol* 1988; **27:** 673–8.
4. Burke RJ. Occupational and life stress and family: conceptual frameworks and research findings. *Int Rev Appl Physiol* 1986; **35:** 347–69.
5. Association of Anaesthetists. *Stress in Anaesthetists.* London: Association of Anaesthetists, 1997.
6. Kureshi J, Rocke AD, Tariq AQ. Perioperative knowledge and anxiety score of patients undergoing surgery. *Middle East J Anesthesiol* 1995; **13:** 325–33.
7. Dodds F. Access to the coping strategies. Managing anxiety in elective surgical patients. *Prof Nurse* 1993; **9:** 45–52.
8. O'Sullivan S, Richardson M. Preoperative interviews: a nursing intervention to reduce patients' anxiety. *Aust J Adv Nurs* 1991; **8:** 3–5.
9. Williams OA. Patient knowledge of operative care. *J R Soc Med* 1993; **86:** 328–31.
10. Vallerand WP, Vallerand AH, Heft M. The effects of postoperative preparatory information on the clinical course following third molar extraction. *J Oral Maxillofac Surg* 1994; **52:** 1165–71.
11. Leske JS. Intraoperative progress reports decrease family members' anxiety. *Assoc Operating Room Nurses J* 1996; **64:** 428–36.
12. Kain ZN, Kosarussavadi B, Hernandez-Conte A, *et al.* Desire for perioperative information in adult patients: a cross sectional study. *J Clin Anesth* 1997; **9:** 467–72.
13. Kain ZN, Mayes LC, Wang SM, *et al.* Parental presence during induction of anesthesia versus sedative premedication: which intervention is more effective? *Anesthesiology* 1998; **89:** 1147–56.
14. Kiefer RT, Weindler J, Ruprecht KW. The endocrine response after oral premedication with low dose midazolam for intraocular surgery in retrobulbar anaesthesia. *Eur J Ophthalmol* 1998; **8:** 239–45.
15. Tusek DL, Church JM, Strong SA, *et al.* Guided imagery: a significant advance in the care of patients undergoing elective colorectal surgery. *Dis Colon Rectum* 1997; **40:** 172–8.
16. Chumbley GM, Hall GM, Salmon P. Patient-controlled analgesia: an assessment by 200 patients. *Anaesthesia* 1998: **53:** 216–21.
17. Egan KJ, Ready LB, Nessly M, Greer BE. Self administration of midazolam for postoperative anxiety: a double blinded study. *Pain* 1992; **49:** 3–8.
18. Augustin P, Hams AA. Effect of music on ambulatory surgery patients' preoperative anxiety. *Assoc Operating Room Nurses J* 1996; **63:** 753–8.
19. Evans MM, Rubio PA. Music: a diversionary therapy. *Todays OR Nurse* 1994; **16:** 17–22.
20. Watt I, Ledingham IMcA. Mortality amongst multiple trauma patients admitted to an intensive therapy unit. *Anaesthesia* 1984; **39:** 973–81.
21. Bion JF. Sedation and analgesia in the intensive care unit. *Hosp Update* 1988; **14:** 1272–86.
22. Gibbons CR, Brown DJ, Shelly MP. Patient memories of and satisfaction with intensive care. *Clin Intensive Care* 1993; **4:** 222–5.
23. Kam PCA, Kam AC, Thompson JF. Noise pollution in the anaesthetic and intensive care environment. *Anaesthesia* 1994; **49:** 982–6.
24. Jones C, Macmillan RR, Griffiths RD. Providing psychological support for patients after critical illness. *Clin Intensive Care* 1994; **5:** 176–9.
25. Leske J S. Anxiety of elective surgical patients' family members. *Assoc Operating Room Nurses J* 1993; **57:** 1091–103.
26. Lepczyk M, Raleigh E H, Rowley C. Timing of preoperative patient teaching. *J Adv Nurs* 1990; **15:** 654–60.
27. Lepczyk M, Raleigh E H, Rowley C. Significant others benefit from preoperative information. *J Adv Nurs* 1990; **15:** 941–5.
28. Vulcan BM, Nikulich-Barrett T. The effect of selected information on mothers' anxiety levels during their children's hospitalisations. *J Paediatr Nurs* 1988; **3:** 97–102.
29. Thompson N, Irwin MG, Gunawardene WMS, Chan L. Pre-operative parental anxiety. *Anaesthesia* 1996; **51:** 1008–12.
30. Karl HW, Pauza KJ, Heyneman N, Tinker DE. Preanesthetic preparation of pediatric outpatients: the role of a videotape for parents. *J Clin Anesth* 1990; **2:** 172–7.

31. Jones C, Griffiths RD. Social support and anxiety levels in relatives of critically ill patients. Link between support networks and physical anxiety. *Br J Intensive Care* 1995; **5:** 44–7.
32. Jones C, Hussey RM, Griffiths RD. Social Support in the ICU? *Br J Intensive Care* 1991; **1:** 66–9.
33. Halm M A, Titler MG, Kleiber C, *et al.* Behavioural responses of family members during critical illness. *Clin Nurs Res* 1993; **2:** 414–37.
34. Hickey M L, Leske JS. Needs of families of critically ill patients. *Crit Care Nurs Clin North Am* 1992; **4:** 645–9.
35. Boumans NPG, Landeweerd JA. Working in an intensive or non-intensive care unit: does it make any difference? *Heart Lung* 1994; **23:** 71–9.
36. Rees D, Cooper CL. Occupational stress in health services workers in the UK. *Stress Med* 1992; **8:** 79–90.
37. Rees D W, Cooper CL. A criterion orientated validation study of the OSI outcome measures on a sample of health service employees. *Stress Med* 1991; **7:** 125–7.
38. Vickers MD, Reeve P. Selection methods in medicine: a case for replacement surgery? *J R Soc Med* 1990; **83:** 541–3.
39. Friedman M, Roseman RH. Type A behaviour pattern: its association with coronary heart disease. *Ann Clin Res* 1971; **3:** 300.
40. Smith WWDA. The anaesthetist's environment. *Proc R Soc Med* 1974; **67:** 987–9.
41. McNamee R, Keen RI, Corkhill CM. Morbidity and early retirement among anaesthetists and other specialists. *Anaesthesia* 1987; **42:** 133–140.
42. Neil HA, Fairer JG, Coleman MP, Thurston A, *et al.* Mortality among male anaesthetists in the UK. *Br Med J* 1987; **295:** 360–2.
43. Greenwell SK. Stress in trainee anaesthetists. *Anaesthesia* 2000; **55:** 203–5.
44. Helliwell PJ. Suicide amongst anaesthetists-in-training. *Anaesthesia* 1983; **38:** 1097.
45. Richings JC, Khara GS, McDowell M. Suicide in young doctors. *Br J Psychol* 1986; **149:** 475–8.
46. Goodfellow A, Varnam R, Rees D, *et al.* Staff stress on the intensive care unit: a comparison of doctors and nurses. *Anaesthesia* 1997; **52:** 1037–41.
47. Guntupalli KK, Fromm RE. Burnout in the internist–intensivist. *Intensive Care Med* 1966; **22:** 625–30.
48. Friedman M, Roseman RH. Type A behaviour pattern: Its association with coronary heart disease. *Ann Clin Res* 1971; **3:** 300.
49. Sexton JB, Thomas EJ, Helmreich RL. Error, stress and teamwork in medicine and aviation: cross sectional surveys. *Br Med J* 2000; **320:** 745–9.
50. Lewis K F, Poppe S, Twomey J, Peltier G. Survey of perceived stressors and coping strategies among burn unit nurses. *Burns* 1990; **16:** 109–12.
51. Adomat R, Killingworth A. Care of the critically ill patient: the impact of stress on the use of touch in the intensive therapy units. *J Adv Nurs* 1994; **19:** 912–22.
52. Coulson J. Stress in doctors. *BMA News Rev* 1996; **April:** 24.
53. Editorial. *Anaesthesia* 1970; **25:** 163–4.
54. Ward CF, Ward GC, Saidman U. Drug abuse in anesthesia training programs. A survey 1970 through 1980. *JAMA* 1983; **250:** 922–5.
55. Everson S, Lynch JW, Chesney MA, *et al.* Interaction of workplace demands and cardiovascular reactivity in progression of carotid atherosclerosis: population based study. *Br Med J* 1997: **314:** 553–8.

83

Bereavement care

CHARLES E GRANGER AND MAIRE P SHELLY

Grief is one of the most disturbing emotions that we can experience. Some of the greatest monuments of human history, and the most enduring works of literature and music, have been created in attempts to alleviate the grief of bereavement, to deny the permanence of death, or to celebrate the memory of the dead. From the pyramids to the Taj Mahal, and from *King Lear* to Mozart's *Requiem*, mankind has tried to find meaning in the chaos of grief, and the emotion that these works can still generate should caution us to pay careful attention to the persisting importance of the grief process in a more secular and scientific age.

A sense of bereavement accompanies any perception of loss, be it death, a physical loss such as after a mastectomy or amputation[1] or psychological loss such as infertility,[2] the loss of career potential, or forced emigration.[3] These are universal experiences, which may be associated with profound physical and psychological consequences, and yet it is only recently that medical schools have started to include the topics of bereavement and the importance of grieving in the medical curriculum. The late arrival of these subjects onto the medical syllabus should not be confused with a lack of importance.

OUR RELATIONSHIP WITH DEATH

In spite of the universality of bereavement and our almost daily involvement in the care of patients with life-threatening disease, most of us remain strangely uninformed – and possibly even somewhat apprehensive – about dealing with the bereaved and the grieving process.[4] The possible reasons for this lack of involvement are legion, but it has been forcefully argued that the progressive ascendance of the scientific process in the development of medicine has led to a change in our relation with death.[5] Once death was depicted as the constant companion to life, or as a force of nature with which one did battle, whereas now death is typified as a failure of medicine or an outrageous intrusion upon our right to a long and healthy life. The diminished importance of the rituals surrounding death has been accompanied by an increasing dislocation between the "social" death of withdrawal from society into hospitals or hospices and the subsequent actual physical death. This progressive medicalization of death has resulted in medical staff having an ever more important role in caring for the newly bereaved, without any corresponding increase in training to meet this role. As a consequence, we are not in a position to provide the support our patients and their families need when they are at their most vulnerable. There is now ample information available to allow us to rectify this deficit.

THE STUDY OF BEREAVEMENT

The first scientific study of bereavement was published by Lindemann in 1944 in a paper which studied the psychology of bereavement in the survivors of a huge fire in a night-club and in the relatives of war casualties.[6] This paper anticipated many themes which have subsequently become the focus of further research, including the symptoms of normal and abnormal grief, the possibility of predicting an abnormal grief reaction in some individuals, the concepts and importance of "grief work" and "anticipatory grief," and the role of psychiatrists in treating "morbid grief."

This first methodical study into the grieving process led to the recognition that grief was a distinct clinical entity, subject to measurable influences by both harmful and helpful external factors. Further research into these factors and into the individual variation in the grief process followed, and attention was directed at trying to alleviate those elements – such as pain, isolation and ignorance – that increased the suffering of the patient and his or her family around the time of death. This approach contributed to the development of the specialty of palliative care and the growth of the hospice movement and, from the methods of pain control developed by these specialists, the subsequent promotion of better pain management throughout the health service.

THE GRIEF PROCESS

Individuals' own experience of grief is unique to them and, fundamentally, unknowable by others.[7] There is, however, some commonality in the process by which grief develops over time during the normal grieving process. The initial descriptions portrayed the grief process as a series of seemingly linked stages, each leading on to the next in a linear fashion, from the first eruption of grief to its eventual resolution. Many different terms and conceptual frameworks have subsequently been used to describe the stages in this process, with the emphasis variously placed on the central role of the family,[8] the importance of cultural and societal rites,[9] or the personal history of the bereaved.[10] What all these different perspectives have in common is the central theme that the personal experience of grief changes over time. The time course over which this transition develops will vary between individuals, but over a period of years the grief process finally evolves into a state of resolution and closure, allowing bereaved individuals to come to terms with their loss, and to concentrate once again on their own needs and personal development.

The normal grief process is, of course, far from linear and sequential. It comprises many conflicting emotions and thoughts that may disappear and reappear over time, coexist, persist for lengthy periods, or occur in pangs. The individual may resist them, suppress them, or succumb to them but, as time goes on, their intensity will slowly wane, until anniversaries or other triggers bring them suddenly back to the fore. The components of this process have been described by many authors[7,11–13] but have been usefully divided into four phases of numbing, yearning, disorganization, and then reorganization.[14] Although these phases describe an apparent sequence of anxiety, waxing and waning anger, pining, and depression followed by adaptation to the new reality, there may be little progress through these stages with time,[15] or the bereaved individual may pass from one to the other nonsequentially or with some abruptness.

Whatever terms are used, the fundamental components of the grief process are the same, and have been described as a series of "grief tasks" which must be completed before the period of grief can be brought to closure.[16] These tasks are, in essence, a combination of looking backwards to what has been lost, sorrow and searching for what has gone, and, intertwined with both, a conflicting urge to look forwards to whatever is to come. To some extent, these two conflicting aspects persist not only throughout the grief process, but also from then on, and the success with which individuals balance these two conflicting impulses determines their success in weathering the trauma of grief and achieving resolution. Far from being unique to humans, similar patterns of grief have been described in animals,[17] but, in contrast to animals, the human expression of grief is overlaid with a highly complex and an individual mosaic of personal beliefs, cultural norms, and religious traditions, which may combine to shape the grieving process in ways a spectator may find difficult to understand.[10]

COMPLICATED GRIEF

Most individuals will manage to work their own way through the grief process without ever needing assistance from outside their family or immediate social contacts. However, in a substantial minority, these immediate supports are either not available or are inadequate for the task. This may occur either when a vulnerable individual is unable to deal with a "normal" bereavement or when the circumstances of the loss are so awful as to try even the most well-adapted individual beyond the limits of tolerance. In either case, if the grieving process is not developing normally, the bereaved individual is said to have developed "complicated grief," with potentially grave implications for his or her own long-term morbidity or mortality. The term "complicated grief" is used here to indicate any bereavement that is not proceeding normally, rather than a precise diagnostic term, although efforts are now being made to define diagnostic criteria.[18] These criteria include features such as preoccupation with the deceased, disbelief in the death with excessive avoidance of reminders of the deceased, prolonged loss of interest in personal activities, and persisting pangs of severe distress more than a year after death has occurred. Other psychological disorders may also occur at the time of bereavement, such as postbereavement depression, anxiety states, or post-traumatic stress disorder; these can usually be differentiated from complicated grief, or from normal bereavement, by the clinical presentation.[15] Postbereavement depression may, of these, be the most common, being evident in up to 25% of bereaved 5 months after the loss occurred and still present in 60% of these patients over 10 months later.[15] The hallmark symptoms of depression, such as the loss of self-esteem, psychomotor retardation, hallucinations, or feelings of guilt not expressly associated with the deceased can help to differentiate this condition from that of complicated grief.[19] When assessing the way in which the bereaved display their grief it is always necessary to try to interpret this in the light of the bereaved individual's own cultural and religious traditions, which may be very different from the Western norms.[20]

In many cases, the development of complicated grief can be anticipated from a knowledge of the personality of the bereaved ("intrinsic factors;" Table 83.1) or from the particular circumstances of the death ("extrinsic factors;" Table 83.2).

Risk factors for complicated grief

The personal risk factors associated with an increased risk of complicated grief are in many cases those that would normally be associated with psychiatric vulnerability.[24] Even in the absence of psychiatric risk factors, two personality traits associated with complicated grief have been described. These are "avoiders," who tend to repress their immediate reaction to bereavement, and "sensitizers," who develop intense grief that may persist or develop into obsessive preoccupation with the deceased.[25] In some cases, however, the link between an increased risk of complicated grief and the circumstances of the bereavement is more obscure.

"Intrinsic" factors

Ambivalence is present to some degree within all relationships. The flux of emotions within a relationship will change over time, but the threat of impending death will usually allow those within the relationship to resolve the ambivalence and achieve some form of acceptance and stability. If a sudden death denies bereaved individuals the opportunity to achieve this resolution prior to their relative's death, they may be left with additional feelings of guilt or unresolved anger to deal with at the start of their bereavement. This combination has been associated with a greater sense of loss and evidence of distress at the time of bereavement, although its association with a long-term complicated grief reaction is less certain.[26]

Dependency may occur either when the bereaved individual had a particularly dependent relationship on the deceased or, by contrast,

Table 83.1 *Intrinsic factors increasing the risk of a poor outcome to bereavement*

Low self-esteem
Previous significant psychiatric or medical disorder
Previous suicide attempt or suicidal threats
Poor social or family support
Ambivalent or dependent relationship with the deceased
Previous unresolved loss
Cultural isolation – for example following emigration
Other simultaneous significant life stresses

Table 83.2 *Extrinsic factors increasing the risk of a poor outcome to bereavement*

Death of a child
Death of a parent during childhood
Sudden or early death
Violent death
Stigmatized death – suicide,[21] alcohol, AIDS
Death for which the bereaved feels some responsibility[22]
Failure to find the body of the deceased[23]
"Unrecognized death," e.g. miscarriage or termination
Grief dysequilibrium
Death of a twin
Multiple death
Insensitively handled death

when he or she had assumed the role of compulsive caregiver. In either case, the survivors are at increased risk of a complicated grief reaction – in the former, they may not believe that they will be able to manage after the death of the caregiver; in the latter, they may suffer a poorly focused loss of self-worth at the same time as their bereavement.[27]

Previous unresolved loss, such as the loss of a parent during childhood or adolescence, may result in a complicated grief reaction during a subsequent bereavement, though the association may not be apparent to the bereaved individual.[28]

Just as many of the "intrinsic" factors associated with complicated grief are intuitive, many of the "extrinsic" factors may also be predicted easily. Of these, the death of a child is the most obvious. Others may be less predictable, but many seem to be associated with the loss of an opportunity for "anticipatory grief" (see below).

"Extrinsic" factors

Death of a child

The loss of a child is almost inconceivably awful.[29] This is obviously true when the child was previously healthy, but it remains true even when the child already suffered from severe illness or significant handicap, or when the loss occurs prior to the child's birth through miscarriage or stillbirth. In these last examples, society's more ambivalent approach toward the death can make it much more difficult for the bereaved parent to grieve properly or even, in the case of a miscarriage, gain recognition that bereavement has occurred.[30]

Bereavement during childhood

The death of a parent during childhood or adolescence is also particularly traumatic and has been linked to the development of psychiatric disorders. The risk of subsequent mental illness is increased up to five-fold,[31] especially following other life stresses, and there is an increased risk of attempted suicide in adulthood.[32] It is therefore of particular importance that appropriate and knowledgeable support is available for bereaved children, and that those who deal with these highly vulnerable individuals are aware of the importance of early intervention in those children for whom a complicated grief process appears more likely.

The traditional approach to a bereaved child seems to be directed at hiding the reality of an actual or approaching death from the child, in the belief that in some way the child is thereby being protected from the associated pain and suffering. This is seldom appropriate. By the age of 5 most children can distinguish between a temporary absence and the permanent separation of death, and can understand that the dead are in some way essentially different from the living.[22] Before this age, any separation from an important individual will evoke anxiety and protest, followed by forms of mourning such as bed-wetting or refusal to eat. Older children become able to understand the physical changes that follow death, and may wish – and should be allowed, in the absence of gross disfigurement at the time of death – to see the body of the deceased. It is more appropriate, therefore, to explain the reality of the approaching death to the child using language and terminology appropriate to the child's age, and avoiding the use of euphemisms, which, rather than soften the blow of the essential news, may simply serve to confuse the child about what is actually happening. Seeing the body – and attending the funeral – has the added advantage that it removes any doubt in the child's mind that the individual has really died, rather than simply "gone away," as well as helping to disabuse the child of what may have been far more frightening imaginings about the appearance of the dead.[22]

Just as the significance of a particular adult's death will be different for different individuals, depending on their relationship with the deceased,[33] so the impact of a child's death on his or her siblings will be affected by their relationship during life and by the way in which the family as a whole deal with the reality of the death.[34] Quite apart from the different dynamics within the family group, children's displays of grief will also be influenced by their age and development. In the very young, grief may present as passivity, whereas older children may exhibit behavioral problems, hallucinations – "seeing ghosts" – or poor progress at school.[22] The child's urge to "protect" a surviving parent from his or her own distress may induce children to hide their grief and give the mistaken impression that they have been relatively unaffected by the death. In reality, some studies suggest that normal bereaved children may retain signs of emotional disturbance for up to 2 years after a death, and in one study 37% of a group of 38 bereaved children had evidence of a major depressive disorder a year after bereavement.[35] Similarly, all that is actually achieved by trying to hide the truth about the terminal illness of a family member is to deny the child the opportunity to prepare for the approaching death, which may serve to increase the severity of the child's subsequent grief process rather than diminish it.[36]

Other extrinsic factors

Stigmatized death, which may occur either when the deceased is perceived to be somehow deserving of their fate or does not "merit" expressions of regret,[37] may reduce the social tolerance of the survivor's expression of grief, or may introduce an unhelpful element of guilt to the grief process. The same difficulties apply if the bereaved individual has suffered a loss that is not apparent to others, such as the loss of an early or concealed pregnancy, even if the loss is due to a deliberate act such as termination of pregnancy.[38]

Grief disharmony has been described in couples following perinatal death, when one partner – usually the woman – is perceived to suffer more acute grief than the other.[39] While some dismiss this suggestion, it is nevertheless true that society places different expectations on the different sexes, which may influence the way in which the individuals express their grief both externally and within the partnership.[40] This disharmony may be so acute as to lead to serious marital difficulties in up to one-third of couples suffering the loss of an infant.[41]

Multiple deaths can mean either a number of deaths occurring within the same family or the death of an individual in an event in which many others have died. In the case of the former, the bereaved may find themselves creating a "hierarchy of loss," so that, for example, the loss of a child may be of much greater significance than the loss of the child's grandparents in the same accident.[42] The consequent particular focus on one death at the expense of another may subsequently make it difficult to mourn, and achieve closure of, the "lesser" death. In the case of one death among many deaths, the individuality of the bereaved may be lost in the enormity of the disaster and the ensuing "public ownership" of the death, and, even though support mechanisms are commonly instituted after such a disaster, these may not be adequate to enable the bereaved to regain "ownership" of the death and the re-establishment of a normal bereavement.

The death of a twin is also associated with an increased risk of a complicated grief process. After a perinatal twin death, there may be conflicting demands on the parents to celebrate the birth of one twin while mourning the death of the other, or a surviving twin may feel pressurized to assume unrealistic expectations to "make up" for the sibling's death.[43]

Consequences of complicated grief

Whatever the particular circumstances of the death, if bereaved individuals are unable to express their grief, or are unable to bring their grief to an eventual resolution ("chronic grief"), they are at significant risk of subsequent physical or psychological morbidity. Although there is no persuasive evidence that uncomplicated bereavement is associated with an increased risk of illness or death in the bereaved, there is increasing evidence that this relationship does exist in complicated grief. A recent study concerning the effects of the loss of a spouse[27] has avoided many of the problems of study design or spousal comorbidity that have troubled earlier work,[44] and demonstrated that if symptoms of severe grief persist for 6 months after death there is an increased probability of significant health problems for the subsequent 18 months, as well as an increased risk of suicide or other symptoms of psychological distress. These findings are supported by other authors.[45]

As knowledge of the risks associated with complicated grief grows, it has been recognized that clinicians should aim to adopt a more proactive approach toward identifying those at the greatest risk.[46] While it is true that in most cases this approach will rely on intuition and consideration of factors such as those above, increasing efforts are being directed at developing objective scales to permit the prediction of a complicated grief reaction from questionnaires or interviews conducted either at the time of the patient's death or after the diagnosis of terminal disease.[12] Some of these scales, such as the Perinatal Grief Scale,[47] are applicable only to specific groups, but many others are of general application to the bereaved, although often these are of more use as research tools than in the day-to-day assessment of the bereaved.[48–50]

Avoiding complicated grief

Complicated grief may be associated with a considerable assortment of significant physical and psychological disorders in the years following bereavement, including an increased risk of heart disease, cancer, and premature death. These represent a serious, but avoidable, threat to the health, well-being, or even life of the bereaved.[51] If these threats are to be avoided, they must first be anticipated. This, in turn, implies that those who deal regularly with the bereaved should have some appreciation of the importance of encouraging a normal bereavement. Important steps in this process are elaborated below.

Anticipatory grief

Death occurring after a period of chronic disease is, predictably enough, associated with a lower incidence of complicated grief than unexpected death. This is not only because the patient has had the opportunity to prepare for death, but also because the family members have had time to prepare themselves mentally for their forthcoming bereavement.[52] This period of "anticipatory grief" can be extremely valuable for the individuals involved, but may be unintentionally lost if a diagnosis of terminal disease is withheld for a period to "protect" patients or their families from bad news. Although patients may have a variable interest in the details of their illness, information can be presented in a way which permits patients to ask for more facts if they wish, without being confronted with information they do not wish to receive. As Kübler-Ross demonstrated, dying patients can benefit greatly from being able to talk through their fears and problems, and may even come to regard their illness as a means to help others if the opportunity is presented to them.[53] Furthermore, dying patients may achieve the same sense of acceptance about their future as is possible for bereaved individuals at the resolution of their grief process.[13]

GIVING BAD NEWS

Medical professionals owe their first duty of confidentiality to their patients. This remains true even when the patient is dying, so patients' wishes should be respected when it comes to informing others about their illness. Although this seldom presents a problem in the context of intensive care, it nevertheless remains true that the critically ill have as much right to privacy as any other patient, whether in response to questions from family members, colleagues, or journalists. It can be easy to forget this fundamental duty when dealing with the victims of newsworthy accidents or illnesses. In the absence of clear instruction to the contrary, however, it often falls to medical staff to inform family members that a patient is not expected to survive. The way in which this news is delivered can play a pivotal role in the course of the bereavement. It is often the "soft" details about how and where the news was given that provide the focus for subsequent distressing images for the bereaved, rather than the "hard" medical details about the cause or circumstances of the patient's death.[29] In particular, due consideration should be given to the following points:

- when to give bad news;
- who gives bad news;
- where to give bad news;
- how to give bad news.

When to give bad news

Bad news should be given as soon as possible, to give family members the time that they will need to prepare themselves for the forthcoming death and to allow them to benefit from anticipatory grief. The need to deliver the news as soon as practical should not, however, be at the cost of delivering bad news if any close family member is absent or when there is insufficient time or information available to deliver the news completely and in an unhurried fashion. The preparation for giving this news should include, if possible, some appreciation of the patient's or family's particular religious or cultural requirements. These may include a resistance against a hospital postmortem or organ donation, or the need to involve the family in washing or laying out their relative after death has occurred, or to arrange burial before the Sabbath.[54]

Who gives bad news

To ensure that information about a poor prognosis carries the stamp of authority, as well as to avoid giving the impression that the outcome might have been different if more experienced staff had been present, bad news should be given by, or in the presence of, the most senior staff involved in the patient's care. It is important that another member of staff is also present when bad news is given, preferably one who has had the time to develop a more personal level of contact with the family than is usually possible for senior medical staff, both to provide comfort to the family and to be a witness to what was said. This role is usually most usefully filled by a member of the nursing staff.[4]

Where to give bad news

Sensitive discussions with the families of the dying or with the newly bereaved should be conducted in an area expressly designed for that purpose, rather than in a room "borrowed" for the event. The room should be private, welcoming, and comfortable, with enough space for a reasonably sized family to collect. A number of minimum comforts should be available, including tea and coffee, a phone, washing facilities, and a room for overnight use. Children's toys should also be available to help emphasize that children should not be excluded from contact with the dying, and the family should be permitted and encouraged to remain in the room, and retain their privacy, once the bad news has been delivered.[55]

How to give bad news

It is important to consider the impact of not just the words we use, but also the message we give with our body language while we are giving bad news to a family. A doctor who informs the family while standing, for instance, may appear to be less involved and approachable than one who gives the same news while sitting down. Equally, if the circumstances of the patient's death are personally distressing it is not necessarily appropriate to try and disguise the distress behind a mask of professional detachment. Indeed, it has been suggested that when families realize that medical staff are also emotionally involved in their relative's survival they are themselves more appreciative of the medical help that is being offered. These are important considerations, as body language is a very potent form of communication: families who have later forgotten the exact detail of what they were told by medical staff may nevertheless clearly remember the way in which they were informed. The choice of words should be equally careful. It is useful initially to establish how much the family already understand about what is going on and what has already been said to them. This may reveal that the family are well aware that their relative is dying, but it will also establish their level of comprehension of the medical situation and give some indication of the sort of language to use when talking to the family. Not infrequently, an early discussion will also serve warning that the family feel that they or their relative have suffered from inadequate care or incorrect advice earlier in the course of their terminal illness. In these circumstances, it is important to accept what the family say at face value, and to resist the temptation to criticize absent colleagues or to attempt to explain away what may be a valid complaint.

Once it is clear how much the family understands, the next step is to put the patient's illness in the context of the earlier symptoms or background health, which will allow the family to begin to understand, if they do not do so already, that the news you have to give is likely to be bad. Then, before delivering the news itself, it is helpful to give a warning such as "I'm afraid I've got some bad news for you." This encourages the family to focus on what you are going to say next. The news itself should be given in as plain language and as short chunks as possible. It is not appropriate to use euphemisms, as these are more often intended to reduce the family's display of grief rather than the intensity of grief they experience. This may reflect more our desire to avoid these emotions than our wish to ease the process for the family. Equally, family members can sometimes make it clear that they do not want to be told everything at once, or in any detail, in which case their wishes should be respected once the essential detail has been given. Most importantly, the bearer of bad news should be honest when dealing with the family, neither encouraging false hope nor implying certainty when doubt exists. This conflict may be most acute when talking to the relatives of a head-injured patient, when the potential outcome may range from death or a persistent vegetative state to a complete or almost complete recovery. In spite of the need to be honest and straightforward, it is nevertheless important to try to moderate the bad news to be given with some element of positivity or planning for the future, such as your ability to avoid any pain or distress for the patient, or your plans for the immediate management of the patient.[56]

Having given the relatives the bad news as truthfully and sensitively as possible, it is appropriate to summarize the main points again, to ensure that the family have understood the significance of what you have told them. It is essential to follow this by inviting the family to ask you any questions that they may have. In many cases, this simple courtesy may reveal areas of quite unexpected misunderstanding, which will give you the opportunity to resolve what might have otherwise become significant grievances.

The way in which families react to bad news may be surprising. In many cases, relatives will have anticipated the news for some time and may even be relieved that some sort of end is within sight. In others, it may represent the final extinction of hope and be greeted with open displays of grief or anger. If this occurs, you should not suggest that you "understand what they are going through," as it is most unlikely that you do, or to try and discourage the relatives from grieving. Overwhelming distress should be acknowledged, rather than just disregarded as a sort of social *faux pas*. The most difficult response to deal with is anger – you should recognize that you are seldom the real target of the anger and should not be drawn into making defensive remarks or, even more importantly, becoming angry yourself. With sensitive handling, anger is usually rapidly dispelled, especially if there is a second member of staff present who has previously got to know the family.

THE AFTERMATH

It is not just the patient's family who are affected by the death of a patient. The nursing and medical staff responsible for the patient's care often feel deeply involved in the patient's fate, and may find it difficult to immediately reapply themselves to other patients. These feelings should be acknowledged and allowed for, rather than suppressed as being in some way "unprofessional" or sentimental.[4,57] Usually, staff will deal with these feelings informally among themselves, but it is important that they also have access to in-house or external support services if necessary. Although they may be used infrequently, these support structures should be available before they are needed, rather than being organized on a sporadic, case-by-case basis.[4] If care is taken to provide these resources, the risk of burn-out or stress-related illness in staff may be significantly reduced.

Support for the bereaved, which may range from sending '*in memoriam*' cards to formal counseling, should be readily available if they are perceived to be at high risk of an abnormal grief reaction. There is good evidence that if an appropriate form of support is provided within a short interval of the patient's death the long-term outcome for the most vulnerable bereaved can be as good as in the case of those who are not at an increased risk of a poor outcome.[58] It is less clear, however, what form of support is the most effective. Often, the general practitioner will be able to provide all the help that is needed, but sometimes a religious figure, a hospital or ICU-based bereavement counseling program or external organizations such as Cruse, Sands, or Compassionate Friends will be more suitable.[4,55] The Citizens' Advice Bureau can usually provide details of the local support structures available.

CONCLUSION

Bereavement is one of the major life stresses. In most cases, the grief process leads to a resolution of grief and a restoration of the normal appetites and interests of life, but in up to one-third of individuals the grief process develops abnormally. The development of an abnormal grief reaction carries significant risks for the mental and physical health of the bereaved. These risks can be minimized if those who deal regularly with the dying and the bereaved are aware of how to give bad news, the importance of the grief process, and the benefit of trying to identify those vulnerable individuals most at risk of and from an abnormal grief reaction. Early recognition of these individuals allows rapid referral to support services and appropriate management to avert the development of an abnormal grief reaction.

Bereavement is a universal experience. Even though death now occurs more frequently in hospital than at home, few hospital doctors have been trained to deal with the dying or the bereaved, and most have little understanding of the grief process or of its importance. The normal grief process encompasses a number of stages, which may occur in an unpredictable order but which finally lead to the stage of resolution and acceptance. If this final stage is not reached, or if the grief process is otherwise disturbed, "complicated grief" is said to have occurred. This may lead the bereaved to suffer significant unnecessary psychological or physical morbidity. The development of complicated grief can be minimized by an awareness of the factors that provoke it. These include the personality and experience of the bereaved and the particular circumstances of the death. It is important to give relatives as much time as possible to prepare for the patient's death, because of the protective effect of "anticipatory grief" on the development of complicated grief. This remains true whether the bereaved are adults or children, and in general it is not appropriate to try and "protect" children from knowledge of the approaching death of a family member.

When giving bad news, careful thought should be given to who gives the news and where and how it is given. Attention to these details will reduce not only the likelihood of complicated grief, but also the stress felt by both the news-giver and the patient's family.

There will inevitably be times when an individual patient's death is particularly traumatic for staff, so support systems should be available to deal with this when it occurs. Staff should feel able to admit to their own distress, and be able to offer time and support to each other when necessary – counseling may be as helpful for bereaved family members as it is for members of staff, and should be available when needed.

REFERENCES

1. Maguire P, Parkes CM. Surgery and loss of body parts. *Br Med J* 1998; **316:** 1086–8.
2. Christie GL. The management of grief in work with infertile couples. *J Assist Reprod Genet* 1997; **14:** 189–91.
3. Dickinson E. Griefs. In: *Emily Dickinson Selected Poems*. New York: Dover Publications, 1990.
4. Granger CE, George C, Shelly MP. The management of bereavement on intensive care units. *Intens Care Med* 1995; **21:** 429–36.
5. Illich I. *Limits to Medicine. Medical Nemesis: The Expropriation of Health.* London: Penguin, 1991.
6. Lindemann E. Symptomatology and management of acute grief. *Am J Psychiatry* 1944; **101:** 141–8.
7. Raphael B. *The Anatomy of Bereavement*. London: Hutchinson, 1984.
8. Kissane DW, McKenzie DP, Bloch S. Family coping and bereavement outcome. *Palliative Med* 1997; **11:** 191–201.
9. O'Gorman SM. Death and dying in contemporary society: an evaluation of current attitudes and the rituals associated with death and dying and their relevance to recent understandings of health and healing. *J Advanc Nurs* 1998; **27:** 1127–35.
10. Schreiber S. Migration, traumatic bereavement and transitional aspects of psychological healing: loss and grief of a refugee woman from Begameder county in Ethiopia. *Br J Med Psychol* 1995; **68:** 135–42.
11. Parkes CM. *Bereavement: Studies of Grief in Adult Life*, 3rd edn. Harmondsworth: Pelican, 1998.
12. Kissane DW, Bloch S, McKenzie M, *et al.* Family grief therapy: a preliminary account of a new model to promote healthy family functioning during palliative care and bereavement. *Psycho-Oncology* 1998; **7:** 14–25.
13. Roddie I. Coming to terms with death. *Br Med J* 1998; **317:** 1737.
14. Bowlby J. *Loss, Sadness and Depression*. Harmondsworth: Penguin, 1981.
15. Rosenzweig A, Prigerson HG, Miller MD, Reynolds CF 3rd. Bereavement and late-life depression: grief and its complications in the elderly. *Annu Rev Med* 1997; **48:** 421–8.
16. Worden J. *Grief Counselling and Grief Therapy: a Handbook for the Mental Health Practitioner*. New York: Springer, 1982.
17. Atkinson E. *Greyfriars Bobby*. Indypublish.com, 2002.
18. Horowitz MJ, Siegel B, Holen A, *et al.* Diagnostic criteria for complicated grief disorder. *Am J Psychiatry* 1997; **154:** 904–10.
19. American Psychiatric Association. *Diagnostic and Statistical Manual of Mental Disorders*. 4th edn. Washington, DC: American Psychiatric Association, 1994.
20. Eisenbruch M. Cross-cultural aspects of bereavement. II. Ethnic and cultural variations in the development of bereavement practices. *Culture Med Psychiatry* 1984; **8:** 315–47.
21. Van Dongen CJ. Experiences of family members after a suicide. *J Family Pract* 1991; **33:** 375–80.
22. Black D. Bereavement in childhood. *Br Med J* 1998; **316:** 931–3.
23. Quirk GJ, Casco L. Stress disorders of families of the disappeared: a controlled study in Honduras. *Soc Sci Med* 1994; **39:** 1675–9.
24. Reed MD. Sudden death and bereavement outcomes: the impact of resources on grief symptomatology and detachment. *Suicide Life-threatening Behav* 1993; **23:** 204–20.
25. Horowitz M. *Stress Response Syndromes*. Northvale, NJ: Aaronson, 1986.
26. Bonnano GA, Notarious CI, Gunzerath L, *et al.* Interpersonal ambivalence, perceived relationship adjustment, and conjugal loss. *J Consult Clin Psychol* 1998; **66:** 1012–22.
27. Prigerson HG, Bierhals AJ, Kasl SV, *et al.* Traumatic grief as a risk factor for mental and physical morbidity. *Am J Psychiatry* 1997; **154:** 616–23.
28. Birtchnell J. Early parent death and mental illness. *Br J Psychiatry* 1970; **116:** 281–8.
29. Awoonor-Renner S. I desperately needed to see my son. *Br Med J* 1991; **302:** 356.
30. Bowlby-West L. The impact of death on the family system. *J Family Ther* 1983; **5:** 279–94.
31. Rutter M. *Children of Sick Parents*. Oxford: Oxford University Press, 1966.
32. Birtchnell J. The relationship between attempted suicide, depression and parent death. *Br J Psychiatry* 1970; **116:** 307–13.
33. Middleton W, Raphael B, Burnett P, Martinek N. A longitudinal study comparing bereavement phenomena in recently bereaved spouses, adult children and parents. *Aust NZ J Psychiatry* 1998; **32:** 235–41.
34. Kissane DW, Bloch S. Family grief. *Br J Psychiatry* 1994; **164:** 728–40.
35. Weller RA, Weller EB, Fristad MA, Bowes JM. Depression in recently bereaved prepubertal children. *Am J Psychiatry* 1991; **148:** 1536–40.
36. Rosenheim E, Reicher R. Informing children about a parent's terminal illness. *J Child Psychol Psychiatry* 1985; **26:** 995–8.
37. Worden JW. Grieving a loss from AIDS. *Hospice J* 1991; **7:** 143–50.
38. Zeanah CH, Dailey JV, Rosenblatt MJ, Saller DN Jr. Do women grieve after terminating pregnancies because of fetal anomalies? A controlled investigation. *Obstet Gynecol* 1993; **82:** 270–5.
39. Benfield DG, Leib SA, Vollman JH. Grief response of parents to neonatal death and parents' participation in deciding care. *Pediatrics* 1978; **62:** 171–7.
40. Hunfeld JA, Mourik MM, Passchier J, Tibboel D. Do couples grieve differently following infant loss? *Psychol Rep* 1996; **79:** 407–10.
41. Forrest GC. Mourning the loss of a new baby. *Bereavement Care* 1983; **2:** 4–5.
42. Davies J. Grieving after a sudden death: the impact of the initial intervention. *Accident Emerg Nurs* 1997; **5:** 181–84.
43. Bryan EM. The death of a twin. *Palliative Med* 1995; **9:** 187–92.
44. Woof WR, Carter YH. The grieving adult and the general practitioner: a literature review in two parts (part 1). *Br J Gen Pract* 1997; **47:** 443–8.
45. Schaefer C, Quesenberry CP Jr, Wi S. Mortality following conjugal bereavement and the effects of a shared environment. *Am J Epidemiol* 1995; **141:** 1142–52.
46. Steen KF. A comprehensive approach to bereavement. *The Nurse Practitioner* 1998; **23:**54–68.
47. Toedter LJ, Lasker JN, Alhadeft JM. The Perinatal Grief Scale: development and initial validation. *Am J Orthopsychiatry* 1988; **58:** 435–49.
48. Weiss RS, Richards TA. A scale for predicting quality of recovery following the death of a partner. *J Personality Soc Psychol* 1997; **72:** 885–91.
49. Prigerson HG, Maciejewski PK, Reynolds CF 3rd. Inventory of Complicated Grief: a scale to measure maladaptive symptoms of loss. *Psychiatry Res* 1995; **59:** 65–79.
50. Burnett P, Middleton W, Raphael B, Martinek N. Measuring core bereavement phenomena. *Psychol Med* 1997; **27:** 49–57.
51. Szanto K, Prigerson HG, Houck P, *et al.* Suicidal ideation in elderly bereaved: the role of complicated grief. *Suicide Life-Threatening Behav* 1997; **27:** 194–207.
52. Byrne GJA, Raphael B. A longitudinal study of bereavement phenomena in recently widowed elderly men. *Psychol Med* 1994; **24:** 411–21.
53. Kübler-Ross E. *On Death and Dying*. London: Tavistock, 1970.
54. Neuberger J. *Caring for Dying People of Different Faiths*, 2nd edn. Oxford: Butterworth Heinemann.
55. *Guidelines for Bereavement Care in Intensive Care Units*. London: The Intensive Care Society, 1998.
56. Baile W, Buckman R. *The Pocket Guide to Communication Skills in Clinical Practice Including Breaking Bad News*. Medical Audio-visual communication Inc. dwc@mavc.com.
57. Tolle SW, Elliot DL, Hickam DH. Physician attitudes and practices at the time of patient death. *Arch Intern Med* 1984; **144:** 2389–91.
58. Parkes CM. Bereavement counselling: does it work? *Br Med J* 1980; **281:** 3–6.

84

Quality assurance

BRIAN J POLLARD

The inclusion of a chapter on aspects of quality, standards, and cost management may initially seem to be out of place in a textbook of anesthesia. Nothing could be further from the truth. Medicine, of which anesthesia is a part of the global picture, has to exist in a cash-limited environment and to share resources with all other aspects of health care. The expectation of patients, doctors, managers, etc. is that health care should be delivered to the highest possible quality standards and should, preferably, be equal for all. In this chapter the important topics will be addressed and set in a context which, hopefully, will make them easier to understand both as stand-alone subjects and together as a whole. The reader should then be better placed to judge the issues of quality assurance and cost management in the world of anesthesia.

QUALITY

The creation of a good definition of quality is very difficult, although everybody is convinced that they know what quality is. Dictionaries give a literal definition which may not be helpful to the anesthesiologist. The definition tends to be given in terms of the degree of excellence or as a measure of "how good or bad the service or product is." More sophisticated definitions are used by experts in specialist subjects. If the dictionary definition is used, a form of comparison or standard against which to measure the quality is required. A standard may or may not be absolute, but may vary with the circumstances. It would be better, therefore, to describe quality in terms of the degree of excellence for a specific purpose. Quality is therefore a relative concept.

CLINICAL GUIDELINES

A change in culture began several years ago, and is still taking place, on the subject of how medicine is best practiced. The days of the individual practitioner "doing it his/her own way" have gone. Teamworking is growing. This change has also been driven by the knowledge that all clinical decisions might be open to scrutiny and form subjects for clinical audit of practice. Clinical freedom still exists but is now more a philosophy than a fact. Much of practice is becoming guideline driven. Clinical guidelines may be defined as "systematically developed statements to assist practitioner and patient decisions about appropriate health care for specific clinical circumstances."[1] Clinical guidelines are a means by which quality can be improved. They are not standards in their own right, but they represent an accepted good way of doing something, and may therefore be used as a quality comparison. Clinical guidelines have been with us for many years. They are not a new concept. The original intention was not to place the clinician in a straightjacket, but rather to assist in encouraging good practice. A factor that is also considered during the development of a set of guidelines is the cost of the treatment in addition to its effectiveness. There was some early antagonism to the introduction of clinical guidelines, driven by a fear of loss of independence and uncertainty about the possible effectiveness of the guidelines. Uncertainty was also expressed as to whether or not guidelines could be easily introduced into routine clinical practice. These fears have proved groundless, and guidelines have entered our everyday practice and led to many improvements. Guidelines for perioperative management of diabetes mellitus and antibiotic prescribing for chest infections are just two such examples which have led to improved patient management and have reduced costs.

To maximize the effectiveness of clinical guidelines, they must be developed in a suitably rigorous manner, by a group of individuals fully conversant with the subject (experts), and include the most up-to-date scientific evidence. The development should not be confined to experts, but advice and input, as necessary, should be obtained from other key groups and organizations such as the relevant national bodies and patient groups. If rigorous scientific evidence is lacking then the best clinical judgment at the time must be used. Potential bias and subjective opinions should be avoided. Clinical guidelines should be aimed at increasing health gains and reducing healthcare costs.[2]

Once developed, the applicability of a guideline to its target and its use and interpretation should be consistent. If two separate anesthesiologists apply them to the same set of clinical circumstances, the same result should be achieved. Some flexibility must be included within a guideline, and this underlies the difference between a guideline and a protocol. The latter describes an exact rigid method of undertaking a sequence of tasks, e.g. dismantling and sterilizing an endoscope. Guidelines must be able to identify or allow exceptions to the recommendations, although the clinician concerned must document why and how the deviation from the guideline has occurred and be able to justify the decision. The guideline needs to be clear and unambiguous in its advice. Finally, the guideline must record the evidence and sources used in its construction, the authorship, and when it is to be reviewed.

Clinical guidelines are difficult to write. They must be correct, as once prepared they will enter the public domain. They may be intended initially for the medical staff of the hospital concerned but will quickly appear outside the intended zone and be present on websites, patient information leaflets, etc. Some guidelines can be expected to be so appropriate that they may be adopted nationally. The existence of guidelines will also be known to patient groups and to their legal advisers. The principle of individual professional freedom which has long been protected by the profession must now be harnessed to best practice. Rapid advances in medical knowledge have made it impossible for any doctor to know in all circumstances the best treatment. It is easy to become out of date.

THE ANESTHESIA RECORD

Everything that takes place during the course of the anesthetic should be recorded on the anesthetic record. This includes all drugs administered with dose and time, together with all interventions which take place. Blood pressure should be recorded repeatedly at preset intervals and, when indicated, oxygen saturation, end-tidal carbon dioxide, inspired oxygen, and vapor concentration should be measured and recorded continuously and other variables such as blood sugar as appropriate. The anesthesia record forms a part of the patient's notes and is a contemporaneous record of events. It is often of no direct interest to other physicians, unless some untoward event took place. It is, of course, of immense interest to subsequent anesthesiologists and also to lawyers. Standard teaching is that, if a patient has had a previous anesthetic, then the record must be examined, if at all possible before each subsequent anesthetic. Therein should be found evidence of any problems, e.g. intubation difficulties and the responses to the drugs given. The anesthesia record is also central to the defense in any legal claim mounted by the patient. If information is missing from the anesthetic record, then the case can be argued quite effectively that such did not take place. The faintest ink is preferred by judges to the strongest memory.

Technology has rapidly advanced to a stage at which there are a number of systems available for automatic measurement and recording of the whole anesthesia process. Some manual input is still required to note events, drugs and doses, etc. All patient vital signs are recorded automatically; however, the automated recording system cannot allow for certain events, such as temporary deliberate interruption of recording. It will faithfully record erroneous readings due to artifacts, and so event markers need to be used to explain any unusual displays or readings. The detailed record of events should not stop once the anesthesia is discontinued but should continue into the postanesthesia recovery area and cease only when the patient leaves to return to the ward. The knowledge of past performance is fundamental in the pursuit of quality. It allows the current situation to be compared with previous experience and adjustments made as necessary.

RISK MANAGEMENT

A risk is a hazard or chance of an undesirable consequence arising from an action. Risk opportunities are all around us, and every one of us takes many risks every day. Most risks (taking a shower, walking the dog, crossing the road, driving to work) are small. Each risk is assessed and managed, and we are therefore all taking risk management actions repeatedly every day, usually without realizing it. The level of risk from any particular activity may be defined but would be defined differently by different individuals depending on circumstances. Clearly, this involves the perception of the risk and its placement in the context of the action involved and the circumstances. The action may then proceed, be cancelled, or an alternative action followed depending on the level of risk versus outcome benefit. In the context of medical practice, risk management involves assessment of the magnitude of risk and its reduction to levels that would be perceived as acceptable to society. To this can be added the caveat that the process should be cost-effective if at all possible.[3]

Risk management covers all aspects of healthcare activity, not simply immediate patient care. There are risk management issues which relate to the hospital buildings, corridors and doorways, beds and ward equipment, car parks, etc. A risk management manager should be appointed to coordinate the management of these risks, supported by a group or committee. Each clinical area should similarly appoint a member of staff to oversee risk management issues in that area. The department of anesthesia is no exception.

The risk associated with anesthesia itself is very difficult to determine because anesthesia is not administered alone to otherwise healthy individuals. Anesthesia is not (currently) of itself therapeutic. It forms a part of a care plan that involves invasive investigation or surgery. The risk from the anesthesia process will be influenced very greatly by the patient's previous medical history and other comorbidities as well as by the current condition requiring surgery. The overall risk has been quantified, and it is generally accepted that the risk of death due to anesthesia alone is approximately 1 in 250 000, although anesthesia may contribute to death in up to 14% of patients.[4]

It is important to consider the expectations of patients. There is an inherent risk in any operation; some may be very hazardous. The risks of the operation should be described to the patient by the surgeon, and most patients can understand the anatomy of the process involved. The possibility of failure is commonly accepted by both patient and surgeon. The anesthetic is different, however. It is not of itself curative and is not understood by the patient (and probably not by the surgeon). Patients do not expect anesthetic failure and will not be tolerant of such failure. Patients perceive anesthesia to be a routine event that is completely safe and incidental, although it can actually be the most hazardous part of the whole procedure. It is difficult to explain to patients that they will be placed into a drug-induced coma, their normal protective reflexes will be abolished, they might be paralyzed (temporarily), and their life will depend upon the normal functioning of a mechanical ventilator operated by a fallible human being.

It is possible to subdivide types of risk which might be encountered (Table 84.1).[5] Those with a direct impact on patient care are clearly the most serious and, in the context of the practice of anesthesia, may prove to be rapidly fatal. Most of the resources should therefore be channeled into ensuring that the risks of anesthesia be prevented or reduced as much as possible. It must always be remembered, however, that many incidences of patient harm arise not from one event but from a series of minor "coincidences," each of which would not of itself cause harm but when taken together do result in damage. Health and safety risks apply to all, staff and patients alike, and it is essential to ensure that these risks are kept to a minimum. It must always be remembered that it is impossible to prevent risks, but it is necessary to limit the possibility of damage from these as far as possible.

Risk management therefore encompasses the identification of risks ("What can go wrong?"), the analysis of the issues concerned ("How often does it go wrong?"), and the prevention of the adverse event occurring ("What can we do to stop it going wrong?") There is one additional step which examines the possible situations that could arise if the risk is incorrectly managed ("What can we do if it still does go wrong?").

Table 84.1 *Types of risk (from Secker Walker[5] with permission)*

Direct	These have a direct impact on patient care, e.g. ventilator disconnection
Indirect	These have an indirect impact on patient care, e.g. power supply failure to operating room lights
Health and safety	This may apply to both staff and patients, e.g. needlestick injury

Adverse incident reporting

Adverse incident reporting constitutes an essential part of a risk management process. It provides information at the first fundamental level. The description and identification of the incident is the first input into the question "What can go wrong?" by seeing at first hand what actually has gone wrong. A more detailed analysis can and should then be undertaken to examine if it has gone wrong before and, if so, when and how often. The incident may need to be categorized, and it may be grouped with other similar ones.

Adverse incident reporting is regarded as a very important part of risk management and quality assurance. One of the fundamental issues is that of persuading staff to report incidents, which most commonly involves completing an adverse incident report form. The first problem is that the amount of paperwork necessary during the average day makes it difficult to persuade individuals to complete yet another form that is not perceived to be of immediate benefit to themselves or to their patient. The second problem is that of blame. Human nature makes us all suspicious of authority. There is a perception that filling in a report form may result in disciplinary action, and it is easy to see how this can arise. If not all members of staff are equally diligent and complete a form for every adverse incident, then an analysis might reveal that members of staff who diligently complete the forms experience more adverse incidents than those who do not. This may be the opposite of reality in that those who have not recorded incidents are, in effect, hiding their higher incident rate. This is viewed by the individual as a personal threat in that his or her job (and hence income and livelihood) may be threatened. An equally valid point is that a high incidence is an opportunity for education and training. It is, however, the fear of reprisal that limits the use of adverse incident reporting.

Attempts have been made to address this issue by introducing anonymity to the reporting process. A remarkable degree of success has been claimed for this process, although there must still be the underlying fear of tracing the report back to its originator. Adverse incident reporting could be regarded as a form of audit of practice. Accurate and complete incident reporting should allow the organization as a whole to reveal the potential and actual risks in the system, their frequency of occurrence, and their danger. This can then be used as a driver toward those procedures or areas of practice that need to be addressed and where working practices need to be examined.

Adverse incident reporting, in order to be effective, should be used correctly and sensibly and be promulgated as a normal part of everyday clinical practice. The reporting form should be simple and straightforward and take a minimum of time to complete. It should be anonymous and not associated with any form of disciplinary process, and education of staff should be undertaken to ensure that forms are fully and accurately completed and used correctly and appropriately.

Critical incident analysis

A particular type of adverse incident is known as a critical incident. Critical incident analysis was a technique originally developed by psychologists as a tool to facilitate studies of human behavior.[6] It was applied specifically to selection, training, and performance of pilots in World War II and allowed an objective approach to performance rather than the previously used subjective approach. It has been applied to the selection of managers, students, and trainees in various businesses with considerable success, and was first applied to anesthesia by Cooper *et al.* in 1978.[7] It is certain, however, that it is still not used to best effect by anesthesiologists.

There are a number of different definitions of a critical incident, but the most commonly used definition is that it is a situation which, if allowed to proceed, would result in harm to the patient. An example might be a disconnection of the anesthetic breathing circuit. The 10 most common critical incidents were listed by Cooper *et al.* in 1984[8] (Table 84.2), and many anesthesiologists will note a familiarity with these as most have occurred in the experience of every anesthesiologist – this author is no exception. I would expect, however, that very few have been the subject of a formal critical incident report on a reporting form. This is partly because of the culture that problems are an everyday hazard and every anesthesiologist is expecting problems, on the lookout for them, and solves them rapidly. A second reason is the fear of reprisal, noted above. The introduction of anonymity, less formality, and less paperwork into a critical incident reporting process might lead to an increase in reporting.

Critical incidents can be analyzed in various ways although two processes are commonly used. These are outcome grading and preventability grading (Table 84.3). The outcome grading analysis is straightforward and readily understandable. The preventability grading is most interesting as this introduces the issue of cost–benefit analysis. The preventability here depends upon the supply of resources. All would doubtless agree that the first two categories should be addressed and if reasonable extra resources will prevent the recurrence of the incident then they should be found. The debate will center around those which are only possibly (not definitely) preventable by the use of current or extra resources. The balance of resources versus preventability has to be determined.

Table 84.2 *The 10 most common critical incidents (from Cooper* et al.[8] *with permission)*

Disconnection	27%
Gas flow errors	22%
Wrong syringe	19%
Wrong gas	15%
Intravenous line disconnection	11%
Laryngoscope failure	11%
Accelerated extubation	10%
Circuit faults	9%
Hypovolemia	9%
Tracheal tube problems	7%

Table 84.3 *Critical incident analysis*

Outcome grading

1. No effect
2. Transient abnormality – unnoticed by patient, e.g. laryngospasm
3. Transient abnormality – full recovery, e.g. postdural puncture headache
4. Potentially permanent not disabling, e.g. damaged tooth at intubation
5. Potentially permanent but disabling, e.g. myocardial infarction, cardiovascular accident
6. Death

Preventability grading

1. Preventable within current resources, e.g. loose laryngoscope bulb not detected on preoperative check
2. Preventable with reasonable extra resources, e.g. no capnograph to detect esophageal intubation
3. Possibly preventable within current resources, e.g. pneumothorax at central venous pressure line insertion due to inadequate training
4. Possibly preventable with reasonably extra resources, e.g. anesthesiologist taken ill, no replacement
5. Not preventable, e.g. anaphylaxis

AUDIT

The Department of Health in the UK in 1989 described audit as "The systematic critical analysis of the quality of medical care, including the procedures used for diagnosis and treatment, the use of resources and the resulting outcome and quality of life for the patient."[9] In reality, the medical profession has always undertaken a process of self-evaluation and group analysis of medical care, it is just that it was not called audit until about 15 years ago. What the rediscovery of the whole process in the late 1980s did, however, was to increase the profile of the process and make it more systematic and structured in application. The process up to that time had existed, but had been undertaken in a more haphazard way. The underlying aim of audit was to improve, maintain, and protect the quality of medical care. The reasoning behind the system went along the lines that the best way to do this would be to regularly and comprehensively review practice. Clearly, however, reviewing practice is only a part of the whole process. There is little point in reviewing current practice and simply filing the results. The findings must be compared with a known (previously defined or newly created) standard to calibrate the practice against that measure. The question must then be asked "Are we achieving the standard, could we do better?" The next obvious step is to introduce appropriate changes which it is anticipated will improve the quality of the care to either achieve or exceed the standard. But one cannot be certain whether or not the change has been successful unless we re-examine the whole process after an interval of time and again compare the situation with respect to the original, or revised, standard. Hence, the whole process of audit is one in which the care process is examined, compared with the standard, changed appropriately and then re-examined. This has been termed the "audit cycle."[10]

Medical audit could be regarded as a form of quality assurance or cost-effectiveness tool. One of the fundamental difficulties with medical audit is the actual measurement of patient outcome. Large variations exist between individual patients in the progress of the same disease process. Some outcomes are very clear-cut, e.g. death, but this is too coarse a standard for routine use in the great majority of cases. It is often necessary therefore to apply audit to surrogate markers or to individual parts of the process. The whole care process is relevant, not just the medical treatment, as it too is likely to have an influence on outcome. This is well illustrated in anesthesia as the mortality rate due to anesthesia is very low and in routine practice the complication rate is also very low. Simple audit of outcome from anesthesia is therefore unlikely to be of great value. The majority of the effort in anesthesia audit therefore tends to be directed toward the process. A periodic review of individual aspects of anesthesia can be a valuable way forward. Although mortality and morbidity following anesthesia is not a fruitful area for local hospital audits, it is a vitally important subject. Local data on perioperative deaths should be examined at regular intervals. This is also addressed on a national scale in the UK by the National Confidential Enquiry into Perioperative Deaths (NCEPOD). A proportion of all deaths occurring within 30 days of surgery are examined in detail; both the surgical and anesthetic factors involved are considered. Publication of the enquiry results should allow a comparative audit between hospital results and national results.

Reviews of adverse events which are not of themselves critical incidents can be a particularly fruitful area for audit. Examples might include unplanned admissions to the high-dependency unit (HDU)/intensive care unit (ICU), canceled operations or cases undertaken between midnight and 7 a.m. These elements of the process can have a significant but indirect bearing on morbidity and outcome.

What to audit? The selection of topics should be a task dedicated to a small group headed by a lead (attending) consultant, although ultimate responsibility lies with the clinical director at departmental level and the medical director at hospital management level (NHS trust). Departmental meetings should be held regularly: one half-day per month for all staff is recommended. All other commitments should be canceled and attendance should be compulsory. The majority of audit is still a local function. The past few years have seen some attempts to extend larger audits throughout regions and also nationally. NCEPOD is one such national body, and the critical care world has the Intensive Care National Audit and Research Centre (ICNARC). Ideally, national audits ought to enable national comparisons between hospitals, and there have been some crude attempts to construct national league tables in the UK. International audits are also theoretically possible and may be more easily achieved in the future with advances in information technology. Accurate comparisons may be complicated by the way in which the separate countries manage their healthcare systems. There are also different drugs and techniques available in different countries, together with cultural differences and differences in patients' expectations .

The revolution in information technology should theoretically have made audit easier and more comprehensive. The sad fact is that this has not happened. Computers have been misused and a great deal of resource wasted in inappropriate systems. In the early days of audit, money was made available for the purchase of hardware and software, much of which proved inadequate for the task for which it was purchased.

RESOURCE MANAGEMENT/COST-EFFECTIVENESS

Considerable advances in medical technology have occurred over the past 20 years. As a result, it is now possible to undertake many complex procedures that were previously impossible. With these procedures has come an increase in cost. In addition, the expectation of society with respect to medical care has progressed at almost the same speed. Only the highest quality of care is now acceptable to society. The concomitant increase in costs requires careful management because we do not live in a society with infinite resources. Even in the USA and Europe, resources are limited and must be effectively managed. The proportion of senior citizens is also increasing, and, as the elderly consume proportionately more of the healthcare resources than do younger people, an increase in the costs will occur. Any restrictions due to cost must not be reflected in a poorer quality of service. The ultimate aim is therefore to maintain and improve quality while maintaining or reducing costs. To put it simply, the treatment has to become more cost-effective.

Resource management has a primary objective, which is the provision of information to healthcare workers and also to those in management to allow them to better manage the finite resources. Data must be collected about patients, their treatment, and outcomes. All these need to be fed into this process. One of the key principles behind recent healthcare reforms in the UK has been to link resource supply to healthcare cost and activity, and the purchaser/provider process has been created to drive this process forward. Certain aspects of this process have, however, led to an increase in costs in unexpected areas. For example, an increase in accountancy and financial management departments has followed the introduction of internal markets within hospitals, i.e. one department charges another for its services. In a number of institutions, departments of anesthesia have been regarded as service providers and the costs have been a charge on surgical purchasers. The service must be costed to allow accurate and appropriate use of resources, although this can of itself be an expensive process. Models have been developed and applied to cost every individual component in the anesthetic process and to allocate these costs to each patient or procedure. Every syringe, needle, ampoule, tube, etc. has a cost. The human resources required to carry out the total costing is considerable and is wasted effort and has been abandoned in favor of a unit cost, which assumes a basic "package" of equipment/disposables/drugs that will be used for an average procedure. This can then be stratified into a number of bands, for example minor, intermediate, major. One of the problems with respect to anesthesia concerns the many variations possible in the use and cost of anesthetic agents. The cost of the inhalational agent, for example, depends not only on the agent itself but on other factors, such as the flow rate of the gases. The commonly accepted method used to calculate these costs is the Dion equation:[11]

$$\text{Cost} = \frac{\text{P} \times \text{F} \times \text{T} \times \text{M} \times \text{C}}{2414 \times \text{D}}$$

where P is vaporizer concentration setting (%), F is the fresh gas flow rate ($\text{L}\,\text{min}^{-1}$), T is the duration of anesthesia (min), M is molecular weight (g), C is the cost of the agent per mL, and D is the density of the liquid agent ($\text{g}\,\text{mL}^{-1}$).There are, however, many inaccuracies in this approach. The most accurate method is to weigh the vaporizer and calculate the actual volume of agent used, but this is technically difficult.

The cost of an anesthetic depends mainly on the staff and capital equipment costs, although consumables (including drugs) feature significantly. A calculation based simply on a fraction of the staff and equipment costs together with the consumables gives only a part of the picture. It is also necessary to introduce a factor that compensates for the duration and complexity of the case. The issue of complexity cannot be easily and simply linked to the surgical complexity. Particularly in larger tertiary centers, the complex comorbidities of some patients may make the anesthetic for a simple operation into a very complex affair. The author recalls one patient who was admitted for closure of an ileostomy, a routine surgical procedure expected to last less than an hour. However, this patient suffered from chronic obstructive airways disease, coronary heart disease, and left ventricular aneurysm, had had two previous coronary artery bypass grafts, and had required a prolonged period of intensive care following his previous surgery. The anesthetic was not as straightforward as the surgery! Duration is easy to measure, and various models incorporating time bands have been proposed. Clearly, these will also have a relation to the anesthetic complexity as a more complicated anesthetic will take longer. A small number of bands, 5–7, is likely to be the optimum. Too few and assessment becomes too coarse; too many and it becomes too cumbersome.

The issue of cost and quality is a potential dilemma for all healthcare workers existing in a cash-limited system. We all strive for the highest possible quality at the lowest possible cost. The equation is difficult to balance. Quality is not easy to measure. Quality is easy to criticize, easy to reduce, but not always easy to increase. Cost is the opposite in many ways as it is relatively easy to measure, easy to increase, and not always easy to reduce. The anesthesiologist represents only a small fraction of the cost of an operation. The majority of the total is composed of the salaries of all those present, the capital equipment and building costs and the surgical instruments purchased, sterilizing and maintenance. Not withstanding the fixed costs, the only method open to the anesthesiologist to reduce costs is to use cheaper drugs and disposables.

Disposables for an "average" anesthetic are principally intravenous cannulae and fluid administration sets, tracheal tube and/or airways, and ECG monitoring electrodes. It is relatively straightforward and reasonable practice to compare the quality, function, and reliability of these items. It is sensible practice to use disposables that are acceptable to the majority. The days of keeping a small stock of a different cannula "because Dr X prefers this type" have gone.

The issue of using cost as a determinant of drug choice is much more difficult. The choice of drug depends on many factors, the most important of which are those pertaining to the patients themselves. The patient's past medical history and present condition are the first consideration, and these may limit the choice of agents. It has been suggested that repeated exposure to the same drug may increase the likelihood of allergic reactions, and any drug must, of course, be avoided if there is a history of allergy to that family of drugs. Some agents are more or less suitable for use in patients at the extremes of age. Finally, any reasonable request by a patient that particular agents should be used or avoided should, if medically safe, be accepted. The postoperative plan or "disposal" of the patient is an additional major factor. The rapid rate of elimination of certain agents, for example, makes them particularly suitable for day-case patients. If the anesthetic techniques require the use of additional agents then the possibility of interactions must be borne in mind. There are particular techniques of anesthesia which are assisted by the use of certain drugs or combinations, e.g. insertion of the laryngeal mask and propofol. The duration of surgery is linked to the nature of the operation and also to the experience of the surgeon and anesthesiologist, and these factors may from time to time suggest a particular choice of drug. Finally, it is appropriate to consider the cost of the drug when all else has been taken into consideration and there is more than one drug available, and with which the anesthesiologist is familiar, for that particular purpose. It is impossible to generalize or to state that there is one agent or technique for any particular situation. Patients differ and apparently similar situations may also be different. The choice of drug may depend on a multitude of factors which need to be considered by each anesthesiologist for each of their patients. Cost is of minor importance only when placed into context with all others.

REGULATION

The regulation and licensing of medical practitioners (and of other healthcare workers) is clearly a quality issue. There are a number of professional bodies, for example in the UK the United Kingdom Central Council (UKCC) for nurses, the General Medical Council (GMC) for medical practitioners, and the General Dental Council (GDC) for dentists. In other countries similar organizations exist either at the national level or at the state level. For very many years, the professions have practiced self-regulation. In the recent past, high-profile legal cases have helped to drive the process toward a more formal activity. Patients put their trust, and often their lives, into the care of a doctor, and it is essential that the doctor is knowledgeable, skilled, and competent. Not only that, but the doctor must also have unimpeachable ethical standards. The GMC in 1995 published a booklet entitled *Good Medical Practice*, and this has been recently updated .[12] This booklet includes advice on good clinical care and relationships with other colleagues and with patients, including consent, confidentiality, and ethical issues. With particular relevance to the subject of quality and regulation of practice, a section is included on keeping up to date and on monitoring performance. "You must keep your knowledge and skills up to date throughout your working life;" "You must work with colleagues to monitor and maintain the quality of the care you provide … ."[12] Clearly, the definitions of good practice will differ between the specialties, and this issue is being addressed by the various royal colleges and other professional bodies. In the UK, the process for regular revalidation of a doctor's medical license including the likelihood of reexamination is being discussed, but it is likely to take several years before revalidation is universally implemented.

A process of regular formal appraisal is being introduced into clinical practice. Many groups in industry and business have undergone regular appraisals for many years. Academic staff of most universities have similarly been subject to regular appraisal. Trainees in the medical profession have been subject to regular appraisal as a part of the training reforms of the past decade. The extension of this process to the consultant medical staff is a logical step. The complexity and the desire to achieve an appropriate and correct approach has delayed its introduction. Careful handling has also been essential as it is perceived as a direct threat by many and as being linked to performance assessment.

Such a view should not have been unexpected and was reinforced by the process being employer led although conducted by professional peers. Appraisal correctly undertaken should be a supportive process.

The above could be considered to be an issue of personal quality control for medical practitioners although driven by guidance from their professional regulatory body. Issues of corporate quality assurance within organizations also exist, and in the UK these are currently addressed by the concept of clinical governance.[13] This was originally intended to form a central plank for a longer term (5–10 years) process to improve quality of care in its entirety throughout the NHS. This is another example of a set of procedures which have been undertaken in various other ways for many years but which have been brought together and formalized. The definitions of clinical governance are many, but it seems to be a generic term bringing together risk management, medical audit, performance assessment, guidelines, and standards and establishing clearer lines of accountability for the maintenance of all of these quality issues.[14] The lines of accountability pass through the hierarchy of the trust (hospital or primary care) and end with the chief executive, who is ultimately accountable. This last point represents a "two-edged sword." Maybe clinicians can rest a little easier knowing that the chief executive will ultimately be held responsible, but, on the other hand, the chief executive will be watching what the clinicians are doing in order to manage his or her own risks effectively. The end result is seen by many as an increasing drive by trust managers (who are usually nonclinicians) to directly influence medical practice and clinical decisions. This dilemma has not yet been fully resolved. No reasonable clinician or manager would consider opposing a measure designed to improve the quality of care. The issue is the manner in which this important matter is being introduced. There is also perceived to be a significant effect on time demands with the introduction of clinical governance. It necessitates the introduction or refinement of standards and guidelines of care and the increasing use of audit and performance monitoring. This reduces the time available for the clinical care of patients and directly conflicts with the desire of all clinicians to simply get on with the job of caring for their patients.

HOW CAN QUALITY BE IMPROVED?

The constant examination and improvement of quality is fundamental to clinical care. Quality should be viewed from the perception of the consumer and not the supplier. It must always be remembered, however, that to achieve excellence in quality depends on the interaction of many individuals and many processes, and that the organization itself must be committed to change before change is possible. The different individuals will also possess different views on what they believe is quality. What is a high-quality anesthetic? The anesthesiologist will put high on the list issues such as no patient's awareness during anesthesia, no postoperative nausea and vomiting, no postoperative pain, no chance of adverse reaction to any drugs. The patient will put high on the list freedom from all risk in addition to those listed by the anesthesiologist. To the surgeon, a high-quality anesthetic produces ideal conditions for surgery and takes zero time to implement.

The problem is that the whole healthcare service was never designed to function in this way. We are working within a cumbersome system that has been in existence for decades and are being asked to alter it by auditing and improving the processes. This is laudable but well nigh impossible. It could be likened to a huge old cargo ship with no power steering and 20 separate steering wheels each in a different room and operated by a different person. The effort to turn the wheels is immense, the amount by which the rudder has moved is not known, and the inertia is such that it will have traveled many miles before any change in course can be detected. The ideal (which is impossible) would be to start again with a new blank sheet of paper. There is an old joke which goes: Question: "Can you direct me to Liverpool?" Reply: "If I were going to Liverpool, I would not start from here." Quality should be designed into a system and not regarded as a late add-on option.

CONCLUSION

Quality, excellence, and cost-effectiveness are all interrelated factors and must be a part of everyday practice in anesthesia. It is clearly the duty of every anesthesiologist to provide a high-quality service. This aim is assisted by the growing number of local, national, and international guidelines for the practice of medicine. As the number of guidelines grows, maintaining current knowledge about them will become a major part in the global need to keep up to date. Last, but by no means least, it is necessary to provide care within the available resources. Care must be as cost-effective as possible without there being any compromise on quality.

REFERENCES

1. Institute of Medicine. *Guidelines for Clinical Practice from Development to Use*. Field MJ, Lohr KN (eds). Washington, DC: National Academic Press,1992.
2. Royal College of General Practitioners. *The Development and Implementation of Clinical Guidelines*. Exeter: Royal College of General Practitioners, 1995.
3. Runciman WB. Risk assessment in the formulation of anaesthetic safety standards. *Eur J Anaesthesiol* 1993; **10:** 26–32.
4. Campling EA, Devlin HB, Lunn JN. *Confidential Enquiry into Perioperative Deaths*. London: The National Confidential Enquiry into Perioperative Deaths, 1987.
5. Secker Walker J. Quality and the management of risk. In: Secker Walker J (ed.) *Quality and Safety in Anaesthesia*. London: BMJ Publishing Group, 1994: 1–17.
6. Flanagan JC. The critical incident technique. *Psychol Bull* 1954; **51:** 327–58
7. Cooper JB, Newbower RS, Long CD, McPeek B. Preventable anesthesia mishaps: a study of human factors. *Anesthesiology* 1978; **49:** 399–406.
8. Cooper JB, Newbower RS, Kitz RJ. An analysis of major errors and equipment failures in anesthesia management: considerations for prevention and detection. *Anesthesiology* 1984; **60:** 34–42.
9. Secretaries of State for Health, Wales, Northern Ireland and Scotland. *Working for Patients*. London: HMSO, 1989.
10. The Royal College of Surgeons of England. *Guidelines to Clinical Audit in Surgical Practice*. London, The Royal College of Surgeons of England, 1987.
11. Dion P. The cost of anaesthetic vapours. *Can J Anesth* 1992; **39:** 633.
12. General Medical Council. *Good Medical Practice*. London: GMC, 2001.
13. Department of Health. *Clinical Governance: Quality in the New NHS*. London: NHS Executive, 1999.
14. Fletcher IR. Clinical governance. *Eur J Anaesthesiol* 2000; **17:** 471–3.

85

Medical ethics and anesthesia

DAVID B WAISEL AND ROBERT D TRUOG

Anesthesiologists face ethical dilemmas daily. These range from the more identifiable, such as how to honor a patient's request to refuse resuscitation in the operating room, to the less obvious but equally important, such as when to use the more expensive, slightly superior, antiemetic.[1] Medical ethics, also known as bioethics, is the discipline that provides the tools necessary to identify, analyze, and manage such problems. When studying bioethics, the reader should (1) seek to recognize ethical dilemmas and high-risk situations, (2) seek to understand and have an approach to common ethical problems, (3) seek insight into different pathways of resolution, and (4) learn when and how to call for help. Rote knowledge of bioethics, as in anesthesiology, is wholly insufficient for providing clinical care or achieving future growth. Medical ethics provides a guide to choosing between two morally compelling actions that appear to conflict.[2] Education in medical ethics gives physicians the tools to use ethical theory and practice to help resolve these unavoidable dilemmas.[3]

INFORMED CONSENT

The cornerstone of the patient–physician relationship is informed consent. Obtaining informed consent is how anesthesiologists acknowledge the responsibility to respect a patient's right to self-determination and to follow a self-chosen plan.[4] This obligation is based on the principle of respect for autonomy.[3] For a decision to be autonomous, a patient must have substantial capacity for intentional action, understanding, and independence from controlling influences. Thus, although it is still important for an anesthesiologist to fulfill the locally defined legal requirements of informed consent, achieving those requirements does not necessarily achieve the spirit of informed consent.

To achieve the ethical sense of informed consent, the anesthesiologist must seek to maximize the ability of the patient to make *substantially* autonomous decisions. It is unreasonable, and ultimately harmful to the concept of informed consent, to expect a patient to be fully informed. This kind of attitude can lead to a view that informed consent is a mythical concept that may never be achieved and is therefore not worth pursuing. A more appropriate goal is to obtain substantial informed consent, which acknowledges that an action may be sufficiently autonomous without complete informed consent.[5]

An analysis of informed consent from the perspective of British and American legal traditions is presented in Chapters 80 and 81.

Components of informed consent

Decision-making capacity

Patients have decision-making capacity if they are capable of making a specific decision at a particular time. Evidence of decision-making capacity includes the ability to understand the situation, to comprehend the relevant information, and to express a preference based on rational, internally consistent reasoning.

Anesthesiologists must often evaluate the decision-making capacity of patients (1) who do not have legal decision-making authority, such as a minor or a legally incompetent patient, (2) whose decision-making capacity is temporarily altered as from preoperative sedation or pain medication, and (3) who have a pre-existing impairment in decision-making capacity. As a general rule, anesthesiologists should permit patients to make decisions to the extent of their capacity. Consider the patient who has received pain or sedation medication. Although ideally patients would not receive psychoactive drugs prior to decision making, this is not always possible. For these patients, the level of impairment varies depending on the medication, the tolerance of the patient to the medication, and the decision to be made. Indeed, some patients have improved decision-making capacity when pain is decreased (consider at which time the parturient receiving a labor epidural may be most capable of making an informed decision).[6] The anesthesiologist needs to use clinical judgment, balancing the medication given and its expected effects and the ability of the patient to show evidence of rational reasoning and understanding, to determine if the patient has the capacity to make the specific decision. In all situations, but particularly when a patient has a pre-existing impairment in decision-making capacity, the anesthesiologist should consider seeking assistance in evaluating the patient from colleagues in ethics consultation, psychiatry, and law. When a patient has temporarily lost decision-making capacity, such as when the patient is anesthetized, anesthesiologists should not implement nonemergent care until after the patient regains decision-making capacity and gives consent. However, in emergencies, such as the need to implement more extensive monitoring, the anesthesiologists should proceed without obtaining informed consent, based on justification as used in emergency situations.

Voluntariness

Physicians should perform procedures only on competent patients who are participating willingly. This issue comes into play most prominently when determining what to do with a patient who may have limited decision-making capacity. This has implications for patients who are in *de facto* positions without choice, such as those with perceived familial or financial pressures. On a daily basis, anesthesiologists compromise voluntariness if they present information in an inappropriate way, by, say, downplaying information to influence an individual to make specific decisions. Censoring the information provided does not permit a patient to make a voluntary decision.

Disclosure

The goal of disclosure is to provide information relevant to the decision maker and the decision to be made. Cataloging a rote list of information does not contribute to this goal, and simply clutters the discussion with extraneous information.[4,7]

One approach to disclosure is to provide disclosure to the level dictated by the practices of the local physician community. This is sometimes known as the professional practice standard or the Bolam principle. The difficulty with this standard is that it does not appear to fulfill the goal of keeping the patient at the center of decision making. This standard is falling out of favor in the UK and the USA.[8]

Another approach is to offer disclosure to the extent that would satisfy the hypothetical reasonable person. This is known as the reasonable person standard or the prudent person test. Information is material if a reasonable person would consider it important for decision making. The trouble is that there is conflicting evidence about what patients consider to be important.[9,10] For example, younger patients may prefer more information than older patients. Gender and other demographic data are not necessarily predictive of what a patient may desire for disclosure. Patients from different cultures desire different information. One benefit of the reasonable person standard is that it is legally accessible. In other words, the requirements should be fairly uniform within a community. The reverse position is that the reasonable person standard does not require the anesthesiologist to individualize the informed consent process.

The ideal option is to tailor the disclosure process to the particular patient's desires. This is known as the subjective person standard. Of course, it may be difficult to determine what particular unusual information the patient wants. This is a difficult legal standard to uphold, because, in essence, a patient can always claim that knowing a certain piece of information would have altered their decision-making process. Nonetheless, the concept of the subjective person standard defines the ideal form of informed consent.

Informed consent discussions should routinely include the specific risks and benefits of each anesthetic option, the complications of instrumentation of the airway, the risks and benefits of invasive monitoring, the presence and use of a fallback plan, and the basis for the anesthesiologist's recommendation. For example, a recommendation might be widely accepted and based on high-quality studies, or it might be controversial and based on personal opinion. Anesthesiologists should also inform the patient whether an individual or an anesthesia care team will be providing anesthesia services, and, if the latter, the names and specific roles (e.g. resident or registrar status) of the team members. The patient should be told about other practical matters, such as the likely sequence of events upon arrival in the surgical unit, who will be with them at the various stops, postoperative pain management, and realistic time estimates.[9–14]

There is some question as to the extent potential complications should be disclosed. Some believe that the most serious but less likely possibilities must be included.[15,16] Others believe that it is more appropriate to discuss the more common risks, and to then offer the decision maker the option of being told about those that are less likely but more dangerous.[9,17,18] This allows the patient to control the extent of disclosure.[7]

On rare occasions, the anesthesiologist's duties to disclosure information may be unwise or even impossible to fulfill. Patients may refuse to receive information, emergency situations may prevent disclosure, and there are times when it is more harmful for the patient to undergo than not to undergo the informed consent process. This last situation is called therapeutic privilege, and holds that a physician may withhold information when this would be "significantly injurious" to the patient. Therapeutic privilege should be used rarely, cautiously, and with hesitation. For example, it may be reasonable to invoke therapeutic privilege when discussing the risk of death with a patient during an active infarction of the myocardium. It would not be reasonable to do the same when discussing the risk of death with the parents of an infant.

Recommendation

Anesthesiologists are obliged to offer an opinion as to which options are preferable and the advantages and disadvantages of each option. By explaining the value judgments behind their opinions, anesthesiologists allow the patient not only to receive the benefit of their expertise, but also to understand the reason for the recommendation. Patients can then decide for themselves which benefits best fit their priorities. Anesthesiologists should conduct the recommendation appropriately. It is appropriate to attempt to persuade the patient by providing information that supports the recommendation. It is not appropriate, however, to manipulate or coerce a patient to make a particular decision. For example, an anesthesiologist may manipulate a patient by not offering general anesthesia for an operation because of a desire to minimize operating room time or a desire to gain experience with regional anesthesia.

Understanding

Patients need to understand the risks and benefits of the proposed procedures, the recommendation made, and why that recommendation has been made. It is difficult to determine if a patient fully understands the informed consent discussion, and, indeed, many patients may not. For instance, in one study, 27% of postoperative surgical patients did not know which organ had been operated upon, and 44% did not know the nature of the procedure.[19] Only 55% of cancer patients could list one of the major complications for chemotherapy within 1 day of signing the consent forms.[20] Preprinted risk-specific consent forms do not necessarily help the patient to remember the risks, and, in fact, patients may sign documents that knowingly they do not understand.[18,21] Patients misunderstand terms that are common to physicians, such as nasogastric tube, fasting, and the purpose of antibiotics.[22] This information should not cause the anesthesiologist to abandon the informed consent process. Instead, this information should spur the anesthesiologist (1) to focus on important information without cluttering the discussion with lists of risks and (2) to attempt to thoroughly educate patients according to their individual needs.

Decision

After considering the information and the anesthesiologist's recommendation, the patient chooses an anesthetic technique. Assuming that it is one that the anesthesiologist considers reasonable, he or she will proceed with that plan. At times, however, a patient may prefer a technique that the anesthesiologist does not recommend.

When a patient refuses an anesthesiologist's recommendation, or requests a technique that the anesthesiologist considers inappropriate, the focus of the conversation moves from informed consent to *informed refusal*. The requirements for an informed refusal are similar to the requirements for informed consent; the patient should be substantially well versed about the risks, benefits, and alternatives before declining. The anesthesiologist should provide additional information concerning the choice to ensure that the patient has all the necessary information. If, in fact, the patient chooses without sufficient information, the anesthesiologist has not fulfilled the obligations of informed refusal. This obligation centers on the anesthesiologist to provide the information and to persuade the patient to hear the information. A patient still may refuse to hear this information. But it is ethically more correct to make a substantial effort to inform the patient than to accept at face value the patient's refusal to be informed. In either case, when a patient chooses a technique that the anesthesiologist believes to be inappropriate, anesthesiologists are not ethically obligated to provide care in nonemergency situations. In most cases, the anesthesiologist should assist in finding the patient a willing caregiver.

Autonomous authorization

The informed consent process concludes with the patient intentionally authorizing the anesthesiologist to perform a specific procedure. This authorization is the expression of the patient's self-determination and is the basis of informed consent. Silent acquiescence is not sufficient evidence of obtaining informed consent. As discussed in the section on informed refusal, respect for autonomy should not be interpreted as "do whatever the patient wants." Only informed patients can give an autonomous authorization, and the anesthesiologist may respect a patient while at the same time refusing to provide care. The informed consent process concludes with the patient authorizing the anesthesiologist to perform a specific procedure.

Issues in informed consent

Emergency situations

Medicine presumes that patients want life-sustaining treatment unless they have declared otherwise. Although this may create ethical problems in certain situations, it is a worthy assumption when considering emergency treatment.[23] As such, the requirement to obtain informed consent to the extent described above is overridden by the exigencies of emergency care. Anesthesiologists should communicate as much information as the time and circumstances permit.

Confusion arises when treatment is needed but there is some evidence that the patient would prefer not to receive treatment. The important ethical distinction is whether the intervention is reversible. When it is reversible, and, for example, in the situation that an unconscious patient arrives in the emergency room needing tracheal intubation and a relative claims that the patient is "DNR" (do not resuscitate) but does not have the proper documentation, the therapy should be instituted. When the preferences are clarified, therapy may be withdrawn if appropriate. The clinicians must ensure that the patient's desires are met even in the face of the relatively slight burden of a temporary intubation, but when the intervention is irreversible, it may be inappropriate to proceed without clarification and documentation of a patient's wishes. For example, consider the Jehovah's Witness who in an emergency needs blood and is unable to communicate his or her preferences for transfusion therapy. Giving blood to a Jehovah's Witness is not a slight, temporary, burden, but creates for this patient a situation in which there is an irreversible loss of a good afterlife. Although emotionally unsettling, the legal and ethical consensus leans toward providing care in these circumstances. This is based on the concept that the refusal of life-sustaining treatment must be unambiguous, either on the basis of refusal by a patient with decision-making capacity or on grounds of a clear and valid advance directive.

Refusing to provide care

Anesthesiologists may refuse to provide care when they disagree for ethical and moral reasons with the proposed procedure. A typical example is an elective termination of pregnancy. Such an anesthesiologist should withdraw from clinical care except in an acute emergency. Some anesthesiologists may be prepared to find a competent and willing replacement but some may find the request to locate an alternative caregiver ethically objectionable.[24]

Physicians may also refuse to provide care if they believe that the patient's choice is inappropriate or likely to result in harm. Determining that an anesthetic choice is inappropriate is a difficult task and should not be invoked lightly or out of convenience. The patient's choice and the resultant risks must be sufficiently extreme to elicit a similar response from at least several other anesthesiologists. In addition, anesthesiologists may and should refuse to provide care when he or she does not feel qualified to provide the care needed. The provision of anesthesia at the extremes of age or in the presence of serious illness is a typical example of a special risk.

Anesthesiologists may refuse care only for reasons based on ethical or moral principles. For example, it is unethical for an anesthesiologist to base refusal to care for patients on factors such as race, gender, or disease status, such as infection with the human immunodeficiency virus (HIV).[25]

Pediatric informed consent

Patients, parents, other surrogate decision makers, and physicians use the concepts of best interests, informed assent, and informed permission to guide decision making in respect of healthcare for minors (Table 85.1).[26] The best interests standard is used when the capacity to apply self-determination is impossible, such as with an infant or a child with severe delay in development. This lack of capacity requires a surrogate decision maker, usually a parent, to select the care that is in the child's best interests. Difficulties may arise in determining who should make the decision and in accepting the assumption that there is always one best choice. Parents who are present and capable of participating in the decision-making process are well suited to be the primary decision makers for their children. This is in part due to society's respect for the concept of the family, and the assumption that parents care greatly for their children. It is also reasonable to assume that the child will incorporate some of the parents' values during growth and maturation, making the values of the parents a practical approximation of the child's future values.[27] For these reasons, parents have extensive leeway in determining what is in a child's best interests. By the same token, there is wide latitude in determining what constitutes acceptable decision making in today's multicultural society. It is often considered that there may be not one best choice, but several reasonable and good choices, depending on how the patient and family weigh benefits and burdens. This is particularly true for complex decisions involving informed consent, end-of-life issues, and confidentiality.[28,29]

Informed assent acknowledges that although most pediatric patients cannot legally consent to medical care (see exceptions below), pediatric patients can and should share in decision making to the extent that their development permits. The participation of children should increase as they grow older and depends on both the patient's maturity and the consequences involved in the decision (Table 85.2).

Pediatric clinicians are moving away from the concept of obtaining informed consent from the parent and are replacing it with the concept of informed permission. Informed permission has the same requirements as informed consent, but it recognizes that the doctrine of informed consent may apply only when individuals make autonomous decision for themselves, and not when surrogates make the decisions.[26] Informed permission provides a way by which this distinction is acknowledged, while still honoring the relations between the surrogate and the patient.

Anesthesiologists should attempt to achieve both informed

Table 85.1 *Elements of consent and assent as defined by the American Academy of Pediatrics, Committee on Bioethics*[26]

Consent

1 Adequate provision of information including the nature of the ailment or condition, the nature of the proposed diagnostic steps or treatment and the probability of their success; the existence and nature of the risks involved; and the existence, potential benefits, and risks of recommended alternative treatments (including the choice of no treatment)
2 Assessment of the patient's understanding of the above information
3 Assessment, if only tacit, of the capacity of the patient or surrogate to make the necessary decisions
4 Assurance, insofar as it is possible, that the patient has the freedom to choose among the medial alternatives without coercion or manipulation

Assent

1 Helping the patient achieve a developmentally appropriate awareness of the nature of his or her condition
2 Telling the patient what he or she can expect with tests and treatment
3 Making a clinical assessment of the patient's understanding of the situation and the factors influencing how he or she is responding (including whether there is inappropriate pressure to accept testing or therapy)
4 Soliciting an expression of the patient's willingness to accept the proposed care

Table 85.2 *Approaches to pediatric consent. This broad outline should be viewed as a guide. Specific circumstances must always be taken into consideration. When children are in the upper range of an age bracket, limited or full inclusion of a higher technique, such as the use of assent for a 6-year-old, may be appropriate*

Age	Decision-making capacity	Techniques
Under 6 years	None	Best interests standard
Ages 6–12 years	Developing	Informed permission Informed assent
Ages 12–18 years	Mostly developed	Informed assent Informed permission
Mature minor	Developed, as legally determined by a judge	Informed consent
Emancipated minor	Developed, as determined by a situation	Informed consent

permission from the parent or surrogate and assent, as appropriate, from the pediatric patient.[26,30] Infants and young children have no decision-making capacity and therefore assent is not a viable option, and anesthesiologists should obtain informed permission from the parent. School-age children are developing decision-making capacity, so anesthesiologists should seek both informed permission from the parent and assent and participatory decision making from the patient. Such situations may include whether to sedate a 6-year-old prior to an inhalation induction, to use an inhalation or intravenous induction of anesthesia in an 8-year-old, and to place an epidural for postoperative analgesia in a 12-year-old. Some adolescents and young adults over 14 years will have developed decision-making capacity and anesthesiologists should try to fulfill the ethical requirements of consent while obtaining assent. Examples may include obtaining consent from a 14-year-old for anesthesia for surgery for scoliosis, and from a 16-year-old for an awake thoracic epidural placement for a pectus repair.

Resolving disagreements in pediatric decision making

Parents and clinicians may disagree about the treatment that is in the best interests of the child. One way to resolve this issue is to define those choices that are unacceptable. The extent to which an anesthesiologist or physician may intervene between a patient and his or her surrogate's decision depends primarily on how harmful the decision is, or may be, to the patient. Criteria that must be used include the amount of harm that may result to the child by the intervention or by its absence, the likelihood of success, and the overall risk-to-benefit ratio.[31] In the practice of anesthesiology, the continuum between unacceptable and acceptable treatment provides clear extremes, but also an ambiguous gray zone. For example, although postoperative epidural pain therapy may be optimal, it is acceptable for the parents to choose to forgo regional analgesia in favor of parenteral analgesia. It is unacceptable, however, for the parent to refuse all forms of pain therapy. Although anesthesiologists must respect the diversity of values in society and the relationship between the parent and the child, decision making that imperils the health of a child needs to be challenged. The anesthesiologist who believes that the parent is choosing an unacceptable treatment should examine the reasons for this judgment, address those concerns, and involve other clinicians, both to offer an assessment of the appropriateness of care and also to engage the parent in discussion.[32] It is a serious issue to accuse a parent of not acting in the child's best interests. It may have significant social, fiscal and familial ramifications. If, however, after exhausting the options the medical staff believe that the parent is making unacceptable treatment decisions, an appropriate report should be submitted to the appropriate child welfare authorities for possible legal action, in accordance with the legal jurisdiction in which the issue arises.

If parents refuse, for a child who lacks capacity, the treatment considered necessary by the clinicians, the best interests standard described above may be invoked. This situation is more difficult to resolve when the minor has significant decision-making capacity and refuses a nonemergency procedure. Anesthesiologists should respect the right of pediatric patients not to assent to a procedure, and should go out of their way to avoid coercing or forcibly making the child accept the procedure. Achieving the patient's assent may necessitate further discussions with the patient, parents, and other providers, and such discussions should be in a place away from the operating room. In cases in which the parent and child disagree, clinicians should seek the assistance of others experienced in conflict resolution to help resolve the dispute with a minimum of rancor.[33] (See The ethics consultation service below.)

Emancipated minor status and mature minor doctrine

Some patients under the age of 18 years have the legal right to consent to treatment.[34,35] The term emancipated minor refers to minors who have been given the global right to make their own healthcare decisions. This status is generally awarded to patients who are married, parents, in the military, or economically independent, and may include patients who are pregnant. The mature minor doctrine holds that minors who have decision-making capacity are legally and ethically capable of giving informed consent in situations as determined by a court. Although particulars vary, the mature minor doctrine in general requires patients to be at least 14 years old, and tends to permit low-risk decisions. The nearer the child is to majority (usually an age of 18 years), the more likely the court is to grant the child the right to consent or withhold consent.[36]

Jehovah's Witness

A Jehovah's Witness believes that blood holds the "life force" and that "anyone who partakes of it shall be 'cut off' from eternal life after death." Patients who hold this belief refuse to accept blood transfusion even to save their lives. Anesthesiologists must therefore be experts in the burgeoning methods by which circulating blood volume and oxygen-carrying capacity may be optimized.[37,38] Anesthesiologists must also be aware that Jehovah's Witnesses do not all apply exactly the same interpretations concerning the prohibition of blood transfusion, and that clinicians must actively clarify what the patient considers acceptable.[39]

Anesthetic techniques designed to reduce blood loss may be used and include deliberate hypotension, deliberate hypothermia, and hemodilution. Most Jehovah's Witnesses accept synthetic colloid solutions, dextran, erythropoietin, desmopressin, and preoperative iron.[40] Some Jehovah's Witnesses accept autologous banked blood or cell saver blood, and some accept blood removed at the beginning of surgery and returned in a closed loop. Although blood components, autologous blood, and banked blood are generally unacceptable, these specifics must be discussed with the patient at the preoperative visit. Documenting acceptable interventions crystallizes the patient's desires and provides legal documentation for the anesthesiologist. Anesthesiologists must be certain that they can fulfill the patient's requests, or they should not agree to provide anesthesia. Indeed, the anesthesiologist and surgeon should provide nonemergent care to the patient only if all parties can agree on the approach to blood management.

Each case involving a Jehovah's Witness must be considered on its own merits. Case law strongly supports the right of the adult patient to refuse blood products. For a patient who is pregnant, a minor or a sole provider, the courts, in some jurisdictions, are more likely to intervene and mandate transfusion.[39]

ISSUES NEAR THE END OF LIFE

Refusal of cardiopulmonary resuscitation

Modern medicine has made the assumption that patients always prefer to be resuscitated. The American Medical Association challenged this assumption in 1974 by endorsing a policy that said in part, "the purpose of cardiopulmonary resuscitation is the prevention of sudden unexpected death. Cardiopulmonary resuscitation is not indicated in cases of terminal irreversible illness where death is not unexpected."[41] Shortly thereafter, policies permitting patients to limit resuscitation were published in the *New England Journal of Medicine*.[42,43] These policies acknowledged the need to protect patients' rights to limit the use of modern-day technology during terminal illness. Since that time, orders permitting refusal of cardiopulmonary resuscitation have undergone many adaptations, addressing recognized and perceived deficits such as documentation, communication, determining whether patients with DNR orders had a right to intensive care therapy and, finally, whether patients having surgical procedures were permitted to define the type of resuscitation received.[44,45]

The right of a patient to reject unwanted therapy in the operating room is now well accepted.[46,47] Before proceeding to the operating room, preoperative DNR orders should be re-evaluated in light of the surgical procedures, the anesthetic options, and the patient's overall goals. Anesthesiologists are then prepared to clarify and document the desired resuscitation status in the operating room by using either the goal-directed approach or the procedure-directed approach.[48]

The goal-directed approach characterizes the patient's preferences in terms of outcome without defining precisely which interventions will be performed.[48,49] The procedure-directed approach considers the patient's goals and then defines which interventions will be performed. Both goal-directed and procedure-directed approaches require the anesthesiologist to make predictions about the outcome of resuscitation. But as the goal-directed approach allows the prediction to be made at the time of resuscitation, it is likely to be more accurate. Clinicians can agree to provide such interventions if the likelihood of success, as defined by the patient, is acceptable, and to refrain from intervention or to stop intervention if the likelihood of success makes the intervention unacceptable (Table 85.3).

Patients may prefer either option. In a sample DNR consent, goal-directed and procedure-directed options may be combined into one form. The sample form lists four options: (1) full resuscitation, (2) a goal-directed order that seems to have the most applicability, (3) a procedure-directed order, and (4) a goal-directed order that the patient and clinicians can tailor. These are explained more fully as:

Option 1: full resuscitation
The patient desires that full resuscitative measures be employed during anesthesia and surgery and in the postanesthesia care unit, regardless of the clinical situation

Option 2: limited resuscitation – defined goal-directed
The patient desires resuscitative efforts during surgery and in the PACU only if the adverse events are believed to be both *temporary* and *reversible*, in the clinical judgment of the attending anesthesiologists and surgeons

Option 3: limited resuscitation – procedure-directed
During anesthesia and surgery the patient refuses the following specific resuscitative interventions [a checklist or summary statement listing desired procedures appears here]

Option 4: limited resuscitation – tailored goal-directed
The patient desires resuscitative efforts during surgery and in the postanesthesia care unit only if, in the clinical judgments of the attending anesthesiologists and surgeons, such resuscitative procedures will support the following goals and values of the patient: [a summary statement appears here]

Clemency and Thompson performed in-depth interviews with 18 terminally ill patients about resuscitative orders in the perioperative period in an attempt to better understand the thoughts of these patients.[50] Patients initiated DNR orders out of a desire to limit the physical, emotional, and financial costs to themselves and their families, and out of a desire not to have a life without quality. The majority of patients would desire treatment that would relieve discomfort, enhance the quality of their lives, or treat an isolated and remediable problem (e.g. a broken leg).

Patients differed on how they wanted their DNR order interpreted for the perioperative period. However, nearly all wanted to have input as to how their DNR orders should be interpreted, and as to whether physicians should use the patients' goals alone or lists of specific interventions. Some wanted to suspend DNR orders – "[The] operating room … is hallowed ground … something special … I want the doctor to do the best he can." Some wanted a procedure-directed order – "My biggest fear … is that some doctors could choose … who is going to live and who is going to die …" "I'd like to spell it out to them … I would want everything to be discussed." Some wanted a goal-directed order. "If [the doctor] … would just talk to me and my family … I would let

Goal directed	Procedure directed
Short-term care: hours	Long-term care: days to months
Operating rooms	Wards
Intimate knowledge of patient	General knowledge of patient
Flexible response	Defined response
A few specified clinicians	Many unspecified clinicians
Narrative or checklist	Checklist

Table 85.3 *A comparison of goal-directed and procedure-directed DNR orders. This comparison illustrates why the more traditional procedure-directed order is well suited for the ward, whereas the goal-directed order takes advantage of the characteristics of operating room care to enable the patient to communicate a more subtle declaration of preferences*

him decide what would be appropriate after he knew my ideas and the order."

Determining a patient's preferences for resuscitation in the operating room may involve both approaches. A procedure-directed approach may facilitate discussion and determine a patient's general preferences while still incorporating a mechanism to include a more aggressive intervention if the likelihood of a successful resuscitation is good. For example, the patient and anesthesiologist may agree to attempt resuscitation should there appear to be an acute reversible process such as ventricular fibrillation after insertion of a central venous catheter, but not attempt at resuscitation if the etiology seems less reversible.

Either approach should include a plan for postoperative care that may include a time-limited trial of intubation and ventilation if consistent with the patient's wishes. Ethical and legal opinion holds that the actions of withholding care and withdrawing care are conceptually equivalent.[51] This statement may feel emotionally to be untrue. Anesthesiologists who are quite comfortable with the decision to withhold treatment often feel great discomfort when asked to withdraw treatment. The withdrawal of treatment may be perceived perceived emotionally to be a proactive action when compared with withholding therapy, which may feel more like a passive action. These interpretations are often due to the honorable but mistaken belief of some physicians that starting a treatment makes them obligated to completing that treatment. Clinician discomforts related to the withdrawal of treatment are often predicated on personal beliefs and values. In fact, the opposite is likely to be true. A physician anesthesiologist should be more concerned about not starting a treatment rather than stopping an ineffective one. Withholding a therapy may require a higher degree of certainty about its probable failure or lack of desirability than withdrawing a therapy that has not achieved its goals. The ethical considerations involved in a decision to withdraw mechanical ventilation should be the same as those involved in a decision not to institute it.

DNR in an emergency situation without time to clarify a patient's wishes is inherently different. The traditional bias of providing treatment in the absence of a clear decision not to treat should hold for the anesthesiologist in the emergency situation. The situation can always be clarified later, and the patient withdrawn from the ventilator if it is determined that the patient would have preferred not to receive the interventions. In short, this "inconvenience" of intervention is worth the greater assurance in not anticipating the unrecorded desire. As discussed above, giving the patient a trial of therapy such as mechanical ventilation is one of the better ways to fulfill a patient's end-of-life desire to be the recipient of resuscitative efforts.[52]

The futility debate: the demand for life-sustaining therapies

The futility debate focuses on whether a therapy should be used when a specified goal is unlikely to be achieved. Anesthesiologists tend to confront this ethical dilemma in two situations. The first is in the intensive care unit, when, for example, families may desire further and extensive therapy for a loved one in the face of extremely low likelihood of success and a high likelihood of pain and discomfort. The second situation is in the operating room when a patient is scheduled for surgery that the anesthesiologist believes is futile. This most often occurs in patients at the extremes of age, such as the very sick neonate or the bedridden octogenarian having a gastric tube inserted.

The ethical goal is to individualize what may be considered futile care by helping individuals to weigh the benefits and burdens of the particular situations.[53,54] Owing to the difference in people's values, expectations, and desires, it is fruitless to attempt to define when a therapy is futile based only on its outcome or likelihood of outcome. Anesthesiologists should be careful not to assume that they fully understand the situation, and if they have this concern they should discuss the problem with the other clinicians involved so that the situation may be clarified. Benefits that are often considered include prolongation of life under certain circumstances, improved quality of life (such as reduction of pain or the ability to leave the hospital), and increased enjoyment of life. Burdens may include intractable pain and suffering, disability, and events that cause a decrement in the quality of life, as viewed by the patient.[31] For example, some patients may value an extra 2 weeks of life, no matter what the burden. Other patients may prefer to forgo the possibility of a longer life because the price required of them is too great.

Good care of the dying patient: palliation, comfort care, and demands for physician aid-in-dying

A good death is likely to include management of pain, aggressive comfort care, maintenance of dignity, a feeling of connectedness, and financial control.[55] One of the ways in which this is achieved is through hospice care, in which an interdisciplinary team brings the patient and family through the end-of-life period and optimizes the time remaining. Hospice care is palliative not curative. It seeks to reduce pain and symptoms by providing medical, emotional, psychologic, and spiritual care to the patient, and by assisting the family to cope with their impending loss and their subsequent grief. Aggressive management of comfort issues enables the patient to focus on more spiritual matters.

Clinicians should ensure that the terminally ill patient is pain free. They must not be afraid that treatment may cause narcotic dependency or hasten death through, perhaps, respiratory depression, but the intention must not be to kill.[56,57] This opinion is rooted in the doctrine of double effect, which places great emphasis upon the intention of the clinician in these cases in which one's actions may have both good and bad effects. The classic example is the administration of morphine to relieve pain in the terminally ill patient near the end of life. Although two possible effects of the morphine are recognized and foreseen (relief of pain as well as respiratory depression), only the good effect (relief of pain) is intended, and thus the caregiver is not held morally culpable if respiratory depression and an earlier death should occur.[58,59] The thrust of the principle is to focus upon the intention of the caregiver in seeking to provide comfort to the terminally ill patient, even though the clinician realizes that a side-effect of the medications could be respiratory depression and an earlier death. If the clinician uses a dose of morphine far in excess of that required to make the patient physically and emotionally comfortable, or if the clinician chooses an agent without pain-relieving properties (e.g. intravenous potassium), then the clinician cannot claim that the intention of the action was focused solely upon relief of the patient's pain and suffering. Indeed, such action may lead to a legal charge of homicide.

Physician aid-in-dying (PAD) includes any act that helps a patient die in response to an informed patient's request.[60] This includes physician-assisted suicide, which means that the physician facilitates the death by making the means, such as medicine, available to the patient. The patient must, however, perform the act of ingestion. Physician-administered euthanasia requires the physician to administer the medication directly. Some believe that there is an ethical distinction between making the medication available and actually administering it. They also believe that by requiring the patient to perform the final act lends some sort of moral safeguard to the procedure. Others, however, do not consider the distinction to be ethically significant, as both require effort and contribution from the physician. Further, they hold that psychologic pressure may defeat any potential safeguards inherent in requiring the patient to self-administer the drug. For the purposes of this discussion, unless otherwise specified, voluntary euthanasia and physician-assisted suicide will be considered together and the term physician-assisted death (PAD) used to denote both. Arguments surrounding PAD center on the interpretations of the principles of respect for autonomy and beneficence, and the possible ramifications of legalization (Table 85.4).[61]

Although physicians in the Netherlands had been practicing PAD for several decades, in 1993 the Dutch parliament granted physicians immunity from prosecution if the competent patient repeatedly requested euthanasia and had suffering that could not be relieved, and the physician reported the true cause of death to the coroner. Two nationwide investigations have been conducted into the Dutch practice of PAD.[62,63] The Remmelink study, in 1990, found that of the 130 000 deaths in the study period, 2700 resulted from PAD; 99% of patients who received PAD were expected to die within 1 month and physicians rejected over two-thirds of patient requests for PAD. In addition to those 2700 cases of PAD, however, the Remmelink study found that an additional 1000 patients had their lives ended by a physician without the explicit request of the patient. Patients requested PAD because of loss of dignity, pain, discomfort, fear of pain and discomfort, dependency, and "tiredness of life." The second study, in 1995, showed similar results. Nearly all the patients who received PAD appeared to have had a short life expectancy. To evaluate individual fear about reporting, regional committees were established in 1998 to evaluate the reported cases. It is too early for this approach to have provided data.[64]

In 1997, Oregon, USA, legalized the Oregon Death With Dignity Act, which permitted terminally ill patients to receive prescriptions in lethal quantities for the purpose of self-administration. It does not permit any other forms of PAD, such as administration of the medication by another person. Twenty-three persons received prescriptions in 1998; 21 used these as of 1999 and the other two were still alive.[65] Primary concerns of the patient were loss of autonomy and loss of control of bodily functions. The financial status of the patient did not seem to play a role in the request for PAD.

Interpretation of this information is not straightforward. One interpretation of the two Dutch studies is that the consistency exhibited over the 5-year period suggests that the Dutch are giving no evidence of increased use in legal terms. Another view, however, is that the interval between the studies has been inadequate to allow assessment of any true increase in use. Concerns remain about those patients who did not explicitly request PAD. Similarly, it is hard to interpret the 1-year information from Oregon.

The future role of the anesthesiologist in PAD is unclear. Some have suggested that anesthesiologists with expertise in pain management and pharmacology are the natural choice for performing PAD, if and when it becomes legalized.[66] Others suggest that the primary care physician, with intimate knowledge of the patient, prognosis, and disease process, should be the physician to provide PAD. The responsibiltiy of anesthesiologists is to ensure the provision of high-quality pain and comfort management.[67] It must also be remembered that legality does not necessarily confer morality. Many great evils have been perpetrated under the guise of the law.

Brain death and organ procurement

The concept of brain death is approximately 30 years old. Until that point, death was always defined as a cessation of heart and lung function. But, following the advances in mechanical ventilation and resuscitation therapy, it became apparent that there were situations in which the brain was dead, even in the presence of heart and lungs that may be kept functioning through medical intervention.

Before testing for brain death, certain conditions must be present to minimize the risk of a mistaken diagnosis. There should be the presence of a known proximate cause, evidence of a compatible central nervous

Table 85.4 *Arguments for and against legalizing physician aid-in-dying*

	Against	For
Autonomy	Requests for PAD are not a true expression of autonomy because: Inadequate patient and physician education about pain and comfort control leads to a choice that is not informed The patient may be depressed or feel like a burden on the family and thus the choice may not be made freely	Since the definition of a good death is personal, people should be allowed to control the circumstances If the burdens of being alive outweigh the benefits, physicians are obligated to permit PAD
Beneficence	Medicine can do a better job of pain and comfort control, thus decreasing the loss of dignity	Physicians can truly be a doctor from cradle to grave
	Permitting PAD will gravely harm the image of physician as healer	Patients will feel supported by physicians during this important time
Legalization	There will be concern about the clinician's impetus for offering euthanasia (e.g. race/gender/socioeconomic status)	Legal safeguards will prevent abuses
	Permitting PAD will discourage physicians from actively seeking solutions to the problems of those near the end of life	
Moral	Permitting PAD will devalue the sanctity of life, thus further nudging society down the slippery slope toward involuntary euthanasia	

system (CNS) catastrophe, absence of a confounding metabolic or toxic disturbance, and the patient should not be hypothermic, hypoxemic, or hypotensive.[68] Brainstem reflexes are then evaluated by examination of pupillary, corneal, and pharyngotracheal reflexes. The presence of brainstem reflexes is not consistent with the diagnosis of brain death. Testing for brainstem function concludes with the performance of the apnea test. Clinicians halt ventilatory support except for a continuous flow of intratracheal oxygen, and observe the patient for respiratory movements. An apnea test does not support the diagnosis of brain death if respiratory movements occur. An apnea test supports the diagnosis of brain death if the patient makes no respiratory movements and the arterial $P_{a}CO_{2}$ increases to greater than 8 kPa (60 mmHg) or increases 2.66 kPa (20 mmHg) over the baseline. A determination of brain death can usually be made after 10 min of apnea.

Movements may occur during the apnea test, which appear to be but are not inconsistent with the diagnosis of brain death. Spinal reflexes originating from below the level of the brainstem may cause limb and shoulder movements, back arching, sweating, and blushing.[69,70] The examination may be repeated 6 h after the initial test before brain death may be definitively diagnosed. The use of electroencephalography, angiography, and transcranial Doppler ultrasonography for the diagnosis or to confirm brain death is controversial.[71,72] Confirmatory tests are not commonly performed except when corroboration is necessary because of an unclear or inadequate clinical examination.

The diagnosis of brain death is disquieting.[73] To the family, the cadaver does not look recognizably different after the diagnosis of brain death. The skin is still warm, the monitor still shows the brightly colored blips of heart rate and blood pressure, and the chest still rhythmically expands and deflates. Family members are further unintentionally misled about the diagnosis by the erroneous use of phrases such as "withdrawing life-support." The term "life-support" may allow the family to infer that the patient will die, that is, not have life, if the support is withdrawn. The linguistic implication is that the patient is alive, and this may complicate the family's acceptance of the diagnosis of death.

Further medical support is necessary to maintain homeostasis for organ procurement or to permit loved ones a limited time to travel to see the cadaver in a more life-like state. Following the diagnosis of brain death, organ procurement officials should be notified so that they may broach the subject of organ donation with the family. In addition to fulfilling the wishes of the donor, the opportunity to donate organs may provide solace to the family by knowing that they are helping an individual in need of a transplantable organ.[74]

Anesthesiologists are responsible for ensuring that the patient is dead before performing organ retrieval.[73] Anesthesiologists should review the tests leading to the diagnosis of brain death to ensure that these were done correctly. A common error is to forget to evaluate the patient for pharmacologically induced neuromuscular paralysis.

There have been recent controversies about the ethics of organ donation using nonheart-beating organ donors (NHBDs).[75,76] In the standard circumstances described above, the patient is declared dead (through brain death criteria) prior to being brought to the operating room. The organs are then retrieved while body homeostasis is maintained through mechanical ventilation, pharmacologic therapy, and other standard resuscitative techniques. In nonheart-beating organ donors, the patient is *not* declared dead prior to being brought to the operating room for organ harvest. In this case, it is determined that the patient has an infinitesimal likelihood of survival and, rather than withdrawing care and letting the patient die outside of the operating room, care is withdrawn in the operating room. After documentation of between 2 and 5 min of pulselessness (depending on the protocol), death is declared, and organ retrieval begins.

The advantages of NHBDs include a possible increase in the number of organs available for donation.[77–79] Some argue that there is no ethically relevant distinction between withdrawing care in the intensive care unit and withdrawing care in the operating room and proceeding rapidly with organ retrieval. Others argue, however, that moving away from the clearer criteria of brain death may leave the system open to abuse, or may at least increase the suspicions of families when they are advised to withdraw care. One of the reasons for an inadequate number of transplantable organs is the perception in some minority groups that they do not benefit from organ donation. This perception, well rooted in a history of abuse in other areas of medicine, creates a cycle: fewer organs are donated, therefore less organs are implanted in members of that group who are more likely to have better matches, leading to fewer organs being donated in that group, longer waiting times, and increased distrust. They argue, then, that minimizing this mistrust will increase the number of organs for transplantation thereby minimizing the need to change the criteria for organ donation.

Other ways of increasing organ donation include the use of donor cards. In practice, however, donor cards are used in conjunction with the family's consent, relegating the cards to little more than evidence to the family that their loved one was, at one point in time, interested in organ donation. In fact, the most effective nonlegislative way to increase organ donation is to raise public awareness so that discussion among family members is increased, and family members can make clear to each other where they stand on organ donation. This clarity minimizes the doubt and anxiety that decision makers may feel.

Legislative initiatives to increase organ donation include the "required request law," presumed consent, and presumed consent with family agreement. In the USA, the "required request law" mandates that hospitals which receive federal monies must ensure that decision makers are asked about organ donation. If patients have not made their wishes clear to their families, decision makers must then try to discern what the deceased would have wanted. In some European countries, presumed consent laws permit organ procurement without any interaction with decision makers. A tempered version, presumed consent with family agreement, asks the decision maker for agreement to the proposed organ harvest. This helps to establish organ donation as normative, while respecting the decision maker's right to refuse organ donation. Presumed consent laws appear to increase organ donation in many situations. However, serious objections have been raised, centering on the rights of a person and family to control the body of a person after death, and excessive or unwarranted government intrusion into privacy. These discussions are part of larger societal issues about the rights and responsibilities of individuals and governments.

OTHER ISSUES

Research ethics

Anesthesiologists, as all physicians, should be diligent in avoiding the many ethical pitfalls involved in performing research. Research ethics is a complex area involving authorship questions, data representation, relations with industry, social responsibility, informed consent, and research design.[80–85] It is particularly helpful to examine perhaps the most notorious event in research, the Tuskegee syphilis experience. Initially designed as a snapshot evaluation of secondary syphilis, the Tuskegee experiment became a 40-year study observing the effects of syphilis on African-American males.[86] These men were lied to in many ways, including being falsely told that they were receiving medical therapy. Furthermore, antibiotics were not offered when their efficacy was recognized.[87] The Tuskegee study became ill focused and incurred patient risk without providing scientific benefit. The Tuskegee experiment continued until 1972 and was pivotal in motivating the formation of the National Commission for the Protection of Human Subjects of Biomedical and Behavioral Research.

Informed consent for research requires the decision makers to be fully informed about the risks, benefits, and alternatives of the proposed research. In addition, patients must be informed that they are free to withdraw from the study at any time without prejudice.[88] Other ethical requirements of research hold. A study must provide quality care for the subject and legitimate options for the nonparticipant. The investigator should have good reason to believe that the study will sufficiently benefit the subject or society as a whole with respect to the incurred risk. A poorly executed study wastes resources and puts subjects at risk, and if published may affect treatment decisions and harm patients. Institutional review boards help to ensure that the above principles are met by monitoring and by safeguarding the quality of the research as well as the informed consent processes.

Obligations of clinicians

Physicians are privileged members of society. These privileges include social standing, excellent remuneration, and the possession of a rationed skill. These skills were not obtained in isolation. The community invested limited resources to develop a medical infrastructure of materials, expertise, and learning opportunities, and also provided a stable society in which to live and study. As such, anesthesiologists have obligations beyond providing quality medical care.[89] Such obligations include participating in local and national governance, training future anesthesiologists, and supporting the advancement of anesthesia knowledge.[90]

Production pressure

Production pressure has been defined as "the internal or external pressure on the anesthesiologist to keep the operating room schedule moving along speedily."[91] Production pressure tends to influence whether anesthesiologists will postpone a case, or will perform clinical and technical duties with inappropriate haste, thus putting their patients at increased risk. Anesthesiologists have an obligation to the patient and themselves to provide care only within their skills, and to recognize when economic and administrative pressures may induce them to do otherwise. Anesthesiologists should attempt to design systems that minimize production pressures.

Another source of production pressure may be from managed care organizations (MCOs). At its best, managed care can encourage preventive care, continuing patient–physician relationships, collaborative relationships among primary care clinicians and specialists, and cost-effective performance improvement programs. At its worst, managed care can result in a mercurial bureaucratic system that prioritizes short-term cost containment, the development of a young and predominantly healthy customer population, and procrastination to avoid paying for expensive care.[92] MCOs accomplish these goals by "managing" or controlling physician and patient behavior through the use of case managers to coordinate care and through financial and administrative incentives to encourage physicians to conserve resources. Standard techniques include gatekeeping devices to control access to specialty care and MCO-specific practice guidelines to limit imaging tests, expensive drugs, and longer stays. Physicians have the obligation to participate in managed care to ensure that it is performed well and should participate in legislative initiatives to curb potential abuses, to work with MCOs to design systems that minimize conflicts of interest, and to actively fight abuses on an individual level. Anesthesiologists should examine MCO contracts for inherent problems, such as compensation through financial incentives, plans that do not have a reasonable or responsive appeals process, and policies that have an undefined physician termination procedure.[93,94]

The sick colleague

Anesthesiologists become ill through licit or illicit substance abuse, fatigue, injury, or increasing age. The most commonly recognized form of impairment is through chemical dependency on controlled substances used in the operating room, including narcotics, benzodiazepines, propofol, and ketamine. If untreated, chemical dependence is a fatal disease.[95]

Colleagues have an ethical responsibility to prevent and detect chemical dependency, and to engage in the treatment of colleagues who have the disease of dependency. This responsibility is rooted in a shared responsibility to ensure that only capable anesthesiologists practice, and in a professional collegiate responsibility to care for one another. Prevention requires active education of both anesthesiologists and their closest relatives about chemical dependency, through conferences, information pamphlets, and educational videos. A reliable accounting system for controlled substances is necessary to keep closer track of these substances, minimizing the opportunity for diversion or first use.[96,97] Prevention also includes establishing a professional environment that helps to minimize those situations which may lead to experimenting with controlled substances and subsequent chemical dependence. Stress from a perceived sense of failure, overwork, unrealized expectations[98] and lack of perspective are often precursors of chemical dependency.

Colleagues and their closest relatives should recognize the characteristics of chemical dependency. The window of time from abuse (the inappropriate use of the drug) to dependency (the physical or psychologic addiction to a drug) varies depending on the potency of the drug but can be very rapid. The characteristics of chemical dependency include rapid and unusual changes in behavior and mood, requests to work alone, and being overly willing to take relief duties, stay late and provide help, especially with cases involving high doses of narcotics. Addicts also have a tendency to care for patients who appear to have postoperative pain out of proportion to the procedure and the charted narcotics. Changes at home include withdrawal from formerly pleasurable activities, reclusive behavior, mood swings, and physical signs of withdrawal.

The process of bringing suspected chemical dependency to the addict's attention and beginning evaluation is known as intervention. Intervention is not ethically quiescent. It may involve manipulation or coercion of individual liberties with the purpose of convincing the physician that he or she does indeed have a problem. It is designed to rescue the physician from this otherwise fatal disease. Intervention is a serious matter that should be undertaken after due consideration and with the greatest of care to preserve the anesthesiologist's rights and dignity.[95]

Intervention is difficult and carries risk, and therefore should include someone with expertise in the area. A typical intervention is designed to bring to the anesthesiologist overwhelming evidence of chemical dependency. A small number of caring colleagues and friends may be required to detail to the anesthesiologist evidence of the addictive behavior, thereby attempting to overcome the addicted physician's natural state of denial. At the same time, given the intense loneliness and "boxed in" feeling that the anesthesiologist is likely to feel, emotional support reaffirming love and respect for the physician and emphasizing the picture of life after treatment is essential. The intervention plan should include the immediate referral to an evaluation center and should include accompaniment at all times until admission. The interval from intervention to evaluation is a risky time in which addicts, faced with "public" acknowledgement of their secret, may rashly hurt themselves. It is for this reason that all efforts should be made to prevent the addict from abruptly leaving the intervention alone.

If treatment is started, and appropriate aftercare implemented, the likelihood of a return to a productive and full life is high. Whether this includes or should include a return to the practice of anesthesia is dependent on the type of addiction, the environment, and the individual, among other things. It is unclear whether anesthesiologists should be encouraged to or be prohibited from returning to anesthesia practice.

Although most of the focus is on chemical dependency on controlled substances, anesthesiologists are susceptible to impairment though other drugs (e.g. alcohol, marijuana), disease (such as worsening eye sight or depression), and the decrement in senses, response time, and vigilance that may accompany fatigue or advanced age. By the same dyad of responsibilities to patients and colleagues, these issues need to be considered and managed in a direct and sympathetic manner.

The ethics consultation service

The ethical dilemmas that occur in the practice of anesthesiology may be difficult for the practitioner to resolve alone. Ethics committees and their consulting services act in an advisory role to help clinicians, patients, and families to resolve ethical dilemmas amicably.[99] Anesthesiologists may find ethics consultation helpful with questions covering informed consent, decision-making capacity, resuscitation decisions, and resolving disagreements among patients, families, and clinicians.[100–102] Following consultations, clinicians feel greater satisfaction in managing cases with ethical conflicts, not only because of their heightened awareness of the expert consulting services available but also because of their increased knowledge and comfort in dealing with these issues.[1,101,103] Ethics committees are also available to consult on policy development and to organize continuing educational programs.

REFERENCES

1. Waisel DB, Truog RD. An introduction to ethics. *Anesthesiology* 1997; **87:** 411–17.
2. Pellegrino ED, Hart RJ, Henderson SR, *et al.* Relevance and utility of courses in medical ethics. *JAMA* 1985; **253:** 49–53.
3. Beauchamp TL, Childress JF. *Principles of Biomedical Ethics*, 4th edn. New York: Oxford University Press, 1994.
4. Hirsh HL. A visitation with informed consent and refusal. In: Wecht CH (ed.). *Legal Medicine 1995.* Charlottesville, VA: Michie, 1995: 147–204.
5. Beauchamp TL. In: Veatch RM (ed.). *Informed Consent, Medical Ethics*, 2nd edn. Sudbury, MA: Jones and Bartlett Publishers, 1997: 185–208.
6. Affleck PJ, Waisel DB, Cusick JM, Van Decar T. Recall of risks following labor epidural analgesia. *J Clin Anesth* 1998; **10:** 141–4.
7. Foley HT, Dornette WHL. Consent and informed consent. In: Dornette WHL (ed.). *Legal Issues in Anesthesia Practice.* Philadelphia: FA Davis Company, 1991: 81–9.
8. Fenwick P, Beran RG. Informed consent: should Bolam be rejected? *Med Law* 1997; **16:** 215–23.
9. Farnill D, Inglis S. Patients' desire for information about anaesthesia: Australian attitudes. *Anaesthesia* 1993; **48:** 162–4.
10. Lonsdale M, Hutchinson GL. Patients' desire for information about anesthesia. *Anaesthesia* 1991; **46:** 410–12.
11. Leigh JM, Walker J, Janaganthan P. Effect of preoperative anaesthetic visit on anxiety. *Br Med J* 1977; **2:** 987–9.
12. Egbert LD, Battit GE, Turndorf H, Beecher HK. The value of the preoperative visit by an anesthetist. *JAMA* 1963; **185:** 535–5.
13. Klock PA, Roizen MF. More or better: educating the patient about the anesthesiologist's role as perioperative physician. *Anesth Analg* 1996; **83:** 671–2.
14. Dawes PJ, Davison P. Informed consent: what do patients want to know? *J R Soc Med* 1994; **87:** 149–52.
15. Kain ZN, Wang SM, Caramico LA, *et al.* Parental desire for perioperative information and informed consent a two-phase study. *Anesth Analg* 1997; **84:** 299–306.
16. Litman RS, Perkins FM, Dawson SC. Parental knowledge and attitudes toward discussing the risk of death from anesthesia. *Anesth Analg* 1993; **77:** 256–60.
17. Lankton JW, Batchelder BM, Ominsky AJ. Emotional responses to detailed risk disclosure for anesthesia, a prospective randomized study. *Anesthesiology* 1977; **46:** 294–6.
18. Waisel DB, Truog RD. The benefits of the explanation of the risks of anesthesia in the day surgery patient. *J Clin Anesth* 1995; **7:** 200–4.
19. Byrne J, Napier A, Cuschieri A. How informed is signed consent? *Br Med J* 1988; **296:** 839–40.
20. Cassileth BR. Informed consent – why are its goals imperfectly realized? *N Engl J Med* 1980; **302:** 896–900.
21. Clark SK, Leighton BL, Seltzer JL. A risk-specific anesthesia consent form may hinder the informed consent process. *J Clin Anesth* 1991; **3:** 11–13.
22. Hume MA, Kennedy B, Asbury AJ. Patient knowledge of anaesthesia and peri-operative care. *Anaesthesia* 1994; **49:** 715–18.
23. Bianco EA, Hirsch HL. Consent to and refusal of medical treatment. In: Sanbar SS, Gibofsky A, Firestone MH, Leblang TR (eds). *Legal Medicine*, 3rd edn. St. Louis: Mosby-Year Book, 1995: 274–96.
24. Dellinger AM, Vickery AM. When staff object to participating in care. *J Health Hosp Law* 1995; **28:** 269–85.
25. Council on Ethical and Judicial Affairs. *Opinion 2.23, HIV Testing, Code of Medical Ethics: Current Opinions with Annotations.* Chicago: American Medical Association, 1997: 61–2.
26. Committee on Bioethics, American Academy of Pediatrics. Informed consent, parental permission, and assent in pediatric practice. *Pediatrics* 1995; **95:** 314–17.
27. President's Commission for the Study of Ethical Problems in Medicine and Biomedical and Behavioral Research. *Deciding to Forgo Life-Sustaining Treatment: Ethical, Medical and Legal Issues in Treatment Decisions.* Washington, DC: US Government Printing Office, 1983.
28. Barker JC. Cultural diversity: changing the context of medical practice. *West J Med* 1992; **157:** 248–54.
29. Orr RD, Marshall PA, Osborn J. Cross-cultural considerations in clinical ethics consultations. *Arch Fam Med* 1995; **4:** 159–64.
30. Midwest Bioethics Center Task Force on Health Care Rights for Minors: health care treatment decision-making guidelines for minors. *Bioethics Forum* 1995; **11 (4):** A1–A16.
31. Committee on Bioethics, American Academy of Pediatrics. Guidelines on forgoing life-sustaining medical treatment. *Pediatrics* 1994; **93:** 532–6.
32. Anderson B, Hall B. Parents' perceptions of decision making for children. *J Law Med Ethics* 1995; **23:** 15–19.
33. Strong C. Respecting the health care decision-making capacity of minors. *Bioethics Forum* 1995; **11** (4): 7–12.
34. Sigman GS, O'Connor C. Exploration for physicians of the mature minor doctrine. *J Pediatr* 1991; **119:** 520–5.
35. Tsai AK, Schafermeyer RW, Kalifon D, *et al.* Evaluation and treatment of minors: reference on consent. *Ann Emerg Med* 1993; **22:** 1211–17.
36. Truog RD. Is "informed right of refusal" the same as "informed consent"? *J Clin Ethics* 1996; **7:** 87–9.
37. Practice guidelines for blood component therapy: A report by the American Society of Anesthesiologists Task Force on Blood Component Therapy. *Anesthesiology* 1996; **84:** 732–47.
38. Weiskopf RB. More on the changing indications for transfusion of blood and blood components during anesthesia. *Anesthesiology* 1996; **84:** 498–501.
39. Rothenberg DM. The approach to the Jehovah's Witness patient. *Anesth Clin North Am* 1990; **8:** 589–607.
40. Benson KT. The Jehovah's Witness patient: considerations for the anesthesiologist. *Anesth Analg* 1989; **69:** 647–56.
41. Standards for cardiopulmonary resuscitation (CPR) and emergency cardiac care (ECC): *JAMA* 1974; **227** (Suppl.): 833–68.
42. Rabkin MT, Gillerman G, Rice NR. Orders not to resuscitate. *N Engl J Med* 1976; **295:** 364–6.
43. Optimal care for hopelessly ill patients. A report of the Clinical Care Committee of the Massachusetts General Hospital. *N Engl J Med* 1976; **295:** 362–4.
44. Cohen CB, Cohen PJ. Do-not-resuscitate orders in the operating room. *N Engl J Med* 1991; **325:** 1879–82.
45. Truog RD. "Do-not-resuscitate" orders during anesthesia and surgery. *Anesthesiology* 1991; **74:** 606–8.
46. Statement of the American College of Surgeons on Advance Directives by Patients. "Do not resuscitate" in the operating room. *Am Coll Surg Bull* 1994; 29.
47. American Society of Anesthesiologists. *Ethical Guidelines for the Anesthesia Care of Patients with Do Not Resuscitate Orders or Other Directives that Limit Treatment.* Park Ridge, IL: House of Delegates, American Society of Anesthesiologists, October 13, 1993.
48. Truog RD, Waisel DB, Burns JP. DNR in the OR: a goal-directed approach. *Anesthesiology* 1999; **90:** 289–95.

49. Bastron RD. Ethical concerns in anesthetic care for patients with do-not-resuscitate orders. *Anesthesiology* 1996; **85:** 1190–3.
50. Clemency MV, Thompson NJ. Do not resuscitate orders in the perioperative period: patient perspectives. *Anesth Analg* 1997; **84:** 859–64.
51. Council on Ethical and Judicial Affairs, American Medical Association. Decisions near the end of life. *JAMA* 1992; **267:** 2229–33.
52. Annas GJ. Nancy Cruzan and the right to die. *N Engl J Med* 1990; **323:** 670–3.
53. The SUPPORT Principal Investigators. A controlled trial to improve care for seriously ill hospitalized patients. The study to understand prognoses and preferences for outcomes and treatments (SUPPORT). *JAMA* 1995; **274:** 1591–8.
54. Tomlinson T, Czlonka D. Futility and hospital policy. *Hastings Cent Rep* 1995; **25(3):** 28–35.
55. Foley KM. Competent care for the dying instead of physician-assisted suicide. *N Engl J Med* 1997; **336:** 54–8.
56. Solomon MZ, O'Donnell L, Jennings B, *et al.* Decisions near the end of life: professional views on life-sustaining treatments. *Am J Public Health* 1993; **83:** 14–23.
57. Practice guidelines for cancer pain management: a report by the American Society of Anesthesiologists Task Force on Pain Management, Cancer Pain Section. *Anesthesiology* 1996; **84:** 1243–57.
58. Quill TE. The ambiguity of clinical intentions. *N Engl J Med* 1993; **329:** 1039–40.
59. Thomson JJ. The trolley problem. In: Parent W (ed.). *Rights, Restrictions, and Risk.* Cambridge: Harvard University Press, 1986: 94–116.
60. Emanuel EJ. Euthanasia: historical, ethical and empiric processes. *Arch Intern Med* 1994; **154:** 1890–1901.
61. Waisel DB, Truog RD. The end-of-life sequence. *Anesthesiology* 1997; **87:** 676–86.
62. van der Maas PJ, van Delden JJM, Pijnenborg L, Looman CWN. Euthanasia and other medical decisions concerning the end of live. *Lancet* 1991; **338:** 669–74.
63. van der Maas PJ, van der Wal G, Haverkate I, *et al.* Euthanasia, physician-assisted suicide, and other medical practices involving the end of life in the Netherlands, 1990–1995. *N Engl J Med* 1996; **335:** 1699–705.
64. Widdershoven GAM. Euthanasia in the Netherlands: some first experiences of evaluation committees. *Hastings Cen Rep* 1999; **29** (4): 47–8.
65. Chin AE, Hedberg K, Higginson GK, Fleming DW. Legalized physician-assisted suicide in Oregon - the first year's experience. *N Engl J Med* 1999; **340:** 577–83.
66. Benrubi GI. Confidentiality in the age of AIDS. *J Reprod Med* 1992; **37:** 969–72.
67. Truog RD, Berde CB. Pain, euthanasia, and anesthesiologists. *Anesthesiology* 1993; **78:** 353–60.
68. Wijdicks EFM. Determining brain death in adults. *Neurology* 1995; **45:** 1003–11.
69. Urasaki E, Tokimura T, Kumai J, *et al.* Preserved spinal dorsal horn potentials in a brain-dead patient with Lazarus' sign. Case report. *J Neurosurg* 1992; **76:** 710–13.
70. Heytens L, Verlooy J, Gheuens J, Bossaert L. Lazarus sign and extensor posturing in a brain-dead patient. Case report. *J Neurosurg* 1989; **71:** 449–51.
71. Buchner H, Schuchardt V. Reliability of electroencephalogram in the diagnosis of brain death. *Eur Neurol* 1990; **30:** 138–41.
72. Grigg MM, Kelly MA, Celesia CG, *et al.* EEG activity after brain death. *Arch Neurol* 1987; **44:** 948–54.
73. Van Norman G. A matter of life and death. What every anesthesiologist should know about the medical, legal, and ethical aspects of declaring brain death. *Anesthesiology* 1999; **91:** 275–87.
74. Raper RF, Fisher MM. Brain death and organ donation – a point of view. *Anaesth Intensive Care* 1995; **23:** 16–19.
75. Fackler JC, Truog RD. Life, death, and solid organ transplantation without brain death. *Crit Care Med* 1993; **21:** S356–7.
76. Truog RD. Is it time to abandon brain death? *Hastings Cent Rep* 1997; **27:** 29–37.
77. Koogler T, Costarino Jr AT. The potential benefits of the pediatric non-heartbeating organ donor. *Pediatrics* 1998; **101:** 1049–52.
78. Evans RW. The actual and potential supply of organ donors in the United States. *Clin Transpl* **1990:** 329–41.
79. Daemen JW, Kootstra G, Wijnen RM, *et al.* Nonheart-beating donors: the Maastricht experience. *Clin Transpl* **1994:** 303–16.
80. Beecher HK. Ethics and clinical research. *N Engl J Med* 1966; **274:** 1354–60.
81. Angell M, Kassirer JP. Clinical research: what should the public believe? *N Engl J Med* 1994; **331:** 189–90.
82. Council on Scientific Affairs and Council on Ethical and Judicial Affairs: conflicts of interest in medical center/industry research relationships. *JAMA* 1990; **263:** 2790–3.
83. Katz J. Ethics and clinical research revisited: a tribute to Henry K Beecher. *Hastings Cen Rep* 1993; **23(5):** 31–9.
84. Lanier WL, Warner MA. New frontiers in anesthesia research: assessing the impact of practice patterns on outcome, health care delivery, and cost. *Anesthesiology* 1993; **78:** 1001–4.
85. Relman AS. Publishing biomedical research: roles and responsibilities. *Hastings Cen Rep* 1990; **20:** 23–7.
86. Caplan AL. When evil intrudes. *Hastings Cen Rep* 1992; **22** (6): 29–32.
87. Edgar H. Outside the community. *Hastings Cen Rep* 1992; **22** (6): 32–5.
88. Montgomery JE, Sneyd JR. Consent to clinical trials in anaesthesia. *Anaesthesia* 1998; **53:** 227–30.
89. Drane JF. *Becoming A Good Doctor: The Place of Virtue and Character in Medical Ethics.* Kansas City: Sheed & Ward, 1988.
90. Waisel DB. Nonpatient care obligations of anesthesiologists. *Anesthesiology* 1999; **91:** 1152–8.
91. Gaba DM, Howard SK, Jump B. Production pressure in the work environment: California anesthesiologists' attitudes and experiences. *Anesthesiology* 1994; **81:** 488–500.
92. Anders G. *Health Against Wealth: HMOs and the Breakdown of Medical Trust.* New York: Houghton Mifflin, 1996.
93. Howe EG. Managed care: "new moves," moral uncertainty, and a radical attitude. *J Clin Ethics* 1995; **6:** 290–305.
94. Committee on Medical Liability, American Academy of Pediatrics. Liability and managed care. *Pediatrics* 1996; **98:** 792–4.
95. Task Force on Chemical Dependence of the Committee on Occupational Health of Operating Room Personnel. *Chemical Dependence in Anesthesiologists: What you Need to Know When you Need to Know it.* Park Ridge, IL: American Society of Anesthesiologists, 1999.
96. Maltby JR, Levy DA, Eagle CJ. Simple narcotic kits for controlled-substance dispensing and accountability. *Can J Anaesth* 1994; **41:** 301–5.
97. Schmidt KA, Schlesinger MD. A reliable accounting system for controlled substances in the operating room. *Anesthesiology* 1993; **78:** 184–90.
98. McCall TB. The impact of long working hours on resident physicians. *N Engl J Med* 1988; **318:** 775.
99. Singer PA, Pellegrino ED, Siegler M. Ethics committees and consultants. *J Clin Ethics* 1990; **1:** 263–7.
100. Simpson KH. The development of a clinical ethics consultation service in a community hospital. *J Clin Ethics* 1992; **3:** 124–30.
101. La Puma J, Stocking CB, Silverstein MD, *et al.* Evaluation and utilization of an ethics consult service. *JAMA* 1988; **260:** 808–11.
102. La Puma J, Stocking CB, Darling CM, Siegler M. Community hospital ethics consultation: evaluation and comparison with a university hospital. *Am J Med* 1992; **92:** 346–51.
103. White BD, Zaner RM. Clinical ethics training for staff physicians: designing and evaluating a model program. *J Clin Ethics* 1993; **4:** 229–35.

86

Epidemiology and effectiveness research

GAVIN M M THOMS, FREDRICK K ORKIN, AND GRETL A McHUGH

This chapter examines three ways in which aspects of epidemiology can assist anesthesiologists to understand the knowledge base of our specialty. Most of the chapter is devoted to exploring methods that help us to formulate and answer research questions. The opening section explores where the foundation stones of our knowledge lie, with a focus on what can be learned from studying deaths and serious adverse events relating to anesthesia. The final section illustrates how anesthesiologists at every level use epidemiologists' techniques in their daily work.

Epidemiology[1–4] is the science concerned with "the occurrence, distribution and determinants of states of health and disease in human groups and populations." It has also been defined as "the study of the distribution and determinants of disease frequency." Typically it involves:[5]

- expertise in a set of methods rather than in a body of knowledge about a patient or disease group, as in much of clinical medicine;
- study of groups (usually comprising human subjects or patients) rather than of individuals;
- making comparisons between groups, often between a study group and a control group, using data on basic demographic details, health status, and histories of exposure to hazards or other suspected causative factors.

Cohen, a Canadian clinical epidemiologist, has explored the type of questions that are important to anesthesiologists which epidemiology can help answer (Table 86.1).[5]

Epidemiologists and anesthesiologists working together have produced a range of contributions to the knowledge base of anesthesia practice, including:

- Descriptions of patterns of disease or some aspect of a health service. Anesthesia examples include descriptions of the patterns of untoward events and anesthesia near misses,[6–9] and a description of pain service provision in the UK.[10]
- Measures of the strength of association between exposure to suspected causative factors and subsequent disease. An anesthesia example is the association between halothane anesthesia and subsequent liver damage.[11]
- Assessments of the effectiveness and cost-effectiveness of treatments of a disease. Anesthesia examples include the effectiveness and economics of different approaches to day-case anesthesia[12] and the growing understanding of costs of anesthesia services.[13,14]
- Explicit evaluations of the strength of evidence relating to a body of medical knowledge. An anesthesia example is the work of the Oxford Pain Relief Unit on the evidence base for pain treatments.[15,16]

HISTORY

The history of epidemiology is several centuries longer than that of anesthesia. Table 86.2 shows some of the major milestones in the history of epidemiology from an anesthesia perspective. It is of special note that John Snow, a renowned epidemiologist, was also one of the founding fathers of anesthesia.

MORTALITY STUDIES

Epidemiologists prefer clear endpoints, the least ambiguous of which is death. Many epidemiology studies have therefore been concerned with quantifying the risk of mortality relating to anesthesia, which has been reported to have decreased 100-fold over the last 50 years.[46,47] Much of this improvement occurred by the mid-1980s, before the advent of modern patient-monitoring standards and pulse oximetry (Fig. 86.1). Whether mortality due to anesthesia has decreased further is unknown, and perhaps unknowable now, because unfeasibly large sample sizes are required to discern true differences in such low rates.[48]

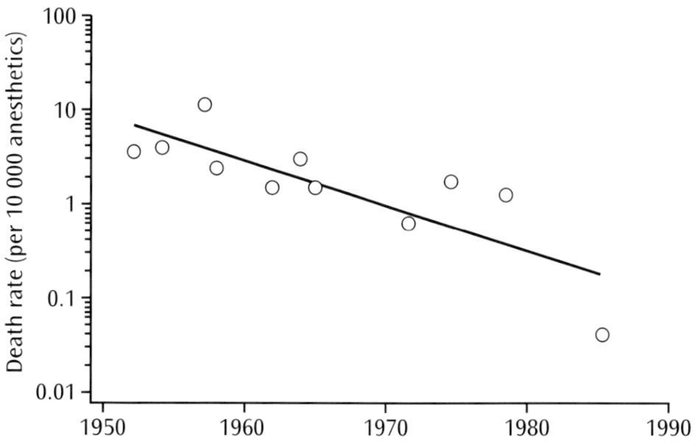

Figure 86.1 *Decreasing mortality primarily attributable to anesthetic management before the advent of patient-monitoring standards and the clinical application of pulse oximetry in the mid-1980s, by publication date of the study, 1952 through 1987.[26,49–62] (Modified after Figure 19.9 in Orkin.[46])*

Table 86.1 *Questions that epidemiology can help answer (adapted from Cohen[5])*

General questions	Specific anesthesia examples
Normality/abnormality: Is a person sick or well?	What is the range of normal responses to anesthetics? What constitutes an abnormal response?
Diagnosis: How accurate are diagnostic tests or strategies used to detect a disease?	How well can you predict which patients will develop malignant hyperthermia and which will not?
Frequency: How often does a disease occur? What are the changes over time?	What is the rate of perioperative reinfarction in those with a past myocardial infarction? Is there an upward or downward trend in incidence?
Risk: What factors are associated with an increased likelihood of disease?	Can we predict which cardiac patients are at highest risk for adverse events?
Prognosis: What is the long-term outlook of having a disease?	What is the long-term outcome for patients with postoperative neurologic deficit?
Treatment: How does treatment change the future course of a disease? Should you replace an old treatment with a new one?	Will using pulse oximeters eliminate or reduce hypoxic events? Should you use isoflurane rather than halothane?
Prevention: Does intervention in people without disease prevent disease from arising?	Should all patients receive antiemetics?
Causation: Which hazards will result in disease when people are exposed to them?	Does halothane cause postoperative liver necrosis?

Some of the mortality studies published in the past 20 years are summarized in Table 86.3. Mortality information is fraught with interpretation problems. Deaths due exclusively to anesthesia are now very rare; and although the occurrence of death is unambiguous, attributing causality is not. Attempts to interpret mortality information have encountered definitional difficulties,[66] can become complicated by issues of blame, and may depend on who is doing the assessing. A working group in 1985 came to a robust "agreed definition,"[67] but this has not been adopted universally. Most authorities now prefer the term "anesthesia-attributable mortality" to "anesthetic death."

Recent reviews of mortality are still beset with definitional uncertainties. Most studies support the notion of a steady downward trend in anesthesia-attributable mortality, while also highlighting lessons for quality of care and for future study design.[47,68–70] One recent study of death associated with anesthetic-related cardiac arrest estimated the risk to be substantially higher than expected. The authors accounted for this by suggesting that mandatory event reporting may have captured more events and using independent evaluators may have resulted in greater attribution to anesthetic management.[65] This is compatible with a general principle that studies focusing on detection of events may be prone to a bias known as ascertainment bias.

Mortality that anesthesia contributes to in part (anesthesia-related mortality) is much more frequent, occurs between 1 in 2000 and 1 in 4000 anesthetics, and may be rising.[53,57,70] Interpretation is difficult, as the background trend is one of an ever-aging population, with deteriorating risk factors such as comorbidity and increasing surgical complexity. Worse outcomes may not therefore represent decreasing standards. The factors leading to death have changed over the years: inadequate preparation and postoperative care have overtaken ventilatory failure and aspiration of gastric contents as the leading factors.[71]

Yet, argument still continues about the apparent steady reduction in anesthesia-attributable mortality.[72] For example, Ross and Tinker, in a careful and thorough analysis of mortality and risk studies in anesthesia, argue against concluding that such a reduction in mortality has definitely occurred.[73] They also note that the vanishingly low mortality directly attributable to anesthesia, resulting from decades of continuing effort by anesthesiologists to improve patient safety, leads to a serious risk of clinicians underestimating the importance of established standards and guidelines.

The "small number" issue requires that other indicators have to be used to evaluate practice standards, such as the routine use of pulse oximetry.[74] Much can be learned to inform quality improvement from an "accident investigation" approach,[70,75] studies of critical incidents and near misses,[6–9] and studies based on the far larger numbers of anesthesia-related deaths, that is perioperative deaths to which anesthesia has been deemed to have contributed in part.[68,76–80]

One such study, a long-running and important initiative in the UK, is the Confidential Enquiry into Perioperative Deaths (CEPOD). This began in 1982 within three National Health Service regions surrounding London and later, as "National CEPOD," developed to cover the entire UK (except Scotland, which has its own system, Scottish Audit of Surgical Mortality – SASM).[58,62,81–93] NCEPOD is a collaboration between anesthesiologists, surgeons, and pathologists, which has published influential reports annually since 1987. There has been a change from the initial purpose of CEPOD, investigating causation of surgical- and anesthesia-related mortality, toward a more practical one: extracting the key lessons for improved quality of medical care. The tone has also changed. Initially there were many critical comments about surgeons' and anesthesiologists' performance and decision making. Latterly the focus has changed to concern about resourcing, provision, and management of services.

Each year's report presents a particular theme, while many recommendations run through the entire series of NCEPOD reports, for example:

- *Supervision*: NCEPOD recommends improvements in levels of supervision; trainee anesthesiologists turning to seniors for advice; and consultant availability.
- *Facilities and organization*: Dedicated emergency operating rooms, emergency operating room staff, and 24-h recovery rooms have been deemed essential. Critical care facilities (high-dependency and intensive care units) appeared inadequate, with many patients who require critical care failing to obtain it. NCEPOD recommends that hospitals admitting emergency surgical patients should be able to provide sufficient critical care services on a 24-h, year-round basis.
- *Decision making*: Decisions regarding resuscitation and surgery have been seen to be flawed, especially in seriously ill patients. Undue pressure to operate often displaced clinical optimization and could be more of a problem than delayed surgery. Terminally ill or moribund patients had surgery that would not have improved their outcome. NCEPOD recommends more involvement of the most senior anesthesiologists in assessing and prioritizing patients in poor physical condition and at high risk of dying.
- *Clinical and educational issues*: Thromboembolic disease and fluid balance, especially in the elderly, have been recurrent problems. The

Table 86.2 *Historic milestones: epidemiology from an anesthesia perspective*

Publication date	Source	Comments
Fifth century BC	Hippocrates[17]	Recognized association between environment and health
1662	Graunt[18]	Quantified and published London's mortality rates
1839	Farr (see Hennekens and Buring)[2]	Compiled causes of death in England and Wales
1855	Snow[19]	Published *On the Mode of Communication of Cholera*
1893	The "Lancet Commission"[20]	Attempted to resolve relative risks of ether and chloroform, without reaching reliable conclusions
1920–46	Morton and Wylie,[21] Mendelson[22]	Characterized pulmonary acid aspiration syndrome, having reviewed large numbers of pregnancy records; leading to improved anesthesia practice
1932–42	Waters,[23] Tovell and Dunn,[24] Rovenstine[25]	Instituted systematic anesthesia record keeping; analyzed local anesthesia practice to improve quality of care
1954	Beecher and Todd[26]	Studied anesthesia-attributable deaths in 600 000 anesthetics; showed relative safety of thiopental (thiopentone); highlighted threefold variation in perioperative mortality rates between hospitals; included some unreliable conclusions (e.g. "inherent toxicity" of curare)
1964	Feinstein[27]	Urged all doctors to demand more scientific underpinning of medical practice
1966	National Halothane Study[28]	Investigated association with hepatic necrosis; highlighted threefold variation in perioperative mortality rates between hospitals, after adjusting for patient risk factors
1969	Sackett[29]	Established major program in critical appraisal skills; pioneered applying literature-based knowledge to physicians' immediate clinical decision making
1972	Cochrane[30]	Noted that clinicians are deluged with unmanageable amounts of information, and that most clinical procedures had never been properly evaluated; advocated more randomized controlled trials across the spectrum of medicine and more reliable, updated systematic reviews of available evidence
1976–87	Scott *et al.*,[31] Flood and Scott[32]	Showed that differences between hospitals in perioperative mortality are partly explained by nonclinical, social, and organizational factors
1977–80	Goldman *et al.*,[33] Leventhal *et al.*[34]	Derived predictive rules for perioperative risk of cardiac complications and respiratory failure, based upon multivariate modeling; ushered in efforts to predict adverse events and provide therapeutic guidance
1986–99	Knaus *et al.*,[35,36] Pronovost *et al.*[37]	Developed predictive scoring for critical care mortality; attributed variation in outcome to a mix of clinical and organizational factors
1988–2002	Cohen *et al.*,[38,39] Cullen *et al.*,[40] Howell *et al.*,[41] Silber *et al.*[42–44]	Quantified multivariate risk for perioperative mortality and complications, using patient, anesthesia, surgery, and hospital data
1999	Cochrane Anaesthesia Review Group[45]	Established headquarters in Copenhagen, linked to regional Cochrane Review Groups throughout the world, conducting and updating systematic reviews and creating a register of methodologically sound controlled trials

Table 86.3 *Recent mortality studies: deaths primarily attributable to anesthesia*

Authors (publication date)	Mortality rate	Details
Lunn and Mushin (1982)[58]	1 in 10 000	Mortality due wholly to anesthesia within 6 days of surgery was judged as 0.9 deaths/10 000 anesthetics in three UK National Health Service districts
Tiret and Hatton (1986)[60]	1 in 13 200	Mortality due wholly to anesthesia in a French study of 198 000 anesthetics between 1978 and 1982. When cases of coma (expected deaths) were added, the rate was 1 in 8000
Holland (1970, 1987)[61,63]	1 in 10 250, falling to 1 in 26 000	Estimates from Australia based on 24–55 deaths between 1960 and 1984; denominators estimated
Buck *et al.* (1987)[62]	1 in 185 000	Mortality in the UK, due wholly to anesthesia in mid-1980s within 30 days of surgery
Eichhorn (1989)[64]	1 in 200 000	Mortality in over 1 million ASA physical status I and II patients anesthetized between 1976 and 1988 in nine affiliated US teaching hospitals
Newland *et al.* (2002)[65]	1 in 18 182	Mortality associated with anesthetic-related cardiac arrest among unselected patients anesthetized between 1989 and 1999 in one US teaching hospital

level of experience of anesthesiologists was often not well matched to the complexity of the cases. NCEPOD recommends better local policies to achieve this matching task, and more multidisciplinary working on quality improvement initiatives.

NCEPOD reports appear to be effective in altering anesthesiologists' attitudes and practice in response to the issues highlighted.[93]

Recent NCEPOD themes have included: changing the way we work,[91] extremes of age,[89] specific operations occurring before death,[88] and the pattern of workload by time of day.[87] Specific recommendations for quality improvement that emerge from these studies include:

- The need for improved record keeping, case notes, and systems for data retrieval. A national specification for case notes is recommended, including a standard audit record for all deaths.
- The need for special skills in effective pain management for the elderly.
- Wider availability of fiberoptic laryngoscopic equipment.
- Attention to the dangers of aortic stenosis, and better provision of echocardiography services.
- Increasing the skills of all doctors and ward nurses in central venous pressure monitoring.
- More regionalization of children's surgery services, to increase expertise available and reduce occasional practice.

National programmes similar to NCEPOD, but on a smaller scale, have been carried out in Germany[94] and The Netherlands.[95]

In contrast, investigators in the USA and Canada have used multivariable modeling of large observational databases to investigate the role of risk factors for specific adverse events[38–40,42–44] and large registries [e.g. American Society of Anesthesiologists' (ASA) Closed Claim Project[96]], which are described later in this chapter.

FORMULATING AND ANSWERING RESEARCH QUESTIONS

The way an epidemiologist approaches a new research question can be divided into three phases. To start with, a problem needs resolving or perhaps a piece of vital knowledge seems to be missing. This phase is characterized by a period spent gathering background facts, literature, and expertise, which are then evaluated to establish what is already known or believed; and what, precisely, is the question that remains to be explored.[97–99] This phase might be typified as being iterative and reflective (Fig. 86.2).

Understanding literature depends on two key skills: defining and carrying out the search, and critically appraising the literature.[100–103]

Literature searching

Electronic databases, on-line and on CD-ROM, form the cornerstone of most modern searching, including MEDLINE (Index Medicus, National Library of Medicine, Washington DC), EMBASE (Excerpta Medica, Reed Elsevier, Amsterdam), CINAHL (Cumulative Index to Nursing and Allied Health Literature, CINAHL Database) and the Science and Social Science Citation Indices (Institute for Scientific Information).

Searching for previous clinical trials can be far more difficult than intuition suggests. A range of searching strategies has been recently published, which shows how the use of different searching terms produces very different results both of relevant and irrelevant material (the "precision" and "sensitivity" characteristics of the search strategy).[102] The National Institutes of Health (NIH) has developed a new Internet-based clinical research trial database that currently contains information on more than 6500 clinical trials (http://clinicaltrials.gov/), and a bibliographic database holding details of many trials is available from the Cochrane Library.[104] In addition, an important review from the Oxford Pain Relief Unit covers literature relating to pain.[16] More anesthesia-specific support is becoming available from the Cochrane Anesthesia Review Group, including access to a clinical trials database relevant to anesthesia and advice on searching for anesthesia-related trials.[45] Electronic databases do not necessarily include all the important publications from health care. Hand-searching may dramatically increase yield of relevant studies and is essential for literature published before 1966.[103,105]

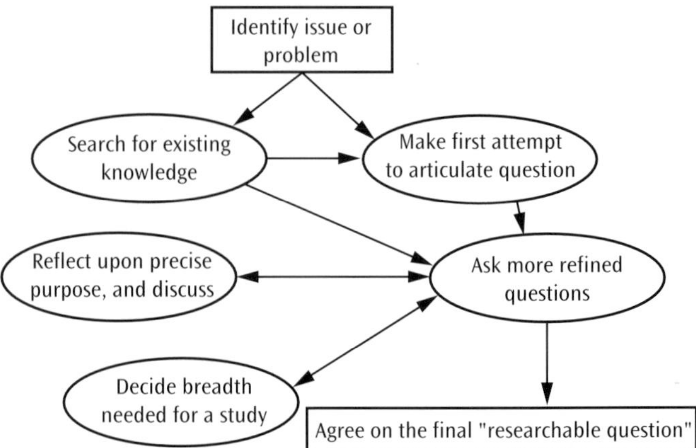

Figure 86.2 *Epidemiologist's approach – phase 1: aims and scope.*

Critical appraisal

Critical appraisal is based on an understanding of research, and involves the systematic scrutiny of the appropriateness of methods, design and conduct of studies, and the conclusions and interpretation drawn. Very helpful guidance is available on critical appraisal of literature.[100,101,106]

The ideal outputs of the first, reflective, stage of the epidemiology process are a broad awareness of the subject and background, a definition of an agreed and negotiated "researchable question," and a defined set of objectives. The first phase will ideally also have identified and brought on board some of the main "stakeholders." The latter include both those who have a positive interest in the outcome of the project that is emerging and, importantly, those, if any, who have the power to make it difficult to carry out, if not included in the project.

By now, the original problem will probably have been redefined. In achieving "researchable question" status, it is likely to be more tightly expressed and more easily quantifiable. Issues to take into account include making the most of existing definitions and data sources, clearly defining the patient group(s) to be studied, identifying selection and exclusion criteria, and making explicit any definitions relating to time and place. An explicit timeline for arriving at the answer is useful.

The second phase of the epidemiologist's approach uses one or more of the many study designs available, to address the question that has emerged as the outcome of phase 1.[1–4,97–99,107,108] This phase involves managing a project, usually involving costly resources (such as researchers and materials), to collect data. Unlike the iterative style of phase 1, the working approach now is one of project management (Fig. 86.3).[109–111]

The third phase of epidemiology's contribution to anesthesia involves extracting the learning. The aim is to apply research findings to the practical day-to-day working of individual professionals, organizations, and those charged with responsibilities relating to policy. This phase is therefore concerned with such issues as:

- determining the key messages that come out of the research findings,[98,99,112] establishing and, if necessary, asserting how robust these findings are;
- distilling and packaging messages for distinct audiences: for clinical practice, for local managers, and for those with policy responsibilities;[97–99,113]
- taking into account the incentives and change devices which have proved successful in influencing the clinical practice patterns of physicians;[114–116]
- finding devices and mechanisms for disseminating information,[117–119] such as publication, education,[120] production and implementation of clinical guidelines,[121–126] conferences, and the use of organizational websites.

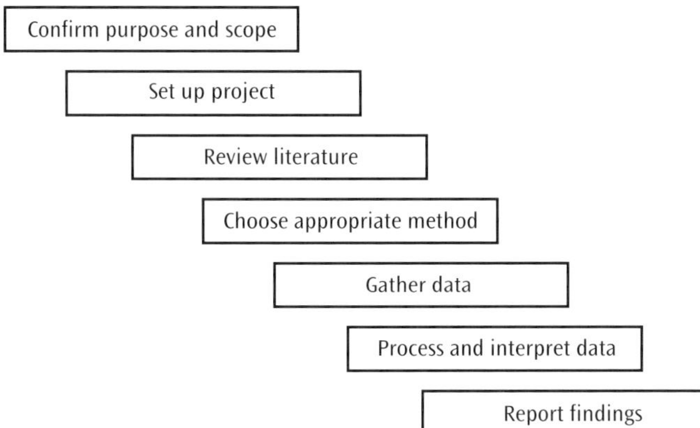

Figure 86.3 *Epidemiologist's approach – phase 2: conducting the research study.*

STUDY DESIGN

Five main study types account for the majority of clinical epidemiologists' work: case studies and case series, cross-sectional, case–control, cohort, and clinical trials. Epidemiologists sometimes classify their armamentarium of study types by intent (descriptive, analytic, or interventional), sometimes by reference to a time dimension (cross-sectional, retrospective, or prospective), sometimes by type of data source (routine or ad hoc), and sometimes by how natural or how artificial the setting is (observational or experimental). Tables 86.4 and 86.5 tie together these potentially confusing nomenclatures, summarize the main types of epidemiology studies, contrast their strengths and weaknesses with those of traditional case study and case series approaches, and outline the kind of findings that emerge from each approach.

Hierarchy of study types

There is a generally agreed hierarchy, ranging from the most robust study, the clinical trial (also the slowest, most costly, and least flexible), to the quickest, the case study (lowest cost and least reliable), as shown in Fig. 86.4. This hierarchy is noteworthy as Cohen[5] (in 1990) noted that, as a specialty, anesthesia appeared to be "...'stuck' in traditional methods such as the use of case reports, case series, anecdotes, and one's 'own experience'."

Cohen's view is supported by a 1988 study of literature of North American anesthesia,[129] which found the following breakdown:

- case reports and case series, 58%;
- cross-sectional and prevalence studies, 1%;
- case–control studies, 3%;
- cohort studies, 8%;
- nonrandomized intervention studies, 13%;
- clinical trials, 18% (many with design problems).

Much of clinical epidemiology is devoted to the effectiveness of treatments and the value of diagnostic tests, processes that constitute so much routine medical care. Our core task of administering anesthesia is arguably neither treatment nor diagnosis, which may go some way to explain the lack of robustness in our literature before recent developments in evidence-based anesthesia.

This quest for highly dependable evidence matters most when establishing drug effectiveness or investigating the potential harm of an interaction, and when emerging knowledge appears to be challenging established medical practice. The most appropriate design for a robust study producing credible findings is widely held to be the randomized clinical trial (RCT), as RCTs measure a difference in impact of an intervention with predetermined precision. However, it is not always possible or appropriate to test every issue by RCT. Simpler descriptive and observational studies are usually needed first. Partly this is to establish the basic facts and generate the key questions for detailed study. Partly it is because the benefit of greater precision is balanced by the disadvantage of focusing only on a very restricted set of issues. Alternatives to the RCT are set out in Table 86.5 and in the later section of this chapter on effectiveness research.

Systematic reviews[16,45,102,104,105,112,130,131] draw on a search for all relevant similar trials, make an explicit assessment of the quality of evidence available, and present the overall picture from all suitable trials considered together. The analysis may be supported by a meta-analysis (of which more details are given later in this chapter).

Much of the impetus for conducting systematic reviews and meta-analyses is the legacy of Archie Cochrane, a British epidemiologist who recognized that healthcare professionals are deluged with an unmanageable amount of information. Calling attention to our great

Table 86.4 *Characteristics of a case study or case series*

Explanation	Advantages	Disadvantages
A descriptive report of a particular patient or group of patients by a clinician. The term also applies to reviews of "cases" that are not people, such as hospitals or services. Case studies and series are considered to be preliminary observations. They may generate hypotheses (about cause and effect for example), but these are tentative and subject to subsequent refutation. However, they are an important starting point for developing a body of knowledge. Snow's 1847 case series[127] helped dispel mistrust of ether anesthesia	Requires few resources	Case definition may be problematic, especially initially, making time series comparisons impossible
	Acts as an important pathway to developing a body of knowledge. The process of description is an essential first step to understanding and can help to clarify events, issues, or objectives. Case studies provide the first building block of much of the knowledge base of medicine	Generally rely heavily on observational skills of the researcher, who may be subject to bias
The investigator setting about a case report or case series requires a working hypothesis, clear aims and objectives, and very clear ideas on what data to collect and how they will be analyzed. The data may involve, for example, clinical procedure details, clinical outcome details, rating or assessment of well-being, rating or assessment of a particular service, testimony from an individual or group	Fits comfortably into the tradition of medical learning and teaching situations	Case studies may appear subjective or unscientific since they are unlikely to contain quantitative data, are not normally subject to statistical analysis, and no comparison group is involved
The problem of observer bias is so large that techniques to minimize this, which have been well described in the context of qualitative research,[97,128] are worth adopting. Studies of this kind may be impossible to repeat and difficult to interpret, so, despite the apparent simplicity, expert advice will often still be required in design and interpretation	The "power of the story" can be an effective contribution to implementing change. Case studies may provide a more effective means of conveying importance of an issue than arguments based on figures alone	Any conclusion must be tentative and qualified with caveats. Generalizability and transferability are very limited. Observations may apply only to specific patients, organizations, or situations

Table 86.5 *Comparison of four basic types of epidemiology studies*

Explanation	Advantages	Disadvantages
Cross-sectional study		
A descriptive study with no comparison group, which surveys current state of health or disease and current information on exposure factors. This is a "snap-shot" of health status, which can be repeated annually or gathered across a very large sample. Many data items can be collected A commonly used tool for planning at government level or for large healthcare organizations	Inexpensive and simple to undertake, and powerful in the sense that the database may be very large and analysis capable of exploring many associations Provides instant indication of the prevalence of disease in a population, possible causative factors, and demographic information. Trends are available from repeated surveys May start the process of hypothesis generation	Generally it is impossible to disentangle cause, effect, and confounding influences Cannot help distinguish between different possible explanations of observed phenomena Not useful in establishing causality
Case–control study		
An observational study, normally retrospective, which selects those patients who have the disease or health state of interest and a suitable number of like subjects who do not have the disease. Past exposure to suspected etiologic factors is compared in the two groups Definition and selection processes for cases and for controls are critically important. Clear inclusion and exclusion criteria are required. The intention is to ensure that bias does not arise from the way cases and controls are selected and managed	Statistically strong, leading to measures such as odds ratio (but not attributable risk). Enables investigation of more than one potentially causative (or risk or preventive) factors at a time. There is a risk of invalidation, though biases can be minimized by careful selection of cases and controls, and careful design Can be carried out relatively quickly. Generally less costly than other epidemiologic studies and fewer subjects are needed than in, for example, cross-sectional studies May be an essential step in making causal or preventive links and generating or strengthening hypotheses Well suited for disease with long incubation periods, e.g. breast cancer or cardiovascular disease, or rare diseases	Susceptible to bias in selection of cases and controls. Recall bias is a major issue. Patients may selectively recall exposure factors of interest, especially if there is widespread awareness about the association under study This and other biases can be impossible to eliminate altogether, and can cast doubt on the findings of even the most elaborate and expensive case–control study Controls may be difficult to identify
Cohort study		
An observational study (normally prospective and sometimes termed "longitudinal") in which people are enlisted who have been (or will be) exposed to the suspected hazard, benefit or cause of illness. This group is followed up over a period of time, sometimes prolonged, along with a group of unexposed people The two groups are then studied for the occurrence of subsequent disease, condition of interest or death	Provides the most direct measurement of the risk of disease developing. Statistical measures used include rates of incidence of the outcome of interest, attributable risk and relative risk. Enables investigation of multiple outcomes Minimal potential for selection bias Provides information about disease etiology	Expensive and time-consuming Controls may be difficult to identify May lose subjects and controls to follow-up, leading to reduction in the value of the study and a source of bias The true determinant of a disease may actually be a hidden (confounding) factor and not the hazard that is under study
Randomized control trial		
An experimental prospective study that randomly allocates comparable subjects into one or more treatment groups and a control group. The intention is that treatment and control groups have similar characteristics (e.g. age spectrum, comorbidity) A further refinement (blinding) aims to ensure that the patient, provider of the treatment, and observer are unaware of group identity until the outcome is known RCTs are generally used to assess efficacy of treatments, but other interventions such as preventive initiatives can also be evaluated Increasingly regarded as the basis for best clinical practice	The gold standard for credible research findings, providing data of high quality Leads to statistical measures such as rates of disease in treated and control groups, relative and attributable risk, numbers needed to treat for each case benefiting Can be used to test service or treatment performance against objectives	Expensive and often difficult to conduct, with major recruitment and management challenges. Long timescales are generally required, and a large sample size may be needed for a definitive finding. Pitfalls include failed randomization, poor blinding, losing patients to follow-up, noncompliance with intervention regimen, and failure to reach desired sample size May be ethically problematic, particularly if there are strongly held beliefs (however unfounded) relating to risks or benefits of a particular intervention (e.g. use of pulmonary artery catheter) Adverse reactions or unexpected events may stop the trial By the end of the trial, medical care may have changed, or the all-important question may have changed May not be generalizable beyond study population

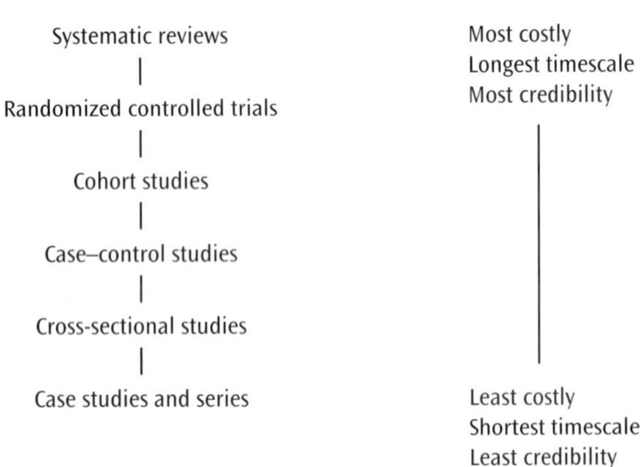

Figure 86.4 *Hierarchy of study types.*

collective ignorance about the effects of health care, he proposed that formal systematic reviews of all relevant RCTs should be undertaken and periodically revised, specialty by specialty.[30]

This Cochrane principle was accepted worldwide, and the Cochrane Centre was established at Oxford in 1992 to develop the International Cochrane Collaboration. This fosters regional Cochrane centers throughout the world, which set up collaborative review groups to undertake systematic reviews. Other Cochrane activities include annual colloquia to agree on methodology, maintenance of a website (http://www.Cochrane.org), and compiling and updating the Cochrane Library's Controlled Trials Register.[104]

For a number of years, there has been a Cochrane Pain, Palliative Care and Supportive Care Collaborative Review Group (http://www.jr2.ox.ac.uk/cochrane). The Cochrane Anesthesia Review Group (http://www.cochrane-anesthesia.suite.dk) was established in 1999 to conduct systematic reviews of clinical trials in anesthesia, perioperative medicine, intensive care medicine, and prehospital, resuscitation, and emergency medicine.

KEY ISSUES IN STUDY DESIGN

Defining a population

The group to be studied must be tightly specified by defining the age, gender, ethnicity, and other characteristics of the subjects. The places of residence, employment, and treatment may be relevant, and details that are to be recorded of the initial patient assessment, intervention, follow-up, and other clinical factors should also be carefully defined. Populations are not always composed of people. For a study of bacterial contamination of intubating bougies, for example, the population is likely to be composed of bougies, anesthetizing rooms, or difficult intubation scenarios.

Drawing a sample

The process of sampling should ensure a true representation of the wider population. Considerations influencing the representativeness of a sample include:[98]

1. *A sampling frame.* This is the list of population members from which the sample will be drawn. Ideally, this list contains the basic identity details of every member of the wider population, in each case entered only once, set out in common format and with an acceptably low error rate. The term sampling strategy is given to the method by which sample members are selected from the sampling frame.
2. *Sample size.* Too small a sample risks failure to demonstrate a real difference where one exists (a type II error) and is a common and important problem in anesthesia studies.[98] Prior calculation of desired sample size is essential. Statistics textbooks[132–135] provide more details on sample size calculations.
3. *Multicenter design.* Sample size considerations may lead one to question the number of patients that can realistically be recruited in one center. It may be necessary to carry out a multicenter trial to achieve sufficient sample size in a reasonable time period. Multicenter design also enables study of outcome determinants associated with facilities of different characteristics.
4. *Response ratio.* This is the proportion of those approached who actually agree to be in the sample. As a certain drop-out rate is expected, an assumption can be made and factored into the project size and timescale. It is vital that this assumption is reconfirmed early in the study when information on actual response ratio emerges.

Detailed accounts of sampling strategies[1,97–99,133] may be valuable for anesthesiologists to refer to when designing research studies. There are four main types: convenience, systematic, random, and stratified.

- *Convenience sampling* is a collective term for selecting those subjects who are easiest to study, "nearest-at-hand," or "likeliest to respond." This type of sampling is not generally regarded as acceptable for reliable quantitative research.
- *Systematic sampling* is one degree more sophisticated and is illustrated by such techniques as selecting every twentieth person from the sampling frame. This may approximate to random sampling if the list is genuinely jumbled, but may well not if there is any logic to the way the list has been assembled, as is often the case.

Convenience sampling and systematic sampling have both been frequently used in anesthesia research but are prone to bias and tend to limit the interpretation and generalization of the findings.

- In *random sampling* all members of the sampling frame are given unique numbers, after which a series of random numbers are generated from a table or computer program, and the subjects with the specified numbers are entered into the sample. The intention is that all subjects have an equal prospect of being selected.
- *Stratified sampling* introduces a refinement to ensure the presence in the final sample of sufficient numbers of subjects with particular characteristics. If an even gender split is critical in the sample, but males are over-represented in the sampling frame, then random selection is made separately within two sampling frames, one male and one female.

Comparison groups

Recruiting a comparison group forms an essential component of many study designs by providing a yardstick against which treatment efficacy or other intervention can be assessed. Ideally, a comparison group is like the group under study in all respects except for the selection criterion, which might be the presence of a specific disease or past exposure to a specific exposure.

In practice, a position must be adopted between inadequate matching and "overmatching," a particular challenge when carrying out case–control studies. Inadequate matching risks an observed difference being wrongly attributed to an intervention or exposure. "Overmatching" risks the possibility of important real differences between groups being missed because the groups have been made too similar.

Use of a historic comparison group rather than a set of specially recruited controls is tempting but not recommended. The argument that pulse oximeter monitoring led to improved outcome was regarded as invalid because so many other improvements in care had occurred over the study period that the benefit could not be attributed to oximetry alone.[136] A trial involving a contemporaneous control group[74] is needed to reach such a conclusion.

DATA QUALITY

Epidemiologists place much emphasis on their data and databases. Completeness and quality of data depend on sustained vigilance; and, as analysis and findings depend on having good data, attentiveness to data quality during the conduct of the study is repaid at the end. Data quality control is needed to ensure that the way the study is carried out and the ways that data are generated and documented are of a high standard. Guidance is available for maximizing data quality and setting up quality assurance systems.[137]

Analysis

The "researchable question" that was originally posed may require only one or two summary statistics to answer, yet there is usually a bewildering quantity of data at the end of the study. Moving too quickly from data collection to statistical analysis can lead to missing key pieces of information or jumping to erroneous conclusions. There are a number of steps involved in logical and robust assessment of study findings, which should be followed:

Confirming the types of variable used

The rules for making sense of findings depend on understanding the nature of the variables used. Continuous variables are common in biologic studies and are those that can assume all possible values along a continuum. They include height, weight, blood pressure, and blood sugar. In contrast, when a variable is discrete, intermediate values have no meaning. Parity and number of previous myocardial infarctions are both examples of discrete numerical variables, as a value of 2.3 would be meaningless.

Two other discrete scales are commonly encountered:

- *Ordinal scales* have a sense of progression, though not of relative magnitude (e.g. cancer staging from I to IV; classification of smoking as none, ex-smoker, light, moderate, or heavy). Two examples especially relevant to anesthesia studies include the ASA Physical Status Classification and the Charlson Comorbidity Score.[138]
- *Nominal scales* have no such inherent order and come in two variants: dichotomous when there are two choices (male or female; alive or dead) or multichotomous (blood group: A, B, AB, or O).

Data reduction and presentation

The first step in taming a sea of data is often to choose a sensible grouping of data values within one or more variables; thus, age may be cut up into 5-year bands. There is no single correct approach to data reduction, and a series of cut-off points and band sizes may need to be tried. Collapsing multiple values into a few manageable categories loses in precision but gains in comprehensibility and insights, and reveals the shape of the distribution. However, if data had been recorded originally in broad categories, it would clearly be impossible to recreate actual values, which might be necessary to carry out a detailed statistical examination of association.

The next step is to prepare a frequency distribution in the form of a table, which may depict findings in a cross-sectional study, or perhaps compare variables of interest among cases and controls.

Using histograms or graphs, taking into account the type of variable is the next step to allow the data to be visually explored and search for patterns before moving on to summary statistics. For detailed statistical tests and advice, readers should refer to standard sources of reference.[132–135] Tests based on proportions, such as chi-square, are appropriate for discrete distributions. Measures of central tendency and of spread are required to characterize continuous distributions. Mean and standard deviation are appropriate for normal distributions, but if the foregoing visual stages show that the distribution is other than normal, other measures of central tendency (median or mode) and spread (e.g. range or interquartile range) are indicated.

Common terms used in epidemiology to express findings

Some of the commonly used means of summarizing findings from epidemiology studies are shown in Table 86.6. Readers will wish to refer to standard textbooks[1–4,97–99,107,108] for details of analytic methods.[108]

INTERPRETATION

Toward the end of a study, the anesthesiologist may have become quite involved and feel close to the work. It is difficult to avoid a feeling of commitment – to the study, its findings, conclusions, and importance. Before the faith in its meaning becomes unshakeable, however, there are several steps to go through to avoid jumping to premature conclusions or believing that a statistically significant finding is significant in any wider sense.

Unfortunately, alternative explanations of apparently important findings are very common in research and take three main forms: the impact of chance; the impact of bias; and the impact of confounding. Each set of influences must be evaluated. For preventive strategies and remedies to deal with these influences and for statistical methods, the reader is referred to standard textbooks.[2,4] The issue of causation also is hedged about with cautions and caveats (see below).

Critical analysis and reflection about alternative explanation of findings is an important part of the scientific method, but overskepticism is also to be guarded against. Studies will always be imperfect, recruitment rates never reach 100%, and alternative explanations of results can never be totally rejected. Yet, it is research that forms the basis of all our knowledge, which in turn informs day-to-day practice and, increasingly, practice that is not evidence based is questioned. This is particularly true of newer techniques and emerging practice, in which the spirit of evaluation appears to be applied most keenly. Furthermore, research does challenge theory from time to time.

Evaluating the impact of chance

Epidemiologists draw conclusions from research through a process of inference – the generalization about a wider population based on a sample. Inherent is the risk that the inference will be flawed through the play of chance; for example, random samples vary from sample to sample. This influence is reduced by investing in large sample sizes, but never totally avoided.

Tests of statistical significance, such as chi-square or *t*-tests, are used to measure the likelihood of findings having arisen by chance alone.[2,132–135] They lead not to a yes or no statement, but to a probability statement, the *P*-value, which expresses the likelihood of achieving a value at least as extreme as that observed through chance alone. *P*-values are useful because essentially they determine the cut-off points for accepting or rejecting the null hypothesis. Confidence intervals can

Table 86.6 *Key terms to express epidemiology findings (drawn largely from Hennekens and Buring,[2] McQuay and Moore,[16] and Sackett* et al.[111])

Term	Purpose (example)	Derivation
Rate	General term for the expression of absolute numbers as a proportion of a suitable denominator (usually the population at risk) and including a time-frame	Number of events, states of interest, or individuals per thousand (or hundred thousand) population per year
Incidence	Measure of frequency of new events (e.g. cases of influenza)	New cases or events occurring during a specified time, per thousand population at risk
Point prevalence	Measure of frequency of chronic disease (e.g. levels of diabetes in the population)	Persons with a disease, per thousand population at risk, at a given time
Period prevalence	Measure of extent of a disease affecting a population during a particular period (e.g. common cold cases per year in the UK)	Episodes of a disease per thousand population at risk, over a specified period of time
Mortality rate	Measure of incidence of death, either from all causes or from specified causes	Number of deaths per thousand population per year
Case fatality ratio (CFR)	Measure of prognosis, representing the proportion of illness episodes that end fatally	Number of persons dying due to a particular disease per thousand with that disease
Standardized mortality ratio (SMR)	Measure for comparing mortality between groups or localities. Standardization is required to allow for the differing age structures (e.g. age-related risk of events) among the population. Values over 100% represent unfavorable mortality	The numerator is the number of actual deaths in a study (from a specific disease or from all causes). The denominator is the "expected" deaths, an imaginary value calculated by assuming the death rate which would have occurred in the study population if the risk of death in each age–sex group had been the same as that in a standard population (such as England and Wales)
Relative risk (RR)	Measure of magnitude of association between exposure and disease. Indicates relative likelihood of developing disease in exposed and unexposed persons	Ratio of the incidence of disease in an exposed group divided by the incidence of disease in a group of unexposed persons
Odds ratio (OR)	Measure of association used to estimate RR in case–control studies when true RR cannot be calculated	Odds of disease in exposed group divided by odds of disease in unexposed group
Attributable risk (or risk difference – AR)	Measure of association used because it takes into account the absolute effect of exposure or nonexposure. Useful in assessing risk pertaining to the individual	Incidence rate of disease in exposed group minus that in unexposed group
Relative risk reduction (RRR)	Measure of relative effectiveness of intervention	(Event rate in control group minus event rate in study group) divided by event rate in control group
Absolute risk reduction (ARR)	Measure of effectiveness of intervention that takes into account the absolute effect. Relevant to treatment decisions for the individual	Event rate in control group minus event rate in study group
Numbers needed to treat (NNT)	Measure of clinical significance of an effective treatment. Represents number needed to be treated to prevent one event	Reciprocal of ARR. Can also be calculated from odds ratios
Numbers needed to harm (NNH)	Measure of harm for effective treatments. Represents numbers treated leading to one adverse event	NNH for major events is an important concept but is rarely made explicit. NNH (for major and for minor events) could be calculated as for NNT above

be more informative, because they show the range within which the true magnitude of effect probably lies and also the effect of sample size. Confidence intervals become smaller, and the estimate becomes more stable, as sample size increases.

A special caution about inferences must be attached to studies in which data are collected on a large number of variables, such as potential risk factors. As the number of variables rises, so does the risk that one will find a statistically significant finding just by chance. Setting a value of $P < 0.05$ connotes that one variable will appear, spuriously, to be "significant" among every 20 tested. The same can be said of a "fishing exercise" in which large datasets are combed for statistical associations. Apart from being methodologically dubious, there is a truism that once the number of variables rises above double figures the chance of finding spurious associations becomes appreciable, and indeed inevitable if hundreds of variables are trawled through.

Evaluating the impact of bias

Biases creep in to research at every stage, from conceptualization, through funding, application, and design, to execution, analysis, and conclusion. The most important types of bias are shown in Table 86.7. Epidemiology study types all have their own susceptibility to particular types of bias. For example, case–control studies are most prone to recall and interviewer bias. Remedies to reduce the impact of bias include greater attention to design, seeking expert opinion before embarking, and having suitable research support and statistical advice. The most effective strategies for keeping bias under control are preventive.

Evaluating the impact of confounding

Sometimes the association between two variables is entirely due to the relation of each to a third – confounding – variable. To confound, a variable must be associated with the exposure factor, be predictive of the disease outcome (independently of the association with the exposure factor), and not be an intermediate link in the chain of causality running from exposure to health consequence.

An example is the association between the carrying of matches and cigarette lighters with respiratory disease. The association is spurious, as a confounding factor (smoking) is more strongly associated with each variable. Subtler confounding can be far harder to identify.

The principle of confounding is easy to grasp, but techniques for exploring and minimizing confounding require reference to standard textbooks[2,4] and may well require expert consultation with an epidemiologist.

Evaluating a possible relation between cause and effect

If an observed association survives the challenges posed by the roles of chance, bias, and confounding, it is then appropriate to evaluate whether

Table 86.7 *Types of bias commonly encountered (modified from Bowling[96])*

Bias	Explanation
Acquiescence response	Respondents more frequently endorse a statement than disagree with its opposite
Apprehension bias	Respondents try to give responses that they believe are expected by the investigator
Ascertainment bias	Undercounting of events of interest
Bias in handling outliers	Unusual or extreme values are inappropriately excluded (or included)
Hawthorne effect (guinea pig or awareness effect)	The research process changes people being studied. Term is also used when the study attracts subjects' interest or leads to behavior or knowledge change attributable to the attention and interest shown
Information bias	Subjects' responses are misclassified owing to error or prejudice
Interviewer bias	The investigator biases respondents (normally unconsciously but occasionally consciously) by virtue of a value system adhered to, by the phrasing of questions, or by using leading questions
Lead time bias	Earlier detection of a medical condition results in a longer period of treatment, creating the appearance of longer survival
Length time bias	Cases with a longer preclinical (presymptomatic) phase of disease appear to have a more favorable prognosis
Measurement biases	Catchall phrase covering errors in measurement, equipment, data collection, and patient recollection. Good design will minimize these or ensure that they cancel each other
Measurement decay	Changes occur in the data gathered or measurement processes over time
Nonresponse bias	Differences exist between characteristics of the group of subjects known to the researcher and the group not known. This extremely important issue reduces effective sample size, but more importantly can lead to unreliable results. It is difficult to deal with once present, as learning more about nonresponders can be impossible, and has to be guarded against proactively. Overlaps with selection bias
Observer bias	The situation recorded differs from the true situation due to observer perception, variation, or prejudice
Publication bias	Investigators are much more likely to submit for publication those studies that show clear differences (and may even exaggerate these differences). Publishers may be unwilling to publish studies, however important, that do not indicate clear associations
Recall bias	Subjects with a particular health outcome report their past exposure differently from those not so affected
Selection bias	Catchall term for differences between those who do and do not take part in a study. Volunteer studies are particularly prone. Overlaps with nonresponse bias
Social desirability bias	Subjects may tend to wish to give a preferred image and present themselves at their best. Particularly afflicts studies on controversial subjects
Systematic error	Term for biases of several kinds when the impact is contamination of the whole or large segments of a study. An example is a difference between two research assistants in their approach to recording data
Total survey error	Term given to the sum of all errors from sampling and data collection processes. In very large surveys this may be explicitly calculated. It may be considered implicitly when assessing whether errors are likely to have compounded or to have canceled each other out

the relation can be judged to be one of cause and effect. Much of the argument above has drawn on information derived from the study itself: its ethos, design, execution, and analysis. Judgments on causality also call on information from other domains, outside the study, and ideally the widest possible range of sources. A set of criteria for causality has been established, building on the work of Sir Austin Bradford Hill.[138] This set of criteria is summarized in Table 86.8.

However, it is important to note that each criterion has weaknesses, alternative explanations are never fully rejected, proving causality may be impossible, and scepticism is to be abandoned only very reluctantly.

EFFECTIVENESS RESEARCH

Effectiveness research extends the population-based perspective of epidemiology to the effectiveness of healthcare interventions in customary medical practice, as opposed to planned experiments. Bridging the gap between what we do and what an intervention actually accomplishes, effectiveness research is also termed outcomes research. Capturing much more than clinical results of care, effectiveness research also includes economic issues and patients' experiences, preferences, and values.[140,141]

This evolving new field seeks to identify which interventions work and at what cost, for which patients or subgroups of patients, when and under what circumstances, why substantial variations in utilization may exist, and what can be done to decrease the variation.

Indeed, the evolution of this field in the past decade reflects growing concern regarding the variation in medical practices for the same medical disorder in different geographic locations. These variations in practice patterns exist usually without commensurate differences in patient benefit and are not explained by organizational and financial arrangements (Fig. 86.5).[142–145] As one might expect, given its broad agenda, the field melds such diverse disciplines as clinical epidemiology, biostatistics, health services research, economics, psychology, pharmacoeconomics, informatics, and organizational theory.

Although prospective experimental designs (e.g. RCT) may be used, effectiveness research develops real-world characterizations of interventions more typically through use of uncontrolled, almost naturalistic observational data. Whereas the elements in a RCT are highly selected to enable a definitive result in the most efficient way, its results often relate poorly to customary clinical practice.[141,146]

Randomization in RCTs engenders administrative complexity and higher cost and does not guarantee balanced study groups, only groups that are alike on average with respect to specific characteristics or equally heterogeneous. Typically, subjects have limited or no comorbidity, unlike the unselected patients treated in customary clinical settings, and trials are usually short in duration rather than longitudinal as in traditional medical care. The comparison intervention may be the standard drug or perhaps a placebo, but the RCT may last so long that the comparator is rendered obsolete. We take for granted that subjects randomly allocated to the intervention group actually receive it, administered in optimal fashion by skilled practitioners who also monitor the treatment carefully. Yet, in the real world, patients do not have equal access to care, especially newest technology,[144] and practitioners differ in skill administering it.[147]

Ethical issues also arise when patients are allocated to a control group and the intervention is commonly believed to be beneficial, even if efficacy is unproved. Underlying this ethical dilemma are the dual physician roles: physician–scientist on behalf of future patients, and caregiver committed to the present physician–patient relationship.[148] Effectiveness research engenders ethical issues of a different sort, in part, because physicians view suspiciously study results based on unfamiliar, often probabilistic methods, and are wary about clinical practice guidelines, based on such data, which may contradict long-held clinical precepts or reasoning.[149,150]

The salient differences between effectiveness research and conventional clinical research are summarized in Table 86.9. Of special note, the strength of each approach is the weakness of the other: clinical research provides unbiased proof of efficacy, but its results are often not generalizable to customary clinical settings, whereas effectiveness research enjoys broad relevance to customary settings, but there may be unknown biases and untreated confounding factor that impair validity.

Given that no approach is fully satisfactory, we gain confidence in the validity of our conclusions when based on research from several studies using different study designs.[151] Although the two approaches are presented here as different undertakings – with clinical research (e.g. RCTs) focused ultimately on the care of individual patients, and effectiveness research emphasizing a population-based, societal perspective – there is a growing expectation that the two approaches will draw closer, if not come under the same heading.[152]

OUTCOMES

Clinicians commonly use *outcome* to mean the clinical results of care, often a narrowly defined group of adverse events (e.g. acute myocardial infarction), and even intermediate states (e.g. myocardial ischemia). Yet, outcomes researchers use the term much more broadly to capture a comprehensive view of an intervention's effectiveness. Such usage is consistent with the original definition of *outcome*:

> A change in a patient's current and future health status that can be attributed to antecedent health care… [which includes] social and psychologic function in addition to the more usual emphasis on the physical and physiologic aspects of performance.[150]

Table 86.8 *Criteria for ascribing causation (drawn largely from Hennekens and Buring,[2] and Bowling[96])*

Criterion	Explanation
Biologic plausibility	Evidence from the biologic sciences shows a credible mechanism
Coherence	Information from other modes of investigation and experimentation and other domains of scientific enquiry are all congruent
Consistency/repeatability	Studies by different investigators at different times and locations, using different but appropriate methods, point to the same conclusion
Dose–response relation	There is a gradient of increasing risk with increasing exposure
Magnitude of association	Stronger associations may be more likely to be causal. Weaker associations are not barred from being causal, but alternative explanations are more likely
Specificity	A cause should lead to a single and not multiple effects
Time sequence	The timing between exposure and consequent disease is known and is congruent with biologic mechanisms

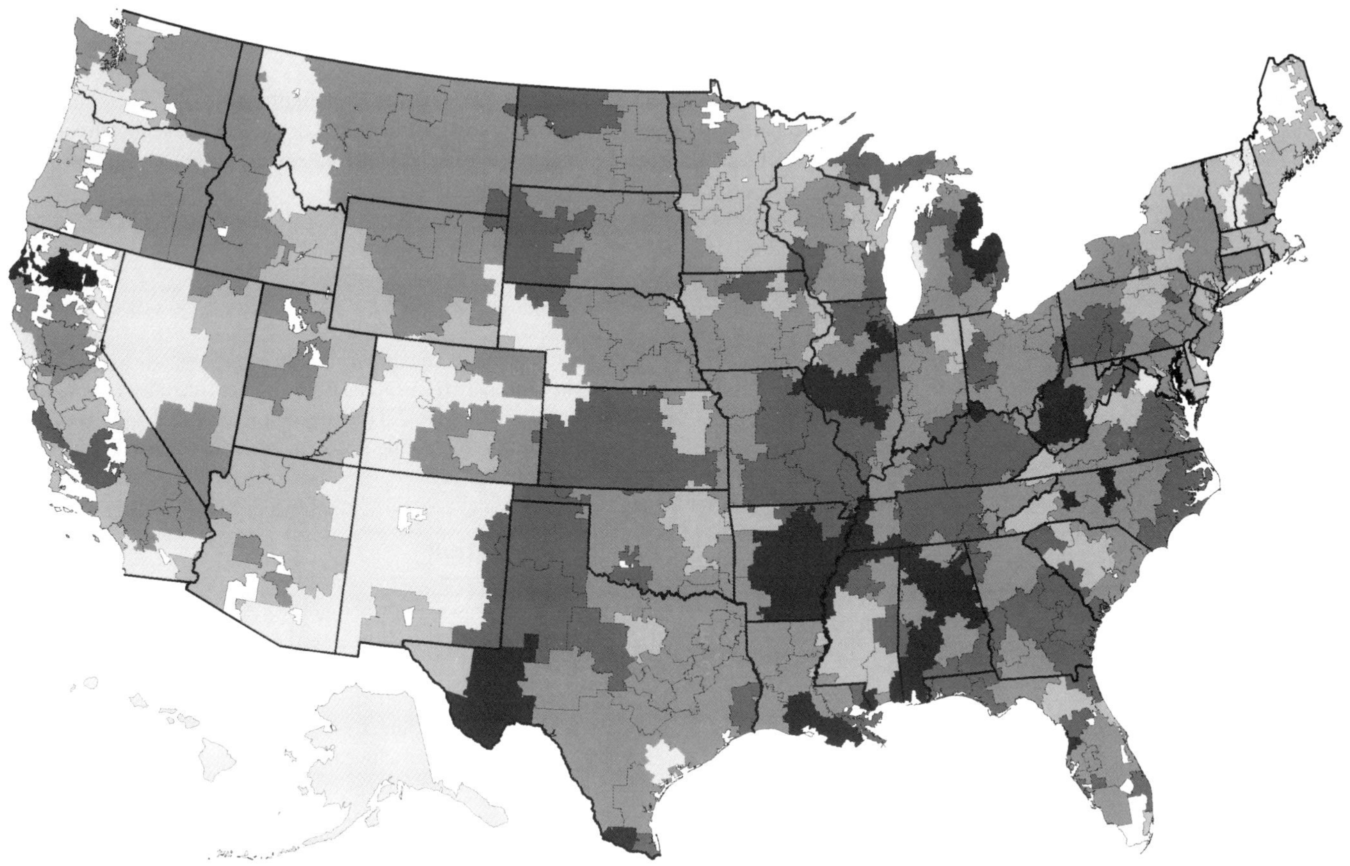

Figure 86.5 *The variation in per capita rates of coronary artery bypass graft (CABG) surgery by hospital referral regions (HRR) across the USA, compared with the national average rate, based on 1995–1996 Medicare data. Overall, there was a 3.5-fold variation in the rate of CABG surgery by HRR. Among the 306 regions, 21 had rates ≥30% higher than the national average, and 19 were >25% below the national average. By HRR, the rate of hospitalization for acute myocardial infarction, a marker for coronary artery disease, and the rate of CABG surgery were uncorrelated. (Reproduced, with permission, from map 5.3, p. 156.[144] ©The Trustees of Dartmouth College.)*

Ratio of Rates of Coronary Artery Bypass Grafting Procedures to the U.S. Average

by Hospital Referral Region (1995-96)

- 1.30 to 1.87 (21)
- 1.10 to < 1.30 (69)
- 0.90 to < 1.10 (126)
- 0.75 to < 0.90 (71)
- 0.50 to < 0.75 (19)
- Not Populated

Table 86.9 *Comparison of effectiveness research and conventional clinical research (modified from Orkin[141])*

	Effectiveness research	Clinical research
What is studied	Effectiveness	Efficacy
Clinical setting	Customary clinical practice	Ideal clinical practice
Caregivers	Customary personnel	Experienced investigator(s)
Study design(s)	Observational study; randomized controlled trial (infrequently)	Randomized controlled trial
Principal measures	Patient-related outcomes[a]	Clinical endpoints
Study subjects	Heterogeneous, usually consecutive	Homogeneous, highly selected
Strength	Relevance to clinical practice	Unbiased proof of efficacy
Weakness	Possible unknown bias(es), confounding	Limited generalizability to other clinical settings, high cost

a. See Table 86.10 for examples.

This broader definition of outcome emphasizes the patient's perspective, including his preferences, expectations, and assessment of the quality of care. Thus, there are several outcomes domains besides clinical outcomes (Table 86.10).

Clinical outcomes

Clinicians are very familiar with the spectrum of clinical outcomes, which range from minor side-effects to major complications and

Table 86.10 *Examples of patient-related outcomes used in effectiveness research (modified from Orkin[141])*

Outcome domain	Patient-related outcomes
Clinical	Clinical endpoints (symptoms, laboratory test values), complications, adverse events, death
Health-related quality of life	Level of function (performance) with regard to physical, psychologic (well-being), social, and role dimensions
Patient satisfaction	Patient-based assessment of care with regard to quality, convenience, information (education), and access
Economic consequences	Utilization of healthcare resources (tests, drugs, procedures)
	Length of stay (hospital, intensive care unit, office)
	Costs (indirect as well as direct); time lost from work (forgone income)

death. Because the incidence of the severe adverse clinical outcomes following anesthesia is low (e.g. 2%), the sample size requirements of related clinical studies are high, often unfeasibly high (Table 86.11). To avoid large, costly studies, one may choose an intermediate or surrogate event (e.g. myocardial ischemia) as an endpoint that is believed to be associated with the outcome of interest (e.g. myocardial infarction) and occurs much more frequently. The countervailing consideration is that the surrogate event may not be closely associated with the outcome of interest (as in the case of intraoperative myocardial ischemia and infarction[153–155]), leading to the need to exercise caution in choosing study endpoints.[156]

Health-related quality of life

Clinicians are familiar with describing patients' functional status using scales, such as the ASA Physical Status Classification.[157] However, consistent with the broad perspective of effectiveness research, other scales and survey instruments are used to capture physical functioning, and social and psychologic well-being, which together characterize health-related quality of life.[158–160] Some of these instruments are condition or disease specific (e.g. visual analog pain rating scale,[161] McGill Pain Questionnaire[162]), whereas others measure general quality of life (e.g. Medical Outcome Study's Short-Form-36 Health Survey[163,164]).

With all such instruments, however, it is the patient rather than the healthcare provider who is the respondent. Many of these scales have been validated, typically for chronic disease, and are described in well-documented compendia.[165–170] Anesthesiologists are beginning to use such scales in the longitudinal evaluation of patients with chronic pain,[171,172] in whom these instruments may prove helpful when assessing the value of different interventions as well as evaluating treatment

Table 86.11 *Sample size requirements in clinical studies given for specified event rates*

Event rate (%)	Sample size per study arm
60	196
50	262
40	376
30	566
20	945
10	2084
5	4361
2.5	9066
2.0	11 192
1.0	22 577
0.5	45 347
0.25	92 434
0.1	227 505

Assumptions: type I error = 5%; type II error = 20% (power = 80%); least important difference = 25%; equal numbers of subjects in each study arm.

results over time. It is incumbent on anesthesiologists to incorporate some of these socially relevant measures in our outcomes research;[48] yet whether such instruments will be sufficiently sensitive to and feasible for the transient and often subtle impairments associated with anesthesia remains to be evaluated.

Patient satisfaction

Rather than an expression of whether the patient liked the caregivers, or a global assessment of the entire anesthetic experience, which is often inextricably intertwined with the surgery, patient satisfaction focuses on whether the care was patient centered. Indeed, most patients find modern health care confusing, frustrating, and even intimidating. They increasingly want a role in clinical decision making and are eager to express preferences for treatment options, where such exist and where appropriate. Thus, assessing patient satisfaction explores whether individual patient preferences were identified and whether they were incorporated into decision making, when possible and appropriate. Were the patient's (reasonable) expectations met? Was the care accessible and convenient? Was appropriate patient education integrated into care? With quality increasingly defined from the consumer's perspective, such questions are becoming especially important. Yet, only recently have patient preferences in relation to anesthesia care attracted scholarly inquiry.[173–176] Clinicians embarking on patient satisfaction surveys will wish to consider the wide range of methods available, and their appropriate use and limitations.[97,98]

Among the dimensions of patient-centered care particularly relevant to anesthesia practice is patient comfort, most notably the treatment of acute postoperative pain. The Picker–Commonwealth telephone survey of more than 6400 recently hospitalized US patients, conducted in 1989, documented that 86% of those with pain described their discomfort as moderate or severe.[177] Even now, 15 years later, much information, including a review of pain services in the UK,[10] suggests that despite the availability of seemingly adequate technology, many patients continue to endure substantial pain.

Economic consequences

Rather than being a tabulation of charges or even costs of care, economic consequences refers to the assessment of the economic burden of the intervention on the patient, on the institution where care is provided, on the healthcare insurer, and, most importantly, on the society that ultimately pays for the care. Instead of merely seeking cost savings, economic analyses increasingly evaluate the efficiency of alternative interventions, as part of a search for greater societal value. There are several types of economic evaluations, with the choice dependent on the particular research problem. Table 86.12 summarizes the salient characteristics of each study type and cites several examples from the anesthesia literature, where they exist.

The simplest type of economic evaluation is cost-minimization

Table 86.12 *Types of economic evaluations*

Evaluation type	Endpoint of study	Measurement of end-point	Compares alternatives	Assumes equivalence of alternatives	Anesthesia literature examples
Cost-minimization	Direct costs	Resources consumed	Yes	Yes	Todd *et al.*,[178] Weiskopf and Eger,[179] Becker and Carrithers[180]
Cost-effectiveness	Effects on health	Lives saved	Yes	No	Fleisher *et al.*,[181] Watcha and Smith,[182] Macario *et al.*[183]
	Indirect costs	Years of life saved			
	Subsequent use of resources	Cases treated			
		Economic			
Cost-utility	Utility of health effects	Quality-adjusted life years (QALYs)	Yes	No	
	Indirect costs	Economic			
	Subsequent use of resources	Economic			
Cost–benefit	Monetary value of outcomes	Economic	No or implied	No	Orkin,[173] Roizin *et al.*[184]

analysis, in which direct costs are compared for two interventions (e.g. thiopental vs. propofol for induction of general anesthesia), and the interventions are assumed to have similar effectiveness. If the interventions actually differ in effectiveness (e.g. shorter sleep time and lower incidence of emetic symptoms with propofol), cost minimization is overly simplistic and likely to mislead.

Frequently confused in colloquial discussions,[185] cost-effectiveness analysis values resources in monetary terms, but at least some outcomes are valued in nonmonetary units (e.g. life years gained, disability days saved). Such evaluations are often summarized with cost-effectiveness ratios (e.g. pounds per life year gained) as a guide to economic efficiency. Yet, the lowest ratio is not necessarily "the best," for social and political considerations may encourage additional spending if the enhanced outcome, albeit more costly, is deemed to have desirable societal benefit.

Cost–utility analysis, a variant of cost-effectiveness analysis, may include outcomes measured in monetary terms, but the respondent's preferences (utilities) for given outcomes are measured and used in the analysis as an adjusting factor. Thus, in a comparison of two interventions (e.g. coronary artery bypass surgery vs. medical therapy for coronary artery disease), survival may be similar, but quality of life following one intervention (e.g. surgery) may be perceived by the patient to be better, resulting in that intervention having more quality-adjusted life-years (QALYs). To date, there have been few attempts to elicit patients' utilities or preferences in relation to anesthetic outcomes.[173,175]

Frequently also invoked erroneously in colloquial discussion, cost–benefit analysis requires that health outcomes be valued solely in monetary terms. As this is rarely possible in health care, this method has few applications outside the realm of national budgeting. One specific exception, the willingness-to-pay method,[173] offers an approach to assessing societal benefit by eliciting the individual's threshold for paying out of pocket (i.e. no reimbursement from government or insurance).

Clearly, economic evaluation of health care outcomes and technology is often more complex than it would appear initially. Indeed, the term health technology assessment has emerged as an encompassing term for the economic evaluations encountered in health care. Fortunately, there are many sources of general[165,186–199] and anesthesia-specific[200–203] guidance. From these sources, one may develop an appreciation of salient considerations when evaluating or planning economic evaluations (Table 86.13).

A special economic focus is achieving more efficient use of operating rooms.[13,14,204] These facilities are among the most costly to operate in both inpatient and outpatient settings due to high labor, supplies, and equipment expenditures. Formal technology assessment enables better decision making, for example on service configuration and quantity to be commissioned, equipment purchasing, and other technology usage decisions.

Disciplines drawn from the management sciences, such as operations management, operations research, and process re-engineering,[205,206] are used in many health service quality improvement initiatives. Anesthesia examples include efforts to decrease delays between surgical cases and to reduce unnecessary quantities of costly materials held in stock in operating room stores.

OBSERVATIONAL DATA

Increasingly, clinical research using RCTs, especially that undertaken by the pharmaceutical and medical equipment industries, includes non-clinical endpoints that relate to health-related quality-of-life and economic considerations.[169] However, because RCTs tend to use restricted, relatively homogeneous study populations and idealized care practices, are costly to undertake, and may have limited general applicability to other healthcare settings, most effectiveness research uses observational data (Table 86.9). Such data may be collected prospectively for the proposed study or may already exist within a database created for some other purpose.

Table 86.13 *Considerations in economic evaluations of healthcare interventions (modified from Watcha and Smith[182])*

1	Be explicit and comprehensive in describing interventions and comparisons of interventions
2	Identify all likely and relevant benefits and risks associated with alternative clinical approaches
3	Focus on costs, not charges (e.g. patient bills)
4	Capture indirect costs (e.g. patients' out-of-pocket losses) as well as direct costs
5	Focus on marginal differences related to alternative approaches, rather than overall costs of care
6	Emphasize real outcomes rather than intermediate or surrogate endpoints whenever feasible
7	Do not lose sight of implications of early "savings" on even more costly events "downstream" in the care process
8	Opt for the lower-cost approach unless value is demonstrated in a higher-cost alternative
9	Discuss all issues of concern to potential users in the study report

Databases are ubiquitous. As a result of the widespread availability of low-cost computer technology, data have been collected for governmental programs (e.g. US Medicare claims, US National Cancer Institute's Cancer Registry), private advocacy (e.g. American Hospital Association's Annual Survey of Hospitals, American Medical Association's Physician Masterfile, ASA Closed Claims Project[96]), and local administrative needs (e.g. a hospital's billing system). Such secondary or administrative data are increasingly used to study quality of care, costs of care, and impact of health policy decisions. Yet, because such data are almost always collected for purposes different from one's proposed research, data elements may be defined differently and are generally of limited quality, detail, and completeness from that desired. Similarly, the patient population reflected in the database may be different or less relevant to the proposed study questions, or the sampling frame may have excluded specific patient types and/or practice sites.[207] Additional technical issues related to large databases include the adequacy and accuracy of the diagnostic and procedural coding, and the level of aggregation (e.g. geographic units, services vs. episodes of care).[207]

Among the better-known databases in US anesthesia is the dataset accrued from the ASA Closed Claims Project,[96] which contains information on patients whose care led to a malpractice liability claim, including a description of those patients, their anesthetic care, their injuries, and disposition of their claims. As the database does not include data from the wider population (for example by sampling from all patients presenting for anesthesia), there is no "denominator." Without similar information on patients not suffering an injury, the database cannot be explored for risk factors for specific adverse events. However, the real value of such registries or case series is the rich descriptions of the individual events, which may give rise to hypotheses and, in turn, more definitive research using population-based databases as well as prospective studies.

There are additional potential problems with observational databases, regardless of whether one uses an available database or creates one's own. Among the most salient data issues is that interventions of interest are unlikely to be distributed randomly, as in an RCT. Indeed, existing medical knowledge, physician judgment, and even socioeconomic factors (some unrelated to the given patient) determine which patients receive which interventions. The decision to use a particular intervention, rather than another, in a given patient or group of patients gives rise to confounding by intention (e.g. one hospital uses general anesthesia for all carotid endarterectomy cases, whereas another uses either general anesthesia or cervical nerve blocks). Similarly, some healthcare providers and facilities may treat patients who are more ill, creating substantial potential confusion when comparing observed outcomes.

RISK ADJUSTMENT FOR OUTCOME COMPARISONS

Clinicians are well aware that patients in poorer health status are likely to have worse clinical (and other) outcomes after anesthesia and surgery.[37–42,208,209] Thus, when the outcomes of two study groups (whose subjects are not allocated randomly) are compared, the observed outcome differences may merely reflect underlying differences in preexisting health status. As the study design is observational and does not control for such differences, the investigator is obliged to incorporate suitable adjustment in the analysis for such uncontrolled factors.

Risk adjustment is the use of statistical methods to "control for" differences among study populations when making outcome comparisons. These methods reduce the effects of confounding factors (e.g. advanced age, poor ASA physical status, high Charlson Comorbidity Score), in an attempt to account for pertinent patient characteristics before making inferences about the effectiveness of an intervention or quality of care. A given outcome is viewed mathematically as a function of a set of predictor variables in an additive model:[210]

$$f(\text{patient characteristics} + \text{treatment effectiveness} + \text{quality of care} + \text{random error}) = \text{outcome}$$

Typically, quality of care is assumed to be the same across study groups, patient characteristics are entered, and regression analysis is used to model the treatment effectiveness. Less commonly, when similar treatment is compared across settings, quality of care is modeled. The particular regression model chosen reflects the type of outcome:

- Multiple linear regression is appropriate for a continuous outcome (e.g. cost of care, length of stay).
- Logistic regression is appropriate for a dichotomous outcome (e.g. survival vs. death) or a polychotomous outcome (e.g. discharged to home, discharge to nursing home, or dead).
- Proportional hazards regression is appropriate for a time-dependent outcome (e.g. length of survival).

There are many nuances in risk adjustment. For example, some continuous data (e.g. cost, length of stay) may require mathematical transformation (e.g. log) to achieve a more normal distribution appropriate to regression models. The field is undergoing rapid evolution.[211,212]

BENCHMARKING

Once study data have been risk-adjusted to reflect underlying patient characteristics, it is appropriate to compare outcome values with those of other practice settings. Not infrequently, large variations become apparent, as noted in the "small-area variation" studies.[142–144] One study identified a low rate of utilization of hospital services in New Haven and high utilization in Boston, without commensurate population differences in health status, begging the question "which rate is right?"[213]

The comparison of outcomes data, including results of care (e.g. mortality) and utilization (e.g. numbers of surgical procedures and physicians, healthcare expenditures, percent compliance with a specific medical practice guideline), across settings or geographic regions gives rise to benchmarking. In the absence of detailed knowledge of precisely how healthcare resources are ultimately translated into high-quality care, an outcomes researcher chooses a particular setting or region as a reference standard, based on its characteristics. For example, when comparing utilization data, one might choose as a "benchmark" a community that appears to have an adequate but not excessive supply of resources. Then, the researcher compares outcomes data values in one or more settings with those of the reference setting, such that the reference setting has a utilization of 1.0 and a setting with 50% greater utilization, 1.5.

The simple standardization procedure underlying benchmarking allows one to consider how much healthcare capacity a country would need if all regions had the benchmark's level of capacity, and how much a given region would have if its capacity were equal to that of the benchmark. Similarly, if the outcome were risk-adjusted mortality, benchmarking would enable the preventable mortality to be estimated if all regions achieved the same outcomes as the reference site.

META-ANALYSIS

Just as there are many observational datasets awaiting study, there are many RCTs calling for further analysis. Some clinical trials have indeterminate results due to inadequate sample size or other technical problems. Sometimes a new research question can be explored with data in existing RCTs. In still other cases, there are multiple RCTs whose results are contradictory. Meta-analysis is an objective, structured, quantitative method that enables the synthesis of the information from existing trials, resulting in greater power and value than any individual RCT.[214–216]

Meta-analysis has a low probability of generating a false-negative inference (a type II error). This methodology is especially helpful in exploring subanalyses, such as those exploring which groups of patients may be particularly susceptible to an intervention that has been demonstrated to have an overall effect.

Among the several applications of meta-analysis to anesthesia care is the study of nitrous oxide as an emetic stimulus: some two dozen RCTs investigating postoperative nausea and vomiting have included the presence or absence of nitrous oxide. However, many of the studies are in conflict over the role of nitrous oxide, with 15 "negative" trials and another four indeterminate trials. Meta-analysis enables aggregation of observed and expected emetic incidences among the disparate studies; and the calculation of a pooled odds ratio summarizing the overall likelihood of emetic symptoms with nitrous oxide use. One meta-analysis found the pooled odds ratio to be 0.63, indicating that omission of nitrous oxide is associated with a substantially lower risk of emetic symptoms, with maximal effect in women.[217]

Although meta-analysis provides a way to trawl for, and make greater use of, available information, the method is potentially problematic. Controversial issues in meta-analysis include multiple opportunities for the introduction of sampling bias (studies with negative results being less likely to be published); variability in data quality across studies; inclusion of analyses lacking robustness (e.g. high probability of false-positive inference or type I error); and influence of outlier values. Moreover, the additional quantification provided by meta-analysis may result in an unwarranted sense of scientific validity undeserved by poor data.[215]

CLINICAL PREDICTION MODELS AND SCORING SYSTEMS

Among the explanations for the variation in medical practice patterns is the paucity of reliable information about how clinical circumstances precisely relate to the occurrence of outcome(s) of interest. As a result, individual practitioners vary in their application of technology (e.g. diagnostic test, testing strategy, drug, dosage) in the same clinical circumstance. An increasingly common way to rationalize medical decision making, and thereby decrease variation in practice patterns, is the use of a clinical prediction rule for the occurrence of the outcome, based on mathematical modeling of the importance of likely clinical predictor variables in an observational dataset.[218]

An early example of a clinical prediction rule relating to anesthesia practice is the Goldman cardiac risk index.[33] The underlying rationale is that the identification of patients at higher risk of developing a severe acute, postoperative cardiac event (e.g. pulmonary edema, cardiac arrest) could lead to specific treatment to enhance health status and thereby decrease the risk. To develop this predictive tool, seemingly important clinical information (e.g. age, myocardial infarction in the past 6 months, presence of S3 gallop or jugular vein distension) was obtained prospectively from those patients suffering such an adverse event. Multivariate statistical techniques, such as those used for risk adjustment (see above), effectively identify the relative importance of the variables in predicting the adverse outcome. Further mathematical manipulation converts variable coefficients (weights) into a set of integers, creating a scoring system that is easy to remember and apply in clinical settings.

A similar clinical prediction rule was developed to identify myasthenic patients likely to suffer respiratory failure after thymectomy via a median sternotomy.[34] The scoring system proved both easy to use and valid when applied to a new set of patients having the same surgery, and using the same criteria for respiratory failure.[219] That the scoring system proved a poor predictor when the surgery and clinical criteria were different[220–222] stresses the importance of the clinical circumstances in defining the model.

Clinical prediction methodologies have been extended to a wide variety of clinical considerations, including predicting patient prognosis in intensive care (e.g. APACHE score),[35,36] specific adverse events and morbidity,[37–42] and important quality problems (e.g. unplanned admission after day-case surgery).[223] Perhaps the real value of clinical prediction rules and scoring systems is not the specific numerical results or mathematical equation, but rather their identification of the important variables to assist physicians in clinical decision making. In turn, this information can be incorporated into clinical practice guidelines, which may decrease variation in practice patterns and ultimately improve quality of care.

EXPERT OPINION

There are still many important areas of medicine and health care where knowledge or clarity is lacking in some important respect, yet there may be no solution at hand from randomized controlled trials and systematic reviews. In such cases, much can be learned by surveying the opinions of those with special skills and knowledge. Research methods that trawl for and amalgamate expert opinion are needed to signpost the way forward.

Group methods can be problematic, as free communication can limit the information that a researcher can obtain, once power, deference, prestige, antagonism, friendships, and loyalties start to play a hand. Research techniques for expert opinion tame the wasteful effects of group dynamics in two distinct ways. Nominal group and Delphi techniques (see below) essentially eliminate group interaction. In contrast, in consensus development and focus groups, group dynamics are allowed to occur and are turned to advantage. In each case, much of the subsequent value depends on the skill, focus, and preparation of the researcher, facilitator, and data-analyst. Clinicians wishing to use any of these qualitative research techniques should first consult the references shown and seek advice from a qualitative researcher.

Nominal group technique

In the nominal group technique,[1,224,225] respondents are asked to clarify their viewpoints and advice on a given topic prior to meeting. The participants then meet and each idea is collected silently and in writing, usually by a facilitator. A group discussion occurs on each idea at a time, so as to clarify matters, but not with the aim of resolving any differences of opinion. Respondents then vote, usually ranking contending ideas in preference order. Further discussion, for clarification only, is allowed before a final vote. The intention is that the facts speak for themselves, but at no stage is the opinion of any one respondent meant to influence the preference of another. Nominal group techniques have been used in the development of quality of life measures.[226]

Delphi technique

The Delphi technique,[1,225,227,228] which has been described as "more of an art than a science," relies on a serial postal or email questionnaire method. The investigator analyses findings from each wave of the survey, tailoring subsequent survey questions in the light of information received. Typically the survey will begin with open-ended questions to obtain ideas or attitudes, then move on to more specific questions. Steps in the process may include: an assessment of the group's judgment and of the variation in their views; a chance for respondents to revise views; casting of votes; and repeated feedback of results with a view to achieving stability or unanimity.

The Delphi technique has been used in anesthesia to develop a malignant hyperthermia clinical grading scale,[229] and to validate definitions and activities important to pain management techniques.[230]

Consensus development panel

This is a broad term for bringing a group of experts together with a facilitator to develop a consensus on a topic. Consensus development conferences have been used extensively (and at high cost) by the National Institutes of Health (NIH) in the USA for a number of topics including pain management;[231] and their use has been reviewed in the UK by the Kings Fund[232] and recently by the NHS Health Technology Assessment Programme.[225] Kosecoff and colleagues[233–235] noted that there was some evidence of convergence of beliefs, less evidence of convergence in practice, and that the methods used needed further development.

Focus groups

A focus group is defined as "a carefully planned discussion designed to obtain perceptions on a defined area of interest in a permissive non-threatening environment."[236] Focus groups provide a way of exploring issues in depth and may lead to generation of hypotheses. The method is useful for examining not only what people think, but how they think and why.[237] It allows researchers to gather data from a number of participants at one sitting, thus eliminating the need for time-consuming face-to-face interviews. Successful focus groups require substantial investment of time and planning, and are best carried out by an experienced facilitator. The composition of the group with respect to age, gender, and ethnicity is carefully matched to the topic.

Capturing the data in a focus group is a major concern: ideally focus groups are tape recorded and later transcribed. The quantity of data that emerges is vast and needs to be analyzed in a systematic way. This can be achieved by content analysis or other qualitative analysis techniques, so that the key themes and concepts emerge.[97,128,236,237] Focus groups have been used in the study of pain experiences and service provision.[10,238,239]

USES OF EPIDEMIOLOGY AND EFFECTIVENESS RESEARCH

Epidemiologists' work significantly impacts on the day-to-day practice of anesthesiologists, whether in the role of clinicians, educators, managers, or clinical leaders. Everyday "users of epidemiology" include:

- *Anesthesiologists working as independent clinical practitioners*, interpreting medical literature, reconciling conflicting advice and guidance in textbooks and journals, using libraries and on-line resources, selecting and using guidelines for care, and minimizing exposure to personal and corporate risk of hazard or litigation.
- *Anesthesiologists in groups* whether at a country or international level, or at the level of the individual hospital, as they work to set quality standards, put in place critical incident programs, design, and implement guidelines, and carry out and interpret audits of local practice.[240]
- *Anesthesiologists as educators and trainers* as they instill and critique practice using a mix of personal experience and observation; and a knowledge base drawn from robust randomized controlled trials and systematic reviews.
- *Anesthesiologists as managers* of anesthesia, pain, critical care, and other services, including operating room suites, as they seek rapid and incisive interpretation of complex information to back up the decision making that the role requires.[241]
- *Anesthesiologists as contributors to policy making at national or local area level* as they use published guidelines, cost and benefit information, and other briefing and advice, to influence decisions that determine resource levels, service configuration, and quantity and quality levels to be provided in our hospitals.

Among the best recent examples of the use of how effectiveness research can be used to modify care processes to improve quality is the work of the Northern New England Cardiovascular Disease Study Group, comprising the region's then five medical centers performing coronary artery bypass grafts. Cardiac surgeons from these sites agreed to develop a common shared database characterizing their practices and results. With the leadership of a clinical epidemiologist, they studied their variation in postoperative mortality, using logistic regression models to adjust for patient risk factors.[242] Surgeons met periodically to review their results, in turn prompting institutional site visits to help them understand how different care processes might underlie the observed variation. They developed hypotheses and tried modifications in practice patterns, in short "tests of change" that are encouraged in improvement programs.[243,244] Through iterative improvement cycles, mortality variation decreased, and overall mortality also decreased 24% from that expected from their multivariate analysis and national data.[245] Although not involved directly in the early improvement efforts, anesthesiologists are now active participants, as this study group continues to explore other opportunities for further improvement.

Myriad other opportunities exist to use effectiveness research to improve care. Among candidate topics are reducing the continuing substantial rate of errors in medical care,[246,247] using technology more selectively, achieving meaningful cost savings without impairing quality of care, and learning how best to respond to patient preferences.

REFERENCES

1. Abramson JH. *Survey Methods in Community Medicine*, 5th edn. Edinburgh: Churchill Livingstone, 1999.
2. Hennekens CH, Buring, JE. *Epidemiology in Medicine.* Boston, MA: Little, Brown, 1987.
3. MacMahon B, Trichopoulos D. *Epidemiology: Principles and Methods*, 2nd edn. Philadelphia, PA: Lippincott Williams & Wilkins, 1997.
4. Rothman KJ, Greenland S. *Modern Epidemiology*, 2nd edn. Philadelphia, PA: Lippincott-Raven, 1998.
5. Cohen MM. Using epidemiology to study adverse outcomes in anaesthesia. *Can J Anaesth* 1990; **37(4):** Sxlv-xlviii.
6. Cooper JB, Newbower RS, Long CD, McPeek B. Preventable anesthesia mishaps: a study of human factors. *Anesthesiology* 1978; **49:** 399–406.
7. Runciman WB, Holland RB. The Australian Incident Monitoring Study. *Anaesth Intensive Care* 1993; **21:** 502–5.
8. Royal College of Anaesthetists. *Report of the National Pilot Critical Incident Study.* London: Royal College of Anaesthetists, 1999.
9. Davies JM. Critical incidents during anaesthesia. In: Healy TEJ, Cohen PJ (eds). *Wiley and Churchill-Davidson's A Practice of Anaesthesia*, 6th edn. London: Edward Arnold, 1995: 924–37.
10. Clinical Standards Advisory Group. *Services for Patients with Pain.* London: Department of Health, 2000.
11. Spence AA. The halothane-liver controversy. In: Lunn J (ed.). *Epidemiology in Anaesthesia: The Techniques of Epidemiology Applied to Anaesthetic Practice.* London: Edward Arnold, 1986: 74–92.
12. Elliot RA, Payne K, Moore JK *et al.* Which anesthetic agents are cost-effective in day surgery? Literature review, national survey of practice and randomised controlled trial. *Healthcare Technol Assess* 2002; **6** (30): 1–264
13. Macario A, Vitez TS, Dunn B, McDonald T. Where are the costs in perioperative care? Analysis of hospital costs and charges for inpatient surgical care. *Anesthesiology* 1995; **83:** 1138–44.

14. Dexter F, Macario A. Does early extubation ("fast-tracking") of coronary artery bypass graft surgery decrease perioperative costs? Appropriate analysis of direct variable costs. *Anesthesiology* 1997; **87:** 181–2.
15. McQuay HJ, Moore RA, Eccleston C, Morley S, *et al.* Systematic Review of Outpatient Services for Chronic Pain Control. *Health Technology Assessment* 1997; **1** (6): 1–135.
16. McQuay HJ, Moore RA. *An Evidence-Based Resource for Pain Relief.* Oxford: University Press, 1998.
17. Hippocrates. On airs, waters, and places. *Med Classics* 1938; **3:** 19.
18. Graunt J. *Natural and Political Observations Made Upon the Bills of Mortality, 1662.* Baltimore, MD: John Hopkins University Press, 1939.
19. Snow J. *On Chloroform and Other Anaesthetics: Their Actions and Administration.* London: John Churchill, 1958.
20. Commission on Anaesthetics. Report of the Lancet Commission appointed to investigate the subject of the administration of chloroform and other anaesthetics from a clinical standpoint. *Lancet* 1893; **1:** 629–38, 693–708, 761–76, 899–914, 971–78, 1111–18, 1236–40, 1479–98.
21. Morton HJV, Wylie WD. Anaesthetic deaths due to regurgitation or vomiting. *Anaesthesia* 1951; **6:** 190–205.
22. Mendelson CL. The aspiration of stomach contents into the lungs during obstetric anesthesia. *Am J Obstet Gynecol* 1946; **52:** 191–205.
23. Waters RM. The evolution of anesthesia: I and II. *Proc Staff Meetings Mayo Clinic* 1942; **17:** 428–40.
24. Tovell RM, Dunn HL. Anesthesia study records. *Anesth Analg* 1932; **11:** 37–41.
25. Rovenstine EA. A method of combining anesthetic and surgical records for statistical purposes. *Anesth Analg* 1934; **13:** 122–8.
26. Beecher HK, Todd DP. A study of the deaths associated with anesthesia and surgery: based on a study of 599 548 anesthesias in ten institutions 1948–1952, inclusive. *Ann Surg* 1954; **140:** 2–34.
27. Feinstein AR. Scientific methodology in clinical medicine (4 parts). *Ann Intern Med* 1964; **61:** 564–79, 757–81, 944–65, 1162–93.
28. Subcommittee on the National Halothane Study of the Committee on Anesthesia, National Academy of Sciences, National Research Council: Summary of the National Halothane Study. Possible association between halothane anesthesia and postoperative hepatic necrosis. *JAMA* 1966; **197:** 775–89.
29. Sackett DL. Clinical epidemiology. *Am J Epidemiol* 1969; **89:** 125–8.
30. Cochrane AL. *Effectiveness and Efficiency: Random Reflections on Health Services.* London: Nuffield Provincial Hospitals Trust, 1972.
31. Scott WR, Forrest Jr WH, Brown BW. Hospital structure and postoperative mortality and morbidity. In: Shortell SM, Brown M (eds). *Organizational Research in Hospitals.* Chicago, IL: Inquiry (Blue Cross Association), 1976: 72–89.
32. Flood AB, Scott WR (eds). *Hospital Structure and Performance.* Baltimore, MD: Johns Hopkins University Press, 1987.
33. Goldman L, Caldera DL, Nussbaum SR, *et al.* Multifactorial index of cardiac risk in noncardiac surgical procedures. *N Engl J Med* 1977; **297:** 845–50.
34. Leventhal SR, Orkin FK, Hirsh RA. Prediction of the need for postoperative mechanical ventilation in myasthenia gravis. *Anesthesiology* 1980; **53:** 26–30.
35. Knaus WA, Draper EA, Wagner DP, Zimmerman JE. An evaluation of outcome from intensive care in major medical centers. *Ann Intern Med* 1986; **104:** 410–18.
36. Knaus WA, Wagner DP, Zimmerman JE, Draper EA. Variations in hospital mortality and length of stay from intensive care. *Ann Intern Med* 1993; **118:** 753–61.
37. Pronovost P, Dorman T, Jenckes M, *et al.* Organizational characteristics of intensive care units related to outcomes of abdominal aortic surgery. *JAMA* 1999; **281:** 1310–17.
38. Cohen MM, Duncan PG, Tate RB. Does anesthesia contribute to operative mortality? *JAMA* 1988; **260:** 2859–61.
39. Cohen MM, Duncan PG. Physical status score and trends in anaesthetic complications. *J Clin Epidemiol* 1988; **41:** 83–90.
40. Cullen DJ, Apolone G, Greenfield S, *et al.* ASA physical status and age predict mortality after three surgical procedures. *Ann Surg* 1994; **220:** 3–9.
41. Howell SJ, Sear YM, Yeates D, *et al.* Risk factors for cardiovascular death after elective surgery under anaesthesia. *Br J Anaesth* 1998; **80:** 14–19.
42. Silber JH, Schwartz JS, Krakauer H, Williams SV. Hospital and patient characteristics associated with death after surgery: A study of adverse occurrence and failure to rescue. *Med Care* 1992; **30:** 615–29.
43. Silber JH, Kennedy SK, Even-Shoshan O, *et al.* Anesthesiologist direction and patient outcomes. *Anesthesiology* 2000; **93:** 152–163.
44. Silber JH, Kennedy SK, Even-Shoshan O, *et al.* Anesthesiologist board certification and patient outcomes. *Anesthesiology* 2002; **96:** 1044–52.
45. Cochrane Anaesthesia Review Group. Denmark: Cochrane collaboration, 1999 (http://www.cochrane-anaesthesia.suite.dk).
46. Orkin FK. Patient monitoring during anesthesia as an exercise in technology assessment. In: Saidman LJ, Smith NT (eds). *Monitoring in Anesthesia,* 3rd edn. Boston, MA: Butterworth-Heinemann, 1993: 439–55.
47. Sigurdsson G, McAteer E. Morbidity and mortality associated with anaesthesia. *Acta Anaesthesiol Scand* 1996; **40:** 1057–63.
48. Orkin FK, Cohen MM, Duncan PG. The quest for meaningful outcomes. *Anesthesiology* 1993; **78:** 417–22.
49. Dornette WHL, Orth OS. Death in the operating room. *Anesth Analg* 1956; **35:** 545–69.
50. Phillips OC, Frazier TM, Graff TD, DeKornfield TJ. The Baltimore Anesthesia Study Commission. A review of 1024 postoperative deaths. *JAMA* 1960; **174:** 2015–19.
51. Schapira M, Kepes ER, Hurwitt ES. An analysis of deaths in the operating room and within 24 hours of surgery. *Anesth Analg* 1960; **39:** 149–57.
52. Dripps RDD, Lamont A, Eckenhoff JE. The role of anesthesia in surgical mortality. *JAMA* 1961; **178:** 261–6.
53. Clifton BS, Hotten WIT. Deaths associated with anaesthesia. *Br J Anaesth* 1963; **35:** 250–9.
54. Memery HN. Anesthesia mortality in private practice. *JAMA* 1965; **194:** 1185–8.
55. Gebbie D. Anaesthesia and death. *Can Anaesth Soc J* 1966; **13:** 390–6.
56. Minuck M. Death in the operating room. *Can Anaesth Soc J* 1967; **14:** 197–204.
57. Bodlander FMS. Deaths associated with anaesthesia. *Br J Anaesth* 1975; **47:** 36–40.
58. Lunn JN, Mushin WW. *Mortality Associated with Anaesthesia.* Oxford: Nuffield Provincial Hospital Trust, 1982.
59. Keenan RL, Boyan CP. Cardiac arrest due to anesthesia: a study of incidence and causes. *JAMA* 1985; **253:** 2373–7.
60. Tiret L, Hatton F. Complications associated with anaesthesia: A prospective survey in France. *Can Anaesth Soc J* 1986; **33:** 336–44.
61. Holland R. Anaesthetic mortality in New South Wales. *Br J Anaesth* 1987; **59:** 834–41.
62. Buck N, Devlin HB, Lunn JN. *Report on the Confidential Enquiry into Perioperative Deaths.* London: Nuffield Provincial Hospitals Trust and the Kings Fund, 1987.
63. Holland R. Special committee investigating deaths under anaesthesia: report in 745 classified cases, 1960–1968. *Med J Aust* 1970; **1:** 573–94.
64. Eichhorn J. Prevention of intraoperative anesthesia accident and related severe injury through safety monitoring. *Anesthesiology* 1989: **70:** 572–7.
65. Newland MC, Ellis SJ, Lydiatt CA, *et al.* Anesthetic-related cardiac arrest and its mortality. *Anesthesiology* 2002; **97:** 108–15.
66. Lunn JN. Mortality studies in quality control. In: Lunn JN (ed.). *Quality of Care in Anaesthetic Practice.* London: Royal Society of Medicine and Macmillan Press Ltd, 1984: 121–38.
67. Lunn JN. Preventable anaesthetic mortality and morbidity (special communication). *Anaesthesia* 1985; **40:** 79.
68. Pederson T. Mortality associated with anaesthesia. In: Aitenhead AR (ed.). Quality Assurance and Risk Management in Anaesthesia. *Baillière's Clinical Anaesthesiology* 1996; **10** (2): 237–50.
69. Duberman SM, Bendixen HH. Mortality, morbidity and risk studies in anaesthesia. In: Lunn JN. *Epidemiology in Anaesthesia: The Techniques of Epidemiology Applied to Anaesthetic Practice.* London: Edward Arnold, 1986: 37–73.
70. Fleisher LH. Risk of anesthesia. In: Miller R (ed.). *Anesthesia,* 5th edn. New York: Churchill Livingstone, 2000: 795–823.
71. Warden JC, Horan BF, Holland R. Morbidity and mortality associated with anaesthesia. *Acta Anaesthesiol Scand* 1997; **41:** 949.
72. Lagasse RA. Anesthesia safety: model or myth? *Anesthesiology* 2002; **97:** 1609–17.
73. Ross AF, Tinker JH. Anesthesia risk. In: Miller R (ed.). *Anesthesia,* 4th edn. New York: Churchill Livingstone, 1994: 791–825.
74. Moller JT, Johannessen NW, Espersen K, *et al.* Randomized evaluation of pulse oximetry in 20 802 patients: II. Perioperative events and postoperative complications. *Anesthesiology* 1993; **78:** 445–53.
75. Eagle CJ, Davies, JM, Reason J. Accident analysis of large-scale technological disasters applied to an anaesthetic complications. *Can J Anaesth* 1992; **39:** 118–22.
76. Forrest JB, Rehder K, Goldsmith CH, *et al.* Multicenter Study of General Anesthesia. I. Design and Patient Demography. *Anesthesiology* 1990; **72:** 252–61.
77. Forrest JB, Rehder K, Cahalan MK, *et al.* Multicentre Study of General Anesthesia. II. Results. *Anesthesiology* 1990; **72:** 262–8.
78. Forrest JB, Rehder K, Cahalan MK, Goldsmith CH. Multicenter Study

of General Anesthesia. III. Predictors of Severe Perioperative Adverse Outcomes. *Anesthesiology* 1992; **76:** 3–15.
79. Harrison GG. Death due to anaesthesia at Groote Schuur Hospital, Cape Town 1956–1987. *SA Med J* 1990; **77:** 416–21.
80. Tikkanen J, Hovi-Viander M. Deaths associated with anaesthesia and surgery in Finland in 1986 compared to 1975. *Acta Anaesthesiol Scand* 1995; **39:** 262–7.
81. Campling EA, Devlin HB, Lunn JN. *The Report of the National Confidential Enquiry into Perioperative Deaths 1989.* London: National Confidential Enquiry into Perioperative Deaths, 1990.
82. Campling EA, Devlin HB, Hoile RW, Lunn JN. *The Report of the National Confidential Enquiry into Perioperative Deaths 1990.* London: National Confidential Enquiry into Perioperative Deaths, 1992.
83. Campling EA, Devlin HB, Hoile RW, Lunn JN. *The Report of the National Confidential Enquiry into Perioperative Deaths 1991/92.* London: National Confidential Enquiry into Perioperative Deaths, 1993.
84. Campling EA, Devlin HB, Hoile RW, Lunn JN. *The Report of the National Confidential Enquiry into Perioperative Deaths 1992/93.* London: National Confidential Enquiry into Perioperative Deaths, 1994.
85. Campling EA, Devlin HB, Hoile RW, Lunn JN. *The Report of the National Confidential Enquiry into Perioperative Deaths 1993/94.* London: National Confidential Enquiry into Perioperative Deaths, 1996.
86. Gallimore SC, Hoile RW, Ingram GS, Sherry KM. *The Report of the National Confidential Enquiry into Perioperative Deaths 1994/95.* London: National Confidential Enquiry into Perioperative Deaths, 1997.
87. Campling EA, Devlin HB, Hoile RW, *et al. Who operates when? A Report by the National Confidential Enquiry into Perioperative Deaths (1 April 1995 to 31 March 1996).* London: National Confidential Enquiry into Perioperative Deaths, 1997.
88. Gray AJG, Hoile RW, Ingram GS, Sherry KM. *The Report of the National Confidential Enquiry into Perioperative Deaths 1996/97.* London: National Confidential Enquiry into Perioperative Deaths, 1998.
89. Callum KG, Gray AJG, Hoile RW, *et al. Extremes of Age: The 1999 Report of the National Confidential Enquiry into Perioperative Deaths (1 April 1997 to 31 March 1998).* London: National Confidential Enquiry into Perioperative Deaths, 1999.
90. Callum KG, Gray Ajg, Hoile RW, *et al. Then and Now. The 2000 Report of the National Enquiry into Perioperative Deaths.* London: National Confidential Enquiry into Perioperative Deaths, 2000.
91. Burke M, Callum KG, Gray AJG, *et al. Changing the Way We Operate. The 2001 Report of the National Confidential Enquiry into Perioperative Deaths.* London: National Confidential Enquiry into Perioperative Deaths, 2001.
92. Lunn JN, Devlin HB. Lessons from the confidential enquiry into perioperative deaths in three NHS regions. *Lancet* 1987; **2:** 1384–6.
93. Derrington MC, Gallimore S. The effect of the National Confidential Enquiry into Perioperative Deaths on clinical practice. *Anaesthesia* 1997; **53:** 3–8.
94. Lunn JN. Perioperative mortality in Germany. *Anaesthetist* 1997; **46:** 369–70.
95. Arbous MS, Grobbee DE, van Kleff JW, Meursing AEE. Dutch case–control study of anaesthesia-related morbidity and mortality. *Anaesthesia* 1998; **53:** 162–8.
96. Cheney FW. The American Society of Anesthesiologists Closed Claims Project: what we have learned, how it has affected practice, and how will it affect practice in the future? *Anesthesiology* 1999; **91:** 552–6.
97. Bowling A. *Research Methods in Health*, 2nd edn. London: Open University Press, 2002.
98. Crombie IK, Davies HT. *Research in Health Care: Design, Conduct and Interpretation of Health Services Research*. London: John Wiley and Sons, 1996.
99. St Leger S, Schnieden H, Walsworth-Bell J. *Evaluating Health Services' Effectiveness.* Milton Keynes: Open University Press, 1992.
100. Crombie IK. *The Pocket Guide to Critical Appraisal.* London: BMJ Publishing Group, 1996.
101. Fowkes FG, Fulton PM. Critical appraisal of published research: introductory guidelines. *BMJ* 1991; **302:** 1136–40.
102. NHS Centre for Reviews and Dissemination. *Undertaking Systematic Reviews of Research on Effectiveness.* University of York: NHS Centre for Reviews and Dissemination, 2001.
103. Dickersin K, Scherer E, Lefebvre C. Identification of relevant studies for systematic reviews. *Br Med J* 1994; **309:** 1286–91.
104. The Cochrane Library. *Cochrane Database of Systematic Reviews*, Issue 3. London: BMJ Publishing Group, 2002.
105. Bender JS, Halpern SH, Thangaroopan M, *et al.* Quality and retrieval of obstetrical anaesthesia randomized controlled trials. *Can J Anaesth* 1997; **44:** 14–18.
106. Guyatt G, Rennie D (eds). *Users' Guides to the Medical Literature: A Manual for Evidence-Based Clinical Practice.* Chicago, IL: AMA Press, 2002.
107. Alderson M. *An Introduction to Epidemiology*. London: Macmillan Press, 1983.
108. Lilienfeld DE, Stolley PD. *Foundations of Epidemiology,* 3rd edn. New York: Oxford University Press, 1994.
109. Krajewski LJ, Ritzman LP. *Operations Management: Strategy and Analysis*, 5th edn. UK: Addison Wesley Longman Higher Education, 1998.
110. Slack N, Chambers S, Harland C, *et al. Operations Management*, 2nd edn. London: Pitman Publishing, 1997.
111. Roberts K, Ludvigsen C. *Project Management for Health Care Professionals.* Oxford: Butterworth-Heinemann, 1998.
112. Sackett DL, Richardson WS, Rosenberg W, Haynes RB. *Evidence-based Medicine. How to Practice and Teach EBM*, 2nd edn. Edinburgh: Churchill Livingstone, 2000.
113. Haynes RB, Sackett DJ, Gray J, *et al.* Transferring evidence from research into practice. I. The role of clinical care research evidence in clinical decisions. *ACP J Club* 1996; **125** (3): A14–16.
114. Lomas J. *Teaching Old (and Not So Old) Docs New Tricks: Effective Ways to Implement Research Findings.* CHEPA Working Paper Series No. 93–94. Hamilton, Canada: Centre for Health Economics and Policy Analysis, 1993.
115. Lomas J. Diffusion, dissemination, and implementation: who should do what? In: Warren KS, Mosteller F (eds). Doing more good than harm: the evaluation of health care interventions. *Ann NY Acad Sci* 1993; **703:** 226–37.
116. Batstone G, Edwards M. Achieving clinical effectiveness: Just another initiative or a real change in working practice? *J Clin Effect* 1996; **1:** 19–21.
117. Haines A, Jones J. Implementing findings of research. *Br Med J* 1994; **308:** 1488–92.
118. Soumerai SB, Avorn J. Principles of educational outreach ("academic detailing") to improve clinical decision making. *JAMA* 1990; **263:** 549–56.
119. Grilli R. Developing recommendations to promote the uptake of research information in clinical practice. *Therapie* 1996; **51:** 265–8.
120. Cheater FM, Closs SJ. The effectiveness of methods of dissemination and implementation of clinical guidelines for nursing practice: a selective review. *Clin Effec Nurs* 1997; **1:** 4–15.
121. Grimshaw J, Freemantle N, Wallace S, *et al.* Developing and implementing clinical practice guidelines. *Quality in Health Care* 1995; **4:** 55–64.
122. Scottish Intercollegiate Guidelines Network (SIGN). Clinical Guidelines. Criteria for Appraisal for National Use. Edinburgh: Royal College of Physicians, 1995.
123. Gupta L, Ward J, Hayward RSA. Future directions for clinical practice guidelines: needs, lead agencies and potential dissemination strategies identified by Australian general practitioners. *Austr New Zealand J Public Health* 1997; **27:** 495–9.
124. Karuza J, Calkins E, Feather J, *et al.* Enhancing physician adoption of practice guidelines. Dissemination of influenza vaccination guideline using a small-group consensus process. *Arch Intern Med* 1995; **155:** 625–32.
125. Feder G, Eccles M, Grol R, *et al.* Using clinical guidelines. *BMJ* 1999; **318:** 728–30.
126. Woolf SH, Grol R, Hutchinson A, *et al.* Potential benefits, limitations and harms of clinical guidelines. *BMJ* 1999; **318:** 527–30.
127. Snow J. *On the Inhalation of Vapour of Ether in Surgical Operations.* London: John Churchill, 1847.
128. Patton MQ. *Qualitative Evaluation and Research Methods*, 3rd edn. Newbury Park: Sage Publication, 2002.
129. Duncan PG, Cohen MM. The literature of anaesthesia: what are we learning? *Can J Anaesth* 1988; **35:** 494–9.
130. Mulrow CD. Rationale for systematic reviews. *Br Med J* 1994; **309:** 597–9.
131. Oxman AD (ed.). *Section VI: Preparing and Maintaining Systematic Reviews. The Cochrane Collaboration Handbook.* Oxford: University of Oxford, 1994: 24–7.
132. Altman DG. *Practical Statistics for Medical Research.* London: Chapman and Hall, 1991.
133. Bland M. *An Introduction to Medical Statistics*, 3rd edn. Oxford: Oxford. University Press, 2000.
134. Fisher DM. Research design and statistics in anesthesia. In: Miller RD (ed.). *Anesthesia*, 5th edn. New York: Churchill Livingstone, 2000: 753–92.
135. Cruickshank S. *Mathematics and Statistics in Anaesthesia.* Oxford: Oxford. University Press, 1998.
136. Orkin FK. Practice standards: the Midas touch or the emperor's new clothes. *Anesthesiology* 1989; **70:** 566–71.

137. Medical Research Council. *MRC Guidelines for Good Clinical Practice in Clinical Trials.* London: Medical Research Council, 1998.
138. Charlson ME, Pompei P, Ales KL, MacKenzie CR. A new method of classifying prognostic comorbidity in longitudinal studies: development and validation. *J Chron Dis* 1987; **40:** 373–83.
139. Hill AB. The environment and disease: association or causation? *Proc R Soc Med* 1965; **58:** 295–300.
140. Clancy CM, Eisenberg JM. Outcomes research: Measuring the end results of health care. *Science* 1998; **282:** 245–6.
141. Orkin FK. Application of outcomes research to clinical decision making in cardiovascular medicine. In: Tuman KJ (ed.). *Outcomes Measurements in Cardiovascular Medicine.* Philadelphia, PA: Lippincott Williams & Wilkins, 1999: 39–66.
142. Wennberg JE, Gittelsohn A. Small area variations in health care delivery: A population-based health information system can guide planning and regulatory decision-making. *Science* 1973; **182:** 1102–8.
143. Wennberg JE, Freeman JL, Shelton RM, Bubolz TA. Hospital use and mortality among Medicare beneficiaries in Boston and New Haven. *N Engl J Med* 1989; **321:** 1168–73.
144. Wennberg JE, Cooper MM (eds). *The Dartmouth Atlas of Health Care 1999.* Chicago, IL: AHA Press, 1999.
145. Fisher ES, Wennberg DE, Stukel TA *et al.* The implications of regional variations in Medicare spending. Part 2: Health outcomes and satisfaction with care. *Ann Intern Med* 2003; **138:** 288–98.
146. Feinstein AR. An additional basic science for clinical medicine. II. The limitations of randomized trials. *Ann Intern Med* 1983; **99:** 544–50.
147. Iberti TJ, Fischer EP, Leibowitz AB, *et al.* A multicenter study of physicians' knowledge of the pulmonary artery catheter. *JAMA* 1990; **264:** 2928–32.
148. Hellman S, Hellman DS. Of mice but not men: problems of the randomized clinical trial. *N Engl J Med* 1991; **324:** 1585–9.
149. Boyle PJ (ed.). *Getting Doctors to Listen: Ethics and Outcomes Data in Context.* Washington DC: Georgetown University Press, 1998.
150. Goodman NW. Anaesthesia and evidence-based medicine. *Anaesthesia* 1998; **53:** 353–68.
151. Shine KI. President's report to the Institute of Medicine: the health sciences, health services research, and the role of the health professions. *Health Serv Res* 1998; **33:** 439–45.
152. Donabedian A. Evaluating the quality of medical care. *Milbank Mem Fund Q* 1966; **44** (Part 2): 166–206.
153. Slogoff S, Keats AS. Does perioperative myocardial ischemia lead to postoperative myocardial infarction? *Anesthesiology* 1985; **62:** 107–14.
154. Mangano DT, Browner WS, Hollenberg M, *et al* and The Study of Perioperative Ischemia Research Group. Association of perioperative myocardial ischemia with cardiac morbidity and mortality in men undergoing noncardiac surgery. *N Engl J Med* 1990; **323:** 1781–8.
155. Raby KE, Barry J, Creager MA, *et al.* Detection and significance of intraoperative and postoperative myocardial ischemia in peripheral vascular surgery. *JAMA* 1992; **268:** 222–7.
156. Fisher DM. Surrogate end points: are they meaningful? *Anesthesiology* 1994; **81:** 795–6.
157. Sakaid M. Grading of patients for surgical procedures. *Anesthesiology* 1941; **2:** 281–4.
158. Guyatt GH, Feeney DH, Patrick DL. Measuring health-related quality of life. *Ann Intern Med* 1993; **118:** 622–9.
159. Wilson IB, Cleary PD. Linking clinical variables with health-related quality of life: a conceptual model of patient outcomes. *JAMA* 1995; **273:** 59–65.
160. Testa MA, Simonson DC. Assessment of quality-of-life outcomes. *N Engl J Med* 1996; **334:** 835–40.
161. Huskisson EC. Measurement of pain. *Lancet* 1974; **2:** 1127–31.
162. Melzack R. The McGill Pain Questionnaire: major properties and scoring methods. *Pain* 1975; **1:** 277–99.
163. Ware Jr JE, Snow KK, Kosinski M, Gandek B. SF-36 *Health Survey: Manual and Interpretation Guide.* Boston, MA: The Health Institute, New England Medical Center, 1993.
164. Stewart AL, Ware Jr JE (eds). *Measuring Functioning and Well-Being: The Medical Outcomes Study Approach.* Durham NC: Duke University Press, 1996.
165. Spilker B (ed.). *Quality of Life and Pharmacoeconomics in Clinical Trials,* 2nd edn. Philadelphia, PA: Lippincott-Raven, 1996.
166. Bowling A. *Measuring Disease: A Review of Disease-Specific Quality of Life Measurement Scales.* Bristol: Open University Press, 1995.
167. McDowell I, Newell C. *Measuring Health: A Guide to Rating Scales and Questionnaires,* 2nd edn. New York: Oxford University Press, 1996.
168. Bowling A. *Measuring Health: A Review of Quality of Life Measurement Scales,* 2nd edn. Bristol: Open University Press, 1997.
169. Frank-Stromborg M, Olsen SJ (eds). *Instruments for Clinical Health Care Research,* 2nd edn. Sudbury: Jones & Bartlett, 1997.
170. Staquet MJ, Hays RD, Fayers PM. *Quality of Life Assessment in Clinical Trials: Methods and Practice.* New York: Oxford University Press, 1998.
171. Lee VC, Rowlingson JC. Defining quality of life in chronic pain. In: Spilker B (ed.). *Quality of Life and Pharmacoeconomics in Clinical Trials,* 2nd edn. Philadelphia, PA: Lippincott-Raven, 1966: 853–64.
172. Rogers WH, Wittink HM, Ashburn MA, *et al.* Using the "TOPS," an outcomes instrument for multidisciplinary outpatient pain treatment. *Pain Med* 2000; **1:** 55–67.
173. Orkin FK. Preferences and willingness to pay for postanesthetic recovery states. *Med Decis Making* 1997: **17:** 543.
174. Fung D, Cohen MM. Measuring patient satisfaction with anesthesia care: a review of current methodology. *Anesth Analg* 1998: **87:** 1089–98.
175. Macario A, Weinger M, Carney S, Kim A. Which clinical anesthesia outcomes are important to avoid? The perspective of patients. *Anesth Analg* 1999; **89:** 652–8.
176. Eberhart LHJ, Morin AM, Wulf H, Geldner G. Patient preference for immediate postoperative recovery. *Br J Anaesth* 2002; **89:** 760–1.
177. Walker J. Enhancing patient comfort. In: Gerteis M, Edgman-Levitan S, Daley J, Delbanco TL (eds). *Through the Patient's Eyes: Understanding and Promoting Patient-Centered Care.* San Francisco: Jossey-Bass, 1993: 119–53.
178. Todd MM, Warner DS, Sokoll MD, *et al.* A prospective, comparative trial of three anesthetics for elective supratentorial craniotomy. *Anesthesiology* 1993; **78:** 1005–20.
179. Weiskopf RB, Eger II EI. Comparing the costs of inhaled anesthetics. *Anesthesiology* 1993; **79:** 1413–18.
180. Becker KE, Carrithers J. Practical methods of cost containment in anesthesia and surgery. *J Clin Anesth* 1994; **6:** 388–99.
181. Fleisher LA, Skolnick ED, Holroyd KJ, Lehmann HP. Coronary artery revascularization before abdominal aortic aneurysm surgery: a decision analytic approach. *Anesth Analg* 1994; **79:** 661–9.
182. Watcha MF, Smith I. Cost effectiveness analysis of antiemetic therapy for ambulatory surgery. *J Clin Anesth* 1994; **6:** 370–7.
183. Macario A, Chang PC, Stempel DB, Brock-Utne J. A cost analysis of the laryngeal mask airway for elective surgery in adult outpatients. *Anesthesiology* 1995; **83:** 250–7.
184. Roizen MF, Schreider B, Austin W, *et al.* Pulse oximetry, capnography and blood gas measurements: reducing cost and improving the quality of care with technology. *J Clin Monit* 1993; **9:** 237–40.
185. Doubilet P, Weinstein MC, McNeil BJ. Use and misuse of the term "cost-effective" in medicine. *N Engl J Med* 1986; **314:** 253–5.
186. Weinstein MC, Stason WB. Foundations of cost-effectiveness analysis for health and medical practices. *N Engl J Med* 1977; **296:** 716–21.
187. Weinstein MC, Fineberg HC (eds). *Clinical Decision Analysis.* Philadelphia, PA: WB Saunders, 1980.
188. Eisenberg JM. Clinical economics: a guide to the economic analysis of clinical practices. *JAMA* 1989; **262:** 2879–86.
189. Detsky AS, Naglie IG. A clinician's guide to cost-effectiveness analysis. *Ann Intern Med* 1990; **113:** 147–54.
190. Luce BR, Elixhauser A. *Standards for Socioeconomic Evaluation of Health Care Products and Services.* New York: Springer-Verlag, 1990.
191. Udvarhelyi IS, Colditz GA, Rai A, Epstein AM. Cost-effectiveness and cost-benefit analyses in the medical literature: are the methods being used correctly? *Ann Intern Med* 1992; **116:** 238–44.
192. Gold MR, Siegel JE, Russell LB, Weinstein MC (eds). *Cost-Effectiveness in Health and Medicine.* New York: Oxford University Press, 1996.
193. Bootman JL, Townsend RJ, McGhan WF (eds). *Principles of Pharmacoeconomics,* 2nd edn. Cincinnati, OH: Harvey Whitney Books, 1996.
194. Drummond MF, O'Brien B, Stoddart GL, Torrance GW. *Methods for the Economic Evaluation of Health Care Programmes,* 2nd edn. New York: Oxford University Press, 1998.
195. Petitti DB. *Meta-analysis, Decision Analysis and Cost-Effectiveness Analysis,* 2nd edn. New York: Oxford University Press, 2000: 17–32, 140–239, 248–50, 259–63, 271–82.
196. Gelijns AC, Halm EA (eds). *Medical Innovation at the Crossroads.* Vol. II. *The Changing Economics of Medical Technology.* Washington DC: National Academy Press, 1991.
197. Gelijns AC (ed.). *Medical Innovation at the Crossroads.* Vol. III. *Technology and Health Care in An Era of Limits.* Washington DC: National Academy Press, 1992.
198. Gelijns AC, Dawkins HV (eds). *Medical Innovation at the Crossroads. Vol IV. Adopting* New *Medical Technology.* Washington DC: National Academy Press, 1994.
199. Hunink M, Glasziou P, Siegel J, *et al. Decision Making in Health and*

Medicine: Integrating Evidence and Values. Cambridge: Cambridge University Press, 2001.

200. Orkin FK. Moving toward value-based anesthesia care. *J Clin Anesth* 1993; **5:** 91–8.
201. Sperry RJ. Principles of economic analysis. *Anesthesiology* 1997; **86:** 1197–1205.
202. Watcha MF, White PF. Economics of anesthetic practice. *Anesthesiology* 1997; **86:** 1170–96.
203. Fleisher LA, Mantha A, Roizen MF. Medical technology assessment: an overview. *Anesth Analg* 1998; **87:** 1271–82.
204. Glenn DM, Macario A. Management of the operating room: a new practice opportunity for anesthesiologists. *Anesthesiol Clin N Am* 1999; **17:** 365–94.
205. Shuman LJ, Speas Jr RD, Young JP (eds). *Operations Research in Health Care: A Critical Analysis*. Baltimore, MD: The Johns Hopkins University Press, 1975.
206. Ozcan YA (ed.). Applications of operations research in health care. *Ann Operations Res* 1996; **67:** 1–285.
207. Connell FA, Diehr P, Hart LG. The use of large data bases in health care studies. *Ann Rev Public Health* 1987; **8:** 51–74.
208. Vacanti CJ, Van Houten RJ, Hill RC. A statistical analysis of the relationship of physical status to postoperative mortality in 68,388 cases. *Anesth Analg* 1970; **49:** 564–6.
209. Marx GF, Mateo CV, Orkin LR. Computer analysis of postanesthetic death. *Anesthesiology* 1973; **39:** 54–8.
210. Iezzoni LI. Risk adjustment for medical effectiveness research: an overview of conceptual and methodological considerations. *J Invest Med* 1995; **43:** 136–50.
211. Iezzoni LI. The risks of risk adjustment. *JAMA* 1997; **278:** 1600–7.
212. Iezzoni LI (ed.). *Risk Adjustment for Measuring Health Outcomes*, 2nd edn. Ann Arbor, MI: Health Administration Press, 1997.
213. Wennberg JE, Freeman JL, Culp WJ. Are hospital services rationed in New Haven or over-utilized in Boston? *Lancet* 1987; **1:** 1185–8.
214. Light RJ, Pillemer DB. *Summing Up: The Science of Reviewing Research*. Cambridge MA: Harvard University Press, 1984.
215. Thacker SB. Meta-analysis: a quantitative approach to research integration. In: Gelijns AC (ed.). *Medical Innovation at the Crossroads*, Vol. I. *Modern Methods of Clinical Investigation*. Washington DC: National Academy Press, 1990: 88–100.
216. Petitti DB. *Meta-analysis, Decision Analysis and Cost-Effectiveness Analysis*, 2nd edn. New York: Oxford University Press, 2000: 13–17, 33–139, 239–47, 264–71, 279–82.
217. Divatia JV, Vaidya JS, Badwe RA, Hawaldar RW. Omission of nitrous oxide during anesthesia reduces the incidence of postoperative nausea and vomiting: a meta-analysis. *Anesthesiology* 1996; **85:** 1055–62.
218. Wasson JH, Sox HC, Neff RK, Goldman L. Clinical prediction rules: Applications and methodologic standards. *N Engl J Med* 1985; **313:** 793–9.
219. Orkin FK, Leventhal SR, Hirsh RA. Respiratory failure following thymectomy. *Ann NY Acad Med* 1981; **377:** 862–3.
220. Grant RP, Jenkins LC. Prediction of the need for postoperative mechanical ventilation in myasthenia gravis. *Can Anaesth Soc J* 1982; **29:** 112–16.
221. Gracey DR, Divertie MB, Howard FM, Payne WS. Postoperative respiratory care after transsternal thymectomy in myasthenia gravis: a three-year experience in 53 patients. *Chest* 1984; **86:** 67–71.
222. Eisenkraft JR, Papatestas AE, Kahn CH, *et al*. Predicting the need for postoperative mechanical ventilation and myasthenia gravis. *Anesthesiology* 1986; **65:** 79–82.
223. Gold BS, Kitz DS, Lecky JH, Nauhaus JM. Unanticipated admission to the hospital following ambulatory surgery. *JAMA* 1989; **262:** 3008–10.
224. Van de Ven AH, Delbecq AI. The effectiveness of nominal, Delphi, and interacting group decision making processes. *Acad Manage J*; **17:** 605–21.
225. Murphy MK, Black NA, Lamping DL, *et al*. Consensus development methods and their use in clinical guideline development. *Health Technol Assess* 1998; **2** (3): 1–88.
226. Lomas J, Pickard L, Mohide A. Patient versus clinician item generation for quality-of-life measures. The case of language-disabled adults. *Med Care* 1987; **25:** 764–9.
227. Pill J. The Delphi method: substance, context, a critique and the annotated bibliography. *Socioecon Planning Sci* 1971; **5:** 57–71.
228. Linstone HA, Turoff M (eds). *The Delphi Method: Techniques and Applications*. Reading, MA: Addison-Wesley Publishing Company, 1979.
229. Larach MG, Localio AR, Allen GC, *et al*. A clinical grading scale to predict malignant hyperthermia susceptibility. *Anesthesiology* 1994; **80:** 771–9.
230. Mobily PR, Herr KA, Kelley LS. Cognitive-behavioural technique to reduce pain: a validation study. *Int J Nurs Stud* 1993; **30:** 537–48.
231. Enger D. Report on the NIH Consensus Development Conferences on Pain. *J Pain Symptom Manage* 1986; **1(3):** 165–7.
232. Stocking B, Jennett B, Spiby J. *Criteria for Change: The history and impact of consensus development conferences in the UK*. London: Kings Fund Centre, 1991.
233. Kosecoff J, Kanouse DE, Rogers WH, *et al*. Effects of the National Institutes of Health Consensus Development Program on physician practice. *J Am Med Assoc* 1987; **258:** 2708–13.
234. Fink A, Kosecoff J, Chassin M, Brook RH. Consensus methods: characteristics and guidelines for use. *Am J Public Health* 1984; **74:** 979–83.
235. McGlynn EA, Kosecoff J, Brook RH. Format and conduct of consensus development conferences. Multination comparison. *Int J Technol Assess Health Care* 1990; **6:** 450–69.
236. Krueger R. *Focus Groups: A Practical Guide for Applied Research*. London: Sage Publications, 1994.
237. Kitzinger J. Introducing focus groups. *Br Med J* 1995; **311:** 299–302.
238. Yates P, Dewar A, Fentiman B. Pain: the views of elderly people living in long-term residential care settings. *J Adv Nurs* 1995; **21:** 667–74.
239. McHugh G, Thoms G. Patient satisfaction with chronic pain management. *Nurs Stand* 2001; **15:** 33–38.
240. Lack JA, White LA, Thoms GM, Rollin AM (eds). *Raising the Standard: A Compendium of Audit Recipes for Continuous Quality Improvement in Anaesthesia*. London: Royal College of Anaesthetists, 2000.
241. Thoms GMM, McHugh GA, Pollard BJ, Moore JK. Anaesthesia clinical directors in the United Kingdom: organisation, objectives and support needs. *Anaesthesia* 1999; **54:** 753–760.
242. O'Connor GT, Plume SK, Olmstead EM, *et al*. Multivariate prediction of in-hospital mortality associated with coronary artery bypass graft surgery. *Circulation* 1992; **85:** 2110–18.
243. Langley GL, Nolan KM, Nolan TW, *et al*. *The Improvement Guide: A Practical Approach to Enhancing Organizational Performance*. San Francisco, CA: Jossey-Bass, 1966.
244. Nelson EC, Batalden PB, Ryer JC (eds). *Clinical Improvement Action Guide*. Oakbrook Terrace, IL: Joint Commission on Accreditation of Healthcare Organizations, 1998.
245. O'Connor GT, Plume SK, Olmstead EM, *et al*. A regional intervention to improve the hospital mortality associated with coronary artery bypass surgery: The Northern New England Cardiovascular Disease Study Group. JAMA 1996; 275: 841–6.
246. Corrigan J, Kohn L, Donaldson M (eds). *To Err is Human: Building a Safer Health System*. Washington DC: National Academy Press, 1999 (http: //books.nap.edu.html/to_err_is_human).
247. Cullen DJ, Bates DW, Leape LL, and the Adverse Drug Event Prevention Study Group. Prevention of adverse drug events: a decade of progress in patient safety. *J Clin Anesth* 2000; **12:** 600–14.

Index

This index is in letter-by-letter order, whereby spaces and hyphens in main entries are excluded from the alphabetization process. Page numbers followed by "f" indicate figures; page numbers followed by "t" indicate tables; page numbers followed by "b" indicate boxes. Page numbers in bold indicate main entries. To save space the following abbreviations have been used:

AED	auditory-evoked potentials
ARDS	acute respiratory distress syndrome
CPB	cardiopulmonary bypass
CPR	cardiopulmonary resuscitation
ECG	electrocardiography
EEG	electroencephalography
IPPV	intermittent positive-pressure ventilation
NSAIDs	nonsteroidal anti-inflammatory drugs
PCA	patient-controlled analgesia
PEEP	positive end-expiratory pressure
PONV	postoperative nausea and vomiting
TENS	transcutaneous electrical nerve stimulation